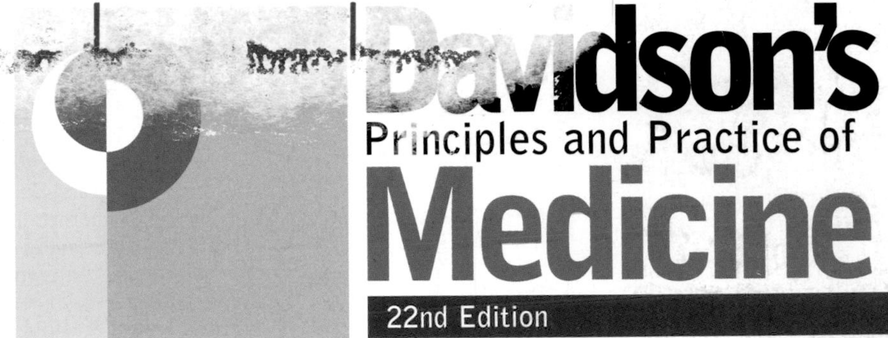
Davidson's
Principles and Practice of
Medicine
22nd Edition

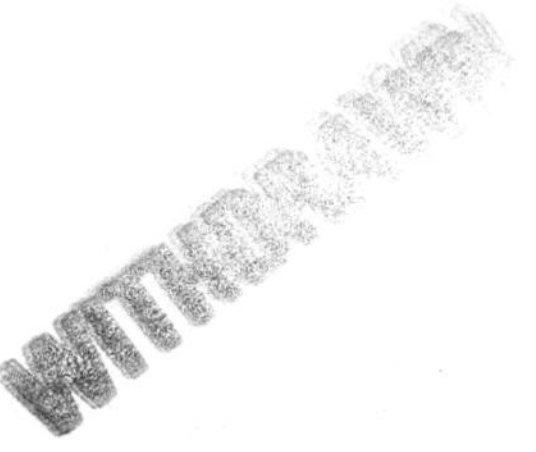
WITHDRAWN

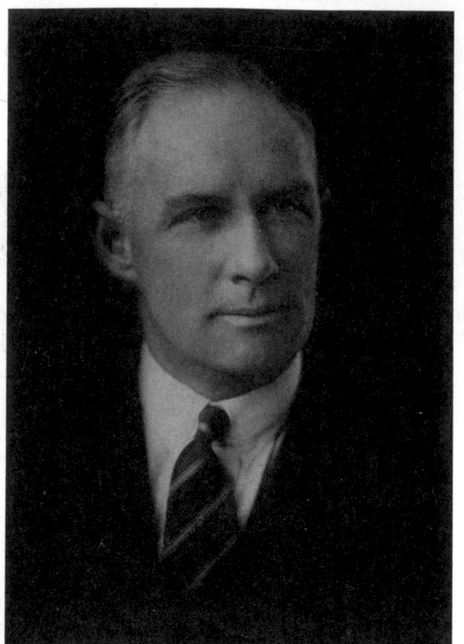

Sir Stanley Davidson (1894–1981)

This famous textbook was the brainchild of one of the great Professors of Medicine of the 20th century. Stanley Davidson was born in Sri Lanka and began his medical undergraduate training at Trinity College, Cambridge; this was interrupted by World War I and later resumed in Edinburgh. He was seriously wounded in battle, and the carnage and shocking waste of young life that he encountered at that time had a profound effect on his subsequent attitudes and values.

In 1930 Stanley Davidson was appointed Professor of Medicine at the University of Aberdeen, one of the first full-time Chairs of Medicine anywhere and the first in Scotland. In 1938 he took up the Chair of Medicine at Edinburgh and was to remain in this post until retirement in 1959. He was a renowned educator and a particularly gifted teacher at the bedside, where he taught that everything had to be questioned and explained. He himself gave most of the systematic lectures in Medicine, which were made available as typewritten notes that emphasised the essentials and far surpassed any textbook available at the time.

Principles and Practice of Medicine was conceived in the late 1940s with its origins in those lecture notes. The first edition, published in 1952, was a masterpiece of clarity and uniformity of style. It was of modest size and price, but sufficiently comprehensive and up to date to provide students with the main elements of sound medical practice. Although the format and presentation have seen many changes in 21 subsequent editions, Sir Stanley's original vision and objectives remain. More than half a century after its first publication, his book continues to inform and educate students, doctors and health professionals all over the world.

Readers may be interested to listen to an interview with Sir Stanley Davidson, which can be found on the Royal College of Physicians of Edinburgh website at: www.rcpe.ac.uk/library-archives/sir-stanley-davidson-1894-1981.

Content Strategist: Laurence Hunter
Content Development Specialist: Wendy Lee
Project Manager: Louisa Talbott
Designer/Design Direction: Miles Hitchen
Illustration Manager: Jennifer Rose

Davidson's Principles and Practice of Medicine

22nd Edition

Edited by

Brian R. Walker BSc MD FRCPE FRSE
Professor of Endocrinology,
University of Edinburgh;
Honorary Consultant Physician,
Royal Infirmary of Edinburgh, UK

Nicki R. Colledge BSc FRCPE
Consultant Physician in Medicine for the Elderly,
Liberton Hospital, Edinburgh,
and Royal Infirmary of Edinburgh;
Honorary Senior Lecturer,
University of Edinburgh, UK

Stuart H. Ralston MD FRCP FMedSci FRSE
Arthritis Research UK Professor of Rheumatology,
University of Edinburgh;
Honorary Consultant Rheumatologist,
Western General Hospital,
Edinburgh, UK

Ian D. Penman BSc MD FRCPE
Consultant Gastroenterologist,
Royal Infirmary of Edinburgh;
Honorary Senior Lecturer,
University of Edinburgh, UK

Illustrations by
Robert Britton

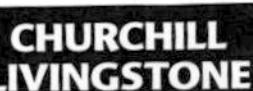

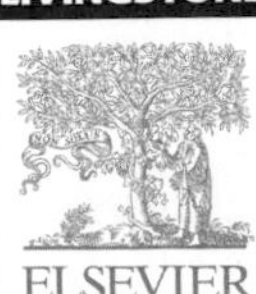

Edinburgh London New York Oxford Philadelphia St Louis Sydney Toronto 2014

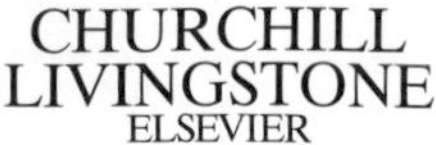

An imprint of Elsevier Limited

First edition 1952
Second edition 1954
Third edition 1956
Fourth edition 1958
Fifth edition 1960
Sixth edition 1962
Seventh edition 1964
Eighth edition 1966
Ninth edition 1968
Tenth edition 1971
Eleventh edition 1974
Twelfth edition 1977
Thirteenth edition 1981
Fourteenth edition 1984
Fifteenth edition 1987
Sixteenth edition 1991
Seventeenth edition 1995
Eighteenth edition 1999
Nineteenth edition 2002
Twentieth edition 2006
Twenty-first edition 2010
Twenty-second edition 2014

Main Edition ISBN-13: 978-0-7020-5035-0
International Edition ISBN-13: 978-0-7020-5047-3
eBook ISBN-13: 978-0-7020-5103-6

British Library Cataloguing in Publication Data
A catalogue record for this book is available from the British Library

Library of Congress Cataloging in Publication Data
A catalog record for this book is available from the Library of Congress

Notices

Knowledge and best practice in this field are constantly changing. As new research and experience broaden our understanding, changes in research methods, professional practices, or medical treatment may become necessary.

Practitioners and researchers must always rely on their own experience and knowledge in evaluating and using any information, methods, compounds, or experiments described herein. In using such information or methods they should be mindful of their own safety and the safety of others, including parties for whom they have a professional responsibility.

With respect to any drug or pharmaceutical products identified, readers are advised to check the most current information provided (i) on procedures featured or (ii) by the manufacturer of each product to be administered, to verify the recommended dose or formula, the method and duration of administration, and contraindications. It is the responsibility of practitioners, relying on their own experience and knowledge of their patients, to make diagnoses, to determine dosages and the best treatment for each individual patient, and to take all appropriate safety precautions.

To the fullest extent of the law, neither the Publisher nor the authors, contributors, or editors, assume any liability for any injury and/or damage to persons or property as a matter of products liability, negligence or otherwise, or from any use or operation of any methods, products, instructions, or ideas contained in the material herein.

Printed in China

Preface

Since *Davidson's Principles and Practice of Medicine* was first published in 1952, over two million copies have been sold and the book has acquired a large following of medical students, doctors and other health professionals all over the world. It has been translated into many languages, most recently Japanese, Russian, Italian and Polish, and has won numerous prizes, the last edition being highly commended in the British Medical Association Book Awards. *Davidson's* has endured because with each new edition it has evolved to provide comprehensive updated information in a concise and easy-to-read format.

From its beginnings, *Davidson's* has sought to explain the basis for medical practice. The integration of 'pre-clinical' science with clinical practice is now a feature of many undergraduate medical curricula, and many students use *Davidson's* from the outset of their medical course. In recognition of this, the first part of the book, 'Principles of Medicine', highlights the mechanisms of health and disease, along with the professional and ethical principles underlying medical practice. Many examples of clinical problems are included to bring the medical sciences to life for the new student and to rejuvenate the interest of the experienced clinician. The second part of the book, 'Practice of Medicine', covers the major medical specialties. Every chapter has been thoroughly revised for this edition to ensure that it reflects the 'cutting edge' of medical knowledge and practice and is pitched at a level of detail to meet the needs of candidates preparing for examination for Membership of the Royal College of Physicians or its equivalents. In recognition of the emerging specialty of Stroke Medicine, this topic is now covered in a separate chapter from Neurological Disease. Surgical approaches to disease management are mentioned in *Davidson's*, but readers are encouraged to consult the sister book, *Principles and Practice of Surgery*, for more details.

Many of the innovations introduced in recent editions have been warmly received. We have retained both a patient-orientated approach, in the ever-popular 'Clinical Examination' overviews and 'Presenting Problems' sections, alongside practical content, in 'Emergency' and 'Practice Point' boxes. Embedding horizontal themes within the book – for example, with the 'In Old Age' and 'In Pregnancy' boxes – has been applauded, and we have extended this approach by adding 'In Adolescence' boxes in relevant chapters; these emphasise key points in managing the transition of patients between paediatric and adult services.

We are proud of *Davidson's* international heritage. As well as recruiting authors from around the globe, particularly for topics such as Infectious Diseases and HIV, we have welcomed new members on to our International Advisory Board. These leading experts from 16 countries provide detailed comments that, along with the feedback received from our global readership, are crucial to our planning of every chapter in each new edition. We have also visited several medical schools on the Indian subcontinent and received invaluable feedback from students and teachers. We have addressed as many of these suggestions as possible in this edition.

Education is achieved by assimilating information from many sources and readers of this book can enhance their learning experience by using complementary resources. The StudentConsult platform continues to provide online access to the text and illustrations of the main edition. The book is also available in various eBook formats. *Davidson's* has had a long-standing association with its sister books, *Macleod's Clinical Examination* (now in its 13th Edition) and *Principles and Practice of Surgery* (now in its 6th Edition). The *Davidson's* 'family' has expanded with the publication of *Davidson's Essentials of Medicine*, a long-requested pocket-size version of the main text; *Davidson's Foundations of Clinical Practice*, a guide to starting work as a junior doctor; *Davidson's 100 Clinical Cases*, which contains cases directly based on the 'Presenting Problems' in the main text; and *Macleod's Clinical Diagnosis*, which describes a systematic approach to differential diagnosis of symptoms and signs. We congratulate the editors and authors of these books for continuing the tradition of concise, easily read and beautifully illustrated texts.

The regular introduction of new authors and editors to *Davidson's* is important to maintain the freshness of each new edition. On this occasion, Dr Ian Penman has joined the editorial team and 18 new authors have contributed material. We all take immense pride in producing an outstanding book for the next generation of doctors, and in continuing the great tradition first established by Sir Stanley Davidson and passed on by all the previous editors and authors, for what remains one of the world's leading textbooks of medicine.

BRW, NRC, SHR, IDP
Edinburgh

Contents

List of presenting problems viii
Contributors x
International Advisory Board xiv
Introduction xvi
Acknowledgements xviii
Figure acknowledgements xix

PART 1 PRINCIPLES OF MEDICINE

1 **Good medical practice** **1**
A.D. Cumming • S.I.R. Noble

2 **Therapeutics and good prescribing** **17**
S. Maxwell

3 **Molecular and genetic factors in disease** **41**
D.R. FitzPatrick • J.R. Seckl

4 **Immunological factors in disease** **71**
S.E. Marshall

5 **Environmental and nutritional factors in disease** **97**
P. Hanlon • M. Byers • J.P.H. Wilding • H.M. Macdonald

6 **Principles of infectious disease** **133**
R.P. Hobson • D.H. Dockrell

7 **Ageing and disease** **165**
M.D. Witham

PART 2 PRACTICE OF MEDICINE

8 **Critical illness** **179**
G.R. Nimmo • T. Walsh

9 **Poisoning** **205**
S.H.L. Thomas • J. White

10 **Medical psychiatry** **231**
M.C. Sharpe • S.M. Lawrie

11 **Oncology** **259**
G.G. Dark • A.R. Abdul Razak

12 **Palliative care and pain** 283
D. Oxenham

13 **Infectious disease** 293
D.H. Dockrell • S. Sundar • B.J. Angus • R.P. Hobson

14 **HIV infection and AIDS** 387
G. Maartens

15 **Sexually transmitted infections** 411
G.R. Scott

16 **Clinical biochemistry and metabolism** 427
M.J. Field • L. Burnett • D.R. Sullivan • P. Stewart

17 **Kidney and urinary tract disease** 461
J. Goddard • A.N. Turner

18 **Cardiovascular disease** 525
D.E. Newby • N.R. Grubb • A. Bradbury

19 **Respiratory disease** 643
P.T. Reid • J.A. Innes

20 **Endocrine disease** 733
M.W.J. Strachan • J. Newell-Price

21 **Diabetes mellitus** 797
E.R. Pearson • R.J. McCrimmon

22 **Alimentary tract and pancreatic disease** 837
I.D. Penman • C.W. Lees

23 **Liver and biliary tract disease** 921
Q.M. Anstee • D.E.J. Jones

24 **Blood disease** 989
H.G. Watson • J.I.O. Craig • L.M. Manson

25 **Rheumatology and bone disease** 1057
S.H. Ralston • I.B. McInnes

26 **Neurological disease** 1137
J.P. Leach • R.J. Davenport

27 **Stroke disease** 1231
P. Langhorne

28 **Skin disease** 1249
S.H. Ibbotson • R.S. Dawe

29 **Laboratory reference ranges** 1307
S.W. Walker

Index 1313

List of presenting problems

These presentations represent the most common reasons for referral to each medical specialty and are described in the 'Presenting Problems' sections of all system-based chapters. The same approach has also been employed in several of the chapters in the 'Principles of Medicine' section, reinforcing the close connection between clinical problems and fundamental mechanisms of disease.

Abnormal investigation results

Acid–base, 443
- Metabolic acidosis, 445
- Metabolic alkalosis, 446
- Mixed abnormalities, 447
- Respiratory acidosis, 447
- Respiratory alkalosis, 447

Blood culture
- Positive, 303

Electrolytes
- Hypercalcaemia, 767
- Hypocalcaemia, 768
- Hyperkalaemia, 442
- Hypokalaemia, 440
- Hypermagnesaemia, 448
- Hypomagnesaemia, 448
- Hypernatraemia, 439
- Hyponatraemia, 437
- Hyperphosphataemia, 449
- Hypophosphataemia, 448

Erythrocyte sedimentation rate
- Raised, 85

Full blood count
- Anaemia, 1001
- Leucocytosis, 1005
- Leucopenia, 1004
- Pancytopenia, 1008
- Polycythaemia, 1003
- Thrombocytopenia, 1007
- Thrombocytosis, 1008

Glucose
- Hyperglycaemia, 808, 818
- Hypoglycaemia, 783, 814

Hormones
- Hyperprolactinaemia, 790
- Hypogonadism, male, 760
- Hypothyroidism, 743
- Thyroid function tests
  - Asymptomatic abnormalities, 745
- Thyrotoxicosis, 740

Lipids, 453
- Hypercholesterolaemia, 453
- Hypertriglyceridaemia, 455
- Mixed hyperlipidaemia, 455
- Rare hyperlipidaemia, 455

Liver function tests, 935

Proteinuria, 476

Radiology
- Adrenal mass, 779
- Incidental pulmonary nodule, 660
- Pituitary tumour, 789

Symptoms and signs

Amenorrhoea, 759

Ascites, 938

Blackouts, 554, 1157

Bleeding
- Gastrointestinal, 853, 942
- Generalised, 201, 1006

Breathlessness, 289, 543, 655

Chest pain, 539, 658

Coma, 198, 1159, 1237

Constipation, 860

Cough, 289, 654

Deafness, 1173

Diarrhoea, 306, 857

Dizziness, 173, 554, 1157, 1167

Dyspepsia, 852

Dysphagia, 851, 1173

Erectile dysfunction, 474

Falls, 172, 554, 1157

Fever, 296
- In immunocompromised host, 301, 396
- In injection drug user, 299
- In neutropenic patient, 302
- With weight loss, 271

Finger clubbing, 271

Gait abnormalities, 1168

Galactorrhoea, 790

Genital problems, 415, 417
- Itch/pain in women, 418
- Itch/rash in men, 415
- Lumps in men, 416
- Lumps in women, 418
- Ulceration in men, 415
- Ulceration in women, 418
- Urethral discharge, 415
- Vaginal discharge, 417

Goitre, 746

Gynaecomastia, 762

Haemoptysis, 658

Hair and nail problems, 1264

Heart murmurs and abnormal heart sounds, 560

Heartburn, 852

Hepatomegaly, 938

Hirsutism, 763

Hypertension, 478

Incontinence
- Faecal, 1174
- Urinary, 175, 472, 1174

Infertility, 761

Jaundice, 936

Lymphadenopathy, 395, 1005

Memory loss, 1161

Movement and coordination problems, 1165, 1237

Nausea, 289, 306, 853
Oedema, 478
Pain, 284
- Abdominal, 418, 861
- Ankle and foot, 1076
- Back, 1072
- Elbow, 1075
- Generalised musculoskeletal, 1071, 1076
- Hand and wrist, 1075
- Headache, 1156, 1237
- Hip, 1075
- Knee, 1075
- Loin, 471
- Multiple joints, 1069
- Neck, 1074
- Regional musculoskeletal, 1074
- Shoulder, 1074
- Single joint, 1069

Palpable mass, 270
Palpitation, 556
Pleural effusion, 661
Psychological
- Abnormal perception, 1167
- Anxiety, 234, 290
- Confusion, agitation, delirium, 173, 237, 238, 290, 1161, 1175
- Delusions, 236, 1175
- Depressed mood, 235, 290, 1175
- Elated mood, 235
- Hallucinations, 236, 1175
- Personality change, 1175

Puberty
- Delayed, 758

Seizures, 1159, 1237
Sensory disturbance, 1164
Skin problems, 1256
- Blisters, 1258
- Colour change, 1263
- Itch (pruritus), 415, 418, 1258
- Leg ulcers, 1262
- Lumps and changing lesions, 1256
- Papulosquamous rashes, 1257
- Photosensitivity, 1260

Sleep disturbance, 1175
Smell disturbance, 1169
Speech disturbance, 1168, 1236
Splenomegaly, 1006
Syncope *see Falls and Blackouts*
Urinary symptoms, 471
- Dysuria, 471
- Frequency, 472
- Haematuria, 474
- Incontinence, 175, 472, 1174
- Nocturia, 472
- Oliguria/anuria, 471
- Polyuria, 472

Visual disturbance, 1169, 1237
Vomiting, 289, 306, 853
Weakness, 290, 1076, 1162, 1236
Weight loss, 271, 290, 396, 859

Syndromes

Adrenal insufficiency, 777
Ageing problems, 176
Alcohol misuse, 240
Allergy, 90
Anaphylaxis, 91, 190
Angioedema, 93
Cardiac arrest, 557
Circulatory failure
- Anaphylaxis, 91, 190
- Shock, 190, 544

Cushing's syndrome, 773
Diabetes mellitus, 808
- Complications, 820
- Hyperosmolarity, 814
- In pregnancy, 817
- In young patients, 818
- Ketoacidosis, 811
- Long-term supervision, 811
- Newly discovered, 808
- Peri-operative, 818

Disseminated intravascular coagulation, 201, 1007
Drug reactions
- Adverse reactions, 175
- Glucocorticoids/corticosteroids, 776

Ectopic hormone production, 271
Fracture, 1071
Gastrointestinal and liver abnormalities in critical illness, 198
Gastrointestinal obstruction in terminal illness, 290
Heart failure, 546
Hepatic encephalopathy, 941
HIV/AIDS manifestations, 395
- Cardiac, 405
- Gastrointestinal, 399
- Haematological, 404
- Liver, 400
- Mucocutaneous, 396
- Neoplasms, 405
- Nervous system, 402
- Ophthalmic, 402
- Renal, 405
- Respiratory, 400
- Rheumatological, 404

Hypopituitarism, 787
Infection manifestations
- In adolescence, 313
- In blood disease, 1008
- In pregnancy, 313
- In the tropics, 308
- Recurrent, 79

Liver failure
- Acute, 932

Malabsorption, 857
Paraneoplastic syndromes, 271
Proctitis, 417
Psychological
- Medically unexplained symptoms, 236
- Psychological factors affecting medical conditions, 240

Renal failure
- Acute, 197, 478
- Chronic, 483

Respiratory failure, 191, 663
Self-harm, 238
Sepsis, 200, 304
Skin
- Acute failure, 1264

Skin manifestations of cancer, 272
Sodium depletion, 432
Sodium excess, 434
Substance misuse, 240
Sudden death, 557
Venous thrombosis, 1008

Contributors

Albiruni Ryan Abdul Razak
MRCPI
Consultant Medical Oncologist, Princess Margaret Cancer Centre, Toronto; Assistant Professor, University of Toronto, Canada

Brian J. Angus
BSc DTM&H FRCP MD FFTM(Glas)
Reader in Infectious Diseases, Nuffield Department of Medicine, University of Oxford; Director, Oxford Centre for Tropical Medicine, UK

Quentin M. Anstee
BSc MBBS PhD MRCP(UK)
Senior Lecturer, Institute of Cellular Medicine, Newcastle University, Newcastle upon Tyne; Honorary Consultant Hepatologist, Freeman Hospital, Newcastle upon Tyne, UK

Andrew W. Bradbury
BSc MBChB(Hons) MD MBA FEBVS(Hon) FRCSE
Sampson Gamgee Professor of Vascular Surgery, Director of Quality Assurance and Enhancement, College of Medical and Dental Sciences, University of Birmingham, UK

Leslie Burnett
MBBS PhD FRCPA FHGSA
Consultant Pathologist, NSW Health, PaLMS Pathology North, Royal North Shore Hospital, Sydney; Clinical Professor in Pathology and Genetic Medicine, Sydney Medical School, University of Sydney, Australia

Mark Byers
OBE FRCGP MCEM MFSEM DA(UK)
General Practitioner, Ministry of Defence, UK

Jenny I.O. Craig
MD FRCPE FRCPath
Consultant Haematologist, Addenbrooke's Hospital, Cambridge, UK

Allan D. Cumming
BSc MD FRCPE
Dean of Students, College of Medicine and Veterinary Medicine, University of Edinburgh, UK

Graham Dark
MBBS FRCP FHEA
Senior Lecturer in Cancer Education, Newcastle University; Consultant Medical Oncologist, Freeman Hospital, Newcastle upon Tyne, UK

Richard J. Davenport
FRCPE DM
Consultant Neurologist, Royal Infirmary of Edinburgh and Western General Hospital, Edinburgh; Honorary Senior Lecturer, University of Edinburgh, UK

Robert S. Dawe
MD FRCPE
Consultant Dermatologist, Ninewells Hospital and Medical School, Dundee; Honorary Clinical Reader, University of Dundee, UK

David Dockrell
MD FRCPI FRCPG FACP
Professor of Infectious Diseases, University of Sheffield, UK

Michael J. Field
AM MD FRACP
Emeritus Professor, Sydney Medical School, University of Sydney, Australia

David R. FitzPatrick
MD FRCPE
Consultant in Clinical Genetics, Royal Hospital for Sick Children, Edinburgh; Professor, University of Edinburgh, UK

Jane Goddard
PhD FRCPE
Consultant Nephrologist, Royal Infirmary of Edinburgh; Part-time Senior Lecturer, University of Edinburgh, UK

Neil R. Grubb
MD FRCP
Consultant Cardiologist, Edinburgh Heart Centre; Honorary Senior Lecturer, University of Edinburgh, UK

Phil Hanlon
BSc MD MPH
Professor of Public Health, University of Glasgow, UK

Richard P. Hobson
PhD MCRP(UK), FRCPath
Consultant Microbiologist, Leeds Teaching Hospitals NHS Trust; Honorary Senior Lecturer, Leeds University, UK

Sally H. Ibbotson
BSc(Hons) MD FRCPE
Clinical Senior Lecturer in Photobiology, University of Dundee; Honorary Consultant Dermatologist, Ninewells Hospital and Medical School, Dundee, UK

J. Alastair Innes
BSc MBChB PhD FRCPE
Consultant Physician, Western General Hospital, Edinburgh; Honorary Reader in Respiratory Medicine, University of Edinburgh, UK

David E. Jones
MA BM BCh PhD FRCP
Professor of Liver Immunology, Institute of Cellular Medicine, Newcastle University, Newcastle upon Tyne; Consultant Hepatologist, Freeman Hospital, Newcastle upon Tyne, UK

Peter Langhorne
PhD FRCPG
Professor of Stroke Care, University of Glasgow; Honorary Consultant, Royal Infirmary, Glasgow, UK

Stephen M. Lawrie
MD(Hons) FRCPsych FRCPE(Hon)
Head, Division of Psychiatry, School of Clinical Sciences, University of Edinburgh; Honorary Consultant Psychiatrist, Royal Edinburgh Hospital, UK

John Paul Leach
MD FRCPG FRCPE
Consultant Neurologist, Institute of Neuroscience, Southern General Hospital, Glasgow; Honorary Associate Clinical Professor, University of Glasgow, UK

Charlie W. Lees
MBBS FRCPE PhD
Consultant Gastroenterologist, Western General Hospital, Edinburgh; Honorary Senior Lecturer, University of Edinburgh, UK

Gary Maartens
MBChB MMed
Consultant Physician, Department of Medicine, Groote Schuur Hospital, Cape Town; Professor of Clinical Pharmacology, University of Cape Town, South Africa

Helen M. Macdonald
BSc(Hons) PhD MSc RNutr(Public Health)
Chair in Nutrition and Musculoskeletal Health, University of Aberdeen, UK

Lynn M. Manson
MD FRCPE FRCPath
Consultant Haematologist, Scottish National Blood Transfusion Service; Honorary Clinical Senior Lecturer, University of Edinburgh, UK

Sara E. Marshall
FRCPE FRCPath PhD
Honorary Consultant Immunologist, NHS Tayside; Professor of Clinical Immunology, University of Dundee, UK

Simon Maxwell
MD PhD FRCP FRCPE FBPharmacolS FHEA
Professor of Student Learning (Clinical Pharmacology and Prescribing), University of Edinburgh; Honorary Consultant Physician, Western General Hospital, Edinburgh, UK

Rory J. McCrimmon
MD FRCPE
Professor of Experimental Diabetes and Metabolism, University of Dundee; Honorary Consultant, Ninewells Hospital and Medical School, Dundee, UK

Iain B. McInnes
FRCP PhD FRSE FMedSci
Muirhead Professor of Medicine and Director of Institute of Infection, Immunity and Inflammation, College of Medical, Veterinary and Life Sciences, University of Glasgow, UK

David E. Newby
FESC FACC FMedSci FRSE
British Heart Foundation John Wheatley Professor of Cardiology, University of Edinburgh; Consultant Cardiologist, Royal Infirmary of Edinburgh, UK

John D. Newell-Price
MA PhD FRCP
Reader in Endocrinology and Honorary Consultant Endocrinologist, Department of Human Metabolism, School of Medicine and Biomedical Science, Sheffield, UK

Graham R. Nimmo
MD FRCPE FFARCSI FFICM
Consultant Physician in Intensive Care Medicine and Clinical Education, Western General Hospital, Edinburgh, UK

Simon I.R. Noble
MBBS MD FRCP Dip Pal Med PGCE
Clinical Senior Lecturer in Palliative Medicine, Cardiff University; Honorary Consultant, Palliative Medicine, Royal Gwent Hospital, Newport, UK

David R. Oxenham
MRCP
Consultant in Palliative Care, Marie Curie Hospice, Edinburgh; Honorary Senior Lecturer, University of Edinburgh, UK

Ewan R. Pearson
PhD FRCPE
Professor of Diabetic Medicine, University of Dundee; Honorary Consultant in Diabetes, Ninewells Hospital and Medical School, Dundee, UK

Ian D. Penman
BSc MD FRCPE
Consultant Gastroenterologist, Royal Infirmary of Edinburgh; Honorary Senior Lecturer, University of Edinburgh, UK

Stuart H. Ralston
MD FRCP FMedSci FRSE
Arthritis Research UK Professor of Rheumatology, University of Edinburgh; Honorary Consultant Rheumatologist, Western General Hospital, Edinburgh, UK

Peter T. Reid
MD FRCPE
Consultant Physician, Western General Hospital, Edinburgh; Honorary Senior Lecturer in Respiratory Medicine, University of Edinburgh, UK

Gordon R. Scott
BSc FRCP
Consultant in Genitourinary Medicine, Chalmers Sexual Health Centre, Edinburgh; Honorary Senior Lecturer, University of Edinburgh, UK

Jonathan R. Seckl
BSc MBBS PhD FRCPE FMedSci FRSE
Professor of Molecular Medicine, Executive Dean (Medicine) and Vice-Principal (Research), University of Edinburgh; Honorary Consultant Physician, Royal Infirmary of Edinburgh, UK

Michael Sharpe
MA MD FRCP FRCPE FRCPsych
Professor of Psychological Medicine, University of Oxford; Honorary Professor, University of Edinburgh; Honorary Consultant in Psychological Medicine, Oxford University Hospitals NHS Trust and Oxford Health NHS Foundation Trust, UK

Peter Stewart
FRACP FRCPA MBA
Clinical Director, Sydney South West Pathology Service; Clinical Associate Professor, University of Sydney, Australia

Mark W.J. Strachan
MD FRCPE
Consultant in Diabetes and Endocrinology, Western General Hospital, Edinburgh; Honorary Professor, University of Edinburgh, UK

David Sullivan
FRACP FRCPA FCSANZ
Clinical Associate Professor, Central Clinical School, Sydney Medical School, University of Sydney, Australia

Shyam Sundar
MD FRCP FNA
Professor of Medicine, Institute of Medical Sciences, Banaras Hindu University, Varanasi, India

Simon H.L. Thomas
BSc MD FRCP FRCPE
Consultant Physician, Newcastle Hospitals NHS Foundation Trust; Professor of Clinical Pharmacology and Therapeutics, Newcastle University, Newcastle upon Tyne, UK

A. Neil Turner
PhD FRCP
Professor of Nephrology, University of Edinburgh; Honorary Consultant Physician, Royal Infirmary of Edinburgh, UK

Simon W. Walker
DM FRCPath FRCPE
Senior Lecturer in Clinical Biochemistry, University of Edinburgh; Honorary Consultant Clinical Biochemist, Royal Infirmary of Edinburgh, UK

Tim Walsh
BSc(Hons) MBChB(Hons) FRCA FRCP FFICM MD MRes
Professor of Critical Care, University of Edinburgh; Honorary Consultant, Royal Infirmary of Edinburgh, UK

Henry Watson
MD FRCPE FRCPath
Consultant Haematologist, Aberdeen Royal Infirmary; Honorary Senior Lecturer, University of Aberdeen, UK

Julian White
MD FACTM
Consultant Clinical Toxinologist and Head of Toxinology, Women's and Children's Hospital, Adelaide; Associate Professor, Department of Paediatrics, University of Adelaide, Australia

John P.H. Wilding
DM FRCP
Professor of Medicine, Head of Department of Obesity and Endocrinology, Institute of Ageing and Chronic Disease, University of Liverpool; Honorary Consultant Physician, University Hospital Aintree, Liverpool, UK

Miles D. Witham
BM BCh PhD FRCPE
Clinical Senior Lecturer in Ageing and Health, University of Dundee; Honorary Consultant Geriatrician, NHS Tayside, Dundee, UK

International Advisory Board

O.C. Abraham
Professor, Department of Medicine, Christian Medical College, Vellore, India

Tofayel Ahmed
Professor of Medicine, Somaj Vittik Medical College, Gono Bishwabidyalay, Dhaka; Professor of Medicine, Pioneer Dental College, Dhaka, Bangladesh

Samar Banerjee
Professor, Department of Medicine, Vivekananda Institute of Medical Sciences and Ramakrishna Mission Seva Pratishthan, Kolkata, India

Matthew A. Brown
Professor of Immunogenetics and Director, University of Queensland Diamantina Institute, Translational Research Institute, University of Queensland, Brisbane, Australia

Khalid I. Bzeizi
Senior Consultant and Head of Hepatology, Prince Sultan Military Medical City, Riyadh, Saudi Arabia

M.K. Daga
Director, Professor of Medicine and In-Charge ICU, Maulana Azad Medical College, New Delhi, India

D. Dalus
Professor and Head, Department of Internal Medicine, Medical College and Hospital, Trivandrum, India

Tapas Das
Professor, Department of Medicine, KPC Medical College and Hospital, Jadavpur, Kolkata, India

Tarun Kumar Dutta
Head, Division of Clinical Haematology; Professor and Head, Department of Medicine, Jawaharlal Institute of Postgraduate Medical Education and Research (JIPMER), Puducherry, India

M. Abul Faiz
Professor of Medicine (Retired), Sir Salimullah Medical College, Mitford, Dhaka, Bangladesh

Albert G. Frauman
Professor of Clinical Pharmacology and Therapeutics, University of Melbourne; Medical Director, Austin Centre for Clinical Studies, Austin Health, Heidelberg, Victoria, Australia

Tsuguya Fukui
President, St Luke's International Hospital, Tokyo, Japan

Hadi A. Goubran
Haematologist, Saskatoon Cancer Centre and Adjunct Professor, College of Medicine, University of Saskatchewan, Canada; Professor of Medicine and Haematology, Cairo University, Egypt

Saman B. Gunatilake
Professor of Medicine, Faculty of Medical Sciences, University of Sri Jayewardenepura, Sri Lanka

Rajiva Gupta
Director and Head, Rheumatology and Clinical Immunology, Medanta - The Medicity, Gurgaon, India

S.M. Wasim Jafri
Alticharn Professor of Medicine, Associate Dean, Aga Khan University, Karachi, Pakistan

Saroj Jayasinghe
Professor, Department of Clinical Medicine, Faculty of Medicine, University of Colombo; Honorary Consultant Physician, National Hospital of Sri Lanka, Colombo, Sri Lanka

A.L. Kakrani
Professor and Head, Department of Medicine, Padmashree Dr D.Y. Patil Medical College and Hospital, Pimpri, Pune, India

Vasantha Kamath
Director–Dean, Karnataka Institute of Medical Sciences (KIMS), Hubli, Karnataka, India

Piotr Kuna
Professor of Medicine, Department of Internal Medicine, Asthma and Allergy, Barlicki University Hospital, Medical University of Lodz, Poland

Introduction

The first section of the book, 'Principles of Medicine', describes the basis on which medicine is practised and the fundamental mechanisms determining health and disease which are relevant to all medical specialties. The second section, 'Practice of Medicine', is devoted to individual medical specialties. Each chapter has been written by experts in the field to provide the level of detail expected of trainees in their discipline. To maintain the book's virtue of being concise, care has been taken to avoid unnecessary duplication between chapters.

The system-based chapters follow a standard format, beginning with an overview of relevant clinical examination, followed by an account of functional anatomy, physiology and investigations, then the common presentations of disease, and details of the individual diseases and treatments of that system. Where appropriate, the chapters in the first section follow a similar format; in chapters which describe the immunological, cellular and molecular basis of disease, this problem-based approach brings the close links between modern medical science and clinical practice into sharp focus.

The methods used to present information are described below.

Clinical examination overviews

The value of good clinical skills is highlighted by a two-page overview of the important elements of the clinical examination at the beginning of most chapters. The left-hand page includes a mannikin to illustrate key steps in examination of the relevant system, beginning with simple observations and progressing in a logical sequence around the body. The right-hand page expands on selected themes and includes tips on examination technique and interpretation of physical signs. These overviews are intended to act as an aide-mémoire and not as a replacement for a detailed text on clinical examination, as provided in the sister title, *Macleod's Clinical Examination*.

Presenting problems

Medical students and junior doctors must not only learn a great many facts about various disorders, but also develop an analytical approach to formulating a differential diagnosis and a plan of investigation for patients who present with particular symptoms or signs. In *Davidson's* this is addressed by incorporating a 'Presenting Problems' section into all system-based chapters. Nearly 300 presentations are included, which represent the most common reasons for referral to each medical specialty. The same approach has been used in several of the chapters in the 'Principles of Medicine' section, to reinforce the close connection between clinical problems and fundamental mechanisms of disease. Many patients present with symptoms such as weight loss, dizziness or breathlessness, which are not specific to a particular system; these are described in the most relevant chapter and cross-referenced elsewhere. A list of presenting problems may be found on pages vii–viii.

Boxes

Boxes are a popular way of presenting information and are particularly useful for revision. They are classified by the type of information they contain, using specific symbols.

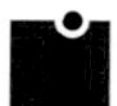

General Information

These include causes, clinical features, investigations, treatments and other useful information.

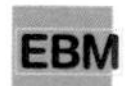

Evidence-based Medicine

Clinicians base their practice on the best available evidence, which needs to be up to date, relevant, authoritative and easily accessible. Over 120 evidence-based medicine (EBM) boxes are included in this edition. They contain recommendations that are supported by evidence obtained from meta-analysis of several randomised controlled trials (RCTs) or one (or more) high-quality RCT, and therefore conform to 'Grade A' criteria, as described in Chapter 1 (p. 8).

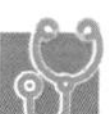

Practice Point

There are many practical skills that students and doctors must learn. These vary from inserting a nasogastric tube to reading an ECG or X-ray, or interpreting investigations such as arterial blood gases or thyroid function tests. 'Practice Point' boxes provide straightforward guidance on how these and many other skills can be acquired and applied.

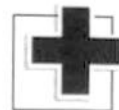

Emergency

These boxes describe management of many of the most common emergencies in medicine.

In Old Age

In most developed countries, older people comprise 20% of the population and are the chief users of health care. While they contract the same diseases as those who are younger, there are often important differences in the way they present and how they are best managed.

Chapter 7, 'Ageing and Disease', concentrates on the principles of managing the frailest group who suffer from multiple comorbidity and disability, and who tend to present with non-specific problems such as falls or delirium. However, many older people also suffer from specific single-organ pathology. 'In Old Age' boxes are thus included in each chapter and describe common presentations, implications of physiological changes of ageing, effects of age on investigations, problems of treatment in old age, and the benefits and risks of intervention in older people.

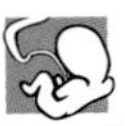

In Pregnancy

Many conditions are different in the context of pregnancy, while some arise only during or shortly after pregnancy. Particular care must be taken with investigations (for example, to avoid radiation exposure to the fetus) and treatment (to avoid the use of drugs which harm the fetus). These issues are highlighted by 'In Pregnancy' boxes distributed throughout the book.

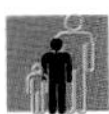

In Adolescence

Although Paediatric Medicine is not covered in *Davidson's*, many chronic disorders begin in childhood and adult physicians often contribute to multidisciplinary teams that manage young patients 'in transition' between paediatric and adult health-care services. This group of patients often presents a particular challenge, due to the physiological and psychological changes that occur in adolescence and which can have a major impact on the disease and its management. Adolescents can be encouraged to take over responsibility from their parents/carers in managing their disease, but are naturally rebellious and often struggle to adhere to the impositions of chronic treatment. To highlight these issues, we have introduced this new box format in the 22nd Edition.

Terminology

Recommended International Non-proprietary Names (rINNs) are used for all drugs, with the exception of adrenaline and noradrenaline. However, British spellings have been retained for drug classes and groups (e.g. amphetamines not amfetamines).

Units of measurement

The International System of Units (SI units) is the recommended means of presentation for laboratory data and has been used throughout *Davidson's*. However, we recognise that many laboratories around the world continue to provide data in non-SI units, so these have been included in the text for the commonly measured analytes. Both SI and non-SI units are also given in Chapter 29, which describes the reference ranges used in Edinburgh's laboratories. It should be appreciated that these reference ranges may vary from those used in other laboratories.

Finding what you are looking for

A contents list is given on the opening page of each chapter. In addition, the book contains numerous cross-references to help readers find their way around, along with an extensive index of over 15 000 subject entries. The online text available on StudentConsult (www.studentconsult.com) allows for detailed searches of the content by keyword. A list of up-to-date reviews and useful websites with links to management guidelines appears at the end of each chapter.

Acknowledgements

We are indebted to former authors who have stepped down from this edition. They include Dr Chris M.C. Allen, Dr Jeffrey K. Aronson, Dr Jane Collier, Professor Martin Dennis, Professor Michael Doherty, Professor B. Miles Fisher, Professor Brian M. Frier, Dr Ian Grant, Professor Christian J. Lueck, Dr Brian McClelland, Dr Kelvin Palmer, Professor Jonathan Rees, Dr Olivia Schofield, Mr Laurence H. Stewart, Dr George Webster and Dr Edmund Wilkins.

We are grateful to members of the International Advisory Board, all of whom provided detailed suggestions which have improved the book. Several members have stepped down and we would like to thank them for their support during the preparation of previous editions. They include Professor Jan D. Bos, Professor Y.C. Chee, Professor W.F. Mollentze, Professor Dato' Tahir Azhar, Professor C.F. Van der Merwe, Dr G. Wittert and Professor M.E. Yeolekar.

Detailed chapter reviews were commissioned to help plan this new edition and we would like to acknowledge all those who assisted, including Dr Sam Alfred, Dr Rustam Al-Shahi Salman, Professor Harry Campbell, Dr Richard Casasola, Dr Gavin Clunie, Professor Michael Eddleston, Dr Catherine Elliot, Professor David Gawkrodger, Professor Jeremy Hall, Dr Amy Hughes, Professor Alan Jardine, Dr Uwe Kornak, Dr Stuart McLellan, Dr Scott Murray, Dr Rak Nandwani, Dr David Patch, Professor Donald Salter, Professor John Simpson, Mr Grant Stewart and Professor Ian Weller.

As part of the publisher's review, students and doctors from medical schools in the UK, Europe, Africa and Asia have provided valuable feedback on this textbook and their comments have helped shape this new edition. We hope we have listed all those who have contributed and apologise if any names have been accidentally omitted. We are indebted to the following for their enthusiastic support: Alessandro Aldera, Sabreen Ali, Syed Hyder Ali, Ashish Kumar Amant, Abdullah Ansaari, Ruhith Ariyapala, James Armstrong, Charu Dutt Arora, Akshay Athreya, Gavin Baillie, Anna Kate Barton, Kapil Battista, Katrina Bell, Andrew Beverstock, B. Bharadwaj, Charlie Billington, Lili Bird, Dwaipayan Biswas, Rudradeep Biswas, Sagnik Biswas, Tamoghna Biswas, Tom Brazel, Mark Karlsson Cairns, Rachel Callaghan, Elizabeth Carr, Richard Cassidy, Yen-Jei Chen, Sudip Chowdhury, Sarah Clay, Danielle Clyde, Andrew Cochrane, Amanda Collins, Guy Conlon, India Cox, Prafulla M. Davangere, Emma Donoghue, Kate Doughty, Jemima Horsley Downie, Simon Durkin, Padmaraj Duvvuri, Ahmad Farooqui, Ruth Fergie, Alice Finlayson, James Fraser, Saad Ahmed Fyyaz, David Gall, Raj Ghoniya, Alice Graham, Paul Gray, Vaibhav Gupta, Vibhuti Gupta, Sarah Guthrie, Ailsa Hamilton, V. Harivanzan, David Haunschmidt, Sandipan Hazra, Francesca Heard, Elizabeth Hird, Bernard Ho, Prerana Huddar, Catherine Humphreys, Adam Hunter, James Hyman, Pankaj Insan, Hemant Iqbal, Neethu Isac, David W. Jack, Ben Jacka, Aasems Jacob, Namrata Joshi, Sonal Sanjay Kadu, Rajdeep Kaur, Amit Kaura, Patrick Kearns, Rahul Khanna, Robert Kimmitt, Omkar Kulkarni, Dinesh Kumar, D. Praveen Kumar, Raghvendra Kumar, Sudhir Kumar, Vishan Lal, Sarah Langlands, Kristina Lee, Jade Liew, Xuxin Lim, Marie-Pier Lirette, Michael Lowe, Stephanie Lua, Jill Macfarlane, Piyush Madaan, Karan Malhotra, Kathryn Maltby, Manu Easow Mathew, Andrew McCulloch, James McDonald, Katy McFadyen, Aaron McLean, Bruce McLintock, Neil McNiven, Sriharsha Merugu, B.N. Mishra, Kevin Mohee, Turlough Montague, Brian Morrissey, Mohammed Abdul Muqeeth, Nikhil Narayanaswamy, Dima Nassif, Vijay Negalur, Anup Netravalkar, Douglas Newlands, Tahseen Nishath, Anna O'Donoghue, Francis O'Hanlon, Anas Onmu, Kate O'Sullivan, Vishal Pandit, Neena Kirit Pankhania, Satvik Patel, Tom Paterson, Abigail Paul, Christopher Pennington, Sinead Philip, Lowri Phillips, Rory Piper, Rachel Poffley, Michael Poon, Gyan Prakash, Harsh Priya, Zara Qureshi, G. Raaja, Adithi S. Raghavan, Arrvind Raghunath, Nidhi Rai, Gomathi Ravula, Chaitanya Reddy, Abhishek Roy, Suhel Abbas Sabunwala, Sanghamitra Samanta, Somya Saxena, Jenna Schafers, Victoria Scott, Sanket Shah, Aitha Shiva, Peng Yong Sim, Ajay Paul Singh, Nikita Nilabh Singh, Kiran Kumar Singuru, Reetu Sinha, Andrew Smith, Amanda Swan, Shabiullah Syyed, Callum Taylor, Iain Tennant, Nailesh Thozanenjan, Jason Ting, Kathleen Tinkler, Prasanna S. Vadhan, Ela Varasi, Siddarth Varshney, Arun Kumar Vasa, Monica Vijayakumar, Andrew Wilson, Vincent Wong, James Wood, Sara Zafar and Jim Zhong.

We would like to extend our thanks to the many readers who contacted us with suggestions for improvements. Their input has been invaluable and is much appreciated; they are unfortunately too numerous to mention individually.

We are grateful to colleagues who have generously provided many of the illustrations that appear in this edition. They are acknowledged on the next page.

We are especially grateful to all those working for Churchill Livingstone, in particular Laurence Hunter, Wendy Lee and Robert Britton, for their endless support and expertise in the shaping, collation and illustration of this edition. We would also like to thank Louisa Talbott for her efficient project management, Susan Boobis for her labours in compiling the extensive index and Ruth Noble for expert proofreading.

BRW, NRC, SHR, IDP
Edinburgh

Figure acknowledgements

Figures reproduced with the publisher's permission are listed at the end of each chapter. We are also grateful to the following individuals and organisations for the loan of illustrations:

Fig. 5.18A Institute of Ophthalmology, Moorfields Eye Hospital, London.

Fig. 6.9 Disc kindly supplied by Charlotte Symes.

Figs 10.4, 10.5AB Dr J. Xuereb.

Fig. 11.5 Dr J. Wilsdon, Freeman Hospital, Newcastle upon Tyne.

Page 294 insets (splinter haemorrhages) Dr Nick Beeching, Royal Liverpool University Hospital; (*Roth's spots*) Prof. Ian Rennie, Royal Hallamshire Hospital, Sheffield. *Page 295* (*streptococcal toxic shock syndrome, meningococcal sepsis, shingles*), *Fig. 13.1 inset* (*cellulitis of the leg*), *Figs 13.6ABD, 13.20, 13.44B, 13.45B, 13.51* Dr Ravi Gowda, Royal Hallamshire Hospital, Sheffield. *Fig. 13.1 insets* (*pulmonary tuberculosis*) Dr Ann Chapman, Royal Hallamshire Hospital, Sheffield; (*empyema, pyogenic liver abscess, diverticular abscess, tuberculous osteomyelitis*) Dr Robert Peck, Royal Hallamshire Hospital, Sheffield. *Fig. 13.3C* Dr Julia Greig, Royal Hallamshire Hospital, Sheffield. *Fig. 13.6C* Dr Rattanaphone Phetsouvanh, Mahosot Hospital, Vientiane, PDR Laos. *Fig. 13.14* Prof. Goura Kudesia, Northern General Hospital, Sheffield. *Fig. 13.29* Institute of Ophthalmology, Moorfields Eye Hospital, London. *Fig. 13.33 insets* (*malaria retinopathy*) Dr Nicholas Beare, Royal Liverpool University Hospital; (*blood films of* P. vivax *and* P. falciparum) Dr Kamolrat Silamut, Mahidol Oxford Research Unit, Bangkok, Thailand. *Fig. 13.41* Dr S. Sundar and Dr H.W. Murray. *Fig. 13.42B* Dr E.E. Zijlstra. *Fig. 13.53* Dr Wendi Bailey, Liverpool School of Tropical Medicine. *Fig. 13.57 insets* (*dimorphic fungi*) Beatriz Gomez and Angela Restrepo, CIB, Medellín, Colombia.

Page 388 inset (*oral hairy leucoplakia*) Audiovisual Dept, St Mary's Hospital, London.

Fig. 15.4 Dr P. Hay, St George's Hospital, London.

Page 463(4AB) Dr G.M. Iadorola and Dr F. Quarello, G. Bosco Hospital, Turin (from www.sin-italia.org/imago/sediment/sed.htm). *Figs 17.1CE, 17.22ACDE* Dr J.G. Simpson, Aberdeen Royal Infirmary. *Figs 17.3AB, 17.4AB, 17.5, 17.25, 17.27, 17.32AB* Dr A.P. Bayliss and Dr P. Thorpe, Aberdeen Royal Infirmary. *Fig. 17.22F–H* Dr R. Herriot. *Fig. 17.23BC* Dr J. Collar, St Mary's Hospital, London. *Fig. 17.29* Dr P. Robinson, St James's University Hospital, Leeds.

Fig. 18.82E Dr T. Lawton. *Fig. 18.83AB* Dr B. Cullen.

Page 644 insets (*idiopathic kyphoscoliosis*) Dr I. Smith, Papworth Hospital, Cambridge; (*serous, mucopurulent and purulent sputum*) Dr J. Foweraker, Papworth Hospital, Cambridge. *Fig. 19.15* Dr P. Sivasothy, Dept of Respiratory Medicine, Addenbrooke's Hospital, Cambridge. *Fig. 19.26B* British Lung Foundation. *Figs 19.36, 19.58, 19.59, 19.66B* Dr William Wallace, Dept of Pathology, Royal Infirmary of Edinburgh. *Fig. 19.41* Adam Hill. *Fig. 19.44* Mr T. Russell and Dr M. Hanson, Dept of Microbiology, NHS Lothian. *Fig. 19.66A* Dr S. Jackson, Western General Hospital, Edinburgh. *Fig. 19.71* Prof N.J. Douglas.

Fig. 20.4 inset (*toxic multinodular goitre*) Dr P.L. Padfield, Western General Hospital, Edinburgh.

Page 798 inset (*exudative maculopathy*), *page 799* (*background and proliferative retinopathy*) Dr A.W. Patrick and Dr I.W. Campbell. *Fig. 21.4 insets* (*normal islet, beta-cell destruction*) Dr A. Foulis, Dept of Pathology, University of Glasgow.

Fig. 22.14A Given Imaging.

Figs 23.10, 23.34, 23.37, 23.43 Dr D. Redhead, Royal Infirmary of Edinburgh.

Fig. 25.6 Dr I. Beggs; *Fig. 25.7* Dr N. McKay.

Page 1138 insets (*winging of scapula, 12th nerve palsy, wasting of thenar eminence*) Dr R.E. Cull, Western General Hospital, Edinburgh. *Figs 26.12A–C, 26.13A–C* Dr D. Collie. *Fig. 26.22C* Dr B. Cullen. *Fig. 26.27* Prof. D.A.S. Compston. *Fig. 26.29* Dr J. Xuereb.

Figs 27.4AB, 27.9AB Dr A. Farrell and Prof. J. Wardlaw. *Fig. 27.5A–D* Dr D. Collie.

A.D. Cumming
S.I.R. Noble

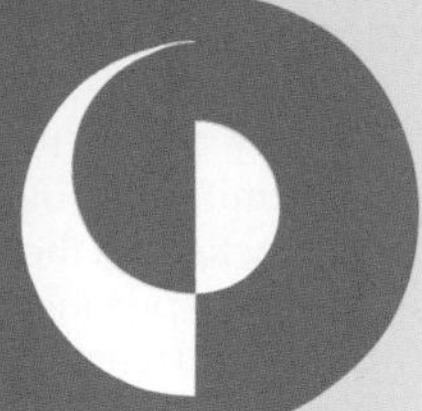

Good medical practice

Medical practice 2
- The doctor–patient relationship 2
- Communication and other clinical skills 4
- Using investigations 4
- Estimating and communicating risk 7
- Clinical decision-making 7
- Practising medicine in low-resource settings 9
- Medical ethics 9
- Medical law 13

Personal and professional development 14

Complementary and alternative medicine 15

Since the time of Hippocrates, the role of the doctor has extended beyond the narrow remit of curing patients of their ailments. Good medical practice, or the art of medicine, hinges on recognising and respecting the breadth of physical, cultural, spiritual, experiential and psychosocial characteristics of each patient, and understanding their impact on the patient's beliefs, attitudes and expectations. Doctors must deliver appropriate care which considers the technical complexities of modern treatment, and at the same time deals with the communication and interpersonal needs of the patient, at a time when he or she may feel most vulnerable. In addition to the diagnosis and treatment of illness, the scope of medicine has expanded to preventing disease through measures such as screening, vaccination and health promotion. Doctors are centrally involved in tackling lifestyle-related issues of the modern world, such as obesity, alcohol excess, cigarette smoking and sexual health.

Medical professionalism has been described in the UK by a Royal College of Physicians working party (2005) as 'a set of values, behaviours and relationships that underpin the trust the public has in doctors'. They stated that doctors should be committed to integrity, compassion, altruism, continuous improvement, excellence, and working in partnership with members of the wider health-care team. They perceived that medical professionalism was relevant to leadership, education, career pathways, appraisal and research.

This chapter outlines how doctors must provide patients and their families with relevant but complex information, discuss management options, and reach appropriate clinical decisions, commensurate with the available resources. It also describes processes to develop, maintain and assure medical professionalism.

MEDICAL PRACTICE

The doctor–patient relationship

The contents of this book are not all based on indisputable contemporary evidence; many reflect wisdom and understanding distilled over hundreds of years and passed from generation to generation of doctors. This perceived wisdom lies at the heart of the way that doctors and patients interact; it demands respect, and if the doctor also displays compassion, sets the scene for the development of trust.

Due to the complexities of many chronic diseases and treatments, and the multifaceted impact of illness on a patient, there is an increasing role for health care to be delivered by a multidisciplinary team (Box 1.1). This model of care recognises the different skills of each allied health professional and focuses patient care beyond surgical procedures or pharmacological manipulation. The doctor usually takes the lead in determining the overall direction of care but must also:

- guide the patient through the unfamiliar landscape, language and customs of clinical care
- interpret, synthesise and convey complex information
- help patients and families to participate fully in the decision-making process.

In many clinical disciplines, doctors from several specialties form a multidisciplinary team in order to formulate a treatment plan. In oncology, for example, this ensures that various modalities of treatment (surgical, oncological and palliative) are considered.

1.1 Members and roles of a multidisciplinary team

Professional	Roles
Doctor	Diagnosis and treatment Overall coordination of care
Specialist nurse	Patient and family support Information-giving
Physiotherapist	Improving physical function Physical rehabilitation
Occupational therapist	Maximising skills and abilities Complex re-enablement
Speech and language therapist	Optimising communication Swallowing assessment
Dietitian	Nutritional advice Parenteral feeding support
Pharmacist	Safe prescribing Complex medicines delivery
Social worker	Coordination of home care Financial advice
Clinical psychologist	Cognitive interventions Psychological support
Pastoral care	Psychological support Spiritual support

The doctor–patient relationship is in itself therapeutic; a successful consultation with a trusted and respected practitioner will have beneficial effects irrespective of any other therapy given. The doctor–patient relationship is multilayered, dynamic and bilateral (Fig. 1.1).

Regulatory bodies, such as the UK General Medical Council, seek to define the medical side of the doctor–patient relationship in terms of the 'Duties of a Doctor' (Box 1.2). It is common for medical schools to require undergraduate students to sign an ethical code of conduct based on statements like this.

Difficulties in the doctor–patient relationship

Regardless of experience and skill, it is inevitable that, at some point in a doctor's career, the doctor–patient relationship will break down. There can be many reasons for this; sometimes, these are beyond the control of the clinician, but often conflict arises when there is a genuine or perceived failure of the doctor to meet one or more of the duties outlined in Box 1.2. It is important to recognise a breakdown in the relationship quickly and, whenever possible, identify the reason. If patients are unhappy with an aspect of their care, they are entitled to a prompt, open, constructive and honest response that includes an explanation and, if appropriate, an apology. It is also important to reassure the patient that the issues raised will not adversely affect their future care.

Often, an acknowledgement that something is wrong and demonstration of a desire to put things right are sufficient to rectify any conflict. However, the longer

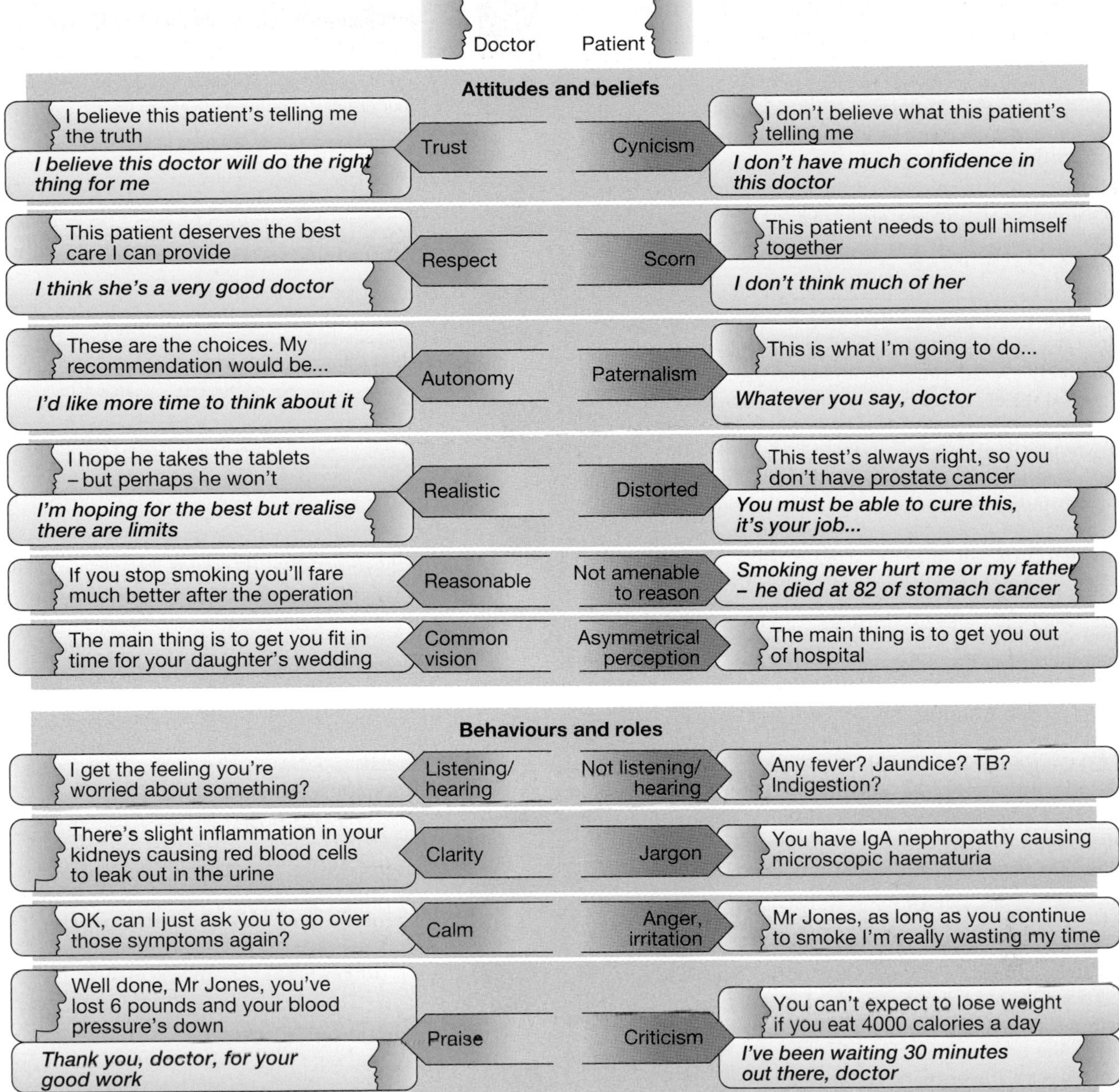

Fig. 1.1 Some aspects of the doctor–patient relationship.

1.2 The duties of a doctor registered with the UK General Medical Council

Patients must be able to trust doctors with their lives and health. To justify that trust you must show respect for human life and make sure your practice meets the standards expected of you in four domains.

Knowledge, skills and performance

- Make the care of your patient your first concern.
- Provide a good standard of practice and care.
  Keep your professional knowledge and skills up to date.
  Recognise and work within the limits of your competence.

Safety and quality

- Take prompt action if you think that patient safety, dignity or comfort is being compromised.
- Protect and promote the health of patients and the public.

Communication, partnership and teamwork

- Treat patients as individuals and respect their dignity.
  Treat patients politely and considerately.
  Respect patients' right to confidentiality.
- Work in partnership with patients.
  Listen to, and respond to, their concerns and preferences.
  Give patients the information they want or need in a way they can understand.
  Respect patients' right to reach decisions with you about their treatment and care.
  Support patients in caring for themselves to improve and maintain their health.
- Work with colleagues in the ways that best serve patients' interests.

Maintaining trust

- Be honest and open and act with integrity.
- Never discriminate unfairly against patients or colleagues.
- Never abuse your patients' trust in you or the public's trust in the profession.

You are personally accountable for your professional practice and must always be prepared to justify your decisions and actions.

one takes to address a problem, the more difficult it becomes to resolve. The patient may continue to be dissatisfied with the doctor and it may be most appropriate for another colleague to take over their care. It is important to reflect on such incidents, to identify whether one would approach a similar challenge differently next time.

Communication and other clinical skills

Communication lies at the heart of good medical practice. The most technically capable clinician will fail in the duty of care if he or she is unable to communicate effectively with patients or relatives, since this is essential for accurate history-taking, information-giving and decision-making. Likewise, the delivery of holistic care requires effective communication with other doctors and members of the multidisciplinary team. Clear and appropriately detailed clinical note-keeping is essential, as are timely and accurate written communications between professionals.

Failures in communication may lead to poor health outcomes, strained working relations, dissatisfaction among patients, their families and health professionals, anger and litigation. The majority of complaints received by health-care professionals could have been avoided by effective communication. Box 1.3 lists some common barriers to good communication.

Developing communication skills to facilitate accurate history-taking and information-giving takes many years and requires frequent personal reflection on previous consultations. A detailed account of history-taking, clinical examination and communication skills is beyond the scope of this chapter but is provided in Davidson's sister book, *Macleod's Clinical Examination*. However, some communication principles are discussed below and these can be applied to most consultations.

The main aim of a medical interview is to establish a factual account of the patient's illness. The clinician must allow the patient to describe the problems without overbearing interrogation, but should try to facilitate the process with appropriate questions (Box 1.4). Techniques such as an unhurried approach, checking prior understanding, making it clear that the interviewer is listening, the use of silence when appropriate, recapping on what has been said, and reflection of key points back to the patient are all important. A major requirement is to express complex information and concepts in language with which the patient can readily engage. Nonverbal communication is equally important. The patient's facial expressions and body language may betray hidden fears. The clinician can help the patient to talk more freely by smiling or nodding appropriately.

Beyond the factual account of symptoms, the clinician should also explore patients' feelings, determine how they interpret their symptoms, unearth their concerns and fears, and explore their expectations before suggesting and agreeing a plan of management. Clinicians should demonstrate understanding, sensitivity and empathy (i.e. imagine themselves in the patient's position). Most patients have more than one concern and will be reluctant to discuss potentially important issues if they feel that the clinician is not interested or is likely to dismiss their complaints as irrational or trivial.

1.3 Some barriers to good communication in health care

The clinician
- Authoritarian or dismissive attitude
- Hurried approach
- Use of jargon
- Inability to speak first language of patient
- No experience of patient's cultural background

The patient
- Anxiety
- Reluctance to discuss sensitive or seemingly trivial issues
- Misconceptions
- Conflicting sources of information
- Cognitive impairment
- Hearing/speech/visual impediment

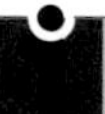

1.4 Communication skills in the medical interview

- **Open questions** allow patients to express their own thoughts and feelings, e.g. 'How have you been since we last saw you?', 'Is there anything else that you want to mention?'
- **Closed questions** are requests for factual information, e.g. 'When did this pain start?'
- **Leading questions** invite specific responses and suggest options, e.g. 'You'll be glad when this treatment is over, won't you?'
- **Reflecting questions** help to develop or expand topics, e.g. 'Can you tell me more about your family?'
- **Active listening** encourages further dialogue, e.g. 'Go on,' 'I see,' 'Hmm' etc.
- **Requesting clarification** encourages further detail, e.g. 'How do mean?', 'In what way?' etc.
- **Summarising** ensures accurate understanding, e.g. 'Tell me if I've got this right.'

Specific communication scenarios, such as breaking bad news or dealing with aggression, require additional targeted strategies (see *Macleod's Clinical Examination*).

While many common clinical conditions can be identified on the basis of the history from the patient, the process of physical examination remains important in most clinical scenarios. Physical examination is an important characteristic of the doctor–patient relationship, at best benefiting from and reinforcing trust, but at worst a focus of complaint when the doctor–patient relationship has not been established or has broken down. Key findings on physical examination pointing to disease in specific body systems are described in the relevant chapters of this book.

Using investigations

Modern medical practice has become dominated by sophisticated and often expensive investigations. It is easy to forget that the judicious use of these tools, and the interpretation of the data that they provide, are crucially dependent on good basic clinical skills. Indeed, a test should only be ordered if it is clear that the result will influence the patient's management and the perceived value of the resulting information exceeds the anticipated discomfort, risk and cost of the procedure. Clinicians should therefore analyse their patient's condition carefully and draw up a provisional management plan before requesting any investigations.

The 'normal' (or reference) range

Although some tests provide qualitative results (present or absent, e.g. faecal occult blood testing, p. 857), most provide quantitative results (i.e. a value on a continuous numeric scale). In order to classify quantitative results as normal or abnormal, it is necessary to define a 'normal range'. Many quantitative measurements in populations exhibit a bell-shaped, or Gaussian, frequency distribution (Fig. 1.2); this is called a 'normal distribution' and is characteristic of biological variables determined by a complex mixture of genetic and environmental factors (e.g. height) and of test results (e.g. plasma sodium concentration). A normal distribution can be described by the mean value (which places the centre of the bell-shaped curve on the x axis) and the standard deviation (SD, which describes the width of the bell-shaped curve). Within each SD away from the mean, there is a fixed percentage of the population. By convention, the 'normal range' is defined as those values which encompass 95% of the population, i.e. the values within 2 SDs above and below the mean. If this convention is used, however, 2.5% of the normal population will have values above, and 2.5% will have values below, the normal range; for this reason, it is more precise to describe 'reference' rather than 'normal' ranges.

'Abnormal' results, i.e. those lying beyond 2 SDs from the mean, may occur either because the person is one of the 2.5% of the normal population whose test result is outside the reference range, or because he or she has a disease characterised by a different result from the test. Test results in 'abnormal' populations also have a bell-shaped distribution with a different mean and SD (see Fig. 1.2). In some diseases, there is typically no overlap between results from the normal and abnormal population (e.g. elevated serum creatinine in renal failure, p. 467). In many diseases, however, there is overlap, sometimes extending into the reference range (e.g. elevated serum thyroxine in toxic multinodular goitre, p. 753). In these circumstances, the greater the difference between the test result and the limits of the reference range, the higher the chance that the person has a disease, but there is a risk that results within the reference range may be 'false negatives' and results outside the reference range may be 'false positives'.

Each time a test is performed in a member of the normal population there is a 5% (1 in 20) chance that the result will be outside the reference range. If two tests are performed, the chance that one of them will be 'abnormal' is 10% (2 in 20), and so on; the chance of an 'abnormal' result increases as more tests are performed, so multiple indiscriminate testing should be avoided.

In practice, reference ranges are usually established by performing the test in a number of healthy volunteers who are assumed to be a random sample of the normal population. Not all populations are the same, however, and while it is common to have different reference ranges for men and women or children and adults, clinicians need to be aware that reference ranges defined either by test manufacturers or even within the local laboratory may have been established in small numbers of healthy young people who are not necessarily representative of their patient population.

For some tests, the clinical decision does not depend on whether or not the patient is a member of the normal population. This commonly applies to quantitative risk factors for future disease. For example, higher plasma total cholesterol levels are associated with a higher risk of future myocardial infarction (p. 583) within the normal population. Although a reference range for cholesterol can be calculated, cholesterol-lowering therapy is commonly recommended for people with values within the reference range; the 'cutoff' value at which therapy is recommended depends upon the presence of other risk factors for cardiovascular disease. The reference range for plasma cholesterol is therefore redundant and the phrase 'normal plasma cholesterol level' is unhelpful. Similar arguments apply for interpretation of values of blood pressure (p. 583), bone mineral density (p. 1065) and so on.

Some quantitative test results are not normally distributed, usually because a substantial proportion of the normal population will have an unrecordably low result (e.g. serum prostate-specific antigen, p. 518), and the distribution cannot be described by mean and SDs. Alternative statistical procedures can be used to calculate 95th centiles, but it is common in these circumstances to use information from normal and abnormal people to identify 'cutoff' values which are associated with a certain risk of disease, as described below.

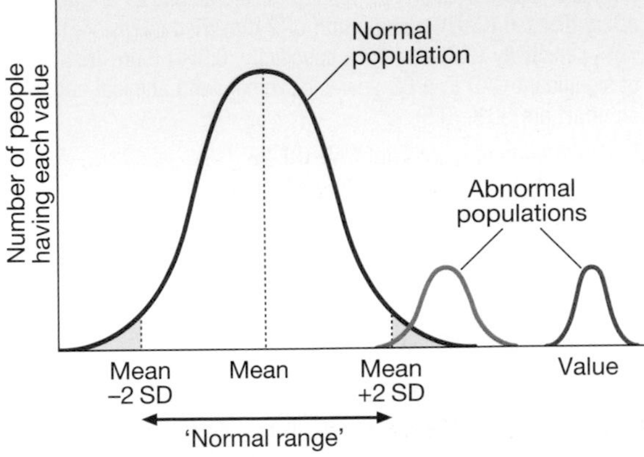

Fig. 1.2 Normal distribution and 'normal' (reference) range. For many tests, the frequency distribution of results in the normal healthy population (red line) is a symmetrical bell-shaped curve. The mean ± 2 standard deviations (SD) encompasses 95% of the normal population and usually defines the 'normal range' (or 'reference range'); 2.5% of the normal population have values above, and 2.5% below, the reference range (shaded areas). For some diseases (blue line), test results overlap with the normal population or even with the reference range. For other diseases (green line), tests may be more reliable because there is no overlap between the normal and abnormal population.

Sensitivity and specificity

No test is completely reliable. All diagnostic tests can produce false positives (an abnormal result in the absence of disease) and false negatives (a normal result in a patient with disease). The diagnostic accuracy of a test can be expressed in terms of its sensitivity and its specificity (Box 1.5).

1.5 The accuracy of diagnostic tests		
	Affected	**Unaffected**
Positive test	True +ve (a)	False +ve (b)
Negative test	False –ve (c)	True –ve (d)
Sensitivity (%) = [a/(a + c)] × 100 Specificity (%) = [d/(b + d)] × 100		
Positive predictive value = a/(a + b) Negative predictive value = d/(c + d)		
Likelihood ratio: positive test = sensitivity/(1 – specificity) negative test = (1 – sensitivity)/specificity		

Sensitivity is defined as the percentage of the test population who are affected by the index condition and test positive for it. In contrast, specificity is defined as the percentage of the test population who are healthy and test negative. A very sensitive test will detect most disease but may generate abnormal findings in healthy people; a negative result will therefore reliably exclude disease but a positive test is likely to require further evaluation. On the other hand, a very specific test may miss significant pathology but is likely to establish the diagnosis, beyond doubt, when the result is positive.

In choosing how a test is used to guide decision-making, there is an inevitable trade-off between emphasising sensitivity versus specificity. For example, defining an exercise electrocardiogram (p. 534) as abnormal if there is at least 0.5 mm ST depression will ensure that very few cases of coronary artery disease are missed but will generate many false-positive tests (high sensitivity, low specificity). On the other hand, a cutoff point of at least 2.0 mm ST depression will detect most cases of important coronary disease with far fewer false-positives. This trade-off can be illustrated by the receiver operating characteristic curve of the test (Fig. 1.3).

Predictive value

The predictive value of a test is determined by its sensitivity and specificity, and can be expressed in several ways. The positive predictive value is the probability that a patient with a positive test has the index condition, while the negative predictive value is the probability that a patient with a negative test does not have the condition (see Box 1.5). The likelihood ratio expresses the odds that a given finding would occur in a patient with, as opposed to a patient without, the index condition (see Box 1.5); as the odds rise above 1, the probability that disease is present rises.

The interpretation and the utility of a test are critically dependent on the circumstances in which it is used. Bayes' theorem dictates that the value of a diagnostic test is determined by the prevalence of the condition in the test population. The probability that a subject has a particular condition (the post-test probability) can be calculated if the pre-test probability and the sensitivity and specificity of the test are known (Box 1.6). A test is most valuable when there is an intermediate pre-test probability of disease. Clinicians seldom have access to such precise information but must appreciate the importance of integrating clinical and laboratory data.

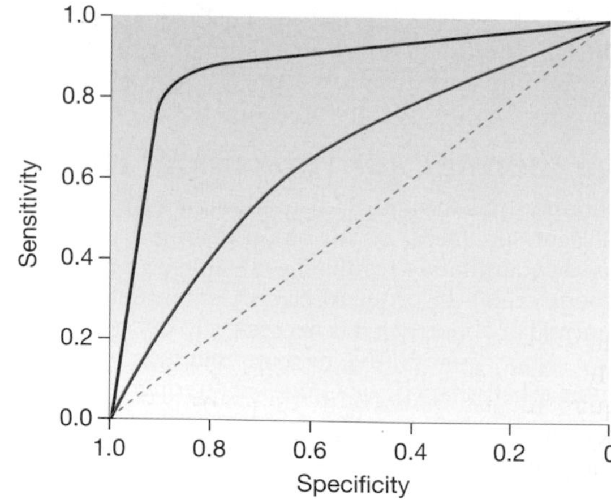

Fig. 1.3 Receiver operating characteristic graphs illustrating the trade-off between sensitivity and specificity for a given test. The curve is generated by 'adjusting' the cutoff values defining normal and abnormal results, calculating the effect on sensitivity and specificity and then plotting these against each other. The closer the curve lies to the top left-hand corner, the more useful the test. The red line illustrates a test with useful discriminant value and the green line illustrates a less useful, poorly discriminant test.

1.6 Bayes' theorem: post-test likelihood of disease

Positive test

$$\text{Post-test probability of disease} = \frac{\text{pre} \times \text{sens}}{(\text{pre} \times \text{sens}) + ((1-\text{sens}) \times (1-\text{spec}))}$$

Negative test

$$\text{Post-test probability of disease} = \frac{\text{pre} \times (1-\text{sens})}{(\text{pre} \times (1-\text{sens})) + ((1-\text{pre}) \times \text{spec})}$$

(pre = pre-test probability of disease; sens = sensitivity; spec = specificity)

Example

Assume: Exercise tolerance testing for the diagnosis of coronary artery disease (CAD) (using cutoff of 2 mm ST depression) has 70% sensitivity (0.7) and 90% specificity (0.9) The pre-test odds of significant CAD in a 65-year-old woman with atypical angina on effort are 50% (0.5)

Post-test odds of significant CAD will be:

$$\text{Positive test } \frac{0.5 \times 0.7}{(0.5 \times 0.7) + (0.3 \times 0.1)} = 92\%$$

$$\text{Negative test } \frac{0.5 \times 0.3}{(0.5 \times 0.3) + (0.5 \times 0.9)} = 25\%$$

In contrast, the pre-test probability of significant coronary disease in a 45-year-old man with typical angina on effort would be 90%, with post-test odds of 95% in the event of a positive exercise test and 75% in the event of a negative test.

Screening

Many health-care systems run screening programmes to detect important (and treatable) disease in apparently healthy but at-risk individuals. These initiatives may be directed towards a single pathology (e.g. mammography for breast cancer, p. 280) or may comprise a battery

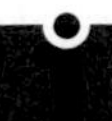

1.7 Factors that influence the cost-effectiveness of screening for a disease

- The prevalence of the disease in the target population
- The cost of the screening test
- The sensitivity and specificity of the screening test
- The availability and effectiveness of treatment
- The cost of not detecting and treating the disease

of tests for a wide range of conditions. Screening inevitably generates a number of false-positive results that require further, potentially expensive and sometimes risky, investigation. This may engender a good deal of anxiety for the patient and create dilemmas for the clinician; for example, it may be difficult to determine how to evaluate minor abnormalities of the liver function tests in an otherwise healthy person (p. 935).

Some of the criteria that must be considered before deciding if the wider costs of a screening programme can be justified are listed in Box 1.7.

Estimating and communicating risk

Medical management decisions are usually made by weighing up the anticipated benefits of a particular procedure or treatment against the potential risks. To allow patients to contribute to the decision-making process, health professionals must be able to explain risk in an accurate and understandable way.

Providing the relevant biomedical facts is seldom sufficient to guide decision-making because a patient's perception of risk is often coloured by emotional, and sometimes irrational, factors. Most patients will have access to information from a wide variety of sometimes conflicting sources, including the Internet, books, magazines, self-help groups, other health-care professionals, friends and family. The clinician must be aware of and sensitive to the way in which these resources influence the individual, while building trust with the patient, clarifying the problem and conveying the key facts.

Research evidence provides statistics but these can be confusing (Box 1.8). Relative risk describes the proportional increase in risk; it is a useful measure of the size of an effect. In contrast, absolute risk describes the actual chance of an event and is what matters to most patients. Terms such as 'common', 'rare', 'probable' and 'unlikely' are elastic. Whenever possible, clinicians should quote numerical information using consistent denominators (e.g. '90 of 100 patients who have this operation feel much better, 1 will die during the operation and 2 will suffer a stroke'). Positive framing ('There is a 99% chance of survival') and negative framing ('There is a 1% chance of death') may both be appropriate. A variety of visual aids can be used to present complex statistical information (Fig. 1.4).

Finally, it is essential to allow the patient to place his or her own weighting on the potential benefits and adverse effects of each course of action. Thus, some patients may choose to sacrifice a good chance of pain relief because they are not prepared to run even a small risk of paralysis, whilst others may opt to proceed with very high-risk spinal surgery because they find their current circumstances intolerable.

1.8 Explaining the risks and benefits of therapy

Would you take a drug once a day for a year to prevent stroke if:

- it reduced your risk of having a stroke by 47%?
- it reduced your chance of suffering a stroke from 0.26% to 0.14%?
- there was one chance in 850 that it would prevent you having a stroke?
- 849 out of 850 patients derived no benefit from the treatment?
- there was a 99.7% chance that you would not have a stroke anyway?

All these statements are derived from the same data and describe an equivalent effect.*

*MRC trial of treatment of mild hypertension (bendroflumethiazide vs placebo). BMJ 1985; 291:97–104.

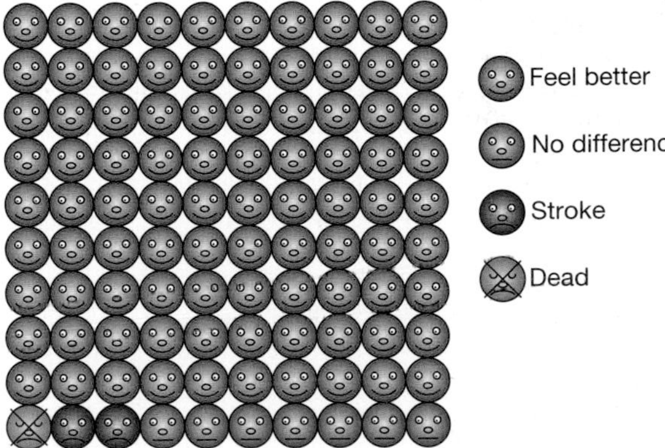

Fig. 1.4 Visual portrayal of benefit and risks. The image refers to an operation that is expected to relieve symptoms in 90% of patients, but cause stroke in 2% and death in 1%. From Edwards, et al. 2002 – see p. 16.

Clinical decision-making

Assimilating symptoms, signs and results of investigations into a diagnosis and then planning treatment are highly complex tasks that require not only factual knowledge but also a highly developed set of skills in decision-making. Diagnostic decision-making is guided by Ockham's razor, originally expressed by the 14th-century Englishman William of Ockham as 'plurality should not be posited without necessity.' In short, all things being equal, the simplest explanation is the best. In practice, clinicians formulate hypotheses about the underlying diagnosis (or shortlist of diagnoses, the 'differential' diagnosis) during the consultation with the patient and refine this hypothesis both by collecting selected additional information and by choosing to ignore other information which they regard as irrelevant, in order to reach the most parsimonious diagnosis.

Decision-making in health care often operates under conditions of uncertainty, where it is uncertain what is wrong with the patient or which treatment is most appropriate. This can lead to variations in how clinicians

1.9 Heuristics in clinical decision-making

Availability

- The probability of an event is estimated based on how easily an individual can recall a similar event, e.g. a doctor judges that a patient has a particular disease because the case reminds him or her of a similar case seen recently
- This can lead to errors, as individuals often recall recent or vivid events more easily, rather than considering the likelihood of an event in the wider population

Representativeness

- The probability of an event is estimated based on how similar (or representative) it is of a wider category of events, e.g. a doctor judges that a patient has a particular disease because the patient's signs and symptoms are 'representative' of that disease
- This can lead to errors, such as neglecting to take into account the prevalence of the disease in a specific patient population

Anchoring and adjustment

- The probability of an event is estimated by taking an initial reference point (anchor) and then adjusting this to reach a final judgement about likelihood, e.g. a doctor judges that the likelihood of a patient having a particular disease is 60%. The doctor collects information (perhaps from diagnostic tests) and re-assesses his or her estimation on the basis of these results to reach a final diagnosis
- This can lead to errors, as final estimations of likelihood are linked to the original anchor, so if this is incorrect, the final judgement is also likely to be inaccurate

make decisions, and subsequently variations in the care that patients receive. Clinicians often employ a process of 'ad hoc' decision-making, where they use some form of global judgement about what might be the best course of action for an individual patient. These ad hoc decisions may be based on a number of factors, including what a clinician has been taught, his or her clinical experience of other patients with that particular disease, or what is common practice within a particular institution. However, such decisions may be governed by heuristics or bias, which may lead to errors. Heuristics are cognitive processes or 'rules of thumb' used unconsciously when making decisions (Box 1.9). Such processes may lead to mistakes, most commonly when there is a lack of evidence to inform practice. Whenever possible, clinical decision-making should be guided by evidence-based medicine.

Evidence-based medicine

Patient treatment should be based on the integration of best research evidence alongside clinical expertise and patient values. The discipline of evidence-based medicine (EBM) came into being in order to introduce a more systematic approach to the use of evidence in making clinical decisions. This was made possible by:

- the development of statistical methods to analyse data systematically
- recognition of the importance of analysing all data, both published and unpublished
- the development of databases of relevant information and systems by which to access such information.

1.10 Categories in evidence-based medicine (EBM)*

Levels of evidence (in descending order of strength)	
Ia	Evidence obtained from meta-analysis of randomised clinical trials
Ib	Evidence obtained from at least one randomised controlled trial
IIa	Evidence obtained from at least one well-designed controlled study without randomisation
IIb	Evidence obtained from at least one other type of well-designed quasi-experimental study
III	Evidence obtained from well-designed non-experimental descriptive studies, such as comparative studies, correlation studies and case studies
IV	Evidence obtained from expert committee reports or opinions and/or clinical experiences of respected authorities
Grades of recommendation	
A	Directly based on level I studies
B	Directly based on level II studies *or* extrapolations from level I studies
C	Directly based on level III studies *or* extrapolations from level I or II studies
D	Directly based on level IV studies *or* extrapolations from level I, II or III studies

*From the Scottish Intercollegiate Guidelines Network (SIGN; see www.sign.ac.uk). This scheme is widely used, although other modified schemes exist.

The principles of EBM are based on the tenet that well-formulated questions about medical management can be answered by:

- conducting high-quality randomised controlled trials
- tracing all the available evidence
- critically appraising the evidence
- applying the evidence to the management of the individual patient.

EBM categorises different types of clinical evidence and ranks them according to their freedom from the various biases that beset medical research. It therefore places greater emphasis on evidence from a meta-analysis of randomised controlled trials than on a series of case reports or expert opinion (Box 1.10).

Guidelines and protocols

The terms 'clinical guidelines' and 'protocols' are often used together, yet they are inherently different.

Guidelines

Clinical guidelines aim to guide clinicians on how to manage specific clinical scenarios using the best available evidence. They have been in existence throughout the history of medicine, although many were based on tradition or authority. A large number of local, national and international bodies have produced guidelines, following a range of different methodologies (see www.evidence.nhs.uk). Some are based on systematic reviews of the medical literature and others on consensus of expert opinion. When considering guidelines, it is important for clinicians to be aware of the strength of the evidence on which the recommendations are based (see Box 1.10).

Properly developed guidelines recognise that medicine is an art as well as a science and that the evidence on which the guidelines are based is, strictly speaking, only applicable to the study population in the trial(s). Clinicians must therefore use their judgement to ascertain whether the recommendations are applicable to the patient in front of them.

Some guidelines are formulated not only from evidence-based best practice but also from cost-effectiveness (see below). An example in the UK is guidance produced by the government-commissioned body, the National Institute for Health and Clinical Excellence (NICE; see www.nice.org.uk). These guidelines recognise that health services have limited resources, and that treatments should be prioritised which offer the greatest improvement in health for the largest number of people per unit of resource.

Protocols

Whilst guidelines recognise the individuality of the patient and help clinicians decide on which action is best, protocols are far more directive and are written to be followed exactly. Protocols usually apply in situations where the clinical decision has already been made and an intervention is then being instigated. Protocols aim to ensure that treatment will be identical, irrespective of where and by whom it is given. For example, a guideline may help a multidisciplinary team decide which modality of treatment is best for someone with lung cancer by evaluating the best evidence alongside the individual psychosocial needs of the patient. However, once a decision has been made in favour of a certain treatment, e.g. chemotherapy, the clinician will be expected to follow a strict protocol outlining dosages, routes of administration and monitoring.

Cost-effectiveness

The best available health care can be expensive. No country can now afford to provide unlimited state-of-the-art medicine for all its citizens. Health-care systems must therefore take account of the cost-effectiveness of the treatments they provide. This can create difficult dilemmas for clinicians, who may be asked to withhold expensive but effective therapies (e.g. implantable defibrillators) from individual patients on the basis that the money will do more good for more patients if it is spent elsewhere (e.g. offering angioplasty to all acute myocardial infarction patients). Assessing the cost-effectiveness of interventions and allocating resources accordingly follows ethical principles such as justice, which are covered in greater detail below.

Quality-adjusted life years

Outcomes from health care can be measured in terms of changes in the quality and quantity of life. Life expectancy is easily defined but quality of life is difficult to measure. Nevertheless, it is possible to construct a continuum between perfect health (score 1), survival with no quality of life (score 0), and states that are perceived to be worse than death (minus score). Quality and quantity of life can then be combined in a measure known as the quality-adjusted life year (QALY). For example, an intervention that results in a patient living an additional 4 years with an average quality of life rated as 0.6 on the continuum would yield 2.4 QALYs (4×0.6). Thus a cost per QALY can be calculated and compared with other interventions (p. 32). This approach is not perfect but offers a means of comparing the cost-effectiveness of a wide range of treatments.

Another useful measure is the disability-adjusted life year (DALY), which is used by the World Health Organization to quantify the overall burden of disease in populations; it cumulatively estimates the number of years lost due to ill health, disability and death.

Practising medicine in low-resource settings

The challenges associated with medical care in low-resource areas cluster in four domains:

- *Prevention versus cure*. Prevention is easier, cheaper and more effective than cure for many diseases. On the other hand, curative medicine is immediate, highly visible and glamorous. This tension is most evident when a disease is common and the benefits of prevention have yet to be realised. The allocation of adequate resources for long-term prevention needs both political will and social acceptance.
- *Acute versus chronic care*. Treating chronic illness can be time-consuming and less immediately gratifying than acute emergency medicine. Facilities for chronic care are therefore accorded a low priority in many health-care systems. Unfortunately, this often results in patients who require long-term care being denied treatment altogether or being managed inappropriately in the acute sector.
- *The ideal versus the possible*. Most medical management guidelines are derived from studies that were conducted in well-resourced health-care systems. In trying to apply this knowledge to the developing world, there are tensions between best practice and what is possible. For example, anticoagulant therapy (p. 1018) may pose risks that were not evident in the studies that underpin guidelines if it is prescribed in areas where reliable laboratories are not available and medications that interact with warfarin are commonly purchased 'over the counter'.
- *Channels of health-care provision*. In developing countries, health care may be delivered through government-run public clinics (usually free or subsidised) or non-governmental organisations (sometimes subsidised but usually privately funded). Many of the available services are too costly for the average patient. There is a need for constructive cooperation between all of the health-care sectors.

The best possible practice is that which can be delivered within the available resources in a specific setting. Compassionate care given with empathy, understanding and good communication is always within the physician's reach, even when resources are inadequate.

Medical ethics

Ethics has been described as the 'science' of morality, and defines systems of moral values. Medical ethics is concerned both with the standards of conduct and competence expected of medical professionals, some of which are captured in legislation, and with the study of moral problems raised by the practice of medicine. Recent advances in biomedical science and their application to clinical care have thrown up many difficult ethical problems. These include human cloning, predictive genetic testing, eugenics, new reproductive technologies, antenatal screening, abortion, priority-setting, under-served populations, brain death, organ transplantation, end-of-life issues, and assisted suicide. Detailed discussion of these is beyond the scope of this chapter but a framework for the application of ethics to medical practice is described.

In general, ethical problems relate to the intentions or motives of those involved, their actions, the consequences of their actions, and the context in which their actions take place. Ethical problems can be analysed in a variety of ways, sometimes leading to different conclusions. To find the best solution, it may be necessary to apply several analytical approaches and attempt to reconcile the conclusions. In modern medical practice, there is not always time to do this systematically. However, the process of applying an ethical framework to a given situation is a key element in clinical decision-making and helps to ensure that a decision is both morally acceptable and legally defensible.

- *Virtue ethics* is concerned with the character of the persons involved and with their actions. Are my intentions (what my actions aim at) and my motives (what moves me to act) good or bad, wise or unwise, sensible or unrealistic, patient-centred or self-centred, and so on? Is the action I propose to take one which would be considered appropriate by a prudent doctor – or by a prudent patient? The focus here is on the characteristics of a virtuous person and the action they would take.
- *Deontological ethics* is concerned with whether a proposed action or course of action, in itself and regardless of its consequences, is right or wrong. Is it ever right or always wrong to kill, to tell a lie, to break a promise? Deontological (from the Greek for 'duty') considerations include rights as well as duties, and omissions as well as acts. An action is right if it is in accordance with an established moral rule or principle.
- *Teleological ethics* (or consequentialism) is concerned with the consequences of a proposed action. Are they likely to be good or bad, in the short term and long term, for the patient, doctor, family and society? What will promote a net balance of good over harm for the individual, as well as 'the greatest good for the greatest number'?

An ethical problem can therefore be addressed by trying to decide what a virtuous person would do, whether an action or course of action is right or wrong in itself, or what its consequences might be. Yet the circumstances in which any decision is made will vary, and what may be right in one context may be wrong in another. *Situation ethics* recognises this, emphasising the need to consider carefully the context (or situation) in which a course of action is chosen.

Ethics is applied to the practice of medicine in three broad areas:

- *Clinical ethics* deals with the relationship between clinicians and patients, as described below.
- *Public health ethics* deals with the health issues of groups of people – the community. Examples include the banning of smoking in public places, where the autonomy of the individual may be coerced for the greater good of the community.
- *Research ethics* deals with issues related to clinical research. This is to ensure not only that research is conducted safely but also that the rights of the participants are paramount. No research can be undertaken unless it has undergone ethical scrutiny.

Principles of clinical ethics

In clinical ethics, four key principles are frequently used to analyse a problem, and often abbreviated to 'autonomy, beneficence, non-maleficence and justice'.

Respect for persons and their autonomy

This respect is a significant aspect of the relationship between patient and doctor. The patient seeks out a doctor based on a desire to attain freedom from a disability or disease which limits his or her ability to exercise autonomy (the power or right of self-determination). Unless the patient is a child, is unconscious or is mentally incapacitated, it is the patient's choice to seek advice. The physician must therefore respect the patient's autonomy. This includes the patient's right to refuse therapy. The doctor must also actively seek to empower the patient with adequate information.

Truth-telling

Telling the truth is essential to generating and maintaining trust between the doctor and the patient. This includes providing information about the nature of the illness, expected outcome and therapeutic alternatives, and answering questions honestly. The facts should not be given 'brutally' but with due sensitivity to appropriate timing and to the patient's capacity to cope with bad news. However, the clinical uncertainties described earlier in the chapter must also be acknowledged. There are two rare situations where the truth may, at least for a time, be withheld:

- If it will cause real harm to the patient (e.g. a depressed patient likely to commit suicide who has to be told that he or she has cancer). This is sometimes called 'therapeutic privilege', since it should be exercised only in the patient's interests, for serious clinical reasons.
- If the patient makes it clear that he or she does not want to hear the bad news (but always bearing in mind that this may be a stage in the patient's adjustment to the condition).

In no case should false information be given, and the physician should always be prepared to justify any decision to withhold relevant information.

Informed consent

This term describes the participation of patients in decisions about their health care. In order to facilitate this, the clinician must provide the patient with an adequate explanation and details of the relevant risks, benefits and uncertainties of each possible course of action. The amount of information to provide will vary, depending on the patient's condition and the complexity of the treatment, and on the physician's assessment of the patient's understanding of the situation. Not all options need be explained, but those that a 'prudent patient' would consider significant should be explored – for example, by open questioning (see Box 1.4, p. 4).

From both a legal and an ethical perspective, the patient retains the right to decide what is in his or her best interests. All adults have decision-making capacity if they can understand the relevant information (which may have to be explained in simple terms), consider the implications of the relevant options, and make a communicable decision. If a patient makes choices that seem irrational or are at variance with professional advice, it does not mean that they lack capacity.

When the patient does lack decision-making capacity, the clinician should always act in the best interests of the patient. In an emergency, consent may be presumed, but only for treatment immediately necessary to preserve the patient's life and health, and if there is no clear evidence that this would be against the previous settled wishes of the patient when competent (for example, blood transfusion in the case of an adult Jehovah's Witness). If the patient has a legally entitled surrogate decision-maker, their consent should be sought if possible. It is also good practice to involve close relatives in decision-making but the hierarchy of surrogate decision-makers will depend on local laws and culture.

Confidentiality

Confidentiality in relation to the management of patient-specific information is important in generating and maintaining trust in the doctor–patient relationship. Health-care teams must take precautions to prevent unauthorised access to patient records, and may disclose patient-identifying information only when the patient has given consent or when required by law. When such information is shared with other health-care professionals in order to optimise patient care, this should be done on a strictly 'need-to-know' basis.

Beneficence

This is the principle of doing good, or acting in another person's best interests. In clinical ethics, the term refers to the good of the individual patient. It means considering the patient's view, as well as the medical view, of his or her own best interests. Situations may arise when there is a conflict between what is good for the individual and what is best for society, but the traditional medical approach is that stated in the Declaration of Geneva (World Medical Association): 'The health of my patient will be my first consideration.'

Non-maleficence

This is the principle of doing no harm: in medicine, the traditional 'primum non nocere'. In balancing beneficence and non-maleficence (benefit versus risk), the clinician must share information with the patient, who can then be helped to make an informed decision.

Justice

In the context of clinical ethics, justice relates primarily to the distribution of medical care and the allocation of resources. In order to distribute health resources justly, the concept of utility – 'greatest good for the greatest number' – must be considered. In the case of individual patients, however, justice is also equated with being 'fair' and 'even-handed'. The concept of fair delivery of health care can be viewed from three perspectives:

- Respect for the *needs* of the individual. Health care is delivered first to those who need it most. This perspective is particularly relevant when need must be assessed by some kind of triage.
- Respect for the *rights* of a person. Everyone who needs health care is entitled to a fair share of the resources available. This perspective is particularly relevant when local or global economic, social, educational or other inequalities prevent or reduce equitable access to health care.
- Respect for *merit*. Health care is delivered on the basis of value judgements, according to financial, political, social or other factors relating to the value of the individual to society. For example, many national leaders have their own personal physician and medical teams. The relevance of this perspective to health care is widely disputed, not least because such value judgements are difficult to make in practice and to defend ethically.

Types of ethical problem

When faced with an ethical problem, it is often helpful to characterise it in terms of certain patterns (Fig. 1.5).

A gap or block

The ideal goal is clearly seen but there are major obstacles to achieving it. The obstacles may be economic or social, or in the belief system of the patient. The obvious answer – to bridge the gap or remove the block – may not be possible within the available time frame and resources. A young boy from a poor family in a developing country, who has Wilson's disease and needs a liver transplant, is an example of an economic block. Some problems of this kind cannot be resolved satisfactorily in the clinical context until or unless they are resolved in the economic or political context.

Priority-setting

The right course of action is clear but prioritisation is necessary and the principles to guide that process have to be defined. A decision to allocate the last bed in intensive care to either an 80-year-old with pneumonia or a 20-year-old with advanced lymphoma is an example. While it is not possible to cover all eventualities, guidelines agreed in advance with stakeholders are helpful.

A moral dilemma

Acting in accordance with one ethical principle may conflict with another ethical principle. This can create a moral dilemma – a choice between two alternatives, neither of which is ethically satisfactory. For example, a physician may decide that a particular mode of therapy is best (principle of beneficence), while the patient makes a different choice (principle of respect for autonomy). Consider artificial feeding by a percutaneous endoscopic gastrostomy (PEG; p. 123). The doctor may be reluctant to see the patient die for lack of nutrition and believe that this is the best route for feeding. The patient may, however, refuse the procedure, based on an informed

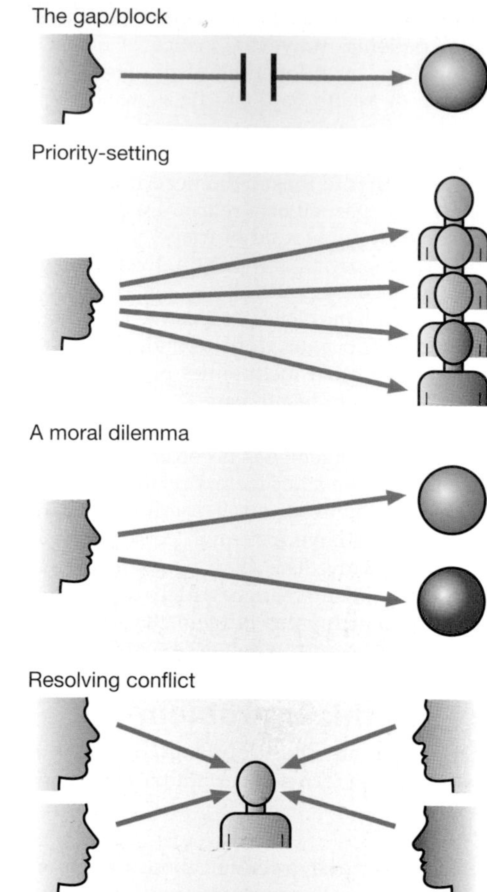

Fig. 1.5 A classification of ethical problems.

assessment of their own quality of life and prospects of recovery. In theory, the dilemma can be resolved only if one of the ethical principles is given priority; ethical analysis (see below) can help to achieve resolution. True moral dilemmas are less common in practice than in theory; apparent dilemmas can often be resolved by good doctor–patient communication.

Resolving conflict

A conflict of opinion may arise between members of the team responsible for care of the patient. For example, doctors in a renal medicine unit providing dialysis therapy (p. 489) may have divergent views on whether this treatment is appropriate for a patient who is elderly with significant comorbidity. Differing views should normally be resolved through discussion; in this example, conflict would usually be resolved in a multidisciplinary team meeting at which discussion of patients approaching end-stage renal failure is routine. However, if this does not work, referral to a decision-making authority allocated in advance (e.g. the clinical director of the service) may be necessary. The challenge then is to ensure consistent and accurate implementation of the decision.

Ethical analysis

Ethical analysis (or moral reasoning) is the process of thinking through ethical problems and reaching a conclusion. It helps the decision-maker to grow personally and professionally, allows communication of the process by which a decision is made, and permits the process to be constructively criticised. When, in everyday practice, time for reflection is limited, knowledge of methods of moral reasoning provides a useful background and aid for decision-making, and is often employed in ways analogous to those of 'the novice-expert shift' (see Box 1.14, p. 14). Some approaches that can be applied are as follows:

- *A principles approach.* This involves analysing an ethical problem in terms of the principles of respect for autonomy, beneficence, non-maleficence and justice. If all of these principles support a particular course of action, then that course of action is probably correct and there may, in fact, no longer be an ethical problem. If, however, different principles suggest different courses of action, this approach has no intrinsic mechanism for deciding which principle has priority. On the other hand, analysing the problem in terms of these principles can help to clarify the nature of the ethical problem and the issues which need to be addressed if the problem is to be resolved.
- *A casuistry (cases) approach.* This uses precedent as a guide to what to do. A case is recalled or imagined which is similar to that under discussion but where the right choice of action/behaviour was obvious. Then the features which make the present case different, if any, are analysed and considered to see if and why they lead to a different conclusion. A variation on this approach, related to virtue ethics, is to imagine what a physician who was particularly skilled or experienced in this type of situation would do, or how a previous patient might have viewed the problem.
- *A perspectives (or narrative) approach.* A perspectives approach involves considering the views of all the stakeholders: the patient, the family or carers, the health-care team, the health service and society. The greater the degree of concordance of these views on a particular outcome, the more likely it is that the decision leading to that outcome is right. A narrative approach is similar but involves listening attentively to the different 'stories' told by the stakeholders about the problem and how they perceive it. Where these stories differ can provide clues to a more nuanced understanding of the problem and how it might be resolved.
- *A counter-argument approach.* A particular course of action is chosen and the best ethical arguments against it are then marshalled and evaluated. This may or may not cause the decision to be reconsidered.
- *Application of rules.* In certain common and clearly defined situations, externally imposed rules (including the law) may require, or guide towards, a specific course of action. This does not obviate the need for ethical analysis. Moreover, any such rules must be reviewed regularly.

While all of these approaches may be useful, it is important to remember that none of them removes the need, on the one hand, for the exercise of judgement and, on the other, for good communication and consensus decision-making. No less important is the

1.11 Ethical analysis: an 'onion-peel' approach

Patient preferences: data gathered from patient and relatives/carers
• What is the quality of life expected after therapy – from the patient's perspective? • If the patient is competent, has he or she been offered options and made choices? • If the patient is not competent, who will make the decisions?
Medical goals: data gathered from literature, guidelines, expert opinion
• What are the prospects of a successful outcome? • What are the best therapeutic options available based on evidence? • Has the therapy been optimised and matched to this individual patient?
Regional issues: data gathered from local sources
• What decisions are most consistent with local laws and with social and cultural values?
Basic ethical principles, type of ethical problem, ethical analysis (see text)
• Consider the basic principles of medical ethics • Consider the type of ethical problem • Choose the ethical analytical approaches to apply to the problem

requirement for all of this to be based on sound and shared information about the clinical and human facts of the case. In this respect, a practical, integrated way of addressing ethical problems is provided by what has been called *an onion-peel approach*, which uses a layered framework to analyse the problem systematically (Box 1.11).

Discussion with colleagues and others is crucial in reaching ethical decisions. Many hospitals have a clinical ethics committee to review difficult decisions. Up-to-date, accurate, valid and reliable data should inform the decision-making progress. Local legal issues must be considered. Once a conclusion has been reached, a strategy to complete the action must be implemented. Post-hoc evaluation of decisions is important, and again is best carried out collectively by an ethics committee or some other means of retrospective review.

A clinical ethics scenario

A 70-year-old man who has chronic obstructive pulmonary disease, hypertension and diabetes mellitus is admitted to hospital with pneumonia. His memory has been deteriorating for 3 years, with a rapid decline in cognition over the last 3 months, and he needs help to carry out activities of daily living. A neurologist has excluded reversible causes of dementia. The patient deteriorates and needs mechanical ventilation. His wife states that he told her (when he was well) that he did not want to be put on 'life support machines' and is therefore opposed to mechanical ventilation. Two of his children fail to confirm this and request active treatment. There is no formal written 'advance directive' on file (pp. 171 and 291). What care should be given?

On the one hand, considered mainly in teleological terms:

The patient is incapable of making an autonomous decision. The closest surrogate indicates that he would have preferred to forego life-sustaining therapy at this stage. (Respect for autonomy might support this.) The consequences of ventilation would probably be to prolong the process of dying (which non-maleficence could argue against) rather than increase his chances of recovery to a good quality of life. Beneficence requires that he receive general care and symptom relief immediately. An appropriate action therefore is not to ventilate the patient but to continue basic medical (fluids, oxygen and antibiotics) and nursing care in a general ward setting in order to optimise patient comfort.

On the other hand, considered in deontological as well as teleological terms:

The present illness is due to a potentially reversible infection. The patient's real preference is uncertain and his family, who have difficulty in looking after him, have expressed differing views. In terms of the duty of a doctor to make the patient's health the first consideration, and of the patient's right to appropriate health care regardless of his age or mental condition, it would therefore be appropriate to institute all possible care, including ventilation on an intensive care unit.

In practice:

The physician responsible for the patient's care should consider the different courses of action suggested, but not determined, by these ethical analyses, explain the reasons for and against each course of action to the patient's family and, if one of them is the patient's legal surrogate, help that person come to a decision. Where there is no legal surrogate, the physician will have to reach a judgement about what is in the patient's best interests, recognising that, while judgement is always fallible, whatever decision is made must be defensible if challenged on ethical or legal grounds. Decisions that are reached on the basis of ethical and moral reasoning will be relatively easy to defend.

In this case, further discussion of the relevant issues with the relatives and other members of the health-care team led to concordance. The patient was treated by artificial ventilation in the intensive care unit for 3 days. He made a good recovery and appeared grateful for the care he had received.

Medical law

The law impinges on medical practice in many ways. Although a description of specific laws in different countries is beyond the scope of this book, it is important for doctors to be familiar with local legislation. Some of the ethical principles described above are captured in legislation, for example, in relation to informed consent (p. 10) and confidentiality (p. 11). Other laws enforce standard requirements for formal procedures, such as death certification. In many countries, regulatory authorities with statutory powers – for example, to license doctors to practise – also impose standards. The distinction and overlap between these domains are illustrated in Box 1.12.

1.12 Some definitions in ethics, law and regulation of medical practice

	Definition	In practice
Ethics	The science of morality; a branch of philosophy concerned with human character and conduct	Morally, what may be the best thing for me to do in this situation?
Law	Rules of action established by authority (normally, a community or state)	What must I do in this situation to avoid breaking the law?
Negligence	Omission of duty and such care for the interests of others as the law may require	What would any 'ordinarily competent' doctor do in this situation?
(Practice) guidance	Direction from another person or body	What do a group of experts say that I should do, supported by the best available evidence (e.g. guidelines, protocols)?
(Clinical) governance	Control, autonomy	What will I and the members of my medical team do, with due regard to ethics, law and practice guidelines?

A high-profile area of overlap between medicine and the law occurs in legal action (litigation) related to processes of care. The latter frequently involves the concept of negligence. In the UK, the 'Bolam test' is often used to define whether medical care is or is not negligent. Care is measured against what any 'ordinarily competent' (or sometimes 'reasonable') doctor would have done in the same situation. In addition to this test, it must also be established that:

- there was a *duty of care* between the doctor and patient (this is usually straightforward)
- there was a *causal link* between any breach of duty and harm to the patient
- the harm was not too *remote* from the episode of care.

PERSONAL AND PROFESSIONAL DEVELOPMENT

Good doctors never stop learning, and continue to develop their knowledge, skills and attributes throughout their working lives, to the benefit of their patients and themselves. Many also participate actively in improving medical knowledge and practice through research. These activities have become an essential component of clinical governance, which is a mechanism for ensuring high standards of clinical care (Box 1.13). Personal and professional development (PPD) requires a reflective and self-directed approach to the study and practice of medicine (Fig. 1.6), and will maximise both lifelong effectiveness and personal satisfaction. Linked to this is the concept of the novice–expert shift (Box 1.14).

PPD begins in the first days at medical school and continues through postgraduate training and subsequent professional practice. Maintaining competence and expertise requires continuous professional development (CPD). In the UK, this is formally regulated by professional bodies such as the Royal Colleges, and is linked to processes of appraisal (Box 1.15) and re-accreditation for established practitioners.

To support this process, outcomes and competences for PPD are being defined at all levels of medical training, including undergraduate and postgraduate study. These sit alongside and complement curricula that focus on discipline-based knowledge and skills. As adult learners, doctors are expected to reflect on their own practice and identify their own particular learning or developmental needs. This recognises that doctors will have different learning needs throughout their career, which will be affected by their current clinical practice, their future career plans and any areas of educational need that have become apparent through the appraisal process.

1.13 Key components in clinical governance

- Continuing education
- Clinical audit
- Clinical effectiveness
- Risk management
- Research and development
- Openness

1.14 The novice–expert shift

- **Novices** use pre-determined methods which they learn
- **Advanced beginners** recognise that these methods are not effective in all circumstances and can adapt them
- **Competent professionals** are able to make conscious, independent choices and can manage and regulate their own practice
- **Proficient professionals** make use of intuition based on experience, and integrate multiple aspects of practice into a holistic model
- **Experts** function largely through 'unconscious competence' and are inseparable from the tasks they undertake

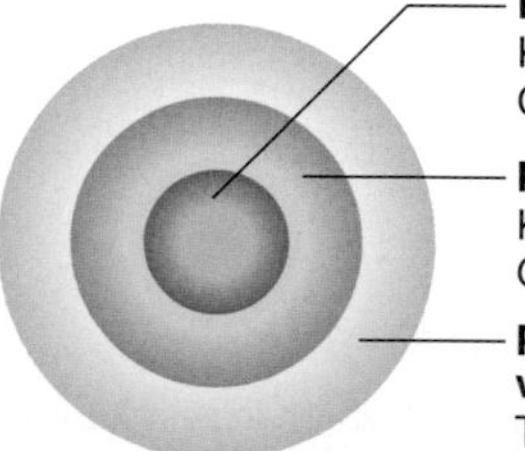

Fig. 1.6 The personal and professional development of a doctor.

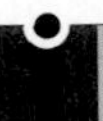

1.15 Some techniques used in the appraisal process

- Formal, structured assessment (e.g. postgraduate examinations)
- 360-degree assessment (surveying colleagues from medicine and other disciplines who work alongside the practitioner)
- Educational supervision and mentoring (a specific colleague has nominated responsibility to guide, and also assess, the practitioner)
- Logbooks (records of work undertaken and outcomes)
- Portfolio-based assessment (the practitioner accumulates a record of educational and clinical experiences, together with evidence of reflective practice)

Each doctor has a duty to ensure that their clinical knowledge and skills are up to date and comparable with their peers. Clinical audit is one method of assessing practice in this context.

Clinical audit

Clinical audit is the process by which the clinical practice of a doctor or medical team and the outcomes of that practice are evaluated against an agreed standard. Where practice fails to meet the standard, changes to practice are implemented; after a period, practice can be re-evaluated to identify any improvement. The continuing evaluation, implementation of change and re-evaluation process is known as the audit loop or cycle (Fig. 1.7). The standard against which practice is measured is usually an externally agreed one, rather than a local one. It is important to know that clinical care is comparable to that delivered elsewhere. For this reason, national standards are the norm in most countries, often set alongside national guidelines which signpost the practice necessary to achieve them. Clinical audit may be conducted by the doctor or team themselves, or by an external body. Outcome measures may include success rates or complication rates of clinical procedures such as surgical operations; process variables such as waiting times for clinical care; or the perspective of patients and relatives. In the UK, all practising clinicians are now expected to participate in audit, and it is an integral part of procedures for appraisal, revalidation and relicensing of doctors.

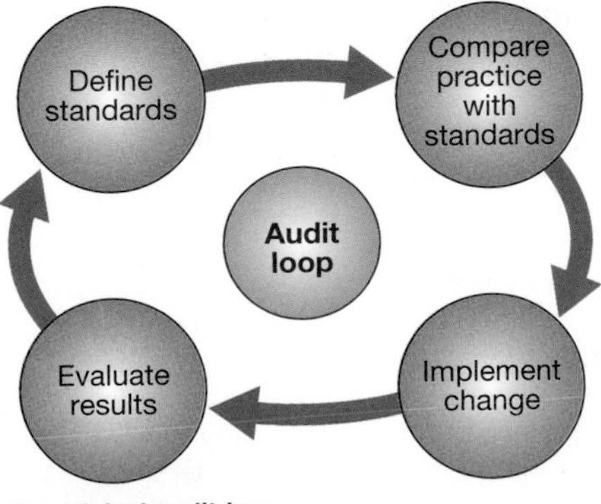

Fig. 1.7 The clinical audit loop.

COMPLEMENTARY AND ALTERNATIVE MEDICINE

Complementary and alternative medicine (CAM) refers to a group of medical and health-care systems, practices and products that are not considered to be part of conventional medicine; as such, the relevant principles and skills are not included in the curricula of conventional medical education programmes. CAM covers an enormous and ever-changing range of activities, from well-established physical therapies such as osteopathy to spiritual measures such as prayer specifically for health. Proponents suggest that CAM focuses on the whole person: their lifestyle, environment, diet, and mental, emotional and spiritual health, as well as physical complaints.

'Complementary medicine' is the term used to describe the use of these treatments in conjunction with conventional medicine (e.g. acupuncture to reduce pain after surgery). 'Alternative medicine' describes their use in place of conventional medicine (e.g. reflexology instead of anti-inflammatory drugs for arthritis). Clearly, most forms of treatment can be used in either way, so the term CAM is often used generically. 'Integrative medicine' describes the use of conventional therapy in combination with one or more complementary therapies.

A variety of different taxonomies are used for CAM therapies. The National Center for Complementary and Alternative Medicine in the USA uses the following classification:

- *Alternative medical systems*. These have their own constructs of theory and practice, often based on ancient historical beliefs. Examples are homeopathy, naturopathy, traditional Chinese medicine and Ayurveda.
- *Mind–body interactions*. These rely on the mind's capacity to influence physical function. Examples are meditation, biofeedback, prayer for healing, mental healing, music therapy and dance.
- *Biologically based therapies*. These involve the use or regulation of an extraneous agent or preparation. Examples include herbal medicine, dietary supplementation and nutritional medicine.
- *Manipulative and body-based methods*. These are based on manipulation or movement of parts of the body. They include osteopathy, chiropractic, reflexology and massage.
- *Energy therapies*. These involve use of energy fields. Examples include qigong, reiki and therapeutic touch.

Some forms of CAM are embedded in the cultural norms of particular social and ethnic groups, e.g. traditional Chinese medicine. In Western society, the use of CAM is extensive. For example, in 2007 in the USA, 38% of the adult population had used some form of CAM in the previous year (males 33.5%, females 42.8%); 12% of children had also used CAM. The most common medical conditions involved were back pain, neck pain, other joint pain/arthritis, anxiety, raised cholesterol, head or chest 'colds', headache, insomnia, stress and depression, and gastrointestinal symptoms.

The popularity of CAM may reflect a lack of confidence in conventional medicine, particularly a belief that it will not help the condition or may cause harm. CAM is often used by cancer patients who have disease which is unresponsive to conventional medicines. In addition, it may reflect the increasing ease of access to information and therapies via the Internet. CAM is often perceived to be completely safe; patients may therefore be willing to experiment with it as a 'no-lose' measure. Many forms of CAM are inherently pleasurable, regardless of any therapeutic benefit.

Safety

Not all CAM therapies are safe; some are toxic in their own right (e.g. dietary supplements containing ephedrine alkaloids, now banned in the USA) and others are harmful if used in combination with conventional treatment (e.g. garlic supplements that interfere with the action of anti-HIV chemotherapy). Others have been associated with rare but serious side-effects, which can be life-threatening (e.g. bowel perforation from coffee enemas, hyponatraemia from noni juice).

There is also a potential for harm when alternative medicine is used to treat serious or life-threatening medical conditions, if the resultant delay in seeking conventional treatment compromises clinical outcome.

On balance, however, the relative safety of most CAM therapies can be regarded as a positive feature; homeopathy is an example.

Evidence

In an era where EBM is the norm, practitioners and advocates of CAM are increasingly challenged to justify these treatments through independent, well-conducted, randomised controlled clinical trials. In some cases, this may be difficult (e.g. the placebo arm of a double-blind trial of acupuncture). In addition, it can be argued that different types and standards of evidence, focusing on patient satisfaction and subjective benefit rather than measurable clinical outcomes, may be more appropriate for CAM. The literature in this area is growing rapidly but, at present, only a minority of CAM therapies are supported by any evidence that would be acceptable for conventional medicine. These are primarily the 'big five' CAM therapies: osteopathy, chiropractic, acupuncture, homeopathy and herbal medicine. Moreover, where such positive evidence does exist, it is often outweighed by negative studies, and limited to a small subset of the clinical conditions for which the treatment is used.

Regulation

Many CAM therapies have professional regulatory frameworks in place and others are following suit. Nevertheless, for many CAM therapies, there is still no established structure of training, certification and accreditation, and practice is effectively open to all. Set against the demanding training and life-long continuous professional development that pertain to conventional medicine, this constitutes an important barrier to integrative medicine.

Integrated health care

There is a considerable impetus behind moves to integrate CAM with conventional medicine and health care at the level of resource allocation, service design, clinical practice, education and research. Almost 50% of general practices in the UK and an increasing number of hospitals offer some form of access to CAM. In many parts of Asia in particular, this kind of medical pluralism is the norm, and patients do not necessarily make a distinction between different systems of health care. Historically, in Western societies, patients using both types of therapy have often experienced conflicting advice and value judgements, poor or absent communication between practitioners, and even hostility or ridicule. They often revert to secrecy, an inherently undesirable and potentially dangerous outcome. Integrated health care aims to understand and remove the barriers that create such dilemmas for patients. It aims to let them exercise their choice of treatment in an open environment characterised by good communication, respect, and due consideration of autonomy, efficacy and risk.

Further information and acknowledgements

Websites

www.dh.gov.uk *UK Department of Health guidance and policy on confidentiality and consent.*

www.evidence.nhs.uk *A UK National Health Service resource providing a searchable library of clinical guidelines from all sources.*

www.gmc-uk.org *UK General Medical Council. Includes access to guidance on professional conduct (Duties of a Doctor, Good Medical Practice) and guidance on medical education, such as 'Tomorrow's Doctors'.*

www.nice.org.uk *National Institute for Health and Clinical Excellence. Includes recommendations for evidence-based treatments.*

www.rcplondon.ac.uk *Royal College of Physicians. Includes access to a working party report: Doctors in Society: Medical Professionalism in a Changing World.*

www.sign.ac.uk *Scottish Intercollegiate Guidelines Network. Includes evidence-based guidelines for clinical practice.*

www.who.int *World Health Organization. Includes information relevant to global health and differences in medical practice.*

Figure acknowledgements

Fig. 1.4 Edwards A, Elwyn G, Mulley A. Explaining risks: turning numerical data into meaningful pictures. BMJ 2002; 324:827–830, reproduced with permission from the BMJ Publishing Group.

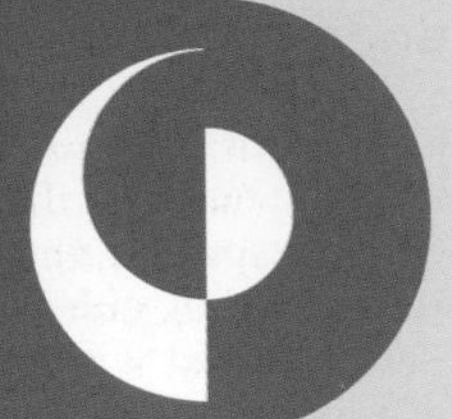

S. Maxwell

Therapeutics and good prescribing

2

Principles of clinical pharmacology 18
- Pharmacodynamics 18
- Pharmacokinetics 21
- Inter-individual variation in drug responses 23

Adverse outcomes of drug therapy 24
- Adverse drug reactions 24
- Drug interactions 28
- Medication errors 29

Drug regulation and management 30
- Drug development and marketing 30
- Managing the use of medicines 31

Prescribing in practice 33
- Decision-making in prescribing 33
- Prescribing in special circumstances 36
- Writing prescriptions 37
- Monitoring drug therapy 39

Prescribing medicines is a major tool used by most doctors to restore or preserve the health of their patients. Medicines contain drugs (the specific chemical substances with pharmacological effects), either alone or in combination, in a formulation mixed with other ingredients. The beneficial effects of medicines must be weighed against their cost and the risks of adverse drug reactions and interactions, often caused by injudicious prescribing decisions and by prescribing errors. The modern prescriber must meet the challenges posed by an increasing number of drugs and formulations available and of indications for prescribing them, and the greater complexity of treatment regimens followed by individual patients ('polypharmacy', a particular challenge in the ageing population). The purpose of this chapter is to elaborate on the principles and practice that underpin good prescribing (Box 2.1).

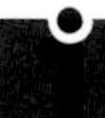

2.1 Steps in good prescribing

- Make a diagnosis
- Consider factors influencing the patient's responses to therapy (age, concomitant drug therapy, renal and liver function etc.)*
- Establish the therapeutic goal*
- Choose the therapeutic approach*
- Choose the drug and its formulation (the 'medicine')
- Choose the dose, route and frequency
- Choose the duration of therapy
- Write an unambiguous prescription (or 'medicatlon order')
- Inform the patient about the treatment and its likely effects
- Monitor treatment effects, both beneficial and harmful
- Review/alter the prescription

*These steps in particular take the patient's views into consideration to establish a therapeutic partnership.

PRINCIPLES OF CLINICAL PHARMACOLOGY

Prescribers need to understand what the drug does to the body (pharmacodynamics) and what the body does to the drug (pharmacokinetics) (Fig. 2.1). Although this chapter is focused on the most common drugs, which are synthetic small molecules, the same principles apply to the increasingly numerous 'biological' therapies (sometimes abbreviated to 'biologics') now in use, which include peptides, proteins, enzymes and monoclonal antibodies (p. 74).

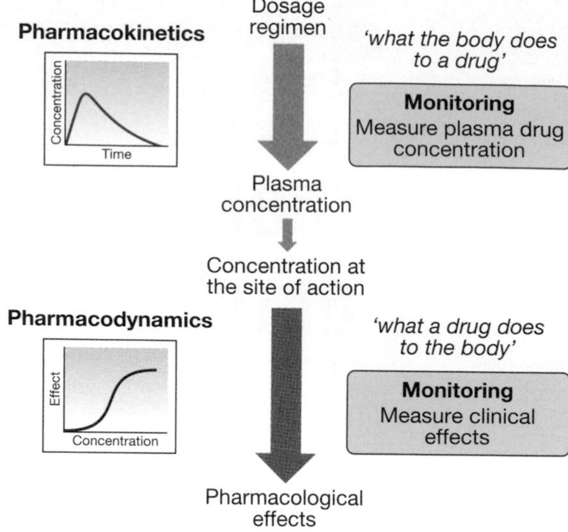

Fig. 2.1 Pharmacokinetics and pharmacodynamics.

Pharmacodynamics

Drug targets and mechanisms of action

Modern drugs are usually discovered by screening compounds for activity either to stimulate or to block the function of a specific molecular target, which is predicted to have a beneficial effect in a particular disease (Box 2.2). Other drugs have useful but less selective chemical properties, such as chelators (e.g. for treatment of iron or copper overload), osmotic agents (used as diuretics in cerebral oedema) or general anaesthetics (that alter the biophysical properties of lipid membranes). The following characteristics of the interaction of drugs with receptors illustrate some of the important determinants of the effects of drugs:

- *Affinity* describes the propensity for a drug to bind to a receptor and is related to the 'molecular fit' and the strength of the chemical bond. Some drug–receptor interactions are *irreversible*, either because the affinity is so strong or because the drug modifies the structure of its molecular target.
- *Selectivity* describes the propensity for a drug to bind to one target rather than another. Selectivity is a relative term, not to be confused with absolute specificity. It is common for drugs targeted at a particular subtype of receptor to exhibit some effect at other subtypes. For example, β-adrenoceptors can be subtyped on the basis of their responsiveness to the endogenous agonist noradrenaline (norepinephrine): the concentration of noradrenaline required to cause bronchodilatation (via β_2-adrenoceptors) is ten times higher than that required to cause tachycardia (via β_1-adrenoceptors). 'Cardioselective' β-blockers have anti-anginal effects on the heart (β_1) but may still cause bronchospasm in the lung (β_2) and are contraindicated for asthmatic patients.
- *Agonists* bind to a receptor to produce a conformational change that is coupled to a biological response. As agonist concentration increases, so does the proportion of receptors occupied, and hence the biological effect. *Partial agonists* activate the receptor, but cannot produce a maximal signalling effect equivalent to that of a full agonist even when all available receptors are occupied.
- *Antagonists* bind to a receptor but do not produce the conformational change that initiates an intracellular signal. A *competitive antagonist* competes with endogenous ligands to occupy receptor binding sites, with the resulting antagonism depending on the relative affinities and concentrations of drug and ligand. *Non-competitive*

2.2 Examples of target molecules for drugs

Drug target	Description	Examples
Receptors		
Channel-linked receptors	Ligand binding controls a linked ion channel, known as 'ligand-gated' (in contrast to 'voltage-gated' channels that respond to changes in membrane potential)	Nicotinic acetylcholine receptor γ-aminobutyric acid (GABA) receptor Sulphonylurea receptor
G-protein-coupled receptors (GPCRs)	Ligand binding affects one of a family of 'G-proteins' that mediate signal transduction either by activating intracellular enzymes (such as adenylate or guanylate cyclase, producing cyclic AMP or GMP, respectively) or by controlling ion channels	Muscarinic acetylcholine receptor β-adrenoceptors Dopamine receptors Serotonin receptors Opioid receptors
Kinase-linked receptors	Ligand binding activates an intracellular protein kinase that triggers a cascade of phosphorylation reactions	Insulin receptor Cytokine receptors
Transcription factor receptors	Intracellular and also known as 'nuclear receptors'; ligand binding promotes or inhibits gene transcription and hence synthesis of new proteins	Steroid receptors Thyroid hormone receptors Vitamin D receptors Retinoid receptors PPARγ and α receptors
Other targets		
Voltage-gated ion channels	Mediate electrical signalling in excitable tissues (muscle and nervous system)	Na^+ channels Ca^{2+} channels
Enzymes	Catalyse biochemical reactions. Drugs interfere with binding of substrate to the active site or of co-factors	Cyclo-oxygenase Angiotensin converting enzyme (ACE) Xanthine oxidase
Transporter proteins	Carry ions or molecules across cell membranes	Serotonin re-uptake transporter Na^+/K^+ ATPase

(AMP = adenosine monophosphate; ATPase = adenosine triphosphatase; GMP = guanosine monophosphate; PPAR = peroxisome proliferator-activated receptor)

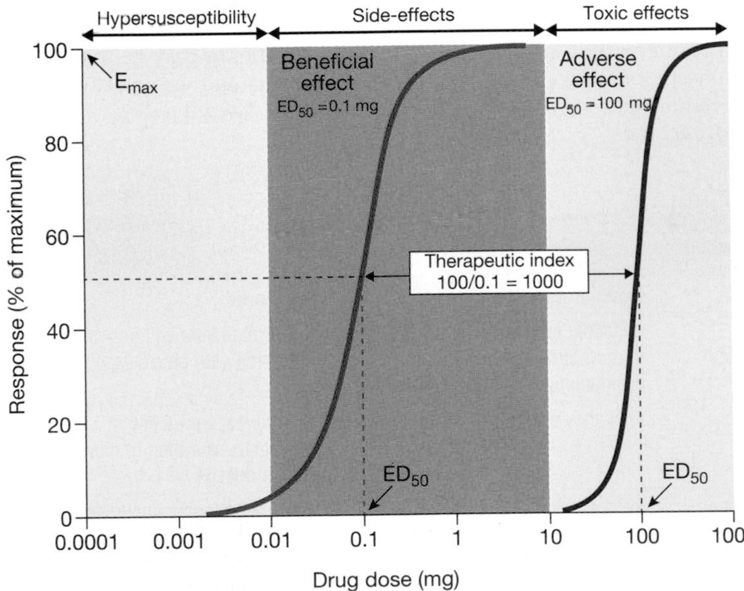

Fig. 2.2 Dose–response curve. The green curve represents the beneficial effect of the drug. The maximum response on the curve is the E_{max} and the dose (or concentration) producing half this value ($E_{max}/2$) is the ED_{50} (or EC_{50}). The red curve illustrates the dose–response relationship for the most important adverse effect of this drug. This occurs at much higher doses; the ratio between the ED_{50} for the adverse effect and that for the beneficial effect is the 'therapeutic index', which indicates how much margin there is for prescribers when choosing a dose that will provide beneficial effects without also causing this adverse effect. Adverse effects that occur at doses above the therapeutic range (yellow area) are normally called 'toxic effects', while those occurring within the therapeutic range are 'side-effects' and those below it are 'hyper-susceptibility effects'.

antagonists inhibit the effect of an agonist by mechanisms other than direct competition for receptor binding with the agonist (e.g. by affecting post-receptor signalling).

Dose–response relationships

Plotting the logarithm of drug dose against drug response typically produces a sigmoidal dose–response curve (Fig. 2.2). Progressive increases in drug dose (which for most drugs is proportional to the plasma drug concentration) produce increasing response, but only within a relatively narrow range of dose; further increases in dose beyond this range produce little extra effect. The following characteristics of the drug response are useful in comparing different drugs:

- *Efficacy* describes the extent to which a drug can produce a target-specific response when all available receptors or binding sites are occupied

(i.e. E_{max} on the dose–response curve). A full agonist can produce the maximum response of which the receptor is capable, while a partial agonist at the same receptor will have lower efficacy. *Therapeutic efficacy* describes the effect of the drug on a desired biological endpoint, and can be used to compare drugs that act via different pharmacological mechanisms (e.g. loop diuretics induce a greater diuresis than thiazide diuretics and therefore have greater therapeutic efficacy).
- *Potency* describes the amount of drug required for a given response. More potent drugs produce biological effects at lower doses, so they have a lower ED_{50}. A less potent drug can still have an equivalent efficacy if it is given in higher doses.

The dose–response relationship varies between patients because of variations in the many determinants of pharmacokinetics and pharmacodynamics. In clinical practice, the prescriber is unable to construct a dose–response curve for each individual patient. Therefore, most drugs are licensed for use within a recommended range of doses that is expected to reach close to the top of the dose–response curve for most patients. However, it is sometimes possible to achieve the desired therapeutic efficacy at doses towards the lower end of, or even below, the recommended range.

Therapeutic index

The adverse effects of drugs are often dose-related in a similar way to the beneficial effects, although the dose–response curve for these adverse effects is normally shifted to the right (see Fig. 2.2). The ratio of the ED_{50} for therapeutic efficacy and for a major adverse effect is known as the 'therapeutic index'. In reality, drugs have multiple potential adverse effects but the concept of therapeutic index is usually reserved for those requiring dose reduction or discontinuation. For most drugs, the therapeutic index is greater than 100 but there are some notable exceptions with therapeutic indices less than 10 (e.g. digoxin, warfarin, insulin, phenytoin, opioids). The doses of such drugs have to be titrated carefully for individual patients to maximise benefits but avoid adverse effects.

Desensitisation and withdrawal effects

Desensitisation refers to the common situation in which the biological response to a drug diminishes when it is given continuously or repeatedly. It may be possible to restore the response by increasing the dose of the drug but, in some cases, the tissues may become completely refractory to its effect.

- *Tachyphylaxis* describes desensitisation that occurs very rapidly, sometimes with the initial dose. This rapid loss of response implies depletion of chemicals that may be necessary for the pharmacological actions of the drug (e.g. a stored neurotransmitter released from a nerve terminal) or receptor phosphorylation.
- *Tolerance* describes a more gradual loss of response to a drug that occurs over days or weeks. This slower change implies changes in receptor numbers or the development of counter-regulatory physiological changes that offset the actions of the drug (e.g. accumulation of salt and water in response to vasodilator therapy).
- *Drug resistance* is a term normally reserved for describing the loss of effectiveness of an antimicrobial (p. 151) or cancer chemotherapy drug.
- In addition to these pharmacodynamic causes of desensitisation, reduced response may be the consequence of lower plasma and tissue drug concentrations as a result of altered *pharmacokinetics* (see below).

2.3 Examples of drugs associated with withdrawal effects

Drug	Symptoms	Signs	Treatment
Alcohol	Anxiety, panic, paranoid delusions, visual and auditory hallucinations	Agitation, restlessness, confusion, tremor, tachycardia, ataxia, disorientation, seizures	Treat immediate withdrawal syndrome with benzodiazepines
Barbiturates, benzodiazepines	Similar to alcohol	Similar to alcohol	Transfer to long-acting benzodiazepine then gradually reduce dosage
Corticosteroids	Weakness, fatigue, decreased appetite, weight loss, nausea, vomiting, diarrhoea, abdominal pain	Hypotension, hypoglycaemia	Prolonged therapy suppresses the hypothalamic–pituitary–adrenal axis and causes adrenal insufficiency requiring corticosteroid replacement. Withdrawal should be gradual after prolonged therapy (p. 776)
Opioids	Rhinorrhoea, sneezing, yawning, lacrimation, abdominal and leg cramping, nausea, vomiting, diarrhoea	Dilated pupils	Transfer addicts to long-acting agonist methadone
Selective serotonin re-uptake inhibitors (SSRIs)	Dizziness, sweating, nausea, insomnia, tremor, confusion, nightmares	Tremor	Reduce SSRIs slowly to avoid withdrawal effects

When drugs induce chemical, hormonal and physiological changes that offset their actions, discontinuation may allow these changes to cause 'rebound' withdrawal effects (Box 2.3).

Pharmacokinetics

Understanding 'what the body does to the drug' (Fig. 2.3) is extremely important for prescribers because this forms the basis on which the optimal route of administration and dose regimen are chosen and explains the majority of inter-individual variation in the response to drug therapy.

Drug absorption and routes of administration

Absorption is the process by which drug molecules gain access to the blood stream. The rate and extent of drug absorption depend on the route of administration (see Fig. 2.3).

Enteral administration

These routes involve administration via the gastrointestinal tract:

- *Oral*. This is the commonest route of administration because it is simple, convenient and readily used by patients to self-administer their medicines. Absorption after an oral dose is a complex process that depends on the drug being swallowed, surviving exposure to gastric acid, avoiding unacceptable food binding, being absorbed across the small bowel mucosa into the portal venous system, and surviving metabolism by gut wall or liver enzymes ('first-pass metabolism'). As a consequence, absorption is frequently incomplete following oral administration. The term 'bioavailability' describes the proportion of the dose that reaches the systemic circulation intact.
- *Buccal, intranasal and sublingual (SL)*. These routes have the advantage of enabling rapid absorption into the systemic circulation without the uncertainties associated with oral administration (e.g. organic nitrates for angina pectoris, triptans for migraine, opioid analgesics).
- *Rectal (PR)*. The rectal mucosa is occasionally used as a site of drug administration when the oral route is compromised because of nausea and vomiting or unconsciousness (e.g. diazepam in status epilepticus).

Parenteral administration

These routes avoid absorption via the gastrointestinal tract and first-pass metabolism in the liver:

- *Intravenous (IV)*. The IV route enables all of a dose to enter the systemic circulation reliably, without any concerns about absorption or first-pass metabolism (i.e. the dose is 100% bioavailable), and rapidly achieve a high plasma concentration. It is ideal for very ill patients when a rapid, certain effect is critical to outcome (e.g. benzylpenicillin for meningococcal meningitis).
- *Intramuscular (IM)*. IM administration is easier to achieve than the IV route (e.g. adrenaline (epinephrine) for acute anaphylaxis) but absorption is less predictable and depends on muscle blood flow.
- *Subcutaneous (SC)*. The SC route is ideal for drugs that have to be administered parenterally because of low oral bioavailability, are absorbed well from subcutaneous fat, and might ideally be injected by patients themselves (e.g. insulin, heparin).
- *Transdermal*. A transdermal patch can enable a drug to be absorbed through the skin and into the circulation (e.g. oestrogens, testosterone, nicotine, nitrates).

Other routes of administration

- *Topical* application of a drug involves direct administration to the site of action (e.g. skin, eye, ear). This has the advantage of achieving sufficient concentration at this site while minimising systemic exposure and the risk of adverse effects elsewhere.
- *Inhaled (INH)* administration allows drugs to be delivered directly to a target in the respiratory tree, usually the small airways (e.g. salbutamol,

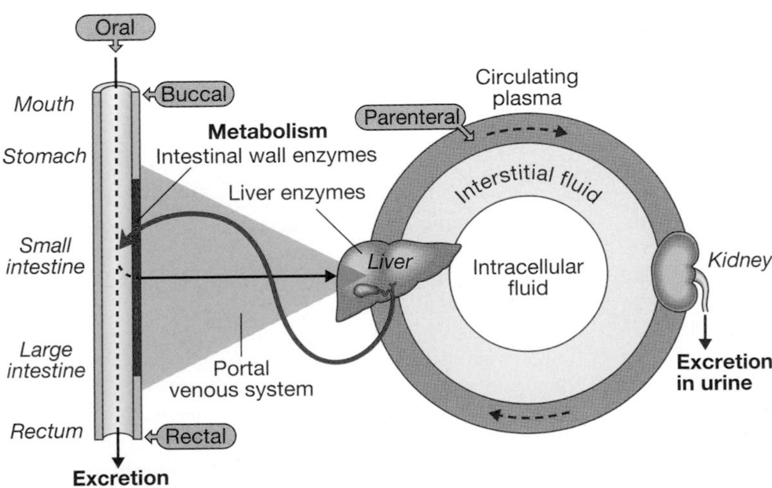

Fig. 2.3 Pharmacokinetics summary. Most drugs are taken orally, are absorbed from the intestinal lumen and enter the portal venous system to be conveyed to the liver, where they may be subject to first-pass metabolism and/or excretion in bile. Active drugs then enter the systemic circulation, from which they may diffuse (or sometimes be actively transported) in and out of the interstitial and intracellular fluid compartments. Drug that remains in circulating plasma is subject to liver metabolism and renal excretion. Drugs excreted in bile may be reabsorbed, creating an enterohepatic circulation. First-pass metabolism in liver is avoided if drugs are administered via the buccal or rectal mucosa, or parenterally (e.g. by intravenous injection).

beclometasone). However, a significant proportion of the inhaled dose may be absorbed from the lung or is swallowed and can reach the systemic circulation. The most common mode of delivery is the metered-dose inhaler but its success depends on some degree of manual dexterity and timing (see Fig. 19.23, p. 670). Patients who find these difficult may use a 'spacer' device to improve drug delivery. A special mode of inhaled delivery is via a nebulised solution created by using pressurised oxygen or air to break up solutions and suspensions into small aerosol droplets that can be directly inhaled from the mouthpiece of the device.

Drug distribution

Distribution is the process by which drug molecules transfer into and out of the blood stream. This is influenced by the drug's molecular size and lipid solubility, the extent to which it binds to proteins in plasma, its susceptibility to drug transporters expressed on cell surfaces, and its binding to its molecular target and to other cellular proteins (which can be irreversible). Most drugs diffuse passively across capillary walls down a concentration gradient into the interstitial fluid until the concentration of free drug molecules in the interstitial fluid is equal to that in the plasma. As drug molecules in the blood are removed by metabolism or excretion, the plasma concentration falls and drug molecules diffuse back from the tissue compartment into the blood, and eventually all will be eliminated. Note that this reverse movement of drug away from the tissues will be prevented if further drug doses are administered and absorbed into the plasma.

Volume of distribution

The apparent volume of distribution (V_d) is the volume into which a drug appears to have distributed following intravenous injection. It is calculated from the equation

$$V_d = D/C_o$$

where D is the amount of drug given and C_0 is the initial plasma concentration (Fig. 2.4A). Drugs that are highly bound to plasma proteins may have a V_d below 10 L (e.g. warfarin, aspirin), while those that diffuse into the interstitial fluid but do not enter cells because they have low lipid solubility may have a V_d between 10 and 30 L (e.g. gentamicin, amoxicillin). It is an 'apparent' volume because those drugs that are lipid-soluble and highly tissue-bound may have a V_d of greater than 100 L (e.g. digoxin, amitriptyline). Drugs with a larger V_d are eliminated more slowly from the body.

Drug elimination

Drug metabolism

Metabolism is the process by which drugs are chemically altered from a lipid-soluble form suitable for absorption and distribution to a more water-soluble form that is necessary for excretion. Some drugs, known as 'pro-drugs', are inactive in the form in which they are administered, but are converted to an active metabolite in vivo.

Phase I metabolism involves oxidation, reduction or hydrolysis to make drug molecules suitable for phase II reactions or for excretion. Oxidation is much the commonest form of phase I reaction and chiefly involves members of the cytochrome P450 family of membrane-bound enzymes in the endoplasmic reticulum of hepatocytes.

Phase II metabolism involves combining phase I metabolites with an endogenous substrate to form an inactive conjugate that is much more water-soluble. Reactions include glucuronidation, sulphation, acetylation or methylation, and conjugation with glutathione. This is necessary to enable renal excretion because lipid-soluble metabolites will simply diffuse back into the body after glomerular filtration (p. 430).

Drug excretion

Excretion is the process by which drugs and their metabolites are removed from the body.

Renal excretion is the usual route of elimination for drugs or their metabolites that are of low molecular weight and sufficiently water-soluble to avoid reabsorption from the renal tubule. Drugs bound to plasma proteins are not filtered by the glomeruli. The pH of the urine is more acidic than that of plasma, so that some drugs (e.g. salicylates) become un-ionised and tend to be reabsorbed. Alkalination of the urine can hasten excretion (e.g. after a salicylate overdose). For some drugs, active secretion into the proximal tubule lumen, rather than glomerular filtration, is the predominant mechanism of excretion (e.g. methotrexate, penicillin).

Faecal excretion is the predominant route of elimination for drugs with high molecular weight, including those that are excreted in the bile after conjugation with glucuronide in the liver, and any drugs that are not absorbed after enteral administration. Molecules of drug or metabolite that are excreted in the bile enter the small intestine, where they may, if they are sufficiently lipid-soluble, be reabsorbed through the gut wall and return to the liver via the portal vein (see Fig. 2.3). This recycling between the liver, bile, gut and portal vein is known as 'enterohepatic circulation' and can significantly prolong the residence of drugs in the body.

Elimination kinetics

The net removal of drug from the circulation results from a combination of drug metabolism and excretion, and is usually described as 'clearance', i.e. the volume of plasma that is completely cleared of drug per unit time.

For most drugs, elimination is a high-capacity process that does not become saturated, even at high dosage. The rate of elimination is therefore directly proportional to the drug concentration because of the 'law of mass action', whereby higher drug concentrations will drive faster metabolic reactions and support higher renal filtration rates. This results in 'first-order' kinetics, when a constant fraction of the drug remaining in the circulation is eliminated in a given time and the decline in concentration over time is exponential (see Fig. 2.4A). This elimination can be described by the drug's half-life ($t_{1/2}$), i.e. the time taken for the plasma drug concentration to halve, which remains constant throughout the period of drug elimination. The significance of this phenomenon for prescribers is that the effect of increasing doses on plasma concentration is predictable – a doubled dose leads to a doubled concentration at all time points.

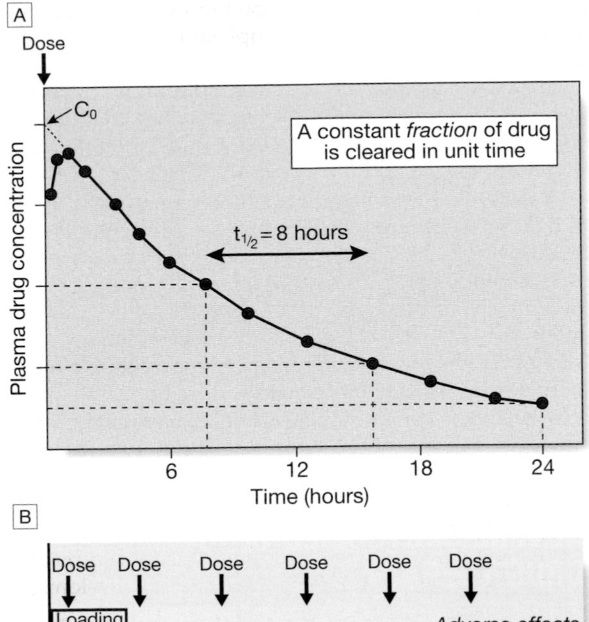

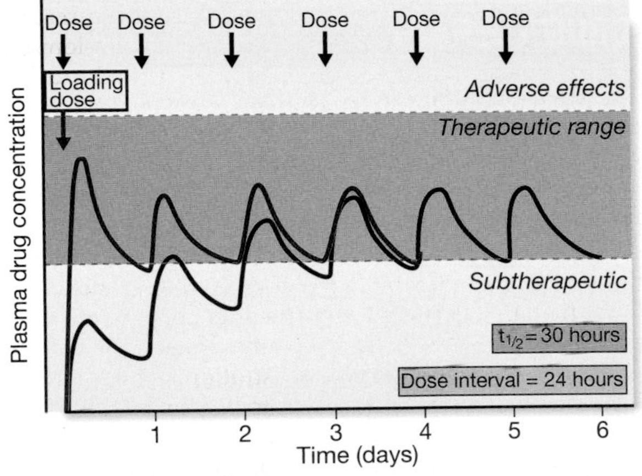

Fig. 2.4 Drug concentrations in plasma following single and multiple drug dosing. **A** In this example of first-order kinetics following a single intravenous dose, the time period required for the plasma drug concentration to halve (half-life, $t_{1/2}$) remains constant throughout the elimination process. **B** After multiple dosing, the plasma drug concentration rises if each dose is administered before the previous dose has been entirely cleared. In this example, the drug's half-life is 30 hours, so that with daily dosing the peak, average and trough concentrations steadily increase as drug accumulates in the body (black line). Steady state is reached after approximately 5 half-lives, when the rate of elimination (the product of concentration and clearance) is equal to the rate of drug absorption (the product of rate of administration and bioavailability). The long half-life in this example means that it takes 6 days for steady state to be achieved and, for most of the first 3 days of treatment, plasma drug concentrations are below the therapeutic range (yellow-shaded area). This problem can be overcome if a larger loading dose (red line) is used to achieve steady state drug concentrations more rapidly.

For a few drugs in common use (e.g. phenytoin, alcohol), elimination capacity is exceeded (saturated) within the usual dose range. This is called 'zero-order' kinetics. Its significance for prescribers is that, if the rate of administration exceeds the maximum rate of elimination, the drug will accumulate progressively, leading to serious toxicity.

Repeated dose regimens

The goal of therapy is usually to maintain drug concentrations within the therapeutic range (see Fig. 2.2) over several days (e.g. antibiotics) or even for months or years (e.g. antihypertensives, lipid-lowering drugs, thyroid hormone replacement therapy). This goal is rarely achieved with single doses, so prescribers have to plan a regimen of repeated doses. This involves choosing the size of each individual dose and the frequency of dose administration.

As illustrated in Figure 2.4B, the time taken to reach drug concentrations within the therapeutic range depends on the half-life of the drug. Typically, with doses administered regularly, it takes approximately 5 half-lives to reach a 'steady state' in which the rate of drug elimination is equal to the rate of drug administration. This applies when starting new drugs and when adjusting doses of current drugs. With appropriate dose selection, steady state drug concentrations will be maintained within the therapeutic range. This is important for prescribers because it means that the effects of a new prescription, or dose titration, for a drug with a long half-life (e.g. digoxin – 36 hours) may not be known for a few days. In contrast, drugs with a very short half-life (e.g. dobutamine – 2 minutes) have to be given continuously by infusion but reach a new steady state within minutes.

For drugs with a long half-life, if it is unacceptable to wait for 5 half-lives until concentrations within the therapeutic range are maintained, then an initial 'loading dose' can be given that is much larger than the maintenance dose, and equivalent to the amount of drug required in the body at steady state. This achieves a peak plasma concentration close to the plateau concentration, which can then be maintained by successive maintenance doses.

'Steady state' actually involves fluctuations in drug concentrations, with peaks just after administration followed by troughs just prior to the next administration. The manufacturers of medicines recommend dosing regimens that predict that, for most patients, these oscillations result in troughs within the therapeutic range and peaks that are not high enough to cause adverse effects. The optimal dose interval is a compromise between convenience for the patient and a constant level of drug exposure. More frequent administration (e.g. 25 mg 4 times daily) achieves a smoother plasma concentration profile than 100 mg once daily but is much more difficult for patients to sustain. A solution to this need for compromise in dosing frequency for drugs with half-lives of less than 24 hours is the use of 'modified-release' formulations. These allow drugs to be absorbed more slowly from the gastrointestinal tract and reduce the oscillation in plasma drug concentration profile, which is especially important for drugs with a low therapeutic index (e.g. levodopa).

Inter-individual variation in drug responses

Prescribers have numerous sources of guidance about how to use drugs appropriately (e.g. dose, route, frequency, duration) for many conditions. However, this advice is based on average dose–response data derived from observations in many individuals. When applying this information to an individual patient, prescribers

2.4 Patient-specific factors that influence pharmacokinetics

Age
- Drug metabolism is low in the fetus and newborn, may be enhanced in young children, and becomes less effective with advancing age
- Drug excretion falls with the age-related decline in renal function

Sex
- Women have a greater proportion of body fat than men, increasing volume of distribution and half-life of lipid-soluble drugs

Body weight
- Obesity increases volume of distribution and half-life of lipid-soluble drugs
- Patients with higher lean body mass have larger body compartments into which drugs are distributed and may require higher doses

Liver function
- Metabolism of most drugs depends on several cytochrome P450 enzymes that are impaired in patients with advanced liver disease
- Hypoalbuminaemia influences the distribution of drugs that are highly protein-bound

Kidney function
- Renal disease and the decline in renal function with ageing may lead to drug accumulation

Gastrointestinal function
- Small intestinal absorption of oral drugs may be delayed by reduced gastric motility
- Absorptive capacity of the intestinal mucosa may be reduced in disease (e.g. Crohn's disease, coeliac disease) or after surgical resection

Food
- Food in the stomach delays gastric emptying and reduces the rate (but not usually the extent) of drug absorption
- Some food constituents bind to certain drugs and prevent their absorption

Smoking
- Tar in tobacco stimulates the oxidation of certain drugs

Alcohol
- Regular alcohol consumption stimulates liver enzyme synthesis, while binge drinking may temporarily inhibit drug metabolism

Drugs
- Drug–drug interactions cause marked variation in pharmacokinetics (see Box 2.11, p. 28)

must take account of inter-individual variability in response. Some of this variability is predictable and good prescribers are able to anticipate it and adjust their prescriptions accordingly to maximise the chances of benefit and minimise harm. Inter-individual variation in responses also mandates that effects of treatment should be monitored (p. 39).

Some inter-individual variation in drug response is accounted for by differences in pharmacodynamics. For example, the beneficial natriuresis produced by the loop diuretic furosemide is often significantly reduced at a given dose in patients with renal impairment, while confusion caused by opioid analgesics is more likely in the elderly. However, differences in pharmacokinetics more commonly account for different drug responses. Examples of factors influencing the absorption, metabolism and excretion of drugs are shown in Box 2.4.

It is hoped that a significant proportion of the inter-individual variation in drug responses can be explained by studying genetic differences in single genes ('pharmacogenetics') (Box 2.5) or the effects of multiple gene variants ('pharmacogenomics'). The aim is to identify those patients most likely to benefit from specific treatments and those most susceptible to adverse effects. In this way, it may be possible to select drugs and dose regimens for individual patients to maximise the benefit:hazard ratio ('personalised medicine').

ADVERSE OUTCOMES OF DRUG THERAPY

The decision to prescribe a drug always involves a judgement of the balance between therapeutic benefits and risk of an adverse outcome. Both prescribers and patients tend to be more focused on the former but a truly informed decision requires consideration of both.

Adverse drug reactions

Some important definitions for the adverse effects of drugs are:
- *Adverse event.* A harmful event that occurs while a patient is taking a drug, irrespective of whether the drug is suspected of being the cause.
- *Adverse drug reaction (ADR).* An unwanted or harmful reaction that is experienced following the administration of a drug or combination of drugs under normal conditions of use and is suspected to be related to the drug. An ADR will usually require the drug to be discontinued or the dose reduced.
- *Side-effect.* Any effect caused by a drug other than the intended therapeutic effect, whether beneficial, neutral or harmful. The term 'side-effect' is often used interchangeably with 'ADR', although the former usually implies an effect that is less harmful, is predictable and may not require discontinuation of therapy (e.g. ankle oedema with vasodilators).
- *Drug toxicity.* Adverse effects of a drug that occur because the dose or plasma concentration has risen above the therapeutic range, either unintentionally or intentionally (drug overdose, see Fig. 2.2, p. 19).
- *Drug abuse.* The misuse of recreational or therapeutic drugs that may lead to addiction or dependence, serious physiological injury (such as liver damage), psychological harm (abnormal behaviour patterns, hallucinations, memory loss) or death (p. 240).

Prevalence of ADRs

ADRs are a common cause of illness, accounting in the United Kingdom (UK) for approximately 3% of consultations in primary care and 7% of emergency

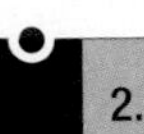

2.5 Examples of pharmacogenetic variations that influence drug response

Genetic variant	Drug affected	Clinical outcome
Pharmacokinetic		
Aldehyde dehydrogenase-2 deficiency	Ethanol	Elevated blood acetaldehyde causes facial flushing and increased heart rate in ~50% of Japanese, Chinese and other Asian populations
Acetylation	Isoniazid, hydralazine, procainamide	Increased responses in slow acetylators, up to 50% of some populations
Oxidation (CYP2D6)	Nortriptyline Codeine	Increased risk of toxicity in poor metabolisers Reduced responses with slower conversion of codeine to more active morphine in poor metabolisers, 10% of European populations Increased risk of toxicity in ultra-fast metabolisers, 3% of Europeans but 40% of North Africans
Oxidation (CYP2C18)	Proguanil	Reduced efficacy with slower conversion to active cycloguanil in poor metabolisers
Oxidation (CYP2C9)	Warfarin	Polymorphisms known to influence dosages
Oxidation (CYP2C19)	Clopidogrel	Reduced enzymatic activation results in reduced antiplatelet effect
Sulphoxidation	Penicillamine	Increased risk of toxicity in poor metabolisers
HLA-B*1502	Carbamazepine	Increased risk of serious dermatological reactions (e.g. Stevens–Johnson syndrome) for 1 in 2000 in Caucasian populations (much higher in some Asian countries)
Pseudocholinesterase deficiency	Suxamethonium (succinylcholine)	Decreased drug inactivation leads to prolonged paralysis and sometimes persistent apnoea requiring mechanical ventilation until the drug can be eliminated by alternate pathways in 1 in 1500 people
Pharmacodynamic		
Glucose-6-phosphate dehydrogenase (G6PD) deficiency	Oxidant drugs including antimalarials (e.g. chloroquine, primaquine)	Risk of haemolysis in G6PD deficiency
Acute intermittent porphyria	Enzyme-inducing drugs	Increased risk of an acute attack
SLC01B1 polymorphism	Statins	Increased risk of rhabdomyolysis
HLA-B*5701 polymorphism	Abacavir	Increased risk of skin hypersensitivity reactions
HLA-B*5801 polymorphism	Allopurinol	Increased risk of rashes in Han Chinese
HLA-B*1502 polymorphism	Carbamazepine	Increased risk of skin hypersensitivity reactions in Han Chinese

(HLA = human leucocyte antigen)

admissions to hospital, and affecting around 15% of hospital inpatients. Many 'disease' presentations are eventually attributed to ADRs, emphasising the importance of always taking a careful drug history (Box 2.6). Factors accounting for the rising prevalence of ADRs are the increasing age of patients, polypharmacy (higher risk of drug interactions), increasing availability of over-the-counter medicines, increase in use of herbal or traditional medicines, and increase in medicines available via the Internet. Risk factors for ADRs are shown in Box 2.7.

ADRs are important because they reduce quality of life for patients, reduce adherence to and therefore efficacy of beneficial treatments, cause diagnostic confusion, undermine the confidence of patients in their health-care professional(s), and consume health-care resources.

Retrospective analysis of ADRs has shown that more than half could have been avoided if the prescriber had taken more care in anticipating the potential hazards of drug therapy. Each year in the UK, non-steroidal anti-inflammatory drug (NSAID) use alone accounts for 65 000 emergency admissions, 12 000 gastrointestinal bleeding episodes and 2000 deaths. In many cases, the patients were at increased risk due to their age, interacting drugs (e.g. aspirin, warfarin) or a past history of peptic ulcer disease. Drugs that commonly cause ADRs are listed in Box 2.8.

Prescribers and their patients ideally want to know the frequency with which ADRs occur for a specific drug. Although this may be well characterised for more common ADRs observed in clinical trials, it is less clear for rarely reported ADRs when the total numbers of reactions and patients exposed are not known. The words used to describe frequency can be misinterpreted by patients, but widely accepted meanings include: *very common* (10% or more), *common* (1–10%), *uncommon* (0.1–1%), *rare* (0.01–0.1%) and *very rare* (0.01% or less).

Classification of ADRs

ADRs have traditionally been classified into two major groups:

- *Type A ('augmented') ADRs*. These are predictable from the known pharmacodynamic effects of the drug, and are dose-dependent, common (detected early in drug development) and usually mild.

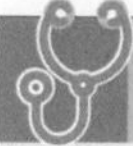

2.6 How to take a drug history

Information from the patient (or carer)

Use language that patients will understand (e.g. 'medicines' rather than 'drugs', which may be mistaken for drugs of abuse) while gathering the following information:

- Current prescribed drugs, including formulations (e.g. modified-release tablets), doses, routes of administration, frequency and timing, duration of treatment
- Other medications that are often forgotten (e.g. over-the-counter drugs, herbal remedies, vitamins)
- Drugs that have been taken in the recent past and reasons for stopping them
- Previous drug hypersensitivity reactions, their nature and time course (e.g. rash, anaphylaxis)
- Previous ADRs, their nature and time course (e.g. muscle aches with simvastatin)
- Adherence to therapy (e.g. 'are you taking your medication regularly?')

Information from the general practitioner (GP) medical records and/or pharmacist

- Up-to-date list of medications
- Previous ADRs
- Last order dates for each medication

Inspection of medicines

- Drugs and their containers (e.g. blister packs, bottles, vials) should be inspected for name, dosage, and the number of dosage forms taken since dispensed

(ADR = adverse drug reaction)

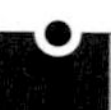

2.7 Risk factors for ADRs

Patient factors

- Elderly age (e.g. low physiological reserve)
- Gender (e.g. ACE inhibitor-induced cough in women)
- Polypharmacy (e.g. drug interactions)
- Genetic predisposition (see Box 2.5)
- Hypersensitivity/allergy (e.g. β-lactam antibiotics)
- Diseases altering pharmacokinetics (e.g. hepatic or renal impairment) or pharmacodynamic responses (e.g. bladder instability)
- Adherence problems (e.g. cognitive impairment)

Drug factors

- Steep dose–response curve (e.g. insulin)
- Low therapeutic index (e.g. digoxin, cytotoxic drugs)

Prescriber factors

- Inadequate understanding of principles of clinical pharmacology
- Inadequate knowledge of the prescribed drug
- Inadequate instructions and warnings provided to patients
- Inadequate monitoring arrangements planned

2.8 Drugs that are common causes of ADRs

Drug or drug class	Common ADRs
ACE inhibitors (e.g. lisinopril)	Renal impairment Hyperkalaemia
Antibiotics (e.g. amoxicillin)	Nausea Diarrhoea
Anticoagulants (e.g. warfarin, heparin)	Bleeding
Antipsychotics (e.g. haloperidol)	Falls Sedation Confusion
Aspirin	Gastrotoxicity (dyspepsia, gastrointestinal bleeding)
Benzodiazepines (e.g. diazepam)	Drowsiness Falls
β-blockers (e.g. atenolol)	Cold peripheries Bradycardia
Calcium channel blockers (e.g. amlodipine)	Ankle oedema
Digoxin	Nausea and anorexia Bradycardia
Diuretics (e.g. furosemide, bendroflumethiazide)	Dehydration Electrolyte disturbance (hypokalaemia, hyponatraemia) Hypotension Renal impairment
Insulin	Hypoglycaemia
NSAIDs (e.g. ibuprofen)	Gastrotoxicity (dyspepsia, gastrointestinal bleeding) Renal impairment
Opioid analgesics (e.g. morphine)	Nausea and vomiting Confusion Constipation

(ACE = angiotensin-converting enzyme; NSAID = non-steroidal anti-inflammatory drug)

Examples include constipation caused by opioids, hypotension caused by antihypertensives and dehydration caused by diuretics.

- *Type B ('bizarre') ADRs*. These are not predictable, are not obviously dose-dependent in the therapeutic range, and are rare (remaining undiscovered until the drug is marketed) and often severe. Patients who experience type B reactions are generally 'hyper-susceptible' because of unpredictable immunological or genetic factors (e.g. anaphylaxis caused by penicillin, peripheral neuropathy caused by isoniazid in poor acetylators).

This simple classification has shortcomings and a more detailed classification based on dose (see Fig. 2.2, p. 19), timing and susceptibility (DoTS) is now used by those analysing ADRs in greater depth (Box 2.9). The AB classification can be extended as a reminder of some other types of ADR:

- *Type C ('chronic/continuous') ADRs*. These occur only after prolonged continuous exposure to a drug. Examples include osteoporosis caused by corticosteroids, retinopathy caused by chloroquine, and tardive dyskinesia caused by phenothiazines.
- *Type D ('delayed') ADRs*. These are delayed until long after drug exposure, making diagnosis difficult. Examples include malignancies that may emerge after immunosuppressive treatment post transplantation (e.g. azathioprine, tacrolimus) and vaginal cancer occurring many years after exposure to diethylstilboestrol.

2.9 DoTS classification of ADRs

Category	Example
Dose	
Below therapeutic dose	Anaphylaxis with penicillin
In the therapeutic dose range	Nausea with morphine
At high doses	Hepatotoxicity with paracetamol
Timing	
With the first dose	Anaphylaxis with penicillin
Early stages of treatment	Hyponatraemia with diuretics
On stopping treatment	Benzodiazepine withdrawal syndrome
Significantly delayed	Clear cell cancer with diethylstilboestrol
Susceptibility	See patient factors in Box 2.7

(INR = international normalised ratio)

- *Type E ('end of treatment') ADRs*. These occur after abrupt drug withdrawal (see Box 2.3, p. 20).

A teratogen is a drug with the potential to affect the development of the fetus in the first 10 weeks of intrauterine life (e.g. phenytoin, warfarin). The thalidomide disaster in the early 1960s highlighted the risk of teratogenicity and led to mandatory testing of all new drugs. Congenital defects in a live infant or aborted fetus should lead to the suspicion of an ADR and a careful exploration of drug exposures (including self-medication and herbal remedies).

Detecting ADRs – pharmacovigilance

Type A ADRs become apparent early in the development of a new drug. However, by the time a new drug is licensed and launched on to a possible worldwide market, hundreds rather than thousands of patients may have been exposed to it, so that rarer but potentially serious type B ADRs may remain undiscovered. Pharmacovigilance is the process of detecting ('signal generation') and evaluating ADRs in order to help prescribers and patients to be better informed about the risks of drug therapy. Drug regulatory agencies may respond to this information by placing restrictions on the licensed indications, reducing the recommended dose range, adding special warnings and precautions for prescribers in the product literature, writing to all health-care professionals, or withdrawing the product from the market.

Voluntary reporting systems allow health-care professionals and patients to report suspected ADRs to the regulatory authorities. A good example is the 'Yellow Card' scheme that was set up in the UK in response to the thalidomide tragedy. Reports are analysed to assess the likelihood that they represent a true ADR (Box 2.10). Although voluntary reporting is a continuously operating and effective early warning system for previously unrecognised rare ADRs, its weaknesses include low reporting rates (only 3% of all ADRs and 10% of serious ADRs are ever reported), an inability to quantify risk (because the ratio of ADRs to prescriptions is unknown), and the influence of prescriber awareness on likelihood of reporting (reporting rates rise rapidly following publicity about potential ADRs).

More systematic approaches to collecting information on ADRs include 'prescription event monitoring', in which a sample of prescribers of a particular drug are issued with questionnaires concerning the clinical outcome for their patients, and the collection of population statistics. Many health-care systems routinely collect patient identifiable data on prescriptions (a surrogate marker of exposure to a drug), health-care events (e.g. hospitalisation, operations, new clinical diagnoses) and other clinical data (e.g. haematology, biochemistry). As these records are linked, with appropriate safeguards for confidentiality and data protection, they are providing a much more powerful mechanism for assessing both the harms and benefits of drugs.

All prescribers will inevitably see patients experiencing ADRs caused by prescriptions written by themselves or their colleagues. It is important that these are recognised early. In addition to the features in Box 2.10, features that should raise suspicion of an ADR and the need to respond (by drug withdrawal, dosage reduction or reporting to the regulatory authorities) include:

- concern expressed by a patient that a drug has harmed him/her
- abnormal clinical measurements (e.g. blood pressure, temperature, pulse, blood glucose and

2.10 TREND analysis of suspected ADRs

Factor	Key question	Comment
***T**emporal relationship*	What is the time interval between the start of drug therapy and the reaction?	Most ADRs occur soon after starting treatment and within hours in the case of anaphylactic reactions
***Re**-challenge*	What happens when the patient is re-challenged with the drug?	Re-challenge is rarely possible because of the need to avoid exposing patients to unnecessary risk
***E**xclusion*	Have concomitant drugs and other non-drug causes been excluded?	ADR is a diagnosis of exclusion following clinical assessment and relevant investigations for non-drug causes
***N**ovelty*	Has the reaction been reported before?	The suspected ADR may already be recognised and mentioned in the SPC approved by the regulatory authorities
***De**-challenge*	Does the reaction improve when the drug is withdrawn or the dose is reduced?	Most, but not all, ADRs improve on drug withdrawal, although recovery may be slow

(SPC = Summary of Product Characteristics)

weight) or laboratory results (e.g. abnormal liver or renal function, low haemoglobin white cell count) while on drug therapy
- new therapy started which could be in response to an ADR (e.g. omeprazole, allopurinol, naloxone)
- the presence of risk factors for ADRs (see Box 2.7).

Drug interactions

A drug interaction has occurred when the administration of one drug increases or decreases the beneficial or adverse responses to another drug. Although the number of potential interacting drug combinations is very large, only a small number are common in clinical practice. Important drug interactions are most likely to occur when the affected drug has a low therapeutic index, steep dose–response curve, high first-pass or saturable metabolism, or single mechanism of elimination.

Mechanisms of drug interactions

Pharmacodynamic interactions occur when two drugs produce additive, synergistic or antagonistic effects at the same drug target (e.g. receptor, enzyme) or physiological system (e.g. electrolyte excretion, heart rate). These are the most common interactions in clinical practice and some important examples are given in Box 2.11.

Pharmacokinetic interactions occur when the administration of a second drug alters the concentration of the first at its site of action. There are numerous potential mechanisms:

- *Absorption interactions.* Drugs that either delay (e.g. anticholinergic drugs) or enhance (e.g. prokinetic drugs) gastric emptying influence the rate of rise in plasma concentration of other drugs but not the total amount of drug absorbed. Drugs that bind to form insoluble complexes or chelates (e.g. aluminium-containing antacids binding with ciprofloxacin) can reduce drug absorption.
- *Distribution interactions.* Co-administration of drugs that compete for protein binding in plasma (e.g. phenytoin and diazepam) can increase the unbound drug concentration, but the effect is usually short-lived due to increased elimination and hence restoration of the pre-interaction equilibrium.
- *Metabolism interactions.* Many drugs rely on metabolism by different isoenzymes of cytochrome P450 (CYP) in the liver. CYP enzyme inducers (e.g. phenytoin, rifampicin) generally reduce plasma concentrations of other drugs, although they may enhance activation of prodrugs. CYP enzyme inhibitors (e.g. clarithromycin, cimetidine, grapefruit

2.11 Common drug interactions

Mechanism	Object drug	Precipitant drug	Result
Pharmaceutical*			
Chemical reaction	Sodium bicarbonate	Calcium gluconate	Precipitation of insoluble calcium carbonate
Pharmacokinetic			
Reduced absorption	Tetracyclines	Calcium, aluminium, and magnesium salts	Reduced tetracycline absorption
Reduced protein binding	Phenytoin	Aspirin	Increased unbound and reduced total phenytoin plasma concentration
Reduced metabolism			
CYP3A4	Terfenadine	Grapefruit juice	Cardiac arrhythmias because of prolonged QT interval (p. 570)
	Warfarin	Clarithromycin	Enhanced anticoagulation
CYP2C19	Phenytoin	Omeprazole	Phenytoin toxicity
CYP2D6	Clozapine	Paroxetine	Clozapine toxicity
Xanthine oxidase	Azathioprine	Allopurinol	Azathioprine toxicity
Monoamine oxidase	Catecholamines	Monoamine oxidase inhibitors	Hypertensive crisis due to monoamine toxicity
Increased metabolism (enzyme induction)	Ciclosporin	St John's wort	Loss of immunosuppression
Reduced renal elimination	Lithium	Diuretics	Lithium toxicity
	Methotrexate	NSAIDs	Methotrexate toxicity
Pharmacodynamic			
Direct antagonism at same receptor	Opiates	Naloxone	Reversal of opiate effects used therapeutically
	Salbutamol	Atenolol	Inhibits bronchodilator effect
Direct potentiation in same organ system	Benzodiazepines	Alcohol	Increased sedation
	ACE inhibitors	NSAIDs	Increased risk of renal impairment
Indirect potentiation	Digoxin	Diuretics	Digoxin toxicity enhanced because of hypokalaemia
	Warfarin	Aspirin, NSAIDs	Increased risk of bleeding because of gastrotoxicity and antiplatelet effects

*Pharmaceutical interactions are related to the formulation of the drugs and occur before drug absorption.

juice) have the opposite effect. Enzyme induction effects usually take a few days to manifest because of the need to synthesise new CYP enzyme, in contrast with the rapid effects of enzyme inhibition.

- *Excretion interactions*. These primarily affect renal excretion. For example, drug-induced reduction in glomerular filtration rate (e.g. diuretic-induced dehydration, ACE inhibitors, NSAIDs) can reduce the clearance and increase the plasma concentration of many drugs, including some with a low therapeutic index (e.g. digoxin, lithium, aminoglycoside antibiotics). Less commonly, interactions may be due to competition for a common tubular organic anion transporter (e.g. methotrexate excretion may be inhibited by competition with NSAIDs).

Avoiding drug interactions

Drug interactions are increasing as patients are prescribed more medicines (polypharmacy). Prescribers can avoid the adverse consequences of drug–drug interactions by taking a careful drug history (see Box 2.6) before prescribing additional drugs, only prescribing for clear indications, and taking special care when prescribing drugs with a narrow therapeutic index (e.g. warfarin). When prescribing an interacting drug is unavoidable, good prescribers will seek further information and anticipate the potential risk. This will allow them to provide special warnings for the patient and arrange for monitoring, either of the clinical effects (e.g. coagulation tests for warfarin) or of plasma concentration (e.g. digoxin).

Medication errors

A medication error is any *preventable* event that may lead to inappropriate medication use or patient harm while the medication is in the control of the health-care professional or patient. Errors may occur in prescribing, dispensing, preparing solutions, administration or monitoring. Many ADRs are considered in retrospect to have been 'avoidable' with more care or forethought; in other words, an adverse event considered by one prescriber to be an unfortunate ADR might be considered by another to be a prescribing error.

Medication errors are very common. Several thousand medication orders are dispensed and administered each day in a medium-sized hospital. Recent UK studies suggest that 7–9% of hospital prescriptions contain an error, and most are written by junior doctors. Common prescribing errors in hospitals include omission of medicines (especially failure to prescribe regular medicines at the point of admission or discharge, i.e. 'medicines reconciliation'), dosing errors, unintentional prescribing and poor use of documentation (Box 2.12).

Most prescription errors result from a combination of failures by the individual prescriber and the health-service systems in which they work (Box 2.13). Health-care organisations increasingly encourage reporting of errors within a 'no blame culture' so that they can be subject to 'root cause analysis' using human error theory (Fig. 2.5). Prevention is targeted at the factors in Box 2.13, and can be supported by prescribers communicating and cross-checking with colleagues (e.g. when calculating doses adjusted for body weight, or planning appropriate monitoring after drug administration), and by health-care systems providing clinical pharmacist support (e.g. for checking the patient's previous medications and current prescriptions) and electronic prescribing (which avoids errors due to illegibility or serious dosing mistakes, and may be combined with a clinical decision support system to take account of patient characteristics and drug history and provide warnings of potential contraindications and drug interactions).

2.12 Hospital prescribing errors

Error type	Approximate % of total
Omission on admission	30
Underdose	11
Overdose	8
Strength/dose missing	7
Omission on discharge	6
Administration times incorrect/missing	6
Duplication	6
Product or formulation not specified	4
Incorrect formulation	4
No maximum dose	4
Unintentional prescribing	3
No signature	2
Clinical contraindication	1
Incorrect route	1
No indication	1
IV instructions incorrect/missing	1
Drug not prescribed but indicated	1
Drug continued for longer than needed	1
Route of administration missing	1
Start date incorrect/missing	1
Risk of drug interaction	< 0.5
Controlled drug requirements incorrect/ missing	< 0.5
Daily dose divided incorrectly	< 0.5
Significant allergy	< 0.5
Drug continued in spite of adverse effects	< 0.5
Premature discontinuation	< 0.5
Failure to respond to out-of-range drug level	< 0.5

Responding when an error is discovered

All prescribers will make errors. When they do, their first duty is to protect the patient's safety. This will involve a clinical review and taking any steps that will reduce harm (e.g. remedial treatment, monitoring, recording the event in the notes, informing colleagues). Patients should be informed if they have been exposed to potential harm. For errors that do not reach the patient, it is the prescriber's duty to report them, so that

2.13 Causes of prescribing errors

Systems factors

- Working hours of prescribers (and others)
- Patient throughput
- Professional support and supervision by colleagues
- Availability of information (medical records)
- Design of prescription forms
- Distractions
- Decision support available
- Checking routines (e.g. clinical pharmacy)
- Reporting and reviewing of incidents

Prescriber factors

Knowledge
- Clinical pharmacology principles
- Drugs in common use
- Therapeutic problems commonly encountered
- Knowledge of workplace systems

Skills
- Taking a good drug history
- Obtaining information to support prescribing
- Communicating with patients
- Numeracy and calculations
- Prescription writing

Attitudes
- Coping with risk and uncertainty
- Monitoring of prescribing
- Checking routines

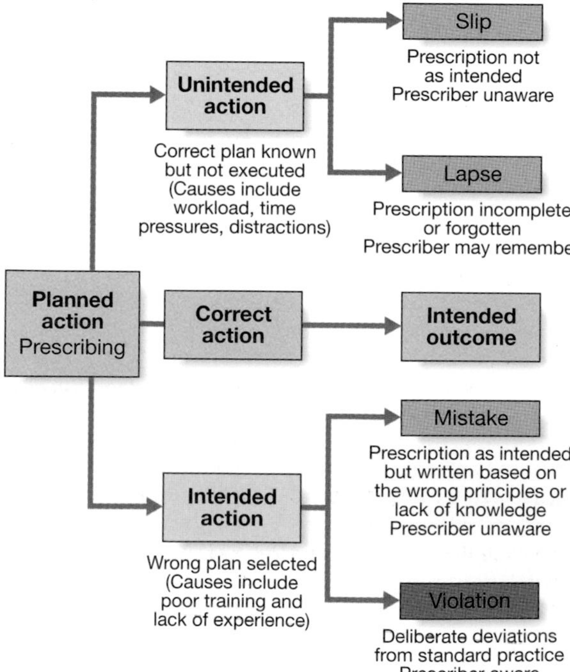

Fig. 2.5 Human error theory. Unintended errors may occur because the prescriber fails to complete the prescription correctly (a slip) (e.g. writes the dose in 'mg' not 'micrograms') or forgets part of the action that is important for success (a lapse) (e.g. forgets to co-prescribe folic acid with methotrexate); prevention requires the system to provide appropriate checking routines. Intended errors occur when the prescriber acts incorrectly due to lack of knowledge (a mistake) (e.g. prescribes atenolol for a patient with known severe asthma because of ignorance about the contraindication); prevention must focus on training the prescriber.

others can learn from the experience, and take the opportunity to reflect on how a similar incident might be avoided in the future.

DRUG REGULATION AND MANAGEMENT

Given the powerful beneficial and potentially adverse effects of drugs, the production and use of medicines are strictly regulated (e.g. by the Food and Drug Administration in the United States (US), Medicines and Healthcare Products Regulatory Agency in the UK, and Central Drugs Standard Control Organisation in India). Regulators are responsible for licensing medicines, monitoring their safety (pharmacovigilance, p. 27), approving clinical trials, and inspecting and maintaining standards of drug development and manufacture.

In addition, because of the high costs of drugs and of their adverse effects, health-care services must prioritise their use in light of the evidence of their benefit and harm, a process referred to as 'medicines management'.

Drug development and marketing

Naturally occurring products have been used to treat illnesses for thousands of years and some remain in common use today. Examples include morphine from the opium poppy (*Papaver somniferum*), digitalis from the foxglove (*Digitalis purpurea*), curare from the bark of a South American tree, and quinine from another bark (*Cinchona* species). Although plants and animals remain a source of discovery, the majority of new drugs come from drug discovery programmes that aim to identify

2.14 Clinical development of new drugs

Phase I
- Healthy volunteers (20–80). These involve initial single-dose, 'first-into-man' studies, followed by repeated-dose studies. They aim to establish the basic pharmacokinetic and pharmacodynamic properties, and short-term safety. Duration: 6–12 months

Phase II
- Patients (100–200). These investigate clinical effectiveness ('proof of concept'), safety and dose–response relationship, often with a surrogate clinical endpoint, in the target patient group to determine the optimal dosing regimen for larger confirmatory studies. Duration: 1–2 years

Phase III
- Patients (100s–1000s). These are large, expensive clinical trials that confirm safety and efficacy in the target patient population, using relevant clinical endpoints. They may be placebo-controlled studies or comparisons with other active compounds. Duration: 1–2 years

Phase IV
- Patients (100s–1000s). These are undertaken after the medicine has been marketed for its first indication to evaluate new indications, new doses or formulations, long-term safety or cost-effectiveness

2.15 Novel therapeutic alternatives to conventional small-molecule drugs

Approaches	Therapeutic indications	Challenges
Monoclonal antibodies: targeting of receptors or other molecules with relatively specific antibodies	Cancer Chronic inflammatory diseases (e.g. rheumatoid arthritis, inflammatory bowel disease)	Selectivity of action Complex manufacturing process
Small interfering RNA (siRNA): inhibits gene expression	Macular degeneration	Delivery to target
Gene therapy: delivery of modified genes that supplement or alter host DNA	Cystic fibrosis Cancer Cardiovascular disease	Delivery to target Adverse effects of delivery vector (e.g. virus)
Stem cell therapy: stem cells differentiate and replace damaged host cells	Parkinson's disease Spinal cord injury Ischaemic heart disease	Delivery to target Immunological compatibility Long-term effects unknown

small-molecule compounds with specific interactions with a molecular target that will induce a predicted biological effect.

The usual pathway for development of these small molecules includes: identifying a plausible molecular target by investigating pathways in disease; screening a large library of compounds for those that interact with the molecular target in vitro; conducting extensive medicinal chemistry to optimise the properties of lead compounds; testing efficacy and toxicity of these compounds in vitro and in animals; and undertaking a clinical development programme (Box 2.14). This process typically takes longer than 10 years and may cost up to $1 billion. Manufacturers have a defined period of exclusive marketing of the drug while it remains protected by an original patent, typically 10–15 years, during which time they must recoup the costs of developing the drug. Meanwhile, competitor companies will often produce similar 'me too' drugs of the same class. Once the drug's patent has expired, 'generic' drug manufacturers may step in to produce cheaper formulations.

The number of new drugs produced by the pharmaceutical industry has declined in recent years. The traditional approach of targeting membrane-bound receptors and enzymes with small molecules (see Box 2.2) is now giving way to new targets such as complex second messenger systems, cytokines, nucleic acids and cellular networks. These require novel therapeutic agents which present new challenges for 'translational medicine', the discipline of converting scientific discoveries into a useful medicine with a well-defined benefit–risk profile (Box 2.15).

Licensing new medicines

New drugs are given a 'market authorisation' based on the evidence of quality, safety and efficacy presented by the manufacturer. The regulator will not only approve the drug but will also take great care to ensure that the accompanying information reflects the evidence that has been presented. The summary of product characteristics (SPC), or 'label', provides detailed information about indications, dosage, adverse effects, warnings, monitoring etc. If approved, drugs can be made available with different levels of restriction:

- *Controlled drug (CD)*. These drugs are subject to strict legal controls on supply and possession, usually due to their abuse potential (e.g. opioid analgesics).
- *Prescription-only medicine (PoM)*. These are only available from a pharmacist and can only be supplied if prescribed by an appropriate practitioner.
- *Pharmacy (P)*. These are only available from a pharmacist but can be supplied without a prescription.
- *General sales list (GSL)*. These medicines may be bought 'over the counter' (OTC) from any shop and without a prescription.

Drug marketing

The marketing activities of the pharmaceutical industry are well resourced and are important in the process of recouping the massive costs of drug development. In some countries, such as the US, it is possible to promote a new drug by direct-to-consumer advertising, although this is illegal in the countries of the European Union. A major focus is on promotion to prescribers via educational events, sponsorship of meetings, adverts in journals, involvement with opinion leaders, and direct contact by company representatives. Such largesse has the potential to cause significant conflicts of interest, and might tempt prescribers to favour one drug over another, even in the face of evidence on effectiveness or cost-effectiveness.

Managing the use of medicines

Many medicines meet the three key regulatory requirements of quality, safety and efficacy. Although prescribers are legally entitled to prescribe any of them, it is desirable to limit the choice so that treatments for specific diseases can be focused on the most effective and cost-effective options, prescribers (and patients) gain familiarity with a smaller number of medicines, and pharmacies can concentrate stocks on them.

The process of ensuring optimal use of available medicines is known as 'medicines management' or 'quality use of medicines'. It involves careful evaluation of the evidence of benefit and harm from using the medicine, an assessment of cost-effectiveness, and support for processes to implement the resulting recommendations.

These activities usually involve both national and local organisations.

Evaluating evidence

The principles of evidence-based medicine are described on page 8. Drugs are often evaluated in high-quality randomised controlled trials, the results of which can be considered by systematic review (Fig. 2.6). Ideally, data are available not only for comparison with placebo but also in 'head-to-head' comparison with alternative therapies. However, trials are conducted in selected patient populations and are not representative of every clinical scenario, so extrapolation to individual patients is not always straightforward.

Clinical trials typically report the percentage reduction in risk of a primary outcome, such as a stroke. However, if the absolute risk of stroke for a given patient is low, then even an apparently substantial percentage reduction in risk may not be worthwhile. As an aid to interpreting the results of clinical trials, it is often helpful to consider the number needed to treat (NNT). For example, in a systematic review of warfarin therapy to prevent stroke in patients with atrial fibrillation, strokes occurred in 133 of 1450 patients given placebo and in 53 of 1450 patients given warfarin. This represents a relative risk of 0.40, i.e. a 60% reduction. It equates to an NNT of 18, i.e. 18 patients would need to be treated for 1 year to prevent 1 stroke; NNT is calculated as the inverse of the difference in absolute rate of stroke = 1/[(133/1450) – (53/1450)]. However, if the absolute risk of stroke were halved, the relative risk reduction with warfarin would still be 60%, but the NNT would increase to 1/[(67/1450) – (27/1450)] = 36, i.e. 36 patients would need to be treated for 1 year to prevent 1 stroke, with a consequent increase in cost and risk of adverse effects compared with benefit. NNT can usefully be applied to assess both benefit (NNT_B) and harm (NNT_H).

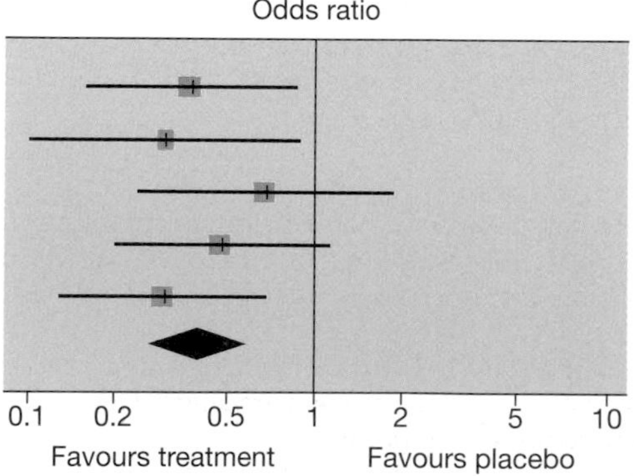

Fig. 2.6 Systematic review of the evidence from randomised controlled clinical trials. This forest plot shows the effect of warfarin compared with placebo on likelihood of stroke in patients with atrial fibrillation in five randomised controlled trials that passed the quality criteria required for inclusion in a meta-analysis. For each trial, the purple box is proportionate to the number of participants. The tick marks show the mean odds ratio, and the black lines indicate its 95% confidence intervals. Note that not all the trials showed statistically significant effects (i.e. the confidence intervals cross 1.0). However, the meta-analysis, represented by the black diamond, confirms a highly significant statistical benefit. The overall odds ratio is approximately 0.4, indicating a mean 60% risk reduction with warfarin treatment in patients with the characteristics of the participants in these trials.

Evaluating cost-effectiveness

New drugs often represent an incremental improvement over the current standard of care but are usually more expensive. The principles for evaluating and comparing cost-effectiveness of treatment are described on page 9. A major challenge is to compare the value of interventions for different clinical outcomes. One method is to calculate the quality-adjusted life years (QALYs) gained if the new drug is used rather than standard treatment. This analysis involves estimating the 'utility' of various health states between 1 (perfect health) and 0 (dead). If the additional costs and any savings are known, then it is possible to derive the incremental cost-effectiveness ratio (ICER) in terms of cost/QALY. These principles are exemplified in Box 2.16. However, there are inherent weaknesses in this kind of analysis: it usually depends on modelling future outcomes well beyond the duration of the clinical trial data that are available; it assumes that QALYs gained at all ages are of equivalent value; and the appropriate standard care against which the new drug should be compared is often uncertain.

These pharmacoeconomic assessments are challenging and resource-intensive, and are undertaken at national level in most countries: for example in the UK by the National Institute for Health and Clinical Excellence (NICE).

Implementing recommendations

Many recommendations about drug therapy are included in clinical guidelines written by an expert group after systematic review of the evidence. As described on page 8, these provide recommendations rather than obligations for prescribers, and are helpful in promoting more consistent and higher-quality

2.16 Cost-effectiveness analysis

A clinical trial lasting 2 years compares two interventions for the treatment of colon cancer:

- Treatment A: standard treatment, cost £1000/year, oral therapy
- Treatment B: new treatment, cost £6000/year, monthly IV infusions often followed by a week of nausea.

The new treatment (B) significantly increases the average time to progression (18 months versus 12 months) and reduces overall mortality (40% versus 60%). The health economist models the survival curves from the trial in order to undertake a cost–utility analysis and concludes that:

- Intervention A: allows a patient to live for 2 extra years at a utility 0.7 = 1.4 QALYs (cost £2000)
- Intervention B: allows a patient to live for 3 extra years at a utility 0.6 = 1.8 QALYs (cost £18 000).

The health economists conclude that Treatment B provides an extra 0.4 QALYs at an extra cost of £16 000, meaning that the ICER = £40 000/QALY. They recommend that the new treatment should not be funded on the basis that their threshold for cost acceptability is £30 000/QALY.

(ICER = incremental cost-effectiveness ratio; QALY = quality-adjusted life year)

prescribing. However, guidelines are often written without concern for cost-effectiveness, and may be limited by the quality of available evidence. Guidelines cannot anticipate the extent of the variation between individual patients who may, for example, have unexpected contraindications to recommended drugs or choose different priorities for treatment. However, when deviating from respected national guidance, prescribers should be able to justify their practice.

Additional recommendations for prescribing are often implemented locally or imposed by bodies responsible for paying for health care. Most health-care units have a drug and therapeutics committee (or equivalent) comprised of senior and junior medical staff, pharmacists and nurses, as well as managers (because of the implications of the committee's work for governance and resources). This group typically develops local prescribing policy and guidelines, maintains a local drug formulary and evaluates requests to use new drugs. The local formulary contains a more limited list than any national formulary (e.g. *British National Formulary*) because the latter lists all licensed medicines that can be prescribed legally, while the former contains only those which the health-care organisation has approved for local use. The local committee may also be involved, with local specialists, in providing explicit protocols for management of clinical scenarios (p. 9).

PRESCRIBING IN PRACTICE

Decision-making in prescribing

Prescribing should be based on a rational approach to a series of challenges (see Box 2.1, p. 18).

Making a diagnosis

Ideally, prescribing should be based on a confirmed diagnosis but, in reality, many prescriptions are based on the balance of probability, taking into account the differential diagnosis (e.g. proton pump inhibitors for post-prandial retrosternal discomfort).

Establishing the therapeutic goal

The goals of treatment are usually clear, particularly when relieving symptoms (e.g. pain, nausea, constipation). Sometimes the goal is less obvious to the patient, especially when aiming to prevent future events (e.g. ACE inhibitors to prevent hospitalisation and extend life in chronic heart failure). Prescribers should be clear about the therapeutic goal against which they will judge success or failure of treatment. It is also important to establish that the value placed on this goal by the prescriber is shared by the patient.

Choosing the therapeutic approach

For many clinical problems, drug therapy is not absolutely mandated. Having taken the potential benefits and harms into account, prescribers must consider whether drug therapy is in the patient's interest and is preferred to no treatment or one of a range of alternatives (e.g. physiotherapy, psychotherapy, surgery). Assessing the balance of benefit and harm is often complicated and depends on various features associated with the patient, disease and drug (Box 2.17).

2.17 Factors to consider when balancing benefits and harms of drug therapy

- Seriousness of the disease or symptom
- Efficacy of the drug
- Seriousness of potential adverse effects
- Likelihood of adverse effects
- Efficacy of alternative drugs or non-drug therapies
- Safety of alternative drugs or non-drug therapies

2

Choosing a drug

For most common clinical indications (e.g. type 2 diabetes, depression), more than one drug is available, often from more than one drug class. Although prescribers often have guidance about which represents the rational choice for the average patient, they still need to consider whether this is the optimal choice for the individual patient. Certain factors may influence the choice of drug:

Absorption. Patients may find some formulations easier to swallow than others or may be vomiting and require a drug available for parenteral administration.

Distribution. Distribution of a drug to a particular tissue sometimes dictates choice (e.g. tetracyclines and rifampicin are concentrated in the bile, and lincomycin and clindamycin in bones).

Metabolism. Drugs that are extensively metabolised should be avoided in severe liver disease (e.g. opioid analgesics).

Excretion. Drugs that depend on renal excretion for elimination (e.g. digoxin, aminoglycoside antibiotics) should be avoided in patients with impaired renal function if suitable alternatives exist.

Efficacy. Prescribers normally choose drugs with the greatest efficacy in achieving the goals of therapy (e.g. proton pump inhibitors rather than histamine$_2$ receptor antagonists). However, it may be appropriate to compromise on efficacy if other drugs are more convenient, safer to use or less expensive.

Avoiding adverse effects. Prescribers should be wary of choosing drugs that are more likely to cause adverse effects (e.g. cephalosporins rather than alternatives for patients allergic to penicillin) or worsen coexisting conditions (e.g. β-blockers as treatment for angina in patients with asthma).

Features of the disease. This is most obvious when choosing antibiotic therapy, which should be based on the known or suspected sensitivity of the infective organism (p. 149).

Severity of disease. The choice of drug should be appropriate to disease severity (e.g. paracetamol for mild pain, morphine for severe pain).

Coexisting diseases may be either an indication or a contraindication to therapy. Hypertensive patients might be prescribed a β-blocker if they also have left ventricular impairment but not if they have asthma.

Avoiding adverse drug interactions. Prescribers should avoid giving combinations of drugs that might interact, either directly or indirectly (see Box 2.11).

Patient adherence to therapy. Prescribers should choose drugs with a simple dosing schedule or easier administration (e.g. the ACE inhibitor enalapril once daily rather than captopril 3 times daily for hypertension).

Cost. Prescribers should choose the cheaper drug if two drugs are of equal efficacy and safety. Even if cost is not a concern for the individual patient, it is important to remember that unnecessary expenditure will ultimately limit choices for other prescribers and patients. Sometimes a more costly drug may be appropriate (e.g. if it yields improved adherence).

Genetic factors. There are already a small number of examples where genotype influences the choice of drug therapy (see Box 2.5).

Choosing a dosage regimen

Prescribers have to choose a dose, route and frequency of administration (dosage regimen) to achieve a steady-state drug concentration that provides sufficient exposure of the target tissue without producing toxic effects. Manufacturers draw up dosage recommendations based on average observations in many patients but the optimal regimen that will maximise the benefit/harm ratio for an individual patient is never certain. Rational prescribing involves treating each prescription as an experiment and gathering sufficient information to amend it if necessary. There are some general principles that should be followed:

Dose titration. Prescribers should generally start with a low dose and titrate this slowly upwards as necessary. This cautious approach is particularly important if the patient is likely to be more sensitive to adverse pharmacodynamic effects (e.g. confusion or postural hypotension in the elderly) or have altered pharmacokinetic handling (e.g. renal or hepatic impairment), and when using drugs with a low therapeutic index (e.g. benzodiazepines, lithium, digoxin). However, there are some exceptions. Some drugs must achieve therapeutic concentration quickly because of the clinical circumstance (e.g. antibiotics, glucocorticoids, carbimazole). When early effect is important but there may be a delay in achieving steady state because of a drug's long half-life (e.g. digoxin, warfarin, amiodarone), an initial loading dose is given prior to establishing the appropriate maintenance dose (see Fig. 2.4, p. 23).

If adverse effects occur, the dose should be reduced or an alternative drug prescribed; in some cases, a lower dose may suffice if it can be combined with another synergistic drug (e.g. the immunosuppressant azathioprine reduces glucocorticoid requirements in patients with inflammatory disease). It is important to remember that the shape of the dose–response curve (see Fig. 2.2, p. 19) means that higher doses may produce little added therapeutic effect and might increase the chances of toxicity.

Route. There are many reasons for choosing a particular route of administration (Box 2.18).

Frequency. Frequency of doses is usually dictated by a manufacturer's recommendation. Less frequent doses are more convenient for patients but result in greater fluctuation between peaks and troughs in drug concentration (see Fig. 2.4, p. 23). This is relevant if the peaks are associated with adverse effects (e.g. dizziness with antihypertensives) or the troughs are associated with troublesome loss of effect (e.g. anti-Parkinsonian drugs). These problems can be tackled either by splitting the dose or by employing a modified-release formulation, if available.

Timing. For many drugs the time of administration is unimportant. However, there are occasionally pharmacokinetic or therapeutic reasons for giving drugs at particular times (Box 2.19).

2.18 Factors influencing the route of drug administration

Reason	Example
Only one route possible	Dobutamine (IV) Gliclazide (oral)
Patient adherence	Phenothiazines and thioxanthenes (2 weekly IM depot injections rather than daily tablets in schizophrenia)
Poor absorption	Furosemide (IV rather than oral, in severe heart failure)
Rapid action	Haloperidol (IM rather than oral, in acute behavioural disturbance)
Vomiting	Phenothiazines (PR or buccal rather than oral, in nausea)
Avoiding first-pass metabolism	Glyceryl trinitrate (SL, in angina pectoris)
Certainty of effect	Amoxicillin (IV rather than oral, in acute chest infection)
Direct access to the site of action (avoiding unnecessary systemic exposure)	Bronchodilators (INH rather than oral, in asthma) Local application of drugs to skin, eyes etc.
Ease of access	Diazepam (PR, if IV access is difficult in status epilepticus) Adrenaline (epinephrine) (IM, if IV access is difficult in acute anaphylaxis)
Comfort	Morphine (SC rather than IV in terminal care)

(IM = intramuscular; INH = by inhalation; IV = intravenous; PR = per rectum; SC = subcutaneous; SL = sublingual)

Formulation. For some drugs there is a choice of formulation, some for use by different routes. Some are easier to ingest, particularly by children (e.g. elixirs). The formulation is important when writing repeat prescriptions for drugs with a low therapeutic index that come in different formulations (e.g. lithium, phenytoin, theophylline). Even if the prescribed dose remains constant, another formulation may differ in its absorption and bioavailability, and hence plasma drug concentration. These are examples of the small number of drugs that should be prescribed by specific brand name rather than 'generic' International Non-proprietary Name (INN).

Duration. Some drugs require a single dose (e.g. thrombolysis post myocardial infarction), while for others the duration of the course of treatment is certain at the outset (e.g. antibiotics). For most, the duration will be largely at the prescriber's discretion and will depend on response and disease progression (e.g. analgesics, antidepressants). For many, the treatment will be long-term (e.g. insulin, antihypertensives, levothyroxine).

Involving the patient

Patients should, whenever possible, be engaged in making choices about drug therapy. Their beliefs and

2.19 Factors influencing the timing of drug therapy

Drug	Recommended timing	Reasons
Diuretics (e.g. furosemide)	Once in the morning	Night-time diuresis undesirable
Statins (e.g. simvastatin)	Once at night	HMG CoA reductase activity is greater at night
Antidepressants (e.g. amitriptyline)	Once at night	Allows adverse effects to occur during sleep
Salbutamol	Before exercise	Reduces symptoms in exercise-induced asthma
Glyceryl trinitrate **Paracetamol**	When required	Relief of acute symptoms only
Regular nitrate therapy (e.g. isosorbide mononitrate)	Eccentric dosing regimen (e.g. twice daily at 8 a.m. and 2 p.m.)	Reduces development of nitrate tolerance by allowing drug-free period each night
Aspirin	With food	Minimises gastrotoxic effects
Alendronate	Once in the morning before breakfast, sitting upright	Minimises risk of oesophageal irritation
Tetracyclines	2 hours before or after food or antacids	Divalent and trivalent cations chelate tetracyclines, preventing absorption
Hypnotics (e.g. temazepam)	Once at night	Maximises therapeutic effect and minimises daytime sedation
Antihypertensive drugs (e.g. amlodipine)	Once in the morning	Blood pressure is higher during the daytime

(HMG CoA = 3-hydroxy-3-methylglutaryl-coenzyme A)

2.20 What patients need to know about their medicines*

Knowledge	Comment
The reason for taking the medicine **How the medicine works**	Reinforces the goals of therapy
How to take the medicine	May be important for the effectiveness (e.g. inhaled salbutamol in asthma) and safety (e.g. alendronate for osteoporosis) of treatment
What benefits to expect	May help to support adherence or prompt review because of treatment failure
What adverse effects might occur	Discuss common and mild effects that may be transient and might not require discontinuation Mention rare but serious effects that might influence the patient's consent
Precautions that improve safety	Explain symptoms to report that might allow serious adverse effects to be averted, monitoring that will be required and potentially important drug–drug interactions
When to return for review	This will be important to enable monitoring

*Many medicines are provided with patient information leaflets, which the patient should be encouraged to read.

expectations affect the goals of therapy and help in judging the acceptable benefit/harm balance when selecting treatments. Very often, patients may wish to defer to the professional expertise of the prescriber. Nevertheless, they play key roles in adherence to therapy and in monitoring treatment, not least by providing early warning of adverse events. It is important that they are provided with the necessary information to understand the choice that has been made, what to expect from the treatment, and any measurements that must be undertaken (Box 2.20).

A major drive to include patients has been the recognition that up to half of the drug doses for chronic preventative therapy are not taken. This is often termed 'non-compliance' but is more appropriately called 'non-adherence', to reflect a less paternalistic view of the doctor–patient relationship; it may or may not be intentional. Non-adherence to the dose regimen reduces the likelihood of benefits to the patient and can be costly in terms of wasted medicines and unnecessary health-care episodes. An important reason may be a failure of concordance with the prescriber about the goals of treatment. A more open and shared decision-making process might resolve any misunderstandings at the outset and foster improved adherence as well as improved satisfaction with health-care services and confidence in prescribers.

Writing the prescription

The culmination of the planning described above is writing an accurate and legible prescription so that the drug will be dispensed and administered as planned (see 'Writing prescriptions' below).

Monitoring treatment effects

Rational prescribing involves monitoring for the beneficial and adverse effects of treatment so that the balance remains in favour of a positive outcome (see 'Monitoring drug therapy' below).

Stopping drug therapy

It is also important to review long-term treatment at regular intervals to assess whether continued treatment is required. Elderly patients are keen to reduce their medication burden and are often prepared to compromise on the original goals of long-term preventative therapy to achieve this.

Prescribing in special circumstances

Prescribing for patients with renal disease

Patients with renal impairment are readily identified by having a low estimated glomerular filtration rate (eGFR < 60 mL/min) based on their serum creatinine, age, sex and ethnic group (p. 466). This group includes a large proportion of elderly patients. If a drug (or its active metabolites) is eliminated predominantly by the kidneys, it will tend to accumulate and so the maintenance dose must be reduced. For some drugs, renal impairment makes patients more sensitive to their adverse pharmacodynamic effects. Examples of drugs that require extra caution in patients with renal disease are listed in Box 2.21.

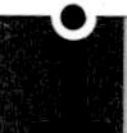

2.21 Some drugs that require extra caution in patients with renal or hepatic disease

Kidney disease	Liver disease
Pharmacodynamic effects enhanced	
ACE inhibitors and ARBs (renal impairment, hyperkalaemia)	Warfarin (increased anticoagulation because of reduced clotting factor synthesis)
Metformin (lactic acidosis)	Metformin (lactic acidosis)
Spironolactone (hyperkalaemia)	Chloramphenicol (bone marrow suppression)
NSAIDs (impaired renal function)	NSAIDs (gastrointestinal bleeding, fluid retention)
Sulphonylureas (hypoglycaemia)	Sulphonylureas (hypoglycaemia)
Insulin (hypoglycaemia)	Benzodiazepines (coma)
Pharmacokinetic handling altered (reduced clearance)	
Aminoglycosides (e.g. gentamicin)	Phenytoin
Vancomycin	Rifampicin
Digoxin	Propranolol
Lithium	Warfarin
Other antibiotics (e.g. ciprofloxacin)	Diazepam
Atenolol	Lidocaine
Allopurinol	Opioids (e.g. morphine)
Cephalosporins	
Methotrexate	
Opioids (e.g. morphine)	

(ARB = angiotensin receptor blocker)

Prescribing for patients with hepatic disease

The liver has a large capacity for drug metabolism and hepatic insufficiency has to be advanced before drug dosages need to be modified. Patients who may have impaired metabolism include those with jaundice, ascites, hypoalbuminaemia, malnutrition or encephalopathy. Hepatic drug clearance may also be reduced in acute hepatitis, in hepatic congestion due to cardiac failure, and if there is intrahepatic arteriovenous shunting (for example, in hepatic cirrhosis). There are no good tests of hepatic drug-metabolising capacity or of biliary excretion, so dosage should be guided by the therapeutic response and careful monitoring for adverse effects. The presence of liver disease also increases the susceptibility to adverse pharmacological effects of drugs. Some drugs that require extra caution in patients with hepatic disease are listed in Box 2.21.

Prescribing for elderly patients

See Box 2.22.

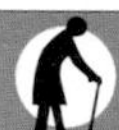

2.22 Prescribing in old age

- **Reduced drug elimination**: partly due to impaired renal function.
- **Increased sensitivity to drug effects**: notably in the brain (leading to sedation or delirium) and as a result of comorbidities.
- **More drug interactions**: largely as a result of polypharmacy.
- **Lower starting doses and slower dose titration**: often required, with careful monitoring of drug effects.
- **Drug adherence**: may be poor because of cognitive impairment, difficulty swallowing (dry mouth) and complex polypharmacy regimens. Supplying medicines in pill organisers (e.g. dosette boxes or calendar blister packs), providing automatic reminders, and regularly reviewing and simplifying the drug regimen can help.
- **Some drugs that require extra caution, and their mechanisms**:
  - Digoxin: increased sensitivity of Na^+/K^+ pump; hypokalaemia due to diuretics; renal impairment favours accumulation → increased risk of toxicity
  - Antihypertensive drugs: reduced baroreceptor function → increased risk of postural hypotension
  - Antidepressants, hypnotics, sedatives, tranquillisers: increased sensitivity of the brain; reduced metabolism → increased risk of toxicity
  - Warfarin: increased tendency to falls and injury and to bleeding from intra- and extracranial sites; increased sensitivity to inhibition of clotting factor synthesis → increased risk of bleeding
  - Clomethiazole, lidocaine, nifedipine, phenobarbital, propranolol, theophylline: metabolism reduced → increased risk of toxicity
  - NSAIDs: poor renal function → increased risk of renal impairment; susceptibility to gastrotoxicity → increased risk of upper gastrointestinal bleeding.

Prescribing for women who are pregnant or breastfeeding

Prescribing in pregnancy should be avoided if possible to minimise the risk of adverse effects in the fetus.

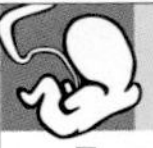

2.23 Prescribing in pregnancy

- **Teratogenesis**: a potential risk, especially when drugs are taken between 2 and 8 weeks of gestation. Common teratogens include retinoids (e.g. isotretinoin), cytotoxic drugs, ACE inhibitors, corticosteroids, antiepileptics and warfarin. If there is inadvertent exposure, then the timing of conception should be established, counselling given and investigations undertaken for fetal abnormalities.
- **Adverse fetal effects in late gestation**: for example, tetracyclines stain growing teeth and bones; sulphonamides displace fetal bilirubin from plasma proteins, potentially causing kernicterus; opioids given during delivery suppress the neonate's respiration.
- **Altered maternal pharmacokinetics**: extracellular fluid volume and V_d increase. Plasma albumin falls but other binding globulins (e.g. for thyroid and steroid hormones) increase. Glomerular filtration increases by approximately 70%, enhancing renal clearance. Placental metabolism contributes to increased clearance, e.g. of thyroxine and corticosteroids.
- **In practice**:
  Avoid any drugs unless the benefit to the mother greatly outweighs the risk to the fetus
  Use drugs for which there is some record of safety
  Use the lowest dose for the shortest time possible
  Choose the least harmful drug if alternatives are available

However, drug therapy in pregnancy may be required either for a pre-existing problem (e.g. epilepsy, asthma, hypothyroidism) or for problems that arise during pregnancy (e.g. morning sickness, anaemia, prevention of neural tube defects, gestational diabetes, hypertension). About 35% of women take drug therapy at least once during pregnancy and 6% take drug therapy during the first trimester (excluding iron, folic acid and vitamins). The most commonly used drugs are simple analgesics, antibacterial drugs and antacids. Some considerations when prescribing in pregnancy are listed in Box 2.23.

Drugs that are excreted in breast milk may cause adverse effects in the baby. Prescribers should always consult the summary of product characteristics for each drug or a reliable formulary when treating a pregnant woman or breastfeeding mother.

Writing prescriptions

A prescription is a means by which a prescriber communicates the intended plan of treatment to the pharmacist who dispenses a medicine and to a nurse or patient who administers it. It should be precise, accurate, clear and legible. The two main kinds of prescription are those written, dispensed and administered in hospital and those written in primary care (in the UK by a GP), dispensed at a community pharmacy and self-administered by the patient. The information supplied must include:

- the date
- identification of the patient
- the name of the drug
- the formulation
- the dose
- the frequency of administration
- the route and method of administration
- the amount to be supplied (primary care only)
- instructions for labelling (primary care only)
- the prescriber's signature.

Prescribing in hospital

Although GP prescribing is increasingly electronic, most hospital prescribing continues to be based around the prescription and administration record (the 'drug chart'). A variety of charts is in use and prescribers must familiarise themselves with the local version. Most contain the following sections:

- *Basic patient information*. Will usually include name, age, date of birth, hospital number and address. These details are often 'filled in' using a sticky addressograph label, but this increases the risk of serious error.
- *Previous adverse reactions/allergies*. Communicates important patient safety information based on a careful drug history and/or the medical record.
- *Other medicines charts*. Notes any other hospital prescription documents that contain current prescriptions being received by the patient (e.g. anticoagulants, insulin, oxygen, fluids).
- *Once-only medications*. For prescribing medicines to be used infrequently, such as single-dose prophylactic antibiotics and other pre-operative medications.
- *Regular medications*. For prescribing medicines to be taken for a number of days or continuously, such as a course of antibiotics, antihypertensive drugs etc.
- *'As required' medications*. For prescribing for symptomatic relief, usually to be administered at the discretion of the nursing staff (e.g. antiemetics, analgesics).

Prescribers should be aware of the risks of prescription error (Box 2.24 and Box 2.13, p. 30), ensure they have considered the rational basis for their prescribing decision described above, and then follow the rules in Box 2.25 in order to write the prescription. It is a basic principle that a prescription will be followed by a judgement as to its success or failure and appropriate changes made, often by discontinuing one prescription and writing another.

Hospital discharge ('to take out') medicines

Most patients will be prescribed a short course of their medicines at discharge. This prescription is particularly important because it usually informs future therapy at the point of transfer of prescribing responsibility to primary care. Great care is required to ensure that this list is accurate and that any hospital medicines to be stopped are not included or are identified as of specified short duration. It is also important that any significant ADRs experienced in hospital are recorded and that any specific monitoring or review is identified.

Prescribing in primary care

Most of the considerations above are equally applicable to primary care (GP) prescriptions. In many health-care systems, community prescribing is electronic, making issues of legibility irrelevant and often providing basic decision support to limit the range of doses that can be written and highlight potential drug interactions.

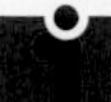

2.24 High-risk prescribing moments

- Trying to amend an active prescription (e.g. altering the dose/timing) – *always avoid and start again*
- Writing up drugs in the immediate presence of more than one prescription chart or set of notes – *avoid*
- Allowing one's attention to be diverted in the middle of completing a prescription – *avoid*
- Prescribing 'high risk' drugs (e.g. anticoagulants, opioids, insulin, sedatives) – *ask for help if necessary*
- Prescribing parenteral drugs – *take care*
- Rushing prescribing (e.g. in the midst of a busy ward round) – *avoid*
- Prescribing unfamiliar drugs – *consult the formulary and ask for help if necessary*
- Transcribing multiple prescriptions from an expired chart to a new one – *take care*
- Writing prescriptions based on information from another source such as a referral letter (the list may contain errors and some of the medicines may be the cause of the patient's illness) – *review the justification for each as if it is a new prescription*
- Writing up 'to take out' drugs (because these will become the patient's regular medication for the immediate future) – *take care and seek advice if necessary*
- Calculating drug doses – *ask a colleague to perform an independent calculation*
- Prescribing sound-alike or look-alike drugs (e.g. chlorphenamine and chlorpromazine) – *take care*

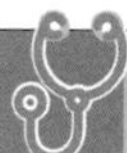

2.25 How to write a drug prescription

- **Write** in block capitals, legibly, with black ballpoint pen. Do not amend what is already written: if a mistake is made, then start again
- Ensure there is clear and unambiguous labelling to **identify the patient.** Write the patient's name, hospital number and date of birth (with age if under 12 years) on every sheet. The patient's weight and height may be required to calculate safe doses for many drugs with narrow therapeutic indices
- Check the **drug sensitivities/allergies** box and obtain further details of the drug history if there are any doubts
- Use the generic **International Non-proprietary Name (INN)** rather than brand name (e.g. write 'SIMVASTATIN', not 'ZOCOR®'). The only exceptions are when variation occurs in the properties of alternative branded formulations (e.g. modified-release preparations of drugs such as lithium, theophylline, phenytoin and nifedipine) or when the drug is a combination product with no generic name (e.g. Kliovance®). Do not use abbreviations, e.g. write 'ISOSORBIDE MONONITRATE' not 'ISMN'
- Write the **drug dose.** The only acceptable abbreviations are 'g' and 'mg'. 'Units' (e.g. of insulin or heparin) and 'micrograms' must always be written in full, never as 'U' or 'µg' (nor 'mcg', nor 'ug'). Avoid decimal points (i.e. 500 mg not 0·5 g) or, if unavoidable, put a '0' in front of it (e.g. '0·5 micrograms' not '·5 micrograms'). Do not use a decimal point for round numbers (e.g. '7 mg' not '7·0 mg'). For liquid preparations write the dose in mg; 'mL' can only be written for a combination product (e.g. Gaviscon® liquid) or if the strength is not expressed in weight (e.g. adrenaline (epinephrine) 1 in 1000). Use numbers/figures (e.g. 1 or 'one') to denote use of a sachet/enema but avoid prescribing numbers of tablets without specifying their strength. Always include the dose of inhaled drugs in addition to stating numbers of 'puffs', as strengths can vary. For some drugs a maximum dose may need to be stated (e.g. colchicine in gout)
- Write the **route and method of administration.** Widely accepted abbreviations are: intravenous – 'IV'; intramuscular – 'IM'; subcutaneous – 'SC'; sublingual – 'SL'; per rectum – 'PR'; per vaginam – 'PV'; nasogastric – 'NG'; inhaled – 'INH'; and topical – 'TOP'. 'ORAL' is preferred to per oram – 'PO'. Never abbreviate 'INTRATHECAL'. Care should be taken in specifying 'RIGHT' or 'LEFT' for eye and ear drops. It may be necessary to specify the method of giving a medicine intravenously (e.g. as a single undiluted bolus injection, or as an infusion in a specified volume of saline over a specified time)
- Indicate the **frequency and timing of administration** clearly. For example: furosemide 40 mg once daily; amoxicillin 250 mg 3 times daily. Widely accepted Latin abbreviations for dose frequency are: once daily – 'OD'; twice daily – 'BD'; 3 times daily – 'TDS'; 4 times daily – 'QDS'; as required – 'PRN'; in the morning – 'OM' (omni mane); at night – 'ON' (omni nocte); and immediately – 'stat'. Alternatives are, for example, 6-hourly and 8-hourly, but these are less precise. The hospital chart usually requires specific times to be identified for regular medicines that coincide with nursing drug rounds. If treatment is for a known time period, cross off subsequent days when the medicine is not required. Similarly, if a drug is not to be given every day, cross off the days when it is not required. For **'as required' medicines** describe the indication, frequency, minimal time interval between doses, and maximum dose in any 24-hour period
- Use the space provided for **added information,** e.g. whether a medicine should be taken with food, type of inhaler device used, and anything else that the drug dispenser should know. State here the times for peak/trough plasma levels for drugs requiring therapeutic monitoring
- **Sign and print your name** clearly so that you can be identified by colleagues. The prescription should be dated
- **Discontinue** a prescription by drawing a vertical line at the point of discontinuation, horizontal lines through the remaining days on the chart, and diagonal lines through the drug details and administration boxes. Sign and date this action and consider writing a supplementary note to explain it (e.g. describing any adverse effect)

Important additional issues more relevant to GP prescribing are:

- *Formulation*. The prescription needs to carry information about the formulation for the dispensing pharmacist (e.g. tablets or oral suspension).
- *Amount to be supplied*. In the hospital the pharmacist will organise this. Elsewhere it must be specified either as the precise number of tablets or as the duration of treatment. Creams and ointments should be specified in grams and lotions in mL.
- *Controlled drugs*. Prescriptions for 'controlled' drugs (e.g. opioid analgesics, with potential for drug abuse) are subject to additional legal requirements. In the UK they must contain the address of the patient and prescriber (not necessary on most hospital forms), the form and the strength of the preparation, and the total quantity of the preparation/number of dose units in both words and figures.
- *'Repeat prescriptions'*. A large proportion of GP prescribing involves 'repeat prescriptions' for chronic medication. These are often generated automatically, although the prescriber remains responsible for regular review and for ensuring that the benefit to harm ratio remains favourable.

Monitoring drug therapy

Prescribers should measure the effects of the drug, both beneficial and harmful, to inform decisions about dose titration (up or down), discontinuation or substitution of treatment. Monitoring can be achieved subjectively by asking the patient about symptoms or more objectively by measuring a clinical effect. Alternatively, if the pharmacodynamic effects of the drug are difficult to assess, then the plasma drug concentration may be measured on the basis that it will be closely related to the effect of the drug (see Fig. 2.2, p. 19).

Clinical and surrogate endpoints

Ideally, clinical endpoints are measured directly and the drug dosage titrated to achieve the therapeutic goal and avoid toxicity (e.g. control of ventricular rate in a patient with atrial fibrillation). Sometimes this is impractical because the clinical endpoint is a future event (e.g. prevention of myocardial infarction by statins or resolution of a chest infection with antibiotics); in these circumstances it may be possible to select a 'surrogate' endpoint that will predict success or failure. This may be an intermediate step in the pathophysiological process (e.g. serum cholesterol as a surrogate for risk of myocardial infarction) or a measurement which follows the pathophysiology even if it is not a key factor in its progression (e.g. serum C-reactive protein as a surrogate for resolution of inflammation in chest infection). Such surrogates are sometimes termed 'biomarkers'.

Plasma drug concentration

The following criteria must be met to justify routine monitoring by plasma drug concentration:

- Clinical endpoints and other pharmacodynamic (surrogate) effects are difficult to monitor.
- The relationship between plasma concentration and clinical effects is predictable.
- The therapeutic index is low. For drugs with a high therapeutic index any variability in plasma concentrations is likely to be irrelevant clinically.

Some examples of drugs that fulfil these criteria are listed in Box 2.26.

Measurement of plasma concentration may be useful in planning adjustments of drug dose and frequency of administration; to explain an inadequate therapeutic

2.26 Drugs commonly monitored by plasma drug concentration

Drug	Half-life (hrs)*	Comment
Digoxin	36	Steady state takes several days to achieve. Samples should be taken 6 hrs post dose. Measurement is useful to confirm the clinical impression of toxicity or non-adherence but clinical effectiveness is better assessed by ventricular heart rate. Risk of toxicity increases progressively at concentrations > 1.5 μg/L, and is likely at concentrations > 3.0 μg/L (toxicity is more likely in the presence of hypokalaemia)
Gentamicin	2	Measure pre-dose trough concentration (should be < 1 μg/mL) to ensure that accumulation (and the risk of nephrotoxicity and ototoxicity) is avoided; see p. 156
Levothyroxine	> 120	Steady state may take up to 6 wks to achieve (p. 743)
Lithium	24	Steady state takes several days to achieve. Samples should be taken 12 hrs post dose. Target range 0.4–1 mmol/L
Phenytoin	24	Measure pre-dose trough concentration (should be 10–20 mg/L) to ensure that accumulation is avoided. Good correlation between concentration and toxicity. Concentration may be misleading in the presence of hypoalbuminaemia
Theophylline (oral)	6	Steady state takes 2–3 days to achieve. Samples should be taken 6 hrs post dose. Target concentration is 10–20 mg/L but its relationship with bronchodilator effect and adverse effects is variable
Vancomycin	6	Measure pre-dose trough concentration (should be 10–15 mg/L) to ensure clinical efficacy and that accumulation and the risk of nephrotoxicity is avoided

*Half-lives vary considerably with different formulations and between patients.

response (by identifying subtherapeutic concentration or incomplete adherence); to establish whether a suspected ADR is likely to be caused by the drug; and to assess and avoid potential drug interactions.

Timing of samples in relation to doses

The concentration of drug rises and falls during the dosage interval (see Fig. 2.4B, p. 23). Measurements made during the initial absorption and distribution phases are unpredictable because of the rapidly changing concentration, so samples are usually taken at the end of the dosage interval (a 'trough' or 'pre-dose' concentration). This measurement is normally made in steady state, which usually takes five half-lives to achieve after the drug is introduced or the dose changed (unless a loading dose has been given).

Interpreting the result

A target range is provided for many drugs, based on average thresholds for therapeutic benefit and toxicity. Inter-individual variability means that these can only be used as a guide. For instance, a patient who describes symptoms that could be consistent with toxicity but has a drug concentration in the top half of the target range should still be suspected of suffering toxic effects. Another important consideration is that some drugs are heavily protein-bound (e.g. phenytoin) but only the unbound drug is pharmacologically active. Therefore, patients with hypoalbuminaemia may have a therapeutic or even toxic concentration of unbound drug, despite a low 'total' concentration.

Further information

Websites

www.bnf.org *The British National Formulary (BNF) is a key reference resource for UK NHS prescribers, with a list of licensed drugs, chapters on prescribing in renal failure, liver disease, pregnancy and during breastfeeding, and appendices on drug interactions*

www.cochrane.org *The Cochrane Collaboration is a leading international collaboration to provide evidence-based reviews (over 4000 so far)*

www.evidence.nhs.uk *NHS Evidence provides a wide range of health information relevant to delivering quality patient care*

www.icp.org.nz *The Interactive Clinical Pharmacology site is designed to increase understanding of principles in clinical pharmacology*

www.medicines.org/emc/ *The electronic Medicines Compendium (eMC) contains up-to-date, easily accessible information about medicines licensed by the UK Medicines and Healthcare Products Regulatory Agency (MHRA) and the European Medicines Agency (EMA)*

www.nice.org.uk *The UK National Institute for Health and Clinical Excellence makes recommendations to the UK NHS on new and existing medicines, treatments and procedures*

www.who.int/medicines/en/ *The World Health Organization Essential Medicines and Pharmaceutical Policies*

D.R. FitzPatrick
J.R. Seckl

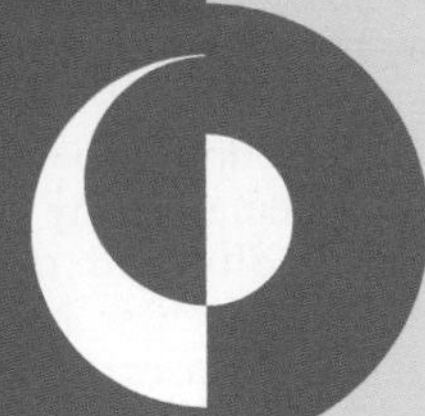

3 Molecular and genetic factors in disease

Functional anatomy and physiology 42

Genetic disease and inheritance 50
- Meiosis 50
- Patterns of disease inheritance 51
- Classes of genetic variant 53
- Consequences of genetic variation 57
- Constitutional genetic disease 58
- Somatic genetic disease 59

Investigation of genetic disease 60
- General principles of diagnosis 60
- Genetic testing in pregnancy and pre-implantation genetic testing 62
- Genetic testing in children 63
- Identifying a disease gene in families 63
- Genetic investigation in populations 64
- Predictive genetic testing 64

Presenting problems in genetic disease 64

Major categories of genetic disease 64
- Inborn errors of metabolism 64
- Neurological disorders 65
- Connective tissue disorders 65
- Learning disability, dysmorphism and malformations 66
- Familial cancer syndromes 66

Genetic counselling 67

Genetics of common diseases 68
- Measuring the genetic contribution to complex disease 68
- Genetic testing in complex disease 69
- Pharmacogenomics 69

Research frontiers in molecular medicine 69
- Gene therapy 69
- Induced pluripotent stem cells and regenerative medicine 69
- Pathway medicine 70

Almost all diseases have a genetic component. In children and young adults in particular, many of the disorders causing long-term morbidity and mortality are genetically determined. The molecular basis of most Mendelian (or 'single-gene') diseases has now been determined, and our understanding of the abnormalities in cell function responsible for the clinical presentation is improving. It has also become clear that variants in many genes contribute to the pathogenesis of several common diseases such as asthma, rheumatoid arthritis and osteoporosis. In this chapter, we review key principles of cell biology, cellular signalling and molecular genetics, with emphasis on the diagnosis and assessment of patients with genetic diseases.

FUNCTIONAL ANATOMY AND PHYSIOLOGY

Cell and molecular biology

All human cell types are derived from a single totipotent stem cell, the zygote (the fertilised ovum). During development, organs and tissues are formed by the integration of four closely regulated cellular processes: cell division, migration, differentiation and programmed cell death. In many adult tissues such as skin, liver and the intestine, these processes continue throughout life, mediated by populations of stem cells that are responsible for tissue maintenance and repair. Cell biology is the study of these processes and of intracellular compartments, called organelles, which maintain cellular homeostasis. Dysfunction of any of these processes may lead to disease.

DNA, chromosomes and chromatin

The nucleus is a membrane-bound compartment found in all cells except erythrocytes and platelets. The human nucleus contains 46 chromosomes, each a single linear molecule of deoxyribonucleic acid (DNA) complexed with proteins to form chromatin. The basic protein unit of chromatin is the nucleosome, comprising 147 base pairs (bp) of DNA wound round a core of four different histone proteins. The vast majority of chromosomal DNA is double-stranded, with the exception of the ends of chromosomes, where 'knotted' domains of single-stranded DNA, called telomeres, are found. Telomeres prevent degradation and accidental fusion of chromosomal DNA.

The genome comprises approximately 3.1 billion bp of DNA. Humans are diploid organisms, meaning that each nucleus contains two copies of the genome, visible microscopically as 22 identical chromosomal pairs – the autosomes – named 1 to 22 in descending size order (see Fig. 3.11, p. 57), and two sex chromosomes (XX in females and XY in males). Each DNA strand consists of a linear sequence of four bases – guanine (G), cytosine (C), adenine (A) and thymine (T) – covalently linked by phosphate bonds. The sequence of one strand of double-stranded DNA determines the sequence of the opposite strand because the helix is held together by hydrogen bonds between adenine and thymine or guanine and cytosine nucleotides.

Genes and transcription

Genes are functional elements on the chromosome that are capable of transmitting information from the DNA template via the production of messenger ribonucleic acid (mRNA) to the production of proteins. The human genome contains an estimated 21 500 genes, although many of these are inactive or silenced in different cell types. For example, although the gene for parathyroid hormone (PTH) is present in every cell, activation of gene expression and production of PTH mRNA is virtually restricted to the parathyroid glands. Genes that are active in different cells undergo transcription, which requires binding of an enzyme called RNA polymerase II to a segment of DNA at the start of the gene termed the promoter. Once bound, RNA polymerase II moves along one strand of DNA, producing an RNA molecule that is complementary to the DNA template. A DNA sequence close to the end of the gene, called the polyadenylation signal, acts as a signal for termination of the RNA transcript (Fig. 3.1). The activity of RNA polymerase II is regulated by transcription factors. These proteins bind to specific DNA sequences at the promoter, or to enhancer elements that may be many thousands of base pairs away from the promoter. A loop in the chromosomal DNA brings the enhancer close to the promoter, enabling the bound proteins to interact.

The human genome encodes approximately 1200 different transcription factors, and mutations in many of these can cause genetic diseases (Fig. 3.2). Mutation of the transcription factor binding sites within promoters or enhancers also causes genetic disease. For example, the blood disorder alpha-thalassaemia can result from loss of an enhancer located more than 100 000 bp from the alpha-globin gene promoter, leading to greatly reduced transcription. Similarly, variation in the promoter of the gene encoding intestinal lactase determines whether or not this is 'shut off' in adulthood, producing lactose intolerance.

The accessibility of promoters to RNA polymerase II depends on the structural configuration of chromatin. Transcriptionally active regions have decondensed (or 'open') chromatin (euchromatin). Conversely, transcriptionally silent regions are associated with densely packed chromatin called heterochromatin. Chemical modification of both the DNA and core histone proteins allows heterochromatic regions to be distinguished from open chromatin. DNA can be modified by addition of a methyl group to cytosine molecules (methylation). In promoter regions, this silences transcription, since methyl cytosines are usually not available for transcription factor binding or RNA transcription. The core histones can also be modified via methylation, phosphorylation, acetylation or sumoylation at specific amino acid residues in a pattern that reflects the functional state of the chromatin; this is called the histone code – reflecting an emerging understanding of the 'rules' by which specific modifications mark transcriptionally activating (trimethylation of lysine 4 on histone H3; acetylation of many histone residues) or silencing (methylation of lysine 9 on histone H4; deacetylation of many histone residues) effects. Such DNA and protein modifications are termed epigenetic, as they do not alter the primary sequence of the DNA code but have biological significance in chromosomal function. Abnormal epigenetic changes are increasingly recognised as

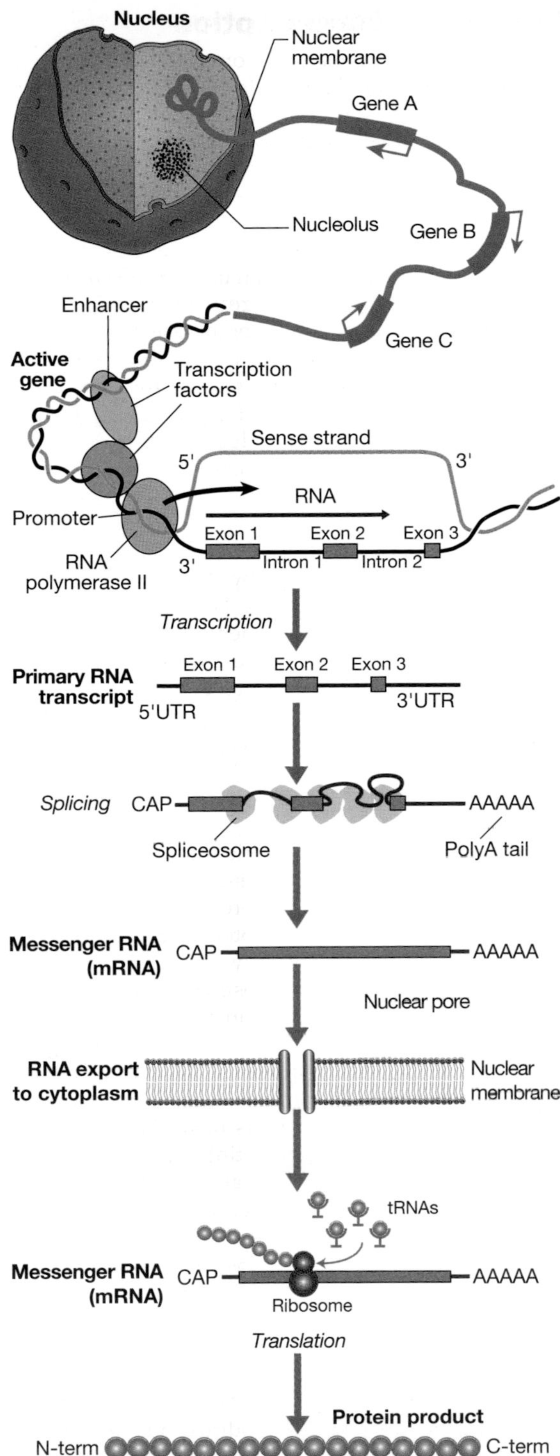

Fig. 3.1 RNA synthesis and its translation into protein. Gene transcription involves binding of RNA polymerase II to the promoter of genes being transcribed with other proteins (transcription factors) that regulate the transcription rate. The primary RNA transcript is a copy of the whole gene and includes both introns and exons, but the introns are removed within the nucleus by splicing and the exons are joined to form the messenger RNA (mRNA). Prior to export from the nucleus, a methylated guanosine nucleotide is added to the 5′ end of the RNA ('cap') and a string of adenine nucleotides is added to the 3′ ('poly A tail'). This protects the RNA from degradation and facilitates transport into the cytoplasm. In the cytoplasm, the mRNA binds to ribosomes and forms a template for protein production.

important events in the progression of cancer, allowing expression of genes which are normally silenced during development to support cancer cell de-differentiation (see Box 3.3, p. 54). They also afford therapeutic targets. For instance, the histone deacetylase inhibitor vorinostat has been successfully used to treat cutaneous T-cell lymphoma, due to the re-expression of genes that had previously been silenced in the tumour. These genes encode transcription factors which promote T-cell cell differentiation as opposed to proliferation, thereby causing tumour regression.

RNA splicing, editing and degradation

Transcription produces an RNA molecule that is a copy of the whole gene, termed the primary or nascent transcript. RNA differs from DNA in three main ways:

- RNA is single-stranded.
- The sugar residue within the nucleotide is ribose, rather than deoxyribose.
- Uracil (U) is used in place of thymine (T).

The nascent RNA molecule then undergoes splicing, to generate the shorter, 'mature' mRNA molecule, which provides the template for protein production. Splicing removes the regions of the nascent RNA molecule that are not required to make protein (intronic regions), and retains and rejoins those segments that are necessary for protein production (exonic regions). Splicing is a highly regulated process that is carried out by a multimeric protein complex called the spliceosome. Following splicing, the mRNA molecule is exported from the nucleus and used as a template for protein synthesis. It should be noted that many genes produce more than one form of mRNA (and thus protein) by a process termed alternative splicing. Different proteins from the same gene can have entirely distinct functions. For example, in thyroid C cells the calcitonin gene produces mRNA encoding the osteoclast inhibitor calcitonin (p. 738), but in neurons the same gene produces an mRNA with a different complement of exons via alternative splicing, which encodes the neurotransmitter calcitonin-gene-related peptide.

The portion of the mRNA molecule that directs synthesis of a protein product is called the open reading frame (ORF). This comprises a contiguous series of three sequential bases (codons), which specify that a particular amino acid should be incorporated into the protein. There are 64 different codons; 61 of these specify incorporation of one of the 20 amino acids, whereas the remaining three codons - UAA, UAG and UGA (stop codons) - cause termination of the growing polypeptide chain. In humans, most ORF start with the amino acid methionine, which is specified by the codon AUG. All mRNA molecules have domains before and after the ORF called the 5′ untranslated region (5′UTR) and 3′UTR, respectively. The start of the 5′UTR contains a cap structure that protects mRNA from enzymatic degradation, and other elements within the 5′UTR are required for efficient translation. The 3′UTR also contains elements that regulate efficiency of translation and mRNA stability, including a stretch of adenine bases known as a polyA tail.

However, there are approximately 4500 genes in humans in which the transcribed RNA molecules do not code for proteins. There are various categories of

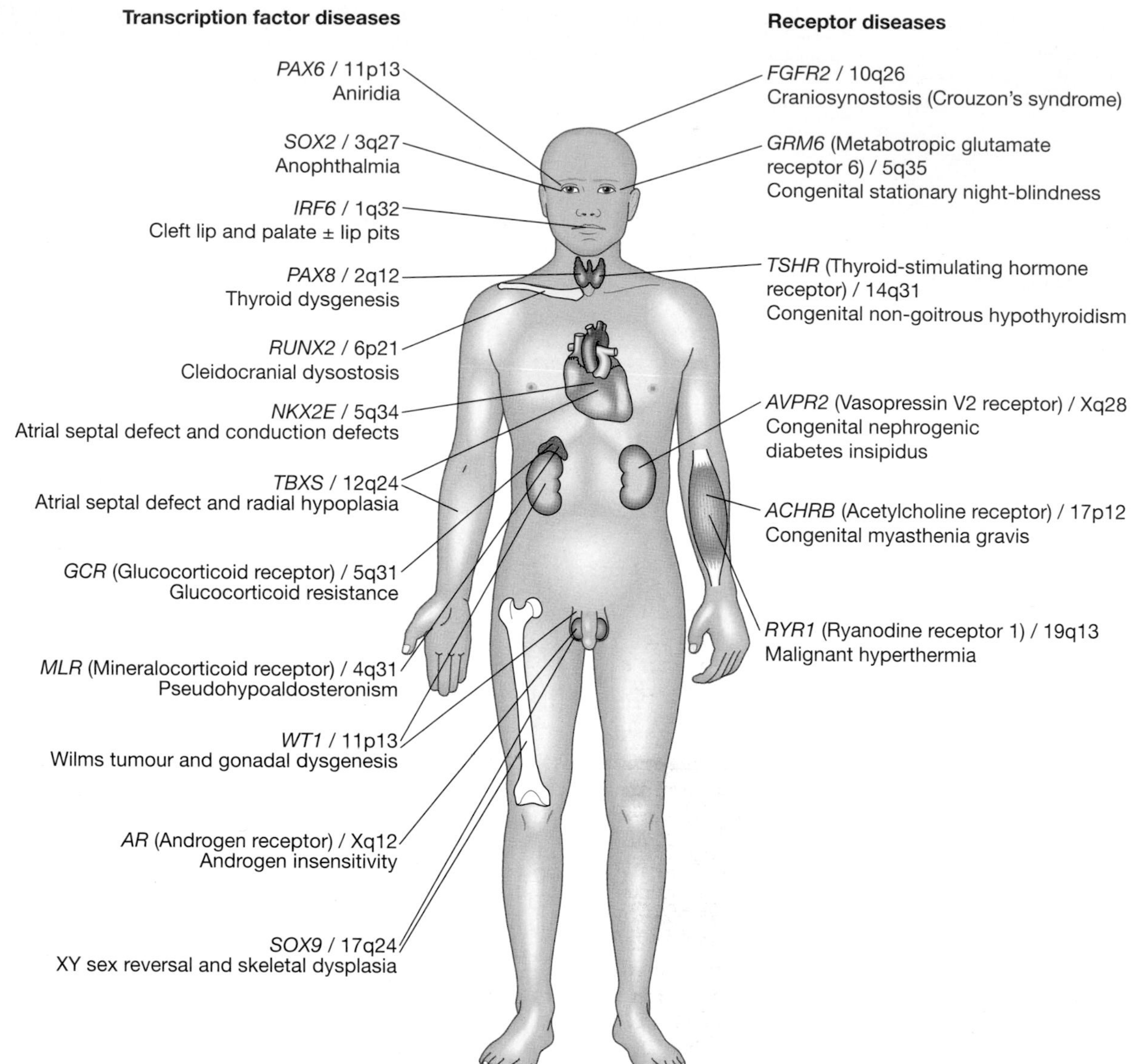

Fig. 3.2 Examples of genetic diseases caused by mutations in genes encoding either transcription factors or receptors.

non-coding RNA (ncRNA), including transfer RNA (tRNA), ribosomal RNA (rRNA), ribozymes and micro-RNA (miRNA). There are more than 1000 miRNAs that bind to various target mRNAs, typically in the 3′UTR, to affect mRNA stability. This usually results in enhanced degradation of the target mRNA, leading to translational gene silencing. Together, miRNAs affect over half of all human genes and have important roles in normal development, cancer and common degenerative disorders. This is the subject of considerable research interest at present.

Translation and protein production

Following splicing and export from the nucleus, mRNAs associate with ribosomes, which are the sites of protein production (see Fig. 3.1). Each ribosome consists of two subunits (40S and 60S), which comprise non-coding rRNA molecules complexed with proteins. During translation, tRNA binds to the ribosome. The tRNAs deliver amino acids to the ribosome so that the newly synthesised protein can be assembled in a stepwise fashion. Individual tRNA molecules bind a specific amino acid and 'read' the mRNA ORF via an 'anti-codon' of three nucleotides that is complementary to the codon in mRNA. A proportion of ribosomes are bound to the membrane of the endoplasmic reticulum (ER), a complex tubular structure that surrounds the nucleus. Proteins synthesised on these ribosomes are translocated into the lumen of the ER, where they undergo folding and processing. From here the protein may be transferred to the Golgi apparatus, where it undergoes post-translational modifications, such as glycosylation (covalent attachment of sugar moieties), to form the mature protein that can be exported into the cytoplasm or packaged into vesicles for secretion. The clinical importance of post-translational modification of proteins is shown by the severe developmental, neurological, haemostatic and soft-tissue abnormalities that occur in patients with mutations of the enzymes that catalyse the addition of chains of sugar moieties to proteins. An example is phosphomannose isomerase deficiency, in which there is a defect in the conversion of fructose-6-phosphate to mannose-6-phosphate. This results in a defect in supply of D-mannose derivatives for glycosylation of a variety of proteins, resulting in a multi-system disorder characterised by protein-losing enteropathy, hepatic fibrosis, coagulopathy and hypoglycaemia. Post-translational modifications can also be disrupted by the synthesis of proteins with abnormal amino acid sequences. For example, the most common mutation in cystic fibrosis (ΔF508) results in an abnormal protein that cannot be exported from the ER and Golgi.

Mitochondria and energy production

The mitochondrion is the main site of energy production within the cell. Mitochondria arose during evolution via the symbiotic association with an intracellular bacterium. They have a distinctive structure with functionally distinct inner and outer membranes. Mitochondria produce energy in the form of adenosine triphosphate (ATP). ATP is mostly derived from the metabolism of glucose and fat (Fig. 3.3). Glucose cannot

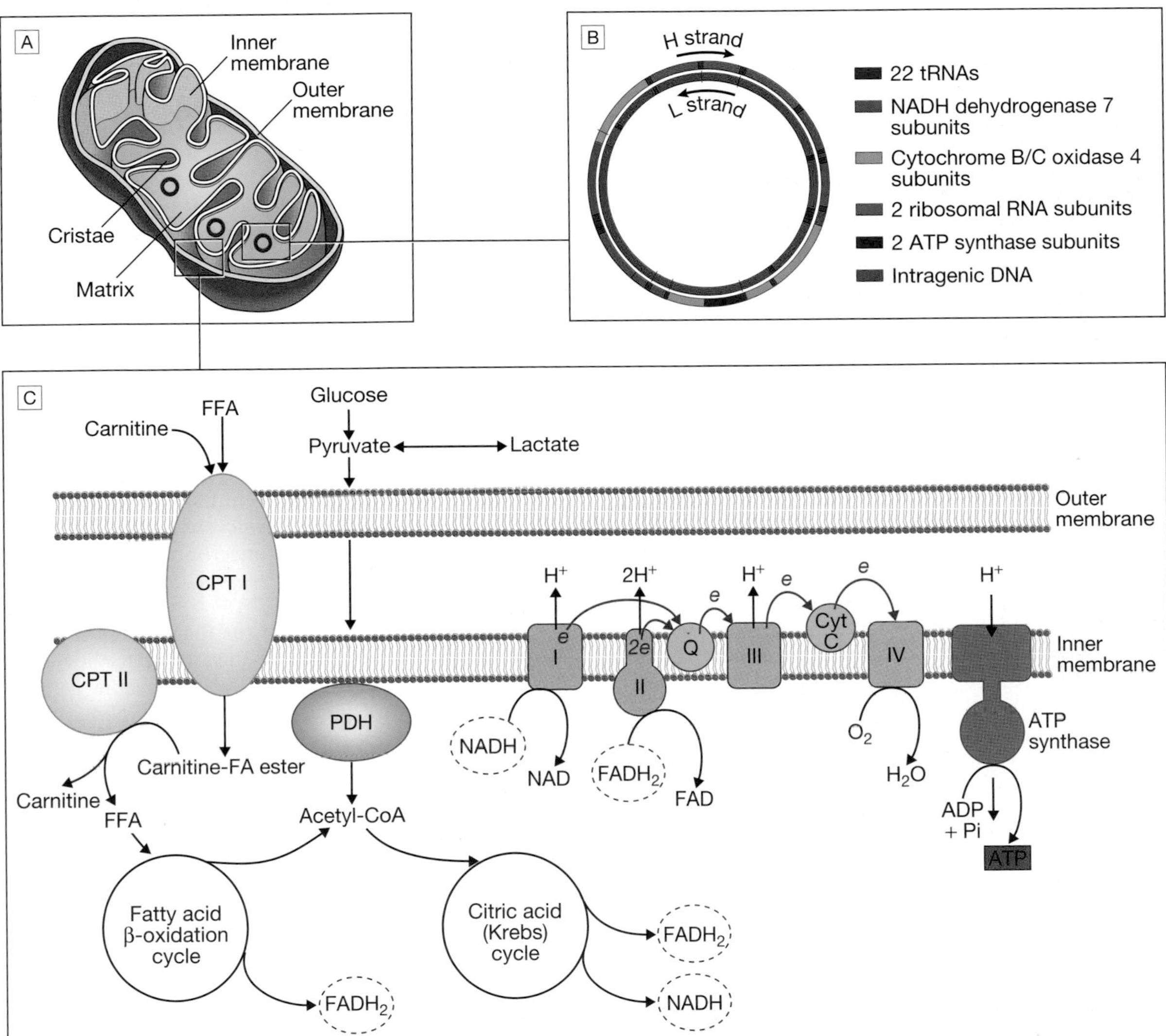

Fig. 3.3 Mitochondria. **A** Mitochondrial structure. There is a smooth outer membrane surrounding a convoluted inner membrane, which has inward projections called cristae. The membranes create two compartments: the inter-membrane compartment, which plays a crucial role in the electron transport chain, and the inner compartment (or matrix), which contains mitochondrial DNA and the enzymes responsible for the citric acid (Krebs) cycle and the fatty acid β-oxidation cycle. **B** Mitochondrial DNA. The mitochondrion contains several copies of a circular double-stranded DNA molecule, which has a non-coding region, and a coding region which encodes the genes responsible for energy production, mitochondrial tRNA molecules and mitochondrial rRNA molecules. ATP = adenosine triphosphate; NADH = nicotinamide adenine dinucleotide. **C** Mitochondrial energy production. Fatty acids enter the mitochondrion conjugated to carnitine by carnitine-palmityl transferase type 1 (CPT I) and, once inside the matrix, are unconjugated by CPT II to release free fatty acids (FFA). These are broken down by the β-oxidation cycle to produce acetyl-CoA. Pyruvate can enter the mitochondrion directly and is metabolised by pyruvate dehydrogenase (PDH) to produce acetyl-CoA. The acetyl-CoA enters the Krebs cycle, leading to the production of NADH and flavine adenine dinucleotide (reduced form) ($FADH_2$), which are used by proteins in the electron transport chain to generate a hydrogen ion gradient across the inter-membrane compartment. Reduction of NADH and $FADH_2$ by proteins I and II respectively releases electrons (e), and the energy released is used to pump protons into the inter-membrane compartment. As these electrons are exchanged between proteins in the chain, more protons are pumped across the membrane, until the electrons reach complex IV (cytochrome oxidase), which uses the energy to reduce oxygen to water. The hydrogen ion gradient is used to produce ATP by the enzyme ATP synthase, which consists of a proton channel and catalytic sites for the synthesis of ATP from ADP. When the channel opens, hydrogen ions enter the matrix down the concentration gradient, and energy is released that is used to make ATP.

enter mitochondria directly but is first metabolised to pyruvate via glycolysis. Pyruvate is then imported into the mitochondrion and metabolised to acetyl-coenzyme A (CoA). Fatty acids are transported into the mitochondria following conjugation with carnitine and are sequentially catabolised by a process called β-oxidation to produce acetyl-CoA. The acetyl-CoA from both pyruvate and fatty acid oxidation is used in the citric acid (Krebs) cycle – a series of enzymatic reactions that produces CO_2, NADH and $FADH_2$. Both NADH and $FADH_2$ then donate electrons to the respiratory chain. Here these electrons are transferred via a complex series of reactions resulting in the formation of a proton gradient across the inner mitochondrial membrane. The gradient is used by an inner mitochondrial membrane protein, ATP synthase, to produce ATP, which is then transported to other parts of the cell. Dephosphorylation of ATP is used to produce the energy required for many cellular processes.

Each mitochondrion contains 2–10 copies of a 16 kilobase (kB) double-stranded circular DNA molecule (mtRNA). mtDNA contains 13 protein-coding genes, all involved in the respiratory chain, and the ncRNA genes required for protein synthesis within the mitochondria (see Fig. 3.3). The mutational rate of mtDNA is relatively high due to the lack of protection by chromatin. Several mtDNA diseases characterised by defects in ATP production have been described. mtDNA diseases are inherited exclusively via the maternal line (see Fig. 3.7, p. 51). This unusual inheritance pattern exists because all mtDNA in an individual is derived from that person's mother via the egg cell, as sperm contribute no mitochondria to the zygote. Mitochondria are most numerous in cells with high metabolic demands, such as muscle, retina and the basal ganglia, and these tissues tend to be the ones most severely affected in mitochondrial diseases (Box 3.1). There are many other mitochondrial diseases that are caused by mutations in nuclear genes, which encode proteins that are then imported into the mitochondrion and are critical for energy production: for example, Leigh's syndrome and complex I deficiency.

Protein degradation

The cell uses several different systems to degrade proteins and other molecules that are damaged, are potentially toxic or have simply served their purpose. The proteasome is the main site of protein degradation within the cell. The first step in proteasomal degradation is ubiquitination – the covalent attachment of a protein called ubiquitin as a side chain to the target protein. Ubiquitination is carried out by a large group of enzymes called E3 ligases, whose function is to recognise specific proteins that should be targeted for degradation by the proteasome. The E3 ligases ubiquitinate their target protein, which is then transported to a large multi-protein complex called the 26S proteasome, where it is degraded. There is mounting evidence that defects in the proteasome contribute to the pathogenesis of many diseases, particularly degenerative diseases of the nervous system like Parkinson's disease and some types of dementia that are characterised by formation of abnormal protein aggregates (inclusion bodies) within neurons. At least one inherited disease, termed Angelman's syndrome, is due to a mutation affecting the UBE3 E3 ligase.

Proteins with complex post-translational modifications are degraded in membrane-bound structures called lysosomes, which have an acidic pH and contain proteolytic enzymes that degrade proteins. There are many inherited defects in lysosomal enzymes that result in failure to degrade intracellular toxic substances. For instance, in Gaucher's disease, mutations of the gene encoding lysosomal (acid) β-glucosidase lead to undigested lipid accumulating in macrophages, producing hepatosplenomegaly and, if severe, deposition in the brain and mental retardation.

Lysosomes are also crucial for the process of autophagy, a process of self-cannibalisation that allows the cell to adapt to periods of starvation by recycling cellular components. Autophagy is triggered by metabolic stress and begins with the formation of a membrane-bound vesicle called the autophagosome, which contains targeted cellular components such as long-lived proteins

3.1 The structure of the respiratory chain complexes and the diseases associated with their dysfunction

Complex	Enzyme	nDNA subunits[1]	mtDNA subunits[2]	Diseases
I	NADH dehydrogenase	38	7	MELAS, bilateral striatal necrosis, LHON, myopathy and exercise intolerance, Parkinsonism, Leigh's disease, exercise myoglobinuria, leucodystrophy/myoclonic epilepsy
II	Succinate dehydrogenase	4	0	Phaeochromocytoma
III	Cytochrome bc_1 complex	10	1	Parkinsonism/MELAS, cardiomyopathy, myopathy, exercise myoglobinuria
IV	Cytochrome c oxidase	10	3	Sideroblastic anaemia, myoclonic ataxia, deafness, myopathy, MELAS, mitochondrial encephalomyopathy, motor neuron disease-like, exercise myoglobinuria
V	ATP synthase	14	2	Leigh's disease, NARP, bilateral striatal necrosis

[1]nDNA subunits
[2]mtDNA subunits = number of different protein subunits in each complex that are encoded in the nDNA and mtDNA respectively.
(LHON = Leber hereditary optic neuropathy; MELAS = myopathy, encephalopathy, lactic acidosis and stroke-like episodes; MERRF = myoclonic epilepsy and ragged red fibres; mtDNA = mitochondrial DNA; NARP = neuropathy, ataxia and retinitis pigmentosa; nDNA = nuclear DNA)

and organelles. The autophagosome then fuses with the lysosome to start the degradation and recycling process. Mutations in proteins that are crucial for formation of the autophagosome lead to neurodegenerative diseases in humans, such as juvenile neuronal ceroid lipofuscinosis (Batten's disease), caused by autosomal recessive mutations in *CLN3*.

Peroxisomes are small, single membrane-bound cytoplasmic organelles containing many different oxidative enzymes such as catalase. Peroxisomes degrade hydrogen peroxide, bile acids and amino acids. However, the β-oxidation of very long-chain fatty acids appears to be their most important function, since mutations in the peroxisomal β-oxidation enzymes (or the proteins that import these enzymes into the peroxisome) result in the same severe congenital disorder as mutations that cause complete failure of peroxisomal biogenesis. This group of disorders is called Zellweger's syndrome (cerebrohepatorenal syndrome) and is characterised by severe developmental delay, seizures, hepatomegaly and renal cysts; the biochemical diagnosis is made on the basis of elevated plasma levels of very long-chain fatty acids.

The cell membrane and cytoskeleton

The cell membrane is a phospholipid bilayer, with hydrophilic surfaces and a hydrophobic core (Fig. 3.4). The cell membrane is, however, much more than a simple wall. Cholesterol-rich 'rafts' float within the membrane, and proteins are anchored to them via the post-translational addition of complex lipid moieties. The membrane also hosts a series of transmembrane proteins that function as receptors, pores, ion channels, pumps and associated energy suppliers. These proteins allow the cell to monitor the extracellular milieu, import crucial molecules for function, and exclude or exchange unwanted substances. Many protein–protein interactions within the cell membrane are highly dynamic, and individual peptides will associate and disassociate to effect specific roles.

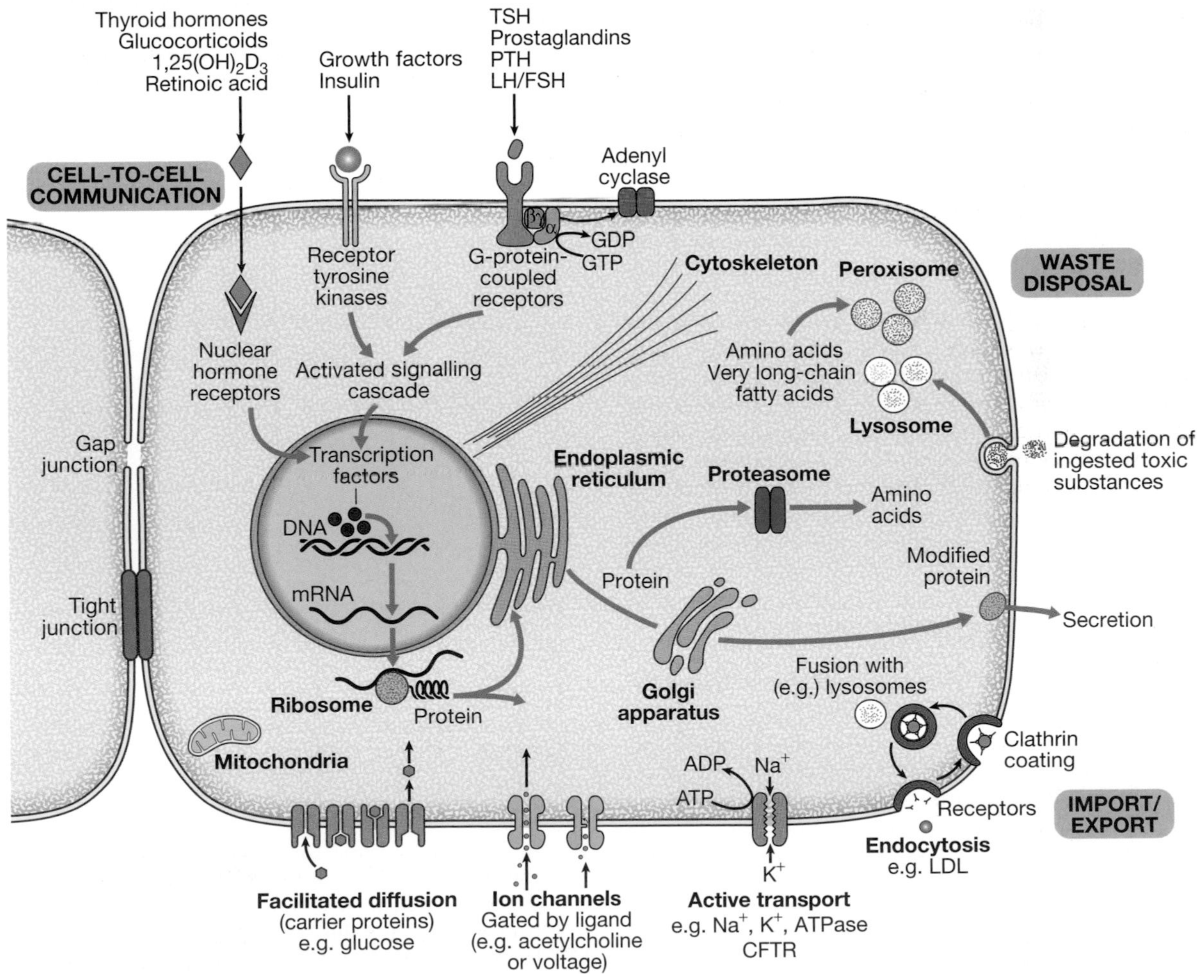

Fig. 3.4 An archetypal human cell. The basic cell components required for function within a tissue: (1) cell-to-cell communication taking place via gap junctions and the various types of receptor that receive signals from the extracellular environment and transduce these into intracellular messengers; (2) the nucleus containing the chromosomal DNA; (3) intracellular organelles, including the mechanisms for proteins and lipid catabolism; (4) the cellular mechanisms for import and export of molecules across the cell membrane. (ABC = ATP-binding cassette transporters; ATP = adenosine triphosphate: cAMP = cyclic adenosine monophosphate; CFTR = cystic fibrosis transmembrane regulator; CREB = cAMP response element-binding protein; GDP/GTP = guanine diphosphate/triphosphate; LDL = low-density lipoproteins; LH/FSH = luteinising hormone/follicle-stimulating hormone; PTH = parathyroid hormone; TSH = thyroid-stimulating hormone)

The cell membrane is permeable to hydrophobic substances, such as anaesthetic gases. Water is able to pass through the membrane via a pore formed by aquaporin proteins; mutations of an aquaporin gene cause congenital nephrogenic diabetes insipidus (p. 794). Most other molecules must be actively transported using either channels or pumps. Channels are responsible for the transport of ions and other small molecules across the cell membrane. They open and close in a highly regulated manner. The cystic fibrosis transmembrane conductance regulator (CFTR) is an example of an ion channel that is responsible for transport of chloride ions across epithelial cell membranes. Mutation of the CFTR chloride channel, highly expressed in the lung and gut, leads to defective chloride transport, producing cystic fibrosis. Pumps are highly specific for their substrate and often use energy (ATP) to drive transport against a concentration gradient.

Endocytosis is a cellular process that allows internalisation of larger complexes and molecules by invagination of plasma membrane to create intracellular vesicles. This process is typically mediated by specific binding of the particle to surface receptors. An important example is the binding of low-density lipoprotein (LDL) cholesterol-rich particles to the LDL receptor (LDLR) in a specialised region of the membrane called a clathrin pit. In some cases of familial hypercholesterolaemia (p. 453), LDLR mutations cause failure of this binding and thus reduce cellular uptake of LDL. Other LDLR mutations change a specific tyrosine in the intracellular tail of the receptor, preventing LDLR from concentrating in clathrin-coated pits and hence impairing uptake of LDL, even though LDLR bound to LDL is present elsewhere in the cell membrane.

The shape and structure of the cell are maintained by the cytoskeleton, which consists of a series of proteins which form microfilaments (actin), microtubules (tubulins) and intermediate filaments (keratins, desmin, vimentin, laminins) that facilitate cellular movement and provide pathways for intracellular transport. Dysfunction of the cytoskeleton may result in a variety of human disorders. For instance, some keratin genes encode intermediate filaments in epithelia. In epidermolysis bullosa simplex (p. 1292), mutations in keratin genes (*KRT5*, *KRT14*) lead to cell fragility, producing the characteristic blistering on mild trauma.

Receptors, cellular communication and intracellular signalling

Several mechanisms exist that allow cells to communicate with one another. Direct communication between adjacent cells occurs through gap junctions. These are pores formed by the interaction of 'hemichannels' in the membrane of adjacent cells. Many diseases are due to mutations in gap junction proteins, including the most common form of autosomal recessive hearing loss (*GJB2*) and the X-linked form of Charcot–Marie–Tooth disease (*GJB1*).

Communication between cells that are not directly in contact with each other occurs through hormones, cytokines and growth factors, which bind to and activate receptors on the target cell. Receptors then bind to various other proteins within the cell termed signalling molecules, which directly or indirectly activate gene expression to produce a cellular response.

There are many different signalling pathways; for example, in nuclear steroid hormone signalling, the ligands (steroid hormones or thyroid hormone) bind to their cognate receptor in the cytoplasm of target cells and the receptor/ligand complex then enters the nucleus, where it acts as a transcription factor to regulate the expression of target genes (Box 3.2). However, the most diverse and abundant types of receptor are located at the cell surface, and these activate gene expression and cellular responses indirectly. Activation of a cell surface receptor by its ligand results in a series of intracellular events, involving a cascade of phosphorylation of specific residues in target proteins by an important group of enzymes called kinases. This cascade typically culminates in phosphorylation and activation of transcription factors, which bind DNA and modulate gene expression.

Figure 3.5 depicts some of the signalling molecules downstream of the tumour necrosis factor (TNF) receptor. On activation of the receptor by the ligand (in this case, TNF), other molecules, including TNF-receptor-associated proteins (TRAFs), are recruited to the intracellular domain of the receptor. These regulate the activity of a kinase termed IKKγ, which in turn regulates activity of two further kinases termed IKKα and IKKβ. These regulate degradation of an inhibitory protein called IκB, which normally binds to the effector protein NFκB, holding it in the cytoplasm. On receptor activation, a signal is transmitted through TRAFs and the IKK proteins to cause phosphorylation and

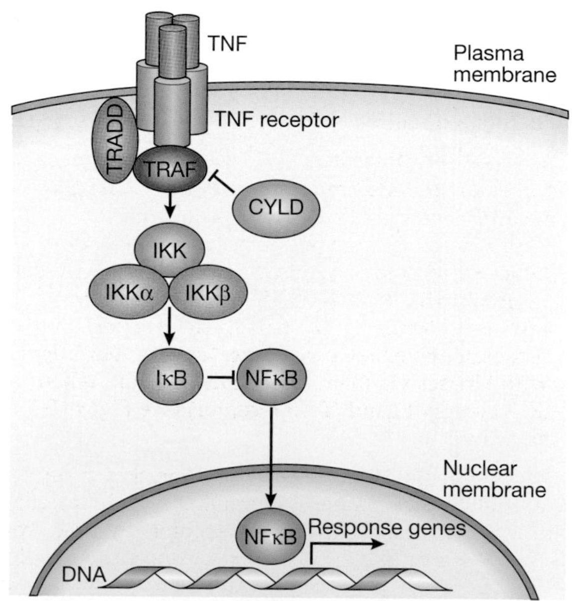

Fig. 3.5 The tumour necrosis factor (TNF) signalling pathway. TNF binds to its receptor, forming a trimeric complex in the cell membrane. Various receptor-associated factors are attracted to the intracellular domain of the receptor, including TNF-receptor-associated protein 6 (TRAF6) and tumour necrosis factor receptor type 1-associated death domain protein (TRADD). These proteins modulate activity of downstream signalling proteins, the most important of which are IKKγ (which in turn modulates activity of IKKα and IKKβ). These proteins cause phosphorylation of IκB, which is targeted for degradation by the proteasome, releasing NFκB, which translocates to the nucleus to activate gene expression. The signalling pathway is further regulated in a negative manner by cylindromatosis (CYLD), which de-ubiquitinates TRAF6, thereby impairing its ability to activate downstream signalling.

3.2 Examples of molecules involved in specific signalling cascades

Receptor	Receptor type	Ligands	Signal transduction	Clinical significance
TNFR1	TNF receptor superfamily	TNF	TRAF2/5, TRADD, IKK, IκB, NFκB, CYLD, RANK	Mediator of inflammatory diseases and immune responses
RANK	TNF receptor superfamily	RANKL	TRAF6, IKK, IκB, NFκB	Regulates bone resorption
Insulin receptor	Receptor tyrosine kinase	Insulin	IRS1, PI3K, PIP3, PKB, PDK1, mTORC2, GSK3	Regulation of energy homeostasis and glucose metabolism
Erythropoietin receptor	Receptor tyrosine kinase	Erythropoietin	JAK2, STAT5, c-Jun, c-Fos, Src PI3K, PIP3, PDK1, PKB	Regulates erythropoiesis
THRα and THRβ	Nuclear receptor superfamily	T3	Ligand/receptor complex	Regulates differentiation and function of many cells and tissues
ERα and ERβ	Nuclear receptor superfamily	Oestrogen	Ligand/receptor complex	Important for fertility, reproduction and bone health
GnRHR	GPCR	GnRH	G_q/G11, PLCbetal, PLA(2), PLD, PKC, MAPK	Regulates fertility
PTHR1	GPCR	PTH, PTHLP	Gs, adenyl cyclase, cAMP, PKA, CREB, G_q/G11, PLC, DAG, IP3, PKC, Ca^{++}	Regulates calcium homeostasis and bone turnover

(cAMP = cyclic adenosine monophosphate; CREB = Ca^{++} intracellular calcium; CYLD = cylindromatosis; DAG = diacylglycerol; ER = (o)estrogen receptor; GnRHR = gonadotrophin releasing hormone receptor; GPCR = G protein-coupled receptor; Gq/G11/Gs = guanine nucleotide binding proteins; GSK3 = glycogen synthetase kinase 3; IκB = inhibitor of kappa B; IKK = I kappa B kinase; IP3 = D-myo-inositol-1,4,5-trisphosphate; IRS1 = insulin receptor substrate 1; JAK2 = Janus activated kinase 2; MAPK = mitogen-activated kinase; mTOR = mammalian target of rapamycin; NFκB = nuclear factor kappa B; PDK1 = phosphoinosotide-dependent kinase 1; PIP3 = phosphoinosotol triphosphate; PI3K = phosphoinosotol 3 kinase; PKA/PKB/PKC = protein kinase A/B/C; PLA/PLC/PLD = phospholipase A/C/D; PTHR1 = parathyroid hormone receptor 1; PTHLP = parathyroid hormone-like protein; RANK = receptor activator of nuclear factor kappa B; STAT5 = signal transducer and activator of transcription; TNF = tumour necrosis factor; TNFR1 = TNF receptor 1; TRAF = TNF receptor-associated factors; TRADD = tumour necrosis factor receptor type 1-associated death domain protein; TRH = thyrotrophin releasing hormone)

degradation of IκB, allowing NFκB to translocate to the nucleus and activate gene expression. The system also has negative regulators, including the cylindromatosis (CYLD) enzyme, which regulates the activity of TRAFs by de-ubiquitination. Other transmembrane receptors can be grouped into:

- ion channel-linked receptors (glutamate and the nicotinic acetylcholine receptor)
- G protein-coupled receptors (GnRH, rhodopsin, olfactory receptors, parathyroid hormone receptor)
- receptors with kinase activity (insulin receptor, erythropoietin receptor, growth factor receptors)
- receptors which have no kinase activity, but interact with kinases via their intracellular domain when activated by ligand (TNF receptor) (see Figure 3.5 and Box 3.2).

Many receptors can signal only when they assemble as a multimeric complex. Mutations which interfere with assembly of the functional receptor multimer can result in disease. For example, mutations of the insulin receptor that inhibit dimerisation lead to childhood insulin resistance and growth failure. Conversely, some fibroblast growth factor receptor 2 (*FGFR2*) gene mutations cause dimerisation in the absence of ligand binding, leading to bone overgrowth and an autosomal dominant form of craniosynostosis called Crouzon's syndrome.

It is becoming clear that specialised projections on the cell surface known as cilia are essential for normal signalling in many tissues. Cilia can be motile or non-motile. Motile cilia are crucial for normal respiratory tract function, with primary ciliary dyskinesia (PCD) resulting in early-onset bronchiectasis due to failure to clear lung secretions. PCD is commonly associated with situs inversus (left–right laterality reversal) as a result of failure of a specific signalling process in very early embryogenesis. Mutations in proteins that are essential for non-motile cilia formation or function are responsible for a large number of autosomal recessive disorders known collectively as ciliopathies, which are commonly associated with intellectual disability, renal cystic dysplasia and retinal degeneration. For example, in the Bardet–Biedl syndrome, mutations in a series of genes encoding ciliary structure cause polydactyly, obesity, hypogonadism, retinitis pigmentosa and renal failure.

Cell division, differentiation and migration

In normal tissues, molecules such as hormones, growth factors and cytokines provide the signal to activate the cell cycle, a controlled programme of biochemical events that culminates in cell division. During the first phase, G1, synthesis of the cellular components necessary to complete cell division occurs. In S phase, the cell produces an identical copy of each chromosome – which carries the cell's genetic information – via a process called DNA replication. The cell then enters G2, when any errors in the replicated DNA are repaired before proceeding to mitosis, in which identical copies of all chromosomes are segregated to the daughter cells. The progression from one phase to the next is tightly controlled by cell cycle checkpoints. For example, the checkpoint between G2 and mitosis ensures that all damaged DNA is repaired prior to segregation of the chromosomes. Failure of these control processes is a crucial driver in the pathogenesis of cancer, as discussed in Chapter 11 (p. 262).

During development, cells must become progressively less like a stem cell and acquire the morphological and biochemical configuration of the tissue to which they will contribute. This process is called differentiation and it is achieved by activation of tissue-specific genes and inactivation or silencing of genes that maintain the cell in a progenitor state. This epigenetic process enables cells containing the same genetic material to have very different structures and functions. The programme of differentiation is often deranged or partially reversed in cancer cells. A similar mechanism allows adult stem cells to maintain and repair tissues. Cell migration is a process that is also necessary for development and wound healing. Migration also requires the activation of a specific set of genes, such as the transcription factor *TWIST*, that give the cell polarity and enable the leading edge of the cell to interact with the extracellular environment to control the speed and direction of travel. Again, this process can be reactivated in cancer cells and is thought to facilitate tumour metastasis.

Cell death, apoptosis and senescence

With the exception of stem cells, human cells have only a limited capacity for cell division. The Hayflick limit is the number of divisions a cell population can go through in culture before division stops and the cell enters a state known as senescence. This 'biological clock' is of great interest in the study of the normal ageing process. Rare human diseases associated with premature ageing, called progeric syndromes, have been very helpful in identifying the importance of DNA repair mechanisms in senescence (p. 168). For example, in Werner syndrome, a DNA helicase (an enzyme that separates the two DNA strands) is mutated, leading to failure of DNA repair and premature ageing. A distinct mechanism of cell death is seen in apoptosis, or programmed cell death.

Apoptosis is an active process that occurs in normal tissues and plays an important role in development, tissue remodelling and the immune response. The signal that triggers apoptosis is specific to each tissue or cell type. This signal activates enzymes, called caspases, which actively destroy cellular components, including chromosomal DNA. This degradation results in cell death, but the cellular corpse contains characteristic vesicles called apoptotic bodies. The corpse is then recognised and removed by phagocytic cells of the immune system, such as macrophages, in a manner that does not provoke an inflammatory response.

A third mechanism of cell death is necrosis. This is a pathological process in which the cellular environment loses one or more of the components necessary for cell viability. Hypoxia is probably the most common cause of necrosis.

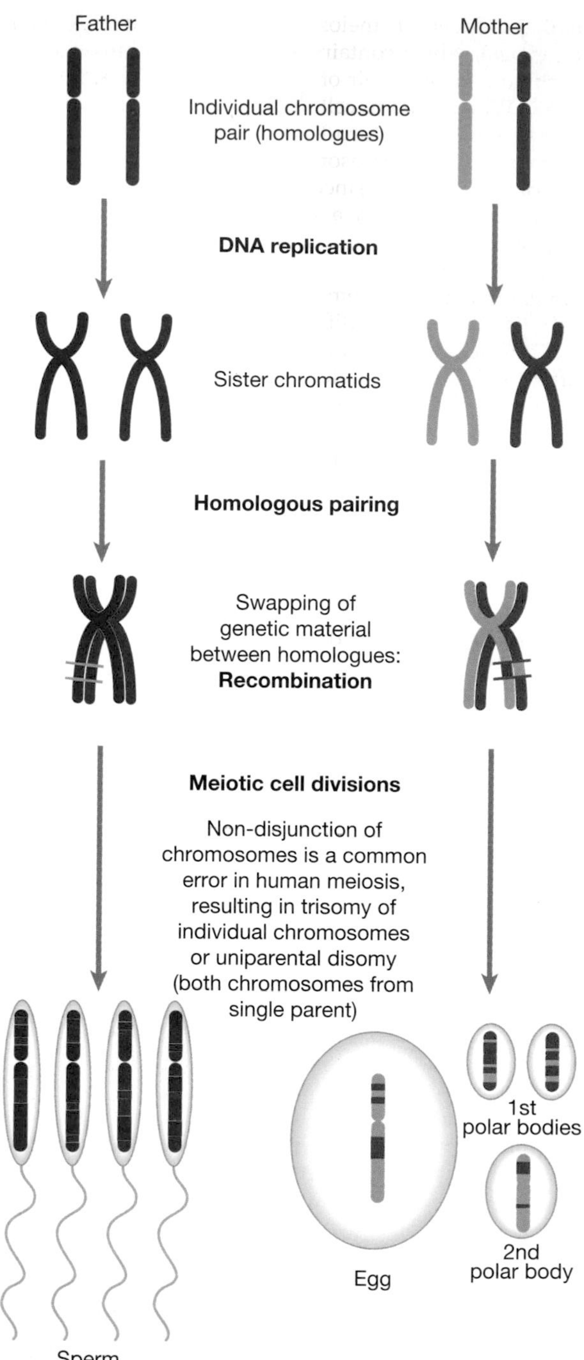

Fig. 3.6 Meiosis and gametogenesis. The main chromosomal stages of meiosis in both males and females. A single homologous pair of chromosomes is represented in different colours. The final step is the production of haploid germ cells. Each round of meiosis in the male results in four sperm cells; in the female, however, only one egg cell is produced, as the other divisions are sequestered on the periphery of the mature egg as peripheral polar bodies.

GENETIC DISEASE AND INHERITANCE

Meiosis

Meiosis is a special form of cell division that only occurs in the post-pubertal testis and the fetal and adult ovary (Fig. 3.6). Meiosis differs from mitosis in two main ways; there are two separate cell divisions and before the first of these there is extensive swapping of genetic material between homologous chromosomes, a process known as recombination. The result of recombination is that each chromosome that a parent passes to his or her offspring is a mix of the chromosomes that the parent inherited from his or her own mother and father. The end products of meiosis are sperm and egg cells (gametes), which contain only 23 chromosomes: one of each homologous pair of autosomes and a sex chromosome. When a sperm cell fertilises the egg, the resulting zygote will thus return to a diploid chromosome complement of 46 chromosomes. The sperm determines the sex of the offspring, since 50% of sperm will carry an X chromosome and 50% a Y chromosome, while each egg cell carries an X chromosome.

The individual steps in meiotic cell division are similar in males and females. However, the timing of the cell divisions is very different (see Fig. 3.6). In females, meiosis begins in fetal life but does not complete until after ovulation. A single meiotic cell division can thus take more than 40 years to complete. In males, meiotic division does not begin until puberty and continues throughout life. In the testes, both meiotic divisions are completed in a matter of days.

Patterns of disease inheritance

Five modes of genetic disease inheritance are discussed below and illustrated in Figures 3.7 and 3.8.

Autosomal dominant inheritance

Autosomal dominant disorders result from a genetic abnormality in one of the two copies (alleles) of a single gene. The risk of an affected individual transmitting an autosomal disease to his or her offspring is 50% for each pregnancy, since half the affected individual gametes (sperm or egg cells) will contain the affected chromosome and half will contain the normal chromosome. However, even within a family, individuals with the same mutation rarely have identical patterns of disease due to variable penetrance and/or expressivity. Penetrance is defined as the proportion of individuals bearing a mutated allele who develop the disease phenotype. The mutation is said to be fully penetrant if all individuals who inherit a mutation develop the disease. Expressivity describes the level of severity of each aspect of the disease phenotype. Neurofibromatosis type 1 (NF1, neurofibromin, 17q11.2) is an example of a disease that is fully (100%) penetrant but which shows extremely variable expressivity. The environmental factors and/or variation in other genes that act as modifiers of the mutated gene's function are mostly unknown. A good example of an environmental influence that can profoundly influence expression of autosomal dominant

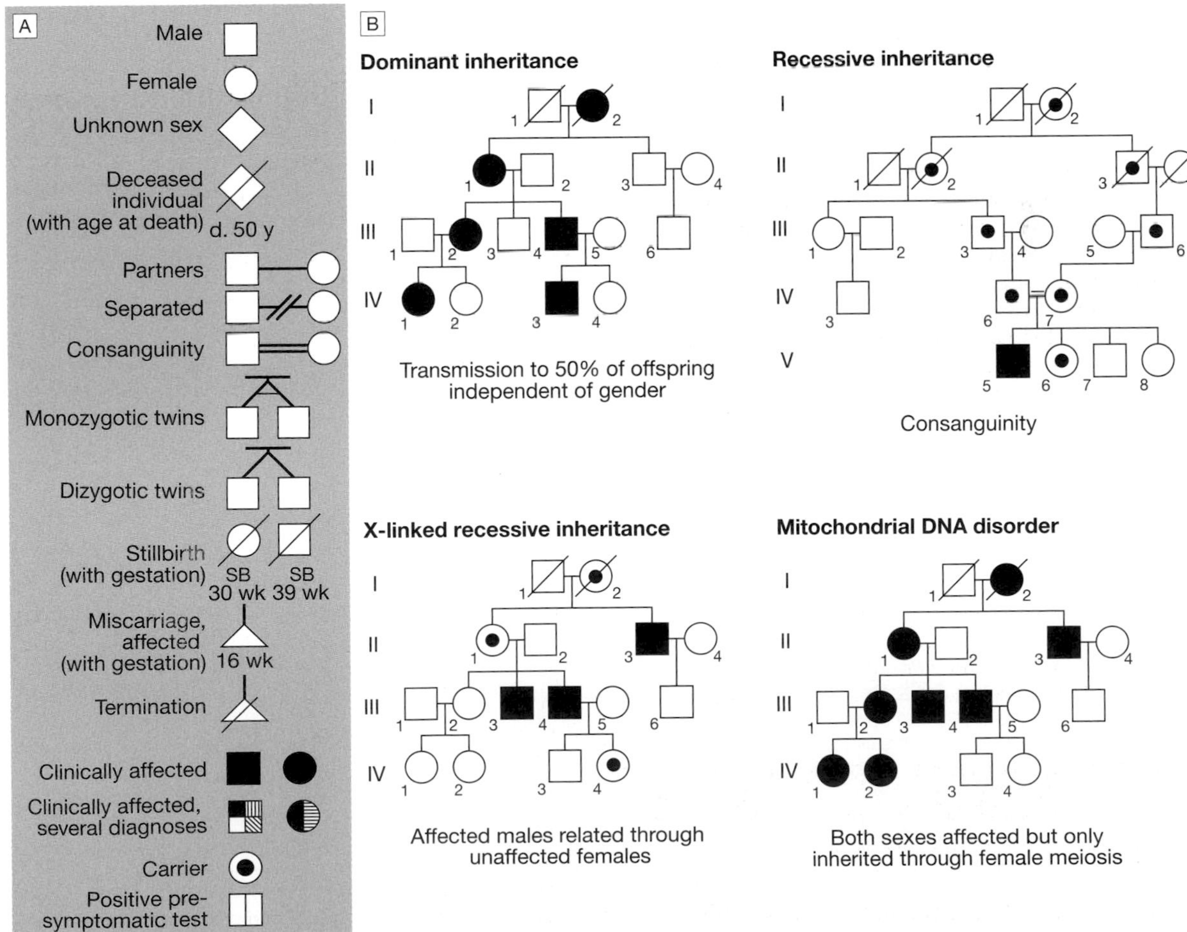

Fig. 3.7 Drawing a pedigree and patterns of inheritance. A The main symbols used to represent pedigrees in diagrammatic form. B The main modes of disease inheritance (see text for details).

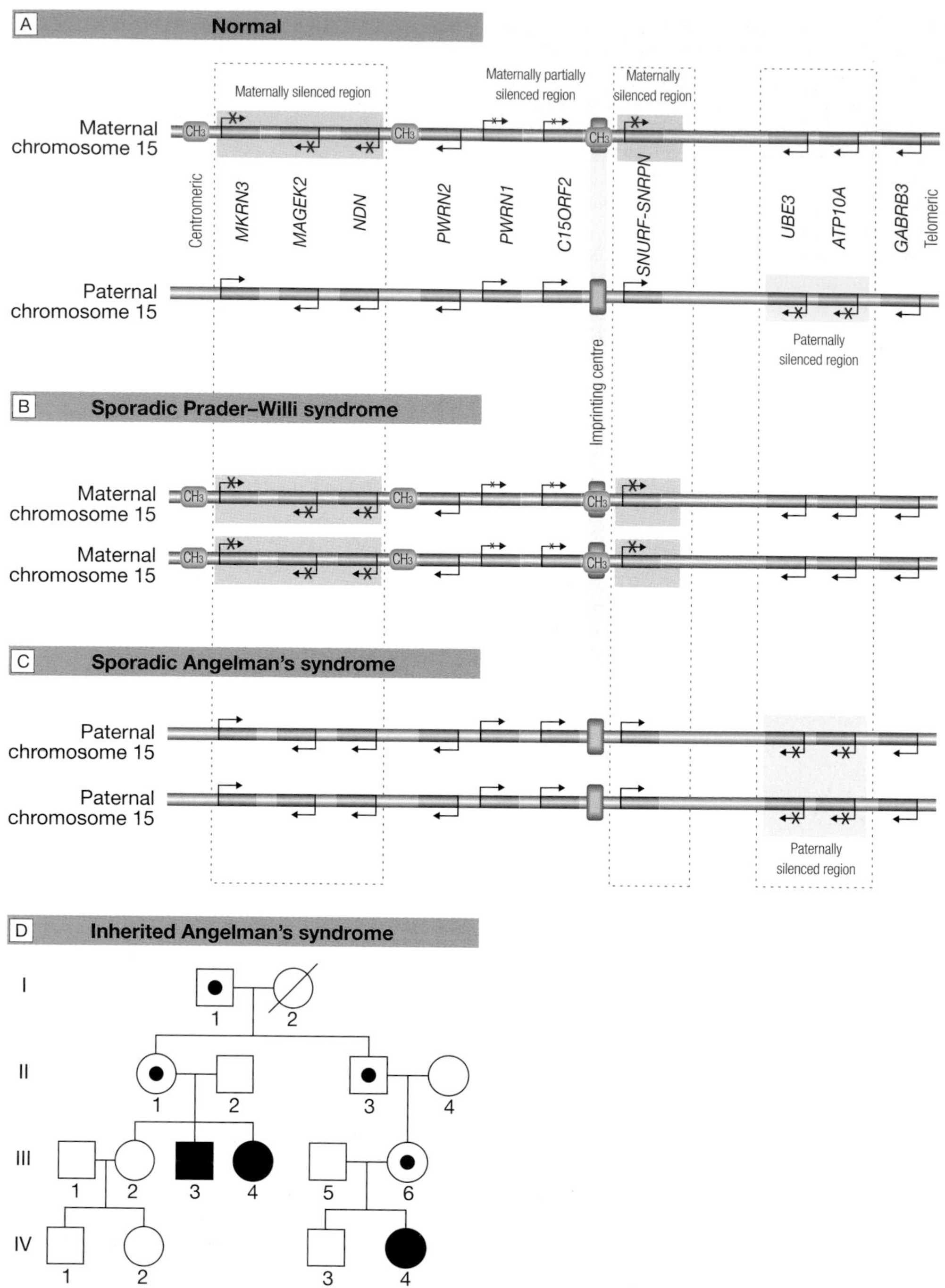

Fig. 3.8 Genomic imprinting and associated diseases. Several regions of the genome exhibit the phenomenon of imprinting, whereby expression of one or a group of genes is influenced by whether the chromosome is derived from the mother or the father; one such region lies on chromosome 15. **A** Normal imprinting. Under normal circumstances, expression of several genes is suppressed (silenced) on the maternal chromosome (red), whereas these genes are expressed normally by the paternal chromosome (blue). However, two genes in the paternal chromosome (*UBE3* and *ATP10A*) are silenced. **B** In sporadic Prader–Willi syndrome, there is a non-disjunction defect on chromosome 15, and both copies of the chromosomal region are derived from the mother (maternal uniparental disomy). In this case, Prader–Willi syndrome occurs because there is loss of function of several paternally expressed genes, including *MKRN3*, *MAGEK2*, *NDN*, *PWRN2*, *C15ORF2* and *SNURF-SNRNP*. **C** In sporadic Angelman's syndrome, both chromosomal regions are derived from the father (paternal uniparental disomy) due to non-disjunction during paternal meiosis. As a result, both copies of the *UBE3* gene are silenced and this causes Angelman's syndrome. Note that the syndrome can also be caused by deletion of this region on the maternal chromosome or a loss-of-function mutation on the maternal copy of *UBE3*, causing an inherited form of Angelman's, as illustrated in panel D. **D** Pedigree of a family with inherited Angelman's syndrome due to a loss-of-function mutation in *UBE3*. Inheriting this mutation from a father causes no disease (because the gene is normally silenced in the paternal chromosome) (see individuals I-1, II-1, II-3, III-6), but the same mutation inherited from the mother causes the syndrome (individuals III-3, III-4, IV-4), as this is the only copy expressed and the *UBE3* gene is mutated.

disease is seen in the triggering of malignant hyperpyrexia by anaesthetic agents in the presence of *RYR1* mutations. Autosomal dominant disorders may be the result of either loss or gain of function of the affected gene. For example, adult polycystic kidney disease type 1 is caused by loss-of-function mutations in *PKD1*, which encodes polycystin I on 16p13.1. Hereditary motor and sensory neuropathy type 1 is caused by increased number of copies (resulting in increased gene dosage) of *PMP22*, encoding peripheral myelin protein 22 on 17p11.2.

Autosomal recessive inheritance

In autosomal recessive disorders, both alleles of a gene must be mutated before the disease is manifest in an individual, and an affected individual must inherit one mutant allele from each parent. What distinguishes autosomal dominant and recessive diseases is that carrying one mutant allele does not produce a disease phenotype. Autosomal recessive disorders are rare in most populations. For example, the most common serious autosomal recessive disorder in the UK is cystic fibrosis, which has a birth incidence of 1:2000. The frequency of autosomal recessive disorders increases with the degree of inbreeding of a population because the risk of inheriting the same mutant allele from both parents (homozygosity) is increased. Genetic risk calculation for a fully penetrant autosomal recessive disorder is straightforward. Each subsequent pregnancy of a couple who have had a previous child affected by an autosomal recessive disorder will have a 25% (1:4) risk of being affected; a healthy individual who has a sibling with an autosomal recessive disorder will have 2/3 chance of being a carrier. The risk of an affected individual having children with the same condition is usually low but is dependent on the carrier rate of the mutant allele in the population.

X-linked inheritance

Genetic diseases caused by mutations on the X chromosome have specific characteristics. X-linked diseases are mostly recessive and restricted to males who carry the mutant allele. This is because males have only one X chromosome, whereas females have two. Thus females who carry a single mutant allele are generally unaffected. Occasionally, female carriers may exhibit signs of an X-linked disease due to a phenomenon called skewed X-inactivation. All female embryos, at about 100 cells in size, stably inactivate one of their two X chromosomes in each cell. This process is random in each cell but if, by chance, there is a disproportionate inactivation of normal X chromosomes carrying the normal allele, then an affected female carrier will be more likely, an extreme example being the rare cases of carrier females affected with Duchenne muscular dystrophy. X-linked recessive disorders have a recognisable pattern of inheritance, with transmission of the disease from carrier females to affected males and absence of father-to-son transmission. The risk of a female carrier having an affected child is 25% (1:4; half of her male offspring). If the carrier status of a woman is unclear, then the risk may be altered by conditional information, as discussed in the autosomal dominant disease section above. Bayes' theorem is commonly used to calculate such modified risks and this is discussed in more detail later in this chapter (p. 68).

Mitochondrial inheritance

The inheritance of mtDNA disorders is characterised by transmission from females, but males and females are generally affected equally. Unlike the other inheritance patterns mentioned above, mitochondrial inheritance has nothing to do with meiosis but reflects the fact that mitochondrial DNA is transmitted by oöcytes. Mitochondrial disorders tend to be very variable in penetrance and expressivity within families, and this is mostly accounted for by the fact that only a proportion of multiple mtDNA molecules within mitochondria contain the causal mutation (the degree of mtDNA heteroplasmy).

Epigenetic inheritance and imprinting

Several chromosomal regions (loci) have been identified where gene repression is inherited in a parent-of-origin-specific manner; these are called imprinted loci. Within these loci the paternal alleles of a gene may be active while the maternal one may be silenced, or vice versa (see Fig. 3.8). Mutations within imprinted loci lead to a very unusual pattern of inheritance in which the phenotype is only manifest if inherited from the parent who contributes the transcriptionally active allele (see Fig. 3.8). Examples of these disorders are given in Box 3.3.

Classes of genetic variant

There are many different classes of variation in the human genome (Figs 3.9 and 3.10). Rare genetic variations that result in a disease are generally referred to as mutations, whereas common variations and those that do not cause disease are referred to as polymorphisms. These different types of variation are further categorised by the size of the DNA segment involved and/or by the mechanism giving rise to the variation.

Nucleotide substitutions

The substitution of one nucleotide for another is the most common type of variation in the human genome. Depending on their frequency and functional consequences, these changes are known as a point mutation or a single nucleotide polymorphism (SNP). They occur by misincorporation of a nucleotide during DNA synthesis or by the action of a chemical mutagen. When these substitutions occur within ORFs of a protein-coding gene, they are further classified into:

- synonymous – resulting in a change in the codon but no change in the amino acid and thus no phenotype
- missense – altering a codon, resulting in an amino acid change in the protein
- nonsense – introducing a premature stop codon, resulting in truncation of the protein
- splicing – occurring at the junction of an intron and an exon, thereby adversely affecting splicing.

Examples of these types of variation are shown in Figures 3.9 and 3.10.

3.3 Epigenetic disease

Disease	Locus	Genes	Notes
Imprinting disorders			
Beckwith–Wiedemann syndrome	11p15	*p57^{KIP2} HASH2, INS2, IGF2, H19*	General 'over-growth', advanced bone age and increased childhood tumours. Some cases due to mutations in *p57^{KIP2}*
Prader–Willi syndrome	15q11–q13	*SNRPN, Necdin* and others	Obesity, hypogonadism and learning disability. Lack of paternal contribution (due to deletion of paternal 15q11–q13, or inheritance of both chromosome 15q11–q13 regions from the mother)
Angelman's syndrome (AS)	15q11–q13	*UBE3A*	Severe mental retardation, ataxia, epilepsy and inappropriate laughing bouts. Due to loss-of-function mutations in the maternal *UBE3A* gene. The neurological phenotype results because most tissues express both maternal and paternal alleles of *UBE3A*, whereas the brain expresses predominantly the maternal allele
Pseudohypoparathyroidism (p. 770)	20q13	*GNAS1*	Inheritance of the mutation from the mother results in hypocalcaemia, hyperphosphataemia, raised parathyroid hormone (PTH) levels, ectopic calcification, obesity, delayed puberty, shortened 4th and 5th metacarpals and ectopic calcification. When the mutation is inherited from the father, PTH, calcium and phosphate levels are normal but the other features are present. These differences are due to the fact that, in the kidney (the main target organ through which PTH regulates serum calcium and phosphate), the paternal allele is silenced and the maternal allele is expressed, whereas both alleles are expressed in other tissues
X-inactivation disorders			
Duchenne muscular dystrophy (DMD) in females	Xp22	*DMD*	If, by chance, a sufficient number of the X chromosomes containing the normal *dystrophin* gene are inactivated in muscle, heterozygous females may rarely develop full-blown DMD. Conversely, if a higher proportion of the disease gene-carrying chromosome is inactivated, a carrier female may test negative on biochemical screening for elevated creatine kinase levels
Epigenetic silencing (oncogenesis)			
Colon cancer	3p21	*MLH1*	Hypermethylation of the promoter results in silencing of *MLH1*, which encodes a DNA repair gene

```
A  DNA      ATG GCC GGG AAG TGT CGT GGT GTT
   mRNA     AUG GCC GGG AAG UGU CGU GGU GUU      Normal
   Protein  Met Ala Gly Lys Cys Arg Gly Val

B  DNA      ATG GCC GGG AAA TGT CGT GGT GTT
   mRNA     AUG GCC GGG AAA UGU CGU GGU GUU      Silent polymorphism
   Protein  Met Ala Gly Lys Cys Arg Gly Val      (no amino acid change)

C  DNA      ATG GCC GGG CAG TGT CGT GGT GTT
   mRNA     AUG GCC GGG CAG UGU CGU GGU GUU      Missense mutation causing
   Protein  Met Ala Gly Gln Cys Arg Gly Val      Lys–Gln amino acid change

D  DNA      ATG GCC GGG GAA GTG TCG TGG TGT T
   mRNA     AUG GCC GGG GAA GUG UCG UGG UGU U    'G' insertion causing
   Protein  Met Ala Gly Gln Val Ser Trp Cys      frameshift mutation

E  DNA      ATG GCC GGG TAG TGT AGT GGT GTT
   mRNA     AUG GCC GGG UAG UGU AGU GGU GUU      Nonsense mutation causing
   Protein  Met Ala Gly  *                       premature termination codon
```

Fig. 3.9 Different types of mutation affecting coding exons. A Normal sequence. B A synonymous nucleotide substitution changing the third base of a codon; the resulting amino acid sequence is unchanged. C A missense mutation in which the nucleotide substitution results in a change in a single amino acid from the normal sequence (AAG) encoding lysine to glutamine (CAG). D Insertion of a G residue (boxed) causes a frameshift mutation, completely altering the amino acid sequence downstream. This usually results in a loss-of-function mutation. E A nonsense mutation resulting in a single nucleotide change from a lysine codon (AAG) to a premature stop codon (TAG).

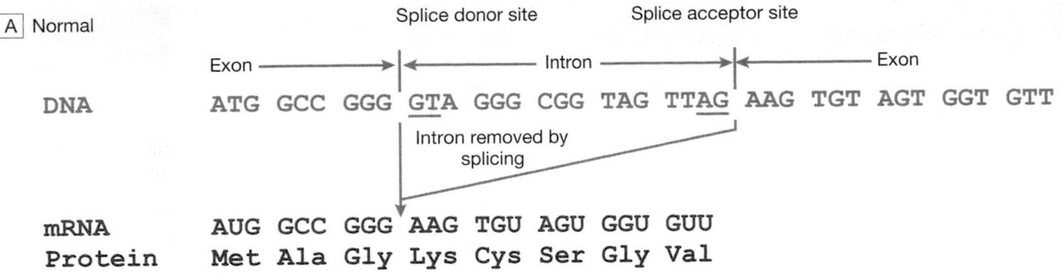

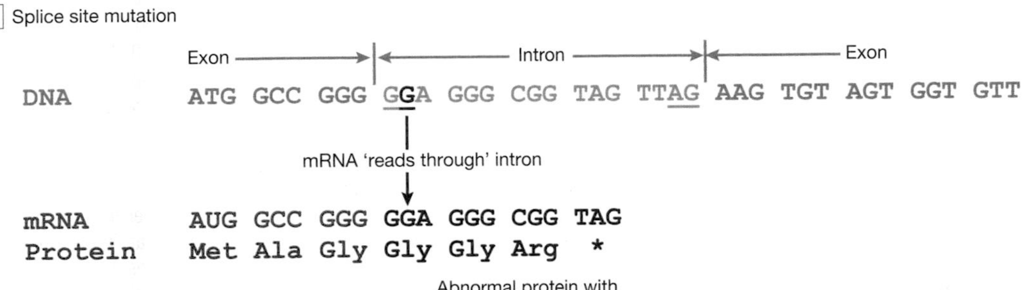

Fig. 3.10 Splice site mutations. **A** The normal sequence is shown, illustrating two exons, and intervening intron (blue) with splice donor (AG) and splice acceptor sites (GT) underlined. Normally, the intron is removed by splicing to give the mature mRNA that encodes the protein. **B** In a splice site mutation the donor site is mutated. As a result, splicing no longer occurs, leading to read-through of the mRNA into the intron, which contains a premature termination codon downstream of the mutation.

Insertions and deletions

One or more nucleotides may be inserted or lost in a DNA sequence, resulting in an insertion/deletion (indel) polymorphism or mutation (see Fig. 3.9). If an indel change affects one or two nucleotides within the ORF of a protein-coding gene, this can have serious consequences because the triple nucleotide sequence of the codons is disrupted, resulting in a frameshift mutation. The effect upon the gene is typically severe because the amino acid sequence is totally disrupted.

Simple tandem repeat mutation

Variations in the length of simple tandem repeats of DNA are thought to arise as the result of slippage of DNA during meiosis and are termed microsatellite (small) or minisatellite (larger) repeats. These repeats are unstable and can expand or contract in different generations. This instability is proportional to the size of the original repeat, in that longer repeats tend to be more unstable. Many microsatellites and minisatellites occur in introns or in chromosomal regions between genes and have no obvious adverse effects. However, some genetic diseases, including Huntington's disease and myotonic dystrophy, are caused by microsatellite repeats, which result in duplication of amino acids within the affected gene product or affect gene expression (Box 3.4).

Copy number variations

Variation in the number of copies of an individual segment of the genome from the usual diploid (two copies) content can be categorised by the size of the segment involved. Rarely, individuals may gain or lose a whole chromosome. Such numerical chromosome anomalies most commonly occur by a process known as meiotic non-dysjunction (Box 3.5). This is the most common cause of Down's syndrome, which results from trisomy (three copies) of chromosome 21.

Large insertions or deletions of chromosomal DNA also occur and are usually associated with learning disability and/or malformations. Such structural chromosomal anomalies arise as the result of two different processes:

- non-homologous end-joining
- non-allelic homologous recombination.

Random double-stranded breaks in DNA are a necessary process in meiotic recombination and also occur during mitosis at a predictable rate. The rate of these breaks is dramatically increased by exposure to ionising radiation. When such breaks occur, they are usually repaired accurately by DNA repair mechanisms within the cell. However, a proportion of breaks undergoes non-homologous end-joining, which results in the joining of two segments of DNA that are not normally contiguous. If the joined fragments are from different chromosomes, this results in a translocation. If they are from the same chromosome, this will result in inversion, duplication or deletion of a chromosomal fragment (Fig. 3.11). Large insertions and deletions may be cytogenetically visible as chromosomal deletions or duplications. If the anomalies are too small to be detected by microscopy, they are termed microdeletions and microduplications. Many microdeletion syndromes have been described and most stem from non-allelic homologous recombination between repeats of highly similar DNA sequences, which results in identical chromosome

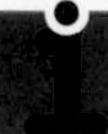

3.4 Diseases associated with triplet and other repeat sequences

	Repeat	No. of repeats		Gene	Gene location	Inheritance
		Normal	Mutant			
Coding repeat expansion						
Huntington's disease	[CAG]	6–34	> 35	*Huntingtin*	4p16	AD
Spinocerebellar ataxia (type 1)	[CAG]	6–39	> 40	*Ataxin*	6p22–23	AD
Spinocerebellar ataxia (types 2, 3, 6, 7)	[CAG]	Various	Various	Various	Various	AD
Dentatorubral-pallidoluysian atrophy	[CAG]	7–25	> 49	*Atrophin*	12p12–13	AD
Machado–Joseph disease	[CAG]	12–40	> 67	*MJD*	14q32	AD
Spinobulbar muscular atrophy	[CAG]	11–34	> 40	Androgen receptor	Xq11–12	XL recessive
Non-coding repeat expansion						
Myotonic dystrophy	[CTG]	5–37	> 50	*DMPK-3′UTR*	19q13	AD
Friedreich's ataxia	[GAA]	7–22	> 200	*Frataxin-intronic*	9q13	AR
Progressive myoclonic epilepsy	$[CCCCGCCCCGCG]_{4-8}$	2–3	> 25	*Cystatin B-5′UTR*	21q	AR
Fragile X mental retardation	[CGG]	5–52	> 200	*FMR1–5′UTR*	Xq27	XL dominant
Fragile site mental retardation 2 (FRAXE)	[GCC]	6–35	> 200	*FMR2*	Xq28	XL, probably recessive

Note The triplet repeat diseases fall into two major groups: those with disease resulting from expansion of $[CAG]_n$ repeats in coding DNA, resulting in multiple adjacent glutamine residues (polyglutamine tracts), and those with non-coding repeats. The latter tend to be longer. Unaffected parents usually display 'pre-mutation' allele lengths that are just above the normal range. (AD/AR = autosomal dominant/recessive; UTR = untranslated region; XL = X-linked)

3.5 Chromosome and contiguous gene disorders

Disease	Locus	Incidence	Clinical features
Numerical chromosomal abnormalities			
Down's syndrome (trisomy 21)	47,XY,+21 or 47,XX+21	1:800	Characteristic facies, IQ usually < 50, congenital heart disease, reduced life expectancy
Edwards' syndrome (trisomy 18)	47,XY,+18 or 47,XX,+18	1:6000	Early lethality, characteristic skull and facies, frequent malformations of heart, kidney and other organs
Patau's syndrome (trisomy 13)	47,XY,+13 or 47, XX,+13	1:15 000	Early lethality, cleft lip and palate, polydactyly, small head, frequent congenital heart disease
Klinefelter's syndrome	47,XXY	1:1000	Phenotypic male, infertility, gynaecomastia, small testes (p. 766)
XYY	47,XYY	1:1000	Usually asymptomatic, some impulse control problems
Triple X syndrome	47,XXX	1:1000	Usually asymptomatic, may have reduced IQ
Turner's syndrome	45,X	1:5000	Phenotypic female, short stature, webbed neck, coarctation of the aorta, primary amenorrhoea (p. 765)
Recurrent deletions, microdeletions and contiguous gene defects			
Di George/ velocardiofacial syndrome	22q11.2	1 in 4000	Cardiac outflow tract defects, distinctive facial appearance, thymic hypoplasia, cleft palate and hypocalcaemia. Major gene seems to be *TBX1* (cardiac defects and cleft palate)
Prader–Willi syndrome	15q11–q13	1:15 000	Distinctive facial appearance, hyperphagia, small hands and feet, distinct behavioural phenotype. Imprinted region, deletions on paternal allele in 70% of cases
Angelman's syndrome	15q11–q13	1:15 000	Distinctive facial appearance, absent speech, EEG abnormality, characteristic gait. Imprinted region, deletions on maternal allele in *UBE3A*
Williams' syndrome	7q11.23	1:10 000	Distinctive facial appearance, supravalvular aortic stenosis, learning disability and infantile hypercalcaemia. Major gene for supravalvular aortic stenosis is *elastin*
Smith–Magenis syndrome	17p11.2	1 in 25 000	Distinctive facial appearance and behavioural phenotype, self-injury and rapid eye movement (REM) sleep abnormalities. Major gene seems to be *RAH*

anomalies – and clinical syndromes – occurring in unrelated individuals (see Fig. 3.11 and Box 3.5).

Polymorphic copy number variants

In addition to the disease-causing structural chromosomal anomalies mentioned above, there are also a considerable number of polymorphic CNVs that exist as common genetic polymorphisms in humans. These involve duplication of large segments of the genome, often containing multiple genes and regulatory elements. These duplications usually result from non-allelic homologous recombination via misalignment of tandem

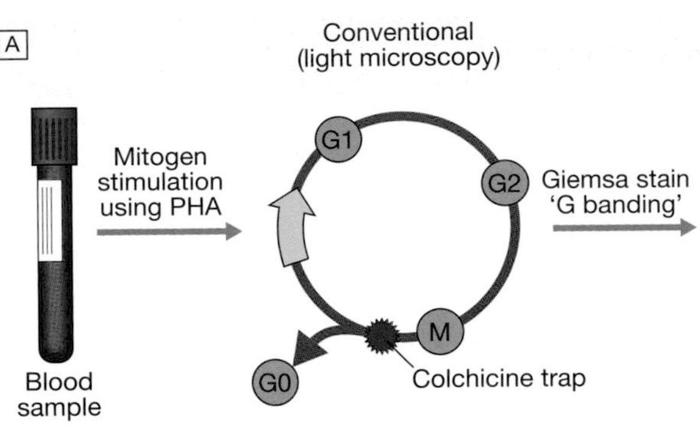

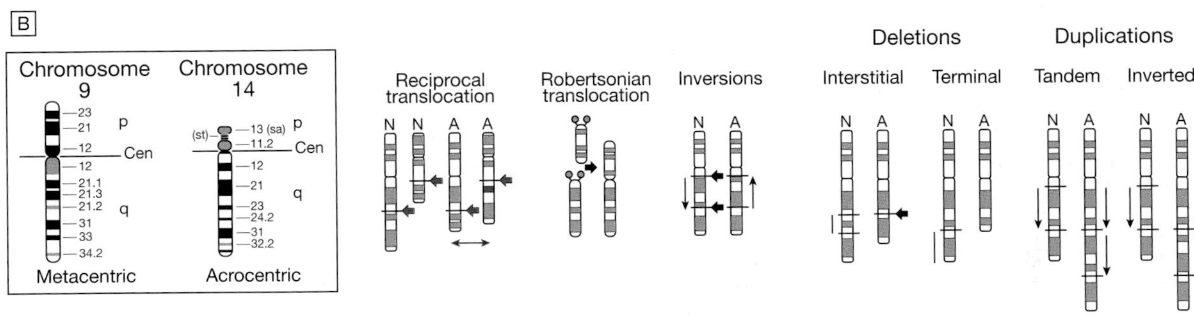

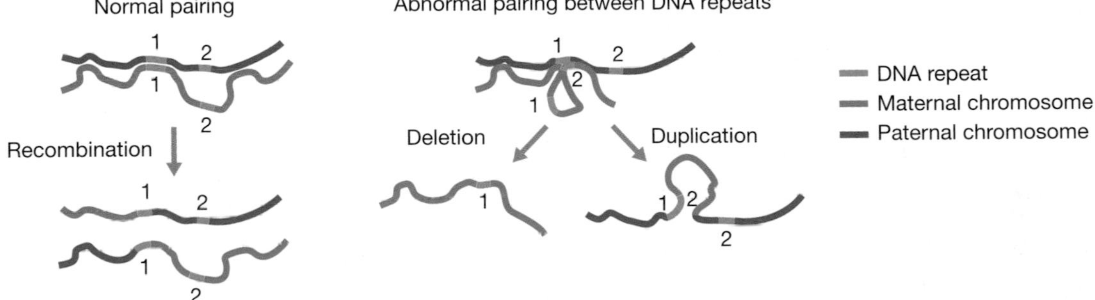

Fig. 3.11 Chromosomal analysis and structural chromosomal disorders. **A** How chromosome analysis is carried out. Starting with a blood sample, the white cells are stimulated to divide by adding the mitogen phytohaemagglutinin (PHA), and colchicine is used to trap the cells in metaphase, which allows the chromosomes to be seen using light microscopy following staining with Giemsa, resulting in a banding pattern. **B** How structural chromosomal anomalies are described. Human chromosomes can be classed as metacentric if the centromere is near the middle, or acrocentric if the centromere is at the end. The bands of each chromosome are given a number, starting at the centromere and working out along the short (p) arm and long (q) arm. Translocations and inversions are balanced structural chromosome anomalies where no genetic material is missing but it is in the wrong order. Translocations can be divided into reciprocal (direct swap of chromosomal material between non-homologous chromosomes) and Robertsonian (fusion of acrocentric chromosomes). Deletions and duplications can also occur due to non-allelic homologous recombination (illustrated in panel C). Deletions are classified as interstitial if they lie within a chromosome, and terminal if the terminal region of the chromosome is affected. Duplications can either be in tandem (where the duplicated fragment is orientated in the correct direction) or inverted (where the duplicated fragment is in the wrong direction). (N = normal; A = abnormal) **C** A common error of meiotic recombination, known as non-allelic homologous recombination, can occur (right panel), resulting in a deletion on one chromosome and a duplication in the homologous chromosome. The error is induced by tandem repeats in the DNA sequences (green), which can misalign and bind to each other, thereby 'fooling' the DNA into thinking the pairing prior to recombination is correct.

repeated DNA elements in the chromosome during recombination (see Fig. 3.11). The consequences of CNV for genetic disease have not been fully explored, although recent studies have shown a strong association between an increased copy number of the gene *FCGR3B* and the risk of systemic lupus erythematosus.

Consequences of genetic variation

Genetic variants can generally be classed into three groups:

- those associated with no detectable change in gene function (neutral variants)
- those which cause a loss of function of the gene product
- those which cause a gain of function of the gene product.

The consequence of an individual mutation depends on many factors, including the mutation type, the nature of the gene product and the position of the variant in the protein. Mutations can have profound effects or subtle effects on gene and cell function (Box 3.6). Variations

3.6 Examples of recessive diseases caused by common genetic variants*

Disease	Inheritance	Gene	Genetic variant	Population frequency
Haemochromatosis	AR	*HFE*	p.Cys282Tyr (p.C282Y; nucleotide c.845G>A) p.His63Asp (p.H63D; nucleotide c.187C>G)	3% 5%
α_1-antitrypsin deficiency	AR	*SERPINA1*	p.Glu342Lys (p.E342K, c.1197G>A)	3%
Spinal muscular atrophy	AR	*SMN1*	Gene deletion by non-allelic homologous recombination	2–3%
Cystic fibrosis	AR	*CFTR*	p.Phe508del (p.F508del aka δF508, c.1521_1523delCTT)	4%

*The genetic variants shown are common in the general population but heterozygotes do not exhibit any evidence of disease. In the homozygous form, however, these variants cause recessive disease due to loss of function of the affected gene.

that have profound effects are responsible for 'classical' genetic diseases, whereas those with subtle effects may contribute to the pathogenesis of complex diseases with a genetic component.

Loss-of-function mutations

These mutations cause the normal function of a protein to be reduced or lost. Deletion of the whole gene is the most extreme example but the same phenotype can be seen with a nonsense or frameshift mutation early in the ORF. Missense mutations that alter a critical domain within the protein can also result in loss of function. In autosomal recessive diseases, mutations that result in no protein function whatsoever are known as null mutations. If loss-of-function mutations result in an autosomal dominant disease, the genetic mechanism is known as haploinsufficiency and indicates that both functional copies of the gene are required for normal cellular function. Mutations in *PKD1* or *PKD2* that cause autosomal dominant adult polycystic kidney disease are mostly loss of function.

Gain-of-function and dominant negative mutations

Gain-of-function and dominant-negative effect mutations are most commonly the result of missense mutation or in-frame deletions but may also be caused by triplet repeat expansion mutations. Gain of function results where a mutation alters the protein structure, causing activation of its normal function, causing it to interact with a novel substrate or causing it to change its normal function. Constitutive activation of fibroblast growth factor receptors by missense mutation, which leads to many disorders such as achondroplasia, is an example of a gain-of-function mutation. Dominant-negative mutations are heterozygous changes that have a more deleterious effect on the protein function than a heterozygous 'null' mutation. For example, heterozygous mutations in *FBN1* cause Marfan's syndrome by the production of a protein with an abnormal amino acid sequence that disrupts the normal assembly of microfibrils. In comparison, complete loss of function of one allele of *FBN1* is usually completely benign.

Polymorphisms

A polymorphism is defined as a change in the nucleotide sequence that exists with a population frequency of more than 1%. Most common polymorphisms are neutral (see below), but some cause subtle changes in gene expression or in protein structure and function (see Box 3.15, p. 69). It is thought that these polymorphisms lead to variations in phenotype within the general population, including variations in susceptibility to common diseases. An example is polymorphism in the gene *SLC2A9* that not only explains a significant proportion of the normal population variation in serum urate concentration but also predisposes 'high-risk' allele carriers to the development of gout. Other examples are listed in Box 3.6.

Neutral variants

The vast majority of variations within the human genome have no discernible effect on the cell or organism. This may be because the variation is non-coding, occurring outside the gene but within an intron, or is within the coding regions of a gene but does not change the amino acid because of a synonymous substitution at the third base of a codon (see Fig. 3.9). Some variations that do change the amino acid may be completely tolerated with regard to protein function.

Evolutionary selection

Genetic variants play an important role in evolutionary selection; some are advantageous to an organism, resulting in positive selection through evolution via improved reproductive fitness. However, variations that decrease reproductive fitness become less common and are excluded through evolution. Given this simple paradigm, it would be tempting to assume that common mutations are all advantageous and all rare mutations are pathogenic. Unfortunately, it is often difficult to classify any common mutation as either advantageous or deleterious – or, indeed, neutral. Mutations that are advantageous in early life and thus enhance reproductive fitness may be deleterious in later life. There may be mutations that are advantageous for survival in particular conditions (for example, famine or pandemic), which may be disadvantageous in more benign circumstances by resulting in a predisposition to obesity or autoimmune disorders. This complexity of balancing selection through evolution is likely to be an important feature of the genetics of common disease.

Constitutional genetic disease

All familial genetic disease is caused by constitutional mutations, which are inherited through the germ line.

However, different mutations in the same gene can have different consequences, depending on the genetic mechanism underlying that disease. About 1% of the population carries constitutional mutations that cause disease.

Allelic heterogeneity

Allelic heterogeneity is where several different mutations cause the same phenotype. This is seen in almost all genetic disease. In familial adenomatous polyposis coli, whole-gene deletions, nonsense mutations, frameshift mutations and some missense mutations result in exactly the same phenotype because they all cause loss of function in the *FAP* gene on chromosome 5q. Many other Mendelian disorders show this phenomenon with loss-of-function mutations, including adult polycystic kidney disease (PKD1, 16p13; PKD2, 4q21). Allelic heterogeneity can also be seen in gain-of-function and dominant-negative mutations. In connective tissue disorders, dominant-negative mutations are almost always missense mutations or in-frame deletions or insertions, since the aberrant protein has to be made for the disease to manifest. In most diseases caused by gain-of-function mutations, allelic heterogeneity is severely restricted. A good example of this is achondroplasia, in which the mutations in *FGFR3* are restricted to a few specific codons that cause constitutive activation of the receptor that is required to cause the disease.

Locus heterogeneity

Locus heterogeneity is where a similar phenotype results from mutations in several different genes. One of the best examples is retinitis pigmentosa, which can occur as the result of mutations in more than 75 genes, each of which has a different chromosomal location.

De novo mutations

Although the vast majority of constitutional mutations are inherited, each gamete will contain mutations that have occurred as a result of meiosis; these are called de novo mutations. Each individual has approximately 70 de novo mutations scattered throughout their genome. This occurs in each generation and is presumably required for evolution to occur. Most are neutral but such mutations may also cause human disease. De novo mutations cause severe congenital disorders such as thanatophoric dysplasia (*FGFR3* gain-of-function mutation), bilateral anophthalmia (*SOX2* haploinsufficiency), campomelic dysplasia (*SOX9* loss of function) (Fig. 3.2) and the severe form of osteogenesis imperfecta (dominant-negative mutations in *COL1A1* or *COL1A2*).

Somatic genetic disease

Somatic mutations are not inherited but instead occur during post-zygotic mitotic cell divisions at any point from embryonic development to late adult life. An example of this phenomenon is polyostotic fibrous dysplasia (McCune–Albright syndrome), in which a somatic mutation in the G_S alpha gene causes constitutive activation of receptor signalling downstream of many G protein-coupled receptors, resulting in focal lesions in the skeleton and endocrine dysfunction (p. 770).

The most important example of human disease caused by somatic mutations is cancer. Here, 'driver' mutations occur within genes that are involved in regulating cell division or apoptosis, resulting in abnormal cell growth and tumour formation. The two general categories of cancer-causing mutation are gain-of-function mutations in growth-promoting genes (oncogenes) and loss-of-function mutations in growth-suppressing genes (tumour suppressor genes). Whichever mechanism is acting, most tumours require an initiating mutation in a single cell that can then escape from normal growth controls. This cell replicates more frequently or fails to undergo programmed death, resulting in clonal expansion. As the size of the clone increases, one or more cells may acquire additional mutations that confer further growth advantage, leading to proliferation of these subclones, which may ultimately lead to aggressive metastatic cancer. The cell's complex self-regulating machinery means that more than one mutation is usually required to produce a malignant tumour (see Fig. 11.3, p. 264). For example, if a mutation results in activation of a growth factor gene or receptor, then that cell will replicate more frequently as a result of autocrine stimulation. However, this mutant cell will still be subject to normal cell cycle checkpoints to promote DNA integrity in its progeny. But if additional mutations in the same cell result in defective cell cycle checkpoints, it will rapidly accumulate further mutations, which may allow completely unregulated growth and/or separation from its matrix and cellular attachments and/or resistance to apoptosis. As cell growth becomes increasingly dysregulated, cells de-differentiate, lose their response to normal tissue environment and cease to ensure appropriate mitotic chromosomal segregation. These processes combine to generate the classical malignant characteristics of disorganised growth, variable levels of differentiation, and numerical and structural chromosome abnormalities. An increase in somatic mutation rate can occur on exposure to external mutagens, such as ultraviolet light or cigarette smoke, or if the cell has defects in DNA repair systems. Cancer therefore affects the fundamental processes of molecular and cell biology.

In many familial cancer syndromes, somatic mutations act together with an inherited mutation to cause cancer. Familial cancer syndromes may be due to loss-of-function mutations in tumour suppressor genes or genes encoding DNA repair enzymes. In DNA repair diseases, the inherited mutations increase the somatic mutation rate. Autosomal dominant mutations in genes encoding components of specific DNA repair systems are relatively common causes of familial colon cancer and breast cancer (e.g. *BRCA1*). Autosomal recessive DNA repair disorders are rare and are associated with almost complete loss of DNA repair enzymes. This is usually associated with a severe multifaceted degenerative disorder with cancer susceptibility as a significant component (e.g. xeroderma pigmentosum, p. 267).

Cancer syndromes are also caused by loss-of-function mutations in tumour suppressor genes. At the cellular level, loss of one functional copy of a tumour suppressor gene does not have any functional consequences, as the cell is protected by the remaining normal copy. However, a somatic mutation affecting the normal allele is likely to occur in one cell at some point during life, resulting in complete loss of tumour suppressor activity and a tumour developing by clonal expansion of that cell. This two-hit mechanism (one inherited, one somatic) for cancer development is known as the Knudsen hypothesis. It explains why tumours may not develop for many years (or ever) in some members of these cancer-prone families. Yet another group of cancer syndromes are the result of gain-of-function mutations in tumour promoter genes (proto-oncogenes).

INVESTIGATION OF GENETIC DISEASE

General principles of diagnosis

Many genetic diseases can be diagnosed by a careful clinical history and examination together with an awareness and knowledge of rare diseases. Although DNA-based diagnostic tools are now widely used, not all diagnostic genetic tests involve analysis of DNA. For example, an electrocardiogram (ECG) can establish the diagnosis in long QT syndrome or a renal ultrasound can detect adult polycystic kidney disease. By definition, all genetic testing (whether DNA-based or not) has implications for both the patient and other members of the family. These issues should be considered before genetic testing is undertaken and a plan should be in place to deliver medical information and support to family members and to organise any relevant downstream investigations.

Constructing a family tree

The family tree – or pedigree – is fundamental to the diagnosis of genetic diseases. The basic symbols and nomenclature used in drawing a pedigree are shown in Figure 3.7 (p. 51). A three-generation family history taken in a routine medical clerking may reveal important genetic information of relevance to the presenting complaint, particularly relating to cancer.

A pedigree should include details from both sides of the family, any history of pregnancy loss or infant death, consanguinity, and details of all medical conditions in family members, including dates of birth and age at death.

It is important to be aware that a diagnosis given by a family member, or even obtained from a death certificate, may be wrong. This is often true in cases of cancer, where 'stomach' may mean any part of the bowel, and 'brain' may refer to secondary deposits or be used where the primary site has not been identified.

Polymerase chain reaction and DNA sequencing

The polymerase chain reaction (PCR) is a fundamental laboratory technique that amplifies targeted sections of the human genome for DNA diagnostic analysis. Almost any tissue can be used to extract DNA for PCR analysis, but most commonly, a sample of peripheral blood is used. PCR is very often used in association with DNA sequencing to determine the exact nucleotide sequence of a specific region of a gene or chromosome. The principles of PCR are shown in Figure 3.12. The technique of DNA sequencing is used for DNA diagnostic analysis in clinical practice. Until recently, most diagnostic DNA laboratories used Sanger sequencing for diagnosis (Fig. 3.13A), but

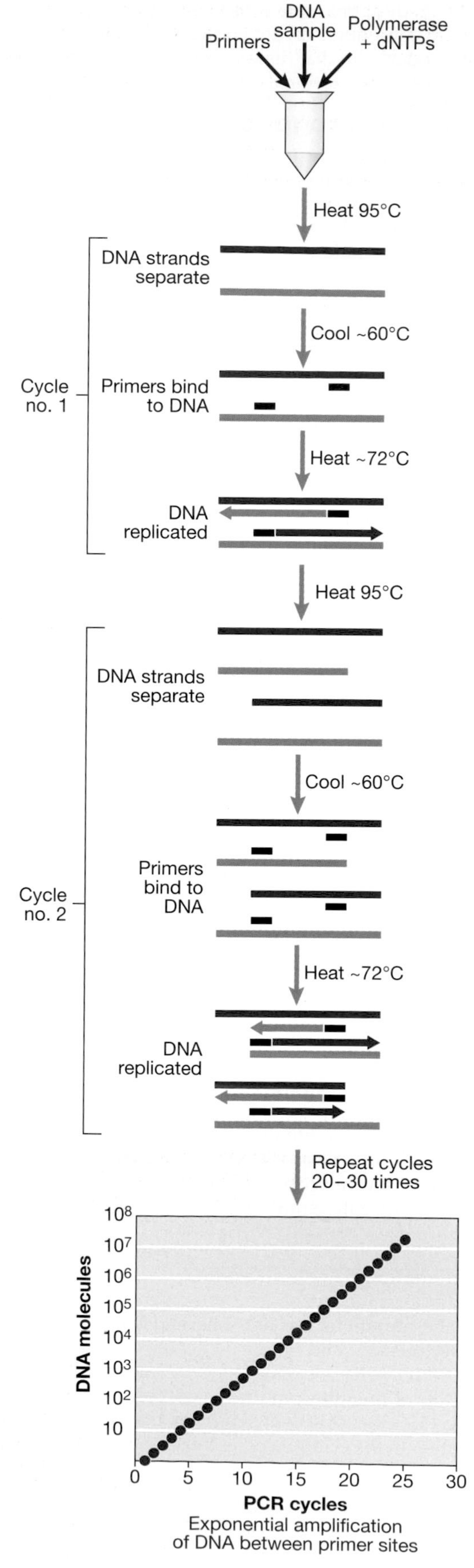

Fig. 3.12 (see opposite) The polymerase chain reaction. The polymerase chain reaction (PCR) involves adding a tiny amount of the patient's DNA to a reaction containing primers (short oligonucleotides 18–21 bp in length, which bind to the DNA flanking the region of interest) and deoxynucleotide phosphates (dATP, dCTP, dGTP, dTTP), which are used to synthesise new DNA and a heat-stable polymerase. The reaction mix is first heated to 95°C, which causes the double-stranded DNA molecules to separate. The reaction is then cooled to 50–60°C, which allows the primers to bind to the target DNA. The reaction is then heated to 72°C, at which point the polymerase starts making new DNA strands. These cycles are repeated 20–30 times, resulting in exponential amplification of the DNA fragment between the primer sites. The resulting PCR products can then be used for further analysis – most commonly DNA sequencing (see Fig. 3.13).

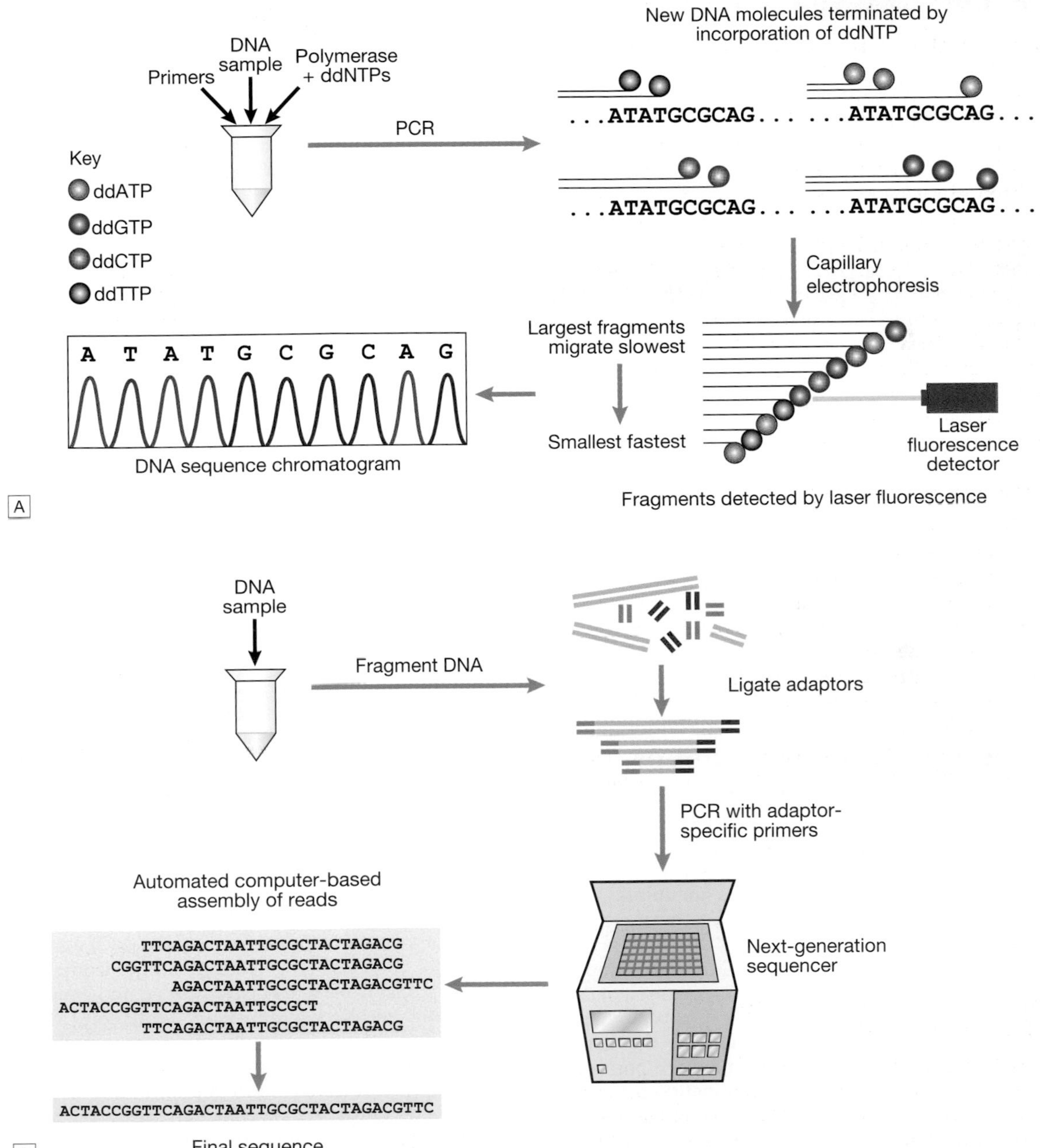

Fig. 3.13 DNA sequencing. A Sanger sequencing of DNA, which is very widely used in DNA diagnostics. This is performed using PCR-amplified fragments of DNA corresponding to the gene of interest. The sequencing reaction is performed using a combination dNTP and fluorescently labelled di-deoxy dNTP (ddATP, ddTTP, ddCTP and ddGTP), which become incorporated into the newly synthesised DNA, causing termination of the chain at that point. The reaction products are then subject to capillary electrophoresis and the different-sized fragments are detected by a laser, producing a sequence chromatogram that corresponds to the target DNA sequence. B Next-generation sequencing. Samples of patient DNA are fragmented and adapters ligated to each end of the fragment. The sequencing reaction is then performed with primers specific for the adaptors, much as described for Sanger sequencing. In next-generation sequencing, however, the reaction products are detected without the need for electrophoresis, and assembled by computer to produce the final sequence read. The absence of electrophoresis allows next-generation sequencing to generate data 100–1000 times faster than Sanger sequencing.

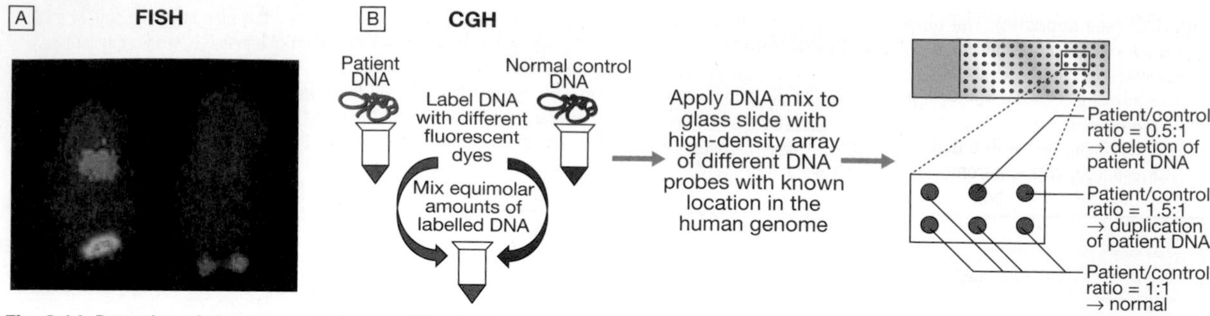

Fig. 3.14 Detection of chromosomal abnormalities by fluorescent in situ hybridisation (FISH) and comparative genomic hybridisation (CGH). **A** An example of FISH analysis showing a pair of homologous metaphase chromosome 22 stained with a blue fluorescent dye. The green spots represent a telomeric probe that has hybridised to both sister chromatids (there are two spots on the right-hand chromosome, whereas on the left the two spots are overlapping). The pink spot shows hybridisation of a probe mapping to band 22q11.2. The left chromosome has a normal signal that is absent on the right. This represents the microdeletion associated with velocardiofacial syndrome on the chromosome on the right. **B** Overview of comparative genomic hybridisation (CGH). Deletions and duplications are detected by looking for deviation from the 1 : 1 ratio of patient and control DNA in a microarray. Ratios in excess of 1 indicate duplications, whereas ratios below 1 indicate deletions.

3.7 Examples of non-DNA-based investigations for common genetic diseases

Disease	Investigation	Page reference
Sickle-cell disease	Haemoglobin electrophoresis	1032
Haemophilia	Clotting factor levels	1051
Hypogammaglobulinaemia	Immunoglobulin levels, complement levels	81
Phenylketonuria	Enzyme assays, amino acid levels	449
Congenital adrenal hyperplasia	Hormone levels, enzyme assays	782
Autosomal dominant polycystic kidney disease	Radiology, renal biopsy	505
Mitochondrial myopathy	Muscle biopsy, enzyme assay	1229
Pseudohypoparathyroidism	Radiology and calcium biochemistry	770

increasingly this is being replaced by next-generation sequencing, which has higher throughput (Fig. 3.13B).

Assessing DNA copy number

For decades, metaphase chromosome analysis by light microscopy has been the mainstay of clinical cytogenetic analysis to detect gain or loss of whole chromosomes or large chromosomal segments (> 4 million bp); such anomalies are collectively known as aneuploidy. More recently, whole-genome microarrays have replaced chromosome analysis, allowing rapid and precise detection of segmental gain or loss of DNA throughout the genome (see Box 3.5, p. 56). Microarrays consist of dense grids of short sequences of DNA (probes) that are complementary to known sequences in the genome (Fig. 3.14B). Each probe is fixed at a known position on the array (often printed on to a specially coated glass slide). The patient's fluorescently labelled DNA sample is hybridised to the array, and results for each probe are read by a laser scanner. This allows a copy number map of the patient's DNA to be constructed and abnormalities to be identified. Many clinically recognisable syndromes are the result of aneuploidy. The specific phenotype associated with individual deletion syndromes is the result of loss of one copy of several adjacent genes – a contiguous gene syndrome (see Box 3.5). Fluorescent in situ hybridisation (FISH, Fig. 3.14A) can be used to confirm specific deletions or duplications on metaphase chromosomes as a follow-up to microarray analysis.

Non-DNA-based methods of assessment

Although DNA-based diagnostic tools are used in the majority of patients with suspected genetic disease, direct analysis of protein function, such as measurement of specific enzyme activity, can also be used to diagnose single-gene disorders. An example of this is the investigation of myopathy thought to be due to defects in mitochondrial complex 1 proteins (Box 3.7). Complex 1 is made up of at least 36 nuclear-encoded and 7 mitochondrial DNA-encoded subunits, and mutations in any of these subunits can cause the disorder, which makes sequence analysis impractical as a first-line clinical test. Conversely, the biochemical measurement of respiratory chain complex I proteins can easily be analysed in muscle biopsies, and this can be diagnostic of a specific mitochondrial cytopathy (see Fig. 3.3, p. 45, and Box 3.1, p. 46).

Genetic testing in pregnancy and pre-implantation genetic testing

Genetic testing may be performed during pregnancy. Invasive tests, such as amniocentesis and chorionic

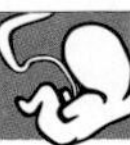

3.8 Some indications for prenatal testing

- Advanced maternal age and a high-risk serum screening result
- A previous child with a detectable chromosome abnormality or a parent with a chromosome abnormality such as a balanced translocation
- A parent or child with a genetic disease for which testing is available
- Abnormal antenatal scan

3.9 Methods used in prenatal testing

Test	Gestation	Comments
Ultrasound	1st trimester onwards	Increased nuchal translucency (an oedematous flap of skin at the base of the neck) for trisomies and Turner's; all major abnormalities such as NTDs, congenital heart disease
Chorionic villus biopsy	From 11 weeks	2% risk of miscarriage; used for early chromosomal, DNA and biochemical analysis; a specialised test
Amniocentesis	From 14 weeks	< 1 % risk of miscarriage; used for chromosomal and some biochemical analysis, e.g. α-fetoprotein for NTD
Cordocentesis	From 19 weeks	2–3% risk of miscarriage; a highly specialised test; used for chromosomal and DNA analysis

(NTD = neural tube defect)

villus sampling, are most often carried out to diagnose conditions that result in early infant death or severe disability. Such tests are only offered after careful explanation of the risks involved. Many couples will use the result of such tests to decide about termination of pregnancy. Some indications for testing are listed in Box 3.8; the methods used are summarised in Boxes 3.9 and 3.10. Non-invasive ultrasound scanning is offered to all pregnant couples and is particularly important if there is a previous history of serious developmental abnormalities. It is now possible to test single cells from a developing human embryo for the presence of deleterious mutations to select unaffected embryos as part of in vitro fertilisation procedures. As the range of tests for genetic diseases increases, demand for prenatal testing and pre-implantation genetic diagnosis is likely to rise. There is considerable ethical debate about the types of disease for which such procedures are appropriate.

Genetic testing in children

Ethical issues often arise with regard to genetic testing of children. For conditions with onset during childhood

EBM 3.10 Screening for Down's syndrome

'Antenatal screening in the first and second trimesters identifies fetuses at risk of Down's syndrome. Tests which currently have sensitivity > 60% and specificity > 95% include:

- *First trimester* (11–14 weeks): nuchal translucency; or nuchal translucency, human chorionic gonadotrophin (hCG) and pregnancy-associated plasma protein-A (PAPP-A)
- *Second trimester* (3–20 weeks): triple test (hCG, α-fetoprotein, unconjugated oestriol, uE3)
- Other combinations are available for use from 11 to 20 weeks.'

For further information: http://publications.nice.org/antenatal-care-cg62

and for which useful medical interventions are available, it is clearly important to test a child. An example of this is neonatal testing for cystic fibrosis, when early therapy reduces disease progression (p. 680), or in multiple endocrine neoplasia type 2B (MEN 2B), when early thyroidectomy prevents medullary thyroid carcinoma (p. 755). However, testing a healthy child for an adult-onset disorder where no benefit from early intervention exists should be avoided. Instead, the child should be left to make his or her own informed decision as an adult.

Identifying a disease gene in families

In families with a genetic disease for which the causative gene is unknown, single nucleotide polymorphisms (SNPs) can be used to track or 'map' disease genes using a technique called genome-wide linkage analysis. Microarray-based techniques allow more than 500 000 SNPs to be typed in a single experiment, and by comparison of the segregation of patterns of contiguous SNPs (called haplotypes) in affected and unaffected individuals, the 'locus' of DNA where the responsible gene resides can be identified. The confidence of association ('linkage') with the disease in question is influenced by the number of subjects studied, the strength of the effect of the gene on the disease, and the closeness of the SNP to the gene in question. The confidence can be expressed as a LoD (logarithm of the odds) score, which is $-\log_{10}$ of the probability (p value) of linkage; by convention, a LoD score of more than 3 ($p < 0.001$) is taken to be statistically significant. Once a locus has been identified, more detailed mapping within the locus can be undertaken and the relevant mutation confirmed by sequencing the relevant gene. Over recent years, next-generation sequencing of every exon in the genome (exome sequencing) has been used as an alternative to linkage analysis in identifying disease-causing mutations in families. Typically affected individuals within the family are sequenced and the results compared with unaffected family members and controls from the general population. For a fully penetrant disorder, the disease-causing mutation will be present in affected individuals and not present in unaffected family members or unrelated controls.

Genetic investigation in populations

Genetic screening may be applied to whole populations. The criteria for the use of population screening are well established; they depend on the incidence of specific conditions in individual populations and on whether an intervention is available to ameliorate the effects of the disease. In the UK, examples include screening for phenylketonuria and cystic fibrosis in the newborn, and prenatal screening for neural tube defects and Down's syndrome in pregnant women (see Box 3.10). Screening for carriers of haemoglobinopathies and Tay–Sachs disease is also carried out in some countries where the incidence of these conditions may be high enough to merit screening the entire population (p. 1031).

Predictive genetic testing

In the absence of symptoms or signs of disease in an individual at risk, a genetic test can be used to determine whether that individual carries the disease-causing mutation. This is known as pre-symptomatic or predictive genetic testing. Predictive tests are usually carried out for adult-onset disorders such as familial cancer syndromes and neurodegenerative disorders such as Huntington's disease (Box 3.11), or when a positive result in children will affect screening and management, such as in familial polyposis coli (p. 911). However, many complicated ethical issues arise with testing of children and such tests should only be carried out by clinicians experienced in their use.

Whilst a negative predictive test is clearly a favourable outcome for the individual concerned, a positive test may have significant negative consequences. These should have been explained fully in the counselling process (see below), and include employment discrimination and psychological effects. Providing this is done, current evidence suggests that serious psychological sequelae are uncommon.

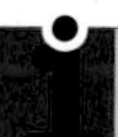

3.11 Predictive testing for Huntington's disease

- Currently, no medical benefit can be derived from knowing pre-symptomatic genetic status. In this situation, predictive testing is not offered to children but is available to capable adults
- Individuals have several reasonably spaced appointments with a genetic counsellor (or medical geneticist or specialist psychiatrist) prior to testing to ensure that the implications of testing are fully understood
- Fully informed patient consent is required prior to testing and individuals must be free to withdraw from testing at any time
- Follow-up support must be available and the result must not be disclosed to any other person without written consent of the tested individual

PRESENTING PROBLEMS IN GENETIC DISEASE

There are many thousands of known single-gene diseases. Individually these are rare, but collectively they are relatively common. This diversity makes clinical genetics a fascinating clinical specialty but it does mean that it is difficult, if not impossible, for any individual clinician to memorise the features associated with all these disorders. It is therefore important to have an awareness of the existence of genetic diseases and some general rules or 'triggers' in mind. Although single-gene disorders can present at any age (Box 3.12) and affect any tissue or organ system, they share some general characteristics:

- positive family history
- early age of onset
- multisystem involvement
- no obvious non-genetic explanation.

It is important to recognise any unusual clinical presentation and to consider genetic disease in the context of the clinical findings and the family history. Publicly accessible online catalogues of Mendelian diseases can be useful sources of potential diagnoses.

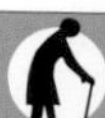

3.12 Genetic disease and counselling in old age

- **Genetic disease**: may present for the first time in elderly patients, e.g. Huntington's disease.
- **Family investigation**: remains essential in the management of genetic disease presenting in old age and referral to clinical genetics services should be considered.

MAJOR CATEGORIES OF GENETIC DISEASE

It is clearly impossible to discuss all Mendelian disease in this chapter, as there are many thousands of single-gene disorders. However, the major categories of genetic disease that are commonly encountered by clinical geneticists in adult practice are discussed below.

Inborn errors of metabolism

Inborn errors of metabolism (IEM) are caused by mutations that disrupt the normal function of a biochemical pathway. A good example is the glycogen storage diseases (see Box 16.23, p. 450), which are caused by mutations in various genes involved in regulating glucose metabolism. Most IEM are due to autosomal or X-linked recessive loss-of-function mutations in genes encoding specific enzymes or enzymatic co-factors. Knowledge of the biochemical pathway involved means that specific blocks have predictable consequences, including deficiency of the end product and build-up of intermediary compounds. Many hundreds of different IEM have been identified and these disorders have contributed a great deal to our understanding of human biochemistry. Most IEM are very rare and some are restricted to paediatric practice; however, a growing number may now present during adult life and some of these are discussed below.

Intoxicating IEM

A subgroup of IEM, termed 'intoxicating IEM', can present as a sudden deterioration in a previously well individual. Such deteriorations are usually precipitated by physiological stress, such as infection, pregnancy, exercise or changes in diet. The intoxication is due to the build-up of intermediary, water-soluble compounds, which will vary according to the pathway involved. For example, in urea cycle disorders ammonia is the toxic substance, whereas in maple syrup urine disease it is branched-chain amino acids. The intoxication is often associated with derangement of the acid–base balance and, if not recognised and treated, will often proceed to multi-organ failure, coma and death. In the porphyrias (Box 16.32, p. 460), the intoxication is caused by a build-up in the metabolites involved in haem synthesis. The diagnosis of these disorders requires specialist biochemical analysis of blood and/or urine. In some disorders, treatment relies on removal of the toxic substance using haemodialysis or chemical conjugation, or prevention of further accumulation by restricting intake of the precursors, such as total protein restriction in urea cycle disorders and avoidance of branched-chain amino-acid intake in maple syrup urine disease. In other disorders, such as the porphyrias, treatment is based on avoiding precipitating factors and supportive care (p. 460).

Mitochondrial disorders

Disorders of energy production are the most common type of IEM presenting in adult life, and some of these disorders have been mentioned in the section on mitochondrial function (see Fig. 3.3, p. 45, and Box 3.1, p. 46). The tissues that are most commonly affected in this group of disorders are those with the highest metabolic energy requirements, such as muscle, heart, retina and brain. Therapy in this group of disorders is based on giving antioxidants and co-factors, such as vitamin C and ubiquinone, that can improve the function of the respiratory chain.

Storage disorders

Storage disorders involve enzyme deficiency in lysosomal degradation pathways. The clinical consequences depend on the specific enzyme involved. For example, Fabry disease, an X-linked recessive deficiency of α-galactosidase A, results in abdominal pain, episodic diarrhoea, renal failure and angiokeratoma. Niemann–Pick disease type C is caused by autosomal recessive loss-of-function mutations in either the *NPC1* or *NPC2* gene. These result in lysosomal cholesterol accumulation, causing hepatosplenomegaly, dysphagia, loss of speech, very early dementia, spasticity and dystonia. An increasing number of storage disorders are treatable with enzyme replacement or substrate depletion therapies, making awareness and diagnosis more important. More details of specific disorders are provided in Chapter 16 (Box 16.24, p. 451).

Neurological disorders

Progressive neurological deterioration is one of the most common presentations of adult genetic disease. These diseases are mostly autosomal dominant and can be grouped into specific neurological syndromes and early-onset forms of well-known, non-Mendelian clinical entities. In the latter group, the best examples would be early-onset familial forms of dementia, Parkinson's disease and motor neuron disease. The triplet repeat disorders cause an interesting group of syndromes and have specific features that are dealt with below.

Huntington's disease

Huntington's disease (HD) is the paradigm of triplet repeat disorders. This condition can present with a movement disorder, weight loss or psychiatric symptoms (depression, addiction, psychosis, dementia), or with a combination of all three. The disease is the result of a $[CAG]_n$ triplet repeat expansion mutation in the *HD* gene on chromosome 4. Since CAG is a codon for glutamine and this mutation is positioned in the ORF, this results in an expansion of a polyglutamine tract in the protein. The mutation probably leads to gain of function, as deletions of the gene do not cause HD. The function of the protein encoded by the *HD* gene is not fully understood, but expansion of the repeat to above the normal range of 3–35 results in neurological disease. In general, the severity of disease and age at onset are related to the repeat length. In HD, atrophy of the caudate nuclei and the putamen is obvious on magnetic resonance imaging (MRI) of the brain, and in later stages cerebral atrophy is also apparent. There is currently no therapy that will alter the progression of the disease, which will often be the cause of the patient's death. Within families there is a tendency for disease severity to increase and age at onset to fall due to further expansion of the repeat, a phenomenon known as anticipation. The mutation is more likely to expand through the male germ line than through female meiosis.

Other triplet repeat disorders

Other progressive neurological disorders caused by triplet repeat expansion mutations in different genes include several forms of autosomal dominant spinocerebellar ataxias, dentatorubral-pallidoluysian atrophy (DRPLA), Machado–Joseph disease and Kennedy disease. These polyglutamine disorders all show intracellular inclusions in affected cells. It is thought that this accumulation may, in itself, be deleterious and is the result of defective protein degradation. Myotonic dystrophy and Friedreich's ataxia are also triplet repeat expansion disorders but the pathogenetic mechanism associated with these diseases is different, as these repeats do not lie within the coding regions of the affected genes.

Connective tissue disorders

Mutations in different types of collagen, fibrillin and elastin make up the majority of connective tissue disorders. The clinical features of these disorders vary, depending on the structural function and tissue distribution of the protein that is mutated. For example, autosomal dominant loss-of-function mutations in the gene encoding elastin cause either supravalvular aortic stenosis, cutis laxa or a combination of both conditions. The most commonly involved systems are:

- *skin* (increased or decreased elasticity, poor wound healing)
- *eyes* (myopia, lens dislocation)
- *blood vessels* (vascular fragility)
- *bones* (osteoporosis, skeletal dysplasia)
- *joints* (hypermobility, dislocation, arthropathy).

Learning disability, dysmorphism and malformations

Congenital global cognitive impairment (also called mental handicap or learning disability) affects about 3% of the population. It is commonly divided into broad categories of mild to moderate (IQ 50–70), moderate to severe (IQ 20–50), and severe to profound (IQ < 20). There are important 'environmental' causes of global cognitive impairment, including:

- *teratogen exposure* during pregnancy (alcohol, anticonvulsants)
- *congenital infections* (cytomegalovirus, rubella, toxoplasmosis, syphilis)
- *the sequelae of prematurity* (intraventricular haemorrhage)
- *birth injury* (hypoxic ischaemic encephalopathy).

Genetic disorders contribute very significantly to the aetiology of global cognitive impairment. Given the complexity of brain development, it is not surprising that global cognitive impairment shows extreme locus heterogeneity. The three most important groups of disorder are reviewed below.

Chromosome disorders

Any significant gain or loss of autosomal chromosomal material (known as aneuploidy) usually results in learning disability and other phenotypic abnormalities (see Fig. 3.11, p. 57). Down's syndrome is the most frequently found and best known of these disorders, and is caused by an increased dosage of genes on chromosome 21. Most cases of Down's syndrome are due to a numerical chromosome abnormality with trisomy of chromosome 21, e.g. 47,XX,+21 or 47,XY,+21. The clinical features are:

- globally delayed development
- characteristic facial appearance
- a significant risk of specific malformations (atrioventricular septal defect, duodenal atresia)
- a predisposition to several late-onset disorders, including hypothyroidism, acute leukaemias and Alzheimer's disease.

Recent surveys have shown that DNA microarray analysis can identify causative structural chromosome abnormalities in 10–25% of cases of significant learning disability. These deletions and duplications are mostly de novo and unique. An interest group of recurrent deletions and duplication caused by non-allelic homologous recombination events has been mentioned above. These result in specific microdeletion or microduplication syndromes, such as:

- *velocardiofacial syndrome* due to deletion of 22q11.2 (learning disability, malformations of the cardiac outflow tract, cleft palate, distinctive facial appearance and immune disorders)
- *Williams' syndrome* due to deletion of 7q11.23 (learning disability, supravalvular aortic stenosis and mild cutis laxa as a result of deletion of the *elastin* gene, distinctive facial appearance and over-friendly, chatty personality).

Dysmorphic syndromes

There are several thousand different dysmorphic syndromes; all are rare but they are characterised by the occurrence of cognitive impairment, malformations and a distinctive facial appearance – or 'gestalt' – associated with various other clinical features. Making the correct diagnosis is important, as it has profound implications on immediate patient management, detection of future complications and assessment of recurrence risks in the family. Clinical examination remains the mainstay of diagnosis and the patient often needs to be evaluated by a clinician who specialises in the diagnosis of these syndromes. The differential diagnosis in dysmorphic syndromes is often very wide and this has resulted in computer-aided diagnosis becoming an established clinical tool. Dysmorphology databases such as POSSUM and LMD have been established that are curated catalogues of the many thousands of known syndrome entities; they can be searched to identify possible explanations of unusual combinations of clinical features. The clinical diagnosis may then be confirmed by specific genetic investigations, as the genetic basis of a wide range of dysmorphic syndromes has been identified.

X-linked mental handicap

X-linked mental handicap (XLMH) accounts for approximately 10% of cases of moderate to severe learning disability. There are over 100 genes on the X chromosome that can cause learning disability but the most common disorder is fragile X syndrome, characterised by a distinctive facial appearance, attention deficit, joint hypermobility, macro-orchism (increased testicular size) and a non-staining gap on the X chromosome on chromosome analysis. Fragile X is caused by a triplet repeat expansion mutation but of a different type from the polyglutamine repeat disorders mentioned above. The repeat in fragile X syndrome is not in the coding region and is a $[CGG]_n$ expansion (see Box 3.4, p. 56). Methylation of the expanded repeat results in silencing of a specific gene called *FMR1*, which encodes an RNA-binding protein.

De novo mutations

Next-generation sequencing technology has made possible trio-based, whole-exome sequencing, in which the affected individual and both of their parents are analysed. It has recently become clear that de novo mutations in the coding regions of one of the many genes that are involved in normal brain development are collectively responsible for severe intellectual disability in at least 25% of affected patients. Trio-exome sequencing is thus likely to become a first-line diagnostic test for such cases in the near future.

Familial cancer syndromes

Most cancers are not inherited but occur as the result of an accumulation of somatic mutations, as discussed previously in this chapter. However, it has been recognised for many decades that some families are prone to one or more specific types of cancer. Affected individuals tend to present with tumours at an early age and are more likely to have multiple primary foci of carcinogenesis.

Retinoblastoma

Patients with autosomal dominant familial retinoblastoma have an inherited mutation in one copy of the *RB* gene, which is a tumour suppressor. This strongly predisposes individuals to the formation of retinoblastoma in one or both eyes. It is possible for more than one primary tumour to form in the same eye and for retinoblastoma to occur in the pineal gland. From a clinical perspective, it is important to screen the eyes and pineal gland of such individuals regularly so that tumours can be treated early and sight preserved. This gene is widely expressed and it is not clear why the retina is the main site of oncogenesis in this syndrome. An increased incidence of osteogenic sarcoma is also seen in affected individuals.

Familial adenomatous polyposis coli

Familial adenomatous polyposis coli (FAP) is an autosomal dominant condition due to inactivation mutations in the *FAP* tumour suppressor gene on 5q. The gene product is thought to modulate a specific signalling cascade (*Wnt* signalling) that regulates cell proliferation. Mutation carriers usually develop many thousands of intestinal polyps in their second and third decades and have a very high risk of malignant change in the colon. Prophylactic colectomy in the third decade is necessary in most cases. Regular screening for polyps in the upper gastrointestinal tract is also recommended.

Li–Fraumeni syndrome

Heterozygous loss-of-function mutations in the gene encoding p53 cause Li–Fraumeni syndrome. Families with this condition have a very significant increased predisposition to early-onset leukaemias, sarcomas, and breast and brain malignancies. Screening for presymptomatic tumours in this condition is very difficult and of unproven benefit, as almost any tissue can be affected.

Hereditary non-polyposis colorectal cancer

Hereditary non-polyposis colorectal cancer (HNPCC) is an autosomal dominant disorder that presents with early-onset familial colon cancer, particularly affecting the proximal colon. Other cancers, such as endometrial cancer, are often observed in affected families. This disorder shows marked locus heterogeneity, as mutations can occur in several different genes encoding proteins involved in DNA mismatch repair.

Familial breast cancer

Familial breast cancer is an autosomal dominant disorder that is most often due to mutations in genes encoding either *BRCA1* or *BRCA2*. Both of these proteins are involved in DNA repair. Individuals who carry a *BRCA1* or *BRCA2* mutation are at high risk of early-onset breast and ovarian tumours, and require regular screening for both of these conditions. Because of the very high risk of cancer, many women who carry these mutations elect to have prophylactic bilateral mastectomy and oophorectomy in the absence of a detectable tumour.

Xeroderma pigmentosum

Xeroderma pigmentosum (XP) is the name given to a group of rare disorders in which there are autosomal recessive defects in DNA repair genes that deal primarily with the effects of non-ionising radiation. The skin is particularly involved, and affected patients develop skin cancers with increased frequency.

GENETIC COUNSELLING

Genetic counselling provides information about the medical and family implications of a specific disease in a clear and non-directive manner. Such counselling aims to help individuals make informed decisions about planning a family, taking part in screening programmes and accepting prophylactic therapies. Genetic counselling may be provided by a medical geneticist, a specialist nurse, or a clinician with particular skills in this area, such as an obstetrician or paediatrician (Box 3.13). Perception of genetic risks clearly depends on perceived hazard. For example, a 5% (or 1:20) risk of genetic disease may be perceived as low if the disease is treatable, but unacceptably high if not.

Specific problems encountered in genetic counselling include:

- accurate assessment of genetic risk
- identification of children at risk of genetic disorders
- the increase in genetic risks associated with consanguinity
- non-paternity as an incidental finding in DNA.

3.13 Clinical genetics services

Component	Role
Medical geneticist	Diagnosis and management of genetic disease, assessment of genetic risk, managing screening programmes, interpretation of genetic test results. Subspecialties include prenatal genetics, dysmorphology (syndrome identification), cancer genetics
Genetic counsellor	Assessing genetic risk, provision of genetic counselling (providing accurate risk information in a comprehensible format), predictive testing for genetic disease and provision of information and support
DNA diagnostic laboratory	Identifying and reporting disease-causing mutations in validated disease genes. Some laboratories also provide linkage analysis to track diseases in families. Laboratories often work in a consortium, as so many different disease genes have now been identified
Cytogenetics laboratory	Identifying pathogenic numerical and structural chromosome anomalies in prenatal, postnatal and oncology samples
Biochemical genetics laboratory	Metabolite and enzymatic-based diagnosis of IEM. Metabolite-based monitoring of treatment of IEM
Newborn screening laboratory	Provision of population-based newborn screening, e.g. PKU, cystic fibrosis, etc.

(IEM = inborn errors of metabolism; PKU = phenylketonuria)

Genetic tests are increasingly used for the diagnosis and prediction of Mendelian disease in a medical context, and such skills will become increasingly important for many clinicians.

Genetic risk is often calculated using Bayes' theorem (Box 1.6, p. 6), which takes prior risk into account to calculate future risk. A simple Bayesian calculation is illustrated here. Consider a woman who is at risk of being a carrier of an X-linked recessive disease. Her grandfather and brother are affected, which makes her mother an obligate gene carrier. Her risk of being a carrier is therefore 50%. However, she has two unaffected sons. This information can be used to modify her risk. The prior probability that she is a carrier is 1:2 and that she is not a carrier also 1:2. The conditional probability that she would have two normal sons if she were a carrier is $1/2 \times 1/2$, i.e. 1/4. If she were not a carrier, the probability of having normal sons is 1. From this, the joint probability for each outcome can be calculated (the prior risk × the conditional risk): $1/2 \times 1/4$ (1/8) for being a carrier and $1/2 \times 1$ (1/2) for not being a carrier. The final risk, or relative probability, for each outcome can then be obtained by dividing the joint probability for that outcome by the sum of the joint probabilities. The probability that she is a carrier is therefore $1/8(1/8 + 1/2) = 1/5$ (20%).

GENETICS OF COMMON DISEASES

Many common disorders, such as diabetes, atherosclerosis, hypertension, cancer, osteoarthritis, inflammatory bowel disease and osteoporosis, have an important genetic component but are not caused by a single mutation. Techniques are now available both to measure the contribution and to identify genes with significant effects. This means that the result of genetic testing is beginning to have an impact on diagnosis, prognosis and therapy for common diseases, and this trend is likely to expand significantly in the years to come. Some of the most useful approaches to clinical interpretation of the genetic aspects of common disorders are outlined below.

Measuring the genetic contribution to complex disease

Genetic contributions to complex disease can be detected and quantified by twin studies and/or by analysing familial clustering. Twin studies use the difference in disease concordance between monozygotic (MZ) and dizygotic (DZ) twins to calculate genetic contribution. MZ twins are genetically identical, whereas DZ twins, like all siblings, are identical for only about 50% of their genetic variation. However, both MZ and DZ twins share an almost identical intrauterine environment and similar postnatal environment. Thus, any evidence of a higher concordance of the disease in MZ compared to DZ twins is assumed to be evidence of genetic contribution. Many common diseases and quantitative traits, such as height, weight, blood pressure and bone mineral density, show higher concordance rates in MZ twins compared to DZ twins. Genetic contributions to common diseases can also be assessed by studying the incidence of the disease in first-degree relatives of affected individuals, as compared with the general population (Fig. 3.15). The difference in incidence is used to calculate a disease risk, which is measured by the λ_s value (Box 3.14).

3.14 Risk to siblings of affected patients for common polygenic diseases

Disease	λ_s
Type 1 diabetes mellitus	15
Systemic lupus erythematosus	10–20
Multiple sclerosis	20–40
Schizophrenia	10
Ischaemic heart disease	4–12

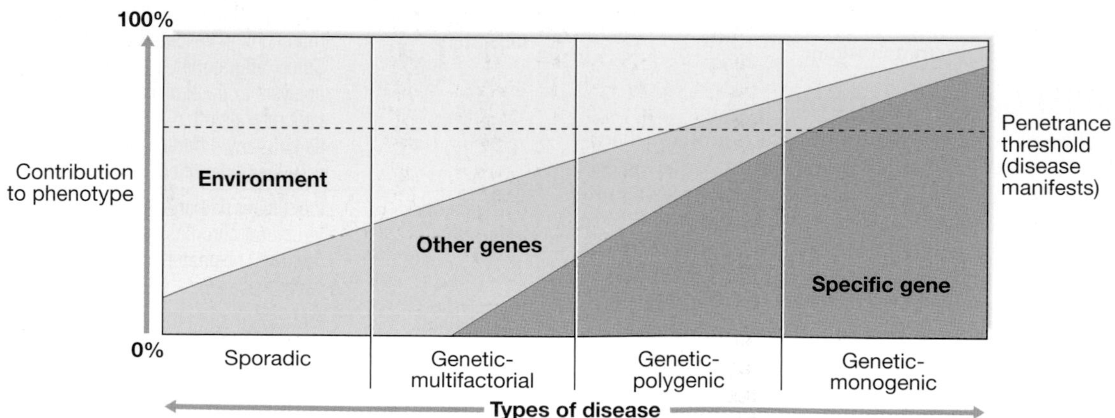

Fig. 3.15 The spectrum of genetic disease: how the genotype influences the phenotype. A particular characteristic or disease in an individual may be due to a specific genetic abnormality (monogenic disease) or may reflect several predisposing genes (polygenic disease). In each case, environmental factors may further influence the phenotype; in their absence, genetic factors alone may be insufficient to allow the disease to develop, resulting in non-penetrance or reduced penetrance (see text).

3.15 Polymorphisms that predispose to common diseases

Disease	Inheritance	No. of loci	Pathways
Colorectal cancer	Polygenic	20	DNA repair enzymes, growth factor signalling pathways, Wnt signalling
Osteoporosis	Polygenic	56	Cytokines, receptors and intracellular signalling molecules in RANK and Wnt pathways. Regulators of stem cell differentiation and bone mineralisation
Systemic lupus erythematosus	Polygenic	60	Cytokines, receptors and intracellular signalling pathways that regulate immune function; complement, intracellular nucleases
Gout	Polygenic	9	Renal solute transporters; regulators of glucose and insulin metabolism

(RANK = receptor activator of nuclear factor κ B)

Genetic testing in complex disease

Most common diseases are determined by interactions between a number of genes and the environment. In this situation, the genetic contribution to disease is termed polygenic. Until recently, very little progress had been made in identifying the genetic variants that predispose to common diseases, but this has been changed by the advent of genome-wide association studies (GWAS). A GWAS typically involves genotyping many (> 500 000) genetic markers spread across the genome in a large group of individuals with the disease and controls. By comparing the genotypes in cases and controls, it is possible to identify regions of the genome and candidate genes that contribute to the disease under study. Some of the candidate genes for common diseases identified by this approach are listed in Box 3.15.

Pharmacogenomics

Pharmacogenomics is the science of dissecting the genetic determinants of drug kinetics and effects using information from the human genome. For more than 50 years, it has been appreciated that polymorphic mutations within genes can affect individual responses to some drugs, such as loss-of-function mutations in *CYP2D6* causing hypersensitivity to debrisoquine, an adrenergic-blocking medication formerly used for the treatment of hypertension, in 3% of the population. This gene is part of a large family of highly polymorphic genes encoding cytochrome P450 proteins, mostly expressed in the liver, which determine the metabolism of a host of specific drugs. Polymorphisms in the *CYP2D6* gene also determine codeine activation, while those in the *CYP2C9* gene affect warfarin inactivation. Polymorphisms in these and other drug metabolic genes determine the persistence of drugs and, therefore, should provide information about dosages and toxicity. At the present time, genetic testing for assessment of drug response is seldom used routinely, but in the future it may be possible to predict the best specific drugs and dosages for individual patients based on genetic profiling: so-called 'personalised medicine'. An example is the enzyme thiopurine methyltransferase (TPMT), which catabolises azathioprine, a drug that is used in the treatment of autoimmune diseases and in cancer chemotherapy. Genetic screening for polymorphic variants of TPMT can be useful in identifying patients who have increased sensitivity to the effects of azathioprine and who can be treated with lower doses than normal.

RESEARCH FRONTIERS IN MOLECULAR MEDICINE

Gene therapy

Replacing or repairing mutated genes (gene therapy) is very difficult in humans. Retroviral-mediated ex vivo replacement of the defective gene in bone marrow cells for the treatment of severe combined immune deficiency syndrome (p. 80) has been partially successful. There have been two major problems with the clinical trials of virally delivered gene therapy conducted to date:

- The random integration of the retroviral DNA (which contains the replacement gene) into the genome has caused leukaemia in some treated children via activation of proto-oncogenes.
- A severe immune response to the viral vector may be induced. It has not yet been possible to use non-viral means to introduce sufficient numbers of copies of replacement genes to produce significant biological effects.

Other therapies for genetic disease include PTC124, a compound that can 'force' cells to read through a mutation that results in a premature termination codon in an ORF with the aim of producing a near-normal protein product. This therapeutic approach could be applied to any genetic disease caused by nonsense mutations.

Induced pluripotent stem cells and regenerative medicine

Adult stem cell therapy has been in wide use for decades in the form of haematopoietic stem cell transplantation. The identification of adult stem cells for other tissues, coupled with the ability to purify and maintain such cells in vitro, now offers exciting therapeutic potential for other diseases. Many different adult cell types can be transdifferentiated to form cells termed induced pluripotent stem cells (iPS cells) with almost all the characteristics of embryonic stem cells. In mammals, iPS cells can be used to regenerate various tissues such as the heart and brain. They have great potential both to develop tissue models of human disease and for regenerative medicine. In mammalian model species, such cells can be taken and used to regenerate differentiated tissue cells, such as in heart and brain.

Pathway medicine

The ability to manipulate pathways that have been altered in genetic disease has tremendous therapeutic potential for Mendelian disease, but a firm understanding of both disease pathogenesis and drug action at a biochemical level is required. An exciting example of this has been the discovery that the vascular pathology associated with Marfan's syndrome is due to the defective fibrillin molecules causing up-regulation of transforming growth factor (TGF)-β signalling in the vessel wall. Losartan is an antihypertensive drug that is marketed as an angiotensin II receptor antagonist. However, it also acts as a partial antagonist of TGF-β signalling and is effective in preventing aortic dilatation in a mouse model of Marfan's syndrome, showing promising effects in early human clinical trials.

Further information

Books and journal articles

Alberts B, Bray D, Hopkin K, et al. Essential cell biology. New York: Garland Science. 3rd edn; 2009.

Read A, Donnai D. New clinical genetics. 2nd edn. Banbury: Scion; 2010.

Strachan T, Read A. Human molecular genetics. 3rd edn. Wilmington: Wiley–Liss; 2003.

Websites

www.bshg.org.uk *British Society for Human Genetics; has report on genetic testing of children.*

www.ensembl.org *Annotated genome databases from multiple organisms.*

www.genome.ucsc.edu *Excellent source of genomic information.*

www.ncbi.nlm.nih.gov *Online Mendelian Inheritance in Man (OMIM).*

S.E. Marshall

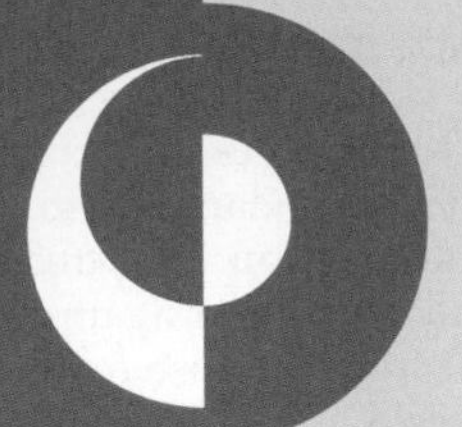

Immunological factors in disease

4

Functional anatomy and physiology of the immune system 72
- The innate immune system 72
- The adaptive immune system 76

Immune deficiency 78
- Presenting problems in immune deficiency 79
  - Recurrent infections 79
- Primary phagocyte deficiencies 79
- Complement pathway deficiencies 79
- Primary deficiencies of the adaptive immune system 80
- Secondary immune deficiencies 82

The inflammatory response 82
- Physiology and pathology of inflammation 82
- Investigations in inflammation 83
- Presenting problems in inflammation 85
  - Unexplained raised ESR 85
- Periodic fever syndromes 85
- Amyloidosis 86

Autoimmune disease 86
- Pathophysiology of autoimmunity 86
- Investigations in autoimmunity 88

Allergy 89
- Pathology of allergy 89
- Presenting problems in allergy 90
  - A general approach to the allergic patient 90
  - Anaphylaxis 91
  - Angioedema 93
- Specific allergies 94
- C1 inhibitor deficiency 94

Transplantation immunology 94
- Transplant rejection 94
- Complications of transplant immunosuppression 95
- Organ donation 96

The immune system has evolved to protect the host from pathogens while minimising damage to self tissue. Despite the ancient observation that recovery from some diseases results in protection against that condition, the existence of the immune system as a functional entity was not recognised until the end of the 19th century. More recently, it has become clear that the immune system not only protects against infection, but also influences healing and governs the responses that can lead to autoimmune diseases. Dysfunction or deficiency of the immune response leads to a wide variety of diseases, involving every organ system in the body.

The aim of this chapter is to provide a general understanding of immunology and how it contributes to human disease. A review of the key components of the immune response is followed by five sections that illustrate the clinical presentation of the most common forms of immune dysfunction. Clinical immunologists are usually involved in managing patients with allergy and immune deficiency. More detailed discussion of individual conditions can be found in the relevant organ-specific chapters of this book.

FUNCTIONAL ANATOMY AND PHYSIOLOGY OF THE IMMUNE SYSTEM

The immune system consists of an intricately linked network of cells, proteins and lymphoid organs that are strategically placed to ensure maximal protection against infection. Immune defences are normally categorised into the innate immune response, which provides immediate protection against an invading pathogen, and the adaptive or acquired immune response, which takes more time to develop but confers exquisite specificity and long-lasting protection.

The innate immune system

Innate defences against infection include anatomical barriers, phagocytic cells, soluble molecules, such as complement and acute phase proteins, and natural killer cells. The innate immune system recognises generic microbial structures present on non-mammalian tissue and can be mobilised within minutes. A specific stimulus will elicit essentially identical responses in different individuals (in contrast with antibody and T-cell responses, which vary greatly between individuals).

Constitutive barriers to infection

The tightly packed, highly keratinised cells of the skin constantly undergo renewal and replacement, which physically limits colonisation by microorganisms. Microbial growth is inhibited by physiological factors, such as low pH and low oxygen tension, and sebaceous glands secrete hydrophobic oils that further repel water and microorganisms. Sweat also contains lysozyme, an enzyme that destroys the structural integrity of bacterial cell walls; ammonia, which has antibacterial properties; and several antimicrobial peptides such as defensins. Similarly, the mucous membranes of the respiratory, gastrointestinal and genitourinary tract provide a constitutive barrier to infection. Secreted mucus acts as a physical barrier to trap invading pathogens, and immunoglobulin A (IgA) prevents bacteria and viruses attaching to and penetrating epithelial cells. As in the skin, lysozyme and antimicrobial peptides within mucosal membranes can directly kill invading pathogens, and additionally lactoferrin acts to starve invading bacteria of iron. Within the respiratory tract, cilia directly trap pathogens and contribute to removal of mucus, assisted by physical manœuvres, such as sneezing and coughing. In the gastrointestinal tract, hydrochloric acid and salivary amylase chemically destroy bacteria, while normal peristalsis and induced vomiting or diarrhoea assist clearance of invading organisms.

Endogenous commensal bacteria provide an additional constitutive defence against infection (p. 136). They compete with pathogenic microorganisms for space and nutrients, and produce fatty acids and bactericidins that inhibit the growth of many pathogens. In addition, commensal bacteria help to shape the immune response by inducing specific regulatory T cells within the intestine (p. 78).

These constitutive barriers are highly effective, but if external defences are breached by a wound or pathogenic organism, the specific soluble proteins and cells of the innate immune system are activated.

Phagocytes

Phagocytes ('eating cells') are specialised cells which ingest and kill microorganisms, scavenge cellular and infectious debris, and produce inflammatory molecules which regulate other components of the immune system. They include neutrophils, monocytes and macrophages, and are particularly important for defence against bacterial and fungal infections.

Phagocytes express a wide range of surface receptors that allow them to identify microorganisms. These pattern recognition receptors include the Toll-like receptors, NOD (nucleotide-oligomerisation domain protein)-like receptors and mannose receptors. They recognise generic molecular motifs not present on mammalian cells, including bacterial cell wall components, bacterial DNA and viral double-stranded RNA. While phagocytes can recognise microorganisms through pattern recognition receptors alone, engulfment of microorganisms is greatly enhanced by opsonisation. Opsonins include acute phase proteins such as C-reactive protein (CRP), antibodies and complement. They bind both to the pathogen and to phagocyte receptors, acting as a bridge between the two to facilitate phagocytosis (Fig. 4.1).

Neutrophils

Neutrophils, also known as polymorphonuclear leucocytes, are derived from the bone marrow (Fig. 4.2). They are short-lived cells with a half-life of 6 hours in the blood stream, and are produced at the rate of approximately 10^{11} cells daily. Their functions are to kill microorganisms directly, facilitate the rapid transit of cells through tissues, and non-specifically amplify the immune response. This is mediated by enzymes contained in granules which also provide an intracellular milieu for the killing and degradation of microorganisms.

The two main types of granule are primary or azurophil granules, and the more numerous secondary or specific granules. Primary granules contain myeloperoxidase and other enzymes important for

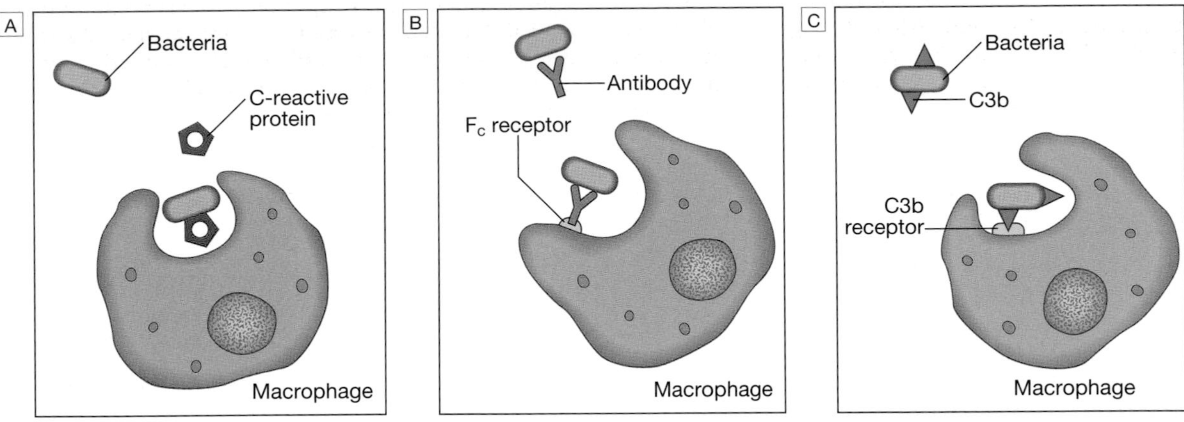

Fig. 4.1 Opsonisation. Phagocytosis of microbial products may be augmented by several opsonins. **A** C-reactive protein. **B** Antibody. **C** Complement fragments.

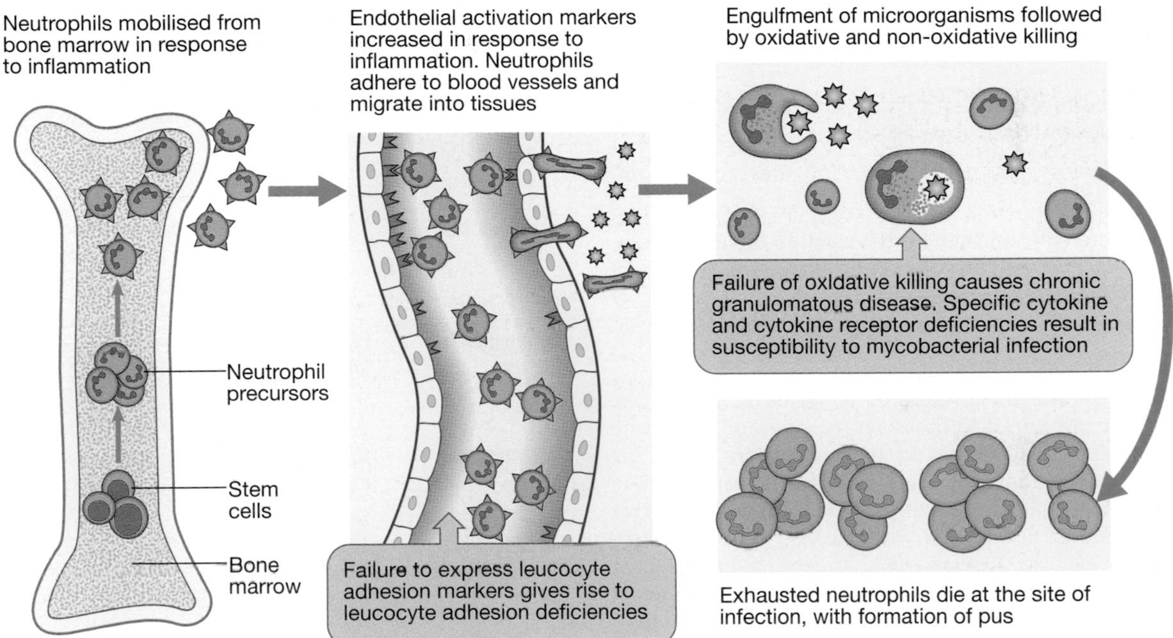

Fig. 4.2 Neutrophil function and dysfunction (green boxes).

intracellular killing and digestion of ingested microbes. Secondary granules are smaller and contain lysozyme, collagenase and lactoferrin, which can be released into the extracellular space. Granule staining becomes more intense in response to infection ('toxic granulation'), reflecting increased enzyme production.

When tissues are changed or damaged, they trigger the local production of inflammatory molecules and cytokines. These stimulate the production and maturation of neutrophils in the bone marrow, and their release into the circulation. The neutrophils are recruited to the inflamed site by chemotactic agents and by activation of local endothelium. Transit of neutrophils through the blood stream is responsible for the rise in leucocyte count that occurs in early infection. Once within infected tissue, activated neutrophils seek out and engulf invading microorganisms. These are initially enclosed within membrane-bound vesicles which fuse with cytoplasmic granules to form the phagolysosome. Within this protected compartment, killing of the organism occurs through a combination of oxidative and non-oxidative killing. Oxidative killing, also known as the respiratory burst, is mediated by the NADPH (nicotinamide adenine dinucleotide phosphate) oxidase enzyme complex. This converts oxygen into reactive oxygen species such as hydrogen peroxide and superoxide that are lethal to microorganisms. When combined with myeloperoxidase, hypochlorous ions ($HOCl^-$, analogous to bleach) are produced, which are highly effective oxidants and antimicrobial agents. Non-oxidative (oxygen-independent) killing occurs through the release of bactericidal enzymes into the phagolysosome. Each enzyme has a distinct antimicrobial spectrum, providing broad coverage against bacteria and fungi.

The process of phagocytosis depletes neutrophil glycogen reserves and is followed by neutrophil cell death. As the cells die, their contents are released and lysosomal enzymes degrade collagen and other components

4.1 Functions of macrophages

Initiation and amplification of the inflammatory response
• Stimulation of the acute phase response • Activation of vascular endothelium • Stimulation of neutrophil maturation and chemotaxis • Stimulation of monocyte chemotaxis
Killing of microorganisms
• Phagocytosis • Microbial killing through oxidative and non-oxidative mechanisms
Clearance, resolution and repair
• Scavenging of necrotic and apoptotic cells • Clearance of toxins and other inorganic debris • Tissue remodelling (elastase, collagenase, matrix proteins) • Down-regulation of inflammatory cytokines • Wound healing and scar formation (interleukin (IL)-1, platelet-derived growth factor, fibroblast growth factor)
Link between innate and adaptive immune system
• Activation of T cells by presenting antigen in a recognisable form • T cell-derived cytokines increase phagocytosis and microbicidal activity of macrophages

of the interstitium, causing liquefaction of closely adjacent tissue. The accumulation of dead and dying neutrophils results in the formation of pus, which, if extensive, may result in abscess formation.

Monocytes and macrophages

Monocytes are the precursors of tissue macrophages. They are produced in the bone marrow and constitute about 5% of leucocytes in the circulation. From the blood stream, they migrate to peripheral tissues, where they differentiate into tissue macrophages and reside for long periods. Specialised populations of tissue macrophages include Kupffer cells in the liver, alveolar macrophages in the lung, mesangial cells in the kidney, and microglial cells in the brain. Macrophages, like neutrophils, are capable of phagocytosis and killing of microorganisms but also play an important role in the amplification and regulation of the inflammatory response (Box 4.1). They are particularly important in tissue surveillance, monitoring their immediate surroundings for signs of tissue damage or invading organisms.

Dendritic cells

Dendritic cells are specialised antigen-presenting cells which are prevalent in tissues in contact with the external environment, such as the skin and mucosa. They can also be found in an immature state in the blood. They sample the environment for foreign particles, and once activated, carry microbial antigens to regional lymph nodes, where they interact with T cells and B cells to initiate and shape the adaptive immune response.

Cytokines

Cytokines are small soluble proteins that act as multipurpose chemical messengers. Examples are listed in Box 4.2. They are produced by cells involved in immune responses and by stromal tissue. More than 100 cytokines have been described, with overlapping, complex roles in intercellular communication. Their clinical importance is demonstrated by the efficacy of 'biological' therapies (often abbreviated to 'biologics') that target specific cytokines (pp. 1102 and 18).

4.2 Some roles for cytokines in regulating the immune response

Cytokine	Source	Actions
Interferon-alpha (IFN-α)	T cells and macrophages	Antiviral activity Activates NK cells, $CD8^+$ T cells and macrophages
Interferon-gamma (IFN-γ)	T cells and NK cells	Increases antimicrobial and antitumour activity of macrophages Regulates cytokine production by T cells and macrophages
Tumour necrosis factor alpha (TNF-α)	Macrophages and NK cells	Pro-inflammatory Increases apoptosis and expression of cytokines and adhesion molecules Directly cytotoxic
Interleukin-1 (IL-1)	Macrophages and neutrophils	Acute phase reactant Stimulates neutrophil recruitment, fever, T-cell and macrophage activation, and immunoglobulin production
Interleukin-2 (IL-2)	T cells	Stimulates proliferation and differentiation of antigen-specific T lymphocytes
Interleukin-4 (IL-4)	$CD4^+$ T cells and mast cells	Stimulates maturation of B and T cells, and production of IgE antibody
Interleukin-6 (IL-6)	Monocytes and macrophages	Acute phase reactant Stimulates maturation of B cells into plasma cells
Interleukin-12 (IL-12)	Monocytes and macrophages	Stimulates IFN-γ and TNF-α release by T cells, activates NK cells

(NK = natural killer)

Complement

The complement system is a group of more than 20 tightly regulated, functionally linked proteins that act to promote inflammation and eliminate invading pathogens. Complement proteins are produced in the liver and are present in the circulation as inactive molecules. When triggered, they enzymatically activate other proteins in a rapidly amplified biological cascade analogous to the coagulation cascade (p. 995).

There are three mechanisms by which the complement cascade may be triggered (Fig. 4.3):

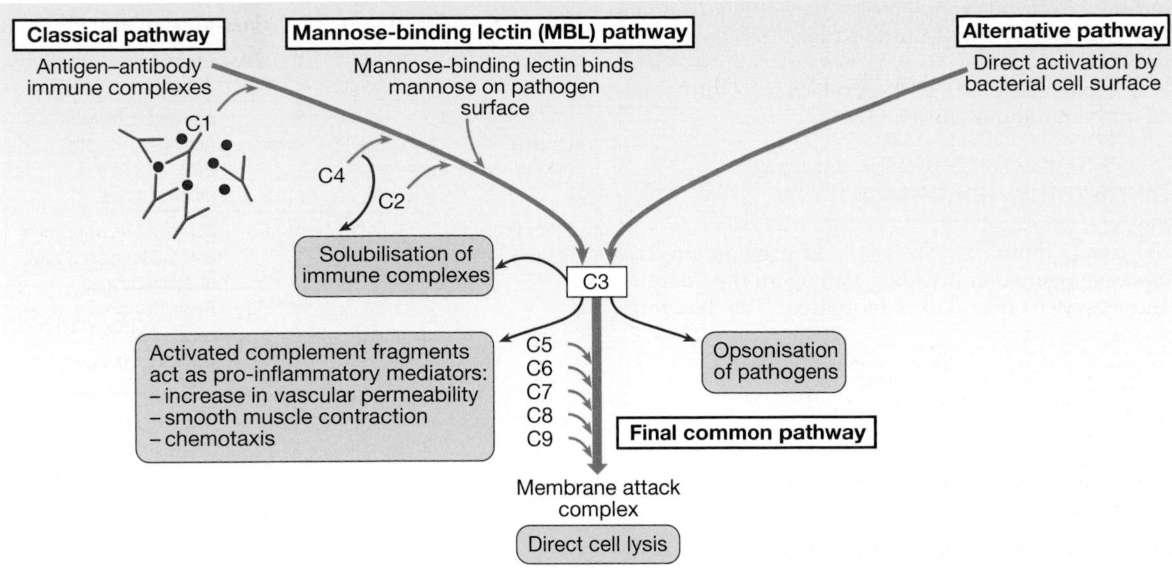

Fig. 4.3 The complement pathway. The activation of C3 is central to complement activation.

- *The alternative pathway* is triggered directly by binding of C3 to bacterial cell wall components, such as lipopolysaccharide of Gram-negative bacteria and teichoic acid of Gram-positive bacteria.
- *The classical pathway* is initiated when two or more IgM or IgG antibody molecules bind to antigen, forming immune complexes. The associated conformational change exposes binding sites on the antibodies for C1. C1 is a multiheaded molecule which can bind up to six antibody molecules. Once two or more 'heads' of a C1 molecule are bound to antibody, the classical cascade is triggered.
- *The lectin pathway* is activated by the direct binding of mannose-binding lectin to microbial cell surface carbohydrates. This mimics the binding of C1 to immune complexes and directly stimulates the classical pathway.

Activation of complement by any of these pathways results in activation of C3. This, in turn, activates the final common pathway, in which the complement proteins C5–C9 assemble to form the membrane attack complex. This can puncture target cell walls, leading to osmotic cell lysis. This step is particularly important in the defence against encapsulated bacteria, such as *Neisseria* spp. and *Haemophilus influenzae*. Complement fragments generated by activation of the cascade can also act as opsonins, rendering microorganisms more susceptible to phagocytosis by macrophages and neutrophils (see Fig. 4.1). In addition, they are chemotactic agents, promoting leucocyte trafficking to sites of inflammation. Some fragments act as anaphylotoxins, binding to complement receptors on mast cells and triggering release of histamine, which increases vascular permeability. The products of complement activation also help to target immune complexes to antigen-presenting cells, providing a link between the innate and the acquired immune systems. Finally, activated complement products dissolve the immune complexes that triggered the cascade, minimising bystander damage to surrounding tissues.

Mast cells and basophils

Mast cells and basophils are bone marrow-derived cells which play a central role in allergic disorders. Mast cells reside predominantly in tissues exposed to the external environment, such as the skin and gut, while basophils are located in the circulation and are recruited into tissues in response to inflammation. Both contain large cytoplasmic granules which contain preformed vasoactive substances such as histamine (see Fig. 4.9, p. 89). Mast cells and basophils express IgE receptors on their cell surface (see Fig. 4.5). On encounter with specific antigen, the cell is triggered to release preformed mediators and synthesise additional mediators, including leukotrienes, prostaglandins and cytokines. These trigger an inflammatory cascade which increases local blood flow and vascular permeability, stimulates smooth muscle contraction, and increases secretion at mucosal surfaces.

Natural killer cells

Natural killer (NK) cells are large granular lymphocytes which play a major role in defence against tumours and viruses. They exhibit features of both the adaptive and innate immune systems: they are morphologically similar to lymphocytes and recognise similar ligands, but they are not antigen-specific and cannot generate immunological memory.

NK cells express a variety of cell surface receptors. Some recognise stress signals, while others recognise the absence of human leucocyte antigen (HLA) molecules on cell surfaces (down-regulation of HLA molecules by viruses and tumour cells is an important mechanism by which they evade T lymphocytes). NK cells can also be activated by binding of antigen–antibody complexes to surface receptors. This physically links the NK cell to its target in a manner analogous to opsonisation, and is known as antibody-dependent cellular cytotoxicity (ADCC).

Activated NK cells can kill their targets in various ways. Pore-forming proteins, such as perforin, induce direct cell lysis, while granzymes are proteolytic enzymes which stimulate apoptosis. In addition, NK cells produce a variety of cytokines, such as tumour necrosis factor (TNF)-α and interferon-γ (IFN-γ), which have direct antiviral and antitumour effects.

The adaptive immune system

If the innate immune system fails to provide effective protection against an invading pathogen, the adaptive immune system (Fig. 4.4) is mobilised. This has three key characteristics:

- It has exquisite specificity and is able to discriminate between very small differences in molecular structure.
- It is highly adaptive and can respond to an unlimited number of molecules.
- It possesses immunological memory, such that subsequent encounters with a particular antigen produce a more effective immune response than the first encounter.

There are two major arms of the adaptive immune response: humoral immunity involves antibodies produced by B lymphocytes; cellular immunity is mediated by T lymphocytes, which release cytokines and kill immune targets. These interact closely with each other and with the innate immune system, to maximise the effectiveness of the response.

Lymphoid organs

- *Primary lymphoid organs.* The primary lymphoid organs are involved in lymphocyte development. They include the bone marrow, where both T and B lymphocytes are derived from haematopoietic stem cells (p. 993) and where B lymphocytes also mature, and the thymus, where T lymphocytes mature.
- *Secondary lymphoid organs.* After maturation, lymphocytes migrate to the secondary lymphoid organs. These include the spleen, lymph nodes and mucosa-associated lymphoid tissue. These organs trap and concentrate foreign substances, and are the major sites of interaction between naïve lymphocytes and microorganisms.

The thymus

The thymus is a bilobed structure organised into cortical and medullary areas. The cortex is densely populated with immature T cells, which migrate to the medulla to undergo selection and maturation. The thymus is most active in the fetal and neonatal period, and involutes after puberty. Failure of thymic development is associated with profound T-cell immune deficiency (p. 80), but surgical removal of the thymus in childhood (usually in the context of major cardiac surgery) is not associated with significant immune dysfunction.

The spleen

The spleen is the largest of the secondary lymphoid organs. It is highly effective at filtering blood and is an important site of phagocytosis of senescent erythrocytes, bacteria, immune complexes and other debris. It is also a major site of antibody synthesis. It is particularly important for defence against encapsulated bacteria, and asplenic individuals are at risk of overwhelming *Streptococcus pneumoniae* and *H. influenzae* infection (see Box 24.40, p. 1028).

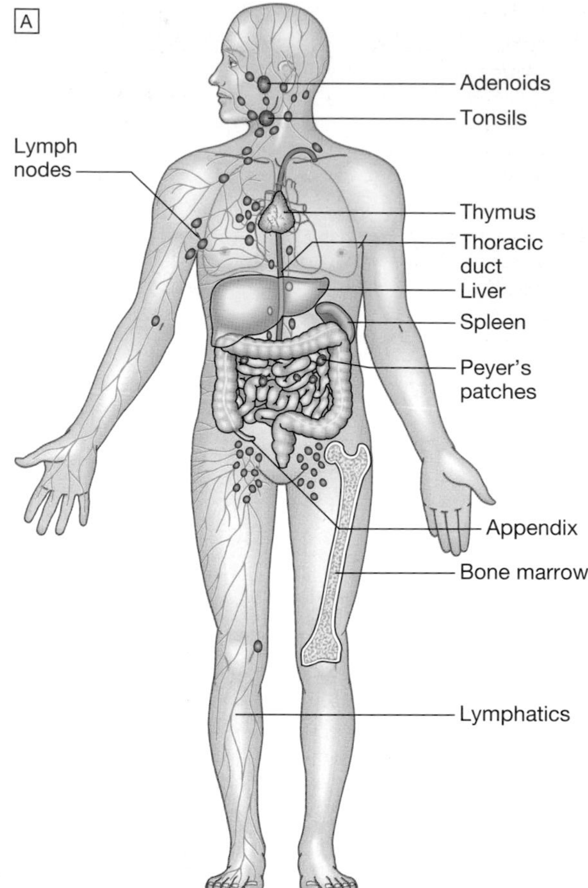

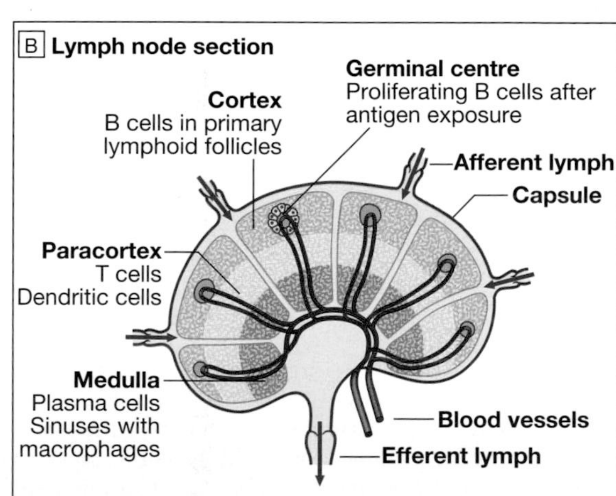

Fig. 4.4 Anatomy of the adaptive immune system. **A** Macroanatomy **B** Anatomy of a lymph node.

Lymph nodes and mucosa-associated lymphoid tissue

Lymph nodes are positioned to maximise exposure to lymph draining from sites of external contact. Their structure is highly organised, as shown in Figure 4.4B.

More diffuse unencapsulated lymphoid cells and follicles are also present on mucosal surfaces: for example, in Peyer's patches in the small intestine.

Lymphatics

Lymphoid tissues are physically connected by a network of lymphatics, which has three major functions: it provides access to lymph nodes, returns interstitial fluid to the venous system, and transports fat from the small intestine to the blood stream (see Fig. 16.14, p. 452). The lymphatics begin as blind-ending capillaries, which come together to form lymphatic ducts. These enter and then leave regional lymph nodes as afferent and efferent ducts respectively. They eventually coalesce and drain into the thoracic duct and thence into the left subclavian vein. Lymphatics may be either deep or superficial, and, in general, follow the distribution of major blood vessels.

Humoral immunity

B lymphocytes

These specialised cells arise in the bone marrow. Mature B lymphocytes (also known as B cells) are found in bone marrow, lymphoid tissue, spleen and, to a lesser extent, the blood stream. They express a unique immunoglobulin receptor on their cell surface (the B-cell receptor), which binds to soluble antigen. Encounters with antigen usually occur within lymph nodes, where, if provided with appropriate signals from nearby T lymphocytes, stimulated antigen-specific B cells respond by proliferating rapidly in a process known as clonal expansion. This is accompanied by a highly complex series of genetic re-arrangements, which generates B-cell populations that express receptors with greater affinity for antigen than the original. These cells differentiate into either long-lived memory cells, which reside in the lymph nodes, or plasma cells, which produce antibody.

Immunoglobulins

Immunoglobulins (Ig) are soluble proteins made up of two heavy and two light chains (Fig. 4.5). The heavy chain determines the antibody class or isotype, i.e. IgG, IgA, IgM, IgE or IgD. Subclasses of IgG and IgA also occur. The antigen is recognised by the antigen-binding regions (F_{ab}) of both heavy and light chains, while the consequences of antibody-binding are determined by the constant region of the heavy chain (F_c) (Box 4.3).

Antibodies can initiate a number of different actions. They facilitate phagocytosis by acting as opsonins (see Fig. 4.1), and can also facilitate cell killing by cytotoxic cells (ADCC, p. 75). Binding of antibodies to antigen can trigger activation of the classical complement pathway (see Fig. 4.3). In addition, antibodies may act directly to neutralise the biological activity of toxins. This is a particularly important feature of IgA antibodies, which act predominantly at mucosal surfaces.

The humoral immune response is characterised by immunological memory: that is, the antibody response to successive exposures to antigen is qualitatively and quantitatively different from that on first exposure. When a previously unstimulated (naïve) B lymphocyte is activated by antigen, the first antibody to be produced is IgM, which appears in the serum after 5–10 days. Depending on additional stimuli provided by T lymphocytes, other antibody classes (IgG, IgA and IgE) are produced 1–2 weeks later. If, some time later, a memory B cell is re-exposed to antigen, the lag time between antigen exposure and the production of antibody is decreased (to 2–3 days), the amount of antibody produced is increased, and the response is dominated by IgG antibodies of high affinity. Furthermore, in contrast

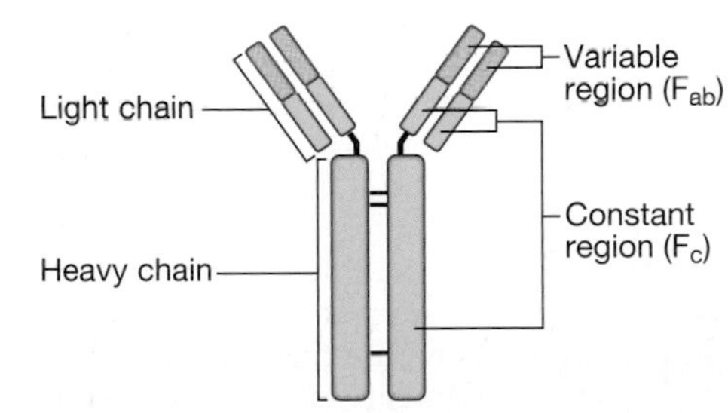

Fig. 4.5 The structure of an immunoglobulin (antibody) molecule.

4.3 Classes and properties of antibody

Antibody/properties	Concentration in adult serum	Complement activation*	Opsonisation
IgG 4 subclasses: IgG1, IgG2, IgG3, IgG4 Distributed equally between blood and extracellular fluid, and transported across placenta IgG2 is the predominant antibody produced against polysaccharides	8.0–16.0 g/L	IgG1 +++ IgG2 + IgG3 +++	IgG1 ++ IgG3 ++
IgA 2 subclasses: IgA1, IgA2 Highly effective at neutralising toxins Particularly important at mucosal surfaces	1.5–4.0 g/L	–	–
IgM Highly effective at agglutinating pathogens	0.5–2.0 g/L	++++	–
IgE Mostly bound to mast cells, basophils and eosinophils Important in allergic disease and defence against parasite infection	0.003–0.04 g/L	–	–
IgD Function unknown	Not detected	–	–

*Refers to activation of the classical complement pathway, also called 'complement fixation'.

to the initial antibody response, secondary antibody responses do not require additional input from T lymphocytes. This allows the rapid generation of highly specific responses on pathogen re-exposure.

Cellular immunity

T lymphocytes (also known as T cells) mediate cellular immunity and are important for defence against viruses, fungi and intracellular bacteria. They also play an important immunoregulatory role, orchestrating and regulating the responses of other components of the immune system. T-lymphocyte precursors arise in bone marrow and are exported to the thymus while still immature (see Fig. 4.6 below). Within the thymus, each cell expresses a T-cell receptor with a unique specificity. These cells undergo a process of stringent selection to ensure that autoreactive T cells are deleted. Mature T lymphocytes leave the thymus and expand to populate other organs of the immune system. It has been estimated that an individual possesses 10^7–10^9 T-cell clones, each with a unique T-cell receptor, ensuring at least partial coverage for any antigen encountered.

T cells respond to protein antigens, but they cannot recognise these in their native form. Instead, intact protein must be processed into component peptides which bind to a structural framework on the cell surface known as HLA (human leucocyte antigen). This process is known as antigen processing and presentation, and it is the peptide/HLA complex which is recognised by individual T cells. While all nucleated cells have the capacity to process and present antigens, specialised antigen-presenting cells include dendritic cells, macrophages and B lymphocytes. HLA molecules exhibit extreme polymorphism; as each HLA molecule has the capacity to present a subtly different peptide repertoire to T lymphocytes, this ensures enormous diversity in recognition of antigens within the population.

T lymphocytes can be segregated into two subgroups on the basis of function and recognition of HLA molecules. These are designated $CD4^+$ and $CD8^+$ T cells, according to the 'cluster of differentiation' (CD) antigen expressed on their cell surface. $CD8^+$ T cells recognise antigenic peptides in association with HLA class I molecules (HLA-A, HLA-B, HLA-C). They kill infected cells directly through the production of pore-forming molecules such as perforin, or by triggering apoptosis of the target cell, and are particularly important in defence against viral infection. $CD4^+$ T cells recognise peptides presented on HLA class II molecules (HLA-DR, HLA-DP and HLA-DQ) and have mainly immunoregulatory functions. They produce cytokines and provide co-stimulatory signals that support the activation of $CD8^+$ T lymphocytes and assist the production of mature antibody by B cells. In addition, their close interaction with phagocytes determines cytokine production by both cell types.

$CD4^+$ lymphocytes can be further subdivided into subsets on the basis of the cytokines they produce:

- Typically, Th1 cells produce IL-2, IFN-γ and TNF-α, and support the development of delayed type hypersensitivity responses (p. 87).
- Th2 cells typically secrete IL-4, IL-5 and IL-10, and promote allergic responses (p. 89).
- A further subset of specialised $CD4^+$ lymphocytes known as regulatory cells are important in immune regulation of other cells and the prevention of autoimmune disease.

IMMUNE DEFICIENCY

The consequences of deficiencies of the immune system include recurrent infections, autoimmunity and susceptibility to malignancy. Immune deficiency may arise through intrinsic defects in immune function, but is much more commonly due to secondary causes, including infection, drug therapy, malignancy and ageing. This chapter gives an overview of the rare primary immune deficiencies. More than a hundred genetically determined deficiencies have been described, most of which present in childhood or adolescence. The clinical manifestations are dictated by the component of the immune system involved (Box 4.4), but there is considerable overlap and redundancy in the immune

4.4 Immune deficiencies and common patterns of infection

	Phagocyte deficiency	Complement deficiency	T-lymphocyte deficiency	Antibody deficiency
Bacteria	*Staphylococcus aureus* *Pseudomonas aeruginosa* *Serratia marcescens* *Burkholderia cenocepacia* *Mycobacterium tuberculosis* Atypical mycobacteria	*Neisseria meningitidis* *Neisseria gonorrhoeae* *Haemophilus influenzae* *Streptococcus pneumoniae*	*Mycobacterium tuberculosis* Atypical mycobacteria	*Haemophilus influenzae* *Streptococcus pneumoniae* *Staphylococcus aureus*
Fungi	*Candida* spp. *Aspergillus* spp.		*Candida* spp. *Aspergillus* spp. *Pneumocystis jirovecii*	
Viruses			Cytomegalovirus (CMV) Enteroviruses Epstein–Barr virus (EBV) Herpes zoster	
Protozoa			*Toxoplasma gondii* Cryptosporidia	*Giardia lamblia*

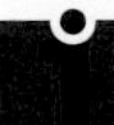

4.5 Warning signs of primary immune deficiency*

The presence of ≥ 2 warning signs may indicate an underlying primary immunodeficiency:
- ≥ 4 new ear infections within 1 yr
- ≥ 2 serious sinus infections within 1 yr
- ≥ 2 mths on antibiotics with little effect
- ≥ 2 pneumonias within 1 yr
- Failure of an infant to gain weight or grow normally
- Recurrent, deep skin or organ abscesses
- Persistent thrush in mouth or fungal infection on skin
- Need for intravenous antibiotics to clear infections
- ≥ 2 deep-seated infections, including septicaemia
- A family history of primary immune deficiency

*Developed by the Jeffrey Modell Foundation (www.info4pi.org/).

network so some diseases do not fall easily into this classification.

Presenting problems in immune deficiency

Recurrent infections

Most patients with an immune deficiency present with recurrent infections. While there is no accepted definition of 'too many' infections, features that may indicate immune deficiency are shown in Box 4.5. Frequent, severe infections or infections caused by unusual organisms or at unusual sites are the most useful indicator.

Baseline investigations include full blood count with white cell differential, acute phase reactants (CRP, see below), renal and liver function tests, urine dipstick, serum immunoglobulins with protein electrophoresis, and total IgE level. Additional microbiological, virological and radiological tests may be appropriate. At this stage, it may be clear which category of immune deficiency should be considered, and specific investigation can be undertaken, as described below.

If an immune deficiency is suspected but has not yet been formally characterised, patients should not receive live vaccines because of the risk of vaccine-induced disease. Discussion with specialists will help determine whether additional preventative measures, such as prophylactic antibiotics, are indicated.

Primary phagocyte deficiencies

Primary phagocyte deficiencies (see Fig. 4.2, p. 73) usually present with recurrent bacterial and fungal infections which may affect unusual sites. Aggressive management of existing infections, including intravenous antibiotics and surgical drainage of abscesses, and long-term prophylaxis with antibacterial and antifungal agents, is required. Specific treatment depends upon the nature of the defect; haematopoietic stem cell transplantation may be considered (p. 1017).

Leucocyte adhesion deficiencies

These are rare disorders of phagocyte migration, when failure to express adhesion molecules on the surface of leucocytes results in their inability to exit the blood stream. They are characterised by recurrent bacterial infections with high blood neutrophil counts but sites of infection lack pus or other evidence of neutrophil infiltration.

Chronic granulomatous disease

This is caused by mutations in the genes encoding the NADPH oxidase enzymes, which results in failure of oxidative killing. The defect leads to susceptibility to catalase-positive organisms, such as *Staphylococcus aureus*, *Burkholderia cenocepacia* and *Aspergillus*. Intracellular killing of mycobacteria is also impaired. Infections most commonly involve the lungs, lymph nodes, soft tissues, bone, skin and urinary tract, and are characterised histologically by granuloma formation.

Defects in cytokines and cytokine receptors

Defects of cytokines such as IFN-γ, IL-12 or their receptors also result in failure of intracellular killing, with particular susceptibility to mycobacterial infections.

Complement pathway deficiencies

Genetic deficiencies of almost all the complement pathway proteins (see Fig. 4.3, p. 75) have been described. Many present with recurrent infection with encapsulated bacteria, particularly *Neisseria* species, reflecting the importance of the membrane attack complex in defence against these bacteria. In addition, genetic deficiencies of the classical complement pathway (C1, C2 and C4) are associated with a high prevalence of autoimmune disease, particularly systemic lupus erythematosus (SLE, p. 1109).

In contrast to other complement deficiencies, mannose-binding lectin deficiency is very common (5% of the northern European population). Complete deficiency may predispose to bacterial infections in the presence of an additional cause of immune compromise, such as premature birth or chemotherapy, but is otherwise well tolerated. Deficiency of the complement regulatory protein Cl inhibitor is not associated with recurrent infections but causes recurrent angioedema (p. 93).

Investigations and management

Complement C3 and C4 are the only complement components that are routinely measured. Screening for complement deficiencies is performed using more specialised functional tests of complement-mediated haemolysis, known as CH50 and AP50 (classical haemolytic pathway 50 and alternative pathway 50). If abnormal, these haemolytic tests should be followed by measurement of individual complement components.

There is no definitive treatment for complement deficiencies. Patients should be vaccinated with meningococcal, pneumococcal and *H. influenzae* B vaccines in order to boost their adaptive immune responses. Lifelong prophylactic penicillin to prevent meningococcal infection is recommended. At-risk family members should also be screened.

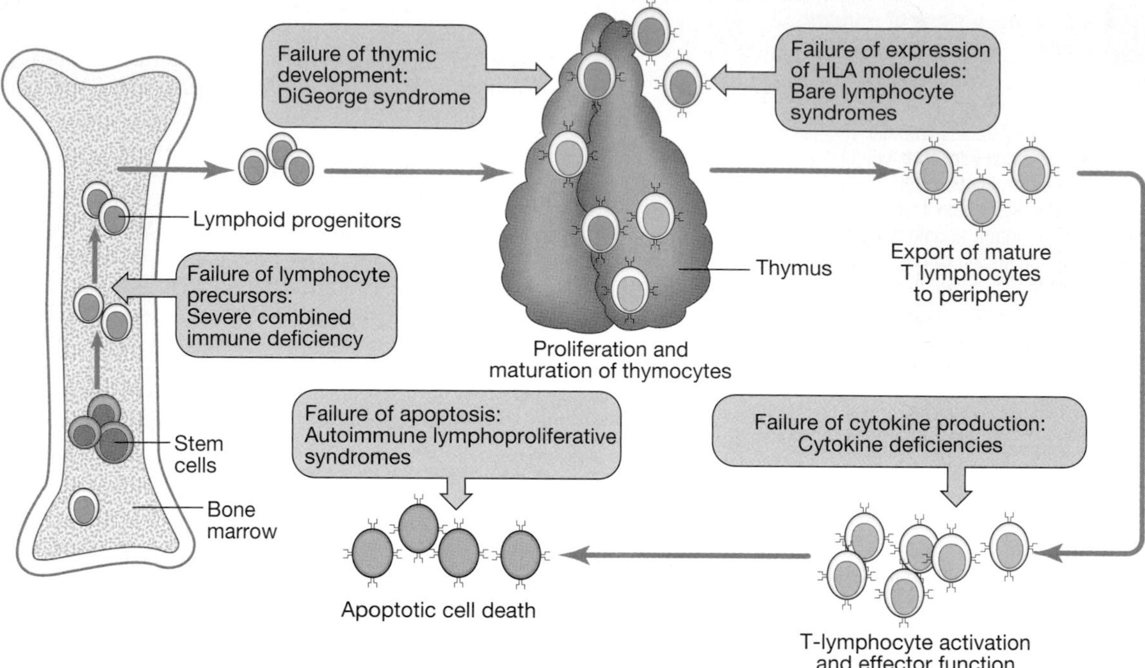

Fig. 4.6 T-lymphocyte function and dysfunction (green boxes).

Primary deficiencies of the adaptive immune system

Primary T-lymphocyte deficiencies

These are characterised by recurrent viral, protozoal and fungal infections (see Box 4.4). In addition, many T-cell deficiencies are associated with defective antibody production because of the importance of T cells in regulating B cells. These disorders generally present in childhood and are illustrated in Figure 4.6.

DiGeorge syndrome

This results from failure of development of the 3rd/4th pharyngeal pouch, usually caused by a deletion of 22q11. It is associated with multiple abnormalities, including congenital heart disease, hypocalcaemia, tracheo-oesophageal fistulae, cleft lip and palate, and absent thymic development. The immune deficiency is characterised by very low numbers of circulating T cells, despite normal development in the bone marrow.

Bare lymphocyte syndromes

These are caused by absent expression of HLA molecules within the thymus. If HLA class I molecules are affected, $CD8^+$ lymphocytes fail to develop, while absent expression of HLA class II molecules affects $CD4^+$ lymphocyte maturation. In addition to recurrent infections, failure to express HLA class I is associated with systemic vasculitis caused by uncontrolled activation of NK cells.

Autoimmune lymphoproliferative syndrome

This is caused by failure of normal lymphocyte apoptosis (p. 50), leading to non-malignant accumulation of autoreactive cells. This results in lymphadenopathy, splenomegaly and a variety of autoimmune diseases.

Investigations and management

The principal tests for T-lymphocyte deficiencies are a total blood lymphocyte count and quantitation of lymphocyte subpopulations by flow cytometry. Serum immunoglobulins should also be measured. Second-line, functional tests of T-cell activation and proliferation may be indicated. Patients in whom T-lymphocyte deficiencies are suspected should be tested for human immunodeficiency (HIV) infection (p. 392).

Anti-*Pneumocystis* and antifungal prophylaxis, and aggressive management of infections, are required. Immunoglobulin replacement may be indicated if antibody production is impaired. Haematopoietic stem cell transplantation (HSCT, p. 1017) may be appropriate.

Combined B- and T-lymphocyte immune deficiencies

Severe combined immune deficiency (SCID) is caused by defects in lymphoid precursors and results in combined failure of B- and T-cell maturation. The absence of an effective adaptive immune response causes recurrent bacterial, fungal and viral infections soon after birth. HSCT (p. 1017) is the only current treatment, although gene therapy is under investigation.

Primary antibody deficiencies

Primary antibody deficiencies (Fig. 4.7) are characterised by recurrent bacterial infections, particularly of the respiratory and gastrointestinal tract. The most common causative organisms are encapsulated bacteria, such as *Strep. pneumoniae* and *H. influenzae*. These disorders may present in infancy, when the protective benefit of transferred maternal immunoglobulin has waned. However, three forms of primary antibody deficiency can also present in adulthood:

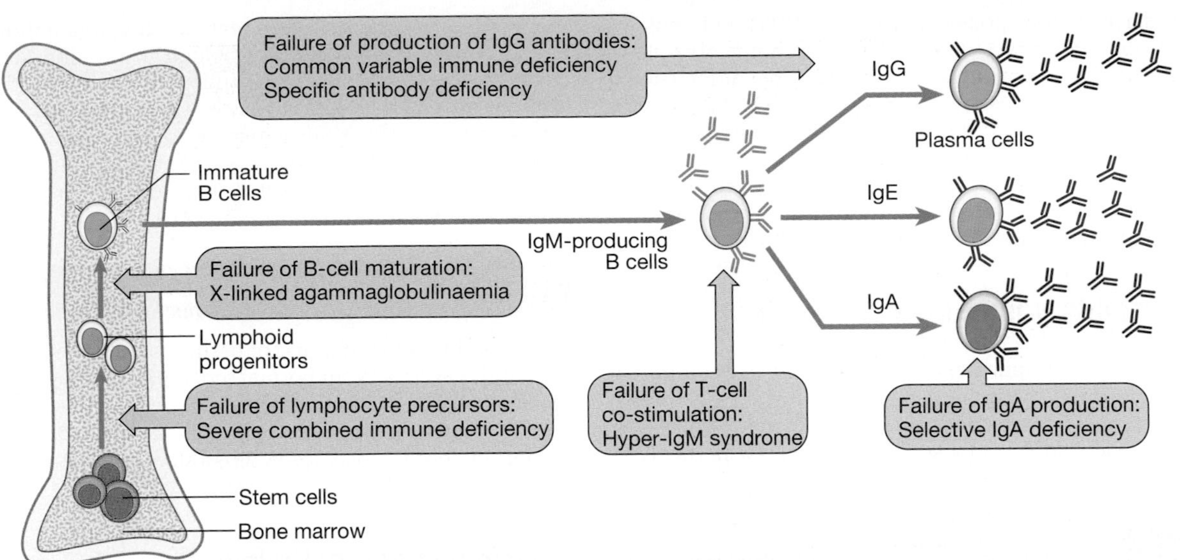

Fig. 4.7 B lymphocytes and primary antibody deficiencies (green boxes).

4.6 Investigation of primary antibody deficiencies

	Serum immunoglobulin concentrations				Blood cell count		
	IgM	**IgG**	**IgA**	**IgE**	**B cells**	**T cells**	**Test immunisation**
Selective IgA deficiency	Normal	Often elevated	Absent	Normal	Normal	Normal	
Common variable immune deficiency	Normal or low	Low	Low or absent	Low or absent	Variable	Variable	No antibody response
Specific antibody deficiency	Normal	Normal	Normal	Normal	Normal	Normal	No antibody response to polysaccharide antigens

- *Selective IgA deficiency* is the most common primary immune deficiency, affecting 1:600 northern Europeans. In most patients, low (< 0.05 g/L) or undetectable IgA is an incidental finding with no clinical sequelae. However, 30% of individuals experience recurrent mild respiratory and gastrointestinal infections. In some patients, there is a compensatory increase in serum IgG levels. Specific treatment is generally not required.
- *Common variable immune deficiency (CVID)* is a heterogeneous primary immune deficiency of unknown cause. It is characterised by low serum IgG levels and failure to make antibody responses to exogenous pathogens. Paradoxically, antibody-mediated autoimmune diseases, such as autoimmune haemolytic anaemia, are common. CVID is also associated with an increased risk of malignancy, particularly lymphoproliferative disease.
- *Specific antibody deficiency or functional IgG antibody deficiency* is a poorly characterised condition which causes defective antibody responses to polysaccharide antigens. Some patients are deficient in antibody subclasses IgG2 and IgG4, and this condition was previously called IgG subclass deficiency.

There is overlap between specific antibody deficiency, IgA deficiency and CVID, and some patients may progress to a more global antibody deficiency over time.

Investigations

Investigations include serum immunoglobulins (Box 4.6), with protein and urine electrophoresis to exclude secondary causes of hypogammaglobulinaemia, and B and T lymphocyte counts in blood by flow cytometry. Specific antibody responses to known pathogens can be assessed by measuring IgG antibodies against tetanus, *H. influenzae* and *Strep. pneumoniae* (most patients will have been exposed to these antigens through infection or immunisation). If specific antibody levels are low, immunisation with the appropriate killed vaccine should be followed by repeat antibody measurement 6–8 weeks later; failure to mount a response indicates a defect in antibody production. These functional tests have superseded IgG subclass quantitation.

Management

With the exception of individuals with selective IgA deficiency, patients with antibody deficiencies require aggressive treatment of infections, and prophylactic antibiotics may be indicated. The mainstay of treatment is life-long immunoglobulin replacement therapy. This is derived from pooled plasma (p. 1011) and contains IgG antibodies to a wide variety of common organisms. Immunoglobulin replacement may be administered either intravenously or subcutaneously, often by the patient, with the aim of maintaining trough IgG levels within the normal range. Immunisation is generally not effective because of the defect in IgG antibody production. As with all primary immune deficiencies, live vaccines should be avoided (p. 148).

Secondary immune deficiencies

Secondary immune deficiencies are much more common than primary immune deficiencies (Box 4.7). Common causes include infections, such as HIV and measles, and cytotoxic and immunosuppressive drugs, particularly those used in the management of transplantation, autoimmunity and cancer. Physiological immune deficiency occurs at the extremes of life; the decline of the immune response in the elderly is known as immune senescence (Box 4.8). Management of secondary immune deficiency is described in the relevant chapters on infectious diseases (Ch. 13), HIV (Ch. 14), oncology (Ch. 11) and haematological disorders (Ch. 24).

4.7 Causes of secondary immune deficiency

Physiological	
• Ageing • Prematurity	• Pregnancy
Infection	
• HIV • Measles	• Mycobacterial infection
Iatrogenic	
• Immunosuppressive therapy • Antineoplastic agents • Corticosteroids	• Stem cell transplantation • Radiation injury • Some anti-epileptic agents
Malignancy	
• B-cell malignancies including leukaemia, lymphoma and myeloma	• Solid tumours • Thymoma
Biochemical and nutritional disorders	
• Malnutrition • Renal insufficiency/dialysis • Diabetes mellitus	• Specific mineral deficiencies, e.g. iron, zinc
Other conditions	
• Burns	• Asplenia/hyposplenism

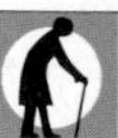

4.8 Ageing and immune senescence

- **T-cell responses**: decline, with reduced delayed type hypersensitivity responses.
- **Antibody production**: decreased for many exogenous antigens. Although autoantibodies are frequently detected, autoimmune disease is less common.
- **Response to vaccination**: reduced, e.g. 30% of healthy older people may not develop protective immunity after influenza vaccination.
- **Allergic disorders and transplant rejection**: less common.
- **Susceptibility to infection**: increased, e.g. community-acquired pneumonia by threefold and urinary tract infection by 20-fold. Latent infections, including tuberculosis and herpes zoster, may be reactivated.
- **Manifestations of inflammation**: may be absent, e.g. lack of pyrexia or leucocytosis.

THE INFLAMMATORY RESPONSE

Inflammation is the response of tissues to injury or infection, and is necessary for normal repair and healing. This section focuses on the generic inflammatory response and its multisystem manifestations. The role of inflammation in specific diseases is illustrated in many other chapters of this book.

Physiology and pathology of inflammation

Acute inflammation

Acute inflammation is the result of rapid and complex interplay between the cells and soluble molecules of the innate immune system. The classical external signs include heat, redness, pain and swelling (calor, rubor, dolor and oedema, Fig. 4.8).

The inflammatory process is initiated by local tissue injury or infection. Damaged epithelial cells produce cytokines and antimicrobial peptides, causing early infiltration of phagocytic cells. As a result, there is production of leukotrienes, prostaglandins, histamine, kinins, anaphylotoxins and inducible nitric oxide synthase within inflamed tissue. The effect is vasodilatation and increased local vascular permeability, which increases trafficking of fluid and cells to the affected tissue. In addition, pro-inflammatory cytokines produced at the site of injury have profound systemic effects. IL-1, TNF-α and IL-6 act on the hypothalamus to raise the temperature set-point, causing fever, and also stimulate the production of acute phase proteins.

Acute phase proteins

Acute phase proteins are produced by the liver in response to inflammatory stimuli and have a wide range of activities. CRP and serum amyloid A may be increased 1000-fold, contributing to host defence and stimulating repair and regeneration. Fibrinogen plays an essential role in wound healing, and α_1-antitrypsin and α_1-antichymotrypsin control the pro-inflammatory cascade by neutralising the enzymes produced by activated neutrophils, preventing widespread tissue destruction. In addition, antioxidants, such as haptoglobin and manganese superoxide dismutase, scavenge for oxygen free radicals, while increased levels of iron-binding proteins, such as ferritin and lactoferrin, decrease the iron available for uptake by bacteria (p. 1023). Immunoglobulins are not acute phase proteins but are often increased in chronic inflammation.

Resolution of inflammation

Resolution of an inflammatory response is crucial for normal healing. This involves active down-modulation

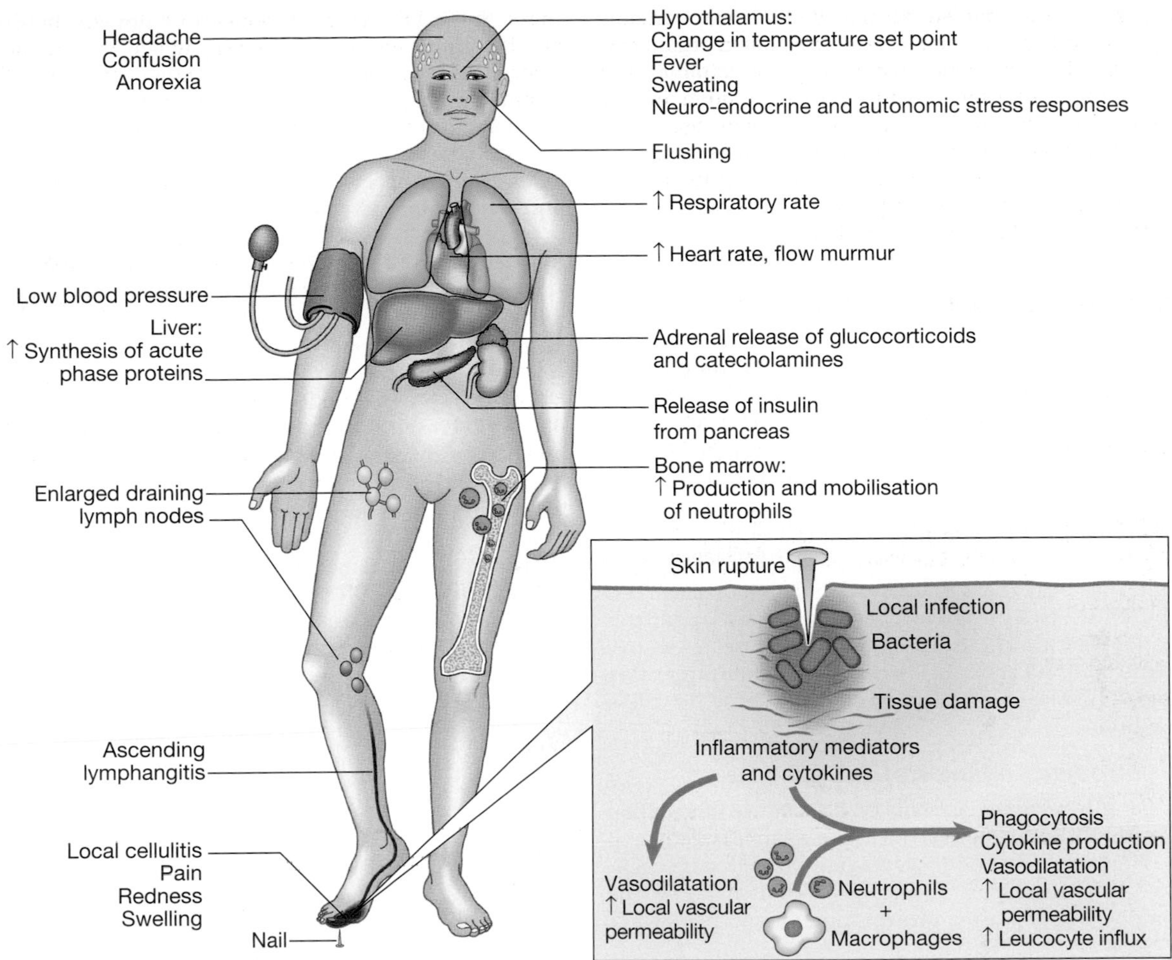

Fig. 4.8 Clinical features of acute inflammation. In this example, the response is to a penetrating injury and infection of the foot.

of inflammatory stimuli and repair of bystander damage to local tissues. Extravasated neutrophils undergo apoptosis and are phagocytosed by macrophages, along with the remains of microorganisms. Macrophages also synthesise collagenase and elastase, which break down local connective tissue and remove debris. Macrophage-derived cytokines, including transforming growth factor (TGF)-β and platelet-derived growth factor, attract fibroblasts and promote synthesis of new collagen, while angiogenic factors stimulate new vessel formation.

Sepsis and septic shock

Septic shock is the clinical manifestation of overwhelming inflammation (p. 190). Failure of normal inhibitory mechanisms results in excessive production of pro-inflammatory cytokines by macrophages, causing hypotension, hypovolaemia, decreased perfusion and tissue oedema. In addition, uncontrolled neutrophil activation causes release of proteases and oxygen free radicals within blood vessels, damaging the vascular endothelium and further increasing capillary permeability. Direct activation of the coagulation pathway combines with endothelial cell disruption to form clots within the damaged vessels. The clinical consequences include cardiovascular collapse, acute respiratory distress syndrome, disseminated intravascular coagulation, multi-organ failure and often death. Septic shock most frequently results from infection with Gram-negative bacteria, because lipopolysaccharide is particularly effective at activating the inflammatory cascade.

Chronic inflammation

In most instances, the development of an active immune response results in either clearance or control of the inflammatory stimulus with minimal local damage. Failure of elimination may result in chronic inflammation. Persisting microorganisms stimulate the ongoing accumulation of neutrophils, macrophages and activated T lymphocytes. If this is associated with local deposition of fibrous connective tissue, a granuloma may form. Granulomas are characteristic of infections such as tuberculosis and leprosy, in which the micro-organism is protected by a robust cell wall which shields it from killing, despite phagocytosis.

Too vigorous or prolonged immune responses may cause bystander tissue damage, known as hypersensitivity responses. The Gell and Coombs classification of hypersensitivity disorders is discussed on page 87.

Investigations in inflammation

Changes associated with inflammation are reflected in many laboratory investigations. Leucocytosis is common, and reflects the transit of activated neutrophils and monocytes to the site of infection. The platelet count may also be increased. The most widely used laboratory measure of acute inflammation is the C-reactive protein (see below). Plasma levels of many other acute phase reactants, including fibrinogen, ferritin and complement components, are increased in response to acute inflammation, while albumin levels are reduced. Chronic inflammation is frequently associated with a normocytic normochromic anaemia of chronic disease (p. 1023).

C-reactive protein

C-reactive protein (CRP) is an acute phase reactant synthesised by the liver, which opsonises invading pathogens. Levels of CRP increase within 6 hours of an inflammatory stimulus and may rise up to 1000-fold. Measurement of CRP provides a direct index of acute inflammation and, because the plasma half-life of CRP is 19 hours, levels fall promptly once the stimulus is removed. Sequential measurement is useful in monitoring disease (Box 4.9). For reasons that remain unclear, some diseases are associated with only minor elevations of CRP, despite unequivocal evidence of active inflammation. These include SLE, systemic sclerosis, ulcerative colitis and leukaemia. However, intercurrent infection does provoke a significant CRP response in these conditions.

Erythrocyte sedimentation rate

In contrast to the CRP, the erythrocyte sedimentation rate (ESR) is an indirect measure of inflammation. It measures how fast erythrocytes fall through anticoagulated blood, and is determined by a combination of the composition of plasma proteins and the morphology of circulating erythrocytes. These factors govern the propensity of red cells to aggregate, which is the major determinant of the ESR. Erythrocytes are inherently negatively charged, and this prevents them clumping together in the blood stream. Plasma proteins are positively charged and an increase in plasma proteins neutralises the surface charge of erythrocytes, overcoming their inherent repulsive forces and causing them to aggregate, or stack like tyres, forming rouleaux. Rouleaux have a higher mass/surface area ratio than single red cells, and therefore sediment faster.

The most common cause of an increased ESR is an acute phase response, which leads to an increase in the concentration of acute phase reactants, including CRP. However, other conditions that do not affect acute phase proteins may alter the composition and concentration of other plasma proteins (see Box 4.9). For example, immunoglobulins comprise a significant proportion of plasma proteins, but do not participate in the acute phase response. Thus, any condition that causes a monoclonal or polyclonal increase in serum immunoglobulins will increase the ESR without a corresponding rise in CRP. In addition, changes in erythrocyte surface area and density influence sedimentation, and abnormal red cell morphology can make rouleaux formation impossible. For these reasons, an inappropriately low ESR occurs in spherocytosis and sickle cell anaemia.

As CRP is a simple and sensitive early indicator of the acute phase response, it is increasingly used in preference to the ESR. If both ESR and CRP are used, any discrepancy should be resolved by assessing the individual determinants of the ESR, i.e. full blood count and blood film, serum immunoglobulins (IgG, IgA and IgM) and protein electrophoresis. The IgE concentration in

4.9 Conditions commonly associated with abnormal CRP and/or ESR

Condition	Consequence	Effect on CRP[1]	Effect on ESR[2]
Acute bacterial, fungal or viral infection	Acute phase response	Increased (range 50–150 mg/L; in severe infections may be > 300 mg/L)	Increased
Necrotising bacterial infection	Profound acute inflammatory response	Increased +++ (may be > 300 mg/L)	Increased
Acute inflammatory diseases, e.g. Crohn's disease, polymyalgia rheumatica	Acute phase response	Increased (range 50–150 mg/L)	Increased
Chronic bacterial or fungal infection, e.g. localised abscess, bacterial endocarditis or tuberculosis	Acute and chronic inflammatory response: increased acute phase proteins with polyclonal increase in immunoglobulins	Increased (range 50–150 mg/L)	Increase disproportionate to CRP
SLE, Sjögren's syndrome	Chronic inflammatory response with polyclonal increase in immunoglobulins	Normal (paradoxically)	Increased
Multiple myeloma	Monoclonal increase in immunoglobulin without acute inflammation	Normal	Increased
Pregnancy, old age, end-stage renal disease	Normal immunoglobulins but increased fibrinogen	Normal	Moderately increased

[1]Reference range < 10 mg/L.
[2]Reference range: adult males < 10 mm/hr, adult females < 20 mm/hr.

plasma is very low and does not contribute significantly to the ESR.

Plasma viscosity

Plasma viscosity is another surrogate measure of plasma protein concentration. Like the ESR, it is affected by the concentration of large plasma proteins, including fibrinogen and immunoglobulins. However, it is not affected by properties of erythrocytes and is generally considered to be more reliable than the ESR.

Presenting problems in inflammation

In most patients presenting with the manifestations of acute inflammation shown in Figure 4.8, it is possible to identify the source of the problem quickly and to assess the consequences, as discussed in other chapters. Systemic manifestations of inflammation include fever (p. 296), leucocytosis (p. 1005) and shock (p. 190).

Unexplained raised ESR

The ESR should not be used to screen asymptomatic patients for the presence of disease. However, in the era of frequent routine laboratory testing, an unexplained raised ESR is a common problem.

Clinical assessment

A comprehensive history and examination are crucial. Extreme elevations in the ESR (> 100 mm/hr) rarely occur in the absence of significant disease (see Box 4.9).

Investigations

Assessing the CRP, serum immunoglobulins and electrophoresis, and urine electrophoresis will help determine whether the elevation in ESR is due to an inflammatory process (see Box 4.9).

A full blood count and film may show a normocytic, normochromic anaemia, which occurs in many chronic diseases. Leucocytosis may reflect infection, inflammatory disease or tissue necrosis. Neutrophilia suggests infection or acute inflammation. Atypical lymphocytes may occur in some chronic infections, such as cytomegalovirus (CMV) and Epstein–Barr virus (EBV).

Abnormalities in liver function suggest either a local infective process (hepatitis, hepatic abscess or biliary sepsis) or systemic disease, including malignancy.

Blood and urine cultures should be performed. It may be relevant to measure antinuclear and antineutrophil cytoplasmic antibodies, and to exclude chronic infections, including HIV and syphilis.

In the unusual circumstances when ESR is elevated but both CRP and immunoglobulins are normal, fibrinogen should be measured. Elevated fibrinogen causes a higher ESR in older people, women, and patients with renal or heart failure, obesity and diabetes mellitus.

Imaging

If indicated by the clinical and laboratory features, a chest X-ray and abdominal computed tomography (CT) scan may identify a source of unknown infection or malignancy. An abdominal and pelvic ultrasound may identify hepatic lesions, abdominal nodes and local intra-abdominal or pelvic abscesses. Magnetic resonance imaging (MRI) is more appropriate for the diagnosis of soft tissue or bone/joint infections. Echocardiography is used to look for vegetations and assess valve function in suspected bacterial endocarditis. White cell scans are rarely indicated but may be useful in identifying the site of pyogenic infection. An isotope bone scan may provide evidence of malignancy or focal bone infection.

Periodic fever syndromes

These rare disorders are characterised by recurrent episodes of fever and systemic inflammation, associated with an elevated acute phase response.

Familial Mediterranean fever

Familial Mediterranean fever (FMF) is the most common of the familial periodic fevers, predominantly affecting Mediterranean people, including Arabs, Turks, Sephardic Jews and Armenians. It results from mutations of the *MEFV* gene, which encodes a protein called pyrin. Pyrin regulates neutrophil-mediated inflammation by indirectly suppressing the production of IL-1. FMF is characterised by recurrent painful attacks of fever associated with peritonitis, pleuritis and arthritis, which last for a few hours to 4 days and which are associated with markedly increased CRP levels. Symptoms resolve completely between episodes. The majority of individuals have their first attack before the age of 20 years. The major complication of FMF is AA amyloidosis (see below). Colchicine significantly reduces the number of febrile episodes in 90% of patients but is ineffective during acute attacks.

Mevalonate kinase deficiency

Mevalonate kinase deficiency (previously known as hyper-IgD syndrome, or HIDS) is an autosomal recessive disorder that causes recurrent attacks of fever, abdominal pain, diarrhoea, lymphadenopathy, arthralgia, skin lesions and aphthous ulceration. Most patients are from Western Europe, particularly the Netherlands and northern France. Mevalonate kinase is involved in the metabolism of cholesterol, but why mutations in its gene cause an inflammatory periodic fever remains unknown. Serum IgD and IgA levels are persistently elevated, and CRP levels are increased during acute attacks. Standard anti-inflammatory drugs (including colchicine and steroids) are ineffective.

TNF receptor-associated periodic syndrome

TNF receptor-associated periodic syndrome (TRAPS), also known as Hibernian fever, is an autosomal dominant syndrome, causing recurrent periodic fever, arthralgia, myalgia, serositis and rashes, which has been reported in many ethnic groups. Attacks may be prolonged (lasting over 1 week). During a typical attack, there is neutrophilia, increased CRP and elevated IgA levels. The diagnosis can be confirmed by low serum levels of the soluble type 1 TNF receptor and by analysis of the *TNFRSF1A* gene. As in FMF, the major complication is amyloidosis, and regular screening for proteinuria is advised. TRAPS responds to systemic corticosteroids and to biological therapies, including soluble TNF receptor therapy and IL-l receptor antagonists (p. 1102).

Amyloidosis

The amyloidoses are a group of acquired and hereditary disorders characterised by extracellular deposition of insoluble proteins (Box 4.10). These complex deposits consist of fibrils of the specific protein involved, linked to glycosaminoglycans, proteoglycans and serum amyloid P (SAP). Protein accumulation may be localised or systemic, and the clinical manifestations depend upon the organ(s) affected. The diagnosis of amyloidosis should be considered in all cases of unexplained nephrotic syndrome (p. 476), cardiomyopathy (p. 636) and peripheral neuropathy (p. 1223).

Diagnosis

The diagnosis is established by biopsy, which may be of an affected organ, rectum or subcutaneous fat. The pathognomonic histological feature is apple-green birefringence of amyloid deposits when stained with Congo red dye and viewed under polarised light. Immunohistochemical staining can identify the type of amyloid fibril present. Quantitative scintigraphy with radio-labelled SAP is a valuable tool in determining the overall load and distribution of amyloid deposits.

Management

The aims of treatment are to support the function of affected organs and, in acquired amyloidosis, to prevent further amyloid deposition through treatment of the primary cause. When the latter is possible, regression of existing amyloid deposits may occur. Liver transplantation may provide definitive treatment in selected patients with hereditary transthyretin amyloidosis.

AUTOIMMUNE DISEASE

Autoimmunity can be defined as the presence of immune responses against self tissue. This may be a harmless phenomenon, identified only by the presence of low titre autoantibodies or autoreactive T cells. However, if these responses cause significant organ damage, this results in autoimmune diseases, which are a major cause of chronic morbidity and disability, affecting up to 1 in 30 adults at some time (Box 4.11).

Pathophysiology of autoimmunity

Immunological tolerance

Autoimmunity results from the failure of immunological tolerance, the process by which the immune system recognises and accepts self tissue. There are a number of mechanisms of immune tolerance. Central tolerance occurs during lymphocyte development, when T and B lymphocytes that recognise self antigens are eliminated before they differentiate into fully immunocompetent cells. This process is most active in fetal life, but

4.10 Amyloid disorders

Disorder	Pathological basis	Predisposing conditions	Other features
Acquired systemic amyloidosis			
Reactive (AA) amyloidosis	Increased production of serum amyloid A as part of prolonged or recurrent acute inflammatory response	Chronic infection (TB, bronchiectasis, chronic abscess, osteomyelitis) Chronic inflammatory diseases (untreated rheumatoid arthritis, FMF)	90% of patients present with non-selective proteinuria or nephrotic syndrome
Light chain amyloidosis (AL)	Increased production of monoclonal light chain	Monoclonal gammopathies, including myeloma, benign gammopathies and plasmacytoma	Restrictive cardiomyopathy, peripheral and autonomic neuropathy, carpal tunnel syndrome, proteinuria, spontaneous purpura, amyloid nodules and plaques. Macroglossia occurs rarely but is pathognomonic. Prognosis is poor
Dialysis-associated (Aβ2M) amyloidosis	Accumulation of circulating β_2-microglobulin due to failure of renal catabolism in kidney failure	Renal dialysis	Carpal tunnel syndrome, chronic arthropathy and pathological fractures secondary to amyloid bone cyst formation. Manifestations occur 5–10 yrs after the start of dialysis
Senile systemic amyloidosis	Normal transthyretin protein deposited in tissues	Age > 70 yrs	Feature of normal ageing (affects > 90% of 90-year-olds). Usually asymptomatic
Hereditary systemic amyloidosis			
> 20 forms of hereditary systemic amyloidosis	Production of protein with an abnormal structure that predisposes to amyloid fibril formation. Most commonly due to mutations in *transthyretin* gene	Autosomal dominant inheritance	Peripheral and autonomic neuropathy, cardiomyopathy Renal involvement unusual 10% of gene carriers are asymptomatic throughout life

(FMF = familial Mediterranean fever)

4.11 The spectrum of autoimmune disease

Type	Disease	Page no.
Organ-specific		
Immune response directed against localised antigens	Graves' disease	747
	Hashimoto's thyroiditis	751
	Addison's disease	777
	Pernicious anaemia	1025
	Type 1 diabetes	803
	Sympathetic ophthalmoplegia	1169
	Multiple sclerosis	1188
	Goodpasture's syndrome	500
	Pemphigus vulgaris	1294
	Bullous pemphigoid	1292
	Idiopathic thrombocytopenic purpura	1050
	Autoimmune haemolytic anaemia	1029
	Myasthenia gravis	1226
	Primary antiphospholipid syndrome	1055
	Rheumatoid arthritis	1096
	Dermatomyositis	1114
	Primary biliary cirrhosis	963
	Autoimmune hepatitis	962
	Sjögren's syndrome	1114
Multisystem		
Immune response directed to widespread target antigens	Systemic sclerosis	1112
	Mixed connective tissue disease	1113
	SLE	1109

continues throughout life as immature lymphocytes are generated. Inevitably some autoreactive cells evade deletion and reach the peripheral tissues, where they are controlled by peripheral tolerance mechanisms. These include suppression of autoreactive cells by regulatory T cells, generation of functional hyporesponsiveness ('anergy') in lymphocytes which encounter antigen in the absence of the co-stimulatory signals that accompany inflammation, and T cell death by apoptosis.

Autoimmune diseases develop when self-reactive lymphocytes escape from these tolerance mechanisms and become activated.

Factors predisposing to autoimmune disease

Autoimmune diseases are much more common in women than in men, for reasons which remain unclear. Most autoimmune diseases have multiple genetic determinants (Box 4.12). Many are associated with variation at specific HLA loci, reflecting the importance of HLA genes in shaping lymphocyte responses. Other important susceptibility genes include those determining cytokine activity, co-stimulation and cell death. Even though some of these associations are the strongest that have been identified in polygenic diseases (p. 68), they have limited predictive value, and are not useful in determining disease risk for individual patients. Several acquired factors can trigger autoimmunity in genetically predisposed individuals, including infection, cigarette smoking and hormone levels. The most widely studied of these is infection, as occurs in acute rheumatic fever following streptococcal infection or reactive arthritis following bacterial infection. A number of mechanisms have been postulated, such as cross-reactivity between the infectious pathogen and self antigens (molecular mimicry), and release of sequestered antigens, which are not usually visible to the immune system, from damaged tissue. Alternatively, infection may result in the production of inflammatory cytokines, which overwhelm the normal control mechanisms that prevent bystander damage. Occasionally, the development of autoimmune disease is a side-effect of drug treatment. For example, the metabolic products of the anaesthetic agent halothane bind to liver enzymes, resulting in a structurally novel protein. This is recognised as a new (foreign) antigen by the immune system, and the autoantibodies and activated T cells directed against it may cause hepatic necrosis.

4.12 Some genetic variations predisposing to autoimmune diseases

Gene	Function	Diseases
HLA complex	Key determinants of antigen presentation to T cells	Most autoimmune diseases
PTPN22	Regulates T- and B-cell receptor signalling	Rheumatoid arthritis, type 1 diabetes, SLE
CTLA4	Important co-stimulatory molecule which transmits inhibitory signals to T cells	Rheumatoid arthritis, type 1 diabetes
TNFRSF1A	Control of TNF network	Multiple sclerosis
ATG5	Autophagy	SLE

Classification of autoimmune diseases

The spectrum of autoimmune diseases is broad. They can be classified by organ involvement (see Box 4.11) or by the predominant mechanism responsible for tissue damage. The Gell and Coombs classification of hypersensitivity is the most widely used, and distinguishes four types of immune response which result in bystander tissue damage (Box 4.13).

- *Type I hypersensitivity* is relevant in allergy but is not associated with autoimmune disease.
- In *type II hypersensitivity*, injury is localised to a single tissue or organ and is mediated by specific autoantibodies.
- *Type III hypersensitivity* is a generalised reaction resulting from immune complex deposition which initiates activation of the classical complement cascade, as well as recruitment and activation of phagocytes and CD4$^+$ lymphocytes. The site of immune complex deposition is determined by the relative amount of antibody, size of the immune complexes, nature of the antigen and local haemodynamics. Generalised deposition of immune complexes gives rise to systemic diseases such as SLE.
- In *type IV hypersensitivity*, activated T cells and macrophages mediate phagocytosis and tissue damage.

4.13 Gell and Coombs classification of hypersensitivity diseases

Type	Mechanism	Example of disease in response to exogenous agent	Example of autoimmune disease
Type I Immediate hypersensitivity	IgE-mediated mast cell degranulation	Allergic disease	None described
Type II Antibody-mediated	Binding of cytotoxic IgG or IgM antibodies to antigens on cell surface causes cell killing	ABO blood transfusion reaction Hyperacute transplant rejection	Autoimmune haemolytic anaemia Idiopathic thrombocytopenic purpura Goodpasture's disease
Type III Immune complex-mediated	IgG or IgM antibodies bind soluble antigen to form immune complexes which trigger classical complement pathway activation	Serum sickness Farmer's lung	SLE
Type IV Delayed type	Activation of T cells and phagocytes	Acute cellular transplant rejection Nickel hypersensitivity	Type 1 diabetes Hashimoto's thyroiditis

Investigations in autoimmunity

Autoantibodies

A number of autoantibodies can be identified in the laboratory and are used in disease diagnosis and monitoring, as discussed elsewhere in this book (e.g. p. 1067). Antibodies are quantified either by titre (the minimal dilution at which the antibody can be detected) or by concentration (in standardised units).

Measures of complement activation

Quantitation of complement components may be useful in the evaluation of immune complex-mediated diseases. Classical complement pathway activation leads to a decrease in circulating (unactivated) C4, and is often also associated with decreased C3 levels. Serial measurement of C3 and C4 is a useful surrogate measure of immune complex formation.

Cryoglobulins

Cryoglobulins are antibodies directed against other immunoglobulins, and which form immune complexes that precipitate in the cold. They are classified into three types on the basis of the properties of the immunoglobulin involved (Box 4.14). Testing for cryoglobulins requires the transport of a serum specimen to the laboratory at 37°C. Cryoglobulins should not be confused with cold agglutinins; the latter are autoantibodies specifically directed against the I/i antigen on the surface of red cells, which can cause intravascular haemolysis in the cold (p. 1030).

4.14 Classification of cryoglobulins

	Type I	Type II	Type III
Immunoglobulin isotype and specificity	Isolated monoclonal IgM paraprotein with no particular specificity	Immune complexes formed by monoclonal IgM paraprotein directed towards constant region of IgG	Immune complexes formed by polyclonal IgM or IgG directed towards constant region of IgG
Prevalence	25%	25%	50%
Disease association	Lymphoproliferative disease, especially Waldenström macroglobulinaemia (p. 1045)	Infection, particularly hepatitis B and hepatitis C; lymphoproliferative disease	Infection, particularly hepatitis B and C; autoimmune disease, including rheumatoid arthritis and SLE
Symptoms	*Hyperviscosity*: Raynaud's phenomenon Acrocyanosis Retinal vessel occlusion Arterial and venous thrombosis	*Small-vessel vasculitis*: Purpuric rash Arthralgia Cutaneous ulceration Hepatosplenomegaly Glomerulonephritis Raynaud's phenomenon	*Small-vessel vasculitis*: Purpuric rash Arthralgia Cutaneous ulceration Hepatosplenomegaly Glomerulonephritis Raynaud's phenomenon
Protein electrophoresis	Monoclonal IgM paraprotein	Monoclonal IgM paraprotein	No monoclonal paraprotein
Rheumatoid factor	Negative	Strongly positive	Strongly positive
Complement	Normal	Decreased C4	Decreased C4

ALLERGY

Allergic diseases are a common and increasing cause of illness, affecting between 15% and 20% of the population at some time. They comprise a range of disorders from mild to life-threatening, and affect many organs. Atopy is the tendency to produce an exaggerated IgE immune response to otherwise harmless environmental substances, while an allergic disease can be defined as the clinical manifestation of this inappropriate IgE immune response.

Pathology of allergy

Normally, the immune system does not make detectable responses to the many environmental substances to which it is exposed daily. However, in an allergic reaction, initial exposure to an otherwise harmless exogenous substance (known as an allergen) triggers the production of specific IgE antibodies by activated B cells (Fig. 4.9). These IgE antibodies bind to the surface of mast cells via high-affinity IgE receptors, a step that is not itself associated with clinical sequelae. However, upon re-exposure, the allergen binds to membrane-bound IgE which activates the mast cells, releasing a variety of mediators (the early phase response, Box 4.15). This type I hypersensitivity reaction is the basis of the symptoms of allergic reactions, which range from sneezing and rhinorrhoea to anaphylaxis (Box 4.16).

In some patients, the early phase response is followed by persistent activation of mast cells, manifest by ongoing swelling and local inflammation. This is known as the late phase reaction and is mediated by basophils, eosinophils and macrophages. Long-standing or recurrent allergic inflammation may give rise to a chronic inflammatory response characterised by a complex infiltrate of macrophages, eosinophils and T lymphocytes, in addition to mast cells and basophils. Once this has been established, inhibition of mast cell mediators with antihistamines is clinically ineffective.

Occasionally, mast cell activation may be non-specifically triggered through other signals, such as neuropeptides, anaphylotoxins and bacterial peptides.

Susceptibility to allergic diseases

The incidence of allergic diseases is increasing. This trend is largely unexplained but one widely held theory is the 'hygiene hypothesis'. This proposes that infections in early life are critically important in maturation of the immune response and bias the immune system against the development of allergies. It is suggested that the high prevalence of allergic disease is the penalty for the decreased exposure to infection that has resulted from improvements in sanitation and health care.

A number of factors predispose to allergic diseases, the strongest of which is a family history. A wide array of genetic determinants of disease susceptibility have been identified, including genes controlling innate immune responses, cytokine production, IgE levels and the ability of the epithelial barrier to protect against environmental agents. Contributory environmental factors include bacterial and viral infection, pollutants and cigarette smoke.

4.15 Products of mast cell degranulation

Mediator	Biological effects
Preformed and stored within granules	
Histamine	Vasodilatation, chemotaxis, bronchoconstriction, increased capillary permeability, increased mucus secretion
Tryptase	Bronchoconstriction, activates complement C3
Eosinophil chemotactic factor	Eosinophil chemotaxis
Neutrophil chemotactic factor	Neutrophil chemotaxis
Synthesised on activation of mast cells	
Leukotrienes	Increase vascular permeability, chemotaxis, mucus secretion, smooth muscle contraction
Prostaglandins	Bronchoconstriction, platelet aggregation, vasodilatation
Thromboxanes	Bronchoconstriction
Platelet-activating factor	Bronchoconstriction, chemotaxis of eosinophils and neutrophils

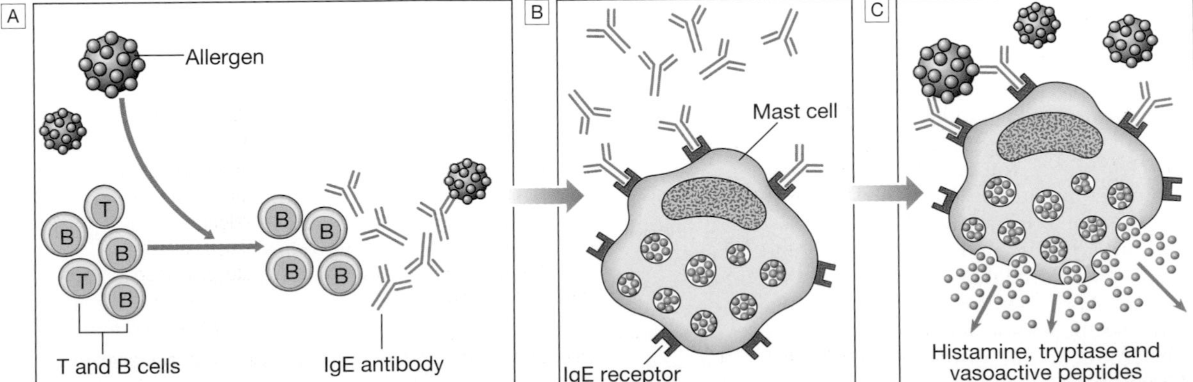

Fig. 4.9 Type I (immediate) hypersensitivity response. **A** After an encounter with allergen, B cells produce IgE antibody against the allergen. **B** Specific IgE antibodies bind to circulating mast cells via high-affinity IgE cell surface receptors. **C** On re-encounter with allergen, the allergen binds to the IgE antibody-coated mast cells. This triggers mast cell activation with release of vasoactive mediators (see Box 4.15).

4.16 Common allergic diseases

• Urticaria	p. 1290
• Angioedema	p. 93
• Atopic dermatitis	p. 1283
• Allergic conjunctivitis	pp. 1105, 1107
• Allergic rhinitis (hay fever)	p. 725
• Allergic asthma	p. 666
• Food allergy	p. 887
• Drug allergy	p. 1303
• Allergy to insect venom	p. 94
• Anaphylaxis	p. 91

Presenting problems in allergy

A general approach to the allergic patient

Common presentations of allergic disease are shown in Box 4.16. This chapter describes the general principles of the approach to the allergic patient and some of the more severe manifestations of allergy.

Clinical assessment

When assessing possible allergic disease, it is important to identify what the patient means by allergy, as up to 20% of the UK population describe themselves as having a food allergy, although fewer than 1% have an IgE-mediated hypersensitivity reaction confirmed on double blind challenge. The nature of symptoms should be established and specific triggers identified, along with the predictability of a reaction, and the time lag between exposure to a potential allergen and onset of symptoms. An allergic reaction usually occurs within minutes of exposure and provokes predictable symptoms (angioedema, urticaria, wheezing and so on). Specific enquiry should be made about other allergic symptoms, past and present, and about family history of allergic disease. Potential allergens in the home and workplace should be identified, and a detailed drug history should always be taken, including compliance, side-effects and the use of complementary therapies.

Investigations

Skin prick tests

These are the mainstay of allergy testing. A droplet of diluted standardised allergen solution is placed on the forearm and the skin is superficially punctured through the droplet with a sterile lancet. After 15 minutes, a positive response is indicated by a local weal and flare response at least 2 mm larger than the negative control. A major advantage of skin prick testing is that patients can clearly see the results, which may be useful in gaining compliance with avoidance measures. Disadvantages include the remote risk of a severe allergic reaction, so resuscitation facilities should be available. Results are unreliable in patients with extensive skin disease. Antihistamines inhibit the magnitude of the response and should be discontinued before testing; corticosteroids do not influence test results.

Specific IgE tests

An alternative to skin prick testing is the quantitation of IgE directed against the putative allergen. The sensitivity and specificity of specific IgE tests (previously known as radioallergosorbent tests, RAST) are lower than skin prick tests. However, IgE tests may be very useful if skin testing is inappropriate: for example, in patients taking antihistamines or those who have severe skin disease or dermatographism. They can also be used to test for cross-reactivity between insect venoms, and post mortem to identify allergens responsible for lethal anaphylaxis.

There is no indication for testing of specific IgG antibodies to allergens in the investigation of allergic diseases.

Supervised exposure to allergen (challenge test)

Allergen challenges are usually performed in specialist centres, and include bronchial provocation testing, nasal challenge and food challenge. These may be particularly useful in the investigation of occupational asthma or food allergy.

Mast cell tryptase

After a systemic allergic reaction, the circulating level of mast cell mediators increases dramatically. Tryptase is the most stable of these and serum levels peak at 1–2 hours. Measurement of serum mast cell tryptase is extremely useful in investigating a possible anaphylactic event. Ideally, measurements should be made at the time of the reaction, and 3 hours and 24 hours later.

Non-specific markers of atopic disease: total serum IgE and eosinophilia

Peripheral blood eosinophilia is common in atopic individuals. However, eosinophilia of more than 20% or an absolute eosinophil count over 1.5×10^9/L should initiate a search for a non-atopic cause (p. 311).

Atopy is the most common cause of elevated total IgE in developed countries. However, there are many other causes, including parasite and helminth infections (pp. 369 and 381), lymphoma (p. 1041), drug reactions and Churg–Strauss vasculitis (p. 1118). Moreover, significant allergic disease can occur despite a normal total IgE level. Thus total IgE quantitation is not indicated in the routine investigation of allergic disease.

Management

- *Avoidance of the allergen* should be rigorously attempted, and the advice of specialist dietitians and occupational physicians may be required.
- *Antihistamines* block histamine H_1 receptors, thereby inhibiting the effects of histamine release. Long-acting, non-sedating preparations are particularly useful for prophylaxis against frequent attacks.
- *Corticosteroids* down-regulate pro-inflammatory cytokine production. They are highly effective in allergic disease and, if used topically, their adverse effects may be minimised.
- *Sodium cromoglicate* stabilises the mast cell membrane, inhibiting release of vasoactive mediators. It is effective as a prophylactic agent in asthma and allergic rhinitis, but has no role in acute attacks. It is poorly absorbed and therefore ineffective in the management of food allergies.
- *Antigen-specific immunotherapy* involves the sequential administration of escalating amounts of dilute allergen over a prolonged period of time. Its mechanism of action is unknown, but it is highly

effective in the prevention of insect venom anaphylaxis, and allergic rhinitis secondary to grass pollen (Box 4.17). The traditional route of administration is via subcutaneous injections, which carry a risk of anaphylaxis and should only be performed in specialised centres. More recently, sublingual immunotherapy has been shown to be effective in the management of moderate grass pollen allergy, and clinical trials of immunotherapy for food allergy are ongoing.
- *Omalizumab*, a monoclonal antibody against IgE, inhibits the binding of IgE to mast cells and basophils. It is effective in moderate and severe allergic asthma and rhinitis.

EBM 4.17 Immunotherapy for allergy

'Immunotherapy is effective for treatment of allergic rhinitis, allergic asthma and stinging insect hypersensitivity. Clinical studies to date do not support the use of allergen immunotherapy for food hypersensitivity, chronic urticaria and/or angioedema.'

- Joint Task Force on Practice Parameters. Ann Allergy Asthma Immunol 2003; 90:1–40.

For further information: www.cochrane.org/cochrane-reviews

- *Preloaded self-injectable adrenaline (epinephrine)* may be life-saving in acute anaphylaxis.

Anaphylaxis

Anaphylaxis is a potentially life-threatening, systemic allergic reaction caused by the release of histamine and other vasoactive mediators from mast cells. The risk of death is increased in patients with pre-existing asthma, particularly if this is poorly controlled, and when treatment with adrenaline (epinephrine) is delayed.

Clinical assessment

The clinical features are shown in Figure 4.10. The severity of a reaction should be assessed; the time between allergen exposure and onset of symptoms provides a guide. Enquiry should be made about potential triggers; if these are not immediately obvious, a detailed history of the previous 24 hours may be helpful. The most common triggers are foods, latex, insect venom and drugs (Box 4.18). A history of previous allergic responses to the offending agent is common. The route of allergen exposure may influence the principal clinical features of a reaction; for example, if an allergen is inhaled, the major symptom is frequently wheezing. Features of anaphylaxis may overlap with the direct toxic effects of drugs and venoms (Ch. 9). Potentiating factors, such as

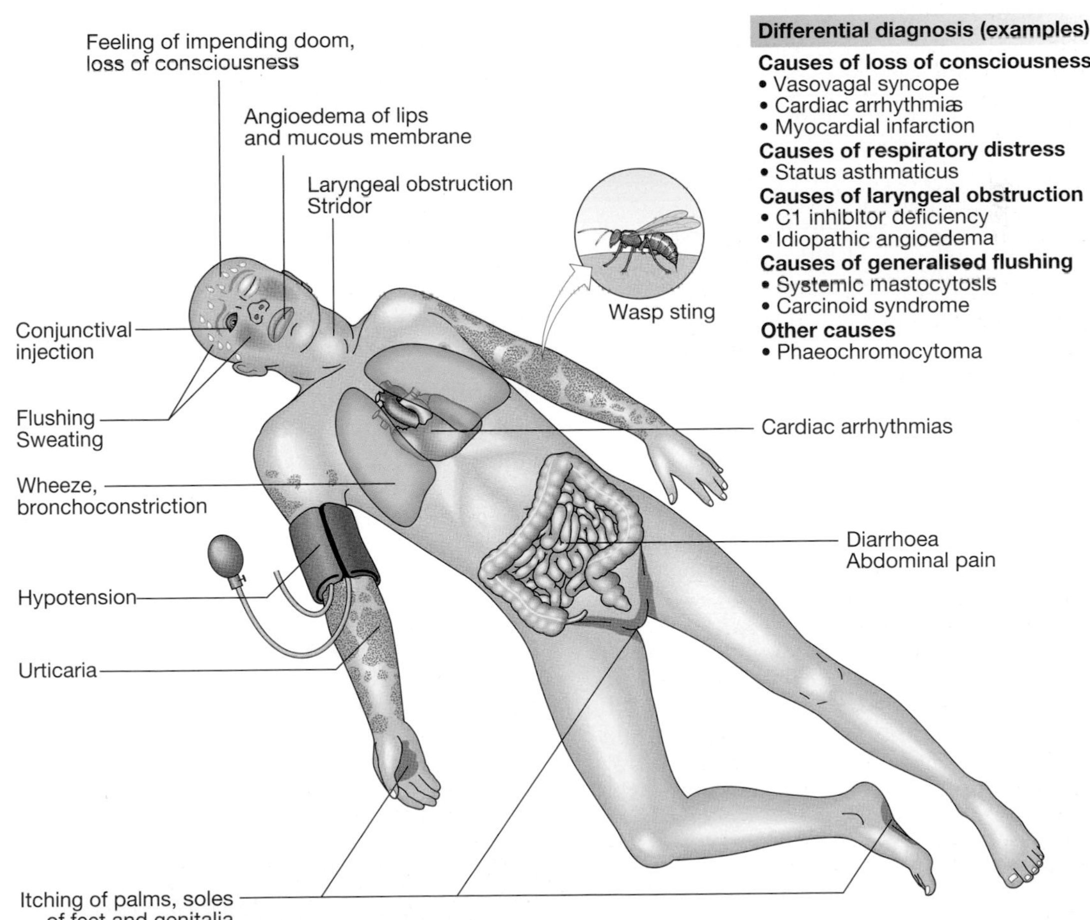

Fig. 4.10 Clinical manifestations of anaphylaxis. In this example, the response is to an insect sting containing venom to which the patient is allergic.

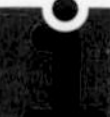

4.18 Common causes of systemic allergic reactions

Anaphylaxis: IgE-mediated mast cell degranulation

Foods
- Peanuts
- Tree nuts
- Fish and shellfish
- Milk
- Eggs
- Soy products

Insect stings
- Bee venom
- Wasp venom

Chemicals, drugs and other foreign proteins
- Intravenous anaesthetic agents, e.g. suxamethonium
- Penicillin and other antibiotics
- Latex

Anaphylactoid: non-IgE-mediated mast cell degranulation

Drugs
- Aspirin and non-steroidal anti-inflammatory drugs (NSAIDs)
- Opiates
- Radiocontrast media

Physical
- Exercise
- Cold

Idiopathic
- No cause is identified in 20% of patients with anaphylaxis

exercise or alcohol, can lower the threshold for an anaphylactic event.

A number of conditions may mimic anaphylaxis (see Fig. 4.10). Anaphylactoid reactions result from the non-specific degranulation of mast cells by drugs, chemicals or other triggers (see Box 4.18), and do not involve IgE antibodies. The clinical presentations are indistinguishable, and in the acute situation discriminating between them is unnecessary. However, this may be important in identifying precipitating factors and appropriate avoidance measures.

Investigations

Measurement of serum mast cell tryptase concentrations is useful to confirm the diagnosis. Specific IgE tests may be preferable to skin prick tests when investigating patients with a history of anaphylaxis.

Management

Anaphylaxis is an acute medical emergency (Box 4.19).

Individuals who have recovered from an anaphylactic event should be referred for specialist assessment. The aim is to identify the trigger factor, to educate the patient regarding avoidance and management of subsequent episodes, and to identify whether specific treatment, such as immunotherapy, is indicated. If the trigger factor cannot be identified or cannot be avoided, recurrence is common. Patients who have previously experienced an anaphylactic event should be prescribed self-injectable adrenaline (epinephrine), and they and their families or carers should be instructed on its use (Box 4.20). The use of a MedicAlert (or similar) bracelet will increase the likelihood that adrenaline will be administered in an emergency. Issues most pertinent to serious allergy in adolescents are shown in Box 4.21.

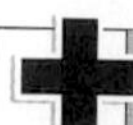

4.19 Emergency management of anaphylaxis

Prevent further contact with allergen
- e.g. Removal of bee sting

Ensure airway patency

Administer *intramuscular* adrenaline (epinephrine) promptly
- Adult dose: 0.3–0.5 mL 1 : 1000 solution
- Acts within minutes
- Repeat at 5–10-min intervals if initial response is inadequate

Administer antihistamines
- e.g. Chlorphenamine 10 mg IM or slow IV injection
- Directly opposes effects of histamine released by activated mast cells

Administer corticosteroids
- e.g. Hydrocortisone 200 mg IV
- Prevents rebound symptoms in severely affected patients

Provide supportive treatments
- e.g. Nebulised β_2-agonists to decrease bronchoconstriction
- Intravenous fluids to restore or maintain blood pressure
- Oxygen

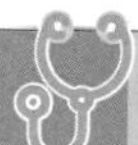

4.20 How to prescribe self-injectable adrenaline (epinephrine)

Prescription of an adrenaline auto-injector is usually initiated by a specialist (e.g. immunologist or allergist)

Indications
- Anaphylaxis to allergens which are difficult to avoid, e.g. insect venom and foods
- Idiopathic anaphylactic reactions
- History of severe localised reactions with high risk of future anaphylaxis, e.g. reaction to trace allergen or likely repeated exposure to allergen
- History of severe localised reactions with high risk of adverse outcome, should anaphylaxis occur, e.g. poorly controlled asthma, lack of access to emergency care

Relative contraindications

Risk of arrhythmia or acute coronary syndrome
- Ischaemic heart disease, uncontrolled hypertension
- Tricyclic antidepressants, monoamine oxidase inhibitors, cocaine use

Key practice points

Patient and family education
- Know when and how to use the device
- Carry the device at all times
- Seek medical assistance immediately after use
- Wear an alert bracelet or necklace
- Include the school in education for young patients

Prescriptions
- Specify the brand of auto-injector, as they have different triggering mechanisms
- Always prescribe two syringes
- Avoid β-blockers, as they may increase the severity of an anaphylactic reaction and reduce the response to adrenaline

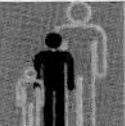

4.21 Allergy in adolescence

- **Resolution of childhood allergy**: most children affected by allergy to milk, egg, soybean or wheat will grow out of their food allergies by adolescence. However, allergies to peanuts, tree nuts, fish and shellfish are frequently life-long.
- **Risk-taking behaviour and fatal anaphylaxis**: serious allergy is increasingly common in adolescents, and this is the highest-risk group for fatal, food-induced anaphylaxis. Food-allergic teenagers are more likely than adults to eat unsafe foods, deny reaction symptoms and delay emergency treatment.
- **Emotional impact of food allergies**: some adolescents neglect to carry a prescribed adrenaline (epinephrine) auto-injector because of the associated nuisance and/or stigma. Surveys of food-allergic teenagers reveal that many take risks because they feel socially isolated by their allergy.

Angioedema

Angioedema is the episodic, localised, non-pitting swelling of submucous or subcutaneous tissues. This most frequently affects the face (Fig. 4.11), extremities and genitalia. Involvement of the larynx or tongue may cause life-threatening respiratory tract obstruction, and oedema of the intestinal mucosa may cause abdominal pain and distension.

In most cases, the underlying mechanism is degranulation of mast cells. However, angioedema may occasionally be mediated by increased local bradykinin concentration (Box 4.22). Differentiating the mechanism of angioedema is important in determining appropriate investigations and treatment.

A

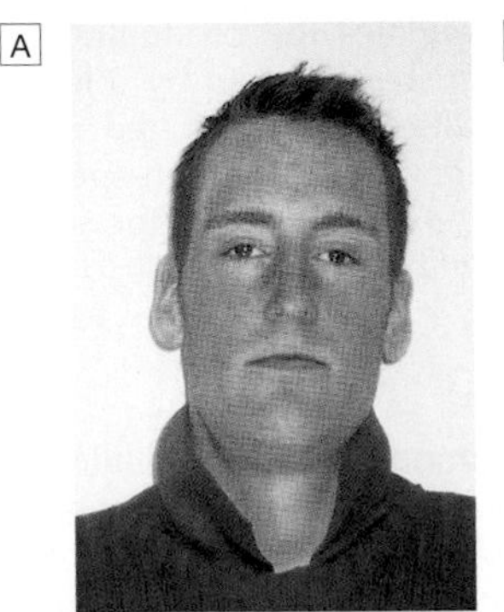

B

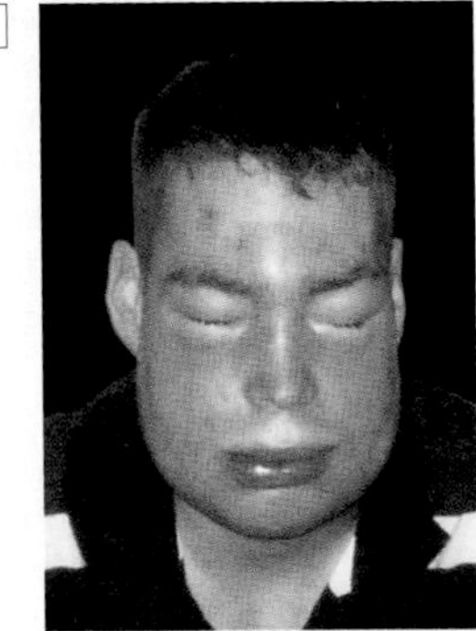

Fig. 4.11 Angioedema. This young man has hereditary angioedema. **A** Normal appearance. **B** During an acute attack. From Helbert 2006 – see p. 96.

4.22 Types of angioedema

	Allergic reaction to specific trigger	Idiopathic angioedema	Hereditary angioedema	ACE-inhibitor associated angioedema
Pathogenesis	IgE-mediated degranulation of mast cells	Non-IgE-mediated degranulation of mast cells	C1 inhibitor deficiency, with resulting increased local bradykinin concentration	Inhibition of breakdown of bradykinin
Key mediator	Histamine	Histamine	Bradykinin	Bradykinin
Prevalence	Common	Common	Rare autosomal dominant disorder	0.1–0.2% of patients treated with ACE inhibitors
Clinical features	Usually associated with urticaria History of other allergies common Follows exposure to specific allergen, e.g. food, animal dander or insect venom	Usually associated with urticaria May be triggered by physical stimuli, such as heat, pressure or exercise Dermatographism common Occasionally associated with infection or thyroid disease	Not associated with urticaria or other features of allergy Does not cause anaphylaxis May cause life-threatening respiratory tract obstruction Can cause severe abdominal pain	Not associated with urticaria Does not cause anaphylaxis Usually affects the head and neck, and may cause life-threatening respiratory tract obstruction Can occur years after the start of treatment
Investigations	Specific IgE tests or skin prick tests	Specific IgE tests and skin prick tests often negative Exclude hypothyroidism	Complement C4 (invariably low in acute attacks) C1 inhibitor levels	No specific investigations
Treatment	Allergen avoidance Antihistamines	Antihistamines are mainstay of treatment and prophylaxis	Unresponsive to antihistamines Attenuated androgens C1 inhibitor concentrate or icatibant for acute attacks	Discontinue ACE inhibitor Avoid angiotensin II receptor blockers
Possible drug causes	Specific drug allergies, e.g. penicillin	NSAIDs Opioids Radiocontrast media		ACE inhibitors Angiotensin II receptor blockers

(ACE = angiotensin-converting enzyme; NSAIDs = non-steroidal anti-inflammatory drugs)

Specific allergies

Insect venom allergy

Local non-IgE-mediated reactions to insect stings are common and may cause extensive swelling around the site lasting as long as 7 days. These usually do not require specific treatment. Toxic reactions to venom after multiple (50–100) simultaneous stings may mimic anaphylaxis. In addition, exposure to large amounts of insect venom frequently stimulates the production of IgE antibodies, and thus may be followed by allergic reactions to single stings. Allergic IgE-mediated reactions vary from mild to life-threatening. Antigen-specific immunotherapy with bee or wasp venom reduces the incidence of recurrent anaphylaxis from 50–60% to 10% but requires treatment for several years (see Box 4.17).

Peanut allergy

Peanut allergy is the most common food-related allergy. More than 50% of patients present before the age of 3 years and some individuals react to their first known exposure to peanuts, possibly because of sensitisation by topical creams. Peanuts are ubiquitous in the Western diet, and every year up to 25% of peanut-allergic individuals will experience a reaction as a result of inadvertent exposure.

Birch oral allergy syndrome

This syndrome is characterised by a combination of birch pollen hay fever and local angioedema after contact with fresh fruit (especially apples), vegetables and nuts. Cooked fruits and vegetables are tolerated without difficulty. It is due to shared or cross-reactive allergens which are destroyed by cooking or digestion, and can be confirmed by skin prick testing using fresh fruit. Severe allergic reactions are unusual.

C1 inhibitor deficiency

Hereditary angioedema

Hereditary angioedema (HAE), also known as inherited C1 inhibitor deficiency, is an autosomal dominant disorder caused by decreased production or activity of C1 inhibitor protein. This complement regulatory protein inhibits spontaneous activation of the classical complement pathway (see Fig. 4.3, p. 75). C1 inhibitor is also a regulatory protein for the kinin cascade, activation of which increases local bradykinin levels and gives rise to local pain and swelling.

In HAE, angioedema may be spontaneous or triggered by local trauma or infection. Multiple parts of the body may be involved, especially the face, extremities, upper airway and gastrointestinal tract. Oedema of the intestinal wall causes severe abdominal pain. The most important complication is laryngeal obstruction, often associated with minor dental procedures, which can be fatal. Episodes of angioedema are self-limiting and usually resolve within 48 hours. Patients with HAE generally present in adolescence, but may go undiagnosed for many years. A family history can be identified in 80% of cases. HAE is not associated with allergic diseases and is specifically not associated with urticaria.

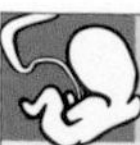

4.23 Immunological diseases in pregnancy

Allergic disease

- **Maternal dietary restrictions during pregnancy or lactation**: current evidence does not support these for prevention of allergic disease.
- **Breastfeeding for at least 4 mths**: prevents or delays the occurrence of atopic dermatitis, cow's milk allergy and wheezing in early childhood, as compared with feeding formula milk containing intact cow's milk protein.

Autoimmune disease

- **Suppressed T cell-mediated immune responses in pregnancy**: autoimmune diseases often improve during pregnancy but flare immediately after delivery. However, an exception is SLE, which is prone to exacerbation in pregnancy.
- **Passive transfer of maternal antibodies**: can mediate autoimmune disease in the fetus and newborn, including SLE, Graves' disease and myasthenia gravis.
- **Antiphospholipid syndrome** (p. 1055): an important cause of fetal loss, intrauterine growth restriction and pre-eclampsia.

Acute episodes are always accompanied by low C4 levels and the diagnosis can be confirmed by C1 inhibitor measurement. Prevention is with modified androgens (e.g. danazol), which increase endogenous production of complement proteins. Severe acute attacks should be treated with purified Cl inhibitor or a bradykinin receptor antagonist (icatibant).

Acquired C1 inhibitor deficiency

This rare disorder is clinically indistinguishable from HAE but presents in late adulthood. It is associated with autoimmune and lymphoproliferative diseases. Treatment of the underlying disorder may induce remission of angioedema.

TRANSPLANTATION IMMUNOLOGY

Transplantation provides the opportunity for definitive treatment of end-stage organ disease. The major complications are graft rejection, drug toxicity and infection consequent on immunosuppression. Transplant survival continues to improve, as a result of the introduction of less toxic immunosuppressive agents and increased understanding of rejection mechanisms.

Haematopoietic stem cell transplantation and its complications are discussed on page 1017.

Transplant rejection

Solid organ transplantation inevitably stimulates an aggressive immune response by the recipient, unless the transplant is between monozygotic twins. The type and severity of the rejection response are determined by the genetic disparity between the donor and recipient, the immune status of the host and the nature of the tissue

4.24 Classification of transplant rejection

Type	Time	Pathological findings	Mechanism	Treatment
Hyperacute rejection	Mins to hrs	Thrombosis, necrosis	Preformed antibody to donor antigens results in complement activation (type II hypersensitivity)	None – irreversible graft loss
Acute vascular rejection	5–30 days	Vasculitis	Antibody and complement activation	Increase immunosuppression
Acute cellular rejection	5–30 days	Cellular infiltration	$CD4^+$ and $CD8^+$ T cells (type IV hypersensitivity)	Increase immunosuppression
Chronic allograft failure	> 30 days	Fibrosis, scarring	Immune and non-immune mechanisms	Minimise drug toxicity, control hypertension and hyperlipidaemia

transplanted (Box 4.24). The most important genetic determinant is the difference between donor and recipient HLA proteins (p. 75). The extensive polymorphism of these proteins means that donor HLA antigens are almost invariably recognised as foreign by the recipient immune system, unless an active attempt has been made to minimise incompatibility.

- *Acute cellular rejection* is the most common form of graft rejection. It is mediated by activated T cells and results in deterioration in graft function. It may cause fever, pain and tenderness over the graft. It is usually amenable to increased immunosuppressive therapy.
- *Hyperacute rejection* results in rapid and irreversible destruction of the graft. It is mediated by pre-existing recipient antibodies against donor HLA antigens, which arise as a result of previous exposure through transplantation, blood transfusion or pregnancy. It is rarely seen in practice, as the use of screening for anti-HLA antibodies and pre-transplant cross-matching ensure prior identification of recipient–donor incompatibility.
- *Acute vascular rejection* is mediated by antibody formed de novo after transplantation. It is more curtailed than the hyperacute response because of the use of intercurrent immunosuppression, but it is also associated with reduced graft survival. Aggressive immunosuppressive therapy is indicated, and physical removal of antibody through plasmapheresis may be effective. Not all post-transplant anti-donor antibodies cause graft damage; their consequences are determined by specificity and ability to trigger other immune components, such as the complement cascade.
- *Chronic allograft failure*, also known as chronic rejection, is a major cause of graft loss. It is associated with proliferation of transplant vascular smooth muscle, interstitial fibrosis and scarring. The pathogenesis is poorly understood but contributing factors include immunological damage caused by subacute rejection, hypertension, hyperlipidaemia and chronic drug toxicity.

Investigations

Pre-transplantation testing

HLA typing determines an individual's HLA polymorphisms and facilitates donor–recipient matching.

Potential transplant recipients are screened for the presence of anti-HLA antibodies using either recombinant HLA proteins or a pool of lymphocytes from individuals with broadly representative HLA types. If antibodies are detected, their specificity is further characterised and the recipient is excluded from receiving a transplant which carries these alleles.

Donor–recipient cross-matching is a functional assay that directly tests whether serum from a recipient (which potentially contains anti-donor antibodies) is able to bind and/or kill donor lymphocytes. It is specific to a prospective donor–recipient pair and is done immediately prior to transplantation. A positive cross-match is a contraindication to transplantation because of the risk of hyperacute rejection.

C4d staining

C4d is a fragment of complement protein C4 (see Fig. 4.3, p. 75). Deposition of C4d in graft capillaries indicates local activation of the classical complement pathway and provides evidence for antibody-mediated damage. This is useful in diagnosis of vascular rejection.

Complications of transplant immunosuppression

The prevention of transplant rejection requires indefinite treatment with immunosuppressive agents. In general, two or more immunosuppressive drugs are used in synergistic combinations in order to minimise drug side-effects (Box 4.25). The major complications of long-term immunosuppression are infection and malignancy.

The risk of some opportunistic infections may be minimised through the use of prophylactic medication (e.g. ganciclovir for CMV prophylaxis and trimethoprim–sulfamethoxazole for *Pneumocystis* prophylaxis). Immunisation with killed vaccines is appropriate, although the immune response may be curtailed. Live vaccines should not be given.

The increased risk of malignancy arises because T-cell suppression results in failure to control viral infections. Virus-associated tumours include lymphoma (associated with EBV), Kaposi's sarcoma (associated with human herpesvirus 8) and skin tumours (associated with human papillomavirus). Immunosuppression is also associated with a small increase in the incidence of common cancers not associated with viral infection

4.25 Immunosuppressive drugs used in transplantation

Drug	Mechanism of action	Major adverse effects
Anti-proliferative agents e.g. azathioprine, mycophenolate mofetil	Inhibit lymphocyte proliferation by blocking DNA synthesis May be directly cytotoxic at high doses	Increased susceptibility to infection Leucopenia Hepatotoxicity
Calcineurin inhibitors e.g. ciclosporin, tacrolimus	Inhibit T-cell signalling; prevent lymphocyte activation and block cytokine transcription	Increased susceptibility to infection Hypertension Nephrotoxicity Diabetogenic (especially tacrolimus) Gingival hypertrophy, hirsutism (ciclosporin)
Corticosteroids	Decrease phagocytosis and release of proteolytic enzymes; decrease lymphocyte activation and proliferation; decrease cytokine production; decrease antibody production	Increased susceptibility to infection Multiple other complications (p. 776)
Anti-T-cell induction agents e.g. anti-thymocyte globulin (ATG)	Antibodies to cell surface proteins deplete or inhibit T cells	Profound non-specific immunosuppression Increased susceptibility to infection

(such as lung, breast and colon cancer), reflecting the importance of T cells in anti-cancer surveillance.

Organ donation

The major problem in transplantation is the shortage of organ donors. Cadaveric organ donors are usually previously healthy individuals who experience brainstem death (p. 1161), frequently as a result of road traffic accidents or cerebrovascular events. However, even if organs were obtained from all potential cadaveric donors, their numbers would be insufficient to meet current needs. An alternative is the use of living donors. Altruistic living donation, usually from close relatives, is widely used in renal transplantation. Living organ donation is inevitably associated with some risk to the donor, and the process is highly regulated to ensure appreciation of the dangers involved. Because of concerns about coercion and exploitation, non-altruistic organ donation (the sale of organs) is illegal in most countries.

Further information and acknowledgements

Websites

www.allergy.org.au *An Australasian site providing information on allergy, asthma and immune diseases.*

www.anaphylaxis.org.uk *Provides information and support for patients with severe allergies.*

www.immunopaedia.org *A South African site designed for health-care providers requiring a general understanding of immunology, providing clinical case studies, articles, links and news, with a particular focus on HIV immunology.*

www.info4pi.org *A US site managed by the non-profit Jeffrey Modell Foundation, which provides extensive information about primary immunodeficiency diseases.*

Figure acknowledgements

Fig. 4.11 Helbert M. Flesh and bones of immunology. Edinburgh: Churchill Livingstone; 2006; copyright Elsevier.

P. Hanlon
M. Byers
J.P.H. Wilding
H.M. Macdonald

Environmental and nutritional factors in disease

5

Principles and investigation of environmental factors in disease 98
- Environmental effects on health 98
- Investigations in environmental health 99
- Preventive medicine 100

Environmental diseases 100
- Alcohol 100
- Smoking 100
- Obesity 101
- Poverty and affluence 101
- Atmospheric pollution 102
- Radiation exposure 102
- Extremes of temperature 103
- High altitude 106
- Under water 108

Nutritional factors and disease 110
- Physiology of nutrition 110
- Clinical assessment and investigation of nutritional status 114

Disorders of altered energy balance 115
- Obesity 115
- Under-nutrition 120

Micronutrients, minerals and their diseases 124
- Vitamins 124
- Inorganic micronutrients 130

PRINCIPLES AND INVESTIGATION OF ENVIRONMENTAL FACTORS IN DISEASE

Environmental effects on health

Health emerges from a highly complex interaction between factors intrinsic to the patient and his or her environment. Many factors within the environment influence health, including aspects of the physical environment, biological environment (bacteria, viruses), built environment and social environment, but these also encompass more distant influences such as the global ecosystem (Fig. 5.1). Environmental changes affect many physiological systems and do not respect boundaries between medical specialties. The specialty of 'public health' in the UK is concerned with the investigation and management of health in communities and populations, but the principles apply in all specialties.

Exposure to infectious agents is a major environmental determinant of health and is described in detail in Chapter 6. This chapter describes the approach to other common environmental factors that influence health.

The hierarchy of systems – from molecules to ecologies

When assessing a patient, a clinician subconsciously considers many levels at which problems may be occurring, including molecular, cellular, tissue, organ and body systems. When the environment's influence on health is being considered, this 'hierarchy of systems' extends beyond the individual to include the family, community, population and ecology. Box 5.1 shows an example of the utility of this concept in describing determinants of coronary heart disease operating at each level of a hierarchy.

Interactions between people and their environment

The hierarchy of systems demonstrates that the clinician should not focus too quickly on the disease process without considering the context. Health is an emergent quality of a complex interaction between many determinants, including genetic inheritance, the physical circumstances in which people live (e.g. housing, air quality, working environment), the social environment (e.g. levels of friendship, support and trust), personal behaviour (smoking, diet, exercise), and access to money and the other resources that give people control over their lives. Health care is not the only determinant – and is usually not the major determinant – of health status in the population.

These systems do not operate in isolation in separate communities. When one group responds to ill health by manipulating its environment, the consequences may be global. For example, an Afghan farmer who starts growing opium for money in order to feed his children influences the environment of a teenager in Europe; in turn, drug misuse in Europe has fostered higher prevalence of blood-borne infectious diseases such as human immunodeficiency virus/acquired immunodeficiency syndrome (HIV/AIDS); in turn, these have spilled out into sexually transmitted disease. This process contributes significantly to the tragedy of the epidemic of HIV/AIDS.

The life course

The determinants of health operate over the whole lifespan. Values and behaviours acquired during childhood and adolescence have a profound influence on

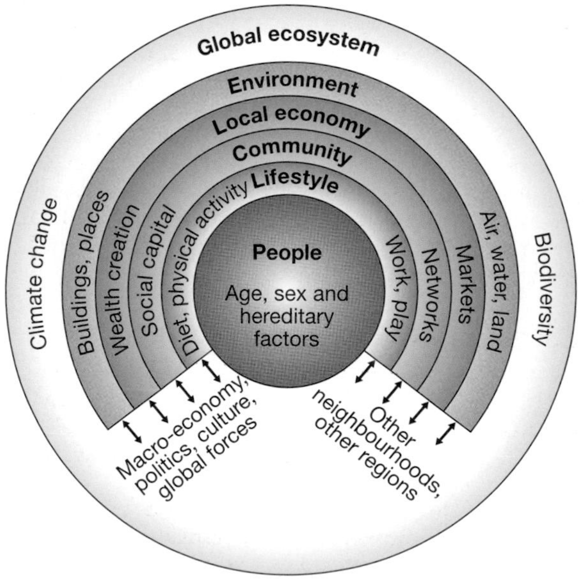

Fig. 5.1 Hierarchy of systems that influence population health. From Rao, et al. 2007 – see p. 132.

5.1 'Hierarchy of systems' applied to ischaemic heart disease

Level in the hierarchy	Example of effect
Molecular	ApoB mutation causing hypercholesterolaemia
Cellular	Foam cells accumulate in vessel wall
Tissue	Atheroma and thrombosis of coronary artery
Organ	Ischaemia and infarction of myocardium
System	Cardiac failure
Person	Limited exercise capacity, impact on employment
Family	Passive smoking, diet
Community	Shops and leisure opportunities
Population	Prevalence of obesity
Society	Policies on smoking, screening for risk factors
Ecology	Agriculture influencing fat content in diet

educational outcomes, job prospects and risk of disease. Attributes such as the ability to form empathetic relationships or assess risk have a strong influence on whether a young person takes up damaging behaviour like smoking, risky sexual activity and drug misuse. Influences on health can even operate before birth.

Individuals with low birth weight have been shown to have a higher prevalence of conditions such as hypertension and type 2 diabetes as young adults and of cardiovascular disease in middle age. It has been suggested that under-nutrition during middle to late gestation permanently 'programmes' cardiovascular and metabolic responses.

This 'life course' perspective highlights the cumulative effect on health of exposures to episodes of illness, adverse environmental conditions and behaviours that damage health. In this way, biological and social risk factors at each stage of life link to form pathways to disease and health.

Investigations in environmental health

Incidence and prevalence

The first task is to establish how common a problem is within the population. This is expressed in two ways (Box 5.2).

- If the problem is a continuing condition (e.g. enlarged spleen due to malaria), then prevalence is the appropriate measurement and is calculated by dividing the number of people with the condition at a specified time by the number of people in the population at risk at that time. Prevalence tends to be higher if the problem is common (many new cases) and/or if it is of longer duration.
- If the problem is an event that occurs at a clear point in time (e.g. fever due to malaria), then incidence is used. Incidence is a measure of the rate at which new cases occur (e.g. confirmed pyrexia with malaria parasites on a blood film) in the population at risk during a defined period of time.

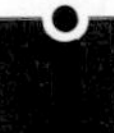

5.2 Calculation of risk using descriptive epidemiology

Prevalence

- The ratio of the number of people with a longer-term disease or condition at a specified time, to the number of people in the population who are at risk

Incidence

- The number of events (new cases or episodes) occurring in the population at risk during a defined period of time

Attributable risk

- The difference between the risk (or incidence) of disease in exposed and non-exposed populations

Attributable fraction

- The ratio of the attributable risk to the incidence

Relative risk

- The ratio of the risk (or incidence) in the exposed population to the risk (or incidence) in the non-exposed population

Variability by time, person and place

The next task is to establish how the problem varies in terms of time, person and place. The incidence may fluctuate throughout the year; for example, malaria occurs in the wet season but not the dry. Observation over longer periods establishes whether a problem is becoming more or less common: malaria may re-emerge due to drug resistance. The next questions are, who are the victims? Are males or females more commonly affected? What is the age pattern? What are the occupations and social positions of those affected? In this example, symptomatic malaria is more common in poorer, rural-dwelling children. Finally, there is the question of variability by place: the prevalence of malaria is dictated by the distribution of *Anopheles* mosquitoes.

Measuring risk

Epidemiology is also concerned with the numerical estimation of risk. This is best illustrated by a simple example. In a rural African town with a population of 5000, disease 'd' is under investigation. The majority of the cases of disease 'd' (300 out of 360) occurred among women and children who use the river, which recently had its flow of water reduced because of a new irrigation scheme. A formal experiment is established to measure risk. The 1000 women and children who use the river are followed up for 1 year and compared to a cohort with a similar age and sex distribution who use standpipes as their source of water.

The incidence (new cases) of disease 'd' in the 1000 exposed to risk 'r' (river water) was 300. The incidence (new cases) of disease 'd' in the 1000 not exposed to risk 'r' was 60. The relative risk is the incidence in the exposed population (300 per 1000 per year) divided by the incidence in the non-exposed population (60 per 1000 per year); 300/60 = 5, meaning that those exposed to the river water are 5 times more likely to contract the disease – their relative risk is 5. The attributable risk of exposure '*r*' for disease 'd' is the incidence in the exposed population (300) minus the incidence in the non-exposed population (60), which is 240 per 1000 per year. The fraction, or proportion, of the disease in the exposed population which can be attributed to risk (r) is called the attributable fraction, in this case (300–60)/300 = 0.8. This means that 80% of the disease can be attributed to exposure to river water.

Establishing cause and effect

Associations between a risk factor and a disease do not prove that the risk factor causes the disease. In the northern hemisphere, both multiple sclerosis and blue eyes are more common but it is implausible that having blue eyes is the cause of multiple sclerosis. Cause and effect can only be proven by more detailed investigation. In the above example, further investigation of the river water will be needed, using the criteria for causation defined in Koch's postulates (for infectious agents, p. 134) or the more generic Bradford Hill criteria.

5

Preventive medicine

There are many examples of epidemiological associations defining causative factors in disease, e.g. the association between cigarette smoking and lung cancer (p. 699). However, as illustrated above, the complexity of the interactions between physical, social and economic determinants of health means that successful prevention is often difficult. Moreover, the life course perspective illustrates that it may be necessary to intervene early in life or even before birth, to prevent important disease in later life. Successful prevention is likely to require many interventions across the life course and at several levels in the hierarchy of systems. The examples below illustrate this principle.

ENVIRONMENTAL DISEASES

The term 'homeostasis' describes the capacity to maintain the internal milieu by adapting to increases or decreases in a given environmental factor. However, there are limits to the coping abilities of any system, at which 'too much' or 'too little' of a given environmental factor will result in ill health. Too many calories lead to obesity, while too few lead to malnutrition. Either involuntarily or deliberately, we expose ourselves to many poisons and hazards. Examples discussed elsewhere include industrial/occupational hazards, such as asbestos (p. 718) and other carcinogens (p. 266). 'Social' poisons, such as tobacco, alcohol and drugs of misuse, also need to be considered (p. 240).

Alcohol

The World Health Organization (WHO) estimates that the harmful use of alcohol results in the death of 2.5 million people annually. Rates of alcohol-related harm vary by place and time but have risen dramatically in the UK, with Scotland showing the highest rates. (Fig. 5.2 demonstrates the climbing rates during the 1990s, since when rates have stabilised at very high levels.) Why did Scotland experience this dramatic increase in alcohol deaths? The most likely explanation is that the environment changed. The price of alcohol fell in real terms and availability increased (more supermarkets sold alcohol and the opening times of public houses were extended). Also, the culture changed in a way that fostered higher levels of consumption and more binge drinking. These changes have caused a trebling of male and a doubling of female deaths due to alcohol. Public, professional and governmental concern has now led to a minimum price being charged for a unit of alcohol, tightening of licensing regulations and curtailment of some promotional activity (e.g. two-for-one offers in bars). Many experts judge that even more aggressive public health measures will be needed to reverse the levels of harm in the community. The approach for individual patients suffering adverse effects of alcohol is described on pages 240 and 252.

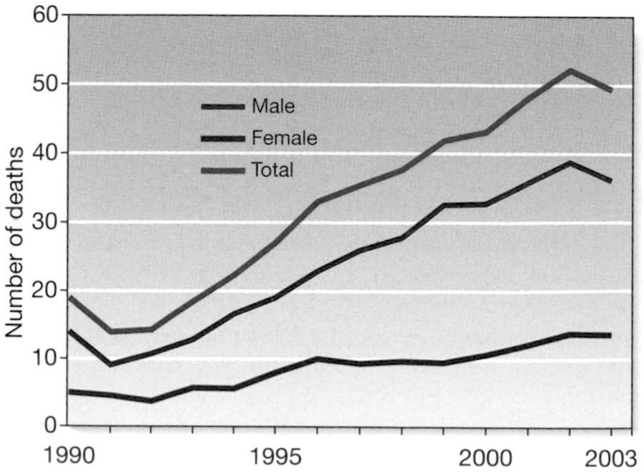

Fig. 5.2 Alcohol-related deaths in Scotland by year and sex (1990–2003). Principal ('underlying') and secondary ('contributing') causes of death. (Source: General Register Office (Scotland))

Smoking

Smoking tobacco dramatically increases the risk of developing many diseases. It is responsible for a substantial majority of cases of lung cancer and chronic obstructive pulmonary disease, and most smokers die either from these respiratory diseases or from ischaemic heart disease. Smoking also causes cancers of the upper respiratory and gastrointestinal tracts, pancreas, bladder and kidney, and increases risks of peripheral vascular disease, stroke and peptic ulceration. Maternal smoking is an important cause of fetal growth retardation. Moreover, there is increasing evidence that passive (or 'secondhand') smoking has adverse effects on cardiovascular and respiratory health.

When the ill-health effects of smoking were first discovered, doctors imagined that warning people about the dangers of smoking would result in them giving up. However, it also took increased taxation of tobacco, banning of advertising and support for smoking cessation to maintain a decline in smoking rates. In several European countries (including the UK), this has culminated in a complete ban on smoking in all public places – legislation that only became possible as the public became convinced of the dangers of secondhand smoke. However, smoking rates remain high in many poorer areas and are increasing amongst young women. In many developing countries, tobacco companies have found new markets and rates are rising. Worldwide, there are approximately 1 billion smokers, and it is estimated by WHO that 6 million die prematurely each year as a result of their habit.

In reality, there is a complex hierarchy of systems that interact to cause smokers to initiate and maintain their habit. At the molecular and cellular levels, nicotine acts on the nervous system to create dependence, so that smokers experience unpleasant effects when they attempt to quit. So, even if they know it is harmful, the role of addiction in maintaining the habit is important. Influences at the personal and social level are just as important. Many individuals bolster their denial of the harmful effects of smoking by focusing on someone they knew personally who smoked until he or she was very old and died peacefully in bed. Such strong counter-examples help smokers to maintain internal beliefs that comfort them when presented with statistical evidence.

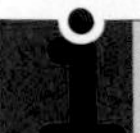

5.3 Methods for smoking cessation*

Smokers who are not motivated to try to stop smoking

- Record smoking status at regular intervals
- Anti-smoking advice
- Encourage change in attitude towards smoking to improve motivation

Motivated light smokers (< 10/day)

- Anti-smoking advice
- Anti-smoking support programme

Motivated heavy smokers (10–15/day)

- As above plus nicotine replacement therapy (NRT) (minimum 8 weeks)

Motivated heavy smokers (> 15/day)

- As above plus bupropion if NRT and behavioural support are unsuccessful and patient remains motivated

*Based on Coleman T. Smoking cessation: integrating recent advances with clinical practice. Thorax 2001; 56:579–582, with permission from the BMJ Publishing Group.

EBM 5.4 Smoking cessation

'Placebo or will-power alone has a ~2% chance of abstinence for ≥ 6 months. This can be increased by the percentage shown by:

- written self-help materials: 1%
- opportunistic advice from doctor: 2%
- face-to-face behavioural support from specialist: 4–7%
- proactive telephone counselling: 2%
- NRT with limited or intensive behavioural support: 5–12%
- bupropion with intensive behavioural support: 9%.'

- Health Education Board for Scotland, Edinburgh; 2000.

Young female smokers are often motivated more by the desire to 'stay thin' or 'look cool' than to avoid an illness in middle life.

Even if a smoker decides to quit, there are a variety of influences in the wider environment that reduce the chances of sustained success, including peer pressure, cigarette advertising, and finding oneself in circumstances where one previously smoked. The tobacco industry works very hard to maintain and expand the smoking habit, and its advertising budget is much greater than that available to health promoters.

Strategies to help individuals quit smoking are outlined in Boxes 5.3 and 5.4. Although the success rates are modest, these interventions are cost-effective and form an important part of the overall anti-tobacco strategy.

Obesity

Obesity is a condition characterised by an excess of body fat. In its simplest terms, obesity can be considered to result from an imbalance between the amount of energy consumed in the diet and the amount of energy expended through exercise and bodily functions. People who are obese are more likely to develop a range of chronic conditions. In 2006, the number of obese and overweight people in the world overtook the numbers who are malnourished and underweight. It would, however, be wrong to focus only on those who are obese because, in countries like the USA and the UK, fat deposition is affecting almost the entire population. The weight distribution of almost the whole population is shifting upwards – the slim are becoming less slim while the fat are getting fatter. In the UK, this translates into a 1-kilogram increase in weight per adult per year (on average over the adult population). It is now widely accepted that we cannot blame the current obesity epidemic on individual behaviour and poor choice, although many current approaches still focus on individuals. The best way, therefore, to understand the current obesity epidemic is to consider humans as 'obesogenic organisms' who, for the first time in their history, find themselves in an obesogenic environment – that is, one where people's circumstances encourage them to eat more and exercise less. This includes the availability of cheap and heavily marketed energy-rich foods, the increase in labour-saving devices (e.g. lifts and remote controls) and the increase in passive transport (cars as opposed to walking, cycling, or walking to public transport hubs). Our physiology was formed a long time ago when food was scarce and we needed large amounts of energy in order to find food and stay alive. We are stuck with the metabolic and behavioural legacy of our evolutionary history – we are organisms that are programmed to eat when we can and preserve energy whenever possible. It is not surprising that we have problems coping with an environment that exerts constant pressure to increase energy intake and to decrease energy expenditure. The rise in obesity suggests that the effects of our obesogenic environment are overriding the biological regulatory mechanisms in more and more people. To combat the health impact of obesity, therefore, we need to help those who are already obese but also develop strategies that impact on the whole population and reverse the obesogenic environment.

Poverty and affluence

The adverse health and social consequences of poverty are well documented: high birth rates, high death rates and short life expectancy (Box 5.5). Typically, with

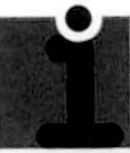

5.5 Examples of effects of financial resources on health

Poverty

- Respiratory disease exacerbated or caused by air pollution
- Exposure to unnecessary hazards in the workplace or living environment
- Poor hygiene causing diarrhoeal diseases and debilitating intestinal parasitic infections
- Malnutrition
- Cardiovascular disease

Affluence

- Physical inactivity
- Alcohol and drug consumption
- High rates of suicide, depression, anxiety and stress
- Sexually transmitted infection
- Obesity

industrialisation, the pattern changes: low birth rates, low death rates and longer life expectancy (Box 5.6). Instead of infections, chronic conditions such as heart disease dominate in an older population. Adverse health consequences of excessive affluence are also becoming apparent. Despite experiencing sustained economic growth for the last 50 years, people in many industrialised countries are not growing any happier and the litany of socioeconomic problems - crime, congestion, inequality - persists. Living in societies that give pride of place to economic growth means that there is constant pressure to contribute by performing ever harder at work and by consuming as much as - or more than - we can afford. As a result, people become stressed and may adopt unhealthy strategies to mitigate their discomfort; they overeat, overshop, or use sex or drugs (legal and illegal) as 'pain-killers'. These behaviours often lead to the problems listed in Box 5.5.

Many countries are now experiencing a 'double burden'. They have large populations still living in poverty who are suffering from problems such as diarrhoea and malnutrition, alongside affluent populations (often in cities) who suffer from chronic illness such as diabetes and heart disease. Recent research suggests that uneven distribution of wealth is a more important determinant of health than the absolute level of wealth; countries with a more even distribution of wealth enjoy longer life expectancies than countries with similar or higher gross domestic products (GDPs) but wider distributions of wealth.

Atmospheric pollution

Emissions from industry, power plants and motor vehicles of sulphur oxides, nitrogen oxides, respirable particles and metals are severely polluting cities and towns in Asia, Africa, Latin America and Eastern Europe. Increased death rates from respiratory and cardiovascular disease occur in vulnerable adults, such as those with established respiratory disease and the elderly, while children experience an increase in bronchitic symptoms. In nations like the UK that have reduced their primary emissions, the new issue of greenhouse gases has emerged. Developing countries also suffer high rates of respiratory disease as a result of indoor pollution caused mainly by heating and cooking combustion.

Carbon dioxide and global warming

Climate change is arguably the world's most important environmental health issue. A combination of increased production of carbon dioxide and habitat destruction, both caused primarily by human activity, seems to be the main cause. The temperature of the globe is rising, climate is being affected, and if the trend continues, sea levels will rise and rainfall patterns will be altered so that both droughts and floods will become more common. These have already claimed millions of lives during the past 20 years and have adversely affected the lives of many more. The economic costs of property damage and the impact on agriculture, food supplies and prosperity have also been substantial. The health impacts of global warming will also include changes in the geographical range of some vector-borne infectious diseases.

Currently, politicians cannot agree on an effective framework of actions to tackle the problem. Meanwhile, the industrialised world continues with lifestyles and levels of waste that are beyond the planet's ability to sustain. Rapidly growing economies in the world's two most populous states, India and China, are going to be a vital part of the unfolding problem or solution.

Radiation exposure

Radiation includes ionising (Box 5.7) and non-ionising radiations (ultraviolet (UV), visible light, laser, infrared and microwave). Whilst global industrialisation and the generation of fluorocarbons have raised concerns about loss of the ozone layer, leading to an increased exposure to UV rays, and disasters such as the Chernobyl and Fukushima nuclear power station explosions have demonstrated the harm of ionising radiation, it is important to remember that it can be harnessed for medical benefit. Ionising radiation is used in X-rays, computed tomography (CT), radionucleotide scans and radiotherapy, and non-ionising UV for therapy in skin diseases and laser therapy for diabetic retinopathy.

Types of ionising radiation

These include charged subatomic alpha and beta particles, uncharged neutrons or high-energy electromagnetic

5.6 Environmental factors in disease in old age

- **Quality of life**: the major goal of public health policy in the young is to prolong lifespan; in old age, quality of life may be more important than its duration.
- **Life course**: the environmental factors that determine life expectancy operate throughout the lifespan and begin before birth.
- **Susceptibility to risk**: decline in many physiological functions increases risks from, for example, extremes of temperature, poverty, pollution and accidents in the home.
- **Reliance on support**: in many societies, financial, family and community support for older people is declining, with increasing risks of social isolation, poverty, malnutrition and neglect.

5.7 Properties of ionising radiations

	Range in air	Range in tissue	Protection
Alpha particles	Few centimetres	No penetration	Paper
Beta particles	Few metres	Few millimetres	Aluminium sheet
X-rays/ gamma rays	Kilometres	Passes through	Lead
Neutrons	Kilometres	Passes through	Concrete or thick polythene

radiations such as X-rays and gamma rays. When they interact with atoms, energy is released and the resulting ionisation can lead to molecular damage. The clinical effects of different forms of radiation depend upon their range in air and tissue penetration (see Box 5.7).

Dosage and exposure

The dose of radiation is based upon the energy absorbed by a unit mass of tissue and is measured in grays (Gy), with 1 Gy representing 1 J/kg. To take account of different types of radiation and variations in the sensitivity of various tissues, weighting factors are used to produce a unit of effective dose, measured in sieverts (Sv). This value reflects the absorbed dose weighted for the damaging effects of a particular form of radiation and is most valuable in evaluating the long-term effects of exposure.

'Background radiation' refers to our exposure to naturally occurring radioactivity (e.g. radon gas and cosmic radiation). This produces an average annual individual dose of approximately 2.6 mSv per year, although this varies according to local geology.

Effects of radiation exposure

Effects on the individual are classified as either deterministic or stochastic.

Deterministic effects

Deterministic (threshold) effects occur with increasing severity as the dose of radiation rises above a threshold level. Tissues with actively dividing cells, such as bone marrow and gastrointestinal mucosa, are particularly sensitive to ionising radiation. Lymphocyte depletion is the most sensitive marker of bone marrow injury, and after exposure to a fatal dose, marrow aplasia is a common cause of death. However, gastrointestinal mucosal toxicity may cause earlier death due to profound diarrhoea, vomiting, dehydration and sepsis. The gonads are highly radiosensitive and radiation may result in temporary or permanent sterility. Eye exposure can lead to cataracts and the skin is susceptible to radiation burns. Irradiation of the lung and central nervous system may induce acute inflammatory reactions, pulmonary fibrosis and permanent neurological deficit respectively. Bone necrosis and lymphatic fibrosis are characteristic following regional irradiation, particularly for breast cancer. The thyroid gland is not inherently sensitive but its ability to concentrate iodine makes it susceptible to damage after exposure to relatively low doses of radioactive iodine isotopes, such as were released from Chernobyl.

Stochastic effects

Stochastic (chance) effects occur with increasing probability as the dose of radiation increases. Carcinogenesis represents a stochastic effect. With acute exposures, leukaemias may arise after an interval of around 2–5 years and solid tumours after an interval of about 10–20 years. Thereafter the incidence rises with time. An individual's risk of developing cancer depends on the dose received, the time to accumulate the total dose and the interval following exposure.

Management of radiation exposure

The principal problems after large-dose exposures are maintenance of adequate hydration, control of sepsis and the management of marrow aplasia. Associated injuries such as thermal burns need specialist management within 48 hours of active resuscitation. Internal exposure to radioisotopes should be treated with chelating agents (such as Prussian blue used to chelate ^{137}-caesium after ingestion). White cell colony stimulation and haematopoietic stem cell transplantation may need to be considered for marrow aplasia.

Extremes of temperature

Thermoregulation

Body heat is generated by basal metabolic activity and muscle movement, and lost by conduction (which is more effective in water than in air), convection, evaporation and radiation (most important at lower temperatures when other mechanisms conserve heat) (Box 5.8). Body temperature is controlled in the hypothalamus, which is directly sensitive to changes in core temperature and indirectly responds to temperature-sensitive neurons in the skin. The normal 'set-point' of core

5.8 Thermoregulation: responses to hot and cold environments

	Mechanism	Hot environment	Cold environment
Heat production	Basal metabolic rate	→	↓ in hypothermia
	Muscle activity	↓ by lethargy	↑ by shivering ↓ in severe hypothermia
Heat loss	Conduction*	↑ by vasodilatation	↓ by vasoconstriction ↑↑ in water < 31°C
	Convection*	↑ by vasodilatation ↓ by lethargy	↓ by vasoconstriction ↑ by wind and movement
	Evaporation*	↑↑ by sweating ↓ by high humidity	↑ by hyperventilation
	Radiation	↑ by vasodilatation	↓ by vasoconstriction (but is the major heat loss in dry cold)

*These losses are dependent on the relative ambient and skin temperatures.

temperature is tightly regulated within 37 ± 0.5°C, which is necessary to preserve the normal function of many enzymes and other metabolic processes. The temperature set-point is increased in response to infection (p. 296).

In a cold environment, protective mechanisms include cutaneous vasoconstriction and shivering; however, any muscle activity that involves movement may promote heat loss by increasing convective loss from the skin, and respiratory heat loss by stimulating ventilation. In a hot environment, sweating is the main mechanism for increasing heat loss. This usually occurs when the ambient temperature rises above 32.5°C or during exercise.

Hypothermia

Hypothermia exists when the body's normal thermal regulatory mechanisms are unable to maintain heat in a cold environment and core temperature falls below 35°C (Fig. 5.3).

Whilst infants are susceptible to hypothermia because of their poor thermoregulation and high body surface area to weight ratio, it is the elderly who are at highest risk (Box 5.9). Hypothyroidism is often a contributory factor in old age, while alcohol and other drugs (e.g. phenothiazines) commonly impede the thermoregulatory response in younger people. More rarely, hypothermia is secondary to glucocorticoid insufficiency, stroke, hepatic failure or hypoglycaemia.

Hypothermia also occurs in healthy individuals whose thermoregulatory mechanisms are intact but insufficient to cope with the intensity of the thermal stress. Typical examples include immersion in cold water, when core temperature may fall rapidly (acute hypothermia), exposure to extreme climates such as during hill walking (subacute hypothermia), and slow-onset hypothermia, as develops in an immobilised older individual (subchronic hypothermia). This classification is important, as it determines the method of rewarming.

Clinical features

Diagnosis is dependent on recognition of the environmental circumstances and measurement of core (rectal) body temperature. Clinical features depend on the degree of hypothermia (see Fig. 5.3).

In a cold patient, it is very difficult to diagnose death reliably by clinical means. It has been suggested that, in extreme environmental conditions, irreversible hypothermia is probably present if there is asystole (no carotid pulse for 1 minute), the chest and abdomen are rigid, the core temperature is below 13°C and serum potassium is > 12 mmol/L. However, in general, resuscitative measures should continue until the core temperature is normal and only then should a diagnosis of brain death be considered (p. 1161).

Investigations

Blood gases, a full blood count, electrolytes, chest X-ray and electrocardiogram (ECG) are all essential investigations. Haemoconcentration and metabolic acidosis are common, and the ECG may show characteristic J waves, which occur at the junction of the QRS complex and the ST segment (Fig. 5.4). Cardiac dysrhythmias, including ventricular fibrillation, may occur. Although the arterial oxygen tension may be normal when measured at room

°C	Definitions	Clinical features
	Heat stroke	**Hot and not sweating** Multiple organ failure, shock Confusion, aggression
40	Heat exhaustion	**Hot and sweating** Dehydration, tachycardia Irritability, fatigue, headache, weakness
37		Tachycardia Vasoconstriction
35	Mild hypothermia	**Cold and shivering** Confusion Dehydration Ataxia
32	Severe hypothermia	**Cold and not shivering** Depressed conscious level Muscle stiffness Failed vasoconstriction Bradycardia, hypotension ECG: J waves, dysrhythmia
28		Coma Absent pupil reflexes May appear dead
23		Loss of corneal reflexes
20		Cardiac standstill

Fig. 5.3 Clinical features of abnormal core temperature. The hypothalamus normally maintains core temperature at 37°C, but this set-point is altered – for example, in fever (pyrexia, p. 296) – and may be lost in hypothalamic disease (p. 785). In these circumstances, the clinical picture at a given core temperature may be different.

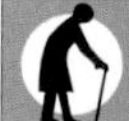

5.9 Thermoregulation in old age

- **Age-associated changes**: impairments in vasomotor function, skeletal muscle response and sweating mean that older people react more slowly to changes in temperature.
- **Increased comorbidity**: thermoregulatory problems are more likely in the presence of pathology such as atherosclerosis and hypothyroidism, and medication such as sedatives and hypnotics.
- **Hypothermia**: may arise as a primary event, but more commonly complicates other acute illness, e.g. pneumonia, stroke or fracture.
- **Ambient temperature**: financial pressures and older equipment may result in inadequate heating during cold weather.

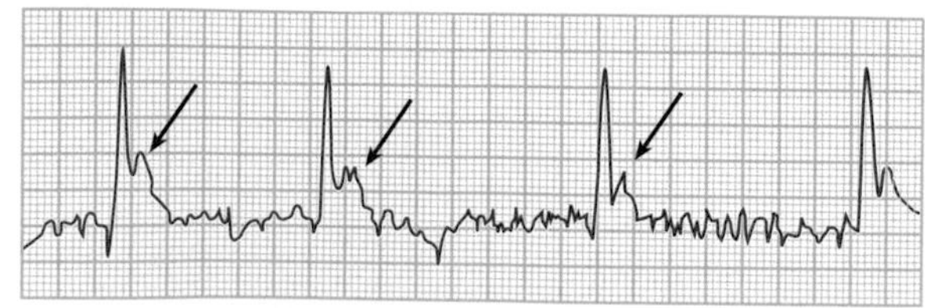

Fig. 5.4 Electrocardiogram showing J waves (arrows) in a hypothermic patient.

temperature, the arterial PO_2 in the blood falls by 7% for each 1°C fall in core temperature. Serum aspartate aminotransferase and creatine kinase may be elevated secondary to muscle damage and the serum amylase is often high due to subclinical pancreatitis. If the cause of hypothermia is not obvious, additional investigations for thyroid and pituitary dysfunction (p. 737), hypoglycaemia (p. 807) and the possibility of drug intoxication (p. 209) should be performed.

Management

Following resuscitation, the objectives of management are to rewarm the patient in a controlled manner while treating associated hypoxia (by oxygenation and ventilation if necessary), fluid and electrolyte disturbance, and cardiovascular abnormalities, particularly dysrhythmias. Careful handling is essential to avoid precipitating the latter. The method of rewarming is dependent not on the absolute core temperature, but on haemodynamic stability and the presence or absence of an effective cardiac output.

Mild hypothermia

Outdoors, continued heat loss is prevented by sheltering the patient from the cold, replacing wet clothing, covering the head and insulating him or her from the ground. Once in hospital, even in the presence of profound hypothermia, if there is an effective cardiac output then forced-air rewarming, heat packs placed in axilla, groin and around the abdomen, inhaled warmed air and correction of fluid and electrolyte disturbances are usually sufficient. Rewarming rates of 1–2°C per hour are effective in leading to a gradual and safe return to physiological normality. Underlying conditions should be treated promptly (e.g. hypothyroidism with triiodothyronine 10 µg IV 3 times daily; p. 743).

Severe hypothermia

In the case of severe hypothermia with cardiopulmonary arrest (non-perfusing rhythm), the aim is to restore perfusion, and rapid rewarming at a rate greater than 2°C per hour is required. This is best achieved by cardiopulmonary bypass or extracorporeal membrane oxygenation. If these are unavailable, then veno–veno haemofiltration, and pleural, peritoneal, thoracic or bladder lavage with warmed fluids are alternatives. Monitoring of cardiac rhythm and arterial blood gases, including H^+ (pH) is essential. Significant acidosis may require correction (p. 445).

Cold injury

Freezing cold injury (frostbite)

This represents the direct freezing of body tissues and usually affects the extremities: in particular, the fingers, toes, ears and face. Risk factors include smoking, peripheral vascular disease, dehydration and alcohol consumption. The tissues may become anaesthetised before freezing and, as a result, the injury often goes unrecognised at first. Frostbitten tissue is initially pale and doughy to the touch and insensitive to pain (Fig. 5.5). Once frozen, the tissue is hard.

Rewarming should not occur until it can be achieved rapidly in a water bath. Give oxygen and aspirin 300 mg as soon as possible. Frostbitten extremities should be rewarmed in warm water at 37–39°C, with antiseptic added. Adequate analgesia is necessary, as rewarming is very painful. Vasodilators such as pentoxifylline (a phosphodiesterase inhibitor) have been shown to improve tissue survival. Once it has thawed, the injured part must not be re-exposed to the cold, and should be dressed and rested. Whilst wound débridement may be necessary, amputations should be delayed for 60–90 days, as good recovery may occur over an extended period.

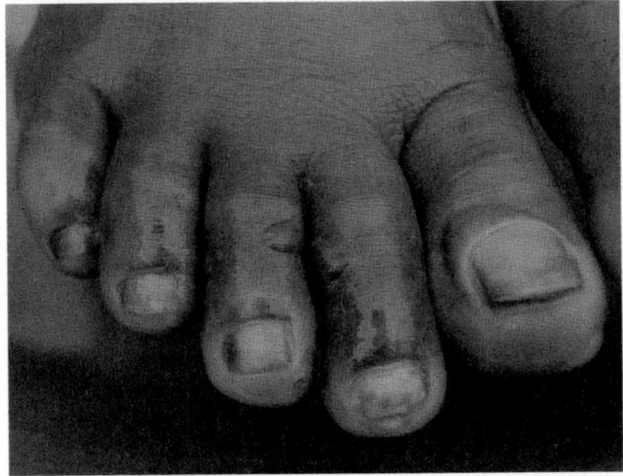

Fig. 5.5 Frostbite in a female Everest sherpa.

Non-freezing cold injury (trench or immersion foot)

This results from prolonged exposure to cold, damp conditions. The limb (usually the foot) appears cold, ischaemic and numb, but there is no freezing of the tissue. On rewarming, the limb appears mottled and thereafter becomes hyperaemic, swollen and painful. Recovery may take many months, during which there may be chronic pain and sensitivity to cold. The pathology remains uncertain but probably involves endothelial injury. Gradual rewarming is associated with less pain than rapid rewarming. The pain and associated paraesthesia are difficult to control with conventional analgesia and may require amitriptyline (50 mg nocte), best instituted early. The patient is at risk of further damage on subsequent exposure to the cold.

Chilblains

Chilblains are tender, red or purplish skin lesions that occur in the cold and wet. They are often seen in horse riders, cyclists and swimmers, and are more common in women than men. They are short-lived, and although painful, not usually serious.

Heat-related illness

When generation of heat exceeds the body's capacity for heat loss, core temperature rises. Non-exertional heat illness (NEHI) occurs with high environmental temperature in those with attenuated thermoregulatory control mechanisms: the elderly, the young, those with comorbidity or those taking drugs that affect thermoregulation (particularly phenothiazines, diuretics and alcohol). Exertional heat illness (EHI), on the other hand, typically develops in athletes when heat production exceeds the body's ability to dissipate it.

5.10 Differential diagnosis in patients with elevated core body temperature

- Heat illness (heat exhaustion, heat stroke)
- Sepsis, including meningitis
- Malaria
- Drug overdose
- Malignant hyperpyrexia
- Thyroid storm (p. 742)

Acclimatisation mechanisms to environmental heat include stimulation of the sweat mechanism with increased sweat volume, reduced sweat sodium content and secondary hyperaldosteronism to maintain body sodium balance. The risk of heat-related illness falls as acclimatisation occurs. Heat illness can be prevented to a large extent by adequate replacement of salt and water, although excessive water intake alone should be avoided because of the risk of dilutional hyponatraemia (p. 437).

A spectrum of illnesses occurs in the heat (see Fig. 5.3). The cause is usually obvious but the differential diagnosis should be considered (Box 5.10).

Heat cramps

These painful muscle contractions occur following vigorous exercise and profuse sweating in hot weather. There is no elevation of core temperature. The mechanism is considered to be extracellular sodium depletion as a result of persistent sweating, exacerbated by replacement of water but not salt. Symptoms usually respond rapidly to rehydration with oral rehydration salts or intravenous saline.

Heat syncope

This is similar to a vasovagal faint (p. 555) and is related to peripheral vasodilatation in hot weather.

Heat exhaustion

Heat exhaustion occurs with prolonged exertion in hot and humid weather, profuse sweating and inadequate salt and water replacement. There is an elevation in core (rectal) temperature to between 37°C and 40°C, leading to the clinical features shown in Figure 5.3. Blood analyses may show evidence of dehydration with mild elevation of the blood urea, sodium and haematocrit. Treatment involves removal of the patient from the heat, and active evaporative cooling using tepid sprays and fanning (strip–spray–fan). Fluid losses are replaced with either oral rehydration mixtures or intravenous isotonic saline. Up to 5 L positive fluid balance may be required in the first 24 hours. Untreated, heat exhaustion may progress to heat stroke.

Heat stroke

Heat stroke occurs when the core body temperature rises above 40°C and is a life-threatening condition. The symptoms of heat exhaustion progress to include headache, nausea and vomiting. Neurological manifestations include a coarse muscle tremor and confusion, aggression or loss of consciousness. The patient's skin feels very hot, and sweating is often absent due to failure of thermoregulatory mechanisms. Complications include hypovolaemic shock, lactic acidosis, disseminated intravascular coagulation, rhabdomyolysis, hepatic and renal failure, and pulmonary and cerebral oedema.

The patient should be resuscitated with rapid cooling by spraying with water, fanning and ice packs in the axillae and groins. Cold crystalloid intravenous fluids are given but solutions containing potassium should be avoided. Over-aggressive fluid replacement must be avoided, as it may precipitate pulmonary oedema or further metabolic disturbance. Appropriate monitoring of fluid balance, including central venous pressure, is important. Investigations for complications include routine haematology and biochemistry, coagulation screen, hepatic transaminases (aspartate aminotransferase and alanine aminotransferase), creatine kinase and chest X-ray. Once emergency treatment is established, heat stroke patients are best managed in intensive care.

With appropriate treatment, recovery from heat stroke can be rapid (within 1–2 hours) but patients who have had core temperatures higher than 40°C should be monitored carefully for later onset of rhabdomyolysis, renal damage and other complications before discharge from hospital. Clear advice to avoid heat and heavy exercise during recovery is important.

High altitude

The physiological effects of high altitude are significant. On Everest, the barometric pressure of the atmosphere falls from sea level by approximately 50% at base camp (5400 m) and approximately 70% at the summit (8848 m). The proportions of oxygen, nitrogen and carbon dioxide in air do not change with the fall in pressure but their partial pressure falls in proportion to barometric pressure (Fig. 5.6). Oxygen tension within the pulmonary alveoli is further reduced at altitude because the partial pressure of water vapour is related to body temperature and not barometric pressure, and so is proportionately greater at altitude, accounting for only 6% of barometric pressure at sea level, but 19% at 8848 m.

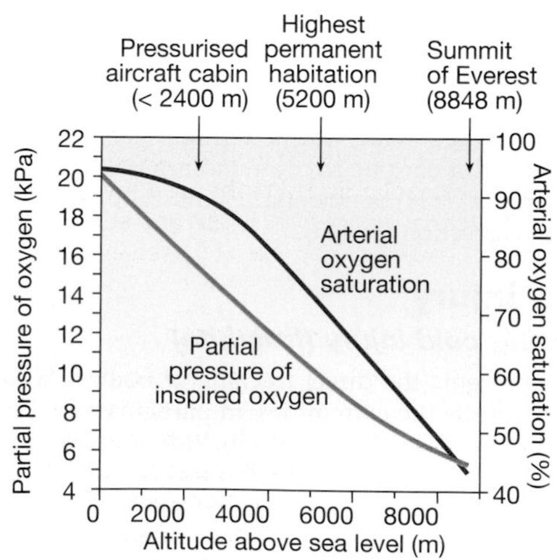

Fig. 5.6 Change in inspired oxygen tension and blood oxygen saturation at altitude. The blue curve shows changes in oxygen availability at altitude and the red curve shows the typical resultant changes in arterial oxygen saturation in a healthy person. Oxygen saturation varies between individuals according to the shape of the oxygen–haemoglobin dissociation curve and the ventilatory response to hypoxaemia. (To convert kPa to mmHg, multiply by 7.5.)

Physiological effects of high altitude

Reduction in oxygen tension results in a fall in arterial oxygen saturation (see Fig. 5.6). This varies widely between individuals, depending on the shape of the sigmoid oxygen–haemoglobin dissociation curve (see Fig. 8.3, p. 183) and the ventilatory response. Acclimatisation to hypoxaemia at high altitude involves a shift in this dissociation curve (dependent on 2,3-diphosphoglycerate (DPG)), erythropoiesis, haemoconcentration, and hyperventilation resulting from hypoxic drive (which is then sustained despite hypocapnia by restoration of cerebrospinal fluid pH to normal in prolonged hypoxia). This process takes several days, so travellers need to plan accordingly.

Illnesses at high altitude

Ascent to altitudes up to 2500 m or travel in a pressurised aircraft cabin is harmless to healthy people. Above 2500 m high-altitude illnesses may occur in previously healthy people, and above 3500 m these become common. Sudden ascent to altitudes above 6000 m, as experienced by aviators, balloonists and astronauts, may result in decompression illness with the same clinical features as seen in divers (see below), or even loss of consciousness. However, most altitude illness occurs in travellers and mountaineers.

Acute mountain sickness

Acute mountain sickness (AMS) is a syndrome comprised principally of headache, together with fatigue, anorexia, nausea and vomiting, difficulty sleeping or dizziness. Ataxia and peripheral oedema may be present. Its aetiology is not fully understood but it is thought that hypoxaemia increases cerebral blood flow and hence intracranial pressure. Symptoms occur within 6–12 hours of an ascent and vary in severity from trivial to completely incapacitating. The incidence in travellers to 3000 m may be 40–50%, depending on the rate of ascent.

Treatment of mild cases consists of rest and simple analgesia; symptoms usually resolve after 1–3 days at a stable altitude, but may recur with further ascent. Occasionally there is progression to cerebral oedema. Persistent symptoms indicate the need to descend but may respond to acetazolamide, a carbonic anhydrase inhibitor that induces a metabolic acidosis and stimulates ventilation; acetazolamide may also be used as prophylaxis if a rapid ascent is planned.

High-altitude cerebral oedema

The cardinal symptoms of high-altitude cerebral oedema (HACE) are ataxia and altered consciousness. This is rare, life-threatening and usually preceded by AMS. In addition to features of AMS, the patient suffers confusion, disorientation, visual disturbance, lethargy and ultimately loss of consciousness. Papilloedema and retinal haemorrhages are common and focal neurological signs may be found.

Treatment is directed at improving oxygenation. Descent is essential and dexamethasone (8 mg immediately and 4 mg 4 times daily) should be given. If descent is impossible, oxygen therapy in a portable pressurised bag may be helpful.

High-altitude pulmonary oedema

High-altitude pulmonary oedema (HAPE) is a life-threatening condition that usually occurs in the first 4 days after ascent above 2500 m. Unlike HACE, HAPE may occur de novo without the preceding signs of AMS. Presentation is with symptoms of dry cough, exertional dyspnoea and extreme fatigue. Later, the cough becomes wet and sputum may be blood-stained. Tachycardia and tachypnoea occur at rest and crepitations may often be heard in both lung fields. There may be profound hypoxaemia, pulmonary hypertension and radiological evidence of diffuse alveolar oedema. It is not known whether the alveolar oedema is a result of mechanical stress on the pulmonary capillaries associated with the high pulmonary arterial pressure, or an effect of hypoxia on capillary permeability. Reduced arterial oxygen saturation is not diagnostic but is a marker for disease progression.

Treatment is directed at reversal of hypoxia with immediate descent and oxygen administration. Nifedipine (20 mg 4 times daily) should be given to reduce pulmonary arterial pressure, and oxygen therapy in a portable pressurised bag should be used if descent is delayed.

Chronic mountain sickness (Monge's disease)

This occurs on prolonged exposure to altitude and has been reported in residents of Colorado, South America and Tibet. Patients present with headache, poor concentration and other signs of polycythaemia. They are cyanosed and often have finger clubbing.

High-altitude retinal haemorrhage

This occurs in over 30% of trekkers at 5000 m. The haemorrhages are usually asymptomatic and resolve spontaneously. Visual defects can occur with haemorrhage involving the macula, but there is no specific treatment.

Venous thrombosis

This has been reported at altitudes over 6000 m. Risk factors include dehydration, inactivity and the cold. The use of the oral contraceptive pill at high altitude should be considered carefully, as this is an additional risk factor.

Refractory cough

A cough at high altitude is common and usually benign. It may be due to breathing dry, cold air and increased mouth breathing, with consequent dry oral mucosa. This may be indistinguishable from the early signs of HAPE.

Air travel

Commercial aircraft usually cruise at 10 000–12 000 m, with the cabin pressurised to an equivalent of around 2400 m. At this altitude, the partial pressure of oxygen is 16 kPa (120 mmHg), leading to a PaO_2 in healthy people of 7.0–8.5 kPa (53–64 mmHg). Oxygen saturation is also reduced, but to a lesser degree (see Fig. 5.6). Although well tolerated by healthy people, this degree of hypoxia may be dangerous in patients with respiratory disease.

Advice for patients with respiratory disease

The British Thoracic Society has published guidance on the management of patients with respiratory disease who want to fly. Specialist pre-flight assessment is advised for all patients who have hypoxaemia (oxygen saturation < 95%) at sea level, and includes spirometry and a hypoxic challenge test with 15% oxygen (performed in hospital). Air travel may have to be avoided or undertaken only with inspired oxygen therapy during the flight. Asthmatic patients should be advised to carry their inhalers in their hand baggage. Following pneumothorax, flying should be avoided while air remains in the pleural cavity, but can be considered after proven resolution or definitive (surgical) treatment.

Advice for other patients

Other circumstances in which patients are more susceptible to hypoxia require individual assessment. These include cardiac dysrhythmia, sickle-cell disease and ischaemic heart disease. Most airlines decline to carry pregnant women after the 36th week of gestation. In complicated pregnancies it may be advisable to avoid air travel at an earlier stage. Patients who have had recent abdominal surgery, including laparoscopy, should avoid flying until all intraperitoneal gas is reabsorbed. Divers should not fly for 24 hours after a dive requiring decompression stops.

Ear and sinus pain due to changes in gas volume are common but usually mild, although patients with chronic sinusitis and otitis media may need specialist assessment. A healthy mobile tympanic membrane visualised during a Valsalva manœuvre usually suggests a patent Eustachian tube.

On long-haul flights, patients with diabetes mellitus may need to adjust their insulin or oral hypoglycaemic dosing according to the timing of in-flight and subsequent meals (p. 825). Advice is available from Diabetes UK and other websites. Patients should be able to provide documentary evidence of the need to carry needles and insulin.

Deep venous thrombosis

Air travellers have an increased risk of venous thrombosis (p. 1008), due to a combination of factors, including loss of venous emptying because of prolonged immobilisation (lack of muscular activity) and reduced barometric pressure on the tissues, together with haemoconcentration as a result of oedema and perhaps a degree of hypoxia-induced diuresis.

Venous thrombosis can probably be prevented by avoiding dehydration and excess alcohol, and exercising muscles during the flight. Without a clear cost–benefit analysis, prophylaxis with aspirin or heparin cannot be recommended routinely, but may be considered in high-risk cases.

Under water

Drowning and near-drowning

Drowning is defined as death due to asphyxiation following immersion in a fluid, whilst near-drowning is defined as survival for longer than 24 hours after suffocation by immersion. Drowning remains a common cause of accidental death throughout the world and is particularly common in young children (Box 5.11). In about 10% of cases, no water enters the lungs and death follows intense laryngospasm ('dry' drowning). Prolonged immersion in cold water, with or without water inhalation, results in a rapid fall in core body temperature and hypothermia (p. 104).

5.11 Most common causes of drowning by age

Infants/young children	
• Domestic baths	• Garden pools
Adolescents	
• Swimming pools	• Rivers, sea, etc.
Adults	
• Water sports, boating, fishing	• Occupational
Older people	
• Domestic baths	

Following inhalation of water, there is a rapid onset of ventilation–perfusion imbalance with hypoxaemia, and the development of diffuse pulmonary oedema. Fresh water is hypotonic and, although rapidly absorbed across alveolar membranes, impairs surfactant function, which leads to alveolar collapse and right-to-left shunting of unoxygenated blood. Absorption of large amounts of hypotonic fluid can result in haemolysis. Salt water is hypertonic and inhalation provokes alveolar oedema, but the overall clinical effect is similar to that of fresh-water drowning.

Clinical features

Those rescued alive (near-drowning) are often unconscious and not breathing. Hypoxaemia and metabolic acidosis are inevitable features. Acute lung injury usually resolves rapidly over 48–72 hours, unless infection occurs (Fig. 5.7). Complications include dehydration, hypotension, haemoptysis, rhabdomyolysis, renal failure and cardiac dysrhythmias. A small number of patients, mainly the more severely ill, progress to develop the acute respiratory distress syndrome (ARDS; p. 192).

Survival is possible after immersion for up to 30 minutes in very cold water, as the rapid development of hypothermia after immersion may be protective, particularly in children. Long-term outcome depends on the severity of the cerebral hypoxic injury and is predicted by the duration of immersion, delay in resuscitation, intensity of acidosis and the presence of cardiac arrest.

Management

Initial management requires cardiopulmonary resuscitation with administration of oxygen and maintenance of the circulation (p. 558). It is important to clear the airway of foreign bodies and protect the cervical spine. Continuous positive airways pressure (CPAP; p. 193) should be considered for spontaneously breathing patients with oxygen saturations below 94%. Observation is required for a minimum of 24 hours. Prophylactic antibiotics are only required if exposure was to obviously contaminated water.

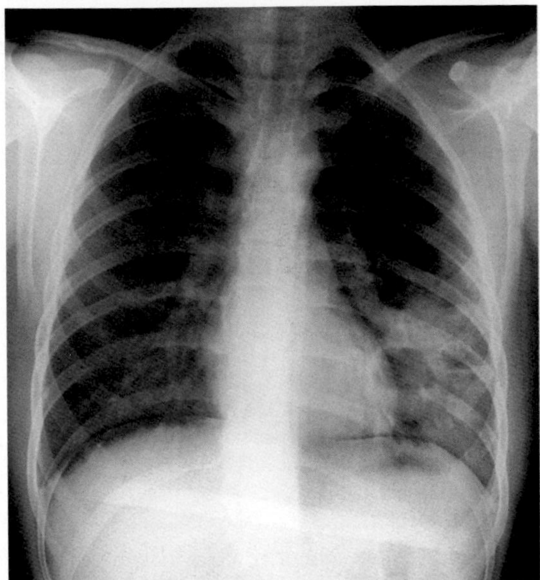

Fig. 5.7 Near-drowning. Chest X-ray of a 39-year-old farmer, 2 weeks after immersion in a polluted freshwater ditch for 5 minutes before rescue. Airspace consolidation and cavities in the left lower lobe reflect secondary staphylococcal pneumonia and abscess formation.

Diving-related illness

The underwater environment is extremely hostile. Other than drowning, most diving illness is related to changes in barometric pressure and its effect on gas behaviour.

Ambient pressure under water increases by 101 kPa (1 atmosphere) for every 10 metres of seawater (msw) depth. As divers descend, the partial pressures of the gases they are breathing increase (Box 5.12), and the blood and tissue concentrations of dissolved gases rise accordingly. Nitrogen is a weak anaesthetic agent, and if the inspiratory pressure of nitrogen is allowed to increase above ~320 kPa (i.e. a depth of approximately 30 msw), it produces 'narcosis', resulting in impairment of cognitive function and manual dexterity, not unlike alcohol intoxication. For this reason, compressed air can only be used for shallow diving. Oxygen is also toxic at inspired pressures above approximately 40 kPa (inducing apprehension, muscle twitching, euphoria, sweating, tinnitus, nausea and vertigo), so 100% oxygen cannot be used as an alternative. For dives deeper than approximately 30 msw, mixtures of oxygen with nitrogen and/or helium are used.

Whilst drowning remains the most common diving-related cause of death, another important group of disorders usually present once the diver returns to the surface: decompression illness (DCI) and barotrauma.

5.12 Physics of breathing compressed air while diving in sea water

Depth	Lung volume	Barometric pressure	PiO_2	PiN_2
Surface	100%	101 kPa (1 atmos)	21 kPa	79 kPa
10 m	50%	202 kPa (2 atmos)	42 kPa	159 kPa
20 m	33%	303 kPa (3 atmos)	63 kPa	239 kPa
30 m	25%	404 kPa (4 atmos)	84 kPa	319 kPa

5.13 Assessment of a patient with decompression illness*

Evolution

- Progressive
- Static
- Relapsing
- Spontaneously improving

Manifestations

- Pain: often large joints, e.g. shoulder ('the bends')
- Neurological: any deficit is possible
- Audiovestibular: vertigo, tinnitus, nystagmus; may mimic inner ear barotrauma
- Pulmonary: chest pain, cough, haemoptysis, dyspnoea; may be due to arterial gas embolism
- Cutaneous: itching, erythematous rash
- Lymphatic: tender lymph nodes, oedema
- Constitutional: headache, fatigue, general malaise

Dive profile

- Depth
- Type of gas used
- Duration of dive

*Information required by diving specialists to decide appropriate treatment. See contact details on page 132.

Clinical features

Decompression illness

This includes decompression sickness (DCS) and arterial gas embolism (AGE). Whilst the vast majority of symptoms of decompression illness present within 6 hours of a dive, they can also be provoked by flying and thus patients may present to medical services at sites far removed from the dive.

Exposure of individuals to increased partial pressures of nitrogen results in additional nitrogen being dissolved in body tissues; the amount dissolved depends on the depth/pressure and on the duration of the dive. On ascent, the tissues become supersaturated with nitrogen, and this places the diver at risk of producing a critical quantity of gas (bubbles) in tissues if the ascent is too fast. The gas so formed may cause symptoms locally, by bubbles passing through the pulmonary vascular bed (Box 5.13) or by embolisation elsewhere. Arterial embolisation may occur if the gas load in the venous system exceeds the lungs' abilities to excrete nitrogen, or when bubbles pass through a patent foramen ovale (present asymptomatically in 25–30% of adults; p. 528). Although DCS and AGE can be indistinguishable, their early treatment is the same.

Barotrauma

During the ascent phase of a dive, the gas in the diver's lungs expands due to the decreasing pressure. The diver must therefore ascend slowly and breathe regularly; if ascent is rapid or the diver holds his/her breath, the expanding gas may cause lung rupture (pulmonary barotrauma). This can result in pneumomediastinum, pneumothorax or AGE due to gas passing directly into the pulmonary venous system. Other air-filled body cavities may be subject to barotrauma, including the ear and sinuses.

Management

The patient is nursed horizontally, and airway, breathing and circulation are assessed. Treatment includes the following:

- *High-flow oxygen* is given by a tight-fitting mask using a rebreathing bag. This assists in the washout of excess inert gas (nitrogen) and may reduce the extent of local tissue hypoxia resulting from focal embolic injury.
- *Fluid replacement* (oral or intravenous) corrects the intravascular fluid loss from endothelial bubble injury and the dehydration associated with immersion. Maintenance of an adequate peripheral circulation is important for the excretion of excess dissolved gas.
- *Recompression* is the definitive therapy. Transfer to a recompression chamber facility may be by surface or air, provided that the altitude remains low (< 300 m) and the patient continues to breathe 100% oxygen. Recompression reduces the volume of gas within tissues and puts nitrogen back into solution.

The majority of patients make a complete recovery with treatment, although a small but significant proportion are left with neurological disability.

NUTRITIONAL FACTORS AND DISEASE

Obtaining adequate nutrition is a fundamental requirement for survival of every individual and species. The politics of food provision for humans are complex, and constitute a prominent factor in wars, natural disasters and the global economy. In recent decades, economic success has been rewarded by plentiful nutrition unknown to previous generations, which has led to a pandemic of obesity and its serious consequences for health. Yet, in many parts of the world, famine and under-nutrition still represent a huge burden. Quality, as well as quantity, of food influences health, with governmental advice on healthy diets maximising fruit and vegetable intakes (Fig. 5.8). Inappropriate diets have been linked with diseases such as coronary heart disease and cancer. Deficiencies of simple vitamins or minerals lead to avoidable conditions such as anaemia due to iron deficiency or blindness due to severe vitamin A deficiency. A proper understanding of nutrition is therefore essential in dealing with the needs of individual patients and to inform the planning of public policy.

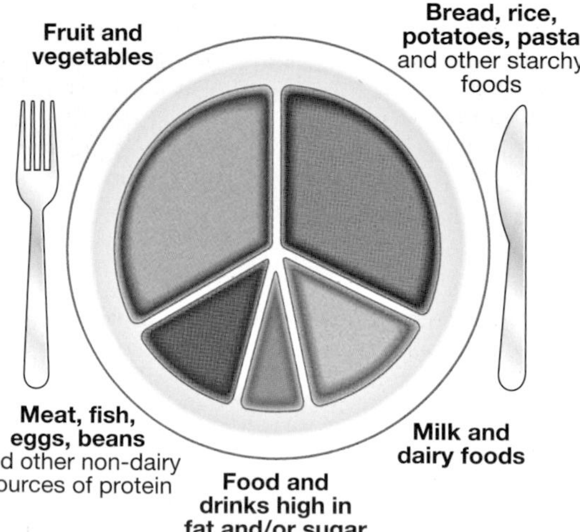

Fig. 5.8 Proportion of key food groups recommended for a healthy, well-balanced diet. Crown copyright – see p. 132.

Physiology of nutrition

Nutrients in the diet can be classified into 'macronutrients', which are eaten in relatively large amounts to provide fuel for energy, and 'micronutrients' (e.g. vitamins and minerals), which do not contribute to energy balance but are required in small amounts because they are not synthesised in the body.

Energy balance

The laws of thermodynamics dictate that energy balance is achieved when energy intake = energy expenditure (Fig. 5.9).

Energy expenditure has several components. The basal metabolic rate (BMR) describes the obligatory energy expenditure required to maintain metabolic functions in tissues and hence sustain life. It is most closely predicted by fat-free mass (i.e. total body mass minus fat mass), which is lower in females and older people (Fig. 5.9B). Extra metabolic energy is consumed during growth, pregnancy and lactation, and when febrile. Metabolic energy is also required for thermal regulation, and expenditure is higher in cold or hot environments. The energy required for digestion of food (diet-induced thermogenesis (DIT); Fig. 5.9D) accounts for approximately 10% of total energy expenditure, with protein requiring more energy than other macronutrients. Another component of energy expenditure is governed by the level of muscular activity, which can vary considerably with occupation and lifestyle (Fig. 5.9C). Physical activity levels are usually defined as multiples of BMR.

Energy intake is determined by the 'macronutrient' content of food. Carbohydrates, fat, protein and alcohol provide fuel for oxidation in the mitochondria to generate energy (as adenosine triphosphate (ATP); p. 45). The energy provided by each of these elements differs:

- carbohydrates (16 kJ/g)
- fat (37 kJ/g)
- protein (17 kJ/g)
- alcohol (29 kJ/g).

Regulation of energy balance

Energy intake and expenditure are highly regulated (Fig. 5.10). A link with reproductive function ensures that pregnancy is most likely to occur during times of nutritional plenty when both mother and baby have a better chance of survival. Improved nutrition is thought to be the reason for the increasingly early onset of puberty in many societies. At the other extreme, anorexia nervosa and excessive exercise can lead to amenorrhoea (p. 255).

Regulation of energy balance is coordinated in the hypothalamus, which receives afferent signals that indicate nutritional status in the short term (e.g. the stomach

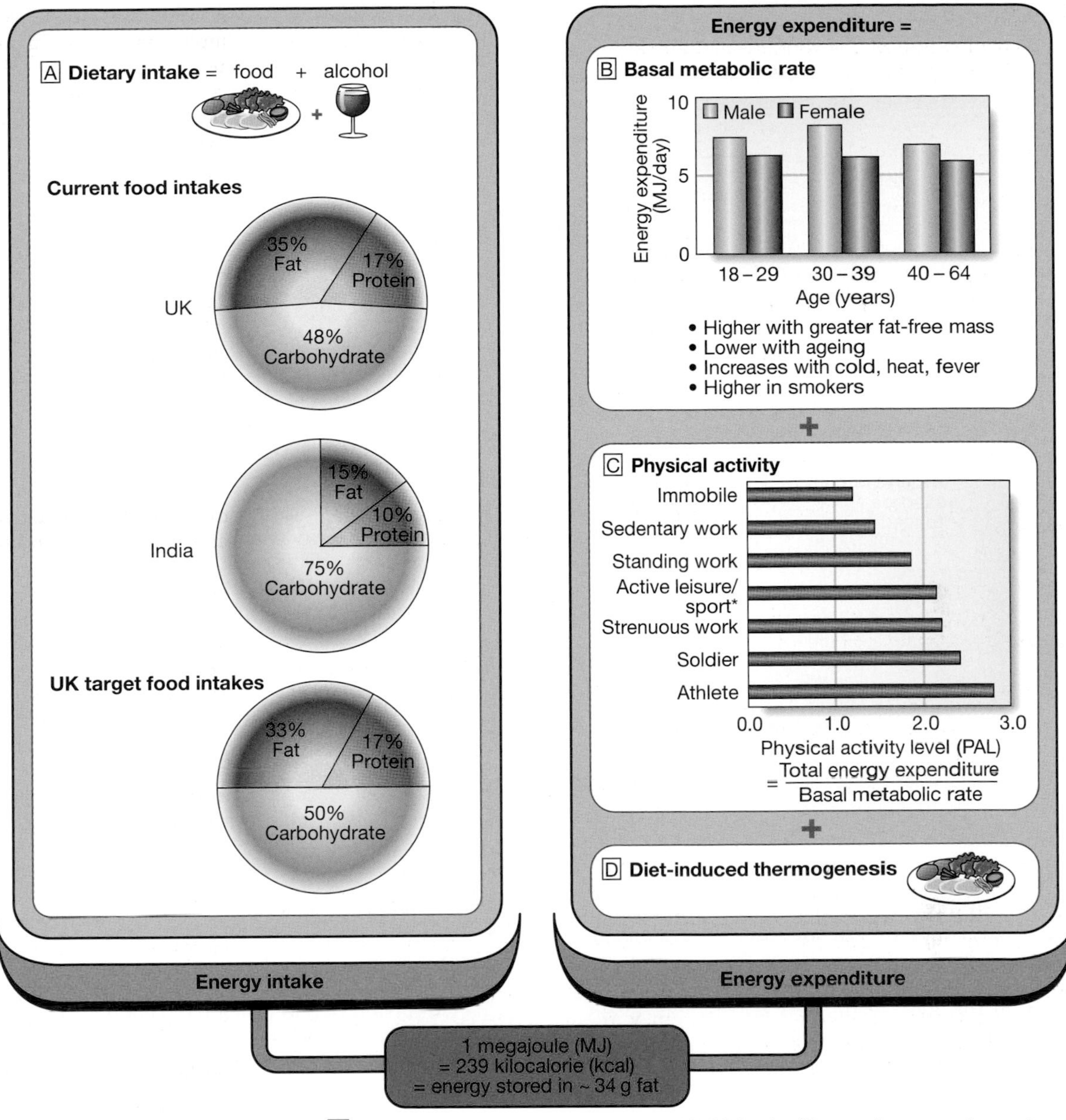

Fig. 5.9 Determinants of energy balance. **A** Energy intake is shown as national averages, highlighting the differences in sources of energy in different countries (but obscuring substantial regional variations). The targets are recommendations as a percentage of food energy only (Source: Dept of Health 1991). For WHO target, see Box 5.17 (p. 114). In the UK, it is assumed that 5% of energy intake will be derived from alcohol. **B** Data for normal basal metabolic rate (BMR) were obtained from healthy men and women in various countries. BMR declines from middle age and is lower in women, even after adjustment for body size because of differences in fat-free mass. **C** Energy is required for movement and activity. Physical activity level (PAL) is the multiple of BMR by which total energy expenditure is increased by activity. **D** Energy is consumed in order to digest food. Leisure or sport activity increases PAL by ~0.3 for each 30–60 minutes of moderate exercise performed 4–5 times per week. The UK population median for PAL is 1.6, with estimates of 1.5 for the 'less active' and 1.8 for the 'more active'.

hormone ghrelin, which falls immediately after eating and rises gradually thereafter, to suppress satiety and signal that it is time for the next meal) and the long term (e.g. the adipose hormone leptin, which increases with growing fat mass and may also link fat mass to reproductive function). The hypothalamus responds with changes in many local neurotransmitters that alter activity in a number of pathways that influence energy balance (see Fig. 5.10), including hormones acting on the pituitary gland (see Fig. 20.2, p. 737), and neural control circuits that connect with the cerebral cortex and autonomic nervous system.

Responses to under- and over-nutrition

These complex regulatory pathways allow adaptation to variations in nutrition. In response to starvation, reproductive function is suppressed, BMR is reduced, and there are profound psychological effects, including energy conservation through lethargy. These adjustments can 'defend' body weight within certain limits.

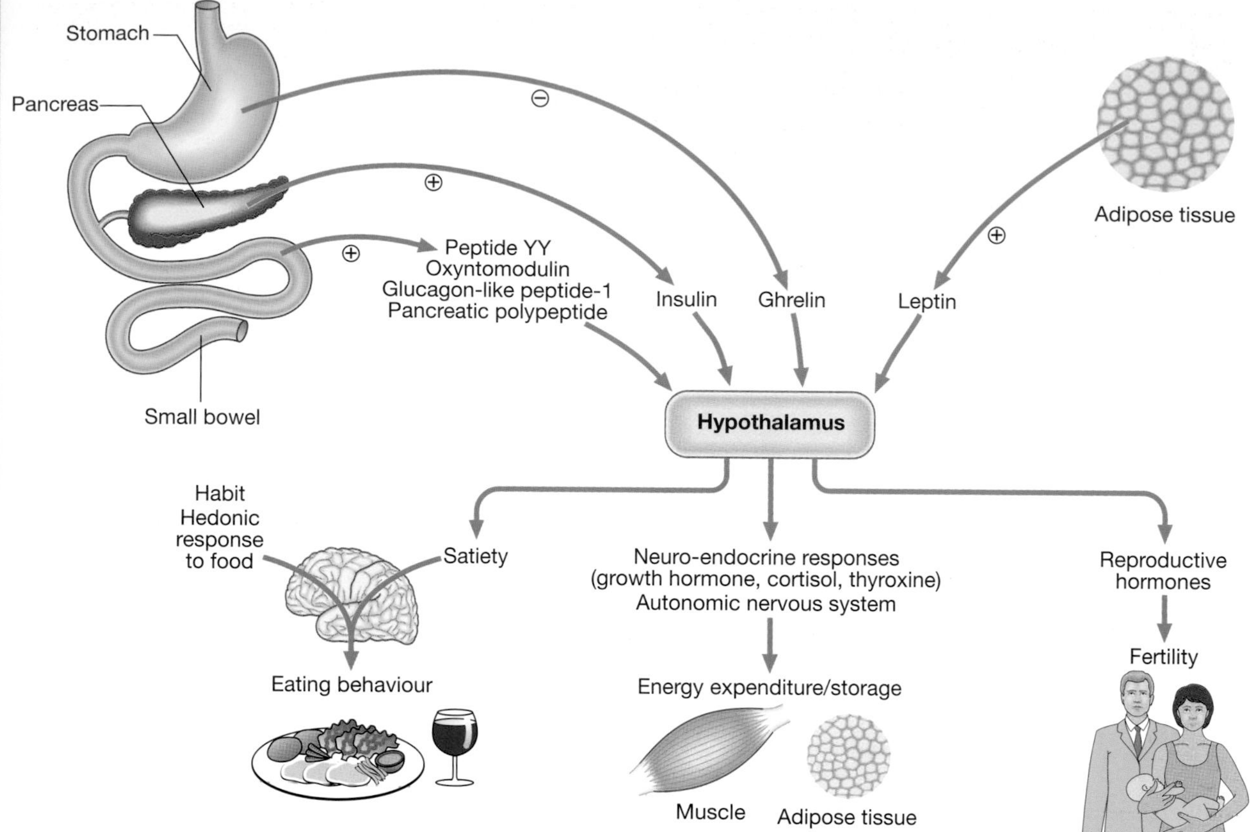

Fig. 5.10 Regulation of energy balance and its link with reproduction. ⊕ indicates factors that are stimulated by eating and induce satiety. ⊖ indicates factors that are suppressed by eating and inhibit satiety.

However, in the low-insulin state of starvation (see Fig. 21.2, p. 801), fuels are liberated from stores initially in glycogen (in liver and muscle), then in triglyceride (lipolysis in adipose tissue, with excess free fatty acid supply to the liver leading to ketosis) and finally in protein (proteolysis in muscle).

In response to over-nutrition, BMR is increased, and extra energy is consumed in the work of carrying increased fat stores, so that body weight is again 'defended' within certain limits. In the high-insulin state of over-nutrition, excess energy is invested in fatty acids and stored as triglycerides; these are deposited principally in adipose tissue but they may also accumulate in the liver (non-alcoholic fatty liver disease; p. 959) and skeletal muscle. In the absence of hypothalamic function (e.g. in those with craniopharyngioma; see Fig. 20.30, p. 794) or in rare patients with mutations in relevant genes (e.g. in leptin or melanocortin-4 receptors), loss of response to satiety signals, together with loss of adaptive changes in energy expenditure, result in relentless weight gain.

Macronutrients (energy-yielding nutrients)

Carbohydrates

Types of carbohydrate and their dietary sources are listed in Box 5.14. The 'available' carbohydrates (starches and sugars) are broken down to monosaccharides before absorption from the gut (p. 842), and supply over half the energy in a normal, well-balanced diet (see Fig. 5.9A). No individual carbohydrate is an essential nutrient, as carbohydrates can be synthesised de novo from glycerol or protein. However, if the available carbohydrate intake is less than 100 g per day, increased lipolysis leads to ketosis (see Fig. 21.5, p. 804).

Dietary guidelines do not restrict the intake of intrinsic sugars in fruit and vegetables or the sugars in milk. However, intake of non-milk extrinsic sugars (sucrose, maltose, fructose), which increase the risk of dental caries and diabetes mellitus, should be limited. Individuals who do not produce lactase ('lactose-intolerant') are advised to avoid or limit dairy products and foods with added lactose. Starches in cereal foods, root foods and legumes provide the largest proportion of energy in most diets around the world. All starches are polymers of glucose, linked by the same 1–4 glycosidic linkages. However, some starches are digested promptly by salivary and then pancreatic amylase, producing rapid delivery of glucose to the blood. Other starches are digested more slowly, either because they are protected in the structure of the food, because of their crystal structure, or because the molecule is unbranched (amylose). These differences are the basis for the 'glycaemic index' of foods. This is the area under the curve of the rise in blood glucose concentration in the 2 hours following ingestion of 50 g carbohydrate, expressed as a percentage of the response to 50 g anhydrous glucose. There is emerging evidence linking high glycaemic index foods with obesity and type 2 diabetes (p. 806).

5.14 Dietary carbohydrates

Class	Components	Examples	Source
Free sugars	Monosaccharides Disaccharides	Glucose, fructose Sucrose, lactose, maltose	Intrinsic: fruits, milks, vegetables Extrinsic (extracted, refined): beet or cane sucrose, high-fructose corn syrup
Short-chain carbohydrates	Oligosaccharides	Maltodextrins, fructo-oligosaccharides	
Starch polysaccharides	Rapidly digestible Slowly digestible Resistant		Cereals (wheat, rice), root vegetables (potato), legumes (lentils, beans, peas)
Non-starch polysaccharides (NSP, dietary fibre)	Fibrous Viscous	Cellulose Hemicellulose Pectins Gums	Plants
Sugar alcohols		Sorbitol, xylitol	Sorbitol: stone fruits (apples, peaches, prunes) Xylitol: maize, berry fruits Both used as low-calorie sugar alternatives

Sugar alcohols (e.g. sorbitol) that are used as replacement sweeteners can cause diarrhoea if eaten in large amounts.

Dietary fibre

Dietary fibre is plant food that is not digested by human enzymes in the gastrointestinal tract. Most dietary fibre is known as the 'non-starch polysaccharides' (NSP) (see Box 5.14). A small percentage of 'resistant' dietary starch may also pass unchanged into the large intestine. Dietary fibre can be broken down by the resident bacteria in the colon to produce short-chain fatty acids. This is essential fuel for the enterocytes and contributes to bowel health. The extent of flatus formed is dependent on the food source.

Some types of NSP, notably the hemicellulose of wheat, increase the water-holding capacity of colonic contents and the bulk of faeces. They relieve simple constipation, appear to prevent diverticulosis and may reduce the risk of cancer of the colon. Other viscous, indigestible polysaccharides like pectin and guar gum are important in the upper gastrointestinal tract, where they slow gastric emptying, contribute to satiety, and reduce bile salt absorption and hence plasma cholesterol concentration.

Fats

Fat has the highest energy density of the macronutrients (37 kJ/g) and excessive consumption may be an insidious cause of obesity (see Fig. 5.9A). Free fatty acids are absorbed in chylomicrons (pp. 450 and 841; see Fig. 22.5, p. 842), allowing access of complex molecules into the circulation. Fatty acid structures are shown in Figure 5.11. The principal polyunsaturated fatty acid (PUFA) in plant seed oils is linoleic acid (18:2 ω6). This and alpha-linolenic acid (18:3 ω3) are the 'essential' fatty acids, which humans cannot synthesise de novo. They undergo further desaturation and elongation, to produce, for example, γ-linolenic acid (18:3 ω6) and arachidonic acid (20:4 ω6). These are precursors of prostaglandins and eicosanoids, and form part of the structure of lipid membranes in all cells. Fish oils are rich in ω3 PUFA (e.g. eicosapentaenoic (20:5 ω3) and docosahexaenoic

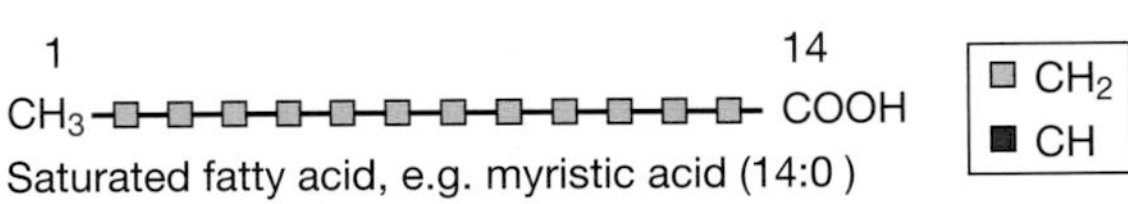

Fig. 5.11 Schematic representation of fatty acids. Standard nomenclature specifies the number of carbon atoms and indicates the number and position of the double bond(s) relative to the methyl ($-CH_3$, ω) end of the molecule after a colon.

(22:6 ω3), which promote the anti-inflammatory cascade of prostaglandin production and occur in the lipids of the human brain and retina. They inhibit thrombosis by competitively antagonising thromboxane A_2 formation. Substituting saturated fat (i.e. from animal sources: butter, ghee or lard) with PUFA in the diet can lower the concentration of circulating low-density lipoprotein (LDL) cholesterol and may help prevent coronary heart disease. High intakes of *trans* fatty acids (TFA) (isomers of the natural *cis* fatty acids) reflect the use of oils that have been partially hydrogenated in the food industry. It is recommended that TFAs are limited to < 2% of the dietary fat intake, as they are associated with cardiovascular disease. Changes in industrial practice in the UK and US have meant that TFA intake is now below 1%, with the residual amounts coming from milk as a result of ruminant digestion.

Cholesterol is also absorbed directly from food in chylomicrons and is an important substrate for steroid and sterol synthesis, but not an important source of energy.

5.15 Amino acids

Essential amino acids	
• Tryptophan	• Valine
• Histidine	• Phenylalanine
• Methionine	• Lysine
• Threonine	• Leucine
• Isoleucine	
Conditionally essential amino acids and their precursors	
• Cysteine: methionine, serine	
• Tyrosine: phenylalanine	
• Arginine: glutamine/glutamate, aspartate	
• Proline: glutamate	
• Glycine: serine, choline	

Proteins

Proteins are made up of some 20 different amino acids, of which nine are 'essential' (Box 5.15), i.e. they cannot be synthesised in humans but are required for synthesis of important proteins. Another group of five amino acids are termed 'conditionally essential', meaning that they can be synthesised from other amino acids, provided there is an adequate dietary supply. The remaining amino acids can be synthesised in the body by transamination, provided there is a sufficient supply of amino groups.

The nutritive or 'biological' value of different proteins depends on the relative proportions of essential amino acids they contain. Proteins of animal origin, particularly from eggs, milk and meat, are generally of higher biological value than proteins of vegetable origin, which are low in one or more of the essential amino acids. However, when two different vegetable proteins are eaten together (e.g. a cereal and a legume), their amino acid contents are complementary and produce an adequate mix, an important principle in vegan diets.

Dietary recommendations for macronutrients

Recommendations for energy intake (Box 5.16) and proportions of macronutrients (Box 5.17) have been calculated to provide a balance of essential nutrients and minimise the risks of excessive refined sugar (dental caries, high glycaemic index/diabetes mellitus), saturated fat or *trans* fat (obesity, coronary heart disease). Recommended dietary fibre intake is based on avoiding risks of colonic disease. The usual recommended protein intake for a healthy man doing light work is 65–100 g/day. The minimum requirement is around 40 g of protein with a high proportion of essential amino acids or a high biological value.

5.16 Daily adult energy requirements in health

	Daily requirements*	
Circumstances	**Females**	**Males**
At rest (basal metabolic rate)	5.4 MJ (1300 kcal)	6.7 MJ (1600 kcal)
Less active	8.0 MJ (1900 kcal)	9.9 MJ (2400 kcal)
Population median	8.8 MJ (2100 kcal)	10.8 MJ (2600 kcal)
More active	9.6 MJ (2300 kcal)	11.8 MJ (2800 kcal)

*These are based on a healthy target body mass index (BMI) of 22.5 kg/m^2. For a female, height is 162 cm and weight 59.0 kg; for a male, height is 175 cm and weight 68.8 kg. Previous average recommendations of 8.1 MJ (1950 kcal, usually rounded up to 2000 kcal) for females and 10.7 MJ (2500 kcal) for males should continue to be used, as these fall within experimental error.

5.17 WHO recommended population macronutrient goals

Nutrient (% of total energy unless indicated)	Target limits for average population intakes: Lower	Upper
Total fat	15	30
Saturated fatty acids	0	10
Polyunsaturated fatty acids	6	10
Trans fatty acids	0	2
Dietary cholesterol (mg/day)	0	300
Total carbohydrate	55	75
Free sugars	0	10
Complex carbohydrate	50	70
Dietary fibre (g/day)		
As non-starch polysaccharides	16	24
As total dietary fibre	27	40
Protein	10	15

Clinical assessment and investigation of nutritional status

The diverse manifestations of inadequate nutrition dictate that its clinical assessment and investigation involve many systems. Energy balance is reflected in body composition, which is most readily assessed by clinical anthropometric measurements. It can also be tested non-invasively by the measurement of body fat by bio-impedance or dual energy X-ray absorptiometry (DEXA) scanning. Abnormal micronutrient status is commonly manifest in clinical signs in the skin and mucous membranes, or in other systems.

A dietary history provides useful information, especially when obtained by a dietitian. A weighed food diary is considered to be the gold standard dietary assessment but is rarely conducted in clinical practice.

Anthropometric measurements

Body mass index (BMI) is useful for categorising under- and over-nutrition. It is the weight in kilograms divided by the height in metres, squared. For example, an adult weighing 70 kg with a height of 1.75 m has a BMI of $70/1.75^2 = 22.9$ kg/m^2. If height cannot be determined (e.g. in older people with kyphosis or in those who cannot stand), a surrogate measure is:

- *the demispan*: measured from the sternal notch to the middle finger; height = 0.73 × (2 × demispan) + 0.43
- *knee height*:

females (60–80 years): height (cm) = (knee height (cm) × 1.91) − (age (years) × 0.17) + 75.00

males (60–80 years): height (cm) = (knee height (cm) × 2.05) + 59.01.

BMI does not discriminate between fat mass and lean body mass and can be increased by muscle mass (e.g. in athletes). Moreover, there are ethnic differences in body fat content; at the same BMI, Asians have more body fat than Europeans. For optimal health, the BMI should be 18.5–24.9 kg/m^2.

An indication of the degree of abdominal obesity is the waist circumference, measured at the level of the umbilicus. Hip circumference can be measured at the level of the greater trochanters; waist:hip ratios show whether the distribution of fat is android or gynoid (see below). Skinfold measurements can be used to calculate body fat content, whereas relative loss of muscle and subcutaneous fat can be estimated by measuring mid-arm circumference (at the middle of the humerus) and skinfold thickness over the triceps (using special callipers); muscle mass is estimated by subtracting triceps skinfold thickness from mid-arm circumference.

DISORDERS OF ALTERED ENERGY BALANCE

Obesity

Obesity is widely regarded as a pandemic, with potentially disastrous consequences for human health. Over one-quarter of adults in the UK were obese (i.e. BMI ≥ 30 kg/m^2) in 2010, compared with 7% prevalence in 1980 and 16% in 1995. Moreover, almost two-thirds of the UK adult population are overweight (BMI ≥ 25 kg/m^2), although there is considerable regional and age group variation. In developing countries, average national rates of obesity are low, but these figures may disguise high rates of obesity in urban communities; for example, nearly one-quarter of women in urban India are overweight.

There is increasing public awareness of the health implications of obesity. Many patients will seek medical help for their obesity, others will present with one of the complications of obesity, and increasing numbers are being identified during health screening examinations.

Complications of obesity

Obesity has adverse effects on both mortality and morbidity (Box 5.18). Changes in mortality are difficult to analyse due to the confounding effects of lower body weight in cigarette smokers and those with other illnesses (such as cancer). However, it is clear that the lowest mortality rates are seen in Europeans in the BMI range 18.5–24 kg/m^2 (and at lower BMI in Asians). It is suggested that obesity at age 40 years can reduce life expectancy by up to 7 years for non-smokers and by 13 years for smokers. Coronary heart disease (Fig. 5.12) is the major cause of death but cancer rates are also increased in the overweight, especially colorectal cancer in males and cancer of the gallbladder, biliary tract, breast, endometrium and cervix in females. Obesity has little effect on life expectancy above 70 years of age, but the obese do spend a greater proportion of their active life disabled. Epidemic obesity has been accompanied by an epidemic of type 2 diabetes (p. 806) and osteoarthritis, particularly of the knee. Although an increased body size results in greater bone density through increased mechanical stress, it is not certain whether this translates to a lower incidence of osteoporotic fractures (p. 1120). Obesity may have profound psychological consequences, compounded by stigmatisation of the obese in many societies.

5.18 Complications of obesity

Risk factors	Outcomes
'Metabolic syndrome' Type 2 diabetes Hypertension Hyperlipidaemia	Coronary heart disease Stroke Diabetes complications
Liver fat accumulation	Non-alcoholic steatohepatitis Cirrhosis
Restricted ventilation	Exertional dyspnoea Obstructive sleep apnoea Obesity hypoventilation syndrome (Pickwickian syndrome)
Mechanical effects of weight	Urinary incontinence Osteoarthritis Varicose veins
Increased peripheral steroid interconversion in adipose tissue	Hormone-dependent cancers (breast, uterus) Polycystic ovarian syndrome (infertility, hirsutism; p. 764)
Others	Psychological morbidity (low self-esteem, depression) Socioeconomic disadvantage (lower income, less likely to be promoted) Gallstones Colorectal cancer Skin infections (groin and submammary candidiasis; hidradenitis)

Body fat distribution

For some complications of obesity, the distribution rather than the absolute amount of excess adipose tissue appears to be important. Increased intra-abdominal fat causes 'central' ('abdominal', 'visceral', 'android' or 'apple-shaped') obesity, which contrasts with subcutaneous fat accumulation causing 'generalised' ('gynoid' or 'pear-shaped') obesity; the former is more common in men and is more closely associated with type 2 diabetes, the metabolic syndrome and cardiovascular disease (see Box 5.18). The key difference between these depots of fat may lie in their vascular anatomy, with intra-abdominal fat draining into the portal vein and thence directly to the liver. Thus many factors that are released from adipose tissue (including free fatty acids; 'adipokines', such as tumour necrosis factor-α, adiponectin and resistin; and steroid hormones) may be at higher concentration in the liver and hence induce insulin resistance and promote type 2 diabetes (p. 805). Recent research has also highlighted the importance of fat deposition within specific organs, especially the

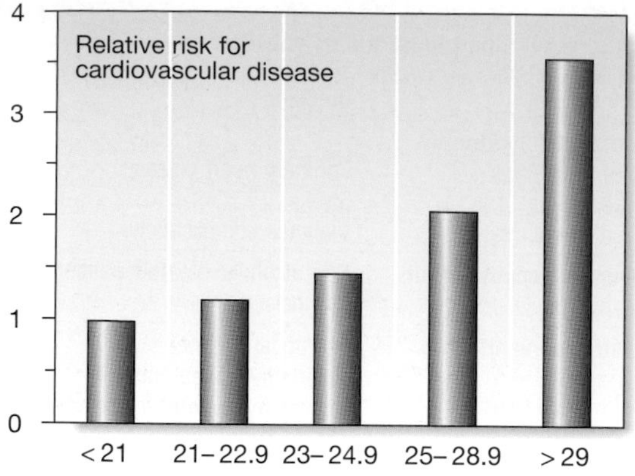

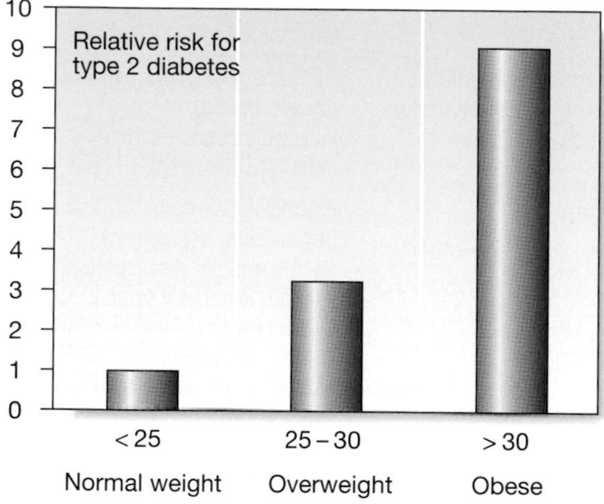

Fig. 5.12 Risks of diabetes and cardiovascular disease in overweight and obese women. Data are from the Nurses' Health Study in the USA, mostly of Caucasian women. In some ethnic groups (e.g. South Asians, Native Americans) and in people with higher waist circumference, the metabolic complications are even more severe at a given level of BMI.

liver, as an important determinant of metabolic risk in the obese.

Aetiology

Accumulation of fat results from a discrepancy between energy consumption and energy expenditure that is too large to be defended by the hypothalamic regulation of BMR. A continuous small daily positive energy balance of only 0.2–0.8 MJ (50–200 kcal; < 10% of intake) would lead to weight gain of 2–20 kg over a period of 4–10 years. Given the cumulative effects of subtle energy excess, body fat content shows 'tracking' with age such that obese children usually become obese adults. Weight tends to increase throughout adult life, as BMR and physical activity decrease (see Fig. 5.9).

The pandemic of obesity reflects changes in both energy intake and energy expenditure (Box 5.19), although both are difficult to measure reliably. The estimated average global daily supply of food energy per person increased from approximately 9.8 MJ (2350 kcal) in the 1960s to approximately 11.7 MJ (2800 kcal) in the 1990s, but its delivery is unequal. For example, in India it is estimated that 5% of the population receives 40% of the available food energy, leading to obesity in the urban population in parallel with persisting under-nutrition in some rural communities. In affluent societies, a significant proportion of this food supply is discarded. In the US, the average daily energy intake of men reportedly rose from 10.2 MJ (2450 kcal) in 1971 to 11.0 MJ (2618 kcal) in 2000. Portion sizes, particularly of energy-dense foods such as drinks with highly refined sugar content and salty snacks, have increased. However, data in the UK suggest that energy intakes have declined (which may in part be due to deliberate restriction or 'dieting'), but this is apparently insufficient to compensate for the decrease in physical activity levels in recent years. Obesity is correlated positively with the number of hours spent watching television, and inversely with levels of physical activity (e.g. stair climbing). It is suggested that minor activities such as fidgeting and chewing gum may contribute to energy expenditure and protect against obesity.

5.19 Some reasons for the increasing prevalence of obesity – the 'obesogenic' environment

Increasing energy intake	
• ↑ Portion sizes • ↑ Snacking and loss of regular meals	• ↑ Energy-dense food (mainly fat) • ↑ Affluence
Decreasing energy expenditure	
• ↑ Car ownership • ↓ Walking to school/work • ↑ Automation; ↓ manual labour	• ↓ Sports in schools • ↑ Time spent on computer games and watching TV • ↑ Central heating

Susceptibility to obesity

Susceptibility to obesity and its adverse consequences undoubtedly varies between individuals. It is not true that obese subjects have a 'slow metabolism', since their BMR is higher than that of lean subjects. Twin and adoption studies confirm a genetic influence on obesity. The pattern of inheritance suggests a polygenic disorder, with small contributions from a number of different genes, together accounting for 25–70% of variation in weight. Recent results from 'genome-wide' association studies of polymorphisms in large numbers of people (p. 53) have identified a handful of genes that influence obesity, some of which encode proteins known to be involved in the control of appetite or metabolism and some of which have unknown function. However, these genes account for less than 5% of the variation in body weight.

A few rare single-gene disorders have been identified that lead to severe childhood obesity. These include mutations of the melanocortin-4 receptor (MC4R), which account for approximately 5% of severe early-onset obesity; defects in the enzymes processing propiomelanocortin (POMC, the precursor for adrenocorticotrophic hormone (ACTH)) in the hypothalamus; and mutations in the leptin gene (see Fig. 5.9). The latter can be treated by leptin injections. Additional genetic conditions in which obesity is a feature include the Prader–Willi (see Box 3.3, p. 54) and Lawrence-Moon-Biedl syndromes.

5.20 Potentially reversible causes of weight gain

Endocrine factors	
• Hypothyroidism • Cushing's syndrome • Insulinoma	• Hypothalamic tumours or injury
Drug treatments	
• Atypical antipsychotics (e.g. olanzapine) • Sulphonylureas, thiazolidinediones, insulin	• Pizotifen • Corticosteroids • Sodium valproate • β-blockers

Reversible causes of obesity and weight gain

In a small minority of patients presenting with obesity, specific causal factors can be identified and treated (Box 5.20). These patients are distinguished from those with idiopathic obesity by their short history, with a recent marked change in the trajectory of their adult weight gain.

Clinical assessment and investigations

In assessing an individual presenting with obesity, the aims are to:

- quantify the problem
- exclude an underlying cause
- identify complications
- reach a management plan.

Severity of obesity can be quantified using the BMI (Box 5.21). A waist circumference of > 102 cm in men or > 88 cm in women indicates that the risk of metabolic and cardiovascular complications of obesity is high.

A dietary history may be helpful in guiding dietary advice, but is notoriously susceptible to under-reporting of food consumption. It is important to consider 'pathological' eating behaviour (such as binge eating, nocturnal eating or bulimia; p. 255), which may be the most important issue to address in some patients. Alcohol is an important source of energy intake and should be considered in detail.

The history of weight gain may help diagnose underlying causes. A patient who has recently gained substantial weight or has gained weight at a faster rate than previously, and is not taking relevant drugs (see Box 5.20), is more likely to have an underlying disorder such as hypothyroidism (p. 743) or Cushing's syndrome (p. 773). All obese patients should have thyroid function tests performed on one occasion, and an overnight dexamethasone suppression test or 24-hour urine free cortisol if Cushing's syndrome is suspected. Monogenic and 'syndromic' causes of obesity are usually only relevant in children presenting with severe obesity.

Assessment of the diverse complications of obesity (see Box 5.18) requires a thorough history, examination and screening investigations. The impact of obesity on the patient's life and work is a major consideration. Assessment of other cardiovascular risk factors is important. Blood pressure should be measured with a large cuff, if required (p. 608). Associated type 2 diabetes and dyslipidaemia are detected by measuring blood glucose or HbA_{1c} and a serum lipid profile, ideally in a fasting morning sample. Elevated serum transaminases occur in patients with non-alcoholic fatty liver disease (p. 959).

5.21 Quantifying obesity with body mass index (weight/height^2)

BMI (kg/m^2)	Classification*	Risk of obesity comorbidity
18.5–24.9	Reference range	Negligible
25.0–29.9	Overweight	Mildly increased
> 30.0	**Obese**	
30.0–34.9	Class I	Moderate
35.0–39.9	Class II	Severe
> 40.0	Class III	Very severe

*Classification of the WHO and International Obesity Task Force. The Western Pacific Region Office of WHO recommends that, amongst Asians, BMI > 23.0 is overweight and > 25.0 is obese.

Management

The health risks of obesity are largely reversible. Interventions proven to reduce weight in obese patients also ameliorate cardiovascular risk factors. Lifestyle advice that lowers body weight and increases physical exercise reduces the incidence of type 2 diabetes (p. 820). Given the high prevalence of obesity and the large magnitude of its risks, population strategies to prevent and reverse obesity are high on the public health priority list for many countries. Initiatives include promoting healthy eating in schools, enhancing walking and cycling options for commuters, and liaising with the food industry to reduce energy and fat content and to label foods appropriately. Unfortunately, 'low-fat' foods are often still energy-dense, and current lifestyles with labour-saving devices, sedentary work and passive leisure activities have much lower energy requirements than the manual labour and household duties of previous generations.

Most patients seeking assistance with obesity are motivated to lose weight but have attempted to do so previously without long-term success. Often weight will have oscillated between periods of successful weight loss and then regain of weight ('recidivism'). These patients may hold misconceptions that they have an underlying disease, inaccurate perceptions of their energy intake and expenditure, and an unrealistic view of the target weight that they would regard as a 'success'. An empathetic explanation of energy balance, which recognises that some individuals are more susceptible to obesity than others and may find it more difficult to lose and sustain body weight loss, is important. Exclusion of underlying 'hormone imbalance' with simple tests is reassuring and shifts the focus on to consideration of energy balance. Appropriate goals for weight loss should be agreed, recognising that the slope of the relationship between obesity and many of its complications becomes steeper with increasing BMI, so that a given amount of weight loss achieves greater risk reduction at higher levels of BMI. A reasonable goal for most patients is to lose 5–10% of body weight.

The management plan will vary according to the severity of the obesity (see Box 5.21) and the associated risk factors and complications. It will also be influenced by availability of resources; health-care providers and regulators have generally been careful not to recommend expensive interventions (especially long-term drug therapy and surgery) for everyone who is overweight. Instead, most guidelines focus resources on short-term interventions in those who have high health risks and comorbidities associated with their obesity, and who have demonstrated their capacity to alter their lifestyle to achieve weight loss (Fig. 5.13).

Lifestyle advice

Behavioural modification to avoid some of the effects of the 'obesogenic' environment (see Box 5.19) is the cornerstone of long-term control of weight. Regular eating patterns and maximising physical activity are advised, with reference to the modest extra activity required to increase physical activity level (PAL) ratios (see Fig. 5.9C, p. 111). Where possible, this should be incorporated in the daily routine (e.g. walking rather than driving to work), since this is more likely to be sustained. Alternative exercise (e.g. swimming) may be considered if musculoskeletal complications prevent walking. Changes in eating behaviour (including food selection, portion size control, avoidance of snacking, regular meals to encourage satiety, and substitution of sugar with artificial sweeteners) should be discussed. Regular support from a dietitian or attendance at a weight loss group may be helpful.

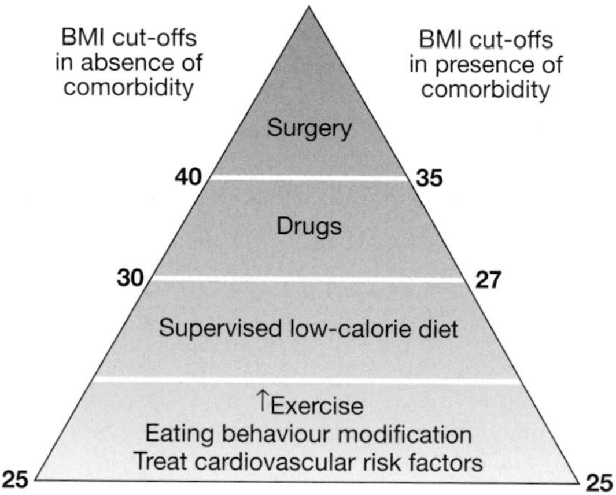

Fig. 5.13 Therapeutic options for obesity. Relevant comorbidities include type 2 diabetes, hypertension, cardiovascular disease, sleep apnoea, and waist circumference > 102 cm in men or 88 cm in women. This is an approximate consensus of the numerous national guidelines, which vary slightly in their recommendations and are revised every few years.

Weight loss diets

In overweight people, adherence to the lifestyle advice given above may gradually induce weight loss. In obese patients, more active intervention is usually required to lose weight before conversion to the 'weight maintenance' advice given above. A significant industry has developed in marketing diets for weight loss. These vary substantially in their balance of macronutrients (Box 5.22), but there is little evidence that they vary in their medium-term (1-year) efficacy. Most involve recommending a reduction of daily total energy intake of –2.5 MJ (600 kcal) from the patient's normal consumption. Modelling data that take into account the reduced energy expenditure as weight is lost suggest that a reduction of energy intake of 100 kJ per day will lead to an eventual bodyweight change of about 1 kg, with half of the weight change being achieved in about 1 year and 95% of the weight change in about 3 years. Weight loss is highly variable, with patient compliance being the major determinant of success. There is some evidence that weight loss diets are most effective in their early weeks, and that compliance is improved by novelty of the diet; this provides some justification for switching to a different dietary regimen when weight loss slows on the first diet. Vitamin supplementation is wise in those diets in which macronutrient balance is markedly disturbed.

In some patients, more rapid weight loss is required, e.g. in preparation for surgery. There is no role for starvation diets, which risk profound loss of muscle mass and the development of arrhythmias (and even sudden death) secondary to elevated free fatty acids, ketosis and deranged electrolytes. Very-low-calorie diets (VLCDs) are recommended for short-term rapid weight loss, producing losses of 1.5–2.5 kg/week, compared to 0.5 kg/week on conventional regimens, but require the supervision of an experienced physician and nutritionist. The composition of the diet should ensure a minimum of 50 g of protein each day for men and 40 g for women to minimise muscle degradation. Energy content should be a minimum of 1.65 MJ (400 kcal) for women of height < 1.73 m, and 2.1 MJ (500 kcal) for all men and for women taller than 1.73 m. Side-effects are a problem in

5.22 Low-calorie diet therapy for obesity

Diet	% carbohydrate	% fat	% protein	Comments
Normal (typical developed country)	50	30	15	
Moderate fat (e.g. Weight Watchers)	60	25	15	Maintains balance in macronutrients and micronutrients while reducing energy-dense fats
Low carbohydrate (e.g. Atkins)	10	60	30	Induction of ketosis may suppress hunger
High protein (e.g. Zone)	43	30	27	Protein has greater satiety effect than other macronutrients
Low fat (e.g. Ornish)	70	13	17	

the early stages and include orthostatic hypotension, headache, diarrhoea and nausea.

Drugs

A huge investment has been made by the pharmaceutical industry in finding drugs for obesity. The side-effect profile has limited the use of many agents, with notable withdrawals from clinical use of sibutramine (increased cardiovascular events) and rimonabant (psychiatric side-effects) in recent years; only one drug, orlistat, is currently licensed for long-term use. A number of other agents are in development, so the situation could change rapidly over the next few years. There is no role for diuretics, or for thyroxine therapy without biochemical evidence of hypothyroidism.

Orlistat inhibits pancreatic and gastric lipases and thereby decreases the hydrolysis of ingested triglycerides, reducing dietary fat absorption by approximately 30%. The drug is not absorbed and adverse side-effects relate to the effect of the resultant fat malabsorption on the gut: namely, loose stools, oily spotting, faecal urgency, flatus and the potential for malabsorption of fat-soluble vitamins. Orlistat is taken with each of the three main meals of the day and the dose can be adjusted (60–120 mg) to minimise side-effects. Its efficacy is shown in Figure 5.14; these effects may be explained because patients taking orlistat adhere better to low-fat diets in order to avoid unpleasant gastrointestinal side-effects.

Drug therapy is usually reserved for patients with high risk of complications from obesity (see Fig. 5.13), and its optimum timing and duration are controversial. Although life-long therapy is advocated for many drugs that reduce risk on the basis of relatively short-term research trials (e.g. drugs for hypertension and osteoporosis), some patients who continue to take anti-obesity drugs tend to regain weight with time; this may partly reflect age-related weight gain, but significant weight gain should prompt reinforcement of lifestyle advice and, if this is unsuccessful, drug therapy should be discontinued (see Fig. 5.14).

Surgery

'Bariatric' surgery is by far the most effective long-term treatment for obesity (see Fig. 5.14 and Box 5.23) and is

5.23 Effectiveness and adverse effects of laparoscopic bariatric surgical procedures

Procedure	Expected weight loss (% excess weight)	Adverse effects
Gastric banding	50–60%	Band slippage, erosion, stricture Port-site infection Mortality < 0.2% in experienced centres
Sleeve gastrectomy	50–60%	Iron deficiency Vitamin B_{12} deficiency Mortality < 0.2% in experienced centres
Roux-en-Y gastric bypass	70–80%	Internal hernia Stomal ulcer Dumping syndrome Hypoglycaemia Iron deficiency Vitamin B_{12} deficiency Vitamin D deficiency Mortality 0.5%
Duodenal switch	Up to 100%	Steatorrhoea Protein-calorie malnutrition Iron deficiency Vitamin B_{12} deficiency Calcium, zinc, copper deficiency Mortality 1%

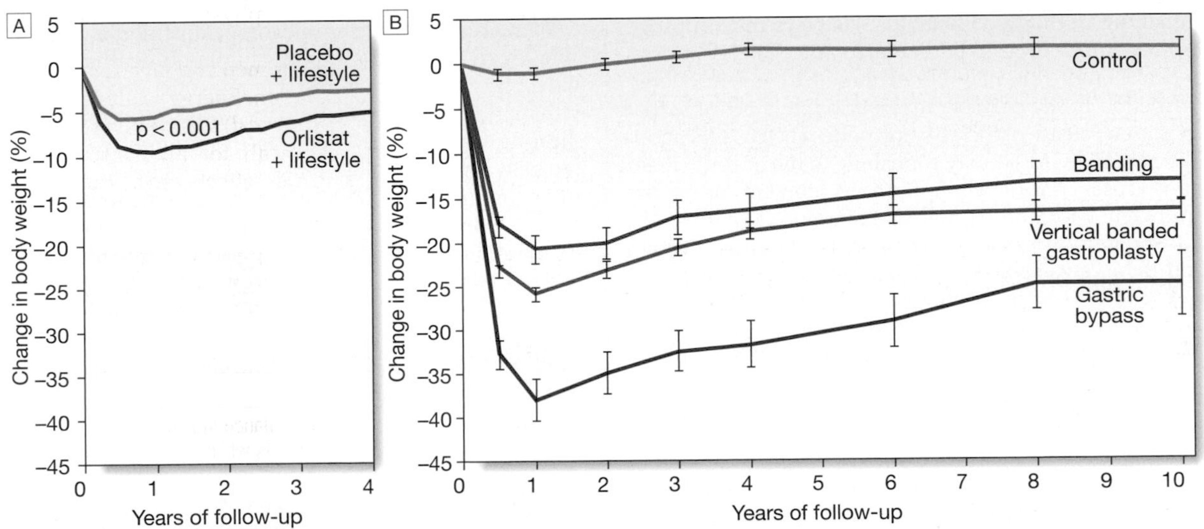

Fig. 5.14 Effects of orlistat and bariatric surgery on weight loss. **A** Data are from Torgerson JS, et al. Diabetes Care 2004; 27:155–161. **B** Data for surgery are from Sjostrom L, et al. New Engl J Med 2004; 351:2683–2693. Each obese subject undergoing surgery was matched with a control subject whose obesity was 'treated' by standard non-operative interventions. Note that the maximum weight loss achieved with orlistat was approximately 11 %; surgery achieves much more substantial and prolonged weight loss.

5

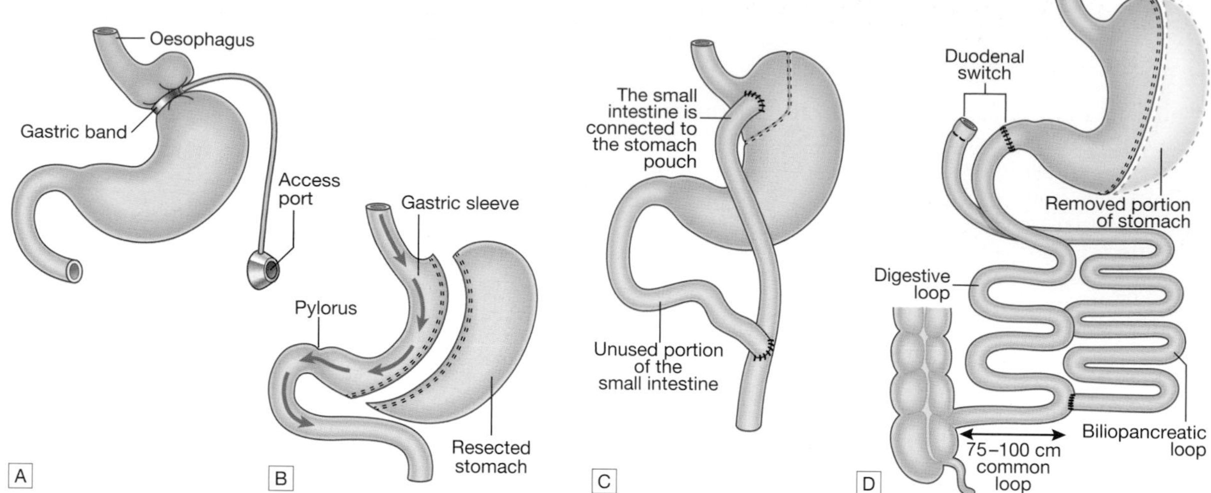

Fig. 5.15 Bariatric surgical procedures. **A** Laparoscopic banding, with the option of a reservoir band and subcutaneous access to restrict the stomach further after compensatory expansion has occurred. **B** Sleeve gastrectomy. **C** Roux-en-Y gastric bypass. **D** Biliopancreatic diversion with duodenal switch.

the only anti-obesity intervention that has been associated with reduced mortality. Bariatric surgery should be contemplated in motivated patients who have very high risks of complications of obesity (see Fig. 5.13), in whom extensive dietary and drug therapy has been insufficiently effective. It is usually reserved for those with severe obesity (BMI > 40 kg/m^2), or those with a BMI > 35 kg/m^2 and significant complications, such as type 2 diabetes or obstructive sleep apnoea. Only experienced specialist surgeons should undertake these procedures, in collaboration with a multidisciplinary team. Several approaches are used (Fig. 5.15) and all can be performed laparoscopically. The mechanism of weight loss may not simply relate to limiting the stomach or absorptive capacity, but rather in disrupting the release of ghrelin from the stomach or promoting the release of other peptides from the small bowel, thereby enhancing satiety signalling in the hypothalamus. Diabetes may improve rapidly after surgery, particularly after gastric bypass, and although this may be attributed to severe energy restriction in the perioperative period, it is possible that increased release of incretin hormones such as glucagon-like peptide (GLP)-1 may contribute to the improvement in glucose control. Complications depend upon the approach. Mortality is low in experienced centres, but post-operative respiratory problems, wound infection and dehiscence, staple leaks, stomal stenosis, marginal ulcers and venous thrombosis may occur. Additional problems may arise at a later stage, such as pouch and distal oesophageal dilatation, persistent vomiting, 'dumping' (p. 875) and micronutrient deficiencies, particularly of folate, vitamin B_{12} and iron, which are of concern especially to women contemplating pregnancy.

Cosmetic surgical procedures may be considered in obese patients after successful weight loss. Apronectomy is usually advocated to remove an overhang of abdominal skin, especially if infected or ulcerated. This operation is of no value for long-term weight reduction if food intake remains unrestricted.

Treatment of additional risk factors

Obesity must not be treated in isolation and other risk factors must be addressed, including smoking, excess alcohol consumption, diabetes mellitus, hyperlipidaemia, hypertension and obstructive sleep apnoea. Treatment of these is discussed in the relevant chapters.

Under-nutrition

Starvation and famine

There remain regions of the world, particularly rural Africa, where under-nutrition due to famine is endemic, the prevalence of BMI < 18.5 kg/m^2 (Box 5.24) in adults is as high as 20%, and growth retardation due to under-nutrition affects 50% of children.

WHO reports that chronic under-nutrition is responsible for more than half of all childhood deaths worldwide. Starvation is manifest as marasmus (malnutrition with marked muscle-wasting), or, when additional complicating mechanisms, such as oxidative stress, come into play, malnourished children can develop kwashiorkor (malnutrition with oedema). Growth retardation is due to deficiency of key nutrients, e.g. protein, zinc, potassium, phosphorus and sulphur. Treatment of these

5.24 Classification of under-nutrition in adults by body mass index (weight/height^2)

BMI (kg/m^2)	Classification
> 20	Adequate nutrition
18.5–20	Marginal
< 18.5	**Under-nutrition**
17–18.4	Mild
16–17	Moderate
< 16	Severe

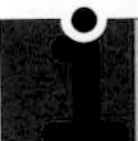

5.25 Causes of under-nutrition and weight loss in adults

Decreased energy intake

- Famine
- Persistent regurgitation or vomiting
- Anorexia, including depression and anorexia nervosa
- Malabsorption (e.g. small intestinal disease)
- Maldigestion (e.g. pancreatic exocrine insufficiency)

Increased energy expenditure

- Increased BMR (thyrotoxicosis, trauma, fever, cancer, cachexia)
- Excessive physical activity (e.g. marathon runners)
- Energy loss (e.g. glycosuria in diabetes)
- Impaired energy storage (e.g. Addison's disease, phaeochromocytoma)

childhood conditions is not discussed in this adult medicine textbook.

In adults, starvation is the result of chronic under-nutrition, i.e. sustained negative energy (calorie) balance. Causes are shown in Box 5.25. Causes of weight loss are considered further on page 859.

Clinical assessment

In starvation, the severity of malnutrition can be assessed by anthropometric measurements, such as BMI (see Box 5.24). Demispan and mid-arm circumference measurements (p. 114) are most useful in monitoring progress during treatment. The clinical features of severe under-nutrition in adults include:

- weight loss
- thirst, craving for food, weakness and feeling cold
- nocturia, amenorrhoea or impotence
- lax, pale, dry skin with loss of turgor and, occasionally, pigmented patches
- cold and cyanosed extremities, pressure sores
- hair thinning or loss (except in adolescents)
- muscle-wasting, best demonstrated by the loss of the temporalis and periscapular muscles and reduced mid-arm circumference
- loss of subcutaneous fat, reflected in reduced skinfold thickness and mid-arm circumference
- hypothermia, bradycardia, hypotension and small heart
- oedema, which may be present without hypoalbuminaemia ('famine oedema')
- distended abdomen with diarrhoea
- diminished tendon jerks
- apathy, loss of initiative, depression, introversion, aggression if food is nearby
- susceptibility to infections (Box 5.26).

Under-nutrition often leads to vitamin deficiencies, especially of thiamin, folate and vitamin C (see below).

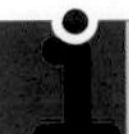

5.26 Infections associated with starvation

- Gastroenteritis and Gram-negative septicaemia
- Respiratory infections, especially bronchopneumonia
- Certain viral diseases, especially measles and herpes simplex
- Tuberculosis
- Streptococcal and staphylococcal skin infections
- Helminthic infestations

Diarrhoea can lead to depletion of sodium, potassium and magnesium. The high mortality rate in famine situations is often due to outbreaks of infection, e.g. typhus or cholera, but the usual signs of infection may not be apparent. In advanced starvation, patients become completely inactive and may assume a flexed, fetal position. In the last stage of starvation, death comes quietly and often quite suddenly. The very old are most vulnerable. All organs are atrophied at necropsy, except the brain, which tends to maintain its weight.

Investigations

In a famine, laboratory investigations may be impractical, but will show that plasma free fatty acids are increased and there is ketosis and a mild metabolic acidosis. Plasma glucose is low but albumin concentration is often maintained because the liver still functions normally. Insulin secretion is diminished, glucagon and cortisol tend to increase, and reverse T_3 replaces normal triiodothyronine (p. 738). The resting metabolic rate falls, partly because of reduced lean body mass and partly because of hypothalamic compensation (see Fig. 5.9, p. 111). The urine has a fixed specific gravity and creatinine excretion becomes low. There may be mild anaemia, leucopenia and thrombocytopenia. The erythrocyte sedimentation rate is normal unless there is infection. Tests of delayed skin hypersensitivity, e.g. to tuberculin, are falsely negative. The electrocardiogram shows sinus bradycardia and low voltage.

Management

Whether in a famine or in wasting secondary to disease, the severity of under-nutrition is graded according to BMI (see Box 5.24). People with mild starvation are in no danger; those with moderate starvation need extra feeding; those who are severely underweight need hospital care.

In severe starvation, there is atrophy of the intestinal epithelium and of the exocrine pancreas, and the bile is dilute. It is critical that the condition is managed by experts. When food becomes available, it should be given by mouth in small, frequent amounts at first, using a suitable formula preparation (Box 5.27). Individual energy requirements can vary by 30%. During rehabilitation, more concentrated formula can be given with additional food that is palatable and similar to the usual staple meal. Salt should be restricted and micronutrient supplements may be essential (e.g. potassium, magnesium, zinc and multivitamins). Between 6.3 and 8.4 MJ/day (1500–2000 kcal/day) will arrest progressive under-nutrition, but additional energy may be required for regain of weight. During refeeding, a weight gain of 5% body weight per month indicates satisfactory progress. Other care is supportive, and includes attention to the skin, adequate hydration, treatment of infections, and careful monitoring of body temperature since thermoregulation may be impaired.

Circumstances and resources are different in every famine, but many problems are non-medical and concern organisation, infrastructure, liaison, politics, procurement, security and ensuring that food is distributed on the basis of need. Lastly, plans must be made for the future for prevention and/or earlier intervention if similar circumstances prevail.

5.27 WHO recommended diets for refeeding

Nutrient (per 100 mL)	F-75 diet[1]	F-100 diet[2]
Energy	315 kJ (75 kcal)	420 kJ (100 kcal)
Protein (g)	0.9	2.9
Lactose (g)	1.3	4.2
Potassium (mmol)	3.6	5.9
Sodium (mmol)	0.9	1.9
Magnesium (mmol)	0.43	0.73
Zinc (mg)	2.0	2.3
Copper (mg)	0.25	0.25
Percentage of energy from		
Protein	5	12
Fat	32	53
Osmolality (osmol/L)	333	419
Dose	170 kJ/kg (40 kcal/kg)	630–920 kJ/kg (150–220 kcal/kg)
Rate of feeding by mouth	2.2 (mL/kg/hr)	Gradual increase in volume, 6 times daily

[1]F-75 is prepared from milk powder (25 g), sugar (70 g), cereal flour (35 g), vegetable oil (27 g) and vitamin and mineral supplements, made up to 1 L with water.
[2]F-100 (1 L) contains milk powder (80 g), sugar (50 g), vegetable oil (60 g) and vitamin and mineral supplements (no cereal).

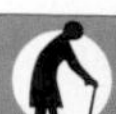

5.28 Energy balance in old age

- **Body composition**: muscle mass is decreased and percentage body fat increased.
- **Energy expenditure**: with the fall in lean body mass, BMR is decreased and energy requirements are reduced.
- **Weight loss**: after weight gain throughout adult life, weight often falls beyond the age of 70 years. This may reflect decreased appetite, loss of smell and taste, and decreased interest in and financial resources for food preparation, especially after loss of a partner.
- **BMI**: less reliable in old age as height is lost (due to kyphosis, osteoporotic crush fractures, loss of intervertebral disc spaces). Alternative measurements include arm demispan and knee height (p. 114), which can be extrapolated to estimate height.

Under-nutrition in hospital

Under-nutrition is a common problem in the hospital setting. In the UK, approximately one-third of patients are affected by moderate or severe under-nutrition on admission. The elderly are particularly at risk (Box 5.28). Once in hospital, many patients lose weight due to factors such as poor appetite, poor dental health, concurrent illness and even being kept 'nil by mouth' for investigations. Under-nutrition is poorly recognised in hospital and has serious consequences. Physical effects include impaired immunity and muscle weakness, which in turn affect cardiac and respiratory function, and delayed wound healing after surgery with increased risks of post-operative infection. The undernourished patient is often apathetic and withdrawn, which may be mistaken for a depressive illness and can affect cooperation with treatment and rehabilitation.

This can be averted with proper monitoring and involvement of an appropriate multidisciplinary team. As a minimum standard, all patients should be weighed on admission to hospital and at least weekly until discharge. A scoring system for identifying patients at nutritional risk is shown in Figure 5.16.

Nutritional support of the hospital patient

Normal diet

As a first step, patients should be encouraged to eat a normal and adequate diet. This is often neglected and there is evidence of substantial wastage in hospital food. In patients at risk of under-nutrition (see Fig. 5.16), quantities eaten should be recorded on a food chart. Hospital staff must identify and overcome barriers to adequate food intake, such as unpalatability of food, cultural and religious factors influencing acceptability of

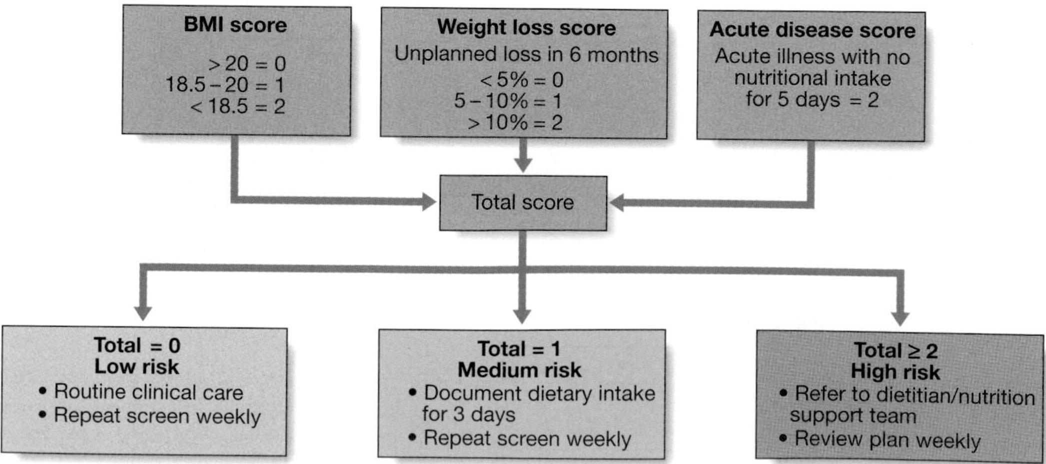

Fig. 5.16 Screening hospitalised patients for risk of malnutrition. Acute illnesses include decompensated liver disease, cancer cachexia or being kept 'nil by mouth'. Adapted from the British Association of Parenteral and Enteral Nutrition Malnutrition Universal Screening Tool' (www.bapen.org.uk).

food, difficulty with hand dexterity (arthritis, stroke), immobility in bed, or poor oral health. Hospital catering departments have an important role in providing acceptable and adequate meals.

Dietary supplements

If sufficient nutritional intake cannot be achieved from normal diet alone, then dietary supplements should be used. These are drinks with high energy and protein content, and are available in cartons as manufactured, flavoured products or are made in the hospital kitchen from milk products and egg. They should be prescribed, and administered by nursing staff, to ensure that they are taken regularly. Dietary supplements do not significantly affect the patient's consumption of normal food.

Enteral tube feeding

Patients who are unable to swallow may require artificial nutritional support: for example, after acute stroke or throat surgery, or when there are long-term neurological problems such as motor neuron disease and multiple sclerosis. The enteral route should always be used if possible, since feeding via the gastrointestinal tract preserves the integrity of the mucosal barrier. This prevents bacteraemia and, in intensive care patients, reduces the risk of multi-organ failure (p. 198).

If the need for artificial nutritional support is thought to be short-term, then feeding is instituted using a fine-bore nasogastric tube. The position of the tube in the stomach must be confirmed before any fluid is administered, as severe respiratory complications can occur if fluid is inadvertently infused into a bronchus (Box 22.48, p. 879). Thereafter, specially prepared liquid feeds are administered either by continuous infusion or using a bolus technique. If the patient fails to absorb the administered feed or vomits it, this may indicate gastric outlet obstruction or gastric stasis, which can be overcome by placing a nasojejunal tube.

If long-term artificial enteral feeding is needed, a percutaneous endoscopic gastrostomy (PEG) should be sited (Fig. 5.17). A PEG tube is more comfortable for the patient, since there is no irritation to the nasal mucosa. The tube is less likely to become displaced or to be pulled out, so the feed can be given more reliably. However, inserting a gastrostomy is an invasive procedure, especially in frail patients with significant comorbidities. It may be complicated by local infection (30%) and inadvertent puncture of other intra-abdominal organs, causing peritonitis and bleeding, so the indication for placement must be carefully considered. It takes approximately 10 days for a fibrous tract to form around the PEG tube. If the PEG is displaced or removed during that time, there is a high risk of peritonitis. If a problem occurs with food absorption, a jejunal extension can be placed through the PEG tube and liquid feed administered directly into the small bowel.

Parenteral nutrition

Intravenous feeding should only be used when enteral feeding is impossible. Parenteral feeding is expensive and carries higher risks of complications. There is little benefit if parenteral feeding is required for less than 1 week.

There are a number of possible routes for parenteral nutrition:

- *Peripheral venous cannula*. This can only be used for low-osmolality solutions due to the development of thrombophlebitis, and is unsuitable for patients with high nutritional requirements.
- *Peripherally inserted cannula (PIC)*. A 20 cm cannula is placed in a mid-arm vein. Once again, hyperosmolar solutions cannot be used.

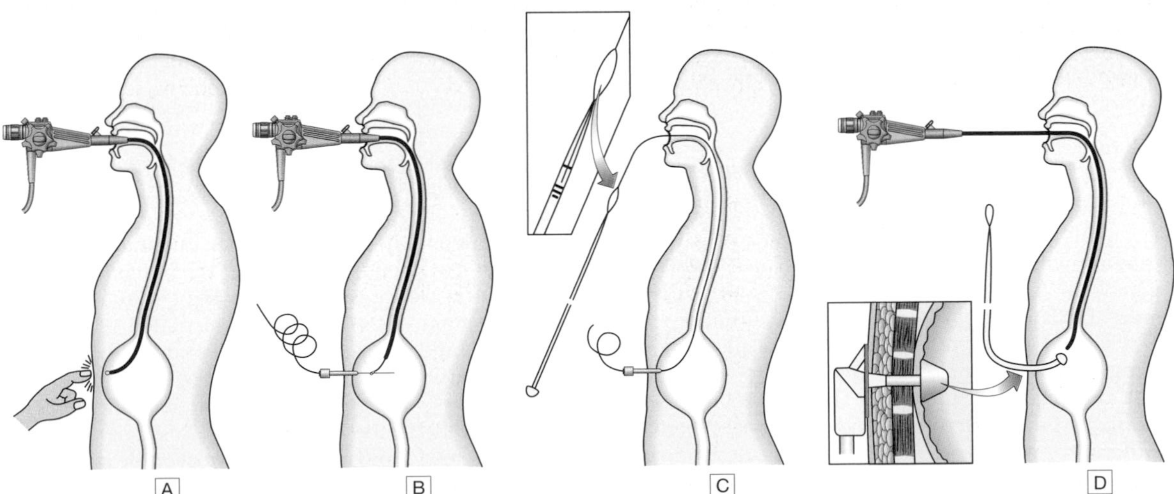

Fig. 5.17 Percutaneous endoscopic gastrostomy (PEG) placement. **A** Finger pressure on the anterior abdominal wall is noted by the endoscopist. **B** Following insertion of a cannula through the anterior abdominal wall into the stomach, a guidewire is threaded through the cannula and grasped by the endoscopic forceps or snare. **C** The endoscope is withdrawn with the guidewire. The gastrostomy tube is then attached to the guidewire. **D** The guidewire and tube are pulled back through the mouth, oesophagus and stomach to exit on the anterior abdominal wall, and the endoscope is repassed to confirm the site of placement of the retention device. The latter closely abuts the gastric mucosa; its position is maintained by an external fixation device (see inset). It is also possible to place PEG tubes using fluoroscopic guidance in patients in whom endoscopy is difficult (radiologically inserted gastrostomy (RIG)).

- *Peripherally inserted central catheter (PICC)*. A 60 cm cannula is inserted into a vein in the antecubital fossa. The distal end lies in a central vein, allowing hyperosmolar solutions to be used.
- *Central line*. The subclavian route is preferred to the internal jugular vein, due to lower infection rates. Hyperosmolar solutions can be used without difficulty. Lines need to be handled with strict aseptic technique, and a single-lumen tube is preferred, to prevent infection.

If access has been gained to a central vein, nutritional support is usually given as an 'all-in-one' mixture. The main energy source is provided by carbohydrate, usually as glucose. The solution also contains amino acids, lipid emulsion, electrolytes, trace elements and vitamins. These are mixed as a large bag in a sterile environment, with the constituents adjusted according to the results of regular blood monitoring. Relevant tests include:

- *daily*: urea and electrolytes, glucose
- *twice* weekly: liver function tests, calcium, phosphate, magnesium
- *weekly*: full blood count, zinc, triglycerides
- *monthly*: copper, selenium, manganese.

If the patient develops fever or other features of septicaemia, it should be assumed to be due to a line infection (p. 200). Blood cultures should be taken, the existing line removed, the tip sent for bacteriological analysis, and a new line inserted.

Refeeding syndrome

When nutritional support is given to an under-nourished patient, there is a rapid conversion from a catabolic to an anabolic state. Administration of carbohydrates stimulates release of insulin, leading to cellular uptake of phosphate, potassium and magnesium, which may provoke significant falls in serum levels. The resulting electrolyte imbalance can have serious consequences, such as cardiac arrhythmias, so careful monitoring is essential. In patients who are thiamin-deficient, Wernicke's encephalopathy can be precipitated by refeeding with carbohydrates (p. 253); this is prevented by administering thiamin before starting nutritional support.

Legal and ethical aspects of artificial nutritional support

The ability to intervene with artificial nutritional support raises many legal and ethical dilemmas (pp. 9 and 291). Starvation will inevitably lead to death, but inability to eat may be part of the terminal stages of a disease process. Difficult decisions are raised by situations such as strokes, which affect swallowing. The instigation of feeding may speed recovery and lead to better functional outcome; on the other hand, feeding might prolong the process of dying in severe stroke. There will be different approaches to these decisions, depending on the local availability of resources as well as legal, cultural and religious influences. Some guidelines are given in Box 5.29.

Cachexia

Cachexia is the weight loss and muscle-wasting associated with chronic illness, which is characteristic of chronic infections such as HIV-AIDS, end-stage organ failure and certain cancers (especially of the lung and upper gastrointestinal tract). Although there is decreased energy intake with loss of appetite, the main cause is thought to be increased metabolic rate through the production of key cytokines and other proteolytic factors.

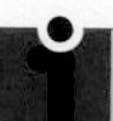

5.29 Ethical and legal considerations in the management of artificial nutritional support*

- Care of the sick involves the duty of providing adequate fluid and nutrients
- Food and fluid should not be withheld from a patient who expresses a desire to eat and drink, unless there is a medical contraindication (e.g. risk of aspiration)
- A treatment plan should include consideration of nutritional issues and should be agreed by all members of the health-care team
- In the situation of palliative care, tube feeding should only be instituted if it is needed to relieve symptoms
- Tube feeding is usually regarded in law as a medical treatment. Like other treatments, the need for such support should be reviewed on a regular basis and changes made in the light of clinical circumstances
- A competent adult patient must give consent for any invasive procedures, including the passage of a nasogastric tube or the insertion of a central venous cannula
- If a patient is unable to give consent, the health-care team should act in that person's best interests, taking into account any wishes previously expressed by the patient and the views of family
- Under certain specified circumstances (e.g. anorexia nervosa), it will be appropriate to provide artificial nutritional support to the unwilling patient

*Based on British Association for Parenteral and Enteral Nutrition guidelines (www.bapen.org.uk).

MICRONUTRIENTS, MINERALS AND THEIR DISEASES

Vitamins

Vitamins are organic substances with key roles in certain metabolic pathways, and are categorised into those that are fat-soluble (vitamins A, D, E and K) and those that are water-soluble (vitamins of the B complex group and vitamin C).

Recommended daily intakes of micronutrients (Box 5.30) vary between countries and the nomenclature has become potentially confusing. In the UK, the 'reference nutrient intake' (RNI) has been calculated as the mean plus two standard deviations (SD) of daily intake in the population, which therefore describes normal intake for 97.5% of the population. The lower reference nutrient intake (LRNI) is the mean minus 2 SD, below which would be considered deficient in most of the population. These dietary reference values (DRV) have superseded the terms RDI (recommended daily intakes) and RDA (recommended daily amounts). Other countries use different terminology. Additional amounts of some micronutrients may be required in pregnancy and lactation (Box 5.31).

Vitamin deficiency diseases are most prevalent in developing countries but still occur in developed

5

5.30 Summary of clinically important vitamins

Vitamin	Sources* Rich	Sources* Important	Reference nutrient intake (RNI)
Fat-soluble			
A (retinol)	Liver	Milk and milk products, eggs, fish oils	700 µg men 600 µg women
D (cholecalciferol)	Fish oils	UV exposure to skin Egg yolks, margarine, fortified cereals	10 µg if > 65 yrs or no sunlight exposure
E (tocopherol)	Sunflower oil	Vegetables, nuts, seed oils	No RNI. Safe intake: 4 mg men 3 mg women
K (phylloquinone, menaquinone)	Green vegetables	Soya oil, menaquinones produced by intestinal bacteria	No RNI. Safe intake: 1 µg/kg
Water-soluble			
B_1 (thiamin)	Pork	Cereals, grains, beans	0.8 mg per 9.68 MJ (2000 kcal) energy intake
B_2 (riboflavin)	Milk	Milk and milk products, breakfast cereals, bread	1.3 mg men 1.1 mg women
B_3 (niacin, nicotinic acid, nicotinamide)	Meat, cereals		17 mg men 13 mg women
B_6 (pyridoxine)	Meat, fish, potatoes, bananas	Vegetables, intestinal microflora synthesis	1.4 mg men 1.2 mg women
Folate	Liver	Green leafy vegetables, fortified breakfast cereals	200 µg
B_{12} (cobalamin)	Animal products	Bacterial colonisation	1.5 µg
Biotin	Egg yolk	Intestinal flora	No RNI. Safe intake: 10–200 µg
C (ascorbic acid)	Citrus fruit	Fresh fruit, fresh and frozen vegetables	40 mg

*Rich sources contain the nutrient in high concentration but are not generally eaten in large amounts; important sources contain less but contribute most because larger amounts are eaten.

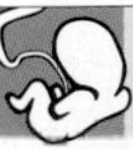

5.31 Nutrition in pregnancy and lactation

- **Energy requirements**: increased in both the mother and fetus, but can be met through reduced maternal energy expenditure.
- **Micronutrient requirements**: adaptive mechanisms ensure increased uptake of minerals in pregnancy, but extra increments of some are required during lactation (see Box 5.33). Additional increments of some vitamins are recommended during pregnancy and lactation:
  - Vitamin A: for growth and maintenance of the fetus, and to provide some reserve (important in some countries to prevent blindness associated with vitamin A deficiency). Teratogenic in excessive amounts.
  - Vitamin D: to ensure bone and dental development in the infant. Higher incidences of hypocalcaemia, hypoparathyroidisim and defective dental enamel have been seen in infants of women not taking vitamin D supplements at > 50° latitude.
  - Folate: to avoid neural tube defects (see Box 5.32).
  - Vitamin B_{12}: in lactation only.
  - Thiamin: to meet increased fetal energy demands.
  - Riboflavin: to meet extra demands.
  - Niacin: in lactation only.
  - Vitamin C: for the last trimester to maintain maternal stores as fetal demands increase.
  - Iodine: in countries with high consumption of staple foods (e.g. brassicas, maize, bamboo shoots) that contain goitrogens (thiocyanates or perchlorates) that interfere with iodine uptake, supplements prevent infants being born with cretinism.

countries. Older people (and alcoholics) are at risk of deficiencies in B vitamins and in vitamins D and C. Nutritional deficiencies in pregnancy can affect either the mother or the developing fetus, and extra increments of vitamins are recommended in the UK (see Boxes 5.31 and 5.32). Darker-skinned individuals living at higher latitude, and those who cover up or do not go outside are at increased risk of vitamin D deficiency due to inadequate sunlight exposure. Dietary supplements are recommended for these 'at-risk' groups. Some nutrient deficiencies are induced by diseases or drugs.

EBM 5.32 Periconceptual folate supplementation and neural tube defects

'Folate supplementation in advance of conception and during the first trimester reduces the incidence of neural tube defects by –70%.'

- De-Regil LM, et al. Effects and safety of periconceptional folate supplementation for preventing birth defects. Cochrane Database of Systematic Reviews, 2010, issue 4. Art. no. CD001056.

For further information: www.cochrane.org/cochrane-reviews

5.33 Biochemical assessment of vitamin status

Nutrient	Biochemical assessments of deficiency or excess
Vitamin A	Serum retinol may be low in deficiency Serum retinyl esters: when vitamin A toxicity is suspected
Vitamin D	Plasma/serum 25-hydroxy vitamin D (25(OH)D): reflects body stores (liver and adipose tissue) Plasma/serum 1,25$(OH)_2$D: difficult to interpret
Vitamin E	Serum tocopherol : cholesterol ratio
Vitamin K	Coagulation assays (e.g. prothrombin time) Plasma vitamin K
Vitamin B_1 (thiamin)	Red blood cell transketolase activity or whole-blood vitamin B_1
Vitamin B_2 (riboflavin)	Red blood cell glutathione reductase activity or whole-blood vitamin B_2
Vitamin B_3 (niacin)	Urinary metabolites: 1-methyl-2-pyridone-5-carboxamide, 1-methylnicotinamide
Vitamin B_6	Plasma pyridoxal phosphate or erythrocyte transaminase activation coefficient
Vitamin B_{12}	Plasma B_{12}: poor measure of overall vitamin B_{12} status but will detect severe deficiency Alternatives (methylmalonic acid and holotranscobalamin) are not used routinely
Folate	Red blood cell folate Plasma folate: reflects recent intake but also detects unmetabolised folic acid from foods and supplements
Vitamin C	Leucocyte ascorbic acid: assesses vitamin C tissue stores Plasma ascorbic acid: reflects recent (daily) intake

Deficiencies of fat-soluble vitamins are seen in conditions of fat malabsorption (e.g. biliary obstruction).

Some vitamins also have pharmacological actions when given at supraphysiological doses, e.g. the use of vitamin A (p. 1282) for acne. Taking vitamin supplements is fashionable in many countries, although there is no evidence of benefit. Toxic effects are most serious with high dosages of vitamins A, B_6 and D.

Investigation of suspected vitamin deficiency or excess may involve biochemical assessment of body stores (Box 5.33). However, measurements in blood should be interpreted carefully in conjunction with the clinical presentation.

Fat-soluble vitamins

Vitamin A (retinol)

Pre-formed retinol is found only in foods of animal origin. Vitamin A can also be derived from carotenes, which are present in green and coloured vegetables and some fruits. Carotenes provide most of the total vitamin A in the UK, and constitute the only supply in vegans. Retinol is converted to several other important molecules:

- *11-cis retinaldehyde* is part of the photoreceptor complex in rods of the retina.
- *Retinoic acid* induces differentiation of epithelial cells by binding to specific nuclear receptors, which induce responsive genes. In vitamin A deficiency, mucus-secreting cells are replaced by keratin-producing cells.
- *Retinoids* are necessary for normal growth, fetal development, fertility, haematopoiesis and immune function.

Globally, the most important consequence of vitamin A deficiency is irreversible blindness in young children. Asia is most notably affected and the problem is being addressed through widespread vitamin A

A

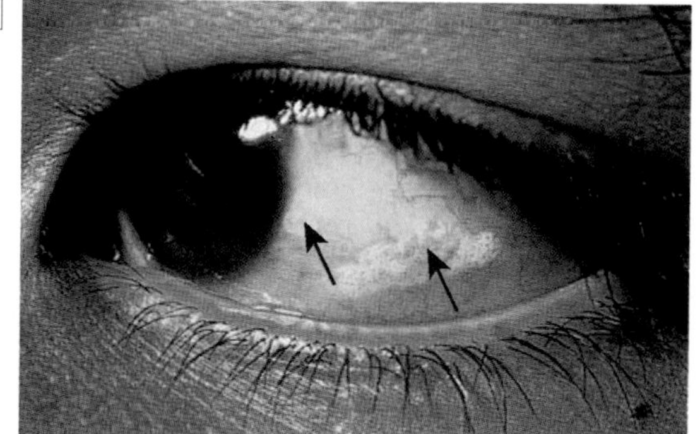

B

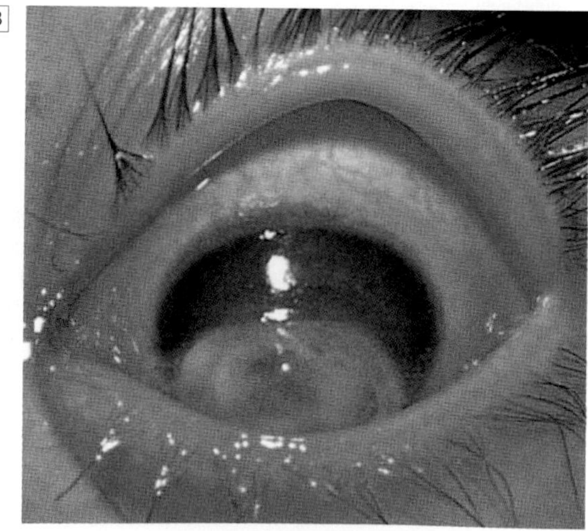

Fig. 5.18 Eye signs of vitamin A deficiency. **A** Bitot's spots in xerophthalmia, showing the white triangular plaques (arrows). **B** Keratomalacia in a 14-month-old child. There is liquefactive necrosis affecting the greater part of the cornea, with typical sparing of the superior aspect. (B) From WHO 1976 – see p. 132.

supplementation programmes. Adults are not usually at risk because liver stores can supply vitamin A when foods containing vitamin A are unavailable.

Early deficiency causes impaired adaptation to the dark (night blindness). Keratinisation of the cornea (xerophthalmia) gives rise to characteristic Bitot's spots, and progresses to keratomalacia, with corneal ulceration, scarring and irreversible blindness (Fig. 5.18). In countries where vitamin A deficiency is endemic, pregnant women should be advised to eat dark-green, leafy vegetables and yellow fruits (to build up stores of retinol in the fetal liver), and infants should be fed the same. WHO is according high priority to prevention in communities where xerophthalmia occurs, giving single prophylactic oral doses of 60 mg retinyl palmitate (providing 200 000 U retinol) to pre-school children. This also reduces mortality from gastroenteritis and respiratory infections.

Repeated moderate or high doses of retinol can cause liver damage, hyperostosis and teratogenicity. Women in countries where deficiency is not endemic are therefore advised not to take vitamin A supplements in pregnancy. Retinol intake may also be restricted in those at risk of osteoporosis. Acute overdose leads to nausea and headache, increased intracranial pressure and skin desquamation. Excessive intake of carotene can cause pigmentation of the skin (hypercarotenosis); this gradually fades when intake is reduced.

Vitamin D

The natural form of vitamin D, cholecalciferol or vitamin D_3, is formed in the skin by the action of UV light on 7-dehydrocholesterol, a metabolite of cholesterol. Few foods contain vitamin D naturally and skin exposure to sunlight is the main source. Moving away from the equator, the intensity of UV light decreases, so that at a latitude above 50° (including northern Europe), vitamin D is not synthesised in winter, and even above 30° there is seasonal variation. The body store accumulated during the summer is consumed during the winter. Vitamin D is converted in the liver to 25-hydroxy vitamin D (25(OH)D), which is further hydroxylated in the kidneys to 1,25-dihydroxy-vitamin D (1,25 $(OH)_2D$), the active form of the vitamin (see Fig. 25.55, p. 1127). 1,25$(OH)_2D$ activates specific intracellular receptors which influence calcium metabolism, bone mineralisation and tissue differentiation. The synthetic form, ergocalciferol, or vitamin D_2, is considered to be less potent than the endogenous D_3.

Recommended dietary intakes aim to prevent rickets and osteomalacia. There is increasing evidence that vitamin D is important for immune and muscle function, and may reduce falls in the elderly (p. 172). Margarines are fortified with vitamin D in the UK, and milk is fortified in some parts of Europe and in North America.

The effects of vitamin D deficiency (calcium deficiency, rickets and osteomalacia) are described on page 1125. An analogue of vitamin D (calcipotriol) is used for treatment of skin conditions such as psoriasis. Excessive doses of cholecalciferol, ergocalciferol or the hydroxylated metabolites cause hypercalcaemia (p. 767).

Vitamin E

There are eight related fat-soluble substances with vitamin E activity. The most important dietary form is α-tocopherol. Vitamin E has many direct metabolic actions:

- It prevents oxidation of polyunsaturated fatty acids in cell membranes by free radicals.
- It helps maintain cell membrane structure.
- It affects DNA synthesis and cell signalling.
- It is involved in the anti-inflammatory and immune systems.

Human deficiency is rare and has only been described in premature infants and in malabsorption. It can cause a mild haemolytic anaemia, ataxia and visual scotomas. Vitamin E intakes are considered safe up to 3200 mg/day (1000-fold greater than recommended intakes). Diets rich in vitamin E are consumed in countries with lower rates of coronary heart disease. However, randomised controlled trials have not demonstrated cardioprotective effects of vitamin E or other antioxidants.

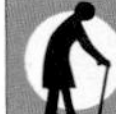

5.34 Vitamin deficiency in old age

- **Requirements**: although energy requirements fall with age, those for micronutrients do not. If dietary intake falls, a vitamin-rich diet is required to compensate.
- **Vitamin D**: levels are commonly low due to reduced dietary intake, decreased sun exposure and less efficient skin conversion. This leads to bone loss and fractures. Supplements should be given to those in institutional care and those with recurrent falls.
- **Vitamin B_{12} deficiency**: a causal relationship with dementia has not been identified, but it does produce neuropsychiatric effects and should be checked in all those with declining cognitive function.

Vitamin K

Vitamin K is supplied in the diet mainly as vitamin K_1 (phylloquinone) in the UK, or as vitamin K_2 (menaquinone) from fermented products in parts of Asia. Vitamin K_2 is also synthesised by bacteria in the colon. Vitamin K is a co-factor for carboxylation reactions: in particular, the production of γ-carboxyglutamate (gla). Gla residues are found in four of the coagulation factor proteins (II, VII, IX and X; p. 997), conferring their capacity to bind to phospholipid surfaces in the presence of calcium. Other important gla proteins are osteocalcin and matrix gla protein, which are important in bone mineralisation.

Vitamin K deficiency leads to delayed coagulation and bleeding. In obstructive jaundice, dietary vitamin K is not absorbed and it is essential to administer the vitamin in parenteral form before surgery. Warfarin and related anticoagulants (p. 1019) act by antagonising vitamin K. Vitamin K is given routinely to newborn babies to prevent haemorrhagic disease. Symptoms of excess have been reported only in infants, with synthetic preparations linked to haemolysis and liver damage.

Water-soluble vitamins

Thiamin (vitamin B_1)

Thiamin is widely distributed in foods of both vegetable and animal origin. Thiamin pyrophosphate (TPP) is a co-factor for enzyme reactions involved in the metabolism of macronutrients (carbohydrate, fat and alcohol), including:

- decarboxylation of pyruvate to acetyl-co-enzyme A, which bridges between glycolysis and the tricarboxylic acid (Krebs) cycle
- transketolase activity in the hexose monophosphate shunt pathway
- decarboxylation of α-ketoglutarate to succinate in the Krebs cycle.

In thiamin deficiency, cells cannot metabolise glucose aerobically to generate energy as ATP. Neuronal cells are most vulnerable, since they depend almost exclusively on glucose for energy requirements. Impaired glucose oxidation also causes an accumulation of pyruvic and lactic acids, which produce vasodilatation and increased cardiac output.

Deficiency – beri-beri

In the developed world, thiamin deficiency is mainly encountered in chronic alcoholics. Poor diet, impaired absorption, storage and phosphorylation of thiamin in the liver, and the increased requirements for thiamin to metabolise ethanol all contribute. In the developing world, deficiency usually arises as a consequence of a diet based on polished rice. The body has very limited stores of thiamin, so deficiency is manifest after only 1 month on a thiamin-free diet. There are two forms of the disease in adults:

- *Dry (or neurological) beri-beri* manifests with chronic peripheral neuropathy and with wrist and/or foot drop, and may cause Korsakoff's psychosis and Wernicke's encephalopathy (p. 253).
- *Wet (or cardiac) beri-beri* causes generalised oedema due to biventricular heart failure with pulmonary congestion.

In dry beri-beri, response to thiamin administration is not uniformly good. However, multivitamin therapy seems to produce some improvement, suggesting that other vitamin deficiencies may be involved. Wernicke's encephalopathy and wet beri-beri should be treated without delay with intravenous vitamin B and C mixture ('Pabrinex', p. 253). Korsakoff's psychosis is irreversible and does not respond to thiamin treatment.

Riboflavin (vitamin B_2)

Riboflavin is required for the flavin co-factors involved in oxidation–reduction reactions. It is widely distributed in animal and vegetable foods. Levels are low in staple cereals but germination increases its content. It is destroyed under alkaline conditions by heat and by exposure to sunlight.

Deficiency is rare in developed countries. It mainly affects the tongue and lips and manifests as glossitis, angular stomatitis and cheilosis. The genitals may be affected, as well as the skin areas rich in sebaceous glands, causing nasolabial or facial dyssebacea. Rapid recovery usually follows administration of riboflavin 10 mg daily by mouth.

Niacin (vitamin B_3)

Niacin encompasses nicotinic acid and nicotinamide. Nicotinamide is an essential part of the two pyridine nucleotides, nicotinamide adenine dinucleotide (NAD) and nicotinamide adenine dinucleotide phosphate (NADP), which play a key role as hydrogen acceptors and donors for many enzymes. Niacin can be synthesised in the body in limited amounts from the amino acid tryptophan.

Deficiency – pellagra

Pellagra was formerly endemic among poor people who subsisted chiefly on maize, which contains niacytin, a form of niacin that the body is unable to utilise. Pellagra can develop in only 8 weeks in individuals eating diets that are very deficient in niacin and tryptophan. It remains a problem in parts of Africa, and is occasionally seen in alcoholics and in patients with chronic small intestinal disease in developed countries. Pellagra can occur in Hartnup's disease, a genetic disorder characterised by impaired absorption of several amino acids, including tryptophan. It is also seen occasionally in carcinoid syndrome (p. 784), when tryptophan is consumed in the excessive production of 5-hydroxytryptamine (5-HT). Pellagra has been called the disease of the three Ds:

- *Dermatitis*. Characteristically, there is erythema resembling severe sunburn, appearing symmetrically over the parts of the body exposed to sunlight, particularly the limbs and especially on the neck, but not the face (Casal's necklace, Fig. 5.19). The skin lesions may progress to vesiculation, cracking, exudation and secondary infection.
- *Diarrhoea*. This is often associated with anorexia, nausea, glossitis and dysphagia, reflecting the presence of a non-infective inflammation that extends throughout the gastrointestinal tract.
- *Dementia*. In severe deficiency, delirium occurs acutely and dementia develops in chronic cases.

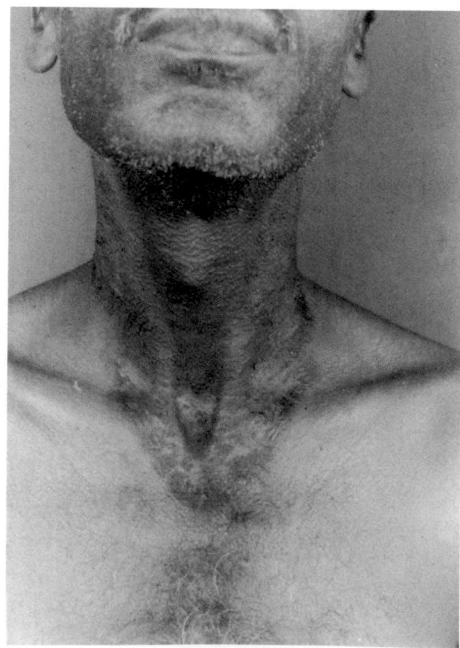

Fig. 5.19 Dermatitis due to pellagra (niacin deficiency). The lesions appear on those parts of the body exposed to sunlight. The classic 'Casal's necklace' can be seen around the neck and upper chest. From Karthikeyan and Thappa 2002 – see p. 132.

Treatment is with nicotinamide, given in a dose of 100 mg 3 times daily orally or parenterally. The response is usually rapid. Within 24 hours, the erythema diminishes, the diarrhoea ceases and a striking improvement occurs in the patient's mental state.

Toxicity

Excessive intakes of niacin may lead to reversible hepatotoxicity. Nicotinic acid is a lipid-lowering agent, but at doses above 200 mg a day gives rise to vasodilatory symptoms ('flushing' and/or hypotension).

Pyridoxine (vitamin B_6)

Pyridoxine, pyridoxal and pyridoxamine are different forms of vitamin B_6 that undergo phosphorylation to produce pyridoxal 5-phosphate (PLP). PLP is the co-factor for a large number of enzymes involved in the metabolism of amino acids. Vitamin B_6 is available in most foods.

Deficiency is rare, although certain drugs, such as isoniazid and penicillamine, act as chemical antagonists to pyridoxine. Pyridoxine administration is effective in isoniazid-induced peripheral neuropathy and some cases of sideroblastic anaemia. Large doses of vitamin B_6 have an antiemetic effect in radiotherapy-induced nausea. Although vitamin B_6 supplements have become popular in the treatment of nausea in pregnancy, carpal tunnel syndrome and premenstrual syndrome, there is no convincing evidence of benefit. Very high doses of vitamin B_6 taken for several months can cause a sensory polyneuropathy.

Biotin

Biotin is a co-enzyme in the synthesis of fatty acids, isoleucine and valine and is also involved in gluconeogenesis. Deficiency results from consuming very large quantities of raw egg whites (> 30% energy intake) because the avidin they contain binds to and inactivates biotin in the intestine. It may also be seen after long periods of total parenteral nutrition. The clinical features of deficiency include scaly dermatitis, alopecia and paraesthesia.

Folate (folic acid)

Folates exist in many forms. The main circulating form is 5-methyltetrahydrofolate. The natural forms are prone to oxidation. Folic acid is the stable synthetic form. Folate works as a methyl donor for cellular methylation and protein synthesis. It is directly involved in DNA and RNA synthesis, and requirements increase during embryonic development.

Folate deficiency may cause three major birth defects (spina bifida, anencephaly and encephalocele) resulting from imperfect closure of the neural tube, which takes place 3–4 weeks after conception. The UK Department of Health advises that women who have experienced a pregnancy affected by a neural tube defect should take 5 mg of folic acid daily from before conception and throughout the first trimester (see Box 5.32, p. 125). All women planning a pregnancy are advised to include good sources of folate in their diet, and to take folate supplements throughout the first trimester. Liver is the richest source of folate but an alternative source (e.g. leafy vegetables) is advised in early pregnancy because of the high vitamin A content of liver (p. 126). Folate deficiency has also been associated with heart disease, dementia and cancer. There is mandatory fortification of flour with folic acid in the US and voluntary fortification of many foods across Europe. There are now concerns that this may contribute to the increased incidence of colon cancer through promotion of the growth of polyps.

Hydroxycobalamin (vitamin B_{12})

Vitamin B_{12} is a co-factor in folate co-enzyme recycling and nerve myelination. Vitamin B_{12} and folate are particularly important in DNA synthesis in red blood cells (p. 1024). The haematological disorders (macrocytic or megaloblastic anaemias) due to their deficiency are discussed on pages 1024–1026. Vitamin B_{12}, but not folate, is needed for the integrity of myelin, so that vitamin B_{12} deficiency is also associated with neurological disease (see Box 24.35, p. 1024).

Neurological consequences of vitamin B_{12} deficiency

In older people and chronic alcoholics, vitamin B_{12} deficiency arises from insufficient intake and/or from malabsorption. Several drugs, including neomycin, can render vitamin B_{12} inactive. Adequate intake of folate maintains erythropoiesis and there is a concern that fortification of foods with folate may mask underlying vitamin B_{12} deficiency. In severe deficiency there is insidious, diffuse and uneven demyelination. It may be clinically manifest as peripheral neuropathy or spinal cord degeneration affecting both posterior and lateral columns ('subacute combined degeneration of the spinal cord'; p. 1222), or there may be cerebral manifestations (resembling dementia) or optic atrophy. Vitamin B_{12} therapy improves symptoms in most cases.

Vitamin C (ascorbic acid)

Ascorbic acid is the most active reducing agent in the aqueous phase of living tissues and is involved in intracellular electron transfer. It takes part in the hydroxylation of proline and lysine in protocollagen to hydroxyproline and hydroxylysine in mature collagen. It is very easily destroyed by heat, increased pH and light, and is very soluble in water; hence many traditional cooking methods reduce or eliminate it. Claims that high-dose vitamin C improves immune function (including resistance to the common cold) and cholesterol turnover remain unsubstantiated.

Deficiency – scurvy

Vitamin C deficiency causes defective formation of collagen with impaired healing of wounds, capillary haemorrhage and reduced platelet adhesiveness (normal platelets are rich in ascorbate) (Fig. 5.20). Precipitants and clinical features of scurvy are shown in Box 5.35. A dose of 250 mg vitamin C 3 times daily by mouth should saturate the tissues quickly. The deficiencies of the patient's diet also need to be corrected and other vitamin supplements given if necessary. Daily intakes of more than 1 g/day have been reported to cause diarrhoea and the formation of renal oxalate stones.

Other dietary organic compounds

There are a number of non-essential organic compounds with purported health benefits such as reducing risk of heart disease or cancer. Groups of compounds such as the flavonoids and phytoestrogens show bioactivity

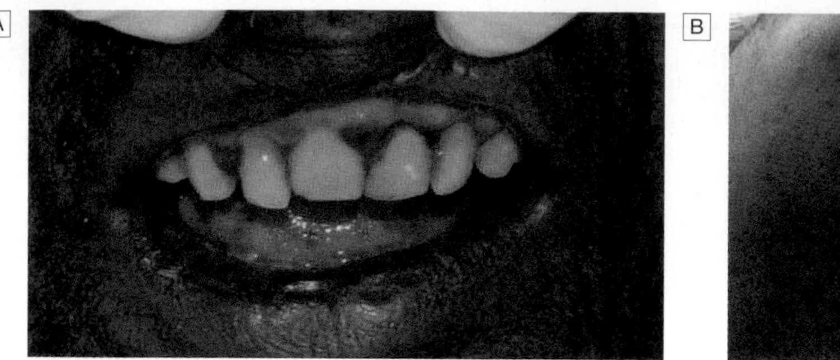

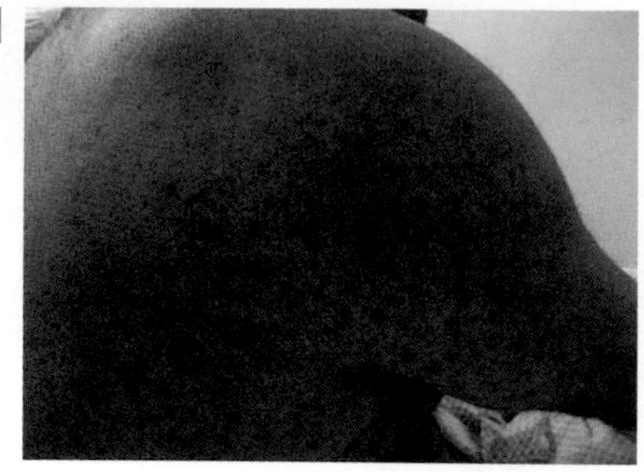

Fig. 5.20 Scurvy. A Gingival swelling and bleeding. B Perifollicular hyperkeratosis. From Ho, et al. 2007 – see p. 132.

5.35 Scurvy – vitamin C deficiency

Precipitants	
Increased requirement	**Dietary deficiency**
• Trauma, surgery, burns, infections • Smoking • Drugs (corticosteroids, aspirin, indometacin, tetracycline)	• Lack of dietary fruit and vegetables for > 2 mths • Infants fed exclusively on boiled milk
Clinical features	
• Swollen gums which bleed easily • Perifollicular and petechial haemorrhages • Ecchymoses	• Haemarthrosis • Gastrointestinal bleeding • Anaemia • Poor wound healing

through their respective antioxidant and oestrogenic or anti-oestrogenic activities. Flavonoids (of which there are a number of different classes of compound) are found in fruit and vegetables, tea and wine; phytoestrogens are found in soy products (with higher intakes in parts of Asia compared to Europe and the US) and pulses. Caffeine from tea and coffee and carbonated beverages affects the nervous system and can improve mental performance in the short term, with adverse effects seen at higher intakes. Intake of non-carbonic organic acids (which are not metabolised to carbon dioxide), e.g. oxalates, may be restricted in individuals prone to kidney stones.

Inorganic micronutrients

A number of inorganic elements are essential dietary constituents for humans (Box 5.36). Deficiency is seen when there is inadequate dietary intake of minerals or excessive loss from the body. Toxic effects have also been observed from self-medication and disordered absorption or excretion. Examples of clinical toxicity include excess of iron (haemochromatosis or haemosiderosis), fluoride (fluorosis; p. 223), copper (Wilson's disease) and selenium (selenosis, seen in parts of China). For most minerals, the available biochemical markers do not accurately reflect dietary intake and dietary assessment is required.

Calcium and phosphorus

Calcium is the most abundant cation in the body and powerful homeostatic mechanisms control circulating ionised calcium levels (pp. 766 and 1126). WHO's dietary guidelines for calcium differ between countries, with higher intakes usually recommended in places with higher fracture prevalence. Between 20 and 30% of calcium in the diet is absorbed, depending on vitamin D status and food source. Calcium requirements depend on phosphorus intakes, with an optimum molar ratio (Ca:P) of 1:1. Excessive phosphorus intakes (e.g. 1–1.5 g/day) with a Ca:P of 1:3 have been shown to cause hypocalcaemia and secondary hyperparathyroidism (p. 768).

Calcium absorption may be impaired in vitamin D deficiency (pp. 766 and 1126) and in malabsorption secondary to small intestinal disease. Calcium deficiency causes impaired bone mineralisation and can lead to osteomalacia in adults. The potential benefits of high calcium intake in osteoporosis are discussed on page 1124. Too much calcium can lead to constipation and toxicity has been observed in 'milk-alkali syndrome' (p. 767).

Dietary deficiency of phosphorus is rare (except in older people with limited diets) since it is present in nearly all foods and phosphates are added to a number of processed foods. Phosphate deficiency in adults occurs:

- in patients with renal tubular phosphate loss (p. 448)
- due to prolonged high dosage of aluminium hydroxide (p. 488)
- sometimes when alcoholics are fed with high-carbohydrate foods
- in patients receiving parenteral nutrition if inadequate phosphate is provided.

Deficiency causes hypophosphataemia (p. 448) and muscle weakness secondary to ATP deficiency.

Iron

Iron is involved in the synthesis of haemoglobin, and is required for the transport of electrons within cells and in a number of enzyme reactions. Non-haem iron in cereals and vegetables is poorly absorbed but makes the greater contribution to overall intake, compared to the well-absorbed haem iron from animal products. Fruits and vegetables containing vitamin C enhance iron absorption, while the tannins in tea reduce it. Dietary calcium reduces iron uptake from the same meal, which

5.36 Summary of clinically important minerals

Mineral	Sources[1] Rich	Important	Reference nutrient intake (RNI)
Calcium	Milk and milk products, tofu	Milk, boned fish, green vegetables, beans	700 mg[2]
Phosphorus	Most foods contain phosphorus Marmite® and dry-roasted peanuts	Milk, cereal products, bread and meat	550 mg[2]
Magnesium	Whole grains, nuts	Unprocessed and wholegrain foods	300 mg men 270 mg women[2]
Iron	Liver, red meat (haem iron)	Non-haem iron from vegetables, wholemeal bread	8.7 mg 14.8 mg women < 50 yrs
Zinc	Red meat, seafood	Dairy produce, wholemeal bread	9.5 mg men 7 mg women[2]
Iodine	Edible seaweeds	Milk and dairy products	140 μg
Selenium	Fish, wheat grown in selenium-rich soils	Fish	75 μg men 60 μg women[2]
Copper	Shellfish, liver	Bread, cereal products, vegetables	1.2 mg[2]
Fluoride	Drinking water, tea		No RNI. Safe intake: 0.5 mg/kg
Potassium	Dried fruit, potatoes, coffee	Fresh fruit, vegetables, milk	3500 mg
Sodium	Table salt, anchovies	Processed foods, bread, bacon	1600 mg

[1]Rich sources contain the nutrient in high concentration but are not generally eaten in large amounts; important sources contain less but contribute most because larger amounts are eaten. [2]Increased amounts are required in women during lactation.

may precipitate iron deficiency in those with borderline iron stores. There is no physiological mechanism for excretion of iron, so homeostasis depends on the regulation of iron absorption (see Fig. 24.20, p. 1022). This is regulated at the level of duodenal enterocytes by hepcidin. The expression of hepcidin (a peptide secreted by hepatocytes in the duodenum) is suppressed when body iron is low, leading to enhanced efflux of iron into the circulation. The normal daily loss of iron is 1 mg, arising from desquamated surface cells and intestinal losses. A regular loss of only 2 mL of blood per day doubles the iron requirement. On average, an additional 20 mg of iron is lost during menstruation, so pre-menopausal women require about twice as much iron as men (and more if menstrual losses are heavy).

The major consequence of iron deficiency is anaemia (p. 1021). This is one of the most important nutritional causes of ill health in all parts of the world. In the UK, it is estimated that 10% women are iron-deficient. Dietary iron overload is occasionally observed and results in iron accumulation in the liver and, rarely, cirrhosis. Haemochromatosis results from an inherited increase in iron absorption (p. 972).

Iodine

Iodine is required for synthesis of thyroid hormones (p. 738). It is present in sea fish, seaweed and most plant foods grown near the sea. The amount of iodine in soil and water influences the iodine content of most foods. Iodine is lacking in the highest mountainous areas of the world (e.g. the Alps and the Himalayas) and in the soil of frequently flooded plains (e.g. Bangladesh).

About a billion people in the world are estimated to have an inadequate iodine intake and hence are at risk of iodine deficiency disorder. Goitre is the most common manifestation, affecting about 200 million people (p. 752).

In those areas where most women have endemic goitre, 1% or more of babies are born with cretinism (characterised by mental and physical retardation). There is a higher than usual prevalence of deafness, slowed reflexes and poor learning in the remaining population. The best way of preventing neonatal cretinism is to ensure adequate levels of iodine during pregnancy. This can be achieved by intramuscular injections with 1–2 mL of iodised poppy seed oil (475–950 mg iodine) to women of child-bearing age every 3–5 years, by administration of iodised oil orally at 6-monthly or yearly intervals to adults and children, or by providing iodised salt for cooking.

Zinc

Zinc is present in most foods of vegetable and animal origin. It is an essential component of many enzymes, including carbonic anhydrase, alcohol dehydrogenase and alkaline phosphatase.

Acute zinc deficiency has been reported in patients receiving prolonged zinc-free parenteral nutrition and causes diarrhoea, mental apathy, a moist, eczematoid dermatitis, especially around the mouth, and loss of hair. Chronic zinc deficiency occurs in dietary deficiency, malabsorption syndromes, alcoholism and its associated hepatic cirrhosis. It causes the clinical features seen in the very rare congenital disorder known as acrodermatitis enteropathica (growth retardation, hair loss and chronic diarrhoea). Zinc deficiency is thought to be responsible for one-third of the world's population not reaching their optimal height. In the Middle East, chronic deficiency has been associated with dwarfism and hypogonadism. In starvation, zinc deficiency causes thymic atrophy, and zinc supplements may accelerate the healing of skin lesions, promote general well-being, improve appetite and reduce the morbidity associated with the under-nourished state, and lower the mortality associated with diarrhoea and pneumonia in children.

Selenium

The family of seleno-enzymes includes glutathione peroxidase, which helps prevent free radical damage to cells, and monodeiodinase, which converts thyroxine to triiodothyronine (p. 738). North American soil has a higher selenium content than European and Asian soil, and the decreasing reliance of Europe on imported American food in recent decades has resulted in a decline in dietary selenium intake.

Selenium deficiency can cause hypothyroidism, cardiomyopathy in children (Keshan's disease) and myopathy in adults. Excess selenium can cause heart disease.

Fluoride

Fluoride helps prevent dental caries, since it increases the resistance of the enamel to acid attack. It is a component of bone mineral and some studies have shown anti-fracture effects at low doses, but excessive intakes may compromise bone structure.

If the local water supply contains more than 1 part per million (ppm) of fluoride, the incidence of dental caries is low. Soft waters usually contain no fluoride, whilst very hard waters may contain over 10 ppm. The benefit of fluoride is greatest when it is taken before the permanent teeth erupt, while their enamel is being laid down. The addition of traces of fluoride (at 1 ppm) to public water supplies is now a widespread practice. Chronic fluoride poisoning is occasionally seen where the water supply contains > 10 ppm fluoride. It can also occur in workers handling cryolite (aluminium sodium fluoride), used in smelting aluminium. Fluoride poisoning is described on page 223. Pitting of teeth is a result of too much fluoride as a child.

Sodium, potassium and magnesium

Western diets are high in sodium due to the sodium chloride (salt) that is added to processed food. In the UK, it is suggested that daily salt intakes are kept well below 6 g. The roles of sodium, potassium and magnesium, along with the disease states associated with abnormal intakes or disordered metabolism, are discussed in Chapter 16.

Other essential inorganic nutrients

These include chloride (a counter-ion to sodium and potassium), cobalt (required for vitamin B_{12}), sulphur (a constituent of methionine and cysteine), manganese (needed for or activates many enzymes) and chromium (necessary for insulin action). Deficiency of chromium presents as hyperglycaemia and has been reported in adults as a rare complication of prolonged parenteral nutrition.

Copper metabolism is abnormal in Wilson's disease (p. 973). Deficiency occasionally occurs but only in young children, causing microcytic hypochromic anaemia, neutropenia, retarded growth, skeletal rarefaction and dermatosis.

Further information and acknowledgements

Websites

www.dh.gov.uk/en/Publichealth/Nutrition/index.htm *UK Department of Health information on food composition and dietary surveys.*

www.diversalertnetwork.org *Advice on the clinical management of diving illness and emergency assistance services.*

www.hpa.org.uk/radiation *The Health Protection Agency provides information and links on all forms of radiation for patients and professionals.*

www.nice.org.uk *NICE guidelines for nutritional support and obesity.*

www.who.int/nutrition *WHO recommendations and intervention programmes for macronutrient- and micronutrient-related diseases.*

www.who.int/topics/global_burden_of_disease/en/ *The WHO global burden of disease project.*

Telephone numbers

- In the UK, two organisations provide advice on the clinical management of diving illness and the availability of the nearest recompression facility:
  - Aberdeen Royal Infirmary +44 (0)845 48 6008 *Hyperbaric doctor on call*
  - Royal Navy +44 (0)7831 151523.
- Outside the UK, contact the Divers Alert Network (DAN; see above).

Figure acknowledgements

Fig. 5.1 Adapted by Rao M, Prasad S, Adshead F, et al. The built environment and health. Lancet 2007; 370:1112, from an original model by Whitehead M, Dahlgren G. What can be done about inequalities in health? Lancet 1991; 338:1059–1063.

Fig. 5.8 Crown copyright. Department of Health in association with the Welsh Government, the Scottish Government and the Food Standards Agency in North Ireland.

Fig. 5.18B WHO. Report of a joint WHO/USAID meeting, vitamin A deficiency and xerophthalmia (WHO technical report series no. 5 W); 1976.

Fig. 5.19 Karthikeyan K, Thappa DM. Pellagra and skin. Int J Dermatol 2002; 41:476–481.

Fig. 5.20AB Ho V, Prinsloo P, Ombiga J. Persistent anaemia due to scurvy. Journal of the New Zealand Medical Association 2007; 120(1262):62. Reproduced with permission.

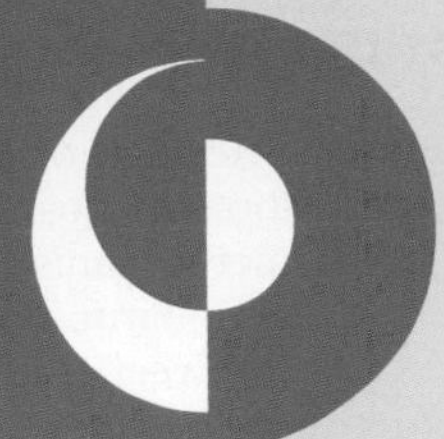

R.P. Hobson
D.H. Dockrell

Principles of infectious disease

6

Infectious agents 134

Normal flora 136

Host–pathogen interactions 137

Investigation of infection 138

Direct detection 139
Culture 140
Specific immunological tests 141
Antimicrobial susceptibility testing 143

Epidemiology of infection 143

Infection prevention and control 145

Health care-acquired infection 145
Outbreaks of infection 147
Immunisation 148

Treatment of infectious diseases 149

Principles of antimicrobial therapy 149
Beta-lactam antibiotics 154
Macrolide and lincosamide antibiotics 156
Ketolides 156
Aminoglycosides 156
Quinolones and fluoroquinolones 157
Glycopeptides 157
Folate antagonists 158
Tetracyclines and glycylcyclines 158
Nitroimidazoles 158
Other antibacterial agents 158
Antifungal agents 159
Antiviral agents 160
Antiparasitic agents 162

Infection is the establishment of foreign organisms, or 'infectious agents', in or on a human host. This may result in colonisation, if the microorganism exists at an anatomical site without causing harm, or infectious disease, when the interaction between the host and microorganism (pathogen) results in illness. In clinical practice, the term 'infection' is often used interchangeably with 'infectious disease'. Most pathogens are microorganisms, although some are multicellular organisms.

The host–pathogen interaction is dynamic and complex. Whilst it is rarely in the microorganism's interest to kill the host (on which it relies for nutrition and protection), the manifestations of disease may aid its dissemination (e.g. diarrhoea, sneezing). Conversely, it is in the host's interests to kill microorganisms likely to cause disease, whilst preserving colonising organisms, which may be beneficial.

Communicable diseases are caused by organisms transmitted between hosts, whereas endogenous diseases are caused by organisms already colonising the host. Cross-infection with colonising organisms (e.g. meticillin-resistant *Staphylococcus aureus*, MRSA) is both communicable and endogenous. Opportunistic infections may be communicable or endogenous and arise only in individuals with impaired host defence. The chain of infection (Fig. 6.1) describes six essential elements for communicable disease transmission.

Despite dramatic advances in hygiene, immunisation and antimicrobial therapy, infectious diseases are still a major cause of disease worldwide. Key challenges remain in tackling infection in resource-poor countries and in the emergence of new infectious agents and antimicrobial-resistant microorganisms. This chapter describes the biological and epidemiological principles of infectious diseases and the general approach to their prevention, diagnosis and treatment. Specific infectious diseases are described in Chapters 13–15 and many of the organ-based chapters.

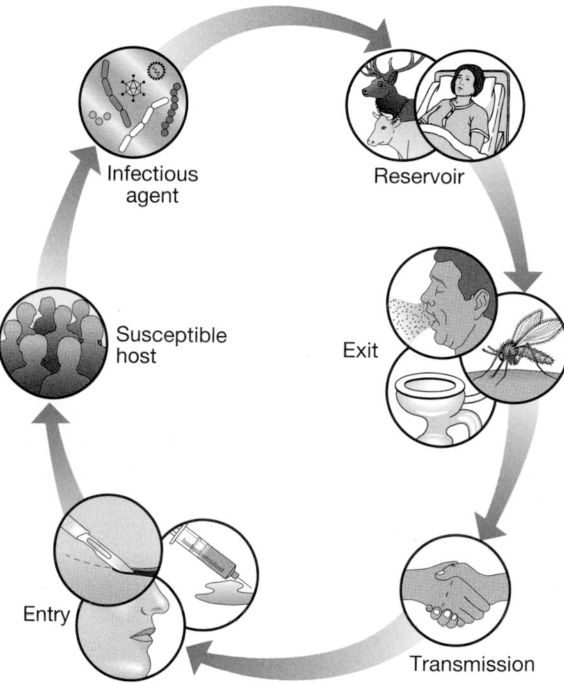

Fig. 6.1 Chain of infection. The infectious agent is the organism that causes the disease. The reservoir is the place where the population of an infectious agent is maintained. The portal of exit is the point from which the infectious agent leaves the reservoir. Transmission is the process by which the infectious agent is transferred from the reservoir to the human host, either directly or via a vector or fomite. The portal of entry is the body site that is first accessed by the infectious agent. Finally, in order for disease to ensue, the person to whom the infectious agent is transmitted must be a susceptible host.

INFECTIOUS AGENTS

The concept of an infectious agent was established by Robert Koch in the 19th century (Box 6.1). Although fulfilment of 'Koch's postulates' became the standard for the definition of an infectious agent, they do not apply to uncultivable organisms (e.g. *Mycobacterium leprae, Tropheryma whipplei)* or members of the normal human flora (e.g. *Escherichia coli, Candida* spp.). The following groups of infectious agents are now recognised.

Prions

Prions are unique amongst infectious agents in that they are devoid of any nucleic acid. They appear to be transmitted by acquisition of a normal mammalian protein (prion protein, PrP^{C}) which is in an abnormal conformation (PrP^{SC}, containing an excess of beta-sheet protein); the abnormal protein inhibits the 26S proteasome, which can degrade misfolded proteins, leading to accumulation of the abnormally configured PrP^{SC} protein instead of normal PrP^{C}. The result is accumulation of protein which forms amyloid in the central nervous system, causing a transmissible spongiform encephalopathy (see Box 13.40, p. 329, and p. 1211).

Viruses

Viruses are incapable of independent replication, instead subverting host cellular processes to ensure synthesis of their nucleic acids and proteins. A virus that infects a bacterium is a bacteriophage (phage). Viruses contain genetic material (genome), which may be single- or double-stranded DNA or RNA. Retroviruses transcribe their RNA into DNA by reverse transcription. An antigenically unique protein coat (capsid) encloses the genome, together forming the nucleocapsid. In many viruses, the nucleocapsid is packaged within a lipid envelope. Enveloped viruses are less able to survive in the environment and are spread by respiratory, sexual or blood-borne routes, including arthropod-based

6.1 Definition of an infectious agent – Koch's postulates

1. The same organism must be present in every case of the disease
2. The organism must be isolated from the diseased host and grown in pure culture
3. The isolate must cause the disease, when inoculated into a healthy, susceptible animal
4. The organism must be re-isolated from the inoculated, diseased animal

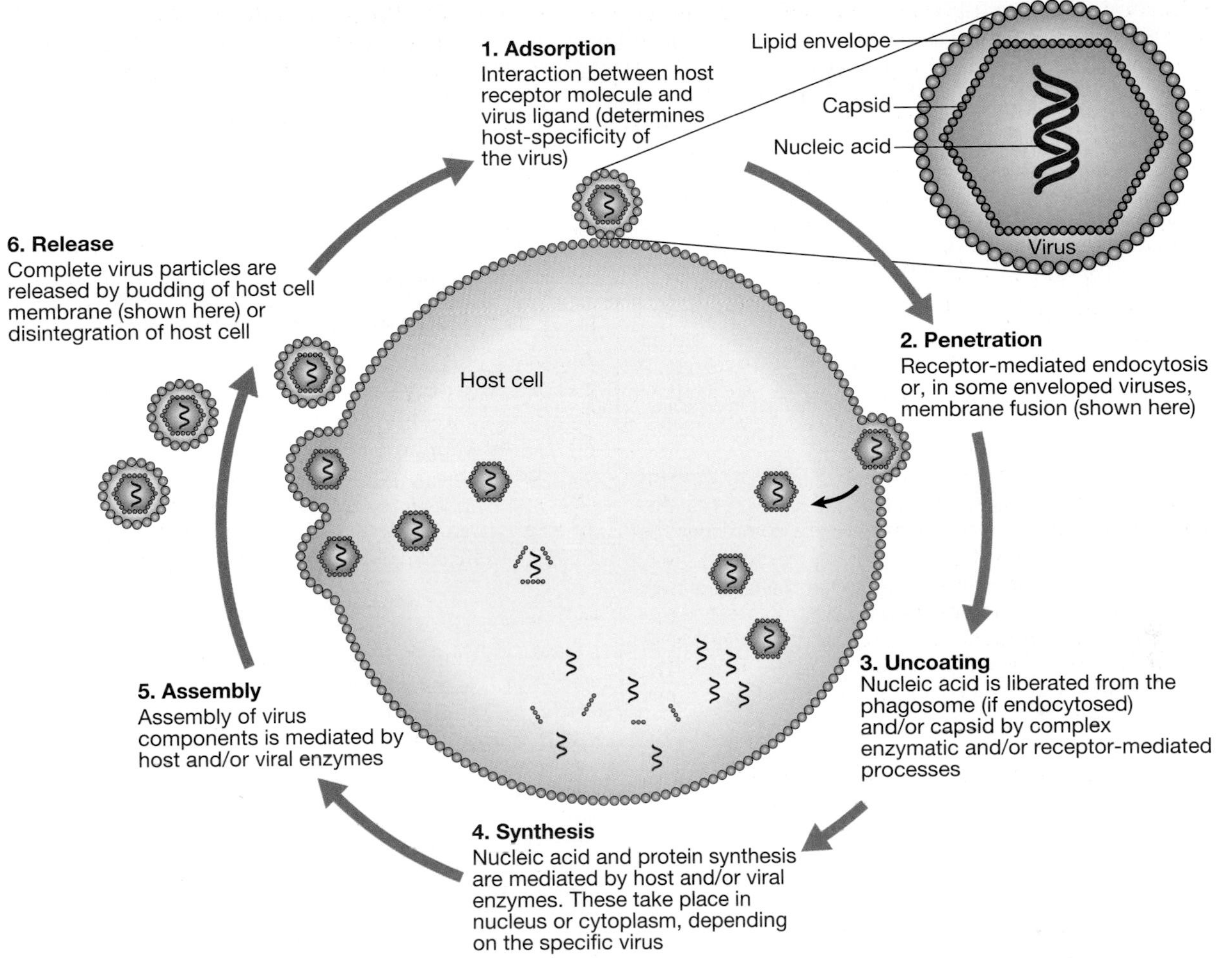

Fig. 6.2 A generic virus life cycle. Life cycle components common to most viruses are host cell attachment and penetration, virus uncoating, nucleic acid and protein synthesis, virus assembly and release. Virus release is achieved either by budding, as illustrated, or by lysis of the cell membrane. Life cycles vary between viruses.

transmission. Non-enveloped viruses survive better in the environment and are predominantly transmitted by faecal–oral or, less often, respiratory routes. A generic virus life cycle is shown in Figure 6.2.

Prokaryotes: bacteria (including mycobacteria and actinomycetes)

Prokaryotic cells are capable of synthesising their own proteins and nucleic acids, and are able to reproduce autonomously, although they lack a nucleus. The bacterial cell membrane is bounded by a peptidoglycan cell wall, which is thick (20–80 nm) in Gram-positive organisms and thin (5–10 nm) in Gram-negative ones. The Gram-negative cell wall is surrounded by an outer membrane containing lipopolysaccharide. Plasmids are rings of extra-chromosomal DNA within bacteria, which can be transferred between organisms. Bacteria may be embedded in a polysaccharide capsule, and motile bacteria are equipped with flagella. Although many prokaryotes are capable of independent existence, some (e.g. *Chlamydia trachomatis*, *Coxiella burnetii*) are obligate intracellular organisms. Bacteria that replicate in artificial culture media are classified and identified using a range of characteristics (Box 6.2), with examples in Figures 6.3 and 6.4.

Eukaryotes: fungi, protozoa and helminths

Eukaryotes contain functional organelles, including nuclei, mitochondria and Golgi apparatus. Eukaryotes involved in human infection include fungi, protozoa (unicellular eukaryotes with a flexible cell membrane, p. 353) and helminths (complex multicellular organisms including nematodes, trematodes and cestodes, p. 369).

Fungi exist as either moulds (filamentous fungi) or yeasts. Dimorphic fungi exist in either form, depending on environmental conditions (see Fig. 13.57, p. 382). The fungal plasma membrane differs from the human cell membrane in that it contains the sterol, ergosterol. Fungi have a cell wall made up of polysaccharides, chitin and manno-proteins. In most fungi, the main structural component of the cell wall is β-1,3-D-glucan, a glucose polymer.

Protozoa and helminths are often referred to as parasites. Many parasites have complex multi-stage life cycles, which involve animal and/or plant hosts in addition to humans.

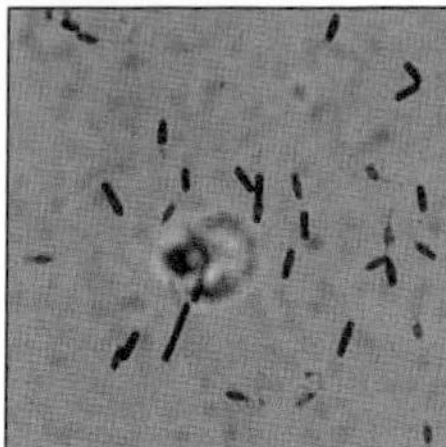

Gram-positive bacilli
- *Clostridium* spp. (shown here)
- *Corynebacterium* spp.
- *Bacillus* spp.

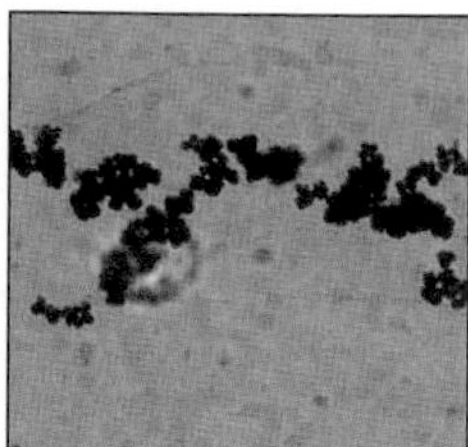

Gram-positive cocci in clusters
- Staphylococci

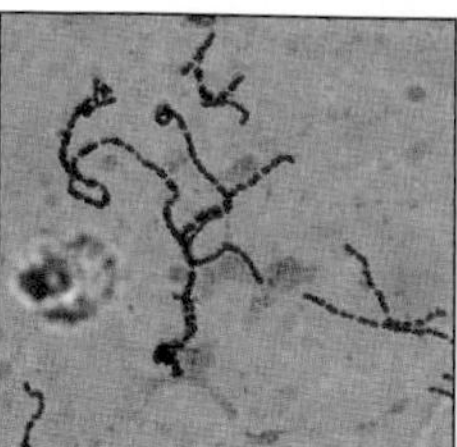

Gram-positive cocci in chains
- Streptococci

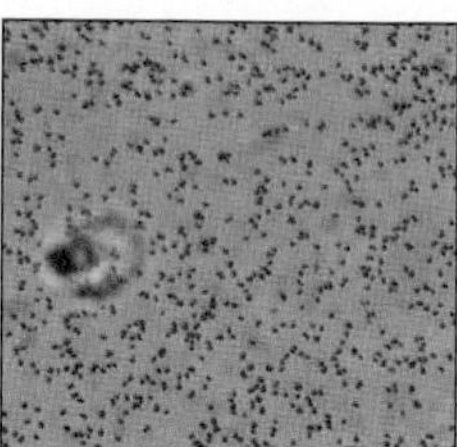

Gram-negative cocci
- *Neisseria* spp. (shown here)
- *Moraxella* spp.

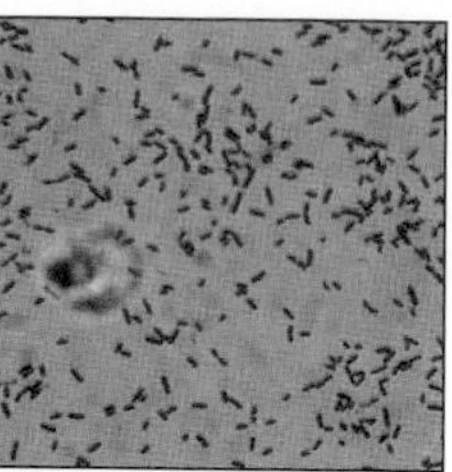

Gram-negative bacilli
- Enterobacteriaceae (shown here)
- *Serratia* spp.
- *Acinetobacter* spp.
- *Bacteroides* spp.

Fig. 6.3 Gram film appearances of bacteria on light microscopy (×100).

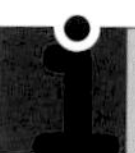

6.2 How bacteria are identified
Gram stain reaction (see Fig. 6.3)
• Gram-positive (thick peptidoglycan layer), Gram-negative (thin peptidoglycan) or unstainable
Microscopic morphology
• Cocci (round cells) or bacilli (elongated cells) • Presence or absence of capsule
Cell association
• Associated in clusters, chains or pairs
Colonial characteristics
• Colony size, shape or colour • Effect on culture media (e.g. β-haemolysis of blood agar in haemolytic streptococci; see Fig. 6.4)
Atmospheric requirements
• Strictly aerobic (requires O_2), strictly anaerobic (requires absence of O_2), facultatively aerobic (grows with or without O_2) or micro-aerophilic (requires reduced O_2)
Biochemical reactions
• Expression of enzymes (oxidase, catalase, coagulase) • Ability to ferment or hydrolyse various biochemical substrates
Motility
• Motile or non-motile
Antibiotic susceptibility
• Identifies organisms with invariable susceptibility (e.g. to optochin in *Streptococcus pneumoniae* or metronidazole in obligate anaerobes)
Matrix-assisted laser desorption/ionisation – time of flight mass spectrometry (MALDI-TOF-MS)
• A rapid technique that identifies bacteria and some fungi from their specific molecular composition
DNA sequencing of bacterial 16s ribosomes
• A highly specific test for definitive identification of organisms in pure culture and in samples from normally sterile sites

NORMAL FLORA

Every human is host to an estimated 10^{13}–10^{14} colonising microorganisms, which constitute the normal flora. Resident flora are able to survive and replicate at a body site, whereas transient flora are present only for short periods.

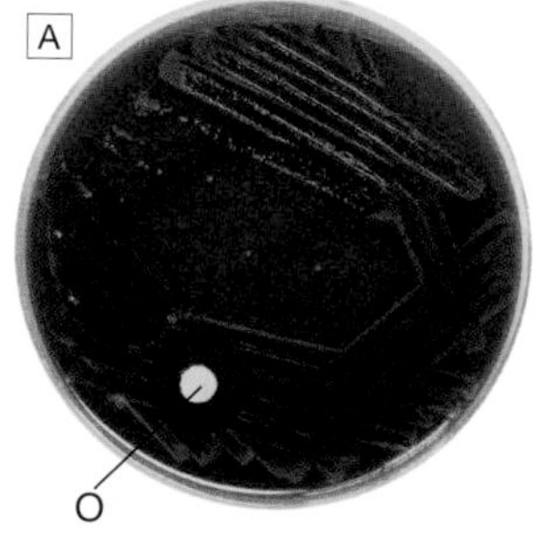

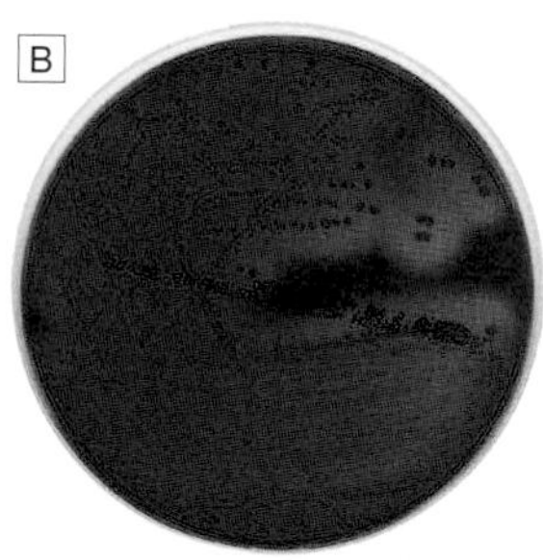

Fig. 6.4 Appearances of α- and β-haemolytic streptococci on blood agar. **A** Alpha-haemolytic streptococci. The colonies cause partial haemolysis, which imparts a green tinge to the agar. The organism shown is *Strep. pneumoniae* from the cerebrospinal fluid of a patient with meningitis (note also the susceptibility to optochin (O), which is another feature used to identify this organism). **B** Beta-haemolytic streptococci. The colonies cause complete haemolysis, which renders the agar transparent. The organism shown is *Strep. pyogenes* (group A β-haemolytic streptococci) from a superficial wound swab.

Knowledge of non-sterile body sites and their normal flora is required to interpret culture results (Fig. 6.5).

The relationship between human host and normal flora is symbiotic, meaning that the organisms are in close proximity, and either mutualistic (both organisms benefit) or commensal (one organism benefits whilst the other derives neither benefit nor harm). The microbiome is the total burden of microorganisms, their genes and environmental interactions; the human microbiome is recognised increasingly as exerting a profound influence over human health and disease.

Maintenance of the normal flora is beneficial to health. For example, lower gastrointestinal tract bacteria synthesise and excrete vitamins (e.g. vitamins K and B_{12}); colonisation with normal flora confers 'colonisation resistance' to infection with pathogenic organisms by altering the local environment (e.g. lowering pH), producing antibacterial agents (e.g. bacteriocins, fatty acids and metabolic waste products), and inducing host antibodies which cross-react with pathogenic organisms.

Conversely, normally sterile body sites must be kept sterile. The mucociliary escalator transports environmental material deposited in the respiratory tract to the nasopharynx. The urethral sphincter prevents flow from the non-sterile urethra to the sterile bladder. Physical barriers, including the skin, lining of the gastrointestinal

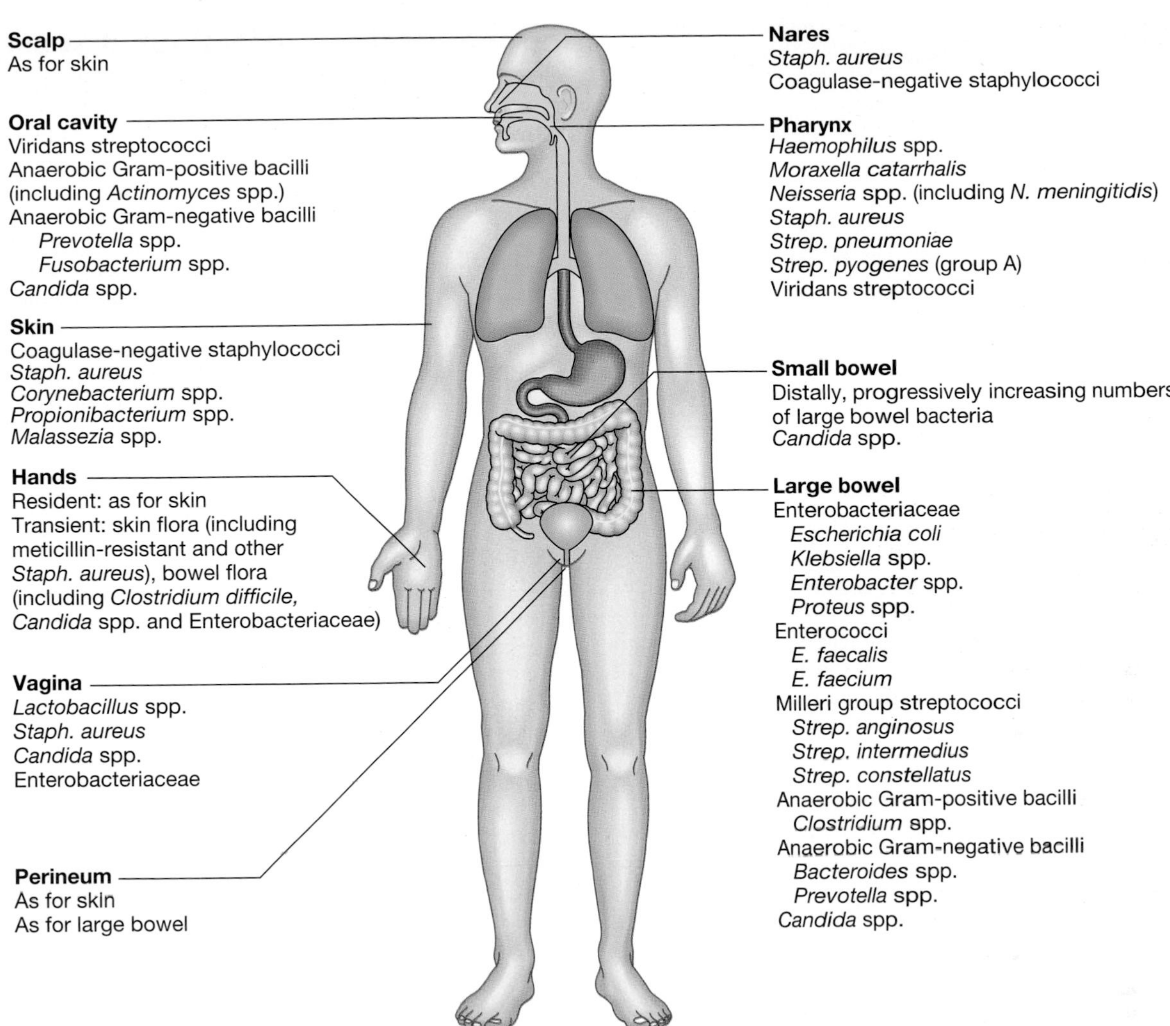

Fig. 6.5 Human non-sterile sites and normal flora in health.

tract and mucous membranes, maintain sterility of the blood stream, peritoneal and pleural cavities, chambers of the eye, subcutaneous tissue and so on.

The normal flora contribute to endogenous disease by either excessive growth at the 'normal' site (overgrowth) or translocation to a sterile site. Overgrowth is exemplified by 'blind loop' syndrome (p. 882), dental caries and vaginal thrush, in which external factors favour overgrowth of specific components of the normal flora. Translocation results from spread along a surface or penetration of a closed barrier: for example, in urinary tract infection caused by perineal/enteric flora, and in surgical site infections, particularly of prosthetic materials, caused by skin flora such as staphylococci. Normal flora also contribute to disease by cross-infection, in which organisms that are colonising one individual cause disease when transferred to another, more susceptible, individual.

HOST–PATHOGEN INTERACTIONS

Pathogenicity is the capability of an organism to cause disease and virulence is the extent to which a pathogen is able to cause disease. Pathogens produce proteins and other factors, termed virulence factors, which interact with host cells to contribute to disease.

- *Primary pathogens* cause disease in a proportion of individuals to whom they are exposed, regardless of their immunological status.
- *Opportunistic pathogens* cause disease only in individuals whose host defences are compromised; for example, by genetic susceptibility or immunosuppressive disease or therapy.

Characteristics of successful pathogens

Successful pathogens have a number of attributes. They compete with host cells and colonising flora by various methods, including sequestration of nutrients, use of metabolic pathways not used by competing bacteria, and production of bacteriocins (small antimicrobial peptides/proteins that kill closely related bacteria). Motility enables pathogens to reach their site of infection, often in sterile sites that colonising bacteria do not reach, such as the distal airway. Many microorganisms, including viruses, use 'adhesins' to attach to host cells at the site of infection. Other pathogens can invade through tissues.

6.3 Exotoxin-mediated bacterial diseases

Disease	Organism
Antibiotic-associated diarrhoea/pseudo-membranous colitis	*Clostridium difficile* (p. 308)
Botulism	*Clostridium botulinum* (p. 1210)
Cholera	*Vibrio cholerae* (p. 344)
Diphtheria	*Corynebacterium diphtheriae* (p. 345)
Haemolytic uraemic syndrome	*Escherichia coli* 0157 (and other strains) (p. 495)
Necrotising pneumonia	*Staphylococcus aureus* (p. 682)
Tetanus	*Clostridium tetani* (p. 1209)
Toxic shock syndrome	*Staphylococcus aureus* (p. 331)

Pathogens may produce toxins, microbial molecules that cause adverse effects on host cells, either at the site of infection, or remotely following carriage through the blood stream. Endotoxin is the lipid A domain of Gram-negative bacterial outer membrane lipopolysaccharide. It is released when bacterial cells are damaged and has generalised inflammatory effects. Exotoxins are proteins released by living bacteria, which often have specific effects on target organs (Box 6.3).

Intracellular pathogens, including viruses, bacteria (e.g. *Salmonella* spp., *Listeria monocytogenes* and *Mycobacterium tuberculosis*), parasites (e.g. *Leishmania* spp.) and fungi (e.g. *Histoplasma capsulatum*), are able to survive in intracellular environments, including after phagocytosis by macrophages.

Pathogenic bacteria express different arrays of genes, depending on environmental stress (pH, iron starvation, O_2 starvation and so on) and anatomical location. In quorum sensing, bacteria communicate with one another to adapt their replication or metabolism according to local population density. Bacteria and fungi may respond to the presence of an artificial surface (e.g. prosthetic device, venous catheter) by forming a biofilm, which is a population of organisms encased in a matrix of extracellular molecules. Biofilm-associated organisms are highly resistant to antimicrobial agents.

Genetic diversity enhances the pathogenic capacity of bacteria. Some virulence factor genes are found on plasmids or in phages and are exchanged between different strains or species. The ability to acquire genes from the gene pool of all strains of the species (the 'bacterial supragenome') increases diversity and the potential for pathogenicity. Viruses exploit their rapid reproduction and potential to exchange nucleic acid with host cells to enhance diversity. Once a strain acquires a particularly effective combination of virulence genes, it may become an epidemic strain, accounting for a large subset of infections in a particular region. This phenomenon accounts for influenza pandemics.

The host response

Innate and adaptive immune and inflammatory responses which humans use to control the normal flora and respond to pathogens are reviewed in Chapter 4.

Pathogenesis of infectious disease

The harmful manifestations of infection are determined by a combination of the virulence factors of the organism and the host response to infection. Despite the obvious benefits of an intact host response, an excessive response is undesirable. Cytokines and antimicrobial factors contribute to tissue injury at the site of infection, and an excessive inflammatory response may lead to hypotension and organ dysfunction (p. 82). The contribution of the immune response to disease manifestations is exemplified by the immune reconstitution inflammatory syndrome (IRIS). This is seen, for example, in human immunodeficiency virus (HIV) infection, post-transplantation neutropenia or tuberculosis (which causes suppression of T-cell function): there is a paradoxical worsening of the clinical condition as the immune dysfunction is corrected, caused by an exuberant but dysregulated inflammatory response.

The febrile response

Thermoregulation (p. 103) is altered in infectious disease. Microbial pyrogens or the endogenous pyrogens released during tissue necrosis stimulate specialised cells such as monocytes/macrophages to release cytokines, including interleukin (IL)-Iβ, tumour necrosis factor-alpha (TNF)-α, IL-6 and interferon (IFN)-γ. Cytokine receptors in the pre-optic region of the anterior hypothalamus activate phospholipase A, releasing arachidonic acid as substrate for the cyclo-oxygenase pathway and producing prostaglandin E_2 (PGE_2), which in turn alters the responsiveness of thermosensitive neurons in the thermoregulatory centre. Rigors occur when the body inappropriately attempts to 'reset' core temperature to a higher level by stimulating skeletal muscle activity and shaking.

The role of the febrile response as a defence mechanism requires further study, but there are data to support the hypothesis that raised body temperature interferes with the replication and/or virulence of pathogens.

INVESTIGATION OF INFECTION

Patients in whom a diagnosis of infectious disease is being considered are investigated with non-specific tests that reflect innate immune and acute phase responses (p. 82), and specific tests, which detect either a micro-organism or the host response to the organism (Box 6.4). Careful sampling increases the likelihood of diagnosis (Box 6.5). Culture results must be interpreted in the context of the normal flora at the sampled site (see Fig. 6.5). The extent to which a microbiological test result supports or excludes a particular diagnosis depends on its statistical performance (e.g. sensitivity, specificity, positive and negative predictive value, p. 5). Sensitivity and specificity vary according to the time between infection and testing, and positive and negative predictive values depend on the prevalence of the condition in the test population. The complexity of test interpretation is illustrated in Figure 6.7 (p. 141), which shows the 'windows of opportunity' afforded by various testing methods. Given this complexity, effective communication between the clinician and the microbiologist is vital to ensure accurate test interpretation.

6.4 Tests used to diagnose infection

Non-specific markers of inflammation/infection
• e.g. Full blood count (FBC), plasma C-reactive protein (CRP), procalcitonin, cell counts in urine or cerebrospinal fluid (CSF), CSF protein and glucose
Direct detection of organisms or organism components
• Microscopy • Detection of organism components (e.g. antigen, toxin) • Nucleic acid amplification (e.g. polymerase chain reaction)
Culture of organisms
• ± Antimicrobial sensitivity testing
Tests of the host's specific immune response
• Antibody detection • Interferon-γ release assays (IGRA)

Direct detection

Direct detection methods provide rapid results and may be applied to organisms that cannot be grown easily on artificial culture media, such as *Chlamydia* spp. They do not usually provide information on antimicrobial susceptibility or the degree to which organisms are related to each other (which is important in the investigation of possible outbreaks), unless relevant specific nucleic acid sequences are detected by polymerase chain reaction (PCR).

Detection of whole organisms

Whole organisms are detected by examination of biological fluids or tissue using a microscope.

- *Bright field microscopy* (in which the test sample is interposed between the light source and the objective lens) uses stains to enhance visual contrast between the organism and its background. Examples include Gram staining of bacteria and Ziehl–Neelsen or auramine staining of acid- and alcohol-fast bacilli (AAFB) in tuberculosis. In histopathological examination of tissue samples, multiple stains are used to demonstrate not only the presence of microorganisms, but also features of disease pathology.
- *Dark field microscopy* (in which light is scattered to make organisms appear bright on a dark background) is used, for example, to examine genital chancre fluid in suspected syphilis.
- *Electron microscopy* may be used to examine stool and vesicle fluid to detect enteric and herpesviruses, respectively, but its use has largely been supplanted by nucleic acid detection (see below).

Detection of components of organisms

Components of microorganisms detected for diagnostic purposes include nucleic acids, cell wall molecules, toxins and other antigens. Commonly used examples include *Legionella pneumophila* serogroup 1 antigen in urine and cryptococcal polysaccharide antigen in cerebrospinal fluid (CSF). Most antigen detection methods

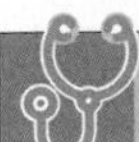

6.5 How to provide samples for microbiological sampling

Communication
• Discuss samples that may require forwarding to another laboratory or processing urgently or by an unusual method with laboratory staff *before* collection • Communication is the most important requirement for good microbiological sampling. If there is doubt about any aspect of sampling, it is far better to discuss it with laboratory staff beforehand than to risk diagnostic delay by inappropriate sampling or sample handling
Indication
• Screening (e.g. collecting 'routine' urine, intravenous cannulae or sputum) in the absence of clinical evidence of infection is rarely appropriate
Container
• Certain tests (e.g. nucleic acid and antigen detection tests) require proprietary sample collection equipment
Collection
• Follow sample collection instructions precisely (e.g. proper collection of mid-stream, terminal and early morning urine samples, skin decontamination prior to blood culture etc.) to increase diagnostic yield
Labelling
• Label sample containers and request forms according to local policies, with demographic identifiers, specimen type and time/date collected • Include clinical details on request forms • Identify samples carrying a high risk of infection (e.g. blood liable to contain a blood-borne virus) with a hazard label
Packaging
• Close sample containers tightly and package securely (usually in sealed plastic bags) • Attach request forms to samples but not in the same compartment (to avoid contamination, should leakage occur)
Storage and transport
• Transport samples to the microbiology laboratory quickly • If pre-transport storage is required, conditions (e.g. refrigeration, incubation, storage at room temperature) vary with sample type • Notify the receiving laboratory prior to arrival of samples, to ensure timely processing

are based on in vitro binding of specific antigen/antibody and are described below (p. 141). However, other methods may be used, such as mouse bioassay for detection of *Clostridium botulinum* toxin or tissue culture cytotoxicity assay for *C. difficile* toxin. In toxin-mediated disease, detection of toxin may be of greater relevance than identification of the organism itself (e.g. stool *C. difficile* toxin).

Nucleic acid amplification tests (NAAT)

Specific sequences of microbial DNA and RNA are identified using a nucleic acid primer which is amplified exponentially by enzymes to generate multiple copies of the specific sequence. The most commonly used amplification method is the polymerase chain reaction (PCR; see Fig. 3.12, p. 60). Reverse transcription (RT) PCR is used to detect RNA from RNA viruses

6

(e.g. hepatitis C virus and HIV-1). The use of fluorescent-labelled primers and probes enables 'real-time' detection of amplified DNA; quantification is based on the principle that the time taken to reach the detection threshold is proportional to the initial number of copies of the target nucleic acid sequence. In multiplex PCR, multiple primer pairs are used to enable detection of several different organisms in a single assay.

Nucleic acid sequencing is also used to assign micro-organisms to specific strains according to their genotype, which may be relevant to treatment and/or prognosis (e.g. in hepatitis C infection, p. 954). Genes that are relevant to pathogenicity (such as toxin genes) or antimicrobial resistance can also be detected. For example, detection of the *mecA* gene is used to screen for MRSA.

NAAT are the most sensitive direct detection methods and are particularly useful when a rapid diagnosis is required. They are used widely in virology, where the possibility of false-positive results from colonising or contaminating organisms is remote, and are applied to blood, respiratory samples, stool and urine. In bacteriology, PCR is used to examine CSF, blood, tissue and genital samples, and multiplex PCR is being developed for use in faeces. PCR is also being used increasingly in mycology and parasitology.

Culture

Microorganisms may be both detected and further characterised by culture from clinical samples (e.g. tissue, swabs and body fluids).

- *In vivo culture* (in a living organism) is not used in routine diagnostic microbiology.
- *Ex vivo culture* (tissue or cell culture) was widely used in the isolation of viruses, but has been largely supplanted by nucleic acid amplification techniques.

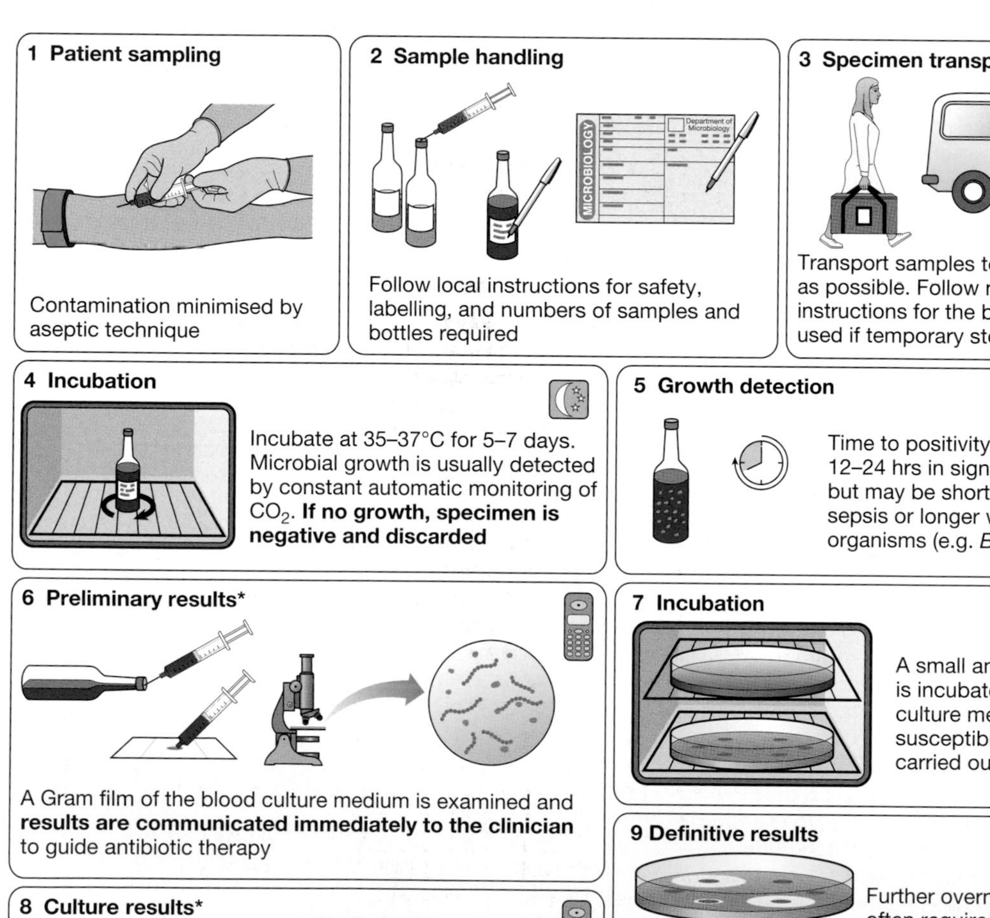

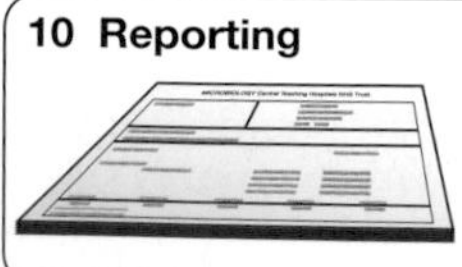

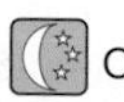

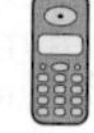

Fig. 6.6 An overview of the processing of blood cultures. *In laboratories equipped with MALDI-TOF (p. 136), rapid definitive organism identification may be achieved at stage 6 and/or stage 8.

- *In vitro culture* (in artificial culture media) of bacteria and fungi is used for definitive identification, to test for antimicrobial susceptibility and to subtype the organism for epidemiological purposes.

However, culture has its limitations. Results are not immediate, even for organisms which are easy to grow, and negative culture rarely excludes infection completely. Organisms such as *Mycobacterium tuberculosis* are inherently slow-growing, typically taking at least 2 weeks to be detectable, even in specialised systems. Certain organisms, such as *Mycobacterium leprae* and *Tropheryma whipplei,* cannot be cultivated on artificial media, and others (e.g. *Chlamydia* spp. and viruses) grow only in ex vivo systems, which are slow and labour-intensive to use.

Blood culture

Rapid microbiological diagnosis is required for bloodstream infection (BSI; Fig. 6.6). To diagnose BSI, a liquid culture medium is inoculated with freshly drawn blood, transported to the microbiology laboratory and incubated in a system that monitors it constantly for products of microbial respiration (mainly CO_2), generally using fluorescence. If growth is detected, organisms are identified and sensitivity testing is performed. Traditionally, identification has been achieved by Gram stain and culture. However, MALDI-TOF (see Box 6.2) is being used increasingly, as it is rapid and inexpensive, and enables identification of organisms directly from the blood-culture medium.

Specific immunological tests

Immunological tests may be used to detect the host response to a specific microorganism, and can enable the diagnosis of infection with organisms that are difficult to detect by other methods or are no longer present in the host. The term 'serology' describes tests carried out on serum, and is used to include both antigen and antibody detection.

Antibody detection

Organism-specific antibody detection is applied mainly to blood (Fig. 6.7). Results are typically expressed as titres: that is, the reciprocal of the highest dilution of the serum at which antibody is detectable (for example, detection at serum dilution of 1:64 gives a titre of 64). 'Seroconversion' is defined as either a change from negative to positive detection or a fourfold rise in titre between acute and convalescent serum samples. An acute sample is usually taken during the first week of disease and the convalescent sample 2–4 weeks later. Earlier diagnosis can be achieved by detection of IgM antibodies, which are produced early in infection (p. 77). A limitation of these tests is that antibody production requires a fully functional host immune system, so there may be false-negative results in immunocompromised patients. Also, other than in chronic infections and with IgM detection, antibody tests usually provide a retrospective diagnosis.

Antibody detection methods are described below (antigen detection methods are also described here as they share similar methodology).

Enzyme-linked immunosorbent assay

The principles of the enzyme-linked immunosorbent assay (ELISA, EIA) are illustrated in Figure 6.8. These assays rely on linking an antibody with an enzyme which generates a colour change on exposure to a chromogenic substrate. Various configurations allow detection of antigens or specific subclasses of immunoglobulin (e.g. IgG, IgM, IgA). ELISA may also be adapted to detect PCR products, using immobilised oligonucleotide hybridisation probe and various detection systems.

Immunoblot (Western blot)

Microbial proteins are separated according to molecular weight by polyacrylamide gel electrophoresis (PAGE) and transferred (blotted) on to a nitrocellulose membrane, which is incubated with patient serum. Binding of specific antibody is detected with an

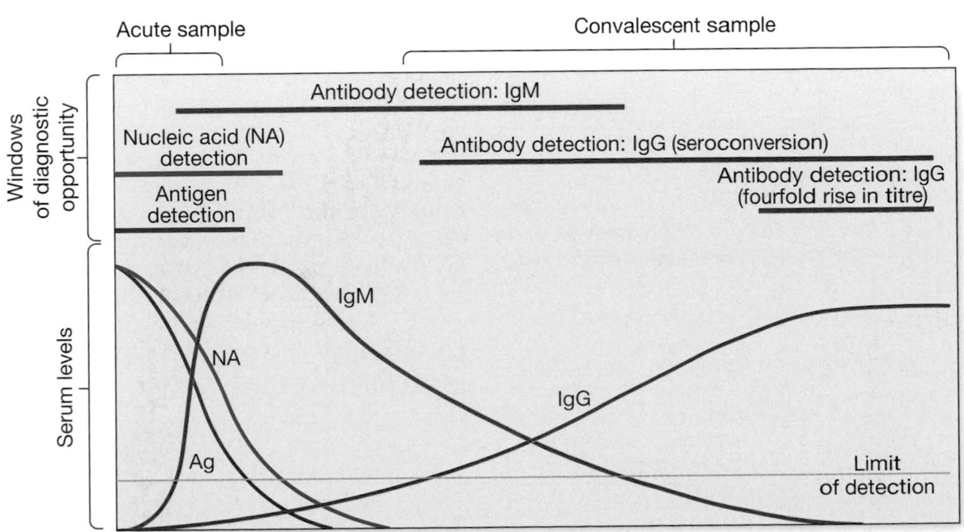

Fig. 6.7 Detection of antigen, nucleic acid and antibody in infectious disease. The acute sample is usually taken during the first week of illness, and the convalescent sample 2–4 weeks later. Detection limits and duration of detectability vary between tests and diseases, although in most diseases immunoglobulin (Ig) M is detectable within the first 1–2 weeks.

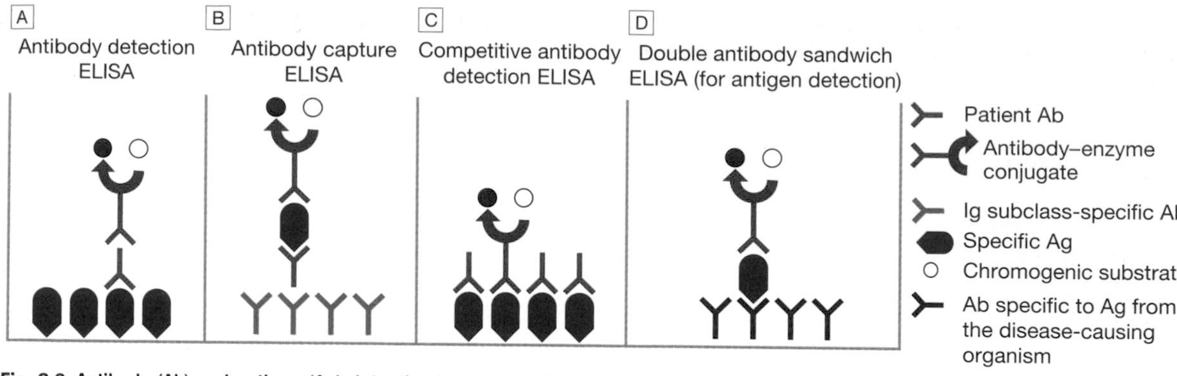

Fig. 6.8 Antibody (Ab) and antigen (Ag) detection by enzyme-linked immunosorbent assay (ELISA). This can be configured in various ways. **A** Patient Ab binds to immobilised specific Ag, and is detected by addition of anti-immunoglobulin–enzyme conjugate and chromogenic substrate. **B** Patient Ab binds to immobilised Ig subclass-specific Ab, and is detected by addition of specific Ag, followed by antibody–enzyme conjugate and chromogenic substrate. **C** Patient Ab and antibody–enzyme conjugate bind to immobilised specific Ag. Magnitude of colour change reaction is inversely proportional to concentration of patient Ab. **D** Patient Ag binds to immobilised Ab, and is detected by addition of antibody–enzyme conjugate and chromogenic substrate. In A, the conjugate Ab is specific for human immunoglobulin. In B–D, it is specific for Ag from the disease-causing organism.

enzyme–anti-immunoglobulin conjugate similar to that used in ELISA, and specificity is confirmed by its location on the membrane. Immunoblotting is a highly specific test, which may be used to confirm the results of less specific tests such as ELISA.

Immunofluorescence assays

Immunofluorescence assays (IFAs) are highly specific. In indirect immunofluorescence, a serum sample is incubated with immobilised antigen (e.g. cells known to be infected with virus on a glass slide) and antibody binding is detected using a fluorescent-labelled anti-human immunoglobulin (the 'secondary' antibody). This method can also detect organisms in clinical samples (usually tissue or centrifuged cells) using a specific antibody in place of patient serum. In direct immunofluorescence, clinical samples are incubated directly with fluorescent-labelled specific antibodies to detect antigen, eliminating the need for secondary antibody.

Complement fixation test

In a complement fixation test (CFT), patient serum is heat-treated to inactivate complement, and added to specific antigen. Any specific antibody present in the serum will complex with the antigen. Complement is then added to the reaction. If antigen–antibody complexes are present, the complement will be 'fixed' (consumed). Sheep erythrocytes, coated with an anti-erythrocyte antibody, are added. The degree of erythrocyte lysis reflects the remaining complement and is inversely proportional to the level of the specific antigen–antibody complexes.

Agglutination tests

When antigens are present on the surface of particles (e.g. cells, latex particles or microorganisms) and cross-linked with antibodies, visible clumping (or 'agglutination') occurs.

- In *direct agglutination*, patient serum is added to a suspension of organisms that express the test antigen. For example, in the Weil–Felix test, host antibodies to various rickettsial species cause agglutination of *Proteus* bacteria because they cross-react with bacterial cell surface antigens.
- In *indirect (passive) agglutination*, specific antigen is attached to the surface of carrier particles which agglutinate when incubated with patient samples that contain specific antibodies.
- In *reverse passive agglutination* (an antigen detection test), the carrier particle is coated with antibody rather than antigen.

Other tests

Immunodiffusion involves antibodies and antigen migrating through gels, with or without the assistance of electrophoresis, and forming insoluble complexes where they meet. The complexes are seen on staining as 'precipitin bands'. Immunodiffusion is used in the diagnosis of endemic mycoses (p. 381) and some forms of aspergillosis (p. 697).

Immunochromatography is used to detect antigen. The system consists of a porous test strip (e.g. a nitrocellulose membrane), at one end of which there is target-specific antibody, complexed with coloured microparticles. Further specific antibody is immobilised in a transverse narrow line some distance along the strip. Test material (e.g. blood or urine) is added to the antibody–particle complexes, which then migrate along the strip by capillary action. If these are complexed with antigen, they will be immobilised by the specific antibody and visualised as a transverse line across the strip. If the test is negative, the antibody–particle complexes will bind to a line of immobilised anti-immunoglobulin antibody placed further along the strip, which acts as a negative control. Immunochromatographic tests are rapid and relatively cheap to perform, and are appropriate for point-of-care testing, e.g. in HIV 1.

Antibody-independent specific immunological tests

Interferon-gamma release assays (IGRA) are being used increasingly to diagnose tuberculosis (p. 692). The principle of the assay is that T lymphocytes of patients infected with *Mycobacterium tuberculosis* (MTB) release IFN-γ when they are exposed to MTB-specific peptides. The absence of these peptides in bacille Calmette–Guérin (BCG; see Box 6.14) vaccine results in IGRA tests being more specific for the diagnosis of tuberculosis infection than the tuberculin skin test (p. 692), because the latter may be positive as a result of previous BCG vaccination.

Antimicrobial susceptibility testing

If growth of microorganisms in culture is inhibited by the addition of an antimicrobial agent, the organism is considered to be susceptible. Bacteriostatic agents cause reversible inhibition of growth and bactericidal agents cause cell death; the terms fungistatic/fungicidal are equivalent for antifungal agents, and virustatic/virucidal for antiviral agents. The lowest concentration of antimicrobial agent at which growth is inhibited is the minimum inhibitory concentration (MIC), and the lowest concentration that causes cell death is the minimum bactericidal concentration (MBC). If the MIC is less than or equal to a predetermined *breakpoint* threshold, the organism is considered susceptible, and if the MIC is greater than the breakpoint, it is resistant.

Breakpoints are determined for each antimicrobial agent from a combination of pharmacokinetic and clinical data. The relationship between in vitro antimicrobial susceptibility and clinical response is complex, as response also depends on immune status, pharmacokinetic variability (p. 21), comorbidities that may influence pharmacokinetics or pharmacodynamics, and antibiotic dosing, as well as MIC/MBC. Thus, susceptibility testing does not guarantee therapeutic success.

Susceptibility testing is most often carried out by disc diffusion (Fig. 6.9). Antibiotic-impregnated filter paper discs are placed on an agar plate containing bacteria. The antibiotic diffuses through the agar, resulting in a concentration gradient centred on the disc. Bacteria are unable to grow where the antibiotic concentration exceeds the MIC, which may therefore be inferred from the size of the zone of inhibition. Susceptibility testing methods using antimicrobials diluted in liquid media are generally more accurate and reproducible, and are used for generating epidemiological data.

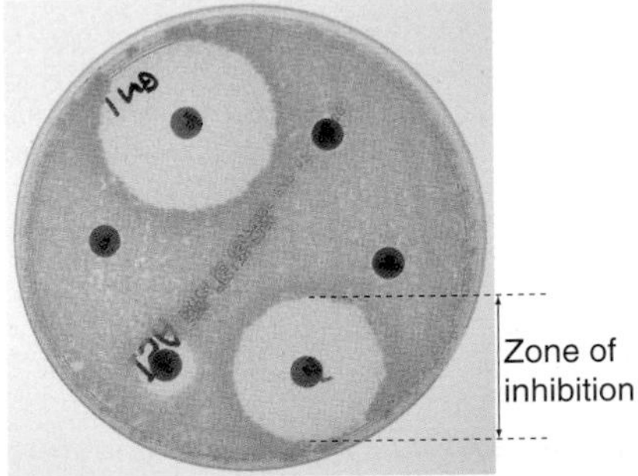

Fig. 6.9 Antimicrobial susceptibility testing by disc diffusion. The test organism is grown as a 'lawn' on an agar plate in the presence of antimicrobial-impregnated discs. The organism is considered susceptible if the diameter of the zone of inhibition exceeds a predetermined threshold.

EPIDEMIOLOGY OF INFECTION

The communicability of infectious disease means that, once a clinician has diagnosed an infectious disease, potential exposure of other patients must be considered. The patient may require treatment in isolation, or an outbreak of disease may need to be investigated in the community (Ch. 5). The approach will be specific to the microorganism involved (Chs 13–15) but the principles are outlined below.

Geographic and temporal patterns of infection

Endemic disease

Endemic disease has a constant presence within a given geographic area or population. The infectious agent may have a reservoir, vector or intermediate host that is geographically restricted, or may itself have restrictive environmental requirements (e.g. temperature range, humidity). The population affected may be geographically isolated, or the disease may be limited to unvaccinated populations. Factors that alter geographical restriction include:

- expansion of an animal reservoir (e.g. Lyme disease from reforestation)
- vector escape (e.g. airport malaria)
- extension of host range (e.g. schistosomiasis from dam construction)
- human migration (e.g. severe acute respiratory syndrome (SARS) coronavirus)
- public health service breakdown (e.g. diphtheria in unvaccinated areas)
- climate change.

Emerging and re-emerging disease

An emerging infectious disease is one that has newly appeared in a population, or has been known for some time but is increasing in incidence or geographic range. If the disease was previously known and thought to have been controlled or eradicated, it is considered to be re-emerging. Many emerging diseases are caused by organisms which infect animals and have undergone adaptations that enable them to infect humans. This is exemplified by HIV, which is believed to have originated in higher primates in Africa. The geographical pattern of some recent emerging and re-emerging infections is shown in Figure 6.10.

Reservoirs of infection

The US Centers for Disease Control (CDC) define a reservoir of infection as 'one or more epidemiologically connected populations or environments in which a pathogen can be permanently maintained, and from which infection is transmitted to a defined target population'. Reservoirs of infection may be human, animal or environmental.

Human reservoirs

Colonised individuals or those with clinical infectious disease may act as reservoirs, e.g. for *Staph. aureus* (including MRSA), which is carried in the nares of 30–40% of humans, and *C. difficile*. For infected humans to act as reservoirs, the infections caused must be long-lasting and/or non-fatal, at least in a proportion of those affected, to enable onward transmission (e.g. tuberculosis, sexually transmitted infections). Humans are the only reservoir for some organisms (e.g. smallpox and measles).

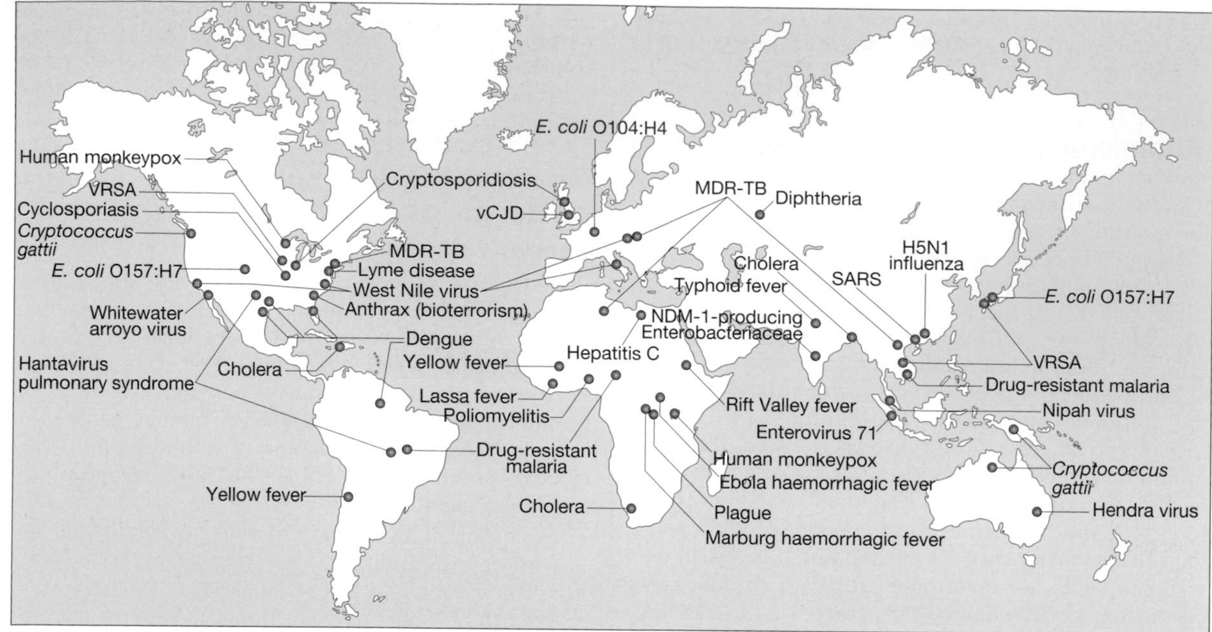

Fig. 6.10 Geographic locations of some infectious disease outbreaks, with examples of emerging and re-emerging diseases. (MDR-TB = multidrug-resistant tuberculosis; SARS = severe acute respiratory syndrome; vCJD = variant Creutzfeldt–Jakob disease; VRSA = vancomycin-resistant *Staph. aureus*) Adapted from Samaranayake 2006 – see p. 164.

Animal reservoirs

The World Health Organization (WHO) defines a zoonosis as 'a disease or infection that is naturally transmissible from vertebrate animals to humans'. The infected animal may be asymptomatic. Zoonotic agents may be transmitted via any of the routes described below. Primary infection with zoonoses may be transmitted onward between humans, causing secondary disease (e.g. Q fever, brucellosis, Ebola).

Environmental reservoirs

Many infective pathogens are acquired from an environmental source. However, some of these are maintained in human or animal reservoirs, with the environment acting only as a conduit for infection.

Transmission of infection

Infectious agents may be transmitted by one or more of the following routes:

- *Respiratory route*: inhalation.
- *Faecal–oral route*: ingestion of infectious material originating from faecal matter.
- *Sexually transmitted infections*: direct contact between mucous membranes.
- *Blood-borne infections*: direct inoculation of infected blood or body fluids.
- *Direct contact*: very few organisms are capable of causing infection by direct contact with intact skin. Most infection by this route requires inoculation or contact with damaged skin.
- *Via a vector or fomite*: the vector/fomite bridges the gap between the infected host or reservoir and the uninfected host. Vectors are animate, and include mosquitoes in malaria and dengue, fleas in plague and humans in MRSA. Fomites are inanimate, and include items such as door handles, water taps, ultrasound probes and so on, which are particularly associated with health care-associated infection.

6.6 Periods of infectivity in childhood infectious diseases[1]

Disease	Infectious period
Chickenpox	From 4 days before[2] until 5 days after appearance of the rash[3]
Measles	From 1–2 days before onset of rash; duration unknown[3]
Mumps	Unknown[4]
Rubella	Unknown, but most infectious during prodromal illness[3]
Scarlet fever	Unknown[5]
Whooping cough	Unknown[5,6]

[1]From Richardson M, Elliman D, Maguire H, et al. Pediatr Infect Dis J 2001; 20:380–388. These recommendations may differ from local or national guidance. [2]Transmission before 48 hrs prior to the onset of rash is rare. [3,4,5]Exclude from contact with non-immune and immunocompromised people for 5 days from [3]onset of rash, [4]onset of parotitis or [5]start of antibiotic treatment. [6]Exclude for 3 weeks if untreated.

The likelihood of infection following transmission of an infectious agent depends on organism factors and host susceptibility. The number of organisms required to cause infection or death in 50% of the exposed population is referred to as the ID_{50} (infectious dose) and LD_{50} (lethal dose), respectively. The incubation period is the time between exposure and development of disease, and the period of infectivity is the period after exposure during which the patient is infectious to others. Knowledge of incubation periods and periods of infectivity is important in controlling the spread of disease, although for many diseases these estimates are imprecise (Boxes 6.6 and 6.7).

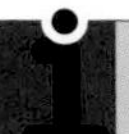

6.7 Incubation periods of important infections[1]

Infection	Incubation period
Short incubation periods	
Anthrax, cutaneous[3]	9 hrs to 2 wks
Anthrax, inhalational[3]	2 days[2]
Bacillary dysentery[5]	1–6 days
Cholera[3]	2 hrs to 5 days
Dengue haemorrhagic fever[6]	3–14 days
Diphtheria[6]	1–10 days
Gonorrhoea[4]	2–10 days
Influenza[5]	1–3 days
Meningococcaemia[3]	2–10 days
Norovirus[1]	1–3 days
SARS coronavirus[3]	2–7 days[2]
Scarlet fever[5]	2–4 days
Intermediate incubation periods	
Amoebiasis[6]	1–4 wks
Brucellosis[4]	5–30 days
Chickenpox[5]	11–20 days
Lassa fever[3]	3–21 days
Malaria[3]	10–15 days
Measles[5]	6–19 days
Mumps[5]	15–24 days
Poliomyelitis[6]	3–35 days
Psittacosis[4]	1–4 wks
Rubella[5]	15–20 days
Typhoid[5]	5–31 days
Whooping cough[5]	5–21 days
Long incubation periods	
Hepatitis A[5]	3–7 wks
Hepatitis B[4]	6 wks to 6 mths
Leishmaniasis, cutaneous[6]	Weeks to months
Leishmaniasis, visceral[6]	Months to years
Leprosy[3]	5–20 yrs
Rabies[4]	2–8 wks[2]
Trypanosoma brucei gambiense infection[6]	Months to years
Tuberculosis[5]	1–12 mths

[1]Incubation periods are approximate and may differ from local or national guidance. [2]Longer incubation periods have been reported.

Reference sources:
[3]WHO. [4]Health Protection Agency (now Health Protection England). [5]Richardson M, Elliman D, Maguire H, et al. Pediatr Infect Dis J 2001; 20:380–388. [6]Centers for Disease Control, USA.

Deliberate release

The deliberate release of infectious agents with the intention of causing disease is known as biological warfare or bioterrorism, depending on the scale and context. Deliberate release incidents have included a 750-person outbreak of *Salmonella typhimurium* by contamination of salads in 1984 (Oregon, USA) and 22 cases of anthrax (five fatal) from the mailing of finely powdered (weaponised) anthrax spores in 2001 (New Jersey, USA). Diseases with high potential for deliberate release include anthrax, plague, tularaemia, smallpox and botulism (through toxin release).

INFECTION PREVENTION AND CONTROL

Infection prevention and control (IPC) describes the measures applied to populations with the aim of breaking the chain of infection (see Fig. 6.1, p. 134).

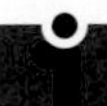

6.8 Measures used in infection prevention and control (IPC)

Institutional

- Handling, storage and disposal of clinical waste
- Containment and safe removal of spilled blood and body fluids
- Cleanliness of environment and medical equipment
- Specialised ventilation (e.g. laminar flow, air filtration, controlled pressure gradients)
- Sterilisation and disinfection of instruments and equipment
- Food hygiene
- Laundry management

Health-care staff

- Education
- Hand hygiene, including hand-washing (see Fig. 6.12)
- Sharps management and disposal
- Use of personal protective equipment (masks, sterile and non-sterile gloves, gowns and aprons)
- Screening health workers for disease (e.g. tuberculosis, hepatitis B virus, MRSA)
- Immunisation and post-exposure prophylaxis

Clinical practice

- Antibiotic stewardship (use only when necessary; avoid drugs known to select multi-resistant organisms or predispose to other infections)
- Aseptic technique (see Box 6.10)
- Perioperative antimicrobial prophylaxis
- Screening patients for colonisation or infection (e.g. MRSA, GRE, CPE)

Response to infections

- Surveillance to detect alert organism (see text) outbreaks and antimicrobial resistance
- Antibiotic chemoprophylaxis to infectious disease contacts, if indicated (see Box 6.19)
- Isolation (see Box 6.9)
- Reservoir control
- Vector control

(CPE = carbapenemase-producing Enterobacteriaceae; GRE = glycopeptide-resistant enterococci; MRSA = meticillin-resistant *Staphyloccus aureus*)

Health care-acquired infection

Admission to a health-care facility in the developed world carries a considerable risk of acquiring infection, estimated by the UK Department of Health as 6–10%. Factors that contribute to health care-acquired infection (HCAI, or nosocomial infection) are shown in Figure 6.11. Many nosocomial bacterial infections are caused by organisms that are resistant to numerous antibiotics (multi-resistant bacteria), including meticillin-resistant *Staph. aureus* (MRSA) (p. 330), extended-spectrum β-lactamase (ESBL)-producing Enterobacteriaceae, glycopeptide-resistant enterococci (GRE) and carbapenemase-producing Enterobacteriaceae (CPE). Other infections of particular concern in hospitals include *C. difficile* (p. 342) and norovirus (p. 327).

IPC measures are described in Box 6.8. The most important infection prevention practice is maintenance of good hand hygiene (Fig. 6.12). Hand decontamination or washing is *mandatory* before and after every patient contact. In most cases, decontamination with alcohol gel

Risk factor	*Acinetobacter* spp.	*Clostridium difficile*	Coagulase-negative staphylococci	Enterococci	Enterobacteriaceae	Environmental Gram-negative bacilli	*Legionella pneumophila*	*Pseudomonas* spp.	*Staph. aureus*	*Strep. pyogenes*	*Stenotrophomonas maltophilia*	Blood-borne infections	Norovirus and other enteric viruses	Respiratory viruses (RSV, rhinovirus, etc.)	Varicella zoster virus	*Aspergillus* spp.	*Candida* spp.
	Bacteria											Viruses				Other	
Antibiotic use, especially broad-spectrum	⬤	•		⬤	⬤			⬤	⬤								•
Contact with health-care staff		•			⬤				⬤	•		•	•	•	•		
Contact with other patients		•			⬤				⬤	•			•	•	•		
Contaminated water supply						•	•	⬤									
Device insertion (prosthetic material, cannulae, shunts, etc.)	⬤		•	⬤	⬤			⬤	⬤		⬤						•
Inadequate cleaning of potential fomites (furniture, shared facilities, medical equipment, etc.)	⬤	•		⬤	⬤	•		⬤	⬤				•				
Receipt of blood products												•					
Surgical procedures					⬤			⬤	⬤	•							
Urinary catheter insertion				⬤	⬤			⬤	⬤								
Building work and dust																•	

• Likely infecting organisms

⬤ Possibility of multi-resistant organisms, e.g. MRSA, GRE, ESBL- or carbapenemase-producing Enterobacteriaceae

Fig. 6.11 Commonly encountered health care-associated infections (HCAI) and the factors that predispose to them. (ESBL = extended spectrum β-lactamases; GRE = glycopeptide-resistant enterococci; MRSA = multidrug-resistant *Staph. aureus*; RSV = respiratory syncytial virus)

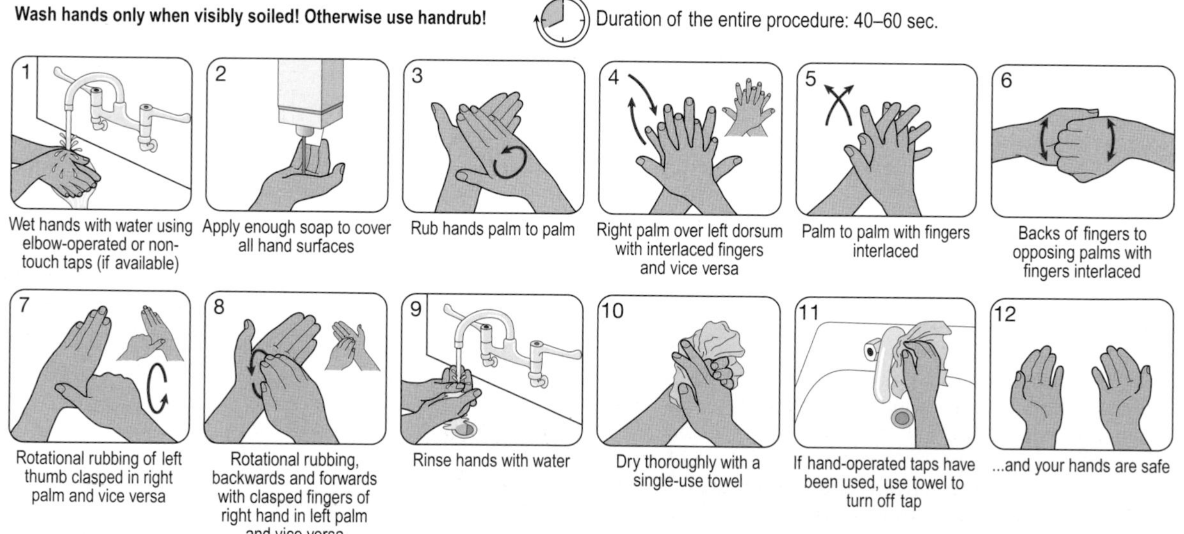

Fig. 6.12 Hand-washing. Good hand hygiene, whether with soap/water or alcohol handrub, includes areas that are often missed, such as fingertips, web spaces, palmar creases and the backs of hands. Adapted from WHO guidance at www.who.int – see p. 164.

is adequate. However, hand-washing (with hot water, liquid soap and complete drying) is required after any procedure that involves more than casual physical contact, or if hands are visibly soiled. In situations where the prevalence of *C. difficile* is high (e.g. a local outbreak), alcohol gel decontamination between patient contacts is inadequate, as it does not kill *C. difficile* spores, and hands must be washed with soap and water.

Some infections necessitate additional measures to prevent cross-infection (Box 6.9). To avoid infection, all

6.9 Types of isolation precaution[1]

Airborne transmission	Contact transmission	Droplet transmission
Precautions		
Negative pressure room with air exhausted externally or filtered N95 masks or personal respirators for staff; avoid using non-immune staff	Private room preferred (otherwise, inter-patient spacing ≥ 1 m) Gloves and gown for staff in contact with patient or contaminated areas	Private room preferred (otherwise, inter-patient spacing ≥ 1 m) Surgical masks for staff in close contact with patient
Infections managed with these precautions		
Measles Tuberculosis, pulmonary or laryngeal, confirmed or suspected	Enteroviral infections in young children (diapered or incontinent) Norovirus[2] *C. difficile* infection Multidrug-resistant organisms (e.g. MRSA, ESBL, GRE, VRSA, penicillin-resistant *Strep. pneumoniae*)[3] Parainfluenza in infants and young children Rotavirus RSV in infants, children and immunocompromised Viral conjunctivitis, acute	Diphtheria, pharyngeal *Haemophilus influenzae* type B infection Herpes simplex virus, disseminated or severe Influenza Meningococcal infection Mumps *Mycoplasma pneumoniae* Parvovirus (erythrovirus) B19 (erythema infectiosum, fifth disease) Pertussis Plague, pneumonic/bubonic Rubella *Strep. pyogenes* (group A), pharyngeal
Infections managed with multiple precautions		
← Smallpox, monkeypox, VZV, (chickenpox or disseminated disease)[4] →		
	← Adenovirus pneumonia	→
←	SARS, viral haemorrhagic fever[2]	→

[1]Recommendations based on 2007 CDC guideline for isolation precautions. May differ from local or national recommendations. [2]Not a CDC recommendation. [3]Subject to local risk assessment. [4]Or in any immunocompromised patient until possibility of disseminated infection excluded.
(ESBL = extended-spectrum β-lactamase; GRE = glycopeptide-resistant enterococci; MRSA = meticillin-resistant *Staph. aureus*; RSV = respiratory syncytial virus; SARS = severe acute respiratory syndrome; VRSA = vancomycin-resistant *Staph. aureus*; VZV = varicella zoster virus)

EBM 6.10 Skin antisepsis prior to insertion of central venous catheters

'Skin preparation with chlorhexidine in 70% isopropyl alcohol is more effective than povidone-iodine or aqueous antiseptic solutions in preventing catheter infections.'

- Pratt RJ, et al. J Hosp Infect 2007; 65S:S1–S64.

invasive procedures must be performed with strict aseptic technique (Box 6.10).

Outbreaks of infection

Descriptive terms are defined in Box 6.11. Confirmation of an infectious disease outbreak usually requires evidence from typing (p. 138) that the causal organisms have identical genotypic characteristics. If this is found not to be the case, the term pseudo-outbreak is used. When an outbreak of infection is suspected, a case definition is agreed. The number of cases that meet the case definition is then assessed by case-finding, using methods ranging from administration of questionnaires to national reporting systems. Case-finding usually includes microbiological testing, at least in the early stages of an outbreak. Temporal changes in cases are noted in order to plot an outbreak curve, and demographic details are collected to identify possible sources of infection. A case control study, in which recent activities (potential exposures) of affected 'cases' are compared to those of unaffected 'controls', may be undertaken to establish the outbreak source, and measures are taken to manage the outbreak and control its spread. Good communication between relevant personnel during and after the outbreak is important to inform practice in future outbreaks.

Surveillance ensures that disease outbreaks are either pre-empted or identified early. In hospitals, staff are made aware of the isolation of alert organisms, which have the propensity to cause outbreaks, and alert conditions, which are likely to be caused by such organisms. Analogous systems are used nationally; many countries publish lists of organisms and diseases, which, if detected (or suspected), must be reported to public health authorities (reportable or notifiable diseases). Reasons for a disease to be classified as reportable are shown in Box 6.12.

Principles of food hygiene

'Food poisoning' (p. 306) is largely preventable by food hygiene measures. The main principles are:

- segregation of uncooked food (which may be contaminated with pathogenic microorganisms) from cooked food
- avoidance of conditions which allow growth of pathogenic bacteria before or after cooking
- adequate bacterial killing during cooking.

Safe storage depends on the temperatures at which food bacteria are inhibited and destroyed (Fig. 6.13).

6.11 Terminology in outbreaks of infection

Term	Definition
Classification of related cases of infectious disease*	
Cluster	An aggregation of cases of a disease which are closely grouped in time and place, and may or may not exceed the expected number
Epidemic	The occurrence of more cases of disease than expected in a given area or among a specific group of people over a particular period of time
Outbreak	Synonymous with epidemic. Alternatively, a localised, as opposed to generalised, epidemic
Pandemic	An epidemic occurring over a very wide area (several countries or continents) and usually affecting a large proportion of the population
Classification of affected patients (cases)	
Index case	The first case identified in an outbreak
Primary cases	Cases acquired from a specific source of infection
Secondary cases	Cases acquired from primary cases
Types of outbreak	
Common source outbreak	Exposure to a common source of infection (e.g. water-cooling tower, medical staff member shedding MRSA). New primary cases will arise until the source is no longer present
Point source outbreak	Exposure to a single source of infection at a specific point in time (e.g. contaminated food at a party). Primary cases will develop disease synchronously
Person-to-person spread	Outbreak with both primary and secondary cases. May complicate point source or common source outbreak

*Adapted from www.cdc.gov.

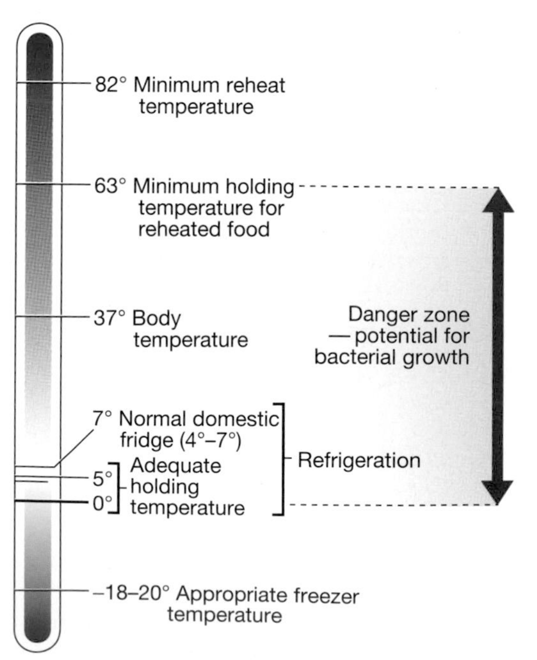

Fig. 6.13 Important temperatures (°C) in food hygiene.

6.12 Reasons for including an infectious disease on a regional/national list of reportable diseases*

Reason for inclusion	Common examples
Endemic/local disease with the potential to spread and/or cause outbreaks	Influenza, *Salmonella*, tuberculosis
Imported disease with the propensity to spread and/or cause outbreaks	Typhoid, cholera (depending on local epidemiology)
Evidence of a possible breakdown in health protection/public health functions	*Legionella*, *Cryptosporidium*
Evidence of a possible breakdown in food safety practices	Botulism, verotoxigenic *E. coli*
Evidence of a possible failure of a vaccination programme	Measles, poliomyelitis, pertussis
Disease with the potential to be a novel or increasing threat to human health	SARS, multi-resistant bacteria
Evidence of expansion of the range of a reservoir/vector	Lyme disease, rabies, West Nile encephalitis
Evidence of possible deliberate release	Anthrax, tularaemia, plague, smallpox, botulism

*Given the different geographic ranges of individual diseases, and wide national variations in public health services, vaccination programmes and availability of resources, reporting regulations vary between regions, states and countries. Many diseases are reportable for more than one reason.

Immunisation

Immunisation may be passive or active. Passive immunisation is achieved by administering antibodies targeted against a specific pathogen. Antibodies are obtained from blood, so confer some of the risks associated with blood products (p. 1012). The protection afforded by passive immunisation is immediate but of short duration (a few weeks or months); it is used to prevent or attenuate infection before or after exposure (Box 6.13).

Vaccination

Active immunisation is achieved by vaccination with whole organisms or organism components (Box 6.14).

Types of vaccine

Whole cell vaccines consist of live or inactivated (killed) microorganisms; component vaccines contain only extracted or synthesised components of microorganisms (e.g. polysaccharides or proteins). Live vaccines contain organisms with attenuated (reduced) virulence, which induce T-lymphocyte and humoral responses (p. 77) and are therefore more immunogenic than inactivated whole cell vaccines. The use of live vaccines in immunocompromised individuals requires careful consideration.

Component vaccines consisting only of polysaccharides, such as the pneumococcal polysaccharide vaccine (PPV), are poor activators of T-lymphocytes, and produce a short-lived antibody response without long-lasting memory. Conjugation of polysaccharide to

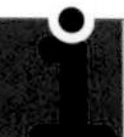

6.13 Indications for post-exposure prophylaxis with immunoglobulins

Human normal immunoglobulin (pooled immunoglobulin)

- Hepatitis A (unvaccinated contacts*)
- Measles (if exposed child has heart or lung disease)

Human specific immunoglobulin

- Hepatitis B (sexual partners, inoculation injuries, infants born to infected mothers)
- Tetanus (high-risk wounds or when immunisation status is incomplete or unknown)
- Rabies
- Chickenpox (immunosuppressed children and adults, pregnant women)

*Active immunisation is preferred if contact is with a patient who is within 1 wk of onset of jaundice.

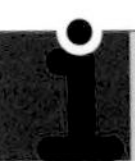

6.14 Vaccines in current clinical use

Live attenuated vaccines

- Measles, mumps, rubella (MMR)
- Oral poliomyelitis (OPV, not used in UK)
- Tuberculosis (bacille Calmette–Guérin, BCG)
- Typhoid (oral typhoid vaccine)
- Varicella zoster virus
- Rotavirus

Inactivated (killed) whole-cell vaccines

- Cholera
- Hepatitis A
- Influenza
- Poliomyelitis (inactivated polio virus, IPV)
- Rabies

Component vaccines

- Anthrax (adsorbed extracted antigens)
- Diphtheria (adsorbed toxoid)
- Hepatitis B (adsorbed recombinant HBsAg)
- *Haemophilus influenzae* type B (conjugated capsular polysaccharide)
- Human papillomavirus (recombinant capsid proteins)
- Meningococcal, quadrivalent A, C, Y, W135 (conjugated capsular polysaccharide)
- Meningococcal, serogroup C (conjugated capsular polysaccharide)
- Pertussis (adsorbed extracted antigens)
- Pneumococcal conjugate (PCV; conjugated capsular polysaccharide, 13 serotypes)
- Pneumococcal polysaccharide (PPV; purified capsular polysaccharide, 23 serotypes)
- Tetanus (adsorbed toxoid)
- Typhoid (purified Vi capsular polysaccharide)

a protein, as in the *Haemophilus influenzae* type B (Hib) vaccine, activates T lymphocytes, which results in a sustained response and immunological memory. Toxoids are bacterial toxins that have been modified to reduce toxicity but maintain antigenicity. Vaccine response can be improved by co-administration with mildly pro-inflammatory adjuvants, such as aluminium hydroxide.

Use of vaccines

Vaccination may be applied to entire populations or to subpopulations at specific risk through travel, occupation or other activities. In ring vaccination, the population immediately surrounding a case or outbreak of infectious disease is vaccinated to curtail further spread. Vaccination is aimed mainly at preventing infectious disease. However, vaccination against human papillomavirus (HPV) was introduced to prevent cervical and other cancers which complicate HPV infection. Vaccination guidelines for individuals are shown in Box 6.15.

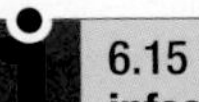

6.15 Guidelines for vaccination against infectious disease

- The principal contraindication to inactivated vaccines is an anaphylactic reaction to a previous dose or a component of the vaccine
- Live vaccines should not be given in the presence of an acute infection, to pregnant women or to the immunosuppressed, unless the immunosuppression is mild and the benefits outweigh the risks
- If two live vaccines are required, they should be given either simultaneously in opposite arms or 4 wks apart
- Live vaccines should not be given for 3 mths after an injection of human normal immunoglobulin (HNI)
- HNI should not be given for 2 wks after a live vaccine
- Hay fever, asthma, eczema, sickle-cell disease, topical corticosteroid therapy, antibiotic therapy, prematurity and chronic heart and lung diseases, including tuberculosis, are not contraindications to vaccination

Vaccination becomes successful once the number of susceptible hosts in a population falls below the level required to sustain continued transmission of the target organism (herd immunity). Naturally acquired smallpox was declared to have been eradicated worldwide in 1980 through mass vaccination. In 1988, the WHO resolved to eradicate poliomyelitis by vaccination; the number of cases worldwide has since fallen from approximately 350 000 per annum to 223 in 2012. Recommended vaccination schedules vary between countries. In addition to standard vaccination schedules, catch-up schedules are specified for individuals who join vaccination programmes later than the recommended age.

TREATMENT OF INFECTIOUS DISEASES

The key components of treating infectious disease are:

- addressing predisposing factors, e.g. diabetes mellitus or known immune deficit (HIV, neutropenia)
- antimicrobial therapy
- adjuvant therapy, e.g. removal of an indwelling catheter (urinary or vascular), abscess drainage or débridement of an area of necrotising fasciitis
- treatment of the consequences of infection, e.g. the systemic inflammatory response syndrome (SIRS; p. 184), inflammation and pain.

For communicable disease, treatment must also take into account contacts of the infected patient, and may include infection prevention and control activities such as isolation, antimicrobial prophylaxis, vaccination and contact tracing.

Principles of antimicrobial therapy

When infection is diagnosed, it is important to start appropriate antimicrobial therapy promptly. The principles underlying the choice of antimicrobial agent(s) are

Clinical diagnosis
Information available:
• Organ system involved
• Endogenous or exogenous infection
• Likely pathogens
Laboratory investigations: microbiological diagnosis
• Infecting organism(s)
• Likely antimicrobial susceptibility
Antimicrobial susceptibility results
• Antimicrobial susceptibility of infecting organism(s)
Level of knowledge of infecting organism(s)
Antimicrobial spectrum of agent(s) used
1 Empiric therapy
Based on:
• Predicted susceptibility of likely pathogens
• Local antimicrobial policies
2 Targeted therapy
Based on:
• Predicted susceptibility of infecting organism(s)
• Local antimicrobial policies
3 Susceptibility-guided therapy
Based on:
• Susceptibility testing results

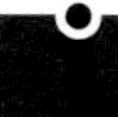

Fig. 6.14 Stages in the selection and refinement of antimicrobial therapy: 'Start Smart – Then Focus'.

discussed below. The process of selecting appropriate antimicrobial therapy has been summarised in UK guidance as 'Start Smart - Then Focus' (Fig. 6.14).

Antimicrobial action and spectrum

Antimicrobial agents kill microorganisms by inhibiting, damaging or destroying a target that is a required component of the organism. The range, or spectrum, of microorganisms that is killed by a particular antimicrobial agent must be considered in selecting therapy. The mechanisms of action of the major classes of antibacterial agent are listed in Box 6.16 and appropriate antibiotic choices for a range of common infecting organisms are shown in Box 6.17. In severe infections and/or immunocompromised patients, it is customary to use bactericidal agents in preference to bacteriostatic agents.

Empiric versus targeted therapy

Empiric antimicrobial therapy is selected to treat a clinical syndrome (e.g. meningitis) before a microbiological diagnosis has been made. Targeted therapy is aimed at the causal pathogen(s) of known antimicrobial sensitivity. 'Start Smart - Then Focus' describes the principle of using appropriate broad-spectrum agents in empiric therapy, followed by narrow-spectrum agents in targeted therapy. Optimum empiric therapy depends on the site of infection, patient characteristics and local antimicrobial resistance patterns. Hospital antibiotic policies are used to guide rational antimicrobial prescribing, maximising efficacy while minimising antimicrobial resistance and cost.

Combination therapy

It is sometimes appropriate to use antimicrobial agents in combination:

- to increase efficacy (e.g. enterococcal endocarditis, where a β-lactam/aminoglycoside combination

6.16 Target and mechanism of action of common antibacterial agents

Aminoglycosides, chloramphenicol, macrolides, lincosamides and streptogramins, oxazolidinones (linezolid)
• Inhibition of bacterial protein synthesis by binding to subunits of bacterial ribosomes
Tetracyclines
• Inhibition of protein synthesis by preventing transfer RNA binding to ribosomes
Beta-lactams
• Inhibition of cell wall peptidoglycan synthesis by competitive inhibition of transpeptidases ('penicillin-binding proteins')
Cyclic lipopeptide (daptomycin)
• Insertion of lipophilic tail into plasma membrane causes depolarisation and cell death
Glycopeptides
• Inhibition of cell wall peptidoglycan synthesis by forming complexes with D-alanine residues on peptidoglycan precursors
Nitroimidazoles
• The reduced form of the drug causes strand breaks in DNA
Quinolones
• Inhibition of DNA replication by binding to DNA topoisomerases (DNA gyrase and topoisomerase IV), preventing supercoiling and uncoiling of DNA
Rifamycins
• Inhibition of DNA synthesis by inhibiting DNA-dependent RNA polymerase
Sulphonamides and trimethoprim
• Inhibition of folate synthesis by dihydropteroate synthase (sulphonamides) and dihydrofolate reductase (trimethoprim) inhibition

6.17 Antimicrobial options for common infecting bacteria

Organism	Antimicrobial options*
Gram-positive organisms	
Enterococcus faecalis	Ampicillin, vancomycin/teicoplanin
Enterococcus faecium	Vancomycin/teicoplanin, linezolid
Glycopeptide-resistant enterococci (GRE)	Linezolid, tigecycline, quinupristin–dalfopristin, daptomycin
MRSA	Clindamycin, vancomycin, rifampicin (never used as monotherapy), linezolid, daptomycin, tetracyclines, tigecycline, co-trimoxazole
Staph. aureus	Flucloxacillin, clindamycin
Strep. pyogenes	Penicillin, clindamycin, erythromycin
Strep. pneumoniae	Penicillin, macrolides, cephalosporins, levofloxacin, vancomycin
Gram-negative organisms	
E. coli, 'coliforms' (enteric Gram-negative bacilli)	Trimethoprim, cefuroxime, ciprofloxacin, co-amoxiclav
Enterobacter spp., *Citrobacter* spp.	Ciprofloxacin, meropenem, ertapenem, aminoglycosides
ESBL-producing Enterobacteriaceae	Ciprofloxacin, meropenem, ertapenem (if sensitive), piperacillin–tazobactam, aminoglycosides, tigecycline
Carbapenemase-producing Enterobacteriaceae	Ciprofloxacin, aminoglycosides, tigecycline, colistin
Haemophilus influenzae	Amoxicillin, co-amoxiclav, macrolides, cefuroxime, cefotaxime, ciprofloxacin
Legionella pneumophila	Azithromycin, levofloxacin, doxycycline
Neisseria gonorrhoeae	Ceftriaxone/cefixime, spectinomycin
Neisseria meningitidis	Penicillin, cefotaxime/ceftriaxone, chloramphenicol
Pseudomonas aeruginosa	Ciprofloxacin, piperacillin–tazobactam, aztreonam, meropenem, aminoglycosides, ceftazidime/cefepime
Salmonella typhi	Ceftriaxone, azithromycin (uncomplicated typhoid), chloramphenicol (resistance common)
Strict anaerobes	
Bacteroides spp.	Metronidazole, clindamycin, co-amoxiclav, piperacillin–tazobactam, meropenem
Clostridium difficile	Metronidazole, vancomycin (oral), fidaxomicin
Clostridium spp.	Penicillin, metronidazole, clindamycin
Fusobacterium spp.	Penicillin, metronidazole, clindamycin
Other organisms	
Chlamydia trachomatis	Azithromycin, doxycycline
Treponema pallidum	Penicillin, doxycycline

*Antibiotic selection depends on multiple factors, including local susceptibility patterns, which vary enormously between geographic areas. There are many appropriate alternatives to those listed.

results in better outcomes than a β-lactam alone)

- when no single agent's spectrum covers all potential pathogens (e.g. in polymicrobial infection or empiric treatment of sepsis)
- to reduce antimicrobial resistance, as the organism would need to develop resistance to multiple agents simultaneously (e.g. antituberculous chemotherapy (p. 693), antiretroviral therapy (ART, p. 407)).

Antimicrobial resistance

Microorganisms have evolved in the presence of naturally occurring antibiotics, and have therefore developed resistance mechanisms (categorised in Fig. 6.15) to all classes of antimicrobial agent (antibiotics and their derivatives). Intrinsic resistance is an innate property of a microorganism, whereas acquired resistance arises by spontaneous mutation or horizontal transfer of genetic material from another organism in a phage or plasmid. Plasmids often encode resistance to multiple antibiotics. For some agents, e.g. penicillins, a degree of resistance occurs in vivo when the bacterial load is high and the molecular target for the antimicrobial is down-regulated (an 'inoculum effect').

The *mecA* gene encodes a low-affinity penicillin-binding protein, which confers resistance to β-lactam antibiotics in staphylococci. Extended spectrum β-lactamases (ESBL) are encoded on plasmids which are transferred relatively easily between bacteria, including Enterobacteriaceae. Plasmid-encoded carbapenemases have been detected in strains of *Klebsiella pneumoniae* (e.g. New Delhi metallo-β-lactamase 1, NDM-1). Strains of MRSA have been described that exhibit intermediate resistance to glycopeptides (GISA) through the development of a relatively impermeable cell wall.

Factors promoting antimicrobial resistance include the inappropriate use of antibiotics (e.g. in viral infections), inadequate dosage or treatment duration, and use

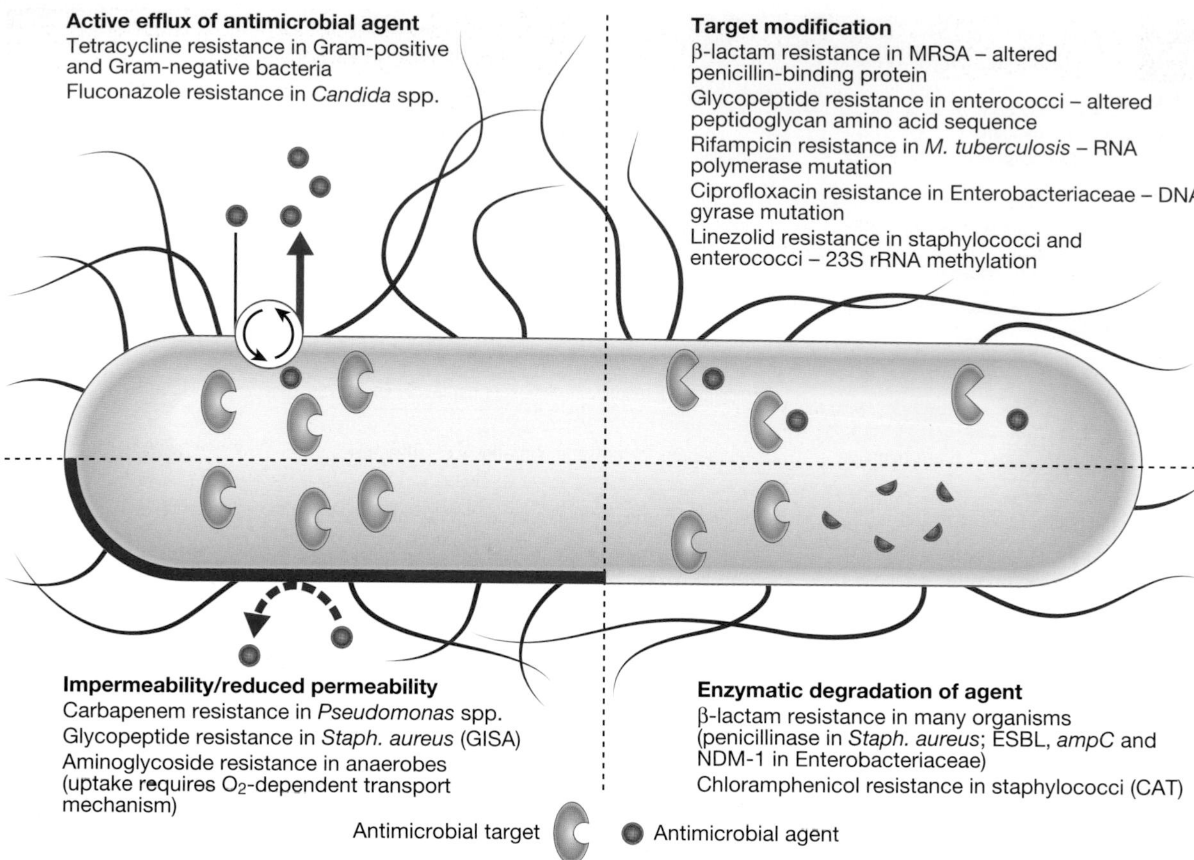

Fig. 6.15 Examples of mechanisms of antimicrobial resistance. (CAT = chloramphenicol acetyltransferase; ESBL = extended spectrum β-lactamases; GISA = glycopeptide-intermediate *Staph. aureus*; MRSA = meticillin-resistant *Staph. aureus*; NDM-1 = New Delhi metallo-β-lactamase 1).

of antimicrobials as growth-promoters in agriculture. However, *any* antimicrobial use exerts a selection pressure that favours the development of resistance. Combination antimicrobial therapy may reduce the emergence of resistance. This is recommended in treatment of patients infected with HIV, which is highly prone to spontaneous mutation (p. 407). Despite use of combination therapy for *M. tuberculosis*, multidrug-resistant tuberculosis (MDR-TB, resistant to isoniazid and rifampicin) and extremely drug-resistant tuberculosis (XDR-TB, resistant to isoniazid and rifampicin, any fluoroquinolone and at least one injectable antimicrobial antituberculous agent) have been reported worldwide and are increasing in incidence (p. 693).

The term post-antibiotic era has been coined to describe a future in which the acquisition of resistance by bacteria will have been so extensive that antibiotic therapy is rendered useless. A more realistic scenario, which is currently being experienced, is a gradual but inexorable progression of resistance, necessitating the use of ever more toxic and expensive antimicrobials.

Duration of therapy

Treatment duration reflects the severity of infection and accessibility of the infected site to antimicrobial agents. For most infections, there is limited evidence available to support a specific duration of treatment (Box 6.18). Depending on the indication, initial intravenous therapy may be switched to oral after fever has settled for approximately 48 hours. In the absence of specific guidance, antimicrobial therapy should be stopped when there is no longer any clinical evidence of infection.

Antimicrobial prophylaxis

Primary prophylaxis is used when there is a risk of infection from a procedure or exposure (Box 6.19). It should be of short duration with minimal adverse effects, and may be combined with passive immunisation (see Box 6.13). Secondary prophylaxis is used in patients who have been treated successfully for an infection but remain predisposed to it. It is used in haemato-oncology patients in the context of fungal infection and in HIV-positive individuals with an opportunistic infection who do not respond to antiretroviral therapy.

Pharmacokinetics and pharmacodynamics

Pharmacokinetics of antimicrobial agents determine whether adequate concentrations are obtained at the sites of infection. Septic patients often have poor gastrointestinal absorption, so the preferred initial route of therapy is intravenous. Knowledge of anticipated antimicrobial drug concentrations at sites of infection is critical. For example, achieving a 'therapeutic' blood level of gentamicin is of little practical use in treating meningitis, as CSF penetration of the drug is poor. Knowledge of routes of antimicrobial elimination is also critical; for instance, urinary tract infection is ideally treated with a drug that is excreted unchanged in the urine.

Pharmacodynamics describes the relationship between antimicrobial concentration and microbial

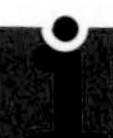

6.18 Duration of antimicrobial therapy for some common infections*

Infection	Duration of therapy
Viral infections	
Herpes simplex encephalitis	2–3 wks
Bacterial infections	
Gonorrhoea	Single dose
Infective endocarditis (streptococcal, native valve)	4 wks ± gentamicin for first 2 wks
Infective endocarditis (prosthetic valve)	≥ 6 wks
Osteomyelitis	4–6 wks
Pneumonia (community-acquired, severe)	10 days (no organism identified), 14–21 days (*Staph. aureus* or *Legionella* spp.)
Septic arthritis	2–4 wks
Urinary tract infection (male)	2 wks
Urinary tract infection, upper (female)	7 days
Urinary tract infection, lower (female)	3 days
Mycobacterial infections	
Tuberculosis (meningeal)	12 mths
Tuberculosis (pulmonary)	6 mths
Fungal infections	
Invasive pulmonary aspergillosis	Until clinical/radiological resolution and reversal of predisposition
Candidaemia (acute disseminated)	2 wks after last positive blood culture and resolution of signs and symptoms

*All recommendations are indicative. Actual duration takes into account predisposing factors, specific organisms and antimicrobial susceptibility, adjuvant therapies, current guidelines and clinical response.

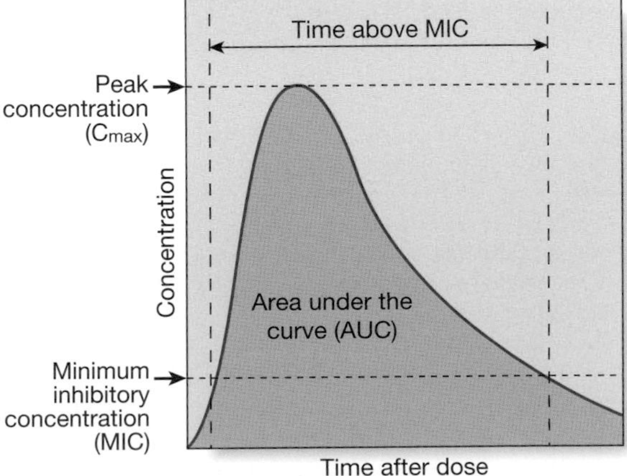

Fig. 6.16 Antimicrobial pharmacodynamics. The curve represents drug concentrations after a single dose of an antimicrobial agent. Factors that determine microbial killing are C_{max} : MIC ratio (concentration-dependent killing), time above MIC (time-dependent killing) and AUC : MIC ratio.

6.19 Recommendations for antimicrobial prophylaxis in adults*

Infection risk	Recommended antimicrobial
Bacterial	
Diphtheria (prevention of secondary cases)	Erythromycin
Gas gangrene (after high amputation or major trauma)	Penicillin or metronidazole
Lower gastrointestinal tract surgery	Cefuroxime + metronidazole, gentamicin + metronidazole, or co-amoxiclav (single dose only)
Meningococcal disease (prevention of secondary cases)	Rifampicin or ciprofloxacin
Rheumatic fever (prevention of recurrence)	Phenoxymethylpenicillin or sulfadiazine
Tuberculosis (prevention of secondary cases)	Isoniazid ± rifampicin
Whooping cough (prevention of secondary cases)	Erythromycin
Viral	
HIV, occupational exposure (sharps injury)	Combination tenofovir/ emtricitabine and lopinavir/ ritonavir. Modified if index case's virus known to be resistant
Influenza A (prevention of secondary cases in adults with chronic respiratory, cardiovascular or renal disease, immunosuppression or diabetes mellitus)	Oseltamivir
Fungal	
Aspergillosis (in high-risk haematology patients)	Itraconazole, voriconazole or posaconazole
Pneumocystis pneumonia (prevention in HIV and other immunosuppressed states)	Co-trimoxazole, pentamidine or dapsone
Protozoal	
Malaria (prevention of travel-associated disease)	Specific antimalarials depend on travel itinerary (p. 357)

*These are based on current UK practice. Recommendations may vary locally or nationally. Antimicrobial prophylaxis for infective endocarditis during dental procedures is not currently recommended in the UK.

killing. For many agents, antimicrobial effect can be categorised as concentration-dependent or time-dependent. The concentration of antimicrobial achieved after a single dose is illustrated in Figure 6.16. The maximum concentration achieved is C_{max} and the measure of overall exposure is the area under the curve (AUC). The efficacy of antimicrobial agents whose killing is concentration-dependent (e.g. aminoglycosides) increases with the amount by which C_{max} exceeds the minimum inhibitory concentration (C_{max}:MIC ratio). For this reason, it has become customary to administer aminoglycosides (e.g. gentamicin) infrequently at high doses (e.g. 7 mg/kg) rather than frequently at low doses. This has the added advantage of minimising toxicity by reducing the likelihood of drug accumulation. Conversely, the β-lactam antibiotics, macrolides and clindamycin exhibit time-dependent killing, and their efficacy depends on C_{max}

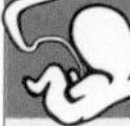

6.20 Antimicrobial agents in pregnancy[1]

Contraindicated

- Chloramphenicol: neonatal 'grey baby' syndrome – collapse, hypotension and cyanosis
- Fluconazole: teratogenic in high doses
- Quinolones: arthropathy in animal studies
- Sulphonamides: neonatal haemolysis and methaemoglobinaemia
- Tetracyclines, glycylcyclines: skeletal abnormalities in animals in 1st trimester; fetal dental discoloration and maternal hepatotoxicity with large parenteral doses in 2nd or 3rd trimesters
- Trimethoprim: teratogenic in 1st trimester

Relatively contraindicated

- Aminoglycosides: potential damage to fetal auditory and vestibular nerves in 2nd and 3rd trimesters
- Metronidazole: avoidance of high dosages is recommended[2]

Not known to be harmful; use only when necessary

- Aciclovir
- Cephalosporins
- Clarithromycin
- Clindamycin
- Erythromycin
- Glycopeptides
- Linezolid
- Meropenem
- Penicillins

[1]Data extracted from Joint Formulary Committee. British National Formulary (online). London: BMJ Group and Pharmaceutical Press; (www.medicinescomplete.com) [accessed on 16 March 2013].
[2]Theoretical risk of teratogenicity, not supported by available clinical evidence.

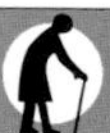

6.21 Problems with antimicrobial therapy in old age

- ***Clostridium difficile* infection**: all antibiotics predispose to some extent, but second- and third-generation cephalosporins and co-amoxiclav especially so.
- **Hypersensitivity reactions**: rise in incidence due to increased previous exposure.
- **Renal impairment**: may be significant in old age, despite 'normal' creatinine levels (p. 467).
- **Nephrotoxicity**: more likely, e.g. first-generation cephalosporins, aminoglycosides.
- **Accumulation of β-lactam antibiotics**: may result in myoclonus, seizures or coma.
- **Reduced gastric acid production**: gastric pH is higher, which causes increased penicillin absorption.
- **Reduced hepatic metabolism**: results in a higher risk of isoniazid-related hepatotoxicity.
- **Quinolones**: associated with confusion and may increase the risk of seizures.

exceeding the MIC for a certain time (which is different for each class of agent). This is reflected in the dosing interval of benzylpenicillin, which is usually given every 4 hours in severe infection (e.g. meningococcal meningitis), and may be administered by continuous infusion. For other antimicrobial agents, the pharmacodynamic relationships are more complex and often less well understood. With some agents, bacterial inhibition persists after antimicrobial exposure (post-antibiotic and post-antibiotic sub-MIC effects).

Therapeutic drug monitoring

Therapeutic drug monitoring is used to confirm that levels of antimicrobial agents with a low therapeutic index (e.g. aminoglycosides) are not excessive, and that levels of agents with marked pharmacokinetic variability (e.g. vancomycin) are adequate. Specific recommendations for monitoring depend on individual clinical circumstances; for instance, different pre- and post-dose levels of gentamicin are recommended, depending on whether it is being used in traditional divided doses, once daily or for synergy in endocarditis (p. 625).

Beta-lactam antibiotics

These antibiotics have a β-lactam ring structure (Fig. 6.17) and exert a bactericidal action by inhibiting enzymes involved in cell wall synthesis (penicillin-binding proteins, PBP). They are classified in Box 6.22.

Pharmacokinetics

- Good drug levels are achieved in lung, kidney, bone, muscle and liver, and in pleural, synovial, pericardial and peritoneal fluids.
- CSF levels are low, except in the presence of inflammation.
- Activity is not inhibited in abscess (e.g. by low pH and PO_2, high protein or neutrophils).
- Beta-lactams are subject to an 'inoculum effect' – activity is reduced in the presence of a high organism burden (PBP expression is down-regulated by high organism density).
- Generally safe in pregnancy (except imipenem/cilastatin).

Adverse effects

Generalised allergy to penicillin occurs in 0.7–10% of cases and anaphylaxis in 0.004–0.015%. A large proportion of patients with infectious mononucleosis develop a rash if given aminopenicillins; this does not imply lasting allergy. The relationship between allergy to penicillin and allergy to cephalosporins depends on the specific cephalosporin used. Although there is significant cross-reactivity with first-generation cephalosporins, cross-reactivity to second- and third-generation cephalosporins is less common. However, avoidance of cephalosporins is recommended in patients who have a type 1 penicillin allergy (p. 89). Cross-reactivity between penicillin and carbapenems is rare (approximately 1%

6.22 Beta-lactam antibiotics

Penicillins

- Natural penicillins: benzylpenicillin, phenoxymethylpenicillin
- Penicillinase-resistant penicillins: meticillin, flucloxacillin, nafcillin, oxacillin
- Aminopenicillins: ampicillin, amoxicillin
- Carboxy- and ureido-penicillins: ticarcillin, piperacillin

Cephalosporins

- See Box 6.23

Monobactams

- Aztreonam

Carbapenems

- Imipenem, meropenem, ertapenem, doripenem

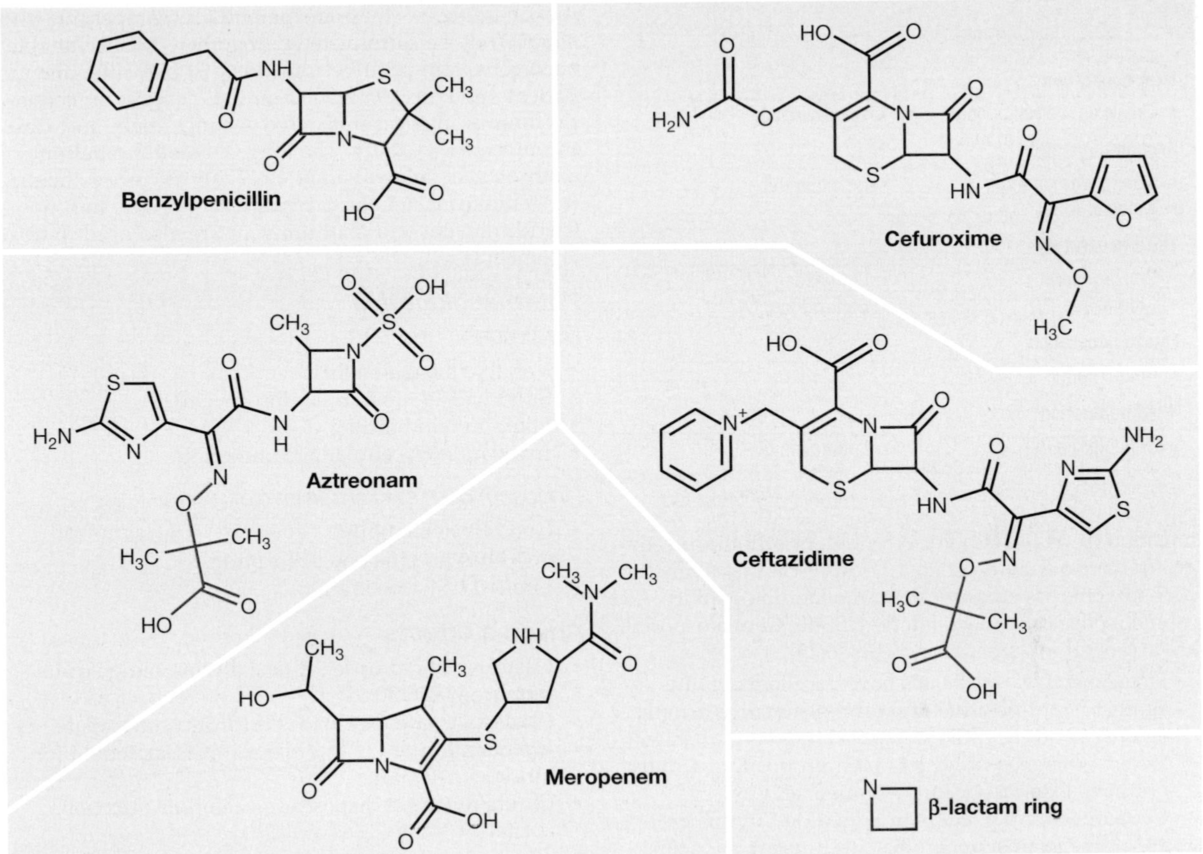

Benzylpenicillin

Cefuroxime

Aztreonam

Ceftazidime

Meropenem

β-lactam ring

Fig. 6.17 Beta-lactam antibiotics. With the exception of aztreonam (monobactam), the β-lactam antibiotics have bicyclic nuclei. This may explain the absence of cross-reaction to aztreonam in penicillin-allergic patients. However, aztreonam and ceftazidime have identical side-chains, so patients with a specific ceftazidime allergy should not be given aztreonam.

by skin-prick testing). Although avoidance of carbapenems is recommended in penicillin-allergic patients, these drugs may be administered if there are no suitable alternatives and appropriate resuscitation facilities are available.

Gastrointestinal upset and diarrhoea are common, and a mild reversible hepatitis is recognised with many β-lactams. Leucopenia, thrombocytopenia and coagulation deficiencies, and interstitial nephritis and potentiation of aminoglycoside-mediated renal damage are also recognised (p. 502). Seizures and encephalopathy have been reported, particularly with high doses in the presence of renal insufficiency. Thrombophlebitis occurs in up to 5% of patients receiving parenteral β-lactams.

Drug interactions

Synergism occurs in combination with aminoglycosides. Ampicillin decreases the biological effect of oral contraceptives and the whole class is significantly affected by concurrent administration of probenecid, producing a 2–4-fold increase in the peak serum concentration.

Penicillins

Natural penicillins are primarily effective against Gram-positive organisms (except staphylococci, most of which produce a penicillinase) and anaerobic organisms. *Strep. pyogenes* has remained sensitive to natural penicillins worldwide. According to the European Antimicrobial Resistance Surveillance Network (EARS-Net), the prevalence of high-level penicillin resistance in *Strep. pneumoniae* in Europe in 2010 was 2.7%. However, the prevalence in individual countries was as high as 33% (Cyprus).

Penicillinase-resistant penicillins are the mainstay of treatment for infections with *Staph. aureus*, other than meticillin-resistant strains (MRSA). However, EARS-Net data from 2010 indicate that almost 1:5 (18.5%) *Staph. aureus* isolates in Europe were MRSA.

Aminopenicillins have the same spectrum of activity as the natural penicillins, with additional Gram-negative cover against Enterobacteriaceae. Amoxicillin has better oral absorption than ampicillin. Unfortunately, resistance to these agents is widespread (54% of *E. coli* Europe-wide in 2010, range 34–83%), so they are no longer appropriate for first-line use in Gram-negative infections. In many organisms, resistance is due to β-lactamase production, which can be overcome by the addition of β-lactamase inhibitors (clavulanic acid or sulbactam).

Carboxypenicillins (e.g. ticarcillin) and ureidopenicillins (e.g. piperacillin) are particularly active against Gram-negative organisms, especially *Pseudomonas* spp. which are resistant to the aminopenicillins. Beta-lactamase inhibitors may be added to extend their spectrum of activity (e.g. piperacillin–tazobactam).

Cephalosporins and cephamycins

Cephalosporins are reliable broad-spectrum agents. Unfortunately, their use is associated with *C. difficile*

6.23 Cephalosporins

First generation	
• Cefalexin, cefradine (oral)	• Cefazolin (IV)
Second generation	
• Cefuroxime (oral/IV) • Cefaclor (oral)	• Cefoxitin (IV)
Third generation	
• Cefixime (oral) • Cefotaxime (IV)	• Ceftriaxone (IV) • Ceftazidime (IV)
Fourth generation	
• Cefepime (IV)	
'Next generation'	
• Ceftobiprole (IV)	• Ceftaroline (IV)

infection (p. 343). With the exception of ceftobiprole, the group has no activity against *Enterococcus* spp. Only the cephamycins have significant anti-anaerobic activity. All cephalosporins are inactivated by ESBL. Cephalosporins are arranged in 'generations' (Box 6.23).

- *First-generation compounds* have excellent activity against Gram-positive organisms and some activity against Gram-negatives.
- *Second-generation drugs* retain Gram-positive activity but have extended Gram-negative activity. Cephamycins (e.g. cefoxitin), included in this group, are active against anaerobic Gram-negative bacilli.
- *Third-generation agents* further improve anti-Gram-negative cover. For some (e.g. ceftazidime), this is extended to include *Pseudomonas* spp. Cefotaxime and ceftriaxone have excellent Gram-negative activity and retain good activity against *Strep. pneumoniae* and β-haemolytic streptococci. Ceftriaxone is administered once daily, and is therefore a suitable agent for outpatient antimicrobial therapy.
- *Fourth-generation agents* have an extremely broad spectrum of activity, including *Pseudomonas* spp., *Staph. aureus* and streptococci.
- *'Next generation' agents* have a third- or fourth-generation spectrum enhanced to include MRSA.

Monobactams

Aztreonam is the only available monobactam. It is excellent against Gram-negative, except ESBL-producing, organisms, but no useful activity against Gram-positive organisms or anaerobes. It is a parenteral-only agent and may be used safely in penicillin-allergic patients.

Carbapenems

These intravenous agents have the broadest antibiotic activity of the β-lactam antibiotics, covering most clinically significant bacteria, including anaerobes.

Macrolide and lincosamide antibiotics

Macrolides (erythromycin, clarithromycin and azithromycin) and lincosamides (lincomycin and clindamycin) are bacteriostatic agents which have related properties. Both classes bind to the same component of the ribosome, so they are potentially competitive and should not be administered together. Macrolides are used for Gram-positive infections in penicillin-allergic patients and in *Mycoplasma* and *Chlamydia* infections. Erythromycin is administered 4 times daily and clarithromycin twice daily. The long intracellular half-life of azithromycin allows single-dose/short-course therapy for genitourinary *Chlamydia/Mycoplasma* spp. infections. Clarithromycin and azithromycin are also used to treat legionellosis.

Pharmacokinetics

Macrolides

- Variable bioavailability.
- Short half-life (except azithromycin).
- High protein binding.
- Excellent intracellular accumulation.

Lincosamides (e.g. clindamycin)

- Good bioavailability.
- Food has no effect on absorption.
- Limited CSF penetration.

Adverse effects

- Gastrointestinal upset, especially in young adults (erythromycin 30%).
- Cholestatic jaundice with erythromycin estolate.
- Prolongation of QT interval on ECG, potential for torsades de pointes.
- Clindamycin predisposes to *C. difficile* infection.

Ketolides

The ketolides were developed in response to the emergence of penicillin and macrolide resistance in respiratory pathogens. Cross-resistance with macrolides is uncommon. Telithromycin is administered orally and has useful activity against common bacterial causes of respiratory infection, as well as *Mycoplasma*, *Chlamydia* and *Legionella* spp.

Aminoglycosides

Aminoglycosides are effective mainly in Gram-negative infections. They act synergistically with β-lactam antibiotics and are particularly useful where β-lactam or quinolone resistance occurs in health care-acquired infections. They cause very little local irritation at injection sites and negligible allergic responses. Oto- and nephrotoxicity must be avoided by monitoring of renal function and drug levels and by use of short treatment regimens. Aminoglycosides are not subject to an inoculum effect (p. 151) and they all exhibit a post-antibiotic effect (p. 153).

Pharmacokinetics

- Negligible oral absorption.
- Hydrophilic, so excellent penetration to extracellular fluid in body cavities and serosal fluids.
- Very poor intracellular penetration (except hair cells in cochlea and renal cortical cells).
- Negligible CSF and corneal penetration.
- Peak plasma levels 30 minutes after infusion.
- Monitoring of therapeutic levels required.

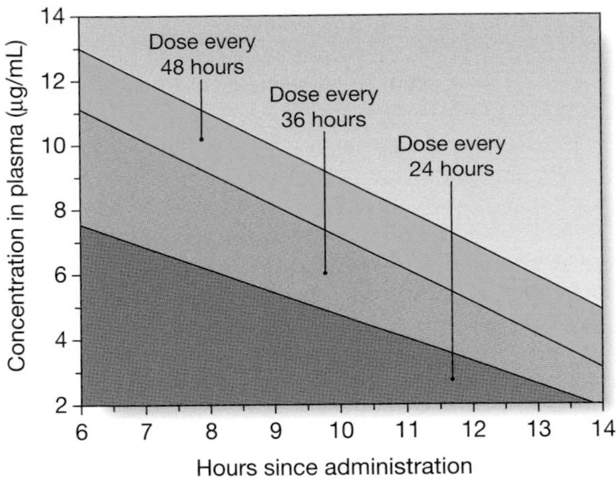

Fig. 6.18 Dosing of aminoglycosides using the Hartford nomogram. The nomogram is used to determine the dose interval for 7 mg doses of gentamicin or tobramycin, using measurements of drug levels in plasma 6–14 hours after a single dose.

Gentamicin dosing

- Except in certain forms of endocarditis, pregnancy, severe burns, end-stage renal disease and paediatric patients, gentamicin is administered at 7 mg/kg body weight. The appropriate dose interval depends on drug clearance, and is determined by reference to the Hartford nomogram (Fig. 6.18).
- In streptococcal and enterococcal endocarditis, gentamicin is used with a cell wall active agent (usually a β-lactam), to provide synergy. The usual dose is 1 mg/kg/day 3 times daily for enterococcal endocarditis and 3 mg/kg once a day for most strains of viridans streptococci. Target pre- and post-dose levels are < 1 mg/L and 3–5 mg/L respectively when gentamicin is dosed 3 times daily.
- When not used once daily or for endocarditis, gentamicin is administered twice or 3 times daily at 3–5 mg/kg/day. Target pre- and post-dose levels are < 1 mg/L and 5–10 mg/L (7–10 mg/L with less sensitive organisms, e.g. *Pseudomonas* spp.) respectively.
- For other aminoglycosides, consult local guidance.

Adverse effects

- Renal toxicity (usually reversible) accentuated by other nephrotoxic agents.
- Cochlear toxicity (permanent) more likely in older people and those with a predisposing mitochondrial gene mutation.
- Neuromuscular blockade after rapid intravenous infusion (potentiated by calcium channel blockers, myasthenia gravis and hypomagnesaemia).

Quinolones and fluoroquinolones

These are effective and generally well-tolerated bactericidal agents. The quinolones have purely anti-Gram-negative activity, whereas the fluoroquinolones are broad-spectrum agents (Box 6.24). Ciprofloxacin has anti-pseudomonal activity but resistance emerges rapidly. In 2010, 21% of *E. coli* isolates were resistant to fluoroquinolones in Europe.

6.24 Quinolones and fluoroquinolones

Agent	Route of administration	Typical antimicrobial spectrum
Quinolones		
Nalidixic acid	Oral	Enteric Gram-negative bacilli (not *Pseudomonas aeruginosa*)
Fluoroquinolones		
Ciprofloxacin	IV/oral	Enteric Gram-negative bacilli, *P. aeruginosa*, *Haemophilus* spp., 'atypical' respiratory pathogens*
Norfloxacin	Oral	(as above)
Ofloxacin	IV/oral/topical	(as above)
Levofloxacin (L-isomer of ofloxacin)	IV/oral	*Haemophilus* spp., *Strep, pneumoniae*, 'atypical' respiratory pathogens*
Moxifloxacin	Oral	*Strep. pneumoniae*, *Staph. aureus*, 'atypical' respiratory pathogens*, Mycobacteria and anaerobes

*'Atypical' pathogens include *Mycoplasma pneumoniae* and *Legionella* spp. Fluoroquinolones have variable activity against *M. tuberculosis and* other mycobacteria.

Pharmacokinetics

- Well absorbed after oral administration but delayed by food, antacids, ferrous sulphate and multivitamins.
- Wide volume of distribution; tissue concentrations twice those in serum.
- Good intracellular penetration, concentrating in phagocytes.

Adverse effects

- Gastrointestinal side-effects in 1–5%.
- Rare skin reactions (phototoxicity).
- Achilles tendon rupture is reported, especially in older people.
- CNS effects (confusion, tremor, dizziness and occasional seizures in 5–12%), especially in older people.
- Reduces clearance of xanthines and theophyllines, potentially inducing insomnia and increased seizure potential.
- Reports of prolongation of QT interval on ECG with newer fluoroquinolones.
- Cases of hypo- or hyperglycaemia in association with gatifloxacin, so glucose monitoring is needed in patients with diabetes or those with severe hepatic dysfunction.
- Ciprofloxacin use is associated with the acquisition of MRSA and emergence of *C. difficile* ribotype 027 (p. 343).

Glycopeptides

Glycopeptides (vancomycin and teicoplanin) are effective against Gram-positive organisms only, and are used against MRSA and ampicillin-resistant enterococci. Some staphylococci and enterococci demonstrate intermediate sensitivity or resistance. Vancomycin use should be restricted to limit emergence of resistant strains. Teicoplanin is not available in all countries. Neither drug is absorbed after oral administration, but vancomycin is used orally to treat *C. difficile* infection.

Pharmacokinetics

Vancomycin

- Administered by slow intravenous infusion, good tissue distribution and short half-life.
- Enters the CSF only in the presence of inflammation.
- Therapeutic monitoring of intravenous vancomycin is recommended, to maintain pre-dose levels of > 10 mg/L (15–20 mg/L in serious staphylococcal infections).

Teicoplanin

- Long half-life allows once-daily dosing.

Adverse effects

- Histamine release due to rapid vancomycin infusion produces a 'red man' reaction (rare with modern preparations).
- Nephrotoxicity is rare, but may occur with concomitant aminoglycoside use, as may ototoxicity.
- Teicoplanin can cause rash, bronchospasm, eosinophilia and anaphylaxis.

Folate antagonists

These bacteriostatic antibiotics interfere with the bacterial synthesis of folic acid from para-aminobenzoic acid. A combination of a sulphonamide and either trimethoprim or pyrimethamine is most commonly used, which interferes with two consecutive steps in the metabolic pathway. Available combinations include trimethoprim/sulfamethoxazole (co-trimoxazole) and pyrimethamine with either sulfadoxine (used to treat malaria) or sulfadiazine (used in toxoplasmosis). Co-trimoxazole in high dosage (120 mg/kg daily in 2–4 divided doses) is the first-line drug for *Pneumocystis jirovecii (carinii)* infection. The clinical use of these agents is limited by adverse effects. Folinic acid should be given if they are used long-term or unavoidably in early pregnancy.

Pharmacokinetics

- Well absorbed orally.
- Sulphonamides are hydrophilic, distributing well to the extracellular fluid.
- Trimethoprim is lipophilic with high tissue concentrations.

Adverse effects

- Trimethoprim is generally well tolerated, with few adverse effects.
- Sulphonamides and dapsone may cause haemolysis in glucose-6-phosphate dehydrogenase deficiency (p. 1029).
- Sulphonamides and dapsone cause skin and mucocutaneous reactions, including Stevens–Johnson syndrome and 'dapsone syndrome' (rash, fever and lymphadenopathy).
- Dapsone causes methaemoglobinaemia and peripheral neuropathy.

Tetracyclines and glycylcyclines

Tetracyclines

Of this mainly bacteriostatic class, the newer drugs doxycycline and minocycline show better absorption and distribution than older ones. Most streptococci and Gram-negative bacteria are now resistant, in part due to use in animals (which is banned in Europe). Tetracyclines are indicated for *Mycoplasma* spp., *Chlamydia* spp., *Rickettsia* spp., *Coxiella* spp., *Bartonella* spp., *Borrelia* spp., *Helicobacter pylori*, *Treponema pallidum* and atypical mycobacterial infections. Minocycline is occasionally used in chronic staphylococcal infections.

Pharmacokinetics

- Best oral absorption is in the fasting state (doxycycline is 100% absorbed unless gastric pH rises).

Adverse effects

- All tetracyclines except doxycycline are contraindicated in renal failure.
- Dizziness with minocycline.
- Binding to metallic ions in bones and teeth causes discoloration (avoid in children and pregnancy) and enamel hypoplasia.
- Phototoxic skin reactions.

Glycylcyclines (tigecycline)

Chemical modification of tetracycline has produced tigecycline, a broad-spectrum, parenteral-only antibiotic with activity against resistant Gram-positive and Gram-negative pathogens, such as MRSA and ESBL (but excluding *Pseudomonas* spp.). Re-analysis of trial data has shown that there was excess mortality following tigecycline treatment compared with comparator antibiotics, so tigecycline should be used only when there are no available alternative agents.

Nitroimidazoles

Nitroimidazoles are highly active against strictly anaerobic bacteria, especially *Bacteroides fragilis*, *C. difficile* and other *Clostridium* spp. They also have significant antiprotozoal activity against amoebae and *Giardia lamblia*.

Pharmacokinetics

- Almost completely absorbed after oral administration (60% after rectal administration).
- Well distributed, especially to brain and CSF.
- Safe in pregnancy.

Adverse effects

- Metallic taste (dose-dependent).
- Severe vomiting if taken with alcohol – 'Antabuse effect'.
- Peripheral neuropathy with prolonged use.

Other antibacterial agents

Anti-tuberculous agents are discussed in detail on page 693.

Chloramphenicol

This is a potent and cheap antibiotic, still widely prescribed throughout the world despite its potential toxicity. Its use is increasingly reserved for severe and life-threatening infections where other antibiotics are either unavailable or impractical. It is bacteriostatic to most organisms but apparently bactericidal to *H. influenzae*, *Strep. pneumoniae* and *Neisseria meningitidis*. It has a very broad spectrum of activity against aerobic and anaerobic organisms, spirochaetes, *Rickettsia*, *Chlamydia* and *Mycoplasma* spp. It also has quite useful activity against anaerobes, such as *B. fragilis*. It competes with macrolides and lincosamides for ribosomal binding sites, so should not be used in combination with these agents. Significant adverse effects are 'grey baby' syndrome in infants (cyanosis and circulatory collapse due to inability to conjugate drug and excrete the active form in urine); reversible dose-dependent bone marrow depression in adults receiving high cumulative doses; and severe aplastic anaemia in 1 in 25 000–40 000 exposures (unrelated to dose, duration of therapy or route of administration).

Daptomycin

Daptomycin is a cyclic lipopeptide with bactericidal activity against Gram-positive organisms (including MRSA and GRE) but not Gram-negatives. It is not absorbed orally, and is used intravenously to treat resistant Gram-positive infections, e.g. soft tissue infections and infective endocarditis, if other options are not available. Treatment can be associated with increased levels of creatine kinase and patients receiving lipid-lowering statins (p. 453) should discontinue these to avoid myopathy.

Fusidic acid

This antibiotic, active against Gram-positive bacteria, is available in intravenous, oral or topical formulations. It is lipid-soluble and distributes well to tissues. However, its antibacterial activity is unpredictable. Fusidic acid is used in combination, typically with antistaphylococcal penicillins, or for MRSA with clindamycin or rifampicin. It interacts with coumarin derivatives and oral contraceptives.

Nitrofurantoin

This drug has very rapid renal elimination and is active against aerobic Gram-negative and Gram-positive bacteria, including enterococci. It is used only for treatment of urinary tract infection, being generally safe in pregnancy and childhood. However, with prolonged use, it can cause eosinophilic lung infiltrates, fever, pulmonary fibrosis, peripheral neuropathy, hepatitis and haemolytic anaemia.

Linezolid

Linezolid is the only currently licensed oxazolidinone antibiotic. It shows excellent oral absorption with good activity against Gram-positive organisms, including MRSA and GRE. It is competitively inhibited by co-administration of chloramphenicol, vancomycin or clindamycin. Common adverse effects include mild gastrointestinal upset and tongue discoloration. Myelodysplasia and peripheral neuropathy can occur with prolonged use. Linezolid has monoamine oxidase inhibitor (MAOI) activity (p. 244), and co-administration with other MAOIs or serotonin re-uptake inhibitors should be avoided, as this may precipitate a serotonin syndrome (neuromuscular effects, autonomic hyperactivity and altered mental status).

Fidaxomicin

Fidaxomicin is an inhibitor of RNA synthesis, which was introduced for the treatment of *C. difficile* infection (CDI) in 2012. In non-severe CDI, it appears to be non-inferior to oral vancomycin and is associated with a lower recurrence rate. Its effectiveness has not been assessed in severe CDI.

Spectinomycin

Chemically similar to the aminoglycosides and given intramuscularly, spectinomycin was developed to treat strains of *N. gonorrhoeae* resistant to β-lactam antibiotics. Unfortunately, resistance to spectinomycin is very common. Its only indication is the treatment of gonococcal urethritis in pregnancy or in patients allergic to β-lactam antibiotics.

Streptogramins

Quinupristin/dalfopristin (supplied as a 30:70% combination) is active against MRSA and GRE (*Enterococcus faecium* but not *E. faecalis*), and its use should be reserved for these organisms. It is available in intravenous formulation only and shows good tissue penetration, but does not cross the blood–brain barrier or the placenta. Significant phlebitis occurs at injection sites and a raised serum creatinine and eosinophilia may occur.

Antifungal agents

See Box 6.25.

Azole antifungals

The azoles (imidazoles and triazoles) inhibit synthesis of ergosterol, a constituent of the fungal cell membrane. Side-effects vary but include gastrointestinal upset, hepatitis and rash. Azoles are inhibitors of cytochrome p450 enzymes, so tend to increase exposure to cytochrome p450-metabolised drugs (p. 28).

Imidazoles

Miconazole, econazole, clotrimazole and ketoconazole are relatively toxic and therefore mainly administered topically. Clotrimazole is used extensively to treat superficial fungal infections. Ketoconazole may be given orally, but causes severe hepatitis in 1:15 000 cases and inhibits enzymes involved in steroid hormone biosynthesis. Triazoles are preferred for systemic administration because of their reduced toxicity.

Triazoles

Fluconazole is effective against yeasts (*Candida* and *Cryptococcus* spp.). It is well absorbed after oral administration, and has a long half-life (approximately 30 hours) and an excellent safety profile. The drug is highly water-soluble and distributes widely to all body sites and tissues, including CSF.

Itraconazole is lipophilic and distributes extensively, including to toenails and fingernails. CSF penetration

6.25 Antifungal agents

Agent	Usual route(s) of administration	Clinically relevant antifungal spectrum
Imidazoles		
Miconazole Econazole Clotrimazole	Topical	*Candida* spp., dermatophytes
Ketoconazole	Topical, oral	*Malassezia* spp., dermatophytes, agents of eumycetoma
Triazoles		
Fluconazole	Oral, IV	Yeasts (*Candida* and *Cryptococcus* spp.)
Itraconazole	Oral, IV	Yeasts, dermatophytes, dimorphic fungi (p. 376), *Aspergillus* spp.
Voriconazole	Oral, IV	Yeasts and most filamentous fungi (excluding mucoraceous moulds)
Posaconazole	Oral	Yeasts and many filamentous fungi (including most mucoraceous moulds)
Echinocandins		
Anidulafungin Caspofungin Micafungin	IV only	*Candida* spp., *Aspergillus* spp. (no activity against *Cryptococcus* spp. or mucoraceous moulds)
Polyenes		
Amphotericin B Nystatin	IV Topical	Yeasts and most dimorphic and filamentous fungi (including mucoraceous moulds)
Others		
Flucytosine	Oral, IV	Yeasts
Griseofulvin	Oral	Dermatophytes
Terbinafine	Topical, oral	Dermatophytes

is poor. Oral absorption is erratic and formulation-dependent, necessitating therapeutic drug monitoring.

Voriconazole is well absorbed (96% oral bioavailability) and used mainly in aspergillosis (p. 697).

Posaconazole is the broadest-spectrum antifungal azole, and the only one with consistent activity against mucoraceous moulds. It is currently available as an oral agent only.

Echinocandins

The echinocandins inhibit β-1,3-glucan synthesis in the fungal cell wall. They have few significant adverse effects. Caspofungin, anidulafungin and micafungin are used to treat systemic candidosis, and caspofungin is also used in aspergillosis.

Polyenes

Amphotericin B (AmB) deoxycholate causes cell death by binding to ergosterol and damaging the fungal cytoplasmic membrane. Its use in resource-rich countries has been largely supplanted by less toxic agents. It is lipophilic, insoluble in water and not absorbed orally. Its long half-life enables once-daily administration. CSF penetration is poor.

Adverse effects include immediate anaphylaxis, other infusion-related reactions and nephrotoxicity. Nephrotoxicity may be sufficient to require dialysis, and occurs in most patients who are adequately dosed. It may be ameliorated by concomitant infusion of normal saline. Irreversible nephrotoxicity occurs with large cumulative doses of AmB.

Nystatin has a similar spectrum of antifungal activity to AmB. Its toxicity limits it to topical use, e.g. in oral and vaginal candidiasis.

Lipid formulations of amphotericin B

Lipid formulations of AmB have been developed to reduce AmB toxicity. They consist of AmB encapsulated in liposomes (liposomal AmB, L-AmB) or complexed with phospholipids (AmB lipid complex, ABLC). The drug becomes active on dissociating from its lipid component. Adverse effects are similar to, but considerably less frequent than, those with AmB deoxycholate, and efficacy is similar. Lipid formulations of AmB are used in invasive fungal disease, as empirical therapy in patients with neutropenic fever (p. 1004), and also in visceral leishmaniasis (p. 362).

Other antifungal agents

Flucytosine

This drug has particular activity against yeasts. When used as monotherapy, resistance develops rapidly, so it should be administered in combination with another antifungal agent. Oral dosing is effective. Adverse effects include myelosuppression, gastrointestinal upset and hepatitis.

Griseofulvin

Griseofulvin has been largely superseded by terbinafine and itraconazole for treatment of dermatophyte infections, except in children, for whom these agents remain largely unlicensed. It demonstrates excellent oral bioavailability and is deposited in keratin precursor cells, which become resistant to fungal invasion. The duration of treatment is 2–4 weeks for tinea corporis/capitis, 4–8 weeks for tinea pedis, and 4–6 months for onychomycosis (fungal nail infections).

Terbinafine

Terbinafine is well absorbed orally, can be given once daily and distributes with high concentration to sebum and skin, with a half-life of more than 1 week. It is used topically for dermatophyte skin infections and orally for onychomycosis. The major adverse reaction is hepatic toxicity (approximately 1:50000 cases). Terbinafine is not recommended for breastfeeding mothers.

Antiviral agents

Most viral infections in immunocompetent individuals resolve without intervention. Antiviral therapy is

6.26 Antiviral agents

Drug	Route(s) of administration	Indications	Significant side-effects
Antiretroviral therapy (ART, p. 403)	Oral	HIV infection (including AIDS)	CNS symptoms, anaemia, lipodystrophy
Anti-herpesvirus agents			
Aciclovir	Topical/oral/IV	Herpes zoster Chickenpox (esp. in immunosuppressed) Herpes simplex infections: encephalitis (IV only), genital tract, oral, ophthalmic	Significant side-effects rare. Hepatitis, renal impairment and neurotoxicity reported rarely
Valaciclovir	Oral	Herpes zoster, herpes simplex	As for aciclovir
Famciclovir	Oral	Herpes zoster, herpes simplex (genital)	As for aciclovir
Penciclovir	Topical	Labial herpes simplex	Local irritation
Ganciclovir	IV	Treatment and prevention of CMV infection in immunosuppressed	Gastrointestinal symptoms, liver dysfunction, neurotoxicity, myelosuppression, renal impairment, fever, rash, phlebitis at infusion sites. Potential teratogenicity
Valganciclovir	Oral	Treatment and prevention of CMV infection in immunosuppressed	As for ganciclovir but neutropenia is predominant
Cidofovir	IV Topical	HIV-associated CMV infections and occasionally other viruses (see text)	Renal impairment, neutropenia
Foscarnet	IV	CMV and aciclovir-resistant HSV and VZV infections in immunosuppressed	Gastrointestinal symptoms, renal impairment, electrolyte disturbances, genital ulceration, neurotoxicity
Anti-influenza agents			
Zanamivir	Inhalation	Influenza A and B	Allergic reactions (very rare)
Oseltamivir	Oral	Influenza A and B	Gastrointestinal side-effects, rash, hepatitis (very rare)
Amantadine, rimantadine	Oral	Influenza A (but see text)	CNS symptoms, nausea
Agents used in viral hepatitis			
Ribavirin	Oral/IV/ inhalation	Hepatitis C infection (with interferons) (oral) Lassa fever (IV) RSV infection in infants (inhalation)	Haemolytic anaemia, cough, dyspnoea, bronchospasm and ocular irritation (when given by inhalation)
Interferon-α, pegylated interferon-α	SC	Chronic hepatitis B and (with ribavirin) hepatitis C	Influenza-like syndrome following dose, gastrointestinal symptoms, hepatitis, myelosuppression
Adefovir dipivoxil, entecavir, lamivudine, telbivudine	Oral	Chronic hepatitis B infection	Generally well tolerated with minimal side-effects Creatine kinase elevation (telbivudine only)
Tenofovir	Oral	Hepatitis B in co-infection with HIV (with other antiretroviral agents)	Minimal side-effects Rarely, nephrotoxicity
Telaprevir	Oral	Hepatitis C genotype 1 with interferon–ribavirin combination treatment	Anaemia, rash, fatigue, nausea and vomiting
Boceprevir	Oral	Hepatitis C genotype 1 with interferon–ribavirin combination treatment	Anaemia, taste disturbance

(CMV = cytomegalovirus; HSV = herpes simplex virus; RSV = respiratory syncytial virus; VZV = varicella zoster virus)

available for a limited number of infections only (Box 6.26 and p. 407).

Antiretroviral agents

These agents, used predominantly against HIV, are discussed in Chapter 14.

Anti-herpesvirus agents

Aciclovir, valaciclovir, penciclovir and famciclovir

Aciclovir, valaciclovir, penciclovir and famciclovir are acyclic analogues of guanosine, which inhibit viral DNA polymerase after being phosphorylated by virus-derived thymidine kinase (TK). Aciclovir is poorly absorbed after oral dosing; better levels are achieved intravenously or by use of the prodrug valaciclovir. Famciclovir is the prodrug of penciclovir. Resistance is mediated by viral kinase or polymerase mutations.

Ganciclovir

Chemical modification of the aciclovir molecule allows preferential phosphorylation by protein kinases of cytomegalovirus (CMV) and other β-herpesviruses (e.g. human herpesvirus (HHV) 6/7) and hence greater inhibition of the DNA polymerase, but at the expense of increased toxicity. Ganciclovir is administered intravenously or as a prodrug (valganciclovir) orally.

Cidofovir

Cidofovir inhibits viral DNA polymerases with potent activity against CMV, including most ganciclovir-resistant CMV. It also has activity against aciclovir-resistant herpes simplex virus (HSV) and varicella zoster virus (VZV), HHV6 and occasionally adenovirus, poxvirus, papillomavirus or polyoma virus, and may be used to treat these infections in immunocompromised hosts.

Foscarnet

This analogue of inorganic pyrophosphate acts as a non-competitive inhibitor of HSV, VZV, HHV6/7 or CMV DNA polymerase. It does not require significant intracellular phosphorylation and so may be effective when HSV or CMV resistance is due to altered drug phosphorylation. It has variable CSF penetration.

Anti-influenza agents

Zanamivir and oseltamivir

These agents inhibit influenza A and B neuraminidase, which is required for release of virus from infected cells (see Fig. 6.2, p. 135). They are used in treatment and prophylaxis of influenza. Administration within 48 hours of disease onset reduces the duration of symptoms by approximately 1–1½ days. In the UK, their use is limited mainly to adults with chronic respiratory or renal disease, significant cardiovascular disease, immunosuppression or diabetes mellitus, during known outbreaks. Peramivir has a distinct chemical structure, which means that it retains activity against some oseltamivir and zanamivir-resistant strains. It has poor oral bioavailability and is being developed as an intravenous or intramuscular formulation. An intravenous formulation of zanamivir is in development for critically ill patients.

Amantadine and rimantadine

These drugs reduce replication of influenza A by inhibition of viral M2 protein ion channel function, which is required for uncoating (see Fig. 6.2, p. 135). Resistance develops rapidly and is widespread, and amantadine and rimantadine should be used only if the prevalence of resistance locally is known to be low. They are no longer recommended for treatment or prophylaxis in the UK or USA, having been superseded by zanamivir and oseltamivir. However, they may still be indicated to treat oseltamivir-resistant influenza A in patients unable to take zanamivir (e.g. ventilated patients).

Agents used against hepatitis viruses

Ribavirin

Ribavirin is a guanosine analogue that inhibits nucleic acid synthesis in a variety of viruses and is used in particular in the treatment of hepatitis C virus.

Lamivudine, adefovir dipivoxil, tenofovir, entecavir and telbivudine

These agents have excellent activity against hepatitis B virus DNA polymerase–reverse transcriptase. They are well tolerated after oral administration but resistance develops with monotherapy. Resistance seems to emerge most rapidly for lamivudine (via the tyrosine–methionine–aspartate–aspartate, or YMDD, mutation) and most slowly for entecavir (multiple mutations required). Organisms resistant to lamivudine are usually also resistant to telbivudine, but not to adefovir/tenofovir. The role of monotherapy for hepatitis B virus is currently a matter for debate, and combination therapy, as used in HIV treatment, is likely to be increasingly employed. Lamivudine and tenofovir are also used against HIV (p. 407).

Telaprevir and boceprevir

A number of antiviral inhibitors of the hepatitis C virus NS3 serine protease or NS5B polymerase are in development. Telaprevir and boceprevir have been licensed for use in chronic hepatitis C virus genotype 1 disease. Addition of these agents to standard interferon–ribavirin combination therapy improves sustained virological response rates. They are prone to drug–drug interactions, including those involving antiretrovirals. Resistance develops to these agents, so they are administered as part of combination treatment.

Interferon-α

The interferons are naturally occurring cytokines that are produced as an early response to viral infection (p. 74). The addition of a polyethylene glycol (PEG) moiety to the molecule significantly enhances pharmacokinetics and efficacy.

Antiparasitic agents

Drugs used against helminths

Benzimidazoles (albendazole, mebendazole)

These agents act by inhibiting both helminth glucose uptake, causing depletion of glycogen stores, and fumarate reductase. Albendazole is used for hookworm, ascariasis, threadworm, *Strongyloides* infection, trichinellosis, *Taenia solium* (cysticercosis) and hydatid disease. Mebendazole is used for hookworm, ascariasis, threadworm and whipworm. The drugs are administered orally. Absorption is relatively poor, but increased by a fatty meal. Significant adverse effects are uncommon.

Bithionol

Bithionol is used to treat fluke infections with *Fasciola hepatica*. It is well absorbed orally. Adverse effects are mild (e.g. nausea, vomiting, diarrhoea, rashes) but relatively common (approximately 30%).

Diethylcarbamazine

Diethylcarbamazine (DEC) is an oral agent used to treat filariasis and loiasis. Treatment of filariasis is often followed by fever, headache, nausea, vomiting, arthralgia and prostration. This is caused by the host response to dying microfilariae, rather than the drug, and may be reduced by pre-treatment with corticosteroids.

Ivermectin

Ivermectin binds to helminth nerve and muscle cell ion channels, causing increased membrane permeability. It is an oral agent, used in *Strongyloides* infection, filariasis and onchocerciasis. Significant side-effects are uncommon.

Niclosamide

Niclosamide inhibits oxidative phosphorylation, causing paralysis of helminths. It is an oral agent, used in *Taenia saginata* and intestinal *T. solium* infection. Systemic absorption is minimal and it has few significant side-effects.

Piperazine

Piperazine inhibits neurotransmitter function, causing helminth muscle paralysis. It is an oral agent, used in ascariasis and threadworm (*Enterobius vermicularis*) infection. Significant adverse effects are uncommon, but include neuropsychological reactions such as vertigo, confusion and convulsions.

Praziquantel

Praziquantel increases membrane permeability to Ca^{++}, causing violent contraction of worm muscle. It is the drug of choice for schistosomiasis, and is also used in *T. saginata*, *T. solium* (cysticercosis) and fluke infections (*Clonorchis*, *Paragonimus*) and in echinococcosis. It is administered orally and is well absorbed. Adverse effects are usually mild and transient, and include nausea and abdominal pain.

Pyrantel pamoate

This agent causes spastic paralysis of helminth muscle through a suxamethonium-like action. It is used orally in ascariasis and threadworm infection. Systemic absorption is poor and adverse effects are uncommon.

Thiabendazole

Thiabendazole inhibits fumarate reductase, which is required for energy production in helminths. It is used orally in *Strongyloides* infection and topically to treat cutaneous larva migrans. Significant adverse effects are uncommon.

Antimalarial agents

Artemisinin (quinghaosu) derivatives

Artemisinin originates from a herb (sweet wormwood, *Artemisia annua*), which was used in Chinese medicine to treat fever. Its derivatives, artemether and artesunate, were developed for use in malaria in the 1970s. Their mechanism of action is unknown. They are used in the treatment, but not prophylaxis, of malaria, usually in combination with other antimalarials, and are effective against strains of *Plasmodium* spp. that are resistant to other antimalarials. Artemether is lipid-soluble and may be administered via intramuscular and oral routes. Artesunate is water-soluble and is administered intravenously or orally. Serious adverse effects are uncommon. Current advice for malaria in pregnancy is that the artemisinin derivatives should be used to treat uncomplicated *falciparum* malaria in the second and third trimesters, but should not be prescribed in the first trimester until more information becomes available.

Atovaquone

Atovaquone inhibits mitochondrial function. It is an oral agent, used for treatment and prophylaxis of malaria, in combination with proguanil (see below), without which it is ineffective. It is also employed in the treatment of mild cases of *Pneumocystis jirovecii (carinii)* pneumonia, where there is intolerance to co-trimoxazole. Significant adverse effects are uncommon.

Folate synthesis inhibitors (proguanil, pyrimethamine–sulfadoxine)

Proguanil inhibits dihydrofolate reductase and is used for malaria prophylaxis. Pyrimethamine–sulfadoxine is used in the treatment of malaria (p. 356).

Quinoline-containing compounds

Chloroquine and quinine are believed to act by intraparasitic inhibition of haem polymerisation, resulting in toxic build-up of intracellular haem. The mechanisms of action of other agents in this group (quinidine, amodiaquine, mefloquine, primaquine, etc.) may differ. They are employed in the treatment and prophylaxis of malaria. Primaquine is used for radical cure of malaria due to *Plasmodium vivax* and *P. ovale* (destruction of liver hypnozoites). Chloroquine is also given for extra-intestinal amoebiasis.

Chloroquine can cause a pruritus sufficient to compromise compliance with therapy. If used in long-term, high-dose regimens, it causes an irreversible retinopathy. Overdosage leads to life-threatening cardiotoxicity. The side-effect profile of mefloquine includes neuropsychiatric effects ranging from mood change, nightmares and agitation to hallucinations and psychosis. Quinine may cause hypoglycaemia and cardiotoxicity, especially when administered parenterally. Primaquine causes haemolysis in people with glucose-6-phosphate dehydrogenase deficiency (p. 1029), which should be excluded before therapy. Chloroquine is considered safe in pregnancy, but mefloquine should be avoided in the first trimester.

Lumefantrine

Lumefantrine is used in combination with artemether to treat uncomplicated *falciparum* malaria, including chloroquine-resistant strains. Its mechanism of action is unknown. Significant adverse effects are uncommon.

Drugs used in trypanosomiasis

Benznidazole

Benznidazole is an oral agent used to treat South American trypanosomiasis (Chagas' disease, p. 360). Significant and common adverse effects include dose-related peripheral neuropathy, purpuric rash and granulocytopenia.

Eflornithine

Eflornithine inhibits biosynthesis of polyamines by ornithine decarboxylase inhibition, and is used in West African trypanosomiasis (*T. brucei gambiense* infection) of the CNS. It is administered as an intravenous infusion 4 times daily, which may be logistically difficult in the geographic areas affected by this disease. Significant adverse effects are common, and include convulsions, gastrointestinal upset and bone marrow depression. Eflornithine is also used (topically) to treat hirsutism (p. 763).

Melarsoprol

This is an arsenical agent, used to treat CNS infections in East and West African trypanosomiasis (*T. brucei rhodesiense* and *gambiense*). It is administered intravenously. Melarsoprol treatment is associated with peripheral neuropathy and reactive arsenical encephalopathy (RAE), which carries a significant mortality.

Nifurtimox

Nifurtimox is administered orally to treat South American trypanosomiasis (Chagas' disease). Gastrointestinal and neurological adverse effects are common.

Pentamidine isetionate

Pentamidine is an inhibitor of DNA replication used in West African trypanosomiasis (*T. brucei gambiense*) and, to a lesser extent, in visceral and cutaneous leishmaniasis. It is also prescribed in *Pneumocystis jirovecii (carinii)* pneumonia. It is administered via intravenous or intramuscular routes. It is a relatively toxic drug, commonly causing rash, renal impairment, profound hypotension (especially on rapid infusion), electrolyte disturbances, blood dyscrasias and hypoglycaemia.

Suramin

Suramin is a naphthaline dye derivative, used to treat East African trypanosomiasis (*T. brucei rhodesiense*). It is administered intravenously. Adverse effects are common, and include rash, gastrointestinal disturbance, blood dyscrasias, peripheral neuropathies and renal impairment.

Other antiprotozoal agents

Pentavalent antimonials

Sodium stibogluconate and meglumine antimoniate inhibit protozoal glycolysis by phosphofructokinase inhibition. They are used parenterally (intravenous or intramuscular) to treat leishmaniasis. Adverse effects include arthralgia, myalgias, raised hepatic transaminases, pancreatitis and ECG changes. Severe cardiotoxicity leading to death is not uncommon.

Diloxanide furoate

This oral agent is used to eliminate luminal cysts following treatment of intestinal amoebiasis, or in asymptomatic cyst excreters. The drug is absorbed slowly (enabling luminal persistence) and has no effect in hepatic amoebiasis. It is a relatively non-toxic drug, the most significant adverse effect being flatulence.

Iodoquinol (di-iodohydroxyquinoline)

Iodoquinol is a quinoline derivative (p. 163) with activity against *Entamoeba histolytica* cysts and trophozoites. It is used orally to treat asymptomatic cyst excreters or, in association with another amoebicide (e.g. metronidazole), to treat extra-intestinal amoebiasis. Long-term use of this drug is not recommended, as neurological adverse effects include optic neuritis and peripheral neuropathy.

Nitazoxanide

Nitazoxanide is an inhibitor of pyruvate–ferredoxin oxidoreductase-dependent anaerobic energy metabolism in protozoa. It is a broad-spectrum agent, active against various nematodes, tapeworms, flukes and intestinal protozoa. Nitazoxanide also has activity against some anaerobic bacteria and viruses. It is administered orally in giardiasis and cryptosporidiosis. Adverse effects are usually mild and involve the gastrointestinal tract (e.g. nausea, diarrhoea and abdominal pain).

Paromomycin

Paromomycin is an aminoglycoside (p. 156) that is used to treat visceral leishmaniasis and intestinal amoebiasis. It is not significantly absorbed when administered orally, and is therefore given orally for intestinal amoebiasis and by intramuscular injection for leishmaniasis. It showed early promise in the treatment of HIV-associated cryptosporidiosis, but subsequent trials have demonstrated that this effect is marginal at best.

Further information and acknowledgements

Websites

http://ecdc.europa.eu *European Centre for Disease Prevention and Control. Data on prevalence of antibiotic resistance in Europe.*

www.cdc.gov *Centers for Disease Control, Atlanta, USA. Provides information on all aspects of communicable disease, including prophylaxis against malaria.*

www.dh.gov.uk *UK Department of Health. The publications section provides current UK recommendations for immunisation.*

www.hpa.org.uk *Health Protection Agency. Provides information on infectious diseases relating mainly to the UK, including community infection control.*

www.idsociety.org *Infectious Diseases Society of America. Publishes up-to-date, evidence-based guidelines.*

www.who.int *World Health Organization. Provides up-to-date information on global aspects of infectious disease, including outbreak updates.*

Figure acknowledgements

Fig. 6.10 Adapted from Samaranayake L. Essential microbiology for dentistry. 3rd edn. Edinburgh: Churchill Livingstone; 2006 (Fig. 1.1); copyright Elsevier.

Fig. 6.12 Based on the 'How to Handwash' URL: http://www.who.int/gpsc/5may/How_To_Handwash_Poster.pdf ©World Health Organization 2009. All rights reserved.

M.D. Witham

7 Ageing and disease

Comprehensive geriatric assessment 166

Demography 168

Functional anatomy and physiology 168
- Biology of ageing 168
- Physiological changes of ageing 169
- Frailty 170

Investigations 170
- Comprehensive geriatric assessment 170
- Decisions about investigation 170

Presenting problems in geriatric medicine 171
- Falls 172
- Dizziness 173
- Delirium 173
- Urinary incontinence 175
- Adverse drug reactions 175
- Other problems in old age 176

Rehabilitation 176

COMPREHENSIVE GERIATRIC ASSESSMENT

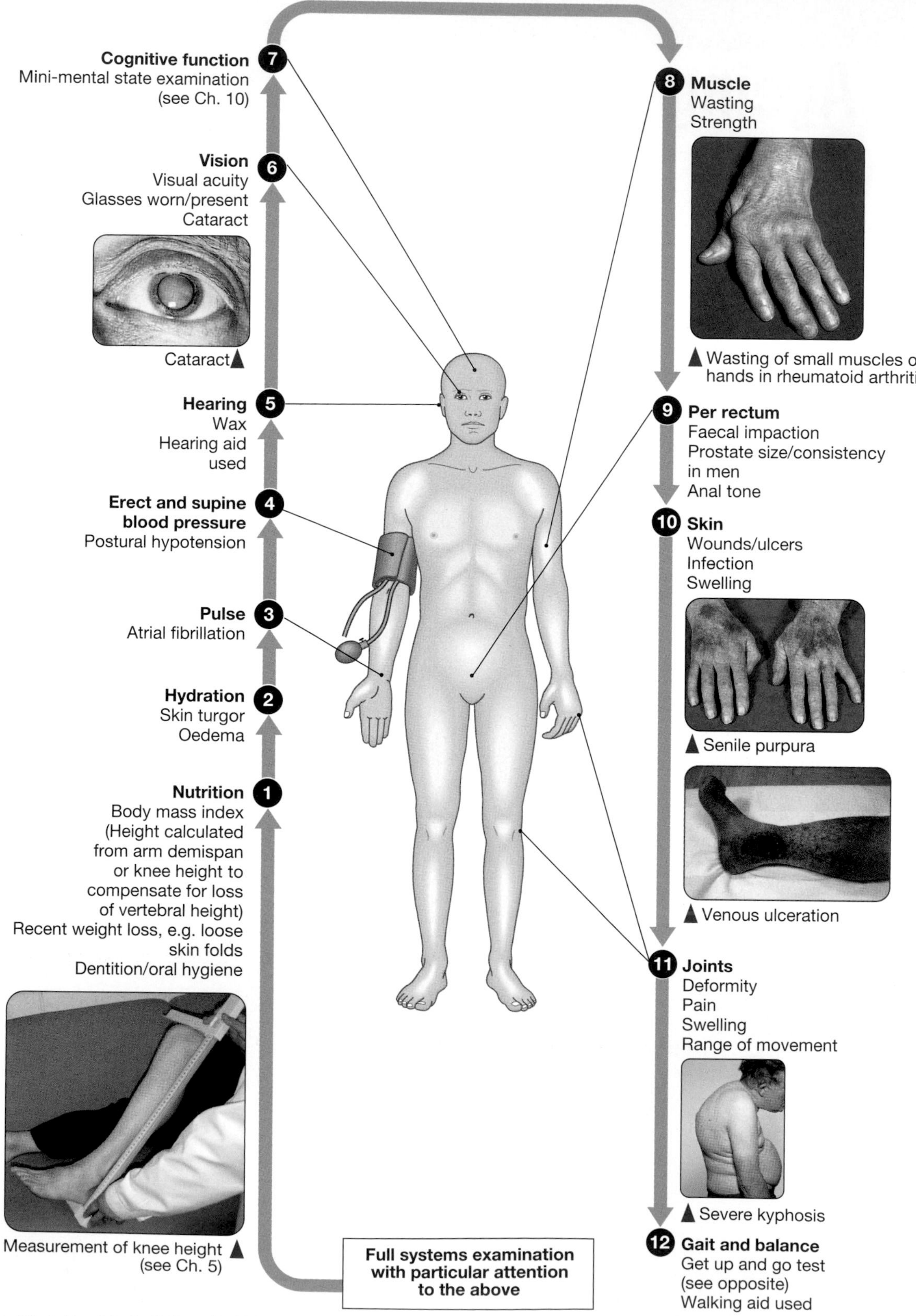

Insets (*Wasted hand, kyphosis*) From Afzal Mir 2003; (*Senile purpura*) Forbes and Jackson 2004; (*Venous ulceration*) Mosti 2012 – see p. 177.

History

- **Slow down** the pace.
- **Ensure the patient can hear**.
- Establish the **speed of onset** of the illness.
- If the presentation is vague, carry out a **systematic enquiry**.
- Obtain full details of:

  all drugs, especially any recent prescription changes

  past medical history, even from many years previously

  usual function

  1. Can the patient walk normally?
  2. Has the patient noticed memory problems?
  3. Can the patient perform all household tasks?
- **Obtain a collateral history**: confirm information with a relative or carer and the general practitioner, particularly if the patient is confused or communication is limited by deafness or speech disturbance.

Examination

- **Thorough** to identify all comorbidities.
- **Tailored to the patient's stamina** and ability to cooperate.
- Include **functional status**:

  cognitive function

  gait and balance

  nutrition

  hearing and vision.

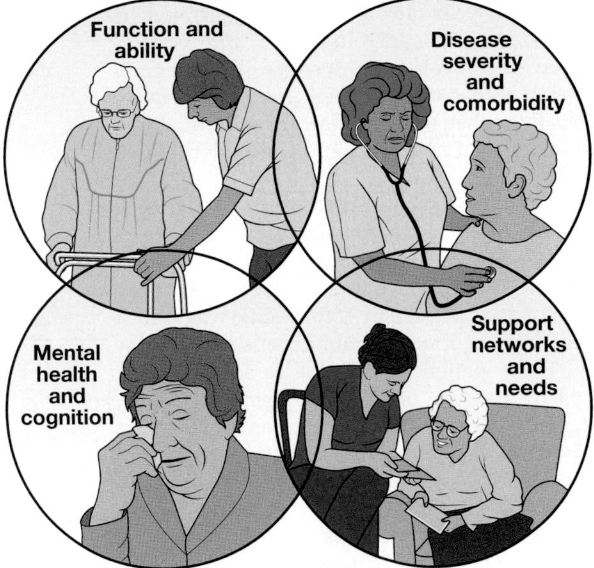

Domains of Comprehensive Geriatric Assessment.

Social assessment

Home circumstances

- Living alone, with another or in a care home.

Activities of daily living (ADL)

- Tasks for which help is needed:

  domestic ADL: shopping, cooking, housework

  personal ADL: bathing, dressing, walking.
- **Informal help**: relatives, friends, neighbours.
- **Formal social services**: home help, meals on wheels.
- Carer stress.

Multidisciplinary team (MDT) roles

Team member	Activity assessed and promoted
Physiotherapist	Mobility, balance and upper limb function
Occupational therapist	ADL, e.g. dressing, cooking Home environment and care needs
Dietitian	Nutrition
Speech and language therapist	Communication and swallowing
Social worker	Care needs and discharge planning, including organisation of institutional care
Nurse	Motivation and initiation of activities; promotion of self-care Education Feeding, continence, skin care Communication with relatives and other professionals Assessment of care needs for discharge
Doctor	Diagnosis and management of medical problems Coordinator of assessment, management and rehabilitation programme

12 Get up and go test

To assess gait and balance, ask the patient to stand up from a sitting position, walk 10 m, turn and go back to the chair. A normal performance takes less than 12 seconds.

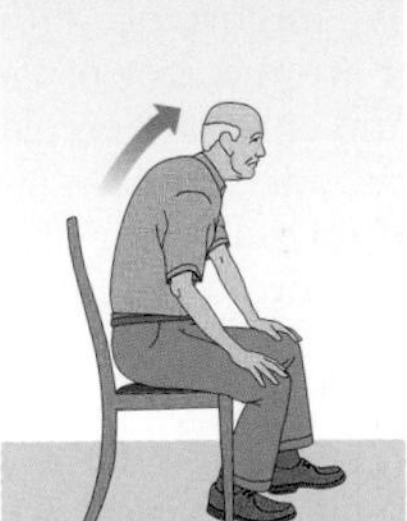

Difficulty rising?

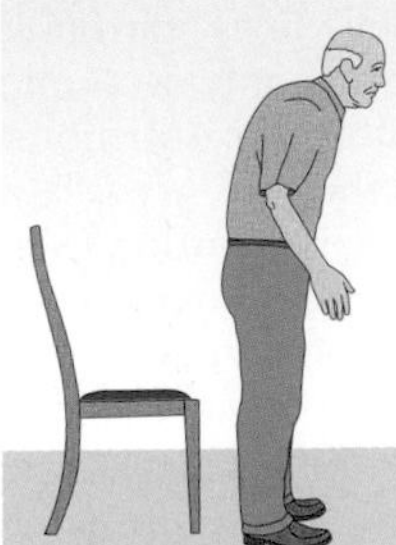

Unsteady on standing?

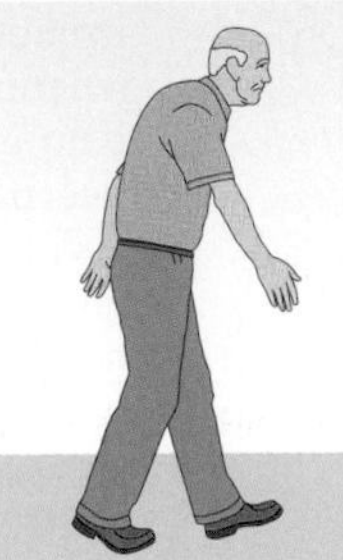

Unsteady gait?

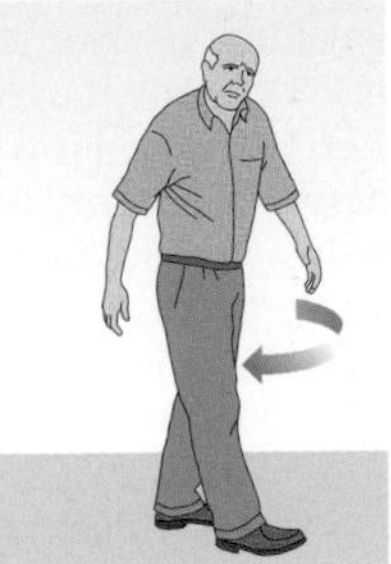

Unsteady on turning?

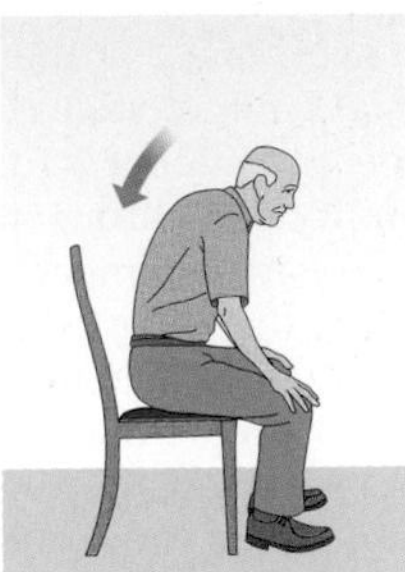

Unsteady on sitting down?

Sweeping demographic change has meant that older people now represent the core practice of medicine in many countries. A good knowledge of the effects of ageing and the clinical problems associated with old age is thus essential in most medical specialties. The older population is extremely diverse; a substantial proportion of 90-year-olds enjoy an active healthy life, while some 70-year-olds are severely disabled by chronic disease. The terms 'chronological' and 'biological' ageing have been coined to describe this phenomenon. Biological rather than chronological age is taken into consideration when making clinical decisions about, for example, the extent of investigation and intervention that is appropriate.

Geriatric medicine is concerned particularly with frail older people, in whom physiological capacity is so reduced that they are incapacitated by even minor illness. They frequently have multiple comorbidities, and acute illness may present in non-specific ways, such as confusion, falls or loss of mobility and day-to-day functioning. These patients are prone to adverse drug reactions, partly because of polypharmacy and partly because of age-related changes in responses to drugs and their elimination (p. 36). Disability is common, but patients' function can often be improved by the interventions of the multidisciplinary team (p. 167).

Older people have been neglected in research terms and, until recently, were rarely included in randomised controlled clinical trials. There is thus little evidence on which to base practice.

7.1 Mean life expectancy in years, UK and India

	Males		Females	
	UK	**India**	**UK**	**India**
At birth	79.1	65.1	83.0	67.2
At 60 years	22.8	16.7	25.5	18.9
At 70 years	15.0	10.9	17.1	12.4
At 80 years	8.7	7.5	9.9	8.0

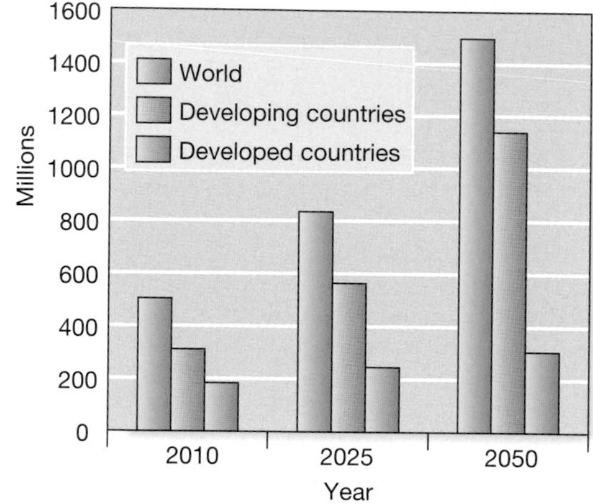

Fig. 7.1 Number of people aged 65 years and over projected in the world population.

DEMOGRAPHY

The demography of developed countries has changed rapidly in recent decades. In the UK, for example, the total population grew by 11% over the last 30 years, but the number of people aged over 65 years rose by 24%. The steepest rise occurred in those aged over 85 – from 600 000 in 1981 to 1.5 million in 2011 – and this number is projected to increase to 2.4 million by 2026, whilst the working-age population (20–64 years) is expected to grow by only 4% between 2011 and 2026. This will have a significant impact on the old-age dependency ratio, i.e. the number of people of working age for each person over retirement age. Young people support older members of the population directly (e.g. through living arrangements) and financially (e.g. through taxation and pension contributions), so the consequences of a reduced ratio are far-reaching. However, many older people support the younger population, through care of children and other older people.

Life expectancy in the developed world is now prolonged, even in old age (Box 7.1); women aged 80 years can expect to live for a further 10 years. However, rates of disability and chronic illness rise sharply with ageing and have a major impact on health and social services. In the UK, the reported prevalence of a chronic illness or disability sufficient to restrict daily activities is around 25% in those aged 50–64, but is 66% in men and 75% in women aged over 85.

Although the proportion of the population aged over 65 years is greater in developed countries, two-thirds of the world population of people aged over 65 live in developing countries at present, and this is projected to rise to 75% in 2025. The rate of population ageing is much faster in developing countries (Fig. 7.1) and so they have less time to adjust to its impact.

FUNCTIONAL ANATOMY AND PHYSIOLOGY

Biology of ageing

Ageing can be defined as a progressive accumulation through life of random molecular defects that build up within tissues and cells. Eventually, despite multiple repair and maintenance mechanisms, these result in age-related functional impairment of tissues and organs.

Many genes probably contribute to ageing, with those that determine durability and maintenance of somatic cell lines particularly important. However, genetic factors only account for around 25% of variance in human lifespan; nutritional and environmental factors determine the rest.

A major contribution to random molecular damage is made by reactive oxygen species produced during the metabolism of oxygen to produce cellular energy. These cause oxidative damage at a number of sites:

- *Nuclear chromosomal DNA*, causing mutations and deletions which ultimately lead to aberrant gene function and potential for malignancy.
- *Telomeres*, which are the protective end regions of chromosomes which shorten with each cell division

because telomerase (which copies the end of the 3′ strand of linear DNA in germ cells) is absent in somatic cells. When telomeres are sufficiently eroded, cells stop dividing. It has been suggested that telomeres represent a 'biological clock' which prevents uncontrolled cell division and cancer. Telomeres are particularly shortened in patients with premature ageing due to Werner's syndrome, in which DNA is damaged due to lack of a helicase.
- *Mitochondrial DNA and lipid peroxidation*, resulting in reduced cellular energy production and ultimately cell death.
- *Proteins* – e.g. those increasing formation of advanced glycosylation end-products from spontaneous reactions between proteins and sugars. These damage structure and function of the affected protein, which becomes resistant to breakdown.

The rate at which damage occurs is malleable and this is where the interplay with environment, particularly nutrition, takes place. There is evidence in some organisms that this interplay is mediated by insulin signalling pathways. Chronic inflammation also plays an important role, again in part by driving the production of reactive oxygen species.

Physiological changes of ageing

The physiological features of normal ageing have been identified by examining disease-free populations of older people, to separate the effects of pathology from those due to time alone. However, the fraction of older people who age without disease ultimately declines to very low levels, so that use of the term 'normal' becomes debatable. There is a marked increase in inter-individual variation in function with ageing; many physiological processes deteriorate substantially when measured across populations, but some individuals show little or no change. This heterogeneity is a hallmark of ageing, meaning that each person must be assessed individually and that one cannot unthinkingly apply the same management to all people of a certain age.

Although some genetic influences contribute to heterogeneity, environmental factors, such as poverty, nutrition, exercise, cigarette smoking and alcohol misuse, play a large part, and a healthy lifestyle should be encouraged even when old age has been reached.

The effects of ageing are usually not enough to interfere with organ function under normal conditions, but reserve capacity is significantly reduced. Some changes

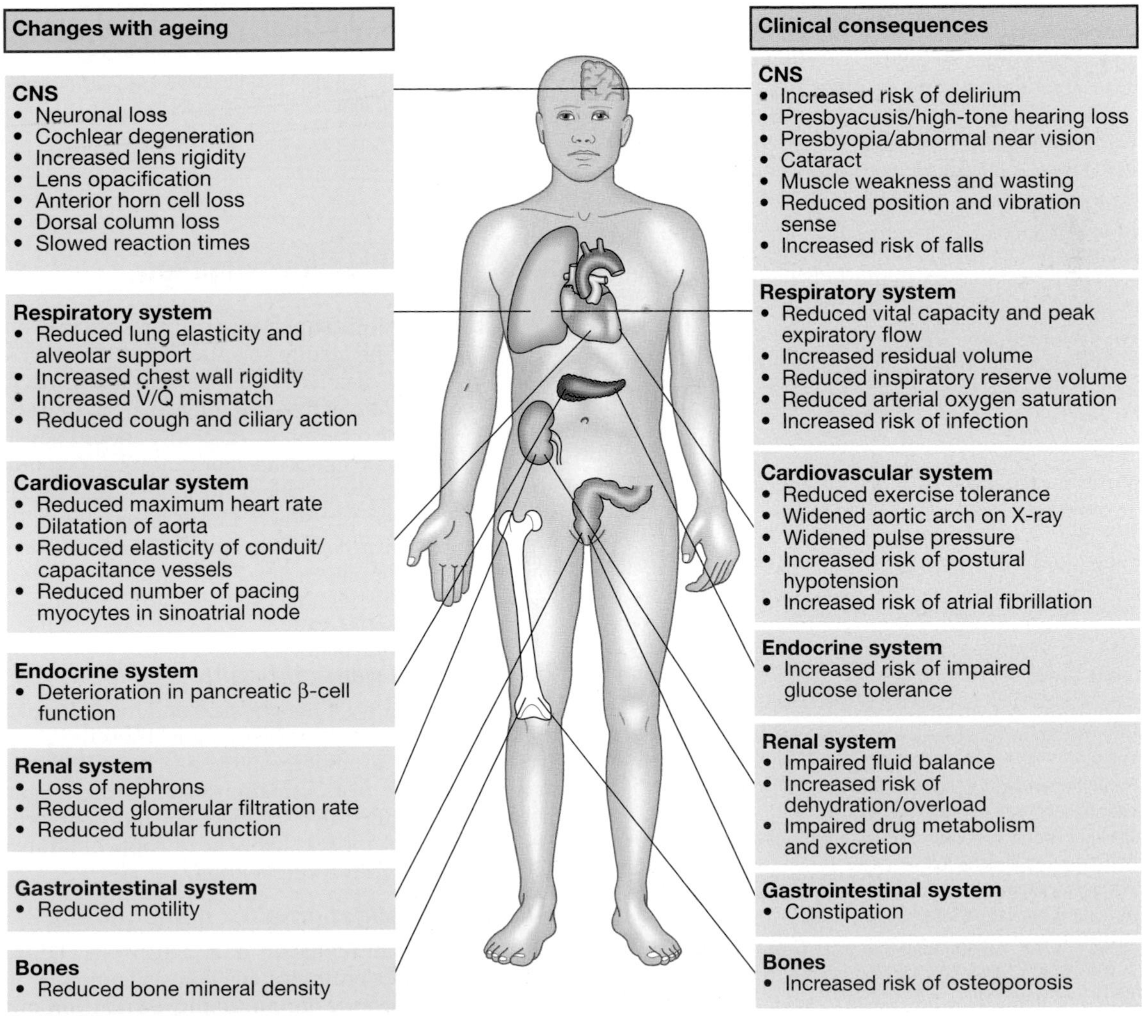

Fig. 7.2 Features and consequences of normal ageing.

of ageing, such as depigmentation of the hair, are of no clinical significance. Figure 7.2 shows many factors that are clinically important.

Frailty

Frailty is defined as the loss of an individual's ability to withstand minor stresses because the reserves in function of several organ systems are so severely reduced that even a trivial illness or adverse drug reaction may result in organ failure and death. The same stresses would cause little upset in a fit person of the same age.

It is important to understand the difference between 'disability', 'comorbidity' and 'frailty'. Disability indicates established loss of function (e.g. mobility; see Box 7.13, p. 176), while frailty indicates increased vulnerability to loss of function. Disability may arise from a single pathological event (such as a stroke) in an otherwise healthy individual. After recovery, function is largely stable and the patient may otherwise be in good health. When frailty and disability coexist, function deteriorates markedly even with minor illness, to the extent that the patient can no longer manage independently. Similarly, comorbidity (the number of diagnoses present) is not equivalent to frailty; it is quite possible to have several diagnoses without major impact on homeostatic reserve.

Unfortunately, the term 'frail' is often used rather vaguely, sometimes to justify a lack of adequate investigation and intervention in older people. However, it can be specifically identified by assessing function in a number of domains. Two main approaches to evaluating frailty exist: measurement of physiological function across a number of domains (e.g. the Fried Frailty score, Box 7.2), or a score based on the number of deficits or problems – for example, the Rockwood score.

Frail older people particularly benefit from a clinical approach that addresses both the precipitating acute illness and their underlying loss of reserves. It may be possible to prevent further loss of function through early intervention; for example, a frail woman with myocardial infarction will benefit from specific cardiac investigation and drug treatment, but may benefit even further from an exercise programme to improve musculoskeletal function, balance and aerobic capacity, with nutritional support to restore lost weight. Establishing a patient's level of frailty also helps inform decisions regarding further investigation and management, and the need for rehabilitation.

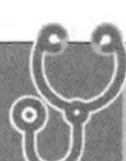

7.2 How to assess a Fried Frailty score

- Handgrip strength in bottom 20% of healthy elderly distribution*
- Walking speed in bottom 20% of healthy elderly distribution*
- Self-reported exhaustion
- Physically inactive
- At least 6 kg weight loss within 1 year

Patient is defined as frail if 3 or more factors are present.

*Varies between populations. Grip cutoff is 30 kg for men, 18 kg for women in US adults; 5 m walk time cutoff is 7 seconds in US adults for both sexes.

INVESTIGATIONS

Comprehensive geriatric assessment

Although not strictly an investigation, one of the most powerful tools in the management of older people is the Comprehensive Geriatric Assessment, which identifies all the relevant factors contributing to their presentation (p. 166). In frail patients with multiple pathology, it may be necessary to perform the assessment in stages to allow for their reduced stamina. The outcome should be a management plan that not only addresses the acute presenting problems, but also improves the patient's overall health and function (Box 7.3).

Comprehensive Geriatric Assessment is performed by a multidisciplinary team (p. 167). Such an approach was pioneered by Dr Marjory Warren at the West Middlesex Hospital in London in the 1930s; her comprehensive assessment and rehabilitation of supposedly incurable, long-term bedridden older people revolutionised the approach of the medical profession to older, frail people and laid the foundations for the modern specialty of geriatric medicine.

EBM 7.3 Comprehensive geriatric assessment

'Inpatient comprehensive geriatric assessment reduces short-term mortality and increases the chance of patients living at home in the long term.'

- Ellis G, Langhorne P. Br Med Bull 2005; 71: 45–59.

Decisions about investigation

Accurate diagnosis is important at all ages but frail older people may not be able to tolerate lengthy or invasive procedures, and diagnoses may be revealed for which patients could not withstand intensive or aggressive treatment. On the other hand, disability should never be dismissed as due to age alone. For example, it would be a mistake to supply a patient no longer able to climb stairs with a stair lift, when simple tests would have revealed osteoarthritis of a hip and vitamin D deficiency, for which appropriate treatment would have restored his or her strength. So how do doctors decide when and how far to investigate?

The patient's general health

Does this patient have the physical and mental capacity to tolerate the proposed investigation? Does he have the aerobic capacity to undergo bronchoscopy? Will confusion prevent her from remaining still in the magnetic resonance imaging (MRI) scanner? The more comorbidities a patient has, the less likely he or she will be able to withstand an invasive intervention.

Will the investigation alter management?

Would the patient be fit for, or benefit from, the treatment that would be indicated if investigation proved positive? The presence of comorbidity is more important than age itself in determining this. When a patient with severe heart failure and a previous disabling stroke presents with a suspicious mass lesion on chest X-ray, detailed investigation and staging may not be appropriate if he is not fit for surgery, radical radiotherapy or chemotherapy. On the other hand, if the same patient presented with dysphagia, investigation of the cause would be important, as he would be able to tolerate endoscopic treatment (for example, to palliate an obstructing oesophageal carcinoma).

The views of the patient and family

Older people may have strong views about the extent of investigation and the treatment they wish to receive, and these should be sought from the outset. If the patient wishes, the views of relatives can be taken into account. If the patient is not able to express a view or lacks the capacity to make decisions because of cognitive impairment or communication difficulties, then relatives' input becomes particularly helpful. They may be able to give information on views previously expressed by the patient or on what the patient would have wanted under the current circumstances. However, families should never be made to feel responsible for difficult decisions.

Advance directives

Advance directives or 'living wills' are statements made by adults at a time when they have the capacity to decide about the interventions they would refuse or accept in the future, should they no longer be able to make decisions or communicate them. An advance directive cannot authorise a doctor to do anything that is illegal and doctors are not bound to provide a specific treatment requested if, in their professional opinion, it is not clinically appropriate. However, any advance refusal of treatment, made when the patient was able to make decisions based on adequate information about their implications, is legally binding in the UK. It must be respected when it clearly applies to the patient's present circumstances and when there is no reason to believe that the patient has changed his or her mind.

PRESENTING PROBLEMS IN GERIATRIC MEDICINE

Characteristics of presenting problems in old age

Problem-based practice is central to geriatric medicine. Most problems are multifactorial and there is rarely a single unifying diagnosis. All contributing factors have to be taken into account and attention to detail is paramount. Two patients who share the same presenting problem may have completely disparate diagnoses. A wide knowledge of adult medicine is required, as disease in any, and often many, of the organ systems has to be managed at the same time. There are a number of features that are particular to older patients.

Late presentation

Many people (of all ages) accept ill health as a consequence of ageing and may tolerate symptoms for lengthy periods before seeking medical advice. Comorbidities may also contribute to late presentation; in a patient whose mobility is limited by stroke, angina may only present when coronary artery disease is advanced, as the patient has been unable to exercise sufficiently to cause symptoms at an earlier stage.

Atypical presentation

Infection may present with delirium and without clinical pointers to the organ system affected. Stroke may present with falls rather than symptoms of focal weakness. Myocardial infarction may present as weakness and fatigue, without the chest pain or dyspnoea. The reasons for these atypical presentations are not always easy to establish. Perception of pain is altered in old age, which may explain why myocardial infarction presents in other ways. The pyretic response is blunted in old age so that infection may not be obvious at first. Cognitive impairment may limit the patient's ability to give a history of classical symptoms.

Acute illness and changes in function

Atypical presentations in frail elderly patients include 'failure to cope', 'found on floor', 'confusion' and 'off feet', but these are *not* diagnoses. The possibility that an acute illness has been the precipitant must always be considered. To establish whether the patient's current status is a change from his or her usual level of function, it helps to ask a relative or carer (by phone if necessary). Investigations aimed at uncovering an acute illness will not be fruitful in a patient whose function has been deteriorating over several months, but are important if function has suddenly changed.

Multiple pathology

Presentations in older patients have a more diverse differential diagnosis because multiple pathology is so common. There are frequently a number of causes for any single problem, and adverse effects from medication often contribute. A patient may fall because of osteoarthritis of the knees, postural hypotension due to diuretic therapy for hypertension, and poor vision due to cataracts. All these factors have to be addressed to prevent further falls, and this principle holds true for most of the common presenting problems in old age.

Approach to presenting problems in old age

For the sake of clarity, the common presenting problems are described individually, but in real life, older patients often present with several at the same time, particularly confusion, incontinence and falls. These share some underlying causes and may precipitate each other.

The approach to most presenting problems in old age can be summarised as follows:

- *Obtain a collateral history.* Find out the patient's usual status (e.g. mobility, cognitive state) from a relative or carer. Call these people by phone if they are not present.
- *Check all medication.* Have there been any recent changes?
- *Search for and treat any acute illness.* See Box 7.4.
- *Identify and reverse predisposing risk factors.* These depend on the presenting problem.

7.4 Screening investigations for acute illness

- Full blood count
- Urea and electrolytes, liver function tests, calcium and glucose
- Chest X-ray
- Electrocardiogram
- C-reactive protein: useful marker for occult infection or inflammatory disease
- Blood cultures if pyrexial

Falls

Around 30% of those over 65 years of age fall each year, this figure rising to more than 40% in those aged over 80. Although only 10–15% of falls result in serious injury, they are the cause of more than 90% of hip fractures in this age group, compounded by the rising prevalence of osteoporosis. Falls also lead to loss of confidence and fear, and are frequently the 'final straw' that makes an older person decide to move to institutional care. Management will vary according to the underlying cause.

Acute illness

Falls are one of the classical atypical presentations of acute illness in frail people. The reduced reserves in older people's neurological function mean that they are less able to maintain their balance when challenged by an acute illness. Suspicion should be high when falls have suddenly occurred over a period of a few days. Common underlying illnesses include infection, stroke, metabolic disturbance and heart failure. Thorough examination and investigation are required (see Box 7.4). It is also important to establish whether any drug which precipitates falls, such as a psychotropic or hypotensive agent, has been started recently. Once the underlying acute illness has been treated, falls may stop.

Blackouts

A proportion of older people who 'fall' have, in fact, had a syncopal episode. A collateral history from a witness is of utmost importance in anyone falling over; people who lose consciousness do not always remember having done so. If loss of consciousness is suggested by the patient or witness, it is important to perform appropriate investigations (pp. 554 and 1157).

Mechanical and recurrent falls

Amongst patients who have tripped or are uncertain how they fell, those who have fallen more than once in the past year and those who are unsteady during a 'get up and go' test (p. 167) require further assessment. Patients with recurrent falls are commonly frail, with multiple medical problems and chronic disabilities. Obviously, such patients may present with a fall resulting from an acute illness or syncope, but they will remain at risk of further falls even when the acute illness has resolved. The risk factors for falls (Box 7.5) should be considered. If problems are identified with muscle strength, balance, vision or cognitive function, the causes of these must be identified by specific investigation, and treatment commenced if appropriate. Careful assessment of the patient's gait may provide important clues to an underlying diagnosis (Box 7.6). Common pathologies identified include cerebrovascular disease (Ch. 27), Parkinson's disease (p. 1195) and osteoarthritis of weight-bearing joints (p. 1081). Osteoporosis risk factors should also be sought and dual energy X-ray absorptiometry (DEXA) bone density scanning considered in all older patients who have recurrent falls, particularly if they have already sustained a fracture (p. 1065).

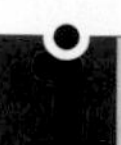

7.5 Risk factors for falls

- Muscle weakness
- History of falls
- Gait or balance abnormality
- Use of a walking aid
- Visual impairment
- Arthritis
- Impaired activities of daily living
- Depression
- Cognitive impairment
- Age over 80 years
- Psychotropic medication

7.6 Abnormal gaits and probable causes

Gait abnormality	Probable cause
Antalgic	Arthropathy
Waddling	Proximal myopathy
Stamping	Sensory neuropathy
Foot drop	Peripheral neuropathy or radiculopathy
Ataxic	Sensory neuropathy or cerebellar disease
Shuffling/festination	Parkinson's disease
Marche à petits pas	Small-vessel cerebrovascular disease
Hemiplegic	Cerebral hemisphere lesion
Apraxic	Bilateral hemisphere lesions

Prevention of falls and fractures

Falls can be prevented by multiple risk factor intervention (Box 7.7). The most effective intervention is balance and strength training by physiotherapists; an alternative with good evidence is tai chi training. An assessment of the patient's home environment for hazards should be undertaken by an occupational therapist, who may also provide personal alarms so that patients can summon help, should they fall again. Rationalising psychotropic medication may help to reduce sedation, although many older patients are reluctant to stop hypnotics. If postural hypotension is present (defined as a drop in blood pressure of > 20 mmHg systolic or > 10 mmHg diastolic pressure on standing from supine), reducing or stopping hypotensive drugs may be helpful. Evidence supporting the efficacy of other interventions for postural hypotension is lacking, but drugs, including fludrocortisone and midodrine, are sometimes used to try to improve dizziness on standing. Simple interventions, such as new glasses to correct visual acuity, and podiatry, can also have a significant impact on function in those who fall.

If osteoporosis is diagnosed, specific drug therapy should be commenced (p. 1122). In patients in institutional care, calcium and vitamin D_3 administration has

EBM 7.7 Evidence-based interventions to prevent falls in older people

- Individualised or group strength and balance training, or tai chi
- Rationalisation of medication, especially psychotropic drugs
- Correction of visual impairment, particularly cataract extraction
- Home environmental hazard assessment and safety education
- Calcium and vitamin D supplementation for those in institutional care

- Gillespie LD, et al. Interventions for preventing falls in older people living in the community. Cochrane Database of Systematic Reviews, 2012, Art. no. CD007146.
- Cameron ID, et al. Interventions for preventing falls in older people in care facilities and hospitals. Cochrane Database of Systematic Reviews, 2010, Art. no. CD005465.

been shown to reduce both falls and fracture rates, through effects on both bone mineral density and neuromuscular function. They are not effective in those with osteoporosis living in the community, in whom bisphosphonates are first-line therapy.

In the UK, government policy and National Institute for Health and Clinical Excellence guidelines (www.nice.org.uk) for falls prevention have led to the development of specific Falls and Fracture Prevention Services in many parts of the country.

Dizziness

Dizziness is very common, affecting at least 30% of those aged over 65 years in community surveys. Dizziness can be disabling in its own right and is also a risk factor for falls. Acute dizziness is relatively straightforward and common causes include:

- hypotension due to arrhythmia, myocardial infarction, gastrointestinal bleed or pulmonary embolism
- onset of posterior fossa stroke
- vestibular neuronitis.

Although older people more commonly present with recurrent dizzy spells and often find it difficult to describe the sensation they experience, the most effective way of establishing the cause(s) of the problem is nevertheless to determine which of the following is predominant (even if more than one is present):

- *lightheadedness*, suggestive of reduced cerebral perfusion
- *vertigo*, suggestive of labyrinthine or brainstem disease (p. 1167)
- *unsteadiness/poor balance*, suggestive of joint or neurological disease.

In lightheaded patients, structural cardiac disease (such as aortic stenosis) and arrhythmia must be considered, but disorders of autonomic cardiovascular control, such as vasovagal syndrome and postural hypotension, are the most common causes in old age. Hypotensive medication may exacerbate these. Further investigation and treatment are described on page 1157.

Vertigo in older patients is most commonly due to benign positional vertigo (p. 1158), but if other brainstem symptoms or signs are present, MRI of the brain is required to exclude a cerebello-pontine angle lesion.

Delirium

Delirium is a syndrome of transient, reversible cognitive dysfunction. It is very common, affecting up to 30% of older hospital inpatients, either at admission or during their hospital stay. It is associated with high rates of mortality, complication and institutionalisation, and with longer lengths of stay. Risk factors are shown in Box 7.8. Its pathophysiology is unclear; it may in part be due to the effect of increased cortisol release in acute illness, or it may reflect a sensitivity of cholinergic neurotransmission to toxic insults. Older terms for delirium, e.g. acute confusion or toxic confusional state, lack diagnostic precision and should be avoided.

Clinical assessment

Assessment has two main goals: firstly, to establish the diagnosis of delirium; and secondly, to identify all of the reversible precipitating factors to allow optimal treatment.

Delirium may be missed unless routine cognitive testing with an Abbreviated Mental Test, CLOX test or mini-mental state examination (MMSE; p. 234) is performed. Delirium often occurs in patients with dementia, and a history from a relative or carer about the onset and course of confusion is needed to distinguish acute from chronic features. The Confusion Assessment Method (Box 7.9) is a useful tool to diagnose delirium accurately and to differentiate the condition from dementia.

More than one of the precipitating causes of delirium (Fig. 7.3) is often present. Symptoms suggestive of a physical illness, such as an infection or stroke, should be elicited. An accurate drug and alcohol history is required, especially to ascertain whether any drugs have been recently stopped or started.

A full physical examination should be performed, noting in particular:

7.8 Risk factors for delirium

Predisposing factors	
• Old age • Dementia • Frailty	• Sensory impairment • Polypharmacy • Renal impairment
Precipitating factors	
• Intercurrent illness • Surgery • Change of environment or ward • Sensory deprivation (e.g. darkness) or overload (e.g. noise) • Medications (e.g. opioids, psychotropics)	• Dehydration • Pain • Constipation • Urinary catheterisation • Acute urinary retention • Hypoxia • Fever • Alcohol withdrawal

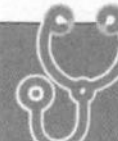

7.9 How to make a diagnosis of delirium: the Confusion Assessment Method (CAM)

Talk to the patient and assess:
• *Cognition* (e.g. MMSE, p. 234). A normal score makes delirium unlikely. • *Inattention.* Can the patient converse with you? If in doubt, give 6–7 digits (between 1 and 9) to remember and repeat back to you; failure suggests inattention. • *Conscious level.* Alert, hyper-alert or drowsy? • *Thinking.* Is speech rambling? Does it make sense? Is the patient hallucinating?
Obtain a collateral history (e.g. from carer, nurse or general practitioner):
• What is the patient normally like? • Has there been a sudden deterioration, e.g. over a few days? • Does confusion fluctuate through the day?
Consider the diagnosis. Delirium is present if there is:
Acute deterioration in cognition, which fluctuates over time **AND** Evidence of inattention **WITH EITHER** Evidence of disorganised thinking **OR** Altered level of consciousness (either drowsy/stupor/coma *or* hyper-alert/agitated/irritable)

- pyrexia and any signs of infection in the chest, skin, urine or abdomen
- oxygen saturation
- signs of alcohol withdrawal, such as tremor or sweating
- any neurological signs.

A range of investigations are needed to identify the common causes (see Fig. 7.3).

Management

Specific treatment of all of the underlying causes must be commenced as quickly as possible. However, the symptoms of delirium also require specific management. To minimise ongoing confusion and disorientation, the environment should be kept well lit and not unduly noisy, with the patient's spectacles and hearing aids in place. Good nursing is needed to preserve orientation, prevent pressure sores and falls, and maintain hydration, nutrition and continence.

The use of sedatives should be kept to a minimum, as they can precipitate delirium. In any case, many confused patients are lethargic and apathetic rather than agitated. Sedation is very much a last resort, and is appropriate only if patients' behaviour is endangering

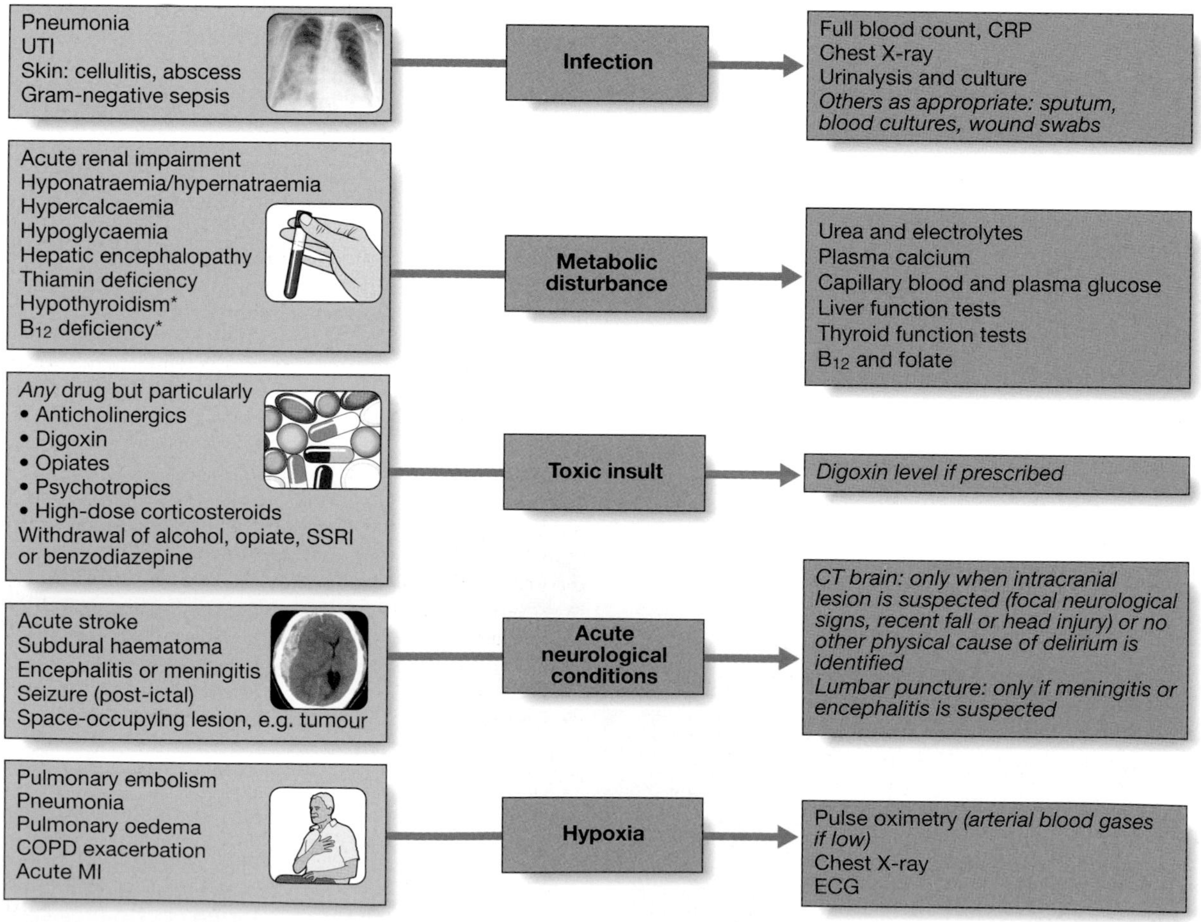

Causes	Category	Investigations
Pneumonia UTI Skin: cellulitis, abscess Gram-negative sepsis	**Infection**	Full blood count, CRP Chest X-ray Urinalysis and culture *Others as appropriate: sputum, blood cultures, wound swabs*
Acute renal impairment Hyponatraemia/hypernatraemia Hypercalcaemia Hypoglycaemia Hepatic encephalopathy Thiamin deficiency Hypothyroidism* B_{12} deficiency*	**Metabolic disturbance**	Urea and electrolytes Plasma calcium Capillary blood and plasma glucose Liver function tests Thyroid function tests B_{12} and folate
Any drug but particularly • Anticholinergics • Digoxin • Opiates • Psychotropics • High-dose corticosteroids Withdrawal of alcohol, opiate, SSRI or benzodiazepine	**Toxic insult**	*Digoxin level if prescribed*
Acute stroke Subdural haematoma Encephalitis or meningitis Seizure (post-ictal) Space-occupying lesion, e.g. tumour	**Acute neurological conditions**	*CT brain: only when intracranial lesion is suspected (focal neurological signs, recent fall or head injury) or no other physical cause of delirium is identified* *Lumbar puncture: only if meningitis or encephalitis is suspected*
Pulmonary embolism Pneumonia Pulmonary oedema COPD exacerbation Acute MI	**Hypoxia**	Pulse oximetry *(arterial blood gases if low)* Chest X-ray ECG

Fig. 7.3 Common causes and investigation of delirium. All investigations are performed routinely, except those in italics. *Tend to present over weeks to months rather than hours to days. The chest X-ray shows consolidation in pneumonia. The CT scan shows a cerebral haemorrhage. (COPD = chronic obstructive pulmonary disease; CRP = C-reactive protein; MI = myocardial infarction; SSRI = selective serotonin re-uptake inhibitor; UTI = urinary tract infection)

themselves or others. Small doses of haloperidol (0.5 mg twice daily) are tried orally first, and the dose increased if the patient fails to respond. Sedation can be given intramuscularly only if absolutely necessary. In those with alcohol withdrawal or Lewy body dementia (p. 252), a reducing course of a benzodiazepine should be prescribed. In other cases, benzodiazepines should be avoided, as they may prolong delirium.

The resolution of delirium in old age may be slow and incomplete. Many patients fail to recover to their pre-morbid level of cognition. Delirium may be the first presentation of an underlying dementia and is also a risk factor for subsequent dementia.

Urinary incontinence

Urinary incontinence is defined as the involuntary loss of urine and comes to medical attention when sufficiently severe to cause a social or hygiene problem. It occurs in all age groups but becomes more prevalent in old age, affecting about 15% of women and 10% of men aged over 65. It may lead to skin damage if severe and can be socially restricting. While age-dependent changes in the lower urinary tract predispose older people to incontinence, it is not an inevitable consequence of ageing and requires investigation and appropriate treatment. Urinary incontinence is frequently precipitated by acute illness in old age and is commonly multifactorial (Fig. 7.4).

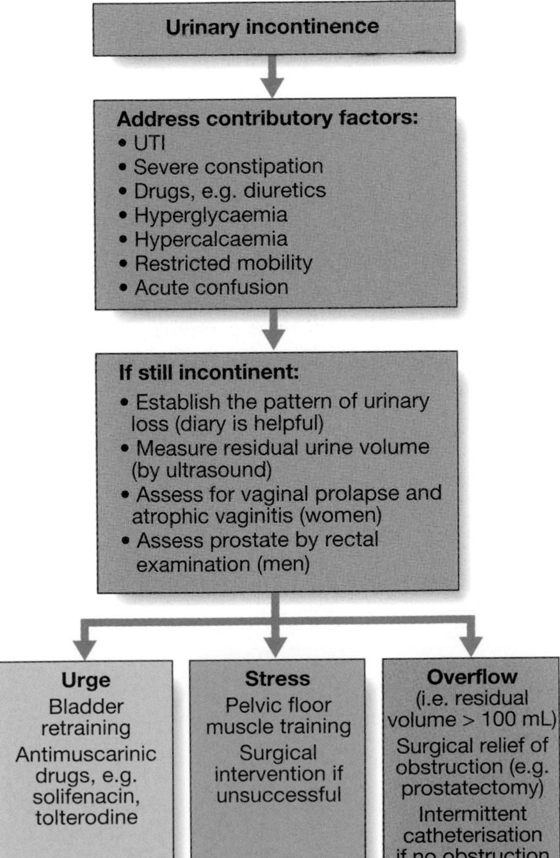

Fig. 7.4 Assessment and management of urinary incontinence in old age. See also page 472 and NICE guideline on the Management of Incontinence in Women: www.nice.org.uk. (UTI = urinary tract infection)

Initial management is to identify and address contributory factors. If incontinence fails to resolve, further diagnosis and management should be pursued, as described on page 472.

- *Urge incontinence* is usually due to detrusor over-activity and results in urgency and frequency.
- *Stress incontinence* is almost exclusive to women and is due to weakness of the pelvic floor muscles, which allows leakage of urine when intra-abdominal pressure rises, e.g. on coughing. It may be compounded by atrophic vaginitis, associated with oestrogen deficiency in old age, which can be treated with oestrogen pessaries.
- *Overflow incontinence* is most commonly seen in elderly men with prostatic enlargement, which obstructs bladder outflow.

In patients with severe stroke disease or dementia, treatment may be ineffective, as frontal cortical inhibitory signals to bladder emptying are lost. A timed/prompted toileting programme may help. Other than in overflow incontinence, urinary catheterisation should never be viewed as first-line management, but may be required as a final resort if the perineal skin is at risk of breakdown or quality of life is affected.

Adverse drug reactions

Adverse drug reactions (ADRs) and the effects of drug interactions are discussed on pages 24–28. They may result in symptoms, abnormal physical signs and altered laboratory test results (Box 7.10). ADRs are the cause of around 5% of all hospital admissions but account for up to 20% of admissions in those aged over 65. This is partly because older people receive many more prescribed drugs than younger people. Polypharmacy has been defined as the use of four or more drugs; this should be avoided if possible, but is not always inappropriate because many conditions, such as hypertension and heart failure, necessitate the use of several drugs, and older people may have several coexisting medical problems (Box 7.11). However, the more drugs that are taken, the greater the risk of an ADR. This risk is compounded by age-related changes in pharmacodynamic and pharmacokinetic factors (pp. 18–21), and by impaired homeostatic mechanisms, such as baroreceptor responses, plasma volume and electrolyte control. Older people are thus especially sensitive to drugs that can cause postural hypotension or volume depletion (see Box 7.10). Non-adherence to drug therapy also rises with the number of drugs prescribed.

The clinical presentations of ADRs are diverse, so for *any* presenting problem in old age the possibility that the patient's medication is a contributory factor should *always* be considered. Failure to recognise this may lead to the use of a further drug to treat the problem, making matters worse, when the better course would be to stop or reduce the dose of the offending drug or to find an alternative.

7.10 Common adverse drug reactions in old age

Drug class	Adverse reaction
NSAIDs	Gastrointestinal bleeding and peptic ulceration Renal impairment
Diuretics	Renal impairment, electrolyte disturbance Gout Hypotension, postural hypotension
Warfarin	Bleeding
ACE inhibitors	Renal impairment, electrolyte disturbance Hypotension, postural hypotension
β-blockers	Bradycardia, heart block Hypotension, postural hypotension
Opiates	Constipation, vomiting Delirium Urinary retention
Antidepressants	Delirium Hyponatraemia (SSRIs) Hypotension, postural hypotension Falls
Benzodiazepines	Delirium Falls
Anticholinergics	Delirium Urinary retention Constipation

(ACE = angiotensin-converting enzyme; NSAID = non-steroidal anti-inflammatory drug; SSRI = selective serotonin re-uptake inhibitor)

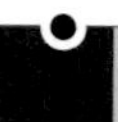

7.11 Factors leading to polypharmacy in old age

- Multiple pathology
- Poor patient education (see Box 2.20, p. 35)
- Lack of routine review of all medications
- Patient expectations of prescribing
- Over-use of drug interventions by doctors
- Attendance at multiple specialist clinics
- Poor communication between specialists

Regular review of medications is important in preventing ADRs. The patient or carer should be asked to bring all medication for review rather than the doctor relying on previous records. Those drugs that are no longer needed or are contraindicated can be discontinued.

Other problems in old age

There is a vast range of other presenting problems in older people and they present to many medical specialties. End-of-life care is an important facet of clinical practice in old age and is discussed on page 290. Relevant sections in other chapters are referenced in Box 7.12.

Within each chapter, 'In Old Age' boxes highlight the areas in which presentation or management differs from that in younger individuals. These are listed on page 178.

7.12 Other presenting problems in old age

• Hypothermia	p. 104
• Under-nutrition	p. 120
• Dementia	p. 250
• Infection	pp. 296 and 306
• Fluid balance problems	p. 439
• Heart failure	p. 546
• Hypertension	p. 606
• Dizziness and blackouts	pp. 554 and 1157
• Atrial fibrillation	p. 564
• Diabetes mellitus	p. 806
• Peptic ulceration	p. 872
• Anaemia	p. 1001
• Painful joints	p. 1069
• Bone disease and fracture	pp. 1120 and 1071
• Stroke	p. 1231

REHABILITATION

Rehabilitation aims to improve the ability of people of all ages to perform day-to-day activities, and to restore their physical, mental and social capabilities as far as possible. Acute illness in older people is often associated with loss of their usual ability to walk or care for themselves, and common disabling conditions such as stroke, fractured neck of femur, arthritis and cardiorespiratory disease become increasingly prevalent with advancing age.

Disability is an interaction between factors intrinsic to the individual and the context in which they live, and both medical and social interventions are needed to address this (Box 7.13). Doctors tend to focus on health conditions and impairments, but patients are more concerned with the effect on their activities and ability to participate in everyday life.

7.13 International classification of functioning and disability

Factor	Intervention required
Health condition Underlying disease, e.g. stroke, osteoarthritis	Medical or surgical treatment
Impairment Symptoms or signs of the condition, e.g. hemiparesis, visual loss	Medical or surgical treatment
Activity limitation Resultant loss of function, e.g. walking, dressing	Rehabilitation, assistance, aids
Participation restriction Resultant loss of social function, e.g. cooking, shopping	Adapted accommodation Social services

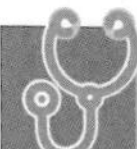

7.14 How to assess rehabilitation needs using the Modified Barthel Index (20-point version)

Mobility
Independent = 3 Needs help = 2 Wheelchair independent = 1 Immobile = 0
Stairs
Independent = 2 Needs help = 1 Unable = 0
Transfers (e.g. from bed to chair)
Independent = 3 Needs minor help = 2 Needs major help = 1 Unable = 0
Bladder
Continent = 2 Occasional incontinence = 1 Incontinent = 0
Bowels
Continent = 2 Occasional incontinence = 1 Incontinent = 0
Grooming
Independent = 1 Needs help = 0
Toilet use
Independent = 2 Needs help = 1 Unable = 0
Feeding
Independent = 2 Needs help = 1 Unable = 0
Dressing
Independent = 2 Needs some help = 1 Completely dependent = 0
Bathing
Independent = 1 Needs help = 0
The total score reflects the degree of dependency; scores of 14 and above are usually consistent with living in the community; scores below 10 suggest the patient is heavily dependent on carers.

The rehabilitation process

Rehabilitation is a problem-solving process focused on improving the patient's physical, psychological and social function. It entails:

- *Assessment.* The nature and extent of the patient's problems can be identified using the framework in Box 7.13. Specific assessment scales, such as the Elderly Mobility Scale or Barthel Index of Activities of Daily Living (Box 7.14), are useful to quantify components of disability, but additional assessment is needed to determine the underlying causes or the interventions required in individual patients.
- *Goal-setting.* Goals should be specific to the patient's problems, realistic, and agreed between the patient and the rehabilitation team.
- *Intervention.* This includes the active treatments needed to achieve the established goals and to maintain the patient's health and quality of life. Interventions include hands-on treatment by therapists using a functional, task-orientated approach to improve day-to-day activities, and also psychological support and education. The emphasis on the type of intervention will be individualised, according to the patient's disabilities, psychological status and progress. The patient and carer(s) must be active participants.
- *Re-assessment.* There is ongoing re-evaluation of the patient's function and progress towards the goals by the rehabilitation team, the patient and the carer. Interventions may be modified as a result.

Multidisciplinary team working

The core rehabilitation team includes all members of the multidisciplinary team (p. 167). Others may be involved, e.g. audiometry to correct hearing impairment, podiatry for foot problems, and orthotics where a prosthesis or splinting is required. Good communication and mutual respect are essential. Regular team meetings allow sharing of assessments, agreement of rehabilitation goals and interventions, evaluation of progress and planning for the patient's discharge home. Rehabilitation is *not* when the doctor orders 'physio' or 'a home visit', and takes no further role.

Rehabilitation outcomes

There is evidence that rehabilitation improves functional outcomes in older people following acute illness, stroke and hip fracture. It also reduces mortality after stroke and hip fracture. These benefits accrue from complex multi-component interventions, but occupational therapy to improve personal ADLs and individualised exercise interventions have now been shown to be effective in improving functional outcome in their own right.

Further information and acknowledgements

Websites

http://profane.co *Prevention of Falls Network Earth: focuses on the prevention of falls and improvement of postural stability in older people.*

www.americangeriatrics.org *American Geriatrics Society. Education, careers vignettes from geriatricians, advocacy and clinical guidelines.*

www.bgs.org.uk *British Geriatrics Society: useful publications on management of common problems in older people and links to other relevant websites.*

www.eugms.org *European Union Geriatric Medicine Society. Research, position papers and educational resources.*

www.iagg.info *International Association of Gerontology and Geriatrics. Promoting care of older people and the science of gerontology globally; research, policy and educational resources.*

www.knowledge.scot.nhs.uk/effectiveolderpeoplecare.aspx *Collates and summarises the Cochrane evidence for best practice in the health care and rehabilitation of frail older people.*

Figure acknowledgements

Page 166 insets (*Wasted hand, kyphosis*) Afzal Mir M. Atlas of clinical diagnosis. 2nd edn. Edinburgh: Saunders; 2003; copyright Elsevier; (*Senile purpura*) Forbes CD, Jackson WF. Clinical medicine. 3rd edn. Edinburgh: Mosby; 2004 (p. 438, Fig. 10.101); copyright Elsevier; (*Venous ulceration*) Giovanni Mosti, Clinics in Plastic Surgery, 2012, 39(3): 269–280, Figure 1; copyright © 2012 Elsevier Inc.; all reproduced with permission.

7.15 Index of 'In Old Age' boxes

Environmental and nutritional factors in disease

- Environmental factors in disease p. 102
- Thermoregulation p. 104
- Energy balance p. 122
- Vitamin deficiency p. 127

Infectious diseases

- Problems with antimicrobial therapy p. 154
- Fever p. 296
- Infectious diarrhoea p. 306

Clinical biochemistry and metabolism

- Hyponatraemia and hypernatraemia p. 439
- Management of hyperlipidaemia p. 458

Kidney and urinary tract disease

- Incontinence p. 473
- Acute kidney injury p. 483
- Renal replacement therapy p. 491
- Urinary infection p. 512

Cardiovascular disease

- Congestive cardiac failure p. 551
- Atrial fibrillation p. 566
- Angina p. 595
- Myocardial infarction p. 599
- Atherosclerotic vascular disease p. 602
- Hypertension p. 610
- Aortic stenosis p. 622
- Endocarditis p. 626

Respiratory disease

- Respiratory function p. 648
- Obstructive pulmonary disease p. 677
- Respiratory infection p. 686
- Interstitial lung disease p. 714
- Thromboembolic disease p. 724
- Pleural disease p. 731

Endocrine disease

- The thyroid gland p. 755
- Gonadal function p. 766
- The parathyroid glands p. 770
- Glucocorticoids p. 779
- Spontaneous hypoglycaemia p. 784
- The pituitary and hypothalamus p. 795

Diabetes mellitus

- Diagnosis of diabetes mellitus p. 806
- Diabetes management p. 828

Alimentary tract and pancreatic disease

- Endoscopy p. 850
- Acute abdominal pain p. 863
- Oral health p. 864
- Gastro-oesophageal reflux disease p. 868
- Peptic ulcer disease p. 875
- Malabsorption p. 883
- Constipation p. 918

Liver and biliary tract disease

- Liver disease p. 980
- Gallbladder disease p. 988

Blood disease

- Haematological investigations p. 1001
- Anaemia p. 1034
- Haematological malignancy p. 1047
- Haemostasis and thrombosis p. 1056

Rheumatology and bone disease

- Use of oral NSAID p. 1079
- Osteoarthritis p. 1085
- Gout p. 1090
- Joint and bone infection p. 1094
- Osteoporosis p. 1124

Neurological disease

- Neurological examination p. 1139
- Dizziness p. 1158
- Epilepsy p. 1185

Other

- Prescribing p. 36
- Genetic disease and counselling p. 64
- Immune senescence p. 82
- The critically ill older patient p. 204
- Poisoning p. 208
- Medical psychiatry p. 238
- Cancer p. 271
- HIV infection p. 410
- Skin changes p. 1254

G.R. Nimmo
T. Walsh

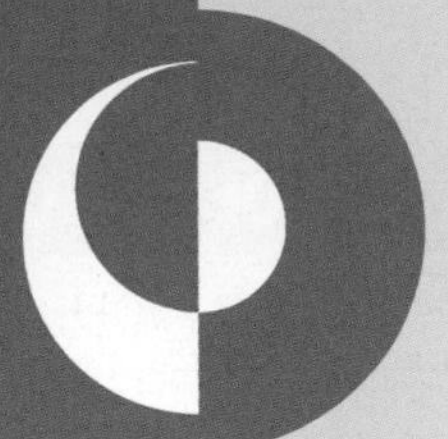

Critical illness 8

Clinical examination of the critically ill patient 180

Physiology of critical illness 182
- Oxygen transport 182
- Cardiovascular component of oxygen delivery: flow 182
- Oxygenation component of oxygen delivery: content 183
- Oxygen consumption 184
- Relationship between oxygen consumption and delivery 184
- Pathophysiology of the inflammatory response 184

Monitoring 185
- Monitoring the circulation 185
- Monitoring respiratory function 187

Recognition of critical illness 188
- Assessment and initial resuscitation of the critically ill patient 188
- Clinical decision-making and referral to critical care 189

Presenting problems/Management of major organ failure 190
- Circulatory failure: 'shock' 190
  - Circulatory support 190
- Respiratory failure and acute respiratory distress syndrome 191
  - Respiratory support 193
- Acute kidney injury 197
  - Renal support 197
- Gastrointestinal and hepatic disturbance 198
  - Gastrointestinal and hepatic support 198
- Neurological failure (coma) 198
  - Neurological support 199
  - Neurological complications in intensive care 199
- Sepsis 200
  - Management 201
- Disseminated intravascular coagulation 201

General principles of critical care management 201
- Daily clinical management in the ICU 202
- Sedation and analgesia 202

Discharge from intensive care 203
- Withdrawal of intensive support 203
- Brainstem death 203

Outcome of intensive care 204
- Scoring systems 204

CLINICAL EXAMINATION OF THE CRITICALLY ILL PATIENT

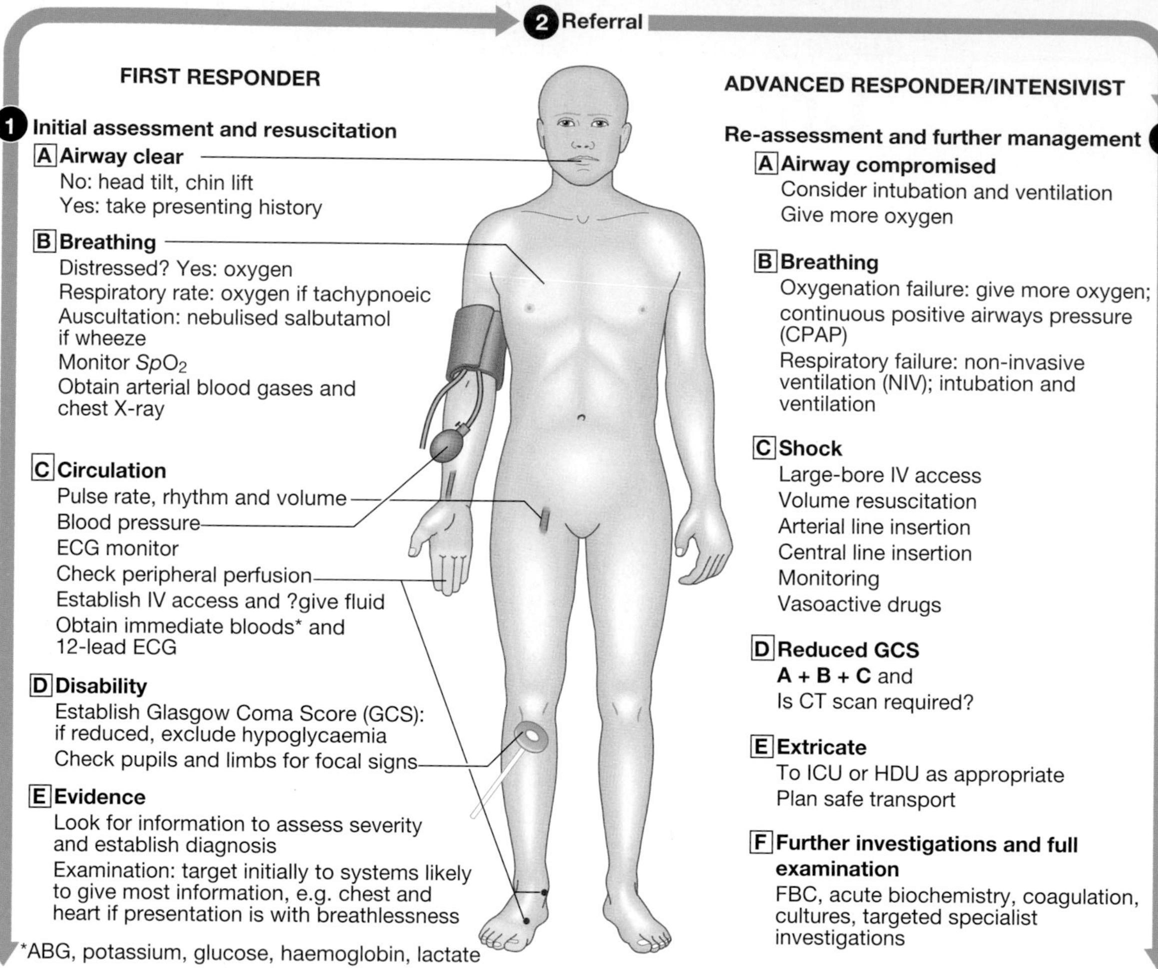

RECOGNISING THE CRITICALLY ILL PATIENT

Respiratory signs

- Respiratory arrest
- Threatened or obstructed airway
- Stridor, intercostal recession, paradoxical breathing (seesaw pattern)
- Respiratory rate < 8 or > 35/min
- Respiratory distress: use of accessory muscles; unable to speak in complete sentences
- SpO_2 < 90% on high-concentration oxygen
- Rising $PaCO_2$ > 7 kPa (52.5 mmHg) or > 2 kPa (> 15 mmHg) above 'normal' with acidosis

Cardiovascular signs

- Cardiac arrest
- Pulse rate < 40 or > 140 bpm
- Systolic blood pressure < 100 mmHg
- Poor peripheral perfusion
- Evidence of inadequate oxygen delivery
  Metabolic acidosis
  Hyperlactataemia
- Poor response to volume resuscitation
- Oliguria < 0.5 mL/kg/hr (check urea, creatinine, K^+)

Neurological signs

- Threatened or obstructed airway
- Absent gag or cough reflex
- Failure to maintain normal PaO_2 and $PaCO_2$
- Failure to obey commands
- GCS < 10
- Sudden fall in level of consciousness (GCS by > 2 points)
- Repeated or prolonged seizures

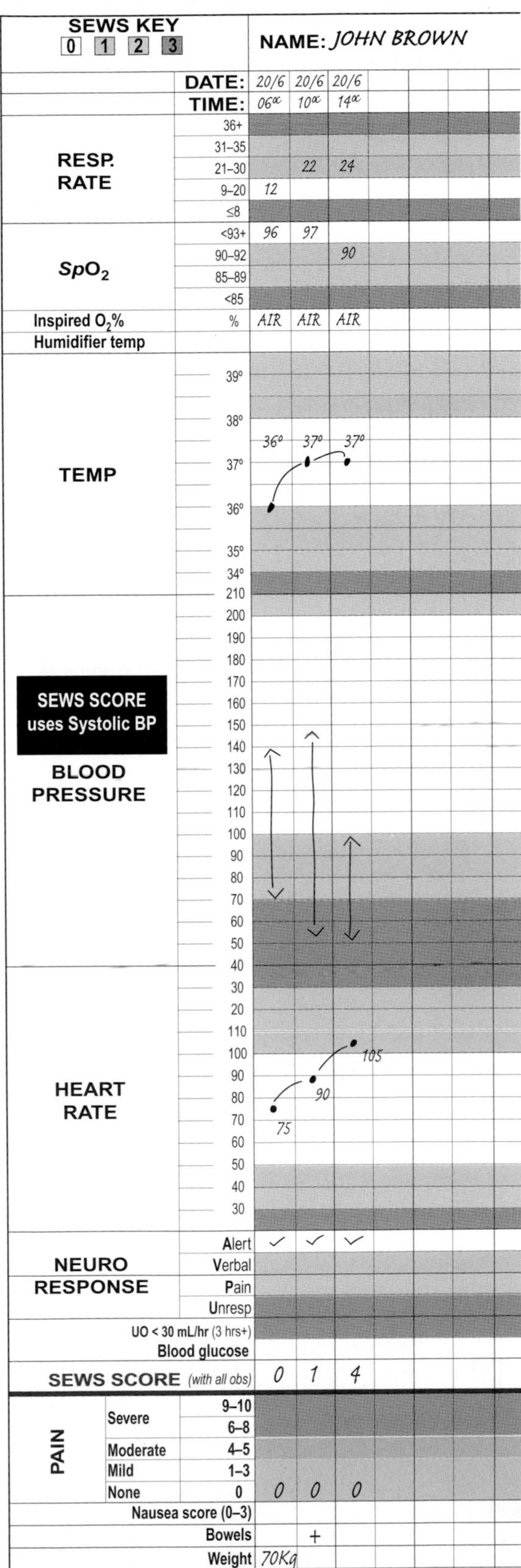

Standard Early Warning System (SEWS) chart. (UO = urine output)

Recognition of critical illness: early warning scores

- Record standard observations:
  - Respiratory rate
  - SpO_2
  - Temperature
  - Blood pressure (BP)
  - Heart rate
  - Neurological response
- Note whether the observation falls in a shaded 'at-risk zone' (see SEWS key)
- Add the points scored and record total SEWS score on chart
- Do not add 'Pain' score to SEWS score

If SEWS score ≥ 4, a doctor should assess the patient within 20 mins.

If SEWS score ≥ 6, a senior doctor should assess the patient within 10 mins.

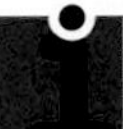

Clinical features of shock

Low-flow shock, e.g. hypovolaemia, cardiogenic shock

- Rapid, shallow respiration
- Cold, clammy skin
- Tachycardia (> 100/min)
- Hypotension (systolic BP < 100 mmHg)
- Drowsiness, confusion, irritability (usually occurs late)
- Oliguria
- Multi-organ failure

Vasodilated shock, e.g. sepsis, anaphylaxis

- Rapid, shallow respiration (very early)
- Warm peripheries*
- Tachycardia (> 100/min)
- Hypotension (systolic BP < 100 mmHg and disproportionately low diastolic BP – early)
- Drowsiness, confusion, irritability (can occur early)
- Oliguria
- Multi-organ failure

*Peripheries may be cool in sepsis with hypovolaemia, or if myocardial depression is present.

A critically ill patient is at imminent risk of death. Recognition, assessment and management of critical illness are thus fundamental to clinical care in any area of medicine. The principle underpinning intensive care is the simultaneous assessment of illness severity and stabilisation of life-threatening physiological abnormalities. The goal is to prevent deterioration and effect improvements as the diagnosis is established, and treatment of the underlying definitive disease process(es) is initiated. Blinkered attention to either resuscitation or diagnosis in isolation results in worse outcomes and increased mortality; the two processes are inextricably interlinked. Appropriate physiological monitoring is required to allow continuing assessment and re-assessment of response to therapy, wherever the clinical environment.

PHYSIOLOGY OF CRITICAL ILLNESS

Oxygen transport

The principal function of the heart, lungs and circulation is the provision of oxygen (and other nutrients) to the various organs and tissues of the body. During this process, carbon dioxide and other metabolic waste products are removed. The rate of supply and removal should match the specific metabolic requirements of the individual tissues. This requires adequate oxygen uptake in the lungs, global matching of delivery and consumption, and regional control of the circulation. Failure to supply sufficient oxygen to meet the metabolic requirements of the tissues is the cardinal feature of circulatory failure or 'shock', and optimisation of tissue oxygen delivery and consumption is the goal of resuscitation.

Atmospheric oxygen moves down a partial pressure gradient from air, through the respiratory tract, from alveoli to arterial blood and then to the capillary beds and cells, diffusing into the mitochondria, where it is utilised at cytochrome a_3 (Fig. 8.1). The movement of oxygen from the left ventricle to the systemic tissue capillaries is known as oxygen delivery (DO_2), and is the product of cardiac output (flow) × arterial oxygen content (CaO_2) The latter is the product of haemoglobin

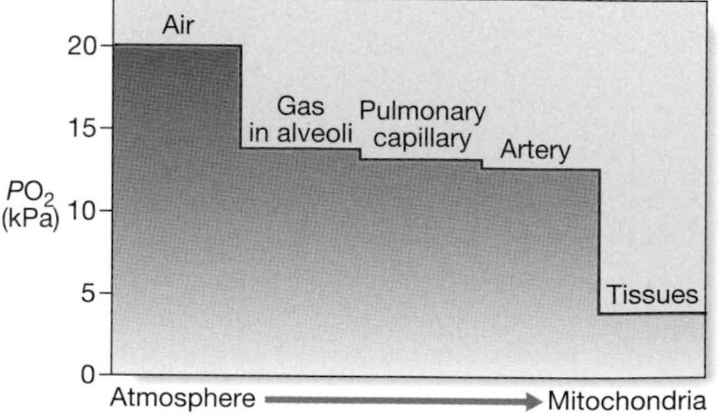

Fig. 8.1 The oxygen cascade in the transport of oxygen from inspired gas to the cell. Gas containing oxygen is entrained into the lungs by inspiratory flow. The partial pressure of O_2 falls as it moves from lungs to blood and then to the tissues. The partial pressure gradient between capillary blood and the intracellular environment is pivotal to oxygen reaching the mitochondria. (PO_2 = oxygen partial pressure (kPa) 1 kPa = 7.5 mmHg).

(Hb) × arterial oxygen saturation of haemoglobin (SaO_2) × 1.34. By increasing cardiac output, arterial oxygen saturation or haemoglobin concentration, DO_2 will be increased.

The regional distribution of oxygen delivery is important. If skin and muscle receive high blood flows but the splanchnic bed does not, the gut will become hypoxic even if overall DO_2 is high.

The movement of oxygen from tissue capillary to cell occurs by diffusion and depends on the gradient of oxygen partial pressures, diffusion distance and the ability of the target cell to take up and use oxygen. Microcirculatory, tissue diffusion and cellular factors thus also influence the oxygen status of the cell.

Cardiovascular component of oxygen delivery: flow

A key determinant of DO_2 is cardiac output, which is determined by the ventricular 'preload' and 'afterload', myocardial contractility and heart rate.

Preload

The atrial filling pressures, or preload, determine the end-diastolic ventricular volume, which, according to Starling's Law and depending on myocardial contractility, defines the force of cardiac contraction and the stroke volume (see Fig. 18.22, p. 547). The principal determinant of preload is venous return, determined by the intravascular volume, venous 'tone' and intrathoracic pressure. This can be measured as the central venous pressure (CVP), as described on page 185 (Box 8.1).

When volume is lost (e.g. in major haemorrhage), venous 'tone' increases and this helps to offset the consequent fall in atrial filling pressure and stroke volume. If the equivalent volume is restored gradually by intravenous fluid administration, the right atrial pressure will return to normal as the intravascular volume is normalised and the reflex increase in venous tone abates. However, if fluid is infused too rapidly, there is insufficient time for the venous and arteriolar tone to fall and pulmonary oedema may occur, even though the intravascular volume has only been restored to the premorbid level.

If the preload is low, volume loading with intravenous fluids is the priority and is the most appropriate means of improving cardiac output and tissue perfusion. The choice of fluid for volume loading is controversial, but as there is no clear advantage of colloid over crystalloid, sodium chloride is used. Fluid challenges of 200–250 mL should be administered rapidly over a couple of minutes, and titrated against heart rate, blood pressure (BP), peripheral circulation, and measurements of CVP (Fig. 8.2). Red cells have traditionally been transfused to

8.1 Central venous pressure measurements

• Normal	0–5 mmHg
• Target (usual) of volume resuscitation	6–10 mmHg
• Normal if ventilated	5–10 mmHg
• Target of volume resuscitation if ventilated	10–15 mmHg

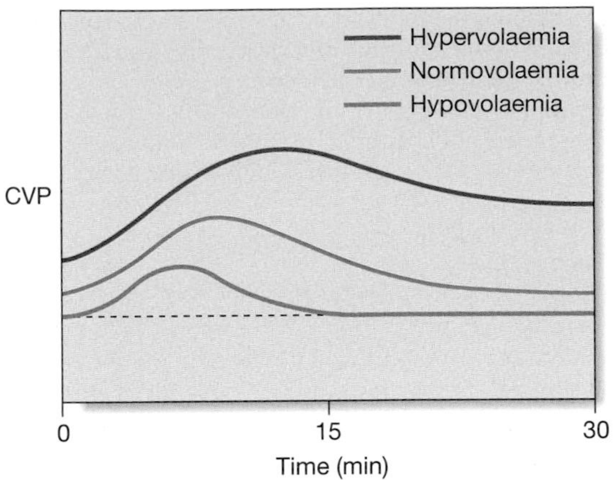

Fig. 8.2 Responses observed in central venous pressure (CVP) after a fluid challenge of 250 mL, depending on the intravascular volume status of the patient.

achieve and maintain a haemoglobin concentration of 100 g/L, but in the absence of significant heart disease, the target is 70–90 g/L (p. 184).

When the preload is high due to excessive intravascular volume or impaired myocardial contractility, removing volume from the circulation by using diuretics or haemofiltration, or increasing the capacity of the vascular bed by using venodilator therapy (glyceryl trinitrate, morphine) often improves stroke volume.

Afterload

Afterload is the tension in the ventricular myocardium during systole, and is determined by the resistance to ventricular outflow, which is a function of the peripheral arteriolar resistance.

Understanding the reciprocal relationship between pressure, flow and resistance is crucial for appropriate circulatory management. High resistances produce lower flows at higher pressures for a given amount of ventricular work. Therefore, a systemic vasodilator (see below) will allow the same cardiac output to be maintained for less ventricular work but with a reduced arterial BP. In hyperdynamic sepsis, the peripheral arteriolar tone and BP are low but the cardiac output is often high; therefore the vasoconstrictor noradrenaline (norepinephrine) is appropriate to restore BP, usually at the price of some reduction in cardiac output.

Myocardial contractility

This determines the stroke volume that the ventricle can generate against a given afterload for a particular preload. The ventricular stroke work is the external work performed by the ventricle with each beat. The relationship between stroke work and filling pressure is shown in Figure 18.22 (p. 547). Myocardial contractility is frequently reduced in critically ill patients due to pre-existing cardiac disease (usually ischaemic), drugs (e.g. β-blockers, verapamil) or to the disease process itself (particularly sepsis, as the associated low diastolic BP may compromise coronary arterial perfusion). It is thus important to maintain satisfactory perfusion and oxygen delivery to all organs at maximum cardiac efficiency, to minimise myocardial ischaemia.

Oxygenation component of oxygen delivery: content

The major determinants of the oxygen content of arterial blood (CaO_2) are the arterial oxygen saturation of haemoglobin (SaO_2) and the haemoglobin concentration. Over 95% of oxygen carried in the blood is bound to haemoglobin.

The oxyhaemoglobin dissociation curve (Fig. 8.3) describes the relationship between the saturation of haemoglobin (SO_2) and the partial pressure (PO_2) of oxygen in the blood. A shift in the curve will influence the uptake and release of oxygen by the haemoglobin molecule. If the curve moves to the right, the haemoglobin saturation will be lower for any given oxygen tension: less oxygen will be taken up in the lungs but more will be released to the tissues. As capillary PCO_2 rises, the curve moves to the right, increasing the unloading of oxygen in the tissues – a phenomenon known as the Bohr effect. Thus a shift to the right increases capillary PO_2 and hence cellular oxygen supply.

Due to the shape of the curve, a small drop in arterial PO_2 (PaO_2) below 8 kPa (60 mmHg) will cause a marked fall in SaO_2.. Its position and the effect of various physicochemical factors are defined by the PO_2 at which 50% of the haemoglobin is saturated (P_{50}), which is normally 3.5 kPa (26 mmHg). The shape of the curve also means that increases in PaO_2 beyond the level that ensures SaO_2 is greater than 90% produce relatively small additional increases in CaO_2 (Fig. 8.3). Thus, in a patient who is both anaemic (Hb 60 g/L or 6 g/dL) and hypoxaemic (SaO_2 75%) when breathing air (fractional inspired oxygen concentration (FiO_2) 20%), supplementary oxygen at FiO_2 40% will increase SaO_2 to 93% and CaO_2 by 24%. However, further increases in FiO_2, while raising PaO_2, cannot produce any further useful increases in SaO_2 or CaO_2. However, increasing haemoglobin to 90 g/L

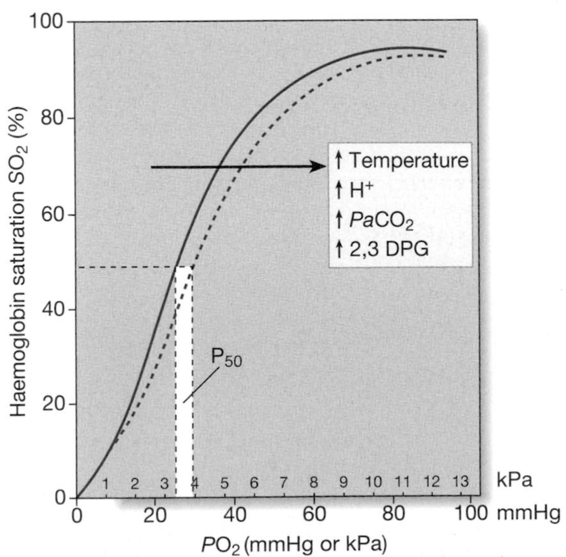

Fig. 8.3 Oxyhaemoglobin dissociation curve: the relationship between oxygen tension (PO_2) and percentage saturation of haemoglobin with oxygen (SO_2). The dotted line illustrates the rightward shift of the curve (i.e. P_{50} increases) caused by increases in temperature, $PaCO_2$, metabolic acidosis and 2,3 diphosphoglycerate (DPG).

(9 g/dL) by blood transfusion will result in a further 50% increase in CaO_2.

Traditionally, the optimum haemoglobin concentration for critically ill patients was considered to be approximately 100 g/L (10 g/dL), representing a balance between maximising the oxygen content of the blood and avoiding regional microcirculatory problems due to increased viscosity. However, improved outcomes have been demonstrated when the haemoglobin is maintained between 70 and 90 g/L (7–9 g/dL). A target haemoglobin of 100 g/L remains appropriate in the elderly and in patients with coronary artery disease, cardiogenic shock, significant aortic stenosis or acute brain trauma.

Oxygen consumption

The sum of the oxygen consumed by the various organs represents the global oxygen consumption (VO_2), and is approximately 250 mL/min for an adult of 70 kg undertaking normal daily activities.

The oxygen saturation in the pulmonary artery, or 'mixed venous oxygen saturation' (SvO_2), is a measure of the oxygen not consumed by the tissues ($DO_2 - VO_2$). The saturation of venous blood from different organs varies considerably; the hepatic venous saturation usually does not exceed 60% but the renal venous saturation may reach 90%, reflecting the difference in the metabolic requirements of these organs, and the oxygen content of the blood delivered to them. The SvO_2 is a flow-weighted average measured in the mixed effluent blood from all perfused tissues, and is influenced by changes in both oxygen delivery (DO_2) and consumption (VO_2). Provided the microcirculation and the mechanisms for cellular oxygen uptake are intact, it can be used to monitor whether global oxygen delivery is adequate to meet overall demand, so its measurement is particularly useful in low-flow situations such as cardiogenic shock. Central venous oxygen saturation ($ScvO_2$) is used in the same way, but as it does not reflect hepatosplanchnic oxygen consumption, it may be less helpful than SvO_2.

The re-oxygenation of the blood that returns to the lungs and the resulting arterial saturation (SaO_2) will depend on how closely pulmonary ventilation and perfusion are matched. If part of the pulmonary blood flow perfuses non-ventilated parts of the lung ('shunting'), the blood entering the left atrium will be desaturated in proportion to the size of the shunt and the level of SvO_2.

Relationship between oxygen consumption and delivery

The tissue oxygen extraction ratio (OER) is 20–25% in a normal individual at rest, but rises as consumption increases or supply diminishes. The maximum OER is approximately 60% for most tissues; at this point, no further increase in extraction can occur and any further increase in oxygen consumption or decline in oxygen delivery will cause tissue hypoxia, anaerobic metabolism and increased lactic acid production. This ultimately results in multiple organ failure and an increased risk of death.

In practice, if there is a metabolic acidosis, hyperlactataemia and/or oliguria that could be due to inadequate oxygen delivery, a therapeutic trial of increased oxygen delivery (while maintaining an adequate BP) may be helpful clinically. If oxygen consumption rises, it can indicate an oxygen debt that is being repaid.

Pathophysiology of the inflammatory response

The mediators and clinical manifestations of the inflammatory response are described on page 82. In critically ill patients, these have important consequences (Box 8.2).

Fever, tachycardia with warm peripheries, tachypnoea and a raised white cell count prompt a diagnosis of sepsis, with the presentation caused by invading microorganisms and their breakdown products. Other conditions, such as pancreatitis, trauma, malignancy, tissue necrosis (e.g. burns), aspiration syndromes, liver failure, blood transfusion and drug reactions, can also present in this way in the absence of infection.

Local inflammation

The body's initial response to a noxious local insult is to produce a local inflammatory response, with sequestration and activation of white blood cells and the release of a

8.2 Terminology in the inflammatory state
Infection
• Invasion of normally sterile tissue by microorganisms
Bacteraemia
• Viable bacteria in the blood
Systemic inflammatory response syndrome (SIRS)
• Defined by the presence of two or more of Respiratory rate > 20/min Heart rate > 90/min White blood count > 12×10^9/L or < 4×10^9/L Temperature > 38.0°C or < 36.0°C $PaCO_2$ < 4.3 kPa (< 32 mmHg) or ventilated • A wide pulse pressure, e.g. 115/42 mmHg, may be an early pointer to systemic sepsis • Cause may be infection or a non-infective condition, e.g. pancreatitis, trauma, cardiopulmonary bypass, vasculitis etc. • Hypothermia and septic neutropenia indicate more severe infection
Sepsis
• Systemic inflammatory response caused by documented infection
Severe sepsis/SIRS
• Sepsis/SIRS with evidence of early organ dysfunction *or* hypotension
Septic/SIRS shock
• Sepsis associated with organ failure *and* hypotension (systolic BP < 90 mmHg or > 40 mmHg fall from baseline) unresponsive to fluid resuscitation
Multiple organ dysfunction syndrome (MODS)
• Development of impaired organ function in a patient with SIRS • Multiple organ failure (MOF) ensues unless there is prompt treatment of the underlying cause and appropriate organ support

variety of mediators to overcome the primary 'insult' and prevent further damage locally or in distant organs.

Normally, a delicate balance is achieved between pro- and anti-inflammatory mediators. However, if the response is excessive, a large array of pro-inflammatory mediators may be released into the circulation (p. 74). The inflammatory and coagulation cascades are intimately linked, as the latter cause not only platelet activation and fibrin deposition, but also activation of leucocytes and endothelial cells. Conversely, leucocyte activation induces tissue factor expression and initiates coagulation pathways. The natural anticoagulants, antithrombin (AT III), activated protein C (APC) and tissue factor pathway inhibitor (TFPI), inhibit pro-inflammatory cytokines. Deficiency of AT III and APC (features of disseminated intravascular coagulation (DIC), p. 1056) facilitates thrombin generation and promotes further endothelial cell dysfunction.

Systemic inflammation

In a severe inflammatory response, systemic release of cytokines and other mediators triggers widespread interaction between the coagulation pathways, platelets, endothelial cells and monocytes, tissue macrophages, and neutrophils. Activated neutrophils express adhesion factors, which make them adhere to and initially roll along the endothelium, before adhering firmly and migrating through the damaged and disrupted endothelium into the extravascular interstitial space (together with fluid and proteins), resulting in tissue oedema and inflammation. A vicious circle of endothelial injury, intravascular coagulation, microvascular occlusion, tissue damage and further release of inflammatory mediators ensues. This can occur in all organs, manifesting in the lungs as acute lung injury and in the kidneys as acute tubular necrosis (ATN). Similar processes probably account for damage to other organs, including the heart.

The endothelium itself produces mediators that control local blood vessel tone. The profound vasodilatation that characterises septic shock and some other acute systemic inflammatory states, such as pancreatitis, results from excessive production of nitric oxide (NO, p. 82), due to activation of inducible NO synthase enzymes.

Systemic inflammatory processes also have important effects on mitochondrial function, resulting in impaired oxidative phosphorylation and aerobic energy generation. This block to oxygen utilisation by cells is sometimes called cytopathic hypoxia. Patients typically have a reduced arteriovenous oxygen difference, a low oxygen extraction ratio, a raised plasma lactate and a paradoxically high mixed venous oxygen saturation (SvO_2), despite normal or supranormal oxygen delivery. This is associated with the development of multiple organ failure (MOF) and reduced survival.

MONITORING

Monitoring in intensive care includes a combination of clinical and automated recordings. Electrocardiogram (ECG), SpO_2 (oxygen saturation), BP and usually CVP recordings are taken at least hourly, using either a 24-hour chart or a computerised system. Urine output measurement requires early catheterisation. All invasive haemodynamic monitoring should be referenced to the mid-axillary line as 'zero'. Clinical monitoring of physical signs, such as respiratory rate, the appearance of the patient, restlessness, conscious level and indices of peripheral perfusion (pale, cold skin; delayed capillary refill in the nailbed), is just as important as a set of blood gases or monitor readings.

Monitoring the circulation

Electrocardiogram

Standard monitors display a single-lead ECG, record heart rate and identify rhythm changes. More sophisticated machines can print out rhythm strips and monitor ST segment shift, which is useful in patients with ischaemic heart disease.

Blood pressure

In critically ill patients, continuous intra-arterial monitoring is necessary using a line placed in the radial artery (or the femoral in vasoconstricted patients or where access is difficult). The brachial artery should be avoided, as it is an end artery of relatively small calibre and occlusion leads to ischaemia of the hand. When there is systemic vasoconstriction, the mean arterial pressure (MAP) may be normal or even high, although the cardiac output is low. Conversely, if there is peripheral vasodilatation, as in sepsis, the MAP may be low, although the cardiac output is high.

Central venous pressure

CVP or right atrial pressure (RAP) is monitored using a catheter inserted via either the internal jugular or the subclavian vein, with the distal end sited in the upper right atrium. The CVP may help in assessing the need for intravascular fluid replacement and the rate at which this should be given (see Box 8.1, p. 182). If the CVP is low in the presence of a low MAP or cardiac output, fluid resuscitation is necessary. However, a raised level does not necessarily mean that the patient is adequately volume-resuscitated. Right heart function, pulmonary artery pressure, intrathoracic pressure and venous 'tone' also influence CVP, and may lead to a raised CVP even when the patient is hypovolaemic (Box 8.3). In addition, positive pressure ventilation raises intrathoracic pressure and causes marked swings in atrial pressures and systemic BP in time with respiration. Pressure measurements should be recorded at end-expiration.

In severe hypovolaemia, the RAP may be sustained by peripheral venoconstriction, and transfusion may initially produce little or no change in the CVP (see Fig. 8.3, p. 183).

Pulmonary artery catheterisation and pulmonary artery 'wedge' pressure

The CVP is usually an adequate guide to the filling pressures of both sides of the heart. However, certain conditions, such as pulmonary hypertension or right ventricular dysfunction, may lead to raised CVP levels even in the presence of hypovolaemia. In these circumstances, it may be appropriate to insert a pulmonary artery flotation catheter (Fig. 8.4) so that pulmonary artery pressure and pulmonary artery 'wedge' pressure

8.3 Factors affecting central venous pressure

Physiological	
• Cardiac function • Blood volume • Venoconstriction	• Intrathoracic pressure
Pathological	
All increase CVP:	
• Superior vena cava occlusion • Chronic obstructive pulmonary disease (COPD)/ cor pulmonale	• Pulmonary embolism • Cardiac tamponade
Interventions	
Increase CVP:	
• Positive pressure ventilation and positive end-expiratory pressure (PEEP)	• Fluid resuscitation • Vasopressors
Reduce CVP:	
• Venodilators	
Artefacts caused by technical problems	
• Line malpositioning: tip in right ventricle, internal jugular line in axillary vein, or subclavian line in internal jugular vein • Transducer not in alignment with phlebostatic axis (mid-axillary line) • Inaccurate calibration of transducer system • Infusion attached to monitoring line • Clot/occlusion in line	

(PAWP), which approximates to left atrial pressure, can be measured.

The mean PAWP normally lies between 6 and 12 mmHg (measured from the mid-axillary line) but in left heart failure it may be grossly elevated, exceeding 30 mmHg. Provided the pulmonary capillary membranes are intact, the optimum PAWP when managing acute circulatory failure in the critically ill patient is generally 12–15 mmHg, because this will ensure good left ventricular filling without risking hydrostatic pulmonary oedema.

Pulmonary artery catheters also allow measurement of cardiac output and sampling of blood from the pulmonary artery ('mixed venous' samples), permitting continuous monitoring of the mixed venous oxygen saturation ($S\bar{v}O_2$) by oximetry. Measurement of $S\bar{v}O_2$ gives an indication of the adequacy of cardiac output (and hence DO_2) in relation to the body's metabolic requirements. It is especially useful in low cardiac output states.

Cardiac output

Measurement of cardiac output is important, particularly when large doses of a vasopressor are being administered, when there is underlying cardiac disease (acute or chronic), and when volume resuscitation and vasoactive drug therapy are not achieving resolution of lactic acidosis or oliguria. It is most accurately measured by indicator dilution methods. Most PA catheters incorporate a heating element, which raises blood temperature at frequent intervals, and the resultant temperature change is detected by a thermistor at the tip of the catheter.

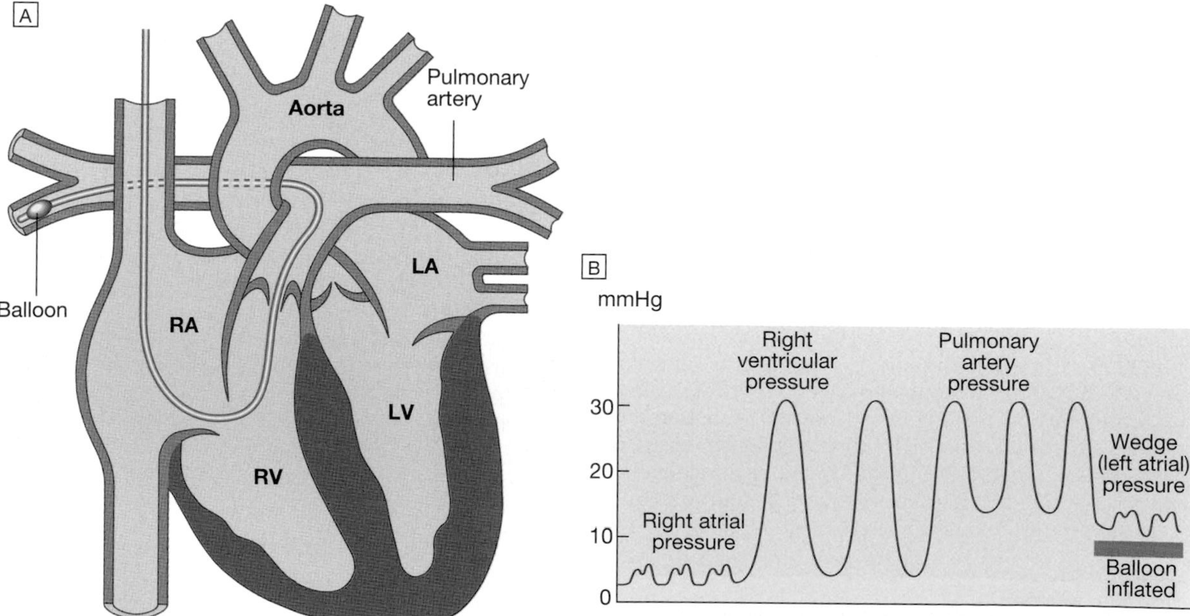

Fig. 8.4 A pulmonary artery catheter. **A** There is a small balloon at the tip of the catheter and pressure can be measured through the central lumen. The catheter is inserted via an internal jugular, subclavian or femoral vein and advanced through the right heart until the tip lies in the pulmonary artery. When the balloon is deflated, the pulmonary artery pressure can be recorded. **B** Advancing the catheter with the balloon inflated will 'wedge' the catheter in the pulmonary artery. Blood cannot then flow past the balloon, so the tip of the catheter will now record the pressure transmitted from the pulmonary veins and left atrium (known as the pulmonary artery wedge pressure), which provides an indirect measure of the left atrial pressure. (LA = left atrium; LV = left ventricle; RA = right atrium; RV = right ventricle).

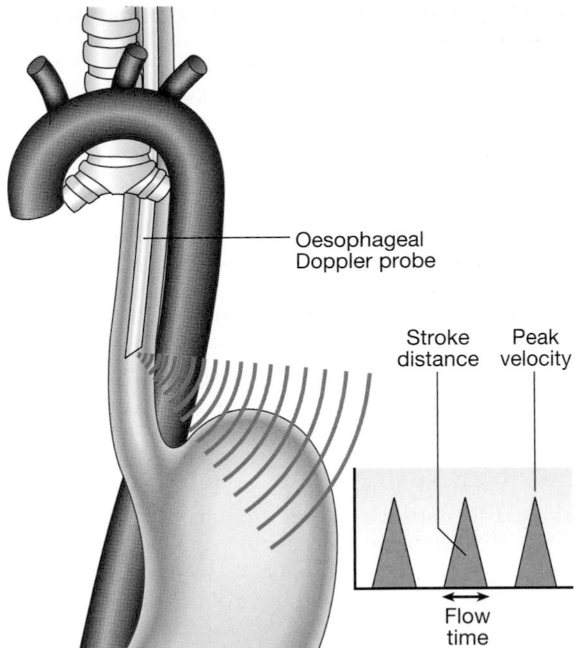

Fig. 8.5 Oesophageal Doppler ultrasonography.

Oesophageal Doppler ultrasonography provides a rapid and useful assessment of volume status and cardiac performance to guide early fluid and vasoactive therapy. A 6 mm probe is inserted into the distal oesophagus, allowing continuous monitoring of the aortic flow signal from the descending aorta (Fig. 8.5). Using the stroke distance (area under the velocity/time waveform) and a correction factor that incorporates the patient's age, height and weight, an estimate of left ventricular stroke volume and hence cardiac output can be made. Peak velocity is an indicator of left ventricular performance, while flow time is an indicator of left ventricular filling and peripheral resistance.

Analysis of arterial pressure waveform is another means of continuously estimating cardiac output, and can be calibrated either by transpulmonary thermodilution (PiCCO) or lithium dilution methods (LidCO). The Vigileo/Flotrac system derives cardiac output from arterial pressure waveform analysis with no external calibration.

Echocardiography

In many centres, echocardiography is increasingly being used for rapid assessment of myocardial function and volume status at the bedside. Continuous transoesophageal echocardiography allows direct assessment of cardiac filling status and ventricular function in real time.

Urine output

This is a sensitive measure of renal perfusion, provided that the kidneys are not damaged (e.g. in ATN) or affected by drugs such as diuretics or dopamine. Output is measured hourly and a lower limit of normal of 0.5 mL/hr/kg body weight is widely used. It reflects renal perfusion over the hours preceding measurement rather than in real time.

Peripheral skin temperature

In general, resuscitation is not complete until the patient's feet are warm and well perfused.

Blood lactate, hydrogen ion and base excess/deficit

Acid–base balance is discussed on page 443. Base excess or deficit is calculated as the difference between the patient's bicarbonate and the normal bicarbonate after the PCO_2 has been maintained in a blood gas machine at 5.33 kPa (40 mmHg). This is particularly useful, as it describes patients' underlying metabolic status independently of their current respiratory status. A metabolic acidosis with base deficit of more than 5 mmol/L requires investigation (p. 445). It often indicates increased lactic acid production in poorly perfused, hypoxic tissues, and impaired lactate metabolism and clearance due to poor hepatic perfusion. Serial lactate measurements may therefore be helpful in monitoring tissue perfusion and response to treatment. Other conditions, such as acute renal failure, ketoacidosis and poisoning, may be the cause, and infusions of large volumes of fluids containing sodium chloride may lead to a hyperchloraemic acidosis.

Monitoring respiratory function

Oxygen saturation

Oxygen saturation (SpO_2) is measured by a probe attached to a finger or earlobe. Spectrophotometric analysis determines the relative proportions of saturated and desaturated haemoglobin. It is unreliable if peripheral perfusion is poor, in the presence of nail polish, excessive movement or high ambient light. It is not useful in carbon monoxide poisoning, as it does not detect carboxy-haemoglobin. If this is suspected, PO_2 must be measured in an arterial blood gas sample. In general, arterial oxygenation is safe if SpO_2 is above 90%. Box 8.4 lists the causes of sudden falls in SpO_2.

Arterial blood gases

Arterial blood gases (ABGs) are measured several times a day in a ventilated patient so that inspired oxygen (FiO_2) and minute volume can be adjusted to achieve the

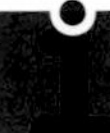

8.4 Causes of sudden changes in oxygen saturation

Patient factors

- Bronchospasm
- Lung collapse due to thick secretions blocking the proximal bronchial tree
- Pneumothorax
- Impaired peripheral perfusion

Equipment factors

- Displacement of the endotracheal tube (extubation, endobronchial intubation)
- Blockage of the endotracheal tube
- Disconnection from the ventilator
- Oxygen supply failure
- Detached probe

desired PaO_2 and $PaCO_2$ respectively. ABG results are also used to monitor disturbances of acid–base balance.

Lung function

In ventilated patients, lung function is monitored by:

- arterial PO_2 taken in relation to the fractional inspired oxygen concentration (PO_2/FiO_2 ratio) and level of end-expiratory pressure
- arterial and end-tidal CO_2, reflecting alveolar ventilation
- airway pressures and tidal volumes, reflecting lung compliance and airways resistance.

Capnography

The CO_2 concentration in inspired gas is zero, but during expiration, after clearing the physiological dead space, it rises progressively to reach a plateau that represents the alveolar or end-tidal CO_2 concentration. This cyclical change in CO_2 concentration, or capnogram, is measured using an infrared sensor inserted between the ventilator tubing and the endotracheal tube (Fig. 8.6). In normal lungs, the end-tidal CO_2 closely mirrors $PaCO_2$, and can be used to assess the adequacy of alveolar ventilation. However, its use is limited as there may be marked discrepancies in the presence of lung disease or impaired pulmonary perfusion (e.g. due to hypovolaemia). In combination with the gas flow and respiratory cycle data from the ventilator, CO_2 production and hence metabolic rate may be calculated. In clinical practice, end-tidal CO_2 is used to confirm correct placement of an endotracheal tube, in the management of head injury, and during the transport of ventilated patients. Continuous measurement of end-tidal CO_2 is important in the minute-to-minute monitoring of any patient ventilated through an endotracheal tube or tracheostomy in the acute setting.

Transcutaneous PCO_2

Monitors that measure transcutaneous PCO_2 are now available with an earlobe probe that incorporates a pulse oximeter and CO_2 electrode. The transcutaneous PCO_2 closely approximates to $PaCO_2$ and gives continuous monitoring. This is useful in patients with no arterial cannula but who require close monitoring: for example, during ventilatory weaning (see below).

RECOGNITION OF CRITICAL ILLNESS

The immediate appearance of the patient yields a wealth of information. Introducing yourself, shaking hands and asking 'How are you?' allow assessment of:

- the airway (for patency and noises, e.g. stridor, snoring, gurgling, none)
- breathing (rate, symmetry, work of breathing, including accessory muscle use, paradoxical chest/abdominal movement or see-saw pattern)
- peripheral circulation (temperature of the extremities)
- conscious level (the response of the patient).

Tachypnoea is often the earliest abnormality to appear and the most sensitive sign of a worsening clinical state, but it is the least well documented. In the UK, the use of early warning scores, such as the Standard Early Warning System chart (SEWS, p. 181), has been adopted to improve the recognition of critical illness. These alert staff to severely ill patients, complement clinical judgement and facilitate the prioritisation of clinical care. A patient with a SEWS score of 4 or more requires urgent review and appropriate interventions. An elevated score correlates with increased mortality.

Assessment and initial resuscitation of the critically ill patient

Airway and breathing

If the patient is talking, the airway is clear and breathing is adequate. A rapid history should be obtained whilst initial assessment is undertaken.

Assess breathing as described above. Supplemental oxygen should be administered to patients who are breathless, tachypnoeic or bleeding, or who have chest pain or reduced conscious level. The clinical status of the patient determines how much oxygen to give, but the critically ill should receive at least 60% oxygen initially. High-concentration oxygen is best given using a mask with a reservoir bag, which, at 15 L/min, can provide nearly 90% oxygen. ABGs should be checked early to assess oxygenation, ventilation ($PaCO_2$) and metabolic state (pH or H^+, HCO_3 and base deficit). Oxygen therapy should be adjusted in light of the ABGs, remembering

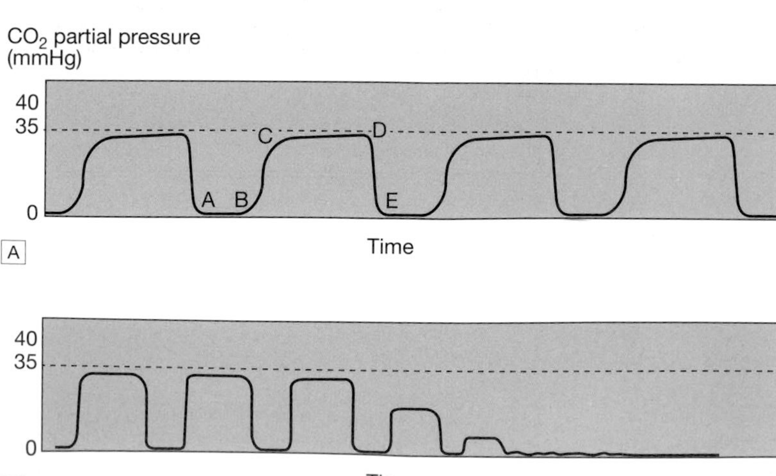

Fig. 8.6 Capnography traces for normal and pathological states. **A** The normal capnogram represents the varying CO_2 level throughout the breath cycle. A–B = baseline, B–C = expiratory upstroke, C–D = expiratory plateau, D = end-tidal concentration, D–E = inspiration. **B** Loss of the capnograph can occur with loss of cardiac output, as well as airway displacement. (1 kPa = 7.5 mmHg)

that oxygen requirements may subsequently increase or decrease. Early application of pulse oximeter monitoring is ideal, although this may not be reliable if the patient is peripherally shut down. Intubation, while often essential, may be hazardous in a patient with cardiorespiratory failure, and full monitoring and resuscitation facilities must be available.

Circulation

The carotid pulse should be sought in the collapsed or unconscious patient, but peripheral pulses checked in the conscious. The radial, brachial, foot and femoral pulses may disappear as shock progresses, and this indicates the severity of circulatory compromise.

Venous access for the administration of drugs and/or fluids is vital but often difficult in sick patients. The gauge of cannula needed is dictated by its purpose. Wide-bore cannulae are required for rapid fluid administration. Ideally, two 16G or larger cannulae should be inserted, one in each arm, in the severely hypovolaemic patient. If the two cannulae are of different sizes, the pulse oximeter should be placed on the same side as the larger one, and the BP cuff on the same side as the smaller one. This facilitates unimpeded volume resuscitation and uninterrupted oxygen saturation monitoring. Pressure infusors and blood warmers should be utilised for rapid, high-volume fluid resuscitation, particularly of blood products. An 18G cannula is adequate for drug administration.

Machine-derived cuff BP measurement is inaccurate at extremes of BP and in tachycardia, especially atrial fibrillation. Manual sphygmomanometer BP readings tend to be more accurate in hypotension. If severe hypotension is not readily corrected with fluid, early consideration should be given to arterial line insertion and vasoactive drug therapy.

Disability

Conscious level should be assessed using the Glasgow Coma Scale (GCS; see Box 26.15, p. 1160). Best eye, verbal and motor responses should be assessed and documented. Appropriate painful stimuli include supraorbital pressure and trapezius pinch. A score of 8 or less denotes coma with associated airway compromise and loss of airway protection, which necessitates intervention. Focal neurological signs may indicate unilateral cerebral pathology. Abnormal pupil size, symmetry or reaction to light may indicate primary cerebral disease or global cerebral insults induced by drugs (e.g. opioids), hypoxia or hypoglycaemia.

Exposure, evidence and examination

'Exposure' indicates the need for targeted clinical examination, and 'evidence' may be gathered from any recent investigations, prescription or monitoring charts.

Clinical decision-making and referral to critical care

During the initial assessment and resuscitation, several decisions must be made (Box 8.5), but particularly whether referral to the critical care service is necessary.

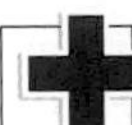

8.5 Clinical decisions in the critically ill

- How ill is the patient?
- How much help is needed and how quickly?
- Where would the patient be best managed?
- When should the patient be moved?
  - All critically ill patients require an appropriately trained escort during transfer
- What is required before transporting the patient?
  - ABCDE resuscitation ± endotracheal intubation and ventilation
  - Monitoring, including invasive arterial ± CVP
  - Volume resuscitation and vasoactive support
  - Imaging/diagnostic processes
- Is specialist involvement required?
  - E.g. transfer to specialist liver, burns, neurosurgical or cardiac surgical units or for specialised investigations
  - The urgency of specialist treatment needs balanced against the patient's condition; it may be necessary to stabilise the patient in the ICU first

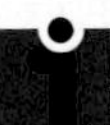

8.6 Admission criteria for intensive care (ICU) and high-dependency units (HDU)

ICU

- Patients requiring/likely to require endotracheal intubation and invasive mechanical ventilatory support
- Patients requiring support of two or more organ systems (e.g. inotropes and haemofiltration)
- Patients with chronic impairment of one or more organ systems (e.g. COPD *or* severe ischaemic heart disease) who require support for acute reversible failure of another organ

HDU

- Patients requiring detailed observation or monitoring that cannot be provided at ward level
  - Direct arterial BP monitoring
  - CVP monitoring
  - Fluid balance
  - Neurological observations, regular GCS recording
- Patients requiring support for a single failing organ system, excluding invasive ventilatory support:
  - CPAP *or* NIV – see p. 193
  - Moderate inotropic or vasopressor support
  - Renal replacement therapy in an otherwise stable patient
- Step down from intensive care

(BP = blood pressure; CPAP = continuous positive airway pressure; COPD = chronic obstructive pulmonary disease; CVP = central venous pressure; GCS = Glasgow Coma Scale; NIV = non-invasive (mask) ventilation)

This requires local knowledge about the clinical areas providing enhanced care, whether intermediate high-dependency or advanced intensive care, and the mechanism of referral.

- *Intensive care units* allow management of the sickest patients who require invasive ventilation, multimodal monitoring and multiple organ system support (Box 8.6).
- *High-dependency care* allows a greater degree of monitoring, physiological support and nursing/medical input than the standard ward, for patients following major surgery, or for the septic patient requiring invasive haemodynamic monitoring and

circulatory support alone, or for the patient with respiratory failure manageable with non-invasive ventilation (NIV) or continuous positive airway pressure (CPAP).

The mechanism of referral to critical care varies between hospitals, and all clinical staff must be aware of the local system and how to access it. Many hospitals have medical emergency or outreach teams that facilitate this. A clear understanding of what is available in critical care and what is achievable allows early referral of appropriate patients, which will improve their survival and reduce length of stay. It prevents referral of patients who have no realistic prospect of meaningful survival, due to either the overwhelming nature of their acute condition or the lack of definitive therapy for the underlying disease process.

PRESENTING PROBLEMS/MANAGEMENT OF MAJOR ORGAN FAILURE

As the diagnosis and management of presenting problems take place simultaneously in critical care, these are described together.

Circulatory failure: 'shock'

The defining feature of 'shock' is a level of oxygen delivery (DO_2) that fails to meet the metabolic requirements of the tissues. 'Shock' is not synonymous with hypotension, which is often a late manifestation. The cardiac output and oxygen delivery may be critically low, even though the BP remains normal, and the underlying problem should be identified and treated before the BP falls. Objective markers of inadequate tissue oxygen delivery, such as increasing base deficit, elevated blood lactate and reduced urine output, can aid earlier identification of shock.

The causes of circulatory failure or 'shock' may be categorised as either low flow or stroke volume, or low peripheral arteriolar resistance (vasodilatation).

Low stroke volume

- *Hypovolaemic:* any condition provoking a major reduction in blood volume, e.g. internal or external haemorrhage, severe burns, salt and water depletion.
- *Cardiogenic:* severe cardiac impairment, e.g. myocardial infarction, acute mitral regurgitation. Subarachnoid haemorrhage may cause catecholamine-mediated myocardial stunning that can result in pulmonary oedema or cardiogenic shock.
- *Obstructive:* obstruction to blood flow around the circulation, e.g. major pulmonary embolism, cardiac tamponade, tension pneumothorax.

Vasodilatation

- *Sepsis/SIRS:* infection or other causes of a systemic inflammatory response that produce widespread endothelial damage with vasodilatation, arteriovenous shunting, microvascular occlusion, capillary leak and tissue oedema.
- *Anaphylactic:* inappropriate vasodilatation triggered by an allergen (e.g. bee sting), often associated with endothelial disruption and capillary leak.
- *Neurogenic:* caused by major brain or spinal injury, which disrupts brainstem and neurogenic vasomotor control. High cervical cord trauma may result in disruption of the sympathetic outflow tracts, leading to inappropriate bradycardia due to a combination of loss of noradrenaline (norepinephrine)-mediated vasoconstriction and adrenaline (epinephrine)-mediated chronotropy. Guillain–Barré syndrome (p. 1224) involves the autonomic as well as the sensorimotor systems, which may result in periods of severe hypo- or hypertension.

Clinical assessment and complications

Clinical features depend on the primary pathophysiology (p. 180). Hypovolaemic, cardiogenic and obstructive causes of circulatory failure produce the 'classical' image of shock with cold peripheries, reduced or absent peripheral pulses, weak central pulses and evidence of a low cardiac output. In early haemorrhagic shock, a narrowed pulse pressure, i.e. a raised diastolic (DBP) and reduced systolic (SBP) blood pressure, such as 105/95 mmHg, indicates the combination of hypovolaemia (reduced stroke volume, hence SBP) and activation of the sympathetic nervous system, with noradrenaline (norepinephrine) inducing vasoconstriction and so raising the DBP.

In contrast, sepsis/SIRS and anaphylactic shock are usually associated with warm peripheries, bounding pulses and features of a high cardiac output. The BP pattern is again distinctive (e.g. 115/42 mmHg), with a low DBP in the early stages due to peripheral vasodilatation, but a normal systolic BP, as the left ventricular afterload is reduced and stroke volume thus maintained, These patients are usually warm peripherally, but in more advanced septic or anaphylactic shock, SBP falls and the peripheries become cool. This is usually due to the hypovolaemia associated with capillary leak and will respond to fluid resuscitation. If there is no improvement with this, myocardial depression may be present.

Neurogenic shock often results in vasodilated hypotension with a paradoxically slow heart rate.

All forms of shock require early identification and treatment because, if inadequate regional tissue perfusion and cellular dysoxia persist, MOF will develop. Early institution of invasive haemodynamic monitoring is required.

Circulatory support

The primary goals (Box 8.7) are to:

- Restore global oxygen delivery (DO_2) by ensuring adequate cardiac output.
- Maintain an MAP that ensures adequate perfusion of vital organs. The target pressure will be patient-specific, depending on pre-morbid factors (e.g. hypertension or coronary artery disease), and may range from 60 to 90 mmHg.

The first objective is to ensure that an 'appropriate' ventricular preload is restored, initially by adequate volume resuscitation. Vasoactive drugs may then have to be considered.

8.7 Immediate management of circulatory collapse

Correct hypoxaemia
• Oxygen therapy • Consider ventilation Intractable hypoxaemia Hypercapnia: $PaCO_2$ > 6.7 kPa (50 mmHg) Respiratory distress Impaired conscious level
Assess circulation
• Heart rate • CVP • BP: direct arterial pressure • Peripheral perfusion
Optimise volume status
• Fluid challenge(s): CVP < 6 mmHg: 250 mL 0.9% saline or colloid CVP > 6 mmHg or poor ventricular function suspected: 100 mL boluses and consider measuring cardiac output by PA catheter or oesophageal Doppler
Optimise haemoglobin concentration
• Transfuse red cells to maintain Hb at 70–90 g/L (or 100 g/L if ischaemic heart disease) • Septic patients can become profoundly anaemic with crystalloid/colloid resuscitation due to haemodilution
Achieve target BP
• Use vasopressor/inotrope once hypovolaemia is corrected
Achieve adequate CO and DO_2
• Inotropic agent if fluid alone is inadequate
Other measures
• Establish monitoring, including invasive measures, at once • Trends in haemodynamics, ABG, H^+, base deficit and lactate guide further treatment

Therapeutic options to optimise cardiac function

If the cardiac output is inadequate and myocardial contractility is poor, the available treatment options are to:

- *Reduce afterload*. Reduction can be achieved by using an arteriolar dilator (e.g. nitrates), but this may be limited by the consequent fall in systemic pressure. A counterpulsation intra-aortic balloon pump offers the ideal physiological treatment because it reduces left ventricular afterload while increasing cardiac output, diastolic pressure and coronary perfusion. It is particularly valuable in treating myocardial ischaemia.
- *Increase preload*. If there is significant impairment of myocardial contractility, giving fluids to increase filling pressures will only produce a small increase in stroke volume and cardiac output, and risks precipitating pulmonary oedema.
- *Improve myocardial contractility*. An inotrope may be required to ensure adequate cardiac output and peripheral blood flow sufficient to secure adequate oxygen delivery. Box 8.8 lists some characteristics of the commonly used vasoactive agents.

8.8 Actions of commonly used vasoactive agents

	Action		
Drug	**Vasoconstrictor**	**Inotrope**	**Chronotrope**
Adrenaline (epinephrine)	++	++	+
Noradrenaline (norepinephrine)	++++	+	(+)
Dobutamine	*	++++	++

*In most patients dobutamine acts as a vasodilator but in some it causes vasoconstriction.

- *Control heart rate and rhythm*. The optimum heart rate is usually between 90 and 110 beats per minute. Correction of low serum potassium and magnesium concentrations should be the first step in treating tachyarrhythmias in the critically ill. Atrial fibrillation is particularly common; intravenous amiodarone (300 mg over 30–60 minutes, followed by 900 mg over 24 hours) can be successful in controlling ventricular rate and in restoring and maintaining sinus rhythm. Other anti-arrhythmic agents are described on page 573.

The management of cardiac tamponade and pulmonary embolism is described on pages 545 and 723, respectively. Circulatory support in the context of sepsis is described below.

Prognosis

If the precipitating cause and accompanying circulatory failure are dealt with promptly, before significant organ failure occurs ('early' shock), the prognosis is good. If not, there is progressive deterioration in organ function and MOF ensues ('late' shock). The mortality of MOF is high and increases with the number of organs that have failed, the duration of organ failure and the patient's age. Failure of four or more organs is associated with a mortality of more than 80%.

Respiratory failure and acute respiratory distress syndrome

Respiratory failure may be the primary problem or could constitute a secondary complication (Box 8.9). The pattern of respiratory failure is classified using ABG analysis:

- *type 1*: hypoxaemia (PaO_2 < 8 kPa (< 60 mmHg) when breathing air) without hypercapnia
- *type 2*: hypoxaemia with hypercapnia ($PaCO_2$ > 6.5 kPa (> 49 mmHg)) due to alveolar hypoventilation.

Acute hypoxaemia results from an increase in ventilation–perfusion mismatch within the lung and this can be caused by almost any pulmonary disease. The most extreme form of mismatch is pulmonary shunting, which occurs when an area of lung is not ventilated at all – for example, due to collapse or consolidation.

8.9 Common causes of respiratory failure in critically ill patients

Type 1 respiratory failure	
• Pneumonia • Pulmonary oedema* • Pulmonary embolism • Pulmonary fibrosis • ARDS* • Aspiration	• Lung collapse*, e.g. retained secretions • Asthma • Pneumothorax • Pulmonary contusion (blunt chest trauma)
Type 2 respiratory failure	
• Reduced respiratory drive*, e.g. drug overdose, head injury • Upper airway obstruction (oedema, infection, foreign body) • Late severe acute asthma	• COPD • Peripheral neuromuscular disease*, e.g. Guillain–Barré syndrome, myasthenia gravis • Flail chest injury • Exhaustion* (includes all type 1 causes)

*Secondary complications of other conditions.
(ARDS = acute respiratory distress syndrome; COPD = chronic obstructive pulmonary disease)

Acute or chronic hypercapnia usually results from alveolar hypoventilation. Causes include:

- central depression of respiratory drive
- impaired nerve transmission between the central nervous system and muscle (especially the diaphragm)
- reduced chest wall movements (including diaphragmatic movements)
- reduced alveolar ventilation due to pathology within the lungs.

The primary respiratory conditions causing acute respiratory failure are detailed in Chapter 19. Critically ill patients may have both type 1 and 2 respiratory failure at some point, and the pattern and severity can change rapidly. Close monitoring and review are thus essential in order to decide which form of respiratory support is required, as this may change rapidly as the patient deteriorates and/or improves. Both the disease causing the illness *and* its effect on the patient's physiology over time must be taken into consideration. A combination of clinical examination and investigation helps to determine the most appropriate interventions (Box 8.10). The best method for assessing hypoxaemia is the ratio of the PaO_2 (measured by blood gas) to the fractional inspired oxygen delivered (PaO_2/FiO_2). This 'PF' ratio is lower, the more severe the disease. For example, a patient receiving 60% oxygen with a PaO_2 of 10.0 kPa (75.2 mmHg) on blood gas has a PF ratio of 10.0/0.6 = 16.7 kPa (125.6 mmHg).

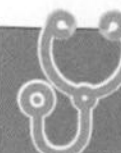

8.10 How to assess respiratory failure

Respiratory pattern
• Inspiratory stridor: typically caused by partial airway obstruction • Tachypnoea: often the first indicator of critical illness • Rapid shallow breathing: indicates more severe respiratory failure • Prolonged expiratory efforts: indicates severe bronchospasm
Conscious level
• Worsening drowsiness or agitation: indicates more severe respiratory failure as a result of hypoxaemia and/or hypercapnia
Pulse oximetry
• Oxygen saturations < 94%: indicate arterial hypoxaemia • Failure to respond to supplemental oxygen therapy, especially FiO_2 > 60%: indicates severe ventilation–perfusion mismatch and/or shunt
Arterial blood gases
• Calculate the PF ratio (see text): lower values indicate more severe disease
Imaging
• Chest X-ray, CT scan or chest ultrasound: information about the underlying pathology and treatable conditions, e.g. pleural effusion

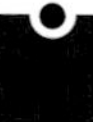

8.11 Conditions predisposing to ARDS

Inhalation (direct)	
• Aspiration of gastric contents • Toxic gases/burn injury	• Pneumonia • Blunt chest trauma • Near-drowning
Blood-borne (indirect)	
• Sepsis • Necrotic tissue (particularly bowel) • Multiple trauma • Pancreatitis • Cardiopulmonary bypass • Drugs (heroin, barbiturates, thiazides)	• Severe burns • Major transfusion reaction • Anaphylaxis • Fat embolism • Carcinomatosis • Obstetric crises (amniotic fluid embolus, eclampsia)

Acute lung injury and the acute respiratory distress syndrome

A range of conditions (Box 8.11) can result in a diffuse acute inflammatory process in the lungs called acute lung injury (ALI); when severe (as defined by hypoxaemia), this is termed the acute respiratory distress syndrome (ARDS; Box 8.12). Inflammation occurs throughout the lungs, affecting both endothelial and epithelial surfaces. Activated neutrophils are sequestered into the lungs and capillary permeability is increased, with damage to type I and II alveolar cells. This results in exudation and accumulation of protein-rich cellular fluid within alveoli and the formation of characteristic 'hyaline membranes'. Local release of cytokines and chemokines by activated macrophages and neutrophils results in progressive recruitment of inflammatory cells. Secondary effects include loss of surfactant and impaired surfactant production.

The net effect is alveolar collapse and reduced lung compliance, which are most marked in dependent regions of the lung, where airspaces become fluid-filled (Fig. 8.7). The combination of loss of surfactant and fluid accumulation makes these areas difficult to ventilate, which results in hypoxaemia due to ventilation–perfusion mismatch and increased pulmonary shunt. ALI and ARDS can be difficult to distinguish from fluid overload or cardiac failure.

8.12 Berlin definition of ARDS

- Onset within 1 week of a known clinical insult, or new or worsening respiratory symptoms
- Bilateral opacities on chest X-ray, not fully explained by effusions, lobar/lung collapse or nodules
- Respiratory failure not fully explained by cardiac failure or fluid overload. Objective assessment (e.g. by echocardiography) must exclude hydrostatic oedema if no risk factor is present
- Impaired oxygenation:
  Mild: 26.6 kPa (200 mmHg) < $PaO_2/FiO_2 \leq$ 39.9 kPa (300 mmHg) with PEEP or CPAP ≤ 5 cmH_2O
  Moderate: 13.3 kPa (100 mmHg) < $PaO_2/FiO_2 \leq$ 26.6 kPa (200 mmHg) with PEEP ≤ 5 cmH_2O
  Severe: $PaO_2/FiO_2 \leq$ 13.3 kPa (100 mmHg) with PEEP ≤ 5 cmH_2O

(CPAP = continuous positive airway pressure; PEEP = positive end expiratory pressure – see text for explanation)

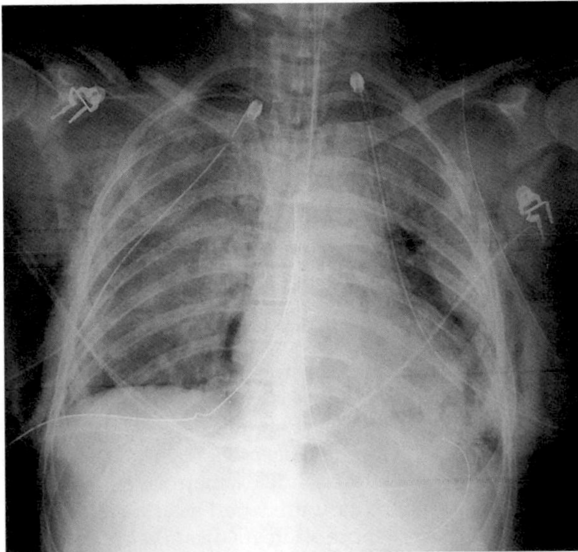

Fig. 8.7 Chest X-ray in acute respiratory distress syndrome (ARDS). Note bilateral lung infiltrates, pneumomediastinum, pneumothoraces with bilateral chest drains, surgical emphysema, and fractures of the ribs, right clavicle and left scapula.

Respiratory support

The aims of respiratory support are to maintain the patency of the airway, correct hypoxaemia and hypercapnia, and reduce the work of breathing.

Oxygen therapy

Oxygen is given to ensure adequate arterial oxygenation (SpO_2 > 90%), initially by facemask or nasal cannulae. The inspired oxygen concentration (FiO_2) is adjusted, depending on pulse oximetry and ABG analysis. If this results in unacceptable hypercapnia, the patient requires some form of mechanical respiratory support. The risk of progressive hypercapnia in patients with chronic obstructive pulmonary disease (COPD) who are dependent on hypoxic drive has been overstated. Hypoxic cerebral damage is irreversible, so the theoretical risks of oxygen toxicity are not relevant if the patient is acutely hypoxaemic, as the maintenance of cerebral oxygenation takes precedence. More detail on oxygen therapy is given on page 664.

Non-invasive respiratory support

Non-invasive respiratory support includes techniques that do not require sedation or an endotracheal or tracheostomy tube. This helps preserve the patient's respiratory muscle activity and reduces complications such as nosocomial infection. It can be used to support selected patients with type 1 or 2 respiratory failure, but the patient's conscious level must be adequate to ensure airway protection from aspiration. Non-invasive respiratory support is classified as continuous positive airway pressure (CPAP) alone or CPAP plus additional support, in the form of pressure applied to the breathing circuit during inspiration (non-invasive ventilation, or NIV).

8

CPAP therapy

CPAP therapy involves the application of a continuous positive airway pressure throughout the patient's breathing cycle, typically between 5 and 10 cmH_2O. CPAP recruits collapsed alveoli and can enhance clearance of alveolar fluid. It is particularly effective for treating pulmonary atelectasis (which may be post-operative) and pulmonary oedema, and helps correct hypoxaemia in some patients with pneumonia, especially the immunocompromised. CPAP therapy is most effective in correcting hypoxaemia in type 1 respiratory failure, but if it improves pulmonary compliance (by clearing fluid or improving lung volume), it can reduce the work of breathing and improve hypercapnia in type 2. However, many patients with the latter require NIV or invasive ventilation. CPAP therapy can be delivered using tight-fitting facial masks, high-flow nasal cannulae, and hoods (Fig. 8.8). Usually, a CPAP mask is tried first, but different systems can be trialled until the most comfortable for the patient is found. Patients must be cooperative,

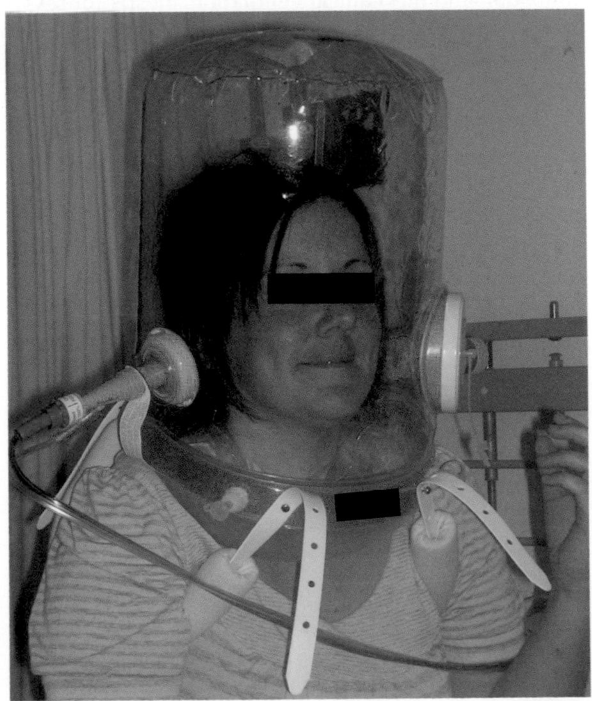

Fig. 8.8 CPAP delivery with a Castar hood.

able to protect their airway, and have the strength to breathe spontaneously and cough effectively. Failure to improve over 24–48 hours, or a further deterioration in conscious level or blood gases, indicates that invasive ventilation should be considered.

Non-invasive ventilation

Non-invasive ventilation (NIV) is ventilatory support by nasal or full facemask. It can be delivered by a simple bi-level (BiPAP) turbine ventilator, which delivers a higher pressure (approximately 15–25 cmH_2O) for inspiration and a lower pressure (4–10 cmH_2O) to allow expiration. If hypoxaemia is severe, a complex ICU ventilator is employed that allows higher oxygen concentrations to be administered. A simple breathing circuit with a leak rather than an expiratory valve is generally used, and ventilation can be spontaneous (triggered by the patient's breaths) or timed (occurring at set intervals and/or frequency). Systems that synchronise with the patient's efforts are better tolerated and more effective. NIV is the first-line therapy in patients with type 2 respiratory failure secondary to acute exacerbation of COPD because it reduces the work of breathing and offloads the diaphragm, allowing it to recover strength. It should be initiated early, especially when severe respiratory acidosis and/or decreased consciousness secondary to hypercapnia are present. Unless there is an improvement in acidosis within 4–6 hours, invasive ventilation is indicated. NIV can also be used to support selected patients with hypercapnia secondary to pulmonary oedema or pneumonia, or during weaning from invasive ventilation, but its effectiveness in these conditions is less certain. As with mask CPAP, NIV requires the patient to be conscious and cooperative.

Emergency endotracheal intubation and mechanical ventilation

Many patients admitted to ICU require endotracheal intubation and mechanical ventilation, mostly for respiratory failure (Boxes 8.13 and 8.14). The final decision to undertake these is based on clinical judgement rather than the results of ABGs in isolation. If possible, the patient's relatives should be given the chance to visit prior to anaesthesia and intubation, as this may be the last opportunity they have to speak together.

In the conscious patient, intubation requires induction of anaesthesia and muscle relaxation, while in more obtunded patients, sedation alone may be adequate. Intubation can be hazardous in the critically ill patient, particularly if there is associated cardiovascular failure. Patients should be pre-oxygenated and cricoid pressure applied, with continuous monitoring of heart rate, ECG and BP (preferably invasively), together with capnography (and subsequently a chest X-ray) to confirm correct endotracheal tube placement. Complications are common, and intubation is ideally performed in a critical care environment, or with expert assistance, resuscitation facilities and appropriate medication immediately available. Hypotension may follow sedation or anaesthesia due to the direct cardiovascular effects of the anaesthetic agent and loss of sympathetic drive. Positive pressure ventilation may compound this by increasing intrathoracic pressure, thereby reducing venous return and thus cardiac output.

8.13 Indications for tracheal intubation and mechanical ventilation

- Protection of airway
- Respiratory arrest or rate < 8 breaths/min
- Tachypnoea > 35 beats/min
- Inability to tolerate oxygen mask/CPAP/NIV, e.g. agitation, confusion
- Removal of secretions
- Hypoxaemia (PaO_2 < 8 kPa (< 60 mmHg); SpO_2 < 90%) despite CPAP with FiO_2 > 0.6
- Hypercapnia if conscious level is impaired or risk of raised intracranial pressure
- Worsening respiratory acidosis
- Vital capacity falling below 1.2 L in patients with neuromuscular disease
- Removing the work of breathing in exhausted patients

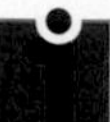

8.14 Conditions requiring mechanical ventilation*

Post-operative

- After major abdominal or cardiac surgery

Respiratory failure

- ARDS
- Pneumonia
- COPD
- Acute severe asthma
- Aspiration
- Smoke inhalation, burns

Circulatory failure

- Low cardiac output: cardiogenic shock
- Pulmonary oedema
- Post-cardiac arrest

Neurological disease

- Coma of any cause
- Status epilepticus
- Drug overdose
- Respiratory muscle failure (see Box 8.9, p. 192)
- Head injury: to avoid hypoxaemia and hypercapnia, and reduce intracranial pressure
- Bulbar abnormalities causing risk of aspiration (e.g. stroke, myasthenia gravis)

Multiple trauma

*Additional considerations:
Metabolic rate: ventilatory requirements rise as metabolic rate increases.
Nutritional reserve: low potassium or phosphate reduces respiratory muscle power.
Abdominal distension due to surgery or tense ascites: causes discomfort and splinting of the diaphragm, compromising spontaneous respiratory effort and promoting bilateral basal lung collapse.

Tracheostomy is usually performed electively when endotracheal intubation is likely to be required for more than 7–10 days (Box 8.15). The timing is determined by individual patient factors and clinical judgement. Tracheostomy is usually carried out percutaneously in the ICU, to avoid transfer to an operating theatre. The passage of a smaller (4.5 mm internal diameter) 'mini-tracheostomy' tube through the cricothyroid membrane is a useful technique for clearing airway secretions in spontaneously breathing patients with a poor cough effort, particularly in the HDU and in post-operative patients.

General considerations in the management of the ventilated/intubated patient

Modern ventilators allow enormous flexibility in the way ventilator support is provided. The terminology used to describe ventilation modes can be confusing,

8.15 Advantages and disadvantages of tracheostomy

Advantages

- Patient comfort
- Improved oral hygiene
- Access for tracheal toilet
- Enables speech with cuff deflated and a speaking valve attached
- Earlier weaning and ICU discharge
- Reduced sedation requirement
- Reduces vocal cord damage

Disadvantages

- Immediate complications: hypoxia, haemorrhage
- Tracheostomy site infection
- Tracheal damage; late stenosis

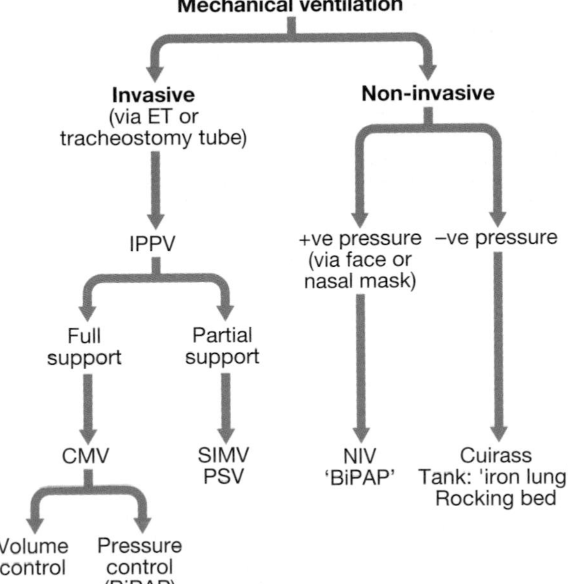

Fig. 8.9 Types of invasive and non-invasive ventilatory support. (BiPAP = bi-level positive airway pressure; CMV = controlled mandatory ventilation; ET = endotracheal; IPPV = intermittent positive pressure ventilation; NIV = non-invasive ventilation; PSV = pressure support ventilation; SIMV = synchronised intermittent mandatory ventilation)

because of subtle differences between modes, and the use of different names by different manufacturers. Figure 8.9 gives a classification of the different types of invasive ventilation support, and Box 8.16 outlines the terminology used and the parameters that are set on any ventilator. The inspired gas should always be humidified and warmed, usually achieved with a heat and moisture exchanger, but occasionally with hot water humidification systems.

Initial settings

Following intubation, the ventilator is set to deliver a safe mandatory mode of ventilation that will achieve oxygenation and carbon dioxide clearance in the majority of patients. Regular re-assessment of the patient's parameters will show if modification is required. Hyperoxia is avoided, as it is associated with adverse outcomes.

8.16 Ventilator parameter settings on initiating mechanical ventilation

Parameter	Setting
FiO_2	Initially set to achieve SpO_2 > 92% based on pulse oximetry Subsequently adjusted to achieve PaO_2 of 8–12 kPa (60.2–90.2 mmHg) on ABGs
Positive end expiratory pressure (PEEP)	The pressure maintained by the ventilator at the end of expiration: important for recruiting and maintaining alveoli for gas exchange Initially set at ~5 cmH_2O, except in patients with severe gas trapping (e.g. acute asthma), but increased in patients with severe hypoxaemia
Tidal volume	Set low in ARDS to minimise pulmonary barotrauma and volutrauma In patients with normal lungs, higher volumes are safe
Respiratory rate	Typically set at 12–15 breaths/min Adjusted according to $PaCO_2$ on ABGs to achieve adequate CO_2 clearance
Mode of ventilation	The safest initial mode is SIMV (see text): synchronises breaths with efforts made by patient, but ventilates at the set rate and tidal volume in the absence of respiratory effort
Breath trigger	Initiates a breath in response to patient's efforts, triggered by flow towards the patient on attempts to breathe Set at the appropriate sensitivity for the patient
Inspired to expired time ratio (I–E ratio)	In most patients, the I–E ratio should be 1:2 to 1:3 Sometimes altered in expiratory airway obstruction (e.g. lengthened in asthma) or difficult oxygenation (e.g. shortened or reversed in ARDS)
Alarms	Disconnection Low or high tidal volumes Low FiO_2 Excessively high or low airway pressures A range of other parameters can also be selected Adjust default settings to optimise safety for the individual patient

Mandatory modes of ventilation

Volume-controlled modes. These are set to deliver a preset tidal volume at a set frequency to guarantee a specified minute ventilation. Synchronised intermittent mandatory ventilation (SIMV) is the most widely used, which also synchronises breaths with any efforts made by the patient. Volume-controlled modes will deliver the set volume, but the pressures generated in the patient's lungs can be excessively high if the pulmonary compliance is low – for example, in ARDS – thus precipitating lung barotrauma or volutrauma, which could cause pneumothorax.

Pressure-controlled modes. These deliver a set pressure for a specified duration. Pressure-controlled ventilation (PCV) and bi-level positive airway pressure ventilation (BiPAP) are examples. The tidal and minute volumes achieved are determined by the pulmonary compliance; in patients with stiff lungs, only small tidal volumes may be achieved, whereas in patients with normal compliance, excessive volumes may result. An advantage of these modes is that airway pressures are controlled, but the effect on blood gases needs to be regularly assessed to identify changes in pulmonary compliance. Tidal volume is a useful safety alarm as it falls with increased resistance, such as with bronchospasm. In difficult-to-ventilate cases, several modes can be attempted sequentially to identify which is most effective.

Weaning or spontaneously breathing modes. Most modern ventilators can detect whether a patient is making breathing efforts, and use a flow trigger to augment each breath. Assisting breathing with additional pressure is more comfortable than fixed tidal volumes and allows sedation to be reduced. The most common mode applies additional pressure during inspiration, assisting the work of breathing and increasing tidal volume. The pressure is removed when the ventilator detects an expiratory effort. These modes are usually called pressure support ventilation (PSV) or assisted spontaneous breathing (ASB).

Mixed modes. Different modes can be applied simultaneously, tailored to meet individual requirements. For example, it is possible to specify a frequency of SIMV or PCV breaths, but also provide PSV for any additional efforts the patient makes.

Advanced ventilation strategies

In patients with severe acute lung disease, especially those resulting in reduced lung compliance such as ARDS, the ventilator can worsen lung injury as a result of overstretch and shearing forces in parts of the lung that continually open and collapse. The aim of advanced ventilation is to minimise further damage due to pressure (barotrauma), volume stretch (volutrauma), and the additional inflammatory mediators released into the body from ongoing lung injury (biotrauma) (Box 8.17). Tidal volumes and airway pressures are kept as low as possible while achieving adequate oxygenation. In many cases, it is best to accept hypercapnia rather than apply higher pressure to clear CO_2. Often, higher levels of positive end expiratory pressure (PEEP) are required to achieve adequate alveolar recruitment and oxygenation.

Several other strategies can be used.

EBM 8.17 Mechanical ventilation in ARDS

- Low tidal volumes (4–6 mL/kg ideal body weight) reduce mortality from ARDS.[1]
- High levels of PEEP should be avoided in patients with less severe ARDS, in whom it may be harmful. In severe ARDS, high level of PEEP to recruit the lungs and improve oxygenation may decrease mortality.[2]
- Early use of neuromuscular relaxing drugs to facilitate mechanical ventilation reduces mortality in severe ARDS.[3]
- Minimised fluid administration and accumulation reduce the duration of mechanical ventilation in ARDS.[4]

- [1]ARDS Clinical Trials Network. N Engl J Med 2000; 342:1301–1308.
- [2]Briel M, et al. JAMA 2010; 303:865–873.
- [3]Papazian L, et al. N Engl J Med 2010; 363:1107–1116.
- [4]ARDS Clinical Trials Network. N Engl J Med 2006; 354:2564–2575.

(PEEP = positive end-expiratory pressure)

Prone ventilation. Oxygenation will often improve in patients turned on their front, as a result of improved lung recruitment and better ventilation–perfusion matching. Prone ventilation has not reduced mortality in controlled trials, but is a useful 'rescue therapy' in cases where oxygenation is difficult.

High-frequency oscillatory ventilation (HFOV). This uses a specialised ventilator to provide gas exchange with high-frequency oscillating gas movements (> 150/min). Conventional breaths and tidal volumes are not set, but effective oxygenation and CO_2 clearance are achieved by adjusting the frequency and power of the oscillations, and the mean airway pressure.

Nitric oxide. Nitric oxide is a very short-acting pulmonary vasodilator. When delivered to the airway, it improves blood flow to ventilated alveoli, thus improving ventilation–perfusion matching. Oxygenation can be improved markedly in some patients but there is evidence that this lasts for only 48 hours, and rebound effects can occur when it is withdrawn. No improvement in mortality has been shown in controlled trials. Its role is limited to rescue therapy when other interventions have failed, and it may be useful in patients with severe pulmonary hypertension.

Extracorporeal membrane oxygenation therapy (ECMO). ECMO involves connecting the patient to an external bypass circuit. Oxygenation and CO_2 clearance are achieved using a membrane oxygenator. The patient's lungs are usually 'rested' and ventilation reduced to low levels. Advances in technology have dramatically improved the safety of these devices, although their use is restricted to specialised centres. Controlled trials indicate improved survival in appropriately selected cases, and patients with severe ARDS should be considered for treatment.

Corticosteroids. There is conflicting evidence regarding the use of steroids as anti-inflammatory agents in acute lung injury. Uncertainty remains about patient selection and the timing of therapy, and use of corticosteroids may be complicated by secondary infection and muscle weakness. However, they are often tried after 7–10 days of ARDS, if the patient remains severely unwell.

Weaning from respiratory support

Patients usually require most mechanical ventilation in the period following intubation when they are most unwell, following which support is gradually reduced as the underlying condition resolves and the patient is able to breathe with less assistance. This is the process of 'weaning' from ventilation. Sufficient support is provided to correct hypoxaemia and hypercapnia, but the level is decreased as quickly as possible to reduce the chance of secondary complications, such as infection and muscle weakness. Rapid weaning, often with reduction in sedation levels (see below), shortens length of ICU stay and improves patient outcomes. Patients who have required long-term ventilatory support for severe lung disease such as ARDS may be unable to sustain even a modest degree of respiratory work initially because of poor lung compliance, high work of breathing and respiratory muscle weakness. They require more prolonged weaning, until respiratory muscle strength improves.

Several criteria can be used to assess whether a patient is ready to start reducing respiratory support (Box 8.18). Approaches include:

8.18 Factors to consider in deciding to wean and extubate a ventilated patient

- Has the original indication for mechanical ventilation resolved?
- Is the patient conscious and able to cough and protect his/her airway?
- Is the circulation stable, without signs of cardiac failure or excessive fluid overload?
- Is gas exchange satisfactory (PaO_2 > 10 kPa (> 75 mmHg) on FiO_2 < 0.5; $PaCO_2$ < 6 kPa (< 45 mmHg))?
- Is analgesia adequate?
- Are any metabolic problems well controlled?

Spontaneous breathing trials (SBTs). These involve removing all respiratory support, typically on a daily basis, and observing how long the patient is able to breathe unassisted. This is particularly effective when linked to sedation breaks. Signs of failure include rapid shallow breathing, hypoxaemia, rising $PaCO_2$, sweating and agitation. Patients who pass an SBT are assessed for extubation.

Progressive reduction in pressure support ventilation. Progressive reduction in the PSV is applied for each breath over a period of hours or days, according to patient response. When patients are strong enough to achieve stable ABGs without distress while receiving minimal or no support, they are likely to be ready for extubation. This can take from several hours to many weeks, according to the severity of illness.

Weaning protocols. The process of weaning is best undertaken as a continuous process. Protocols that empower nursing staff to initiate and progress weaning within agreed guidelines reduce ventilation times. Patients requiring prolonged mechanical ventilation typically require individualised weaning plans, with regular periods of training followed by rest, to enable respiratory muscles to regain strength.

The timing of extubation relies on clinical judgement. Patients must have stable ABGs with resolution of hypoxaemia and hypercapnia despite withdrawal of ventilator support. Conscious level must be adequate to protect the airway, comply with physiotherapy, and cough. The need for re-intubation following extubation is associated with poorer outcomes.

Acute kidney injury

Acute kidney injury (AKI) is defined as an abrupt and sustained decrease in kidney function (Box 8.19). AKI in the critically ill patient is often due to pre-renal problems such as hypovolaemia, hypotension and ischaemia resulting in reduced renal DO_2. However, it may also be due to acute tubular necrosis (ATN, p. 479), which may result from ischaemia, or nephrotoxicity caused by chemical or bacterial toxins, or a combination of these. Potentially nephrotoxic drugs include non-steroidal anti-inflammatory drugs (NSAIDs), angiotensin-converting enzyme (ACE) inhibitors, angiotensin II receptor antagonists, radiological contrast media and some antibiotics.

Oliguria (< 0.5 mL/kg/hr for several hours) is an important early sign of systemic problems in critical illness. It requires investigation and early intervention to correct hypoxaemia, hypovolaemia, hypotension and renal hypoperfusion. Successful resuscitation is associated with restoration of good urine output, an improving acid–base balance and correction of plasma potassium, urea and creatinine.

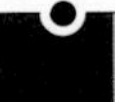

8.19 Diagnostic criteria for acute kidney injury*

An abrupt (within 48 hrs) decline in kidney function defined as:

- An absolute increase in serum creatinine of ≥ 26.4 μmol/L (0.3 mg/dL)
- A percentage increase in serum creatinine of ≥ 50% (1.5-fold from baseline)
- A reduction in urine output (documented oliguria of < 0.5 mL/kg for > 6 consecutive hrs)

*Mehta R, et al. http://ccforum.eom/content/11/2/R31.

Oliguria is an integral part of the normal stress response to major surgery, and care should be taken not to overfill the post-operative patient who has oliguria but is otherwise well from a cardiovascular and biochemical point of view.

Renal support

Sepsis is frequently implicated in the development of AKI, and the source must be promptly identified and adequately treated. Obstruction of the renal tract (including catheter blockage) should always be excluded and is most easily identified with abdominal ultrasound. It must be relieved at once. Acute glomerulonephritis and vasculitis must also be considered, and appropriate specialist referral, with investigations such as urine microscopy and immunopathological tests (p. 480), carried out early.

The mainstay of management is aggressive haemodynamic resuscitation to achieve normovolaemia, normotension and an appropriate cardiac output. There is little evidence that specific treatments aimed at inducing a diuresis, such as low-dose dopamine, furosemide or mannitol, have any renoprotective action or other benefit in restoring renal function.

If renal function cannot be restored following resuscitation, renal replacement therapy (p. 488) is indicated (Box 8.20). The preferred renal replacement therapy in ICU patients is pumped venovenous haemofiltration. This is associated with fewer osmotic fluid shifts and hence greater haemodynamic stability than haemodialysis. It is carried out using a double-lumen central venous catheter placed percutaneously. Haemofiltration should

8.20 Indications for renal replacement therapy

- Hyperkalaemia: potassium > 6 mmol/L despite medical treatment
- Fluid overload: pulmonary oedema
- Metabolic acidosis: H^+ > 56 nmol/L (pH < 7.25)
- Uraemia:
  - Urea > 30–35 mmol/L (180–210 mg/dL)
  - Creatinine > 600 μmol/L (> 6.78 mg/dL)
- Drug removal in overdose
- Sepsis: tentative evidence for mediator removal

be continuous in the early phase of treatment. Intermittent treatment may be used when the patient is recovering from the primary insult and return of normal renal function is expected. Provided the precipitating cause can be successfully treated, renal failure due to ATN usually recovers between 5 days and several weeks later.

Survival rates from MOF, including AKI, have been around 50% for many years, but modern haemofiltration techniques are being shown to produce better outcomes.

Gastrointestinal and hepatic disturbance

Gastrointestinal symptoms, such as nausea, vomiting and large nasogastric aspirates, may be the earliest signs of regional circulatory failure, and when associated with a tender, distended, silent abdomen, indicate that this is the probable site of the primary pathology. The gut has a rapid cell turnover rate and fasting alone can produce marked changes in mucosal structure and function. In hypovolaemia and frank shock states, splanchnic vasoconstriction produces gut mucosal ischaemia, damaging the mucosal barrier and allowing toxins to enter the portal circulation and lymphatics. Splanchnic ischaemia may contribute to the progression of MOF, possibly as a source of bacteraemia or systemic inflammation. Manifestations of MOF within the gastrointestinal tract include loss of gastric acid production, erosive gastritis, stress ulceration, bleeding, ischaemia, pancreatitis and acalculous cholecystitis. These occur less frequently when adequate circulatory resuscitation occurs early. Ischaemic bowel is difficult to diagnose in the critically ill patient, but in the context of otherwise unexplained lactic acidosis, hyperkalaemia and coagulopathy, abdominal imaging by contrast-enhanced computed tomography (CT) and laparotomy should be considered.

Three distinctive hepatic dysfunction syndromes can occur in the critically ill:

- *Shock liver or ischaemic hepatitis* results from extreme hepatic tissue hypoxia and is characterised by centrilobular hepatocellular necrosis. Transaminase levels are often massively raised (> 1000–5000 U/L) at an early stage, followed by moderate hyperbilirubinaemia (< 100 μmol/L or < 5.8 mg/dL). There is often associated hypoglycaemia, coagulopathy and lactic acidosis. Following successful resuscitation, hepatic function generally returns to normal.
- *Hyperbilirubinaemia* (*'ICU jaundice'*) frequently develops following trauma or sepsis, particularly if there is inadequate control of the inflammatory process. There is a marked rise in bilirubin (predominantly conjugated), but only mild elevation of transaminase and alkaline phosphatase. This results from failure of bilirubin transport within the liver and produces the histological appearance of intrahepatic cholestasis. Extrahepatic cholestasis must be excluded by abdominal ultrasound and potentially hepatotoxic drugs should be stopped. Treatment is non-specific and should include early institution of enteral feeding. Therapy that compromises splanchnic blood flow, particularly high doses of vasoconstrictor agents, should be avoided.
- *Transaminitis* is most commonly due to drug toxicity: for example, antibiotics.

Gastrointestinal and hepatic support

Early institution of enteral nutrition is the most effective strategy for protecting the gut mucosa and providing nutritional support. The optimum use of enteral nutrition involves simple protocols that initiate nutrition as early as possible, and progressively increase feeding volumes until nutritional targets are met. Current evidence supports early enteral nutrition using standard feeds, with the addition of prokinetic agents such as metoclopramide or low-dose erythromycin when gastric aspirates are high. The evidence for early supplementation with total parenteral nutrition (TPN) is weak, and it is not routinely indicated until enteral feeding attempts have been unsuccessful for approximately 7 days. Nutritional support is further considered on page 122.

Hyperglycaemia is common during critical illness and is associated with poor outcomes. Tight glycaemic control, using insulin infusions, has been studied in several controlled trials in the critically ill. The benefit was greatest in surgical patients at low risk of death, but the risk-to-benefit profile in the mixed critically ill population is uncertain. Inadvertent hypoglycaemia is associated with adverse patient outcomes. In most ICUs, the current target is for modestly elevated blood glucose concentrations: for example, 5.5–8 mmol/L (100–144 mg/dL).

Stress ulcer prophylaxis is best achieved with H_2-receptor antagonists (e.g. ranitidine), which are both safe and effective. Although stress ulcer bleeding is rare with modern resuscitation, evidence supports routine use in mechanically ventilated patients and those with renal failure or coagulopathy. H_2-receptor antagonists are associated with an increased incidence of nosocomial pneumonia, and treatment should be stopped following extubation in the absence of other indications. Withdrawal can also be considered when full enteral nutrition has been established, unless the patient has a history of peptic ulcer disease. Proton pump inhibitors are only required in upper gastrointestinal bleeding due to ulceration, and they should also be continued when the patient has been taking them long-term.

The management of liver failure is discussed on page 934.

Neurological failure (coma)

Impaired consciousness or coma is often an early feature of severe systemic illness (Box 8.21). Prompt assessment of consciousness level and management of airway, breathing and circulation are essential to prevent further brain injury, to allow diagnosis and to permit definitive treatment to be instituted. Any patient with confusion or reduced conscious level should have blood sugar measured and hypoglycaemia corrected.

Impairment of conscious level is graded using the Glasgow Coma Scale (GCS, p. 1160), which is also used to monitor progress. A targeted neurological examination is very important. Pupil size and reaction to light,

8.21 Causes of coma

Systemic causes	
Cerebral hypoxia or hypercapnia	
• Respiratory failure	
Cerebral ischaemia	
• Cardiac arrest	• Hypotension
Metabolic disturbance	
• Diabetes mellitus	• Uraemia
Hypoglycaemia	• Hepatic failure
Ketoacidosis	• Hypothermia
Hyperosmolar coma	• Drugs
• Hyponatraemia	• Sepsis
• Myxoedema coma	
Primary neurological causes	
Trauma	
• Cerebral contusion	• Subdural haematoma
• Extradural haematoma	
Infection	
• Cerebral abscess	• Meningitis
• Encephalitis	
Cerebrovascular disease	
• Intracerebral haemorrhage	• Cerebral venous sinus thrombosis
• Brainstem infarction	
• Subarachnoid haemorrhage	
Cerebral tumour	
Epilepsy	
Hydrocephalus	

presence or absence of neck stiffness, focal neurological signs and evidence of other organ impairment should be noted. After cardiorespiratory stability is achieved, the cause of the coma must be sought from the history (family, witness, general practitioner), examination and investigation, particularly CT of brain. The possibility of drug overdose should always be considered.

Neurological support

A diverse range of neurological conditions require management in the ICU. These include not only the various causes of coma, but also spinal cord injury, peripheral neuromuscular disease and prolonged seizures. The goals are to:

- protect the airway, if necessary by endotracheal intubation
- provide respiratory support to correct hypoxaemia and hypercapnia
- treat circulatory problems, e.g. neurogenic pulmonary oedema in subarachnoid haemorrhage, autonomic disturbances in Guillain–Barré syndrome, and spinal shock following high spinal cord injuries
- manage acute brain injury with control of raised intracranial pressure (ICP)
- manage status epilepticus using anaesthetic agents such as thiopental or propofol.

The aim of management in acute brain injury is to optimise cerebral oxygen delivery by maintaining a normal arterial oxygen content and a cerebral perfusion pressure of more than 60 mmHg. Avoiding secondary insults to the brain, such as hypoxaemia and hypotension, improves outcome. ICP rises in acute brain injury as a result of haematoma, contusions, oedema or ischaemic swelling. Raised ICP causes direct damage to the cerebral cortex and, as a result of downward pressure on the brainstem, indirect damage by reducing cerebral perfusion pressure, thereby threatening cerebral blood flow and oxygen delivery:

8.22 Strategies to control intracranial pressure

- Prevent coughing with sedation, analgesia and occasionally paralysis
- Nurse with 30° head-up tilt and avoid excessive flexion of the head or pressure around the neck that may impair cerebral venous drainage
- Control epileptiform activity with appropriate anticonvulsant therapy: an electroencephalogram (EEG) may be necessary to ensure that this is achieved
- Maintain blood glucose between 5.5 and 8 mmol/L (99–144 mg/dL)
- Aim for a core body temperature of between 36 and 37°C
- Maintain sodium > 140 mmol/L using IV 0.9% saline
- Avoid volume depletion or overload
- Ventilate aiming to reduce the $PaCO_2$ to 4–4.5 kPa (~30–34 mmHg) for the first 24 hrs
- Osmotic diuretic: mannitol 20% 100–200 mL (0.25–0.5 g/kg), coupled with volume replacement
- Hypnotic infusion: thiopental, titrated to 'burst suppression' on EEG
- Surgery: drainage of haematoma or ventricles; lobectomy, decompressive craniectomy

Cerebral perfusion pressure (CPP) = mean BP − ICP

ICP is measured by pressure transducers that are inserted directly into the brain tissue. The normal upper limit for ICP is 15 mmHg and management should be directed at keeping it below 20 mmHg (Box 8.22). Sustained pressures of more than 30 mmHg are associated with a poor prognosis.

CPP should be maintained above 60 mmHg by ensuring adequate fluid replacement and, if necessary, by treating hypotension with a vasopressor such as noradrenaline (norepinephrine).

Complex neurological monitoring must be combined with frequent clinical assessment of GCS, pupil response to light, and focal neurological signs. The motor response to pain is an important prognostic sign. No response or extension of the upper limbs is associated with severe injury, and unless there is improvement within a few days, prognosis is very poor. A flexor response is encouraging and indicates that a good outcome is still possible.

Neurological complications in intensive care

Neurological complications may occur as a result of systemic critical illness. Sepsis may be associated both with an encephalopathy characterised by delirium, and with cerebral oedema and loss of vasoregulation. Hypotension and coagulopathy may provoke cerebral infarction or haemorrhage. Neurological examination is very difficult if patients are sedated or paralysed, and it is important to stop sedation regularly to re-assess their underlying level of consciousness. If there is evidence of a focal neurological deficit or a markedly declining level of consciousness, CT of brain should be performed.

Critical illness polyneuropathy is another potential complication in patients with sepsis and MOF. It is due to peripheral nerve axonal loss and can result in areflexia, gross muscle wasting and failure to wean from the ventilator, thus prolonging the duration of intensive care. Recovery can take many weeks.

Sepsis

Sepsis can occur in many clinical situations. It may be due to a primary infection (e.g. pneumonia) or it may be the result of clinical interventions for other conditions (e.g. immunosuppressive drugs, chemotherapy, invasive lines). Patients who are in hospital are at increased risk of certain specific infections, such as meticillin-resistant *Staphylococcus aureus* (MRSA). Sepsis usually originates from a localised infection that progresses to an uncontrolled systemic response. It can rapidly lead to acute physiological deterioration with the risk of MOF and death. Early identification of sepsis and appropriate intervention with oxygen, fluids, antibiotics, and more advanced resuscitation where indicated, has been shown to improve survival.

The incidence of sepsis is thought to be increasing, possibly as a result of a growing elderly population, increased use of invasive surgery, higher bacterial resistance, and greater numbers of immunocompromised patients. Important comorbidities and risk factors for sepsis are shown in Box 8.23. These conditions not only increase risk of development of sepsis but also can exaggerate the severity of the process. However, sepsis can affect healthy people at any age.

Box 8.24 gives the common sites of infection in critically ill patients and appropriate investigations to consider. Any pathogen, including aerobic Gram-positive and negative bacteria, anaerobes and fungi, may cause sepsis but in nearly 45% of cases microbiological confirmation of the organism is lacking.

Any or all of the features of SIRS (see Box 8.2, p. 184) may be present, together with an obvious focus of infection, such as purulent sputum with chest X-ray shadowing, or erythema around an intravenous line. However, severe sepsis may present with unexplained hypotension (i.e. septic shock), and the speed of onset may mimic a major pulmonary embolus or myocardial infarction.

Nosocomial infections are an increasing problem in critical care units. Risk factors are similar to those in Box 8.23, but also include prolonged ICU stay, invasive ventilation and stress ulcer prophylaxis with H_2 antagonists. Cross-infection is a major concern, particularly with MRSA, multidrug-resistant Gram-negative organisms and *Clostridium difficile*. If cross-infection occurs frequently, it should prompt a review of the unit's infection

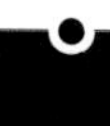

8.23 Risk factors for sepsis

- Diabetes mellitus
- Immunodeficiency
- Trauma
- Burns
- Alcohol and substance abuse
- Chronic disease (heart, lungs, kidneys, liver)
- Haematological disorders
- Recent surgery/invasive procedure
- Invasive lines: intravenous or arterial, urinary catheters, nasogastric tubes

8.24 Sites of infection in critically ill patients

Sites of infection	Investigations and comments
Major	
Intravenous lines (particularly central)	If the patient develops sepsis, replace any lines that have not been changed for > 4 days
Lungs	High risk of nosocomial pneumonia in intubated patients. After ICU stay > 3–4 days, particularly if antibiotics are given, the nasopharynx becomes colonised with Gram-negative bacteria, which migrate to the lower respiratory tract. Prophylaxis with parenteral and enteral antibiotics (selective decontamination of the digestive tract) reduces the incidence of nosocomial pneumonia
Abdomen	Consider intra-abdominal abscess or necrotic gut in patients who have had abdominal surgery Pancreatitis, acute cholecystitis or perforated peptic ulcer may develop as a complication of critical illness. Ultrasound, CT, aspiration of collections of fluid/pus and laparotomy may be required
Urinary tract	Urine culture (but this is a relatively unusual source in unexplained sepsis)
Other	
Heart valves	Transthoracic or transoesophageal echocardiogram
Meninges	Lumbar puncture after checking coagulation and platelet count
Joints and bones	X-ray, gallium or technetium white cell scan
Nasal sinuses, ears, retropharyngeal space	Clinical examination, plain X-ray, CT
Genitourinary tract (particularly post-partum)	PV examination, ultrasound
Gastrointestinal tract	PR examination, stool culture, *Clostridium difficile* toxin, sigmoidoscopy

control policies (p. 145). Limiting antibiotic use helps to prevent the emergence of multidrug-resistant bacteria.

Management

Prompt resuscitation, with early cultures, administration of appropriate antibiotics and eradication of the source of infection (if necessary by surgical drainage), is required (Box 8.25). Antibiotics should have a spectrum wide enough to cover probable causative organisms, based on the likely site of infection, whether community-acquired or nosocomial, previous antibiotic therapy and known local resistance patterns.

Other investigations required include:

- cultures of sputum, intravascular lines, urine and any wound discharge
- ABGs and coagulation profile
- urinalysis and chest X-ray.

Only 10% of ICU patients with a clinical diagnosis of 'septic' shock will have positive blood cultures, due to prior antibiotic treatment and the fact that an inflammatory state is not always due to infection. More specific investigations are driven by the history and examination (see Box 8.24).

The haemodynamic changes in septic shock are very variable and not specific for the Gram status of the infecting organism. The first feature is often tachypnoea and the early stages are frequently dominated by hypotension with relative volume depletion due to vasodilatation. Sufficient intravenous fluid should be given to ensure that the intravascular volume is not the limiting factor in determining global oxygen delivery. The type of fluid that should be administered and what constitutes 'adequate' volume resuscitation remain controversial. The response to therapy is crucial when deciding this and is frequently unpredictable, so rigid protocols cannot be used. Depending on haemoglobin concentration, blood or synthetic colloid should be given as 100–200 mL boluses to assess BP response to volume (see Fig. 8.2, p. 183).

Although ventricular function is frequently impaired, the characteristically low systemic vascular resistance (SVR) usually ensures a high cardiac output (once the patient is adequately volume-resuscitated), albeit with low BP.

The choice of the most appropriate vasoactive drug to use should be based on a full assessment of the circulation and the different inotropic, dilating or constricting properties of these drugs (see Box 8.8, p. 191). In most cases, a vasoconstrictor such as noradrenaline (norepinephrine) is necessary to increase SVR and BP, while an inotrope (dobutamine) may be necessary to maintain cardiac output. In the later stages of severe sepsis, the fundamental problem is at the microcirculatory level. Oxygen uptake and utilisation are impaired due to failure of the regional distribution of flow and direct cellular toxicity despite adequate global oxygen delivery. Tissue oxygenation may be improved and aerobic metabolism sustained by reducing demand, i.e. metabolic rate (Box 8.26). This can be achieved with sedatives and muscle relaxants (see below).

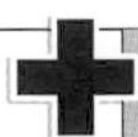

8.25 Immediate management of severe sepsis

- Give high-concentration oxygen
- Take blood cultures
- Give intravenous antibiotics (appropriate to likely organism)
- Volume-resuscitate
- Measure Hb and lactate
- Measure urine output
- Control source of infection

8.26 Factors increasing the metabolic rate in critical illness

- Fever
- Sepsis
- Trauma
- Burns
- Sympathetic activation due to pain, shivering or agitation
- Surgery
- Drugs, e.g. β-blockers, amphetamines, tricyclics
- Nursing procedures, visitors or physiotherapy

Corticosteroids

Assessment of the pituitary–adrenal axis is difficult in the critically ill but in some series up to 30% of patients have adrenal insufficiency, as assessed by a short Synacthen test (p. 778). Corticosteroid replacement therapy is controversial. Recent evidence suggests that, although it is associated with earlier resolution of shock, it has no effect on survival.

Disseminated intravascular coagulation

Also known as consumptive coagulopathy, disseminated intravascular coagulation (DIC) is an acquired disorder of haemostasis (p. 1055); it is common in critically ill patients and often heralds the onset of MOF. It is characterised by an increase in prothrombin time, partial thromboplastin time and fibrin degradation products, and a fall in platelets and fibrinogen. The clinically dominant feature may be widespread bleeding from vascular access points, gastrointestinal tract, bronchial tree and surgical wound sites, or widespread microvascular and even macrovascular thrombosis. Management is supportive with infusions of fresh frozen plasma and platelets, while the underlying cause is treated.

GENERAL PRINCIPLES OF CRITICAL CARE MANAGEMENT

Essential aspects of the management of critically ill patients on admission to the ICU are shown in Box 8.27.

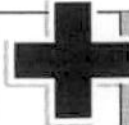

8.27 Management of patients on admission to ICU

- Handover from transferring team to ICU staff
- Full clinical assessment
- Ongoing resuscitation/stabilisation
- Establishment of monitoring
- Review of medical and social history
- Communication with and explanation to relatives
- Investigations to establish or confirm the definitive diagnosis
- Formulation and implementation of a management plan

8

Daily clinical management in the ICU

Regular clinical examination is essential to identify any changes in a patient's condition. Detailed clinical examination is performed at least daily, with additional focused and systematic assessment on ward rounds at least twice daily. Ward rounds are also an opportunity to ensure the reliable application of evidence-based measures to reduce complications; the mnemonic FAST HUG provides a useful checklist of feeding, analgesia, sedation, thromboprophylaxis, head of bed elevation, ulcer prophylaxis, glucose control.

Patient review should include:

- Review of progress reports from nursing and medical staff, and any specialist opinions.
- Review of 24-hour charts.
- Examination: general (including skin, line sites, wounds etc.).
- System reviews:
  Cardiovascular: haemodynamics, fluids and inotropes
  Respiratory: ventilator settings and ABGs
  Gastrointestinal: nutrition (calorie, protein intake, route), nasogastric aspirate and bowel function
  Renal: urine output, overall fluid balance, urea and electrolytes, and renal replacement therapy
  Neurological: sedation level, GCS and pupil responses.
- Laboratory results: haematology, coagulation and biochemistry.
- Microbiology: temperature, white blood count, line sites and other possible sources of infection, results of cultures, antibiotic therapy.
- Drug therapy: review with pharmacist, consider adverse effects and interactions, and identify drugs that can be discontinued. Medicines required for long-term conditions should be continued in the context of the acute illness. An accurate record of the patient's usual medicines must be obtained.
- Imaging: review X-rays and other specialist investigations with radiologists.
- Monitoring: are all measures still required? In particular, remove central venous catheters, arterial lines and peripheral venous catheters as soon as no longer needed, in order to avoid infection.
- Management plan: formulate an integrated plan, with specific goals for each organ system and goals for the patient, e.g. mobilising out of bed. Involve the family in the patient's care.

Sedation and analgesia

Intensive care is an extremely stressful experience for the patient, with pain, discomfort and anxiety related to endotracheal intubation, invasive monitoring and other procedures.

Most patients require sedation and analgesia to ensure comfort, relieve anxiety, and allow tolerance of an endotracheal tube, mechanical ventilation and invasive procedures. Some conditions, especially severe neurological conditions that cause brain swelling and raised ICP, require deep sedation to reduce tissue oxygen requirements and protect organs from ischaemic damage. Excessive sedation is common in ICU patients, and is associated with longer ICU stays, a higher prevalence of delirium, prolonged requirement for mechanical ventilation, and more ICU-acquired infections. The optimally sedated patient is comfortable and tolerates treatments, but is awake and lucid.

8.28 Richmond Agitation Sedation Scale (RASS)

Score	Term	Description
+4	Combative	Overtly combative, or violent or immediate danger to staff
+3	Very agitated	Pulls on/removes tubes or catheters, or aggressive to staff
+2	Agitated	Frequent non-purposeful movement or patient–ventilator dyssynchrony
+1	Restless	Anxious or apprehensive but no aggressive or vigorous movements
0	Alert and calm	
–1	Drowsy	Not fully alert but sustained awakening (>10 secs) with eye opening/contact to voice
–2	Light sedation	Brief awakening (< 10 secs) with eye contact to voice
–3	Moderate sedation	Movement but no eye contact to voice
–4	Deep sedation	Movement to physical stimulation but no response to voice
–5	Unrousable	No response to voice or physical stimulation

Sedation and analgesia are usually provided via continuous infusions of sedative and/or analgesic drugs. As many critically ill patients have impaired liver and renal function, the potential for drugs to accumulate is high and the patient's sedation must be regularly monitored. The sedative agents used ideally have predictable short half-lives that are not affected by liver or renal impairment. Short-acting intravenous agents, such as propofol, are usually employed. Analgesia can be provided using morphine infusions, but in patients with MOF, especially renal failure, active metabolites can accumulate. Opiates such as fentanyl or alfentanil, which are not renally metabolised or excreted, are commonly chosen.

Sedation is monitored via clinical sedation scales (Box 8.28) that record responses to voice and physical stimulation. Regular use of these to adjust sedation is associated with a shorter ICU stay. Many ICUs also have a daily 'sedation break', when all sedation is stopped in appropriate cases for a period, in order to re-assess the patient. This approach reduces the chance of oversedation and shortens ICU stay.

Muscle relaxants

Muscle relaxants are avoided whenever possible in ICU patients. Their use is associated with a higher prevalence of critical illness neuropathy and myopathy, resulting in muscle weakness. Sedation use also tends to be higher when muscle relaxants are employed. They are required to facilitate endotracheal intubation and to facilitate ventilation in patients with critical oxygenation and/or poor lung compliance. Patients with critically increased ICP often receive intravenous infusions of muscle relaxant drugs such as atracurium, to help control it and to prevent coughing and high intrathoracic pressures, which increase ICP.

Delirium

Delirium is extremely common in critically ill patients. It often becomes apparent as sedation is reduced and stopped. About 60–80% of patients have hypoactive delirium, which is often missed unless formal testing is undertaken. Between 5 and 10% of patients have agitated delirium, and 10–20% a mixed pattern. Delirium of any type is associated with poorer outcome. Management is focused on reducing or avoiding precipitating factors, such as benzodiazepines and metabolic disturbances. Patients with agitated delirium should be managed with haloperidol in 2.5 mg increments, rather than additional sedatives. Some sedative drugs are associated with a lower incidence of delirium, such as α_2-adrenergic agonists (clonidine and dexmedetomidine). These have a central sedative action and can be useful in difficult cases. There is no evidence that pharmacological interventions are useful as prophylaxis or in hypoactive delirium. Additional information about diagnosis and management of delirium is given on page 1161.

8.29 Common problems after ICU discharge

Physical

- Fatigue: almost universal and can last for many weeks
- Breathlessness
- Muscle weakness: a combination of muscle wasting from inadequate nutritional intake, muscle breakdown associated with inflammation/infection, and damage to nerves and muscle associated with severe systemic illness (critical illness polyneuropathy and polymyopathy – p. 1230)
- Altered taste and poor appetite: can result in weight loss
- Joint stiffness
- Itch
- Hair loss

Psychological

- Anxiety
- Depression
- Traumatic memories: including delusional memories (often unpleasant), dreams, flashbacks and hyperarousal. Worse in more severe and prolonged illness, more prolonged deep sedation and after delirium. Recovery occurs over weeks/months, but can persist and affect quality of life

DISCHARGE FROM INTENSIVE CARE

Discharge is appropriate when the original indication for admission has resolved and the patient has sufficient physiological reserve to continue recovery without the facilities of intensive care. Many ICUs and HDUs function as combined units, which allows stepdown to HDU care without a change of clinical team. Critically ill patients often have complex medical histories, multiple ongoing medical problems, and family and social issues. Many also have the emotional problems associated with survival from a life-threatening event or illness. Discharge from the ICU is stressful for patients and families, and communication with the clinical team accepting responsibility is vital. A key issue is that nursing care changes from one-to-one or one-to-two to much lower staffing levels. Discharges from ICU/HDU to standard wards should take place within normal working hours to ensure adequate medical and nursing support and detailed handover, as discharge outside normal working hours (and early discharge) are associated with higher ICU re-admission rates and increased mortality.

The receiving team should be provided with a written summary, including relevant recent investigations, and the critical care team should remain available for advice. Many ICU teams provide an outreach service to furnish advice and ensure continuity. Irrespective of the reason for admission to the ICU, many patients suffer problems (Box 8.29). These can last from weeks to many months and require ongoing support and rehabilitation.

Withdrawal of intensive support

Withdrawal of support must be considered when it is clear that the patient has no realistic prospect of recovery or of surviving with a quality of life that he or she would value. In these situations, intensive care will only prolong the dying process and is therefore futile. When intensive support is withdrawn, management remains active and is aimed at allowing the patient to die with dignity and as free from distress as possible (p. 290). Patients' views are paramount and increasing use is being made of advance directives or 'living wills'. Communication with the patient, if possible, and with the family, the referring clinicians, and between members of the critical care team is crucial (p. 165). Failure in this area causes stress and unrealistic expectations, damages working relations and leads to subsequent unhappiness, anger and litigation.

Brainstem death

Recent advances in the resuscitation and intensive care management of brain-injured patients have inevitably increased the survival of patients who remain ventilated on ICU, in whom progression of brain injury results in brainstem death. The preconditions for considering brainstem death and the criteria for establishing the diagnosis are listed on page 1160.

When the formal criteria for brainstem death are met, it is clearly inappropriate to continue supporting life with mechanical ventilation, and the possibility of organ donation should be considered. All intensive care clinicians have a responsibility to approach relatives to seek consent for organ donation, provided there is no contraindication to their use. This can be very difficult, but is easier if the patient carried an organ donor card or was registered with an organisation such as the UK Organ Donor Register. In the UK, each region has a team of specialist nurses in organ donation who provide help with the process and with care of the potential organ donor.

OUTCOME OF INTENSIVE CARE

The measure used most widely to assess outcome from intensive care is mortality. Mortality is strongly influenced by the case mix of an ICU (the type of patients and their illness severity at admission). Typically, about 20% of ICU patients will die during their ICU stay despite treatment, and about 30% will die before leaving hospital. Some factors associated with higher mortality are shown in Box 8.30. Mortality in patients requiring HDU care is much lower. Many patients have pre-existing illnesses prior to ICU admission, which, combined with the effect of the illness that resulted in ICU admission and the subsequent complications, means that many who survive the ICU admission have reduced life expectancy compared to those of similar age in the general population. The long-term physical and psychological effects of critical illness can mean that surviving patients have a reduced quality of life for many months or years. Families often carry a heavy burden of care after critical illness. Many patients do not regain pre-illness health and may be unable to work, resulting in economic and social hardship.

Scoring systems

Admission and discharge criteria vary between ICUs, so it is important to define the characteristics of the patients admitted (case mix) in order to assess the effects of the care provided on the outcome achieved. Two systems are widely used to measure severity of illness:

- *'APACHE' II*: Acute Physiology Assessment and Chronic Health Evaluation
- *'SAPS'* 2: Simplified Acute Physiology Score.

These scores include assessment of certain admission characteristics (e.g. age and pre-existing organ dysfunction) and a variety of routine physiological measurements (e.g. temperature, BP, GCS) that reflect the response of the patient to his or her illness (Box 8.31). Patient age is included in many scoring systems (Box 8.32). When combined with the admission diagnosis, scoring systems have been shown to correlate well with the risk of hospital death. Such outcome predictions can never be 100% accurate and should be viewed as only one of many factors to be considered when deciding whether or not further intervention is appropriate.

Predicted mortality figures by diagnosis have been calculated from large databases generated from a range of ICUs. These allow a particular unit to evaluate its performance compared to the reference ICUs by calculating standardised mortality ratios (SMRs) for each diagnostic group, by dividing observed mortality by predicted mortality.

A value of unity indicates the same performance as the reference ICUs, while a value less than 1 indicates a better than predicted outcome. If a unit has a high SMR in a certain diagnostic category, it should prompt investigation into the management of patients with that diagnosis, in order to identify aspects of care that could be improved.

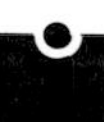

8.30 Factors associated with higher mortality from critical illness

- Older age
- Significant pre-existing comorbidities, especially liver disease, severe cardiorespiratory disease, malignancy, immunosuppression and chronic renal failure
- Poor pre-existing nutritional state and/or general physical condition
- Higher illness severity at ICU admission, measured with the APACHE or SAPS score (see text)
- Worse or multiple acute organ failures during ICU (especially shock, respiratory failure and acute renal failure)

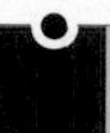

8.31 Uses of critical care scoring systems

- Comparison of the performance of different units
- Assessment of new therapies
- Assessment of changes in unit policies and management guidelines
- Measurement of the cost-effectiveness of care

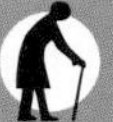

8.32 The critically ill older patient

- **ICU demography**: increasing numbers of critically ill older patients are admitted to the ICU; more than 50% of patients in many general ICUs are over 65 years old.
- **Outcome**: affected to some extent by age, as reflected in APACHE II, but age should not be used as the sole criterion for withholding or withdrawing ICU support.
- **Cardiopulmonary resuscitation (CPR)**: successful hospital discharge following in-hospital CPR is rare in patients over 70 years old in the presence of significant chronic disease.
- **Functional independence**: tends to be lost during an ICU stay and prolonged rehabilitation may subsequently be necessary.
- **Specific problems**:
  Skin fragility and ulceration
  Poor muscle strength: difficulty in weaning from ventilator and in mobilising
  Delirium: compounded by sedatives and analgesics
  High prevalence of underlying nutritional deficiency.

Further information

Websites

www.adqi.net *Evidence-based appraisal and consensus recommendations for diagnosis, treatment and research in acute kidney injury.*

www.esicm.org *European Society of Intensive Care Medicine: guidelines, recommendations, consensus conference reports.*

www.ics.ac.uk *Intensive Care Society: clinical guidelines and standards for intensive care.*

www.icudelirium.org *Information on delirium and sedation in intensive care patients.*

www.scottishintensivecare.org.uk/education/index.htm *On-line tutorials, educational materials for learners and teaching support materials for educators.*

www.sicsebm.org.uk *Intensive care evidence-based medicine website. Reviews and critical appraisal of topics.*

www.survivingsepsis.org *Surviving Sepsis website.*

S.H.L. Thomas
J. White

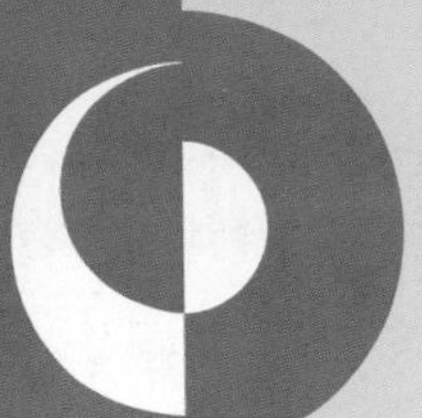

Poisoning 9

Comprehensive evaluation of the poisoned patient 206

Evaluation of the envenomed patient 207

General approach to the poisoned patient 208
- Triage and resuscitation 208
- Clinical assessment and investigations 209
- Psychiatric assessment 210
- General management 210

Poisoning by specific pharmaceutical agents 212
- Analgesics 212
- Antidepressants 213
- Cardiovascular medications 214
- Antimalarials 215
- Iron 216
- Antipsychotic drugs 216
- Antidiabetic agents 216

Drugs of misuse 216
- Cannabis 216
- Benzodiazepines 217
- Stimulants and entactogens 217
- Gammahydroxybutyrate and gamma butyrolactone 218
- d-Lysergic acid diethylamide 218
- Opioids 219
- Body packers and body stuffers 219

Chemicals and pesticides 219
- Carbon monoxide 219
- Organophosphorus insecticides and nerve agents 220
- Carbamate insecticides 222
- Methanol and ethylene glycol 222
- Aluminium and zinc phosphide 223

Environmental poisoning and illness 223
- Arsenism 223
- Fluorosis 223

Substances less commonly taken in overdose 224

Envenoming 224
- Venom 225
- Venomous animals 225
- Clinical effects 226
- Management 226

COMPREHENSIVE EVALUATION OF THE POISONED PATIENT

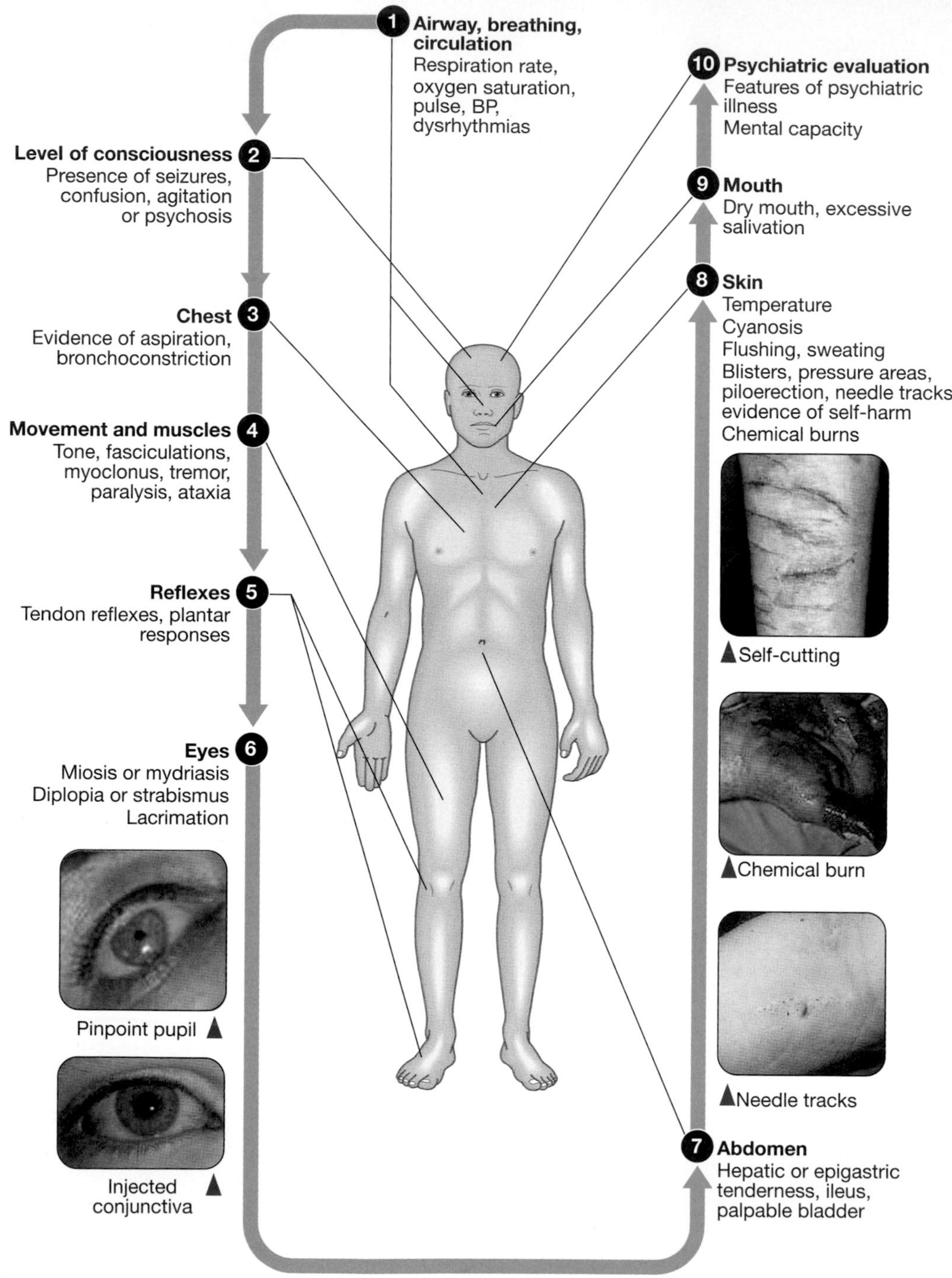

Insets (*Self-cutting*) From Douglas, et al. 2005; (*Burn*) www.firewiki.net; (*Needle tracks*) www.deep6inc.com; (*Pupil*) drugrecognition.com; (*Conjunctiva*) knol.google.com – see p. 230.

Taking a history in poisoning

- What toxin(s) have been taken and how much?
- What time were they taken and by what route?
- Has alcohol or any drug of misuse been taken as well?
- Obtain details from witnesses of the circumstances of the overdose (e.g. family, friends ambulance personnel)
- Ask the general practitioner for background and details of prescribed medication
- Assess suicide risk (full psychiatric evaluation when patient has physically recovered)
- Assess capacity to make decisions about accepting or refusing treatment
- Establish past medical history, drug history and allergies, social and family history
- Record all information carefully

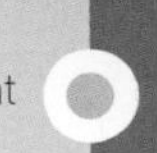
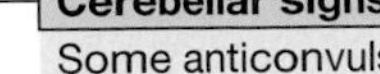

Pupil size
Small: opioids, clonidine, organophosphorus compounds
Large: tricyclic antidepressants, amphetamines, cocaine

Respiratory rate
Reduced: opioids, benzodiazepines
Increased: salicylates

Blood pressure
Hypotension: tricyclic antidepressants, haloperidol
Hypertension: cocaine, α-adrenoceptor agonists

Right upper quadrant /renal angle tenderness
Paracetamol hepatotoxicity, renal toxicity

Epigastric tenderness
NSAIDs, salicylates

Rhabdomyolysis
Amphetamines, caffeine

Cerebellar signs
Some anticonvulsants, alcohol

Extrapyramidal signs
Phenothiazines, haloperidol, metoclopramide

Cyanosis
Any CNS depressant drug or agent (N.B. consider methaemoglobinaemia caused by dapsone, amyl nitrite)

Heart rate
Tachycardia or tachyarrhythmias: tricyclic antidepressants, theophylline, digoxin, antihistamines
Bradycardia or bradyarrhythmias: digoxin, β-blockers, calcium channel blockers, opioids

Needle tracks
Drugs of misuse: opioids etc.

Body temperature
Hyperthermia and sweating: ecstasy, serotonin re-uptake inhibitors, salicylates
Hypothermia: any CNS depressant drug, opioids, chlorpromazine

Clinical signs of poisoning by pharmaceutical agents and drugs of misuse.

EVALUATION OF THE ENVENOMED PATIENT

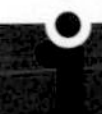

Assessment of type and extent of envenoming

Neurotoxic paralysis
- 'Sleepy' or drooping eyelids
- Difficulty swallowing, dysarthria and drooling
- Limb weakness
- Respiratory distress

Excitatory neurotoxicity
- Sweating, salivation, piloerection
- Tingling around mouth or tongue, muscle twitching
- Dyspnoea (pulmonary oedema)

Myolysis
- Muscle pain or weakness

Coagulopathy
- Blood oozing from bite site and/or gums
- Bruising
- Melaena, haematemesis

Local effects
- Pain, sweating, blistering, bruising etc.

Taking a history in envenoming

- When was the patient exposed to a bite/sting?
- Was the organism causing it seen and what did it look like (size, colour)?
- What were the circumstances (on land, in water etc.)?
- Was there more than one bite/sting?
- What first aid was used, when and for how long?
- What symptoms has the patient had (local and systemic)?
- Are there symptoms suggesting systemic envenoming (paralysis, myolysis, coagulopathy etc.)?
- Past medical history and medications?
- Past exposure to antivenom/venom and allergies?

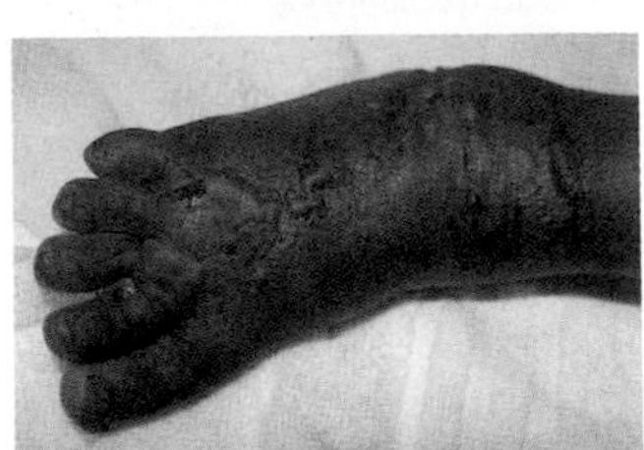
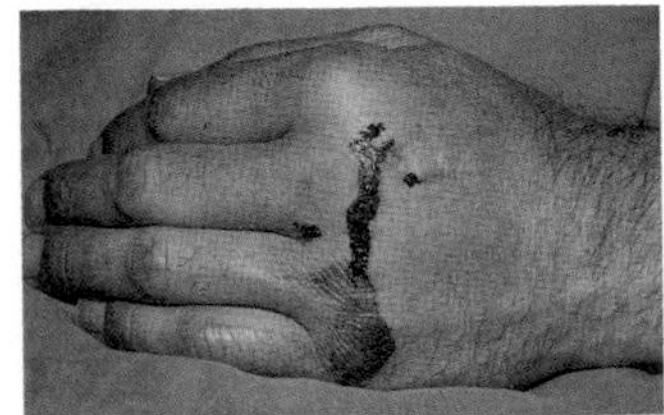
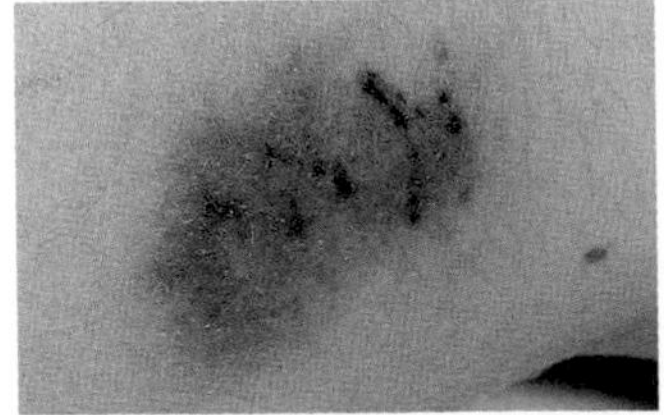

Bites showing puncture marks, blistering, bruising and bleeding.

Acute poisoning is common, accounting for about 1% of hospital admissions in the UK. Common or otherwise important substances involved are shown in Box 9.1. In developed countries, the most frequent cause is intentional drug overdose in the context of self-harm and usually involves prescribed or 'over-the-counter' medicines. Accidental poisoning is also common, especially in children and the elderly (Box 9.2). Toxicity also may occur as a result of alcohol or recreational substance use, or following occupational or environmental exposure. Poisoning is a major cause of death in young adults, but most deaths occur before patients reach medical attention, and mortality is much lower than 1% in those admitted to hospital.

In developing countries, the frequency of self-harm is more difficult to estimate. Household and agricultural products, such as pesticides and herbicides, are more freely available, are common sources of poisoning and are associated with a much higher case fatality. In China and South-east Asia, pesticides account for about 300 000 suicides each year.

GENERAL APPROACH TO THE POISONED PATIENT

A general approach is shown on pages 206–207.

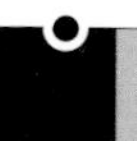

9.1 Important substances involved in poisoning

In the UK

- Analgesics: paracetamol and non-steroidal anti-inflammatory drugs (NSAIDs)
- Antidepressants: tricyclic antidepressants (TCAs), selective serotonin re-uptake inhibitors (SSRIs) and lithium
- Cardiovascular agents: β-blockers, calcium channel blockers and cardiac glycosides
- Drugs of misuse: opiates, benzodiazepines, stimulants (e.g. amphetamines, MDMA, cocaine)
- Carbon monoxide
- Alcohol

In South and South-east Asia

- Organophosphorus and carbamate insecticides
- Aluminium and zinc phosphide
- Oleander
- Snake venoms
- Antimalarial drugs: chloroquine
- Antidiabetic medication

9.2 Poisoning in old age

- **Aetiology**: commonly results from accidental poisoning (e.g. due to confusion or dementia) or drug toxicity as a consequence of impaired renal or hepatic function or drug interaction. Toxic prescription medicines are more likely to be available.
- **Psychiatric illness**: self-harm is less common than in younger adults but more frequently associated with depression and other psychiatric illness, as well as chronic illness and pain. There is a higher risk of subsequent suicide.
- **Severity of poisoning**: increased morbidity and mortality result from reduced renal and hepatic function, reduced functional reserve, increased sensitivity to sedative agents and frequent comorbidity.

Triage and resuscitation

Patients who are seriously poisoned must be identified early so that appropriate management is not delayed. Triage involves:

- immediate assessment of vital signs
- identifying the poison(s) involved and obtaining adequate information about them
- identifying patients at risk of further attempts at self-harm and removing any remaining hazards.

Those with possible external contamination with chemical or environmental toxins should undergo appropriate decontamination (Fig. 9.1). Critically ill patients must be resuscitated (p. 180).

The Glasgow Coma Scale (GCS) is commonly employed to assess conscious level, although it has not been specifically validated in poisoned patients. The AVPU (alert/verbal/painful/unresponsive) scale is also a rapid and simple method. An electrocardiogram (ECG) should be performed and cardiac monitoring instituted in all patients with cardiovascular features or where exposure to potentially cardiotoxic substances is suspected. Patients who may need antidotes should be weighed when this is feasible, so that appropriate weight-related doses can be prescribed.

Substances that are unlikely to be toxic in humans should be identified so that inappropriate admission and intervention are avoided (Box 9.3).

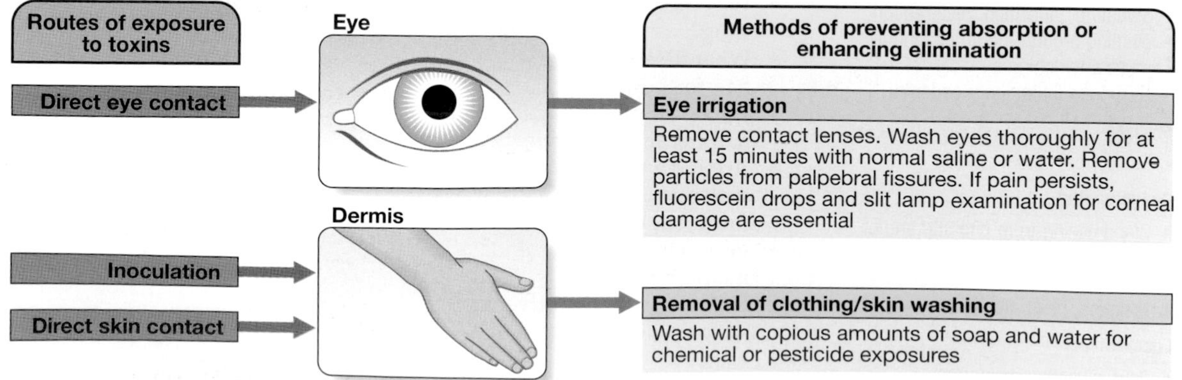

Fig. 9.1 Methods of external decontamination.

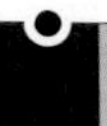

9.3 Substances of very low toxicity

- Writing/educational materials
- Decorating products
- Cleaning/bathroom products (except dishwasher tablets, which are corrosive)
- Pharmaceuticals: oral contraceptives, most antibiotics (but not tetracyclines and antituberculous drugs), H_2-blockers, proton pump inhibitors, emollients and other skin creams, baby lotion
- Miscellaneous: plasticine, silica gel, household plants, plant food

Clinical assessment and investigations

History and examination are described on page 206. Occasionally, patients may be unaware or confused about what they have taken, or may exaggerate (or less commonly underestimate) the size of the overdose, but rarely mislead medical staff deliberately. In regions of the world where self-poisoning is illegal, patients may be reticent about giving a history.

Toxic causes of abnormal physical signs are shown on page 207. The patient may have a cluster of clinical features ('toxidrome') suggestive of poisoning with a particular drug type, e.g. anticholinergic, serotoninergic (see Box 9.11, p. 213), stimulant, sedative, opioid (see Box 9.12, p. 217) or cholinergic (see Box 9.14, p. 221) feature clusters. Poisoning is a common cause of coma, especially in younger people, but it is important to exclude other potential causes (p. 1159), unless the aetiology is certain.

Urea, electrolytes and creatinine should be measured in all patients with suspected systemic poisoning. Arterial blood gases should be checked in those with significant respiratory or circulatory compromise, or when poisoning with substances likely to affect acid–base status is suspected (Box 9.4). Calculation of anion and osmolar gaps may help to inform diagnosis and management (Box 9.5).

For a limited number of specific substances, management may be facilitated by measurement of the amount of toxin in the blood (Box 9.6). Qualitative urine screens for potential toxins, including near-patient testing kits, have a limited clinical role.

9.4 Causes of acidosis in the poisoned patient

Cause	Normal lactate*	High lactate
Toxic	Salicylates Methanol Ethylene glycol Paraldehyde	Metformin Iron Cyanide Sodium valproate Carbon monoxide
Other	Renal failure Ketoacidosis Severe diarrhoea	Shock

*Unless circulatory shock is present, when it will be high in any case.

9.5 Anion and osmolal gaps in poisoning

	Anion gap	Osmolal gap
Calculation	$[Na^+ + K^+] - [Cl^- + HCO_3^-]$	[Osm (measured)] [2 × Na + Urea + Glucose (all mmol/L)][1]
Reference range	12–16 mmol/L	< 10 mOsm/kg
Common toxic causes of elevation[2]	Ethanol Ethylene glycol Methanol Salicylates Iron Cyanide	Ethanol Ethylene glycol Methanol

[1]Osm (measured) stands for measured osmolality. For non-SI units, the corresponding formula is [Osm (measured)] – [2 × Na (meq/L) + Urea/2.8 (mg/dL) + Glucose/18 (mg/dL)].
[2]Box 16.19 (p. 445) gives non-toxic causes.

9.6 Laboratory analysis in poisoning

Organophosphates
- Plasma cholinesterase is reduced more rapidly but is less specific than red cell cholinesterase (p. 222)
- Antidote use should not be delayed pending results

Carboxyhaemoglobin
- > 20% indicates significant carbon monoxide exposure

Digoxin
- Therapeutic range usually 1–2 ng/mL (1.28–2.46 mmol/L)
- Concentrations > 4 ng/mL (5.12 mmol/L) usually associated with toxicity, especially with chronic poisoning

Ethanol
- Toxicity at concentrations > 1.8 g/L

Iron
- Take sample ≥ 4 hrs after overdose or if clinical signs of toxicity
- Concentrations > 5 mg/L suggest severe toxicity

Lithium
- Take sample ≥ 6 hrs after overdose or if clinical signs of toxicity
- Usual therapeutic range 0.4–1.0 mmol/L

Methaemoglobin
- Poisoning with nitrites, benzocaine, dapsone, chloroquine and aniline dyes is associated with methaemoglobinaemia
- Concentrations > 20% may require treatment with methylthioninium chloride (methylene blue)

Paracetamol
- Take sample ≥ 4 hrs after overdose
- Use nomogram to determine need for antidotal treatment (see Fig. 9.2, p. 212)

Salicylate
- Take sample ≥ 2 hrs (symptomatic patients) or 4 hrs (asymptomatic patients) after overdose
- Concentrations > 500 mg/L suggest serious toxicity
- Repeat after 2 hrs if severe toxicity is suspected

Theophylline
- Take sample ≥ 4 hrs after overdose or if clinical signs of toxicity
- Repeat after 2 hrs if severe toxicity is suspected
- Concentrations > 60 mg/L suggest severe toxicity

Psychiatric assessment

All patients presenting with deliberate drug overdose should undergo psychiatric evaluation by a health professional with appropriate training prior to discharge (p. 238). This should take place once the patient has recovered from any features of poisoning, unless there is an urgent issue, such as uncertainty about their capacity to decline medical treatment.

General management

Patients presenting with eye/skin contamination should undergo local decontamination procedures (see Fig. 9.1).

Gastrointestinal decontamination

Patients who have ingested potentially life-threatening quantities of toxins may be considered for gastrointestinal decontamination if poisoning has been recent (Box 9.7). Induction of emesis using ipecacuanha is no longer recommended.

Activated charcoal

Given orally as slurry, activated charcoal absorbs toxins in the bowel as a result of its large surface area. If given sufficiently early, it can prevent absorption of an important proportion of the ingested dose of toxin. Efficacy decreases with time and current guidelines do not advocate use more than 1 hour after overdose in most circumstances (see Box 9.7). However, use after a longer interval may be reasonable when a delayed-release preparation has been taken or when gastric emptying may be delayed. Some toxins do not bind to activated charcoal (Box 9.8) so it will not affect their absorption. In patients with impaired swallowing or a reduced level of consciousness, activated charcoal, even via a nasogastric tube, carries a risk of aspiration pneumonitis, which can be reduced (but not eliminated) by protecting the airway with a cuffed endotracheal tube.

EBM 9.7 Use of gastric decontamination methods

'Single-dose activated charcoal may be considered if a patient has ingested a potentially toxic amount of a poison (known to be adsorbed to charcoal) up to 1 hr previously.'[1]

'Multiple-dose activated charcoal should be considered only if a patient has ingested a life-threatening amount of carbamazepine, dapsone, phenobarbital, quinine or theophylline.'[2]

'Gastric lavage should not be employed routinely, if ever, in the management of poisoned patients.'[3]

'Whole bowel irrigation should be considered for:
- poisoning with sustained-release or emetic-coated drugs
- patients who have ingested substantial amounts of iron (as morbidity is high and other options are limited)
- removal of ingested packets of illicit drugs.

- American Academy of Clinical Toxicology and European Association of Poison Centres and Clinical Toxicologists Joint Position Statements on Gastric Decontamination Methods:
- [1]Clin Toxicol 2005; 43:61–87.
- [2]Clin Toxicol 1999; 37:731–751.
- [3]Clin Toxicol 2004; 42:933–943.
- [4]J Toxicol Clin Toxicol 2004; 42:843–42854.

9.8 Substances poorly adsorbed by activated charcoal

Medicines	
• Iron	• Lithium
Chemicals	
• Acids*	• Mercury
• Alkalis*	• Methanol
• Ethanol	• Petroleum distillates*
• Ethylene glycol	

*Gastric lavage contraindicated.

Multiple doses of oral activated charcoal (50 g 6 times daily in an adult) may enhance the elimination of some drugs at any time after poisoning and are recommended for serious poisoning with some substances (see Box 9.7). This interrupts enterohepatic circulation or reduces the concentration of free drug in the gut lumen, to the extent that drug diffuses from the blood back into the bowel to be absorbed on to the charcoal: so-called 'gastrointestinal dialysis'. A laxative is generally given with the charcoal to reduce the risk of constipation or intestinal obstruction by charcoal 'briquette' formation in the gut lumen.

Evidence suggests that single or multiple doses of activated charcoal do not improve clinical outcomes after poisoning with pesticides or oleander.

Gastric aspiration and lavage

Gastric aspiration and/or lavage is very infrequently indicated in acute poisoning, as it is no more effective than activated charcoal and complications are common, especially aspiration. Use may be justified for life-threatening overdoses of some substances that are not absorbed by activated charcoal (see Box 9.8).

Whole bowel irrigation

This is occasionally indicated to enhance the elimination of ingested packets of illicit drugs or slow-release tablets such as iron and lithium that are not absorbed by activated charcoal. It involves the administration of large quantities of osmotically balanced polyethylene glycol and electrolyte solution (1–2 L/hr for an adult), usually by a nasogastric tube, until the rectal effluent is clear. Contraindications include inadequate airway protection, haemodynamic instability, gastrointestinal haemorrhage, obstruction or ileus. Whole bowel irrigation may precipitate nausea and vomiting, abdominal pain and electrolyte disturbances.

Urinary alkalinisation

Urinary excretion of weak acids and bases is affected by urinary pH, which changes the extent to which they are ionised. Highly ionised molecules pass poorly through lipid membranes and therefore little tubular reabsorption occurs and urinary excretion is increased. If the urine is alkalinised (pH > 7.5) by the administration of sodium bicarbonate (e.g. 1.5 L of 1.26% sodium bicarbonate over 2 hrs), weak acids (e.g. salicylates, methotrexate and the herbicides 2,4-dichlorophenoxyacetic acid and mecoprop) are highly ionised, resulting in enhanced urinary excretion.

Urinary alkalinisation is currently recommended for patients with clinically significant salicylate poisoning when the criteria for haemodialysis are not met (see below). It is also sometimes used for poisoning with methotrexate. Complications include alkalaemia, hypokalaemia and occasionally alkalotic tetany (p. 447). Hypocalcaemia may occur but is rare.

Haemodialysis and haemoperfusion

These techniques can enhance the elimination of poisons that have a small volume of distribution and a long half-life after overdose, and are appropriate when poisoning is sufficiently severe to justify invasive elimination methods. The toxin must be small enough to cross the dialysis membrane (haemodialysis) or must bind to activated charcoal (haemoperfusion) (Box 9.9). Haemodialysis may also correct acid-base and metabolic disturbances associated with poisoning (p. 209).

9.9 Poisons effectively eliminated by haemodialysis or haemoperfusion

Haemodialysis	
• Ethylene glycol • Isopropanol • Methanol	• Salicylates • Sodium valproate • Lithium
Haemoperfusion	
• Theophylline • Phenytoin • Carbamazepine	• Phenobarbital • Amobarbital

Lipid emulsion therapy

Lipid emulsion therapy, or 'lipid rescue', is being used increasingly for the management of poisoning with lipid-soluble agents, such as local anaesthetics, tricyclic antidepressants, calcium channel blockers and lipid-soluble β-blockers such as propranolol. It involves intravenous infusion of 20% lipid emulsion (e.g. Intralipid®) at an initial dose of 1.5 mL/kg, followed by a continued infusion of 0.25 mL/kg/min until there is clinical improvement. It is thought that lipid-soluble toxins partition into the intravenous lipid, reducing target tissue concentrations. The elevated myocardial concentration of free fatty acid induced by Intralipid administration may also have beneficial effects on myocardial metabolism and performance by counteracting the inhibition of myocardial fatty acid oxidation produced by local anaesthetics and some other cardiotoxins. This reverses cardiac depression by enabling increased ATP synthesis and energy production. Animal studies have suggested efficacy and case reports of use in human poisoning have also been encouraging, with recovery of circulatory collapse reported in cases where other treatment modalities have been unsuccessful. No controlled trials of this technique have been performed, however, and as a result, its efficacy remains uncertain.

9.10 Complications of poisoning and their management

	Examples of causative agents	Management
Coma	Sedative agents	Appropriate airway protection and ventilatory support Pressure area and bladder care Identification and treatment of aspiration pneumonia
Seizures	NSAIDs Anticonvulsants TCAs Theophylline	Appropriate airway and ventilatory support IV benzodiazepine (e.g. diazepam 10–20 mg, lorazepam 2–4 mg) Correction of hypoxia, acid–base and metabolic abnormalities
Acute dystonias	Typical antipsychotics Metoclopramide	Procyclidine, benzatropine or diazepam
Hypotension		
Due to vasodilatation	Vasodilator antihypertensives Anticholinergic agents TCAs	IV fluids Vasopressors (rarely indicated; p. 191)
Due to myocardial suppression	β-blockers Calcium channel blockers TCAs	Optimisation of volume status Inotropic agents (p. 191)
Ventricular tachycardia		
Monomorphic, associated with QRS prolongation	Sodium channel blockers	Correction of electrolyte and acid–base abnormalities and hypoxia Sodium bicarbonate
Torsades de pointes, associated with QT_c prolongation	Anti-arrhythmic drugs (quinidine, amiodarone, sotalol) Antimalarials Organophosphate insecticides Antipsychotic agents Antidepressants Antibiotics (erythromycin)	Magnesium sulphate, 2 g IV over 1–2 mins, repeated if necessary

9

Supportive care

For most poisons, antidotes and methods to accelerate elimination are inappropriate, unavailable or incompletely effective. Outcome is dependent on appropriate nursing and supportive care, and on treatment of complications (Box 9.10). Patients should be monitored carefully until the effects of any toxins have dissipated.

Antidotes

Antidotes are available for some poisons and work by a variety of mechanisms: for example, by specific antagonism (isoprenaline for β-blockers), chelation (desferrioxamine for iron) or reduction (methylene blue for dapsone). The use of some antidotes is described in the management of specific poisons below.

POISONING BY SPECIFIC PHARMACEUTICAL AGENTS

Analgesics

Paracetamol

Paracetamol (acetaminophen) is the drug most commonly used in overdose in the UK. Toxicity results from formation of an intermediate reactive metabolite that binds covalently to cellular proteins, causing cell death. This results in hepatic and occasionally renal failure. In therapeutic doses, the toxic intermediate metabolite is detoxified in reactions requiring glutathione, but in overdose, glutathione reserves become exhausted.

Management

Management is summarised in Figure 9.2. Activated charcoal may be used in patients presenting within 1 hour. Antidotes for paracetamol act by replenishing hepatic glutathione and should be administered to all patients with paracetamol concentrations above the 'treatment line' provided on paracetamol poisoning nomograms. Acetylcysteine given intravenously (or orally in some countries) is highly efficacious if administered within 8 hours of the overdose. However, since efficacy declines thereafter, administration should not be delayed in patients presenting after 8 hours to await a paracetamol blood concentration result. The antidote can be stopped if the paracetamol concentration is shown to be below the nomogram treatment line.

The most important adverse effect of acetylcysteine is related to dose-related histamine release, the 'anaphylactoid' reaction, which causes itching and urticaria, and in occasional severe cases, bronchospasm and hypotension. Most cases can be managed by temporary discontinuation of acetylcysteine and administration of an antihistamine.

An alternative antidote is methionine 2.5 g orally (adult dose) every 4 hours to a total of 4 doses, but this is less effective, especially after delayed presentation. If a patient presents more than 15 hours after ingestion, liver function tests, prothrombin time (or international normalised ratio – INR), renal function tests and a venous bicarbonate should be measured, the antidote started, and a poisons information centre or local liver unit contacted for advice if results are abnormal. An

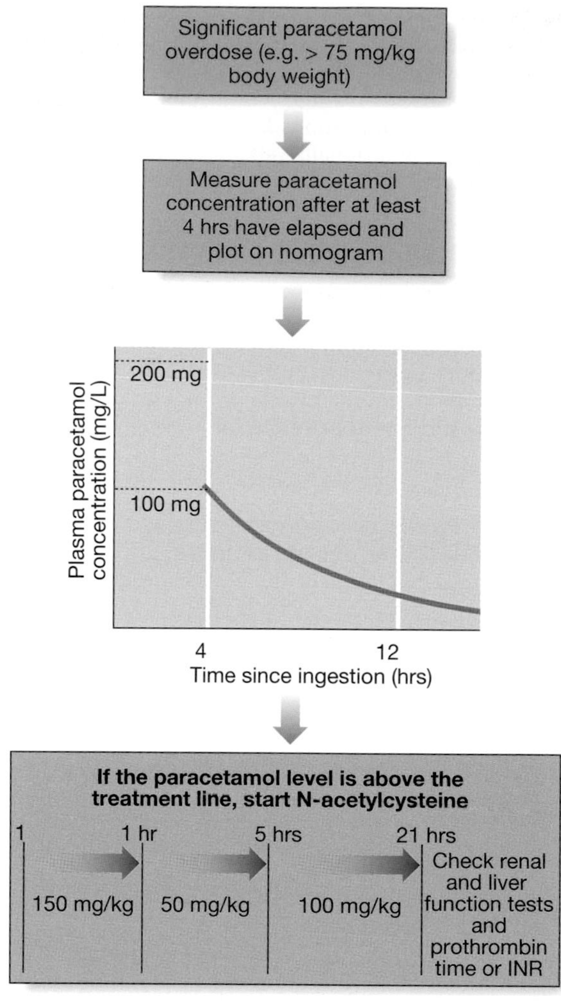

Fig. 9.2 The management of a paracetamol overdose.

arterial blood gas sample should be taken in patients with severe liver function abnormalities; metabolic acidosis indicates severe poisoning. Liver transplantation should be considered in individuals who develop life-threatening liver failure due to paracetamol poisoning (p. 932).

If multiple ingestions of paracetamol have taken place over several hours or days (i.e. a staggered overdose), acetylcysteine may be indicated. Recommended thresholds for treatment vary between countries.

Salicylates (aspirin)

Clinical features

Salicylate overdose commonly causes nausea, vomiting, sweating, tinnitus and deafness. Direct stimulation of the respiratory centre produces hyperventilation and respiratory alkalosis. Peripheral vasodilatation with bounding pulses and profuse sweating occurs in moderately severe poisoning. Serious salicylate poisoning is associated with metabolic acidosis, hypoprothrombinaemia, hyperglycaemia, hyperpyrexia, renal failure, pulmonary oedema, shock and cerebral oedema. Agitation, confusion, coma and fits may occur, especially in children. Toxicity is enhanced by acidosis, which increases salicylate transfer across the blood–brain barrier.

Management

Activated charcoal should be administered if the patient presents within 1 hour. Multiple doses of activated charcoal may enhance salicylate elimination but currently are not routinely recommended.

The plasma salicylate concentration should be measured at least 2 (in symptomatic patients) or 4 hours (asymptomatic patients) after overdose and repeated in suspected serious poisoning, since concentrations may continue to rise some hours after overdose. In adults, concentrations above 500 mg/L and 700 mg/L suggest serious and life-threatening poisoning respectively, although clinical status is more important than the salicylate concentration in assessing severity.

Dehydration should be corrected carefully, as there is a risk of pulmonary oedema, and metabolic acidosis should be identified and treated with intravenous sodium bicarbonate (8.4%), once plasma potassium has been corrected. Urinary alkalinisation is indicated for adults with salicylate concentrations above 500 mg/L.

Haemodialysis is very effective at removing salicylate and correcting acid–base and fluid balance abnormalities, and should be considered when serum concentrations are above 700 mg/L in adults with severe toxic features, or when there is renal failure, pulmonary oedema, coma, convulsions or refractory acidosis.

Non-steroidal anti-inflammatory drugs

Clinical features

Overdose of most non-steroidal anti-inflammatory drugs (NSAIDs) usually causes little more than minor abdominal discomfort, vomiting and/or diarrhoea, but convulsions can occur occasionally, especially with mefenamic acid. Coma, prolonged seizures, apnoea, liver dysfunction and renal failure can occur after substantial overdose but are rare. Features of toxicity are unlikely to develop in patients who are asymptomatic more than 6 hours after overdose.

Management

Electrolytes, liver function tests and a full blood count should be checked in all but the most trivial cases. Activated charcoal may be given if the patient presents sufficiently early. Symptomatic treatment for nausea and gastrointestinal irritation may be necessary.

Antidepressants

Tricyclic antidepressants

Tricyclic antidepressants (TCAs) are used frequently in overdose and carry a high morbidity and mortality relating to their sodium channel-blocking, anticholinergic and α-adrenoceptor-blocking effects.

Clinical features

Anticholinergic effects are common (Box 9.11). Life-threatening complications are frequent, including convulsions, coma, arrhythmias (ventricular tachycardia, ventricular fibrillation and, less commonly, heart block) and hypotension, which results from inappropriate vasodilatation or impaired myocardial contractility. Serious complications appear to be more common with dosulepin and amitriptyline.

9.11 Anticholinergic and serotonergic feature clusters

	Anticholinergic	Serotonin syndrome
Common causes	Benzodiazepines Antipsychotics TCAs Antihistamines Scopolamine Benzatropine Belladonna Jimson weed Mushrooms (some)	SSRIs Monoamine oxidase inhibitors (MAOIs) TCAs Amphetamines Buspirone Bupropion (especially in combination)
Clinical features		
Cardiovascular	Tachycardia, hypertension	Tachycardia, hyper- or hypotension
CNS	Confusion, hallucinations, sedation	Confusion, delirium, hallucinations, sedation, coma
Muscle	Myoclonus	Shivering, tremor, myoclonus, raised creatine kinase
Temperature	Fever	Fever
Eyes	Diplopia, mydriasis	Normal pupil size
Abdomen	Ileus, palpable bladder	Diarrhoea, vomiting
Mouth	Dry	
Skin	Flushing, hot, dry	Flushing, sweating
Complications	Seizures	Seizures Rhabdomyolysis Renal failure Metabolic acidosis Coagulopathies

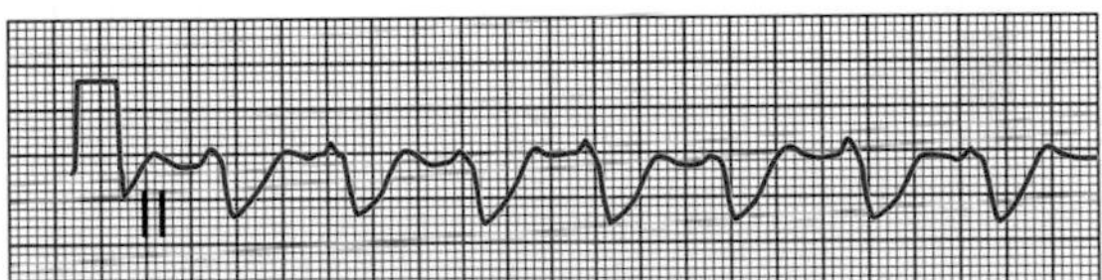

Fig 9.3 ECG in severe tricyclic antidepressant poisoning. This rhythm strip shows a broad QRS complex due to impaired conduction.

Management

Activated charcoal should be administered if the patient presents within 1 hour. All patients with possible TCA overdose should have a 12-lead ECG and ongoing cardiac monitoring for at least 6 hours. Prolongation of the QRS interval (especially if > 0.16 s) indicates severe sodium channel blockade and is associated with an increased risk of arrhythmia (Fig. 9.3). QT interval prolongation may also occur. Arterial blood gases should be measured in suspected severe poisoning.

In patients with arrhythmias, significant QRS or QT prolongation or acidosis, intravenous sodium bicarbonate (50 mL of 8.4% solution) should be administered and repeated to correct pH. The correction of the acidosis and the sodium loading that result is often associated with rapid improvement in ECG features and arrhythmias. Hypoxia and electrolyte abnormalities should also be corrected. Anti-arrhythmic drugs should only be given on specialist advice. Prolonged convulsions should be treated with intravenous benzodiazepines (see Box 9.10). There is anecdotal evidence of benefit from lipid emulsion therapy in severe intractable poisoning.

Selective serotonin and noradrenaline re-uptake inhibitors

Selective serotonin re-uptake inhibitors (SSRIs) are a group of antidepressants that include fluoxetine, paroxetine, fluvoxamine, sertraline, citalopram and escitalopram. They are increasingly used to treat depression, partly because they are less toxic in overdose than TCAs. A related group of compounds termed serotonin-noradrenaline reuptake inhibitors (SNRIs), such as venlafaxine and duloxetine, are also in common use and are sometimes taken in overdose.

Clinical features and management

Overdose of SSRIs may produce nausea and vomiting, tremor, insomnia and sinus tachycardia. Agitation, drowsiness and convulsions occur infrequently and may be delayed for several hours after ingestion. Occasionally, features of serotonin syndrome may develop (see Box 9.11), especially if SSRIs are taken in combination or with other serotonergic agents. Cardiac arrhythmias occur infrequently and most patients require supportive care only. The toxic effects of SNRIs are similar but tachycardia, hypertension or hypotension and ECG changes (QRS and QT prolongation) may be more prominent and hypoglycaemia can also occur.

Lithium

Severe lithium toxicity is uncommon after intentional overdose and is more often encountered in patients taking therapeutic doses as the result of interactions with drugs such as diuretics or NSAIDs that can cause dehydration or renal impairment, or because an excessive dose has been prescribed. Severe toxicity is more common with acute overdose in patients taking chronic therapy ('acute on chronic' poisoning).

Clinical features

Nausea, diarrhoea, polyuria, dizziness and tremor may progress to muscular weakness, drowsiness, confusion, myoclonus, fasciculations, choreoathetosis and renal failure. Coma, convulsions, ataxia, cardiac dysrhythmias such as heart block, blood pressure disturbances and renal failure may all occur in severe poisoning.

Management

Activated charcoal is ineffective. Gastric lavage is of theoretical benefit if used early after overdose, but lithium tablets are likely to remain intact in the stomach and may be too large for aspiration via a lavage tube. Some advocate whole bowel irrigation after substantial overdose but efficacy is unknown.

Lithium concentrations should be measured immediately in symptomatic patients or after at least 6 hours in asymptomatic patients following acute overdose. Adequate hydration should be maintained with intravenous fluids. Convulsions should be treated as in Box 9.10.

In patients with features suggesting severe toxicity associated with high lithium concentrations (e.g. > 4.0 mmol/L after chronic or 'acute on chronic' poisoning, or > 7.5 mmol/L after acute poisoning), haemodialysis should be considered. Lithium concentrations are reduced substantially during dialysis but rebound increases occur after discontinuation, and multiple sessions may be required.

Cardiovascular medications

Beta-adrenoceptor blockers

These have negative inotropic and chronotropic effects. Some have additional properties that may increase toxicity, such as blockade of sodium channels with propranolol, acebutolol and carvedilol, and blockade of potassium channels with sotalol.

Clinical features

The major features of toxicity are bradycardia and hypotension. Heart block, pulmonary oedema and cardiogenic shock occur in severe poisoning. Beta-blockers with sodium channel-blocking effects may cause seizures, confusion and coma, while sotalol may be associated with repolarisation abnormalities (including QT_c prolongation) and torsades de pointes (p. 570).

Management

Intravenous fluids may reverse hypotension but care is required to avoid pulmonary oedema. Bradycardia and hypotension may respond to high doses of atropine (up to 3 mg in an adult). The adrenoceptor agonist isoprenaline may also be effective but high doses are often needed. Glucagon (5–10 mg over 10 mins, then 1–5 mg/hr by infusion), which counteracts the effect of β-blockers by stimulating intracellular production of cyclic adenosine monophosphate (cAMP), is now more commonly used. In severe cases, 'hyperinsulinaemia euglycaemic therapy' has been used, as described under calcium channel blockers. Lipid emulsion therapy may have a role in severe poisoning with lipid-soluble agents such as propranolol, carvedilol and oxprenolol.

Calcium channel blockers

Calcium channel blockers are highly toxic in overdose because of their inhibitory effects on L-type calcium channels. Dihydropyridines, such as nifedipine or amlodipine, affect vascular smooth muscle in particular, resulting in vasodilatation, whereas diltiazem and verapamil, which are used in the treatment of arrhythmias, have predominantly cardiac effects, including bradycardia and reduced myocardial contractility.

Clinical features

The usual presentation is with hypotension due to vasodilatation or myocardial depression. Bradycardias and heart block may also occur, especially with verapamil and diltiazem. Gastrointestinal disturbances, confusion, metabolic acidosis, hyperglycaemia and hyperkalaemia may also be present.

Management

Hypotension should be corrected with intravenous fluids, taking care to avoid pulmonary oedema. Persistent hypotension may respond to intravenous calcium gluconate (10 mg IV over 5 mins, repeated as required). Isoprenaline and glucagon may also be useful. Successful use of intravenous insulin with glucose (10–20%

dextrose with insulin initially at 0.5–2.0 U/kg/hr, increasing to 5–10 U/kg/hr according to clinical response), so-called 'hyperinsulinaemia euglycaemic therapy', has been reported in patients unresponsive to other strategies. The mechanism of action remains to be fully elucidated, but in states of shock myocardial metabolism switches from use of free fatty acids to glucose. Calcium channel blocker poisoning is also associated with hypoinsulinaemia and insulin resistance, impeding glucose uptake by myocytes. High doses of insulin inhibit lipolysis and increase glucose uptake and the efficiency of glucose utilisation. Cardiac pacing may be needed for severe unresponsive bradycardias or heart block. Lipid emulsion therapy has been used in severe poisoning with apparent benefit, although evidence is largely anecdotal.

Digoxin and oleander

Poisoning with digoxin is usually accidental, arising from prescription of an excessive dose, impairment of renal function or drug interactions. In South Asia, deliberate self-poisoning with yellow oleander (*Thevetia peruviana*), which contains cardiac glycosides, is common.

Clinical features

Characteristic cardiac effects of toxicity are tachyarrhythmias (either atrial or ventricular) and bradycardias, with or without atrioventricular block. Ventricular bigeminy is common and atrial tachycardia with evidence of atrioventricular block is highly suggestive of the diagnosis. Severe poisoning is associated with hyperkalaemia. Non-cardiac features include confusion, headache, nausea, vomiting, diarrhoea and (rarely) altered colour vision.

Management

Activated charcoal is commonly administered to patients presenting within 1 hour of ingestion of an acute overdose, although evidence of benefit is lacking. Urea, electrolytes and creatinine should be measured, a 12-lead ECG performed and cardiac monitoring instituted. Hypoxia, hypokalaemia (sometimes associated with concurrent diuretic use), hypomagnesaemia and acidosis increase the risk of arrhythmias and should be corrected. Significant bradycardias may respond to atropine, although temporary pacing is sometimes needed. Ventricular arrhythmias may respond to intravenous magnesium (see Box 9.10). If available, digoxin-specific antibody fragments should be administered when there are severe ventricular arrhythmias or unresponsive bradycardias. This antidote has been shown to be effective for both digitalis and yellow oleander poisoning.

Antimalarials

Chloroquine

Chloroquine is highly toxic in overdose and quantities of 5 g or more of chloroquine base are likely to be fatal in an adult.

Clinical features

Features of toxicity occur within 1 hour of ingestion and include nausea, vomiting, agitation, drowsiness, hypokalaemia, acidosis, headaches and blurred vision. Coma, convulsions and hypotension may occur in severe poisoning. ECG changes indicating conduction and repolarisation delay (prolonged QRS and QT_c intervals) occur and are associated with ventricular tachycardia (including torsades de pointes), ventricular fibrillation and sudden death.

Management

Activated charcoal should be given to all patients presenting within 1 hour of ingestion of chloroquine in amounts greater than 15 mg/kg. Cardiac rhythm should be monitored and dysrhythmias managed as outlined in Box 9.10. The arterial pH should be corrected, but hypokalaemia is thought to have a protective effect and should not be corrected in the first 8 hours after poisoning. High-dose diazepam (2 mg/kg body weight IV over 30 mins followed by an infusion of 2 mg/kg/hr) has been suggested to have a protective effect, especially if given in the early stages of severe chloroquine poisoning, but evidence is limited as yet. One controlled trial did not show beneficial effects on the ECG. Diazepam therapy requires intubation and mechanical ventilation to avoid pulmonary aspiration.

Quinine

Quinine salts are widely used for treating malaria and leg cramps. Deaths have been reported with ingestion of as little as 1.5 g in an adult and 900 mg in a child.

Clinical features

Features of toxicity include nausea, vomiting, tremor, tinnitus and deafness. Hypotension, haemolysis, renal failure, ataxia, convulsions and coma are features of serious poisoning. Conduction and repolarisation delay results in prolonged QRS and QT_c intervals on the ECG, and ventricular tachycardia (including torsades de pointes), ventricular fibrillation and sudden death may occur. Quinine-induced retinal photoreceptor cell toxicity may result in blurred vision and impaired colour perception. This usually develops a few hours after overdose and progresses to constriction of the visual field, scotoma and complete blindness associated with pupillary dilatation and unresponsiveness to light. Fundoscopy may show retinal artery spasm, disc pallor and retinal oedema. Although visual loss can be permanent, some degree of recovery, especially of central vision, often occurs over several weeks.

Management

Multiple-dose activated charcoal should be commenced in patients who have taken quinine in amounts greater than 15 mg/kg. Gastric lavage should be considered in patients who have taken a substantial overdose who present within 1 hour. All patients should have a 12-lead ECG and cardiac monitoring, and their urea, electrolytes and glucose checked. Dysrhythmias, hypotension, seizures and coma should be managed as outlined in Box 9.10.

There are no effective treatments for the visual effects of quinine. Stellate ganglion block and retrobulbar or intravenous injections of vasodilators such as nitrates were previously used but are ineffective, as are haemodialysis and haemoperfusion.

Iron

Overdose with iron can cause severe and sometimes fatal poisoning. The toxicity of individual iron preparations is related to their elemental iron content.

Clinical features

Early clinical features include gastrointestinal disturbance with the passage of grey or black stools. Hyperglycaemia and leucocytosis may occur. Haematemesis, rectal bleeding, drowsiness, convulsions, coma, metabolic acidosis and cardiovascular collapse may occur in severe poisoning.

Early symptoms may improve or even resolve within 6–12 hours, but hepatocellular necrosis may develop 12–24 hours after overdose and occasionally progresses to hepatic failure. Gastrointestinal strictures are late complications of iron poisoning.

Management

Gastric lavage may be considered in patients presenting within 1 hour of life-threatening overdose but efficacy has not been established. Activated charcoal is ineffective since iron is not bound. Serum iron concentration should be measured (see Box 9.6, p. 209). The antidote desferrioxamine chelates iron and should be administered immediately in patients with severe features, without waiting for serum iron concentrations to be available. Symptomatic patients with high serum iron concentrations (e.g. > 5 mg/L) should also receive desferrioxamine. Desferrioxamine may cause hypotension, allergic reactions and occasionally pulmonary oedema. Otherwise, treatment is supportive and directed at complications.

Antipsychotic drugs

Antipsychotic drugs (p. 248) are often prescribed for patients at high risk of self-harm or suicide, and are commonly encountered in overdose.

Clinical features

Drowsiness, tachycardia and hypotension are frequently found. Anticholinergic features (see Box 9.11) and acute dystonias, such as oculogyric crisis, torticollis and trismus, may occur after overdose with typical antipsychotics like haloperidol or chlorpromazine. QT interval prolongation and torsades de pointes can occur with typical antipsychotics such as thioridazine and haloperidol, as well as atypical antipsychotics like quetiapine, amisulpride and ziprasidone. Convulsions may occur with both groups of agent.

Management

Activated charcoal may be of benefit if given within 1 hour of overdose. Cardiac monitoring should be undertaken for at least 6 hours. Management is largely supportive, with treatment directed at complications (see Box 9.10, p. 211).

Antidiabetic agents

Antidiabetic agents commonly causing toxicity in overdose include sulphonylureas such as chlorpropamide, glibenclamide, gliclazide, glipizide and tolbutamide; biguanides like metformin and phenformin; and insulins. Overdose may also be encountered with some of the newer antidiabetic drugs, such as thiazolidinediones (pioglitazone), meglinides (nateglinide, repaglinide) and dipeptidyl peptidase (DPP)-IV inhibitors (sitagliptin).

Clinical features

Sulphonylureas, meglitinides and parenteral insulin cause hypoglycaemia when taken in overdose, although insulin is non-toxic if ingested by mouth. The duration of hypoglycaemia depends on the half-life or release characteristics of the preparation and may be prolonged over several days with long-acting agents such as chlorpropamide, insulin zinc suspension or insulin glargine.

Features of hypoglycaemia include nausea, agitation, sweating, aggression and behavioural disturbances, confusion, tachycardia, hypothermia, drowsiness, coma or convulsions (p. 814). Permanent neurological damage can occur if hypoglycaemia is prolonged. Hypoglycaemia can be diagnosed using bedside glucose strips but venous blood should also be sent for laboratory confirmation.

Metformin is uncommonly associated with hypoglycaemia. Its major toxic effect in overdose is lactic acidosis, which can have a high mortality, and is particularly common in older patients and those with renal or hepatic impairment, or when ethanol is co-ingested. Other features of metformin overdose are nausea and vomiting, diarrhoea, abdominal pain, drowsiness, coma, hypotension and cardiovascular collapse.

There is limited experience of overdose involving thiazolidinediones and DPP-IV inhibitors, but significant hypoglycaemia is unlikely.

Management

Activated charcoal should be considered for all patients who present within 1 hour of ingestion of a substantial overdose of an oral hypoglycaemic agent. Venous blood glucose and urea and electrolytes should be measured and tests repeated regularly. Hypoglycaemia should be corrected using oral or intravenous glucose (50 mL of 50% dextrose); an infusion of 10–20% dextrose may be required to prevent recurrence. Intramuscular glucagon can be used as an alternative, especially if intravenous access is unavailable. Failure to regain consciousness within a few minutes of normalisation of the blood glucose can indicate that a central nervous system (CNS) depressant has also been ingested, the hypoglycaemia has been prolonged, or that the coma has another cause (e.g. cerebral haemorrhage or oedema).

Arterial blood gases should be taken after metformin overdose to assess the extent of acidosis. If present, plasma lactate should be measured and acidosis should be corrected with intravenous sodium bicarbonate (250 mL 1.26% solution or 50 mL 8.4% solution, repeated as necessary). In severe cases, haemodialysis or haemodiafiltration is used.

DRUGS OF MISUSE

Cannabis

Cannabis is derived from the dried leaves and flowers of *Cannabis sativa*. When it is smoked, the onset of effect occurs within 10–30 minutes, whereas after ingestion

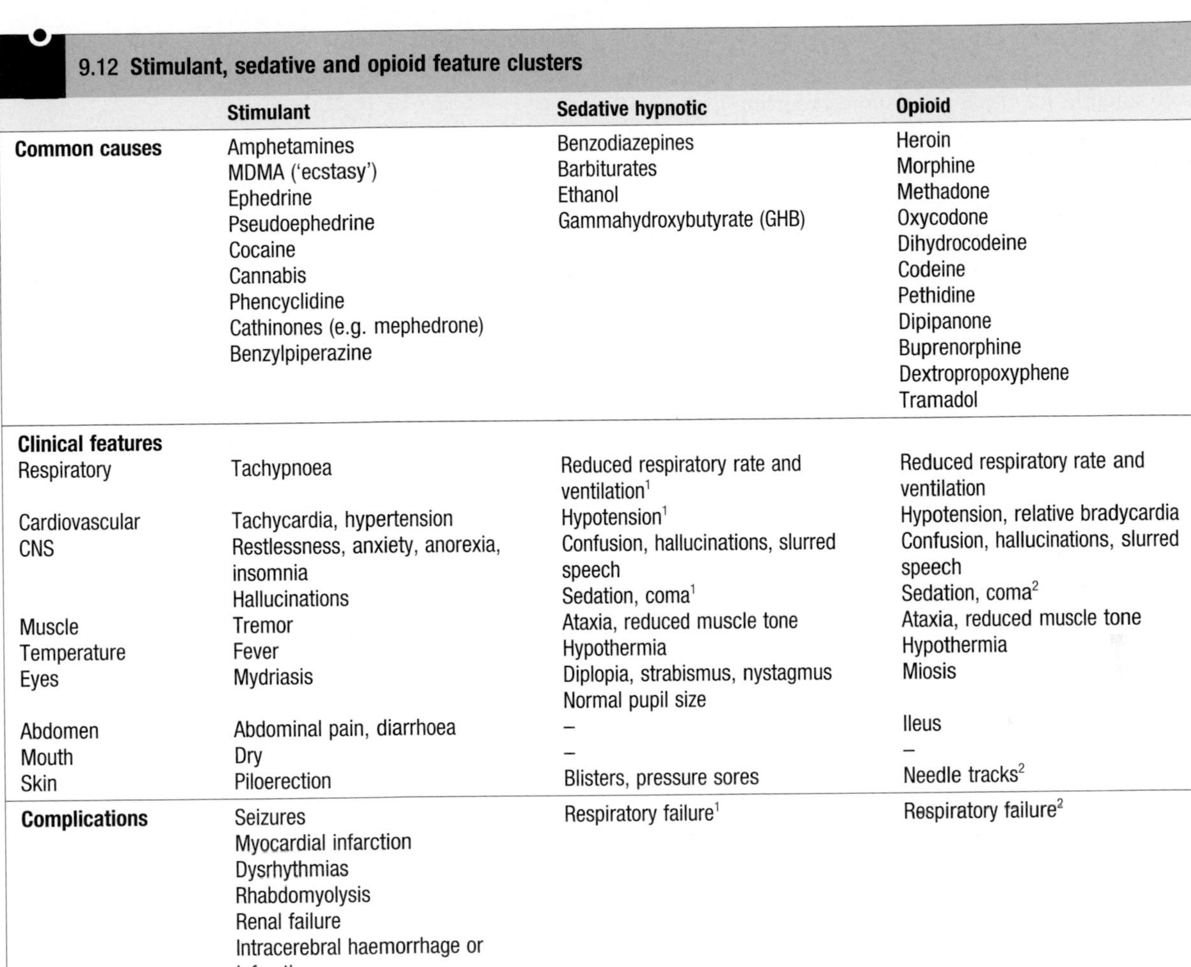

9.12 Stimulant, sedative and opioid feature clusters

	Stimulant	Sedative hypnotic	Opioid
Common causes	Amphetamines MDMA ('ecstasy') Ephedrine Pseudoephedrine Cocaine Cannabis Phencyclidine Cathinones (e.g. mephedrone) Benzylpiperazine	Benzodiazepines Barbiturates Ethanol Gammahydroxybutyrate (GHB)	Heroin Morphine Methadone Oxycodone Dihydrocodeine Codeine Pethidine Dipipanone Buprenorphine Dextropropoxyphene Tramadol
Clinical features			
Respiratory	Tachypnoea	Reduced respiratory rate and ventilation[1]	Reduced respiratory rate and ventilation
Cardiovascular	Tachycardia, hypertension	Hypotension[1]	Hypotension, relative bradycardia
CNS	Restlessness, anxiety, anorexia, insomnia Hallucinations	Confusion, hallucinations, slurred speech Sedation, coma[1]	Confusion, hallucinations, slurred speech Sedation, coma[2]
Muscle	Tremor	Ataxia, reduced muscle tone	Ataxia, reduced muscle tone
Temperature	Fever	Hypothermia	Hypothermia
Eyes	Mydriasis	Diplopia, strabismus, nystagmus Normal pupil size	Miosis
Abdomen	Abdominal pain, diarrhoea	–	Ileus
Mouth	Dry	–	–
Skin	Piloerection	Blisters, pressure sores	Needle tracks[2]
Complications	Seizures Myocardial infarction Dysrhythmias Rhabdomyolysis Renal failure Intracerebral haemorrhage or infarction	Respiratory failure[1]	Respiratory failure[2]

[1]Especially barbiturates. [2]IV use.

the onset is 1–3 hours later. The duration of effect is 4–8 hours. Cannabis produces euphoria, perceptual alterations and conjunctival injection, followed by enhanced appetite, relaxation and occasionally hypertension, tachycardia, slurred speech and ataxia. High doses may produce anxiety, confusion, hallucinations and psychosis (Box 9.12). Psychological dependence is common but tolerance and withdrawal symptoms are unusual. Long-term use is thought to increase the lifetime risk of developing schizophrenia. Ingestion or smoking of cannabis rarely results in serious poisoning and supportive treatment is all that is required.

Benzodiazepines

Benzodiazepines may be prescribed or used illicitly. They are of low toxicity when taken alone in overdose but can enhance CNS depression when taken with other sedative agents, including alcohol. They may also cause significant toxicity in the elderly and those with chronic lung or neuromuscular disease.

Clinical features

Clinical features of toxicity include drowsiness, ataxia and confusion (see Box 9.12). Respiratory depression and hypotension may occur with severe poisoning in susceptible groups, especially after intravenous administration of short-acting agents.

Management

Activated charcoal may be useful after ingestion in susceptible patients or after mixed overdose, if given within 1 hour. Conscious level, respiratory rate and oxygen saturation should be monitored for at least 6 hours after substantial overdose.

The specific benzodiazepine antagonist flumazenil increases conscious level in patients with overdose but carries a risk of seizures, and is contraindicated in patients co-ingesting proconvulsant agents such as TCAs and in those with a history of seizures.

Stimulants and entactogens

This group includes amphetamines, ecstasy, cathinones such as mephedrone, piperazines and cocaine. These are sympathomimetic and serotonergic amines; as a result, they have clinical features of poisoning that overlap (see Box 9.12).

Cocaine

Cocaine is available as a water-soluble hydrochloride salt suitable for nasal inhalation ('snorting'), or as an insoluble free base ('crack' cocaine) that, unlike the hydrochloride salt, vaporises at high temperature and can be smoked, giving a more rapid and intense effect. Cocaine hydrochloride is usually purchased as a white crystalline powder, and crack cocaine in 'rocks'.

Clinical features

Effects appear rapidly after inhalation and especially after smoking. Sympathomimetic stimulant effects are common (see Box 9.12). Serious complications usually occur within 3 hours of use and include coronary artery spasm, which may result in myocardial ischaemia or infarction, even in patients with normal coronary arteries. This may lead to hypotension, cyanosis and ventricular arrhythmias. Cocaine toxicity should be considered in young adults who present with ischaemic chest pain. Hyperpyrexia may be associated with rhabdomyolysis, acute renal failure and disseminated intravascular coagulation.

Management

All patients should be observed with ECG monitoring for a minimum of 4 hours. A 12-lead ECG should be performed. Abnormalities are common, including ST segment elevation, which may occur even in the absence of myocardial infarction. Troponin T estimations are the most sensitive and specific markers of myocardial damage. Benzodiazepines and intravenous nitrates are useful for managing patients with chest pain or hypertension, but β-blockers are best avoided because of the risk of unopposed α-adrenoceptor stimulation. Coronary angiography should be considered in patients with myocardial infarction or acute coronary syndromes. Acidosis should be corrected. Physical cooling measures may be required for hyperthermia (p. 105).

Amphetamines and cathinones

These include amphetamine sulphate ('speed'), methylamphetamine ('crystal meth'), 3,4-methylenedioxymethamphetamine (MDMA, 'ecstasy') and mephedrone. Tolerance is common, leading regular users to seek progressively higher doses.

Clinical features

Toxic features usually appear within a few minutes of use and last 4–6 hours, or substantially longer after a large overdose. Sympathomimetic stimulant and serotonergic effects are common (see Boxes 9.11 and 9.12). A proportion of ecstasy users develop hyponatraemia as a result of excessive water drinking and inappropriate antidiuretic hormone secretion. Muscle rigidity, pain and bruxism (clenching of the jaw) may occur. Hyperpyrexia, rhabdomyolysis, metabolic acidosis, acute renal failure, disseminated intravascular coagulation, hepatocellular necrosis, acute respiratory distress syndrome (ARDS) and cardiovascular collapse have all been described following MDMA use but are rare. Cerebral infarction and haemorrhage have been reported, especially after intravenous amphetamine use.

Management

Management is supportive and directed at complications (see Box 9.10, p. 211).

Gammahydroxybutyrate and gamma butyrolactone

Gamma hydroxybuterate (GHB) and gamma butyrolactone (GBL) are sedative agents with psychedelic and body-building effects. They are easily manufactured from commonly available industrial chemicals, including 1,4 butanediol, which is metabolised to GHB in vivo and has similar effects after ingestion. GHB solution is drunk by users, who titrate the dose until the desired effects are achieved.

Clinical features

Toxic features are those of a sedative hypnotic (see Box 9.12). Nausea, diarrhoea, vertigo, tremor, myoclonus, extrapyramidal signs, euphoria, bradycardia, convulsions, metabolic acidosis, hypokalaemia and hyperglycaemia may also occur. As the drug may be produced in batches and shared amongst a number of individuals, several patients may present with coma at the same time. The sedative effects are potentiated by other CNS depressants, such as alcohol, benzodiazepines, opioids and neuroleptics. Coma usually resolves spontaneously and abruptly within a few hours but may occasionally persist for several days. Dependence may develop in regular users, who may experience severe prolonged withdrawal effects if use is discontinued abruptly.

Management

Activated charcoal is recommended within 1 hour for ingestion of GHB in amounts greater than 20 mg/kg. Urea, electrolytes and glucose should be measured in all but the most trivial of cases. All patients should be observed for a minimum of 2 hours, with monitoring of blood pressure, heart rate, respiratory rate and oxygenation. Patients who remain symptomatic should be observed in hospital until symptoms resolve, but require supportive care only. Withdrawal may require treatment with high doses of benzodiazepines.

d-Lysergic acid diethyamide

d-Lysergic acid diethylamide (LSD) is a synthetic hallucinogen usually ingested as small squares of impregnated absorbent paper (often printed with a distinctive design) or as 'microdots'. The drug causes perceptual effects, such as heightened visual awareness of colours, distortion of images, and hallucinations that may be pleasurable or terrifying ('bad trip') and associated with panic, confusion, agitation or aggression. Dilated pupils, hypertension, pyrexia and metabolic acidosis may occur and psychosis may sometimes last several days.

Patients with psychotic reactions or CNS depression should be observed in hospital, preferably in a quiet, dimly lit room to minimise external stimulation. Where sedation is required, diazepam is the drug of choice. Antipsychotics should be avoided if possible, as they may precipitate cardiovascular collapse or convulsions.

Opioids

Commonly encountered opioids are shown in Box 9.12. Toxicity may result from misuse of illicit drugs such as heroin or after overdose of medicinal opiates such as dextropropoxyphene. Intravenous use of heroin or morphine gives a rapid, intensely pleasurable experience, often accompanied by heightened sexual arousal. Physical dependence occurs within a few weeks of regular high-dose injection; as a result, the dose is escalated and the user's life becomes increasingly centred on obtaining and taking the drug. Withdrawal, which can start within 12 hours, presents with intense craving, rhinorrhoea, lacrimation, yawning, perspiration, shivering, piloerection, vomiting, diarrhoea and abdominal cramps. Examination reveals tachycardia, hypertension, mydriasis and facial flushing.

Accidental overdose with prescribed strong opioid preparations is common, especially in the elderly.

Clinical features

These are shown in Box 9.12. Needle tracks may be visible in intravenous drug misusers and drug-related paraphernalia may be found amongst their possessions. Severe poisoning results in respiratory depression, hypotension, non-cardiogenic pulmonary oedema and hypothermia, leading to respiratory arrest or aspiration of gastric contents. Dextropropoxyphene (the opioid component of co-proxamol) may cause cardiac conduction effects, particularly QRS prolongation, ventricular arrhythmias and heart block, and has been withdrawn in the UK and other countries. Methadone may cause QT_c prolongation and torsades de pointes.

Symptoms of opioid poisoning can be prolonged for up to 48 hours after use of long-acting agents such as methadone, dextropropoxyphene and oxycodone.

Management

The airway should be cleared and, if necessary, respiratory support and oxygen given. Oxygen saturation monitoring and measurement of arterial blood gases should be performed. Prompt use of the specific opioid antagonist naloxone (0.4–2 mg IV in an adult, repeated if necessary) may obviate the need for intubation, although excessive doses may precipitate acute withdrawal in chronic opiate users. An infusion may be required in some cases because the half-life of the antidote is short compared to that of most opiates, especially those with prolonged elimination. Patients must be monitored for at least 6 hours after the last naloxone dose. Other complications of naloxone therapy include fits and ventricular arrhythmias, although these are rare. Box 9.10 (p. 211) describes the management of coma, fits and hypotension. Non-cardiogenic pulmonary oedema does not usually respond to diuretic therapy, and continuous positive airways pressure (CPAP) or positive end-expiratory pressure (PEEP) ventilatory support (p. 193) may be required.

Body packers and body stuffers

Body packers ('mules') attempt to smuggle illicit drugs (usually cocaine, heroin or amphetamines) by ingesting multiple small packages wrapped in several layers of clingfilm or in condoms. Body stuffers are those who

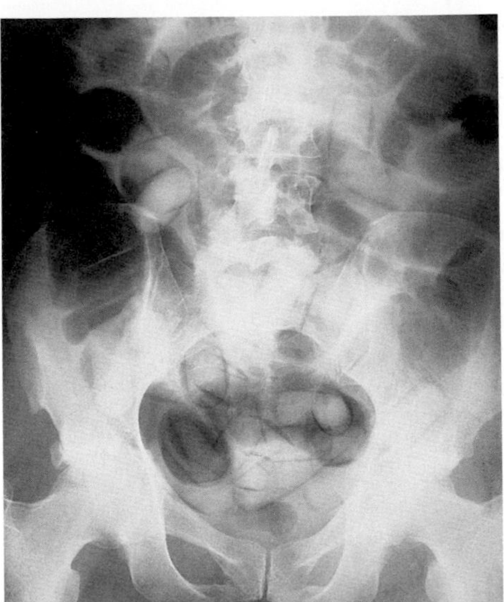

Fig. 9.4 Abdominal X-ray of a body packer showing multiple drug-filled condoms.

have ingested unpackaged or poorly wrapped substances, often to avoid arrest. Both groups are at risk of severe toxicity if the packages rupture. This is more likely for body stuffers, who may start to develop symptoms of poisoning within 8 hours of ingestion. The risk of poisoning depends on the quality of the wrapping, and the amount and type of drug ingested. Cocaine, for example, presents a much higher risk than heroin because of its high toxicity and lack of a specific antidote.

Patients suspected of body packing or stuffing should be admitted for observation. A careful history taken in private is important, but for obvious reasons patients may withhold details of the drugs involved. The mouth, rectum and vagina should be examined as possible sites for concealed drugs. A urine toxicology screen performed at intervals may provide evidence of leakage, although positive results may reflect earlier recreational drug use. Packages may be visible on plain abdominal films (Fig. 9.4), but this is not always the case, and ultrasound and computed tomography (CT) are more sensitive methods of visualisation. One of these (preferably CT) should be performed in all suspected body packers.

Antimotility agents are often used by body packers to prevent premature passage of packages, so it can take a number of days for packages to pass spontaneously; during this period the carrier is at risk from package rupture. Whole bowel irrigation is commonly used to accelerate passage and is continued until all packages have passed. Surgery may be required for mechanical bowel obstruction or when evolving clinical features suggest package rupture, especially with cocaine.

CHEMICALS AND PESTICIDES

Carbon monoxide

Carbon monoxide (CO) is a colourless, odourless gas produced by faulty appliances burning organic fuels. It is also present in vehicle exhaust fumes and sometimes in smoke from house fires. It causes toxicity by binding with haemoglobin and cytochrome oxidase, which reduces tissue oxygen delivery and inhibits cellular respiration. It is a common cause of death by poisoning and most patients who die of CO poisoning do so before reaching hospital.

Clinical features

Early clinical features of acute severe carbon monoxide poisoning include headache, nausea, irritability, weakness and tachypnoea. Because these are non-specific, the correct diagnosis will not be obvious if the exposure is occult, such as from a faulty domestic appliance. Subsequently, ataxia, nystagmus, drowsiness and hyperreflexia may develop, progressing to coma, convulsions, hypotension, respiratory depression, cardiovascular collapse and death. Myocardial ischaemia may occur and results in arrhythmias or myocardial infarction. Cerebral oedema is common and rhabdomyolysis may lead to myoglobinuria and renal failure. In those who recover from acute toxicity, longer-term neuropsychiatric effects are common, such as personality change, memory loss and concentration impairment. Extrapyramidal effects, urinary or faecal incontinence, and gait disturbance may also occur. Poisoning during pregnancy may cause fetal hypoxia and intrauterine death.

Management

Patients should be removed from exposure as soon as possible and resuscitated as necessary. Oxygen should be administered in as high a concentration as possible via a tightly fitting facemask, as this reduces the half-life of carboxyhaemoglobin from 4–6 hours to about 40 minutes. Measurement of carboxyhaemoglobin is useful for confirming exposure (see Box 9.6, p. 209) but levels do not correlate well with the severity of poisoning, partly because concentrations fall rapidly after removal of the patient from exposure, especially if supplemental oxygen has been given.

An ECG should be performed in all patients with acute poisoning, especially those with pre-existing heart disease. Arterial blood gas analysis should be checked in those with serious poisoning. Oxygen saturation readings by pulse oximetry are misleading since both carboxyhaemoglobin and oxyhaemoglobin are measured. Excessive intravenous fluid administration should be avoided, particularly in the elderly, because of the risk of pulmonary and cerebral oedema. Convulsions should be controlled with diazepam.

Hyperbaric oxygen therapy is controversial. At 2.5 atmospheres it reduces the half-life of carboxyhaemoglobin to about 20 minutes and increases the amount of dissolved oxygen by a factor of 10, but systematic reviews have shown no improvement in clinical outcomes. The logistical difficulties of transporting sick patients to hyperbaric chambers and managing them therein should not be underestimated.

Organophosphorus insecticides and nerve agents

Organophosphorus (OP) compounds (Box 9.13) are widely used as pesticides, especially in developing countries. The case fatality rate following deliberate ingestion of OP pesticides in developing countries in Asia is 5–20%.

9.13 Organophosphorus compounds

Nerve agents	
• G agents: sarin, tabun, soman	• V agents: VX,VE
Insecticides	
Dimethyl compounds	**Diethyl compounds**
• Dichlorvos	• Chlorpyrifos
• Fenthion	• Diazinon
• Malathion	• Parathion-ethyl
• Methamidophos	• Quinalphos

Nerve agents developed for chemical warfare are derived from OP insecticides but are much more toxic. They are commonly classified as G (originally synthesised in Germany) or V ('venomous') agents. The 'G' agents, such as tabun, sarin and soman, are volatile, absorbed by inhalation or via the skin, and dissipate rapidly after use. 'V' agents, such as VX, are contact poisons unless aerosolised, and contaminate ground for weeks or months.

The toxicology and management of nerve agent and pesticide poisoning are similar.

Mechanism of toxicity

OP compounds phosphonylate the active site of acetylcholinesterase (AChE), inactivating the enzyme and leading to the accumulation of acetylcholine (ACh) in cholinergic synapses (Fig. 9.5). Spontaneous hydrolysis of the OP–enzyme complex allows reactivation of the enzyme. However, loss of a chemical group from the OP–enzyme complex prevents further enzyme reactivation, a process termed 'ageing'. After ageing has taken place, new enzyme needs to be synthesised before function can be restored. The rate of ageing is an important determinant of toxicity and is more rapid with dimethyl compounds (3.7 hours) than diethyl (31 hours), and especially rapid after exposure to nerve agents (soman in particular), which cause ageing within minutes.

Clinical features and management

OP poisoning causes an acute cholinergic phase, which may occasionally be followed by the intermediate syndrome or organophosphate-induced delayed polyneuropathy (OPIDN). The onset, severity and duration of poisoning depend on the route of exposure and agent involved. Cholinergic features may be prolonged over several weeks with some lipid-soluble agents.

Acute cholinergic syndrome

The acute cholinergic syndrome usually starts within a few minutes of exposure. Nicotinic or muscarinic features may be present (Box 9.14). Vomiting and profuse diarrhoea are typical following oral ingestion. Bronchoconstriction, bronchorrhoea and salivation may cause severe respiratory compromise. Miosis is characteristic and the presence of muscle fasciculations strongly suggests the diagnosis, although this feature is often absent, even in serious poisoning. Subsequently, the patient may develop generalised flaccid paralysis which can affect respiratory and ocular muscles and result in respiratory failure. Ataxia, coma and convulsions may

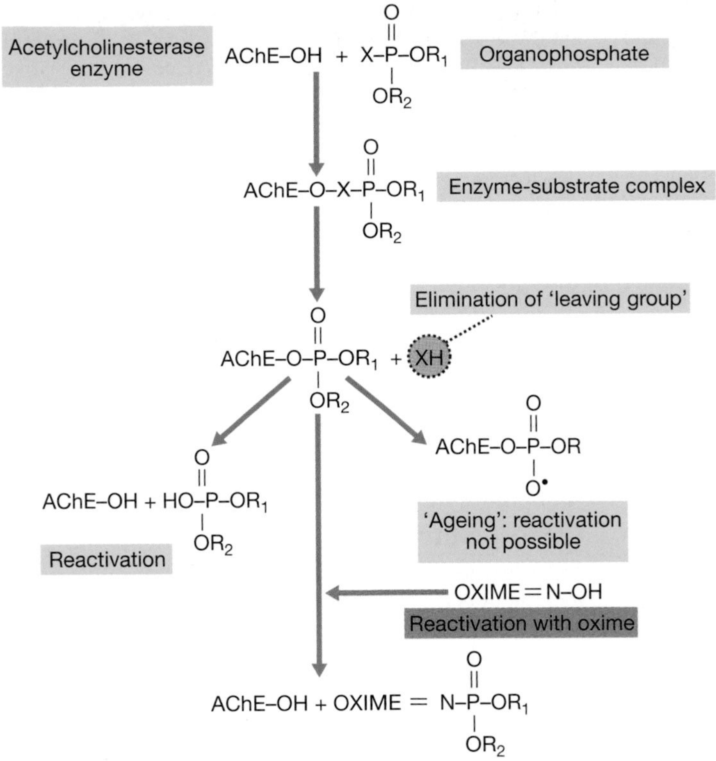

Fig. 9.5 Mechanism of toxicity of organophosphorus compounds and treatment with oxime.

9.14 Cholinergic features in poisoning*

	Cholinergic muscarinic	Cholinergic nicotinic
Respiratory	Bronchorrhoea, bronchoconstriction	Reduced ventilation
Cardiovascular	Bradycardia, hypotension	Tachycardia, hypertension
CNS	Confusion	–
Muscle	–	Fasciculation, paralysis
Temperature	Fever	–
Eyes	Diplopia, mydriasis	Lacrimation, miosis
Abdomen	Ileus, palpable bladder	Vomiting, profuse diarrhoea
Mouth	Dry	Salivation
Skin	Flushing, hot, dry	Sweating
Complications	Seizures	Seizures

*Both muscarinic and nicotinic features occur in OP poisoning. Nicotinic features occur in nicotine poisoning and black widow spider bites. Cholinergic features are sometimes seen with some mushrooms.

occur. In severe poisoning, cardiac repolarisation abnormalities and torsades de pointes may occur. Other early complications of OP poisoning include extrapyramidal features, pancreatitis, hepatic dysfunction and pyrexia.

Management

The airway should be cleared of excessive secretions, breathing and circulation assessed, high-flow oxygen administered and intravenous access obtained. In the event of external contamination, further exposure should be prevented, contaminated clothing and contact lenses removed, the skin washed with soap and water, and the eyes irrigated. Gastric lavage or activated charcoal may be considered if the patient presents within 1 hour of ingestion. Convulsions should be treated as described in Box 9.10 (p. 211). The ECG, oxygen saturation, blood gases, temperature, urea and electrolytes, amylase and glucose should be monitored closely.

Early use of sufficient doses of atropine is potentially life-saving in patients with severe toxicity. Atropine reverses ACh-induced bronchospasm, bronchorrhoea, bradycardia and hypotension. When the diagnosis is uncertain, a marked increase in heart rate associated with skin flushing after a 1 mg intravenous dose makes OP poisoning unlikely. In OP poisoning, atropine should be administered in doses of 0.6–2 mg IV, repeated every 10–25 mins until secretions are controlled, the skin is dry and there is a sinus tachycardia. Large doses may be needed but excessive doses may cause anticholinergic effects (see Box 9.11, p. 213).

In patients requiring atropine, an oxime such as pralidoxime chloride (or obidoxime), if available, should also be administered, as this may reverse or prevent muscle weakness, convulsions or coma, especially if given rapidly after exposure. The pralidoxime dose for an adult is 2 g IV over 4 mins, repeated 4–6 times daily. Oximes work by reactivating AChE that has not undergone 'ageing' and are therefore less effective with dimethyl compounds and nerve agents, especially soman. Oximes may provoke hypotension, especially if administered rapidly.

Ventilatory support should be instituted before the patient develops respiratory failure (p. 193).

Benzodiazepines may be used to reduce agitation and fasciculations, treat convulsions and sedate patients during mechanical ventilation.

Exposure is confirmed by measurement of plasma (butyrylcholinesterase) or red blood cell cholinesterase activity. These correlate poorly with the severity of clinical features, although values are usually less than 10% in severe poisoning, 20–50% in moderate poisoning and > 50% in subclinical poisoning.

The acute cholinergic phase usually lasts 48–72 hours, with most patients requiring intensive cardiorespiratory support and monitoring.

The intermediate syndrome

About 20% of patients with OP poisoning develop weakness that spreads rapidly from the ocular muscles to those of the head and neck, proximal limbs and the muscles of respiration, resulting in ventilatory failure. This 'intermediate syndrome' (IMS) generally develops quite rapidly between 1 and 4 days after exposure, often after resolution of the acute cholinergic syndrome, and may last 2–3 weeks. There is no specific treatment but supportive care, including maintenance of airway and ventilation, should be provided if necessary.

Organophosphate-induced delayed polyneuropathy

Organophosphate-induced delayed polyneuropathy (OPIDN) is a rare complication that usually occurs 2–3 weeks after acute exposure. It is a mixed sensory/motor polyneuropathy, especially affecting long myelinated neurons, and appears to result from inhibition of enzymes other than AChE. It is a feature of poisoning with some OPs such as trichlorocresylphosphate, but is less common with nerve agents,. Early clinical features are muscle cramps followed by numbness and paraesthesiae, proceeding to flaccid paralysis of the lower and subsequently the upper limbs. Paralysis of the lower limbs is associated with foot drop and a high-stepping gait, progressing to paraplegia. Paralysis of the arms leads to wrist drop. Sensory loss may also be present but is variable. Initially, tendon reflexes are reduced or lost but mild spasticity may develop later.

There is no specific therapy for OPIDN. Regular physiotherapy may limit deformity caused by muscle-wasting. Recovery is often incomplete and may be limited to the hands and feet, although substantial functional recovery after 1–2 years may occur, especially in younger patients.

Carbamate insecticides

Carbamate insecticides such as aldicarb, carbofuran and methomyl inhibit a number of tissue esterases, including AChE. The mechanism of action, clinical features and management are similar to those of OP compounds. However, clinical features tend to be less severe and of shorter duration, because the carbamate–AChE complex dissociates quickly, with a half-life of 30–40 minutes, and does not undergo ageing. Also, carbamates penetrate the CNS poorly. OPIDN and IMS are not common features of carbamate poisoning. Pancreatitis has been reported as a sequel, and deaths have occurred.

Atropine may be given intravenously in frequent small doses (0.6–2.0 mg IV for an adult) until signs of atropinisation develop. Diazepam may be used to relieve anxiety. The use of oximes is unnecessary.

Methanol and ethylene glycol

Ethylene glycol (1,2-ethanediol) is found in antifreeze, brake fluids and, in lower concentrations, windscreen washes. Methanol is present in some antifreeze products and commercially available industrial solvents, and in low concentrations in some screen washes and methylated spirits. It may also be an adulterant of illicitly produced alcohol. Both are rapidly absorbed after ingestion. Although methanol and ethylene glycol are not of high intrinsic toxicity, they are converted via alcohol dehydrogenase to toxic metabolites that are largely responsible for their clinical effects (Fig. 9.6).

Clinical features

Early features with either methanol or ethylene glycol include ataxia, drowsiness, dysarthria and nystagmus, often associated with vomiting. As the toxic metabolites are formed, metabolic acidosis, tachypnoea, coma and seizures may develop.

Toxic effects of ethylene glycol include ophthalmoplegia, cranial nerve palsies, hyporeflexia and myoclonus. Renal pain and acute tubular necrosis occur because of precipitation of calcium oxalate in the kidneys. Hypocalcaemia, hypomagnesaemia and hyperkalaemia are common.

Features of methanol poisoning include headache, confusion and vertigo. Visual impairment and photophobia develop, associated with optic disc and retinal oedema and impaired pupil reflexes. Blindness may be permanent, although some recovery may occur over several months. Pancreatitis and abnormal liver function have also been reported.

Management

Urea, electrolytes, chloride, bicarbonate, glucose, calcium, magnesium, albumin and plasma osmolarity and arterial blood gases should be measured in all

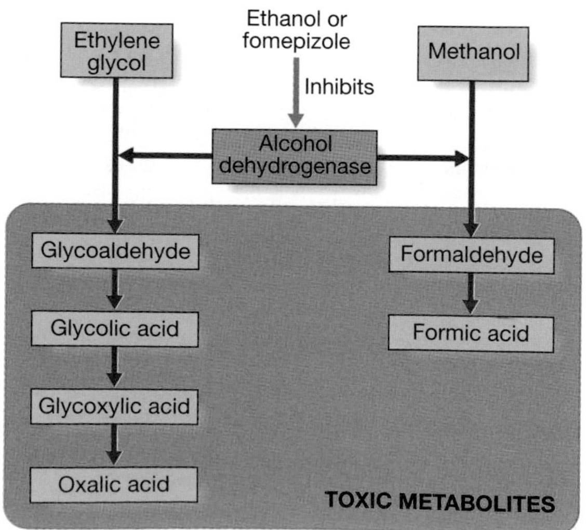

Fig. 9.6 Metabolism of methanol and ethylene glycol.

patients with suspected methanol or ethylene glycol toxicity. The osmolal and anion gaps should be calculated (see Box 9.5, p. 209). Initially, poisoning is associated with an increased osmolar gap, but as toxic metabolites are produced, an increased anion gap associated with metabolic acidosis will develop. The diagnosis can be confirmed by measurement of ethylene glycol or methanol concentrations, but assays are not widely available.

An antidote, either ethanol or fomepizole, should be administered to all patients with suspected significant exposure while awaiting the results of laboratory investigations. These block alcohol dehydrogenase and delay the formation of toxic metabolites until the parent drug is eliminated in the urine or by dialysis. The antidote should be continued until ethylene glycol or methanol concentrations are undetectable. Metabolic acidosis should be corrected with sodium bicarbonate (e.g. 250 mL of 1.26% solution, repeated as necessary). Convulsions should be treated with an intravenous benzodiazepine. In ethylene glycol poisoning, hypocalcaemia should only be corrected if there are severe ECG features or seizures occur, since this may increase calcium oxalate crystal formation.

Haemodialysis or haemodiafiltration should be used in severe poisoning, especially if renal failure is present or there is visual loss in the context of methanol poisoning. It should be continued until acute toxic features are no longer present and ethylene glycol or methanol concentrations are no longer detectable.

Aluminium and zinc phosphide

These rodenticides and fumigants are a common means of self-poisoning in northern India. The mortality rate for aluminium phosphide ingestion has been estimated at 60%; zinc phosphide ingestion appears less toxic, at about 2%. When ingested, both compounds react with gastric acid to form phosphine, a potent pulmonary and gastrointestinal toxicant. Clinical features include severe gastrointestinal disturbances, chest tightness, cough and breathlessness progressing to ARDS and respiratory failure, tremor, paraesthesiae, convulsions, coma, tachycardia, metabolic acidosis, electrolyte disturbances, hypoglycaemia, myocarditis, liver and renal failure, and leucopenia. Just a few tablets can be fatal.

Detection of phosphine in the exhaled air or stomach aspirate using either a silver nitrate-impregnated strip or specific phosphine detector tube is diagnostic, but gas chromatography provides the most sensitive indicator. Treatment is supportive and directed at correcting electrolyte abnormalities and treating complications; there is no specific antidote. Early gastric lavage is sometimes used, often with vegetable oil to reduce the release of toxic phosphine, but the benefit is uncertain.

ENVIRONMENTAL POISONING AND ILLNESS

Arsenism

Chronic arsenic exposure from drinking water has been reported in many countries, especially India, Bangladesh, Nepal, Thailand, Taiwan, China, Mexico and South America, where a large proportion of the drinking water (ground water) has a high arsenic content, placing large population groups at risk. The World Health Organization (WHO) guideline value for arsenic content in tube well water is 10 μg/L.

Health effects associated with chronic exposure to arsenic in drinking water are shown in Box 9.15. In exposed individuals, high concentrations of arsenic are present in bone, hair and nails. Specific treatments are of no benefit in chronic arsenic toxicity and recovery from the peripheral neuropathy may never be complete. The emphasis should be on the prevention of exposure to arsenic in drinking water.

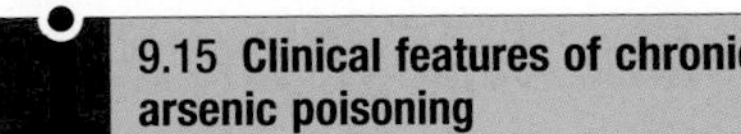

9.15 Clinical features of chronic arsenic poisoning

Gastrointestinal tract
• Anorexia, vomiting, weight loss, diarrhoea, increased salivation, metallic taste
Neurological
• Peripheral neuropathy (sensory and motor) with muscle wasting and fasciculation, ataxia
Skin
• Hyperpigmentation, palmar and plantar keratosis, alopecia, multiple epitheliomas, Mee's lines (transverse white lines on finger nails)
Eyes
• Conjunctivitis, corneal necrosis and ulceration
Bone marrow
• Aplastic anaemia
Other
• Low-grade fever, vasospasm and gangrene, jaundice, hepatomegaly, splenomegaly
Increased risk of malignancy
• Lung, liver, bladder, kidney, larynx and lymphoid system

Fluorosis

Fluoride poisoning can result either from exposure to excessive quantities of fluoride (> 10 ppm) in drinking water or from industrial exposure to fluoride dust and consumption of brick teas. Clinical features include yellow staining and pitting of permanent teeth, osteosclerosis, soft tissue calcification, deformities (e.g. kyphosis) and joint ankylosis. Changes in the bones of the thoracic cage may lead to rigidity that causes dyspnoea on exertion. Very high doses of fluoride may cause abdominal pain, nausea, vomiting, seizures and muscle spasm. In calcium-deficient children, the toxic effects of fluoride manifest even at marginally high exposures to fluoride.

In endemic areas, such as Jordan, Turkey, Chile, India, Bangladesh, China and Tibet, fluorosis is a major public health problem. The maximum impact is seen in communities engaged in physically strenuous agricultural or industrial activities. Dental fluorosis is endemic in East Africa and some West African countries.

SUBSTANCES LESS COMMONLY TAKEN IN OVERDOSE

Boxes 9.16 and 9.17 respectively give an overview of the clinical features and management for some substances that are less often encountered in overdose.

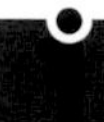

9.16 Clinical features associated with substances taken less commonly in overdose

Anticonvulsants	
Carbamazepine, phenytoin • Cerebellar signs • Convulsions • Cardiac arrhythmias • Coma	**Sodium valproate** • Coma • Metabolic acidosis
Isoniazid	
• Peripheral neuropathy	• Convulsions
Theophylline	
• Cardiac arrhythmias • Convulsions	• Coma
Corrosives and bleach	
• Injuries to stomach (esp. acids) and oesophagus (esp. alkali)	• GI perforation and late strictures • Aspiration pneumonitis
Lead, e.g. chronic occupational exposure, leaded paint, water contaminated by lead pipes, use of kohl cosmetics	
• Abdominal pain • Microcytic anaemia with basophilic stippling • Headache and encephalopathy	• Motor neuropathy • Nephrotoxicity • Hypertension • Hypocalcaemia
Petroleum distillates, white spirit, kerosene	
• Vomiting	• Aspiration pneumonitis
Paraquat	
• Progressive respiratory fibrosis with respiratory failure	• Buccal ulceration • Renal failure
Organochlorines, e.g. DDT, lindane, dieldrin, endosulfan	
• Nausea, vomiting • Agitation • Fasciculation • Paraesthesiae (face, extremities) • Convulsions • Coma	• Respiratory depression • Cardiac arrhythmias • Hyperthermia • Rhabdomyolysis • Pulmonary oedema • Disseminated intravascular coagulation
Pyrethroid insecticides, e.g. cypermethrin, permethrin, imiprothrin	
• Skin contact: dermatitis, skin paraesthesiae • Eye contact: lacrimation, photophobia and oedema of the eyelids • Inhalation: dyspnoea, nausea, headaches	• Ingestion: epigastric pain, nausea, vomiting, headache, coma, convulsions, pulmonary oedema
Anticoagulant rodenticides, (e.g. brodifacoum, bromodialone) and warfarin	
• Abnormal bleeding (prolonged)	

9.17 Specific management of poisoning by substances taken less commonly in overdose

Anticonvulsants
Carbamazepine, phenytoin • Multiple-dose activated charcoal (carbamazepine) **Sodium valproate** • Haemodialysis for severe poisoning
Isoniazid
• Activated charcoal • IV pyridoxine
Theophylline
• Multiple-dose activated charcoal
Corrosives and bleach
• Gastric lavage and neutralising chemicals are contraindicated • Chest X-ray to exclude perforation • Consider early endoscopy or Gastrografin studies to assess extent of damage and need for surgery
Lead
• Prevent further exposure • Measure blood lead concentration, full blood count and blood film, urea and electrolytes, liver function tests and calcium • Abdominal X-ray in children to detect pica • Bone X-ray for 'lead lines' • Chelation therapy with dimercaprol, DMSA, DMPS or sodium calcium edetate for severe poisoning (esp. in children)
Petroleum distillates, white spirit, kerosene
• Gastric lavage contraindicated • Activated charcoal ineffective • Oxygen and nebulised bronchodilators • Chest X-ray to assess pulmonary effects
Paraquat
• Urine screen for paraquat • Multiple-dose activated charcoal • Check blood paraquat concentration and compare with survival curve for prognosis
Organochlorines
• Activated charcoal (with nasogastric aspiration for liquid preparations) within 1 hour of ingestion • Cardiac monitoring
Pyrethroid insecticides
• Symptomatic and supportive care • Washing contaminated skin makes irritation worse
Anticoagulant rodenticides and warfarin
• Monitor INR/prothrombin time • Vitamin K_1 by slow IV injection if coagulopathy • Fresh frozen plasma or specific clotting factors for bleeding
(DMPS = 2,3-dimercapto-1-propane sulphonate; DMSA = 2,3-dimercaptosuccinic acid)

ENVENOMING

Envenoming occurs when a venomous animal injects sufficient venom by a bite or a sting into a prey item or perceived predator to cause deleterious local and/or systemic effects. Venomous animals generally use their venom to acquire and in some cases predigest prey, with defensive use a secondary function. Accidental encounters between venomous animals and humans are frequent, particularly in the rural tropics, where millions of cases of venomous bites and stings occur annually. Globally, an increasing number of exotic venomous animals are kept privately, so cases of envenoming may present to hospitals where doctors have insufficient knowledge to manage potentially complex presentations. Doctors everywhere should thus be aware of the basic principles of management of envenoming and how to seek expert support.

Venom

Venom is a complex mixture of diverse components, often with several separate toxins that can cause adverse effects in humans, and each potentially capable of multiple effects (Box 9.18). Venom is produced at considerable metabolic cost, so is used sparingly; thus only some bites/stings by venomous animals result in significant envenoming, the remainder being 'dry bites'. The concept of dry bites is important in understanding approaches to management.

Venomous animals

There are many animal groups that contain venomous species (Box 9.19). The epidemiology estimates shown reflect the importance of snakes and scorpions as causes of severe or lethal envenoming. Social insect stings from bees and wasps may also cause lethal anaphylaxis. Other venomous animals may commonly envenom humans but cause mostly non-lethal effects. A few rarely envenom humans, but have a high potential for severe or lethal envenoming. These include box jellyfish, cone shells, blue-ringed octopus, paralysis ticks and Australian funnel web spiders. Within any given group, particularly snakes, there may be a wide range of clinical presentations. Some are described here but for a more detailed discussion of the types of

9.18 Key venom effects*

Venom component	Clinical effects	Type of venomous animal
Neurotoxin		
Paralytic	Flaccid paralysis	Some snakes, paralysis ticks, cone shells, blue-ringed octopus
Excitatory	Neuroexcitation: autonomic storm, cardiotoxicity, pulmonary oedema	Some scorpions, spiders, jellyfish
Myotoxins	Systemic or local myolysis	Some snakes
Cardiotoxins	Direct or indirect cardiotoxicity; cardiac collapse, shock	Some snakes, scorpions, spiders, and jellyfish
Haemostasis system toxins	Vary from rapid coagulopathy and bleeding to thrombosis, deep venous thrombosis and pulmonary emboli	Many snakes and a few scorpions Brazilian caterpillars
Nephrotoxins	Renal damage	Some snakes, multiple bee, wasp stings
Necrotoxins	Local tissue injury/necrosis, shock	Some snakes, a few scorpions, spiders, jellyfish and stingrays
Allergic toxins	Induce acute allergic response (direct and indirect)	Almost all venoms but particularly those of social insects (bees, wasps, ants)

*All venom components have lethal potential.

9.19 Venomous animals and human envenoming

Phyla	Principal venomous animal groups	Estimated number of human cases/year	Estimated number of human deaths/year
Chordata	Snakes	> 2.5 million	> 100 000
	Spiny fish	? > 100 000	Close to 0
	Stingrays	? > 100 000	? < 10
Arthropoda	Scorpions	> 1 million	? < 5000
	Spiders	? > 100 000	? < 100
	Paralysis ticks	? > 1000	? < 10
	Insects	? > 1 million	? > 1000*
Mollusca	Cone shells	? < 1000	? < 10
	Blue-ringed octopus	? < 100	? < 10
Coelenterata	Jellyfish	? > 1 million	? < 10

*Social insect stings cause death by anaphylaxis rather than primary venom toxicity, except for massive multiple sting attacks.

9

venomous animal, their venoms and effects on humans see www.toxinology.com.

Clinical effects

With the exception of dry bites where no significant effects occur, venomous bites/stings can result in three broad classes of effect.

Local effects

These vary from trivial to severe (Box 9.20). There may be minimal or no local effects with some snakebites (not even pain), yet lethal systemic envenoming may still be present. For other species, local effects predominate over systemic, and for some species such as snakes, both are important.

General systemic effects

By definition, these are non-specific (see Box 9.20). Shock is an important complication of major local envenoming by some snake species and, if inadequately treated, can prove lethal, especially in children.

Specific systemic effects

These are important in both diagnosis and treatment.

- *Neurotoxic flaccid paralysis* can develop very rapidly, progressing from mild weakness to full respiratory paralysis in less than 30 minutes (blue-ringed octopus bite, cone shell sting), or may develop far more slowly, over hours (some snakes) to days (paralysis tick). For neurotoxic snakes, the cranial nerves are usually involved first, with ptosis a common initial sign (Fig. 9.7). From this, paralysis may extend to the limbs, with weakness and loss of deep tendon reflexes, then respiratory paralysis.
- *Excitatory neurotoxins* cause an 'autonomic storm', with profuse sweating, variable cardiac effects and cardiac failure, sometimes with pulmonary oedema (notably Australian funnel web spider bite, some scorpions such as Indian red scorpion). This type of envenoming can be rapidly fatal (many scorpions, funnel web spiders), or may cause distressing symptoms but constitute a lesser risk of death (widow spiders, banana spiders).

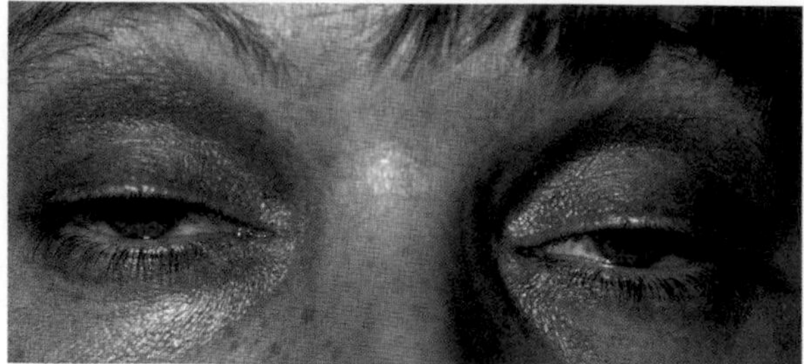

Fig. 9.7 Ptosis following neurotoxin envenomation.

- *Myotoxicity* can initially be silent, then present with generalised muscle pain, tenderness, myoglobinuria and huge rises in serum creatine kinase (CK). Secondary renal failure can precipitate potentially lethal hyperkalaemic cardiotoxicity.
- *Cardiotoxicity* is often secondary, but symptoms and signs are non-specific in most cases.
- *Haemostasis system toxins* cause a variety of effects, depending on the type of toxin, and the specific features can be diagnostic. Coagulopathy may present as bruising and bleeding from the bite site, gums and intravenous sites. Surgical interventions are high-risk in such cases. Other venoms cause thrombosis, usually presenting as deep venous thrombosis (DVT), pulmonary embolus or stroke (particularly Caribbean/Martinique vipers).
- *Renal damage* in envenoming is mostly secondary, although some species such as Russell's vipers can cause primary renal damage. The presentation is similar in both cases, with changes in urine output (polyuria, oliguria or anuria) or rises in creatinine and urea. In cases with intravascular haemolysis, secondary renal damage is likely. The clinical effects of specific animals in different regions of the world are shown in Boxes 9.21–9.23.

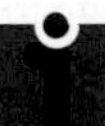

9.20 Local and systemic effects of envenoming

Local effects	
• Pain • Sweating • Swelling • Erythema • Bleeding and bruising	• Blistering • Necrosis • Major direct tissue trauma (e.g. stingray injuries)
Non-specific systemic effects	
• Headache • Nausea • Vomiting and diarrhoea • Abdominal pain • Hypertension or hypotension	• Tachycardia or bradycardia • Dizziness • Collapse • Convulsions • Shock • Cardiac arrest

Management

It is important to determine an accurate diagnosis and the degree of risk, so that severe and potentially lethal cases are identified quickly and managed as a priority. With correct care, even severe cases are treatable, but delays in initiating effective treatment can severely compromise outcome. Expert advice should thus be sought at the earliest opportunity.

First aid

Pre-hospital first aid (Box 9.24) can be critical in major envenoming. It depends on the type of envenoming, but the key principles are to:

- support vital systems
- delay or prevent the onset of envenoming
- avoid harmful 'treatments' such as electric shock, cut and suck, tourniquets, and cryotherapy in snakebite.

Many preventable deaths occur prior to hospital transfer when ineffective cardiorespiratory resuscitation is given to patients with respiratory paralysis or cardiac arrest/failure, which can occur due to either primary envenoming or an anaphylactic reaction (p. 91).

9.21 Important venomous animals in Asia

Scientific name[1]	Common name	Clinical effects	Antivenom/antidote/treatment
Indian subcontinent			
Bungarus spp. (E)	Kraits	Flaccid paralysis[2,3], myolysis[4], hyponatraemia[4]	Indian PV or specific
Naja spp. (E)	Cobras	Flaccid paralysis[3], local necrosis/ blistering, shock	Indian PV or specific
Ophiophagus hannah (E)	King cobra	Flaccid paralysis[3], local necrosis, shock	Indian PV or specific
Echis spp. (Vv)	Saw-scaled vipers	Procoagulant coagulopathy, local necrosis/blistering, renal failure	Indian PV or specific
Daboia russelli (Vv)	Russell's viper	Procoagulant coagulopathy, local necrosis/blistering, myolysis, renal failure, shock, flaccid paralysis[2]	Indian PV or specific
Hypnale spp. (Vc)	Hump-nosed vipers	Procoagulant coagulopathy, shock, renal failure	Try Indian PV
Trimeresurus[4] spp. (Vc)	Green pit vipers	Procoagulant coagulopathy, local necrosis, shock	Indian PV or specific
Mesobuthus spp. (Sc)	Indian scorpions	Neuroexcitation, cardiotoxicity	Indian specific AV, prazosin
East Asia			
Bungarus spp. (E)	Kraits	Flaccid paralysis[2,3]	Specific AV from country
Naja spp. (E)	Cobras (some spitters)	Flaccid paralysis[3], local necrosis/ blistering, shock	Specific AV from country
Ophiophagus hannah (E)	King cobra	Flaccid paralysis[3], local necrosis, shock	King cobra AV
Calloselasma rhodostoma (Vc)	Malayan pit viper	Procoagulant coagulopathy, local necrosis/blistering, renal failure, shock	Specific AV from country
Daboia russelli (Vv)	Russell's viper	Procoagulant coagulopathy, local necrosis/blistering, renal failure, shock	Specific AV from country
Gloydius (Vc)	Mamushis, pit vipers	Procoagulant coagulopathy, local necrosis/blistering, shock, renal failure, flaccid paralysis[2]	Specific AV from country
Trimeresurus[5] (Vc)	Green pit vipers, habus	Procoagulant coagulopathy, local necrosis/blistering, shock	Specific AV from country

[1]Family names: A = Atractaspididae; C = 'Colubridae' (mostly 'non-venomous'; family subject to major taxonomic revisions); E = Elapidae (all venomous); Sc = scorpions; Vc = Viperidae crotalinae (New World and Asian vipers); Vv = Viperidae viperinae (Old World vipers). [2]Pre-synaptic. [3]Post-synaptic. [4]Only reported so far for *B. candidus* and *B. multicinctus*. [5]Genus is subject to major taxonomic change (split into at least eight genera).
(AV = antivenom; PV = polyvalent)
More information is available from WHO-SEARO Guidelines for the management of snakebite and www.toxinology.com.

Diagnosis

Envenoming is usually obvious but might not be on some occasions. Humans may be bitten or stung by an unseen organism, or may not be aware of a bite or sting having occurred at all. In such cases the patient may present with a variety of symptoms but with no linking history to indicate envenoming. Accordingly, envenoming should be considered as a possible diagnosis in cases of unexplained paralysis, myotoxicity, coagulopathy, nephrotoxicity, cardiotoxicity, pulmonary oedema, necrosis, collapse and convulsions.

History, examination and laboratory findings help to confirm or exclude a diagnosis of envenoming and to determine its extent. It is also important to obtain a description of the organism if possible. Multiple bites or stings are more likely to cause major envenoming. Ask for specific symptoms and search for specific signs that may indicate the type and extent of envenoming (p. 207).

Specific tests for venom are currently only commercially available for Australian snakebite but are likely to be developed for snakebite in other regions. They are not available for other types of envenoming, where venom concentrations are low. For snakebite, a screen for envenoming includes full blood count, coagulation screen, urea and electrolytes, creatinine, CK and ECG. Lung function tests, peripheral oximetry or arterial blood gases may be indicated in cases with potential or established respiratory failure. In areas without access to routine laboratory tests, the whole-blood clotting time (using a glass test tube) is a valuable test for coagulopathy. A derivative of this, the 20-minute whole-blood clotting test is useful (a few millilitres of venous blood are placed in a glass vessel and checked for clotting at 20 minutes).

If patients state that they have been bitten by a particular species, ensure this is accurate. Private keepers of venomous animals may not have accurate

9.22 Important venomous animals in the Americas and Australia

Scientific name[1]	Common name	Clinical effects	Antivenom/antidote/treatment
North America			
Crotalus spp. (Vc)	Rattlesnakes	Procoagulant coagulopathy, local necrosis/ blistering (flaccid paralysis[2] rare)	CroFab AV® or Bioclon Antivipmyn AV®
Sistrurus spp. (Vc)	Massasaugas	Procoagulant coagulopathy, local necrosis/ blistering, shock	CroFab AV® or Bioclon Antivipmyn AV®
Agkistrodon spp. (Vc)	Copperheads and moccasins	Procoagulant coagulopathy, local necrosis/ blistering, shock	CroFab AV® or Bioclon Antivipmyn AV®
Micrurus spp. (E)	Coral snakes	Flaccid paralysis[3]	Bioclon Coralmyn AV®
Latrodectus mactans	Widow spider	Neuroexcitation	MSD Widow spider AV®
Centruroides sculpturatus	Arizona bark scorpion	Neuroexcitation	Bioclon Anascorp AV®
Central and South America			
Crotalus spp. (Vc)	Rattlesnakes	Flaccid paralysis[2], myolysis, procoagulant coagulopathy, shock, renal failure	Specific AV from country
Bothrops spp. (Vc)	Lancehead vipers	Procoagulant coagulopathy, local necrosis/ blistering, shock, renal failure	Specific AV from country
Bothriechis spp. (Vc)	Eyelash pit vipers	Shock, pain and swelling	Specific AV from country
Lachesis spp. (Vc)	Bushmasters	Procoagulant coagulopathy, shock, renal failure, local necrosis/blistering	Specific AV from country
Micrurus spp. (E)	Coral snakes	Flaccid paralysis[2,3], myolysis, renal failure	Specific AV from country
Tityus serrulatus	Brazilian scorpion	Neuroexcitation, shock	Instituto Butantan scorpion AV®
Loxosceles spp.	Recluse spiders	Local necrosis	Instituto Butantan spider AV®
Phoneutria nigriventer	Banana spider	Neuroexcitation, shock	Instituto Butantan spider AV®
Potamotrygon, Dasyatis spp.	Freshwater stingrays	Necrosis of bite area, shock, severe pain and oedema	No available AV; good wound care
Australia			
Pseudonaja spp. (E)	Brown snakes	Procoagulant coagulopathy, renal failure, flaccid paralysis[2] (rare)	CSL brown snake AV® or PVAV
Notechis spp. (E)	Tiger snakes	Procoagulant coagulopathy, myolysis, flaccid paralysis[2,3], renal failure	CSL tiger snake AV® or PVAV
Oxyuranus spp. (E)	Taipans	Procoagulant coagulopathy, flaccid paralysis[2,3], myolysis, renal failure	CSL taipan AV® or PVAV
Acanthophis spp. (E)	Death adders	Flaccid paralysis[3]	CSL death adder AV® or PVAV
Pseudechis spp.	Black and mulga snakes	Anticoagulant coagulopathy, myolysis, renal failure	CSL black snake AV® or PVAV
Enhydrina schistosa	Sea snakes (all species globally)	Flaccid paralysis and/or myolysis	CSL sea snake AV®
Atrax, Hadronyche spp.	Funnel web spiders	Neuroexcitation, shock	CSL funnel web spider AV®
Latrodectus hasseltii	Red back spider	Neuroexcitation, pain and sweating	CSL red back spider AV®
Chironex fleckeri	Box jellyfish	Neuroexcitation, cardiotoxicity, local necrosis	CSL box jellyfish AV®
Synanceia spp.	Stonefish	Severe local pain	CSL stonefish AV®

[1]For family name, see Box 9.21. [2]Pre-synaptic. [3]Post-synaptic. (CSL = CSL Ltd, Melbourne, producer of Australian antivenoms)

knowledge of what they are keeping, and misidentification of a snake, scorpion or spider can have dire consequences if the wrong antivenom is used.

Treatment

Envenoming is managed on two levels, which must be delivered in tandem:

- supportive management of the organ systems affected and of the whole patient
- treating the effects with specific treatments/ antidotes (usually antivenom).

For a snakebite by a potentially lethal species such as Russell's viper, the patient might have local effects with oedema, blistering, necrosis, and resultant fluid shifts causing shock, and at the same time have systemic effects such as intractable vomiting, coagulopathy, paralysis and secondary renal failure. Specific treatment with antivenom will be required to reverse

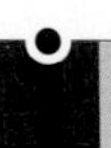

9.23 Important venomous animals in Africa and Europe

Scientific name[1]	Common name	Clinical effects	Antivenom/antidote/treatment
Africa			
Naja spp. (E)	Cobras		
	Non-spitters	Flaccid paralysis[3] ± local necrosis/blistering	South African PV or Sanofi Pasteur FavAfrica AV®
	Spitters	Local necrosis/blistering (flaccid paralysis[3] uncommon)	South African PV or Sanofi Pasteur FavAfrica AV®
Dendroaspis spp. (E)	Mambas	Mamba neurotoxin flaccid paralysis and muscle fasciculation, shock, necrosis (uncommon)	South African PV or Sanofi Pasteur FavAfrica AV®
Hemachatus haemachatus (E)	Rinkhals	Flaccid paralysis[3], local necrosis, shock	South African PV
Atheris spp. (Vv)	Bush vipers	Procoagulant coagulopathy, shock, pain and swelling	No available AV (can try South African AV)
Bitis spp. (Vv)	Puff adders etc.	Procoagulant coagulopathy, shock, cardiotoxicity, local necrosis/blistering	South African PV or Sanofi Pasteur FavAfrica AV®
Causus spp. (Vv)	Night adders	Pain and swelling	No available AV
Echis spp. (Vv)	Carpet vipers	Procoagulant coagulopathy, shock, renal failure, local necrosis/blistering	Specific anti-*Echis* AV for species/geographic region or Sanofi Pasteur FavAfrica AV®
Cerastes spp. (Vv)	Horned desert vipers	Procoagulant coagulopathy, local necrosis, shock	Specific or polyspecific AV covering *Cerastes* from country of origin
Dispholidus typus (C)	Boomslang	Procoagulant coagulopathy, shock	Boomslang AV
Androctonus spp.	North African scorpions	Neuroexcitation	Specific scorpion AV (Algeria, Tunisia, Sanofi Pasteur Scorpifav®)
Leiurus quinquestriatus	Yellow scorpion	Neuroexcitation, shock	Specific scorpion AV (Algeria, Tunisia, Sanofi Pasteur Scorpifav®)
Europe			
Vipera spp. (Vv)	Vipers and adders	Shock, local necrosis/blistering, procoagulant coagulopathy (flaccid paralysis[2] rare)	ViperaTab AV® or Zagreb AV® or SanofiPasteur Viperfav AV®

[1]For family name, see Box 9.21. [2]Pre-synaptic. [3]Post-synaptic.
More information is available from WHO Guidelines for the prevention and clinical management of snakebite in Africa and www.toxinology.com.

9.24 First aid for envenoming

Method	Situations where indicated
Immobilisation of bitten limb	All snakebites
Pressure bandage and immobilisation of bitten limb	Non-necrotic snakebites (Australian snakes, sea snakes, some cobras, king cobra, kraits, coral snakes, mambas, a few vipers, Australian funnel web spiders, blue-ringed octopus, cone shell)
Local heat (hot water immersion or shower, to 45°C)	Venomous fish stings, stingray injuries, jellyfish stings (except possibly box jellyfish)
Staunching local bleeding	Traumatic injury with significant bleeding (some stingray injuries)
Cardiorespiratory support	Cardiac or respiratory impairment and particularly if respiratory paralysis is developing (some snakes, paralysis ticks, blue-ringed octopus, cone shells)
No specific first aid	Widow and recluse spider bites

the coagulopathy, and may prevent worsening of the paralysis and reduce the vomiting, but will not greatly affect the local tissue damage or the renal failure or shock. The latter will require intravenous fluid therapy, possibly respiratory support, renal dialysis and local wound care, possibly including antibiotics.

Each animal will cause a particular pattern of envenoming, requiring a tailored response. Listing all of these is beyond the scope of this chapter (see Further information below). Pulse, blood pressure, pulse oximetry and urine output should be monitored in all cases.

Antivenom

This is the most important tool in treating envenoming. It is made by hyperimmunising an animal, usually horses, to produce antibodies against venom. Once refined, these bind to venom toxins and render them inactive or allow their rapid clearance. Antivenom is only available for certain venomous animals and cannot reverse all types of envenoming. With a few exceptions, it should be given intravenously, with adrenaline (epinephrine) ready in case of anaphylaxis. It should only be used when clearly indicated, and indications will vary between animals. It is critical that the correct antivenom is used at the appropriate dose. Doses vary widely between antivenoms; those recommended for North American antivenoms are not applicable to those elsewhere. In some situations (such as the Indian subcontinent), pre-treatment with subcutaneous adrenaline may reduce the chance of anaphylaxis to antivenom.

Antivenom can sometimes reverse post-synaptic neurotoxic paralysis (α-bungarotoxin-like neurotoxins) but will not usually reverse established pre-synaptic paralysis (β-bungarotoxin-like neurotoxins), so should be given before major paralysis has occurred. Coagulopathy is best reversed by antivenom, but even after all venom is neutralised, there may be a delay of hours before normal coagulation is restored. More antivenom should not be given because coagulopathy has failed to normalise fully in the first 1–3 hours (except in very particular circumstances). Thrombocytopenia may persist for days, despite antivenom. The role of antivenom in reversing established myolysis and renal failure is uncertain. Antivenom may help limit local tissue effects/injury in the bitten limb, but this is quite variable and time-dependent. Neuroexcitatory envenoming can respond very well to antivenom (Australian funnel web spider bites; Mexican, South American, Indian scorpion stings), but there is controversy about the effectiveness of antivenom for some species (some North African and Middle Eastern scorpions). The role of antivenom in limiting local venom effects, including necrosis, is also controversial; it is most likely to be effective when given early.

All patients receiving antivenom are at risk of both early and late adverse reactions, including anaphylaxis (early; not always IgE-related) and serum sickness (late).

Other treatments

Anticholinesterases are used as an adjunctive treatment for post-synaptic paralysis.

Prazosin (an α-adrenoceptor antagonist) is used in the management of hypertension or pulmonary oedema in scorpion sting cardiotoxicity, particularly for Indian red scorpion stings, though antivenom is now the preferred treatment.

Antibiotics are not routinely required for most bites/stings, though a few animals regularly cause significant wound infection/abscess, such as some South American pit vipers and stingrays. Tetanus is a risk in some bites or stings, such as snakebite, but intramuscular toxoid should not be given until any coagulopathy is reversed.

Mechanical ventilation (p. 194) is vital for established respiratory paralysis that will not reverse with antivenom, and may be required for prolonged periods - up to several months in some cases.

Follow-up

Cases with significant envenoming and those receiving antivenom should be followed up to ensure that any complications have resolved and to identify any delayed envenoming.

Further information and acknowledgements

Books and journal articles

Meier J, White J. Handbook of clinical toxicology of animal venoms and poisons. Boca Raton: CRC; 1995.

Thomas SH, Watson ID, on behalf of the National Poisons Information Service and Association of Clinical Biochemists. Laboratory analyses for poisoned patients. Annals of Clinical Biochemistry 2002; 39:328–339.

White J. Snakebite and spiderbite: management guidelines for South Australia; 2007.

WHO Regional Office for Africa. Guidelines for the prevention and clinical management of snakebite in Africa; 2010.

WHO-SEARO. Guidelines for the management of snakebites (for SE Asia); 2010.

The last three documents can be accessed via www.toxinology.org/Links.htm.

Websites

http://curriculum.toxicology.wikispaces.net/ *Free access to educational material related to poisoning.*

www.toxbase.org *Toxbase, the clinical toxicology database of the UK National Poisons Information Service. Free for UK health professionals but registration is required. Access for overseas users by special arrangement.*

www.toxinology.com *Women's and Children's Hospital Adelaide Toxinology Department.*

www.toxnet.nlm.nih.gov *US National Library of Medicine's Toxnet: a hazardous substances databank, including Toxline for references to literature on drugs and other chemicals.*

www.who.int/gho/phe/chemical safety/poisons centres/en/ *World directory of poisons centres held by the WHO, including interactive map and contact details.*

Figure acknowledgements

Page 206 insets (*Self-cutting*) Douglas G, Nicol F, Robertson C. Macleod's clinical examination. 11th edn. Edinburgh: Churchill Livingstone; 2005 (p. 48, Fig. 2.16); copyright Elsevier. (*Chemical burn*) www.firewiki.net. (*Needle tracks*) www.deep6inc.com. (*Pinpoint pupil*) http://drugrecognition.com/images. (*Injected conjunctiva*) http://knol.google.com.

M.C. Sharpe
S.M. Lawrie

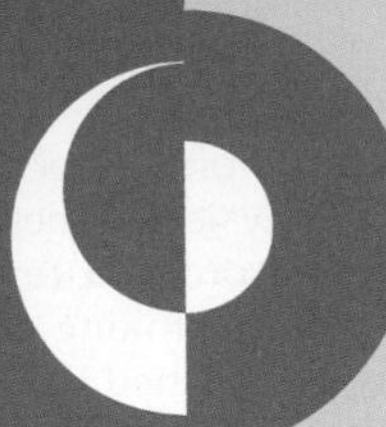

Medical psychiatry 10

Classification of psychiatric disorders 232

Epidemiology of psychiatric disorders 232

Aetiology of psychiatric disorders 232

Diagnosing psychiatric disorders 233

Presenting problems in psychiatric illness 234
- Anxiety symptoms 234
- Depressed mood 235
- Elated mood 235
- Medically unexplained somatic symptoms 236
- Delusions and hallucinations 236
- Disturbed and aggressive behaviour 237
- Confusion 238
- Self-harm 238
- Alcohol misuse 240
- Substance misuse 240
- Psychological factors affecting medical conditions 240

Treating psychiatric disorders 240
- Biological treatments 240
- Psychological treatments 241
- Social interventions 242

Psychiatric disorders 242
- Stress-related disorders 242
- Anxiety disorders 242
- Mood disorders 243
- Somatoform disorders 245
- Factitious disorders and malingering 247
- Schizophrenia 247
- Delirium, dementia and other organic disorders 250
- Alcohol misuse and dependence 252
- Substance misuse disorder 254
- Personality disorders 255
- Eating disorders 255
- Puerperal disorders 256

Psychiatry and the law 257

Psychiatric disorders have traditionally been considered as 'mental' rather than as 'physical' illnesses. This is because they manifest with disordered functioning in the areas of emotion, perception, thinking and memory, and/or have had no clearly established biological basis. However, as research identifies abnormalities of the brain in an increasing number of psychiatric disorders and an important role for psychological and behavioural factors in many medical illnesses, a clear distinction between mental and physical illness has become increasingly questionable. We therefore refer to psychiatric disorders simply to mean those conditions traditionally regarded as the province of psychiatry.

CLASSIFICATION OF PSYCHIATRIC DISORDERS

There are two main classifications of psychiatric disorders in current use:

- the American Psychiatric Association's Diagnostic and Statistical Manual (4th edition), or DSM-IV
- the World Health Organization's International Classification of Disease (10th edition), known as ICD-10.

The two systems are similar; here we use the ICD-10 classification (Box 10.1).

EPIDEMIOLOGY OF PSYCHIATRIC DISORDERS

Psychiatric disorders are amongst the most common of all human illnesses. The relative frequency of each varies with the setting (Box 10.2). In the general population, depression, anxiety disorders and adjustment disorders are most common (10%) and psychosis is rare (1–2%); in acute medical wards of general hospitals, organic disorders such as delirium (20–30%) are prevalent; in specialist general psychiatric services, psychoses are the most common disorders.

AETIOLOGY OF PSYCHIATRIC DISORDERS

The aetiology of psychiatric disorders is multifactorial, with a combination of biological, psychological and social causes. Each of these factors may play a role in predisposing to, precipitating or perpetuating the disorder (Box 10.3).

Biological factors

Genetic

Genetic factors play a predisposing role in many psychiatric disorders, including schizophrenia and bipolar

10.1 Classification of psychiatric disorders

Stress-related disorders
- Acute stress disorder
- Adjustment disorder
- Post-traumatic stress disorder

Anxiety disorders
- Generalised anxiety
- Phobic anxiety
- Panic disorder
- Obsessive-compulsive disorder

Affective (mood) disorders
- Depressive disorder
- Mania and bipolar disorder

Schizophrenia and delusional disorders

Substance misuse disorders
- Alcohol
- Drugs

Organic disorders
- Acute, e.g. delirium
- Chronic, e.g. dementia

Disorders of adult personality and behaviour
- Personality disorder
- Factitious disorder

Eating disorders
- Anorexia nervosa
- Bulimia nervosa

Somatoform disorders
- Somatisation disorder
- Dissociative (conversion) disorder
- Pain disorder
- Hypochondriasis
- Body dysmorphic disorder
- Somatoform autonomic dysfunction

Neurasthenia

Puerperal mental disorders

10.2 Prevalence of psychiatric disorders by medical setting

	Medical/surgical			
	General practice	Outpatients	Inpatients	Psychiatric services
Adjustment disorders	++	++	+++	++
Depression/anxiety	++	++	+++	+++
Alcohol abuse	++	++	+++	+++
Personality disorders	++	++	++	+++
Somatoform disorders	+	+++	++	+
Delirium	–	–	+++	–
Psychosis	–	–	–	+++

(– rare; + uncommon; ++ common; +++ very common)

10.3 Classification of aetiological factors in psychiatric disorders

Predisposing
• Increase susceptibility to psychiatric disorder • Established in utero or in childhood • Operate throughout patient's lifetime (e.g. genetic factors, congenital defects, disturbed family background, chronic physical illness)
Precipitating
• Trigger an episode of illness • Determine its time of onset (e.g. stressful life events, acute physical illness)
Perpetuating
• Delay recovery from illness (e.g. lack of social support, chronic physical illness)

affective disorder. However, whilst some disorders such as Huntington's disease are due to mutations in a single gene, the genetic contribution to most psychiatric disorders is polygenic in nature and mediated by the combined effects of several genetic variants, each with modest effects and modulated by environmental factors.

Brain structure and function

Brain structure is grossly normal in most psychiatric disorders, although abnormalities may be observed in some conditions, such as generalised atrophy in Alzheimer's disease and enlarged ventricles with a slight decrease in brain size in schizophrenia. The functioning of the brain, however, is commonly altered with, for example, changes in neurotransmitters such as dopamine, noradrenaline (norepinephrine) and 5-hydroxytryptamine (5-HT, serotonin), and differences in activity of specific areas of the brain, as seen on functional brain scans.

Psychological and behavioural factors

Early environment

Early childhood adversity, such as emotional deprivation or abuse, predisposes to psychiatric disorders such as depression and eating disorders in adulthood.

Personality

The relationship between personality and psychiatric disorder can be difficult to assess because the development of psychiatric disorder can change a patient's personality. However, some personality types predispose the individual to develop psychiatric disorder; for example, a depressive personality increases the risk of depression. A disordered personality may also perpetuate a psychiatric disorder once it is established, leading to a poorer prognosis.

Behaviour

A person's behaviour may predispose to the development of a disorder (e.g. excess alcohol intake leading to dependence, and dieting to anorexia) or perpetuate it, as in persistent avoidance of the feared situation in phobias.

Social and environmental factors

Social isolation

The lack of a close, confiding relationship predisposes to some psychiatric disorders such as depression. The reduced social support resulting from having a psychiatric disorder may also act to perpetuate it.

Stressors

Social and environmental stressors often play an important role in precipitating psychiatric disorder in those who are predisposed. For example, trauma in post-traumatic stress disorder, losses (such as bereavement) in depression, and events perceived as threatening (such as potential loss of employment) in anxiety.

DIAGNOSING PSYCHIATRIC DISORDERS

Psychiatric assessment differs from a standard medical assessment in the following ways:

- There is greater emphasis on the history.
- It includes a systematic examination of the patient's thinking, emotion and behaviour (mental state).
- It commonly includes the routine interviewing of an informant (usually a relative or friend who knows the patient), especially when the illness affects the patient's ability to give an accurate history.

Because of its greater complexity, a full psychiatric history (Box 10.4) and detailed mental state examination (MSE) may take an hour or more. However, a brief mental state examination, usually taking no more than a few minutes (see below), should be part of the assessment of *all* patients, not merely those deemed to be 'psychiatric'.

Psychiatric interview

The aims of the interview are to:

- establish a therapeutic relationship with the patient
- elicit the symptoms, history and background information (see Box 10.4)
- examine the mental state
- provide information, reassurance and advice.

Whilst some aspects of the patient's mental state may be observed whilst the history is being taken, specific enquiries for important features should always be made.

Mental state examination

General appearance and behaviour

Any abnormalities of alertness or motor behaviour, such as restlessness or retardation, are noted. The level of consciousness should be determined, especially in the assessment of possible delirium.

Speech

Speed and fluency should be observed, including slow (retarded) speech and word-finding difficulty. 'Pressure of speech' describes rapid speech that is difficult to interrupt.

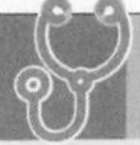

10.4 How to structure a psychiatric interview

Presenting problem

Reason for referral
- Why the patient has been referred and by whom

Presenting complaints
- The patient should be asked to describe the main problems for which help is requested and what he or she wants the doctor to do

History of present illness
- The patient should be asked to describe the course of the illness from when symptoms were first noticed
- The interviewer asks direct questions to determine the nature, duration and severity of symptoms, and any associated factors

Background

Family history
- Description of parents and siblings, and a record of any mental illness in relatives

Personal history
- Birth history, major events in childhood, education, occupational history, relationship(s), marriage, children, current social circumstances

Previous medical and psychiatric history
- Previous health, accidents and operations
- Use of alcohol, tobacco and other drugs
- Direct questions may be needed concerning previous psychiatric history since this may not be volunteered: 'Have you ever been treated for depression or nerves?' or 'Have you ever suffered a nervous breakdown?'

Previous personality
- The patterns of behaviour and thinking that characterise a person, including their relationships with other people and reactions to stress
- The most useful information may be obtained from an informant who has known the patient well for many years

Mood

This can be judged by facial expression, posture and movements. Patients should also be asked if they feel sad or depressed and if they lack ability to experience pleasure (anhedonia). Are they anxious, worried or tense? Is mood elevated with excess energy and a reduced need for sleep, as in mania?

Thoughts

The content of thought can be elicited by asking 'What are your main concerns?' Is thinking negative, guilty or hopeless, suggesting depression? Are there thoughts of self-harm? If so, enquiry should be made about plans. Is he or she excessively worried about many things, suggesting anxiety? Does the patient think that he or she is especially powerful, important or gifted (grandiose thoughts), suggesting mania?

The form of thinking may also be abnormal. In schizophrenia, patients may display loosened associations between ideas, making it difficult to follow their train of thought. There may also be abnormalities of thought possession, when patients experience the intrusion of alien thoughts into their mind or the broadcasting of their own thoughts to other people (p. 247).

Abnormal beliefs

A delusion is a false belief, out of keeping with a patient's cultural background, which is held with conviction despite evidence to the contrary (p. 236).

Abnormal perceptions

Illusions are abnormal perceptions of real stimuli. Hallucinations are sensory perceptions which occur in the absence of external stimuli: for example, hearing voices when no one is present (p. 237).

Cognitive function

The Mini-Mental State Examination (MMSE) is a useful screening questionnaire to detect cognitive impairment. A score of less than 24 out of 30 typically suggests cognitive impairment. The Addenbrooke's Cognitive Examination – Revised (ACE-R) provides a more comprehensive assessment. A brief clinical assessment is as follows:

- *Memory.* Registration of memories is tested by asking the patient to repeat simple new information, such as a name and address, immediately after hearing it. Short-term memory is assessed by asking him or her to repeat it after an interval of 1–2 minutes, during which time the patient's attention should be diverted elsewhere. Long-term memory is assessed by gauging the recall of previous events.
- *Concentration.* Serial 7s is a test in which the patient is asked to subtract 7 from 100 and then 7 from the answer, and so on.
- *Orientation.* This is assessed by asking the patient about place – his or her exact location; time – what day, date, month and year it is now; and person – details of personal identity, such as name, date of birth, marital status and address.
- *Intellectual ability.* This can be gauged from the history of the patient's educational background and attainments but can also be assessed during the interview from the patient's speech, vocabulary and grasp of the interviewer's questions.

Note that the degree of cognitive impairment in delirium typically fluctuates over time, and consequently may be missed by a single assessment.

Patients' own understanding of their symptoms ('insight')

Patients should be asked what they think their symptoms are due to, and whether they warrant treatment. Lack of insight refers to a failure to accept that one is ill and/or in need of treatment, and is characteristic of acute psychosis.

PRESENTING PROBLEMS IN PSYCHIATRIC ILLNESS

Anxiety symptoms

Anxiety may be transient, persistent, episodic or limited to specific situations. The symptoms of anxiety are both psychological and somatic (Box 10.5). The differential diagnosis of anxiety is shown in Box 10.6. Most anxiety is part of a transient adjustment to stressful events: adjustment disorders (p. 242). Other more persistent forms of anxiety are described in detail on page 242.

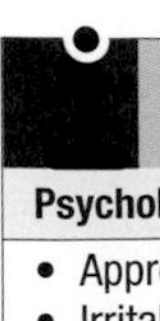

10.5 Symptoms of anxiety disorder

Psychological	
• Apprehension	• Fear of impending disaster
• Irritability	• Poor concentration
• Worry	• Depersonalisation
Somatic	
• Palpitations	• Frequent desire to pass urine
• Fatigue	• Chest pain
• Tremor	• Initial insomnia
• Dizziness	• Breathlessness
• Sweating	• Headache
• Diarrhoea	

10.6 Differential diagnosis of anxiety

- Normal response to threat
- Adjustment disorder
- Generalised anxiety disorder
- Panic disorder
- Phobic disorder
- Organic (medical) cause
  - Hyperthyroidism
  - Paroxysmal arrhythmias
  - Phaeochromocytoma
  - Alcohol and benzodiazepine withdrawal
  - Hypoglycaemia
  - Temporal lobe epilepsy

Anxiety may occasionally be a manifestation of a medical condition such as thyrotoxicosis (see Box 10.6).

Depressed mood

Depressive disorder is common, with a prevalence of approximately 5% in the general population. Depression is at least twice as common in the medically ill. It is important to note that depression has physical as well as mental symptoms (Box 10.7). The diagnosis of depression in the medically ill, who may have physical symptoms of disease, relies on detection of the core psychological symptoms of low mood and anhedonia.

Differential diagnosis

Depressive disorder must be differentiated from an adjustment disorder with depressed mood (p. 242). Adjustment disorders are common, self-limiting reactions to adversity, including physical illness, which are transient and require only general support. Depressive disorders (p. 243) are characterised by a more severe and persistent disturbance of mood and require specific treatment. In some cases, depression may occur as a result of a direct effect of a medical condition or its treatment on the brain, when it is referred to as an 'organic mood disorder' (Box 10.8).

Suicide

Depression is the major risk factor for suicide. Other risk factors are shown in Box 10.9. When depression is suspected, tactful enquiry should always be made into suicidal thoughts and plans. Asking about suicide does not increase the risk of it occurring, whereas failure to enquire denies the opportunity to prevent it.

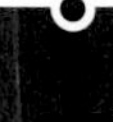

10.7 Symptoms of depressive disorders

Psychological	
• Depressed mood	• Loss of interest
• Reduced self-esteem	• Loss of enjoyment (anhedonia)
• Pessimism	• Suicidal thinking
• Guilt	
Somatic	
• Reduced appetite	• Loss of libido
• Weight change	• Bowel disturbance
• Disturbed sleep	• Motor retardation (slowing of activity)
• Fatigue	

10.8 Organic mood disorders*

Neurological
- Cerebrovascular disease
- Cerebral tumour
- Multiple sclerosis
- Parkinson's disease
- Huntington's disease
- Alzheimer's disease
- Epilepsy

Endocrine
- Hypothyroidism
- Hyperthyroidism
- Cushing's syndrome
- Addison's disease
- Hyperparathyroidism

Malignant disease

Infections
- Infectious mononucleosis
- Herpes simplex
- Brucellosis
- Typhoid
- Toxoplasmosis

Connective tissue disease
- Systemic lupus erythematosus

Drugs
- Phenothiazines
- Phenylbutazone
- Corticosteroids, oral contraceptives
- Interferon

*Diseases that may cause organic affective disorders by direct action on the brain.

10.9 Risk factors for suicide

- Psychiatric illness (depressive illness, schizophrenia)
- Older age
- Male sex
- Living alone
- Unemployment
- Recent bereavement, divorce or separation
- Chronic physical ill health
- Drug or alcohol misuse
- Suicide note written
- History of previous attempts (especially if a violent method was used)

Elated mood

Elation, or euphoria, is the converse of depression and is characteristic of mania. It may manifest as infectious joviality, over-activity, lack of sleep and appetite, undue optimism, over-talkativeness, irritability, and recklessness in spending and sexual behaviour. When elated mood is severe, psychotic symptoms are often evident, such as delusions of grandeur (e.g. believing erroneously that one is royalty). Elevated mood is much less common than depressed mood, and in medical settings is often secondary to drug or alcohol misuse, an organic disorder or medical treatment. Where none of these applies, the patient may have a bipolar disorder (p. 244).

Medically unexplained somatic symptoms

Patients commonly present to doctors with physical symptoms. Whilst these symptoms may be an expression of a medical condition, they often are not. They may then be referred to as 'medically unexplained symptoms' (MUS). MUS are very common in patients attending general medical outpatient clinics. Almost any symptom can be medically unexplained, e.g.:

- pain (including back, chest, abdominal and headache)
- fatigue
- dizziness
- fits, 'funny turns' and feelings of weakness.

Patients with MUS may receive a medical diagnosis of a so-called functional somatic syndrome, such as irritable bowel syndrome (Box 10.10), and may also merit a psychiatric diagnosis on the basis of the same symptoms. The most frequent psychiatric diagnoses associated with MUS are anxiety or depressive disorders. When these are absent, a diagnosis of somatoform disorder may be appropriate (Box 10.11).

Differential diagnosis

The main medical differential diagnosis for MUS is from symptoms of a medical disease. Diagnostic difficulties are most likely with unusual presentations of common diseases and with rare diseases. MUS are commonly an expression of depression and anxiety. A medical and psychiatric assessment should be completed in all cases (Fig. 10.1).

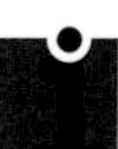

10.10 Functional somatic syndromes

- Gastroenterology: irritable bowel syndrome, functional dyspepsia
- Gynaecology: premenstrual syndrome, chronic pelvic pain
- Rheumatology: fibromyalgia
- Cardiology: atypical or non-cardiac chest pain
- Respiratory medicine: hyperventilation syndrome
- Infectious diseases: chronic (post-viral) fatigue syndrome
- Neurology: tension headache, non-epileptic attacks
- Dentistry: temporomandibular joint dysfunction, atypical facial pain
- Ear, nose and throat: globus syndrome
- Allergy: multiple chemical sensitivity

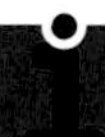

10.11 Psychiatric diagnoses for medically unexplained somatic symptoms

- Hypochondriasis: predominant concern about disease
- Somatisation: predominant concern about symptoms
- Somatic presentation of depression and anxiety
- Simple somatoform disorders: small number of symptoms
- Somatisation disorder (Briquet's syndrome): chronic multiple symptoms
- Conversion disorder: loss of function
- Body dysmorphic disorder: dislike of body parts

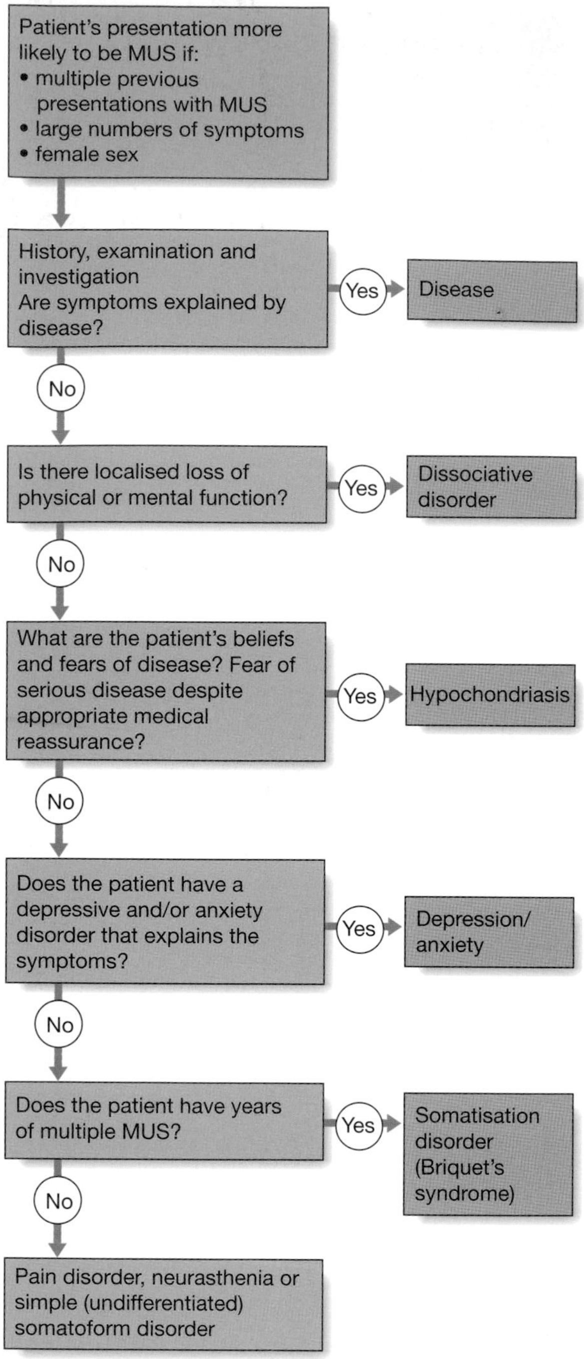

Patient's presentation more likely to be MUS if:
- multiple previous presentations with MUS
- large numbers of symptoms
- female sex

↓

History, examination and investigation
Are symptoms explained by disease? — Yes → Disease

No ↓

Is there localised loss of physical or mental function? — Yes → Dissociative disorder

No ↓

What are the patient's beliefs and fears of disease? Fear of serious disease despite appropriate medical reassurance? — Yes → Hypochondriasis

No ↓

Does the patient have a depressive and/or anxiety disorder that explains the symptoms? — Yes → Depression/ anxiety

No ↓

Does the patient have years of multiple MUS? — Yes → Somatisation disorder (Briquet's syndrome)

No ↓

Pain disorder, neurasthenia or simple (undifferentiated) somatoform disorder

Fig. 10.1 Diagnosis of medically unexplained symptoms (MUS).

Delusions and hallucinations

Delusions

Various types of delusion are identified on the basis of their content. They may be:

- persecutory, such as a conviction that others are out to get me

- hypochondriacal, such as an unfounded conviction that one has cancer
- grandiose, such as a belief that one has special powers or status
- nihilistic, e.g. 'My head is missing', 'I have no body', 'I am dead'.

Delusions should be differentiated from over-valued ideas, which are strongly held but not fixed.

Hallucinations

These are perceptions without external stimuli. They can occur in any sensory modality, most commonly visual or auditory. Typical examples are hearing voices when no one else is present, or seeing 'visions'. Hallucinations have the quality of ordinary perceptions and are perceived as originating in the external world, not in the patient's own mind (when they are termed pseudo-hallucinations). Those occurring when falling asleep ('hypnagogic') and on waking ('hypnopompic') are not pathological. Hallucinations should be distinguished from illusions, which are misperceptions of real external stimuli (such as mistaking a shrub for a person in poor light).

Differential diagnosis

Agitation, terror or the fear of being thought 'mad' may make patients unable or unwilling to volunteer or describe their abnormal beliefs or experiences. Careful and tactful enquiry is therefore required. The nature of hallucinations can be important diagnostically; for example, 'running commentary' voices that discuss the patient are strongly associated with schizophrenia. In general, auditory hallucinations suggest schizophrenia, while hallucinations in other sensory modalities, especially vision but also taste and smell, suggest an 'organic psychosis' such as delirium or temporal lobe epilepsy.

Hallucinations and delusions often co-occur; if their content is consistent with coexisting emotional symptoms, they are described as 'mood-congruent'. Thus, patients with severely depressed mood may believe themselves responsible for all the evils in the world, and hear voices saying 'You're worthless. Go and kill yourself.' In this case, the diagnosis of depressive psychosis is made on the basis of the congruence of different phenomena (mood, delusion and hallucination). Incongruence between hallucinations, delusions and mood suggests schizophrenia.

Where hallucinations and delusions arise within disturbed consciousness and impaired cognition, the diagnosis is usually an organic disorder, most commonly delirium and/or dementia (p. 244). This differential diagnosis is made by assessing the nature, extent and time course of any cognitive disturbances, and by investigating for underlying causes.

Disturbed and aggressive behaviour

Disturbed and aggressive behaviour is common in general hospitals, especially in emergency departments. Most behavioural disturbance arises not from medical or psychiatric illness, but from alcohol intoxication, reaction to the situation and personality characteristics. The key principles of management are, first, to establish control of the situation rapidly and thereby ensure the safety of the patient and others, and, second, to assess the cause of the disturbance in order to remedy it. Establishing control requires the presence of an adequate number of trained staff, an appropriate physical environment and sometimes sedation (Fig. 10.2). Hospital security staff and sometimes the assistance of the police may be required. In all cases, the staff approach is important; a calm, non-threatening manner expressing understanding of the patient's concerns is often all that is required to defuse potential aggression (Box 10.12).

If sedating drugs are required, antipsychotic drugs, such as haloperidol, and benzodiazepines, such as diazepam, are commonly used. The choice of drug, dose, route and rate of administration will depend on the

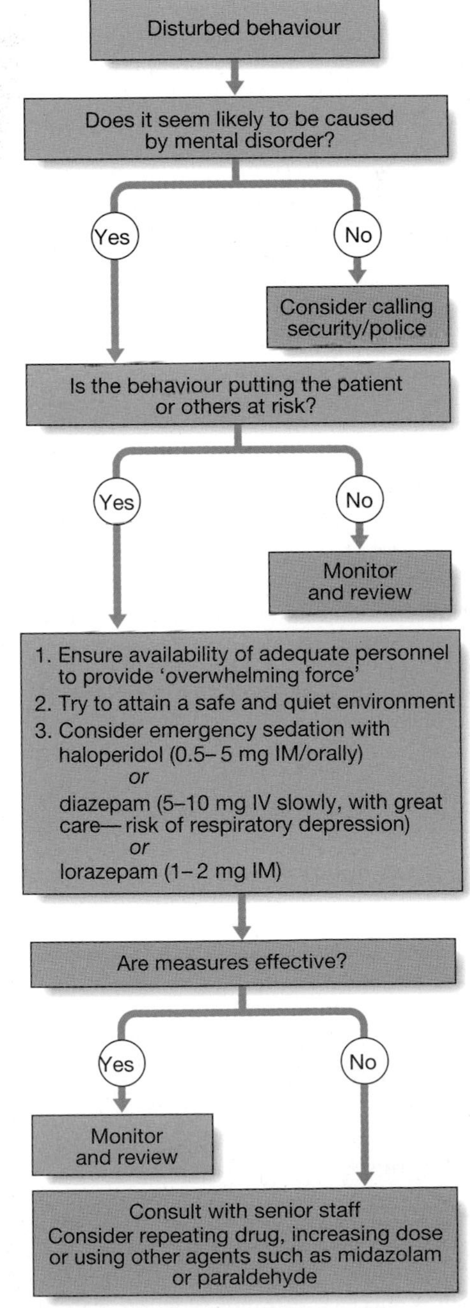

Fig. 10.2 Acute management of disturbed behaviour.

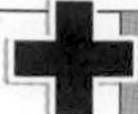

10.12 Psychiatric emergencies

- Intervene as necessary to reduce the risk of harm to the patient and to others
- Adopt a calm, non-threatening approach
- Arrange availability of other staff and parenteral medication
- Consider diagnostic possibilities of drug intoxication, acute psychosis and delirium
- Involve friends and relatives as appropriate

patient's age, sex and physical health, as well as the likely cause of the disturbed behaviour. The benefits of sedation must be balanced against the associated risks, however. Haloperidol can cause acute dystonias, including oculogyric crises, while the benzodiazepines can precipitate respiratory depression in patients with lung disease, and encephalopathy in those with liver disease. Thus, for a frail elderly woman with emphysema and delirium, sedation may be achieved with a low dose (0.5 mg) of oral haloperidol, while for a strong young man with an acute psychotic episode, at least 10 mg of intravenous diazepam and a similar dose of haloperidol may be needed. A parenterally administered anticholinergic agent, such as procyclidine, should be available to treat extrapyramidal effects arising from haloperidol, and flumazenil (p. 217) to reverse respiratory depression if large doses of benzodiazepines are used.

Differential diagnosis

Many factors may contribute to disturbed behaviour. When the patient is cooperative, these are best determined at interview. Other sources of information about the patient include medical and psychiatric records, and discussion with nursing staff, family members and other informants, including the patient's general practitioner. The following information should be sought:

- psychiatric, medical (especially neurological) and criminal history
- current psychiatric and medical treatment
- alcohol and drug misuse
- recent stressors
- the time course and accompaniments of the current episode in terms of mood, belief and behaviour.

Observation of the patient's behaviour may also yield useful clues. Do they appear to be responding to hallucinations? Are they alert or variably drowsy and confused? Are there physical features suggestive of drug or alcohol misuse or withdrawal? Are there new injuries or old scars, especially on the head? Do they smell of alcohol or solvents? Do they bear the marks of drug injection? Are they unwashed and unkempt, suggesting a gradual development of their condition?

If the person has an acute psychiatric disorder, then admission to a psychiatric facility may be indicated. If a medical cause is likely, psychiatric transfer is usually inappropriate and the patient should be managed in a medical setting, with whatever nursing and security support is required. Where it is clear that there is no medical or psychiatric illness, the person should be removed from the hospital, to police custody if necessary.

Measures such as restraint, sedation, the investigation and treatment of medical problems, and psychiatric transfer all raise legal as well as medical issues (p. 257). In most countries, including the UK, common law confers upon doctors the right, and indeed the duty, to intervene against a patient's wishes in cases of acute behavioural disturbance, if this is necessary to protect the patient or other people. Many countries, such as the UK, also have specific mental health legislation that may be used to detain patients.

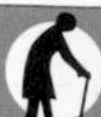

10.13 Medical psychiatry in old age

- **Organic psychiatric disorders**: especially common, so cognitive function should always be assessed; if impaired, an associated medical condition or adverse drug effect should be suspected.
- **Disturbed behaviour**: delirium is the most common cause.
- **Depression**: common. Just because a person is old and frail does not mean that depression is 'to be expected' and that it should not be treated.
- **Self-harm**: associated with an increased risk of completed suicide.
- **Medically unexplained symptoms**: common and often associated with depressive disorder.
- **Loneliness, poverty and lack of social support**: must be taken into consideration in management decisions.

Confusion

This is a vague term used to describe a range of primarily cognitive problems, including disturbances in perception, belief and behaviour. 'Confusion' usually presents as a problem when it becomes clear that the patient cannot comply with medical care; they may repeatedly wander off the ward, pull out essential cannulae and catheters, and hit nurses. The methods of assessment of cognitive function range from simple screening questions to detailed psychometric testing. All doctors should be able to undertake a brief cognitive assessment, as outlined above (p. 233).

Differential diagnosis

A history from the patient and informants is essential to establish the time course, variability and functional consequences of any cognitive deficit. Mental state examination is necessary to seek evidence of associated mood disorder, hallucinations, delusions or behavioural abnormalities, and physical examination to identify any relevant medical conditions. The assessment should seek to distinguish between:

- organic disorders such as delirium, dementia, and focal deficits secondary to brain lesions
- psychiatric disorders such as depressive pseudodementia and dissociative disorder
- malingering (p. 247).

Further investigation will usually be needed to identify the specific causes of any cognitive impairment identified (see Box 10.32, p. 250, and p. 209).

Self-harm

Self-harm (SH) is a common reason for presentation to medical services. The term 'attempted suicide' is potentially misleading, as most such patients are not unequivocally trying to kill themselves. Most cases of SH involve overdose, of either prescribed or non-prescribed drugs (Ch. 9). Less common methods include asphyxiation, drowning, hanging, jumping from a height or in front of a moving vehicle, and the use of firearms. Methods that carry a high chance of being fatal are more likely to be associated with serious psychiatric disorder. Self-cutting is common and often repetitive, but rarely leads to contact with medical services.

The incidence of SH varies over time and between countries. In the UK, the lifetime prevalence of suicidal ideation is 15% and that of acts of SH is 4%. SH is more common in women than men, and in young adults than the elderly. (In contrast, completed suicide is more common in men and the elderly (see Box 10.9).) There is a higher incidence of self-harm among lower socioeconomic groups, particularly those living in crowded, socially deprived urban areas. There is also an association with alcohol misuse, child abuse, unemployment and recently broken relationships.

Differential diagnosis

The main differential diagnosis is from accidental poisoning and so-called 'recreational' overdose in drug users. It must be remembered that SH is not a diagnosis but a presentation, and may be associated with any psychiatric diagnosis, the most common being adjustment disorder, substance and alcohol misuse, depressive disorder and personality disorder. In many cases, however, no psychiatric diagnosis can be made.

Initial management

A thorough psychiatric and social assessment should be attempted in all cases (Fig. 10.3), although some patients will discharge themselves before this can take place. The need for psychiatric assessment should not, however, delay urgent medical or surgical treatment, and may need to be deferred until the patient is well enough for interview. The purpose of the psychiatric assessment is to:

- establish the short-term risk of suicide
- identify potentially treatable problems, whether medical, psychiatric or social.

Topics to be covered when assessing a patient are listed in Box 10.14. The history should include events occurring immediately before and after the act, and especially any evidence of planning. The nature and severity of any current psychiatric symptoms must be assessed, along with the personal and social supports available to the patient outside hospital.

Most SH patients have depressive and anxiety symptoms on a background of chronic social and personal difficulties and alcohol misuse but no psychiatric disorder. They do not usually require psychotropic

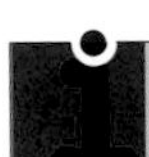

10.14 Assessment of patients after self-harm

Current attempt

- Patient's account
- Degree of intent at the time: preparations, plans, precautions against discovery, note
- Method used, particularly whether violent
- Degree of intent now
- Symptoms of psychiatric illness

Background

- Previous attempts and their outcome
- Family and personal history
- Social support
- Previous response to stress
- Extent of drug and alcohol misuse

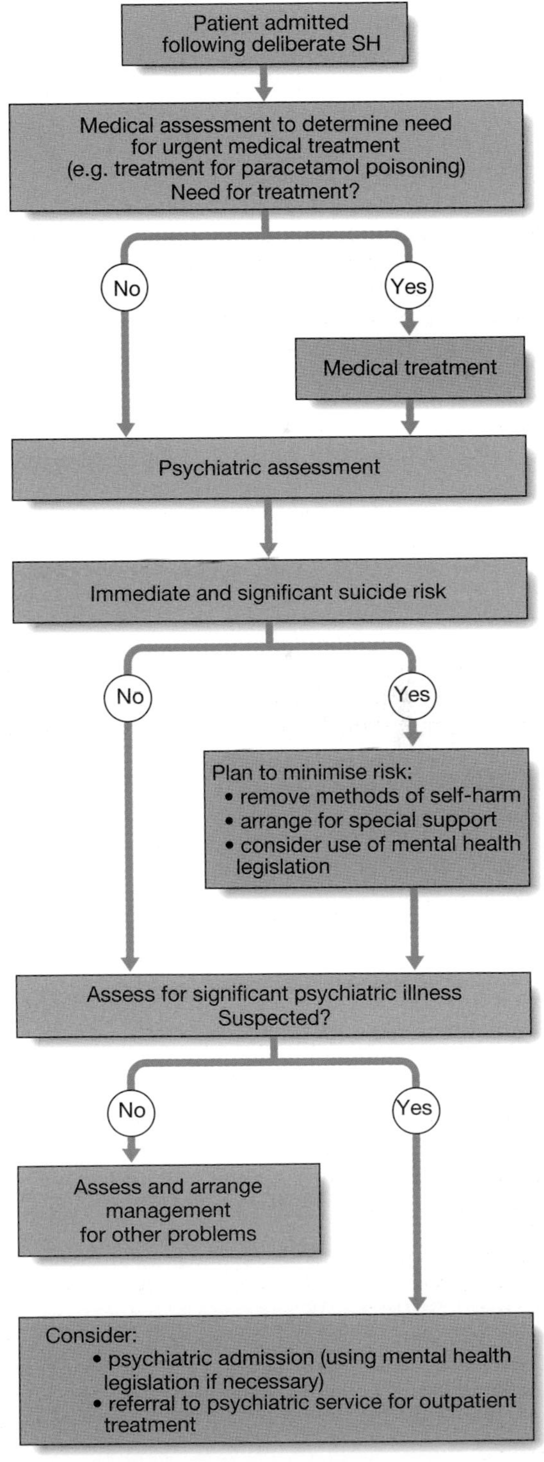

Fig. 10.3 Assessment of patients admitted following self-harm (SH).

medication or specialised psychiatric treatment but may benefit from personal support and practical advice from a GP, social worker or community psychiatric nurse. Admission to a psychiatric ward is necessary only for persons who:

- have an acute psychiatric disorder
- are at high risk of suicide
- need temporary respite from intolerable circumstances
- require further assessment of their mental state.

Approximately 20% of SH patients make a repeat attempt during the following year and 1–2% kill themselves. Factors associated with suicide after an episode of SH are listed in Box 10.9.

Alcohol misuse

Misuse of alcohol is a major problem worldwide. It presents in a multitude of ways, which are discussed further on page 252 and in Box 10.35 (p. 253). In many cases, the link to alcohol will be all too obvious; in others, it may not be. Denial and concealment of alcohol intake are common. In the assessment of alcohol intake, the patient should be asked to describe a typical week's drinking, quantified in terms of units of alcohol (1 unit contains approximately 8 g alcohol and is the equivalent of half a pint of beer, a single measure of spirits or a small glass of wine). Drinking becomes hazardous at levels above 21 units weekly for men and 14 units weekly for women. The history from the patient may need corroboration by the GP, earlier medical records and family members. The mean cell volume (MCV) and γ-glutamyl transferase (GGT) may be raised, but are abnormal in only half of problem drinkers; consequently, normal results on these tests do not exclude an alcohol problem. When abnormal, these measures may be helpful in challenging denial and monitoring treatment response. The prevention and management of alcohol-related problems are discussed on page 253.

Substance misuse

The misuse of drugs of all kinds is also widespread. As well as the general headings listed for alcohol problems in Box 10.35 (p. 253), there are two additional sets of problems associated with drug misuse:

- problems linked with the route of administration, such as intravenous injection
- problems arising from pressure applied to doctors to prescribe the misused substances (Box 10.15).

Assessment and management are described on page 254.

Psychological factors affecting medical conditions

Psychological factors may influence the presentation, management and outcome of medical conditions. Specific factors are shown in Box 10.16. The most common psychiatric diagnoses in the medically ill are anxiety and depressive disorders. Often these appear understandable as adjustments to illness and its treatment; however, if the anxiety and depression are severe and persistent, they may complicate the management of the medical condition and active management is required. Anxiety may present as an increase in somatic symptoms such as breathlessness, tremor or palpitations, or as the avoidance of medical treatment. It is most common in those facing difficult or painful treatments, deterioration of their illness or death. Depression may manifest as increased physical symptoms such as pain or fatigue and disability, as well as with depressed mood and loss of interest and pleasure. It is most common in patients who have suffered actual or anticipated losses, such as receiving a terminal diagnosis or undergoing disfiguring surgery.

Treatment is by psychological and/or pharmacological therapies, as described below. Care is required when prescribing psychotropic drugs to the medically ill in order to avoid exacerbation of the medical condition and harmful interactions with other prescribed drugs.

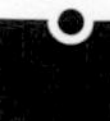

10.15 Substance misuse: additional presenting problems

Complications arising from the route of use

Intravenous
- Local: abscesses, cellulitis, thrombosis
- Systemic: bacterial (endocarditis), viral (hepatitis, human immunodeficiency virus (HIV))

Nasal ingestion
- Erosion of nasal septum, epistaxis

Smoking
- Oral, laryngeal and lung cancer

Inhalation
- Burns, chemical pneumonitis, rashes

Pressure to prescribe misused substance
- Manipulation, deceit and threats
- Factitious description of illness
- Malingering

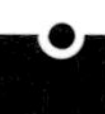

10.16 Risk factors for psychological problems associated with medical conditions

- Previous history of depression or anxiety
- Lack of social support
- New diagnosis of a serious medical condition
- Deterioration of or failure of treatment for medical condition
- Unpleasant, disabling or disfiguring treatment
- Change in medical care, e.g. discharge from hospital
- Impending death

TREATING PSYCHIATRIC DISORDERS

The multifactorial origin of most psychiatric disorders means that there are multiple potential targets for treatment.

Biological treatments

These aim to relieve psychiatric disorder by modifying brain function. The main biological treatments are psychotropic drugs. These are widely used for various

10.17 Classification of commonly used psychotropic drugs

Action	Main groups	Clinical use
Antipsychotic	Phenothiazines Butyrophenones Second-generation antipsychotics	Schizophrenia Bipolar mania Acute confusion
Antidepressant	Tricyclics and related drugs	Depression/anxiety Obsessive-compulsive disorder
	Monoamine oxidase inhibitors	Depression/anxiety
	Serotonin and noradrenergic re-uptake inhibitors	Depression/anxiety Obsessive-compulsive disorder
Mood-stabilising	Lithium (Semi-)Sodium valproate	Treatment and prophylaxis of bipolar disorder
Anti-anxiety	Benzodiazepines	Anxiety/insomnia (short term) Alcohol withdrawal (short term)
	β-adrenoceptor antagonists	Anxiety (somatic symptoms)

purposes; a pragmatic classification is set out in Box 10.17. It should be noted that some drugs have applications to more than one condition; for example, antidepressants are also widely used in the treatment of anxiety *and* chronic pain. The specific subgroups of psychotropic drugs are discussed in the sections on the appropriate disorders.

Electroconvulsive therapy (ECT) entails producing a convulsion by the administration of high-voltage, brief, direct-current impulses to the head while the patient is anaesthetised and paralysed by muscle relaxant. If properly administered, it is remarkably safe, has few side-effects, and is of proven efficacy for severe depressive illness. There may be amnesia for events occurring a few hours before ECT (retrograde) and after it (anterograde). Pronounced amnesia can occur but is infrequent and difficult to distinguish from the effects of severe depression. Surgery to the brain (psychosurgery) has a very limited place and then only in the treatment of severe chronic psychiatric illness resistant to other measures.

Psychological treatments

These treatments are useful in many psychiatric disorders and also in non-psychiatric conditions. They are based on talking with patients, either individually or in groups. Sometimes discussion is supplemented by 'homework' or tasks to complete between treatment sessions. Psychological treatments take a number of forms based on the duration and frequency of contact, the specific techniques applied and their underlying theory.

General or supportive psychotherapy

This should be part of all medical treatment. It involves empathic listening to the patient's account of their symptoms and associated fears and concerns, followed by the sympathetic provision of accurate information that addresses these.

Cognitive therapy

This therapy is based on the observation that some psychiatric disorders are associated with systematic errors

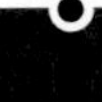

10.18 The negative cognitive triad associated with depression

- Negative view of self, e.g. 'I am no good'
- Negative view of current life experiences, e.g. 'The world is an awful place'
- Negative view of the future, e.g. 'The future is hopeless'

in the patient's conscious thinking: for example, a tendency to interpret events in a negative way or see them as unduly threatening. A triad of 'cognitive errors' has been described in depression (Box 10.18). Cognitive therapy aims to help patients to identify such cognitive errors and to learn how to challenge them. It is widely used for depression, anxiety and eating and somatoform disorders, and also increasingly in psychoses.

Behaviour therapy

This is a practically orientated form of treatment, in which patients are assisted in changing unhelpful behaviour: for example, helping patients to implement carefully graded exposure to the feared stimulus in phobias.

Cognitive behaviour therapy

Cognitive behaviour therapy (CBT) combines the methods of behaviour therapy and cognitive therapy. It is the most widely available and extensively researched psychological treatment.

Problem-solving therapy

This is a simplified brief form of CBT, which helps patients actively tackle problems in a structured way (Box 10.19). It is of benefit in mild to moderate depression, and can be delivered by non-psychiatric doctors and nurses after appropriate training.

Psychodynamic psychotherapy

This treatment, also known as 'interpretive psychotherapy', was pioneered by Freud, Jung and Klein, amongst others. It is based upon the theory that early life experience generates powerful but unconscious motivations. Psychotherapy aims to help the patient to

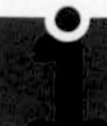

10.19 Stages of problem-solving therapy

- Define and list problems
- Choose one to work on
- List possible solutions
- Evaluate these and choose the best
- Try it out
- Evaluate the result
- Repeat until problems are resolved

become aware of these unconscious factors on the assumption that, once identified, their negative effects are reduced. The relationship between therapist and patient is used as a therapeutic tool to identify issues in patients' relationships with others, particularly parents, which may be replicated or transferred to their relationship with the therapist. Explicit discussion of this relationship (transference) is the basis for the treatment, which traditionally requires frequent sessions over a period of months or even years.

Interpersonal psychotherapy

Interpersonal psychotherapy (IPT) is a specific form of brief psychotherapy that focuses on patients' current interpersonal relationships and is an effective treatment for mild to moderate depression.

Social interventions

Some adverse social factors, such as unemployment, may not be readily amenable to intervention, but others, such as access to benefits and poor housing, may be. Patients can be helped to address these problems themselves by being taught problem-solving. Befrienders and day centres can reduce social isolation, benefits advisers can ensure appropriate financial assistance, and medical recommendations can be made to local housing departments to help patients obtain more appropriate accommodation.

PSYCHIATRIC DISORDERS

Stress-related disorders

Acute stress reaction

Following a stressful event such as a serious medical diagnosis or a major accident, some people develop a characteristic pattern of symptoms. These include a sense of bewilderment, anxiety, anger, depression, altered activity and withdrawal. The symptoms are transient and usually resolve completely within a few days.

Adjustment disorder

A more common psychological response to a major stressor is a less severe but more prolonged emotional reaction. The predominant symptom is usually depression and/or anxiety, which is insufficiently persistent or intense to merit a diagnosis of depressive or anxiety disorder. There may also be anger, aggressive behaviour and associated excessive alcohol use. Symptoms develop within a month of the onset of the stress, and their duration and severity reflect the course of the underlying stressor.

Grief reactions following bereavement are a particular type of adjustment disorder. They manifest as a brief period of emotional numbing, followed by a period of distress lasting several weeks, during which sorrow, tearfulness, sleep disturbance, loss of interest and a sense of futility are common. Perceptual distortions may occur, including misinterpreting sounds as the dead person's voice. 'Pathological grief' describes a grief reaction that is abnormally intense or persistent.

Management and prognosis

Ongoing contact with and support from a doctor or other who can listen, reassure, explain and advise are often all that is needed. Most patients do not require psychotropic medication, although benzodiazepines reduce arousal in acute stress reactions and can aid sleep in adjustment disorders. Psychotherapy may be helpful for patients with abnormal grief reactions. These conditions usually resolve with time but can develop into depressive or anxiety disorders and require treating as such.

Post-traumatic stress disorder

Post-traumatic stress disorder (PTSD) is a protracted response to a stressful event of an exceptionally threatening or catastrophic nature. Examples of such events include natural disasters, terrorist activity, serious accidents and witnessing violent deaths. PTSD may also sometimes occur after distressing medical treatments. There is usually a delay ranging from a few days to several months between the traumatic event and the onset of symptoms. Typical symptoms are recurrent intrusive memories (flashbacks) of the trauma, as well as sleep disturbance, especially nightmares (usually of the traumatic event) from which the patient awakes in a state of anxiety, symptoms of autonomic arousal, emotional blunting and avoidance of situations that evoke memories of the trauma. Anxiety and depression are often associated and excessive use of alcohol or drugs frequently complicates the clinical picture.

Management and prognosis

Immediate counselling for those who have survived a major trauma is only likely to benefit those who request it. The main aims are to provide support, direct advice and the opportunity for emotional catharsis. In established PTSD, structured psychological approaches (CBT, eye movement desensitisation and reprocessing (EMDR), and stress management) are effective. Antidepressant drugs are moderately effective. The condition runs a fluctuating course, with most patients recovering within 2 years. In a small proportion, the symptoms become chronic.

Anxiety disorders

These are characterised by the emotion of anxiety, worrisome thoughts, avoidance behaviour and the somatic symptoms of autonomic arousal. Anxiety disorders are divided into three main subtypes: phobic, paroxysmal (panic) and generalised (Box 10.20). The nature and prominence of the somatic symptoms often lead the

10.20 Classification of anxiety disorders

	Phobic anxiety disorder	Panic disorder	Generalised anxiety disorder
Occurrence	Situational	Paroxysmal	Persistent
Behaviour	Avoidance	Escape	Agitation
Cognitions	Fear of situation	Fear of symptoms	Worry
Symptoms	On exposure	Episodic	Persistent

patient to present initially to medical services. Anxiety may be stress-related and phobic anxiety may follow an unpleasant incident. Patients with anxiety often also have depression.

Phobic anxiety disorder

A phobia is an abnormal or excessive fear of an object or situation, which leads to avoidance of it (such as excessive fear of dying in an air crash leading to avoidance of flying). A generalised phobia of going out alone or being in crowded places is called agoraphobia. Phobic responses can develop to medical procedures such as venepuncture.

Panic disorder

Panic disorder describes repeated attacks of severe anxiety, which are not restricted to any particular situation or circumstances. Somatic symptoms such as chest pain, palpitations and paraesthesiae in lips and fingers are common. The symptoms are in part due to involuntary over-breathing (hyperventilation). Patients with panic attacks often fear that they are suffering from a serious illness such as a heart attack or stroke, and seek emergency medical attention. Panic disorder is often associated with agoraphobia.

Generalised anxiety disorder

This is a chronic anxiety state associated with uncontrollable worry. The associated somatic symptoms of muscle tension and bowel disturbance often lead to a medical presentation.

Management of anxiety disorders

Psychological treatment

Explanation and reassurance are essential, especially when patients fear they have a serious medical condition. Specific treatment may be needed. Treatments include relaxation, graded exposure (desensitisation) to feared situations for phobic disorders, and CBT.

Drug treatment

Antidepressants are the drugs of choice. Benzodiazepines are useful in the short term but long-term use can lead to dependence. A β-blocker such as propranolol can help when somatic symptoms are prominent.

Obsessive-compulsive disorder

Obsessive-compulsive disorder (OCD) is characterised by obsessive thoughts, which are recurrent, unwanted and usually anxiety-provoking, but recognised as one's own; and by compulsions, which are repeated acts performed to relieve the anxiety. An example is repeated hand-washing related to thoughts of contamination. The differential diagnosis is normal checking behaviour and delusional beliefs about thought possession. Unlike other anxiety disorders, which are more common in women, OCD is equally common in men and women.

Management and prognosis

OCD usually responds to some degree to antidepressant drugs (SSRIs; see Box 10.17) and to CBT, which helps patients expose themselves to the feared thought or situation without performing the anxiety-relieving compulsions. However, relapses are common and the condition often becomes chronic.

Mood disorders

Mood or affective disorders include:

- *unipolar depression*: one or more episodes of low mood and associated symptoms
- *bipolar disorder*: episodes of elevated mood interspersed with episodes of depression
- *dysthymia*: chronic low-grade depressed mood without sufficient other symptoms to count as 'clinically significant' or 'major' depression.

Depression

Major depressive disorder has a prevalence of 5% in the general population and approximately 10–20% in chronically ill medical outpatients. It is a major cause of disability and suicide. If comorbid with a medical condition, depression magnifies disability, diminishes adherence to medical treatment and rehabilitation, and may even shorten life expectancy.

Aetiology

There is a genetic predisposition to depression, especially when of early onset. The number and identity of the genes are largely unknown but the serotonin transporter gene is a candidate. Adversity and emotional deprivation early in life also predispose to depression. Depressive episodes are often, but not always, triggered by stressful life events (especially those that involve loss), including medical illnesses. Associated biological factors include hypofunction of monoamine neurotransmitter systems (5-HT and noradrenaline (norepinephrine)) and abnormal hypothalamo-pituitary-adrenal axis (HPA) regulation, which results in elevated cortisol levels that do not suppress with dexamethasone. Exclusion of Cushing's syndrome is described on page 773.

Diagnosis

The symptoms are listed in Box 10.7 (p. 235). Depression may be mild, moderate or severe. It may also be episodic, recurrent or chronic. It can be both a complication of a medical condition and a cause of MUS (see below), so physical examination is essential; an associated medical condition should always be considered (Box 10.21).

Management and prognosis

There is evidence that both drug and psychological treatments work in depression. In practice, the choice is

10.21 Pointers to an organic cause for psychiatric disorder

- Late age of onset of psychiatric illness
- No previous history of psychiatric illness
- No family history of psychiatric illness
- No apparent psychological precipitant

determined by patient preference and local availability. Severe depression complicated by psychosis, dehydration or suicide risk may require ECT.

Drug treatment

Antidepressant drugs are effective in patients whose depression is secondary to medical illness, as well as those in whom it is the primary problem (Box 10.22). These agents are all effective in moderate and severe depression. Commonly used antidepressants are shown in Box 10.23.

- *Tricyclic antidepressants (TCAs).* These agents inhibit the *re-uptake* of the amines noradrenaline (norepinephrine) and 5-HT at synaptic clefts. The therapeutic effect is noticeable within a week or two. Side-effects, such as sedation, anticholinergic effects, postural hypotension, lowering of the seizure threshold and cardiotoxicity, can be troublesome during this period. TCAs may be dangerous in overdose and in people who have coexisting heart disease, glaucoma and prostatism.
- *Selective serotonin re-uptake inhibitors (SSRIs).* These are less cardiotoxic and less sedative than TCAs, and have fewer anticholinergic effects. They are safer in overdose, but can still cause headache, nausea, anorexia and sexual dysfunction. They can also interact with other drugs increasing serotonin to produce 'serotonin syndrome'. This is a rare syndrome of neuromuscular hyperactivity, autonomic hyperactivity and agitation, and potentially seizures, hyperthermia, confusion and even death.
- *Newer antidepressants.* A variety is available, including venlafaxine, mirtazapine and duloxetine. They have slightly different modes of action and adverse effects but are generally no more effective than the agents listed above.
- *Monoamine oxidase inhibitors (MAOIs).* These drugs increase the availability of neurotransmitters at synaptic clefts by inhibiting *metabolism* of noradrenaline (norepinephrine) and 5-HT. They are now rarely prescribed in the UK, since they can cause potentially dangerous interactions with drugs such as amphetamines, and foods rich in tyramine such as cheese and red wine. This is due to accumulation of amines in the systemic circulation, causing a potentially fatal hypertensive crisis.

EBM 10.22 Antidepressants in the medically ill

'Antidepressants are efficacious and safe in the treatment of depression occurring in the context of chronic physical health problems. The selective serotonin re-uptake inhibitors are probably the antidepressants of first choice, given their demonstrable effect on quality of life and their apparent safety in cardiovascular disease.'

- Taylor D, et al. B J Psych 2011; 198:179–188.

10.23 Antidepressant drugs

Group	Drug	Usual dose*
Tricyclics	Amitriptyline Imipramine Dosulepin Clomipramine	75–150 mg daily 75–150 mg daily 75–150 mg daily 75–150 mg daily
Selective serotonin re-uptake inhibitors (SSRIs)	Citalopram Escitalopram Fluoxetine Fluvoxamine Sertraline Paroxetine	20–40 mg daily 10–20 mg daily 20–60 mg daily 100–300 mg daily 50–100 mg daily 20–50 mg daily
Monoamine oxidase inhibitors (MAOIs)	Phenelzine Tranylcypromine Moclobemide	45–90 mg daily 20–40 mg daily 300–600 mg daily
Noradrenergic re-uptake inhibitors and SSRIs	Venlafaxine	75–375 mg daily
Noradrenergic and specific serotonergic inhibitor	Mirtazapine	15–45 mg daily

*Higher doses may be required: see guidelines.

These different classes of antidepressant have similar efficacy and about three-quarters of patients respond to treatment. Successful treatment requires the patient to take an appropriate dose of an effective drug for an adequate period. For patients who do not respond, a proportion will do so if changed to another antidepressant. The patient's progress must be monitored and, after recovery, treatment should be continued for at least 6–12 months to reduce the high risk of relapse. The dose should then be tapered off over several weeks to avoid discontinuation symptoms. SIGN (www.sign.ac.uk) and NICE (www.nice.org.uk) have published treatment guidelines.

Psychological treatments

Both CBT and interpersonal therapy are as effective as antidepressants for mild to moderate depression. Antidepressant drugs are, however, preferred for severe depression. Drug and psychological treatments can be used in combination.

Over 50% of people who have had one depressive episode and over 90% of people who have had three or more episodes will have another. The risk of suicide in an individual who has had a depressive disorder is ten times greater than in the general population.

Bipolar disorder

Bipolar disorder is an episodic disturbance with interspersed periods of depressed and elevated mood; the latter is known as hypomania when mild or short-lived, or mania when severe or chronic. The lifetime risk of developing bipolar disorder is approximately 1–2%. Onset is usually in the twenties, and men and women are equally affected. In DSM-IV, bipolar disorder has been divided into two types:

- *Bipolar I disorder* has a clinical course characterised by one or more manic episodes or mixed episodes. Often individuals have also had one or more major depressive episodes.
- *Bipolar II disorder* features depressive episodes that are more frequent and more intense than manic episodes, but there is a history of at least one hypomanic episode.

Aetiology

Bipolar disorder is strongly heritable (approximately 70%). Relatives of patients have an increased incidence of both bipolar and unipolar affective disorder. Life events, such as physical illness, sleep deprivation and medication, may play a role in triggering episodes.

Diagnosis

The diagnosis is based on clear evidence of episodes of depression and mania. Isolated episodes of hypomania or mania do occur but they are usually preceded or followed by an episode of depression. Psychosis may occur in both the depressive and the manic phases, with delusions and hallucinations that are usually in keeping with the mood disturbance. This is described as an affective psychosis. Patients who present with symptoms of both bipolar disorder and schizophrenia may be given a diagnosis of schizoaffective disorder. A clinical picture of recurrent depression with one or more episodes of hypomania may be referred to as type 2 bipolar disorder.

Management and prognosis

Depression should be treated as described above. However, if antidepressants are prescribed, they should be combined with a mood-stabilising drug (see below) to avoid 'switching' the patients into (hypo)mania. Manic episodes and psychotic symptoms usually respond well to antipsychotic drugs (see Box 10.30, p. 249).

Prophylaxis to prevent recurrent episodes of depression and mania with mood-stabilising agents is important. The main drugs used are lithium and sodium valproate. Olanzapine, quetiapine and risperidone are increasingly used. Caution must be exercised when stopping these drugs, as a relapse may follow.

- *Lithium carbonate* is the drug of choice. It is also used for acute mania, and in combination with a tricyclic as an adjuvant treatment for resistant depression. It has a narrow therapeutic range, so regular blood monitoring is required to maintain a serum level of 0.5–1.0 mmol/L. Toxic effects include nausea, vomiting, tremor and convulsions. With long-term treatment, weight gain, hypothyroidism, increased calcium and parathormone, nephrogenic diabetes insipidus (p. 794) and renal failure can occur. Thyroid and renal function should be checked before treatment is started and regularly thereafter. Lithium may be teratogenic, and should not be prescribed during the first trimester of pregnancy.
- *Sodium valproate (an anticonvulsant) and olanzapine (an antipsychotic)* are both used as prophylaxis in bipolar disorder, usually as a second-line alternative to lithium. Valproate conveys a high risk of birth defects and should also not be used in women of child-bearing age. Olanzapine can cause significant weight gain. (For a list of the adverse effects of antipsychotic drugs, see Box 10.31.)

The relapse rate of bipolar disorder is high, although patients may be perfectly well between episodes. After one episode the annual average risk of relapse is about 10–15%, which doubles after more than three episodes. There is a substantially increased lifetime risk of suicide of 5–10%.

Somatoform disorders

The essential feature of these disorders is that the somatic symptoms are not explained by a medical condition (medically unexplained symptoms), nor better diagnosed as part of a depressive or anxiety disorder. Several syndromes are described within this category; there is considerable overlap between them in both aetiology and clinical presentation.

Aetiology

The cause of somatoform disorders is incompletely understood but contributory factors include depression and anxiety, the erroneous interpretation of somatic symptoms as evidence of disease, excessive concern with physical illness and a tendency to seek medical care. A family history or previous history of a particular condition may have shaped the patient's beliefs about illness. Doctors may exacerbate the problem, either by dismissing the complaints as non-existent or by over-emphasising the possibility of disease.

Somatisation disorder

Somatisation disorder (Briquet's syndrome) is characterised by the occurrence of chronic multiple somatic symptoms for which there is no physical cause. Symptoms start in early adult life and may be referred to any part of the body. The disorder is much more common in women. Common complaints include pain, vomiting, nausea, headache, dizziness, menstrual irregularities and sexual dysfunction. Patients may undergo a multitude of negative investigations and unhelpful operations, particularly hysterectomy and cholecystectomy. There is no proven treatment but minimisation of iatrogenic harm from multiple investigations and attempts at medical treatment is important.

Hypochondriacal disorder

Patients with this condition, also known as health anxiety, have a strong fear or belief that they have a serious, often fatal, disease and that fear persists despite appropriate medical reassurance. They are typically highly anxious and seek many medical opinions and investigations in futile but repeated attempts to relieve their fears. Treatment with CBT may be helpful. The condition may become chronic.

In a small proportion of cases, the conviction that disease is present reaches delusional intensity. The best-known example is that of parasitic infestation ('delusional parasitosis'), which leads patients to consult dermatologists. Antipsychotic medication may be effective in such cases.

Body dysmorphic disorder

This describes a preoccupation with bodily shape or appearance, with the belief that one is disfigured in some way (previously known as dysmorphophobia). People with this condition may make inappropriate requests for cosmetic surgery. CBT or antidepressants may be helpful. The belief in disfigurement may sometimes be delusional, in which case antipsychotic drugs may help.

Somatoform autonomic dysfunction

This describes somatic symptoms referable to bodily organs that are largely under the control of the autonomic nervous system. The most common examples involve the cardiovascular system ('cardiac neurosis'), respiratory system (psychogenic hyperventilation) and gut (psychogenic vomiting and irritable bowel syndrome). Antidepressant drugs and CBT may be helpful.

Somatoform pain disorder

This describes severe, persistent pain that cannot be adequately explained by a medical condition. Antidepressant drugs (especially tricyclics and dual action drugs such as duloxetine and mirtazapine) are helpful, as are some of the anticonvulsant drugs, particularly carbamazepine, gabapentin and pregabalin. CBT and multidisciplinary pain management teams are also useful.

Chronic fatigue syndrome

Chronic fatigue syndrome (CFS) is also referred to as neurasthenia. It is characterised by excessive fatigue after minimal physical or mental exertion, poor concentration, dizziness, muscular aches and sleep disturbance. This pattern of symptoms may follow a viral infection such as infectious mononucleosis, influenza or hepatitis. Symptoms overlap with those of depression and anxiety. There is good evidence that many patients improve with carefully graded exercise and with CBT, as long as the benefits of such treatment are carefully explained.

Dissociative (conversion) disorder

Dissociative disorder refers to a loss or distortion of neurological functioning that is not fully explained by organic disease. Psychological functions commonly affected include conscious awareness and memory. Physical functions affected (conversion) include changes in sensory or motor function that may mimic lesions in the motor or sensory nervous system (Box 10.24). The aetiology of dissociation is unknown. There is an association with adverse childhood experiences, including physical and sexual abuse. Organic disease may both facilitate dissociative mechanisms and provide a model for symptoms; thus, for example, non-epileptic seizures often occur in those with epilepsy. CBT may be of benefit. Coexisting depression should be treated with CBT or antidepressant drugs.

General management for medically unexplained symptoms

The management of the various syndromes of medically unexplained complaints described above is based on general principles (Box 10.25).

Reassurance

Patients should be asked what they are most worried about. Clearly, it may be unwise to state categorically that the patient does not have any disease, as that is difficult to establish with certainty. However, it can be emphasised that the probability of having a disease is low. If patients repeatedly ask for reassurance about the same health concern despite reassurance, they may have hypochondriasis.

Explanation

Patients need a positive explanation for their symptoms. It is unhelpful to say that symptoms are psychological or 'all in the mind'. Rather, a term such as 'functional' (meaning that the symptoms represent a reversible disturbance of bodily function) may be more acceptable. When possible, it is useful to describe a plausible physiological mechanism that is linked to psychological factors such as stress and implies that the symptoms are reversible. For example, in irritable bowel syndrome, psychological stress results in increased activation of the autonomic nervous system, which leads to constriction of smooth muscle in the gut wall, which in turn causes pain and bowel disturbance.

Advice

This should focus on how to overcome factors perpetuating the symptoms: for example, by resolving stressful social problems or by practising relaxation. The doctor can offer to review progress, to prescribe (for example) an antidepressant drug and, if appropriate, to refer for physiotherapy or psychological treatments such as CBT. The attitudes of relatives may need to be addressed if they have adopted an over-protective role, unwittingly reinforcing the patient's disability.

Drug treatment

Antidepressant drugs are often helpful, even if the patient is not depressed (Box 10.26).

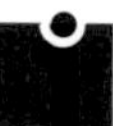

10.24 Common presentations of dissociative (conversion) disorder

- Gait disturbance
- Loss of function in limbs
- Aphonia
- Non-epileptic seizures
- Sensory loss
- Blindness

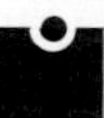

10.25 General management principles for medically unexplained symptoms

- Take a full sympathetic history
- Exclude disease but avoid unnecessary investigation or referral
- Seek specific treatable psychiatric syndromes
- Demonstrate to patients that you believe their complaints
- Establish a collaborative relationship
- Give a positive explanation for the symptoms, including but not over-emphasising psychological factors
- Encourage a return to normal functioning

EBM 10.26 Antidepressants for medically unexplained somatic symptoms

'There is evidence for the efficacy of antidepressant drugs for patients with medically unexplained symptoms.'

- Sumathipala A. Psychosom Med 2007; 69:889–900.

EBM 10.27 CBT for medically unexplained somatic symptoms

'CBT is consistently effective (11 of 13 trials) across a spectrum of somatoform disorders. Also, a psychiatric consultation letter to the primary care physician about strategies for managing the somatising patient seems to improve physical functioning and reduce costs.'

- Kroenke K. Psychosom Med 2007; 69:881–888.

Psychological treatment

There is evidence for the effectiveness of CBT (Box 10.27). Other psychological treatments such as IPT may also have a role.

Rehabilitation

Where there is chronic disability, particularly in dissociative (conversion) disorder, conventional physical rehabilitation may be the best approach.

Shared care with the GP

Ongoing planned care is required for patients with chronic intractable symptoms, especially those of somatisation disorder. Review by the same specialist, interspersed with visits to the same GP, is probably the best way to avoid unnecessary multiple re-referral for investigation, to ensure that treatable aspects of the patient's problems, such as depression, are actively managed, and to prevent the GP from becoming demoralised.

Factitious disorder and malingering

It is important to distinguish somatoform disorders from factitious disorder and malingering.

Factitious disorder

This describes the repeated and deliberate production of the signs or symptoms of disease to obtain medical care. It is uncommon. An example is the dipping of thermometers into hot drinks to fake a fever. The disorder feigned is usually medical but can be a psychiatric illness, with false reports of hallucinations or symptoms of depression.

Münchausen's syndrome

This refers to a severe chronic form of factitious disorder. Patients are usually older and male, with a solitary, peripatetic lifestyle in which they travel widely, sometimes visiting several hospitals in one day. Although the condition is rare, such patients are memorable because they present so dramatically. The history can be convincing enough to persuade doctors to undertake investigations or initiate treatment, including exploratory surgery. It may be possible to trace the patient's history and show that he has presented similarly elsewhere, often changing name several times. Some emergency departments hold lists of such patients.

Management is by gentle but firm confrontation with clear evidence of the fabrication of illness, together with an offer of psychological support. Treatment is usually declined but recognition of the condition may help to avoid further iatrogenic harm.

Malingering

Malingering is a description of behaviour, not a psychiatric diagnosis. It refers to the deliberate and conscious simulation of signs of disease and disability. Patients have motives that are clear to them but which they conceal from doctors. Examples include the avoidance of burdensome responsibilities (such as work or court appearances) or the pursuit of financial gain (fraudulent claims for benefits or compensation). Malingering can be hard to detect at clinical assessment, but is suggested by evasion or inconsistency in the history.

Schizophrenia

Schizophrenia is a psychosis characterised by delusions, hallucinations and lack of insight. Acute schizophrenia may present with disturbed behaviour, marked delusions, hallucinations and disordered thinking, or with insidious social withdrawal and other so-called negative symptoms and less obvious delusions and hallucinations. The prevalence is similar worldwide at about 1% and the disorder is more common in men. The children of one affected parent have approximately a 10% risk of developing the illness, but this rises to 50% if an identical twin is affected. The usual age of onset is the mid-twenties.

Aetiology

There is a strong genetic contribution, probably involving many susceptibility genes, each of small effect. The best candidates, such as *disrupted in schizophrenia-1* (*DISC1*) and *neuregulin-1* (*NRG1*), have supportive linkage, association, animal model and basic neurobiological evidence. Environmental risk factors include obstetric complications and urban birth. Brain imaging techniques have identified subtle structural abnormalities, including an enlargement of the lateral ventricles and an overall decrease in brain size (by about 3% on average), with relatively greater reduction in temporal lobe volume (5–10%). Episodes of acute schizophrenia may be precipitated by social stress and also by cannabis, which increase dopamine turnover and sensitivity. Consequently, schizophrenia is now viewed as a neurodevelopmental disorder, caused by abnormalities of brain development associated with genetic predisposition and early environmental influences, but precipitated by later triggers.

Diagnosis

Schizophrenia usually presents with an acute episode and progresses to a chronic state. Acute schizophrenia should be suspected in any individual with bizarre behaviour accompanied by delusions and hallucinations that are not due to organic brain disease or substance misuse. The diagnosis is made on clinical grounds, with

10.28 Symptoms of schizophrenia

First-rank symptoms of acute schizophrenia
• A = Auditory hallucinations – second- or third-person/écho de la pensée • B = Broadcasting, insertion/withdrawal of thoughts • C = Controlled feelings, impulses or acts ('passivity' experiences/phenomena) • D = Delusional perception (a particular experience is bizarrely interpreted)
Symptoms of chronic schizophrenia (negative symptoms)
• Flattened (blunted) affect • Apathy and loss of drive (avolition) • Social isolation/withdrawal (autism) • Poverty of speech (alogia) • Poor self-care

investigations used principally to rule out organic brain disease. The characteristic clinical features are listed in Box 10.28. Hallucinations are typically auditory, although they can occur in any sensory modality. They commonly involve voices from outside the head that talk to or about the person. Sometimes the voices repeat the person's thoughts. Patients may also describe 'passivity of thought', experienced as disturbances in the normal privacy of thinking – for example, the delusional belief that their thoughts are being 'withdrawn' from them, perhaps 'broadcast' to others, and/or alien thoughts being 'inserted' into their mind. Other characteristic symptoms are delusions of control: believing that one's emotions, impulses or acts are controlled by others. Another phenomenon is delusional perception, a delusion that arises suddenly alongside a normal perception (e.g. 'I saw the moon and I immediately knew he was evil'). Many other, less specific symptoms may occur, including thought disorder, as manifest by incomprehensible speech and abnormalities of movement, such as those in which the patient can become immobile or adopt awkward postures for prolonged periods (catatonia).

The main differential diagnosis of schizophrenia (Box 10.29) is:

- *Other functional psychoses*, particularly psychotic depression and mania, in which delusions and hallucinations are congruent with a marked mood disturbance (negative in depression and grandiose in mania). If features of schizophrenia and affective disorder coexist in equal measure, a diagnosis of schizoaffective disorder is made. Schizophrenia must also be differentiated from specific delusional disorders that are not associated with the other typical features of schizophrenia.
- *Organic psychoses*, including delirium, in which there is impairment of consciousness and loss of orientation (not found in schizophrenia), typically with visual hallucinations, and drug misuse, the latter particularly in young people. Schizophrenia must also be differentiated from other organic psychoses such as temporal lobe epilepsy, in which olfactory and gustatory hallucinations may occur.

Many of those who experience acute schizophrenia go on to develop a chronic state in which the acute,

10.29 Differential diagnosis of schizophrenia

Alternative diagnosis	Distinguishing features
Other functional psychoses	
Delusional disorders	Absence of specific features of schizophrenia
Psychotic depression	Prominent depressive symptoms
Manic episode	Prominent manic symptoms
Schizoaffective disorder	Mood and schizophrenia symptoms both prominent
Puerperal psychosis	Acute onset after childbirth
Organic disorders	
Drug-induced psychosis	Evidence of drug or alcohol misuse
Side-effects of prescribed drugs	Levodopa, methyldopa, corticosteroids, antimalarial drugs
Temporal lobe epilepsy	Other evidence of seizures
Delirium	Visual hallucinations; impaired consciousness
Dementia	Age; established cognitive impairment
Huntington's disease	Family history; choreiform movements; dementia

so-called positive symptoms resolve, or at least do not dominate the clinical picture, leaving so-called negative symptoms that include blunt affect, apathy, social isolation, poverty of speech and poor self-care. Patients with chronic schizophrenia may also manifest positive symptoms, particularly when under stress, and it can be difficult for those who do not know the patient to judge whether or not these are signs of an acute relapse.

Management

First-episode schizophrenia usually requires admission to hospital because patients lack the insight that they are ill and are unwilling to accept treatment. In some cases, they may be at risk of harming themselves or others. Subsequent acute relapses and chronic schizophrenia are now usually managed in the community.

Drug treatment

Antipsychotic agents are effective against the positive symptoms of schizophrenia in the majority of cases. They take 2–4 weeks to be maximally effective but have some beneficial effects shortly after administration. Treatment is then ideally continued to prevent relapse. In a patient with a first episode of schizophrenia, this will usually be for 1–2 years, but in patients with multiple episodes, treatment may be required for many years. The benefits of prolonged treatment must be weighed against the adverse effects, which include extrapyramidal side-effects (EPSE) like acute dystonic reactions (which may require treatment with parenteral anticholinergics), akathisia, Parkinsonism and tardive dyskinesia (abnormal movements, commonly of the face, over which the patient has no voluntary control). For long-term use, antipsychotic agents are often given in slow-release (depot) injected form to improve patient adherence.

10.30 Antipsychotic drugs

Group	Drug	Dose range
Phenothiazines	Chlorpromazine	100–1000 mg daily
Butyrophenones	Haloperidol	5–30 mg daily
Thioxanthenes	Flupentixol decanoate	20–200 mg fortnightly (depot injection)
Diphenylbutylpiperidines	Pimozide	4–30 mg daily
Substituted benzamides	Sulpiride	200–1800 mg daily
Dibenzodiazepines*	Clozapine	200–900 mg daily
Benzisoxazole*	Risperidone	2–16 mg daily
Thienobenzodiazepines*	Olanzapine	5–20 mg daily
Dibenzothiazepines	Quetiapine	25–800 mg daily

*Second-generation antipsychotics.

10.31 Side-effects of antipsychotic drugs

Weight gain due to increased appetite

Effects due to dopamine blockade*
- Acute dystonia
- Akathisia (motor restlessness)
- Parkinsonism
- Tardive dyskinesia
- Gynaecomastia
- Galactorrhoea

Effects due to cholinergic blockade
- Dry mouth
- Blurred vision
- Impotence
- Constipation
- Urinary retention

Hypersensitivity reactions
- Blood dyscrasias (neutropenia with clozapine)
- Cholestatic jaundice
- Photosensitive dermatitis

Ocular complications (long-term use)
- Corneal and lens opacities

*Less severe with clozapine, quetiapine and olanzapine, possibly because of strong 5-HT-blocking effect and relatively weak dopamine blockade.

A number of antipsychotic agents are available (Box 10.30). These may be divided into conventional (typical, first-generation) drugs such as chlorpromazine and haloperidol, and newer or atypical (also so-called novel or second-generation) drugs such as clozapine. All are believed to work by blocking D_2 dopamine receptors in the brain. Patients who have not responded to conventional drugs may respond to newer agents, which are also less likely to produce unwanted EPSE but do tend to cause greater weight gain and metabolic disturbances such as dyslipidaemia. Clozapine can also cause an agranulocytosis and consequently requires regular monitoring of the white blood cell count, initially on a weekly basis. Details of the side-effects of antipsychotic drugs are listed in Box 10.31.

Serious adverse effects of antipsychotic drugs include:

- *Neuroleptic malignant syndrome*, which is a rare but serious condition. It is characterised by fever, tremor and rigidity, autonomic instability and confusion. Characteristic laboratory findings are an elevated creatinine phosphokinase and leucocytosis. Antipsychotic medication must be stopped immediately and supportive therapy provided, often in an intensive care unit. Treatment includes ensuring hydration and reducing hyperthermia. Dantrolene sodium and bromocriptine may be helpful. Mortality is 20% untreated and 5% with treatment.
- *Prolongation of the QT_c interval*, which may be associated with ventricular tachycardia, torsades de pointes and sudden death. Treatment is by stopping the drug, monitoring the electrocardiogram (ECG) and treating serious arrhythmias (p. 562).

Psychological treatment

Psychological treatment, including general support for the patient and his or her family, is now seen as an essential component of management. CBT may help patients to cope with symptoms. There is evidence that personal and/or family education, when given as part of an integrated treatment package, reduces the rate of relapse.

Social treatment

After an acute episode of schizophrenia has been controlled by drug therapy, social rehabilitation may be required. Recurrent illness is likely to cause disruption to patients' relationships and their ability to manage their accommodation and occupation; consequently, they may need help to obtain housing and employment. A graded return to employment and sometimes a period of supported accommodation are required.

Patients with chronic schizophrenia have particular difficulties and may need long-term, supervised accommodation. This now tends to be in sheltered or hostel accommodation in the community. Patients may also benefit from sheltered employment if they are unable to participate effectively in the labour market. Ongoing contact with a health worker allows monitoring for signs of relapse, sometimes as part of a multidisciplinary team working to agreed plans (the 'care programme approach'). Partly because of a tendency to inactivity, smoking and a poor diet, patients with chronic schizophrenia are at increased risk of cardiovascular disease, diabetes and stroke, and require proactive medical as well as psychiatric care.

Prognosis

About one-quarter of those who develop an acute schizophrenic episode have a good outcome. One-third develop chronic, incapacitating schizophrenia, and the remainder largely recover after each episode but suffer relapses. Most will not work or live independently. Prophylactic treatment with antipsychotic drugs reduces the rate of relapse in the first 2 years after an episode of schizophrenia from 50% to 10%. Schizophrenia is associated with suicide, with up to 1 in 10 patients taking their own lives.

Delirium, dementia and other organic disorders

Delirium, dementia and other organic disorders could be considered to be medical conditions rather than psychiatric disorders, as they are a result of reduced brain function; they are, however, included in psychiatric classifications and are sometimes misdiagnosed because they often manifest with disturbed behaviour.

Delirium

Delirium is common in acute medical settings, especially in the elderly and patients in high-dependency and intensive care units. Aetiology, assessment and management are described in Chapters 7 and 26.

Dementia

Dementia is a clinical syndrome characterised by a loss of previously acquired intellectual function in the absence of impairment of arousal, and affects 5% of those over 65 and 20% of those over 85. It is defined as a global impairment of cognitive function, and is typically progressive and non-reversible. Although memory is most affected in the early stages, deficits in visuospatial function, language ability, concentration and attention gradually become apparent. There are many causes (Box 10.32) but Alzheimer's disease and diffuse vascular disease are the most common. Rarer causes of dementia should be actively sought in younger patients and those with short histories.

Aetiology

Dementia may be divided into 'cortical' and 'subcortical' types, depending on the clinical features. Many of the primary degenerative diseases that cause dementia have characteristic features that may allow a specific diagnosis during life. Creutzfeldt–Jakob disease, for example, is usually relatively rapidly progressive (over months), is associated with myoclonus, and demonstrates characteristic abnormalities on electroencephalogram (EEG). The more slowly progressive dementias are more difficult to distinguish during life, but fronto-temporal dementia typically presents with focal (temporal or frontal lobe) dysfunction, and Lewy body dementia may present with visual hallucinations. The course may also help to distinguish types of dementia, as it may be gradual (as in Alzheimer's disease) or step-wise (as in vascular dementia).

Clinical features

The usual presentation is with a disturbance of personality or memory dysfunction. A careful history is essential

10.32 Causes of dementia

Type	Common	Unusual	Rare
Vascular	Diffuse small-vessel disease	Amyloid angiopathy Multiple emboli	Cerebral vasculitis
Degenerative/ inherited	Alzheimer's disease	Fronto-temporal dementia (including Pick's disease) Leucodystrophies Huntington's disease Wilson's disease Dystrophia myotonica Cortical Lewy body disease Progressive supranuclear palsy Others (e.g. cortico-basal degeneration)	Mitochondrial encephalopathies
Neoplastic (p. 1193)	Secondary deposits	Primary cerebral tumour	Paraneoplastic syndrome (limbic encephalitis)
Inflammatory	–	Multiple sclerosis	Sarcoidosis
Traumatic	Chronic subdural haematoma Post-head injury	Punch-drunk syndrome	–
Hydrocephalus (p. 1216)		Communicating/non-communicating 'normal pressure' hydrocephalus	–
Toxic/nutritional	Alcohol	Thiamin deficiency B_{12} deficiency	Anoxia/carbon monoxide poisoning Heavy metal poisoning
Infective	–	Syphilis HIV	Post-encephalitic Whipple's disease Subacute sclerosing panencephalitis
Prion diseases (p. 1211)	–	Sporadic Creutzfeldt–Jakob disease (CJD)	Variant CJD Kuru Gerstmann–Sträussler–Scheinker disease

and it is important to interview both the patient and a close family member. Simple bedside tests such as the MMSE (p. 234), are useful in assessing the nature and severity of the cognitive deficit, although a more intensive neuropsychological assessment may sometimes be required, especially if there is diagnostic uncertainty. It is important to exclude a focal brain lesion. This is done by determining that there is cognitive disturbance in more than one area. Mental state assessment is important to seek evidence of depression, which may coexist with or occasionally cause apparent cognitive impairment.

Investigations

The aim is to seek treatable causes and to estimate prognosis. This is done using a standard set of investigations (Box 10.33). Imaging of the brain can exclude potentially treatable structural lesions, such as hydrocephalus, cerebral tumour or chronic subdural haematoma, though the only abnormality usually seen is that of generalised atrophy. If the initial tests are negative, more invasive investigations, such as lumbar puncture or, rarely, brain biopsy, may be indicated.

Management

This is directed at addressing treatable causes, and providing support for patient and carers if no specific treatment exists. If the diagnosis is Alzheimer-type dementia, anticholinesterase inhibitors and memantine may arrest progression for a time. Treating vascular risk factors may slow deterioration in vascular dementia. Psychotropic drugs may help where there is associated disturbance of sleep, perception or mood, but should be used with care because of an increased mortality in patients who have been treated long-term with these agents. Sedation is not a substitute for good care for patients and carers or, in the later stages, attentive residential nursing care. In the UK, incapacity and mental health legislation may be required to manage patients' financial and domestic affairs, as well as to determine their safe placement.

10.33 Initial investigation of dementia

In most patients

- Imaging of head (computed tomography (CT) and/or magnetic resonance imaging (MRI))
- Blood tests
  - Full blood count, erythrocyte sedimentation rate
  - Urea and electrolytes, glucose
  - Calcium, liver function tests
  - Thyroid function tests
  - Vitamin B_{12}
  - Venereal Diseases Research Laboratory (VDRL) test
  - ANA, anti-dsDNA
- Chest X-ray
- EEG

In selected patients

- Lumbar puncture
- HIV serology
- Brain biopsy

Alzheimer's disease

Alzheimer's disease is the most common cause of dementia, but is rare under the age of 45 years.

Aetiology

Genetic factors play an important role and about 15% of cases are familial. Familial cases fall into two main groups: early-onset disease with autosomal dominant inheritance and a later-onset group whose inheritance is polygenic. Mutations in several genes have been described. The inheritance of one of the alleles of apolipoprotein ε (apo ε4) is associated with an increased risk of developing the disease (2–4 times higher in heterozygotes and 6–8 times in homozygotes). Its presence is, however, neither necessary nor sufficient for the development of the disease, so screening for its presence is not clinically useful. The brain in Alzheimer's disease is macroscopically atrophic, particularly the cerebral cortex and hippocampus. Histologically, the disease is characterised by the presence of senile plaques and neurofibrillary tangles in the cerebral cortex. Histochemical staining demonstrates significant quantities of amyloid in the plaques (Fig. 10.4), which typically stain positive for the protein ubiquitin, involved in targeting unwanted or damaged proteins for degradation. This has led to the suggestion that the disease may be due to defects in the ability of neuronal cells to degrade unwanted proteins. Many different neurotransmitter abnormalities have also been described. In particular, there is impairment of cholinergic transmission, although

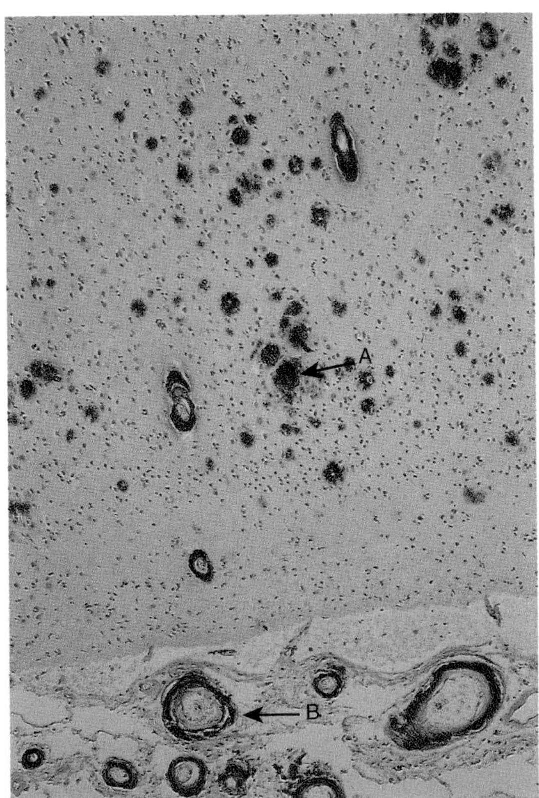

Fig. 10.4 Alzheimer's disease. Section of neocortex stained with polyclonal antibody against βA4 peptide showing amyloid deposits in plaques in brain substance (arrow A) and in blood vessel walls (arrow B).

10

abnormalities of noradrenaline, 5-HT, glutamate and substance P have also been described.

Clinical features

The key clinical feature is impairment of the ability to remember new information. Hence, patients present with gradual impairment of memory, usually in association with disorders of other cortical functions. Short-term and long-term memory are both affected, but defects in the former are usually more obvious. Later in the course of the disease, typical features include apraxia, visuo-spatial impairment and aphasia. In the early stages of the disease, patients may notice these problems, but as the disease progresses it is common for patients to deny that there is anything wrong (anosognosia). In this situation, patients are often brought to medical attention by their carers. Depression is commonly present. Occasionally, patients become aggressive, and the clinical features can be made acutely worse by intercurrent physical disease.

Investigations and management

Investigation is aimed at excluding treatable causes of dementia (see Box 10.32), as histological confirmation of the diagnosis usually occurs only after death. There is no known treatment, though anticholinesterases such as donepezil, rivastigmine and galantamine, and the NMDA receptor antagonist, memantine, have been shown to be of some benefit. Management consists largely of providing a familiar environment for the patient and support for the carers. Many patients are depressed, and treatment with antidepressant medication may be helpful.

Fronto-temporal dementia

This term encompasses a number of different syndromes, including Pick's diseases and primary progressive aphasia. Patients may present with personality change due to frontal lobe involvement or with language disturbance due to temporal lobe involvement. These diseases are much rarer than Alzheimer's disease. Histological examination of the brain reveals argyrophilic cytoplasmic inclusion bodies of tau (τ) protein rather than the ubiquitin as in Alzheimer's disease (Fig. 10.5). Memory is relatively preserved in the early stages. There is no specific treatment.

Lewy body dementia

This is a neurodegenerative disorder clinically characterised by dementia and signs of Parkinson's disease. The cognitive state often fluctuates and there is a high incidence of visual hallucinations. Affected individuals are particularly sensitive to the side-effects of anti-Parkinsonian medication and also to antipsychotic drugs. The condition is associated with accumulation of abnormal protein aggregates in neurons that contain the protein α-synuclein in association with other proteins including ubiquitin (see Fig. 26.29, p. 1195). The condition is often inherited and mutations in the α-synuclein and β-synuclein genes have been identified in affected patients. There is no specific treatment but anticholinesterase agents may well be helpful.

Alcohol misuse and dependence

Alcohol consumption associated with social, psychological and physical problems constitutes misuse. The criteria for alcohol dependence, a more restricted term, are shown in Box 10.34. Approximately one-quarter of male patients in general hospital medical wards in the UK have a current or previous alcohol problem.

Aetiology

Availability of alcohol and social patterns of use appear to be the most important factors. Genetic factors predispose to dependence. The majority of alcoholics do not have an associated psychiatric disorder, but a few drink heavily in an attempt to relieve anxiety or depression.

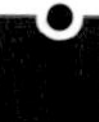

10.34 Criteria for alcohol dependence

- Narrowing of the drinking repertoire
- Priority of drinking over other activities (salience)
- Tolerance of effects of alcohol
- Repeated withdrawal symptoms
- Relief of withdrawal symptoms by further drinking
- Subjective compulsion to drink
- Reinstatement of drinking behaviour after abstinence

A

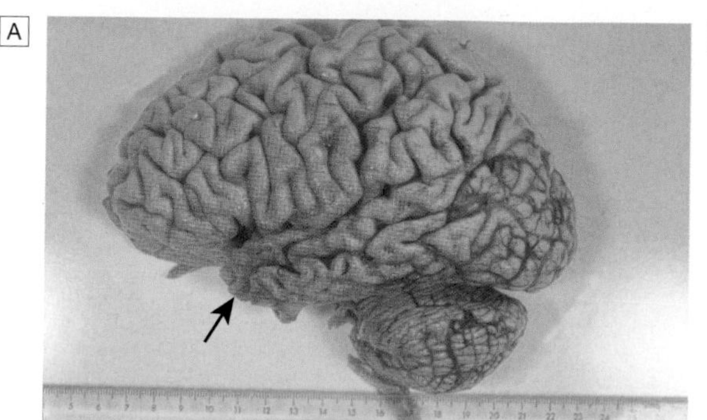

B

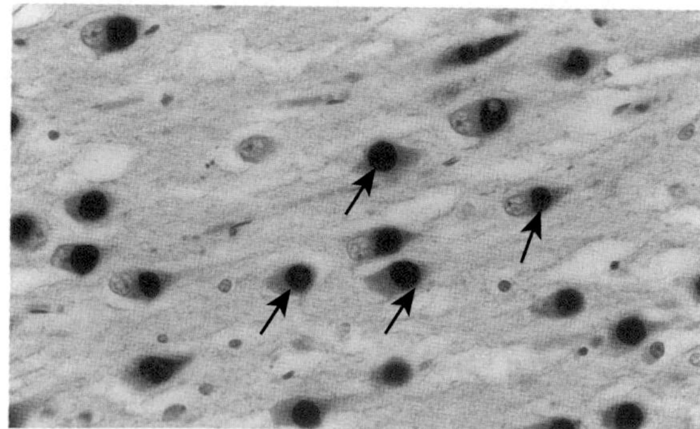

Fig. 10.5 Fronto-temporal dementia. **A** Lateral view of formalin-fixed brain from a patient who died of Pick's disease, showing gyral atrophy of frontal and parietal lobes and a more severe degree of atrophy affecting the anterior half of the temporal lobe (arrow). **B** High power (× 200) of hippocampal pyramidal layer, prepared with monoclonal anti-tau antibody. Many neuronal cell bodies contain sharply circumscribed, spherical cytoplasmic inclusion bodies (Pick bodies).

Diagnosis

Alcohol misuse may emerge during the patient's history, although patients may minimise their intake. It may also present via its effects on one or more aspects of the patient's life, listed below. Alcohol dependence commonly presents with withdrawal in those admitted to hospital, as they can no longer maintain their high alcohol intake in this setting.

Complications of chronic alcohol misuse

- *Social problems* include absenteeism from work, unemployment, marital tensions, child abuse, financial difficulties and problems with the law, such as violence and traffic offences.
- *Depression* is common. Alcohol has a direct depressant effect and heavy drinking creates numerous social problems. Attempted and completed suicide are associated with alcohol misuse.
- *Anxiety* is relieved by alcohol in the short term. People who are socially anxious may consequently use alcohol in this way and may develop dependence. Conversely, alcohol withdrawal increases anxiety.
- *Alcoholic hallucinosis* is a rare condition in which alcoholic individuals experience auditory hallucination in clear consciousness.
- *Alcohol withdrawal* is described in Box 10.35. Symptoms usually become maximal about 2–3 days after the last drink and can include seizures ('rum fits').
- *Delirium tremens* is a form of delirium associated with severe alcohol withdrawal. It has a significant mortality and morbidity (see Box 10.35).

Effects on the brain

The familiar features of drunkenness are ataxia, slurred speech, emotional incontinence and aggression. Very heavy drinkers may experience periods of amnesia for events that occurred during bouts of intoxication, termed 'alcoholic blackouts'. Established alcoholism may lead to alcoholic dementia, a global cognitive impairment resembling Alzheimer's disease, but which does not progress and may even improve if the patient becomes abstinent. Indirect effects on behaviour can result from head injury, hypoglycaemia and encephalopathy (p. 941).

A rare but important effect of chronic alcohol misuse is the Wernicke–Korsakoff syndrome. This organic brain disorder results from damage to the mamillary bodies, dorsomedial nuclei of the thalamus and adjacent areas of periventricular grey matter caused by a deficiency of thiamin (vitamin B_1), which most commonly results from long-standing heavy drinking and an inadequate diet. It can also arise from malabsorption or even protracted vomiting. Without prompt treatment (see below), the acute presentation of Wernicke's encephalopathy (nystagmus, ophthalmoplegia, ataxia and confusion) can progress to the irreversible deficits of Korsakoff's syndrome (severe short-term memory deficits and confabulation, and also reduced red blood cell transketolase). In those who die in the acute stage, microscopic examination of the brain shows hyperaemia, petechial haemorrhages and astrocytic proliferation.

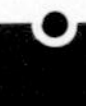

10.35 Consequences of chronic alcohol misuse

Acute intoxication

- Emotional and behavioural disturbance
- Medical problems: hypoglycaemia, aspiration of vomit, respiratory depression
- Complication of other medical problems
- Accidents, injuries sustained in fights

Withdrawal phenomena

- Psychological symptoms: restlessness, anxiety, panic attacks
- Autonomic symptoms: tachycardia, sweating, pupil dilatation, nausea, vomiting
- Delirium tremens: agitation, hallucinations, illusions, delusions
- Seizures

Harmful use

Medical consequences

- Neurological: peripheral neuropathy, cerebellar degeneration, cerebral haemorrhage, dementia
- Hepatic: fatty change and cirrhosis, liver cancer
- Gastrointestinal: oesophagitis, gastritis, pancreatitis, oesophageal cancer, Mallory–Weiss syndrome, malabsorption, oesophageal varices
- Respiratory: pulmonary tuberculosis, pneumonia
- Skin: spider naevi, palmar erythema, Dupuytren's contractures, telangiectasias
- Cardiac: cardiomyopathy, hypertension
- Musculoskeletal: myopathy, fractures
- Endocrine and metabolic: pseudo-Cushing's syndrome, hypoglycaemia, gout
- Reproductive: hypogonadism, fetal alcohol syndrome, infertility

Psychiatric and cerebral consequences

- Depression
- Alcoholic hallucinosis
- Alcoholic 'blackouts'
- Wernicke's encephalopathy: nystagmus, ophthalmoplegia, ataxia, confusion
- Korsakoff's syndrome: short-term memory deficits, confabulation

Effects on other organs

These are protean and virtually any organ can be involved (see Box 10.35). These effects are discussed in detail in the relevant chapters.

Management and prognosis

For the person misusing alcohol, provision of clear information from a doctor about the harmful effects of alcohol and the safe levels of consumption is often all that is needed. In more serious cases, patients may have to be advised to alter leisure activities or change jobs to help them to reduce their consumption. Psychological treatment is used for patients who have recurrent relapses and is usually available at specialised centres. Support to stop drinking is also provided by voluntary organisations, such as Alcoholics Anonymous (AA) in the UK.

Alcohol withdrawal syndromes can be prevented, or treated once established, with benzodiazepines. Large doses may be required (e.g. diazepam 20 mg 4 times daily), tailed off over a period of 5–7 days as symptoms subside. Prevention of the Wernicke–Korsakoff syndrome requires the immediate use of high doses of thiamine, which is initially given parenterally in the form of Pabrinex (two vials 3 times daily for 48 hours) and then orally (100 mg 3 times daily). There is no treatment for Korsakoff's syndrome once it has arisen. The risk of side-effects, such as respiratory depression with benzodiazepines and anaphylaxis with Pabrinex, is small when weighed against the risks of no treatment.

Acamprosate (666 mg 3 times daily) may help to maintain abstinence by reducing the craving for alcohol. Disulfiram (200–400 mg daily) can be given as a deterrent to patients who have difficulty resisting the impulse to drink after becoming abstinent. It blocks the metabolism of alcohol, causing acetaldehyde to accumulate. When alcohol is consumed, an unpleasant reaction follows, with headache, flushing and nausea. Disulfiram is always an adjunct to other treatments, especially supportive psychotherapy. Treatment with antidepressants may be required if depression is severe or does not resolve with abstinence. Antipsychotics (e.g. chlorpromazine 100 mg 3 times daily) are needed for alcoholic hallucinosis. Although such treatment may be successful, there is a high relapse rate.

Chronic alcohol misuse greatly increases the risk of death from accidents, disease and suicide (p. 100).

Substance misuse disorder

Dependence on and misuse of both illegal and prescribed drugs is a major problem worldwide. Drugs of misuse are described in detail in Chapter 9. They can be grouped as follows.

Sedatives

These commonly give rise to physical dependence, the manifestations of which are tolerance and a withdrawal syndrome. Drugs include benzodiazepines, opiates (including morphine, heroin, methadone and dihydrocodeine) and barbiturates (now rarely prescribed). Overdosage with opiates and benzodiazepines can be fatal, primarily as a result of respiratory depression (Ch. 9). Withdrawal from opiates is notoriously unpleasant, and withdrawal from benzodiazepines (Box 10.36) and barbiturates may cause seizures.

Intravenous opiate users are prone to bacterial infections, hepatitis B (p. 950), hepatitis C (p. 954) and HIV infection (Ch. 14) through needle contamination. Accidental overdose is common, mainly because of the varied and uncertain potency of illicit supplies of the drug. The withdrawal syndrome, which can start within 12 hours of last use, presents with intense craving, rhinorrhoea, lacrimation, yawning, perspiration, shivering, piloerection, vomiting, diarrhoea and abdominal cramps. Examination reveals tachycardia, hypertension, mydriasis and facial flushing.

10.36 Benzodiazepine withdrawal symptoms

- Anxiety
- Heightened sensory perception
- Hallucinations
- Epileptic seizures
- Ataxia
- Paranoid delusions

Stimulants

Stimulant drugs include amphetamines and cocaine. They are less dangerous than the sedatives in overdose, although they can cause cardiac and cerebrovascular problems through their pressor effects. Physical dependence syndromes do not arise, but withdrawal causes a rebound lowering in mood and can give rise to an intense craving for further use, especially in any form of drug with a rapid onset and offset of effect, such as crack cocaine. Chronic ingestion can cause a paranoid psychosis similar to schizophrenia. A 'toxic psychosis' (delirium) can occur with high levels of consumption, and tactile hallucinations (formication) may be prominent.

Hallucinogens

The hallucinogens are a disparate group of drugs that cause prominent sensory disturbances. They include cannabis, ecstasy, lysergic acid diethylamide (LSD) and *Psilocybin* (magic mushrooms). A toxic confusional state can occur after heavy cannabis consumption. Acute psychotic episodes are well recognised, especially in those with a family or personal history of psychosis, and there is evidence that prolonged heavy use increases the risk of developing schizophrenia. Paranoid psychoses have been reported in association with ecstasy. A chronic psychosis has also been reported after regular LSD use.

Organic solvents

Solvent inhalation (glue sniffing) is popular in some adolescent groups. Solvents produce acute intoxication characterised by euphoria, excitement, dizziness and a floating sensation. Further inhalation leads to loss of consciousness; death can occur from the direct toxic effect of the solvent, or from asphyxiation if the substance is inhaled from a plastic bag.

Aetiology

Many of the aetiological factors for alcohol misuse also apply to drug dependence. The main factors are cultural pressures, particularly within a peer group, and availability of a drug. In the case of some drugs, medical over-prescribing (for example, of synthetic opiates) has increased their availability, but there has also been a relative decline in the price of illegal drugs. Most drug users take a range of drugs – so-called polydrug misuse.

Diagnosis

As with alcohol, the diagnosis either may be apparent from the history, or may only be made once the patient presents with a complication. Drug screening of samples of urine or blood can be valuable in confirming the diagnosis, especially if the patient persists in denial.

Management and prognosis

The first step is to determine whether patients wish to stop using the drug. If they do not, they can still benefit from advice about how to minimise harm from their habit: for example, how to obtain and use clean needles for those who inject. For those who are physically dependent on sedative drugs, substitute prescribing (using methadone, for example, in opiate dependence) may help stabilise their lives sufficiently to allow a gradual reduction in dosage until they reach abstinence. Some specialist units offer inpatient detoxification. For details of the medical management of overdose, see Chapter 9.

The drug lofexidine, a centrally acting α-agonist, can be useful in treating the autonomic symptoms of opiate withdrawal, as can clonidine, although this carries a risk of hypotension and is best used by specialists. Long-acting opiate antagonists, such as naltrexone, may also have a place, again in specialist hands, in blocking the euphoriant effects of the opiate, thereby reducing addiction.

In some cases, complete opiate withdrawal is not successful and the patient functions better if maintained on regular doses of oral methadone as an outpatient. This decision to prescribe long-term methadone should only be taken by a specialist, and carried out under long-term supervision at a specialist drug treatment centre.

Substitute prescribing is neither necessary nor possible for the hallucinogens and stimulants, but the principles of management are the same as those that should accompany prescribing for the sedatives. These include identifying problems associated with the drug misuse that may serve to maintain it, and intervening where possible. Intervention may be directed at physical illness, psychiatric comorbidity, social problems or family disharmony.

Relapsing patients and those with complications should be referred to specialist drug misuse services. Support can also be provided by self-help groups and voluntary bodies, such as Narcotics Anonymous in the UK.

Personality disorders

Personality refers to the set of characteristics and behavioural traits that best describes an individual's patterns of interaction with the world. The intensity of particular traits varies from person to person, although many, such as shyness or irritability, are displayed to some degree by most people.

A personality disorder (PD) is diagnosed when an individual's personality causes persistent and severe problems for the person or for others. For example, anxiety may be so pronounced that the individual rarely ventures into any situation where he or she fears scrutiny. Antisocial traits, such as disregard for the well-being of others and a lack of guilt concerning the adverse effects of one's actions on others, if pronounced, may lead to damage to others and to criminal acts.

PD is classified into several subtypes (such as emotionally unstable, antisocial or schizotypal), depending on the particular behavioural traits in question. A patient who meets diagnostic criteria for one subtype commonly meets criteria for two or three others. As allocation to one particular subtype gives little guidance to management or prognosis, classification is of limited value. PD commonly accompanies other psychiatric conditions, making treatment of the latter more difficult and therefore affecting their prognosis.

Aetiology

Some personality disorders appear to have an inherited aspect (especially paranoid and schizotypal types) but most are more clearly related to an unsatisfactory upbringing and adverse childhood experiences.

Management and prognosis

Personality disorders usually persist throughout life and are not readily treated. However, they often become less extreme with age. Treatment options are limited but there is some evidence that emotionally unstable PD may also respond to dialectical behavioural therapy (an intensive type of CBT). Anxious (avoidant) and obsessional (anankastic) PD may benefit from prescription of anxiolytic drugs, while paranoid/schizotypal PD may benefit from treatment with low doses of antipsychotic agents.

Eating disorders

There are two well-defined eating disorders, anorexia nervosa (AN) and bulimia nervosa (BN); they share some overlapping features. Ninety per cent of cases are female. There is a much higher prevalence of abnormal eating behaviour in the population that does not meet diagnostic criteria for AN or BN. In developed societies, obesity is arguably a much greater problem but is usually considered to be more a disorder of lifestyle or physiology than a psychiatric disorder.

Anorexia nervosa

There is marked weight loss, arising from food avoidance, often in combination with bingeing, purging, excessive exercise, or the use of diuretics and laxatives. Body image is profoundly disturbed so that, despite emaciation, patients still feel overweight and are terrified of weight gain. These preoccupations are intense and pervasive, and the false beliefs may be held with a conviction approaching the delusional. Anxiety and depressive symptoms are common accompaniments. Downy hair (lanugo) may develop on the back, forearms and cheeks. Extreme starvation is associated with a wide range of physiological and pathological bodily changes. All organ systems may be affected, although the most serious problems are cardiac and skeletal (Box 10.37).

Aetiology

This is unknown but probably includes genetic and environmental factors, including, in many societies, the social pressure on women to be thin.

Diagnosis

The condition usually emerges in adolescence, with a marked female preponderance. Diagnostic criteria are shown in Box 10.38. Differential diagnosis is from other causes of weight loss, including psychiatric disorders such as depression, and medical conditions such as inflammatory bowel disease, malabsorption, hypopituitarism and cancer. The diagnosis is based on a pronounced fear of fatness despite being thin, and on the absence of alternative causes of weight loss.

Management and prognosis

The aims of management are to ensure patient's physical well-being, whilst helping them to gain weight by addressing the beliefs and behaviours that maintain the

10.37 Medical consequences of eating disorders

Cardiac
• ECG abnormalities: T wave inversion, ST depression and prolonged QT_c interval • Arrhythmias, including profound sinus bradycardia and ventricular tachycardia
Haematological
• Anaemia, thrombocytopenia and leucopenia
Endocrine
• Pubertal delay or arrest • Growth retardation and short stature • Amenorrhoea • Sick euthyroid state
Metabolic
• Uraemia • Renal calculi • Osteoporosis
Gastrointestinal
• Constipation • Abnormal liver function tests

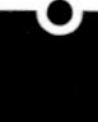

10.38 Diagnostic criteria for eating disorders

Anorexia nervosa
• Weight loss of at least 15% of total body weight (or body mass index ≤ 17.5) • Avoidance of high-calorie foods • Distortion of body image so that patients regard themselves as fat even when grossly underweight • Amenorrhoea for at least 3 months
Bulimia nervosa
• Recurrent bouts of binge eating • Lack of self-control over eating during binges • Self-induced vomiting, purgation or dieting after binges • Weight maintained within normal limits

low weight. Treatment is usually given on an outpatient basis, inpatient treatment being indicated only if weight loss is intractable and severe (for example, less than 65% of normal), or if there is a risk of death from medical complications or from suicide. There is a limited evidence base for treatment, although CBT and family therapy are commonly used. Psychotropic drugs are of little benefit except in those with clear-cut comorbid depressive disorder.

Weight gain is best achieved in a collaborative fashion. Compulsory admission and refeeding (including tube feeding) are very occasionally resorted to when patients are at risk of death and other measures have failed. Whilst this may produce a short-term improvement in weight, it probably does not change long-term prognosis. About 20% of patients with AN have a good outcome, a further 20% develop a chronic intractable disorder and the rest have an intermediate outcome. There is a long-term mortality rate of 10–20%, either due to the complications of starvation or from suicide.

Bulimia nervosa

In BN, patients are usually at or near normal weight (unlike in AN), but display a morbid fear of fatness associated with disordered eating behaviour. They recurrently embark on eating binges, often followed by corrective measures such as self-induced vomiting. The prevalence is similar to or slightly greater than that of AN, but only a small proportion of sufferers reach treatment services.

Diagnosis

BN usually begins later in adolescence than AN, and is even more predominantly a female malady. Diagnostic criteria are shown in Box 10.38. Physical signs of repeated self-induced vomiting include pitted teeth (from gastric acid), calluses on knuckles ('Russell's sign') and parotid gland enlargement. There are many associated physical complications, including the dental and oesophageal consequences of repeated vomiting, as well as electrolyte abnormalities, cardiac arrhythmias and renal problems (see Box 10.37).

Management and prognosis

CBT achieves both short-term and long-term improvements. Guided self-help and interpersonal psychotherapy may also be of value. There is also evidence for benefit from the SSRI, fluoxetine, although high doses (60 mg daily) and long courses (1 year) may be required; this appears to be independent of the antidepressant effect.

Bulimia does not carry the mortality associated with AN, and few sufferers develop anorexia. At 10-year follow-up, approximately 10% are still unwell, 20% have a subclinical degree of BN, and the remainder have recovered.

Puerperal disorders

There are three common psychiatric disorders that occur after childbirth. When managing these conditions, it is important always to consider both the mother and the baby, and their relationship (Box 10.39).

Post-partum blues

These are characterised by irritability, labile mood and tearfulness. Most women are affected to some degree. Symptoms begin soon after childbirth, peak on about the fourth day and then resolve. They may be related to hormonal or psychological changes associated with childbirth. No treatment is required, other than to reassure the mother.

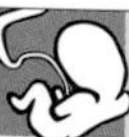

10.39 Psychiatric illness and pregnancy

- Always consider the effects of psychiatric disorder and treatment on mother, fetus and neonate
- Lithium, carbamazepine and valproate are significant teratogens, so minimise their use
- Most cases of post-partum low mood ('blues') are transient
- However, persistent low mood may indicate depressive illness
- Puerperal psychosis usually requires psychiatric admission

Post-partum depression

This occurs in 10–15% of women and within a month of delivery. Women with a previous history of depression are at risk. Explanation and reassurance are important. The usual psychological and drug treatments for depression should be considered, as well as practical help with childcare. If hospital admission is required, it should ideally be to a mother and baby unit. Further episodes of depression, both after childbirth and in response to other stressors, are likely.

Puerperal psychosis

This has its onset in the first 2 weeks after childbirth. It is a rare but serious complication affecting about 1 in 500 women and usually takes the form of a manic or depressive psychosis. There is an association with a personal or familial history of bipolar disorder. Delirium is rare with modern obstetric management but should still be considered in the differential diagnosis. Admission to a psychiatric mother and baby unit may be required. Management depends on the type of psychosis that presents. In addition, it is important to consider the welfare of the baby, especially if the mother has ideas of harming it. If so, the risk to the baby must be assessed and, if necessary, the baby temporarily removed. Most women recover but are at an increased (25%) risk of puerperal psychosis with the next pregnancy, and a 50% lifetime risk.

PSYCHIATRY AND THE LAW

Medicine takes place in a legal framework, made up of legislation (statute law) drafted by parliament or other governing bodies, and common law (case law) built up from court judgements over time. Psychiatry is similar to other branches of medicine in the applicability of common law but differs in that patients with psychiatric disorders can also be subject to legislative requirements to remain in hospital or to undergo treatments they refuse, such as the administration of antipsychotic drugs to a patient with acute schizophrenia who lacks insight, and whose symptoms and/or behaviour pose a risk to himself/herself or to others.

The UK has three different Mental Health Acts, covering England and Wales, Scotland, and Northern Ireland, and all of these have recently been revised. Other countries may have very different provisions. It is important for practitioners to be familiar with the relevant provisions that apply in their jurisdictions and are likely to arise in the clinical settings in which they work.

All the countries that make up the UK have also introduced Incapacity Acts in recent years, with detailed provisions covering medical treatments for patients incapable of consenting, whether this incapacity arises from physical or mental illness. In general, the guiding principle in British law is that people should be free to make their own decisions about medical treatment, except where their ability to decide is impaired by mental illness or physical incapacity, and where there are clear risks to the health and safety of themselves or others. Any restrictions or compulsions applied should be the minimum necessary, and they should only be applied for as long as is necessary; there should also be provisions for appeals and oversight.

Further information

Books

Harrison P, Geddes J, Sharpe M. Lecture notes on psychiatry. 10th edn. Oxford: Blackwell Science; 2010.

Johnstone EC, Owens DGC, Lawrie SM, et al (eds). Companion to psychiatric studies. 8th edn. Edinburgh: Churchill Livingstone; 2009.

Websites

http://cebmh.warne.ox.ac.uk/cebmh/ *Website of the Centre for Evidence-based Mental Health.*

www.depressionalliance.org *Information on depression.*

www.niaaa.nih.gov/ *Information on alcoholism.*

www.rcpsych.ac.uk/info/index.htm *Royal College of Psychiatrists: mental health information.*

www.who.int/mental_health/ *WHO website on mental health and brain disorders.*

G.G. Dark
A.R. Abdul Razak

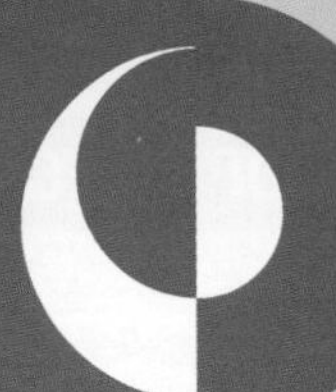

Oncology 11

Clinical examination of the cancer patient 260

The ten hallmarks of cancer 262

Environmental and genetic determinants of cancer 266

Investigations 268
- Histology 268
- Imaging 269
- Biochemical markers 269

Presenting problems in oncology 269
- Palpable mass 270
- Weight loss and fever 271
- Finger clubbing 271
- Ectopic hormone production 271
- Neurological paraneoplastic syndromes 271
- Cutaneous manifestations of cancer 272

Emergency complications of cancer 272

Metastatic disease 274

Therapeutics in oncology 276
- Surgical treatment 276
- Systemic chemotherapy 276
- Radiation therapy 277
- Hormone therapy 278
- Immunotherapy 278
- Biological therapies 278

Specific cancers 279
- Breast cancer 279
- Ovarian cancer 280
- Endometrial cancer 281
- Cervical cancer 281
- Head and neck tumours 281
- Carcinoma of unknown origin 282

CLINICAL EXAMINATION OF THE CANCER PATIENT

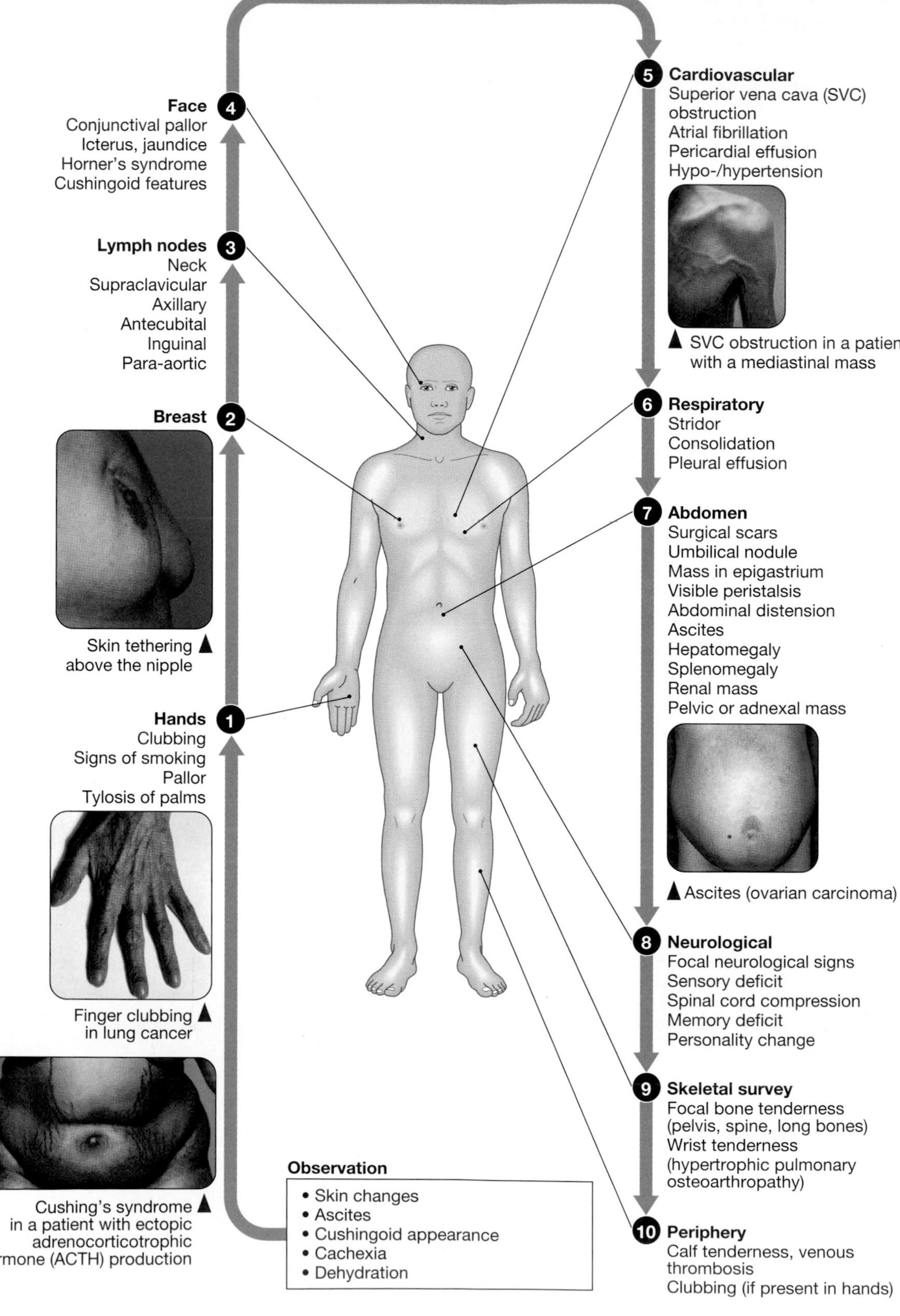

Skin tethering above the nipple

Finger clubbing in lung cancer

Cushing's syndrome in a patient with ectopic adrenocorticotrophic hormone (ACTH) production

SVC obstruction in a patient with a mediastinal mass

Ascites (ovarian carcinoma)

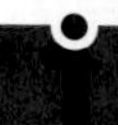

Examination of the skin

Important features of skin lesions that should alert suspicion include:

- Asymmetry: irregular shape
- Bleeding
- Border: not a smooth edge
- Colour: uneven, variegated or changing colour
- Diameter: > 6 mm in diameter or growing
- Itching or pain in a pre-existing mole

7 Abdominal examination

- Are there scars from previous surgery?
- Is the umbilicus everted, suggesting ascites?
- Is there a firm nodule at the umbilicus due to ovarian or gastric cancer metastasis, causing a Sister Mary Joseph's nodule?
- Is there smooth hepatomegaly – possibly primary liver cancer or heart failure?
- Is the liver firm or knobbly, suggesting metastasis?
- Is the ascites too tense to demonstrate hepatomegaly?
- Are other masses palpable in the abdomen?
- Are there signs of obstruction or paralytic ileus with absence of bowel sounds?
- Palpate for inguinal nodes (occasionally involved in ovarian cancer)
- Percuss for flank dullness and shifting dullness
- Perform vaginal and rectal examinations to detect adnexal or rectal masses

3 Examination of the lymph nodes

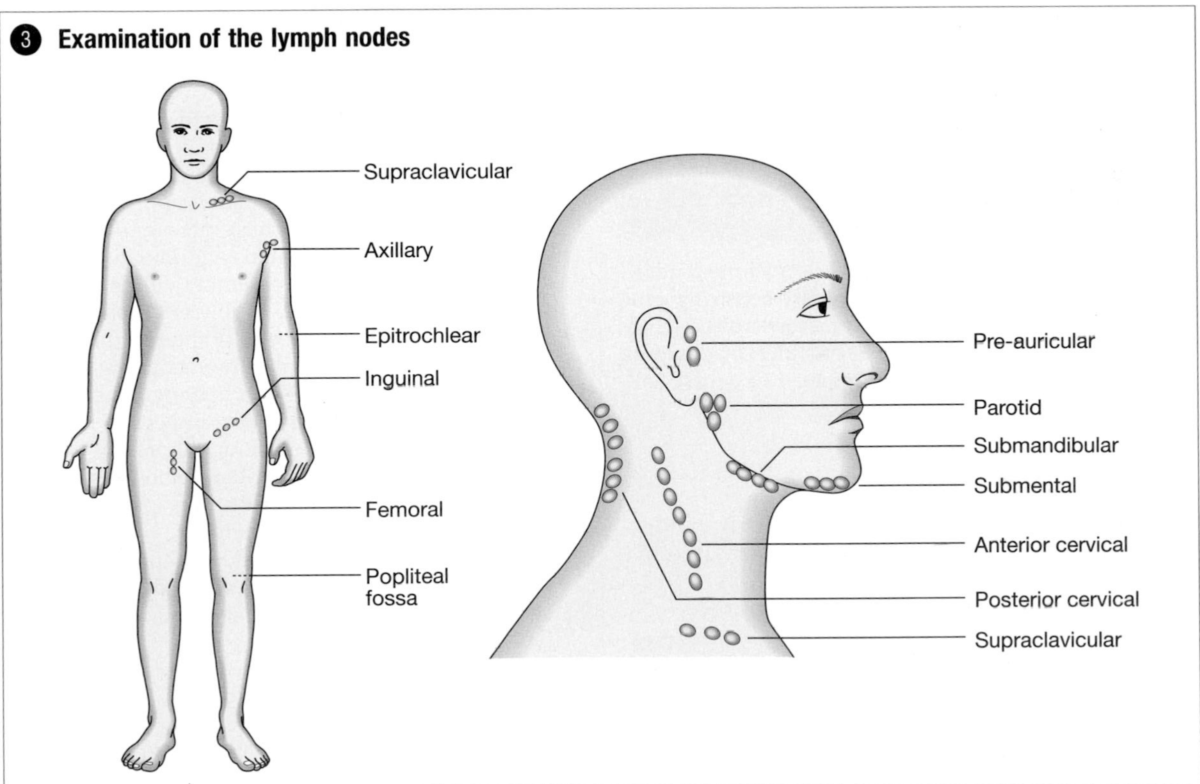

5 Superior vena cava obstruction

- Venous distension of neck
- Elevated but non-pulsatile jugular venous pulse
- Venous distension of chest wall
- Facial oedema
- Cyanosis
- Plethora of face
- Oedema of arms

5 Pericardial effusion

- Tachycardia
- Falling blood pressure
- Rising jugular venous pressure
- Muffled heart sounds
- Kussmaul's sign

6 Malignant pleural effusions

Large right pleural effusion

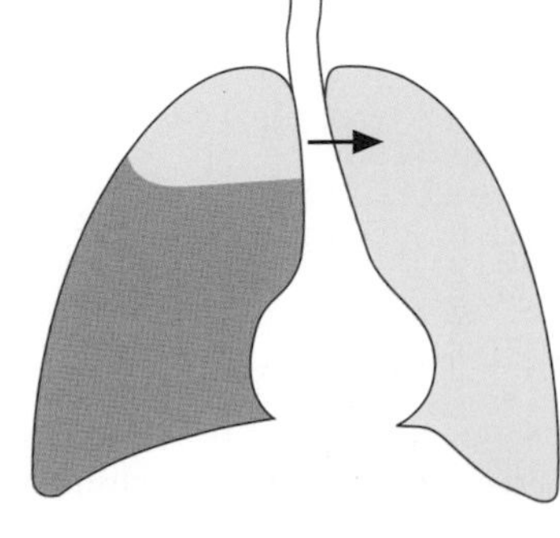

Inspection
Tachypnoea
Palpation
↓Expansion on R
Trachea and apex may be moved to L
Percussion
Stony dull
R mid- and lower zones
Auscultation
Absent breath sounds and diminished or absent vocal resonance R base
Crackles above effusion

Cancer is a significant global health-care problem, with an estimated worldwide incidence of 10 million new cases per year, 46% of which are in developed countries. Mortality is high, with more than 7 million deaths per year. The global costs and socioeconomic impact are considerable. The most common solid organ malignancies arise in the lung, breast and gastrointestinal tract (Fig. 11.1), but the most common form worldwide is skin cancer. Tobacco is a major factor in the aetiology of 30% of cancers, including those of the lung, nasopharynx, bladder and kidney, and these could be prevented by smoking cessation. Diet and alcohol contribute to a further 30% of cancers, including those of the stomach, colon, oesophagus, breast and liver. Lifestyle modification could reduce these if steps were taken to avoid animal fat and red meat, reduce alcohol, increase fibre, fresh fruit and vegetable intake, and avoid obesity. Infections account for a further 15% of cancers, including those of the cervix, stomach, liver, nasopharynx and bladder, and some of these could be prevented by infection control and vaccination.

THE TEN HALLMARKS OF CANCER

The formation and growth of cancer constitute a multistep process, during which sequentially occurring gene mutations result in the formation of a cancerous cell. For cells to initiate carcinogenesis successfully, they require key characteristics, collectively referred to as the hallmarks of cancer.

1. Genome instability and mutation

Random genetic mutations occur continuously throughout all cells of the body and very rarely confer a selective advantage on single cells, allowing overgrowth and dominance in local tissue environments. Multistep carcinogenesis results from successive clonal expansions of pre-malignant cells, each expansion being triggered by acquisition of a random enabling genetic mutation. Under normal circumstances, cellular DNA repair mechanisms are so effective that almost all spontaneous mutations are corrected without producing phenotypic changes, keeping the overall mutation rates very low. In cancer cells, the accumulation of mutations can be accelerated by compromising the surveillance systems that normally monitor genomic integrity and force genetically damaged cells into either senescence or apoptosis. Therefore, they can become more sensitive to mutagenic actions or develop DNA repair mechanism failure.

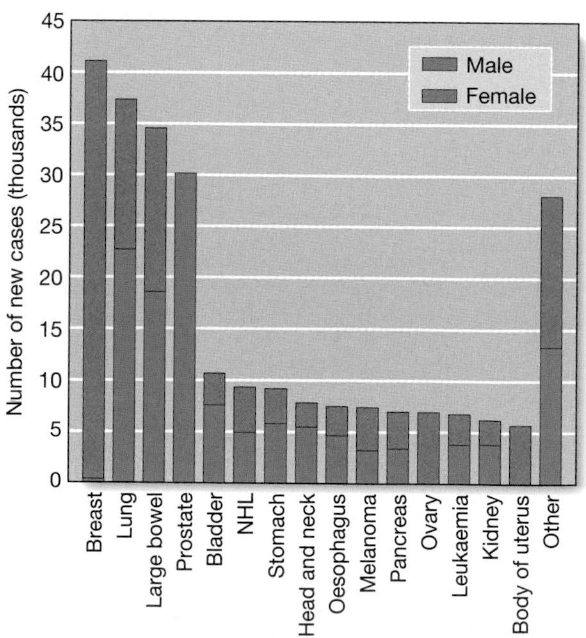

Fig. 11.1 The most commonly diagnosed cancers in the UK. (NHL = non-Hodgkin lymphoma) Statistics from Cancer Research UK website (http://info.cancerresearchuk.org).

2. Resisting cell death

There are three principal mechanisms through which cell death occurs in healthy tissues:

- *Apoptosis* is programmed cell death and is frequently found at markedly reduced rates in cancers, particularly those of high grade or those resistant to treatment. The cellular apoptotic system has regulatory elements which sense intrinsic and extrinsic pro-apoptotic signals and initiate a cascade of proteolysis and cell disassembly with nuclear fragmentation, chromosomal condensation, and shrinking of the cell with loss of intercellular contact, followed by cellular fragmentation and the formation of apoptotic bodies that are phagocytosed by neighbouring cells. The most important regulator of apoptosis is the *TP53* tumour suppressor gene, often described as the 'guardian of the genome', as it is able to induce apoptosis in response to sufficient levels of genomic damage. The largest initiator of apoptosis via *TP53* is cellular injury, particularly due to DNA damage from chemotherapy, oxidative damage and ultraviolet (UV) radiation.
- *Autophagy* is a catabolic process during which cellular constituents are degraded by lysosomal machinery within the cell. It is an important physiological mechanism, which usually occurs at low levels in cells but can be induced in response to environmental stresses, particularly radiotherapy and cytotoxic chemotherapy, which induce elevated levels of autophagy that are cytoprotective for malignant cells, thus impeding rather than perpetuating the killing actions of these stress situations. Severely stressed cancer cells have been shown to shrink via autophagy to a state of reversible dormancy.
- *Necrosis* is the premature death of cells and is characterised by the release of cellular contents into the local tissue microenvironment, in marked contrast to apoptosis, where cells are disassembled in a step-by-step fashion and the resulting cellular fragments phagocytosed. Necrotic cell death results in the recruitment of inflammatory immune cells, promotion of angiogenesis, cellular proliferation and tissue invasion. Necrotic cells also release stimulatory factors, which promote proliferation of neighbouring cells and can promote rather than inhibit carcinogenesis.

3. Sustaining proliferative signalling

Cancer cells can sustain proliferation beyond what would be expected for normal cells; this is typically due to growth factors, which are able to bind to cell surface-bound receptors that activate an intracellular tyrosine kinase-mediated signalling cascade, ultimately leading to changes in gene expression and promoting cellular proliferation and growth. Sustained proliferative capacity can result from over-production of growth factor ligands or receptors and production of structurally altered receptors, which can signal in the absence of ligand binding and activation of intracellular signalling pathway components so that signalling is no longer ligand-dependent.

The cell cycle

The cell cycle is comprised of four ordered, strictly regulated phases referred to as G_1 (gap 1), S (DNA synthesis), G_2 (gap 2) and M (mitosis) (Fig. 11.2). Normal cells grown in culture will stop proliferating and enter a quiescent state called G_0 once they become confluent or are deprived of serum or growth factors. The first gap phase (G_1) prior to the initiation of DNA synthesis represents the period of commitment that separates M and S phases as cells prepare for DNA duplication. Cells in G_0 and G_1 are receptive to growth signals, but once they have passed a restriction point, they are committed to enter DNA synthesis (S phase). Cells demonstrate arrest at different points in G_1 in response to different inhibitory growth signals. Mitogenic signals promote progression through G_1 to S phase, utilising phosphorylation of the retinoblastoma gene product (pRb). Following DNA synthesis, there is a second gap phase (G_2) prior to mitosis (M), allowing cells to repair errors that have occurred during DNA replication and thus preventing propagation of these errors to daughter cells. Although the duration of individual phases may vary, depending on cell and tissue type, most adult cells are in a G_0 state at any one time.

Cell cycle regulation

The cell cycle is orchestrated by a number of molecular mechanisms, most importantly by cyclins and cyclin-dependent kinases (CDKs). Cyclins bind to CDKs, and are regulated by both activating and inactivating phosphorylation, with two main checkpoints at G_1/S and G_2/M transition. The genes that inhibit progression play an important part in tumour prevention and are referred to as tumour suppressor genes (e.g. *TP53, TP21, TP16* genes). The products of these genes deactivate the cyclin–CDK complexes and are thus able to halt the cell cycle. The complexity of cell cycle control is susceptible to dysregulation, which may produce a malignant phenotype.

11

Stimulation of the cell cycle

Many cancer cells produce growth factors, which drive their own proliferation by a positive feedback known as autocrine stimulation. Examples include transforming growth factor-alpha (TGF-α) and platelet-derived growth factor (PDGF). Other cancer cells express growth factor receptors at increased levels due to gene amplification or express abnormal receptors that are permanently activated. This results in abnormal cell growth in response to physiological growth factor stimulation or even in the absence of growth factor stimulation (ligand-independent signalling). The epidermal growth factor receptor (EGFR) is often over-expressed in lung and gastrointestinal tumours and the HER2/neu receptor is frequently over-expressed in breast cancer. Both receptors activate the Ras–Raf–MAP kinase pathway, causing cell proliferation.

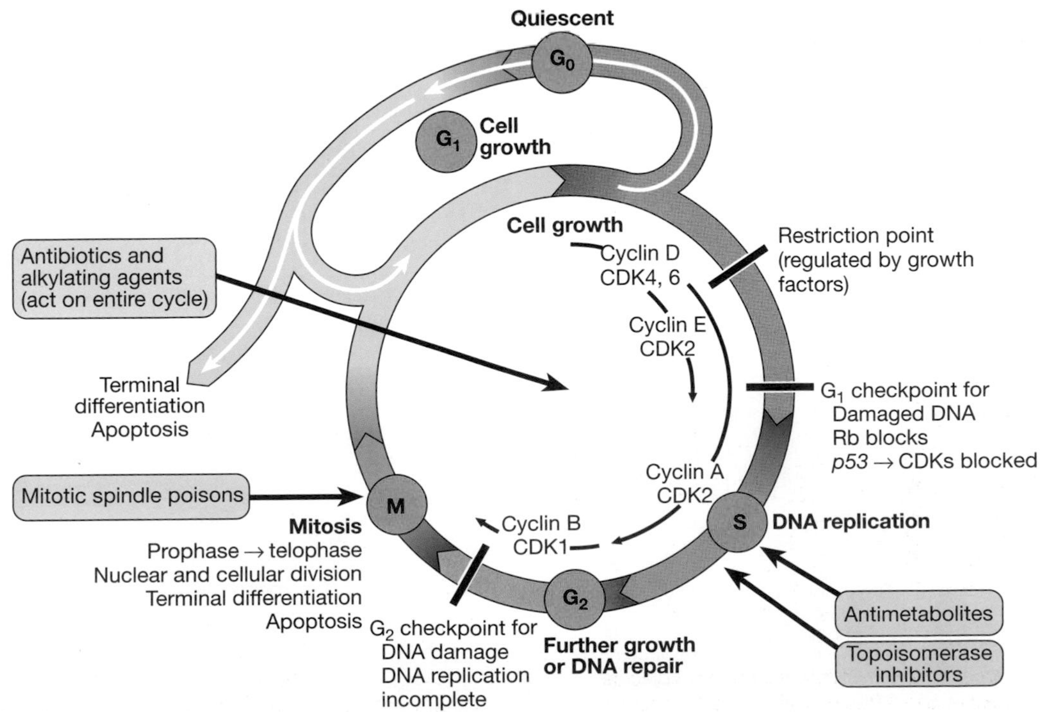

Fig. 11.2 The cell cycle and sites of action of chemotherapeutic agents. (Rb = retinoblastoma gene; CDK = cyclin-dependent kinase)

4. Evading growth suppressors

In healthy tissues, cell-to-cell contact in dense cell populations acts as an inhibitory factor on proliferation. This contact inhibition is typically absent in many cancer cell populations. Growth-inhibitory factors can modulate the cell cycle regulators and produce activation of the CDK inhibitors, causing inhibition of the CDKs. Mutations within inhibitory proteins are common in cancer. Loss of restriction by disruption of pRb regulation can be found in human tumours, which produces a loss of restraint on transition from G_1 to S phase of the cell cycle. Disruption of *p53* function will have downstream effects on *p21* that alter the coordination of DNA repair with cycle arrest and that result in the affected cell accumulating genomic defects. Down-regulation of *p21* and *p27*, which can be found in tumours with normal *p53* function, correlates notably with high tumour grade and poor prognosis.

5. Enabling replicative immortality

For cancer cells to evolve into macroscopic tumours, they need to acquire the ability for unlimited proliferation. Telomeric DNA sequences, which protect and stabilise chromosomal ends, play a central role in conferring this limitless replicative potential. During replication of normal cells, telomeres shorten progressively as small fragments of telomeric DNA are lost with successive cycles of replication. This shortening process is thought to represent a mitotic clock and eventually prevents the cell from dividing further. Telomerase, a specialised polymerase enzyme, adds nucleotides to telomeres, allowing continued cell division and thus preventing premature arrest of cellular replication. The telomerase enzyme is almost absent in normal cells but is expressed at significant levels in many human cancers.

6. Inducing angiogenesis

All cancers require a functional vascular network to ensure continued growth and will be unable to grow beyond 1 mm^3 without stimulating the development of a vascular supply. Tumours require sustenance in the form of nutrients and oxygen, as well as an ability to evacuate metabolic waste products and carbon dioxide. This entails the development of new blood vessels, which is termed angiogenesis (Figs 11.3 and 11.4).

Angiogenesis is dependent on the production of angiogenic growth factors, of which vascular endothelial growth factor (VEGF) and platelet-derived endothelial growth factor (PDGF) are the best characterised. During tumour progression, an angiogenic switch is activated and remains on, causing normally quiescent vasculature to sprout new vessels continually that help sustain expanding tumour growth. Angiogenesis is governed by a balance of pro-angiogenic stimuli and angiogenesis inhibitors, such as thrombospondin (TSP)-1, which binds to transmembrane receptors on endothelial cells and evokes suppressive signals.

A number of cells can contribute to the maintenance of a functional tumour vasculature and therefore sustain angiogenesis. These include pericytes and a variety of bone marrow-derived cells such as macrophages, neutrophils, mast cells and myeloid progenitors.

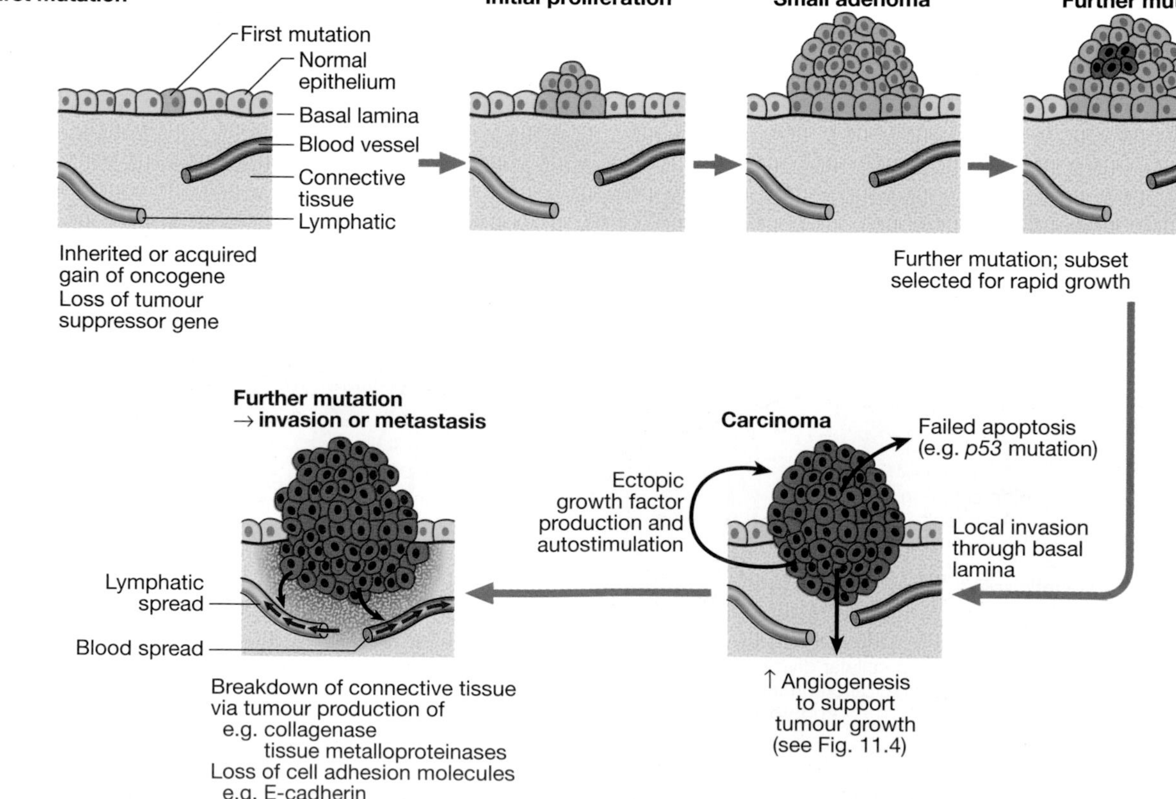

Fig. 11.3 Oncogenesis. The multistep origin of cancer, showing events implicated in cancer initiation, progression, invasion and metastasis.

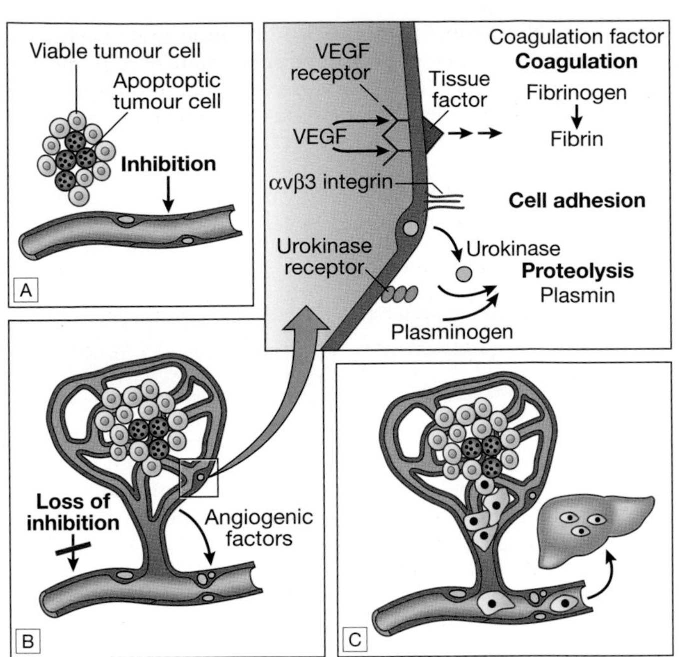

Fig. 11.4 Angiogenesis, invasion and metastasis. **A** For any cancer to grow beyond 1 mm^3 it must evoke a blood supply. **B** New vessel formation results from the release of angiogenic factors by the tumour cells and loss of inhibition of the endothelial cells. **C** The loss of cellular adhesion and disruption of the extracellular matrix allow cells to extravasate into the blood stream and metastasise to distant sites.

7. Activating invasion and metastasis

Invasion and metastasis are complex processes involving multiple discrete steps; it begins with local tissue invasion, followed by infiltration of nearby blood and lymphatic vessels by cancer cells. Malignant cells are eventually transported through haematogenous and lymphatic spread to distant sites within the body, where they form micrometastases that will eventually grow into macroscopic metastatic lesions (see Fig. 11.3).

Cadherin-1 (CDH1) is a calcium-dependent cell–cell adhesion glycoprotein that facilitates assembly of organised cell sheets in tissues, and increased expression is recognised as an antagonist of invasion and metastasis. In situ tumours usually retain cadherin-1 production, whereas loss of cadherin-1 production due to down-regulation or occasional mutational inactivation of CDH1 has been observed in human cancers, supporting the theory that CDH1 plays a key role in suppression of invasion and metastasis.

Cross-talk between cancer cells and cells of the surrounding stromal tissue is involved in the acquired capability for invasive growth and metastasis. Mesenchymal stem cells in tumour stroma have been found to secrete CCL5, a protein chemokine that helps recruit leucocytes into inflammatory sites. With the help of particular T-cell-derived cytokines (interleukin (IL)-2 and interferon (IFN)-γ), CCL5 induces proliferation and activation of natural killer cells and then acts reciprocally on cancer cells to stimulate invasive behaviour. Macrophages at the tumour periphery can foster local invasion by supplying matrix-degrading enzymes such as metalloproteinases and cysteine cathepsin proteases.

8. Reprogramming energy metabolism

Under aerobic conditions, oxidative phosphorylation functions as the main metabolic pathway for energy production; cells process glucose, first to pyruvate via glycolysis and thereafter to carbon dioxide in the mitochondria. Whilst under anaerobic conditions, glycolysis is favoured to produce adenosine triphosphate (ATP). Cancer cells can reprogramme their glucose metabolism to limit energy production to glycolysis, even in the presence of oxygen. This has been termed 'aerobic glycolysis'. Up-regulation of glucose transporters, such as GLUT1, is the main mechanism through which aerobic glycolysis is achieved.

This reprogramming of energy metabolism appears paradoxical, as overall energy production from glycolysis is significantly lower (18-fold) than that from oxidative phosphorylation. One explanation may be that the increased production of glycolytic intermediates can be fed into various biosynthetic pathways, including those that generate the nucleosides and amino acids, necessary for the production of new cells.

9. Tumour-promoting inflammation

Almost all tumours show infiltration with immune cells on pathological investigation and historically this finding was thought to represent an attempt of the immune system to eradicate the cancer. It is now clear that tumour-associated inflammatory responses promote tumour formation and cancer progression.

Cytokines are able to alter blood vessels to permit migration of leucocytes (mainly neutrophils), in order to permeate from the blood vessels into the tissue, a process known as extravasation. Migration across the endothelium occurs via the process of diapedesis, where chemokine gradients stimulate adhered leucocytes to move between endothelial cells and pass through the basement membrane into the surrounding tissues. Once within the tissue interstitium, leucocytes bind to extracellular matrix proteins via integrins and CD44 to prevent their loss from the site.

As well as cell-derived mediators, several acellular biochemical cascade systems consisting of pre-formed plasma proteins act in parallel to initiate and propagate the inflammatory response. These include the complement system activated by bacteria, and the coagulation and fibrinolytic systems activated by necrosis, and also in burns and trauma, as well as cancer. Other bioactive molecules, such as growth factors and pro-angiogenic factors, may be released by inflammatory immune cells into the surrounding tumour microenvironment. In particular, the release of reactive oxygen species, which are actively mutagenic, will accelerate the genetic evolution of surrounding cancer cells, enhancing growth and contributing to cancer progression.

10. Evading immune destruction

The immune system operates as a significant barrier to tumour formation and progression, and the ability to escape from immunity is a hallmark of cancer development. Cancer cells continuously shed surface antigens into the circulatory system, prompting an immune response that includes cytotoxic T cell, natural killer cell and macrophage production. The immune system is thought to provide continuous surveillance, with resultant elimination of cells that undergo malignant transformation.

However, deficiencies in the development or function of CD8+ cytotoxic T lymphocytes, CD4+ Th1 helper T cells, or natural killer cells can each lead to a demonstrable increase in cancer incidence. Also, highly immunogenic cancer cells may evade immune destruction by disabling components of the immune system. This is done through recruitment of inflammatory cells, including regulatory T cells and myeloid-derived suppressor cells, both actively immunosuppressive against the actions of cytotoxic lymphocytes (see Fig. 4.6, p. 80).

Cancers develop and progress when there is loss of recognition by the immune system, lack of susceptibility due to escape from immune cell action and induction of immune dysfunction, often via inflammatory mediators.

ENVIRONMENTAL AND GENETIC DETERMINANTS OF CANCER

The majority of cancers do not have a single cause but rather are the result of a complex interaction between genetic factors and exposure to environmental carcinogens. These are often tumour type-specific but some general principles do apply.

Environmental factors

Environmental triggers for cancer have mainly been identified through epidemiological studies that examine patterns of distribution of cancers in patients in whom age, sex, presence of other illnesses, social class, geography and so on differ. Sometimes, these give strong

11.1 Environmental factors that predispose to cancer

Environmental aetiology	Processes	Diseases
Occupational exposure (see also ultraviolet and radiation)	Dye and rubber manufacturing (aromatic amines) Asbestos mining, construction work, shipbuilding (asbestos) Vinyl chloride (PVC) manufacturing Petroleum industry (benzene)	Bladder cancer Lung cancer and mesothelioma Liver angiosarcoma Acute leukaemia
Chemicals	Chemotherapy (e.g. melphalan, cyclophosphamide)	Acute myeloid leukaemia
Cigarette smoking	Exposure to carcinogens from inhaled smoke	Lung and bladder cancer
Viral infection	Epstein–Barr virus Human papillomavirus Hepatitis B and C viruses	Burkitt's lymphoma and nasopharyngeal cancer Cervical cancer Hepatocellular carcinoma
Bacterial infection	*Helicobacter pylori*	Gastric mucosa-associated lymphoid tissue (MALT) lymphomas, gastric cancer
Parasitic infection	Liver fluke *(Opisthorchis sinensis)* *Schistosoma haematobium*	Cholangiocarcinoma Squamous cell bladder cancer
Dietary factors	Low-roughage/high-fat content diet High nitrosamine intake Aflatoxin from contamination of *Aspergillus flavus*	Colonic cancer Gastric cancer Hepatocellular cancer
Radiation	Ultraviolet (UV) exposure Nuclear fallout following explosion (e.g. Hiroshima) Diagnostic exposure (e.g. computed tomography (CT)) Occupational exposure (e.g. beryllium and strontium mining) Therapeutic radiotherapy	Basal cell carcinoma Melanoma Non-melanocytic skin cancer Leukaemia Solid tumours, e.g. thyroid Cholangiocarcinoma following thorotrast usage Lung cancer Medullary thyroid cancer Sarcoma
Inflammatory diseases	Ulcerative colitis	Colon cancer
Hormonal	Use of diethylstilbestrol Oestrogens	Vaginal cancer Endometrial cancer Breast cancer

pointers to the molecular or cellular causes of the disease, such as the association between aflatoxin production within contaminated food supplies and hepatocellular carcinomas. However, for many solid cancers, such as breast and colorectal, there is evidence of a multifactorial pathogenesis, even when there is a principal environmental cause (Box 11.1).

Smoking is now established beyond all doubt as a major cause of lung cancer, but there are obviously additional predisposing factors since not all smokers develop cancer. Similarly, most carcinomas of the cervix are related to infection with human papillomavirus (HPV subtypes 16 and 18). For carcinomas of the bowel and breast, there is strong evidence of an environmental component. For example, the risk of breast cancer in women of Far Eastern origin remains relatively low when they first migrate to a country with a Western lifestyle, but rises in subsequent generations to approach that of the resident population of the host country. The precise environmental factor that causes this change is unclear, but may include diet (higher intake of saturated fat and/or dairy products), reproductive patterns (later onset of first pregnancy) and lifestyle (increased use of artificial light and shift in diurnal rhythm).

Genetic factors

A number of inherited cancer syndromes are recognised that account for 5–10% of all cancers (Box 11.2). Their molecular basis is discussed in Chapter 3, but in general they result from inherited mutations in genes that regulate cell growth, cell death and apoptosis. Examples include the *BRCA1*, *BRCA2* and *AT* (ataxia telangiectasia) genes that cause breast and some other cancers, the *FAP* gene that causes bowel cancer, and the *Rb* gene that causes retinoblastoma. Although carriers of these gene mutations have a greatly elevated risk of cancer, none has 100% penetrance and additional modulating factors, both genetic and environmental, are likely to be operative. Exploration of a possible genetic contribution is a key part of cancer management, especially with regard to ascertaining the risk for an affected patient's offspring.

11

11.2 Inherited cancer predisposition syndromes

Syndrome	Malignancies	Inheritance	Gene
Ataxia telangiectasia	Leukaemia, lymphoma, ovarian, gastric, brain, colon	AR	*AT*
Breast/ovarian	Breast, ovarian, colonic, prostatic, pancreatic	AD	*BRCA1, BRCA2*
Bloom's syndrome	Leukaemia, tongue, oesophageal, colonic, Wilms' tumour	AR	*BLM*
Cowden's syndrome	Breast, thyroid, gastrointestinal tract, pancreatic	AD	*PTEN*
Familial adenomatous polyposis	Colonic, upper gastrointestinal tract	AD	*APC, MUTYH*
Fanconi anaemia	Leukaemia, oesophageal, skin, hepatoma	AR	*FACA, FACC, FACD*
Gorlin's syndrome	Basal cell skin, brain	AD	*PTCH*
Hereditary non-polyposis colon cancer (HNPCC)	Colonic, endometrial, ovarian, pancreatic, gastric	AD	*MSH2, MLH1, MSH6, PMS1, PMS2*
Li–Fraumeni syndrome	Sarcoma, breast, osteosarcoma, leukaemia, glioma, adrenocortical	AD	*TP53*
Melanoma	Melanoma	AD	*CDK2 (TP16)*
Multiple endocrine neoplasia (MEN)-1	Pancreatic islet cell, pituitary adenoma, parathyroid adenoma and hyperplasia	AD	*MEN1*
MEN-2	Medullary thyroid, phaeochromocytoma, parathyroid hyperplasia	AD	*RET*
Neurofibromatosis 1	Neurofibrosarcoma, phaeochromocytoma, optic glioma	AD	*NF1*
Neurofibromatosis 2	Vestibular schwannoma	AD	*NF2*
Papillary renal cell cancer syndrome	Renal cell cancer	AD	*MET*
Peutz–Jeghers syndrome	Colonic, ileal, breast, ovarian	AD	*STK11*
Prostate cancer	Prostate	AD	*HPC1*
Retinoblastoma	Retinoblastoma, osteosarcoma	AD	*RB1*
von Hippel–Lindau syndrome	Haemangioblastoma of retina and CNS, renal cell, phaeochromocytoma	AD	*VHL*
Wilms' tumour	Nephroblastoma, neuroblastoma, hepatoblastoma, rhabdomyosarcoma	AD	*WT1*
Xeroderma pigmentosum	Skin, leukaemia, melanoma	AR	*XPA, XPC, XPD (ERCC2), XPF*

(AD = autosomal dominant; AR = autosomal recessive)

INVESTIGATIONS

When a patient is suspected of having cancer, a full history should be taken; specific questions should be included as to potential risk factors such as smoking and occupational exposures. A thorough clinical examination is also essential to identify sites of metastases, and to discover any other conditions that may have a bearing on the management plan. In order to make a diagnosis and to plan the most appropriate management, information is needed on:

- the type of tumour
- the extent of disease, as assessed by staging investigations
- the patient's general condition and any comorbidity.

The overall fitness of a patient is often assessed by the Eastern Cooperative Oncology Group (ECOG) performance scale (Box 11.3). The outcome for patients with a performance status of 3 or 4 is worse in almost all malignancies than for those with a status of 0–2, and this has a strong influence on the approach to treatment in the individual patient.

The process of staging determines the extent of the tumour; it entails clinical examination, imaging and in some cases surgery, to establish the extent of disease involvement. The outcome is recorded using a standard staging classification that allows comparisons to be made between different groups of patients. Therapeutic decisions and prognostic predictions can then be made using the evidence base for the disease. One of the most commonly used systems is the T (tumour), N (regional lymph nodes), M (metastatic sites) approach of the International Union against Cancer (UICC, Box 11.4). For some tumours, such as colon cancer, the Dukes system (p. 914) is used rather than the UICC classification.

11.3 Eastern Cooperative Oncology Group (ECOG) performance status scale

0	Fully active, able to carry on all usual activities without restriction and without the aid of analgesics
1	Restricted in strenuous activity but ambulatory and able to carry out light work or pursue a sedentary occupation. This group also contains patients who are fully active, as in grade 0, but only with the aid of analgesics
2	Ambulatory and capable of all self-care but unable to work. Up and about more than 50% of waking hours
3	Capable of only limited self-care, confined to bed or chair more than 50% of waking hours
4	Completely disabled, unable to carry out any self-care and confined totally to bed or chair

11.4 TNM classification

Extent of primary tumour*	
TX	Not assessed
T0	No tumour
T1, T2, T3, T4	Increases in primary tumour size or depth of invasion
Increased involvement of nodes*	
NX	Not assessed
N0	No nodal involvement
N1, N2/3	Increases in involvement
Presence of metastases	
MX	Not assessed
M0	Not present
M1	Present

*Exact criteria for size and region of nodal involvement have been defined for each anatomical site.

Histology

Histological analysis of a biopsy or resected specimen is pivotal in clinching the diagnosis and in deciding on the best form of management. The results of histological analysis are most informative when combined with knowledge of the clinical picture; therefore biopsy results should be reviewed and discussed within the context of a multidisciplinary team meeting.

Light microscopy

Examination of tumour samples by light microscopy remains the core method of cancer diagnosis and, in cases where the primary site is unclear, may also give clues to the origin of the tumour:

- Signet-ring cells favour a gastric primary.
- Presence of melanin favours melanoma.
- Mucin is common in gut/lung/breast/endometrial cancers, but particularly common in ovarian cancer and rare in renal cell or thyroid cancers.
- Psammoma bodies are a feature of ovarian cancer (mucin +) and thyroid cancer (mucin –).

Immunohistochemistry

Immunohistochemical (IHC) staining for tumour markers can provide useful diagnostic information and can help with treatment decisions. Commonly used examples of IHC in clinical practice include:

- *Oestrogen (ER) and progesterone (PR) receptors.* Positive results indicate that the tumour may be sensitive to hormonal manipulation.
- *Alpha-fetoprotein (AFP)* and *human chorionic gonadotrophin (hCG) ± placental alkaline phosphatase (PLAP).* These favour germ-cell tumours.
- *Prostate-specific antigen (PSA)* and *prostatic acid phosphatase (PAP).* These favour prostate cancer.
- *Carcinoembryonic antigen (CEA), cytokeratin* and *epithelial membrane antigen (EMA).* These favour carcinomas.
- *HER2 receptor.* Breast cancers that have high levels of expression of HER2 indicate that the tumour may respond to trastuzumab (herceptin), an antibody directed against the HER2 receptor.

The pattern of immunoglobulin, T-cell receptor and cluster designation (CD) antigen expression on the surface is also helpful in the diagnosis and classification of lymphomas. This can be achieved by IHC staining of biopsy samples or flow cytometry.

Electron microscopy

Electron microscopy (EM) can sometimes be of diagnostic value. Examples include the visualisation of melanosomes in amelanotic melanoma and dense core granules in neuro-endocrine tumours. EM may also help to distinguish adenocarcinoma from mesothelioma, as the ultrastructural properties of these two diseases are different (mesothelioma appears to have long, narrow, branching microvilli while adenocarcinomas appear to have short, stubby microvilli). EM is also useful for differentiating spindle-cell tumours (sarcomas, melanomas, squamous cell cancers) from small round-cell tumours, again due to their ultra-structural differences.

Cytogenetic analysis

Some tumours demonstrate typical chromosomal changes that help in diagnosis. The utilisation of fluorescent in situ hybridisation (FISH) techniques can be useful in Ewing's sarcoma and peripheral neuroectodermal tumours where there is a translocation between chromosome 11 and 22–t(11; 22)(q24; q12). In some cases, gene amplification can also be detected via FISH (e.g. determining over-expression of HER2/neu).

Imaging

Imaging plays a critical role in oncology, not only in locating the primary tumour, but also in staging the disease. The imaging modality employed depends primarily on the site of the disease and likely patterns of spread, but usually more than one modality is required.

Radiography

Plain radiographs remain part of the initial workup, but have a limited role in defining disease extent and have been superseded by more sophisticated techniques.

Ultrasound

Ultrasound is useful in characterising lesions within the liver, kidney, pancreas and reproductive organs. It can be used for guiding biopsies of tumours in breast and liver. Endoscopic ultrasound is helpful in staging upper gastrointestinal and pancreatic cancers; it involves a special endoscope with an ultrasound probe attached.

Computerised tomography

Computerised tomography (CT) is a key investigation in cancer patients and is particularly useful in imaging the thorax and abdomen. With some modern scanners it is possible to visualise the bowel, and sometimes detection of colorectal adenomas and cancer is feasible.

Magnetic resonance imaging

Magnetic resonance imaging (MRI) has a high resolution and because of this is the preferred technique for brain imaging. It is also used to image structures within the pelvis and is widely employed for staging of rectal, cervical and prostate cancers.

Positron emission tomography

Positron emission tomography (PET) visualises metabolic activity of tumour cells and is widely used, often in combination with CT (PET-CT), to evaluate patients with various cancers, including lung cancer and lymphoma (Fig. 11.5). It can accurately assess the severity and spread of cancer by detecting tumour metabolic activity following injection of small amounts of radioactive tracers such as fluorodeoxyglucose (FDG). In addition to having a role in diagnosis, PET can also be used in some patients to assess treatment response.

A
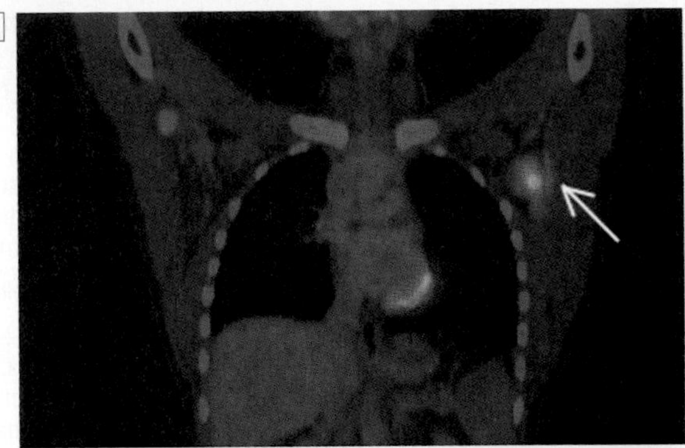

B
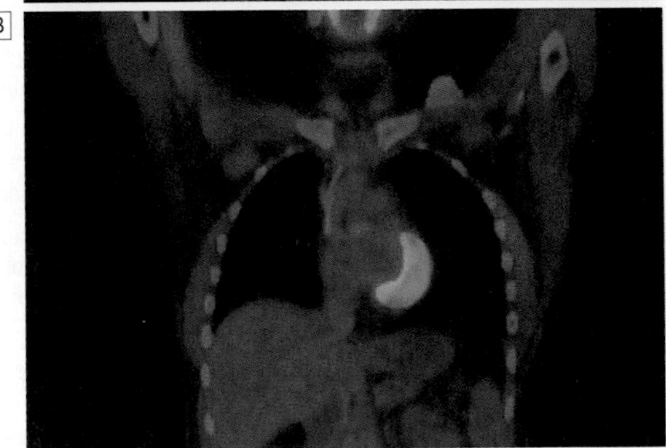

Fig. 11.5 PET-CT images. **A** There is a neoplastic lesion in the left axilla, evidenced by the increased uptake of FDG traces. **B** Imaging after chemotherapy, demonstrating that the abnormal uptake has disappeared and indicating a response to treatment.

Biochemical markers

Many tumours produce substances called tumour markers, which can be used in diagnosis and surveillance. Some are useful in population screening, diagnosis, prognostication, treatment monitoring, detection of relapse and imaging of metastasis. Unfortunately, most tumour markers are not sufficiently sensitive or specific to be used in isolation and need to be interpreted in the context of the other clinical features. However, some can be used for antibody-directed therapy or imaging, where they have a greater role in diagnosis. Tumour markers in routine use are outlined in Box 11.5.

PRESENTING PROBLEMS IN ONCOLOGY

In the early stages of cancer development, the number of malignant cells is small and the patient is usually asymptomatic. With tumour progression, localised signs or symptoms develop due to mass effects and/or invasion of local tissues. With further progression, symptoms may occur at distant sites as a result of metastatic disease or from non-metastatic manifestations due to

11.5 Commonly used serum tumour markers

Name	Natural occurrence	Tumours
Alpha-fetoprotein (AFP)	Glycoprotein found in yolk sac and fetal liver tissue. Transient elevation in liver diseases. Has a role in screening during pregnancy for the detection of neural tube defects and Down's syndrome	Ovarian non-seminomatous germ cell tumours (80%), testicular teratoma (80%), hepatocellular cancer (50%)
Calcitonin	32 amino acid peptide from C cells of thyroid. Used to screen for MEN-2	Medullary cell carcinoma of thyroid
Cancer antigen 125 (CA-125)	Differentiation antigen of coelomic epithelium (Muller's duct). Raised in any cause of ascites, pleural effusion or heart failure. Can be raised in inflammatory conditions	Ovarian epithelial cancer (75%), gastrointestinal cancer (10%), lung cancer (5%) and breast cancer (5%)
CA-19.9	A mucin found in epithelium of fetal stomach, intestine and pancreas. It is eliminated exclusively via bile and so any degree of cholestasis can cause levels to rise	Pancreatic cancer (80%), mucinous tumour of the ovary (65%), gastric cancer (30%), colon cancer (30%)
Carcinoembryonic antigen (CEA)	Glycoprotein found in intestinal mucosa during embryonic and fetal life. Elevated in smokers, cirrhosis, chronic hepatitis, ulcerative colitis, pneumonia	Colorectal cancer, particularly with liver metastasis, gastric cancer, breast cancer, lung cancer, mucinous cancer of the ovary
Human chorionic gonadotrophin (hCG)	Glycoprotein hormone, 14KD α subunit and 24KD β subunit from placental syncytiotrophoblasts. Used for disease monitoring in hydatidiform mole and as the basis of a pregnancy test	Choriocarcinoma (100%), hydatidiform moles (97%), ovarian non-seminomatous germ cell tumours (50–80%), seminoma (15%)
Placental alkaline phosphatase (PLAP)	Isoenzyme of alkaline phosphatase	Seminoma (40%), ovarian dysgerminoma (50%)
Prostate-specific antigen (PSA)	Glycoprotein member of human kallikrein gene family. PSA is a serine protease that liquefies semen in excretory ducts of prostate. Can be elevated in benign prostatic hypertrophy and prostatitis	Prostate cancer (95%)
Thyroglobulin	Matrix protein for thyroid hormone synthesis in normal thyroid follicles	Papillary and follicular thyroid cancer
β-2-microglobulin	A human leucocyte antigen (HLA) common fragment present on surface of lymphocytes, macrophages and some epithelial cells. Can be elevated in autoimmune disease and renal glomerular disease	Non-Hodgkin's lymphoma, myeloma

11.6 Local features of malignant disease

Symptom	Typical site or possible tumour
Haemorrhage	Stomach, colon, bronchus, endometrium, bladder, kidney
Lump	Breast, lymph node (any site), testicle
Bone pain or fracture	Bone (primary sarcoma, secondary metastasis from breast, prostate, bronchus, thyroid, kidney)
Skin abnormality	Melanoma, basal cell carcinoma (rodent ulcer)
Ulcer	Oesophagus, stomach, anus, skin
Dysphagia	Oesophagus, bronchus, gastric
Increasing constipation, abdominal discomfort or pain	Colon, rectum, ovary
Airway obstruction, stridor, cough, recurrent infection	Bronchus, thyroid
Odynophagia, early satiety, vomiting	Bronchus, stomach, oesophagus, colon, rectum
Abdominal swelling (ascites)	Ovary, stomach, pancreas

production of biologically active hormones by the tumour or as the result of an immune response to the tumour. The possible presentations are summarised in Boxes 11.6 and 11.7, and common presenting features discussed below. Although the incidence of cancer increases with patient age, the approach to investigation and management is similar at all ages (Box 11.8).

Palpable mass

A palpable mass detected by the patient or physician may be the first sign of cancer. Primary tumours of the thyroid, breast, testis and skin are often detected in this way, whereas palpable lymph nodes in the neck, groin

11.7 Non-metastatic manifestations of malignant disease

Feature	Common cancer site associations
Weight loss and anorexia	Lung, gastrointestinal tract
Fatigue	Any
Hypercalcaemia	Myeloma, breast, kidney
Prothrombotic tendency	Ovary, pancreas, gastrointestinal tract
SIADH **Ectopic ACTH**	Small cell lung cancer
Lambert–Eaton myasthenia-like syndrome	Small cell lung cancer
Subacute cerebellar degeneration	Small cell lung cancer, ovarian cancer
Acanthosis nigricans	Stomach, oesophagus
Dermatomyositis/ polymyositis	Stomach, lung

(ACTH = adrenocorticotrophic hormone; SIADH = syndrome of inappropriate antidiuretic hormone secretion)

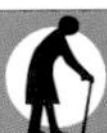

11.8 Cancer in old age

- **Incidence**: around 50% of cancers occur in the 15% of the population aged over 65 years.
- **Screening**: women aged over 65 in the UK are not invited to breast cancer screening but can request it. Uptake is low despite increasing incidence with age.
- **Presentation**: may be later for some cancers. When symptoms are non-specific, patients (and their doctors) may initially attribute them to age alone.
- **Life expectancy**: an 80-year-old woman can expect to live 8 years, so cancer may still shorten life and an active approach remains appropriate.
- **Prognosis**: histology, stage at presentation and observation for a brief period are better guides to outcome than age.
- **Rate of progression**: malignancy may have a more indolent course. This is poorly understood but may be due to reduced effectiveness of angiogenesis with age, inhibiting the development of metastases.
- **Response to treatment**: equivalent to that in younger people – well documented for a range of cancers and for surgery, radiotherapy, chemotherapy and hormonal therapy.
- **Treatment selection**: chronological age is of minor importance compared to comorbid illness and patient choice. Although older patients can be treated effectively and safely, aggressive intervention is not appropriate for all. Symptom control may be all that is possible or desired by the patient.

or axilla may indicate secondary spread of tumour. Hepatomegaly may be the first sign of primary liver cancer or tumour metastasis, whereas skin cancer may present as an enlarging or changing pigmented lesion.

Weight loss and fever

Unintentional weight loss is a characteristic feature of advanced cancer, but can be due to other causes such as thyrotoxicosis, chronic inflammatory disease and chronic infective disorders. Fever can occur in any cancer secondary to infection, but may be a primary feature in Hodgkin's disease, lymphoma, leukaemia, renal cancer and liver cancer. The presence of unexplained weight loss or fever warrants investigation to exclude the presence of occult malignancy.

Finger clubbing

Finger clubbing is a characteristic feature of lung cancer, and especially non-small cell lung cancer, although benign causes are recognised. It is often part of the wider process of hypertrophic osteoarthropathy in which there is periosteal new bone formation and arthritis due to increased levels of prostaglandin E. The diagnosis is primarily clinical, but X-rays show periosteal reaction and an isotope bone scan shows increased tracer update in the affected digits.

Ectopic hormone production

In some cases, the first presentation of cancer is with a metabolic abnormality due to ectopic production of hormones by tumour cells, including insulin, ACTH, ADH, fibroblast growth factor (FGF) 23, erythropoietin and parathyroid hormone-related protein (PTHrP). This can result in a wide variety of presentations, as summarised in Box 11.9. Further details on presentation and management of ACTH- and ADH-producing tumours are given on page 776, and of FGF23-producing tumours on page 1128. The management of hypercalcaemia associated with malignancy is discussed on page 273.

11.9 Ectopic hormone production by tumours

Hormone	Consequence	Tumours
ADH	Hyponatraemia	SCLC
ACTH	Cushing's syndrome	SCLC
FGF-23	Hypophosphataemic osteomalacia	Mesenchymal tumours
Insulin	Hypoglycaemia	Insulinoma
Erythropoietin	Polycythaemia	Kidney, hepatoma, cerebellar haemangioblastoma, uterine fibroids
PTHrP	Hypercalcaemia	NSCLC (squamous cell), breast, kidney

(ACTH = adrenocorticotrophic hormone; ADH = antidiuretic hormone; FGF = fibroblast growth factor; NSCLC = non-small cell lung cancer; PTHrP = parathyroid hormone-related protein; SCLC = small cell lung cancer)

Neurological paraneoplastic syndromes

These form a group of conditions associated with cancer thought to be due to an immunological response to the tumour that results in damage to the nervous system or muscle. The cancers most commonly implicated are those of the lung (small cell and non-small cell), pancreas, breast, prostate, ovary and lymphoma.

- *Peripheral neuropathy* results from axonal degeneration or demyelination.
- *Encephalomyelitis* can present with diverse symptoms, depending on which region of the brain is involved. Lumbar puncture shows raised protein in the cerebrospinal fluid (CSF) and a pleocytosis, predominantly that of lymphocytes. In some centres, flow cytometry of the CSF is also used to detect carcinomatous cells. MRI shows meningeal enhancement, particularly at the level of the brain stem, and anti-Hu antibodies may be detectable in serum. Encephalomyelitis is due to perivascular inflammation and selective neuronal degeneration. Most cases are caused by small cell lung cancer (75%).
- *Cerebellar degeneration* may be the presenting feature of an underlying malignancy and presents with rapid onset of cerebellar ataxia. Diagnosis is by MRI or CT, which may show cerebellar atrophy. Patients with these neurological paraneoplastic syndromes may be found to have circulating anti-Yo, Tr and Hu antibodies, but these are not completely specific and negative results do not exclude the diagnosis.
- *Retinopathy* is a rare complication of cancer and presents with blurred vision, episodic visual loss and impaired colour vision. If left untreated, it may lead to blindness. The diagnosis should be suspected if the electroretinogram is abnormal and anti-retinal antibodies are detected.
- *Lambert–Eaton syndrome* (LEMS) is due to underlying cancer in about 60% of cases. It presents with proximal muscle weakness that improves on exercise and is caused by the development of antibodies to pre-synaptic calcium channels (p. 1227). The diagnosis is made by electromyelogram (EMG), which shows a low-amplitude compound muscle action potential that enhances to near normal following exercise.
- *Dermatomyositis* or *polymyositis* may be the first presentation of some cancers. Clinical features and management of these conditions are discussed on page 1114.

Cutaneous manifestations of cancer

Many cancers can present with skin manifestations that are not due to metastases:

- *Pruritus* may be a presenting feature of lymphoma, leukaemia and CNS tumours.
- *Acanthosis nigricans* may precede cancers by many years and is particularly associated with gastric cancer.
- *Vitiligo* may be associated with malignant melanoma, and is possibly due to an immune response to melanocytes.
- *Pemphigus* may occur in lymphoma, Kaposi's sarcoma and thymic tumours.
- *Dermatitis herpetiformis* associated with coeliac disease may precede tumour development by many years, and is associated with gastrointestinal lymphoma.

The clinical features and management of these skin conditions is discussed in Chapter 28.

EMERGENCY COMPLICATIONS OF CANCER

Spinal cord compression

Spinal cord compression complicates 5% of cancers and is most common in myeloma, prostate, breast and lung cancers that involve bone. Cord compression often results from posterior extension of a vertebral body mass but intrathecal spinal cord metastases can cause similar signs and symptoms.

Clinical features

The earliest sign is back pain, particularly on coughing and lying flat. Subsequently, sensory changes develop in dermatomes below the level of compression and motor weakness distal to the block occurs. Finally, sphincter disturbance, causing urinary retention and bowel incontinence, is observed. Involvement of the lumbar spine may cause conus medullaris or cauda equina compression (Box 11.10). Physical examination reveals findings consistent with an upper motor neuron lesion, but lower motor neuron findings may predominate early on or in cases of nerve root compression.

Management

Spinal cord compression is a medical emergency and should be treated with analgesia and high-dose steroid therapy (Box 11.11). Neurosurgical treatment produces superior outcome and survival compared to radiotherapy alone, and should be considered first for all patients. Radiotherapy is used for the remaining patients and selected tumour types when the cancer is likely to be radiosensitive. The prognosis varies considerably, depending on tumour type, but the degree of neurological dysfunction at presentation is the strongest predictor of outcome irrespective of the underlying diagnosis.

11.10 Comparison of features of neurological deficit

Clinical feature	Spinal cord	Conus medullaris	Cauda equina
Weakness	Symmetrical and profound	Symmetrical and variable	Asymmetrical, may be mild
Reflexes	Increased (or absent) knee and ankle reflexes with extensor plantar reflex	Increased knee reflex, decreased ankle reflex, extensor plantar reflex	Decreased knee and ankle reflexes with flexor plantar reflex
Sensory loss	Symmetrical, sensory level	Symmetrical, saddle distribution	Asymmetrical, radicular pattern
Sphincters	Late loss	Early loss	Often spared
Progression	Rapid	Variable	Variable

11.11 Management of suspected spinal cord compression

- Confirm diagnosis with urgent MRI scan
- Administer high-dose steroids
  - Dexamethasone 16 mg IV stat
  - Dexamethasone 8 mg twice daily orally
- Ensure adequate analgesia
- Refer for surgical decompression or urgent radiotherapy

Ambulation can be preserved in more than 80% of patients who are ambulatory at presentation, but neurological function is seldom regained in patients with established deficits such as paraplegia.

Superior vena cava obstruction

Superior vena cava obstruction (SVCO) is a common complication of cancer that can occur through extrinsic compression or intravascular blockage. The most common causes of extrinsic compression are lung cancer, lymphoma and metastatic tumours. Patients with cancer can also develop SVCO due to intravascular blockage in association with a central catheter or thrombophilia secondary to the tumour.

Clinical features

The typical presentation is with oedema of the arms and face, distended neck and arm veins and dusky skin coloration over the chest, arms and face. Collaterals may develop over a period of weeks and the flow of blood in the collaterals helps to confirm the diagnosis. Headache secondary to cerebral oedema arising from the backflow pressure may also occur and tends to be aggravated by bending forward, stooping or lying down. The severity of symptoms is related to the rate of obstruction and the development of a venous collateral circulation. Accordingly, symptoms may develop rapidly or gradually. Clinical features are summarised in Box 11.12.

Investigations and management

The investigation of choice is CT of the thorax since it can clinch the diagnosis and distinguish between extra- and intravascular causes. A biopsy should be obtained when the tumour type is unknown because tumour type has a major influence on treatment. CT of the brain may be indicated if cerebral oedema is suspected. Tumours that are exquisitely sensitive to chemotherapy, such as germ cell tumours and lymphoma, can be treated with chemotherapy alone, but for most other tumours mediastinal radiotherapy is required. This relieves symptoms within 2 weeks in 50–90% of patients. In most centres, stenting is now increasingly favoured over radiotherapy, as it produces rapid results and can be repeated with reasonable effectiveness. This technique is particularly useful when dealing with tumours that are relatively chemo- or radio-resistant, such as non-small cell lung cancer or carcinoma of unknown primary. Where possible, these measures should be followed by treatment of the primary tumour, as long-term outcome is strongly dependent on the prognosis of the underlying cancer.

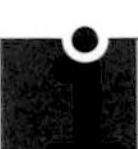

11.12 Common symptoms and physical findings in superior vena cava obstruction*

Symptoms	
• Dyspnoea (63%) • Facial swelling and head fullness (50%) • Cough (24%)	• Arm swelling (18%) • Chest pain (15%) • Dysphagia (9%)
Physical findings	
• Venous distension of neck (66%) • Venous distension of chest wall (54%)	• Facial oedema (46%) • Cyanosis (20%) • Plethora of face (19%) • Oedema of arms (14%)

*Percentage of patients affected.

Hypercalcaemia

Hypercalcaemia is the most common metabolic disorder in patients with cancer and has a prevalence of 15–20 cases per 100 000 persons. The incidence is highest in myeloma and breast cancer (approximately 40%), intermediate in non-small cell lung cancer, and uncommon in colon, prostate and small cell lung carcinomas. It is most commonly due to over-production of PTHrP, which binds to the PTH receptor and elevates serum calcium by stimulating osteoclastic bone resorption and increasing renal tubular reabsorption of calcium.

Clinical features

The symptoms of hypercalcaemia are often non-specific and may mimic those of the underlying malignancy. They include drowsiness, confusion, nausea and vomiting, constipation, polyuria, polydipsia and dehydration.

Investigations and management

The diagnosis is made by measuring serum total calcium and adjusting for albumin. It is especially important to correct for albumin in cancer because hypoalbuminaemia is common and total calcium values underestimate the level of ionised calcium. The principles of management are outlined in Box 11.13.

Patients should initially be treated with intravenous 0.9% saline to improve renal function and increase urinary calcium excretion. This alone often results in clinical improvement. Concurrently, intravenous bisphosphonates should be given to inhibit bone resorption. Calcitonin acts rapidly to increase calcium excretion and to reduce bone resorption and can be combined with fluid and bisphosphonate therapy for the first 24–48 hours in patients with life-threatening hypercalcaemia. Bisphosphonates will usually reduce the serum calcium levels to normal within 5 days, but if not, treatment can be repeated. The duration of action is up to 4 weeks and repeated therapy can be given at 3–4-weekly intervals as an outpatient. Hypercalcaemia is frequently a sign of tumour progression and the patient requires further investigation to establish disease status and review of the anti-cancer therapy.

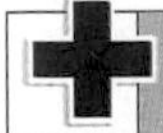

11.13 Medical management of severe hypercalcaemia

- IV 0.9% saline 2–4 L/day
- Zoledronic acid 4 mg IV *or* pamidronate 60–90 mg IV
- IM/SC calcitonin 100 U 3 times daily for first 24–48 hours in life-threatening hypercalcaemia

Neutropenic fever

Neutropenia is a common complication of malignancy. It is usually secondary to chemotherapy but may occur with radiotherapy if large amounts of bone marrow are irradiated; it may also be a component of pancytopenia due to malignant infiltration of the bone marrow. Neutropenic fever is defined as a pyrexia of 38°C for over 1 hour in a patient with a neutrophil count $< 1.0 \times 10^9/L$. The risk of sepsis is related to the severity and duration of neutropenia and the presence of other risk factors such as intravenous or bladder catheters. Neutropenic fever is an emergency in cancer patients as, if left untreated, it can result in septicaemia with a high mortality rate.

Clinical features

The typical presentation is with high fever and affected patients are often non-specifically unwell. Examination is usually unhelpful in defining a primary source of the infection. Hypotension is an adverse prognostic feature and may progress to systemic circulatory shutdown and organ failure.

Investigations and management

An infection screen should be performed to include blood cultures (both peripheral and from central lines), urine culture, chest X-ray, and swabs for culture (throat, central line, wound). High-dose intravenous antibiotics should then be commenced, pending the results of cultures. Typical first-line empirical therapy consists of an anti-pseudomonal β-lactam (ceftazidime, cefotaxime or meropenem), or a combination of an aminoglycoside and a broad-spectrum penicillin with anti-pseudomonal activity (gentamicin and piperacillin), but this may need adjusting on the basis of local hospital policy and antibiotic resistance patterns. Metronidazole should be added if anaerobic infection is suspected, and flucloxacillin or vancomycin or teicoplanin where Gram-positive infection is suspected (for example, in patients with central lines). If there is no response after 36–48 hours, treatment with amphotericin B or voriconazole should be considered to cover fungal infection. Antibiotics should be adjusted according to culture results, though these are often negative. Other supportive therapy, including intravenous fluids, inotrope therapy, ventilation or haemofiltration, may be required.

METASTATIC DISEASE

Metastatic disease is the major cause of death in cancer patients and the principal cause of morbidity. For the majority, the aim of treatment is palliative, but treatment of a solitary metastasis can occasionally be curative.

Brain metastases

Brain metastases occur in 10–30% of adults and 6–10% of children with cancer, and are an increasingly important cause of morbidity. Tumours that typically metastasise to the brain are shown in Box 11.14. Most involve the brain parenchyma but can also affect the cranial nerves, the blood vessels and other intracranial structures. In cases of solitary metastasis to the brain, the use of surgery and adjuvant radiotherapy has been shown to increase survival. However, practices vary for patients with more advanced brain metastases. In these cases, median survival without treatment is approximately 1 month. Steroids can increase survival to 2–3 months and whole-brain radiotherapy improves survival to 3–6 months, but the true efficacy of these interventions has not been proven adequately in a randomised trial setting. Patients with brain metastases as the only manifestation of an undetected primary tumour have a more favourable prognosis, with an overall median survival of 13.4 months. Tumour type also influences prognosis; breast cancer patients have a better prognosis than those with other types of tumour, and those with colorectal carcinoma tend to have a poorer prognosis.

11.14 Primary tumour sites that metastasise to brain

Primary tumour	Patients (%)
Lung	48
Breast	15
Melanoma	9
Colon	5
Other known primary	13
Unknown primary	11

Clinical features

Presentation is with headaches (40–50%), focal neurological dysfunction (20–40%), cognitive dysfunction (35%), seizures (10–20%) and papilloedema (< 10%).

Investigations and management

The diagnosis can be confirmed by CT or contrast-enhanced MRI. Treatment options include high-dose steroids (dexamethasone 4 mg 4 times daily) for tumour-associated oedema, anticonvulsants for seizures, whole-brain radiotherapy, and chemotherapy. Surgery may be considered for single sites of disease and can be curative; stereotactic radiotherapy may also be considered for solitary site involvement where surgery is not possible.

Lung metastases

These are common in breast cancer, colon cancer and tumours of the head and neck. The presentation is usually with a lesion on chest X-ray or CT. Solitary lesions require investigation, as single metastases can be difficult to distinguish from a primary lung tumour. Patients with two or more pulmonary nodules can be assumed to have metastases. The approach to treatment depends on the extent of disease in the lung and elsewhere. For solitary lesions, surgery should be considered with a generous wedge resection. Radiotherapy, chemotherapy or endocrine therapy can be used as systemic treatment and is dependent on the underlying primary cancer diagnosis.

Liver metastases

Metastatic cancer in the liver can represent the sole or life-limiting component of disease for many with colorectal cancer, ocular melanoma, neuro-endocrine tumours and, less commonly, other tumour types. The most common clinical presentations are with right upper quadrant pain due to stretching of the liver capsule, jaundice, deranged liver function tests or an abnormality detected on imaging. In selected cases, resection of the metastasis can be contemplated. In colorectal cancer, successful resection of a metastasis improves 5-year survival from 3% to 30–40%. Other techniques, such as chemoembolisation or radiofrequency ablation, can also be used, provided the number and size of metastases remain small. If these are not feasible, symptoms may respond to systemic chemotherapy.

Bone metastases

Bone is the third most common organ involved by metastasis, after lung and liver. Bone metastases are a major clinical problem in patients with myeloma and breast or prostate cancers, but other tumours that commonly metastasise to bone include those of the kidney and thyroid. Bone metastases are an increasing management problem in other tumour types that do not classically target bone, due to the prolonged survival of patients generally. Accordingly, effective management of bony metastases has become a focus in the treatment of patients with many incurable cancers.

Clinical features

The main presentations are with pain, pathological fractures and spinal cord compression (p. 272). The pain tends to be progressive and worst at night, and may be partially relieved by activity, but subsequently becomes more constant in nature and is exacerbated by movement. Most pathological fractures occur in metastatic breast cancer (53%); other tumour types associated with fracture include the kidney (11%), lung (8%), thyroid (5%), lymphoma (5%) and prostate (3%).

Investigations and management

The most sensitive way of detecting bone metastases is by isotope bone scan. This can have false-positive results in healing bone, particularly as a flare response following treatment and false-negative results occur in multiple myeloma due to suppression of osteoblast activity. Therefore plain X-ray films are preferred for any sites of bone pain, as lytic lesions may not be detected by a bone scan. In patients with a single lesion, it is especially important to perform a biopsy to obtain a tissue diagnosis, since primary bone tumours may look very similar to metastases on X-ray.

The main goals of management are:

- pain relief
- preservation and restoration of function
- skeletal stabilisation
- local tumour control (e.g. relief of tumour impingement on normal structure).

Surgical intervention may be warranted where there is evidence of skeletal instability (e.g. anterior or posterior spinal column fracture) or an impending fracture (e.g. large lytic lesion on a weight-bearing bone with more than 50% cortical involvement). Intravenous bisphosphonates (pamidronate, zoledronic acid or ibandronate) are widely used for bone metastases and are effective at improving pain and in reducing further skeletal related events, such as fractures and hypercalcaemia (Box 11.15). In certain types of cancer, such as breast and prostate, hormonal therapy may be effective. Radiotherapy, in the form of external beam therapy or systemic radionucleotides (strontium treatment), can also be useful for these patients. In some settings (e.g. breast carcinoma), chemotherapy may also be used in the management of bony metastases.

EBM 11.15 Use of bisphosphonates in bony metastases

'The use of bisphosphonates in cancer patients with bony metastases results in decreased pain and a decrease in skeletal-related events.'

- Dennis K, et al. J Rad Oncol; epub 17 July 2012; 1(1): DOI: 10.1007/s13566-012-0058-3.
- Dror Michaelson M, Smith MR. J Clin Oncol 2005; 23(32): 8219–8224.

Malignant pleural effusion

This is a common complication of cancer and 40% of all pleural effusions are due to malignancy. The most common causes are lung and breast cancers, and the presence of an effusion indicates advanced and incurable disease. The presentation may be with dyspnoea, cough or chest discomfort, which can be dull or pleuritic in nature. Diagnosis and management of ascites is discussed on p. 938.

Investigations and management

Pleural aspirate is the key investigation and may show the presence of malignant cells. Malignant effusions are commonly blood-stained and are exudates with a raised fluid to serum lactate dehydrogenase (LDH) ratio (> 0.6) and a raised fluid to serum protein ratio (> 0.5). Treatment should focus on palliation of symptoms and be tailored to the patient's physical condition and prognosis. Aspiration alone may be an appropriate treatment in frail patients with a limited life expectancy (Box 11.16). Those who present with malignant pleural effusion as the initial manifestation of breast cancer, small cell lung cancer, germ cell tumours or lymphoma should

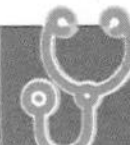

11.16 How to aspirate a malignant pleural effusion

- Ask the patient to sit up and lean forward slightly.
- Identify a suitable site for aspiration. Typically, this should be in the mid-scapular line, below the top of the fluid level and above the diaphragm.
- Confirm that the site is below the fluid level by reviewing the chest X-ray and percussing the chest.
- Infiltrate the skin and the intercostal space immediately above the rib below with 1% lidocaine.
- As you advance the needle, aspirate at each step prior to injecting the local anaesthetic.
- On reaching the pleural cavity, you should be able to aspirate pleural fluid; when you do, note the depth of the needle.
- Insert a thoracentesis needle into the pleural space by advancing it along the same track as was used for the local anaesthetic and connect it to a three-way tap and container to collect the fluid.
- Drain the pleural effusion, to a maximum of 1.5 L. If the effusion is larger than this, repeat the procedure on further occasions as necessary.
- Consider using ultrasound-guided placement of a drainage catheter if the effusion proves difficult to drain.
- Permanent drains can be useful for some patients with recurrent effusions where pleurodesis is not possible.

11

have the fluid aspirated and should be given systemic chemotherapy to try to treat disease in the pleural space. Treatment options for patients with recurrent pleural effusion include pleurodesis, pleurectomy and pleuroperitoneal shunt. Ideally, pleurodesis should be attempted once effusions recur after initial drainage.

THERAPEUTICS IN ONCOLOGY

Anti-cancer therapy may be either curative or palliative, and this distinction influences the approach to management of individual patients. The goal of treatment should be recorded in the medical notes.

- *Palliative chemotherapy* is the most common treatment and is primarily used to treat patients with metastasis. The goal is an improvement in symptoms with a focus on improving quality of life, and any survival increments are secondary. As a result, the treatment should be well tolerated and should aim to minimise adverse effects.
- *Adjuvant chemotherapy* is given after an initial intervention that is designed to cyto-reduce the tumour bulk and remove all macroscopic disease. Chemotherapy is then given with the intention of eradicating the micrometastatic disease that remains. The focus is on achieving an improvement in disease-free and overall survival.
- *Neoadjuvant chemotherapy* or primary medical therapy is where chemotherapy is administered first before a planned cyto-reductive procedure. This can result in a reduced requirement for surgery, increase the likelihood of successful debulking, reduce the duration of hospitalisation and improve the fitness of the patient prior to interval debulking. This approach has the same goals as adjuvant treatment but creates an opportunity for translational research to measure responses to treatment and correlate with subsequent specimens removed at the time of surgery.
- *Chemoprevention* is the use of pharmacological agents to prevent cancer developing in patients identified as being at particular risk. Therefore the agents used aim to modify risk and, as such, should not have significant adverse effects.

Surgical treatment

Surgery has a pivotal role in the management of cancer. There are three main situations in which it is necessary.

Biopsy

In the vast majority of cases, a histological or cytological diagnosis of cancer is necessary, and tissue will also provide important information such as tumour type and differentiation, to assist subsequent management. Cytology can be obtained with fine needle aspiration but a biopsy is usually preferred. This can be a core biopsy, an image-guided biopsy or an excision biopsy.

Excision

The main curative management of most solid cancers is surgical excision. In early, localised cases of colorectal, breast and lung cancer, cure rates are high with surgery. There is increasing evidence that outcome is related to surgical expertise, and most multidisciplinary teams include surgeons experienced in the management of a particular cancer. There are some cancers for which surgery is one of two or more options for primary management, and the role of the multidisciplinary team is to recommend appropriate treatment for a specific patient. Examples include prostate and transitional cell carcinoma of the bladder, in which radiotherapy and surgery may be equally effective.

Palliation

Surgical procedures are often the quickest and most effective way of palliating symptoms. Examples include the treatment of faecal incontinence with a defunctioning colostomy; fixation of pathological fractures and decompression of spinal cord compression; and the treatment of fungating skin lesions by 'toilet' surgery. A more specialist role for surgery is in resection of residual masses after chemotherapy and, in very selected cases, resection of metastases.

Systemic chemotherapy

Chemotherapeutic drugs are classified by their mode of action. They have the greatest activity in proliferating cells and this provides the rationale for their use in the treatment of cancer. Chemotherapeutic agents are not specific for cancer cells, however, and the side-effects of treatment are a result of their anti-proliferative actions in normal tissues such as the bone marrow, skin and gut.

Combination therapy

In order to overcome drug resistance and to limit the side-effects of different drugs, chemotherapy is most commonly given as a combination of agents. Combinations usually include drugs from different classes, with the aim of targeting several pathways and gaining maximum therapeutic effect. Drugs are conventionally given by intravenous injection every 3–4 weeks, allowing enough time for the patient to recover from short-term toxic effects before the next dose. Between four and eight such cycles of treatment are usually given in total. More recently, other strategies have been developed. For example, 5-fluorouracil (5-FU), which has a very short half-life, has increased efficacy when given by continuous intravenous infusion, using a semi-permanent in-dwelling intravenous catheter. However, the use of such catheters is not without risk and the potential of oral 5-FU is now being explored, using precursors such as capecitabine. Schedules of administration at weekly or 2-weekly intervals have also found their place in the management of both solid and haematological malignancies. Each tumour type has specific regimens that are used at various stages of the disease.

Mode of administration

Most drugs have to be given intravenously, and many are vesicant or locally irritant if there is an extravasation. Chemotherapy should be administered into a vein in which the infusion is free-flowing to minimise the risk of extravasation. A few patients require central venous catheters due to the nature of their treatment or poor vascular access. Patients who receive chemotherapy through a peripheral line must be carefully observed, and the chemotherapy stopped at the first sign of any extravasation. Chemotherapy is potentially dangerous to the person giving the therapy, because cytotoxics are carcinogenic and teratogenic. In view of this, policies must be in place for the use of gloves and aprons and for the safe disposal of syringes containing cytotoxics. Other oral chemotherapeutic agents have been developed over the past 30 years, although not many have replaced their intravenous counterparts.

Adverse effects

Most cytotoxics have a narrow therapeutic window or index and can have significant adverse effects, as shown in Figure 11.6. Considerable supportive therapy is often required to enable patients to tolerate therapy and achieve benefit. Nausea and vomiting are common, but with modern antiemetics, regimens such as the combination of dexamethasone and highly selective 5-hydroxytryptamine (5-HT_3) receptor antagonists like ondansetron, most patients now receive chemotherapy without any significant problems. Myelosuppression is common to almost all cytotoxics. This not only limits the dose of drug, but also can cause life-threatening complications. The risk of neutropenia can be reduced with the use of specific growth factors that accelerate the re-population of myeloid precursor cells. The most commonly employed is granulocyte–colony-stimulating factor (G-CSF), which is widely used in conjunction with chemotherapy regimens that induce a high rate of neutropenia. More recently, it has also been used to 'accelerate' the administration of chemotherapy, enabling standard doses to be given at shorter intervals where the rate-limiting factor has been the time taken for the peripheral neutrophil count to recover. Accelerated chemotherapy regimens have now been demonstrated to offer therapeutic advantages in small cell lung cancer, lymphoma and possibly breast cancer.

Radiation therapy

Radiation therapy (radiotherapy) involves treating the cancer with ionising radiation; for certain localised cancers it may be curative. Ionising radiation can be delivered by radiation emitted from the decay of radioactive isotopes or by high-energy radiation beams, usually X-rays. Three methods are usually employed:

- *Teletherapy*: application from a distance by a linear accelerator.
- *Brachytherapy*: direct application of a radioactive source on to or into a tumour. This allows the delivery of a very high, localised dose of radiation and is integral to the management of localised

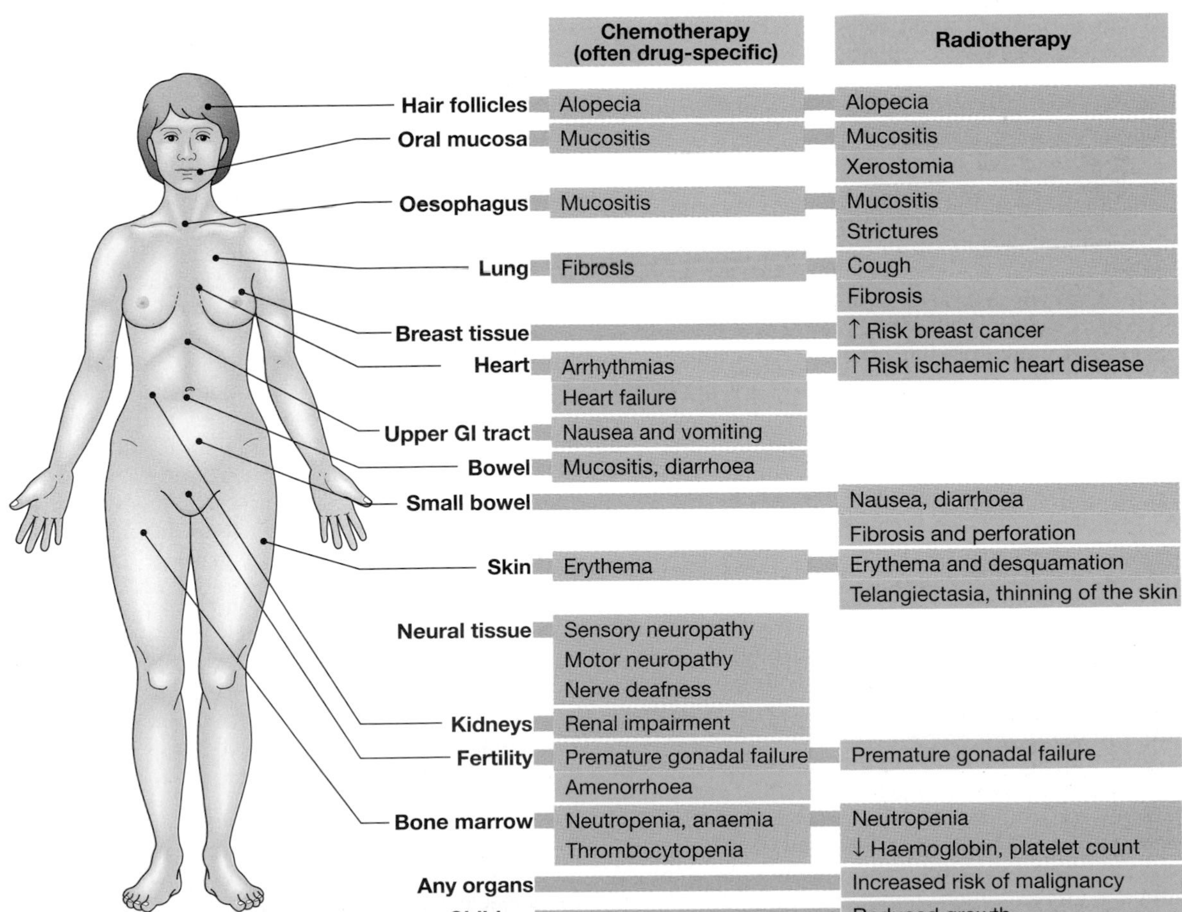

Fig. 11.6 Adverse effects of chemotherapy and radiotherapy. Acute effects are shown in pink and late effects in blue.

cancers of the head and neck and cancer of the cervix and endometrium.

- *Intravenous injection of a radioisotope*: such as ^{131}iodine for cancer of the thyroid and ^{89}strontium for the treatment of bone metastases from prostate cancer.

The majority of treatments are now delivered by linear accelerators; these produce electron or X-ray beams of high energy that are used to target tumour tissue. Whatever the method of delivery, the biological effect of ionising radiation is to cause lethal and sublethal damage to DNA. Since normal tissues are also radiosensitive, treatment has to be designed to maximise exposure of the tumour and minimise exposure of normal tissues. This is now possible with modern imaging techniques such as CT and MRI, which allow better visualisation of normal and tumour tissue. In addition, techniques such as conformal radiotherapy, where shaped rather than conventional square or rectangular beams are used, allow much more precise targeting of therapy to the tumour, and reduce the volume of normal tissue irradiated by up to 40% compared to non-conformal techniques.

Biological differences between normal and tumour tissues are also used to obtain therapeutic gain. Fundamental to this is fractionation, which entails delivering the radiation as a number of small doses on a daily basis. This allows normal cells to recover from irradiation damage but recovery occurs to a lesser degree in malignant cells. Fractionation regimens vary from centre to centre but radical treatments given with curative intent are often delivered in 20–30 fractions given daily, 5 days a week over 4–6 weeks. Radiotherapy can also be extremely useful for the alleviation of symptoms, and for palliative treatments such as this a smaller number of fractions (1–5) is usually adequate.

Both normal and malignant tissues vary widely in their sensitivity to radiotherapy. Germ cell tumours and lymphomas are extremely radiosensitive and relatively low doses are adequate for cure, but most cancers require doses close to or beyond that which can be tolerated by adjacent normal structures. Normal tissue also varies in its radiosensitivity, the central nervous system, small bowel and lung being amongst the most sensitive. The side-effects of radiotherapy (see Fig. 11.6) depend on the normal tissues treated, their radiosensitivity and the dose delivered.

Adverse effects

An acute inflammatory reaction commonly occurs towards the end of most radical treatments and is localised to the area treated. For example, skin reactions are common with breast or chest wall radiotherapy, and proctitis and cystitis with treatment to the bladder or prostate. These acute reactions settle over a period of a few weeks after treatment, assuming normal tissue tolerance has not been exceeded. Late effects of radiotherapy develop 6 weeks or more after treatment and occur in 5–10% of patients. Examples include brachial nerve damage and subcutaneous fibrosis after breast cancer treatment, and shrinkage and fibrosis of the bladder after treatment for bladder cancer. There is a risk of inducing cancer after radiotherapy, which varies depending on the site treated and whether the patient has had other treatment such as chemotherapy.

Hormone therapy

Hormone therapy is most commonly used in the treatment of breast cancer and prostate cancer. Breast tumours that are positive for expression of the oestrogen receptor (ER) respond well to anti-oestrogen therapy, and assessment of ER status is now standard in the diagnosis of breast cancer. Several drugs are now available that reduce oestrogen levels or block the effects of oestrogen on the receptor. When targeted appropriately, adjuvant hormone therapy reduces the risk of relapse and death at least as much as chemotherapy, and in advanced cases can induce stable disease and remissions that may last months to years, with acceptable toxicity. Hormonal manipulation may be effective in other cancers. In prostate cancer, hormonal therapy (e.g. luteinising hormone releasing hormone (LHRH) analogues such as goserelin and/or anti-androgens such as bicalutamide) aimed at reducing androgen levels can provide good long-term control of advanced disease, but there is no convincing evidence that it is an effective therapy following potentially curative surgery. Progestogens are active in the treatment of endometrial and breast cancer. In the metastatic setting, progestogen use (e.g. megestrol acetate) is associated with response rates of 20–40% in endometrial cancer. In breast cancer, progestogens are used in patients whose disease has progressed with conventional anti-oestrogen therapy. Their exact mechanism in this setting is not fully understood.

Immunotherapy

A profound stimulus to the patient's immune system can sometimes alter the natural history of a malignancy, and the discovery of interferons was the impetus for much research. Although solid tumours show little benefit, interferons are active in melanoma and lymphoma, and there is evidence that they are beneficial as adjuvants (after surgery and chemotherapy respectively) to delay recurrence. Whether interferon-induced stimulation of the immune system is capable of eradicating microscopic disease remains unproven. More powerful immune responses can be achieved with potent agents like interleukin-2 (IL-2), but the accompanying systemic toxicity is a problem still to be overcome. The most striking example of successful immunotherapy is that with rituximab, an antibody against the common B-cell antigen CD20. It increases complete response rates and improves survival in diffuse large cell non-Hodgkin's lymphoma when combined with chemotherapy, and is also effective in palliating advanced follicular non-Hodgkin's lymphoma (p. 1043).

Biological therapies

Advances in knowledge about the molecular basis of cancer have resulted in the development of a new generation of treatments to block the signalling pathways responsible for the growth of specific tumours. This has created the potential to target cancer cells more selectively, with reduced toxicity to normal tissues. Some examples are discussed below, but in the years to come many more such agents will come into clinical use, with the potential to revolutionise our approach to some cancers.

Gefitinib/erlotinib

These agents inhibit the activity of the epidermal growth factor receptor, which is over-expressed in many solid tumours. However, the drugs' activity does not depend on the amount of receptor over-expression but on factors such as gene copy number and mutation status.

Imatinib

Imatinib was developed to inhibit the *BCR-ABL* gene product, tyrosine kinase, that is responsible for chronic myeloid leukaemia (p. 1039), and it does this extremely effectively. It is also active in gastrointestinal stromal tumour (GIST), a type of sarcoma that has over-expression of another cell surface tyrosine kinase, c-kit. This agent has good tolerability and is particularly useful in GIST, where conventional chemotherapy is less effective.

Bevacizumab

This is a humanised monoclonal antibody that inhibits vascular endothelial growth factor A (VEGF-A), a key stimulant of angiogenesis in tumours. This has activity in colorectal, lung, breast, renal and ovarian cancers, although the licence was subsequently revoked for breast cancer; while bevacizumab slows the rate of progression of metastatic breast cancer, it had little impact on survival or improved quality of life.

Trastuzumab

Trastuzumab (herceptin) targets the HER2 receptor, an oncogene that is over-expressed in around one-third of breast cancers and in a number of other solid tumours. It is effective as a single-agent therapy, but also improves survival in patients with advanced breast cancer when used in conjunction with chemotherapy. Unfortunately, trastuzumab can induce cardiac failure by an unknown biological mechanism, especially in combination with doxorubicin.

SPECIFIC CANCERS

The diagnosis and management of cancers are discussed in more detail elsewhere in the book (Box 11.17). Here we discuss the clinical features, pathogenesis and management of common tumours that are not covered elsewhere.

11.17 Specific cancers covered in other chapters

Bladder cancer	p. 516
Colorectal cancer	p. 910
Familial cancer syndromes	p. 66
Gastric cancer	p. 877
Hepatocellular carcinoma	p. 966
Leukaemia	p. 1035
Lung cancer	p. 699
Lymphoma	p. 1041
Mesothelioma	p. 719
Myeloma	p. 1046
Oesophageal cancer	p. 870
Pancreatic cancer	p. 895
Prostate cancer	p. 517
Renal cancer	p. 515
Seminoma	p. 518
Skin cancer	p. 1269
Teratoma	p. 518
Thyroid cancer	p. 754

Breast cancer

Globally, the incidence of breast cancer is only second to that of lung cancer and the disease represents the leading cause of cancer-related deaths among women. Invasive ductal carcinoma with or without ductal carcinoma in situ (DCIS) is the most common histology, accounting for 70%, whilst invasive lobular carcinoma accounts for most of the remaining cases. DCIS constitutes 20% of breast cancers detected by mammography screening. It is multifocal in one-third of women and has a high risk of becoming invasive (10% at 5 years following excision only). Pure DCIS does not cause lymph node metastases, although these are found in 2% of cases where nodes are examined, owing to undetected invasive cancer. Lobular carcinoma in situ (LCIS) is a predisposing risk factor for developing cancer in either breast (7% at 10 years). The survival for breast cancer by stage is outlined in Box 11.18.

11.18 Five-year survival rates for breast cancer by stage

Tumour stage	Stage definition	5-year survival (%)
Stage I	Tumour < 2 cm, no lymph nodes	96
Stage II	Tumour 2–5 cm, and/or mobile axillary lymph nodes	81
Stage III	Chest wall or skin fixation, and/or fixed axillary lymph nodes	52
Stage IV	Metastasis	18

Pathogenesis

Both genetic and hormonal factors play a role; about 5–10% of breast cancers are hereditary and occur in patients with mutations of *BRCA1*, *BRCA2*, *AT* or *TP53* genes. Prolonged oestrogen exposure associated with early menarche, late menopause and use of hormone replacement therapy (HRT) has been associated with an increased risk. Other risk factors include obesity, alcohol intake, nulliparity and late first pregnancy. There is no definite evidence linking use of the contraceptive pill to breast cancer.

Clinical features

Breast cancer usually presents as a result of mammographic screening or as a palpable mass with nipple discharge in 10% and pain in 7% of patients. Less common presentations include inflammatory carcinoma with diffuse induration of the skin of the breast, and this confers an adverse prognosis. Around 40% of patients will have axillary nodal disease, with likelihood correlating with increasing size of the primary tumour. Distant metastases are infrequently present at diagnosis and the most common sites of spread are: bone (70%), lung (60%), liver (55%), pleura (40%), adrenals (35%), skin (30%) and brain (10–20%).

Investigations

Following clinical examination, patients should have imaging with mammography or ultrasound evaluation and a biopsy using fine needle aspiration for cytology or core biopsy for histology. Histological assessment should be carried out to assess tumour type and to determine oestrogen and progesterone receptor (ER/PR) status and HER2 status. If distant spread is suspected, CT of the thorax and abdomen and an isotope bone scan are required.

Management

Surgery is the mainstay of treatment for most patients, and this can range from a lumpectomy, where only the tumour is removed, to mastectomy, where the whole breast is removed. Lymph node sampling is performed at the time of surgery. Adjuvant radiotherapy is given to reduce the risk of local recurrence to 4–6%. Adjuvant hormonal therapy improves disease-free and overall survival in pre- and post-menopausal patients who have tumours that express ER. Patients at low risk, with tumours that are small and ER-positive, only require adjuvant hormonal therapy with tamoxifen. Patients with tumours that are ER-positive and who are pre-menopausal should receive an LHRH analogue. Aromatase inhibitors also have benefit in this setting and are still under investigation.

Adjuvant chemotherapy is considered for patients at higher risk of recurrence. Factors that increase the risk of recurrence include a tumour of greater than 1 cm, tumour that is ER-negative or the presence of involved axillary lymph nodes. Such patients should be offered adjuvant chemotherapy, which improves disease-free and overall survival (Box 11.19). The role of adjuvant treatment has been studied by meta-analyses and data support the use of adjuvant trastuzumab, a humanised monoclonal antibody to HER2, in addition to standard chemotherapy for women with early HER2-positive breast cancer.

Metastatic disease management includes radiotherapy to palliate painful bone metastases and second-line endocrine therapy with aromatase inhibitors, which inhibit peripheral oestrogen production in adrenal and adipose tissues. Advanced ER-negative disease may be treated with combination chemotherapy.

EBM 11.19 Use of adjuvant chemotherapy and endocrine therapy in early breast cancer

'The use of anthracycline-based chemotherapy reduces the annual breast cancer rate from 38% to 20%, while the adjuvant use of tamoxifen for 5 years in early breast cancer for patients with ER-positive disease reduces the annual breast cancer death rate by 31%.'

- Early Breast Cancer Trialists Collaborative Group (EBCTCG). Lancet 4 Feb 2012; 379(9814):432–444.

Ovarian cancer

Ovarian cancer is the most common gynaecological tumour in Western countries. Most ovarian cancers are epithelial in origin (90%), and up to 7% of women with ovarian cancer have a positive family history. Patients often present late in ovarian cancer with vague abdominal discomfort, low back pain, bloating, altered bowel habit and weight loss. Occasionally, peritoneal deposits are palpable as an omental 'cake' and nodules in the umbilicus (Sister Mary Joseph nodules).

Pathogenesis

Genetic and environmental factors play a role. The risk of ovarian cancer is increased in patients with *BRCA1* or *BRCA2* mutations, and Lynch type II families (a subtype of hereditary non-polyposis colon cancer (HNPCC)) have ovarian, endometrial, colorectal and gastric tumours due to mutations of mismatch repair enzymes. Advanced age, nulliparity, ovarian stimulation and Caucasian descent all increase the risk of ovarian cancer, whilst suppressed ovulation appears to protect, so pregnancy, prolonged breastfeeding and the contraceptive pill have all been shown to reduce the risk of ovarian cancer.

Investigations

Initial workup for patients with suspected ovarian malignancy includes imaging in the form of ultrasound and CT. Serum levels of the tumour marker CA-125 are often measured. Surgery plays a key role in the diagnosis, staging and treatment of ovarian cancer, and in early cases, palpation of viscera, intraoperative washing and biopsies are generally performed to define disease extent.

Management

In early disease, surgery followed by adjuvant chemotherapy with carboplatin, or carboplatin plus paclitaxel, is the treatment of choice. Surgery should include removal of the tumour along with total hysterectomy, bilateral salpingo-oophorectomy, and omentectomy. Even in advanced disease, surgery is undertaken to debulk the tumour and is followed by adjuvant chemotherapy, typically using carboplatin and paclitaxel. Bevacizumab is indicated for patients with high-grade tumours that are suboptimally debulked or those with a more aggressive biological pattern. Monitoring for relapse is achieved through a combination of serum CA-125 and clinical examination with CT imaging for those with suspected relapse. Second-line chemotherapy is aimed at improving symptoms and should not be used for CA-125 elevation only in the absence of symptoms. Treatments can include further platinum/

paclitaxel combination, liposomal doxorubicin or topotecan. These regimens are associated with a response rate of 10–40%. The best responses are observed in patients with a treatment-free interval of more than 12 months.

Endometrial cancer

Endometrial cancer accounts for 4% of all female malignancies, producing a 1 in 73 lifetime risk. The majority of patients are post-menopausal, with a peak incidence at 50–60 years of age. Mortality from endometrial cancer is currently falling. The most common presentation is with post-menopausal bleeding, which often results in detection of the disease before distant spread has occurred.

Pathogenesis

Oestrogen plays an important role in the pathogenesis of endometrial cancer, and factors that increase the duration of oestrogen exposure, such as nulliparity, early menarche, late menopause and unopposed HRT, increase the risk. Endometrial cancer is 10 times more common in obese women, and this is thought to be due to elevated levels of oestrogens.

Investigations

The diagnosis is confirmed by endometrial biopsy.

Management

Surgery is the treatment of choice and is also used for staging. A hysterectomy and bilateral salpingo-oophorectomy are performed with peritoneal cytology and, in some cases, lymph node dissection. Where the tumour extends beyond the inner 50% of the myometrium, involves the cervix and local lymph nodes, or there is lymphovascular space invasion, adjuvant pelvic radiotherapy is recommended. Chemotherapy and hormonal therapies have not demonstrated a sufficient survival advantage to be recommended for routine use in the adjuvant setting but have a role in recurrent disease.

Cervical cancer

This is the second most common gynaecological tumour worldwide. The incidence is decreasing in developed countries but continues to rise in developing nations. Cervical cancer is the leading cause of death from gynaecological cancer. The most common presentation is with an abnormal smear test, but with locally advanced disease the presentation is with vaginal bleeding, discomfort, discharge or symptoms attributable to involvement of adjacent structures, such as bladder, or rectal or pelvic wall. Occasionally, patients present with distant metastases to bone and lung.

Pathogenesis

There is a strong association between cervical cancer and sexual activity that includes sex at a young age and multiple sexual partners. Infection with HPV has an important causal role, and this has underpinned the introduction of programmes to immunise teenagers against HPV in an effort to prevent the later development of cervical cancer (p. 425).

Investigations

Diagnosis is made by smear or cone biopsy. Dilatation and curettage is also used diagnostically, with cystoscopy and flexible sigmoidoscopy if there are symptoms referable to the bladder, colon or rectum. In contrast to other gynaecological malignancies, cervical cancer is a clinically staged disease. MRI is often used to characterise the primary tumour. A routine chest X-ray should be obtained to help rule out pulmonary metastasis. CT of the abdomen and pelvis is performed to look for metastasis in the liver and lymph nodes and to exclude hydronephrosis and hydroureter.

Management

This depends on the stage of disease. Pre-malignant disease can be treated with laser ablation or diathermy, whereas in microinvasive disease a large loop excision of the transformation zone (LLETZ) or a simple hysterectomy is employed. Invasive but localised disease requires radical surgery, while chemotherapy and radiotherapy, including brachytherapy, may be given as primary treatment, especially in patients with adverse prognostic features such as bulky or locally advanced disease, or lymph node or parametrium invasion. In metastatic disease, cisplatin-based chemotherapy may be beneficial in improving symptoms but does not improve survival significantly.

Head and neck tumours

Head and neck cancers are typically squamous tumours that arise in the nasopharynx, hypopharynx and larynx. They are most common in elderly males, but now occur with increasing frequency in a younger cohort, as well as in women, especially where oropharyngeal cancers are concerned. The rising incidence of oropharyngeal cancers, especially in the developed world, is thought to be secondary to HPV infection. Presentation depends on the location of the primary tumour and the extent of disease. For example, early laryngeal cancers may present with hoarseness, while more extensive local disease may present with pain due to invasion of local structures or with a lump in the neck. Patients who present late often have pulmonary symptoms, as this is the most common site of distant metastases (Box 11.20).

Pathogenesis

The tumours are strongly associated with a history of smoking and excess alcohol intake, but other recognised risk factors include Epstein–Barr virus for nasopharyngeal cancer and HPV infection for oropharyngeal tumours.

Investigations

Careful inspection of the primary site is required as part of the staging process, and most patients will require endoscopic evaluation and examination under anaesthesia. Tissue biopsies should be taken from the most accessible site. CT of the primary site and the thorax is the

11.20 Common presenting features by location in head and neck cancer

Hypopharynx	
• Dysphagia • Odynophagia	• Referred otalgia • Enlarged lymph nodes
Mouth	
• Non-healing ulcers	• Ipsilateral otalgia
Nasal cavity and sinuses	
• Discharge (bloody) or obstruction	
Nasopharynx	
• Nasal discharge or obstruction • Conduction deafness • Atypical facial pain	• Diplopia • Hoarse voice • Horner's syndrome
Oropharynx	
• Dysphagia • Pain	• Otalgia
Salivary gland	
• Painless swelling	• Facial nerve palsy

investigation of choice for visualising the tumour, while MRI may be useful in certain cases.

Management

Generally speaking, the majority of patients with early or locally advanced disease are treated with curative intent. In localised disease where there is no involvement of the lymph nodes, long-term remission can be achieved in up to 90% of patients with surgery or radiotherapy. The choice of surgery versus radiotherapy often depends on patient preference, as surgical treatment can be mutilating with an adverse cosmetic outcome. Patients with lymph node involvement or metastasis are treated with a combination of surgery and radiotherapy (often with chemotherapy as a radiosensitising agent – proven agents include cisplatin or cetuximab), and this produces long-term remission in approximately 60–70% of patients. Recurrent or metastatic tumour may be palliated with further surgery or radiotherapy to aid local control, and systemic chemotherapy has a response rate of around 20–30%. Second malignancies are common (3% per year) following successful treatment for primary disease, and all patients should be encouraged to give up smoking and drinking alcohol to lower their risk.

Carcinoma of unknown origin

Some patients are found to have evidence of metastatic disease at their initial presentation prior to diagnosis of a primary site. In many cases, a subsequent biopsy reveals adenocarcinoma but the primary site is not always clear.

Investigations

In this situation, there is a temptation to investigate the patient endlessly in order to determine the original primary site. However, there is a compromise between exhaustive investigation and obtaining sufficient information to plan appropriate management. For all patients, histological examination of an accessible site of metastasis is required. The architecture of the tissue can assist the pathologist in determining the likely primary site, and therefore it is better to perform a biopsy rather than fine needle aspiration. The greater volume of tissue also permits the use of immunohistochemistry. Extensive imaging to search for the primary is rarely indicated; a careful history to identify symptoms and risk factors (including familial) will often permit a judicious choice of imaging.

Management

Management of the patient will depend on that person's circumstances, as well as on the site(s) involved and the likely primary sites. The overriding principle is to ensure that a curable diagnosis has not been overlooked. For example, lung metastases from a testicular teratoma do not preclude cure; nor do one or two liver metastases from a colorectal cancer. Early discussion with an oncologist within a multidisciplinary team is essential and avoids unnecessary investigation; for example, a single hCG-based pregnancy test in a young man with lung metastases might confirm the presence of a teratoma and allow rapid administration of potentially curative chemotherapy. Treatment should not necessarily wait for a definitive diagnosis; appropriate analgesia, radiotherapy and surgical palliation can all be helpful. Some patients remain free of cancer for some years after resection of a single metastasis of an adenocarcinoma of unknown primary, justifying this approach in selected patients.

In those with no obvious primary, systemic chemotherapy may achieve some reduction in tumour burden and alleviation of symptoms, but long-term survival is rare.

Further information

Books and journal articles

Cassidy J, Bissett D, Spence R, Payne M. Oxford handbook of oncology. 3rd edn. Oxford: Oxford University Press; 2010.

Hanahan D, Weinberg RA. The hallmarks of cancer: the next generation. Cell 2011; 144:646–674.

Tobias J, Hochhauser D. Cancer and its management. 6th edn. Wiley-Blackwell; 2010.

Websites

http://info.cancerresearchuk.org/cancerstats/ *A wide range of cancer statistics that can be sorted by type or geographical location.*

www.cancer.org *American Cancer Society: clinical practice guidelines.*

D. Oxenham

12 Palliative care and pain

Principles of palliative care 284

Presenting problems in palliative care 284

Pain 284
Breathlessness 289
Cough 289
Nausea and vomiting 289
Gastrointestinal obstruction 290
Weight loss and general weakness 290
Anxiety and depression 290
Delirium and terminal agitation 290

Death and dying 290

Talking about and planning towards dying 290
Diagnosing dying 291
Management 291
Ethical issues at the end of life 291

PRINCIPLES OF PALLIATIVE CARE

Palliative care is the active total care of patients with far advanced, rapidly progressive and ultimately fatal disease. Its focus is quality of life rather than cure, and it encompasses a distinct body of knowledge and skills that all good physicians must possess to allow them to care effectively for patients at the end of life. In palliative care, there is a fundamental change of emphasis in decision-making away from a focus on prolonging life towards decisions that balance comfort and the individual's wishes with treatments that might prolong life. There is a growing recognition that the principles of, and some specific interventions developed in the palliative care of patients with cancer are equally applicable to other conditions. The principles of palliative care may therefore be applied not only to cancer but also to any chronic disease state.

Palliative care is often seen as a means of managing distress and symptoms in patients with cancer, where metastatic disease has been diagnosed and death is seen as inevitable. In other illnesses, the challenge is recognising when patients have entered this phase of their illness, as there are fewer clear markers and the course of the illness is much more variable.

Different chronic disease states progress at different rates, allowing some general trajectories of illness or dying to be defined (Fig. 12.1). These trajectories are useful in helping decision-making in individual patients and also in planning services.

Traditionally, palliative care has been associated with cancer because the latter is typified by a progressive decline in function which was more predictable than in many other diseases. This 'rapid decline' trajectory is the best-recognised pattern need for palliative care and many traditional hospice services are designed to meet the needs of people on this trajectory: for example, motor neuron disease, or AIDS where antiretroviral therapy (ART) is not available. With the improvements in management of malignant disease, this is no longer so true for all patients with cancer, whose illness may follow an erratic or intermittent decline trajectory.

Many chronic diseases, such as advanced chronic obstructive pulmonary disease (COPD) and intractable congestive heart failure, carry as high a burden of symptoms as cancer, as well as psychological and family distress. The 'palliative phase' of these illnesses may be more difficult to identify because of periods of relative stability interspersed with acute episodes of severe illness. However, it is still possible to recognise those patients whose care may benefit from a palliative approach. The challenge is that symptom management needs to be delivered at the same time as treatment for acute exacerbations. This leads to difficult decisions as to the balance between symptom relief and aggressive management of the underlying disease. The starting point of need for palliative care in these conditions is the point at which consideration of comfort and individual values becomes important in decision-making, often alongside management of the underlying disease.

The third major trajectory is categorised by years of poor function and frailty before a relatively short terminal period; it is exemplified by dementia, but is also increasingly true for patients with many different chronic illnesses. As medical advances extend survival, this mode of dying is being experienced by increasing numbers of people. The main challenge lies in providing nursing care and ensuring that plans are agreed for the time when medical intervention is no longer beneficial.

In a situation where death is inevitable and foreseeable, palliative care balances the 'standard textbook' approach with the wishes and values of the patient and a realistic assessment of the benefits of medical interventions. This often results in a greater focus on comfort, symptom control and support for patient and family, and may enable withdrawal of interventions that are ineffective or burdensome. Commonly, the outcome is less certain. In many cases, there is a substantial risk that the patient will die but there may be a small chance of improvement with further treatment. In these circumstances, it is often (but not always) correct and helpful to share this information with the patient so that better decisions can be made about further care.

The principles of palliative care are being used increasingly in many different diseases so that death can be managed effectively and compassionately. Palliative management of the most common symptoms is discussed in the next section.

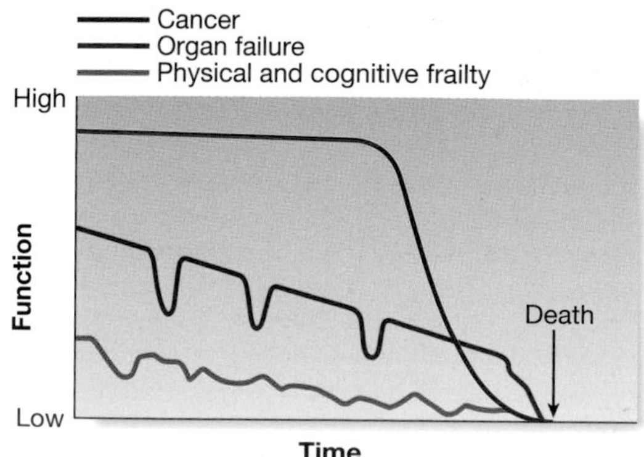

Fig. 12.1 Archetypal trajectories of dying. From Murray, et al. 2005 – see p. 292.

PRESENTING PROBLEMS IN PALLIATIVE CARE

Pain

The International Association for the Study of Pain (IASP) has defined pain as 'an unpleasant sensory and emotional experience associated with actual or potential tissue damage or described in terms of such damage'. It follows that each patient's experience and expression of pain are different, and that severity of pain does not correlate with the degree of tissue damage. Effective pain treatment facilitates recovery from injury or surgery, aids rapid recovery of function, and may minimise chronic pain and disability. Unfortunately, the delivery of effective pain relief is often impeded by factors such as poor assessment and concerns about the use of opioid analgesia.

12.1 Features of neuropathic pain

- Burning, stabbing or pulsing pain
- Spontaneous pain, without ongoing tissue damage
- Pain in an area of sensory loss
- Presence of a major neurological deficit
- Pain in response to non-painful stimuli: 'allodynia'
- Increased pain in response to painful stimuli: 'hyperalgesia'
- Unpleasant abnormal sensations: 'dysaesthesias'
- Poor relief from opioids alone

12.2 Types of pain

Type of pain	Features	Management options
Bone pain	Tender area over bone Possible pain on movement	Non-steroidal anti-inflammatory drugs (NSAIDs) Bisphosphonates Radiotherapy
Increased intracranial pressure	Headache, worse in the morning, associated with vomiting and occasionally confusion	Corticosteroids Radiotherapy Codeine
Abdominal colic	Intermittent, severe, spasmodic, associated with nausea or vomiting	Antispasmodics Hyoscine butylbromide
Liver capsule pain	Right upper quadrant abdominal pain, often associated with tender enlarged liver Responds poorly to opioids	Corticosteroids
Neuropathic pain	See Box 12.1	Anticonvulsants: Gabapentin Pregabalin Carbamazepine Antidepressants Amitriptyline Duloxetine Ketamine
Ischaemic pain	Diffuse severe aching pain associated with evidence of poor perfusion Responds poorly to opioids	NSAIDs Ketamine
Incident pain	Episodic pain usually related to movement or bowel spasm	Intermittent short-acting opioids Nerve block

Pain classification and mechanisms

Pain can be classified into two types:

- *Nociceptive*: due to direct stimulation of peripheral nerve endings by a noxious stimulus such as trauma, burns or ischaemia.
- *Neuropathic*: due to dysfunction of the pain perception system within the peripheral or central nervous system as a result of injury, disease or surgical damage, such as continuing pain experienced from a limb which has been amputated (phantom limb pain). This should be identified early (Box 12.1) because it is more difficult to treat once established.

The pain perception system (p. 1147) is not a simple hard-wired circuit of nerves connecting tissue pain receptors to the brain, but a dynamic system in which a continuing pain stimulus can cause central changes that lead to an increase in pain perception. This plasticity (changeability) applies to all the peripheral and central components of the pain pathway. Early and appropriate treatment of pain reduces the potential for chronic undesirable changes to develop.

Assessment and measurement of pain

Accurate assessment of the patient is the first step in providing good analgesia.

History and measurement of pain

A full pain history should be taken, to establish its causes and the underlying diagnoses. Patients may have more than one pain; for example, bone and neuropathic pain may both arise from skeletal metastases (Box 12.2).

A diagram of the body on which the patient can mark the pain site can be helpful. When asked to score pain, patients consistently rate it higher than health professionals and should, if able, always be asked to rate pain themselves. Methods include:

- *Verbal rating scale.* Different verbal descriptions are used to rate pain – 'no pain', 'mild pain', 'moderate pain' and 'severe pain'.
- *Visual analogue scale.* A question is used, such as 'Over the past 24 hours, how would you rate your pain, if 0 is no pain and 10 is the worst pain you could imagine?'
- *Behavioural rating scale.* It can be particularly difficult to decide whether a patient with cognitive impairment is suffering pain. A variety of measures are available which use observed behaviours, such as agitation and withdrawn posture, to assess levels of pain. Commonly used scales include Abbey and Dolorplus. Changes in behavioural rating pain scores can indicate whether drug measures have been successful.

Regular recording of formal pain assessment and patient-rated pain scores improves pain management and reduces the time taken to achieve pain control.

Psychological aspects of chronic pain

Perception of pain is influenced by many factors other than the painful stimulus, and pain cannot therefore be easily classified as wholly physical or psychogenic in any individual (Fig. 12.2). Patients who suffer chronic pain will be affected emotionally and, conversely, emotional distress can exacerbate physical pain (p. 240). Full assessment for symptoms of anxiety and depression is essential to effective pain management.

Examination

This should include careful assessment of the painful area, looking for signs of neuropathic pain (see Box 12.1) or bony tenderness suggestive of bone metastases. In

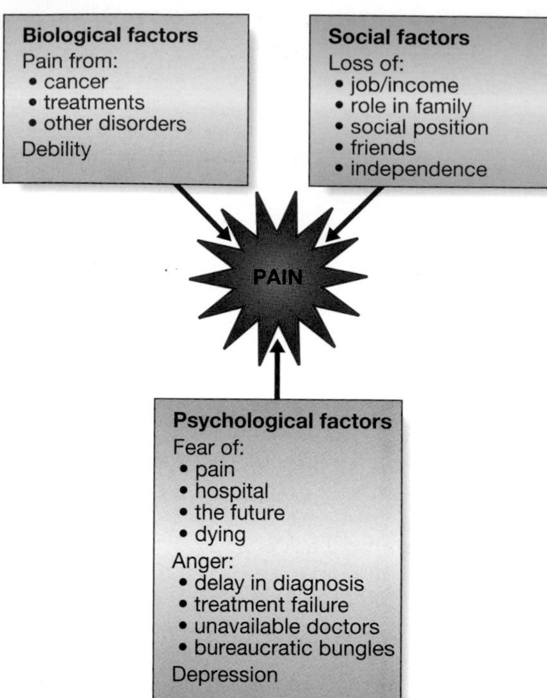

Fig. 12.2 Components of pain.

patients with cancer, it should not be assumed that all pains are due to the cancer or its metastases.

Appropriate investigations

Investigations should be directed towards diagnosis of an underlying cause, remembering that treatable conditions are possible even in patients with advanced disease. Imaging may be indicated, such as plain X-ray for fracture or magnetic resonance imaging (MRI) for spinal cord compression.

Management of pain

Many of the principles of pain management apply to any painful condition. There are, however, distinct differences between management of acute, chronic and palliative pain. Acute pain post-surgery or following trauma should be controlled with medication without causing unnecessary side-effects or risk to the patient. Chronic, non-malignant pain is more difficult and it may be impossible to relieve completely. In the management of chronic pain there is a greater emphasis on non-pharmacological treatments and on enabling the patient to live with pain. Strong opioids may help chronic pain but need to be used with caution after full assessment. They are used more readily in patients with a poorer prognosis.

Two-thirds of patients with cancer experience moderate or severe pain, and a quarter will have three or more different pains. Many of these are of mixed aetiology and 50% of pain from cancer has a neuropathic element. Careful evaluation to identify the likely pain mechanism facilitates appropriate treatment (see Box 12.2). It is vital that the patient's concerns about opioids are explored. Patients should be reassured that, when they are used for pain, psychological dependence and tolerance are extremely rare (Box 12.3).

12.3 Opioid myths

Myth	Fact
Pain is inevitable in cancer and many other diseases	**Pain can usually be controlled**
Opioids should be avoided because of dangerous side-effects	**Opioids can cause side-effects and sometimes the therapeutic window is narrow. However, side-effects are treatable and reversible**
The use of opioids commonly leads to addiction	**Addiction is very rare in patients who have pain and no previous history of addiction**
Taking opioids leads to more rapid decline and earlier death	**Opioids do not cause organ damage or other serious harm when used appropriately**

Nearly all types of pain respond to morphine to some degree. Some are completely opioid-responsive but others, such as neuropathic and ischaemic pain, are relatively unresponsive. Opioid-unresponsive or poorly responsive pain will only be relieved by opioids at a dose which causes significant side-effects. In these situations, effective pain relief may only be achieved with the use of adjuvant analgesics (see below).

Pharmacological treatments

Non-opioids

- *Paracetamol.* This is often effective for mild to moderate pain. For severe pain, it is inadequate alone, but is a useful and well-tolerated adjunct.
- *NSAIDs.* These are effective in the treatment of mild to moderate pain, and are also useful adjuncts in the treatment of severe pain. Adverse effects may be serious, especially in the elderly (p. 175).

Weak opioids

Codeine and dihydrocodeine are weak opioids. They have lower analgesic efficacy than strong opioids and a ceiling dose. They are effective for mild to moderate pain.

Strong opioids

Immediate-release (IR) oral morphine takes about 20 minutes to have an effect and usually provides pain relief for 4 hours. Most patients with continuous pain should be prescribed IR oral morphine every 4 hours initially, as this will provide continuous pain relief over the whole 24-hour period. Controlled-release (CR) morphine lasts for 12 or 24 hours but takes longer to provide analgesia.

The WHO analgesic ladder

The basic principle of the WHO ladder (Fig. 12.3) is that analgesia which is appropriate for the degree of pain should be prescribed. If pain is severe or remains poorly controlled, strong opioids should be prescribed and increased as indicated by the patient's need for additional analgesia (opioid titration).

A patient with mild pain is started on a non-opioid analgesic drug, such as paracetamol 1 g 4 times daily (step 1). If the maximum recommended dose is not

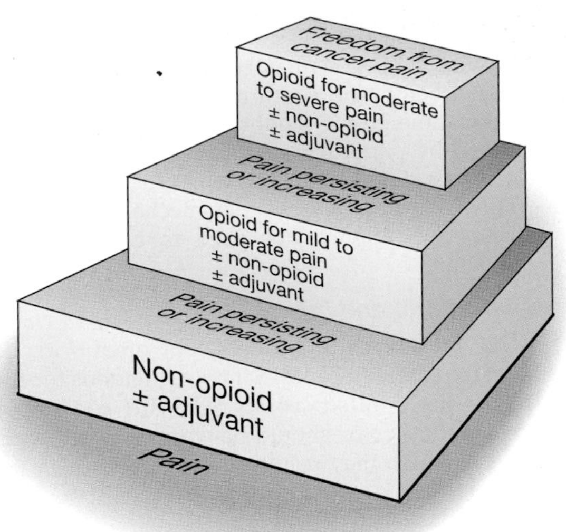

Fig. 12.3 The WHO analgesic ladder. From WHO 1996 – see p. 292.

sufficient or the patient has moderate pain, a weak opioid, such as codeine 60 mg 4 times daily, should be added (step 2). If adequate pain relief is still not achieved with the maximum recommended dosages or if the patient has severe pain, a strong opioid is substituted for the weak opioid (step 3). It is important not to move 'sideways' (change from one drug to another of equal potency) on a particular step of the ladder. All patients with severe pain should receive a full trial of strong opioids with appropriate adjuvant analgesia, as described below.

In addition to the regular dose, an extra dose of IR morphine should be prescribed 'as required' for when the patient has pain that is not controlled by the regular prescription (breakthrough pain). This should be one-sixth of the total 24-hour dose of opiate. The frequency of breakthrough doses should be dictated by their efficacy and any side-effects, rather than by a fixed time interval. A patient may require breakthrough analgesia as frequently as hourly if pain is severe, but this should lead to early review of the regular prescription. The patient and/or carer should note the timing of any breakthrough doses and the reason for them. These should be reviewed daily and the regular 4-hourly dose increased for the next 24 hours on the basis of:

- frequency of and reasons for breakthrough analgesia
- degree and acceptability of side-effects.

The regular dose should be increased by adding the total of the breakthrough doses over the previous 24 hours, unless there are significant problems with unacceptable side-effects. When the correct dose has been established, a CR preparation can be prescribed, usually twice daily.

Worldwide, the most effective and appropriate route of administration is oral, though transdermal preparations of strong opioids (usually fentanyl) are useful in certain situations, such as in patients with dysphagia or those who are reluctant to take tablets on a regular basis. Diamorphine is a highly soluble strong opioid used for subcutaneous infusions, particularly in the last few days of life, but is only available in certain countries.

12.4 Opioid side-effects

Side-effect	Management
Constipation	Regular laxative, such as co-danthramer or co-danthrusate (starting dose 2 capsules daily and titrate as needed) Opiates can be co-prescribed with oral naloxone
Dry mouth	Frequent sips of iced water, soft white paraffin to lips, chlorhexidine mouthwashes twice daily, sugar-free gum, water or saliva sprays
Nausea/ vomiting	Oral haloperidol 0.5–1 mg at night, oral metoclopramide 10 mg 3 times daily or oral domperidone 10 mg 3 times daily If constant, haloperidol or levomepromazine may be given parenterally to break the nausea cycle
Sedation	Explanation very important Symptoms usually settle in a few days Avoid other sedating medication where possible Ensure appropriate use of adjuvant analgesics which can have an opioid-sparing effect May require alternative opioid

Common side-effects of opioids are shown in Box 12.4. Nausea and vomiting occur initially but usually settle after a few days. Confusion and drowsiness are dose-related and reversible. In acute dosing, respiratory depression can occur but this is rare in those on regular opioids.

Opioid toxicity

All patients will develop dose-related side-effects, such as nausea, drowsiness, confusion or myoclonus; this is termed opiate toxicity. The dose at which this occurs varies from 10 to 5000 mg of morphine, depending on the patient and the type of pain. When opiates are being titrated, side-effects should be assessed regularly. The earliest side-effects are often visual hallucinations (often a sense of movement at the periphery of vision) and a distinct myoclonic movement. Pain should be re-assessed to ensure that appropriate adjuvants are being used. Parenteral rehydration is often helpful to speed up excretion of active metabolites of morphine. The dose of opioid may need to be reduced or changed to an alternative strong opiate.

Different opioids have different side-effect profiles in different people. If a patient develops side-effects, switching to an alternative strong opioid may be helpful. Options include oxycodone, transdermal fentanyl, alfentanil, hydromorphone and occasionally methadone, any of which may produce a better balance of benefit against side-effects. Fentanyl and alfentanil have no renally excreted active metabolites and may be particularly useful in patients with renal failure. Pethidine is used in acute pain management but not for chronic or cancer pain because of its short half-life and ceiling dose.

It is important to be very careful when switching opiates, as it is easy to make calculation mistakes and prescribe too much or too little.

Adjuvant analgesics

An adjuvant analgesic is a drug with a primary indication other than pain but which provides analgesia in some painful conditions and may enhance the effect of the primary analgesic. At each step of the WHO analgesic ladder, an adjuvant analgesic should be considered, the choice depending on the type of pain (Boxes 12.5 and 12.6).

Non-pharmacological and complementary treatments

Radiotherapy

Radiotherapy can improve pain from bone metastases and may be considered for cancer in other sites (see Box 12.2).

Physiotherapy

This helps to alleviate pain and restore function, through active mobilisation and specific physiotherapy techniques, such as spinal manipulation, massage, application of heat or cold, and exercise. Immediate application of cold with ice packs can reduce subsequent swelling and inflammation after a direct injury.

Psychological techniques

These include simple relaxation, hypnosis, cognitive behavioural therapies and biofeedback (pp. 240–241), which train the patient to use coping strategies and behavioural techniques. This is often more relevant in chronic non-malignant pain than in cancer pain.

EBM 12.5 Treatment of neuropathic pain

'Tricyclic antidepressants, a variety of anticonvulsants, and gabapentin are effective treatments for neuropathic pain.'

- Guideline 106. Scottish Intercollegiate Guidelines Network; 2008.

For further information: www.sign.ac.uk

Stimulation therapies

Acupuncture (Fig. 12.4) has been used successfully in Eastern medicine for centuries. It causes release of endogenous analgesics (endorphins) within the spinal cord. It can be particularly effective in pain related to muscle spasm. Transcutaneous electrical nerve stimulation (TENS) may have a similar mechanism of action to acupuncture and can be used in both acute and chronic pain.

Herbal medicine and homeopathy

These are widely used for pain, but often with little evidence for efficacy (p. 15). Safety regulations for these treatments are limited, compared with conventional drugs, and the doctor should be wary of unrecognised side-effects which may result.

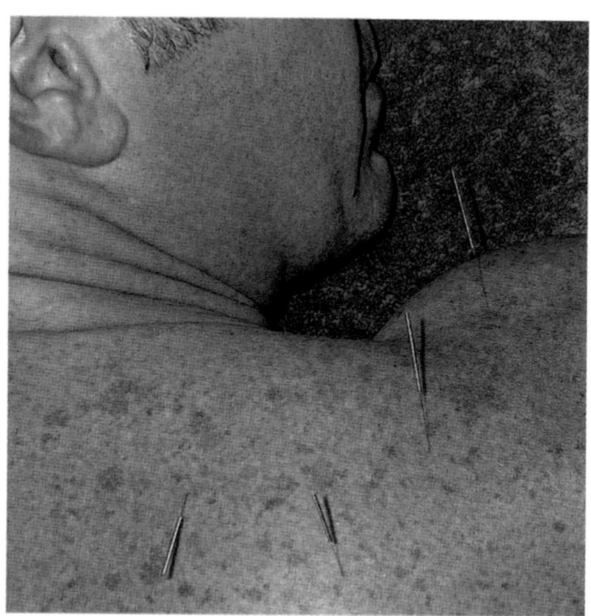

Fig. 12.4 Acupuncture.

12.6 Adjuvant analgesics

Drug	Example	Indications	Side-effects*
NSAIDs	Diclofenac	Bone metastases, soft tissue infiltration, liver pain, inflammatory pain	Gastric irritation and bleeding, fluid retention, headache; caution in renal impairment
Corticosteroids	Dexamethasone 8–16 mg per day, titrated to lowest dose that controls pain	Raised intracranial pressure, nerve compression, soft tissue infiltration, liver pain	Gastric irritation if used together with NSAID, fluid retention, confusion, Cushingoid appearance, candidiasis, hyperglycaemia
Anticonvulsants	Evidence strongest for: Gabapentin, Pregabalin, Duloxetine	Neuropathic pain of any aetiology	Mild sedation, tremor, confusion
Tricyclic antidepressants	Amitriptyline	Neuropathic pain of any aetiology	Sedation, dizziness, confusion, dry mouth, constipation, urinary retention; avoid in cardiac disease
NMDA blockers	Ketamine	Severe neuropathic pain (only under specialist supervision)	Confusion, anxiety, agitation, hypertension

*In old age, all drugs can cause confusion.
(NMDA = N-methyl-D-aspartate)

Breathlessness

The sensation of breathlessness is the result of a complex interaction between different factors at the levels of production (the pathophysiological cause), perception (the severity of breathlessness perceived by the patient) and expression (the symptoms expressed by an individual patient). A patient's perception and expression of breathlessness can be significantly improved, even if there is no reversible 'cause' (Box 12.7). Assessment and treatment should therefore be targeted at modifying these factors, particularly when there is no reversible pathophysiology.

Clearly reversible causes of breathlessness (p. 655) should be identified and managed, but investigation and treatment should be appropriate to the prognosis and stage of disease. A therapeutic trial of corticosteroids (dexamethasone 8 mg for 5 days) and/or nebulised salbutamol may be helpful.

Breathlessness may be worsened by specific anxieties and beliefs; these should be explored. Many people with heart failure are concerned that exertional breathlessness will lead to worsening of their heart condition. Patients with advanced disease have specific panic-breathlessness cycles in which breathlessness leads to panic, which leads to worsening breathlessness and worsening panic. These should be identified and explained to the patient. Many fear that they will die during one of these episodes, and explanation of the panic cycle can be very reassuring. Another frequently expressed fear is that breathlessness will continue to worsen until it is continuous and unbearable, leading to a distressing and undignified death. Reassurance should again be given that this is uncommon and can be effectively managed with opioids and benzodiazepines.

A rapidly acting benzodiazepine, such as sublingual lorazepam, or non-drug measures, such as relaxation techniques, may help panic-breathlessness cycles. Attention to energy conservation (thinking clearly about using limited energy reserves sensibly) and pacing of activity is also extremely helpful. Physiotherapists are good at this and should be involved in developing an individual plan for each patient.

Perception of breathlessness may also be improved by night-time or regular morphine, or by regular benzodiazepines.

Oxygen does not help breathlessness unless the patient is hypoxic. An electric fan, piped air or an open window can be as effective as oxygen in patients who are breathless but not hypoxic. The patient's, family's or even professional beliefs about the benefits and need for oxygen may be the main reason for its apparent efficacy in non-hypoxic patients who feel less breathless when using oxygen.

EBM 12.7 Palliative treatment of breathlessness

'Interventions based on psychosocial support, breathing control and coping strategies can help patients to cope with the symptom of breathlessness and reduce physical and emotional distress.'

- Bredin M, et al. BMJ 1999; 318:901.

Cough

Cough can be a troubling symptom in cancer and other illnesses such as motor neuron disease, cardiac failure and COPD. There are many possible causes (p. 654). Management should focus on treating the underlying condition if possible. If this fails to bring about the desired response, antitussives, such as codeine linctus, are sometimes effective, particularly for cough at night.

Nausea and vomiting

The presentation of nausea and vomiting differs, depending on the underlying cause, of which there are many (p. 853). Large-volume vomiting with little nausea is common in intestinal obstruction, whereas constant nausea with little or no vomiting is often due to metabolic abnormalities or drugs. Vomiting related to raised intracranial pressure is worse in the morning.

Different receptors are activated, depending on the cause or causes of the nausea (Fig. 12.5). For example, dopamine receptors in the chemotactic trigger zone in the fourth ventricle are stimulated by metabolic and drug causes of nausea, whereas gastric irritation stimulates histamine receptors in the vomiting centre via the vagus nerve.

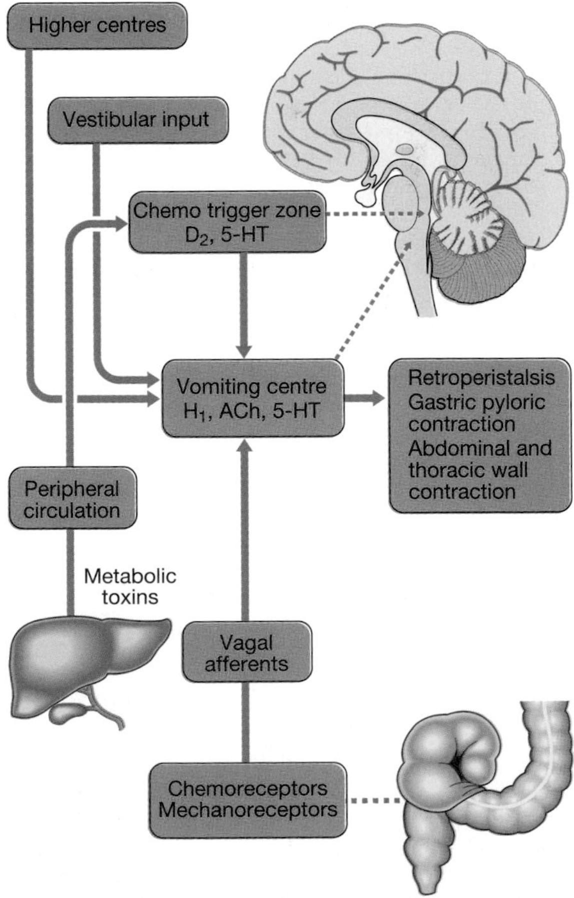

Fig. 12.5 Mechanisms of nausea. (ACh = acetylcholine; D_2 = dopamine; 5-HT = 5-hydroxytryptamine, serotonin; H_1 = histamine)

12.8 Receptor site activity of antiemetic drugs

Area	Receptors	Drugs
Chemo trigger zone	Dopamine$_2$ 5-HT	Haloperidol Metoclopramide
Vomiting centre	Histamine$_1$ Acetylcholine	Cyclizine Levomepromazine Hyoscine
Gut (gastric stasis)		Metoclopramide
Gut distension (vagal stimulation)	Histamine$_1$	Cyclizine
Gut (chemoreceptors)	5-HT	Levomepromazine

Reversible causes, such as hypercalcaemia and constipation, should be treated appropriately. Drug-induced causes should be considered and the offending drugs stopped if possible. As different classes of antiemetic drug act at different receptors, antiemetic therapy should be based on a careful assessment of the probable causes and a rational decision to use a particular class of drug (Box 12.8). The subcutaneous route is often required initially to overcome gastric stasis and poor absorption of oral medicines.

Gastrointestinal obstruction

Gastrointestinal obstruction is a frequent complication of intra-abdominal cancer. Patients may have multiple levels of obstruction and symptoms may vary greatly in nature and severity. Surgical mortality is high in patients with advanced disease and obstruction should normally be managed without surgery.

The key to effective management is to address the presenting symptoms - colic, abdominal pain, nausea, vomiting, intestinal secretions - individually or in combination, using drugs which do not cause or worsen other symptoms. This can be problematic when a specific treatment worsens another symptom. Cyclizine improves nausea and colic responds well to anticholinergic agents, such as hyoscine butylbromide, but both slow gut motility. Nausea will improve with metoclopramide, although this is contraindicated in the presence of colic because of its prokinetic effect. There is some evidence that corticosteroids (dexamethasone 8 mg) can shorten the length of obstructive episodes. Somatostatin analogues, such as octreotide, will reduce intestinal secretions and therefore large-volume vomits. Occasionally, a nasogastric tube is required to reduce gaseous or fluid distension.

Weight loss and general weakness

Patients with cancer lose weight due to an alteration of metabolism by the tumour known as the cancer cachexia syndrome. NSAIDs and megestrol may be helpful in early-stage disease but are unlikely to be effective in advanced cancer. Corticosteroids can temporarily boost appetite and general well-being, but may cause false weight gain by promoting fluid retention. Their benefits need to be weighed against the risk of side-effects.

Anxiety and depression

Depression is common in palliative care but diagnosis is more difficult, as the physical symptoms of depression are similar to those of advanced disease. Anxiety and depression may still respond to treatment with a combination of drugs and psychotherapeutic approaches (p. 243). Citalopram and mirtazapine are better tolerated in patients with advanced disease. It should not be assumed that depression is an 'understandable' consequence of the patient's situation.

Delirium and terminal agitation

Many patients become confused or agitated in the last days of life. It is important to identify and treat potentially reversible causes (pp. 173 and 280), unless the patient is too close to death for this to be feasible. Early diagnosis and effective management of delirium are extremely important. As in other palliative situations, it may not be possible to identify and treat the underlying cause, and the focus of management may be to ensure comfort. It is important to distinguish between behavioural change due to pain and that due to delirium, as opioids will improve one and worsen the other.

The management of delirium is detailed on page 174. It is important, even in palliative care to treat delirium with antipsychotic medicines such as haloperidol rather than regard it as distress or anxiety and use benzodiazepines only.

DEATH AND DYING

Talking about and planning towards dying

There have been dramatic improvements in medical treatment and care of patients with cancer and other illnesses over recent years, but the inescapable fact remains that everyone will die at some time. Planning for death is not required for people who die suddenly but should be actively considered in patients with chronic diseases when the death is considered to be foreseeable or inevitable. Doctors rarely know exactly when a patient will die but we are often aware that the risk of dying is increasing and that medical interventions are unlikely to prolong life or improve function. Many people wish their doctors to be honest about this situation to allow them time to think ahead, make plans and address practical issues. A smaller number do not wish to discuss future deterioration or death; this avoidance of discussion should be respected.

For doctors, it is helpful to understand an individual's wishes and values about medical interventions at this time, as this can help guide decisions about ceilings of intervention. Some interventions will not work in patients with far advanced disease. It is useful to distinguish between those that will not work (a medical decision) and those that do not confer sufficient benefit to be worthwhile (a decision that can only be reached with a patient's involvement and consent). A common example of this would be decisions about not attempting cardiopulmonary resuscitation.

In general, people wish for a dignified and peaceful death and most prefer to die at home. Families also are grateful for the chance to prepare themselves for the death of a relative, by timely and gentle discussion with their doctor or other health professionals. Early discussion and effective planning improve the chances that an individual's wishes will be achieved.

Diagnosing dying

When patients with cancer become bed-bound, semi-comatose, unable to take tablets and only able to take sips of water, with no reversible cause, they are likely to be dying and many will have died within 2 days. Patients with other conditions also reach a stage where death is predictable and imminent. Doctors are sometimes poor at recognising this, and should be alert to the views of other members of the multidisciplinary team. A clear decision that the patient is dying should be agreed and recorded.

Management

Once the conclusion has been reached that a patient is going to die in the next few days, there is a significant shift in management (Box 12.9). Symptom control, relief of distress and care for the family become the most important elements of care. Medication and investigation are only justifiable if they contribute to these ends. When patients can no longer drink because they are dying, intravenous fluids are usually not necessary and may cause worsening of bronchial secretions. Medicines should always be prescribed for the relief of symptoms. For example, morphine or diamorphine may be used to control pain, levomepromazine to control nausea, haloperidol to treat confusion, diazepam or midazolam to treat distress, and hyoscine hydrobromide to reduce respiratory secretions. Side-effects, such as drowsiness, may be acceptable if the principal aim of relieving distress is achieved. It is important to discuss and agree the aims of care with the patient's family.

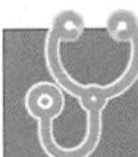

12.9 How to manage a patient who is dying

Patient and family awareness
• Assess patient's and family's awareness of the situation • Ensure family understands plan of care
Medical interventions
• Stop non-essential medications that do not contribute to symptom control • Stop inappropriate investigations and interventions, including routine observations
Resuscitation
• Complete Do Not Attempt Cardiopulmonary Resuscitation (DNACPR) form • Deactivate implantable defibrillator
Symptom control
• Ensure availability of parenteral medication for symptom relief
Support for family
• Make sure you have contact details for family, that you know when they want to be contacted and that they are aware of the facilities available to them
Religious and spiritual needs
• Make sure any particular wishes are identified and followed
Ongoing assessment
• Family's awareness of condition • Management of symptoms • Need for parenteral hydration
Care after death
• Make sure family know what they have to do • Notify other appropriate health professionals

Ethical issues at the end of life

In Europe, between 25 and 50% of all deaths are associated with some form of decision which may affect the length of a patient's life. The most common form of decision involves withdrawing or withholding further treatment: for example, not treating a chest infection in a patient who is clearly dying from advanced cancer. It is important to have a framework for considering such decisions (such as the four ethical principles: autonomy, beneficence, non-maleficence and justice, p. 10), which balances degrees of importance when there is conflict: for example, when a patient wishes to receive treatment which a doctor believes will be ineffective or which may cause harm. A decision has to be taken as to which principle is most important: whether it is better to respect a patient's wishes, even if it causes harm, or to reduce the risk of harm but not accede to those wishes.

A futile treatment is one which has no chance of achieving worthwhile benefit: that is, the treatment cannot achieve a result that the patient would consider, now or in the future, to be worthwhile. Doctors are not required to institute futile treatments, such as resuscitation, in the event of cardiac arrest in a patient with terminal cancer.

Incapacity and advance directives

Patients' wishes are very important in Western medical ethics, although other cultures emphasise the views of the family. If a patient is unable to express his or her view because of communication or cognitive impairment, that person lacks 'capacity'. In order to decide what the patient would have wished, as much information as possible should be gained about any previously expressed wishes, along with the views of relatives and other health professionals.

An advance directive is a previously recorded, written document of a patient's wishes (p. 171). It should carry the same weight in decision-making as a patient's contemporaneously expressed wishes, but may not be sufficiently specific to be used in a particular clinical situation. The legal framework for decision-making varies in different countries.

Hydration

Deciding whether to give intravenous fluids can be difficult when a patient is very unwell and the prognosis is uncertain. If a patient is clearly dying and has a prognosis of a few days, rehydration may cause harm by increasing bronchial secretions, and will not benefit the patient by prolonging life. A patient with a major stroke, who is unable to swallow but expected to survive the event, will develop renal impairment and thirst if not given fluids and should be hydrated. Each decision should be individual and discussed with the patient's family.

Euthanasia

In the UK and Europe, between 3 and 6% of dying patients ask a doctor to end their life. Many of these requests are transient; some are associated with poor control of physical symptoms or a depressive illness. All expressions of a wish to die are an opportunity to help the patient discuss and address unresolved issues and problems.

Reversible causes, such as pain or depression, should be treated. Sometimes, patients may choose to discontinue life-prolonging treatments, such as diuretics or anticoagulation, following discussion and the provision of adequate alternative symptom control. However, there remain a small number of patients who have a sustained, competent wish to end their lives, despite good control of physical symptoms. Euthanasia is now permitted or legal in some countries but remains illegal in many others; public ethical and legal debate over this issue is likely to continue.

Further information and acknowledgements

Websites

www.anaesthetist.com/ *Information on pain physiology and acute management of pain.*

www.helpthehospices.org.uk/clip/index.htm *Useful online tutorials on all aspects of palliative symptom control.*

www.palliativecareguidelines.scot.nhs.uk *Regularly reviewed, evidence-based clinical guidelines.*

www.palliativedrugs.co.uk *Information for health professionals about the use of drugs in palliative care. It highlights drugs given for unlicensed indications or by unlicensed routes, and the administration of multiple drugs by continuous subcutaneous infusion.*

Figure acknowledgements

Fig. 12.1 Reproduced from Murray SA, Kendall M, Boyd K, et al. Illness trajectories and palliative care. BMJ 2005; 330:7498; reproduced with permission from the BMJ Publishing Group.

Fig. 12.3 WHO. Cancer pain relief. 2nd edn. Geneva: WHO; 1996.

D.H. Dockrell
S. Sundar
B.J. Angus
R.P. Hobson

Infectious disease

13

Clinical examination of patients with infectious disease 294

Presenting problems in infectious diseases 296

Fever 296
Positive blood culture 303
Sepsis 304
Acute diarrhoea and vomiting 306
Infections acquired in the tropics 308
Infections in adolescence 313
Infections in pregnancy 313

Viral infections 314

Systemic viral infections with exanthem 314
Systemic viral infections without exanthem 319
Viral infections of the skin 325
Gastrointestinal viral infections 327
Respiratory viral infections 328
Viral infections with neurological involvement 328
Viral infections with rheumatological involvement 329

Prion diseases 329

Bacterial infections 329

Bacterial infections of the skin, soft tissues and bones 329
Systemic bacterial infections 333
Gastrointestinal bacterial infections 341
Respiratory bacterial infections 345
Bacterial infections with neurological involvement 347
Mycobacterial infections 347
Rickettsial and related intracellular bacterial infections 350
Chlamydial infections 353

Protozoal infections 353

Systemic protozoal infections 353
Leishmaniasis 362
Gastrointestinal protozoal infections 367

Infections caused by helminths 369

Intestinal human nematodes 369
Tissue-dwelling human nematodes 372
Zoonotic nematodes 375
Trematodes (flukes) 376
Cestodes (tapeworms) 378

Ectoparasites 381

Fungal infections 381

Superficial mycoses 381
Subcutaneous mycoses 381
Systemic mycoses 383

CLINICAL EXAMINATION OF PATIENTS WITH INFECTIOUS DISEASE

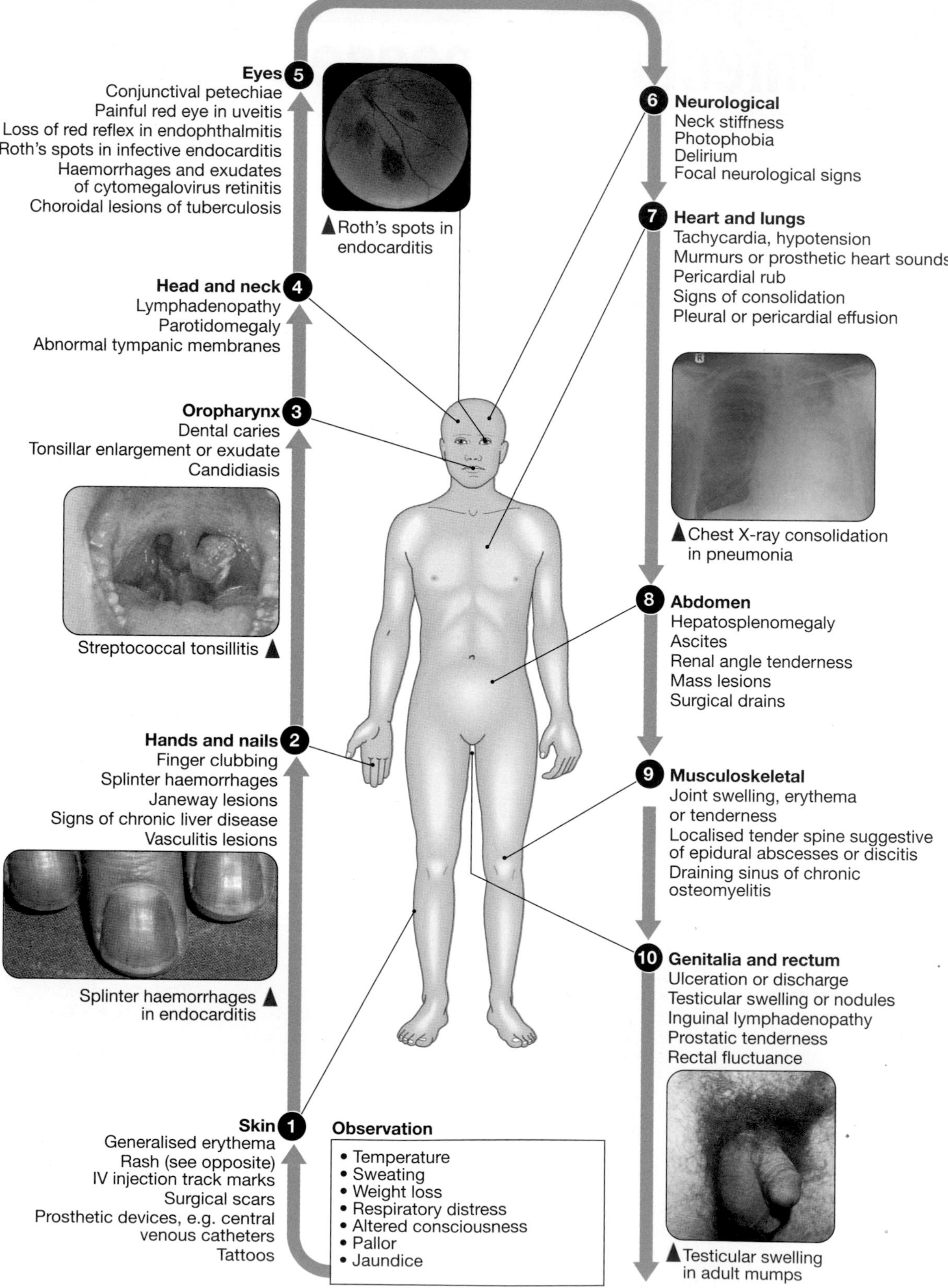

Fever

- *Documentation of fever.* 'Feeling hot' or sweaty does not necessarily signify fever. Fever is diagnosed only when a body temperature of over 38.0°C has been recorded. Axillary and aural measurement is less accurate than oral or rectal. Outpatients may be trained to keep a temperature chart.
- *Rigors.* Shivering (followed by excessive sweating) occurs with a rapid rise in body temperature from any cause.
- *Night sweats.* These are associated with particular infections (e.g. tuberculosis, infective endocarditis), but sweating from any cause is worse at night.
- *Excessive sweating.* Alcohol, anxiety, thyrotoxicosis, diabetes mellitus, acromegaly, lymphoma and excessive environmental heat all cause sweating without temperature elevation.
- *Recurrent fever.* There are various causes, e.g. *Borrelia recurrentis*, bacterial abscess.
- *Accompanying features.*
  HEADACHE. Severe headache and photophobia, although characteristic of meningitis, may accompany other infections.
  DELIRIUM. Mental confusion during fever is more common in young children or the elderly.
  MUSCLE PAIN. Myalgia may occur with viral infections, such as influenza, and with septicaemia, including meningococcal sepsis.
  SHOCK. Shock may accompany severe infections and sepsis (Ch. 8).

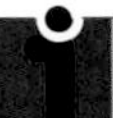

History-taking in suspected infectious disease*

Presenting complaint
- Diverse manifestations of infectious disease make accurate assessment of features and duration critical; e.g. fever and cough lasting 2 days imply an acute respiratory tract infection but suggest TB if they last 2 months

Review of systems
- Must be comprehensive

Past medical history
- Define the 'host' and likelihood of infection(s)
- Include surgical and dental procedures involving prosthetic materials
- Document previous infections

Medication history
- Include non-prescription drugs, use of antimicrobials and immunosuppressive drugs
- Identify medicines which interact with antimicrobials

Allergy history
- Esp. to antimicrobials, noting allergic manifestation (e.g. rash versus anaphylaxis)

Family and contact history
- Note infections and their time course
- Sensitively explore exposure to key infections, e.g. TB and HIV-1

Travel history
- Include countries visited and where previously resident (relevant to exposure and likely vaccination history, e.g. likelihood of BCG vaccination in childhood)

Occupation
- e.g. Anthrax in leather tannery workers

Recreational pursuits
- e.g. Leptospirosis in canoeists and windsurfers

Animal exposures
- Include pets, e.g. dog exposure and hydatid disease

Dietary history
- Consider undercooked meats, shellfish, unpasteurised dairy products or well water
- Establish who else was exposed, e.g. to food-borne pathogens

History of intravenous drug injection or receipt of blood products
- Risks for blood-borne viruses, e.g. HIV-1, and HBV and HCV

Sexual history
- Explore in a confidential and non-threatening way (Ch. 15); remember that the most common mechanism of HIV-1 transmission is heterosexual contact (Ch. 14)

Vaccination history and use of prophylactic medicines
- Consider occupation- or age-related vaccines
- In a traveller or infection-predisposed patient, establish compliance with prophylactic treatments

*Always consider non-infectious aetiologies in the differential diagnosis.
(HBV/HCV = hepatitis B/C virus; HIV-1 = human immunodeficiency virus-1; TB = tuberculosis)

1 Skin lesions in infectious diseases

- Diffuse erythema, e.g. A
- Migrating erythema, e.g. enlarging rash of erythema migrans in Lyme disease (see Fig. 13.20, p. 335)
- Purpuric or petechial rashes, e.g. B
- Macular or papular rashes, e.g. primary infection with HIV (Box 14.8, p. 395)
- Vesicular or blistering rash, e.g. C
- Erythema multiforme (Fig. 28.48 and Box 28.41, p. 1302)
- Nodules or plaques, e.g. Kaposi's sarcoma (p. 384)
- Erythema nodosum (D and Box 28.42, p. 1303)

A
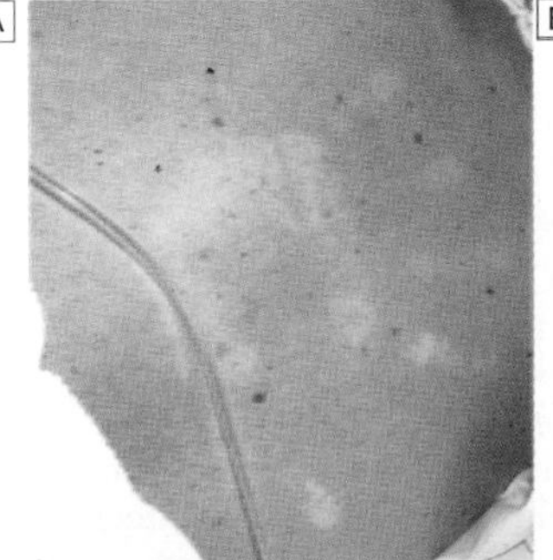
Streptococcal toxic shock syndrome

B
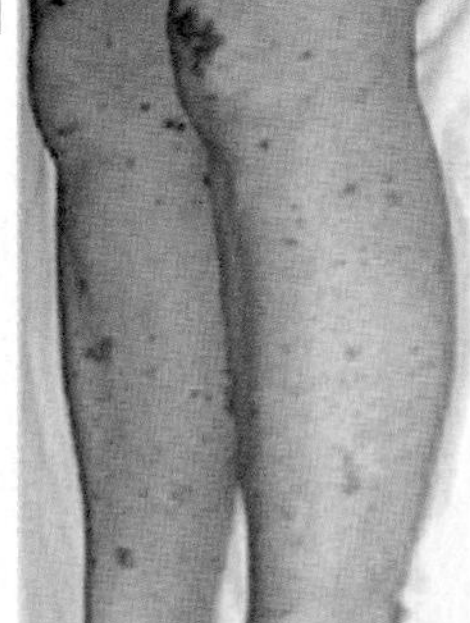
Meningococcal sepsis

C
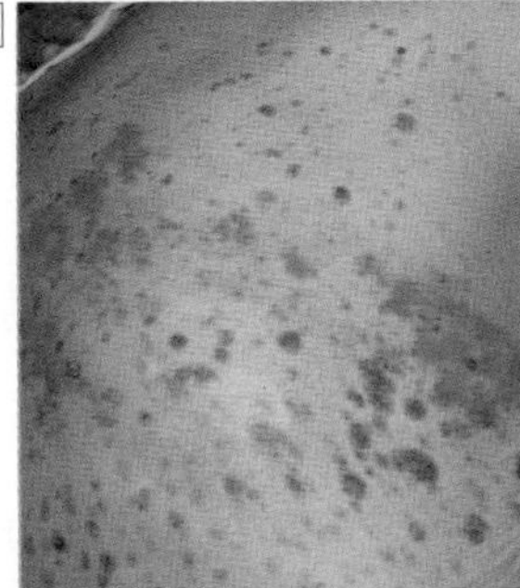
Shingles

D
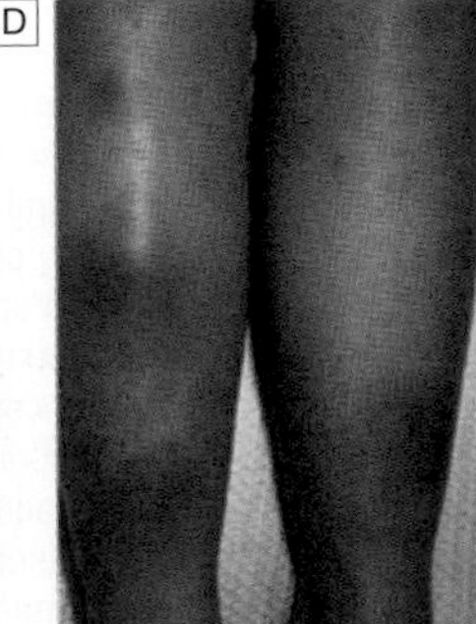
Erythema nodosum

The principles of infection and its investigation and therapy are described in Chapter 6. This chapter and the following ones on human immunodeficiency virus/acquired immunodeficiency syndrome (HIV/AIDS) and sexually transmitted infection (STI) describe the approach to patients with potential infectious disease, the individual infections and the resulting syndromes.

PRESENTING PROBLEMS IN INFECTIOUS DISEASES

Infectious diseases present with myriad clinical manifestations. Many of these are described either in other chapters of this book or below.

Fever

'Fever' implies an elevated core body temperature of more than 38.0°C (p. 138). Fever is a response to cytokines and acute phase proteins (pp. 74 and 82) and occurs in infections and in non-infectious conditions.

Clinical assessment

The differential diagnosis is very broad so clinical features are used to guide the most appropriate investigations. The systematic approach described on pages 294–295 should be followed. Box 13.1 describes the assessment of elderly patients.

Investigations

If the clinical features do not suggest a specific infection, then initial investigations should include:

- a full blood count (FBC) with differential, including eosinophil count
- urea and electrolytes, liver function tests (LFTs), blood glucose and muscle enzymes
- inflammatory markers, erythrocyte sedimentation rate (ESR) and C-reactive protein (CRP)
- a test for antibodies to HIV-1 (p. 392)
- autoantibodies, including antinuclear antibodies (ANA)

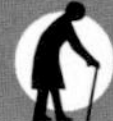

13.1 Fever in old age

- **Temperature measurement**: fever may be missed because oral temperatures are unreliable. Rectal measurement may be needed but core temperature is increasingly measured using eardrum reflectance.
- **Acute confusion**: common with fever, especially in those with underlying cerebrovascular disease or dementia.
- **Prominent causes of pyrexia of unknown origin**: include tuberculosis and intra-abdominal abscesses, complicated urinary tract infection and infective endocarditis. Non-infective causes include polymyalgia rheumatica/temporal arteritis and tumours. A smaller fraction of cases remain undiagnosed than in young people.
- **Pitfalls in the elderly**: conditions such as cerebrovascular accident or thromboembolic disease can cause fever but every effort must be made to exclude concomitant infection.
- **Common infectious diseases in the very frail** (e.g. nursing home residents): pneumonia, urinary infection, soft tissue infection and gastroenteritis.

- chest X-ray and electrocardiogram (ECG)
- urinalysis and urine culture
- blood culture (p. 140)
- throat swab for culture
- other specimens, as indicated by history and examination, e.g. wound swab; sputum culture; stool culture, microscopy for ova and parasites, and *Clostridium difficile* toxin assay; if relevant, malaria films on 3 consecutive days or a malaria rapid diagnostic test (antigen detection, p. 355).

Subsequent investigations in patients with HIV-related (p. 396), immune-deficient (p. 301), nosocomial or travel-related (p. 309) pyrexia and in individuals with associated symptoms or signs of involvement of the respiratory, gastrointestinal or neurological systems are described elsewhere.

Management

Fever and its associated systemic symptoms can be treated with paracetamol, and by tepid sponging to cool the skin. Replacement of salt and water is important in patients with drenching sweats. Further management is focused on the underlying cause.

Fever with localising symptoms or signs

In most patients, the site of infection is apparent after clinical evaluation (p. 294), and the likelihood of infection is reinforced by investigation results (e.g. neutrophilia with raised ESR and CRP in bacterial infections). Not all apparently localising symptoms are reliable, however; headache, breathlessness and diarrhoea can occur in sepsis without localised infection in the central nervous system (CNS), respiratory tract or gastrointestinal tract. Careful interpretation of the clinical features is vital (e.g. severe headache associated with photophobia, rash and neck stiffness suggests meningitis, whereas moderate headache with cough and rhinorrhoea is consistent with a viral upper respiratory tract infection).

Common infections that present with fever are shown in Figure 13.1. Further investigation and management are specific to the cause, but may include empirical antimicrobial therapy (p. 149) pending confirmation of the microbiological diagnosis.

Pyrexia of unknown origin

Pyrexia of unknown origin (PUO) is defined as a temperature persistently above 38.0°C for more than 3 weeks, without diagnosis, despite initial investigation during 3 days of inpatient care or after more than two outpatient visits. Subsets of PUO are described by medical setting: HIV-1 related, immune-deficient or nosocomial. Up to one-third of cases of PUO remain undiagnosed.

Clinical assessment

Major causes of PUO are outlined in Box 13.2. Rare causes, such as periodic fever syndromes (p. 85), should be considered in those with a positive family history. Children and younger adults are more likely to have infectious causes – in particular, viral infections. Older adults are more likely to have certain infectious and non-infectious causes (see Box 13.1). Detailed history and examination should be repeated at regular intervals

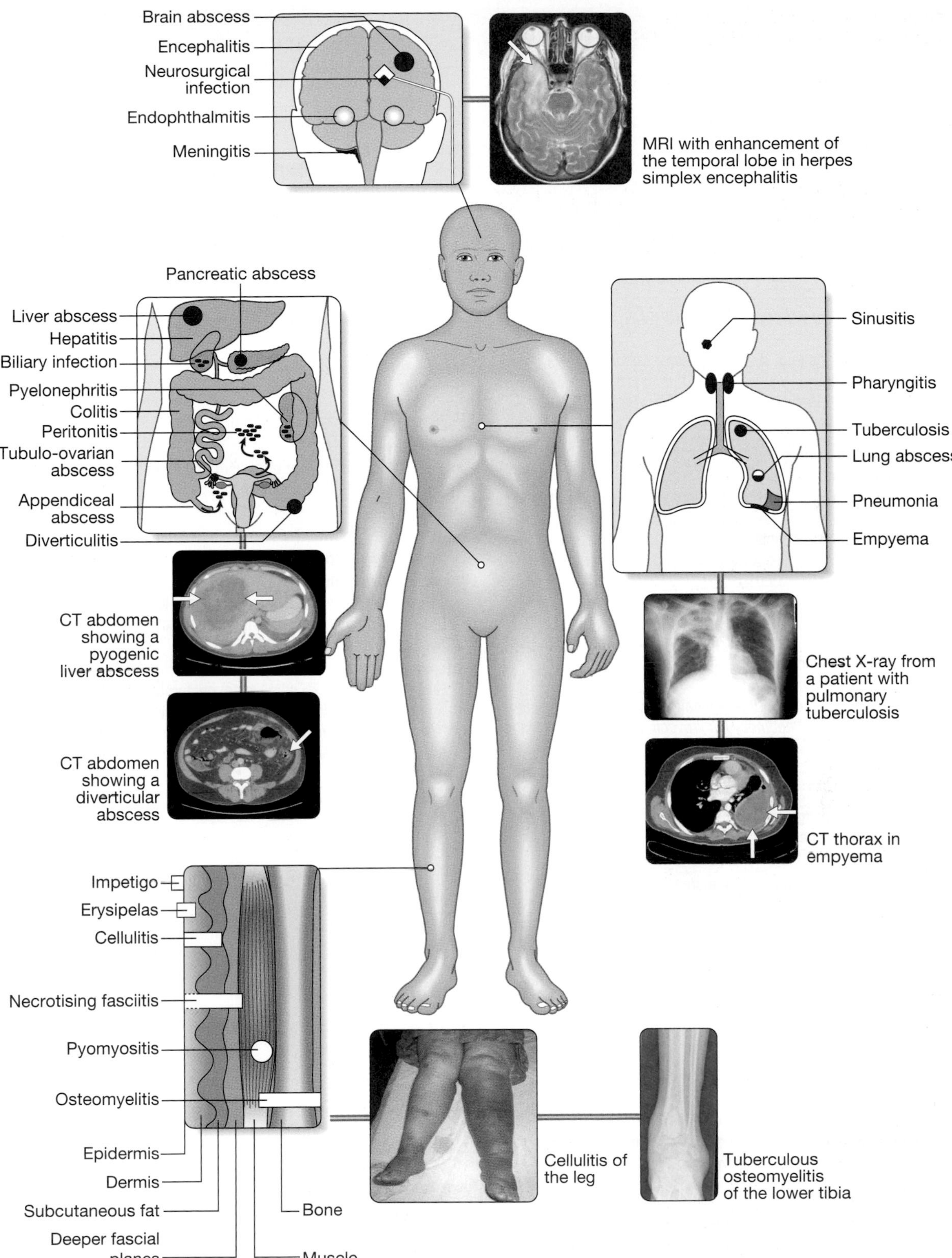

Fig. 13.1 Common infectious syndromes presenting with fever and localised features. Major causes are grouped by approximate anatomical location and include central nervous system infection; respiratory tract infections; abdominal, pelvic or urinary tract infections; and skin and soft tissue infections (SSTI) or osteomyelitis. For each site of infection, particular syndromes and their common causes are described elsewhere in the book. The causative organisms vary, depending on host factors, which include whether the patient has lived or resided in a tropical country or particular geographical location, has acquired the infection in a health-care environment or is immunocompromised.

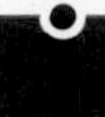

13.2 Aetiology of pyrexia of unknown origin (PUO)

Infections (~30%)

Specific locations
- Abscesses: hepatobiliary*, diverticular*, urinary tract* (including prostate), pulmonary, CNS
- Infections of oral cavity (including dental), head and neck (including sinuses)
- Bone and joint infections
- Infective endocarditis*

Specific organisms
- Tuberculosis (particularly extrapulmonary)*
- HIV-1 infection
- Other viral infections (cytomegalovirus (CMV), Epstein–Barr virus (EBV))
- Fungal infections (e.g. *Aspergillus* spp., *Candida* spp. or dimorphic fungi)
- Infections with fastidious organisms (e.g. *Bartonella* spp., *Tropheryma whipplei*)

Specific patient groups
- Imported infections
  Malaria, dengue, rickettsial infections, *Brucella* spp., amoebic liver abscess, enteric fevers, *Leishmania* spp. (southern Europe, India, Africa and Latin America), *Burkholderia pseudomallei* (South-east Asia), HIV and respiratory tract infections
- Nosocomial infections
  Infections related to prosthetic materials and surgical procedures
- HIV-positive individuals
  Acute retroviral syndrome
  AIDS-defining infections (disseminated *Mycobacterium avium* complex (DMAC), *Pneumocystis jirovecii (carinii)* pneumonia, CMV and others)

Malignancy (~20%)

Haematological malignancy
- Lymphoma*, leukaemia and myeloma

Solid tumours
- Renal, liver, colon, stomach, pancreas, kidney

Connective tissue disorders (~15%)

Older adults
- Temporal arteritis/polymyalgia rheumatica*

Younger adults
- Still's disease (juvenile rheumatoid arthritis)*
- Systemic lupus erythematosus (SLE)
- Vasculitic disorders (including polyarteritis nodosa, rheumatoid disease with vasculitis and granulomatosis with polyangiitis (also known as Wegener's granulomatosis))
- Polymyositis
- Behçet's disease

Geographically restricted
- Rheumatic fever

Miscellaneous (~20%)

Cardiovascular
- Atrial myxoma, aortitis, aortic dissection

Respiratory
- Sarcoidosis, pulmonary embolism and other thromboembolic disease, extrinsic allergic alveolitis

Gastrointestinal
- Inflammatory bowel disease, granulomatous hepatitis, alcoholic liver disease, pancreatitis

Endocrine/metabolic
- Thyrotoxicosis, thyroiditis, hypothalamic lesions, phaeochromocytoma, adrenal insufficiency, hypertriglyceridaemia

Haematological
- Haemolytic anaemia, paroxysmal nocturnal haemoglobinuria, thrombotic thrombocytopenic purpura, myeloproliferative disorders, Castleman's disease, graft-versus-host disease (after allogeneic haematopoietic stem cell transplantation)

Inherited
- Familial Mediterranean fever and periodic fever syndromes

Drug reactions*
- e.g. Antibiotic fever, drug hypersensitivity reactions etc.

Factitious fever

Idiopathic (~15%)

*Most common causes within each group.

to detect emerging features (e.g. rashes, signs of infective endocarditis (p. 625) or features of vasculitis). In men, the prostate should be considered as a potential source of infection.

Clinicians should be alert to the possibility of factitious fever, in which high temperature recordings are engineered by the patient (Box 13.3).

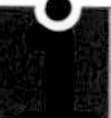

13.3 Clues to the diagnosis of factitious fever

- A patient who looks well
- Bizarre temperature chart with absence of diurnal variation and/or temperature-related changes in pulse rate
- Temperature > 41°C
- Absence of sweating during defervescence
- Normal ESR and CRP despite high fever
- Evidence of self-injection or self-harm
- Normal temperature during supervised (observed) measurement

Investigations

If initial investigation of fever (see above) is negative, a series of further microbiological and non-microbiological investigations should be considered (Boxes 13.4 and 13.5). These will usually include:

- induced sputum or other specimens for mycobacterial stains and culture
- serological tests
- imaging of the abdomen by ultrasonography or computed tomography (CT)
- echocardiography.

Lesions identified on imaging should usually be biopsied in order to seek evidence of relevant pathogens by culture, histopathology or nucleic acid detection. The chance of a successful diagnosis is greatest if procedures for obtaining and transporting the correct samples in the appropriate media are carefully planned in advance;

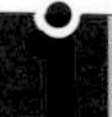

13.4 Microbiological investigation of PUO

Microscopy
- Blood for atypical lymphocytes (EBV, CMV, HIV-1, hepatitis viruses or *Toxoplasma gondii*), trypanosomiasis, malaria, *Borrelia* spp.
- Respiratory samples for mycobacteria, fungi
- Stool for ova, cysts and parasites
- Biopsy for light microscopy (bacteria, mycobacteria, fungi, *Leishmania* and other parasites) and/or electron microscopy (viruses, protozoa (e.g. microsporidia) and other fastidious organisms (e.g. *T. whipplei*))
- Urine for white or red blood cells, schistosome ova, mycobacteria (early morning urine × 3)

Culture
- Aspirates and biopsies (e.g. joint, deep abscess, debrided tissues)
- Blood, including prolonged culture and special media conditions
- Sputum for mycobacteria
- Cerebrospinal fluid (CSF)
- Gastric aspirate for mycobacteria
- Stool
- Swabs
- Urine ± prostatic massage in older men

Antigen detection
- Blood, e.g. HIV p24 antigen, cryptococcal antigen, *Histoplasma* antigen (restricted availability) and *Aspergillus* galactomannan enzyme-linked immunosorbent assay (ELISA)
- CSF for cryptococcal antigen
- Bronchoalveolar lavage fluid for *Aspergillus* galactomannan
- Nasopharyngeal aspirate/throat swab for respiratory viruses
- Urine, e.g. for *Legionella* antigen

Nucleic acid detection
- Blood for *Bartonella* spp. and viruses
- CSF for viruses and key bacteria (meningococcus, pneumococcus)
- Nasopharyngeal aspirate/throat swab for respiratory viruses
- Bronchoalveolar lavage fluid, e.g. for respiratory viruses
- Tissue specimens, e.g. for *Tropheryma whipplei*
- Urine, e.g. for *Chlamydia trachomatis*, *Neisseria gonorrhoeae*
- Stool, e.g. for norovirus, rotavirus

Immunological tests
- Serology (antibody detection) for viruses, dimorphic fungi and some bacteria and protozoa
- Interferon-γ release assay for diagnosis of tuberculosis

Note This list does not apply to every patient with a PUO. Appropriate tests should be selected in a stepwise manner, according to specific predisposing factors, epidemiological exposures and local availability, and should be discussed with a microbiologist.

this requires discussion between the clinical team, the radiologist or surgeon performing the procedure, and the local microbiologist and histopathologist. Liver biopsy may be justified, e.g. to identify idiopathic granulomatous hepatitis, if there are biochemical or radiological abnormalities. Bone marrow biopsies have a diagnostic yield of up to 15%, most often revealing haematological malignancy, myelodysplasia or tuberculosis, and also identifying brucellosis, typhoid fever or visceral leishmaniasis. Bone marrow should be sent for culture, as well as microscopy. Laparoscopy is occasionally undertaken with biopsy of abnormal tissues. Splenic

13.5 Additional investigations in PUO

Serological tests for connective tissue disorders
- Autoantibody screen
- Complement levels
- Immunoglobulins
- Cryoglobulins

Echocardiography

Ultrasound of abdomen

CT/MRI of thorax, abdomen and/or brain

Imaging of the skeletal system
- Plain X-rays
- CT/MRI spine
- Isotope bone scan

Labelled white cell scan

Positron emission tomography (PET)/single photon emission computed tomography (SPECT)

Biopsy
- Bronchoscopy and lavage ± transbronchial biopsy
- Lymph node aspirate or biopsy
- Biopsy of radiological lesion
- Biopsy of liver
- Bone marrow aspirate and biopsy
- Lumbar puncture
- Laparoscopy and biopsy
- Temporal artery biopsy

aspiration in specialist centres is the diagnostic test of choice for suspected visceral leishmaniasis. Temporal artery biopsy should be considered in patients over the age of 50 years, even in the absence of physical signs or a raised ESR. 'Blind' biopsy of other structures in the absence of localising signs, or laboratory or radiology results is unhelpful.

Prognosis

The overall mortality of PUO is 30–40%, mainly attributable to malignancy in older patients. If no cause is found, the long-term mortality is low and fever often settles spontaneously.

Fever in the injection drug-user

Intravenous injection of recreational drugs is widespread in many parts of the world (p. 240). Infective organisms are introduced by non-sterile (often shared) injection equipment (Fig. 13.2), and infection is facilitated by immunodeficiency due to malnutrition or the toxic effects of drugs. The risks increase with prolonged drug use and injection into large veins of the groin and neck because of progressive thrombosis of superficial peripheral veins. The most common causes of fever are soft tissue or respiratory infections.

Clinical assessment

The history should address the following risk factors:

- *Site of injection.* Femoral vein injection is associated with vascular complications such as deep venous thrombosis (50% of which are septic) and accidental arterial injection with false aneurysm formation or a compartment syndrome due to swelling within the fascial sheath. Local complications include iliopsoas abscess, and septic arthritis of the hip joint or sacroiliac joint. Injection of the jugular vein can be

13

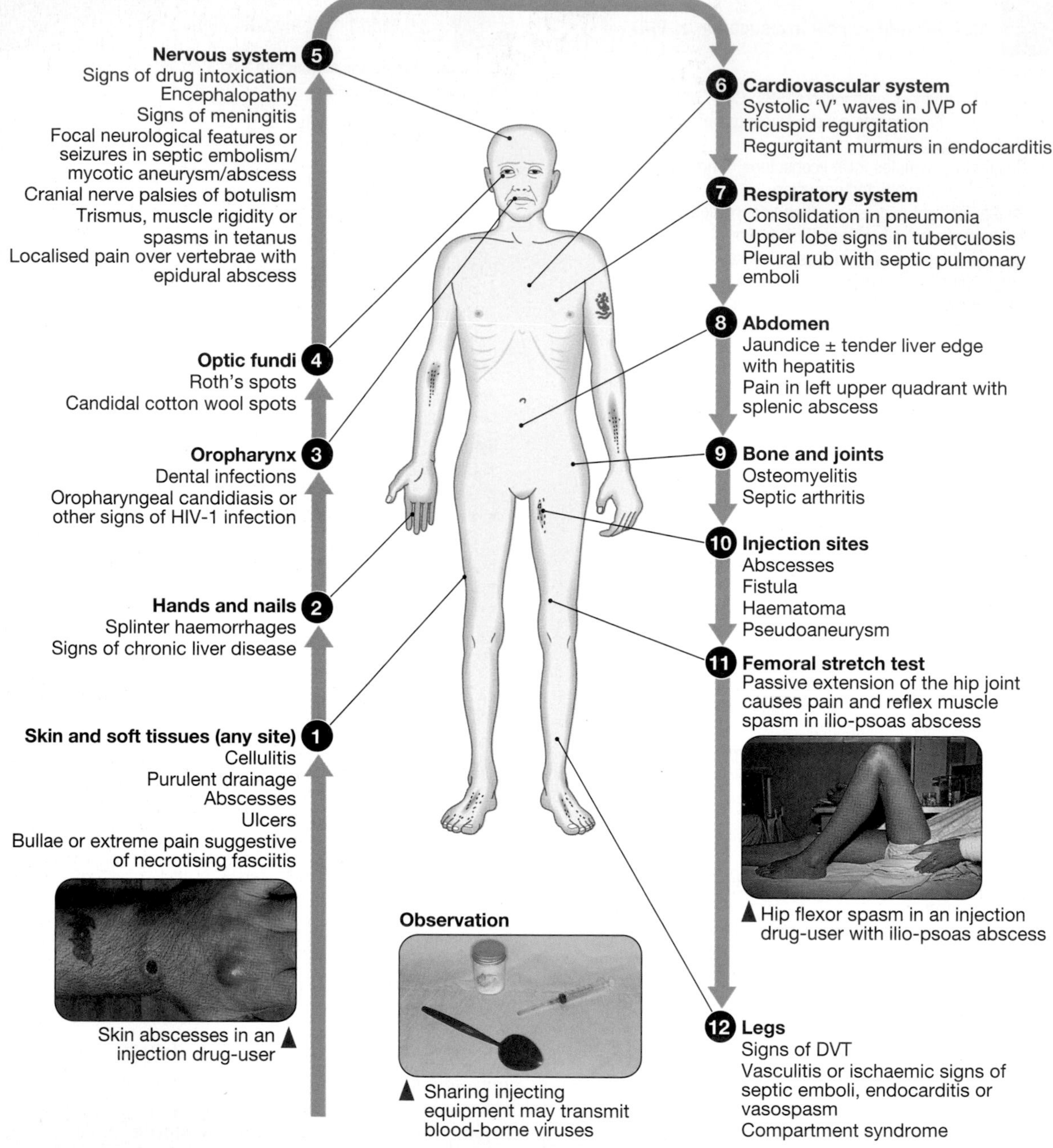

Fig. 13.2 Fever in the injection drug-user: key features of clinical examination. Full examination (p. 294) is required but features most common amongst injection drug-users are shown here. (DVT = deep venous thrombosis; JVP = jugular venous pulse)

associated with cerebrovascular complications. Subcutaneous and intramuscular injection has been related to infection by clostridial species, the spores of which contaminate heroin. *Clostridium novyi* causes a local lesion with significant toxin production, leading to shock and multi-organ failure. Tetanus, wound botulism and gas gangrene also occur.

- *Technical details of injection.* Sharing of needles and other injecting paraphernalia (including spoons and filters) greatly increases the risk of blood-borne virus infection (e.g. HIV-1, hepatitis B or C virus). Some users lubricate their needles by licking them prior to injection, thus introducing mouth organisms (e.g. anaerobic streptococci, *Fusobacterium* spp. and *Prevotella* spp). Contamination of commercially available lemon juice, used to dissolve heroin before injection, has been associated with blood-stream infection with *Candida* spp.
- *Substances injected.* Injection of cocaine is associated with a variety of vascular complications. Certain formulations of heroin have been linked with particular infections, e.g. wound botulism with black tar heroin. Drugs are often mixed with other substances, e.g. talc.
- *Blood-borne virus status.* Results of previous HIV-1 and hepatitis virus tests or vaccinations for hepatitis viruses should be recorded.

- *Surreptitious use of antimicrobials.* Addicts may use antimicrobials to self-treat infections, masking initial blood culture results.

Key findings on clinical examination are shown in Figure 13.2. It can be difficult to distinguish the effects of infection from the effects of drugs or drug withdrawal (excitement, tachycardia, sweating, marked myalgia, confusion). Stupor and delirium may result from drug administration but may also indicate meningitis or encephalitis. Non-infected venous thromboembolism is also common in this group.

Investigations

The initial investigations are as for any fever (see above), including a chest X-ray and blood cultures. Since blood sampling may be difficult, contamination is often a problem. Echocardiography to detect infective endocarditis should be performed in all injection drug-users with: bacteraemia due to *Staphylococcus aureus* or other organisms associated with endocarditis (Fig. 13.3A); thromboembolic phenomena; or a new or previously undocumented murmur. Endovascular infection should also be suspected if lung abscesses or pneumatocoeles are detected radiologically. Additional imaging should be focused on sites of injection or of localising symptoms and signs (Fig. 13.3B). Any pathological fluid collections should be sampled.

Urinary toxicology tests may suggest a non-infectious cause of the presenting complaint. While being investigated, all injection drug-users should be offered testing for infection with hepatitis B and C virus and HIV-1.

Microbiological results are crucial in guiding therapy. Injection drug-users may have more than one infection. Skin and soft tissue infections are most often due to *Staph. aureus* or streptococci, and sometimes to *Clostridium* spp. or anaerobes. Pulmonary infections are most often due to the common pathogens causing community-acquired pneumonia, tuberculosis or septic emboli (Fig. 13.3C). Endocarditis with septic emboli commonly involves *Staph. aureus* and viridans streptococci, but *Pseudomonas aeruginosa* and *Candida* spp. are also encountered.

Management

Empirical therapy of fever in the injection drug-user includes an antistaphylococcal penicillin (e.g. flucloxacillin) or, if meticillin-resistant *Staph. aureus* (MRSA) is prevalent in the community, a glycopeptide (e.g. vancomycin). Once a particular pathogen is identified, specific therapy is commenced, with modification when antimicrobial susceptibility is available. In injection drug-users, right-sided endocarditis due to *Staph. aureus* is customarily treated with high-dose intravenous flucloxacillin. In left-sided *Staph. aureus* endocarditis, aminoglycoside therapy may be added. Right-sided endocarditis caused by MRSA is usually treated with 4 weeks of vancomycin plus gentamicin for the first week. Specialist advice should be sought.

For localised infections of the skin and soft tissues, oral therapy with agents active against staphylococci, streptococci and anaerobes is appropriate (e.g. flucloxacillin plus co-amoxiclav or clindamycin). Non-adherence with prescribed antimicrobial regimens leads to a high rate of relapse for all infections in this patient group.

A
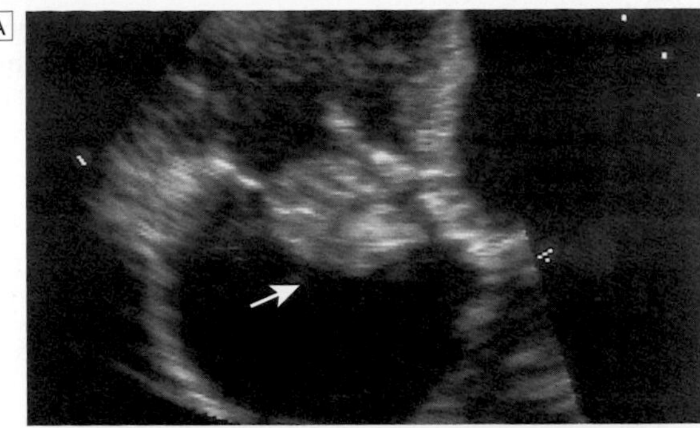
B
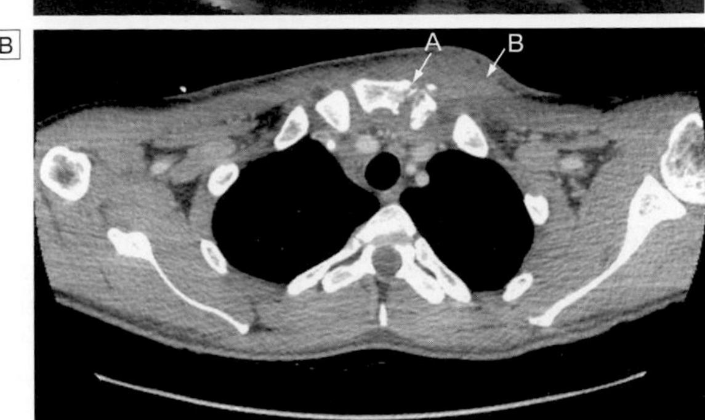

C
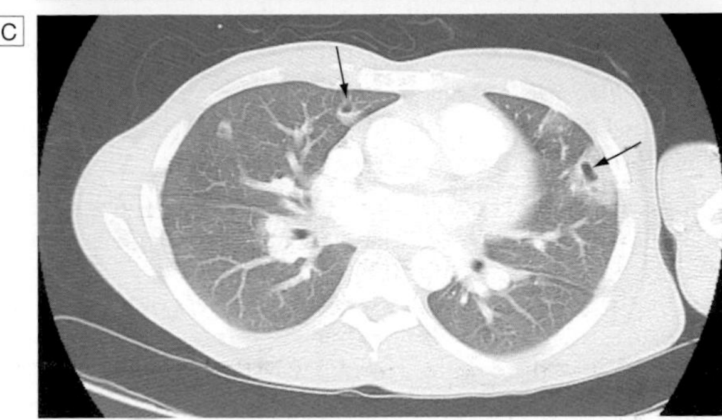

Fig. 13.3 Causes of fever in injection drug-users. **A** Endocarditis: large vegetation on the tricuspid valve (arrow). **B** Septic arthritis of the left sternoclavicular joint (arrow A) (note the erosion of the bony surfaces at the sternoclavicular joint) with overlying soft tissue collection (arrow B). **C** CT of the thorax showing *Staph. aureus* endocarditis of the tricuspid valve and haemoptysis, showing multiple embolic lesions with cavitation (arrows).

Fever in the immunocompromised host

Immunocompromised hosts include those with congenital immunodeficiency (p. 78), HIV infection (Ch. 14) and iatrogenic immunosuppression induced by chemotherapy (p. 276), transplantation (p. 95) or immunosuppressant medicines, including high-dose corticosteroids. Metabolic abnormalities, such as under-nutrition or hyperglycaemia, may also contribute. Multiple elements of the immune system are potentially compromised. A patient may have impaired neutrophil function from chemotherapy, impaired T-cell and/or B-cell responses due to underlying malignancy, T-cell and phagocytosis defects due to corticosteroids, mucositis from chemotherapy and an impaired skin barrier due to insertion of a central venous catheter.

Fever may result from infectious or from non-infectious causes, including drugs, vasculitis, neoplasm, organising pneumonitis, lymphoproliferative disease, graft-versus-host disease (in recipients of haematopoietic stem cell transplants; p. 1017) or Sweet's syndrome (reddish nodules or plaques with fever and leucocytosis, in association with haematological malignancy).

Clinical assessment

The following should be addressed in the history:

- Identification of the immunosuppressant factors, and nature of the immune defect.
- Any past infections and their treatment. Infections may recur and antimicrobial resistance may have been acquired in response to prior therapy.
- Exposure to infections, including opportunistic infections that would not cause disease in an immunocompetent host.
- Prophylactic medicines and vaccinations administered.

Examination should include inspection of the normal physical barriers provided by skin and mucosal surfaces and, in particular, central venous catheters, the mouth, sinuses, ears and perianal area (digital rectal examination should be avoided). Disseminated infections can manifest as cutaneous lesions. The areas around fingernails and toenails should also be inspected closely.

Investigations

Initial screening tests are as described above (p. 296). Immunocompromised hosts often have decreased inflammatory responses leading to attenuation of physical signs, such as neck stiffness with meningitis, radiological features and laboratory findings, such as leucocytosis. Chest CT scan should be considered in addition to chest X-ray when respiratory symptoms occur. Abdominal imaging may also be warranted, particularly if there is right lower quadrant pain, which may indicate typhlitis (inflammation of the caecum) in neutropenic patients. Blood cultures from a central venous catheter, urine cultures, and stool cultures if diarrhoea is present are also recommended.

Nasopharyngeal aspirates are sometimes diagnostic, as immunocompromised hosts may shed respiratory viruses for prolonged periods. Skin lesions should be biopsied if nodules are present, and investigation should include fungal stains. Useful molecular techniques include polymerase chain reaction (PCR) for CMV and *Aspergillus* spp. DNA, and antigen assays (e.g. cryptococcal antigen (CrAg) for *Cryptococcus neoformans*, and galactomannan for *Aspergillus* spp. in blood or *Legionella pneumophila* type 1 in urine). Antibody detection is rarely useful in immunocompromised patients. Patients with respiratory signs or symptoms should be considered for bronchoscopy in order to obtain bronchoalveolar lavage fluid to detect pathogens, including *Pneumocystis jirovecii* (*carinii*), as well as bacteria, fungi and viruses.

Neutropenic fever

Neutropenic fever is strictly defined as a neutrophil count of less than $0.5 \times 10^9/L$ (p. 1004) and a single axillary temperature above 38.5°C or three recordings above 38.0°C over a 12-hour period, although the infection risk increases progressively as the neutrophil count drops below $1.0 \times 10^9/L$. Patients with neutropenia are particularly prone to bacterial or fungal infection. Gram-positive organisms are the most common pathogens, particularly in association with in-dwelling catheters.

EBM 13.6 Treatment of neutropenic fever

'Broad spectrum β-lactam monotherapy is as effective as β-lactam-aminoglycoside combination therapy for neutropenic fever in many settings.'

- Paul M, et al. BMJ 2003; 326:1111.
- Del Favero A, et al. Clin Infect Dis 2001; 33:1295–1301.

Empirical broad-spectrum antimicrobial therapy is commenced as soon as neutropenic fever occurs and cultures have been obtained. The most common regimens for neutropenic sepsis are broad-spectrum penicillins, such as piperacillin–tazobactam IV. Although aminoglycosides are commonly used in combination, routine use is not supported by trial data (Box 13.6). If fever has not resolved after 3–5 days, empirical antifungal therapy (e.g. caspofungin) is added (p. 159). An alternative antifungal strategy is to use azole prophylaxis in high-risk patients and markers of early fungal infection, such as galactomannan antigen, to guide initiation of antifungal treatment (a 'pre-emptive approach').

Post-transplantation fever

Fever in transplant recipients may be due to infection, episodes of graft rejection in solid organ transplant recipients, or graft-versus-host disease following haematopoietic stem cell transplantation (HSCT; p. 1017).

Infections in solid transplant recipients are grouped according to the time of onset (Box 13.7). Those in the first month are related to the underlying condition or surgical complications. Those occurring 1–6 months after transplantation are characteristic of impaired T-cell function. Risk factors for CMV infection have

13.7 Infections in transplant recipients

Time post-transplantation	Infections
Solid organ recipients	
0–1 mth	Bacterial or fungal infections related to the underlying condition or surgical complications
1–6 mths	CMV, other opportunistic infections (e.g. *Pneumocystis jirovecii* pneumonia)
> 6 mths	Bacterial pneumonia, other bacterial community-acquired infections, shingles, cryptococcal infection, PTLD
Myeloablative haematopoietic stem cell transplant recipients	
Pre-engraftment (typically 0–4 wks)	Bacterial and fungal infections, respiratory viruses or HSV reactivation
Post-engraftment	
Early (< 100 days)	CMV, *Pneumocystis jirovecii* pneumonia, moulds or other opportunistic infections
Late (> 100 days)	Community-acquired bacterial infections, shingles, CMV, PTLD

(CMV = cytomegalovirus; HSV = herpes simplex virus; PTLD = post-transplant lymphoproliferative disorder)

been identified and patients commonly receive either prophylaxis or intensive monitoring involving regular testing for CMV DNA by PCR and early initiation of anti-CMV therapy using intravenous ganciclovir or oral valganciclovir if tests become positive.

Following HSCT, infections in the first 4 weeks are more common in patients receiving a myeloablative conditioning regimen (see Box 13.7). Later infections are more common if an allogeneic procedure is performed.

Post-transplant lymphoproliferative disorder (PTLD) is an Epstein–Barr virus (EBV)-associated lymphoma that can complicate transplantation, particularly when primary EBV infection occurs after transplantation.

13.8 Common causes of blood-stream infection

Community-acquired	
• *Staph. aureus*, including MRSA • *Streptococcus pneumoniae*	• Other streptococci • *Escherichia coli*
Nosocomial	
• *Staph. aureus*, including MRSA • Coagulase-negative staphylococci	• Enterococci, including VRE • Gram-negative bacteria • *Candida* spp.

(MRSA = meticillin-resistant *Staph. aureus*; VRE = vancomycin-resistant enterococci)

Positive blood culture

Blood-stream infection (BSI) or bacteraemia is a frequent presentation of infection. This can be community-acquired or may arise in hospital ('nosocomial'). The most common causes are shown in Box 13.8. In immunocompromised hosts, a wider range of microorganisms may be isolated, e.g. fungi in neutropenic hosts.

Primary bacteraemia refers to cases in which the site of infection is unknown; this applies in approximately 10% of community-acquired cases and approximately 30% of nosocomial cases, and is more common in *Staph. aureus* bacteraemias. In community-acquired *Staph. aureus* bacteraemia, 20–30% of cases are associated with infectious endocarditis and up to 10% are due to osteomyelitis. Peripheral and central venous catheters are an important source of nosocomial BSI.

BSI has an associated mortality of 15–40%, depending on the setting, host and microbial factors.

Clinical assessment

The history should determine the setting in which BSI has occurred. Host factors predisposing to infection include skin disease, diabetes mellitus, injection drug use, the presence of a central venous, urinary or haemodialysis catheter, and surgical procedures, especially those involving the implantation of prosthetic materials (in particular, endovascular prostheses).

Physical examination should focus on signs of endocarditis (p. 625), evidence of bone or joint infection (tenderness or restriction of movement), and abdominal or flank tenderness. Central venous catheters should be examined for erythema or purulence at the exit site. Particularly in cases with *Candida* spp. infection or suspected infectious endocarditis, fundoscopy after pupil dilatation should be performed.

Investigations

Positive blood cultures may be caused by contaminants. When isolated from only one bottle, or from all bottles from one venesection, coagulase-negative staphylococci often represent contamination. Repeated isolation of this organism, however, should raise suspicion of infective endocarditis or, in a patient with any form of prosthetic material, prosthesis infection. Viridans streptococci occasionally cause transient non-significant bacteraemia or blood culture contamination but, in view of their association with infective endocarditis, significant infection must always be sought clinically. *Bacillus* spp. ('aerobic spore bearers') and *Clostridium* spp. often represent incidental transient bacteraemia or contamination, but certain species (e.g. *C. septicum*) may be genuine pathogens.

Further investigations are influenced by the causative organism and setting. Initial screening tests are similar to those for fever (p. 296) and should include chest X-ray, urine culture and, in many cases, ultrasound or other imaging of the abdomen. Imaging should also include any areas of bone or joint pain and any prosthetic material, e.g. a prosthetic joint or an aortic graft.

Echocardiography should be considered for those patients with BSI who have valvular heart disease or clinical features of endocarditis (p. 625), those whose cultures reveal an organism that is a common cause of endocarditis (e.g. *Staph. aureus*, viridans streptococci or enterococci), those in whom multiple blood cultures are positive for the same organism, and those with rapid positive result on culture. The sensitivities of transthoracic echocardiography (TTE) and transoesophageal echocardiography (TOE) for the detection of vegetations are 50–90% and over 95%, respectively. Therefore, if TTE is negative, TOE should be performed (Box 18.115, p. 627).

Certain rare causes of BSI have specific associations that warrant further investigation. *Strep. bovis* (biotype I, *Strep. gallolyticus*) endocarditis and *C. septicum* BSI are both associated with colonic carcinoma and their isolation is an indication for colonoscopy.

Management

BSI requires antimicrobial therapy and attention to the source of infection, including surgical drainage if appropriate. Two weeks of therapy may be sufficient for *Staph. aureus* BSI from central and peripheral venous catheter infections when the source is identified and removed, for uncomplicated skin and soft tissue infections, and for uncomplicated right-sided infective endocarditis. Other *Staph. aureus* BSIs are usually treated for 4–6 weeks.

Central venous catheter infections

Infections of central venous catheters typically involve the catheter lumen and are associated with fever, positive blood cultures and, in some cases, signs of purulence or exudate at the site of insertion. Infection is more common in temporary catheters inserted into the groin or jugular vein than those in the subclavian vein. Tunnelled catheters, e.g. Hickman catheters, may also develop tunnel site infections.

Staphylococci account for 70–90% of catheter infections, with coagulase-negative staphylococci more common than *Staph. aureus*. Other causes include enterococci and Gram-negative bacilli. Unusual Gram-negative organisms, such as *Citrobacter freundii* and *Pseudomonas fluorescens*, cause pseudo-outbreaks and raise the possibility of non-sterile infusion equipment or infusate. *Candida* spp. are a common cause of line infections, particularly in association with total parenteral nutrition. Non-tuberculous mycobacteria may cause tunnel infections.

Investigations and management

In bacteraemic patients with fever and no other obvious source of infection, a catheter infection is likely. Local evidence of erythema, purulence or thrombophlebitis supports the diagnosis. However, microbiological confirmation is essential (p. 140). Catheter-related infection is suggested by higher colony counts or shorter time to positivity in blood cultures obtained through the catheter than in peripheral blood cultures. If the line is removed, a semi-quantitative culture of the tip should confirm the presence of 15 or more colony-forming units, but this is retrospective and does not detect luminal infection.

For coagulase-negative staphylococcal line infections, the options are to remove the line or, particularly in the case of tunnelled catheters, to treat empirically with a glycopeptide antibiotic, e.g. vancomycin, with or without the use of antibiotic-containing lock therapy to the catheter for approximately 14 days. For *Staph. aureus* infection, the chance of curing an infection with the catheter in situ is low and the risks from infection are high. Therefore, unless the risks of catheter removal outweigh the benefits, treatment involves catheter removal, followed by 14 days of antimicrobial therapy; the same applies to infections with *Candida* spp. or *Bacillus* spp.

Infection prevention is a key component of the management of vascular catheters. Measures include strict attention to hand hygiene, optimal siting, full aseptic technique on insertion and subsequent interventions, skin antisepsis with chlorhexidine and isopropyl alcohol, daily assessment of catheter sites (e.g. with visual infusion phlebitis (VIP) score (p. 330)), and daily consideration of the continuing requirement for catheterisation. The use of catheters impregnated with antimicrobials such as chlorhexidine or silver is advocated in some settings.

Sepsis

Sepsis is discussed on page 200. It describes patients with evidence of infection and signs of the systemic inflammatory response syndrome (SIRS), which entails two of: temperature over 38°C or under 36°C; pulse rate more than 90 beats per minute; respiratory rate over 20 breaths per minute or PCO_2 below 4.3 kPa (32.5 mmHg); and white blood cell count over 12 or below 4×10^9/L (Box 8.2, p. 184). Septic shock describes sepsis plus hypotension (systolic blood pressure below 90 mmHg systolic or a fall of more than 40 mmHg from baseline that is not responsive to fluid challenge or due to another cause). It may be complicated by multi-organ failure and requires intensive care unit admission.

Sepsis largely results from host responses to microbial lipopolysaccharide, peptidoglycans, lipoproteins or

13.9 Causes of sepsis

Infection	Setting
Bacterial	
Staph. aureus, coagulase-negative staphylococci	Bacteraemia may be associated with endocarditis, intravascular cannula infection, or skin or bone foci
Streptococcus pneumoniae	Invasive pneumococcal disease, usually with pneumonia or meningitis
Other streptococci	Invasive streptococcal disease, especially necrotising fasciitis Viridans streptococci in neutropenic host with severe mucositis
Staphylococcal or streptococcal toxic shock syndrome	Toxin-mediated, blood cultures negative; clues include erythrodermic rash and epidemiological setting
Enterococci	Most often with abdominal focus
Neisseria meningitidis	Sepsis in children or young adults with petechial rash and/or meningitis
E. coli, other Gram-negative bacteria	Urinary or biliary tract infection, or other abdominal infections
Pseudomonas aeruginosa, multidrug-resistant Gram-negative bacteraemia	Nosocomial infection
Yersinia pestis	In plague
Burkholderia pseudomallei	Endemic in areas of Thailand; more likely to involve patients with diabetes mellitus or immunocompromised
Capnocytophaga canimorsus	Associated with dog bites and asplenic individuals
C. difficile	Severe colitis, particularly in the elderly
Polymicrobial infection with Gram-negatives and anaerobes	Bowel perforation
Mycobacterium tuberculosis, *M. avium complex* (MAC)	HIV-positive or immunocompromised with miliary TB or disseminated MAC
Fungal	
Candida spp.	Line infection or post-operative complication, nosocomial or immunocompromised host
Histoplasma capsulatum, other dimorphic fungi	Immunocompromised host
Parasitic	
Falciparum malaria	Malaria with high-level parasitaemia and multi-organ failure or as a complication of bacterial superinfection
Babesia microti	Asplenic individual
Strongyloides stercoralis hyperinfection syndrome	Gram-negative infection complicating *Strongyloides* infection in immunocompromised host

superantigens, and there are many infectious causes (Box 13.9). The results of blood cultures and known host factors guide initial investigations. Patients who are immunocompromised may have a broader range of causal pathogens which may be harder to culture, including mycobacteria and fungi. In any individual who has recently visited the tropics, malaria must also be considered.

Severe skin and soft tissue infections

Skin and soft tissue infections (SSTIs) are an important cause of sepsis. Cases can be classified as in Box 13.10, according to the clinical features and microbiological findings. In some cases, severe systemic features may be out of keeping with mild local features.

Necrotising fasciitis

In necrotising fascitis, cutaneous erythema and oedema progress to bullae or areas of necrosis. Unlike in cellulitis, pain may be disproportionately intense in relation to the visible cutaneous features. The infection spreads quickly along the fascial plane. Type 1 necrotising fasciitis is a mixed infection with Gram-negative bacteria and anaerobes, often seen post-operatively in diabetic or immunocompromised hosts. Subcutaneous gas may be present. Type 2 necrotising fasciitis is caused by group A or other streptococci. Approximately 60% of cases are associated with streptococcal toxic shock syndrome (p. 331).

Necrotising fasciitis is a medical emergency, requiring immediate surgical débridement with inspection of the involved muscle groups, in addition to antimicrobial therapy (Fig. 13.4). Empiric treatment is with broad-spectrum agents (e.g. piperacillin–tazobactam plus clindamycin and ciprofloxacin; meropenem monotherapy; or third-generation cephalosporin plus metronidazole). Hyperbaric oxygen therapy may be considered for polymicrobial infection. Group A streptococcal infection is treated with benzylpenicillin plus clindamycin, and often immunoglobulin.

Gas gangrene

Although *Clostridium* spp. may colonise or contaminate wounds, no action is required unless there is evidence of spreading infection. Infection may be limited to tissue that is already damaged (anaerobic cellulitis) or involve healthy muscle (gas gangrene).

In anaerobic cellulitis, usually that due to *C. perfringens* or to other strains infecting devitalised tissue following a wound, gas forms locally and extends along tissue planes but bacteraemia does not occur. Prompt surgical débridement of devitalised tissue and therapy with penicillin or clindamycin is usually effective.

Gas gangrene (clostridial myonecrosis) is defined as acute invasion of healthy living muscle undamaged by previous trauma, and is most commonly caused by *C. perfringens*. In at least 70% of cases, it follows deep penetrating injury sufficient to create an anaerobic (ischaemic) environment and allow clostridial introduction and proliferation. Severe pain at the site of the injury progresses rapidly over 18–24 hours. Skin colour changes from pallor to bronze/purple discoloration and the skin is tense, swollen, oedematous and exquisitely tender. Gas in tissues may be obvious, with crepitus on clinical examination, or visible on X-ray, CT or ultrasound. Signs of systemic toxicity develop rapidly, with high leucocytosis, multi-organ dysfunction, raised creatine kinase and evidence of disseminated intravascular coagulation and haemolysis. Antibiotic therapy with high-dose intravenous penicillin and clindamycin is recommended, coupled with aggressive surgical débridement of the affected tissues. Alternative agents include cephalosporins and metronidazole. Hyperbaric oxygen has a putative but controversial role.

Other SSTIs

'Synergistic gangrene' is a combined infection with anaerobes and other bacteria (*Staph. aureus* or Gram-negatives). When this affects the genital/perineal area, it is known as 'Fournier's gangrene'. Severe gangrenous cellulitis in immunocompromised hosts may involve Gram-negative bacteria or fungi. *Entamoeba histolytica* can cause soft tissue necrosis following abdominal surgery in areas of the world where infection is common. Contact with shellfish in tropical areas and regions such as the Gulf of Mexico can lead to infection with *Vibrio vulnificus*, which causes soft tissue necrosis and bullae. Patients with chronic liver disease are particularly susceptible.

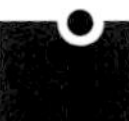

13.10 Severe necrotising soft tissue infections

- Necrotising fasciitis (primarily confined to subcutaneous fascia and fat)
- Clostridial anaerobic cellulitis (confined to skin and subcutaneous tissue)
- Non-clostridial anaerobic cellulitis
- Progressive bacterial synergistic gangrene (*Staph. aureus* + micro-aerophilic streptococcus) ('Meleney's gangrene', primarily confined to skin)
- Pyomyositis (discrete abscesses within individual muscle groups)
- Clostridial myonecrosis (gas gangrene)
- Anaerobic streptococcal myonecrosis (non-clostridial infection mimicking gas gangrene)
- Group A streptococcal necrotising myositis

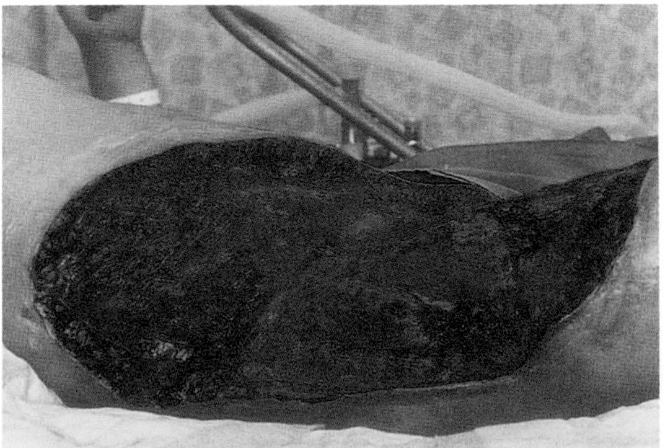

Fig. 13.4 Excision following necrotising fasciitis in an injection drug-user.

Acute diarrhoea and vomiting

Acute diarrhoea (p. 857), sometimes with vomiting, is the predominant symptom in infective gastroenteritis (Box 13.11). Acute diarrhoea may also be a symptom of other infectious and non-infectious diseases (Box 13.12). Stress, whether psychological or physical, can also produce loose stools.

The World Health Organization (WHO) estimates that there are more than 1000 million cases of acute diarrhoea annually in developing countries, with 3–4 million deaths, half of these in infants and children. In developed countries, diarrhoea remains an important problem and the elderly are most vulnerable (Box 13.13). The majority of episodes are due to infections spread by the faecal–oral route and transmitted either on fomites, on contaminated hands, or in food or water. Measures such as the provision of clean drinking water, appropriate disposal of human and animal sewage, and the application of simple principles of food hygiene can all limit gastroenteritis.

The clinical features of food-borne gastroenteritis vary. Some organisms (*Bacillus cereus*, *Staph. aureus* and *Vibrio cholerae*) elute exotoxins which cause vomiting and/or so-called 'secretory' diarrhoea (watery diarrhoea without blood or faecal leucocytes, reflecting small bowel dysfunction). In general, the time from ingestion to the onset of symptoms is short and, other than dehydration, little systemic upset occurs. Other organisms, such as *Shigella* spp., *Campylobacter* spp. and enterohaemorrhagic *E. coli* (EHEC), may directly invade the mucosa of the small bowel or produce cytotoxins that cause mucosal ulceration, typically affecting the terminal small bowel and colon. The incubation period is longer and more systemic upset occurs, with prolonged bloody diarrhoea. *Salmonella* spp. are capable of invading enterocytes, and of causing both a secretory response and invasive disease with systemic features. This is seen with *Salmonella typhi* and *S. paratyphi* (enteric fever), and, in the immunocompromised host, with non-typhoidal *Salmonella* spp.

Clinical assessment

The history should address foods ingested (Box 13.14), duration and frequency of diarrhoea, presence of blood or steatorrhoea, abdominal pain and tenesmus, and whether other people have been affected. Fever and bloody diarrhoea suggest an invasive, colitic, dysenteric process. An incubation period of less than 18 hours suggests toxin-mediated food poisoning, and longer than 5 days suggests diarrhoea caused by protozoa or helminths. Person-to-person spread suggests certain infections, such as shigellosis or cholera.

Examination includes assessment of the degree of dehydration by skin turgor, pulse and blood pressure measurement. The urine output and ongoing stool losses should be monitored.

13.11 Causes of infectious gastroenteritis

Toxin in food: < 6 hrs incubation
- *Bacillus cereus* (p. 341)
- *Staph. aureus* (p. 341)
- *Clostridium* spp. enterotoxin (p. 342)

Bacterial: 12–72 hrs incubation
- Enterotoxigenic *E. coli* (ETEC, p. 342)
- Shiga toxin-producing *E. coli* (EHEC, p. 343)*
- Enteroinvasive *E. coli* (EIEC, p. 342)*
- *Vibrio cholerae* (p. 344)
- *Salmonella* (p. 342)
- *Shigella** (p. 345)
- *Campylobacter** (p. 342)
- *C. difficile** (p. 343)

Viral: short incubation
- Rotavirus (p. 327)
- Norovirus (p. 327)

Protozoal: long incubation
- Giardiasis (p. 368)
- *Cryptosporidium* (pp. 369 and 399)
- Microsporidiosis (p. 399)
- Amoebic dysentery (p. 367)*
- Isosporiasis (p. 399)

*Associated with bloody diarrhoea.

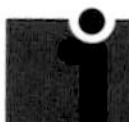

13.12 Differential diagnosis of acute diarrhoea and vomiting

Infectious causes
- Gastroenteritis
- *C. difficile* infection (p. 343)
- Acute diverticulitis (p. 916)
- Sepsis (p. 304)
- Pelvic inflammatory disease (p. 418)
- Meningococcaemia (p. 1201)
- Pneumonia (especially 'atypical disease', p. 682)
- Malaria (p. 353)

Non-infectious causes

Gastrointestinal
- Inflammatory bowel disease (p. 897)
- Bowel malignancy (p. 910)
- Overflow from constipation (p. 917)
- Enteral tube feeding

Metabolic
- Diabetic ketoacidosis (p. 811)
- Thyrotoxicosis (p. 740)
- Uraemia (p. 483)
- Neuroendocrine tumours releasing (e.g.) VIP or 5-HT

Drugs and toxins
- NSAIDs
- Cytotoxic agents
- Antibiotics
- Proton pump inhibitors
- Dinoflagellates (p. 308)
- Plant toxins (p. 308)
- Heavy metals (p. 308)
- Ciguatera fish poisoning (p. 308)
- Scombrotoxic fish poisoning (p. 308)

(5-HT = 5-hydroxytryptamine, serotonin; NSAID = non-steroidal anti-inflammatory drugs; VIP = vasoactive intestinal peptide)

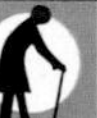

13.13 Infectious diarrhoea in old age

- **Incidence**: not increased but the impact is greater.
- **Mortality**: most deaths due to gastroenteritis in the developed world are in adults aged over 70. Most are presumed to be caused by dehydration leading to organ failure.
- ***C. difficile* infection (CDI)**: more common, especially in hospital and nursing home settings, usually following antibiotic exposure.

13.14 Foods associated with infectious illness, including gastroenteritis

Raw seafood	
• Norovirus • *Vibrio* spp.	• Hepatitis A
Raw eggs	
• *Salmonella* spp.	
Undercooked meat or poultry	
• *Salmonella* spp. • *Campylobacter* spp.	• EHEC • *C. perfringens*
Unpasteurised milk or juice	
• *Salmonella* spp. • *Campylobacter* spp.	• EHEC • *Y. enterocolitica*
Unpasteurised soft cheeses	
• *Salmonella* spp. • *Campylobacter* spp. • ETEC	• *Y. enterocolitica* • *L. monocytogenes*
Home-made canned goods	
• *C. botulinum*	
Raw hot dogs, pâté	
• *L. monocytogenes*	

Investigations

These include stool inspection for blood and microscopy for leucocytes, and also an examination for ova, cysts and parasites if the history indicates former tropical residence or travel. Stool culture should be performed and *C. difficile* toxin sought. FBC and serum electrolytes indicate the degree of inflammation and dehydration. In a malarious area, a blood film for malaria parasites should be obtained. Blood and urine cultures and a chest X-ray may identify alternative sites of infection, particularly if the clinical features suggest a syndrome other than gastroenteritis.

Management

All patients with acute, potentially infective diarrhoea should be appropriately isolated to minimise person-to-person spread of infection. If the history suggests a food-borne source, public health measures must be implemented to identify the source and to establish whether other linked cases exist (p. 147).

Fluid replacement

Replacement of fluid losses in diarrhoeal illness is crucial and may be life-saving.

Although normal daily fluid intake in an adult is only 1–2 L, there is considerable additional fluid movement in and out of the gut in secretions (Fig. 22.7, p. 843). Altered gut resorption with diarrhoea can result in substantial fluid loss, e.g. 10–20 L of fluid may be lost in 24 hours in cholera. The fluid lost in diarrhoea is isotonic, so both water and electrolytes need to be replaced. Absorption of electrolytes from the gut is an active process requiring energy. Infected mucosa is capable of very rapid fluid and electrolyte transport if carbohydrate is available as an energy source. Oral rehydration solutions (ORS) therefore contain sugars, as well as water and electrolytes (Box 13.15). ORS can be just as effective as intravenous replacement fluid, even in the management of cholera. In mild to moderate gastroenteritis, adults should be encouraged to drink fluids and, if possible, continue normal dietary food intake. If this is impossible, e.g. due to vomiting, intravenous fluid administration will be required. In very sick patients, or those with cardiac or renal disease, monitoring of urine output and central venous pressure may be necessary.

13.15 Composition of oral rehydration solution and other replacement fluids*

Fluid	Na	K	Cl	Energy
WHO	90	20	80	54
Dioralyte	60	20	60	71
Pepsi®	6.5	0.8	–	400
7UP®	7.5	0.2	–	320
Apple juice	0.4	26	–	480
Orange juice	0.2	49	–	400
Breast milk	22	36	28	670

*mmol/L for electrolyte and kcal/L for energy components.

The volume of fluid replacement required should be estimated based on the following considerations.

- *Replacement of established deficit.* After 48 hours of moderate diarrhoea (6–10 stools per 24 hours), the average adult will be 2–4 L depleted from diarrhoea alone. Associated vomiting will compound this. Adults with this symptomatology should therefore be given rapid replacement of 1–1.5 L, either orally (ORS) or by intravenous infusion (normal saline), within the first 2–4 hours of presentation. Longer symptomatology or more persistent/severe diarrhoea rapidly produces fluid losses comparable to diabetic ketoacidosis and is a metabolic emergency requiring active intervention.
- *Replacement of ongoing losses.* The average adult's diarrhoeal stool accounts for a loss of 200 mL of isotonic fluid. Stool losses should be carefully charted and an estimate of ongoing replacement fluid calculated. Commercially available rehydration sachets are conveniently produced to provide 200 mL of ORS; one sachet per diarrhoea stool is an appropriate estimate of supplementary replacement requirements.
- *Replacement of normal daily requirement.* The average adult has a daily requirement of 1–1.5 L of fluid in addition to the calculations above. This will be increased substantially in fever or a hot environment.

Antimicrobial agents

In non-specific gastroenteritis, antibiotics have been shown to shorten symptoms by only 1 day in an illness usually lasting 1–3 days. This benefit, when related to the potential for the development of antimicrobial resistance or side-effects, does not justify treatment, except if there is systemic involvement, a host with immunocompromise or significant comorbidity.

Evidence suggests that, in EHEC infections, the use of antibiotics may make the complication of haemolytic uraemic syndrome (HUS; p. 495) more likely due to increased toxin release. Antibiotics should therefore not be used in this condition.

Conversely, antibiotics are indicated in *Sh. dysenteriae* infection and in invasive salmonellosis – in particular, typhoid fever. Antibiotics may also be advantageous in cholera epidemics, reducing infectivity and controlling the spread of infection.

Antidiarrhoeal, antimotility and antisecretory agents

These agents are not usually recommended in acute infective diarrhoea. Loperamide, diphenoxylate and opiates are potentially dangerous in dysentery in childhood, causing intussusception. Antisecretory agents, such as bismuth and chlorpromazine, may be effective but can cause significant sedation. They do not reduce stool fluid losses, although the stools may appear more bulky. Adsorbents, such as kaolin or charcoal, have little effect.

Non-infectious causes of food poisoning

Whilst acute food poisoning and gastroenteritis are most frequently caused by bacteria or their toxins, a number of non-infectious causes must be considered in the differential diagnosis.

Plant toxins

Legumes and beans produce oxidants which are toxic to people with glucose-6-phosphate dehydrogenase (G6PD) deficiency (p. 1029). Consumption produces headache, nausea and fever, progressing to potentially severe haemolysis, haemoglobinuria and jaundice (favism). Red kidney beans, if incompletely cooked, cause acute abdominal pain and diarrhoea from their lectin content. Adequate cooking abolishes this.

Alkaloids develop in potato tubers exposed to light, causing green discoloration. Ingestion induces acute vomiting and anticholinesterase-like activity.

Fungi and mushrooms of the *Psilocybe* spp. produce hallucinogens. Many fungal species induce a combination of gastroenteritis and cholinergic symptoms of blurred vision, salivation, sweating and diarrhoea. *Amanita phalloides* ('death cap') causes acute abdominal cramps and diarrhoea, followed by inexorable hepatorenal failure, often fatal.

Chemical toxins

Paralytic shellfish toxin

Saxitoxin from dinoflagellates, responsible for 'red tides', is concentrated in bivalve molluscs, e.g. mussels, clams, oysters, cockles and scallops. Consumption produces gastrointestinal symptoms within 30 minutes, followed by perioral paraesthesia and even respiratory paralysis. The UK water authorities ban the harvesting of molluscs at times of the year associated with excessive dinoflagellate numbers.

Ciguatera fish poisoning

Warm-water coral reef fish acquire ciguatoxin from dinoflagellates in their food chain. Consumption produces gastrointestinal symptoms 1–6 hours later, with associated paraesthesiae of the lips and extremities, distorted temperature sensation, myalgia and progressive flaccid paralysis. Autonomic dysfunction with hypotension may occur. In the South Pacific and Caribbean, there are 50 000 cases per year, with a case fatality of 0.1%. The gastrointestinal symptoms resolve rapidly but the neuropathic features may persist for months.

Scombrotoxic fish poisoning

Under poor storage conditions, histidine in scombroid fish – tuna, mackerel, bonito, skipjack and the canned dark meat of sardines – may be converted by bacteria to histamine and other chemicals. Consumption produces symptoms within minutes, with flushing, burning, sweating, urticaria, pruritus, headache, colic, nausea and vomiting, diarrhoea, bronchospasm and hypotension. Management is with salbutamol and antihistamines. Occasionally, intravenous fluid replacement is required.

Heavy metals

Thallium and cadmium can cause acute vomiting and diarrhoea resembling staphylococcal enterotoxin poisoning.

Antimicrobial-associated diarrhoea

Antimicrobial-associated diarrhoea (AAD) is a common complication of antimicrobial therapy, especially with broad-spectrum agents. It is most common in the elderly but can occur at all ages. Although the specific mechanism is unknown in most AAD, *C. difficile* is implicated in 20–25% of cases and is the most common cause amongst patients with evidence of colitis. Infection is diagnosed by detection of *C. difficile* toxins and is usually treated with metronidazole or vancomycin (p. 343). *C. perfringens* is a rarer cause which usually remains undiagnosed, and *Klebsiella oxytoca* is an occasional cause of antibiotic-associated haemorrhagic colitis.

Infections acquired in the tropics

Recent decades have seen unprecedented increases in long-distance business and holiday travel, as well as extensive migration. Although certain diseases retain their relatively fixed geographical distribution, being dependent on specific vectors or weather conditions, many travel with their human hosts and some may then be transmitted to other people. This means that the pattern of infectious diseases seen in each country changes constantly, and travel history and information on countries previously lived in, particularly during childhood, are crucial.

In general, the diversity of infectious diseases is greater in tropical than in temperate countries, and people in temperate countries have immunity to a narrower range of infections, reflecting less exposure in childhood and less ongoing boosting of immunity later in life, so that the most common travel-associated infections are those which are acquired by residents of temperate countries during visits to the tropics. In addition, those who have lived in tropical areas may lose immunity when they move to temperate countries and become susceptible when visiting their homeland.

Most travel-associated infections can be prevented. Pre-travel advice is tailored to the destination and the traveller (Box 13.16). It includes avoidance of insect bites (using at least 20% diethyltoluamide (DEET)), sun protection (sunscreen with a sun protection factor (SPF) of at least 15), food and water hygiene ('Boil it, cook it, peel

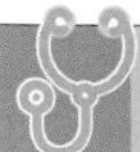

13.16 How to assess health needs in travellers before departure*

- Destination
- Personal details, including previous travel experience
- Dates of trip
- Itinerary and purpose of trip
- Personal medical history, including pregnancy, medication and allergies (e.g. to eggs, vaccines, antibiotics)
- Past vaccinations
  Childhood schedule followed? Diphtheria, tetanus, pertussis, polio, *N. meningitidis* type C, *Haemophilus influenzae* B (HiB)
  Travel-related? Typhoid, yellow fever, hepatitis A, hepatitis B, meningococcal ACW135Y, rabies, Japanese B encephalitis, tick-borne encephalitis
- Malaria prophylaxis: questions influencing the choice of antimalarial drugs are destination, past experience with antimalarials, history of epilepsy or psychiatric illness

*Further information is available at www fitfortravel.nhs.uk/

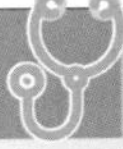

13.17 How to obtain a history from travellers to the tropics with fever

Questions	Factors to ascertain
Countries visited and dates of travel	Relate travel to known outbreaks of infection or antimicrobial resistance
Determine the environment visited	Travel to rural environments, forests, rivers or lakes
Clarify where the person slept	Sleeping in huts, use of bed nets, sleeping on the ground
Establish what he/she was doing	Exposure to people with medical illness, animals, soil, lakes, rivers
History of insect bites	Type of insect responsible, circumstances (location, time of day etc.), preventive measures
Dietary history	Ingestion of uncooked foods, salads and vegetables, meats (especially if undercooked), shellfish, molluscs, unpasteurised dairy products, unbottled water and sites at which food prepared
Sexual history	History of sexual intercourse with commercial sex workers, local population
Malaria prophylaxis	Type of prophylaxis
Vaccination history	Receipt of pre-travel vaccines and appropriateness to area visited
History of any treatments received while abroad	Receipt of medicines, local remedies, blood transfusions or surgical procedures

it or forget it!'), how to respond to travellers' diarrhoea (seek medical advice if bloody or lasts more than 48 hours) and, if relevant, safe sex (condom use).

Fever in travellers recently in the tropics

Presentation with unexplained fever is common in travellers who are visiting or have recently travelled to tropical areas. Frequent final diagnoses in such patients are

13.18 Specific exposures and causes of fever in the tropics

Exposure	Infection or disease
Mosquito bite	Malaria, dengue fever, Chikungunya, filariasis, tularaemia
Tsetse fly bite	African trypanosomiasis
Tick bite	Rickettsial infections, including typhus, Lyme disease, tularaemia, Crimean–Congo haemorrhagic fever, Kyasanur forest disease, babesiosis, tick-borne encephalitis
Louse bite	Typhus
Flea bite	Plague
Sandfly bite	Leishmaniasis, arbovirus infection
Reduviid bug	Chagas' disease
Animal contact	Q fever, brucellosis, anthrax, plague, tularaemia, viral haemorrhagic fevers, rabies
Fresh-water swimming	Schistosomiasis, leptospirosis, *Naegleria fowleri*
Exposure to soil	Inhalation: dimorphic fungi Inhalation or inoculation: *Burkholderia pseudomallei* Inoculation (most often when barefoot): hookworms, *Strongyloides stercoralis*
Raw or undercooked fruit and vegetables	Enteric bacterial infections, hepatitis A or E virus, *Fasciola hepatica*, *Toxocara* spp., *Echinococcus granulosus* (hydatid disease), *Entamoeba histolytica*
Undercooked pork	*Taenia solium* (cysticercosis)
Crustaceans or molluscs	Paragonimiasis, gnathostomiasis, *Angiostrongylus cantonensis* infection, hepatitis A virus, cholera
Unpasteurised dairy products	Brucellosis, salmonellosis, abdominal tuberculosis, listeriosis
Untreated water	Enteric bacterial infections, giardiasis, *Cryptosporidium* spp. (chronic in immunocompromised), hepatitis A or E virus

malaria, typhoid fever, viral hepatitis and dengue fever. Travellers to West Africa may have viral haemorrhagic fevers (VHF), such as Lassa fever, Crimean–Congo haemorrhagic fever, Marburg and Ebola (see Box 13.39, p. 325). Those to South-east Asia may have avian influenza (H5N1), which requires special isolation precautions.

Clinical assessment

The approach to unexplained fever is described above and key questions are listed in Box 13.17. Medicines purchased in some countries may have reduced efficacy, e.g. for malaria prophylaxis. Consult reliable up-to-date sources about resistance to antimalarial drugs in the country visited. Vaccinations against yellow fever and hepatitis A and B are sufficiently effective to virtually exclude these infections. Oral and injectable typhoid vaccinations are 70–90% effective.

The differential diagnosis is guided by the clinical scenario, presence of specific exposures (Box 13.18) and the incubation period (Box 13.19). *Falciparum* malaria

13.19 Incubation times and illnesses in travellers*

< 2 wks

Non-specific fever

- Malaria
- Chikungunya
- Dengue
- Scrub typhus
- Spotted group rickettsiae
- Acute HIV
- Acute hepatitis C virus
- *Campylobacter*
- Salmonellosis
- Shigellosis
- East African trypanosomiasis
- Leptospirosis
- Relapsing fever
- Influenza
- Yellow fever

Fever and coagulopathy (usually thrombocytopenia)

- Malaria
- VHF
- Meningococcaemia
- Enteroviruses
- Leptospirosis and other bacterial pathogens associated with coagulopathy

Fever and CNS involvement

- Malaria
- Typhoid fever
- Rickettsial typhus (epidemic caused by *Rickettsia prowazekii*)
- Meningococcal meningitis
- Arboviral encephalitis
- East African trypanosomiasis
- Other causes of encephalitis or meningitis
- Angiostrongyliasis
- Rabies

Fever and pulmonary involvement

- Influenza
- Pneumonia, including *Legionella* pneumonia
- Acute histoplasmosis
- Acute coccidioidomycosis
- Q fever
- SARS

Fever and rash

- Viral exanthems (rubella, measles, varicella, mumps, HHV-6, enteroviruses
- Chikungunya
- Dengue
- Spotted or typhus group rickettsiosis
- Typhoid fever
- Parvovirus B19
- HIV-1

2–6 wks

- Malaria
- Tuberculosis
- Hepatitis A, B, C and E viruses
- Visceral leishmaniasis
- Acute schistosomiasis
- Amoebic liver abscess
- Leptospirosis
- African trypanosomiasis
- VHF
- Q fever
- Acute American trypanosomiasis
- Viral causes of mononucleosis syndromes

> 6 wks

- Non-*falciparum* malaria
- Tuberculosis
- Hepatitis B and E viruses
- HIV-1
- Visceral leishmaniasis
- Filariasis
- Onchocerciasis
- Schistosomiasis
- Amoebic liver abscess
- Chronic mycoses
- African trypanosomiasis
- Rabies
- Typhoid fever

*Adapted from Traveller's Health Yellow Book, CDC Health Information for International Travel 2008.
(HHV-6 = human herpes virus-6; SARS = severe acute respiratory syndrome; VHF = viral haemorrhagic fever)

tends to present between 7 and 28 days after exposure in an endemic area. VHF, dengue and rickettsial infection can usually be excluded if more than 21 days have passed between leaving the area and onset of illness.

13.20 Investigation of tropically acquired acute fever without localising signs

Features on FBC	Further investigations
Neutrophil leucocytosis	
Bacterial sepsis	Blood culture
Leptospirosis	Culture of blood and urine, serology
Borreliosis (tick- or louse-borne relapsing fever)	Blood film
Amoebic liver abscess	Ultrasound
Normal white cell count and differential	
Typhoid fever	Blood and stool culture
Typhus	Serology
Arboviral infection	Serology (PCR and viral culture)
Lymphocytosis	
Viral fevers	Serology
Infectious mononucleosis	Monospot test
Rickettsial fevers	Serology

(PCR = polymerase chain reaction)

Clinical examination is summarised on page 294. Particular attention should be paid to the skin, throat, eyes, nail beds, lymph nodes, abdomen and heart. Patients may be unaware of tick bites or eschars (p. 350). Body temperature should be measured at least twice daily.

Investigations and management

Initial investigations should start with thick and thin blood films for malaria parasites, FBC, urinalysis and chest X-ray if indicated. Box 13.20 lists diagnoses and investigations to consider in unexplained acute fever.

Management is directed at the underlying cause. In patients with suspected VHF (p. 324), strict infection control measures with isolation and barrier nursing are implemented to prevent contact with the patient's body fluids. The risk of VHF should be determined using epidemiological risk factors and clinical signs (Fig. 13.5), and further management undertaken as described on page 324.

Diarrhoea acquired in the tropics

Gastrointestinal illness is the most common infection amongst visitors to the tropics, with *Salmonella* spp., *Campylobacter* spp. and *Cryptosporidium* spp. infections prevalent worldwide (Box 13.21). Typhoid, paratyphoid, *Shigella* spp. and *Entamoeba histolytica* (amoebiasis) are usually encountered in visitors to the Indian subcontinent or sub-Saharan and southern Africa.

The approach to patients with acute diarrhoea is described on page 306. The benefits of treating travellers' diarrhoea with antimicrobials are marginal (Box 13.22). The differential diagnosis of diarrhoea persisting for more than 14 days is wide (Box 22.21, p. 857). Parasitic and bacterial causes, tropical malabsorption, inflammatory bowel disease and neoplasia should all be considered. Box 13.23 lists causes encountered particularly in visitors to the tropics. The work-up should include tests for parasitic causes of chronic diarrhoea,

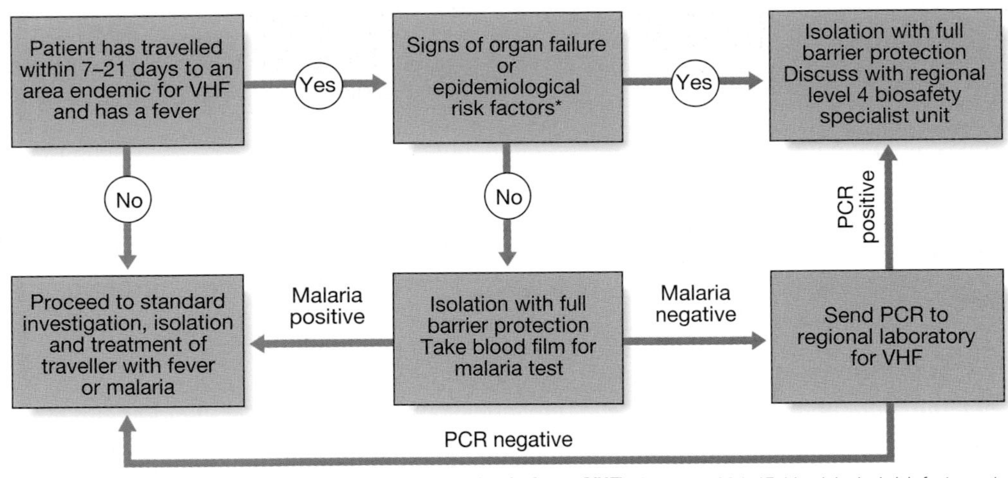

Fig. 13.5 Approach to the patient with suspected viral haemorrhagic fever (VHF). See page 324. *Epidemiological risk factors: staying with a febrile individual, caring for a sick individual, or contact with body fluids from a suspected human or animal case of VHF. (PCR = polymerase chain reaction)

13

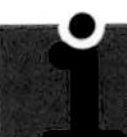

13.21 Most common causes of travellers' diarrhoea

- Enterotoxigenic *E. coli* (ETEC)
- *Shigella* spp.
- *Campylobacter jejuni*
- *Salmonella* spp.
- *Plesiomonas shigelloides*
- Non-cholera *Vibrio* spp.
- *Aeromonas* spp.

EBM 13.22 Antimicrobials in travellers' diarrhoea

'Antimicrobials reduce the duration of acute non-bloody diarrhoea.'

- de Bruyn G, et al. Antibiotic treatment for travellers' diarrhoea. Cochrane Database of Systematic Reviews, 2000, issue 3. Art. no. CD002242.

For further information: www.cochrane.org/cochrane-reviews

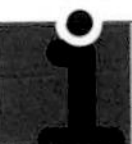

13.23 Causes of chronic diarrhoea acquired in the tropics

- *Giardia lamblia*
- Strongyloidiasis
- Enteropathic *E. coli*
- HIV enteropathy
- Intestinal flukes
- Tropical sprue
- Chronic intestinal schistosomiasis
- Chronic calcific pancreatitis
- Hypolactasia (primary and secondary)

e.g. examination of stool and duodenal aspirates for ova and parasites, and serological investigation.

Tropical sprue is a malabsorption syndrome (p. 882) with no defined aetiology. It was typically associated with a long period of residence in the tropics or with overland travel but is now rarely seen. *Giardia lamblia* infection may progress to a malabsorption syndrome that mimics tropical sprue. If no cause is found, empirical treatment for *Giardia lamblia* infection with metronidazole is often helpful.

HIV-1 has now emerged as a major cause of chronic diarrhoea. This may be due to HIV enteropathy or infection with agents such as *Cryptosporidium* spp., *Isospora belli* or microsporidia (p. 399). However, many other causes of chronic AIDS-associated diarrhoea seen in the developed world are less common in tropical settings, e.g. CMV or disseminated *Mycobacterium avium* complex infections.

Eosinophilia acquired in the tropics

Eosinophilia occurs in a variety of haematological, allergic and inflammatory conditions discussed on p. 1004. It may also arise in HIV-1 and human T-cell lymphotropic virus (HTLV)-1 infection. However, eosinophils are important in the immune response to parasitic infections, in particular those involving parasites with a tissue migration phase. In the context of travel to or residence in the tropics, a patient with an eosinophil count of more than 0.4×10^9/L should be investigated for both non-parasitic (Box 24.9, p. 1004) and parasitic causes (Box 13.24).

The response to parasite infections is often different when travellers to and residents of endemic areas are compared. Travellers often have recent and light infections associated with eosinophilia. Residents have often been infected for a long time, have evidence of chronic pathology and no longer have eosinophilia.

Clinical assessment

A history of travel to known endemic areas for schistosomiasis, onchocerciasis and the filariases will indicate possible causes. Assessment should establish how long patients have spent in endemic areas and the history should address all the elements in Box 13.17.

Physical signs or symptoms that suggest a parasitic cause for eosinophilia include transient rashes (schistosomiasis or strongyloidiasis), fever (Katayama syndrome – p. 377), pruritus (onchocerciasis) or migrating subcutaneous swellings (loiasis, gnathostomiasis) (see Box 13.24). Paragonimiasis can give rise to haemoptysis and the migratory phase of intestinal nematodes or lymphatic filariasis may cause cough, wheezing and transient pulmonary infiltrates. Schistosomiasis induces transient respiratory symptoms with infiltrates in the acute stages and, when eggs reach the pulmonary vasculature in chronic infection, can result in shortness of breath with features of right heart failure due to pulmonary hypertension. Fever and hepatosplenomegaly are seen in schistosomiasis, *Fasciola hepatica* infection and

13.24 Parasite infections that cause eosinophilia

Infestation	Pathogen	Clinical syndrome with eosinophilia
Strongyloidiasis	*Strongyloides stercoralis*	Larva currens
Soil-transmitted helminthiases		
Hookworm	*Necator americanus*	Anaemia
	Ancylostoma duodenale	Anaemia
Ascariasis	*Ascaris lumbricoides*	Löffler's syndrome
Toxocariasis	*Toxocara canis*	Visceral larva migrans
Schistosomiasis	*Schistosoma haematobium*	Katayama fever
	S. mansoni, S. japonicum	Chronic infection
Filariases		
Loiasis	*Loa loa*	Skin nodules
Wuchereria bancrofti	*W. bancrofti*	Lymphangitis, lymphadenopathy, orchitis, intermittent bouts of cellulitis, lymphoedema and elephantiasis
Brugia malayi	*B. malayi*	Brugian elephantiasis similar but typically less severe than that caused by *W. bancrofti*
Mansonella perstans	*M. perstans*	Asymptomatic infection, occasionally subconjunctival nodules
Onchocerciasis	*Onchocerca volvulus*	Visual disturbance, dermatitis
Other nematode infections	*Trichinella spiralis*	Myositis
Cestode infections	*Taenia saginata, T. solium*	Usually asymptomatic; eosinophilia associated with migratory phase
	Echinococcus granulosus	Lesions in liver or other organ; eosinophilia associated with leakage from cyst
Liver flukes	*Fasciola hepatica*	Hepatic symptoms; eosinophilia associated with migratory phase
	Clonorchis sinensis	As for fascioliasis
	Opisthorchis felineus	As for fascioliasis
Lung fluke	*Paragonimus westermani*	Lung lesions

toxocariasis (visceral larva migrans). Intestinal worms, such as *Ascaris lumbricoides* and *Strongyloides stercoralis*, can cause abdominal symptoms, including intestinal obstruction and diarrhoea. In the case of heavy infestation with *Ascaris*, this may be due to fat malabsorption and there may be associated nutritional deficits. *Schistosoma haematobium* can cause haematuria or haematospermia. *Toxocara* spp. can give rise to choroidal lesions with visual field defects. *Angiostrongylus cantonensis* and gnathostomiasis induce eosinophilic meningitis, and the hyperinfection syndrome caused by *Strongyloides stercoralis* in immunocompromised hosts induces meningitis due to Gram-negative bacteria. Myositis is a feature of trichinellosis and cysticercosis, while periorbital oedema is found in trichinellosis.

Investigations

The diagnosis of a parasitic infestation requires direct visualisation of adult worms, larvae or ova. Serum antibody detection may not distinguish between active and past infection and is often unhelpful in those born in endemic areas. Radiological investigations may provide circumstantial evidence of parasite infestation. Box 13.25 describes initial investigations for eosinophilia.

Management

A specific diagnosis guides therapy. In the absence of a specific diagnosis, many clinicians will give an empirical course of praziquantel if the individual has been potentially exposed to schistosomiasis, or with albendazole/ivermectin if strongyloidiasis or intestinal nematodes are likely causes.

13.25 Initial investigation of eosinophilia

Investigation	Pathogens sought
Stool microscopy	Ova, cysts and parasites
Terminal urine	Ova of *Schistosoma haematobium*
Duodenal aspirate	Filariform larvae of *Strongyloides*, liver fluke ova
Day bloods	Microfilariae *Brugia malayi, Loa loa*
Night bloods	Microfilariae *Wuchereria bancrofti*
Skin snips	*Onchocerca volvulus*
Slit lamp examination	*Onchocerca volvulus*
Serology	Schistosomiasis, filariasis, strongyloidiasis, hydatid, trichinosis etc.

Skin conditions acquired in the tropics

Community-based studies in the tropics consistently show that skin infections (bacterial and fungal), scabies and eczema are the most common skin problems (Box 13.26). Scabies and eczema are discussed on pages 1280 and 1283. Cutaneous leishmaniasis and onchocerciasis have defined geographical distributions (pp. 365 and 374). In travellers, secondarily infected insect bites, pyoderma, cutaneous larva migrans and non-specific dermatitis are common.

13.26 Rash in tropical travellers/residents

Maculopapular rash	• Dengue • HIV-1 • Typhoid	• *Spirillum minus* • Rickettsial infections • Measles
Petechial or purpuric rash	• Viral haemorrhagic fevers • Yellow fever • Meningococcal sepsis	• Leptospirosis • Rickettsial spotted fevers • Malaria
Vesicular rash	• Monkeypox • Insect bites	• Rickettsial pox
Urticarial rash	• Katayama fever (schistosomiasis) • *Toxocara* spp.	• *Strongyloides stercoralis* • Fascioliasis
Ulcers	• Leishmaniasis • *Mycobacterium ulcerans* (Buruli ulcer) • Dracunculosis • Anthrax • Rickettsial eschar	• Tropical ulcer (*Fusobacterium ulcerans* and *Treponema vincentii*) • Ecthyma (staphylococci, streptococci)
Papules	• Scabies • Insect bites • Prickly heat	• Ringworm • Onchocerciasis
Nodules or plaques	• Leprosy • Chromoblastomycosis • Dimorphic fungi • Trypanosomiasis • Onchocerciasis	• Myiasis (larvae of Tumbu or botfly) • Tungiasis (*Tunga penetrans*)
Migratory linear rash	• Cutaneous larva migrans (dog hookworms)	• *Strongyloides stercoralis*
Migratory papules/nodules	• *Loa loa* • Gnathosomiasis	• Schistosomiasis
Thickened skin	• Mycetoma (fungi/*Nocardia* spp.)	• Elephantiasis (filariasis)

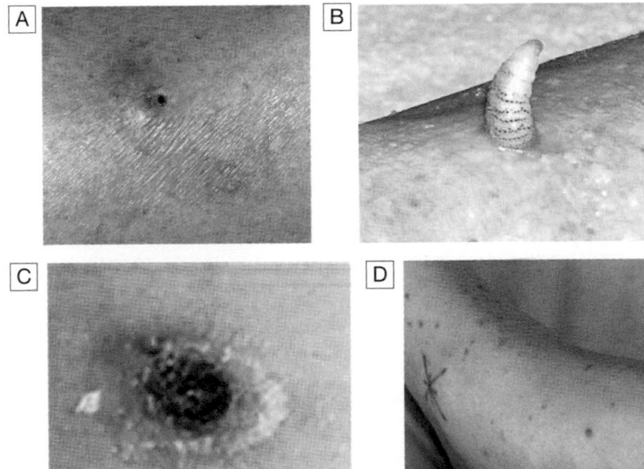

Fig. 13.6 Examples of skin lesions in patients with fever in the tropics. **A** Subcutaneous nodule due to botfly infection. **B** Emerging larva after treatment with petroleum jelly. **C** Eschar of scrub typhus. **D** Rat bite fever.

During the investigation of skin lesions, enquiry should be made about habitation, activities undertaken and regions visited (see Box 13.17). Examples of skin lesions in tropical disease are shown in Figure 13.6.

Skin biopsies are helpful in diagnosing aetiology. Culture of biopsy material may be needed to diagnose bacterial, fungal, parasitic and mycobacterial infections.

Infections in adolescence

Particular issues of relevance in adolescent patients are shown in Box 13.27.

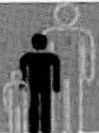

13.27 Key issues in infectious diseases in adolescence

- **Common infectious syndromes**: include infectious mononucleosis, bacterial pharyngitis, whooping cough, pneumonia, staphylococcal skin and soft tissue infections, urinary tract infections, acute gastroenteritis.
- **Life-threatening infections**: include meningococcal meningitis and bacterial sepsis.
- **Sexually transmitted infections**: include HIV-1, hepatitis B virus and chlamydia. These may reflect either voluntary sexual activity or sexual coercion/abuse.
- **Travel-related infections**: diarrhoea, malaria etc. are relatively common.
- **Infections in susceptible groups**: patients with cystic fibrosis, congenital immunodeficiency, acute leukaemia and other adolescent malignancies are vulnerable to specific groups of infections.
- **Infections requiring prolonged antimicrobial use**: adherence to chronic therapy is challenging, for both oral (antituberculous or antiretroviral) and systemic (osteomyelitis, septic arthritis or post-operative infections) treatments. Outpatient antimicrobial therapy is preferred to minimise hospitalisation.
- **Vaccination**: engagement with age-specific vaccine programmes should be ensured, e.g. for human papillomavirus.
- **Risk reduction**: education relating to sexual health and alcohol and recreational drug usage is important.

Infections in pregnancy

Box 13.28 shows some of the infections encountered in pregnancy.

13.28 Infections during pregnancy

Infection	Consequence	Prevention and management
Rubella	Congenital malformation	Vaccination of non-immune mothers
Cytomegalovirus	Neonatal infection, congenital malformation	Limited prevention strategies
Varicella zoster virus	Neonatal infection, congenital malformation, severe infection in mother	VZ immune globulin (see Box 13.34, p. 318), or aciclovir if exposure > 4 days previously
Herpes simplex virus	Congenital or neonatal infection	Aciclovir and consideration of caesarean section for mothers who shed HSV from genital tract at time of delivery. Aciclovir for infected neonates
Hepatitis B virus	Chronic infection of neonate	Hepatitis B immune globulin and active vaccination of newborn
HIV-1	Chronic infection of neonate	Antiretrovirals for mother and infant and consideration of caesarean section if HIV-1 viral load detectable. Avoidance of breastfeeding
Parvovirus B19	Congenital infection	Avoid individuals with acute infection if pregnant
Measles	More severe infection in mother and neonate	Immunisation of mother
Dengue	Neonatal dengue if mother has infection < 5 wks prior to delivery	Vector (mosquito) control
Syphilis	Congenital malformation	Serological testing in pregnancy with prompt treatment of infected mothers
Neisseria gonorrhoeae* and *Chlamydia trachomatis	Neonatal conjunctivitis (*ophthalmia neonatorum*, p. 422)	Treatment of infection in mother and neonate
Listeriosis	Neonatal meningitis or bacteraemia, bacteraemia or PUO in mother	Avoidance of unpasteurised cheeses and other dietary sources
Brucellosis	Possibly increased incidence of fetal loss	Avoidance of unpasteurised dairy products
Group B streptococcal infection	Neonatal meningitis and sepsis. Sepsis in mother after delivery	Risk- or screening-based antimicrobial prophylaxis in labour (recommendations vary between countries)
Toxoplasmosis	Congenital malformation	Diagnosis and prompt treatment of cases, avoidance of undercooked meat while pregnant
Malaria	Fetal loss, intrauterine growth retardation, severe malaria in mother	Avoidance of insect bites. Intermittent preventative treatment during pregnancy to decrease incidence in high-risk countries

VIRAL INFECTIONS

Systemic viral infections with exanthem

Childhood exanthems are characterised by fever and widespread rash. Maternal antibody gives protection for the first 6–12 months of life and infection occurs thereafter. Comprehensive immunisation programmes have dramatically reduced the number of paediatric infections but incomplete uptake results in infections in later life.

Measles

The WHO has set the objective of eradicating measles globally using the live attenuated vaccine. However, vaccination of more than 95% of the population is required to prevent outbreaks. Natural illness produces life-long immunity.

Clinical features

Infection is by respiratory droplets with an incubation period of 6–19 days. A prodromal illness, 1–3 days before the rash, occurs, with upper respiratory symptoms, conjunctivitis and the presence of the pathognomonic Koplik's spots, small white spots surrounded by erythema on the buccal mucosa (Fig. 13.7A). As natural antibody develops, the maculopapular rash appears, spreading from the face to the extremities (Fig. 13.7B). Generalised lymphadenopathy and diarrhoea are common. Complications are more common in older children and adults, and include otitis media, bacterial pneumonia, transient hepatitis and clinical encephalitis (approximately 0.1% of cases). A rare late complication is subacute sclerosing panencephalitis (SSPE), which occurs up to 7 years after infection. Diagnosis is clinical (although this has become unreliable in areas where measles is no longer common) and by detection of antibody (serum IgM, seroconversion or salivary IgM).

Measles is a serious disease in the malnourished, vitamin-deficient or immunocompromised, in whom the typical rash may be missing and persistent infection with a giant cell pneumonitis or encephalitis may occur. In tuberculosis infection, measles suppresses cell-mediated immunity and may exacerbate disease; for this reason, measles vaccination should be deferred until after commencing antituberculous treatment. Measles does not cause congenital malformation but may be more severe in pregnant women.

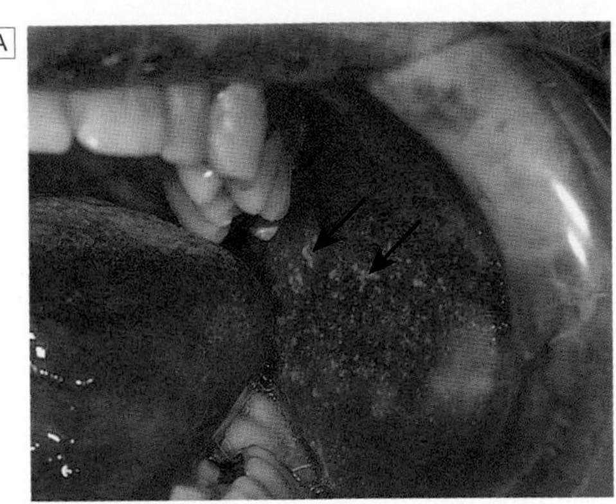

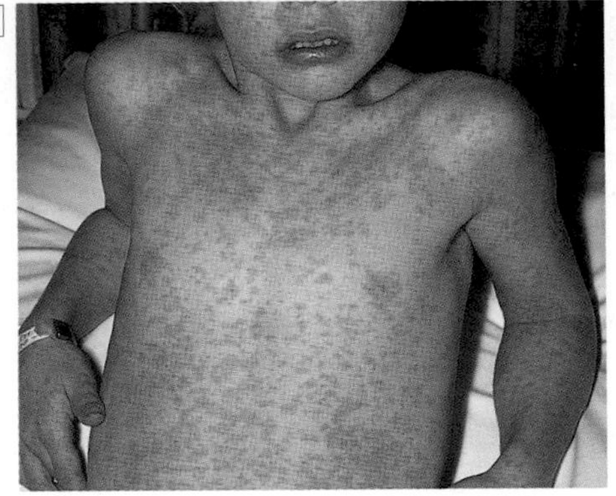

Fig. 13.7 Measles. **A** Koplik's spots (arrows) seen on buccal mucosa in the early stages of clinical measles. **B** Typical measles rash.

Mortality clusters at the extremes of age, averaging 1:1000 in developed countries and up to 1:4 in developing countries. Death usually results from a bacterial superinfection, occurring as a complication of measles, most often pneumonia, diarrhoeal disease or noma/cancrum oris, a gangrenous stomatitis. Death may also result from complications of measles encephalitis.

Management and prevention

Normal immunoglobulin attenuates the disease in the immunocompromised (regardless of vaccination status) and in non-immune pregnant women, but must be given within 6 days of exposure. Vaccination can be used in outbreaks and vitamin A may improve the outcome in uncomplicated disease. Antibiotic therapy is reserved for bacterial complications. All children aged 12–15 months should receive measles vaccination (as combined measles, mumps and rubella (MMR), a live attenuated vaccine), and a further MMR dose at age 4 years.

Rubella (German measles)

Rubella causes exanthem in the non-immunised.

Clinical features

Rubella is spread by respiratory droplet, with infectivity from up to 10 days before to 2 weeks after the onset of the rash. The incubation period is 15–20 days. In childhood, most cases are subclinical, although clinical features may include fever, maculopapular rash spreading from the face, and lymphadenopathy. Complications are rare but include thrombocytopenia and hepatitis. Encephalitis and haemorrhage are occasionally reported. In adults, arthritis involving hands or knees is relatively common, especially in women.

If transplacental infection takes place in the first trimester or later, persistence of the virus is likely and severe congenital disease may result (Box 13.29). Even if normal at birth, the infant has an increased incidence of other diseases developing later, e.g. diabetes mellitus.

Diagnosis

Laboratory confirmation of rubella is required if there has been contact with a pregnant woman. This is achieved either by detection of rubella IgM in serum or by IgG seroconversion. In the exposed pregnant woman, absence of rubella-specific IgG confirms the potential for congenital infection.

13.29 Rubella infection: risk of congenital malformation

Stage of gestation	Likelihood of malformations
1–2 mths	65–85% chance of illness, multiple defects/spontaneous abortion
3 mths	30–35% chance of illness, usually a single congenital defect (most frequently deafness, cataract, glaucoma, mental retardation or congenital heart disease, especially pulmonary stenosis or patent ductus arteriosus)
4 mths	10% risk of congenital defects, most commonly deafness
> 20 wks	Occasional deafness

Prevention

All children should be immunised with MMR, as above for measles. In view of the risks of congenital rubella syndrome, all women of child-bearing age should also be tested for rubella and vaccinated if seronegative.

Parvovirus B19

Parvovirus B19 causes exanthem and other clinical syndromes. Some 50% of children and 60–90% of adults are seropositive. Most infections are spread by the respiratory route, although spread via contaminated blood is also possible. The virus has particular tropism for red cell precursors.

Clinical features

Many infections are subclinical. Clinical manifestations result after an incubation period of 14–21 days (Box 13.30). The classic exanthem (erythema infectiosum) is preceded by a prodromal fever and coryzal symptoms. A 'slapped cheek' rash is characteristic but the rash is very variable (Fig. 13.8). In adults, polyarthropathy is common. Infected individuals have a transient block in erythropoiesis for a few days, which is of no clinical consequence, except in individuals with increased red cell turnover due to haemoglobinopathy or haemolytic anaemia. These individuals develop an acute anaemia which may be severe (transient aplastic crisis; p. 1032). Erythropoiesis usually recovers spontaneously after 10–14 days. Immunocompromised individuals,

13.30 Clinical features of parvovirus B19 infection

Affected age group	Clinical manifestations
Fifth disease (erythema infectiosum)	
Small children	Three clinical stages: a 'slapped cheek' appearance, followed by a maculopapular rash progressing to a reticulate eruption on the body and limbs, then a final stage of resolution. Often the child is quite well throughout
Gloves and socks syndrome	
Young adults	Fever and an acral purpuric eruption with a clear margin at the wrists and ankles. Mucosal involvement also occurs
Arthropathies	
Adults and occasionally children	Symmetrical small-joint polyarthropathy. In children it tends to involve the larger joints in an asymmetrical distribution
Impaired erythropoiesis	
Adults, those with haematological disease, the immunosuppressed	Mild anaemia; in an individual with an underlying haematological abnormality can precipitate transient aplastic crisis, or in the immunocompromised a more sustained but often milder pure red cell aplasia
Hydrops fetalis	
Transplacental fetal infection	Asymptomatic or symptomatic maternal infection can cause fetal anaemia with an aplastic crisis, leading to non-immune hydrops fetalis and spontaneous abortion

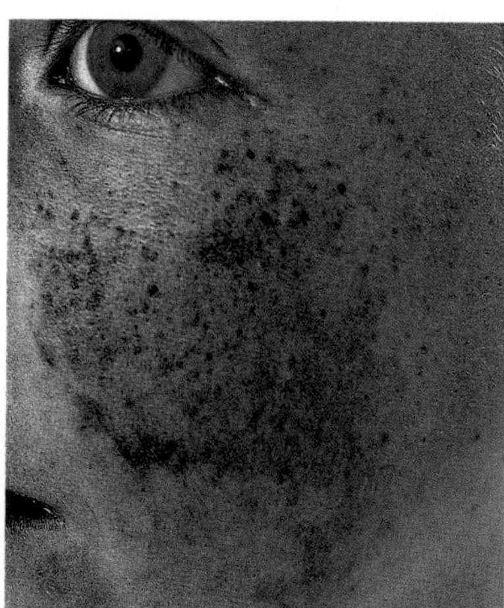

Fig. 13.8 Slapped cheek syndrome. The typical facial rash of parvovirus B19 infection.

including those with congenital immunodeficiency or AIDS, can develop a more sustained block in erythropoiesis in response to the chronic viraemia that results from their inability to clear the infection. Infection during the first two trimesters of pregnancy can result in intrauterine infection and impact on fetal bone marrow; it causes 10–15% of non-immune (non-Rhesus-related) hydrops fetalis, a rare complication of pregnancy.

Diagnosis

IgM to parvovirus B19 suggests recent infection but may persist for months and false positives occur. Seroconversion to IgG positivity confirms infection but in isolation a positive IgG is of little diagnostic utility. Detection of parvovirus B19 DNA in blood is particularly useful in immunocompromised patients. Giant pronormoblasts or haemophagocytosis may be demonstrable in the bone marrow.

Management

Infection is usually self-limiting. Symptomatic relief for arthritic symptoms may be required. Severe anaemia requires transfusion. Persistent viraemia in immunocompromised hosts may require immunoglobulin therapy to clear the virus.

Pregnant women should avoid contact with cases of parvovirus B19 infection; if they are exposed, serology should be performed to establish whether they are non-immune.

Passive prophylaxis with normal immunoglobulin has been suggested for non-immune pregnant women exposed to infection but there are limited data to support this recommendation. The pregnancy should be closely monitored by ultrasound scanning, so that hydrops fetalis can be treated by fetal transfusion.

Human herpesvirus 6 and 7

Human herpesvirus 6 (HHV-6) is a lymphotropic virus that causes a childhood viral exanthem (exanthem subitum), rare cases of an infectious mononucleosis-like syndrome and infection in the immunocompromised host. Infection is almost universal, with approximately 95% of children acquiring this virus by 2 years of age. Transmission is via saliva.

HHV-7 is very closely related to HHV-6, and is believed to be responsible for a proportion of cases of exanthem subitum. Like HHV-6, HHV-7 causes an almost universal infection in childhood, with subsequent latent infection and occasional infection in the immunocompromised host.

Clinical features

Exanthem subitum is also known as roseola infantum or sixth disease (Box 13.31). A high fever is followed by a maculopapular rash as the fever resolves. Fever and/or febrile convulsions may also occur without a rash. Rarely, older children or adults may develop an infectious mononucleosis-like illness, hepatitis or rash. In the immunocompromised, infection is rare but can cause fever, rash, hepatitis, pneumonitis, cytopenia or encephalitis.

Diagnosis and management

Exanthem subitum is usually a clinical diagnosis but can be confirmed by antibody and/or DNA detection. The disease is self-limiting. Treatment with ganciclovir or foscarnet is used in immunocompromised hosts infected with HHV-6.

Chickenpox (varicella)

Varicella zoster virus (VZV) is a dermotropic and neurotropic virus that produces primary infection, usually in childhood, which may reactivate in later life. VZV is spread by aerosol and direct contact. It is highly

13.31 Herpesvirus infections

Virus	Infection
***Herpesvirus hominis* (herpes simplex, HSV)**	
HSV-1 (p. 325)	Herpes labialis ('cold sores') Stomatitis, pharyngitis Corneal ulceration Finger infections ('whitlows') Eczema herpeticum Encephalitis
HSV-2 (p. 325)	Genital ulceration and neonatal infection (acquired during vaginal delivery) Acute meningitis or transverse myelitis. Rarely, encephalitis
Varicella zoster virus (VZV) (p. 316)	Chickenpox (varicella) Shingles (herpes zoster)
Cytomegalovirus (CMV) (p. 321)	Congenital infection Infectious mononucleosis (heterophile antibody-negative) Hepatitis Disease in immunocompromised patients: retinitis, encephalitis, pneumonitis, hepatitis, enteritis Fever with abnormalities in haematological parameters
Epstein–Barr virus (EBV) (p. 320)	Infectious mononucleosis Burkitt's and other lymphomas Nasopharyngeal carcinoma Oral hairy leucoplakia (AIDS patients) Other lymphomas
Human herpesvirus 6 and 7 (HHV-6, HHV-7)	Exanthem subitum Disease in immunocompromised patients
Human herpesvirus 8 (HHV-8) (p. 326)	Kaposi's sarcoma, primary effusion lymphoma, multicentric Castleman's disease

infectious to non-immune individuals. Disease in children is usually well tolerated. Manifestations are more severe in adults, pregnant women and the immunocompromised.

Clinical features

The incubation period is 11–20 days, after which a vesicular eruption begins (Fig. 13.9), often on mucosal surfaces first, followed by rapid dissemination in a centripetal distribution (most dense on trunk and sparse on limbs). New lesions occur every 2–4 days and each crop is associated with fever. The rash progresses from small pink macules to vesicles and pustules within 24 hours. Infectivity lasts from up to 4 days (but usually 48 hours) before the lesions appear until the last vesicles crust over. Due to intense itching, secondary bacterial infection from scratching is the most common complication of primary chickenpox. Self-limiting cerebellar ataxia and encephalitis are rare complications.

Adults, pregnant women and the immunocompromised are at increased risk of visceral involvement, which presents as pneumonitis, hepatitis or encephalitis. Pneumonitis can be fatal and is more likely to occur in smokers. Maternal infection in early pregnancy carries a 3% risk of neonatal damage with developmental abnormalities of eyes, CNS and limbs. Chickenpox within 5 days of delivery leads to severe neonatal varicella with visceral involvement and haemorrhage.

Diagnosis

Diagnosis is primarily clinical, by recognition of the rash. If necessary, this can be confirmed by detection of antigen (direct immunofluorescence) or DNA (PCR) of aspirated vesicular fluid. Serology is used to identify seronegative individuals at risk of infection.

Management and prevention

The benefits of antivirals for uncomplicated primary VZV infection in children are marginal and treatment is not required (Box 13.32). Antivirals are, however, used for uncomplicated chickenpox when the patient presents within 24–48 hours of onset of vesicles, in all patients with complications, and in those who are immunocompromised, including pregnant women, regardless of duration of vesicles (Box 13.33). More severe disease, particularly in immunocompromised hosts, requires initial parenteral therapy. Immunocompromised patients may have prolonged viral shedding and may require prolonged treatment until all lesions crust over.

EBM 13.32 Aciclovir for chickenpox/shingles

'Aciclovir shortens symptoms in chickenpox by an average of 1 day. In shingles, aciclovir reduces pain by 10 days and the risk of post-herpetic neuralgia by 8%. Aciclovir is therefore cost-effective in shingles but not chickenpox.'

- Nathwani D, et al. Infect Dis Clin Prac 1995; 4:138–145.
- Trying SK. Arch Fam Med; 2000; 9:863–869.

A

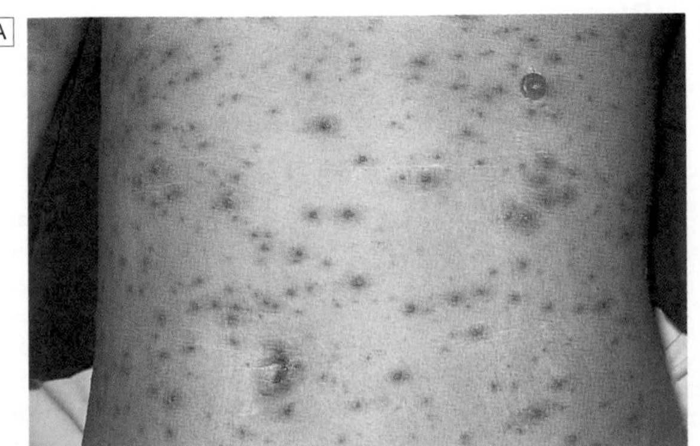

B

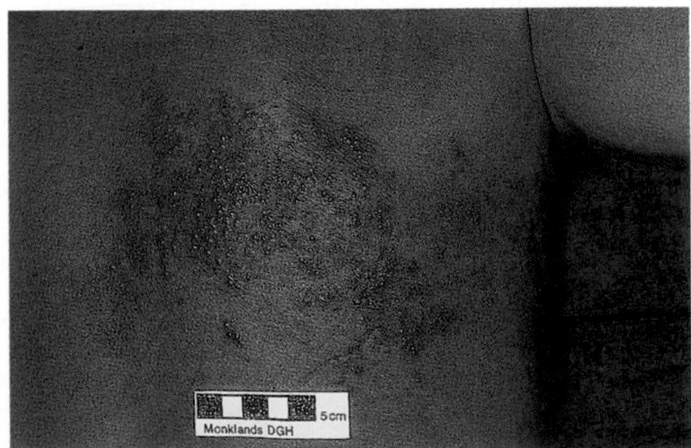

Fig. 13.9 Varicella zoster virus infection. A Chickenpox. B Shingles in a thoracic dermatome.

13.33 Therapy for herpes simplex and varicella zoster virus infection

Disease state	Treatment options
Primary genital HSV	Famciclovir 250 mg 3 times daily for 7–10 days Valaciclovir 1 g twice daily for 7–10 days Oral aciclovir 200 mg 5 times daily or 400 mg 3 times daily for 7–10 days
Severe and preventing oral intake	Aciclovir 5 mg/kg 3 times daily IV until patient can tolerate oral therapy
Recurrent genital HSV-1 or 2	Oral aciclovir 200 mg 5 times daily or 400 mg 3 times daily for 5 days Famciclovir 125 mg twice daily for 5 days Valaciclovir 500 mg twice daily for 3–5 days or 2 g twice daily for 1 day. Shorter durations increasingly favoured
Primary or recurrent oral HSV	Usually no treatment If required, usually short duration, e.g. valaciclovir 2 g twice daily for 1 day
Mucocutaneous HSV infection in immunocompromised host	Aciclovir 5 mg/kg 3 times daily IV for 7–10 days Oral aciclovir 400 mg 4 times daily for 7–10 days Famciclovir 500 mg 3 times daily for 7–10 days Valaciclovir 1 g twice daily for 7–10 days
Chickenpox in adult or child	Oral aciclovir 800 mg 5 times daily for 5 days Famciclovir 500 mg 3 times daily for 5 days Valaciclovir 1 g 3 times daily for 5 days
Immunocompromised host/pregnant woman	Aciclovir 5 mg/kg 3 times daily IV until patient is improving, then complete therapy with oral therapy until all lesions crusting over
Shingles	Treatment and doses as for chickenpox but duration typically 7–10 days
Visceral involvement (non-CNS) in HSV	Aciclovir IV 5 mg/kg 3 times daily for 14 days
Visceral involvement (non-CNS) in VZV	Aciclovir IV 5 mg/kg 3 times daily for 7 days
Severe complications (encephalitis, disseminated infection)	Aciclovir IV 10 mg/kg 3 times daily (up to 20 mg/kg in neonates) for 14–21 days
HSV disease suppression	Aciclovir 400 mg twice daily Famciclovir 250 mg twice daily Valaciclovir 500 mg daily

13.34 Indications for varicella zoster immunoglobulin (VZIG) in adults

An adult should satisfy all three of the following conditions:

1. Significant contact

Contact with chickenpox (any time from 48 hrs before the rash until crusting of lesions) or zoster (exposed, disseminated or, with immunocompromised contacts, localised zoster; between development of the rash until crusting) defined as:

- Prolonged household contact, sharing a room for ≥ 15 mins or face-to-face contact (includes direct contact with zoster lesions)
- Hospital contact with chickenpox in another patient, health-care worker or visitor
- Intimate contact (e.g. touching) with person with shingles lesions
- Newborn whose mother develops chickenpox no more than 5 days before delivery or 2 days after delivery

2. Susceptible contact

- Individual with no history of chickenpox, ideally confirmed by negative test for VZV IgG

3. Predisposition to severe chickenpox

- Immunocompromised due to disease (e.g. acute leukaemia, HIV, other primary or secondary immunodeficiency)
- Medically immunosuppressed (e.g. following solid organ transplant; current or recent (< 6 mths) cytotoxic chemotherapy or radiotherapy; current or recent (< 3 mths) high-dose corticosteroids; haematopoietic stem cell transplant)
- Pregnant (any stage)
- Infants: newborn whose mother has had chickenpox as above; premature infants < 28 wks

Human VZ immunoglobulin (VZIG) is used to attenuate infection in people who have had significant contact with VZV, are susceptible to infection (i.e. have no history of chickenpox or shingles and are seronegative for VZV IgG) and are at risk of severe disease (e.g. immunocompromised, steroid-treated or pregnant) (Box 13.34). Ideally, VZIG should be given within 7 days of exposure, but it may attenuate disease even if given up to 10 days afterwards. Susceptible contacts who develop severe chickenpox after receiving VZIG should be treated with aciclovir.

A live, attenuated VZV vaccine is available and in routine use in the USA and other countries, but in the UK its use has been restricted to non-immune health-care workers and household contacts of immunocompromised individuals. Children receive one dose after 1 year of age and a second dose at 4–6 years of age; seronegative adults receive two doses at least 1 month apart. The vaccine may also be used prior to planned iatrogenic immunosuppression, e.g. before transplant.

Shingles (herpes zoster)

After initial infection, VZV persists in latent form in the dorsal root ganglion of sensory nerves and can reactivate in later life.

Clinical features

Burning discomfort occurs in the affected dermatome, where discrete vesicles appear 3–4 days later. This is associated with a brief viraemia, which can produce distant satellite 'chickenpox' lesions. Occasionally, paraesthesia occurs without rash ('zoster sine herpete'). Severe disease, a prolonged duration of rash, multiple dermatomal involvement or recurrence suggests underlying immune deficiency, including HIV. Chickenpox may be contracted from a case of shingles but not vice versa.

Although thoracic dermatomes are most commonly involved (Fig. 13.9B), the ophthalmic division of the trigeminal nerve is also frequently affected; vesicles may appear on the cornea and lead to ulceration. This condition can lead to blindness and urgent ophthalmology review is required. Geniculate ganglion involvement causes the Ramsay Hunt syndrome of facial palsy, ipsilateral loss of taste and buccal ulceration, plus a rash in the external auditory canal. This may be mistaken for Bell's palsy (p. 1163). Bowel and bladder dysfunction occur with sacral nerve root involvement. The virus occasionally causes cranial nerve palsy, myelitis or encephalitis. Granulomatous cerebral angiitis is a cerebrovascular complication that leads to a stroke-like syndrome in association with shingles, especially in an ophthalmic distribution.

Post-herpetic neuralgia causes troublesome persistence of pain for 1–6 months or longer, following healing of the rash. It is more common with advanced age.

Management

Early therapy with aciclovir or related agents has been shown to reduce both early- and late-onset pain, especially in patients over 65 years (see Box 13.32). Post-herpetic neuralgia requires aggressive analgesia, along with agents such as amitriptyline 25–100 mg daily or gabapentin (commencing at 300 mg daily and building slowly to 300 mg twice daily or more). Capsaicin cream (0.075%) may be helpful. Although controversial, corticosteroids have not been demonstrated to reduce post-herpetic neuralgia to date.

Enteroviral exanthems

Coxsackie or echovirus infections can lead to a maculopapular eruption or roseola-like rash that occurs after fever falls. Enteroviral infections are discussed further under viral infections of the skin (see below).

Systemic viral infections without exanthem

Other systemic viral infections present with features other than a rash suggestive of exanthem. Rashes may occur in these conditions but differ from those seen in exanthems or are not the primary presenting feature.

Mumps

Mumps is a systemic viral infection characterised by swelling of the parotid glands. Infection is endemic worldwide and peaks at 5–9 years of age. Vaccination has reduced the incidence in children but incomplete coverage and waning immunity with time have led to outbreaks in young adults. Infection is spread by respiratory droplets.

Clinical features

The median incubation period is 19 days, with a range of 15–24 days. Classical tender parotid enlargement, which is bilateral in 75%, follows a prodrome of pyrexia and headache (Fig. 13.10). Meningitis complicates up to 10% of cases. The CSF reveals a lymphocytic pleocytosis or, less commonly, neutrophils. Rare complications include encephalitis, transient hearing loss, labyrinthitis, electrocardiographic abnormalities, pancreatitis and arthritis.

A 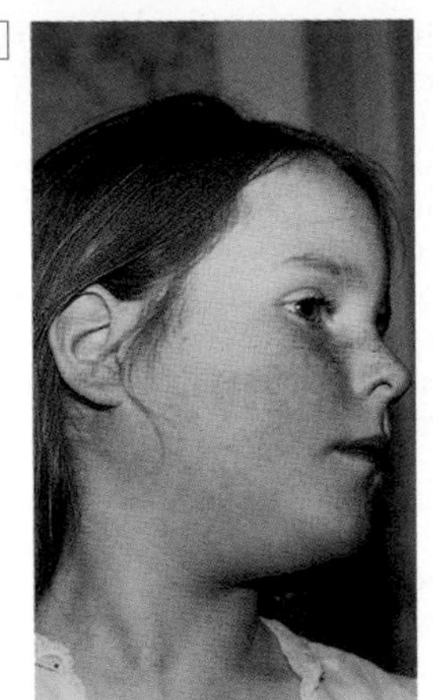

B 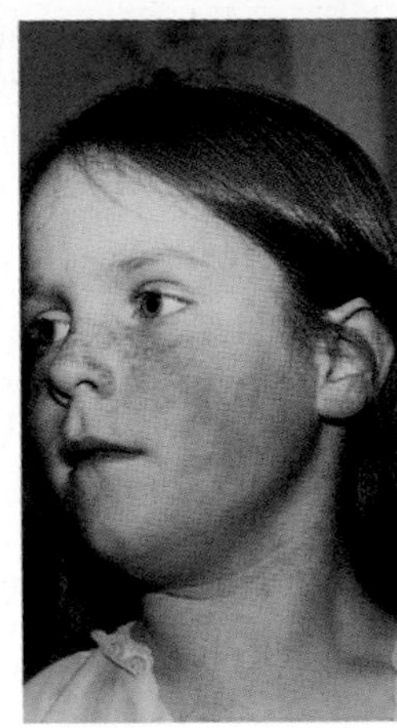

Fig. 13.10 Typical unilateral mumps. A Note the loss of angle of the jaw on the affected (right) side. B Comparison showing normal (left) side.

Approximately 25% of post-pubertal males with mumps develop epididymo-orchitis but, although testicular atrophy occurs, sterility is unlikely. Oophoritis is less common. Abortion may occur if infection takes place in the first trimester of pregnancy. Complications may occur in the absence of parotitis.

Diagnosis

The diagnosis is usually clinical. In atypical presentations without parotitis, serology for mumps-specific IgM or IgG seroconversion (four-fold rise in IgG convalescent titre) confirms the diagnosis. Virus can also be cultured from urine in the first week of infection or detected by PCR in urine, saliva or CSF.

Management and prevention

Treatment is with analgesia. There is no evidence that corticosteroids are of value for orchitis. Mumps vaccine is one of the components of the combined MMR vaccine.

Influenza

Influenza is an acute systemic viral infection that primarily affects the respiratory tract; it carries a significant mortality. It is caused by influenza A virus or, in milder form, influenza B virus. Infection is seasonal, and variation in the haemagglutinin (H) and neuraminidase (N) glycoproteins on the surface of the virus leads to disease of variable intensity each year. Minor changes in haemagglutinin are known as 'genetic drift', whereas a switch in the haemagglutinin or neuraminidase antigen is termed 'genetic shift'. Nomenclature of influenza strains is based on these glycoproteins, e.g. H1N1, H3N2 etc. Genetic shift results in the circulation of a new influenza strain within a community to which few people are immune, potentially initiating an influenza epidemic or pandemic in which there is a high attack rate and there may be increased disease severity.

Clinical features

After an incubation period of 1–3 days, uncomplicated disease leads to fever, malaise and cough. Viral pneumonia may occur, although pulmonary complications are most often due to superinfection with *Strep. pneumoniae*, *Staph. aureus* or other bacteria. Rare extrapulmonary manifestations include myositis, myocarditis, pericarditis and neurological complications (Reye's syndrome in children, encephalitis or transverse myelitis). Mortality is greatest in the elderly, those with medical comorbidities and pregnant women. Recently, polymorphisms in the gene encoding an antiviral protein, interferon-induced transmembrane protein 3 (IFITM3), have been associated with more severe influenza.

Diagnosis

Acute infection is diagnosed by viral antigen or RNA detection in a nasopharyngeal sample. The disease may also be diagnosed retrospectively by serology.

Management and prevention

Management involves early microbiological identification of cases and good infection control, with an emphasis on hand hygiene and preventing dissemination of infection by coughing and sneezing. Administration of neuraminidase inhibitor, oral oseltamivir (75 mg twice daily) or inhaled zanamivir (10 mg twice daily) for 5 days, can reduce the severity of symptoms if started within 48 hours of symptom onset (or possibly later in immunocompromised individuals). These agents have superseded routine use of amantadine and rimantadine. Antiviral drugs can also be used as prophylaxis in high-risk individuals during the 'flu' season. Resistance can emerge to all of these agents and so updated local advice should be followed.

Prevention relies on seasonal vaccination of the elderly and of individuals with chronic medical illnesses which place them at increased risk of the complications of influenza, such as chronic cardiopulmonary diseases or immune compromise, as well as their health-care workers. The vaccine composition changes each year to cover the 'predicted' seasonal strains but vaccination may fail when a new pandemic strain emerges.

Avian influenza

Avian influenza is caused by transmission of avian influenza A viruses to humans. Avian viruses, such as H5N1, possess alternative haemagglutinin antigens to seasonal influenza strains. Most cases have had contact with sick poultry, predominantly in South-east Asia, and person-to-person spread has been limited to date. Infections with H5N1 viruses have been severe, with enteric features and respiratory failure. Treatment depends on the resistance pattern but often involves oseltamivir. Vaccination against seasonal 'flu' does not adequately protect against avian influenza. There is a concern that adaptation of an avian strain to allow effective person-to-person transmission is likely to lead to a global pandemic of life-threatening influenza.

Swine influenza

Occasional cases of influenza are transmitted from pigs to humans. Re-assortment of swine, avian and human influenza strains can occur in pigs. Sometimes this can lead to an outbreak of swine 'flu' in humans, as occurred in 2009, when an outbreak of H1N1 influenza spread around the world from Mexico.

Infectious mononucleosis and Epstein–Barr virus

Infectious mononucleosis (IM) is a clinical syndrome characterised by pharyngitis, cervical lymphadenopathy, fever and lymphocytosis. It is most often caused by Epstein–Barr virus (EBV) but other infections can produce a similar clinical syndrome (Box 13.35).

EBV is a gamma herpesvirus. In developing countries, subclinical infection in childhood is virtually universal. In developed countries, primary infection may be delayed until adolescence or early adult life. Under these circumstances, about 50% of infections result in typical IM. The virus is usually acquired from asymptomatic excreters via saliva, either by droplet infection or environmental contamination in childhood, or by kissing among adolescents and adults. EBV is not highly contagious and isolation of cases is unnecessary.

Clinical features

EBV infection has a prolonged and undetermined incubation period, followed in some cases by a prodrome of fever, headache and malaise. This is succeeded by IM with severe pharyngitis, which may include tonsillar exudates and non-tender anterior and posterior cervical lymphadenopathy. Palatal petechiae, periorbital oedema, splenomegaly, inguinal or axillary lymphadenopathy, and macular, petechial or erythema multiforme rashes may occur. In most cases, fever resolves over 2 weeks, and fatigue and other abnormalities settle over a further few weeks. Complications are listed in Box 13.36. Death is rare but can occur due to respiratory obstruction, haemorrhage from splenic rupture or thrombocytopenia, or encephalitis.

The diagnosis of EBV infection outside the usual age in adolescence and young adulthood is more challenging. In children under 10 years the illness is mild and short-lived, but in adults over 30 years of age it can be severe and prolonged. In both groups, pharyngeal symptoms are often absent. EBV may present with jaundice, as a PUO or with a complication.

Long-term complications of EBV infection

Lymphoma complicates EBV infection in immunocompromised hosts, and some forms of Hodgkin's disease are EBV-associated (p. 1042). The endemic form of Burkitt's lymphoma complicates EBV infection in areas of sub-Saharan Africa where *falciparum* malaria is endemic. Nasopharyngeal carcinoma is a geographically restricted tumour seen in China and Alaska that is associated with EBV infection. X-linked lymphoproliferative (Duncan's) syndrome is a familial lymphoproliferative disorder that follows primary EBV infection in boys without any other history of immunodeficiency; it is due to mutation of the *SAP* gene, causing failure of T-cell and NK-cell activation and inability to contain EBV infection.

13.35 Causes of infectious mononucleosis syndrome

- Epstein–Barr virus infection
- Cytomegalovirus
- Human herpesvirus-6 or 7
- HIV-1 primary infection (p. 394)
- Toxoplasmosis

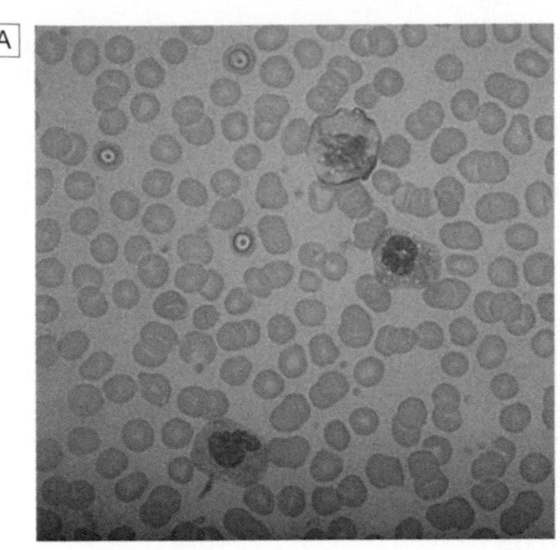

Fig. 13.11 Features of infectious mononucleosis. **A** Atypical lymphocytes in peripheral blood. **B** Skin reaction to ampicillin.

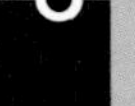

13.36 Complications of Epstein–Barr virus infection

Common	
• Severe pharyngeal oedema • Antibiotic-induced rash (80–90% with ampicillin) • Hepatitis (80%)	• Prolonged post-viral fatigue (10%) • Jaundice (< 10%)
Uncommon	
Neurological	
• Cranial nerve palsies • Polyneuritis	• Transverse myelitis • Meningoencephalitis
Haematological	
• Haemolytic anaemia	• Thrombocytopenia
Renal	
• Abnormalities on urinalysis	• Interstitial nephritis
Cardiac	
• Myocarditis • ECG abnormalities	• Pericarditis
Rare	
• Ruptured spleen • Respiratory obstruction • Agranulocytosis	• X-linked lymphoproliferative syndrome
EBV-associated malignancy	
• Nasopharyngeal carcinoma • Burkitt's lymphoma • Hodgkin's disease (certain subtypes only)	• Primary CNS lymphoma • Lymphoproliferative disease in immunocompromised

Investigations

Atypical lymphocytes are common in EBV infection but also occur in other causes of IM, acute retroviral syndrome with HIV infection, viral hepatitis, mumps and rubella (Fig. 13.11A). A 'heterophile' antibody is present during the acute illness and convalescence, which is detected by the Paul–Bunnell or 'Monospot' test. Sometimes antibody production is delayed, so an initially negative test should be repeated. However, many children and 10% of adolescents with IM do not produce heterophile antibody at any stage.

Specific EBV serology confirms the diagnosis. Acute infection is characterised by IgM antibodies against the viral capsid, antibodies to EBV early antigen and the initial absence of antibodies to EBV nuclear antigen (anti-EBNA). Seroconversion of anti-EBNA at approximately 1 month after the initial illness may confirm the diagnosis in retrospect. CNS infections may be diagnosed by detection of viral DNA in cerebrospinal fluid.

Management

Treatment is largely symptomatic. If a throat culture yields a β-haemolytic streptococcus, penicillin should be given. Administration of ampicillin or amoxicillin in this condition commonly causes an itchy macular rash and should be avoided (Fig. 13.11B). When pharyngeal oedema is severe, a short course of corticosteroids, e.g. prednisolone 30 mg daily for 5 days, may help. Current antiviral drugs are not active against EBV.

Return to work or school is governed by physical fitness rather than laboratory tests; contact sports should be avoided until splenomegaly has resolved because of the danger of splenic rupture. Unfortunately, about 10% of patients with IM suffer a chronic relapsing syndrome.

Cytomegalovirus

Cytomegalovirus (CMV), like EBV, circulates readily among children. A second period of virus acquisition occurs among teenagers and young adults, peaking between the ages of 25 and 35 years, rather later than with EBV infection. CMV infection is persistent, and is characterised by subclinical cycles of active virus replication and by persistent low-level virus shedding. Most post-childhood infections are therefore acquired from asymptomatic excreters who shed virus in saliva, urine, semen and genital secretions. Sexual transmission and oral spread are common among adults, but infection may also be acquired by women caring for children with asymptomatic infections.

Clinical features

Most post-childhood CMV infections are subclinical, although some young adults develop an IM-like syndrome and some have a prolonged influenza-like illness lasting 2 weeks or more. Physical signs resemble those of IM, but in CMV infections hepatomegaly is more common, while lymphadenopathy, splenomegaly, pharyngitis and tonsillitis occur less often. Jaundice is uncommon and usually mild. Complications include meningoencephalitis, Guillain–Barré syndrome, autoimmune haemolytic anaemia, thrombocytopenia, myocarditis and skin eruptions, such as ampicillin-induced rash. Immunocompromised patients can develop hepatitis, oesophagitis, colitis, pneumonitis, retinitis, encephalitis and polyradiculitis.

Women who develop a primary CMV infection during pregnancy have about a 40% chance of passing CMV to the fetus, causing congenital infection and disease at any stage of gestation. Features include petechial rashes, hepatosplenomegaly and jaundice; 10% of infected infants will have long-term CNS sequelae, such as microcephaly, cerebral calcifications, chorioretinitis and deafness. Infections in the newborn usually are asymptomatic or have features of an IM-like illness, although some studies suggest that subtle sequelae affecting hearing or mental development may occur.

Investigations

Atypical lymphocytosis is not as prominent as in EBV infection and heterophile antibody tests are negative. LFTs are often abnormal, with an alkaline phosphatase level raised out of proportion to transaminases. Serological diagnosis depends on the detection of CMV-specific IgM antibody plus a four-fold rise or seroconversion of IgG. In the immunocompromised, antibody detection is unreliable and detection of CMV in an involved organ by PCR, culture or histopathology establishes the diagnosis. A positive culture of CMV in the blood may be useful in transplant populations but not in HIV-positive individuals, since in HIV infection CMV reactivates at regular intervals, but these episodes do not correlate well with episodes of clinical disease. Detection of CMV in urine is not helpful in diagnosing infection, except in neonates, since CMV is intermittently shed in the urine throughout life following infection.

Management

Only symptomatic treatment is required in the immunocompetent patient. Immunocompromised individuals are treated with ganciclovir 5 mg/kg IV twice daily or with oral valganciclovir 900 mg twice daily for at least 14 days. Foscarnet or cidofovir is also used in CMV treatment of immunocompromised patients who are resistant to or intolerant of ganciclovir-based therapy.

Dengue

Dengue is a febrile illness caused by a flavivirus transmitted by mosquitoes. It is endemic in Asia, the Pacific, Africa and the Americas (Fig. 13.12). Approximately 50 million infections occur annually and dengue is the most rapidly spreading mosquito-borne viral illness. The principal vector is the mosquito *Aedes aegypti*, which breeds in standing water; collections of water in containers, water-based air coolers and tyre dumps are a good environment for the vector in large cities. *Aedes albopictus* is a vector in some South-east Asian countries. There are four serotypes of dengue virus, all producing a similar clinical syndrome; type-specific immunity is life-long, but immunity against the other serotypes lasts only a few months. Dengue haemorrhagic fever (DHF) and dengue shock syndrome (DSS) occur in individuals who are immune to one dengue virus serotype and are then infected with another. Prior immunity results in increased uptake of virus by cells expressing the antibody Fc receptor and increased T-cell activation with resultant cytokine release, causing capillary leak and disseminated intravascular coagulation (DIC, pp. 201 and 1055).

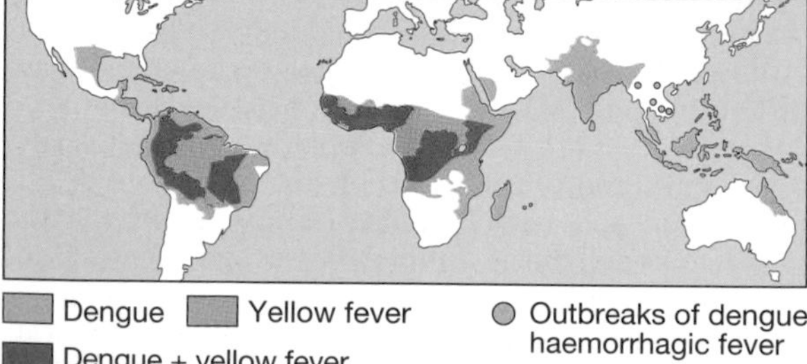

Fig. 13.12 Endemic zones of yellow fever and dengue. From Halstead 1997 – see p. 386.

Clinical features

Clinical features of dengue fever are listed in Box 13.37. Asymptomatic infections are common, particularly in children, but the disease is more severe in infants and the elderly. The initial febrile phase is frequently followed by a rash as the fever settles. Laboratory features include leucopenia, neutropenia, thrombocytopenia and elevated alanine aminotransferase (ALT) or aspartate aminotransferase (AST). Many symptomatic infections run an uncomplicated course, but complications or a protracted convalescence may ensue.

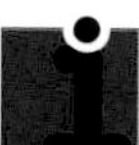

13.37 Clinical features of dengue fever

Incubation period
• 2–7 days
Prodrome
• 2 days of malaise and headache
Acute onset
• Fever, backache, arthralgias, headache, generalised pains ('break-bone fever'), pain on eye movement, lacrimation, scleral injection, anorexia, nausea, vomiting, pharyngitis, upper respiratory tract symptoms, relative bradycardia, prostration, depression, hyperaesthesia, dysgeusia, lymphadenopathy
Fever
• Continuous or 'saddle-back', with break on 4th or 5th day and then recrudescence; usually lasts 7–8 days
Rash
• Initial flushing faint macular rash in first 1–2 days. Maculopapular, scarlet morbilliform blanching rash from days 3–5 on trunk, spreading centrifugally and sparing palms and soles, onset often with fever defervescence. May desquamate on resolution or give rise to petechiae on extensor surfaces
Convalescence
• Slow and may be associated with prolonged fatigue syndrome, arthralgia or depression
Complications
• Dengue haemorrhagic fever and disseminated intravascular coagulation • Dengue shock syndrome • Hepatitis, cerebral haemorrhage or oedema, encephalitis, cranial nerve palsies, rhabdomyolysis, myocarditis • Vertical transmission if infection within 5 wks of delivery

The period 3–7 days after onset of fever is termed the 'critical' phase, during which signs of DHF or DSS may develop. In mild forms, petechiae occur in the arm when a blood pressure cuff is inflated to a point between systolic and diastolic blood pressure and left for 5 minutes (the positive 'tourniquet test') – a non-specific test of capillary fragility and thrombocytopenia. As the extent of capillary leak increases, there may be a raised haematocrit, tachycardia and hypotension, pleural effusions and ascites. This may progress to metabolic acidosis and multi-organ failure, including acute respiratory distress syndrome (ARDS, p. 192). Minor (petechiae, ecchymoses, epistaxis) or major (gastrointestinal or cerebrovascular) haemorrhage may occur.

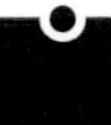

13.38 WHO-proposed clinical definition of dengue

Probable dengue
• Exposure in an endemic area • Fever • Two of: Nausea/vomiting Rash Aches/pains Positive tourniquet test Leucopenia Any warning sign *Laboratory confirmation important* *Needs regular medical observation and instruction in the warning signs* *If there are no warning signs, need for hospitalisation is influenced by age, comorbidities, pregnancy and social factors*
Dengue with warning signs
• Probable dengue plus one of: Abdominal pain or tenderness Persistent vomiting Signs of fluid accumulation, e.g. pleural effusion or ascites Mucosal bleed Lethargy Hepatomegaly > 2 cm Rapid increase in haematocrit with fall in platelet count *Needs medical intervention, e.g. intravenous fluid*
Severe dengue
• Severe plasma leakage leading to: Shock (dengue shock syndrome) Fluid accumulation with respiratory distress • Severe haemorrhagic manifestations, e.g. GI haemorrhage • Severe organ involvement: Liver AST or ALT ≥ 1000 U/L CNS: impaired consciousness Cardiomyopathy Other organs, e.g. renal impairment *Needs emergency medical treatment and specialist care with intensive care input*
Adapted from http://www.who.int/csr/disease/dengue/en/ (ALT = alanine aminotransferase; AST = aspartate aminotransferase)

Diagnosis

In endemic areas, mild dengue must be distinguished from other viral infections. The WHO recently revised its clinical classification of dengue and is evaluating the usefulness of these categories in guiding diagnosis and treatment (Box 13.38). The diagnosis can be confirmed by seroconversion of IgM or a fourfold rise in IgG antibody titres. Serological tests may detect cross-reacting antibodies against other flaviviruses, including yellow fever vaccine. IgM/IgG ratios may be used to distinguish primary from secondary infection. Isolation of dengue virus from blood or detection of dengue virus RNA by PCR (p. 139) is available in specialist laboratories. Commercial enzyme-linked immunosorbent assay (ELISA) kits to detect the NS1 viral antigen, although less sensitive than PCR, are becoming more widely available in endemic areas.

Management and prevention

Treatment is supportive, emphasising fluid replacement and appropriate management of shock and organ dysfunction. With intensive care support, mortality rates are 1% or less. Aspirin should be avoided due to bleeding risk. Corticosteroids have not been shown to help. No existing antivirals are effective.

Breeding places of *Aedes* mosquitoes should be abolished and the adults destroyed by insecticides. There is no licensed vaccine available.

Yellow fever

Yellow fever is a haemorrhagic fever of the tropics, caused by a flavivirus. It is a zoonosis of monkeys in West and Central African, and South and Central American tropical rainforests, where it may cause devastating epidemics (see Fig. 13.12). Transmission is by tree-top mosquitoes *Aedes africanus* (Africa) and *Haemagogus* spp. (America). The infection is introduced to humans either by infected mosquitoes when trees are felled, or by monkeys raiding human settlements. In towns, yellow fever may be transmitted between humans by *Aedes aegypti*, which breeds efficiently in small collections of water. The distribution of this mosquito is far wider than that of yellow fever, and more widespread infection is a continued threat.

Yellow fever causes approximately 200 000 infections each year, mainly in sub-Saharan Africa, and the number is increasing. Overall mortality is around 15%, although this varies widely. Humans are infectious during the viraemic phase, which starts 3–6 days after the bite of the infected mosquito and lasts for 4–5 days.

Clinical features

After an incubation period of 3–6 days, yellow fever is often a mild febrile illness lasting less than 1 week, with headache, myalgia, conjunctival erythema and bradycardia. This is followed by fever resolution (defervescence), but in some cases, fever recurs after a few hours to days. In more severe disease, fever recrudescence is associated with lower back pain, abdominal pain and somnolence, prominent nausea and vomiting, bradycardia and jaundice. Liver damage and DIC lead to bleeding with petechiae, mucosal haemorrhages and gastrointestinal bleeding. Shock, hepatic failure, renal failure, seizures and coma may ensue.

Diagnosis

The differential diagnosis includes malaria, typhoid, viral hepatitis, leptospirosis, haemorrhagic fevers and aflatoxin poisoning. Diagnosis of yellow fever can be confirmed by viral isolation from blood in the first 24 days of illness, the presence of IgM or a fourfold rise in IgG antibody titre. Leucopenia is characteristic. Liver biopsy should be avoided in life due to the risk of fatal bleeding. Post-mortem features, such as acute mid-zonal necrosis and Councilman bodies with minimal inflammation in the liver, are suggestive but not specific. Immunohistochemistry for viral antigens improves specificity.

Management and prevention

Treatment is supportive, with meticulous attention to fluid and electrolyte balance, urine output and blood pressure. Blood transfusions, plasma expanders and peritoneal dialysis may be necessary. Patients should be isolated, as their blood and body products may contain virus particles.

A single vaccination with a live attenuated vaccine gives full protection for at least 10 years. Potential side-effects include hypersensitivity, encephalitis and systemic features of yellow fever (viscerotropic disease) caused by the attenuated virus. Vaccination is not recommended in people who are significantly immunosuppressed. The risk of vaccine side-effects must be balanced against the risk of infection for less immunocompromised hosts, pregnant women and older patients. An internationally recognised certificate of vaccination is sometimes necessary when crossing borders.

Viral haemorrhagic fevers

Viral haemorrhagic fevers (VHF) are zoonoses caused by several different viruses (Box 13.39). They are geographically restricted and occur in rural settings or in health-care facilities. All of these viral illnesses, except Ebola and Marburg, have mild self-limiting forms.

Serological surveys have shown that Lassa fever is widespread in West Africa and may lead to up to 500 000 infections annually. Mortality overall may be low, as 80% of cases are asymptomatic, but in hospitalised cases mortality averages 15%. Ebola outbreaks have occurred at a rate of approximately one per year, involving up to a few hundred cases. The largest outbreaks have been in the Democratic Republic of Congo, Uganda and Sudan. Marburg has been documented less frequently, with outbreaks in the Democratic Republic of Congo and Uganda, but the largest outbreak to date involved 163 cases in Angola in 2005. Mortality rates of Ebola and Marburg are high.

VHF have extended into Europe, with an outbreak of Congo–Crimean haemorrhagic fever in Turkey in 2006, and cases of haemorrhagic fever with renal syndrome in the Balkans and Russia. These conditions remain very rare in the UK, with about one case of Lassa fever arriving in the country every 2 years.

Kyasanur forest disease is a tick-borne VHF currently confined to a small focus in Karnataka, India; there are about 500 cases annually. Monkeys are the principal hosts, but with forest felling, there are fears that this disease will increase.

New outbreaks and new agents are identified sporadically. In 2008, Lujo virus, a novel arenavirus, caused an outbreak of VHF involving a woman from Zambia and several health-care workers associated with her care, and had 80% fatality. Details on recent disease outbreaks can be found at the WHO website (www.who.int).

Clinical features

VHF present with non-specific fever, malaise, body pains, sore throat and headache. On examination, conjunctivitis, throat injection, an erythematous or petechial rash, haemorrhage, lymphadenopathy and bradycardia may be noted. The viruses cause endothelial dysfunction with the development of capillary leak. Bleeding is due to endothelial damage and platelet dysfunction. Hypovolaemic shock and ARDS may develop (p. 192).

Haemorrhage is a late feature of VHF and most patients present with earlier features. In Lassa fever, joint and abdominal pain is prominent. A macular blanching rash may be present but bleeding is unusual, occurring in only 20% of hospitalised patients. Encephalopathy may develop and deafness affects 30% of survivors.

The clue to the viral aetiology comes from the travel and exposure history. Travel to an outbreak area, activity in a rural environment and contact with sick individuals or animals within 21 days all increase the risk of VHF. Enquiry should be made about insect bites, hospital visits and attendance at ritual funerals (Ebola virus infection). For Lassa fever, retrosternal pain, pharyngitis and proteinuria have a positive predictive value of 80% in West Africa.

Investigations and management

Non-specific findings include leucopenia, thrombocytopenia and proteinuria. In Lassa fever, an AST > 150 U/L is associated with a 50% mortality. It is important to exclude other causes of fever, especially malaria, typhoid and respiratory tract infections. Most patients suspected of having a VHF in the UK turn out to have malaria.

The diagnosis of VHF must be considered in all febrile individuals who present within 21 days of leaving an endemic area or who present with haemorrhage or organ failure. A febrile patient from an endemic area within the incubation period, who has specific epidemiological risk factors (see Fig. 13.5, p. 311) or who has signs of organ failure or haemorrhage, should be treated as being at high risk of VHF; appropriate infection control measures must be implemented and the patient transferred to a centre with biosafety level (BSL) 4 facilities. Individuals with a history of travel within 21 days and fever, but without the relevant epidemiological features or signs of VHF, are classified as medium-risk and should have an initial blood sample tested to exclude malaria. If this is negative, relevant specimens (blood, throat swab, urine and pleural fluid, if available) are collected and sent to an appropriate reference laboratory for nucleic acid detection (PCR), virus isolation, and serology. If patients are still felt to be at significant risk of VHF or if infection is confirmed, they should be transferred to a specialised high-security infectious disease unit. All further laboratory tests should be performed at BSL4. Transport requires an ambulance with BSL3 facilities.

13.39 Viral haemorrhagic fevers

Disease	Reservoir	Transmission	Incubation period	Geography	Mortality rate	Clinical features of severe disease[1]
Lassa fever	Multimammate rats (*Mastomys natalensis*)	Urine from rat Body fluids from patients	6–21 days	West Africa	15%	Haemorrhage, shock, encephalopathy, ARDS (responds to ribavirin) Deafness in survivors
Ebola fever	Undefined (?bats)	Body fluids from patients Handling infected primates	2–21 days	Central Africa Outbreaks as far north as Sudan	25–90%	Haemorrhage, hepatic and renal failure
Marburg fever	Undefined	Body fluids from patients Handling infected primates	3–9 days	Central Africa Outbreak in Angola	25–90%	Haemorrhage, diarrhoea, encephalopathy, orchitis
Yellow fever	Monkeys	Mosquitoes	3–6 days	See Fig. 13.12	~15%	Hepatic failure, renal failure, haemorrhage
Dengue	Humans	*Aedes aegypti*	2–7 days	See Fig. 13.12	< 10%[2]	Haemorrhage, shock
Crimean–Congo haemorrhagic fever	Small vertebrates Domestic and wild animals	*Ixodes* tick Body fluids	1–3 days up to 9 days 3–6 days up to 13 days	Africa, Asia, Eastern Europe	30%	Encephalopathy, haemorrhage, hepatic or renal failure, ARDS
Rift Valley fever	Domestic livestock	Contact with animals, mosquito or other insect bites	2–6 days	Africa, Arabian peninsula	1%	Haemorrhage, blindness, meningoencephalitis (complications only in a minority)
Kyasanur fever	Monkeys	Ticks	3–8 days	Karnataka State, India	5–10%	Haemorrhage, pulmonary oedema, neurological features, iridokeratitis in survivors
Bolivian and Argentinian haemorrhagic fever (Junin and Machupo viruses)	Rodents (*Calomys* spp.)	Urine, aerosols Body fluids from case (rare)	5–19 days (3–6 days for parenteral)	South America	15–30%	Haemorrhage, shock, cerebellar signs (may respond to ribavirin)
Haemorrhagic fever with renal syndrome (Hantaan fever)	Rodents	Aerosols from faeces	5–42 days (typically 14 days)	Northern Asia, northern Europe, Balkans	5%	Acute renal impairment, cerebrovascular accidents, pulmonary oedema, shock (hepatic failure and haemorrhagic features only in some variants)

[1]All potentially have circulatory failure. [2]Mortality of uncomplicated and haemorrhagic dengue fever, respectively.

In addition to general supportive measures, ribavirin is given intravenously (100 mg/kg, then 25 mg/kg daily for 3 days and 12.5 mg/kg daily for 4 days) when Lassa fever or South American haemorrhagic fevers are suspected.

Prevention

Ribavirin has been used as prophylaxis in close contacts in Lassa fever but there are no formal trials of its efficacy.

Viral infections of the skin

Herpes simplex virus 1 and 2

Herpes simplex viruses (HSV) cause recurrent mucocutaneous infection; HSV-1 typically involves the mucocutaneous surfaces of the head and neck (Fig. 13.13), whilst HSV-2 predominantly involves the genital mucosa (pp. 415 and 418), although there is overlap (see Box 13.31, p. 317). The seroprevalence of HSV-1 is 30–100%, varying by socioeconomic status, while that of HSV-2 is 20–60%. Infection is acquired by inoculation of viruses shed by an infected individual on to a mucosal surface in a susceptible person. The virus infects sensory and autonomic neurons and establishes latent infection in the nerve ganglia. Primary infection is followed by episodes of reactivation throughout life.

Clinical features

Primary HSV-1 or 2 infection is more likely to be symptomatic later in life, causing gingivostomatitis, pharyngitis or painful genital tract lesions. The primary

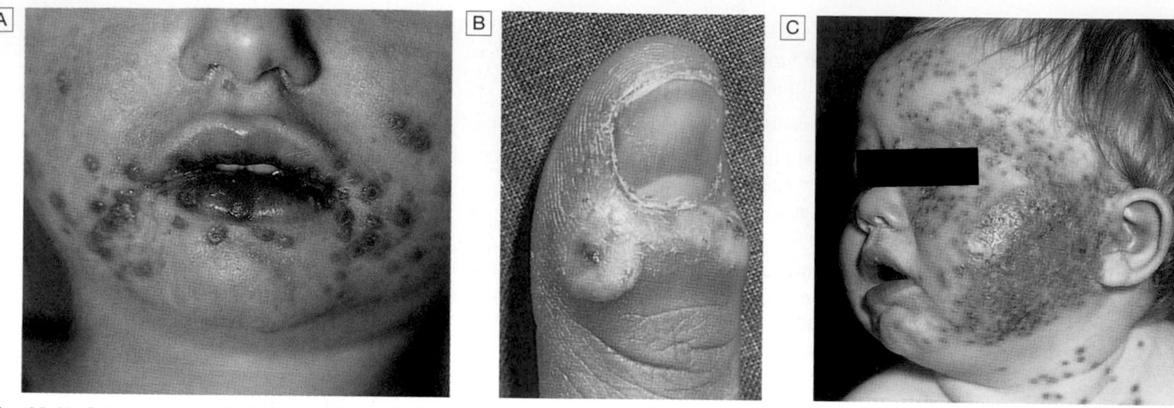

Fig. 13.13 Cutaneous manifestations of herpes simplex virus-1 (HSV-1). **A** Acute HSV-1. There were also vesicles in the mouth – herpetic stomatitis. **B** Herpetic whitlow. **C** Eczema herpeticum. HSV-1 infection spreads rapidly in eczematous skin.

attack may be associated with fever and regional lymphadenopathy.

Recurrence

Recurrent attacks occur throughout life, most often in association with concomitant medical illness, menstruation, mechanical trauma, immunosuppression, psychological stress or, for oral lesions, ultraviolet light exposure. HSV reactivation in the oral mucosa produces the classical 'cold sore' or 'herpes labialis'. Prodromal hyperaesthesia is followed by rapid vesiculation, pustulation and crusting. Recurrent HSV genital disease is a common cause of recurrent painful ulceration (pp. 415 and 418). An inoculation lesion on the finger gives rise to a paronychia termed a 'whitlow' in contacts of patients with herpetic lesions (Fig. 13.13B). It was formerly seen in health-care workers and dentists, but is prevented by protective gloves.

Complications

Disseminated cutaneous lesions can occur in individuals with underlying dermatological diseases, such as eczema (eczema herpeticum) (Fig. 13.13C). Herpes keratitis presents with pain and blurring of vision; characteristic dendritic ulcers are visible on slit-lamp examination and may produce corneal scarring and permanent visual impairment.

Primary HSV-2 can cause meningitis or transverse myelitis. HSV is the leading cause of sporadic viral encephalitis (p. 1205); this serious complication may occur following either primary or secondary disease, usually with HSV-1. A haemorrhagic necrotising temporal lobe cerebritis produces temporal lobe epilepsy and altered consciousness/coma. Without treatment, mortality is 80%. HSV is also implicated in the pathogenesis of Bell's palsy with a lower motor neuron VII nerve palsy, although antivirals have not been demonstrated to improve outcome.

Neonatal HSV disease is usually associated with primary infection of the mother at term (see Box 13.28, p. 314). In excess of two-thirds of cases develop disseminated disease with cutaneous lesions, hepatitis, pneumonitis and frequently encephalitis.

Immunocompromised hosts can develop visceral disease with oesophagitis, hepatitis, pneumonitis, encephalitis or retinitis.

Diagnosis

Differentiation from other vesicular eruptions is achieved by demonstration of virus in vesicular fluid, usually by direct immunofluorescence or PCR. HSV encephalitis is diagnosed by a positive PCR for HSV in CSF. Serology is of limited value, only confirming whether an individual has had previous infection.

Management

The acyclic antivirals are the treatment of choice for HSV infection (see Box 13.33, p. 318). Therapy of localised disease must commence in the first 48 hours of clinical disease (primary or recurrent); thereafter it is unlikely to influence clinical outcome. Oral lesions in an immunocompetent individual may be treated with topical aciclovir. All severe manifestations should be treated, regardless of the time of presentation. Suspicion of HSV encephalopathy is an indication for immediate empirical antiviral therapy. Aciclovir resistance is encountered occasionally in immunocompromised hosts, in which case foscarnet is the treatment of choice.

Human herpesvirus 8

Human herpesvirus 8 (HHV-8) (see Box 13.31, p. 317) causes Kaposi's sarcoma in both AIDS-related and endemic non-AIDS-related forms (p. 397). HHV-8 is spread via saliva, and men who have sex with men have increased incidence of infection. Seroprevalence varies widely, being highest in sub-Saharan Africa. HHV-8 also causes two rare haematological malignancies: primary effusion lymphoma and multicentric Castleman's disease. Current antivirals are not effective.

Enterovirus infections

Hand, foot and mouth disease

This systemic infection is usually caused by Coxsackie viruses or occasionally echoviruses. It affects children and occasionally adults, resulting in local or household outbreaks, particularly in the summer months. A relatively mild illness with fever and lymphadenopathy develops after an incubation period of approximately 10 days; 2–3 days later, a painful papular or vesicular rash appears on palmoplantar surfaces of hands and feet, with associated oral lesions on the buccal mucosa and tongue that ulcerate rapidly. A papular erythematous rash may appear on buttocks and thighs. Antiviral treatment is not available and management consists of symptom relief with analgesics.

Herpangina

This infection, caused by Coxsackie viruses, primarily affects children and teenagers in the summer months. It is characterised by a small number of vesicles at the soft/hard palate junction, often associated with high fever, an extremely sore throat and headache. The lesions are short-lived, rupturing after 2–3 days and rarely persisting for more than 1 week. Treatment is with analgesics if required. Culture of the virus from vesicles or DNA detection by PCR differentiates herpangina from HSV.

Poxviruses

These DNA viruses are rare but potentially important pathogens.

Smallpox (variola)

This severe disease, which has high mortality, was eradicated worldwide by a global vaccination programme. Interest in the disease has re-emerged due to its potential as a bioweapon. The virus is spread by the respiratory route or contact with lesions, and is highly infectious.

The incubation period is 7–17 days. A prodrome with fever, headache and prostration leads, in 1–2 days, to the rash, which develops through macules and papules to vesicles and pustules, worst on the face and distal extremities. Lesions in one area are all at the same stage of development with no cropping (unlike chickenpox). Vaccination can lead to a modified course of disease with milder rash and lower mortality.

If a case of smallpox is suspected, national public health authorities must be contacted. Electron micrography (like Fig. 13.14) and DNA detection tests (PCR) are used to confirm smallpox or, using specific primers, an alternative poxvirus.

Monkeypox

Despite the name, the animal reservoirs for this virus are probably small squirrels and rodents. It causes a rare zoonotic infection in communities in the rainforest belt of Central Africa, producing a vesicular rash that is indistinguishable from smallpox, but differentiated by the presence of lymphadenopathy. Little person-to-person transmission occurs. Outbreaks outside Africa have been linked to importation of African animals as exotic pets. Diagnosis is by electron micrography and/or DNA detection (PCR).

Cowpox

Humans in contact with infected cows develop large vesicles, usually on the hands or arms and associated with fever and regional lymphadenitis. The reservoir is thought to be wild rodents, and the virus also produces symptomatic disease in cats and a range of other animals.

Vaccinia virus

This laboratory strain is the basis of the existing vaccine to prevent smallpox. Widespread vaccination is no longer recommended due to the likelihood of local spread from the vaccination site (potentially life-threatening in those with eczema (eczema vaccinatum) or immune deficiency) and of encephalitis. However, vaccination may still be recommended for key medical staff.

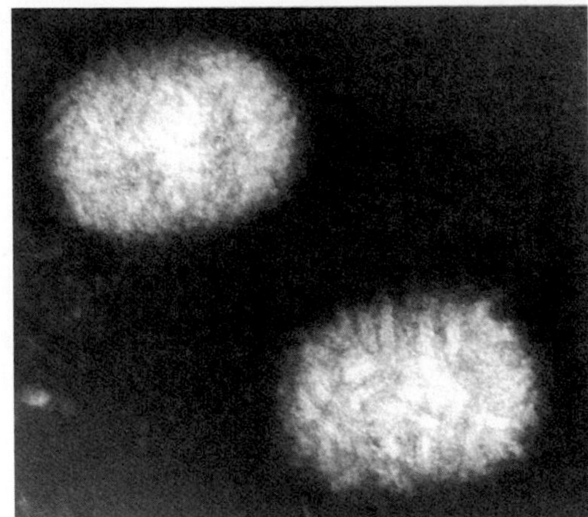

Fig. 13.14 Electron micrograph of molluscum contagiosum, a poxvirus.

Other poxviruses: orf and molluscum contagiosum

See page 1279 and Figure 13.14.

Gastrointestinal viral infections

Norovirus (Norwalk agent)

Norovirus is the most common cause of infectious gastroenteritis in the UK and causes outbreaks in closed communities, such as long-stay hospital wards, cruise ships and military camps. Food handlers may also transmit this virus, which is relatively resistant to decontamination procedures. The incubation period is 24–48 hours. High attack rates and prominent vomiting are characteristic. Diagnosis is by electron microscopy, antigen or DNA detection (PCR) in stool samples. The virus is highly infectious and cases should be isolated and environmental surfaces cleaned with detergents and disinfected with bleach.

Astrovirus

Astroviruses cause diarrhoea in small children and occasionally in immunocompromised adults.

Rotavirus

Rotaviruses are the major cause of diarrhoeal illness in young children worldwide and cause 10–20% of deaths due to gastroenteritis in developing countries. There are winter epidemics in developed countries, particularly in nurseries. Adults are less often infected but those in close contact with cases may develop disease. The virus infects enterocytes, causing decreased surface absorption. The incubation period is 48 hours and patients present with watery diarrhoea, vomiting, fever and abdominal pain. Dehydration is prominent. Diagnosis is aided by commercially available enzyme immunoassay kits, which require fresh or refrigerated stool samples. Immunity develops to natural infection. Monovalent and multivalent vaccines have been licensed in many countries and have now demonstrated efficacy in large trials in Africa and the Americas. Increased rates of intussusception were observed with early rotavirus vaccines, but the benefits of the recently licensed vaccines outweigh this risk.

Hepatitis viruses (A–E)

See Chapter 23.

Other viruses

Adenoviruses are frequently identified from stool culture and implicated as a cause of diarrhoea in children. They have also been linked to cases of intussusception.

Respiratory viral infections

These infections are described on page 681.

Adenoviruses, rhinoviruses and enteroviruses (Coxsackie viruses and echoviruses) often produce non-specific symptoms. Parainfluenza and respiratory syncytial viruses cause upper respiratory tract disease, croup and bronchiolitis in small children and pneumonia in the immunocompromised. Respiratory syncytial virus also causes pneumonia in nursing home residents and may be associated with nosocomial pneumonia. In recent years, metapneumovirus and bocavirus have been identified as causes of upper and occasionally lower respiratory tract infection. They may also cause pneumonia in immunosuppressed individuals, such as recipients of allogeneic haematopoietic stem cell transplants. The severe acute respiratory syndrome (SARS) caused by the SARS coronavirus emerged as a major respiratory pathogen during an outbreak in 2002–2003, with 8000 cases and 10% mortality (p. 683). In 2012, a novel coronavirus, distantly related to the SARS coronavirus, caused several deaths connected with pneumonia and acute renal failure in patients originating from the Middle East.

Viral infections with neurological involvement

See also page 1205.

Japanese B encephalitis

This flavivirus is an important cause of endemic encephalitis in Japan, China, Russia, South-east Asia, India and Pakistan; outbreaks also occur elsewhere. There are 10 000–20 000 cases reported to the WHO annually. Pigs and aquatic birds are the virus reservoirs and transmission is by mosquitoes. Exposure to rice paddies is a recognised risk factor.

Clinical features

The incubation period is 4–21 days. Most infections are subclinical in childhood and 1% or less of infections lead to encephalitis. Initial systemic illness with fever, malaise and anorexia is followed by photophobia, vomiting, headache and changes in brainstem function. Neurological features other than encephalitis include meningitis, seizures, cranial nerve palsies, flaccid or spastic paralysis, and extrapyramidal features. Mortality with neurological disease is 25%. Most children die from respiratory failure with infection of brainstem nuclei. Approximately 50% of survivors are left with neurological sequelae.

Investigations, management and prevention

Other infectious causes of encephalitis should be excluded (p. 1205). There is neutrophilia and often hyponatraemia. CSF analysis reveals lymphocytosis and elevated protein. Serological testing may be helpful and there is a CSF antigen test.

Treatment is supportive, anticipating and treating complications. Vaccination for travellers to endemic areas during the monsoon period is effective prophylaxis. Some endemic countries include this vaccination in their childhood schedules.

West Nile virus

This flavivirus has emerged as an important cause of neurological disease in an area that extends from Australia, India and Russia through Africa and Southern Europe and across to North America. The disease has an avian reservoir and a mosquito vector. The elderly are at increased risk of neurological disease.

Clinical features

Most infections are asymptomatic. After 2–6 days' incubation, a mild febrile illness and arthralgia constitute the most common clinical presentation. A prolonged incubation may be seen in immunocompromised individuals. Children may develop a maculopapular rash. Neurological disease is seen in 1% and is characterised by encephalitis, meningitis or asymmetric flaccid paralysis with 10% mortality.

Diagnosis and management

Diagnosis is by serology or detection of viral RNA in blood or CSF. Serological tests may show cross-reactivity with other flaviviruses, including vaccine strains. Treatment is supportive.

Enterovirus 71

Enterovirus 71 has caused outbreaks around the globe of enteroviral disease with hand, foot and mouth disease (p. 326) and aseptic meningitis. Some cases have been complicated by encephalitis with flaccid paralysis or by brainstem involvement and death. The virus can be isolated from vesicle fluid, stool or CSF, and viral RNA can be detected in CSF by reverse transcription (RT-)PCR.

Nipah virus encephalitis

In 1999, a newly discovered paramyxovirus in the Hendra group, the Nipah virus, caused an epidemic of encephalitis amongst Malaysian pig farmers. Infection is through direct contact with pig secretions. Mortality is around 30%. Antibodies to the Hendra virus are present in 76% of cases.

Human T-cell lymphotropic virus type I

Human T-cell lymphotropic virus type I (HTLV-1) is a retrovirus which causes chronic infection with development of adult T-cell leukaemia/lymphoma or HTLV-1-associated myelopathy (HAM) in a subset of those infected (p. 1043). It is found mainly in Japan, the Caribbean, Central and South America, and the Seychelles.

HAM or tropical spastic paraparesis occurs in less than 5% of those with chronic infection, and presents with gait disturbance, spasticity of the lower extremities, urinary incontinence, impotence and sensory disturbance. Myositis and uveitis may also occur with HTLV-1 infection. Serology confirms the diagnosis. Treatment is usually supportive for asymptomatic patients but can include zidovudine and interferon-alfa for leukaemia. The role of antivirals in other settings including HAM is being investigated.

Viral infections with rheumatological involvement

Rheumatological syndromes characterise a variety of viral infections ranging from exanthems, such as rubella and parvovirus B19 (p. 315), to blood-borne viruses, such as HBV and HIV-1.

Chikungunya virus

Chikungunya is an alphavirus that causes fever, rash and arthropathy. It is found principally in Africa and Asia, including India. Humans and non-human primates are the main reservoir and the main vector is the *Aedes aegypti* mosquito. Cases occur in epidemics on a background of sporadic cases. In 2007, an outbreak extended as far north as Italy.

The incubation period is 2–12 days. A period of fever may be followed by an afebrile phase and then recrudescence of fever. Children may develop a maculopapular rash. Adults are susceptible to arthritis, which causes early morning pain and swelling, most often in the small joints. Arthritis can persist for months and may become chronic in individuals who are positive for human leucocyte antigen (HLA)-B27. Related alphaviruses causing similar syndromes include Sindbis virus (Scandinavia and Africa), O'nyong-nyong virus (Central Africa), Ross River virus (Australia) and Mayaro virus (Caribbean and South America).

Diagnosis is by serology but cross-reactivity between alphaviruses occurs. Treatment is symptomatic.

PRION DISEASES

Prions (p. 134) cause transmissible spongiform encephalopathies in humans, sheep, cows and cats (Box 13.40 and p. 1211). The prion protein is not inactivated by cooking or conventional sterilisation, and transmission is thought to occur by consumption of infected CNS tissue or by inoculation (e.g. via depth EEG electrodes, corneal grafts, cadaveric dura mater grafts and pooled cadaveric growth hormone preparations). The same diseases can occur in an inherited form, due to mutations in the PrP gene.

The apparent transmission of bovine spongiform encephalopathy (BSE) to humans following an outbreak of BSE in the UK beginning in the late 1980s has caused great concern, leading to precautionary measures in the UK, such as leucodepletion of all blood used for transfusion, and the mandatory use of disposable surgical instruments wherever possible for tonsillectomy, appendicectomy and ophthalmological procedures.

13.40 Prion diseases affecting humans

Disease	Mechanism
Creutzfeldt–Jakob disease	
Sporadic	Spontaneous PrP^{c} to PrP^{Sc} conversion or somatic mutation
Familial	Mutations in the PrP gene
Variant	Infection from bovine spongiform encephalopathy
Gerstmann–Sträussler–Scheinker disease	Mutations in the PrP gene
Fatal familial insomnia	Mutations in the PrP gene
Sporadic fatal insomnia	Spontaneous PrP^{c} to PrP^{Sc} conversion or somatic mutation
Kuru	Cannibalism

BACTERIAL INFECTIONS

Bacterial infections of the skin, soft tissues and bones

Most infections of the skin, soft tissues and bone are caused by either staphylococci (mainly *Staph. aureus*) or streptococci (mainly *Strep. pyogenes*). Clinical manifestations are also described in Chapters 25 and 27.

Staphylococcal infections

Staphylococci are usually found colonising the anterior nares and skin. Traditionally, staphylococci were divided into two groups according to their ability to produce coagulase, an enzyme that converts fibrinogen to fibrin in rabbit plasma, causing it to clot. *Staph. aureus* is coagulase-positive, and most other species coagulase-negative. The coagulase test is now less commonly undertaken, with identification of *Staph. aureus* often achieved by other methods.

Staph. aureus is the main cause of staphylococcal infections. *Staph. intermedius* is another coagulase-positive staphylococcus, which causes infection following dog bites. Among coagulase-negative organisms, *Staph. epidermidis* is the predominant commensal organism of the skin, and can cause severe infections in those with central venous catheters or implanted prosthetic materials. *Staph. saprophyticus* is part of the normal vaginal flora and causes urinary tract infections in sexually active young women. Others implicated in human infections include *Staph. lugdunensis*, *Staph. schleiferi*, *Staph. haemolyticus* and *Staph. caprae*. Coagulase-negative staphylococci are not usually identified to species level.

Staphylococci are particularly dangerous if they gain access to the blood stream, having the potential to cause disease in many sites (Fig. 13.15). In any patient with staphylococcal bacteraemia, especially injection drug-users, the possibility of endocarditis must be considered (p. 625). Growth of *Staph. aureus* in blood cultures should not be dismissed as a 'contaminant' unless all possible underlying sources have been excluded and repeated

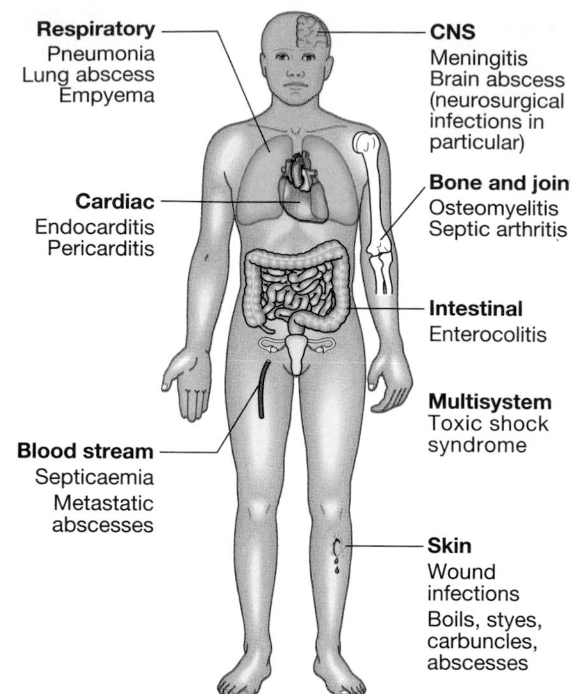

Fig. 13.15 Infections caused by *Staphylococcus aureus.*

blood culture is negative. Any evidence of spreading cellulitis indicates the urgent need for an antistaphylococcal antibiotic, such as flucloxacillin. This is particularly true for mid-facial cellulitis, which can result in cavernous sinus thrombophlebitis.

In addition, *Staph. aureus* can cause severe systemic disease due to the effects of toxin produced at superficial sites in the absence of tissue invasion by bacteria.

Skin infections

Staphylococcal infections cause ecthyma, folliculitis, furuncles, carbuncles, bullous impetigo and the scalded skin syndrome (pp. 1275–1276). They may also be involved in necrotising infections of the skin and subcutaneous tissues (p. 305).

Wound infections

Many wound infections are caused by staphylococci, which may significantly prolong post-operative hospital stays (Fig. 13.16A). Prevention involves careful attention to hand hygiene, skin preparation and aseptic technique, and the use of topical and systemic antibiotic prophylaxis.

Treatment is by drainage of any abscesses plus adequate dosage of antistaphylococcal antibiotics. These should be instituted early, particularly if prosthetic implants of any kind have been inserted.

Cannula-related infection

Staphylococcal infection associated with cannula sepsis (Fig. 13.16B and p. 304) and thrombophlebitis is an important and, unfortunately, extremely common reason for morbidity following hospital admission. The Visual Infusion Phlebitis (VIP) score is a useful way of monitoring cannulae (Box 13.41). Staphylococci have a predilection for plastic, rapidly forming a biofilm which remains as a source of bacteraemia as long as the plastic is in situ. Local poultice application may relieve symptoms but cannula removal and antibiotic treatment with flucloxacillin (or a glycopeptide if MRSA is suspected) are necessary if there is any suggestion of spreading infection.

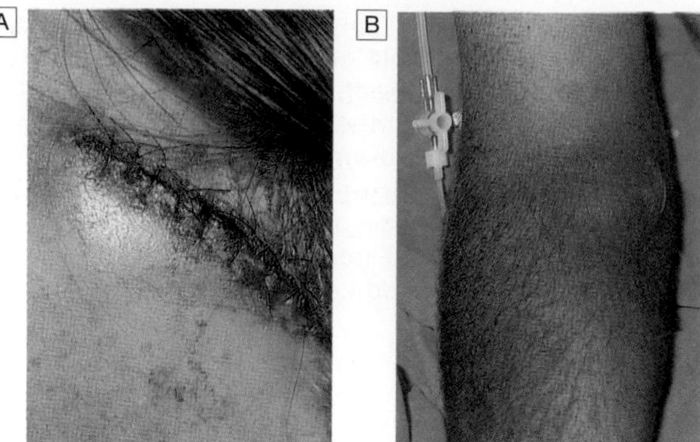

Fig. 13.16 Manifestations of skin infection with *Staph. aureus.* **A** Wound infection. **B** Cannula-related infection.

13.41 How to assess an intravenous cannula using the Visual Infusion Phlebitis score (VIP)*

Clinical features	Score	Assessment and management
IV site appears healthy	0	**No signs of phlebitis** Observe cannula
One of the following is evident: Slight pain near IV site Slight redness near IV site	1	**Possible first signs of phlebitis** Observe cannula
Two of the following are evident: Pain near IV site Erythema Swelling	2	**Early stage of phlebitis** Resite cannula
ALL of the following are evident and extensive: Pain along path of cannula Erythema Induration	3	**Medium stage of phlebitis** Resite cannula Consider treatment
ALL of the following are evident and extensive: Pain along path of cannula Erythema Induration Palpable venous cord	4	**Advanced stage of phlebitis or start of thrombophlebitis** Resite cannula Consider treatment
ALL of the following are evident: Pain along path of cannula Erythema Induration Palpable venous cord Pyrexia	5	**Advanced stage of thrombophlebitis** Initiate treatment Resite cannula

*Adapted from Jackson A. Nursing Times 1997; 94:68–71.

Meticillin-resistant Staph. aureus

Resistance to meticillin, due to a penicillin-binding protein mutation, has been recognised in *Staph. aureus* for more than 30 years. The recognition of resistance to vancomycin/teicoplanin (glycopeptides) in either glycopeptide intermediate *Staph. aureus* (GISA) or, rarely, vancomycin-resistant (VRSA) strains threatens the ability to manage serious infections produced by such organisms. Meticillin-resistant *Staph. aureus* (MRSA) is now a major worldwide health care-acquired pathogen, accounting for up to 40% of staphylococcal bacteraemia in developed countries. Community-acquired MRSA (c-MRSA) currently accounts for 50% of all MRSA infections in the USA. These organisms have also acquired other virulence factors, such as Panton–Valentine leukocidin (PVL), which can cause rapidly fatal infection in young people. Clinicians must be aware of the potential danger of these infections and be prepared to take whatever appropriate infection control measures are locally advised (p. 145).

Treatment options for MRSA are shown in Box 6.17 (p. 151). Treatment should always be based on the results of antimicrobial susceptibility testing, since resistance to all these agents occurs. Milder MRSA infections may be treated with clindamycin, tetracyclines or co-trimoxazole. Glycopeptides, linezolid and daptomycin are reserved for treatment of more severe infections. PVL-producing *Staph. aureus* infections should be treated with protein-inhibiting antibiotics (clindamycin, linezolid).

Staphylococcal toxic shock syndrome

Staphylococcal toxic shock syndrome (TSS) is a serious and life-threatening disease associated with infection by *Staph. aureus*, which produces a specific toxin (toxic shock syndrome toxin 1, TSST1). It was commonly seen in young women in association with the use of highly absorbent intravaginal tampons but can occur with any *Staph. aureus* infection involving a relevant toxin-producing strain. The toxin acts as a 'superantigen', triggering significant T-helper cell activation and massive cytokine release.

TSS has an abrupt onset with high fever, generalised systemic upset (myalgia, headache, sore throat and vomiting), a generalised erythematous blanching rash resembling scarlet fever, and hypotension. It rapidly progresses over a matter of hours to multisystem involvement with cardiac, renal and hepatic compromise, leading to death in 10–20%. Recovery is accompanied at 7–10 days by desquamation (Fig. 13.17).

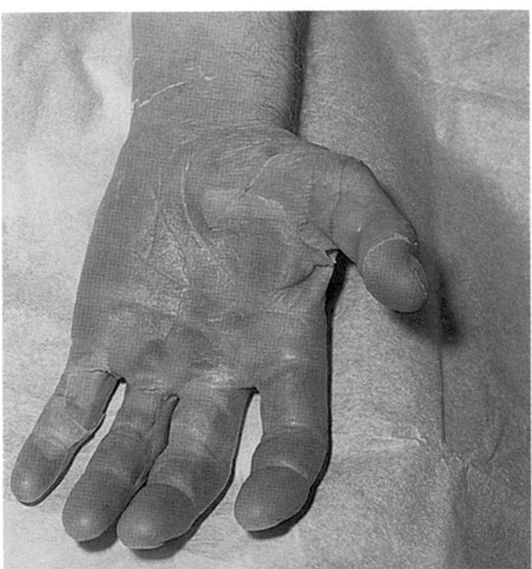

Fig. 13.17 Full-thickness desquamation after staphylococcal toxic shock syndrome.

The diagnosis is clinical and may be confirmed in menstrual cases by vaginal examination, the finding of a retained tampon, and microbiological examination by Gram stain demonstrating typical staphylococci. Subsequent culture and demonstration of toxin production are confirmatory.

Management

Treatment is with immediate and aggressive fluid resuscitation and an intravenous antistaphylococcal antibiotic (flucloxacillin or vancomycin), usually with the addition of a protein synthesis inhibitor (e.g. clindamycin) to inhibit toxin production. Intravenous immunoglobulin is occasionally added in the most severe cases on the basis of efficacy in streptococcal toxic shock. Women who recover should be advised not to use tampons for at least 1 year and should also be warned that, due to an inadequate antibody response to TSST1, the condition can recur.

Streptococcal infections

Streptococci are nasopharyngeal and gut commensals, which appear as Gram-positive cocci in chains (Fig. 6.3, p. 136). They are classified by the haemolysis they produce on blood agar (Fig. 6.4, p. 136) and by their serotypes (Box 13.42). Some streptococci (e.g. *Strep. milleri* group) defy simple classification.

Skin presentations of streptococcal infections

Group A streptococci (GAS) are the major cause of cellulitis, erysipelas and impetigo (pp. 1275 and 1277). Groups C and G streptococci cause cellulitis, in elderly, diabetic or immunocompromised patients in particular. Group B streptococcal (GBS) infection is an increasing problem at the extremes of age.

Streptococcal scarlet fever

Group A (or occasionally groups C and G) streptococci causing pharyngitis, tonsillitis or other infection may lead to scarlet fever, if the infecting strain produces a streptococcal pyrogenic exotoxin. Common in school-age children, scarlet fever can occur in young adults who have contact with young children. A diffuse erythematous rash occurs, which blanches on pressure (Fig. 13.18A), classically with circumoral pallor. The tongue, initially coated, becomes red and swollen ('strawberry tongue' - Fig. 13.18B). The disease lasts about 7 days, the rash disappearing in 7–10 days, followed by a fine desquamation. Residual petechial lesions in the antecubital fossa may be seen ('Pastia's sign' - Fig. 13.18C).

Treatment involves active therapy for the underlying infection (benzylpenicillin or orally available penicillin) plus symptomatic measures.

Streptococcal toxic shock syndrome

This is associated with severe group A (or occasionally group C or G) streptococcal skin infections producing one of a variety of toxins, such as pyogenic exotoxin A. Like staphylococcal toxic shock syndrome toxin (see above), these act as superantigens, stimulating a dramatic cytokine response. Initially, an influenza-like illness occurs with, in 50% of cases, signs of localised infection, most often involving the skin and soft tissues. A faint erythematous rash, mainly on the chest, rapidly

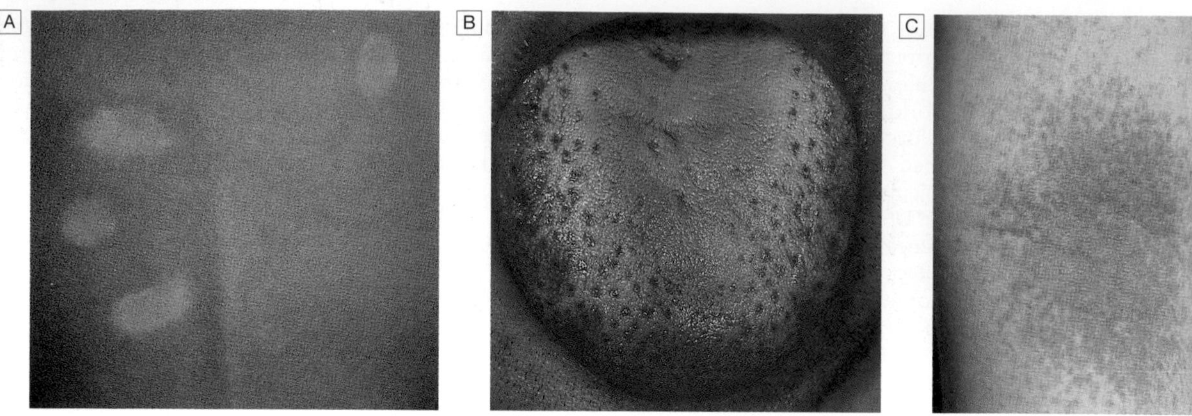

Fig. 13.18 Clinical features of scarlet fever. **A** Characteristic rash with blanching on pressure. **B** 'Strawberry tongue'. **C** Pastia's sign: a petechial rash in the cubital fossa.

13.42 Streptococcal and related infections

β-haemolytic group A (*Strep. pyogenes*)	
• Skin and soft tissue infection (including erysipelas, impetigo, necrotising fasciitis) • Streptococcal toxic shock syndrome	• Puerperal sepsis • Scarlet fever • Glomerulonephritis • Rheumatic fever • Bone and joint infection • Tonsillitis
β-haemolytic group B (*Strep. agalactiae*)	
• Neonatal infections, including meningitis • Septicaemia	• Female pelvic infections • Cellulitis
β-haemolytic group C (various zoonotic streptococci)	
• Septicaemia • Cellulitis	• Pharyngitis
α, β- or non-haemolytic group D enterococci (*E. faecalis/faecium*)	
• Endocarditis • Intra-abdominal infections	• Urinary tract infection
α, β- or non-haemolytic group D streptococci (*Strep. bovis*)	
• Endocarditis • Septicaemia	• Liver abscess • Brain abscess
β-haemolytic group G streptococci	
• Septicaemia • Cellulitis	• Liver abscess
α-haemolytic viridans group (*Strep. mitis, sanguis, mutans, salivarius*)	
• Septicaemia in immunosuppressed	• Endocarditis
α-haemolytic optochin-sensitive (*Strep. pneumoniae*)	
• Pneumonia • Meningitis • Endocarditis • Otitis media	• Septicaemia • Spontaneous bacterial peritonitis
Anaerobic streptococci (*Peptostreptococcus* spp.)	
• Peritonitis • Dental infections	• Liver abscess • Pelvic inflammatory disease
N.B. All streptococci can cause septicaemia.	

progresses to circulatory shock. Without aggressive management, multi-organ failure will develop.

Fluid resuscitation must be undertaken, with parenteral antistreptococcal antibiotic therapy, usually with benzylpenicillin and a protein inhibitor, such as clindamycin, to inhibit toxin production. Intravenous immunoglobulin is usually administered in addition. If necrotising fasciitis is present, it should be treated as described on page 305 with urgent débridement.

Treponematoses

Syphilis

This disease is described on page 419.

Endemic treponematoses

Yaws

Yaws is a granulomatous disease, mainly involving the skin and bones; it is caused by *Treponema pertenue*, morphologically and serologically indistinguishable from the causative organisms of syphilis and pinta. It is important to establish the geographical origin and sexual history of patients to exclude a false-positive syphilis serology due to the endemic treponemal infections. Between 1950 and 1960, WHO campaigns treated over 60 million people and eradicated yaws from many areas, but the disease has persisted patchily throughout the tropics; there was resurgence in the 1980s and 1990s in West and Central Africa and the South Pacific.

Organisms are transmitted by bodily contact from a patient with infectious yaws through minor abrasions of the skin of another patient, usually a child. After an incubation period of 3–4 weeks, a proliferative granuloma containing numerous treponemes develops at the site of inoculation. This primary lesion is followed by secondary eruptions. In addition, there may be hypertrophic periosteal lesions of many bones, with underlying cortical rarefaction. Lesions of late yaws are characterised by destructive changes which closely resemble the osteitis and gummas of tertiary syphilis and which heal with much scarring and deformity. Investigations and management are outlined in Box 13.43.

The disease disappears with improved housing and cleanliness. In few fields of medicine have

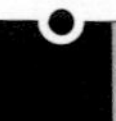

13.43 Diagnosis and treatment of yaws, pinta and bejel
Diagnosis of early stages
• Detection of spirochaetes in exudate of lesions by dark ground microscopy
Diagnosis of latent and early stages
• Positive serological tests, as for syphilis (see Box 15.8, p. 421)
Treatment of all stages
• Single intramuscular injection of 1.2 g long-acting (e.g. benzathine) benzylpenicillin

chemotherapy and improved hygiene achieved such dramatic success as in the control of yaws.

Pinta and bejel

These two treponemal infections occur in poor rural populations with low standards of domestic hygiene, but are found in separate parts of the world. They have features in common, notably that they are transmitted by contact, usually within the family and not sexually, and in the case of bejel, through common eating and drinking utensils. Their diagnosis and management are as for yaws (see Box 13.43).

- *Pinta.* Pinta is probably the oldest of the human treponemal infections. It is found only in South and Central America, where its incidence is declining. The infection is confined to the skin. The early lesions are scaly papules or dyschromic patches on the skin. The late lesions are often depigmented and disfiguring.
- *Bejel.* Bejel is the Middle Eastern name for non-venereal syphilis, which has a patchy distribution across sub-Saharan Africa, the Middle East, Central Asia and Australia. It has been eradicated from Eastern Europe. Transmission is most commonly from the mouth of the mother or child and the primary mucosal lesion is seldom seen. The early and late lesions resemble those of secondary and tertiary syphilis (pp. 419–420) but cardiovascular and neurological disease is rare.

Tropical ulcer

Tropical ulcer is due to a synergistic bacterial infection caused by a fusobacterium (*F. ulcerans*, an anaerobe) and *Treponema vincentii.* It is common in hot, humid regions. The ulcer is most common on the lower legs and develops as a papule that rapidly breaks down to a sharply defined, painful ulcer. The base of the ulcer has a foul slough. Penicillin and metronidazole are useful in the early stages but rest, elevation and dressings are the mainstays of treatment.

Buruli ulcer

This ulcer is caused by *Mycobacterium ulcerans* and occurs widely in tropical rainforests. In 1999, a survey in Ghana found 6500 cases; there are an estimated 10 000 cases in West Africa as a whole.

The initial lesion is a small subcutaneous nodule on the arm or leg. This breaks down to form a shallow, necrotic ulcer with deeply undermined edges, which extends rapidly. Healing may occur after 6 months, but granuloma formation and the accompanying fibrosis cause contractures and deformity. Clumps of acid-fast bacilli can be detected in the ulcer floor.

A combination of rifampicin and streptomycin can cure the infection. Infected tissue should be removed surgically. Health campaigns in Ghana have successfully focused on early removal of the small, pre-ulcerative nodules.

Systemic bacterial infections

Brucellosis

Brucellosis is an enzootic infection (i.e. endemic in animals). Although six species of *Brucella* Gram-negative bacilli are known, only four are important to humans: *B. melitensis* (goats, sheep and camels in Europe, especially the Mediterranean basin, the Middle East, Africa, India, Central Asia and South America), *B. abortus* (cattle, mainly in Africa, Asia and South America), *B. suis* (pigs in South Asia) and *B. canis* (dogs). *B. melitensis* causes the most severe disease; *B. suis* is often associated with abscess formation.

13

Infected animals may excrete *Brucella* spp. in their milk for prolonged periods, and human infection is acquired by ingesting contaminated dairy products (especially unpasteurised milk), uncooked meat or offal. Animal urine, faeces, vaginal discharge and uterine products may act as sources of infection through abraded skin or via splashes and aerosols to the respiratory tract and conjunctiva.

Clinical features

Brucella spp. are intracellular organisms that survive for long periods within the reticulo-endothelial system. This explains many of the clinical features, including the chronicity of disease and tendency to relapse, even after antimicrobial therapy.

Acute illness is characterised by a high swinging temperature, rigors, lethargy, headache, joint and muscle pains, and scrotal pain. Occasionally, there is delirium, abdominal pain and constipation. Physical signs are non-specific, e.g. enlarged lymph nodes. Enlargement of the spleen may lead to hypersplenism and thrombocytopenia.

Localised infection (Fig. 13.19), which occurs in about 30% of patients, is more likely if diagnosis and treatment are delayed.

Diagnosis

Definitive diagnosis depends on the isolation of the organism. Blood cultures are positive in 75–80% of infections caused by *B. melitensis* and 50% of those caused by *B. abortus*. Bone marrow culture should not be used routinely but may increase the diagnostic yield, particularly if antibiotics have been given before specimens are taken. CSF culture in neurobrucellosis is positive in about 30% of cases. The laboratory should be alerted to a suspected diagnosis of brucellosis, as the organism has a propensity for infecting laboratory workers and must be cultured at an enhanced containment level.

Serology may also aid diagnosis. In endemic areas, a single high antibody titre of more than 1/320 or a four-fold rise in titre is needed to support a diagnosis of acute infection. The test usually takes several weeks to become

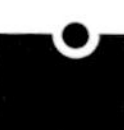

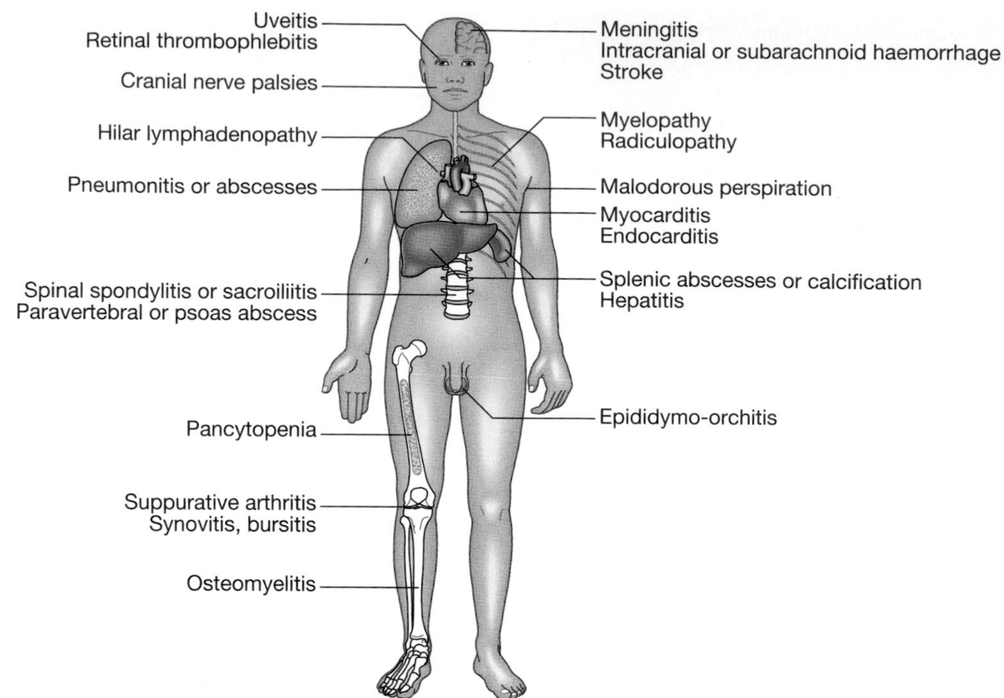

Fig. 13.19 Clinical features of brucellosis.

13.44 Treatment of brucellosis

Adults with non-localised disease
• Doxycycline 100 mg twice daily orally for 6 wks *plus* gentamicin 5 mg/kg IV once daily for 7 days *or* • Doxycycline 100 mg twice daily *plus* rifampicin 600–900 mg orally once daily for 6 wks
Bone disease
• Doxycycline 100 mg twice daily plus rifampicin 600–900 mg once daily orally for 6 wks *plus* gentamicin 5 mg/kg IV once daily for 7 days *or* • Ciprofloxacin 750 mg twice daily orally plus rifampicin 600–900 mg orally once daily for 3 mths
Neurobrucellosis
• Doxycycline 100 mg twice daily *plus* rifampicin 600–900 mg orally once daily for 6 wks *plus* ceftriaxone 2 g IV twice daily until CSF is clear (though susceptibility should be confirmed because sensitivity to third-generation cephalosporins varies amongst strains)
Endocarditis
• Almost always needs surgical intervention *plus* • Doxycycline 100 mg twice daily, rifampicin 600–900 mg orally once daily and co-trimoxazole 5 mg/kg of trimethoprim component for 6 mths *plus* gentamicin 5 mg/kg IV once daily for 2–4 wks
Pregnancy
• Rifampicin 600–900 mg orally once daily and co-trimoxazole 5 mg/kg of trimethoprim component for 4 wks, but caution in last week of pregnancy due to displacement of bilirubin from albumin by drugs and risk of kernicterus to the fetus

positive but should eventually detect 95% of acute infections.

Management

Aminoglycosides show synergistic activity with tetracyclines against brucellae. Treatment regimens for different forms of brucellosis are outlined in Box 13.44.

Borrelia infections

Borrelia are flagellated spirochaetal bacteria which infect humans after bites from ticks or lice. They cause a variety of human infections worldwide (Box 13.45).

Lyme disease

Lyme disease (named after the town of Old Lyme in Connecticut, USA) is caused by *B. burgdorferi,* which occurs in the USA, Europe, Russia, China, Japan and Australia. In Europe, two additional genospecies are also encountered, *B. afzelii* and *B. garinii.* The reservoir of infection is ixodid (hard) ticks that feed on a variety of large mammals, particularly deer. Birds may spread ticks over a wide area. The organism is transmitted to humans via the bite of infected ticks; larval, nymphal and adult forms are all capable of spreading infection.

Ehrlichiosis is a common co-infection with Lyme disease (*Anaplasma phagocytophila,* human granulocytic anaplasmosis (HGA); *Ehrlichia chaffeensis,* human monocytic ehrlichiosis (HME)).

Clinical features

There are three stages of disease. Progression may be arrested at any stage.

- *Early localised disease.* The characteristic feature is a skin reaction around the site of the tick bite, known as erythema migrans (Fig. 13.20). Initially, a red

13.45 Clinical diseases caused by *Borrelia* spp.

Species	Vector	Geographic distribution
Lyme disease		
B. burgdorferi sensu stricto	Tick: *Ixodes scapularis*	Northern and eastern USA
	I. pacificus	Western USA
B. afzelii	*I. ricinus*	Europe
	I. persulcatus	Asia
B. garinii	*I. ricinus*	Europe
	I. persulcatus	Asia
Louse-borne relapsing fever		
B. recurrentis	Human louse: *Pediculus humanus corporis*	Worldwide
Tick-borne relapsing fever		
B. hermsii	Tick: *Ornithodoros hermsii*	Western North America
B. turicatae	*O. turicatae*	Southwestern North America and northern Mexico
B. venezuelensis	*O. rudis*	Central America and northern South America
B. hispanica	*O. erraticus*	Iberian peninsula and northwestern Africa
B. crocidurae	*O. erraticus*	North Africa and Mediterranean region
B. duttonii	*O. moubata*	Central, eastern and southern Africa
B. persica	*O. tholozani*	Western China, India, central Asia, Middle East
B. latyschewii	*O. tartakovskyi*	Tajikistan, Uzbekistan

'bull's eye' macule or papule appears 2–30 days after the bite. It then enlarges peripherally with central clearing, and may persist for months. Atypical forms are fairly common. The lesion is not pathognomonic of Lyme disease since similar lesions can occur after tick bites in areas where Lyme disease does not occur. Other acute manifestations, such as fever, headache and regional lymphadenopathy, may develop with or without the rash.

- *Early disseminated disease*. Dissemination occurs via the blood stream and lymphatics. There may be a systemic reaction with malaise, arthralgia, and occasionally metastatic areas of erythema migrans (see Fig. 13.20). Neurological involvement may follow weeks or months after infection. Common features include lymphocytic meningitis, cranial nerve palsies (especially unilateral or bilateral facial nerve palsy) and peripheral neuropathy. Radiculopathy, often painful, may present a year or more after initial infection. Carditis, sometimes accompanied by atrioventricular conduction defects, is not uncommon in the USA but appears to be rare in Europe.
- *Late disease*. Late manifestations include arthritis, polyneuritis and encephalopathy. Prolonged arthritis, particularly affecting large joints, and brain parenchymal involvement causing neuropsychiatric abnormalities may occur, but are rare in the UK. Acrodermatitis chronica atrophicans is an uncommon late complication seen more frequently in Europe than North America. Doughy, patchy discoloration occurs on the peripheries, eventually leading to shiny atrophic skin. The lesions are easily mistaken for those of peripheral vascular disease. In patients from an endemic area or with risk factors, who have facial nerve palsy, Lyme disease should be considered.

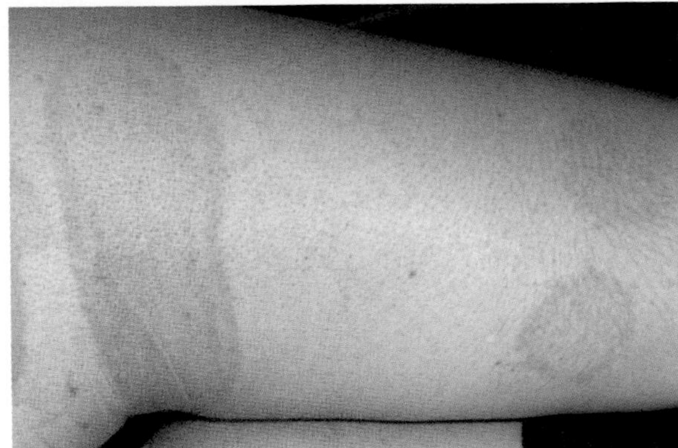

Fig. 13.20 Rash of erythema migrans in Lyme disease with metastatic secondary lesions.

13

Diagnosis

The diagnosis of early Lyme borreliosis is often clinical. Culture from biopsy material is not generally available, has a low yield, and may take longer than 6 weeks. Antibody detection is frequently negative early in the course of the disease, but sensitivity increases to 90–100% in disseminated or late disease. Immunofluorescence or ELISA can give false-positive reactions in a number of conditions, including other spirochaetal infections, infectious mononucleosis, rheumatoid arthritis and systemic lupus erythematosus (SLE). Immunoblot (Western blot) techniques are more specific and, although technically demanding, should be used to confirm the diagnosis. Microorganism DNA detection by PCR has been applied to blood, urine, CSF, and biopsies of skin and synovium.

Management

Recent evidence suggests that asymptomatic patients with positive antibody tests should not be treated. However, erythema migrans always requires therapy because organisms may persist and cause progressive disease, even if the skin lesions resolve. Standard therapy consists of a 14-day course of doxycycline (200 mg daily) or amoxicillin (500 mg 3 times daily). Some 15% of patients with early disease will develop a mild Jarisch–Herxheimer reaction (JHR) during the first 24 hours of therapy (p. 421). In pregnant women and small children, or in those allergic to amoxicillin and doxycycline, 14-day treatment with cefuroxime axetil (500 mg twice daily) or erythromycin (250 mg 4 times daily) may be used.

Disseminated disease and arthritis require therapy for a minimum of 28 days. Arthritis may respond poorly, and prolonged or repeated courses may be necessary. Neuroborreliosis is treated with parenteral β-lactam antibiotics for 3–4 weeks; the cephalosporins may be superior to penicillin in this situation.

Prevention

Protective clothing and insect repellents should be used in tick-infested areas. Since the risk of borrelial transmission is lower in the first few hours of a blood feed, prompt removal of ticks is advisable. Unfortunately, larval and nymphal ticks are tiny and may not be noticed. Where risk of transmission is high, a single 200 mg dose of doxycycline, given within 72 hours of exposure, has been shown to prevent erythema migrans. A recombinant OspA vaccine was developed but withdrawn due to side-effects.

Louse-borne relapsing fever

The human body louse, *Pediculus humanus*, causes itching. Borreliae (*B. recurrentis*) are liberated from infected lice when they are crushed during scratching, which also inoculates the borreliae into the skin. The disease occurs worldwide, with epidemic relapsing fever most often seen in Central/East Africa and South America.

The borreliae multiply in the blood, where they are abundant in the febrile phases, and invade most tissues, especially the liver, spleen and meninges. Hepatitis and thrombocytopenia are common.

Clinical features

Onset is sudden with fever. The temperature rises to 39.5–40.5°C, accompanied by a tachycardia, headache, generalised aching, injected conjunctivae (Fig. 13.21) and, frequently, a petechial rash, epistaxis and herpes labialis. As the disease progresses, the liver and spleen frequently become tender and palpable, and jaundice is common. There may be severe serosal and intestinal haemorrhage, mental confusion and meningism. The fever ends in crisis between the 4th and 10th days, often associated with profuse sweating, hypotension, and circulatory and cardiac failure. There may be no further fever but, in a proportion of patients, after an afebrile period of about 7 days, there are one or more relapses, which are usually milder and less prolonged. In the absence of specific treatment, the mortality rate is up to 40%, especially among the elderly and malnourished.

Investigations and management

The organisms are demonstrated in the blood during fever either by dark ground microscopy of a wet film or in Wright–Giemsa stained thick and thin films.

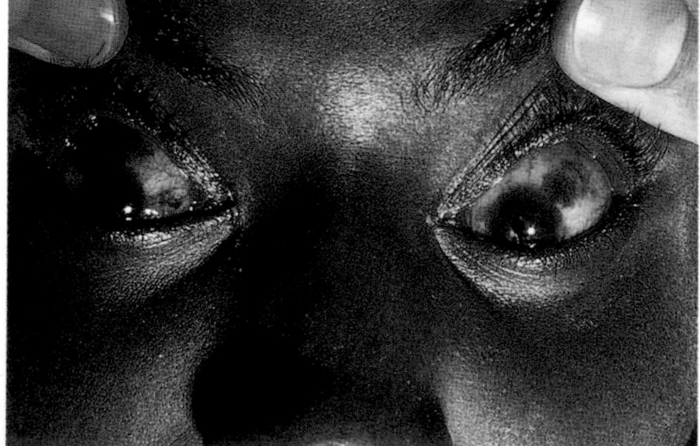

Fig. 13.21 Louse-borne relapsing fever. Injected conjunctivae.

The problems of treatment are to eradicate the organism, to minimise the severe JHR which inevitably follows successful chemotherapy, and to prevent relapses. The safest treatment is procaine penicillin 300 mg IM, followed the next day by 0.5 g tetracycline. Tetracycline alone is effective and prevents relapse, but may give rise to a worse reaction. Doxycycline 200 mg once orally in place of tetracycline has the advantage of also being curative for typhus, which often accompanies epidemics of relapsing fever. JHR is best managed in a high-dependency unit with expert nursing and medical care.

The patient, clothing and all contacts must be freed from lice, as in epidemic typhus.

Tick-borne relapsing fever

Soft ticks (*Ornithodoros* spp.) transmit *B. duttonii* (and several other borrelia species) through saliva while feeding on their host. People sleeping in mud houses are at risk, as the tick hides in crevices during the day and feeds on humans during the night. Rodents are the reservoir in all parts of the world except East Africa, where humans are the reservoir. Clinical manifestations are similar to those seen with the louse-borne disease, but spirochaetes are detected in fewer patients on dark field microscopy. A 7-day course (due to a higher relapse rate than in louse-borne relapsing fever) of treatment with either tetracycline (500 mg 4 times daily) or erythromycin (500 mg 4 times daily) is needed.

Leptospirosis

Microbiology and epidemiology

Leptospirosis is one of the most common zoonotic diseases, favoured by a tropical climate and flooding during the monsoon but occurring worldwide. Leptospires are tightly coiled, thread-like organisms about 5–7 μm in length, which are actively motile; each end is bent into a hook. *Leptospira interrogans* is pathogenic for humans. The genus can be separated into more than 200 serovars (subtypes) belonging to 23 serogroups.

Leptospirosis appears to be ubiquitous in wildlife and in many domestic animals. The organisms persist indefinitely in the convoluted tubules of the kidney and are shed into the urine in massive numbers, but infection is asymptomatic in the host. The most frequent hosts are rodents, especially the common rat (*Rattus norvegicus*). Particular leptospiral serogroups are associated with characteristic animal hosts; for example, *L. icterohaemorrhagiae* is the classical parasite of rats and *L. canicola* of dogs. There is nevertheless considerable overlap in host–serogroup associations.

Leptospires can enter their human hosts through intact skin or mucous membranes, but entry is facilitated by cuts and abrasions. Prolonged immersion in contaminated water will also favour invasion, as the spirochaete can survive in water for months. Leptospirosis is common in the tropics and also in freshwater sports enthusiasts.

Clinical features

After a relatively brief bacteraemia, invading organisms are distributed throughout the body, mainly in kidneys, liver, meninges and brain. The incubation period averages 1–2 weeks. Four main clinical syndromes can be discerned and clinical features can involve multiple different organ systems (Fig. 13.22).

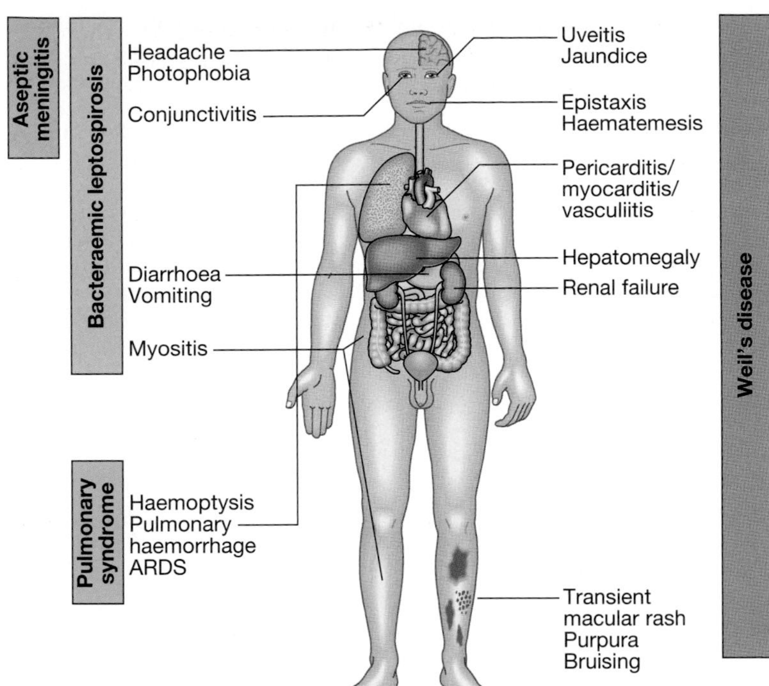

Fig. 13.22 Clinical syndromes of leptospirosis. (ARDS = acute respiratory distress syndrome)

Bacteraemic leptospirosis

Bacteraemia with any serogroup can produce a non-specific illness with high fever, weakness, muscle pain and tenderness (especially of the calf and back), intense headache and photophobia, and sometimes diarrhoea and vomiting. Conjunctival congestion is the only notable physical sign. The illness comes to an end after about 1 week, or else merges into one of the other forms of infection.

Aseptic meningitis

Classically associated with *L. canicola* infection, this illness is very difficult to distinguish from viral meningitis. The conjunctivae may be congested but there are no other differentiating signs. Laboratory clues include a neutrophil leucocytosis, abnormal LFTs, and the occasional presence of albumin and casts in the urine.

Icteric leptospirosis (Weil's disease)

Fewer than 10% of symptomatic infections result in severe icteric illness. Weil's disease is a dramatic life-threatening event, characterised by fever, haemorrhages, jaundice and renal impairment. Conjunctival hyperaemia is a frequent feature. The patient may have a transient macular erythematous rash, but the characteristic skin changes are purpura and large areas of bruising. In severe cases there may be epistaxis, haematemesis and melaena, or bleeding into the pleural, pericardial or subarachnoid spaces. Thrombocytopenia, probably related to activation of endothelial cells with platelet adhesion and aggregation, is present in 50% of cases. Jaundice is deep and the liver is enlarged, but there is usually little evidence of hepatic failure or encephalopathy. Renal failure, primarily caused by impaired renal perfusion and acute tubular necrosis, manifests as oliguria or anuria, with the presence of albumin, blood and casts in the urine.

Weil's disease may also be associated with myocarditis, encephalitis and aseptic meningitis. Uveitis and iritis may appear months after apparent clinical recovery.

Pulmonary syndrome

This syndrome has long been recognised in the Far East, and has been described during an outbreak of leptospirosis in Nicaragua. It is characterised by haemoptysis, patchy lung infiltrates on chest X-ray, and respiratory failure. Total bilateral lung consolidation and ARDS (p. 192) with multi-organ dysfunction may develop, with a high mortality (over 50%).

Diagnosis

A polymorphonuclear leucocytosis is accompanied in severe infection by thrombocytopenia and elevated blood levels of creatine kinase. In jaundiced patients, there is hepatitis and the prothrombin time may be prolonged. The CSF in leptospiral meningitis shows a variable cellular response, a moderately elevated protein level and normal glucose content. Acute renal failure due to interstitial nephritis is common.

In the tropics, dengue, malaria, typhoid fever, scrub typhus and hantavirus infection are important differential diagnoses.

Definitive diagnosis of leptospirosis depends upon isolation of the organism, serological tests or the detection of specific DNA. In general, however, it is probably under-diagnosed.

- Blood cultures are most likely to be positive if taken before the tenth day of illness. Special media are required and cultures may have to be incubated for several weeks.
- Leptospires appear in the urine during the second week of illness, and in untreated patients may be recovered on culture for several months.

- Serological tests are diagnostic if seroconversion or a fourfold increase in titre is demonstrated. The microscopic agglutination test (MAT) is the test of choice and can become positive by the end of the first week. IgM ELISA and immunofluorescent techniques are, however, easier to perform, while rapid immunochromatographic tests are specific but of only moderate sensitivity in the first week of illness.
- Detection of leptospiral DNA by PCR is possible in blood in early symptomatic disease, and in urine from the eighth day of illness and for many months thereafter.

Management and prevention

The general care of the patient is critically important. Blood transfusion for haemorrhage and careful attention to renal failure, the usual cause of death, are especially important. Renal failure is potentially reversible with adequate support, such as dialysis. The optimal antimicrobial regimen has not been established. Most infections are self-limiting. Therapy with either oral doxycycline (100 mg twice daily for 1 week) or intravenous penicillin (900 mg 4 times daily for 1 week) is effective but may not prevent the development of renal failure. Parenteral ceftriaxone (1 g daily) is as effective as penicillin. A Jarisch–Herxheimer reaction may occur during treatment but is usually mild. Uveitis is treated with a combination of systemic antibiotics and local corticosteroids. There is no role for the routine use of corticosteroids in the management of leptospirosis.

Trials in military personnel have shown that infection with *L. interrogans* can be prevented by taking prophylactic doxycycline 200 mg weekly.

Plague

Plague is caused by *Yersinia pestis*, a small Gram-negative bacillus that is spread between rodents by their fleas. If domestic rats become infected, infected fleas may bite humans. Hunters and trappers can contract plague from handling rodents. In the late stages of human plague, *Y. pestis* may be expectorated and spread between humans by droplets, causing 'pneumonic plague'.

Epidemics of plague, such as the 'Black Death', have occurred since ancient times. It is often said that the first sign of plague is the appearance of dead rats. Plague foci are widely distributed throughout the world, including the USA; human cases are reported from about ten countries per year (Fig. 13.23).

Y. pestis is a potential bioweapon because of its capacity for mass production and aerosol transmission, and the high fatality rate associated with pneumonic plague.

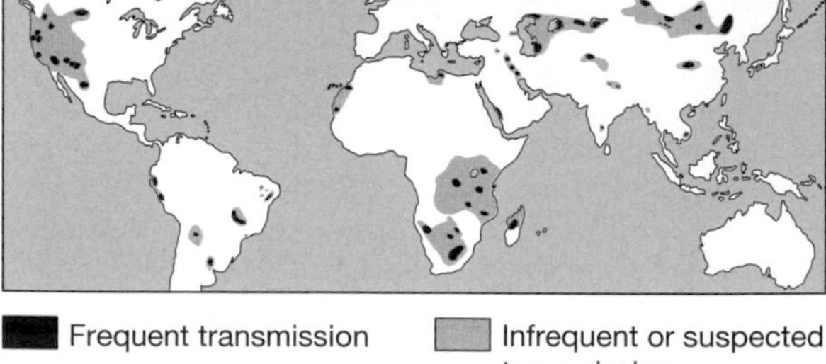

Fig. 13.23 Foci of the transmission of plague. Reproduced by permission of WHO.

Clinical features

Organisms inoculated through the skin are taken rapidly to the draining lymph nodes, where they elicit a severe inflammatory response that may be haemorrhagic. If the infection is not contained, septicaemia ensues and necrotic, purulent or haemorrhagic lesions develop in many organs. Oliguria and shock follow, and disseminated intravascular coagulation may result in widespread haemorrhage. Inhalation of *Y. pestis* causes alveolitis. The incubation period is 3–6 days, but shorter in pneumonic plague.

Bubonic plague

In this, the most common form of the disease, onset is usually sudden, with a rigor, high fever, dry skin and severe headache. Soon, aching and swelling at the site of the affected lymph nodes begin. The groin is the most common site of this 'bubo', made up of the swollen lymph nodes and surrounding tissue. Some infections are relatively mild but, in the majority of patients, toxaemia quickly increases, with a rapid pulse, hypotension and mental confusion. The spleen is usually palpable.

Septicaemic plague

Those not exhibiting a bubo usually deteriorate rapidly and have a high mortality. The elderly are more prone to this form of illness. The patient is toxic and may have gastrointestinal symptoms, such as nausea, vomiting, abdominal pain and diarrhoea. DIC may occur, manifested by bleeding from various orifices or puncture sites, along with ecchymoses. Hypotension, shock, renal failure and ARDS may lead to further deterioration. Meningitis, pneumonia and expectoration of blood-stained sputum containing *Y. pestis* may complicate septicaemic, or occasionally bubonic, plague.

Pneumonic plague

Following primary infection in the lung, the onset of disease is very sudden, with cough and dyspnoea. The patient soon expectorates copious blood-stained, frothy, highly infective sputum, becomes cyanosed and dies. Chest radiology reveals bilateral infiltrates which may be nodular and progress to an ARDS-like picture.

Investigations

The organism may be cultured from blood, sputum and bubo aspirates. For rapid diagnosis, Gram, Giemsa and Wayson's stains (the latter containing methylene blue) are applied to smears from these sites. *Y. pestis* is seen as bipolar staining coccobacilli, sometimes referred to as having a 'safety pin' appearance. Smears are also subjected to antigen detection by immunofluorescence, using *Y. pestis* F1 antigen-specific antibodies. The diagnosis may be confirmed by seroconversion or a single high titre (> 128) of anti-F1 antibodies in serum. DNA detection by PCR is under evaluation.

Plague is a notifiable disease under international health regulations (p. 147).

Management

If the diagnosis is suspected on clinical and epidemiological grounds, treatment must be started as soon as, or even before, samples have been collected for laboratory diagnosis. Streptomycin (1 g twice daily) or gentamicin (1 mg/kg 3 times daily) is the drug of choice. Tetracycline (500 mg 4 times daily) and chloramphenicol (12.5 mg/kg 4 times daily) are alternatives. Fluoroquinolones (ciprofloxacin and levofloxacin) may be as effective, but there is less clinical experience. Treatment may also be needed for acute circulatory failure, DIC and hypoxia.

Prevention and infection control

Rats and fleas should be controlled. In endemic areas, people should avoid handling and skinning wild animals. The patient should be isolated for the first 48 hours or until clinical improvement begins. Attendants must wear gowns, masks and gloves. Exposed symptomatic or asymptomatic people who have been in close contact with a patient with pneumonic plague should receive post-exposure antibiotic prophylaxis (doxycycline 100 mg or ciprofloxacin 500 mg twice daily) for 7 days.

A formalin-killed vaccine is available for those at occupational risk but offers little protection against pneumonic plague. A recombinant subunit vaccine (protein antigens F1 + V) is in development.

Listeriosis

Listeria monocytogenes is an environmental Gram-positive bacillus which can contaminate food. Outbreaks have been associated with raw vegetables, soft cheeses, undercooked chicken, fish, meat and pâtés. The bacterium demonstrates 'cold enrichment', outgrowing other contaminating bacteria during refrigeration. Although food-borne outbreaks of gastroenteritis have been reported in immunocompetent individuals, *Listeria* causes more significant invasive infection, especially in pregnancy, the elderly (over 55 years) and the immunocompromised.

In pregnancy, in addition to systemic symptoms of fever and myalgia, listeriosis causes chorioamnionitis, fetal deaths, abortions and neonatal infection. In other susceptible individuals, it causes systemic illness due to bacteraemia without focal symptoms. Meningitis, similar to other bacterial meningitis but with normal CSF glucose, is the next most common presentation; CSF usually shows increased neutrophils but occasionally only the mononuclear cells are increased (p. 1201).

Investigations and management

Diagnosis is made by blood and CSF culture. The organism grows readily in culture media.

The most effective regimen consists of a combination of an intravenous aminopenicillin (amoxicillin or ampicillin) plus an aminoglycoside. A sulfamethoxazole/trimethoprim combination can be used in those with penicillin allergy. Cephalosporins are of no use in this infection, as the organism is inherently resistant, an important consideration when empirically treating meningitis.

Proper treatment of foods before eating is the key to preventing listeriosis. Pregnant women are advised to avoid high-risk products, including soft cheeses.

Typhoid and paratyphoid (enteric) fevers

Typhoid and paratyphoid fevers, which are transmitted by the faecal–oral route, are important causes of fever in India, sub-Saharan Africa and Latin America. Elsewhere, they are relatively rare. Enteric fevers are caused by infection with *Salmonella typhi* and *S. paratyphi* A and B. After a few days of bacteraemia, the bacilli localise, mainly in the lymphoid tissue of the small intestine, resulting in typical lesions in the Peyer's patches and follicles. These swell at first, then ulcerate and usually heal. After clinical recovery, about 5% of patients become chronic carriers (i.e. continue to excrete the bacteria after 1 year); the bacilli may live in the gallbladder for months or years and pass intermittently in the stool and, less commonly, in the urine.

Clinical features

Typhoid fever

Clinical features are outlined in Box 13.46. The incubation period is typically about 10–14 days but can be longer, and the onset may be insidious. The temperature rises in a stepladder fashion for 4 or 5 days with malaise, increasing headache, drowsiness and aching in the limbs. Constipation may be caused by swelling of lymphoid tissue around the ileocaecal junction, although in children diarrhoea and vomiting may be prominent early in the illness. The pulse is often slower than would be expected from the height of the temperature, i.e. a relative bradycardia.

At the end of the first week, a rash may appear on the upper abdomen and on the back as sparse, slightly raised, rose-red spots, which fade on pressure. It is usually visible only on white skin. Cough and epistaxis occur. Around the 7th–10th day, the spleen becomes palpable. Constipation is then succeeded by diarrhoea and abdominal distension with tenderness. Bronchitis and delirium may develop. If untreated, by the end of the second week the patient may be profoundly ill.

Paratyphoid fever

The course tends to be shorter and milder than that of typhoid fever and the onset is often more abrupt with acute enteritis. The rash may be more abundant and the intestinal complications less frequent.

Complications

These are given in Box 13.47. Haemorrhage from, or a perforation of, the ulcerated Peyer's patches may occur at the end of the second week or during the third week of the illness. A drop in temperature to normal or subnormal levels may be falsely reassuring in patients with intestinal haemorrhage. Additional complications may

13.46 Clinical features of typhoid fever

First week	
• Fever • Headache • Myalgia • Relative bradycardia	• Constipation • Diarrhoea and vomiting in children
End of first week	
• Rose spots on trunk • Splenomegaly • Cough	• Abdominal distension • Diarrhoea
End of second week	
• Delirium, complications, then coma and death (if untreated)	

13.47 Complications of typhoid fever	
Bowel	
• Perforation	• Haemorrhage
Septicaemic foci	
• Bone and joint infection • Meningitis	• Cholecystitis
Toxic phenomena	
• Myocarditis	• Nephritis
Chronic carriage	
• Persistent gallbladder carriage	

involve almost any viscus or system because of the septicaemia present during the first week. Bone and joint infection is common in children with sickle-cell disease.

Investigations

In the first week, diagnosis may be difficult because, in this invasive stage with bacteraemia, the symptoms are those of a generalised infection without localising features. A white blood count may be helpful, as there is typically a leucopenia. Blood culture is the most important diagnostic method. The faeces contain the organism more frequently in the second and third weeks.

Management

Antibiotic therapy must be guided by in vitro sensitivity testing. Chloramphenicol (500 mg 4 times daily), ampicillin (750 mg 4 times daily) and co-trimoxazole (2 tablets or IV equivalent twice daily) are losing their effect due to resistance in many areas of the world, especially India and South-east Asia. The fluoroquinolones are the drugs of choice (e.g. ciprofloxacin 500 mg twice daily) if the organism is susceptible, but resistance is common, especially in the Indian subcontinent and also in the UK. Extended-spectrum cephalosporins (ceftriaxone and cefotaxime) are useful alternatives but have a slightly increased treatment failure rate. Azithromycin (500 mg once daily) is an alternative when fluoroquinolone resistance is present but has not been validated in severe disease. Treatment should be continued for 14 days. Pyrexia may persist for up to 5 days after the start of specific therapy. Even with effective chemotherapy, there is still a danger of complications, recrudescence of the disease and the development of a carrier state.

Chronic carriers were formerly treated for 4 weeks with ciprofloxacin but may require an alternative agent and duration, as guided by antimicrobial sensitivity testing. Cholecystectomy may be necessary.

Prevention

Improved sanitation and living conditions reduce the incidence of typhoid. Travellers to countries where enteric infections are endemic should be inoculated with one of the three available typhoid vaccines (two inactivated injectable and one oral live attenuated).

Tularaemia

Tularaemia is primarily a zoonotic disease of the northern hemisphere. It is caused by a highly infectious Gram-negative bacillus, *Francisella tularensis*. *F. tularensis* is passed transovarially (ensuring transmission from parent to progeny) in ticks, which allows persistence in nature without the absolute requirement for an infected animal reservoir. It is a potential weapon for bioterrorism. Wild rabbits, rodents, and domestic dogs or cats are some of the many potential reservoirs, and ticks, mosquitoes or other biting flies are the vectors.

Infection is introduced either through an arthropod or animal bite or via contact with infected animals, soil or water through skin abrasions. This results in the most common 'ulceroglandular' variety of the disease (70–80%), characterised by skin ulceration with regional lymphadenopathy. There is also a purely 'glandular' form. Alternatively, inhalation of the infected aerosols may result in pulmonary tularaemia, presenting as pneumonia. Rarely, the portal of entry of infection may be the conjunctiva, leading to a nodular, ulcerated conjunctivitis with regional lymphadenopathy (an 'oculoglandular' form).

Investigations and management

Demonstration of a single high titre (≥ 1:160) or a fourfold rise in 2–3 weeks in the tularaemia tube agglutination test confirms the diagnosis. Bacterial yield from the lesions is extremely poor. DNA detection methods to enable rapid diagnosis are in development.

Treatment consists of a 7–10-day course of parenteral aminoglycosides, streptomycin (7.5–10 mg/kg twice daily) or gentamicin (1.7 mg/kg 3 times daily). *F. tularensis* is not susceptible to most other antibiotics.

Melioidosis

Melioidosis is caused by *Burkholderia pseudomallei*, a saprophyte found in soil and water (rice paddy fields). Infection is by inoculation or inhalation, leading to bacteraemia, which is followed by the formation of abscesses in the lungs, liver and spleen. Patients with diabetes, renal stones, thalassaemia or severe burns are particularly susceptible. The disease is most common in South India, East Asia and northern Australia, and carries a significant mortality. Disease may present many years or decades after the initial exposure.

Clinical features

There is high fever, prostration and sometimes diarrhoea, with signs of pneumonia and enlargement of the liver and spleen. The chest X-ray resembles that of acute caseous tuberculosis. In more chronic forms, multiple abscesses occur in subcutaneous tissue and bone, and profound wasting is a major problem.

Investigations and management

Culture of blood, sputum or pus may yield *B. pseudomallei*. Indirect haemagglutination testing can be helpful in travellers; however, most people in endemic areas are seropositive.

In the acute illness, prompt treatment, without waiting for confirmation by culture, may be life-saving. Ceftazidime 100 mg/kg (2 g 3 times daily), imipenem 50 mg/kg (1 g 4 times daily) or meropenem (0.5–1 g 3 times daily) is given for 2–3 weeks. This is followed by maintenance therapy of doxycycline 200 mg daily, plus co-trimoxazole (sulfamethoxazole 1600 mg plus trimethoprim 320 mg twice daily) for a minimum of 12 weeks. Abscesses should be drained surgically.

Actinomycete infections

Nocardiosis

Nocardiosis is an uncommon Gram-positive bacterial infection caused by aerobic actinomycetes of the genus *Nocardia* found in the soil. Infection occurs most frequently by direct traumatic inoculation or occasionally via inhalation or ingestion. Nocardiosis can result in localised cutaneous ulcers or nodules, most often in the lower limbs. Chronic destructive infection in tropical countries can result in actinomycetoma, involving soft tissues with occasional penetration to the bone. Actinomycetoma may also be caused by other bacteria, and a similar clinical syndrome, termed eumycetoma, is caused by fungi (p. 382). Systemic *Nocardia* infection, most likely in immunocompromised individuals, results in suppurative disease with lung and brain abscesses.

On microscopy, *Nocardia* spp. appear as long, filamentous, branching Gram-positive rods which are also weakly acid-fast. They are easily grown in culture but require prolonged incubation.

Treatment is guided by susceptibility testing. Systemic infection typically requires combinations of ceftriaxone, meropenem, amikacin and co-trimoxazole, often for 6–12 months or longer. Abscesses are drained surgically when this is feasible. Localised cutaneous infection is usually treated with a single agent for 1–3 months.

Actinomycetoma is also treated with prolonged antibiotic combinations. There is no universal consensus on the most appropriate drug or combination. The usual combination is streptomycin and dapsone, with dapsone replaced by co-trimoxazole in cases with intolerance or refractory disease. Success has also been reported with co-trimoxazole plus amikacin, with rifampicin added in difficult cases and to prevent recurrence.

Actinomyces israelii

Actinomyces israelii can cause deep infection in the head and neck, and also suppurating disease in the pelvis associated with intrauterine contraceptive devices (IUCDs). Treatment is usually with penicillin or doxycycline.

Gastrointestinal bacterial infections

The differential diagnosis and approach to patients presenting with acute gastroenteritis are described on page 306.

Staphylococcal food poisoning

Staph. aureus transmission takes place via the hands of food handlers to foodstuffs such as dairy products, including cheese, and cooked meats. Inappropriate storage of these foods allows growth of the organism and production of one or more heat-stable enterotoxins which cause the symptoms.

Nausea and profuse vomiting develop within 1–6 hours. Diarrhoea may not be marked. The toxins that cause the syndrome act as 'superantigens', inducing a significant neutrophil leucocytosis that may be clinically misleading. Superantigens are secreted proteins (exotoxins) that exhibit highly potent lymphocyte-transforming (mitogenic) activity directed towards T lymphocytes. Most cases settle rapidly but severe dehydration can occasionally be life-threatening.

Antiemetics and appropriate fluid replacement are the mainstays of treatment. Suspect food should be cultured for staphylococci and demonstration of toxin production. The public health authorities should be notified if food vending is involved.

Bacillus cereus food poisoning

Ingestion of the pre-formed heat-stable exotoxins of *B. cereus* causes rapid onset of vomiting and some diarrhoea within hours of food consumption, which resolves within 24 hours. Fried rice and freshly made sauces are frequent sources; the organism grows and produces enterotoxin during storage (Fig. 13.24). If viable bacteria are ingested and toxin formation takes place within the gut lumen, then the incubation period is longer (12–24 hours) and watery diarrhoea and cramps are the predominant symptoms. The disease is self-limiting but can be quite severe.

Rapid and judicious fluid replacement and appropriate notification of the public health authorities are all that is required.

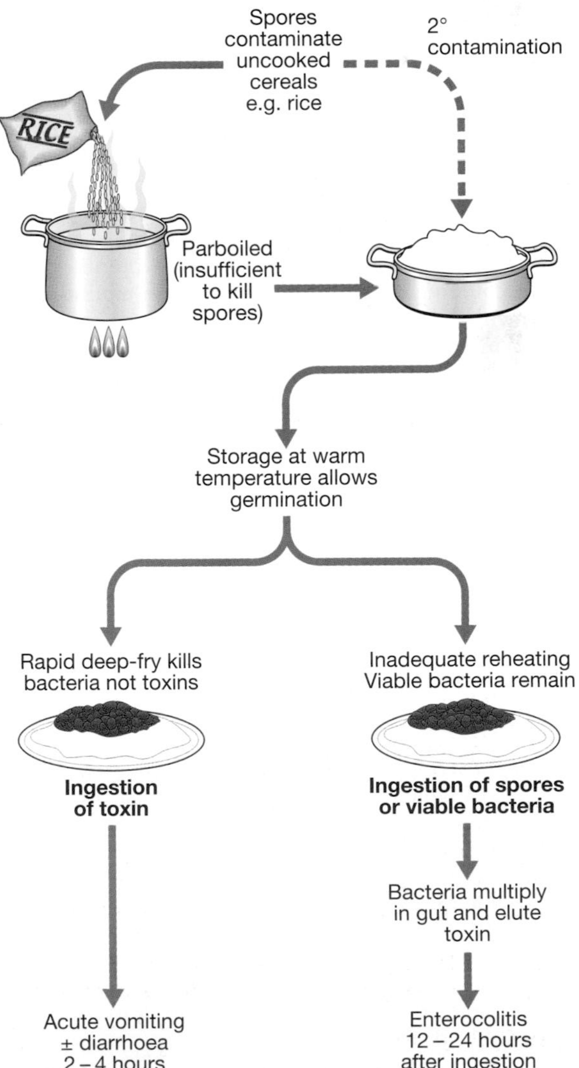

Fig. 13.24 *Bacillus cereus* food poisoning.

Clostridium perfringens food poisoning

Spores of *C. perfringens* are widespread in the guts of large animals and in soil. If contaminated meat products are incompletely cooked and stored in anaerobic conditions, *C. perfringens* spores germinate and viable organisms multiply to give large numbers. Subsequent reheating of the food causes heat-shock sporulation of the organisms, during which they release an enterotoxin. Symptoms (diarrhoea and cramps) occur some 6–12 hours following ingestion. The illness is usually self-limiting.

Clostridial enterotoxins are potent and most people who ingest them will be symptomatic. 'Point source' outbreaks, in which a number of cases all become symptomatic following ingestion, classically occur after school or canteen lunches where meat stews are served.

Clostridial necrotising enteritis (CNE) or pigbel is an often-fatal type of food poisoning caused by a β-toxin of *C. perfringens*, type C. The toxin is normally inactivated by certain proteases or by normal cooking. Pigbel is more likely in protein malnutrition or in the presence of trypsin inhibitors, either in foods such as sweet potatoes or during infection with *Ascaris* sp. roundworms.

Campylobacter jejuni infection

This infection is essentially a zoonosis, although contaminated water may be implicated, as the organism can survive for many weeks in fresh water. The most common sources of the infection are chicken, beef and contaminated milk products. There has been an association with pet puppies. *Campylobacter* infection is now the most common cause of bacterial gastroenteritis in the UK, accounting for some 100 000 cases per annum, most of which are sporadic.

The incubation period is 2–5 days. Colicky abdominal pain, which may be quite severe and mimic surgical pathology, occurs with nausea, vomiting and significant diarrhoea, frequently containing blood. The majority of *Campylobacter* infections affect fit young adults and are self-limiting after 5–7 days. About 10–20% will have prolonged symptomatology, occasionally meriting treatment with antibiotics such as erythromycin, as many organisms are resistant to ciprofloxacin.

Approximately 1% of cases will develop bacteraemia and possible distant foci of infection. *Campylobacter* spp. have been linked to Guillain–Barré syndrome and post-infectious reactive arthritis (pp. 1224 and 1107).

Salmonella spp. infection

Salmonella serotypes other than *S. typhi* and *S. paratyphi* (p. 339), of which there are more than 2000, are subdivided into five distinct subgroups which produce gastroenteritis. They are widely distributed throughout the animal kingdom. Two serotypes are most important worldwide: *S. enteritidis* phage type 4 and *S. typhimurium* dt.104. The latter may be resistant to commonly used antibiotics such as ciprofloxacin. Some strains have a clear relationship to particular animal species, e.g. *S. arizonae* and pet reptiles. Transmission is by contaminated water or food, particularly poultry, egg products and related fast foods, direct person-to-person spread or the handling of exotic pets such as salamanders, lizards or turtles. The incidence of *Salmonella* enteritis is falling in the UK due to an aggressive culling policy in broiler chicken stocks, coupled with vaccination.

EBM 13.48 Antibiotics in *Salmonella* gastroenteritis

'In otherwise healthy adults or children with non-severe *Salmonella* diarrhoea, antibiotics have no clinical benefit over placebo, increase side-effects and prolong *Salmonella* detection.'

- Sirinavin S, Garner P. Antibiotics for treating salmonella gut infections. Cochrane Database of Systematic Reviews, 1999, issue 1. Art. no.: CD001167.

For further information: www.cochrane.org/cochrane-reviews

The incubation period of *Salmonella* gastroenteritis is 12–72 hours and the predominant feature is diarrhoea, sometimes with passage of blood. Vomiting may be present at the outset. Approximately 5% of cases are bacteraemic. Reactive (post-infective) arthritis occurs in approximately 2%.

Antibiotics are not indicated for uncomplicated *Salmonella* gastroenteritis (Box 13.48). However, evidence of bacteraemia is a clear indication for antibiotic therapy, as salmonellae are notorious for persistent infection and often colonise endothelial surfaces such as an atherosclerotic aorta or a major blood vessel. Mortality, as with other forms of gastroenteritis, is higher in the elderly (see Box 13.13, p. 306).

Escherichia coli infection

Many serotypes of *E. coli* are present in the human gut at any given time. Production of disease depends on either colonisation with a new or previously unrecognised strain, or the acquisition by current colonising bacteria of a particular pathogenicity factor for mucosal attachment or toxin production. Travel to unfamiliar areas of the world allows contact with different strains of endemic *E. coli* and the development of travellers' diarrhoea. Enteropathogenic strains may be found in the gut of healthy individuals and, if these people move to a new environment, close contacts may develop symptoms.

At least five different clinico-pathological patterns of diarrhoea are associated with specific strains of *E. coli* with characteristic virulence factors.

Enterotoxigenic E. coli

Enterotoxigenic *E. coli* (ETEC) cause the majority of cases of travellers' diarrhoea in developing countries, although there are other causes (see Box 13.21, p. 311). The organisms produce either a heat-labile or a heat-stable enterotoxin, causing marked secretory diarrhoea and vomiting after 1–2 days' incubation. The illness is usually mild and self-limiting after 3–4 days. Antibiotics, such as ciprofloxacin, have been used to limit the duration of symptoms (see Box 13.22, p. 311) but are of questionable value.

Entero-invasive E. coli

Illness caused by entero-invasive *E. coli* (EIEC) is very similar to *Shigella* dysentery (p. 345) and is caused by invasion and destruction of colonic mucosal cells. No enterotoxin is produced. Acute watery diarrhoea, abdominal cramps and some scanty blood-staining of the stool are common. The symptoms are rarely severe and are usually self-limiting.

Enteropathogenic E. coli

Enteropathogenic *E. coli* (EPEC) organisms are very important in infant diarrhoea. They are able to attach to the gut mucosa, inducing a specific 'attachment and effacement' lesion, and causing destruction of microvilli and disruption of normal absorptive capacity. The symptoms vary from mild non-bloody diarrhoea to quite severe illness, but without bacteraemia.

Entero-aggregative E. coli

Entero-aggregative *E. coli* (EAEC) strains adhere to the mucosa but also produce a locally active enterotoxin and demonstrate a particular 'stacked brick' aggregation to tissue culture cells when viewed by microscopy. They have been associated with prolonged diarrhoea in children in South America, South-east Asia and India.

Enterohaemorrhagic E. coli

A number of distinct 'O' serotypes of *E. coli* possess both the genes necessary for adherence (see 'EPEC' above) and plasmids encoding for two distinct enterotoxins (verotoxins) which are identical to the toxins produced by *Shigella* ('shiga toxins 1 and 2'). *E. coli* O157:H7 is perhaps the best-known of these verotoxin-producing *E. coli* (VTEC), but others, including types O126 and O11, are also implicated. In 2011, an outbreak of food-borne illness linked to fenugreek seeds occurred in Germany and was due to *E. coli* O104:H4, an EAEC strain that had acquired genes encoding shiga toxin 2a. Although the incidence of enterohaemorrhagic *E. coli* (EHEC) is considerably lower than that of *Campylobacter* and *Salmonella* infection, it is increasing in the developing world.

The reservoir of infection is in the gut of herbivores. The organism has an extremely low infecting dose (10–100 organisms). Runoff water from pasture lands where cattle have grazed, which is used to irrigate vegetable crops, as well as contaminated milk, meat products (especially hamburgers which have been incompletely cooked), lettuce, radish shoots and apple juice, have all been implicated as sources (Fig. 13.25).

The incubation period is between 1 and 7 days. Initial watery diarrhoea becomes frankly and uniformly blood-stained in 70% of cases and is associated with severe and often constant abdominal pain. There is little systemic upset, vomiting or fever.

Enterotoxins have both a local effect on the bowel and a distant effect on particular body tissues, such as glomerular apparatus, heart and brain. The potentially life-threatening haemolytic uraemic syndrome (HUS, p. 495) occurs in 10–15% of sufferers from this infection, arising 5–7 days after the onset of symptoms. It is most likely at the extremes of age, is heralded by a high peripheral leucocyte count, and may be induced, particularly in children, by antibiotic therapy.

HUS is treated by dialysis if necessary and may be averted by plasma exchange. Antibiotics should be avoided since they can stimulate toxin release.

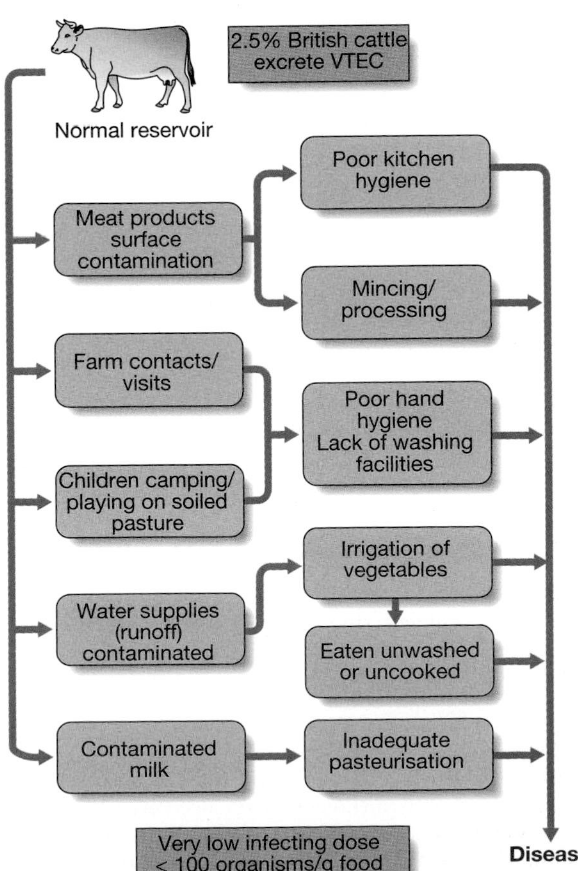

Fig. 13.25 Verocytotoxigenic *E. coli* (VTEC) infections.

Clostridium difficile infection

C. difficile is the most commonly diagnosed cause of antibiotic-associated diarrhoea (p. 308), and is an occasional constituent of the normal intestinal flora. *C. difficile* is capable of producing two toxins (A and B). *C. difficile* infection (CDI) usually follows antimicrobial therapy, which alters the composition of the gastrointestinal flora and may result in colonisation with *C. difficile* if the patient is exposed to *C. difficile* spores. The combination of toxin production and the ability to produce environmentally stable spores accounts for the clinical features and transmissibility of CDI. A hypervirulent strain of *C. difficile*, ribotype 027, has emerged, which produces more toxin than other *C. difficile* strains and thus more severe disease.

Clinical features

Disease manifestations range from diarrhoea to life-threatening pseudomembranous colitis. Around 80% of cases occur in people over 65 years of age, many of whom are frail with comorbid diseases. Symptoms usually begin in the first week of antibiotic therapy but can occur at any time up to 6 weeks after treatment has finished. The onset is often insidious, with lower abdominal pain and diarrhoea which may become profuse and watery. The presentation may resemble acute ulcerative colitis with bloody diarrhoea, fever and even toxic dilatation and perforation. Ileus is also seen in pseudomembranous colitis.

Investigations

C. difficile can be isolated from stool culture in 30% of patients with antibiotic-associated diarrhoea and over 90% of those with pseudomembranous colitis, but also from 5% of healthy adults and up to 20% of elderly patients in residential care. The diagnosis of CDI

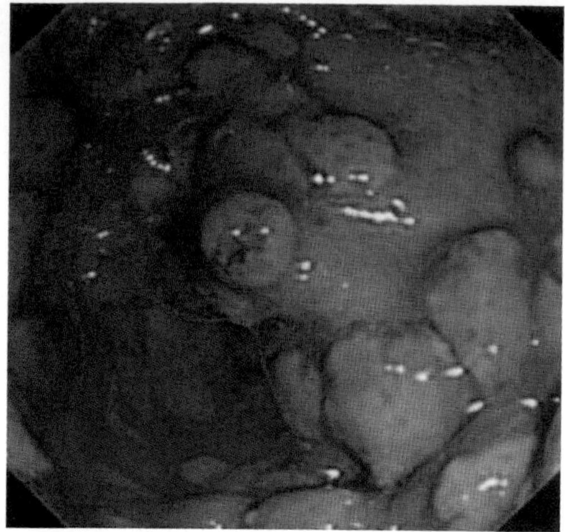

Fig. 13.26 ***Clostridium difficile*** **infection. Colonoscopic view showing numerous adherent 'pseudomembranes' on the mucosa.**

therefore rests on detection of toxins A or B in the stool. Current practice in the UK is to screen stool from patients with a compatible clinical syndrome by detection either of glutamate dehydrogenase (GDH), an enzyme produced by *C. difficile*, or of *C. difficile* nucleic acid (e.g. by PCR); if screening is positive, a *C. difficile* toxin ELISA or a tissue culture cytotoxicity assay is performed.

The rectal appearances at sigmoidoscopy may be characteristic, with erythema, white plaques or an adherent pseudomembrane (Fig. 13.26). Appearances may also resemble those of ulcerative colitis. In some cases, the rectum is spared and abnormalities are observed in the proximal colon. Patients who are ill may require abdominal and erect chest X-rays to exclude perforation or toxic dilatation. CT may be useful when the diagnosis is in doubt.

Management

The precipitating antibiotic should be stopped and the patient should be isolated. Supportive therapy with intravenous fluids and resting of the bowel is often needed. CDI is treated with antibiotics. The options for first-line therapy are metronidazole (500 mg orally 3 times daily for 10 days) or vancomycin (125 mg orally 4 times daily for 7–10 days). Although vancomycin is more effective than metronidazole against hypervirulent *C. difficile* strains (e.g. ribotype 027), it is more expensive and may drive the emergence of vancomycin resistance in other organisms (e.g. enterococci, *Staph. aureus*). For these reasons, some authorities reserve its use for relapse (15–30% of patients), failure of initial response or severe infection. A new agent, fidaxomicin, is associated with a lower relapse rate than vancomycin. Intravenous immunoglobulin and/or corticosteroids are sometimes given in the most severe or refractory cases and faecal transplantation is also emerging as a therapy in relapsing patients. Surgical intervention is sometimes needed and needs to be considered early in severe cases.

Yersinia enterocolitica infection

This organism, commonly found in pork, causes mild to moderate gastroenteritis and can produce significant mesenteric adenitis after an incubation period of 3–7 days. It predominantly causes disease in children but adults may also be affected. The illness resolves slowly, with 10–30% of cases complicated by persistent arthritis or Reiter's syndrome (p. 1107).

Cholera

Cholera, caused by *Vibrio cholerae* serotype O1, is the archetypal toxin-mediated bacterial cause of acute watery diarrhoea. The enterotoxin activates adenylate cyclase in the intestinal epithelium, inducing net secretion of chloride and water. *V. cholerae* O1 has two biotypes, classical and El Tor, and each of these has two distinct serotypes, Inaba and Ogawa. Following its origin in the Ganges valley, devastating epidemics have occurred, often in association with large religious festivals, and pandemics have spread worldwide. The seventh pandemic, due to the El Tor biotype, began in 1961 and spread via the Middle East to become endemic in Africa. In 1990, it reached Peru and spread throughout South and Central America. Since 2005, numbers of cases of cholera have been increasing. There are recurrent outbreaks and epidemics in Africa, often related to flooding. El Tor is more resistant to commonly used antimicrobials than classical *Vibrio*, and causes prolonged carriage in 5% of infections. A new classical toxigenic strain, serotype O139, established itself in Bangladesh in 1992 and started a new pandemic.

Infection spreads via the stools or vomit of symptomatic patients or of the much larger number of subclinical cases. Organisms survive for up to 2 weeks in fresh water and 8 weeks in salt water. Transmission is normally through infected drinking water, shellfish and food contaminated by flies, or on the hands of carriers.

Clinical features

Severe diarrhoea without pain or colic begins suddenly and is followed by vomiting. Following the evacuation of normal gut faecal contents, typical 'rice water' material is passed, consisting of clear fluid with flecks of mucus. Classical cholera produces enormous loss of fluid and electrolytes, leading to intense dehydration with muscular cramps. Shock and oliguria develop but mental clarity remains. Death from acute circulatory failure may occur rapidly unless fluid and electrolytes are replaced. Improvement is rapid with proper treatment.

The majority of infections, however, cause mild illness with slight diarrhoea. Occasionally, a very intense illness, 'cholera sicca', occurs, with loss of fluid into dilated bowel, killing the patient before typical gastrointestinal symptoms appear. The disease is more dangerous in children.

Diagnosis and management

Clinical diagnosis is easy during an epidemic. Otherwise, the diagnosis should be confirmed bacteriologically. Stool dark-field microscopy shows the typical 'shooting star' motility of *V. cholerae*. Rectal swab or stool cultures allow identification. Cholera is notifiable under international health regulations.

Maintenance of circulation by replacement of water and electrolytes is paramount (p. 307). Ringer-Lactate is the best fluid for intravenous replacement. Vomiting usually stops once the patient is rehydrated, and fluid should then be given orally up to 500 mL hourly. Early intervention with oral rehydration solutions that include resistant starch, based on either rice or cereal, shortens the duration of diarrhoea and improves prognosis. Total fluid requirements may exceed 50 L over a period of 2–5 days. Accurate records are greatly facilitated by the use of a 'cholera cot', which has a reinforced hole under the patient's buttocks, beneath which a graded bucket is placed.

Three days treatment with tetracycline 250 mg 4 times daily, a single dose of doxycycline 300 mg or ciprofloxacin 1 g in adults reduces the duration of excretion of *V. cholerae* and the total volume of fluid needed for replacement.

Prevention

Strict personal hygiene is vital and drinking water should come from a clean piped supply or be boiled. Flies must be denied access to food. Parenteral vaccination with a killed suspension of *V. cholerae* provides some protection. Oral vaccines containing killed *V. cholerae* and the B subunit of cholera toxin are available but are of limited efficacy.

In epidemics, public education and control of water sources and population movement are vital. Mass single-dose vaccination and treatment with tetracycline are valuable. Disinfection of discharges and soiled clothing, and scrupulous hand-washing by medical attendants reduce the danger of spread.

Vibrio parahaemolyticus infection

This marine organism produces a disease similar to enterotoxigenic *E. coli* (see above). It is acquired from raw seafood and is very common where ingestion of such food is widespread (e.g. Japan). After an incubation period of approximately 20 hours, explosive diarrhoea, abdominal cramps and vomiting occur. Systemic symptoms of headache and fever are frequent but the illness is self-limiting after 4–7 days. Rarely, a severe septicaemic illness arises; in this case, *V. parahaemolyticus* can be isolated using specific halophilic culture.

Bacillary dysentery (shigellosis)

Shigellae are Gram-negative rods, closely related to *E. coli,* that invade the colonic mucosa. There are four main groups: *Sh. dysenteriae, flexneri, boydii* and *sonnei.* In the tropics, bacillary dysentery is usually caused by *Sh. flexneri,* whilst in the UK most cases are caused by *Sh. sonnei.* Shigellae are often resistant to multiple antibiotics, especially in tropical countries. The organism only infects humans and its spread is facilitated by its low infecting dose of around 10 organisms.

Spread may occur via contaminated food or flies, but transmission by unwashed hands after defecation is by far the most important factor. Outbreaks occur in mental hospitals, residential schools and other closed institutions, and dysentery is a constant accompaniment of wars and natural catastrophes, which bring crowding and poor sanitation in their wake. *Shigella* infection may spread rapidly amongst men who have sex with men.

Clinical features

Disease severity varies from mild *Sh. sonnei* infections that may escape detection to more severe *Sh. flexneri* infections, while those due to *Sh. dysenteriae* may be fulminating and cause death within 48 hours.

In a moderately severe illness, the patient complains of diarrhoea, colicky abdominal pain and tenesmus. Stools are small, and after a few evacuations contain blood and purulent exudate with little faecal material. Fever, dehydration and weakness occur, with tenderness over the colon. Arthritis or iritis may occasionally complicate bacillary dysentery (Reiter's syndrome, p. 1107), associated with HLA-B27.

Management and prevention

Oral rehydration therapy or, if diarrhoea is severe, intravenous replacement of water and electrolyte loss is necessary. Antibiotic therapy with ciprofloxacin (500 mg twice daily for 3 days) is effective in known shigellosis and appropriate in epidemics. The use of antidiarrhoeal medication should be avoided.

The prevention of faecal contamination of food and milk and the isolation of cases may be difficult, except in limited outbreaks. Hand-washing is very important.

Respiratory bacterial infections

Most of these infections are described in Chapter 19.

Diphtheria

Infection with *Corynebacterium diphtheriae* occurs most commonly in the upper respiratory tract and is usually spread by droplet infection. Infection may also complicate skin lesions, especially in those who misuse alcohol. The organisms remain localised at the site of infection but release of a soluble exotoxin damages the heart muscle and the nervous system.

Diphtheria has been eradicated from many parts of the world by mass vaccination using a modified exotoxin but remains important in areas where vaccination has been incomplete, e.g. in Russia and South-east Asia. The disease is notifiable in all countries of Europe and North America, and international guidelines have been issued by the WHO for the management of infection.

Clinical features

The average incubation period is 2–4 days. The disease begins insidiously with a sore throat (Box 13.49). Despite modest fever, there is usually marked tachycardia. The diagnostic feature is the 'wash-leather' elevated, greyish-green membrane on the tonsils. It has a well-defined edge, is firm and adherent, and is surrounded by a zone of inflammation. There may be swelling of the neck ('bull neck') and tender enlargement of the lymph nodes. In the mildest infections, especially in the presence of a high degree of immunity, a membrane may never appear and the throat is merely slightly inflamed.

13.49 Clinical features of diphtheria

Acute infection
• Membranous tonsillitis • *or* Nasal infection • *or* Laryngeal infection • *or* Skin/wound/conjunctival infection (rare)
Complications
• Laryngeal obstruction or paralysis • Myocarditis • Peripheral neuropathy

With anterior nasal infection there is nasal discharge, frequently blood-stained. In laryngeal diphtheria, a husky voice and high-pitched cough signal potential respiratory obstruction requiring urgent tracheostomy. If infection spreads to the uvula, fauces and nasopharynx, the patient is gravely ill.

Death from acute circulatory failure may occur within the first 10 days. Late complications arise as a result of toxin action on the heart or nervous system. About 25% of survivors of the early toxaemia may later develop myocarditis with arrhythmias or cardiac failure. These are usually reversible, with no permanent damage other than heart block in survivors.

Neurological involvement occurs in 75% of cases. After tonsillar or pharyngeal diphtheria, it usually starts after 10 days with palatal palsy. Paralysis of accommodation often follows, manifest by difficulty in reading small print. Generalised polyneuritis with weakness and paraesthesia may follow in the next 10–14 days. Recovery from such neuritis is always ultimately complete.

Management

A clinical diagnosis of diphtheria must be notified to the public health authorities and the patient sent urgently to a specialist infectious diseases unit. Treatment should begin once appropriate swabs have been taken before waiting for microbiological confirmation.

Diphtheria antitoxin is produced from hyperimmune horse serum. It neutralises circulating toxin but has no effect on toxin already fixed to tissues, so it must be injected intramuscularly without awaiting the result of a throat swab. However, reactions to this foreign protein include a potentially lethal immediate anaphylactic reaction (p. 91) and a 'serum sickness' with fever, urticaria and joint pains, which occurs 7–12 days after injection. A careful history of previous horse serum injections or allergic reactions should be taken and a small test injection of serum should be given half an hour before the full dose in every patient. Adrenaline (epinephrine) solution must be available to deal with any immediate type of reaction (0.5–1.0 mL of 1/1000 solution IM). An antihistamine is also given. In a severely ill patient, the risk of anaphylactic shock is outweighed by the mortal danger of diphtheritic toxaemia, and up to 100 000 U of antitoxin are injected intravenously if the test dose has not given rise to symptoms. For disease of moderate severity, 16 000–40 000 U IM will suffice, and for mild cases 4000–8000 U.

Penicillin (1200 mg 4 times daily IV) or amoxicillin (500 mg 3 times daily) should be administered for 2 weeks to eliminate *C. diphtheriae*. Patients allergic to penicillin can be given erythromycin. Due to poor immunogenicity of primary infection, all sufferers should be immunised with diphtheria toxoid following recovery.

Patients must be managed in strict isolation and attended by staff with a clearly documented immunisation history until three swabs 24 hours apart are culture-negative.

Prevention

Active immunisation should be given to all children. If diphtheria occurs in a closed community, contacts should be given erythromycin, which is more effective than penicillin in eradicating the organism in carriers.

All contacts should also be immunised or given a booster dose of toxoid. Booster doses are required every 10 years to maintain immunity.

Pneumococcal infection

Strep. pneumoniae (the pneumococcus) is the leading cause of community-acquired pneumonia globally (p. 682) and one of the leading causes of infection-related mortality. Otitis media, meningitis and sinusitis are also frequently due to *Strep. pneumoniae*. Occasional patients present with bacteraemia without obvious focus. Asplenic individuals are at risk of fulminant pneumococcal disease with purpuric rash.

Increasing rates of penicillin resistance have been reported around the world for *Strep. pneumoniae*, although they remain relatively low in the UK. Strains with high-level resistance causing meningitis require treatment with glycopeptides rather than with penicillins or cephalosporins. Macrolide resistance is also increasing. Newer quinolones are also used but rates of resistance are rising.

Vaccination of infants with the protein conjugate pneumococcal vaccine decreases *Strep. pneumoniae* infection in infants and in their relatives. The polysaccharide pneumococcal vaccine is used in individuals predisposed to *Strep. pneumoniae* infection and the elderly, but only modestly reduces pneumococcal bacteraemia and does not prevent pneumonia. All asplenic individuals should receive vaccination against *Strep. pneumoniae*.

Anthrax

Anthrax is an endemic zoonosis in many countries; it causes human disease following inoculation of the spores of *Bacillus anthracis*. *B. anthracis* was the first-recognised bacterial pathogen described by Koch and became the model pathogen for 'Koch's postulates' (Box 6.1, p. 134). It is a Gram-positive organism with a central spore. The spores can survive for years in soil. Infection is commonly acquired from contact with animals, particularly herbivores. The ease of production of *B. anthracis* spores makes this infection a candidate for biological warfare or bioterrorism. *B. anthracis* produces a number of toxins which mediate the clinical features of disease.

Clinical features

These depend on the route of entry of the anthrax spores.

Cutaneous anthrax

This skin lesion is associated with occupational exposure to anthrax spores during processing of hides and bone products. It accounts for the vast majority of clinical cases. Animal infection is a serious problem in Africa, India, Pakistan and the Middle East.

Spores are inoculated into exposed skin. A single lesion develops as an irritable papule on an oedematous haemorrhagic base. This progresses to a depressed black eschar. Despite extensive oedema, pain is infrequent.

Gastrointestinal anthrax

This is associated with the ingestion of contaminated meat products. The caecum is the seat of the infection, which produces nausea, vomiting, anorexia and fever, followed in 2–3 days by severe abdominal pain and bloody diarrhoea. Toxaemia and death can develop rapidly thereafter.

Inhalational anthrax

This form of the disease is extremely rare but has been associated with bioterrorism. Without rapid and aggressive therapy at the onset of symptoms, the mortality is 50–90%. Fever, dyspnoea, cough, headache and symptoms of septicaemia develop 3–14 days following exposure. Typically, the chest X-ray shows only widening of the mediastinum and pleural effusions, which are haemorrhagic. Meningitis may occur.

Management

B. anthracis can be cultured from skin swabs from lesions. Skin lesions are readily curable with early antibiotic therapy. Treatment is with ciprofloxacin (500 mg twice daily) until penicillin susceptibility is confirmed; the regimen can then be changed to benzylpenicillin with doses up to 2.4 g IV given 6 times daily or phenoxymethylpenicillin 500–1000 mg 4 times daily administered for 10 days. The addition of an aminoglycoside may improve the outlook in severe disease. In view of concerns about concomitant inhalational exposure, particularly in the era of bioterrorism, a further 2-month course of ciprofloxacin 500 mg twice daily or doxycycline 100 mg twice daily orally is added. Prophylaxis with ciprofloxacin (500 mg twice daily) is recommended for anyone at high risk of exposure to anthrax spores.

Bacterial infections with neurological involvement

Infections affecting the CNS, including bacterial meningitis, botulism and tetanus, are described on page 1201.

Mycobacterial infections

Tuberculosis is predominantly, although by no means exclusively, a respiratory disease and is described on page 688.

Leprosy

Leprosy (Hansen's disease) is a chronic granulomatous disease affecting skin and nerves, and is caused by *Mycobacterium leprae*, a slow-growing mycobacterium which cannot be cultured in vitro. The clinical manifestations are determined by the degree of the patient's cell-mediated immunity (CMI, p. 78) towards *M. leprae* (Fig. 13.27). High levels of CMI with elimination of leprosy bacilli produces tuberculoid leprosy, whereas absent CMI results in lepromatous leprosy. The complications of leprosy are due to nerve damage, immunological reactions and bacillary infiltration. Leprosy patients are frequently stigmatised and using the word 'leper' is inappropriate.

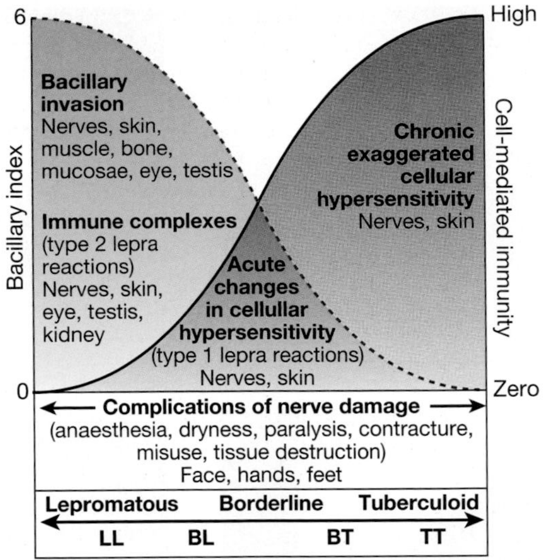

Fig. 13.27 Leprosy: mechanisms of damage and tissue affected. Mechanisms under the broken line are characteristic of disease near the lepromatous end of the spectrum, and those under the solid line are characteristic of the tuberculoid end. They overlap in the centre where, in addition, instability predisposes to type 1 lepra reactions. At the peak in the centre, neither bacillary growth nor cell-mediated immunity has the upper hand (BL = borderline lepromatous; BT = borderline tuberculoid). Based on Bryceson and Pfaltzgraff 1990 – see p. 386.

Epidemiology and transmission

Some 4 million people have leprosy and around 750 000 new cases are detected annually. About 70% of the world's leprosy patients live in India, with the disease endemic in Brazil, Indonesia, Mozambique, Madagascar, Tanzania and Nepal.

Untreated lepromatous patients discharge bacilli from the nose. Infection occurs through the nose, followed by haematogenous spread to skin and nerve. The incubation period is 2–5 years for tuberculoid cases and 8–12 years for lepromatous cases. Leprosy incidence peaks at 10–14 years, and is more common in males and in those with close household exposure to leprosy cases.

Pathogenesis

M. leprae has a predilection for infecting Schwann cells and skin macrophages. In tuberculoid leprosy, effective CMI controls bacillary multiplication ('paucibacillary') but organised epithelioid granulomas are formed. In lepromatous leprosy, there is abundant bacillary multiplication ('multibacillary'), e.g. in Schwann cells and perineurium. Between these two extremes is a continuum, varying from patients with moderate CMI (borderline tuberculoid) to patients with little cellular response (borderline lepromatous).

In addition, immunological reactions to the infection occur as the immune response develops and the antigenic stimulus from the bacilli varies, particularly in borderline patients. Delayed hypersensitivity reactions produce type 1 (reversal) reactions, while immune complexes contribute to type 2 (erythema nodosum leprosum) reactions.

HIV/leprosy co-infected patients have typical lepromatous and tuberculoid leprosy skin lesions and typical leprosy histology and granuloma formation. Surprisingly, even with low circulating CD4 counts, tuberculoid leprosy may be observed and there is not an obvious shift to lepromatous leprosy.

Clinical features

Box 13.50 gives the cardinal features of leprosy. Types of leprosy are compared in Box 13.51.

- *Skin.* The most common skin lesions are macules or plaques. Tuberculoid patients have few,

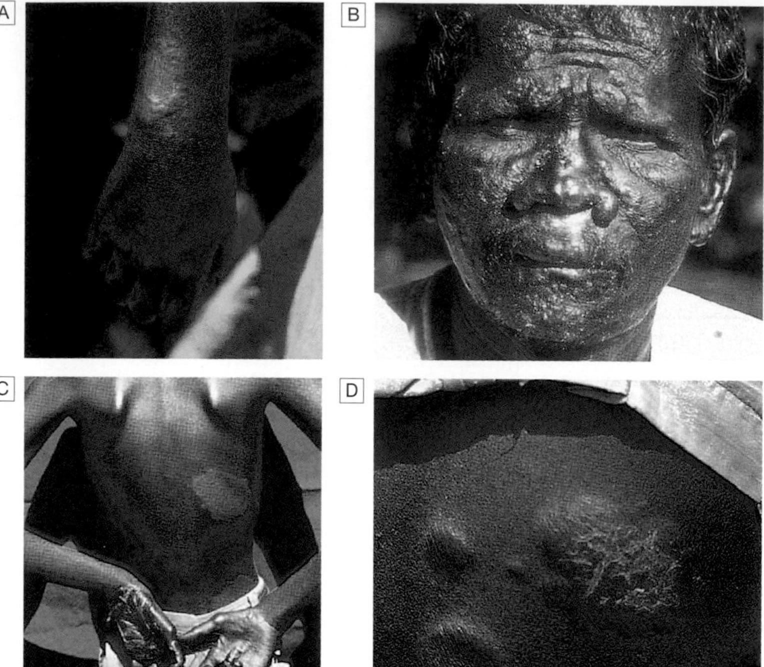

Fig. 13.28 Clinical features of leprosy. **A** Tuberculoid leprosy. Single lesion with a well-defined active edge and anaesthesia within the lesion. **B** Lepromatous leprosy. Widespread nodules and infiltration, with loss of the eyebrows. This man also has early collapse of the nose. **C** Borderline tuberculoid leprosy with severe nerve damage. This boy has several well-defined, hypopigmented, macular, anaesthetic lesions. He has severe nerve damage affecting both ulnar and median nerves bilaterally and has sustained severe burns to his hands. **D** Reversal (type 1) reactions. Erythematous, oedematous lesions.

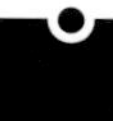

13.50 Cardinal features of leprosy

- Skin lesions, typically anaesthetic at tuberculoid end of spectrum
- Thickened peripheral nerves
- Acid-fast bacilli on skin smears or biopsy

hypopigmented lesions (Fig. 13.28A). In lepromatous leprosy, papules, nodules or diffuse infiltration of the skin occur. The earliest lesions are ill defined; gradually, the skin becomes infiltrated and thickened. Facial skin thickening leads to the characteristic leonine facies (Fig. 13.28B).

- *Anaesthesia.* In skin lesions, the small dermal sensory and autonomic nerve fibres are damaged, causing local sensory loss and loss of sweating within that area. Anaesthesia may also occur in the distribution of a damaged large peripheral nerve. A 'glove and stocking' sensory neuropathy is also common in lepromatous leprosy.
- *Nerve damage.* Peripheral nerve trunks are affected at 'sites of predilection'. These are the ulnar (elbow), median (wrist), radial (humerus), radial cutaneous (wrist), common peroneal (knee), posterior tibial and sural nerves (ankle), facial nerve (zygomatic arch) and great auricular nerve (posterior triangle of the neck). Damage to peripheral nerve trunks produces characteristic signs with regional sensory loss and muscle dysfunction (Fig. 13.28C). All these nerves should be examined for enlargement and tenderness and tested for motor and sensory function. The CNS is not affected.
- *Eye involvement.* Blindness is a devastating complication for a patient with anaesthetic hands and feet. Eyelid closure is impaired when the facial

13.51 Clinical characteristics of the polar forms of leprosy

Clinical and tissue-specific features	Lepromatous	Tuberculoid
Skin and nerves		
Number and distribution	Widely disseminated	One or a few sites, asymmetrical
Skin lesions		
Definition		
Clarity of margin	Poor	Good
Elevation of margin	Never	Common
Colour		
Dark skin	Slight hypopigmentation	Marked hypopigmentation
Light skin	Slight erythema	Coppery or red
Surface	Smooth, shiny	Dry, scaly
Central healing	None	Common
Sweat and hair growth	Impaired late	Impaired early
Loss of sensation	Late	Early and marked
Nerve enlargement and damage	Late	Early and marked
Bacilli (bacterial index)	Many (5 or 6+)	Absent (0)
Natural history	Progressive	Self-healing
Other tissues	Upper respiratory mucosa, eye, testes, bones, muscle	None
Reactions	Immune complexes (type 2)	Cell-mediated (type 1)

nerve is affected. Damage to the trigeminal nerve causes anaesthesia of the cornea and conjunctiva. The cornea is then susceptible to trauma and ulceration.

- *Other features.* Many organs can be affected. Nasal collapse occurs secondary to bacillary destruction of the bony nasal spine. Diffuse infiltration of the testes causes testicular atrophy and the acute orchitis that occurs with type 2 reactions. This results in azoospermia and hypogonadism.

Leprosy reactions

Leprosy reactions (Box 13.52) are events superimposed on the cardinal features shown in Box 13.50.

- *Type 1 (reversal) reactions.* These occur in 30% of borderline patients (BT, BB or BL) and are delayed hypersensitivity reactions. Skin lesions become erythematous (Fig. 13.28D). Peripheral nerves become tender and painful, with sudden loss of nerve function. These reactions may occur spontaneously, after starting treatment and also after completion of multidrug therapy.
- *Type 2 (erythema nodosum leprosum, ENL) reactions.* These are partly due to immune complex deposition and occur in BL and LL patients who produce antibodies and have a high antigen load. They manifest with malaise, fever and crops of small pink nodules on the face and limbs. Iritis and episcleritis are common. Other signs are acute neuritis, lymphadenitis, orchitis, bone pain, dactylitis, arthritis and proteinuria. ENL may continue intermittently for several years.

Borderline cases

In borderline tuberculoid (BT) cases, skin lesions are more numerous than in tuberculoid (TT) cases, and there is more severe nerve damage and a risk of type 1 reactions. In borderline leprosy (BB) cases, skin lesions are numerous and vary in size, shape and distribution; annular lesions are characteristic and nerve damage is variable. In borderline lepromatous (BL) cases, there are widespread small macules in the skin and widespread nerve involvement; both type 1 and type 2 reactions occur.

Pure neural leprosy (i.e. without skin lesions) occurs principally in India and accounts for 10% of patients. There is asymmetrical involvement of peripheral nerve trunks and no visible skin lesions. On nerve biopsy, all types of leprosy have been found.

Investigations

The diagnosis is clinical, made by finding a cardinal sign of leprosy and supported by finding acid-fast bacilli in slit-skin smears or typical histology in a skin biopsy. Slit-skin smears are obtained by scraping dermal material on to a glass slide. The smears are then stained for acid-fast bacilli, the number counted per high-power field and a score derived on a logarithmic scale (0–6): the bacterial index (BI). Smears are useful for confirming the diagnosis and monitoring response to treatment. Neither serology nor PCR testing for *M. leprae* DNA is sensitive or specific enough for diagnosis.

Management

The principles of treatment are outlined in Box 13.53. All leprosy patients should be given multidrug treatment (MDT) with an approved first-line regimen (Box 13.54).

13.52 Reactions in leprosy

	Lepra reaction type 1 (reversal)	Lepra reaction type 2 (erythema nodosum leprosum)
Mechanism	Cell-mediated hypersensitivity	Immune complexes
Clinical features	Painful tender nerves, loss of function Swollen skin lesions New skin lesions	Tender papules and nodules; may ulcerate Painful tender nerves, loss of function Iritis, orchitis, myositis, lymphadenitis Fever, oedema
Management	Prednisolone 40 mg, reducing over 3–6 mths[1]	Moderate: prednisolone 40 mg daily Severe: thalidomide[2] or prednisolone 40–80 mg daily, reducing over 1–6 mths; local if eye involved[3]

[1]Indicated for any new impairment of nerve or eye function.
[2]Contraindicated in women who may become pregnant.
[3]1% hydrocortisone drops or ointment and 1% atropine drops.

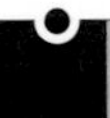

13.53 Principles of leprosy treatment

- Stop the infection with chemotherapy
- Treat reactions
- Educate the patient about leprosy
- Prevent disability
- Support the patient socially and psychologically

13.54 Modified WHO-recommended multidrug therapy (MDT) regimens in leprosy

Type of leprosy[1]	Monthly supervised treatment	Daily self-administered treatment	Duration of treatment[2]
Paucibacillary	Rifampicin 600 mg	Dapsone 100 mg	6 mths
Multibacillary	Rifampicin 600 mg Clofazimine 300 mg	Clofazimine 50 mg Dapsone 100 mg	12 mths
Paucibacillary single-lesion	Ofloxacin 400 mg Rifampicin 600 mg Minocycline 100 mg		Single dose

[1]Classification uses the bacillary index (BI) in slit-skin smears or, if BI is not available, the number of skin lesions:
- paucibacillary single-lesion leprosy (one skin lesion)
- paucibacillary (2–5 skin lesions)
- multibacillary (> 5 skin lesions).

[2]Studies from India have shown that multibacillary patients with an initial BI > 4 need longer treatment, for at least 24 mths.

Rifampicin is a potent bactericidal for *M. leprae* but should always be given in combination with other antileprotics, since a single-step mutation can confer resistance. Dapsone is bacteriostatic. It commonly causes mild haemolysis and rarely anaemia. Clofazimine is a red, fat-soluble crystalline dye, weakly bactericidal for *M. leprae*. Skin discoloration (red to purple-black) and ichthyosis are troublesome side-effects, particularly on pale skins. New drugs that are bactericidal for *M. leprae* have been identified, notably the fluoroquinolones pefloxacin and ofloxacin, minocycline and clarithromycin. These agents are now established second-line drugs. Minocycline causes a grey pigmentation of skin lesions.

Although single-dose treatment is less effective than the conventional 6-month treatment for paucibacillary leprosy, it is an operationally attractive field regimen and has been recommended for use by the WHO.

Lepra reactions are treated as shown in Box 13.52. Chloroquine can also be used.

Patient education

Educating leprosy patients about their disease is vital. Patients should be reassured that, after 3 days of chemotherapy, they are not infectious and can lead a normal social life. It should be emphasised that gross deformities are not inevitable.

Patients with anaesthetic hands or feet need to take special care to avoid and treat burns and other minor injuries. Good footwear is important. Physiotherapy may be required to maintain range of movement of affected muscles and neighbouring joints.

Prognosis

Untreated, tuberculoid leprosy has a good prognosis; it may self-heal and peripheral nerve damage is limited. Lepromatous leprosy (LL) is a progressive condition with high morbidity if untreated.

After treatment, the majority of patients, especially those who have no nerve damage at the time of diagnosis, do well, with resolution of skin lesions. Borderline patients are at risk of developing type 1 reactions, which may result in devastating nerve damage.

Prevention and control

The previous strategy of centralised leprosy control campaigns has now been superseded by integrated programmes, with primary health-care workers in many countries now responsible for case detection and provision of MDT. It is not yet clear how successful this will be, especially in the time-consuming area of disability prevention.

BCG vaccination has been shown to give good but variable protection against leprosy; adding killed *M. leprae* to BCG does not enhance protection.

Rickettsial and related intracellular bacterial infections

Rickettsial fevers

The rickettsial fevers are the most common tick-borne infections. It is important to ask potentially infected patients about contact with ticks, lice or fleas. There are two main groups of rickettsial fevers: spotted fevers and typhus (Box 13.55).

Pathogenesis

The rickettsiae are intracellular Gram-negative organisms which parasitise the intestinal canal of arthropods. Infection is usually conveyed to humans through the skin from the excreta of arthropods, but the saliva of some biting vectors is infected. The organisms multiply in capillary endothelial cells, producing lesions in the skin, CNS, heart, lungs, liver, kidneys and skeletal muscles. Endothelial proliferation, associated with a perivascular reaction, may cause thrombosis and purpura. In epidemic typhus, the brain is the target organ; in scrub typhus, the cardiovascular system and lungs in particular are attacked. An eschar, a black necrotic crusted sore, is often found in tick- and mite-borne typhus (see Fig. 13.6C, p. 313). This is due to vasculitis following immunological recognition of the inoculated organism. Regional lymph nodes often enlarge.

Spotted fever group

Rocky Mountain spotted fever

Rickettsia rickettsii is transmitted by tick bites. It is widely distributed and increasing in western and south-eastern states of the USA and also in Central and South America. The incubation period is about 7 days. The rash appears on about the third or fourth day of illness, looking at first like measles, but in a few hours a typical maculopapular eruption develops. The rash spreads in 24–48 hours from wrists, forearms and ankles to the back, limbs and chest, and then to the abdomen, where it is least pronounced. Larger cutaneous and subcutaneous haemorrhages may appear in severe cases. The liver and spleen become palpable. At the extremes of life, the mortality is 2–12%.

Other spotted fevers

R. conorii (boutonneuse fever) and *R. africae* (African tick fever) cause Mediterranean and African tick typhus, which also occurs on the Indian subcontinent. The incubation period is approximately 7 days. Infected ticks may be picked up by walking on grasslands, or dogs may bring ticks into the house. Careful examination might reveal a diagnostic eschar, and the maculopapular rash on the trunk, limbs, palms and soles. There may be delirium and meningeal signs in severe infections but recovery is usual. *R. africae* can be associated with multiple eschars. Some cases, particularly those with *R. africae*, present without rash ('spotless spotted fever'). Other spotted fevers are shown in Box 13.55.

Typhus group

Scrub typhus fever

Scrub typhus is caused by *Orientia tsutsugamushi* (formerly *Rickettsia tsutsugamushi*), transmitted by mites. It occurs in the Far East, Myanmar, Pakistan, Bangladesh, India, Indonesia, the South Pacific islands and Queensland, particularly where patches of forest cleared for plantations have attracted rats and mites.

In many patients, one eschar or more develops, surrounded by an area of cellulitis (see Fig. 13.6C, p. 313) and enlargement of regional lymph nodes. The incubation period is about 9 days.

Mild or subclinical cases are common. The onset of symptoms is usually sudden, with headache (often retro-orbital), fever, malaise, weakness and cough. In severe illness, the general symptoms increase, with

13.55 Features of rickettsial infections

Disease	Organism	Reservoir	Vector	Geographical area	Rash	Gangrene	Target organs	Mortality
Spotted fever group								
Rocky Mountain spotted fever	*R. rickettsii*	Rodents, dogs, ticks	*Ixodes* tick	North, Central and South America	Morbilliform Haemorrhagic	Often	Bronchi, myocardium, brain, skin	2–12%[2]
Boutonneuse fever	*R. conorii*	Rodents, dogs, ticks	*Ixodes* tick	Mediterranean, Africa, South-west Asia, India	Maculopapular	–	Skin, meninges	2.5%[3]
Siberian tick typhus	*R. siberica*	Rodents, birds, domestic animals, ticks	Various ticks	Siberia, Mongolia, northern China	Maculopapular	–	Skin, meninges	Rare[3]
Australian tick typhus	*R. australis*	Rodents, ticks	Ticks	Australia	Maculopapular	–	Skin, meninges	Rare[3]
Oriental spotted fever	*R. japonica*	Rodents, dogs, ticks	Ticks	Japan	Maculopapular	–	Skin, meninges	Rare[3]
African tick bite fever[1]	*R. africae*	Cattle, game, ticks	*Ixodes* tick	South Africa	Can be spotless	–	Skin, meninges	Rare[3]
Typhus group								
Scrub typhus	*Orientia tsutsugamushi*	Rodents	*Trombicula* mite	South-east Asia	Maculopapular	Unusual	Bronchi, myocardium, brain, skin	Rare[3]
Epidemic typhus	*R. prowazekii*	Humans	Louse	Worldwide	Morbilliform Haemorrhagic	Often	Brain, skin, bronchi, myocardium	Up to 40%
Endemic typhus	*R. typhi*	Rats	Flea	Worldwide	Slight	–	–	Rare[3]

[1]Eschar at bite site and local lymphadenopathy. [2]Highest in adult males. [3]Except in infants, older people and the debilitated.

apathy and prostration. An erythematous maculopapular rash often appears on about the 5th–7th day and spreads to the trunk, face and limbs, including the palms and soles, with generalised painless lymphadenopathy. The rash fades by the 14th day. The temperature rises rapidly and continues as a remittent fever (i.e. the difference between maximum and minimum temperature exceeds 1°C), remaining above normal with sweating until it falls on the 12th–18th day. In severe infection, the patient is prostrate with cough, pneumonia, confusion and deafness. Cardiac failure, renal failure and haemorrhage may develop. Convalescence is often slow and tachycardia may persist for some weeks.

Epidemic (louse-borne) typhus

Epidemic typhus is caused by *R. prowazekii* and is transmitted by infected faeces of the human body louse, usually through scratching the skin. Patients suffering from epidemic typhus infect the lice, which leave when the patient is febrile. In conditions of overcrowding, the disease spreads rapidly. It is prevalent in parts of Africa, especially Ethiopia and Rwanda, and in the South American Andes and Afghanistan. Large epidemics have occurred in Europe, usually as a sequel to war. The incubation period is usually 12–14 days.

There may be a few days of malaise but the onset is more often sudden, with rigors, fever, frontal headaches, pains in the back and limbs, constipation and bronchitis. The face is flushed and cyanotic, the eyes are congested and the patient becomes confused. The rash appears on the 4th–6th day. In its early stages, it disappears on pressure but soon becomes petechial with subcutaneous mottling. It appears first on the anterior folds of the axillae, sides of the abdomen or backs of hands, then on the trunk and forearms. The neck and face are seldom affected. During the second week, symptoms increase in severity. Sores develop on the lips. The tongue becomes dry, brown, shrunken and tremulous. The spleen is palpable, the pulse feeble and the patient stuporous and delirious. The temperature falls rapidly at the end of the second week and the patient recovers gradually. In fatal cases, the patient usually dies in the second week from toxaemia, cardiac or renal failure, or pneumonia.

Endemic (flea-borne) typhus

Flea-borne or 'endemic' typhus caused by *R. typhi* is endemic worldwide. Humans are infected when the faeces or contents of a crushed flea, which has fed on an infected rat, are introduced into the skin. The incubation period is 8–14 days. The symptoms resemble those of a mild louse-borne typhus. The rash may be scanty and transient.

Investigation of rickettsial infection

Routine blood investigations are not diagnostic but malaria must be excluded by blood film examination in most cases, and there is usually hepatitis and thrombocytopenia. Diagnosis is made on clinical grounds and response to treatment, and may be confirmed by antibody detection or PCR in specialised laboratories. Differential diagnoses include malaria, typhoid, meningococcal sepsis and leptospirosis.

Management of rickettsial fevers

The different rickettsial fevers vary greatly in severity but all respond to tetracycline 500 mg 4 times daily, doxycycline 200 mg daily or chloramphenicol 500 mg 4 times daily for 7 days. Louse-borne typhus and scrub typhus can be treated with a single dose of 200 mg doxycycline, repeated for 2–3 days to prevent relapse. Chloramphenicol- and doxycycline-resistant strains of *O. tsutsugamushi* have been reported from Thailand and patients here may need treatment with rifampicin.

Nursing care is important, especially in epidemic typhus. Sedation may be required for delirium and blood transfusion for haemorrhage. Relapsing fever and typhoid are common intercurrent infections in epidemic typhus, and pneumonia in scrub typhus. They must be sought and treated. Convalescence is usually protracted, especially in older people.

To prevent rickettsial infection, lice, fleas, ticks and mites need to be controlled with insecticides.

Q fever

Q fever occurs worldwide and is caused by the rickettsia-like organism *Coxiella burnetii*, an obligate intracellular organism that can survive in the extracellular environment. Cattle, sheep and goats are important reservoirs and the organism is transmitted by inhalation of aerosolised particles. An important characteristic of *C. burnetii* is its antigenic variation, called phase variation, due to a change of lipopolysaccharide (LPS). When isolated from animals or humans, *C. burnetii* expresses phase I antigen and is very infectious (a single bacterium is sufficient to infect a human). In culture, there is an antigenic shift to the phase II form, which is not infectious. This antigenic shift can be measured and is valuable for the differentiation of acute and chronic Q fever.

Clinical features

The incubation period is 3–4 weeks. The initial symptoms are non-specific with fever, headache and chills; in 20% of cases, a maculopapular rash occurs. Other presentations include pneumonia and hepatitis. Chronic Q fever may present with osteomyelitis, encephalitis and endocarditis.

Investigations and management

Diagnosis is usually serological and the stage of the infection can be distinguished by isotype tests and phase-specific antigens. Phase I and II IgM titres peak at 4–6 weeks. In chronic infections, IgG titres to phase I and II antigens may be raised.

Prompt treatment of acute Q fever with doxycycline reduces fever duration. Treatment of Q fever endocarditis is problematic, requiring prolonged therapy with doxycycline and rifampicin or ciprofloxacin with hydroxychloroquine; even then, organisms are not always eradicated. Valve surgery is often required (p. 629).

Bartonellosis

This group of diseases are caused by intracellular Gram-negative bacilli closely related to the rickettsiae, which have been discovered to be important causes of 'culture-negative' endocarditis. They are found in many domestic pets, such as cats, although for several the host is ill defined (Box 13.56). The principal human pathogens are *Bartonella quintana*, *B. henselae* and *B. bacilliformis*. *Bartonella* infections are associated with the following:

- *Trench fever*. This is a relapsing fever with severe leg pain and is caused by *B. quintana*. The disease is not fatal but is very debilitating.
- *Bacteraemia and endocarditis in the homeless*. Endocarditis due to *B. quintana* or *henselae* is associated with severe damage to the heart valves.
- *Cat scratch disease*. *B. henselae* causes this common benign lymphadenopathy in children and young adults. A vesicle or papule develops on the head, neck or arms after a cat scratch. The lesion resolves spontaneously but there may be regional lymphadenopathy that persists for up to 4 months before also resolving spontaneously.
- *Bacillary angiomatosis*. This is an HIV-associated disease caused by *B. quintana* or *henselae* (p. 398).
- *Oroya fever and verruga peruana* (*Carrion's disease*). This is endemic in areas of Peru. It is a biphasic disease caused by *B. bacilliformis* and is transmitted by sandflies of the genus *Phlebotomus*. Fever, haemolytic anaemia and microvascular thrombosis with end-organ ischaemia are features. It is frequently fatal if untreated.

Investigations and management

Bartonellae can be grown from the blood but this requires prolonged incubation using enriched media. Serum antibody detection is possible.

Bartonella species are susceptible to β-lactams, rifampicin, erythromycin and tetracyclines. Antibiotic use is guided by clinical need. Cat scratch disease usually

13.56 Clinical diseases caused by *Bartonella* spp.

Reservoir	Vector	Organism	Disease
Cats	Flea	*B. henselae*	**Cat scratch disease, bacillary angiomatosis, endocarditis**
Undefined	Lice	*B. quintana*	**Trench fever, bacillary angiomatosis, endocarditis**
Undefined	Sandfly	*B. bacilliformis*	**Carrion's disease: Oroya fever and verruga peruana**
Undefined	Flea	*B. rochalimae*	**Fever, rash, anaemia, splenomegaly**

resolves spontaneously but *Bartonella* endocarditis requires valve replacement and combination antibiotic therapy.

Chlamydial infections

These are listed in Box 13.57 and are also described in Chapters 15 and 19.

Trachoma

Trachoma is a chronic keratoconjunctivitis caused by *Chlamydia trachomatis*, and is the most common cause of avoidable blindness. The classic trachoma environment is dry and dirty, causing children to have eye and nose discharges. Transmission occurs through flies, on fingers and within families. In endemic areas, the disease is most common in children.

Pathology and clinical features

The onset is usually insidious. Infection may be asymptomatic, lasts for years, may be latent over long periods and may recrudesce. The conjunctiva of the upper lid is first affected with vascularisation and cellular infiltration. Early symptoms include conjunctival irritation and blepharospasm. The early follicles are characteristic (Fig. 13.29), but clinical differentiation from conjunctivitis due to other viruses may be difficult. Scarring causes inversion of the lids (entropion) so that the lashes rub against the cornea (trichiasis). The cornea becomes vascularised and opaque. The problem may not be detected until vision begins to fail.

13.57 Chlamydial infections

Organism	Disease caused
Chlamydia trachomatis	Trachoma Lymphogranuloma venereum (see Box 15.12, p. 424) Cervicitis, urethritis, proctitis (p. 422)
Chlamydia psittaci	Psittacosis (Box 19.42, p. 683)
Chlamydophila (Chlamydia) pneumoniae	Atypical pneumonia (Box 19.42, p. 683) Acute/chronic sinusitis

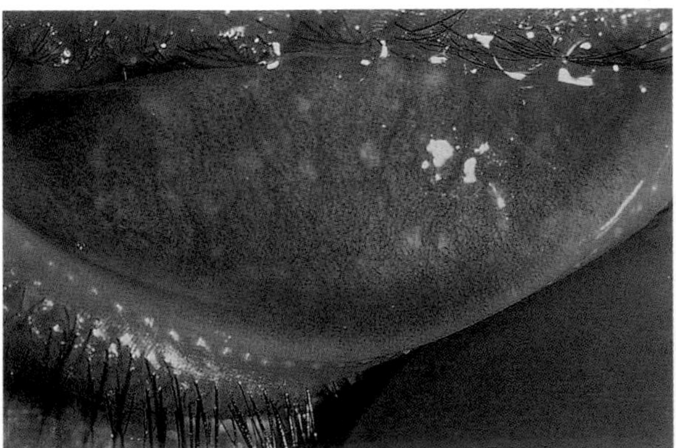

Fig. 13.29 Trachoma. Trachoma is characterised by hyperaemia and numerous pale follicles.

Investigations and management

Intracellular inclusions may be demonstrated in conjunctival scrapings by staining with iodine or immunofluorescence. Chlamydia may be isolated in chick embryo or cell culture.

A single dose of azithromycin (20 mg/kg) has been shown to be superior to 6 weeks of tetracycline eye ointment twice daily for individuals in mass treatment programmes. Deformity and scarring of the lids, and corneal opacities, ulceration and scarring require surgical treatment after control of local infection.

Prevention

Personal and family cleanliness should be improved. Proper care of the eyes of newborn and young children is essential. Family contacts should be examined. The WHO is promoting the SAFE strategy for trachoma control (surgery, antibiotics, facial cleanliness and environmental improvement).

PROTOZOAL INFECTIONS

Protozoa are responsible for many important infectious diseases. They can be categorised according to whether they cause systemic or local infection. Trichomoniasis is described on page 417.

Systemic protozoal infections

Malaria

Malaria in humans is caused by *Plasmodium falciparum, P. vivax, P. ovale, P. malariae* and the predominantly simian parasite, *P. knowlesi*. It is transmitted by the bite of female anopheline mosquitoes and occurs throughout the tropics and subtropics at altitudes below 1500 metres (Fig. 13.30). Recent estimates have put the number of episodes of clinical malaria at 515 million cases per year, with two-thirds of these occurring in sub-Saharan Africa, especially amongst children and pregnant women. Following previous WHO-sponsored campaigns focusing on prevention and effective treatment, the incidence of malaria was greatly reduced between 1950 and 1960, but since 1970 there has been resurgence. Furthermore, *P. falciparum* has now become resistant to chloroquine and sulfadoxine-pyrimethamine, initially in South-east Asia and now throughout Africa. The WHO's Millennium Development Goal 6 aims to halt the spread of the disease by 2015, and its 'Roll Back Malaria' campaign was designed to halve mortality by 2010 by utilising the 'best evidence' vector and disease control methods, such as artemisinin combination therapy (ACT).

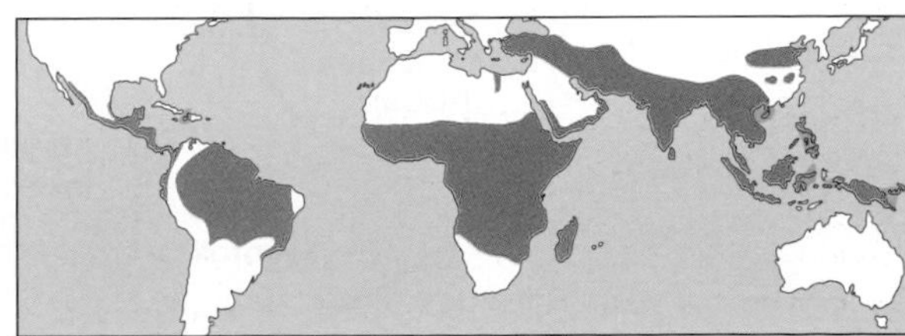

Fig. 13.30 Distribution of malaria. (For up-to-date information see the Malaria Atlas Project (MAP): www.map.ox.ac.uk)

Travellers are susceptible to malaria (p. 309). Due to increased travel, over 2000 cases are imported annually into the UK. Most are due to *P. falciparum*, usually from Africa, and of these 1% die because of late diagnosis. Immigrants returning home after visiting family and friends overseas but who have long-term residence in the UK are particularly at risk. They have lost their partial immunity and do not realise that they should be taking malaria prophylaxis. A few people living near airports in Europe have acquired malaria from accidentally imported mosquitoes.

Pathogenesis

Life cycle of the malarial parasite

The female anopheline mosquito becomes infected when it feeds on human blood containing gametocytes, the sexual forms of the malarial parasite (Figs 13.31 and 13.32). Development in the mosquito takes from 7 to 20 days, and results in sporozoites accumulating in the salivary glands and being inoculated into the human blood stream. Sporozoites disappear from human blood within half an hour and enter the liver. After some days, merozoites leave the liver and invade red blood cells, where further asexual cycles of multiplication take place, producing schizonts. Rupture of the schizont releases more merozoites into the blood and causes fever, the periodicity of which depends on the species of parasite.

P. vivax and *P. ovale* may persist in liver cells as dormant forms, hypnozoites, capable of developing into merozoites months or years later. Thus the first attack of clinical malaria may occur long after the patient has left the endemic area, and the disease may relapse after treatment if drugs that kill only the erythrocytic stage of the parasite are given.

P. falciparum and *P. malariae* have no persistent exo-erythrocytic phase but recrudescence of fever may result from multiplication of parasites in red cells which have not been eliminated by treatment and immune processes (Box 13.58).

Pathology

Red cells infected with malaria are prone to haemolysis. This is most severe with P. *falciparum*, which invades red cells of all ages but especially young cells; *P. vivax* and *P. ovale* invade reticulocytes, and *P. malariae*

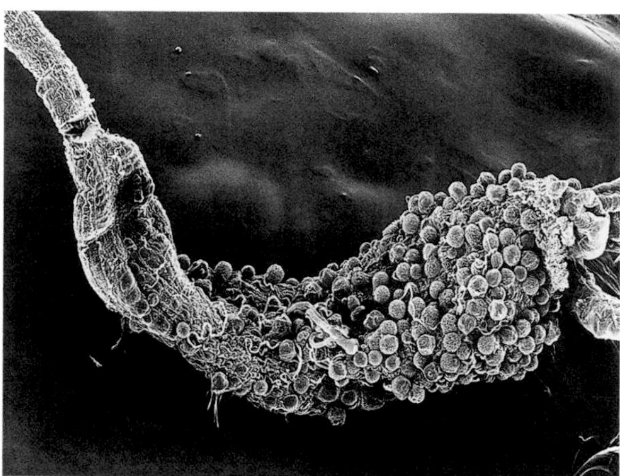

Fig. 13.31 Scanning electron micrograph of *P. falciparum* oöcysts lining an anopheline mosquito's stomach.

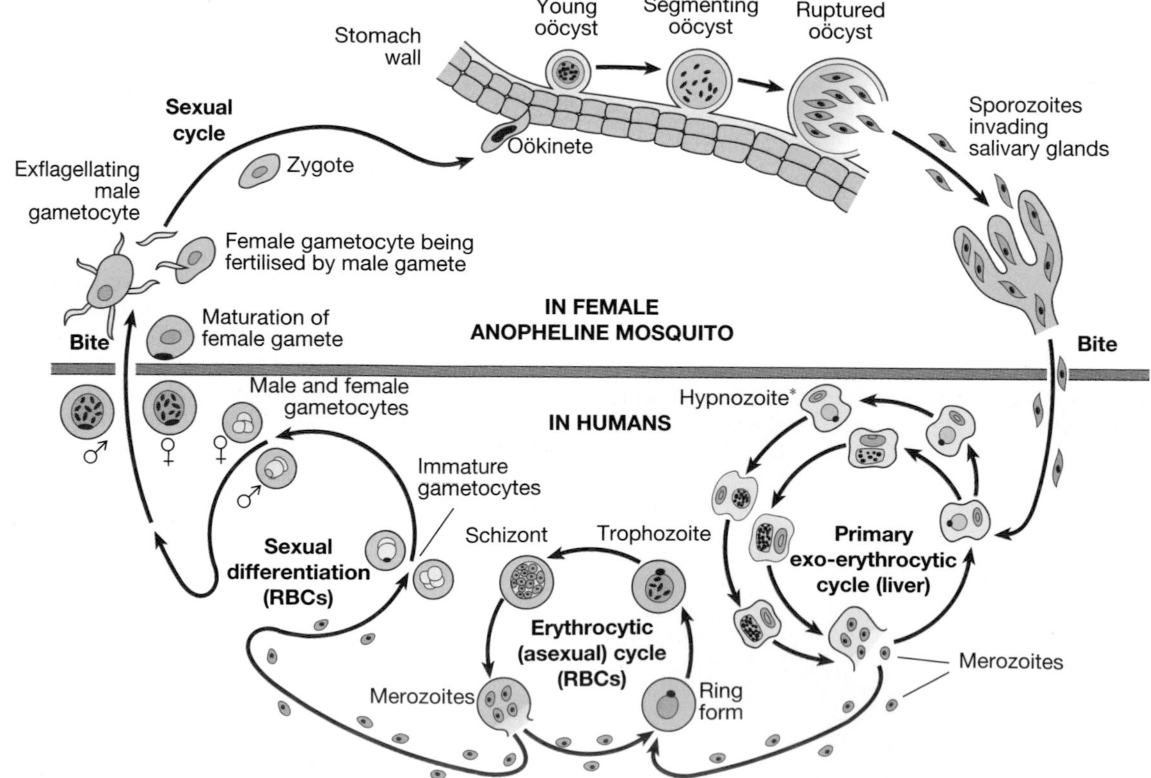

Fig. 13.32 Malarial parasites: life cycle. Hypnozoites(*) are present only in *P. vivax* and *P. ovale* infections. (RBC = red blood cell)

13.58 Relationships between life cycle of parasite and clinical features of malaria

Cycle/ feature	*P. vivax, P. ovale*	*P. malariae*	*P. falciparum*
Pre-patent period (minimum incubation)	8–25 days	15–30 days	8–25 days
Exo-erythrocytic cycle	Persistent as hypnozoites	Pre-erythrocytic only	Pre-erythrocytic only
Asexual cycle	48 hrs synchronous	72 hrs synchronous	< 48 hrs asynchronous
Fever periodicity	Alternate days	Every third day	None
Delayed onset	Common	Rare	Rare
Relapses	Common up to 2 yrs	Recrudescence many years later	Recrudescence up to 1 yr

normoblasts, so that infections remain lighter. Anaemia may be profound and is worsened by dyserythropoiesis, splenomegaly and depletion of folate stores.

In *P. falciparum* malaria, red cells containing trophozoites adhere to vascular endothelium in post-capillary venules in brain, kidney, liver, lungs and gut by the formation of 'knob' proteins. They also form 'rosettes' and rouleaux with uninfected red cells. The vessels become congested, resulting in widespread organ damage which is exacerbated by rupture of schizonts, liberating toxic and antigenic substances (see Fig. 13.32).

P. falciparum has influenced human evolution, with the appearance of protective mutations such as sickle-cell (HbS; p. 1032), thalassaemia (p. 1034), G6PD deficiency (p. 1029) and HLA-B53. *P. falciparum* does not grow well in red cells that contain haemoglobin F, C or especially S. Haemoglobin S heterozygotes (AS) are protected against the lethal complications of malaria. *P. vivax* cannot enter red cells that lack the Duffy blood group; therefore many West Africans and African-Americans are protected.

Clinical features

The clinical features of malaria are non-specific and the diagnosis must be suspected in anyone returning from an endemic area who has features of infection.

P. falciparum *infection*

This is the most dangerous of the malarias and patients are either 'killed or cured'. The onset is often insidious, with malaise, headache and vomiting. Cough and mild diarrhoea are also common. The fever has no particular pattern. Jaundice is common due to haemolysis and hepatic dysfunction. The liver and spleen enlarge and may become tender. Anaemia develops rapidly, as does thrombocytopenia.

A patient with *falciparum* malaria, apparently not seriously ill, may rapidly develop dangerous complications (Fig. 13.33 and Box 13.59). Cerebral malaria is manifested by confusion, seizures or coma, usually without localising signs. Children die rapidly without any special symptoms other than fever. Immunity is impaired in pregnancy and the parasite can preferentially bind to a placental protein known as chondroitin sulphate A. Abortion and intrauterine growth retardation from parasitisation of the maternal side of the placenta are frequent. Previous splenectomy increases the risk of severe malaria.

P. vivax *and* P. ovale *infection*

In many cases, the illness starts with several days of continued fever before the development of classical bouts of fever on alternate days. Fever starts with a rigor. The patient feels cold and the temperature rises to about 40°C. After half an hour to an hour, the hot or flush phase begins. It lasts several hours and gives way to profuse perspiration and a gradual fall in temperature. The cycle is repeated 48 hours later. Gradually, the spleen and liver enlarge and may become tender. Anaemia develops slowly. Relapses are frequent in the first 2 years after leaving the malarious area and infection may be acquired from blood transfusion.

P. malariae *infection*

This is usually associated with mild symptoms and bouts of fever every third day. Parasitaemia may persist for many years, with the occasional recrudescence of fever or without producing any symptoms. Chronic *P. malariae* infection causes glomerulonephritis and long-term nephrotic syndrome in children.

Investigations

Giemsa-stained thick and thin blood films should be examined whenever malaria is suspected. In the thick film, erythrocytes are lysed, releasing all blood stages of the parasite. This, as well as the fact that more blood is used in thick films, facilitates the diagnosis of low-level parasitaemia. A thin film is essential to confirm the diagnosis, to identify the species of parasite and, in *P. falciparum* infections, to quantify the parasite load (by counting the percentage of infected erythrocytes). *P. falciparum* parasites may be very scanty, especially in patients who have been partially treated. With *P. falciparum*, only ring forms are normally seen in the early stages (see Fig. 13.33); with the other species, all stages of the erythrocytic cycle may be found. Gametocytes appear after about 2 weeks, persist after treatment and are harmless, except that they are the source by which more mosquitoes become infected.

Immunochromatographic tests for malaria antigens, such as OptiMal® (which detects the *Plasmodium* lactate dehydrogenase of several species) and ParasightF® (which detects the *P. falciparum* histidine-rich protein 2), are extremely sensitive and specific for *falciparum* malaria but less so for other species. They should be used in parallel with blood film examination but are especially useful where the microscopist is less experienced in examining blood films (e.g. in the UK). The QBC Malaria Test is a fluorescence microscopy-based malaria diagnostic test which is also widely used.

DNA detection (PCR) is used mainly in research and is useful for determining whether a patient has a recrudescence of the same malaria parasite or a re-infection with a new parasite.

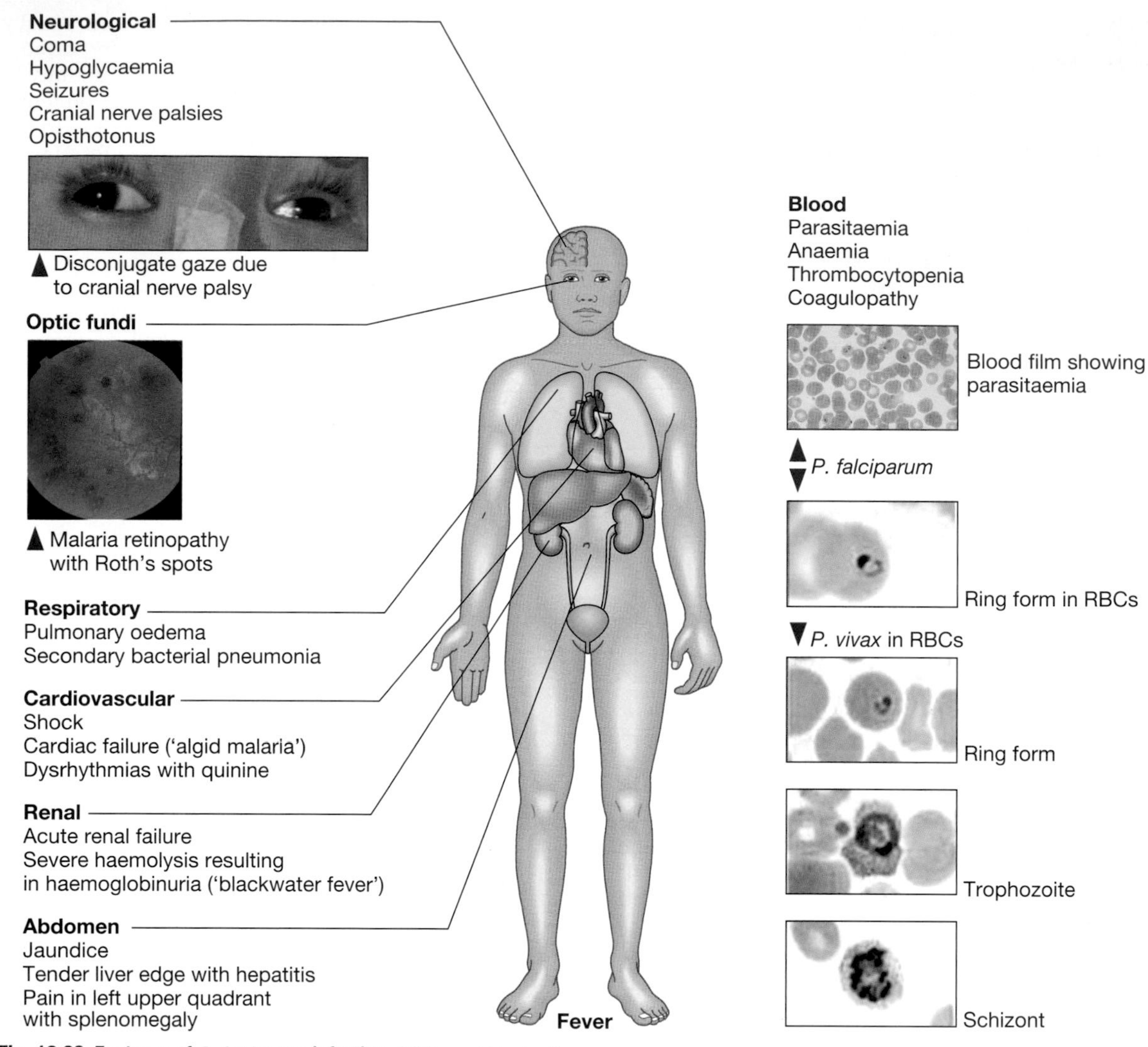

Fig. 13.33 Features of *P. falciparum* infection. (RBC = red blood cell)

Management

Mild P. falciparum *malaria*

Since *P. falciparum* is now resistant to chloroquine and sulfadoxine-pyrimethamine (Fansidar) almost worldwide, an artemisinin-based treatment is recommended. Co-artemether (CoArtem® or Riamet®) contains artemether and lumefantrine and is given as 4 tablets at 0, 8, 24, 36, 48 and 60 hours. Alternatives are quinine by mouth (600 mg of quinine salt 3 times daily for 5–7 days), together with or followed by either doxycycline (200 mg once daily for 7 days) or clindamycin (450 mg 3 times daily for 7 days) or atovaquone-proguanil (Malarone®, 4 tablets once daily for 3 days). Doxycycline should not be used in pregnancy and artemether should be avoided in early pregnancy.

WHO policy in Africa is moving towards always using artemisinin-based combination therapy (ACT), e.g. co-artemether or artesunate-amodiaquine. In India and other areas, artesunate (200 mg orally daily for 3 days) and mefloquine (1 g orally on day 2 and 500 mg orally on day 3) may be used. Unfortunately, artemisinin resistance has now been reported in Cambodia.

Complicated P. falciparum *malaria*

Severe malaria should be considered in any non-immune patient with a parasite count greater than 2% and is a medical emergency (see Box 13.59). Management includes early and appropriate antimalarial chemotherapy, active treatment of complications, correction of fluid, electrolyte and acid–base balance, and avoidance of harmful ancillary treatments.

The treatment of choice is intravenous artesunate given as 2.4 mg/kg IV at 0, 12 and 24 hours and then once daily for 7 days. However, as soon as the patient has recovered sufficiently to swallow tablets, oral artesunate 2 mg/kg once daily is given instead of intravenous therapy, to complete a total cumulative dose of 17–18 mg/kg. Rectal administration of artesunate is also being developed to allow administration in remote rural areas.

Quinine salt can also be used and is started with a loading dose infusion of 20 mg/kg over 4 hours, up to a maximum of 1.4 g. This is followed by maintenance doses of 10 mg/kg quinine salt given as 4-hour infusions 2–3 times daily, up to a maximum of 700 mg per dose,

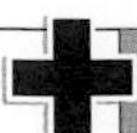

13.59 Severe manifestations/complications of *falciparum* malaria and their immediate management

Coma (cerebral malaria)
- Maintain airway
- Nurse on side
- Exclude other treatable causes of coma (e.g. hypoglycaemia, bacterial meningitis)
- Avoid harmful ancillary treatments such as corticosteroids, heparin and adrenaline (epinephrine)
- Intubate if necessary

Hyperpyrexia
- Tepid sponging, fanning, cooling blanket
- Antipyretic drug (paracetamol)

Convulsions
- Maintain airway
- Treat promptly with diazepam or paraldehyde injection

Hypoglycaemia
- Measure blood glucose
- Give 50% dextrose injection followed by 10% dextrose infusion (glucagon may be ineffective)

Severe anaemia (packed cell volume < 15%)
- Transfuse fresh whole blood or packed cells if pathogen screening of donor blood is available

Acute pulmonary oedema
- Nurse at 45°, give oxygen, venesect 250 mL of blood, give diuretic, stop intravenous fluids
- Intubate and add PEEP/CPAP (p. 193) in life-threatening hypoxaemia
- Haemofilter

Acute renal failure
- Exclude pre-renal causes
- Fluid resuscitation if appropriate
- Peritoneal dialysis (haemofiltration or haemodialysis if available)

Spontaneous bleeding and coagulopathy
- Transfuse screened fresh whole blood (cryoprecipitate/fresh frozen plasma and platelets if available)
- Vitamin K injection

Metabolic acidosis
- Exclude or treat hypoglycaemia, hypovolaemia and Gram-negative septicaemia
- Fluid resuscitation
- Give oxygen

Shock ('algid malaria')
- Suspect Gram-negative septicaemia
- Take blood cultures
- Give parenteral antimicrobials
- Correct haemodynamic disturbances

Aspiration pneumonia
- Give parenteral antimicrobial drugs
- Change position
- Physiotherapy
- Give oxygen

Hyperparasitaemia
- Consider exchange or partial exchange transfusion, manual or haemophoresis (e.g. > 10% of circulating erythrocytes parasitised in non-immune patient with severe disease)

Specific therapy
- Intravenous artesunate
- Mefloquine should be avoided due to increased risk of post-malaria neurological syndrome

From WHO. Severe falciparum malaria. In: Severe and complicated malaria. 3rd edn. Trans Roy Soc Trop Med Hyg 2000; 94 (suppl. 1): S1–41.

until the patient can take drugs orally. The loading dose should *not* be given if the patient has received quinine, quinidine or mefloquine during the previous 24 hours. Patients should be monitored by ECG, with special attention to QRS duration and QT interval. Mefloquine should not be used for severe malaria since no parenteral form is available.

Exchange transfusion has not been tested in randomised controlled trials but may be beneficial for non-immune patients with persisting high parasitaemias (> 10% circulating erythrocytes).

*Management of non-*falciparum *malaria*

P. vivax, *P. ovale* and *P. malariae* infections should be treated with oral chloroquine: 600 mg chloroquine base, followed by 300 mg base in 6 hours, then 150 mg base twice daily for 2 more days. Some chloroquine resistance has been reported from Indonesia.

Late relapses can be prevented by prescribing antimalarial drugs in suppressive doses. However, 'radical cure' is now achieved in most patients with *P. vivax* or *P. ovale* malaria using a course of primaquine (15 mg daily for 14 days), which destroys the hypnozoite phase in the liver. Haemolysis may develop in those who are G6PD-deficient. Cyanosis due to the formation of methaemoglobin in the red cells is more common but not dangerous.

Prevention

Clinical attacks of malaria may be preventable with chemoprophylaxis using chloroquine, atovaquone plus proguanil (Malarone), doxycycline or mefloquine. Box 13.60 gives the recommended doses for protection of the non-immune. The risk of malaria in the area to be visited and the degree of chloroquine resistance guide the recommendations for prophylaxis. Updated recommendations are summarised at www.fitfortravel.nhs.uk. Fansidar should not be used for chemoprophylaxis, as deaths have occurred from agranulocytosis or Stevens–Johnson syndrome (p. 1302). Mefloquine is useful in areas of multiple drug resistance, such as East and Central Africa and Papua New Guinea. Experience shows it to be safe for at least 2 years, but there are several contraindications to its use (see Box 13.60).

Expert advice is required for individuals unable to tolerate the first-line agents listed or in whom they are contraindicated. Mefloquine should be started 2–3 weeks before travel to give time for assessment of

13.60 Chemoprophylaxis of malaria[1]

Antimalarial tablets	Adult prophylactic dose	Regimen
Chloroquine resistance high		
Mefloquine[2]	250 mg weekly	Started 2–3 wks before travel and continued until 4 wks after
or Doxycycline[3,4]	100 mg daily	Started 1 wk before and continued until 4 wks after travel
or Malarone[4]	1 tablet daily	From 1–2 days before travel until 1 wk after return
Chloroquine resistance absent		
Chloroquine[5] *and*	300 mg base weekly	Started 1 wk before and continued until 4 wks after travel
proguanil	100–200 mg daily	

[1]Choice of regimen is determined by area to be visited, length of stay, level of malaria transmission, level of drug resistance, presence of underlying disease in the traveller and concomitant medication taken.
[2]Contraindicated in the first trimester of pregnancy, lactation, cardiac conduction disorders, epilepsy, psychiatric disorders; may cause neuropsychiatric disorders.
[3]Causes photosensitisation and sunburn if high-protection sunblock is not used.
[4]Avoid in pregnancy.
[5]British preparations of chloroquine usually contain 150 mg base, French preparations 100 mg base and American preparations 300 mg base.

EBM 13.61 Prevention of malaria

Insecticide-treated bed nets (ITNs)

'Five randomised controlled clinical trials provided strong evidence that widespread use of ITNs reduces overall mortality by about one-fifth in Africa. For every 1000 children aged 1–5 years protected, approximately 5.5 lives can be saved every year. In Africa, full ITN coverage could prevent 370 000 child deaths per year.'

Electronic mosquito repellents (EMRs)

'EMRs are not effective.'

Intermittent preventive treatment in pregnancy

'Antimalarial drugs reduce antenatal parasitaemia and fever in pregnant women living in areas with endemic malaria. For women in their first or second pregnancy, this reduces the instances of severe antenatal anaemia, antenatal parasitaemia and perinatal deaths, and increases birth weight.'

Intermittent preventive treatment in children

'Antimalarial drugs reduce clinical malaria, severe anaemia and hospital admissions. Effects on mortality and on health, if prophylaxis is stopped, are unknown.'

- Gamble C, et al. (2007) PLoS Med 2007; 4(3):e107.
- Enayati A, et al. Electronic mosquito repellents for preventing mosquito bites and malaria infection. Cochrane Database of Systematic Reviews, 2007, issue 2. Art. no.: CD005434.
- Garner P, Gülmezoglu AM. Drugs for preventing malaria in pregnant women. Cochrane Database of Systematic Reviews, 2006, issue 4. Art. no.: CD000169.
- Chandramohan D, et al. BMJ 2005; 331(7519):727–733.

For further information: www.cochrane.org/cochrane-reviews

side-effects. Chloroquine should not be taken continuously as a prophylactic for more than 5 years without regular ophthalmic examination, as it may cause irreversible retinopathy. Pregnant and lactating women may take proguanil or chloroquine safely.

Prevention also involves advice about the use of high-percentage diethyltoluamide (DEET), covering up extremities when out after dark, and sleeping under permethrin-impregnated mosquito nets (Box 13.61).

Malaria control in endemic areas

There are major initiatives under way to reduce malaria in endemic areas and it is estimated that these would be cost-effective, even at a cost of $3 billion per year. Successful programmes have involved a combination of vector control, including indoor residual spraying, use of long-lasting insecticide-treated bed nets (ITNs) and intermittent preventative therapy (IPT; repeated dose of prophylactic drugs in high-risk groups, such as children and pregnant women) (see Box 13.61).

Development of a fully protective malaria vaccine is still some way off, which is not surprising, considering that natural immunity is incomplete and not long-lived. There is, however, some evidence that vaccination can reduce the incidence of severe malaria in populations. Trial vaccines are being evaluated in Africa.

Babesiosis

This is caused by a tick-borne intra-erythrocytic protozoon parasite. There are more than 100 species of *Babesia*, all of which have an animal reservoir, typically either rodents or cattle, and are transmitted to humans via the tick vector *Ixodes scapularis*. Most cases of babesiosis in the USA are due to *B. microti* and most in Europe to *B. divergens*. Patients present with fever and malaise 1–4 weeks after a tick bite. Illness may be complicated by haemolytic anaemia. Severe illness is seen in splenectomised patients. The diagnosis is made by blood-film examination. Treatment is with quinine and clindamycin.

African trypanosomiasis (sleeping sickness)

African sleeping sickness is caused by trypanosomes (Fig. 13.34) conveyed to humans by the bites of infected tsetse flies, and is unique to sub-Saharan Africa (Fig. 13.35). There has been a more than 60% decline in the incidence of sleeping sickness across Africa since 1990 due to better control measures. *Trypanosoma brucei gambiense* trypanosomiasis has a wide distribution in West and Central Africa and accounts for 90% of reported cases. *T. brucei rhodesiense* trypanosomiasis is found in parts of East and Central Africa. In West Africa, transmission is mainly at the riverside, where the fly rests in the shade of trees; no animal reservoir has been identified for *T. gambiense*. *T. rhodesiense* has a large reservoir in numerous wild animals and transmission takes place in the shade of woods bordering grasslands. Rural populations earning their livelihood from agriculture, fishing and animal husbandry are susceptible. Local

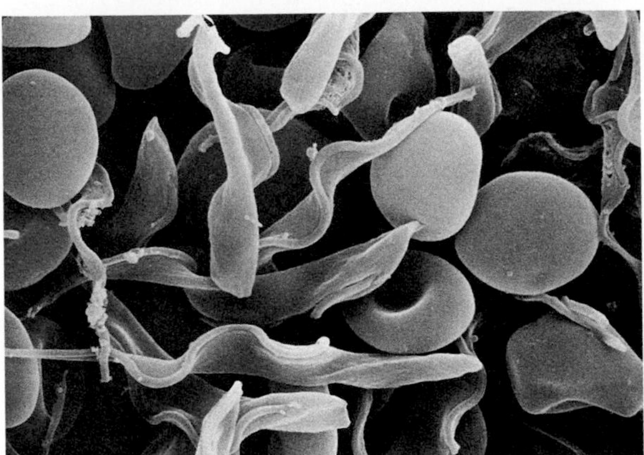

Fig. 13.34 Trypanosomiasis. Scanning electron micrograph showing trypanosomes swimming among erythrocytes.

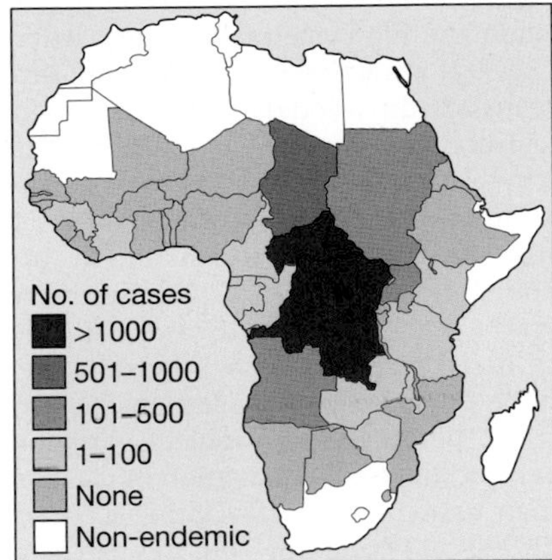

Fig. 13.35 Distribution of human African trypanosomiasis. From Simarro, et al. 2011 – see p. 386. Data are from 2009.

people and tourists visiting forests infested with tsetse flies and animal reservoirs may become infected.

Clinical features

A bite by a tsetse fly is painful and commonly becomes inflamed, but if trypanosomes are introduced, the site may again become painful and swollen about 10 days later ('trypanosomal chancre') and the regional lymph nodes enlarge ('Winterbottom's sign'). Within 2–3 weeks of infection, the trypanosomes invade the blood stream. The disease is characterised by an early haemato-lymphatic stage and a late encephalitic stage, in which the parasite crosses the blood–brain barrier and chronic encephalopathy develops.

Rhodesiense *infections*

In these infections, the disease is more acute and severe than in *gambiense* infections, so that, within days or a few weeks, the patient is usually severely ill and may have developed pleural effusions and signs of myocarditis or hepatitis. There may be a petechial rash. The patient may die before there are signs of involvement of the CNS. If the illness is less acute, drowsiness, tremors and coma develop.

Gambiense *infections*

The distinction between early and late stages may not be apparent in *gambiense* infections. The disease usually runs a slow course over months or years, with irregular bouts of fever and enlargement of lymph nodes. These are characteristically firm, discrete, rubbery and painless, and are particularly prominent in the posterior triangle of the neck. The spleen and liver may become palpable. After some months without treatment, the CNS is invaded. This is shown clinically by headache and changed behaviour, blunting of higher mental functions, insomnia by night and sleepiness by day, mental confusion and eventually tremors, pareses, wasting, coma and death.

Investigations

Trypanosomiasis should be considered in any febrile patient from an endemic area. In *rhodesiense* infections, thick and thin blood films, stained as for the detection of malaria, will reveal trypanosomes. The trypanosomes may be seen in the blood or from puncture of the primary lesion in the earliest stages of *gambiense* infections, but it is usually easier to demonstrate them by aspiration of a lymph node. Concentration methods include buffy coat microscopy and miniature anion exchange chromatography.

Due to the cyclical nature of parasitaemia, the diagnosis is often made by demonstration of antibodies using a simple, rapid screening card agglutination trypanosomiasis test (CATT), followed by parasitological confirmation. If the CNS is affected, the cell count ($> 20 \times 10^9$ leucocytes per litre) and protein content of the CSF are increased and the glucose is diminished. A very high level of serum IgM or the presence of IgM in the CSF is suggestive of trypanosomiasis. Recognition of CNS involvement is critical, as failure to treat it might be fatal.

Management

Unfortunately, therapeutic options for African trypanosomiasis are limited and most of the antitrypanosomal drugs are toxic and expensive. The prognosis is good if treatment is begun early, before the brain has been invaded. At this stage, intravenous suramin, after a test dose of 100–200 mg, should be given for *rhodesiense* infections (1 g on days 1, 3, 7, 14 and 21). For *gambiense* infections, intramuscular or intravenous pentamidine 4 mg/kg for 10 days is given (Box 13.62).

13.62 Drugs used to treat human African trypanosomiasis

***Gambiense* trypanosomiasis**

Stage 1
- First-line: pentamidine
- Second-line: eflornithine or melarsoprol

Stage 2
- First-line: eflornithine
- Second-line: melarsoprol

***Rhodesiense* trypanosomiasis**

Stage 1
- First-line: suramin
- Second-line: melarsoprol

Stage 2
- First-line: melarsoprol
- Second-line: nifurtimox combined with melarsoprol

Once the nervous system is affected, treatment with melarsoprol (an arsenical) is effective for both East and West African diseases. It is used in a dose of 2–3.6 mg/kg/day IV for the first course and 3.6 mg/kg/day thereafter. Three 3-day treatment courses are given, separated by 7 days and by 10–21 days. Melarsoprol should be given with prednisolone 1 mg/kg up to 40 mg started 1–2 days before, continued during and tapered after treatment to reduce side-effects. Treatment-related mortality with melarsoprol is 4–12% due to reactive encephalopathy. For CNS infections due to *gambiense*, eflornithine (DFMO), an irreversible inhibitor of ornithine decarboxylase (100 and 150 mg/kg IV 4 times daily for 14 days for adults and children, respectively), is considered to be a safer and cost-effective option. Combinations of eflornithine (400 mg daily for 7 days) with oral nifurtimox (15 mg/kg daily for 15 days) have been shown to decrease relapses, deaths and drug toxicity.

Prevention

In endemic *gambiense* areas, various measures may be taken against tsetse flies, and field teams help to detect and treat early human infection. In *rhodesiense* areas, control is difficult.

American trypanosomiasis (Chagas' disease)

Chagas' disease occurs widely in South and Central America. The cause is *Trypanosoma cruzi*, transmitted to humans from the faeces of a reduviid (triatomine) bug, in which the trypanosomes have a cycle of development before becoming infective to humans. These bugs live in wild forests in crevices, burrows and palm trees. The *Triatoma infestans* bug has become domesticated in the Southern Cone countries (Argentina, Brazil, Chile, Paraguay and Uruguay). It lives in the mud and wattle walls and thatched roofs of simple rural houses, and emerges at night to feed and defecate on the sleeping occupants. Infected faeces are rubbed in through the conjunctiva, mucosa of mouth or nose, or abrasions of the skin. Over one hundred species of mammal, domestic, peridomestic and wild, may serve as reservoirs of infection. In some areas, blood transfusion accounts for about 5% of cases. Congenital transmission occasionally occurs.

Pathology

The trypanosomes migrate via the blood stream, develop into amastigote forms in the tissues and multiply intracellularly by binary fission. In the acute phase (primarily cell-mediated), inflammation of parasitised as well as non-parasitised cardiac muscles and capillaries occurs, resulting in acute myocarditis. In the chronic phase, focal myocardial atrophy, signs of chronic passive congestion and thromboembolic phenomena, cardiomegaly and apical cardiac aneurysm are salient findings. In the digestive form of disease, focal myositis and discontinuous lesions of the intramural myenteric plexus, predominantly in the oesophagus and colon, are seen.

Clinical features

Acute phase

Clinical manifestations of the acute phase are seen in only 1–2% of individuals who are infected before the age of 15 years. Young children (1–5 years) are most commonly affected. The entrance of *T. cruzi* through an abrasion produces a dusky-red firm swelling and enlargement of regional lymph nodes. A conjunctival lesion, although less common, is characteristic; the unilateral firm, reddish swelling of the lids may close the eye and constitutes 'Romaña's sign'. In a few patients, an acute generalised infection soon appears, with a transient morbilliform or urticarial rash, fever, lymphadenopathy and enlargement of the spleen and liver. In a small minority of patients, acute myocarditis and heart failure or neurological features, including personality changes and signs of meningoencephalitis, may be seen. The acute infection may be fatal to infants.

Chronic phase

About 50–70% of infected patients become seropositive and develop an indeterminate form when no parasitaemia is detectable. They have a normal lifespan with no symptoms, but are a natural reservoir for the disease and maintain the life cycle of parasites. After a latent period of several years, 10–30% of chronic cases develop low-grade myocarditis, and damage to conducting fibres causes a cardiomyopathy characterised by cardiac dilatation, arrhythmias, partial or complete heart block and sudden death. In nearly 10% of patients, damage to Auerbach's plexus results in dilatation of various parts of the alimentary canal, especially the colon and oesophagus, so-called 'mega' disease. Dilatation of the bile ducts and bronchi is also a recognised sequela. Autoimmune processes may be responsible for much of the damage. There are geographical variations of the basic pattern of disease. Reactivation of Chagas' disease can occur in patients with HIV if the CD4 count falls lower than 200 cells/mm^3 (p. 393); this can cause space-occupying lesions with a presentation similar to *Toxoplasma* encephalitis, encephalitis, meningoencephalitis or myocarditis.

Investigations

T. cruzi is easily detectable in a blood film in the acute illness. In chronic disease, it may be recovered in up to 50% of cases by xenodiagnosis, in which infection-free, laboratory-bred reduviid bugs are allowed to feed on the patient; subsequently, the hind gut or faeces of the bug are examined for parasites. Parasite DNA detection by PCR in the patient's blood is a highly sensitive method for documentation of infection and, in addition, can be employed in faeces of bugs used in xenodiagnosis tests to improve sensitivity. Antibody detection is also highly sensitive.

Management and prevention

Parasiticidal agents are used to treat the acute phase, congenital disease and early chronic phase (within 10 years of infection). Nifurtimox is given orally. The dose, which has to be carefully supervised to minimise toxicity while preserving parasiticidal activity, is 10 mg/kg divided into three equal doses, daily orally for 60–90 days. The paediatric dose is 15 mg/kg daily. Cure rates of 80% in acute disease are obtained. Benznidazole is an alternative, given at a dose of 5–10 mg/kg daily orally, in two divided doses for 60 days; children receive 10 mg/kg daily. Both nifurtimox and benznidazole are toxic, with adverse reaction rates of 30–55%. Specific drug treatment of the chronic form is now increasingly favoured, but, in the cardiac or digestive 'mega' diseases, it does not reverse established tissue damage. Surgery may be needed.

Preventative measures include improving housing and destruction of reduviid bugs by spraying of houses with insecticides. Blood donors should be screened.

Toxoplasmosis

Toxoplasma gondii is an intracellular parasite. The sexual phase of the parasite's life cycle (Fig. 13.36) occurs in the small intestinal epithelium of the domestic cat. Oöcysts are shed in cat faeces and are spread to intermediate hosts (pigs, sheep and also humans) through widespread contamination of soil. Oöcysts may survive in moist conditions for weeks or months. Once they are ingested, the parasite transforms into rapidly dividing tachyzoites through cycles of asexual multiplication. This leads to the formation of microscopic tissue cysts containing bradyzoites, which persist for the lifetime of the host. Cats become infected or re-infected by ingesting tissue cysts in prey such as rodents and birds.

Human acquisition of infection occurs via oöcyst-contaminated soil, salads and vegetables, or by the ingestion or tasting of raw or undercooked meats containing tissue cysts. Sheep, pigs and rabbits are the most common meat sources. Outbreaks of toxoplasmosis have been linked to the consumption of unfiltered water. In developed countries, toxoplasmosis is the most common protozoal infection; around 22% of adults in the UK are seropositive. Most primary infections are subclinical; however, toxoplasmosis is thought to account for about 15% of heterophile antibody-negative glandular fever (p. 320). In India or Brazil, approximately 40–60% of pregnant females are seropositive for *T. gondii*. In HIV-1 infection (p. 402), toxoplasmosis is an important opportunistic infection with considerable morbidity and mortality. Generalised toxoplasmosis has been described after accidental laboratory infection with highly virulent strains.

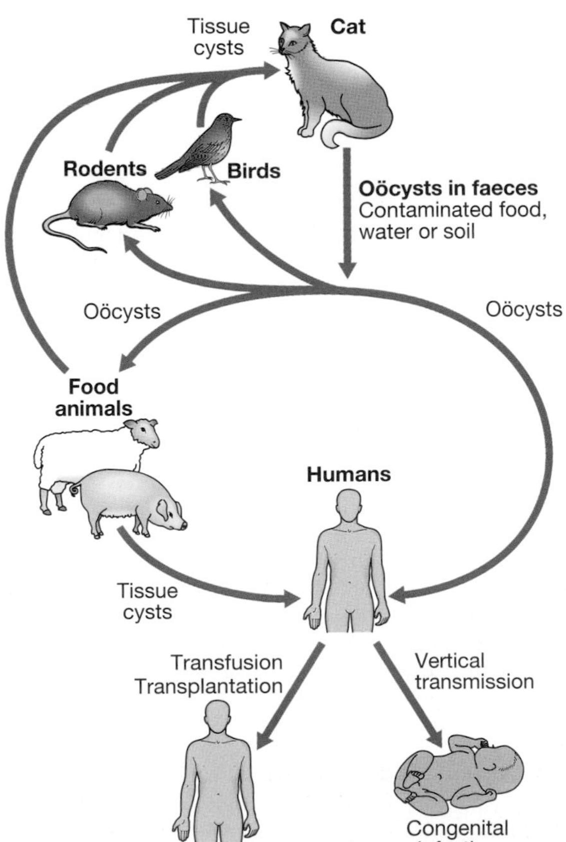

Fig. 13.36 Life cycle of *Toxoplasma gondii.*

Clinical features

In most immunocompetent individuals, including children and pregnant women, the infection goes unnoticed. In approximately 10% of patients, it causes a self-limiting illness, most common in adults aged 25–35 years. The most common presenting feature is painless lymphadenopathy, either local or generalised. In particular, the cervical nodes are involved, but mediastinal, mesenteric or retroperitoneal groups may be affected. The spleen is seldom palpable. Most patients have no systemic symptoms, but some complain of malaise, fever, fatigue, muscle pain, sore throat and headache. Complete resolution usually occurs within a few months, although symptoms and lymphadenopathy tend to fluctuate unpredictably and some patients do not recover completely for a year or more. Very infrequently, patients may develop encephalitis, myocarditis, polymyositis, pneumonitis or hepatitis. Retinochoroiditis (Fig. 13.37) is nearly always the result of congenital infection but has also been reported in acquired disease.

Congenital toxoplasmosis

Acute toxoplasmosis, mostly subclinical, affects 0.3–1% of pregnant women, with an approximately 60% transmission rate to the fetus, which rises with increasing gestation. Seropositive females infected 6 months before conception have no risk of fetal transmission. Congenital disease affects approximately 40% of infected fetuses, and is more likely and more severe with infection early in gestation (see Box 13.28, p. 314). Many fetal infections are subclinical at birth but long-term sequelae include retinochoroiditis, microcephaly and hydrocephalus.

Investigations

In contrast to immunocompromised patients, in whom the diagnosis often requires direct detection of parasites, serology is often used in immunocompetent individuals.

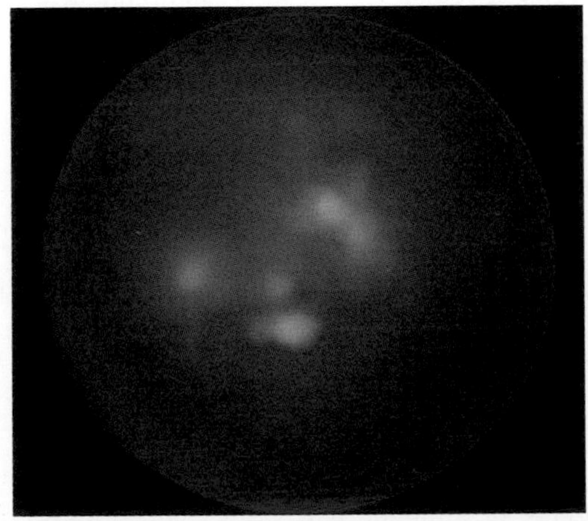

Fig. 13.37 Retinochoroiditis due to toxoplasmosis.

The Sabin–Feldman dye test (indirect fluorescent antibody test), which detects IgG antibody, is most commonly used. Recent infection is indicated by a fourfold or greater increase in titre when paired sera are tested in parallel. Peak titres of 1/1000 or more are reached within 1–2 months of the onset of infection, and the dye test then becomes an unreliable indicator of recent infection. The detection of significant levels of *Toxoplasma*-specific IgM antibody may be useful in confirming acute infection. A false-positive result or persistence of IgM antibodies for years after infection makes interpretation difficult; however, negative IgM antibodies virtually rule out acute infection.

During pregnancy, it is critical to differentiate between recent and past infection; the presence of high-avidity IgG antibodies excludes infection acquired in the preceding 3–4 months.

If necessary, the presence of *Toxoplasma* organisms in a lymph node biopsy can be sought by staining sections histochemically with *T. gondii* antiserum, or by the use of PCR to detect *Toxoplasma*-specific DNA.

Management

In immunocompetent subjects, uncomplicated toxoplasmosis is self-limiting and responds poorly to antimicrobial therapy. Treatment with pyrimethamine, sulfadiazine and folinic acid is therefore usually reserved for rare cases of severe or progressive disease, and for infection in immunocompromised patients.

In a pregnant woman with an established recent infection, spiramycin (3 g daily in divided doses) should be given until term. Once fetal infection is established, treatment with sulfadiazine and pyrimethamine plus calcium folinate is recommended (spiramycin does not cross the placental barrier). The cost/benefit of routine *Toxoplasma* screening and treatment in pregnancy is being debated in many countries. There is insufficient evidence to determine the effects on mother or baby of current antiparasitic treatment for women who seroconvert in pregnancy.

Leishmaniasis

Leishmaniasis is caused by unicellular, flagellate, intracellular protozoa belonging to the genus *Leishmania* (order Kinetoplastidae). There are 21 leishmanial species that cause several diverse clinical syndromes, which can be placed into three broad groups:

- visceral leishmaniasis (VL, kala-azar)
- cutaneous leishmaniasis (CL)
- mucosal leishmaniasis (ML).

Epidemiology and transmission

Although most clinical syndromes are caused by zoonotic transmission of parasites from animals (chiefly canine and rodent reservoirs) to humans through phlebotomine sandfly vectors (Fig. 13.38A), humans are the only known reservoir (anthroponotic) in major VL foci in the Indian subcontinent and for transmission of leishmaniasis between injection drug-users (Fig. 13.38B and C). Leishmaniasis occurs in approximately 100 countries around the world, with an estimated annual incidence of 2 million new cases (500 000 for VL and 1.5 million for CL).

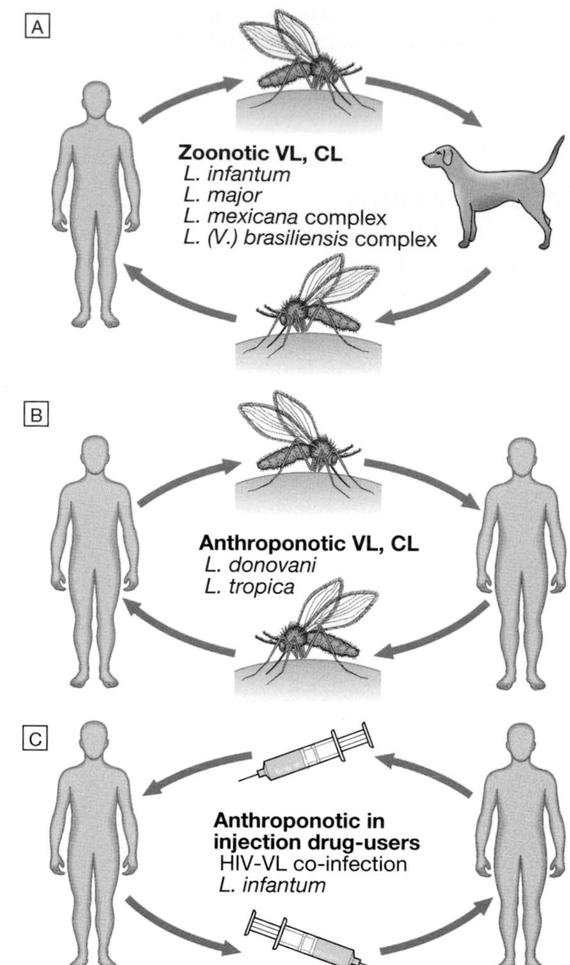

Fig. 13.38 Transmission of leishmaniasis. **A** Zoonotic transmission. **B** Anthroponotic transmission. **C** Anthroponotic transmission in the injection drug-user.

The life cycle of *Leishmania* is shown in Figure 13.39. Flagellar promastigotes (10–20 μm) are introduced by the feeding female sandfly. The promastigotes are taken up by neutrophils, which undergo apoptosis and are then engulfed by macrophages, in which the parasites transform into amastigotes (2–4 μm; Leishman–Donovan body). These multiply, ultimately causing lysis of the macrophages and infection of other cells. Sandflies pick up amastigotes when feeding on infected patients or animal reservoirs. In the sandfly, the parasite transforms into a flagellar promastigote, which multiplies by binary fission in the gut of the vector and migrates to the proboscis to infect a new host.

Sandflies live in hot and humid climates in the cracks and crevices of mud or straw houses and lay eggs in organic matter. People living in such conditions are more prone to acquiring the disease. Female sandflies bite during the night and preferentially feed on animals; humans are incidental hosts.

Visceral leishmaniasis (kala-azar)

VL is caused by the protozoon *Leishmania donovani* complex (comprising *L. donovani*, *L. infantum* and *L. chagasi*). India, Sudan, Bangladesh and Brazil account for 90% of cases of VL, while other affected regions include

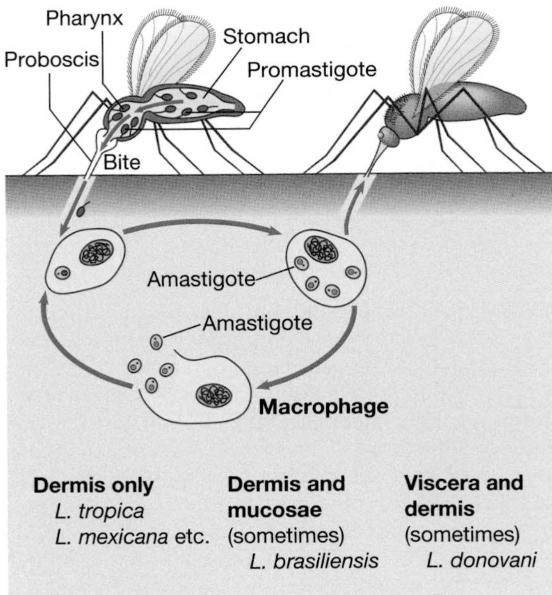

Fig. 13.39 Life cycle of *Leishmania*. From Knight 1982 – see p. 386.

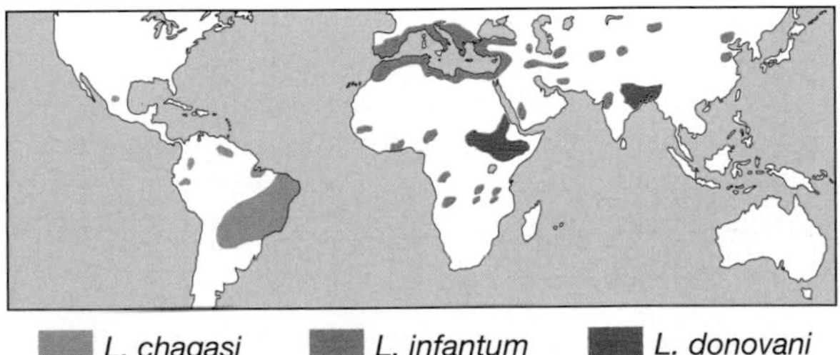

Fig. 13.40 World distribution of visceral leishmaniasis.

the Mediterranean, East Africa, China, Arabia, Israel and other South American countries (Fig. 13.40). In addition to sandfly transmission, VL has also been reported to follow blood transfusion, and disease can present unexpectedly in immunosuppressed patients – for example, after renal transplantation and in HIV infection.

The great majority of people infected remain asymptomatic. In visceral diseases, the spleen, liver, bone marrow and lymph nodes are primarily involved.

Clinical features

In the Indian subcontinent, adults and children are equally affected; elsewhere, VL is mainly a disease of small children and infants, except in adults with HIV co-infection. The incubation period ranges from weeks to months (occasionally several years).

The first sign of infection is high fever, usually accompanied by rigor and chills. Fever intensity decreases over time, and patients may become afebrile for intervening periods ranging from weeks to months. This is followed by a relapse of fever, often of lesser intensity. Splenomegaly develops quickly in the first few weeks and becomes massive as the disease progresses. Moderate hepatomegaly occurs later. Lymphadenopathy is seen in the majority of cases in Africa, the Mediterranean and South America, but is rare in the Indian subcontinent. Blackish discoloration of the skin, from which the disease derived its name, kala-azar (the Hindi word for 'black fever'), is a feature of advanced illness and is now rarely seen. Pancytopenia is a common feature. Moderate to severe anaemia develops rapidly, and can result in congestive cardiac failure and associated clinical features. Thrombocytopenia, often compounded by hepatic dysfunction, may result in bleeding from the retina, gastrointestinal tract and nose. In advanced illness, hypoalbuminaemia may manifest as pedal oedema, ascites and anasarca (gross generalised oedema and swelling).

As the disease advances, there is profound immunosuppression and secondary infections are very common. These include tuberculosis, pneumonia, severe amoebic or bacillary dysentery, gastroenteritis, herpes zoster and chickenpox. Skin infections, boils, cellulitis and scabies are common. Without adequate treatment, most patients with clinical VL die.

Investigations

Pancytopenia is the most dominant feature, with granulocytopenia and monocytosis. Polyclonal hypergammaglobulinaemia, chiefly IgG followed by IgM, and hypoalbuminaemia are seen later.

Demonstration of amastigotes (Leishman–Donovan bodies) in splenic smears is the most efficient means of diagnosis, with 98% sensitivity (Fig. 13.41); however, it carries a risk of serious haemorrhage in inexperienced hands. Safer methods, such as bone marrow or lymph node smears, are not as sensitive. Parasites may be demonstrated in buffy coat smears, especially in immunosuppressed patients. Sensitivity can be improved by culturing the aspirate material or by PCR for DNA detection and species identification, but these tests can only be performed in specialised laboratories.

Serodiagnosis, by ELISA or immunofluorescence antibody test, is employed in developed countries. In endemic regions, a highly sensitive direct agglutination test using stained promastigotes and an equally efficient rapid immunochromatographic k39 strip test have become popular. These tests remain positive for several months after cure has been achieved, so do not predict

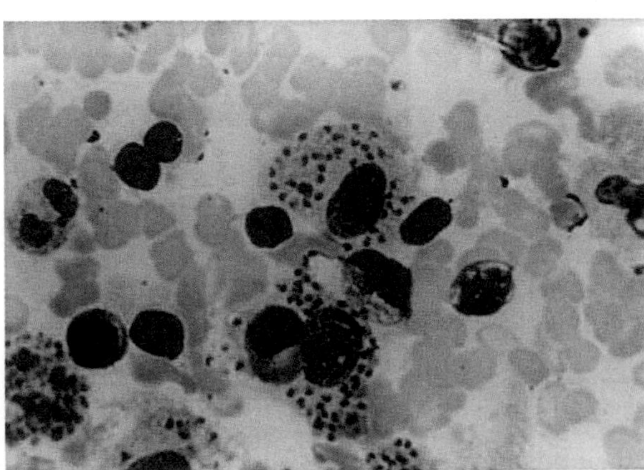

Fig. 13.41 Splenic smear showing numerous intracellular, and a few extracellular, amastigotes.

response to treatment or relapse. The vast majority of people exposed to the parasite do not develop clinical illness but may have positive serological tests thereafter. Formal gel (aldehyde) or other similar tests based on the detection of raised globulin have limited value and should not be employed for the diagnosis of VL.

Differential diagnosis

This includes malaria, typhoid, tuberculosis, schistosomiasis and many other infectious and neoplastic conditions, some of which may coexist with VL. Fever, splenomegaly, pancytopenia and non-response to antimalarial therapy may provide clues before specific laboratory diagnosis is made.

Management

Pentavalent antimonials

Antimony (Sb) compounds were the first drugs to be used for the treatment of leishmaniasis and remain the mainstay of treatment in most parts of the world. The exception is the Indian subcontinent, especially Bihar state, where almost two-thirds of cases are refractory to Sb treatment. Traditionally, pentavalent antimony is available as sodium stibogluconate (100 mg/mL) in English-speaking countries and meglumine antimoniate (85 mg/mL) in French-speaking ones. The daily dose is 20 mg/kg body weight, given either intravenously or intramuscularly for 28–30 days. Side-effects are common and include arthralgias, myalgias, raised hepatic transaminases, pancreatitis (especially in patients co-infected with HIV) and ECG changes (T wave inversion and reduced amplitude). Severe cardiotoxicity, manifest by concave ST segment elevation, prolongation of QT_c greater than 0.5 msec, and ventricular dysrhythmias, is not uncommon. The incidence of cardiotoxicity and death can be very high with improperly manufactured Sb.

Amphotericin B

Amphotericin B deoxycholate, given once daily or on alternate days at a dose of 0.75–1.00 mg/kg for 15–20 doses, is used as the first-line drug in many regions where there is a significant level of Sb unresponsiveness. It has a cure rate of nearly 100%. Infusion-related side-effects, e.g. high fever with rigor, thrombophlebitis, diarrhoea and vomiting, are extremely common. Serious adverse events, such as renal or hepatic toxicity, hypokalaemia and thrombocytopenia, are not uncommon.

Lipid formulations of amphotericin B (p. 160) are less toxic. AmBisome is approved by the US Food and Drug Administration and is first-line therapy in Europe for VL. Drug doses vary according to geographical location. In the Indian subcontinent, a total dose of 10 or 15 mg/kg, administered in a single dose or as multiple doses over several days, respectively, is considered adequate, whereas in Africa 14–18 mg, and in South America and Europe 21–24 mg, in divided doses, typically spread over 10 days, is needed for immunocompetent patients. High daily doses of the lipid formulations are well tolerated, and in one study a single dose of 10 mg/kg of AmBisome cured 96% of Indian patients. AmBisome has been made available at a preferential low price for developing countries, and greater use of this drug for treatment of VL is expected.

EBM 13.63 Combination therapy for visceral leishmaniasis

'In India, combinations of a single dose of liposomal amphotericin B (AmBisome, 5 mg/kg) with either 7 days of miltefosine or 10 days of paromomycin, or 10 days each of miltefosine and paromomycin, cured at least 97% of patients.'

'In Sudan, a combination of 17 days of antimony (Sb) with paromomycin produces a similar rate of cure (> 90%) to conventional treatment with 30 days of antimony.'

- Sundar S, et al. Lancet 2011; 377:477–486.
- Musa A, et al. PLoS NTD 2012; e1674.

Other drugs

The oral drug miltefosine, an alkyl phospholipid, has been approved in several countries for the treatment of VL. A daily dose of 50 mg (patient's body weight < 25 kg) to 100 mg (≥ 25 kg), or 2.5 mg/kg body weight for children, for 28 days cures over 90% of patients. Side-effects include mild to moderate vomiting and diarrhoea, and rarely skin allergy or renal or liver toxicity. Since it is a teratogenic drug, it cannot be used in pregnancy; female patients are advised not to become pregnant for the duration of treatment and 3 months thereafter, because of its half-life of nearly 1 week.

Paromomycin is an aminoglycoside that has undergone trials in India and Africa, and is highly effective if given intramuscularly at 11 mg/kg body weight of paromomycin base, daily for 3 weeks. No significant auditory or renal toxicity is seen. The drug has been approved in India for the treatment of VL.

Pentamidine isethionate was used to treat Sb-refractory patients with VL. However, declining efficacy and serious side-effects, such as type 1 diabetes mellitus, hypoglycaemia and hypotension, have led to it being abandoned.

Multidrug therapy of VL is likely to be used increasingly to prevent emergence of drug resistance (Box 13.63).

Response to treatment

A good response results in abatement of fever, a feeling of well-being, gradual decrease in spleen size, weight gain and recovery of blood counts. Patients should be followed regularly for a period of 6–12 months, as a small minority may experience a relapse of the disease during this period, irrespective of the treatment regimen.

HIV–visceral leishmaniasis co-infection

HIV-induced immunosuppression (Ch. 14) increases the risk of contracting VL 100–1000 times. Most cases of HIV–VL co-infection have been reported from Spain, France, Italy and Portugal. Antiretroviral therapy (ART) has led to a remarkable decline in the incidence of VL co-infection in Europe. However, numbers are increasing in Africa (mainly Ethiopia), Brazil and in the Indian subcontinent.

Although the clinical triad of fever, splenomegaly and hepatomegaly is found in the majority of co-infected patients, those with low CD4 count may have atypical clinical presentations, posing a diagnostic challenge. VL may present with gastrointestinal involvement (stomach, duodenum or colon), ascites, pleural or pericardial effusion, or involvement of lungs, tonsil, oral mucosa or skin. Diagnostic principles remain the same as those in non-HIV patients. Parasites are numerous and easily demonstrable, even in buffy coat preparations. Sometimes amastigotes are found in unusual sites, such as bronchoalveolar lavage fluid, pleural fluid or biopsies of the gastrointestinal tract. Immunofluorescence, Western blot, ELISA and other serological tests used singly have low sensitivity. DNA detection by PCR of the blood or its buffy coat are at least 95% sensitive, and accurately track recovery and relapse.

Treatment of VL with HIV co-infection is essentially the same as in immunocompetent patients but there are some differences in outcome. Conventional amphotericin B (0.7 mg/kg/day for 28 days) may be more effective in achieving initial cure than Sb (20 mg/kg/day for 28 days). Using high-dose liposomal amphotericin B (4 mg/kg on days 1–5, 10, 17, 24, 31 and 38), a high cure rate is possible. However, these co-infected patients have a tendency to relapse within 1 year. For prevention of relapse, maintenance chemotherapy with monthly liposomal amphotericin B is useful.

Post-kala-azar dermal leishmaniasis

After treatment and apparent recovery from the visceral disease in India and Sudan, some patients develop dermatological manifestations due to local parasitic infection.

Clinical features

In India, dermatological changes occur in a small minority of patients 6 months to at least 3 years after the initial infection. They are seen as macules, papules, nodules (most frequently) and plaques, which have a predilection for the face, especially the area around the chin. The face often appears erythematous (Fig. 13.42A). Hypopigmented macules can occur over all parts of the body and are highly variable in extent and location. There are no systemic symptoms and no spontaneous healing.

In Sudan, approximately 50% of patients with VL develop post-kala-azar dermal leishmaniasis (PKDL), experiencing skin manifestations concurrently with VL or within the following 6 months. In addition to the dermatological features described above, a measles-like micropapular rash (Fig. 13.42B) may be seen all over the body. In Sudan, children are more frequently affected than in India. Spontaneous healing occurs in about three-quarters of cases within 1 year.

Investigations and management

The diagnosis is clinical, supported by demonstration of scanty parasites in lesions by slit-skin smear and culture. Immunofluorescence and immunohistochemistry may demonstrate the parasite in skin tissues. In the majority of patients, serological tests (direct agglutination test or k39 strip tests) are positive.

Treatment of PKDL is difficult. In India, Sb for 120 days, several courses of amphotericin B infusions, or miltefosine for 12 weeks is required. In Sudan, Sb for 2 months is considered adequate. In the absence of a physical handicap, most patients are reluctant to complete the treatment. PKDL patients are a human reservoir, and focal outbreaks have been linked to patients with PKDL in areas previously free of VL.

Prevention and control

Sandflies are extremely sensitive to insecticides, and vector control through insecticide spray is very important. Mosquito nets or curtains treated with insecticides will keep out the tiny sandflies. In endemic areas with zoonotic transmission, infected or stray dogs should be destroyed.

In areas with anthroponotic transmission, early diagnosis and treatment of human infections, to reduce the reservoir and control epidemics of VL, is extremely important. Serology is useful in diagnosis of suspected cases in the field. No vaccine is currently available.

Cutaneous and mucosal leishmaniasis

Cutaneous leishmaniasis

CL (oriental sore) occurs in both the Old World and the New World (the Americas). Transmission is described on page 362.

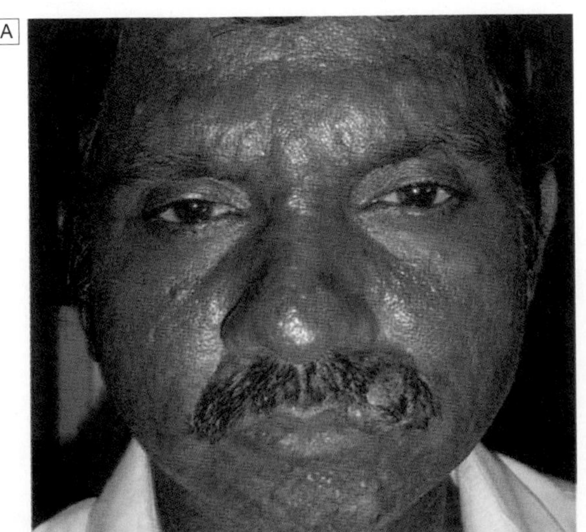

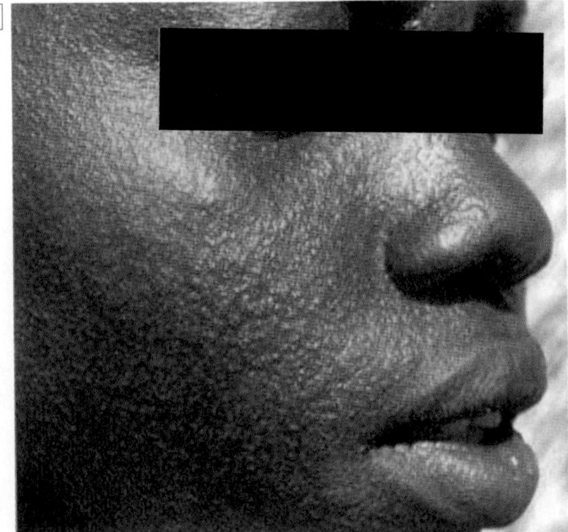

Fig. 13.42 Post-kala-azar dermal leishmaniasis. **A** In India, with macules, papules, nodules and plaques. From Sundar S, et al. 2006 – see p. 386. **B** In Sudan, with micronodular rash.

In the Old World, CL is mild. It is found around the Mediterranean basin, throughout the Middle East and Central Asia as far as Pakistan, and in sub-Saharan West Africa and Sudan (Fig. 13.43). The causative organisms for Old World zoonotic CL are *L. major*, *L. tropica* and *L. aethiopica* (Box 13.64). Anthroponotic CL is caused by *L. tropica*, and is confined to urban or suburban areas of the Old World. Afghanistan is currently the biggest focus, but infection is endemic in Pakistan, the western deserts of India, Iran, Iraq, Syria and other areas of the Middle East. In recent years, there has been an increase in the incidence of zoonotic CL in both the Old and the New World due to urbanisation and deforestation which led to peridomestic transmission (in and around human dwellings).

New World CL is a more significant disease, which may disfigure the nose, ears and mouth, and is caused by the *L. mexicana* complex (comprising *L. mexicana*, *L. amazonensis* and *L. venezuelensis*) and by the *Viannia* subgenus *L. (V.) brasiliensis* complex (comprising *L. (V.) guyanensis*, *L. (V.) panamensis*, *L. (V.) brasiliensis* and *L. (V.) peruviana*).

13.64 Types of Old World cutaneous leishmaniasis

Leishmania spp.	Host	Clinical features
L. tropica	Dogs	Slow evolution, less severe
L. major	Gerbils, desert rodents	Rapid necrosis, wet sores
L. aethiopica	Hyraxes	Solitary facial lesions with satellites

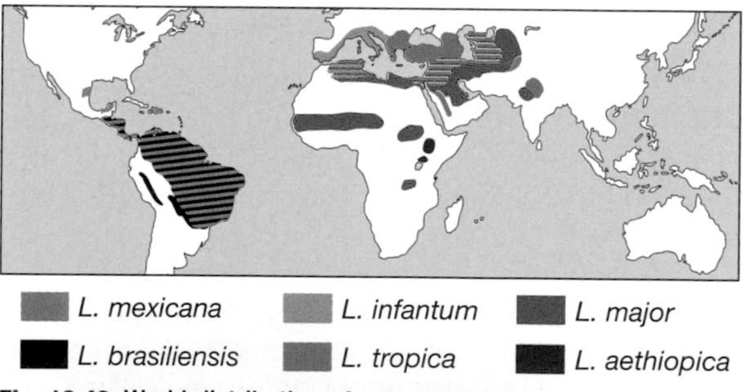

Fig. 13.43 World distribution of cutaneous leishmaniasis.

CL is commonly imported and should be considered in the differential diagnosis of an ulcerating skin lesion, especially in travellers who have visited endemic areas of the Old World or forests in Central and South America.

Pathogenesis

Inoculated parasites are taken up by dermal macrophages, in which they multiply and form a focus for lymphocytes, epithelioid cells and plasma cells. Self-healing may occur with necrosis of infected macrophages, or the lesion may become chronic with ulceration of the overlying epidermis, depending upon the aetiological pathogen.

Clinical features

The incubation period is typically 2–3 months (range 2 weeks to 5 years). In all types of CL, the common feature is development of a papule followed by ulceration of the skin with raised borders, usually at the site of the bite of the vector. Lesions, single or multiple, start as small red papules that increase gradually in size, reaching 2–10 cm in diameter. A crust forms, overlying an ulcer with a granular base (Fig. 13.44). These ulcers develop a few weeks or months after the bite. There can be satellite lesions, especially in *L. major* and occasionally in *L. tropica* infections. Regional lymphadenopathy, pain, pruritus and secondary bacterial infections may occur.

Clinically, lesions of *L. mexicana* and *L. peruviana* closely resemble those seen in the Old World, but lesions on the pinna of the ear are common, and are chronic and destructive. *L. mexicana* is responsible for chiclero ulcers, the self-healing sores of Mexico.

If immunity is good, there is usually spontaneous healing in *L. tropica*, *L. major* and *L. mexicana* lesions. In some patients with anergy to *Leishmania*, the skin lesions of *L. aethiopica*, *L. mexicana* and *L. amazonensis* infections progress to the development of diffuse CL; this is characterised by spread of the infection from the initial ulcer, usually on the face, to involve the whole body in the form of non-ulcerative nodules. Occasionally, in *L. tropica* infections, sores that have apparently healed relapse persistently (recidivans or lupoid leishmaniasis).

Mucosal leishmaniasis

The *Viannia* subgenus extends widely from the Amazon basin as far as Paraguay and Costa Rica, and is

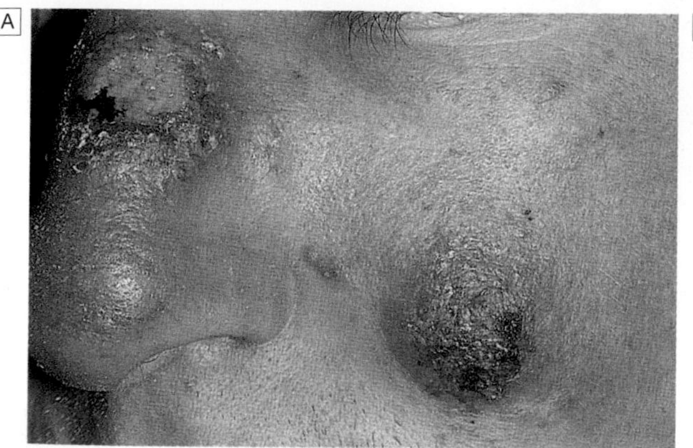

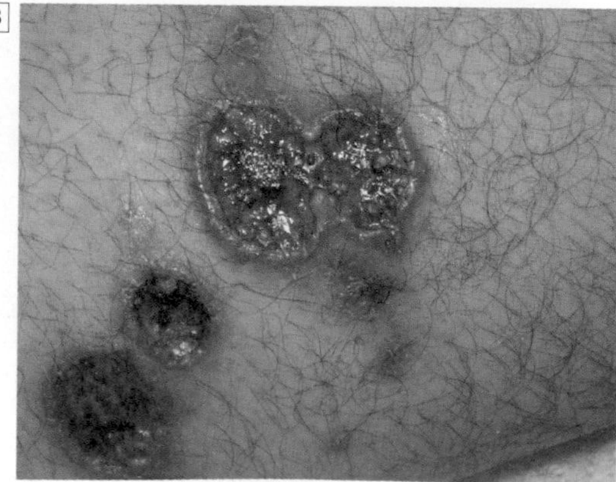

Fig. 13.44 Cutaneous leishmaniasis. **A** Papule. **B** Ulcer.

responsible for deep sores and ML. In *L. (V.) brasiliensis* complex infections, cutaneous lesions may be followed by mucosal spread of the disease simultaneously or even years later. Young men with chronic lesions are particularly at risk, and between 2% and 40% of infected persons develop 'espundia', metastatic lesions in the mucosa of the nose or mouth. This is characterised by thickening and erythema of the nasal mucosa, typically starting at the junction of the nose and upper lip. Later, ulceration develops. The lips, soft palate, fauces and larynx may also be invaded and destroyed, leading to considerable suffering and deformity. There is no spontaneous healing, and death may result from severe respiratory tract infections due to massive destruction of the pharynx.

Investigations in CL and ML

CL is often diagnosed on the basis of the lesions' clinical characteristics. However, parasitological confirmation is important because clinical manifestations may be mimicked by other infections. Amastigotes can be demonstrated on a slit-skin smear with Giemsa staining; alternatively, they can be cultured from the sores early during the infection. Parasites seem to be particularly difficult to isolate from sores caused by *L. brasiliensis*, responsible for the vast majority of cases in Brazil. Touch preparations from biopsies and histopathology usually have a low sensitivity. Culture of fine needle aspiration material has been reported to be the most sensitive method.

ML is more difficult to diagnose parasitologically. The leishmanin skin test measures delayed-type hypersensitivity to killed *Leishmania* organisms. A positive test is defined as induration of more than 5 mm 48 hours after intradermal injection. The test is positive, except in diffuse CL and during active VL. PCR is used increasingly for diagnosis and speciation, which is useful in selecting therapy.

Management of CL and ML

Small lesions may self-heal or are treated by freezing with liquid nitrogen or curettage. There is no ideal antimicrobial therapy. Treatment should be individualised on the basis of the causative organism, severity of the lesions, availability of drugs, tolerance of the patient for toxicity, and local resistance patterns.

In CL, topical application of paromomycin 15% plus methylbenzethonium chloride 12% is beneficial. Intralesional antimony (Sb: 0.2–0.8 mL/lesion) up to 2 g seems to be rapidly effective in suitable cases; it is well tolerated and economic, and is safe in patients with cardiac, liver or renal diseases.

In ML, and in CL when the lesions are multiple or in a disfiguring site, it is better to treat with parenteral Sb in a dose of 20 mg/kg/day (usually given for 20 days for CL and 28 days for ML), or with conventional or liposomal amphotericin B (see treatment of VL above). Sb is also indicated to prevent the development of mucosal disease, if there is any chance that a lesion acquired in South America is due to an *L. brasiliensis* strain. Refractory CL or ML should be treated with an amphotericin B preparation.

Other regimens may be effective. Two to four doses of pentamidine (2–4 mg/kg), administered on alternate days, are effective in New World CL caused by *L. guyanensis*. In ML, 8 injections of pentamidine (4 mg/kg on alternate days) cure the majority of patients. Ketoconazole (600 mg daily for 4 weeks) has shown some potential against *L. mexicana* infection. In Saudi Arabia, fluconazole (200 mg daily for 6 weeks) reduced healing times and cured 79% of patients with CL caused by *L. major*. In India, itraconazole (200 mg daily for 6 weeks) produced good results in CL.

Prevention of CL and ML

Personal protection against sandfly bites is important. No effective vaccine is yet available.

Gastrointestinal protozoal infections

Amoebiasis

Amoebiasis is caused by *Entamoeba histolytica*, which is spread between humans by its cysts. It is one of the leading parasitic causes of morbidity and mortality in the tropics and is occasionally acquired in other countries, such as the UK. Two non-pathogenic *Entamoeba* species (*E. dispar* and *E. moshkovskii*) are morphologically identical to *E. histolytica*, and are distinguishable only by molecular techniques, isoenzyme studies or monoclonal antibody typing. However, only *E. histolytica* causes amoebic dysentery or liver abscess. The life cycle of the amoeba is shown in Figure 13.45A.

Pathology

Cysts of *E. histolytica* are ingested in water or uncooked foods contaminated by human faeces. Infection may also be acquired through anal/oral sexual practices. In the colon, trophozoite forms emerge from the cysts. The parasite may invade the mucous membrane of the large bowel, producing lesions that are maximal in the caecum but found as far down as the anal canal. These are flask-shaped ulcers, varying greatly in size and surrounded by healthy mucosa. A localised granuloma (amoeboma), presenting as a palpable mass in the rectum or a filling defect in the colon on radiography, is a rare complication which should be differentiated from colonic carcinoma. Amoebic ulcers may cause severe haemorrhage but rarely perforate the bowel wall.

Amoebic trophozoites can emerge from the vegetative cyst from the bowel and be carried to the liver in a portal venule. They can multiply rapidly and destroy the liver parenchyma, causing an abscess (see also p. 956). The liquid contents at first have a characteristic pinkish colour, which may later change to chocolate-brown (like anchovy sauce).

Cutaneous amoebiasis, though rare, causes progressive genital, perianal or peri-abdominal surgical wound ulceration.

Clinical features

Intestinal amoebiasis – amoebic dysentery

Most amoebic infections are asymptomatic. The incubation period of amoebiasis ranges from 2 weeks to many years, followed by a chronic course with abdominal pains and two or more unformed stools a day. Offensive diarrhoea alternating with constipation, and blood or mucus in the stool, are common. There may be abdominal pain, especially right lower quadrant (which may simulate acute appendicitis). A dysenteric presentation

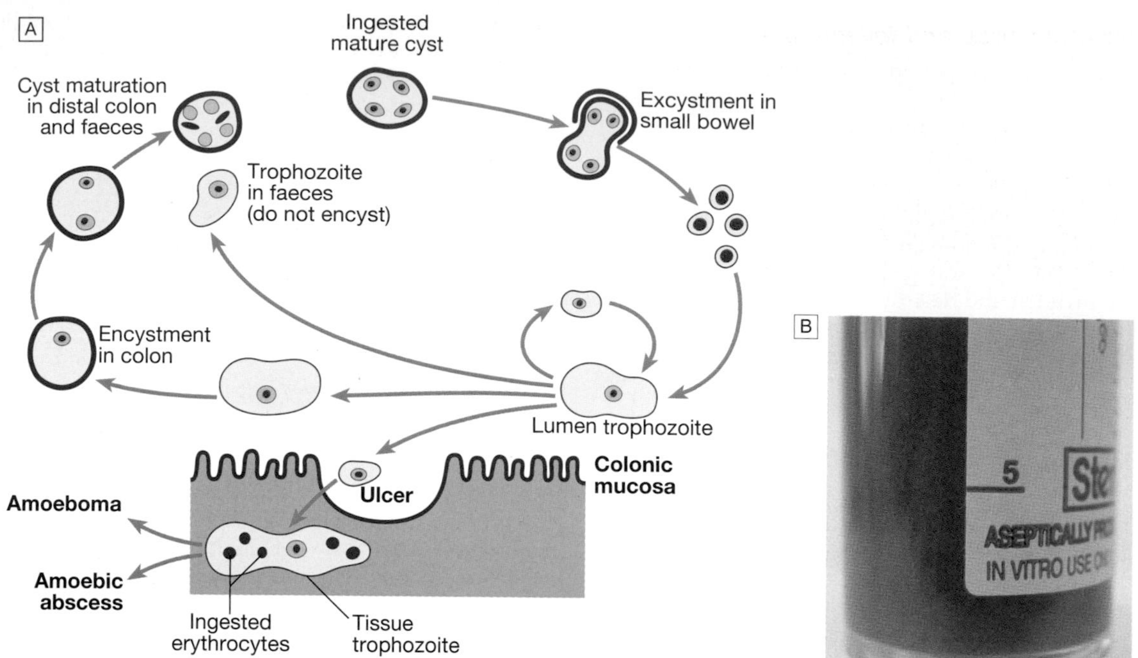

Fig. 13.45 Amoebiasis. A The life cycle of *Entamoeba histolytica*. From Knight 1982 – see p. 386. B The chocolate-brown appearance of aspirated material from an amoebic liver abscess.

with passage of blood, simulating bacillary dysentery or ulcerative colitis, occurs particularly in older people, in the puerperium and with superadded pyogenic infection of the ulcers.

Amoebic liver abscess

The abscess is usually found in the right hepatic lobe. There may not be associated diarrhoea. Early symptoms may be local discomfort only and malaise; later, a swinging temperature and sweating may develop, usually without marked systemic symptoms or associated cardiovascular signs. An enlarged, tender liver, cough and pain in the right shoulder are characteristic, but symptoms may remain vague and signs minimal. A large abscess may penetrate the diaphragm and rupture into the lung, from where its contents may be coughed up through a hepaticobronchial fistula. Rupture into the pleural or peritoneal cavity, or rupture of a left lobe abscess in the pericardial sac, is less common but more serious.

Investigations

The stool and any exudate should be examined at once under the microscope for motile trophozoites containing red blood cells. Movements cease rapidly as the stool preparation cools. Several stools may need to be examined in chronic amoebiasis before cysts are found. Sigmoidoscopy may reveal typical flask-shaped ulcers, which should be scraped and examined immediately for *E. histolytica*. In endemic areas, one-third of the population are symptomless passers of amoebic cysts.

An amoebic abscess of the liver is suspected on clinical grounds; there is often a neutrophil leucocytosis and a raised right hemidiaphragm on chest X-ray. Confirmation is by ultrasonic scanning. Aspirated pus from an amoebic abscess has the characteristic anchovy sauce or chocolate-brown appearance but only rarely contains free amoebae (Fig. 13.45B).

Serum antibodies are detectable by immunofluorescence in over 95% of patients with hepatic amoebiasis and intestinal amoeboma, but in only about 60% of dysenteric amoebiasis. DNA detection by PCR has been shown to be useful in diagnosis of *E. histolytica* infections but is not generally available.

Management

Intestinal and early hepatic amoebiasis responds quickly to oral metronidazole (800 mg 3 times daily for 5–10 days) or other long-acting nitroimidazoles like tinidazole or ornidazole (both in doses of 2 g daily for 3 days). Nitazoxanide (500 mg twice daily for 3 days) is an alternative drug. Either diloxanide furoate or paromomycin, in doses of 500 mg orally 3 times daily for 10 days after treatment, should be given to eliminate luminal cysts.

If a liver abscess is large or threatens to burst, or if the response to chemotherapy is not prompt, aspiration is required and is repeated if necessary. Rupture of an abscess into the pleural cavity, pericardial sac or peritoneal cavity necessitates immediate aspiration or surgical drainage. Small serous effusions resolve without drainage.

Prevention

Personal precautions against contracting amoebiasis consist of not eating fresh, uncooked vegetables or drinking unclean water.

Giardiasis

Infection with *Giardia lamblia* is found worldwide and is common in the tropics. It particularly affects children, tourists and immunosuppressed individuals, and is the parasite most commonly imported into the UK. In cystic form, it remains viable in water for up to 3 months and infection usually occurs by ingesting contaminated water. Its flagellar trophozoite form attaches to the duodenal and jejunal mucosa, causing inflammation.

Clinical features and investigations

After an incubation period of 1–3 weeks, there is diarrhoea, abdominal pain, weakness, anorexia, nausea and vomiting. On examination, there may be abdominal distension and tenderness.

Stools obtained at 2–3-day intervals should be examined for cysts. Duodenal or jejunal aspiration by endoscopy gives a higher diagnostic yield. The 'string test' may be used, in which one end of a piece of string is passed into the duodenum by swallowing and retrieved after an overnight fast; expressed fluid is then examined for the presence of *G. lamblia* trophozoites. A number of stool antigen detection tests are available. Jejunal biopsy specimens may show *G. lamblia* on the epithelial surface.

Management

Treatment is with a single dose of tinidazole 2 g, metronidazole 400 mg 3 times daily for 10 days, or nitazoxanide 500 mg orally twice daily for 3 days.

Cryptosporidiosis

Cryptosporidium spp. are coccidian protozoal parasites of humans and domestic animals. Infection is acquired by the faecal–oral route through contaminated water supplies. The incubation period is approximately 7–10 days and is followed by watery diarrhoea and abdominal cramps. The illness is usually self-limiting, but in immunocompromised patients, especially those with HIV, the illness can be devastating, with persistent severe diarrhoea and substantial weight loss (p. 399).

Cyclosporiasis

Cyclospora cayetanensis is a globally distributed coccidian protozoal parasite of humans. Infection is acquired by ingestion of contaminated water. The incubation period is approximately 2–11 days and is followed by acute onset of diarrhoea with abdominal cramps, which may remit and relapse. Although usually self-limiting, the illness may last as long as 6 weeks, with significant associated weight loss and malabsorption, and is more severe in immunocompromised individuals. Diagnosis is by detection of oöcysts on faecal microscopy. Treatment may be necessary in a few cases, and the agent of choice is co-trimoxazole 960 mg twice daily for 7 days.

INFECTIONS CAUSED BY HELMINTHS

Helminths (from the Greek *helmins*, meaning worm) include three groups of parasitic worm (Box 13.65), large multicellular organisms with complex tissues and organs.

Intestinal human nematodes

Diseases are caused by adult nematodes living in the human gut. There are two types:

- the hookworms, which have a soil stage in which they develop into larvae that then penetrate the host
- a group of nematodes which survive in the soil merely as eggs that have to be ingested for their life cycle to continue.

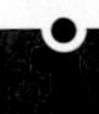

13.65 Classes of helminth that parasitise humans

Nematodes or roundworms
• Intestinal human nematodes: *Ancylostoma duodenale, Necator americanus, Strongyloides stercoralis, Ascaris lumbricoides, Enterobius vermicularis, Trichuris trichiura*
• Tissue-dwelling human nematodes: *Wuchereria bancrofti, Brugia malayi, Loa loa, Onchocerca volvulus, Dracunculus medinensis, Mansonella perstans, Dirofilaria immitis*
• Zoonotic nematodes: *Trichinella spiralis*
Trematodes or flukes
• Blood flukes: *Schistosoma haematobium, S. mansoni, S. japonicum, S. mekongi, S. intercalatum*
• Lung flukes: *Paragonimus* spp.
• Hepatobiliary flukes: *Clonorchis sinensis, Fasciola hepatica, Opisthorchis felineus*
• Intestinal flukes: *Fasciolopsis buski*
Cestodes or tapeworms
• Intestinal tapeworms: *Taenia saginata, T. solium, Diphyllobothrium latum, Hymenolepis nana*
• Tissue-dwelling cysts or worms: *Taenia solium, Echinococcus granulosus*

The geographical distribution of hookworms is limited by the larval requirement for warmth and humidity. Soil-transmitted nematode infections can be prevented by avoidance of faecal soil contamination (adequate sewerage disposal) or skin contact (wearing shoes), and by strict personal hygiene.

Ancylostomiasis (hookworm)

Ancylostomiasis is caused by parasitisation with *Ancylostoma duodenale* or *Necator americanus*. The complex life cycle is shown in Figure 13.46. The adult hookworm is 1 cm long and lives in the duodenum and upper jejunum. Eggs are passed in the faeces. In warm, moist, shady soil, the larvae develop into rhabditiform and then the infective filariform stages; they then penetrate human skin and are carried to the lungs. After entering the alveoli, they ascend the bronchi, are swallowed and mature in the small intestine, reaching maturity 4–7 weeks after infection. The worms attach themselves to the mucosa of the small intestine by their buccal capsule (Fig. 13.47) and withdraw blood. The mean daily loss of blood from one *A. duodenale* is 0.15 mL and from *N. americanus* 0.03 mL.

Hookworm infection is one of the main causes of anaemia in the tropics and subtropics. *A. duodenale* is endemic in the Far East and Mediterranean coastal regions, and is also present in Africa, while *N. americanus* is endemic in West, East and Central Africa, and Central and South America, as well as in the Far East.

Clinical features

An allergic dermatitis, usually on the feet (ground itch), may be experienced at the time of infection. The passage of the larvae through the lungs in a heavy infection causes a paroxysmal cough with blood-stained sputum, associated with patchy pulmonary consolidation and eosinophilia. When the worms have reached the small intestine, vomiting and epigastric pain resembling peptic ulcer disease may occur. Sometimes, frequent loose stools are passed. The degree of iron and protein

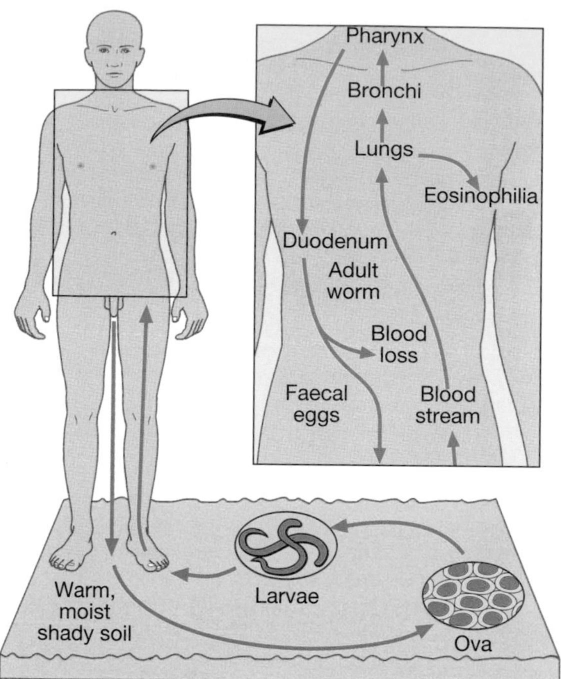

Fig. 13.46 Ancylostomiasis. Life cycle of *Ancylostoma.*

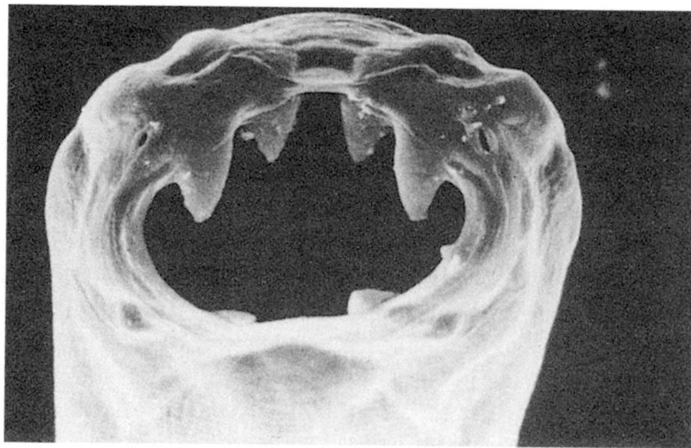

Fig. 13.47 *Ancylostoma duodenale.* Electron micrograph showing the ventral teeth. From Gibbons 1986 – see p. 386.

deficiency which develops depends not only on the load of worms but also on the nutrition of the patient and especially on the iron stores. Anaemia with high-output cardiac failure may result. The mental and physical development of children may be retarded in severe infection.

Investigations

There is eosinophilia. The characteristic ovum can be recognised in the stool. If hookworms are present in numbers sufficient to cause anaemia, faecal occult blood testing will be positive and many ova will be present.

Management

A single dose of albendazole (400 mg) is the treatment of choice. Alternatively, mebendazole 100 mg twice daily for 3 days may be used. Anaemia and heart failure associated with hookworm infection respond well to oral iron, even when severe; blood transfusion is rarely required.

Strongyloidiasis

Strongyloides stercoralis is a very small nematode (2 mm × 0.4 mm) which parasitises the mucosa of the upper part of the small intestine, often in large numbers, causing persistent eosinophilia. The eggs hatch in the bowel but only larvae are passed in the faeces. In moist soil, they moult and become the infective filariform larvae. After penetrating human skin, they undergo a development cycle similar to that of hookworms, except that the female worms burrow into the intestinal mucosa and submucosa. Some larvae in the intestine may develop into filariform larvae, which may then penetrate the mucosa or the perianal skin and lead to autoinfection and persistent infection. Patients with *Strongyloides* infection persisting for more than 35 years have been described. Strongyloidiasis occurs in the tropics and subtropics, and is especially prevalent in the Far East.

Clinical features

These are shown in Box 13.66. The classic triad of symptoms consists of abdominal pain, diarrhoea and urticaria. Cutaneous manifestations, either urticaria or larva currens (a highly characteristic pruritic, elevated, erythematous lesion advancing along the course of larval migration), are characteristic and occur in 66% of patients.

Systemic strongyloidiasis (the *Strongyloides* hyperinfection syndrome), with dissemination of larvae throughout the body, occurs in association with immune suppression (intercurrent disease, HIV and HTLV-1 infection, corticosteroid treatment). Patients present with severe, generalised abdominal pain, abdominal distension and shock. Massive larval invasion of the lungs causes cough, wheeze and dyspnoea; cerebral involvement has manifestations ranging from subtle neurological signs to coma. Gram-negative sepsis frequently complicates the picture.

Investigations

There is eosinophilia. Serology (ELISA) is helpful but definitive diagnosis depends upon finding the larvae. The faeces should be examined microscopically for motile larvae; excretion is intermittent and so repeated examinations may be necessary. Larvae can also be found in jejunal aspirate or detected using the string test (p. 369). Larvae may also be cultured from faeces.

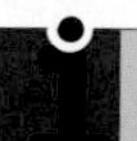

13.66 Clinical features of strongyloidiasis
Penetration of skin by infective larvae
• Itchy rash
Presence of worms in gut
• Abdominal pain, diarrhoea, steatorrhoea, weight loss
Allergic phenomena
• Urticarial plaques and papules, wheezing, arthralgia
Autoinfection
• Transient itchy, linear, urticarial weals across abdomen and buttocks (larva currens)
Systemic (super)infection
• Diarrhoea, pneumonia, meningoencephalitis, death

Management

A course of two doses of ivermectin (200 µg/kg), administered on successive days, is effective. Alternatively, albendazole is given orally in a dose of 15 mg/kg body weight twice daily for 3 days. A second course may be required. For the *Strongyloides* hyperinfection syndrome, ivermectin is given at 200 µg/kg for 5–7 days.

Ascaris lumbricoides (roundworm)

This pale yellow nematode is 20–35 cm long. Humans are infected by eating food contaminated with mature ova. *Ascaris* larvae hatch in the duodenum, migrate through the lungs, ascend the bronchial tree, are swallowed and mature in the small intestine. This tissue migration can provoke both local and general hypersensitivity reactions, with pneumonitis, eosinophilic granulomas, bronchial asthma and urticaria.

Clinical features

Intestinal ascariasis causes symptoms ranging from occasional vague abdominal pain through to malnutrition. The large size of the adult worm and its tendency to aggregate and migrate can result in obstructive complications. Tropical and subtropical areas are endemic for ascariasis, and in these areas it causes up to 35% of all intestinal obstructions, most commonly in the terminal ileum. Obstruction can be complicated further by intussusception, volvulus, haemorrhagic infarction and perforation. Other complications include blockage of the bile or pancreatic duct and obstruction of the appendix by adult worms.

Investigations

The diagnosis is made microscopically by finding ova in the faeces. Adult worms are frequently expelled rectally or orally. Occasionally, the worms are demonstrated radiographically by a barium examination. There is eosinophilia.

Management

A single dose of albendazole (400 mg), pyrantel pamoate (11 mg/kg; maximum 1 g), ivermectin (150–200 µg/kg) or mebendazole (100 mg twice daily for 3 days) is effective for intestinal ascariasis. Patients should be warned that they might expel numerous whole, large worms. Obstruction due to ascariasis should be treated with nasogastric suction, piperazine and intravenous fluids.

Prevention

Community chemotherapy programmes have been used to reduce *Ascaris* infection. The whole community can be treated every 3 months for several years. Alternatively, schoolchildren can be targeted; treating them lowers the prevalence of ascariasis in the community.

Enterobius vermicularis (threadworm)

This helminth is common throughout the world and affects mainly children. After the ova are swallowed, development takes place in the small intestine, but the adult worms are found chiefly in the colon.

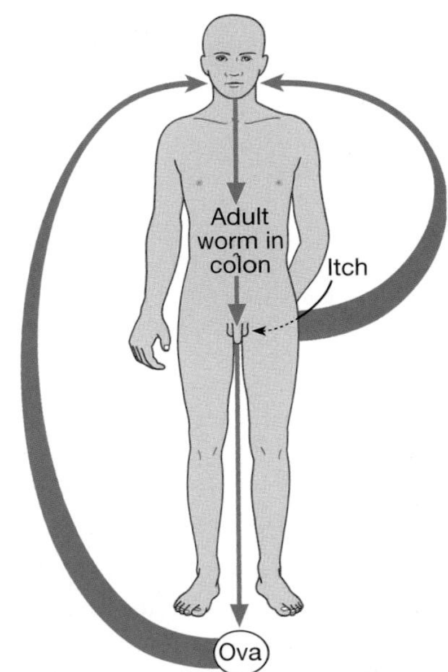

Fig. 13.48 Threadworm. Life cycle of *Enterobius vermicularis.*

Clinical features

The gravid female worm lays ova around the anus, causing intense itching, especially at night. The ova are often carried to the mouth on the fingers and so re-infection or human-to-human infection takes place (Fig. 13.48). In females, the genitalia may be involved. The adult worms may be seen moving on the buttocks or in the stool.

Investigations

Ova are detected by applying the adhesive surface of cellophane tape to the perianal skin in the morning. This is then examined on a glass slide under the microscope. A perianal swab, moistened with saline, is an alternative sampling method.

Management

A single dose of mebendazole (100 mg), albendazole (400 mg), pyrantel pamoate (11 mg/kg) or piperazine (4 g) is given and may be repeated after 2 weeks to control auto-reinfection. If infection recurs in a family, each member should be treated as above. During this period all nightclothes and bed linen are laundered. Fingernails must be kept short and hands washed carefully before meals. Subsequent therapy is reserved for those family members who develop recurrent infection.

Trichuris trichiura (whipworm)

Infections with whipworm are common all over the world under unhygienic conditions. Infection is contracted by the ingestion of earth or food contaminated with ova which have become infective after lying for 3 weeks or more in moist soil. The adult worm is 3–5 cm long and has a coiled anterior end resembling a whip. Whipworms inhabit the caecum, lower ileum, appendix, colon and anal canal. There are usually no symptoms, but intense infections in children may cause persistent diarrhoea or rectal prolapse, and growth retardation. The diagnosis is readily made by identifying ova in faeces. Treatment is with mebendazole in doses of

100 mg twice daily or albendazole 400 mg daily for 3 days for patients with light infections, and for 5–7 days for those with heavy infections.

Tissue-dwelling human nematodes

Filarial worms are tissue-dwelling nematodes. The larval stages are inoculated by biting mosquitoes or flies, each specific to a particular filarial species. The larvae develop into adult worms (2–50 cm long) which, after mating, produce millions of microfilariae (170–320 μm long) that migrate in blood or skin. The life cycle is completed when the vector takes up microfilariae while feeding on humans. In the insect, ingested microfilariae develop into infective larvae for inoculation in humans, normally the only host.

Disease is due to the host's immune response to the worms (both adult and microfilariae), particularly dying worms, and its pattern and severity vary with the site and stage of each species (Box 13.67). The worms are long-lived; microfilariae survive 2–3 years and adult worms 10–15 years. The infections are chronic and worst in individuals constantly exposed to re-infection.

Lymphatic filariasis

Infection with the filarial worms *Wuchereria bancrofti* and *Brugia malayi* is associated with clinical outcomes ranging from subclinical infection to hydrocele and elephantiasis.

W. bancrofti is transmitted by night-biting culicine or anopheline mosquitoes in most areas (Fig. 13.49). The adult worms, 4–10 cm in length, live in the lymphatics, and the females produce microfilariae which circulate in large numbers in the peripheral blood, usually at night. The infection is widespread in tropical Africa, on the North African coast, in coastal areas of Asia, Indonesia and northern Australia, the South Pacific islands, the West Indies and also in North and South America.

B. malayi usually causes less severe disease than *W. bancrofti* and is transmitted by *Mansonia* or *Anopheles* mosquitoes in Indonesia, Borneo, Malaysia, Vietnam, South China, South India and Sri Lanka.

Pathology

Several factors contribute to the pathogenesis of lymphatic filariasis. Toxins released by the adult worm cause lymphangiectasia; this dilatation of the lymphatic vessels leads to lymphatic dysfunction and the chronic clinical manifestations of lymphatic filariasis, lymphoedema and hydrocele. Death of the adult worm results in acute filarial lymphangitis. The filariae are symbiotically infected with rickettsia-like bacteria (*Wolbachia* spp.), and release of lipopolysaccharide from these bacteria contributes to inflammation. Lymphatic obstruction persists after death of the adult worm. Secondary bacterial infections cause tissue destruction. The host response to microfilariae is central to the pathogenesis of tropical pulmonary eosinophilia.

13.67 Pathogenicity of filarial infections depending on site and stage of worms

Worm species	Adult worm	Microfilariae
Wuchereria bancrofti* and *Brugia malayi	Lymphatic vessels+++	Blood− Pulmonary capillaries++
Loa loa	Subcutaneous+	Blood+
Onchocerca volvulus	Subcutaneous+	Skin+++ Eye+++
Mansonella perstans	Retroperitoneal−	Blood−
Mansonella streptocerca	Skin+	Skin++

(+++ severe; ++ moderate; + mild; – rarely pathogenic)

Clinical features

Acute filarial lymphangitis presents with fever, pain, tenderness and erythema along the course of inflamed lymphatic vessels. Inflammation of the spermatic cord, epididymis and testis is common. The whole episode lasts a few days but may recur several times a year. Temporary oedema becomes more persistent and regional lymph nodes enlarge. Progressive enlargement, coarsening, corrugation, fissuring and bacterial infection of the skin and subcutaneous tissue develop gradually, causing irreversible 'elephantiasis'. The scrotum may reach an enormous size. Chyluria and chylous effusions are milky and opalescent; on standing, fat globules rise to the top.

The acute lymphatic manifestations of filariasis must be differentiated from thrombophlebitis and infection. The oedema and lymphatic obstructive changes must be distinguished from congestive cardiac failure, malignancy, trauma and idiopathic abnormalities of the lymphatic system. Silicates absorbed from volcanic soil can also cause non-filarial elephantiasis.

Tropical pulmonary eosinophilia is a complication seen mainly in India and is likely to be due to microfilariae trapped in the pulmonary capillaries and destroyed

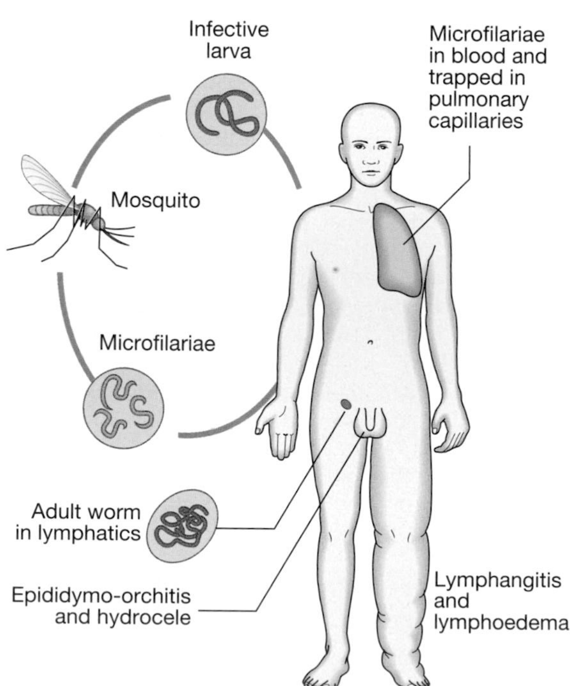

Fig. 13.49 ***Wuchereria bancrofti* and *Brugia malayi*.** Life cycle of organisms and pathogenesis of lymphatic filariasis.

by allergic inflammation. Patients present with paroxysmal cough, wheeze and fever. If untreated, this may progress to debilitating chronic interstitial lung disease.

Investigations

In the earliest stages of lymphangitis, the diagnosis is made on clinical grounds, supported by eosinophilia and sometimes by positive filarial serology. Filarial infections cause the highest eosinophil counts of all helminthic infections.

Microfilariae can be found in the peripheral blood at night, and either are seen moving in a wet blood film or are detected by microfiltration of a sample of lysed blood. They are usually present in hydrocele fluid, which may occasionally yield an adult filaria. By the time elephantiasis develops, microfilariae become difficult to find. Calcified filariae may sometimes be demonstrable by radiography. Movement of adult worms can be seen on scrotal ultrasound. PCR-based tests for detection of *W. bancrofti* and *B. malayi* DNA from blood have been developed.

Indirect fluorescence and ELISA detect antibodies in over 95% of active cases and 70% of established elephantiasis. The test becomes negative 1–2 years after cure. Serological tests cannot distinguish the different filarial infections. Highly sensitive and specific immunochromatographic card tests for detection of circulating *W. bancrofti* antigen are now commercially available; fingerprick blood taken at any time of the day can be used for these.

In tropical pulmonary eosinophilia, serology is strongly positive and IgE levels are massively elevated, but circulating microfilariae are not found. The chest X-ray shows miliary changes or mottled opacities. Pulmonary function tests show a restrictive picture.

Management

Treatment of the individual is aimed at reversing and halting disease progression. Diethylcarbamazine (DEC, 2 mg/kg orally 3 times daily for 12 days, or as a single dose) kills microfilariae and adult worms. Most adverse effects seen with DEC treatment are due to the host response to dying microfilariae, and the reaction intensity is directly proportional to the microfilarial load. The main symptoms are fever, headache, nausea, vomiting, arthralgia and prostration. These usually occur within 24–36 hours of the first dose of DEC. Antihistamines or corticosteroids may be required to control these allergic phenomena. Combining albendazole (400 mg) with ivermectin (200 μg/kg) in a single dose, with or without DEC (300 mg), is also highly effective in clearing the parasites. Treatment of *Wolbachia* with doxycycline (200 mg/day) for 4–8 weeks provides additional benefit by eliminating the bacteria; this leads to interruption of parasite embryogenesis. For tropical pulmonary eosinophilia, DEC for 14 days is the treatment of choice.

Chronic lymphatic pathology

Experience in India and Brazil shows that active management of chronic lymphatic pathology can alleviate symptoms. Patients should be taught meticulous skin care of their lymphoedematous limbs to prevent secondary bacterial and fungal infections. Tight bandaging, massage and bed rest with elevation of the affected limb may help to control the lymphoedema. Prompt diagnosis and antibiotic therapy of bacterial cellulitis are important in preventing further lymphatic damage and worsening of existing elephantiasis. Plastic surgery may be indicated in established elephantiasis. Great relief can be obtained by removal of excess tissue but recurrences are probable unless new lymphatic drainage is established. Hydroceles and chyluria can be repaired surgically.

Prevention

Treatment of the whole population in endemic areas with annual single-dose DEC (6 mg/kg), either alone or in combination with albendazole or ivermectin, can reduce filarial transmission. This mass treatment should be combined with mosquito control programmes.

Loiasis

Loiasis is caused by infection with the filaria *Loa loa*. The disease is endemic in forested and swampy parts of Western and Central Africa. The adult worms, 3–7 cm × 4 mm, chiefly parasitise the subcutaneous tissue of humans, releasing larval microfilariae into the peripheral blood in the daytime. The vector is *Chrysops*, a forest-dwelling, day-biting fly.

The host response to *Loa loa* is usually absent or mild, so that the infection may be harmless. From time to time a short-lived, inflammatory, oedematous swelling (a Calabar swelling) is produced around an adult worm. Heavy infections, especially when treated, may cause encephalitis.

Clinical features

The infection is often symptomless. The incubation period is commonly over a year but may be just 3 months. The first sign is usually a Calabar swelling, an irritating, tense, localised swelling that may be painful, especially if it is near a joint. The swelling is generally on a limb; it measures a few centimetres in diameter but sometimes is more diffuse and extensive. It usually disappears after a few days but may persist for 2 or 3 weeks. A succession of such swellings may appear at irregular intervals, often in adjacent sites. Sometimes, there is urticaria and pruritus elsewhere. Occasionally, a worm may be seen wriggling under the skin, especially that of an eyelid, and may cross the eye under the conjunctiva, taking many minutes to do so.

Investigations

Diagnosis is by demonstrating microfilariae in blood taken during the day, but they may not always be found in patients with Calabar swellings. Antifilarial antibodies are positive in 95% of patients and there is massive eosinophilia. Occasionally, a calcified worm may be seen on X-ray.

Management

DEC (see above) is curative, in a dose of 9–12 mg/kg daily, continued for 21 days. Treatment may precipitate a severe reaction in patients with a heavy microfilaraemia characterised by fever, joint and muscle pain, and encephalitis; microfilaraemic patients should be given corticosteroid cover.

Prevention

Protection is afforded by building houses away from trees and by having dwellings wire-screened. Protective clothing and insect repellents are also useful. DEC in a dose of 5 mg/kg daily for 3 days each month is partially protective.

Onchocerciasis (river blindness)

Onchocerciasis is the result of infection by the filarial *Onchocerca volvulus*. The infection is conveyed by flies of the genus *Simulium*, which breed in rapidly flowing, well-aerated water. Adult flies inflict painful bites during the day, both inside and outside houses. While feeding, they pick up the microfilariae, which mature into the infective larva and are transmitted to a new host in subsequent bites. Humans are the only known hosts (Fig. 13.50).

Onchocerciasis is endemic in sub-Saharan Africa, Yemen and a few foci in Central and South America. It is estimated that 17.7 million people are infected, of whom 500000 are visually impaired and 270000 blind. Due to onchocerciasis, huge tracts of fertile land lie virtually untilled, and individuals and communities are impoverished.

Pathology

After inoculation of larvae by a bite from an infected fly, the worms mature in 2–4 months and live for up to 17 years in subcutaneous and connective tissues. At sites of trauma, over bony prominences and around joints, fibrosis may form nodules around adult worms, which otherwise cause no direct damage. Innumerable microfilariae, discharged by the female *O. volvulus*, move actively in these nodules and in the adjacent tissues, are widely distributed in the skin, and may invade the eye. Live microfilariae elicit little tissue reaction, but dead ones may cause severe allergic inflammation, leading to hyaline necrosis and loss of collagen and elastin. Death of microfilariae in the eye causes inflammation and may lead to blindness.

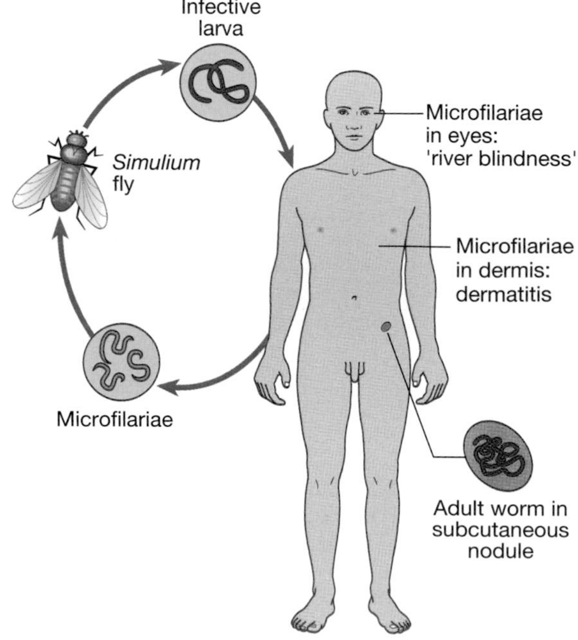

Fig. 13.50 ***Onchocerca volvulus.*** Life cycle of organism and pathogenesis of onchocerciasis.

Clinical features

The infection may remain symptomless for months or years. The first symptom is usually itching, localised to one quadrant of the body and later becoming generalised and involving the eyes. Transient oedema of part or all of a limb is an early sign, followed by papular urticaria spreading gradually from the site of infection. This is difficult to see on dark skins, in which the most common signs are papules excoriated by scratching, spotty hyperpigmentation from resolving inflammation, and more chronic changes of a rough, thickened or inelastic, wrinkled skin. Both infected and uninfected superficial lymph nodes enlarge and may hang down in folds of loose skin in the groin. Hydrocele, femoral hernias and scrotal elephantiasis can occur. Firm subcutaneous nodules of more than 1 cm in diameter (onchocercomas) occur in chronic infection.

Eye disease is most common in highly endemic areas and is associated with chronic heavy infections and nodules on the head. Early manifestations include itching, lacrimation and conjunctival injection. These cause conjunctivitis, sclerosing keratitis with pannus formation, uveitis which may lead to glaucoma and cataract, and, less commonly, choroiditis and optic neuritis. Classically, 'snowflake' deposits are seen in the edges of the cornea.

Investigations

The finding of nodules or characteristic lesions of the skin or eyes in a patient from an endemic area, associated with eosinophilia, is suggestive. Skin snips or shavings, taken with a corneoscleral punch or scalpel blade from calf, buttock and shoulder, are placed in saline under a cover slip on a microscope slide and examined after 4 hours. Microfilariae are seen wriggling free in all but the lightest infections. Slit-lamp examination may reveal microfilariae moving in the anterior chamber of the eye or trapped in the cornea. A nodule may be removed and incised, showing the coiled, thread-like adult worm.

Filarial antibodies may be detected in up to 95% of patients. Several promising rapid strip tests based on antibody or antigen detection are under clinical evaluation. When there is a strong suspicion of onchocerciasis but tests are negative, a provocative Mazzotti test, in which administration of 0.5–1.0 mg/kg of DEC exacerbates pruritus or dermatitis, strongly suggests onchocerciasis.

Management

Ivermectin, in a single dose of 100–200 μg/kg, repeated several times at 3-monthly intervals to prevent relapses, is recommended. It kills microfilariae and has minimal toxicity. In the rare event of a severe reaction causing oedema or postural hypotension, prednisolone 20–30 mg may be given daily for 2 or 3 days. Ivermectin has little macrofilaricidal effect so that, 1 year after ivermectin treatment, skin microfilarial densities regain at least 20% of pre-treatment levels; repeated treatments are required for the lifespan of the adult worm. Eradication of *Wolbachia* with doxycycline (100 mg daily for 6 weeks) prevents worm reproduction.

Prevention

Mass treatment with ivermectin is practised. It reduces morbidity in the community and slows the progression of eye disease, but it does not clear worm infection. *Simulium* can be destroyed in its larval stage by the application of insecticide to streams. Long trousers, skirts and sleeves discourage the fly from biting.

Dracunculiasis (Guinea worm)

Infestation with the Guinea worm *Dracunculus medinensis* manifests itself when the female worm, over a metre long, emerges from the skin. Humans are infected by ingesting a small crustacean, *Cyclops*, which inhabits wells and ponds, and contains the infective larval stage of the worm. The worm was widely distributed across Africa and the Middle East, but after a successful eradication programme is now seen only in sub-Saharan Africa.

Management and prevention

Traditionally, the protruding worm is extracted by winding it out gently over several days on a matchstick. The worm must never be broken. Antibiotics for secondary infection and prophylaxis of tetanus are also required.

A global elimination campaign is based on the provision of clean drinking water and eradication of water fleas from drinking water. The latter is being achieved by simple filtration of water through a plastic mesh filter and chemical treatment of water supplies.

Other filariases

Mansonella perstans

This filarial worm is transmitted by the midges *Culicoides austeni* and *C. grahami*. It is common throughout equatorial Africa as far south as Zambia, and also in Trinidad and parts of northern and eastern South America.

M. perstans has never been proven to cause disease but it may be responsible for a persistent eosinophilia and occasional allergic manifestations. *M. perstans* is resistant to ivermectin and DEC, and the infection may persist for many years.

Dirofilaria immitis

This dog heart worm infects humans, causing skin and lung lesions. It is not uncommon in the USA, Japan and Australia.

Zoonotic nematodes

Trichinosis (trichinellosis)

Trichinella spiralis is a nematode that parasitises rats and pigs, and is only transmitted to humans if they eat partially cooked infected pork, usually as sausage or ham. Bear meat is another source. Symptoms result from invasion of intestinal submucosa by ingested larvae, which develop into adult worms, and the secondary invasion of striated muscle by fresh larvae produced by these adult worms. Outbreaks have occurred in the UK, as well as in other countries where pork is eaten.

Clinical features

The clinical features of trichinosis are determined by the larval numbers. A light infection with a few worms may be asymptomatic; a heavy infection causes nausea and diarrhoea 24–48 hours after the infected meal. A few days later, the symptoms associated with larval invasion predominate: there is fever and oedema of the face, eyelids and conjunctivae; invasion of the diaphragm may cause pain, cough and dyspnoea; and involvement of the muscles of the limbs, chest and mouth causes stiffness, pain and tenderness in affected muscles. Larval migration may cause acute myocarditis and encephalitis. An eosinophilia is usually found after the second week. An intense infection may prove fatal but those who survive recover completely.

Investigations

Commonly, a group of people who have eaten infected pork from a common source develop symptoms at about the same time. Biopsy from the deltoid or gastrocnemius muscle after the third week of symptoms may reveal encysted larvae. Serological tests are also helpful.

Management

Treatment is with albendazole (400 mg twice daily for 8–14 days) or mebendazole (200–400 mg three times daily for 3 days, followed by 400–500 mg three times daily for 10 days). Given early in the infection, this may kill newly formed adult worms in the submucosa and thus reduce the number of larvae reaching the muscles. Corticosteroids are necessary to control the serious effects of acute inflammation.

Cutaneous larva migrans

Cutaneous larva migrans (CLM) is the most common linear lesion seen in travellers (Fig. 13.51). Intensely pruritic, linear, serpiginous lesions result from the larval migration of the dog hookworm (*Ancylostoma caninum*). The track moves across the skin at a rate of 2–3 cm/day. This contrasts with the rash of *Strongyloides* (p. 370), which is fast-moving and transient. Although the larvae of dog hookworms frequently infect humans, they do not usually develop into the adult form. The most common site for CLM is the foot but elbows, breasts and buttocks may be affected. Most patients with CLM have recently visited a beach where the affected part was exposed. The diagnosis is clinical. Treatment may be

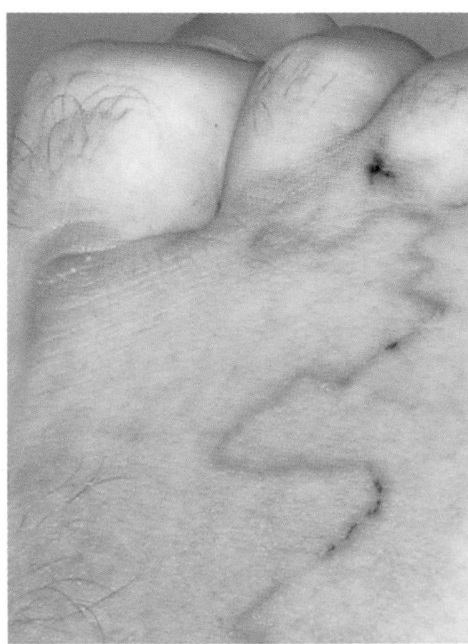

Fig. 13.51 Cutaneous larva migrans.

local with 12-hourly application of 15% thiabendazole cream, or systemic with a single dose of albendazole (400 mg) or ivermectin (150–200 μg/kg).

Trematodes (flukes)

These leaf-shaped worms are parasitic to humans and animals. Their complex life cycles may involve one or more intermediate hosts, often freshwater molluscs.

Schistosomiasis

Schistosomiasis is one of the most important causes of morbidity in the tropics. There are five species of the genus *Schistosoma* which commonly cause disease in humans: *S. haematobium*, *S. mansoni*, *S. japonicum*, *S. mekongi* and *S. intercalatum*. *S. haematobium* was discovered by Theodor Bilharz in Cairo in 1861 and the disease is sometimes called bilharzia or bilharziasis. Schistosome eggs have been found in Egyptian mummies dated 1250 BC.

The life cycle is shown in Figure 13.52A. The ovum is passed in the urine or faeces of infected individuals and gains access to fresh water, where the ciliated miracidium inside it is liberated; it enters its intermediate host, a species of freshwater snail, in which it multiplies. Large numbers of fork-tailed cercariae are then liberated into the water, where they may survive for 2–3 days. Cercariae can penetrate the skin or the mucous membrane of the mouth of humans. They transform into schistosomulae and moult as they pass through the lungs; thence they are carried by the blood stream to the liver, and so to the portal vein, where they mature. The male worm is up to 20 mm in length and the more slender cylindrical female, usually enfolded longitudinally by the male, is rather longer (Fig. 13.52B). Within 4–6 weeks of infection, they migrate to the venules draining the pelvic viscera, where the females deposit ova.

Pathology

This depends on the species and the stage of infection (Box 13.68). Most disease is due to the passage of eggs through mucosa and to the granulomatous reaction to eggs deposited in tissues. The eggs of *S. haematobium* pass mainly through the wall of the bladder, but may also involve rectum, seminal vesicles, vagina, cervix and uterine tubes. *S. mansoni* and *S. japonicum* eggs pass mainly through the wall of the lower bowel or are carried to the liver. The most serious, although rare, site of ectopic deposition of eggs is in the CNS. Granulomas are composed of macrophages, eosinophils, and epithelioid and giant cells around an ovum. Later, there is fibrosis and eggs calcify, often in sufficient numbers to become radiologically visible. Eggs of *S. haematobium* may leave the vesical plexus and be carried directly to the lung. Those of *S. mansoni* and *S. japonicum* may also reach the lungs after the development of portal hypertension and consequent portasystemic collateral circulation. In both circumstances, egg deposition in the pulmonary vasculature, and the resultant host response, can lead to the development of pulmonary hypertension.

Clinical features

Recent travellers, especially those overlanding through Africa, may present with allergic manifestations and eosinophilia; residents of schistosomiasis-endemic areas are more likely to present with chronic urinary tract pathology or portal hypertension.

During the early stages of infection, there may be itching lasting 1–2 days at the site of cercarial penetration

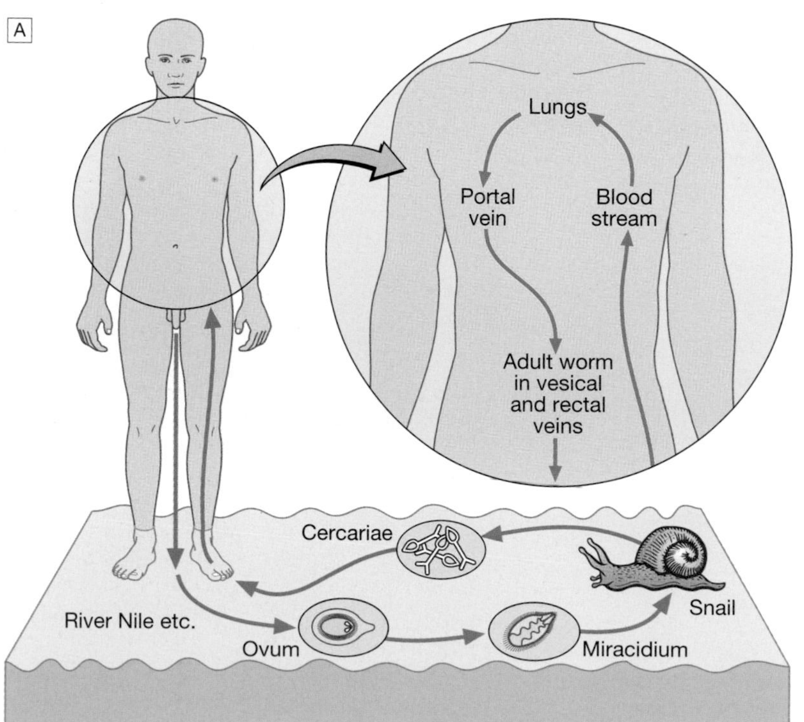

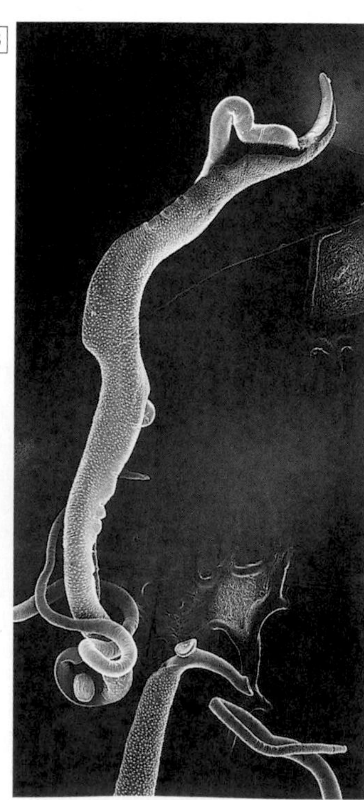

Fig. 13.52 ***Schistosoma.*** **A** Life cycle. **B** Scanning electron micrograph of adult schistosome worms, showing the larger male worm embracing the thinner female.

13.68 Pathogenesis of schistosomiasis

Time	*S. haematobium*	*S. mansoni* and *S. japonicum*
Cercarial penetration		
Days	Papular dermatitis at site of penetration	As for *S. haematobium*
Larval migration and maturation		
Weeks	Pneumonitis, myositis, hepatitis, fever, 'serum sickness', eosinophilia, seroconversion	As for *S. haematobium*
Early egg deposition		
Months	Cystitis, haematuria	Colitis, granulomatous hepatitis, acute portal hypertension
	Ectopic granulomatous lesions: skin, CNS etc.	As for *S. haematobium*
	Immune complex glomerulonephritis	
Late egg deposition		
Years	Fibrosis and calcification of ureters, bladder: bacterial infection, calculi, hydronephrosis, carcinoma	Colonic polyposis and strictures, periportal fibrosis, portal hypertension
	Pulmonary granulomas and pulmonary hypertension	As for *S. haematobium*

('swimmer's itch'). After a symptom-free period of 3–5 weeks, acute schistosomiasis (Katayama syndrome) may present with allergic manifestations, such as urticaria, fever, muscle aches, abdominal pain, headaches, cough and sweating. On examination, hepatomegaly, splenomegaly, lymphadenopathy and pneumonia may be present. These allergic phenomena may be severe in infections with *S. mansoni* and *S. japonicum*, but are rare with *S. haematobium*. The features subside after 1–2 weeks.

Chronic schistosomiasis is due to egg deposition and occurs months to years after infection. The symptoms and signs depend upon the intensity of infection and the species of infecting schistosome (see Box 13.68).

Schistosoma haematobium

Humans are the only natural hosts of *S. haematobium*, which is highly endemic in Egypt and East Africa, and occurs throughout Africa and the Middle East (Fig. 13.53). Infection can be acquired after a brief exposure, such as swimming in freshwater lakes in Africa.

Painless terminal haematuria is usually the first and most common symptom. Frequency of micturition follows, due to bladder neck obstruction. Later, the disease may be complicated by frequent urinary tract infections, bladder or ureteric stone formation, hydronephrosis, and ultimately renal failure with a contracted calcified bladder. Pain is often felt in the iliac fossa or in the loin, and radiates to the groin. In several endemic areas, there is a strong epidemiological association of *S. haematobium* infection with squamous cell carcinoma of the bladder. Disease of the seminal vesicles may lead to haemospermia. Females may develop schistosomal papillomas of the vulva, and schistosomal lesions of the cervix may be mistaken for cancer. Intestinal symptoms may follow involvement of the bowel wall. Ectopic worms cause skin or spinal cord lesions.

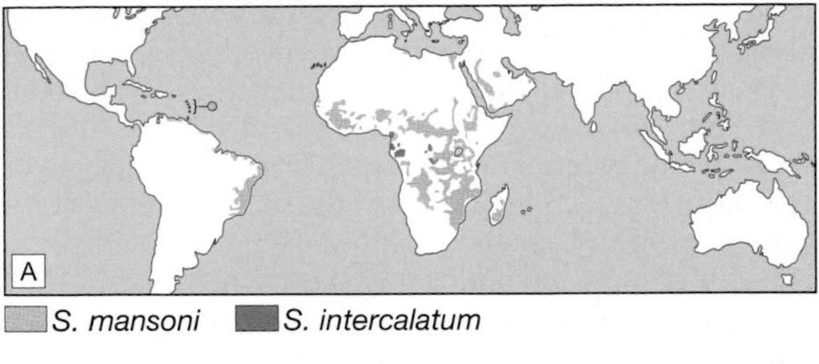

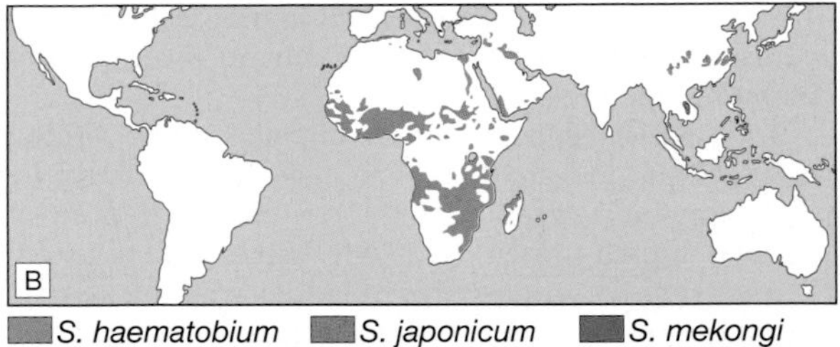

Fig. 13.53 Geographical distribution of schistosomiasis. From Cook 1995 – see p. 386.

The severity of *S. haematobium* infection varies greatly, and many with a light infection are asymptomatic. However, as adult worms can live for 20 years or more and lesions may progress, these patients should always be treated.

Schistosoma mansoni

S. mansoni is endemic throughout Africa, the Middle East, Venezuela, Brazil and the Caribbean (see Fig. 13.53).

Characteristic symptoms begin 2 months or more after infection. They may be slight, no more than malaise, or consist of abdominal pain and frequent stools which contain blood-stained mucus. With severe advanced disease, increased discomfort from rectal polyps may be experienced. The early hepatomegaly is reversible, but portal hypertension may cause massive splenomegaly, fatal haematemesis from oesophageal varices, or progressive ascites (p. 938). Liver function is initially preserved because the pathology is fibrotic rather than cirrhotic. *S. mansoni* and other schistosome infections predispose to the carriage of *Salmonella*, in part because *Salmonella* may attach to the schistosomes and in part because shared antigens on schistosomes may induce immunological tolerance to *Salmonella*.

Schistosoma japonicum, S. mekongi *and* S. intercalatum

In addition to humans, the adult worm of *S. japonicum* infects the dog, rat, field mouse, water buffalo, ox, cat, pig, horse and sheep. Although other *Schistosoma* spp. can infect species other than humans, the non-human reservoir seems to be particularly important in transmission for *S. japonicum* but not for *S. haematobium* or *S. mansoni*. *S. japonicum* is prevalent in the Yellow River and Yangtze–Jiang basins in China, where the infection is a major public health problem. It also has a focal distribution in the Philippines, Indonesia and Thailand (see Fig. 13.53). The related *S. mekongi* occurs in Laos, Thailand and Myanmar, and *S. intercalatum* in West and Central Africa.

The pathology of *S. japonicum* is similar to that of *S. mansoni*, but as this worm produces more eggs, the lesions tend to be more extensive and widespread. The clinical features resemble those of severe infection with *S. mansoni*, with added neurological features. The small and large bowel may be affected, and hepatic fibrosis with splenic enlargement is usual. Deposition of eggs or worms in the CNS, especially in the brain or spinal cord, causes symptoms in about 5% of infections, notably epilepsy, blindness, hemiplegia or paraplegia.

Investigations

There is marked eosinophilia. Serological tests (ELISA) are useful as screening tests but remain positive after chemotherapeutic cure.

In *S. haematobium* infection, dipstick urine testing shows blood and albumin. The eggs can be found by microscopic examination of the centrifuged deposit of terminal stream urine (Fig. 13.54). Ultrasound is useful for assessing the urinary tract; bladder wall thickening, hydronephrosis and bladder calcification can be detected. Cystoscopy reveals 'sandy' patches, bleeding mucosa and later distortion.

In a heavy infection with *S. mansoni* or *S. japonicum*, the characteristic egg with its lateral spine can usually be found in the stool. When the infection is light or of long duration, a rectal biopsy can be examined. Sigmoidoscopy may show inflammation or bleeding. Biopsies should be examined for ova.

Management

The object of specific treatment is to kill the adult schistosomes and so stop egg-laying. Praziquantel (20 mg/kg orally twice daily for 1 day) is the drug of choice for all forms of schistosomiasis. The drug produces parasitological cure in 80% of treated individuals and over 90% reduction in egg counts in the remainder. Side-effects are uncommon but include nausea and abdominal pain. Praziquantel therapy in early infection reverses pathologies such as hepatomegaly and bladder wall thickening and granulomas.

Surgery may be required to deal with residual lesions such as ureteric stricture, small fibrotic urinary bladders, or granulomatous masses in the brain or spinal cord. Removal of rectal papillomas by diathermy or by other means may provide symptomatic relief.

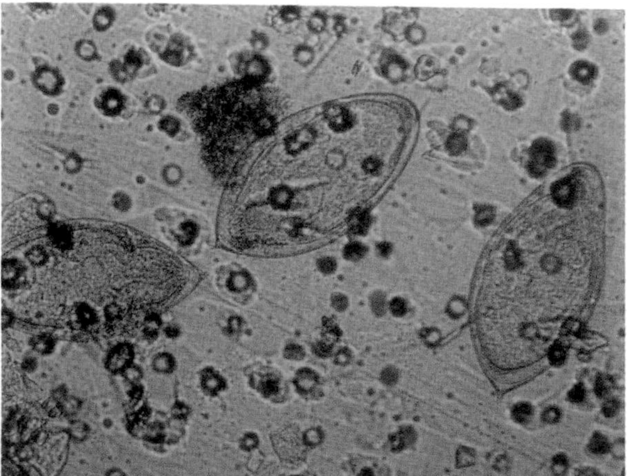

Fig. 13.54 Ova of *Schistosoma haematobium* in urine. Note the terminal spike.

Prevention

So far, no satisfactory single means of controlling schistosomiasis has been established. The life cycle is terminated if the ova in urine or faeces are not allowed to contaminate fresh water containing the snail host. The provision of latrines and of a safe water supply, however, remains a major problem in rural areas throughout the tropics. Furthermore, *S. japonicum* has so many hosts besides humans that latrines would be of little avail. Annual mass treatment of the population helps prevent *S. haematobium* and *S. mansoni* infection, but this method has so far had little success with *S. japonicum*. Targeting the intermediate host, the snail, presents many difficulties and has not, on its own, proved successful on any scale. For personal protection, contact with infected water must be avoided.

Liver flukes

Liver flukes infect at least 20 million people and remain an important public health problem in many endemic areas. They are associated with abdominal pain, hepatomegaly and relapsing cholangitis. *Clonorchis sinensis* is a major aetiological agent of bile duct cancer. The three major liver flukes have similar life cycles and pathologies, as outlined in Box 13.69.

Other flukes of medical importance include lung and intestinal flukes (see Box 13.65, p. 369).

Cestodes (tapeworms)

Cestodes are ribbon-shaped worms which inhabit the intestinal tract. They have no alimentary system and absorb nutrients through the tegumental surface. The anterior end, or scolex, has suckers for attaching to the host. From the scolex, a series of progressively developing segments arise, the proglottides, which may continue to show active movements when shed. Cross-fertilisation takes place between segments. Ova, present in large numbers in mature proglottides, remain viable for weeks, and during this period, they may be consumed by the intermediate host. Larvae liberated from the ingested ova pass into the tissues, forming larval cysticerci.

Tapeworms cause two distinct patterns of disease, either intestinal infection or systemic cysticercosis (Fig. 13.55). *Taenia saginata* (beef tapeworm), *Taenia asiatica* and *Diphyllobothrium latum* (fish tapeworm) cause only intestinal infection, following human ingestion of intermediate hosts that contain cysticerci (the larval stage of the tapeworm). *Taenia solium* causes intestinal infection if a cysticerci-containing intermediate host is ingested, and cysticercosis (systemic infection from larval migration) if ova are ingested. *Echinococcus granulosus* (dog tapeworm) does not cause human intestinal infection, but causes hydatid disease (which is analogous to cysticercosis) following ingestion of ova and subsequent larval migration.

Intestinal tapeworm

Humans acquire tapeworm by eating undercooked beef infected with the larval stage of *T. saginata*, undercooked pork containing the larval stage of *T. solium* or *T. asiatica*, or undercooked freshwater fish containing larvae of *D. latum*. Usually, only one adult tapeworm is present in the gut but up to ten have been reported. The ova of all

13.69 Diseases caused by flukes in the bile duct

	Clonorchiasis	Opisthorchiasis	Fascioliasis
Parasite	*Clonorchis sinensis*	*Opisthorchis felineus*	*Fasciola hepatica*
Other mammalian hosts	Dogs, cats, pigs	Dogs, cats, foxes, pigs	Sheep, cattle
Mode of spread	Ova in faeces, water	As for *C. sinensis*	Ova in faeces on to wet pasture
1st intermediate host	Snails	Snails	Snails
2nd intermediate host	Freshwater fish	Freshwater fish	Encysts on vegetation
Geographical distribution	Far East, especially S. China	Far East, especially NE Thailand	Cosmopolitan, including UK
Pathology	*E. coli* cholangitis, abscesses, biliary carcinoma	As for *C. sinensis*	Toxaemia, cholangitis, eosinophilia
Symptoms	Often symptom-free, recurrent jaundice	As for *C. sinensis*	Unexplained fever, tender liver, may be ectopic, e.g. subcutaneous fluke
Diagnosis	Ova in stool or duodenal aspirate	As for *C. sinensis*	As for *C. sinensis*, also serology
Prevention	Cook fish	Cook fish	Avoid contaminated watercress
Treatment	Praziquantel 25 mg/kg 3 times daily for 2 days	As for *C. sinensis* but for 1 day only	Triclabendazole 10 mg/kg single dose; repeat treatment may be required*

*In the UK, available from the Hospital for Tropical Diseases, London.

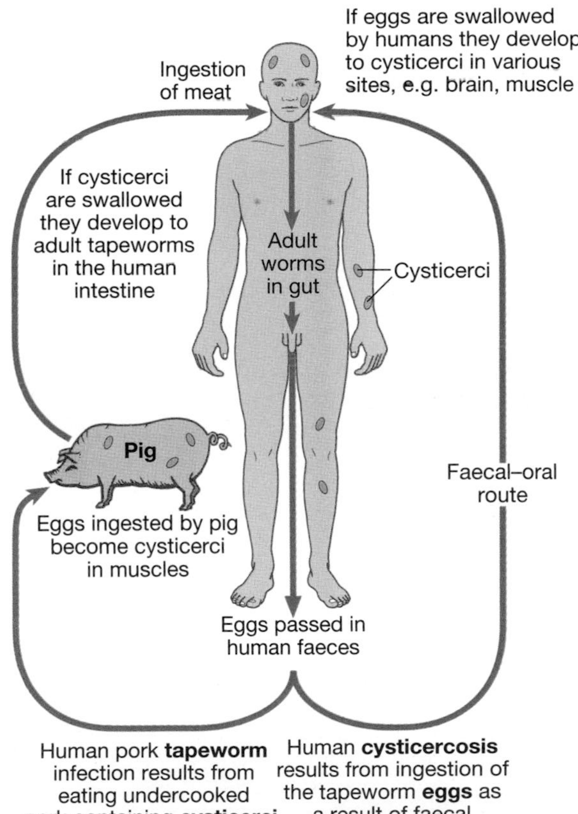

Fig. 13.55 Cysticercosis. Life cycle of *Taenia solium.*

the three *Taenia* are indistinguishable microscopically. However, examination of scolex and proglottides can differentiate: *T. solium* has a rostellum and two rows of hooklets on the scolex, and discharges multiple proglottides (3–5) attached together with lower degrees of uterine branching (approximately 10); *T. saginata* has only four suckers in its scolex, and discharges single proglottids with greater uterine branching (up to 30); *T. asiatica* has a rostellum without hooks on its scolex, and is difficult to differentiate from *T. saginata*, except that there are fewer uterine branches (16–21).

Taenia saginata

Infection with *T. saginata* occurs in all parts of the world. The adult worm may be several metres long and produces little or no intestinal upset in human beings, but knowledge of its presence, by noting segments in the faeces or on underclothing, may distress the patient. Ova may be found in the stool. Praziquantel is the drug of choice; niclosamide or nitazoxanide is an alternative. Prevention depends on efficient meat inspection and the thorough cooking of beef.

Taenia solium

T. solium, the pork tapeworm, is common in central Europe, South Africa, South America and parts of Asia. It is not as large as *T. saginata*. The adult worm is found only in humans following the eating of undercooked pork containing cysticerci. Intestinal infection is treated with praziquantel (5–10 mg/kg) or niclosamide (2 g), both as a single dose, or alternatively with nitazoxanide (500 mg twice daily for 3 days). These are followed by a mild laxative (after 1–2 hours) to prevent retrograde intestinal autoinfection. Cooking pork well prevents intestinal infection. Great care must be taken while attending a patient harbouring an adult worm to avoid ingestion of ova or segments.

Taenia asiatica

T. asiatica is a newly recognised species of *Taenia*, restricted to Asia. It is acquired by eating uncooked meat or viscera of pigs. Clinical features and treatment are similar to those of *T. saginata*.

Cysticercosis

Human cysticercosis is acquired by ingesting *T. solium* tapeworm ova, from either contaminated fingers or food (see Fig. 13.55). The larvae are liberated from eggs in the stomach, penetrate the intestinal mucosa and are carried to many parts of the body, where they develop and form cysticerci, 0.5–1 cm cysts that contain the head of a young worm. They do not grow further or migrate. Common locations are the subcutaneous tissue, skeletal muscles and brain.

Clinical features

When superficially placed, cysts can be palpated under the skin or mucosa as pea-like ovoid bodies. Here they cause few or no symptoms, and will eventually die and become calcified.

Heavy brain infections, especially in children, may cause features of encephalitis. More commonly, however, cerebral signs do not occur until the larvae die, 5–20 years later. Epilepsy, personality changes, staggering gait or signs of hydrocephalus are the most common features.

Investigations

Calcified cysts in muscles can be recognised radiologically. In the brain, however, less calcification takes place and larvae are only occasionally visible by plain X-ray; usually CT or MRI will show them. Epileptic fits starting in adult life suggest the possibility of cysticercosis if the patient has lived in or travelled to an endemic area. The subcutaneous tissue should be palpated and any nodule excised for histology. Radiological examination of the skeletal muscles may be helpful. Antibody detection is available for serodiagnosis.

Management and prevention

Albendazole, 15 mg/kg daily for a minimum of 8 days, has now become the drug of choice for parenchymal neurocysticercosis. Praziquantel is another option, 50 mg/kg in three divided doses daily for 10 days. Prednisolone, 10 mg 3 times daily, is also given for 14 days, starting 1 day before the albendazole or praziquantel. In addition, anti-epileptic drugs should be given until the reaction in the brain has subsided. Operative intervention is indicated for hydrocephalus. Studies from India and Peru suggest that most small, solitary cerebral cysts will resolve without treatment.

Echinococcus granulosus (*Taenia echinococcus*) and hydatid disease

Dogs are the definitive hosts of the tiny tapeworm *E. granulosus*. The larval stage, a hydatid cyst, normally occurs in sheep, cattle, camels and other animals that are infected from contaminated pastures or water. By handling a dog or drinking contaminated water, humans may ingest eggs (Fig. 13.56). The embryo is liberated from the ovum in the small intestine and gains access to the blood stream and thus to the liver. The resultant cyst grows very slowly, sometimes intermittently. It is composed of an enveloping fibrous pericyst, laminated hyaline membrane (ectocyst) and inner germinal layers (endocyst) which gives rise to daughter cysts, or germinating cystic brood capsule in which larvae (protoscolices) develop. Over time, some cysts may calcify and become non-viable. The disease is common in the Middle East, North and East Africa, Australia and Argentina. Foci of infection persist in the UK in rural Wales and Scotland. *E. multilocularis*, which has a cycle between foxes and voles, causes a similar but more severe

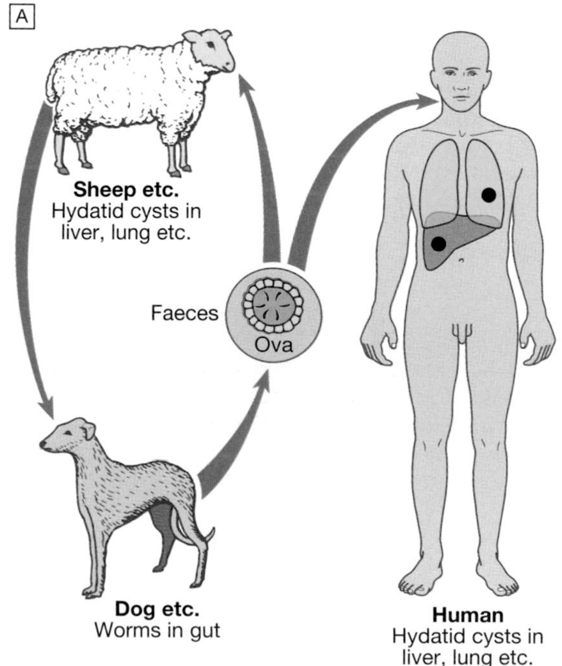

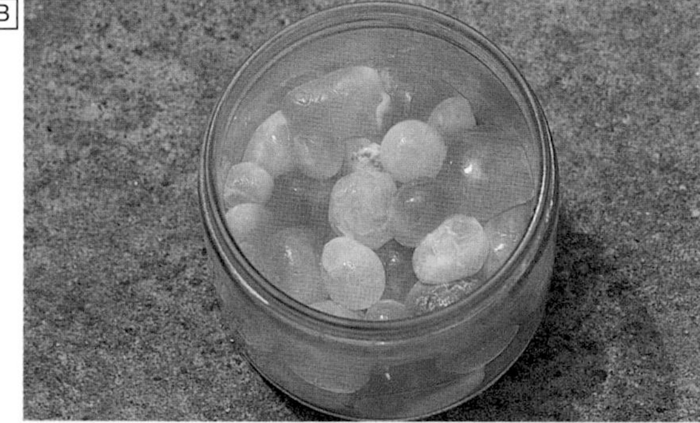

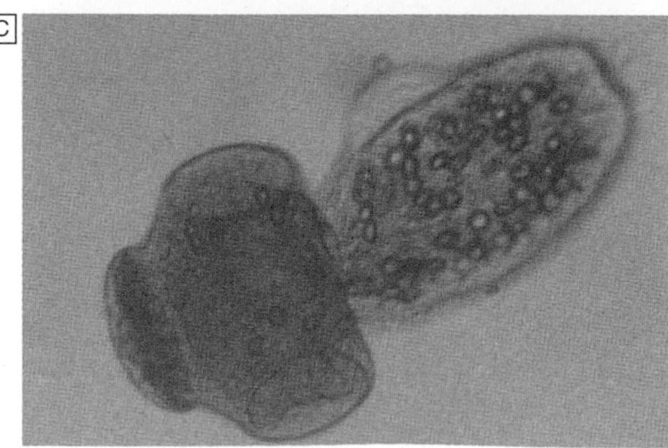

Fig. 13.56 Hydatid disease. **A** Life cycle of *Echinococcus granulosus.* **B** Daughter cysts removed at surgery. **C** Within the daughter cysts are the protoscolices.

infection, 'alveolar hydatid disease', which invades the liver like cancer.

Clinical features

A hydatid cyst is typically acquired in childhood and may, after growing for some years, cause pressure symptoms. These vary, depending on the organ or tissue involved. In nearly 75% of patients with hydatid disease, the right lobe of the liver is invaded and contains a single cyst (p. 956). In others, a cyst may be found in lung, bone, brain or elsewhere.

Investigations

The diagnosis depends on the clinical, radiological and ultrasound findings in a patient who has lived in close contact with dogs in an endemic area. Complement fixation and ELISA are positive in 70–90% of patients.

Management and prevention

Hydatid cysts should be excised wherever possible. Great care is taken to avoid spillage and cavities are sterilised with 0.5% silver nitrate or 2.7% sodium chloride. Albendazole (400 mg twice daily for 3 months) should also be used. The drug is now often combined with PAIR (percutaneous puncture, aspiration, injection of scolicidal agent and re-aspiration) to good effect. Praziquantel (20 mg/kg twice daily for 14 days) also kills protoscolices perioperatively.

Prevention is difficult in situations where there is a close association with dogs and sheep. Personal hygiene, satisfactory disposal of carcasses, meat inspection and deworming of dogs can greatly reduce the prevalence of disease.

Other tapeworms

There are many other cestodes whose adult or larval stages may infect humans. Sparganosis is a condition in which an immature worm develops in humans, usually subcutaneously, as a result of eating or applying to the skin the secondary or tertiary intermediate host.

ECTOPARASITES

Ectoparasites only interact with the outermost surfaces of the host; see also page 1280.

Jiggers (tungiasis)

This is widespread in tropical America and Africa, and is caused by the sand flea *Tunga penetrans*. The pregnant flea burrows into the skin around toes and produces large numbers of eggs. The burrows are intensely irritating and the whole inflammatory nodule should be removed with a sterile needle. Secondary infection of tunga lesions is common.

Myiasis

Myiasis is due to skin infestation with larvae of the South American botfly, *Dermatobia hominis*, or the African Tumbu fly, *Cordylobia anthropophaga*. The larvae develop in a subcutaneous space with a central sinus. This orifice is the air source for the larvae, and periodically the larval respiratory spiracles protrude through the sinus. Patients with myiasis feel movement within the larval burrow and can experience intermittent sharp, lancinating pains. Myiasis is diagnosed clinically and should be suspected with any furuncular lesion accompanied by pain and a crawling sensation in the skin. The larva may be suffocated by blocking the respiratory orifice with petroleum jelly and gently removing it with tweezers. Secondary infection of myiasis is remarkably infrequent and rapid healing follows removal of intact larvae.

FUNGAL INFECTIONS

Fungal infections, or mycoses, are classified as superficial, subcutaneous or systemic (deep), depending on the degree of invasion of the host. They are also classified by the kind of fungus that causes the infection, which may be a filamentous fungus (mould) or a yeast, or may vary between these two forms, depending on the environmental conditions (dimorphic fungi; Fig. 13.57).

13

Superficial mycoses

Superficial cutaneous fungal infections caused by dermatophyte fungi are described in Chapter 28.

Candidiasis (thrush)

Superficial candidiasis is caused by *Candida* spp., mainly *C. albicans.* Manifestations include oropharyngeal (pp. 864 and 399) and vaginal candidiasis ('thrush'), intertrigo and chronic paronychia. Superficial candidiasis often follows antibiotic therapy. Intertrigo is characterised by inflammation in skin folds with surrounding 'satellite lesions'. Chronic paronychia is associated with frequent wetting of the hands. Superficial candidiasis is treated mainly with topical azoles (p. 159), oral azoles being reserved for refractory or recurrent disease. Severe oropharyngeal and oesophageal candidiasis is a consequence of CD4+ T lymphocyte depletion/dysfunction, as in HIV infection (p. 399). Recurrent vaginal or penile candidiasis may be a manifestation of diabetes mellitus. Rarely, mutations in the autoimmune regulator gene, *AIRE*, cause a syndrome of chronic mucocutaneous candidiasis (p. 796).

Subcutaneous mycoses

Chromoblastomycosis

Chromoblastomycosis is a predominantly tropical or subtropical fungal disease caused by environmental dematiaceous (dark-pigmented) fungi, most commonly *Fonsecaea pedrosoi*. Other causes include *F. compacta, Cladophialophora carrionii* and *Phialophora verrucosa*. The disease is a cutaneous/subcutaneous mycosis acquired by traumatic inoculation. Consequently, the most commonly affected areas are the foot, ankle and lower leg. Lesions may start several months after the initial injury, and medical attention is often sought several years later. The initial lesion is a papule. Further papules develop, and coalesce to form irregular plaques. Nodular lesions may produce a characteristic 'cauliflower' appearance.

Diagnosis is by histopathological examination of infected material, which shows dematiaceous, rounded, thick-walled 'sclerotic bodies' with septa at right angles

Filamentous fungi (moulds)	Dimorphic fungi	Yeasts
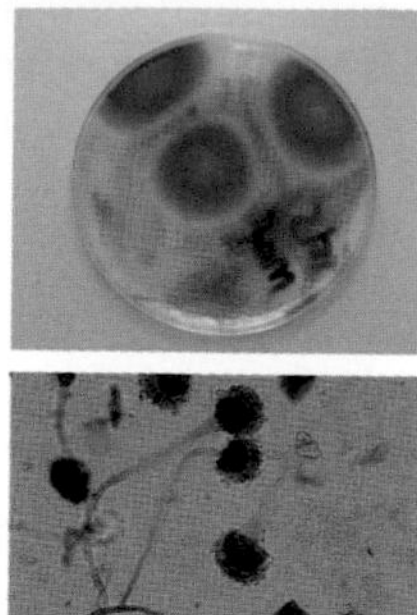	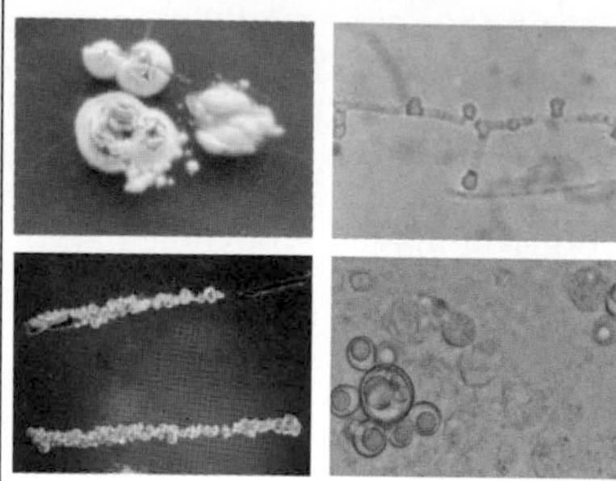	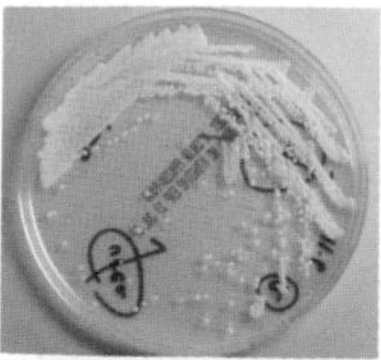 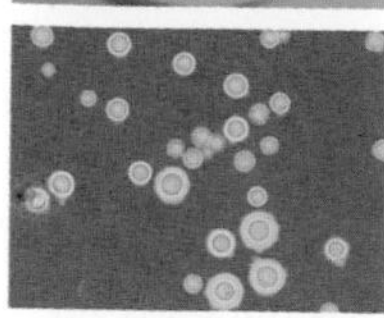
Characterised by the production of elongated, cylindrical, often septate cells (hyphae) and conidia (spores)	Exist in filamentous (top) or yeast (bottom) form, depending on environmental conditions	Characterised by the production of oval or round cells, which reproduce by binary fission (budding)
Examples: • *Aspergillus* spp. (*A. fumigatus* shown here) • *Fusarium* spp. • Dermatophyte fungi (*Tricophyton* spp., *Microsporum* spp. etc.) • Mucorales	Examples: • *Histoplasma capsulatum, Coccidioides immitis, Paracoccidioides brasiliensis* (shown here), *Blastomyces dermatidis* • *Sporothrix schenkii* • *Penicillium marneffei* • *Malassezia* spp.	Examples: • *Candida* spp.* • *Cryptococcus* spp. (*C. neoformans* shown here)

Fig. 13.57 Classification of medically important fungi. Fungal classification is based on simple morphological characteristics. *Pneumocystis jirovecii* (*carinii*) is morphologically distinct from other fungi and does not fit into this classification. *Although *Candida albicans* exists in a number of forms, including filamentous (hyphae and pseudohyphae), it is generally encountered in its yeast form, so is classified in this category.

to each other. The aetiological agent is confirmed by culture. Many therapeutic approaches have been explored, including antifungal agents, cryosurgery and surgical excision, alone or in combination, but the optimal therapy is unknown. Of the antifungal agents, itraconazole and terbinafine are considered to be the most effective. However, posaconazole has also been used with a good outcome.

Mycetoma

Mycetoma is a chronic suppurative infection of the deep soft tissues and bones, most commonly of the limbs but also of the abdominal or chest wall or head. It is caused by either aerobic or anaerobic branching Gram-positive bacilli, *Actinomycetales* (actinomycetoma – 60%, p. 135), or by true fungi, Eumycetes (eumycetoma – 40%). Many fungi cause eumycetomas, the most common being *Madurella mycetomatis, M. grisea, Leptosphaeria senegalensis* and *Scedosporium apiospermum*. Actinomycetomas are caused by *Actinomadura, Nocardia* and *Streptomyces* spp. Both groups produce characteristically coloured grains, the colour depending on the organism (black grains – eumycetoma, red and yellow grains – actinomycetoma, white grains – either). The disease occurs mostly in the tropics and subtropics.

Clinical features

The disease is acquired by inoculation (e.g. from a thorn) and most commonly affects the foot (Madura foot). Mycetoma begins as a painless swelling at the implantation site, which becomes chronic and progressive, grows and spreads steadily within the soft tissues, eventually extending into bone. Nodules develop under the epidermis and these rupture, revealing sinuses through which grains (fungal colonies) may be discharged. Sinuses heal with scarring, while fresh sinuses appear elsewhere. Deeper tissue invasion and bone involvement are less rapid and extensive in eumycetoma than actinomycetoma. There is little pain and usually no fever or lymphadenopathy, but there is progressive disability.

Investigations

Diagnosis is confirmed by demonstration of fungal grains in pus, and/or histopathological examination of tissue. Culture is necessary for species identification and susceptibility testing. Serological tests are not available.

Management

Eumycetoma is usually treated with a combination of surgery and antifungal therapy. Antifungal susceptibility testing, if available, is recommended, although clinical outcome does not necessarily correspond to in vitro test results. Itraconazole and ketoconazole (both 200–400 mg/day) are used most commonly. Success has also been reported with terbinafine monotherapy, and refractory cases have responded to both voriconazole and posaconazole. Amphotericin B is not generally considered effective. Therapy is continued for 6–12 months or longer. In extreme cases, amputation may be required. Management of actinomycetoma is described on page 341.

Phaeohyphomycosis

Phaeohyphomycoses are a heterogenous group of fungal diseases caused by a large number (more than 70) of dematiaceous fungi. In phaeohyphomycosis, the tissue form of the fungus is predominantly mycelial (filamentous), as opposed to eumycetoma (grain) or chromoblastomycosis (sclerotic body). Disease may be superficial, subcutaneous or deep. The most serious manifestation is cerebral phaeohyphomycosis, which presents with a ring-enhancing, space-occupying cerebral lesion. Optimal therapy for this condition has not been established, but treatment usually consists of neurosurgical intervention and antifungal (usually triazole) therapy. Causative agents are *Cladophialophora bantiana*, *Fonsecaea* spp. and *Rhinocladiella mackenziei*, which occurs in the Middle East and is usually fatal.

Sporotrichosis

Sporotrichosis is caused by *Sporothrix schenckii*, a dimorphic fungal saprophyte of plants in tropical and subtropical regions. Disease is caused by dermal inoculation of the fungus, usually from a thorn (occasionally from a cat scratch). In fixed cutaneous sporotrichosis, a subcutaneous nodule develops at the site of infection and subsequently ulcerates, with a purulent discharge. The disease may then spread along the cutaneous lymphatic channels, resulting in multiple cutaneous nodules along their route, which ulcerate and discharge (lymphocutaneous sporotrichosis). Rarer forms of disease are seen: for example, in patients with cutaneous disease presenting with arthritis. Later, draining sinuses may form. Pulmonary sporotrichosis occurs as a result of inhalation of the conidia, and manifests itself as chronic cavitary fibronodular disease with haemoptysis and constitutional symptoms. Disseminated disease may occur, especially in patients with HIV.

Investigations

Typical yeast forms detected on histology of the biopsy confirm the diagnosis but are rarely seen; the fungus can be grown from the specimen in culture. A latex agglutination test is available to detect *S. schenkii* antibodies in serum.

Management

Cutaneous and lymphocutaneous disease is treated with oral itraconazole (200–400 mg daily, prescribed as the oral solution, which has better bio-availability than the capsule formulation) for 3–6 months. Alternative agents include a saturated solution of potassium iodide (SSKI, given orally), initiated with 5 drops and increased to 40–50 drops 3 times daily, or terbinafine (500 mg twice daily). Localised hyperthermia may be used in pregnancy (to avoid azole use). Osteoarticular disease requires a longer course of therapy (at least 12 months). Severe or life-threatening disease is treated with amphotericin B (lipid formulation preferred).

Systemic mycoses

Aspergillosis

Aspergillosis is an opportunistic systemic mycosis, which affects predominantly the respiratory tract. It is described on page 697.

Candidiasis

Systemic candidiasis is an opportunistic mycosis caused by *Candida* spp. The most common cause is *C. albicans*. Other agents include *C. dubliniensis*, *C. glabrata*, *C. krusei*, *C. parapsilosis* and *C. tropicalis*. Species distribution varies geographically. *Candida* species identification often enables prediction of susceptibility to fluconazole: *C. krusei* is universally resistant, many *C. glabrata* isolates have reduced susceptibility or are resistant, and other species are mostly susceptible. Candidiasis is usually an endogenous disease that originates from oropharyngeal, genitourinary or skin colonisation, although nosocomial spread has been reported.

Syndromes of systemic candidiasis

Acute disseminated candidiasis

This usually presents as candidaemia (isolation of *Candida* spp. from the blood). The main predisposing factor is the presence of a central venous catheter. Other major factors include recent abdominal surgery, total parenteral nutrition (TPN), recent antibiotic therapy and localised *Candida* colonisation. Up to 40% of cases will have ophthalmic involvement, with characteristic retinal 'cotton wool' exudates. As this is a sight-threatening condition, candidaemic patients should be assessed by detailed ophthalmoscopy. Skin lesions (non-tender pink/red nodules) may be seen. Although predominantly a disease of intensive care and surgical patients, acute disseminated candidiasis and/or *Candida* endophthalmitis is seen occasionally in injection drug-users, thought to be due to candidal contamination of citric acid or lemon juice used to dissolve heroin.

Chronic disseminated candidiasis (hepatosplenic candidiasis)

In this condition, a neutropenic patient has a persistent fever, despite antibacterial therapy. The fever persists, even though there is neutrophil recovery, and is associated with the development of abdominal pain, raised alkaline phosphatase and multiple lesions in abdominal organs (e.g. liver, spleen and/or kidneys) on radiological imaging. Chronic disseminated candidiasis is a form of immune reconstitution syndrome (p. 138) in patients recovering from neutropenia and usually lasts for several months, despite appropriate therapy.

Other manifestations

Renal tract candidiasis, osteomyelitis, septic arthritis, peritonitis, meningitis and endocarditis are all well recognised, and are usually sequelae of acute disseminated disease. Diagnosis and treatment of these conditions require specialist mycological advice.

Management

Blood cultures positive for *Candida* spp. must never be ignored. Acute disseminated candidiasis is treated with antifungal therapy, removal of any in-dwelling central venous catheter (whether known to be the source of infection or not) and removal of any known source. Current evidence suggests that candidaemia should be treated initially with an echinocandin (p. 160), with subsequent adjustment (usually to IV or oral fluconazole) guided by clinical response, species identification and susceptibility testing. Treatment should continue for a minimum of 14 days. Other appropriate therapies include voriconazole and amphotericin B formulations.

Chronic disseminated candidiasis requires prolonged treatment over several months with fluconazole or other agents, depending on species and clinical response. The duration of the condition may be reduced by adjuvant therapy with systemic corticosteroids.

Cryptococcosis

Cryptococcosis is a systemic mycosis caused by two environmental yeast species, *Cr. neoformans* and *Cr. gattii*. *Cr. neoformans* is distributed worldwide and is primarily an opportunistic pathogen, most commonly associated with HIV infection. *Cr. gattii* is a primary pathogen with a widespread distribution that includes Australasia, Africa, Canada (Vancouver Island) and the north-western USA.

Cryptococcosis is acquired by inhalation of yeasts. These may disseminate to any organ, most commonly the CNS and skin. The manifestations of *Cr. neoformans* are most severe in immunocompromised individuals. Conversely, *Cr. gattii* causes severe disease most often in immunocompetent hosts. Disseminated cryptococcosis (sepsis with cryptococci present in the blood stream or at multiple sites) is largely restricted to immunocompromised patients. CNS manifestations of cryptococcosis include meningitis (p. 403) and cryptococcoma (Fig. 13.58), the latter more likely with *Cr. gattii* infection. Manifestations of pulmonary cryptococcosis range from severe pneumonia (in immunocompromised patients) to asymptomatic disease with single or multiple pulmonary nodules, sometimes exhibiting cavitation (in immunocompetent patients). Cryptococcal nodules may mimic other causes of lung pathology, such as tuberculosis or malignancy, and diagnosis is often made by histopathology and/or culture.

Treatment of severe cryptococcosis is the same as for cryptococcal meningitis (p. 403). Mild pulmonary disease is usually treated with fluconazole, although, for asymptomatic nodules, resection of the lesions is likely to be sufficient. Relevant guidelines (e.g. www.idsociety.org) should be consulted.

A

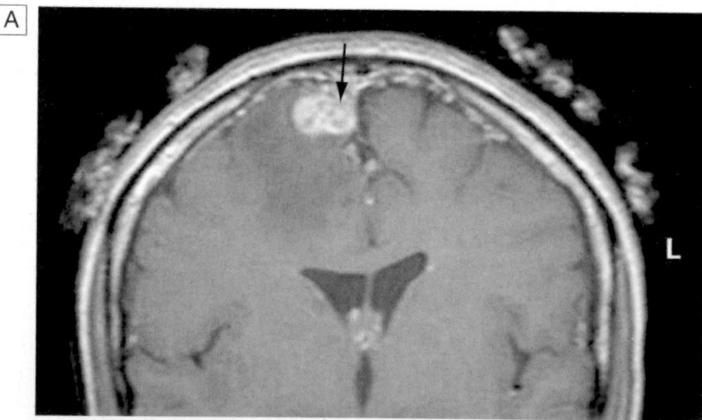

B

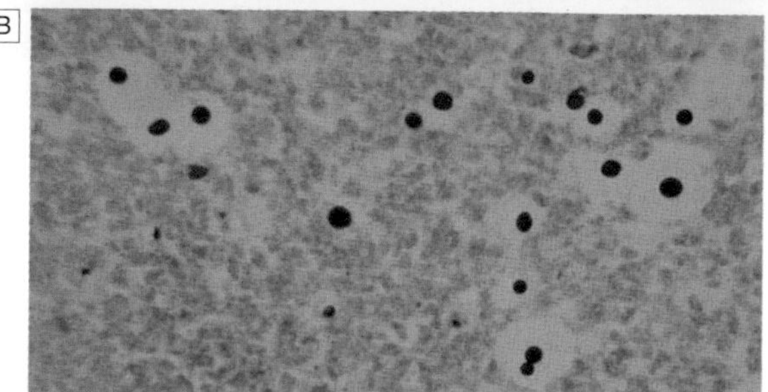

Fig. 13.58 Cryptococcal disease. A 23-year-old HIV-positive male developed headache and left-sided weakness. **A** MRI scan of the brain showed a space-occupying lesion (arrow) with surrounding oedema. **B** Histopathological examination of the lesion stained with Grocott's silver stain showed encapsulated yeasts. *Cryptococcus neoformans* was cultured.

A

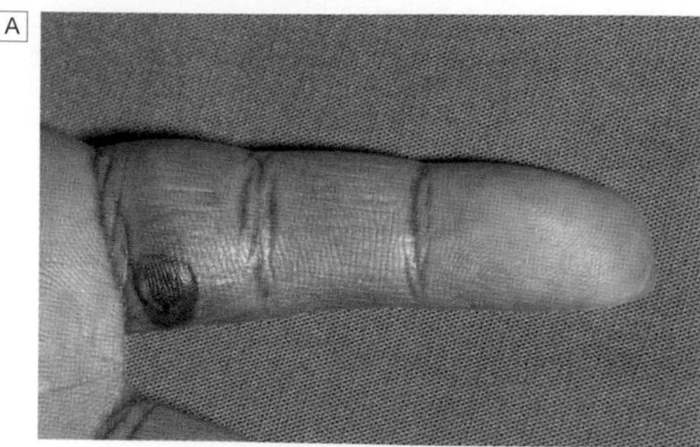

B

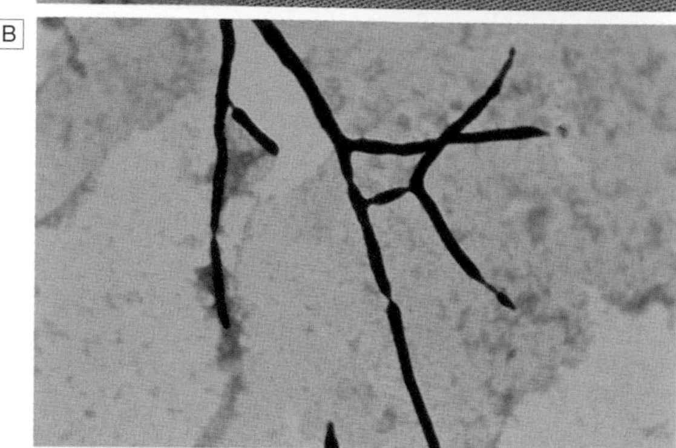

Fig. 13.59 *Fusarium* infection. A patient presented with fever and skin nodules after developing neutropenia secondary to haematopoietic stem cell transplantation and chemotherapy for relapsed leukaemia. *Fusarium solani* was cultured from skin lesions and blood cultures. **A** Tender, erythematous papules/nodules on upper arm. **B** Gram stain of *Fusarium* in blood culture medium.

Fusariosis

Fusarium spp. cause disseminated disease in patients with profound or prolonged neutropenia. The disease presents with antibiotic-resistant fever and evidence of dissemination (e.g. skin nodules, endophthalmitis, septic arthritis, pulmonary disease; Fig. 13.59). In contrast to *Aspergillus* spp., *Fusarium* spp. is often recovered from blood cultures. Treatment is challenging because of resistance to several antifungal agents. Voriconazole, posaconazole and lipid-formulated amphotericin B are the most commonly used antifungal agents.

Mucormycosis

Mucormycosis is a severe but uncommon opportunistic systemic mycosis caused by a number of 'mucoraceous' moulds, most commonly *Lichtheimia* (formerly *Absidia*) spp., *Rhizomucor* spp., *Mucor* spp. and *Rhizopus* spp. Disease patterns include rhinocerebral/craniofacial, pulmonary, cutaneous and systemic disease. All are characterised by the rapid development of severe tissue necrosis, which is almost always fatal if left untreated. The most common predisposing factors are profound immunosuppression from neutropenia and/or haematopoietic stem cell transplantation, uncontrolled diabetes mellitus, iron chelation therapy with desferrioxamine and severe burns.

Definitive diagnosis is by culture, but histopathological confirmation is required as the fungi may be environmental contaminants. Treatment requires a combination of antifungal therapy and surgical débridement, with correction of predisposing factor(s) if possible. High-dose lipid-formulated amphotericin B is used most commonly. Posaconazole is active against many mucoraceous moulds in vitro and may be used as a second-line agent or as oral 'step-down' therapy.

Penicillium marneffei infection

P. marneffei is a thermally dimorphic pathogen (filamentous in environmental conditions and yeast at body temperature), which causes disease in South-east Asia, mainly in association with HIV infection (although immunocompetent patients may also be infected). Acquisition is most likely to be by inhalation of environmental spores, with primary lung infection followed by haematogenous dissemination. A generalised papular rash, which progresses to widespread necrosis and ulceration, is a characteristic feature. Skin lesions may resemble those of molluscum contagiosum. Diagnosis is by histopathology and/or culture of respiratory secretions, blood or any infected clinical material (e.g. skin lesions, bone marrow, biopsies). Recommended treatment is with an amphotericin B formulation followed by itraconazole (in severe infection), or with itraconazole alone.

Histoplasmosis

Histoplasmosis is a primary systemic mycosis caused by the dimorphic fungus *Histoplasma capsulatum*. *H. capsulatum* var. *capsulatum* is endemic to east-central USA (especially the Mississippi and Ohio river valleys), parts of Canada, Latin America, the Caribbean, East and South-east Asia, and Africa. It occurs sporadically in Australia and India, and is very rare in Europe. *H. capsulatum* var. *duboisii* is found in West Africa and Madagascar. Genetic analysis suggests that *H. capsulatum* may, in fact, be made up of several different species, and its taxonomy is under review.

Habitat

The primary reservoir of *H. capsulatum* is soil enriched by bird and bat droppings, in which the fungus remains viable for many years. Infection is by inhalation of dust from such soil. Natural infections are found in bats, which represent a secondary reservoir of infection (via bat faeces). Histoplasmosis is a specific hazard for explorers of caves and people who clear out bird (including chicken) roosts.

Pathology

The organism is inhaled in the form of conidia (spores) or hyphal fragments and transforms to the yeast phase during infection. Conidia or yeasts are phagocytosed by alveolar macrophages and neutrophils, and this may be followed by haematogenous dissemination to any organ. Subsequent development of a T-lymphocyte response brings the infection under control, resulting in a latent state in most exposed individuals.

Clinical features

Disease severity depends on the quantity of spores inhaled and the immune status of the host. In most cases, infection is asymptomatic. Pulmonary symptoms are the most common disease presentation, with fever, non-productive cough and an influenza-like illness. Erythema nodosum, myalgia and joint pain are common, and chest radiography may reveal a pneumonitis with hilar or mediastinal lymphadenopathy.

Patients with pre-existing lung disease, such as chronic obstructive pulmonary disease (COPD) or emphysema, may develop chronic pulmonary histoplasmosis. The predominant features of this condition, which may easily be mistaken for tuberculosis, are fever, cough, dyspnoea, weight loss and night sweats. Radiological findings include fibrosis, nodules, cavitation and hilar/mediastinal lymphadenopathy.

Disease caused by *H. capsulatum* var. *duboisii* presents more commonly with papulonodular and ulcerating lesions of the skin and underlying subcutaneous tissue and bone (sometimes referred to as 'African histoplasmosis'). Multiple lesions of the ribs are common and the bones of the limbs may be affected. Lung involvement is relatively rare. Radiological examination may show rounded foci of bone destruction, sometimes associated with abscess formation. Other disease patterns include a visceral form with liver and splenic invasion, and disseminated disease.

Acute disseminated histoplasmosis is seen in association with immunocompromise, including HIV infection. Features include fever, pancytopenia, hepatosplenomegaly, lymphadenopathy and often a papular skin eruption. Chronic disseminated disease presents with fever, anorexia and weight loss. Cutaneous and mucosal lesions, lymphadenopathy, hepatosplenomegaly and meningitis may also develop.

Investigations

In areas where the disease occurs, histoplasmosis should be suspected in every undiagnosed infection in which there are pulmonary signs, enlarged lymph nodes, hepatosplenomegaly or characteristic cutaneous/bony lesions. Radiological examination in long-standing cases may show calcified lesions in the lungs, spleen or other organs. In the more acute phases of the disease, single or multiple soft pulmonary shadows with enlarged tracheobronchial nodes are seen on chest X-ray.

Laboratory diagnosis is by direct detection (histopathology or antigen detection), culture and serology; although antigen detection is the most effective method, it is not widely available. Antibody is detected by complement fixation testing or immunodiffusion; the pattern of antibody production is complex and the results require specialist interpretation. *Histoplasma* antigen may be detectable in blood or urine. Culture is definitive but slow (up to 12 weeks). Histopathology may show characteristic intracellular yeasts. Diagnosis of subcutaneous or bony infection is mainly by histopathological examination and/or culture.

Management

Mild pulmonary disease does not require treatment. However, if prolonged, it may be treated with itraconazole. More severe pulmonary disease is treated with an amphotericin B formulation for 2 weeks, followed by itraconazole for 12 weeks, with methylprednisolone added for the first 2 weeks of therapy if there is hypoxia or ARDS. Chronic pulmonary histoplasmosis is treated with itraconazole (prescribed as the oral solution) for 12–24 months, and disseminated histoplasmosis with an amphotericin B formulation followed by itraconazole. Lipid formulations of amphotericin B are preferred, but their use is subject to availability. Treatment should be guided by current evidence-based guidelines (e.g.

Infectious Diseases Society of America practice guidelines: www.idsociety.org). In subcutaneous and bone infection, patterns of remission and relapse are more common than cure. A solitary bony lesion may require local surgical treatment only.

Coccidioidomycosis

This is a primary systemic mycosis caused by the dimorphic fungi *Coccidioides immitis* and *C. posadasii*, found in the south-western USA, and Central and South America. The disease is acquired by inhalation of conidia (arthrospores). In 60% of cases it is asymptomatic, but in the remainder it affects the lungs, lymph nodes and skin. Rarely (in approximately 0.5%), it may spread haematogenously to bones, adrenal glands, meninges and other organs.

Pulmonary coccidioidomycosis has two forms: primary and progressive. If symptomatic, primary coccidioidomycosis presents with cough, fever, chest pain, dyspnoea and (commonly) arthritis and a rash (erythema multiforme). Progressive disease presents with systemic upset (e.g. fever, weight loss, anorexia) and features of lobar pneumonia, and may resemble tuberculosis.

Coccidioides meningitis (which may be associated with CSF eosinophils) is the most severe disease manifestation; it is fatal if untreated, and requires life-long suppressive therapy with antifungal azoles.

Investigations and management

Diagnosis is by direct detection (histopathological examination of infected tissue), culture of infected tissue or fluids, or antibody detection. IgM may be detected after 1–3 weeks of disease by precipitin tests. IgG appears later and is detected with the complement fixation test. Change in IgG titre may be used to monitor clinical progress.

Treatment depends on specific disease manifestations, and ranges from regular clinical re-assessment without antifungal therapy (in mild pulmonary, asymptomatic cavitary or single nodular disease) to high-dose treatment with an antifungal azole, which may be continued indefinitely (e.g. in meningitis). Amphotericin B is used in diffuse pneumonia, disseminated disease and, intrathecally, in meningitis. Posaconazole has been used successfully in refractory disease.

Paracoccidioidomycosis

This is a primary systemic mycosis caused by inhalation of the dimorphic fungus *Paracoccidioides brasiliensis*, which is restricted to South America. The disease affects the lungs, mucous membranes (painful destructive ulceration in 50% of cases), skin, lymph nodes and adrenal glands (hypoadrenalism). Diagnosis is by microscopy and culture of lesions, and antibody detection. Oral itraconazole solution (200 mg/day) has demonstrated 98% efficacy and is currently the treatment of choice (mean duration 6 months). Ketoconazole, fluconazole and voriconazole have also been used, as have long (2–3-year) courses of sulphonamides. Amphotericin B may be used in severe or refractory disease, followed by an azole or sulphonamide.

Blastomycosis

Blastomyces dermatitidis is a dimorphic fungus endemic to restricted parts of North America, mainly around the Mississippi and Ohio rivers. Very occasionally, it is reported from Africa. The disease usually presents as a chronic pneumonia similar to pulmonary tuberculosis. Bones, skin and the genitourinary tract may also be affected. Diagnosis is by culture of the organism or identification of the characteristic yeast form in a clinical specimen. Antibody detection is rarely helpful. Treatment is with amphotericin B (severe disease) or itraconazole.

Further information and acknowledgements

Websites

www.britishinfection.org *British Infection Society. Source of general information on communicable diseases.*

www.cdc.gov *Centers for Disease Control, USA. Source of general information about infectious diseases.*

www.fitfortravel.nhs.uk *Scottish site with valuable information for travellers.*

www.hpa.org.uk *Health Protection Agency. Information on infectious diseases in the UK.*

www.idsociety.org *Infectious Diseases Society of America. Source of general information relating to infectious diseases and of authoritative practice guidelines.*

www.who.int *World Health Organization. Invaluable links on travel medicine with updates on outbreaks of infections, changing resistance patterns and vaccination requirements.*

Figure acknowledgements

Fig. 13.12 Reproduced from Halstead SB. Dengue. Medicine 1997; 25:1 and Monath TP Yellow fever. Medicine 1997; 25:1. Copyright Elsevier and Dr TP Monath.

Fig. 13.23 Reproduced by permission of WHO.

Fig. 13.27 Based on Bryceson ADM, Pfaltzgraff RE. Leprosy. 3rd edn. Edinburgh: Churchill Livingstone; 1990; copyright Elsevier.

Fig. 13.35 Simarro PP, Diarra A, Ruiz Postigo JA, et al. The human African trypanosomiasis control and surveillance programme of the World Health Organization 2000–2009: the way forward. PLoS Negl Trop Dis 2011; 5(2): e1007. doi 10.1371/journal.pntd.0001007.

Figs 13.39 and 13.45A Knight R. Parasitic disease in man. Edinburgh: Churchill Livingstone; 1982; copyright Elsevier.

Fig. 13.42A Sundar S, Kumar K, Chakravarty J, et al. Cure of antimony-unresponsive Indian post-kala-azar dermal leishmaniasis with oral miltefosine. Trans R Soc Trop Med Hyg 2006; 100(7):698–700.

Fig. 13.47 Gibbons LM. SEM guide to the morphology of nematode parasites of vertebrates. Farnham Royal, Slough: Commonwealth Agricultural Bureau International; 1986.

Fig. 13.53 Cook GC, ed. Manson's tropical diseases. 20th edn. London: WB Saunders; 1995; copyright Elsevier.

G. Maartens

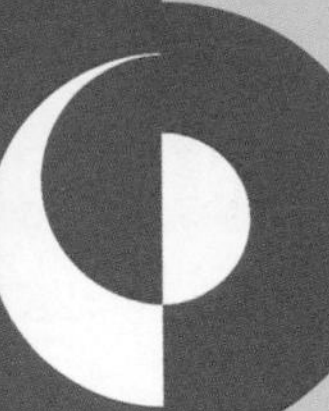

HIV infection and AIDS

14

Clinical examination in HIV disease 388

Epidemiology 390
- Global epidemic and regional patterns 390
- Modes of transmission 390

Virology and immunology 391

Diagnosis and investigations 392
- Diagnosing HIV infection 392
- Viral load and CD4 counts 393

Natural history and staging of HIV 394

Presenting problems in HIV infection 395
- Lymphadenopathy 395
- Weight loss 396
- Fever 396
- Mucocutaneous disease 396
- Gastrointestinal disease 399
- Hepatobiliary disease 400
- Respiratory disease 400
- Nervous system and eye disease 402
- Rheumatological disease 404
- Haematological abnormalities 404
- Renal disease 405
- Cardiac disease 405
- HIV-related cancers 405

Prevention of opportunistic infections 405
- Preventing exposure 405
- Chemoprophylaxis 406
- Immunisation 407

Antiretroviral therapy 407
- ART complications 408
- ART in special situations 409
- Prevention of HIV 410

CLINICAL EXAMINATION IN HIV DISEASE

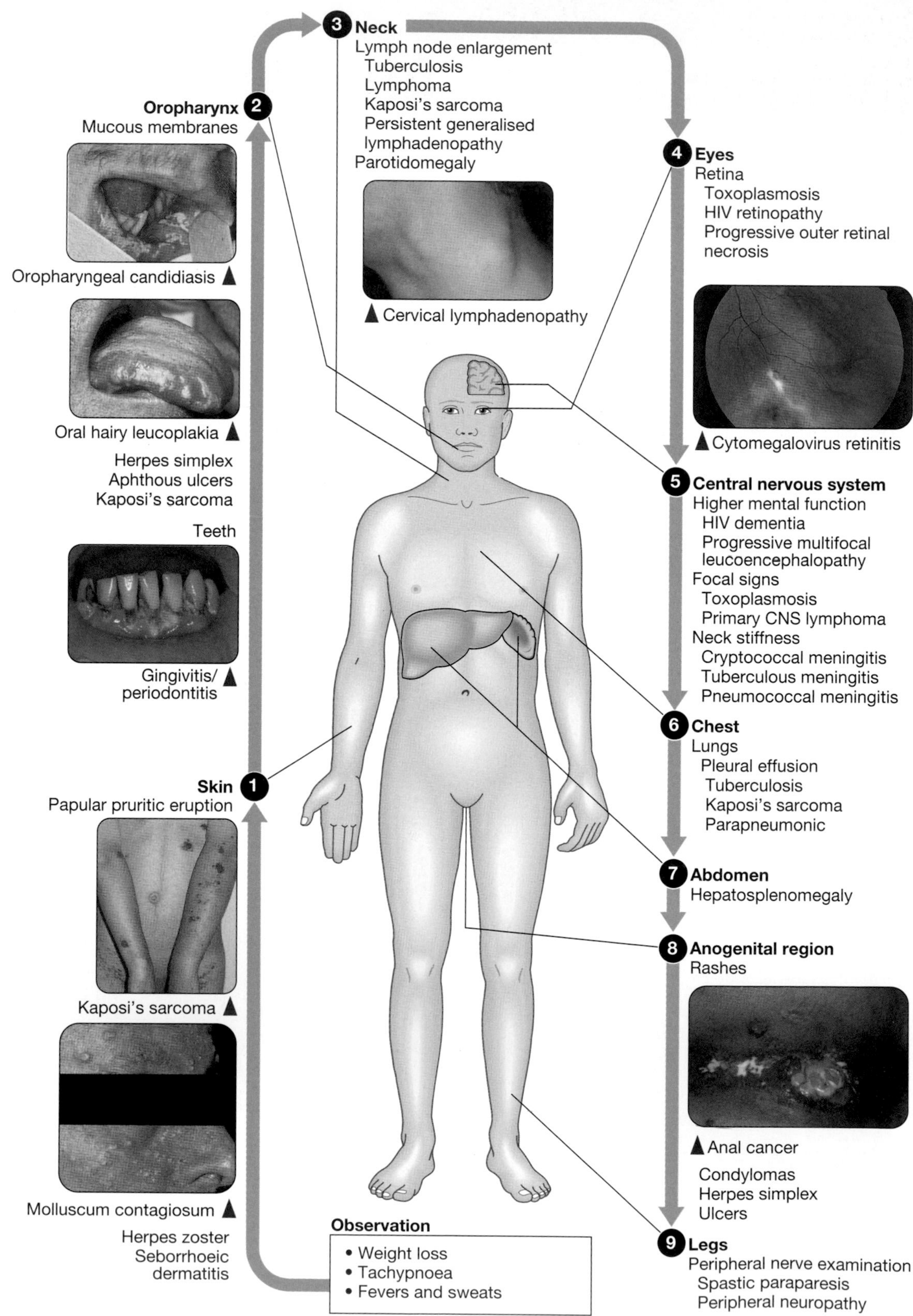

HIV clinical staging classifications

<table>
<tr><th>World Health Organization (WHO) clinical stage
(used in low- and middle-income countries)</th><th>Centers for Disease Control (CDC) clinical categories
(used in high-income countries)</th></tr>
<tr><td>Stage 1
Asymptomatic
Persistent generalised lymphadenopathy</td><td>Category A
Primary HIV infection
Asymptomatic
Persistent generalised lymphadenopathy</td></tr>
<tr><td>Stage 2
Unexplained moderate weight loss (< 10% of body weight)
Recurrent upper respiratory tract infections
Herpes zoster
Angular cheilitis
Recurrent oral ulceration
Papular pruritic eruptions
Seborrhoeic dermatitis
Fungal nail infections</td><td rowspan="2">Category B
Bacillary angiomatosis
Candidiasis, oropharyngeal (thrush)
Candidiasis, vulvovaginal; persistent, frequent or poorly responsive to therapy
Cervical dysplasia (moderate or severe)/cervical carcinoma in situ
Constitutional symptoms, such as fever (38.5°C) or diarrhoea lasting > 1 mth
Oral hairy leucoplakia
Herpes zoster, involving two distinct episodes or more than one dermatome
Idiopathic thrombocytopenic purpura
Listeriosis
Pelvic inflammatory disease, particularly if complicated by tubo-ovarian abscess
Peripheral neuropathy</td></tr>
<tr><td>Stage 3
Unexplained severe weight loss (> 10% of body weight)
Unexplained chronic diarrhoea for > 1 mth
Unexplained persistent fever (> 37.5°C for > 1 mth)
Persistent oral candidiasis
Oral hairy leucoplakia
Pulmonary tuberculosis
Severe bacterial infections
Acute necrotising ulcerative stomatitis, gingivitis or periodontitis
Unexplained anaemia (< 80 g/L (8 g/dL)), neutropenia (< 0.5 × 10^9/L) and/or chronic thrombocytopenia (< 50 × 10^9/L)</td></tr>
<tr><td>Stage 4</td><td>Category C</td></tr>
<tr><td colspan="2">Candidiasis of oesophagus, trachea, bronchi or lungs
Cervical carcinoma – invasive
Cryptococcosis – extrapulmonary
Cryptosporidiosis, chronic (> 1 mth)
Cytomegalovirus disease (outside liver, spleen and nodes)
Herpes simplex chronic (> 1 mth) ulcers or visceral
HIV encephalopathy
HIV wasting syndrome
Isosporiasis, chronic (> 1 mth)
Kaposi's sarcoma
Lymphoma (cerebral or B-cell non-Hodgkin)
Mycobacterial infection, non-tuberculous, extrapulmonary or disseminated
Mycosis – disseminated endemic (coccidiodomycosis or histoplasmosis)
Pneumocystis pneumonia
Pneumonia, recurrent bacterial
Progressive multifocal leucoencephalopathy
Toxoplasmosis – cerebral
Tuberculosis – extrapulmonary (CDC includes pulmonary)
Septicaemia, recurrent (including non-typhoidal Salmonella) (CDC only includes Salmonella)</td></tr>
<tr><td>Symptomatic HIV-associated nephropathy*
Symptomatic HIV-associated cardiomyopathy*
Leishmaniasis, atypical disseminated*</td><td></td></tr>
<tr><td colspan="2">*These conditions are in WHO stage 4 but not in CDC category C.</td></tr>
</table>

EPIDEMIOLOGY

The acquired immunodeficiency syndrome (AIDS) was first recognised in 1981, although the earliest documented case of HIV infection has been traced to a blood sample from the Democratic Republic of Congo in 1959. AIDS is caused by the human immunodeficiency virus (HIV), which progressively impairs cellular immunity. The origin of HIV is a zoonotic infection with simian immunodeficiency viruses (SIV) from African primates, probably first infecting local hunters. SIVs do not cause disease in their natural primate hosts. HIV-1 was transmitted from chimpanzees and HIV-2 from sooty mangabey monkeys. HIV-1 is the cause of the global HIV pandemic, while HIV-2, which causes a similar illness to HIV-1 but progresses more slowly and is less transmissible, is restricted mainly to western Africa. It has been estimated from mutation rates of SIV and HIV that both HIV-1 and HIV-2 first infected humans about 100 years ago.

There are three groups of HIV-1 representing three separate transmission events from chimpanzees: M ('major', worldwide distribution), O ('outlier') and N ('non-major and non-outlier'). Groups O and N are restricted to West Africa. Group M consists of nine subtypes: A–D, F–H, J and K (subtypes E and I were subsequently shown to be recombinants of other subtypes). Globally, subtype C (Africa and India) accounts for half of strains and appears to be more readily transmitted. Subtype B predominates in Western Europe, the Americas and Australia. In Europe, the prevalence of non-B subtypes is increasing because of migrants (predominantly from Africa). Subtypes A and D are associated with slower and faster disease progression respectively.

Global epidemic and regional patterns

In 2011 it was estimated that there were 34.2 million people living with HIV/AIDS, 2.5 million new infections and 1.7 million deaths (Fig. 14.1). Globally, new infections have declined by 20% over the last 10 years. Not all regions have experienced reductions in new infections and the dominant modes of transmission also vary regionally (Box 14.1). Expanding access to combination antiretroviral therapy (ART) has resulted in a 24% decline in global AIDS-related deaths since the peak in 2005. The improved life expectancy on ART has resulted in an increase in the number of people living with HIV. Despite these encouraging epidemiological data, HIV remains an important cause of death globally and has caused over 30 million deaths since the epidemic started. HIV has had a devastating effect in sub-Saharan Africa, particularly in southern African where average life expectancy of the general population fell to below 40 years.

Modes of transmission

HIV is transmitted by sexual contact, by exposure to blood (e.g. injection drug use, occupational exposure in

14.1 Regional HIV incidence and transmission, 2001–2011

Region	HIV incidence	Dominant transmission
Sub-Saharan Africa	Decreasing	Heterosexual
South, South-east and East Asia	Decreasing	IDU, heterosexual
Oceania	Decreasing	Heterosexual
Caribbean	Decreasing	Heterosexual
Latin America	Stable	MSM
North America	Stable	MSM
Western and Central Europe	Stable	MSM
Eastern Europe and Central Asia	Increasing	IDU
Middle East and North Africa	Increasing	IDU, MSM

(IDU = intravenous drug users; MSM = men who have sex with men)

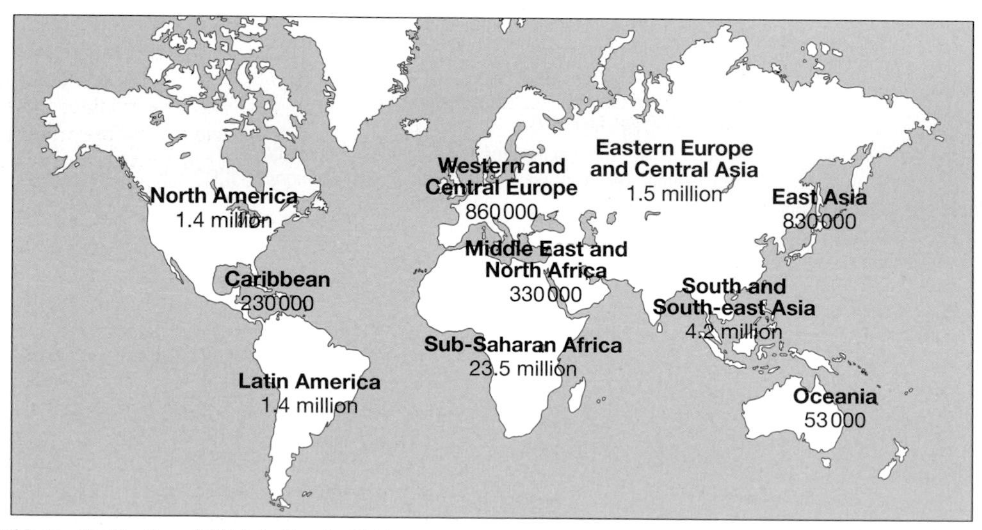

Fig. 14.1 Worldwide distribution of HIV infection in 2011.

health-care workers) and blood products, or to infants of HIV-infected mothers (who may be infected in utero, perinatally or via breastfeeding). Worldwide, the major route of transmission is heterosexual. The risk of contracting HIV after exposure to infected body fluid is dependent on the integrity of the exposed site, the type and volume of fluid, and the level of viraemia in the source person. The approximate transmission risk after exposure is given in Box 14.2. Factors that increase the risk of transmission are listed in Box 14.3.

A high proportion of patients with haemophilia in high-income countries had been infected through contaminated blood products by the time HIV antibody screening was adopted in 1985. Routine screening of blood and blood products for HIV infection using antibody and antigen tests (or polymerase chain reaction, PCR) has virtually eliminated this as a mode of transmission. However, the World Health Organization (WHO) estimates that, because of the lack of adequate screening facilities in resource-poor countries, 5–10% of blood transfusions globally are with HIV-infected blood.

14.2 Risk of HIV transmission after single exposure to an HIV-infected source

HIV exposure	Approximate risk
Sexual	
Vaginal intercourse: female to male	0.05%
Vaginal intercourse: male to female	0.1%
Anal intercourse: insertive	0.05%
Anal intercourse: receptive	0.5%
Oral intercourse: insertive	0.005%
Oral intercourse: receptive	0.01%
Blood exposure	
Blood transfusion	90%
Intravenous drug users sharing needles	0.67%
Percutaneous needle stick injury	0.3%
Mucous membrane splash	0.09%
Mother to child	
Vaginal delivery	15%
Breastfeeding (per month)	0.5%

14.3 Factors increasing the risk of transmission of HIV

Common to all transmission categories
- High viral load

Sexual transmission
- STIs, especially genital ulcers
- Cervical ectopy
- Rectal or vaginal lacerations
- Menstruation
- Uncircumcised male partner
- Depot intramuscular progesterone contraceptive use

Injection drug use transmission
- Sharing equipment
- Linked commercial sex
- Intravenous use
- Concomitant cocaine use
- Incarceration

Occupational transmission
- Deep injury
- Visible blood on device
- Needle was in a blood vessel

Vertical transmission
- Older gestational age
- Prolonged rupture of membranes

(STIs = sexually transmitted infections)

VIROLOGY AND IMMUNOLOGY

HIV is an enveloped ribonucleic acid (RNA) retrovirus from the lentivirus family. After mucosal exposure, HIV is transported to the lymph nodes via dendritic cells, where infection becomes established. This is followed by viraemia and dissemination to lymphoid organs, which are the main sites of viral replication.

Each mature virion has a lipid membrane lined by a matrix protein that is studded with glycoprotein (gp) 120 and gp41 spikes. The inner cone-shaped protein core (p24) houses two copies of the single-stranded RNA genome and viral enzymes. The HIV genome consists of three characteristic retroviral genes – *gag* (encodes a polyprotein that is processed into structural proteins, including p24), *pol* (codes for the enzymes reverse transcriptase, integrase and protease) and *env* (codes for envelope proteins gp120 and gp41) – as well as six regulatory genes (*vif*, *vpr*, *vpu*, *nef*, *tat* and *rev*).

HIV can only infect cells bearing the CD4 receptor; these are T-helper lymphocytes, monocyte–macrophages, dendritic cells, and microglial cells in the central nervous system (CNS). Entry into the cell commences with binding of gp120 to the CD4 receptor (stage 1, Fig. 14.2), which results in a conformational change in gp120 that permits binding to one of two chemokine co-receptors (CXCR4 or CCR5: stage 2). The chemokine co-receptor CCR5 is utilised during initial infection, but later on the virus may adapt to use CXCR4. Individuals who are homozygous for the CCR5 delta 32 mutation do not express CCR5 on CD4 cells and are immune to HIV infection. Chemokine receptor binding is followed by membrane fusion and cellular entry involving gp41 (stage 3). After penetrating the cell and uncoating, a deoxyribonucleic acid (DNA) copy is transcribed from the RNA genome by the reverse transcriptase (RT) enzyme (stage 4) that is carried by the infecting virion. Reverse transcription is an error-prone process and multiple mutations arise with ongoing replication, which results in considerable viral genetic heterogeneity. Viral DNA is transported into the nucleus and integrated within the host cell genome by the integrase enzyme (stage 5). Integrated virus is known as proviral DNA and persists for the life of the cell. Cells infected with proviral HIV DNA produce new virions only if they undergo cellular activation, resulting in the transcription of viral messenger RNA (mRNA) copies (stage 6), which are then translated into viral peptide chains (stage 7). The precursor polyproteins are then cleaved by the viral protease enzyme to form new viral structural proteins and enzymes (stage 8). These then migrate to the cell surface and are assembled using the host cellular apparatus to produce infectious viral particles, which bud from the cell surface, incorporating the host cell membrane into the viral envelope (stage 9). The mature virion then infects other CD4 cells and the process is repeated. CD4 lymphocytes that are replicating HIV have a very short

Stage	Steps in replication	Drug targets
1	Attachment to CD4 receptor	
2	Binding to co-receptor CCR5 or CXCR4	CCR5/CXCR4 receptor inhibitors
3	Fusion	Fusion inhibitors
4	Reverse transcription	Nucleoside and non-nucleoside reverse transcriptase inhibitors
5	Integration	Integrase inhibitors
6	Transcription	
7	Translation	
8	Cleavage of polypeptides and assembly	Protease inhibitors
9	Viral release	

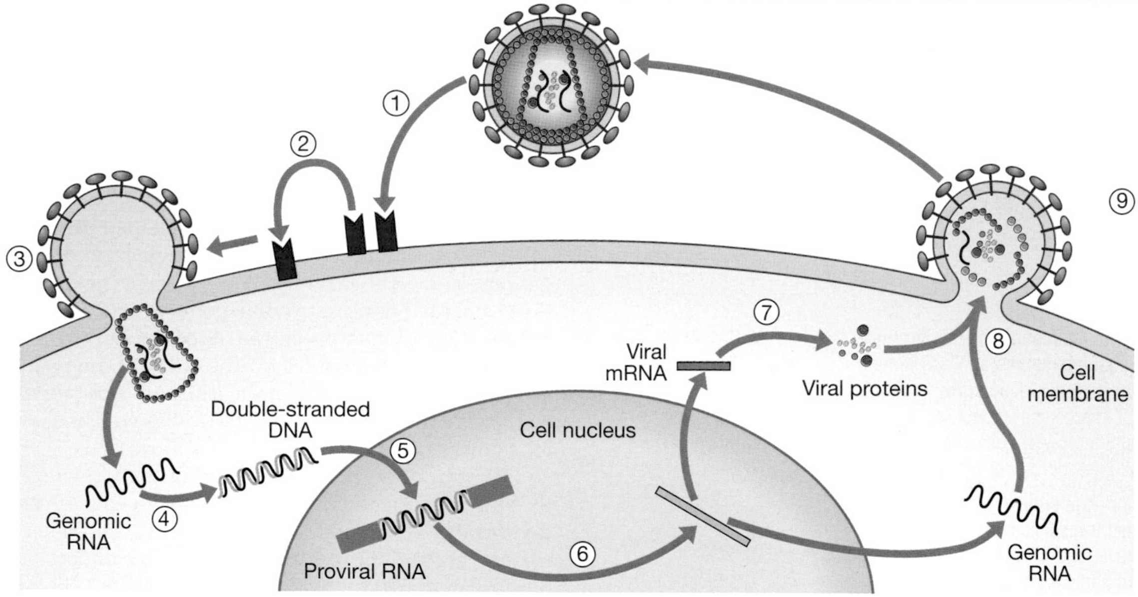

Fig. 14.2 Life cycle of HIV.

survival time of about 1 day. It has been estimated that in asymptomatic HIV-infected people, more than 10^{10} virions are produced and 10^9 CD4 lymphocytes destroyed each day.

A small percentage of T-helper lymphocytes enter a post-integration latent phase. Latently infected cells are important as sanctuary sites from antiretroviral drugs, which only act on replicating virus. Current ART is unable to eradicate HIV infection due to the persistence of proviral DNA in long-lived latent CD4 cells. Novel HIV eradication strategies are being devised to target latently infected cells.

The host immune response to HIV infection is both humoral, with the development of antibodies to a wide range of antigens, and cellular, with a dramatic expansion of HIV-specific CD8 cytotoxic T lymphocytes, resulting in a CD8 lymphocytosis and reversal of the usual CD4:CD8 ratio. CD8 cytotoxic T lymphocytes kill activated CD4 cells that are replicating HIV, but not latently infected CD4 cells. HIV evades destruction despite this vigorous immune response in part because the highly conserved regions of gp120 and gp41 that are necessary for viral attachment and entry are covered by highly variable protein loops that change over time as a result of mutations selected for by the immune response. The initial peak of viraemia in primary infection settles to a plateau phase of persistent chronic viraemia. With time, there is gradual attrition of the T-helper lymphocyte population and, as these cells are pivotal in orchestrating the immune response, the patient becomes susceptible to opportunistic diseases. The predominant opportunist infections in HIV-infected people are the consequences of impaired cell-mediated rather than antibody-mediated immunity (e.g. mycobacteria, herpesviruses). However, there is also a B lymphocyte defect with impaired antibody production to new antigens and dysregulated antibody production with a polyclonal increase in gamma globulins, resulting in an increased risk of infection with encapsulated bacteria, notably *Streptococcus pneumoniae*.

DIAGNOSIS AND INVESTIGATIONS

Diagnosing HIV infection

Globally, the trend is towards universal HIV testing, rather than testing patients at high risk or those with manifestations of HIV infection only. However, in the UK, testing is still targeted (Box 14.4). HIV is diagnosed by detecting host antibodies either by using rapid point-of-care tests or in the laboratory, where enzyme-linked immunosorbent assay (ELISA) tests are usually done. Most tests detect antibodies to both HIV-1 and HIV-2. A positive antibody test from two different immunoassays is sufficient to confirm infection. Western blot assays can also be used to confirm infection, but they are expensive

14.4 HIV testing in the UK
Settings where recommended to all
• Genitourinary medicine or sexual health clinics • Antenatal services • Termination of pregnancy services • Drug dependency programmes • Services for those with hepatitis B, hepatitis C, tuberculosis and lymphoma
Patients routinely offered and recommended testing
• All those presenting with a possible primary HIV infection or where HIV enters the differential diagnosis • All with an STI • All sexual partners of an HIV-positive individual • All MSM and female sexual contacts of MSM • All with a history of injecting drug use • All from a country of high HIV prevalence • All who report sexual contact abroad or in the UK with individuals from a country of high HIV prevalence (> 1%)
Settings where testing should be considered, in areas where HIV prevalence in the local population is > 2 in 1000 population
• All registering with a general practice • All general medical admissions
Groups in whom testing is routinely performed
• Blood donors • Dialysis patients • Organ transplant donors and recipients

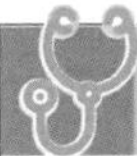

14.5 How to carry out pre-test counselling
• Discuss meaning of positive and negative test results • Realise importance of maintaining confidentiality • Identify person to whom positive result could be disclosed • Explore knowledge and explain natural history of HIV • Discuss transmission and risk reduction • Assess coping strategy • Explain test procedure • Obtain informed consent

and sometimes yield indeterminate results. Screening tests often include a test for p24 antigen in addition to antibodies, in order to detect patients with primary infection before the antibody response occurs. Nucleic acid amplification tests (usually PCR) to detect HIV-RNA are used to diagnose infections in infants of HIV-infected mothers, who carry maternal antibodies to HIV for up to 15 months irrespective of whether they are infected, and to diagnose primary infection before antibodies have developed. (PCR is more sensitive than p24 antigen detection, but p24 is more widely available.)

The purpose of HIV testing is not simply to identify infected individuals, but also to educate people about prevention and transmission of the virus. Counselling is essential both before HIV testing and after the result is obtained (Boxes 14.5 and 14.6). There are major advantages to using rapid point-of-care HIV tests in that pre- and post-test counselling can be done at the same visit. Counselling should always be given in the client's home language.

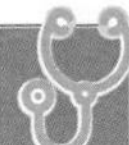

14.6 How to carry out post-test counselling
Test result negative
• Discuss transmission and need for behaviour modification • Advise second test 3 mths after last exposure
Test result positive
• Explain meaning of result • Organise medical follow-up • Assess coping strategy • Stress importance of disclosure • Explain value of antiretroviral therapy • Provide written information and useful Internet resources • Discuss confidentiality issues • Organise emotional and practical support (provide names/phone numbers) • Facilitate notification of sexual partners

14.7 Baseline investigations	
• CD4 count • Viral load • Hepatitis B surface antigen • Hepatitis C antibody (injection drug users) • Liver function tests • Full blood count • Urinalysis and serum creatinine	• Syphilis serology • Cervical smear in women • Serum cryptococcal antigen (if CD4 < 100) • Tuberculin skin test • STI screen

A number of baseline investigations should be done at the initial medical evaluation (Box 14.7). The extent of these investigations will depend on the resources available.

Viral load and CD4 counts

CD4 counts

CD4 lymphocyte counts are usually determined by flow cytometry, but cheaper methods have been developed for low-income countries. The CD4 count is the most clinically useful laboratory indicator of the degree of immune suppression and is used, together with clinical staging, in decisions to start ART and prophylaxis against opportunistic infections, and in the differential diagnosis of clinical problems.

The CD4 count varies by up to 20% from day to day and is also transiently reduced by intercurrent infections. Due to this variability, major therapeutic decisions should not be taken on the basis of a single count. This is particularly important when ART is being initiated in patients who do not fulfil the clinical criteria to start ART. The percentage of lymphocytes that are CD4+, rather than the absolute count, is routinely used in paediatrics, as the normal CD4 counts in infants and young children are much higher. In adults, the CD4 percentage is occasionally useful when evaluating significant reductions in an individual's CD4 count, which may be associated with transient lymphopenia due to intercurrent infection or pregnancy. In this case, the CD4 percentage will be unchanged.

14

The normal CD4 count is > 500 cells/mm^3. The rate of decline in CD4 count is highly variable. People with CD4 counts between 200 and 500 cells/mm^3 have a low risk of developing major opportunistic infections. Morbidity due to inflammatory dermatoses, herpes zoster, oral candidiasis, tuberculosis, bacterial pneumonia and HIV-related immune disorders (e.g. immune thrombocytopenia) becomes increasingly common as CD4 counts decline. Once the count is below 200 cells/mm^3, there is severe immune suppression and a high risk of AIDS-defining conditions. It is important to note that patients can be asymptomatic despite very low CD4 counts and that major opportunistic diseases occasionally present with high CD4 counts.

The CD4 count should be performed every 3–6 months in patients not yet eligible for ART and is usually done at similar intervals in patients on ART, together with measurement of the viral load.

Viral load

The level of viraemia is measured by quantitative PCR of HIV-RNA, known as the viral load. Determining the viral load is important for monitoring responses to ART (p. 407) and also has some prognostic value before starting ART. However, many low-income countries are unable to afford viral load measurements. People with high viral loads (e.g. > 100 000 copies/mL) experience more rapid declines in CD4 count, while those with low viral loads (< 1000 copies/mL) usually have slow or even no decline in CD4 counts. There is little point in repeated measurements of viral load before starting ART, as viral loads remain at a relatively stable plateau after primary infection (Fig. 14.3).

Transient increases in viral load occur with intercurrent infections and immunisations, so the test should be done at least 2 weeks afterwards. Viral load results vary because of assay variability and fluctuations within patients. Only changes in viral load of more than 0.5 $\log_{10}$ copies/mL are considered clinically significant. The same laboratory and viral load test manufacturer should be used for follow-up tests in individual patients if possible.

NATURAL HISTORY AND STAGING OF HIV

Clinical staging of patients should be done at the initial medical examination, as it provides prognostic information and is a key criterion for initiating ART and prophylaxis against opportunistic infections. Two clinical staging systems are used internationally (p. 389). In both systems, patients are staged according to the most severe manifestation and do not improve their classification. For example, a patient who is asymptomatic following a major opportunistic disease (AIDS) remains at stage 4 or category C of the WHO and CDC systems respectively, and never reverts to earlier stages. Finally, patients do not always progress steadily through all stages and may present with AIDS, having previously been asymptomatic.

Primary infection

Primary infection is symptomatic in more than 50% of cases, but the diagnosis is often missed. The incubation period is usually 2–4 weeks after exposure. The duration of symptoms is variable, but is seldom longer than 2 weeks. The clinical manifestations (Box 14.8) resemble a glandular fever-type illness, but the presence of maculo-papular rash or mucosal ulceration strongly suggests primary HIV infection rather than the other viral causes of glandular fever (p. 320). In infectious mononucleosis due to other viruses, rashes generally only occur if aminopenicillins are given. Atypical lymphocytosis occurs less frequently than in Epstein–Barr virus (EBV) infection. Transient lymphopenia, including CD4 lymphocytes, is found in most cases (see Fig. 14.3), which may result in opportunistic infections, notably oropharyngeal candidiasis. Major opportunistic infections like *Pneumocystis jirovecii* pneumonia (PJP) may rarely occur. Thrombocytopenia and moderate elevation of liver enzymes are commonly present. The differential diagnosis of primary HIV includes acute EBV, primary cytomegalovirus (CMV) infection, rubella, primary toxoplasmosis and secondary syphilis.

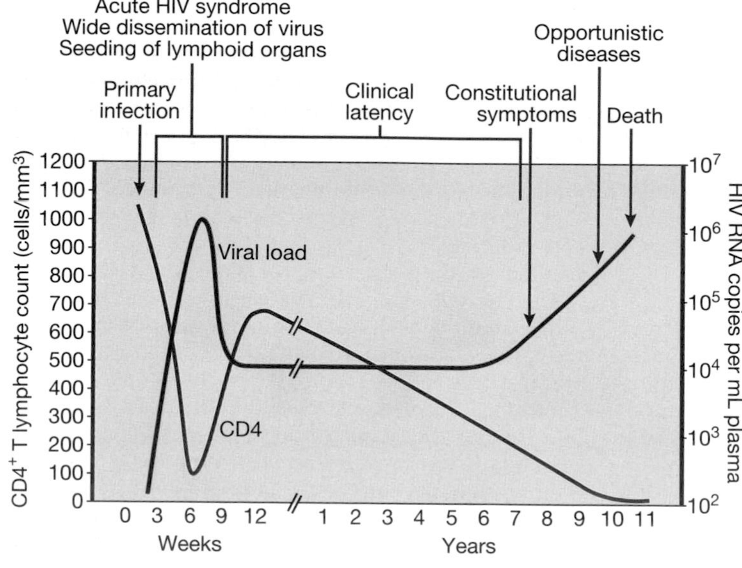

Fig. 14.3 Virological and immunological progression of untreated HIV infection.

14.8 Clinical features of primary infection

• Fever	• Diarrhoea
• Maculo-papular rash	• Headache
• Pharyngitis	• Oral and genital ulceration
• Lymphadenopathy	• Meningo-encephalitis
• Myalgia/arthralgia	• Bell's palsy

Early diagnosis is made by detecting HIV-RNA on PCR or p24 antigenaemia. The appearance of specific anti-HIV antibodies in serum (seroconversion) occurs 2–12 weeks after the development of symptoms. The window period during which antibody tests may be false-negative is prolonged when post-exposure prophylaxis has been used.

Asymptomatic infection

A prolonged period of clinical latency follows primary infection, during which infected individuals are asymptomatic. Persistent generalised lymphadenopathy with nodes typically < 2 cm diameter is a common finding. Eventually the lymph nodes regress, with destruction of node architecture as disease advances.

Viraemia peaks during primary infection and then drops as the immune response develops, to reach a plateau about 3 months later. The level of viraemia post-seroconversion is a predictor of the rate of decline in CD4 counts, which is highly variable and explained in part by genetic factors affecting the immune response. The median time from infection to the development of AIDS in adults is about 9 years (see Fig. 14.3). A small proportion of untreated HIV-infected people are long-term non-progressors with CD4 counts in the reference range for 10 years or more. Some long-term non-progressors have undetectable viral loads and are known as 'elite controllers'.

Minor HIV-associated disorders

A wide range of disorders indicating some impairment of cellular immunity occur in most patients before they develop AIDS (CDC category B or WHO stages 2 and 3). Careful examination of the mouth is important when patients are being followed up, as oral candidiasis and oral hairy leucoplakia are common and important conditions that require initiation of ART and prophylaxis against opportunistic infections, irrespective of the CD4 count.

Acquired immunodeficiency syndrome

AIDS is defined by the development of specified opportunistic infections, cancers and severe manifestations of HIV itself (p. 389). CDC category C is the most widely used definition of AIDS. WHO updated its classification more recently and added a few conditions of similar prognosis to its stage 4 disease. Box 14.9 outlines the correlation between CD4 count and HIV-related diseases.

PRESENTING PROBLEMS IN HIV INFECTION

HIV itself is associated with a wide variety of clinical manifestations, and opportunistic diseases add many more. All body systems can be affected by HIV. The CD4 count is useful in differential diagnosis (see Box 14.9): opportunistic diseases that may present at higher CD4 counts become increasingly common as CD4 counts decline, so the CD4 count helps to rule out certain disorders. For example, in a patient with a pulmonary infiltrate and a CD4 count of 350 cells/mm^3, pulmonary tuberculosis is a likely diagnosis and *Pneumocystis* infection is very unlikely, but if the patient's CD4 count is 50 cells/mm^3, both *Pneumocystis* and tuberculosis are likely.

Globally, tuberculosis is the most common cause of morbidity and mortality in HIV-infected patients. Tuberculosis should be considered in the differential diagnosis of most presenting problems in patients from communities where tuberculosis is common.

14.9 CD4 count and risk of common HIV-associated diseases

< 500 cells/mm^3	
• Tuberculosis • Bacterial pneumonia • Herpes zoster • Oropharyngeal candidiasis • Non-typhoid salmonellosis	• Kaposi's sarcoma • Non-Hodgkin lymphoma • HIV-associated idiopathic thrombocytopenic purpura
< 200 cells/mm^3	
• *Pneumocystis jirovecii* pneumonia • Chronic herpes simplex ulcers • Oesophageal candidiasis	• *Isospora belli* diarrhoea • HIV wasting syndrome • HIV-associated dementia • Peripheral neuropathy • Endemic mycoses
< 100 cells/mm^3	
• Cerebral toxoplasmosis • Cryptococcal meningitis • Cryptosporidiosis and microsporidiosis • Primary CNS lymphoma • Cytomegalovirus	• Disseminated *Mycobacterium avium* complex (MAC) • Progressive multifocal leucoencephalopathy

Lymphadenopathy

Persistent generalised lymphadenopathy due to HIV is described above under asymptomatic infection. Lymphadenopathy may also be due to malignancy (Kaposi's sarcoma or lymphoma) or infections, especially tuberculosis, which is an extremely common cause in low- and middle-income countries. Rapid enlargement of a node, asymmetric enlargement or lymphadenopathy associated with constitutional symptoms (even if the nodes are symmetrical) warrants further investigation. Tuberculous lymph nodes often undergo extensive caseous necrosis, causing them to become fluctuant, and inexperienced clinicians often inappropriately perform incision and drainage. Lymphoma typically presents with large nodes that are not fluctuant. Lymph node needle aspiration (using a wide-bore needle such as 19G) should be undertaken for microscopy. One slide should be air-dried and sent for staining for acid-fast bacilli, which has about a 70% yield in tuberculosis. The other slide should be fixed and sent for cytology. If caseous liquid is

14

aspirated, this should be sent for mycobacterial culture. If needle aspiration is unhelpful, or if lymphoma or Kaposi's sarcoma is suspected, excision biopsy should be performed.

Weight loss

Weight loss is a very common finding in advanced HIV infection. The HIV wasting syndrome is an AIDS-defining condition and is defined as weight loss of more than 10% of body weight, plus either unexplained chronic diarrhoea (lasting > 1 month) or chronic weakness and unexplained prolonged fever (lasting > 1 month). This is a diagnosis of exclusion. If the weight loss is rapid (more than 1 kg a month), then major opportunistic infections or cancers become more likely. Painful oral conditions and nausea from drugs contribute by limiting intake. Depression is very common and can cause significant weight loss. Measurement of C-reactive protein is helpful in the work-up of weight loss, as this is markedly raised with most opportunistic diseases but not with HIV itself. Erythrocyte sedimentation rate (ESR) is elevated by HIV infection and is therefore not useful. The presence of fever or diarrhoea is helpful in the differential diagnosis (Fig. 14.4).

Fever

Fever is a very common presenting feature. Common causes of prolonged fever with weight loss are listed in Figure 14.4. Non-typhoid *Salmonella* bacteraemia, which commonly presents with fever in low-income countries, presents without diarrhoea in about 50% of patients. Pyrexia of unknown origin (PUO) in HIV infection is defined as temperature over 38°C with no cause found after 4 weeks in outpatients or 3 days in inpatients, and initial investigations such as chest X-rays, urinalysis and blood cultures will have failed to identify the cause. HIV itself can present with prolonged fever, but this is a diagnosis of exclusion, as a treatable cause will be found in most patients. Abdominal imaging, preferably by computed tomography (CT), should be requested. Abdominal nodes (especially if they are hypodense in the centre) or splenic microabscesses strongly suggest tuberculosis. Mycobacterial (or 'lytic') blood cultures, which can also detect fungi, should be performed. Bone marrow aspirate and trephine biopsy are helpful if the full blood count shows cytopenias. Liver biopsy may be helpful if the liver enzymes are elevated, but is invasive and seldom necessary. Mycobacterial and fungal stains and cultures should be done on all biopsies. Chest X-rays should be repeated after about a week, as micronodular or interstitial infiltrates may have become apparent (see p. 401 for differential diagnosis).

Tuberculosis is by far the most common cause of PUO in low- and middle-income countries, and in these settings an early trial of empiric therapy is warranted after cultures have been sent. In high-income countries, disseminated *Mycobacterium avium* complex (MAC) infection is an important cause of PUO, often with diarrhoea and splenomegaly. Disseminated endemic mycoses (histoplasmosis, coccidiodomycosis and penicilliosis) present with PUO, often with papular skin eruptions. Skin biopsy for histology and fungal culture is often diagnostic.

Mucocutaneous disease

The skin and mouth must be carefully examined, as mucocutaneous manifestations are extremely common in HIV and many prognostically important conditions can be diagnosed by simple inspection. The differential diagnosis of dermatological conditions is simplified by categorising disorders according to the lesion type (Box 14.10). Some common dermatological diseases, notably psoriasis, are exacerbated by HIV. The risk of drug

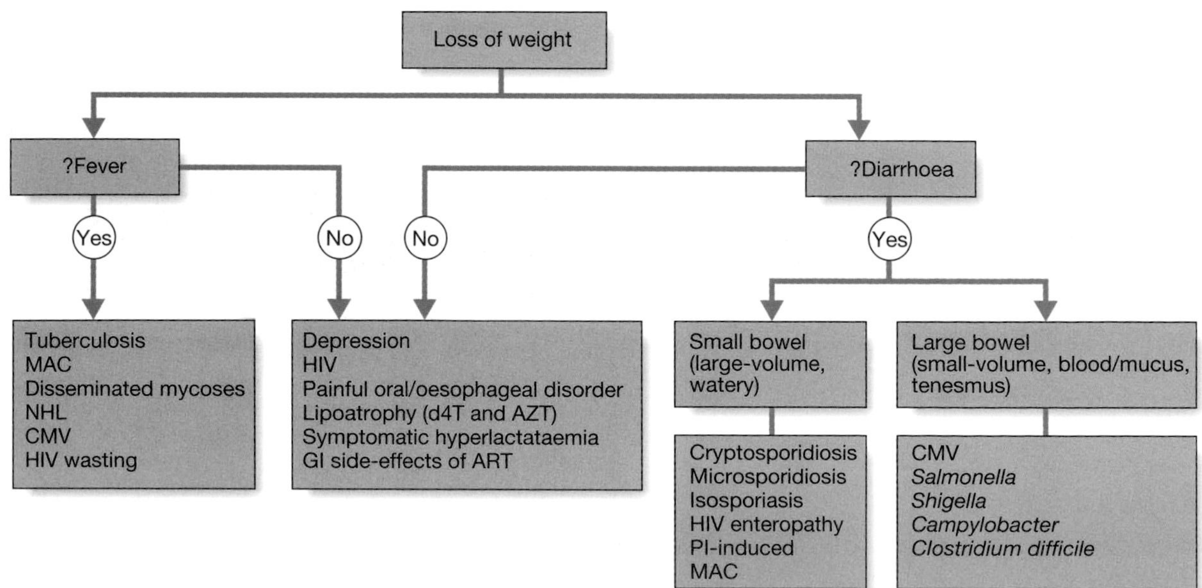

Fig. 14.4 Presentation and differential diagnosis of weight loss. (AZT = zidovudine; CMV = cytomegalovirus; d4T = stavudine; KS = Kaposi's sarcoma; MAC = *Mycobacterium avium* complex; NHL = non-Hodgkin lymphoma; PI = protease inhibitor)

14.10 Differential diagnosis of skin conditions by lesion type

Scaly rashes	
• Seborrhoeic dermatitis • Psoriasis* (exacerbated by HIV) • Tinea corporis*	• Dry skin/icthyosis • Norwegian scabies* • Drug rashes*
Pruritic papules	
• Pruritic papular eruption ('itchy red bump disease')	• Eosinophilic folliculitis • Scabies*
Papules and nodules (non-pruritic)	
• Molluscum contagiosum* • Secondary syphilis • Kaposi's sarcoma • Bacillary angiomatosis • Cryptococcosis	• Warts* • Disseminated endemic mycoses (histoplasmosis, coccidiodomycosis and penicilliosis)
Blisters	
• Herpes simplex • Herpes zoster • Fixed drug eruptions	• Drug rashes (especially toxic epidermal necrolysis)
Mucocutaneous ulcers	
• Ecthyma • Herpes simplex • Aphthous ulcers (minor and major)	• Histoplasmosis • Drug rashes (Stevens–Johnson syndrome)
Hyperpigmentation	
• Post-inflammatory (especially pruritic papular eruption)	• Zidovudine • Emtricitabine (palms and soles)

*See Chapter 28 for more information.

rashes is greatly increased in HIV-infected patients. Skin biopsy should be taken, and sent for histology and culture for mycobacteria and fungi in patients with unusual rashes or if there are constitutional symptoms coinciding with the development of the rash.

Seborrhoeic dermatitis

Seborrhoeic dermatitis is very common in HIV. The severity increases as the CD4 count falls. It presents as scaly red patches, typically in the nasolabial folds and in hairy areas. Fungal infections are thought to play a role in the pathogenesis of this condition. It responds well to a combined topical antifungal and steroid. Selenium sulphide shampoo is helpful for scalp involvement.

Herpes simplex infections

Recurrences of herpes simplex infection are very common and primarily affect the nasolabial and anogenital areas (Fig. 14.5). As immune suppression worsens, the ulcers take longer to heal and become more extensive. Ulcers that persist for more than 4 weeks are AIDS-defining. The diagnosis is clinical, but PCR of vesicle fluid or from ulcer swabs may be diagnostic with unusual presentations. Response to a course of aciclovir or a related drug is good, but relapses are common. Frequent relapses that persist despite ART should be treated with aciclovir 400 mg twice daily for 6–12 months.

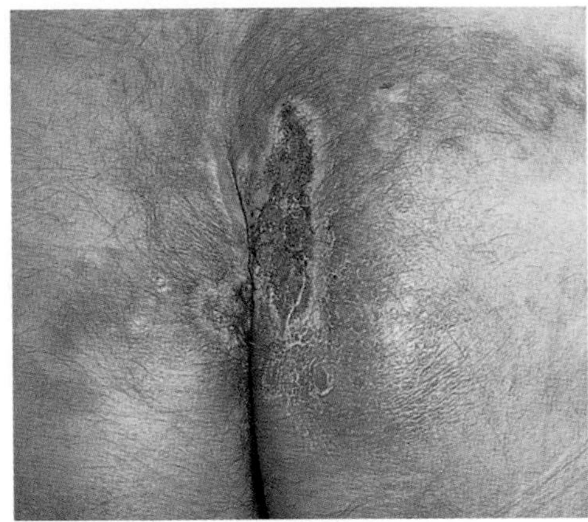

Fig. 14.5 Severe mucocutaneous herpes simplex. Chronic anogenital or perioral ulcers are very common in advanced HIV infection.

14

Herpes zoster

This usually presents with a pathognomonic vesicular rash on an erythematous base in a dermatomal distribution (p. 318). The median CD4 count at the first episode of zoster is 350 cells/mm^3. In patients with advanced disease, the rash may be multidermatomal and recurrent episodes may occur. Disseminated zoster is rare. In HIV-infected patients, zoster is generally more extensive, has a longer duration, and there is a higher risk of developing post-herpetic neuralgia. High doses of aciclovir or its congeners should be given for all cases with active disease, irrespective of the time since the onset of the rash. Post-herpetic neuralgia is difficult to manage. Analgesic adjuvants, e.g. amitriptyline and pregabalin, should be commenced in all patients with prolonged pain. Topical capsaicin has modest efficacy.

Kaposi's sarcoma

Kaposi's sarcoma (KS) is a spindle-cell tumour of lympho-endothelial origin. All forms of KS are due to sexually transmitted human herpesvirus 8, also known as KS-associated herpesvirus. KS occurs in four patterns:

- classic KS: rare, indolent and restricted largely to elderly Mediterranean or Jewish men
- endemic KS: occurs in sub-Saharan Africa, is more aggressive, presents at earlier ages than classic KS, and affects men more than women
- KS in patients on immunosuppressant drugs: usually transplant recipients, who experience disseminated disease
- AIDS-associated KS.

In Africa, the male:female ratio of AIDS-associated KS is much lower than is seen with endemic KS, but men are still more affected than women despite the fact that the seroprevalence of human herpesvirus 8 is the same in both sexes.

AIDS-associated KS is always a multicentric disease. Early mucocutaneous lesions are macular and may be difficult to diagnose. Subsequently, lesions become papular or nodular, and may ulcerate. KS lesions typically have a red–purple colour (Fig. 14.6 and p. 388), but may become hyperpigmented, especially in dark-skinned patients. As the disease progresses, the skin

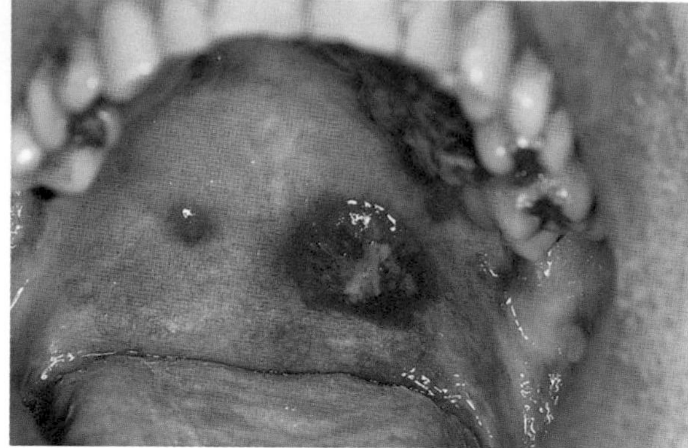

Fig. 14.6 Oral Kaposi's sarcoma. A full examination is important to detect disease that may affect the palate, gums, fauces or tongue.

lesions become more numerous and larger. Lymphoedema is common, as lymphatic vessels are infiltrated. KS also commonly spreads to lymph nodes and viscerally, especially to the lungs and gastrointestinal tract. Visceral disease occasionally occurs in the absence of mucocutaneous involvement. B symptoms of fever, night sweats and weight loss may occur.

KS may respond to ART. Chemotherapy should be reserved for those patients who fail to remit on ART, or given together with ART if there are poor prognostic features such as visceral involvement, oedema, ulcerated lesions and B symptoms.

Bacillary angiomatosis

Bacillary angiomatosis is a bacterial infection caused by *Bartonella henselae* or *B. quintana*. Skin lesions range from solitary superficial red–purple lesions resembling Kaposi's sarcoma or pyogenic granuloma, to multiple subcutaneous nodules or plaques. Lesions are painful and may bleed or ulcerate. The infection may become disseminated with fevers, lymphadenopathy and hepatosplenomegaly. Diagnosis is made by biopsy of a lesion and Warthin–Starry silver staining, which reveals aggregates of bacilli. Treatment with doxycycline or azithromycin is effective.

Papular pruritic eruption

Papular pruritic eruption ('itchy red bump disease') is an intensely itchy, symmetrical rash affecting the trunk and extremities. It thought to be due to an allergic reaction to insect bites. In sub-Saharan Africa, it is the most common skin manifestation of HIV. Post-inflammatory hyperpigmentation is common. Topical steroids, emollients and antihistamines are useful but response is variable. Measures to reduce insect bites are logical, but difficult to implement in low-income settings.

Drug rashes

Cutaneous hypersensitivity to drugs is said to occur 100 times more frequently in HIV infection. The most common type is an erythematous maculo-papular rash, which may be scaly. The drugs most commonly associated with rashes are sulphonamides and non-nucleoside reverse transcriptase inhibitors (NNRTIs – see below). Severe, life-threatening features of drug rashes include blistering (when this affects more than 30% of surface area it is known as toxic epidermal necrolysis), involvement of mucous membranes (Stevens–Johnson syndrome, pp. 1264 and 1302), or systemic involvement with fever or organ dysfunction (especially hepatitis, which is often delayed for a few days after the rash develops). Because sulphonamides are important in the treatment and prophylaxis of opportunistic infections, rechallenge or desensitisation is often attempted in patients who have previously experienced rashes, provided the reaction was not life-threatening. Details of rashes caused by ART are given below.

Oral conditions

Oropharyngeal candidiasis is very common. It is nearly always caused by *C. albicans* (p. 381), but other azole-resistant *Candida* species may be selected for if there have been repeated courses of azole drugs. Pseudomembranous candidiasis is the most common manifestation, with white patches on the buccal mucosa (p. 388) that can be scraped off to reveal a red raw surface. Erythematous candidiasis is more difficult to diagnose and presents with a reddened mucosa and a smooth shiny tongue. Angular cheilitis due to *Candida* is a common manifestation. Topical antifungals are usually effective. Antifungal lozenges and gentian violet are both more effective than antifungal solutions. Systemic azole therapy, usually fluconazole, should be given if topical therapy fails or if there are oesophageal symptoms.

Oral hairy leucoplakia (p. 388) appears as corrugated white plaques running vertically on the side of the tongue, and is virtually pathognomonic of HIV disease. It is usually asymptomatic and is due to EBV. If high doses of aciclovir or a related drug are given for varicella zoster virus infections, the lesions may temporarily regress.

Oral ulcers are common. Herpetiform oral ulcers occur in primary infection. Herpes simplex typically affects the nasolabial area, but may cause oral ulcers. In early disease, minor aphthous ulcers are common. In advanced disease, giant aphthous ulcers occur. These destroy tissue, are painful and need to be differentiated from herpes simplex and CMV ulcers by biopsy. They respond to systemic steroids. Histoplasmosis (p. 385) is an uncommon cause of oral ulcers, usually associated with constitutional symptoms. Finally, superficial oral ulcers may occur as part of the Stevens–Johnson syndrome, usually caused by sulphonamides or NNRTIs.

KS often involves the mouth, especially the hard palate (see above and Fig. 14.6). Nodular oral lesions are associated with a worse prognosis.

Gingivitis is very common. Good oral hygiene and regular dental checkups are important. Acute necrotising ulcerative gingivitis and periostitis (p. 388) can result in loss of teeth; they should be treated with a course of metronidazole and a dental referral should be made.

Nail disorders

Fungal infections (onychomycosis, p. 1280) are very common and often involve multiple nails. Blue discoloration of nails is common and may be due to HIV or to the antiretroviral drug zidovudine.

Gastrointestinal disease

Oesophageal diseases

Oesophageal candidiasis (Fig. 14.7) is the most common cause of pain on swallowing (odynophagia), dysphagia and regurgitation. Concomitant oral candidiasis is present in about 70% of patients. Systemic azole therapy, e.g. fluconazole 200 mg daily for 14 days, is usually curative, but relapses are common. Patients whose oesophageal symptoms fail to respond to azoles should be investigated with oesophagoscopy. Major aphthous ulceration and CMV ulcers are the most likely causes and need to be differentiated by biopsy. Occasionally, herpes simplex oesophagitis or obstructive KS is responsible.

Diarrhoea

Chronic diarrhoea is a very common presenting problem in patients with advanced HIV, especially in areas where there is no access to safe water. It is a major cause of wasting. The differential diagnosis of diarrhoea depends on whether the presentation is with large- or small-bowel symptoms (see Fig. 14.4, p. 396). The presentation and aetiology of acute diarrhoea are similar to those in HIV-uninfected patients.

Large-bowel diarrhoea

Acute diarrhoea caused by the bacterial enteric pathogens *Campylobacter*, *Shigella* and *Salmonella* occurs more frequently than in HIV-uninfected people and the illness is more severe. Bacteraemia is much more common, notably due to non-typhoid *Salmonella*. Diarrhoea caused by *Clostridium difficile* should be considered if there has been prior exposure to antibiotics, as is often the case in patients with symptomatic HIV.

CMV colitis presents with chronic large-bowel symptoms and fever in patients with CD4 counts below 100 cells/mm^3. On colonoscopy, ulcers are seen, mostly involving the left side of the colon. Biopsy of ulcers shows typical 'owl's-eye' inclusion bodies.

Small-bowel diarrhoea

Chronic small-bowel diarrhoea may be due to HIV enteropathy, but this is a diagnosis of exclusion. It typically presents with chronic watery diarrhoea and wasting without fever. Infection with one of three unicellular organisms is responsible for most cases: cryptosporidiosis, microsporidiosis and isosporiasis (Box 14.11). All three are intracellular parasites that invade enterocytes. If the diagnosis is not made by stool microscopy on at least two specimens, a duodenal biopsy should be performed (Fig. 14.8). Electron microscopy is essential for speciation of microsporidia.

14.11 Common causes of chronic watery diarrhoea

	Cryptosporidiosis	Microsporidiosis	Isosporiasis
Organism	Protozoan	Fungus	Protozoan
Species	*Cryptosporidium parvum* *C. hominis*	*Encephalitozoon bieneusi* *E. intestinalis*, etc.	*Isospora belli*
Animal host	Multiple	Multiple	No
Distribution	Global	Global	Tropics
Stool examination	Acid-fast stain	Trichrome stain PCR	Acid-fast stain
Specific treatment	No established therapy	Albendazole (some species)	Co-trimoxazole

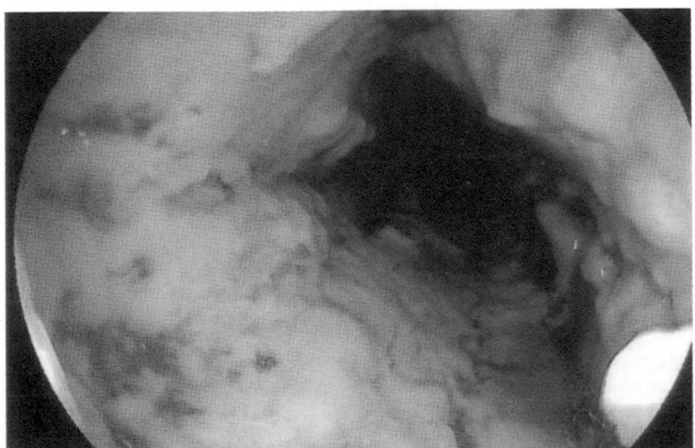

Fig. 14.7 Oesophageal candidiasis. Endoscopy showing typical pseudomembranous candidiasis.

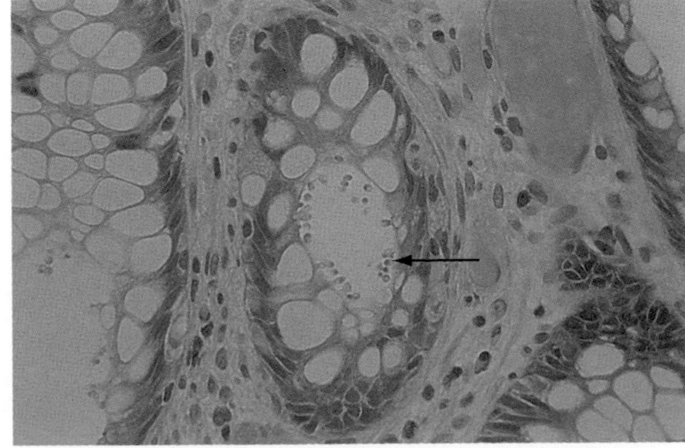

Fig. 14.8 Cryptosporidiosis. Duodenal biopsy may be necessary to confirm cryptosporidiosis or microsporidiosis. Arrow indicates an öocyst.

14

About 40% of patients with disseminated MAC infections have watery diarrhoea. Unlike in cryptosporidiosis, microsporidiosis and isosporiasis, fever is a prominent feature of MAC infection. Intestinal tuberculosis typically involves the ileocaecal area and may present with fever and diarrhoea, but the diarrhoea is seldom profuse.

Hepatobiliary disease

Chronic viral hepatitis

Hepatitis B and/or C (HBV and HCV) co-infection is common in HIV-infected people due to shared risk factors for transmission. The natural history of both HBV and HCV is altered by HIV co-infection. In the ART era, chronic liver disease from viral hepatitis has emerged as a major cause of morbidity and mortality. HBV and HCV are further described on pages 950 and 954.

Hepatitis B

HBV infection is common in several groups of people at risk of HIV infection: residents of low- and middle-income countries, injection drug users, haemophiliacs and MSM. HIV co-infection increases HBV viraemia, is associated with less elevation of transaminase (presumably due to immune suppression), and increases the risk of liver fibrosis and hepatoma. Several NRTIs (lamivudine, emtricitabine and tenofovir) are also effective against HBV. HBV status should be checked at baseline in all HIV-infected patients. Treatment with anti-HBV drugs should be considered for all patients who have active HBV replication (HBeAg-positive or HBV DNA > 2000 U/mL) and/or evidence of inflammation or fibrosis on liver biopsy. This is best achieved by starting an ART regimen that includes tenofovir with either lamivudine or emtricitabine. Interferon is seldom used, but may be considered in patients with CD4 counts above 500 cells/mm^3. A flare of hepatitis may be associated with improved immune function after starting ART or discontinuing antiretrovirals that have anti-HBV activity. There is an increased risk of antiretroviral hepatotoxicity.

Hepatitis C

HCV infection is extremely common in injection drug users and haemophiliacs. HIV co-infection increases HCV viraemia and increases the risk of liver fibrosis and hepatoma. Treatment for HCV should preferably be deferred in patients with low CD4 counts until the CD4 count has risen to 350 cells/mm^3 or more. As with HBV, a flare of hepatitis may be associated with improved immune function after starting ART, and there is an increased risk of antiretroviral hepatotoxicity. Response to anti-HCV therapy is similar to that seen in HIV-uninfected people, but there is more toxicity and there are important drug–drug interactions between several antiretrovirals and both ribavirin and the newer HCV protease inhibitors.

HIV cholangiopathy

HIV cholangiopathy, a form of secondary sclerosing cholangitis (p. 965), is seen in patients with severe immune suppression. In some patients, co-existing intestinal infection with CMV, cryptosporidiosis or microsporidiosis is present, but it is uncertain if these organisms play an aetiological role. Papillary stenosis is common and is amenable to cautery via endoscopic retrograde cholangiopancreatography (ERCP), which provides symptomatic relief. Acalculous cholecystitis is a common complication of cholangiopathy. ART may improve the condition.

Respiratory disease

Pulmonary disease is very common and is the major reason for hospital admission. More than 90% of patients who are admitted for respiratory diseases will have either bacterial pneumonia, pulmonary tuberculosis or *Pneumocystis jirovecii* pneumonia (PJP). PJP is more common in high-income countries, while tuberculosis is more common in low- and middle-income countries. An approach to the differential diagnosis of all three conditions is given in Box 14.12.

Pneumocystis jirovecii pneumonia

The key presenting feature of PJP is progressive dyspnoea. Dry cough and fever are common. The chest X-ray typically shows a bilateral interstitial infiltrate spreading out from the hilar regions (Fig. 14.9), but may be normal initially. High-resolution CT scan is more sensitive than chest X-ray, usually showing typical 'ground-glass' interstitial infiltrates. Pneumatocoeles may occur and may rupture, resulting in a pneumothorax. The diagnosis is made with silver stains, PCR or immunofluorescence of broncho-alveolar lavage or induced sputum. Treatment is with high-dose co-trimoxazole, together with adjunctive steroids if the patient is hypoxic.

Pulmonary tuberculosis

Tuberculosis is the most common cause of admission in countries with a high tuberculosis incidence. Pulmonary tuberculosis in patients with mild immune suppression typically presents as in HIV-uninfected patients, with a chronic illness and apical pulmonary cavities (p. 688). However, in patients with CD4 counts below 200 cells/mm^3, there are four important differences in the clinical presentation of pulmonary tuberculosis.

14.12 Characteristic features of bacterial pneumonia, PJP and pulmonary TB

	Bacterial pneumonia	PJP	Pulmonary TB
Duration	Acute	Subacute	Variable
Dyspnoea	Common	Prominent	Occasional
White cell count	Increased	Normal	Variable
Chest X-ray			
Infiltrate	Consolidation	Interstitial	Variable
Bilateral infiltrate	Occasional	Yes	Common
Effusion	Occasional	No	Common
Nodes	Uncommon	No	Common
C-reactive protein	Markedly increased	Variable	Increased

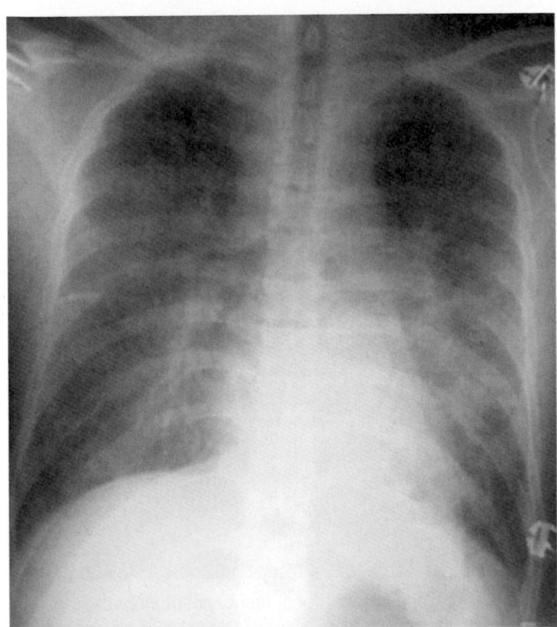

Fig. 14.9 *Pneumocystis* pneumonia: typical chest X-ray appearance. Note the interstitial bilateral infiltrate.

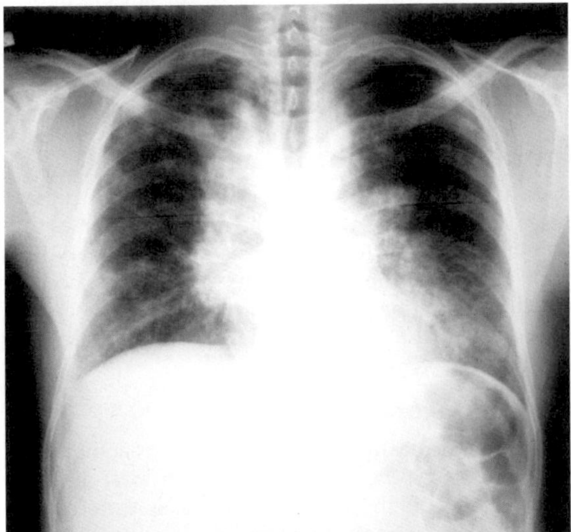

Fig. 14.10 Chest X-ray of pulmonary tuberculosis in advanced HIV infection. Lower-zone infiltrates and hilar or mediastinal nodes in a patient with a CD4 count of less than 200 cells/mm^3.

- Tuberculosis progresses more rapidly, with a subacute or even acute presentation. Therefore the diagnosis needs to be made and therapy commenced promptly. A trial of empirical therapy is often started while awaiting the results of mycobacterial cultures.
- The chest X-ray appearance alters: cavities are rarely seen, pulmonary infiltrates are no longer predominantly in apical areas, and pleural effusions and hilar or mediastinal lymphadenopathy are common (Fig. 14.10). A normal chest X-ray is not unusual in symptomatic patients with tuberculosis confirmed on sputum culture. These atypical findings can result in delayed or missed diagnosis.
- Sputum smears, which are positive in most HIV-uninfected adults with pulmonary tuberculosis, are negative in more than half of patients. The main reason for this is the absence of pulmonary cavities.
- Many patients have disseminated tuberculosis, sometimes with a classic miliary pattern on chest X-ray, but more commonly presenting with pulmonary and extrapulmonary tuberculosis. The most common sites of concomitant extrapulmonary tuberculosis are the pleura and lymph nodes. Acid-fast bacilli are more often found on wide-needle aspirate of nodes than on sputum (p. 395). Pleural aspirate showing a lymphocytic exudate suggests tuberculosis as a likely cause and pleural biopsy will usually confirm the diagnosis.

Tuberculosis in HIV-infected patients responds well to standard short-course therapy (p. 693).

Bacterial pneumonia

The incidence of bacterial pneumonia is increased about 100-fold by HIV infection. The severity, likelihood of bacteraemia, risk of recurrent pneumonia, and mortality are all increased compared with HIV-uninfected patients. The aetiology is similar to that of community-acquired pneumonia in HIV-uninfected patients with co-morbidity: *S. pneumoniae* is the commonest, followed by *Haemophilus influenzae*, enterobacteriaceae (e.g. *Klebsiella pneumoniae*) and *Staphylococcus aureus*. The prevalence of atypical bacteria in HIV-infected patients with pneumonia is probably similar to that in the general population, but the data are limited. Treatment is with a broad-spectrum β-lactam (e.g. ceftriaxone, amoxicillin-clavulanate), with the addition of a macrolide if the pneumonia is severe.

Uncommon bacteria causing pneumonia include *Pseudomonas aeruginosa, Nocardia* (which mimics tuberculosis) and *Rhodococcus equi* (which can cause pulmonary cavities).

Miscellaneous causes of pulmonary infiltrates

Pulmonary cryptococcosis may present as a component of disseminated disease or be limited to the lungs. The chest X-ray appearances are variable. Cryptococcomas occur less commonly than in HIV-uninfected people. The commonest radiographic pattern seen in HIV infection is patchy consolidation, often with small areas of cavitation resembling tuberculosis. Pleural involvement is rare. The endemic mycoses (histoplasmosis, coccidioidomycosis and penicilliosis) often also cause non-specific pulmonary infiltrates.

Lymphoid interstitial pneumonitis is a slowly progressive disorder with a diffuse reticulonodular infiltrate. It is caused by a benign polyclonal lymphocytic interstitial infiltrate and is part of the diffuse infiltrative lymphocytosis syndrome (DILS – see p. 404). Patients may have other features of DILS, notably parotidomegaly.

Kaposi's sarcoma often spreads to the lungs. Typical chest X-ray appearances are large, irregular nodules, linear reticular pattern and pleural effusions. Bronchoscopy is diagnostic.

Nervous system and eye disease

The central and peripheral nervous systems are commonly involved in HIV, either as a direct consequence of HIV infection or due to opportunistic diseases. Presentations are outlined in Figure 14.11.

Cognitive impairment

HIV-associated neurocognitive disorders

HIV is a neurotropic virus and invades the CNS early during infection. Meningo-encephalitis may occur at seroconversion. About 50% of HIV-infected people have abnormal neuropsychiatric testing, the proportion increasing with declining CD4 counts. The term HIV-associated neurocognitive disorders (HAND) describes a spectrum of disorders: asymptomatic neurocognitive impairment (which is the most common), minor neurocognitive disorder and HIV-associated dementia (also called HIV encephalopathy). Dementia occurs in late disease and is a subcortical dementia characterised by impairment of executive function, psychomotor retardation and impaired memory. There is no diagnostic test for HIV-associated dementia. CT or magnetic resonance imaging (MRI) shows diffuse cerebral atrophy out of keeping with age. It is important to exclude depression, cryptococcal meningitis and neurosyphilis. ART usually improves HIV-associated dementia, but milder forms of HAND often persist.

Progressive multifocal leucoencephalopathy

Progressive multifocal leucoencephalopathy (PML) is a progressive disease that presents with stroke-like episodes and cognitive impairment. Vision is often impaired due to involvement of the occipital cortex. PML is caused by the JC virus. A combination of characteristic appearances on MRI (Fig. 14.12) and detection of JC virus DNA in the cerebrospinal fluid (CSF) by PCR is diagnostic. No specific treatment exists and prognosis remains poor despite ART.

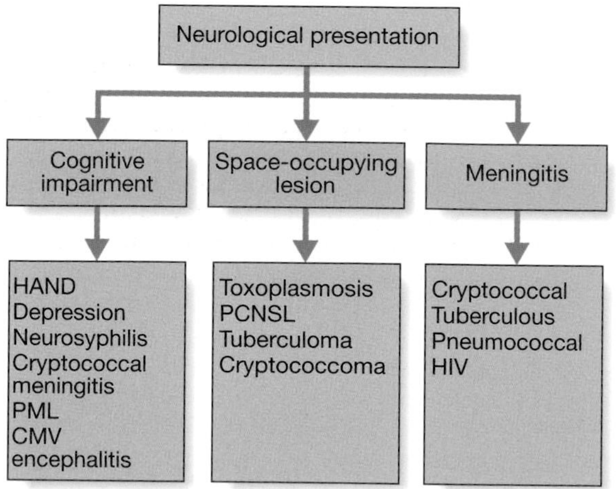

Fig. 14.11 Presentation and differential diagnosis of HIV-related neurological disorders. (CMV = cytomegalovirus; HAND = HIV-associated neurocognitive disorder; PCNSL = primary CNS lymphoma; PML = progressive multifocal leucoencephalopathy; TB = tuberculosis)

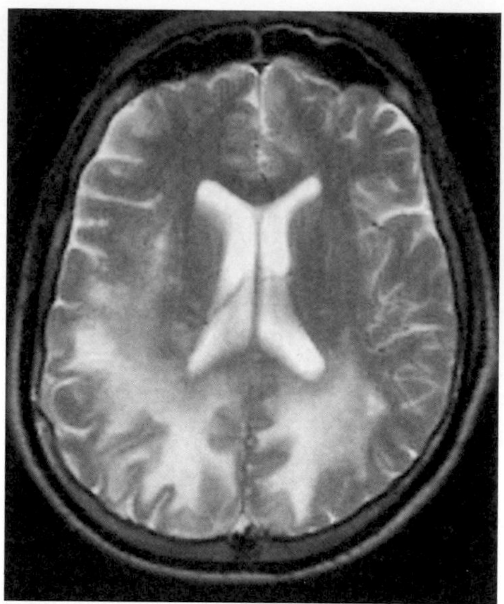

Fig. 14.12 Progressive multifocal leucoencephalopathy. Non-enhancing white-matter lesions without surrounding oedema are seen.

CMV encephalitis

This presents with behavioural disturbance, cognitive impairment and a reduced level of consciousness. Focal signs may also occur. Detection of CMV DNA in the CSF supports the diagnosis. Response to anti-CMV therapy is poor.

Space-occupying lesions

Space-occupying lesions in AIDS patients typically present over days to weeks. The most common cause is toxoplasmosis. As toxoplasmosis responds rapidly to therapy, a trial of anti-toxoplasmosis therapy should be given to all patients presenting with space-occupying lesions while the results of diagnostic tests are being awaited.

Cerebral toxoplasmosis

Cerebral toxoplasmosis is caused by reactivation of residual *Toxoplasma gondii* cysts from past infection, which results in the development of space-occupying lesions. The characteristic findings on imaging are multiple space-occupying lesions with ring enhancement on contrast and surrounding oedema (Fig. 14.13). *Toxoplasma* serology shows evidence of previous exposure (positive immunoglobulin (Ig)G antibodies). The standard therapy for toxoplasmosis is sulfadiazine with pyrimethamine, together with folinic acid, to reduce the risk of bone marrow suppression. However, co-trimoxazole has been shown to be as effective and less toxic, and is also more widely available. Response to a trial of therapy is usually diagnostic, with clinical improvement in 1–2 weeks and shrinkage of lesions on imaging in 2–4 weeks. Definitive diagnosis is by brain biopsy but this is seldom necessary.

Primary CNS lymphoma (PCNSL)

Primary CNS lymphomas (PCNSLs) are high-grade B-cell lymphomas associated with EBV infection. Characteristically, imaging demonstrates a single,

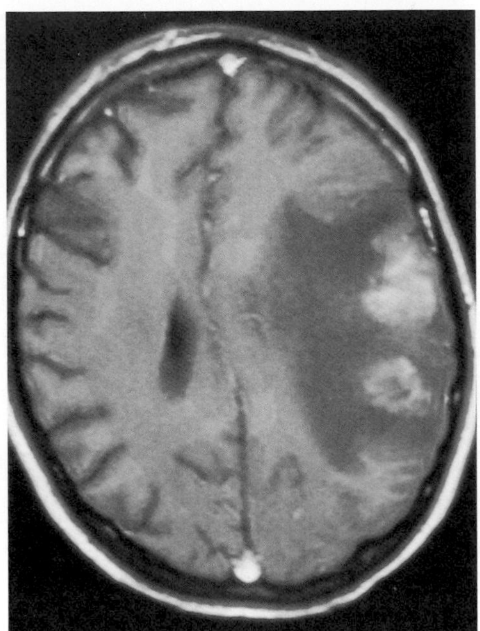

Fig. 14.13 Cerebral toxoplasmosis. Multiple ring-enhancing lesions with surrounding oedema are characteristic.

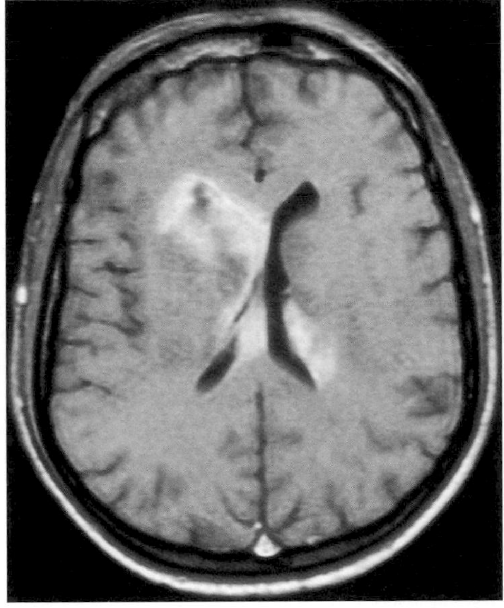

Fig. 14.14 Primary CNS lymphoma. A single enhancing periventricular lesion with moderate oedema is typical.

homogeneously enhancing, periventricular lesion with surrounding oedema (Fig. 14.14). If it is considered safe to perform a lumbar puncture, PCR for EBV DNA in the CSF has a high sensitivity and specificity for PCNSL. Brain biopsy is definitive, but carries a risk of morbidity and may be non-diagnostic in up to one-third. The prognosis is very poor.

Tuberculoma

Lesions resemble toxoplasmosis on imaging, except that oedema tends to be less marked and single lesions occur more commonly. There may be evidence of tuberculosis elsewhere. The CSF may show features consistent with tuberculous meningitis. Response to antituberculosis therapy is slow and paradoxical expansion of lesions despite therapy is not uncommon.

Stroke

There is a higher incidence of stroke in patients with HIV disease. Atherosclerosis is accelerated by HIV-associated inflammation and by some antiretroviral drugs. HIV vasculopathy with occlusion can cause a stroke. The aetiology is thought to be a vasculitis. It is important to exclude tuberculous meningitis and meningovascular syphilis in all patients who present with a stroke.

Meningitis

Cryptococcal meningitis

Cryptococcus neoformans is the most common cause of meningitis in AIDS patients. Patients usually present subacutely with headache, vomiting and mild confusion. Neck stiffness is present in less than half. CSF pleocytosis is often mild or even absent, and protein and glucose concentrations are variable. It is important to request CSF cryptococcal antigen tests in all HIV-infected patients undergoing lumbar puncture, as this test has a sensitivity and specificity of almost 100%. Treatment is with amphotericin B (plus flucytosine if available) for 2 weeks, followed by fluconazole. Raised intracranial pressure is common and should be treated with repeated therapeutic lumbar punctures, removing sufficient CSF to reduce pressure to less than 20 cmH_2O. (Most experts would be reluctant to withdraw more than 30 mL at a time.)

Tuberculous meningitis

The presentation and CSF findings of tuberculous meningitis are similar to those in HIV-uninfected patients (p. 1201), except that concomitant tuberculosis at other sites is more common in HIV infection.

Peripheral nerve disease

HIV infection causes axonal degeneration, resulting in a sensorimotor peripheral neuropathy in about one-third of AIDS patients. The incidence is increased with lower CD4 counts, older age and increased height. Sensory symptoms predominate. Treatment involves foot care, analgesia and analgesic adjuvants. ART has minimal effect on halting or reversing the process. The NRTIs stavudine and didanosine can cause drug-induced peripheral neuropathy, which is typically more painful and more rapidly progressive than HIV neuropathy. It may remit if the offending drug is withdrawn early.

Acute inflammatory demyelinating polyneuropathy is an uncommon manifestation, usually occurring in primary infection. It resembles Guillain–Barré syndrome (p. 1224), except that CSF pleocytosis is more prominent. Mononeuritis may also occur, commonly involving the facial nerve.

Myelopathy and radiculopathy

Globally, the most common cause of myelopathy in HIV infection is cord compression from tuberculous spondylitis. Vacuolar myelopathy is seen in advanced disease and is due to HIV. It presents with a slowly progressive paraparesis with no sensory level. MRI of the spine is normal, but is an important investigation to exclude other causes. Most patients have concomitant HIV-associated dementia.

CMV polyradiculitis presents with painful legs, progressive flaccid paraparesis, saddle anaesthesia, absent reflexes and sphincter dysfunction. CSF shows a neutrophil pleocytosis (which is unusual for a viral infection), and the detection of CMV DNA by PCR confirms the diagnosis. Despite treatment with ganciclovir or valganciclovir, functional recovery is poor.

Psychiatric disease

Significant psychiatric morbidity is very common and is a major risk factor for poor adherence. Reactive depression is the most common disorder. Diagnosis is often difficult, as many patients have concomitant HAND. Substance misuse is common in many groups of people at risk of HIV. Some forms of ART can cause psychiatric adverse effects and these are detailed on page 409.

Retinopathy

CMV retinitis presents with painless, progressive visual loss in patients with severe immune suppression. On fundoscopy the vitreous is clear. Haemorrhages and exudates are seen in the retina (p. 388), often with sheathing of vessels ('frosted branch angiitis'). The disease usually starts unilaterally, but progressive bilateral involvement occurs in most untreated patients. Diagnosis is usually clinical, but if there is doubt, demonstrating CMV DNA by PCR of vitreous fluid is diagnostic. Treatment with ganciclovir or valganciclovir stops progression of the disease, but vision does not recover. Some patients may develop immune recovery uveitis in response to ART, with intraocular inflammation, macular oedema and cataract formation that requires prompt treatment with oral and intraocular corticosteroids to prevent visual loss.

Three other conditions may mimic CMV retinitis. Like CMV, they all occur in patients with CD4 counts below 100 cells/mm^3. Ocular toxoplasmosis typically presents with a vitritis and retinitis without retinal haemorrhages. HIV retinopathy is a microangiopathy that causes cotton wool spots, which are not sight-threatening. Varicella zoster virus can cause rapidly progressive outer retinal necrosis.

Rheumatological disease

The immune dysregulation associated with HIV infection may result in autoantibody formation, usually in low titres. Mild arthralgias and a fibromyalgia-like syndrome are common in HIV-infected people.

Arthritis

HIV can cause a seronegative arthritis, which resembles rheumatoid arthritis. A more benign oligoarthritis may also occur. Reactive arthritis and Reiter's syndrome are more severe in HIV infection (Ch. 25).

Diffuse infiltrative lymphocytosis syndrome

Diffuse infiltrative lymphocytosis syndrome (DILS) is a benign disorder involving polyclonal CD8 lymphocytic

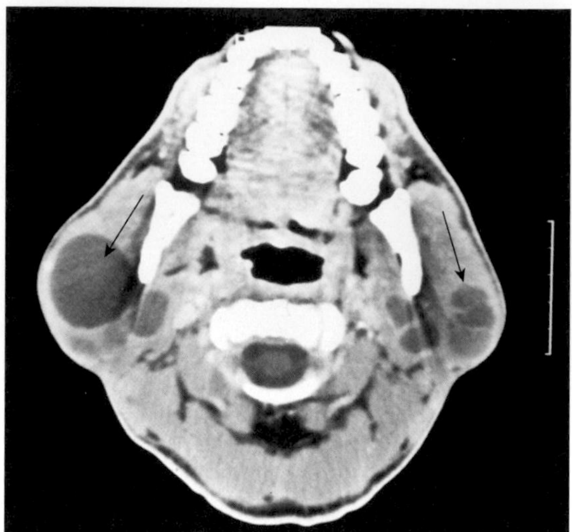

Fig. 14.15 CT scan of parotid glands showing multiple cysts (arrows) in a patient with the diffuse infiltrative lymphocytosis syndrome.

infiltration of tissues, which has some features in common with Sjögren's syndrome (p. 1114). It is linked to human leucocyte antigen (HLA)-DRB1. Most patients have a CD8 lymphocytosis. DILS usually presents in patients with mild immune suppression. The most common manifestation is bilateral parotid gland enlargement; the glands are often massive, with lymphoepithelial cysts on histology (Fig. 14.15). Other salivary glands may also be enlarged. Sicca symptoms are common but usually mild. Lymphocytic interstitial pneumonitis is the most common manifestation outside the salivary glands. Generalised lymphadenopathy with nodes, larger than those seen with persistent generalised lymphadenopathy of HIV, may occur. Hepatitis, mononeuritis, polyarthritis and polymyositis may also occur. The manifestations outside the salivary glands usually respond to steroids. The parotid glands are treated for cosmetic reasons but surgery is best avoided. Aspiration of parotid cysts and instillation of a sclerosant are of some benefit. Low-dose irradiation has also been used successfully. DILS may regress on ART but response is variable.

Haematological abnormalities

Disorders of all three major cell lines may occur in HIV. In advanced disease, haematopoiesis is impaired due to the direct effect of HIV and by cytokines. Pancytopenia may occur as a consequence of HIV but it is important to exclude a disorder infiltrating the bone marrow, such as mycobacterial or fungal infections, or lymphoma.

Anaemia

Normochromic, normocytic anaemia is very common in advanced HIV disease. Opportunistic diseases may cause anaemia of chronic disease (e.g. tuberculosis) or marrow infiltration (e.g. MAC, tuberculosis, lymphoma, fungi). Anaemia is a common adverse effect of zidovudine, which also causes a macrocytosis. Red cell aplasia is rare and may be caused either by parvovirus B19 infection or by lamivudine.

Neutropenia

Isolated neutropenia is occasionally due to HIV but is nearly always caused by drug toxicity (e.g. zidovudine, co-trimoxazole, ganciclovir).

Thrombocytopenia

Mild thrombocytopenia is common in HIV-infected people. The most common disorder causing severe thrombocytopenia is immune-mediated platelet destruction resembling idiopathic thrombocytopenic purpura (p. 1050). This responds to steroids or intravenous immunoglobulin, together with ART. Splenectomy should be avoided if possible because it further increases the risk of infection with encapsulated bacteria. Severe thrombocytopenia with a microangiopathic anaemia also occurs in a thrombotic thrombocytopenic purpura-like illness (p. 1056), which seems to have a better prognosis than the classical disease. Transient thrombocytopenia is common in primary infection.

Renal disease

Acute renal failure is common, usually due to acute infection or nephrotoxicity of drugs (e.g. tenofovir, p. 481), amphotericin B). HIV-associated nephropathy (HIVAN) is the most important cause of chronic renal failure and is seen most frequently in patients of African descent and those with low CD4 counts. Progression to end-stage renal failure is more rapid than with most other causes of chronic renal failure, and renal size may be preserved even when it is severe. HIVAN usually presents with nephrotic syndrome, chronic renal failure or a combination of both. ART has some effect in slowing progression of HIVAN. Other important HIV-associated renal diseases include HIV immune complex kidney diseases and thrombotic microangiopathy. With the overall improvement in life expectancy from ART, conditions such as diabetes mellitus, hypertension and vascular disease add to the burden of chronic kidney disease. Outcomes of renal transplantation are good in patients on ART.

Cardiac disease

HIV-associated cardiomyopathy resembles idiopathic dilated cardiomyopathy (p. 636) but progresses more rapidly. ART may improve cardiac failure but does not reverse established cardiomyopathy. Pericardial disease due to opportunistic diseases is not uncommon. Globally, the most common cause is tuberculous pericardial effusions. Tuberculous constrictive pericarditis is less common than in HIV-uninfected people. Kaposi's sarcoma and lymphoma may cause pericardial effusions. Septic pericarditis, usually due to *S. pneumoniae*, is uncommon.

HIV is associated with an increased risk of myocardial infarction due to accelerated atherogenesis caused by the inflammatory state. Certain protease inhibitors (p. 407) that cause dyslipidaemia have been associated with an increased risk of myocardial infarction.

14.13 Approximate incidence ratio of virus-related cancers compared to the general population

Viral cancers	Incidence ratio
Human herpesvirus 8-related	
Kaposi's sarcoma	3600
Epstein–Barr virus-related	
Non-Hodgkin lymphoma	80
Hodgkin lymphoma	10
Human papillomavirus-related	
Cervical cancer	6
Vulval cancer	6
Anal cancer	30
Penile cancer	4
Hepatitis B/C virus-related	
Hepatoma	5

HIV-related cancers

The AIDS-defining cancers are Kaposi's sarcoma (see above), cervical cancer and non-Hodgkin lymphoma (NHL – p. 1043). NHL may occur at any CD4 count but is more commonly seen below 200 cells/mm^3. Almost all NHL are B-cell tumours and most are stage 4 when the patient presents. Long-term remission rates of about 50% can be achieved with NHL in AIDS patients using ART and chemotherapy (including the anti-B-cell monoclonal antibody rituximab if it is a B-cell tumour).

The incidence of a number of other cancers induced by viruses is also increased in HIV-infected people (Box 14.13). Regular cytological examination of the cervix, and of the anus in people who practise anal sex, should be performed to detect pre-malignant lesions, which are easier to treat. In general, the incidence of cancers that are not induced by viruses is similar to that in the general population.

PREVENTION OF OPPORTUNISTIC INFECTIONS

The best way to prevent opportunistic infections is to improve the CD4 count with ART. However, infections continue to occur in the ART era; CD4 counts take time to improve if ART is initiated in patients with profound immune suppression, immune reconstitution on ART is often suboptimal, and CD4 counts may decline because antiretroviral resistance develops.

Preventing exposure

The best method for avoiding infection is to prevent exposure to the infectious agent. However, this is only possible for a few opportunistic infections. The pathogenesis of several of these is thought to be reactivation of latent/dormant infection after prior exposure – examples include herpes simplex virus, zoster, CMV and toxoplasmosis. Preventing exposure to some of these infections is thus only of benefit if exposure has not already occurred.

Safe water and food

Cryptosporidiosis, microsporidiosis and isosporiasis may be water-borne. If there is no access to safe water, then water should be boiled before drinking. Food-borne illnesses are also important in HIV infection, notably *Salmonella* species. *Toxoplasma* exposure is related to eating raw or undercooked meat. People living with HIV infection need to be informed about food hygiene and the importance of adequately cooked meat.

Tuberculosis

Preventing exposure to tuberculosis is important when there is an infectious case in the household, in clinics and in hospitals. Adequate ventilation, masks and safe coughing procedures reduce the risk of exposure.

Malaria vector control

All HIV-infected individuals living in malarious areas should practise vector control, as malaria occurs more frequently and is more severe in HIV-infected people. The most cost-effective way to achieve this is by using insecticide-impregnated bed nets. Other modalities of vector control that are of benefit to the community, such as reducing standing water and spraying with residual insecticides and larvicides, should also be implemented.

Safer sex

HIV-infected individuals should practise safer sex in order to reduce the transmission of HIV. Even if their partners are HIV-infected, condoms should be used, as HIV mutants that are more virulent or have developed antiretroviral drug resistance can be transmitted. Safer sex will also lower the risk of acquiring herpes simplex virus and human herpesvirus 8.

Pets

Toxoplasma gondii can be acquired from kittens or cat litter, and people living with HIV infection should avoid handling either. Cryptosporidiosis can be transmitted from animals, and patients should be advised to wash their hands after handling animals.

Chemoprophylaxis

Chemoprophylaxis is the use of antimicrobial agents to prevent infections. Primary prophylaxis is used to prevent opportunistic infections that have not yet occurred. Secondary prophylaxis is used to prevent recurrence of opportunistic infections because many may recur after an initial response to therapy. Secondary prophylaxis (Box 14.14) can be discontinued when ART results in immune reconstitution, with CD4 counts increasing to over 200 cells/mm^3, but for CMV and MAC, prophylaxis can be stopped if CD4 counts increase to more than 100 cells/mm^3.

14.14 Secondary prophylaxis of opportunistic infections

Infection	Drug regimen
Pneumocystis jirovecii pneumonia	Co-trimoxazole 960 mg daily
Toxoplasmosis	Co-trimoxazole 960 mg daily
Cryptococcosis	Fluconazole 200 mg daily
Cytomegalovirus infection	Valganciclovir 900 mg daily
Mycobacterium avium complex	Clarithromycin 500 mg twice daily + Ethambutol 800 mg daily
Isospora belli infection	Co-trimoxazole 960 mg daily

14.15 Opportunistic infections reduced by co-trimoxazole

- *Pneumocystis jirovecii* pneumonia
- Cerebral toxoplasmosis
- Bacterial pneumonia
- Bacteraemia
- Isosporiasis
- Malaria

Co-trimoxazole primary prophylaxis

Co-trimoxazole reduces the incidence of a number of opportunistic infections (Box 14.15), as well as hospitalisation and mortality rates. The indications for initiating co-trimoxazole are either clinical evidence of immune suppression (WHO clinical stages 3 or 4) or laboratory evidence of immune suppression (CD4 count below 200 cells/mm^3). In low-income countries, there is considerable morbidity from infectious diseases (including malaria) in earlier HIV disease, and the WHO recommends initiating co-trimoxazole at a CD4 count of less than 350 cells/mm^3, or at WHO stages 2–4. The recommended dose of co-trimoxazole is 960 mg daily, but trials have shown that half this dose is as effective and may be associated with less toxicity. Co-trimoxazole prophylaxis can be discontinued when CD4 counts increase to more than 200 cells/mm^3 on ART.

Co-trimoxazole prophylaxis is well tolerated. The most common side-effect is hypersensitivity, causing a maculo-papular rash. If therapy is discontinued, desensitisation or rechallenge under antihistamine cover should be attempted, unless the rash was accompanied by systemic symptoms or mucosal involvement. Prophylactic doses of co-trimoxazole can also cause neutropenia, but this is very uncommon and routine monitoring of blood counts is not necessary. If co-trimoxazole cannot be tolerated, then dapsone 100 mg daily should be substituted. Dapsone is equally effective at reducing the incidence of *P. jirovecii* pneumonia, but has little or no effect on reducing the other opportunistic infections prevented by co-trimoxazole.

Isoniazid preventive therapy

Isoniazid preventive therapy (IPT) has been shown to reduce the risk of tuberculosis only in HIV-infected patients with a positive tuberculin skin test, which should be done in all patients at baseline. There is no CD4 count or clinical threshold for starting or stopping IPT. In HIV infection, induration of 5 mm or more on a Mantoux test is regarded as positive. It is important to rule out active tuberculosis before starting IPT, and symptom screening has been shown to be adequate to achieve this (Box 14.16). The usual duration of IPT is

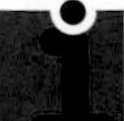

14.16 Symptom screen for tuberculosis before isoniazid preventive therapy

All of the following must be absent:

- Active cough
- Weight loss
- Night sweats
- Fever

EBM 14.17 Duration of isoniazid preventive therapy

'Thirty-six months' isoniazid prophylaxis was more effective for prevention of tuberculosis than 6-month prophylaxis in individuals with HIV infection, and chiefly benefited those who were tuberculin skin test-positive.'

- Samandari T, et al. Lancet 2011; 377:1588–1598.

6 months but this does not provide long-term reduction in the risk of tuberculosis. Continuation for 36 months has been shown to be much more effective (Box 14.17).

Mycobacterium avium complex

In high-income countries, a macrolide (azithromycin or clarithromycin) is recommended to prevent MAC in patients with a CD4 count below 50 cells/mm^3. This can be discontinued once the CD4 count has risen to over 100 cells/mm^3 on ART.

Immunisation

There are significant problems associated with vaccination in HIV infection. First, vaccination with live organisms is contraindicated in patients with severe immune suppression, as this may result in disease from the attenuated organisms. Second, immune responses to vaccination are impaired in HIV-infected patients. If the CD4 count is below 200 cells/mm^3, then immune responses to immunisation are very poor. Therefore it is preferable to wait until the CD4 count has increased to more than 200 cells/mm^3 on ART before immunisation is given. All patients should be given a conjugate pneumococcal vaccine (not the polysaccharide vaccine, which has been shown to be harmful) and annual influenza vaccination. Hepatitis B vaccination should be given to those who are not immune.

ANTIRETROVIRAL THERAPY

ART that is capable of suppressing viral replication has been available since 1996. ART has transformed HIV from a progressive illness with a fatal outcome into a chronic manageable disease (Box 14.18).

The goals of ART are to:

- reduce the viral load to an undetectable level for as long as possible
- improve the CD4 count to over 200 cells/mm^3 so that severe HIV-related disease is unlikely
- improve the quantity and quality of life without unacceptable drug toxicity
- reduce HIV transmission.

EBM 14.18 Life expectancy on ART

'A mathematical model predicted that people with HIV who can access ART will have life expectancy shortened by only 7 or 10.5 years, depending on whether ART is started early (CD4 count 432) or late (CD4 count 140) respectively.'

- Nakagawa F, et al. AIDS 2012; 26:335–343.

14.19 Commonly used antiretroviral drugs

Classes	Drugs
Nucleoside reverse transcriptase inhibitors (NRTIs)	Abacavir, emtricitabine, lamivudine, tenofovir, zidovudine
Non-nucleoside reverse transcriptase inhibitors (NNRTIs)	Efavirenz, nevirapine, etravirine
Protease inhibitors (PIs)	Atazanavir, darunavir, lopinavir
Integrase inhibitors	Raltegravir
Chemokine receptor inhibitor	Maraviroc

Many of the antiretroviral drugs which were used initially have been largely abandoned because of toxicity or poor efficacy. The drugs that are currently most commonly used are shown in Box 14.19, and their targets in the HIV life cycle in Figure 14.2 (p. 392).

Selecting antiretroviral regimens

The standard combination antiretroviral regimens are two NRTIs together with an NNRTI, protease inhibitor (PI) or integrase inhibitor. Dual NRTI combinations are usually emtricitabine or lamivudine (they are closely related and so are never combined) together with one of abacavir, tenofovir or zidovudine. It is possible to construct effective regimens without NRTIs if there is intolerance or resistance to the NRTIs. Currently used PIs should always be administered with ritonavir, which itself is a PI that is toxic in therapeutic doses. Low doses of ritonavir dramatically increase the concentrations and elimination half-lives of other PIs by inhibiting their metabolism by cytochrome P450. This increases drug exposure, thereby prolonging the PI's half-life, allowing reduction in pill burden and dosing frequency, and so optimising adherence.

Most guidelines from high-income countries allow clinicians to choose a starting regimen of dual NRTIs combined with an NNRTI, or a PI or an integrase inhibitor, as these three regimens have similar efficacy. Subsequent ART regimen switches for virological failure are guided by the results of resistance testing (p. 408). For low- and middle-income countries, the WHO recommends a public health approach to using ART with standardised first-line (NNRTI plus dual NRTIs) and second-line (ritonavir-boosted PI plus dual NRTIs) regimens. NNRTIs are preferred by the WHO in first-line regimens, as they are cheaper than PIs and better tolerated. Furthermore, NNRTIs need to be given with two fully active NRTIs because they have a low genetic barrier to resistance (see below), whereas PI-containing regimens are effective even when there are some mutations conferring resistance to the NRTIs. Therefore PIs in second-line regimens are preferable in settings where resistance testing is unavailable. The public health approach to using ART can be implemented by nurses and has been successfully implemented in resource-poor settings.

Criteria for starting ART

The 2010 WHO guidelines recommend starting ART in adults with either a CD4 count below 350 cells/mm^3 or clinical stage 3–4. Other international guidelines are very similar, but criteria are updated regularly and it is likely that starting ART at higher CD4 counts will be recommended in the near future. HIV-infected partners in serodiscordant couples should commence ART irrespective of their CD4 count or clinical stage to reduce the risk of transmission to the uninfected partner (Box 14.20). Other categories of patients who should start ART earlier include those with chronic liver disease from viral hepatitis, non-AIDS malignancies, and conditions requiring long-term immunosuppressant therapy.

It is seldom necessary to start ART urgently. Several consultations are required to give patients insight into the need for life-long ART, to stress the importance of adherence, and to formulate a personal treatment plan. Disclosure of HIV status, joining support groups and using patient-nominated treatment supporters should be encouraged, as these have been shown to improve adherence. Management of depression and substance abuse is also important.

EBM 14.20 When should ART be started?

'In serodiscordant couples, early initiation of ART reduced rates of sexual transmission of HIV-1 by 96%, and led to a 41% reduction in the combined end point of major clinical events or death.'

- Cohen MS, et al. N Engl J Med 2011; 365:493–505.

Monitoring efficacy

The most important measure of ART efficacy is the viral load. A baseline viral load should be measured prior to initiating treatment. The viral load should be repeated 4–8 weeks after starting a new ART regimen when the count should show at least a tenfold decrease. Thereafter it should be checked every 3–6 months. After 6 months of ART, the viral load should be suppressed, defined as below the limit of detection of the assay (usually less than 50 copies/mL), and this is achieved in 80–90% of patients. Failure of ART is defined by the viral load becoming detectable after suppression. (In most guidelines a threshold is used – typically more than 400 or more than 1000 copies/mL.) Adherence support should be enhanced if virological failure is detected, and the viral load repeated to confirm failure before switching to a new ART regimen.

CD4 counts are generally monitored every 3–6 months together with the viral load. Typically, the CD4 count increases rapidly in the first month, followed by a more gradual increase. In the first year, the count typically increases by 100–150 cells/mm^3, and about 80 cells/mm^3 per annum thereafter until the reference range is reached, provided the viral load is suppressed. If ART is stopped, the CD4 count rapidly falls to the baseline value before ART was commenced. For countries where viral load monitoring is unavailable, the WHO has defined immunological failure as a fall in CD4 count to baseline, or a 50% fall from peak on ART, or persistent count below 100 cells/mm^3. However, CD4 responses are highly variable: in about 15–30% of patients the CD4 count does not increase despite virological suppression, and in a similar proportion of patients the CD4 response is good despite the presence of virological failure. Therefore it is not surprising that both unnecessary switches to second-line ART and continuation of failing first-line ART regimens (which will increase the number of resistance mutations) are common in settings where viral load monitoring is not available.

Antiretroviral resistance

Reverse transcription is error-prone, generating a large number of mutations. If the viral load is suppressed on ART, viral replication is suppressed and resistance mutations will not be selected. If ART is taken and there is ongoing replication, due to either resistant mutations or suboptimal adherence, mutations conferring resistance to antiretroviral drugs will be selected. Antiretroviral drugs differ in their ability to select for resistant mutations. Some drugs (e.g. emtricitabine, lamivudine, efavirenz, nevirapine) have a low genetic barrier to resistance, rapidly selecting for a single mutation conferring high-level resistance. PIs and some NRTIs (e.g. zidovudine) select for resistance mutations slowly, and multiple resistant mutations often need to accumulate before the drug's efficacy is lost. Patients who develop antiretroviral resistance may transmit resistant virus to others and will eventually develop clinical failure.

Antiretroviral resistance is assessed by sequencing the relevant viral genes to detect mutations that are known to confer resistance. The resistant proviral DNA is archived in latent CD4 cells and will re-emerge rapidly on exposure to the antiretroviral. The patient must therefore be taking ART when the test is performed, as otherwise the wild-type virus will predominate and resistant mutations will not be detected. In regions where resistance testing is affordable, it is recommended at baseline (to detect primary resistance) and at every confirmed virological failure, in order to select the most appropriate antiretrovirals in a new regimen.

ART complications

Immune reconstitution inflammatory syndrome

Immune reconstitution inflammatory syndrome (IRIS) is a common (15–20%) early complication of ART, especially in patients who start it with CD4 counts below 50 cells/mm^3. IRIS presents either with paradoxical deterioration of an existing opportunistic disease (including infections that are responding to appropriate therapy) or with the unmasking of a new infection. The clinical presentation of IRIS events is often characterised by an exaggerated immune response, with pronounced inflammatory features. For example, patients with CMV retinitis developing IRIS on ART develop a uveitis; and inflammatory haloes occur around KS lesions. Paradoxical tuberculosis IRIS events are common and it is important to exclude multidrug resistance, which could be responsible for the deterioration. IRIS is associated with a mortality of around 5%, but this is higher when it complicates CNS infections.

The management of IRIS is to continue ART and to ensure that the opportunistic disease is adequately treated. Symptomatic treatments are helpful. Corticosteroids are often used for more severe IRIS manifestations, but they should not be given to patients with KS, as this can result in rapid progression of KS lesions.

Lipodystrophy

Long-term use of ART may cause changes in body fat distribution. This can present either with fat accumulation (e.g. visceral fat, breast enlargement, 'buffalo hump') or with subcutaneous fat loss ('lipoatrophy' – Fig 14.16) or with both fat loss and accumulation. The thymidine analogue NRTIs (stavudine and, to a lesser extent, zidovudine) are associated with fat loss. Switching to the non-thymidine NRTIs abacavir or tenofovir will result in very gradual improvement of lipoatrophy.

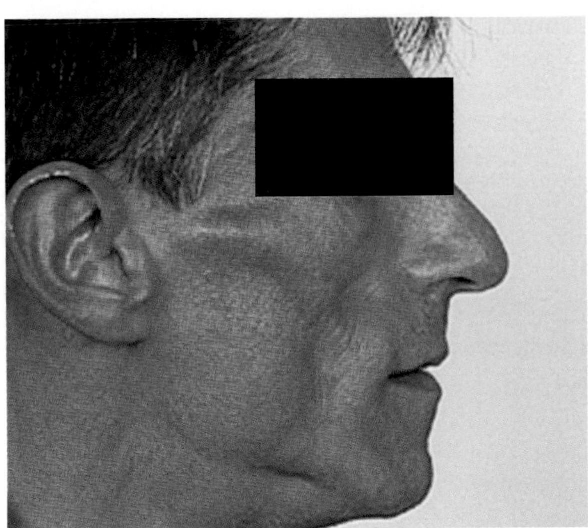

Fig. 14.16 Fat loss complicating long-term use of the thymidine analogue NRTIs stavudine and zidovudine.

Previously, PIs were thought to be the cause of fat accumulation. However, recent studies have shown that all classes of antiretrovirals are associated with fat gain to the same extent. Furthermore, longitudinal studies comparing HIV-uninfected people with HIV-infected people on long-term ART show that the extent and distribution of fat gain are similar. These data suggest that fat gain is a consequence of treating HIV rather than a side-effect of ART.

Rashes

These are common but must be differentiated from the other causes described above. The NRTI abacavir typically causes a systemic hypersensitivity reaction, which is HLA-associated. HLA-B*5701 has a 100% negative predictive value for abacavir hypersensitivity. HLA testing should be done before abacavir is given and the drug should not be prescribed for people who are HLA-B*5701-positive. This is rare in people of African descent. Rechallenge must never be attempted after abacavir hypersensitivity, as fatal reactions may occur.

Drug rashes are very common with NNRTIs. When the NNRTI rash is mild and not accompanied by systemic involvement, the suspected drug is often continued and antihistamines are administered. The rash usually resolves. If it worsens or if systemic features develop, the NNRTI should be discontinued.

Other adverse effects

The NNRTI efavirenz causes insomnia, agitation, euphoria or dysphoria in many patients, but tolerance to its neuropsychiatric effects develops in a few weeks in most. The NRTI zidovudine can cause anaemia and neutropenia, and tenofovir may cause nephrotoxicity. PIs are associated with dyslipidaemias and may increase the risk of myocardial infarction.

ART in special situations

Pregnancy

All pregnant women should routinely be recommended for HIV testing at an early stage in pregnancy, with rapid tests for those presenting in or just after labour. The CD4 count falls by about 25% during pregnancy due to haemodilution. The course of HIV disease progression is not altered by pregnancy. Pre-ART, the rate of mother-to-child transmission was 15–40%, with rates being influenced by several factors (see Box 14.3, p. 391).

ART has dramatically reduced the risk of mother-to-child transmission of HIV to less than 1%. All pregnant women who qualify for ART for their own health should start treatment at the beginning of the second trimester. If they have severe disease, they should start ART in the first trimester. Two ART strategies are currently used to prevent mother-to-child transmission for women who do not yet require ongoing ART: commence standard ART and discontinue at delivery or after weaning; or zidovudine monotherapy, usually started at 28 weeks, augmented with single-dose nevirapine at delivery. The latter approach is widely used in low- and middle-income countries. A randomised controlled trial is under way in order to assess which strategy is more effective.

Caesarean section is associated with a lower risk of mother-to-child transmission than vaginal delivery, but the mode of delivery does not affect transmission risk if the viral load is suppressed on ART.

HIV is also transmitted by breastfeeding. In high-income countries, exclusive formula feeding is generally recommended. However in resource-poor settings, formula feeding is associated with a risk of infant morbidity and mortality, which may negate the benefit of not transmitting HIV to the infant. Furthermore, providing antiretrovirals to the infant (usually nevirapine monotherapy) while they are breastfeeding has been shown to reduce the risk of transmission. Therefore breastfeeding is now encouraged in resource-poor settings. Infants should be exclusively breastfed for the first

6 months, as mixed feeding (with formula or solids) is associated with a higher risk of transmission.

Diagnosis of HIV in infancy requires the detection of HIV RNA by PCR as maternal antibodies to HIV, which persist for up to 15 months, will give a false-positive result on antibody assays. PCR should ideally be carried out within 6 weeks of birth to facilitate early ART initiation, which is recommended for all infants irrespective of their CD4 percentage or clinical stage. If the baby is breastfed, the PCR should be repeated 2 weeks after weaning.

Post-exposure prophylaxis

Post-exposure prophylaxis (PEP) is recommended when the risk is deemed to be significant after a careful risk assessment, in both occupational and non-occupational settings. The first dose should be given as soon as possible, preferably within 6–8 hours. There is no point in starting PEP after 72 hours. Most guidelines recommend dual NRTIs for low-risk exposures, with the addition of either a PI or efavirenz in high-risk exposures (see Boxes 14.2 and 14.3, p. 391). Tenofovir together with emtricitabine is the most widely used dual NRTI combination, as it is well tolerated and well studied in pre-exposure prophylaxis trials. PEP should not be given if the exposed person is HIV-infected. HIV antibody testing should be performed at 6, 12 and 24 weeks after exposure.

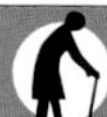

14.21 HIV infection in old age

- **Epidemiology**: the HIV-infected population is ageing due to the life-prolonging effects of ART.
- **Immunity**: age-related decline increases the risk of infections. CD4 counts decline more rapidly as age increases over 40 years, resulting in faster disease progression. CD4 responses to ART decrease with increasing age.
- **Dementia**: HIV causes cerebral atrophy and neurocognitive disorders; therefore dementia is more common and more severe than in the HIV-uninfected elderly.
- **Vascular disease**: HIV is associated with an increased risk, exacerbated by some antiretrovirals that increase the risk of vascular disease by causing dyslipidaemia or insulin resistance.
- **Polypharmacy**: treating co-morbidities is complex due to the many drug interactions with antiretrovirals.

Prevention of HIV

An effective HIV vaccine remains elusive due to the extensive genetic diversity of HIV and the lack of a safe attenuated virus. Measures for the prevention of HIV transmission are shown in Box 14.22.

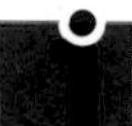

14.22 Prevention measures for HIV transmission

Sexual

- Sex education programmes in schools
- Easily accessible voluntary counselling and testing centres
- Promotion of safer sex practices (delaying sexual debut, condom use, fewer sexual partners)
- Effective ART treatment of HIV-infected individuals
- Pre-exposure prophylaxis for high-risk groups
- Male circumcision

Parenteral

- Blood product transmission: donor questionnaire, routine screening of donated blood
- Injection drug use: education, needle/syringe exchange, avoidance of 'shooting galleries', methadone maintenance programmes

Perinatal

- Routine 'opt-out' antenatal HIV antibody testing
- Measures to reduce vertical transmission (p. 409)

Occupational

- Education/training: universal precautions, needlestick injury avoidance
- Post-exposure prophylaxis

Further information

Websites with updated clinical guidelines

http://www.aidsinfo.nih.gov/guidelines/
http://www.bhiva.org/ClinicalGuidelines.aspx
http://www.who.int/hiv/pub/guidelines/en/

G.R. Scott

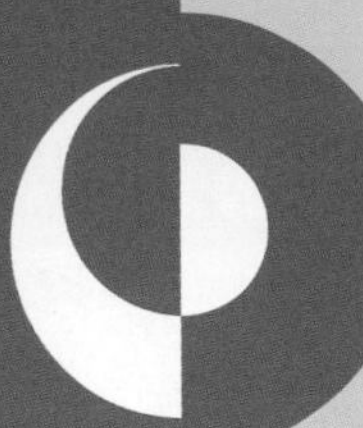

Sexually transmitted infections 15

Clinical examination in men 412

Clinical examination in women 413

Approach to patients with a suspected STI 414

Presenting problems in men 415

Urethral discharge 415
Genital itch and/or rash 415
Genital ulceration 415
Genital lumps 416
Proctitis in men who have sex with men 417

Presenting problems in women 417

Vaginal discharge 417
Lower abdominal pain 418
Genital ulceration 418
Genital lumps 418
Chronic vulval pain and/or itch 418

Prevention of STI 419

Sexually transmitted bacterial infections 419

Syphilis 419
Gonorrhoea 422
Chlamydial infection 423
Other sexually transmitted bacterial infections 423

Sexually transmitted viral infections 423

Genital herpes simplex 423
Human papillomavirus and anogenital warts 425
Molluscum contagiosum 426
Viral hepatitis 426

CLINICAL EXAMINATION IN MEN

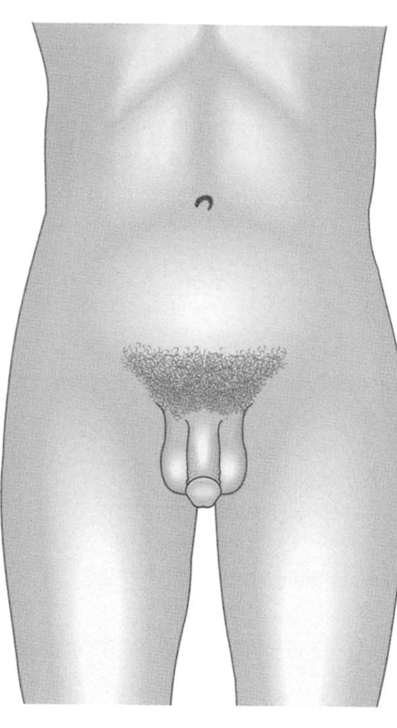

Observation

- Mouth
- Eyes
- Joints
- Skin:
  Rash of secondary syphilis
  Scabies
  Manifestations of HIV infection (Ch. 14)

1 Inguinal glands
Significant enlargement

2 Skin around groin and scrotum
Warts
Tinea cruris

3 Pubic area
Pthirus pubis (crab louse)

4 Scrotal contents
Abnormal masses or tenderness (epididymo-orchitis)

5 Skin of penis
(Retract prepuce if present)
Genital warts
Ulcers
Be aware of normal anatomical features such as coronal papillae, or prominent sebaceous or parafrenal glands

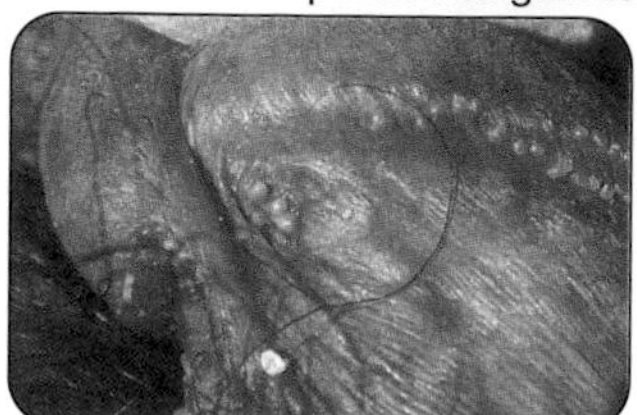

Coronal papillae ▲

6 Urethral meatus
▼ Discharge

7 Perianal area
(Men who have sex with men, and heterosexual men)
▼ Warts

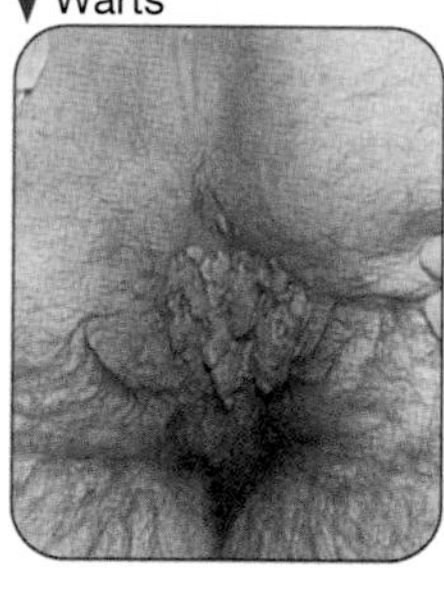

8 Rectum
(men who have sex with men practising receptive anal intercourse)

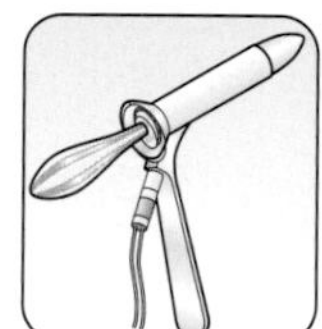

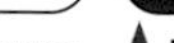

▲ Proctoscope

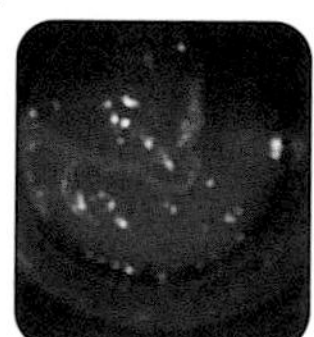

▲ Proctitis

Investigations for STIs in heterosexual males

- First void urine (FVU)* is the specimen of choice for the combined nucleic acid amplification test (NAAT) for gonorrhoea and chlamydia
- Alternatively, for gonorrhoea, a urethral swab plated directly on a selective medium such as modified New York City (MNYC), or sent in an appropriate transport medium, can be cultured to allow for assessment of antimicrobial sensitivities
- Serological test for syphilis (STS), e.g. enzyme immunoassay (EIA) for antitreponemal immunoglobulin (Ig) G antibody
- Human immunodeficiency virus (HIV) test (see note)

*A urethral swab can be submitted if the patient is unable to pass urine.

Investigations for STIs in men who have sex with men

- FVU,* and pharyngeal and rectal swabs for combined NAAT for gonorrhoea and chlamydia
- STS (repeat testing may be necessary in the event of negative test results in the first few weeks following exposure)
- Serological tests for hepatitis A/B (with a view to vaccination if seronegative)
- HIV test (see note)

*A urethral swab can be submitted if the patient is unable to pass urine.

HIV testing

It should always be standard practice to offer HIV testing as part of screening for STI (sexually transmitted infection) because the benefits of early diagnosis outweigh other considerations. Extensive pre-test counselling is not required in most instances, but it is important to establish efficient pathways for referral of patients at high risk for whom the clinician wishes specialist support, and for those diagnosed as HIV-positive.

CLINICAL EXAMINATION IN WOMEN

Labia majora and minora 4
Ulcers
Vulvitis
Warts ▼

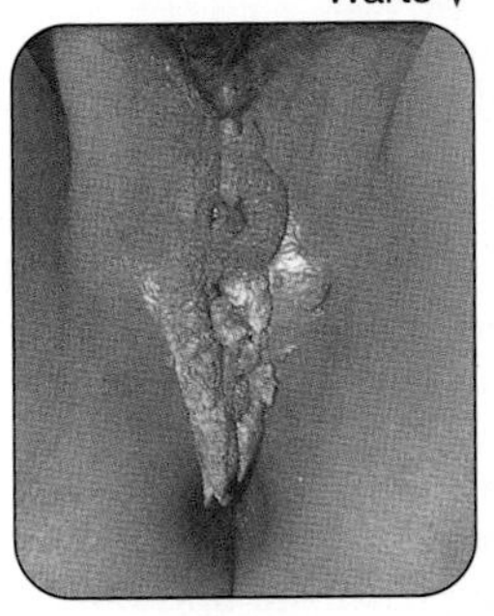

Pubic area 3
Pthirus pubis (crab louse) ▼

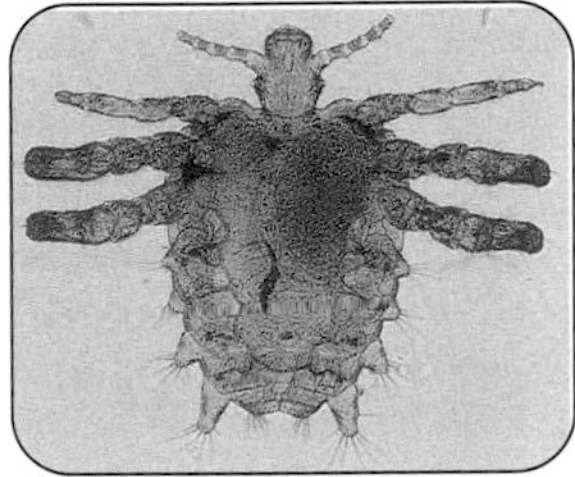

Inguinal glands 2
Significant enlargement

Abdomen 1
Abnormal masses or tenderness

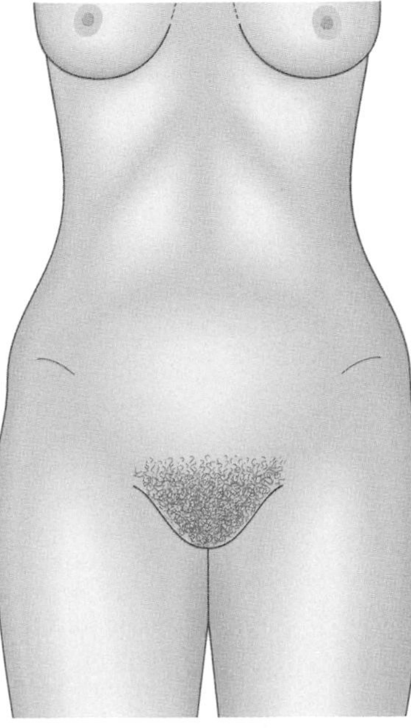

Observation
- Mouth
- Eyes
- Joints
- Skin:
  Rash of secondary syphilis
  Scabies
  Manifestations of HIV infection (Ch. 14)

5 **Perineum and perianal skin**
Warts
Ulcers

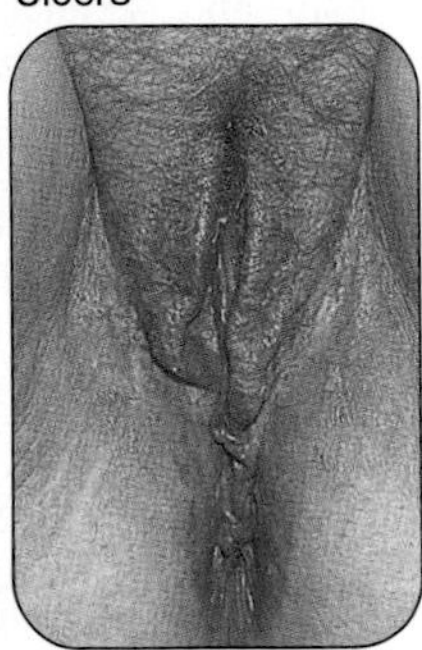

▲ Inflammation

6 **Vagina and cervix**
Abnormal discharge
Warts
Ulcers
Inflammation
In women with lower abdominal pain, bimanual examination for adnexal tenderness (pelvic inflammatory disease)

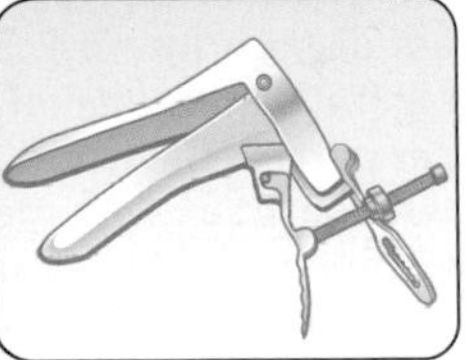

▲ Speculum

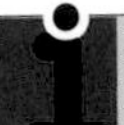

Investigations for STIs in women

- Clinician-obtained cervical or vaginal swab, or self-taken vaginal swab for combined NAAT for gonorrhoea and chlamydia
- Alternatively, for gonorrhoea, cervical and urethral swabs plated directly on a selective medium such as MNYC, or sent in appropriate transport medium, can be cultured to allow for assessment of antimicrobial sensitivities
- Wet mount for microscopy or high vaginal swab (HVS) for culture of *Trichomonas*
- STS, e.g. EIA for antitreponemal IgG antibody
- HIV test (see note)

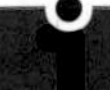

Management goals in suspected STI

- Relief of any symptoms
- Screening for treatable STI that may not be causing symptoms
- Tracing and treatment of sexual contacts who may also be infected
- Advice to reduce risk of infection in the future

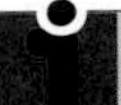

Those at particular risk from STIs*

- Sex workers, male and female
- Clients of sex workers
- Men who have sex with men
- Injecting drug users (sex for money or drugs) and their partners
- Frequent travellers

*Adapted from WHO/UNAIDS, 1997.

Insets on pp. 412–413 (*Perianal warts, coronal papillae, mucopus, inflammation*) – see p. 426.

Sexually transmitted infections (STIs) are a group of contagious conditions whose principal mode of transmission is by intimate sexual activity involving the moist mucous membranes of the penis, vulva, vagina, cervix, anus, rectum, mouth and pharynx, along with their adjacent skin surfaces. A wide range of infections may be sexually transmitted, including syphilis, gonorrhoea, human immunodeficiency virus (HIV), genital herpes, genital warts, chlamydia and trichomoniasis. Bacterial vaginosis and genital candidiasis are not regarded as STIs, although they are common causes of vaginal discharge in sexually active women. Chancroid, lymphogranuloma venereum (LGV) and granuloma inguinale are usually seen in tropical countries. Hepatitis viruses A, B, C and D (p. 948) may be acquired sexually, as well as by other routes.

The World Health Organization estimates that 448 million curable STIs (*Trichomonas vaginalis, Chlamydia trachomatis*, gonorrhoea and syphilis) occur world-wide each year. In the UK in 2010, the most common treatable STIs diagnosed were chlamydia (more than 200 000 cases) and gonorrhoea (19 000 cases). Genital warts are the second most common complaint seen in genito-urinary medicine (GUM) departments. In addition to causing morbidity themselves, STIs may increase the risk of transmitting or acquiring HIV infection (Ch. 14).

As coincident infection with more than one STI is seen frequently, GUM clinics routinely offer a full set of investigations at the patient's first visit (pp. 412–413), regardless of the reason for attendance. In other settings, less comprehensive investigation may be appropriate.

The extent of the examination largely reflects the likelihood of HIV infection or syphilis. Most heterosexuals in the UK are at such low risk of these infections that routine extragenital examination is unnecessary. This is not the case in parts of the world where HIV is endemic, or for men who have sex with men (MSM) in the UK. In other words, the extent of the examination is determined by the sexual history (Box 15.1).

APPROACH TO PATIENTS WITH A SUSPECTED STI

Patients concerned about the possible acquisition of an STI are often anxious. Staff must be friendly, sympathetic and reassuring; they should have the ability to put patients at ease, whilst emphasising that clinic attendance is confidential. The history focuses on genital symptoms, with reference to genital ulceration, rash, irritation, pain, swelling and urinary symptoms, especially dysuria. In men, the clinician should ask about urethral discharge, and in women, vaginal discharge, pelvic pain or dyspareunia. Enquiry about general health should include menstrual and obstetric history, cervical cytology, recent medication, especially with antimicrobial or antiviral agents, previous STI and allergy. Immunisation status for hepatitis A and B should be noted, as should information about recreational drug use and alcohol intake.

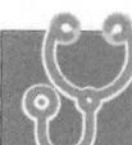

15.1 How to take a sexual history

- In your lifetime, have your sexual partners been male, female or both?
- Do you have a regular sexual partner at present?
- If yes:
  - How long have you been together?
  - When did you last have sex with anyone else?
- If no:
  - When did you last have sex?
  - Was this a regular or a casual partner?
- Do/did you use a condom?

A detailed sexual history is imperative (see Box 15.1), as this informs the clinician of the degree of risk for certain infections, as well as specific sites that should be sampled; for example, rectal samples should be taken from men who have had unprotected anal sex with other men. Sexual partners, whether male or female, and casual or regular, should be recorded. Sexual practices – insertive or receptive vaginal, anal, orogenital or oro-anal – should be noted, as should choice of contraception for women, and condom use for both sexes.

STI during pregnancy

Many STIs can be transmitted from mother to child in pregnancy, either transplacentally or during delivery. Possible outcomes are highlighted in Box 15.2.

STI in children

The presence of an STI in a child may be indicative of sexual abuse, although vertical transmission may explain some presentations in the first 2 years. In an older child and in adolescents, STI may be the result of voluntary

15.2 Possible outcomes of STI in pregnancy

Organism	Mode of transmission	Outcome for fetus/neonate	Outcome for mother
Treponema pallidum	Transplacental	Ranges from no effect to severe stigmata or miscarriage/stillbirth	None directly relating to the pregnancy
Neisseria gonorrhoeae	Intrapartum	Severe conjunctivitis	Possibility of ascending infection postpartum
Chlamydia trachomatis	Intrapartum	Conjunctivitis, pneumonia	Possibility of ascending infection postpartum
Herpes simplex	Usually intrapartum, but transplacental infection may occur rarely	Ranges from no effect to severe disseminated infection	Rarely, primary infection during 2nd/3rd trimesters becomes disseminated, with high maternal mortality
Human papillomaviruses	Intrapartum	Anogenital warts or laryngeal papillomas are very rare	Warts may become more florid during pregnancy, but usually regress postpartum

sexual activity. Specific issues regarding the management of STI and other infections in adolescence are discussed in Box 13.27 (p. 313).

PRESENTING PROBLEMS IN MEN

Urethral discharge

In the UK the most important causes of urethral discharge are gonorrhoea and chlamydia. In a significant minority of cases, tests for both of these infections are negative, a scenario often referred to as non-specific urethritis (NSU). Some of these cases may be caused by *Trichomonas vaginalis*, herpes simplex virus (HSV), mycoplasmas or ureaplasmas. A small minority seem not to have an infectious aetiology.

Gonococcal urethritis usually causes symptoms within 7 days of exposure. The discharge is typically profuse and purulent. Chlamydial urethritis has an incubation period of 1–4 weeks, and tends to result in milder symptoms than gonorrhoea; there is overlap, however, and microbiological confirmation should always be sought.

Investigations

A presumptive diagnosis of urethritis can be made from a Gram-stained smear of the urethral exudate (Fig. 15.1), which will demonstrate significant numbers of polymorphonuclear leucocytes (≥ 5 per high-power field). A working diagnosis of gonococcal urethritis is made if Gram-negative intracellular diplococci (GNDC) are seen; if no GNDC are seen, a label of NSU is applied.

If microscopy is not available, urine samples and/or swabs should be taken and empirical antimicrobials prescribed. A first-void urine (FVU) sample should be submitted for a combined nucleic acid amplification test (NAAT) for gonorrhoea and chlamydia; a urethral swab is an alternative if the patient cannot pass urine. When gonorrhoea is suspected, a urethral swab should be sent for culture and antimicrobial sensitivities of *Neisseria gonorrhoeae*. Tests for other potential causes of urethritis are not performed routinely.

A swab should also be taken from the pharynx because gonococcal infection here is not reliably eradicated by single-dose therapy. In MSM, swabs for gonorrhoea and chlamydia should be taken from the rectum.

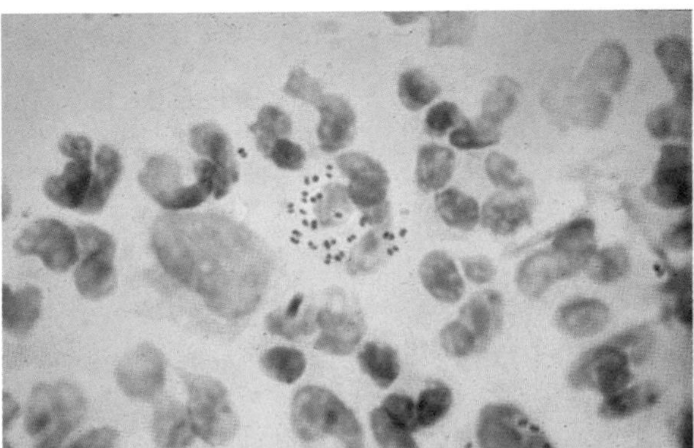

Fig. 15.1 A Gram-stained urethral smear from a man with gonococcal urethritis. Gram-negative diplococci are seen within polymorphonuclear leucocytes.

Management

This depends on local epidemiology and the availability of diagnostic resources. Treatment is often presumptive, with prescription of multiple antimicrobials to cover the possibility of gonorrhoea and/or chlamydia. This is likely to include a single-dose treatment for gonorrhoea, which is desirable because it eliminates the risk of non-adherence. The recommended agents for treating gonorrhoea vary according to local antimicrobial resistance patterns (p. 422). Appropriate treatment for chlamydia (p. 423) should also be prescribed because concurrent infection is present in up to 50% of men with gonorrhoea. Non-gonococcal, non-chlamydial urethritis is treated as for chlamydia.

Patients should be advised to avoid sexual contact until it is confirmed that any infection has resolved and, whenever possible, recent sexual contacts should be traced. The task of contact tracing – also called partner notification – is best performed by trained nurses based in GUM clinics; it is standard practice in the UK to treat current sexual partners of men with gonococcal or non-specific urethritis without waiting for microbiological confirmation.

If symptoms clear, a routine test of cure is not necessary, but patients should be re-interviewed to confirm that there was no immediate vomiting or diarrhoea after treatment, that there has been no risk of re-infection, and that traceable partners have sought medical advice.

Genital itch and/or rash

Patients may present with many combinations of penile/genital symptoms, which may be acute or chronic, and infectious or non-infectious. Box 15.3 provides a guide to diagnosis.

Balanitis refers to inflammation of the glans penis, often extending to the under-surface of the prepuce, in which case it is called balanoposthitis. Tight prepuce and poor hygiene may be aggravating factors. Candidiasis is sometimes associated with immune deficiency, diabetes mellitus, and the use of broad-spectrum antimicrobials, corticosteroids or antimitotic drugs. Local saline bathing is usually helpful, especially when no cause is found.

Genital ulceration

The most common cause of ulceration is genital herpes. Classically, multiple painful ulcers affect the glans, coronal sulcus or shaft of penis (Fig. 15.2), but solitary lesions occur rarely. Perianal ulcers may be seen in MSM. The diagnosis is made by gently scraping material from lesions and sending this in an appropriate transport medium for culture or detection of HSV DNA by polymerase chain reaction (PCR). Increasingly, laboratories will also test for *Treponema pallidum* by PCR.

In the UK, the possibility of syphilis or any other ulcerating STI is much less likely unless the patient is an MSM and/or has had a sexual partner from a region where tropical STIs are more common. The classic lesion

15.3 Differential diagnosis of genital itch and/or rash in men

Likely diagnosis	Acute or chronic	Itch	Pain	Discharge (non-urethral)	Specific characteristics	Diagnostic test	Treatment
Subclinical urethritis	Either	±	–	±	Often intermittent	Gram stain and urethral swabs	As for urethral discharge
Candidiasis	Acute	✓	–	White	Postcoital	Microscopy	Antifungal cream, e.g. clotrimazole
Anaerobic (erosive) balanitis	Acute	±	–	Yellow	Offensive	Microscopy	Saline bathing ± metronidazole
***Pthirus pubis* ('crab lice') infection**	Either	✓	–	–	Lice and nits seen attached to pubic hairs	Can be by microscopy, but usually visual	According to local policy – often permethrin
Lichen planus (p. 1289)	Either	±	–	–	Violaceous papules ± Wickham's striae	Clinical	None or mild topical corticosteroid, e.g. hydrocortisone
Lichen sclerosus	Chronic	±	–	–	Ivory-white plaques, scarring	Clinical or biopsy	Strong topical corticosteroid, e.g. clobetasol
Plasma cell balanitis of Zoon	Chronic	✓	–	±	Shiny, inflamed circumscribed areas	Clinical or biopsy	Strong topical corticosteroid, e.g. clobetasol
Dermatoses, e.g. eczema or psoriasis	Either	✓	–	–	Similar to lesions elsewhere on skin	Clinical	Mild topical corticosteroid, e.g. hydrocortisone
Genital herpes	Acute	±	✓	–	Atypical ulcers are not uncommon	Swab for HSV PCR	Oral antiviral, e.g. aciclovir
Circinate balanitis	Either	–	–	–	Painless erosions with raised edges; usually as part of Reiter's syndrome (p. 1107)	Clinical	Mild topical steroid, e.g. hydrocortisone

(HSV PSR = herpes simplex virus polymerase chain reaction)

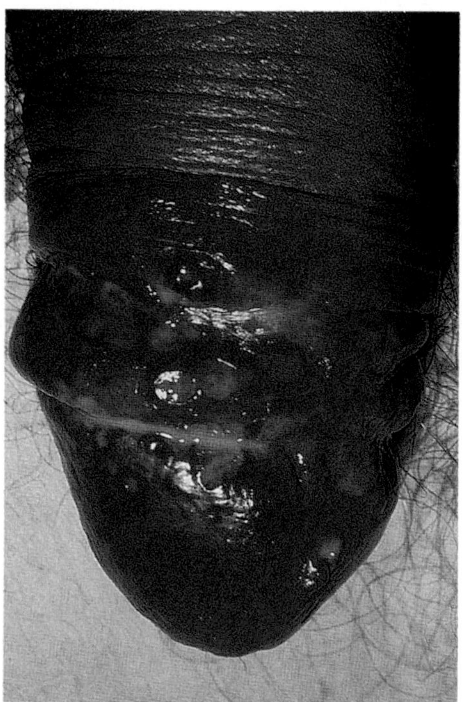

Fig. 15.2 Penile herpes simplex (HSV-2) infection.

of primary syphilis (chancre) is single, painless and indurated; however, multiple lesions are seen rarely and anal chancres are often painful. Diagnosis is made in GUM clinics by dark-ground microscopy and/or PCR on a swab from a chancre, but in other settings by serological tests for syphilis (p. 420). Other rare infective causes seen in the UK include varicella zoster virus (p. 316) and trauma with secondary infection. Tropical STI, such as chancroid, LGV and granuloma inguinale, are described in Box 15.12 (p. 424). Inflammatory causes include Stevens–Johnson syndrome (pp. 1264 and 1302), Behçet's syndrome (p. 1107) and fixed drug reactions. In older patients, malignant and pre-malignant conditions, such as squamous cell carcinoma and erythroplasia of Queyrat (intra-epidermal carcinoma), should be considered.

Genital lumps

The most common cause of genital 'lumps' is warts (p. 425). These are classically found in areas of friction during sex, such as the parafrenal skin and prepuce of the penis. Warts may also be seen in the urethral meatus, and less commonly on the shaft or around the base of the penis. Perianal warts are surprisingly common in men who do not have anal sex.

The differential diagnosis includes molluscum contagiosum and skin tags. Adolescent boys may confuse normal anatomical features such as coronal papillae (p. 412), parafrenal glands or sebaceous glands (Fordyce spots) with warts.

Proctitis in men who have sex with men

STIs that may cause proctitis in MSM include gonorrhoea, chlamydia, herpes and syphilis. The substrains of *Chlamydia trachomatis* that cause LGV (L1–3) have been associated with outbreaks of severe proctitis in Northern Europe, including the UK. Symptoms include mucopurulent anal discharge, rectal bleeding, pain and tenesmus.

Examination may show mucopus and erythema with contact bleeding (p. 412). In addition to the diagnostic tests on page 412, a PCR test for HSV and a request for identification of the LGV substrain should be arranged if chlamydial infection is detected. Treatment is directed at the individual infections (see below).

MSM may also present with gastrointestinal symptoms from infection with organisms such as *Entamoeba histolytica* (p. 367), *Shigella* spp. (p. 345), *Campylobacter* spp. (p. 342) and *Cryptosporidium* spp. (p. 369).

PRESENTING PROBLEMS IN WOMEN

Vaginal discharge

The natural vaginal discharge may vary considerably, especially under differing hormonal influences such as puberty, pregnancy or prescribed contraception. A sudden or recent change in discharge, especially if associated with alteration of colour and/or smell, or vulval itch/irritation, is more likely to indicate an infective cause than a gradual or long-standing change.

Local epidemiology is particularly important when assessing possible causes. In the UK, most cases of vaginal discharge are not sexually transmitted, being due to either candidal infection or bacterial vaginosis (BV). World-wide, the most common treatable STI causing vaginal discharge is trichomoniasis; other possibilities include gonorrhoea and chlamydia. HSV may cause increased discharge, although vulval pain and dysuria are usually the predominant symptoms. Non-infective causes include retained tampons, malignancy and/or fistulae.

Speculum examination often allows a relatively accurate diagnosis, with appropriate treatment to follow (Box 15.4). If the discharge is homogeneous and off-white in colour, vaginal pH is greater than 4.5, and Gram stain microscopy reveals scanty or absent lactobacilli with significant numbers of Gram-variable organisms, some of which may be coating vaginal squamous cells (so-called Clue cells, Fig. 15.3), the likely diagnosis is BV. If there is vulval and vaginal erythema, the discharge is curdy in nature, vaginal pH is less than 4.5, and Gram stain microscopy reveals fungal spores and pseudohyphae, the diagnosis is candidiasis. Trichomoniasis tends to cause a profuse yellow or green discharge and is usually associated with significant vulvovaginal inflammation. Diagnosis is made by observing motile

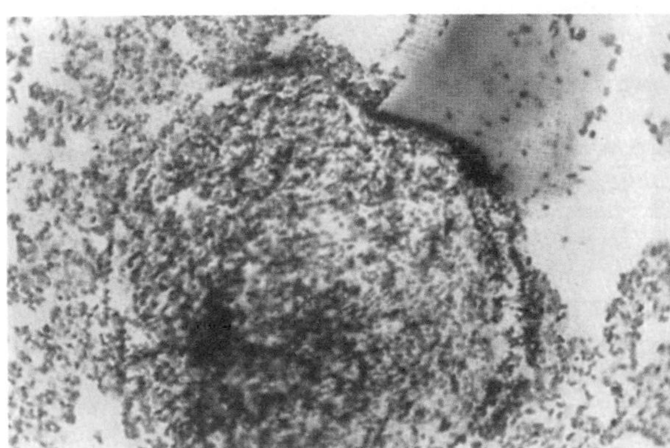

Fig. 15.3 Gram stain of a Clue cell from a patient with bacterial vaginosis. The margin of this vaginal epithelial cell is obscured by a coating of anaerobic organisms. From McMillan, et al. 2002 – see p. 426.

15.4 Infections that cause vaginal discharge

Cause	Clinical features	Treatment (in pregnancy seek specialist advice)
Candidiasis	Vulval and vaginal inflammation Curdy white discharge adherent to walls of vagina Low vaginal pH	Clotrimazole[1] 500 mg pessary once at night and clotrimazole cream twice daily *or* Econazole[1] pessary 150 mg for 3 nights and econazole cream twice daily (topical creams for 7 days) *or* Fluconazole[2] 150 mg orally stat
Trichomoniasis	Vulval and vaginal inflammation Frothy yellow/green discharge	Metronidazole[3] 400 mg twice daily orally for 5–7 days *or* Metronidazole[3] 2 g orally as a single dose
Bacterial vaginosis	No inflammation White homogeneous discharge High vaginal pH	Metronidazole[3] 2 g stat or 400 mg twice daily orally for 5–7 days Metronidazole[3] vaginal gel 0.75% daily for 5 days Clindamycin[1,4] vaginal cream 2% daily for 7 days
Streptococcal/staphylococcal infection	Purulent vaginal discharge	Choice of antibiotic depends on sensitivity tests

[1]Clotrimazole, econazole and clindamycin damage latex condoms and diaphragms. [2]Avoid in pregnancy and breastfeeding.
[3]Avoid alcoholic drinks until 48 hours after finishing treatment. Avoid high-dose regimens in pregnancy or breastfeeding.
[4]Pseudomembranous colitis has been reported with the use of clindamycin cream.

flagellate protozoa on a wet-mount microscopy slide of vaginal material.

If examination reveals the discharge to be cervical in origin, the possibility of chlamydial or gonococcal infection is increased and appropriate cervical or vaginal swabs should be taken (p. 413). In addition, Gram stain of cervical and urethral material may reveal GNDC, allowing presumptive treatment for gonorrhoea to be given. If gonococcal cervicitis is suspected, swabs should also be taken from the pharynx and rectum; infections at these sites are not reliably eradicated by single-dose therapy and a test of cure will therefore be required.

GUM clinics in the UK may offer sexually active women presenting with vaginal discharge an STI screen (p. 413). In other settings, such as primary care or gynaecology, testing for chlamydia and gonorrhoea may be considered in young women (< 25 years old), those who have changed partner recently, and those not using a barrier method of contraception, even if a non-STI cause of discharge is suspected clinically.

Treatment of infections causing vaginal discharge is shown in Box 15.4.

Lower abdominal pain

Pelvic inflammatory disease (PID, infection or inflammation of the Fallopian tubes and surrounding structures) is part of the extensive differential diagnosis of lower abdominal pain in women, especially those who are sexually active. The possibility of PID is increased if, in addition to acute/subacute pain, there is dyspareunia, abnormal vaginal discharge and/or bleeding. There may also be systemic features, such as fever and malaise. On examination, lower abdominal pain is usually bilateral, and vaginal examination reveals adnexal tenderness with or without cervical excitation. Unfortunately, a definitive diagnosis can only be made by laparoscopy. A pregnancy test should be performed (as well as the diagnostic tests on p. 413) because the differential diagnosis includes ectopic pregnancy.

Broad-spectrum antibiotics, including those active against gonorrhoea and chlamydia, such as ofloxacin and metronidazole, should be prescribed if PID is suspected, along with appropriate analgesia. Delaying treatment increases the likelihood of adverse sequelae, such as abscess formation, and tubal scarring that may lead to ectopic pregnancy or infertility. Hospital admission may be indicated for severe symptoms.

Genital ulceration

The most common cause of ulceration is genital herpes. Classically, multiple painful ulcers affect the introitus, labia and perineum, but solitary lesions occur rarely. Inguinal lymphadenopathy and systemic features, such as fever and malaise, are more common than in men. Diagnosis is made by gently scraping material from lesions and sending this in an appropriate transport medium for culture or detection of HSV DNA by PCR. Increasingly, laboratories will also test such samples for *Treponema pallidum* by PCR. In the UK, the possibility of any other ulcerating STI is unlikely unless the patient has had a sexual partner from a region where tropical STIs are more common (see Box 15.12, p. 424).

Inflammatory causes include lichen sclerosus, Stevens–Johnson syndrome (pp. 1264 and 1302), Behçet's syndrome (p. 1119) and fixed drug reactions. In older patients, malignant and pre-malignant conditions, such as squamous cell carcinoma, should be considered.

Genital lumps

The most common cause of genital 'lumps' is warts. These are classically found in areas of friction during sex, such as the fourchette and perineum. Perianal warts are surprisingly common in women who do not have anal sex.

The differential diagnosis includes molluscum contagiosum, skin tags and normal papillae or sebaceous glands.

Chronic vulval pain and/or itch

Women may present with a range of chronic symptoms that may be intermittent or continuous (Box 15.5).

Recurrent candidiasis may lead to hypersensitivity to candidal antigens, with itch and erythema becoming more prominent than increased discharge. Effective

15.5 Chronic vulval pain and/or itch

Likely diagnosis	Itch	Pain	Specific characteristics	Diagnostic test	Treatment
Candidiasis	✓	±	Usually cyclical	Microscopy	Oral antifungal, e.g. fluconazole 150 mg
Lichen planus	±	–	Violaceous papules ± Wickham's striae	Clinical	No treatment, or mild topical corticosteroid, e.g. hydrocortisone
Lichen sclerosus	±	–	Ivory-white plaques, scarring ± labial resorption	Clinical or biopsy	Strong topical corticosteroid, e.g. clobetasol
Vestibulitis	–	✓	Dyspareunia common, pain on touching erythematous area	Clinical	Refer to specialist vulva clinic
Vulvodynia	–	✓	Pain usually neuropathic in nature	Clinical	Refer to specialist vulva clinic
Dermatoses, e.g. eczema or psoriasis	✓	–	Similar to lesions elsewhere on skin	Clinical	Mild topical corticosteroid, e.g. hydrocortisone
Genital herpes	±	✓	Atypical ulcers are not uncommon	Swab for HSV PCR	Oral antiviral, e.g. aciclovir

treatment may require regular oral antifungals, e.g. fluconazole 150 g once every 2–4 weeks plus a combined antifungal/corticosteroid cream such as Daktacort or Canesten HC.

PREVENTION OF STI

Case-finding

Early diagnosis and treatment facilitated by active case-finding will help to reduce the spread of infection by limiting the period of infectivity; tracing and treating sexual partners will also reduce the risk of re-infection. Unfortunately, the majority of individuals with an STI are asymptomatic and therefore unlikely to seek medical attention. Improving access to diagnosis in primary care or non-medical settings, especially through opportunistic testing, may help. However, the impact of medical intervention through improved access alone is likely to be small.

Changing behaviour

The prevalence of STIs is driven largely by sexual behaviour. Primary prevention encompasses efforts to delay the onset of sexual activity and limit the number of sexual partners thereafter. Encouraging the use of barrier methods of contraception will also help to reduce the risk of transmitting or acquiring STIs. This is especially important in the setting of 'sexual concurrency', where sexual relationships overlap.

Unfortunately, there is contradictory evidence as to which (if any) interventions can reduce sexual activity. Knowledge alone does not translate into behaviour change, and broader issues, such as poor parental role modelling, low self-esteem, peer group pressure in the context of the increased sexualisation of our societies, gender power imbalance and homophobia, all need to be addressed. Throughout the world there is a critical need to enable women to protect themselves from undisciplined and coercive male sexual activity. Economic collapse and the turmoil of war regularly lead to situations where women are raped or must turn to prostitution to feed themselves and their children, and an inability to negotiate safe sex increases their risk of acquiring STI, including HIV.

SEXUALLY TRANSMITTED BACTERIAL INFECTIONS

Syphilis

Syphilis is caused by infection, through abrasions in the skin or mucous membranes, with the spirochaete *Treponema pallidum.* In adults the infection is usually sexually acquired; however, transmission by kissing, blood transfusion and percutaneous injury has been reported. Transplacental infection of the fetus can occur.

The natural history of untreated syphilis is variable. Infection may remain latent throughout, or clinical features may develop at any time. The classification of syphilis is shown in Box 15.6. All infected patients should be treated. Penicillin remains the drug of choice for all stages of infection.

Acquired syphilis

Early syphilis

Primary syphilis

The incubation period is usually between 14 and 28 days, with a range of 9–90 days. The primary lesion or chancre (Fig. 15.4) develops at the site of infection, usually in the genital area. A dull red macule develops, becomes papular and then erodes to form an indurated ulcer (chancre). The draining inguinal lymph nodes may become moderately enlarged, mobile, discrete and rubbery. The chancre and the lymph nodes are both painless and non-tender, unless there is concurrent or secondary infection. Without treatment, the chancre will resolve within 2–6 weeks to leave a thin atrophic scar.

Chancres may develop on the vaginal wall and on the cervix. Extragenital chancres are found in about 10% of patients, affecting sites such as the finger, lip, tongue, tonsil, nipple, anus or rectum. Anal chancres often resemble fissures and may be painful.

Secondary syphilis

This occurs 6–8 weeks after the development of the chancre, when treponemes disseminate to produce a multisystem disease. Constitutional features, such as mild fever, malaise and headache, are common. Over 75% of patients present with a rash on the trunk and limbs that may later involve the palms and soles; this is initially macular but evolves to maculopapular or papular forms, which are generalised, symmetrical and non-irritable. Scales may form on the papules later. The rash affects the trunk and proximal limbs, and characteristically involves the palms, soles and face. Lesions

15.6 Classification of syphilis

Stage	Acquired	Congenital
Early	Primary Secondary Latent	Clinical and latent
Late	Latent Benign tertiary Cardiovascular Neurosyphilis	Clinical and latent

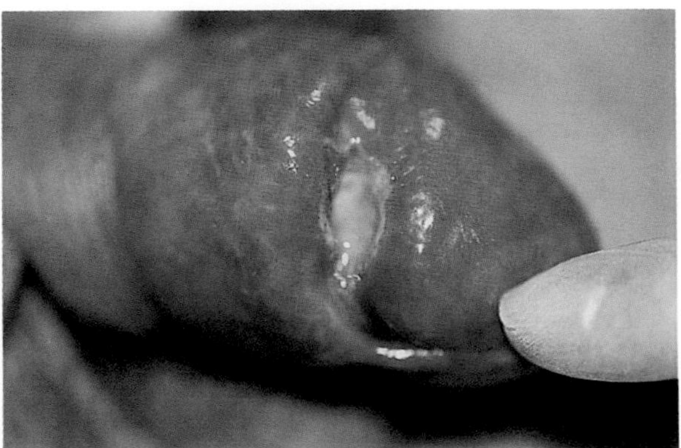

Fig. 15.4 Primary syphilis. A painless ulcer (chancre) is shown in the coronal sulcus of the penis. This is usually associated with inguinal lymphadenopathy.

15

are red, changing to a 'gun-metal' grey as they resolve. Without treatment, the rash may last for up to 12 weeks. Condylomata lata (papules coalescing to plaques) may develop in warm, moist sites such as the vulva or perianal area. Generalised non-tender lymphadenopathy is present in over 50% of patients. Mucosal lesions, known as mucous patches, may affect the genitalia, mouth, pharynx or larynx and are essentially modified papules, which become eroded. Rarely, confluence produces characteristic 'snail track ulcers' in the mouth.

Other features, such as meningitis, cranial nerve palsies, anterior or posterior uveitis, hepatitis, gastritis, glomerulonephritis or periostitis, are sometimes seen. Neurological involvement may be more common in HIV-positive patients.

The differential diagnosis of secondary syphilis can be extensive, but in the context of a suspected STI, primary HIV infection is the most important alternative condition to consider (see Ch. 14). Non-STI conditions that mimic the rash include psoriasis, pityriasis rosea, scabies, allergic drug reaction, erythema multiforme and tinea versicolor.

The clinical manifestations of secondary syphilis will resolve without treatment but relapse may occur, usually within the first year of infection. Thereafter, the disease enters the phase of latency.

Latent syphilis

This phase is characterised by the presence of positive syphilis serology or the diagnostic cerebrospinal fluid (CSF) abnormalities of neurosyphilis in an untreated patient with no evidence of clinical disease. It is divided into early latency (within 2 years of infection), when syphilis may be transmitted sexually, and late latency, when the patient is no longer sexually infectious. Transmission of syphilis from a pregnant woman to her fetus, and rarely by blood transfusion, is possible for several years following infection.

Late syphilis

Late latent syphilis

This may persist for many years or for life. Without treatment, over 60% of patients might be expected to suffer little or no ill health. Coincidental prescription of antibiotics for other illnesses, such as respiratory tract or skin infections, may treat latent syphilis serendipitously.

Benign tertiary syphilis

This may develop between 3 and 10 years after infection but is now rarely seen in the UK. Skin, mucous membranes, bone, muscle or viscera can be involved. The characteristic feature is a chronic granulomatous lesion called a gumma, which may be single or multiple. Healing with scar formation may impair the function of the structure affected. Skin lesions may take the form of nodules or ulcers, whilst subcutaneous lesions may ulcerate with a gummy discharge. Healing occurs slowly, with the formation of characteristic tissue paper scars. Mucosal lesions may occur in the mouth, pharynx, larynx or nasal septum, appearing as punched-out ulcers. Of particular importance is gummatous involvement of the tongue, healing of which may lead to leucoplakia with the attendant risk of malignant change. Gummas of the tibia, skull, clavicle and sternum have been described, as has involvement of the brain, spinal cord, liver, testis and, rarely, other organs. Resolution of active disease should follow treatment, though some tissue damage may be permanent. Paroxysmal cold haemoglobinuria (p. 1031) may be seen.

Cardiovascular syphilis

This may present many years after initial infection. Aortitis, which may involve the aortic valve and/or the coronary ostia, is the key feature. Clinical features include aortic incompetence, angina and aortic aneurysm (p. 603). The condition typically affects the ascending aorta and sometimes the aortic arch; aneurysm of the descending aorta is rare. Treatment with penicillin will not correct anatomical damage and surgical intervention may be required.

Neurosyphilis

This may also take years to develop. Asymptomatic infection is associated with CSF abnormalities in the absence of clinical signs. Meningovascular disease, tabes dorsalis and general paralysis of the insane constitute the symptomatic forms (p. 1209). Neurosyphilis and cardiovascular syphilis may coexist and are sometimes referred to as quaternary syphilis.

Congenital syphilis

Congenital syphilis is rare where antenatal serological screening is practised. Antisyphilitic treatment in pregnancy treats the fetus, if infected, as well as the mother.

Treponemal infection may give rise to a variety of outcomes after 4 months of gestation, when the fetus becomes immunocompetent:

- miscarriage or stillbirth, prematurely or at term
- birth of a syphilitic baby (a very sick baby with hepatosplenomegaly, bullous rash and perhaps pneumonia)
- birth of a baby who develops signs of early congenital syphilis during the first few weeks of life (Box 15.7)
- birth of a baby with latent infection who either remains well or develops congenital syphilis/stigmata later in life (see Box 15.7).

Investigations in adult cases

Treponema pallidum may be identified in serum collected from chancres, or from moist or eroded lesions in secondary syphilis using a dark-field microscope, a direct fluorescent antibody test or PCR.

The serological tests for syphilis are listed in Box 15.8. Many centres use treponemal EIAs for IgG and IgM antibodies to screen for syphilis. EIA for antitreponemal IgM becomes positive at approximately 2 weeks, whilst non-treponemal tests become positive about 4 weeks after primary syphilis. All positive results in asymptomatic patients must be confirmed by repeat tests.

Biological false positive reactions occur occasionally; these are most commonly seen with Venereal Diseases Research Laboratory (VDRL) or rapid plasma reagin (RPR) tests (when treponemal tests will be negative). Acute false-positive reactions may be associated with infections, such as infectious mononucleosis, chickenpox and malaria, and may also occur in pregnancy. Chronic false-positive reactions may be associated with autoimmune diseases. False-negative results for non-treponemal tests may be found in secondary syphilis

15.7 Clinical features of congenital syphilis

Early congenital syphilis (neonatal period)	
• Maculopapular rash • Condylomata lata • Mucous patches • Fissures around mouth, nose and anus • Rhinitis with nasal discharge (snuffles)	• Hepatosplenomegaly • Osteochondritis/periostitis • Generalised lymphadenopathy • Choroiditis • Meningitis • Anaemia/thrombocytopenia
Late congenital syphilis	
• Benign tertiary syphilis • Periostitis • Paroxysmal cold haemoglobinuria • Neurosyphilis	• 8th nerve deafness • Interstitial keratitis • Clutton's joints (painless effusion into knee joints)
Stigmata	
• Hutchinson's incisors (anterior–posterior thickening with notch on narrowed cutting edge) • Mulberry molars (imperfectly formed cusps/deficient dental enamel) • High arched palate • Maxillary hypoplasia • Saddle nose (following snuffles) • Rhagades (radiating scars around mouth, nose and anus following rash) • Salt and pepper scars on retina (from choroiditis) • Corneal scars (from interstitial keratitis) • Sabre tibia (from periostitis) • Bossing of frontal and parietal bones (healed periosteal nodes)	

because extremely high antibody levels can prevent the formation of the antibody–antigen lattice necessary for the visualisation of the flocculation reaction (the prozone phenomenon).

In benign tertiary and cardiovascular syphilis, examination of CSF should be considered because asymptomatic neurological disease may coexist. The CSF should also be examined in patients with clinical signs of neurosyphilis (p. 1209) and in both early and late congenital syphilis. Positive STS may be found in patients who are being investigated for neurological disease, especially dementia. In many instances, the serology reflects previous infection unrelated to the presenting complaint, especially when titres are low. Examination of CSF is occasionally necessary.

Chest X-ray, electrocardiogram (ECG) and echocardiogram are useful in the investigation of cardiovascular syphilis. Biopsy may be required to diagnose gumma.

Endemic treponematoses, such as yaws, endemic (non-venereal) syphilis (bejel) and pinta (pp. 332–333), are caused by treponemes that are morphologically indistinguishable from *T. pallidum* and cannot be differentiated by serological tests. A VDRL or RPR test may help to elucidate the correct diagnosis because adults with late yaws usually have low titres.

Investigations in suspected congenital syphilis

Passively transferred maternal antibodies from an adequately treated mother may give rise to positive serological tests in her baby. In this situation, non-treponemal tests should become negative within 3–6 months of birth. A positive EIA test for antitreponemal IgM suggests early congenital syphilis. A diagnosis of congenital syphilis mandates investigation of the mother, her partner and any siblings.

15.8 Serological tests for syphilis

Non-treponemal (non-specific) tests
• Venereal Diseases Research Laboratory (VDRL) test • Rapid plasma reagin (RPR) test
Treponemal (specific) antibody tests
• Treponemal antigen-based enzyme immunoassay (EIA) for IgG and IgM • *T. pallidum* haemagglutination assay (TPHA) • *T. pallidum* particle agglutination assay (TPPA) • Fluorescent treponemal antibody-absorbed (FTA-ABS) test

Management

Penicillin is the drug of choice. Currently, a single dose of 2.4 megaunits of intramuscular benzathine penicillin is recommended for early syphilis (< 2 years' duration), with three doses at weekly intervals being recommended in late syphilis. Doxycycline is indicated for patients allergic to penicillin, except in pregnancy (see below). Azithromycin is a further alternative. All patients must be followed up to ensure cure, and partner notification is of particular importance. Resolution of clinical signs in early syphilis with declining titres for non-treponemal tests, usually to undetectable levels within 6 months for primary syphilis and 12–18 months for secondary syphilis, is an indicator of successful treatment. Specific treponemal antibody tests may remain positive for life. In patients who have had syphilis for many years there may be little serological response following treatment.

Pregnancy

Penicillin is the treatment of choice in pregnancy. Erythromycin stearate can be given if there is penicillin hypersensitivity, but crosses the placenta poorly; the newborn baby must therefore be treated with a course of penicillin and consideration given to retreating the mother. Some specialists recommend penicillin desensitisation for pregnant mothers so that penicillin can be given during temporary tolerance. The author has successfully prescribed ceftriaxone 250 mg IM for 10 days in this situation. Babies should be treated in hospital with the help of a paediatrician.

Treatment reactions

- *Anaphylaxis.* Penicillin is a common cause; on-site facilities should be available for management (p. 91).
- *Jarisch–Herxheimer reaction.* This is an acute febrile reaction that follows treatment and is characterised by headache, malaise and myalgia; it resolves within 24 hours. It is common in early syphilis and rare in late syphilis. Fetal distress or premature labour can occur in pregnancy. The reaction may also cause worsening of neurological (cerebral artery occlusion) or ophthalmic (uveitis, optic neuritis) disease, myocardial ischaemia (inflammation of the coronary ostia) and laryngeal stenosis (swelling of a gumma). Prednisolone

10–20 mg orally three times daily for 3 days is recommended to prevent the reaction in patients with these forms of the disease; antisyphilitic treatment can be started 24 hours after introducing corticosteroids. In high-risk situations it is wise to initiate therapy in hospital.
- *Procaine reaction.* Fear of impending death occurs immediately after the accidental intravenous injection of procaine penicillin and may be associated with hallucinations or fits. Symptoms are short-lived, but verbal assurance and sometimes physical restraint are needed. The reaction can be prevented by aspiration before intramuscular injection to ensure the needle is not in a blood vessel.

Gonorrhoea

Gonorrhoea is caused by infection with *Neisseria gonorrhoeae* and may involve columnar epithelium in the lower genital tract, rectum, pharynx and eyes. Transmission is usually the result of vaginal, anal or oral sex. Gonococcal conjunctivitis may be caused by accidental infection from contaminated fingers. Untreated mothers may infect babies during delivery, resulting in ophthalmia neonatorum (Fig. 15.5). Infection of children beyond the neonatal period usually indicates sexual abuse.

Clinical features

The incubation period is usually 2–10 days. In men the anterior urethra is commonly infected, causing urethral discharge and dysuria, but symptoms are absent in about 10% of cases. Examination will usually show a mucopurulent or purulent urethral discharge. Rectal infection in MSM is usually asymptomatic but may present with anal discomfort, discharge or rectal bleeding. Proctoscopy may reveal either no abnormality, or clinical evidence of proctitis (see p. 417) such as inflamed rectal mucosa and mucopus.

In women, the urethra, paraurethral glands/ducts, Bartholin's glands/ducts or endocervical canal may be infected. The rectum may also be involved either due to contamination from a urogenital site or as a result of anal sex. Occasionally, the rectum is the only site infected.

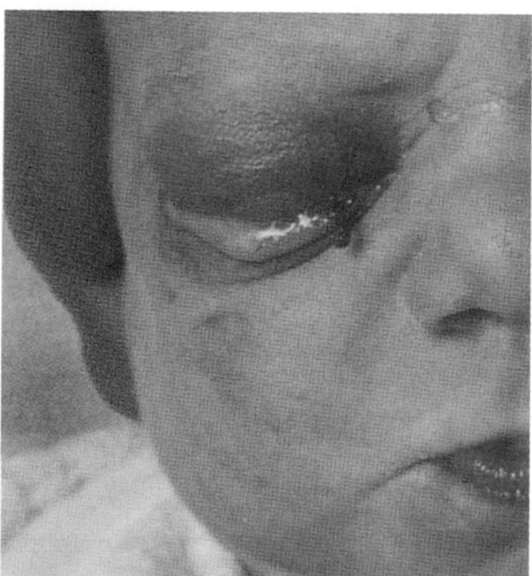

Fig. 15.5 Gonococcal ophthalmia neonatorum. From McMillan and Scott 2000 – see p. 426.

About 80% of women who have gonorrhoea are asymptomatic. There may be vaginal discharge or dysuria but these symptoms are often due to additional infections, such as chlamydia (see below), trichomoniasis or candidiasis, making full investigation essential (p. 413). Lower abdominal pain, dyspareunia and intermenstrual bleeding may be indicative of PID. Clinical examination may show no abnormality, or pus may be expressed from urethra, paraurethral ducts or Bartholin's ducts. The cervix may be inflamed, with mucopurulent discharge and contact bleeding.

Pharyngeal gonorrhoea is the result of receptive orogenital sex and is usually symptomless. Gonococcal conjunctivitis is an uncommon complication, presenting with purulent discharge from the eye(s), severe inflammation of the conjunctivae and oedema of the eyelids, pain and photophobia. Gonococcal ophthalmia neonatorum presents similarly with purulent conjunctivitis and oedema of the eyelids. Conjunctivitis must be treated urgently to prevent corneal damage.

Disseminated gonococcal infection (DGI) is seen rarely, and typically affects women with asymptomatic genital infection. Symptoms include arthritis of one or more joints, pustular skin lesions and fever. Gonococcal endocarditis has been described.

Investigations

Gram-negative diplococci may be seen on microscopy of smears from infected sites (see Fig. 15.1, p. 415). Pharyngeal smears are difficult to analyse due to the presence of other diplococci, so the diagnosis must be confirmed by culture or NAAT.

Management of adults

Emerging resistance is making it increasingly difficult to cure gonorrhoea with a single oral dose of

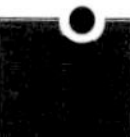

15.9 Treatment of uncomplicated anogenital gonorrhoea

Uncomplicated infection

- Ceftriaxone 500 mg IM *or*
- Cefixime 400 mg stat *or*
- Ciprofloxacin 500 mg orally stat[1],[2] *or*
- Ofloxacin 400 mg orally stat[1],[2] *or*
- Amoxicillin 3 g *plus* probenecid 1 g orally stat[3]

Quinolone resistance

- Ceftriaxone 500 mg IM stat *or*
- Spectinomycin 2 g IM stat[4]

Pregnancy and breastfeeding

- Ceftriaxone 500 mg IM stat *or*
- Cefixime 400 mg stat *or*
- Amoxicillin 3 g *plus* probenecid 1 g orally stat[3] *or*
- Spectinomycin 2 g IM stat[4]

Pharyngeal gonorrhoea

- Ceftriaxone 500 mg IM stat *or*
- Cefixime 400 mg stat *or*
- Ciprofloxacin 500 mg[1],[2] orally stat *or*
- Ofloxacin 400 mg[1,2] orally stat

[1]Contraindicated in pregnancy and breastfeeding.
[2]If prevalence of quinolone resistance for *N. gonorrhoeae* < 5%.
[3]If prevalence of penicillin resistance for *N. gonorrhoeae* < 5%.
[4]May only be available in specialist clinics.

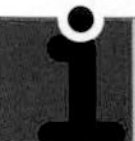

15.10 Complications of delayed therapy in gonorrhoea

- Acute prostatitis
- Epididymo-orchitis
- Bartholin's gland abscess
- PID (may lead to infertility or ectopic pregnancy)
- Disseminated gonococcal infection

antimicrobials, and recommended treatment in the UK has changed to intramuscular ceftriaxone 500 mg. The alternatives listed in Box 15.9 are less likely to be effective.

Longer courses of antibiotics are required for complicated infection. Partner(s) of patients with gonorrhoea should be seen as soon as possible. Delay in treatment may lead to complications (Box 15.10).

Chlamydial infection

Chlamydial infection in men

Chlamydia is transmitted and presents in a similar way to gonorrhoea; however, urethral symptoms are usually milder and may be absent in over 50% of cases. Conjunctivitis is also milder than in gonorrhoea; pharyngitis does not occur. The incubation period varies from 1 week to a few months. Without treatment, symptoms may resolve but the patient remains infectious for several months. Complications, such as epididymo-orchitis and Reiter's syndrome, or sexually acquired reactive arthropathy (SARA, p. 1107), are rare. Sexually transmitted pathogens, such as chlamydia or gonococci, are usually responsible for epididymo-orchitis in men aged less than 35 years, whereas bacteria such as Gram-negative enteric organisms are more commonly implicated in older men.

Treatments for chlamydia are listed in Box 15.11. NSU is treated identically. The partner(s) of men with chlamydia should be treated, even if laboratory tests for chlamydia are negative. Investigation is not mandatory but serves a useful epidemiological purpose; moreover, positive results encourage further attempts at contact-tracing.

Chlamydial infection in women

The cervix and urethra are commonly involved. Infection is asymptomatic in about 80% of patients but may cause vaginal discharge, dysuria and intermenstrual and/or postcoital bleeding. Lower abdominal pain and dyspareunia are features of PID. Examination may reveal mucopurulent cervicitis, contact bleeding from the cervix, evidence of PID or no obvious clinical signs. Treatment options are listed in Box 15.11. The patient's male partner(s) should be investigated and treated.

Some infections may clear spontaneously but others persist. PID, with the risk of tubal damage and subsequent infertility or ectopic pregnancy, is a rare but important long-term complication. Other complications include perihepatitis, chronic pelvic pain, conjunctivitis and Reiter's syndrome or SARA. Perinatal transmission may lead to ophthalmia neonatorum and/or pneumonia in the neonate.

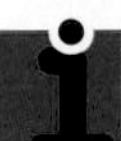

15.11 Treatment of chlamydial infection

Standard regimens

- Azithromycin 1 g orally as a single dose[1] *or*
- Doxycycline 100 mg twice daily orally for 7 days[2]

Alternative regimens

- Erythromycin 500 mg four times daily orally for 7 days *or* 500 mg twice daily for 2 weeks *or*
- Ofloxacin 200 mg twice daily orally for 7 days[2]

[1]Safety in pregnancy and breastfeeding has not been fully assessed.
[2]Contraindicated in pregnancy and breastfeeding.

Other sexually transmitted bacterial infections

Chancroid, granuloma inguinale and LGV as causes of genital ulcers in the tropics are described in Box 15.12. LGV is also a cause of proctitis in MSM (p. 417).

15

SEXUALLY TRANSMITTED VIRAL INFECTIONS

Genital herpes simplex

Infection with herpes simplex virus type 1 (HSV-1) or type 2 (HSV-2) produces a wide spectrum of clinical problems (p. 325), and may facilitate HIV transmission. Infection is usually acquired sexually (vaginal, anal, oro-genital or oro-anal), but perinatal transmission to the neonate may also occur. Primary infection at the site of HSV entry, which may be symptomatic or asymptomatic, establishes latency in local sensory ganglia. Recurrences, either symptomatic or asymptomatic viral shedding, are a consequence of HSV reactivation. The first symptomatic episode is usually the most severe. Although HSV-1 is classically associated with orolabial herpes and HSV-2 with anogenital herpes, HSV-1 now accounts for more than 50% of anogenital infections in the UK.

Clinical features

The first symptomatic episode presents with irritable vesicles that soon rupture to form small, tender ulcers on the external genitalia (see Figs 15.6 and 15.2, p. 416). Lesions at other sites (e.g. urethra, vagina, cervix, perianal area, anus or rectum) may cause dysuria, urethral or vaginal discharge, or anal, perianal or rectal pain. Constitutional symptoms, such as fever, headache and malaise, are common. Inguinal lymph nodes become enlarged and tender, and there may be nerve root pain in the 2nd and 3rd sacral dermatomes.

Extragenital lesions may develop at other sites, such as the buttock, finger or eye, due to auto-inoculation. Oropharyngeal infection may result from orogenital sex. Complications, such as urinary retention due to autonomic neuropathy, and aseptic meningitis, are occasionally seen.

First episodes usually heal within 2–4 weeks without treatment; recurrences are usually milder and of shorter duration than the initial attack. They occur more often

15.12 Salient features of lymphogranuloma venereum, chancroid and granuloma inguinale (Donovanosis)

Infection and distribution	Organism	Incubation period	Genital lesion	Lymph nodes	Diagnosis	Management
Lymphogranuloma venereum (LGV)						
E/W Africa, India, SE Asia, S America, Caribbean	*Chlamydia trachomatis* types L1, 2, 3	3–30 days	Small, transient, painless ulcer, vesicle, papule; often unnoticed	Tender, usually unilateral, matted, suppurative bubo; inguinal/femoral nodes involved[1]	Serological tests for L1–3 serotypes; swab from ulcer or bubo pus for *Chlamydia*	Doxycycline[2] twice daily orally for 21 days *or* Erythromycin 500 mg four times daily orally
Chancroid						
Africa, Asia, Central and S America	*Haemophilus ducreyi* (short Gram-negative bacillus)	3–10 days	Single or multiple painful ulcers with ragged undermined edges	As above but unilocular, suppurative bubo; inguinal nodes involved in ~50%	Microscopy and culture of scrapings from ulcer or pus from bubo	Azithromycin[3] 1 g orally once *or* Ceftriaxone 250 mg IM once *or* Ciprofloxacin[2] 500 mg twice daily orally for 3 days
Granuloma inguinale						
Australia, Caribbean, India, S Africa, S America, Papua New Guinea	*Klebsiella granulomatis* (Donovan bodies)	3–40 days	Ulcers or hypertrophic granulomatous lesions; usually painless[4]	Initial swelling of inguinal nodes, then spread of infection to form abscess or ulceration through adjacent skin	Microscopy of cellular material for intracellular bipolar-staining Donovan bodies	Azithromycin[3] 1 g weekly orally or 500 mg daily orally *or* Doxycycline[2] 100 mg twice daily orally *or* Ceftriaxone 1 g IM daily

[1]The genito-ano-rectal syndrome is a late manifestation of LGV. [2]Doxycycline and ciprofloxacin are contraindicated in pregnancy and breastfeeding.
[3]The safety of azithromycin in pregnancy and breastfeeding has not been fully assessed. [4]Mother-to-baby transmission of granuloma inguinale may rarely occur.
N.B. Partners of patients with LGV, chancroid and granuloma inguinale should be investigated and treated, even if asymptomatic.

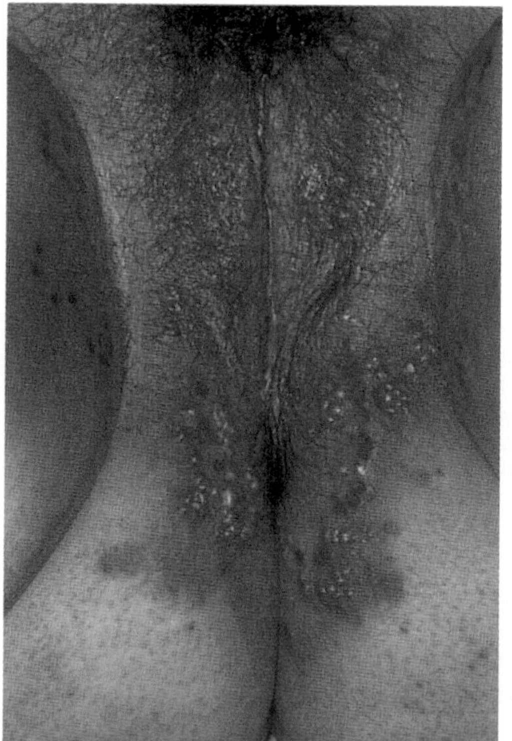

Fig. 15.6 Herpetic ulceration of the vulva. From McMillan and Scott 2000 – see p. 426.

in HSV-2 infection and their frequency tends to decrease with time. Prodromal symptoms, such as irritation or burning at the subsequent site of recurrence, or neuralgic pains affecting buttocks, legs or hips, are commonly seen. The first symptomatic episode may be a recurrence of a previously undiagnosed primary infection. Recurrent episodes of asymptomatic viral shedding are important in the transmission of HSV.

Diagnosis

Swabs are taken from vesicular fluid or ulcers for detection of DNA by PCR, or tissue culture and typing as either HSV-1 or 2. Electron microscopy of such material will only give a presumptive diagnosis, as herpes group viruses appear similar. Type-specific antibody tests are available but are not sufficiently accurate for general use.

Management

First episode

The following 5-day oral regimens are all recommended and should be started within 5 days of the beginning of the episode, or whilst lesions are still forming:

- aciclovir 200 mg five times daily
- famciclovir 250 mg three times daily
- valaciclovir 500 mg twice daily.

Analgesia may be required and saline bathing can be soothing. Treatment may be continued for longer than 5 days if new lesions develop. Occasionally, intravenous therapy may be indicated if oral therapy is poorly tolerated or aseptic meningitis occurs.

Catheterisation via the suprapubic route is advisable for urinary retention due to autonomic neuropathy because the transurethral route may introduce HSV into the bladder.

Recurrent genital herpes

Symptomatic recurrences are usually mild and may require no specific treatment other than saline bathing. For more severe episodes, patient-initiated treatment at onset, with one of the following 5-day oral regimens, should reduce the duration of the recurrence:

- aciclovir 200 mg five times daily
- famciclovir 125–250 mg twice daily
- valaciclovir 500 mg twice daily.

In a few patients, treatment started at the onset of prodromal symptoms may abort recurrence.

Suppressive therapy may be required for patients with frequent recurrences, especially if these occur at intervals of less than 4 weeks. Treatment should be given for a minimum of 1 year before stopping to assess recurrence rate. About 20% of patients will experience reduced attack rates thereafter, but for those whose recurrences remain unchanged, resumption of suppressive therapy is justified. Aciclovir 400 mg twice daily is most commonly prescribed.

Management in pregnancy

If her partner is known to be infected with HSV, a pregnant woman with no previous anogenital herpes should be advised to protect herself during sexual intercourse because the risk of disseminated infection is increased in pregnancy. Consistent condom use during pregnancy may reduce transmission of HSV. Genital herpes acquired during the first or second trimester of pregnancy is treated with aciclovir as clinically indicated. Although aciclovir is not licensed for use in pregnancy in the UK, there is considerable clinical evidence to support its safety. Third-trimester acquisition of infection has been associated with life-threatening haematogenous dissemination and should be treated with aciclovir.

Vaginal delivery should be routine in women who are symptomless in late pregnancy. Caesarean section is sometimes considered if there is a recurrence at the beginning of labour, although the risk of neonatal herpes through vaginal transmission is very low. Caesarean section is often recommended if primary infection occurs after 34 weeks because the risk of viral shedding is very high in labour.

Human papillomavirus and anogenital warts

Human papillomavirus (HPV) DNA typing has demonstrated over 90 genotypes (p. 1278), of which HPV-6, HPV-11, HPV-16 and HPV-18 most commonly infect the genital tract through sexual transmission. It is important to differentiate between the benign genotypes (HPV-6 and 11) that cause anogenital warts, and genotypes such as 16 and 18 that are associated with dysplastic conditions and cancers of the genital tract but are not a cause of benign warts. All genotypes usually result in subclinical infection of the genital tract rather than clinically obvious lesions affecting penis, vulva, vagina, cervix, perineum or anus.

Clinical features

Anogenital warts caused by HPV may be single or multiple, exophytic, papular or flat. Perianal warts (p. 412), whilst being more commonly found in MSM, are also found in heterosexual men and in women. Rarely, a giant condyloma (Buschke–Löwenstein tumour) develops with local tissue destruction. Atypical warts should be biopsied. In pregnancy, warts may dramatically increase in size and number, making treatment difficult. Rarely, they are large enough to obstruct labour and, in this case, delivery by Caesarean section will be required. Rarely, perinatal transmission of HPV leads to anogenital warts, or possibly laryngeal papillomas, in the neonate.

Management

The use of condoms can help prevent the transmission of HPV to non-infected partners, but HPV may affect parts of the genital area not protected by condoms. Vaccination against HPV infection has been introduced and is in routine use in several countries. There are two types of vaccine:

- *A bivalent vaccine* (Cervarix®) offers protection against HPV types 16 and 18, which account for approximately 75% of cervical cancers in the UK.
- *A quadrivalent vaccine* (Gardasil®) offers additional protection against HPV types 6 and 11, which account for over 90% of genital warts.

Both types of vaccine have been shown to be highly effective in the prevention of cervical intra-epithelial neoplasia in young women, and the quadrivalent vaccine has also been shown to be highly effective in protecting against HPV-associated genital warts (Box 15.13). It is currently recommended that HPV vaccination should be administered prior to the onset of sexual activity, typically at age 11–13, in a course of three injections. In the UK, only girls are offered vaccination, and it should be noted that this approach will not protect HPV transmission for MSM. As neither vaccine protects against all oncogenic types of HPV, cervical screening programmes will still be necessary.

A variety of treatments are available for established disease, including the following:

- *Podophyllotoxin, 0.5% solution or 0.15% cream* (contraindicated in pregnancy), applied twice daily for 3 days, followed by 4 days' rest, for up to 4 weeks is suitable for home treatment of external warts.

EBM 15.13 HPV vaccination and precancerous cervical intra-epithelial neoplasia

'Prophylactic HPV vaccination in women aged 15–25 years is highly effective at preventing precancerous cervical intra-epithelial neoplasia in young women who have not previously been infected with HPV.'

- Garland SM, et al. New Engl J Med 2007; 356:1928–1943.
- Paavonen J, et al. Lancet 2007; 369:2161–2170.

15

- *Imiquimod* cream (contraindicated in pregnancy), applied 3 times weekly (and washed off after 6–10 hours) for up to 16 weeks, is also suitable for home treatment of external warts.
- *Cryotherapy* using liquid nitrogen to freeze warty tissue is suitable for external and internal warts but often requires repeated clinic visits.
- *Hyfrecation* – electrofulguration that causes superficial charring – is suitable for external and internal warts. Hyfrecation results in smoke plume which contains HPV DNA and has the potential to cause respiratory infection in the operator/patient. Masks should be worn during the procedure and adequate extraction of fumes should be provided.
- *Surgical removal.* Refractory warts, especially pedunculated perianal lesions, may be excised under local or general anaesthesia.

Molluscum contagiosum

Infection by molluscum contagiosum virus, both sexual and non-sexual, produces flesh-coloured umbilicated hemispherical papules usually up to 5 mm in diameter after an incubation period of 3–12 weeks (Fig. 15.7). Larger lesions may be seen in HIV infection (p. 388). Lesions are often multiple and, once established in an individual, may spread by auto-inoculation. They are found on the genitalia, lower abdomen and upper thighs when sexually acquired. Facial lesions are highly suggestive of underlying HIV infection. Diagnosis is made on clinical grounds and by expression of the central core, in which the typical pox-like viral particles can be seen on electron microscopy (differentiating molluscum contagiosum from genital warts). Typically, lesions persist for an average of 2 years before spontaneous resolution occurs. Treatment regimens are therefore cosmetic; they include cryotherapy, hyfrecation, topical applications of 0.15% podophyllotoxin cream (contraindicated in pregnancy) or expression of the central core.

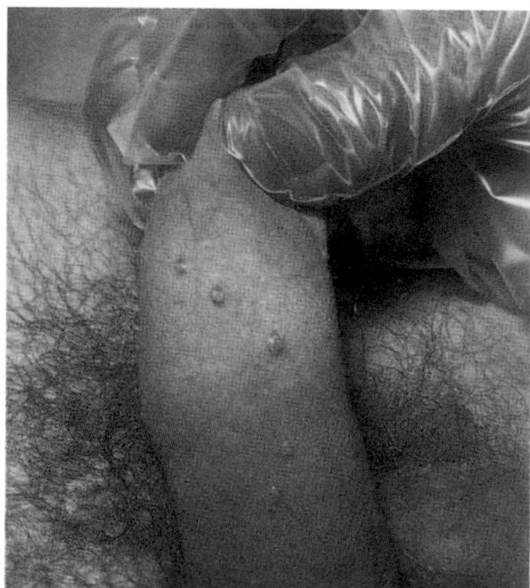

Fig. 15.7 Molluscum contagiosum of the shaft of the penis. From McMillan and Scott 2000 – see right.

Viral hepatitis

The hepatitis viruses A–D (p. 948) may be sexually transmitted:

- *Hepatitis A (HAV).* Insertive oro-anal sex, insertive digital sex, insertive anal sex and multiple sexual partners have been linked with HAV transmission in MSM. HAV transmission in heterosexual men and women is also possible through oro-anal sex.
- *Hepatitis B (HBV).* Insertive oro-anal sex, anal sex and multiple sexual partners are linked with HBV infection in MSM. Heterosexual transmission of HBV is well documented and commercial sex workers are at particular risk. Hepatitis D (HDV) may also be sexually transmitted.
- *Hepatitis C (HCV).* Sexual transmission of HCV is well documented in MSM, but less so in heterosexuals. Sexual transmission is less efficient than for HBV.

The sexual partner(s) of patients with HAV and HBV should be seen as soon as possible and offered immunisation where appropriate. Patients with HAV should abstain from all forms of unprotected sex until non-infectious. Those with HBV should likewise abstain from unprotected sex until they are non-infectious or until their partners have been vaccinated successfully. No active or passive immunisation is available for protection against HCV but the consistent use of condoms is likely to protect susceptible partners. Active immunisation against HAV and HBV should be offered to susceptible people at risk of infection. Many STI clinics offer HAV immunisation to MSM along with routine HBV immunisation; a combined HAV and HBV vaccine is available.

Further information and acknowledgements

Books and journal articles

Clutterbuck D. Specialist training in sexually transmitted infections and HIV. London: Mosby; 2004.

Low N, Aral S, Cassell J (eds). Global aspects of STI and HIV. Sexually Transmitted Infections 2007; 83:501–589.

McMillan A, Young H, Ogilvie MM, Scott GR. Clinical practice in sexually transmissible infections. London: Saunders; 2002.

Rogstad KE (ed.). ABC of sexually transmitted infections, 6th edn. Oxford: Wiley-Blackwell; 2011.

Website

www.bashh.org/guidelines *Updates on treatment of all STIs.*

Figure acknowledgements

Page 412 inset (Perianal warts), Figs 15.5, 15.6, 15.7 McMillan A, Scott GR. Sexually transmitted infections: a colour guide. Edinburgh: Churchill Livingstone; 2000; copyright Elsevier.

Page 412 insets (Coronal papillae, mucopus), page 413 inset (Inflammation), Fig. 15.3 McMillan A, Young H, Ogilvie MM, Scott GR. Clinical practice in sexually transmissible infections. Edinburgh: Saunders; 2002; copyright Elsevier.

M.J. Field
L. Burnett
D.R. Sullivan
P. Stewart

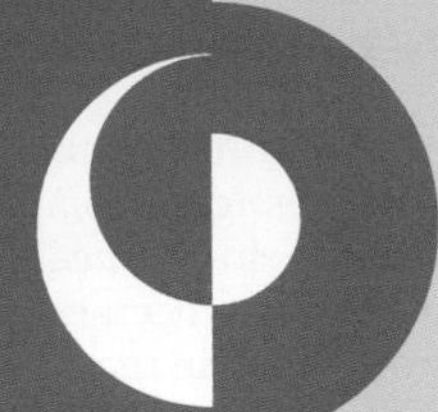

Clinical biochemistry and metabolism 16

Biochemical investigations 428

Integrated water and electrolyte balance 429
- Water and electrolyte distribution 429
- Investigation of water and electrolytes 429

Disorders of sodium balance 430
- Functional anatomy and physiology of renal sodium handling 430
- Presenting problems in disorders of sodium balance 432
  - Sodium depletion 432
  - Sodium excess 434
- Diuretic therapy 434

Disorders of water balance 436
- Functional anatomy and physiology of renal water handling 436
- Presenting problems in disorders of water balance 437
  - Hyponatraemia 437
  - Hypernatraemia 439

Disorders of potassium balance 439
- Functional anatomy and physiology of renal potassium handling 440
- Presenting problems in disorders of potassium balance 440
  - Hypokalaemia 440
  - Hyperkalaemia 442

Disorders of acid–base balance 443
- Functional anatomy and physiology of acid–base homeostasis 443
- Presenting problems in disorders of acid–base balance 444
  - Metabolic acidosis 445
  - Metabolic alkalosis 446
  - Respiratory acidosis 447
  - Respiratory alkalosis 447
  - Mixed acid-base disorders 447

Disorders of divalent ion metabolism 447
- Functional anatomy and physiology of magnesium metabolism 447
- Presenting problems in disorders of magnesium metabolism 448
  - Hypomagnesaemia 448
  - Hypermagnesaemia 448
- Functional anatomy and physiology of phosphate metabolism 448
- Presenting problems in disorders of phosphate metabolism 448
  - Hypophosphataemia 448
  - Hyperphosphataemia 449

Disorders of amino acid metabolism 449

Disorders of carbohydrate metabolism 449

Disorders of complex lipid metabolism 450

Disorders of blood lipids and lipoproteins 450
- Functional anatomy, physiology and investigation of lipid metabolism 450
- Presenting problems in disorders of lipids 453

Disorders of haem synthesis – the porphyrias 458

There is a worldwide trend towards increased use of laboratory-based diagnostic investigations, and biochemical investigations in particular. In the health-care systems of developed countries, it has been estimated that 60–70% of all critical decisions taken in regard to patients, and over 90% of data stored in electronic medical records systems, involve a laboratory service or result.

This chapter covers a diverse group of disorders affecting adults not considered elsewhere in this book, whose primary manifestation is in abnormalities of biochemistry laboratory results, or whose underlying pathophysiology involves disturbance in specific biochemical pathways.

BIOCHEMICAL INVESTIGATIONS

There are three broad reasons why a clinician may request a biochemical laboratory investigation:

- to screen an asymptomatic subject for the presence of disease
- to assist in diagnosis of a patient's presenting complaint
- to monitor changes in test results, as a marker of disease progression or response to treatment.

Contemporary medical practice has become increasingly reliant on laboratory investigation, and in particular, on biochemical investigation. This has been associated with extraordinary improvements in the analytical capacity and speed of laboratory instrumentation and the following operational trends:

- Large central biochemistry laboratories feature extensive use of automation and information technology. Specimens are transported from clinical areas to the laboratory using high-speed transport systems (such as pneumatic tubes) and identified with machine-readable labels (such as bar codes). Laboratory instruments have been miniaturised and integrated with robot transport systems to enable multiple rapid analyses of a single sample. Statistical process control techniques are used to assure the quality of analytical results, and increasingly to monitor other aspects of the laboratory, such as the time taken to complete the analysis ('turn-around time').
- Point-of-care testing (POCT) brings selected laboratory analytical systems into clinical areas, to the patient's bedside or even connected to an individual patient. These systems allow the clinician to receive results almost instantaneously for immediate treatment of the patient, although often with less precision or at greater cost than using a central laboratory.
- The diversity of analyses has widened considerably with the introduction of many techniques borrowed from the chemical or other industries (Box 16.1).

Good medical practice involves the appropriate ordering of laboratory investigations and correct

16.1 Range of analytical modalities used in the clinical biochemistry laboratory

Analytical modality	Analyte	Typical applications
Ion-selective electrodes	Blood gases, electrolytes (e.g. Na, K, Cl)	Point-of-care testing (POCT) High-throughput analysers
Colorimetric chemical reaction or coupled enzymatic reaction	Simple mass or concentration measurement (e.g. creatinine, phosphate) Simple enzyme activity	High-throughput analysers
Ligand assay (usually immunoassay)	Specific proteins Hormones Drugs	Increasingly available for POCT or high-throughput analysers
Chromatography: gas chromatography (GC), high-pressure liquid chromatography (HPLC), thin-layer chromatography (TLC)	Organic compounds	Therapeutic drug monitoring (TDM)
Mass spectroscopy (MS)		Drug screening (e.g. drugs of misuse) Vitamins Biochemical metabolites
Spectrophotometry, turbidimetry, nephelometry, fluorimetry	Haemoglobin derivatives Specific proteins Immunoglobulins	Xanthochromia Lipoproteins Paraproteins
Electrophoresis	Proteins Some enzymes	Paraproteins Isoenzyme analysis
Atomic absorption (AA) **Inductively coupled plasma/mass spectroscopy (ICP-MS)**	Trace elements and metals	Quantitation of heavy metals
Molecular diagnostics	Nucleic acid quantification and/or sequence	Inherited and somatic cell mutations (Ch. 3) Genetic polymorphisms (Ch. 3) Variations in rates of drug metabolism (Ch. 2) Microbial diagnosis (Ch. 6)

interpretation of test results. The key principles, including the concepts of sensitivity and specificity, are described on page 5. Reference ranges for laboratory results are provided in Chapter 29. Many laboratory investigations can be subject to variability arising from incorrect patient preparation (for example, in the fasting or fed state), timing of sample collection (for example, in relation to diurnal variation of hormone levels, or dosage regimens for therapeutic agents), analytical factors (for example, serum versus plasma; use of the correct anticoagulant, or POCT versus central analysis) or artefact (for example, taking a venous sample proximal to the site of an intravenous infusion). It is therefore important for clinical and laboratory staff to communicate effectively and for clinicians to follow local recommendations concerning collection and transport of samples in the appropriate container and with appropriate labelling.

INTEGRATED WATER AND ELECTROLYTE BALANCE

One of the most common uses of the clinical biochemistry laboratory is to monitor electrolyte and acid–base status. The diverse clinical consequences of these biochemical disorders are illustrated in Box 16.2. Some whole-body electrolyte disturbances (notably of sodium) result in major clinical problems with minimal disturbance in measured biochemical parameters. However, these will also be considered for convenience here.

Before considering individual electrolytes and acid-base balance, it is important to review the relationships between them.

Water and electrolyte distribution

The following basic concepts are relevant to understanding the origin, consequences and therapy of many of the fluid and electrolyte disturbances discussed.

In a typical adult male, total body water (TBW) is approximately 60% of body weight (somewhat more for infants and less for women). For an average individual, TBW is about 40 L. Approximately 25 L is located inside cells (the intracellular fluid or ICF), while the remaining 15 L is in the extracellular fluid (ECF) compartment (Fig. 16.1). Most of the ECF (approximately 12 L) is interstitial fluid, which is within the tissues but outside cells, whereas the remainder (about 3 L) is in the plasma compartment.

16.2 Manifestations of disordered water, electrolyte and acid–base status

Primary disturbance	Altered physiology	Clinical effect
Sodium	ECF volume	Circulatory changes
Water	ECF osmolality	Cerebral changes
Potassium	Action potential in excitable tissues	Neuromuscular weakness, cardiac effects
Hydrogen ion	Acid–base balance (pH)	Altered tissue function, respiratory compensation
Magnesium	Cell membrane stability	Neuromuscular, vascular and cardiac effects
Phosphate	Cellular energetics	Widespread tissue effects

(ECF = extracellular fluid)

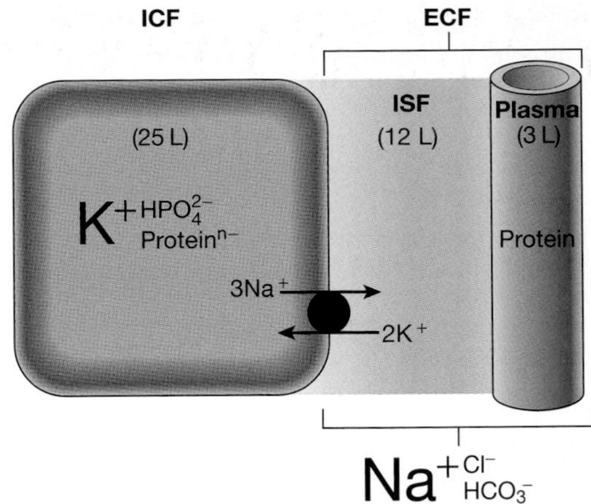

Fig. 16.1 Normal distribution of body water and electrolytes. Schematic representation of volume (L = litres) and composition (dominant ionic species only shown) of the intracellular fluid (ICF) and extracellular fluid (ECF) in a 70 kg male. The main difference in composition between the plasma and interstitial fluid (ISF) is the presence of appreciable concentrations of protein in the plasma but not the ISF.

Figure 16.1 illustrates some of the major differences in composition between the main body fluid compartments. The dominant cation in the ICF is potassium, while the dominant cation in the ECF is sodium. Phosphates and negatively charged proteins constitute the major intracellular anions, while chloride and, to a lesser extent, bicarbonate dominate the ECF anions. An important difference between the plasma and interstitial compartments of the ECF is that only plasma contains significant concentrations of protein.

The major force maintaining the difference in cation concentration between the ICF and ECF is the sodium–potassium pump (Na,K-activated ATPase), which is present in all cell membranes. Maintenance of the cation gradients across cell membranes is essential for many cell processes, including the excitability of conducting tissues such as nerve and muscle. The difference in protein content between the plasma and the interstitial fluid compartment is maintained by the impermeability of the capillary wall to protein. This protein concentration gradient (the colloid osmotic, or oncotic, pressure of the plasma) contributes to the balance of forces across the capillary wall that favour fluid retention within the plasma compartment.

Investigation of water and electrolytes

The most common biochemical test in plasma is called the urea and electrolytes (U&E) test in some parts of the world, and the electrolytes/urea/creatinine (EUC) in others. A guide to its interpretation is shown in Box 16.3. Because the blood consists of both intracellular (red cell) and extracellular (plasma) components, it is important

16

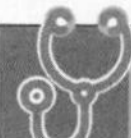

16.3 How to interpret 'U&Es' (urea and electrolytes) or 'EUC' (electrolytes/urea/creatinine) results

Na^+ (sodium)
• Largely reflects reciprocal changes in body water content • See 'Hypernatraemia' and 'Hyponatraemia', pp. 437 and 439
K^+ (potassium)
• May reflect K shifts in and out of cells • Low levels usually mean excessive losses (gastrointestinal or renal) • High levels usually mean renal dysfunction • See 'Hypokalaemia' and 'Hyperkalaemia', pp. 440 and 442
Cl^- (chloride)
• Generally changes in parallel with plasma Na • Low in metabolic alkalosis • High in some forms of metabolic acidosis
HCO_3^- (bicarbonate)
• Abnormal in acid–base disorders • See Box 16.18, p. 445
Urea
• Increased with a fall in glomerular filtration rate (GFR), reduced renal perfusion or urine flow rate, and in high protein intake or catabolic states • See page 466
Creatinine
• Increased with a fall in GFR, in individuals with high muscle mass, and with some drugs • See Fig. 17.2, p. 467

to avoid haemolysis during or after collection of the sample, which causes contamination of the plasma compartment by intracellular elements, particularly potassium. Blood should not be drawn from an arm into which an intravenous infusion is being given, to avoid contamination by the infused fluid. Repeated measurements of plasma electrolytes are frequently necessary when abnormalities have been detected and corrective therapy instituted.

Since the kidney maintains the constancy of body fluids by adjusting urine volume and composition, it is frequently helpful to obtain a sample of urine ('spot' specimen or 24-hour collection) at the time of blood analysis. An example of the use of urine biochemistry is given for the differential diagnosis of hyponatraemia in Box 16.14 (p. 438).

DISORDERS OF SODIUM BALANCE

Functional anatomy and physiology of renal sodium handling

Since the great majority of the body's sodium content is located in the ECF, where it is by far the most abundant cation, total body sodium is a principal determinant of ECF volume. Regulation of sodium excretion by the kidney is crucially important in maintaining normal ECF volume, and plasma volume, in the face of wide variations in sodium intake, which typically may range between 50 and 250 mmol/day.

The functional unit for renal excretion is the nephron (Fig. 16.2). Blood undergoes ultrafiltration in the

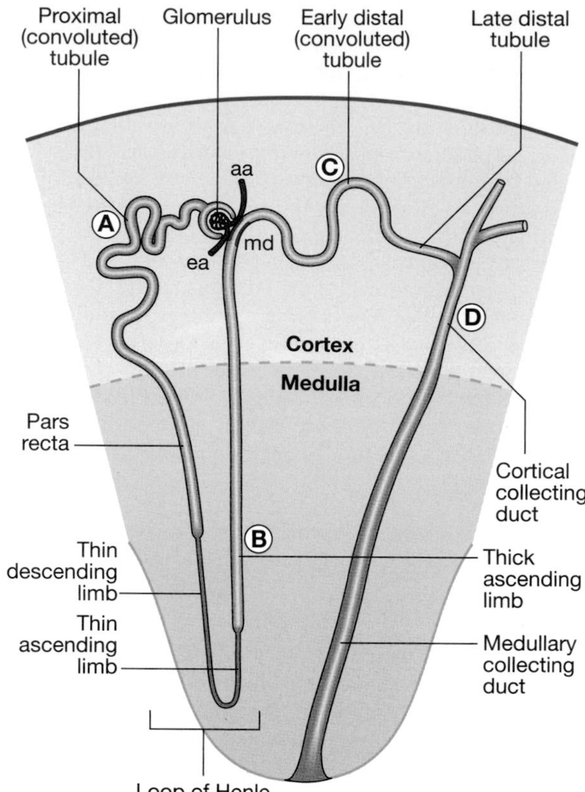

Fig. 16.2 The nephron. Letters A–D refer to tubular segments shown in more detail in Figure 16.3. (aa = afferent arteriole; ea = efferent arteriole; md = macula densa)

glomerulus, generating a fluid that is free from cells and protein and which resembles plasma in its electrolyte composition. This is then delivered into the renal tubules, where reabsorption of water and various electrolytes occurs (more detail on the structure and function of the glomerulus is given in Ch. 17). The glomerular filtration rate (GFR) is approximately 125 mL/min (equivalent to 180 L/day) in a typical adult. Over 99% of this filtered fluid is reabsorbed into the blood in the peritubular capillaries during its passage through successive segments of the nephron, largely as a result of tubular reabsorption of sodium. The processes mediating this sodium reabsorption, and the factors that regulate it, are key to understanding clinical disturbances and pharmacological interventions.

Nephron segments

At least four different functional segments of the nephron can be defined in terms of their mechanism for sodium reabsorption (Fig. 16.3).

Proximal tubule

This is responsible for the reabsorption of some 65% of the filtered sodium load. The cellular mechanisms are complex but some of the key features are shown in Figure 16.3A. Filtered sodium in the luminal fluid enters the cell via several sodium transporters in the apical membrane that couple sodium transport to the entry of glucose, amino acid, phosphate and other organic molecules. Entry of sodium into the tubular cells at this site is also linked to secretion of H^+ ions, through the

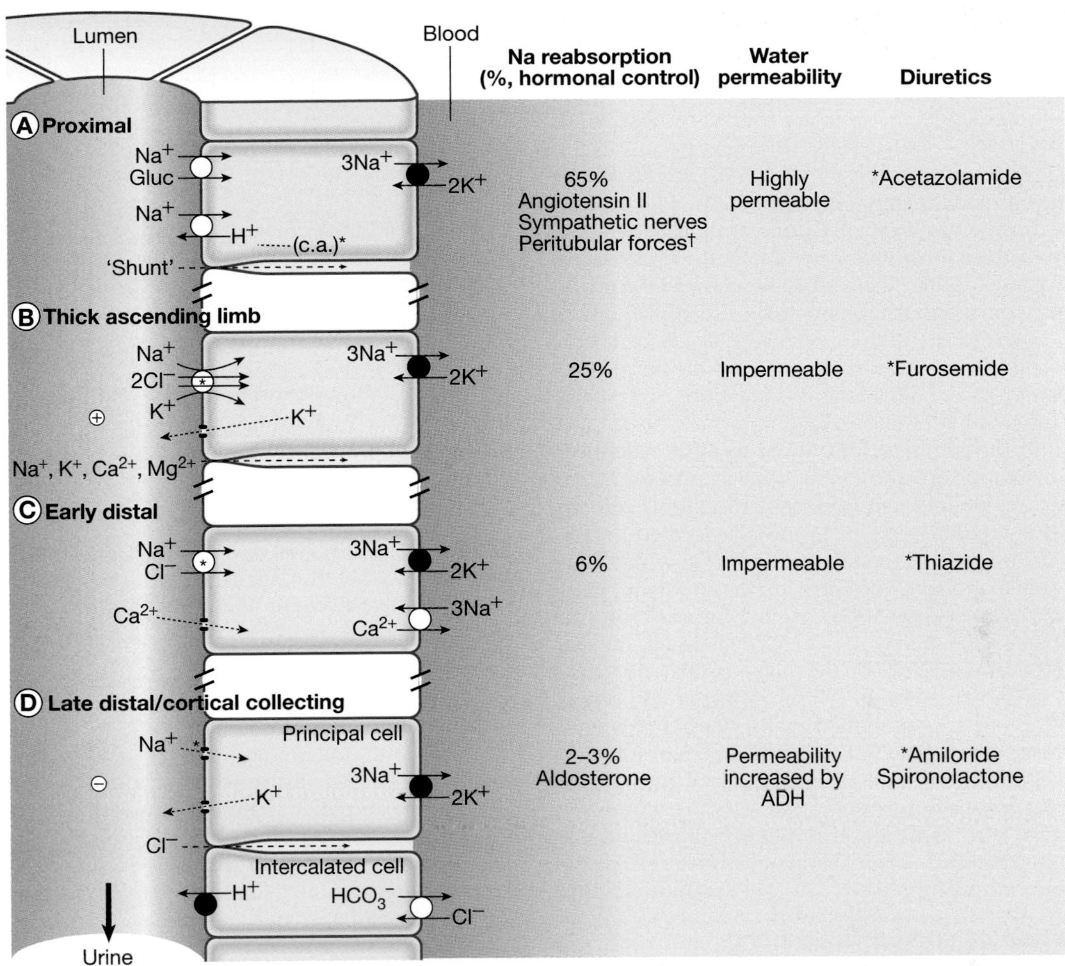

Fig. 16.3 Principal transport mechanisms in segments of the nephron. See text for further details. The apical membrane of the tubular cells is the side facing the lumen, and the basolateral membrane is the side facing the blood. Black circles indicate primary active transport pumps; open circles are carrier molecules without direct linkage to adenosine triphosphate (ATP) hydrolysis. *Site of diuretic action in each segment. †Peritubular forces refers to the hydrostatic and oncotic pressures in the peritubular capillaries. (ADH = antidiuretic hormone; c.a. = carbonic anhydrase)

sodium–hydrogen exchanger (NHE-3). Intracellular H^+ ions are generated within tubular cells from the breakdown of carbonic acid, which is produced from carbon dioxide and water under the influence of carbonic anhydrase. Large numbers of Na,K-ATPase pumps are present on the basolateral membrane of tubular cells that transport sodium from the cells into the blood. In addition, a large component of the transepithelial flux of sodium, water and other dissolved solutes occurs through the gaps *between* the cells (the 'shunt' pathway). Overall, fluid and electrolyte reabsorption is almost isotonic in this segment, as water reabsorption is matched very closely to sodium fluxes. A component of this water flow also passes *through* the cells, via aquaporin-1 (AQP-1) water channels, which are not sensitive to hormonal regulation.

The loop of Henle

The thick ascending limb of the loop of Henle (Fig. 16.3B) reabsorbs a further 25% of the filtered sodium but is impermeable to water, resulting in dilution of the luminal fluid. Again, the primary driving force for sodium reabsorption is the Na,K-ATPase on the basolateral cell membrane, but in this segment sodium enters the cell from the lumen via a specific carrier molecule, the Na,K,2Cl co-transporter ('triple co-transporter', or NKCC2), which allows electroneutral entry of these ions into the renal tubular cell. Some of the potassium accumulated inside the cell recirculates across the apical membrane back into the lumen through a specific potassium channel (ROMK), providing a continuing supply of potassium to match the high concentrations of sodium and chloride available in the lumen. A small positive transepithelial potential difference exists in the lumen of this segment relative to the interstitium, and this serves to drive cations such as sodium, potassium, calcium and magnesium between the cells, forming a reabsorptive shunt pathway.

Early distal tubule

Some 6% of filtered sodium is reabsorbed in the early distal tubule (also called distal convoluted tubule) (Fig. 16.3C), again driven by the activity of the basolateral Na,K-ATPase. In this segment, entry of sodium into the cell from the luminal fluid is via a sodium–chloride co-transport carrier (NCCT). This segment is also impermeable to water, resulting in further dilution of the luminal fluid. There is no significant transepithelial flux of potassium in this segment, but calcium is reabsorbed through the mechanism shown in Figure 16.3C: a basolateral sodium–calcium exchanger leads to low intracellular concentrations of calcium, promoting calcium entry from the luminal fluid through a calcium channel.

Late distal tubule and collecting ducts

The late distal tubule and cortical collecting duct are anatomically and functionally continuous (Fig. 16.3D). Here, sodium entry from the luminal fluid occurs via the epithelial sodium channel (ENaC) through which sodium passes alone, generating a substantial lumen-negative transepithelial potential difference. This sodium flux into the tubular cells is balanced by secretion of potassium and hydrogen ions into the lumen and by reabsorption of chloride ions. Potassium is accumulated in the cell by the basolateral Na,K-ATPase, and passes into the luminal fluid down its electrochemical gradient, through an apical potassium channel (ROMK). Chloride ions pass largely between cells. Hydrogen ion secretion is mediated by an H^+-ATPase located on the luminal membrane of the intercalated cells, which constitute approximately one-third of the epithelial cells in this nephron segment. This part of the nephron has a variable permeability to water, depending on the availability of antidiuretic hormone (ADH, or vasopressin) in the circulation. All ion transport processes in this segment are stimulated by the steroid hormone aldosterone, which can increase sodium reabsorption in this segment to a maximum of 2–3% of the filtered sodium load.

Less than 1% of sodium reabsorption occurs in the medullary collecting duct, where it is inhibited by atrial natriuretic peptide (ANP) and brain natriuretic peptide (BNP).

Regulation of sodium transport

A large number of interrelated mechanisms serve to maintain whole body sodium balance and hence ECF volume by matching urinary sodium excretion to sodium intake (Fig. 16.4).

Important sensing mechanisms include volume receptors in the cardiac atria and the intrathoracic veins, as well as pressure receptors located in the central arterial tree (aortic arch and carotid sinus) and the afferent arterioles within the kidney. A further afferent signal is generated within the kidney itself; the enzyme renin is released from specialised smooth muscle cells in the walls of the afferent and efferent arterioles, at the point where they make contact with the early distal tubule (at the macula densa) to form the juxtaglomerular apparatus. Renin release is stimulated by:

- reduced perfusion pressure in the afferent arteriole
- increased sympathetic nerve activity
- decreased sodium chloride concentration in the distal tubular fluid.

Renin released into the circulation activates the effector mechanisms for sodium retention, which are components of the renin–angiotensin–aldosterone (RAA) system (see Fig. 20.17, p. 771). Renin acts on the peptide substrate, angiotensinogen (manufactured in the liver), producing angiotensin I in the circulation. This in turn is cleaved by angiotensin-converting enzyme (ACE) into angiotensin II, largely in the pulmonary capillary bed. Angiotensin II has multiple actions: it stimulates proximal tubular sodium reabsorption and release of aldosterone from the zona glomerulosa of the adrenal

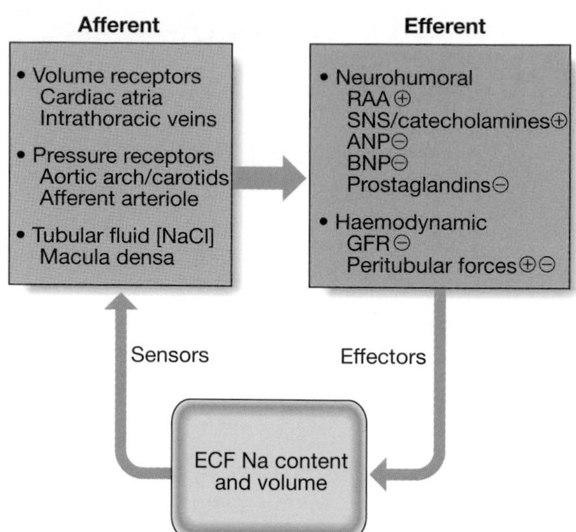

Fig. 16.4 Mechanisms involved in the regulation of sodium transport. (ANP = atrial natriuretic peptide; BNP = brain natriuretic peptide; ECF = extracellular fluid; GFR = glomerular filtration rate; RAA = renin–angiotensin–aldosterone system; SNS = sympathetic nervous system. ⊕ indicates an effect to stimulate Na reabsorption and hence reduce Na excretion, while ⊖ indicates an effect to inhibit Na reabsorption and hence increase Na excretion)

cortex, and causes vasoconstriction of small arterioles. Aldosterone amplifies sodium retention by its action on the cortical collecting duct. The net effect is to restore ECF volume and blood pressure towards normal, thereby correcting the initiating hypovolaemic stimulus.

The sympathetic nervous system also increases sodium retention, both through haemodynamic mechanisms (afferent arteriolar vasoconstriction and GFR reduction) and by direct stimulation of proximal tubular sodium reabsorption. Other humoral mediators, such as the natriuretic peptides, inhibit sodium reabsorption, contributing to natriuresis during periods of sodium and volume excess. Hypovolaemia also has haemodynamic effects that reduce GFR and alter the peritubular physical forces around the proximal tubule, thereby decreasing sodium excretion. Conversely, increased renal perfusion in hypervolaemia and hypertension results in a compensatory increase in sodium excretion.

Presenting problems in disorders of sodium balance

When the balance of sodium intake and excretion is disturbed, any tendency for plasma sodium concentration to change is usually corrected by the osmotic mechanisms controlling water balance (p. 436). As a result, disorders in sodium balance present chiefly as alterations in the ECF volume, resulting in hypovolaemia or oedema, rather than as an alteration in plasma sodium concentration. Clinical manifestations of altered volume are illustrated in Box 16.4.

Sodium depletion

Aetiology and clinical assessment

Sodium depletion can occur occasionally under extreme environmental conditions due to inadequate intake of

16.4 Clinical features of hypovolaemia and hypervolaemia

	Hypovolaemia	Hypervolaemia
Symptoms	Thirst Dizziness on standing Weakness	Ankle swelling Abdominal swelling Breathlessness
Signs	Low JVP Postural hypotension Tachycardia Dry mouth Reduced skin turgor Reduced urine output Weight loss Confusion, stupor	Peripheral oedema Raised JVP Pulmonary crepitations Pleural effusion Ascites Weight gain Hypertension (sometimes)

(JVP = jugular venous pressure)

16.5 Causes of sodium and water depletion

Mechanism	Examples
Inadequate intake	Environmental deprivation, inadequate therapeutic replacement
Gastrointestinal sodium loss	Vomiting, diarrhoea, nasogastric suction, external fistula
Skin sodium loss	Excessive sweating, burns
Renal sodium loss	Diuretic therapy, mineralocorticoid deficiency, tubulointerstitial disease
Internal sequestration*	Bowel obstruction, peritonitis, pancreatitis, crush injury

*A cause of circulatory volume depletion, although total body sodium and water may be normal or increased.

salt, but it is much more commonly due to pathological losses of sodium-containing fluids (Box 16.5). Loss of whole blood, as in acute haemorrhage, is also an obvious cause of hypovolaemia, and elicits the same mechanisms for the conservation of sodium and water.

The diagnosis of hypovolaemia is based on characteristic symptoms and signs (see Box 16.4) in the context of a relevant precipitating illness. Supportive evidence may be obtained from the clinical biochemistry laboratory. Although plasma sodium concentration may not be reduced if salt and water are lost in equal proportions, a number of other parameters are altered during appropriate renal, hormonal and haemodynamic responses to hypovolaemia. During the early stages of hypovolaemia, GFR is maintained while urinary flow rate is reduced as a consequence of activation of sodium- and water-retaining mechanisms in the nephron. Thus, plasma creatinine, which reflects GFR, may be relatively normal, but the plasma urea concentration is typically elevated, since urea excretion is affected by both GFR and urine flow rate. Plasma uric acid may also rise, reflecting activation of compensatory proximal tubular reabsorption. With avid retention of sodium and water, the urine osmolality increases while the urine sodium concentration falls. Under these circumstances, sodium excretion may fall to less than 0.1% of the filtered sodium load.

Management

Management of sodium and water depletion has two main components:

- treat the cause where possible, to stop ongoing salt and water losses
- replace the salt and water deficits, and provide ongoing maintenance requirements, usually by intravenous fluid replacement when depletion is severe.

Intravenous fluid therapy

Box 16.6 shows the daily maintenance requirements for water and electrolytes in a typical adult, and Box 16.7 summarises the composition of some widely available intravenous fluids. The choice of fluid and the rate of administration depend on the clinical circumstances, as assessed at the bedside and from laboratory data, and as described in Box 16.8.

In the absence of normal oral intake (as in a fasting or post-operative patient in hospital), maintenance quantities of fluid, sodium and potassium should be provided. If any deficits or continuing pathological losses are identified, additional fluid and electrolytes will be required. In prolonged periods of fasting (more than a few days), attention also needs to be given to providing sufficient caloric and nutritional intake to prevent excessive catabolism of body energy stores (p. 120).

The choice of intravenous fluid therapy in the treatment of significant hypovolaemia relates to the concepts in Figure 16.1 (p. 429). If fluid containing neither sodium nor protein is given, it will distribute in the body fluid compartments in proportion to the normal distribution of total body water. Thus, giving 1 L of 5% dextrose will contribute relatively little (approximately 3/40 of the infused volume) towards expansion of the plasma volume. This makes 5% dextrose ineffective at restoring the circulation and perfusion of vital organs. Intravenous infusion of an isotonic (normal) saline solution, on the other hand, results in more effective expansion of the extracellular fluid, although a minority of the infused volume (some 3/15) will contribute to plasma volume.

16.6 Basic daily water and electrolyte requirements

	Requirement per kg	Typical 70 kg adult
Water	35–45 mL/kg	2.5–3.0 L/day
Sodium	1.5–2 mmol/kg	100–140 mmol/day
Potassium	1.0–1.5 mmol/kg	70–100 mmol/day

16.7 Composition of some isotonic intravenous fluids

Fluid	D-glucose	Calories	Na^+ (mmol/L)	Cl^- (mmol/L)	Other (mmol/L)
5% dextrose	50 g	200	0	0	0
Normal (0.9%) saline	0	0	154	154	0
Hartmann's solution	0	0	131	111	K^+ 5 Ca^{2+} 2 $Lactate^-$ 29

16

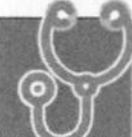

16.8 How to assess fluid and electrolyte balance in hospitalised patients

Step 1: assess clinical volume status

- Examine patient for signs of hypovolaemia or hypervolaemia (see Box 16.4)
- Check daily weight change

Step 2: review fluid balance chart

- Check total volumes IN and OUT on previous day (IN–OUT is positive by ~400 mL in normal balance, reflecting insensible fluid losses of ~800 mL and metabolic water generation of ~400 mL)
- Check cumulative change in daily fluid balance over previous 3–5 days
- Correlate chart figures with weight change and clinical volume status to estimate net fluid balance

Step 3: assess ongoing pathological process

- Check losses from gastrointestinal tract and surgical drains
- Estimate increased insensible losses (e.g. in fever) and internal sequestration ('third space')

Step 4: check plasma U&Es (see Box 16.3)

- Check plasma Na as marker of relative water balance
- Check plasma K as a guide to extracellular K balance
- Check HCO_3 as a clue to acid–base disorder
- Check urea and creatinine to monitor renal function

Step 5: prescribe appropriate IV fluid replacement therapy

- Replace basic water and electrolytes each day (see Box 16.6)
- Allow for anticipated oral intake and pathological fluid loss
- Adjust amounts of water (if IV, usually given as isotonic 5% dextrose), sodium and potassium according to plasma electrolyte results

EBM 16.9 Albumin infusions in hypovolaemia

'For patients with hypovolaemia there is no evidence that albumin reduces mortality when compared with cheaper alternatives such as saline.'

- Roberts I et al. Human albumin solution for resuscitation and volume expansion in critically ill patients. Cochrane Database of Systematic Reviews, 2011, issue 11. Art. no.: CD001208.

Carrying this reasoning further, it might be expected that a solution containing plasma proteins would be largely retained within the plasma, thus maximally expanding the circulating fluid volume and improving tissue perfusion. However, recent clinical studies have not shown any overall advantage of infusions containing albumin in the treatment of acute hypovolaemia (Box 16.9). Resuscitation fluids containing synthetic colloids such as carbohydrate polymers should not be used in the acute resuscitation of volume-depleted patients since they offer no benefit over crystalloids and are associated with increased mortality (see Box 17.21, p. 482).

Sodium excess

Aetiology and clinical assessment

In patients with normal cardiac and renal function, excessive intakes of salt and water are compensated for by increased excretion and do not lead to clinically obvious features of sodium and water overload. However, patients with cardiac, renal or hepatic disease frequently present with signs and symptoms of sodium excess (Fig. 16.5). This does not always involve an increase in circulating blood volume, since the excess fluid often leaks out of the capillaries to expand the interstitial compartment of the ECF, especially in diseases like nephrotic syndrome and chronic liver disease that cause hypoalbuminaemia. Important causes of sodium excess are shown in Box 16.10.

16.10 Causes of sodium and water excess

Mechanism	Examples
Impaired renal function (Ch. 17)	Primary renal disease
Primary hyperaldosteronism* (p. 780)	Conn's syndrome
Secondary hyperaldosteronism (see Fig. 16.5)	Congestive cardiac failure Cirrhotic liver disease Nephrotic syndrome Protein-losing enteropathy Malnutrition Idiopathic/cyclical oedema Renal artery stenosis*

*Conditions in this table *other than* primary hyperaldosteronism and renal artery stenosis are typically associated with generalised oedema.

Peripheral oedema is the most common physical sign of ECF volume expansion (p. 478). The three most common systemic disorders associated with sodium and fluid overload are cardiac failure, cirrhosis and nephrotic syndrome. In each of these, sodium retention is largely a secondary response to circulatory insufficiency caused by the primary disorder, as illustrated in Figure 16.5. The pathophysiology is different in renal failure, when the primary cause of volume expansion is the profound reduction in GFR impairing sodium and water excretion, and secondary tubular mechanisms are of lesser importance. Further detail on each of these conditions is given in other chapters of this book.

Management

The management of ECF volume overload involves a number of components:

- specific treatment directed at the underlying cause, such as ACE inhibitors in heart failure and corticosteroids in minimal change nephropathy
- restriction of dietary sodium (to 50–80 mmol/day) to match the diminished excretory capacity
- treatment with diuretics.

Diuretic therapy

Diuretics are important in the treatment of conditions of ECF expansion due to salt and water retention and in hypertension (p. 606). They act by inhibiting sodium reabsorption at various locations along the nephron (see Fig. 16.3, p. 431). Their potency and adverse effects relate to their mechanism and site of action.

Mechanisms of action

In the proximal tubule, carbonic anhydrase inhibitors such as acetazolamide inhibit the intracellular production of H^+ ions, thereby reducing the fraction of sodium reabsorption that is exchanged for H^+ by the apical

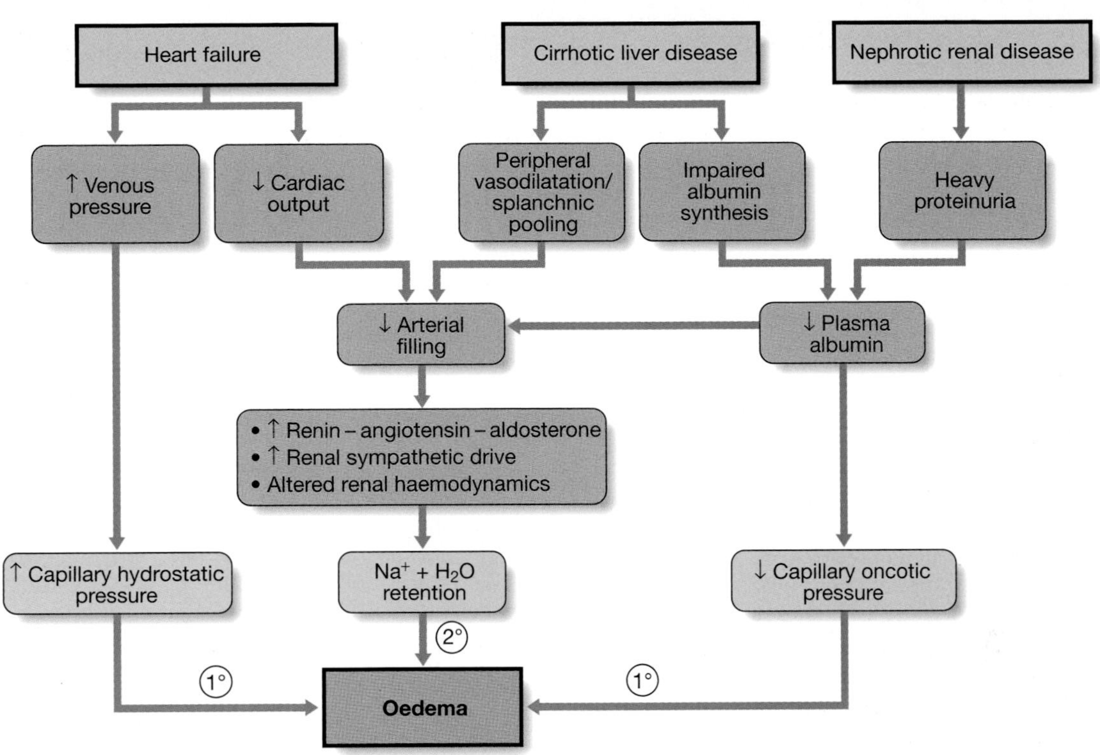

Fig. 16.5 Secondary mechanisms causing sodium excess and oedema in cardiac failure, cirrhosis and nephrotic syndrome. Primary renal retention of Na and water may also contribute to oedema formation when GFR is significantly reduced (see Box 16.10 and p. 478).

membrane sodium–hydrogen exchanger. These drugs have limited usefulness, however, since only a small fraction of proximal sodium reabsorption uses this mechanism, and much of the sodium that is not reabsorbed can be reabsorbed by downstream segments of the nephron.

In the thick ascending limb of the loop of Henle, loop diuretics such as furosemide inhibit sodium reabsorption by blocking the action of the apical membrane Na,K,2Cl co-transporter. Because this segment reabsorbs a large fraction of the filtered sodium, these drugs are potent diuretics, and are commonly used in diseases associated with significant oedema.

In the early distal tubule, thiazides inhibit sodium reabsorption by blocking the sodium–chloride co-transporter in the apical membrane. Since this segment reabsorbs a much smaller fraction of the filtered sodium, these are less potent than loop diuretics, but are widely used in the treatment of hypertension and less severe oedema.

All diuretic drugs acting in the proximal, loop and early distal segments cause excretion not only of sodium (and with it water), but also of potassium. This occurs largely as a result of delivery of increased amounts of sodium to the late distal/cortical collecting ducts, where sodium reabsorption is associated with excretion of potassium, and is amplified if circulating aldosterone levels are high. By contrast, drugs acting to inhibit sodium reabsorption in the late distal/cortical collecting duct segment are associated with reduced potassium secretion, and are described as 'potassium-sparing'. One target of drug action in this segment is the apical sodium channel in the principal cells (see Fig. 16.3), which is blocked by drugs such as amiloride and triamterene. Another is the mineralocorticoid receptor, to which binding of aldosterone is blocked by spironolactone and eplerenone.

An important feature of the most commonly used diuretic drugs (furosemide, thiazides and amiloride) is that they act on their target transport molecules from the luminal side of the tubular epithelium. Since they are highly protein-bound in the plasma, very little reaches the urinary fluid by glomerular filtration, but there are active transport mechanisms for secreting organic acids and bases, including these drugs, across the proximal tubular wall into the lumen, resulting in adequate drug concentrations being delivered to later tubular segments. This secretory process may be impaired by certain other drugs, and also by accumulated organic anions as occurs in chronic renal failure and chronic liver failure, leading to resistance to diuretics.

Osmotic diuretics act independently of specific transport mechanism. They are freely filtered at the glomerulus but are not reabsorbed by any part of the tubular system. They retain fluid osmotically within the tubular lumen and limit the extent of sodium reabsorption in multiple segments. Mannitol is the most commonly used osmotic diuretic. It is given by intravenous infusion to achieve short-term diuresis in conditions such as cerebral oedema.

Clinical use of diuretics

In the selection of a diuretic drug for hypertension or oedema disorders, the following principles should be observed:

- Use the minimum effective dose.
- Use for as short a period of time as necessary.
- Monitor regularly for adverse effects.

16.11 Adverse effects of loop-acting and thiazide diuretics

Renal side-effects	
• Hypovolaemia • Hyponatraemia • Hypokalaemia • Metabolic alkalosis	• Hyperuricaemia • Hypomagnesaemia • Hypercalciuria (loop) • Hypocalciuria (thiazide)
Metabolic side-effects	
• Glucose intolerance/ hyperglycaemia	• Hyperlipidaemia
Miscellaneous side-effects	
• Hypersensitivity reactions • Erectile dysfunction	• Acute pancreatitis/ cholecystitis (thiazides)

The choice of diuretic will be determined by the required potency, the presence of coexistent conditions, and the anticipated side-effect profile.

Adverse effects encountered with the most commonly used classes of diuretic (loop drugs and thiazide drugs) are summarised in Box 16.11. Volume depletion and electrolyte disorders commonly occur, as predicted from their mechanism of action. The metabolic side-effects listed are rarely of clinical significance and may reflect effects on K^+ channels that influence insulin secretion (p. 800). Since most drugs from these classes are sulphonamides, there is a relatively high incidence of hypersensitivity reactions, and occasional idiosyncratic side-effects in a variety of organ systems.

The side-effect profile of the potassium-sparing diuretics differs in a number of important respects from that of other diuretics. The disturbances in potassium, magnesium and acid–base balance are in the opposite direction, so that normal or increased levels of potassium and magnesium are found in the blood, and there is a tendency to metabolic acidosis, especially when renal function is impaired.

Diuretic resistance is encountered under a variety of circumstances, including impaired renal function, activation of sodium-retaining mechanisms, impaired oral bioavailability (for example, in patients with gastrointestinal disease) and decreased renal blood flow. In these circumstances, short-term intravenous therapy with a loop-acting agent such as furosemide may be useful. Combinations of diuretics administered orally may also increase potency. Either a loop or a thiazide drug can be combined with a potassium-sparing drug, and all three classes can be used together for short periods, with carefully supervised clinical and laboratory monitoring.

DISORDERS OF WATER BALANCE

Daily water intake can vary from about 500 mL to several litres a day. While a certain amount of water is lost through the stool, sweat and the respiratory tract ('insensible losses', approximately 800 mL/day), and some water is generated by oxidative metabolism ('metabolic water', approximately 400 mL/day), the kidneys are chiefly responsible for adjusting water excretion to maintain constancy of body water content and body fluid osmolality (reference range 280–295 mmol/kg).

Functional anatomy and physiology of renal water handling

While regulation of total ECF volume is largely achieved through renal control of sodium excretion, mechanisms also exist to allow for the excretion of a 'pure' water load when water intake is high, and for retention of water when access is restricted.

These functions are largely achieved by the loop of Henle and the collecting ducts. The counter-current configuration of flow in adjacent limbs of the loop (see Fig. 16.2, p. 430), involves osmotic movement of water from the descending limbs and reabsorption of solute from neighbouring ascending limbs, to set up a gradient of osmolality from isotonic (like plasma) in the renal cortex to hypertonic (around 1200 mmol/kg) in the inner part of the medulla. At the same time, the fluid emerging from the thick ascending limb is hypotonic compared to plasma, because it has been diluted by the reabsorption of sodium, but not water, from the thick ascending limb and early distal tubule. As this dilute fluid passes from the cortex through the collecting duct system to the renal pelvis, it traverses the medullary interstitial gradient of osmolality set up by the operation of the loop of Henle, and water is reabsorbed.

Further changes in the urine osmolality on passage through the collecting ducts depend on the circulating level of antidiuretic hormone (ADH), which is released by the posterior pituitary gland under conditions of increased plasma osmolality or hypovolaemia (Ch. 20).

- When water intake is high and plasma osmolality is normal or low-normal, ADH levels are suppressed and the collecting ducts remain impermeable to water. The luminal fluid osmolality remains low, resulting in the excretion of a dilute urine (minimum osmolality approximately 50 mmol/kg in a healthy young person).
- When water intake is restricted and plasma osmolality is high, or in the presence of plasma volume depletion, ADH levels rise. This causes water permeability of the collecting ducts to increase through binding of ADH to the V2 receptor, which enhances collecting duct water permeability through the insertion of aquaporin (AQP-2) channels into the luminal cell membrane. This results in osmotic reabsorption of water along the entire length of the collecting duct, with maximum urine osmolality approaching that in the medullary tip (up to 1200 mmol/kg).

Parallel to these changes in ADH release are changes in water-seeking behaviour triggered by the sensation of thirst, which also becomes activated as plasma osmolality rises.

In summary, for adequate dilution of the urine there must be:

- adequate solute delivery to the loop of Henle and early distal tubule
- normal function of the loop of Henle and early distal tubule
- absence of ADH in the circulation.

If any of these processes is faulty, water retention and hyponatraemia may result.

Conversely, to achieve concentration of the urine there must be:

- adequate solute delivery to the loop of Henle
- normal function of the loop of Henle
- ADH release into the circulation
- ADH action on the collecting ducts.

Failure of any of these steps may result in inappropriate water loss and hypernatraemia.

Presenting problems in disorders of water balance

Disturbances in body water balance, in the absence of changes in sodium balance, alter plasma sodium concentration and hence plasma osmolality. When extracellular osmolality changes abruptly, water flows rapidly across cell membranes with resultant cell swelling (during hypo-osmolality) or shrinkage (during hyper-osmolality). Cerebral function is very sensitive to such volume changes, particularly brain swelling during hypo-osmolality, which can lead to an increase in intracerebral pressure and reduced cerebral perfusion.

Hyponatraemia

Aetiology and clinical assessment

Hyponatraemia (plasma Na < 135 mmol/L) is a common electrolyte abnormality, which is often asymptomatic but which can also be associated with profound disturbances of cerebral function, manifesting as anorexia, nausea, vomiting, confusion, lethargy, seizures and coma. The likelihood of symptoms occurring is related more to the speed at which electrolyte abnormalities develop rather than their severity. When plasma osmolality falls rapidly, water flows into cerebral cells, which become swollen and ischaemic. However, when hyponatraemia develops gradually, cerebral neurons have time to respond by reducing intracellular osmolality, through excreting potassium and reducing synthesis of intracellular organic osmolytes (Fig. 16.6). The osmotic gradient favouring water movement into the cells is thus reduced and symptoms are avoided.

The causes of hyponatraemia are best categorised according to any associated changes in the ECF volume (Box 16.12). In all cases, there is retention of water relative to sodium, and it is clinical examination rather than the biochemical results that gives a clue to the underlying cause.

Artefactual causes of hyponatraemia should also be considered. These can occur in the presence of severe hyperlipidaemia or hyperproteinaemia, when the aqueous fraction of the plasma specimen is reduced because of the volume occupied by the macromolecules (although this artefact is dependent on the assay technology). Transient hyponatraemia may also occur due to osmotic shifts of water out of cells during hyperosmolar states caused by acute hyperglycaemia or by mannitol infusion.

Hyponatraemia with hypovolaemia

Patients who have hyponatraemia in association with a sodium deficit ('depletional hyponatraemia') have clinical features of hypovolaemia (see Box 16.4, p. 433) and supportive laboratory findings, including low urinary

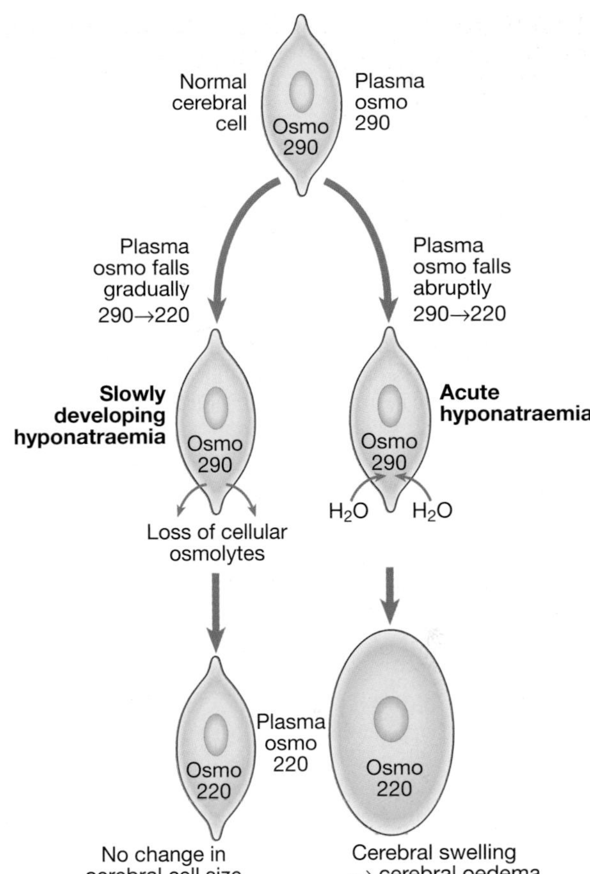

Fig. 16.6 Hyponatraemia and the brain. Numbers represent osmolality (osmo) in mmol/kg.

16.12 Causes of hyponatraemia

Volume status	Examples
Hypovolaemic (sodium deficit with a relatively smaller water deficit)	Renal sodium losses Diuretic therapy (especially thiazides) Adrenocortical failure Gastrointestinal sodium losses Vomiting Diarrhoea Skin sodium losses Burns
Euvolaemic (water retention alone)	Primary polydipsia Excessive electrolyte-free water infusion SIADH Hypothyroidism
Hypervolaemic (sodium retention with relatively greater water retention)	Congestive cardiac failure Cirrhosis Nephrotic syndrome Chronic renal failure (during free water intake)

(SIADH = syndrome of inappropriate antidiuretic hormone secretion; see Box 16.13).

sodium concentration (< 30 mmol/L) and elevated plasma renin activity. The cause of sodium loss is usually apparent; common examples are shown in Box 16.12.

Hyponatraemia with euvolaemia

Patients in this group (dilutional hyponatraemia) have no major disturbance of body sodium content and are clinically euvolaemic. Excess body water may be the result of abnormally high intake, either orally (primary polydipsia) or as a result of medically infused fluids (as intravenous dextrose solutions, or by absorption of sodium-free bladder irrigation fluid after prostatectomy).

Water retention also occurs in the syndrome of inappropriate secretion of ADH (SIADH). In this condition, an endogenous source of ADH (either cerebral or tumour-derived) promotes water retention by the kidney in the absence of an appropriate physiological stimulus (Box 16.13). The clinical diagnosis requires the patient to be euvolaemic, with no evidence of cardiac, renal or hepatic disease potentially associated with hyponatraemia. Other non-osmotic stimuli that cause release of ADH (pain, stress, nausea) should also be excluded. Supportive laboratory findings are shown in Box 16.13. In this situation, plasma concentrations of sodium, chloride, urea and uric acid are low with a correspondingly reduced osmolality. Urine osmolality, which should physiologically be maximally dilute (approximately 50 mmol/kg) in the face of low plasma osmolality, is higher than at least 100 mmol/kg and indeed is typically higher than the plasma osmolality. The urine sodium concentration is typically high (> 30 mmol/L), consistent with euvolaemia and lack of compensatory factors promoting sodium retention.

Hyponatraemia with hypervolaemia

In this situation, excess water retention is associated with sodium retention and volume expansion, as in heart failure, liver disease or kidney disease.

Investigations

Plasma and urine electrolytes and osmolality (Box 16.14) are usually the only tests required to classify the hyponatraemia. Doubt about clinical signs of ECF volume may be resolved with measurement of plasma renin activity.

16.13 Syndrome of inappropriate antidiuretic hormone secretion (SIADH): causes and diagnosis

Causes

- Tumours
- CNS disorders: stroke, trauma, infection, psychosis, porphyria
- Pulmonary disorders: pneumonia, tuberculosis, obstructive lung disease
- Drugs: anticonvulsants, psychotropics, antidepressants, cytotoxics, oral hypoglycaemic agents, opiates
- Idiopathic

Diagnosis

- Low plasma sodium concentration (typically < 130 mmol/L)
- Low plasma osmolality (< 270 mmol/kg)
- Urine osmolality not minimally low (typically > 150 mmol/kg)
- Urine sodium concentration not minimally low (> 30 mmol/L)
- Low-normal plasma urea, creatinine, uric acid
- Exclusion of other causes of hyponatraemia (see Box 16.12)
- Appropriate clinical context (above)

16.14 Urine Na and osmolality in the differential diagnosis of hyponatraemia*

Urine Na (mmol/L)	Urine osmolality (mmol/kg)	Possible diagnoses
Low (< 30)	Low (< 100)	Primary polydipsia Malnutrition Beer excess
Low	High (> 150)	Salt depletion Hypovolaemia
High (> 40)	Low	Diuretic action (acute phase)
High	High	SIADH Cerebral salt-wasting Adrenal insufficiency

*Urine analysis may give results of indeterminate significance, and in this case the diagnosis depends on a comprehensive clinical assessment.

Measurement of ADH is not generally helpful in distinguishing between these categories of hyponatraemia. This is because ADH is activated both in hypovolaemic states and in most chronic hypervolaemic states, as the impaired circulation in those disorders activates ADH release through non-osmotic mechanisms. Indeed, these disorders may have higher circulating ADH levels than patients with SIADH. The only disorders listed in Box 16.12 in which ADH is suppressed are primary polydipsia and iatrogenic water intoxication, where the hypo-osmolar state inhibits ADH release from the pituitary.

Management

The treatment of hyponatraemia is critically dependent on its rate of development, severity and underlying cause. If hyponatraemia has developed rapidly (over hours to days), and there are signs of cerebral oedema such as obtundation or convulsions, sodium levels should be restored to normal rapidly by infusion of hypertonic (3%) sodium chloride. A common approach is to give an initial bolus of 100 mL, which may be repeated once or twice over the initial hours of observation, depending on the neurological response and rise in plasma sodium.

On the other hand, rapid correction of hyponatraemia that has developed slowly (over weeks to months) can be hazardous, since brain cells adapt to slowly developing hypo-osmolality by reducing the intracellular osmolality, thus maintaining normal cell volume (see Fig. 16.6). Under these conditions, an abrupt increase in extracellular osmolality can lead to water shifting out of neurons, abruptly reducing their volume and causing them to detach from their myelin sheaths. The resulting 'myelinolysis' can produce permanent structural and functional damage to mid-brain structures, and is generally fatal. The rate of correction of the plasma Na concentration in chronic asymptomatic hyponatraemia should not exceed 10 mmol/L/day, and an even slower rate is generally safer.

The underlying cause should be treated. For hypovolaemic patients, this involves controlling the source of sodium loss, and administering intravenous saline if clinically warranted. Patients with dilutional hyponatraemia generally respond to fluid restriction in the range of 600–1000 mL/day, accompanied where possible by withdrawal of the precipitating stimulus (such as drugs causing SIADH). If the response of plasma sodium is inadequate, treatment with demeclocycline (600–900 mg/day) may be of value by enhancing water excretion, through its inhibitory effect on responsiveness to ADH in the collecting duct. An effective alternative for subjects with persistent hyponatraemia due to prolonged SIADH is oral urea therapy (30–45 g/day), which provides a solute load to promote water excretion. Where available, oral vasopressin receptor antagonists such as tolvaptan may be used to block the ADH-mediated component of water retention in a range of hyponatraemic conditions. Hypervolaemic patients with hyponatraemia need treatment of the underlying condition, accompanied by cautious use of diuretics in conjunction with strict fluid restriction. Potassium-sparing diuretics may be particularly useful in this context where there is significant secondary hyperaldosteronism.

Hypernatraemia

Aetiology and clinical assessment

Just as hyponatraemia represents a failure of the mechanisms for diluting the urine during free access to water, so hypernatraemia (plasma Na > 148 mmol/L) reflects inadequate concentration of the urine in the face of restricted water intake. This can be due to failure to generate an adequate medullary concentration gradient (low GFR states, loop diuretic therapy), but more commonly it is due to failure of the ADH system, either because of pituitary damage (central or 'cranial' diabetes insipidus, p. 794) or because the collecting duct cells are unable to respond to circulating ADH (nephrogenic diabetes insipidus).

Patients with hypernatraemia generally have reduced cerebral function, either as a primary problem or as a consequence of the hypernatraemia itself, which results in dehydration of neurons and brain shrinkage. In the presence of an intact thirst mechanism and preserved capacity to obtain and ingest water, hypernatraemia may not progress very far. If adequate water is not obtained, dizziness, confusion, weakness and ultimately coma and death can result.

The causes of hypernatraemia are best grouped according to the associated disturbance, if any, in total body sodium content (Box 16.15). It is important to remember that hypernatraemia may be iatrogenic, and to reiterate that, whatever the underlying cause, sustained or severe hypernatraemia generally reflects an impaired thirst mechanism or responsiveness to thirst.

Management

Treatment of hypernatraemia depends on both the rate of development and the underlying cause. If there is reason to think that the condition has developed rapidly, neuronal shrinkage may be acute and relatively rapid correction may be attempted. This can be achieved by infusing an appropriate volume of intravenous fluid (isotonic 5% dextrose or hypotonic 0.45% saline) at an initial rate of 50–70 mL/hour. However, in older, institutionalised patients it is more likely that the disorder has developed slowly, and extreme caution should be exercised in lowering plasma sodium to avoid the risk of cerebral oedema. Where possible, the underlying cause should also be addressed (see Box 16.15).

16.15 Causes of hypernatraemia

Volume status	Examples
Hypovolaemic (sodium deficit with a relatively greater water deficit)	Renal sodium losses Diuretic therapy (especially osmotic diuretic, or loop diuretic during water restriction) Glycosuria (HONK, p. 814) Gastrointestinal Na losses Colonic diarrhoea Skin sodium losses Excessive sweating
Euvolaemic (water deficit alone)	Diabetes insipidus (central or nephrogenic) (p. 794)
Hypervolaemic (sodium retention with relatively less water retention)	Enteral or parenteral feeding IV or oral salt administration Chronic renal failure (during water restriction)

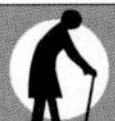

16.16 Hyponatraemia and hypernatraemia in old age

- **Decline in GFR:** older patients are predisposed to both hyponatraemia and hypernatraemia, mainly because, as GFR declines with age, the capacity of the kidney to dilute or concentrate the urine is impaired.
- **Hyponatraemia:** occurs when free water intake continues in the presence of a low dietary salt intake and/or diuretic drugs (particularly thiazides).
- **ADH release:** water retention is aggravated by any condition that stimulates ADH release, especially heart failure. Moreover, the ADH response to non-osmotic stimuli may be brisker in older subjects. Appropriate water restriction may be a key part of management.
- **Hypernatraemia:** occurs when water intake is inadequate, due to physical restrictions preventing access to drinks and/or blunted thirst. Both are frequently present in patients with advanced dementia or following a severe stroke.
- **Dietary salt:** hypernatraemia is aggravated if dietary supplements or medications with a high sodium content (especially effervescent preparations) are administered. Appropriate prescription of fluids is a key part of management.

Elderly patients are predisposed, in different circumstances, to both hyponatraemia and hypernatraemia, and a high index of suspicion of these electrolyte disturbances is appropriate in elderly patients with recent alterations in behaviour (Box 16.16).

DISORDERS OF POTASSIUM BALANCE

Potassium is the major intracellular cation (see Fig. 16.1, p. 429), and the steep concentration gradient for potassium across the cell membrane of excitable cells plays an important part in generating the resting membrane potential and allowing the propagation of the action potential that is crucial to normal functioning of nerve, muscle and cardiac tissues. Control of body potassium balance is described below.

Changes in the distribution of potassium between the ICF and ECF compartments can alter plasma potassium concentration, without any overall change in total body potassium content. Potassium is driven into the cells by extracellular alkalosis and by a number of hormones, including insulin, catecholamines (through the β_2 receptor) and aldosterone. Any of these factors can produce hypokalaemia, whereas extracellular acidosis, lack of insulin, and insufficiency or blockade of catecholamines or aldosterone can cause hyperkalaemia due to efflux of potassium from the intracellular compartment.

Functional anatomy and physiology of renal potassium handling

In the steady state, the kidneys excrete some 90% of the daily intake of potassium, typically 80–100 mmol/day. Potassium is freely filtered at the glomerulus; around 65% is reabsorbed in the proximal tubule and a further 25% in the thick ascending limb of the loop of Henle. Little potassium is transported in the early distal tubule but a significant secretory flux of potassium into the urine occurs in the late distal tubule and cortical collecting duct to ensure that the amount removed from the blood is proportional to the ingested load.

The mechanism for potassium secretion in the distal parts of the nephron is shown in Figure 16.3D (p. 431). Movement of potassium from blood to lumen is dependent on active uptake across the basal cell membrane by the Na,K-ATPase, followed by diffusion of potassium through a luminal membrane potassium channel (ROMK) into the tubular fluid. The electrochemical gradient for potassium movement into the lumen is contributed to both by the high intracellular potassium concentration and by the negative luminal potential difference relative to the blood.

A number of factors influence the rate of potassium secretion. Luminal influences include the rate of sodium delivery and fluid flow through the late distal tubule and cortical collecting ducts. This is a major factor responsible for the increased potassium loss that accompanies diuretic treatment. Agents interfering with the generation of the negative luminal potential also impair potassium secretion, and this is the basis of reduced potassium secretion associated with potassium-sparing diuretics such as amiloride. Factors acting on the blood side of this tubular segment include plasma potassium and pH, such that hyperkalaemia and alkalosis both enhance potassium secretion directly. However, the most important factor in the acute and chronic adjustment of potassium secretion to match metabolic potassium load is aldosterone.

As shown in Figure 16.7, a negative feedback relationship exists between the plasma potassium concentration and aldosterone. In addition to its regulation by the renin–angiotensin system (see Fig. 20.19, p. 771), aldosterone is released from the adrenal cortex in direct response to an elevated plasma potassium. Aldosterone then acts on the kidney to enhance potassium secretion, hydrogen secretion and sodium reabsorption, in the late distal tubule and cortical collecting ducts. The resulting increased excretion of potassium maintains plasma potassium within a narrow range (3.3–4.7 mmol/L). Factors that reduce angiotensin II levels may indirectly affect potassium balance by blunting the rise in aldosterone that would otherwise be provoked by hyperkalaemia. This accounts for the increased risk of hyperkalaemia during therapy with ACE inhibitors and related drugs.

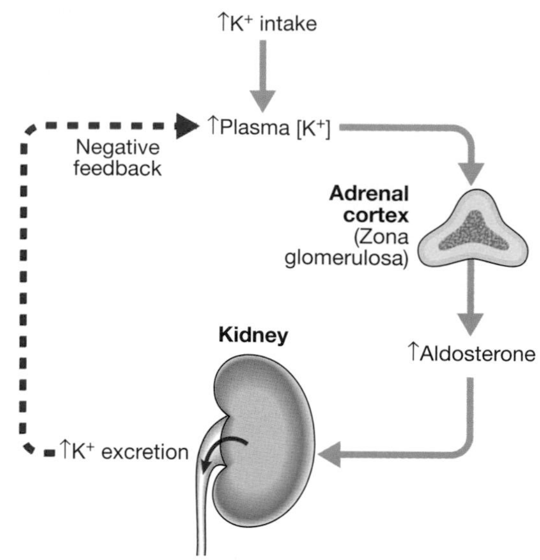

Fig. 16.7 Feedback control of plasma potassium concentration.

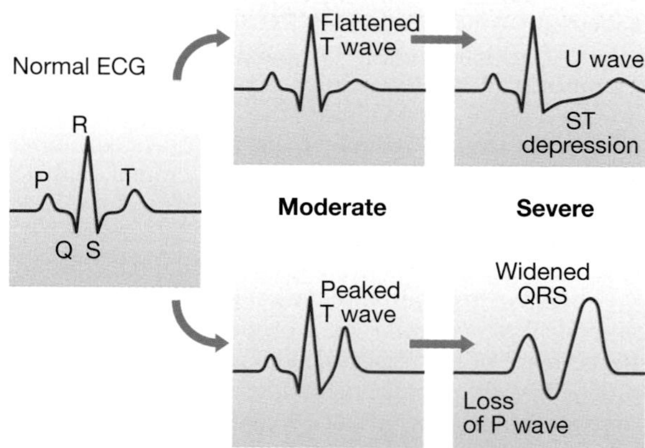

Fig. 16.8 The ECG in hypokalaemia and hyperkalaemia.

Presenting problems in disorders of potassium balance

Hypokalaemia

Aetiology and clinical assessment

Patients with mild hypokalaemia (plasma K 3.0–3.3 mmol/L) are generally asymptomatic, but more profound reductions in plasma potassium often lead to muscular weakness and associated tiredness. Ventricular ectopic beats or more serious arrhythmias may occur and the arrhythmogenic effects of digoxin may be potentiated. Typical ECG changes occur, affecting the T wave in particular (Fig. 16.8). Functional bowel obstruction may occur due to paralytic ileus. Long-standing hypokalaemia causes renal tubular damage (hypokalaemic nephropathy) and interferes with the tubular response to ADH (acquired nephrogenic diabetes insipidus), resulting in polyuria and polydipsia.

The main causes of hypokalaemia and an approach to the differential diagnosis are shown in Figure 16.9.

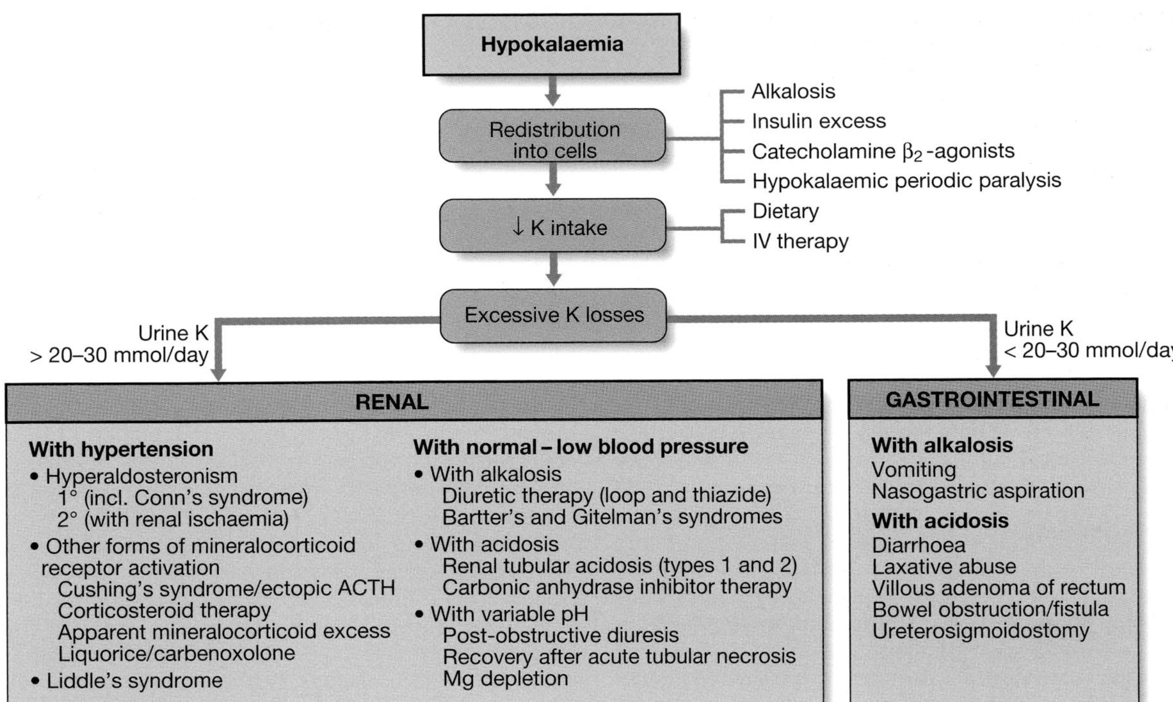

Fig. 16.9 Diagnostic decision tree for hypokalaemia. (ACTH = adrenocorticotrophic hormone)

Redistribution of potassium into cells should be considered, since correction of the factors involved (see above) may be sufficient to correct the plasma concentration. An inadequate intake of potassium can contribute to hypokalaemia but is unlikely to be the only cause, except in extreme cases. Generally, hypokalaemia is indicative of abnormal potassium loss from the body, either through the kidney or the gastrointestinal tract. When there is no obvious clinical clue to which pathway is involved, measurement of urinary potassium may be helpful; if the kidney is the route of potassium loss, the urine potassium is high (> 30 mmol/day), whereas if potassium is being lost through the gastrointestinal tract, the kidney retains potassium, resulting in a lower urinary potassium (generally < 20 mmol/day). It should be noted, however, that if gastrointestinal fluid loss is also associated with hypovolaemia, activation of the renin–angiotensin–aldosterone system may occur, causing increased loss of potassium in the urine.

Renal causes of hypokalaemia can be divided into those with and those without hypertension. Hypokalaemia in the presence of hypertension may be due to increased aldosterone secretion in Conn's syndrome (p. 780) or a genetic defect affecting sodium channels in the distal nephron (Liddle's syndrome). Excessive intake of liquorice or treatment with carbenoxolone may result in a similar clinical picture, due to inhibition of the renal 11βHSD2 enzyme, which inactivates cortisol in peripheral tissues.

If blood pressure is normal or low, hypokalaemia can be classified according to the associated change in acid–base balance. Inherited defects in tubular transport should be suspected when hypokalaemia occurs in association with alkalosis, provided that diuretic use has been excluded. One such disease is Bartter's syndrome, in which sodium reabsorption in the thick ascending limb of Henle is defective, usually due to a loss-of-function mutation of the NKCC2 transporter. The clinical and biochemical features are similar to chronic treatment with furosemide. In Gitelman's syndrome there is a loss-of-function mutation affecting the NCCT transporter in the early distal tubule. The clinical and biochemical features are similar to chronic thiazide treatment. Note that while both Bartter's and Gitelman's syndromes are characterised by hypokalaemia and hypomagnesaemia, urinary calcium excretion is increased in Bartter's syndrome but decreased in Gitelman's syndrome, analogous to the effects of the loop and thiazide diuretics, respectively, on calcium transport (see Box 16.11, p. 436).

If hypokalaemia occurs in the presence of a normal blood pressure and metabolic acidosis, renal tubular acidosis (proximal or 'classical' distal) should be suspected (p. 446).

When hypokalaemia is due to potassium wasting through the gastrointestinal tract, the cause is usually obvious clinically. In some cases, when there is occult induction of vomiting, the hypokalaemia is characteristically associated with metabolic alkalosis, due to loss of gastric acid. If, however, potassium loss has occurred through the surreptitious use of aperients, the hypokalaemia is generally associated with metabolic acidosis. In both cases, urinary potassium excretion is low unless there is significant extracellular volume depletion, which can raise urinary potassium levels by stimulating aldosterone production.

Investigations

Measurement of plasma electrolytes, bicarbonate, urine potassium and sometimes of plasma calcium and magnesium is usually sufficient to establish the diagnosis. If the diagnosis remains unclear, plasma renin should be measured. Levels are low in patients with primary hyperaldosteronism (p. 780) and other forms of mineralocorticoid excess, but raised in other causes of hypokalaemia.

The cause of hypokalaemia may remain unclear despite the above investigations when urinary potassium measurements are inconclusive and the history is incomplete or unreliable. Many such cases are associated with metabolic alkalosis, and in this setting the measurement of urine chloride concentration can be helpful. A low urine chloride (< 30 mmol/L) is characteristic of vomiting (spontaneous or self-induced, in which chloride is lost in HCl in the vomit), while a urine chloride > 40 mmol/L suggests diuretic therapy (acute phase) or a tubular disorder such as Bartter's or Gitelman's syndrome. Differentiation between occult diuretic use and primary tubular disorders can be achieved by performing a screen of urine for diuretic drugs.

Management

Treatment of hypokalaemia involves first determining the cause and then correcting this where possible. If the problem is mainly one of redistribution of potassium into cells, reversal of this (for example, correction of alkalosis) may be sufficient to restore plasma potassium without providing supplements. In most cases, however, some form of potassium replacement will be required. This can generally be achieved with slow-release potassium chloride tablets, but in more acute circumstances intravenous potassium chloride may be necessary. The rate of administration depends on the severity of hypokalaemia and the presence of cardiac or neuromuscular complications, but should generally not exceed 10 mmol of potassium per hour. In patients with severe, life-threatening hypokalaemia, the concentration of potassium in the infused fluid may be increased to 40 mmol/L if a peripheral vein is used, but higher concentrations must be infused into a large 'central' vein with continuous cardiac monitoring.

In the less common situation where hypokalaemia occurs in the presence of systemic acidosis, alkaline salts of potassium, such as potassium bicarbonate, can be given by mouth. If magnesium depletion is also present, replacement of magnesium may also be required for hypokalaemia to be corrected since low cell magnesium can enhance the mechanism for tubular potassium secretion, causing ongoing urinary losses. In some circumstances, potassium-sparing diuretics, such as amiloride, can assist in the correction of hypokalaemia, hypomagnesaemia and metabolic alkalosis, especially when loop or thiazide diuretics are the underlying cause.

Hyperkalaemia

Aetiology and clinical assessment

Hyperkalaemia can present with progressive muscular weakness, but sometimes there are no symptoms until cardiac arrest occurs. The typical ECG changes are shown in Figure 16.8. Peaking of the T wave is an early ECG sign, but widening of the QRS complex presages a dangerous cardiac arrhythmia.

Hyperkalaemia may occur either because of redistribution of potassium between the ICF and ECF or because intake exceeds excretion. It is also important to remember that hyperkalaemia can also be artefactual due to in vitro haemolysis of blood specimens. An approach to defining the underlying cause of hyperkalaemia is shown in Figure 16.10. Redistribution of potassium from the ICF to the ECF may occur in the presence of systemic acidosis, or when the circulating levels of insulin, catecholamines and aldosterone are reduced or when the effects of these hormones are blocked (p. 440). High potassium intake may contribute to hyperkalaemia, but is seldom the only explanation unless renal excretion mechanisms are impaired.

Impaired excretion of potassium into the urine may be associated with a reduced GFR, as in acute kidney injury or chronic kidney disease. Acute kidney injury can be associated with severe hyperkalaemia when there is a concomitant potassium load, such as in rhabdomyolysis or in sepsis, particularly when acidosis is present. In chronic kidney disease, adaptation to moderately elevated plasma potassium levels commonly occurs. However, acute rises in potassium triggered by excessive dietary intake, hypovolaemia or drugs (see below) may occur and destabilise the situation.

Hyperkalaemia can also develop when tubular potassium secretory processes are impaired, even if the GFR is well maintained. In some cases, this is due to low levels of aldosterone, as occurs in Addison's disease or with ACE inhibitor therapy. Another cause is hyporeninaemic hypoaldosteronism where the renin–angiotensin system is inactivated. This condition typically occurs in association with diabetic nephropathy with neuropathy, and is thought to be due to impaired β-adrenergic stimulation of renin release. Other causes include angiotensin receptor antagonists, non-steroidal anti-inflammatory drugs (NSAIDs) and β-blocking drugs. In another group of conditions, tubular potassium secretion is impaired as the result of aldosterone resistance. This can occur in a variety of diseases in which there is inflammation of the tubulointerstitium, such as systemic lupus erythematosus; following renal transplantation; during treatment with potassium-sparing diuretics; and in a number of inherited disorders of tubular transport.

In all conditions of aldosterone deficiency or aldosterone resistance, hyperkalaemia may be associated with acid retention, giving rise to the pattern of hyperkalaemic distal ('type 4') renal tubular acidosis (p. 446).

Investigations

Measurement of electrolytes, creatinine and bicarbonate, when combined with clinical assessment, usually provides the explanation for hyperkalaemia. In aldosterone deficiency, plasma sodium concentration is characteristically low, although this can occur in many causes of hyperkalaemia. Addison's disease should be excluded unless there is an obvious alternative diagnosis, as described on page 777.

Management

Treatment of hyperkalaemia depends on its severity and the rate of development. In the absence of neuromuscular symptoms or ECG changes, reduction of potassium intake and correction of underlying abnormalities may be sufficient. However, in acute and/or severe hyperkalaemia (plasma K > 6.5–7.0 mmol/L) more urgent measures must be taken (Box 16.17).

If ECG changes are present, the first step should be infusion of 10 mL 10% calcium gluconate to stabilise conductive tissue membranes (calcium has the opposite

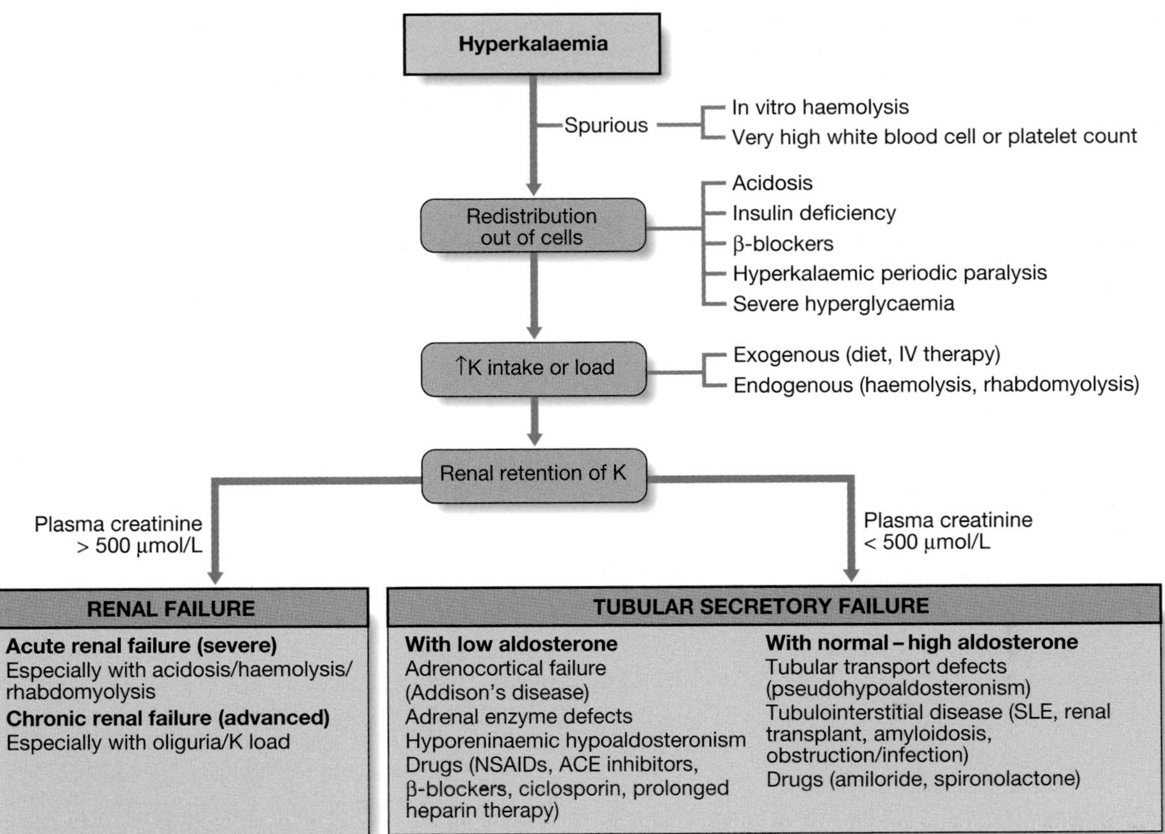

Fig. 16.10 Diagnostic decision tree for hyperkalaemia. Creatinine of 500 µmol/L = 5.67 mg/dL.

16.17 Treatment of severe hyperkalaemia

Objective	Therapy
Stabilise cell membrane potential[1]	IV calcium gluconate (10 mL of 10% solution)
Shift K into cells	Inhaled β_2-adrenoceptor agonist (e.g. salbutamol) IV glucose (50 mL of 50% solution) and insulin (5 U Actrapid®) IV sodium bicarbonate[2]
Remove K from body	IV furosemide and normal saline[3] Ion-exchange resin (e.g. Resonium®) orally or rectally Dialysis

[1]If ECG changes suggestive of hyperkalaemia (K typically > 7 mmol/L)
[2]If acidosis present. [3]If adequate residual renal function.

effect to potassium on conduction of an action potential). Measures to shift potassium from the ECF to the ICF should also be taken, as they generally act rapidly and may avert arrhythmias. Ultimately, a means of removing potassium from the body is generally necessary. When renal function is reasonably preserved, loop diuretics (accompanied by intravenous saline if hypovolaemia is present) may be effective; in established renal failure, ion-exchange resins acting through the gastrointestinal tract and urgent dialysis may be required.

DISORDERS OF ACID–BASE BALANCE

The pH of the arterial plasma is normally 7.40, corresponding to a H^+ concentration of 40 nmol/L. An increase in H^+ concentration corresponds to a decrease in pH. Under normal circumstances, H^+ concentrations do not vary outside the range of 36–44 nmol/L (pH 7.44–7.36), but abnormalities of acid–base balance occur in a wide range of diseases.

Functional anatomy and physiology of acid–base homeostasis

A variety of physiological mechanisms maintain pH of the ECF within narrow limits. The first is the action of blood and tissue buffers, of which the most important involves reaction of H^+ ions with bicarbonate to form carbonic acid, which, under the influence of the enzyme carbonic anhydrase (CA), dissociates to form CO_2 and water:

$$CO_2 + H_2O \underset{CA}{\rightleftharpoons} H_2CO_3 \rightleftharpoons H^+ + HCO_3^-$$

This buffer system is important because bicarbonate is present at relatively high concentration in ECF (21–28 mmol/L), and two of its key components are under physiological control: CO_2 by the lungs, and bicarbonate by the kidneys. These relationships are illustrated in Figure 16.11 (a form of the Henderson–Hasselbalch equation).

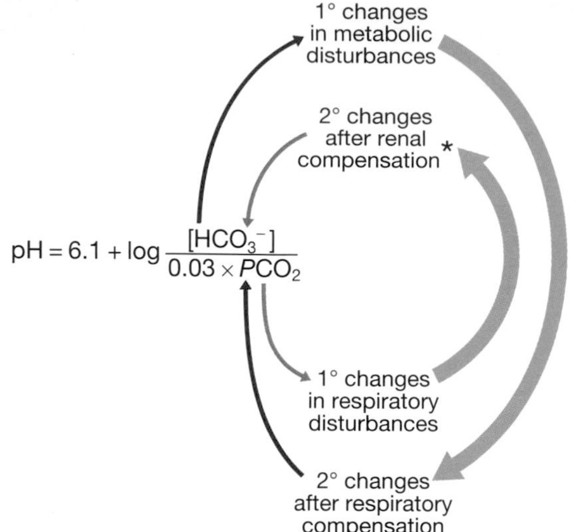

Fig. 16.11 Relationship between pH, PCO_2 (in mmHg) and plasma bicarbonate concentration (in mmol/L). *Note that changes in HCO_3^- concentration are also part of the renal correction for sustained metabolic acid–base disturbances as long as the kidney itself is not the cause of the primary disturbance.

Respiratory compensation for acid–base disturbances can occur quickly. In response to acid accumulation, pH changes in the brainstem stimulate ventilatory drive, serving to reduce PCO_2 and increase pH (p. 653). Conversely, systemic alkalosis leads to inhibition of ventilation, causing a rise in PCO_2 and reduction in pH, although it should be noted that this mechanism has limited capacity to change pH because hypoxia provides an alternative stimulus to drive ventilation.

The kidney provides a third line of defence against disturbances of arterial pH. When acid accumulates due to chronic respiratory or metabolic (non-renal) causes, the kidney has the long-term capacity to enhance urinary excretion of acid, effectively increasing the plasma bicarbonate.

Renal control of acid–base balance

Regulation of acid–base balance occurs at several sites in the kidney. The proximal tubule reabsorbs some 85% of the filtered bicarbonate ions, through the mechanism for H^+ secretion illustrated in Figure 16.3A (p. 431). This is dependent on the enzyme carbonic anhydrase both in the cytoplasm of the proximal tubular cells and on the luminal surface of the brush border membranes. The system has a high capacity but does not lead to significant acidification of the luminal fluid.

Distal nephron segments have an important role in determining net acid excretion by the kidney. In the intercalated cells of the cortical collecting duct and the outer medullary collecting duct cells, acid is secreted into the lumen by an H^+-ATPase. This excreted acid is generated in the tubular cell from the hydration of CO_2 to form carbonic acid, which dissociates into an H^+ ion secreted luminally, and a bicarbonate ion that passes across the basolateral membrane into the blood. The secreted H^+ ions contribute to the reabsorption of any residual bicarbonate present in the luminal fluid, but also contribute net acid for removal from the body, bound to a variety of urinary buffers, of which phosphate and ammonia are the most important. Filtered phosphate (HPO_4^{2-}) combines with H^+ in the distal tubular lumen to form dihydrogen phosphate ($H_2PO_4^-$), which is excreted in the urine with sodium. Ammonia (NH_3) is generated within tubular cells by deamination of the amino acid glutamine by the enzyme glutaminase. The NH_3 then reacts with secreted H^+ in the tubular lumen to form ammonium (NH_4^+), which becomes trapped in the luminal fluid and is excreted with chloride ions.

These two mechanisms remove approximately 1 mmol/kg of hydrogen ions from the body per day, which equates to the non-volatile acid load arising from the metabolism of dietary protein. The slightly alkaline plasma pH of 7.4 (H^+ 40 nmol/L) that is maintained during health can be accounted for by the kidney's ability to generate an acidic urine (pH typically 5–6), in which the net daily excess of metabolic acid produced by the body can be excreted.

Presenting problems in disorders of acid–base balance

Patients with disturbances of acid–base balance may present clinically either with the effects of tissue malfunction due to disturbed pH (such as altered cardiac and central nervous system function), or with secondary changes in respiration as a response to the underlying metabolic change (such as Kussmaul respiration during metabolic acidosis). The clinical picture is often dominated by the cause of the acid–base change, such as uncontrolled diabetes mellitus or primary lung disease. Frequently the acid–base disturbance only becomes evident when the venous plasma bicarbonate concentration is noted to be abnormal, or when a full arterial blood gas analysis shows abnormalities in pH, PCO_2 or bicarbonate. The 'base excess' or 'base deficit' can also be calculated from these data. This is the difference between the patient's bicarbonate level and the normal bicarbonate, measured in vitro with the PCO_2 adjusted to 5.33 kPa (40 mmHg). Calculation of the base excess or deficit is particularly useful in patients with combined respiratory and metabolic disorders (p. 187).

The most common patterns of abnormality in blood gas parameters are shown in Box 16.18. (Note that the terms acidosis and alkalosis strictly refer to the underlying direction of the acid–base change, while acidaemia and alkalaemia more correctly refer to the net change present in the blood). Interpretation of arterial blood gases is also described on page 653.

In metabolic disturbances, respiratory compensation is almost immediate, so that the predicted compensatory change in PCO_2 is achieved soon after the onset of the metabolic disturbance. In respiratory disorders, on the other hand, a small initial change in bicarbonate occurs as a result of chemical buffering of CO_2, largely within red blood cells, but over days and weeks the kidney achieves further compensatory changes in bicarbonate concentration as a result of long-term adjustments in acid secretory capacity. When the clinically obtained acid–base parameters do not accord with the predicted compensation shown, a mixed acid–base disturbance should be suspected (p. 447).

16.18 Principal patterns of acid–base disturbance

Disturbance	Blood H^+	Primary change	Compensatory response	Predicted compensation
Metabolic acidosis	> 40[1]	HCO_3^- < 24 mmol/L	PCO_2 < 5.33 kPa[2]	PCO_2 fall in kPa = 0.16 × HCO_3^- fall in mmol/L
Metabolic alkalosis	< 40[1]	HCO_3^- > 24 mmol/L	PCO_2 > 5.33 kPa[2,3]	PCO_2 rise in kPa = 0.08 × HCO_3^- rise in mmol/L
Respiratory acidosis	> 40[1]	PCO_2 > 5.33 kPa[2]	HCO_3^- > 24 mmol/L	Acute: HCO_3^- rise in mmol/L = 0.75 × PCO_2 rise in kPa Chronic: HCO_3^- rise in mmol/L = 2.62 × PCO_2 rise in kPa
Respiratory alkalosis	< 40[1]	PCO_2 < 5.33 kPa[2]	HCO_3^- < 24 mmol/L	Acute: HCO_3^- fall in mmol/L = 1.50 × PCO_2 fall in kPa Chronic: HCO_3^- fall in mmol/L = 3.75 × PCO_2 fall in kPa

[1]H^+ of 40 nmol/L = pH of 7.40. [2]PCO_2 of 5.33 kPa = 40 mmHg. [3]PCO_2 does not rise above 7.33 kPa (55 mmHg) because hypoxia then intervenes to drive respiration.

Metabolic acidosis

Aetiology and assessment

Metabolic acidosis occurs when an acid other than carbonic acid (due to CO_2 retention) accumulates in the body, resulting in a fall in the plasma bicarbonate. The pH fall that would otherwise occur is blunted by hyperventilation, resulting in a reduced PCO_2. If the kidneys are intact and the primary cause of acidosis is not renal in origin, the kidney can gradually increase acid secretion over days to weeks and restore a new steady state.

Two patterns of metabolic acidosis are recognised (Box 16.19), depending on the nature of the accumulating acid:

- In *pattern A*, when a mineral acid such as hydrochloric acid accumulates, or when there is a primary loss of bicarbonate buffer from the ECF, there is no addition to the plasma of a new acidic anion. In this case, the 'anion gap' (calculated as the difference between the main measured cations (Na^+ + K^+) and the anions (Cl^- + HCO_3^-)) is normal, since the plasma chloride increases to replace the depleted bicarbonate levels. This 'gap' is normally around 12–16 mmol/L (12–16 meq/L) and is made up of anions such as phosphate, sulphate and multiple negative charges on plasma protein molecules. Normal anion gap metabolic acidosis (pattern A) is usually due either to bicarbonate loss in diarrhoea, where the clinical diagnosis is generally obvious, or to renal tubular acidosis (see below).
- In *pattern B*, an accumulating acid is accompanied by its corresponding anion, which adds to the unmeasured anion gap, while the chloride concentration remains normal. The cause is usually apparent from associated clinical features such as uncontrolled diabetes mellitus, renal failure or shock, or may be suggested by associated symptoms, such as visual complaints in methanol poisoning (p. 222). It is noteworthy that a number of causes of increased anion gap acidosis are associated with alcoholism, including starvation ketosis, lactic acidosis and intoxication by methanol or ethylene glycol.

16.19 Causes of metabolic acidosis

Disorder	Mechanism
A. Normal anion gap	
Ingestion or infusion of inorganic acid	Therapeutic infusion of or poisoning with NH_4Cl, HCl
Gastrointestinal HCO_3 loss	Loss of HCO_3 in diarrhoea, small bowel fistula, urinary diversion procedure
Renal tubular acidosis (RTA)	Urinary loss of HCO_3 in proximal RTA; impaired tubular acid secretion in distal RTA
B. Increased anion gap	
Endogenous acid load	
Diabetic ketoacidosis	Accumulation of ketones[1] with hyperglycaemia (p. 811)
Starvation ketosis	Accumulation of ketones without hyperglycaemia (p. 800)
Lactic acidosis	Shock, liver disease, drugs
Renal failure	Accumulation of organic acids
Exogenous acid load	
Aspirin poisoning	Accumulation of salicylate[2]
Methanol poisoning	Accumulation of formate
Ethylene glycol poisoning	Accumulation of glycolate, oxalate

[1]Ketones include acid anions acetoacetate and β-hydroxybutyrate (p. 802). [2]Salicylate poisoning is also associated with respiratory alkalosis due to direct ventilatory stimulation.

Lactic acidosis

The diagnosis of lactic acidosis can be confirmed by the measurement of plasma lactate, which is increased over the normal maximal level of 2 mmol/L (20 mg/dL) by as much as tenfold. Two types of lactic acidosis have been defined:

- *type 1*, due to tissue hypoxia and peripheral generation of lactate, as in patients with circulatory failure and shock
- *type 2*, due to impaired metabolism of lactate, as in liver disease or by a number of drugs and toxins, including metformin, which inhibit lactate metabolism (p. 823).

Renal tubular acidosis

Renal tubular acidosis (RTA) should be suspected when there is a hyperchloraemic acidosis with a normal anion gap and no evidence of gastrointestinal disturbance. The urine pH is inappropriately high (> 5.5) in the presence of systemic acidosis. RTA can be caused by a defect in one of three processes: impaired bicarbonate reabsorption in the proximal tubule (proximal RTA); impaired acid secretion in the late distal tubule or cortical collecting duct intercalated cells (classical distal RTA); or impaired sodium reabsorption in the late distal tubule or cortical collecting duct, which is associated with reduced secretion of both potassium and H^+ ions (hyperkalaemic distal RTA).

Various subtypes of RTA are recognised and the most common causes are shown in Box 16.20. The inherited forms of RTA are due to mutations in the genes that regulate acid or bicarbonate transport in the renal tubules (see Fig. 16.3, p. 431). However, RTA is often an acquired disorder and in these circumstances the metabolic acidosis may serve as an early clue to the underlying diagnosis.

Sometimes distal RTA is 'incomplete' and the plasma bicarbonate concentration is normal under resting conditions. However, in incomplete distal RTA the urine pH fails to fall below 5.3 after an acid challenge test, involving the ingestion of ammonium chloride sufficient to lower the plasma bicarbonate.

A number of features allow differentiation of types of RTA. Proximal RTA is frequently associated with urinary wasting of amino acids, phosphate and glucose (Fanconi's syndrome), as well as bicarbonate and potassium. Patients with this disorder can lower the urine pH when the acidosis is severe and plasma bicarbonate levels have fallen below 16 mmol/L since distal H^+ secretion mechanisms are intact. In the classical form of distal RTA, however, acid accumulation is relentless and progressive, resulting in mobilisation of calcium from bone and consequent osteomalacia with hypercalciuria, renal stone formation and nephrocalcinosis. Potassium is also lost in classical distal RTA, while it is retained in hyperkalaemic distal RTA.

16.20 Causes of renal tubular acidosis

Proximal renal tubular acidosis	
• Inherited Fanconi's syndrome Cystinosis Wilson's disease • Paraproteinaemia Myeloma • Amyloidosis • Hyperparathyroidism	• Heavy metal toxicity Lead, cadmium and mercury poisoning • Drugs Carbonic anhydrase inhibitors Ifosfamide
Classical distal renal tubular acidosis	
• Inherited • Autoimmune diseases Systemic lupus erythematosus Sjögren's syndrome	• Hyperglobulinaemia • Toxins and drugs Toluene Lithium Amphotericin
Hyperkalaemic distal renal tubular acidosis	
• Hypoaldosteronism (primary or secondary) • Obstructive nephropathy • Renal transplant rejection	• Drugs Amiloride Spironolactone

Management

The first step in management of metabolic acidosis is to identify and correct the underlying cause when possible (see Box 16.19). This may involve controlling diarrhoea, treating diabetes mellitus, correcting shock, stopping drugs that might cause the condition, or using dialysis to remove toxins. Since metabolic acidosis is frequently associated with sodium and water depletion, resuscitation with intravenous fluids is often needed. Use of intravenous bicarbonate in this setting is controversial. Because rapid correction of acidosis can induce hypokalaemia or a fall in plasma ionised calcium, the use of bicarbonate infusions is best reserved for situations where the underlying disorder cannot be readily corrected and acidosis is severe (H^+ > 100 nmol/L, pH < 7.00) or associated with evidence of tissue dysfunction.

The acidosis in RTA can sometimes be controlled by treating the underlying cause (see Box 16.20), but supplements of sodium and potassium bicarbonate are usually also necessary in types 1 and 2 RTA to achieve a target plasma bicarbonate level of above 18 mmol/L and normokalaemia. In type 4 RTA, loop diuretics, thiazides or fludrocortisone (as appropriate to the underlying diagnosis) may be effective in correcting the acidosis and the hyperkalaemia.

Metabolic alkalosis

Aetiology and clinical assessment

Metabolic alkalosis is characterised by an increase in the plasma bicarbonate concentration and the plasma pH (see Box 16.18). There is a compensatory rise in PCO_2 due to hypoventilation but this is limited by the need to avoid hypoxia. The causes are best classified by the accompanying changes in ECF volume.

Hypovolaemic metabolic alkalosis is the most common pattern. This can be caused by sustained vomiting, in which acid-rich fluid is lost directly from the body, or by treatment with loop diuretics or thiazides. In the case of sustained vomiting, loss of gastric acid is the immediate cause of the alkalosis, but several factors act to sustain or amplify this in the context of volume depletion (Fig. 16.12). Loss of sodium and fluid leads to hypovolaemia and secondary hyperaldosteronism, triggering proximal sodium bicarbonate reabsorption and additional acid secretion by the distal tubule. Hypokalaemia occurs due to potassium loss in the vomitus and by the kidney as the result of secondary hyperaldosteronism, and itself is a stimulus to acid secretion. Additionally, the compensatory rise in PCO_2 further enhances tubular acid secretion. The net result is sustained metabolic alkalosis with an inappropriately acid urine, which cannot be corrected until the deficit in circulating volume has been replaced.

Normovolaemic (or hypervolaemic) metabolic alkalosis occurs when bicarbonate retention and volume expansion occur simultaneously. Classical causes include primary hyperaldosteronism (Conn's syndrome, p. 780), Cushing's syndrome (p. 773) and corticosteroid therapy (p. 776). Occasionally, overuse of antacid salts for treatment of dyspepsia produces a similar pattern.

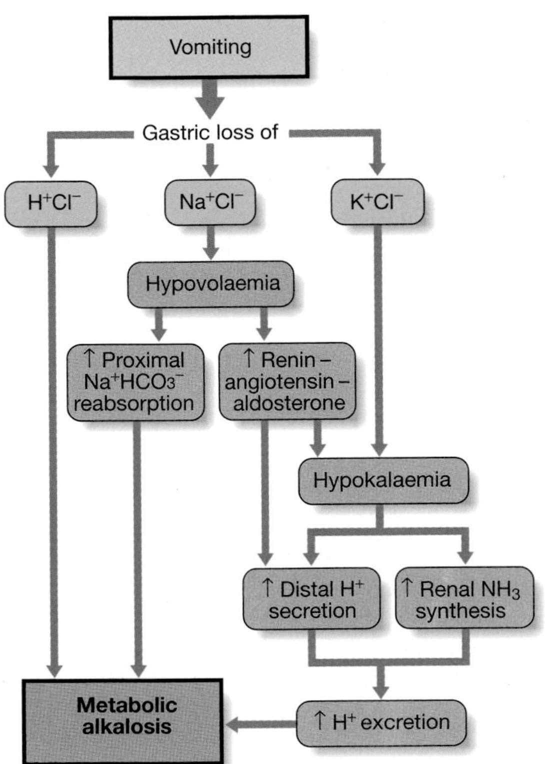

Fig. 16.12 Generation and maintenance of metabolic alkalosis during prolonged vomiting. Loss of H^+Cl^- generates metabolic alkalosis, which is maintained by renal changes.

Clinically, apart from manifestations of the underlying cause, there may be few symptoms or signs related to alkalosis itself. When the rise in systemic pH is abrupt, plasma ionised calcium falls and signs of increased neuromuscular irritability, such as tetany, may develop (p. 768).

Management

Metabolic alkalosis with hypovolaemia can be corrected by intravenous infusions of 0.9% saline with potassium supplements. This reverses the secondary hyperaldosteronism and allows the kidney to excrete the excess alkali in the urine.

In metabolic alkalosis with normal or increased volume, treatment should focus on management of the underlying endocrine cause (Ch. 20).

Respiratory acidosis

Respiratory acidosis occurs when there is accumulation of CO_2 due to type II respiratory failure (p. 663). This results in a rise in the PCO_2, with a compensatory increase in plasma bicarbonate concentration, particularly when the disorder is of long duration and the kidney has fully developed its capacity for increased acid excretion.

This acid–base disturbance can arise from lesions anywhere along the neuromuscular pathways from the brain to the respiratory muscles that result in impaired ventilation. It can also arise during intrinsic lung disease if there is significant mismatching of ventilation and perfusion.

Clinical features are primarily those of the underlying cause of the respiratory disorder such as paralysis, chest wall injury or chronic obstructive lung disease, but the CO_2 accumulation may itself lead to drowsiness that further depresses respiratory drive.

Management involves correction of causative factors where possible, but ultimately ventilatory support may be necessary.

Respiratory alkalosis

Respiratory alkalosis develops when there is a period of sustained hyperventilation, resulting in a reduction of PCO_2 and increase in plasma pH. If the condition is sustained, renal compensation occurs, such that tubular acid secretion is reduced and the plasma bicarbonate falls.

Respiratory alkalosis is usually of short duration, occurring in anxiety states or as the result of over-vigorous assisted ventilation. It can be prolonged in the context of pregnancy, pulmonary embolism, chronic liver disease, and ingestion of certain drugs such as salicylates that directly stimulate the respiratory centre in the brainstem.

Clinical features are those of the underlying cause but agitation associated with perioral and digital tingling may also occur, due to a reduction in ionised calcium concentrations because of increased binding of calcium to albumin as the result of the alkalosis. In severe cases, Trousseau's sign and Chvostek's sign may be positive, and tetany or seizures may develop (p. 768).

Management involves correction of identifiable causes, reduction of anxiety, and a period of rebreathing into a closed bag to allow CO_2 levels to rise.

Mixed acid–base disorders

It is not uncommon for more than one disturbance of acid–base metabolism to be present at the same time in the same patient: for example, respiratory acidosis due to narcotic overdose with metabolic alkalosis due to vomiting. In these situations, the arterial pH will represent the net effect of all primary and compensatory changes. Indeed, the pH may be normal, but the presence of underlying acid–base disturbances can be gauged from concomitant abnormalities in the PCO_2 and bicarbonate concentration.

In assessing these disorders, all clinical influences on the patient's acid–base status should be identified, and reference should be made to the table of predicted compensation given in Box 16.18. If the compensatory change is discrepant from the rules of thumb provided, more than one disturbance of acid–base metabolism may be suspected.

DISORDERS OF DIVALENT ION METABOLISM

The present section excludes discussion of calcium disorders, which are considered in Chapters 20 (pp. 767–770) and 25 (p. 1125).

Functional anatomy and physiology of magnesium metabolism

Like potassium, magnesium is mainly an intracellular cation. It is important to the function of many enzymes, including the Na,K-ATPase, and can regulate both potassium and calcium channels. Its overall effect is to stabilise excitable cell membranes.

Renal handling of magnesium involves filtration of free plasma magnesium at the glomerulus (about 70% of the total) with extensive reabsorption (50–70%) in the loop of Henle, and other parts of the proximal and distal renal tubule. Magnesium reabsorption is also enhanced by parathyroid hormone (PTH).

Presenting problems in disorders of magnesium metabolism

Hypomagnesaemia

Aetiology and clinical assessment

Hypomagnesaemia exists when plasma magnesium concentrations are below the reference range of 0.75–1.0 mmol/L (1.5–2.0 meq/L). This is usually a reflection of magnesium depletion (Box 16.21), which can be caused by excessive magnesium loss from the gastrointestinal tract (notably in chronic diarrhoea) or the kidney (during prolonged use of loop diuretics). Excessive alcohol ingestion can cause magnesium depletion through both gut and renal losses. Some inherited tubular transport disorders, such as Gitelman's syndrome, can also result in urinary magnesium wasting (p. 440).

Hypomagnesaemia is frequently associated with hypocalcaemia, probably because magnesium is required for the normal secretion of PTH in response to a fall in serum calcium, and because hypomagnesaemia causes end-organ resistance to PTH. The clinical features of hypomagnesaemia and hypocalcaemia are similar in that tetany, cardiac arrhythmias (notably torsades de pointes, p. 570), central nervous excitation and seizures, vasoconstriction and hypertension may all occur. Magnesium depletion is also associated (through uncertain mechanisms) with hyponatraemia and hypokalaemia, which may contribute to some of the clinical manifestations.

16.21 Causes of hypomagnesaemia

Mechanism	Examples
Inadequate intake	Starvation Malnutrition (esp. alcoholism) Parenteral alimentation
Excessive losses	
Gastrointestinal	Prolonged vomiting/nasogastric aspiration Chronic diarrhoea/laxative abuse Malabsorption Small bowel bypass surgery Fistulae
Urinary	Diuretic therapy (loop, thiazide) Alcohol Tubulotoxic drugs (gentamicin, cisplatin) Volume expansion (e.g. primary hyperaldosteronism) Diabetic ketoacidosis Post-obstructive diuresis Recovery from acute tubular necrosis Inherited tubular transport defect (Bartter's syndrome, Gitelman's syndrome Primary renal magnesium wasting)
Miscellaneous	Acute pancreatitis Foscarnet therapy Proton pump inhibitor therapy (prolonged) Hungry bone syndrome Diabetes mellitus

Management

The underlying cause should be identified and treated where possible. When symptoms are present, the treatment of choice is intravenous magnesium chloride at a rate not exceeding 0.5 mmol/kg in the first 24 hours. When intravenous access is not available, magnesium sulphate can be given intramuscularly. Oral magnesium salts have limited effectiveness due to poor absorption and may cause diarrhoea. If hypomagnesaemia is due to diuretic treatment, adjunctive use of a potassium-sparing agent can also help by reducing magnesium loss into the urine.

Hypermagnesaemia

This is a much less common abnormality than hypomagnesaemia. Predisposing conditions include acute kidney injury and chronic kidney disease, and adrenocortical insufficiency. The condition is generally precipitated in patients at risk by an increased intake of magnesium, or through the use of magnesium-containing medications, such as antacids, laxatives and enemas.

Clinical features include bradycardia, hypotension, reduced consciousness and respiratory depression.

Management involves ceasing all magnesium-containing drugs and reducing dietary magnesium intake, improving renal function if possible, and promoting urinary magnesium excretion using a loop diuretic with intravenous hydration, if residual renal function allows. Calcium gluconate may be given intravenously to ameliorate cardiac effects. Dialysis may be necessary in patients with poor renal function.

Functional anatomy and physiology of phosphate metabolism

Inorganic phosphate (mainly present as HPO_4^{2-}) is intimately involved in cell energy metabolism, intracellular signalling and bone and mineral balance (Ch. 25). The normal plasma concentration is 0.8–1.4 mmol/L (2.48–4.34 mg/dL). It is freely filtered at the glomerulus and approximately 65% is reabsorbed by the proximal tubule, via an apical sodium–phosphate co-transport carrier. A further 10–20% is reabsorbed in the distal tubules, leaving a fractional excretion of some 10% to pass into the urine, usually as $H_2PO_4^-$. Proximal reabsorption is decreased by PTH, fibroblast growth factor 23 (FGF-23), volume expansion, osmotic diuretics and glucose infusion.

Presenting problems in disorders of phosphate metabolism

Hypophosphataemia

The causes of hypophosphataemia are shown in Box 16.22. Phosphate may redistribute into cells during

16.22 Causes of hypophosphataemia

Mechanism	Examples
Redistribution into cells	Refeeding after starvation Respiratory alkalosis Treatment for diabetic ketoacidosis
Inadequate intake or absorption	Malnutrition Malabsorption Chronic diarrhoea Phosphate binders (antacids) Vitamin D deficiency or resistance
Increased renal excretion	Hyperparathyroidism ECF volume expansion with diuresis Osmotic diuretics Fanconi's syndrome Familial hypophosphataemic rickets Tumour-induced hypophosphataemic rickets

periods of increased energy utilisation (such as refeeding after a period of starvation) and during systemic alkalosis. However, severe hypophosphataemia usually represents an overall body deficit due to either inadequate intake or absorption through the gut, or excessive renal losses, most notably in primary hyperparathyroidism (p. 769) or as the result of acute plasma volume expansion, osmotic diuresis and diuretics acting on the proximal renal tubule. Less common causes include inherited defects of proximal sodium–phosphate co-transport and tumour-induced osteomalacia due to ectopic production of the hormone FGF-23 (p. 1125).

The clinical manifestations of phosphate depletion are wide-ranging, reflecting the involvement of phosphate in many aspects of metabolism. Defects appear in the blood (impaired function and survival of all cell lines), skeletal muscle (weakness, respiratory failure), cardiac muscle (congestive cardiac failure), smooth muscle (ileus), central nervous system (decreased consciousness, seizures and coma) and bone (osteomalacia in severe prolonged hypophosphataemia, p. 1125).

Management involves administering oral phosphate supplements and high-protein/high-dairy dietary supplements that are rich in naturally occurring phosphate. Intravenous treatment with sodium or potassium phosphate salts can be used in critical situations, but there is a risk of precipitating hypocalcaemia and metastatic calcification.

Hyperphosphataemia

Phosphate accumulation is usually the result of acute kidney injury or chronic kidney disease (pp. 768 and 483, and p. 768). Phosphate excretion is also reduced in hypoparathyroidism and pseudohypoparathyroidism (p. 770). Redistribution of phosphate from cells into the plasma can also be a contributing factor in the 'tumour lysis' syndrome and in catabolic states. Phosphate accumulation is aggravated in any of these conditions if the patient takes phosphate-containing preparations or inappropriate vitamin D therapy.

The clinical features relate to hypocalcaemia and metastatic calcification, particularly in chronic renal failure with tertiary hyperparathyroidism (when a high calcium–phosphate product occurs).

If renal function is normal, intravenous normal saline should be given to promote phosphate excretion. Hyperphosphataemia in patients with renal failure should be treated with dietary phosphate restriction and the use of oral phosphate binders (p. 486).

DISORDERS OF AMINO ACID METABOLISM

Congenital disorders of amino acid metabolism usually present in the neonatal period and may involve life-long treatment regimens. However, some disorders, particularly those involved in amino acid transport, may not present until later in life.

Phenylketonuria

Phenylketonuria (PKU) is inherited as an autosomal recessive disorder caused by loss-of-function mutations in the *PAH* gene, which encodes phenylalanine hydroxylase, an enzyme required for degradation of phenylalanine. As a result, phenylalanine accumulates at high levels in the neonate's blood, causing mental retardation.

The diagnosis of PKU is almost always made by routine neonatal screening (p. 64). Treatment involves life-long adherence to a low-phenylalanine diet. Early and adequate dietary treatment prevents major mental retardation, although there may still be a slight reduction in IQ.

Homocystinuria

Homocystinuria is an autosomal recessive disorder caused by loss-of-function mutations in the *CBS* gene, which encodes cystathionine beta-synthase. The enzyme deficiency causes accumulation of homocysteine and methionine in the blood. Many cases of homocystinuria are diagnosed through newborn screening programmes.

Clinical manifestations are wide-ranging and involve the eyes (ectopia lentis – displacement of the lens), central nervous system (mental retardation, delayed developmental milestones, seizures, psychiatric disturbances), skeleton (resembling Marfan's syndrome, and also with generalised osteoporosis), vascular system (thrombotic lesions of arteries and veins) and skin (hypopigmentation).

Treatment is dietary, involving a methionine-restricted, cystine-supplemented diet, as well as large doses of pyridoxine.

DISORDERS OF CARBOHYDRATE METABOLISM

The most common disorder of carbohydrate metabolism is diabetes mellitus, which is discussed in Chapter 21. There are also some rare inherited defects.

Galactosaemia

Galactosaemia is caused by loss-of-function mutations in the *GALT* gene, which encodes galactose-1-phosphate uridyl transferase. It is usually inherited as an autosomal recessive disorder. The neonate is unable to metabolise galactose, one of the hexose sugars contained in lactose.

Vomiting or diarrhoea usually begins within a few days of ingestion of milk, and the neonate may become jaundiced. Failure to thrive is the most common clinical presentation. The classic form of the disease results in hepatomegaly, cataracts and mental retardation, and fulminant infection with *Escherichia coli* is a frequent complication. Treatment involves life-long avoidance of galactose- and lactose-containing foods.

The widespread inclusion of galactosaemia in newborn screening programmes has resulted in the identification of a number of milder variants.

Glycogen storage diseases

Glycogen storage diseases (GSD, or glycogenoses) result from an inherited defect in one of the many enzymes responsible for the formation or breakdown of glycogen, a complex carbohydrate that can be broken down quickly to release glucose during exercise or between meals.

There are several major types of GSD, which are classified by a number, by the name of the defective enzyme or eponymously after the physician who first described the condition (Box 16.23). Most forms of GSD are inherited as autosomal recessive disorders.

A diagnosis of GSD is made on the basis of the symptoms, physical examination and results of biochemical tests. Occasionally, a muscle or liver biopsy is required to confirm the enzyme defect. Different types of GSD present at different ages, and some may require life-long modifications of diet and lifestyle.

DISORDERS OF COMPLEX LIPID METABOLISM

Complex lipids are key components of the cell membrane (p. 47) that are normally catabolised in organelles called lysosomes. The lysosomal storage diseases are a heterogeneous group of disorders caused by loss-of-function mutations in various lysosomal enzymes (Box 16.24), resulting in an inability to break down complex glycolipids or other intracellular macromolecules. These disorders have diverse clinical manifestations, typically including mental retardation. Some can be treated with enzyme replacement therapy, while others (such as Tay–Sachs disease) can be prevented through community participation in genetic carrier screening programmes (p. 64).

DISORDERS OF BLOOD LIPIDS AND LIPOPROTEINS

The three most important classes of lipid are cholesterol, which is composed of hydrocarbon rings; triglycerides (TG), which are esters composed of glycerol linked to three long-chain fatty acids; and phospholipids, which are composed of a hydrophobic 'tail' consisting of two long-chain fatty acids linked through glycerol to a hydrophilic head containing a phosphate group. Phospholipids are present in cell membranes and are important signalling molecules.

Despite their poor water solubility, lipids need to be absorbed from the gastrointestinal tract and transported throughout the body. This is achieved by incorporating lipids within lipoproteins. Plasma cholesterol and TG are clinically important because they are major treatable risk factors for cardiovascular disease, whilst severe hypertriglyceridaemia also predisposes to acute pancreatitis.

Functional anatomy, physiology and investigation of lipid metabolism

Lipids are transported and metabolised by apolipoproteins, which combine with lipids to form spherical or disc-shaped lipoproteins, consisting of a hydrophobic core and a less hydrophobic coat (Fig. 16.13). The structure of some apolipoproteins also enables them to act as enzyme co-factors or cell receptor ligands. Variations in lipid and apolipoprotein composition result in distinct classes of lipoprotein that perform specific metabolic functions.

Processing of dietary lipid

The intestinal absorption of dietary lipid is described on page 841 (see also Fig. 16.14). Enterocytes lining the gut extract monoglyceride and free fatty acids from micelles and re-esterify them into TG, which are combined with a truncated form of apolipoprotein B (Apo B48) as it is synthesised. Intestinal cholesterol derived from dietary

16.23 Glycogen storage diseases

Type	Eponym	Enzyme deficiency	Clinical features and complications
I	Von Gierke	Glucose-6-phosphatase	Childhood presentation, hypoglycaemia, hepatomegaly
II	Pompe	α-glucosidase (acid maltase)	Classical presentation in infancy, muscle weakness (may be severe)
III	Cori	Glycogen debrancher enzyme	Childhood presentation, hepatomegaly, mild hypoglycaemia
IV	Andersen	Brancher enzyme	Presentation in infancy, severe muscle weakness (may affect heart), cirrhosis
V	McArdle	Muscle glycogen phosphorylase	Exercise-induced fatigue and myalgia
VI	Hers	Liver phosphorylase	Mild hepatomegaly
VII	Tarui	Muscle phosphofructokinase	Exercise-induced fatigue and myalgia
IX*		Liver phosphorylase kinase	Mild hepatomegaly
0		Hepatic glycogen synthase	Fasting hypoglycaemia, post-prandial hyperglycaemia

*Note that type VIII has been merged into type IX and no longer exists as a separate entity.

16.24 Lysosomal storage diseases

Lysosomal storage disease	Clinical features	Enzyme deficiency	Human enzyme replacement therapy
Fabry disease	Variable age of onset Neurological (pain in extremities) Dermatological (hypohidrosis, angiokeratomas) Cerebrovascular (renal, cardiac, central nervous system)	α-galactosidase A	In clinical practice
Gaucher disease (various types)	Splenic and liver enlargement, with variable severity of disease Some types also have neurological involvement	Glucocerebrosidase	In clinical practice for some types
Mucopolysaccharidosis (MPS) (various types, including Hurler's, Hunter's, Sanfilippo's and Morquio's syndromes)	Vary with syndrome. Can cause mental retardation, skeletal and joint abnormalities, abnormal facies, obstructive respiratory diseases and recurrent respiratory infections	Each MPS type has a different enzyme deficiency	In clinical practice for some types; clinical trials under way for other types
Niemann–Pick disease	Most common presentation is as a progressive neurological disorder, accompanied by organomegaly Some variants do not have neurological symptoms	Acid sphingomyelinase	Clinical trials planned for some types
GM2-gangliosidosis (various types, including Tay–Sachs and Sandhoff diseases)	Severe progressive neurological disorder. Sandhoff disease also characterised by organomegaly	Hexosaminidase A, B	

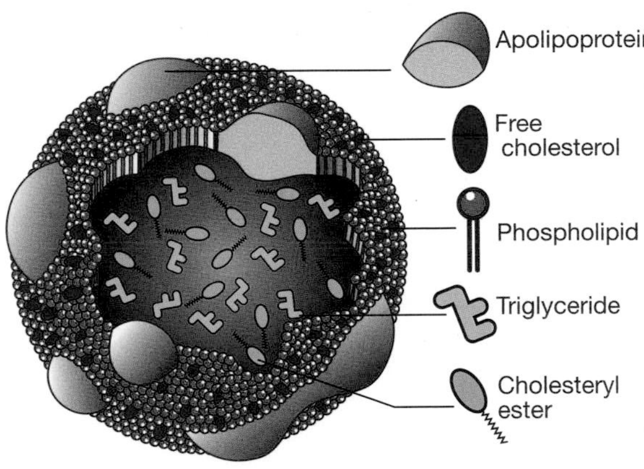

Fig. 16.13 Structure of lipoproteins.

and biliary sources is also absorbed via a specific intestinal membrane transporter termed NPC1L1. This produces chylomicrons containing TG and cholesterol ester that are secreted basolaterally into lymphatic lacteals and carried to the circulation through the thoracic duct. Upon entering the blood stream, nascent chylomicrons are modified by further addition of apolipoproteins. Chylomicron TG are hydrolysed by lipoprotein lipase located on the endothelium of tissue capillary beds. This releases fatty acids that are used locally for energy production or stored as TG in muscle or fat. The residual 'remnant' chylomicron particle is avidly cleared by low-density lipoprotein (LDL)-receptors in the liver, which recognise Apo E on the remnant lipoproteins. Complete absorption of dietary lipids takes about 6–10 hours, so chylomicrons are usually undetectable in the plasma after a 12-hour fast.

The main dietary determinants of plasma cholesterol concentrations are the intake of saturated and trans-unsaturated fatty acids, which reduce LDL-receptor activity (see below). Dietary cholesterol has surprisingly little effect on fasting cholesterol levels. Plant sterols and drugs that inhibit cholesterol absorption are effective because they also reduce the re-utilisation of biliary cholesterol. The dietary determinants of plasma TG concentrations are complex since excessive intake of carbohydrate, fat or alcohol may all contribute to increased plasma TG by different mechanisms.

Endogenous lipid synthesis

In the fasting state, the liver is the major source of plasma lipids (see Fig. 16.14). The liver may acquire lipids by uptake, synthesis or conversion from other macronutrients. These lipids are transported to other tissues by secretion of very low-density lipoproteins (VLDL), which are rich in TG but differ from chylomicrons in that they contain full-length Apo B100. Following secretion into the circulation, VLDL undergo metabolic processing similar to that of chylomicrons. Hydrolysis of VLDL TG releases fatty acids to tissues and converts VLDL into 'remnant' particles, referred to as intermediate-density lipoproteins (IDL). Most IDL are rapidly cleared by LDL receptors in the liver, but some are processed by hepatic lipase, which converts the particle to an LDL by removing TG and most materials other than Apo B100, and free and esterified cholesterol.

The LDL particles act as a source of cholesterol for cells and tissues (see Fig. 16.14). LDL cholesterol is internalised by receptor-mediated endocytosis via the LDL receptor. Delivery of cholesterol via this pathway down-regulates further expression of the LDL receptor gene and reduces the synthesis and activity of

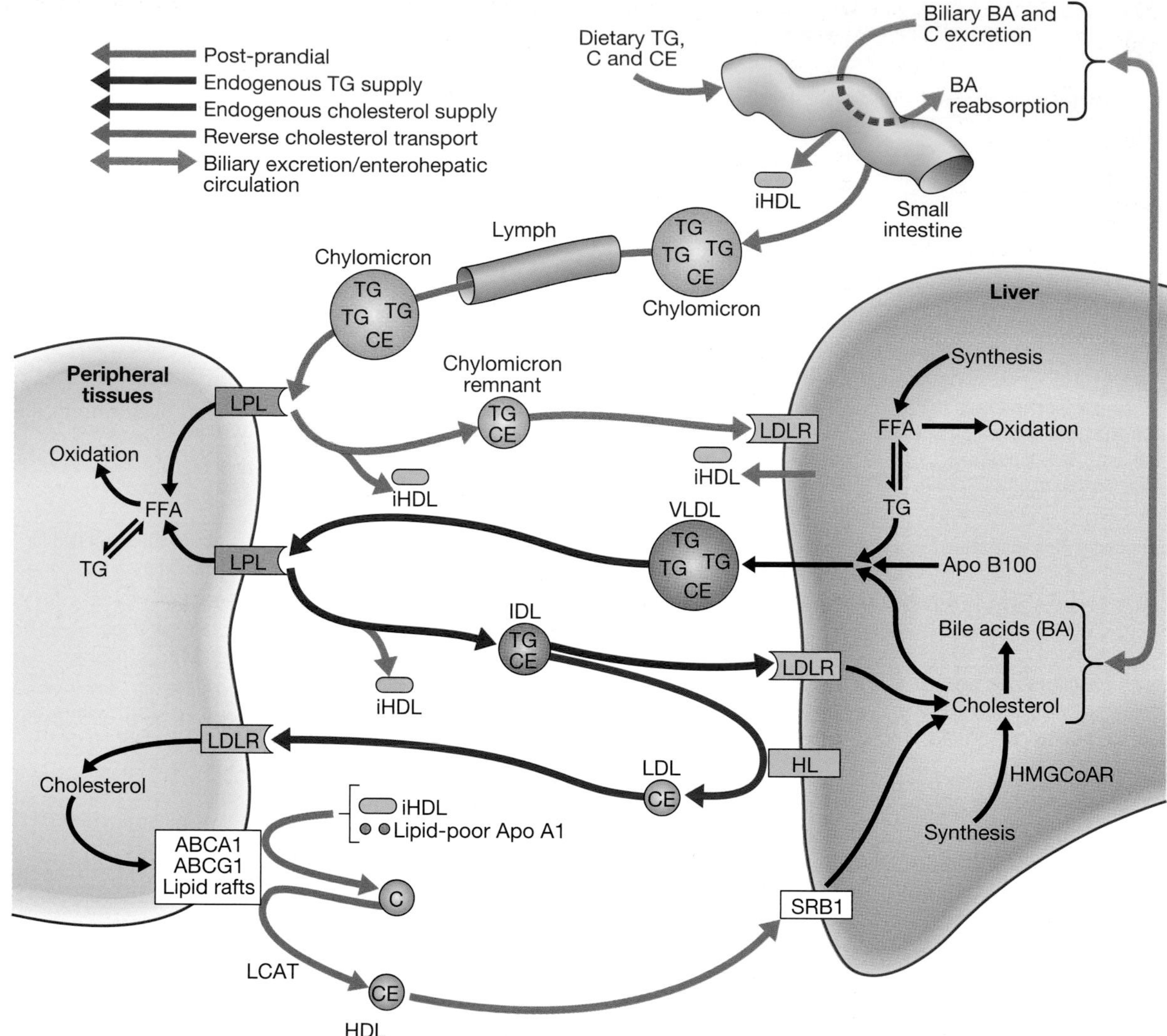

Fig. 16.14 Absorption, transport and storage of lipids. Pathways of lipid transport are shown; in addition, cholesterol ester transfer protein exchanges triglyceride and cholesterol ester between VLDL/chylomicrons and HDL/LDL, and free fatty acids released from peripheral lipolysis can be taken up in the liver. (ABCA1/ABCG1 = ATP-binding cassette A1/G1; Apo = apolipoprotein; BA = bile acids; C = cholesterol; CE = cholesterol ester; FFA = free fatty acids; HDL = mature high-density lipoprotein; HL = hepatic lipase; HMGCoAR = hydroxy-methyl-glutaryl-coenzyme A reductase; IDL = intermediate-density lipoprotein; iHDL = immature high-density lipoprotein; LCAT = lecithin cholesterol acyl transferase; LDL = low-density lipoprotein; LDLR = low-density lipoprotein receptor (Apo B100 receptor); LPL = lipoprotein lipase; SRB1 = scavenger receptor B1; TG = triglyceride; VLDL = very low-density lipoprotein)

the rate-limiting enzyme for cholesterol synthesis, HMGCoA reductase. This negative feedback loop, together with the modulation of cholesterol esterification, controls the intracellular free cholesterol level within a narrow range.

Reverse cholesterol transport

Peripheral tissues are further guarded against excessive cholesterol accumulation by high-density lipoproteins (HDL; see Fig. 16.14). Lipid-poor Apo A1 (derived from the liver, intestine and the outer layer of chylomicrons and VLDL) accepts cellular cholesterol and phospholipid from a specific membrane transporter known as the ATP-binding cassette A1 (ABCA1). This produces small HDL that are able to accept more free cholesterol from cholesterol-rich regions of the cell membrane known as 'rafts' via another membrane transporter (ABCG1). The cholesterol that has been accepted by these small HDL is esterified by lecithin cholesterol acyl transferase (LCAT), thus maintaining an uptake gradient and remodelling the particle into a mature spherical HDL. These HDL release their cholesterol to the liver and other cholesterol-requiring tissues via the scavenger receptor B1 (SRB1).

The cholesterol ester transfer protein (CETP) in plasma allows transfer of cholesterol from HDL or LDL to VLDL or chylomicrons in exchange for TG. When TG is elevated, the action of CETP may reduce HDL cholesterol and remodel LDL into 'small, dense' LDL particles that appear to be more atherogenic in the blood vessel wall. Animal species that lack CETP are resistant to atherosclerosis.

Lipids and cardiovascular disease

Plasma lipoprotein levels are major modifiable risk factors for cardiovascular disease. Increased levels of atherogenic lipoproteins (especially LDL, but also IDL, lipoprotein(a) and possibly chylomicron remnants) contribute to the development of atherosclerosis (p. 579). Increased plasma concentration and reduced diameter favour subendothelial accumulation of these lipoproteins. Following chemical modifications such as oxidation, Apo B-containing lipoproteins are no longer cleared by normal mechanisms. They trigger a self-perpetuating inflammatory response during which they are taken up by macrophages to form foam cells, a hallmark of atherosclerotic lesions. These processes also have an adverse effect on endothelial function.

Conversely, HDL removes cholesterol from the tissues to the liver, where it is metabolised and excreted in bile. HDL may also counteract some components of the inflammatory response, such as the expression of vascular adhesion molecules by the endothelium. Consequently, low HDL cholesterol levels, which are often associated with TG elevation, also predispose to atherosclerosis.

Lipid measurement

Abnormalities of lipid metabolism most commonly come to light following routine blood testing. Measurement of plasma cholesterol alone is not sufficient for comprehensive assessment. Levels of total cholesterol (TC), triglyceride (TG) and HDL cholesterol (HDL-C) need to be obtained after a 12-hour fast to permit accurate calculation of LDL cholesterol (LDL-C) according to the Friedewald formula (LDL-C = TC − HDL-C − (TG/2.2) mmol/L; or LDL-C = TC − HDL-C − (TG/5) mg/dL). The formula becomes unreliable when TG levels exceed 4 mmol/L (350 mg/dL). Other risk markers, such as NHDL-C (non-HDL-C, calculated as the difference between TC and HDL-C levels) or Apo B, may assess risk of cardiovascular disease more accurately than LDL-C when TG levels are increased. Furthermore, non-fasting samples are often used to guide therapeutic decisions since they are unaffected in terms of TC and measured LDL-C, albeit that they differ from fasting samples in terms of TG, HDL-C and, to some extent, calculated LDL-C. Consideration must be given to confounding factors, such as recent illness, after which cholesterol, LDL and HDL levels temporarily decrease in proportion to severity. Results that will affect major decisions, such as initiation of drug therapy, should be confirmed with a repeat measurement.

Elevated levels of TG are common in obesity, diabetes and insulin resistance (Chs 5 and 21), and are frequently associated with low HDL and increased 'small, dense' LDL. Under these circumstances, LDL-C may underestimate risk. This is one situation in which measurement of Apo B may provide additional useful information.

Presenting problems in disorders of lipids

Lipid measurements are usually performed for the following reasons:

- screening for primary or secondary prevention of cardiovascular disease
- investigation of patients with clinical features of lipid disorders (Fig. 16.15) and their relatives
- monitoring of response to diet, weight control and medication.

Aetiology and clinical assessment

The first step is to consider the effect of other diseases and drugs (Box 16.25). Overt or subclinical hypothyroidism (p. 743) may cause hypercholesterolaemia, and so measurement of thyroid function is warranted in most cases, even in the absence of typical symptoms and signs.

Once secondary causes are excluded, primary lipid abnormalities may be diagnosed. Primary lipid abnormalities can be classified according to the predominant lipid problem: hypercholesterolaemia, hypertriglyceridaemia or mixed hyperlipidaemia (Box 16.26). Although single-gene disorders are encountered in all three categories, most cases are due to multiple-gene (polygenic) loci interacting with environmental factors. Clinical consequences of dyslipidaemia vary somewhat between these causes (see Fig. 16.15).

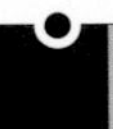

16.25 Causes of secondary hyperlipidaemia

Secondary hypercholesterolaemia	
Moderately common	
• Hypothyroidism • Pregnancy • Cholestatic liver disease	• Drugs (diuretics, ciclosporin, corticosteroids, androgens, antiretroviral agents)
Less common	
• Nephrotic syndrome • Anorexia nervosa	• Porphyria • Hyperparathyroidism
Secondary hypertriglyceridaemia	
Common	
• Diabetes mellitus (type 2) • Chronic renal disease • Abdominal obesity • Excess alcohol	• Hepatocellular disease • Drugs (β-blockers, retinoids, corticosteroids, anti-retroviral agents)

Predominant hypercholesterolaemia

Polygenic hypercholesterolaemia is the most common cause of a mild to moderate increase in LDL-C (see Box 16.26). Physical signs, such as corneal arcus and xanthelasma, may be found in this as well as other forms of lipid disturbance (see Fig. 16.15). The risk of cardiovascular disease is proportional to the degree of LDL-C (or Apo B) elevation, but is modified by other major risk factors, particularly low HDL-C.

Familial hypercholesterolaemia (FH) causes moderate to severe hypercholesterolaemia and has a prevalence of at least 0.2% in most populations. It is usually caused by a loss-of-function mutation in the LDL receptor gene, which results in an autosomal dominant pattern of inheritance. A similar syndrome can arise with loss-of-function mutations in the ligand-binding domain of Apo B100 or gain-of-function mutations in the *PCSK9* gene. The latter increases the activity of the PCSK9 protein, which is a sterol-sensitive protease that targets the LDL receptor for degradation. Causative mutations can be detected in one of these three genes by genetic testing in about 70% of patients with FH. Most patients with these types of FH have LDL levels that are approximately twice as high as in normal

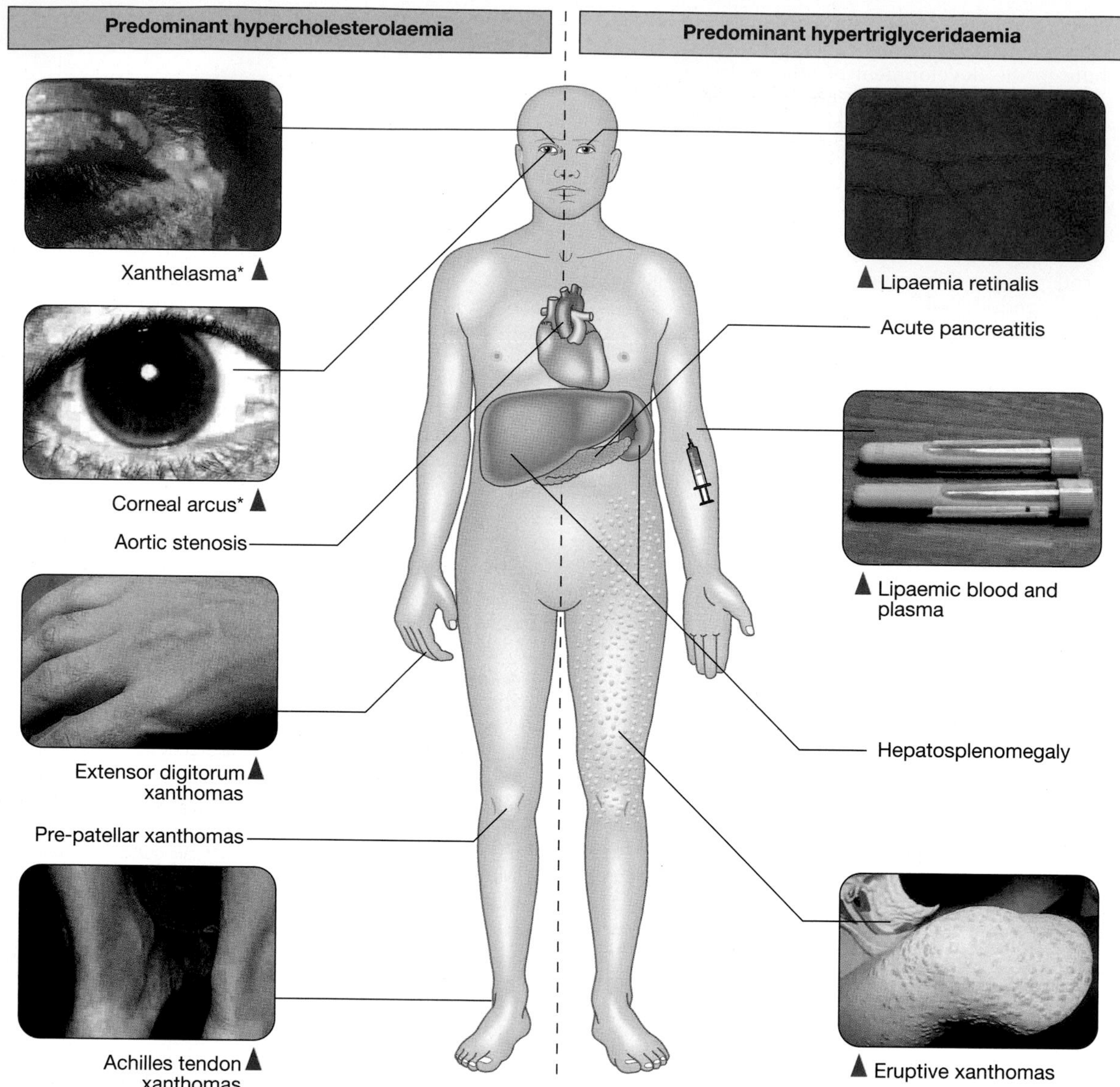

Fig. 16.15 Clinical manifestations of hyperlipidaemia. *Note that xanthelasma and corneal arcus may be non-specific, especially in later life.

16.26 Classification of hyperlipidaemia

Disease	Elevated lipid results	Elevated lipoprotein	CHD risk	Pancreatitis risk
Predominant hypercholesterolaemia				
Polygenic (majority)	TC ± TG	LDL ± VLDL	+	–
Familial hypercholesterolaemia (LDL receptor defect, defective Apo B100, increased function of PCSK-9)	TC ± TG	LDL ± VLDL	+++	–
Hyperalphalipoproteinaemia	TC ± TG	HDL	–	–
Predominant hypertriglyceridaemia				
Polygenic (majority)	TG	VLDL ± LDL	Variable	+
Lipoprotein lipase deficiency	TG >> TC	Chylo	?	+++
Familial hypertriglyceridaemia	TG > TC	VLDL ± Chylo	?	++
Mixed hyperlipidaemia				
Polygenic (majority)	TC + TG	VLDL + LDL	Variable	+
Familial combined hyperlipidaemia*	TC and/or TG	LDL and/or VLDL	++	+
Dysbetalipoproteinaemia*	TC and/or TG	IDL	+++	+

+ = slightly increased risk; ++ = increased risk; +++ = greatly increased risk.
*Familial combined hyperlipidaemia and dysbetalipoproteinaemia may also present as predominant hypercholesterolaemia or predominant hypertriglyceridaemia.
(CHD = coronary heart disease; Chylo = chylomicrons; TC = total cholesterol; TG = triglycerides)

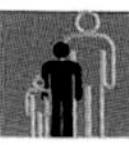

16.27 Familial hypercholesterolaemia in adolescence

- **Statin treatment**: may be required from the age of about 10. It does not compromise normal growth and maturation.
- **Tobacco**: patients should be strongly advised to avoid this.

subjects of the same age and gender. Affected subjects suffer from severe hypercholesterolaemia and premature cardiovascular disease. FH may be accompanied by xanthomas of the Achilles or extensor digitorum tendons (see Fig. 16.15), which are strongly suggestive of FH. The onset of corneal arcus before age 40 is also suggestive of this condition. Identification of an index case of FH (the first case of FH in a family) should trigger genetic and biochemical screening of other family members, which is a cost-effective method for case detection. Affected individuals should be managed from childhood (Box 16.27).

Homozygous FH may occur in populations in which there is a 'founder' effect or consanguineous marriage, resulting in more extensive xanthomas and precocious cardiovascular disease in childhood. Hyperalphalipoproteinaemia refers to increased levels of HDL-C. In the absence of an increase in LDL-C, this condition does not cause cardiovascular disease, so it should not be regarded as pathological.

Familial combined hyperlipidaemia, and dysbetalipoproteinaemia, may present with the pattern of predominant hypercholesterolaemia (see 'Mixed hyperlipidaemia' below).

Predominant hypertriglyceridaemia

Polygenic hypertriglyceridaemia is the most common cause of a raised TG level (see Box 16.26). Other common causes include excess alcohol intake, medications (such as β-blockers and retinoids), type 2 diabetes, impaired glucose tolerance, central obesity or other manifestations of insulin resistance (p. 805) and impaired absorption of bile acids. It is often accompanied by post-prandial hyperlipidaemia and reduced HDL-C, both of which may contribute to cardiovascular risk. Excessive intake of alcohol or dietary fat, or other exacerbating factors may precipitate a massive increase in TG levels, which, if they exceed 10 mmol/L (880 mg/dL), may pose a risk of acute pancreatitis.

Inherited forms of hypertriglyceridaemia also occur. Loss-of-function mutations in the *LPL* gene, which encodes lipoprotein lipase, or the *APOC2* gene, which encodes the Apo C2 protein that acts as a co-factor for lipoprotein lipase, may cause recessively inherited forms of hypertriglyceridaemia. These mutations cause massive hypertriglyceridaemia that is not readily amenable to drug treatment. It often presents in childhood and is associated with episodes of acute abdominal pain and pancreatitis. In common with other causes of severe hypertriglyceridaemia, it may result in hepatosplenomegaly, lipaemia retinalis and eruptive xanthomas (see Fig. 16.15).

Familial hypertriglyceridaemia may also be inherited in a dominant manner due to mutations in the *APOA5* gene, which encodes Apo A5 – a co-factor that is essential for lipoprotein lipase activity. This disorder may be associated with high levels of TG that predispose to cardiovascular disease and pancreatitis.

Familial combined hyperlipidaemia, and dysbetalipoproteinaemia, may present with the pattern of predominant hypertriglyceridaemia (see 'Mixed hyperlipidaemia', below).

Mixed hyperlipidaemia

It is difficult to define quantitatively the distinction between predominant hyperlipidaemias and mixed hyperlipidaemia. The term 'mixed' usually implies the presence of hypertriglyceridaemia, as well as an increase in LDL or IDL. Treatment of massive hypertriglyceridaemia may improve TG faster than cholesterol, thus temporarily mimicking mixed hyperlipidaemia.

Primary mixed hyperlipidaemia is usually polygenic and, like predominant hypertriglyceridaemia, often occurs in association with type 2 diabetes, impaired glucose tolerance, central obesity or other manifestations of insulin resistance (p. 805). Both components of mixed hyperlipidaemia may contribute to the risk of cardiovascular disease.

Familial combined hyperlipidaemia is a term used to identify an inherited tendency towards the overproduction of atherogenic Apo B-containing lipoproteins. It results in elevation of cholesterol, TG or both in different family members at different times. It is associated with an increased risk of cardiovascular disease but it does not produce any pathognomonic physical signs. In practice, this relatively common condition is substantially modified by factors such as age and weight. It may not be a monogenic condition, but rather one end of a heterogeneous spectrum that overlaps insulin resistance (p. 805).

Dysbetalipoproteinaemia (also referred to as type 3 hyperlipidaemia, broad-beta dyslipoproteinaemia or remnant hyperlipidaemia) involves accumulation of roughly equimolar levels of cholesterol and TG. It is caused by homozygous inheritance of the Apo E2 allele, which is the isoform least avidly recognised by the LDL receptor. In conjunction with other exacerbating factors, such as obesity and diabetes, it leads to accumulation of atherogenic IDL and chylomicron remnants. Premature cardiovascular disease is common and it may also result in the formation of palmar xanthomas, tuberous xanthomas or tendon xanthomas.

Rare dyslipidaemias

Several rare disturbances of lipid metabolism have been described (Box 16.28). They provide important insights into lipid metabolism and its impact on risk of cardiovascular disease.

Fish eye disease, Apo A1 Milano and LCAT deficiency demonstrate that very low HDL levels do not necessarily cause cardiovascular disease, but Apo A1 deficiency, and possibly Tangier disease, demonstrate that low HDL-C can be atherogenic under some circumstances. Autosomal recessive FH and *PCSK9* gain-of-function mutations reveal the importance of proteins that chaperone the LDL receptor. Sitosterolaemia and cerebrotendinous xanthomatosis demonstrate that sterols other than cholesterol can cause xanthomas and cardiovascular disease, while *PCSK9* loss-of-function mutations, abetalipoproteinaemia and hypobetalipoproteinaemia suggest that low levels of Apo B-containing lipoproteins reduce the risk of cardiovascular disease. The only adverse health outcomes associated with

16.28 Miscellaneous and rare forms of hyperlipidaemia

Condition	Lipoprotein pattern	CVD risk
Tangier disease	Very low HDL, low TC	+
Apo A1 deficiency	Very low HDL	++
Apo A1 Milano	Very low HDL	–
Fish eye disease	Very low HDL, high TG	–
LCAT deficiency	Very low HDL, high TG	?
Autosomal recessive FH	Very high LDL	++
Sitosterolaemia	High plant sterols including sitosterol	+
Cerebrotendinous xanthomatosis	Bile acid defect (cholestanol accumulation)	+

+ = slightly increased risk; ++ = increased risk.
(CVD = cardiovascular disease; FH = familial hypercholesterolaemia; HDL = high-density lipoprotein; LCAT = lecithin cholesterol acyl transferase; TC = total cholesterol; TG = triglycerides)

extremely low plasma lipid levels in the latter two conditions are attributable to fat-soluble vitamin deficiency, or impaired transport of lipid from intestine or liver.

Management of dyslipidaemia

Lipid-lowering therapies have a key role in the secondary and primary prevention of cardiovascular diseases (p. 581). Assessment of absolute risk, treatment of all modifiable risk factors and optimisation of lifestyle, especially diet and exercise, are central to management in all cases.

Patients with the greatest absolute risk of cardiovascular disease will derive the greatest absolute benefit from treatment. Public health organisations recommend thresholds for the introduction of lipid-lowering therapy based on the identification of patients in very high-risk categories, or those calculated to be at high absolute risk according to algorithms or tables such as the Joint British Societies Coronary Risk Prediction Chart (see Fig. 18.62, p. 582). These tables, which are based on large epidemiological studies, should be recalibrated for the local population, if possible. In general, patients who have cardiovascular disease, diabetes mellitus, chronic renal impairment, familial hypercholesterolaemia or an absolute risk of cardiovascular disease of greater than 20% in the ensuing 10 years are arbitrarily regarded as having sufficient risk to justify drug treatment.

Public health organisations also recommend target levels for patients receiving drug treatment. High-risk patients should aim for HDL-C > 1 mmol/L (38 mg/dL) and fasting TG < 2 mmol/L (approximately 180 mg/dL), whilst target levels for LDL-C have been reduced from 2.5 to 2.0 mmol/L (76 mg/dL) or less. In general, total cholesterol should be < 5 mmol/L (190 mg/dL) during treatment, and < 4 mmol/L (approximately 150 mg/dL) in high-risk patients and in secondary prevention of cardiovascular disease.

Non-pharmacological management

Patients with lipid abnormalities should receive medical advice and, if necessary, dietary counselling to:

- reduce intake of saturated and trans-unsaturated fat to less than 7–10% of total energy
- reduce intake of cholesterol to < 250 mg/day
- replace sources of saturated fat and cholesterol with alternative foods, such as lean meat, low-fat dairy products, polyunsaturated spreads and low glycaemic index carbohydrates
- reduce energy-dense foods such as fats and soft drinks, whilst increasing activity and exercise to maintain or lose weight
- increase consumption of cardioprotective and nutrient-dense foods, such as vegetables, unrefined carbohydrates, fish, pulses, nuts, legumes, fruit, etc.
- adjust alcohol consumption, reducing intake if excessive or if associated with hypertension, hypertriglyceridaemia or central obesity
- achieve additional benefits with supplementary intake of foods containing lipid-lowering nutrients such as n-3 fatty acids, dietary fibre and plant sterols.

The response to diet is usually apparent within 3–4 weeks but dietary adjustment may need to be introduced gradually. Although hyperlipidaemia in general, and hypertriglyceridaemia in particular, can be very responsive to these measures, LDL-C reductions are often only modest in routine clinical practice. Explanation, encouragement and persistence are often required to induce patient compliance. Even minor weight loss can substantially reduce cardiovascular risk, especially in centrally obese patients (p. 116).

All other modifiable cardiovascular risk factors should be assessed and treated. If possible, intercurrent drug treatments that adversely affect the lipid profile should be replaced.

Pharmacological management

The main diagnostic categories provide a useful framework for management and the selection of first-line pharmacological treatment (Fig. 16.16).

Predominant hypercholesterolaemia

Predominant hypercholesterolaemia can be treated with one or more of the cholesterol-lowering drugs:

Statins. These reduce cholesterol synthesis by inhibiting the HMGCoA reductase enzyme. The reduction in cholesterol synthesis up-regulates activity of the LDL receptor, which increases clearance of LDL and its precursor, IDL, resulting in a secondary reduction in LDL synthesis. Statins reduce LDL-C by up to 60%, reduce TG by up to 40% and increase HDL-C by up to 10%. They also reduce the concentration of intermediate metabolites such as isoprenes, which may lead to other effects such as suppression of the inflammatory response. There is clear evidence of protection against total and coronary mortality, stroke and cardiovascular events across the spectrum of CVD risk (Box 16.29).

Statins are generally well tolerated and serious side-effects are rare (well below 2%). Liver function test abnormalities and muscle problems, such as myalgia, asymptomatic increase in creatine kinase (CK), myositis and, infrequently, rhabdomyolysis, are the most common. Side-effects are more likely in patients who are elderly, debilitated or receiving other drugs that interfere with statin degradation, which usually involves cytochrome P450 3A4 or glucuronidation.

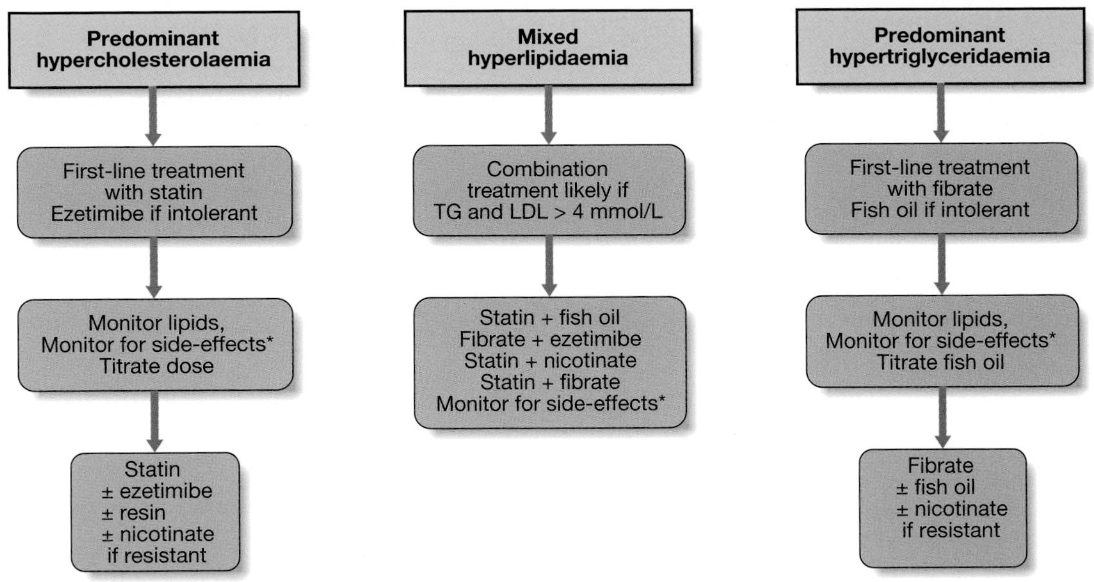

Fig. 16.16 Flow chart for the drug treatment of hyperlipidaemia. *Interrupt treatment if CK is more than 5–10 times the upper limit of normal, or if elevated with muscle symptoms, or if ALT is more than 2–3 times the upper limit. To convert TG in mmol/L to mg/dL, multiply by 88. To convert LDL-C in mmol/L to mg/dL, multiply by 38. (ALT = alanine aminotransferase; CK = creatine kinase)

EBM 16.29 Benefits of using statins to treat patients with hypercholesterolaemia

'Meta-analysis of major randomised controlled clinical trials involving over 130 000 subjects receiving statins for approximately 5 years showed a reduced risk of a major cardiovascular event of 21% (95% confidence interval 19–23%) per 1 mmol/L reduction in LDL-C, irrespective of age, gender, baseline LDL-C or intercurrent cardiovascular disease. Relative risk reduction was equally favourable in the subjects with the lowest risk.'

- Cholesterol Treatment Trialists Collaborators. Lancet 2012; 380:581–590.

Cholesterol absorption inhibitors. The only licensed drug in this class is ezetimibe, which inhibits activity of the intestinal mucosal transporter NPC1L1 that absorbs dietary and biliary cholesterol. Depletion of hepatic cholesterol up-regulates hepatic LDL receptor activity. This mechanism of action is synergistic with the effect of statins. Monotherapy with the standard 10 mg/day dose reduces LDL-C by 15–20%. Slightly greater (17–25%) incremental LDL-C reduction occurs when ezetimibe is added to statins. Ezetimibe is well tolerated, and evidence of a beneficial effect on cardiovascular disease endpoints may be inferred from a trial of combination therapy with simvastatin. Plant sterol-supplemented foods, which also reduce cholesterol absorption, lower LDL-C by 7–15%.

Bile acid sequestering resins. Drugs in this class include colestyramine, colestipol and colesevelam. These prevent the reabsorption of bile acids, thereby increasing de novo bile acid synthesis from hepatic cholesterol. As with ezetimibe, the resultant depletion of hepatic cholesterol up-regulates LDL receptor activity and reduces LDL-C in a manner that is synergistic with the action of statins. Resins reduce LDL-C and modestly increase HDL-C, but may increase TG. They are safe but may interfere with bioavailability of other drugs. Colesevelam has fewer gastrointestinal effects than older preparations that are less well tolerated. Development of specific inhibitors of the intestinal bile acid transporter may further improve tolerability of this class of agent.

Nicotinic acid. Pharmacological doses reduce peripheral fatty acid release with the result that VLDL and LDL decline whilst HDL-C increases. Randomised clinical trials have been inconsistent regarding effects on atherosclerosis and cardiovascular events. Side-effects include flushing, gastric irritation, liver function disturbances, and exacerbation of gout and hyperglycaemia. Slow-release formulations and low-dose aspirin may reduce flushing. Combination therapy with the prostaglandin D2 receptor inhibitor laropiprant to reduce flushing further is being evaluated.

Combination therapy. In many patients, treatment of predominant hypercholesterolaemia can be achieved by diet plus the use of a statin in sufficient doses to achieve target LDL-C levels. Patients who do not reach LDL targets on the highest tolerated statin dose, or who are intolerant of statins, may receive ezetimibe, plant sterols, nicotinic acid or resins. Ezetimibe and resins are safe and effective in combination with a statin, but nicotinic acid with a statin requires a greater level of caution because the risk of side-effects is slightly increased.

Predominant hypertriglyceridaemia

Predominant hypertriglyceridaemia can be treated with one of the TG-lowering drugs (see Fig. 16.16).

Fibrates. These stimulate peroxisome proliferator activated receptor (PPAR) alpha, which controls the expression of gene products that mediate the metabolism of TG and HDL. As a result, synthesis of fatty acids, TG and VLDL is reduced, whilst that of lipoprotein lipase, which catabolises TG, is enhanced. In addition, production of Apo A1 and ATP binding cassette A1 is up-regulated, leading to increased reverse cholesterol transport via HDL. Consequently, fibrates reduce TG by up to 50%

and increase HDL-C by up to 20%, but LDL-C changes are variable.

Fewer large-scale trials have been conducted with fibrates than with statins and the results are less conclusive, but reduced rates of cardiovascular disease have been reported with fibrate therapy in the subgroup of patients with low HDL-C levels and elevated TG (e.g. TG > 2.3 mmol/L (200 mg/dL)). Fibrates are usually well tolerated but share a similar side-effect profile to statins. In addition, they may increase the risk of cholelithiasis and prolong the action of anticoagulants. Accumulating evidence suggests that they may also have a protective effect against diabetic microvascular complications.

Highly polyunsaturated long-chain n-3 fatty acids. These include eicosapentaenoic acid (EPA) and docosahexaenoic acid (DHA), which comprise approximately 30% of the fatty acids in fish oil. EPA and DHA are potent inhibitors of VLDL TG formation. Intakes of greater than 2 g n-3 fatty acid (equivalent to 6 g of most forms of fish oil) per day lower TG in a dose-dependent fashion. Up to 50% reduction in TG may be achieved with 15 g fish oil per day. Changes in LDL-C and HDL-C are variable. Fish oil fatty acids have also been shown to inhibit platelet aggregation and improve cardiac arrhythmia in animal models. Dietary and pharmacological trials suggest that n-3 fatty acids may reduce mortality from coronary heart disease. Fish oils appear to be safe and well tolerated.

Patients with predominant hypertriglyceridaemia who do not respond to lifestyle intervention can be treated with fibrates, fish oil or nicotinic acid, depending on individual response and tolerance. If target levels are not achieved, the fibrates and fish oil or nicotinic acid can be combined. Massive hypertriglyceridaemia may require more aggressive limitation of dietary fat intake (< 10–20% energy as fat). Any degree of insulin deficiency should be corrected because insulin is required for optimal activity of lipoprotein lipase. The initial target for patients with massive hypertriglyceridaemia is TG < 10 mmol/L (880 mg/dL), to reduce the risk of acute pancreatitis.

Mixed hyperlipidaemia

Mixed hyperlipidaemia can be difficult to treat. Statins alone are less effective first-line therapy once fasting TG exceeds around 4 mmol/L (350 mg/dL). Fibrates are first-line therapy for dysbetalipoproteinaemia, but they may not control the cholesterol component in other forms of mixed hyperlipidaemia. Combination therapy is often required. Effective combinations include: statin plus fish oil when TG is not too high; fibrate plus ezetimibe; statin plus nicotinic acid; or statin plus fibrate. The risk of myopathy is increased with gemfibrozil, but fenofibrate is relatively safe in this regard.

Monitoring of therapy

The effect of drug therapy should be assessed after 6 weeks (12 weeks for fibrates). At this point, it is prudent to review side-effects, lipid response (see target levels above), CK and liver function tests. During longer-term follow-up, compliance with drug treatment, diet and exercise should be assessed, with monitoring of weight, blood pressure and lipid levels. The presence of cardiovascular symptoms or signs should be noted and absolute cardiovascular risk assessed periodically. It is not necessary to perform routine checks of CK and liver function unless symptoms occur, or if statins are used in combination with fibrates, nicotinic acid or other drugs that may interfere with their clearance. If myalgia or weakness occurs in association with CK elevation over 5–10 times the upper limit of normal, or if sustained alanine aminotransferase (ALT) elevation more than 2–3 times the upper limit of normal occurs that is not accounted for by fatty liver (p. 959), treatment should be discontinued and alternative therapy sought.

The principles of the management of dyslipidaemia can be applied broadly, but the objectives of treatment in the elderly (Box 16.30) and the safety of pharmacological therapy in pregnancy (Box 16.31) warrant special consideration.

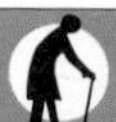

16.30 Management of hyperlipidaemia in old age

- **Prevalence of atherosclerotic cardiovascular disease**: greatest in old age.
- **Associated cardiovascular risk**: lipid levels become less predictive, as do other risk factors apart from age itself.
- **Benefit of statin therapy**: maintained up to the age of 80 years but evidence is lacking beyond this.
- **Life expectancy and statin therapy**: lives saved by intervention are associated with shorter life expectancy than in younger patients, and so the impact of statins on quality-adjusted life years is smaller in old age.

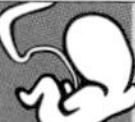

16.31 Dyslipidaemia in pregnancy

- **Lipid metabolism**: lipid and lipoprotein levels increase during pregnancy. This includes an increase in LDL-C, which resolves post-partum. Remnant dyslipidaemia and hypertriglyceridaemia may be exacerbated during pregnancy.
- **Treatment**: dyslipidaemia is rarely thought to warrant urgent treatment so pharmacological therapy is usually contraindicated when conception or pregnancy is anticipated. Teratogenicity has been reported with systemically absorbed agents, and non-absorbed agents may interfere with nutrient bioavailability.
- **Monitoring**: cardiovascular disease is very unlikely amongst women of child-bearing age, but is possible in women with severe risk factor profiles or familial hypercholesterolaemia, when pre-conception cardiovascular review can be considered to ensure that the patient will be able to withstand the demands of pregnancy and labour.

DISORDERS OF HAEM SYNTHESIS – THE PORPHYRIAS

The porphyrias are a group of disorders caused by inherited abnormalities in the haem biosynthetic pathway (Fig. 16.17). Most of the described forms are due to partial enzyme deficiencies with a dominant mode of inheritance. They are commonly classified as either hepatic or erythropoietic, depending on whether the major site of excess porphyrin production is in the liver or in the red cell.

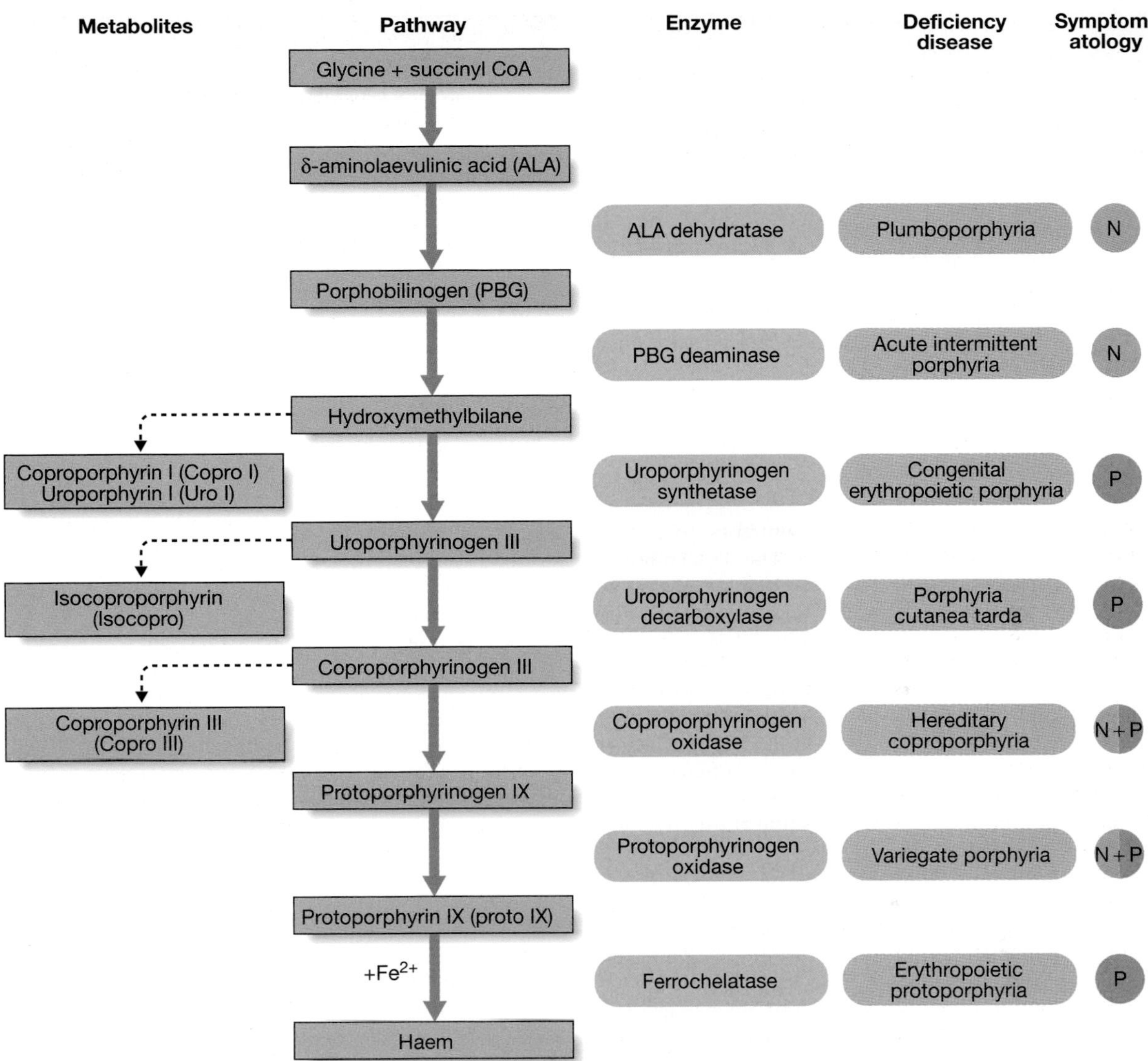

Fig. 16.17 Haem biosynthetic pathway and enzyme defects responsible for the porphyrias. (N = neurovisceral; P = photosensitive)

The porphyrias show a low penetrance in the order of 25%. Environmental factors are important in disease expression in some forms. In the most common of these conditions, porphyria cutanea tarda (PCT), these include alcohol, iron accumulation, exogenous oestrogens and exposure to various chemicals. Many cases are associated with hepatitis C infection and this should always be screened for on presentation.

Clinical features

The clinical features of porphyria fall into two broad categories, photosensitivity and acute neurovisceral syndrome. The enzyme defects responsible for the diseases are shown in Figure 16.17.

Photosensitive skin manifestations, attributable to excess production and accumulation of porphyrins in the skin, cause pain, erythema, bullae, skin erosions, hirsutism and hyperpigmentation, and occur predominantly on areas of the skin that are exposed to sunlight (p. 1260). The skin also becomes sensitive to damage from minimal trauma.

The other pattern of presentation is with an acute neurological syndrome. This presents with acute abdominal pain together with features of autonomic dysfunction such as tachycardia, hypertension and constipation. Neuropsychiatric manifestations, hyponatraemia due to inappropriate ADH release (p. 438), and an acute neuropathy may also occur (p. 1223). The neuropathy is usually motor and may, in severe cases, progress to respiratory failure.

There is no proven explanation for the episodic nature of the attacks in porphyria, which can relapse and remit or follow a prolonged and unremitting course. Sometimes, specific triggers can be identified, such as alcohol, fasting, or drugs such as anticonvulsants, sulphonamides, oestrogen and progesterone. The oral contraceptive pill is a common precipitating factor. In a significant number, no precipitant can be identified.

Diagnosis

The diagnosis of porphyria and classification into the various forms have traditionally relied on the pattern of

16.32 Diagnostic biochemical findings in the porphyrias

Condition	Elevated porphyrins and precursors		
	Blood	**Urine**	**Faeces**
ALA dehydratase deficiency (plumboporphyria)	Proto IX*	ALA, Copro III*	
Acute intermittent porphyria (AIP)		ALA, PBG	
Congenital erythropoietic porphyria (CEP)	Uro I	Uro I	Copro I
Porphyria cutanea tarda (PCT)		Uro I	Isocopro
Hereditary coproporphyria (HCP)		ALA, PBG, Copro III	Copro III
Variegate porphyria (VP)		ALA, PBG, Copro III	Proto IX
Erythropoietic protoporphyria (EPP)	Proto IX		Proto IX

*The paradoxical rise in coproporphyrin III (Copro III) and protoporphyrin (Proto) in this very rare condition is poorly understood.
Refer to Figure 16.17 for metabolic pathways.

the porphyrins and porphyrin precursors found in blood, urine and faeces (Box 16.32). This is a straightforward diagnosis at clinical presentation when the metabolites are significantly elevated, but this is not always the case in asymptomatic individuals.

More recently, measurement of the enzymes that are deficient in the various porphyrias has provided further diagnostic information (for example, PBG deaminase activity in red blood cells to diagnose acute intermittent porphyria). However, there is often considerable overlap between enzyme activities in affected and normal subjects. Furthermore, some of the enzymes occur in the mitochondria, for which it is more difficult to obtain suitable specimens for analysis. All the genes of the haem biosynthetic pathway have now been characterised. This has made it possible to identify affected individuals in families by genetic testing, a significant advance considering that penetrance of porphyria is low.

Metabolite excretory patterns are always grossly abnormal during an acute attack or in the presence of cutaneous manifestations of porphyria and are diagnostic of the particular porphyria. A normal metabolite profile under these circumstances effectively excludes porphyria. Metabolites usually remain abnormal for long periods after an acute attack, and in some individuals never return to normal. The diagnosis is not so straightforward in patients who are in remission, or in asymptomatic individuals with a positive family history. Neurological porphyria rarely manifests before puberty, nor can it be readily diagnosed from metabolite patterns after the menopause. In these circumstances, genetic testing for disease-specific mutations can now clarify the situation.

Management

For patients predisposed to neurovisceral attacks, general management includes avoidance of any agents known to precipitate acute porphyria. Specific management includes intravenous glucose, as provision of 5000 kilojoules per day can, in some cases, terminate acute attacks through a reduction in ALA synthetase activity, leading to reduced ALA synthesis. More recently, administration of haem (in various forms such as haematin or haem arginate) has been shown to reduce metabolite excretory rates, relieve pain and accelerate recovery. Cyclical acute attacks in women sometimes respond to suppression of the menstrual cycle using gonadotrophin-releasing hormone analogues. In rare cases with frequent prolonged attacks or attacks intractable to treatment, liver transplantation has been effective.

There are few specific or effective measures to treat the photosensitive manifestations. The primary goal is to avoid sun exposure and skin trauma. Barrier sun creams containing zinc or titanium oxide are the most effective products. New colourless creams containing nanoparticle formulations have improved patient acceptance. Beta-carotene is used in some patients with erythropoietic porphyria with some efficacy. Afamelanotide, a synthetic analogue of alpha-melanocyte stimulating hormone (α-MSH), has also been shown to provide protection in erythropoietic protoporphyria. In porphyria cutanea tarda, a course of venesections to remove iron can result in long-lasting clinical and biochemical remission, especially if exposure to identified precipitants, such as alcohol or oestrogens, is reduced. Alternatively, a prolonged course of low-dose chloroquine therapy is also effective.

Further information

Websites

http://emedicine.medscape.com *The Nephrology link on this site contains a useful compendium of articles.*

www.lipidsonline.org *Summarises management strategies for dyslipidaemia.*

www.ncbi.nlm.nih.gov *The link to OMIM (Online Mendelian Inheritance in Man) provides updated information on the genetic basis of metabolic disorders.*

www.porphyria-europe.com and www.drugs-porphyria.org *Excellent resources on drug safety in porphyria.*

J. Goddard
A.N. Turner

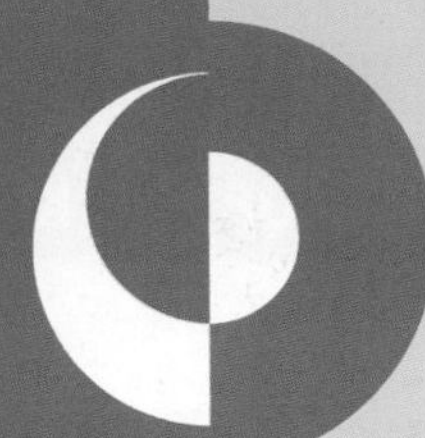

Kidney and urinary tract disease 17

Clinical examination of the kidney and urinary tract 462

Functional anatomy and physiology 464

Investigation of renal and urinary tract disease 466
- Glomerular filtration rate 466
- Urinalysis 468
- Blood tests 468
- Imaging 468
- Renal biopsy 471

Presenting problems in renal and urinary tract disease 471
- Dysuria 471
- Loin pain 471
- Oliguria/anuria 471
- Polyuria 472
- Nocturia 472
- Frequency 472
- Urinary incontinence 472
- Erectile dysfunction 474
- Haematuria 474
- Proteinuria and nephrotic syndrome 476
- Oedema 478
- Hypertension 478

Acute kidney injury 478

Chronic kidney disease 483

Renal replacement therapy 488
- Preparing for renal replacement therapy 489
- Conservative treatment 490
- Haemodialysis 490
- Haemofiltration 491
- Haemodiafiltration 492
- Peritoneal dialysis 492
- Renal transplantation 492

Renal vascular diseases 494
- Renal artery stenosis 494
- Acute renal infarction 495
- Diseases of small intrarenal vessels 495

Glomerular diseases 497
- Glomerulonephritis 498
- Inherited glomerular diseases 502

Tubulo-interstitial diseases 502
- Acute interstitial nephritis 502
- Chronic interstitial nephritis 503
- Reflux nephropathy 504
- Papillary necrosis 505
- Sickle-cell nephropathy 505

Cystic diseases of the kidney 505

Renal stone disease 507

Isolated defects of tubular function 510

Diseases of the collecting system and ureters 510
- Congenital abnormalities 510
- Retroperitoneal fibrosis 511

Infections of the urinary tract 511

Benign prostatic enlargement 514
- Prostatitis 515

Tumours of the kidney and urinary tract 515
- Renal adenocarcinoma 515
- Urothelial tumours 516
- Prostate cancer 517
- Testicular tumours 518
- Inherited tumour syndromes affecting the renal tract 519

Renal involvement in systemic conditions 519

Pregnancy and renal disease 520

Kidney disease in adolescence 521

Drugs and the kidney 522

CLINICAL EXAMINATION OF THE KIDNEY AND URINARY TRACT

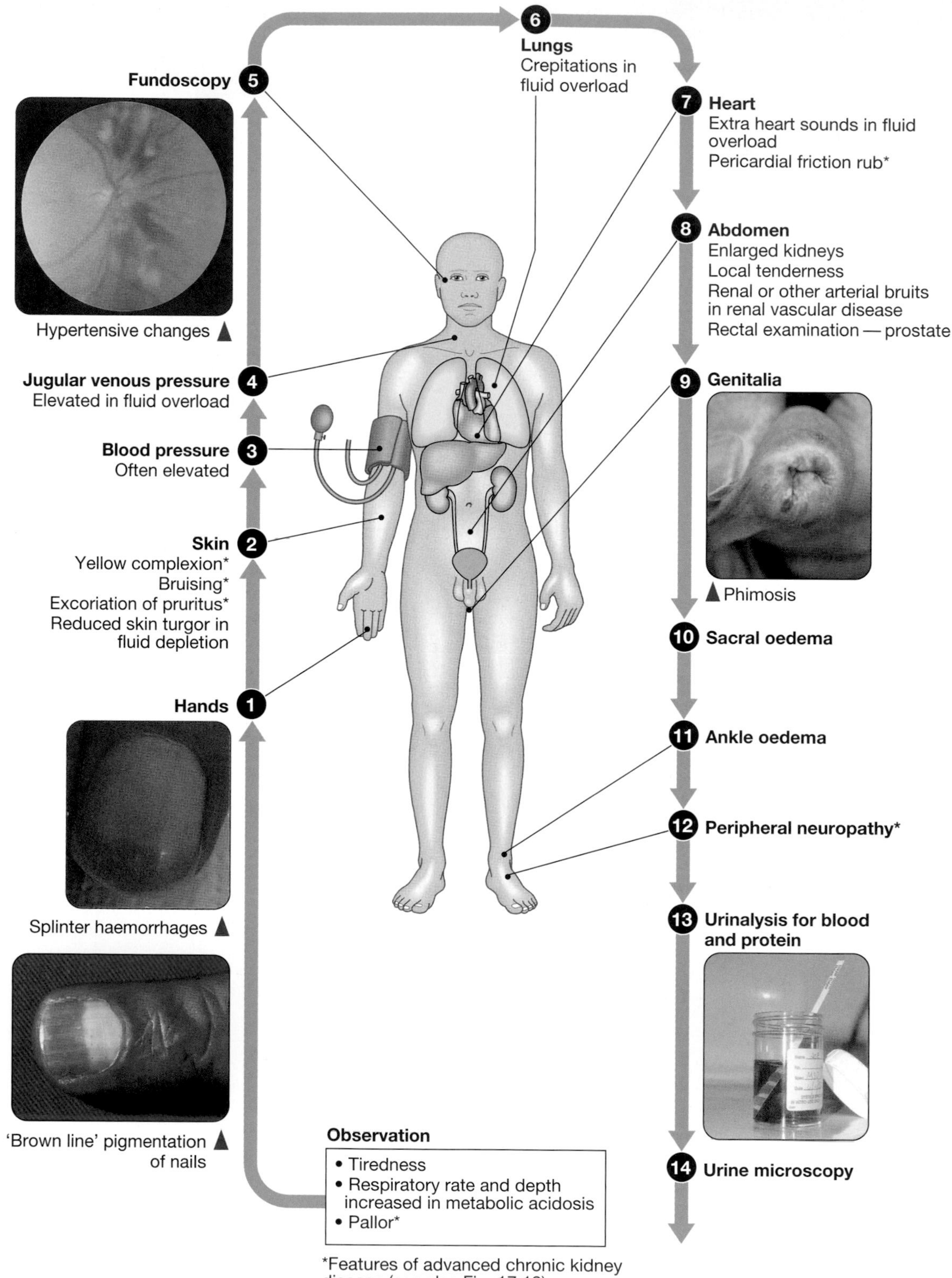

*Features of advanced chronic kidney disease (see also Fig. 17.13)

Many diseases of the kidney and urinary tract are clinically silent, at least in the early stages. Accordingly, it is common for these conditions to first be detected by routine blood tests or on dipstick testing of the urine. Several important abnormalities can also be picked up on physical examination, however, as summarised below.

1

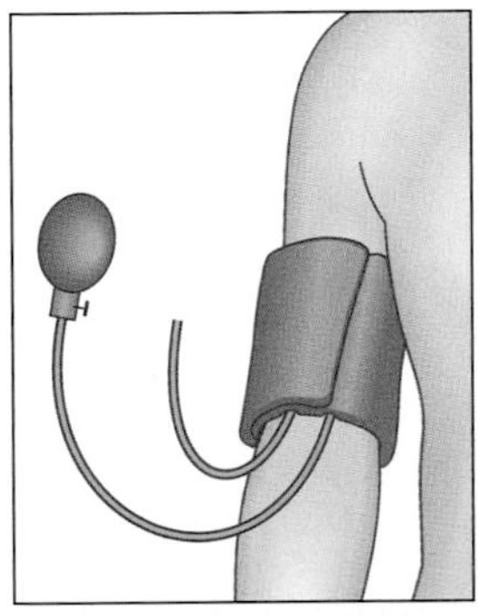

Blood pressure measurements

2

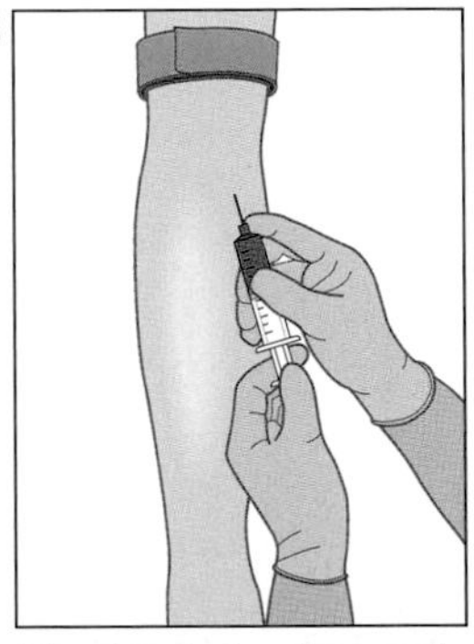

Blood tests for abnormal creatinine and electrolytes

3

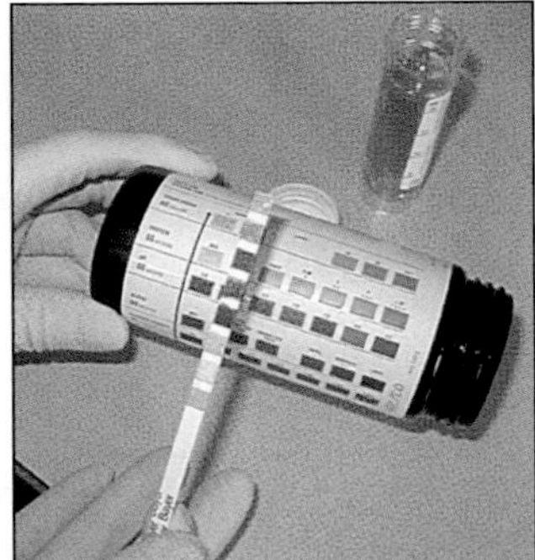

Dipstick testing for protein, blood, nitrate and leucocytes

4

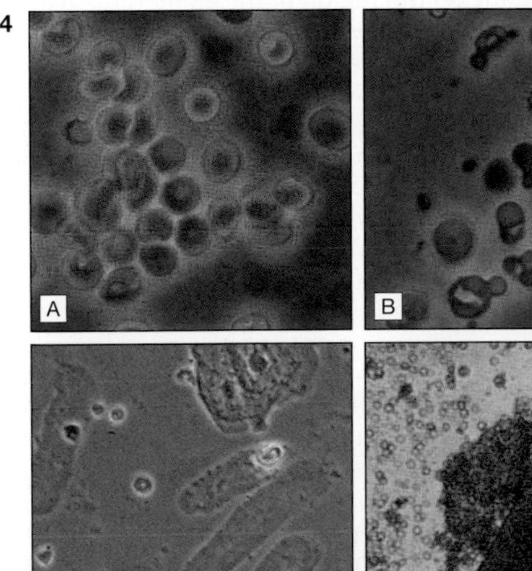

Urine microscopy. A Erythrocytes due to bleeding from lower in the urinary tract (x400). B Dysmorphic erythrocytes due to glomerular inflammation (x400). C Hyaline casts (arrows), in normal urine (×160). D Erythrocytes and a red cell cast (arrow) in glomerulonephritis (x100). Panels A–C are phase contrast images; D is a bright field image.

5

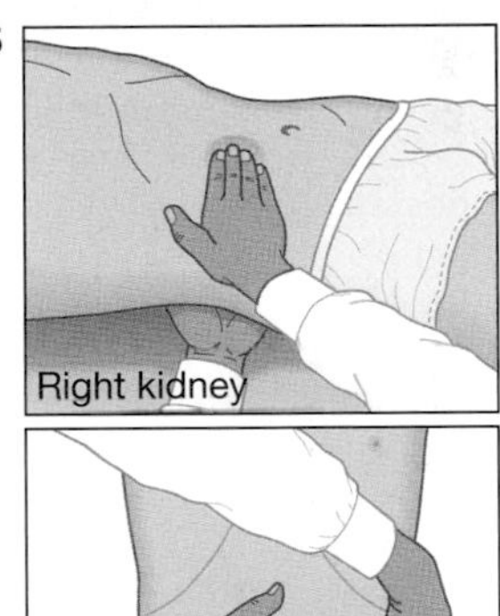

Abdominal examination for palpable kidneys

6

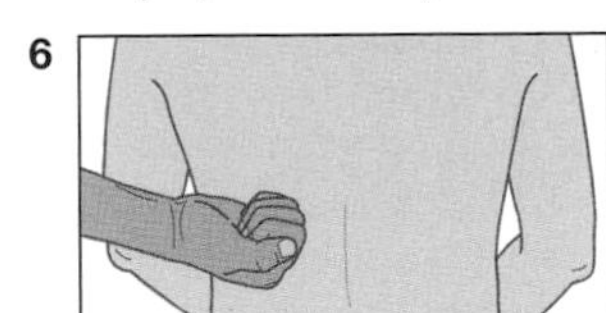

Percussing for tenderness in renal angle

7

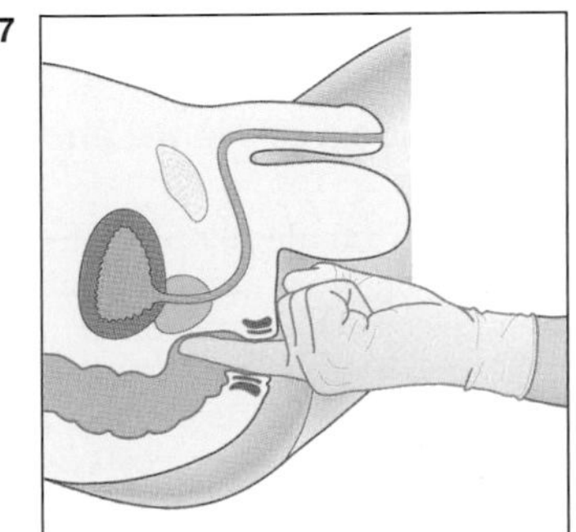

Digital rectal examination for prostate enlargement

8

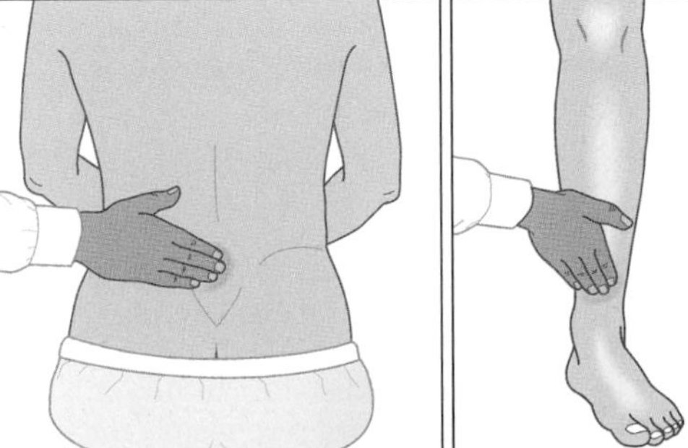

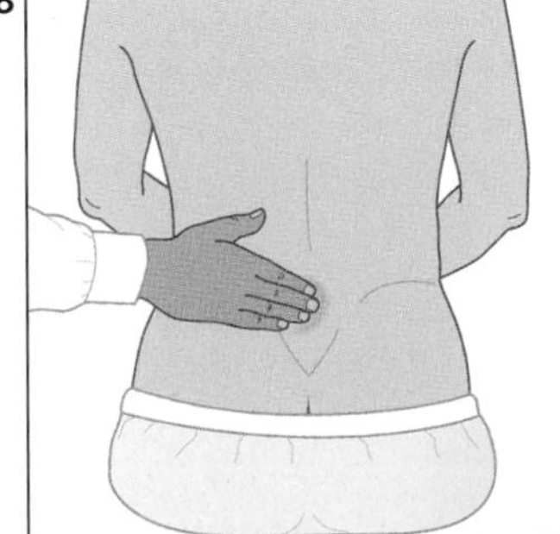

Checking sacrum and ankles for pitting oedema

Inset (Dipstick): From Pitkin J, et al. 2003 – see p. 523.

This chapter describes the disorders of the kidneys and urinary tract that are commonly encountered in routine practice, as well as giving an overview of the highly specialised field of renal replacement therapy. Disorders of renal tubular function, which may cause alterations in electrolyte and acid–base balance, are described in Chapter 16.

FUNCTIONAL ANATOMY AND PHYSIOLOGY

The kidneys

The kidneys play a central role in excretion of many metabolic breakdown products, including ammonia, urea and creatinine from protein, and uric acid from nucleic acids, drugs and toxins. They also regulate fluid and electrolyte balance. This is achieved by making large volumes of an ultrafiltrate of plasma (120 mL/min, 170 L/day) at the glomerulus, and selectively reabsorbing components of this ultrafiltrate at points along the nephron. The rates of filtration and reabsorption are controlled by many hormonal and haemodynamic signals.

The kidneys also regulate acid–base homeostasis, calcium and phosphate homeostasis, vitamin D metabolism and production of red blood cells. They are important in regulating blood pressure. Renin is secreted from the juxtaglomerular apparatus in response to reduced afferent arteriolar pressure, stimulation of sympathetic nerves, and changes in sodium content of fluid in the distal convoluted tubule at the macula densa, and is the first step in the generation of angiotensin II and aldosterone release, which in turn regulate systemic vasoconstriction and extracellular volume.

Each kidney is approximately 11–14 cm in length in healthy adults; they are located retroperitoneally on either side of the aorta and inferior vena cava between the 12th thoracic and 3rd lumbar vertebra (Fig. 17.1A). The right kidney is usually a few centimetres lower because the liver lies above it. Both kidneys rise and descend several centimetres with respiration.

The kidneys have a rich blood supply and receive approximately 20–25% of cardiac output through the renal arteries, which arise from the abdominal aorta. The renal arteries undergo various subdivisions within the kidney, eventually forming interlobular arteries that run through the renal cortex. These eventually give rise to afferent glomerular arterioles that supply individual nephrons, which are the functional units of the kidney. The efferent arteriole, leading from the glomerulus, supplies the distal nephron and medulla in a 'portal' circulation (Fig. 17.1B).

The nephron

Healthy kidneys contain approximately 1 million individual nephrons. Each nephron consists of a glomerulus, which is responsible for ultrafiltration of blood, a proximal renal tubule, a loop of Henle, a distal renal tubule and a collecting duct, which together are responsible for selective reabsorption of water and electrolytes that have been filtered at the glomerulus (see Fig. 16.2, p. 430). Under normal circumstances, more than 99% of the 170 litres of glomerular filtrate that is produced each day is reabsorbed in the tubules. The remainder passes through the collecting ducts of multiple nephrons and drains into the renal pelvis and ureters.

The glomerulus

The glomerulus comprises a tightly packed loop of capillaries supplied by an afferent arteriole and drained by an efferent arteriole. It is surrounded by a cup-shaped extension of the proximal tubule termed Bowman's capsule, which is comprised of epithelial cells. Blood that enters the glomerulus undergoes ultrafiltration across the glomerular basement membrane (GBM), which is formed by fusion of the basement membranes of tubular epithelial and vascular endothelial cells (Fig. 17.1C and D). The glomerular capillary endothelial cells contain pores (fenestrae), through which circulating molecules can pass to reach the underlying GBM. Glomerular epithelial cells (podocytes) have multiple long foot processes which interdigitate with those of the adjacent epithelial cells (Fig. 17.1E). As well as maintaining a selective barrier to filtration, podocytes are involved in regulating turnover of the GBM. Mesangial cells lie in the central region of the glomerulus. They have contractile properties similar to those of vascular smooth muscle cells but also have macrophage-like properties.

Under normal circumstances, the glomerulus is impermeable to proteins the size of albumin (67 kDa) or larger, while proteins of 20 kDa or smaller are filtered freely. The ability of molecules between 20 and 67 kDa to pass through the GBM is variable and depends on the size (smaller molecules are filtered more easily) and charge (positively charged molecules are filtered more easily). Very little lipid is filtered by the glomerulus.

Filtration pressure at the glomerulus is normally maintained at a constant level, in the face of wide variations in systemic blood pressure and cardiac output, by alterations in muscle tone within the afferent and efferent arterioles. This is known as autoregulation. When there is a reduction in renal perfusion pressure, renin is released by specialised smooth muscle cells in the juxtaglomerular apparatus. Renin cleaves angiotensinogen to release angiotensin I, which is further cleaved by angiotensin-converting enzyme (ACE) to produce angiotensin II (Fig. 17.1D). This restores glomerular perfusion pressure in the short term by causing vasoconstriction of the efferent arterioles within the kidney and by inducing systemic vasoconstriction to increase blood pressure and thus renal perfusion pressure. In the longer term, angiotensin II increases plasma volume by stimulating aldosterone release, which enhances sodium reabsorption by the renal tubules (see Fig. 20.17, p. 771).

Renal tubules, loop of Henle and collecting ducts

The proximal renal tubule, loop of Henle, distal renal tubule and collecting ducts are responsible for reabsorption of water, electrolytes and other solutes, as well as regulating acid–base balance, as described in detail on page 430 and in Figure 16.3. They also play a key role in regulating calcium homeostasis by converting 25-hydroxyvitamin D to the active metabolite 1,25-dihydroxyvitamin D (p. 1126). Failure of this process contributes to the pathogenesis of hypocalcaemia and bone disease which occurs in chronic kidney disease (CKD, p. 483). Fibroblast-like cells that lie in the interstitium of the renal cortex are responsible for production

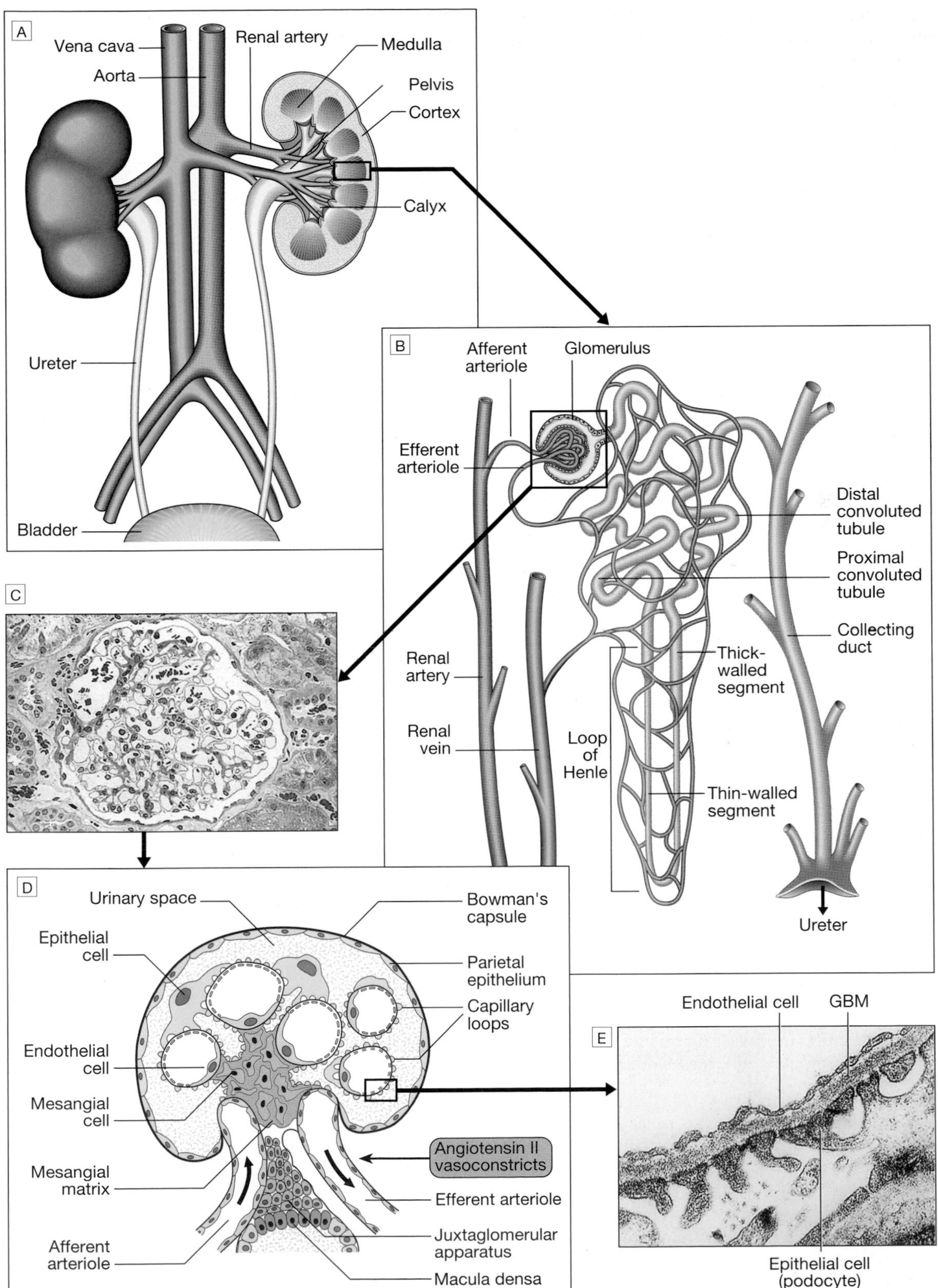

Fig. 17.1 Functional anatomy of the kidney. **A** Anatomical relationships of the kidney. **B** A single nephron. For the functions of different segments, see Figures 16.2 and 16.3 (pp. 430 and 431). **C** Histology of a normal glomerulus. **D** Schematic cross-section of a glomerulus, showing five capillary loops, to illustrate structure and show cell types. **E** Electron micrograph of the filtration barrier. (GBM = glomerular basement membrane)

of erythropoietin, which in turn is required for production of red blood cells. Erythropoietin synthesis is regulated by oxygen tension; anaemia and hypoxia increase production, whereas polycythaemia and hyperoxia inhibit it. Failure of erythropoietin production plays an important role in the pathogenesis of anaemia in CKD.

Ureters and bladder

The ureters drain urine from the renal pelvis (Fig. 17.1A) and deliver it to the bladder, a muscular organ that lies anteriorly in the lower part of the pelvis, just behind the pubic bone. The function of the bladder is to store and then release urine during micturition. The bladder is richly innervated. Sympathetic nerves arising from T10–L2 relay in the pelvic ganglia to cause relaxation of the detrusor muscle and contraction of the bladder neck (both via α-adrenoceptors), thereby preventing release of urine from the bladder. The distal sphincter mechanism is innervated by somatic motor fibres from sacral segments S2–4, which reach the sphincter either by the pelvic plexus or via the pudendal nerves. Afferent sensory impulses pass to the cerebral cortex, from where reflex-increased sphincter tone and suppression of detrusor contraction inhibit micturition until it is appropriate. Conversely, parasympathetic nerves arising from S2–4 stimulate detrusor contraction, promoting micturition.

The micturition cycle has a storage (filling) phase and a voiding (micturition) phase. During the filling phase, the high compliance of the detrusor muscle allows the bladder to fill steadily without a rise in intravesical pressure. As bladder volume increases, stretch receptors in its wall cause reflex bladder relaxation and increased sphincter tone. At approximately 75% bladder capacity, there is a desire to void. Voluntary control is now exerted over the desire to void, which disappears temporarily. Compliance of the detrusor allows further increase in capacity until the next desire to void. Just how often this desire needs to be inhibited depends on many factors, not the least of which is finding a suitable place in which to void.

The act of micturition is initiated first by voluntary and then by reflex relaxation of the pelvic floor and distal sphincter mechanism, followed by reflex detrusor contraction. These actions are coordinated by the pontine micturition centre. Intravesical pressure remains greater than urethral pressure until the bladder is empty.

The prostate gland

The prostate gland is situated at the base of the bladder, surrounding the proximal urethra. Exocrine glands within the prostate produce fluid, which comprises about 20% of the volume of ejaculated seminal fluid and is rich in zinc and proteolytic enzymes. The remainder of the ejaculate is formed in the seminal vesicles and bulbo-urethral glands, with spermatozoa arising from the testes.

Smooth muscle fibres within the prostate, which are under sympathetic control, play a role in controlling urine flow through the bulbar urethra, and also contract at orgasm to move seminal fluid through ejaculatory ducts into the bulbar urethra (emission). Contraction of the bulbocavernosus muscle (via a spinal muscle reflex) then ejaculates the semen out of the urethra.

The penis

Blood flow into the corpus cavernosum of the penis is controlled by sympathetic nerves from the thoracolumbar plexus, which maintain smooth muscle contraction. In response to afferent input from the glans penis and from higher centres, pelvic splanchnic parasympathetic nerves actively relax the cavernosal smooth muscle via neurotransmitters such as nitric oxide, acetylcholine, vasoactive intestinal polypeptide (VIP) and prostacyclin, with consequent dilatation of the lacunar space. At the same time, draining venules are compressed, trapping blood in the lacunar space with consequent elevation of pressure and erection (tumescence) of the penis.

INVESTIGATION OF RENAL AND URINARY TRACT DISEASE

Glomerular filtration rate

The glomerular filtration rate (GFR) is the rate at which fluid passes into nephrons after filtration and is a measure of renal function. It is proportionate to body

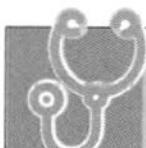

17.1 How to estimate glomerular filtration rate (GFR)

Measuring GFR

- Direct measurement using labelled EDTA or inulin
- Creatinine clearance (CrCl)
  Minor tubular secretion of creatinine causes CrCl to exaggerate GFR when renal function is poor, and can be affected by drugs (e.g. trimethoprim, cimetidine)
  Needs 24-hr urine collection (inconvenient and often unreliable)

$$\text{CrCl (mL/min)} = \frac{\text{urine creatinine concentration } (\mu\text{mol / L}) \times \text{volume (mL)}}{\text{plasma creatinine concentration } (\mu\text{mol/L}) \times \text{time (min)}}$$

Estimating GFR with equations

- Cockcroft and Gault equation
  Reasonably accurate at normal to moderately impaired renal function
  Estimates CrCl, not GFR
  Requires patient weight

$$\text{CrCl} = \frac{(140 - \text{age in yrs}) \times \text{lean body weight (kg)} \times (1.22 \text{ males or } 1.04 \text{ females})}{\text{serum creatinine } (\mu\text{mol/L})}$$

- The Modification of Diet in Renal Disease (MDRD) study equation (see www.renal.org/eGFR)
  Performs better than Cockcroft and Gault at low GFR
  Requires knowledge of age and sex only
  Can be reported automatically by laboratories
  For limitations, see Box 17.2

$$\text{eGFR} = 186^* \times (\text{creatinine in } \mu\text{mol/L}/88.4)^{-1.154} \times (\text{age in yrs})^{-0.203} \times (0.742 \text{ if female}) \times (1.21 \text{ if black})$$

- No equations perform well in unusual circumstances, such as extremes of body (and muscle) mass or in acutely unwell patients (see Box 17.2)

*A correction factor, either a value recommended by the laboratory/assay manufacturer or a default value of 186; see www.renal.org/ckd. To convert creatinine in mg/dL to µmol/L, multiply by 88.4.

size and the reference range is usually expressed after correction for body surface area as 120 ± 25 mL/min/1.73 m^2. The GFR may be measured directly by injecting and measuring the clearance of compounds such as inulin or radiolabelled ethylenediaminetetracetic acid, which are completely filtered at the glomerulus and are not secreted or reabsorbed by the renal tubules (Box 17.1). However, this is not performed routinely and is usually reserved for special circumstances, such as the assessment of renal function in potential live kidney donors. Instead, GFR is usually indirectly assessed in clinical practice by measuring serum levels of endogenously produced compounds that are excreted by the kidney. The most widely used is serum creatinine, which is produced by muscle at a constant rate, is almost completely filtered at the glomerulus, and is not reabsorbed. Although creatinine is secreted to a small degree by the proximal tubule, this is only usually significant in terms of GFR estimation in severe renal impairment, where it accounts for a larger proportion of the creatinine excreted. Accordingly, provided muscle mass remains constant, changes in serum creatinine concentrations closely reflect changes in GFR, although the reference range for creatinine is wide due to the fact that muscle mass varies widely between different individuals (Fig. 17.2). Several methods have been developed with which to estimate GFR from serum

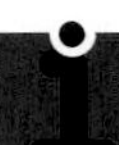

17.2 Limitations of eGFR

- It is only an estimate, least reliable at extremes of body composition (malnourished, amputees) and in hospital inpatients (as it was derived from outpatients)
- Confidence intervals are wide (90% of patients will have eGFR within 30% of their measured GFR, and 98% within 50%)
- Values are consistent in individuals, so changes mean more than absolute values
- Creatinine level must be stable over days; eGFR is not valid in assessing acute kidney injury
- It tends to underestimate normal or near-normal function, so slightly low values should not be over-interpreted. Many laboratories report only up to > 60 mL/min/1.73 m^2 for this reason
- In the elderly, who constitute the majority of those with low eGFR, there is controversy about categorising people as having chronic kidney disease (CKD; Box 17.3) on the basis of eGFR alone, particularly at stage 3A, since there is little evidence of adverse outcomes when eGFR is > 50 unless there is also proteinuria
- eGFR is not valid in under-18s or during pregnancy
- The equation was originally validated in US patients and eGFR for any given creatinine was 21% higher in blacks. Performance in other racial groups is under investigation

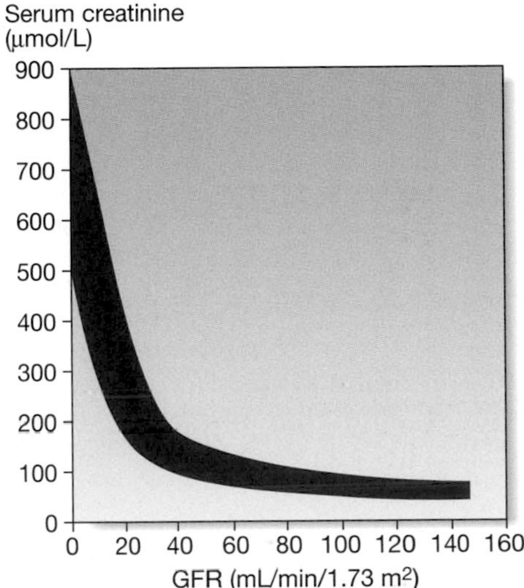

Fig. 17.2 Serum creatinine and the glomerular filtration rate (GFR). The inverse reciprocal relationship between GFR and serum creatinine is shown for a group of patients with renal disease. The red band indicates the range of values obtained. Note that some individuals have a GFR as low as 30–40 mL/min without serum creatinine rising out of the reference range.

17.3 Stages of chronic kidney disease (CKD)

Stage[1]	Definition[2]	Description	Prevalence[3]	Clinical presentation[4]
1	Kidney damage with normal or high GFR (> 90)	Mild CKD	6.5%	Asymptomatic
2	Kidney damage and GFR 60–89			Asymptomatic
3A[5]	GFR 45–59	Moderate CKD	4.5%	Usually asymptomatic
3B[5]	GFR 30–44			Anaemia in some patients at 3B Most are non-progressive or progress very slowly
4	GFR 15–29	Severe CKD	0.4%	First symptoms often at GFR < 20 Electrolyte problems likely as GFR falls
5	GFR < 15 or on dialysis	Kidney failure		Significant symptoms and complications usually present Dialysis initiation varies but usually at GFR < 10

[1]Stages of CKD 1–5 were originally defined by the US National Kidney Foundation Kidney Disease Quality Outcomes Initiative 2002.
[2]Kidney damage means pathological abnormalities or markers of damage, including abnormalities in urine tests or imaging studies. Two GFR values 3 mths apart are required to assign a stage. All GFR values are mL/min/1.73 m^2.
[3]From the NHANES III study of > 15 000 US adults (Am J Kid Dis 2003; 41:1–12).
[4]For further information, see page 483.
[5]3A/3B split recommended for UK in 2007/8, plus a suffix P, indicating presence of proteinuria (albumin:creatinine ratio (ACR) > 30 or protein:creatinine ratio (PCR) > 50 mg/mmol), e.g. 3 Ap, in view of the prognostic importance of proteinuria.

creatinine measurements (see Box. 17.1) but the most widely used is the MDRD equation, which is now the accepted standard for assessing estimated GFR (eGFR). Although the eGFR has several limitations (Box 17.2), its routine reporting by laboratories has increased recognition of moderate kidney damage and encouraged early deployment of protective therapies (Box 17.3).

A potentially more accurate assessment of GFR can be obtained by collection of a 24-hour urine sample and relating serum creatinine levels to urinary creatinine excretion (see Box 17.1).

Urinalysis

Screening for the presence of blood, protein, glucose, ketones, nitrates and leucocytes and to assess pH and osmolality of urine can be achieved by dipstick testing (p. 474). Urine microscopy (p. 463) or flow cytometry can detect erythrocytes, which are indicative of bleeding from the urogenital tract (anywhere from kidney to tip of penis); dysmorphic erythrocytes, which suggest the presence of nephritis; red cell casts, indicative of glomerular disease; and crystals, which may be observed in patients with renal stone disease. It should be noted that calcium oxalate and urate crystals can sometimes be found in normal urine that has been left to stand, due to crystal formation ex vivo. The presence of leucocytes and bacteria in urine is indicative of renal tract infection. White cell casts are strongly suggestive of pyelonephritis. Urine pH can provide diagnostic information in the assessment of renal tubular acidosis (p. 446). Urine collection over a 24-hour period can be performed to measure excretion of solutes, such as calcium, oxalate and urate, in patients with recurrent renal stone disease (p. 507). Proteinuria can also be measured on 24-hour collections but is usually now quantified by protein/creatinine ratio on spot urine samples.

Other dynamic tests of tubular function, including concentrating ability (p. 794), ability to excrete a water load (p. 438) and ability to excrete acid (p. 426), and calculation of fractional calcium, phosphate or sodium excretion, are valuable in some circumstances. The fractional excretion of these ions can be calculated by the general formula: (urine concentration of analyte × serum creatinine) / (serum concentration of analyte × urinary creatinine). For example, familial benign hypercalcaemia is characterised by a very low fractional excretion of calcium (p. 770), and hypophosphataemic rickets (p. 1128) by an increased fractional excretion of phosphate. Calculation of fractional excretion of sodium (FENa) can help differentiate volume depletion, when the tubules are avidly conserving sodium (FENa typically < 1.0), from acute tubular necrosis, when the tubules are damaged and are less able to conserve sodium (FENa typically > 1.0).

Blood tests

Haematology

A normochromic normocytic anaemia is common in CKD and is due in part to deficiency of erythropoietin and bone marrow suppression secondary to toxins retained in CKD. Other causes of anaemia include iron deficiency from urinary tract bleeding, and haemolytic anaemia secondary to disorders such as haemolytic uraemic syndrome (HUS) and thrombotic thrombocytopenic purpura (TTP). Other abnormalities may be observed that reflect underlying disease processes, such as neutrophilia and raised erythrocyte sedimentation rate (ESR) in vasculitis or sepsis; lymphopenia and raised ESR in systemic lupus erythematosus (SLE); and fragmented red cells in HUS and TTP.

Biochemistry

Abnormalities of routine biochemistry are common in renal disease. Serum levels of creatinine may be raised, reflecting reduced GFR (see above), although serum creatinine values can remain within the reference range in patients with reduced muscle mass, even when the GFR has fallen by more than 50%. Serum levels of urea are often increased in kidney disease but this analyte has limited value as a measure of GFR since levels increase with protein intake, following gastrointestinal haemorrhage and in catabolic states. Conversely, urea levels may be reduced in patients with liver failure or anorexia and in malnourished patients, independently of changes in renal function. Serum calcium tends to be reduced and phosphate increased in CKD, in association with high parathyroid hormone (PTH) levels caused by reduced production of $1,25(OH)_2D$ by the kidney (secondary hyperparathyroidism). In some patients, this may be accompanied by raised serum alkaline phosphatase levels, which are indicative of renal osteodystrophy. Other biochemical abnormalities may be observed that reflect underlying disease processes, such as raised glucose and HbA_{1c} levels in diabetes mellitus (p. 807) and raised levels of C-reactive protein (CRP) in sepsis and vasculitis.

Immunology

Antinuclear antibodies, antibodies to extractable nuclear antigens and anti-double-stranded DNA antibodies may be detected in patients with renal disease secondary to SLE (p. 1109). Antineutrophil cytoplasmic antibodies (ANCA) may be detected in patients with glomerulonephritis secondary to systemic vasculitis (p. 1115), as may antibodies to GBM in patients with Goodpasture's syndrome (p. 497) and low levels of complement in SLE, systemic vasculitis and HUS.

Imaging

Ultrasound

Renal ultrasound is a valuable non-invasive technique that is indicated to assess renal size and to investigate patients who are suspected of having obstruction of the urinary tract (Fig. 17.3) or renal tumours, cysts or stones. It is often the only method required for renal imaging and has the advantage of showing other abdominal, pelvic and retroperitoneal pathology. Ultrasound can also be used to provide images of the prostate gland and bladder, and to estimate the completeness of emptying in patients with suspected bladder outflow obstruction. Ultrasonography may show increased density of the renal cortex with loss of distinction between cortex and medulla, which is characteristic of CKD. Doppler

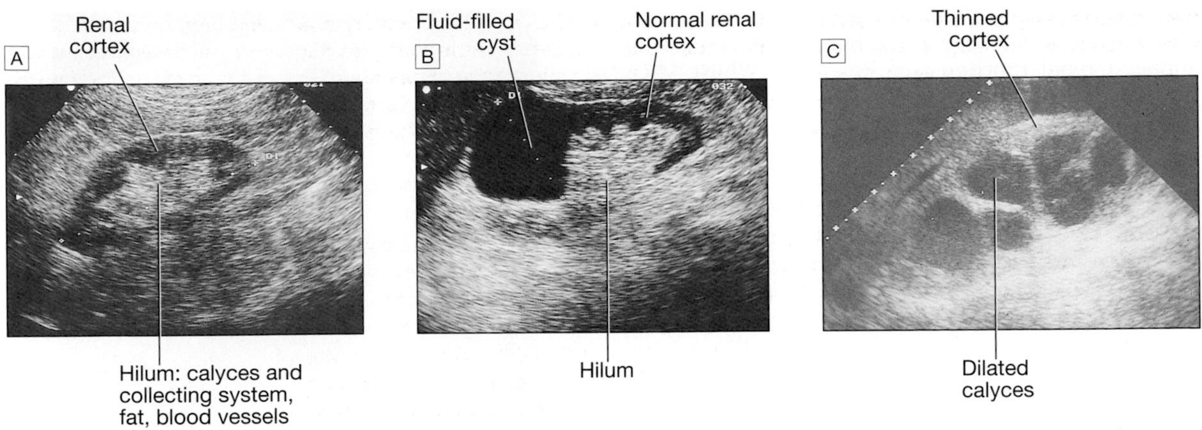

Fig. 17.3 Renal ultrasound. **A** Normal kidney. The normal cortex is less echo-dense (blacker) than the adjacent liver. **B** A simple cyst occupies the upper pole of an otherwise normal kidney. **C** The renal pelvis and calyces are dilated by a chronic obstruction to urinary outflow. The thinness and increased density of the remaining renal cortex indicate chronic changes.

imaging can be used to study blood flow in extrarenal and larger intrarenal vessels and can assess the resistivity index, which is the ratio of peak systolic and diastolic velocity. This is influenced by the resistance to flow through small intrarenal arteries and may be elevated in various diseases, including acute glomerulonephritis and rejection of a renal transplant. High peak velocities can also occur in severe renal artery stenosis. However, renal ultrasound is operator-dependent, the stored images convey only a fraction of the dynamic information gained during the investigation, and the results are often less clear in obese patients.

Computed tomography

Computed tomography urography (CTU) is used to evaluate cysts and mass lesions in the kidney or filling defects within the collecting systems. It usually entails an initial scan without contrast medium, and subsequent scans following injection of contrast to obtain a nephrogram image and images during the excretory phases. This technique gives more information than intravenous urography (IVU) but entails a substantially larger radiation dose. Contrast enhancement is particularly useful for characterising mass lesions within the kidney and differentiating benign from malignant lesions (see Fig. 17.32A, p. 516). Computed tomography without contrast (CT) gives clear definition of retroperitoneal anatomy regardless of obesity and is superior to ultrasound in this respect. Non-contrast CT of kidneys, ureters and bladder (CTKUB) is the method of choice for demonstrating stones within the kidney or ureter.

Computed tomography and angiography

This technique (CT-angiography) involves performing computed tomography, following an intravenous injection of contrast medium, to obtain images of the renal vasculature. It produces high-quality images of the main renal vessels and is of value in patients who have suffered renal trauma and those with haemorrhage from the renal tract, and in the investigation of renal artery stenosis. Other vascular structures, such as angiomyolipomas and aneurysms, can also be detected. Drawbacks include the fact that relatively large doses of contrast medium are required, which can cause renal dysfunction, and that the radiation dose is significant (Box 17.4).

17.4 Renal complications of radiological investigations

Contrast nephrotoxicity

- Acute deterioration in renal function, sometimes life-threatening, commencing < 48 hrs after administration of IV radiographic contrast media

Risk factors

- Pre-existing renal impairment
- Use of high-osmolality, ionic contrast media and repetitive dosing in short time periods
- Diabetes mellitus
- Myeloma

Prevention

- Provide hydration with free oral fluids plus IV isotonic saline 500 mL, then 250 mL/hr during procedure
- Avoid nephrotoxic drugs; withhold non-steroidal anti-inflammatory drugs (NSAIDs). Omit metformin for 48 hrs after the procedure, in case renal impairment occurs
- *N*-acetylcysteine may provide some protection but data are conflicting
- If the risks are high, consider alternative methods of imaging

Cholesterol atheroembolism

- Typically follows days to weeks after intra-arterial investigations or interventions (p. 496)

Nephrogenic sclerosing fibrosis after MRI contrast agents

- Chronic progressive sclerosis of skin, deeper tissues and other organs, associated with gadolinium-based contrast agents
- Only reported in patients with renal impairment, typically on dialysis or with GFR < 15 mL/min/1.73 m^2, but caution is advised in patients with GFR < 30 mL/min/1.73 m^2

Magnetic resonance imaging

Magnetic resonance imaging (MRI) offers excellent resolution and gives good distinction between different tissue types (see Fig. 17.26, p. 506). It is very useful for local staging of prostate, bladder and penile cancers. Magnetic resonance angiography (MRA) provides an alternative to CT-angiography for imaging renal vessels but involves administration of gadolinium-based contrast media, which may carry risks for patients with impaired renal function (see Box 17.4). Whilst MRA gives good images of the main renal vessels, stenosis of small branch arteries may be missed.

Renal arteriography

Renal arteriography involves taking X-rays following an injection of contrast medium directly into the renal artery. The main indication is to investigate renal artery stenosis (p. 494) or haemorrhage. Renal angiography can often be combined with therapeutic balloon dilatation or stenting of the renal artery and can be used to occlude bleeding vessels and arteriovenous fistulae by the insertion of thin platinum wires (coils). These curl up within the vessel and promote thrombosis, thereby securing haemostasis.

Intravenous urography

Intravenous urography (IVU) involves taking serial plain X-rays immediately before and after an intravenous injection of contrast medium. It has largely been replaced by ultrasound, CTKUB and CTU for most renal imaging purposes but remains a useful method of viewing the renal papillae, stones and urothelial malignancies (Fig. 17.4). The initial X-rays may show the renal outlines (if perinephric fat and bowel gas shadows allow), as well as radio-opaque calculi and calcification within the renal tract. Early films taken 1 minute after injection can be used to assess renal perfusion, whereas films at later time points provide images of the collecting system, ureters and bladder. The disadvantages of this technique are the need for an injection, dependence on adequate renal function, and exposure to irradiation and contrast medium (see Box 17.4).

Pyelography

Pyelography involves direct injection of contrast medium into the collecting system from above or below. It offers the best views of the collecting system and upper tract, and is sometimes used to identify the cause of urinary tract obstruction (p. 472). Antegrade pyelography requires the insertion of a fine needle into the pelvicalyceal system under ultrasound or radiographic control. This approach is much more difficult and hazardous in a non-obstructed kidney. In the presence of obstruction, percutaneous nephrostomy drainage can be established, and often stents can be passed through any obstruction. Retrograde pyelography can be performed by inserting catheters into the ureteric orifices at cystoscopy (Fig. 17.5).

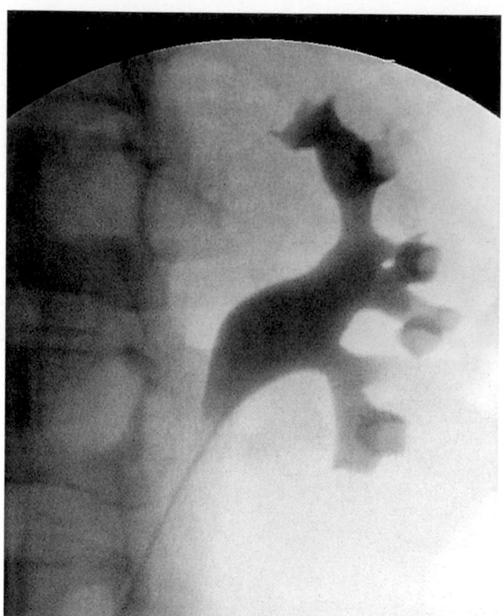

Fig. 17.5 Retrograde pyelography. The best views of the normal collecting system are shown by pyelography. A catheter has been passed into the left renal pelvis at cystoscopy. The anemone-like calyces are sharp-edged and normal.

Radionuclide studies

These are functional studies requiring the injection of gamma ray-emitting radiopharmaceuticals that are taken up and excreted by the kidney, a process that can be monitored by an external gamma camera.

Dynamic radionucleotide studies are performed with mercaptoacetyltriglycine labelled with technetium (^{99m}Tc-MAG3), which is filtered by the glomerulus and excreted into the urine. Imaging following ^{99m}Tc-MAG3 injection can provide valuable information about the perfusion of each kidney but is not a reliable method for identifying renal artery stenosis. In patients with significant obstruction of the outflow tract, ^{99m}Tc-MAG3

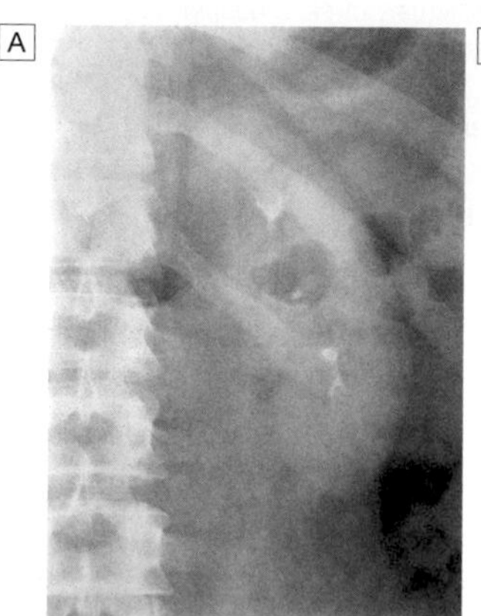

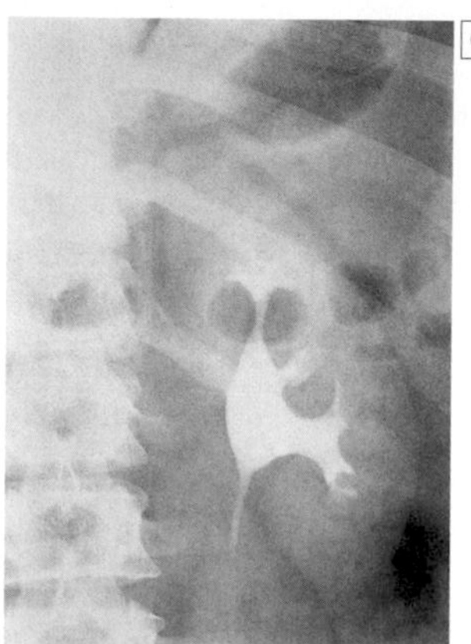

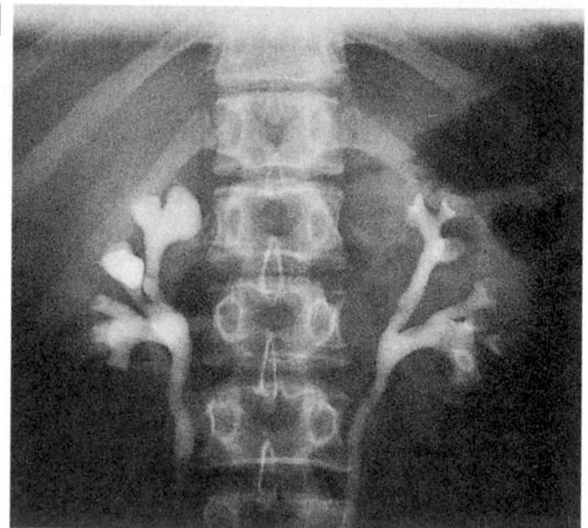

Fig. 17.4 Intravenous urography (IVU). **A** Normal nephrogram phase at 1 minute. **B** Normal collecting system at 5 minutes. **C** Bilateral reflux nephropathy (and chronic pyelonephritis), showing clubbing of the calyces that is particularly marked in the upper right pole.

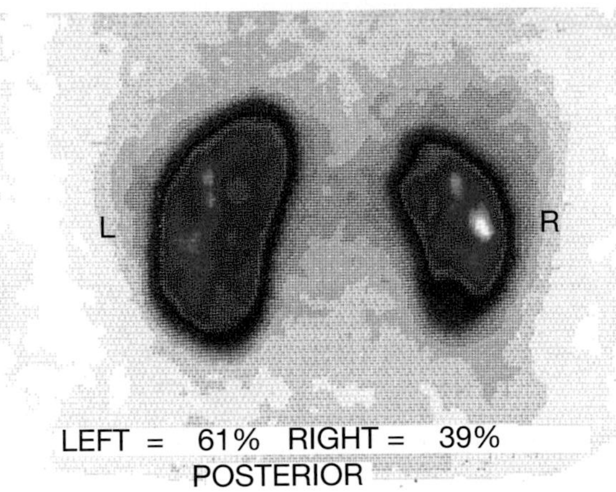

Fig. 17.6 DMSA isotope renogram. A posterior view is shown of a normal left kidney and a small right kidney (with evidence of cortical scarring at upper and lower poles) that contributes only 39% of total renal function.

persists in the renal pelvis and a loop diuretic fails to accelerate its disappearance. This can be useful in determining the functional significance of a 'baggy' or equivocally obstructed collecting system without undertaking pyelography.

Formal measurements of GFR can be made by radionuclide studies following the injection of diethylenetriamine pentacetic acid (^{99m}Tc-DPTA).

Static radionucleotide studies are performed with dimercaptosuccinic acid labelled with technetium (^{99m}Tc-DMSA), which is taken up by proximal tubular cells. Following intravenous injection, images of the renal cortex are obtained that show the shape, size and relative function of each kidney (Fig. 17.6). This is a sensitive method for demonstrating cortical scarring in reflux nephropathy and a way of assessing the individual function of each kidney.

Radionuclide bone scanning following the injection of methylene diphosphonate (^{99m}Tc-MDP) is indicated to assess the presence and extent of bone metastases in men with advanced prostate cancer (p. 517).

Renal biopsy

Renal biopsy is used to establish the nature and extent of renal disease in order to judge the prognosis and need for treatment (Box 17.5). The procedure is performed transcutaneously with ultrasound or contrast radiography guidance to ensure accurate needle placement into a renal pole. Light microscopy, electron microscopy and immunohistological assessment of the specimen may all be required.

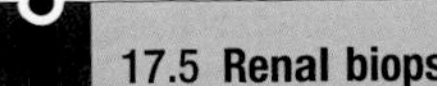

17.5 Renal biopsy

Indications
- Acute kidney injury that is not adequately explained
- CKD with normal-sized kidneys
- Nephrotic syndrome or glomerular proteinuria in adults
- Nephrotic syndrome in children that has atypical features or is not responding to treatment
- Isolated haematuria or proteinuria with renal characteristics or associated abnormalities

Contraindications
- Disordered coagulation or thrombocytopenia. Aspirin and other antiplatelet agents increase bleeding risk
- Uncontrolled hypertension
- Kidneys < 60% predicted size
- Solitary kidney* (except transplants)

Complications
- Pain, usually mild
- Bleeding into urine, usually minor but may produce clot colic and obstruction
- Bleeding around the kidney, occasionally massive and requiring angiography with intervention, or surgery
- Arteriovenous fistula, rarely significant clinically

*Relative contraindication.

PRESENTING PROBLEMS IN RENAL AND URINARY TRACT DISEASE

Dysuria

Dysuria refers to painful urination, often described as burning, scalding or stinging, and commonly accompanied by suprapubic pain. It is often associated with frequency of micturition and a feeling of incomplete emptying of the bladder. By far the most common cause is urinary tract infection, as described on page 511. Other diagnoses that need to be considered in patients with dysuria include sexually transmitted infections (p. 411) and bladder stones (p. 507).

Loin pain

Loin pain is often caused by musculoskeletal disease but can be a manifestation of renal tract disease; in the latter case, it may arise from renal stones, ureteric stones, renal tumours, acute pyelonephritis and urinary tract obstruction. Acute loin pain radiating anteriorly and often to the groin is termed renal colic. When combined with haematuria, this is typical of ureteric obstruction due to calculi (p. 507). When loin pain is precipitated by a large fluid intake (Dietl's crisis), upper urinary tract obstruction caused by a congenital abnormality of the pelviureteric junction (PUJ, p. 510) is often responsible.

Oliguria/anuria

Oliguria is defined as being present when less than 300 mL urine is passed per day, whereas anuria is deemed to exist when less than 50 mL urine is passed per day.

The volume of urine produced represents a balance between the amount of fluid that is filtered at the glomerulus and that reabsorbed by the renal tubules. When GFR is low, urine volumes may still be normal if tubular reabsorption is also reduced; hence urine volume alone is a poor indicator of kidney disease. Oliguria and anuria may be caused by a reduction in urine production, as in pre-renal acute kidney injury, when GFR is reduced but tubular homeostatic mechanisms increase reabsorption to conserve salt and water. A high solute load or associated tubular dysfunction may, however, produce normal or high urine volumes in such cases until the pre-renal insult becomes severe and GFR is markedly reduced, such as occurs in diabetic ketoacidosis with marked glycosuria. Urine volumes are variable in acute kidney injury due to intrinsic renal disease, but a rapid decline in urine volume may be observed in patients with bilateral renal infarction, in those with a single functioning kidney, and in those with rapidly progressive glomerulonephritis.

Obstruction of the renal tract can also produce oliguria and anuria, but to do so, obstruction must be complete and occur distal to the bladder neck, be bilateral, or be unilateral on the side of a single functioning kidney. If an obstruction is not relieved, the pressure will be transmitted back to the nephrons, causing GFR to fall.

Patients with oliguria and anuria should be assessed clinically to look for evidence of hypotension or volume depletion; of bladder enlargement; and of phimosis or meatal stenosis.

The presence of pain that is exacerbated by a fluid load suggests an acute obstruction of the renal tract, and its characteristics may be of value in reaching a diagnosis. Obstruction at the bladder neck is associated with lower midline abdominal discomfort due to bladder dilatation, whereas ureteric obstruction typically presents as loin pain radiating to the groin. Obstructions at the level of the renal pelvis may present as flank pain. Chronic obstruction rarely produces pain but may give rise to a dull ache. Unilateral ureteric obstruction may not lead to any noticeable reduction in urine output, whereas bilateral ureteric obstruction will result in oliguria or anuria. Urethral strictures should be considered as a possible cause, especially in patients with a history of instrumentation of the renal tract. Urethral valves should also be considered, especially in the paediatric population.

The presence of bladder enlargement in a middle-aged or elderly man suggests benign or malignant enlargement of the prostate gland as a potential cause of oliguria or anuria (pp. 515 and 517). It is important to note that about 50% of cases of acute urinary retention are seen after general anaesthesia, particularly in patients with pre-existing prostatic enlargement. Partial obstruction can be associated with a normal or even high urine volume due to chronic tubular injury, which causes loss of tubular concentrating ability. This chronic tubular injury can also produce a type 1 renal tubular acidosis (p. 446). Over time, even partial obstruction can cause tubular atrophy and irreversible renal failure.

All patients with oliguria or anuria should have routine biochemistry and haematology checked. Catheterisation should be performed so that urine volumes can be accurately monitored and the urine analysed for evidence of proteinuria and red cell casts, which may be found in patients with glomerulonephritis and systemic diseases such as vasculitis or SLE. Isolated haematuria may be indicative of an obstructive uropathy secondary to urinary calculi (p. 507) or tumours affecting the renal tract. If oliguria persists without any other clear explanation, ultrasound examination should be undertaken promptly to look for evidence of obstruction. Rarely, however, the urinary tract may not be particularly dilated in patients with acute kidney injury due to obstruction because of lack of urine production.

Management of oliguria and anuria should be directed at the underlying cause. While relief of obstruction is usually accompanied by a rapid return of renal function, tubular function may be impaired, resulting in polyuria and failure to conserve electrolytes.

Polyuria

Polyuria is defined as a urine volume in excess of 3 L/day. Various underlying conditions, both renal and extrarenal, may be responsible, as outlined in Box 17.6.

Investigation of polyuria includes measurement of urea, creatinine and electrolytes, glucose, calcium and albumin. A 24-hour urine collection may be helpful to confirm the severity of polyuria and the presence of nocturnal polyuria. Investigation and management of suspected diabetes insipidus are described on page 794.

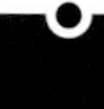

17.6 Causes of polyuria

- Excess fluid intake
- Hyperglycaemia
- Cranial diabetes insipidus
- Nephrogenic diabetes insipidus
  - Lithium
  - Diuretics
  - Interstitial nephritis
  - Hypokalaemia
  - Hypercalcaemia

Nocturia

Nocturia is defined as waking up at night to void urine. It may be a consequence of polyuria but may also result from increased fluid intake or diuretic use in the late evening. Nocturia also occurs in CKD, and in prostatic enlargement when it is associated with poor stream, hesitancy, incomplete bladder emptying, terminal dribbling and urinary frequency due to partial urethral obstruction (p. 515). Nocturia may also occur in sleep disturbance without functional abnormalities of the urinary tract.

Frequency

Frequency describes micturition more often than a patient's expectations. It may be a consequence of polyuria, when urine volume is normal or high, but is also found in patients with dysuria and prostatic diseases, when the urine volume is low.

Urinary incontinence

Urinary incontinence is defined as any involuntary leakage of urine. It may occur in patients with a normal urinary tract, as the result of dementia or poor mobility, or transiently during an acute illness or hospitalisation,

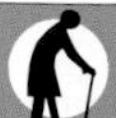

17.7 Incontinence in old age

- **Prevalence**: urinary incontinence affects 15% of women and 10% of men aged over 65 years.
- **Cause**: incontinence may be transient and due to an acute confusional state, urinary infection, medication (such as diuretics), faecal impaction or restricted mobility, and these should be treated before embarking on further specific investigation.
- **Detrusor over-activity**: established incontinence in old age is most commonly due to detrusor over-activity, which may be caused by damage to central inhibitory centres or local detrusor muscle abnormalities.
- **Catheterisation**: poor manual dexterity or cognitive impairment may necessitate the help of a carer to assist with intermittent catheterisation.

especially in older people (Box 17.7). Diuretics, alcohol and caffeine may worsen incontinence.

Pathophysiology

As urine accumulates in the bladder during the storage phase, the sphincter tone gradually increases, but there are no significant changes in vesical pressure, detrusor pressure or intra-abdominal pressure. During voiding, intravesical pressure increases, due to detrusor contraction, and the sphincter relaxes, allowing urine to flow from the bladder until it is empty. Clinical disorders associated with incontinence are connected with various abnormalities in this cycle and these are discussed in more detail below.

Stress incontinence

This occurs because passive bladder pressure exceeds the urethral pressure, due to either poor pelvic floor support or a weak urethral sphincter. Most often, there is an element of both. Stress incontinence is very common in women and seen most frequently following childbirth. It is rare in men and usually follows surgery to the prostate. The presentation is with incontinence during coughing, sneezing or exertion. In women, perineal inspection may reveal leakage of urine when the patient coughs.

Urge incontinence

This usually occurs because of detrusor overactivity, which produces an increased bladder pressure that overcomes the urethral sphincter. Urgency with or without incontinence may also be driven by a hypersensitive bladder resulting from urinary tract infection or a bladder stone. Detrusor overactivity is usually idiopathic, other than in patients with neurological conditions such as spina bifida or multiple sclerosis, in which case it is neurogenic (p. 1174). The incidence of urge incontinence increases with age, occurring in 10-15% of the population aged over 65 years and around 50% of patients requiring nursing home care. It is also seen in men with lower urinary tract obstruction and most often remits after the obstruction is relieved.

Continual incontinence

This is suggestive of a fistula, usually between the bladder and vagina (vesicovaginal), or the ureter and vagina (ureterovaginal). It is most common following gynaecological surgery but is also seen in patients with gynaecological malignancy or post-radiotherapy. In parts of the world where obstetric services are scarce, prolonged obstructed labour can be a common cause of vesicovaginal fistulae. Continual incontinence may also be seen in infants with congenital ectopic ureters. Occasionally, stress incontinence is so severe that the patient leaks continuously.

Overflow incontinence

This occurs when the bladder becomes chronically overdistended and may be associated with acute kidney injury (high-pressure chronic urinary retention). It is most commonly seen in men with benign prostatic enlargement or bladder neck obstruction (p. 514), but may arise in either sex as a result of failure of the detrusor muscle (atonic bladder). The latter may be idiopathic but more commonly is the result of damage to the pelvic nerves, either from surgery (commonly, hysterectomy or rectal excision), trauma or infection, or from compression of the cauda equina by disc prolapse, trauma or tumour. Incontinence due to prostatic enlargement can be regarded as a type of overflow incontinence.

Post-micturition dribble

This is very common in men, even in the relatively young. It is due to a small amount of urine becoming trapped in the U-bend of the bulbar urethra, which leaks out when the patient moves. It is more pronounced if associated with a urethral diverticulum or urethral stricture. It may occur in females with a urethral diverticulum and may mimic stress incontinence.

Clinical assessment

Patients should be encouraged to keep a voiding diary, including the measured volume voided, frequency of voiding, precipitating factors and associated features, such as urgency, since this can be of diagnostic value. The patient should be assessed for evidence of cognitive impairment and mobility. A neurological assessment should be performed to detect disorders such as multiple sclerosis that may affect the nervous supply of the bladder, and the lumbar spine should be inspected for features of spina bifida occulta. Perineal sensation and anal sphincter tone should be assessed. Rectal examination is needed to assess the prostate in men and to exclude faecal impaction as a cause of incontinence. Genital examination should be done to identify phimosis and paraphimosis in men, and vaginal mucosal atrophy, cystoceles or rectoceles in women.

Investigations

Urinalysis and culture should be performed in all patients. Ultrasound examination can be helpful in identifying patients with overflow incontinence who have incomplete bladder emptying, as they may reveal a significant amount of fluid in the bladder (> 100 mL) post-micturition. Urine flow rates and full urodynamic assessment by cystometrography may be required to diagnose the type of incontinence and are indicated in selected cases when the diagnosis is unclear on clinical grounds. An IVU should be performed in patients with continual incontinence who are suspected of having a fistula. Imaging with MRI is indicated when a urethral diverticulum is suspected.

Management

Females with stress incontinence respond well to physiotherapy. The mainstay of treatment for urge incontinence is bladder retraining, which involves teaching patients to hold more urine voluntarily in their bladder, assisted by anticholinergic medication. Surgery may be required in patients who have severe daytime incontinence despite conservative treatment. The treatment of incontinence secondary to fistula formation is surgical. Patients with overflow incontinence due to bladder obstruction should be treated surgically or with long-term catheterisation (intermittent or continuous). Incontinence secondary to neurological diseases can be treated by intermittent self-catheterisation.

Erectile dysfunction

Causes of erectile failure are shown in Box 17.8. Vascular, neuropathic and psychological causes are most common. With the exception of diabetes mellitus, endocrine causes are relatively uncommon and are characterised by loss of libido, as well as erectile dysfunction. Erectile dysfunction and reduced libido occur in over 50% of men with advanced CKD or on dialysis. Erectile dysfunction is a markedly under-diagnosed problem. It is important to discuss matters frankly with the patient, and to establish whether there are associated features of hypogonadism (p. 760) and if erections occur at any other time. If the patient has erections on wakening, vascular and neuropathic causes are much less likely and a psychological cause should be suspected.

Investigations

Blood should be taken for glucose, prolactin, testosterone, luteinising hormone (LH) and follicle-stimulating hormone (FSH). A number of further tests are available but are rarely employed because they do not usually influence management. These include nocturnal tumescence monitoring (using a plethysmograph placed around the shaft of the penis overnight) to establish whether blood supply and nerve function are sufficient to allow erections to occur during sleep; intracavernosal injection of prostaglandin E1 to test the adequacy of blood supply; internal pudendal artery angiography; and tests of autonomic and peripheral sensory nerve conduction.

17.8 Causes of erectile dysfunction

With reduced libido

- Hypogonadism
- Depression

With intact libido

- Psychological problems, including anxiety
- Vascular insufficiency (atheroma)
- Neuropathic causes (diabetes mellitus, alcohol excess, multiple sclerosis)
- Drugs (β-blockers, thiazide diuretics)

Management

First-line therapy is usually with oral phosphodiesterase type 5 inhibitors, such as sildenafil, which elevate cyclic guanosine monophosphate (cGMP) levels in vascular smooth muscle cells of the corpus cavernosum, causing vasodilatation and penile erection. Co-administration of these drugs with nitric oxide donors, such as glycerol trinitrate, is contraindicated because of the risk of severe hypotension. Other treatments for impotence include self-administered intracavernosal injection or urethral administration of prostaglandin E1; vacuum devices which achieve an erection that is maintained by a tourniquet around the base of the penis; and prosthetic implants, either of a fixed rod or an inflatable reservoir. Psychotherapy involving the patient and sexual partner may be helpful for psychological problems. Erectile dysfunction associated with peripheral neuropathy and vascular disease is difficult to treat. If hypogonadism is detected, it should be managed as described on page 760.

Haematuria

Healthy individuals may have occasional red blood cells in the urine (up to 12 500 cells/mL), but the presence of macroscopic haematuria (visible to the naked eye) or non-visible haematuria on dipstick testing (15 000–20 000 cells/mL or more) is indicative of significant bleeding from somewhere in the urinary tract (Fig. 17.7) and demands further assessment. First, it is important to confirm the presence of blood cells in the urine by microscopy (p. 463), since dipstick tests can also be positive in the presence of free haemoglobin or myoglobin. Microscopy not only confirms the diagnosis but may also be helpful in establishing the cause of bleeding (Box 17.9). Other causes of red or dark urine may sometimes be confused with haematuria but produce negative dipstick tests and microscopy (Box 17.10). Positive tests may also occur during menstruation, infection or strenuous exercise. Investigation

17.9 Interpretation of dipstick-positive haematuria

Dipstick test positive	Urine microscopy	Suggested cause
Haematuria	White blood cells	Infection
	Abnormal epithelial cells	Tumour
	Red cell casts Dysmorphic erythrocytes (phase contrast microscopy)	Glomerular bleeding*
Haemoglobinuria	No red cells	Intravascular haemolysis
Myoglobinuria (brown urine)	No red cells	Rhabdomyolysis

*Glomerular bleeding implies that the GBM is ruptured. It can occur physiologically following very strenuous exertion but usually indicates intrinsic renal disease and is an important feature of the nephritic syndrome (see Box 17.12).

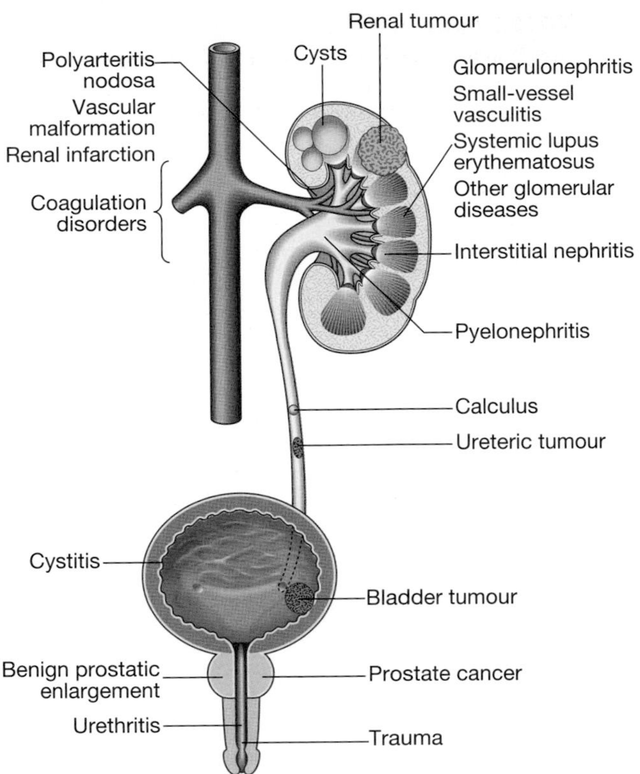

Fig. 17.7 Causes of haematuria.

17.10 Dipstick-negative dark urine

Cause	Urine colour
Food dyes	
Acanthocyanins	Red
Drugs	
Phenolphthalein	Pink when alkaline
Senna/other anthaquinones	Orange
Rifampicin	Orange
Levodopa	Darkens on standing
Porphyria	Darkens on standing
Alkaptonuria	Darkens on standing
Bilirubinuria	
Obstructive jaundice	Dark Dipstick-positive for bilirubin, negative for haemoglobin

17.11 Nephritic and nephrotic syndromes

Nephritic syndrome[1]

- Haematuria (red or brown urine)
- Oedema and generalised fluid retention
- Hypertension
- Oliguria

Nephrotic syndrome[2]

- Overt proteinuria: usually > 3.5 g/24 hrs (urine may be frothy)
- Hypoalbuminaemia (< 30 g/L)
- Oedema and generalised fluid retention
- Intravascular volume depletion with hypotension, or intravascular expansion with hypertension, may occur

[1]The complete form is classically seen in post-infectious glomerulonephritis, may occur in acute IgA nephropathy, and occasionally occurs in other types of glomerulonephritis. The presence of one or more features is common to many types of glomerular disease.
[2]Classically seen in non-inflammatory and subacute inflammatory/proliferative glomerular disorders (see Fig. 17.21, p. 497).

of haematuria is always required, as even non-visible haematuria can be caused by malignancy.

Glomerular bleeding is characteristic of inflammatory, destructive or degenerative processes that disrupt the GBM and may cause microscopic or macroscopic haematuria. In glomerulonephritis, one or more other features of the 'nephritic syndrome' (Box 17.11) may be present but the full syndrome is rare (p. 497). Other benign causes include thin basement membrane disease (p. 502) and vascular malformations.

Visible haematuria is most likely to be caused by tumour, which can affect any part of the urogenital tract (p. 515 and Box 17.12). Other common causes of visible haematuria are urine infection and stones. Investigation of haematuria (Fig. 17.8), whether non-visible or visible, should be directed first at the exclusion of an anatomical bleeding lesion, such as malignancy (see Box 17.12). If haematuria occurs with proteinuria and other clinical features of kidney disease (see Box 17.11), inflammatory

EBM 17.12 Haematuria and urothelial malignancy

'Macroscopic haematuria has a positive predictive value of 83% for bladder cancer and 22% for all urothelial tumours, rising to 41% in patients over the age of 40.'

- Buntinx F, et al. Fam Pract 1997; 14(1):63–68.

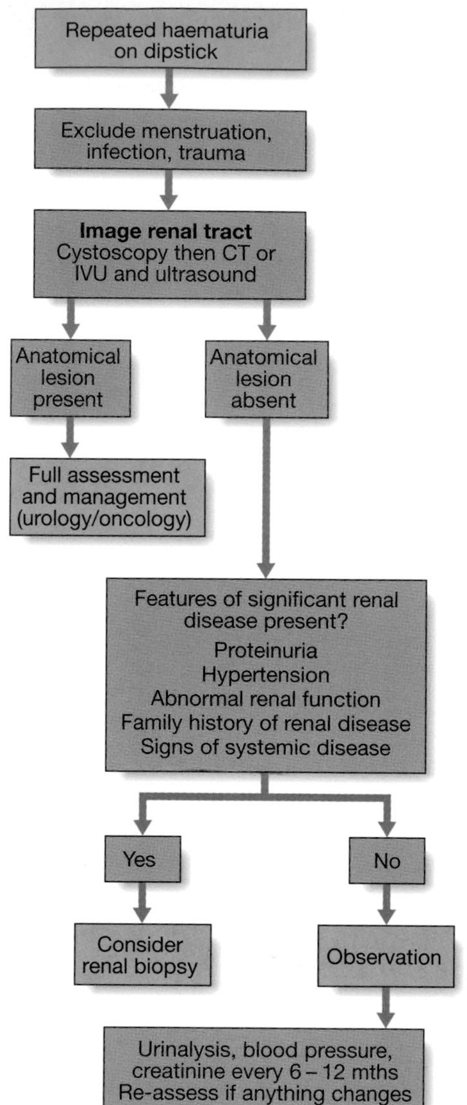

Fig. 17.8 Investigation of haematuria.

renal disease (p. 497) should be considered and a renal biopsy may be indicated. Where there are no features of significant kidney disease, and malignancy and renal stones have been excluded, it may be appropriate to manage the patient by observation with periodic review, although occasionally these individuals develop significant overt renal disease during follow-up. Management of haematuria should be directed at the underlying cause.

Proteinuria and nephrotic syndrome

Whilst moderate amounts of low-molecular-weight protein pass through the healthy GBM, these proteins are normally reabsorbed by receptors on tubular cells. In healthy individuals, less than 150 mg of protein is excreted in the urine each day. A proportion of this is Tamm–Horsfall protein, secreted by the renal tubules. The presence of larger amounts of protein is usually indicative of significant renal disease (Box 17.13).

17.13 Quantifying proteinuria in random urine samples

ACR[1]	PCR[2]	Typical dipstick results[3]	Significance
< 3.5 (female) < 2.5 (male)		–	Normal
~3.5–15		–	Microalbuminuria
~15–50	~15–50	+ to ++	Dipsticks positive; equivalent to 24-hr protein excretion < 0.5 g
50–200	> 250	++ to +++	Glomerular disease more likely
> 200	> 300	+++ to ++++	Nephrotic range: always glomerular disease, equivalent to 24-hr protein excretion > 3 g

[1]Urinary albumin (mg/L)/urine creatinine (mmol/L). [2]Urine protein (mg/L)/urine creatinine (mmol/L). (If urine creatinine is measured in mg/dL, reference values for PCR and ACR can be derived by dividing by 11.31.) [3]Dipstick results are affected by urine concentration and are occasionally weakly positive on normal samples.

Clinical assessment

Proteinuria is usually asymptomatic and is often picked up by urinalysis. Transient proteinuria can occur after vigorous exercise, during fever, in heart failure and in patients with urinary tract infection. Patients should be assessed for the presence of these conditions and urine testing repeated once the potential trigger has been treated or resolved. So-called orthostatic proteinuria may arise in the absence of renal disease. This occurs only during the day, in association with an upright posture, and the first morning sample is negative. Typically, less than 1 g protein per day is excreted. Orthostatic proteinuria is regarded as a benign disorder which does not require treatment. Large amounts of protein make urine froth easily and this may be noticed by the patient. Very large amounts can cause nephrotic syndrome, which presents with oedema (Boxes 17.11 and 17.14). In adults, this predominantly affects the lower limbs but extends to the genitalia and lower abdomen as it becomes more severe. The upper limbs and face may be more affected on waking in the morning. In children, ascites occurs early and oedema is often seen only in the face. Blood volume may be normal, reduced or increased. Renal sodium retention is an early and universal feature; the mechanisms of this are shown in Figure 16.5 (p. 435).

Microalbuminuria refers to the urinary excretion of small amounts of albumin. The consistent presence of albumin in the urine is abnormal and is clinically important in identifying the very early stages of glomerular disease, as occurs in conditions like diabetic nephropathy (p. 830). Because significant renal damage has already taken place before standard dipstick tests become positive, patients with diabetes mellitus should be screened regularly for microalbuminuria. Persistent microalbuminuria has also been associated with an increased risk of atherosclerosis and cardiovascular

17.14 Consequences of the nephrotic syndrome and their management

Feature	Mechanism	Consequence	Management
Hypoalbuminaemia	Urinary protein losses exceed synthetic capacity of liver	Reduced oncotic pressure Oedema	Treat underlying cause
Avid sodium retention	Secondary hyper-aldosteronism Additional poorly characterised intrarenal mechanisms	Oedema	Diuretics and a low-sodium diet*
Hypercholesterolaemia	Non-specific increase in lipoprotein synthesis by liver in response to low oncotic pressure	High rate of atherosclerosis	Statins, ezetimibe
Hypercoagulability	Relative loss of inhibitors of coagulation (antithrombin III, protein C and S) and increase in liver synthesis of procoagulant factors	Venous thromboembolism	Consider prophylaxis in chronic or severe nephrotic syndrome
Infection	Hypogammaglobulinaemia due to urinary loss of immunoglobulins	Pneumococcal and meningococcal infection	Consider vaccination

*Severe nephrotic syndrome may need very large doses of combinations of diuretics acting on different parts of the nephron (e.g. loop diuretic plus thiazide plus amiloride). In occasional patients with hypovolaemia, intravenous salt-poor albumin infusions may help to establish a diuresis, although efficacy is controversial. Over-diuresis risks secondary impairment of renal function through hypovolaemia.

17

mortality but neither the mechanism of proteinuria nor an explanation for this association has been established.

Investigations

All patients with persistent proteinuria should have the amount of protein quantified to guide further investigations (Fig. 17.9). Since quantification by 24-hour urine collection is often inaccurate, the protein : creatinine ratio (PCR) in a spot sample of urine is preferred. This makes an allowance for the variable degree of urinary dilution and can be used to extrapolate to 24-hour values (see Box 17.13). Changes in PCR also give valuable information about the progression of renal disease in CKD. It is possible to measure 24-hour albumin excretion or albumin : creatinine ratio (ACR), but this requires a more expensive immunoassay and is usually reserved for detection of the early stages of diabetic nephropathy (p. 830). When assessing protein excretion by analysis of spot urine samples, greater consistency can be achieved by using first morning urine samples but this is not essential for routine clinical use.

It is sometimes helpful to identify the type of protein in the urine. Low-molecular-weight proteins may appear in the urine in quantities greater than 150 mg/day. This is usually assessed by measurement of specific low-molecular-weight proteins, such as β_2-microglobulin (molecular weight 12 kDa). Large amounts of small proteins in the urine suggest renal tubular damage and are referred to as tubular proteinuria. This rarely exceeds 1.5–2 g/24 hours (maximum PCR 150–200 mg/mmol). When more than 2 g protein per day is being excreted, glomerular disease is likely and this is an indication for renal biopsy. The diseases that cause nephrotic syndrome all affect the glomerulus (see Fig. 17.21, p. 497), either directly, by damaging podocytes, or indirectly, by causing scarring or by depositing exogenous material such as amyloid into the glomerulus. A notable exception is in children, when heavy proteinuria and nephrotic syndrome are most commonly caused by minimal change glomerulonephritis. In this case, renal biopsy is not usually required unless the patient fails to respond to high-dose corticosteroid therapy.

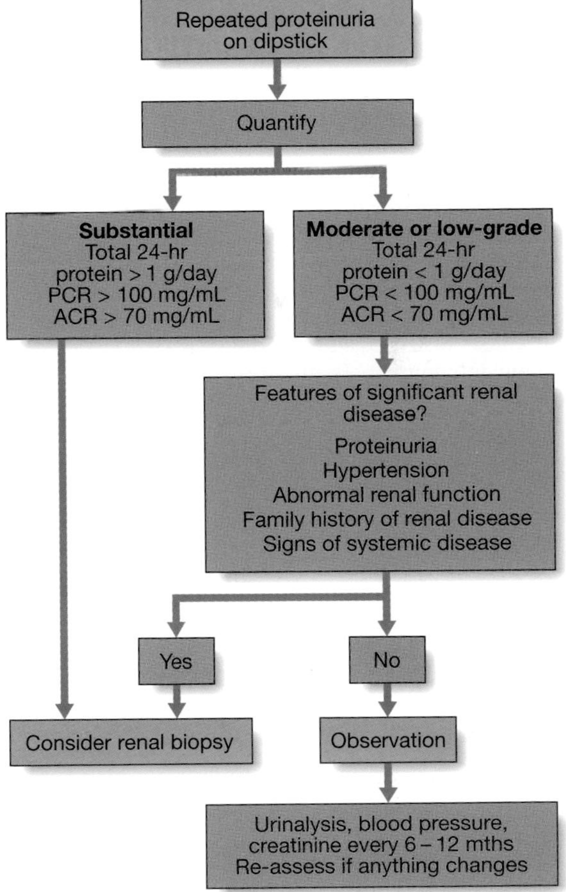

Fig. 17.9 Investigation of proteinuria. (ACR = albumin : creatinine ratio; PCR = protein : creatinine ratio.)

Free immunoglobulin light chains (molecular weight 25 kDa) are filtered freely at the glomerulus and can be identified as 'Bence Jones protein' in fresh urine samples. Bence Jones protein is poorly identified by dipstick tests and so specific immunodetection methods are required. This may occur in AL amyloidosis (p. 86) and in B-cell disorders, but is particularly important as a marker for myeloma (p. 1046).

Management

Management of proteinuria should be directed at the underlying cause. This may involve immunosuppressive therapy in glomerulonephritis and supportive management for nephrotic syndrome (Box 17.14).

Oedema

Oedema is caused by an excessive accumulation of fluid within the interstitial space. Clinically, this can be detected by persistence of an indentation in tissue following pressure on the affected area (pitting oedema). Non-pitting oedema is typical of lymphatic obstruction and may also occur as the result of excessive matrix deposition in tissues – for example, in hypothyroidism (p. 743) or scleroderma (p. 1112). There are various possible causes (Box 17.15). Pitting oedema tends to accumulate in the ankles during the day and improves overnight as the interstitial fluid is reabsorbed. In developed countries, the most common causes of oedema are local venous problems and heart failure (p. 546), but it is important to identify other causes.

Clinical assessment

The ankles and lower parts of the leg are typically affected first but oedema can be restricted to the sacrum in bed-bound patients. With increasing severity, oedema spreads to affect the upper parts of the legs, the genitalia and abdomen. Ascites is common and often an earlier feature in children or young adults, and in liver disease. Pleural effusions are common and can be a feature of any cause of generalised oedema. Facial oedema on waking is common. Features of intravascular volume depletion (tachycardia, postural hypotension) may occur when oedema is due to decreased oncotic pressure or increased capillary permeability. If oedema is localised – for example, to one ankle but not the other, then venous thrombosis, inflammation or lymphatic disease should be suspected.

Investigations

The cause of oedema is usually apparent from the history and examination of the cardiovascular system and abdomen. Blood should be taken for measurement of urea and electrolytes and serum albumin, and the urine tested for protein. Further imaging of the liver, heart or kidneys may be indicated, based on history and clinical examination. Where ascites or pleural effusions occur in isolation, aspiration of fluid with measurement of protein and glucose, and microscopy for cells, will usually help to clarify the diagnosis in differentiating a transudate (typical of oedema) from an exudate (more suggestive of local pathology, p. 662).

Management

Mild oedema usually responds to a thiazide or a low dose of a loop diuretic, such as furosemide or bumetanide. In nephrotic syndrome, renal failure and severe cardiac failure, very large doses of diuretics, sometimes in combination, may be required to achieve a negative sodium and fluid balance. In resistant cases, restriction of sodium intake and fluid intake may be required. Diuretics are not helpful in the treatment of oedema caused by venous or lymphatic obstruction or by increased capillary permeability. Specific causes of oedema, such as venous thrombosis, should be treated.

17.15 Causes of oedema

Increased total extracellular fluid	
• Congestive heart failure • Renal failure	• Liver disease
High local venous pressure	
• Deep venous thrombosis or venous insufficiency	• Pregnancy • Pelvic tumour
Low plasma oncotic pressure/serum albumin	
• Nephrotic syndrome • Liver failure	• Malnutrition/malabsorption
Increased capillary permeability	
• Leakage of proteins into the interstitium, reducing the osmotic pressure gradient which draws fluid into the lymphatics and blood • Infection/inflammation • Severe sepsis • Calcium channel blockers	
Lymphatic obstruction	
• Infection: filariasis, lymphogranuloma venereum (pp. 372 and 424)	• Malignancy • Radiation injury • Congenital abnormality

Hypertension

Hypertension is a very common feature of renal disease. Additionally, the presence of hypertension identifies a population at risk of developing CKD and current recommendations are that patients on antihypertensive medication should have renal function checked annually. Control of hypertension is very important in patients with renal impairment because of its close relationship with further decline of renal function (p. 486) and because of the exaggerated cardiovascular risk associated with CKD. Pathophysiology and management are discussed on pages 606–613.

ACUTE KIDNEY INJURY

Acute kidney injury (AKI), also referred to as acute renal failure, describes the situation where there is a sudden and often reversible loss of renal function, which develops over days or weeks and is usually accompanied by a reduction in urine volume. Approximately 7% of all hospitalised patients and 20% of acutely ill patients develop signs of AKI. In uncomplicated AKI, such as that due to haemorrhage or drugs, mortality is low, even when renal replacement therapy is required. In AKI associated with serious infection and multiple organ failure, mortality is 50–70% and the outcome is usually determined by the severity of the underlying disorder and other complications, rather than by renal failure itself.

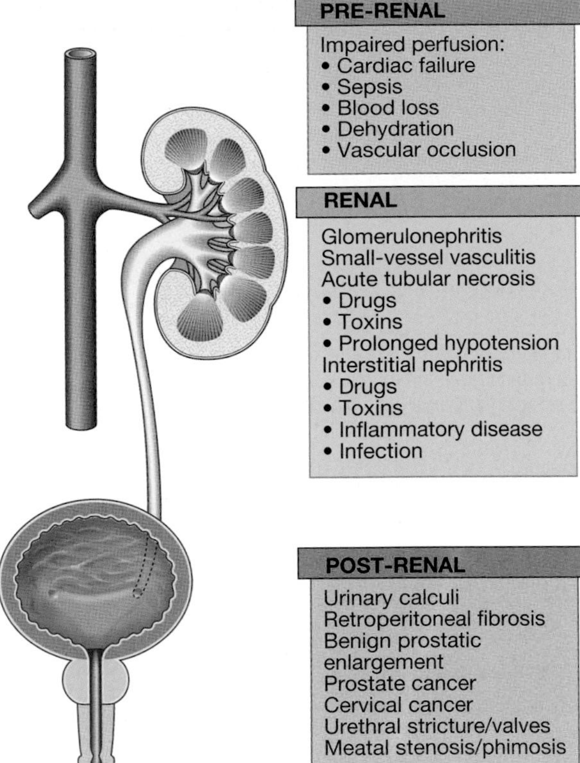

Fig. 17.10 Causes of acute kidney injury.

Pathophysiology

There are many causes of AKI and it is frequently multifactorial. It is often classified into three subtypes: 'pre-renal', when perfusion to the kidney is reduced; 'renal', when the primary insult affects the kidney itself; and 'post-renal', when there is obstruction to urine flow at any point from the tubule to the urethra (Fig. 17.10). In pre-renal AKI, the kidney becomes damaged as the result of hypoperfusion, leading to acute tubular necrosis. Histologically, the kidney shows inflammatory changes, focal breaks in the tubular basement membrane and interstitial oedema. Dead tubular cells may also be shed into the tubular lumen, leading to tubular obstruction. Although tubular cell damage is the dominant feature under the microscope, there may also be profound alterations in the renal microcirculation. Renal AKI may be caused by nephrotoxic drugs (p. 522), which can cause acute tubular necrosis and a similar histological picture to pre-renal AKI or interstitial nephritis. The other common cause is glomerulonephritis, in which there is direct inflammatory damage to the glomeruli (p. 498). Post-renal AKI occurs as the result of obstruction to the renal tract, with kidney damage arising as the result of back pressure. Anaemia is common in AKI and may occur as the result of blood loss, haemolysis or decreased erythropoiesis. In established AKI, there is an increased risk of bleeding and spontaneous gastrointestinal haemorrhage due to the uraemia.

Clinical features

Early recognition and intervention is important in AKI; all emergency admissions to hospital should have renal function, blood pressure, temperature and pulse checked on arrival and should undergo a risk assessment for the likelihood of developing AKI. This includes looking at coexisting diseases such as diabetes, vascular disease and liver disease, which make AKI more likely, as well as gathering information on drug treatments such as ACE inhibitors and NSAIDs, which may be associated with renal dysfunction. If a patient is found to have a high serum creatinine, it is important to establish whether this is an acute or acute-on-chronic phenomenon, or a sign of chronic kidney disease. Previous measurements of renal function can be of great value in differentiating these possibilities. Patients with AKI need to be assessed quickly to determine the likely underlying cause. Investigations that are required in all cases are shown in Box 17.16. Additional investigations that are required in some cases, depending on the clinical picture are shown in Box 17.17. The diagnosis of pre-renal AKI is usually obvious clinically (see below). Various criteria have been proposed to classify AKI and to help identify high-risk patients, guide treatment and provide information regarding prognosis. The most commonly used are the KDIGO and RIFLE criteria (Box 17.18), which use serum creatinine and urine output as biomarkers of kidney function.

Pre-renal AKI

Patients with pre-renal AKI are typically hypotensive and tachycardic with signs of poor peripheral perfusion, such as delayed capillary return. Tachycardia and postural hypotension (a fall in blood pressure of > 20/10 mmHg from lying to standing) are valuable signs of early hypovolaemia. Many patients with sepsis initially present with poor peripheral perfusion, as mentioned above, but then show evidence of peripheral vasodilatation once they have undergone initial resuscitation with intravenous fluids. However, this is accompanied by relative underfilling of the arterial tree and the kidney responds as it would to absolute hypovolaemia, with renal vasoconstriction leading to AKI with acute tubular necrosis. Biochemical assessment in pre-renal AKI usually reveals evidence of a metabolic acidosis and hyperkalaemia. It is important to note that pre-renal AKI may also occur without systemic hypotension, particularly in patients taking NSAIDs or ACE inhibitors. The cause of the hypotension is usually obvious clinically, but concealed blood loss can occur into the gastrointestinal tract, following trauma (particularly where there are fractures of the pelvis or femur), and into the pregnant uterus. Large volumes of intravascular fluid may also be lost into tissues after crush injuries or burns, and in severe inflammatory skin diseases or sepsis.

Renal AKI

Factors that can help differentiate the various causes of renal and post-renal AKI are summarised in Box 17.19. Patients with glomerulonephritis usually demonstrate significant haematuria and proteinuria and may have clinical manifestations of an underlying disease, such as SLE or systemic vasculitis. Although blood tests, including an immunological screen, should be performed to clarify the diagnosis in glomerulonephritis, a renal biopsy is usually required. Drug-induced acute interstitial nephritis is harder to spot but should be suspected in a previously well patient if there is an acute

17.16 Investigation of patients with established acute kidney injury

Initial test	Interpretation and further tests
Urea and creatinine	Compare to previous results. Chronically abnormal in CKD (see Box 17.26)
Electrolytes	If potassium > 6 mmol/L, treat urgently (p. 442)
Calcium and phosphate	Low calcium and high phosphate may indicate CKD (see Box 17.26) Calcium low in rhabdomyolysis: measure creatine kinase Hypercalcaemia in myeloma
Albumin	Low albumin in nephrotic syndrome (see urinalysis below) Low albumin in sepsis: take blood cultures
Full blood count **Clotting screen**	Anaemia may indicate CKD (see Box 17.26) or myeloma (see Box 17.17) Anaemia and fragmented RBC on blood film with raised LDH in thrombotic microangiopathy Low platelets and abnormal coagulation in DIC, including in sepsis: take blood cultures
C-reactive protein	ESR is misleading in renal failure High CRP may indicate sepsis or inflammatory disease
Urinalysis	Less reliable in an oliguric catheterised patient Seek earlier results if possible Marked haematuria suggests glomerulonephritis, tumour of renal tract or bleeding disorder Heavy proteinuria suggests glomerular disease: measure PCR or ACR
Urine microscopy	Casts or dysmorphic red cells suggest glomerulonephritis Leucocytes suggest infection/interstitial nephritis Crystals may be observed in drug-induced or uric acid nephropathy
Renal ultrasound	Hydronephrosis ± enlarged bladder in urinary tract obstruction: consider PSA and further imaging of urinary tract Small kidneys suggest CKD (see Box 17.26) Asymmetric kidneys suggest renovascular or developmental disease: consider renal artery imaging
Cultures	Culture blood, urine, sputum, wounds as appropriate Treat all infections
Chest X-ray	Pulmonary oedema in fluid overload Globular heart in pericardial (uraemic) effusion: perform echocardiogram 'Bat wing' appearance with normal heart size (± low Hb) may suggest pulmonary haemorrhage: measure CO transfer factor Fibrotic change in systemic inflammatory disease with lung and kidney involvement: request pulmonary function and high-resolution CT
Serology	HIV and hepatitis serology is urgent if dialysis is needed
ECG	If patient is > 40 yrs or has electrolyte abnormalities or risk of cardiac disease

(ACR = albumin:creatinine ratio; CKD = chronic kidney disease; CRP = C-reactive protein; DIC = disseminated intravascular coagulation; ESR = erythrocyte sedimentation rate; Hb = haemoglobin; LDH = lactate dehydrogenase; PCR = protein:creatinine ratio; PSA = prostate-specific antigen; RBC = red blood cells)

17.17 Clinical features and investigations of specific causes of acute kidney injury

Possibility	Consider
Vascular occlusion Aorta, or renal artery to single kidney; pointers include newly missing pulses, complete anuria	Urgent arteriography Doppler ultrasound
Malignant hypertension BP very high; RBC fragments on blood film and haemolysis	Examine optic fundi for typical features Check previous BP readings
Scleroderma Sclerodactyly, other features of scleroderma, severe hypertension	Autoantibodies to extractable nuclear antigens Imaging for involvement of other organs (p. 1112)
Systemic inflammatory disease Multi-organ involvement, rash and evidence of glomerular disease Differential diagnosis includes infection, especially endocarditis or tuberculosis	Complement (see Box 17.40), ANCA, ANF, anti-GBM antibodies, cryoglobulins and tissue biopsy Cultures, echocardiogram

Continued

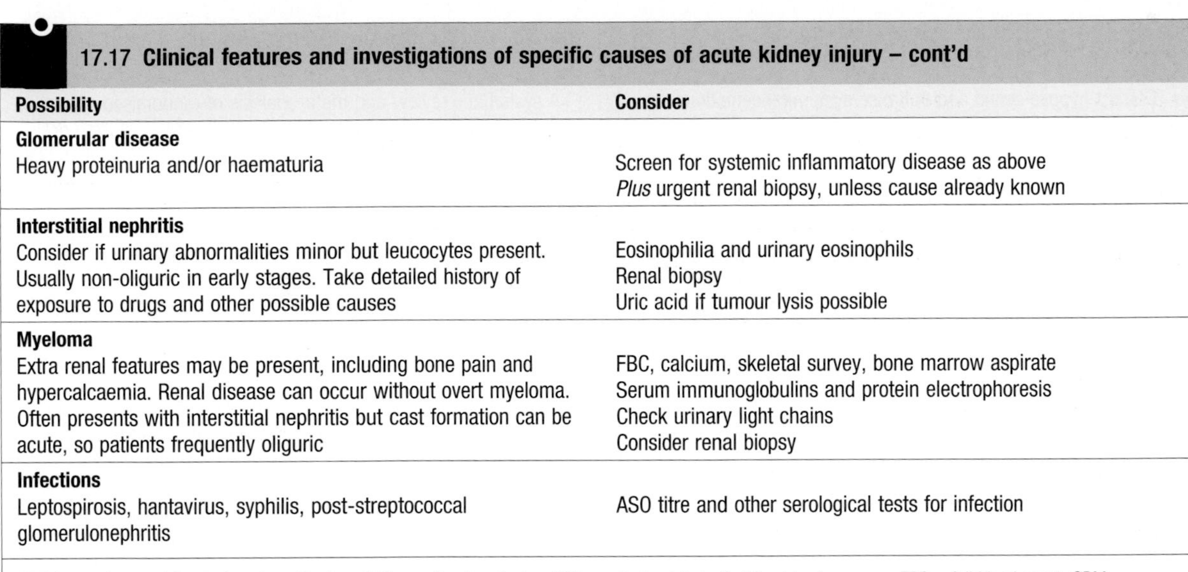

17.17 Clinical features and investigations of specific causes of acute kidney injury – cont'd

Possibility	Consider
Glomerular disease Heavy proteinuria and/or haematuria	Screen for systemic inflammatory disease as above *Plus* urgent renal biopsy, unless cause already known
Interstitial nephritis Consider if urinary abnormalities minor but leucocytes present. Usually non-oliguric in early stages. Take detailed history of exposure to drugs and other possible causes	Eosinophilia and urinary eosinophils Renal biopsy Uric acid if tumour lysis possible
Myeloma Extra renal features may be present, including bone pain and hypercalcaemia. Renal disease can occur without overt myeloma. Often presents with interstitial nephritis but cast formation can be acute, so patients frequently oliguric	FBC, calcium, skeletal survey, bone marrow aspirate Serum immunoglobulins and protein electrophoresis Check urinary light chains Consider renal biopsy
Infections Leptospirosis, hantavirus, syphilis, post-streptococcal glomerulonephritis	ASO titre and other serological tests for infection

(ANCA = antineutrophil cytoplasmic antibodies; ANF = antinuclear factor; ASO = anti-streptolysin O; BP = blood pressure; FBC = full blood count; GBM = glomerular basement membrane; RBC = red blood cells)

17.18 Criteria for acute kidney injury

KDIGO (Kidney disease: improving global outcomes)	RIFLE (Risk, injury, failure, loss, end-stage)
Stage 1: serum creatinine increase > 1.5–1.9-fold, urine production of < 0.5 mL/kg/hr for 6–12 hrs	= Risk
Stage 2: serum creatinine increase > 2.0–2.9-fold, urine production of < 0.5 mL/kg/hr for ≥ 12 hrs	= Injury
Stage 3: serum creatinine increase > 3.0-fold, urine production of < 0.3 mL/kg/hr for ≥ 24 hrs or absolute anuria for ≥ 12 hrs, or absolute serum creatinine > 354 μmol/L with an acute rise of > 44 μmol/L	= Failure
	Loss: persistent AKI, or complete loss of kidney function for > 4 wks
	End-stage renal disease: need for renal replacement therapy for > 3 mths

deterioration of renal function coinciding with introduction of a new drug treatment. Drugs that are commonly implicated include gentamicin, omeprazole, cisplatin and amphotericin B.

Post-renal AKI

Patients should be examined clinically to look for evidence of bladder enlargement and should also undergo imaging with ultrasound to detect evidence of obstruction above the level of the bladder. Post-renal AKI is usually accompanied by hydronephrosis, but this can be absent if the ureters are affected by fibrosis or malignancy, or if obstruction of the renal tract occurs in combination with a renal disorder such as acute tubular necrosis that causes reduced urinary flow.

17.19 Acute kidney injury in a haemodynamically stable, non-septic patient

Urinary tract obstruction

- Suggested by a history of loin pain, haematuria, renal colic or difficulty in micturition but often clinically silent
- Can usually be excluded by renal ultrasound: essential in any patient with unexplained AKI
- Prompt relief of the obstruction restores renal function

Drugs and toxins

- Poisoning, paraphenylenediamine hair dye, snake bite, paraquat, paracetamol, herbal medicines, *Cortinarius* mushrooms
- Therapeutic agents: direct toxicity (aminoglycosides, amphotericin, tenofovir); or haemodynamic effects (NSAIDs, ACE inhibitors), often with other factors. Phosphate crystallisation after IV administration or from bowel preparation
- Sometimes associated with systemic vasculitis, systemic lupus erythematosus (SLE) and Goodpasture's (anti-GBM) disease
- Useful blood tests include: antineutrophil cytoplasmic antibodies (ANCA), antinuclear antibodies (ANA), anti-GBM antibodies, complement, immunoglobulins
- Renal biopsy shows aggressive glomerular inflammation, usually with crescent formation

Acute interstitial nephritis

- Usually caused by an adverse drug reaction
- Characterised by small amounts of blood and protein in urine, often with leucocyturia
- Kidneys are normal size
- Requires cessation of drug and often prednisolone treatment

Management

Management options common to all forms of AKI are discussed in more detail below and summarised in Box 17.20.

17.20 Management of acute kidney injury

- Correct hypovolaemia and optimise systemic haemodynamic status with inotropic drugs if necessary
- Administer glucose and insulin to correct hyperkalaemia if K^+ > 6.5 mmol/L
- Consider administering sodium bicarbonate (100 mmol) to correct acidosis if pH < 7.0 (> 100 nmol/L)
- Discontinue potentially nephrotoxic drugs and reduce doses of therapeutic drugs according to level of renal function
- Match fluid intake to urine output plus an additional 500 mL to cover insensible losses once patient is euvolaemic
- Measure body weight on a regular basis as a guide to fluid requirements
- Ensure adequate nutritional support
- Administer proton pump antagonists to reduce the risk of upper gastrointestinal bleeding
- Screen for intercurrent infections and treat promptly if present

Haemodynamic status

If hypovolaemia is present, it should be corrected by replacement of intravenous fluid or blood; excessive administration of fluid should be avoided, since this can worsen outcome in AKI due to the development of pulmonary oedema. Monitoring of the central venous pressure may be of value in determining the rate of administration of fluid in these circumstances. Balanced salt solutions, such as Hartmann's or Ringer's lactate, may be preferable to isotonic (0.9%) saline when large volumes of fluid resuscitation are required, in order to avoid hyperchloraemic acidosis, but whether this substantially influences outcome remains unclear. Administration of hydroxyethyl starch solutions should be avoided, since they have been associated with higher rates of established AKI (Box 17.21). Critically ill patients may require inotropic drugs to restore an effective blood pressure but clinical trials do not support a specific role for low-dose dopamine (Box 17.22).

Hyperkalaemia and acidosis

Hyperkalaemia is common, particularly in patients with sepsis, burns, haemolysis or metabolic acidosis (p. 442). If serum K^+ concentration is > 6.5 mmol/L, this should be treated immediately, as described in Box 16.17 (p. 443), to prevent life-threatening cardiac arrhythmias. Metabolic acidosis develops unless prevented by loss of hydrogen ions through vomiting or aspiration of gastric contents. Severe acidosis can be ameliorated with sodium bicarbonate if volume status allows. Restoration of blood volume will correct acidosis by restoring kidney function. Infusions of sodium bicarbonate (50 mL of 8.4%) may also be used, if acidosis is severe, to reduce life-threatening hyperkalaemia.

Cardiopulmonary complications

Pulmonary oedema (Fig. 17.11) may result from the administration of excessive amounts of fluids relative to urine output and because of increased pulmonary capillary permeability. If pulmonary oedema is present and urine output cannot be rapidly restored, treatment with dialysis may be required to remove excess fluid. Temporary respiratory support may also be necessary with continuous positive airways pressure (CPAP) or intermittent positive pressure ventilation (IPPV). Once initial resuscitation has been performed, fluid intake should be matched to urine output plus 500 mL to cover insensible losses, unless diarrhoea is present, in which case additional fluids might be required.

EBM 17.21 Colloid resuscitation fluids in the critically ill

'A systematic review and meta-analysis of randomised controlled trials comparing hydroxyethyl starch (HES) with crystalloid or albumin solutions in the resuscitation of critically ill patients with sepsis revealed that, in trials with a low risk of bias, HES was associated with increased mortality (relative risk 1.11. 95% confidence interval 1.0–1.23), a greater requirement for renal replacement therapy (1.36 [1.03–1.80]) and more serious adverse events (1.30 [1.02–1.67]).'

- Haase N, et al. BMJ 2103; 346:f839.

EBM 17.22 Low-dose dopamine in acute kidney injury

'Dopamine at low, "renal" doses has been used in the belief that it may increase renal blood flow in critically ill patients (as it does in normal individuals) and prevent AKI. However, meta-analysis of clinical trials does not support its use in patients with, or at risk of, acute kidney injury.'

- Friedrich JO, et al. Ann Intern Med 2005; 142(7):510–524.

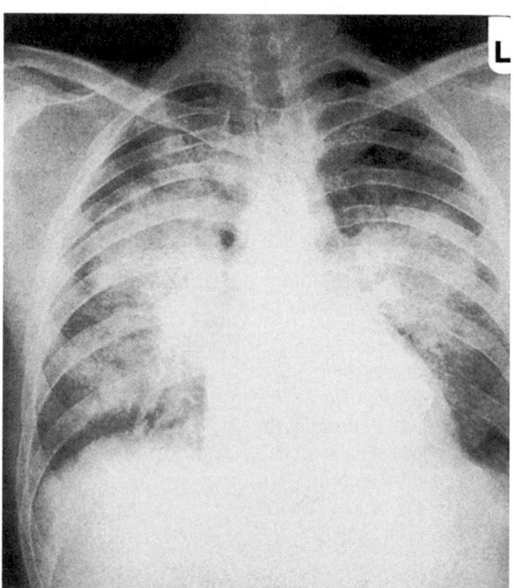

Fig. 17.11 Pulmonary oedema in acute kidney injury. The appearances are indistinguishable from left ventricular failure but the heart size is usually normal. Blood pressure is often high.

Electrolyte disturbances

Electrolyte disturbances, such as dilutional hyponatraemia, may occur if the patient has continued to drink freely despite oliguria or has received inappropriate amounts of intravenous dextrose. They can be avoided by paying careful attention to fluid balance and by giving intravenous fluids slowly. Modest hypocalcaemia is common but rarely requires treatment. Serum phosphate levels are usually high but may fall to dangerously low levels in patients on daily or continuous dialysis or haemofiltration, necessitating phosphate replacement.

Dietary measures

Adequate nutritional support should be ensured and it is important to give sufficient amounts of energy and adequate amounts of protein; high protein intake should be avoided. This is particularly important in patients with sepsis and burns who are hypercatabolic. Enteral or parenteral nutrition may be required (p. 123).

Infection

Patients with AKI are at substantial risk of intercurrent infection because humoral and cellular immune mechanisms are depressed. Regular clinical examination, supplemented by microbiological investigation where appropriate, is required to diagnose infection. If infection is discovered, it should be treated promptly according to standard principles (Ch. 6).

Medications

Patients with drug-induced acute tubular necrosis (see Fig. 17.24B, p. 503) or drug-induced acute interstitial nephritis should have the offending drug withdrawn. Additionally, vasoactive drugs, such as NSAIDs and ACE inhibitors, should be discontinued, as they may prolong AKI. H_2-receptor antagonists should be given to prevent gastrointestinal bleeding. Other drug treatments should be reviewed and the doses adjusted if necessary, to take account of renal function. Non-essential drug treatments should be stopped.

Immunosuppression

Patients with glomerulonephritis may require immunosuppressive drugs (p. 498), plasma infusion and plasma exchange (p. 501).

Renal tract obstruction

In post-renal AKI, the obstruction should be relieved as soon as possible. This may involve catheterisation in urethral obstruction, or correction of ureteric obstruction with a ureteric stent or percutaneous nephrostomy.

Renal replacement therapy

Conservative management can be successful in AKI with meticulous attention to fluid balance, electrolytes and nutrition, but renal replacement therapy (RRT) may be required in patients who are not showing signs of recovery with these measures. Typically, the decision to start RRT is driven by hyperkalaemia, fluid overload or acidosis. Severe uraemia with pericarditis and neurological signs (uraemic encephalopathy) is uncommon in AKI but, when present, is a strong indication for RRT. No specific cut-off values for serum urea or creatinine have been identified at which RRT should be commenced, and clinical trials of earlier versus later RRT in unselected patients with AKI have not shown differences in outcome. Furthermore, RRT can be a risky intervention in patients with comorbidity, since it requires the placement of large intravenous catheters that may become infected and can also represent a major haemodynamic challenge in unstable patients. Accordingly, the decision to institute RRT should be made on an individual basis, taking account of the potential risks and benefits, comorbidity and other aspects of the patient's care, including an assessment of whether early or delayed recovery is likely. The two main options for RRT in AKI are haemodialysis and high-volume haemofiltration, or the hybrid approach of haemodiafiltration. Peritoneal dialysis is also an option if haemodialysis is not available (p. 490).

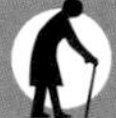

17.23 Acute kidney injury in old age

- **Physiological change**: nephrons decline in number with age and average GFR falls progressively.
- **Creatinine**: as muscle mass falls with age, less creatinine is produced each day. Serum creatinine can be misleading as a guide to renal function.
- **Renal tubular function**: declines with age, leading to loss of urinary concentrating ability.
- **Drugs**: increased drug prescription in older people (diuretics, ACE inhibitors and NSAIDs) may contribute to risk of AKI.
- **Causes**: infection, renal vascular disease, prostatic obstruction, hypovolaemia and severe cardiac dysfunction are common.
- **Mortality**: rises with age, primarily because of comorbid conditions.

Recovery from AKI

This is usually heralded by a gradual return of urine output and a steady improvement in plasma biochemistry. During recovery, there is often a diuretic phase in which urine output increases rapidly and remains excessive for several days before returning to normal. This may be due in part to tubular damage and to temporary loss of the medullary concentration gradient. This gradient plays a key role in concentrating urine in the collecting duct, and depends on continued delivery of filtrate to the ascending limb of the loop of Henle and active tubular transport. After a few days, urine volume falls to normal as the concentrating mechanism and tubular reabsorption are restored. During the recovery phase of AKI, it may be necessary to provide supplements of sodium chloride, sodium bicarbonate, potassium chloride and sometimes phosphate temporarily, to compensate for increased urinary losses.

CHRONIC KIDNEY DISEASE

Chronic kidney disease (CKD), previously termed chronic renal failure, refers to an irreversible deterioration in renal function which usually develops over a period of years (see Box 17.3, p. 467). Initially, it is manifest only as a biochemical abnormality but, eventually, loss of the excretory, metabolic and endocrine functions of the kidney leads to the clinical symptoms and signs of renal failure, collectively referred to as uraemia. When death is likely without RRT (CKD stage 5), it is called end-stage renal disease or failure (ESRD or ESRF).

Epidemiology

The social and economic consequences of CKD are considerable. In most countries, estimates of the prevalence of CKD stage 3–5 (eGFR < 60) are around 5–7%, mostly affecting people aged 65 years and above. The prevalence of CKD in hypertension, diabetes and vascular disease is substantially higher, and targeted screening for CKD should be considered in these and other high-risk groups. The great majority of patients with earlier CKD (stages 1–3) never develop ESRD, which is fortunate, given the numbers (see Box 17.3).

Pathophysiology

Common causes of CKD are shown in Box 17.24. In many cases, the underlying diagnosis is unclear, especially among the large number of elderly patients with moderate GFR reductions (stage 3 CKD; see Box 17.3), in whom the additional information gained from a biopsy would not alter treatment. Many patients diagnosed at a late stage have bilateral small kidneys; renal biopsy is rarely undertaken in this group since it is more risky, less likely to provide a histological diagnosis because of the severity of damage, and unlikely to alter management.

17.24 Common causes of end-stage renal failure

Disease	Proportion	Comments
Congenital and inherited	5%	Polycystic kidney disease, Alport's syndrome
Renovascular disease	5%	Mostly atheromatous, may be more common
Hypertension	5–20%	Causality controversial, much may be renal disease
Glomerular diseases	10–20%	IgA nephropathy is most common
Interstitial diseases	20–30%	Often drug-induced
Systemic inflammatory diseases	5–10%	Systemic lupus erythematosus, vasculitis
Diabetes mellitus	20–40%	Large racial and geographical differences
Unknown	5–20%	

Clinical features

The typical presentation is with a raised urea and creatinine found during routine blood tests, frequently accompanied by hypertension, proteinuria or anaemia. The rate of change in renal function varies between patients but is relatively constant for an individual and provides useful prognostic information. A plot of GFR, or of the reciprocal of the plasma creatinine concentration against time (Fig. 17.12), can demonstrate whether a patient has a stable GFR over time, predict when ESRF will be reached if decline is progressive, and can detect any unexpected worsening of kidney disease. It can also be used to monitor the success of interventions.

General symptoms

Most patients with slowly progressive disease are asymptomatic until GFR falls below 30 mL/min/1.73 m^2 (stage 4 or 5) and some can remain asymptomatic with much lower GFR values than this. An early symptom is nocturia, due to the loss of concentrating ability and increased osmotic load per nephron, but this is non-specific. When GFR falls below 15–20 mL/min/1.73 m^2, symptoms and signs are common and can affect almost all body systems (Fig. 17.13). They typically include tiredness or breathlessness, which may, in part, be related to renal anaemia, pruritus, anorexia, weight loss, nausea and vomiting. With further deterioration in renal function, patients may suffer hiccups, experience unusually deep respiration related to metabolic acidosis (Kussmaul's respiration), and develop muscular twitching, fits, drowsiness and coma.

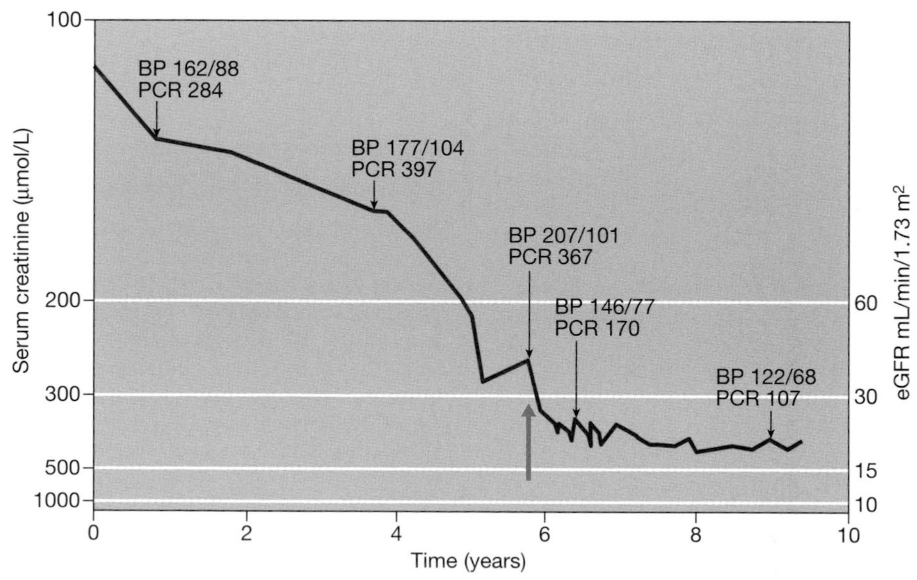

Fig. 17.12 Plot of the reciprocal of serum creatinine concentration against time in a patient with type 1 diabetes mellitus. After approximately 6 years of monitoring (blue arrow), he entered an aggressive treatment programme aimed at optimising blood pressure (BP) and glycaemic control. The reduction in blood pressure was accompanied by a fall in proteinuria (protein : creatinine ratio, PCR; mg/mmol) and a stabilisation in renal function.

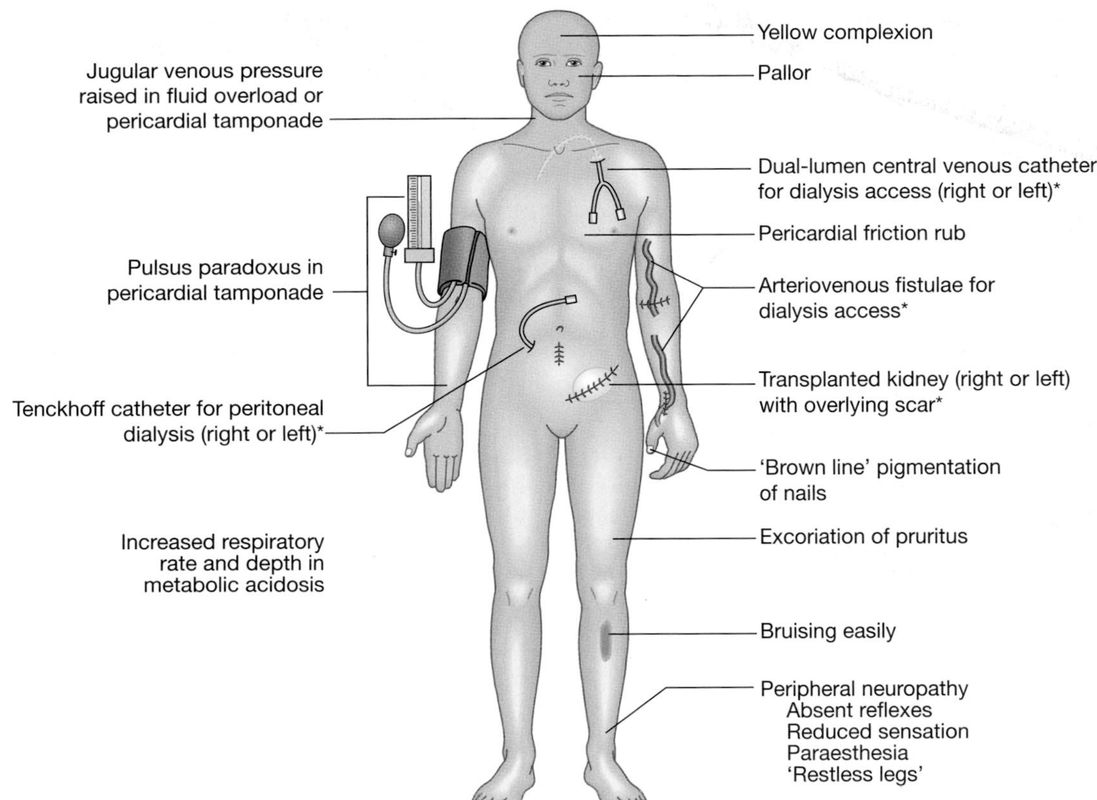

Fig. 17.13 Physical signs in advanced chronic kidney disease. (*Features of renal replacement therapy)

Immune dysfunction

Cellular and humoral immunity is impaired in advanced CKD and there is increased susceptibility to infections, the second most common cause of death in dialysis patients, after cardiovascular disease. Many infections are associated with access devices but some are common infections, such as pneumonia.

Haematological

There is an increased bleeding tendency in advanced CKD, which manifests as cutaneous ecchymoses and mucosal bleeds. Platelet function is impaired and bleeding time prolonged. Adequate dialysis partially corrects the bleeding tendency in those with severe uraemia, but these patients are at significantly increased risk of complications from all anticoagulants, including those that are required during dialysis. Anaemia is common and is due in part to reduced erythropoietin production. Haemoglobin can be as low as 50–70 g/L in CKD stage 5, although it is often less severe or absent in patients with polycystic kidney disease. Several mechanisms are implicated, as summarised in Box 17.25.

17.25 Causes of anaemia in chronic kidney disease

- Deficiency of erythropoietin
- Toxic effects of uraemia on marrow precursor cells
- Reduced red cell survival
- Increased blood loss due to capillary fragility and poor platelet function
- Reduced intake, absorption and utilisation of dietary iron

Electrolyte abnormalities

Patients with CKD often develop electrolyte abnormalities and metabolic acidosis (p. 445). Fluid retention is common in advanced CKD and disproportionate fluid retention may occur in milder disease, sometimes leading to episodic pulmonary oedema. This is particularly associated with renal artery stenosis. Conversely, some patients with tubulo-interstitial disease can develop 'salt-wasting' disease and may require a high sodium and water intake, including supplements of sodium salts, to prevent fluid depletion and worsening of renal function. Acidosis is common. Although it is usually asymptomatic, it may be associated with increased tissue catabolism and decreased protein synthesis, and may exacerbate bone disease and the rate of decline in renal function.

Endocrine function

A number of hormonal abnormalities may also be observed. In both genders, there is loss of libido related, at least in part, to hypogonadism as a consequence of hyperprolactinaemia (p. 790). The half-life of insulin is prolonged in CKD due to reduced tubular metabolism of insulin but there is also insulin resistance and reduced appetite. Because of this, insulin requirements are unpredictable in diabetic patients in advanced CKD.

Neurological and muscle function

Generalised myopathy may occur due to a combination of poor nutrition, hyperparathyroidism, vitamin D deficiency and disorders of electrolyte metabolism. Muscle cramps are common. The 'restless leg syndrome', in which the patient's legs are jumpy during the night, may be troublesome. Both sensory and motor neuropathy can arise, presenting as paraesthesia and foot drop, respectively, but appear late during the course of CKD. They are now unusual, given the widespread availability of RRT; if present, they can often improve once dialysis is established.

Cardiovascular disease

The risk of cardiovascular disease is substantially increased in patients with CKD stage 3 or worse (GFR < 60 mL/min/1.73 m^2) and those with proteinuria or microalbuminuria. Left ventricular hypertrophy may occur, secondary to hypertension, and may account for the increased risk of sudden death (presumed to be caused by dysrhythmias) in this patient group. Pericarditis may complicate untreated or inadequately treated ESRD and cause pericardial tamponade or constrictive pericarditis. Medial vascular calcification is common and may be due, in part, to the high serum phosphate levels which are present in stage 3b CKD and above. Hyperphosphataemia may also contribute to the itching that arises in advanced CKD and probably contributes in an important way to the increased risk of cardiovascular disease. Reflecting this fact, serum fibroblast growth factor 23 (FGF23) levels (which increase in response to serum phosphate - see below) are an independent predictor of mortality in CKD.

Metabolic bone disease

Disturbances of calcium and phosphate metabolism are almost universal in advanced CKD, and various types of metabolic bone disease may also occur, including osteitis fibrosa cystica, osteomalacia and osteoporosis (Fig. 17.14). The sequence of events that leads to renal bone disease is complex. There is impaired conversion of 25-hydroxyvitamin D to its active metabolite, 1,25-dihydroxyvitamin D, due in part to renal tubular cell damage and elevated FGF23 levels. The reduced 1,25-dihydroxyvitamin D levels impair intestinal absorption of calcium, thereby causing hypocalcaemia, which leads in turn to increased PTH production by the parathyroid glands. Serum phosphate levels also start to rise because of the reduction in GFR. This leads to increased production of the hormone FGF23 from osteocytes (p. 1061). The FGF23 promotes phosphate excretion, thereby compensating in part for the reduced glomerular filtration of phosphate. This homeostatic response eventually fails, however, as renal failure progresses and hyperphosphataemia develops. The raised levels of serum phosphate complex with calcium in the extracellular space, causing ectopic calcification in blood vessels and other tissues. Patients with CKD commonly develop parathyroid gland hypertrophy and secondary hyperparathyroidism. In some cases, tertiary hyperparathyroidism supervenes, due to autonomous production of PTH by the enlarged parathyroid glands; this presents with hypercalcaemia. The histological picture in renal bone disease is complex. In osteitis fibrosa cystica, there is increased bone turnover due to the high levels of PTH, whereas low bone turnover (adynamic bone disease) may be observed in patients who have been over-treated with vitamin D metabolites.

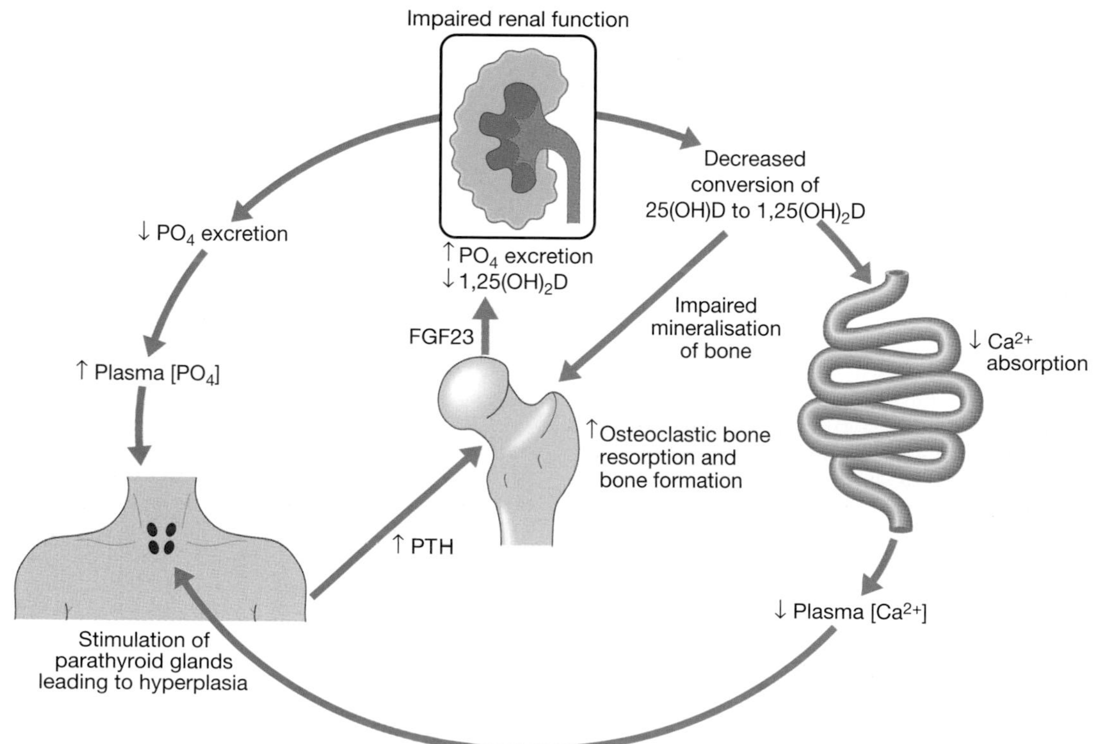

Fig. 17.14 Pathogenesis of renal osteodystrophy. Low 1,25(OH)$_2$D levels cause calcium malabsorption and this, combined with high phosphate levels, causes hypocalcaemia, which increases PTH production by the parathyroid glands. The raised level of PTH increases osteoclastic bone resorption and bone formation. Although production of FGF23 from osteocytes also increases, promoting phosphate excretion, this is insufficient to prevent hyperphosphataemia in advanced CKD.

17.26 Suggested investigations in chronic kidney disease

Initial tests	Interpretation
Urea and creatinine	To assess stability/progression: compare to previous results
Urinalysis and quantification of proteinuria	Haematuria and proteinuria may indicate cause. Proteinuria indicates risk of progressive CKD requiring preventive ACE inhibitor or ARB therapy
Electrolytes	To identify hyperkalaemia and acidosis
Calcium, phosphate, parathyroid hormone and 25(OH)D	Assessment of renal osteodystrophy
Albumin	Low albumin: consider malnutrition, inflammation
Full blood count (± Fe, ferritin, folate, B_{12})	If anaemic, exclude common non-renal explanations then manage as renal anaemia
Lipids, glucose ± HbA_{1c}	Cardiovascular risk high in CKD: treat risk factors aggressively
Renal ultrasound	Only if there are urinary symptoms (to exclude obstruction) or progressive CKD. Small kidneys suggest chronicity. Asymmetric renal size suggests renovascular or developmental disease
Hepatitis and HIV serology	If dialysis or transplant is planned. Hepatitis B vaccination recommended if seronegative
ECG	If patient is > 40 yrs or hyperkalaemic, or there are risk factors for cardiac disease
Other tests	Consider relevant tests from Boxes 17.16 and 17.17 (p. 480), especially if the cause of CKD is unknown

(ACE = angiotensin-converting enzyme; ARB = angiotensin II receptor blocker)

Osteomalacia can occur with over-treatment of hyperphosphataemia (p. 449).

Investigations

The recommended investigations in patients with CKD are shown in Box 17.26. Their main aims are:

- to identify the underlying cause where possible, since this may influence the treatment
- to identify reversible factors that may worsen renal function, such as hypertension, urinary tract obstruction, nephrotoxic drugs, and salt and water depletion
- to screen for complications of CKD, such as anaemia and renal osteodystrophy
- to screen for cardiovascular risk factors.

Referral to a nephrologist is appropriate for patients with potentially treatable underlying disease and those who are likely to progress to ESRD. Suggested referral criteria are listed in Box 17.27.

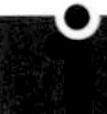

17.27 Criteria for referral of chronic kidney disease patients to a nephrologist

- Age < 40 years
- Stage 4 CKD or worse (eGFR < 30 mL/min/1.73 m^2)
- Rapid deterioration in renal function[1]
- Significant proteinuria (PCR > 100 mg/mmol or ACR > 70 mg/mmol)
- Significant haematuria[2]

[1]Fall in eGFR > 5 mL/min/1.73 m2/yr or > 10 mL/min/1.73 m2 over 5 yrs.
[2]After exclusion of urinary tract infection and urological abnormalities such as stones and tumours.

Management

The aims of management in CKD are to prevent or slow further renal damage; to limit the adverse physiological effects of renal impairment on the skeleton and on haematopoiesis; to treat risk factors for cardiovascular disease; and to prepare for RRT, if appropriate (p. 489).

Antihypertensive therapy

Lowering of blood pressure slows the rate at which renal function declines in CKD, independently of the agent used (Box 17.28), and has additional benefits in lowering the risk of hypertensive heart failure, stroke and peripheral vascular disease, as well as reducing proteinuria (see below). No threshold for beneficial effects has been identified and any reduction of blood pressure appears to be beneficial. Various targets have been suggested, such as 130/80 mmHg for uncomplicated CKD, and 125/75 mmHg for CKD complicated by significant proteinuria of more than 1 g/day (PCR > 100 mg/mmol or ACR > 70 mg/mmol). Achieving these blood pressure targets often requires multiple drugs, and therapeutic success may be limited by adverse effects and poor compliance.

Reduction of proteinuria

There is a clear relationship between the degree of proteinuria and the rate of progression of renal disease, and strong evidence that reducing proteinuria reduces the risk of progression. Angiotensin-converting enzyme (ACE) inhibitors and angiotensin II receptor blockers (ARBs) reduce proteinuria and retard the progression of CKD (Box 17.28). These effects are partly due to the reduction in blood pressure but there is evidence for a specific beneficial effect in patients with proteinuria (PCR > 50 mg/mmol or ACR > 30 mg/mmol) and those with incipient or overt diabetic nephropathy. In addition, ACE inhibitors have been shown to reduce the risk of cardiovascular events and all-cause mortality in CKD. Treatment with ACE inhibitors and ARBs may be accompanied by an immediate reduction in GFR when treatment is initiated, due to a reduction in glomerular perfusion pressure. Treatment can be continued so long

EBM 17.28 Lowering blood pressure in chronic kidney disease

'A meta-analysis of randomised controlled trials, including over 50 000 patients, showed that the risk of progression to end-stage renal disease (ESRD) was reduced as blood pressure was lowered. Patients with the greatest reduction in blood pressure (–6.9 mmHg; 95% confidence interval –9.1 to –4.8) had a relative risk of ESRD of 0.74 (0.59–0.92).'

'Angiotensin-converting enzyme inhibitors and angiotensin II receptor blockers reduce proteinuria and slow the progression of CKD in hypertensive patients to a greater extent than can be explained by the reduction in blood pressure alone.'

- Casas JP, et al. Lancet 2005; 366:2026–2033.
- Scottish Intercollegiate Guidelines Network 103. Diagnosis and management of chronic kidney disease.

For further information: www.sign.ed.ac.uk

EBM 17.29 Effects of lipid-lowering therapy in chronic kidney disease

'The SHARP trial of lipid-lowering in patients with CKD studied approximately 9500 patients aged 40 years or more, with a median follow-up of 4.9 years. The combination of ezetimibe 10 mg and simvastatin 20 mg reduced major atherosclerotic events by 17%, compared to placebo in patients not on dialysis (approximately 6000) ($p < 0.01$) and by 10% in patients on dialysis (not significant), although there was no overall benefit for mortality.'

- Baigent C, et al. Lancet 2011; 377:2181–2192.

as the reduction in GFR is less than 20% and is not progressive. Accordingly ACE inhibitors and/or ARBs should be prescribed to all patients with diabetic nephropathy and those with proteinuria, irrespective of whether or not hypertension is present, providing that hyperkalaemia does not occur.

Dietary and lifestyle interventions

There is experimental evidence that restricting dietary protein can reduce progression of CKD in animal models but the results are less clear-cut in humans. All patients with stage 4 and 5 CKD should be given dietetic advice aimed at preventing excessive consumption of protein, ensuring adequate calorific intake and limiting potassium and phosphate intake. Severe protein restriction is not recommended. All patients should be advised to stop smoking, since there is evidence that this slows the decline in renal function in addition to reducing cardiovascular risk. Exercise and weight loss may also reduce proteinuria and have beneficial effects on cardiovascular risk profile.

Lipid-lowering therapy

Hypercholesterolaemia is almost universal in patients with significant proteinuria, and increased triglyceride levels are also common in patients with CKD. Lipid lowering has been shown to reduce vascular events in non-dialysis CKD patients (Box 17.29). There is some evidence that control of dyslipidaemia with statins may slow the rate of progression of renal disease.

Treatment of anaemia

Anaemia is common in patients with a GFR below 30 mL/min/1.73 m^2 and contributes to many of the non-specific symptoms of CKD. Recombinant human erythropoietin is effective in correcting the anaemia of CKD and improving the associated morbidity. Erythropoietin treatment does not influence mortality, however, and correcting haemoglobin to normal levels may carry some extra risk, including hypertension and thrombosis (including thrombosis of the arteriovenous fistulae used for haemodialysis). The target haemoglobin is usually between 100 and 120 g/L (10–20 g/dL). Erythropoietin is less effective in the presence of iron deficiency, active inflammation or malignancy, and in patients with aluminium overload, which may occur in dialysis.

Maintaining fluid and electrolyte balance

Patients with evidence of fluid retention should have dietary sodium intake limited to about 100 mmol/day, but often loop diuretics may also be required to treat fluid overload. If hyperkalaemia occurs, drug therapy should be reviewed, to reduce or stop potassium-sparing diuretics, ACE inhibitors and ARBs. Correction of acidosis may be helpful, and limiting potassium intake to about 70 mmol/day may be necessary in late CKD. Potassium-binding resins, such as calcium resonium, may be useful in the short term but should not be used chronically. The plasma bicarbonate should be maintained above 22 mmol/L by giving sodium bicarbonate supplements (starting dose of 1 g 3 times daily, increasing as required). If the increased sodium intake induces hypertension or oedema, calcium carbonate (up to 3 g daily) may be used as an alternative, since this has the advantage of also binding dietary phosphate.

Renal bone disease

Treatment should be initiated with active vitamin D metabolites (either 1-α-hydroxyvitamin D or 1,25-dihydroxyvitamin D) in patients who are found to have hypocalcaemia or serum PTH levels more than twice the upper limit of normal. The dose should be adjusted to try to reduce PTH levels to between 2 and 4 times the upper limit of normal to avoid over-suppression of bone turnover and adynamic bone disease, but care must be exercised in order to avoid hypercalcaemia. Hyperphosphataemia should be treated by dietary restriction of foods with high phosphate content (milk, cheese, eggs and protein-rich foods) and by the use of phosphate-binding drugs. Various drugs are available, including calcium carbonate, aluminium hydroxide, lanthanum carbonate and polymer-based phosphate binders such as sevelamer. The aim is to maintain serum phosphate values at 1.8 mmol/L (5.6 mg/dL) or below if possible, but many of these drugs are difficult to take and compliance may be a problem.

Parathyroidectomy may be required for the treatment of tertiary hyperparathyroidism. An alternative is to employ calcimimetic agents, such as cinacalcet, which bind to the calcium-sensing receptor and reduce PTH secretion. They have a place if parathyroidectomy is unsuccessful or not possible.

RENAL REPLACEMENT THERAPY

Renal replacement therapy (RRT) may be required on a temporary basis in patients with AKI or on a permanent basis for those with CKD secondary to the many different types of renal disease discussed in this chapter.

Since the advent of long-term RRT in the 1960s, the numbers of patients with ESRD who are kept alive by dialysis and transplantation have increased considerably. For example, in the UK, there was a 3.3% increase per year between 2005 and 2010. By the end of 2010, over 51 000 patients (832 per million) were on RRT, and the incidence of new patients starting RRT was 107 per million of the adult population. Whilst these numbers have been relatively steady over the last few years in the UK, they are still rising in the USA. The median age of patients starting RRT in the UK is now 65 years and 24% have a primary renal diagnosis of diabetic nephropathy. There are variations in the numbers of patients receiving RRT in different countries due to differences in the incidence of predisposing disease, as well as differences in medical practice. For example, in the USA, incidence rates for RRT in 2010 were about three times higher than in the UK at 348 per million population, and prevalence rates more than twice as high at 1752 per million population. Nearly half of these patients had a primary diagnosis of diabetes mellitus.

At the present time, RRT is commenced in about 1 in 10 000 of the general population in the UK each year. Of patients starting dialysis in 2010, about 68% were still being treated with haemodialysis 3 months later – 18% by peritoneal dialysis, 8% by renal transplant (often before dialysis has been initiated) – and 6% had died or stopped treatment. Of prevalent patients established on RRT, about 48% had been transplanted, 44% were maintained on haemodialysis (approximately 1.5% on home haemodialysis) and 8% were on peritoneal dialysis.

Following initiation of dialysis in the UK, the survival is 84% at 1 year and 50% after 5 years. Mortality is strongly influenced by age; patients over 65 have a 76% survival at 1 year and 29% survival at 5 years, whereas corresponding figures for patients aged less than 65 are 91% and 71%, respectively. Although many young patients without extrarenal disease lead normal and active lives on RRT, those aged 30–34 have a mortality rate 25 times higher than age-matched controls. Comorbid conditions, such as diabetes mellitus (47% 5-year survival versus 66% for non-diabetics starting at age 45–64 years) and generalised vascular disease, also have a strong influence on mortality.

The aim of RRT is to replace the excretory functions of the kidney, and to maintain normal electrolyte concentrations and fluid balance. Various options are available, including haemodialysis, haemofiltration, haemodiafiltration, peritoneal dialysis and renal transplantation, and each of these is discussed in more detail below.

Preparing for renal replacement therapy

It is crucial that patients who are known to have progressive CKD are prepared well in advance for the institution of RRT. This involves ensuring that they are referred to a nephrologist in a timely manner, as those who are referred late, when they are either at the stage of or very close to requiring dialysis (about 20% of referrals in the UK), tend to have poorer outcomes. It is often possible to predict when RRT will be required from serial measurements of serum creatinine in patients with progressive CKD (see Box 17.3, p. 467). In such patients, preparations for the initiation of RRT should be started at least 12 months before the predicted start date.

At the present time, the average eGFR at the time of initiating RRT in the UK is about 8 mL/min/1.73 m^2 but there is wide variation. Since there is no evidence that early initiation of RRT improves outcome, the overall aim is to commence RRT by the time symptoms of CKD have started to appear but before serious complications have occurred. Preparation for RRT involves providing the patient with psychological and social support, assessing home circumstances and discussing the various choices of treatment (Fig. 17.15). Depression is common in patients who are on or approaching RRT, and support from the renal multidisciplinary team should be provided for both them and their relatives, to explain and help them adapt to the changes to lifestyle that may be necessary once RRT starts; this may help to reduce their anxieties about these changes.

Several decisions need to be taken in discussion with the patient and their family. The first is to decide whether RRT is an appropriate choice or whether conservative treatment might be preferable (p. 490). This is especially relevant in older people with significant comorbidity. For those that decide to go ahead with RRT, there are further choices between haemodialysis and peritoneal dialysis (Box 17.30), between hospital and home treatment, and on referral for renal transplantation.

17.30 Comparison of haemodialysis and peritoneal dialysis

Haemodialysis	Peritoneal dialysis
Efficient; 4 hrs three times per wk is usually adequate	Less efficient; 4 exchanges per day are usually required, each taking 30–60 mins (continuous ambulatory peritoneal dialysis) or 8–10 hrs each night (automated peritoneal dialysis)
2–3 days between treatments	A few hours between treatments
Requires visits to hospital (although home treatment is possible for some patients)	Performed at home
Requires adequate venous circulation for vascular access	Requires an intact peritoneal cavity without major scarring from previous surgery
Careful compliance with diet and fluid restrictions required between treatments	Diet and fluid less restricted
Fluid removal compressed into treatment periods; may cause symptoms and haemodynamic instability	Slow continuous fluid removal, usually asymptomatic
Infections related to vascular access may occur	Peritonitis and catheter-related infections may occur
Patients are usually dependent on others	Patients can take full responsibility for their treatment

17

A Haemodialysis

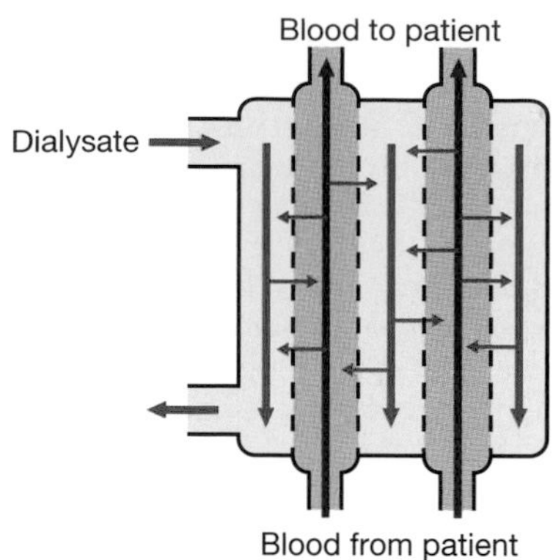

B Haemofiltration

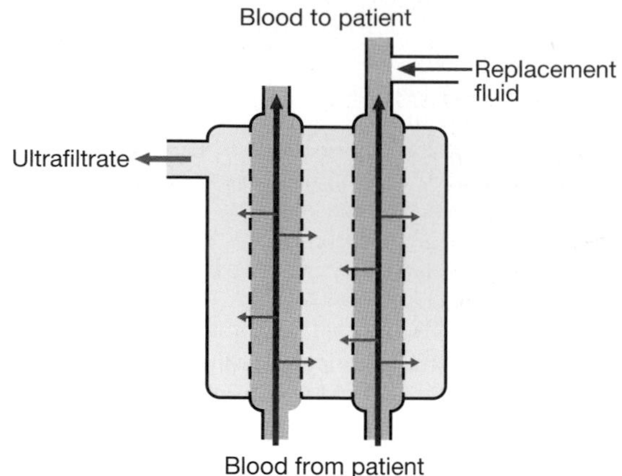

C Peritoneal dialysis

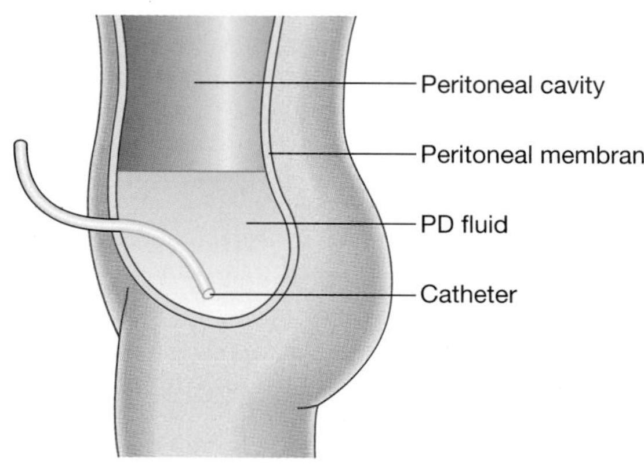

D Transplantation

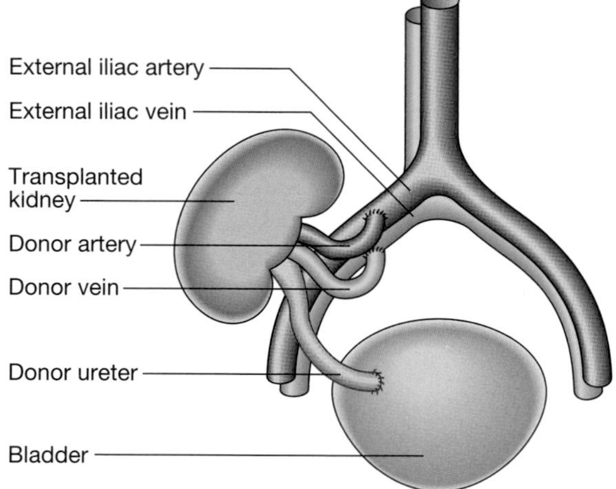

Fig. 17.15 Options for renal replacement therapy. **A** In haemodialysis, there is diffusion of solutes from blood to dialysate across a semi-permeable membrane down a concentration gradient. **B** In haemofiltration, both water and solutes are filtered across a porous semipermeable membrane by a pressure gradient. Replacement fluid is added to the filtered blood before it is returned to the patient. **C** In peritoneal dialysis (PD), fluid is introduced into the abdominal cavity using a catheter. Solutes diffuse from blood across the peritoneal membrane to PD fluid down a concentration gradient and water diffuses through osmosis (see text for details). **D** In transplantation, the blood supply of the transplanted kidney is anastomosed to the internal iliac vessels and the ureter to the bladder. The transplanted kidney replaces all functions of the failed kidney.

Conservative treatment

In older patients with multiple comorbidities, conservative treatment of stage 5 CKD, aimed at limiting the adverse symptomatic effects of ESRD without commencing RRT, is increasingly viewed as a positive choice (Box 17.31). Current evidence suggests that survival of these patients without dialysis can be similar or only slightly shorter than that of patients who undergo RRT, but they avoid the hospitalisation and interventions associated with dialysis. Patients are offered full medical, psychological and social support to optimise and sustain their existing renal function and to treat complications, such as anaemia, for as long as possible, with appropriate palliative care in the terminal phase of their disease. Many of these patients enjoy a good quality of life for several years. It is also appropriate to discontinue dialysis treatment, with the consent of the patient, and to offer conservative therapy and palliative care when quality of life on dialysis is inadequate.

Haemodialysis

Haemodialysis is the most common form of RRT in ESRD and is also used in AKI. Haemodialysis involves gaining access to the circulation, either through an arteriovenous fistula, a central venous catheter or an arteriovenous shunt, such as a Scribner shunt. The patient's blood is pumped through a haemodialyser, which allows bidirectional diffusion of solutes between blood and the dialysate across a semipermeable membrane down a concentration gradient (Fig. 17.15A). The composition of the dialysate can be varied to achieve the desired gradient and fluid can be removed by applying negative pressure to the dialysate side.

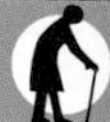

17.31 Renal replacement therapy in old age

- **Quality of life**: age itself is not a barrier to good quality of life on RRT.
- **Coexisting cardiovascular disease**: older people are more sensitive to fluid balance changes, predisposing to hypotension during dialysis with rebound hypertension between dialyses. A failing heart cannot cope with fluid overload, and pulmonary oedema develops easily.
- **Provision of treatment**: often only hospital-provided haemodialysis is suitable and older patients require more medical and nursing time.
- **Survival on dialysis**: difficult to predict for an individual patient, but old age plus substantial comorbidity are associated with poor median survival.
- **Withdrawal from dialysis**: a common cause of death in older patients with comorbid disease.
- **Transplantation**: relative risks of surgery and immunosuppression, and limited organ availability exclude most older people from transplantation.
- **Conservative therapy**: without dialysis but with adequate support; is an appropriate option for patients at high risk of complications from dialysis, who have a limited prognosis and little hope of functional recovery.

Haemodialysis in AKI

Haemodialysis offers the best rate of small solute clearance in AKI, as compared with other techniques such as haemofiltration, but should be started gradually because of the risk of confusion and convulsions due to cerebral oedema (dialysis disequilibrium). Typically, 1–2 hours of dialysis is prescribed initially but, subsequently, patients with AKI who are haemodynamically stable can be treated by 4–5 hours of haemodialysis on alternate days, or 2–3 hours every day. During dialysis, it is standard practice to anticoagulate patients with heparin but the dose may be reduced if there is a bleeding risk. Epoprostenol can be used as an alternative but carries a risk of hypotension. For short dialyses and in patients with abnormal clotting, it may be possible to avoid anticoagulation altogether. In AKI, dialysis is performed through a large-bore, dual-lumen catheter inserted into the femoral or internal jugular vein. Subclavian lines are avoided where possible, as thromboses or stenoses here will compromise the ability to form a functioning fistula in the arm if the patient fails to recover renal function and needs chronic dialysis.

Haemodialysis in CKD

In CKD, vascular access for haemodialysis is gained by formation of an arteriovenous fistula, usually in the forearm, up to a year before dialysis is contemplated. After 4–6 weeks, increased pressure transmitted from the artery to the vein leading from the fistula causes distension and thickening of the vessel wall (arterialisation). Large-bore needles can then be inserted into the vein to provide access for each haemodialysis treatment. Figure 17.16 shows a patient undergoing haemodialysis through such a fistula. Preservation of arm veins is thus very important in patients with progressive renal disease who may require haemodialysis in the future. If this access is not possible, venous or Gortex grafts may be fashioned or plastic catheters in central veins can be used for short-term access. These may be tunnelled under the skin to reduce infection risk. All patients must be screened in advance for hepatitis B, hepatitis C and human immunodeficiency virus (HIV), and vaccinated against hepatitis B if they are not immune. All dialysis units should have segregation facilities for hepatitis B-positive patients, given its easy transmissibility. Patients with hepatitis C and HIV are less infectious and can be treated satisfactorily using machine segregation and standard infection control measures.

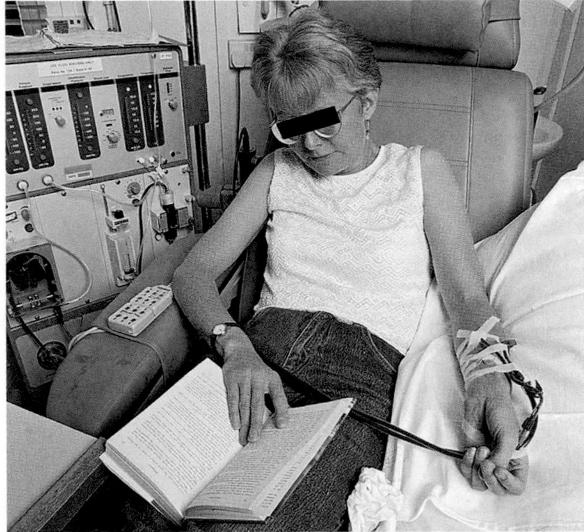

Fig. 17.16 Haemodialysis. A patient receiving haemodialysis through a forearm subcutaneous (Brescia–Cimino) fistula. She subsequently received a live related transplant.

Haemodialysis is usually carried out for 3–5 hours three times weekly, either at home or in an outpatient dialysis unit. The intensity and frequency of dialysis should be adjusted to achieve a reduction in urea during dialysis (urea reduction ratio) of over 65%. Most patients notice an improvement in symptoms during the first 6 weeks of treatment. Plasma urea and creatinine are lowered by each treatment but do not return to normal. The intensity of dialysis can be increased by escalating the number of standard sessions to four or more per week; by performing short, frequent dialysis sessions of 2–3 hours 5–7 times per week; or by performing nocturnal haemodialysis, when low blood-pump speeds and single-needle dialysis are used for approximately 8 hours overnight 5–6 times per week.

More frequent dialysis and nocturnal dialysis can achieve better fluid balance and electrolyte control than standard dialysis and, in particular, better control of serum phosphate levels. Studies are currently in progress to determine whether these different modes of dialysis improve clinical outcome. Box 17.32 summarises some of the problems related to haemodialysis.

Haemofiltration

This technique is principally used in the treatment of AKI. Water and solutes are filtered from blood across a porous semipermeable membrane under a pressure gradient. Replacement fluid of a suitable electrolyte composition is added to the blood after it exits from the haemofilter. If removal of fluid is required, then less

17.32 Problems with haemodialysis

Problem	Clinical features	Cause	Treatment
Hypotension during dialysis	Sudden ↓BP; often leg cramps; sometimes chest pain	Fluid removal and hypovolaemia	Saline infusion; exclude cardiac ischaemia; quinine may help cramp
Cardiac arrhythmias	Hypotension, sometimes chest pain	Potassium and acid–base shifts	Check K^+ and arterial blood gases; review dialysis prescription; stop dialysis
Haemorrhage	Blood loss (overt or occult); hypotension	Anticoagulation Venous needle disconnection	Stop dialysis; seek source; consider heparin-free treatment
Air embolism	Circulatory collapse; cardiac arrest	Disconnected or faulty lines and equipment malfunction	Stop dialysis
Dialyser hypersensitivity	Acute circulatory collapse	Allergic reaction to dialysis membrane or sterilisant	Stop dialysis; change to different artificial kidney
Between treatments			
Pulmonary oedema	Breathlessness	Fluid overload	Ultrafiltration ± dialysis
Systemic sepsis	Rigors; fever; ↓BP	Usually involves vascular access devices (catheter or fistula)	Blood cultures; antibiotics

fluid is added back than is removed (Fig. 17.15B). Haemofiltration may be either intermittent or continuous, and typically 1–2 litres of filtrate is replaced per hour (equivalent to a GFR of 15–30 mL/min); higher rates of filtration may be of benefit in patients with sepsis and multi-organ failure. In continuous arteriovenous haemofiltration (CAVH), the extracorporeal blood circuit is driven by the arteriovenous pressure difference, but poor filtration rates and clotting of the filter are common and this treatment has fallen out of favour. Continuous venovenous haemofiltration (CVVH) is pump-driven, providing a reliable extracorporeal circulation. Issues concerning anticoagulation are similar to those for haemodialysis, but may be more problematic because longer or continuous anticoagulation is necessary.

Haemodiafiltration

This technique combines haemodialysis with approximately 20–30 litres of ultrafiltration (with replacement of filtrate) over a 3–5-hour treatment. It uses a large-pore membrane and combines the improved middle-molecule clearance of haemofiltration with the higher small-solute clearance of haemodialysis. It is sometimes used in the treatment of AKI but is increasingly favoured in the treatment of CKD. It is more expensive than haemodialysis, however, and the long-term benefits are not yet established.

Peritoneal dialysis

Peritoneal dialysis is principally used in the treatment of CKD. It requires the insertion of a permanent Silastic catheter into the peritoneal cavity (Fig. 17.15C). Two types are in common use. In continuous ambulatory peritoneal dialysis (CAPD), about 2 litres of sterile, isotonic dialysis fluid are introduced and left in place for approximately 4–6 hours. Metabolic waste products diffuse from peritoneal capillaries into the dialysis fluid down a concentration gradient. The fluid is then drained and fresh dialysis fluid introduced, in a continuous four-times-daily cycle. The inflow fluid is rendered hyperosmolar by the addition of glucose or glucose polymer; this results in net removal of fluid from the patient during each cycle, due to diffusion of water from the blood through the peritoneal membrane down an osmotic gradient (ultrafiltration). The patient is mobile and able to undertake normal daily activities. Automated peritoneal dialysis (APD) is similar to CAPD but uses a mechanical device to perform the fluid exchanges during the night, leaving the patient free, or with only a single exchange to perform, during the day.

CAPD is particularly useful in children, as a first treatment in adults with residual renal function, and as a treatment for elderly patients with cardiovascular instability. The long-term use of peritoneal dialysis may be limited by episodes of bacterial peritonitis and damage to the peritoneal membrane, including sclerosing peritonitis, but some patients have been treated successfully for more than 10 years. Box 17.33 summarises some of the problems related to CAPD treatment.

Renal transplantation

Renal transplantation offers the best chance of long-term survival in ESRD, and is the most cost-effective treatment. Transplantation can restore normal kidney function and correct all the metabolic abnormalities of CKD but requires long-term immunosuppression with its attendant risks (see below). All patients with ESRD should be considered for transplantation, unless there are contraindications (Box 17.34).

Kidney grafts may be taken from a cadaver in the UK after brain death (51%) or circulatory death (11%), or from a living donor (38%). As described on page 94, matching of a donor to a specific recipient is strongly influenced by immunological factors, since graft rejection is the major cause of transplant failure. Compatibility of ABO blood group between donor and recipient is usually required and the degree of matching for major histocompatibility (MHC) antigens, particularly HLA-DR, influences the incidence of rejection. Immediately prior to transplantation, tests should be performed for

17.33 Problems with continuous ambulatory peritoneal dialysis

Problem	Clinical features	Cause	Treatment
Peritonitis	Cloudy drainage fluid; abdominal pain and systemic sepsis are variable	Usually entry of skin contaminants via catheter; bowel organisms less common	Culture of peritoneal dialysis fluid Intraperitoneal antibiotics, tobramycin, vancomycin Catheter removal sometimes required
Catheter exit site infection	Erythema and pus around exit site	Usually skin organisms	Antibiotics; sometimes surgical drainage
Ultrafiltration failure	Fluid overload	Damage to peritoneal membrane, leading to rapid transport of glucose and loss of osmotic gradient	Replace glucose with synthetic, poorly absorbed polymers for some exchanges (icodextrin)
Peritoneal membrane failure	Inadequate clearance of urea etc.	Scarring/damage to peritoneal membrane	Increase exchange volumes; consider automated peritoneal dialysis or switch to haemodialysis
Sclerosing peritonitis	Intermittent bowel obstruction Malnutrition	Unknown; typically occurs after many years	Switch to haemodialysis (may still progress) Surgery and tamoxifen may be used

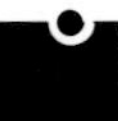

17.34 Contraindications to renal transplantation

Absolute

- Active malignancy: a period of at least 2 yrs of complete remission recommended for most tumours
- Active vasculitis or recent anti-GBM disease
- Severe heart disease
- Severe occlusive aorto-iliac vascular disease

Relative

- Age: while practice varies, transplants are not routinely offered to very young children (< 1 yr) or older people (> 75 yrs)
- High risk of disease recurrence in the transplant kidney
- Disease of the lower urinary tract: in patients with impaired bladder function, an ileal conduit may be considered
- Significant comorbidity

antibodies against HLA antigens and for antibodies that can bind to lymphocytes of the donor (p. 95). Positive tests predict early rejection. Although some ABO- and HLA-incompatible transplants are now possible, this involves appropriate preparation with pre-transplant plasma exchange and/or immunosuppression, so that recipient antibodies to the donor's tissue are reduced to acceptably low levels. This option is generally only available for living donor transplants because of the preparation required. Paired exchanges, in which a donor–recipient pair which has compatibility issues, either blood group or HLA, is computer-matched with another pair to overcome the mismatch, are also used to help increase the number of successful transplants that can be performed.

During the transplant operation, the kidney is placed in the pelvis; the donor vessels are usually anastomosed to the recipient's internal iliac artery and vein, and the donor ureter anastomosed to the bladder (Fig. 17.15D). The failed kidneys are usually left in place. Peri-operative problems include:

- *Fluid balance.* Careful matching of input to output is required. Patients can be very polyuric in the initial period after transplantation.
- *Primary graft non-function.* Causes include hypovolaemia, preservation injury/acute tubular necrosis during storage and transfer, other pre-existing renal damage, hyperacute rejection, vascular occlusion and urinary tract obstruction.
- *Sepsis.* In addition to risks of sepsis associated with any operation, there is an increased risk due to the uraemia and immunosuppression.

Once the graft begins to function, near-normal biochemistry is usually achieved within days to weeks. The median eGFR of patients in the UK receiving a deceased donor transplant at 1 year is 51 mL/min/1.73 m^2.

All transplant patients require regular life-long follow-up to monitor renal function and immunosuppression. Life-long immunosuppressive therapy (see Box 4.25, p. 96) is required to prevent rejection but needs to be more intensive in the early post-transplantation period, when the risk is highest. A common regimen is triple therapy with prednisolone; ciclosporin or tacrolimus; and azathioprine or mycophenolate mofetil. Sirolimus (rapamycin) is an alternative that can be introduced later. Antibodies to deplete or modulate specific lymphocyte populations are increasingly used; targeting the lymphocyte interleukin (IL)-2 receptor is particularly effective for preventing rejection. Acute rejection is usually treated, in the first instance, by short courses of high-dose corticosteroids, such as methylprednisolone 500 mg IV on 3 consecutive days. Other therapies, such as antilymphocyte antibodies, intravenous immunoglobulin and plasma exchange, can be used for episodes of acute rejection that do not respond to high-dose corticosteroids.

Complications of immunosuppression include infections and malignancy (p. 95). Approximately 50% of white patients develop skin malignancy by 15 years after transplantation.

The prognosis after kidney transplantation is good. Recent UK statistics for transplants from cadaver donors indicate 96% patient survival and 93% graft survival at 1 year, and 88% patient survival and 84% graft survival at 5 years. Even better figures are obtained with living donor transplantation (91% graft survival at 5 years).

Advances in immunosuppression have greatly improved results from using genetically unrelated donors, such as spouses.

RENAL VASCULAR DISEASES

Diseases which affect renal blood vessels may cause renal ischaemia, leading to acute or chronic kidney disease or secondary hypertension. The rising prevalence of atherosclerosis and diabetes mellitus in ageing populations has made renovascular disease an important cause of ESRD.

Renal artery stenosis

Renal artery stenosis is a relatively uncommon disorder, which presents clinically with hypertension. It has been estimated to occur in about 2% of unselected patients with hypertension but may affect up to 4% of older patients with hypertension who have evidence of atherosclerotic disease elsewhere. Most cases of renal artery stenosis are caused by atherosclerosis but fibromuscular dysplasia involving the vessel wall may be responsible in younger patients. Rare causes include vasculitis, thromboembolism and aneurysms of the renal artery.

Pathophysiology

Renal artery stenosis results in a reduction in renal perfusion pressure, which activates the renin–angiotensin system, leading to increased circulating levels of angiotensin II. This provokes vasoconstriction and increases aldosterone production by the adrenal, causing sodium retention by the renal tubules. Significant reduction of renal blood flow occurs when there is greater than 70% narrowing of the artery, and this is commonly associated with a dilated region more distally (post-stenotic dilatation). Atherosclerosis is the most common cause. The characteristic lesion is an ostial stenosis that is associated with atherosclerosis within the aorta and affects other major branches, particularly the iliac vessels. The picture is often complicated by small-vessel disease in affected kidneys, which may be related to subclinical atheroemboli or other vascular disease. As the stenosis becomes more severe, global renal ischaemia leads to shrinkage of the affected kidney and may cause renal failure (ischaemic nephropathy). However, the progression of stenosis is not easily predictable, and many patients die from coronary, cerebral or other vascular disease rather than renal failure.

In younger patients, fibromuscular dysplasia is a more likely cause of renal artery stenosis. This is an uncommon disorder of unknown cause. It is characterised by hypertrophy of the media (medial fibroplasia), which narrows the artery but rarely leads to total occlusion. It may be associated with disease in other arteries; for example, those who have carotid artery dissections are more likely to have renal arteries with this appearance. It most commonly presents with hypertension in patients aged 15–30 years, and women are affected more frequently than men. Irregular narrowing (beading) may occur in the distal renal artery and this sometimes extends into the intrarenal branches of the vessel. Rarely, renal artery stenosis may occur as a complication of large-vessel vasculitis, such as Takayasu's arteritis and polyarteritis nodosa (pp. 1116 and 1117). Untreated, atheromatous renal artery stenosis is thought to progress to complete arterial occlusion in about 15% of cases. This figure increases with more severe degrees of stenosis. If the progression is gradual, collateral vessels may develop and some function may be preserved, preventing infarction and loss of kidney structure. Conversely, at least 85% of patients with renal artery stenosis will not develop progressive renal impairment, and indeed, in many patients, the stenosis may be haemodynamically insignificant and not responsible for coexisting essential hypertension. Unfortunately, methods of predicting which patients are at risk of progression or who will respond to treatment are still imperfect.

Clinical features

Renal artery stenosis can present in various ways (Box 17.35), including hypertension, renal failure (with bilateral disease), a deterioration in renal function when ACE inhibitors or ARBs are used, or acute pulmonary oedema. Although many patients experience a slight drop in GFR when commencing these drugs, an increase in serum creatinine of 25% or more raises the possibility of renal artery stenosis. Acute pulmonary oedema is particularly characteristic of bilateral renovascular disease. It is associated with severe hypertension, occurring without other obvious cause in patients with normal or only mildly impaired renal function. Clinical evidence of generalised vascular disease may be observed, particularly in the legs, in older patients with atherosclerotic renal artery stenosis. Clinical features associated with an increased risk of renal artery stenosis in hypertensive patients are summarised in Box 17.35. The presence of one or more of these features should prompt investigation for possible renal artery stenosis, as described below, provided that intervention is being contemplated to improve renal perfusion.

Investigations

When appropriate, imaging of the renal vasculature with either CT angiography or MR angiography should be performed to confirm the diagnosis (Fig. 17.17). Both give good views of the main renal arteries, the vessels predominantly involved and the most amenable to intervention. Biochemical testing may reveal impaired renal function and an elevated plasma renin activity, sometimes with hypokalaemia due to hyperaldosteronism. Ultrasound may also reveal a discrepancy in size between the two kidneys. While these investigations

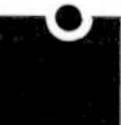

17.35 Presentation and clinical features of renal artery stenosis

Renal artery stenosis is more likely if:

- hypertension is severe, of recent onset or difficult to control
- kidneys are asymmetrical in size
- flash pulmonary oedema occurs repeatedly*
- there is peripheral vascular disease of the lower limbs
- there is renal impairment*
- renal function has deteriorated on ACE inhibitors or angiotensin II receptor blockers

*Particularly with bilateral disease.

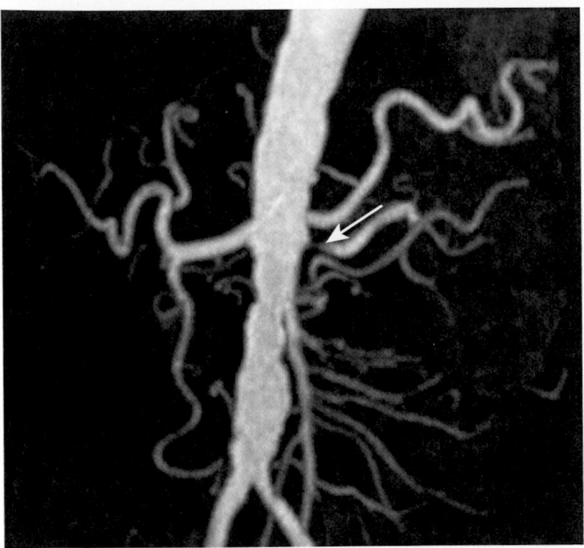

Fig. 17.17 Renal artery stenosis. A magnetic resonance angiogram following injection of contrast. The abdominal aorta is severely irregular and atheromatous. The left renal artery is stenosed (arrow).

provide supportive information, they are insufficiently sensitive or specific to be of value in diagnosis of renovascular disease in hypertensive patients.

Management

The first-line management in patients with renal artery stenosis is medical therapy with antihypertensive drugs, supplemented, where appropriate, by statins and low-dose aspirin in those with atherosclerotic disease. Interventions to correct the vessel narrowing should be considered in young patients (age below 40) suspected of having renal artery stenosis; those in whom blood pressure cannot easily be controlled with antihypertensive agents; those who have a history of 'flash' pulmonary oedema or accelerated phase (malignant) hypertension; and those in whom renal function is deteriorating. The most commonly used technique is angioplasty. The best results are obtained in non-atheromatous fibromuscular dysplasia, where correction of the stenosis has a high chance of success in improving blood pressure and protecting renal function. Angioplasty and stenting can sometimes be successful in atherosclerotic disease but randomised trials have produced no convincing evidence for overall benefit in terms of renal function or blood pressure control (Box 17.36). The risks of angioplasty and stenting include renal artery occlusion, renal infarction, and atheroemboli (p. 496) from manipulations in a severely diseased aorta. Small-vessel disease distal to the stenosis may preclude substantial functional recovery.

EBM 17.36 Stenting for renal artery stenosis

'The ASTRAL trial compared medical therapy to revascularisation in 806 patients with atherosclerotic renal disease and found substantial risks but no evidence of a worthwhile clinical benefit from revascularisation over 5 years of follow-up. Specifically, there was no statistical difference in blood pressure or rate of change of renal function between the groups, but serious complications associated with revascularisation occurred in 23 patients, including 2 deaths and 3 amputations of toes or limbs.'

- ASTRAL Investigators. N Engl J Med 2009; 361:1953–1962.

Acute renal infarction

This is an uncommon condition that occurs as the result of sudden occlusion of the renal arteries. The presentation is typically with loin pain of acute onset, usually in association with haematuria detected on dipstick testing or urine microscopy, but pain may be absent in some cases. Severe hypertension is common but not universal, presumably because some residual renal perfusion is required to generate renin release. Blood levels of lactate dehydrogenase (LDH) and CRP are commonly raised. The condition may be caused by local atherosclerosis (atheroembolic) or by thromboemboli from a distant source, where occlusion may occur in branch arteries distal to the main renal artery. This can cause multiple infarcts within the renal parenchyma of both kidneys, which may be visualised by CT scanning. If occlusion of the main renal arteries is bilateral or if there is occlusion of a single functioning kidney, the presentation is with AKI and the patient is typically anuric. Patients with bilateral occlusion usually have evidence of widespread vascular disease and may show evidence of aortic occlusion, with absent femoral pulses and reduced lower limb perfusion. Management is largely supportive, and includes anticoagulation if a source of thromboembolism is an identified source. It is sometimes possible to carry out stenting of an acutely blocked main renal artery to try to restore renal blood flow and kidney function.

Diseases of small intrarenal vessels

A number of conditions are associated with acute damage and occlusion of small blood vessels (arterioles and capillaries) in the kidney (Box 17.37). They are often found in conjunction with similar changes elsewhere in the body. A common feature of these syndromes is microangiopathic haemolytic anaemia, in which haemolysis and red cell fragmentation arise as consequences of damage incurred to red blood cells during passage through the abnormal vessels.

Haemolytic uraemic syndrome

Haemolytic uraemic syndrome (HUS) is characterised by thrombotic microangiopathy that causes damage to

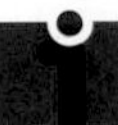

17.37 Microvascular disorders associated with acute renal damage

- Thrombotic microangiopathy (haemolytic uraemic syndrome and thrombotic thrombocytopenic purpura)
  - Associated with verotoxin-producing *E. coli*
  - Other (familial, drugs, cancer)
- Disseminated intravascular coagulation
- Malignant hypertension
- Small-vessel vasculitis
- Systemic sclerosis (scleroderma)
- Atheroemboli ('cholesterol' emboli)

endothelial cells of the microcirculation. This is accompanied by swelling of the endothelial cells, increased platelet adherence and intravascular thrombosis. There is a marked reduction in the platelet count and anaemia, with features of intravascular haemolysis (p. 1026), such as a raised unconjugated bilirubin level, raised levels of LDH and decreased circulating levels of haptoglobin. A reticulocytosis is often seen. The kidney microcirculation tends to be most affected in HUS, with involvement of other organs (including the brain) in more severe cases. The most common cause of classical HUS is infection associated with organisms that produce enterotoxins called verotoxins: so-called diarrhoea-positive HUS (D+HUS). In about 10% of cases, however, no infective cause can be identified and this is termed atypical HUS.

The organisms most commonly implicated in D+HUS are enterohaemorrhagic *Escherichia coli* (p. 342). The O157:H7 serotype is the best known but other serotypes that produce verotoxins can also be responsible. Although these bacteria live as commensals in the gut of cattle and other domestic livestock, they can cause haemorrhagic diarrhoea in humans when the infection is contracted from contaminated food products, water or other infected individuals. In a proportion of cases, verotoxin produced by the organisms enters the circulation and binds to specific glycolipid receptors that are expressed on the surface of microvascular endothelial cells. In developed countries, D+HUS is now the most common cause of AKI in children. Recovery is good in most patients but sometimes RRT may be required for up to 14 days. No other specific treatments have been shown to help the renal lesion.

Atypical HUS is subclassified into familial and sporadic subtypes but both are associated with abnormalities of the complement system. Up to 70% of sporadic cases are associated with the development of autoantibodies to complement factor H, whereas the inherited forms are due to mutations in various genes that encode components of the complement cascade, including factor H (*CFH*), factor B (*CFB*) and complement component 3 (*C3*). The penetrance of familial HUS is incomplete, indicating that environmental triggers are also involved, but the nature of these triggers is poorly understood. Management of atypical HUS involves supportive care, optimising fluid and electrolyte balance, transfusion and RRT if necessary. Infusion of fresh frozen plasma can be helpful (presumably by replacing complement components), as can plasma exchange (presumably by removing pathogenic autoantibodies). Recently, impressive results have been reported with the anti-C5 monoclonal antibody, eculizumab, which binds to C5, thereby preventing activation of the terminal complement cascade.

Thrombotic thrombocytopenic purpura

Like HUS, thrombotic thrombocytopenic purpura (TTP) is characterised by thrombotic microangiopathy, which causes damage to endothelial cells of the microcirculation. This leads to swelling of the endothelial cells, increased platelet adherence and intravascular thrombosis. In contradistinction to HUS, the brain is more commonly affected in TTP and involvement of the kidney is usually less prominent. TTP is an autoimmune disorder caused by antibodies against ADAMTS-13, which is involved in regulating platelet aggregation. More details are provided on page 1056.

Disseminated intravascular coagulation

This may occur as a complication of a range of illnesses and can be accompanied by multi-organ failure and renal failure. Pathogenesis and management are discussed in more detail on pages 201 and 1055.

Systemic sclerosis

Renal involvement is a serious complication of systemic sclerosis, which is more likely to occur in diffuse cutaneous systemic sclerosis (DCSS) than in limited cutaneous systemic sclerosis (LCSS). The renal lesion is caused by intimal cell proliferation and luminal narrowing of intrarenal arteries and arterioles. There is intense intrarenal vasospasm and plasma renin activity is markedly elevated. Renal involvement usually presents clinically with severe hypertension, microangiopathic features and progressive oliguric renal failure (scleroderma renal crisis). Use of ACE inhibitors to control the hypertension has improved the 1-year survival from 20% to 75% but about 50% of patients continue to require RRT. Onset or acceleration of the syndrome after stopping ACE inhibitors is now well described.

Cholesterol emboli

These present with renal impairment, haematuria, proteinuria and sometimes eosinophilia with inflammatory features that can mimic a small-vessel vasculitis. The symptoms are provoked by showers of cholesterol-containing microemboli, arising in atheromatous plaques in major arteries. The diagnosis should be suspected when these clinical features occur in patients with widespread atheromatous disease, who have undergone interventions such as surgery or arteriography. It may also be precipitated by anticoagulants and thrombolytic agents. On clinical examination, signs of large-vessel disease and microvascular occlusion in the lower limbs (ischaemic toes, livedo reticularis) are common but not invariable (Fig. 17.18). There is no specific treatment.

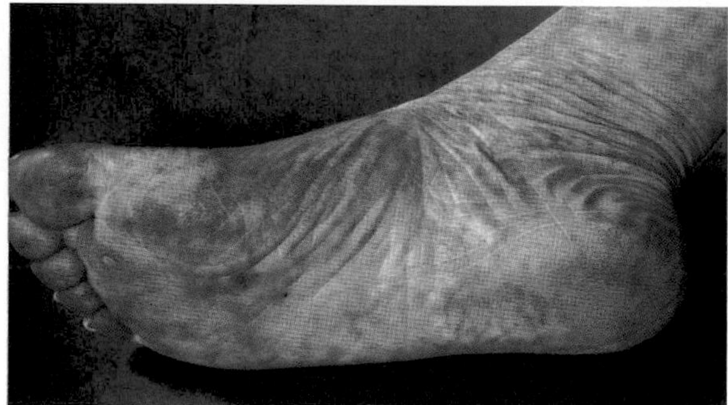

Fig. 17.18 The foot of a patient who suffered extensive atheroembolism following coronary artery stenting.

Small-vessel vasculitis

Renal disease caused by small-vessel vasculitis usually affects the glomeruli, as described in the next section and on page 519.

Accelerated phase hypertension

Accelerated phase hypertension (p. 609) is deemed to exist when it is associated with acute damage to renal and other arterioles. It is often symptomatic, with headache, impaired vision and renal impairment (Fig. 17.19). Physical examination reveals severe hypertension with evidence of hypertensive retinopathy. Papilloedema is almost always present. Clinical features of microangiopathy, such as fragmented red cells and anaemia, may be present and, in the absence of a previous history, it may be difficult to distinguish patients with accelerated phase hypertension from those with HUS and hypertension. Most patients respond to effective control of blood pressure, although renal function is permanently lost in 20% of cases.

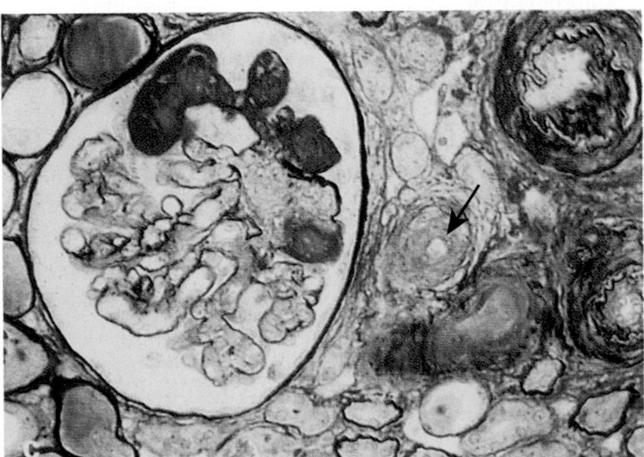

Fig. 17.19 Glomerular capillary thrombosis in malignant hypertension. Similar changes occur in thrombotic microangiopathy. The adjacent arteriole (arrow) shows gross intimal thickening. From Beutler and Koomans 1977 – see p. 523.

GLOMERULAR DISEASES

Glomerular diseases account for a significant proportion of acute and chronic kidney disease. There are many causes of glomerular damage, including immunological injury, inherited diseases such as Alport's syndrome

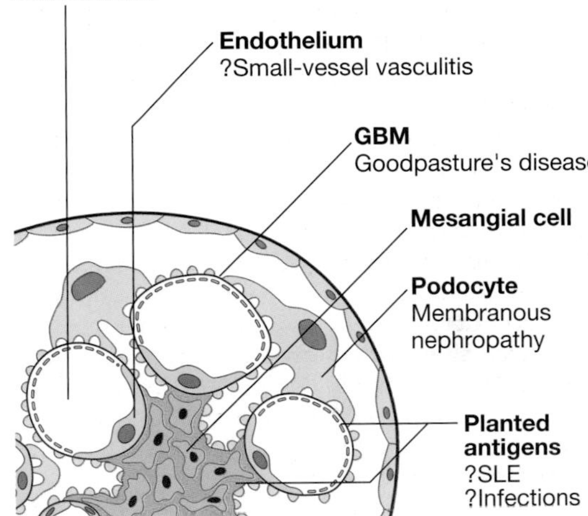

Fig. 17.20 Cells of the glomerulus and targets of immunity and autoimmunity. Antibodies and antigen–antibody (immune) complexes are described according to their site of deposition: subepithelial, between podocyte and GBM; intramembranous, within the GBM; subendothelial, between endothelial cell and GBM; and mesangial, within the mesangial matrix. (GBM = glomerular basement membrane; SLE = systemic lupus erythematosus)

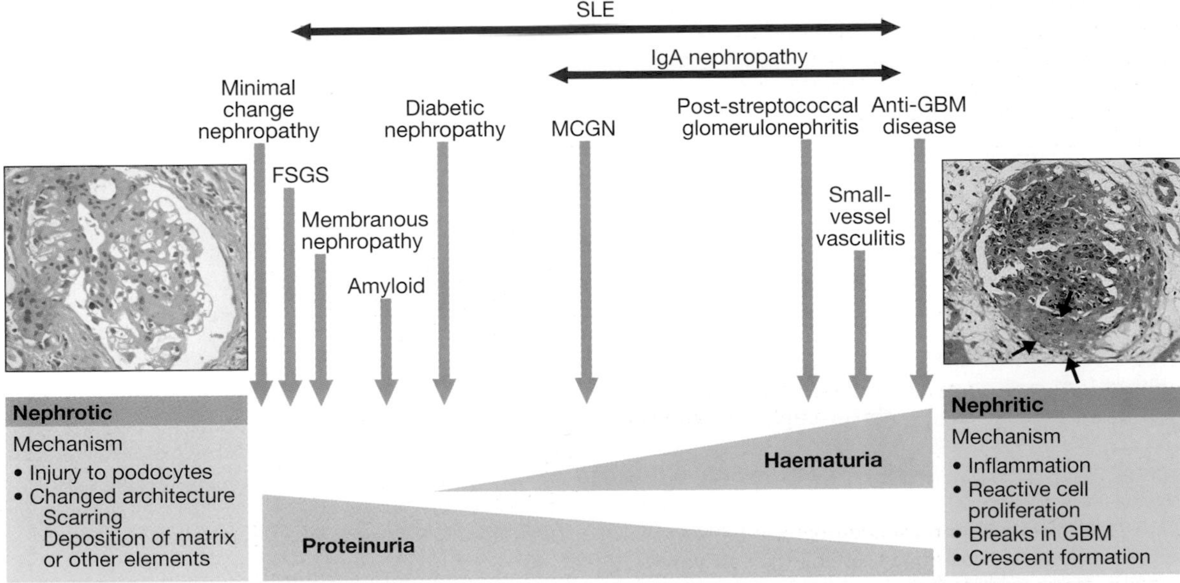

Fig. 17.21 Spectrum of glomerular diseases. At one extreme, specific injury to podocytes or structural alteration of the glomerulus affecting podocyte function (for example, by scarring or deposition of excess matrix or other material) causes proteinuria and nephrotic syndrome (see Box 17.11, p. 475). The histology to the left shows diabetic nephropathy. At the other end of the spectrum, inflammation leads to cell damage and proliferation, breaks form in the GBM and blood leaks into urine. In its extreme form, with acute sodium retention and hypertension, such disease is labelled nephritic syndrome. The histology to the right shows a glomerulus with many extra nuclei from proliferating intrinsic cells, and influx of inflammatory cells shows crescent formation (arrows) in response to severe post-infectious glomerulonephritis. (FSGS = focal and segmental glomerulosclerosis; MCGN = mesangiocapillary glomerulonephritis)

17

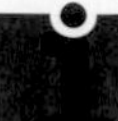

17.38 Clinical and laboratory features of glomerular injury

- Leakage of cells and macromolecules across the glomerular filtration barrier
  - Proteinuria: characteristic of diseases that affect the podocyte, scarring and deposition of foreign material
  - Haematuria: characteristic of inflammatory and destructive processes
- Impaired renal function and reduced GFR
- Hypertension

(p. 502), metabolic diseases such as diabetes mellitus (p. 830), and deposition of abnormal proteins such as amyloid in the glomeruli. The cell types of the glomerulus that may be the target of injury are shown in Figure 17.20. The response of the glomerulus to injury and hence the predominant clinical features vary according to the nature of the insult (Fig. 17.21). Clinical and laboratory features common to many glomerular diseases are shown in Box 17.38. Most patients with glomerular disease do not present acutely and are asymptomatic until abnormalities are detected on routine screening of blood or urine samples.

Glomerulonephritis

Glomerulonephritis literally means 'inflammation of glomeruli'. The term is used to describe all types of glomerular disease, even though some of these (such as minimal change nephropathy) are not associated with inflammation.

Most types of glomerulonephritis are immunologically mediated and several respond to immunosuppressive drugs. Deposition of antibody occurs in many types of glomerulonephritis (Box 17.39) but, frequently, the presumed mechanisms involve cellular immunity, which is more difficult to investigate. Although deposition of circulating immune complexes was previously thought to be a common mechanism, it now seems that most granular deposits of immunoglobulin are formed 'in situ' by antibodies which complex with glomerular antigens, or with other extraneous antigens derived from viruses and bacteria that have become deposited in the glomeruli (see Fig. 17.20).

Glomerulonephritis is generally classified in terms of the histopathological appearances, as summarised in Box 17.39 and Figure 17.22. The most common subtypes are discussed in more detail below.

Minimal change nephropathy

Minimal change disease occurs at all ages but accounts for nephrotic syndrome (see Box 17.11, p. 475) in most children and about one-quarter of adults. It is caused by reversible dysfunction of podocytes. The presentation is with proteinuria or nephrotic syndrome, which typically remits with high-dose corticosteroid therapy (1 mg/kg prednisolone for 6 weeks). Some patients who respond incompletely or relapse frequently need maintenance

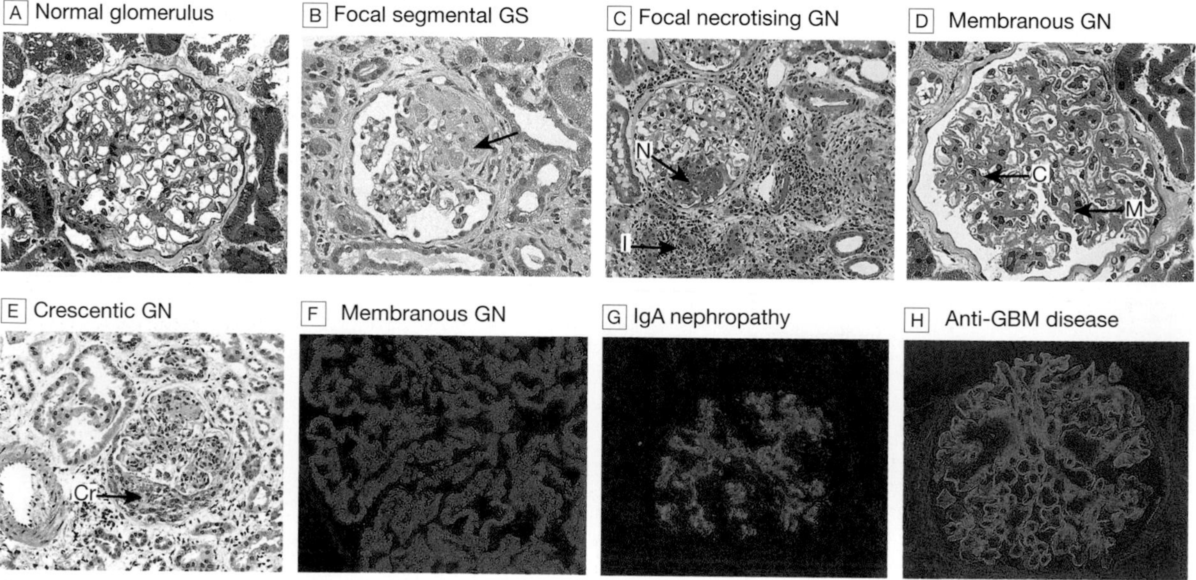

Fig. 17.22 Histopathology of glomerular disease. (A–E light microscopy) A A normal glomerulus. Note the open capillary loops and thinness of their walls – 'should look as if you could cut yourself on them'. **B** Focal segmental glomerulosclerosis (GS). The portion of the glomerulus arrowed shows loss of capillary loops and cells, which are replaced by matrix. **C** Focal necrotising glomerulonephritis (GN). A portion of the glomerulus (N = focal necrotising lesion) is replaced by bright pink material with some 'nuclear dust'. Neutrophils may be seen elsewhere in the glomerulus. There is surrounding interstitial inflammation (I). This is most commonly associated with small-vessel vasculitis and may progress to crescentic nephritis (see **E**). **D** Membranous glomerulonephritis. The capillary loops (C) are thickened (compare with the normal glomerulus) and there is expansion of the mesangial regions by matrix deposition (M). However, there is no gross cellular proliferation or excess of inflammatory cells. **E** Crescentic glomerulonephritis. The lower part of Bowman's space is occupied by a semicircular formation ('crescent', Cr) of large pale cells, compressing the glomerular tuft. This is seen in aggressive inflammatory glomerulonephritis. **Antibody deposition in the glomerulus.** (**F–H direct immunofluorescence**) **F** Granular deposits of IgG along the basement membrane in a subepithelial pattern, typical of membranous GN. **G** Immunoglobulin A (IgA) deposits in the mesangium, as seen in IgA nephropathy. **H** Ribbon-like linear deposits of anti-GBM antibodies along the glomerular basement membrane in Goodpasture's disease. The glomerular structure is well preserved in all of these examples.

17.39 Glomerulonephritis: types, associations and causes

Histology	Immune deposits	Pathogenesis	Associations	Comments
Minimal change				
Normal, except on electron microscopy, where fusion of podocyte foot processes is seen (a non-specific finding)	None	Unknown	Atopy HLA-DR7 Drugs	Acute and often severe nephrotic syndrome Good response to corticosteroids Dominant cause of idiopathic nephrotic syndrome in childhood
Focal segmental glomerulosclerosis (FSGS)				
Segmental scars in some glomeruli No acute inflammation Podocyte foot process fusion seen in primary FSGS with nephrotic syndrome	Non-specific trapping in focal scars	Unknown; in some, circulating factors increase glomerular permeability Injury to podocytes may be a common feature	Healing of previous local glomerular injury HIV infection Heroin misuse Morbid obesity	*Primary FSGS* presents as idiopathic nephrotic syndrome but is less responsive to treatment than minimal change; may progress to renal impairment, can recur after transplantation *Secondary FSGS* presents with variable proteinuria and outcome
Focal segmental glomerulonephritis				
Segmental inflammation and/or necrosis in some glomeruli ± crescent formation	Variable according to cause, but typically negative (or 'pauci-immune')	Small-vessel vasculitis	Primary or secondary small-vessel vasculitis	Often occurs in systemic disease. Responds to treatment with corticosteroids and immunosuppressants Check ANCA, ANA
Membranous glomerulonephritis				
Thickening of GBM Progressing to increased matrix deposition and glomerulosclerosis	Granular subepithelial IgG	Antibodies to a podocyte surface antigen, with complement-dependent podocyte injury	HLA-DR3 (for idiopathic) Drugs Mercury, heavy metals Hepatitis B virus Malignancy	Usually idiopathic; common cause of adult idiopathic nephrotic syndrome One-third progress; may respond to corticosteroids and immunosuppressants
IgA nephropathy				
Increased mesangial matrix and cells Focal segmental nephritis in acute disease	Mesangial IgA	Unknown	Usually idiopathic Liver disease	Common disease with a range of presentations, usually including haematuria and hypertension
Mesangiocapillary glomerulonephritis				
Immunoglobulin type	Immunoglobulins	Deposition of circulating immune complexes or 'planted' antigens	Infections, autoimmunity, or monoclonal immunoglobulin-related	Most common pattern found in association with subacute bacterial infection, but also with Cryoglobulinaemia ± hepatitis C virus, and others
Complement type	Complement components	Complement abnormalities, inherited or acquired. Dense deposit disease is associated with abnormal activation of the alternative complement pathway	Complement gene mutations C3 nephritic factor and partial lipodystrophy	In dense deposit disease, intramembranous deposits No proven treatments
Post-infection				
Diffuse proliferation of endothelial and mesangial cells Infiltration by neutrophils and macrophages ± crescent formation	Subendothelial	Immune response to streptococcal infection with presumed cross-reactive epitopes	Streptococcal and other infections	Now rare in developed countries Presents with severe sodium and fluid retention, hypertension, haematuria, oliguria Usually resolves spontaneously

Continued

17.39 Glomerulonephritis: types, associations and causes – cont'd

Histology	Immune deposits	Pathogenesis	Associations	Comments
Goodpasture's disease				
Usually crescentic nephritis	Linear IgG along GBM	Autoantibodies to α3 chain of type IV collagen in the GBM	HLA-DR15 (previously known as DR2)	Associated with lung haemorrhage but either may occur alone Treat with corticosteroids, cyclophosphamide and plasma exchange
Lupus nephritis				
Almost any histological type	Always positive and often profuse Pattern varies according to type	Some anti-DNA antibodies also bind to glomerular targets	Complement deficiencies Complement consumption	Variable presentation, sometimes as renal disease alone without systemic features Responds to cytotoxic therapy in addition to prednisolone

(ANCA = antineutrophil cytoplasmic antibodies; ANA = antinuclear antibody; HLA = human leucocyte antigen)

corticosteroids, cytotoxic therapy or other agents. Minimal change disease does not progress to CKD but can present with problems related to the nephrotic syndrome and complications of treatment.

Focal segmental glomerulosclerosis

Primary focal segmental glomerulosclerosis (FSGS) (Fig. 17.22B) can occur in all age groups. In some patients, FSGS can have specific causes, such as HIV infection, podocyte toxins and massive obesity, but in most cases the underlying cause is unknown (primary FSGS). Patients with primary FSGS present with massive proteinuria and idiopathic nephrotic syndrome. Histological analysis shows sclerosis affecting segments of the glomeruli, which may also show positive staining for deposits of C3 and IgM on immunofluorescence. Since FSGS is a focal process, abnormal glomeruli may not be seen on renal biopsy if only a few are sampled, leading to an initial diagnosis of minimal change nephropathy. Juxtamedullary glomeruli are more likely to be affected in early disease. Although nephrotic syndrome is typical, some patients present with the histological features of FSGS but less proteinuria. In these patients, the focal scarring may reflect healing of previous focal glomerular injury, such as HUS, cholesterol embolism or vasculitis. These examples of secondary FSGS have different course and treatments.

Primary FSGS can respond to high-dose corticosteroid therapy (0.5–2.0 mg/kg/day) but most patients show little or no response. Immunosuppressive drugs, such as ciclosporin, cyclophosphamide and mycophenolate mofetil, have also been used but their efficacy is uncertain. Progression to CKD is common in patients who do not respond to steroids and the disease frequently recurs after renal transplantation, with an almost immediate return of proteinuria following transplant in some cases.

Membranous glomerulonephritis

Membranous glomerulonephritis, also known as membranous nephropathy, is the most common cause of nephrotic syndrome in adults. It is caused by antibodies (usually autoantibodies) directed at antigen(s) expressed on the surface of podocytes. Recent studies suggest that one such antigen is the M-type phospholipase A_2 receptor 1. A proportion of cases are associated with other causes, such as heavy metal poisoning, drugs, infections and tumours (see Box 17.39 and Fig. 17.22D and F) but most are idiopathic. Approximately one-third of patients with idiopathic membranous glomerulonephritis undergo spontaneous remission; one-third remain in a nephrotic state, and one-third go on to develop CKD. Short-term treatment with high doses of corticosteroids and cyclophosphamide may improve both the nephrotic syndrome and the long-term prognosis. However, because of the toxicity of these regimens, many nephrologists reserve such treatment for those with severe nephrotic syndrome or deteriorating renal function.

IgA nephropathy

This is one of the most common types of glomerulonephritis and can present in many ways (Fig. 17.22G). Haematuria is the earliest sign and is almost universal, and hypertension is also very common. Proteinuria can also occur but is usually a later feature. In many cases, there is slowly progressive loss of renal function leading to ESRD. Clinical presentations are protean and vary with age. A particular hallmark of IgA nephropathy in young adults is the occurrence of acute self-limiting exacerbations, often with gross haematuria, in association with minor respiratory infections. This may be so acute as to resemble acute post-infectious glomerulonephritis, with fluid retention, hypertension and oliguria with dark or red urine. Characteristically, the latency from clinical infection to nephritis is short: a few days or less. Asymptomatic presentations dominate in older adults, with haematuria, hypertension and loss of GFR. Occasionally, IgA nephropathy progresses rapidly and crescent formation may be seen. The response to immunosuppressive therapy is usually poor. The management of less acute disease is largely directed towards the control of blood pressure in an attempt to prevent or retard progressive renal disease. There is some evidence for additional benefit from several months of high-dose corticosteroid treatment in high-risk disease, but no strong evidence for other immunosuppressive agents. Other therapies are under investigation.

Henoch–Schönlein purpura

This condition most commonly occurs in children but can also be observed in adults. It is characterised by a systemic vasculitis that often arises in response to an infectious trigger. The presentation is with a characteristic petechial rash typically affecting buttocks and lower legs, and abdominal pain due to the occurrence of vasculitis involving the gastrointestinal tract. The presence of glomerulonephritis is usually indicated by the occurrence of haematuria. When Henoch–Schönlein purpura occurs in older children or adults, the glomerulonephritis is usually more prominent and less likely to resolve completely. Renal biopsy shows mesangial IgA deposition and appearances that are indistinguishable from acute IgA nephropathy. Treatment is supportive in nature; in most patients, the prognosis is good, with spontaneous resolution, but some, particularly adults, progress to develop ESRD.

Mesangiocapillary glomerulonephritis

Mesangiocapillary glomerulonephritis (MCGN), also known as membranoproliferative glomerulonephritis (MPGN), is characterised by an increase in mesangial cellularity with thickening of glomerular capillary walls and subendothelial deposition of immune complexes and/or components of the complement pathway. The typical presentation is with proteinuria and haematuria. Several underlying causes have been identified, as summarised in Box 17.39. It can be classified into two main subtypes. The first is characterised by deposition of immunoglobulins within the glomeruli. This subtype is associated with chronic infections, autoimmune diseases and monoclonal gammopathy. The second is characterised by deposition of complement in the glomeruli and is associated with inherited or acquired abnormalities in the complement pathway. Within this category is so-called 'dense deposit disease', which is typified by deposition of electron-dense deposits within the GBM. A third subtype is recognised, in which neither immunoglobulins nor complement are deposited in the glomeruli. This is associated with healing following thrombotic microangiopathies, such as HUS and TTP.

Treatment of MCGN associated with immunoglobulin deposits consists of identifying and treating the underlying disease, if possible, and the use of immunosuppressive drugs such as mycophenolate mofetil or cyclophosphamide. There is no specific treatment for MCGN associated with deposition of complement in the glomeruli or for dense deposit disease.

Infection-related glomerulonephritis

Glomerulonephritis may occur in connection with infections of various types, including subacute bacterial endocarditis. The most common histological pattern in bacterial infection is mesangiocapillary glomerulonephritis, often associated with extensive immunoglobulin deposition in the glomeruli with evidence of complement consumption (low serum C3, Box 17.40). In the developed world, hospital-acquired infections with various organisms are a common cause of these syndromes.

17.40 Causes of glomerulonephritis associated with low serum complement

- Post-infection glomerulonephritis
- Subacute bacterial infection: especially endocarditis
- Systemic lupus erythematosus
- Cryoglobulinaemia
- Mesangiocapillary glomerulonephritis, usually complement type

Worldwide, glomerulonephritis more commonly follows hepatitis B, hepatitis C, schistosomiasis, leishmaniasis, malaria and other chronic infections. Infection with HIV may be associated with FSGS (see above), particularly in people of African descent.

Post-streptococcal glomerulonephritis

This is a specific subtype of post-infectious glomerulonephritis. It is much more common in children than adults but is now rare in the developed world. The latency is usually about 10 days after a throat infection or longer after skin infection, suggesting an immune mechanism rather than direct infection. An acute nephritis of varying severity occurs. Sodium retention, hypertension and oedema are particularly pronounced. There is also reduction of GFR, proteinuria, haematuria and reduced urine volume. Characteristically, this gives the urine a red or smoky appearance. As in other causes of post-infectious glomerulonephritis, serum concentrations of C3 and C4 are typically reduced, reflecting complement consumption (see Box 17.40), and evidence of streptococcal infection may be found. Renal function begins to improve spontaneously within 10–14 days, and management by fluid and sodium restriction with diuretic and hypotensive agents is usually adequate. Remarkably, the renal lesion in almost all children and many adults seems to resolve completely, despite the severity of the glomerular inflammation and proliferation seen histologically.

Rapidly progressive glomerulonephritis

Rapidly progressive glomerulonephritis (also known as crescentic glomerulonephritis) is characterised by rapid loss of renal function over days to weeks. Renal biopsy shows crescentic lesions, often associated with necrotising lesions within the glomerulus, termed focal segmental (necrotising) glomerulonephritis. It is typically seen in Goodpasture's disease, where the underlying cause is the development of antibodies to the glomerular basement membrane (anti-GBM antibodies), and in small-vessel vasculitides (pp. 519 and 1115). It can also be observed in SLE (pp. 520 and 1109) and occasionally IgA and other nephropathies. Rapid-onset disease may be associated with relatively little proteinuria (see Fig. 17.21). Management depends on the underlying cause but immunosuppressive drugs are often required. Patients with anti-GBM disease should be treated with plasma exchange combined with corticosteroids and immunosuppressants. Patients

17

with renal involvement secondary to ANCA-associated vasculitis and SLE should also be treated with corticosteroids and immunosuppressants, as described on pages 1118 and 1112.

Inherited glomerular diseases

Alport's syndrome

A number of uncommon diseases may involve the glomerulus in childhood, but the most important one affecting adults is Alport's syndrome. Most cases arise from a mutation or deletion of the *COL4A5* gene on the X chromosome, which encodes type IV collagen, resulting in inheritance as an X-linked recessive disorder (p. 53). Mutations in *COL4A3* or *COL4A4* genes are less common and cause autosomal recessive disease. The accumulation of abnormal collagen results in a progressive degeneration of the GBM (Fig. 17.23). Affected patients progress from haematuria to ESRD in their late teens or twenties. Female carriers of *COL4A5* mutations usually have haematuria but less commonly develop significant renal disease. Some other basement membranes containing the same collagen isoforms are similarly involved, notably in the cochlea, so that Alport's syndrome is associated with sensorineural deafness and ocular abnormalities.

ACE inhibitors may slow but not prevent loss of kidney function. Patients with Alport's syndrome are good candidates for RRT, as they are young and usually otherwise healthy. They can develop an immune response to the normal collagen antigens present in the GBM of the donor kidney and, in a small minority, anti-GBM disease develops and destroys the allograft.

Thin glomerular basement membrane disease

In thin glomerular basement membrane disease there is glomerular bleeding, usually only at the microscopic or dipstick level, without associated hypertension, proteinuria or a reduction in GFR. The glomeruli appear normal by light microscopy but, on electron microscopy, the GBM is abnormally thin. The condition may be familial and some patients are carriers of Alport mutations. This does not appear to account for all cases, and in many patients the cause is unclear. Monitoring of these patients is advisable, as proteinuria may develop in some and there seems to be an increased rate of progressive CKD in the long term.

TUBULO-INTERSTITIAL DISEASES

These diseases primarily affect the renal tubules and interstitial components of the renal parenchyma. They are characterised by tubular dysfunction with electrolyte abnormalities, moderate levels of proteinuria and varying degrees of renal impairment. Acute tubular necrosis falls into this category but this is described separately on page 479, since it usually presents with AKI.

Acute interstitial nephritis

Acute interstitial nephritis (AIN) is characterised by acute inflammation affecting the tubulo-interstitium of the kidney. It is commonly drug-induced but can be caused by other factors, such as renal toxins, and can complicate a variety of systemic diseases and infections (Box 17.41).

Clinical features

The clinical presentation is typically with renal impairment but, in some patients with drug-induced acute interstitial nephritis, there may be signs of a generalised drug hypersensitivity reaction with fever, rash and eosinophilia. Proteinuria is generally modest (PCR < 100 mg/mmol) and tubular in type (p. 476). The urine may contain red and white blood cells but is sterile on

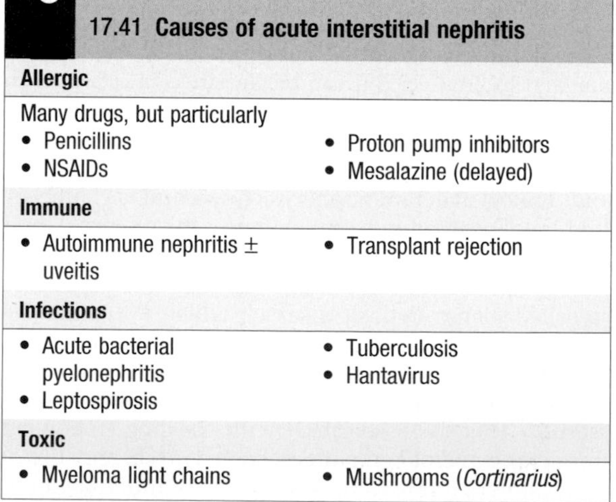

17.41 Causes of acute interstitial nephritis

Allergic	
Many drugs, but particularly • Penicillins • NSAIDs	• Proton pump inhibitors • Mesalazine (delayed)
Immune	
• Autoimmune nephritis ± uveitis	• Transplant rejection
Infections	
• Acute bacterial pyelonephritis • Leptospirosis	• Tuberculosis • Hantavirus
Toxic	
• Myeloma light chains	• Mushrooms (*Cortinarius*)

A

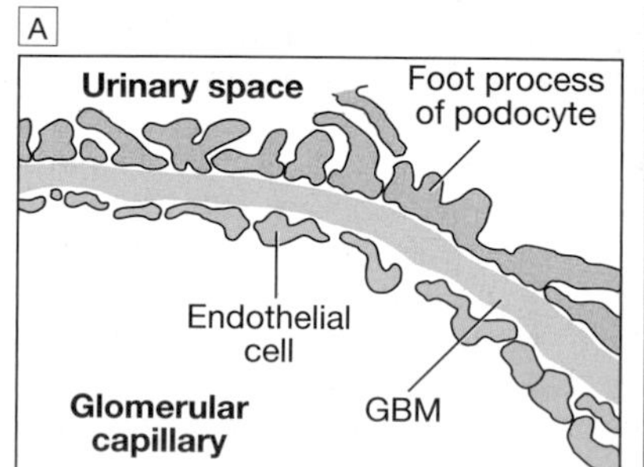

B

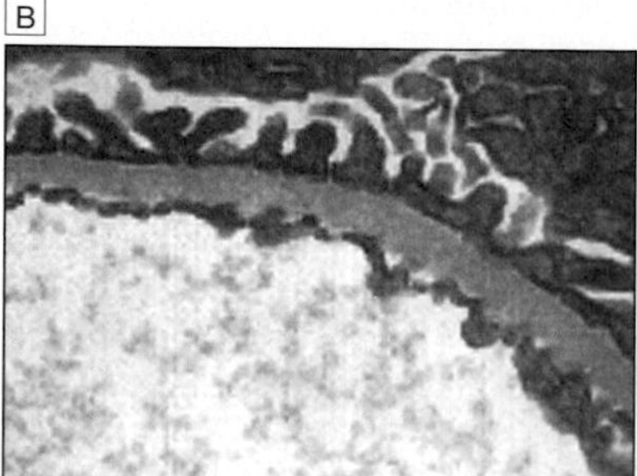

C

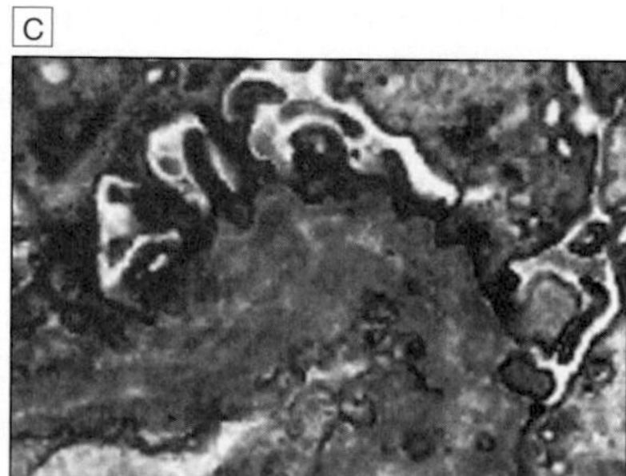

Fig. 17.23 Alport's syndrome. A Diagrammatic structure of the normal GBM. B The normal GBM (electron micrograph) contains mostly the tissue-specific (α3, α4 and α5) chains of type IV collagen. C In Alport's syndrome, this network is disrupted and replaced by α1 and α2 chains. Although the GBM appears structurally normal in early life, in time thinning appears, progressing to thickening, splitting and degeneration.

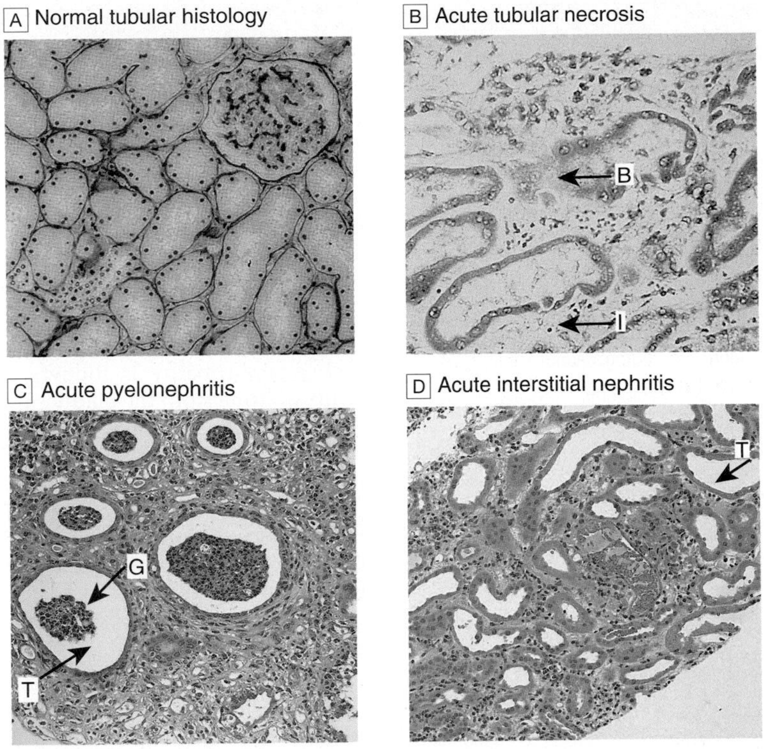

A Normal tubular histology

B Acute tubular necrosis

C Acute pyelonephritis

D Acute interstitial nephritis

Fig. 17.24 Tubular histopathology. **A** Normal tubular histology. The tubules are back to back. Brush borders can be seen on the luminal borders of cells in the proximal tubule. **B** Acute tubular necrosis. There are scattered breaks (B) in tubular basement membranes, swelling and vacuolation of tubular cells, and, in places, apoptosis and necrosis of tubular cells with shedding of cells into the lumen. During the regenerative phase, there is increased tubular mitotic activity. The interstitium (I) is oedematous and infiltrated by inflammatory cells. The glomeruli (not shown) are relatively normal, although there may be endothelial cell swelling and fibrin deposition. **C** Acute bacterial pyelonephritis. A widespread inflammatory infiltrate that includes many neutrophils is seen. Granulocyte casts (G) are forming within some dilated tubules (T). Other tubules are scarcely visible because of the extent of the inflammation and damage. **D** Acute (allergic) interstitial nephritis. In this patient who received an NSAID, an extensive mononuclear cell infiltrate (no neutrophils) involving tubules (T) is seen. This inflammation does not involve the glomeruli (not shown). Sometimes eosinophils are prominent. Transplant rejection looks similar to this.

culture. Eosinophils are present in up to 70% of patients but this is a non-specific finding. Many patients are not oliguric, despite moderately severe renal impairment, and AIN should always be considered in patients with non-oliguric AKI. There may be a rapid deterioration of renal function in some cases of drug-induced AIN, causing the condition to be mistaken for rapidly progressive glomerulonephritis.

Investigations

Renal biopsy is usually required to confirm the diagnosis (Fig. 17.24). This typically shows evidence of intense inflammation, with infiltration of the tubules and interstitium by polymorphonuclear leucocytes, and lymphocytes. Eosinophils may also be observed, especially in drug-induced AIN. The degree of chronic inflammation in a biopsy is a useful predictor of the eventual outcome for renal function.

Management

Some patients with drug-induced AIN recover following withdrawal of the drug alone, but high-dose corticosteroids (prednisolone 1 mg/kg/day) accelerate recovery and may prevent long-term scarring. Dialysis is sometimes necessary but is usually only short-term. Other specific causes (see Box 17.41) should be treated, if possible.

Chronic interstitial nephritis

Chronic interstitial nephritis (CIN) is characterised by renal dysfunction with fibrosis and infiltration of the renal parenchyma by lymphocytes, plasma cells and macrophages, in association with tubular damage.

Pathophysiology

The disease may follow on from acute interstitial nephritis that does not resolve, or may be associated with ingestion of various toxins and drugs, or with metabolic and chronic inflammatory diseases, as summarised in Box 17.42. In many patients, CIN presents at a late stage and no underlying cause can be identified. Toxins that have been associated with CIN include those contained within the plant *Aristolochia clematitis*. These are probably responsible for the severe nephrotoxicity that can be associated with treatment with herbal medicines in Asia. There is some evidence that these toxins are also responsible for Balkan nephropathy, which affects isolated rural communities in Bosnia, Bulgaria, Croatia, Romania and Serbia. The nephropathy is commonly linked with tumours of the collecting system and is probably due to the mutagenic effects of the plant toxin on the urothelial epithelium. Ingestion of mushrooms within the *Cortinarius* genus can cause a devastating and irreversible renal tubular toxicity. The typical scenario is when a

17.42 Causes of chronic interstitial nephritis

Acute interstitial nephritis	
• Any of the causes of AIN, if persistent (see Box 17.41)	
Glomerulonephritis	
• Varying degrees of interstitial inflammation occur in association with most types of inflammatory glomerulonephritis	
Immune/inflammatory	
• Sarcoidosis • Sjögren's syndrome • Chronic transplant rejection	• Systemic lupus erythematosus, primary autoimmune
Toxic	
• *Aristolochia* in herbal medicines • Lead	• Balkan nephropathy • Mushrooms (*Cortinarius*)
Drugs	
• All drugs causing AIN • Tenofovir • Lithium toxicity	• Analgesic nephropathy • Ciclosporin, tacrolimus
Infection	
• Consequence of severe pyelonephritis	
Congenital/developmental	
• Vesico-ureteric reflux: associated but causation not clear • Renal dysplaslas: often associated with reflux • Inherited: now well recognised but mechanisms unclear • Other: Wilson's disease, medullary sponge kidney, sickle-cell nephropathy	
Metabolic and systemic diseases	
• Calcium phosphate crystallisation after excessive phosphate administration (e.g. phosphate enemas in patients with CKD) • Hypokalaemia • Hyperoxaluria	

patient mistakes a poisonous mushroom for an edible type. It is encountered occasionally in Scandinavia and Scotland.

Clinical features

Most patients with CIN present in adult life with CKD, hypertension and small kidneys. The CKD is often moderate (stage 3) but, because of tubular dysfunction, electrolyte abnormalities are typically more severe, resulting in hyperkalaemia and acidosis. Urinalysis abnormalities are non-specific. A minority of patients present with salt-losing nephropathy, characterised by hypotension, polyuria and features of sodium and water depletion. Patients with CIN have an impairment of urine-concentrating ability and sodium conservation, which puts them at risk of AKI due to salt and water depletion during an acute illness. Renal tubular acidosis (p. 446) may complicate CIN but is seen most often in myeloma, sarcoidosis, cystinosis, amyloidosis and Sjögren's syndrome.

Management

Management is supportive in nature, with correction of acidosis and hyperkalaemia; replacement of fluid and electrolytes, as required; and RRT if irreversible renal damage has occurred.

Reflux nephropathy

This condition, which was previously known as chronic pyelonephritis, is a specific type of chronic interstitial nephritis (see previous section) associated with vesico-ureteric reflux (VUR) in early life and with the appearance of scars in the kidney, as demonstrated by various imaging techniques. About 12% of patients in Europe requiring treatment for ESRD may have this disorder but diagnostic criteria are imprecise.

Pathophysiology

Reflux nephropathy is thought to be due to chronic reflux of urine from the bladder into the ureters, in association with recurrent urinary tract infection (UTI) in childhood. It was previously assumed that ascending infection was necessary for progressive renal damage in patients with VUR, but there is evidence to suggest that renal scars can occur, even in the absence of infection. Furthermore, epidemiological surveys and controlled trials have found that efforts to correct VUR by using surgical or other means are ineffective in halting progression of the disease.

Susceptibility to VUR has a genetic component and may be associated with renal dysplasia and other congenital abnormalities of the urinary tract. It can be connected with outflow obstruction, usually caused by urethral valves, but usually occurs with an apparently normal bladder.

Clinical features

Usually, the renal scarring and dilatation are asymptomatic and the patient may present at any age with hypertension (sometimes severe), proteinuria or features of CKD. There may be no history of overt UTI. However, symptoms arising from the urinary tract may be present and include frequency of micturition, dysuria and aching lumbar pain. VUR may occur in children but diminishes as the child grows, and usually has disappeared by adulthood. Urinalysis often shows the presence of leucocytes and moderate proteinuria (usually < 1 g/24 hrs) but these are not invariable. The risk of renal stone formation is increased. A number of women first present with hypertension and/or proteinuria in pregnancy. Children and adults with small or unilateral renal scars have a good prognosis, provided renal growth is normal. With significant unilateral scars there is usually compensatory hypertrophy of the contralateral kidney. In patients with more severe bilateral disease, prognosis is related to the severity of renal dysfunction, hypertension and proteinuria. If the serum creatinine is normal and hypertension and proteinuria are absent, then the long-term prognosis is usually good.

Investigations

Renal scarring can be detected by ultrasound but it has poor sensitivity and is only capable of detecting major defects and excluding significant obstruction. Radionuclide DMSA scans are more sensitive (see Fig. 17.6, p. 471), and longitudinal imaging by MRI or CT may be useful in assessing progression. Abnormalities may be unilateral or bilateral and of any grade of severity. Gross scarring of the kidneys, commonly at the poles, is seen, with reduced kidney size and narrowing of the cortex

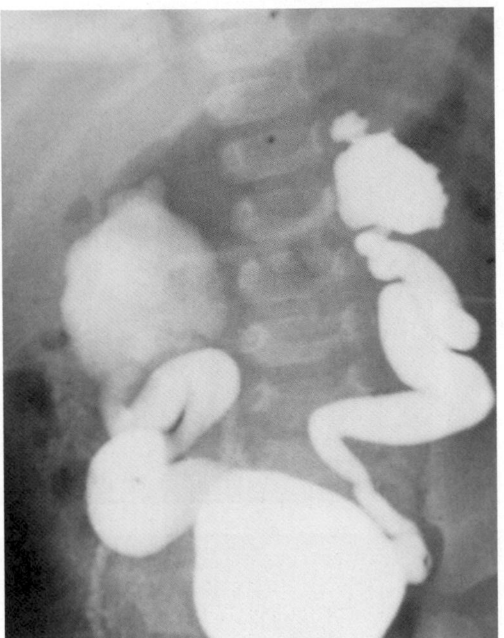

Fig. 17.25 Vesico-ureteric reflux (grade IV) shown by micturating cystogram. The bladder has been filled with contrast medium through a urinary catheter. After micturition, there was gross VUR into widely distended ureters and pelvicalyceal systems.

and medulla. Renal scars may be juxtaposed to dilated calyces. In patients who develop heavy proteinuria and hypertension, renal biopsies show glomerulomegaly and focal glomerulosclerosis, probably as a secondary response to reduced nephron numbers. Radionuclide techniques can also be used to demonstrate VUR as an alternative to micturating cystourethrography (MCUG; the bladder is filled with contrast media through a urinary catheter and images are taken during and after micturition – Fig. 17.25). However, as surgical intervention for VUR has declined in popularity (see below), this type of imaging is used less often.

Management

Infection, if present, should be treated (Box 17.43); if recurrent, it should be prevented with prophylactic therapy, as described for UTI (p. 512). If recurrent pyelonephritis occurs in an abnormal kidney with minimal function, nephrectomy may be indicated. Occasionally, hypertension is cured by the removal of a diseased kidney when the disease is predominantly or entirely unilateral.

As most childhood reflux tends to disappear spontaneously and trials have shown small or no benefits from anti-reflux surgery, such intervention is now less common.

EBM 17.43 Prophylactic antibiotics and vesico-ureteric reflux

'Prophylactic antibiotics reduce recurrences of UTI but there is no evidence that they protect against further renal scarring or dysfunction.'

- Smellie JM, et al. Lancet 2001; 357:1329–1333.

For further information: www.clinicalevidence.org

Papillary necrosis

The renal papillae lie within a hypertonic environment in the renal medulla, at the end of the vasa recta. They are susceptible to ischaemic damage because of this and can undergo necrosis when their vascular supply is impaired as the result of diabetes mellitus and sickle-cell disease or with long-term ingestion of NSAID. The condition may occasionally occur in other diseases. There is an association with pyelonephritis but it is difficult to determine whether this is a cause of papillary necrosis or a complication. The clinical presentation is variable. Some patients are asymptomatic and clinically silent, whereas others present with renal colic and renal impairment as necrosed papillae slough off and cause ureteric obstruction. Urinalysis may be normal but, more frequently haematuria and sterile pyuria are present. Significant proteinuria is unusual, unless there is renal failure. The imaging method of choice to make the diagnosis is pyelography. Management is based on relieving obstruction, where present, and withdrawal of the offending drugs.

Sickle-cell nephropathy

The longer survival of patients with sickle-cell disease (p. 1033) means that a high proportion now live to develop chronic complications of microvascular occlusion. In the kidney, these changes are most pronounced in the medulla, where the vasa recta are the site of sickling because of hypoxia and hypertonicity. Loss of urinary concentrating ability and polyuria are the earliest changes; distal renal tubular acidosis and impaired potassium excretion are typical. Papillary necrosis may also occur (see above). A minority of patients develop ESRD. This is managed according to the usual principles, but response to recombinant erythropoietin is poor due to the haemoglobinopathy. Patients with sickle trait have an increased incidence of unexplained microscopic haematuria.

CYSTIC DISEASES OF THE KIDNEY

It is common to encounter patients with a single renal cyst or even multiple ones as an incidental finding, especially in those aged 50 years and over. Usually, these cysts are of no clinical consequence and are asymptomatic, but occasionally they can cause pain or haematuria. In addition, several specific diseases are recognised as being caused by the formation of multiple renal cysts. These are discussed in more detail below.

Adult polycystic kidney disease

Adult polycystic kidney disease (PKD) is a common condition, with a prevalence of approximately 1:1000, and is inherited as an autosomal dominant trait. Small cysts lined by tubular epithelium develop from infancy or childhood and enlarge slowly and irregularly. The surrounding normal kidney tissue is compressed and progressively damaged. Mutations in the *PKD1* gene account for 85% of cases and *PKD2* for about 15%. ESRD occurs in approximately 50% of patients with *PKD1*

17.44 Adult polycystic kidney disease: common clinical features

- Vague discomfort in loin or abdomen due to increasing mass of renal tissue
- Acute loin pain or renal colic due to haemorrhage into a cyst
- Hypertension
- Haematuria (with little or no proteinuria)
- Urinary tract or cyst infections
- Renal failure

mutations, with a mean age of onset of 52 years, but in a minority of patients with *PKD2* mutations, with a mean age of onset of 69 years. It has been estimated that between 5% and 10% of patients on RRT have adult PKD.

Clinical features

Common clinical features are shown in Box 17.44. Affected subjects are usually asymptomatic until later life but hypertension usually occurs from the age of 20 onwards. One or both kidneys may be palpable and the surface may feel nodular. About 30% of patients with PKD also have hepatic cysts (see Fig. 23.38, p. 970) but disturbance of liver function is rare. Sometimes (almost always in women) this causes massive and symptomatic hepatomegaly, usually concurrent with renal enlargement but occasionally with only minor renal involvement. Berry aneurysms of cerebral vessels are an associated feature and about 10% of patients have a subarachnoid haemorrhage. This feature appears to be largely restricted to certain families (and presumably specific mutations). Mitral and aortic regurgitation is frequent but rarely severe, and colonic diverticula and abdominal wall hernias may occur.

Investigations

The diagnosis is usually based on family history, clinical findings and ultrasound examination. Ultrasound examination demonstrates cysts in approximately 95% of affected patients over the age of 20 and is the screening method of choice but may not detect small developing cysts in younger subjects. Cysts may also be identified by other imaging modalities, such as MRI (Fig. 17.26). It is now possible to make a molecular diagnosis by mutation screening of *PDK1* or *PDK2* but this is seldom used in routine clinical practice. Screening for intracranial aneurysms is not generally indicated but can be done by MR angiography in families with a history of subarachnoid haemorrhage. The yield of screening is low, however, and the risk–benefit ratio of intervention in asymptomatic aneurysms in this disease is not clear.

Management

Good control of blood pressure is important because cardiovascular morbidity and mortality are so common in renal disease, but there is no evidence that control of moderate hypertension retards the development of renal failure in PKD, in contrast to the evidence for glomerular diseases. There is some evidence that the vasopressin V2 receptor antagonist, tolvaptan, can slow cyst formation in some patients but its place in treatment has yet to be established.

Patients with PKD are usually good candidates for dialysis and transplantation. Sometimes kidneys are so large that one or both have to be removed to make space for a renal transplant. Otherwise, unless they are a source of pain or infection, they are usually left in situ.

A

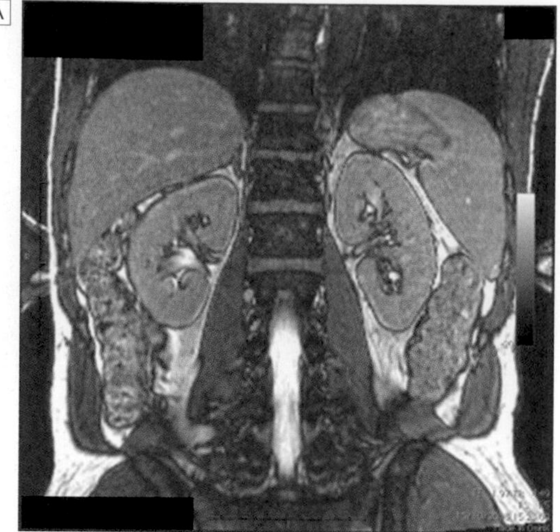

B

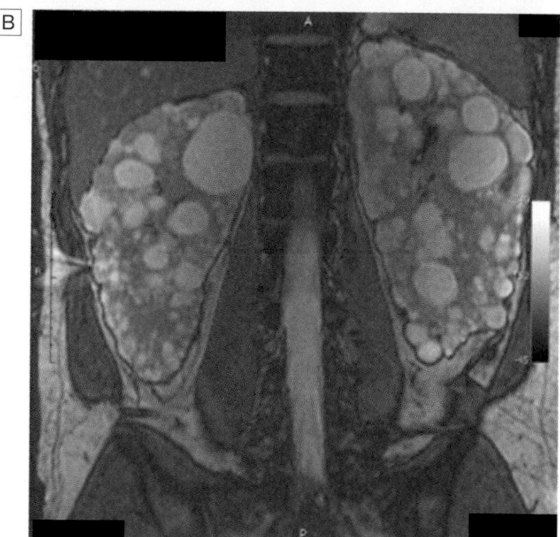

Fig. 17.26 MRI images of the kidneys. **A** Normal kidneys. **B** Polycystic kidneys; although the kidney enlargement is extreme, this patient had only slightly reduced GFR.

Medullary sponge kidney disease

Medullary sponge kidney is characterised by cysts confined to papillary collecting ducts. The disease is not inherited and its cause is unknown. Patients usually present as adults with renal stones. These are often recurrent, and preventive measures (p. 509) need to be implemented if so, but the prognosis is generally good. The diagnosis is made by ultrasound or IVU (Fig. 17.27). Contrast medium is seen to fill dilated or cystic tubules, which are sometimes calcified.

Medullary cystic kidney disease

This is a heterogenous group of inherited disorders, known as nephronophthisis in children. Small cortical cysts are associated with progressive destruction of the nephron. The childhood variants are characterised by thirst and polyuria due to nephrogenic diabetes insipidus, often with a family history of similar disease. Sometimes, affected patients are 'salt-losing', which

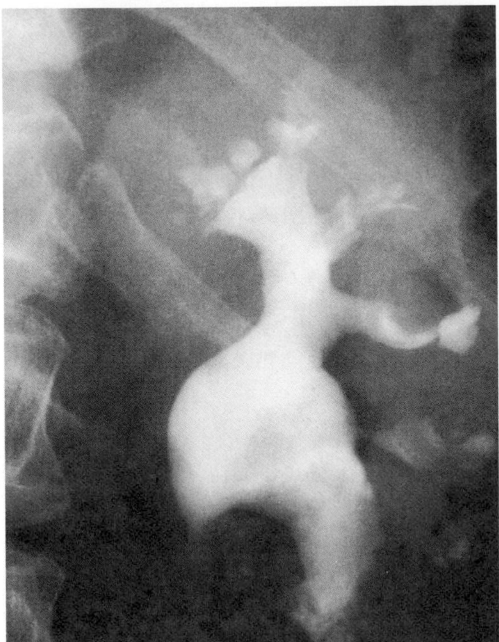

Fig. 17.27 Medullary sponge kidney. Intravenous urogram showing contrast medium filling both the collecting system and cavities arising from collecting ducts, especially within papillae of the upper pole. The cavities have been likened to bunches of grapes. A plain abdominal X-ray may show calcification in the same regions.

aggravates the degree of renal failure. Even when they are treated appropriately, serious renal failure is usual. Several of these conditions are associated with retinal dystrophies and brain or other abnormalities. The genetic basis of these disorders is emerging; several genes are involved.

Other cystic diseases

A number of other rarer inherited cystic diseases are recognised that have some similarities to PKD but distinct genetic causes. Multicystic dysplastic kidneys are often unilateral and are a developmental abnormality found in children. Most of these seem to involute during growth, leaving a solitary kidney in adults. Acquired cystic kidney disease can develop in patients with a very long history of renal failure, including those who have had many years of dialysis. It is associated with increased erythropoietin production and sometimes with the development of renal cell carcinoma.

RENAL STONE DISEASE

Renal stone disease is common, affecting individuals of all countries and ethnic groups. In the UK, the prevalence is about 1.2%, with a lifetime risk of developing a renal stone at age 60–70 of about 7% in men. In some regions, the risk is higher, most notably in countries like Saudi Arabia, where the lifetime risk of developing a renal stone in men aged 60–70 is just over 20%.

Pathophysiology

Urinary calculi consist of aggregates of crystals, usually containing calcium or phosphate in combination with small amounts of proteins and glycoproteins. The most common types are summarised in Box 17.45. A number of risk factors have been identified for renal stone formation (Box 17.46). In developed countries, however, most calculi occur in healthy young men, in whom investigations reveal no clear predisposing cause. Renal stones vary greatly in size. There may be particles like sand anywhere in the urinary tract, or large round stones in the bladder. In developing countries, bladder stones are common, particularly in children. In developed countries, the incidence of childhood bladder stones is low; renal stones in adults are more common. Staghorn calculi fill the whole renal pelvis and branch into the calyces (Fig. 17.28); they are usually associated with infection and composed largely of struvite. Deposits of calcium may be present throughout the renal parenchyma, giving rise to fine calcification within it (nephrocalcinosis), especially in patients with renal tubular acidosis, hyperparathyroidism, vitamin D intoxication and healed renal tuberculosis. Cortical nephrocalcinosis may occur in areas of cortical necrosis, typically after AKI in pregnancy or other severe AKI.

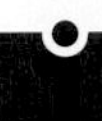

17.45 Composition of renal stones

Calcium oxalate[1]	60%
Calcium phosphate	15%
Uric acid	10%
Magnesium ammonium phosphate (struvite)[2]	15%
Cystine and others	1%

[1]Stones often contain small amounts of calcium phosphate.
[2]Associated with urine infection.

17.46 Predisposing factors for kidney stones

Environmental and dietary causes

- Low urine volumes: high ambient temperatures, low fluid intake
- Diet: high protein, high sodium, low calcium
- High sodium excretion
- High oxalate excretion
- High urate excretion
- Low citrate excretion

Acquired causes

- Hypercalcaemia of any cause (p. 767)
- Ileal disease or resection (increases oxalate absorption and urinary excretion)
- Renal tubular acidosis type I (distal, p. 446)

Congenital and inherited causes

- Familial hypercalciuria
- Medullary sponge kidney
- Cystinuria
- Renal tubular acidosis type I (distal)
- Primary hyperoxaluria

Clinical features

The clinical presentation is highly variable. Most patients with renal stone disease are asymptomatic, whereas others present with pain, haematuria, UTI or urinary tract obstruction. A common presentation is with acute

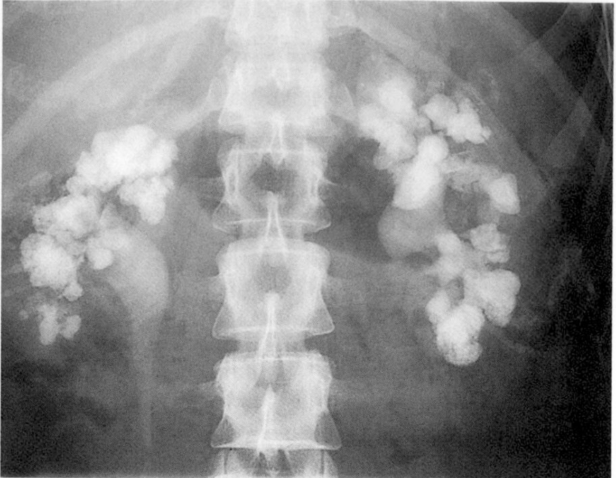

Fig. 17.28 Radio-opaque bilateral staghorn calculi visible during intravenous urography. The intravenous pyelogram demonstrates that, while some dye is being excreted by the right kidney, there is little function on the left.

loin pain radiating to the anterior abdominal wall, together with haematuria: a symptom complex termed renal or ureteric colic. This is most commonly caused by ureteric obstruction by a calculus but the same symptoms can occur in association with a sloughed renal papilla, tumour or blood clot. The patient is suddenly aware of pain in the loin, which radiates round the flank to the groin and often into the testis or labium, in the sensory distribution of the first lumbar nerve. The pain steadily increases in intensity to reach a peak in a few minutes. The patient is restless and generally tries unsuccessfully to obtain relief by changing position or pacing the room. There is pallor, sweating and often vomiting. Frequency, dysuria and haematuria may occur. The intense pain usually subsides within 2 hours but may continue unabated for hours or days. It is usually constant during attacks, although slight fluctuations in severity may be seen. Subsequent to an attack of renal colic, intermittent dull pain in the loin or back may persist for several hours.

Investigations

Patients with symptoms of renal colic should be investigated to determine whether or not a stone is present, to identify its location and to assess whether it is causing obstruction. About 90% of stones contain calcium and these can be visualised on plain abdominal X-ray but CTKUB is the gold standard for diagnosing a stone within the kidney or ureter, as 99% are visible using this method. Alternatively, an IVU can be performed. The advantage of CTKUB over IVU is that it is more sensitive and can identify non-radio-opaque stones, such as those containing uric acid and cystine. When the stone is in the ureter, an IVU shows delayed excretion of contrast from the kidney, and a ureter that is dilated down as far as the stone (Fig. 17.29). Ultrasound can show stones within the kidney and dilatation of the renal pelvis and ureter if the stone is obstructing urine flow; it is useful in unstable patients or young women, in whom exposure to ionising radiation is undesirable.

A minimum set of investigations (Box 17.47) should be performed in patients with a first renal stone. The yield of more detailed investigation is low, and hence usually reserved for young patients, those with recurrent or multiple stones, or those with complicated or unexpected presentations. Chemical analysis of stones is often helpful in defining the underlying cause. Since most stones pass spontaneously through the urinary tract, urine should be sieved for a few days after an episode of colic in order to collect the calculus for analysis.

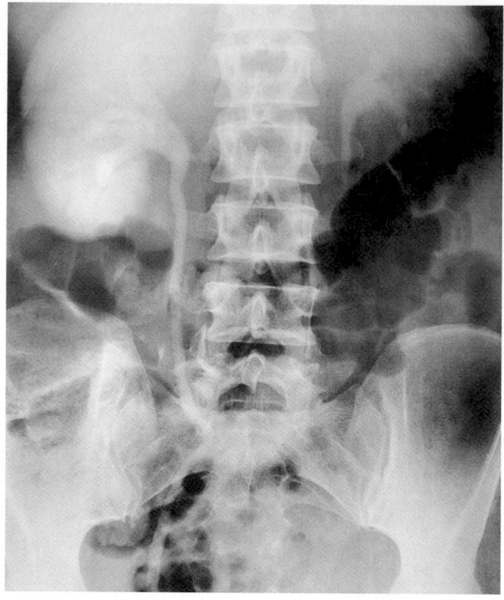

Fig. 17.29 Unilateral ureteric obstruction. Intravenous urogram of a patient with a stone (not visible) at the lower end of the right ureter. This film, taken 2 hours post-contrast injection, demonstrates persistence of contrast medium in the right kidney, pelvicalyceal system and ureter, whereas only a small amount remains visible in the normal left pelvicalyceal system.

17.47 Investigations for renal stones

Sample	Test	First stone	Recurrent stone
Stone	Chemical composition[1]		✓
Blood	Calcium	✓	✓
	Phosphate	✓	✓
	Uric acid	✓	✓
	Urea and electrolytes	✓	✓
	Bicarbonate	✓	✓
	Parathyroid hormone[2]		(✓)
Urine	Dipstick test for protein, blood, glucose	✓	✓
	Amino acids		✓
24-hr urine	Urea		✓
	Creatinine clearance		✓
	Sodium		✓
	Calcium		✓
	Oxalate		✓
	Uric acid		✓

[1]The most valuable test if a stone can be obtained.
[2]Only if serum calcium or urinary calcium excretion high.

Management

The immediate treatment of renal colic is with analgesia and antiemetics. Renal colic is often unbearably painful and demands powerful analgesia; diclofenac orally or as a suppository (100 mg) is often very effective, followed by morphine (10–20 mg) or pethidine (100 mg) intramuscularly. Around 90% of stones of less than 4 mm diameter pass spontaneously, but only 10% of stones bigger than 6 mm, and these may require endoscopic surgical intervention (see below). Patients with renal stones are at high risk of infection; if surgery is contemplated, it should be covered with appropriate antibiotics. Immediate action is required if infection occurs in the stagnant urine proximal to the stone (pyonephrosis), and in patients with a solitary kidney who develop anuria in association with a stone in the ureter.

Stones that do not pass spontaneously through the urinary tract may need to be removed surgically or fragmented by extracorporeal shock wave lithotripsy (ESWL), in which shock waves generated outside the body are focused on the stone, breaking it into small pieces that can pass easily down the ureter. The indications for intervention to remove stones from the renal tract are summarised in Box 17.48. Procedures vary, depending on the site (Fig. 17.30).

Measures to prevent further stone formation are guided by the investigations in Box 17.47. Some general principles apply to almost every patient with calcium-containing stones (Box 17.49). More specific measures

17.48 Indications for intervention to remove stones from the urinary tract

Clinical presentation	Procedure
Obstruction and/or anuria	Emergency PCNL or stent
Pyonephrosis associated with stone	Emergency PCNL or stent
Stone in a patient with solitary kidney	Urgent PCNL, stent, ESWL or ureteroscopy*
Severe pain and persistence of stone in renal tract	Urgent PCNL, stent, ESWL or ureteroscopy*
Pain and persistence of stone in renal tract	Elective PCNL, ESWL or ureteroscopy*

*Procedure depends on site of stone – see Fig. 17.30. (ESWL = extracorporeal shock wave lithotripsy; PCNL = percutaneous nephrolithotomy)

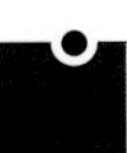

17.49 Measures to prevent calcium stone formation

Diet

Fluid
- At least 2 L output per day (intake 3–4 L): check with 24-hr urine collections
- Intake distributed throughout the day (especially before bed)

Sodium
- Restrict intake

Protein
- Moderate, not high

Calcium
- Maintain good calcium intake (calcium forms an insoluble salt with dietary oxalate, lowering oxalate absorption and excretion)
- Avoid calcium supplements separate from meals (increase calcium excretion without reducing oxalate excretion)

Oxalate
- Avoid foods that are rich in oxalate (spinach, rhubarb)

Drugs

Thiazide diuretics
- Reduce calcium excretion
- Valuable in recurrent stone-formers and hypercalciuria

Allopurinol
- If urate excretion high (unproven except for urate stones)

Avoid
- Vitamin D supplements (increase calcium absorption and excretion)
- Vitamin C supplementation (increases oxalate excretion)

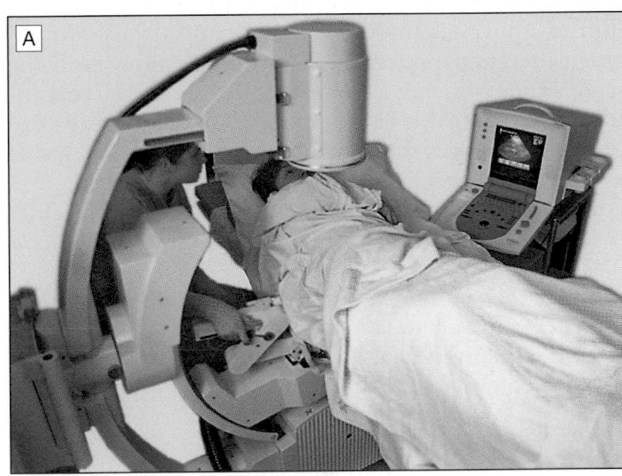

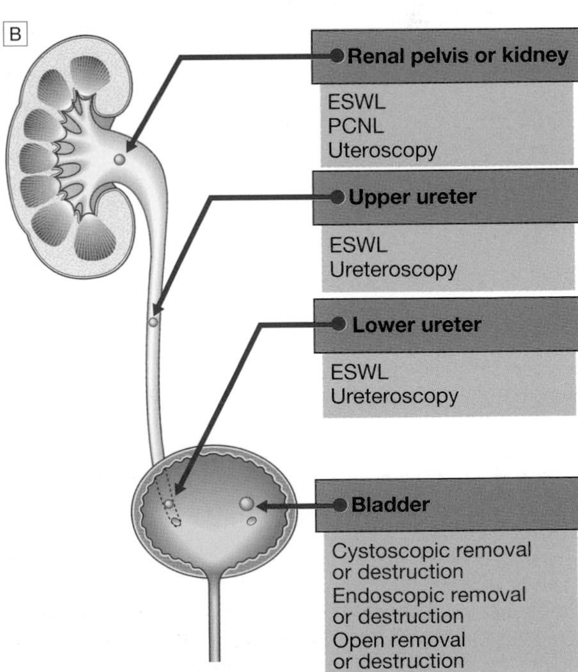

Fig. 17.30 Options for removal of urinary stones. **A** A patient undergoing extracorporeal shock wave lithotripsy (ESWL). **B** The procedures that are used for removal of stones in the urinary tract, shown in relation to the site of the stone. Very rarely, open or laparoscopic surgery may be necessary for removal of stones in the upper renal tract, if other methods fail. (PCNL = percutaneous nephrolithotomy)

17

apply to some types. Urate stones can be prevented by allopurinol, but its role in patients with calcium stones and high urate excretion is uncertain. Stones formed in cystinuria can be reduced by penicillamine therapy. It may also be helpful to attempt to alkalinise the urine with sodium bicarbonate, as a high pH discourages urate and cystine stone formation.

ISOLATED DEFECTS OF TUBULAR FUNCTION

An increasing number of disorders have been identified that are caused by specific defects in transporter molecules expressed in renal tubular cells. Only the most common are mentioned here. Renal glycosuria is a benign autosomal recessive defect of tubular reabsorption of glucose, caused by mutations of the sodium/glucose co-transporter *SGLT2*. Glucose appears in the urine in the presence of a normal blood glucose concentration. Cystinuria is a rare condition, in which reabsorption of filtered cystine, ornithine, arginine and lysine is defective. It is caused by mutations in the *SLC3A1* amino acid transporter gene. The high concentration of cystine in urine leads to cystine stone formation (p. 507).

Other uncommon tubular disorders include hereditary hypophosphataemic rickets (pp. 127 and 1128), in which reabsorption of filtered phosphate is reduced; nephrogenic diabetes insipidus (p. 794), in which the tubules are resistant to the effects of vasopressin; and Bartter's and Gitelman's syndromes, in which there is sodium-wasting and hypokalaemia (p. 440).

The term 'Fanconi syndrome' is used to describe generalised proximal tubular dysfunction. The condition typically presents with low blood phosphate and uric acid, glycosuria, amino aciduria and proximal renal tubular acidosis. In addition to the causes of interstitial nephritis described above, some congenital metabolic disorders are associated with Fanconi syndrome, notably Wilson's disease, cystinosis and hereditary fructose intolerance.

Renal tubular acidosis describes the common endpoint of a variety of diseases affecting distal (classical or type 1) or proximal (type 2) renal tubular function. These syndromes are described on page 446.

DISEASES OF THE COLLECTING SYSTEM AND URETERS

Congenital abnormalities

Various congenital anomalies of the urinary tract can occur (Fig. 17.31); they affect more than 10% of infants. If not immediately lethal, they can lead to complications in later life, including obstructive nephropathy and CKD.

Single kidneys

About 1 in 500 infants is born with only one kidney. Although this is usually compatible with normal life, it may be associated with other abnormalities.

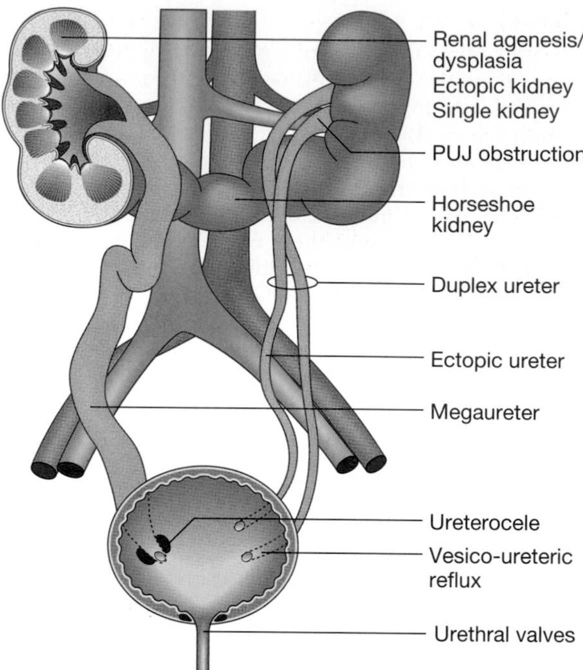

Fig. 17.31 Congenital abnormalities of the urinary tract.

Ureterocele

A ureterocele occurs behind a pin-hole ureteric orifice when the intramural part of the ureter dilates and bulges into the bladder. It can become very large and cause lower urinary tract obstruction. Incision of the pin-hole opening relieves the obstruction.

Ectopic ureters and duplex kidneys

Ectopic ureters occur with congenital duplication of one or both kidneys (duplex kidneys). Developmentally, the ureter has two main branches and, if this arrangement persists, the two ureters of the duplex kidneys may drain separately into the bladder. The lower pole moiety enters the bladder superiorly and laterally, while the upper pole moiety enters the bladder inferomedially to the lower pole moiety ureter or, more rarely, the vagina or seminal vesicle. The lower pole moiety has an ineffective valve mechanism, so that urine passes up the ureter on voiding (vesico-ureteric reflux, p. 504), whereas the upper pole moiety is often associated with a ureterocele.

Obstructive megaureter

In primary obstructive megaureter, there is dilatation of the ureter in all but its terminal segment without obvious cause and without vesico-ureteric reflux. Radiographic and pressure/flow studies may be needed to determine whether there is obstruction to urine flow. Narrowing of the ureter and re-implantation may be necessary.

Pelvi-ureteric junction obstruction

This causes idiopathic hydronephrosis and results from a functional obstruction at the junction of the ureter and renal pelvis. The abnormality is likely to be congenital and is often bilateral. It can be seen in very young children but gross hydronephrosis may present at any age. The common presentation is ill-defined renal pain or ache, exacerbated by drinking large volumes of liquid (Dietl's crisis). Rarely, it is asymptomatic. The diagnosis is often suspected after ultrasound or IVU, and can be confirmed with a ^{99m}Tc-MAG3 renogram followed by diuretic. Treatment is surgical excision of the PUJ and re-anastomosis (pyeloplasty), which can now be performed laparoscopically. Less invasive alternatives are also possible, including balloon dilatation and endoscopic pyelotomy, but are generally less effective.

Retroperitoneal fibrosis

Fibrosis of the retroperitoneal connective tissues may encircle and compress the ureter(s), causing obstruction. The fibrosis is most commonly idiopathic, but can represent a reaction to infection, radiation or aortic aneurysm, or be caused by cancer or a drug reaction – methysergide, for example. Patients usually present with ill-defined symptoms of ureteric obstruction. Typically, there is an acute-phase response (high CRP and ESR). Imaging with UVI or CT shows ureteric obstruction with medial deviation of the ureters. Idiopathic retroperitoneal fibrosis responds well to corticosteroids and may respond more slowly to tamoxifen, but ureteric stenting is often necessary to relieve obstruction. Failure to improve indicates the need for surgery (ureterolysis) both to relieve obstruction and to exclude malignancy.

INFECTIONS OF THE URINARY TRACT

In health, bacterial colonisation is confined to the lower end of the urethra and the remainder of the urinary tract is sterile (see Ch. 6). The urinary tract can become infected with various bacteria but the most common is *E. coli* derived from the gastrointestinal tract. The most common presenting problem is cystitis with urethritis (generally referred to as urinary tract infection) but this is only part of a spectrum of severity (Box 17.50).

Urinary tract infection

Urinary tract infection (UTI) is the term used to describe acute urethritis and cystitis caused by a microorganism. It is a common disorder accounting for 1–3% of consultations in general medical practice. The prevalence of UTI in women is about 3% at the age of 20, increasing by about 1% in each subsequent decade. In males, UTI is uncommon, except in the first year of life and in men over 60, when it may complicate bladder outflow obstruction.

Pathophysiology

Urine is an excellent culture medium for bacteria; in addition, the urothelium of susceptible persons may have more receptors, to which virulent strains of *E. coli* become adherent. In women, the ascent of organisms into the bladder is easier than in men; the urethra is shorter and the absence of bactericidal prostatic secretions may be relevant. Sexual intercourse may cause minor urethral trauma and transfer bacteria from the perineum into the bladder. Instrumentation of the bladder may also introduce organisms. Multiplication of organisms then depends on a number of factors, including the size of the inoculum and virulence of the bacteria. Conditions that predispose to UTI are shown in Box 17.51.

17.50 The spectrum of presentations of urinary tract infection

- Asymptomatic bacteriuria
- Symptomatic acute urethritis and cystitis
- Acute pyelonephritis (p. 513)
- Acute prostatitis (p. 515)
- Septicaemia (usually Gram-negative bacteria)

17.51 Risk factors for urinary tract infection

Incomplete bladder emptying

- Bladder outflow obstruction
  - Benign prostatic enlargement
  - Prostate cancer
  - Urethral stricture
  - Vesico-ureteric reflux
- Uterine prolapse
- Neurological problems
  - Multiple sclerosis
  - Spina bifida
  - Diabetic neuropathy

Foreign bodies

- Urethral catheter or ureteric stent
- Urolithiasis

Loss of host defences

- Atrophic urethritis and vaginitis in post-menopausal women
- Diabetes mellitus

Clinical features

Typical features of cystitis and urethritis include:

- abrupt onset of frequency of micturition and urgency
- scalding pain in the urethra during micturition (dysuria)
- suprapubic pain during and after voiding
- intense desire to pass more urine after micturition, due to spasm of the inflamed bladder wall (strangury)
- urine that may appear cloudy and have an unpleasant odour
- microscopic or visible haematuria.

Systemic symptoms are usually slight or absent. However, infection in the lower urinary tract can spread (see Box 17.50); acute pyelonephritis is suggested by prominent systemic symptoms with fever, rigors, vomiting, hypotension and loin pain, guarding or tenderness, and may be an indication for hospitalisation. Only about 30% of patients with acute pyelonephritis have associated symptoms of cystitis or urethritis. Prostatitis is suggested by perineal or suprapubic pain, pain on ejaculation and prostatic tenderness on rectal examination.

The differential diagnosis of lower urinary tract symptoms includes urethritis due to sexually transmitted disease, notably chlamydia (p. 422) or Reiter's syndrome (p. 1107). Some patients, usually female, have symptoms suggestive of urethritis and cystitis but no bacteria are cultured from the urine (the 'urethral syndrome'). Possible explanations include infection with organisms not readily cultured by ordinary methods (such as *Chlamydia* and certain anaerobes), intermittent or low-count bacteriuria, reaction to toiletries or disinfectants, symptoms related to sexual intercourse, or post-menopausal atrophic vaginitis.

The differential diagnosis of acute pyelonephritis includes pyelonephrosis, acute appendicitis, diverticulitis, cholecystitis, salpingitis, ruptured ovarian cyst or ectopic pregnancy. In pyelonephrosis due to upper urinary tract obstruction, patients may become extremely ill, with fever, leucocytosis and positive blood cultures. With a perinephric abscess, there is marked pain and tenderness, and often bulging of the loin on the affected side. Urinary symptoms may be absent in this situation and urine testing negative, containing neither pus cells nor organisms.

Investigations

An approach to investigation is shown in Box 17.52. In an otherwise healthy woman with a single lower urinary tract infection, urine culture prior to treatment is not mandatory. Investigation is necessary, however, in patients with recurrent infection or after failure of initial treatment, during pregnancy, or in patients susceptible to serious infection, such as the immunocompromised, those with diabetes or an indwelling catheter, and older people (Box 17.53). The diagnosis can be made from the combination of typical clinical features and abnormalities on urinalysis. Most urinary pathogens can reduce nitrate to nitrite, and neutrophils and nitrites can usually be detected in symptomatic infections by urine dipstick tests for leucocyte esterase and nitrite, respectively. The absence of both nitrites and leucocyte esterase in the urine makes UTI unlikely. Interpretation of bacterial counts in the urine, and of what is a 'significant' culture result, is based on probabilities. Urine taken by suprapubic aspiration should be sterile, so the presence of any organisms is significant. If the patient has symptoms and there are neutrophils in the urine, a small number of organisms is significant. In asymptomatic patients, more than 10^5 organisms/mL is usually regarded as significant (asymptomatic bacteriuria, see below).

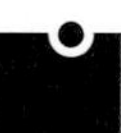

17.52 Investigation of patients with urinary tract infection

All patients
• Dipstick* estimation of nitrite, leucocyte esterase and glucose • Microscopy/cytometry of urine for white blood cells, organisms • Urine culture
Infants, children, and anyone with fever or complicated infection
• Full blood count; urea, electrolytes, creatinine • Blood cultures
Pyelonephritis; males; children; women with recurrent infections
• Renal tract ultrasound or CT • Pelvic examination in women, rectal examination in men
Continuing haematuria or other suspicion of bladder lesion
• Cystoscopy

*May substitute for microscopy and culture in simple uncomplicated infection.

17.53 Urinary infection in old age

- **Prevalence of asymptomatic bacteriuria**: rises with age. Amongst the most frail in institutional care it rises to 40% in women and 30% in men.
- **Decision to treat**: treating asymptomatic bacteriuria does not improve chronic incontinence or decrease mortality or morbidity from symptomatic urinary infection. It risks adverse effects from the antibiotic and promoting the emergence of resistant organisms.
- **Source of infection**: the urinary tract is the most frequent source of bacteraemia in older patients admitted to hospital.
- **Incontinence**: new or increased incontinence is a common presentation of UTI in older women.
- **Treatment**: post-menopausal women with acute lower urinary tract symptoms may require longer than 3 days' therapy.

Typical organisms causing UTI in the community include *E. coli* derived from the gastrointestinal tract (about 75% of infections), *Proteus* spp., *Pseudomonas* spp., streptococci and *Staphylococcus epidermidis*. In hospital, *E. coli* still predominates, but *Klebsiella* or streptococci are more common. Certain strains of *E. coli* have a particular propensity to invade the urinary tract.

Investigations to detect underlying predisposing factors for UTI are used selectively, most commonly in children, men or patients with recurrent infections (see Box 17.52).

Management

Antibiotics are recommended in all cases of proven UTI (Box 17.54). If urine culture has been performed, treatment may be started while awaiting the result. For infection of the lower urinary tract, treatment for 3 days is the norm and is less likely to induce significant alterations in bowel flora than more prolonged therapy. Trimethoprim is the usual choice for initial treatment; however, between 10% and 40% of organisms causing UTI are resistant to trimethoprim, the lower rates being seen in community-based practice. Nitrofurantoin, quinolone antibiotics such as ciprofloxacin and norfloxacin, and cefalexin are also generally effective. Co-amoxiclav or amoxicillin should only be used when the organism is known to be sensitive. Penicillins and cephalosporins are safe to use in pregnancy but trimethoprim, sulphonamides, quinolones and tetracyclines should be avoided.

In more severe infection, antibiotics should be continued for 7–14 days. Seriously ill patients may require intravenous therapy with a cephalosporin, quinolone or gentamicin for a few days (see Box 17.54), later switching to an oral agent.

A fluid intake of at least 2 L/day is usually recommended, although this is not based on evidence and may make symptoms of dysuria worse.

Persistent or recurrent UTI

If the causative organism persists on repeat culture despite treatment, or if there is re-infection with any organism after an interval, then an underlying cause is more likely to be present (see Box 17.51) and more detailed investigation is justified (see Box 17.52). In women, recurrent infections are common and

17.54 Antibiotic regimens for urinary tract infection in adults[1]

Scenario	Drug	Regimen	Duration	Comment
Cystitis				
First choice	Trimethoprim	200 mg twice daily	3 days	7–10 days in men
Second choices[1]	Amoxicillin	250 mg 3 times daily		
	Nitrofurantoin	50 mg 4 times daily		
	Cefalexin	250 mg 4 times daily		
	Ciprofloxacin	100 mg twice daily		
In pregnancy	Co-amoxiclav	250/125 mg 3 times daily	7 days	Avoid trimethoprim and quinolones during pregnancy
	Cefalexin	250 mg 4 times daily		
	Amoxicillin	250 mg 3 times daily		
Prophylactic therapy				
First choice	Trimethoprim	100 mg at night	Continuous	
Second choices[1]	Nitrofurantoin	50 mg at night		
	Co-amoxiclav	250/125 mg at night		
Pyelonephritis				
First choice	Co-amoxiclav	500/125 mg 3 times daily	14 days	Admit to hospital if no response within 24 hrs
	Ciprofloxacin	500 mg twice daily	7 days	
Second choice	Gentamicin[2]	Adjust dose according to renal function and serum levels	14 days	Switch to appropriate oral agent as soon as possible
	Cefuroxime	150–1500 mg 3 times daily		
Epididymo-orchitis				
First choice	Ciprofloxacin	500 mg twice daily	14 days	Refer to genito-urinary department to exclude *N. gonorrhoeae*
Acute prostatitis				
First choice	Trimethoprim	200 mg twice daily	28 days	
Second choice	Ciprofloxacin	500 mg twice daily		

[1]In all cases, the choice of drug should take locally determined antibiotic resistance patterns into account. [2]See Hartford nomogram (p. 157).

17.55 Prophylactic measures to be adopted by women with recurrent urinary infections

- Fluid intake of at least 2 L/day
- Regular complete emptying of bladder
- Good personal hygiene
- Emptying of bladder before and after sexual intercourse
- Cranberry juice may be effective

investigation is only justified if infections are frequent (three or more per year) or unusually severe. Recurrent UTI, particularly in the presence of an underlying cause, may result in permanent renal damage, whereas uncomplicated infections rarely (if ever) do so (see chronic reflux nephropathy, p. 504).

If an underlying cause cannot be treated, suppressive antibiotic therapy (see Box 17.54) can be used to prevent recurrence and reduce the risk of septicaemia and renal damage. Urine should be cultured at regular intervals; a regime of two or three antibiotics in sequence, rotating every 6 months, is often used in an attempt to reduce the emergence of resistant organisms. Other simple measures may help to prevent recurrence (Box 17.55).

Asymptomatic bacteriuria

This is defined as more than 10^5 organisms/mL in the urine of apparently healthy asymptomatic patients. Approximately 1% of children under the age of one, 1% of schoolgirls, 0.03% of schoolboys and men, 3% of non-pregnant adult women and 5% of pregnant women have asymptomatic bacteriuria. It is increasingly common in those aged over 65. There is no evidence that this condition causes renal scarring in adults who are not pregnant and have a normal urinary tract and, in general, treatment is not indicated. However, up to 30% will develop symptomatic infection within 1 year. Treatment is required in infants, pregnant women and those with urinary tract abnormalities.

Catheter-related bacteriuria

In patients with a urethral catheter, bacteriuria increases the risk of Gram-negative bacteraemia fivefold. Bacteriuria is common, however, and almost universal during long-term catheterisation. Treatment is usually avoided in asymptomatic patients, as this may promote antibiotic resistance. Careful sterile insertion technique is important, and the catheter should be removed as soon as it is not required.

Acute pyelonephritis

The kidneys are infected in a minority of patients with UTI. Acute renal infection (pyelonephritis) presents as a classic triad of loin pain, fever and tenderness over the kidneys. The renal pelvis is inflamed and small abscesses are often evident in the renal parenchyma (see Fig. 17.24C, p. 503).

Renal infection is almost always caused by organisms ascending from the bladder, and the bacterial profile is the same as for lower urinary tract infection (p. 512). Rarely, bacteraemia may give rise to renal or perinephric abscesses, most commonly due to staphylococci. Predisposing factors, such as cysts or renal scarring, facilitate infection.

Rarely, acute pyelonephritis is associated with papillary necrosis. Fragments of renal papillary tissue are passed per urethra and can be identified histologically. They may cause ureteric obstruction and, if this occurs bilaterally or in a single kidney, it may lead to AKI. Predisposing factors include diabetes mellitus, chronic urinary obstruction, analgesic nephropathy and sickle-cell disease. A necrotising form of pyelonephritis with gas formation, 'emphysematous pyelonephritis', is occasionally seen in patients with diabetes mellitus. Xanthogranulomatous pyelonephritis is a chronic infection that can resemble renal cell cancer. It is usually associated with obstruction, is characterised by accumulation of foamy macrophages and generally requires nephrectomy. Infection of cysts in polycystic kidney disease (p. 505) calls for prolonged antibiotic treatment.

Appropriate investigations are shown in Box 17.52 and management is described above and in Box 17.54. Intravenous rehydration may be needed in severe cases. If complicated infection is suspected or response to treatment is not prompt, urine should be recultured and renal tract ultrasound performed to exclude urinary tract obstruction or a perinephric collection. If obstruction is present, drainage by a percutaneous nephrostomy or ureteric stent should be considered.

Tuberculosis

Tuberculosis of the kidney and renal tract is secondary to tuberculosis elsewhere (p. 688) and is the result of blood-borne infection. Initially, lesions develop in the renal cortex; these may ulcerate into the renal pelvis and involve the ureters, bladder, epididymis, seminal vesicles and prostate. Calcification in the kidney and stricture formation in the ureter are typical.

Clinical features may include symptoms of bladder involvement (frequency, dysuria); haematuria (sometimes macroscopic); malaise, fever, night sweats, lassitude and weight loss; loin pain; associated genital disease; and chronic renal failure as a result of urinary tract obstruction or destruction of kidney tissue.

Neutrophils are present in the urine but routine urine culture may be negative ('sterile pyuria'). Special techniques of microscopy and culture may be required to identify tubercle bacilli and are most usefully performed on early morning urine specimens. Bladder involvement should be assessed by cystoscopy. Radiology of the urinary tract and a chest X-ray to look for pulmonary tuberculosis are mandatory. Anti-tuberculous chemotherapy follows standard regimes (p. 693). Surgery to relieve urinary tract obstruction or to remove a very severely infected kidney may be required.

BENIGN PROSTATIC ENLARGEMENT

Benign prostatic enlargement (BPE) is extremely common. It has been estimated that about half of all men aged 80 years and over will have lower urinary tract symptoms associated with BPE. Benign prostatic hyperplasia (BPH) is the histological abnormality that underlies BPE.

Pathophysiology

The prostate gland increases in volume by 2.4 cm^3 per year on average from 40 years of age. The process begins in the peri-urethral (transitional) zone and involves both glandular and stromal tissue to a variable degree. The cause is unknown, although BPE does not occur in patients with hypogonadism, suggesting that hormonal factors may be important.

Clinical features

The primary symptoms of BPE arise because of difficulty in voiding urine due to obstruction of the urethra by the prostate; they consist of hesitancy, poor urinary flow and a sensation of incomplete emptying. Other symptoms include urinary frequency, urgency of micturition and urge incontinence, although these are not specific to BPE. Some patients present suddenly with acute urinary retention, when they are unable to micturate and develop a painful distended bladder. This is often precipitated by excessive alcohol intake, constipation and prostatic infection. Severity of symptoms can be ascertained by using the International Prostate Symptom Score questionnaire (IPSS, Box 17.56), which serves as a valuable starting point for assessment of the patient. Once a baseline value is established, any improvement or deterioration may be monitored on subsequent visits. The IPSS may be combined with a quality of life score, in which patients are asked the following question 'If you were to spend the rest of your life with your

17.56 The International Prostate Symptom Score (IPSS)

Symptom	Question	Example score
Straining	How often have you had to push or strain to begin urination?	1
Urgency	How often have you found it difficult to postpone urination?	2
Hesitancy	How often have you found that you stopped and started again several times when you urinated?	1
Incomplete emptying	How often have you had a sensation of not emptying your bladder completely after you finished urinating?	3
Frequency	How often have you had to urinate again less than 2 hours after you finished urinating?	1
Weak stream	How often have you had a weak urinary stream?	2
Nocturia	How many times did you most typically get up to urinate from the time you went to bed at night until the time you got up in the morning?	1
Total score		11

0 = not at all; 1 = less than one-fifth of the time; 2 = less than half the time; 3 = about half of the time; 4 = more than half of the time; 5 = almost always

A score of 0–1 indicates mild symptoms, 8–19 moderate symptoms and 20–35 severe symptoms. In the example shown, the patient had moderate symptoms.

urinary condition the way it is now, how would you feel about that?' Responses range from 0 (delighted) to 6 (terrible).

Patients may also present with chronic urinary retention. Here, the bladder slowly distends due to inadequate emptying over a long period of time. Patients with chronic retention can also develop acute retention: so-called acute-on-chronic retention. This condition is characterised by pain-free bladder distension, which may result in hydroureter, hydronephrosis and renal failure (high-pressure chronic retention). On digital rectal examination, patients with BPE have evidence of prostatic enlargement with a smooth prostate gland. Abdominal examination may also reveal evidence of bladder enlargement in patients with urinary retention.

Investigations

The diagnosis of BPE is a clinical one but flow rates can be accurately measured with a flow meter, and prostate volume by transrectal ultrasound scan (TRUS). Objective assessment of obstruction is possible by urodynamics but this is seldom required. If symptoms or signs, such as a palpable bladder, nocturnal enuresis, recurrent urinary tract infections or a history of renal stones, are present, renal function should be assessed; if it is abnormal, screening should be conducted for evidence of obstructive nephropathy by ultrasound examination.

Management

Patients who present with acute retention require urgent treatment and should undergo immediate catheterisation to relieve the obstruction. Those with mild to moderate symptoms can be treated by medication (Boxes 17.57 and 17.58). The first-line treatments are α_{1A}-adrenoceptor blockers such as tamsulosin, which reduce the tone of smooth muscle cells in the prostate and bladder neck, thereby reducing the obstruction. The 5α-reductase inhibitors, finasteride and dutasteride, inhibit conversion of testosterone to the more potent dihydrotestosterone in the prostate and so cause the prostate to shrink. This class of drugs is indicated in patients with an estimated prostate size of more than 30 g or a prostate specific antigen (PSA) of more than 1.4 μg/L. Patients who fail to respond to a single drug may be treated with a combination of α-blockers and 5α-reductase inhibitors, since this is more efficacious than either agent alone. Symptoms that are resistant to medical therapy require surgical treatment to remove some of the prostate tissue that is causing urethral obstruction. This is usually achieved by transurethral resection of the prostate (TURP) but enucleation of the prostate by holmium laser is equally effective and has potentially fewer complications. Open surgery is rarely needed, unless the gland is very large.

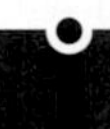

17.57 Treatment for benign prostatic enlargement

Medical

- Prostate < 30 g: α-adrenoceptor blockers
- Prostate > 30 g: 5α-reductase inhibitors ± α-adrenoceptor blockers

Surgical

- Transurethral resection of prostate (TURP)
- Holmium laser enucleation
- Open prostatectomy

EBM 17.58 Medical management of benign prostatic enlargement

'Oral α-adrenoceptor blockers produce rapid improvement in urinary flow in 60–70% of patients. The 5α-reductase inhibitor, finasteride, causes slow shrinkage of large prostate glands with improvement in symptoms.'

- Clifford GM, et al. Eur Urol 2000; 38:2–19.
- Boyle R, et al. Urology 2001; 58:717–722.

Prostatitis

This condition is due to inflammation of the prostate gland. Acute or chronic bacterial prostatitis can be caused by infection with the same bacteria that are associated with UTI (p. 511) but prostatitis can also be 'non-bacterial', in which case no organism can be cultured from the urine. This is also known as chronic pelvic pain syndrome. Clinical features of prostatitis include frequency, dysuria, painful ejaculation, perineal or groin pain, difficulty passing urine and, in acute disease, considerable systemic disturbance. The prostate is enlarged and tender. Bacterial prostatitis is confirmed by a positive culture from urine or from urethral discharge obtained after prostatic massage, and the treatment of choice is trimethoprim or a quinolone antibiotic. A 4–6-week course is required (see Box 17.54). Treatment of chronic pelvic pain syndrome is challenging but some patients respond to a combination of α-blockers, NSAIDs and amitriptyline.

TUMOURS OF THE KIDNEY AND URINARY TRACT

Several malignant tumours can affect the kidney and urinary tract, including renal adenocarcinoma, bladder carcinoma, prostate carcinoma, and tumours of the testis and penis. The urogenital tract can also be affected by benign tumours and secondary tumour deposits, which can cause obstructive uropathy.

Renal adenocarcinoma

Renal adenocarcinoma is by far the most common malignant tumour of the kidney in adults, making up 2.5% of all adult cancers, with a prevalence of 16 cases per 100 000 population. It is twice as common in males as in females. The peak incidence is between 65 and 75 years of age and it is uncommon before 40. The tumour arises from renal tubular cells. Haemorrhage and necrosis give the cut surface a characteristic mixed golden-yellow and red appearance (Fig. 17.32B). Microscopically, clear cell carcinomas are the most common histological subtype (85%), with papillary, chromophobe and collecting duct tumours making up the remaining 15%. With clear cell

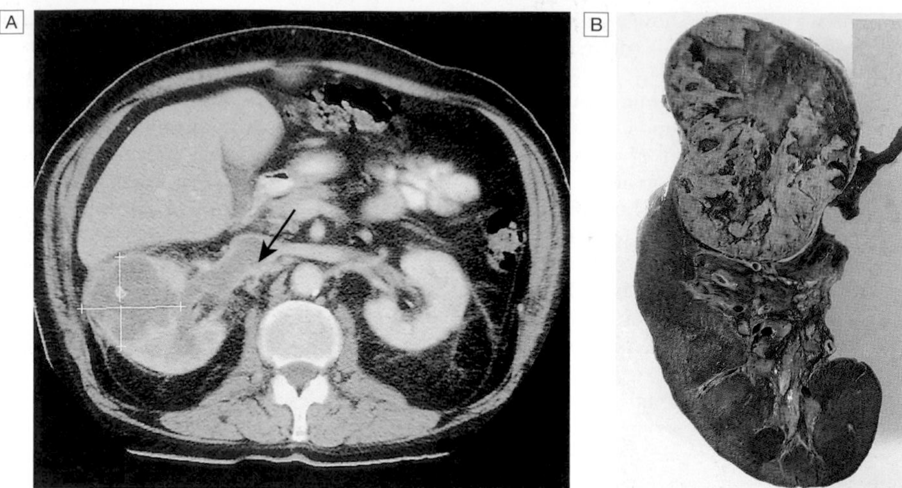

Fig. 17.32 Renal adenocarcinoma. **A** In this CT, the right kidney is expanded by a low-density tumour, which fails to take up contrast material. Tumour is shown extending into the renal vein and inferior vena cava (arrow). **B** Pathology specimen showing typical necrosis.

carcinomas, there is early spread of the tumour into the renal pelvis, causing haematuria, and along the renal vein, often extending into the inferior vena cava. Direct invasion of perinephric tissues is common. Lymphatic spread to para-aortic nodes occurs, while blood-borne metastases (which may be solitary) most commonly develop in the lungs, bone and brain.

Clinical features

In 50% of patients, asymptomatic renal tumours are identified as an incidental finding during imaging investigations carried out for other reasons. Amongst symptomatic patients, about 60% present with haematuria, 40% with loin pain and 25% with a mass; about 10% present with a triad of pain, haematuria and a mass. A remarkable range of systemic effects may be present, including fever, raised ESR, polycythaemia, disorders of coagulation, hypercalcaemia, and abnormalities of plasma proteins and liver function tests. The patient may present with pyrexia of unknown origin or, rarely, with neuropathy. Some of these systemic effects are caused by secretion of products by the tumour, such as renin, erythropoietin, PTH-related protein (PTHrP) and gonadotrophins. The effects disappear when the tumour is removed but may re-appear when metastases develop, and so can be used as markers of tumour activity.

Investigations

Ultrasound is the investigation of first choice and allows differentiation between solid tumour and simple renal cysts. If the results are suggestive of a tumour, contrast-enhanced CT of the abdomen and chest should be performed for staging (see Fig. 17.32A). For tumours more than 3 cm in diameter with no evidence of metastatic spread and when the nature of the lesion is uncertain, ultrasound or CT-guided biopsy may be used to avoid nephrectomy for benign disease.

Management

Radical nephrectomy that includes the perirenal fascial envelope and ipsilateral para-aortic lymph nodes is the treatment of choice. Nephrectomy is commonly performed laparoscopically, with equivalent outcomes to open surgery. Partial nephrectomy is recommended for tumours of 4 cm or less, as there is a lower incidence of cardiac and renal morbidity. Patients at high operative risk, who have small tumours, may also be treated percutaneously by cryoablation or radiofrequency ablation. Surgery may also play a role in the treatment of solitary metastases, since these can remain single for long periods and excision may be worthwhile.

Renal adenocarcinoma is resistant to most chemotherapeutic agents. For many years, cytokine therapy with interferon and interleukin-2 was used in metastatic renal cancer but, in recent years, two new classes of targeted drugs have been introduced and are now the mainstay of therapy. These are the tyrosine kinase inhibitors, sunitinib and pazopanib, and the mammalian target of rapamycin (mTOR) inhibitors, temsirolimus and everolimus.

In previous years, patients who presented with distant metastases were treated with cytoreductive nephrectomy, in which nephrectomy was coupled with systemic cytokine treatment, since this was shown to improved survival as compared with either treatment in isolation. It is, at present, unclear whether this survival benefit still prevails with the newer agents mentioned above.

Studies that antedate the introduction of these new agents show that, if the tumour is confined to the kidney, 5-year survival is 75%, but this falls to 5% when there are distant metastases.

Urothelial tumours

Tumours arising from the transitional epithelium of the renal tract can affect the renal pelvis, ureter, bladder or urethra. They are rare under the age of 40, affect males about 3–4 times as commonly as females, and account for about 3% of all malignant tumours. The bladder is by far the most frequently affected site. Although almost all tumours are transitional cell carcinomas, squamous carcinoma may occur in urothelium that has undergone metaplasia, usually following chronic inflammation or irritation due to stones or schistosomiasis. The

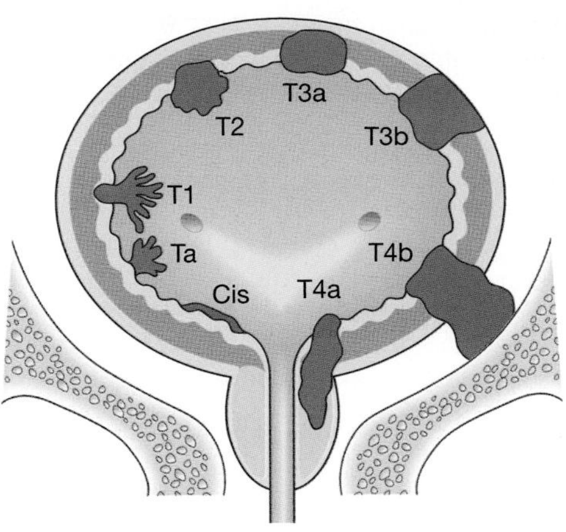

Fig. 17.33 Transitional cell carcinoma of the bladder. Stages are shown from carcinoma in situ (Cis) to invasive tumour progressing beyond the bladder and prostate (T4b).

appearance of a transitional cell tumour ranges from a delicate papillary structure with relatively good prognosis to a solid ulcerating mass in more aggressive disease (Fig. 17.33).

Pathophysiology

Risk factors include cigarette smoking and exposure to industrial carcinogens like aromatic amines, aniline dyes and aldehydes. Chronic inflammatory processes, such as schistosomiasis and chronic bladder stones, predispose to squamous carcinomas by causing squamous metaplasia.

Clinical features

More than 80% of patients present with painless, visible haematuria. It should be assumed that such bleeding is from a tumour until proven otherwise (p. 474). Tumours of the ureter or bladder may also cause symptoms of obstruction, depending on the site of involvement, and tumours of the bladder present with dysuria or storage symptoms. Physical examination is usually unremarkable, except in patients with very advanced disease, when bimanual examination may reveal a palpable mass.

Investigations

Cystoscopy (usually flexible cystoscopy under a local anaesthetic) is mandatory to evaluate the bladder in cases of haematuria or suspected bladder cancer. Imaging of the upper urinary tract (CT urogram is the gold standard but IVU and renal ultrasound are also acceptable) is also important to rule out abnormalities of the kidney, ureters and renal pelvis in patients with haematuria. If a suspicious defect is seen on CTU or IVU in the ureter or renal pelvis, a retrograde ureteropyelogram, ureteroscopy and biopsy are required. If evidence of a solid invasive urothelial tumour is found, CT of the abdomen, pelvis and chest should be performed as a staging procedure.

Management

Most bladder tumours are low-grade superficial lesions that can be successfully treated endoscopically by transurethral resection of the tumour. Intravesical chemotherapy with mitomycin C is usually administered as a one-off treatment post resection to prevent tumour recurrence, or may be given as a prolonged course to treat multiple low-grade bladder tumours. Patients with carcinoma in situ have a high risk of progression to invasive cancer. These patients often respond well to intravesical bacille Calmette–Guérin (BCG) treatment but more radical treatment may also be needed if this is unsuccessful. Following initial treatment and endoscopic clearance of bladder tumours, regular check cystoscopies are required to look for evidence of recurrence. Patients with recurrences of superficial disease can usually be treated by further resection and diathermy, but if this is unsuccessful, a cystectomy may be needed.

The management of invasive bladder tumours involves radical cystectomy with urinary diversion into an incontinent ileal conduit or a continent catheterisable bowel pouch; the latter is usually reserved for patients under the age of 70 years.

The prognosis of bladder tumours depends on tumour stage and grade. About 5% of patients with low-grade superficial bladder cancer progress to develop invasion of the bladder muscle, compared with about 50% of those with high-grade superficial bladder cancers. Overall, the 5-year survival for patients with muscle-invasive bladder cancer of either grade is about 50–70%.

Transitional cell carcinoma of the renal pelvis and ureter is usually treated by open or laparoscopic nephroureterectomy, but if the tumour is solitary and low-grade, it can be treated endoscopically.

Prostate cancer

Prostate cancer is the most common malignancy in men in the UK, with a prevalence of 105 per 100 000 population. It is also common in northern Europe and the USA (particularly in the black population) but is rare in China and Japan. It rarely occurs before the age of 50 and has a mean age at presentation of 70 years.

Pathophysiology

Prostate cancers tend to arise within the peripheral zone of the prostate and almost all are adenocarcinomas. Metastatic spread to pelvic lymph nodes occurs early and metastases to bone, mainly the lumbar spine and pelvis, are common. Genetic factors are known to play an important role in pathogenesis, and multiple predisposing loci have been found to predispose to the disease in genome-wide association studies. A family history of prostate cancer greatly increases a man's chances of developing the disease. It seems likely that the differences in incidence between different ethnic groups may be explained by genetic factors.

Clinical features

Most patients either are asymptomatic or present with lower urinary tract symptoms indistinguishable from benign prostatic enlargement. On digital rectal examination (DRE), the prostate may feel nodular and stony-hard, and the median sulcus may be lost, but up to 45% of tumours are impalpable. Symptoms and signs due to metastases are much less common at the initial presentation but may include back pain, weight loss, anaemia and obstruction of the ureters.

Investigations

Measurement of PSA levels in a peripheral blood sample, together with DRE, is the cornerstone of diagnosis. Prior to a PSA test, men should be given careful counselling about the limitations of the test: namely, a normal level does not exclude prostate cancer; a high value does not confirm the diagnosis but will open a discussion about biopsy. The need for radical treatment of localised prostate cancer is still not established; radical treatments have significant potential morbidity and mortality; and early identification and treatment of prostate cancer may save lives. Current evidence suggests that population-based screening for prostate cancer with PSA is of limited value, due in part to the fact that over 1000 patients would need to be screened to cure one man of prostate cancer. Individuals suspected of having prostate cancer, based on an elevated PSA and/or abnormal DRE, should undergo transrectal ultrasound-guided prostate biopsies. About 40% of patients with a serum PSA of 4.0–10 ug/L or more will have prostate cancer on biopsy, although 25% patients with a PSA of less than 4 ng/mL may also have prostate cancer. Occasionally, a small focus of tumour is found incidentally in patients undergoing transurethral resection of the prostate for benign hyperplasia. If the diagnosis of prostate cancer is confirmed, staging should be performed by pelvic MRI to assess the presence and extent of local involvement. An isotope bone scan should be carried out if distant metastases are suspected (rare if the PSA is below 20 ng/mL); very high levels of serum PSA (> 100 ng/mL) almost always indicate distant bone metastases. Following diagnosis, serial assessment of PSA levels is useful for monitoring response to treatment and disease progression.

Management

Tumour confined to the prostate is potentially curable by radical prostatectomy, radical radiotherapy or brachytherapy (implantation of small radioactive particles into the prostate). These options should only be considered in patients with more than 10 years' life expectancy. Patients who are found to have small foci of tumour do not require specific treatment but should be followed up periodically with PSA, DRE and a schedule of biopsies; this is known as active surveillance. Prostatic cancer, like breast cancer, is sensitive to steroid hormones; metastatic prostate cancer is treated by androgen depletion, involving either surgery (orchidectomy) or, more commonly, androgen-suppressing drugs (Box 17.59). Androgen receptor blockers, such as bicalutamide or cyproterone acetate, may also prevent tumour cell growth. Gonadotrophin-releasing hormone (GnRH) analogues, such as goserelin, continuously occupy pituitary receptors, preventing them from responding to the GnRH pulses that normally stimulate luteinising hormone (LH) and follicle-stimulating hormone (FSH) release. This initially causes an increase in testosterone before producing a prolonged reduction, and for this reason the initial dose must be covered with an androgen receptor blocker to prevent a tumour flare.

EBM 17.59 Hormone manipulation in prostate cancer

'Reducing circulating testosterone levels (either by castration or by medication) results in a 70% initial response rate. Additional androgen blockade produces a small increase in survival but with poorer quality of life.'

- Huggins C, et al. Arch Surg 1941; 43:209.
- Huggins C. Cancer Res 1967; 27:1925–1930.
- Schmitt B, et al. Maximal androgen blockade for advanced prostate cancer. Cochrane Database of Systematic Reviews, 1999, issue 2. Art. no. CD001526.

For further information: www.cochrane.org/cochrane-reviews

A small proportion of patients fail to respond to endocrine treatment. A larger number respond for a year or two but then the disease progresses. Chemotherapy with docetaxel can then be effective and provide a modest (around 3 months) survival advantage. Radiotherapy is useful for localised bone pain but the basis of treatment remains pain control by analgesia (p. 286). Provided that patients do not die of another cause, the 10-year survival rate of patients with tumours localised to the prostate is 95%, but if metastases are present, this falls to 10%. Life expectancy is not reduced in patients with small foci of tumour.

Testicular tumours

Testicular tumours are uncommon, with a prevalence of 5 cases per 100 000 population. They occur mainly in young men aged between 20 and 40 years. They often secrete α-fetoprotein (AFP) and β-human chorionic gonadotrophin (β-hCG), which are useful biochemical markers for both diagnosis and prognosis. Seminoma and teratoma account for 85% of all tumours of the testis. Leydig cell tumours are less common.

Seminomas arise from seminiferous tubules and represent a relatively low-grade malignancy. Metastases can occur through lymphatic spread, however, and typically involve the lungs.

Teratomas arise from primitive germinal cells and tend to occur at a younger age than seminomas. They may contain cartilage, bone, muscle, fat and a variety of other tissues, and are classified according to the degree of differentiation. Well-differentiated tumours are the least aggressive; at the other extreme, trophoblastic teratoma is highly malignant. Occasionally, teratoma and seminoma occur together.

Leydig cell tumours are usually small and benign but secrete oestrogens, leading to presentation with gynaecomastia (p. 762).

Clinical features and investigations

The common presentation is incidental discovery of a painless testicular lump, although some patients complain of a testicular ache.

All suspicious scrotal lumps should be imaged by ultrasound. Serum levels of AFP and β-hCG are elevated in extensive disease. Oestradiol may be elevated, suppressing luteinising hormone (LH), follicle-stimulating hormone (FSH) and testosterone. Accurate staging is based on CT of the lungs, liver and retroperitoneal area.

Management and prognosis

The primary treatment is surgical orchidectomy. Subsequent treatment depends on the histological type and stage. Radiotherapy is the treatment of choice for early-stage seminoma. Teratoma confined to the testes may be managed conservatively, but more advanced cancers are treated with chemotherapy, usually the combination of bleomycin, etoposide and cisplatin. Follow-up is by CT and assessment of AFP and β-hCG. Retroperitoneal lymph node dissection is now only performed for residual or recurrent nodal masses.

The 5-year survival rate for patients with seminoma is 90–95%. For teratomas, the 5-year survival varies between 60% and 95%, depending on tumour type, stage and volume.

Inherited tumour syndromes affecting the renal tract

Some uncommon autosomal dominantly inherited conditions are associated with multiple renal tumours in adult life. In tuberous sclerosis (p. 1302), replacement of renal tissue by multiple angiomyolipomas (tubers) may occasionally cause renal failure in adults. Other organs affected include the skin (adenoma sebaceum on the face) and brain (causing seizures and mental retardation). The von Hippel–Lindau syndrome (p. 1216) is connected with multiple renal cysts, renal adenomas and renal adenocarcinoma. Other organs affected include the central nervous system (haemangioblastomas) and the adrenals (phaeochromocytoma).

RENAL INVOLVEMENT IN SYSTEMIC CONDITIONS

The kidneys may be directly involved in a number of multisystem diseases or secondarily affected by diseases of other organs. Involvement may be at a pre-renal, renal (glomerular or interstitial) or post-renal level. Many of the diseases are described in other sections of this chapter or in other chapters of the book.

Diabetes mellitus

Diabetes mellitus is the most common cause of CKD in developed countries. In patients with diabetes, there is a steady advance from microalbuminuria to dipstick-positive proteinuria, and a progression to renal failure, as described on page 830. Few patients require renal biopsy to establish the diagnosis, but atypical features or progression should lead to suspicion that an alternative condition could be present.

Management with ACE inhibitors and other hypotensive agents to slow progression is described on page 831 and has been dramatically effective. In some patients, proteinuria may be eradicated and progression completely halted, even if renal function is abnormal.

Hepatic–renal disease

Severe hepatic dysfunction may cause a haemodynamically mediated type of renal failure, hepatorenal syndrome, described on page 940. Patients with chronic liver disease are also predisposed to develop AKI (acute tubular necrosis) in response to relatively minor insults, including bleeding and infection. Such patients are often difficult to treat by dialysis and have a poor prognosis. Where treatment is justified – for example, if there is a good chance of recovery or of a liver transplant – slow or continuous treatments are less likely to precipitate or exacerbate hepatic encephalopathy. IgA nephropathy (p. 500) is more common in patients with liver disease.

Pulmonary-renal syndrome

The pulmonary–renal syndrome is a dramatic presentation with renal and respiratory failure that is not explained by excess intravascular fluid or by severe pneumonia; it occurs in Goodpasture's (anti-GBM) disease and small-vessel vasculitis (see below). There are some other uncommon causes of a similar syndrome, including poisoning with the herbicide paraquat.

Malignant diseases

The kidney may be affected in many different ways in patients with malignant disease (Box 17.60). Direct involvement of the kidneys or other parts of the urinary tract can occur, causing obstructive uropathy, and glomerulonephritis may occur, presumably as the result of an immunological reaction to the tumour. Hypercalcaemia can be caused by parathyroid hormone-related protein (PTHrP) production by tumours, whereas treatment of leukaemia and lymphoma can sometimes be complicated by interstitial nephritic and acute kidney injury due to uric acid release from necrotic tumour cells. Finally, in myeloma and other monoclonal gammopathies, renal impairment can occur as the result of the nephrotoxic effects of immunoglobulin light chains released by the tumour.

17.60 Renal effects of malignancies

Direct involvement	
• Renal adenocarcinoma • Urothelial tumours	• Cervical carcinoma • Lymphoma
Immune reaction	
• Glomerulonephritis*	
Metabolic consequences	
• Hypercalcaemia	• Uric acid nephropathy
Remote effects of tumour products	
• Light chains in myeloma	

*Especially membranous nephropathy.

Systemic vasculitis

Small-vessel vasculitis (p. 1115) commonly affects the kidneys, with rapid and profound impairment of glomerular function. Histologically, there is a focal inflammatory glomerulonephritis, usually with focal necrosis (see Box 17.39, p. 499, and Fig. 17.22, p. 498) and often with crescentic changes. Typically, the patient is systemically unwell with an acute phase response, weight loss and arthralgia. In some patients, pulmonary haemorrhage may occur, which can be life-threatening. In others, it presents as a kidney-limited disorder, with

EBM 17.61 Role of rituximab in ANCA-associated vasculitis

'The RAVE study compared the effectiveness of rituximab and oral cyclophosphamide for inducing remission in 197 patients with ANCA-associated vasculitis with renal and/or pulmonary involvement. Both groups received high-dose glucocorticoids. The rituximab-based regimen was non-inferior to the cyclophosphamide-based regimen at inducing remission and was superior in patients with a history of relapsing disease. Rituximab was equally effective as cyclophosphamide in the treatment of major renal disease and alveolar haemorrhage. There were no significant differences between the treatment groups with respect to glucocorticoid dose or adverse events.'

- Stone JH. N Engl J Med 2010; 363(3):221–232.

rapidly deteriorating renal function and crescentic nephritis.

The most important cause is antineutrophil cytoplasmic antibody (ANCA)-positive vasculitis (p. 1118). Two subtypes are recognised. Microscopic polyangiitis (MPA) typically presents with glomerulonephritis and pulmonary haemorrhage, along with gastrointestinal involvement and neuropathy, whereas polyangiitis with granulomatosis (also known as Wegener's granulomatosis) typically presents with glomerulonephritis and granulomatous lesions affecting the nasal passages and lungs. Serological testing for myeloperoxidase (MPO) and proteinase 3 (PR3) is usually positive but these antibodies are not specific and a biopsy of affected tissue should be obtained if possible to confirm the diagnosis.

The standard treatment of glomerulonephritis associated with systemic vasculitis is high-dose glucocorticoids combined with pulse cyclophosphamide, or mycophenolate mofetil (p. 1118). Recent studies indicate that rituximab (p. 1103), when combined with high-dose steroids, is as effective as oral cyclophosphamide and high-dose steroids in the treatment of ANCA-associated vasculitis (Box 17.61). Plasma exchange can offer additional benefit in patients with progressive renal damage who are not responding adequately to immunosuppressive therapy.

Glomerulonephritis secondary to vasculitis may rarely also be seen in rheumatoid arthritis, SLE and cryoglobulinaemia, although SLE usually involves the kidney in different ways (see below).

Medium- to large-vessel vasculitis, such as polyarteritis nodosa, p. 1117), does not cause glomerulonephritis but can cause hypertension, renal infarction or haematuria if the renal vessels are involved.

Systemic lupus erythematosus

Subclinical renal involvement, with low-level haematuria and proteinuria but minimally impaired or normal renal function, is common in systemic lupus erythematosus (SLE). Usually, this is due to glomerular disease, although interstitial nephritis may also occur, particularly in patients with overlap syndromes such as mixed connective tissue disease and Sjögren's syndrome (p. 499 and Figure 17.21 (p. 497)).

Almost any histological pattern of glomerular disease can be observed in SLE and the clinical presentation ranges from florid, rapidly progressive glomerulonephritis to nephrotic syndrome. The most common presentation is with subacute disease and inflammatory features (haematuria, hypertension, variable renal impairment), accompanied by heavy proteinuria that often reaches nephrotic levels. In severely affected patients, the most common histological pattern is a proliferative glomerulonephritis with substantial deposits of immunoglobulins on immunofluorescence. Randomised controlled trials have shown that the risk of ESRD in lupus nephritis is significantly reduced by high-dose steroids administered in combination with cyclophosphamide, usually given as regular intravenous pulses. More recently, it has been shown that the combination of corticosteroids and mycophenolate mofetil is as effective as corticosteroids and cyclophosphamide, at least in short-term studies.

Many patients with SLE who develop ESRD go into remission, possibly because of immunosuppression related to the ESRD. Patients with ESRD caused by SLE are usually good candidates for dialysis and transplantation. Although it may recur in renal allografts, the immunosuppression required to prevent allograft rejection usually controls the SLE too.

PREGNANCY AND RENAL DISEASE

Pregnancy has important physiological effects on the renal system. Some diseases are more common in pregnancy, the manifestations of others are modified during pregnancy, and a few diseases, such as pre-eclampsia, are unique to pregnancy.

Physiological adaptations begin in the first few weeks. Peripheral vascular resistance declines, blood volume, cardiac output and GFR increase, and there is usually a reduction in blood pressure and plasma creatinine and urea values in the first trimester. Baseline blood pressure and urine testing from the first antenatal clinic visit are valuable if problems arise later.

Infections

Pyelonephritis is more common during pregnancy, perhaps because of dilatation of the urinary collecting system and ureters. It is important to treat asymptomatic bacteriuria during pregnancy, since this can progress to pyelonephritis, which, in turn, can trigger premature labour (Box 17.62 and p. 513).

Glomerular diseases

Proteinuria caused by glomerular disease is usually exacerbated, and nephrotic syndrome may develop

EBM 17.62 Treatment of asymptomatic bacteriuria in pregnancy

'Antibiotic therapy for asymptomatic bacteriuria reduces the incidence of pyelonephritis (risk ratio (RR) 0.23, 95% confidence interval (CI) 0.13–0.41) and is also associated with a reduction in the incidence of low-birthweight babies (RR 0.66, 95% CI 0.49–0.89), but does not affect the incidence of preterm delivery.'

- Smaill F, Vazquez JC. Antibiotics for asymptomatic bacteriuria in pregnancy. Cochrane Database of Systematic Reviews, 2007, issue 2. Art. no. CD000490.

For further information: www.cochrane.org/cochrane-reviews

without any alteration in the underlying disease activity in individuals who had only slight proteinuria before pregnancy. This further increases the risk of venous thromboembolism, the leading cause of maternal deaths in developed countries.

Autoimmune diseases

Systemic autoimmune diseases typically are relatively quiescent during pregnancy but tend to relapse in the first few weeks and months following delivery. Pre-existing renal disease increases the fetal and maternal risk involved in pregnancy, to a degree dependent on the level of renal function, proteinuria and hypertension. Patients with such diseases who may become pregnant should be aware of the associated risks. During pregnancy, therapy should not usually be stopped, but blood pressure targets may be modified and agents altered to those of proven safety.

Pre-eclampsia

Pre-eclampsia is a systemic disorder that occurs in or near the third trimester of pregnancy (triplets > twins > singleton). The cause is unknown, although a number of risk factors have been identified (Box 17.63).

Clinical features

Pre-eclampsia is traditionally defined by the triad of oedema, proteinuria and hypertension. However, oedema is common in late pregnancy, proteinuria is a late sign and, while hypertension is usually present, it may be relative, mild or even absent. Furthermore, all these features occur in pre-existing renal disease exacerbated by pregnancy.

It is important to distinguish pre-eclampsia from pre-existing renal disease, since this affects management. Pre-eclampsia presents progressively, increasing risks to mother and fetus, which can be reversed almost immediately by early delivery. In contrast, continuing the pregnancy for as long as possible in patients with pre-existing renal disease, may permit delivery of a healthier, more mature baby. Proteinuria and hypertension in the first trimester of pregnancy suggest pre-existing renal disease.

Management

The only effective management for pre-eclampsia is delivery. The role of antiplatelet therapy (low-dose aspirin) remains controversial. Hypertension is a consequence and not the cause of the disorder, and treatment is only justified to lower it from severe and immediately dangerous levels (> 150–160/100–110 mmHg). Treating lower levels has been shown to confer no benefit and exposes the fetus to additional drugs. If life-threatening complications are not present and the baby is immature, corticosteroids may be given to induce maturation of fetal lungs, and delivery postponed while mother and baby are closely observed. Magnesium sulphate reduces the incidence of eclamptic convulsions.

Acute kidney injury

Maternal AKI may occur in almost any of the pre-eclamptic syndromes. Worldwide, a more important cause of AKI is septic abortion, when the uterus becomes infected because of retained products of conception or poor sterility in an often illegally induced abortion. Renal function is usually recoverable, but AKI in pregnancy is particularly prone to progress to cortical necrosis, with incomplete or total failure to recover renal function.

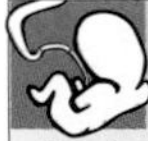

17.63 Pre-eclampsia and related diseases in pregnancy

Clinical syndromes

- Eclampsia: severe hypertension, encephalopathy and fits
- Disseminated intravascular coagulation
- Thrombotic microangiopathy: may also occur post-partum (post-partum haemolytic uraemic syndrome)
- Acute fatty liver of pregnancy
- 'HELLP' syndrome: haemolysis, elevated liver enzymes, low platelets (thrombotic microangiopathy with abnormal liver function)

Risk factors

- First pregnancy
- First pregnancy with a new partner or long inter-pregnancy interval
- Pre-eclampsia in previous pregnancies
- Age < 20 yrs or > 35 yrs
- Multiple pregnancy (triplets > twins > singleton)
- Pre-existing hypertension
- Pre-existing renal disease

Clinical signs

- Hypertension
- Proteinuria
- Oedema
- Evidence of the clinical syndromes listed above

Investigations

- Uric acid levels increased (before renal impairment apparent)
- Platelets decreased
- Reduced GFR (late)
- Fetus small for dates and growing slowly
- Fetal distress (late)

KIDNEY DISEASE IN ADOLESCENCE

Many causes of renal failure present during infancy or childhood, such as congenital urological malformations and inherited disorders like cystinosis and autosomal recessive polycystic kidney disease. The consequences continue throughout the patient's life and the situation often arises whereby patients transition from paediatric to adult nephrology services. Some of the issues and challenges surrounding this transition are summarised in Box 17.64.

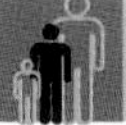

17.64 Kidney disease in adolescence

- **Adherence**: young adults moving from parental supervision may become disengaged. There may also be reduced adherence to prophylactic and therapeutic treatment.
- **Adverse events**: there is an increased risk of transplant loss and other adverse events in young adults on RRT.
- **Management**: joint clinics should be established with the paediatric team to facilitate transfer to regional specialist clinics.

17

DRUGS AND THE KIDNEY

Drug-induced renal disease

The kidney is susceptible to damage by drugs because it is the route of excretion of many water-soluble compounds, including drugs and their metabolites. Some may reach high concentrations in the renal cortex as a result of proximal tubular transport mechanisms. Others are concentrated in the medulla by the operation of the countercurrent system. The same applies to certain toxins.

Toxic renal damage may occur by a variety of mechanisms (Box 17.65). Very commonly, drugs contribute to the development of acute tubular necrosis as one of multiple insults. Numerically, reactions to NSAIDs and ACE inhibitors are the most important. Haemodynamic renal impairment, acute tubular necrosis and allergic reactions are usually reversible if recognised early enough. Other types, however, especially those associated with extensive fibrosis, are less likely to be reversible.

NSAIDs

Impairment of renal function may develop in patients on NSAID, since prostaglandins play an important role in regulating renal blood flow. This is particularly likely in patients with other disorders, such as heart failure, cirrhosis, sepsis and pre-existing renal impairment. In addition, idiosyncratic immune reactions may occur, causing minimal change nephrotic syndrome (p. 498) and acute interstitial nephritis (p. 502). Analgesic nephropathy (p. 504) is now a rare complication of long-term use.

ACE inhibitors

These abolish the compensatory angiotensin II-mediated vasoconstriction of the glomerular efferent arteriole that takes place in order to maintain glomerular perfusion pressure distal to a renal artery stenosis and in renal hypoperfusion (see Fig. 17.1, p. 465). Monitoring of renal function before and after initiation of therapy is essential.

17.65 Mechanisms and examples of drug-induced renal disease/dysfunction

Mechanism	Drug or toxin	Comments
Haemodynamic	NSAIDs	Reduced renal blood flow due to inhibition of prostaglandin synthesis
	ACE inhibitors	Reduce efferent glomerular arteriolar tone. Toxic in the presence of renal artery stenosis and other conditions of renal hypoperfusion
	Radiographic contrast media	Multifactorial aetiology may include intense vasoconstriction
Acute tubular necrosis	Aminoglycosides, amphotericin	In most examples, there is evidence of direct tubular toxicity but haemodynamic and other factors probably contribute
	Paracetamol overdose	May occur with or without serious hepatotoxicity
	Radiographic contrast media	May be secondary to precipitation in tubules. Furosemide is a co-factor
Loss of tubular/collecting duct function	Lithium	Dose-related, partially reversible loss of concentrating ability.
	Cisplatin	Occurs at lower exposures than cause acute tubular necrosis
	Aminoglycosides, amphotericin	
Glomerulonephritis (immune-mediated)	Penicillamine, gold	Membranous nephropathy
	Penicillamine	Crescentic or focal necrotising glomerulonephritis in association with ANCA and systemic small-vessel vasculitis
	NSAIDs	Minimal change nephropathy
Interstitial nephritis (immune-mediated)	NSAIDs, penicillins, proton pump inhibitors, many others	Acute interstitial nephritis
Interstitial nephritis (toxicity)	Lithium	As a consequence of acute toxicity. Otherwise controversial
	Ciclosporin, tacrolimus	The major problem with these drugs
Interstitial nephritis (with papillary necrosis)	Various NSAIDs (p. 505)	Ischaemic damage secondary to NSAID effects on renal blood flow
Tubular obstruction (crystal formation)	Aciclovir	Crystals of the drug form in tubules. Aciclovir is now more common than the original example of sulphonamides
	Chemotherapy	Uric acid crystals form as a consequence of tumour lysis (typically, a first-dose effect in haematological malignancy)
Nephrocalcinosis	Oral sodium phosphate-containing bowel cleansing agents	Precipitation of calcium phosphate occurring in 1–4% and exacerbated by volume depletion. Usually mild but damage can be irreversible
Retroperitoneal fibrosis	Ergolinic dopamine agonists (cabergoline), methysergide*, practolol*	Idiopathic is more common (p. 511)

*These drugs are no longer in use in the UK.

Prescribing in renal disease

Many drugs and drug metabolites are excreted by the kidney and so the presence of renal impairment alters the required dose and frequency (p. 36).

Further information and acknowledgements

Websites

www.edren.org *Renal Unit, Royal Infirmary of Edinburgh; information about individual diseases, protocols for immediate in-hospital management and more.*

www.edrep.org/resources *Educational resources.*

www.nephron.com *The links under 'Physicians' include useful urology pages, eGFR and other calculators, and other resources.*

www.renal.org/ckd *UK Renal Association; current UK guidelines on the detection, referral and management of chronic kidney disease.*

www.uroweb.org/guidelines *European Association of Urology guidelines. Current European guidelines on the management of all common urological conditions.*

Figure acknowledgements

Page 463 inset (Dipstick): Pitkin J, Peattie AB, Magowan BA. Obstetrics and Gynaecology: An Illustrated Colour Text. Edinburgh: Churchill Livingstone; 2003.

Fig. 17.19 Beutler JJ, Koomans HA. Malignant hypertension: still a challenge. Nephrol Dial Transplant 1977; 12:2019–2023; photograph courtesy of Prof PJ Slootweg, University Hospital, Utrecht. By permission of Oxford University Press.

17

D.E. Newby
N.R. Grubb
A. Bradbury

Cardiovascular disease 18

Clinical examination of the cardiovascular system 526

Functional anatomy and physiology 528
- Anatomy 528
- Physiology 530

Investigation of cardiovascular disease 532
- Electrocardiogram 532
- Cardiac biomarkers 535
- Chest X-ray 535
- Echocardiography (echo) 536
- Computed tomographic imaging 537
- Magnetic resonance imaging 537
- Cardiac catheterisation 538
- Electrophysiology study 539
- Radionuclide imaging 539

Presenting problems in cardiovascular disease 539
- Chest pain 539
- Breathlessness (dyspnoea) 543
- Acute circulatory failure (cardiogenic shock) 544
- Heart failure 546
- Syncope and presyncope 554
- Palpitation 556
- Cardiac arrest and sudden cardiac death 557
- Abnormal heart sounds and murmurs 560

Disorders of heart rate, rhythm and conduction 562
- Sinoatrial nodal rhythms 563
- Atrial tachyarrhythmias 564
- 'Supraventricular' tachycardias 567
- Ventricular tachyarrhythmias 569
- Atrioventricular and bundle branch block 571
- Anti-arrhythmic drug therapy 573
- Therapeutic procedures 577

Atherosclerosis 579

Coronary artery disease 583
- Stable angina 583
- Acute coronary syndrome 589
- Cardiac risk of non-cardiac surgery 600

Vascular disease 600
- Peripheral arterial disease 600
- Diseases of the aorta 603
- Hypertension 607

Diseases of the heart valves 613
- Rheumatic heart disease 614
- Mitral valve disease 616
- Aortic valve disease 620
- Tricuspid valve disease 624
- Pulmonary valve disease 625
- Infective endocarditis 625
- Valve replacement surgery 629

Congenital heart disease 629

Diseases of the myocardium 636
- Myocarditis 636
- Cardiomyopathy 636
- Specific diseases of heart muscle 638
- Cardiac tumours 639

Diseases of the pericardium 639

CLINICAL EXAMINATION OF THE CARDIOVASCULAR SYSTEM

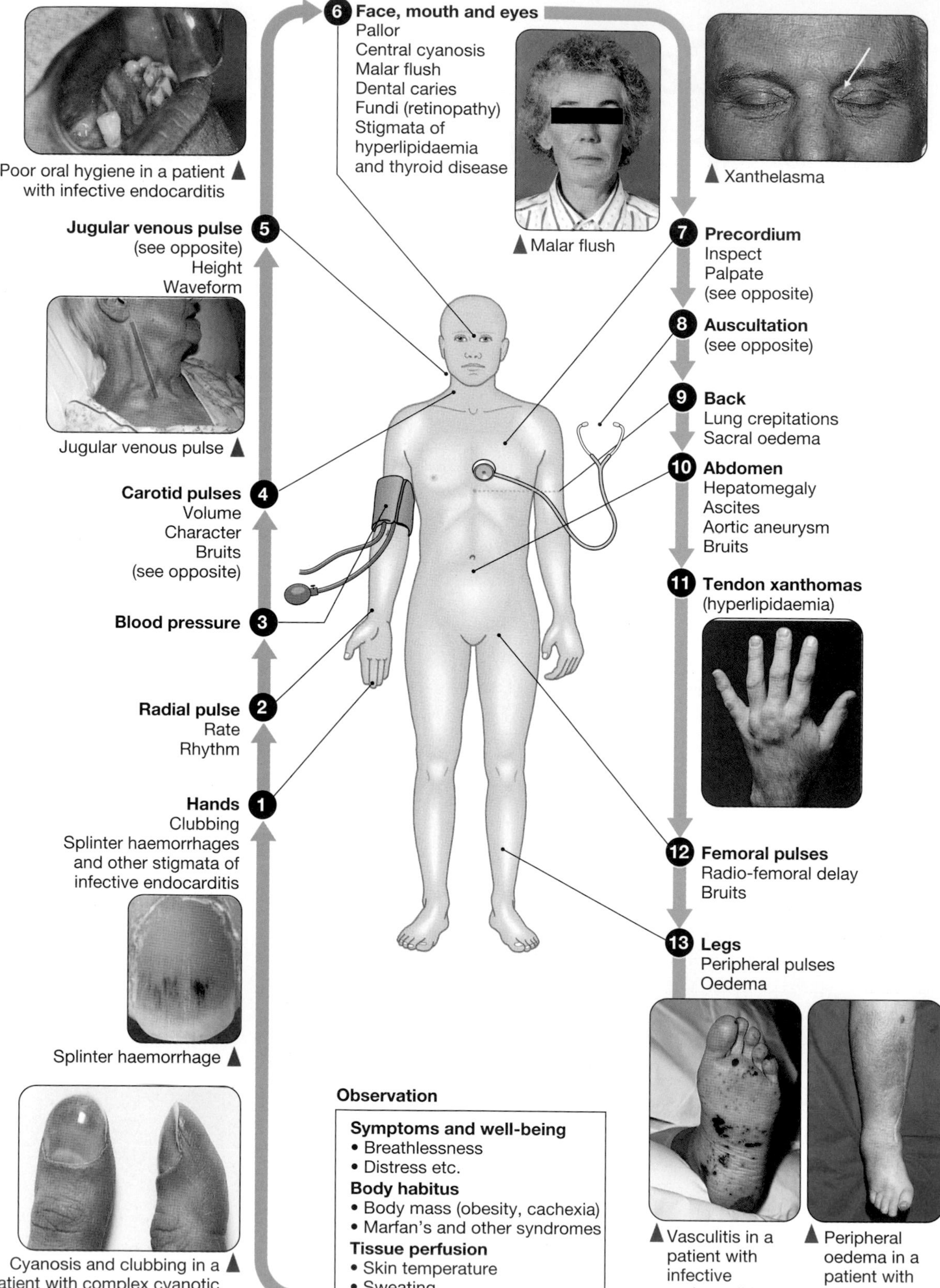

Insets (Splinter haemorrhage, jugular venous pulse, malar flush, tendon xanthomas) From Newby and Grubb 2005 – see p. 641.

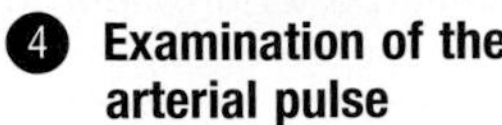

4 Examination of the arterial pulse

- The character of the pulse is determined by stroke volume and arterial compliance, and is best assessed by palpating a major artery, such as the carotid or brachial artery.
- Aortic regurgitation, anaemia, sepsis and other causes of a large stroke volume typically produce a bounding pulse with a high amplitude and wide pulse pressure (panel A).
- Aortic stenosis impedes ventricular emptying and may cause a slow-rising, weak and delayed pulse (panel A).
- Normal sinus rhythm produces a pulse that is regular in time and force. Arrhythmias may cause irregularity. Atrial fibrillation produces a pulse that is irregular in time and volume (panel B).

A

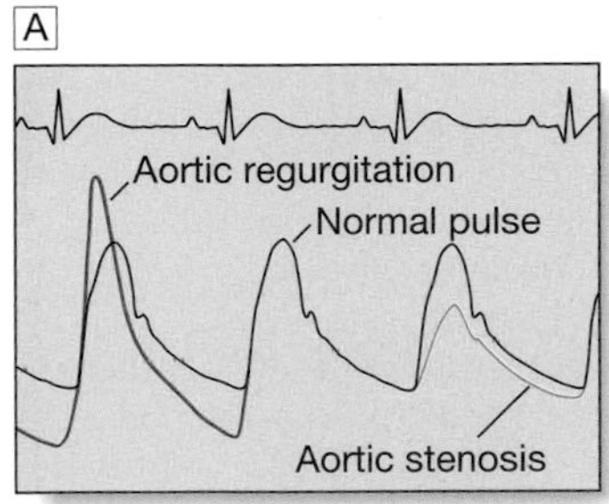

B

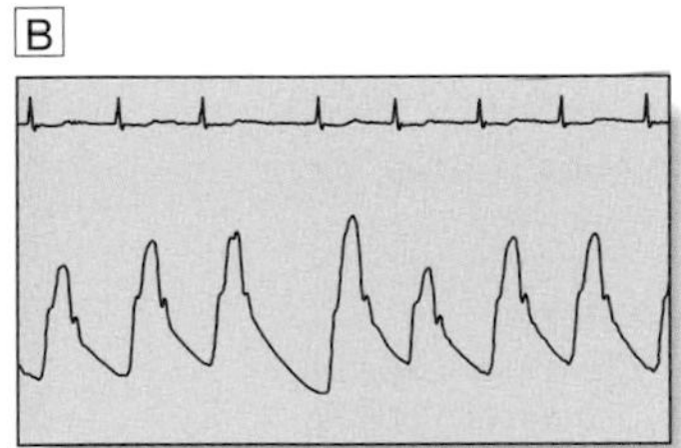

Waveform of the arterial pulse.
A Aortic regurgitation (red line) and stenosis (blue line). B Atrial fibrillation.

5 Examination of the jugular venous pulse

The internal jugular vein, superior vena cava and right atrium are in continuity, so the height of the jugular venous pulsation reflects right atrial pressure. When the patient is placed at 45°, with the head supported and turned a few degrees to the left, the jugular venous pulse is visible along the line of the sternocleidomastoid muscle (see opposite).

- The height of the jugular venous pulse is determined by right atrial pressure and is therefore elevated in right heart failure and reduced in hypovolaemia.
- If the jugular venous pulse is not easily seen, it may be highlighted by gentle pressure on the abdomen.
- In normal sinus rhythm, the two venous peaks, the *a* and *v* waves, approximate to atrial and ventricular systole respectively.
- The *x* descent reflects atrial relaxation and apical displacement of the tricuspid valve ring. The *y* descent reflects atrial emptying early In diastole. These signs are subtle.
- Tricuspid regurgitation produces giant *v* waves that coincide with ventricular systole.

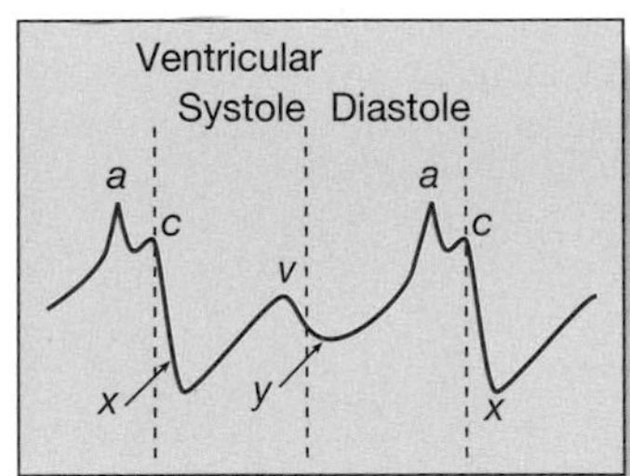

Waveform of the jugular venous pulse.

Distinguishing venous/arterial pulsation in the neck

- Venous pulse has two peaks in each cardiac cycle; the arterial pulse has one peak.
- The height of the venous pulse varies with respiration (falls on inspiration) and position.
- Abdominal compression causes the venous pulse to rise.
- Venous pulse is not palpable and can be occluded by light pressure.

7 Palpation of the precordium

Technique

- Place fingertips over apex (1) to assess for position and character. Place heel of hand over left sternal edge (2) for a parasternal heave or 'lift'. Assess for the presence of thrills in all areas, including the aortic and pulmonary areas (3).

Common abnormalities of the apex beat

- Volume overload, such as mitral or aortic regurgitation: displaced, forceful
- Pressure overload, such as aortic stenosis, hypertension: discrete, thrusting
- Dyskinetic, such as left ventricular aneurysm: displaced, incoordinate

Other abnormalities

- Palpable S1 (tapping apex beat: mitral stenosis)
- Palpable P2 (severe pulmonary hypertension)
- Left parasternal heave or 'lift' felt by heel of hand (right ventricular hypertrophy)
- Palpable thrill (aortic stenosis)

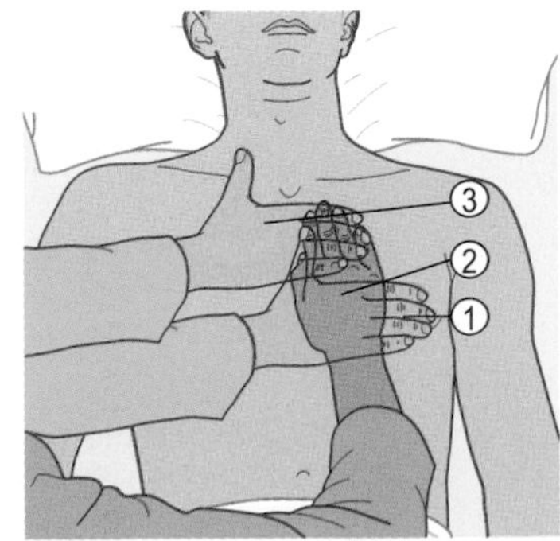

Palpation of the precordium.

8 Auscultation of the heart

- Use the diaphragm to examine at the apex, lower left sternal edge (tricuspid area) and upper left (pulmonary area) and right (aortic area) sternal edges.
- Use the bell to examine low-pitched noises, particularly at the apex for mid-diastolic murmurs.
- Time the sounds and murmurs by feeling the carotid pulse; systolic murmurs are synchronous with the pulse.
- Listen for radiation of systolic murmurs, over the base of the neck (aortic stenosis) and in the axilla (mitral incompetence).
- Listen over the left sternal border with the patient sitting forward (aortic incompetence), then at the apex with the patient rolled on to the left side (mitral stenosis).

The haemodynamic effects of respiration are discussed on page 532.
See page 560 for analysis and interpretation of heart sounds and murmurs.

Cardiovascular disease is the most frequent cause of adult death in the Western world; in the UK, one-third of men and one-quarter of women will die as a result of ischaemic heart disease. In many developed countries, the incidence of ischaemic heart disease has been falling for the last two or three decades, but it is rising in Eastern Europe and Asia. Cardiovascular disease may thus soon become the leading cause of death on all continents. Strategies for the treatment and prevention of heart disease can be highly effective and have been subjected to rigorous evaluation. The evidence base for the treatment of cardiovascular disease is stronger than for almost any other disease group.

Valvular heart disease is common, but the aetiology varies in different parts of the world. On the Indian subcontinent and in Africa, it is predominantly due to rheumatic fever, whereas calcific aortic valve disease is the most common problem in developed countries.

Prompt recognition of the development of heart disease is limited by two key factors. Firstly, it is often latent; coronary artery disease can proceed to an advanced stage before the patient notices any symptoms. Secondly, the diversity of symptoms attributable to heart disease is limited, so different pathologies may frequently present with the same symptoms.

FUNCTIONAL ANATOMY AND PHYSIOLOGY

Anatomy

The heart acts as two serial pumps that share several electrical and mechanical components. The right heart circulates blood to the lungs where it is oxygenated, and the left heart receives this and circulates it to the rest of the body (Fig. 18.1). The atria are thin-walled structures that act as priming pumps for the ventricles, which provide most of the energy to the circulation. Within the mediastinum, the atria are situated posteriorly and the left atrium (LA) sits anterior to the oesophagus and descending aorta. The interatrial septum separates the two atria. In 20% of adults, a patent foramen ovale is found; this communication in the fetal circulation between the right and left atria normally closes at birth (p. 629). The right atrium (RA) receives blood from the superior and inferior venae cavae and the coronary sinus. The LA receives blood from four pulmonary veins, two from each of the left and right lungs. The ventricles are thick-walled structures, adapted to circulating blood through large vascular beds under pressure. The atria and ventricles are separated by the annulus fibrosus, which forms the skeleton for the atrioventricular (AV) valves and which electrically insulates the atria from the ventricles. The right ventricle (RV) is roughly triangular in shape and extends from the annulus fibrosus to near the cardiac apex, which is situated to the left of the midline. Its anterosuperior surface is rounded and convex, and its posterior extent is bounded by the interventricular septum, which bulges into the chamber. Its upper extent is conical, forming the conus arteriosus or outflow tract, from which the pulmonary artery arises. The RV sits anterior to, and to the right of, the left ventricle (LV). The LV is more conical in shape and in cross-section is nearly circular. It extends from the LA to the apex of the heart. The LV myocardium is normally around 10 mm thick (c.f. RV thickness of 2–3 mm) because it pumps blood at a higher pressure.

The normal heart occupies less than 50% of the transthoracic diameter in the frontal plane, as seen on a chest X-ray. On the patient's left, the cardiac silhouette is formed by the aortic arch, the pulmonary trunk, the left atrial appendage and the LV. On the right, the RA is joined by superior and inferior venae cavae, and the lower right border is made up by the RV (Fig. 18.2). In disease states or congenital cardiac abnormalities, the

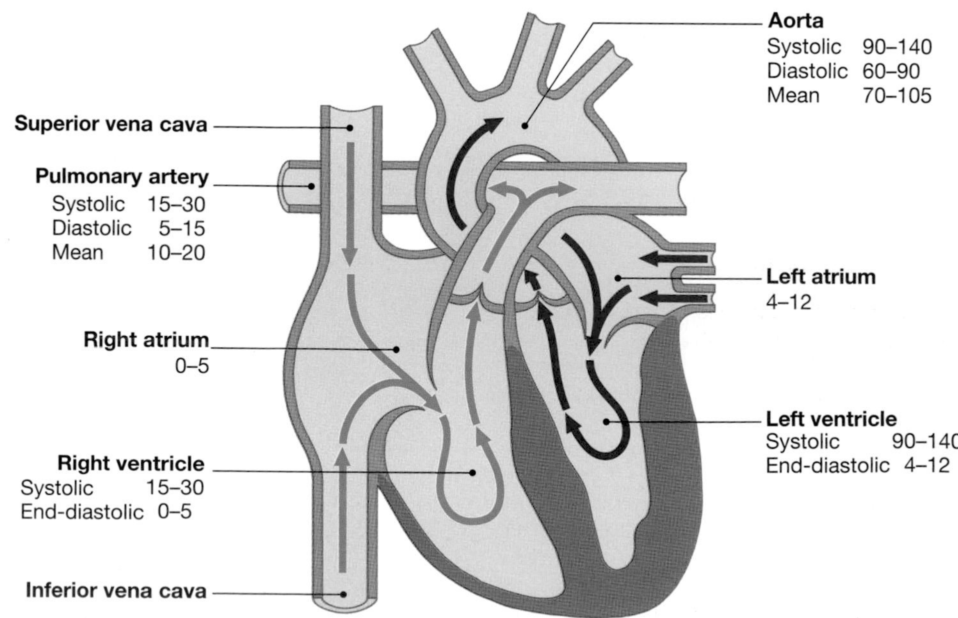

Fig. 18.1 Direction of blood flow through the heart. The blue arrows show deoxygenated blood moving through the right heart to the lungs. The red arrows show oxygenated blood moving from the lungs to the systemic circulation. The normal pressures are shown for each chamber in mmHg.

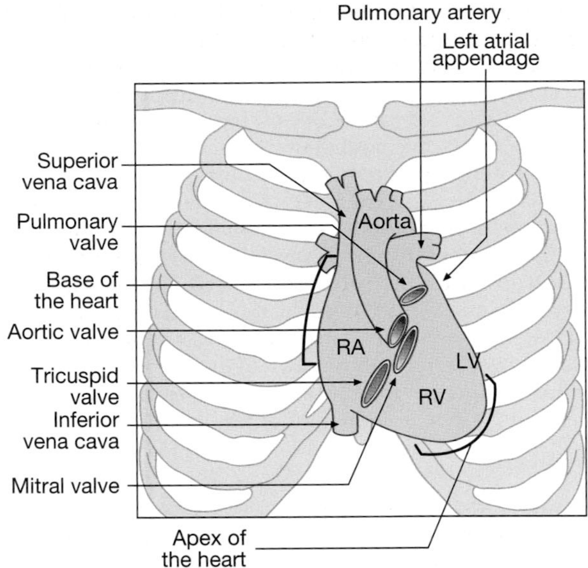

Fig. 18.2 Surface anatomy of the heart. The positions of the major cardiac chambers and heart valves are shown.

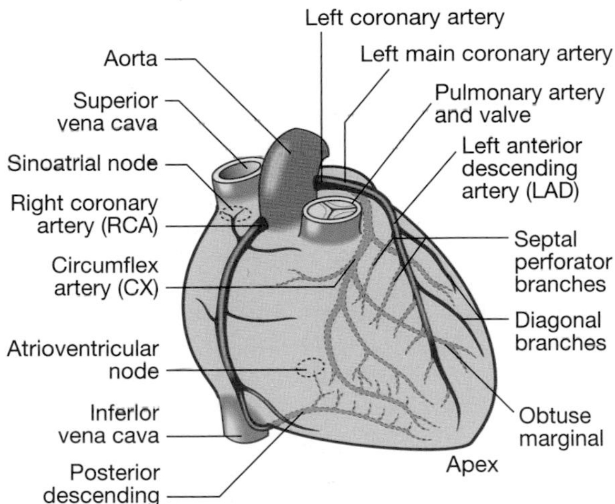

Fig. 18.3 The coronary arteries. Diagram of the anterior view.

silhouette may change as a result of hypertrophy or dilatation.

The coronary circulation

The left main and right coronary arteries arise from the left and right sinuses of the aortic root, distal to the aortic valve (Fig. 18.3). Within 2.5 cm of its origin, the left main coronary artery divides into the left anterior descending artery (LAD), which runs in the anterior interventricular groove, and the left circumflex artery (CX), which runs posteriorly in the atrioventricular groove. The LAD gives branches to supply the anterior part of the septum (septal perforators) and the anterior, lateral and apical walls of the LV. The CX gives marginal branches that supply the lateral, posterior and inferior segments of the LV. The right coronary artery (RCA) runs in the right atrioventricular groove, giving branches that supply the RA, RV and inferoposterior aspects of the LV. The posterior descending artery runs in the posterior interventricular groove and supplies the inferior part of the interventricular septum. This vessel is a branch of the RCA in approximately 90% of people (dominant right system) and is supplied by the CX in the remainder (dominant left system). The coronary anatomy varies greatly from person to person and there are many 'normal variants'.

The RCA supplies the sinoatrial (SA) node in about 60% of individuals and the AV node in about 90%. Proximal occlusion of the RCA therefore often results in sinus bradycardia and may also cause AV nodal block. Abrupt occlusions in the RCA, due to coronary thrombosis, result in infarction of the inferior part of the LV and often the RV. Abrupt occlusion of the LAD or CX causes infarction in the corresponding territory of the LV, and occlusion of the left main coronary artery is usually fatal.

The venous system follows the coronary arteries but drains into the coronary sinus in the atrioventricular groove, and then to the RA. An extensive lymphatic system drains into vessels that travel with the coronary vessels and then into the thoracic duct.

Conducting system of the heart

The SA node is situated at the junction of the superior vena cava and RA (Fig. 18.4). It comprises specialised atrial cells that depolarise at a rate influenced by the autonomic nervous system and by circulating catecholamines. During normal (sinus) rhythm, this depolarisation wave propagates through both atria via sheets of atrial myocytes. The annulus fibrosus forms a conduction barrier between atria and ventricles, and the only pathway through it is the AV node. This is a midline structure, extending from the right side of the interatrial septum, penetrating the annulus fibrosus anteriorly. The AV node conducts relatively slowly, producing a necessary time delay between atrial and ventricular contraction. The His–Purkinje system is comprised of the bundle of His extending from the AV node into the interventricular septum, the right and left bundle branches passing along the ventricular septum and into the respective ventricles, the anterior and posterior fascicles

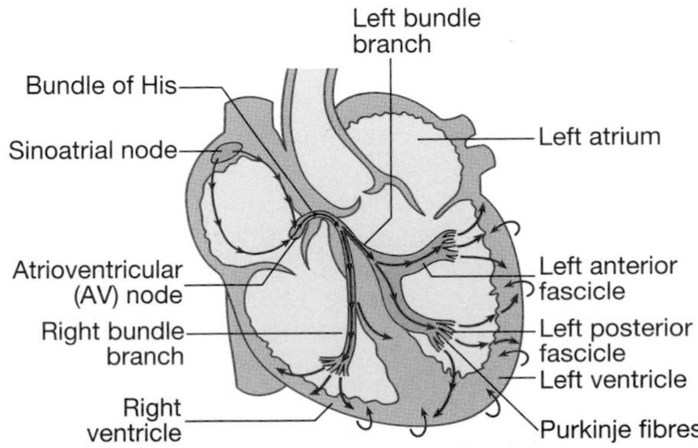

Fig. 18.4 The cardiac conduction system. Depolarisation starts in the sinoatrial node and spreads through the atria (blue arrows), and then through the atrioventricular node (black arrows). Depolarisation then spreads through the bundle of His and the bundle branches to reach the ventricular muscle (red arrows). Repolarisation spreads from epicardium to endocardium (green arrows).

of the left bundle branch, and the smaller Purkinje fibres that ramify through the ventricular myocardium. The tissues of the His–Purkinje system conduct very rapidly and allow near-simultaneous depolarisation of the entire ventricular myocardium.

Nerve supply of the heart

The heart is innervated by both sympathetic and parasympathetic fibres. Adrenergic nerves from the cervical sympathetic chain supply muscle fibres in the atria and ventricles and the electrical conducting system. Positive inotropic and chronotropic effects are mediated by β_1-adrenoceptors, whereas β_2-adrenoceptors predominate in vascular smooth muscle and mediate vasodilatation. Parasympathetic pre-ganglionic fibres and sensory fibres reach the heart through the vagus nerves. Cholinergic nerves supply the AV and SA nodes via muscarinic (M2) receptors. Under resting conditions, vagal inhibitory activity predominates and the heart rate is slow. Adrenergic stimulation, associated with exercise, emotional stress, fever and so on, causes the heart rate to increase. In disease states, the nerve supply to the heart may be affected. For example, in heart failure the sympathetic system may be up-regulated, and in diabetes mellitus the nerves themselves may be damaged (autonomic neuropathy, p. 831) so that there is little variation in heart rate.

Physiology

The circulation

The RA receives deoxygenated blood from the superior and inferior venae cavae and discharges blood to the RV, which in turn pumps it into the pulmonary artery. Blood passes through the pulmonary arterial and alveolar capillary bed, where it is oxygenated, then drains via four pulmonary veins into the LA. This, in turn, fills the LV, which delivers blood into the aorta (see Fig. 18.1). During ventricular contraction (systole), the tricuspid valve in the right heart and the mitral valve in the left heart close, and the pulmonary and aortic valves open. In diastole, the pulmonary and aortic valves close, and the two AV valves open. Collectively, these atrial and ventricular events constitute the cardiac cycle of filling and ejection of blood from one heartbeat to the next.

Myocardial contraction

Myocardial cells (myocytes) are about 50–100 µm long; each cell branches and interdigitates with adjacent cells. An intercalated disc permits electrical conduction via gap junctions, and mechanical conduction via the fascia adherens, to adjacent cells (Fig. 18.5A). The basic unit of contraction is the sarcomere (2 µm long), which is aligned to those of adjacent myofibrils, giving a striated appearance due to the Z-lines (Fig. 18.5B and C). Actin filaments are attached at right angles to the Z-lines and interdigitate with thicker parallel myosin filaments. The cross-links between actin and myosin molecules contain myofibrillar adenosine triphosphatase (ATPase), which breaks down adenosine triphosphate (ATP) to provide the energy for contraction (Fig. 18.5E). Two chains of actin molecules form a helical structure, with a second molecule, tropomyosin, in the grooves of the actin helix, and a further molecule complex, troponin, attached to every seventh actin molecule (Fig. 18.5D).

During the plateau phase of the action potential, calcium ions enter the cell and are mobilised from the sarcoplasmic reticulum. They bind to troponin and thereby precipitate contraction by shortening of the sarcomere through the interdigitation of the actin and myosin molecules. The force of cardiac muscle contraction, or inotropic state, is regulated by the influx of calcium ions through 'slow calcium channels'. The extent to which the sarcomere can shorten determines stroke volume of the ventricle. It is maximally shortened in response to powerful inotropic drugs or marked exercise. However, the enlargement of the heart seen in heart failure is due to slippage of the myofibrils and adjacent cells rather than lengthening of the sarcomere.

Cardiac output

Cardiac output is the product of stroke volume and heart rate. Stroke volume is the volume of blood ejected in each cardiac cycle (see Fig. 18.36, p. 561), and is dependent upon end-diastolic volume and pressure (preload), myocardial contractility and systolic aortic pressure (afterload). Stretch of cardiac muscle (from increased end-diastolic volume) causes an increase in the force of contraction, producing a greater stroke volume: Starling's Law of the heart (see Fig. 18.22, p. 547).

The contractile state of the myocardium is controlled by neuro-endocrine factors, such as adrenaline (epinephrine), and can be influenced by inotropic drugs and their antagonists. The response to a physiological change or to a drug can be predicted on the basis of its combined influence on preload, afterload and contractility (see Fig. 18.26, p. 551).

Blood flow

Blood passes from the heart through the large central elastic arteries into muscular arteries before encountering the resistance vessels, and ultimately the capillary bed, where there is exchange of nutrients, oxygen and waste products of metabolism. The central arteries, such as the aorta, are predominantly composed of elastic tissue with little or no vascular smooth muscle cells. When blood is ejected from the heart, the compliant aorta expands to accommodate the volume of blood before the elastic recoil sustains blood pressure (BP) and flow following cessation of cardiac contraction. This 'Windkessel effect' prevents excessive rises in systolic BP whilst sustaining diastolic BP, thereby reducing cardiac afterload and maintaining coronary perfusion. These benefits are lost with progressive arterial stiffening: a feature of ageing and advanced renal disease.

Passing down the arterial tree, vascular smooth muscle cells progressively play a greater role until the resistance arterioles are encountered. Although all vessels contribute, the resistance vessels (diameter 50–200 µm) provide the greatest contribution to systemic vascular resistance, with small changes in radius having a marked influence on blood flow; resistance is proportional to the fourth power of the radius (Poiseuille's Law). The tone of these resistance vessels is tightly regulated by humoral, neuronal and mechanical factors. Neurogenic constriction operates via α-adrenoceptors on vascular smooth muscle, and dilatation

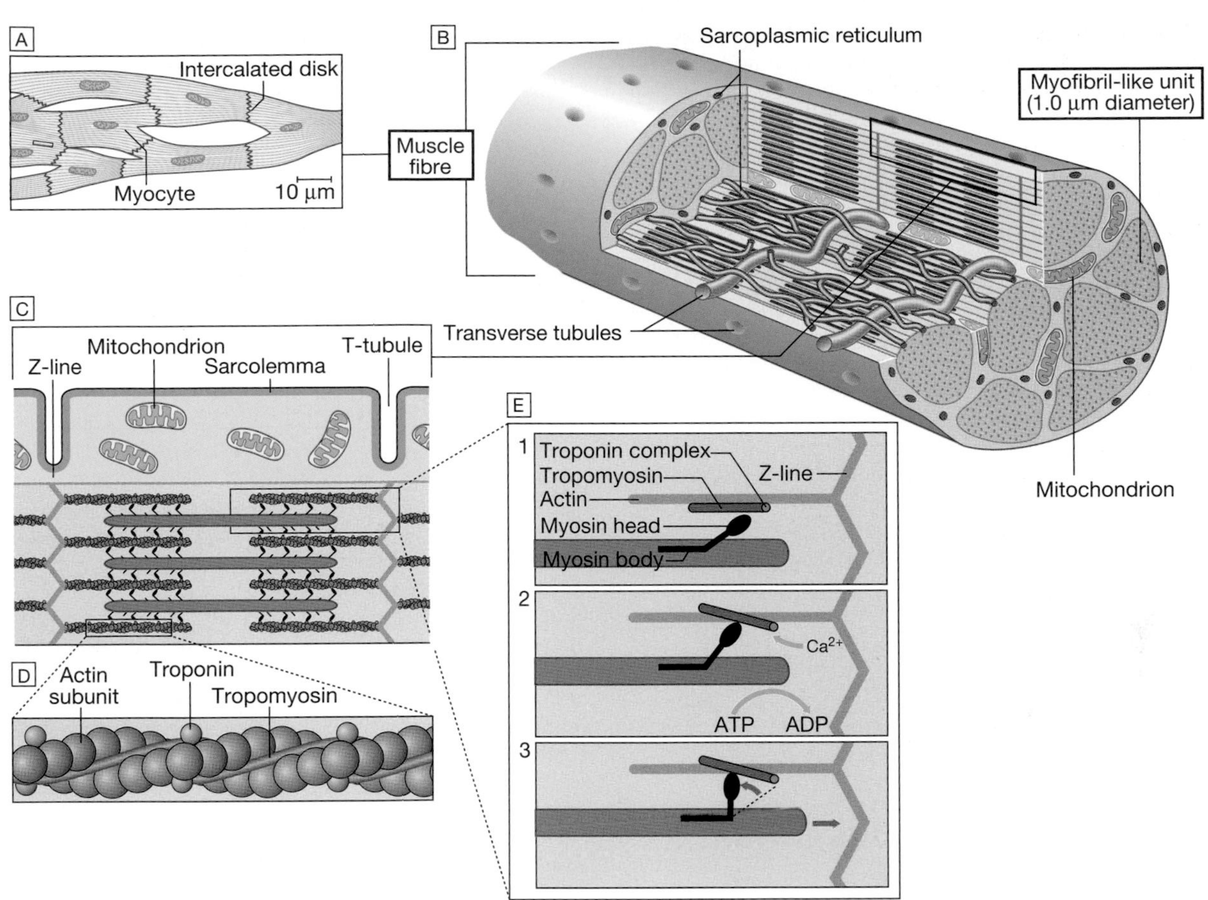

Fig. 18.5 Schematic of myocytes and the contraction process within a muscle fibre. **A** Myocytes are joined together through intercalated discs. **B** Within the myocytes, myofibrils are composed of longitudinal and transverse tubules extending from the sarcoplasmic reticulum. **C** The expanded section shows a schematic of an individual sarcomere with thick filaments composed of myosin and thin filaments composed primarily of actin. **D** Actin filaments are composed of troponin, tropomyosin and actin subunits. **E** The three stages of contraction, resulting in shortening of the sarcomere. (1) The actin-binding site is blocked by tropomyosin. (2) ATP-dependent release of calcium ions, which bind to troponin, displacing tropomyosin. The binding site is exposed. (3) Tilting of the angle of attachment of the myosin head, resulting in fibre shortening. (ADP = adenosine diphosphate; ATP = adenosine triphosphate)

via muscarinic and β_2-adrenoceptors. In addition, systemic and locally released vasoactive substances influence tone; vasoconstrictors include noradrenaline (norepinephrine), angiotensin II and endothelin-1, whereas adenosine, bradykinin, prostaglandins and nitric oxide are vasodilators. Resistance to blood flow rises with viscosity and is mainly influenced by red cell concentration (haematocrit).

Coronary blood vessels receive sympathetic and parasympathetic innervation. Stimulation of α-adrenoceptors causes vasoconstriction; stimulation of β_2-adrenoceptors causes vasodilatation; the predominant effect of sympathetic stimulation in coronary arteries is vasodilatation. Parasympathetic stimulation also causes modest dilatation of normal coronary arteries. As a result of vascular regulation, an atheromatous narrowing (stenosis) in a coronary artery does not limit flow, even during exercise, until the cross-sectional area of the vessel is reduced by at least 70%.

Endothelial function

The endothelium plays a vital role in the control of vascular homeostasis. It synthesises and releases many vasoactive mediators that cause vasodilatation, including nitric oxide, prostacyclin and endothelium-derived hyperpolarising factor, and vasoconstriction, including endothelin-1 and angiotensin II. A balance exists whereby the release of such factors contributes to the maintenance and regulation of vascular tone and BP. Damage to the endothelium may disrupt this balance and lead to vascular dysfunction, tissue ischaemia and hypertension.

The endothelium also has a major influence on key regulatory steps in the recruitment of inflammatory cells and on the formation and dissolution of thrombus. Once activated, the endothelium expresses surface receptors such as E-selectin, intercellular adhesion molecule type 1 (ICAM-1) and platelet endothelial cell adhesion molecule type 1 (PECAM-1), which mediate rolling, adhesion and migration of inflammatory leucocytes into the subintima. The endothelium also stores and releases the multimeric glycoprotein, von Willebrand factor, which promotes thrombus formation by linking platelet adhesion to denuded surfaces, especially in the arterial vasculature. In contrast, once intravascular thrombus forms, tissue plasminogen activator is rapidly released from a dynamic storage pool within the endothelium to induce fibrinolysis and thrombus dissolution. These processes are critically involved in the development and progression of atherosclerosis, and endothelial function and injury are seen as central to the pathogenesis of many cardiovascular disease states.

Effects of respiration

There is a fall in intrathoracic pressure during inspiration that tends to promote venous flow into the chest, producing an increase in the flow of blood through the right heart. However, a substantial volume of blood is sequestered in the chest as the lungs expand; the increase in the capacitance of the pulmonary vascular bed usually exceeds any increase in the output of the right heart and therefore there is a reduction in the flow of blood into the left heart during inspiration. In contrast, expiration is accompanied by a fall in venous return to the right heart, a reduction in the output of the right heart, a rise in the venous return to the left heart (as blood is squeezed out of the lungs) and an increase in the output of the left heart (Box 18.1).

18.1 Haemodynamic effects of respiration

	Inspiration	Expiration
Jugular venous pressure	Falls	Rises
Blood pressure	Falls (up to 10 mmHg)	Rises
Heart rate	Accelerates	Slows
Second heart sound	Splits*	Fuses*

*Inspiration prolongs RV ejection, delaying P_2, and shortens LV ejection, bringing forward A_2; expiration produces the opposite effects.

Pulsus paradoxus

This term is used to describe the exaggerated fall in BP during inspiration that is characteristic of cardiac tamponade (pp. 545 and 640) and severe airways obstruction. In airways obstruction, it is due to accentuation of the change in intrathoracic pressure with respiration. In cardiac tamponade, compression of the right heart prevents the normal increase in flow through the right heart on inspiration, which exaggerates the usual drop in venous return to the left heart and produces a marked fall in BP (> 10 mmHg fall during inspiration).

INVESTIGATION OF CARDIOVASCULAR DISEASE

Specific investigations may be required to confirm a diagnosis of cardiac disease. Basic tests, such as electrocardiography, chest X-ray and echocardiography, can be performed in an outpatient clinic or at the bedside. Procedures such as cardiac catheterisation, radionuclide imaging, computed tomography (CT) and magnetic resonance imaging (MRI) require specialised facilities.

Electrocardiogram

The electrocardiogram (ECG) is used to assess cardiac rhythm and conduction. It provides information about

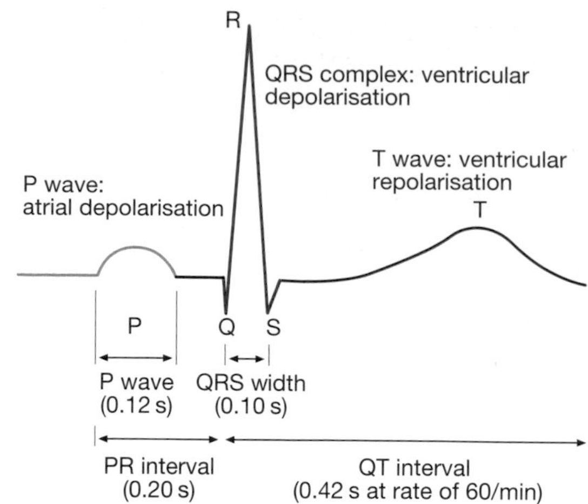

Fig. 18.6 The electrocardiograph. The components correspond to depolarisation and repolarisation, as depicted in Figure 18.4. The upper limit of the normal range for each interval is given in brackets.

chamber size and is the main test used to assess for myocardial ischaemia and infarction.

The basis of an ECG recording is that the electrical depolarisation of myocardial tissue produces a small dipole current which can be detected by electrode pairs on the body surface. These signals are amplified and either printed or displayed on a monitor (Fig. 18.6). During sinus rhythm, the SA node triggers atrial depolarisation, producing a P wave. Depolarisation proceeds slowly through the AV node, which is too small to produce a depolarisation wave detectable from the body surface. The bundle of His, bundle branches and Purkinje system are then activated, initiating ventricular myocardial depolarisation, which produces the QRS complex. The muscle mass of the ventricles is much larger than that of the atria, so the QRS complex is larger than the P wave. The interval between the onset of the P wave and the onset of the QRS complex is termed the 'PR interval' and largely reflects the duration of AV nodal conduction. Injury to the left or right bundle branch delays ventricular depolarisation, widening the QRS complex. Selective injury of one of the left fascicles (hemiblock, p. 573) affects the electrical axis. Repolarisation is slower and spreads from the epicardium to the endocardium. Atrial repolarisation does not cause a detectable signal but ventricular repolarisation produces the T wave. The QT interval represents the total duration of ventricular depolarisation and repolarisation.

The standard 12-lead ECG

The 12-lead ECG (Box 18.2) is generated from ten physical electrodes that are attached to the skin. One electrode is attached to each limb and six electrodes are attached to the chest. In addition, the left arm, right arm and left leg electrodes are attached to a central terminal acting as an additional virtual electrode in the centre of the chest (the right leg electrode acts as an earthing electrode). The twelve 'leads' of the ECG refer to recordings made from pairs or sets of these electrodes. They comprise three groups: three dipole limb leads, three augmented voltage limb leads and six unipole chest leads.

Leads I, II and III are the dipole limb leads and refer to recordings obtained from pairs of limb electrodes.

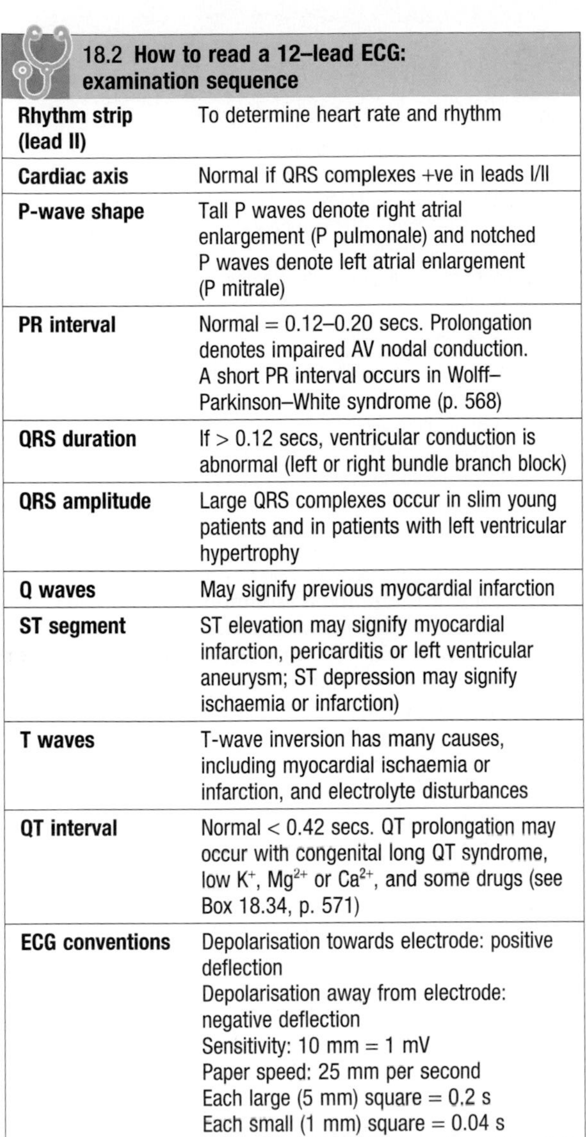

18.2 How to read a 12-lead ECG: examination sequence

Rhythm strip (lead II)	To determine heart rate and rhythm
Cardiac axis	Normal if QRS complexes +ve in leads I/II
P-wave shape	Tall P waves denote right atrial enlargement (P pulmonale) and notched P waves denote left atrial enlargement (P mitrale)
PR interval	Normal = 0.12–0.20 secs. Prolongation denotes impaired AV nodal conduction. A short PR interval occurs in Wolff–Parkinson–White syndrome (p. 568)
QRS duration	If > 0.12 secs, ventricular conduction is abnormal (left or right bundle branch block)
QRS amplitude	Large QRS complexes occur in slim young patients and in patients with left ventricular hypertrophy
Q waves	May signify previous myocardial infarction
ST segment	ST elevation may signify myocardial infarction, pericarditis or left ventricular aneurysm; ST depression may signify ischaemia or infarction)
T waves	T-wave inversion has many causes, including myocardial ischaemia or infarction, and electrolyte disturbances
QT interval	Normal < 0.42 secs. QT prolongation may occur with congenital long QT syndrome, low K^+, Mg^{2+} or Ca^{2+}, and some drugs (see Box 18.34, p. 571)
ECG conventions	Depolarisation towards electrode: positive deflection Depolarisation away from electrode: negative deflection Sensitivity: 10 mm = 1 mV Paper speed: 25 mm per second Each large (5 mm) square = 0.2 s Each small (1 mm) square = 0.04 s Heart rate = 1500/RR interval (mm) (i.e. 300 ÷ number of large squares between beats)

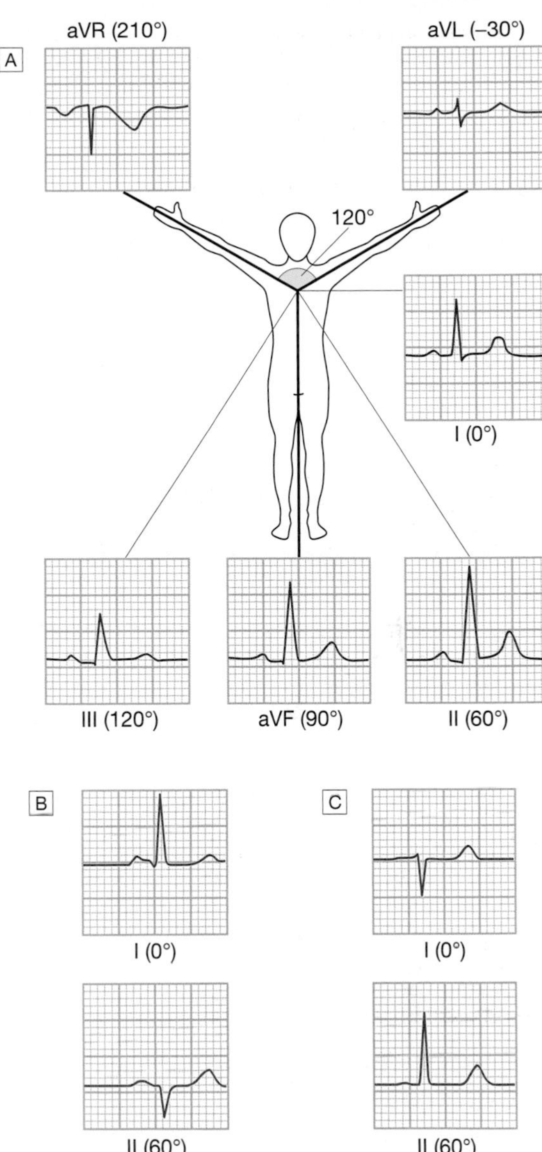

Fig. 18.7 The appearance of the ECG from different leads in the frontal plane. **A** Normal. **B** Left axis deviation, with negative deflection in lead II and positive in lead I. **C** Right axis deviation, with negative deflection in lead I and positive in lead II.

Lead I records the signal between the right (negative) and left (positive) arms. Lead II records the signal between the right arm (negative) and left leg (positive). Lead III records the signal between the left arm (negative) and left leg (positive). These three leads thus record electrical activity along three different axes in the frontal plane. Leads aVR, aVL and aVF are the augmented voltage limb leads. These record electrical activity between a limb electrode and a modified central terminal. For example, lead aVL records the signal between the left arm (positive) and a central (negative) terminal, formed by connecting the right arm and left leg electrodes (Fig. 18.7). Similarly augmented signals are obtained from the right arm (aVR) and left leg (aVF). These leads also record electrical activity in the frontal plane, with each lead 120° apart. Lead aVF thus examines activity along the axis +90°, and lead aVL along the axis –30°, and so on.

When depolarisation moves towards a positive electrode, it produces a positive deflection in the ECG; depolarisation in the opposite direction produces a negative deflection. The average vector of ventricular depolarisation is known as the frontal cardiac axis. When the vector is at right angles to a lead, the depolarisation in that lead is equally negative and positive (isoelectric). In Figure 18.7A, the QRS complex is isoelectric in aVL, negative in aVR and most strongly positive in lead II; the main vector or axis of depolarisation is therefore 60°. The normal cardiac axis lies between –30° and +90°. Examples of left and right axis deviation are shown in Figures 18.7B and C.

There are six chest leads, V_1–V_6, derived from electrodes placed on the anterior and lateral left side of the chest, over the heart. Each lead records the signal between the corresponding chest electrode (positive) and the central terminal (negative). Leads V_1 and V_2 lie approximately over the RV, V_3 and V_4 over the

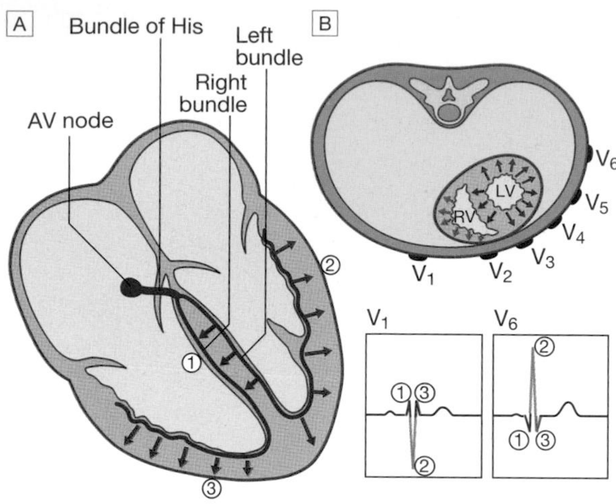

Fig. 18.8 The sequence of activation of the ventricles. **A** Activation of the septum occurs first (red arrows), followed by spreading of the impulse through the LV (blue arrows) and then the RV (green arrows). **B** Normal electrocardiographic complexes from leads V_1 and V_6.

interventricular septum, and V_5 and V_6 over the LV (Fig. 18.8). The LV has the greater muscle mass and contributes the major component of the QRS complex.

The shape of the QRS complex varies across the chest leads. Depolarisation of the interventricular septum occurs first and moves from left to right; this generates a small initial negative deflection in lead V_6 (Q wave) and an initial positive deflection in lead V_1 (R wave). The second phase of depolarisation is activation of the body of the LV, which creates a large positive deflection or R wave in V_6 (with reciprocal changes in V_1). The third and final phase involves the RV and produces a small negative deflection or S wave in V_6.

The ECG in ischaemia and infarction

When an area of the myocardium is ischaemic or undergoing infarction, repolarisation and depolarisation become abnormal relative to the surrounding myocardium. In transmural infarction, there is initial ST segment elevation (the current of injury) in the leads facing or overlying the infarct; Q waves (negative deflections) will then appear as the entire thickness of the myocardial wall becomes electrically neutral relative to the adjacent myocardium. The changes occurring in infarction are described in more detail on page 589, and shown in Figures 18.71–18.74 (pp. 592–593). In myocardial ischaemia, the ECG typically shows ST segment depression and/or T-wave inversion; it is usually the subendocardium that most readily becomes ischaemic. Other conditions, such as left ventricular hypertrophy and electrolyte disturbances, can cause similar ST and T-wave changes.

Exercise (stress) ECG

Exercise electrocardiography is used to detect myocardial ischaemia during physical stress and is helpful in the diagnosis of coronary artery disease. A 12-lead ECG is recorded during exercise on a treadmill or bicycle ergometer. The limb electrodes are placed on the shoulders and hips rather than the wrists and ankles. The

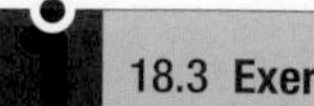

18.3 Exercise testing

Indications

- To confirm the diagnosis of angina
- To evaluate stable angina
- To assess prognosis following myocardial infarction
- To assess outcome after coronary revascularisation, e.g. coronary angioplasty
- To diagnose and evaluate the treatment of exercise-induced arrhythmias

High-risk findings

- Low threshold for ischaemia (i.e. within stage 1 or 2 of the Bruce Protocol)
- Fall in BP on exercise
- Widespread, marked or prolonged ischaemic ECG changes
- Exercise-induced arrhythmia

Bruce Protocol is the most commonly used for testing. BP is recorded and symptoms assessed throughout the test. Common indications for exercise testing are shown in Box 18.3. A test is 'positive' if anginal pain occurs, BP falls or fails to increase, or if there are ST segment shifts of more than 1 mm (see Fig. 18.64, p. 584). Exercise testing is useful in confirming the diagnosis in patients with suspected angina, and in such patients has good sensitivity and specificity (see Box 18.3). False-negative results can occur in patients with coronary artery disease, and some patients with a positive test will not have coronary disease (false-positive). It is an unreliable population screening tool because, in low-risk individuals (e.g. asymptomatic young or middle-aged women), an abnormal response is more likely to represent a false-positive than a true positive test.

Stress testing is contraindicated in the presence of acute coronary syndrome, decompensated heart failure and severe hypertension.

Ambulatory ECG

Continuous (ambulatory) ECG recordings can be obtained using a portable digital recorder. These devices usually provide limb lead ECG recordings only, and can record for between 1 and 7 days. Ambulatory ECG recording is principally used in the investigation of patients with suspected arrhythmia, such as those with intermittent palpitation, dizziness or syncope. For these patients, a 12-lead ECG provides only a snapshot of the cardiac rhythm and is unlikely to detect an intermittent arrhythmia, so a longer period of recording is useful (see Fig. 18.39, p. 563). These devices can also be used to assess rate control in patients with atrial fibrillation, and are sometimes used to detect transient myocardial ischaemia using ST segment analysis. For patients with more infrequent symptoms, small, patient-activated ECG recorders can be issued for several weeks until a symptom episode occurs. The patient places the device on the chest to record the rhythm during the episode. With some devices, the recording can be transmitted to hospital via telephone. Implantable 'loop recorders' resemble a leadless pacemaker and are implanted subcutaneously. They have a lifespan of 1–3 years and are used to investigate patients with infrequent but potentially serious symptoms, such as syncope.

Cardiac biomarkers

Plasma or serum biomarkers can be measured to assess myocardial dysfunction and ischaemia.

Brain natriuretic peptide

This is a 32-amino acid peptide and is secreted by the LV along with an inactive 76-amino acid N-terminal fragment (NT-proBNP). The latter is diagnostically more useful, as it has a longer half-life. It is elevated principally in conditions associated with left ventricular systolic dysfunction, and may aid the diagnosis and assess prognosis and response to therapy in patients with heart failure (p. 546).

Cardiac troponins

Troponin I and troponin T are structural cardiac muscle proteins (see Fig. 18.5, p. 531) that are released during myocyte damage and necrosis, and represent the cornerstone of the diagnosis of acute myocardial infarction (MI, p. 593). However, modern assays are extremely sensitive and some have a normal reference range and can detect very low levels of myocardial damage, so that elevated plasma troponin concentrations are seen in other acute conditions, such as pulmonary embolus, septic shock and acute pulmonary oedema. The diagnosis of MI therefore relies on the patient's clinical presentation (see Box 18.61, p. 590).

Chest X-ray

This is useful for determining the size and shape of the heart, and the state of the pulmonary blood vessels and lung fields. Most information is given by a postero-anterior (PA) projection taken in full inspiration. Antero-posterior (AP) projections are convenient when patient movement is restricted but result in magnification of the cardiac shadow.

An estimate of overall heart size can be made by comparing the maximum width of the cardiac outline with the maximum internal transverse diameter of the thoracic cavity. 'Cardiomegaly' is the term used to describe an enlarged cardiac silhouette where the 'cardiothoracic ratio' is greater than 0.5. It can be caused by chamber dilatation, especially left ventricular dilatation, or by a pericardial effusion. Artefactual cardiomegaly may be due to a mediastinal mass or pectus excavatum (p. 731), and cannot be reliably assessed from an AP film. Cardiomegaly is not a sensitive indicator of left ventricular systolic dysfunction since the cardiothoracic ratio is normal in many affected patients (false-negative) and also lacks specificity with many patients with apparent cardiomegaly having normal echocardiograms (false-positive).

Dilatation of individual cardiac chambers can be recognised by the characteristic alterations to the cardiac silhouette:

- Left atrial dilatation results in prominence of the left atrial appendage, creating the appearance of a straight left heart border, a double cardiac shadow to the right of the sternum, and widening of the angle of the carina (bifurcation of the trachea) as the left main bronchus is pushed upwards (Fig. 18.9).

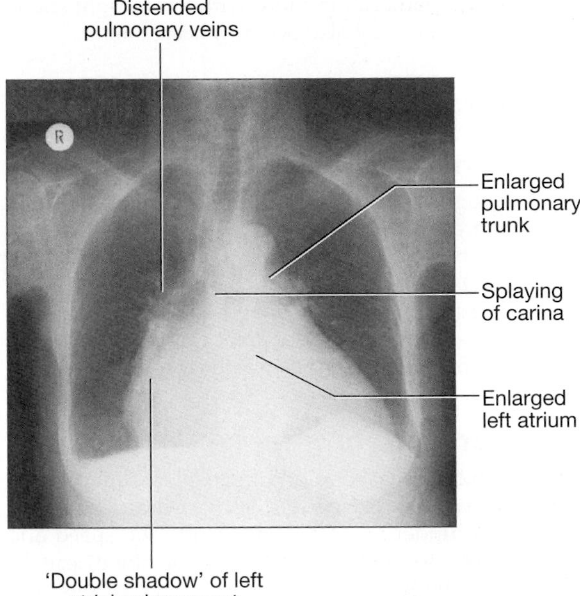

Fig. 18.9 Chest X-ray of a patient with mitral stenosis and regurgitation indicating enlargement of the LA and prominence of the pulmonary artery trunk.

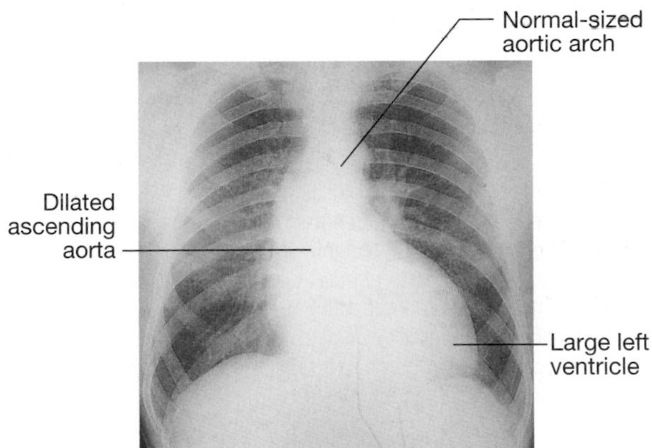

Fig. 18.10 Chest X-ray of a patient with aortic regurgitation, left ventricular enlargement and dilatation of the ascending aorta.

- Right atrial enlargement projects from the right heart border towards the right lower lung field.
- Left ventricular dilatation causes prominence of the left heart border and enlargement of the cardiac silhouette. Left ventricular hypertrophy produces rounding of the left heart border (Fig. 18.10).
- Right ventricular dilatation increases heart size, displaces the apex upwards and straightens the left heart border.

Lateral or oblique projections may be useful for detecting pericardial calcification in patients with constrictive pericarditis (p. 641) or a calcified thoracic aortic aneurysm, as these abnormalities may be obscured by the spine on the PA view.

The lung fields on the chest X-ray may show congestion and oedema in patients with heart failure (see Fig. 18.25, p. 550), and an increase in pulmonary blood flow ('pulmonary plethora') in those with left-to-right shunt. Pleural effusions may also occur in heart failure.

Echocardiography (echo)

Two-dimensional echocardiography

Echocardiography, or cardiac ultrasound, is obtained by placing an ultrasound transducer on the chest wall to image the heart structures as a real-time, two-dimensional 'slice'. This permits the rapid assessment of cardiac structure and function. Left ventricular wall thickness and ejection fraction can be estimated. Common indications for echocardiography are shown in Box 18.4.

Doppler echocardiography

This depends on the Doppler principle that sound waves reflected from moving objects, such as intracardiac red blood cells, undergo a frequency shift. The speed and direction of the red cells, and thus of blood, can be detected in the heart chambers and great vessels. The greater the frequency shift, the faster the blood is moving. The derived information can be presented either as a plot of blood velocity against time for a particular point in the heart (Fig. 18.11) or as a colour overlay on a two-dimensional real-time echo picture (colour-flow Doppler, Fig. 18.12). Doppler echocardiography can be used to detect valvular regurgitation, where the direction of

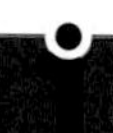

18.4 Common indications for echocardiography

- Assessment of left ventricular function
- Diagnosis and quantification of severity of valve disease
- Identification of vegetations in endocarditis
- Identification of structural heart disease in atrial fibrillation, cardiomyopathies or congenital heart disease
- Detection of pericardial effusion
- Identification of structural heart disease or intracardiac thrombus in systemic embolism

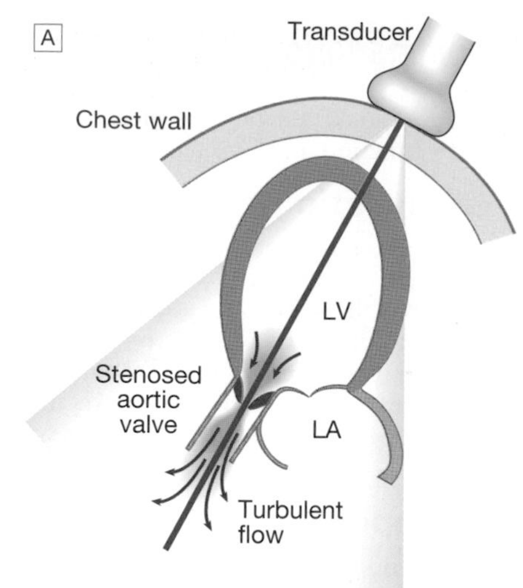

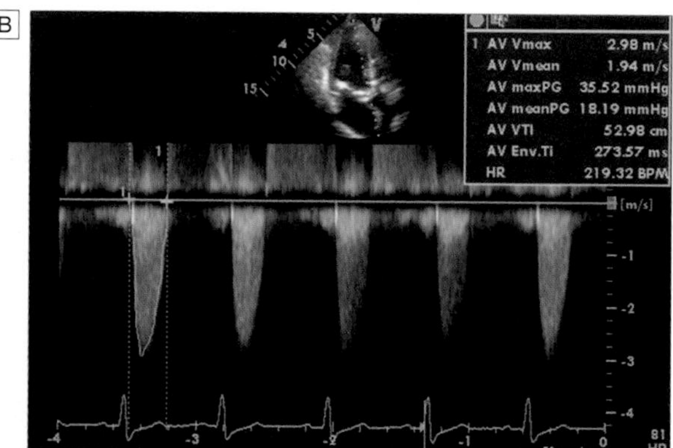

Fig. 18.11 Doppler echocardiography in aortic stenosis. **A** The aortic valve is imaged and a Doppler beam passed directly through the left ventricular outflow tract and the aorta into the turbulent flow beyond the stenosed valve. **B** The velocity of the blood cells is recorded to determine the maximum velocity and hence the pressure gradient across the valve. In this example, the peak velocity is approximately 450 cm/sec (4.5 m/sec), indicating severe aortic stenosis (peak gradient of 81 mmHg).

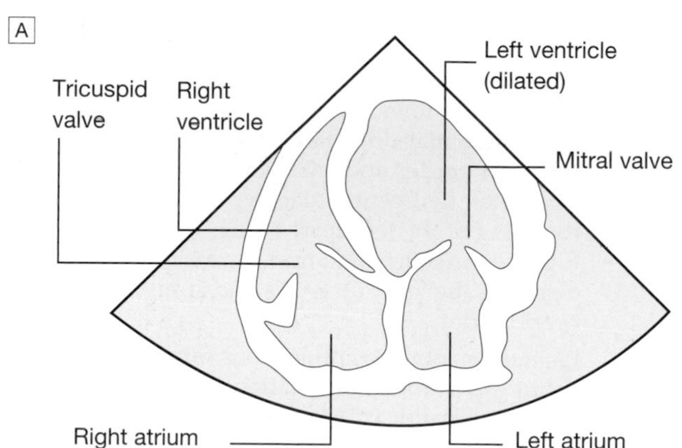

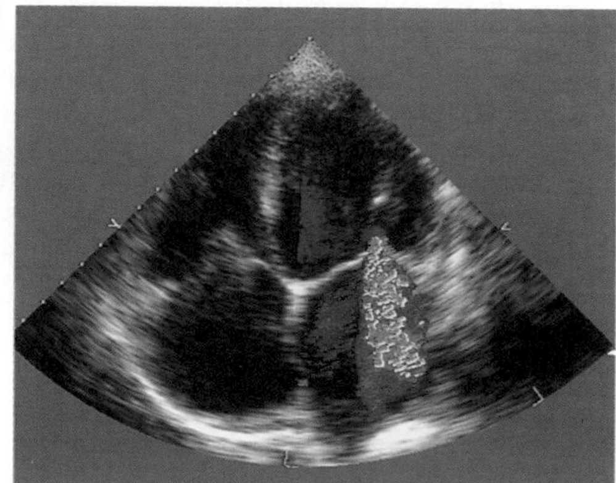

Fig. 18.12 Echocardiographic illustration of the principal cardiac structures in the 'four-chamber' view. **A** The major chambers and valves. **B** Colour-flow Doppler has been used to demonstrate mitral regurgitation: a flame-shaped (yellow/blue) turbulent jet into the left atrium.

blood flow is reversed and turbulence is seen, and is also used to detect high pressure gradients associated with stenosed valves. For example, the normal resting systolic flow velocity across the aortic valve is approximately 1 m/sec; in the presence of aortic stenosis, this is increased as blood accelerates through the narrow orifice. In severe aortic stenosis, the peak aortic velocity may be increased to 5 m/sec (see Fig. 18.11). An estimate of the pressure gradient across a valve or lesion is given by the modified Bernoulli equation:

$$\textbf{Pressure gradient (mmHg)} = 4 \times (\textbf{peak velocity in m/sec})^2$$

Advanced techniques include three-dimensional echocardiography, intravascular ultrasound (defines vessel wall abnormalities and guides coronary intervention), intracardiac ultrasound (provides high-resolution images) and tissue Doppler imaging (quantifies myocardial contractility and diastolic function).

Transoesophageal echocardiography

Transthoracic echocardiography sometimes produces poor images, especially if the patient is overweight or has obstructive airways disease. Some structures are difficult to visualise in transthoracic views, such as the left atrial appendage, pulmonary veins, thoracic aorta and interatrial septum. Transoesophageal echocardiography (TOE) uses an endoscope-like ultrasound probe which is passed into the oesophagus under light sedation and positioned behind the LA. This produces high-resolution images, which makes the technique particularly valuable for investigating patients with prosthetic (especially mitral) valve dysfunction, congenital abnormalities (e.g. atrial septal defect), aortic dissection, infective endocarditis (vegetations that are too small to be detected by transthoracic echocardiography) and systemic embolism (intracardiac thrombus or masses).

Stress echocardiography

Stress echocardiography is used to investigate patients with suspected coronary artery disease who are unsuitable for exercise stress testing, such as those with mobility problems or pre-existing bundle branch block. A two-dimensional echo is performed before and after infusion of a moderate to high dose of an inotrope, such as dobutamine. Myocardial segments with poor perfusion become ischaemic and contract poorly under stress, showing as a wall motion abnormality on the scan. Stress echocardiography is sometimes used to examine myocardial viability in patients with impaired left ventricular function. Low-dose dobutamine can induce contraction in 'hibernating' myocardium; such patients may benefit from bypass surgery or percutaneous coronary intervention.

Computed tomographic imaging

Computed tomography (CT) is useful for imaging the cardiac chambers, great vessels, pericardium, and mediastinal structures and masses. Multidetector scanners can acquire up to 320 slices per rotation, allowing very high-resolution imaging. CT is often performed using a timed injection of X-ray contrast to produce clear images of blood vessels and associated pathologies. Contrast scans are very useful for imaging the aorta in suspected aortic dissection (see Fig. 18.82, p. 607), and the pulmonary arteries and branches in suspected pulmonary embolism (p. 721).

Some centres use cardiac CT scans for quantification of coronary artery calcification, which may serve as an index of cardiovascular risk. However, modern multidetector scanning allows non-invasive coronary angiography (Fig. 18.13) with a spatial resolution approaching that of conventional coronary arteriography and at a lower radiation dose. CT coronary angiography is particularly useful in the initial elective assessment of patients with chest pain and a low or intermediate likelihood of disease, since its negative predictive value is very high: that is, excluding the presence of coronary artery disease. Modern volume scanners are also able to assess myocardial perfusion, often at the same sitting.

Magnetic resonance imaging

Magnetic resonance imaging (MRI) requires no ionising radiation and can be used to generate cross-sectional images of the heart, lungs and mediastinal structures. It provides better differentiation of soft tissue structures than CT but is poor at demonstrating calcification. MRI scans need to be 'gated' to the ECG, allowing the scanner to produce moving images of the heart and mediastinal structures throughout the cardiac cycle. MRI is very

A
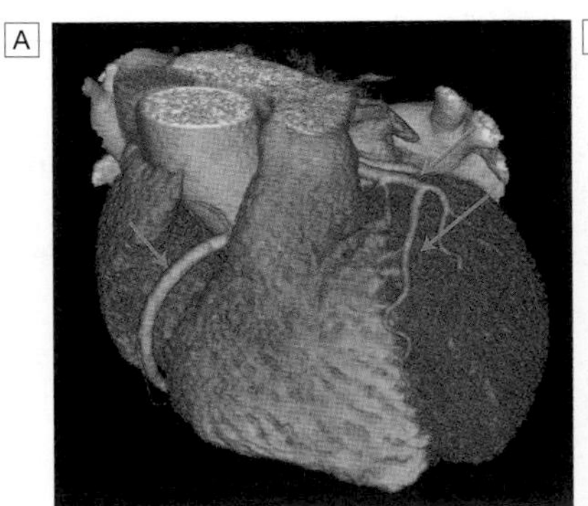
B
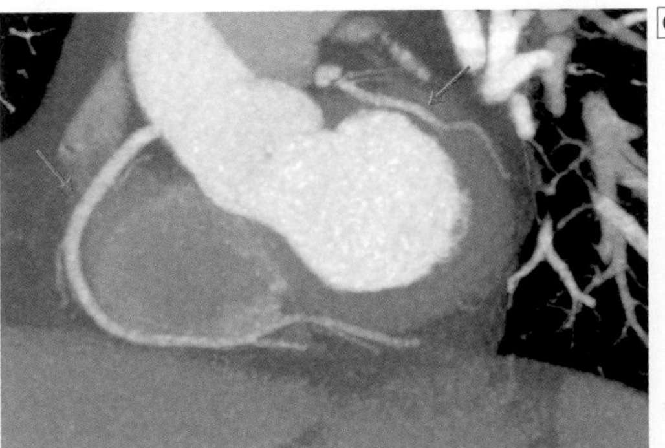
C
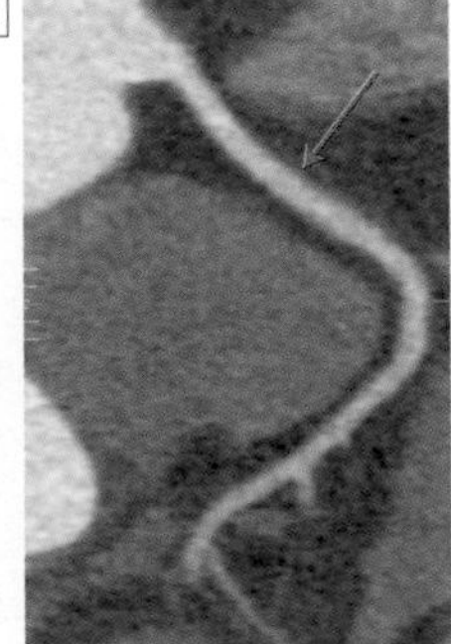

Fig. 18.13 Computed tomography coronary angiography demonstrating normal coronary arteries (arrows).

useful for imaging the aorta, including suspected dissection (see Fig. 18.81, p. 606), and can define the anatomy of the heart and great vessels in patients with congenital heart disease. It is also useful for detecting infiltrative conditions affecting the heart.

Physiological data can be obtained from the signal returned from moving blood, which allows quantification of blood flow across regurgitant or stenotic valves. It is also possible to analyse regional wall motion in patients with suspected coronary disease or cardiomyopathy. The RV is difficult to assess using echocardiography because of its retrosternal position but is readily visualised with MRI.

MRI can also be employed to assess myocardial perfusion and viability. When a contrast agent, such as gadolinium, is injected, areas of myocardial hypoperfusion can be identified with better spatial resolution than nuclear medicine techniques. Later redistribution of this contrast, so-called delayed enhancement, can be used to identify myocardial scarring and fibrosis (Fig. 18.14). This can help in selecting patients for revascularisation procedures, or in identifying those with myocardial infiltration such as that seen with sarcoid heart disease and right ventricular dysplasia.

Cardiac catheterisation

This involves passage of a preshaped catheter via a vein or artery into the heart under X-ray guidance, which allows the measurement of pressure and oxygen saturation in the cardiac chambers and great vessels, and the performance of angiograms by injecting contrast media into a chamber or blood vessel.

Left heart catheterisation involves accessing the arterial circulation, usually via the radial artery, to allow catheterisation of the aorta, LV and coronary arteries. Coronary angiography is the most widely performed procedure, in which the left and right coronary arteries are selectively cannulated and imaged, providing information about the extent and severity of coronary stenoses, thrombus and calcification (Fig. 18.15). This permits

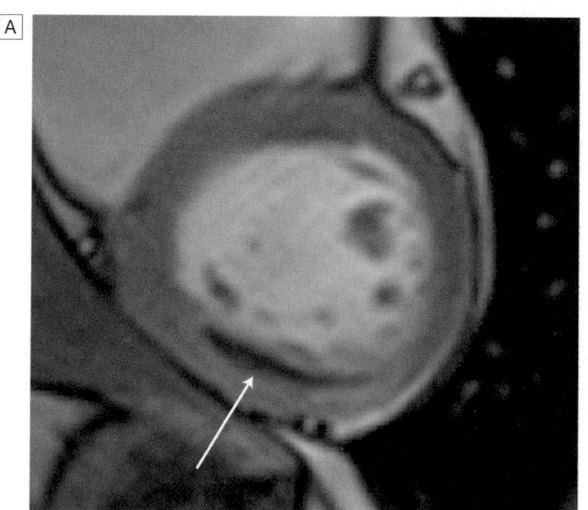

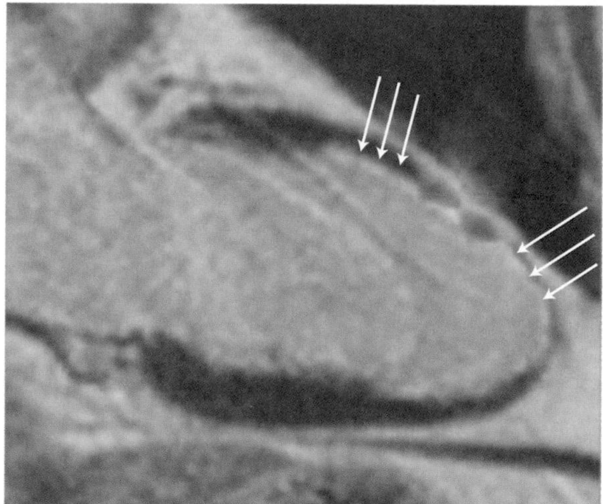

Fig. 18.14 Cardiac magnetic resonance imaging. **A** Recent inferior myocardial infarction with black area of microvascular obstruction (arrow). **B** Old anterior myocardial infarction with large area of subendocardial delayed gadolinium enhancement (white area, arrows).

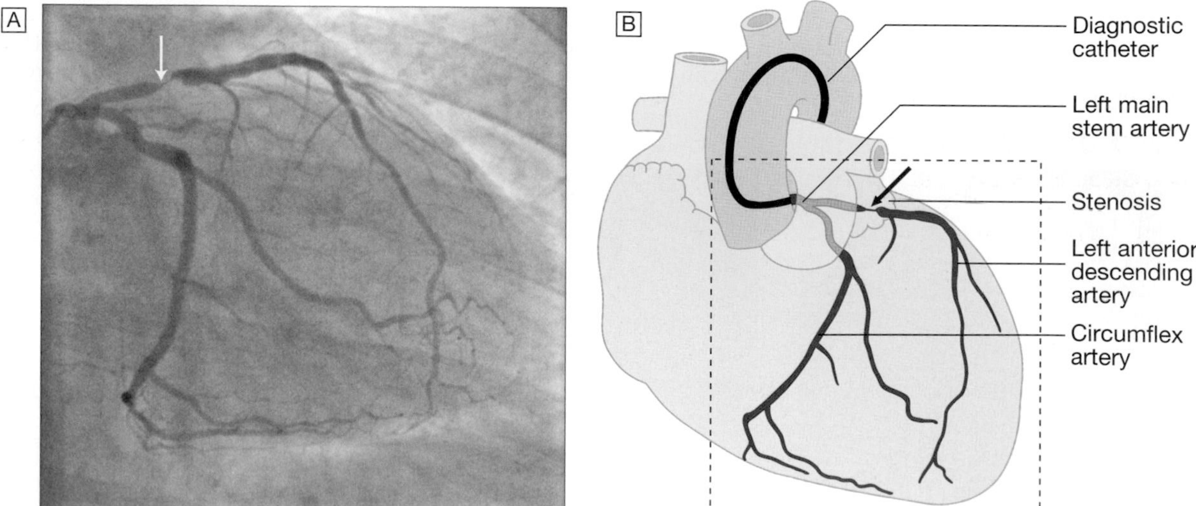

Fig. 18.15 The left anterior descending and circumflex coronary arteries with a stenosis in the left anterior descending vessel. **A** Coronary artery angiogram. **B** Schematic of the vessels and branches.

planning of percutaneous coronary intervention and coronary artery bypass graft surgery. Left ventriculography can be performed during the procedure to determine the size and function of the LV and to demonstrate mitral regurgitation. Aortography defines the size of the aortic root and thoracic aorta, and can help quantify aortic regurgitation. Left heart catheterisation is a day-case procedure and is relatively safe, with serious complications occurring in fewer than 1 in 1000 cases.

Right heart catheterisation is used to assess right heart and pulmonary artery pressures, and to detect intracardiac shunts by measuring oxygen saturations in different chambers. For example, a step up in oxygen saturation from 65% in the RA to 80% in the pulmonary artery is indicative of a large left-to-right shunt that might be due to a ventricular septal defect. Cardiac output can also be measured using thermodilution techniques. Left atrial pressure can be measured directly by puncturing the interatrial septum from the RA with a special catheter. For most purposes, however, a satisfactory approximation to left atrial pressure can be obtained by 'wedging' an end-hole or balloon catheter in a branch of the pulmonary artery. Swan–Ganz balloon catheters are often used to monitor pulmonary 'wedge' pressure as a guide to left heart filling pressure in critically ill patients (p. 186).

Electrophysiology study

Patients with known or suspected arrhythmia are investigated by percutaneous placement of electrode catheters into the heart via the femoral and neck veins. Electrophysiology study (EPS) is most commonly performed to evaluate patients for catheter ablation, normally done during the same procedure. It is occasionally used for risk stratification of patients suspected of being at risk of ventricular arrhythmias.

Radionuclide imaging

The availability of gamma-emitting radionuclides with a short half-life has made it possible to study cardiac function non-invasively. Two techniques are available, although their use is declining due to the availability of equivalent or superior imaging techniques that have lower or no exposure to ionising radiation.

Blood pool imaging

The isotope is injected intravenously and mixes with the circulating blood. A gamma camera detects the amount of radiation-emitting blood in the heart at different phases of the cardiac cycle, thereby permitting the calculation of ventricular ejection fractions. It also allows the assessment of the size and 'shape' of the cardiac chambers.

Myocardial perfusion imaging

This technique involves obtaining scintiscans of the myocardium at rest and during stress after the administration of an intravenous radioactive isotope, such as ^{99}technetium tetrofosmin (see Fig. 18.65, p. 585). More sophisticated quantitative information is obtained with positron emission tomography (PET), which can also be used to assess myocardial metabolism, but this is only available in a few centres.

PRESENTING PROBLEMS IN CARDIOVASCULAR DISEASE

Cardiovascular disease gives rise to a relatively limited range of symptoms. Differential diagnosis depends on careful analysis of the factors that provoke symptoms, the subtle differences in how they are described by the patient, the clinical findings and appropriate investigations. A close relationship between symptoms and exercise is the hallmark of heart disease. The New York Heart Association (NYHA) functional classification is used to grade disability (Box 18.5).

Chest pain

Chest pain is a common presentation of cardiac disease but can also be a manifestation of anxiety or disease of the respiratory, musculoskeletal or gastrointestinal systems (see Box 18.6 below). Some patients deny 'pain' in favour of 'discomfort' but the significance remains the same.

Characteristics of cardiac pain

Several key characteristics help to distinguish cardiac pain from that of other causes (Fig. 18.16). Diagnosis may be difficult and it is helpful to classify pain as typical, atypical or non-cardiac chest pain, based on the balance of evidence (Fig. 18.17).

- *Site.* Cardiac pain is typically located in the centre of the chest because of the derivation of the nerve supply to the heart and mediastinum.

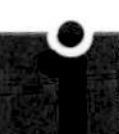

18.5 New York Heart Association (NYHA) functional classification

• **Class I**	No limitation during ordinary activity
• **Class II**	Slight limitation during ordinary activity
• **Class III**	Marked limitation of normal activities without symptoms at rest
• **Class IV**	Unable to undertake physical activity without symptoms; symptoms may be present at rest

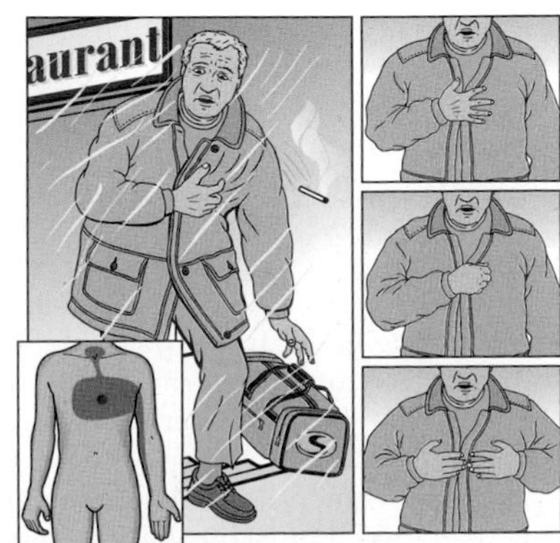

Fig. 18.16 Typical ischaemic cardiac pain. Characteristic hand gestures used to describe cardiac pain. Typical radiation of pain is shown in the schematic.

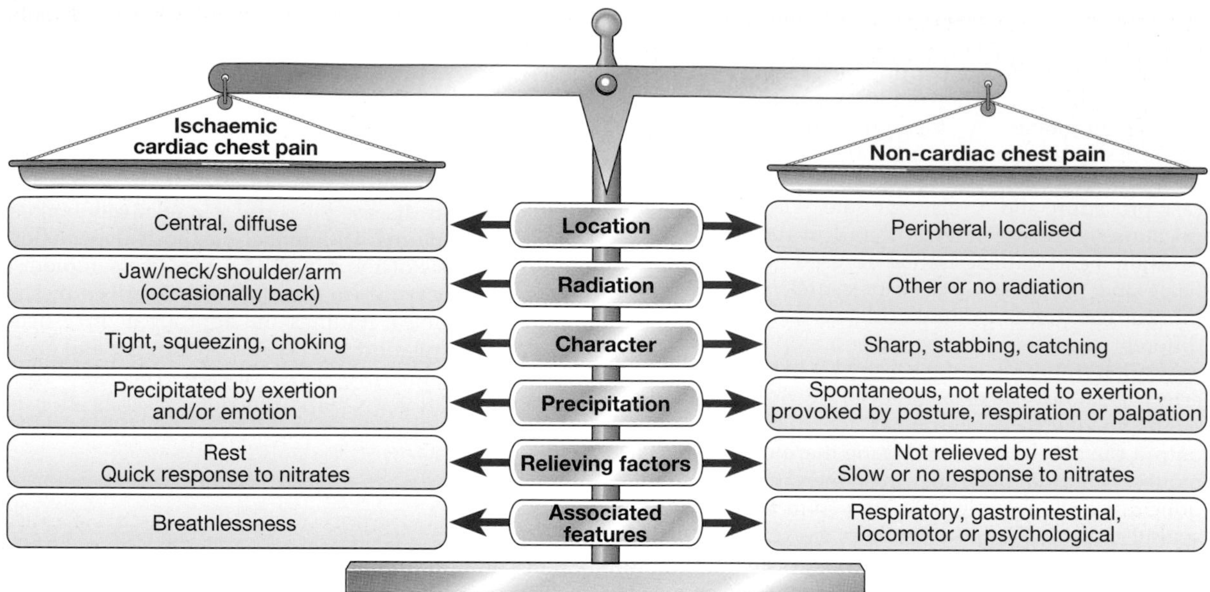

Fig. 18.17 Identifying ischaemic cardiac pain: the 'balance' of evidence.

- *Radiation.* Ischaemic cardiac pain may radiate to the neck, jaw, and upper or even lower arms. Occasionally, cardiac pain may be experienced only at the sites of radiation or in the back. Pain situated over the left anterior chest and radiating laterally is unlikely to be due to cardiac ischaemia and may have many causes, including pleural or lung disorders, musculoskeletal problems and anxiety.
- *Character.* Cardiac pain is typically dull, constricting, choking or 'heavy', and is usually described as squeezing, crushing, burning or aching but not sharp, stabbing, pricking or knife-like. The sensation can be described as breathlessness. Patients often emphasise that it is a discomfort rather than a pain. They typically use characteristic hand gestures (e.g. open hand or clenched fist) when describing ischaemic pain (see Fig. 18.16).
- *Provocation.* Anginal pain occurs during (not after) exertion and is promptly relieved (in less than 5 minutes) by rest. The pain may also be precipitated or exacerbated by emotion but tends to occur more readily during exertion, after a large meal or in a cold wind. In crescendo or unstable angina, similar pain may be precipitated by minimal exertion or at rest. The increase in venous return or preload induced by lying down may also be sufficient to provoke pain in vulnerable patients (decubitus angina). The pain of MI may be preceded by a period of stable or unstable angina but often occurs de novo. In contrast, pleural or pericardial pain is usually described as a 'sharp' or 'catching' sensation that is exacerbated by breathing, coughing or movement. Pain associated with a specific movement (bending, stretching, turning) is likely to be musculoskeletal in origin.
- *Onset.* The pain of MI typically takes several minutes or even longer to develop; similarly, angina builds up gradually in proportion to the intensity of exertion. Pain that occurs after rather than during exertion is usually musculoskeletal or psychological in origin. The pain of aortic dissection, massive pulmonary embolism or pneumothorax is usually very sudden or instantaneous in onset.
- *Associated features.* The pain of MI, massive pulmonary embolism or aortic dissection is often accompanied by autonomic disturbance, including sweating, nausea and vomiting. Breathlessness, due to pulmonary congestion arising from transient ischaemic left ventricular dysfunction, is often a prominent and occasionally the dominant feature of MI or angina (angina equivalent). Breathlessness may also accompany any of the respiratory causes of chest pain and can be associated with cough, wheeze or other respiratory symptoms. Gastrointestinal disorders, such as gastro-oesophageal reflux, peptic ulceration or biliary colic, may present with chest pain but effort-related 'indigestion' is usually due to heart disease.

Differential diagnosis of chest pain

Common causes of chest pain are listed in Box 18.6.

Psychological aspects of chest pain

Emotional distress is a common cause of atypical or non-cardiac chest pain. This diagnosis should be considered if there are features of anxiety and the pain lacks a predictable relationship with exercise. However, the prospect of heart disease is a frightening experience, particularly when it has been responsible for the death of a close friend or relative; psychological and organic features therefore often coexist. Anxiety may amplify the effects of organic disease and can create a very confusing picture. Patients who believe they are suffering from heart disease are sometimes afraid to take exercise and this may make it difficult to establish their true effort tolerance; assessment may also be complicated by the impact of physical deconditioning.

Myocarditis and pericarditis

Pain is characteristically felt retrosternally, to the left of the sternum, or in the left or right shoulder, and typically varies in intensity with movement and the phase of respiration. The pain is described as 'sharp' and may 'catch' the patient during inspiration, coughing or lying flat; there may be a history of a prodromal viral illness.

Mitral valve prolapse

Sharp left-sided chest pain that is suggestive of a musculoskeletal problem may be a feature of mitral valve prolapse (p. 618).

Aortic dissection

This pain is severe, sharp and tearing, is often felt in or penetrating through to the back, and is typically very abrupt in onset (p. 605). The pain follows the path of the dissection.

Oesophageal pain

This can mimic the pain of angina very closely, is sometimes precipitated by exercise and may be relieved by nitrates. However, it is usually possible to elicit a history relating chest pain to supine posture or eating, drinking or oesophageal reflux. It often radiates to the interscapular region and dysphagia may be present.

Bronchospasm

Patients with reversible airways obstruction, such as asthma, may describe exertional chest tightness that is relieved by rest. This may be difficult to distinguish from ischaemic chest tightness. Bronchospasm may be associated with wheeze, atopy and cough (p. 654).

Musculoskeletal chest pain

This is a common problem that is very variable in site and intensity but does not usually fall into any of the patterns described above. The pain may vary with posture or movement of the upper body and is sometimes accompanied by local tenderness over a rib or costal cartilage. There are numerous causes, including arthritis, costochondritis, intercostal muscle injury and Coxsackie viral infection (epidemic myalgia or Bornholm disease). Many minor soft tissue injuries are related to everyday activities, such as driving, manual work and sport. The differential diagnosis of peripheral or pleural chest pain is discussed on page 658.

18.6 Common causes of chest pain

Anxiety/emotion	
Cardiac	
• Myocardial ischaemia (angina) • MI	• Pericarditis • Mitral valve prolapse
Aortic	
• Aortic dissection	• Aortic aneurysm
Oesophageal	
• Oesophagitis • Oesophageal spasm	• Mallory–Weiss syndrome
Lungs/pleura	
• Bronchospasm • Pulmonary infarct • Pneumonia • Tracheitis • Pneumothorax	• Pulmonary embolism • Malignancy • Tuberculosis • Connective tissue disorders (rare)
Musculoskeletal	
• Osteoarthritis • Rib fracture/injury • Costochondritis (Tietze's syndrome)	• Intercostal muscle injury • Epidemic myalgia (Bornholm disease)
Neurological	
• Prolapsed intervertebral disc	• Herpes zoster • Thoracic outlet syndrome

Initial evaluation of suspected cardiac pain

A careful history is crucial in determining whether pain is cardiac or not. Although the physical findings and subsequent investigations may help to confirm the diagnosis, they are of more value in determining the nature and extent of any underlying heart disease, the risk of a serious adverse event, and the best course of management.

Stable angina

Effort-related chest pain is the hallmark of angina pectoris or 'choking in the chest' (Fig. 18.18). The reproducibility, predictability and relationship to physical exertion (and occasionally emotion) of the chest pain are

	Stable angina	Acute coronary syndrome
Pathophysiology	• Fixed stenosis • Stable fibrous plaque	• Dynamic stenosis • Ruptured or inflamed plaque
Clinical features	• Demand-led ischaemia • Related to effort • Predictable • Symptoms over long term	• Supply-led ischaemia • Symptoms at rest • Unpredictable • Symptoms over short term • Frequent or nocturnal symptoms
Risk assessment	• Symptoms on minimal exertion • Exercise testing Duration of exercise Degree of ECG changes Abnormal BP response • CT coronary angiogram	• ECG changes at rest • ECG changes with symptoms • Elevation of troponin

Fig. 18.18 Pathophysiology, clinical features and risk assessment of patients with stable or unstable coronary heart disease.

the most important features. The duration of symptoms should be noted because patients with recent-onset angina are at greater risk than those with long-standing and unchanged symptoms.

Physical examination is often normal but may reveal evidence of risk factors (e.g. xanthoma indicating hyperlipidaemia), left ventricular dysfunction (e.g. dyskinetic apex beat, gallop rhythm), other manifestations of arterial disease (e.g. bruits, signs of peripheral vascular disease) and unrelated conditions that may exacerbate angina (e.g. anaemia, thyroid disease). Stable angina is usually a symptom of coronary artery disease but may be a manifestation of other forms of heart disease, particularly aortic valve disease and hypertrophic cardiomyopathy. In patients with angina in whom a murmur is found, echocardiography should be performed.

A full blood count, fasting blood glucose, lipids, thyroid function tests and a 12-lead ECG are the most important baseline investigations. Exercise testing may confirm the diagnosis and also identify high-risk patients

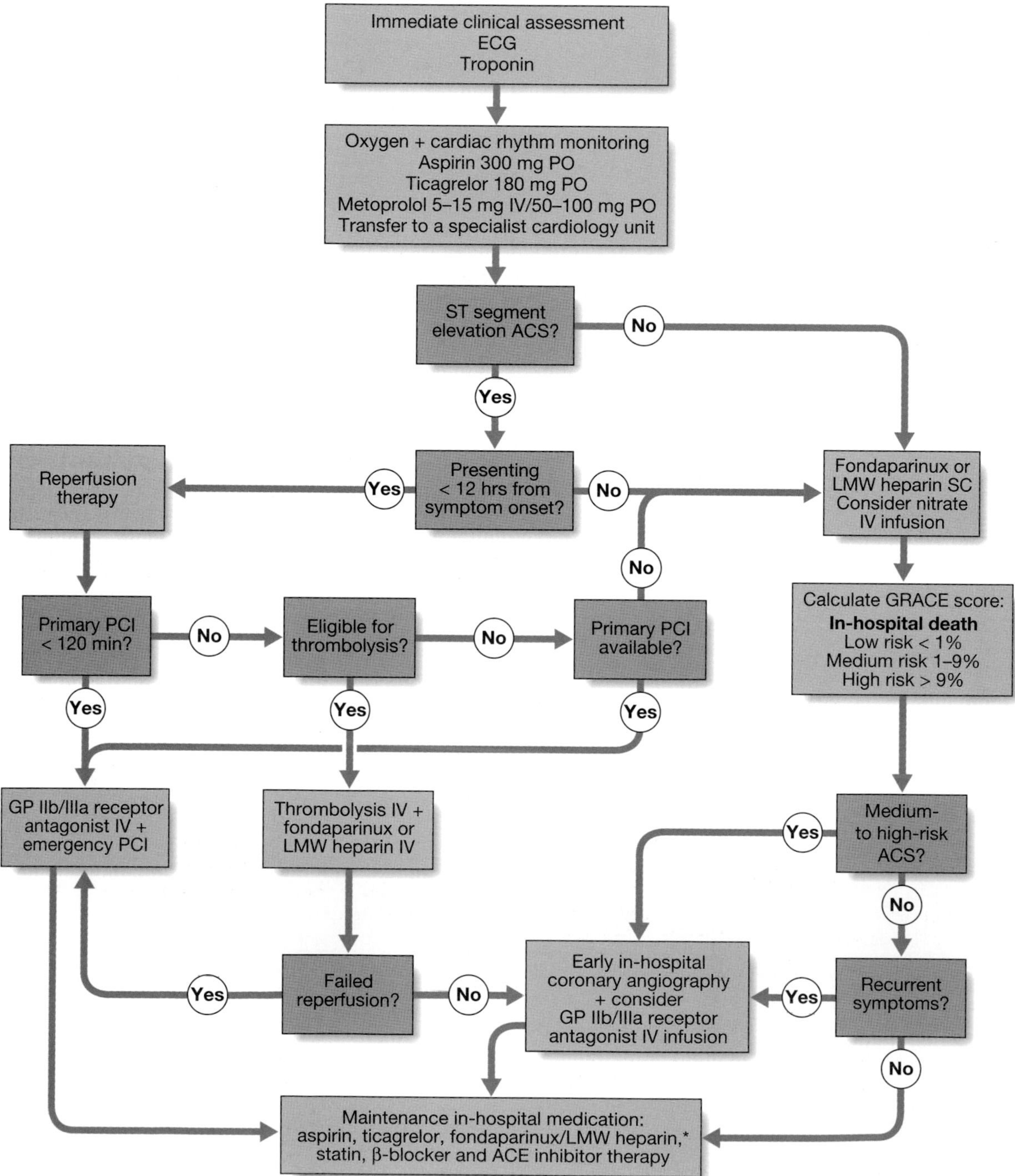

Fig. 18.19 Summary of treatment for acute coronary syndrome (ACS). *Not required following PCI. Amended from SIGN 93. For details of the GRACE score, see Figure 18.70, p. 591 (ACE = angiotensin-converting enzyme; GP = glycoprotein; LMW = low molecular weight; PCI = percutaneous coronary intervention). From SIGN 93 – see p. 641.

who require further investigation and treatment (p. 534). CT coronary angiography is very useful to exclude the presence of coronary artery disease where doubt exists.

Acute coronary syndromes

Prolonged, severe cardiac chest pain may be due to unstable angina (which comprises recent-onset limiting angina, rapidly worsening or crescendo angina, and angina at rest) or acute MI; these are known collectively as the acute coronary syndromes. Although there may be a history of antecedent chronic stable angina, an episode of chest pain at rest is often the first presentation of coronary artery disease. Diagnosis depends on analysis of the character of the pain and its associated features. Physical examination may reveal signs of important comorbidity, such as peripheral or cerebrovascular disease, autonomic disturbance (pallor or sweating) and complications (arrhythmia or heart failure).

Patients presenting with symptoms consistent with an acute coronary syndrome require urgent evaluation because there is a high risk of avoidable complications, such as sudden death and MI. Signs of haemodynamic compromise (hypotension, pulmonary oedema), ECG changes (ST segment elevation or depression) and biochemical markers of cardiac damage, such as elevated troponin I or T, are powerful indicators of short-term risk. A 12-lead ECG is mandatory and is the most useful method of initial triage (Fig. 18.19). The release of markers such as creatine kinase, troponin and myoglobin is relatively slow (p. 593) but can help guide immediate management and treatment.

If the diagnosis is unclear, patients with a suspected acute coronary syndrome should be observed in hospital. Repeated ECG recordings are valuable, particularly if obtained during an episode of pain. Plasma troponin concentrations should be measured at presentation and, if normal, repeated 6–12 hours after the onset of symptoms or hospital admission. New ECG changes or an elevated plasma troponin concentration confirm the diagnosis of an acute coronary syndrome. The subsequent management is described on page 593.

If the pain has not recurred, troponin concentrations are not elevated and there are no new ECG changes, the patient may be discharged from hospital. At this stage, an exercise test or CT coronary angiogram may help diagnose underlying coronary artery disease.

Breathlessness (dyspnoea)

Dyspnoea of cardiac origin may vary in severity from an uncomfortable awareness of breathing to a frightening sensation of 'fighting for breath'. The sensation of dyspnoea originates in the cerebral cortex and is described in detail on page 655.

There are several causes of cardiac dyspnoea: acute left heart failure, chronic heart failure, arrhythmia and angina equivalent (Box 18.7). The assessment and treatment of heart failure is described on pages 548–553, and arrhythmias on pages 562–571.

18.7 Some causes of dyspnoea

Acute dyspnoea	Chronic exertional dyspnoea
Cardiovascular system	
*Acute pulmonary oedema	*Congestive cardiac failure Myocardial ischaemia
Respiratory system	
*Acute severe asthma *Acute exacerbation of COPD *Pneumothorax *Pneumonia *Pulmonary embolus ARDS Inhaled foreign body (especially in a child) Lobar collapse Laryngeal oedema (e.g. anaphylaxis)	*COPD *Chronic asthma Chronic pulmonary thromboembolism Bronchial carcinoma Interstitial lung diseases: sarcoidosis, fibrosing alveolitis, extrinsic allergic alveolitis, pneumoconiosis Lymphatic carcinomatosis Large pleural effusion(s)
Others	
Metabolic acidosis (e.g. diabetic ketoacidosis, lactic acidosis, uraemia, overdose of salicylates, ethylene glycol poisoning) Hyperventilation	Severe anaemia Obesity

*Common cause. (ARDS = acute respiratory distress syndrome; COPD = chronic obstructive pulmonary disease)

Acute left heart failure

Acute left heart failure may be triggered by a major event, such as MI, in a previously healthy heart, or by a relatively minor event, such as the onset of atrial fibrillation, in a diseased heart. An increase in the left ventricular diastolic pressure causes the pressure in the LA, pulmonary veins and pulmonary capillaries to rise. When the hydrostatic pressure of the pulmonary capillaries exceeds the oncotic pressure of plasma (about 25–30 mmHg), fluid moves from the capillaries into alveoli. This stimulates respiration through a series of autonomic reflexes, producing rapid shallow respiration. Congestion of the bronchial mucosa may cause wheeze (cardiac asthma).

Acute pulmonary oedema is a terrifying experience because of the sensation of 'fighting for breath'. Sitting upright or standing may provide some relief by helping to reduce congestion at the apices of the lungs. The patient may be unable to speak and is typically distressed, agitated, sweaty and pale. Respiration is rapid, with recruitment of accessory muscles, coughing and wheezing. Sputum may be profuse, frothy and blood-streaked or pink. Extensive crepitations and rhonchi are usually audible in the chest and there may also be signs of right heart failure.

Chronic heart failure

Chronic heart failure is the most common cardiac cause of chronic dyspnoea. Symptoms may first present on moderate exertion, such as walking up a steep hill, and may be described as a difficulty in 'catching my breath'. As heart failure progresses, the dyspnoea is provoked by less exertion and, ultimately, the patient may be breathless walking from room to room, washing, dressing or trying to hold a conversation. Other symptoms may include:

- *Orthopnoea*. Lying down increases the venous return to the heart and provokes breathlessness. Patients may prop themselves up with pillows to prevent this.

- *Paroxysmal nocturnal dyspnoea*. In patients with severe heart failure, fluid shifts from the interstitial tissues of the peripheries into the circulation within 1–2 hours of lying down. Pulmonary oedema supervenes, causing the patient to wake and sit upright, profoundly breathless.
- *Cheyne–Stokes respiration*. This cyclical pattern of respiration is due to impaired responsiveness of the respiratory centre to carbon dioxide and occurs in severe left ventricular failure. The pattern of slowly diminishing respiration, leading to apnoea, followed by progressively increasing respiration and hyperventilation, may be accompanied by a sensation of breathlessness and panic during the period of hyperventilation. The Cheyne–Stokes cycle length is a function of the circulation time. The condition can also occur in diffuse cerebral atherosclerosis, stroke or head injury, and may be exaggerated by sleep, barbiturates and opiates.

Arrhythmia

Any arrhythmia may cause breathlessness but usually only does so if the heart is structurally abnormal, such as with the onset of atrial fibrillation in a patient with mitral stenosis.

Angina equivalent

Breathlessness is a common feature of angina. Patients will sometimes describe chest tightness as 'breathlessness'. However, myocardial ischaemia may also induce true breathlessness by provoking transient left ventricular dysfunction or heart failure. When breathlessness is the dominant or sole feature of myocardial ischaemia, it is known as 'angina equivalent'. A history of chest tightness, the close correlation with exercise, and objective evidence of myocardial ischaemia from stress testing may all help to establish the diagnosis.

Acute circulatory failure (cardiogenic shock)

'Shock' is used to describe the clinical syndrome that develops when there is critical impairment of tissue perfusion due to some form of acute circulatory failure. There are numerous causes of shock, described in detail on page 190. The important features and causes (Fig. 18.20) of acute heart failure or cardiogenic shock are described here.

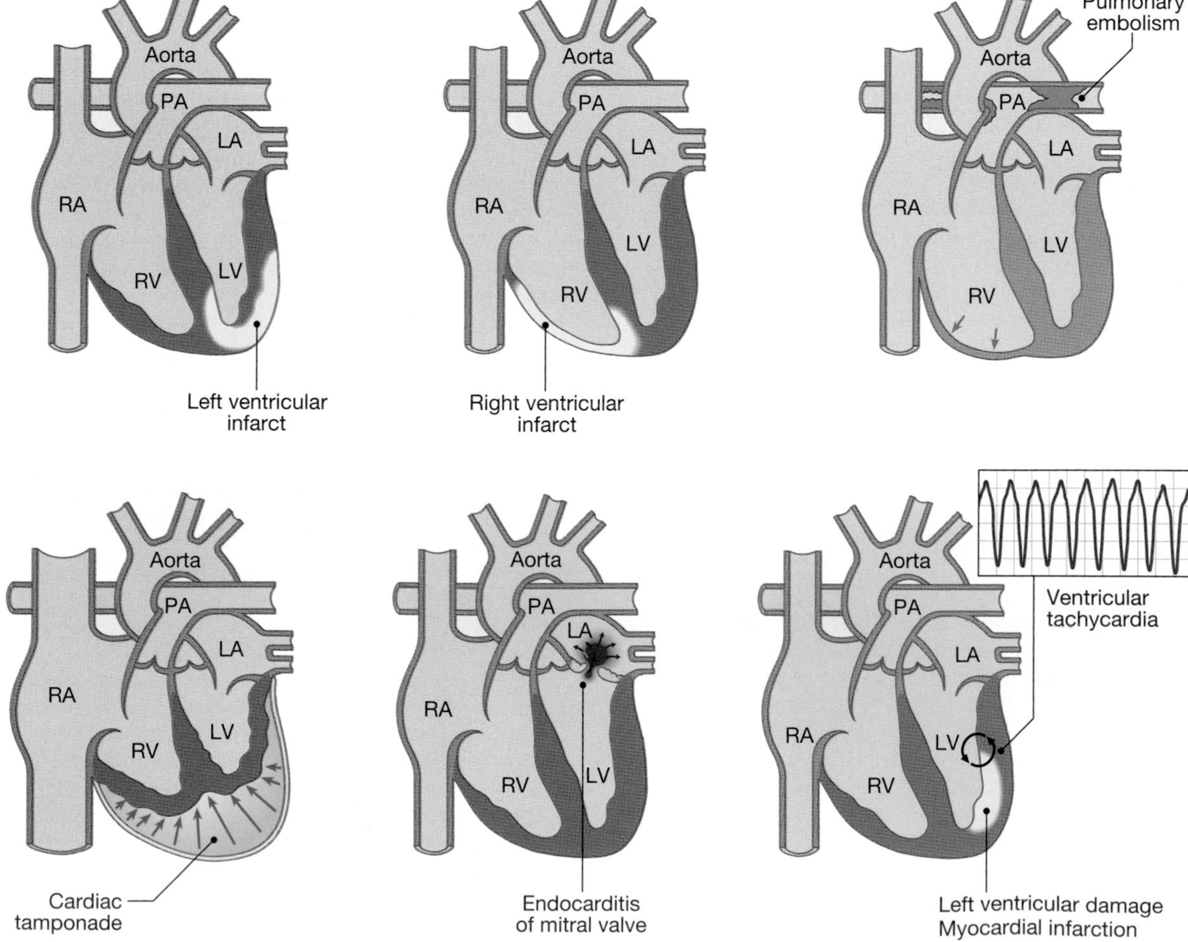

Fig. 18.20 Some common causes of cardiogenic shock.

Myocardial infarction

Shock in acute MI is due to left ventricular dysfunction in more than 70% of cases. However, it may also be due to infarction of the RV and a variety of mechanical complications, including tamponade (due to infarction and rupture of the free wall), an acquired ventricular septal defect (due to infarction and rupture of the septum) and acute mitral regurgitation (due to infarction or rupture of the papillary muscles).

Severe myocardial systolic dysfunction causes a fall in cardiac output, BP and coronary perfusion pressure. Diastolic dysfunction causes a rise in left ventricular end-diastolic pressure, pulmonary congestion and oedema, leading to hypoxaemia that worsens myocardial ischaemia. This is further exacerbated by peripheral vasoconstriction. These factors combine to create the 'downward spiral' of cardiogenic shock (Fig. 18.21).

Hypotension, oliguria, confusion and cold, clammy peripheries are the manifestations of a low cardiac output, whereas breathlessness, hypoxaemia, cyanosis and inspiratory crackles at the lung bases are typical features of pulmonary oedema. A chest X-ray (see Fig. 18.25, p. 550) may reveal signs of pulmonary congestion when clinical examination is normal. If necessary, a Swan–Ganz catheter can be used to measure the pulmonary artery wedge pressure and to guide fluid replacement. The findings can be used to categorise patients with acute MI into four haemodynamic subsets (Box 18.8). Those with cardiogenic shock should be considered for immediate coronary revascularisation.

The viable myocardium surrounding a fresh infarct may contract poorly for a few days and then recover. This phenomenon is known as myocardial stunning and means that acute heart failure should be treated intensively because overall cardiac function may subsequently improve.

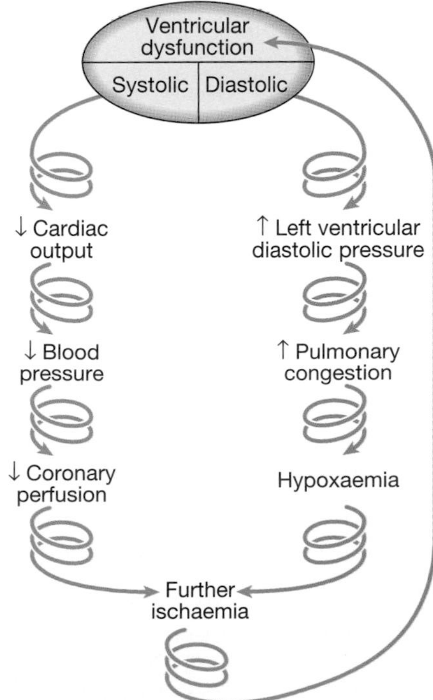

Fig. 18.21 The downward spiral of cardiogenic shock.

18.8 Acute myocardial infarction: haemodynamic subsets

Cardiac output	Pulmonary oedema: No	Pulmonary oedema: Yes
Normal	Good prognosis and requires no treatment for heart failure	Due to moderate left ventricular dysfunction. Treat with vasodilators and diuretics
Low	Due to right ventricular dysfunction or concomitant hypovolaemia. Give fluid challenge and consider pulmonary artery catheter to guide therapy	Extensive MI and poor prognosis. Consider intra-aortic balloon pump, vasodilators, diuretics and inotropes

Acute massive pulmonary embolism

This may complicate leg or pelvic vein thrombosis and usually presents with sudden collapse. The clinical features and treatment are discussed on page 721. Bedside echocardiography may demonstrate a small, underfilled, vigorous LV with a dilated RV; it is sometimes possible to see thrombus in the right ventricular outflow tract or main pulmonary artery. CT pulmonary angiography usually provides a definitive diagnosis.

Cardiac tamponade

This is due to a collection of fluid or blood in the pericardial sac, compressing the heart; the effusion may be small and is very occasionally less than 100 mL. Sudden deterioration (Box 18.9) may be due to bleeding into the pericardial space. Tamponade may complicate any form of pericarditis but can be caused by malignant disease. Other causes include trauma and rupture of the free wall of the myocardium following MI.

An ECG may show features of the underlying disease, such as pericarditis or acute MI. When there is a large pericardial effusion, the ECG complexes are small and there may be electrical alternans: a changing axis with alternate beats caused by the heart swinging from side to side in the pericardial fluid. A chest X-ray shows an enlarged globular heart but can look normal. Echocardiography is the best way of confirming the diagnosis

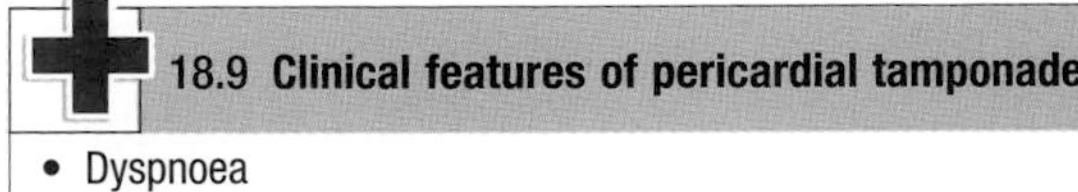

18.9 Clinical features of pericardial tamponade

- Dyspnoea
- Collapse
- Tachycardia
- Hypotension
- Gross elevation of the JVP
- Soft heart sounds with an early third heart sound
- Pulsus paradoxus (a large fall in BP during inspiration, when the pulse may be impalpable)
- Kussmaul's sign (a paradoxical rise in the JVP during inspiration)

(JVP = jugular venous pressure)

and helps to identify the optimum site for aspiration of the fluid. Prompt recognition of tamponade is important because the patient usually responds dramatically to percutaneous pericardiocentesis (p. 640) or surgical drainage.

Valvular heart disease

Acute left ventricular failure and shock may be due to the sudden onset of aortic regurgitation, mitral regurgitation or prosthetic valve dysfunction (Box 18.10).

The clinical diagnosis of acute valvular dysfunction is sometimes difficult. Murmurs are often unimpressive because there is usually a tachycardia and a low cardiac output. Transthoracic echocardiography will establish the diagnosis in most cases; however, transoesophageal echocardiography is sometimes required, especially in patients with prosthetic mitral valves.

Patients with acute valve failure usually require cardiac surgery and should be referred for urgent assessment in a cardiac centre.

Aortic dissection may lead to shock by causing aortic regurgitation, coronary dissection, tamponade or blood loss (p. 605).

Management of shock

This is discussed in detail on page 190.

18.10 Causes of acute valve failure

Aortic regurgitation
- Aortic dissection
- Infective endocarditis

Mitral regurgitation
- Papillary muscle rupture due to acute MI
- Infective endocarditis
- Rupture of chordae due to myxomatous degeneration

Prosthetic valve failure
- Mechanical valves: fracture, jamming, thrombosis, dehiscence
- Biological valves: degeneration with cusp tear

Heart failure

Heart failure describes the clinical syndrome that develops when the heart cannot maintain adequate output, or can do so only at the expense of elevated ventricular filling pressure. In mild to moderate forms of heart failure, cardiac output is normal at rest and only becomes impaired when the metabolic demand increases during exercise or some other form of stress. In practice, heart failure may be diagnosed when a patient with significant heart disease develops the signs or symptoms of a low cardiac output, pulmonary congestion or systemic venous congestion.

Almost all forms of heart disease can lead to heart failure. An accurate aetiological diagnosis (Box 18.11) is

18.11 Mechanisms of heart failure

Cause	Examples	Features
Reduced ventricular contractility	MI (segmental dysfunction)	In coronary artery disease, 'akinetic' or 'dyskinetic' segments contract poorly and may impede the function of normal segments by distorting their contraction and relaxation patterns
	Myocarditis/cardiomyopathy (global dysfunction)	Progressive ventricular dilatation
Ventricular outflow obstruction (pressure overload)	Hypertension, aortic stenosis (left heart failure) Pulmonary hypertension, pulmonary valve stenosis (right heart failure)	Initially, concentric ventricular hypertrophy allows the ventricle to maintain a normal output by generating a high systolic pressure. Later, secondary changes in the myocardium and increasing obstruction lead to failure with ventricular dilatation and rapid clinical deterioration
Ventricular inflow obstruction	Mitral stenosis, tricuspid stenosis	Small, vigorous ventricle, dilated hypertrophied atrium. Atrial fibrillation is common and often causes marked deterioration because ventricular filling depends heavily on atrial contraction
Ventricular volume overload	Ventricular septal defect Right ventricular volume overload (e.g. atrial septal defect) Increased metabolic demand (high output)	Dilatation and hypertrophy allow the ventricle to generate a high stroke volume and help to maintain a normal cardiac output. However, secondary changes in the myocardium lead to impaired contractility and worsening heart failure
Arrhythmia	Atrial fibrillation	Tachycardia does not allow for adequate filling of the heart, resulting in reduced cardiac output and back pressure
	Tachycardia cardiomyopathy	Incessant tachycardia causes myocardial fatigue
	Complete heart block	Bradycardia limits cardiac output, even if stroke volume is normal
Diastolic dysfunction	Constrictive pericarditis	Marked fluid retention and peripheral oedema, ascites, pleural effusions and elevated jugular veins
	Restrictive cardiomyopathy	Bi-atrial enlargement (restrictive filling pattern and high atrial pressures). Atrial fibrillation may cause deterioration
	Left ventricular hypertrophy and fibrosis	Good systolic function but poor diastolic filling
	Cardiac tamponade	Hypotension, elevated jugular veins, pulsus paradoxus, poor urine output

important because treatment of the underlying cause may reverse heart failure or prevent its progression.

Heart failure is most common in the elderly. The prevalence of heart failure rises from 1% in those aged 50–59 years to over 10% in those aged 80–89 years. In the UK, most patients admitted to hospital with heart failure are more than 70 years old; they remain hospitalised for a week or more and may be left with chronic disability. The most common aetiology is coronary artery disease and myocardial infarction.

Although the outlook depends, to some extent, on the underlying cause of the problem, untreated heart failure carries a poor prognosis; approximately 50% of patients with severe heart failure due to left ventricular dysfunction will die within 2 years, because of either pump failure or malignant ventricular arrhythmias.

Pathophysiology

Cardiac output is determined by preload (the volume and pressure of blood in the ventricles at the end of diastole), afterload (the volume and pressure of blood in the ventricles during systole) and myocardial contractility; this is the basis of Starling's Law (Fig. 18.22).

In patients without valvular disease, the primary abnormality is impairment of ventricular myocardial function, leading to a fall in cardiac output. This can occur because of impaired systolic contraction, impaired diastolic relaxation, or both. This activates counter-regulatory neurohumoral mechanisms that, in normal physiological circumstances, would support cardiac function but, in the setting of impaired ventricular function, can lead to a deleterious increase in both afterload and preload (Fig. 18.23). A vicious circle may be established because any additional fall in cardiac output will cause further neurohumoral activation and increasing peripheral vascular resistance.

Stimulation of the renin–angiotensin–aldosterone system leads to vasoconstriction, sodium and water retention, and sympathetic nervous system activation. This is mediated by angiotensin II, a potent constrictor of arterioles, in both the kidney and the systemic circulation (see Fig. 18.23). Activation of the sympathetic nervous system may initially sustain cardiac output through increased myocardial contractility (inotropy) and heart rate (chronotropy). Prolonged sympathetic stimulation also causes negative effects, including cardiac myocyte apoptosis, hypertrophy and focal myocardial necrosis. Sympathetic stimulation also causes peripheral vasoconstriction and arrhythmias. Sodium and water retention is promoted by the release of aldosterone, endothelin-1 (a potent vasoconstrictor peptide with marked effects on the renal vasculature) and, in severe heart failure, antidiuretic hormone (ADH). Natriuretic peptides are released from the atria in response to atrial stretch, and act as physiological antagonists to the fluid-conserving effect of aldosterone.

After MI, cardiac contractility is impaired and neurohumoral activation causes hypertrophy of non-infarcted segments, with thinning, dilatation and expansion of the

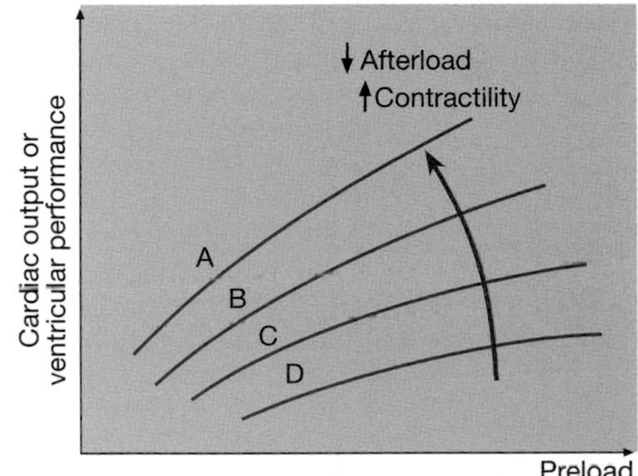

Fig. 18.22 Starling's Law. Normal (A), mild (B), moderate (C) and severe (D) heart failure. Ventricular performance is related to the degree of myocardial stretching. An increase in preload (end-diastolic volume, end-diastolic pressure, filling pressure or atrial pressure) will therefore enhance function; however, overstretching causes marked deterioration. In heart failure, the curve moves to the right and becomes flatter. An increase in myocardial contractility or a reduction in afterload will shift the curve upwards and to the left (green arrow).

18

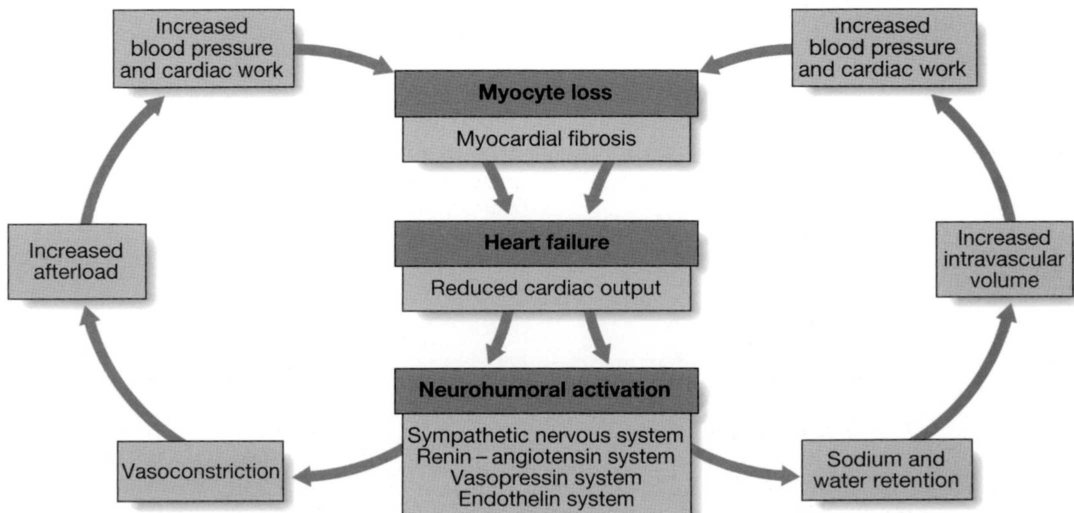

Fig. 18.23 Neurohumoral activation and compensatory mechanisms in heart failure. There is a vicious circle in progressive heart failure.

infarcted segment (remodelling; see Fig. 18.77, p. 597). This leads to further deterioration in ventricular function and worsening heart failure.

Pulmonary and peripheral oedema occurs because of high left and right atrial pressures, respectively; this is compounded by sodium and water retention, caused by impairment of renal perfusion and by secondary hyperaldosteronism.

Types of heart failure

Left, right and biventricular heart failure

The left side of the heart comprises the functional unit of the LA and LV, together with the mitral and aortic valves; the right heart comprises the RA, RV, and tricuspid and pulmonary valves.

- *Left-sided heart failure.* There is a reduction in left ventricular output and an increase in left atrial and pulmonary venous pressure. An acute increase in left atrial pressure causes pulmonary congestion or pulmonary oedema; a more gradual increase in left atrial pressure, as occurs with mitral stenosis, leads to reflex pulmonary vasoconstriction, which protects the patient from pulmonary oedema. This increases pulmonary vascular resistance and causes pulmonary hypertension, which can, in turn, impair right ventricular function.
- *Right-sided heart failure.* There is a reduction in right ventricular output and an increase in right atrial and systemic venous pressure. Causes of isolated right heart failure include chronic lung disease (cor pulmonale), pulmonary embolism and pulmonary valvular stenosis.
- *Biventricular heart failure.* Failure of the left and right heart may develop because the disease process, such as dilated cardiomyopathy or ischaemic heart disease, affects both ventricles or because disease of the left heart leads to chronic elevation of the left atrial pressure, pulmonary hypertension and right heart failure.

Diastolic and systolic dysfunction

Heart failure may develop as a result of impaired myocardial contraction (systolic dysfunction) but can also be due to poor ventricular filling and high filling pressures stemming from abnormal ventricular relaxation (diastolic dysfunction). The latter is caused by a stiff, non-compliant ventricle and is commonly found in patients with left ventricular hypertrophy. Systolic and diastolic dysfunction often coexist, particularly in patients with coronary artery disease.

High-output failure

A large arteriovenous shunt, beri-beri (p. 128), severe anaemia or thyrotoxicosis can occasionally cause heart failure due to an excessively high cardiac output.

Acute and chronic heart failure

Heart failure may develop suddenly, as in MI, or gradually, as in progressive valvular heart disease. When there is gradual impairment of cardiac function, several compensatory changes may take place.

The term 'compensated heart failure' is sometimes used to describe the condition of those with impaired cardiac function, in whom adaptive changes have prevented the development of overt heart failure. A minor event, such as an intercurrent infection or development of atrial fibrillation, may precipitate overt or acute heart failure (Box 18.12). Acute left heart failure occurs, either de novo or as an acute decompensated episode, on a background of chronic heart failure: so-called acute-on-chronic heart failure.

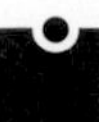

18.12 Factors that may precipitate or aggravate heart failure in pre-existing heart disease

- Myocardial ischaemia or infarction
- Intercurrent illness, e.g. infection
- Arrhythmia, e.g. atrial fibrillation
- Inappropriate reduction of therapy
- Administration of a drug with negative inotropic (β-blocker) or fluid-retaining properties (NSAIDs, corticosteroids)
- Pulmonary embolism
- Conditions associated with increased metabolic demand, e.g. pregnancy, thyrotoxicosis, anaemia
- IV fluid overload, e.g. post-operative IV infusion

(NSAIDs = non-steroidal anti-inflammatory drugs)

Clinical assessment

Acute left heart failure

Acute de novo left ventricular failure presents with a sudden onset of dyspnoea at rest that rapidly progresses to acute respiratory distress, orthopnoea and prostration. The precipitant, such as acute MI, is often apparent from the history.

The patient appears agitated, pale and clammy. The peripheries are cool to the touch and the pulse is rapid. Inappropriate bradycardia or excessive tachycardia should be identified promptly, as this may be the precipitant for the acute episode of heart failure. The BP is usually high because of sympathetic nervous system activation, but may be normal or low if the patient is in cardiogenic shock.

The jugular venous pressure (JVP) is usually elevated, particularly with associated fluid overload or right heart failure. In acute de novo heart failure, there has been no time for ventricular dilatation and the apex is not displaced. A 'gallop' rhythm, with a third heart sound, is heard quite early in the development of acute left-sided heart failure. A new systolic murmur may signify acute mitral regurgitation or ventricular septal rupture. Auscultatory findings in pulmonary oedema are crepitations at the lung bases, or throughout the lungs if pulmonary oedema is severe. Expiratory wheeze often accompanies this.

Acute-on-chronic heart failure will have additional features of long-standing heart failure (see below). Potential precipitants, such as an upper respiratory tract infection or inappropriate cessation of diuretic medication, should be identified.

Chronic heart failure

Patients with chronic heart failure commonly follow a relapsing and remitting course, with periods of stability and episodes of decompensation, leading to worsening symptoms that may necessitate hospitalisation. The clinical picture depends on the nature of the underlying heart disease, the type of heart failure that it has evoked, and the neurohumoral changes that have developed (see Box 18.11 and Fig. 18.24).

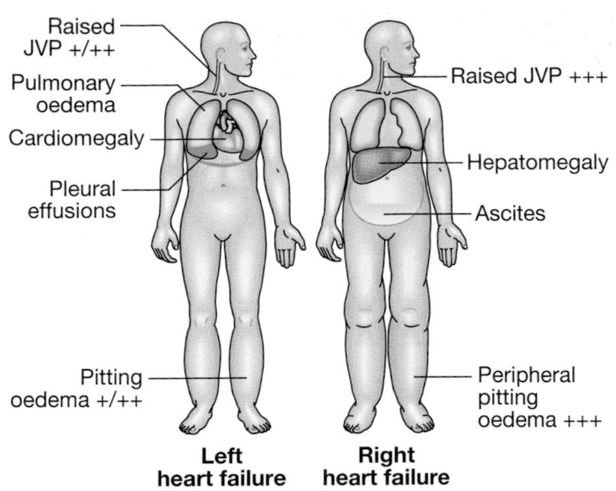

Fig. 18.24 Clinical features of left and right heart failure. (JVP = jugular venous pressure)

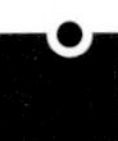

18.13 Differential diagnosis of peripheral oedema

- Cardiac failure: right or combined left and right heart failure, pericardial constriction, cardiomyopathy
- Chronic venous insufficiency: varicose veins
- Hypoalbuminaemia: nephrotic syndrome, liver disease, protein-losing enteropathy; often widespread, can affect arms and face
- Drugs:
  Sodium retention: fludrocortisone, NSAIDs
  Increasing capillary permeability: nifedipine, amlodipine
- Idiopathic: women > men
- Chronic lymphatic obstruction

Low cardiac output causes fatigue, listlessness and a poor effort tolerance; the peripheries are cold and the BP is low. To maintain perfusion of vital organs, blood flow is diverted away from skeletal muscle and this may contribute to fatigue and weakness. Poor renal perfusion leads to oliguria and uraemia.

Pulmonary oedema due to left heart failure presents as above and with inspiratory crepitations over the lung bases. In contrast, right heart failure produces a high JVP with hepatic congestion and dependent peripheral oedema. In ambulant patients, the oedema affects the ankles, whereas, in bed-bound patients, it collects around the thighs and sacrum. Ascites or pleural effusion may occur (see Fig. 18.24). Heart failure is not the only cause of oedema (Box 18.13).

Chronic heart failure is sometimes associated with marked weight loss (cardiac cachexia), caused by a combination of anorexia and impaired absorption due to gastrointestinal congestion, poor tissue perfusion due to a low cardiac output, and skeletal muscle atrophy due to immobility.

Complications

In advanced heart failure, the following may occur:

- *Renal failure* is caused by poor renal perfusion due to low cardiac output and may be exacerbated by diuretic therapy, angiotensin-converting enzyme (ACE) inhibitors and angiotensin receptor blockers.
- *Hypokalaemia* may be the result of treatment with potassium-losing diuretics or hyperaldosteronism caused by activation of the renin–angiotensin system and impaired aldosterone metabolism due to hepatic congestion. Most of the body's potassium is intracellular and there may be substantial depletion of potassium stores, even when the plasma concentration is in the reference range.
- *Hyperkalaemia* may be due to the effects of drugs which promote renal resorption of potassium, in particular the combination of ACE inhibitors (or angiotensin receptor blockers) and mineralocorticoid receptor antagonists. These effects are amplified if there is renal dysfunction due to low cardiac output or atherosclerotic renal vascular disease.
- *Hyponatraemia* is a feature of severe heart failure and is a poor prognostic sign. It may be caused by diuretic therapy, inappropriate water retention due to high ADH secretion, or failure of the cell membrane ion pump.
- *Impaired liver function* is caused by hepatic venous congestion and poor arterial perfusion, which frequently cause mild jaundice and abnormal liver function tests; reduced synthesis of clotting factors can make anticoagulant control difficult.
- *Thromboembolism.* Deep vein thrombosis and pulmonary embolism may occur due to the effects of a low cardiac output and enforced immobility. Systemic emboli occur in patients with atrial fibrillation or flutter, or with intracardiac thrombus complicating conditions such as mitral stenosis, MI or left ventricular aneurysm.
- *Atrial and ventricular arrhythmias* are very common and may be related to electrolyte changes (e.g. hypokalaemia, hypomagnesaemia), the underlying cardiac disease, and the pro-arrhythmic effects of sympathetic activation. Atrial fibrillation occurs in approximately 20% of patients with heart failure and causes further impairment of cardiac function. Sudden death occurs in up to 50% of patients with heart failure and is often due to a ventricular arrhythmia. Frequent ventricular ectopic beats and runs of non-sustained ventricular tachycardia are common findings in patients with heart failure and are associated with an adverse prognosis.

Investigations

Serum urea, creatinine and electrolytes, haemoglobin, thyroid function, ECG and chest X-ray may help to establish the nature and severity of the underlying heart disease and detect any complications. Brain natriuretic peptide (BNP) is elevated in heart failure and is a marker of risk; it is useful in the investigation of patients with breathlessness or peripheral oedema.

Echocardiography is very useful and should be considered in all patients with heart failure in order to:

- determine the aetiology
- detect hitherto unsuspected valvular heart disease, such as occult mitral stenosis, and other conditions that may be amenable to specific remedies
- identify patients who will benefit from long-term drug therapy, e.g. ACE inhibitors (see below).

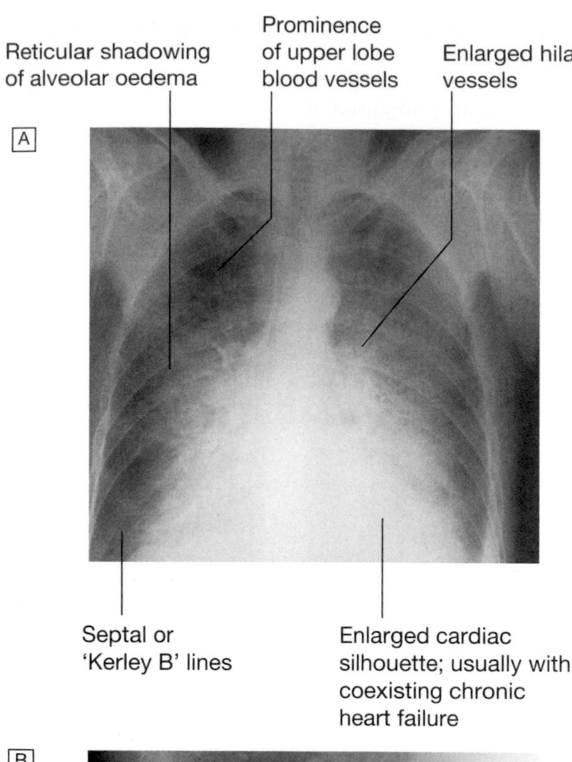

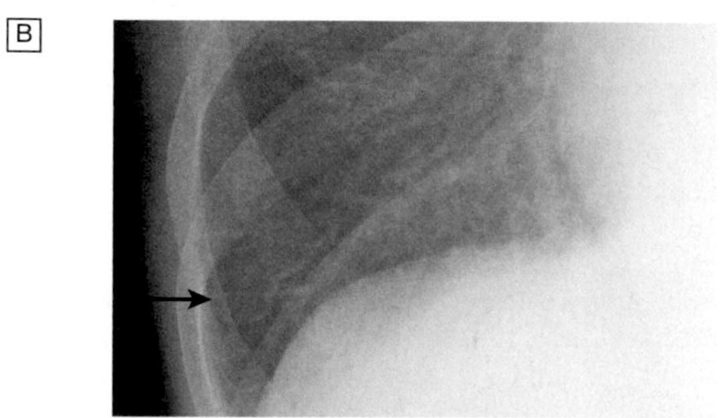

Fig. 18.25 Radiological features of heart failure. A Chest X-ray of a patient with pulmonary oedema. B Enlargement of lung base showing septal or 'Kerley B' lines (arrow).

Chest X-ray

High pulmonary venous pressure in left-sided heart failure first shows on the chest X-ray (Fig. 18.25) as an abnormal distension of the upper lobe pulmonary veins (with the patient in the erect position). The vascularity of the lung fields becomes more prominent, and the right and left pulmonary arteries dilate. Subsequently, interstitial oedema causes thickened interlobular septa and dilated lymphatics. These are evident as horizontal lines in the costophrenic angles (septal or 'Kerley B' lines). More advanced changes due to alveolar oedema cause a hazy opacification spreading from the hilar regions, and pleural effusions.

Management of acute pulmonary oedema

This is an acute medical emergency:

- Sit the patient up to reduce pulmonary congestion.
- Give oxygen (high-flow, high-concentration). Non-invasive positive pressure ventilation (continuous positive airways pressure (CPAP) of 5–10 mmHg) by a tight-fitting facemask results in a more rapid clinical improvement.
- Administer nitrates, such as IV glyceryl trinitrate (10–200 µg/min or buccal glyceryl trinitrate 2–5 mg, titrated upwards every 10 minutes), until clinical improvement occurs or systolic BP falls to less than 110 mmHg.
- Administer a loop diuretic, such as furosemide (50–100 mg IV).

The patient should initially be kept rested, with continuous monitoring of cardiac rhythm, BP and pulse oximetry. Intravenous opiates must be used sparingly in distressed patients, as they may cause respiratory depression and exacerbation of hypoxaemia and hypercapnia.

If these measures prove ineffective, inotropic agents may be required to augment cardiac output, particularly in hypotensive patients. Insertion of an intra-aortic balloon pump may be beneficial in patients with acute cardiogenic pulmonary oedema and shock.

Management of chronic heart failure

General measures

Education of patients and their relatives about the causes and treatment of heart failure can help adherence to a management plan (Box 18.14). Some patients may need to weigh themselves daily, as a measure of fluid load, and adjust their diuretic therapy accordingly. Treatment of the underlying cause of heart failure (e.g. coronary artery disease) is important to prevent its progression.

Drug therapy

Cardiac function can be improved by increasing contractility, optimising preload or decreasing afterload (see Fig. 18.23). Drugs that reduce preload are appropriate in patients with high end-diastolic filling pressures and evidence of pulmonary or systemic venous congestion. Those that reduce afterload or increase myocardial

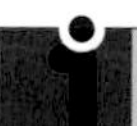

18.14 General measures for the management of heart failure

Education
• Explanation of nature of disease, treatment and self-help strategies
Diet
• Good general nutrition and weight reduction for the obese • Avoidance of high-salt foods and added salt, especially for patients with severe congestive heart failure
Alcohol
• Moderation or elimination of alcohol consumption. Alcohol-induced cardiomyopathy requires abstinence
Smoking
• Cessation
Exercise
• Regular moderate aerobic exercise within limits of symptoms
Vaccination
• Consider influenza and pneumococcal vaccination

contractility are more useful in patients with signs and symptoms of a low cardiac output.

Diuretic therapy

In heart failure, diuretics produce an increase in urinary sodium and water excretion, leading to reduction in blood and plasma volume (p. 434). Diuretic therapy reduces preload and improves pulmonary and systemic venous congestion. It may also reduce afterload and ventricular volume, leading to a fall in ventricular wall tension and increased cardiac efficiency.

Although a fall in preload (ventricular filling pressure) tends to reduce cardiac output, the 'Starling curve' in heart failure is flat, so there may be a substantial and beneficial fall in filling pressure with little change in cardiac output (see Figs 18.22 and 18.26). Nevertheless, excessive diuretic therapy may cause an undesirable fall in cardiac output, especially in patients with a marked diastolic component to their heart failure. This leads to hypotension, lethargy and renal failure.

In some patients with severe chronic heart failure, particularly if there is associated renal impairment, oedema may persist, despite oral loop diuretic therapy. In such patients, an intravenous infusion of furosemide (5–10 mg/hr) may initiate a diuresis. Combining a loop diuretic with a thiazide diuretic (e.g. bendroflumethiazide 5 mg daily) may prove effective, but this can cause an excessive diuresis.

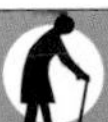

18.15 Congestive cardiac failure in old age

- **Incidence**: rises with age and affects 5–10% of those in their eighties.
- **Common causes**: coronary artery disease, hypertension and calcific degenerative valvular disease.
- **Diastolic dysfunction**: often prominent, particularly in those with a history of hypertension.
- **ACE inhibitors**: improve symptoms and mortality but are more frequently associated with postural hypotension and renal impairment than in younger patients.
- **Loop diuretics**: usually required but may be poorly tolerated in those with urinary incontinence and men with prostate enlargement.

Cardiac output or ventricular performance

Normal

Heart failure

C

B

A

Forward failure
Fatigue

Preload

Backward failure
Dyspnoea/oedema

Fig. 18.26 The effect of treatment on ventricular performance curves in heart failure. Diuretics and venodilators (A), angiotensin-converting enzyme (ACE) inhibitors and mixed vasodilators (B), and positive inotropic agents (C).

Mineralocorticoid receptor antagonists, such as spironolactone and eplerenone, are potassium-sparing diuretics that are of particular benefit in patients with heart failure with severe left ventricular systolic dysfunction. They may cause hyperkalaemia, particularly when used with an ACE inhibitor. They improve long-term clinical outcome in patients with severe heart failure or heart failure following acute MI.

Angiotensin-converting enzyme inhibition therapy

Angiotensin-converting enzyme (ACE) inhibition therapy interrupts the vicious circle of neurohumoral activation that is characteristic of moderate and severe heart failure by preventing the conversion of angiotensin I to angiotensin II, thereby preventing peripheral vasoconstriction, activation of the sympathetic nervous system (Fig. 18.27), and salt and water retention due to aldosterone release. These drugs also prevent the undesirable activation of the renin–angiotensin system caused by diuretic therapy.

In moderate and severe heart failure, ACE inhibitors can produce a substantial improvement in effort tolerance and in mortality. They can also improve outcome and prevent the onset of overt heart failure in patients with poor residual left ventricular function following MI (Box 18.16).

ACE inhibitors can cause symptomatic hypotension and impairment of renal function, especially in patients with bilateral renal artery stenosis or those with pre-existing renal disease. An increase in serum potassium concentration may occur that can offset hypokalaemia associated with loop diuretic therapy. Short-acting ACE inhibitors can cause marked falls in BP, particularly in the elderly or when started in the presence of hypotension, hypovolaemia or hyponatraemia. In stable patients without hypotension (systolic BP over 100 mmHg), ACE inhibitors can usually be safely started in the community. However, in other patients, it is usually advisable to withhold diuretics for 24 hours before starting treatment with a small dose of a long-acting agent, preferably given at night (Box 18.17). Renal function and serum potassium must be monitored and should be checked 1–2 weeks after starting therapy.

EBM 18.16 ACE inhibitors and treatment of chronic heart failure

'ACE inhibitors in chronic heart failure due to ventricular dysfunction reduce mortality and re-admission rates; average NNT_B for 3 years to prevent 1 death = 26 and for the combined endpoint of death or re-admission = 19.'

- Flather M, et al. Lancet 2000; 355:1575–1581.

For further information: www.sign.ac.uk/guidelines/fulltext/95/contents.html

Angiotensin receptor blocker therapy

Angiotensin receptor blockers (ARBs; see Box 18.17) act by blocking the action of angiotensin II on the heart, peripheral vasculature and kidney. In heart failure, they produce beneficial haemodynamic changes that are similar to the effects of ACE inhibitors (see Fig. 18.27) but are generally better tolerated. They have comparable effects on mortality and are a useful alternative for patients who cannot tolerate ACE inhibitors (Box 18.18).

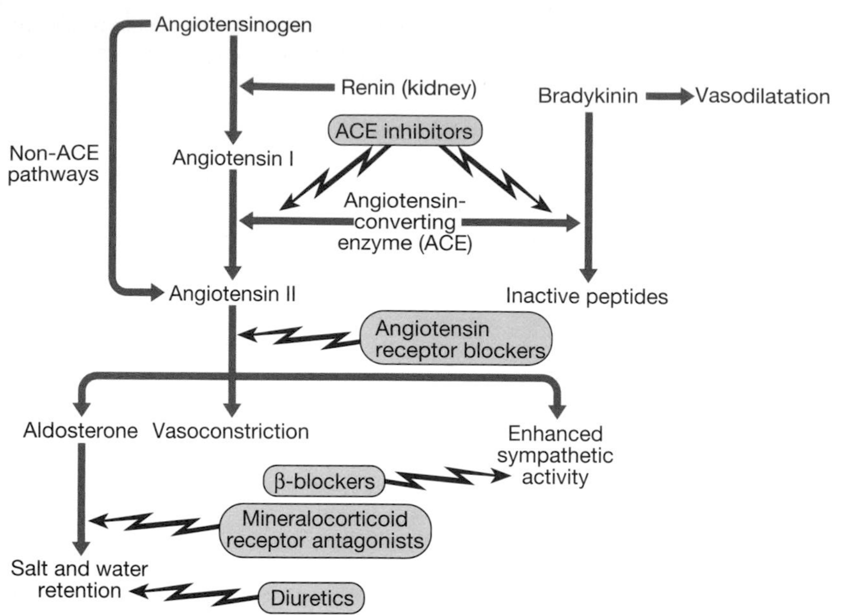

Fig. 18.27 Neurohumoral activation and sites of action of drugs used in the treatment of heart failure.

18.17 ACE inhibitor and angiotensin receptor blocker (ARB) dosages in heart failure

	Starting dose	Target dose
ACE inhibitors		
Enalapril	2.5 mg twice daily	10 mg twice daily
Lisinopril	2.5 mg daily	20 mg daily
Ramipril	1.25 mg daily	10 mg daily
Angiotensin receptor blockers		
Losartan	25 mg daily	100 mg daily
Candesartan	4 mg daily	32 mg daily
Valsartan	40 mg daily	160 mg daily

EBM 18.18 Angiotensin receptor blockers (ARBs) and chronic heart failure

'Compared with ACE inhibitors, ARBs are better tolerated and have similar efficacy in reducing cardiovascular events. ARBs reduce cardiovascular morbidity and mortality in patients with symptomatic heart failure who are intolerant of ACE inhibitors. NNT_B for 5 years to prevent 1 death or hospitalisation for heart failure = 8. The addition of an ARB to an ACE inhibitor produces further additional benefit. NNT_B for 5 years to prevent 1 death or hospitalisation for heart failure = 16.'

- Granger CB, et al. Lancet 2003; 362:772–776.
- McMurray JJV, et al. Lancet 2003; 362:767–771.

Unfortunately, they share all the more serious adverse effects of ACE inhibitors, including renal dysfunction and hyperkalaemia. ARBs are normally used as an alternative to ACE inhibitors, but the two can be combined in patients with resistant or recurrent heart failure.

Vasodilator therapy

These drugs are valuable in chronic heart failure, when ACE inhibitor or ARB drugs are contraindicated (e.g. in severe renal failure). Venodilators, such as nitrates, reduce preload, and arterial dilators, such as hydralazine, reduce afterload (see Fig. 18.26). Their use is limited by pharmacological tolerance and hypotension.

EBM 18.19 Beta-blockers and treatment of chronic heart failure

'Adding oral β-blockers gradually in small incremental doses to standard therapy, including ACE inhibitors, in people with heart failure reduces the rate of death or hospital admission. NNT_B for 1 year to prevent 1 death = 21.'

- Lechat P, et al. Circulation 1998; 98:1184–1191.
- Shibata MC, et al. Eur J Heart Fail 2001; 34:351–357.

For further information: www.escardio.org

Beta-adrenoceptor blocker therapy

Beta-blockade helps to counteract the deleterious effects of enhanced sympathetic stimulation and reduces the risk of arrhythmias and sudden death. When initiated in standard doses, they may precipitate acute-on-chronic heart failure, but when given in small incremental doses (e.g. bisoprolol started at a dose of 1.25 mg daily, and increased gradually over a 12-week period to a target maintenance dose of 10 mg daily), they can increase ejection fraction, improve symptoms, reduce the frequency of hospitalisation and reduce mortality in patients with chronic heart failure (Box 18.19). Beta-blockers are more effective at reducing mortality than ACE inhibitors: relative risk reduction of 33% versus 20%, respectively.

Ivabradine

Ivabradine acts on the I_f inward current in the SA node, resulting in reduction of heart rate. It reduces hospital admission and mortality rates in patients with heart failure due to moderate or severe left ventricular systolic impairment. In trials, its effects were most marked in patients with a relatively high heart rate (over 77/min), so ivabradine is best suited to patients who cannot take β-blockers or in whom the heart rate remains high despite β-blockade. It is ineffective in patients in atrial fibrillation.

Digoxin

Digoxin (p. 576) can be used to provide rate control in patients with heart failure and atrial fibrillation. In patients with severe heart failure (NYHA class III–IV, see Box 18.5, p. 539), digoxin reduces the likelihood of hospitalisation for heart failure, although it has no effect on long-term survival.

Amiodarone

This is a potent anti-arrhythmic drug (p. 576) that has little negative inotropic effect and may be valuable in patients with poor left ventricular function. It is only effective in the treatment of symptomatic arrhythmias, and should not be used as a preventative agent in asymptomatic patients.

Implantable cardiac defibrillators and resynchronisation therapy

Patients with symptomatic ventricular arrhythmias and heart failure have a very poor prognosis. Irrespective of their response to anti-arrhythmic drug therapy, all should be considered for implantation of a cardiac defibrillator because it improves survival (p. 579). In patients with marked intraventricular conduction delay, prolonged depolarisation may lead to uncoordinated left ventricular contraction. When this is associated with severe symptomatic heart failure, cardiac resynchronisation therapy should be considered. Here, both the LV and RV are paced simultaneously (Fig. 18.28) to generate a more coordinated left ventricular contraction and improve cardiac output. This is associated with improved symptoms and survival.

Coronary revascularisation

Coronary artery bypass surgery or percutaneous coronary intervention may improve function in areas of the myocardium that are 'hibernating' because of inadequate blood supply, and can be used to treat carefully selected patients with heart failure and coronary artery disease. If necessary, 'hibernating' myocardium can be identified by stress echocardiography and specialised nuclear or MR imaging.

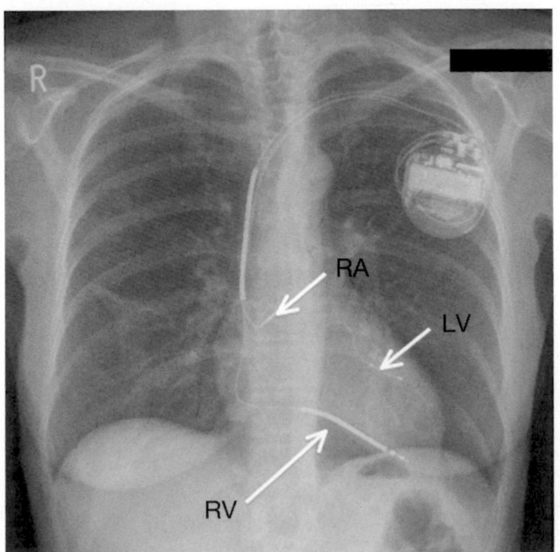

Fig. 18.28 Chest X-ray of a biventricular pacemaker and defibrillator (cardiac resynchronisation therapy). The right ventricular lead (RV) is in position in the ventricular apex and is used for both pacing and defibrillation. The left ventricular lead (LV) is placed via the coronary sinus, and the right atrial lead (RA) is placed in the right atrial appendage; both are used for pacing only.

Heart transplantation

Cardiac transplantation is an established and successful treatment for patients with intractable heart failure. Coronary artery disease and dilated cardiomyopathy are the most common indications. The introduction of ciclosporin for immunosuppression (p. 96) has improved survival, which is around 80% at 1 year. The use of transplantation is limited by the efficacy of modern drug and device therapies, as well as the availability of donor hearts, so it is generally reserved for young patients with severe symptoms despite optimal therapy.

Conventional heart transplantation is contraindicated in patients with pulmonary vascular disease due to long-standing left heart failure, complex congenital heart disease (e.g. Eisenmenger's syndrome) or primary pulmonary hypertension because the RV of the donor heart may fail in the face of high pulmonary vascular resistance. However, heart–lung transplantation can be successful in patients with Eisenmenger's syndrome. Lung transplantation has been used for primary pulmonary hypertension.

Although cardiac transplantation usually produces a dramatic improvement in the recipient's quality of life, serious complications may occur:

- *Rejection*. In spite of routine therapy with ciclosporin A, azathioprine and corticosteroids, episodes of rejection are common and may present with heart failure, arrhythmias or subtle ECG changes; cardiac biopsy is often used to confirm the diagnosis before starting treatment with high-dose corticosteroids.
- *Accelerated atherosclerosis*. Recurrent heart failure is often due to progressive atherosclerosis in the coronary arteries of the donor heart. This is not confined to patients who underwent transplantation for coronary artery disease and is probably a manifestation of chronic rejection. Angina is rare because the heart has been denervated.
- *Infection*. Opportunistic infection with organisms such as cytomegalovirus or *Aspergillus* remains a major cause of death in transplant recipients.

Ventricular assist devices

Because of the limited supply of donor organs, ventricular assist devices (VADs) have been employed as:

- a bridge to cardiac transplantation
- potential long-term therapy
- short-term restoration therapy following a potentially reversible insult, e.g. viral myocarditis.

VADs assist cardiac output by using a roller, centrifugal or pulsatile pump that, in some cases, is implantable and portable. They withdraw blood through cannulae inserted in the atria or ventricular apex and pump it into the pulmonary artery or aorta. They are designed not only to unload the ventricles but also to provide support to the pulmonary and systemic circulations. Their more widespread application is limited by high complication rates (haemorrhage, systemic embolism, infection, neurological and renal sequelae), although some improvements in survival and quality of life have been demonstrated in patients with severe heart failure.

Syncope and presyncope

The term 'syncope' refers to sudden loss of consciousness due to reduced cerebral perfusion. 'Presyncope' refers to lightheadedness in which the individual thinks he or she may black out. Syncope affects around 20% of the population at some time and accounts for more than 5% of hospital admissions. Dizziness and presyncope are very common in old age (p. 173). Symptoms are disabling, undermine confidence and independence, and can affect an individual's ability to work or to drive. There are three principal mechanisms that underlie recurrent presyncope or syncope:

- *cardiac syncope* due to mechanical cardiac dysfunction or arrhythmia
- *neurocardiogenic syncope*, in which an abnormal autonomic reflex causes bradycardia and/or hypotension
- *postural hypotension*, in which physiological peripheral vasoconstriction on standing is impaired, lead to hypotension.

Loss of consciousness can also be caused by non-cardiac pathology, such as epilepsy, cerebrovascular ischaemia or hypoglycaemia (Fig. 18.29).

Differential diagnosis

History-taking, from the patient or a witness, is the key to establishing a diagnosis. Attention should be paid to potential triggers (e.g. medication, exertion, posture), the victim's appearance (e.g. colour, seizure activity), the duration of the episode and the speed of recovery (Box 18.20). Cardiac syncope is usually sudden but can be associated with premonitory lightheadedness, palpitation or chest discomfort. The blackout is usually brief and recovery rapid. Neurocardiogenic syncope will often be associated with a situational trigger, and the patient may experience flushing, nausea and malaise for several minutes afterwards. Patients with seizures do not exhibit pallor, may have abnormal movements, usually take more than 5 minutes to recover and are often confused. A history of rotational vertigo is suggestive of a labyrinthine or vestibular disorder (p. 1167). The pattern and description of the patient's symptoms should indicate the probable mechanism and help to determine subsequent investigations (Fig. 18.30). Postural hypotension is normally obvious from the history, with presyncope or, less commonly, syncope, occurring within a few seconds of standing.

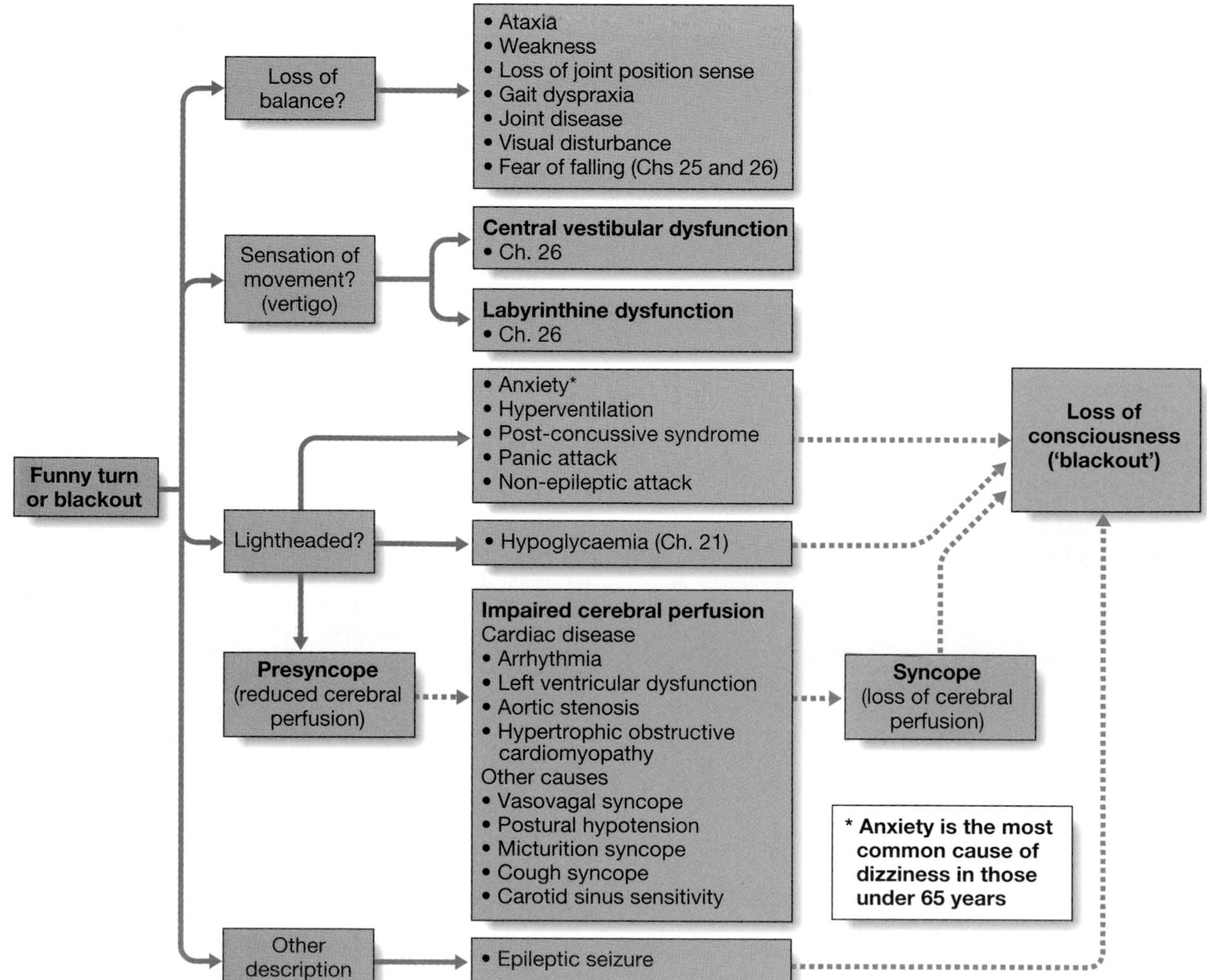

Fig. 18.29 The differential diagnosis of syncope and presyncope.

18.20 Typical features of cardiac syncope, vasovagal syncope and seizures

	Cardiac syncope	Neurocardiogenic syncope	Seizures
Premonitory symptoms	Often none Lightheadedness Palpitation Chest pain Breathlessness	Nausea Lightheadedness Sweating	Confusion Hyperexcitability Olfactory hallucinations 'Aura'
Unconscious period	Extreme 'death-like' pallor	Pallor	Prolonged (> 1 min) unconsciousness Motor seizure activity* Tongue-biting Urinary incontinence
Recovery	Rapid recovery (< 1 min) Flushing	Slow Nausea Lightheadedness	Prolonged confusion (> 5 mins) Headache Focal neurological signs

***N.B.** Cardiac syncope can also cause convulsions by inducing cerebral anoxia.

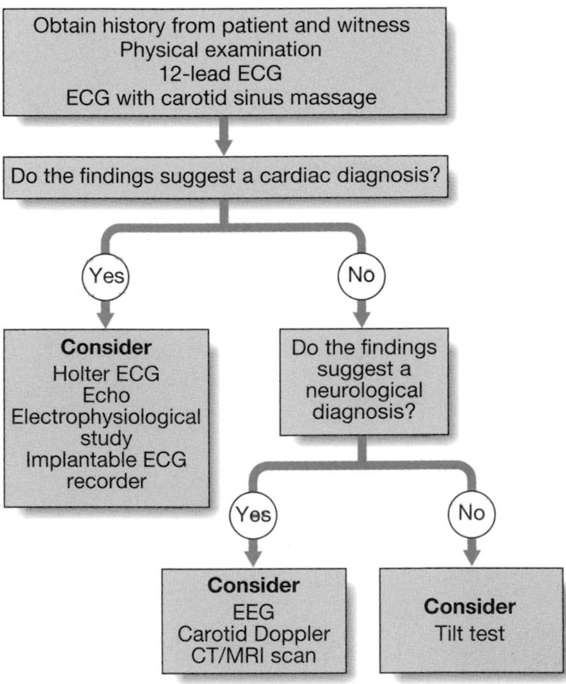

Fig. 18.30 A simple guide to the investigation and diagnosis of recurrent presyncope and syncope.

Cardiac syncope

Arrhythmia

Lightheadedness may occur with many arrhythmias, but blackouts (Stokes–Adams attacks, p. 572) are usually due to profound bradycardia or malignant ventricular tachyarrhythmias. The 12-lead ECG may show evidence of conducting system disease (e.g. sinus bradycardia, atrioventricular block, bundle branch block or axis deviation), which would predispose a patient to bradycardia, but the key to establishing a diagnosis is to obtain an ECG recording *while symptoms are present*. Since minor rhythm disturbances are common, especially in old age, symptoms must occur at the same time as a recorded arrhythmia before a diagnosis can be made. Ambulatory ECG recordings are helpful only if symptoms occur several times per week. Patient-activated ECG recorders are useful for examining the rhythm in patients with recurrent dizziness but are not useful in assessing sudden blackouts. When these investigations fail to establish a cause in patients with presyncope or syncope, an implantable ECG recorder can be sited subcutaneously over the upper left chest. This device continuously records the cardiac rhythm and will activate automatically if extreme bradycardia or tachycardia occurs. The ECG memory can also be tagged by the patient, using a hand-held activator. Stored ECGs can be accessed by the implanting centre, using a telemetry device in a clinic, or using a home monitoring system via an online link.

Structural heart disease

Severe aortic stenosis and hypertrophic obstructive cardiomyopathy can lead to lightheadedness or syncope on exertion. This is caused by profound hypotension due to a fall in cardiac output, or failure to increase output during exertion, coupled with exercise-induced peripheral vasodilatation. Severe coronary artery disease can produce the same symptoms because of ischaemic left ventricular dysfunction. Exertional arrhythmias also occur in these patients.

Neurocardiogenic syncope

This encompasses a family of syndromes in which bradycardia and/or hypotension occur because of a series of abnormal autonomic reflexes. The two main conditions are hypersensitive carotid sinus syndrome and malignant vasovagal syncope.

Situational syncope

This is the collective name given to some variants of neurocardiogenic syncope that occur in the presence of identifiable triggers (e.g. cough syncope, micturition syncope).

Vasovagal syncope

This is normally triggered by a reduction in venous return due to prolonged standing, excessive heat or a large meal. It is mediated by the Bezold–Jarisch reflex, in which a combination of sympathetic activation, and reduced venous return due to an impaired vasoconstrictor response to standing, leads to vigorous contraction of relatively under-filled ventricles. This stimulates ventricular mechanoreceptors, producing parasympathetic (vagal) activation and sympathetic withdrawal, causing bradycardia, vasodilatation or both. Head-up tilt-table testing is a provocation test used to establish the diagnosis, and involves positioning the patient supine on a padded table that is then tilted to an angle of 60–70° for up to 45 minutes, while the ECG and BP responses are monitored. A positive test is characterised by bradycardia (cardio-inhibitory response) and/or hypotension (vasodepressor response) associated with typical symptoms. Initial management involves lifestyle modification (salt supplementation and avoiding prolonged standing, dehydration or missing meals). In resistant cases, drug therapy can be tried, although efficacy is inconsistent in clinical trials. Fludrocortisone (causes sodium and water retention and expands plasma volume), disopyramide (a vagolytic agent) or midodrine (a vasoconstrictor α-adrenoceptor agonist) may be helpful. Beta-blockers (inhibit the initial sympathetic activation) are seldom effective and are rarely used. In patients with resistant vasovagal syncope in which bradycardia is the predominant response, a dual-chamber pacemaker can be useful. Patients with a urinary sodium excretion of less than 170 mmol/day may respond to salt loading.

Hypersensitive carotid sinus syndrome

Hypersensitive carotid sinus syndrome (HCSS) causes presyncope or syncope because of reflex bradycardia and vasodilatation. Carotid baroreceptors are involved in BP regulation and are activated by increased BP, resulting in a vagal discharge that causes a compensatory drop in BP. In HCSS, the baroreceptor is sensitive to external pressure (e.g. during neck movement or if a tight collar is worn), so that pressure over the carotid artery causes an inappropriate and intense vagal discharge. The diagnosis can be established by monitoring the ECG and BP during carotid sinus pressure. This manœuvre should not be attempted in patients with a carotid bruit or with a history of cerebrovascular disease because of the risk of embolic stroke. A positive cardio-inhibitory response is defined as a sinus pause of 3 seconds or more; a positive vasodepressor response is defined as a fall in systolic BP of more than 50 mmHg. Carotid sinus pressure will produce positive findings in about 10% of elderly individuals but less than 25% of these experience spontaneous syncope. Symptoms should not therefore be attributed to HCSS unless they are reproduced by carotid sinus pressure. Dual-chamber pacemaker implantation usually prevents syncope in patients with the more common cardio-inhibitory response.

Postural hypotension

This is caused by a failure of normal postural compensatory mechanisms. Relative hypovolaemia (often due to excessive diuretic therapy), sympathetic degeneration (diabetes mellitus, Parkinson's disease, ageing) and drug therapy (vasodilators, antidepressants) can all cause or aggravate the problem. Treatment is often ineffective; however, withdrawing unnecessary medication and advising the patient to wear graduated elastic stockings and to get up slowly may be helpful. Fludrocortisone, which can expand blood volume through sodium and water retention, may be of value.

Palpitation

Palpitation is a very common and sometimes frightening symptom. Patients use the term to describe many sensations, including an unusually erratic, fast, slow or forceful heart beat, or even chest pain or breathlessness. Initial evaluation should concentrate on determining its likely mechanism, and whether or not there is significant underlying heart disease.

A detailed description of the sensation is essential and patients should be asked to describe their symptoms clearly, or to demonstrate the sensation of rhythm by tapping with their hand. A provisional diagnosis can usually be made on the basis of a thorough history (Box 18.21 and Fig. 18.31). The diagnosis should be confirmed by an ECG recording during an episode using an ambulatory ECG monitor or a patient-activated ECG recorder.

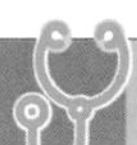

18.21 How to evaluate palpitation

- Is the palpitation continuous or intermittent?
- Is the heart beat regular or irregular?
- What is the approximate heart rate?
- Do symptoms occur in discrete attacks?
  Is the onset abrupt? How do attacks terminate?
- Are there any associated symptoms?
  e.g. Chest pain, lightheadedness, polyuria (a feature of supraventricular tachycardia, p. 567)
- Are there any precipitating factors, e.g. exercise, alcohol?
- Is there a history of structural heart disease, e.g. coronary artery disease, valvular heart disease?

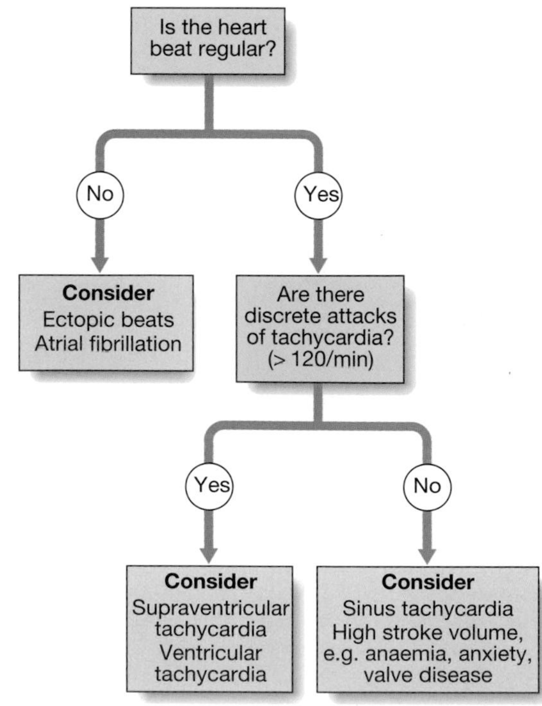

Fig. 18.31 A simple approach to the diagnosis of palpitation.

Recurrent but short-lived bouts of an irregular heart beat are usually due to atrial or ventricular extrasystoles (ectopic beats). Some patients will describe the experience as a 'flip' or a 'jolt' in the chest, while others report dropped or missed beats. Extrasystoles are often more frequent during periods of stress or debility; they can be triggered by alcohol or nicotine.

Episodes of a pounding, forceful and relatively fast (90–120 / min) heart beat are a common manifestation of anxiety. These may also reflect a hyperdynamic circulation, such as anaemia, pregnancy and thyrotoxicosis, and can occur in some forms of valve disease (e.g. aortic regurgitation). Discrete bouts of a very rapid (over 120/min) heart beat are more likely to be due to a paroxysmal tachyarrhythmia. Supraventricular and ventricular tachycardias may present in this way. In contrast, episodes of atrial fibrillation typically present with irregular and usually rapid palpitation.

Palpitation is usually benign and, even if the patient's symptoms are due to an arrhythmia, the outlook is good if there is no underlying structural heart disease. Most cases are due to an awareness of the normal heart beat, a sinus tachycardia or benign extrasystoles, in which case an explanation and reassurance may be all that is required. Palpitation associated with presyncope or syncope may reflect more serious structural or electrical disease and should be investigated without delay.

The diagnosis and management of individual arrhythmias are considered on pages 562–579.

Cardiac arrest and sudden cardiac death

Cardiac arrest describes the sudden and complete loss of cardiac output due to asystole, ventricular tachycardia or fibrillation, or loss of mechanical cardiac contraction (pulseless electrical activity). The clinical diagnosis is based on the victim being unconscious and pulseless; breathing may take some time to stop completely after cardiac arrest. Death is virtually inevitable, unless effective treatment is given promptly.

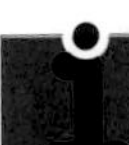

18.22 Causes of sudden arrhythmic death

Coronary artery disease (85%)

- Myocardial ischaemia
- Acute MI
- Prior MI with myocardial scarring

Structural heart disease (10%)

- Aortic stenosis (p. 620)
- Hypertrophic cardiomyopathy (p. 637)
- Dilated cardiomyopathy (p. 636)
- Arrhythmogenic right ventricular dysplasia (p. 638)
- Congenital heart disease (p. 629)

No structural heart disease (5%)

- Long QT syndrome (p. 570)
- Brugada syndrome (p. 571)
- Wolff–Parkinson–White syndrome (p. 568)
- Adverse drug reactions (torsades de pointes, p. 570)
- Severe electrolyte abnormalities

Sudden cardiac death is usually caused by a catastrophic arrhythmia and accounts for 25–30% of deaths from cardiovascular disease, claiming an estimated 70 000–90 000 lives each year in the UK. Many of these deaths are potentially preventable. Arrhythmias complicate many types of heart disease and can sometimes occur in the absence of recognisable structural abnormalities (causes are listed in Box 18.22). Sudden death less often occurs because of an acute mechanical catastrophe such as cardiac rupture or aortic dissection (pp. 597 and 605).

Coronary artery disease is the most common condition leading to cardiac arrest. Ventricular fibrillation or ventricular tachycardia is common in the first few hours of MI and many victims die before medical help is sought. Up to one-third of people developing MI die before reaching hospital, emphasising the importance of educating the public to recognise symptoms and to seek medical help quickly. Acute myocardial ischaemia (in the absence of infarction) can also cause these arrhythmias, although less commonly. Patients with a history of previous MI may be at risk of sudden arrhythmic death, especially if there is extensive left ventricular scarring and impairment, or if there is ongoing myocardial ischaemia. In these patients, the risk is reduced by the treatment of heart failure with β-blockers and ACE inhibitors, and by coronary revascularisation. For some patients, the risk of sudden death is reduced by the implantation of a cardiac defibrillator (p. 579).

Aetiology of cardiac arrest

Cardiac arrest may be caused by ventricular fibrillation, pulseless ventricular tachycardia, asystole or pulseless electrical activity.

Ventricular fibrillation and pulseless ventricular tachycardia

These are the most common and most easily treatable cardiac arrest rhythms. Ventricular fibrillation produces rapid, ineffective, uncoordinated movement of the ventricles, which therefore produces no pulse. The ECG (Fig. 18.32) shows rapid, bizarre and irregular ventricular complexes. Ventricular tachycardia (p. 569) can cause cardiac arrest if the ventricular rate is so rapid that effective mechanical contraction and relaxation cannot occur, especially in the presence of severe left ventricular impairment. It may degenerate into ventricular fibrillation. Defibrillation will restore cardiac output in more than 80% of patients, if delivered immediately. However, the chances of survival fall by at least 10% with each minute's delay, and by more if basic life support is not given (see below); thus provision of these is the key to survival.

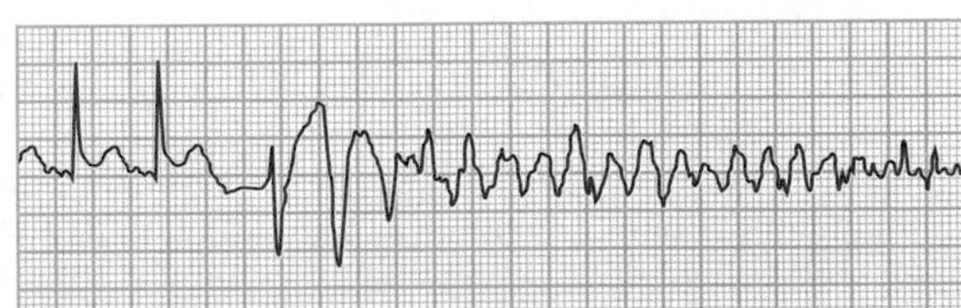

Fig. 18.32 Ventricular fibrillation. A bizarre chaotic rhythm, initiated in this case by two ventricular ectopic beats in rapid succession.

18

Asystole

This occurs when there is no electrical activity within the ventricles and is usually due to failure of the conducting tissue or massive ventricular damage complicating MI. A precordial thump, external cardiac massage, or administration of intravenous atropine or adrenaline (epinephrine) may restore cardiac activity. When due to conducting tissue failure, permanent pacemaker implantation will be required if the individual survives.

Pulseless electrical activity

This occurs when there is no effective cardiac output despite the presence of organised electrical activity. It may be caused by reversible conditions, such as hypovolaemia, cardiac tamponade or tension pneumothorax (see Fig. 18.35 below), but is often due to a catastrophic event, such as cardiac rupture or massive pulmonary embolism, and therefore carries an extremely poor prognosis.

Management of cardiac arrest

The Chain of Survival

This term refers to the sequence of events that is necessary to maximise the chances of a cardiac arrest victim surviving (Fig. 18.33). Survival is most likely if all links in the chain are strong: that is, if the arrest is witnessed, help is called immediately, basic life support is administered by a trained individual, the emergency medical services respond promptly, and defibrillation is achieved within a few minutes. Good training in both basic and advanced life support is essential and should be maintained by regular refresher courses. In recent years, public access defibrillation has been introduced in places of high population density, particularly where traffic congestion may impede the response of emergency services, such as railway stations, airports and sports stadia. Designated individuals can respond to a cardiac arrest using basic life support and an automated external defibrillator.

Basic life support

Basic life support (BLS) encompasses manœuvres that aim to maintain a low level of circulation until more definitive treatment with advanced life support can be given. The ABCDE approach to management of the collapsed patient should be followed: prompt assessment and restoration of the Airway, maintenance of ventilation using rescue Breathing ('mouth-to-mouth' breathing), maintenance of the Circulation using chest compressions; Disability, in resuscitated patients, refers to assessment of neurological status, and Exposure entails removal of clothes to enable defibrillation, auscultation of the chest, and assessment for a rash caused by anaphylaxis, injuries or so on (Fig. 18.34). Chest compression-only ('hands-only') CPR is easier for members of the public to learn and administer, and is now advocated in public education campaigns.

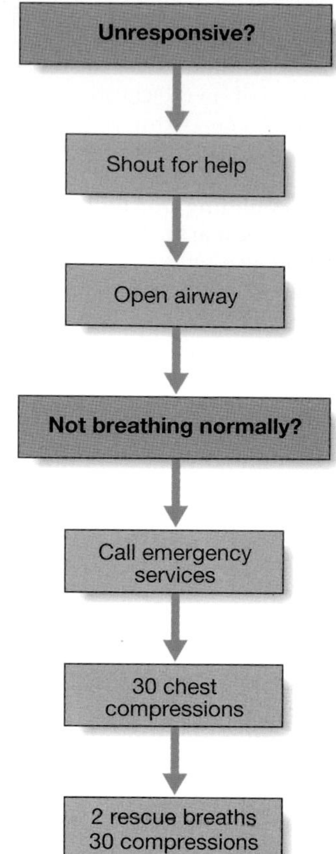

Fig. 18.34 Algorithm for adult basic life support. For further information see www.resus.org.uk. From Resuscitation Council (UK) guidelines – see p. 641.

Advanced life support (ALS)

ALS (Fig. 18.35) aims to restore normal cardiac rhythm by defibrillation when the cause of cardiac arrest is due to a tachyarrhythmia, or to restore cardiac output by correcting other reversible causes of cardiac arrest. ALS can also involve administration of intravenous drugs to

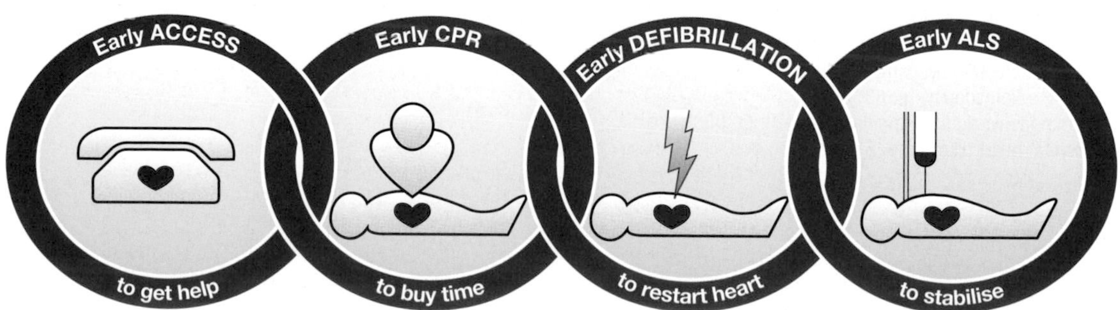

Fig. 18.33 The Chain of Survival in cardiac arrest. (ALS = advanced life support; CPR = cardiopulmonary resuscitation)

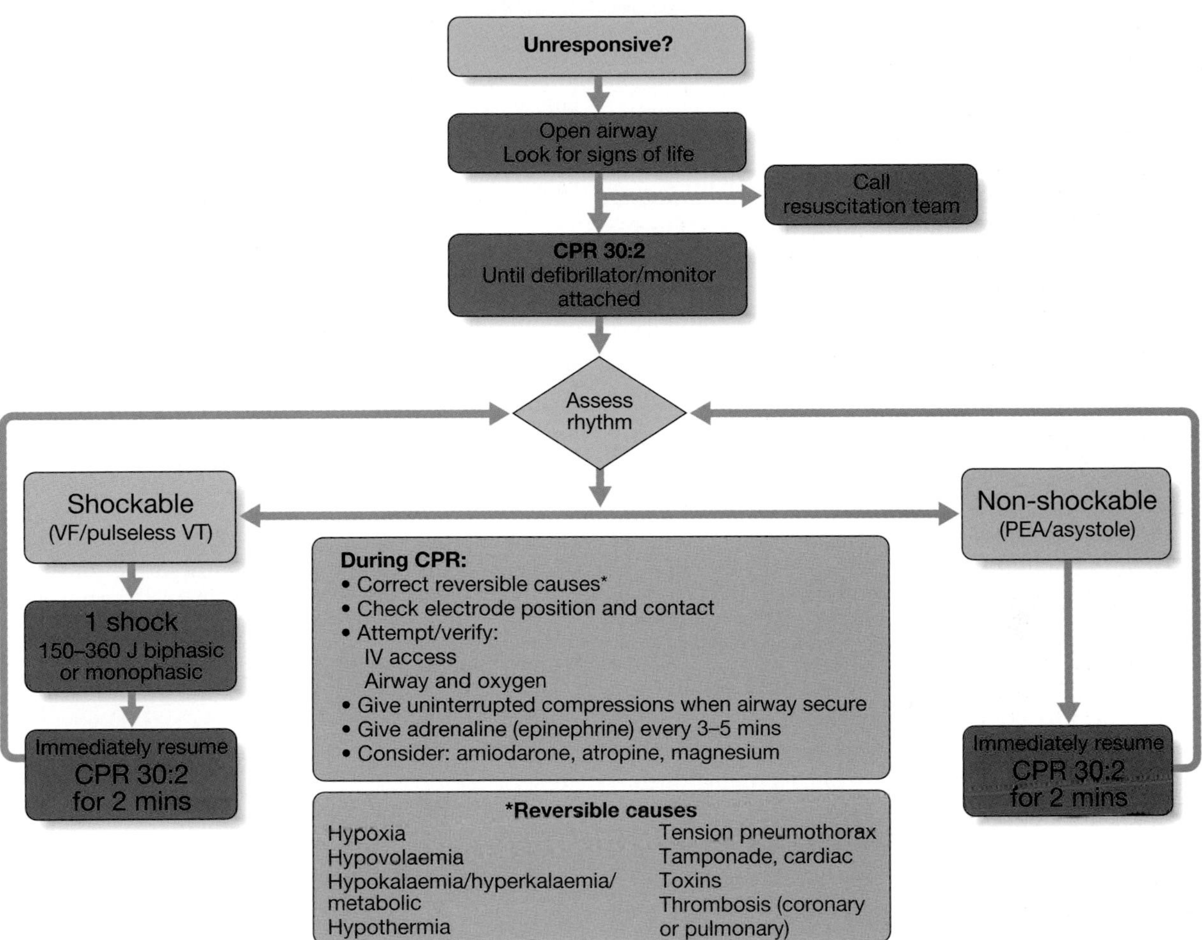

Fig. 18.35 Algorithm for adult advanced life support. For further information see www.resus.org.uk (CPR = cardiopulmonary resuscitation: PEA = pulseless electrical activity; VF = ventricular fibrillation; VT = pulseless ventricular tachycardia) From Resuscitation Council (UK) guidelines – see p. 641.

support the circulation, and endotracheal intubation to ventilate the lungs.

If cardiac arrest is witnessed, a precordial thump may sometimes convert ventricular fibrillation or tachycardia to normal rhythm, but this is futile if cardiac arrest has lasted longer than a few seconds. The priority is to assess the patient's cardiac rhythm by attaching a defibrillator or monitor. Ventricular fibrillation or pulseless ventricular tachycardia is treated with immediate defibrillation. Defibrillation is more likely to be effective if a biphasic shock defibrillator is used, where the polarity of the shock is reversed midway through its delivery. Defibrillation is usually administered using a 150-Joule biphasic shock, and CPR resumed immediately for 2 minutes without attempting to confirm restoration of a pulse, because restoration of mechanical cardiac output rarely occurs immediately after successful defibrillation. If, after 2 minutes, a pulse is not restored, a further biphasic shock of 150–200 joules is given. Thereafter, additional biphasic shocks of 150–200 joules are given every 2 minutes after each cycle of cardiopulmonary resuscitation (CPR). During resuscitation, adrenaline (epinephrine, 1 mg IV) should be given every 3–5 minutes and consideration given to the use of intravenous amiodarone, especially if ventricular fibrillation or ventricular tachycardia re-initiates after successful defibrillation.

Ventricular fibrillation of low amplitude, or 'fine VF', may mimic asystole. If asystole cannot be confidently diagnosed, the patient should be treated for VF and defibrillated. If an electrical rhythm is observed that would be expected to produce a cardiac output, 'pulseless electrical activity' is present. Pulseless electrical activity is treated by continuing CPR and adrenaline (epinephrine) administration whilst seeking such causes. Asystole is treated similarly, with the additional support of atropine and sometimes external or transvenous pacing in an attempt to generate an electrical rhythm.

There are many potentially reversible causes of cardiac arrest and the main causes can be easily remembered as a list of four Hs and four Ts (see Fig. 18.35).

Survivors of cardiac arrest

Patients who survive a cardiac arrest caused by acute MI need no specific treatment beyond that given to those recovering from an uncomplicated infarct, since their prognosis is similar (p. 599). Those with reversible causes, such as exercise-induced ischaemia or aortic stenosis, should have the underlying cause treated if possible. Survivors of ventricular tachycardia or ventricular fibrillation arrest in whom no reversible cause can be identified may be at risk of another episode, and should be considered for an implantable cardiac defibrillator (p. 579) and anti-arrhythmic drug therapy.

Abnormal heart sounds and murmurs

The first indication of heart disease may be the discovery of an abnormal sound on auscultation (Box 18.23). This may be incidental – for example, during a routine childhood examination – or may be prompted by symptoms of heart disease. Clinical evaluation is helpful, and is supported by more detailed evaluation of the abnormal sound or murmur using echocardiography.

Is the sound cardiac?

Additional heart sounds and murmurs demonstrate a consistent relationship to a specific part of the cardiac cycle but extracardiac sounds (e.g. pleural rub or venous hum) do not. Pericardial friction produces a characteristic scratching noise (a pericardial 'rub'), which may have two components corresponding to atrial and ventricular systole, and may vary with posture and respiration.

Is the sound pathological?

Pathological sounds and murmurs are the product of turbulent blood flow or rapid ventricular filling due to abnormal loading conditions. Some added sounds are physiological but may also occur in pathological conditions; for example, a third sound is common in young people and in pregnancy but is also a feature of heart failure (see Box 18.23). Similarly, a systolic murmur due to turbulence across the right ventricular outflow tract may occur in hyperdynamic states (e.g. anaemia, pregnancy), but may also be due to pulmonary stenosis or an intracardiac shunt leading to volume overload of the RV (e.g. atrial septal defect).

Benign murmurs do not occur in diastole (Box 18.24), and systolic murmurs that radiate or are associated with a thrill are almost always pathological.

Auscultatory evaluation of a heart murmur

Timing, intensity, location, radiation and quality are all useful clues to the origin and nature of a heart murmur (Box 18.25). Radiation of a murmur is determined by the direction of turbulent blood flow and is only detectable when there is a high-velocity jet, such as in mitral regurgitation (radiation from apex to axilla) or aortic stenosis (radiation from base to neck). Similarly, the pitch and quality of the sound can help to distinguish the murmur,

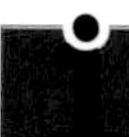

18.24 Features of a benign or innocent heart murmur

- Soft
- Mid-systolic
- Heard at left sternal edge
- No radiation
- No other cardiac abnormalities

18.23 Normal and abnormal heart sounds

Sound	Timing	Characteristics	Mechanisms	Variable features
First heart sound (S1)	Onset of systole	Usually single or narrowly split	Closure of mitral and tricuspid valves	Loud: hyperdynamic circulation (anaemia, pregnancy, thyrotoxicosis); mitral stenosis Soft: heart failure; mitral regurgitation
Second heart sound (S2)	End of systole	Split on inspiration Single on expiration (p. 532)	Closure of aortic and pulmonary valve A_2 first P_2 second	Fixed wide splitting with atrial septal defect Wide but variable splitting with delayed right heart emptying (e.g. right bundle branch block) Reversed splitting due to delayed left heart emptying (e.g. left bundle branch block)
Third heart sound (S3)	Early in diastole, just after S2	Low pitch, often heard as 'gallop'	From ventricular wall due to abrupt cessation of rapid filling	Physiological: young people, pregnancy Pathological: heart failure, mitral regurgitation
Fourth heart sound (S4)	End of diastole, just before S1	Low pitch	Ventricular origin (stiff ventricle and augmented atrial contraction) related to atrial filling	Absent in atrial fibrillation A feature of severe left ventricular hypertrophy (e.g. hypertrophic cardiomyopathy)
Systolic clicks	Early or mid-systole	Brief, high-intensity sound	Valvular aortic stenosis Valvular pulmonary stenosis Floppy mitral valve Prosthetic heart sounds from opening and closing of normally functioning mechanical valves	Click may be lost when stenotic valve becomes thickened or calcified Prosthetic clicks lost when valve obstructed by thrombus or vegetations
Opening snap (OS)	Early in diastole	High pitch, brief duration	Opening of stenosed leaflets of mitral valve Prosthetic heart sounds	Moves closer to S2 as mitral stenosis becomes more severe. May be absent in calcific mitral stenosis

18.25 How to assess a heart murmur

When does it occur?	Time the murmur using heart sounds, carotid pulse and the apex beat. Is it systolic or diastolic? Does the murmur extend throughout systole or diastole or is it confined to a shorter part of the cardiac cycle?
How loud is it? (intensity)	Grade 1: very soft (only audible in ideal conditions) Grade 2: soft Grade 3: moderate Grade 4: loud with associated thrill Grade 5: very loud Grade 6: heard without stethoscope N.B. Diastolic murmurs are sometimes graded 1–4
Where is it heard best? (location)	Listen over the apex and base of the heart, including the aortic and pulmonary areas
Where does it radiate?	Listen at the neck, axilla or back
What does it sound like? (pitch and quality)	Pitch is determined by flow (high pitch indicates high-velocity flow) Is the intensity constant or variable?

such as the 'blowing' murmur of mitral regurgitation or the 'rasping' murmur of aortic stenosis.

The position of a murmur in relation to the cardiac cycle is crucial and should be assessed by timing it with the heart sounds, carotid pulse and apex beat (Figs 18.36 and 18.37).

Systolic murmurs

Ejection systolic murmurs are associated with ventricular outflow tract obstruction and occur in mid-systole with a crescendo–decrescendo pattern, reflecting the changing velocity of blood flow (Box 18.26). Pansystolic murmurs maintain a constant intensity and extend from the first heart sound throughout systole to the second heart sound, sometimes obscuring it. They occur when blood leaks from a ventricle into a low-pressure chamber at an even or constant velocity. Mitral regurgitation, tricuspid regurgitation and ventricular septal defect are the only causes of a pansystolic murmur. Late systolic murmurs are unusual but may occur in mitral valve prolapse, if the mitral regurgitation is confined to late systole, and hypertrophic obstructive cardiomyopathy, if dynamic obstruction occurs late in systole.

Diastolic murmurs

These are due to accelerated or turbulent flow across the mitral or tricuspid valves. They are low-pitched noises that are often difficult to hear and should be evaluated with the bell of the stethoscope. A mid-diastolic murmur may be due to mitral stenosis (located at the apex and axilla), tricuspid stenosis (located at the left sternal edge), increased flow across the mitral valve (e.g. the to-and-fro murmur of severe mitral regurgitation) or increased flow across the tricuspid valve (e.g. left-to-right shunt through a large atrial septal defect). Early diastolic murmurs have a soft, blowing quality with a

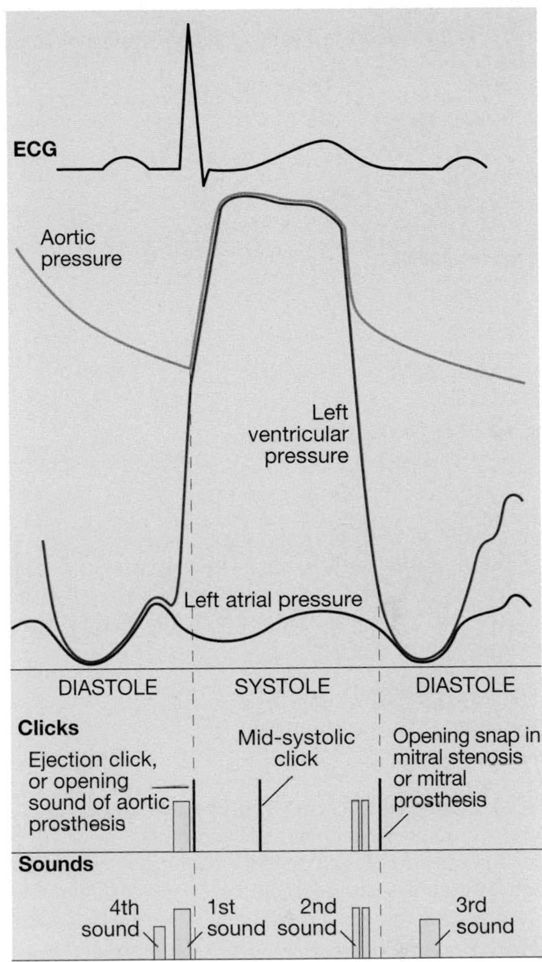

Fig. 18.36 The relationship of the cardiac cycle to the ECG, the left ventricular pressure wave and the position of heart sounds.

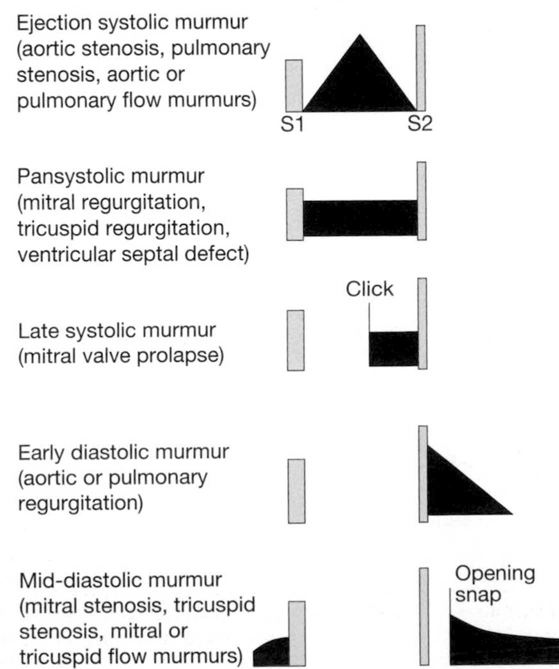

Fig. 18.37 The timing and pattern of cardiac murmurs.

18

18.26 Features of some common systolic murmurs

Condition	Timing and duration	Quality	Location and radiation	Associated features
Aortic stenosis	Mid-systolic	Loud, rasping	Base and left sternal edge, radiating to suprasternal notch and carotids	Single second heart sound Ejection click (in young patients) Slow rising pulse Left ventricular hypertrophy (pressure overload)
Mitral regurgitation	Pansystolic	Blowing	Apex, radiating to axilla	Soft first heart sound Third heart sound Left ventricular hypertrophy (volume overload)
Ventricular septal defect (VSD)	Pansystolic	Harsh	Lower left sternal edge, radiating to whole precordium	Thrill Biventricular hypertrophy
Benign	Mid-systolic	Soft	Left sternal edge, no radiation	No other signs of heart disease

decrescendo pattern and should be evaluated with the diaphragm of the stethoscope. They are due to regurgitation across the aortic or pulmonary valves and are best heard at the left sternal edge, with the patient sitting forwards in held expiration.

Continuous murmurs

These result from a combination of systolic and diastolic flow (e.g. persistent ductus arteriosus), and must be distinguished from extracardiac noises such as bruits from arterial shunts, venous hums (high rates of venous flow in children) and pericardial friction rubs.

The characteristics of specific valve defects and congenital anomalies are described on pages 613 and 629.

DISORDERS OF HEART RATE, RHYTHM AND CONDUCTION

The heart beat is normally initiated by an electrical discharge from the sinoatrial (sinus) node. The atria and ventricles then depolarise sequentially as electrical depolarisation passes through specialised conducting tissues (see Fig. 18.4, p. 529). The sinus node acts as a pacemaker and its intrinsic rate is regulated by the autonomic nervous system; vagal activity decreases the heart rate, and sympathetic activity increases it via cardiac sympathetic nerves and circulating catecholamines.

If the sinus rate becomes unduly slow, another, more distal part of the conducting system may assume the role of pacemaker. This is known as an escape rhythm and may arise in the atrioventricular (AV) node or His bundle (junctional rhythm) or the ventricles (idioventricular rhythm).

A cardiac arrhythmia is a disturbance of the electrical rhythm of the heart. Arrhythmias are often a manifestation of structural heart disease but may also occur because of abnormal conduction or depolarisation in an otherwise healthy heart. A heart rate of more than 100/min is called a tachycardia, and a heart rate of less than 60/min is called a bradycardia.

There are three main mechanisms of tachycardia:

- *Increased automaticity.* The tachycardia is produced by repeated spontaneous depolarisation of an ectopic focus, often in response to catecholamines.
- *Re-entry.* The tachycardia is initiated by an ectopic beat and sustained by a re-entry circuit (Fig. 18.38). Most tachyarrhythmias are due to re-entry.
- *Triggered activity.* This can cause ventricular arrhythmias in patients with coronary artery disease. It is a form of secondary depolarisation arising from an incompletely repolarised cell membrane.

Bradycardia may be due to:

- *Reduced automaticity,* e.g. sinus bradycardia.
- *Blocked or abnormally slow conduction,* e.g. AV block.

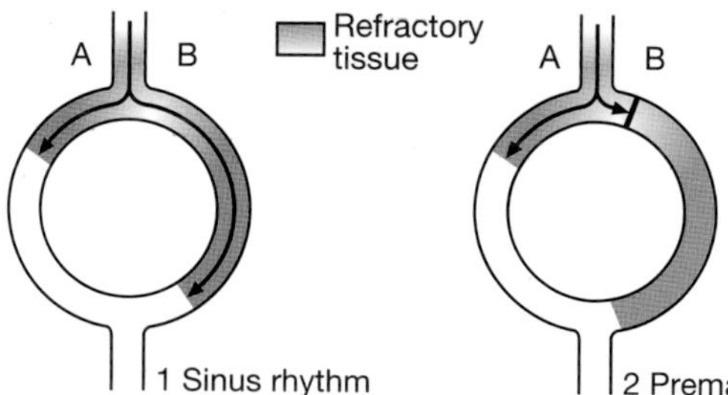

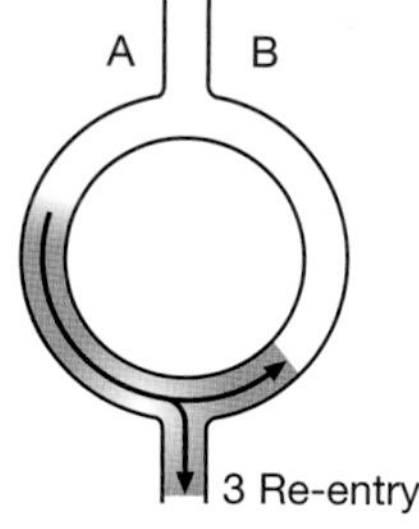

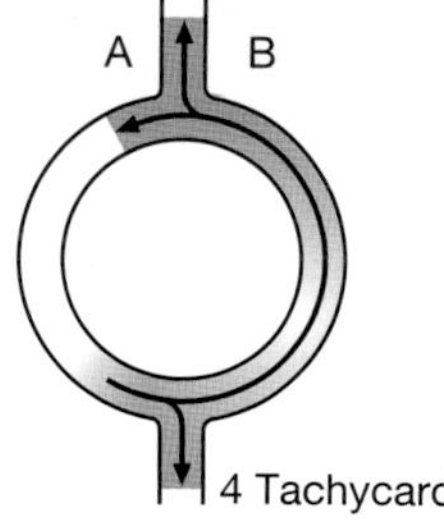

Fig. 18.38 The mechanism of re-entry. Re-entry can occur when there are two alternative pathways with different conducting properties (e.g. the AV node and an accessory pathway, or an area of normal and an area of ischaemic tissue). Here, pathway A conducts slowly and recovers quickly, while pathway B conducts rapidly and recovers slowly. (1) In sinus rhythm, each impulse passes down both pathways before entering a common distal pathway. (2) As the pathways recover at different rates, a premature impulse may find pathway A open and B closed. (3) Pathway B may recover while the premature impulse is travelling selectively down pathway A. The impulse can then travel retrogradely up pathway B, setting up a closed loop or re-entry circuit. (4) This may initiate a tachycardia that continues until the circuit is interrupted by a change in conduction rates or electrical depolarisation.

An arrhythmia may be 'supraventricular' (sinus, atrial or junctional) or ventricular in origin. Supraventricular rhythms usually produce narrow QRS complexes because the ventricles are depolarised in their normal sequence via the AV node and bundle of His. In contrast, ventricular rhythms produce broad, bizarre QRS complexes because the ventricles are activated in an abnormal sequence. Occasionally, however, a supraventricular rhythm can produce broad or wide QRS complexes due to coexisting bundle branch block or the presence of an additional atrioventricular connection (accessory pathway, see below).

Bradycardias cause symptoms that reflect low cardiac output: fatigue, lightheadedness and syncope. Tachycardias cause rapid palpitation, dizziness, chest discomfort or breathlessness. Extreme tachycardias can cause syncope because the heart is unable to contract or relax properly at extreme rates. Extreme bradycardias or tachycardias can precipitate sudden death or cardiac arrest.

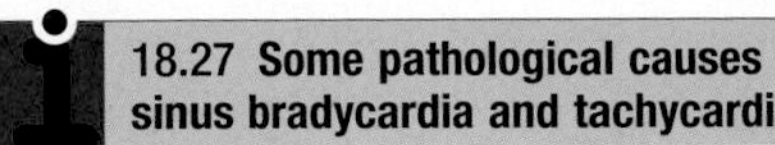

18.27 Some pathological causes of sinus bradycardia and tachycardia

Sinus bradycardia

- MI
- Sinus node disease (sick sinus syndrome)
- Hypothermia
- Hypothyroidism
- Cholestatic jaundice
- Raised intracranial pressure
- Drugs, e.g. β-blockers, digoxin, verapamil

Sinus tachycardia

- Anxiety
- Fever
- Anaemia
- Heart failure
- Thyrotoxicosis
- Phaeochromocytoma
- Drugs, e.g. β-agonists (bronchodilators)

Sinoatrial nodal rhythms

Sinus arrhythmia

Phasic alteration of the heart rate during respiration (the sinus rate increases during inspiration and slows during expiration) is a consequence of normal parasympathetic nervous system activity and can be pronounced in children. Absence of this normal variation in heart rate with breathing or with changes in posture may be a feature of autonomic neuropathy (p. 831).

Sinus bradycardia

A sinus rate of less than 60/min may occur in healthy people at rest and is a common finding in athletes. Some pathological causes are listed in Box 18.27. Asymptomatic sinus bradycardia requires no treatment. Symptomatic acute sinus bradycardia usually responds to intravenous atropine 0.6–1.2 mg. Patients with recurrent or persistent symptomatic sinus bradycardia should be considered for pacemaker implantation.

Sinus tachycardia

This is defined as a sinus rate of more than 100/min, and is usually due to an increase in sympathetic activity associated with exercise, emotion, pregnancy or pathology (see Box 18.27). Young adults can produce a rapid sinus rate, up to 200/min, during intense exercise.

Sinoatrial disease (sick sinus syndrome)

Sinoatrial disease can occur at any age but is most common in older people. The underlying pathology involves fibrosis, degenerative changes or ischaemia of the SA (sinus) node. The condition is characterised by a variety of arrhythmias (Box 18.28) and may present with palpitation, dizzy spells or syncope, due to intermittent tachycardia, bradycardia, or pauses with no atrial or ventricular activity (SA block or sinus arrest) (Fig. 18.39).

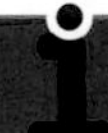

18.28 Common features of sinoatrial disease

- Sinus bradycardia
- Sinoatrial block (sinus arrest)
- Paroxysmal atrial fibrillation
- Paroxysmal atrial tachycardia
- Atrioventricular block

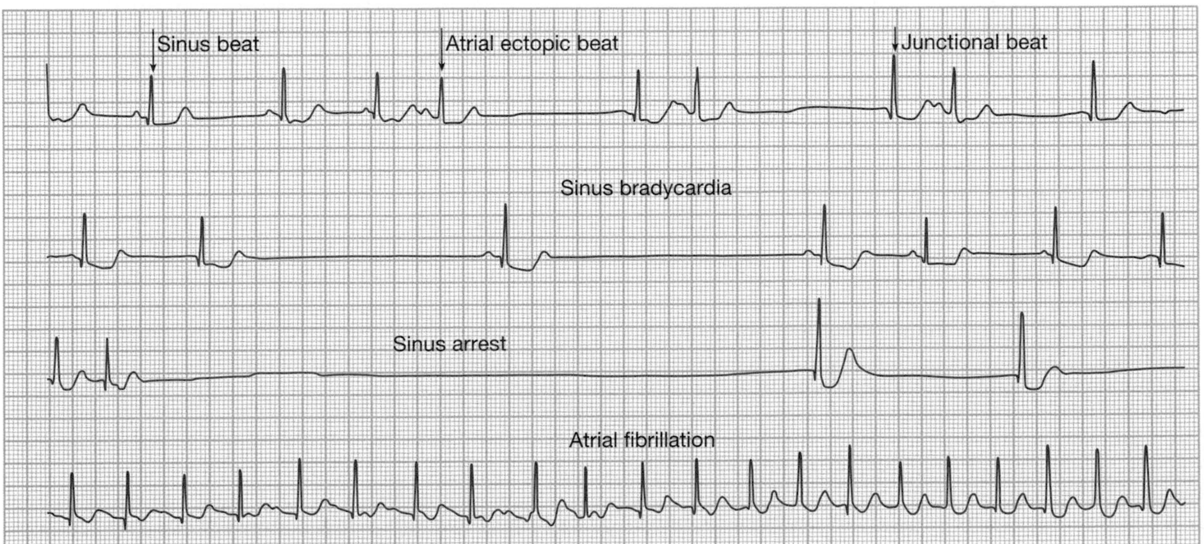

Fig. 18.39 Sinoatrial disease (sick sinus syndrome). A continuous rhythm strip from a 24-hour ECG tape recording illustrating periods of sinus rhythm, atrial ectopics, junctional beats, sinus bradycardia, sinus arrest and paroxysmal atrial fibrillation.

A permanent pacemaker may benefit patients with troublesome symptoms due to spontaneous bradycardias, or those with symptomatic bradycardias induced by drugs required to prevent tachyarrhythmias. Atrial pacing may prevent episodes of atrial fibrillation. Pacing improves symptoms but not prognosis, and is not indicated in patients who are asymptomatic.

Atrial tachyarrhythmias

Atrial ectopic beats (extrasystoles, premature beats)

These usually cause no symptoms but can give the sensation of a missed beat or an abnormally strong beat. The ECG (Fig. 18.40) shows a premature but otherwise normal QRS complex; if visible, the preceding P wave has a different morphology because the atria activate from an abnormal site. In most cases, these are of no consequence, although very frequent atrial ectopic beats may herald the onset of atrial fibrillation. Treatment is rarely necessary but β-blockers can be used if symptoms are intrusive.

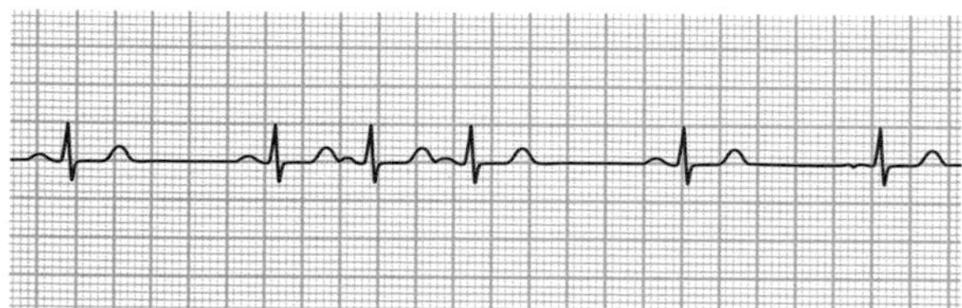

Fig. 18.40 Atrial ectopic beats. The first, second and fifth complexes are normal sinus beats. The third, fourth and sixth complexes are atrial ectopic beats with identical QRS complexes and abnormal (sometimes barely visible) P waves.

Atrial tachycardia

Atrial tachycardia may be a manifestation of increased atrial automaticity, sinoatrial disease or digoxin toxicity. It produces a narrow-complex tachycardia with abnormal P-wave morphology, sometimes associated with AV block if the atrial rate is rapid. It may respond to β-blockers, which reduce automaticity, or class I or III anti-arrhythmic drugs (see Box 18.38, p. 575). The ventricular response in rapid atrial tachycardias may be controlled by AV node-blocking drugs. Catheter ablation (p. 577) can be used to target the ectopic site and should be offered as an alternative to anti-arrhythmic drugs in patients with recurrent atrial tachycardia.

Atrial flutter

Atrial flutter is characterised by a large (macro) re-entry circuit, usually within the right atrium encircling the tricuspid annulus. The atrial rate is approximately 300/min, and is usually associated with 2:1, 3:1 or 4:1 AV block (with corresponding heart rates of 150, 100 or 75/min). Rarely, in young patients, every beat is conducted, producing a rate of 300/min and, potentially, haemodynamic compromise. The ECG shows saw-toothed flutter waves (Fig. 18.41). When there is regular 2:1 AV block, it may be difficult to identify flutter waves that are buried in QRS complexes and T waves. Atrial flutter should always be suspected when there is a narrow-complex tachycardia of 150/min. Carotid sinus pressure or intravenous adenosine may help to establish the diagnosis by temporarily increasing the degree of AV block and revealing flutter waves (Fig. 18.42).

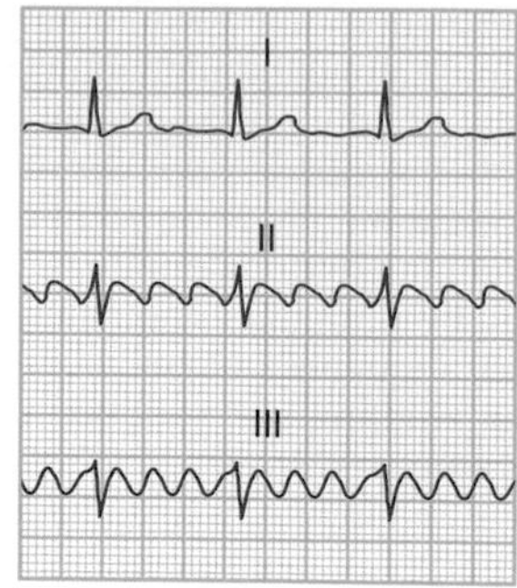

Fig. 18.41 Atrial flutter. Simultaneous recording showing atrial flutter with 3:1 AV block; flutter waves are only visible in leads II and III.

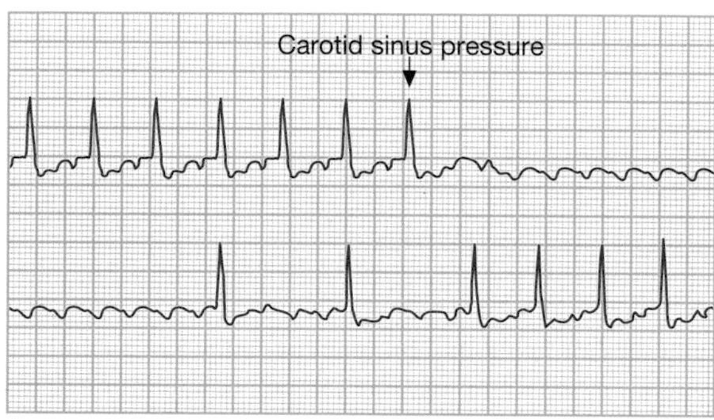

Fig. 18.42 Carotid sinus pressure in atrial flutter: continuous trace. The diagnosis of atrial flutter with 2:1 block was established when carotid sinus pressure produced temporary AV block, revealing the flutter waves.

Management

Digoxin, β-blockers or verapamil can control the ventricular rate (pp. 574–576). However, in many cases, it may be preferable to try to restore sinus rhythm by direct current (DC) cardioversion or by using intravenous amiodarone. Beta-blockers or amiodarone can also be used to prevent recurrent episodes of atrial flutter. Although flecainide can also be used for acute treatment or prophylaxis, it should be avoided because there is a risk of slowing the flutter circuit and facilitating 1:1 AV nodal conduction. This can cause a paradoxical tachycardia and haemodynamic compromise. If used, it should always be prescribed along with an AV node-blocking drug, such as a β-blocker. Catheter ablation offers a 90% chance of complete cure and is the treatment of choice for patients with persistent symptoms.

Atrial fibrillation

Atrial fibrillation (AF) is the most common sustained cardiac arrhythmia, with an overall prevalence of 0.5% in the adult population of the UK. The prevalence rises with age, affecting 1% of those aged 60–64 years, increasing to 9% of those aged over 80 years. AF is a complex arrhythmia characterised by both abnormal automatic firing and the presence of multiple interacting re-entry

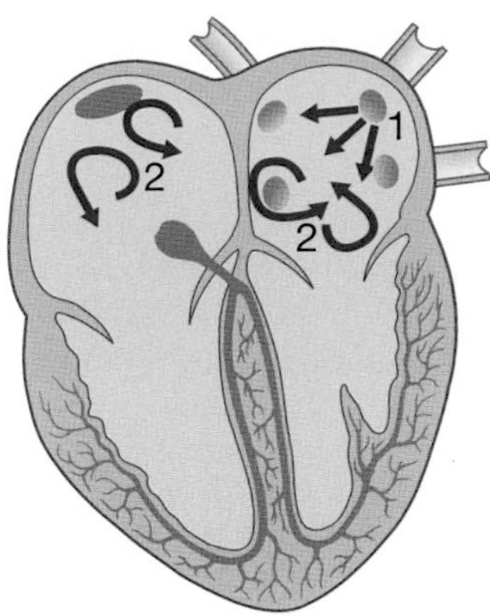

Fig. 18.43 Mechanisms initiating atrial fibrillation. (1) Ectopic beats, often arising from the pulmonary veins, trigger atrial fibrillation. (2) Re-entry within the atria maintains atrial fibrillation, with multiple interacting re-entry circuits operating simultaneously.

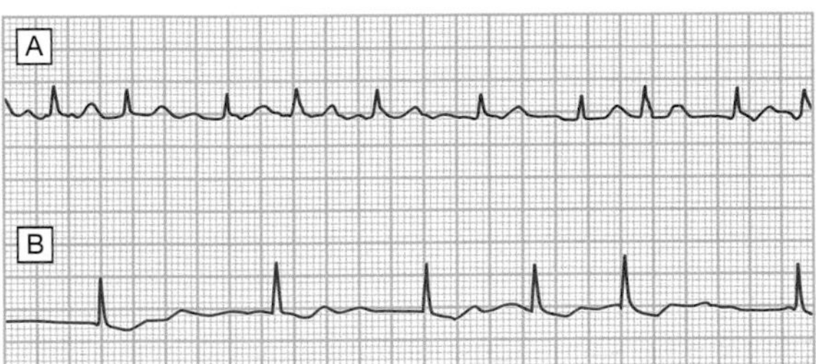

Fig. 18.44 Two examples of atrial fibrillation. The QRS complexes are irregular and there are no P waves. **A** There is usually a fast ventricular rate, e.g. between 120 and 160/min, at the onset of atrial fibrillation. **B** In chronic atrial fibrillation, the ventricular rate may be much slower, due to the effects of medication and AV nodal fatigue.

circuits looping around the atria. Episodes of atrial fibrillation are initiated by rapid bursts of ectopic beats arising from conducting tissue in the pulmonary veins or from diseased atrial tissue. AF becomes sustained because of re-entrant conduction within the atria or sometimes because of continuous ectopic firing (Fig. 18.43). Re-entry is more likely to occur in atria that are enlarged, or in which conduction is slow (as is the case in many forms of heart disease). During episodes of AF, the atria beat rapidly but in an uncoordinated and ineffective manner. The ventricles are activated irregularly at a rate determined by conduction through the AV node. This produces the characteristic 'irregularly irregular' pulse. The ECG (Fig. 18.44) shows normal but irregular QRS complexes; there are no P waves but the baseline may show irregular fibrillation waves.

AF can be classified as paroxysmal (intermittent episodes which self-terminate within 7 days), persistent (prolonged episodes that can be terminated by electrical or chemical cardioversion) or permanent. In patients with AF seen for the first time, it can be difficult to identify which of these is present. Unfortunately for many patients, paroxysmal AF will become permanent as the underlying disease process that predisposes to AF progresses. Electrophysiological changes occur in the atria within a few hours of the onset of AF that tend to maintain fibrillation: electrical remodelling. When AF persists for a period of months, structural remodelling occurs, with atrial fibrosis and dilatation that further predispose to AF. Thus early treatment of AF will prevent re-initiation of the arrhythmia.

18.29 Common causes of atrial fibrillation

- Coronary artery disease (including acute MI)
- Valvular heart disease, especially rheumatic mitral valve disease
- Hypertension
- Sinoatrial disease
- Hyperthyroidism
- Alcohol
- Cardiomyopathy
- Congenital heart disease
- Chest infection
- Pulmonary embolism
- Pericardial disease
- Idiopathic (lone atrial fibrillation)

AF may be the first manifestation of many forms of heart disease (Box 18.29), particularly those that are associated with enlargement or dilatation of the atria. Alcohol excess, hyperthyroidism and chronic lung disease are also common causes of AF, although multiple aetiological factors often coexist, such as the combination of alcohol, hypertension and coronary artery disease. About 50% of all patients with paroxysmal AF and 20% of patients with persistent or permanent AF have structurally normal hearts; this is known as 'lone atrial fibrillation'.

AF can cause palpitation, breathlessness and fatigue. In patients with poor ventricular function or valve disease, it may precipitate or aggravate cardiac failure because of loss of atrial function and heart rate control. A fall in BP may cause lightheadedness, and chest pain may occur with underlying coronary artery disease. In older patients, AF may not be associated with a rapid ventricular rate and is thus often asymptomatic, in which case it is usually discovered as a result of a routine examination or ECG.

AF is associated with significant morbidity and a twofold increase in mortality (mainly because of its association with other underlying heart disease). By far the most disabling consequence is its association with stroke and systemic embolism. Careful assessment, risk stratification and therapy can markedly improve prognosis.

Management

Assessment of patients with newly diagnosed AF includes a full history, physical examination, 12-lead ECG, echocardiogram and thyroid function tests. Additional investigations may be needed to determine the nature and extent of any underlying heart disease. Biochemical evidence of hyperthyroidism is found in a small minority of patients with otherwise unexplained AF.

When AF complicates an acute illness (e.g. chest infection, pulmonary embolism), effective treatment of the primary disorder will often restore sinus rhythm. Otherwise, the main objectives are restoration of sinus rhythm (when possible), prevention of recurrent AF, optimisation of the heart rate during periods of AF, reduction of the risk of thromboembolism, and treatment of underlying cardiac disease.

Paroxysmal atrial fibrillation

Occasional attacks that are well tolerated do not necessarily require treatment. Beta-blockers are normally

18

used as first-line therapy if symptoms are troublesome, and are particularly useful for treating patients with AF associated with coronary artery disease, hypertension and cardiac failure. Beta-blockers reduce the ectopic firing that normally initiates AF. Class Ic drugs (see Box 18.38, p. 575), such as propafenone or flecainide, are also effective at preventing episodes but should not be given to patients with coronary artery disease or left ventricular dysfunction. Flecainide is usually prescribed along with a rate limiting β-blocker because it occasionally precipitates atrial flutter. Class III drugs can also be used; amiodarone is the most effective agent for preventing AF but its side-effects restrict its use to patients in whom other measures fail. Dronedarone is an effective alternative, but is contraindicated in patients with heart failure or significant left ventricular impairment. Digoxin and verapamil are not effective drugs for preventing paroxysms of AF, although they do limit the heart rate when AF occurs by blocking the AV node. In patients with AF in whom anti-arrhythmic drug therapy is ineffective or causes side-effects, catheter ablation can be considered. Ablation is used to disconnect the pulmonary veins from the LA electrically, preventing ectopic triggering of AF. In addition, lines of conduction block can be created within the atria to prevent re-entry. Ablation prevents AF in approximately 75% of patients with prior drug-resistant episodes, although a repeat procedure is sometimes required before this is achieved. Ablation for AF is an attractive treatment for patients in whom drugs are ineffective or poorly tolerated but it is associated with a risk of cardiac tamponade, stroke and other complications.

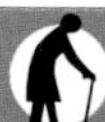

18.30 Atrial fibrillation in old age

- **Prevalence**: rises with age, reaching 9% in those over 80 yrs of age.
- **Symptoms**: sometimes asymptomatic but often accompanied by diastolic heart failure.
- **Hyperthyroidism**: atrial fibrillation may emerge as the dominant feature of otherwise silent or occult hyperthyroidism.
- **Cardioversion**: followed by high rates (~70% at 1 yr) of recurrent atrial fibrillation.
- **Stroke**: atrial fibrillation is an important cause of cerebral embolism, found in 15% of all stroke patients and 2–8% of those with transient ischaemic attacks (TIAs).
- **Anticoagulation**: although the risk of thromboembolism rises, the hazards of anticoagulation also become greater with age because of increased comorbidity, particularly cognitive impairment and falls.
- **Target INR**: if anticoagulation is recommended in those over 75 yrs, care should be taken to maintain an INR below 3.0 because of the increased risk of intracranial haemorrhage.
- **Direct thrombin (e.g. dabigatran) and factor Xa (e.g. rivaroxaban) inhibitors**: alternatives to warfarin. No blood monitoring is required, there are fewer drug interactions, and fixed dosing may aid compliance. Dabigatran dose is reduced from 150 mg twice daily to 110 mg twice daily in the over-eighties or if creatinine clearance is less than 30 mL/min. Rivaroxaban dose is reduced from 20 mg once daily to 15 mg once daily if creatinine clearance is 30–49 mL/min, and contraindicated if below 30 mL/min.

Persistent and permanent atrial fibrillation

There are two options for treating persistent AF:

- *rhythm control:* attempting to restore and maintain sinus rhythm
- *rate control:* accepting that AF will be permanent and using treatments to control the ventricular rate and to prevent embolic complications.

Rhythm control. An attempt to restore sinus rhythm is particularly appropriate if the arrhythmia causes troublesome symptoms and if there is a modifiable or treatable underlying cause. Electrical cardioversion (p. 577) is initially successful in three-quarters of patients but relapse is frequent (25–50% at 1 month and 70–90% at 1 year). Attempts to restore and maintain sinus rhythm are most successful if AF has been present for less than 3 months, the patient is young and there is no important structural heart disease.

Immediate cardioversion, after administration of intravenous heparin, is appropriate if AF has been present for under 48 hours. In stable patients with no history of structural heart disease, intravenous flecainide (2 mg/kg over 30 mins, maximum dose 150 mg) can be used for pharmacological cardioversion and will restore sinus rhythm in 75% of patients within 8 hours. In patients with structural or ischaemic heart disease, intravenous amiodarone can be given via a central venous catheter. Electrical cardioversion, using a DC shock, is an alternative and is often effective when drugs fail. In other situations, DC cardioversion should be deferred until the patient has been established on warfarin, with an international normalised ratio (INR) of more than 2.0 for a minimum of 4 weeks, and any underlying problems, such as hypertension or alcohol excess, have been eliminated. Anticoagulation should be maintained for at least 3 months following successful cardioversion. If AF recurs, further cardioversion may be appropriate but consideration should be given to pretreatment with amiodarone to reduce the risk of recurrence. Catheter ablation is sometimes used to help restore and maintain sinus rhythm in resistant cases, but is a less effective treatment than for paroxysmal AF.

Rate control. If sinus rhythm cannot be restored, treatment should be directed at maintaining an appropriate heart rate. Digoxin, β-blockers and rate-limiting calcium antagonists, such as verapamil or diltiazem (pp. 574–576), reduce the ventricular rate by increasing the degree of AV block. This alone may produce a striking improvement in cardiac function, particularly in patients with mitral stenosis. Beta-blockers and rate-limiting calcium antagonists are more effective than digoxin at controlling the heart rate during exercise and have additional benefits in patients with hypertension or structural heart disease. Combination therapy (e.g. digoxin and atenolol) is often advisable but rate-limiting calcium channel antagonists should not be used with β-blockers because of the risk of bradycardia.

In exceptional cases, poorly controlled and symptomatic AF can be treated by deliberately inducing complete AV nodal block with catheter ablation; a permanent pacemaker must be implanted beforehand. This is known as the 'pace and ablate' strategy.

Prevention of thromboembolism

Loss of atrial contraction and left atrial dilatation cause stasis of blood in the LA and may lead to thrombus

18.31 CHA_2DS_2-VAS_c stroke risk scoring system for non-valvular atrial fibrillation

	Parameter	Score
C	Congestive heart failure	1 point
H	Hypertension history	1 point
A_2	Age ≥ 75 yrs	2 points
D	Diabetes mellitus	1 point
S_2	Previous stroke or TIA	2 points
V	Vascular disease	1 point
A	Age 65–74 yrs	1 point
S_c	Sex category female	1 point
	Maximum total score	9 points

Annual stroke risk

0 points = 0% (no prophylaxis required)

1 point = 1.3% (oral anticoagulant or aspirin recommended)

2+ points = > 2.2% (oral anticoagulant recommended)

European Society of Cardiology Clinical Practice Guidelines: Atrial Fibrillation (Management of) 2010 and Focused Update (2012). Eur Heart J 2012; 33:2719–2747.

formation in the left atrial appendage. This predisposes patients to stroke and other forms of systemic embolism. The annual risk of stroke in patients with AF (Box 18.31) is influenced by many factors, and in each patient a decision has to be made about the risk of stroke versus the risk of anticoagulation.

Several large randomised trials have shown that treatment with adjusted-dose warfarin (target INR 2.0–3.0) reduces the risk of stroke by about two-thirds, at the cost of an annual risk of bleeding of 1–1.5%, whereas treatment with aspirin reduces the risk of stroke by only one-fifth, is associated with significant bleeding risk and, although still included in European guidelines, has a very limited role. Warfarin is thus indicated for patients with AF who have specific risk factors for stroke. In intermittent AF, the risk of stroke is only loosely related to the frequency and duration of AF episodes, so stroke prevention guidelines do not distinguish between those with paroxysmal, persistent and permanent AF.

An assessment of the risk of embolism helps to define the possible benefits of antithrombotic therapy (see Box 18.31), which must be balanced against its potential hazards. Risk stratification is based on clinical factors using the CHA_2DS_2-VAS_C scoring system. Echocardiographic assessment (e.g. left atrial size) is of limited value in predicting stroke risk and is mainly used to identify associated structural disease. Oral anticoagulation is indicated in patients at moderate or high risk of stroke, unless there is an unacceptable bleeding risk. The choice of oral anticoagulant is widening (Box 18.32). Until recently, warfarin was the treatment of choice, mandating regular blood testing, with a target INR of 2.0–3.0. The direct thrombin inhibitor, dabigatran, is the first novel oral anticoagulant drug shown to be as effective and safe as warfarin at stroke prevention in AF. No blood monitoring is required and there are few drug interactions. For all anticoagulant drugs, comorbid conditions that may be complicated by bleeding, such as peptic ulcer, uncontrolled hypertension, alcohol misuse, frequent falls, poor drug compliance and potential drug interactions, are all relative contraindications. In warfarin-treated patients, anticoagulation can be reversed by administering vitamin K or clotting factors, but there are no current antidotes for the direct thrombin inhibitors. Young patients (under 65 years) with no evidence of structural heart disease have a very low risk of stroke and may not require oral anticoagulation.

EBM 18.32 Anticoagulation in atrial fibrillation

'Anticoagulation with warfarin reduces the risk of ischaemic stroke in non-rheumatic atrial fibrillation by about 62% (absolute risk reduction 2.7% for primary prevention and 8.4% for secondary prevention).

Newer anticoagulants, such as the direct thrombin inhibitor, dabigatran, and the factor Xa inhibitors, apixaban and rivaroxaban, appear to have better efficacy and safety profiles than warfarin. They are most effective in patients who have poorly controlled anticoagulation with warfarin or those who are unable to take warfarin.'

- Hart RG, et al. Ann Intern Med 1999; 131:492–501.
- Connolly S, et al. N Engl J Med 2009; 361:1139–1151.
- Granger CB, et al. N Engl J Med 2011; 365:981–992.

For further information: www.nice.org.uk/CG36
www.clinicaltrials.gov (numbers NCT00262600 and NCT00412984)

'Supraventricular' tachycardias

The term 'supraventricular tachycardia' (SVT) is commonly used to describe regular tachycardias that have a similar appearance on ECG. These are usually associated with a narrow QRS complex and are characterised by a re-entry circuit or automatic focus involving the atria. The term SVT is misleading, as, in many cases, the ventricles also form part of the re-entry circuit, such as in patients with AV re-entrant tachycardia.

Atrioventricular nodal re-entrant tachycardia

Atrioventricular nodal re-entrant tachycardia (AVNRT) is due to re-entry in a circuit involving the AV node and its two right atrial input pathways: a superior 'fast' pathway and an inferior 'slow' pathway (see Fig. 18.46A below). This produces a regular tachycardia with a rate of 120–240/min. It tends to occur in the absence of structural heart disease and episodes may last from a few seconds to many hours. The patient is usually aware of a rapid, very forceful, regular heart beat and may experience chest discomfort, lightheadedness or breathlessness. Polyuria, mainly due to the release of atrial natriuretic peptide, is sometimes a feature. The ECG (Fig. 18.45) usually shows a tachycardia with normal

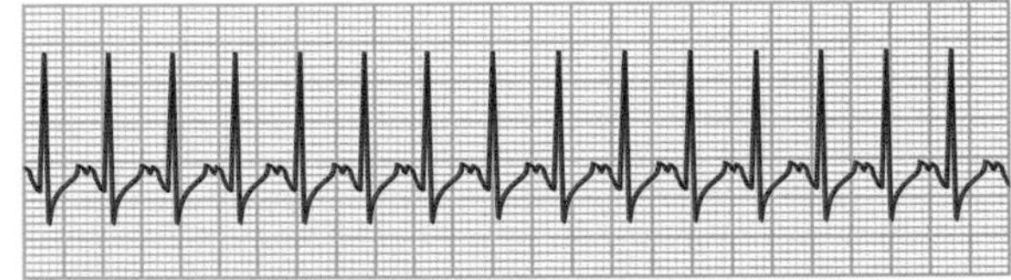

Fig. 18.45 Supraventricular tachycardia. The rate is 180/min and the QRS complexes are normal.

QRS complexes but occasionally there may be rate-dependent bundle branch block.

Management

Treatment is not always necessary. However, an episode may be terminated by carotid sinus pressure or by the Valsalva manœuvre. Adenosine (3–12 mg rapidly IV in incremental doses until tachycardia stops) or verapamil (5 mg IV over 1 min) will restore sinus rhythm in most cases. Intravenous β-blocker or flecainide can also be used. In rare cases, when there is severe haemodynamic compromise, the tachycardia should be terminated by DC cardioversion (p. 577).

In patients with recurrent SVT, catheter ablation (p. 577) is the most effective therapy and will permanently prevent SVT in more than 90% of cases. Alternatively, prophylaxis with oral β-blocker, verapamil or flecainide may be used but commits predominantly young patients to long-term drug therapy and can create difficulty in female patients, as these drugs are normally avoided during pregnancy.

Wolff–Parkinson–White syndrome and atrioventricular re-entrant tachycardia

Here, an abnormal band of conducting tissue connects the atria and ventricles. This 'accessory pathway' comprises rapidly conducting fibres which resemble Purkinje tissue, in that they conduct very rapidly and are rich in sodium channels. In around half of cases, this pathway only conducts in the retrograde direction (from ventricles to atria) and thus does not alter the appearance of the ECG in sinus rhythm. This is known as a concealed accessory pathway. In the rest, the pathway also conducts antegradely (from atria to ventricles) so AV conduction in sinus rhythm is mediated via both the AV node and the accessory pathway, distorting the QRS complex. Premature ventricular activation via the pathway shortens the PR interval and produces a 'slurred' initial deflection of the QRS complex, called a delta wave (Fig. 18.46B). This is known as a manifest accessory pathway. As the AV node and accessory pathway have different conduction speeds and refractory periods, a re-entry circuit can develop, causing tachycardia (Fig. 18.46C); when associated with symptoms, the condition is known as Wolff–Parkinson–White syndrome. The ECG during this tachycardia is almost indistinguishable from that of AVNRT (Fig. 18.46A). Carotid sinus pressure or intravenous adenosine can terminate the tachycardia. If atrial fibrillation occurs, it may produce a dangerously rapid ventricular rate because the accessory pathway lacks the rate-limiting properties of the AV node (Fig. 18.46D). This is known as pre-excited atrial fibrillation and may cause collapse, syncope and even death. It should be treated as an emergency, usually with DC cardioversion.

Catheter ablation is first-line treatment in symptomatic patients and is nearly always curative. Alternatively, prophylactic anti-arrhythmic drugs, such as

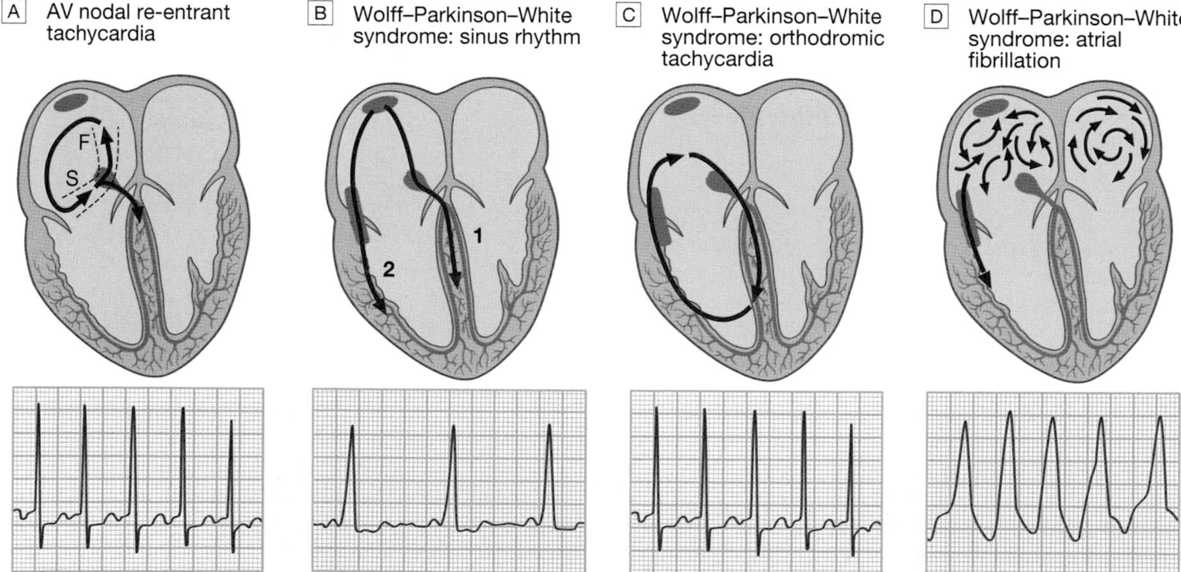

Fig. 18.46 AV nodal re-entrant tachycardia (AVNRT) and Wolff–Parkinson–White (WPW) syndrome. **A** AV node re-entrant tachycardia. The mechanism of AVNRT occurs via two right atrial AV nodal input pathways: the slow (S) and fast (F) pathways. Antegrade conduction occurs via the slow pathway; the wavefront enters the AV node and passes into the ventricles, at the same time re-entering the atria via the fast pathway.

In WPW syndrome, there is a strip of accessory conducting tissue that allows electricity to bypass the AV node and spread from the atria to the ventricles rapidly and without delay. When the ventricles are depolarised through the AV node, the ECG is normal, but when the ventricles are depolarised through the accessory conducting tissue, the ECG shows a very short PR interval and a broad QRS complex. **B** Sinus rhythm. In sinus rhythm, the ventricles are depolarised through (1) the AV node and (2) the accessory pathway, producing an ECG with a short PR interval and broadened QRS complexes; the characteristic slurring of the upstroke of the QRS complex is known as a delta wave. The degree of pre-excitation (the proportion of activation passing down the accessory pathway) and therefore the ECG appearances may vary a lot, and at times the ECG can look normal. **C** Orthodromic tachycardia. This is the most common form of tachycardia in WPW. The re-entry circuit passes antegradely through the AV node and retrogradely through the accessory pathway. The ventricles are therefore depolarised in the normal way, producing a narrow-complex tachycardia that is indistinguishable from other forms of SVT. **D** Atrial fibrillation. In this rhythm, the ventricles are largely depolarised through the accessory pathway, producing an irregular broad-complex tachycardia which is often more rapid than the example shown.

flecainide or propafenone (p. 574), can be used to slow conduction in, and prolong the refractory period of, the accessory pathway. Long-term drug therapy is not the preferred treatment for most patients and amiodarone should not be used, as its side-effect profile cannot be justified and ablation is safer and more effective. Digoxin and verapamil shorten the refractory period of the accessory pathway and should not be used.

Ventricular tachyarrhythmias

Ventricular ectopic beats (extrasystoles, premature beats)

QRS complexes in sinus rhythm are normally narrow because the ventricles are activated rapidly and simultaneously via the His–Purkinje system. The complexes of ventricular ectopic beats (VEBs) are premature, broad and bizarre because the ventricles are activated sequentially rather than simultaneously. The complexes may be unifocal (identical beats arising from a single ectopic focus) or multifocal (varying morphology with multiple foci, Fig. 18.47). 'Couplet' and 'triplet' are the terms used to describe two or three successive ectopic beats. A run of alternating sinus and ventricular ectopic beats is known as ventricular 'bigeminy'. Ectopic beats produce a low stroke volume because left ventricular contraction occurs before filling is complete. The pulse is therefore irregular, with weak or missed beats (see Fig. 18.47). Patients are usually asymptomatic but may complain of an irregular heart beat, missed beats or abnormally strong beats (due to the increased output of the post-ectopic sinus beat). The significance of VEBs depends on the presence or absence of underlying heart disease.

Ventricular ectopic beats in otherwise healthy subjects

VEBs are frequently found in healthy people and their prevalence increases with age. Ectopic beats in patients with otherwise normal hearts are more prominent at rest and disappear with exercise. Treatment is not necessary, unless the patient is highly symptomatic, in which case β-blockers or, in some situations, catheter ablation can be used. VEBs are sometimes a manifestation of otherwise subclinical heart disease, such as coronary artery disease or cardiomyopathy. There is no evidence that anti-arrhythmic therapy improves prognosis but the discovery of very frequent VEBs should prompt investigations, such as an echocardiogram (looking for structural heart disease) and an exercise stress test (to detect underlying ischaemic heart disease).

Ventricular ectopic beats associated with heart disease

Frequent VEBs often occur during acute MI but need no treatment. Persistent, frequent (over 10/hr) VEBs in patients who have survived the acute phase of MI indicate a poorer long-term outcome. Other than β-blockers, anti-arrhythmic drugs do not improve and may even worsen prognosis.

VEBs are common in patients with heart failure of any cause, including cardiomyopathy. While they are associated with an adverse prognosis, this is not improved by anti-arrhythmic drugs. Effective treatment of the heart failure may suppress the ectopic beats.

VEBs are also a feature of digoxin toxicity, and may occur as 'escape beats' in patients with bradycardia. Treatment is that of the underlying condition.

Ventricular tachycardia

Ventricular tachycardia (VT) occurs most commonly in the settings of acute MI, chronic coronary artery disease, and cardiomyopathy. It occurs when there is extensive ventricular disease, such as impaired left ventricular function or a left ventricular aneurysm. In these settings, VT may cause haemodynamic compromise or degenerate into ventricular fibrillation (p. 557). It is caused by abnormal automaticity or triggered activity in ischaemic tissue, or by re-entry within scarred ventricular tissue. Patients may complain of palpitation or symptoms of low cardiac output, e.g. dizziness, dyspnoea or syncope. The ECG shows tachycardia and broad, abnormal QRS complexes with a rate of more than 120/min (Fig. 18.48). VT may be difficult to distinguish from SVT with bundle branch block or pre-excitation (WPW syndrome). Features in favour of a diagnosis of VT are listed in Box 18.33. A 12-lead ECG (Fig. 18.49) or electrophysiology

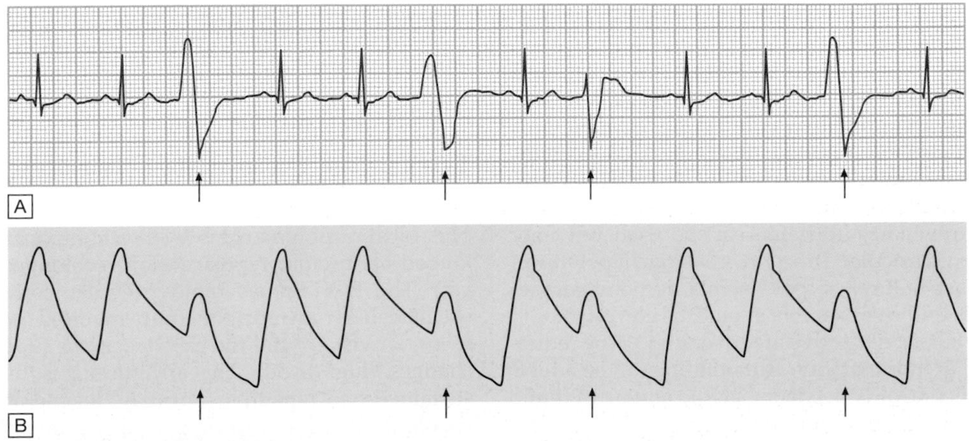

Fig. 18.47 Ventricular ectopic beats. **A** There are broad, bizarre QRS complexes (arrows) with no preceding P wave in between normal sinus beats. Their configuration varies, so these are multifocal ectopics. **B** A simultaneous arterial pressure trace is shown. The ectopic beats result in a weaker pulse (arrows), which may be perceived as a 'dropped beat'.

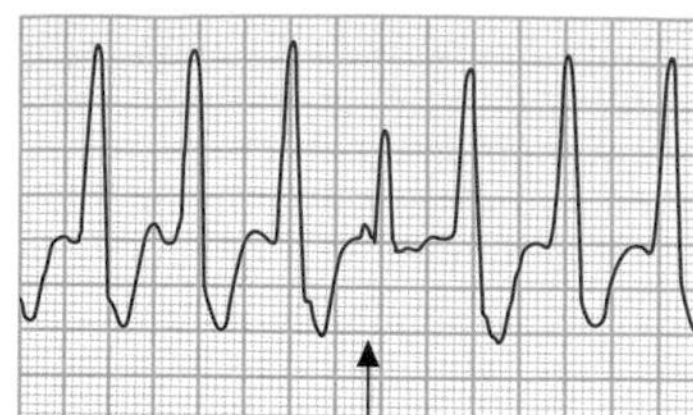

Fig. 18.48 Ventricular tachycardia: fusion beat (arrow). In ventricular tachycardia, there is independent atrial and ventricular activity. Occasionally, a P wave is conducted to the ventricles through the AV node, producing a normal sinus beat in the middle of the tachycardia (a capture beat); more commonly, however, the conducted impulse fuses with an impulse from the tachycardia (a fusion beat). This can only occur when there is AV dissociation and is therefore diagnostic of ventricular tachycardia.

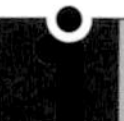

18.33 Features more in keeping with ventricular tachycardia

- History of MI
- AV dissociation (pathognomonic)
- Capture/fusion beats (pathognomonic; see Fig. 18.48)
- Extreme left axis deviation
- Very broad QRS complexes (> 140 ms)
- No response to carotid sinus massage or IV adenosine

study (p. 539) may help establish the diagnosis. When there is doubt, it is safer to manage the problem as VT.

Patients recovering from MI sometimes have periods of idioventricular rhythm ('slow' VT) at a rate only slightly above the preceding sinus rate and below 120/min. These episodes often reflect reperfusion of the infarct territory and may be a good sign. They are usually self-limiting and asymptomatic, and do not require treatment. Other forms of sustained VT will require treatment, often as an emergency.

VT occasionally occurs in patients with otherwise healthy hearts ('normal heart VT'), usually because of abnormal automaticity in the right ventricular outflow tract or one of the fascicles of the left bundle branch. The prognosis is good and catheter ablation can be curative.

Management

Prompt action to restore sinus rhythm is required and should usually be followed by prophylactic therapy. Synchronised DC cardioversion is the treatment of choice if systolic BP is less than 90 mmHg. If the arrhythmia is well tolerated, intravenous amiodarone may be given as a bolus, followed by a continuous infusion (p. 576). Intravenous lidocaine can be used but may depress left ventricular function, causing hypotension or acute heart failure. Hypokalaemia, hypomagnesaemia, acidosis and hypoxaemia should be corrected.

Beta-blockers are effective at preventing VT by reducing ventricular automaticity. Amiodarone can be added if additional control is needed. Class Ic anti-arrhythmic drugs should not be used for prevention of VT in patients with coronary artery disease or heart failure because they depress myocardial function and can be pro-arrhythmic (increase the likelihood of a dangerous

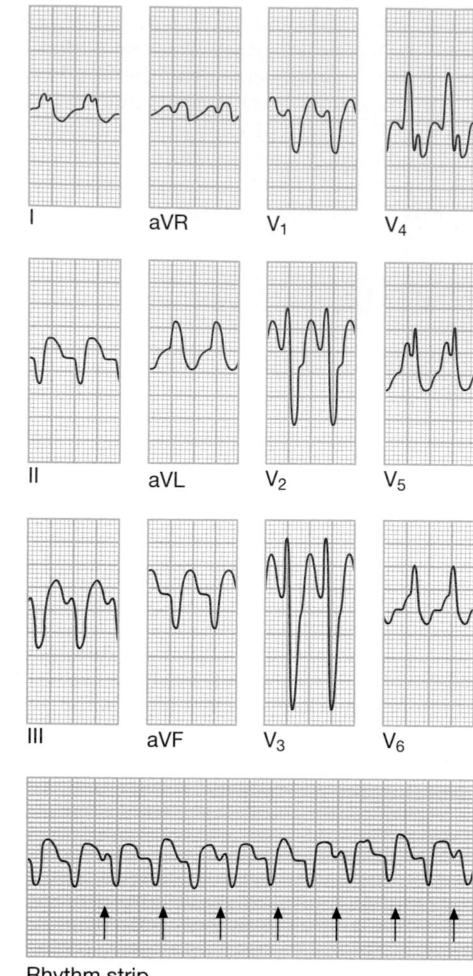

Fig. 18.49 Ventricular tachycardia: 12-lead ECG. There are typically very broad QRS complexes and marked left axis deviation. There is also AV dissociation; some P waves are visible and others are buried in the QRS complexes (arrows).

arrhythmia). In patients at high risk of arrhythmic death (e.g. those with poor left ventricular function, or where VT is associated with haemodynamic compromise), the use of an implantable cardiac defibrillator is recommended (p. 579). Rarely, surgery (e.g. aneurysm resection) or catheter ablation can be used to interrupt the arrhythmia focus or circuit in patients with VT associated with a myocardial infarct scar.

Torsades de pointes (ventricular tachycardia)

This form of polymorphic VT is a complication of prolonged ventricular repolarisation (prolonged QT interval). The ECG shows rapid irregular complexes that oscillate from an upright to an inverted position and seem to twist around the baseline as the mean QRS axis changes (Fig. 18.50). The arrhythmia is usually non-sustained and repetitive, but may degenerate into ventricular fibrillation. During periods of sinus rhythm, the ECG will usually show a prolonged QT interval (> 0.43 s in men, > 0.45 s in women when corrected to a heart rate of 60/min).

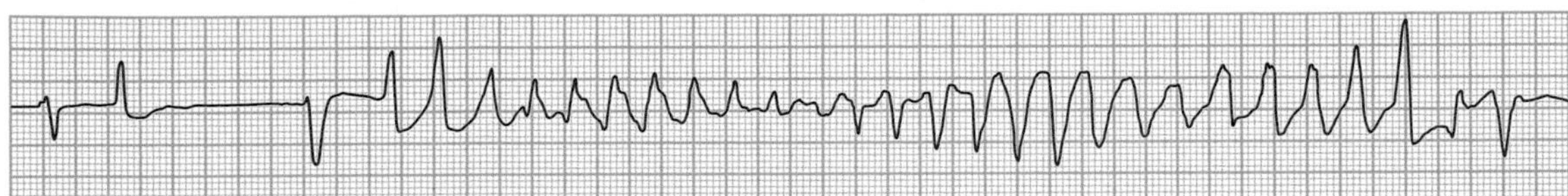

Fig. 18.50 Torsades de pointes. A bradycardia with a long QT interval is followed by polymorphic ventricular tachycardia that is triggered by an R on T ectopic.

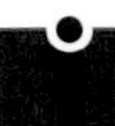

18.34 Causes of long QT interval and torsades de pointes
Bradycardia
• Bradycardia compounds other factors that cause torsades de pointes
Electrolyte disturbance
• Hypokalaemia • Hypomagnesaemia • Hypocalcaemia
Drugs
• Disopyramide, flecainide (and other class Ia, Ic anti-arrhythmic drugs, p. 574) • Sotalol, amiodarone (and other class III anti-arrhythmic drugs) • Amitriptyline (and other tricyclic antidepressants) • Chlorpromazine (and other phenothiazines) • Erythromycin (and other macrolides) ... and many more
Congenital syndromes
• Long QT1: gene affected *KCNQI*: K^+ channel, 30–35% • Long QT2: gene affected *HERG*: K^+ channel, 25–30% • Long QT3: gene affected *SCNSA*: Na^+ channel, 5–10% • Long QT4–12: rare

Some of the common causes are listed in Box 18.34. The arrhythmia is more common in women and is often triggered by a combination of aetiological factors (e.g. QT-prolonging medications and hypokalaemia). The congenital long QT syndromes are a family of genetic disorders that are characterised by mutations in genes that code for cardiac sodium or potassium channels. Long QT syndrome subtypes have different triggers, which are important when counselling patients. Adrenergic stimulation (e.g. exercise) is a common trigger in long QT type 1, and a sudden noise (e.g. an alarm clock) may trigger arrhythmias in long QT type 2. Arrhythmias are more common during sleep in type 3.

Treatment should be directed at the underlying cause. Intravenous magnesium (8 mmol over 15 mins, then 72 mmol over 24 hrs) should be given in all cases. Atrial pacing will usually suppress the arrhythmia through rate-dependent shortening of the QT interval. Intravenous isoprenaline is a reasonable alternative to pacing but should be avoided in patients with the congenital long QT syndromes.

Long-term therapy may not be necessary if the underlying cause can be removed. Beta-blockers are effective at preventing syncope in patients with congenital long QT syndrome. Some patients, particularly those with extreme QT interval prolongation (> 500 ms) or certain high-risk genotypes should be considered for implantation of a defibrillator. Left stellate ganglion block may be of value in patients with resistant arrhythmias.

The Brugada syndrome is a related genetic disorder that may present with polymorphic VT or sudden death. It is characterised by a defect in sodium channel function and an abnormal ECG (right bundle branch block and ST elevation in V_1 and V_2 but not usually prolongation of the QT interval). The only known effective treatment is an implantable defibrillator.

Atrioventricular and bundle branch block

Atrioventricular block

Atrioventricular conduction is influenced by autonomic activity. AV block can therefore be intermittent and only evident when the conducting tissue is stressed by a rapid atrial rate. Accordingly, atrial tachyarrhythmias are often associated with AV block (see Fig. 18.44, p. 565).

First-degree atrioventricular block

In this condition, AV conduction is delayed and so the PR interval is prolonged (> 0.20 s; Fig. 18.51). It rarely causes symptoms.

Second-degree atrioventricular block

In this, dropped beats occur because some impulses from the atria fail to conduct to the ventricles.

In Mobitz type I second-degree AV block (Fig. 18.52), there is progressive lengthening of successive PR intervals, culminating in a dropped beat. The cycle then repeats itself. This is known as the Wenckebach phenomenon and is usually due to impaired conduction in the AV node itself. The phenomenon may be physiological and is sometimes observed at rest or during sleep in athletic young adults with high vagal tone.

In Mobitz type II second-degree AV block (Fig. 18.53), the PR interval of the conducted impulses remains constant but some P waves are not conducted. This is usually caused by disease of the His–Purkinje system and carries a risk of asystole.

In 2:1 AV block (Fig. 18.54), alternate P waves are conducted, so it is impossible to distinguish between Mobitz type I and type II block.

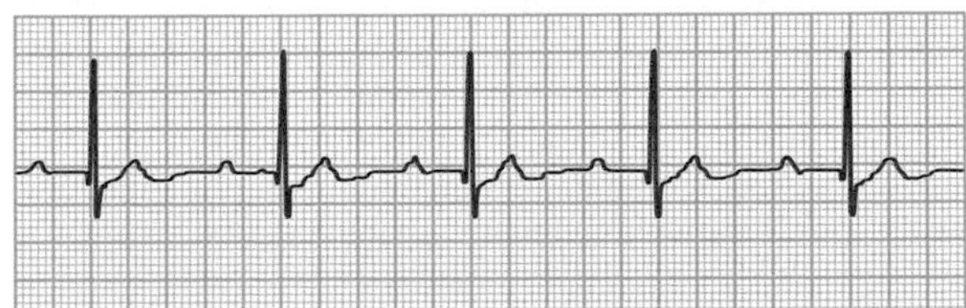

Fig. 18.51 First-degree AV block. The PR interval is prolonged and measures 0.26 s.

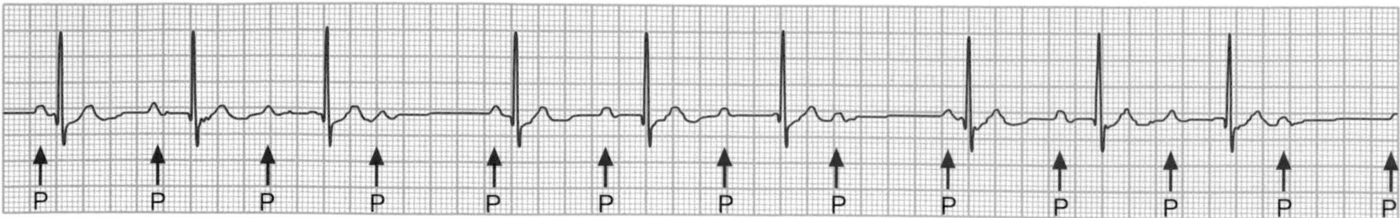

Fig. 18.52 Second-degree AV block (Mobitz type I – Wenckebach's phenomenon). The PR interval progressively increases until a P wave is not conducted. The cycle then repeats itself. In this example, conduction is at a ratio of 4:3, leading to groupings of three ventricular complexes in a row.

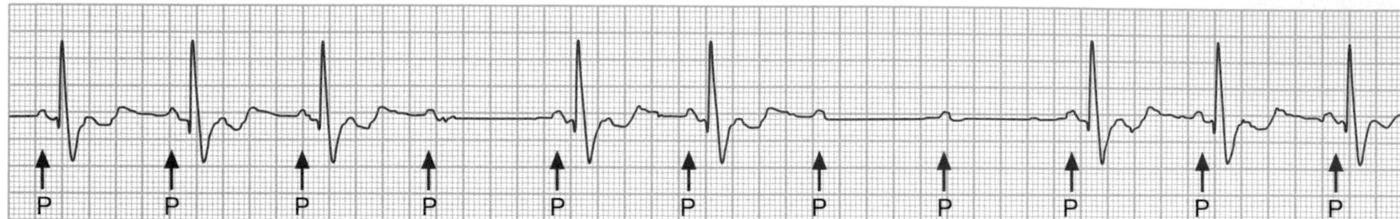

Fig. 18.53 Second-degree AV block (Mobitz type II). The PR interval of conducted beats is normal but some P waves are not conducted. The constant PR interval distinguishes this from Wenckebach's phenomenon.

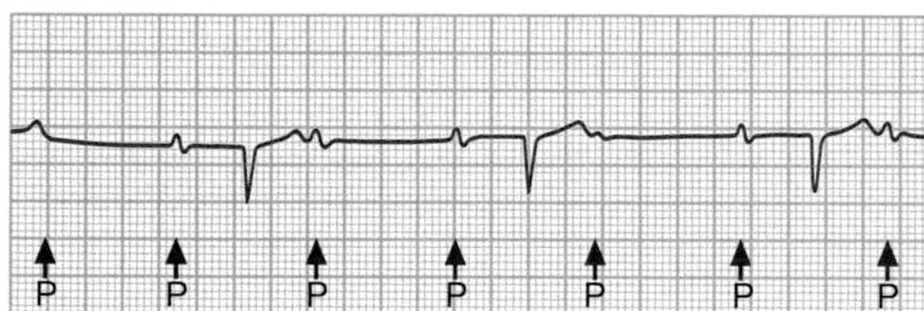

Fig. 18.54 Second-degree AV block with fixed 2:1 block. Alternate P waves are not conducted. This may be due to Mobitz type I or II block.

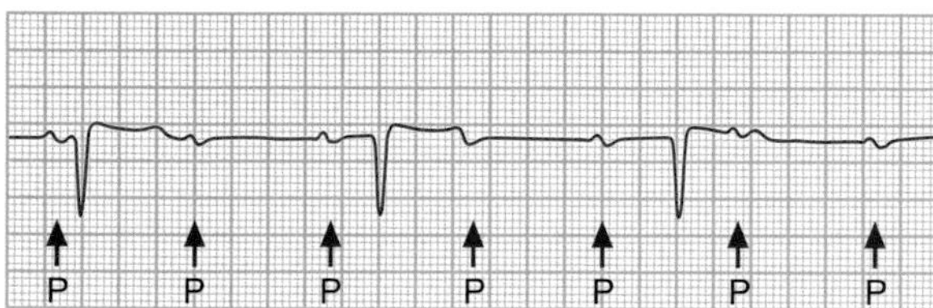

Fig. 18.55 Complete (third-degree) AV block. There is complete dissociation of atrial and ventricular complexes. The atrial rate is 80/min and the ventricular rate is 38/min.

Third-degree (complete) atrioventricular block

When AV conduction fails completely, the atria and ventricles beat independently (AV dissociation, Fig. 18.55). Ventricular activity is maintained by an escape rhythm arising in the AV node or bundle of His (narrow QRS complexes) or the distal Purkinje tissues (broad QRS complexes). Distal escape rhythms tend to be slower and less reliable.

Complete AV block (Box 18.35) produces a slow (25–50/min), regular pulse that, except in the case of congenital complete AV block, does not vary with exercise. There is usually a compensatory increase in stroke volume, producing a large-volume pulse. Cannon waves may be visible in the neck and the intensity of the first heart sound varies due to the loss of AV synchrony.

Stokes–Adams attacks

Episodes of ventricular asystole may complicate complete heart block or Mobitz type II second-degree AV block, or occur in patients with sinoatrial disease (see Fig. 18.39, p. 563). This may cause recurrent syncope or 'Stokes–Adams' attacks.

A typical episode is characterised by sudden loss of consciousness that occurs without warning and results in collapse. A brief anoxic seizure (due to cerebral ischaemia) may occur if there is prolonged asystole. There is pallor and a death-like appearance during the attack, but when the heart starts beating again, there is a characteristic flush. Unlike in epilepsy, recovery is rapid. Sinoatrial disease and neurocardiogenic syncope (p. 555) may cause similar symptoms.

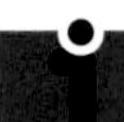

18.35 Aetiology of complete AV block

Congenital

Acquired

- Idiopathic fibrosis
- MI/ischaemia
- Inflammation
  Acute (e.g. aortic root abscess in infective endocarditis)
  Chronic (e.g. sarcoidosis, p. 709; Chagas' disease, p. 360)
- Trauma (e.g. cardiac surgery)
- Drugs (e.g. digoxin, β-blocker)

Management

Atrioventricular block complicating acute myocardial infarction

Acute inferior MI is often complicated by transient AV block because the right coronary artery (RCA) supplies the AV node. There is usually a reliable escape rhythm and, if the patient remains well, no treatment is required. Symptomatic second- or third-degree AV block may respond to atropine (0.6 mg IV, repeated as necessary) or, if this fails, a temporary pacemaker. In most cases, the AV block will resolve within 7–10 days.

Second- or third-degree AV heart block complicating acute anterior MI indicates extensive ventricular damage involving both bundle branches and carries a poor prognosis. Asystole may ensue and a temporary pacemaker should be inserted promptly. If the patient presents with asystole, IV atropine (3 mg) or IV isoprenaline (2 mg in 500 mL 5% dextrose, infused at 10–60 mL/hr) may help to maintain the circulation until a temporary pacing electrode can be inserted. External (transcutaneous) pacing can provide effective temporary rhythm support.

Chronic atrioventricular block

Patients with symptomatic bradyarrhythmias associated with AV block should receive a permanent pacemaker (see below). Asymptomatic first-degree or Mobitz type I second-degree AV block (Wenckebach phenomenon) does not require treatment but may be an indication of serious underlying heart disease. A permanent pacemaker is usually indicated in patients with asymptomatic Mobitz type II second- or third-degree AV heart block because of the risk of asystole and sudden death. Pacing improves prognosis.

Bundle branch block and hemiblock

Conduction block in the right or left bundle branch can occur as a result of many pathologies, including ischaemic or hypertensive heart disease or cardiomyopathies (Box 18.36). Depolarisation proceeds through a slow myocardial route in the affected ventricle rather than through the rapidly conducting Purkinje tissues that constitute the bundle branches. This causes delayed conduction into the LV or RV, broadens the QRS complex (≥ 0.12 s) and produces the characteristic alterations in QRS morphology (Figs 18.56 and 18.57). Right bundle branch block (RBBB) can occur in healthy people but left

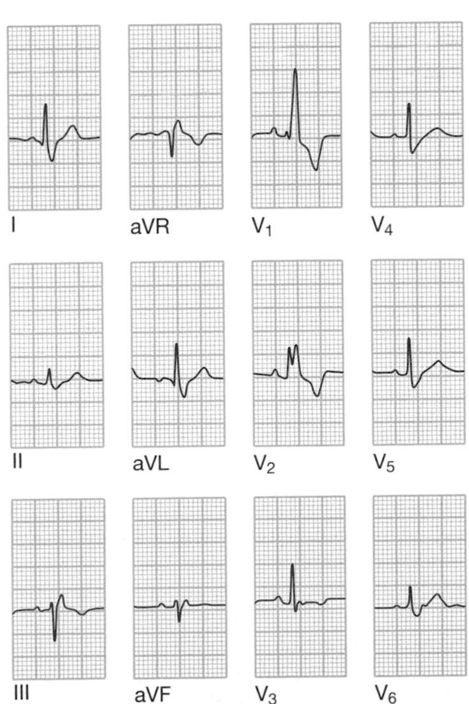

Fig. 18.56 Right bundle branch block. Note the wide QRS complexes with 'M'-shaped configuration in leads V, and V_2 and a wide S wave in lead I.

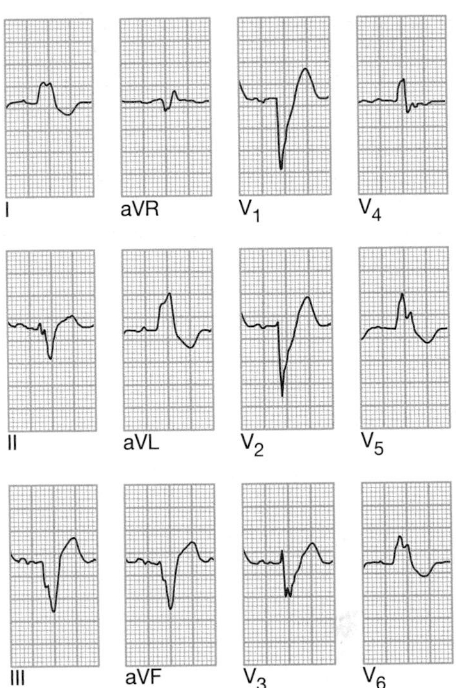

Fig. 18.57 Left bundle branch block. Note the wide QRS complexes with loss of the Q wave or septal vector in lead I and 'M'-shaped QRS complexes in V_5 and V_6.

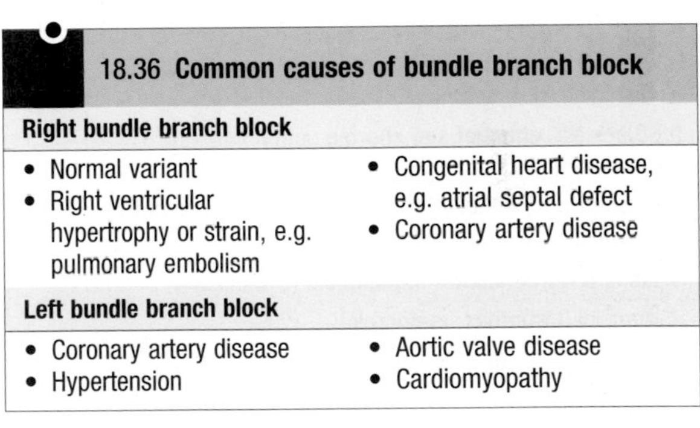

18.36 Common causes of bundle branch block

Right bundle branch block	
• Normal variant • Right ventricular hypertrophy or strain, e.g. pulmonary embolism	• Congenital heart disease, e.g. atrial septal defect • Coronary artery disease
Left bundle branch block	
• Coronary artery disease • Hypertension	• Aortic valve disease • Cardiomyopathy

bundle branch block (LBBB) often signifies important underlying heart disease.

The left bundle branch divides into an anterior and a posterior fascicle. Damage to the conducting tissue at this point (hemiblock) does not broaden the QRS complex but alters the mean direction of ventricular depolarisation (mean QRS axis), causing left axis deviation in left anterior hemiblock and right axis deviation in left posterior hemiblock (see Fig. 18.7, p. 533). The combination of right bundle branch block and left anterior or posterior hemiblock is known as bifascicular block.

Anti-arrhythmic drug therapy

Classification

Anti-arrhythmic drugs may be classified according to their mode or site of action (Box 18.37 and Fig. 18.58).

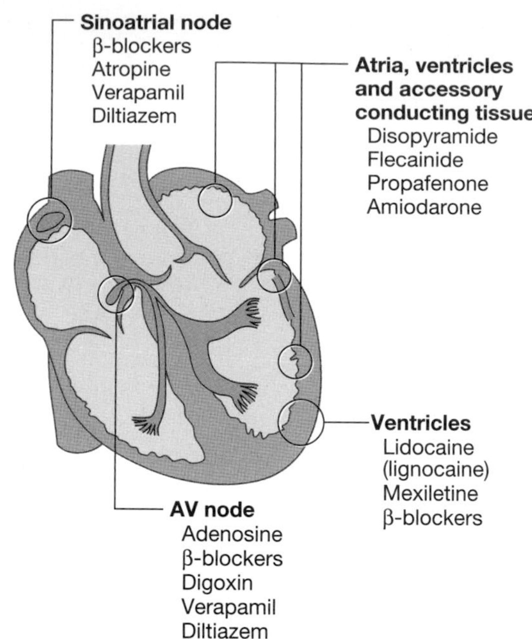

Fig. 18.58 Classification of anti-arrhythmic drugs by site of action.

18.37 Classification of anti-arrhythmic drugs by effect on the intracellular action potential

Class I: membrane-stabilising agents (sodium channel blockers)
(a) Block Na^+ channel and prolong action potential • Quinidine, disopyramide **(b) Block Na^+ channel and shorten action potential** • Lidocaine, mexiletine **(c) Block Na^+ channel with no effect on action potential** • Flecainide, propafenone
Class II: β-adrenoceptor antagonists (β-blockers)
• Atenolol, bisoprolol, metoprolol
Class III: drugs whose main effect is to prolong the action potential
• Amiodarone, dronedarone, sotalol
Class IV: slow calcium channel blockers
• Verapamil, diltiazem
N.B. Some drugs (e.g. digoxin, ivabradine and adenosine) have no place in this classification, while others have properties in more than one class: e.g. amiodarone, which has actions in all four classes.

Identification of ion channel subtypes has led to refinement of drug classifications, according to the specific mechanisms targeted. The Vaughan-Williams classification is a simple system but is convenient for describing the main mode of action of anti-arrhythmic drugs (Box 18.38) that should be used following guiding principles (Box 18.39). Anti-arrhythmic drugs can also be more accurately categorised by referring to the cardiac ion channels and receptors on which they act.

Class I drugs

Class I drugs act principally by suppressing excitability and slowing conduction in atrial or ventricular muscle. They block sodium channels, of which there are several types in cardiac tissue. These drugs should generally be avoided in patients with heart failure because they depress myocardial function, and class Ia and Ic drugs are often pro-arrhythmic.

Class Ia drugs

These prolong cardiac action potential duration and increase the tissue refractory period. They are used to prevent both atrial and ventricular arrhythmias.

Disopyramide. An effective drug but causes anticholinergic side-effects, such as urinary retention, and can precipitate glaucoma. It can depress myocardial function and should be avoided in cardiac failure.

Quinidine. Now rarely used, as it increases mortality and causes gastrointestinal upset.

Class Ib drugs

These shorten the action potential and tissue refractory period. They act on channels found predominantly in ventricular myocardium and so are used to treat or prevent ventricular tachycardia and ventricular fibrillation.

Lidocaine. Must be given intravenously and has a very short plasma half-life.

Mexiletine. Can be given intravenously or orally, but has many side-effects (see Box 18.38).

Class Ic drugs

These affect the slope of the action potential without altering its duration or refractory period. They are used mainly for prophylaxis of atrial fibrillation but are effective in prophylaxis and treatment of supraventricular or ventricular arrhythmias. They are useful for WPW syndrome because they block conduction in accessory pathways. They should not be used as oral prophylaxis in patients with previous MI because of pro-arrhythmia.

Flecainide. Effective for prevention of atrial fibrillation, and an intravenous infusion may be used for pharmacological cardioversion of atrial fibrillation of less than 24 hours' duration. It should be prescribed along with an AV node-blocking drug, such as a β-blocker, to prevent pro-arrhythmia.

Propafenone. Also has some β-blocker (class II) properties. Important interactions with digoxin, warfarin and cimetidine have been described.

Class II drugs

This group comprises the β-adrenoceptor antagonists (β-blockers). These agents reduce the rate of SA node depolarisation and cause relative block in the AV node, making them useful for rate control in atrial flutter and atrial fibrillation. They can be used to prevent supraventricular and ventricular tachycardia. They reduce myocardial excitability and the risk of arrhythmic death in patients with coronary artery disease and heart failure.

'Non-selective' β-blockers. Act on both β_1 and β_2 receptors. $Beta_2$ blockade causes side-effects, such as bronchospasm and peripheral vasoconstriction. *Propranolol* is non-selective and is subject to extensive first-pass metabolism in the liver. The effective oral dose is therefore unpredictable and must be titrated after treatment is started with a small dose. Other non-selective drugs include *nadolol* and *carvedilol.*

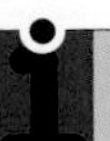

18.38 The main uses, dosages and side-effects of the most widely used anti-arrhythmic drugs

Drug	Main uses	Route	Dose (adult)	Important side-effects
Class I				
Disopyramide	Prevention and treatment of atrial and ventricular tachyarrhythmias	IV	2 mg/kg at 30 mg/min, then 0.4 mg/kg/hr (max 800 mg/day)	Myocardial depression, hypotension, dry mouth, urinary retention
		Oral	300–800 mg daily in divided dosage	
Lidocaine	Treatment and short-term prevention of VT and VF	IV	Bolus 50–100 mg, 4 mg/min for 30 mins, then 2 mg/min for 2 hrs, then 1 mg/min for 24 hrs	Myocardial depression, confusion, convulsions
Mexiletine	Prevention and treatment of ventricular tachyarrhythmias	IV	Loading dose: 100–250 mg at 25 mg/min, then 250 mg in 1 hr, then 250 mg in 2 hrs	Myocardial depression, gastrointestinal irritation, confusion, dizziness, tremor, nystagmus, ataxia
		Oral	Maintenance therapy: 0.5 mg/min, 200–250 mg 3 times daily	
Flecainide	Prevention and treatment of atrial and ventricular tachyarrhythmias	IV	2 mg/kg over 10 mins, then 1.5 mg/kg/hr for 1 hr, then 0.1 mg/kg/hr	Myocardial depression, dizziness
		Oral	50–100 mg twice daily	
Propafenone	Prevention and treatment of atrial and ventricular tachyarrhythmias	Oral	150 mg 3 times daily for 1 wk, then 300 mg twice daily	Myocardial depression, dizziness
Class II				
Atenolol	Treatment and prevention of SVT and AF Prevention of VEs and exercise-induced VT	IV	2.5 mg at 1 mg/min, repeated at 5-min intervals (max 10 mg)	Myocardial depression, bradycardia, bronchospasm, fatigue, depression, nightmares, cold peripheries
		Oral	25–100 mg daily	
Bisoprolol		Oral	2.5–10 mg daily	
Metoprolol		IV	5 mg over 2 mins to a maximum of 15 mg	
Class III				
Amiodarone	Serious or resistant atrial and ventricular tachyarrhythmias	IV	5 mg/kg over 20–120 mins, then up to 15 mg/kg/24 hrs	Photosensitivity, skin discoloration, corneal deposits, thyroid dysfunction, alveolitis, nausea and vomiting, hepatotoxicity, peripheral neuropathy, torsades de pointes; potentiates digoxin and warfarin
		Oral	Initially 600–1200 mg/day, then 100–400 mg daily	
Dronedarone	Paroxysmal atrial fibrillation	Oral	400 mg twice daily	Renal and hepatic dysfunction requiring regular blood monitoring
Sotalol	Atrial fibrillation, rarely ventricular tachyarrhythmias	IV	10–20 mg slowly	Can cause torsades de pointes
		Oral	40–160 mg twice daily	
Class IV				
Verapamil	Treatment of SVT, control of AF	IV	5–10 mg over 30 secs	Myocardial depression, hypotension, bradycardia, constipation
		Oral	40–120 mg 3 times daily or 240 mg SR daily	
Other				
Atropine	Treatment of bradycardia and/or hypotension due to vagal overactivity	IV	0.6–3 mg	Dry mouth, thirst, blurred vision, atrial and ventricular extrasystoles
Adenosine	Treatment of SVT, aid to diagnosis in unidentified tachycardia	IV	3 mg over 2 secs, followed if necessary by 6 mg, then 12 mg at intervals of 1–2 mins	Flushing, dyspnoea, chest pain Avoid in asthma
Digoxin	Treatment and prevention of SVT, rate control of AF	IV	Loading dose: 0.5–1 mg (total), 0.5 mg over 30 mins, then 0.25–0.5 mg 3–6 times daily, to maximum total of 1 mg, assessing response before each additional dose	Gastrointestinal disturbance, xanthopsia, arrhythmias (see Box 18.41)
		Oral	0.5 mg 4 times daily for 2 doses, then 0.125–0.25 mg daily	

(AF = atrial fibrillation; SR = sustained-release formulation; SVT = supraventricular tachycardia; VE = ventricular ectopic; VF = ventricular fibrillation; VT = ventricular tachycardia)

18.39 Anti-arrhythmic drugs: principles of use

Anti-arrhythmic drugs are potentially toxic and should be used carefully according to the following principles:

- Many arrhythmias are benign and do not require specific treatment
- Precipitating or causal factors should be corrected if possible, e.g. excess alcohol or caffeine consumption, myocardial ischaemia, hyperthyroidism, acidosis, hypokalaemia and hypomagnesaemia
- If drug therapy is required, it is best to use as few drugs as possible
- In difficult cases, programmed electrical stimulation (electrophysiological study) may help to identify the optimum therapy
- When managing life-threatening arrhythmias, it is essential to ensure that prophylactic treatment is effective. Ambulatory monitoring and exercise testing may be of value
- Patients on long-term anti-arrhythmic drugs should be reviewed regularly and attempts made to withdraw therapy if the factors which precipitated the arrhythmias are no longer operative
- For patients with recurrent SVT, radiofrequency ablation is often preferable to long-term drug therapy

'Cardioselective' β-blockers. Act mainly on myocardial β_1 receptors and are relatively well tolerated. *Bisoprolol* and *metoprolol* are examples of cardioselective β-blockers.

Sotalol. A racemic mixture of two isomers with non-selective β-blocker (mainly l-sotalol) and class III (mainly d-sotalol) activity. It may cause torsades de pointes.

Class III drugs

Class III drugs act by prolonging the plateau phase of the action potential, thus lengthening the refractory period. These drugs are very effective at preventing atrial and ventricular tachyarrhythmias. They cause QT interval prolongation and can predispose to torsades de pointes and ventricular tachycardia (p. 570), especially in patients with other predisposing risk factors (see Box 18.34, p. 571).

Amiodarone. The principal drug in this class, although both disopyramide and sotalol have class III activity. Amiodarone is a complex drug that also has class I, II and IV activity. It is probably the most effective drug currently available for controlling paroxysmal atrial fibrillation. It is also used to prevent episodes of recurrent ventricular tachycardia, particularly in patients with poor left ventricular function or those with implantable defibrillators (to prevent unnecessary DC shocks). Amiodarone has a very long tissue half-life (25–110 days). An intravenous or oral loading regime is often used to achieve therapeutic tissue concentrations rapidly. The drug's effects may last for weeks or months after treatment has been stopped. Side-effects are common (up to one-third of patients), numerous and potentially serious. Drug interactions are also common (see Box 18.38).

Dronedarone. A related drug that has a short tissue half-life and fewer side-effects. It has recently been shown to be effective at preventing episodes of atrial flutter and fibrillation. It is contraindicated in patients with permanent atrial fibrillation, or if there is heart failure or left ventricular impairment, because it increases mortality. Regular liver function test monitoring is required.

Class IV drugs

These block the 'slow calcium channel', which is important for impulse generation and conduction in atrial and nodal tissue, although it is also present in ventricular muscle. Their main indications are prevention of supraventricular tachycardia (by blocking the AV node) and rate control in patients with atrial fibrillation.

Verapamil. The most widely used drug in this class. Intravenous verapamil may cause profound bradycardia or hypotension, and should not be used in conjunction with β-blockers.

Diltiazem. Has similar properties.

Other anti-arrhythmic drugs

Atropine sulphate (0.6 mg IV, repeated if necessary to a maximum of 3 mg). Increases the sinus rate and SA and AV conduction, and is the treatment of choice for severe bradycardia or hypotension due to vagal overactivity. It is used for initial management of symptomatic brady-arrhythmias complicating inferior MI, and in cardiac arrest due to asystole. Repeat dosing may be necessary because the drug disappears rapidly from the circulation after parenteral administration. Side-effects are listed in Box 18.38.

Adenosine. Must be given intravenously. It produces transient AV block lasting a few seconds. It is used to terminate supraventricular tachycardias when the AV node is part of the re-entry circuit, or to help establish the diagnosis in difficult arrhythmias, such as atrial flutter with 2:1 AV block (see Fig. 18.41, p. 564) or broad-complex tachycardia (Boxes 18.38 and 18.40). Adenosine is given as an intravenous bolus, initially 3 mg over 2 seconds (see Box 18.38). If there is no response after 1–2 minutes, 6 mg should be given; if necessary, after another 1–2 minutes, the maximum dose of 12 mg may be given. Patients should be warned to expect short-lived and sometimes distressing flushing, breathlessness and chest pain. Adenosine can cause bronchospasm and should be avoided in asthmatics; its effects are greatly potentiated by dipyridamole and inhibited by theophylline and other xanthines.

18.40 Response to intravenous adenosine

Arrhythmia	Response
Supraventricular tachycardia	Termination
Atrial fibrillation, atrial flutter	Transient AV block
Ventricular tachycardia	No effect

Digoxin. A purified glycoside from the European foxglove, *Digitalis lanata,* which slows conduction and prolongs the refractory period in the AV node. This effect helps to control the ventricular rate in atrial fibrillation and may interrupt supraventricular tachycardias involving the AV node. Digoxin also shortens refractory periods and enhances excitability and conduction in other parts of the heart (including accessory conduction pathways). It may therefore increase atrial and ventricular ectopic activity and can lead to more complex atrial

18.41 Digoxin toxicity

Extracardiac manifestations	
• Anorexia, nausea, vomiting • Diarrhoea	• Altered colour vision (xanthopsia)
Cardiac manifestations	
• Bradycardia • Multiple ventricular ectopics • Ventricular bigeminy (alternate ventricular ectopics)	• Atrial tachycardia (with variable block) • Ventricular tachycardia • Ventricular fibrillation

and ventricular tachyarrhythmias. Digoxin is largely excreted by the kidneys, and the maintenance dose (see Box 18.38) should be reduced in children, older people and those with renal impairment. It is widely distributed and has a long tissue half-life (36 hours), so that effects may persist for several days. Measurement of plasma digoxin concentration helps identify digoxin toxicity or under-treatment (Box 18.41).

Therapeutic procedures

External defibrillation and cardioversion

The heart can be completely depolarised by passing a sufficiently large electrical current through it from an external source. This will interrupt any arrhythmia and produce a brief period of asystole that is usually followed by the resumption of sinus rhythm. Defibrillators deliver a DC, high-energy, short-duration shock via two large electrodes or paddles coated with conducting jelly or a gel pad, positioned over the upper right sternal edge and the apex. Modern units deliver a biphasic shock, during which the shock polarity is reversed mid-shock. This reduces the total shock energy required to depolarise the heart.

Electrical cardioversion

This is the termination of an organised rhythm, such as atrial fibrillation or ventricular tachycardia, with a synchronised shock, usually under general anaesthesia. The shock is delivered immediately after detection of the R wave because, if it is applied during ventricular repolarisation (on the T wave), it may provoke ventricular fibrillation. High-energy shocks may cause chest wall pain post-procedure, so, if there is no urgency, it is appropriate to begin with a lower-amplitude shock (e.g. 50 joules), going on to larger shocks if necessary. Patients with atrial fibrillation or flutter of more than 48 hours' duration are at risk of left atrial appendage thrombus, and thus systemic embolism after cardioversion. In such cases, cardioversion should be delayed until effective anticoagulation has been given for at least 4 weeks.

Defibrillation

This is the delivery of an unsynchronised shock during a cardiac arrest caused by ventricular fibrillation. The precise timing of the discharge is not important in this situation. In ventricular fibrillation and other emergencies, the energy of the first and second shocks should be 150 joules and thereafter up to 200 joules; there is no need for an anaesthetic, as the patient is unconscious.

Catheter ablation

Catheter ablation therapy is the treatment of choice for patients with supraventricular tachycardia or atrial flutter, and is a useful treatment for some patients with atrial fibrillation or ventricular arrhythmias (Fig. 18.59). A series of catheter electrodes are inserted into the heart via the venous system and are used to record the activation sequence of the heart in sinus rhythm, during tachycardia and after pacing manœuvres. Once the arrhythmia focus or circuit is identified (e.g. an accessory pathway in WPW syndrome), a catheter is used to ablate the culprit tissue using heat (via radiofrequency current) or sometimes by freezing (cryoablation). The procedure takes approximately 1–4 hours and does not require a general anaesthetic. The patient may experience some discomfort during the ablation itself. Serious complications are rare (< 1%) but include inadvertent complete heart block requiring pacemaker implantation, and cardiac tamponade. For many arrhythmias, radiofrequency ablation is very attractive because it offers the prospect of a lifetime cure, thereby eliminating the need for long-term drug therapy.

The technique has revolutionised the management of many arrhythmias and is now the treatment of choice for AVNRT and AV re-entrant (accessory pathway) tachycardias, when it is curative in over 90% of cases. Focal atrial tachycardias and atrial flutter can also be eliminated by radiofrequency ablation, although some patients subsequently experience episodes of atrial fibrillation. The applications of the technique are expanding and it can now be used to treat some forms of ventricular tachycardia. Catheter ablation techniques are also used to prevent atrial fibrillation. This involves ablation at two sites: the ostia of the pulmonary veins, from which ectopic beats may trigger paroxysms of arrhythmia, and in the LA itself, where re-entry circuits maintain atrial fibrillation, once established. This is effective at reducing episodes of atrial fibrillation in

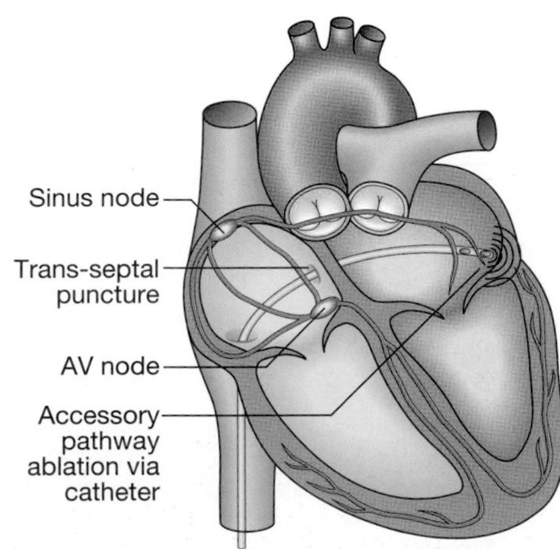

Fig. 18.59 Radiofrequency ablation.

18

around 70–80% of younger patients with structurally normal hearts, and tends to be reserved for patients with drug-resistant atrial fibrillation.

In patients with permanent atrial fibrillation and poor rate control, in whom drugs are ineffective or are not tolerated, rate control can be achieved by: (i) implantation of a permanent pacemaker, followed by (ii) ablation of the AV node to induce complete AV block and bradycardia, thus allowing the pacemaker to assume control of the heart rate.

Temporary pacemakers

Temporary pacing involves delivery of an electrical impulse into the heart to initiate tissue depolarisation and to trigger cardiac contraction. This is achieved by inserting a bipolar pacing electrode via the internal jugular, subclavian or femoral vein and positioning it at the apex of the RV, using fluoroscopic imaging. The electrode is connected to an external pacemaker with an adjustable energy output and pacing rate. The ECG of right ventricular pacing is characterised by regular broad QRS complexes with a left bundle branch block pattern. Each complex is immediately preceded by a 'pacing spike' (Fig. 18.60). Nearly all pulse generators are used in the 'demand' mode, so that the pacemaker will only operate if the heart rate falls below a preset level. Occasionally, temporary atrial or dual-chamber pacing (see below) is used.

Temporary pacing may be indicated in the management of transient AV block and other arrhythmias complicating acute MI or cardiac surgery, to maintain the rhythm in other situations of reversible bradycardia (i.e. due to metabolic disturbance or drug overdose), or as a bridge to permanent pacing. Complications include pneumothorax, brachial plexus or subclavian artery injury, local infection or septicaemia (usually *Staphylococcus aureus*), and pericarditis. Failure of the system may be due to lead displacement or a progressive increase in the threshold (exit block) caused by tissue oedema. Complication rates increase with time and so a temporary pacing system should ideally not be used for more than 7 days.

Transcutaneous pacing is administered by delivering an electrical stimulus through two large adhesive gel pad electrodes placed over the apex and upper right sternal edge, or over the anterior and posterior chest. It is easy and quick to set up, but causes discomfort because it induces forceful pectoral and intercostal muscle contraction. Modern external cardiac defibrillators often incorporate a transcutaneous pacing system that can be used during an emergency until transvenous pacing is established.

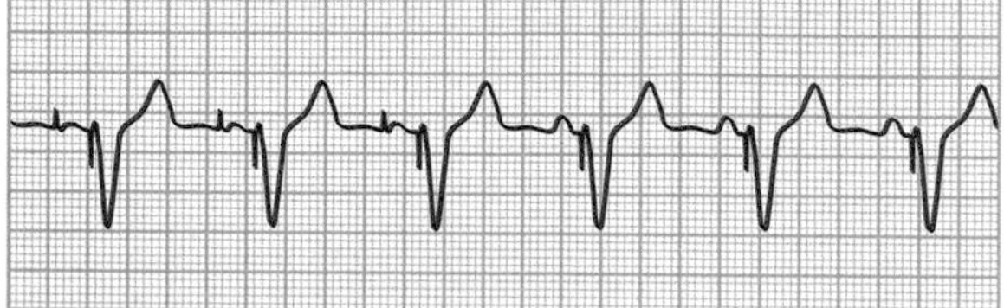

Fig. 18.60 Dual-chamber pacing. The first three beats show atrial and ventricular pacing with narrow pacing spikes in front of each P wave and QRS complex. The last four beats show spontaneous P waves with a different morphology and no pacing spike; the pacemaker senses or tracks these P waves and maintains AV synchrony by pacing the ventricle after an appropriate interval.

Permanent pacemakers

Permanent pacemakers are small, flat, metal devices that are implanted under the skin, usually in the pectoral area. They contain a battery, a pulse generator, and programmable electronics that allow adjustment of pacing and memory functions. Pacing electrodes (leads) can be placed via the subclavian or cephalic veins into the RV (usually at the apex), the right atrial appendage or, to maintain AV synchrony, both.

Permanent pacemakers are programmed using an external programmer via a wireless telemetry system. Pacing rate, output, timing and other parameters can be adjusted. This allows the device to be set to the optimum settings to suit the patient's needs. Pacemakers store useful diagnostic data about the patient's heart rate trends and the occurrence of tachyarrhythmias, such as ventricular tachycardia.

Single-chamber atrial pacing is used in patients with sinoatrial disease without AV block (the pacemaker acts as an external sinus node). Single-chamber ventricular pacing is used in patients with continuous atrial fibrillation and bradycardia. Dual-chamber pacing is most often used in patients with second- or third-degree AV block; here, the atrial electrode is used to detect spontaneous atrial activity and trigger ventricular pacing (see Fig. 18.60), thereby preserving AV synchrony and allowing the ventricular rate to increase, together with the sinus node rate, during exercise and other forms of stress. Dual-chamber pacing has many advantages over ventricular pacing; these include superior haemodynamics, leading to a better effort tolerance, a lower prevalence of atrial arrhythmias in patients with sinoatrial disease, and avoidance of 'pacemaker syndrome' (a fall in BP and dizziness precipitated by loss of AV synchrony).

A code is used to signify the pacing mode (Box 18.42). For example, a system that paces the atrium, senses the atrium and is inhibited if it senses spontaneous activity is designated AAI. Most dual-chamber pacemakers are programmed to a mode termed DDD; in this case, ventricular pacing is triggered by a sensed sinus P wave and inhibited by a sensed spontaneous QRS complex. A fourth letter, 'R', is added if the pacemaker has a rate response function (e.g. AAIR = atrial demand pacemaker with rate response function). Rate-responsive pacemakers are used in patients with chronotropic incompetence, who are unable to increase their heart rate during exercise. These devices have a sensor that triggers an increase in heart rate in response to movement or increased respiratory rate. The sensitivity of

18.42 International generic pacemaker code

Chamber paced	Chamber sensed	Response to sensing
0 = none	0 = none	0 = none
A = atrium	A = atrium	T = triggered
V = ventricle	V = ventricle	I = inhibited
D = both	D = both	D = both

the sensor is programmable, as is the maximum paced heart rate.

Early complications of permanent pacing include pneumothorax, cardiac tamponade, infection and lead displacement. Late complications include infection (which usually necessitates removing the pacing system), erosion of the generator or lead, chronic pain related to the implant site, and lead fracture due to mechanical fatigue.

Implantable cardiac defibrillators

In addition to the functions of a permanent pacemaker, implantable cardiac defibrillators (ICDs) can also detect and terminate life-threatening ventricular tachyarrhythmias. ICDs are larger than pacemakers mainly because of the need for a large battery and capacitor to enable cardioversion or defibrillation. ICD leads are similar to pacing leads but have one or two shock coils along the length of the lead, used for delivering defibrillation. ICDs treat ventricular tachyarrhythmias using overdrive pacing, cardioversion or defibrillation. They are implanted in a similar manner to pacemakers and carry a similar risk of complications. In addition, patients can be prone to psychological problems and anxiety, particularly if they have experienced repeated shocks from their device.

The evidence-based indications for ICD implantation are shown in Box 18.43. These can be divided into 'secondary prevention' indications, when patients have already had a potentially life-threatening ventricular arrhythmia, and 'primary prevention' indications, when patients are considered to be at significant future risk of arrhythmic death. ICDs may be used prophylactically in selected patients with inherited conditions associated with a high risk of sudden cardiac death, such as long QT syndrome (p. 571), hypertrophic cardiomyopathy and arrhythmogenic right ventricular dysplasia (pp. 637 and 638). ICD treatment is expensive and so the indications for which the devices are routinely implanted depend on the health-care resources available.

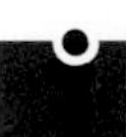

18.43 Key indications for ICD therapy

Primary prevention

- After MI, if LV ejection fraction < 30%
- Mild to moderate symptomatic heart failure on optimal drug therapy, with LV ejection fraction < 35%

Secondary prevention

- Survivors of ventricular fibrillation or ventricular tachycardia cardiac arrest not due to transient or reversible cause
- Ventricular tachycardia with haemodynamic compromise or significant LV impairment (LV ejection fraction < 35%)

Cardiac resynchronisation therapy

Cardiac resynchronisation therapy (CRT) is a treatment for selected patients with heart failure, in whom cardiac function is further impaired by the presence of left bundle branch block. This conduction defect is associated with left ventricular dys-synchrony (poorly coordinated left ventricular contraction) and can aggravate heart failure in susceptible patients. CRT systems have an additional lead that is placed via the coronary sinus into one of the veins on the epicardial surface of the LV (see Fig. 18.28, p. 553). Simultaneous septal and left ventricular epicardial pacing resynchronises left ventricular contraction. These devices improve effort tolerance, reduce heart failure symptoms (Box 18.44), and are more effective in patients in sinus rhythm than in those with atrial fibrillation. Most devices are also defibrillators (CRT-D) because many patients with heart failure are predisposed to ventricular arrhythmias. CRT-pacemakers (CRT-P) are used in patients considered to be at relatively low risk of these arrhythmias.

EBM 18.44 Cardiac resynchronisation therapy (CRT) for heart failure

'CRT improves symptoms and quality of life, and reduces mortality in patients with moderate to severe (NYHA class III–IV) heart failure who are in sinus rhythm, with left bundle branch block and LV ejection fraction ≤ 35%. CRT also prevents heart failure progression in similar patients with mild (NYHA class I–II) heart failure symptoms.'

- Cardiac Resynchronisation-Heart Failure (CARE-HF) Study. Cleland J, et al. N Engl J Med 2005; 352:1539–1549.
- COMPANION Study. Bristow MR, et al. N Engl J Med 2004; 350:2140–2150.
- MADIT-CRT study. Moss AJ, et al. N Engl J Med 2009; 361:1329–1338.

ATHEROSCLEROSIS

Atherosclerosis can affect any artery in the body. When it occurs in the heart, it may cause angina, MI and sudden death; in the brain, stroke and transient ischaemic attack (TIA); and in the limbs, claudication and critical limb ischaemia. Occult coronary artery disease is common in those who present with other forms of atherosclerotic vascular disease, such as intermittent claudication or stroke, and is an important cause of morbidity and mortality in these patients.

Pathophysiology

Atherosclerosis is a progressive inflammatory disorder of the arterial wall that is characterised by focal lipid-rich deposits of atheroma that remain clinically silent until they become large enough to impair tissue perfusion, or until ulceration and disruption of the lesion result in thrombotic occlusion or distal embolisation of the vessel. These mechanisms are common to the entire vascular tree, and the clinical manifestations of atherosclerosis depend upon the site of the lesion and the vulnerability of the organ supplied.

Atherosclerosis begins early in life. Abnormalities of arterial function have been detected among high-risk children and adolescents, such as cigarette smokers and those with familial hyperlipidaemia or hypertension. Early lesions have been found in the arteries of victims of accidental death in the second and third decades of life. Nevertheless, clinical manifestations often do not appear until the sixth, seventh or eighth decade.

Early atherosclerosis

Fatty streaks tend to occur at sites of altered arterial shear stress, such as bifurcations, and are associated with abnormal endothelial function. They develop when inflammatory cells, predominantly monocytes, bind to

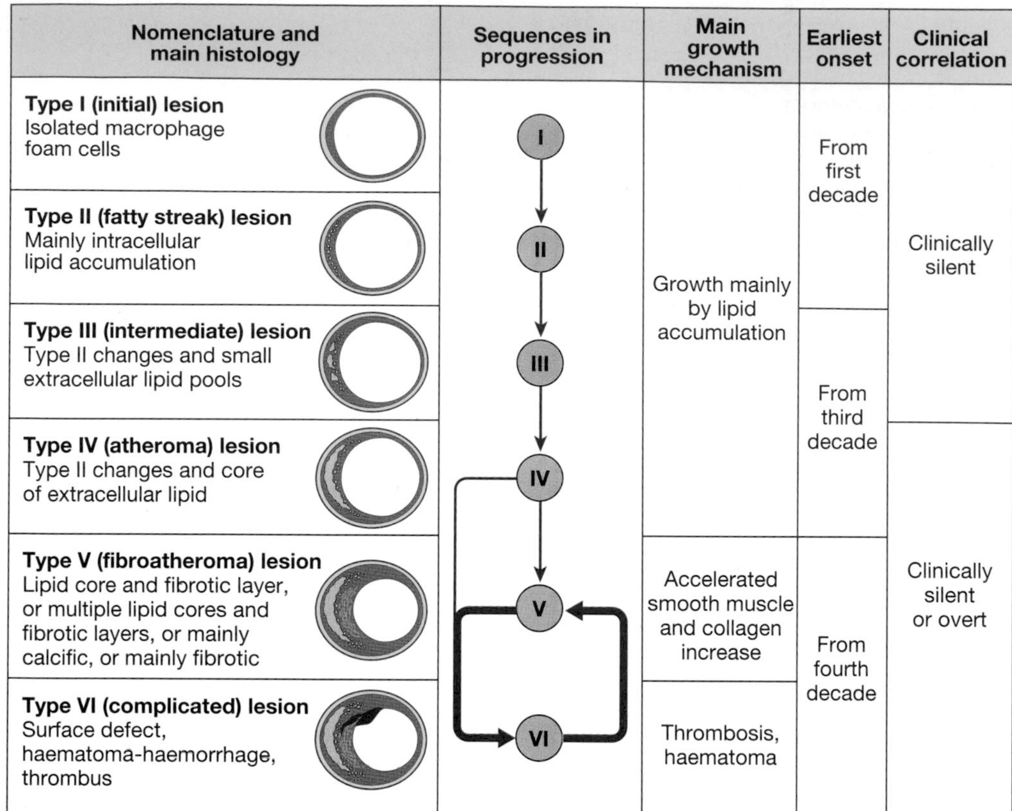

Nomenclature and main histology	Sequences in progression	Main growth mechanism	Earliest onset	Clinical correlation
Type I (initial) lesion Isolated macrophage foam cells	I	Growth mainly by lipid accumulation	From first decade	Clinically silent
Type II (fatty streak) lesion Mainly intracellular lipid accumulation	II			
Type III (intermediate) lesion Type II changes and small extracellular lipid pools	III		From third decade	
Type IV (atheroma) lesion Type II changes and core of extracellular lipid	IV			Clinically silent or overt
Type V (fibroatheroma) lesion Lipid core and fibrotic layer, or multiple lipid cores and fibrotic layers, or mainly calcific, or mainly fibrotic	V	Accelerated smooth muscle and collagen increase	From fourth decade	
Type VI (complicated) lesion Surface defect, haematoma-haemorrhage, thrombus	VI	Thrombosis, haematoma		

Fig. 18.61 The six stages of atherosclerosis. American Heart Association classification. From Stary, et al. 1995 – see p. 641.

receptors expressed by endothelial cells, migrate into the intima, take up oxidised low-density lipoprotein (LDL) particles and become lipid-laden macrophages or foam cells. Extracellular lipid pools appear in the intimal space when foam cells die and release their contents (Fig. 18.61). In response to cytokines and growth factors produced by activated macrophages, smooth muscle cells migrate from the media of the arterial wall into the intima, and change from a contractile to a repair phenotype in an attempt to stabilise the atherosclerotic lesion. If this is successful, the lipid core will be covered by smooth muscle cells and matrix, producing a stable atherosclerotic plaque that will remain asymptomatic until it becomes large enough to obstruct arterial flow.

Advanced atherosclerosis

In an established atherosclerotic plaque, macrophages mediate inflammation and smooth muscle cells promote repair. If inflammation predominates, the plaque becomes active or unstable and may be complicated by ulceration and thrombosis. Cytokines, such as interleukin-1, tumour necrosis factor-alpha, interferon-gamma, platelet-derived growth factors, and matrix metalloproteinases are released by activated macrophages; they cause the intimal smooth muscle cells overlying the plaque to become senescent and collagen cross-struts within the plaque to degrade. This results in thinning of the protective fibrous cap, making the lesion vulnerable to mechanical stress that ultimately causes erosion, fissuring or rupture of the plaque surface (see Fig. 18.61). Any breach in the integrity of the plaque will expose its contents to blood and will trigger platelet aggregation and thrombosis that extend into the atheromatous plaque and the arterial lumen. This type of plaque event may cause partial or complete obstruction at the site of the lesion or distal embolisation resulting in infarction or ischaemia of the affected organ. This common mechanism underlies many of the acute manifestations of atherosclerotic vascular disease, such as acute lower limb ischaemia, MI and stroke.

The number and complexity of arterial plaques increase with age and with risk factors (see below) but the rate of progression of individual plaques is variable. There is a complex and dynamic interaction between mechanical wall stress and atherosclerotic lesions. 'Vulnerable' plaques are characterised by a lipid-rich core, a thin fibrocellular cap, speckled calcification and an increase in inflammatory cells that release specific enzymes to degrade matrix proteins. In contrast, stable plaques are typified by a small lipid pool, a thick fibrous cap, heavy calcification and plentiful collagenous cross-struts. Fissuring or rupture tends to occur at sites of maximal mechanical stress, particularly the margins of an eccentric plaque, and may be triggered by a surge in BP, such as during exercise or emotional stress. Surprisingly, the majority of plaque events are subclinical and heal spontaneously, although this may allow thrombus to be incorporated into the lesion, producing plaque growth and further obstruction to flow.

Atherosclerosis may induce complex changes in the media that lead to arterial remodelling. Some arterial segments may slowly constrict (negative remodelling), whilst others may gradually enlarge (positive remodelling). These changes are important because they may amplify or minimise the degree to which atheroma encroaches into the arterial lumen.

Risk factors

The role and relative importance of many risk factors for the development of coronary, peripheral and cerebrovascular disease have been defined in experimental animal studies, epidemiological studies and clinical interventional trials. Key factors have emerged but do not explain all the risk, and unknown factors may account for up to 40% of the variation in risk from one person to the next.

The impact of genetic risk is illustrated by twin studies; a monozygotic twin of an affected individual has an eightfold increased risk and a dizygotic twin a fourfold increased risk of dying from coronary artery disease, compared to the general population.

The effect of risk factors is multiplicative rather than additive. People with a combination of risk factors are at greatest risk and so assessment should take account of all identifiable risk factors. It is important to distinguish between relative risk (the proportional increase in risk) and absolute risk (the actual chance of an event). Thus, a man of 35 years with a plasma cholesterol of 7 mmol/L (approximately 170 mg/dL), who smokes 40 cigarettes a day, is relatively much more likely to die from coronary disease within the next decade than a non-smoking woman of the same age with a normal cholesterol, but the absolute likelihood of his dying during this time is still small (high relative risk, low absolute risk).

- *Age and sex*. Age is the most powerful independent risk factor for atherosclerosis. Pre-menopausal women have lower rates of disease than men, although this sex difference disappears after the menopause. However, hormone replacement therapy has no role in the primary or secondary prevention of coronary artery disease, and isolated oestrogen therapy may cause an increased cardiovascular event rate.
- *Family history*. Atherosclerotic vascular disease often runs in families, due to a combination of shared genetic, environmental and lifestyle factors. The most common inherited risk characteristics (hypertension, hyperlipidaemia, diabetes mellitus) are polygenic. A 'positive' family history is present when clinical problems in first-degree relatives occur at relatively young age, such as below 50 years for men and below 55 years for women.
- *Smoking*. This is probably the most important avoidable cause of atherosclerotic vascular disease. There is a strong, consistent and dose-linked relationship between cigarette smoking and coronary artery disease, especially in younger (< 70 years) individuals.
- *Hypertension* (see below). The incidence of atherosclerosis increases as BP rises, and this excess risk is related to both systolic and diastolic BP, as well as pulse pressure. Antihypertensive therapy reduces cardiovascular mortality, stroke and heart failure.
- *Hypercholesterolaemia* (p. 453). Risk rises with increasing serum cholesterol concentrations. Lowering serum total and LDL cholesterol concentrations reduces the risk of cardiovascular events, including death, MI, stroke and coronary revascularisation.
- *Diabetes mellitus*. This is a potent risk factor for all forms of atherosclerosis and is often associated with diffuse disease that is difficult to treat. Insulin resistance (normal glucose homeostasis with high levels of insulin) is associated with obesity and physical inactivity, and is a risk factor for coronary artery disease (p. 805). Glucose intolerance accounts for a major part of the high incidence of ischaemic heart disease in certain ethnic groups, e.g. South Asians.
- *Haemostatic factors*. Platelet activation and high plasma fibrinogen concentrations are associated with an increased risk of coronary thrombosis. Antiphospholipid antibodies are associated with recurrent arterial thromboses (p. 1055).
- *Physical activity*. Physical inactivity roughly doubles the risk of coronary artery disease and is a major risk factor for stroke. Regular exercise (brisk walking, cycling or swimming for 20 minutes two or three times a week) has a protective effect that may be related to increased serum high-density lipoprotein (HDL) cholesterol concentrations, lower BP, and collateral vessel development.
- *Obesity* (p. 115). Obesity, particularly if central or truncal, is an independent risk factor, although it is often associated with other adverse factors, such as hypertension, diabetes mellitus and physical inactivity.
- *Alcohol*. Alcohol consumption is associated with reduced rates of coronary artery disease. Excess alcohol consumption is associated with hypertension and cerebrovascular disease.
- *Other dietary factors*. Diets deficient in fresh fruit, vegetables and polyunsaturated fatty acids are associated with an increased risk of cardiovascular disease. The introduction of a Mediterranean-style diet reduces cardiovascular events. However, dietary supplements, such as vitamin C and E, beta-carotene, folate and fish oils, do not reduce cardiovascular events and, in some cases, have been associated with harm.
- *Personality*. Certain personality traits are associated with an increased risk of coronary disease. Nevertheless, there is little or no evidence to support the popular belief that stress is a major cause of coronary artery disease.
- *Social deprivation*. Health inequalities have a major influence on cardiovascular disease. The impact of established risk factors is amplified in patients who are socially deprived and current guidelines recommend that treatment thresholds should be lowered for them.

Primary prevention

Two complementary strategies can be used to prevent atherosclerosis in apparently healthy but at-risk individuals: population and targeted strategies.

The population strategy aims to modify the risk factors of the whole population through diet and lifestyle advice, on the basis that even a small reduction in

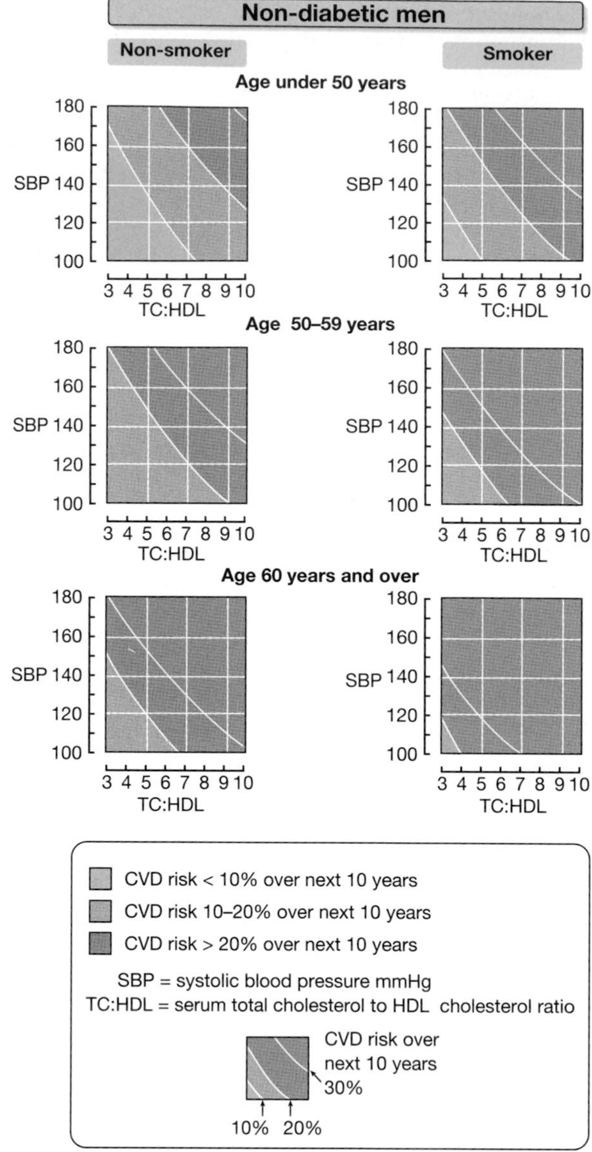

Fig. 18.62 Example of cardiovascular risk prediction chart for non-diabetic men. Cardiovascular risk is predicted from the patient's age, sex, smoking habit, BP and cholesterol ratio. The ratio of total to high-density lipoprotein (HDL) cholesterol can be determined in a non-fasting blood sample. Where HDL cholesterol concentration is unknown, it should be assumed to be 1 mmol/L; the lipid scale should be used as total serum cholesterol. Current guidelines suggest initiation of primary prevention in individuals with a 10-year cardiovascular risk ≥ 20%. Patients with diabetes mellitus should be assumed to have a 10-year cardiovascular risk of ≥ 20% and receive secondary prevention therapy. Modified charts exist for women. For further details, see www.who.int/cardiovascular_diseases/guidelines/Pocket_GL_information/en/index.html. From Joint British Societies Cardiovascular Risk Prediction Chart – see p. 641.

- To estimate an individual's absolute 10-year risk of developing cardiovascular disease (CVD), choose the panel for the appropriate gender, smoking status and age. Within this, define the level of risk from the point where the coordinates for systolic blood pressure (SBP) and ratio of the total to high-density lipoprotein (HDL)-cholesterol cross.
- Highest-risk individuals (red areas) are those whose 10-year CVD risk exceeds 20%, which is approximately equivalent to a 10-year coronary artery disease risk of > 15%. As a minimum, those with CVD risk > 30% (shown by the line within the red area) should be targeted and treated now. When resources allow, others with a CVD risk > 20% should be targeted progressively.
- The chart also assists in identification of individuals with a moderately high 10-year CVD risk, in the range of 10–20% (orange area) and those in whom it is < 10% (green area).
- Smoking status should reflect lifetime exposure to tobacco. For further information, see www.bhf.org.uk

18.45 Population advice to prevent coronary disease

- Do not smoke
- Take regular exercise (minimum of 20 mins, three times/wk)
- Maintain 'ideal' body weight
- Eat a mixed diet rich in fresh fruit and vegetables
- Aim to get no more than 10% of energy intake from saturated fat

smoking or average cholesterol, or modification of exercise and diet will produce worthwhile benefits (Box 18.45). Some risk factors for atheroma, such as obesity and smoking, are also associated with a higher risk of other diseases and should be actively discouraged through public health measures. Legislation restricting smoking in public places is associated with reductions in rates of MI.

The targeted strategy aims to identify and treat high-risk individuals, who usually have a combination of risk factors and can be identified by using composite scoring systems (Fig. 18.62). It is important to consider the absolute risk of atheromatous cardiovascular disease that an individual is facing before contemplating specific antihypertensive or lipid-lowering therapy because this will help to determine whether the possible benefits of intervention are likely to outweigh the expense, inconvenience and possible side-effects of treatment. For example, a 65-year-old man with an average BP of 150/90 mmHg, who smokes and has diabetes mellitus, a total:HDL cholesterol ratio of 8 and left ventricular hypertrophy on ECG, will have a 10-year risk of coronary artery disease of 68% and a 10-year risk of any cardiovascular event of 90%. Lowering his cholesterol will reduce these risks by 30% and lowering his BP will produce a further 20% reduction; both would obviously be worthwhile. Conversely, a 55-year-old woman who has an identical BP, is a non-smoker, does not have diabetes mellitus and has a normal ECG and a total:HDL cholesterol ratio of 6 has a much better outlook, with a predicted coronary artery disease risk of 14% and cardiovascular risk of 19% over the next 10 years. Although lowering her cholesterol and BP would also reduce risk by 30% and 20% respectively, the value of either or both treatments is questionable.

Secondary prevention

Patients who already have evidence of atheromatous vascular disease are at high risk of future cardiovascular events and should be offered treatments and measures to improve their outlook. The energetic correction of modifiable risk factors, particularly smoking, hypertension and hypercholesterolaemia, is particularly important because the absolute risk of further vascular events is high. All patients with coronary artery disease should be given statin therapy, irrespective of their serum cholesterol concentration (Box 18.46). BP should be treated to a target of 140/85 mmHg or lower (p. 610). Aspirin and ACE inhibitors are of benefit in patients with evidence of vascular disease (Boxes 18.47 and 18.48). Beta-blockers benefit patients with a history of MI (see below) or heart failure.

Many clinical events offer an unrivalled opportunity to introduce effective secondary preventive measures; patients who have just survived an MI or undergone bypass surgery are usually keen to help themselves and may be particularly receptive to lifestyle advice, such as dietary modification and smoking cessation.

EBM 18.46 Use of statins in prevention of atherosclerotic disease

Primary prevention

'In patients *without evidence of coronary disease* but with high serum cholesterol concentrations, cholesterol-lowering with statins does not lower mortality but does prevent coronary events (angina and MI).'

Secondary prevention

'In patients *with established coronary disease* (MI or angina), statin therapy can safely reduce the 5-year incidence of all-cause death, as well as major coronary events, coronary revascularisation and stroke. Benefit depends on the overall risk of the study population but the NNT_B for 5 years to prevent 1 death ranges from 10 to 90.'

- Cholesterol Treatment Trialists' Collaborators. Lancet 2005; 366:1267–1277.

For further information: www.sign.ac.uk/guidelines/fulltext/93-97/index.html

EBM 18.47 ACE inhibitors and secondary prevention of atherosclerotic disease

'ACE inhibitor therapy reduces the risk of death, MI and stroke in patients with atherosclerotic vascular disease without apparent left ventricular systolic dysfunction or heart failure. NNT_B to avoid 1 event over 4 years ranges from 6 to 50, depending upon the level of cardiovascular risk.'

- HOPE trial. N Engl J Med 2000; 342:145–153.
- EUROPA trial. Lancet 2003; 362:782–788.

EBM 18.48 Aspirin and secondary prevention in atherosclerotic vascular disease

'In patients with established coronary artery disease, peripheral vascular disease or thrombotic stroke, aspirin is effective in reducing morbidity and mortality (non-fatal MI, stroke and cardiovascular death). In patients at high risk of future vascular events, the overall risk reduction is 22%.'

- Antithrombotic Trialist Collaboration. BMJ 2002; 324:71–86.

For further information: www.clinicalevidence.org

CORONARY ARTERY DISEASE

Coronary artery disease (CAD) is the most common form of heart disease and the single most important cause of premature death in Europe, the Baltic states, Russia, North and South America, Australia and New Zealand. By 2020, it is estimated that it will be the major cause of death in all regions of the world.

In the UK, 1 in 3 men and 1 in 4 women die from CAD, an estimated 330 000 people have a myocardial infarct each year, and approximately 1.3 million people have angina. The death rates from CAD in the UK are amongst the highest in Western Europe (more than 140 000 people) but are falling, particularly in younger age groups; in the last 10 years, CAD mortality has fallen by 42% among UK men and women aged 16–64. However, in Eastern Europe and much of Asia, the rates of CAD are rapidly rising.

Disease of the coronary arteries is almost always due to atheroma and its complications, particularly thrombosis (Box 18.49). Occasionally, the coronary arteries are involved in other disorders such as aortitis, polyarteritis and other connective tissue disorders.

18.49 Coronary artery disease: clinical manifestations and pathology

Clinical problem	Pathology
Stable angina	Ischaemia due to fixed atheromatous stenosis of one or more coronary arteries
Unstable angina	Ischaemia caused by dynamic obstruction of a coronary artery due to plaque rupture or erosion with superimposed thrombosis
Myocardial infarction	Myocardial necrosis caused by acute occlusion of a coronary artery due to plaque rupture or erosion with superimposed thrombosis
Heart failure	Myocardial dysfunction due to infarction or ischaemia
Arrhythmia	Altered conduction due to ischaemia or infarction
Sudden death	Ventricular arrhythmia, asystole or massive myocardial infarction

Stable angina

Angina pectoris is the symptom complex caused by transient myocardial ischaemia and constitutes a clinical syndrome rather than a disease. It may occur whenever there is an imbalance between myocardial oxygen supply and demand (Box 18.50). Coronary atheroma is by far the most common cause of angina, although the symptom may be a manifestation of other forms of heart disease, particularly aortic valve disease and hypertrophic cardiomyopathy

Clinical features

The history is the most important factor in making the diagnosis (p. 539). Stable angina is characterised by central chest pain, discomfort or breathlessness that is

18.50 Factors influencing myocardial oxygen supply and demand

Oxygen demand: cardiac work

- Heart rate
- BP
- Myocardial contractility
- Left ventricular hypertrophy
- Valve disease, e.g. aortic stenosis

Oxygen supply: coronary blood flow

- Duration of diastole
- Coronary perfusion pressure (aortic diastolic minus coronary sinus or right atrial diastolic pressure)
- Coronary vasomotor tone
- Oxygenation
  Haemoglobin
  Oxygen saturation

N.B. Coronary blood flow occurs mainly in diastole.

18.51 Activities precipitating angina

Common

- Physical exertion
- Cold exposure
- Heavy meals
- Intense emotion

Uncommon

- Lying flat (decubitus angina)
- Vivid dreams (nocturnal angina)

precipitated by exertion or other forms of stress (Box 18.51), and is promptly relieved by rest (see Figs 18.17 and 18.18, pp. 540 and 541). Some patients find the discomfort comes when they start walking, and that later it does not return despite greater effort ('warm-up angina').

Physical examination is frequently unremarkable but should include a careful search for evidence of valve disease (particularly aortic), important risk factors (e.g. hypertension, diabetes mellitus), left ventricular dysfunction (cardiomegaly, gallop rhythm), other manifestations of arterial disease (carotid bruits, peripheral vascular disease) and unrelated conditions that may exacerbate angina (anaemia, thyrotoxicosis).

Investigations

Resting ECG

The ECG may show evidence of previous MI but is often normal, even in patients with severe coronary artery disease. Occasionally, there is T-wave flattening or inversion in some leads, providing non-specific evidence of myocardial ischaemia or damage. The most convincing ECG evidence of myocardial ischaemia is the demonstration of reversible ST segment depression or elevation, with or without T-wave inversion, at the time the patient is experiencing symptoms (whether spontaneous or induced by exercise testing).

Exercise ECG

An exercise tolerance test (ETT) is usually performed using a standard treadmill or bicycle ergometer protocol (p. 534) while monitoring the patient's ECG, BP and general condition. Planar or down-sloping ST segment depression of 1 mm or more is indicative of ischaemia (Fig. 18.63). Up-sloping ST depression is less specific and often occurs in normal individuals.

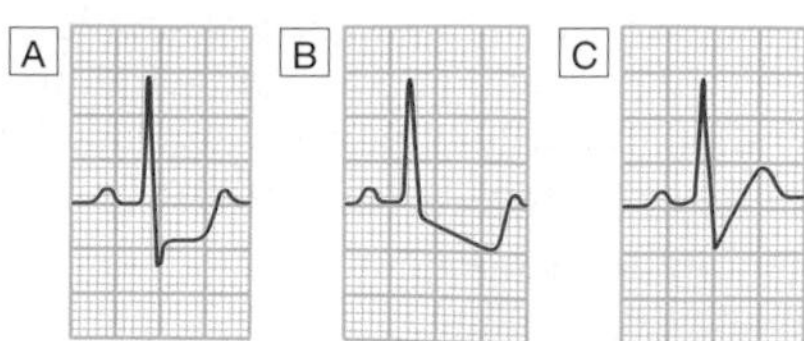

Fig. 18.63 Forms of exercise-induced ST depression. **A** Planar ST depression is usually indicative of myocardial ischaemia. **B** Down-sloping depression also usually indicates myocardial ischaemia. **C** Up-sloping depression may be a normal finding.

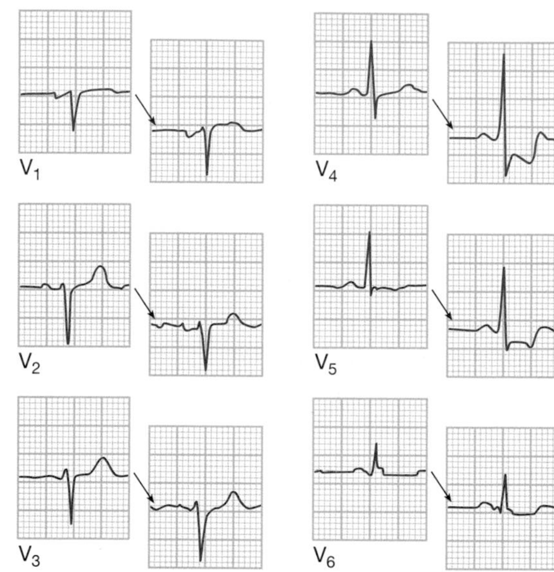

Fig. 18.64 A positive exercise test (chest leads only). The resting 12-lead ECG shows some minor T-wave changes in the inferolateral leads but is otherwise normal. After 3 minutes' exercise on a treadmill, there is marked planar ST depression in leads V_4 and V_5 (right offset). Subsequent coronary angiography revealed critical three-vessel coronary artery disease.

18.52 Risk stratification in stable angina

High risk	Low risk
Post-infarct angina	Predictable exertional angina
Poor effort tolerance	Good effort tolerance
Ischaemia at low workload	Ischaemia only at high workload
Left main or three-vessel disease	Single-vessel or two-vessel disease
Poor LV function	Good LV function

N.B. Patients may fall between these categories.

Exercise testing is also a useful means of assessing the severity of coronary disease and identifying high-risk individuals (Box 18.52). For example, the amount of exercise that can be tolerated and the extent and degree of any ST segment change (Fig. 18.64) provide a useful guide to the likely extent of coronary disease. Exercise testing is not infallible and may produce false-positive results in the presence of digoxin therapy, left ventricular hypertrophy, bundle branch block or WPW syndrome. The predictive accuracy of exercise testing is lower in women than in men. The test should be classed as inconclusive (rather than negative) if the patient cannot achieve an adequate level of exercise because of locomotor or other non-cardiac problems.

Other forms of stress testing

- *Myocardial perfusion scanning.* This may be helpful in the evaluation of patients with an equivocal or uninterpretable exercise test and those who are unable to exercise (p. 539). It entails obtaining scintiscans of the myocardium at rest and during stress (either exercise testing or pharmacological stress, such as a controlled infusion of dobutamine), after the administration of an intravenous radioactive isotope, such as ^{99}technetium tetrofosmin. Thallium and tetrofosmin are taken up by viable perfused myocardium. A perfusion defect present during stress but not at rest provides evidence of reversible myocardial ischaemia (Fig. 18.65), whereas a persistent perfusion defect seen during both phases of the study is usually indicative of previous MI.
- *Stress echocardiography.* This is an alternative to myocardial perfusion scanning and can achieve similar predictive accuracy. It uses transthoracic echocardiography to identify ischaemic segments of myocardium and areas of infarction (p. 537). The former characteristically exhibit reversible defects in contractility during exercise or pharmacological stress, and the latter do not contract at rest or during stress.

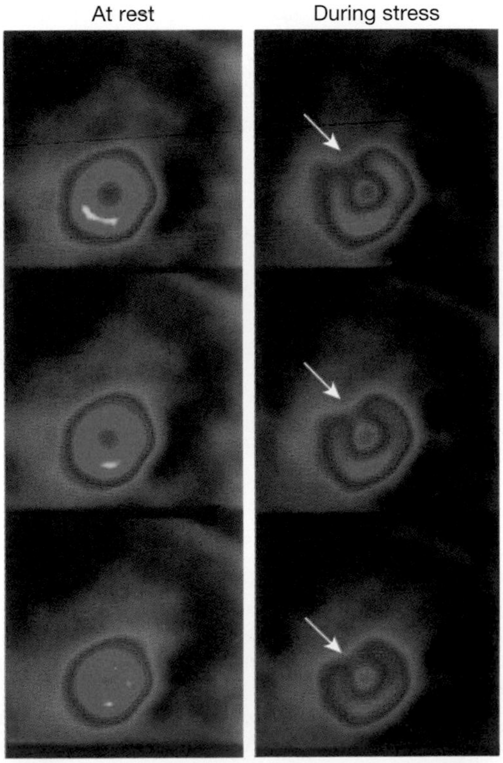

At rest | During stress

Fig. 18.65 A myocardial perfusion scan showing reversible anterior myocardial ischaemia. The images are cross-sectional tomograms of the LV. The resting scans (left) show even uptake of the ^{99}technetium-labelled tetrofosmin and look like doughnuts. During stress (e.g. a dobutamine infusion), there is reduced uptake of technetium, particularly along the anterior wall (arrows), and the scans look like crescents (right).

Coronary arteriography

This provides detailed anatomical information about the extent and nature of coronary artery disease (see Fig. 18.15, p. 538), and is usually performed with a view to coronary artery bypass graft (CABG) surgery or percutaneous coronary intervention (PCI) (pp. 587 and 588). In some patients, diagnostic coronary angiography may be indicated when non-invasive tests have failed to establish the cause of atypical chest pain. The procedure is performed under local anaesthesia and requires specialised radiological equipment, cardiac monitoring and an experienced operating team.

Management: general measures

The management of angina pectoris involves:

- a careful assessment of the likely extent and severity of arterial disease
- the identification and control of risk factors such as smoking, hypertension and hyperlipidaemia
- the use of measures to control symptoms
- the identification of high-risk patients for treatment to improve life expectancy.

Symptoms alone are a poor guide to the extent of coronary artery disease. Stress testing is therefore advisable in all patients who are potential candidates for revascularisation. An algorithm for the investigation and treatment of patients with stable angina is shown in Figure 18.66.

Management should start with a careful explanation of the problem and a discussion of the potential lifestyle and medical interventions that may relieve symptoms and improve prognosis (Box 18.53). Anxiety and misconceptions often contribute to disability; for example, some patients avoid all forms of exertion because they believe that each attack of angina is a 'mini heart attack' that results in permanent damage. Effective management of these psychological factors can make a huge difference to the patient's quality of life.

Antiplatelet therapy

Low-dose (75 mg) aspirin reduces the risk of adverse events such as MI and should be prescribed for all patients with coronary artery disease indefinitely (see Box 18.48). Clopidogrel (75 mg daily) is an equally effective antiplatelet agent that can be prescribed if aspirin causes troublesome dyspepsia or other side-effects.

18.53 Advice to patients with stable angina

- Do not smoke
- Aim for ideal body weight
- Take regular exercise (exercise up to, but not beyond, the point of chest discomfort is beneficial and may promote collateral vessels)
- Avoid severe unaccustomed exertion, and vigorous exercise after a heavy meal or in very cold weather
- Take sublingual nitrate before undertaking exertion that may induce angina

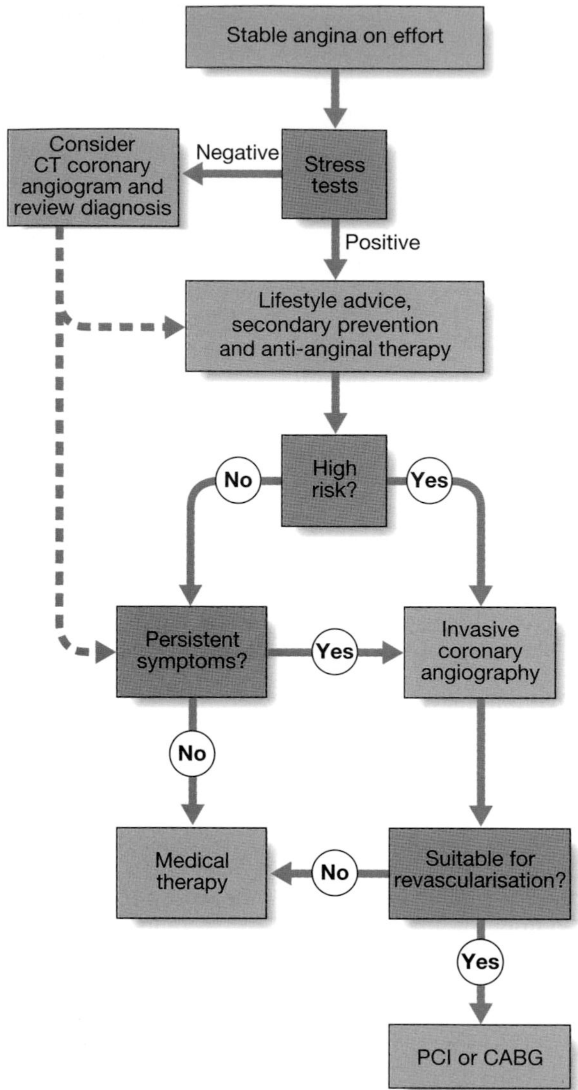

Fig. 18.66 A scheme for the investigation and treatment of stable angina on effort. The selection of percutaneous coronary intervention (PCI) or coronary artery bypass grafting (CABG) depends upon patient choice, coronary artery anatomy and extent of coronary artery disease. In general, left main stem and three-vessel coronary artery disease should be treated by CABG surgery.

Anti-anginal drug treatment

Five groups of drug are used to help relieve or prevent the symptoms of angina: nitrates, β-blockers, calcium antagonists, potassium channel activators and an I_f channel antagonist.

Nitrates

These drugs act directly on vascular smooth muscle to produce venous and arteriolar dilatation. Their beneficial effects are due to a reduction in myocardial oxygen demand (lower preload and afterload) and an increase in myocardial oxygen supply (coronary vasodilatation). Sublingual glyceryl trinitrate (GTN), administered from a metered-dose aerosol (400 μg per spray) or as a tablet (300 or 500 μg), will relieve an attack of angina in 2–3 minutes. Side-effects include headache, symptomatic hypotension and, rarely, syncope.

18.54 Duration of action of some nitrate preparations

Preparation	Peak action	Duration of action
Sublingual GTN	4–8 mins	10–30 mins
Buccal GTN	4–10 mins	30–300 mins
Transdermal GTN	1–3 hrs	Up to 24 hrs
Oral isosorbide dinitrate	45–120 mins	2–6 hrs
Oral isosorbide mononitrate	45–120 mins	6–10 hrs

(GTN = glyceryl trinitrate)

Patients should be encouraged to use the drug prophylactically before taking exercise that is liable to provoke symptoms. Sublingual GTN has a short duration of action (Box 18.54); however, a variety of alternative nitrate preparations can provide a more prolonged therapeutic effect. GTN can be given transcutaneously as a patch (5–10 mg daily), or as a slow-release buccal tablet (1–5 mg 4 times daily). GTN undergoes extensive first-pass metabolism in the liver and is ineffective when swallowed. Other nitrates, such as isosorbide dinitrate (10–20 mg 3 times daily) and isosorbide mononitrate (20–60 mg once or twice daily), can be given by mouth. Headache is common but tends to diminish if the patient perseveres with the treatment. Continuous nitrate therapy can cause pharmacological tolerance. This can be avoided by a 6–8-hour nitrate-free period, best achieved at night when the patient is inactive. If nocturnal angina is a predominant symptom, long-acting nitrates can be given at the end of the day.

Beta-blockers

These lower myocardial oxygen demand by reducing heart rate, BP and myocardial contractility, but they may provoke bronchospasm in patients with asthma. The properties and side-effects of β-blockers are discussed on page 599.

In theory, non-selective β-blockers may aggravate coronary vasospasm by blocking the coronary artery β_2-adrenoceptors and so a once-daily cardioselective preparation is used (e.g. slow-release metoprolol 50–200 mg daily, bisoprolol 5–15 mg daily). Beta-blockers should not be withdrawn abruptly as rebound effects may precipitate dangerous arrhythmias, worsening angina or MI: the β-blocker withdrawal syndrome.

Calcium channel antagonists

These drugs inhibit the slow inward current caused by the entry of extracellular calcium through the cell membrane of excitable cells, particularly cardiac and arteriolar smooth muscle, and lower myocardial oxygen demand by reducing BP and myocardial contractility.

Dihydropyridine calcium antagonists, such as nifedipine and nicardipine, often cause a reflex tachycardia. This may be counterproductive and it is best to use them in combination with a β-blocker. In contrast, verapamil and diltiazem are particularly suitable for patients who are not receiving a β-blocker (e.g. those with airways obstruction) because they slow SA node firing, inhibit conduction through the AV node and

18.55 Calcium channel antagonists used for the treatment of angina

Drug	Dose	Feature
Nifedipine	5–20 mg 3 times daily*	May cause marked tachycardia
Nicardipine	20–40 mg 3 times daily	May cause less myocardial depression than the other calcium antagonists
Amlodipine	2.5–10 mg daily	Ultra-long-acting
Verapamil	40–80 mg 3 times daily*	Commonly causes constipation; useful anti-arrhythmic properties (p. 576)
Diltiazem	60–120 mg 3 times daily*	Similar anti-arrhythmic properties to verapamil

*Once- or twice-daily slow-release preparations are available.

tend to cause a bradycardia. Calcium channel antagonists reduce myocardial contractility and can aggravate or precipitate heart failure. Other unwanted effects include peripheral oedema, flushing, headache and dizziness (Box 18.55).

Potassium channel activators

These have arterial and venous dilating properties but do not exhibit the tolerance seen with nitrates. Nicorandil (10–30 mg twice daily orally) is the only drug in this class currently available for clinical use.

I_f channel antagonist

Ivabradine is the first of this class of drug. It induces bradycardia by modulating ion channels in the sinus node. In contrast to β-blockers and rate-limiting calcium antagonists, it does not have other cardiovascular effects. It appears to be safe to use in patients with heart failure.

Although each of these anti-anginal drugs is superior to placebo in relieving the symptoms of angina, there is little evidence that one group is more effective than another. It is conventional to start therapy with low-dose aspirin, a statin, sublingual GTN and a β-blocker, and then add a calcium channel antagonist or a long-acting nitrate later, if needed. The goal is the control of angina with minimum side-effects and the simplest possible drug regimen. There is little evidence that prescribing multiple anti-anginal drugs is of benefit, and revascularisation should be considered if an appropriate combination of two or more drugs fails to achieve an acceptable symptomatic response.

Invasive treatment

Percutaneous coronary intervention

Percutaneous coronary intervention (PCI) is performed by passing a fine guidewire across a coronary stenosis under radiographic control and using it to position a balloon, which is then inflated to dilate the stenosis (Fig. 18.67). A coronary stent is a piece of coated metallic 'scaffolding' that can be deployed on a balloon and used to maximise and maintain dilatation of a stenosed vessel. The routine use of stents in appropriate vessels reduces

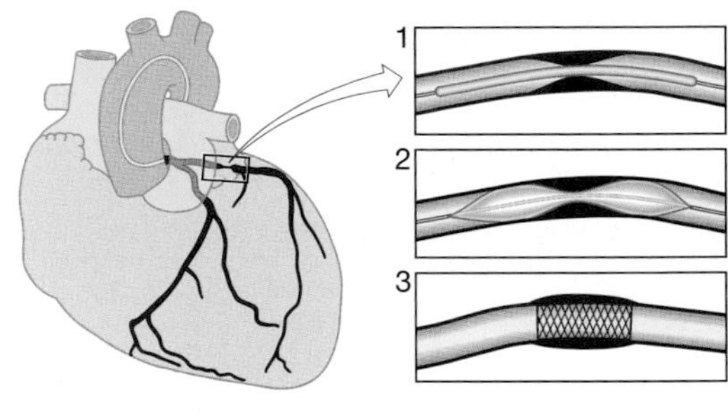

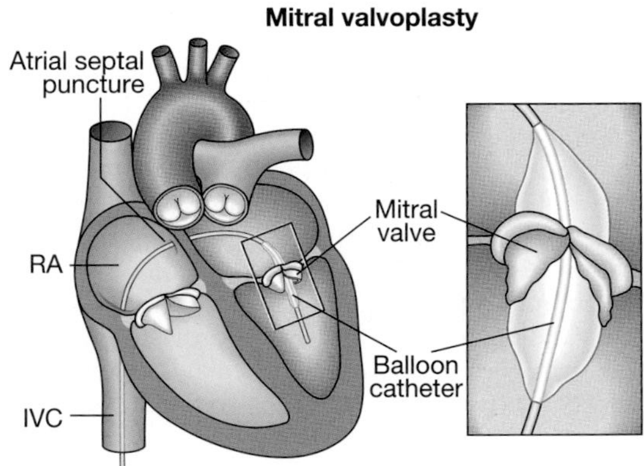

Fig. 18.67 Vascular and valvular balloon dilatations.

EBM 18.56 Angioplasty and intracoronary stents in angina

'In comparison with simple balloon angioplasty, intracoronary stents afford superior acute and long-term clinical and angiographic results, with lower rates of re-stenosis (e.g. 17% vs 40%) and recurrent angina (13% vs 30%). Re-stenosis rates are reduced even further (< 10%) with drug-eluting stents.'

- Stettler C, et al. BMJ 2008; 337:a1331.

For further information: http://guidance.nice.org.uk/TA152

both acute complications and the incidence of clinically important re-stenosis (Box 18.56 and Fig. 18.76, p. 595).

PCI provides an effective symptomatic treatment but definitive evidence that it improves survival in patients with chronic stable angina is lacking. It is mainly used in single- or two-vessel disease. Stenoses in bypass grafts can be dilated, as well as those in the native coronary arteries. The technique is often used to provide palliative therapy for patients with recurrent angina after CABG. Coronary surgery is usually the preferred option in patients with three-vessel or left main stem disease, although recent trials have demonstrated that PCI is also feasible in such patients.

The main acute complications of PCI are occlusion of the target vessel or a side branch by thrombus or a loose flap of intima (coronary artery dissection), and consequent myocardial damage. This occurs in about 2–5% of procedures and can often be corrected by deploying a stent; however, emergency CABG is sometimes required. Minor myocardial damage, as indicated by elevation of sensitive intracellular markers (troponins, p. 535), occurs

EBM 18.57 Percutaneous coronary intervention vs medical therapy in stable angina

'PCI is more effective than medical therapy in alleviating angina pectoris and improving exercise tolerance but does not reduce mortality. It carries risks of procedure-related MI, emergency CABG and repeat procedures for re-stenosis.'

- Weintraub WS, et al. N Engl J Med 2008; 359(7):677–687.

For further information: www.nice.org.uk/CG126

in up to 10% of cases. The main long-term complication of PCI is re-stenosis (Box 18.57), in up to one-third of cases. This is due to a combination of elastic recoil and smooth muscle proliferation (neo-intimal hyperplasia) and tends to occur within 3 months. Stenting substantially reduces the risk of re-stenosis, probably because it allows the operator to achieve more complete dilatation in the first place. Drug-eluting stents reduce this risk even further by allowing an antiproliferative drug, e.g. sirolimus or paclitaxel, to elute slowly from the coating and prevent neo-intimal hyperplasia and in-stent re-stenosis. There is an increased risk of late stent thrombosis with drug-eluting stents, although the absolute risk is small (< 0.5%). Recurrent angina (affecting up to 15–20% of patients receiving an intracoronary stent at 6 months) may require further PCI or bypass grafting.

The risk of complications and the likely success of the procedure are closely related to the morphology of the stenoses, the experience of the operator and the presence of important comorbidity, e.g. diabetes, peripheral arterial disease. A good outcome is less likely if the target lesion is complex, long, eccentric or calcified, lies on a bend or within a tortuous vessel, involves a branch or contains acute thrombus.

In combination with aspirin and heparin, adjunctive therapy with potent platelet inhibitors, such as clopidogrel or glycoprotein IIb/IIIa receptor antagonists, improves the outcome of PCI, with lower short- and long-term rates of death and MI.

Coronary artery bypass grafting

The internal mammary arteries, radial arteries or reversed segments of the patient's own saphenous vein can be used to bypass coronary artery stenoses (Fig. 18.68). This usually involves major surgery under cardiopulmonary bypass but, in some cases, grafts can be applied to the beating heart: 'off-pump' surgery. The operative mortality is approximately 1.5% but risks are higher in elderly patients, those with poor left ventricular function and those with significant comorbidity, such as renal failure.

Approximately 90% of patients are free of angina 1 year after CABG surgery, but fewer than 60% of patients are asymptomatic after 5 or more years. Early postoperative angina is usually due to graft failure arising from technical problems during the operation, or poor 'run-off' due to disease in the distal native coronary vessels. Late recurrence of angina may be due to progressive disease in the native coronary arteries or graft degeneration. Fewer than 50% of vein grafts are patent 10 years after surgery. However, arterial grafts have a much better long-term patency rate, with more than 80% of internal mammary artery grafts patent at

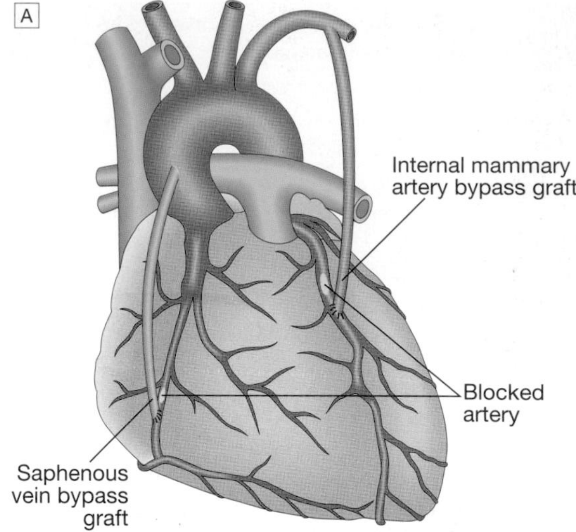

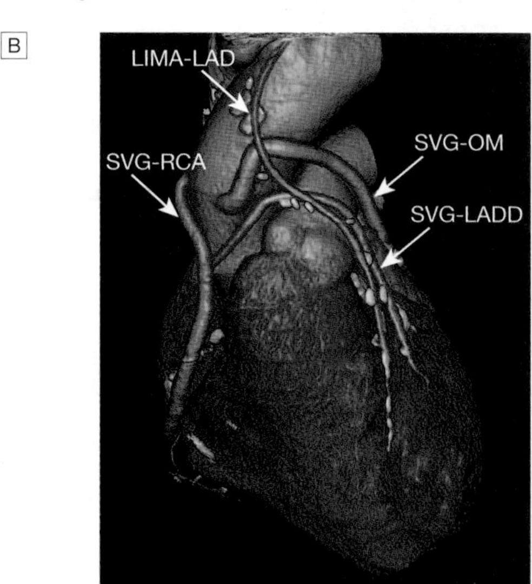

Fig. 18.68 Coronary artery bypass graft surgery. **A** Narrowed or stenosed arteries are bypassed using saphenous vein grafts connected to the aorta or by utilising the internal mammary artery. **B** Three-dimensional reconstruction of multidetector CT of the heart. The image shows the patent saphenous vein grafts (SVG) to the right coronary artery (RCA), obtuse marginal branch (OM) and diagonal branch (LADD), and left internal mammary artery graft (LIMA) to the left anterior descending (LAD) coronary artery.

10 years. This has led many surgeons to consider total arterial revascularisation during CABG surgery. Aspirin (75–150 mg daily) and clopidogrel (75 mg daily) both improve graft patency, and one or other should be prescribed indefinitely, if well tolerated. Intensive lipid-lowering therapy slows the progression of disease in the native coronary arteries and bypass grafts, and reduces clinical cardiovascular events. There is substantial excess cardiovascular morbidity and mortality in patients who continue to smoke after bypass grafting. Persistent smokers are twice as likely to die in the 10 years following surgery than those who give up at surgery.

CABG improves survival in symptomatic patients with left main stem stenosis or three-vessel coronary disease (i.e. involving LAD, CX and right coronary arteries, Box 18.58) or two-vessel disease involving the

EBM 18.58 Coronary artery bypass grafting for stable angina

'CABG is superior to medical treatment for at least 10 years after surgery in terms of survival. Greatest benefit occurs in those with a significant stenosis in the left main coronary artery or those with three-vessel disease and impaired ventricular function.'

- Yusuf S, et al. Lancet 1994; 344:563–570.
- Davies RF, et al. Circulation 1997; 95:2037–2043.

For further information: www.sign.ac.uk/guidelines/fulltext/96/index.html

18.59 Comparison of PCI and CABG

	PCI	CABG
Death	< 0.5%	< 1.5%
Myocardial infarction*	2%	10%
Hospital stay	12–36 hrs	5–8 days
Return to work	2–5 days	6–12 wks
Recurrent angina	15–20% at 6 mths	10% at 1 yr
Repeat revascularisation	10–20% at 2 yrs	2% at 2 yrs
Neurological complications	Rare	Common (see text)
Other complications	Emergency CABG Vascular damage related to access site	Diffuse myocardial damage Infection (chest, wound) Wound pain

*Defined as CK-MB > 2 × normal, p. 589.

EBM 18.60 Comparison of PCI and CABG surgery in stable angina

'Systematic reviews and meta-analyses have found similar rates of death and MI, and similar quality of life. PCI is associated with a greater need for repeat procedures, although this has been halved by the introduction of intracoronary stent implantation. For patients with multi-vessel disease or diabetes, CABG appears to confer better survival rates at 4–5 years.'

- Serruys PW, et al. N Engl J Med 2009; 360:961–972.

For further information: www.nice.org.uk/CG126

proximal LAD coronary artery. Improvement in survival is most marked in those with impaired left ventricular function or positive stress testing prior to surgery and in those who have undergone left internal mammary artery grafting.

Neurological complications are common, with a 1–5% risk of peri-operative stroke. Between 30% and 80% of patients develop short-term cognitive impairment that typically resolves within 6 months. There are also reports of long-term cognitive decline that may be evident in more than 30% of patients at 5 years. PCI and CABG are compared in Boxes 18.59 and 18.60.

Prognosis

Symptoms are a poor guide to prognosis; nevertheless, the 5-year mortality of patients with severe angina (NYHA class III or IV, p. 539) is nearly double that of patients with mild symptoms. Exercise testing and other forms of stress testing are much more powerful predictors of mortality; for example, in one study, the 4-year mortality of patients with stable angina and a negative exercise test was 1%, compared to more than 20% in those with a strongly positive test.

In general, the prognosis of coronary artery disease is related to the number of diseased vessels and the degree of left ventricular dysfunction. A patient with single-vessel disease and good left ventricular function has an excellent outlook (5-year survival > 90%), whereas a patient with severe left ventricular dysfunction and extensive three-vessel disease has a poor prognosis (5-year survival < 30%) without revascularisation. Spontaneous symptomatic improvement due to the development of collateral vessels is common.

Angina with normal coronary arteries

Approximately 10% of patients who report stable angina on effort will have angiographically normal coronary arteries. Many of these patients are women and the mechanism of their symptoms is often difficult to establish. It is important to review the original diagnosis and explore other potential causes.

Coronary artery spasm

Vasospasm in coronary arteries may coexist with atheroma, especially in unstable angina (see below); in less than 1% of cases, vasospasm may occur without angiographically detectable atheroma. This is sometimes known as variant angina, and may be accompanied by spontaneous and transient ST elevation on the ECG (Prinzmetal's angina). Calcium channel antagonists, nitrates and other coronary vasodilators are the most useful therapeutic agents but may be ineffective.

Syndrome X

The constellation of typical angina on effort, objective evidence of myocardial ischaemia on stress testing, and angiographically normal coronary arteries is sometimes known as syndrome X. This disorder is poorly understood but carries a good prognosis and may respond to treatment with anti-anginal therapy.

Acute coronary syndrome

Acute coronary syndrome is a term that encompasses both unstable angina and myocardial infarction (MI). It is characterised by new-onset or rapidly worsening angina (crescendo angina), angina on minimal exertion or angina at rest in the absence of myocardial damage. In contrast, MI occurs when symptoms occur at rest and there is evidence of myocardial necrosis, as demonstrated by an elevation in cardiac troponin or creatine kinase-MB isoenzyme (Box 18.61).

An acute coronary syndrome may present as a new phenomenon or against a background of chronic stable angina. The culprit lesion is usually a complex

18.61 Universal definition of myocardial infarction

Criteria for acute myocardial infarction
The term acute myocardial infarction (MI) should be used when there is evidence of myocardial necrosis in a clinical setting consistent with acute myocardial ischaemia. Under these conditions, any one of the following criteria meets the diagnosis for MI: • Detection of a rise and/or fall of cardiac biomarker values (preferably cardiac troponin (cTn)), with at least one value above the 99th centile upper reference limit (URL) and with at least one of the following: 1. Symptoms of ischaemia 2. New or presumed new significant ST segment–T wave (ST–T) changes or new left bundle branch block (LBBB) 3. Development of pathological Q waves in the ECG 4. Imaging evidence of new loss of viable myocardium or new regional wall motion abnormality 5. Identification of an intracoronary thrombus by angiography or post-mortem • Cardiac death with symptoms suggestive of myocardial ischaemia and presumed new ischaemic ECG changes or new LBBB, but death occurred before cardiac biomarkers were obtained, or before cardiac biomarker values would be increased • Percutaneous coronary intervention (PCI)-related MI is arbitrarily defined by elevation of cTn values (> 5 × 99th centile URL) in patients with normal baseline values (≤ 99th centile URL) or a rise of cTn values > 20% if the baseline values are elevated and are stable or falling. In addition, either (i) symptoms suggestive of myocardial ischaemia, or (ii) new ischaemic ECG changes, or (iii) angiographic findings consistent with a procedural complication, or (iv) imaging demonstration of new loss of viable myocardium or new regional wall motion abnormality are required • Stent thrombosis associated with MI when detected by coronary angiography or post-mortem in the setting of myocardial ischaemia and with a rise and/or fall of cardiac biomarker values with at least one value above the 99th centile URL • Coronary artery bypass grafting (CABG)-related MI is arbitrarily defined by elevation of cardiac biomarker values (> 10 × 99th centile URL) in patients with normal baseline cTn values (≤ 99th centile URL). In addition, either (i) new pathological Q waves or new LBBB, or (ii) angiographic documented new graft or new native coronary artery occlusion, or (iii) imaging evidence of new loss of viable myocardium or new regional wall motion abnormality
Criteria for prior myocardial infarction
Any one of the following criteria meets the diagnosis for prior MI: • Pathological Q waves with or without symptoms in the absence of non-ischaemic causes • Imaging evidence of a region of loss of viable myocardium that is thinned and fails to contract, in the absence of a non-ischaemic cause Pathological findings of a prior MI
Adapted from Thygesen K, et al. Eur Heart J 2012;33:2251–2267.

ulcerated or fissured atheromatous plaque with adherent platelet-rich thrombus and local coronary artery spasm (see Fig. 18.61, p. 580). This is a dynamic process whereby the degree of obstruction may either increase, leading to complete vessel occlusion, or regress due to the effects of platelet disaggregation and endogenous fibrinolysis. In acute MI, occlusive thrombus is almost always present at the site of rupture or erosion of an atheromatous plaque. The thrombus may undergo spontaneous lysis over the course of the next few days, although, by this time, irreversible myocardial damage has occurred. Without treatment, the infarct-related artery remains permanently occluded in 20–30% of patients. The process of infarction progresses over several hours (Fig. 18.69) and most patients present when it is still possible to salvage myocardium and improve outcome.

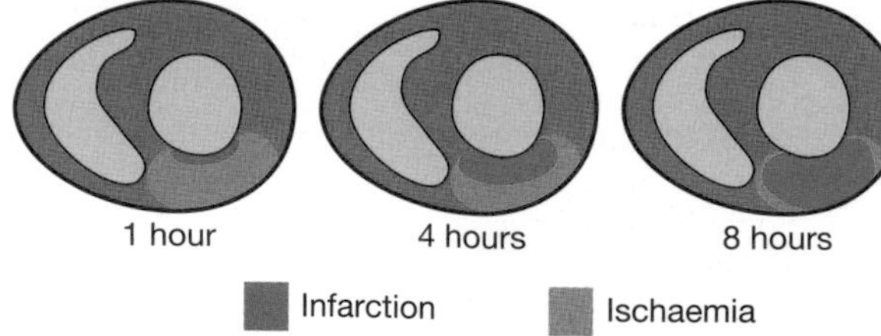

Fig. 18.69 The time course of MI. The relative proportion of ischaemic, infarcting and infarcted tissue slowly changes over a period of 12 hours. In the early stages of MI, a significant proportion of the myocardium in jeopardy is potentially salvageable.

Clinical features

Pain is the cardinal symptom of an acute coronary syndrome but breathlessness, vomiting and collapse are common features (Box 18.62). The pain occurs in the same sites as angina but is usually more severe and lasts longer; it is often described as a tightness, heaviness or constriction in the chest. In acute MI, the pain can be excruciating, and the patient's expression and pallor may vividly convey the seriousness of the situation.

Most patients are breathless and, in some, this is the only symptom. Indeed, MI may pass unrecognised. Painless or 'silent' MI is particularly common in older patients or those with diabetes mellitus. If syncope

18.62 Clinical features of acute coronary syndromes

Symptoms
• Prolonged cardiac pain: chest, throat, arms, epigastrium or back • Anxiety and fear of impending death • Nausea and vomiting • Breathlessness • Collapse/syncope
Physical signs
• Signs of sympathetic activation: pallor, sweating, tachycardia • Signs of vagal activation: vomiting, bradycardia • Signs of impaired myocardial function Hypotension, oliguria, cold peripheries Narrow pulse pressure Raised JVP Third heart sound Quiet first heart sound Diffuse apical impulse Lung crepitations • Signs of tissue damage: fever • Signs of complications: e.g. mitral regurgitation, pericarditis

occurs, it is usually due to an arrhythmia or profound hypotension. Vomiting and sinus bradycardia are often due to vagal stimulation and are particularly common in patients with inferior MI. Nausea and vomiting may also be caused or aggravated by opiates given for pain relief. Sometimes infarction occurs in the absence of physical signs.

Sudden death, from ventricular fibrillation or asystole, may occur immediately and often within the first hour. If the patient survives this most critical stage, the liability to dangerous arrhythmias remains, but diminishes as each hour goes by. It is vital that patients know not to delay calling for help if symptoms occur. The development of cardiac failure reflects the extent of myocardial ischaemia and is the major cause of death in those who survive the first few hours.

Diagnosis and risk stratification

The differential diagnosis is wide and includes most causes of central chest pain or collapse (pp. 540 and 554). The assessment of acute chest pain depends heavily on an analysis of the character of the pain and its associated features, evaluation of the ECG, and serial measurements of biochemical markers of cardiac damage, such as troponin I and T. A 12-lead ECG is mandatory and defines the initial triage, management and treatment (see Fig. 18.19, p. 542). Patients with ST-segment elevation or new bundle branch block require emergency reperfusion therapy (see below). In patients with acute coronary syndrome without ST-segment elevation, the ECG may show transient or persistent ST–T wave changes, including ST depression and T-wave inversion.

Approximately 12% of patients will die within 1 month and a fifth within 6 months of the index event. The risk markers that are indicative of an adverse prognosis include recurrent ischaemia, extensive ECG changes at rest or during pain, the release of biochemical markers (creatine kinase or troponin), arrhythmias, recurrent ischaemia and haemodynamic complications (e.g. hypotension, mitral regurgitation) during episodes of ischaemia. Risk stratification is important because it guides the use of more complex pharmacological and interventional treatment (Figs 18.70 and 18.19 (p. 542)).

1. Find points for each predictive factor

Killip class	Points	SBP (mmHg)	Points	Heart rate (beats/min)	Points	Age (years)	Points	Serum creatinine level (μmol/L)	Points
I	0	≤ 80	58	≤ 50	0	≤ 30	0	0–34	1
II	20	80–99	53	50–69	3	30–39	8	35–70	4
III	39	100–119	43	70–89	9	40–49	25	71–105	7
IV	59	120–139	34	90–109	15	50–59	41	106–140	10
		140–159	24	110–149	24	60–69	58	141–176	13
		160–199	10	150–199	38	70–79	75	177–353	21
		≥ 200	0	≥ 200	46	80–89	91	≥ 353	28
						≥ 90	100		

Other risk factors	Points
Cardiac arrest at admission	39
ST-segment deviation	28
Elevated cardiac enzyme levels	14

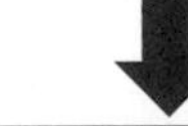

2. Sum points for all predictive factors

Killip class + SBP + Heart rate + Age + Creatinine level + Cardiac arrest at admission + ST-segment deviation + Elevated cardiac enzyme levels = Total points

3. Look up risk corresponding to total points

Total points	≤ 60	70	80	90	100	110	120	130	140	150	160	170	180	190	200	210	220	230	240	≤ 250
Probability of in-hospital death (%)	≤ 0.2	0.3	0.4	0.6	0.8	1.1	1.6	2.1	2.9	3.9	5.4	7.3	9.8	13	18	23	29	36	44	≤ 52

Examples

A patient has Killip class II, SBP of 99 mmHg, heart rate of 100 beats/min, is 65 years of age, has a serum creatinine level of 76 μmol/L, did not have a cardiac arrest at admission but did have ST-segment deviation and elevated enzyme levels. His score would be: 20 + 53 + 15 + 58 + 7 + 0 + 28 + 14 = 195. This gives about a 16% risk of having an in-hospital death.

Similarly, a patient with Killip class I, SBP of 80 mmHg, heart rate of 60 beats/min, who is 55 years of age, has a serum creatinine level of 30 μmol/L, and no risk factors would have the following score: 0 + 58 + 3 + 41 + 1 = 103. This gives about a 0.9% risk of having an in-hospital death.

Fig. 18.70 Risk stratification in the acute coronary syndrome: the GRACE score. Killip class refers to a categorisation of the severity of heart failure based on easily obtained clinical signs. The main clinical features are as follows: class I = no heart failure; class II = crackles audible halfway up the chest; class III = crackles heard in all the lung fields; class IV = cardiogenic shock (SBP = systolic blood pressure). From SIGN 93 – see p. 641.

Investigations

Electrocardiography

The ECG is central to confirming the diagnosis but may be difficult to interpret if there is bundle branch block or previous MI. The initial ECG may be normal or non-diagnostic in one-third of cases. Repeated ECGs are important, especially where the diagnosis is uncertain or the patient has recurrent or persistent symptoms.

The earliest ECG change is usually ST-segment deviation. With proximal occlusion of a major coronary artery, ST-segment elevation (or new bundle branch block) is seen initially, with later diminution in the size of the R wave and, in transmural (full-thickness) infarction, development of a Q wave. Subsequently, the T wave becomes inverted because of a change in ventricular repolarisation; this change persists after the ST segment has returned to normal. These sequential features (Fig. 18.71) are sufficiently reliable for the approximate age of the infarct to be deduced.

In non-ST segment elevation acute coronary syndrome, there is partial occlusion of a major vessel or complete occlusion of a minor vessel, causing unstable angina or partial-thickness (subendocardial) MI. This is usually associated with ST-segment depression and T-wave changes. In the presence of infarction, this may be accompanied by some loss of R waves in the absence of Q waves (Fig. 18.72).

The ECG changes are best seen in the leads that 'face' the ischaemic or infarcted area. When there has been anteroseptal infarction, abnormalities are found in one or more leads from V_1 to V_4, while anterolateral infarction produces changes from V_4 to V_6, in aVL and in lead I. Inferior infarction is best shown in leads II, III and aVF, while, at the same time, leads I, aVL and the anterior chest leads may show 'reciprocal' changes of ST depression (Figs 18.73–18.74). Infarction of the posterior

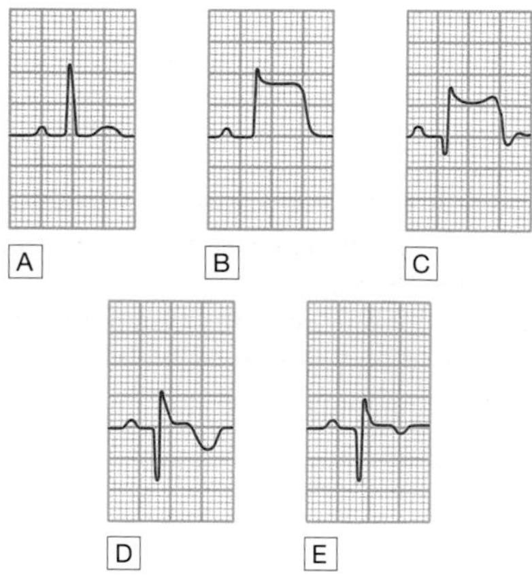

Fig. 18.71 The serial evolution of ECG changes in transmural MI. A Normal ECG complex. B Acute ST elevation ('the current of injury'). C Progressive loss of the R wave, developing Q wave, resolution of the ST elevation and terminal T-wave inversion. D Deep Q wave and T-wave inversion. E Old or established infarct pattern; the Q wave tends to persist but the T-wave changes become less marked. The rate of evolution is very variable but, in general, stage B appears within minutes, stage C within hours, stage D within days and stage E after several weeks or months. This should be compared with the 12-lead ECGs in Figures 18.72–18.74.

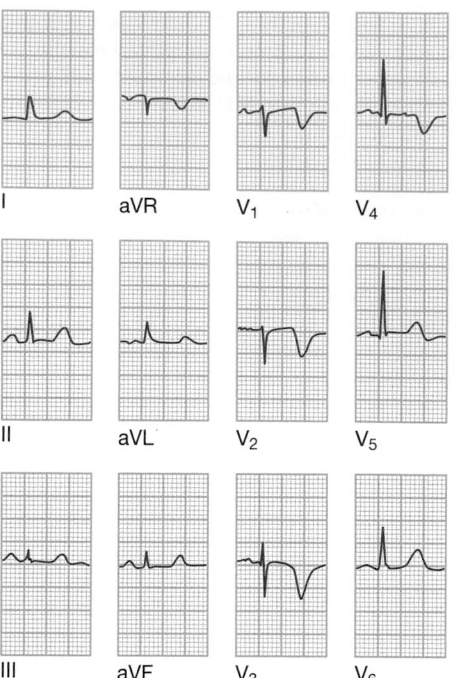

Fig. 18.72 Recent anterior non-ST elevation (subendocardial) MI. This ECG demonstrates deep symmetrical T-wave inversion, together with a reduction in the height of the R wave in leads V_1, V_2, V_3 and V_4.

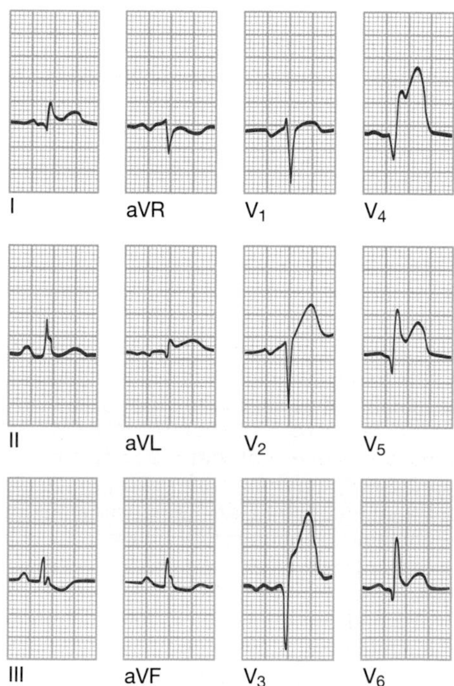

Fig. 18.73 Acute transmural anterior MI. This ECG was recorded from a patient who had developed severe chest pain 6 hours earlier. There is ST elevation in leads I, aVL, V_2, V_3, V_4, V_5 and V_6, and there are Q waves in leads V_3, V_4 and V_5. Anterior infarcts with prominent changes in leads V_2, V_3 and V_4 are sometimes called 'anteroseptal' infarcts, as opposed to anterolateral' infarcts, in which the ECG changes are predominantly found in V_4, V_5 and V_6.

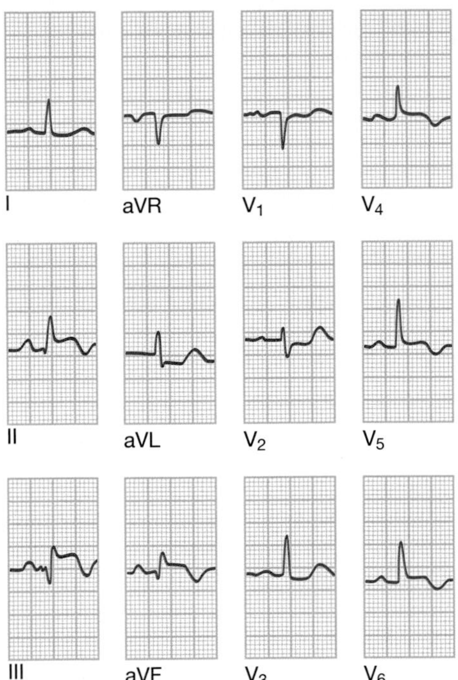

Fig. 18.74 Acute transmural inferolateral MI. This ECG was recorded from a patient who had developed severe chest pain 4 hours earlier. There is ST elevation in the inferior leads II, III and aVF and the lateral leads V_4, V_5 and V_6. There is also 'reciprocal' ST depression in leads aVL and V_2.

wall of the LV does not cause ST elevation or Q waves in the standard leads, but can be diagnosed by the presence of reciprocal changes (ST depression and a tall R wave in leads V_1–V_4). Some infarctions (especially inferior) also involve the RV. This may be identified by recording from additional leads placed over the right precordium.

Plasma cardiac biomarkers

In unstable angina, there is no detectable rise in cardiac biomarkers or enzymes, and the initial diagnosis is made from the clinical history and ECG only. In contrast, MI causes a rise in the plasma concentration of enzymes and proteins that are normally concentrated within cardiac cells. These biochemical markers are creatine kinase (CK), a more sensitive and cardio-specific isoform of this enzyme (CK-MB), and the cardio-specific proteins, troponins T and I (p. 535). Admission and serial (usually daily) estimations are helpful because it is the change in plasma concentrations of these markers that confirms the diagnosis of MI (Fig. 18.75 and Box 18.61).

CK starts to rise at 4–6 hours, peaks at about 12 hours and falls to normal within 48–72 hours. CK is also present in skeletal muscle, and a modest rise in CK (but not CK-MB) may sometimes be due to an intramuscular injection, vigorous physical exercise or, particularly in older people, a fall. Defibrillation causes significant release of CK but not CK-MB or troponins. The most sensitive markers of myocardial cell damage are the cardiac troponins T and I, which are released within 4–6 hours and remain elevated for up to 2 weeks.

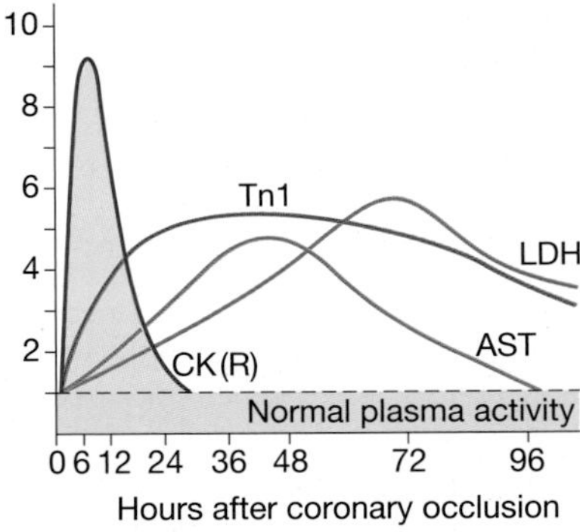

Fig. 18.75 Changes in plasma cardiac biomarker concentrations after MI. Creatine kinase (CK) and troponin I (Tn I) are the first to rise, followed by aspartate aminotransferase (AST) and then lactate (hydroxybutyrate) dehydrogenase (LDH). In patients treated with reperfusion therapy, a rapid rise in plasma creatine kinase (curve CK (R)) occurs, due to a washout effect.

Other blood tests

A leucocytosis is usual, reaching a peak on the first day. The erythrocyte sedimentation rate (ESR) and C-reactive protein (CRP) are also elevated.

Chest X-ray

This may demonstrate pulmonary oedema that is not evident on clinical examination (see Fig. 18.25, p. 550). The heart size is often normal but there may be cardiomegaly due to pre-existing myocardial damage.

Echocardiography

This is useful for assessing ventricular function and for detecting important complications, such as mural thrombus, cardiac rupture, ventricular septal defect, mitral regurgitation and pericardial effusion.

Immediate management: the first 12 hours

Patients should be admitted urgently to hospital because there is a significant risk of death or recurrent myocardial ischaemia during the early unstable phase, and appropriate medical therapy can reduce the incidence of these by at least 60%. The essentials of the immediate in-hospital management of acute coronary syndrome are shown in Figure 18.19 (p. 542).

Patients are usually managed in a dedicated cardiac unit, where the necessary expertise, monitoring and resuscitation facilities can be concentrated. If there are no complications, the patient can be mobilised from the second day and discharged after 3–5 days.

Analgesia

Adequate analgesia is essential, not only to relieve distress but also to lower adrenergic drive and thereby reduce vascular resistance, BP, infarct size and susceptibility to ventricular arrhythmias. Intravenous opiates (initially, morphine sulphate 5–10 mg or diamorphine 2.5–5 mg) and antiemetics (initially, metoclopramide 10 mg) should be administered, and titrated by giving repeated small aliquots until the patient is comfortable. Intramuscular injections should be avoided because the clinical effect may be delayed by poor skeletal muscle perfusion, and a painful haematoma may form following thrombolytic or antithrombotic therapy.

Antithrombotic therapy

Antiplatelet therapy

In patients with acute coronary syndrome, oral administration of 75–325 mg aspirin daily improves survival, with a 25% relative risk reduction in mortality. The first tablet (300 mg) should be given orally within the first 12 hours and therapy should be continued indefinitely if there are no side-effects. In combination with aspirin, the early (within 12 hours) use of clopidogrel (600 mg, followed by 150 mg daily for 1 week and 75 mg daily thereafter) confers a further reduction in ischaemic events (Box 18.63). In patients with an acute coronary syndrome, with or without ST-segment elevation, ticagrelor (180 mg, followed by 90 mg twice daily) is more effective than clopidogrel in reducing vascular death, MI or stroke, and all-cause death, without affecting overall major bleeding risk.

Glycoprotein IIb/IIIa receptor antagonists, such as tirofiban and abciximab, block the final common pathway of platelet aggregation and are potent inhibitors of platelet-rich thrombus formation. They are of particular benefit in patients with acute coronary syndromes who undergo PCI (Box 18.64), those with recurrent ischaemia and those at particularly high risk, such as patients with diabetes mellitus or an elevated troponin concentration.

Anticoagulants

Anticoagulation reduces the risk of thromboembolic complications, and prevents re-infarction in the absence of reperfusion therapy or after successful thrombolysis (Box 18.65). Anticoagulation can be achieved using unfractionated heparin, fractioned (low-molecular-weight) heparin or a pentasaccharide. Comparative clinical trials suggest that the pentasaccharides (subcutaneous fondaparinux 2.5 mg daily) have the best safety and efficacy profile, with low-molecular-weight heparin (subcutaneous enoxaparin 1 mg/kg twice daily) being a reasonable alternative. Anticoagulation should be continued for 8 days or until discharge from hospital or coronary revascularisation.

A period of treatment with warfarin should be considered if there is persistent atrial fibrillation or evidence of extensive anterior infarction, or if echocardiography shows mobile mural thrombus, because these patients are at increased risk of systemic thromboembolism.

EBM 18.63 Oral antiplatelet agents in acute coronary syndromes

'Aspirin alone (75–325 mg/day) reduces the risk of death, MI and stroke in acute coronary syndromes ($NNT_B = 20–25$). Although the addition of clopidogrel to aspirin reduces recurrent ischaemic events, ticagrelor (90 mg twice daily) is more effective than clopidogrel and causes a further reduction in these events ($NNT_B = 60$), including all-cause mortality ($NNT_B = 85$).'

- Antithrombotic Trialists Collaboration. BMJ 2002; 324:71–86.
- The Study of Platelet Inhibition and Patient Outcomes (PLATO) trial investigators. N Engl J Med 2009; 361:1045–1057.

For further information: www.acc.org

EBM 18.64 Intravenous glycoprotein IIb/IIIa inhibitors in acute coronary syndromes

'In patients with acute coronary syndromes, antiplatelet treatment with IV glycoprotein IIb/IIIa inhibitors reduces the combined endpoint of death or MI. Most benefit is seen in the context of percutaneous coronary intervention, but there is no convincing evidence of benefit in patients who are treated without revascularisation (NNT_B (death or MI at 30 days) = 100; NNT_B (death, MI or revascularisation at 30 days) = 63).'

- Boersma E, et al. Lancet 2002; 359:189–198.

For further information: www.sign.ac.uk/guidelines/fulltext/93/index.html

EBM 18.65 Anticoagulation in acute coronary syndromes

'Aspirin plus low-molecular-weight heparin is more effective than aspirin alone in reducing the combined endpoint of death, MI, refractory angina and urgent need for revascularisation. In comparison to low-molecular-weight heparin, the pentasaccharide, fondaparinux (2.5 mg SC), is associated with lower bleeding rates and better overall survival.'

- Antman EM, et al. for the TIMI IIB (Thrombolysis in Myocardial Infarction) and ESSENCE (Efficacy and Safety of Subcutaneous Enoxaparin in Non-Q-wave Coronary Events) Investigators. TIMI IIB-ESSENCE meta-analysis. Circulation 1999; 100:1602–1608.
- Elkelboom JW, et al. Lancet 2000; 355:1936–1942.
- Yusuf S, et al. N Engl J Med 2006; 354:1464–1476.

For further information: www.acc.org

Anti-anginal therapy

Sublingual glyceryl trinitrate (300–500 μg) is a valuable first-aid measure in unstable angina or threatened infarction, and intravenous nitrates (glyceryl trinitrate 0.6–1.2 mg/hr or isosorbide dinitrate 1–2 mg/hr) are useful for the treatment of left ventricular failure and the relief of recurrent or persistent ischaemic pain.

Intravenous β-blockers (e.g. atenolol 5–10 mg or metoprolol 5–15 mg given over 5 mins) relieve pain, reduce arrhythmias and improve short-term mortality in patients who present within 12 hours of the onset of symptoms (see Fig. 18.19). However, they should be avoided if there is heart failure (pulmonary oedema), hypotension (systolic BP < 105 mmHg) or bradycardia (heart rate < 65/min).

A dihydropyridine calcium channel antagonist (e.g. nifedipine or amlodipine) can be added to the β-blocker if there is persistent chest discomfort but may cause tachycardia if used alone. Because of their rate-limiting action, verapamil and diltiazem are the calcium channel antagonists of choice if a β-blocker is contraindicated.

Reperfusion therapy

Non-ST segment elevation acute coronary syndrome

Immediate emergency reperfusion therapy has no demonstrable benefit in patients with non-ST segment elevation MI and thrombolytic therapy may be harmful. Selected medium- to high-risk patients do benefit from in-hospital coronary angiography and coronary revascularisation but this does not need to take place in the first 12 hours.

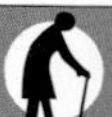

18.66 Angina in old age

- **Incidence**: coronary artery disease increases in and affects women almost as often as men.
- **Comorbid conditions**: anaemia and thyroid disease are common and may worsen angina.
- **Calcific aortic stenosis**: common and should be sought in all old people with angina.
- **Atypical presentations**: when myocardial ischaemia occurs, age-related changes in myocardial compliance and diastolic relaxation can cause the presentation to be with symptoms of heart failure, such as breathlessness, rather than with chest discomfort.
- **Angioplasty and coronary artery bypass surgery**: provide symptomatic relief, although with an increased procedure-related morbidity and mortality. Outcome is determined by the number of diseased vessels, severity of cardiac dysfunction and the number of concomitant diseases, as much as age itself.

ST segment elevation acute coronary syndrome

Immediate reperfusion therapy restores coronary artery patency, preserves left ventricular function and improves survival. Successful therapy is associated with pain relief, resolution of acute ST elevation and, sometimes, transient arrhythmias (e.g. idioventricular rhythm).

Primary percutaneous coronary intervention (PCI). This is the treatment of choice for ST segment elevation MI (Figs 18.19 and 18.76). Outcomes are best when it is used in combination with glycoprotein IIb/IIIa receptor antagonists and intracoronary stent implantation. In comparison to thrombolytic therapy, it is associated with a greater reduction in the risk of death, recurrent MI or stroke (Box 18.67). The universal use of primary PCI has been limited by availability of the necessary resources to provide this highly specialised emergency service. Thus, intravenous thrombolytic therapy remains the first-line reperfusion treatment in many hospitals, especially those in rural or remote areas. When primary PCI cannot be achieved within 2 hours of diagnosis, thrombolytic therapy should be administered.

Thrombolysis. The appropriate use of thrombolytic therapy can reduce hospital mortality by 25–50% and this survival advantage is maintained for at least 10 years (Box 18.68). The benefit is greatest in those patients who receive treatment within the first few hours: 'minutes mean muscle'.

Alteplase (human tissue plasminogen activator, or tPA) is a genetically engineered drug that is given over 90 minutes (bolus dose of 15 mg, followed by 0.75 mg/kg body weight but not exceeding 50 mg, over 30 mins, and then 0.5 mg/kg body weight but not exceeding 35 mg, over 60 mins). Its use is associated with better survival rates than other thrombolytic agents, such as streptokinase, but carries a slightly higher risk of intracerebral bleeding (10 per 1000 increased survival, but 1 per 1000 more non-fatal stroke).

Analogues of tPA, such as tenecteplase (TNK) and reteplase (rPA), have a longer plasma half-life than alteplase and can be given as an intravenous bolus. TNK is as effective as alteplase at reducing death and MI, whilst conferring similar intracerebral bleeding risks. However, other bleeding and transfusion risks are lower and the practical advantages of bolus administration provide opportunities for prompt treatment in the emergency department or in the pre-hospital setting. rPA is administered as a double bolus and also produces a similar outcome to that achieved with alteplase, although some of the bleeding risks appear slightly higher.

An overview of all large randomised trials confirms that thrombolytic therapy reduces short-term mortality in patients with MI if given within 12 hours of the onset

A

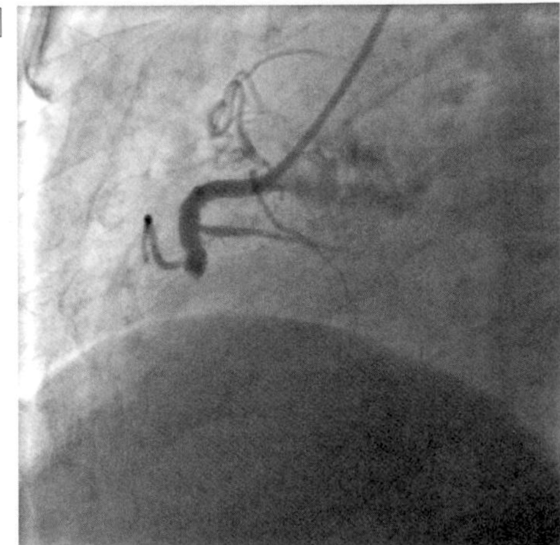

B

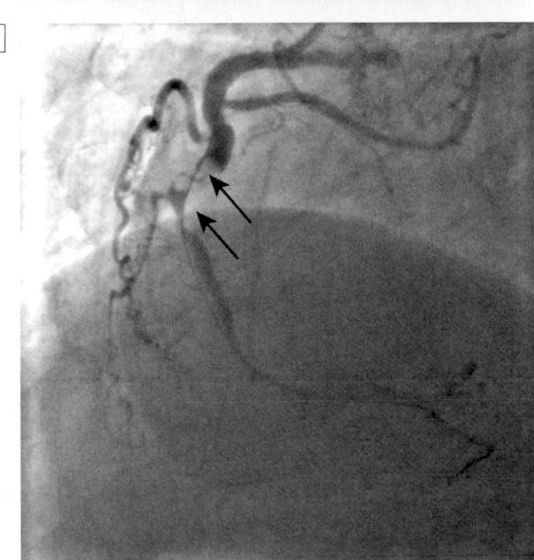

C

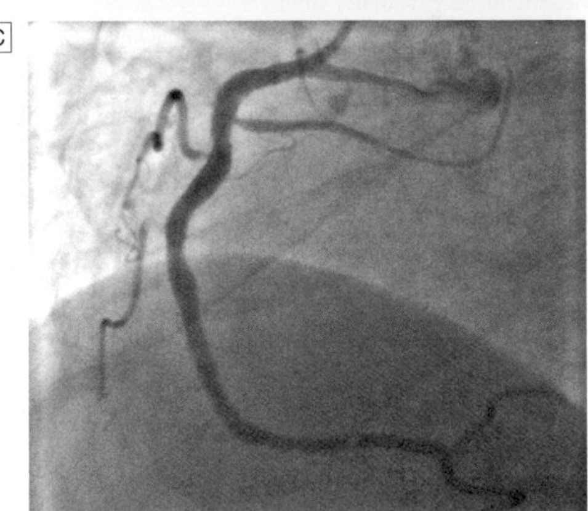

Fig. 18.76 Primary PCI. **A** Acute right coronary artery occlusion. **B** Initial angioplasty demonstrates a large thrombus filling defect (arrows). **C** Complete restoration of normal flow following intracoronary stenting.

EBM 18.67 Primary PCI in acute ST segment elevation MI

'Primary PCI is more effective than thrombolysis for the treatment of acute MI. Death, non-fatal re-infarction and stroke are reduced from 14% with thrombolytic therapy to 8% with primary PCI ($NNT_B = 33$ for death and 9 for recurrent ischaemia).'

- Keeley EC, et al. Lancet 2003; 361:13–20.

For further information: www.acc.org
www.sign.ac.uk/guidelines/fulltext/93/index.html

EBM 18.68 Thrombolytic treatment in acute ST segment elevation MI

'Prompt thrombolytic treatment (within 12 hours, and particularly within 6 hours, of the onset of symptoms) reduces mortality in patients with acute MI and ECG changes of ST elevation or new bundle branch block ($NNT_B = 56$). Intracranial haemorrhage is more common in people given thrombolysis, with 1 additional stroke for every 250 people treated.'

- Fibrinolytic Therapy Trialists' (FTT) Collaborative Group. Lancet 1994; 343:311–322.
- Collins R. N Engl J Med 1997; 336:847–860.

For further information: www.escardio.org

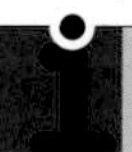

18.69 Relative contraindications to thrombolytic therapy: potential candidates for primary PCI

- Active internal bleeding
- Previous subarachnoid or intracerebral haemorrhage
- Uncontrolled hypertension
- Recent surgery (within 1 mth)
- Recent trauma (including traumatic resuscitation)
- High probability of active peptic ulcer
- Pregnancy

of symptoms and the ECG shows bundle branch block or characteristic ST segment elevation of more than 1 mm in the limb leads or 2 mm in the chest leads (see Box 18.68). Thrombolysis appears to be of little net benefit and may be harmful in those who present more than 12 hours after the onset of symptoms and in those with a normal ECG or ST depression. In patients with ST elevation or bundle branch block, the absolute benefit of thrombolysis plus aspirin is approximately 50 lives saved per 1000 patients treated within 6 hours, and 40 lives saved per 1000 treated between 7 and 12 hours after the onset of symptoms. The benefit is greatest for patients treated within the first 2 hours.

The major hazard of thrombolytic therapy is bleeding. Cerebral haemorrhage causes 4 extra strokes per 1000 patients treated, and the incidence of other major bleeds is between 0.5% and 1%. Accordingly, the treatment should be withheld if there is a significant risk of serious bleeding (Box 18.69).

For some patients, thrombolytic therapy is contraindicated or fails to achieve coronary arterial reperfusion (see Fig. 18.19, p. 542). Early emergency PCI may then be considered, particularly where there is evidence of cardiogenic shock.

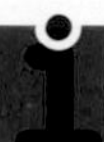

18.70 Common arrhythmias in acute coronary syndrome

• Ventricular fibrillation	• Atrial fibrillation
• Ventricular tachycardia	• Atrial tachycardia
• Accelerated idioventricular rhythm	• Sinus bradycardia (particularly after inferior MI)
• Ventricular ectopics	• Atrioventricular block

Complications of acute coronary syndrome

Complications are seen in all forms of acute coronary syndrome, although the frequency and extent vary with the severity of ischaemia and infarction. Major mechanical and structural complications are seen only with significant, often transmural, MI.

Arrhythmias

Many patients with acute coronary syndrome have some form of arrhythmia (Box 18.70). In the majority of cases this is transient and of no haemodynamic or prognostic importance. Pain relief, rest and the correction of hypokalaemia may help prevent arrhythmias. Diagnosis and management of arrhythmias are discussed in detail on pages 562–579.

Ventricular fibrillation

This occurs in 5–10% of patients who reach hospital and is thought to be the major cause of death in those who die before receiving medical attention. Prompt defibrillation restores sinus rhythm and is life-saving. The prognosis of patients with early ventricular fibrillation (within the first 48 hours) who are successfully and promptly resuscitated is identical to that of patients who do not suffer ventricular fibrillation.

Atrial fibrillation

This is common but frequently transient, and usually does not require emergency treatment. However, if it causes a rapid ventricular rate with hypotension or circulatory collapse, prompt cardioversion by immediate synchronised DC shock is essential. In other situations, digoxin or a β-blocker is usually the treatment of choice. Atrial fibrillation (due to acute atrial stretch) is often a feature of impending or overt left ventricular failure, and therapy may be ineffective if heart failure is not recognised and treated appropriately. Anticoagulation is required if atrial fibrillation persists.

Bradycardia

This does not usually require treatment, but if there is hypotension or haemodynamic deterioration, atropine (0.6–1.2 mg IV) may be given. AV block complicating inferior infarction is usually temporary and often resolves following reperfusion therapy. If there is clinical deterioration due to second-degree or complete AV block, a temporary pacemaker should be considered. AV block complicating anterior infarction is more serious because asystole may suddenly supervene; a prophylactic temporary pacemaker should be inserted (p. 578).

Ischaemia

Patients who develop recurrent angina at rest or on minimal exertion following an acute coronary syndrome are at high risk and should be considered for prompt coronary angiography with a view to revascularisation. Patients with dynamic ECG changes and ongoing pain should be treated with intravenous glycoprotein IIb/IIIa receptor antagonists. Patients with resistant pain or marked haemodynamic changes should be considered for intra-aortic balloon counterpulsation and emergency coronary revascularisation.

Post-infarct angina occurs in up to 50% of patients treated with thrombolysis. Most patients have a residual stenosis in the infarct-related vessel, despite successful thrombolysis, and this may cause angina if there is still viable myocardium downstream. For this reason, all patients who have received successful thrombolysis should be considered for early (within the first 6–24 hours) coronary angiography with a view to coronary revascularisation.

Acute circulatory failure

Acute circulatory failure usually reflects extensive myocardial damage and indicates a bad prognosis. All the other complications of MI are more likely to occur when acute heart failure is present. The assessment and management of heart failure complicating acute MI are discussed in detail on page 545.

Pericarditis

This only occurs following infarction and is particularly common on the second and third days. The patient may recognise that a different pain has developed, even though it is at the same site, and that it is positional and tends to be worse or sometimes only present on inspiration. A pericardial rub may be audible. Opiate-based analgesia should be used. Non-steroidal (NSAIDs) and steroidal anti-inflammatory drugs may increase the risk of aneurysm formation and myocardial rupture in the early recovery period, and so should be avoided.

The post-MI syndrome (Dressler's syndrome) is characterised by persistent fever, pericarditis and pleurisy, and is probably due to autoimmunity. The symptoms tend to occur a few weeks or even months after the infarct and often subside after a few days; prolonged or severe symptoms may require treatment with high-dose aspirin, NSAIDs or even corticosteroids.

Mechanical complications

Part of the necrotic muscle in a fresh infarct may tear or rupture, with devastating consequences:

- *Rupture of the papillary muscle* can cause acute pulmonary oedema and shock due to the sudden onset of severe mitral regurgitation, which presents with a pansystolic murmur and third heart sound. In the presence of severe regurgitation, the murmur may be quiet or absent. The diagnosis is confirmed by echocardiography and emergency valve replacement may be necessary. Lesser degrees of mitral regurgitation due to papillary muscle dysfunction are common and may be transient.
- *Rupture of the interventricular septum* causes left-to-right shunting through a ventricular septal defect. This usually presents with sudden haemodynamic deterioration accompanied by a new loud pansystolic murmur radiating to the right sternal border, but may be difficult to distinguish from acute mitral regurgitation. However, patients with an acquired ventricular septal defect tend to develop right heart failure rather than pulmonary oedema. Doppler echocardiography and right heart catheterisation will confirm the diagnosis. Without prompt surgery, the condition is usually fatal.
- *Rupture of the ventricle* may lead to cardiac tamponade and is usually fatal (p. 545), although it may rarely be possible to support a patient with an incomplete rupture until emergency surgery is performed.

Embolism

Thrombus often forms on the endocardial surface of freshly infarcted myocardium. This can lead to systemic embolism and occasionally causes a stroke or ischaemic limb. Venous thrombosis and pulmonary embolism may occur but have become less common with the use of prophylactic anticoagulants and early mobilisation.

Impaired ventricular function, remodelling and ventricular aneurysm

Acute transmural MI is often followed by thinning and stretching of the infarcted segment (infarct expansion). This leads to an increase in wall stress with progressive dilatation and hypertrophy of the remaining ventricle (ventricular remodelling, Fig. 18.77). As the ventricle dilates, it becomes less efficient and heart failure may supervene. Infarct expansion occurs over a few days and weeks but ventricular remodelling can take years. ACE inhibitor therapy reduces late ventricular remodelling and can prevent the onset of heart failure (p. 551).

A left ventricular aneurysm develops in approximately 10% of patients with MI and is particularly common when there is persistent occlusion of the infarct-related vessel. Heart failure, ventricular arrhythmias, mural thrombus and systemic embolism are all recognised complications of aneurysm formation. Other features include a paradoxical impulse on the chest wall, persistent ST elevation on the ECG, and sometimes an unusual bulge from the cardiac silhouette on the chest X-ray. Echocardiography is diagnostic. Surgical removal

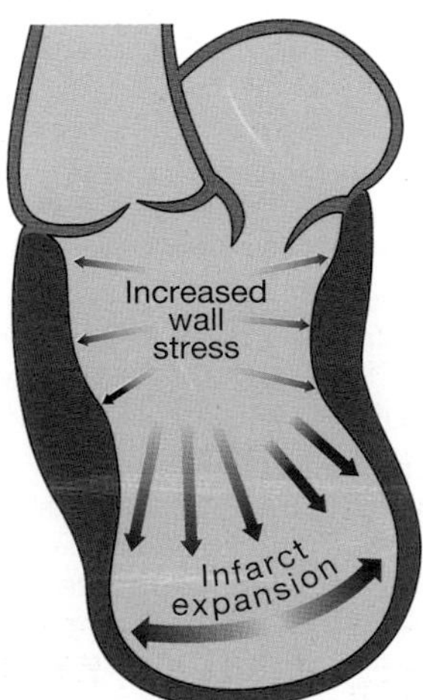

Fig. 18.77 Infarct expansion and ventricular remodelling. Full-thickness MI causes thinning and stretching of the infarcted segment (infarct expansion), which leads to increased wall stress with progressive dilatation and hypertrophy of the remaining ventricle (ventricular remodelling).

18

of a left ventricular aneurysm carries a high morbidity and mortality but is sometimes necessary.

Later in-hospital management

Late management of MI is summarised in Box 18.71.

Risk stratification and further investigation

Simple clinical tools can be used to identify medium- to high-risk patients. The GRACE score (see Fig. 18.70, p. 591) is a simple method of calculating early mortality that can help guide which patients should be selected for intensive therapy, and specifically early inpatient coronary angiography.

The prognosis of patients who have survived an acute coronary syndrome is related to the extent of residual myocardial ischaemia, the degree of myocardial damage and the presence of ventricular arrhythmias.

Left ventricular function

The degree of left ventricular dysfunction can be crudely assessed from physical findings (tachycardia, third heart sound, crackles at the lung bases, elevated venous pressure and so on), ECG changes and chest X-ray (size of the heart and presence of pulmonary oedema). Formal assessment with echocardiography should, however, be undertaken in the early recovery phase.

Ischaemia

Patients with early ischaemia following an acute coronary syndrome should undergo coronary angiography with a view to revascularisation. Low-risk patients without spontaneous ischaemia should undergo an exercise tolerance test approximately 4 weeks after the acute coronary syndrome. This will help to identify those individuals with residual myocardial ischaemia who require further investigation, and may help to boost the confidence of the remainder.

If the exercise test is negative and the patient has a good effort tolerance, the outlook is good, with a 1–4% chance of an adverse event in the next 12 months. In contrast, patients with residual ischaemia in the form of chest pain or ECG changes at low exercise levels are at high risk, with a 15–25% chance of suffering a further ischaemic event in the next 12 months.

18.71 Late management of MI

Risk stratification and further investigation (see text)

Lifestyle modification
- Diet (weight control, lipid-lowering, 'Mediterranean diet')
- Cessation of smoking
- Regular exercise

Secondary prevention drug therapy
- Antiplatelet therapy (aspirin and/or clopidogrel)
- β-blocker
- ACE inhibitor/ARB
- Statin
- Additional therapy for control of diabetes and hypertension
- Mineralocorticoid receptor antagonist

Rehabilitation

Devices
- Implantable cardiac defibrillator (high-risk patients)

(ACE = angiotensin-converting enzyme; ARB = angiotensin receptor blocker)

Arrhythmias

The presence of ventricular arrhythmias during the convalescent phase of acute coronary syndrome may be a marker of poor ventricular function and may herald sudden death. Although empirical anti-arrhythmic treatment is of no value and is even hazardous, selected patients may benefit from electrophysiological testing and specific anti-arrhythmic therapy (including implantable cardiac defibrillators, p. 579).

Recurrent ventricular arrhythmias are sometimes manifestations of myocardial ischaemia or impaired left ventricular function and may respond to appropriate treatment directed at the underlying problem.

Lifestyle and risk factor modification

Smoking

The 5-year mortality of patients who continue to smoke cigarettes is double that of those who quit smoking at the time of their acute coronary syndrome. Giving up smoking is the single most effective contribution a patient can make to his or her future. The success of smoking cessation can be increased by supportive advice and pharmacological therapy (p. 100).

Hyperlipidaemia

The importance of lowering serum cholesterol following acute coronary syndrome has been demonstrated in large-scale randomised trials. Lipids should be measured within 24 hours of presentation because there is often a transient fall in cholesterol in the 3 months following infarction. HMG CoA reductase enzyme inhibitors ('statins', p. 456) can produce marked reductions in total (and LDL) cholesterol and reduce the subsequent risk of death, re-infarction, stroke and the need for revascularisation (see Box 18.46, p. 583). Irrespective of serum cholesterol concentrations, all patients should receive statin therapy after acute coronary syndrome, but those with serum LDL cholesterol concentrations above 3.2 mmol/L (~120 mg/dL) benefit from more intensive therapy, such as atorvastatin 80 mg daily.

Other risk factors

Maintaining an ideal body weight, eating a Mediterranean-style diet, taking regular exercise, and achieving good control of hypertension and diabetes mellitus may all improve the long-term outlook.

Mobilisation and rehabilitation

The necrotic muscle of an acute myocardial infarct takes 4–6 weeks to be replaced with fibrous tissue and it is conventional to restrict physical activities during this period. When there are no complications, the patient can mobilise on the second day, return home in 3–5 days and gradually increase activity, with the aim of returning to work in 4–6 weeks. The majority of patients may resume driving after 4–6 weeks, although, in most countries, vocational driving licence holders (e.g. heavy goods and public service vehicles) require special assessment.

Emotional problems, such as denial, anxiety and depression, are common and must be addressed. Many patients are severely and even permanently incapacitated as a result of the psychological effects of acute coronary syndrome rather than the physical ones, and all benefit from thoughtful explanation, counselling and reassurance at every stage of the illness. Many patients mistakenly believe that 'stress' was the cause of their heart attack and may restrict their activity inappropriately. The patient's spouse or partner will also require emotional support, information and counselling. Formal rehabilitation programmes, based on graded exercise protocols with individual and group counselling, are often very successful and, in some cases, have been shown to improve the long-term outcome.

Secondary prevention drug therapy

Aspirin and clopidogrel

Low-dose aspirin therapy reduces the risk of further infarction and other vascular events by approximately 25% and should be continued indefinitely if there are no unwanted effects. Clopidogrel should be given in combination with aspirin for at least 3 months. If patients are intolerant of long-term aspirin, clopidogrel is a suitable alternative.

Beta-blockers

Continuous treatment with an oral β-blocker reduces long-term mortality by approximately 25% among the survivors of acute MI (Box 18.72). Unfortunately, a minority of patients do not tolerate β-blockers because of bradycardia, AV block, hypotension or asthma. Patients with heart failure, irreversible chronic obstructive pulmonary disease or peripheral vascular disease derive similar, if not greater secondary preventative benefits from β-blocker therapy if they can tolerate it, so it should be tried. The secondary preventative role of β-blockers in patients with unstable angina is unknown.

ACE inhibitors

Several clinical trials have shown that long-term treatment with an ACE inhibitor (e.g. enalapril 10 mg twice daily or ramipril 2.5–5 mg twice daily) can counteract ventricular remodelling, prevent the onset of heart failure, improve survival, reduce recurrent MI and avoid rehospitalisation. The benefits are greatest in those with overt heart failure (clinical or radiological) but extend to patients with asymptomatic left ventricular dysfunction and those with preserved left ventricular function. They should therefore be considered in all patients with acute coronary syndrome. Caution must be exercised in hypovolaemic or hypotensive patients because the introduction of an ACE inhibitor may exacerbate hypotension and impair coronary perfusion. In patients intolerant of ACE inhibitors, angiotensin receptor blockers (e.g. valsartan 40–160 mg twice daily or candesartan 4–16 mg daily) are alternatives and are better tolerated.

Patients with acute MI and left ventricular dysfunction (ejection fraction < 35%) and either pulmonary oedema or diabetes mellitus further benefit from additional mineralocorticoid receptor antagonism (e.g. eplerenone 25–50 mg daily).

Coronary revascularisation

Most low-risk patients stabilise with aspirin, clopidogrel, anticoagulation and anti-anginal therapy, and can be rapidly mobilised. In the absence of recurrent symptoms, low-risk patients do not benefit from routine coronary angiography. Coronary angiography should be considered with a view to revascularisation in all patients at moderate or high risk, including those who fail to settle on medical therapy, those with extensive ECG changes, those with an elevated plasma troponin and those with severe pre-existing stable angina. This often reveals disease that is amenable to PCI or urgent CABG. In these cases, coronary revascularisation is associated with short- and long-term benefits, including reductions in MI and death.

Device therapy

Implantable cardiac defibrillators are of benefit in preventing sudden cardiac death in patients who have severe left ventricular impairment (ejection fraction ≤ 30%) after MI (p. 579).

Prognosis

In almost one-quarter of all cases of MI, death occurs within a few minutes without medical care. Half the deaths occur within 24 hours of the onset of symptoms and about 40% of all affected patients die within the first month. The prognosis of those who survive to reach hospital is much better, with a 28-day survival of more than 85%. Patients with unstable angina have a mortality of approximately half that of those patients with MI.

Early death is usually due to an arrhythmia and is independent of the extent of MI. However, late outcomes are determined by the extent of myocardial damage, and unfavourable features include poor left ventricular function, AV block and persistent ventricular arrhythmias. The prognosis is worse for anterior than for inferior infarcts. Bundle branch block and high

EBM 18.72 Beta-blockers in secondary prevention after MI

'Beta-blockers reduce the risk of overall mortality (NNT_B = 48), sudden death (NNT_B = 63) and non-fatal re-infarction (NNT_B = 56) after MI. The greatest benefit is seen in those at highest risk, and about one-quarter of patients suffer adverse events.'

- Freemantle N, et al. BMJ 1999; 318:1730–1737.

For further information: www.sign.ac.uk/guidelines/fulltext/93/index.html

18.73 Myocardial infarction in old age

- **Atypical presentation**: often with anorexia, fatigue or weakness rather than chest pain.
- **Case fatality**: rises steeply. Hospital mortality exceeds 25% in those over 75 yrs old, which is five times greater than that seen in those aged less than 55 yrs.
- **Survival benefit of treatments**: not influenced by age. The absolute benefit of evidence-based treatments may therefore be greatest in older people.
- **Hazards of treatments**: rise with age (e.g. increased risk of intracerebral bleeding after thrombolysis) and are due partly to increased comorbidity.
- **Quality of evidence**: older patients, particularly those with significant comorbidity, were under-represented in many of the randomised controlled clinical trials that helped to establish the treatment of MI. The balance of risk and benefit for many treatments (e.g. thrombolysis, primary percutaneous transluminal coronary angiography) in frail older people is therefore uncertain.

cardiac marker levels both indicate extensive myocardial damage. Old age, depression and social isolation are also associated with a higher mortality.

Of those who survive an acute attack, more than 80% live for a further year, about 75% for 5 years, 50% for 10 years and 25% for 20 years.

Cardiac risk of non-cardiac surgery

Non-cardiac surgery, particularly major vascular, abdominal or thoracic surgery, can precipitate serious peri-operative cardiac complications, such as MI and death, in patients with coronary artery and other forms of heart disease. Careful pre-operative cardiac assessment may help to determine the balance of benefit versus risk on an individual basis, and identify measures that minimise the operative risk (Box 18.74).

A hypercoagulable state is part of the normal physiological response to surgery, and may promote coronary thrombosis leading to an acute coronary syndrome in the early post-operative period. Patients with a history of recent PCI or acute coronary syndrome are at greatest risk and, whenever possible, elective non-cardiac surgery should be avoided for 3 months after such an event. Antiplatelet agents, statins and β-blockers reduce the risk of peri-operative MI in patients with coronary artery disease and, where possible, should be prescribed throughout the peri-operative period.

Careful attention to fluid balance during and after surgery is particularly important in patients with impaired left ventricular function and valvular heart disease because antidiuretic hormone is released as part of the normal physiological response to surgery and, in these circumstances, the overzealous administration of intravenous fluids can easily precipitate heart failure. Patients with severe valvular heart disease, particularly aortic stenosis and mitral stenosis, are also at increased risk because they may not be able to increase their cardiac output in response to the stress of surgery.

Atrial fibrillation may be triggered by hypoxia, myocardial ischaemia or heart failure, and is a common post-operative complication in patients with pre-existing heart disease. It usually terminates spontaneously when the precipitating factors have been eliminated, but digoxin or β-blockers can be prescribed to control the heart rate.

18.74 Major risk factors for cardiac complications of non-cardiac surgery

- Recent (< 6 mths) MI or unstable angina
- Severe coronary artery disease: left main stem or three-vessel disease
- Severe stable angina on effort
- Severe left ventricular dysfunction
- Severe valvular heart disease (especially aortic stenosis)

VASCULAR DISEASE

Peripheral arterial disease

In developed countries, almost all peripheral arterial disease (PAD) is due to atherosclerosis (p. 579) and so shares common risk factors with coronary artery disease: namely, smoking, diabetes mellitus, hyperlipidaemia and hypertension. As with coronary artery disease, plaque rupture is responsible for the most serious manifestations of PAD, and not infrequently occurs in a plaque that hitherto has been asymptomatic.

Approximately 20% of middle-aged (55–75 years) people in the UK have PAD but only one-quarter of them will have symptoms. The clinical manifestations depend upon the anatomical site, the presence or absence of a collateral supply, the speed of onset and the mechanism of injury (Box 18.75).

18.75 Factors influencing the clinical manifestations of peripheral arterial disease

Anatomical site

Cerebral circulation
- TIA, amaurosis fugax, vertebrobasilar insufficiency

Renal arteries
- Hypertension and renal failure

Mesenteric arteries
- Mesenteric angina, acute intestinal ischaemia

Limbs (legs ≫ arms)
- Intermittent claudication, critical limb ischaemia, acute limb ischaemia

Collateral supply

- In a patient with a complete circle of Willis, occlusion of one carotid artery may be asymptomatic
- In a patient without cross-circulation, stroke is likely

Speed of onset

- Where PAD develops slowly, a collateral supply will develop
- Sudden occlusion of a previously normal artery is likely to cause severe distal ischaemia

Mechanism of injury

Haemodynamic
- Plaque must reduce arterial diameter by 70% ('critical stenosis') to reduce flow and pressure at rest. On exertion (e.g. walking), a much lesser stenosis may become 'critical'. This mechanism tends to have a relatively benign course due to collateralisation

Thrombotic
- Occlusion of a long-standing critical stenosis may be asymptomatic due to collateralisation. However, acute rupture and thrombosis of a non-haemodynamically significant plaque usually has severe consequences

Atheroembolic
- Symptoms depend upon embolic load and size
- Carotid (TIA, amaurosis fugax or stroke) and peripheral arterial (blue toe/finger syndrome) plaque are common examples

Thromboembolic
- Usually secondary to atrial fibrillation
- The consequences are usually dramatic, as the thrombus load is often large and occludes a major, previously healthy, non-collateralised artery suddenly and completely

(TIA = transient ischaemic attack)

Chronic lower limb arterial disease

PAD affects the leg eight times more often than the arm. The lower limb arterial tree comprises the aorto-iliac ('inflow'), femoro-popliteal and infra-popliteal ('outflow') segments. One or more segments may be affected in a variable and asymmetric manner. Lower limb ischaemia presents as two distinct clinical entities: intermittent claudication (IC) and critical limb ischaemia (CLI). The presence and severity of ischaemia can be determined by clinical examination (Box 18.76) and measurement of the ankle–brachial pressure index (ABPI), which is the ratio between the (highest systolic) ankle and brachial blood pressures. In health, the ABPI is over 1.0, in IC typically 0.5–0.9 and in CLI usually below 0.5.

Intermittent claudication

This term describes ischaemic pain affecting the muscles of the leg upon walking. The pain is usually felt in the calf because the disease most commonly affects the superficial femoral artery. However, the pain may be felt in the thigh or buttock if the iliac arteries are involved. Typically, the pain comes on after a reasonably constant 'claudication distance' and rapidly subsides on stopping walking. Resumption of walking leads to a return of the pain. Most patients describe a cyclical pattern of exacerbation and resolution due to the progression of disease and the subsequent development of collaterals.

Approximately 5% of middle-aged men report IC. Provided patients comply with 'best medical therapy' (BMT, Box 18.77), only 1–2% per year will deteriorate to a point where amputation and/or revascularisation are required. However, the annual mortality rate exceeds 5%, 2–3 times higher than in an equivalent non-claudicant population. This is because IC is nearly always found in association with widespread atherosclerosis, so that most claudicants succumb to MI or stroke. The mainstay of treatment is BMT, including (preferably supervised) exercise therapy. The peripheral vasodilator, cilostazol, has been shown to improve walking distance. Intervention with angioplasty, stenting, endarterectomy or bypass is usually only considered after BMT has been given at least 6 months to effect symptomatic improvement, and then only in patients who are severely disabled or whose livelihood is threatened by their disability.

Critical limb ischaemia

This is defined as rest (night) pain, requiring opiate analgesia, and/or tissue loss (ulceration or gangrene), present for more than 2 weeks, in the presence of an ankle BP of less than 50 mmHg (Fig. 18.78). Rest pain only, with ankle pressures above 50 mmHg, is known as subcritical limb ischaemia (SCLI). The term severe limb ischaemia (SLI) is used to describe both CLI and SCLI. Whereas IC is usually due to single-segment plaque, SLI is always due to multilevel disease.

Many patients with SLI have not previously sought medical advice for IC, principally because they have other comorbidity that prevents them from walking to a point where claudication pain might develop. In contrast to patients with IC, those with SLI are at high risk of losing their limb, and sometimes their life, in a matter of weeks or months without surgical bypass or endovascular revascularisation by angioplasty or stenting. Treatment is difficult, however, because patients

18.76 Clinical features of chronic lower limb ischaemia

- Pulses: diminished or absent
- Bruits: denote turbulent flow but bear no relationship to the severity of the underlying disease
- Reduced skin temperature
- Pallor on elevation and rubor on dependency (Buerger's sign)
- Superficial veins that fill sluggishly and empty ('gutter') upon minimal elevation
- Muscle-wasting
- Skin and nails: dry, thin and brittle
- Loss of hair

18.77 Best medical therapy (BMT) for peripheral arterial disease*

- Smoking cessation
- Regular exercise (30 mins of walking, three times per week)
- Antiplatelet agent (aspirin 75 mg or clopidogrel 75 mg daily)
- Reduction of cholesterol (diet and statin therapy)
- Diagnosis and treatment of diabetes mellitus (all should have fasting glucose measured)
- Diagnosis and treatment of frequently associated conditions (e.g. hypertension, anaemia, heart failure)

*All patients with any manifestation of PAD should be considered for BMT.

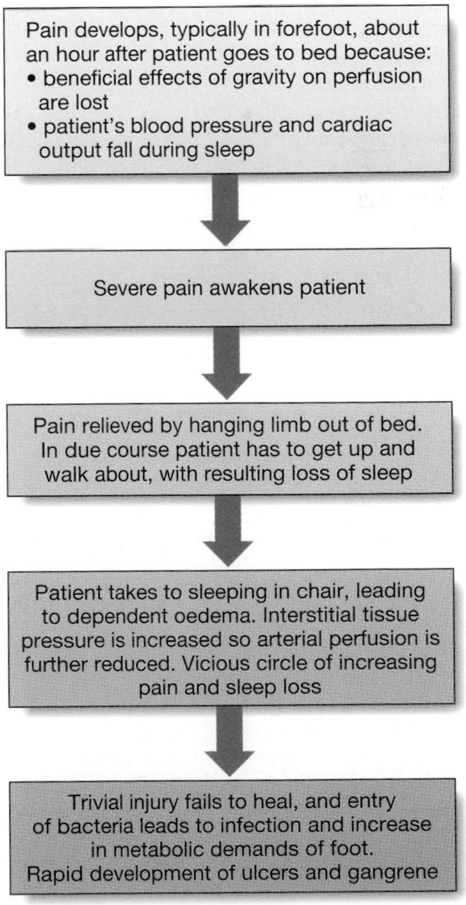

Pain develops, typically in forefoot, about an hour after patient goes to bed because:
- beneficial effects of gravity on perfusion are lost
- patient's blood pressure and cardiac output fall during sleep

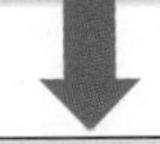

Severe pain awakens patient

Pain relieved by hanging limb out of bed. In due course patient has to get up and walk about, with resulting loss of sleep

Patient takes to sleeping in chair, leading to dependent oedema. Interstitial tissue pressure is increased so arterial perfusion is further reduced. Vicious circle of increasing pain and sleep loss

Trivial injury fails to heal, and entry of bacteria leads to infection and increase in metabolic demands of foot. Rapid development of ulcers and gangrene

Fig. 18.78 Progressive night pain and the development of tissue loss.

have extensive and severe (often bilateral) end-stage disease, are usually elderly and nearly always have significant multisystem comorbidity. Imaging is performed using duplex ultrasonography, MRI or CT with intravenous injection of contrast agents. Intra-arterial digital subtraction angiography (IA-DSA) is usually reserved for those undergoing endovascular revascularisation.

Diabetic vascular disease

Approximately 5–10% of patients with PAD have diabetes but this proportion increases to 30–40% in those with SLI. Diabetes does not cause obstructive microangiopathy at the capillary level, as previously thought, and so is not a contraindication to lower limb revascularisation. Nevertheless, the 'diabetic foot' does pose a number of particular problems (Box 18.78 and p. 833). If the blood supply is adequate, then dead tissue can be excised in the expectation that healing will occur, provided infection is controlled and the foot is protected from pressure. However, if significant ischaemia is also present, the priority is to revascularise the foot if possible. Sadly, many diabetic patients present late with extensive tissue loss, which accounts for the high amputation rate.

18.78 Diabetic vascular disease: the 'diabetic foot'

Feature	Difficulty
Arterial calcification	Spuriously high ABPI due to incompressible ankle vessels. Inability to clamp arteries for the purposes of bypass surgery. Resistant to angioplasty
Immunocompromise	Prone to rapidly spreading cellulitis, gangrene and osteomyelitis
Multisystem arterial disease	Coronary and cerebral arterial disease increase the risks of intervention
Distal disease	Diabetic vascular disease has a predilection for the calf vessels. Although vessels in the foot are often spared, performing a satisfactory bypass or angioplasty to these small vessels is a technical challenge
Sensory neuropathy	Even severe ischaemia and/or tissue loss may be completely painless. Diabetic patients often present late with extensive destruction of the foot. Loss of proprioception leads to abnormal pressure loads and worsens joint destruction (Charcot joints)
Motor neuropathy	Weakness of the long and short flexors and extensors leads to abnormal foot architecture, abnormal pressure loads, callus formation and ulceration
Autonomic neuropathy	Leads to a dry foot deficient in sweat that normally lubricates the skin and is antibacterial. Scaling and fissuring create a portal of entry for bacteria. Abnormal blood flow in the bones of the ankle and foot may also contribute to osteopenia and bony collapse

(ABPI = ankle–brachial pressure index)

Buerger's disease (thromboangiitis obliterans)

This is an inflammatory obliterative arterial disease that is distinct from atherosclerosis and usually presents in young (20–30 years) male smokers. It is most common in those from the Mediterranean and North Africa. It characteristically affects distal arteries, giving rise to claudication in the feet or rest pain in the fingers or toes. Wrist and ankle pulses are absent but brachial and popliteal pulses are present. Disease also affects the veins, giving rise to superficial thrombophlebitis. It often remits if the patient stops smoking; sympathectomy and prostaglandin infusions may be helpful. Major limb amputation is the most frequent outcome if patients continue to smoke.

Chronic upper limb arterial disease

In the arm, the subclavian artery is the most common site of disease, which may manifest as:

- *Arm claudication* (rare).
- *Atheroembolism* (blue finger syndrome). Small emboli lodge in digital arteries and may be confused with Raynaud's phenomenon (see below) but, in this case, the symptoms are unilateral. Failure to make the diagnosis may eventually lead to amputation.
- *Subclavian steal.* When the arm is used, blood is 'stolen' from the brain via the vertebral artery. This leads to vertebro-basilar ischaemia, which is characterised by dizziness, cortical blindness and/or collapse. Where possible, subclavian artery disease is treated by means of angioplasty and stenting, as surgery (e.g. carotid–subclavian bypass) can be difficult.

Raynaud's phenomenon and Raynaud's disease

Cold (and emotional) stimuli may trigger vasospasm, leading to the characteristic sequence of digital pallor due to vasospasm, cyanosis due to deoxygenated blood, and rubor due to reactive hyperaemia.

Primary Raynaud's phenomenon (or disease)

This affects 5–10% of young women aged 15–30 years in temperate climates and may be familial. It does not

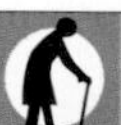

18.79 Atherosclerotic vascular disease in old age

- **Prevalence**: related almost exponentially to age in developed countries, although atherosclerosis is not considered part of the normal ageing process.
- **Statin therapy**: no role in the primary prevention of atherosclerotic disease in those over 75 yrs but reduces cardiovascular events in those with established vascular disease, albeit with no reduction in overall mortality.
- **Presentation in the frail**: frequently with advanced multisystem arterial disease, along with a host of other comorbidities.
- **Intervention in the frail**: in those with extensive disease and limited life expectancy, the risks of surgery may outweigh the benefits, and symptomatic care is all that should be offered.

progress to ulceration or infarction, and significant pain is unusual. The underlying cause is unclear. No investigation is necessary. The patient should be reassured and advised to avoid exposure to cold. Long-acting nifedipine may be helpful but sympathectomy is not indicated.

Secondary Raynaud's phenomenon (or syndrome)

This occurs in older people in association with connective tissue disease (most commonly systemic sclerosis or CREST syndrome, p. 1112), vibration-induced injury (from the use of power tools) and thoracic outlet obstruction (e.g. cervical rib). Unlike primary disease, it is often associated with fixed obstruction of the digital arteries, fingertip ulceration, and necrosis and pain. The fingers must be protected from cold and trauma, infection requires treatment with antibiotics, and surgery should be avoided if possible. Vasoactive drugs have no clear benefit. Sympathectomy helps for a year or two. Prostacyclin infusions are sometimes beneficial.

Acute limb ischaemia

This is most frequently caused by acute thrombotic occlusion of a pre-existing stenotic arterial segment, thromboembolism, and trauma that may be iatrogenic. Apart from paralysis (inability to wiggle toes/fingers) and paraesthesia (loss of light touch over the dorsum of the foot/hand), the so-called 'Ps of acute ischaemia' (Box 18.80) are non-specific for ischaemia and/or inconsistently related to its severity. Pain on squeezing the calf indicates muscle infarction and impending irreversible ischaemia.

All patients with suspected acutely ischaemic limbs must be discussed immediately with a vascular surgeon; a few hours can make the difference between death/amputation and complete recovery of limb function. If there are no contraindications (for example, acute aortic dissection or trauma, particularly head injury), an intravenous bolus of heparin (3000–5000 U) should be administered to limit propagation of thrombus and protect the collateral circulation. Distinguishing thrombosis from embolism is frequently difficult but is important because treatment and prognosis are different (Box 18.81). Acute limb ischaemia due to thrombosis in situ can usually be treated medically in the first instance with intravenous heparin (target activated partial thromboplastin time (APTT) 2.0–3.0), antiplatelet agents, high-dose statins, intravenous fluids to avoid dehydration, correction of anaemia, oxygen and sometimes prostaglandins, such as iloprost. Careful monitoring is required. Embolism will normally result in extensive tissue necrosis within 6 hours unless the limb is revascularised. The indications for thrombolysis, if any, remain controversial. Irreversible ischaemia mandates early amputation or palliative care.

18.80 Symptoms and signs of acute limb ischaemia

Symptoms/signs	Comment
Pain Pallor Pulselessness	May be absent in complete acute ischaemia, and can be present in chronic ischaemia
Perishing cold	Unreliable, as the ischaemic limb takes on the ambient temperature
Paraesthesia Paralysis	Important features of impending irreversible ischaemia

18.81 Acute limb ischaemia: distinguishing features of embolism and thrombosis in situ

Clinical features	Embolism	Thrombosis in situ
Severity	Complete (no collaterals)	Incomplete (collaterals)
Onset	Seconds or minutes	Hours or days
Limb	Leg 3:1 arm	Leg 10:1 arm
Multiple sites	Up to 15%	Rare
Embolic source	Present (usually atrial fibrillation)	Absent
Previous claudication	Absent	Present
Palpation of artery	Soft, tender	Hard, calcified
Bruits	Absent	Present
Contralateral leg pulses	Present	Absent
Diagnosis	Clinical	Angiography
Treatment	Embolectomy, warfarin	Medical, bypass, thrombolysis
Prognosis	Loss of life > loss of limb	Loss of limb > loss of life

Cerebrovascular/renovascular disease and ischaemic gut injury

See Ch. 27 and pp. 494 and 909.

Diseases of the aorta

Aneurysm, dissection and aortitis are the main pathologies (Fig. 18.79).

Aortic aneurysm

This is an abnormal dilatation of the aortic lumen; a true aneurysm involves all the layers of the wall, whereas a false aneurysm does not.

Aetiology and types of aneurysm

Non-specific aneurysms

Why some patients develop occlusive vascular disease, some develop aneurysmal vascular disease and some develop both in response to atherosclerosis risk factors remains unclear. Unlike occlusive disease, aneurysmal disease tends to run in families and genetic factors are undoubtedly important. The most common site for 'non-specific' aneurysm formation is the infrarenal abdominal aorta. The suprarenal abdominal aorta and a variable length of the descending thoracic aorta may be affected in 10–20% of patients but the ascending aorta is usually spared.

Marfan's syndrome

This disorder of connective tissue is inherited as an autosomal dominant trait and is caused by mutations in the

18

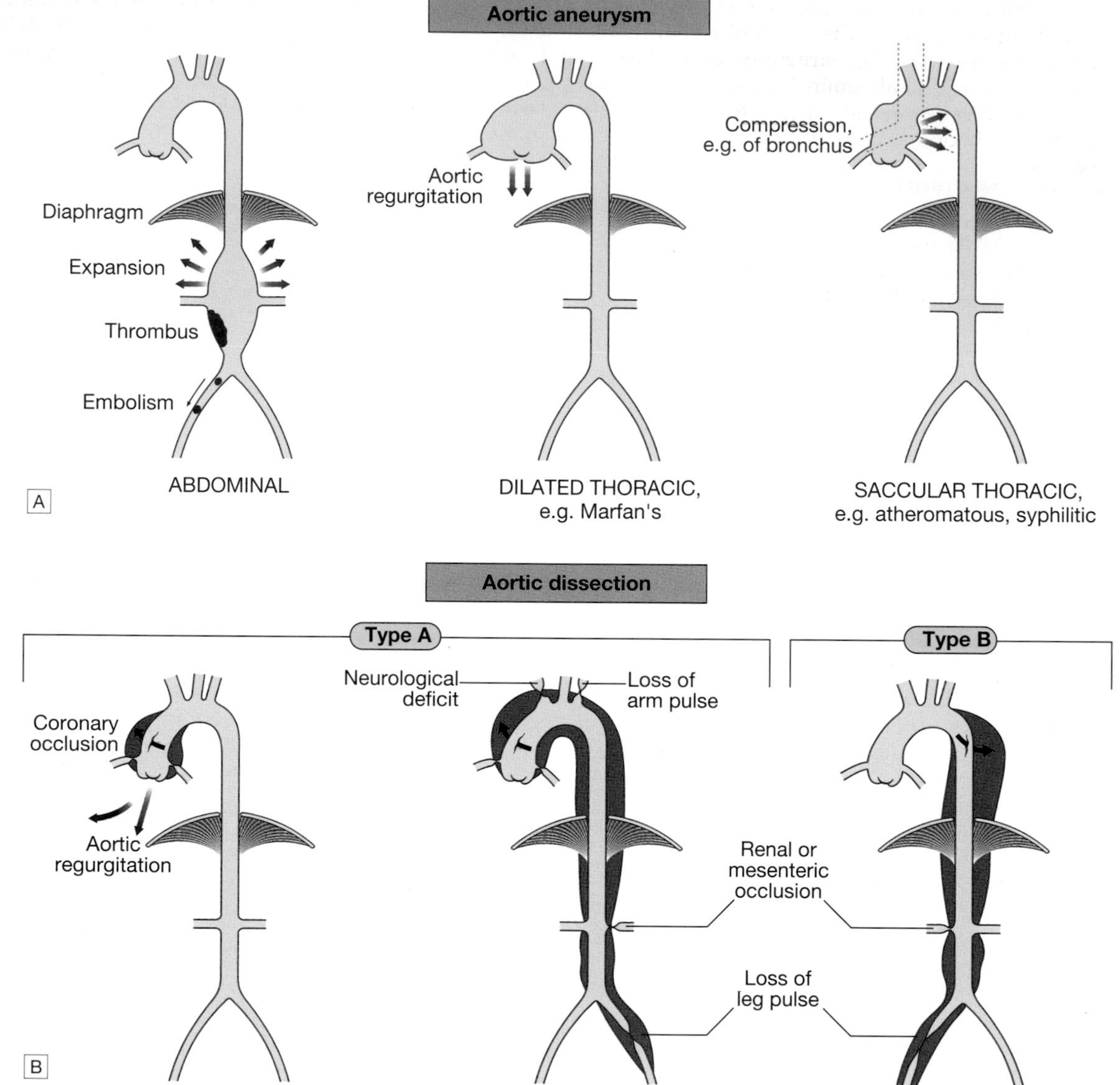

Fig. 18.79 Types of aortic disease and their complications. **A** Types of aortic aneurysm. **B** Types of aortic dissection.

fibrillin gene on chromosome 15. Affected systems include the skeleton (arachnodactyly, joint hypermobility, scoliosis, chest deformity and high arched palate), the eyes (dislocation of the lens) and the cardiovascular system (aortic disease and mitral regurgitation). Weakening of the aortic media leads to aortic root dilatation, regurgitation and dissection (see below). Pregnancy is particularly hazardous. Chest X-ray, echocardiography, MRI or CT may detect aortic dilatation at an early stage and can be used to monitor the disease.

Treatment with β-blockers reduces the rate of aortic dilatation and the risk of rupture. Elective replacement of the ascending aorta may be considered in patients with evidence of progressive aortic dilatation but carries a mortality of 5–10%.

Aortitis

Syphilis is a rare cause of aortitis that characteristically produces saccular aneurysms of the ascending aorta containing calcification. Other rare conditions associated with aortitis include Takayasu's disease (p. 1116), Reiter's syndrome (p. 1107), giant cell arteritis and ankylosing spondylitis (pp. 1105 and 1117).

Thoracic aortic aneurysms

These may produce chest pain, aortic regurgitation, compressive symptoms such as stridor (trachea, bronchus) and hoarseness (recurrent laryngeal nerve), and superior vena cava syndrome (see Fig. 18.79A). If they erode into adjacent structures, e.g. aorto-oesophageal fistula, massive bleeding occurs.

Abdominal aortic aneurysms

Abdominal aortic aneurysms (AAAs) are present in 5% of men aged over 60 years and 80% are confined to the infrarenal segment. Men are affected three times more commonly than women. AAAs can present in a number of ways (Box 18.82). The usual age at presentation is 65–75 years for elective presentations and 75–85 years for emergency presentations. Ultrasound is the best way of establishing the diagnosis and of following up patients with asymptomatic aneurysms that are not yet large enough to warrant surgical repair. CT provides more accurate information about the size and extent of the aneurysm, the surrounding structures and whether there is any other intra-abdominal pathology. It is the standard pre-operative investigation but is not suitable for surveillance because of cost and radiation dose.

Management. Until an asymptomatic AAA has reached a maximum of 5.5 cm in diameter, the risks of surgery generally outweigh the risks of rupture (Box 18.83). All symptomatic AAAs should be considered for repair, not only to rid the patient of symptoms but also because pain often predates rupture. Distal embolisation is a strong indication for repair, regardless of size, because otherwise limb loss is common. Most patients with a ruptured AAA do not survive to reach hospital, but if they do and surgery is thought to be appropriate, there must be no delay in getting them to the operating theatre to clamp the aorta.

Open AAA repair has been the treatment of choice in both the elective and the emergency settings, and entails replacing the aneurysmal segment with a prosthetic (usually Dacron) graft. The 30-day mortality for this procedure is approximately 5–8% for elective asymptomatic AAA, 10–20% for emergency symptomatic AAA and 50% for ruptured AAA. However, patients who survive the operation to leave hospital have a long-term survival which approaches that of the normal population. Increasingly, endovascular aneurysm repair (EVAR), using a stent-graft introduced via the femoral arteries in the groin, is replacing open surgery. It is cost-effective and likely to become the treatment of choice for infrarenal AAA. It is possible to treat many suprarenal and thoraco-abdominal aneurysms by EVAR too.

In the UK, a national screening programme for men over 65 years of age has been introduced using ultrasound scanning. For every 10 000 men scanned, 65 ruptures are prevented and 52 lives saved.

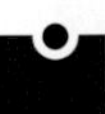

18.82 Abdominal aortic aneurysm: common presentations

Incidental

- On physical examination, plain X-ray or, most commonly, abdominal ultrasound
- Even large AAAs can be difficult to feel, so many remain undetected until they rupture
- Studies are currently under way to determine whether screening will reduce the number of deaths from rupture (see Box 18.83)

Pain

- In the central abdomen, back, loin, iliac fossa or groin

Thromboembolic complications

- Thrombus within the aneurysm sac may be a source of emboli to the lower limbs
- Less commonly, the aorta may undergo thrombotic occlusion

Compression

- Surrounding structures such as the duodenum (obstruction and vomiting) and the inferior vena cava (oedema and deep vein thrombosis)

Rupture

- Into the retroperitoneum, the peritoneal cavity or surrounding structures (most commonly the inferior vena cava, leading to an aortocaval fistula)

EBM 18.83 Population screening and prevention of ruptured abdominal aortic aneurysm

'Ultrasound screening for AAA in men aged 65–75 years, with surgical repair of those AAAs that are bigger than 5.5 cm, are rapidly growing or become symptomatic, reduces the community incidence of rupture by approximately 50% and is cost-effective.'

- MASS Study Group. Lancet 2002; 360:1531–1539.
- MASS Study Group. BMJ 2002; 352:1135.

For further information: www.mrc-bsu.cam.ac.uk

Aortic dissection

A breach in the integrity of the aortic wall allows arterial blood to enter the media, which is then split into two layers, creating a 'false lumen' alongside the existing or 'true lumen' (see Fig. 18.79B). The aortic valve may be damaged and the branches of the aorta may be compromised. Typically, the false lumen eventually re-enters the true lumen, creating a double-barrelled aorta, but it may also rupture into the left pleural space or pericardium with fatal consequences.

The primary event is often a spontaneous or iatrogenic tear in the intima of the aorta; multiple tears or entry points are common. Other dissections are triggered by primary haemorrhage in the media of the aorta, which then ruptures through the intima into the true lumen. This form of spontaneous bleeding from the vasa vasorum is sometimes confined to the aortic wall, when it may present as a painful intramural haematoma.

Aortic disease and hypertension are the most important aetiological factors but other conditions may also be implicated (Box 18.84). Chronic dissections may lead to aneurysmal dilatation of the aorta, and thoracic aneurysms may be complicated by dissection. It can therefore be difficult to identify the primary pathology.

The peak incidence is in the sixth and seventh decades but dissection can occur in younger patients, usually in association with Marfan's syndrome, pregnancy or trauma; men are twice as frequently affected as women.

Aortic dissection is classified anatomically and for management purposes into type A and type B (see Fig. 18.79B), involving or sparing the ascending aorta, respectively. Type A dissections account for two-thirds of cases and frequently also extend into the descending aorta.

18.84 Factors that may predispose to aortic dissection

- Hypertension (in 80%)
- Aortic atherosclerosis
- Non-specific aortic aneurysm
- Aortic coarctation (p. 632)
- Collagen disorders (e.g. Marfan's syndrome, Ehlers–Danlos syndrome)
- Fibromuscular dysplasia
- Previous aortic surgery (e.g. CABG, aortic valve replacement)
- Pregnancy (usually third trimester)
- Trauma
- Iatrogenic (e.g. cardiac catheterisation, intra-aortic balloon pumping)

(CABG = coronary artery bypass grafting)

Clinical features

Involvement of the ascending aorta typically gives rise to anterior chest pain, and involvement of the descending aorta to intrascapular pain. The pain is typically described as 'tearing' and very abrupt in onset; collapse is common. Unless there is major haemorrhage, the patient is invariably hypertensive. There may be asymmetry of the brachial, carotid or femoral pulses and signs of aortic regurgitation. Occlusion of aortic branches may cause MI (coronary), stroke (carotid) paraplegia (spinal), mesenteric infarction with an acute abdomen (coeliac and superior mesenteric), renal failure (renal) and acute limb (usually leg) ischaemia.

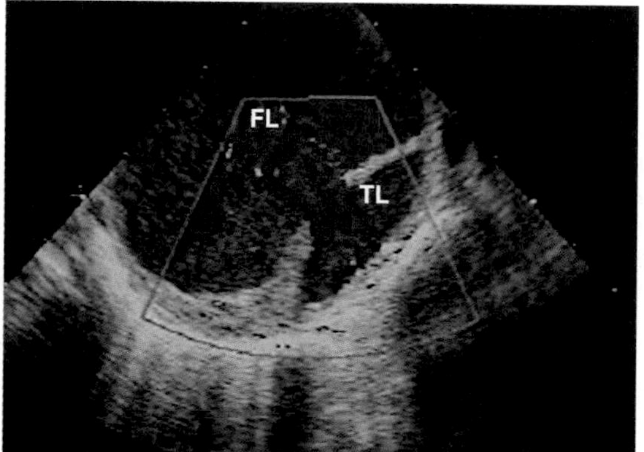

Fig. 18.80 Echocardiograms from a patient with a chronic aortic dissection. Colour flow Doppler shows flow from the larger false lumen (FL) into the true lumen (TL), characteristic of chronic disease.

Investigations

The chest X-ray characteristically shows broadening of the upper mediastinum and distortion of the aortic 'knuckle', but these findings are variable and are absent in 10% of cases. A left-sided pleural effusion is common. The ECG may show left ventricular hypertrophy in patients with hypertension, or rarely changes of acute MI (usually inferior). Doppler echocardiography may

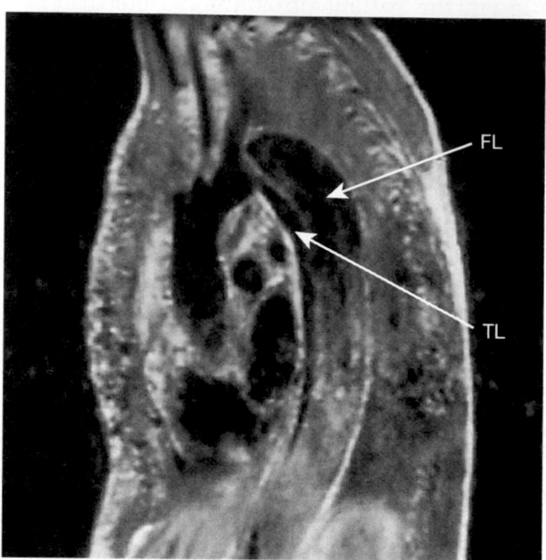

Fig. 18.81 Sagittal view of an MRI scan from a patient with longstanding aortic dissection, illustrating a biluminal aorta. There is sluggish flow in the false lumen (FL), accounting for its grey appearance. (TL = true lumen)

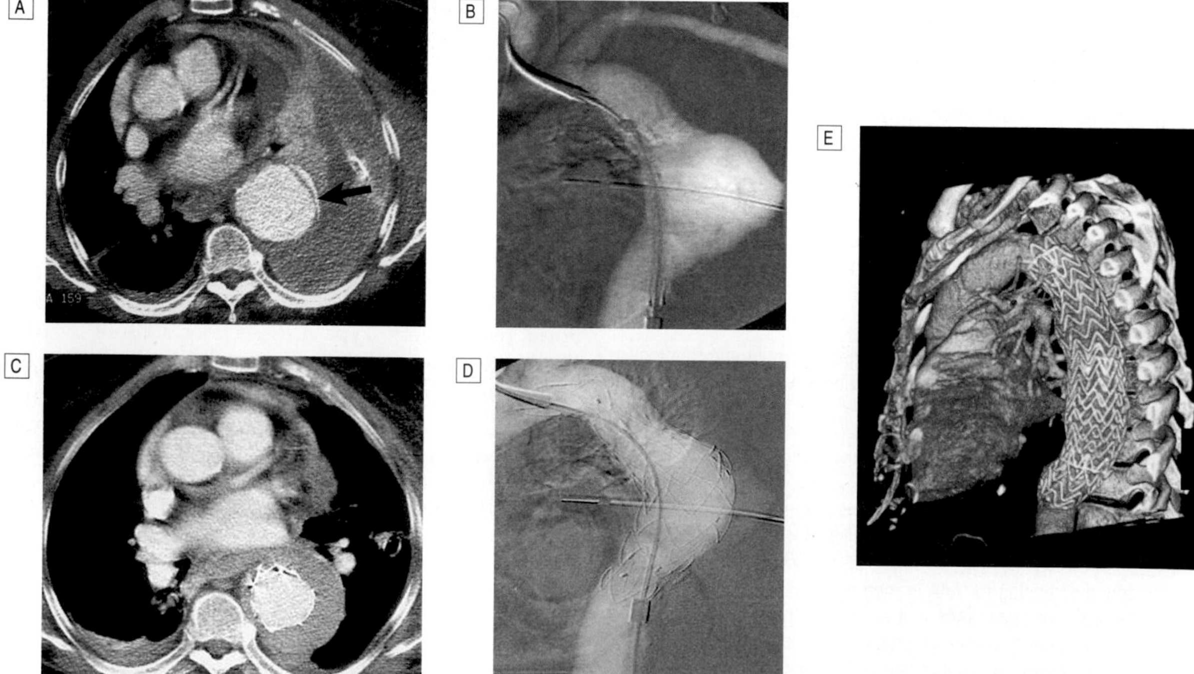

Fig. 18.82 Images from a patient with an acute type B aortic dissection that had ruptured into the left pleural space and was repaired by deploying an endoluminal stent graft. **A** CT scan illustrating an intimal flap (arrow) in the descending aorta and a large pleural effusion. **B** Aortogram illustrating aneurysmal dilatation; a stent graft has been introduced from the right femoral artery and is about to be deployed. **C** CT scan after endoluminal repair. The pleural effusion has been drained but there is a haematoma around the descending aorta. **D** Aortogram illustrating the stent graft. **E** Three-dimensional reconstruction of aortic stent graft.

show aortic regurgitation, a dilated aortic root and, occasionally, the flap of the dissection. Transoesophageal echocardiography is particularly helpful because transthoracic echocardiography can only provide images of the first 3–4 cm of the ascending aorta (Fig. 18.80). CT and MRI angiography (Figs 18.81 and 18.82) are both highly specific and sensitive.

Management

The early mortality of acute dissection is approximately 1–5% per hour and so treatment is urgently required. Initial management comprises pain control and antihypertensive treatment. Type A dissections require emergency surgery to replace the ascending aorta. Type B aneurysms are treated medically unless there is actual or impending external rupture, or vital organ (gut, kidneys) or limb ischaemia, as the morbidity and mortality associated with surgery are very high. The aim of medical management is to maintain a mean arterial pressure (MAP) of 60–75 mmHg to reduce the force of the ejection of blood from the LV. First-line therapy is with β-blockers; the additional α-blocking properties of labetalol make it especially useful. Rate-limiting calcium channel blockers, such as verapamil or diltiazem, are used if β-blockers are contraindicated. Sodium nitroprusside may be considered if these fail to control BP adequately.

Percutaneous or minimal access endoluminal repair is sometimes possible and involves either 'fenestrating' (perforating) the intimal flap so that blood can return from the false to the true lumen (so decompressing the former), or implanting a stent graft placed from the femoral artery (see Fig. 18.82).

Hypertension

Within any population, blood pressure values occur within a continuum, and are determined by mechanical, hormonal and environmental factors. Any definition of hypertension therefore utilises arbitrary threshold values within this continuum. Systemic BP rises with age, and the incidence of cardiovascular disease (particularly stroke and coronary artery disease) is closely related to average BP at all ages, even when BP readings are within the so-called 'normal range'.

The cardiovascular risks associated with BP depend upon the combination of risk factors in an individual, such as age, gender, weight, physical activity, smoking, family history, serum cholesterol, diabetes mellitus and pre-existing vascular disease. Thus a practical definition of hypertension is 'the level of BP at which the benefits of treatment outweigh the costs and hazards'. The British Hypertension Society classification is provided in Box 18.85 and is consistent with those defined by the European Society of Hypertension and the World Health Organization–International Society of Hypertension.

18.85 Definition of hypertension

Category	Systolic BP (mmHg)	Diastolic BP (mmHg)
BP		
Optimal	< 120	< 80
Normal	< 130	85
High normal	130–139	85–89
Hypertension		
Grade 1 (mild)	140–159	90–99
Grade 2 (moderate)	160–179	100–109
Grade 3 (severe)	≥ 180	> 110
Isolated systolic hypertension		
Grade 1	140–159	< 90
Grade 2	≥ 160	< 90

18.86 Causes of secondary hypertension

Alcohol

Obesity

Pregnancy (pre-eclampsia)

Renal disease (Ch. 17)
- Parenchymal renal disease, particularly glomerulonephritis
- Renal vascular disease
- Polycystic kidney disease

Endocrine disease (Ch. 20)
- Phaeochromocytoma
- Cushing's syndrome
- Primary hyperaldosteronism (Conn's syndrome)
- Glucocorticoid-suppressible hyperaldosteronism
- Hyperparathyroidism
- Acromegaly
- Primary hypothyroidism
- Thyrotoxicosis
- Congenital adrenal hyperplasia due to 11-β-hydroxylase or 17-α-hydroxylase deficiency
- Liddle's syndrome (p. 441)
- 11-β-hydroxysteroid dehydrogenase deficiency

Drugs
- e.g. Oral contraceptives containing oestrogens, anabolic steroids, corticosteroids, NSAIDs, carbenoxolone, sympathomimetic agents

Coarctation of the aorta (p. 632)

Aetiology

In more than 95% of cases, a specific underlying cause of hypertension cannot be found. Such patients are said to have essential hypertension. The pathogenesis is not clearly understood. Many factors may contribute to its development, including renal dysfunction, peripheral resistance vessel tone, endothelial dysfunction, autonomic tone, insulin resistance and neurohumoral factors. Hypertension is more common in some ethnic groups, particularly African Americans and Japanese, and approximately 40–60% is explained by genetic factors. Important environmental factors include a high salt intake, heavy consumption of alcohol, obesity, lack of exercise and impaired intrauterine growth. There is little evidence that 'stress' causes hypertension.

In about 5% of cases, hypertension can be shown to be a consequence of a specific disease or abnormality leading to sodium retention and/or peripheral vasoconstriction (secondary hypertension, Box 18.86).

Approach to newly diagnosed hypertension

Hypertension is predominantly an asymptomatic condition and the diagnosis is usually made at routine examination or when a complication arises. A BP check is advisable every 5 years in adults.

The objectives of the initial evaluation of a patient with high BP readings are:

- to obtain accurate, representative BP measurements
- to identify contributory factors and any underlying cause (secondary hypertension)
- to assess other risk factors and quantify cardiovascular risk
- to detect any complications (target organ damage) that are already present
- to identify comorbidity that may influence the choice of antihypertensive therapy.

These goals are attained by a careful history, clinical examination and some simple investigations.

Measurement of blood pressure

A decision to embark upon antihypertensive therapy effectively commits the patient to life-long treatment, so BP readings must be as accurate as possible.

Measurements should be made to the nearest 2 mmHg, in the sitting position with the arm supported, and repeated after 5 minutes' rest if the first recording is high (Box 18.87). To avoid spuriously high readings in obese subjects, the cuff should contain a bladder that encompasses at least two-thirds of the arm circumference.

Home and ambulatory BP recordings

Exercise, anxiety, discomfort and unfamiliar surroundings can all lead to a transient rise in BP. Sphygmomanometry, particularly when performed by a doctor, can cause an unrepresentative surge in BP which has been termed 'white coat' hypertension, and as many as 20% of patients with apparent hypertension in the clinic may have a normal BP when it is recorded by automated devices used at home. The risk of cardiovascular disease in these patients is less than that in patients with sustained hypertension but greater than that in normotensive subjects.

A series of automated ambulatory BP measurements obtained over 24 hours or longer provides a better profile than a limited number of clinic readings and correlates more closely with evidence of target organ damage than casual BP measurements. Treatment thresholds and targets (see Box 18.93, p. 611) must be adjusted downwards, however, because ambulatory BP readings are systematically lower (approximately 12/7 mmHg) than clinic measurements. The average ambulatory daytime (not 24-hour or night-time) BP should be used to guide management decisions.

Patients can measure their own BP at home using a range of commercially available semi-automatic devices. The value of such measurements is less well established and is dependent on the environment and timing of the readings measured. Home or ambulatory BP measurements are particularly helpful in patients with unusually labile BP, those with refractory hypertension, those who may have symptomatic hypotension, and those in whom white coat hypertension is suspected.

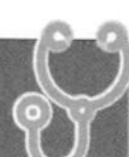

18.87 How to measure blood pressure

- Use a machine that has been validated, well maintained and properly calibrated
- Measure sitting BP routinely, with additional standing BP in elderly and diabetic patients and those with possible postural hypotension
- Remove tight clothing from the arm
- Support the arm at the level of the heart
- Use a cuff of appropriate size (the bladder must encompass more than two-thirds of the arm)
- Lower the pressure slowly (2 mmHg per second)
- Read the BP to the nearest 2 mmHg
- Use phase V (disappearance of sounds) to measure diastolic BP
- Take two measurements at each visit

History

Family history, lifestyle (exercise, salt intake, smoking habit) and other risk factors should be recorded. A careful history will identify those patients with drug- or alcohol-induced hypertension and may elicit the symptoms of other causes of secondary hypertension, such as phaeochromocytoma (paroxysmal headache, palpitation and sweating, p. 781) or complications such as coronary artery disease (e.g. angina, breathlessness).

Examination

Radio-femoral delay (coarctation of the aorta; see Fig. 18.97, p. 632), enlarged kidneys (polycystic kidney disease), abdominal bruits (renal artery stenosis) and the characteristic facies and habitus of Cushing's syndrome are all examples of physical signs that may help to identify causes of secondary hypertension (see Box 18.86). Examination may also reveal features of important risk factors, such as central obesity and hyperlipidaemia (tendon xanthomas and so on). Most abnormal signs are due to the complications of hypertension.

Non-specific findings may include left ventricular hypertrophy (apical heave), accentuation of the aortic component of the second heart sound, and a fourth heart sound. The optic fundi are often abnormal (see Fig. 18.83 below) and there may be evidence of generalised atheroma or specific complications, such as aortic aneurysm or peripheral vascular disease.

Target organ damage

The adverse effects of hypertension on the organs can often be detected clinically.

Blood vessels

In larger arteries (> 1 mm in diameter), the internal elastic lamina is thickened, smooth muscle is hypertrophied and fibrous tissue is deposited. The vessels dilate and become tortuous, and their walls become less compliant. In smaller arteries (< 1 mm), hyaline arteriosclerosis occurs in the wall, the lumen narrows and aneurysms may develop. Widespread atheroma develops and may lead to coronary and cerebrovascular disease, particularly if other risk factors (e.g. smoking, hyperlipidaemia, diabetes) are present.

These structural changes in the vasculature often perpetuate and aggravate hypertension by increasing peripheral vascular resistance and reducing renal blood flow, thereby activating the renin–angiotensin–aldosterone axis (p. 547).

Hypertension is a major risk factor in the pathogenesis of aortic aneurysm and aortic dissection.

Central nervous system

Stroke is a common complication of hypertension and may be due to cerebral haemorrhage or infarction. Carotid atheroma and TIAs are more common in hypertensive patients. Subarachnoid haemorrhage is also associated with hypertension.

Hypertensive encephalopathy is a rare condition characterised by high BP and neurological symptoms, including transient disturbances of speech or vision, paraesthesiae, disorientation, fits and loss of consciousness. Papilloedema is common. A CT scan of the brain often shows haemorrhage in and around the basal ganglia; however, the neurological deficit is usually reversible if the hypertension is properly controlled.

Retina

The optic fundi reveal a gradation of changes linked to the severity of hypertension; fundoscopy can, therefore, provide an indication of the arteriolar damage occurring elsewhere (Box 18.88).

'Cotton wool' exudates are associated with retinal ischaemia or infarction, and fade in a few weeks (Fig. 18.83A). 'Hard' exudates (small, white, dense deposits of lipid) and microaneurysms ('dot' haemorrhages) are more characteristic of diabetic retinopathy (see Fig. 21.12, p. 829). Hypertension is also associated with central retinal vein thrombosis (Fig. 18.83B).

18.88 Hypertensive retinopathy

• **Grade 1**	Arteriolar thickening, tortuosity and increased reflectiveness ('silver wiring')
• **Grade 2**	Grade 1 plus constriction of veins at arterial crossings ('arteriovenous nipping')
• **Grade 3**	Grade 2 plus evidence of retinal ischaemia (flame-shaped or blot haemorrhages and 'cotton wool' exudates)
• **Grade 4**	Grade 3 plus papilloedema

Heart

The excess cardiac mortality and morbidity associated with hypertension are largely due to a higher incidence of coronary artery disease. High BP places a pressure load on the heart and may lead to left ventricular hypertrophy with a forceful apex beat and fourth heart sound. ECG or echocardiographic evidence of left ventricular hypertrophy is highly predictive of cardiovascular complications and therefore particularly useful in risk assessment.

Atrial fibrillation is common and may be due to diastolic dysfunction caused by left ventricular hypertrophy or the effects of coronary artery disease.

Severe hypertension can cause left ventricular failure in the absence of coronary artery disease, particularly when renal function, and therefore sodium excretion, are impaired.

Kidneys

Long-standing hypertension may cause proteinuria and progressive renal failure (p. 478) by damaging the renal vasculature.

A

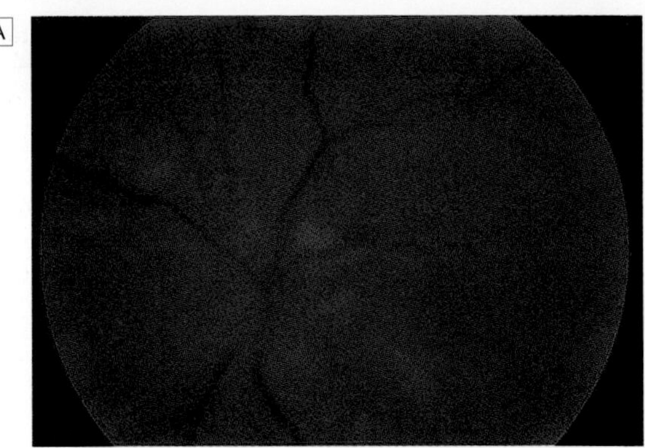

B

Fig. 18.83 Retinal changes in hypertension. **A** Grade 4 hypertensive retinopathy showing swollen optic disc, retinal haemorrhages and multiple cotton wool spots (infarcts). **B** Central retinal vein thrombosis showing swollen optic disc and widespread fundal haemorrhage, commonly associated with systemic hypertension.

'Malignant' or 'accelerated' phase hypertension

This rare condition may complicate hypertension of any aetiology and is characterised by accelerated microvascular damage with necrosis in the walls of small arteries and arterioles ('fibrinoid necrosis') and by intravascular thrombosis. The diagnosis is based on evidence of high BP and rapidly progressive end organ damage, such as retinopathy (grade 3 or 4), renal dysfunction (especially proteinuria) and/or hypertensive encephalopathy (see above). Left ventricular failure may occur and, if this is untreated, death occurs within months.

Investigations

All hypertensive patients should undergo a limited number of investigations (Box 18.89). Additional investigations are appropriate in selected patients (Box 18.90).

Management

Quantification of cardiovascular risk

The sole objective of antihypertensive therapy is to reduce the incidence of adverse cardiovascular events, particularly coronary artery disease, stroke and heart failure. Randomised controlled trials have demonstrated that antihypertensive therapy can reduce the incidence of stroke and, to a lesser extent, coronary artery disease (Box 18.91). The relative benefits (approximately 30% reduction in risk of stroke and 20% reduction in risk of coronary artery disease) are similar in all patient groups,

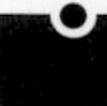

18.89 Hypertension: investigation of all patients

- Urinalysis for blood, protein and glucose
- Blood urea, electrolytes and creatinine
  N.B. Hypokalaemic alkalosis may indicate primary hyperaldosteronism but is usually due to diuretic therapy
- Blood glucose
- Serum total and HDL cholesterol
- Thyroid function tests
- 12-lead ECG (left ventricular hypertrophy, coronary artery disease)

(HDL = high-density lipoprotein)

18.90 Hypertension: investigation of selected patients

- Chest X-ray: to detect cardiomegaly, heart failure, coarctation of the aorta
- Ambulatory BP recording: to assess borderline or 'white coat' hypertension
- Echocardiogram: to detect or quantify left ventricular hypertrophy
- Renal ultrasound: to detect possible renal disease
- Renal angiography: to detect or confirm presence of renal artery stenosis
- Urinary catecholamines: to detect possible phaeochromocytoma (p. 781)
- Urinary cortisol and dexamethasone suppression test: to detect possible Cushing's syndrome (p. 773)
- Plasma renin activity and aldosterone: to detect possible primary aldosteronism (p. 780)

so the absolute benefit of treatment (total number of events prevented) is greatest in those at highest risk. For example, to extrapolate from the Medical Research Council (MRC) Mild Hypertension Trial (1985), 566 young patients would have to be treated with bendroflumethiazide for 1 year to prevent 1 stroke, while in the MRC trial of antihypertensive treatment in the elderly (1992), 1 stroke was prevented for every 286 patients treated for 1 year.

A formal estimate of absolute cardiovascular risk, which takes account of all the relevant risk factors, may help to determine whether the likely benefits of therapy will outweigh its costs and hazards. A variety of risk algorithms are available for this purpose (see Fig. 18.62, p. 582). Most of the excess morbidity and mortality associated with hypertension is attributable to coronary artery disease and many treatment guidelines are therefore based on estimates of the 10-year coronary artery disease risk. Total cardiovascular risk can be estimated by multiplying coronary artery disease risk by 4/3 (i.e. if coronary artery disease risk is 30%, cardiovascular risk is 40%). The value of this approach can be illustrated by comparing the two hypothetical cases on page 582.

Threshold for intervention

Systolic BP and diastolic BP are both powerful predictors of cardiovascular risk. The British Hypertension Society management guidelines therefore utilise both readings, and treatment should be initiated if they exceed the given threshold (Fig. 18.84).

EBM 18.91 Benefit of antihypertensive drug therapy

'Diuretics or β-blockers have been shown to reduce the risk of coronary artery disease by 16%, stroke by 38%, cardiovascular death by 21% and all causes of mortality by 13%. The effects of ACE inhibitors and calcium antagonists are similar. NNT_B varies greatly, according to the absolute baseline risk of cardiovascular disease.'

- Blood Pressure Lowering Treatment Trialists' Collaboration. Lancet 2003; 362:1527–1535.

Patients with diabetes or cardiovascular disease are at particularly high risk and the threshold for initiating antihypertensive therapy is therefore lower (≥ 140/90 mmHg) in these patient groups. The thresholds for treatment in the elderly are the same as for younger patients (Box 18.92).

Treatment targets

The optimum BP for reduction of major cardiovascular events has been found to be 139/83 mmHg, and even lower in patients with diabetes mellitus. Moreover, reducing BP below this level causes no harm. The targets suggested by the British Hypertension Society (Box 18.93) are ambitious. Primary care strategies have been devised to improve screening and detection of hypertension that, in the past, remained undetected in up to half of affected individuals. Application of new guidelines should help establish patients on appropriate treatment, and allow step-up if lifestyle modification and first-line drug therapy fail to control patients' BP.

Patients taking antihypertensive therapy require follow-up at 3-monthly intervals to monitor BP, minimise side-effects and reinforce lifestyle advice.

Non-drug therapy

Appropriate lifestyle measures may obviate the need for drug therapy in patients with borderline hypertension, reduce the dose and/or the number of drugs required in patients with established hypertension, and directly reduce cardiovascular risk.

Correcting obesity, reducing alcohol intake, restricting salt intake, taking regular physical exercise and increasing consumption of fruit and vegetables can all lower BP. Moreover, quitting smoking, eating oily fish and adopting a diet that is low in saturated fat may produce further reductions in cardiovascular risk.

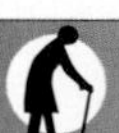

18.92 Hypertension in old age

- **Prevalence**: affects more than half of all people over the age of 60 yrs (including isolated systolic hypertension).
- **Risks**: hypertension is the most important risk factor for MI, heart failure and stroke in older people.
- **Benefit of treatment**: absolute benefit from therapy is greatest in older people (at least up to age 80 yrs).
- **Target BP**: similar to that for younger patients.
- **Tolerance of treatment**: antihypertensives are tolerated as well as in younger patients.
- **Drug of choice**: low-dose thiazides but, in the presence of coexistent disease (e.g. gout, diabetes), other agents may be more appropriate.

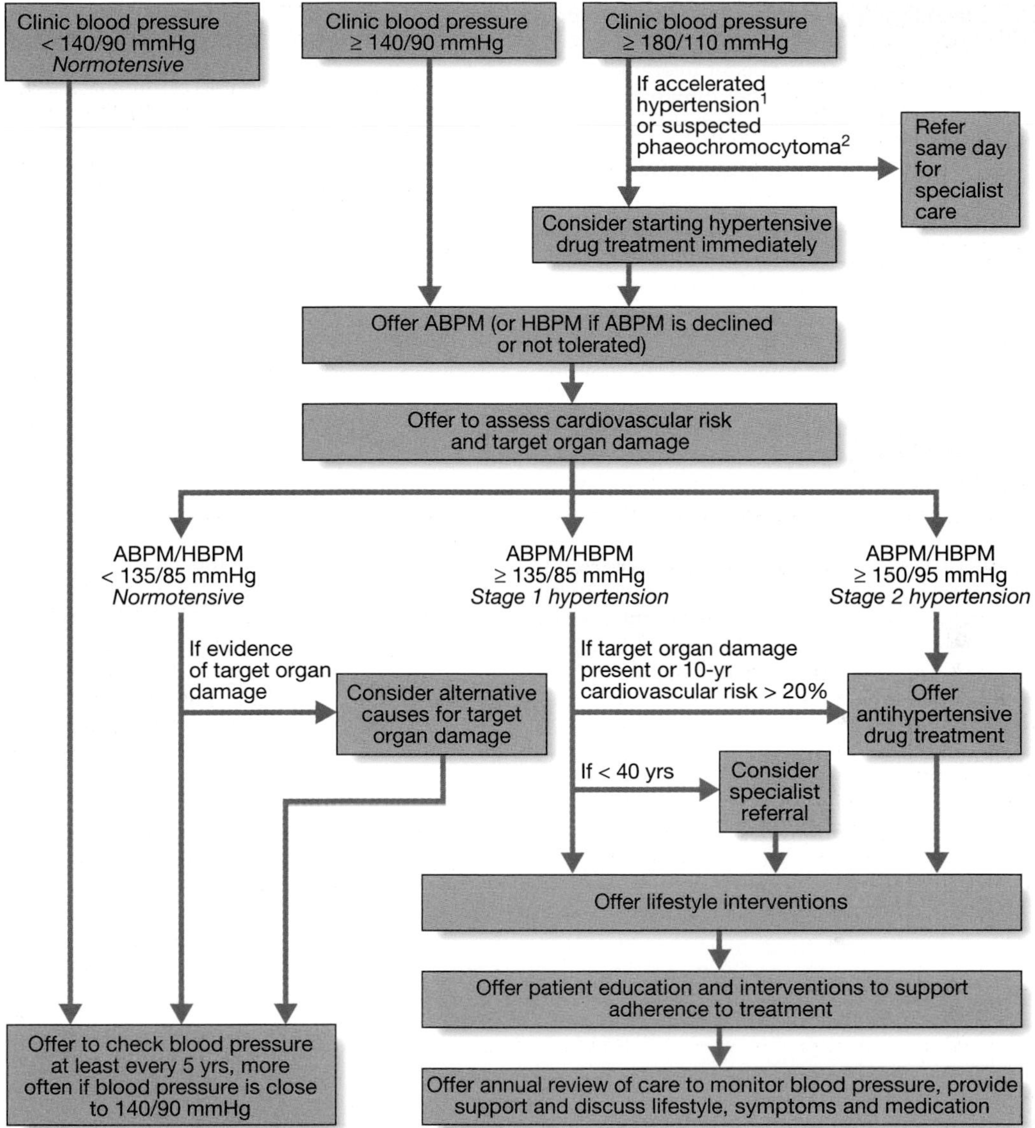

Fig. 18.84 Management of hypertension: British Hypertension Society guidelines. [1]Signs of papilloedema or retinal haemorrhage. [2]Labile or postural hypotension, headache, palpitations, pallor and diaphoresis (ABPM = ambulatory blood pressure monitoring; HBPM = home blood pressure monitoring). From NICE Clinical Guideline 127 – see p. 641.

18.93 Optimal target blood pressures[1]

Age	Clinic BP (mmHg)	Ambulatory or home BP (mmHg)[2]
< 80 yrs	< 140/90	< 135/85
≥ 80 yrs	< 150/90	< 140/85

[1]Both systolic and diastolic values should be attained.
[2]Average BP during waking hours.

Antihypertensive drugs

Thiazide and other diuretics. The mechanism of action of these drugs is incompletely understood and it may take up to a month for the maximum effect to be observed. An appropriate daily dose is 2.5 mg bendroflumethiazide or 0.5 mg cyclopenthiazide. More potent loop diuretics, such as furosemide (40 mg daily) or bumetanide (1 mg daily), have few advantages over thiazides in the treatment of hypertension, unless there is substantial renal impairment or they are used in conjunction with an ACE inhibitor.

ACE inhibitors. ACE inhibitors (e.g. enalapril 20 mg daily, ramipril 5–10 mg daily or lisinopril 10–40 mg daily) inhibit the conversion of angiotensin I to angiotensin II and are usually well tolerated. They should be used with particular care in patients with impaired renal function or renal artery stenosis because they can reduce the filtration pressure in the glomeruli and precipitate renal failure. Electrolytes and creatinine should be checked before and 1–2 weeks after commencing therapy. Side-effects include first-dose hypotension, cough, rash, hyperkalaemia and renal dysfunction.

Angiotensin receptor blockers. Angiotensin receptor blockers (e.g. irbesartan 150–300 mg daily, valsartan

40–160 mg daily) block the angiotensin II type I receptor and have similar effects to ACE inhibitors; however, they do not cause cough and are better tolerated.

Calcium channel antagonists. The dihydropyridines (e.g. amlodipine 5–10 mg daily, nifedipine 30–90 mg daily) are effective and usually well-tolerated antihypertensive drugs that are particularly useful in older people. Side-effects include flushing, palpitations and fluid retention. The rate-limiting calcium channel antagonists (e.g. diltiazem 200–300 mg daily, verapamil 240 mg daily) can be useful when hypertension coexists with angina but they may cause bradycardia. The main side-effect of verapamil is constipation.

Beta-blockers. These are no longer used as first-line antihypertensive therapy, except in patients with another indication for the drug (e.g. angina). Metoprolol (100–200 mg daily), atenolol (50–100 mg daily) and bisoprolol (5–10 mg daily) preferentially block cardiac β_1-adrenoceptors, as opposed to the β_2-adrenoceptors that mediate vasodilatation and bronchodilatation.

Labetalol and carvedilol. Labetalol (200 mg–2.4 g daily in divided doses) and carvedilol (6.25–25 mg twice daily) are combined β- and α-adrenoceptor antagonists which are sometimes more effective than pure β-blockers. Labetalol can be used as an infusion in malignant phase hypertension (see below).

Other drugs. A variety of vasodilators may be used. These include the α_1-adrenoceptor antagonists (α-blockers), such as prazosin (0.5–20 mg daily in divided doses), indoramin (25–100 mg twice daily) and doxazosin (1–16 mg daily), and drugs that act directly on vascular smooth muscle, such as hydralazine (25–100 mg twice daily) and minoxidil (10–50 mg daily). Side-effects include first-dose and postural hypotension, headache, tachycardia and fluid retention. Minoxidil also causes increased facial hair and is therefore unsuitable for female patients.

Choice of antihypertensive drug

Trials that have compared thiazides, calcium antagonists, ACE inhibitors and angiotensin receptor blockers have not shown consistent differences in outcome, efficacy, side-effects or quality of life. Beta-blockers, which previously featured as first-line therapy in guidelines, have a weaker evidence base (see Box 18.91). The choice of antihypertensive therapy is initially dictated by the patient's age and ethnic background, although cost and convenience will influence the exact drug and preparation used. Response to initial therapy and side-effects guides subsequent treatment. Comorbid conditions also have an influence on initial drug selection (Box 18.94); for example, a β-blocker might be the most appropriate treatment for a patient with angina. Thiazide diuretics and dihydropyridine calcium channel antagonists are the most suitable drugs for treatment in older people.

Although some patients can be treated with a single antihypertensive drug, a combination of drugs is often required to achieve optimal BP control (Fig. 18.85). Combination therapy may be desirable for other reasons; for example, low-dose therapy with two drugs may produce fewer unwanted effects than treatment with the maximum dose of a single drug. Some drug combinations have complementary or synergistic actions; for example, thiazides increase activity of the renin–angiotensin system, while ACE inhibitors block it.

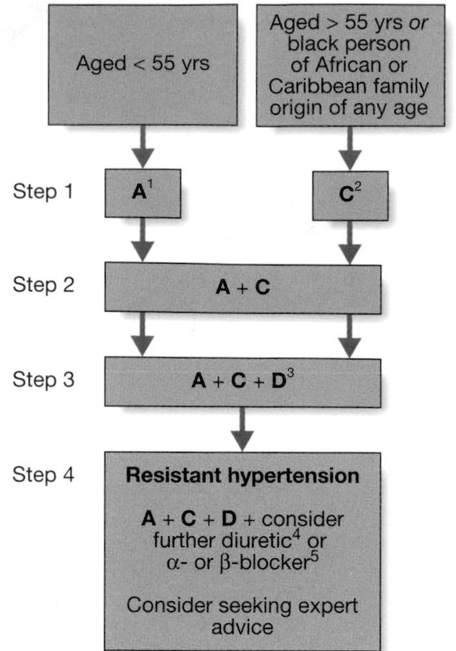

Fig. 18.85 Antihypertensive drug combinations. Black patients are those of African or Caribbean descent, and not mixed-race, Asian or Chinese patients. [1]A = ACE inhibitor or consider angiotensin II receptor blocker (ARB); choose a low-cost ARB. [2]C = calcium channel blocker (CCB); a CCB is preferred but consider a thiazide-like diuretic if a CCB is not tolerated or the person has oedema, evidence of heart failure or a high risk of heart failure. [3]D = thiazide-type diuretic. [4]Consider a low dose of spironolactone or higher doses of a thiazide-like diuretic. At the time of publication by NICE (August 2011), spironolactone did not have a UK marketing authorisation for this indication. Informed consent should be obtained and documented. [5]Consider an α- or β-blocker if further diuretic therapy is not tolerated, or is contraindicated or ineffective. From NICE Clinical Guideline 127 – see p. 641.

Emergency treatment of accelerated phase or malignant hypertension

In accelerated phase hypertension, lowering BP too quickly may compromise tissue perfusion (due to altered autoregulation) and can cause cerebral damage, including occipital blindness, and precipitate coronary or renal insufficiency. Even in the presence of cardiac failure or hypertensive encephalopathy, a controlled reduction to a level of about 150/90 mmHg over a period of 24–48 hours is ideal.

In most patients, it is possible to avoid parenteral therapy and bring BP under control with bed rest and oral drug therapy. Intravenous or intramuscular labetalol (2 mg/min to a maximum of 200 mg), intravenous glyceryl trinitrate (0.6–1.2 mg/hr), intramuscular hydralazine (5 or 10 mg aliquots repeated at half-hourly intervals) and intravenous sodium nitroprusside (0.3–1.0 μg/kg body weight/min) are all effective but require careful supervision, preferably in a high-dependency unit.

Refractory hypertension

The common causes of treatment failure in hypertension are non-adherence to drug therapy, inadequate therapy, and failure to recognise an underlying cause, such as

18.94 The influence of comorbidity on the choice of antihypertensive drug therapy

Class of drug	Compelling indications	Possible indications	Caution	Compelling contraindications
α-blockers	Benign prostatic hypertrophy	–	Postural hypotension, heart failure[1]	Urinary incontinence
ACE inhibitors	Heart failure Left ventricular dysfunction, post-MI or established coronary artery disease Type 1 diabetic nephropathy Secondary stroke prevention[4]	Chronic renal disease[2] Type 2 diabetic nephropathy	Renal impairment[2] Peripheral vascular disease[3]	Pregnancy Renovascular disease[2]
Angiotensin II receptor blockers	ACE inhibitor intolerance Type 2 diabetic nephropathy Hypertension with left ventricular hypertrophy Heart failure in ACE-intolerant patients, after MI	Left ventricular dysfunction after MI Intolerance of other antihypertensive drugs Proteinuric renal disease, chronic renal disease[2] Heart failure	Renal impairment[2] Peripheral vascular disease[3]	Pregnancy
β-blockers	MI, angina Heart failure[5]	–	Heart failure[5] Peripheral vascular disease Diabetes (except with coronary artery disease)	Asthma or chronic obstructive pulmonary disease Heart block
Calcium channel blockers (dihydropyridine)	Older patients, isolated systolic hypertension	Angina	–	–
Calcium channel blockers (rate-limiting)	Angina	Older patients	Combination with β-blockade	Atrioventricular block, heart failure
Thiazides or thiazide-like diuretics	Older patients, isolated systolic hypertension, heart failure, secondary stroke prevention	–	–	Gout[6]

[1]In heart failure when used as monotherapy. [2]ACE inhibitors or angiotensin II receptor blockers may be beneficial in chronic renal failure and renovascular disease but should be used with caution, close supervision and specialist advice when there is established and significant renal impairment. [3]Caution with ACE inhibitors and angiotensin II receptor blockers in peripheral vascular disease because of association with renovascular disease. [4]In combination with a thiazide or thiazide-like diuretic. [5]β-blockers are used increasingly to treat stable heart failure but may worsen acute heart failure. [6]Thiazides or thiazide-like diuretics may sometimes be necessary to control BP in people with a history of gout, ideally used in combination with allopurinol.

renal artery stenosis or phaeochromocytoma; of these, the first is by far the most prevalent. There is no easy solution to compliance problems but simple treatment regimens, attempts to improve rapport with the patient and careful supervision may all help.

Adjuvant drug therapy

- *Aspirin*. Antiplatelet therapy is a powerful means of reducing cardiovascular risk but may cause bleeding, particularly intracerebral haemorrhage, in a small number of patients. The benefits are thought to outweigh the risks in hypertensive patients aged 50 years or over who have well-controlled BP and either target organ damage, diabetes or a 10-year coronary artery disease risk of at least 15% (or 10-year cardiovascular disease risk of at least 20%).
- *Statins*. Treating hyperlipidaemia can produce a substantial reduction in cardiovascular risk. These drugs are strongly indicated in patients who have established vascular disease, or hypertension with a high (at least 20% in 10 years) risk of developing cardiovascular disease (p. 583).

DISEASES OF THE HEART VALVES

A diseased valve may be narrowed (stenosed) or may fail to close adequately, and thus permit regurgitation of blood. 'Incompetence' is a less precise term for regurgitation or reflux, and should be avoided. Box 18.95 gives the principal causes of valve disease.

Doppler echocardiography is the most useful technique for assessing valvular heart disease (p. 536) but may also detect minor and even 'physiological' abnormalities, e.g. trivial mitral regurgitation. Disease of the heart valves may progress with time and selected patients require regular review every 1 or 2 years, to ensure that deterioration is detected before complications, such as heart failure, ensue. Patients with valvular heart disease are susceptible to bacterial endocarditis, which can be prevented by good dental hygiene. The routine use of

18.95 Principal causes of valve disease

Valve regurgitation	
• Congenital • Acute rheumatic carditis • Chronic rheumatic carditis • Infective endocarditis • Valve ring dilatation (e.g. dilated cardiomyopathy)	• Syphilitic aortitis • Traumatic valve rupture • Senile degeneration • Damage to chordae and papillary muscles (e.g. MI)
Valve stenosis	
• Congenital • Rheumatic carditis	• Senile degeneration

antibiotic prophylaxis at times of bacteraemia, e.g. dental extraction, is no longer recommended.

Rheumatic heart disease

Acute rheumatic fever

Incidence and pathogenesis

Acute rheumatic fever usually affects children (most commonly between 5 and 15 years) or young adults, and has become very rare in Western Europe and North America. However, it remains endemic in parts of Asia, Africa and South America, with an annual incidence in some countries of more than 100 per 100 000, and is the most common cause of acquired heart disease in childhood and adolescence.

The condition is triggered by an immune-mediated delayed response to infection with specific strains of group A streptococci, which have antigens that may cross-react with cardiac myosin and sarcolemmal membrane protein. Antibodies produced against the streptococcal antigens cause inflammation in the endocardium, myocardium and pericardium, as well as the joints and skin. Histologically, fibrinoid degeneration is seen in the collagen of connective tissues. Aschoff nodules are pathognomonic and occur only in the heart. They are composed of multinucleated giant cells surrounded by macrophages and T lymphocytes, and are not seen until the subacute or chronic phases of rheumatic carditis.

Clinical features

Acute rheumatic fever is a multisystem disorder that usually presents with fever, anorexia, lethargy and joint pain, 2–3 weeks after an episode of streptococcal pharyngitis. There may, however, be no history of sore throat. Arthritis occurs in approximately 75% of patients. Other features include rashes, carditis and neurological changes (Fig. 18.86). The diagnosis, made using the revised Jones criteria (Box 18.96), is based upon two or more major manifestations, or one major and two or more minor manifestations, along with evidence of preceding streptococcal infection. Only about 25% of patients will have a positive culture for group A streptococcus at the time of diagnosis because there is a latent period between infection and presentation. Serological evidence of recent infection with a raised antistreptolysin O (ASO) antibody titre is helpful. A presumptive diagnosis of acute rheumatic fever can be made without

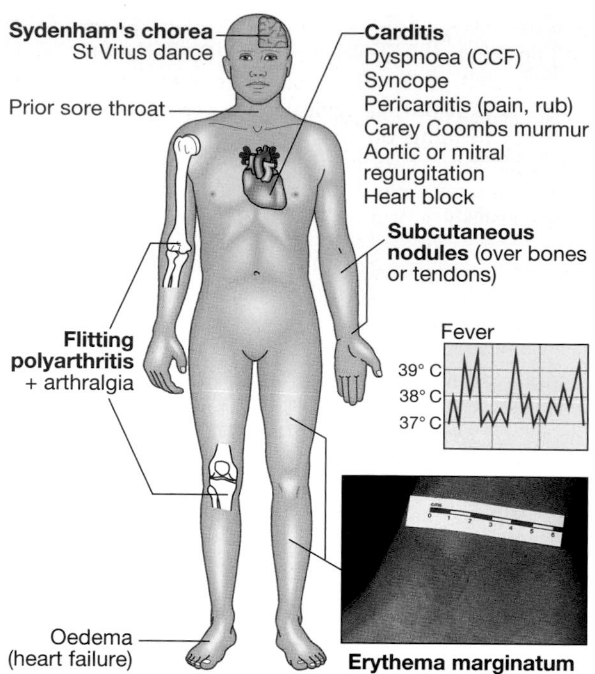

Fig. 18.86 Clinical features of rheumatic fever. Bold labels indicate Jones major criteria (CCF = congestive cardiac failure). *Inset (Erythema marginatum)* From Savin et al. 1997 – see p. 641.

18.96 Jones criteria for the diagnosis of rheumatic fever

Major manifestations	
• Carditis • Polyarthritis • Chorea	• Erythema marginatum • Subcutaneous nodules
Minor manifestations	
• Fever • Arthralgia • Previous rheumatic fever	• Raised ESR or CRP • Leucocytosis • First-degree AV block
Plus	
• Supporting evidence of preceding streptococcal infection: recent scarlet fever, raised antistreptolysin O or other streptococcal antibody titre, positive throat culture	
N.B. Evidence of recent streptococcal infection is particularly important if there is only one major manifestation.	

evidence of preceding streptococcal infection in cases of isolated chorea or pancarditis, if other causes for these have been excluded. In cases of established rheumatic heart disease or prior rheumatic fever, a diagnosis of acute rheumatic fever can be made based only on the presence of multiple minor criteria and evidence of preceding group A streptococcal pharyngitis.

Carditis

A 'pancarditis' involves the endocardium, myocardium and pericardium to varying degrees. Its incidence declines with increasing age, ranging from 90% at 3 years to around 30% in adolescence. It may manifest as breathlessness (due to heart failure or pericardial effusion), palpitations or chest pain (usually due to pericarditis or pancarditis). Other features include tachycardia, cardiac enlargement and new or changed murmurs. A soft systolic murmur due to mitral regurgitation is very common. A soft mid-diastolic murmur (the Carey Coombs murmur) is typically due to valvulitis, with nodules forming on the mitral valve leaflets. Aortic regurgitation occurs in 50% of cases but the tricuspid and pulmonary valves are rarely involved. Pericarditis may cause chest pain, a pericardial friction rub and precordial tenderness. Cardiac failure may be due to myocardial dysfunction or valvular regurgitation. ECG changes commonly include ST and T wave changes. Conduction defects sometimes occur and may cause syncope.

Arthritis

This is the most common major manifestation and occurs early when streptococcal antibody titres are high. An acute painful asymmetric and migratory inflammation of the large joints typically affects the knees, ankles, elbows and wrists. The joints are involved in quick succession and are usually red, swollen and tender for between a day and 4 weeks. The pain characteristically responds to aspirin; if not, the diagnosis is in doubt.

Skin lesions

Erythema marginatum occurs in less than 5% of patients. The lesions start as red macules that fade in the centre but remain red at the edges, and occur mainly on the trunk and proximal extremities but not the face. The resulting red rings or 'margins' may coalesce or overlap (see Fig. 18.86). Subcutaneous nodules occur in 5–7% of patients. They are small (0.5–2.0 cm), firm and painless, and are best felt over extensor surfaces of bone or tendons. They typically appear more than 3 weeks after the onset of other manifestations and therefore help to confirm rather than make the diagnosis. Other systemic manifestations are rare but include pleurisy, pleural effusion and pneumonia.

Sydenham's chorea (St Vitus dance)

This is a late neurological manifestation that appears at least 3 months after the episode of acute rheumatic fever, when all the other signs may have disappeared. It occurs in up to one-third of cases and is more common in females. Emotional lability may be the first feature and is typically followed by purposeless, involuntary, choreiform movements of the hands, feet or face. Speech may be explosive and halting. Spontaneous recovery usually occurs within a few months. Approximately one-quarter of affected patients will go on to develop chronic rheumatic valve disease.

Investigations

The ESR and CRP are useful for monitoring progress of the disease (Box 18.97). Positive throat swab cultures are obtained in only 10–25% of cases. ASO titres are normal in one-fifth of adult cases of rheumatic fever and most cases of chorea. Echocardiography typically shows mitral regurgitation with dilatation of the mitral annulus and prolapse of the anterior mitral leaflet, and may also show aortic regurgitation and pericardial effusion.

Management of the acute attack

A single dose of benzyl penicillin (1.2 million U IM) or oral phenoxymethylpenicillin (250 mg 4 times daily for 10 days) should be given on diagnosis to eliminate any residual streptococcal infection. If the patient is penicillin-allergic, erythromycin or a cephalosporin can be used. Treatment is then directed towards limiting cardiac damage and relieving symptoms.

18.97 Investigations in acute rheumatic fever

Evidence of a systemic illness (non-specific)
• Leucocytosis, raised ESR and CRP
Evidence of preceding streptococcal infection (specific)
• Throat swab culture: group A β-haemolytic streptococci (also from family members and contacts)
• Antistreptolysin O antibodies (ASO titres): rising titres, or levels of > 200 U (adults) or > 300 U (children)
Evidence of carditis
• Chest X-ray: cardiomegaly; pulmonary congestion
• ECG: first- and rarely second-degree AV block; features of pericarditis; T-wave inversion; reduction in QRS voltages
• Echocardiography: cardiac dilatation and valve abnormalities

Bed rest and supportive therapy

Bed rest is important, as it lessens joint pain and reduces cardiac workload. The duration should be guided by symptoms, along with temperature, leucocyte count and ESR, and should be continued until these have settled. Patients can then return to normal physical activity but strenuous exercise should be avoided in those who have had carditis.

Cardiac failure should be treated as necessary. Some patients, particularly those in early adolescence, develop a fulminant form of the disease with severe mitral regurgitation and, sometimes, concomitant aortic regurgitation. If heart failure in these cases does not respond to medical treatment, valve replacement may be necessary and is often associated with a dramatic decline in rheumatic activity. AV block is seldom progressive and pacemaker insertion rarely needed.

Aspirin

This usually relieves the symptoms of arthritis rapidly and a response within 24 hours helps confirm the diagnosis. A reasonable starting dose is 60 mg/kg body weight/day, divided into six doses. In adults, 100 mg/kg per day may be needed up to the limits of tolerance or a maximum of 8 g per day. Mild toxicity includes nausea, tinnitus and deafness; vomiting, tachypnoea and acidosis are more serious. Aspirin should be continued until the ESR has fallen, and then gradually tailed off.

Corticosteroids

These produce more rapid symptomatic relief than aspirin and are indicated in cases with carditis or severe arthritis. There is no evidence that long-term steroids are beneficial. Prednisolone (1.0–2.0 mg/kg per day in divided doses) should be continued until the ESR is normal, and then tailed off.

Secondary prevention

Patients are susceptible to further attacks of rheumatic fever if another streptococcal infection occurs, and long-term prophylaxis with penicillin should be given as benzathine penicillin (1.2 million U IM monthly), if compliance is in doubt, or oral phenoxymethylpenicillin (250 mg twice daily). Sulfadiazine or erythromycin may be used if the patient is allergic to penicillin; sulphonamides prevent infection but are not effective in the eradication of group A streptococci. Further attacks of rheumatic fever are unusual after the age of 21, when treatment may be stopped. However, it should be extended if an attack has occurred in the last 5 years, or if the patient lives in an area of high prevalence or has an occupation (e.g. teaching) with high exposure to streptococcal infection. In those with residual heart disease, prophylaxis should continue until 10 years after the last episode or 40 years of age, whichever is later. Long-term antibiotic prophylaxis prevents another attack of acute rheumatic fever but does not protect against infective endocarditis.

Chronic rheumatic heart disease

Chronic valvular heart disease develops in at least half of those affected by rheumatic fever with carditis. Two-thirds of cases occur in women. Some episodes of rheumatic fever pass unrecognised and it is only possible to elicit a history of rheumatic fever or chorea in about half of all patients with chronic rheumatic heart disease.

The mitral valve is affected in more than 90% of cases; the aortic valve is the next most frequently involved, followed by the tricuspid and then the pulmonary valve. Isolated mitral stenosis accounts for about 25% of all cases, and an additional 40% have mixed mitral stenosis and regurgitation. Valve disease may be symptomatic during fulminant forms of acute rheumatic fever but may remain asymptomatic for many years.

Pathology

The main pathological process in chronic rheumatic heart disease is progressive fibrosis. The heart valves are predominantly affected but involvement of the pericardium and myocardium may contribute to heart failure and conduction disorders. Fusion of the mitral valve commissures and shortening of the chordae tendineae may lead to mitral stenosis with or without regurgitation. Similar changes in the aortic and tricuspid valves produce distortion and rigidity of the cusps, leading to stenosis and regurgitation. Once a valve has been damaged, the altered haemodynamic stresses perpetuate and extend the damage, even in the absence of a continuing rheumatic process.

Mitral valve disease

Mitral stenosis

Aetiology and pathophysiology

Mitral stenosis is almost always rheumatic in origin, although in older people it can be caused by heavy calcification of the mitral valve apparatus. There is also a rare form of congenital mitral stenosis.

In rheumatic mitral stenosis, the mitral valve orifice is slowly diminished by progressive fibrosis, calcification of the valve leaflets, and fusion of the cusps and subvalvular apparatus. The flow of blood from LA to LV is restricted and left atrial pressure rises, leading to pulmonary venous congestion and breathlessness. There is dilatation and hypertrophy of the LA, and left ventricular filling becomes more dependent on left atrial contraction.

Any increase in heart rate shortens diastole when the mitral valve is open and produces a further rise in left atrial pressure. Situations that demand an increase in cardiac output also increase left atrial pressure, so exercise and pregnancy are poorly tolerated.

The mitral valve orifice is normally about 5 cm^2 in diastole and may be reduced to 1 cm^2 in severe mitral stenosis. Patients usually remain asymptomatic until the stenosis is less than 2 cm^2. Reduced lung compliance, due to chronic pulmonary venous congestion, contributes to breathlessness, and a low cardiac output may cause fatigue.

Atrial fibrillation due to progressive dilatation of the LA is very common. Its onset often precipitates pulmonary oedema because the accompanying tachycardia and loss of atrial contraction lead to marked haemodynamic deterioration with a rapid rise in left atrial pressure. In contrast, a more gradual rise in left atrial pressure tends to cause an increase in pulmonary vascular resistance, which leads to pulmonary hypertension that may protect the patient from pulmonary oedema. Pulmonary hypertension leads to right ventricular hypertrophy and dilatation, tricuspid regurgitation and right heart failure.

Fewer than 20% of patients remain in sinus rhythm; many of these have a small fibrotic LA and severe pulmonary hypertension.

Clinical features

Effort-related dyspnoea is usually the dominant symptom (Box 18.98). Exercise tolerance typically diminishes very slowly over many years and patients often do not appreciate the extent of their disability. Eventually, symptoms occur at rest. Acute pulmonary oedema or pulmonary hypertension can lead to haemoptysis. All patients with mitral stenosis, and particularly those with atrial fibrillation, are at risk from left atrial thrombosis and systemic thromboembolism. Prior to the advent of anticoagulant therapy, emboli caused one-quarter of all deaths.

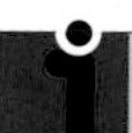

18.98 Clinical features (and their causes) in mitral stenosis

Symptoms

- Breathlessness (pulmonary congestion)
- Fatigue (low cardiac output)
- Oedema, ascites (right heart failure)
- Palpitation (atrial fibrillation)
- Haemoptysis (pulmonary congestion, pulmonary embolism)
- Cough (pulmonary congestion)
- Chest pain (pulmonary hypertension)
- Thromboembolic complications (e.g. stroke, ischaemic limb)

Signs

- Atrial fibrillation
- Mitral facies
- Auscultation
  - Loud first heart sound, opening snap
  - Mid-diastolic murmur
- Crepitations, pulmonary oedema, effusions (raised pulmonary capillary pressure)
- RV heave, loud P_2 (pulmonary hypertension)

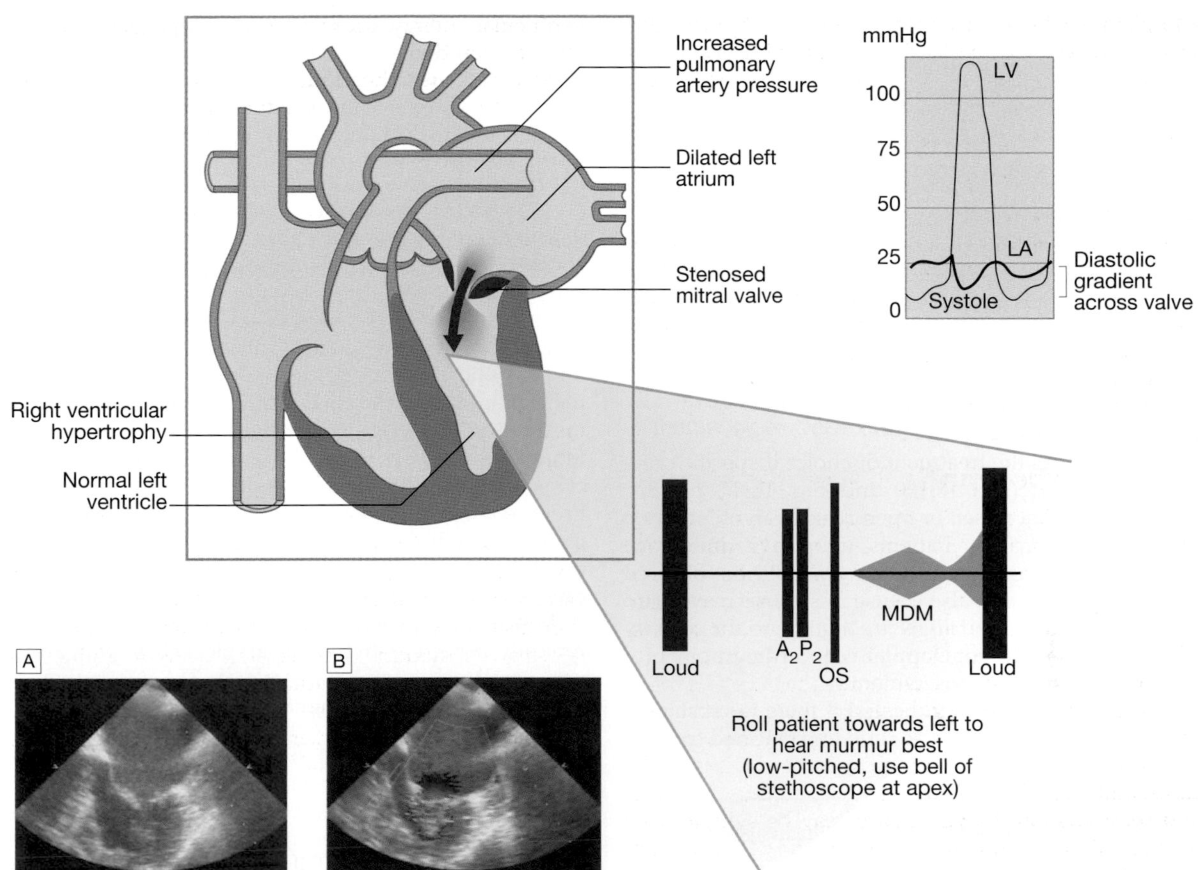

Fig. 18.87 Mitral stenosis: murmur and the diastolic pressure gradient between LA and LV. (Mean gradient is reflected by the area between LA and LV in diastole.) The first heart sound is loud, and there is an opening snap (OS) and mid-diastolic murmur (MDM) with pre-systolic accentuation. **A** Echocardiogram showing reduced opening of the mitral valve in diastole. **B** Colour Doppler showing turbulent flow.

The physical signs of mitral stenosis are often found before symptoms develop and their recognition is of particular importance in pregnancy. The forces that open and close the mitral valve increase as left atrial pressure rises. The first heart sound (S1) is therefore loud and can be palpable (tapping apex beat). An opening snap may be audible and moves closer to the second sound (S2) as the stenosis becomes more severe and left atrial pressure rises. However, the first heart sound and opening snap may be inaudible if the valve is heavily calcified.

Turbulent flow produces the characteristic low-pitched mid-diastolic murmur and sometimes a thrill (Fig. 18.87). The murmur is accentuated by exercise and during atrial systole (pre-systolic accentuation). Early in the disease, a pre-systolic murmur may be the only auscultatory abnormality but, in patients with symptoms, the murmur extends from the opening snap to the first heart sound. Coexisting mitral regurgitation causes a pansystolic murmur that radiates towards the axilla.

Pulmonary hypertension may ultimately lead to right ventricular hypertrophy and dilatation with secondary tricuspid regurgitation, which causes a systolic murmur and giant '*v* waves' in the venous pulse.

Investigations

The ECG may show either atrial fibrillation or bifid P waves (P mitrale) associated with left atrial hypertrophy (Box 18.99). A typical chest X-ray is shown in Figure 18.9 (p. 535). Doppler echocardiography provides the definitive evaluation of mitral stenosis (see Fig. 18.87). Cardiac catheterisation is used to assess coexisting conditions.

18.99 Investigations in mitral stenosis

ECG	
• Right ventricular hypertrophy: tall R waves in V_1–V_3	• P mitrale or atrial fibrillation
Chest X-ray	
• Enlarged LA and appendage	• Signs of pulmonary venous congestion
Echo	
• Thickened immobile cusps • Reduced valve area • Enlarged LA	• Reduced rate of diastolic filling of LV
Doppler	
• Pressure gradient across mitral valve	• Pulmonary artery pressure • Left ventricular function
Cardiac catheterisation	
• Coronary artery disease • Pulmonary artery pressure	• Mitral stenosis and regurgitation

Management

Patients with minor symptoms should be treated medically. Intervention by balloon valvuloplasty, mitral valvotomy or mitral valve replacement should be considered if the patient remains symptomatic despite medical treatment or if pulmonary hypertension develops.

Medical management

This consists of anticoagulation to reduce the risk of systemic embolism, ventricular rate control (digoxin, β-blockers or rate-limiting calcium antagonists) in atrial fibrillation, and diuretic therapy to control pulmonary congestion. Antibiotic prophylaxis against infective endocarditis is no longer routinely recommended.

Mitral balloon valvuloplasty and valve replacement

Valvuloplasty is the treatment of choice if specific criteria are fulfilled (Box 18.100 and Fig. 18.67, p. 587), although surgical closed or open mitral valvotomy is an acceptable alternative. Patients who have undergone mitral valvuloplasty or valvotomy should be followed up at 1–2-yearly intervals because re-stenosis may occur. Clinical symptoms and signs are a guide to the severity of mitral re-stenosis but Doppler echocardiography provides a more accurate assessment.

Valve replacement is indicated if there is substantial mitral reflux or if the valve is rigid and calcified (p. 629).

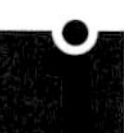

18.100 Criteria for mitral valvuloplasty*

- Significant symptoms
- Isolated mitral stenosis
- No (or trivial) mitral regurgitation
- Mobile, non-calcified valve/subvalve apparatus on echo
- LA free of thrombus

*For comprehensive guidelines on valvular heart disease, see www.acc.org

Mitral regurgitation

Aetiology and pathophysiology

Rheumatic disease is the principal cause in countries where rheumatic fever is common, but elsewhere, including in the UK, other causes are more important (Box 18.101). Mitral regurgitation may also follow mitral valvotomy or valvuloplasty.

Chronic mitral regurgitation causes gradual dilatation of the LA with little increase in pressure and therefore relatively few symptoms. Nevertheless, the LV dilates slowly and the left ventricular diastolic and left atrial pressures gradually increase as a result of chronic volume overload of the LV. In contrast, acute mitral regurgitation causes a rapid rise in left atrial pressure (because left atrial compliance is normal) and marked symptomatic deterioration.

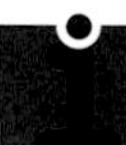

18.101 Causes of mitral regurgitation

- Mitral valve prolapse
- Dilatation of the LV and mitral valve ring (e.g. coronary artery disease, cardiomyopathy)
- Damage to valve cusps and chordae (e.g. rheumatic heart disease, endocarditis)
- Ischaemia or infarction of the papillary muscle
- Myocardial infarction

Mitral valve prolapse

This is also known as 'floppy' mitral valve and is one of the more common causes of mild mitral regurgitation (Fig. 18.88). It is caused by congenital anomalies or degenerative myxomatous changes, and is sometimes a feature of connective tissue disorders such as Marfan's syndrome (p. 603).

In its mildest forms, the valve remains competent but bulges back into the atrium during systole, causing a mid-systolic click but no murmur. In the presence of a regurgitant valve, the click is followed by a late systolic murmur, which lengthens as the regurgitation becomes more severe. A click is not always audible and the physical signs may vary with both posture and respiration. Progressive elongation of the chordae tendineae leads to increasing mitral regurgitation, and if chordal rupture occurs, regurgitation suddenly becomes severe. This is rare before the fifth or sixth decade of life.

Mitral valve prolapse is associated with a variety of typically benign arrhythmias, atypical chest pain and a very small risk of embolic stroke or TIA. Nevertheless, the overall long-term prognosis is good.

Other causes of mitral regurgitation

Mitral valve function depends on the chordae tendineae and their papillary muscles; dilatation of the LV distorts the geometry of these and may cause mitral regurgitation (see Box 18.101). Dilated cardiomyopathy and heart failure from coronary artery disease are common causes of so-called 'functional' mitral regurgitation. Endocarditis is an important cause of acute mitral regurgitation.

Clinical features

Symptoms depend on how suddenly the regurgitation develops (Box 18.102). Chronic mitral regurgitation produces a symptom complex that is similar to that of mitral stenosis, but sudden-onset mitral regurgitation usually presents with acute pulmonary oedema.

The regurgitant jet causes an apical systolic murmur (see Fig. 18.88), which radiates into the axilla and may be accompanied by a thrill. Increased forward flow through the mitral valve causes a loud third heart sound

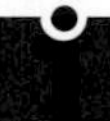

18.102 Clinical features (and their causes) in mitral regurgitation

Symptoms

- Dyspnoea (pulmonary venous congestion)
- Fatigue (low cardiac output)
- Palpitation (atrial fibrillation, increased stroke volume)
- Oedema, ascites (right heart failure)

Signs

- Atrial fibrillation/flutter
- Cardiomegaly: displaced hyperdynamic apex beat
- Apical pansystolic murmur ± thrill
- Soft S1, apical S3
- Signs of pulmonary venous congestion (crepitations, pulmonary oedema, effusions)
- Signs of pulmonary hypertension and right heart failure

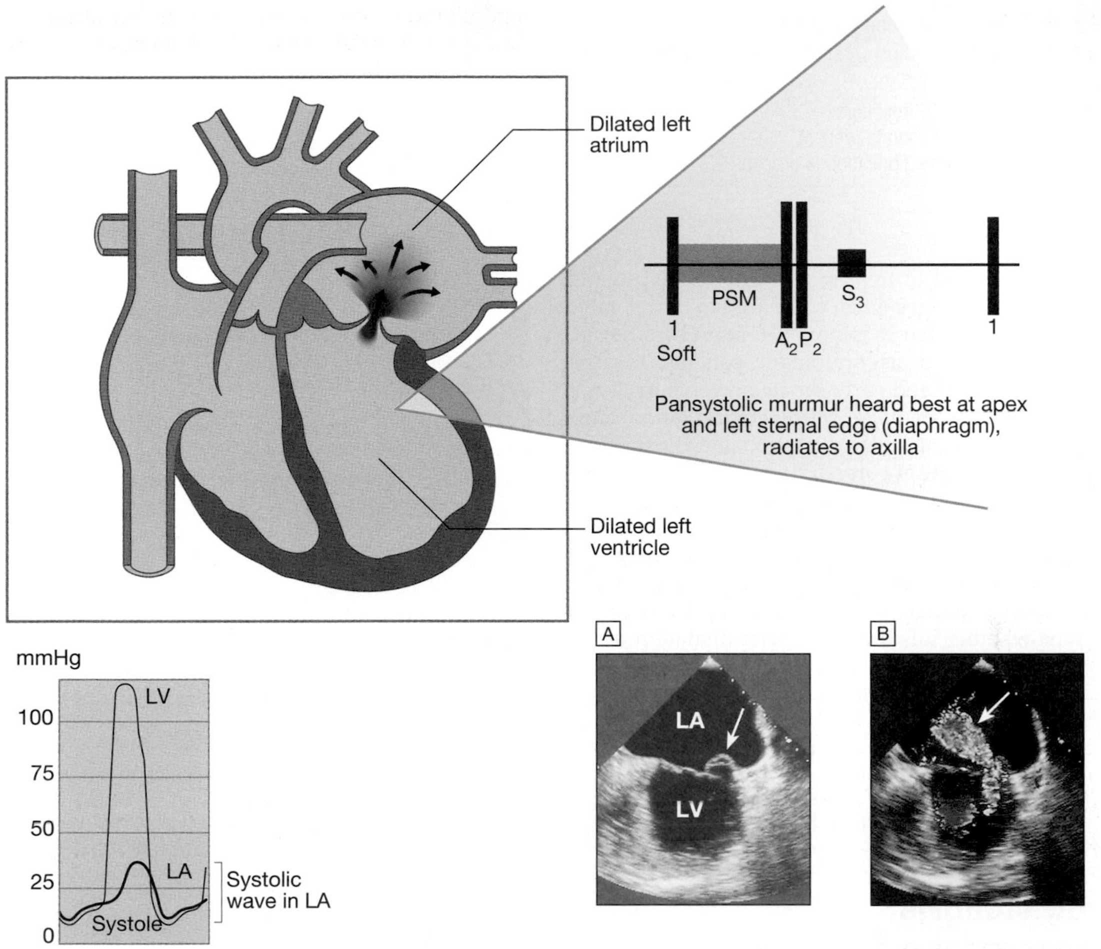

Fig. 18.88 Mitral regurgitation: murmur and systolic wave in left atrial pressure. The first sound is normal or soft and merges with a pansystolic murmur (PSM) extending to the second heart sound. A third heart sound occurs with severe regurgitation. **A** A transoesophageal echocardiogram shows mitral valve prolapse, with one leaflet bulging towards the LA (arrow). **B** This results in a jet of mitral regurgitation on colour Doppler (arrow).

and even a short mid-diastolic murmur. The apex beat feels active and rocking due to left ventricular volume overload and is usually displaced to the left as a result of left ventricular dilatation.

Investigations

Atrial fibrillation is common, as a consequence of atrial dilatation. At cardiac catheterisation (Box 18.103), the severity of mitral regurgitation can be assessed by left ventriculography and by the size of the *v* (systolic) waves in the left atrial or pulmonary artery wedge pressure trace.

Management

Mitral regurgitation of moderate severity can be treated medically (Box 18.104). In all patients with mitral regurgitation, high afterload may worsen the degree of regurgitation, and hypertension should be treated with vasodilators, such as ACE inhibitors. Patients should be reviewed at regular intervals because worsening symptoms, progressive cardiomegaly or echocardiographic evidence of deteriorating left ventricular function are indications for mitral valve replacement or repair. Mitral

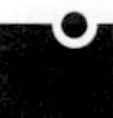

18.103 Investigations in mitral regurgitation

ECG
• Left atrial hypertrophy (if not in atrial fibrillation) • Left ventricular hypertrophy
Chest X-ray
• Enlarged LA • Enlarged LV • Pulmonary venous congestion • Pulmonary oedema (if acute)
Echo
• Dilated LA, LV • Dynamic LV (unless myocardial dysfunction predominates) • Structural abnormalities of mitral valve (e.g. prolapse)
Doppler
• Detects and quantifies regurgitation
Cardiac catheterisation
• Dilated LA, dilated LV, mitral regurgitation • Pulmonary hypertension • Coexisting coronary artery disease

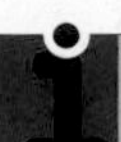

18.104 Medical management of mitral regurgitation
• Diuretics • Vasodilators, e.g. ACE inhibitors • Digoxin if atrial fibrillation is present • Anticoagulants if atrial fibrillation is present

valve repair is used to treat mitral valve prolapse and offers many advantages when compared to mitral valve replacement, such that it is now advocated for severe regurgitation, even in asymptomatic patients, because results are excellent and early repair prevents irreversible left ventricular damage. Mitral regurgitation often accompanies the ventricular dilatation and dysfunction that are concomitants of coronary artery disease. If such patients are to undergo coronary bypass graft surgery, it is common practice to repair the valve and restore mitral valve function by inserting an annuloplasty ring to overcome annular dilatation and to bring the valve leaflets closer together. It can be difficult, however, to determine whether it is the ventricular dilatation or the mitral regurgitation that is the predominant problem. If ventricular dilatation is the underlying cause of mitral regurgitation, then mitral valve repair or replacement may actually worsen ventricular function, as the ventricle can no longer empty into the low-pressure LA.

Aortic valve disease

Aortic stenosis

Aetiology and pathophysiology

The likely aetiology depends on the age of the patient (Box 18.105). In congenital aortic stenosis, obstruction is present from birth or becomes apparent in infancy. With bicuspid aortic valves, obstruction may take years to develop as the valve becomes fibrotic and calcified. The aortic valve is the second most frequently affected by rheumatic fever and, commonly, both the aortic and mitral valves are involved. In older people, a structurally normal tricuspid aortic valve may be affected by fibrosis and calcification, in a process that is histologically similar to that of atherosclerosis affecting the arterial wall. Haemodynamically significant stenosis develops slowly, typically occurring at 30–60 years in those with rheumatic disease, 50–60 in those with bicuspid aortic valves and 70–90 in those with degenerative calcific disease.

Cardiac output is initially maintained at the cost of a steadily increasing pressure gradient across the aortic valve. The LV becomes increasingly hypertrophied and coronary blood flow may then be inadequate; patients may therefore develop angina, even in the absence of concomitant coronary disease. The fixed outflow obstruction limits the increase in cardiac output required on exercise. Eventually, the LV can no longer overcome the outflow tract obstruction and pulmonary oedema supervenes. In contrast to patients with mitral stenosis, which tends to progress very slowly, those with aortic stenosis typically remain asymptomatic for many years but deteriorate rapidly when symptoms develop, and death usually ensues within 3–5 years of these.

18.105 Causes of aortic stenosis
Infants, children, adolescents
• Congenital aortic stenosis • Congenital subvalvular aortic stenosis • Congenital supravalvular aortic stenosis
Young adults to middle-aged
• Calcification and fibrosis of congenitally bicuspid aortic valve • Rheumatic aortic stenosis
Middle-aged to elderly
• Senile degenerative aortic stenosis • Calcification of bicuspid valve • Rheumatic aortic stenosis

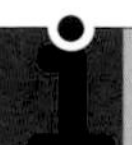

18.106 Clinical features of aortic stenosis	
Symptoms	
• Mild or moderate stenosis: usually asymptomatic • Exertional dyspnoea • Angina	• Exertional syncope • Sudden death • Episodes of acute pulmonary oedema
Signs	
• Ejection systolic murmur • Slow-rising carotid pulse • Thrusting apex beat (LV pressure overload)	• Narrow pulse pressure • Signs of pulmonary venous congestion (e.g. crepitations)

Clinical features

Aortic stenosis is commonly picked up in asymptomatic patients at routine clinical examination but the three cardinal symptoms are angina, breathlessness and syncope (Box 18.106). Angina arises because of the increased demands of the hypertrophied LV working against the high-pressure outflow tract obstruction, leading to a mismatch between oxygen demand and supply, but may also be due to coexisting coronary artery disease, especially in old age, when it affects over 50% of patients. Exertional breathlessness suggests cardiac decompensation as a consequence of the excessive pressure overload placed on the LV. Syncope usually occurs on exertion when cardiac output fails to rise to meet demand, leading to a fall in BP.

The characteristic clinical signs of severe aortic stenosis are shown in Box 18.106. A harsh ejection systolic murmur radiates to the neck, with a soft second heart sound, particularly in those with calcific valves. The murmur is often likened to a saw cutting wood and may (especially in older patients) have a musical quality like the 'mew' of a seagull (Fig. 18.89). The severity of aortic stenosis may be difficult to gauge clinically, as older patients with a non-compliant 'stiff' arterial system may have an apparently normal carotid upstroke in the presence of severe aortic stenosis. Milder degrees of stenosis may be difficult to distinguish from aortic sclerosis, in which the valve is thickened or calcified but not obstructed. A careful examination should be made for other valve lesions, particularly in rheumatic heart disease, when there is frequently concomitant mitral valve disease.

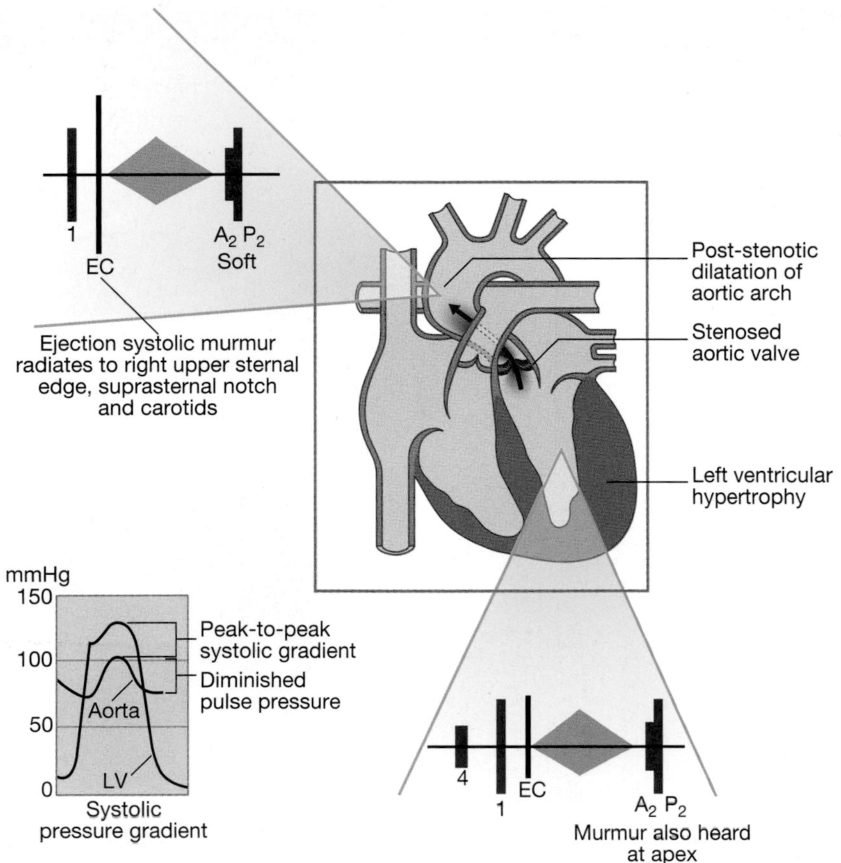

Fig. 18.89 Aortic stenosis. Pressure traces show the systolic gradient between LV and aorta. The 'diamond-shaped' murmur is heard best with the diaphragm in the aortic outflow and also at the apex. An ejection click (EC) may be present in young patients with a bicuspid aortic valve but not in older patients with calcified valves. Aortic stenosis may lead to left ventricular hypertrophy with a fourth sound at the apex and post-stenotic dilatation of the aortic arch. Figure 18.11 (p. 536) shows the typical Doppler signal with aortic stenosis.

18.107 Investigations in aortic stenosis

ECG
• Left ventricular hypertrophy (usually) • Left bundle branch block
Chest X-ray
• May be normal; sometimes enlarged LV and dilated ascending aorta on PA view, calcified valve on lateral view
Echo
• Calcified valve with restricted opening, hypertrophied LV (see Fig. 18.91)
Doppler
• Measurement of severity of stenosis • Detection of associated aortic regurgitation
Cardiac catheterisation
• Mainly to identify associated coronary artery disease • May be used to measure gradient between LV and aorta

Investigations

In advanced cases, ECG features of hypertrophy (Box 18.107) are often gross (Fig. 18.90), and down-sloping ST segments and T inversion ('strain pattern') are seen in leads reflecting the LV. Nevertheless, especially in old age, the ECG can be normal, despite severe stenosis. Echocardiography demonstrates restricted valve opening (Fig. 18.91) and Doppler assessment permits calculation of the systolic gradient across the aortic valve, from which the severity of stenosis can be assessed (see Fig. 18.11, p. 536). In patients with an impaired LV, velocities across the aortic valve may be diminished because of a reduced stroke volume, while when aortic regurgitation is present, velocities are increased because of an increased stroke volume. In these circumstances, aortic valve area calculated from Doppler measurements is a more accurate assessment of severity. CT and MRI are useful in assessing the degree of valve calcification and stenosis, respectively, but are rarely necessary.

Management

Irrespective of the severity of valve stenosis, patients with asymptomatic aortic stenosis have a good immediate prognosis and conservative management is appropriate. Such patients should be kept under review, as the development of angina, syncope, symptoms of low cardiac output or heart failure has a poor prognosis and is an indication for prompt surgery. In practice, patients with moderate or severe stenosis are evaluated every 1–2 years with Doppler echocardiography to detect progression in severity; this is more rapid in older patients with heavily calcified valves.

Patients with symptomatic severe aortic stenosis should have prompt aortic valve replacement. Old age

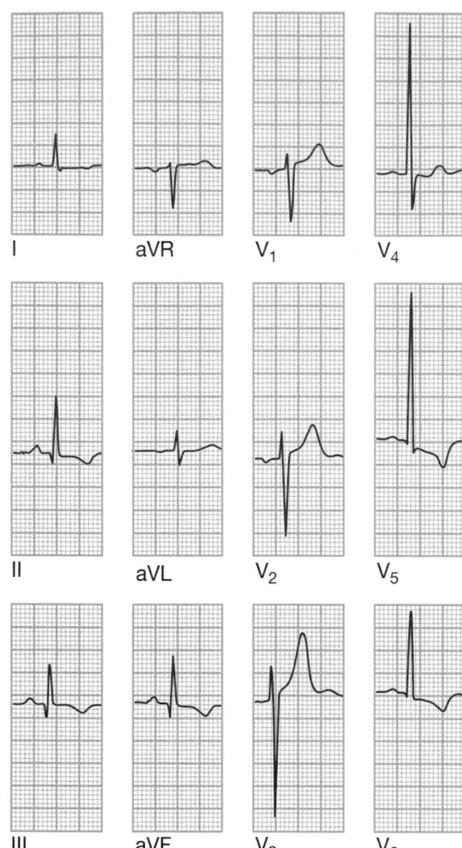

Fig. 18.90 Left ventricular hypertrophy. QRS complexes in limb leads have increased amplitude with a very large R wave in V_6 and S wave in V_2. There is ST depression and T-wave inversion in leads II, III, aVF, V_5 and V_6: a 'left ventricular strain' pattern.

18.108 Aortic stenosis in old age

- **Incidence**: the most common form of valve disease affecting the very old.
- **Symptoms**: a common cause of syncope, angina and heart failure in the very old.
- **Signs**: because of increasing stiffening in the central arteries, low pulse pressure and a slow rising pulse may not be present.
- **Surgery**: can be successful in those aged 80 yrs or more in the absence of comorbidity, but with a higher operative mortality. The prognosis without surgery is poor once symptoms have developed.
- **Valve replacement type**: a biological valve is often preferable to a mechanical one because this obviates the need for anticoagulation, and the durability of biological valves usually exceeds the patient's anticipated life expectancy.

is not a contraindication to valve replacement and results are very good in experienced centres, even for those in their eighties (Box 18.108). Delay exposes the patient to the risk of sudden death or irreversible deterioration in ventricular function. Some patients with severe aortic stenosis deny symptoms, and if this could be due to a sedentary lifestyle, a careful exercise test may reveal symptoms on modest exertion. Aortic balloon

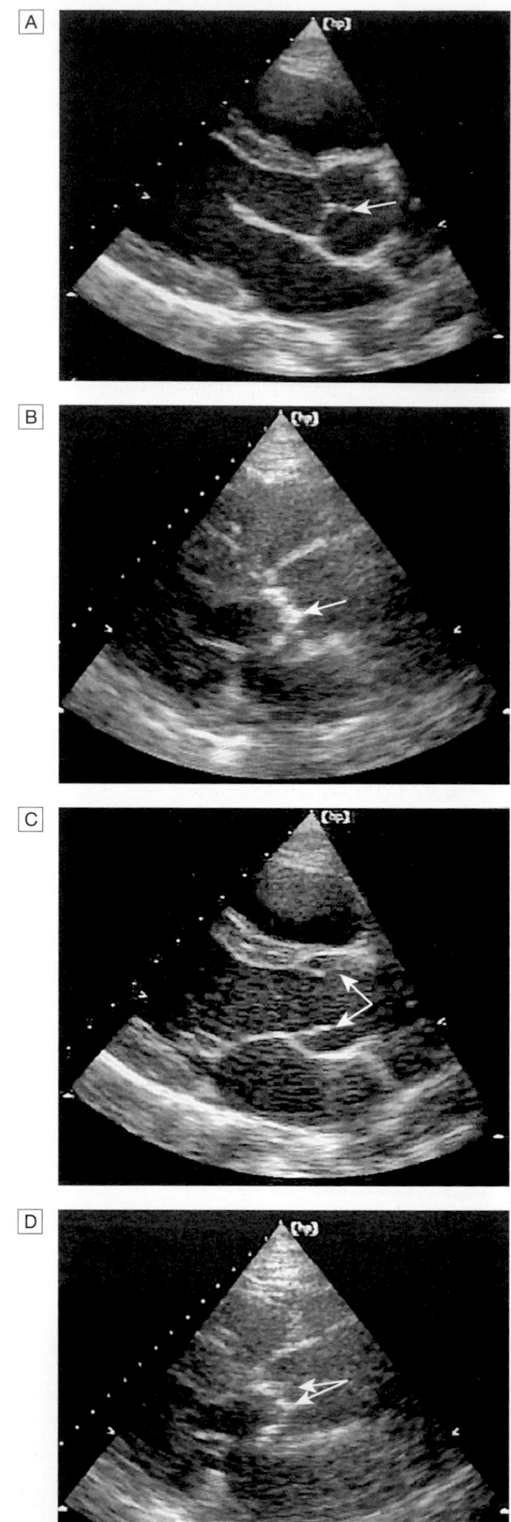

Fig. 18.91 Two-dimensional echocardiogram comparing a normal subject with a patient with calcific aortic stenosis. **A** Normal subject in diastole; the aortic leaflets are closed and thin, and a point of coaptation is seen (arrow). **B** Calcific aortic stenosis in diastole; the aortic leaflets are thick and calcified (arrow). **C** Normal in systole; the aortic leaflets are open (arrows). **D** Calcific aortic stenosis in systole; the thickened leaflets have barely moved (arrows). From Newby and Grubb 2005 – see p. 641.

valvuloplasty is useful in congenital aortic stenosis but is of no value in older patients with calcific aortic stenosis.

Anticoagulants are only required in patients who have atrial fibrillation or those who have had a valve replacement with a mechanical prosthesis.

Aortic regurgitation

Aetiology and pathophysiology

This condition is due to disease of the aortic valve cusps or dilatation of the aortic root (Box 18.109). The LV dilates and hypertrophies to compensate for the regurgitation. The stroke volume of the LV may eventually be doubled or trebled, and the major arteries are then conspicuously pulsatile. As the disease progresses, left ventricular diastolic pressure rises and breathlessness develops.

Clinical features

Until the onset of breathlessness, the only symptom may be an awareness of the heart beat (Box 18.110), particularly when lying on the left side, which results from the increased stroke volume. Paroxysmal nocturnal dyspnoea is sometimes the first symptom, and peripheral oedema or angina may occur. The characteristic murmur is best heard to the left of the sternum during held expiration (Fig. 18.92); a thrill is rare. A systolic murmur due to the increased stroke volume is common and does not

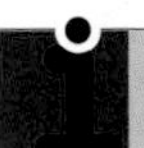

18.109 Causes of aortic regurgitation

Congenital
• Bicuspid valve or disproportionate cusps
Acquired
• Rheumatic disease • Infective endocarditis • Trauma • Aortic dilatation (Marfan's syndrome, aneurysm, dissection, syphilis, ankylosing spondylitis)

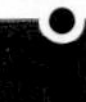

18.110 Clinical features of aortic regurgitation

Symptoms

Mild to moderate aortic regurgitation
- Often asymptomatic
- Awareness of heart beat, 'palpitations'

Severe aortic regurgitation
- Breathlessness
- Angina

Signs

Pulses
- Large-volume or 'collapsing' pulse
- Low diastolic and increased pulse pressure
- Bounding peripheral pulses
- Capillary pulsation in nail beds: Quincke's sign
- Femoral bruit ('pistol shot'): Duroziez's sign
- Head nodding with pulse: de Musset's sign

Murmurs
- Early diastolic murmur
- Systolic murmur (increased stroke volume)
- Austin Flint murmur (soft mid-diastolic)

Other signs
- Displaced, heaving apex beat (volume overload)
- Pre-systolic impulse
- Fourth heart sound
- Crepitations (pulmonary venous congestion)

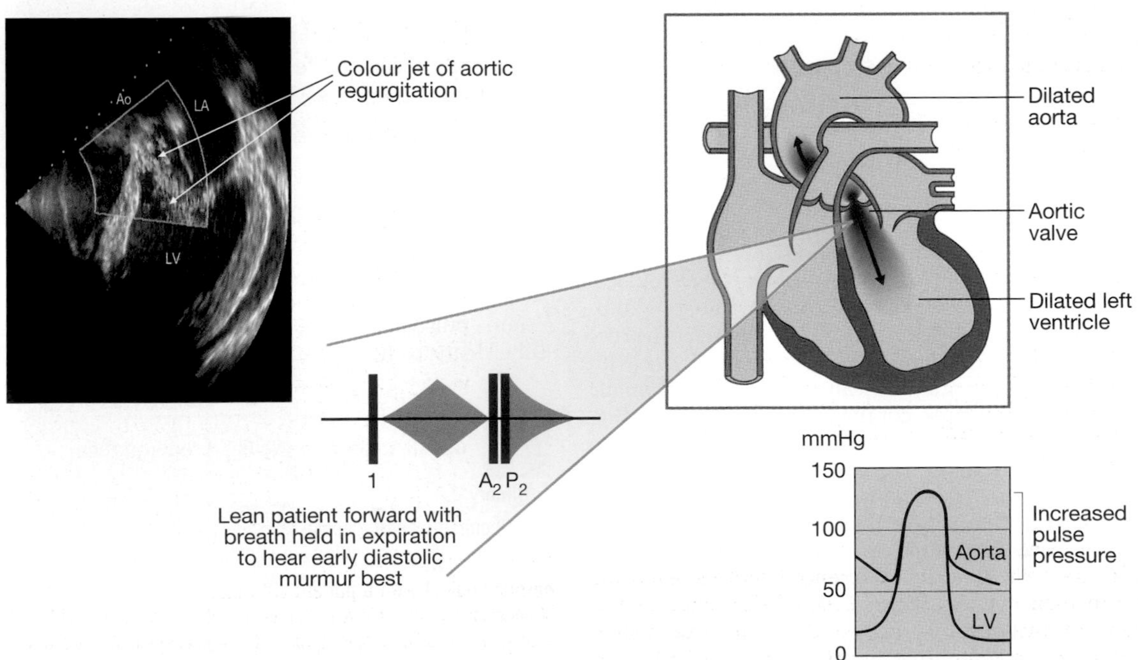

Fig. 18.92 Aortic regurgitation. The early diastolic murmur is best heard at the left sternal edge and may be accompanied by an ejection systolic ('to and fro') murmur. The aortic arch and LV may become dilated. **A** Doppler echocardiogram with the regurgitant jet (arrows). *Inset (Colour Doppler echo)* From Newby and Grubb 2005 – see p. 641.

18

necessarily indicate stenosis. The regurgitant jet causes fluttering of the mitral valve and, if severe, causes partial closure of the anterior mitral leaflet, leading to functional mitral stenosis and a soft mid-diastolic (Austin Flint) murmur.

In acute severe regurgitation (e.g. perforation of aortic cusp in endocarditis), there may be no time for compensatory left ventricular hypertrophy and dilatation to develop and the features of heart failure may predominate. In this situation, the classical signs of aortic regurgitation may be masked by tachycardia and an abrupt rise in left ventricular end-diastolic pressure; thus, the pulse pressure may be near normal and the diastolic murmur may be short or even absent.

Investigations

Regurgitation is detected by Doppler echocardiography (Box 18.111). In severe acute aortic regurgitation, the rapid rise in left ventricular diastolic pressure may cause premature mitral valve closure. Cardiac catheterisation and aortography can help in assessing the severity of regurgitation, and dilatation of the aorta and the presence of coexisting coronary artery disease. MRI is useful in assessing the degree and extent of aortic dilatation.

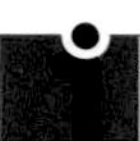

18.111 Investigations in aortic regurgitation

ECG	
• Initially normal, later left ventricular hypertrophy and T-wave inversion	
Chest X-ray	
• Cardiac dilatation, maybe aortic dilatation • Features of left heart failure	
Echo	
• Dilated LV • Hyperdynamic LV • Doppler detects reflux	• Fluttering anterior mitral leaflet
Cardiac catheterisation (may not be required)	
• Dilated LV • Aortic regurgitation	• Dilated aortic root

Management

Treatment may be required for underlying conditions, such as endocarditis or syphilis. Aortic valve replacement is indicated if aortic regurgitation causes symptoms, and this may need to be combined with aortic root replacement and coronary bypass surgery. Those with chronic aortic regurgitation can remain asymptomatic for many years because compensatory ventricular dilatation and hypertrophy occur, but should be advised to report the development of any symptoms of breathlessness or angina. Asymptomatic patients should also be followed up annually with echocardiography for evidence of increasing ventricular size. If this occurs or if the end-systolic dimension increases to 55 mm or more, then aortic valve replacement should be undertaken. Systolic BP should be controlled with vasodilating drugs, such as nifedipine or ACE inhibitors. There is conflicting evidence regarding the need for aortic valve replacement in asymptomatic patients with severe aortic regurgitation. When aortic root dilatation is the cause of aortic regurgitation (e.g. Marfan's syndrome), aortic root replacement is usually necessary.

Tricuspid valve disease

Tricuspid stenosis

Aetiology

Tricuspid stenosis is usually rheumatic in origin and is rare in developed countries. Tricuspid disease occurs in fewer than 5% of patients with rheumatic heart disease and then nearly always in association with mitral and aortic valve disease. Tricuspid stenosis and regurgitation are features of the carcinoid syndrome (p. 784).

Clinical features and investigations

Although the symptoms of mitral and aortic valve disease predominate, tricuspid stenosis may cause symptoms of right heart failure, including hepatic discomfort and peripheral oedema.

The main clinical feature is a raised JVP with a prominent *a* wave, and a slow *y* descent due to the loss of normal rapid right ventricular filling (p. 527). There is also a mid-diastolic murmur, best heard at the lower left or right sternal edge. This is generally higher-pitched than the murmur of mitral stenosis and is increased by inspiration. Right heart failure causes hepatomegaly with pre-systolic pulsation (large *a* wave), ascites and peripheral oedema. On Doppler echocardiography, the valve has similar appearances to those of rheumatic mitral stenosis.

Management

In patients who require surgery to other valves, either the tricuspid valve is replaced or valvotomy is performed at surgery. Balloon valvuloplasty can be used to treat rare cases of isolated tricuspid stenosis.

Tricuspid regurgitation

Aetiology, clinical features and investigations

Tricuspid regurgitation is common, and is most frequently 'functional' as a result of right ventricular dilatation (Box 18.112).

Symptoms are usually non-specific, with tiredness related to reduced forward flow, and oedema and hepatic enlargement due to venous congestion. The most prominent sign is a 'giant' *v* wave in the jugular venous pulse (a *cv* wave replaces the normal *x* descent). Other features include a pansystolic murmur at the left

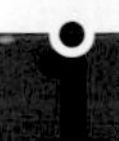

18.112 Causes of tricuspid regurgitation

Primary
• Rheumatic heart disease • Endocarditis, particularly in injection drug-users • Ebstein's congenital anomaly (see Box 18.123, p. 635)
Secondary
• Right ventricular dilatation due to chronic left heart failure ('functional tricuspid regurgitation') • Right ventricular infarction • Pulmonary hypertension (e.g. cor pulmonale)

sternal edge and a pulsatile liver. Echocardiography may reveal dilatation of the RV. If the valve has been affected by rheumatic disease, the leaflets will appear thickened and, in endocarditis, vegetations may be seen. Ebstein's anomaly (see Box 18.123, p. 635) is a congenital abnormality in which the tricuspid valve is displaced towards the right ventricular apex, with consequent enlargement of the RA. It is commonly associated with tricuspid regurgitation.

Management

Tricuspid regurgitation due to right ventricular dilatation often improves when the cause of right ventricular overload is corrected, with diuretic and vasodilator treatment of congestive cardiac failure. Patients with a normal pulmonary artery pressure tolerate isolated tricuspid reflux well, and valves damaged by endocarditis do not usually need to be replaced. Patients undergoing mitral valve replacement, who have tricuspid regurgitation due to marked dilatation of the tricuspid annulus, benefit from valve repair with an annuloplasty ring to bring the leaflets closer together. Those with rheumatic damage may require tricuspid valve replacement.

Pulmonary valve disease

Pulmonary stenosis

This can occur in the carcinoid syndrome but is usually congenital, in which case it may be isolated or associated with other abnormalities, such as Fallot's tetralogy (p. 634).

The principal finding on examination is an ejection systolic murmur, loudest at the left upper sternum and radiating towards the left shoulder. There may be a thrill, best felt when the patient leans forward and breathes out. The murmur is often preceded by an ejection sound (click). Delay in right ventricular ejection may cause wide splitting of the second heart sound. Severe pulmonary stenosis is characterised by a loud harsh murmur, an inaudible pulmonary closure sound (P_2), an increased right ventricular heave, prominent *a* waves in the jugular pulse, ECG evidence of right ventricular hypertrophy, and post-stenotic dilatation in the pulmonary artery on the chest X-ray. Doppler echocardiography is the definitive investigation.

Mild to moderate isolated pulmonary stenosis is relatively common and does not usually progress or require treatment. Severe pulmonary stenosis (resting gradient > 50 mmHg with a normal cardiac output) is treated by percutaneous pulmonary balloon valvuloplasty or, if this is not available, by surgical valvotomy. Long-term results are very good. Post-operative pulmonary regurgitation is common but benign.

Pulmonary regurgitation

This is rare in isolation and is usually associated with pulmonary artery dilatation due to pulmonary hypertension. It may complicate mitral stenosis, producing an early diastolic decrescendo murmur at the left sternal edge that is difficult to distinguish from aortic regurgitation (Graham Steell murmur). The pulmonary hypertension may be secondary to other disease of the left side of the heart, primary pulmonary vascular disease or Eisenmenger's syndrome (p. 631). Trivial pulmonary regurgitation is a frequent finding in normal individuals and has no clinical significance.

Infective endocarditis

This is caused by microbial infection of a heart valve (native or prosthetic), the lining of a cardiac chamber or blood vessel, or a congenital anomaly (e.g. septal defect). The causative organism is usually a bacterium, but may be a rickettsia, chlamydia or fungus.

Pathophysiology

Infective endocarditis typically occurs at sites of pre-existing endocardial damage, but infection with particularly virulent or aggressive organisms (e.g. *Staphylococcus aureus*) can cause endocarditis in a previously normal heart; staphylococcal endocarditis of the tricuspid valve is a common complication of intravenous drug misuse. Many acquired and congenital cardiac lesions are vulnerable to endocarditis, particularly areas of endocardial damage caused by a high-pressure jet of blood, such as ventricular septal defect, mitral regurgitation and aortic regurgitation, many of which are haemodynamically insignificant. In contrast, the risk of endocarditis at the site of haemodynamically important low-pressure lesions, such as a large atrial septal defect, is minimal.

Infection tends to occur at sites of endothelial damage because they attract deposits of platelets and fibrin that are vulnerable to colonisation by blood-borne organisms. The avascular valve tissue and presence of fibrin and platelet aggregates help to protect proliferating organisms from host defence mechanisms. When the infection is established, vegetations composed of organisms, fibrin and platelets grow and may become large enough to cause obstruction or embolism. Adjacent tissues are destroyed and abscesses may form. Valve regurgitation may develop or increase if the affected valve is damaged by tissue distortion, cusp perforation or disruption of chordae. Extracardiac manifestations, such as vasculitis and skin lesions, are due to emboli or immune complex deposition. Mycotic aneurysms may develop in arteries at the site of infected emboli. At autopsy, infarction of the spleen and kidneys and, sometimes, an immune glomerulonephritis are found.

Microbiology

Over three-quarters of cases are caused by streptococci or staphylococci. The *viridans* group of streptococci (*Streptococcus mitis, Strep. sanguis*) are commensals in the upper respiratory tract that may enter the blood stream on chewing or teeth-brushing, or at the time of dental treatment, and are common causes of subacute endocarditis (Box 18.113). Other organisms, including *Enterococcus faecalis, E. faecium* and *Strep. bovis*, may enter the blood from the bowel or urinary tract. *Strep. milleri* and *Strep. bovis* endocarditis is associated with large-bowel neoplasms.

Staph. aureus has now overtaken streptococci as the most common cause of acute endocarditis. It originates from skin infections, abscesses or vascular access sites (e.g. intravenous and central lines), or from intravenous drug use. It is highly virulent and invasive, usually producing florid vegetations, rapid valve destruction and abscess formation. Other causes of acute endocarditis include *Strep. pneumoniae* and *Strep. pyogenes*.

18.113 Microbiology of infective endocarditis

Pathogen	Of native valve (n = 280)	In IV drug users (n = 87)	Of prosthetic valve Early (n = 15)	Of prosthetic valve Late (n = 72)
Staphylococci	124 (44%)	60 (69%)	10 (67%)	33 (46%)
Staph. aureus	106 (38%)	60 (69%)	3 (20%)	15 (21%)
Coagulase-negative	18 (6%)	0	7 (47%)	18 (25%)
Streptococci	86 (31%)	7 (8%)	0	25 (35%)
Oral	59 (21%)	3 (3%)	0	19 (26%)
Others (non-enterococcal)	27 (10%)	4 (5%)	0	6 (8%)
***Enterococcus* spp.**	21 (8%)	2 (2%)	1 (7%)	5 (7%)
HACEK group (see text)	12 (4%)	0	0	1 (1%)
Polymicrobial	6 (2%)	8 (9%)	0	1 (1%)
Other bacteria	12 (4%)	4 (5%)	0	2 (3%)
Fungi	3 (1%)	2 (2%)	0	0
Negative blood culture	16 (6%)	4 (5%)	4 (27%)	5 (7%)

Adapted from Moreillon P, Que YA. Lancet 2004; 363:139–149.

Post-operative endocarditis after cardiac surgery may affect native or prosthetic heart valves or other prosthetic materials. The most common organism is a coagulase-negative staphylococcus (*Staph. epidermidis*), a normal skin commensal. There is frequently a history of wound infection with the same organism. *Staph. epidermidis* occasionally causes endocarditis in patients who have not had cardiac surgery, and its presence in blood cultures may be erroneously dismissed as contamination. Another coagulase-negative staphylococcus, *Staph. lugdenensis,* causes a rapidly destructive acute endocarditis that is associated with previously normal valves and multiple emboli. Unless accurately identified, it may also be overlooked as a contaminant.

In Q fever endocarditis due to *Coxiella burnetii*, the patient often has a history of contact with farm animals. The aortic valve is usually affected and there may also be hepatitis, pneumonia and purpura. Life-long antibiotic therapy may be required.

Gram-negative bacteria of the so-called HACEK group (*Haemophilus* spp., *Actinobacillus actinomycetemcomitans, Cardiobacterium hominis, Eikenella* spp. and *Kingella kingae*) are slow-growing, fastidious organisms that are only revealed after prolonged culture and may be resistant to penicillin.

Brucella is associated with a history of contact with goats or cattle and often affects the aortic valve.

Yeasts and fungi (*Candida, Aspergillus*) may attack previously normal or prosthetic valves, particularly in immunocompromised patients or those with indwelling intravenous lines. Abscesses and emboli are common, therapy is difficult (surgery is often required) and mortality is high. Concomitant bacterial infection may be present.

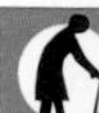

18.114 Endocarditis in old age

- **Symptoms and signs**: may be non-specific, e.g. confusion, weight loss, malaise and weakness, and the diagnosis may not be suspected.
- **Common causative organisms**: often enterococci (from the urinary tract) and *Strep. bovis* (from a colonic source).
- **Morbidity and mortality**: much higher.

Incidence

The incidence of infective endocarditis in community-based studies ranges from 5 to 15 cases per 100 000 per annum. More than 50% of patients are over 60 years of age (Box 18.114). In a large British study, the underlying condition was rheumatic heart disease in 24% of patients, congenital heart disease in 19%, and other cardiac abnormalities (e.g. calcified aortic valve, floppy mitral valve) in 25%. The remaining 32% were not thought to have a pre-existing cardiac abnormality.

Clinical features

Endocarditis can take either an acute or a more insidious 'subacute' form. However, there is considerable overlap because the clinical pattern is influenced not only by the organism, but also by the site of infection, prior antibiotic therapy and the presence of a valve or shunt prosthesis. The subacute form may abruptly develop acute life-threatening complications, such as valve disruption or emboli.

Subacute endocarditis

This should be suspected when a patient with congenital or valvular heart disease develops a persistent fever, complains of unusual tiredness, night sweats or weight loss, or develops new signs of valve dysfunction or heart failure. Less often, it presents as an embolic stroke or peripheral arterial embolism. Other features (Fig. 18.93) include purpura and petechial haemorrhages in the skin and mucous membranes, and splinter haemorrhages under the fingernails or toe nails. Osler's nodes are painful tender swellings at the fingertips that are probably the product of vasculitis; they are rare. Digital clubbing is a late sign. The spleen is frequently palpable; in *Coxiella* infections, the spleen and the liver may be considerably enlarged. Microscopic haematuria is common. The finding of any of these features in a patient with persistent fever or malaise is an indication for re-examination to detect hitherto unrecognised heart disease.

Acute endocarditis

This presents as a severe febrile illness with prominent and changing heart murmurs and petechiae. Clinical stigmata of chronic endocarditis are usually absent. Embolic events are common, and cardiac or renal failure may develop rapidly. Abscesses may be detected on echocardiography. Partially treated acute endocarditis behaves like subacute endocarditis.

Post-operative endocarditis

This may present as an unexplained fever in a patient who has had heart valve surgery. The infection usually involves the valve ring and may resemble subacute or

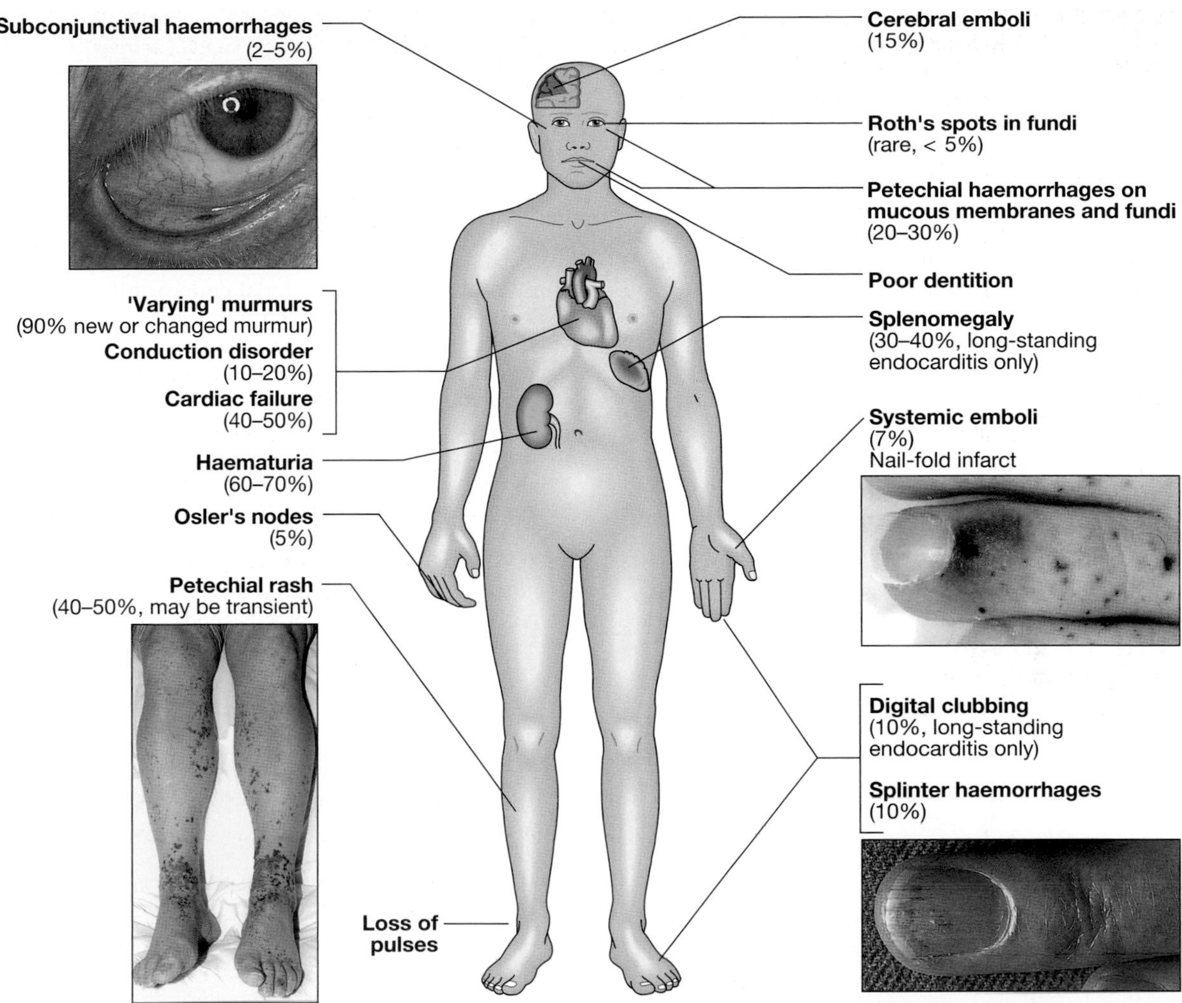

Fig. 18.93 Clinical features which may be present in endocarditis. *Insets (Petechial rash, nail-fold infarct)* From Newby and Grubb 2005 – see p. 641.

acute endocarditis, depending on the virulence of the organism. Morbidity and mortality are high and redo surgery is often required. The range of organisms is similar to that seen in native valve disease, but when endocarditis occurs during the first few weeks after surgery, it is usually due to infection with a coagulase-negative staphylococcus that was introduced during the peri-operative period. A clinical diagnosis of endocarditis can be made on the presence of two major, one major and three minor, or five minor criteria (Box 18.115).

Investigations

Blood culture is the crucial investigation because it may identify the infection and guide antibiotic therapy. Three to six sets of blood cultures should be taken prior to commencing therapy and should not wait for episodes of pyrexia. The first two specimens will detect bacteraemia in 90% of culture-positive cases. Aseptic technique is essential and the risk of contaminants should be minimised by sampling from different venepuncture sites. An in-dwelling line should not be used to take cultures. Aerobic and anaerobic cultures are required.

Echocardiography is key for detecting and following the progress of vegetations, for assessing valve damage

18.115 Diagnosis of infective endocarditis (modified Duke criteria)

Major criteria
Positive blood culture • Typical organism from two cultures • Persistent positive blood cultures taken > 12 hrs apart • Three or more positive cultures taken over > 1 hr **Endocardial involvement** • Positive echocardiographic findings of vegetations • New valvular regurgitation
Minor criteria
• Predisposing valvular or cardiac abnormality • Intravenous drug misuse • Pyrexia ≥ 38°C • Embolic phenomenon • Vasculitic phenomenon • Blood cultures suggestive: organism grown but not achieving major criteria • Suggestive echocardiographic findings
Definite endocarditis = two major, or one major and three minor, or five minor Possible endocarditis = one major and one minor, or three minor

and for detecting abscess formation. Vegetations as small as 2–4 mm can be detected by transthoracic echocardiography, and even smaller ones (1–1.5 mm) can be visualised by transoesophageal echocardiography (TOE), which is particularly valuable for identifying abscess formation and investigating patients with prosthetic heart valves. Vegetations may be difficult to distinguish in the presence of an abnormal valve; the sensitivity of transthoracic echo is approximately 65% but that of TOE is more than 90%. Failure to detect vegetations does not exclude the diagnosis.

Elevation of the ESR, a normocytic normochromic anaemia, and leucocytosis are common but not invariable. Measurement of serum CRP is more reliable than the ESR in monitoring progress. Proteinuria may occur and microscopic haematuria is usually present.

The ECG may show the development of AV block (due to aortic root abscess formation) and occasionally infarction due to emboli. The chest X-ray may show evidence of cardiac failure and cardiomegaly.

Management

The case fatality of bacterial endocarditis is approximately 20% and even higher in those with prosthetic valve endocarditis and those infected with antibiotic-resistant organisms. A multidisciplinary approach, with cooperation between the physician, surgeon and microbiologist, increases the chance of a successful outcome. Any source of infection should be removed as soon as possible; for example, a tooth with an apical abscess should be extracted.

Empirical treatment depends on the mode of presentation, the suspected organism, and whether the patient has a prosthetic valve or penicillin allergy (Box 18.116). If the presentation is acute, flucloxacillin and gentamicin are recommended, while for a subacute or indolent presentation, benzyl penicillin and gentamicin are preferred. In those with penicillin allergy, a prosthetic valve or suspected meticillin-resistant *Staph. aureus* (MRSA) infection, triple therapy with vancomycin, gentamicin and oral rifampicin should be considered. Following identification of the causal organism, determination of the minimum inhibitory concentration (MIC) for the organism is essential to guide antibiotic therapy.

A 2-week treatment regimen may be sufficient for fully sensitive strains of *Strep. viridans* and *Strep. bovis*, provided specific conditions are met (Box 18.117). For the empirical treatment of bacterial endocarditis, penicillin plus gentamicin is the regimen of choice for most patients; when staphylococcal infection is suspected, however, vancomycin plus gentamicin is recommended.

Cardiac surgery (débridement of infected material and valve replacement) is advisable in a substantial proportion of patients, particularly those with *Staph. aureus* and fungal infections (Box 18.118). Antimicrobial therapy must be started before surgery.

Prevention

Until recently, antibiotic prophylaxis was routinely given to people at risk of infective endocarditis undergoing interventional procedures. However, as this has not been proven to be effective and the link between

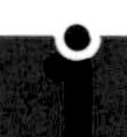

18.117 Conditions for the short-course treatment of *Strep. viridans/bovis* endocarditis

- Native valve infection
- MIC ≤ 0.1 mg/L
- No adverse prognostic factors (e.g. heart failure, aortic regurgitation, conduction defect)
- No evidence of thromboembolic disease
- No vegetations > 5 mm diameter
- Clinical response within 7 days

18.116 Antimicrobial treatment of common causative organisms in infective endocarditis

			Duration	
Organism	**Antimicrobial**	**Dose**	**Native valve**	**Prosthetic valve**
Viridans* streptococci and *Strep. bovis				
MIC ≤ 0.1 mg/L	Benzyl penicillin IV	1.2 g 6 times daily	4 wks[1]	6 wks
	and gentamicin IV	1 mg/kg 2–3 times daily	2 wks	2 wks
MIC > 0.1 to < 0.5 mg/L	Benzyl penicillin IV	1.2 g 6 times daily	4 wks	6 wks
	and gentamicin IV	1 mg/kg 2–3 times daily	2 wks	4–6 wks
MIC ≥ 0.5 mg/L	Benzyl penicillin IV	1.2 g 6 times daily	4 wks	6 wks
	and gentamicin IV	1 mg/kg 2–3 times daily	4 wks	4–6 wks
Enterococci				
Ampicillin-sensitive	Ampicillin IV	2 g 6 times daily	4 wks	6 wks
	and gentamicin IV[2]	1 mg/kg 2–3 times daily	4 wks	6 wks
Ampicillin-resistant	Vancomycin IV	1 g twice daily	4 wk	6 wks
	and gentamicin IV[2]	1 mg/kg 2–3 times daily	4 wks	6 wks
Staphylococci				
Penicillin-sensitive	Benzyl penicillin IV	1.2 g 6 times daily	4 wks	6 wks
Penicillin-resistant Meticillin-sensitive	Flucloxacillin IV	2 g 6 times daily (< 85 kg 6-hourly)	4 wks	6 wks[3]
Penicillin-resistant Meticillin-resistant	Vancomycin IV and gentamicin IV	1 g twice daily 1 mg/kg 3 times daily	4 wks 4 wks	6 wks[3] 6 wks[3]

[1]When conditions in Box 18.117 are met, 2 wks of benzyl penicillin. [2]In high-level gentamicin resistance, consider streptomycin. [3]Consider additional rifampicin 300–600 mg twice daily orally for 2 wks. (MIC = minimum inhibitory concentration)

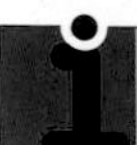

18.118 Indications for cardiac surgery in infective endocarditis

- Heart failure due to valve damage
- Failure of antibiotic therapy (persistent/uncontrolled infection)
- Large vegetations on left-sided heart valves with evidence or 'high risk' of systemic emboli
- Abscess formation

N.B. Patients with prosthetic valve endocarditis or fungal endocarditis often require cardiac surgery.

episodes of infective endocarditis and interventional procedures has not been demonstrated, antibiotic prophylaxis is no longer offered routinely for defined interventional procedures.

Valve replacement surgery

Diseased heart valves can be replaced with mechanical or biological prostheses. The three most commonly used types of mechanical prosthesis are the ball and cage, tilting single disc and tilting bi-leaflet valves. All generate prosthetic sounds or clicks on auscultation. Pig or allograft valves mounted on a supporting stent are the most commonly used biological valves. They generate normal heart sounds. All prosthetic valves used in the aortic position produce a systolic flow murmur.

All mechanical valves require long-term anticoagulation because they can cause systemic thromboembolism or may develop valve thrombosis or obstruction (Box 18.119); the prosthetic clicks may become inaudible if the valve malfunctions. Biological valves have the advantage of not requiring anticoagulants to maintain proper function; however, many patients undergoing valve replacement surgery, especially mitral valve replacement, will have atrial fibrillation that requires anticoagulation anyway. Biological valves are less durable than mechanical valves and may degenerate 7 or more years after implantation, particularly when used in the mitral position. They are more durable in the aortic position and in older patients, so are particularly appropriate for patients over 65 undergoing aortic valve replacement.

Symptoms or signs of unexplained heart failure in a patient with a prosthetic heart valve may be due to valve dysfunction, and urgent assessment is required. Biological valve dysfunction is usually associated with the development of a regurgitant murmur.

18.119 Prosthetic heart valves: optimal anticoagulant control

Mechanical valves	Target INR
Ball and cage (e.g. Starr–Edwards) Tilting disc (e.g. Bjork–Shiley)	3.5
Bi-leaflet (e.g. St Jude)	3.0
Biological valves with atrial fibrillation	2.5

CONGENITAL HEART DISEASE

Congenital heart disease usually manifests in childhood but may pass unrecognised and not present until adult life. Defects that are well tolerated, such as atrial septal defect, may cause no symptoms until adult life or may be detected incidentally on routine examination or chest X-ray. Congenital defects that were previously fatal in childhood can now be corrected, or at least partially, so that survival to adult life is the norm. Such patients remain well for many years but subsequently re-present in later life with related problems such as arrhythmia or ventricular dysfunction (Box 18.120).

18.120 Presentation of congenital heart disease throughout life

Birth and neonatal period	
• Cyanosis	• Heart failure
Infancy and childhood	
• Cyanosis • Heart failure • Arrhythmia	• Murmur • Failure to thrive
Adolescence and adulthood	
• Heart failure • Murmur • Arrhythmia • Cyanosis due to shunt reversal (Eisenmenger's syndrome)	• Hypertension (coarctation) • Late consequences of previous cardiac surgery, e.g. arrhythmia, heart failure

The fetal circulation

Understanding the fetal circulation helps clarify how some forms of congenital heart disease occur. The fetus has only a small flow of blood through the lungs, as it does not breathe in utero. The fetal circulation allows oxygenated blood from the placenta to pass directly to the left side of the heart through the foramen ovale without having to flow through the lungs, and also from the pulmonary artery into the aorta via the ductus arteriosus (Fig. 18.94).

Congenital defects may arise if the changes from fetal circulation to the extrauterine circulation are incomplete. Atrial septal defects occur at the site of the foramen ovale. A patent ductus arteriosus may remain if it fails to close after birth. Failure of the aorta to develop at the point of the aortic isthmus and where the ductus arteriosus attaches can lead to coarctation of the aorta.

In fetal development, the heart develops as a single tube which folds back on itself and then divides into two separate circulations. Failure of septation can lead to some forms of atrial and ventricular septal defect. Failure of alignment of the great vessels with the ventricles contributes to transposition of the great arteries, tetralogy of Fallot and truncus arteriosus.

Aetiology and incidence

The incidence of haemodynamically significant congenital cardiac abnormalities is about 0.8% of live births (Box 18.121). Maternal infection or exposure to drugs or toxins may cause congenital heart disease. Maternal rubella infection is associated with persistent ductus arteriosus, pulmonary valvular and/or artery stenosis, and atrial septal defect. Maternal alcohol misuse is associated with septal defects, and maternal lupus erythematosus with congenital complete heart block. Genetic or chromosomal abnormalities, such as Down's syndrome, may cause septal defects, and gene defects have also

18

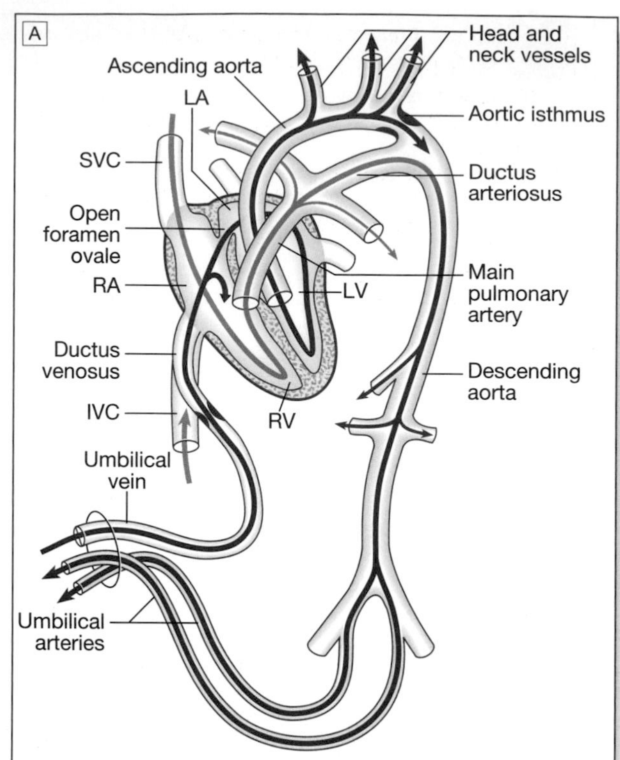

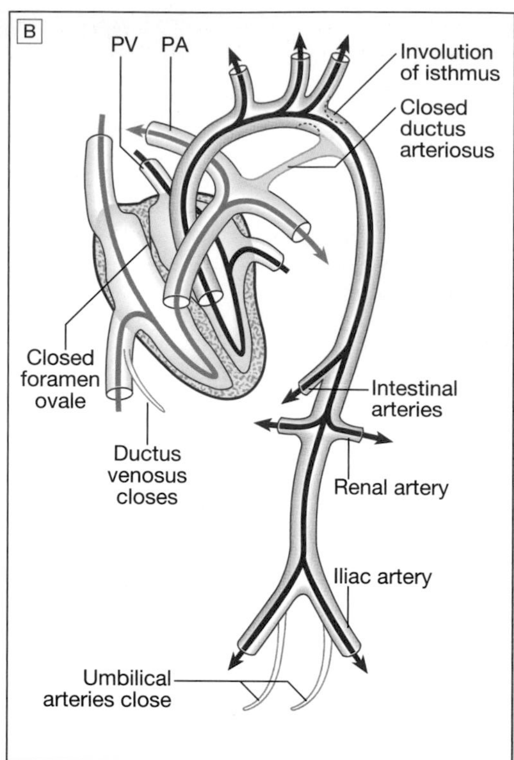

Fig. 18.94 Changes in the circulation at birth. A In the fetus, oxygenated blood comes through the umbilical vein where it enters the inferior vena cava via the ductus venosus (red). The oxygenated blood streams from the RA through the open foramen ovale to the LA and via the LV into the aorta. Venous blood from the superior vena cava (blue) crosses under the main blood stream into the RA and then, partly mixed with oxygenated blood (purple), into the RV and pulmonary artery. The pulmonary vasculature has a high resistance and so little blood passes to the lungs; most blood passes through the ductus arteriosus to the descending aorta. The aortic isthmus is a constriction in the aorta that lies in the aortic arch before the junction with the ductus arteriosus and limits the flow of oxygen-rich blood to the descending aorta. This configuration means that less oxygen-rich blood is supplied to organ systems that take up their function mainly after birth, e.g. the kidneys and intestinal tract. B At birth, the lungs expand with air and pulmonary vascular resistance falls, so that blood now flows to the lungs and back to the LA. The left atrial pressure rises above right atrial pressure and the flap valve of the foramen ovale closes. The umbilical arteries and the ductus venosus close. In the next few days, the ductus arteriosus closes under the influence of hormonal changes (particularly prostaglandins) and the aortic isthmus expands (IVC = inferior vena cava; LA = left atrium; LV = left ventricle; PA = pulmonary artery; PV = pulmonary vein; RA = right atrium; RV = right ventricle; SVC = superior vena cava). Adapted from Drews 1995 – see p. 641.

18.121 Incidence and relative frequency of congenital cardiac malformations

Lesion	% of all congenital heart defects
Ventricular septal defect	30
Atrial septal defect	10
Patent ductus arteriosus	10
Pulmonary stenosis	7
Coarctation of aorta	7
Aortic stenosis	6
Tetralogy of Fallot	6
Complete transposition of great arteries	4
Others	20

been identified as leading to specific abnormalities, such as Marfan's syndrome (p. 603) and DiGeorge's (deletion in chromosome 22q) syndrome.

Clinical features

Symptoms may be absent, or the child may be breathless or fail to attain normal growth and development. Some

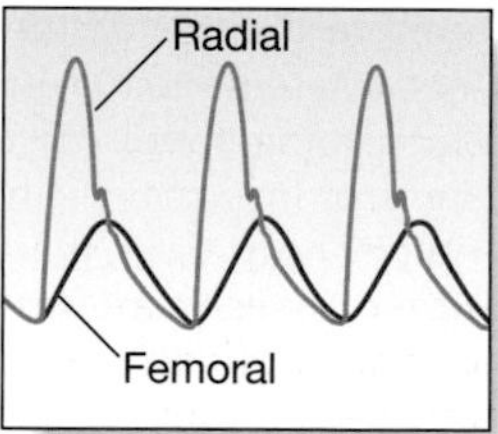

Fig. 18.95 Radiofemoral delay. The difference in pulse pressures is shown.

defects are not compatible with extrauterine life, or are so only for a short time. Clinical signs vary with the anatomical lesion. Murmurs, thrills or signs of cardiomegaly may be present. In coarctation of the aorta, radiofemoral delay may be noted (Fig. 18.95) and some female patients have the features of Turner's syndrome (p. 765). Features of other congenital conditions, such as Marfan's syndrome or Down's syndrome, may also be apparent. Cerebrovascular accidents and cerebral abscesses may complicate severe cyanotic congenital disease.

Early diagnosis is important because many types of congenital heart disease are amenable to surgery, but this opportunity is lost if secondary changes, such as irreversible pulmonary hypertension, occur.

Central cyanosis and digital clubbing

Central cyanosis of cardiac origin occurs when desaturated blood enters the systemic circulation without passing through the lungs (i.e. a right-to-left shunt). In the neonate, the most common cause is transposition of the great arteries, in which the aorta arises from the RV and the pulmonary artery from the LV in association with a ventricular septal defect. In older children, cyanosis is usually the consequence of a ventricular septal defect combined with severe pulmonary stenosis (tetralogy of Fallot) or with pulmonary vascular disease (Eisenmenger's syndrome). Prolonged cyanosis is associated with finger and toe clubbing (p. 526).

Growth retardation and learning difficulties

These may occur with large left-to-right shunts at ventricular or great arterial level, and also with other defects, especially if they form part of a genetic syndrome. Major intellectual impairment is uncommon in children with isolated congenital heart disease; however, minor learning difficulties can occur and may complicate cardiac surgery if cerebral perfusion is compromised.

Syncope

In the presence of increased pulmonary vascular resistance or severe left or right ventricular outflow obstruction, exercise may provoke syncope as systemic vascular resistance falls but pulmonary vascular resistance rises, worsening right-to-left shunting and cerebral oxygenation. Syncope can also occur because of associated arrhythmias.

Pulmonary hypertension and Eisenmenger's syndrome

Persistently raised pulmonary flow (e.g. with left-to-right shunt) causes increased pulmonary resistance followed by pulmonary hypertension. Progressive changes, including obliteration of distal vessels, occur and are irreversible. Central cyanosis appears and digital clubbing develops. The chest X-ray shows enlarged central pulmonary arteries and peripheral 'pruning' of the pulmonary vessels. The ECG shows right ventricular hypertrophy. If severe pulmonary hypertension develops, a left-to-right shunt may reverse, resulting in right-to-left shunt and marked cyanosis (Eisenmenger's syndrome), which may be more apparent in the feet and toes than in the upper part of the body: differential cyanosis. This is more common with large ventricular septal defects or persistent ductus arteriosus than with atrial septal defects. Patients with Eisenmenger's syndrome are at particular risk from abrupt changes in afterload that exacerbate right-to-left shunting, such as vasodilatation, anaesthesia and pregnancy.

Pregnancy

During pregnancy, there is a 50% increase in plasma volume, a 40% increase in whole blood volume and a similar increase in cardiac output, so problems may arise in women with congenital heart disease (Box 18.122). Many with palliated or untreated disease will tolerate pregnancy well, however. Pregnancy is particularly hazardous in the presence of conditions associated with cyanosis or severe pulmonary hypertension; maternal mortality in patients with Eisenmenger's syndrome is more than 50%.

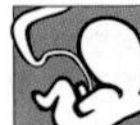

18.122 Pregnancy in women with congenital heart disease

- **Obstructive lesions** (e.g. severe aortic stenosis): poorly tolerated and associated with significant maternal morbidity and mortality.
- **Cyanotic conditions** (e.g. Eisenmenger's syndrome): especially poorly tolerated and pregnancy should be avoided.
- **Surgically corrected disease**: patients often tolerate pregnancy well.
- **Children of patients with congenital heart disease**: 2–5% will be born with cardiac abnormalities, especially if the mother is affected.

Persistent ductus arteriosus

Aetiology

During fetal life, before the lungs begin to function, most of the blood from the pulmonary artery passes through the ductus arteriosus into the aorta (see Fig. 18.94). Normally, the ductus closes soon after birth but sometimes fails to do so. Persistence of the ductus is associated with other abnormalities and is more common in females.

Since the pressure in the aorta is higher than that in the pulmonary artery, there will be a continuous arterio-venous shunt, the volume of which depends on the size of the ductus. As much as 50% of the left ventricular output is recirculated through the lungs, with a consequent increase in the work of the heart (Fig. 18.96).

Clinical features

With small shunts there may be no symptoms for years but, when the ductus is large, growth and development may be retarded. Usually, there is no disability in infancy

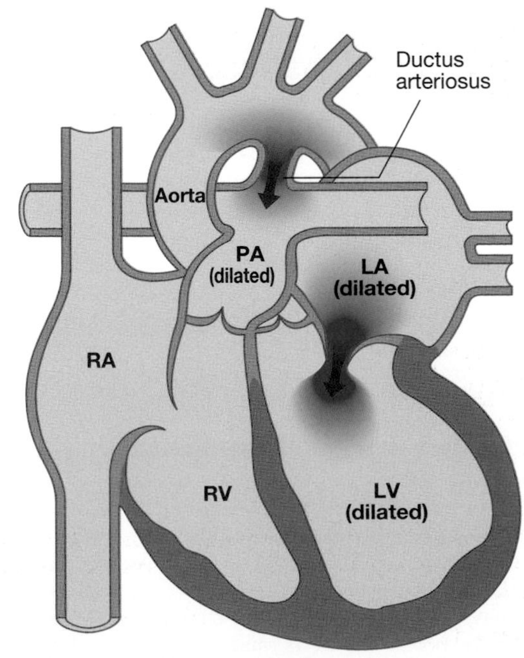

Fig. 18.96 Persistent ductus arteriosus. There is a connection between the aorta and the pulmonary artery with left-to-right shunting.

but cardiac failure may eventually ensue, dyspnoea being the first symptom. A continuous 'machinery' murmur is heard with late systolic accentuation, maximal in the second left intercostal space below the clavicle (see Fig. 18.96). It is frequently accompanied by a thrill. Pulses are increased in volume.

A large left-to-right shunt in infancy may cause a considerable rise in pulmonary artery pressure and sometimes this leads to progressive pulmonary vascular damage. Enlargement of the pulmonary artery may be detected radiologically. The ECG is usually normal.

Persistent ductus with reversed shunting

If pulmonary vascular resistance increases, pulmonary artery pressure may rise until it equals or exceeds aortic pressure. The shunt through the defect may then reverse, causing Eisenmenger's syndrome. The murmur becomes quieter, may be confined to systole or may disappear. The ECG shows evidence of right ventricular hypertrophy.

Management

A patent ductus is closed at cardiac catheterisation with an implantable occlusive device. Closure should be undertaken in infancy if the shunt is significant and pulmonary resistance not elevated, but this may be delayed until later childhood in those with smaller shunts, for whom closure remains advisable to reduce the risk of endocarditis.

Pharmacological treatment in the neonatal period

When the ductus is structurally intact, a prostaglandin synthetase inhibitor (indometacin or ibuprofen) may be used in the first week of life to induce closure. However, in the presence of a congenital defect with impaired lung perfusion (e.g. severe pulmonary stenosis and left-to-right shunt through the ductus), it may be advisable to improve oxygenation by keeping the ductus open with prostaglandin treatment. Unfortunately, these treatments do not work if the ductus is intrinsically abnormal.

Coarctation of the aorta

Aetiology

Narrowing of the aorta occurs in the region where the ductus arteriosus joins the aorta, i.e. at the isthmus just below the origin of the left subclavian artery (see Fig. 18.94). The condition is twice as common in males and occurs in 1 in 4000 children. It is associated with other abnormalities, most frequently bicuspid aortic valve and 'berry' aneurysms of the cerebral circulation (p. 1246). Acquired coarctation of the aorta is rare but may follow trauma or occur as a complication of a progressive arteritis (Takayasu's disease, p. 1116).

Clinical features and investigations

Aortic coarctation is an important cause of cardiac failure in the newborn but symptoms are often absent when it is detected in older children or adults. Headaches may occur from hypertension proximal to the coarctation, and occasionally weakness or cramps in the legs may result from decreased circulation in the lower part of the body. The BP is raised in the upper body but normal or low in the legs. The femoral pulses are weak and delayed in comparison with the radial pulse (see Fig. 18.95). A systolic murmur is usually heard posteriorly, over the coarctation. There may also be an ejection click and systolic murmur in the aortic area due to a bicuspid aortic valve. As a result of the aortic narrowing, collaterals form; they mainly involve the periscapular, internal mammary and intercostal arteries, and may result in localised bruits.

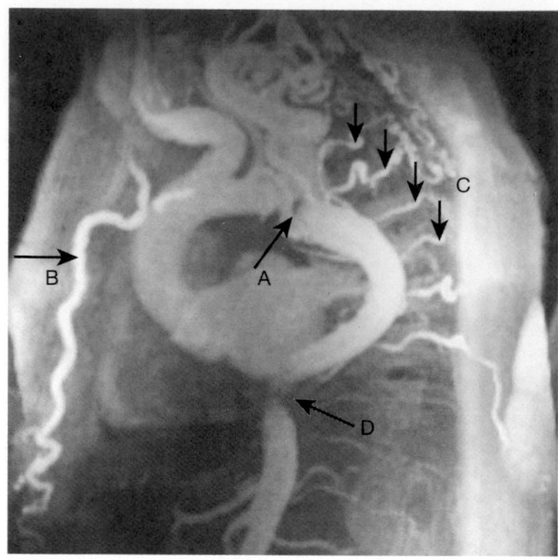

Fig. 18.97 MRI scan of coarctation of the aorta. The aorta is severely narrowed just beyond the arch at the start of the descending aorta (arrow A). Extensive collaterals have developed; a large internal mammary artery (arrow B) and several intercostal arteries (arrows C) are shown. Unusually, in this case, there is also a coarctation of the abdominal aorta (arrow D).

The chest X-ray in early childhood is often normal but later may show changes in the contour of the aorta (indentation of the descending aorta, '3 sign') and notching of the under-surfaces of the ribs from collaterals. MRI is the best imaging method. (Fig. 18.97). The ECG may show evidence of left ventricular hypertrophy, which can be confirmed by echocardiography.

Management

In untreated cases, death may occur from left ventricular failure, dissection of the aorta or cerebral haemorrhage. Surgical correction is advisable in all but the mildest cases. If this is carried out sufficiently early in childhood, persistent hypertension can be avoided. Patients repaired in late childhood or adult life often remain hypertensive or develop recurrent hypertension later on. Recurrence of stenosis may occur as the child grows and this may be managed by balloon dilatation and sometimes stenting. The latter may be used as the primary treatment. Coexistent bicuspid aortic valve, which occurs in over 50% of cases, may lead to progressive aortic stenosis or regurgitation, and also requires long-term follow-up.

Atrial septal defect

Aetiology

Atrial septal defect is one of the most common congenital heart defects and occurs twice as frequently in females. Most are 'ostium secundum' defects, involving the fossa ovalis that, in utero, was the foramen ovale (see Fig. 18.94). 'Ostium primum' defects result from a defect

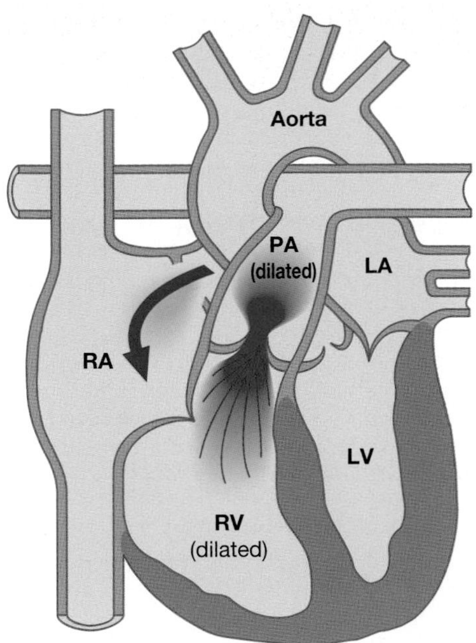

Fig. 18.98 Atrial septal defect. Blood flows across the atrial septum (arrow) from left to right. The murmur is produced by increased flow velocity across the pulmonary valve, as a result of left-to-right shunting and a large stroke volume. The density of shading is proportional to velocity of blood flow.

in the atrioventricular septum and are associated with a 'cleft mitral valve' (split anterior leaflet).

Since the normal RV is more compliant than the LV, a large volume of blood shunts through the defect from the LA to the RA, and then to the RV and pulmonary arteries (Fig. 18.98). As a result, there is gradual enlargement of the right side of the heart and of the pulmonary arteries. Pulmonary hypertension and shunt reversal sometimes complicate atrial septal defect, but are less common and tend to occur later in life than with other types of left-to-right shunt.

Clinical features and investigations

Most children are asymptomatic for many years and the condition is often detected at routine clinical examination or following a chest X-ray. Dyspnoea, chest infections, cardiac failure and arrhythmias, especially atrial fibrillation, are other possible manifestations. The characteristic physical signs are the result of the volume overload of the RV:

- wide, fixed splitting of the second heart sound: wide because of delay in right ventricular ejection (increased stroke volume and right bundle branch block) and fixed because the septal defect equalises left and right atrial pressures throughout the respiratory cycle
- a systolic flow murmur over the pulmonary valve.

In children with a large shunt, there may be a diastolic flow murmur over the tricuspid valve. Unlike a mitral flow murmur, this is usually high-pitched.

The chest X-ray typically shows enlargement of the heart and the pulmonary artery, as well as pulmonary plethora. The ECG usually shows incomplete right bundle branch block because right ventricular depolarisation is delayed as a result of ventricular dilatation

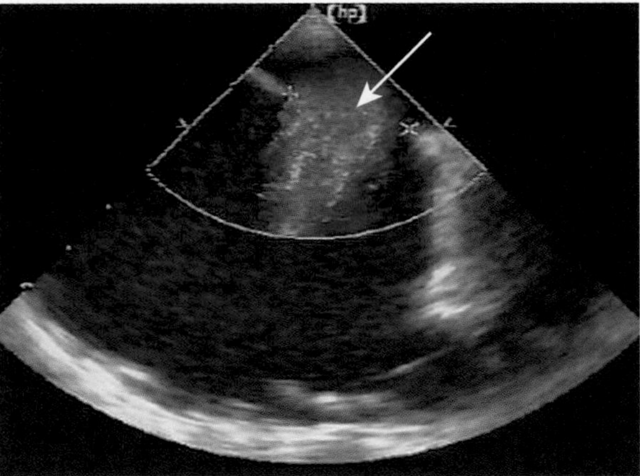

Fig. 18.99 Transoesophageal echocardiogram of an atrial septal defect. The defect is clearly seen (arrow) between the LA above and RA below. Doppler colour-flow imaging shows flow (blue) across the defect.

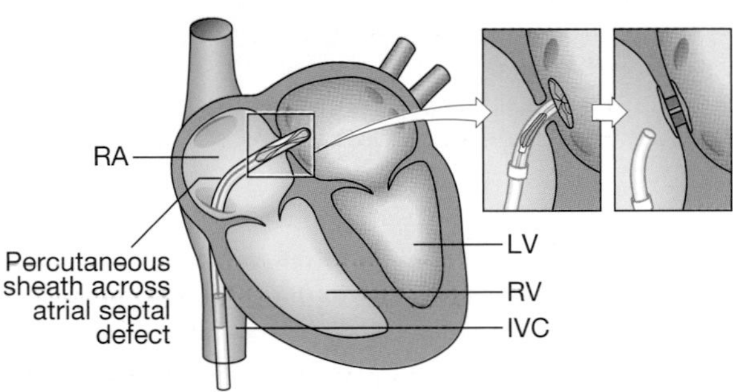

Fig. 18.100 Percutaneous close of atrial septal defect. The closure device is delivered across the inter-atrial septum and a disc deployed on either side to seal the defect.

(with a 'primum' defect, there is also left axis deviation). Echocardiography can directly demonstrate the defect and typically shows RV dilatation, RV hypertrophy and pulmonary artery dilatation. The precise size and location of the defect can be shown by transoesophageal echocardiography (Fig. 18.99).

Management

Atrial septal defects in which pulmonary flow is increased 50% above systemic flow (i.e. flow ratio of 1.5:1) are often large enough to be clinically recognisable and should be closed surgically. Closure can also be accomplished at cardiac catheterisation using implantable closure devices (Fig. 18.100). The long-term prognosis thereafter is excellent, unless pulmonary hypertension has developed. Severe pulmonary hypertension and shunt reversal are both contraindications to surgery.

Ventricular septal defect

Aetiology

Congenital ventricular septal defect occurs as a result of incomplete septation of the ventricles. Embryologically, the interventricular septum has a membranous and a muscular portion, and the latter is further divided into inflow, trabecular and outflow portions. Most congenital defects are 'perimembranous', i.e. at the junction of the membranous and muscular portions.

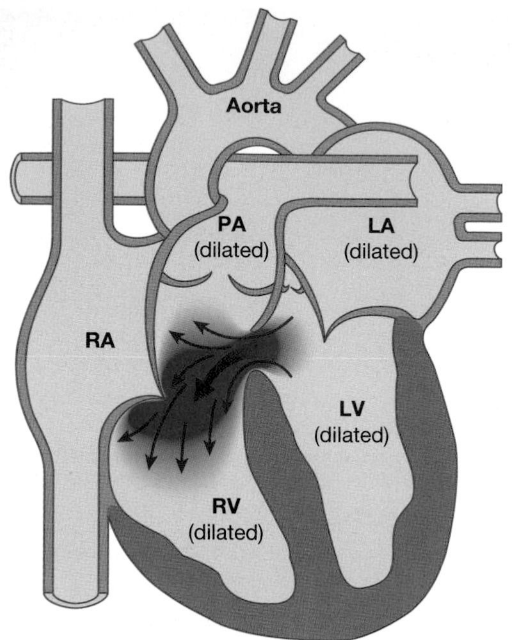

Fig. 18.101 Ventricular septal defect. In this example, a large left-to-right shunt (arrows) has resulted in chamber enlargement.

Ventricular septal defects are the most common congenital cardiac defect, occurring once in 500 live births. The defect may be isolated or part of complex congenital heart disease. Acquired ventricular septal defect may result from rupture as a complication of acute MI or, rarely, from trauma.

Clinical features

Flow from the high-pressure LV to the low-pressure RV during systole produces a pansystolic murmur, usually heard best at the left sternal edge but radiating all over the precordium (Fig. 18.101). A small defect often produces a loud murmur (maladie de Roger) in the absence of other haemodynamic disturbance. Conversely, a large defect produces a softer murmur, particularly if pressure in the RV is elevated. This may be found immediately after birth, while pulmonary vascular resistance remains high, or when the shunt is reversed in Eisenmenger's syndrome.

Congenital ventricular septal defect may present as cardiac failure in infants, as a murmur with only minor haemodynamic disturbance in older children or adults, or, rarely, as Eisenmenger's syndrome. In a proportion of infants, the murmur gets quieter or disappears due to spontaneous closure of the defect.

If cardiac failure complicates a large defect, it is usually absent in the immediate postnatal period and only becomes apparent in the first 4–6 weeks of life. In addition to the murmur, there is prominent parasternal pulsation, tachypnoea and indrawing of the lower ribs on inspiration. The chest X-ray shows pulmonary plethora and the ECG shows bilateral ventricular hypertrophy.

Management and prognosis

Small ventricular septal defects require no specific treatment. Cardiac failure in infancy is initially treated medically with digoxin and diuretics. Persisting failure is an indication for surgical repair of the defect. Percutaneous closure devices are under development.

Doppler echocardiography helps to predict the small septal defects that are likely to close spontaneously. Eisenmenger's syndrome is avoided by monitoring for signs of rising pulmonary resistance (serial ECG and echocardiography) and carrying out surgical repair, when appropriate. Surgical closure is contraindicated in fully developed Eisenmenger's syndrome when heart–lung transplantation may be the only effective treatment.

Except in Eisenmenger's syndrome, long-term prognosis is very good in congenital ventricular septal defect. Many patients with Eisenmenger's syndrome die in the second or third decade of life, but a few survive to the fifth decade without transplantation.

Tetralogy of Fallot

The RV outflow obstruction is most often subvalvular (infundibular) but may be valvular, supravalvular or a combination of these (Fig. 18.102). The ventricular septal defect is usually large and similar in aperture to the aortic orifice. The combination results in elevated right ventricular pressure and right-to-left shunting of cyanotic blood across the ventricular septal defect.

Aetiology

The embryological cause is abnormal development of the bulbar septum that separates the ascending aorta from the pulmonary artery, and which normally aligns and fuses with the outflow part of the interventricular septum. The defect occurs in about 1 in 2000 births and is the most common cause of cyanosis in infancy after the first year of life.

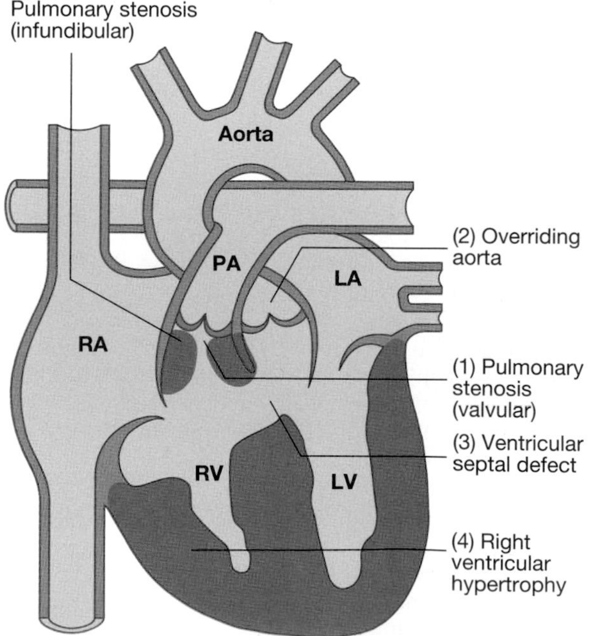

Fig. 18.102 Tetralogy of Fallot. The tetralogy comprises (1) pulmonary stenosis, (2) overriding of the ventricular septal defect by the aorta, (3) a ventricular septal defect and (4) right ventricular hypertrophy.

Clinical features

Children are usually cyanosed but this may not be the case in the neonate because it is only when right ventricular pressure rises to equal or exceed left ventricular pressure that a large right-to-left shunt develops. The subvalvular component of the RV outflow obstruction is dynamic and may increase suddenly under adrenergic stimulation. The affected child suddenly becomes increasingly cyanosed, often after feeding or a crying attack, and may become apnoeic and unconscious. These attacks are called 'Fallot's spells'. In older children, Fallot's spells are uncommon but cyanosis becomes increasingly apparent, with stunting of growth, digital clubbing and polycythaemia. Some children characteristically obtain relief by squatting after exertion, which increases the afterload of the left heart and reduces the right-to-left shunting: Fallot's sign. The natural history before the development of surgical correction was variable but most patients died in infancy or childhood.

On examination, the most characteristic feature is the combination of cyanosis with a loud ejection systolic murmur in the pulmonary area (as for pulmonary stenosis). However, cyanosis may be absent in the newborn or in patients with only mild right ventricular outflow obstruction ('acyanotic tetralogy of Fallot').

Investigations and management

The ECG shows right ventricular hypertrophy and the chest X-ray shows an abnormally small pulmonary artery and a 'boot-shaped' heart. Echocardiography is diagnostic and demonstrates that the aorta is not continuous with the anterior ventricular septum.

The definitive management is total correction of the defect by surgical relief of the pulmonary stenosis and closure of the ventricular septal defect. Primary surgical correction may be undertaken prior to the age of 5 years. If the pulmonary arteries are too hypoplastic, then palliation in the form of a Blalock–Taussig shunt may be performed, with an anastomosis created between the pulmonary artery and subclavian artery. This improves pulmonary blood flow and pulmonary artery development, and may facilitate later definitive correction.

The prognosis after total correction is good, especially if the operation is performed in childhood. Follow-up is needed to identify residual shunting, recurrent pulmonary stenosis and arrhythmias. An implantable defibrillator is sometimes recommended in adulthood.

Other causes of cyanotic congenital heart disease

There are other causes of cyanotic congenital heart disease (Box 18.123) and echocardiography is usually the definitive diagnostic procedure, supplemented, if necessary, by cardiac catheterisation.

Grown-up congenital heart disease

There are increasing numbers of children who have had surgical correction of congenital defects and who may have further problems as adults. The transition period between paediatric and adult care needs to be managed in a carefully planned manner, addressing many diverse aspects of care (Box 18.124). Those who have undergone correction of coarctation of the aorta may develop

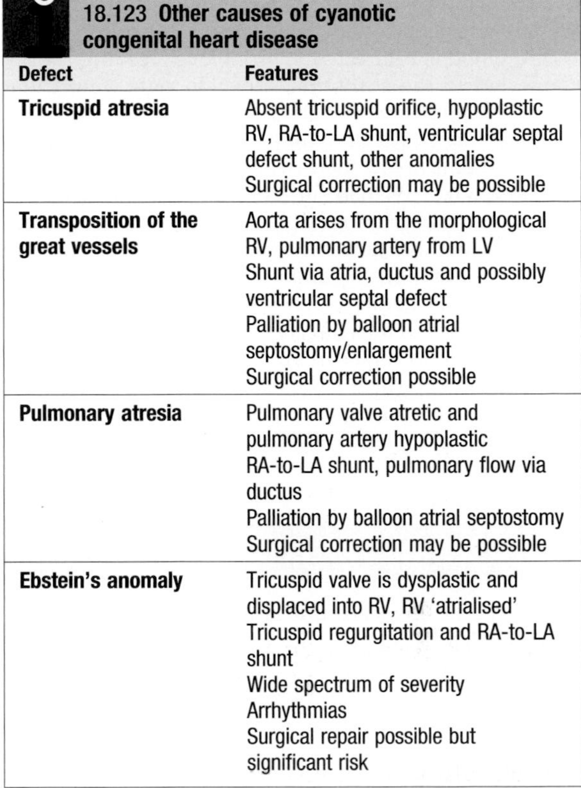

18.123 Other causes of cyanotic congenital heart disease

Defect	Features
Tricuspid atresia	Absent tricuspid orifice, hypoplastic RV, RA-to-LA shunt, ventricular septal defect shunt, other anomalies Surgical correction may be possible
Transposition of the great vessels	Aorta arises from the morphological RV, pulmonary artery from LV Shunt via atria, ductus and possibly ventricular septal defect Palliation by balloon atrial septostomy/enlargement Surgical correction possible
Pulmonary atresia	Pulmonary valve atretic and pulmonary artery hypoplastic RA-to-LA shunt, pulmonary flow via ductus Palliation by balloon atrial septostomy Surgical correction may be possible
Ebstein's anomaly	Tricuspid valve is dysplastic and displaced into RV, RV 'atrialised' Tricuspid regurgitation and RA-to-LA shunt Wide spectrum of severity Arrhythmias Surgical repair possible but significant risk

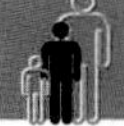

18.124 Congenital heart disease in adolescence

- **Patients**: a heterogeneous population with residual disease and sequelae that vary according to the underlying lesion and in severity; each patient must be assessed individually.
- **Management plan**: should be agreed with the patient and include a 'cardiac destination'.
- **Risks of surgery**: non-cardiac surgery, e.g. for associated congenital abnormalities, carries increased risks and needs to be planned, with careful pre-operative assessment. Risks include thrombosis, embolism from synthetic shunts or patches, and volume overload from fluid shifts. Operative approaches should address cosmetic concerns, e.g. abdominal generator implantation may be less unsightly.
- **Exercise**: patients with mild or repaired defects can undertake moderately vigorous exercise but those with complex defects, cyanosis, ventricular dysfunction or arrhythmias require specialist evaluation and individualised advice regarding exercise.
- **Genetics**: 10–15% have a genetic basis and this should be assessed to understand the impact it may have for the patient's own future children. A family history, genetic evaluation of syndromic versus non-syndromic disorders and, sometimes, cytogenetics are required.
- **Education and employment**: may be adversely affected and occupational activity levels need to be assessed.
- **End of life**: some adolescents with complex disorders may misperceive and think they have been cured; transition to adult services may be the first time they receive information about mortality. Expectations on life expectancy need to be managed and adolescents are often willing to engage with this and play a role in decision-making.

hypertension in adult life. Those with transposition of the great arteries who have had a 'Mustard' repair, where blood is redirected at atrial level, leaving the RV connected to the aorta, may develop right ventricular failure in adult life. The RV is unsuited for function at systemic pressures and may begin to dilate and fail when patients are in their twenties or thirties.

Those who have had surgery involving the atria may develop atrial arrhythmias, and those who have ventricular scars may develop ventricular arrhythmias and need consideration for implantation of an implantable cardiac defibrillator. Such patients require careful follow-up from the teenage years throughout adult life, so that problems can be identified early and appropriate medical or surgical treatment instituted. The management of patients with grown-up congenital heart disease ('GUCH') is complex and has developed as a cardiological subspecialty.

DISEASES OF THE MYOCARDIUM

Although the myocardium is involved in most types of heart disease, the terms 'myocarditis' and 'cardiomyopathy' are usually reserved for conditions that primarily affect the heart muscle.

Myocarditis

This is an acute inflammatory condition that can have an infectious, toxic or autoimmune aetiology. Myocarditis can complicate many infections in which inflammation may be due directly to infection of the myocardium or the effects of circulating toxins. Viral infections are the most common causes, such as Coxsackie (35 cases per 1000 infections) and influenza A and B (25 cases per 1000 infections) viruses. Myocarditis may occur several weeks after the initial viral symptoms and susceptibility is increased by corticosteroid treatment, immunosuppression, radiation, previous myocardial damage and exercise. Some bacterial and protozoal infections may be complicated by myocarditis; for example, approximately 5% of patients with Lyme disease (*Borrelia burgdorferi*, p. 334) develop myopericarditis, which is often associated with AV block. Toxic aetiologies include drugs, which may directly injure the myocardium (e.g. cocaine, lithium and anti-cancer drugs, such as doxorubicin) or which may cause a hypersensitivity reaction and associated myocarditis (e.g. penicillins and sulphonamides, lead and carbon monoxide). Occasionally, autoimmune conditions, such as systemic lupus erythematosus and rheumatoid arthritis, are associated with myocarditis.

Clinical features and investigations

Myocarditis can be classified by four distinct clinical presentations:

- *Fulminant myocarditis* follows a viral prodrome or influenza-like illness, and results in severe heart failure or cardiogenic shock.
- *Acute myocarditis* presents over a longer period with heart failure; it can lead to dilated cardiomyopathy.
- *Chronic active myocarditis* is rare and associated with chronic myocardial inflammation.
- *Chronic persistent myocarditis* is characterised by focal myocardial infiltrates and can cause chest pain and arrhythmia without necessarily causing ventricular dysfunction.

In myocarditis, ECG changes are common but non-specific. Biochemical markers of myocardial injury (e.g. troponin I and T, creatine kinase) may be elevated in the early phases. Echocardiography may reveal left ventricular dysfunction that is sometimes regional (due to focal myocarditis), and cardiac MRI may show diagnostic patterns of myocardial inflammation or infiltration. Endomyocardial biopsy is sometimes used to confirm the diagnosis.

Management and prognosis

In most patients, myocarditis is self-limiting and the immediate prognosis is good. However, death may occur due to a ventricular arrhythmia or rapidly progressive heart failure. Myocarditis has been reported as a cause of sudden and unexpected death in young athletes. Some forms of myocarditis may lead to chronic low-grade myocarditis or dilated cardiomyopathy (see below); for example, in Chagas' disease (p. 360), the patient frequently recovers from the acute infection but goes on to develop a chronic dilated cardiomyopathy 10 or 20 years later.

Specific antimicrobial therapy may be used if a causative organism has been identified; this is rare, however, and in most cases only supportive therapy is available. Treatment for cardiac failure or arrhythmias may be required and patients should be advised to avoid intense physical exertion because there is some evidence that this can induce potentially fatal ventricular arrhythmias. There is no evidence for any benefit from treatment with corticosteroids and immunosuppressive agents. Rarely cardiac transplantation or temporary circulatory support with a mechanical ventricular assist device is required.

Cardiomyopathy

Cardiomyopathies are diseases of the myocardium, and are classified according to their structural and functional presentation (Fig. 18.103). They can be inherited or have infective, toxic or idiopathic aetiologies.

Dilated cardiomyopathy

This is characterised by dilatation and impaired contraction of the LV and often the RV. Left ventricular mass is increased but wall thickness is normal or reduced (see Fig. 18.103). Dilatation of the valve rings can lead to 'functional' mitral and tricuspid incompetence. Histological changes are variable but include myofibrillary loss, interstitial fibrosis and T-cell infiltrates. The differential diagnosis includes ventricular dysfunction due to coronary artery disease, and a diagnosis of dilated cardiomyopathy should only be made when this has been excluded.

The pathogenesis is not clear but dilated cardiomyopathy probably encompasses a heterogenous group of conditions. Alcohol may be an important cause in some patients. At least 25% of cases are inherited as an autosomal dominant trait and a variety of single-gene mutations have been identified. Most of these mutations

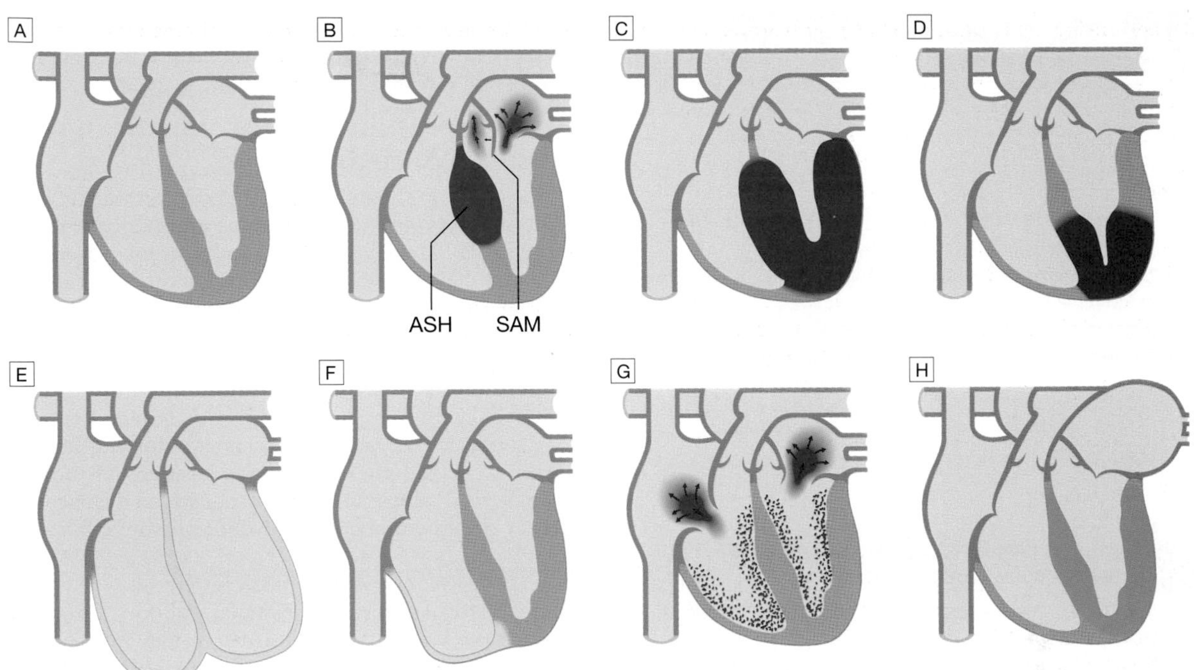

Fig. 18.103 Types of cardiomyopathy. A Normal heart. B Hypertrophic cardiomyopathy: asymmetric septal hypertrophy (ASH) with systolic anterior motion of the mitral valve (SAM), causing mitral reflux and dynamic left ventricular outflow tract obstruction. C Hypertrophic cardiomyopathy: concentric hypertrophy. D Hypertrophic cardiomyopathy: apical hypertrophy. E Dilated cardiomyopathy. F Arrhythmogenic right ventricular cardiomyopathy. G Obliterative cardiomyopathy. H Restrictive cardiomyopathy.

affect proteins in the cytoskeleton of the myocyte (e.g. dystrophin, lamin A and C, emerin and metavinculin) and many are associated with minor skeletal muscle abnormalities. Most of the X-linked inherited skeletal muscular dystrophies (e.g. Becker and Duchenne, p. 1228) are associated with cardiomyopathy. Finally, a late autoimmune reaction to viral myocarditis is thought to be the cause in a substantial subgroup of patients with dilated cardiomyopathy; a similar mechanism is thought to be responsible for the heart muscle disease that occurs in up to 10% of patients with advanced HIV infection.

In North America and Europe, symptomatic dilated cardiomyopathy has an incidence of 20 per 100 000 and a prevalence of 38 per 100 000. Men are affected more than twice as often as women. Most patients present with heart failure or are found to have the condition during routine investigation. Arrhythmia, thromboembolism and sudden death may occur at any stage; sporadic chest pain is a surprisingly frequent symptom. The ECG usually shows non-specific changes but echocardiography and cardiac MRI are useful in establishing the diagnosis. Treatment is aimed at controlling the resulting heart failure. Although some patients remain well for many years, the prognosis is variable and cardiac transplantation may be indicated. Patients with dilated cardiomyopathy and moderate or severe heart failure may be at risk of sudden arrhythmic death. This risk is substantially reduced by rigorous medical therapy with β-blockers and angiotensin receptor antagonists. Some patients may be considered for implantation of a cardiac defibrillator and/or cardiac resynchronisation therapy (p. 579).

Hypertrophic cardiomyopathy

This is the most common form of cardiomyopathy, with a prevalence of approximately 100 per 100 000. It is characterised by inappropriate and elaborate left ventricular hypertrophy with malalignment of the myocardial fibres and myocardial fibrosis. The hypertrophy may be generalised or confined largely to the interventricular septum (asymmetric septal hypertrophy, see Fig. 18.103) or other regions (e.g. apical hypertrophic cardiomyopathy, a variant which is common in the Far East).

Heart failure may develop because the stiff non-compliant ventricles impede diastolic filling. Septal hypertrophy may also cause dynamic left ventricular outflow tract obstruction (hypertrophic obstructive cardiomyopathy, HOCM) and mitral regurgitation due to abnormal systolic anterior motion of the anterior mitral valve leaflet. Effort-related symptoms (angina and breathlessness), arrhythmia and sudden death are the dominant clinical presentations.

Hypertrophic cardiomyopathy is a genetic disorder, usually with autosomal dominant transmission, a high degree of penetrance and variable expression. In most patients, it is due to a single point mutation in one of the genes that encode sarcomeric contractile proteins. There are three common groups of mutation with different phenotypes. Beta-myosin heavy chain mutations are associated with elaborate ventricular hypertrophy. Troponin mutations are associated with little, and sometimes even no, hypertrophy but marked myocardial fibre disarray, an abnormal vascular response (e.g. exercise-induced hypotension) and a high risk of sudden death. Myosin-binding protein C mutations tend to

18.125 Clinical features of hypertrophic cardiomyopathy

Symptoms

- Angina on effort
- Dyspnoea on effort
- Syncope on effort
- Sudden death

Signs

- Jerky pulse*
- Palpable left ventricular hypertrophy
- Double impulse at the apex (palpable fourth heart sound due to left atrial hypertrophy)
- Mid-systolic murmur at the base*
- Pansystolic murmur (due to mitral regurgitation) at the apex

*Signs of left ventricular outflow tract obstruction may be augmented by standing up (reduced venous return), inotropes and vasodilators (e.g. sublingual nitrate).

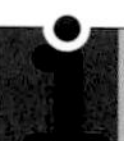

18.126 Risk factors for sudden death in hypertrophic cardiomyopathy

- A history of previous cardiac arrest or sustained ventricular tachycardia
- Recurrent syncope
- An adverse genotype and/or family history
- Exercise-induced hypotension
- Non-sustained ventricular tachycardia on ambulatory ECG monitoring
- Marked increase in left ventricular wall thickness

present late in life and are often associated with hypertension and arrhythmia.

Symptoms and signs are similar to those of aortic stenosis, except that, in hypertrophic cardiomyopathy, the character of the arterial pulse is jerky (Box 18.125).

The ECG is abnormal and shows features of left ventricular hypertrophy with a wide variety of often bizarre abnormalities (e.g. pseudo-infarct pattern, deep T-wave inversion). Echocardiography is diagnostic, although the diagnosis may be difficult when another cause of left ventricular hypertrophy is present (e.g. physical training – athletes' heart, hypertension) but the degree of hypertrophy is greater than expected. Genetic testing may facilitate diagnosis and, in some cases, is helpful in screening relatives of affected individuals.

The natural history is variable but clinical deterioration is often slow. The annual mortality from sudden death is 2–3% among adults and 4–6% in children and adolescents (Box 18.126). Sudden death typically occurs during or just after vigorous physical activity; indeed, hypertrophic cardiomyopathy is the most common cause of sudden death in young athletes. Ventricular arrhythmias may be responsible for many of these.

Beta-blockers, rate-limiting calcium antagonists (e.g. verapamil) and disopyramide can help to relieve symptoms and sometimes prevent syncopal attacks; however, there is no pharmacological treatment that is definitely known to improve prognosis. Arrhythmias are common and often respond to treatment with amiodarone. Outflow tract obstruction can be improved by partial surgical resection (myectomy) or by iatrogenic infarction of the basal septum (septal ablation) using a catheter-delivered alcohol solution. An implantable cardiac defibrillator should be considered in patients with clinical risk factors for sudden death (see Box 18.126). Digoxin and vasodilators may increase outflow tract obstruction and should be avoided.

Arrhythmogenic right ventricular cardiomyopathy

In this condition, patches of the right ventricular myocardium are replaced with fibrous and fatty tissue (see Fig. 18.102). It is inherited as an autosomal dominant trait and has a prevalence of approximately 10 per 100 000. The dominant clinical problems are ventricular arrhythmias, sudden death and right-sided cardiac failure. The ECG typically shows a slightly broadened QRS complex and inverted T waves in the right precordial leads. MRI is a useful diagnostic tool and is used, along with the 12-lead ECG and ambulatory ECG monitoring, to screen the first-degree relatives of affected individuals. Patients at high risk of sudden death can be offered an implantable cardiac defibrillator.

Restrictive cardiomyopathy

In this rare condition, ventricular filling is impaired because the ventricles are 'stiff' (see Fig. 18.102). This leads to high atrial pressures with atrial hypertrophy, dilatation and, later, atrial fibrillation. Amyloidosis is the most common cause in the UK, although other forms of infiltration (e.g. glycogen storage diseases), idiopathic perimyocyte fibrosis and a familial form of restrictive cardiomyopathy do occur. Diagnosis can be very difficult and requires complex Doppler echocardiography, CT or MRI, and endomyocardial biopsy. Treatment is symptomatic but the prognosis is usually poor and transplantation may be indicated.

Obliterative cardiomyopathy

This is a rare form of restrictive cardiomyopathy, involving the endocardium of one or both ventricles; it is characterised by thrombosis and fibrosis, with gradual obliteration of the ventricular cavities (e.g. endomyocardial fibroelastosis, see Fig. 18.103). The mitral and tricuspid valves become regurgitant. Heart failure and pulmonary and systemic embolism are prominent features. It can sometimes be associated with eosinophilia (e.g. eosinophilic leukaemia, Churg–Strauss syndrome, p. 1118). In tropical countries, the disease can be responsible for up to 10% of cardiac deaths. Mortality is high: 50% at 2 years. Anticoagulation and antiplatelet therapy are used, and diuretics may help symptoms of heart failure. Surgery (tricuspid and/or mitral valve replacement with decortication of the endocardium) may be helpful in selected cases.

Specific diseases of heart muscle

Many forms of specific heart muscle disease produce a clinical picture that is indistinguishable from dilated cardiomyopathy (e.g. connective tissue disorders, sarcoidosis, haemochromatosis, alcoholic heart muscle disease, Box 18.127). In contrast, amyloidosis and eosinophilic heart disease produce symptoms and signs similar to those found in restrictive or obliterative cardiomyopathy, whereas the heart disease associated with Friedreich's ataxia (p. 1199) can mimic hypertrophic cardiomyopathy.

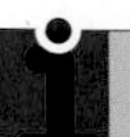

18.127 Specific diseases of heart muscle

Infections
• Viral, e.g. Coxsackie A and B, influenza, HIV • Bacterial, e.g. diphtheria, *Borrelia burgdorferi* • Protozoal, e.g. trypanosomiasis
Endocrine and metabolic disorders
• Diabetes, hypo- and hyperthyroidism, acromegaly, carcinoid syndrome, phaeochromocytoma, inherited storage diseases
Connective tissue diseases
• Systemic sclerosis, systemic lupus erythematosus, polyarteritis nodosa
Infiltrative disorders
• Haemochromatosis, haemosiderosis, sarcoidosis, amyloidosis
Toxins
• Doxorubicin, alcohol, cocaine, irradiation
Neuromuscular disorders
• Dystrophia myotonica, Friedreich's ataxia

Treatment and prognosis are determined by the underlying disorder. Abstention from alcohol may lead to a dramatic improvement in patients with alcoholic heart muscle disease.

Cardiac tumours

Primary cardiac tumours are rare (< 0.2% of autopsies) but the heart and mediastinum may be the sites of metastases. Most primary tumours are benign (75%) and, of these, the majority are myxomas. The remainder are fibromas, lipomas, fibroelastomas and haemangiomas.

Atrial myxoma

Myxomas most commonly arise in the LA as single or multiple polypoid tumours, attached by a pedicle to the interatrial septum. They are usually gelatinous but may be solid and even calcified, with superimposed thrombus.

On examination, the first heart sound is usually loud, and there may be a murmur of mitral regurgitation with a variable diastolic sound (tumour 'plop') due to prolapse of the mass through the mitral valve. The tumour can be detected incidentally on echocardiography, or following investigation of pyrexia, syncope, arrhythmias or emboli. Occasionally, the condition presents with malaise and features suggestive of a connective tissue disorder, including a raised ESR.

Treatment is by surgical excision. If the pedicle is removed, fewer than 5% of tumours recur.

DISEASES OF THE PERICARDIUM

The normal pericardial sac contains about 50 mL of fluid, similar to lymph, which lubricates the surface of the heart. The pericardium limits distension of the heart, contributes to the haemodynamic interdependence of the ventricles, and acts as a barrier to infection. Nevertheless, congenital absence of the pericardium does not result in significant clinical or functional limitations.

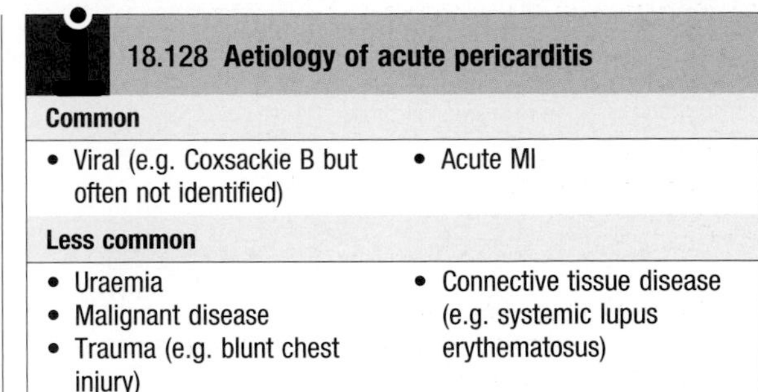

18.128 Aetiology of acute pericarditis

Common	
• Viral (e.g. Coxsackie B but often not identified)	• Acute MI
Less common	
• Uraemia • Malignant disease • Trauma (e.g. blunt chest injury)	• Connective tissue disease (e.g. systemic lupus erythematosus)
Rare (in UK)	
• Bacterial infection • Rheumatic fever	• Tuberculosis

Acute pericarditis

Aetiology

Pericardial inflammation may be due to a number of pathologies (Box 18.128) but sometimes remains unexplained. Pericarditis and myocarditis often coexist, and all forms of pericarditis may produce a pericardial effusion (see below) that, depending on the aetiology, may be fibrinous, serous, haemorrhagic or purulent.

A fibrinous exudate may eventually lead to varying degrees of adhesion formation, whereas serous pericarditis often produces a large effusion of turbid, straw-coloured fluid with a high protein content.

A haemorrhagic effusion is often due to malignant disease, particularly carcinoma of the breast or bronchus, and lymphoma.

Purulent pericarditis is rare and may occur as a complication of septicaemia, by direct spread from an intrathoracic infection, or from a penetrating injury.

Clinical features

The characteristic pain of pericarditis is retrosternal, radiates to the shoulders and neck, and is typically aggravated by deep breathing, movement, a change of position, exercise and swallowing. A low-grade fever is common. A pericardial friction rub is a high-pitched superficial scratching or crunching noise, produced by movement of the inflamed pericardium, and is diagnostic of pericarditis; it is usually heard in systole but may also be audible in diastole and frequently has a 'to-and-fro' quality.

Investigations and management

The ECG shows ST elevation with upward concavity (Fig. 18.104) over the affected area, which may be widespread. PR interval depression is a very specific indicator of acute pericarditis. Later, there may be T-wave inversion, particularly if there is a degree of myocarditis.

The pain is usually relieved by aspirin (600 mg 6 times daily) but a more potent anti-inflammatory agent, such as indometacin (25 mg 3 times daily), may be required. Colchicine or corticosteroids may suppress symptoms but there is no evidence that they accelerate cure.

In viral pericarditis, recovery usually occurs within a few days or weeks but there may be recurrences (chronic relapsing pericarditis). Purulent pericarditis requires

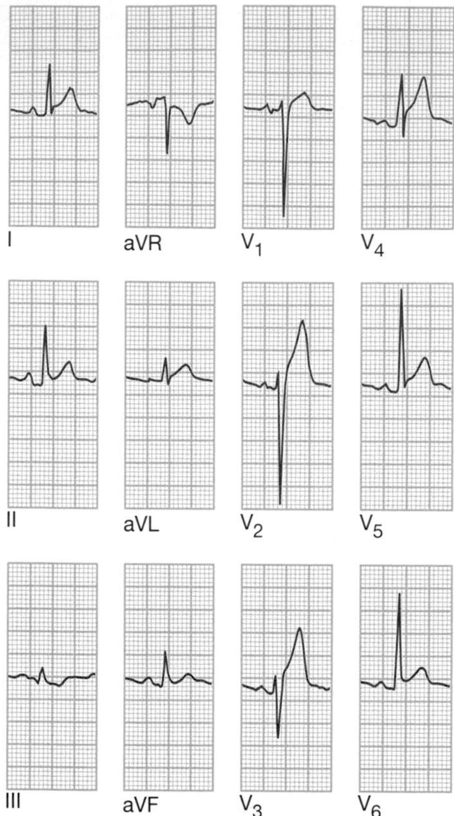

Fig. 18.104 ECG in viral pericarditis. Widespread ST elevation (leads I, II, aVL and V_1–V_6) is shown. The upward concave shape of the ST segments (see leads II and V_6) and the unusual distribution of changes (involving anterior and inferior leads) help to distinguish pericarditis from acute MI.

treatment with antimicrobial therapy, pericardiocentesis and, if necessary, surgical drainage.

Pericardial effusion

If a pericardial effusion develops, there is sometimes a sensation of retrosternal oppression. An effusion is difficult to detect clinically. The heart sounds may become quieter, although a friction rub is not always abolished.

The QRS voltages on the ECG are often reduced in the presence of a large effusion. The QRS complexes may alternate in amplitude due to a to-and-fro motion of the heart within the fluid-filled pericardial sac (electrical alternans). The chest X-ray may show an increased size of the cardiac silhouette and, when there is a large effusion, this has a globular appearance. Echocardiography is the definitive investigation and is used to monitor the size of the effusion and its effect on cardiac function (Fig. 18.105).

Cardiac tamponade

This term is used to describe acute heart failure due to compression of the heart by a large or rapidly developing effusion, and is described in detail on page 545. Typical physical findings are of a markedly raised JVP, hypotension, pulsus paradoxus (p. 532) and oliguria. Atypical presentations may occur when the effusion is loculated as a result of previous pericarditis or cardiac surgery.

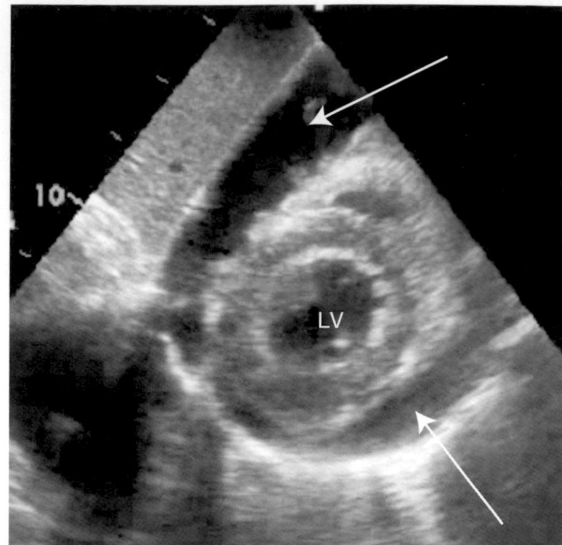

Fig. 18.105 Pericardial effusion: echocardiogram (apical view). Short axis view of the heart showing a large circumferential pericardial effusion (arrows). (LV = left ventricle)

Pericardial aspiration (pericardiocentesis)

Aspiration of a pericardial effusion is indicated for diagnostic purposes or for the treatment of cardiac tamponade. A needle is inserted under echocardiographic guidance medial to the cardiac apex or below the xiphoid process, directed upwards towards the left shoulder. The route of choice will depend on the experience of the operator, the shape of the patient and the position of the effusion. A few millilitres of fluid aspirated through the needle may be sufficient for diagnostic purposes but pericardial drainage is needed for symptom relief.

Complications of pericardiocentesis include arrhythmias, damage to a coronary artery, and bleeding with exacerbation of tamponade as a result of injury to the RV. When tamponade is due to cardiac rupture or aortic dissection, pericardial aspiration may precipitate further potentially fatal bleeding and, in these situations, emergency surgery is the treatment of choice. A viscous, loculated or recurrent effusion may also require formal surgical drainage.

Tuberculous pericarditis

Tuberculous pericarditis may complicate pulmonary tuberculosis but may also be the first manifestation of the infection. In Africa, a tuberculous pericardial effusion is a common feature of AIDS (p. 405).

The condition typically presents with chronic malaise, weight loss and a low-grade fever. An effusion usually develops and the pericardium may become thick and unyielding, leading to pericardial constriction or tamponade. An associated pleural effusion is often present.

The diagnosis may be confirmed by aspiration of the fluid and direct examination or culture for tubercle bacilli. Treatment requires specific antituberculous chemotherapy (p. 693); in addition, a 3-month course of prednisolone (initial dose 60 mg a day, tapering down rapidly) improves outcome.

Chronic constrictive pericarditis

Constrictive pericarditis is due to progressive thickening, fibrosis and calcification of the pericardium. In effect, the heart is encased in a solid shell and cannot fill properly. The calcification may extend into the myocardium, so there may also be impaired myocardial contraction. The condition often follows an attack of tuberculous pericarditis but can also complicate haemopericardium, viral pericarditis, rheumatoid arthritis and purulent pericarditis. It is often impossible to identify the original insult.

Clinical features and management

The symptoms and signs of systemic venous congestion are the hallmarks of constrictive pericarditis. Atrial fibrillation is common and there is often dramatic ascites and hepatomegaly (Box 18.129). Breathlessness is not a prominent symptom because the lungs are seldom congested.

The condition is sometimes overlooked but should be suspected in any patient with unexplained right heart failure and a small heart. A chest X-ray, which may show pericardial calcification (Fig. 18.106), and echocardiography often help to establish the diagnosis. CT scanning is useful for imaging the pericardial calcification.

Constrictive pericarditis is often difficult to distinguish from restrictive cardiomyopathy and the final diagnosis may depend on complex echo–Doppler studies and cardiac catheterisation. Surgical resection of the diseased pericardium can lead to a dramatic improvement but carries a high morbidity with disappointing results in up to 50% of patients.

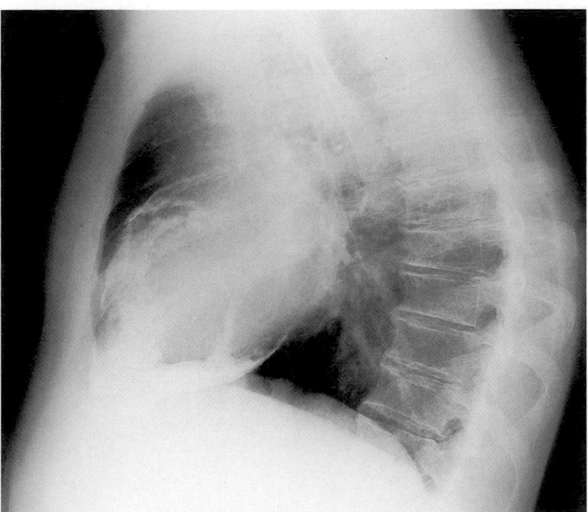

Fig. 18.106 Lateral chest X-ray from a patient with severe heart failure due to chronic constrictive pericarditis. There is heavy calcification of the pericardium.

18.129 Clinical features of constrictive pericarditis

- Fatigue
- Rapid, low-volume pulse
- Elevated JVP with a rapid *y* descent
- Kussmaul's sign (a paradoxical rise in the JVP during inspiration)
- Loud early third heart sound or 'pericardial knock'
- Hepatomegaly
- Ascites
- Peripheral oedema
- Pulsus paradoxus (excessive fall in BP during inspiration): present in some cases

Further information and acknowledgements

Websites

www.acc.org *American College of Cardiology (ACC): free access to guidelines for the evaluation and management of many cardiac conditions.*

www.americanheart.org *American Heart Association (AHA): free access to all the ACC/AHA/ESC guidelines, AHA scientific statements and fact sheets for patients.*

www.escardio.org *European Society of Cardiology (ESC): free access to guidelines for the diagnosis and management of many cardiac conditions, and to educational modules.*

Figure acknowledgements

Page 526 insets (Splinter haemorrhage, jugular venous pulse, malar flush, tendon xanthomas), Fig. 18.91, 18.92 inset (Doppler echo), 18.93 insets (Petechial rash, nail-fold infarct) Newby D, Grubb N. Cardiology: an illustrated colour text. Edinburgh: Churchill Livingstone; 2005; copyright Elsevier.

Figs 18.19, 18.70 Scottish Intercollegiate Guidelines Network (SIGN) 93; Feb 2007; pp. 42 (annex 1) and 47 (annex 4).

Figs 18.34, 18.35 Resuscitation Council (UK) guidelines.

Fig. 18.61 Stary HC, et al. Circulation 1995; 92:1355–1374. © 1995 American Heart Association.

Fig. 18.62 Joint British Societies Cardiovascular Risk Prediction Chart, reproduced with permission from the University of Manchester.

Figs 18.84, 18.85 From NICE Clinical Guideline 127, Hypertension; August 2011.

Fig. 18.86 inset (Erythema marginatum) Savin JA, Hunter JAA, Hepburn NC. Skin signs in clinical medicine. London: Mosby–Wolfe; 1997; copyright Elsevier.

Fig. 18.94 Adapted from Drews U. Colour atlas of embryology. Stuttgart: Georg Thieme; 1995 (Fig. 6.9, p. 299).

P.T. Reid
J.A. Innes

Respiratory disease 19

Clinical examination of the respiratory system 644

Functional anatomy and physiology 646

Investigation of respiratory disease 649
- Imaging 649
- Endoscopic examination 651
- Immunological and serological tests 652
- Microbiological investigations 652
- Respiratory function testing 652

Presenting problems in respiratory disease 654
- Cough 654
- Breathlessness 655
- Chest pain 658
- Haemoptysis 658
- The incidental pulmonary nodule 660
- Pleural effusion 661
- Respiratory failure 663

Obstructive pulmonary diseases 666
- Asthma 666
- Chronic obstructive pulmonary disease 673
- Bronchiectasis 678
- Cystic fibrosis 680

Infections of the respiratory system 681
- Upper respiratory tract infection 681
- Pneumonia 682
- Tuberculosis 688
- Respiratory diseases caused by fungi 697

Tumours of the bronchus and lung 699
- Primary tumours of the lung 699
- Secondary tumours of the lung 704
- Tumours of the mediastinum 705

Interstitial and infiltrative pulmonary diseases 706
- Diffuse parenchymal lung disease 706
- Lung diseases due to systemic inflammatory disease 711
- Pulmonary eosinophilia and vasculitides 713
- Lung diseases due to irradiation and drugs 714
- Rare interstitial lung diseases 714

Occupational and environmental lung disease 715
- Occupational airway disease 715
- Pneumoconiosis 716
- Asbestos-related lung and pleural diseases 718
- Lung diseases due to organic dusts 719
- Occupational lung cancer 720
- Occupational pneumonia 720

Pulmonary vascular disease 721
- Venous thromboembolism 721
- Pulmonary hypertension 724

Diseases of the upper airway 725
- Diseases of the nasopharynx 725
- Sleep-disordered breathing 725
- Laryngeal disorders 727
- Tracheal disorders 728

Pleural disease 728
- Pneumothorax 728

Diseases of the diaphragm and chest wall 731
- Disorders of the diaphragm 731
- Deformities of the chest wall 731

CLINICAL EXAMINATION OF THE RESPIRATORY SYSTEM

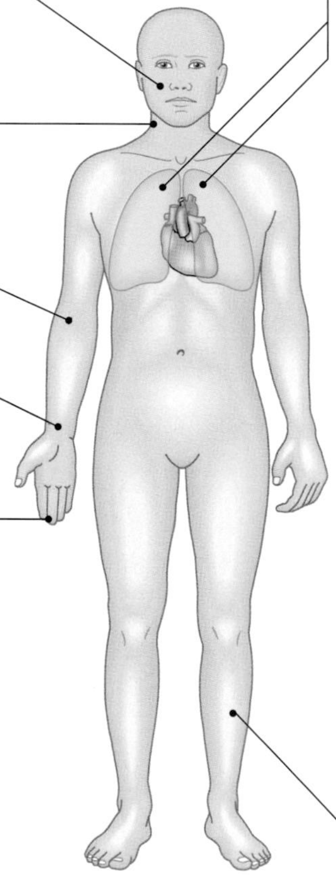

Thorax 6–9
(see opposite)

Face, mouth and eyes 5
Pursed lips
Central cyanosis
Anaemia
Horner's syndrome
(Ch. 26)

Jugular venous pulse 4
Elevated
Pulsatile

Blood pressure 3
Arterial paradox

Radial pulse 2
Rate
Rhythm

Hands 1
Digital clubbing
Tar staining
Peripheral cyanosis
Signs of occupation
CO_2 retention flap

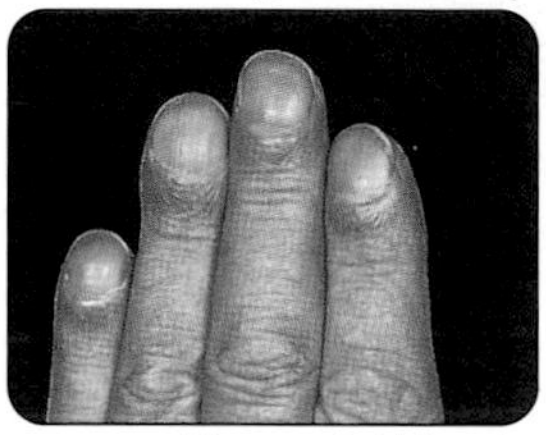

▲ Finger clubbing

Inspection 6
Deformity
(e.g. pectus excavatum)
Scars
Intercostal indrawing
Symmetry of expansion
Hyperinflation
Paradoxical rib movement
(low flat diaphragm)

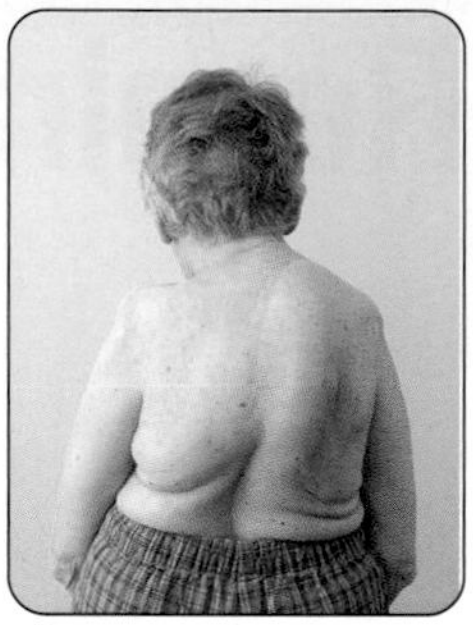

▲ Idiopathic kyphoscoliosis

7 **Palpation**
From the front:
Trachea central
Cricosternal distance
Cardiac apex displaced
Expansion
From behind:
Cervical lymphadenopathy
Expansion

8 **Percussion**
Resonant or dull
'Stony dull' (effusion)

9 **Auscultation**
Breath sounds:
normal, bronchial, louder or softer
Added sounds:
wheezes, crackles, rubs
Spoken voice (vocal resonance):
absent (effusion), increased (consolidation)
Whispered voice:
whispering pectoriloquy

10 **Leg oedema**
Cor pulmonale
Venous thrombosis

Observation

- Respiratory rate
- Cachexia, fever, rash
- Sputum (see below)
- Fetor
- Locale
  Oxygen delivery (mask, cannulae)
  Nebulisers
  Inhalers

Sputum

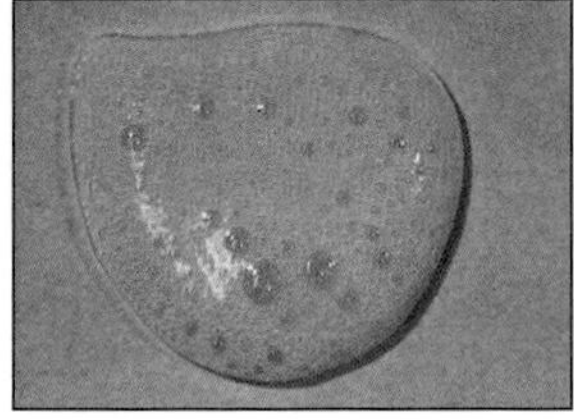
▲ Serous/frothy/pink
Pulmonary oedema

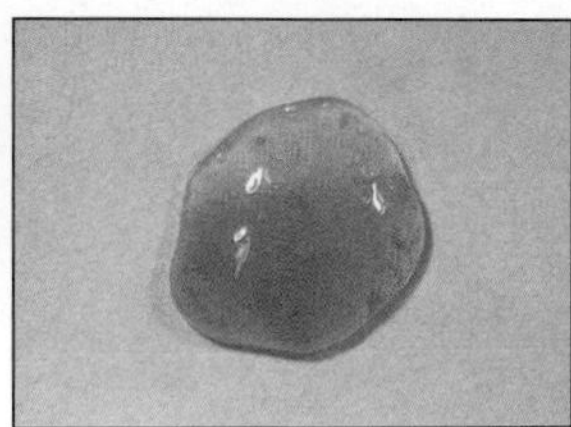
▲ Mucopurulent
Bronchial or pneumonic infection

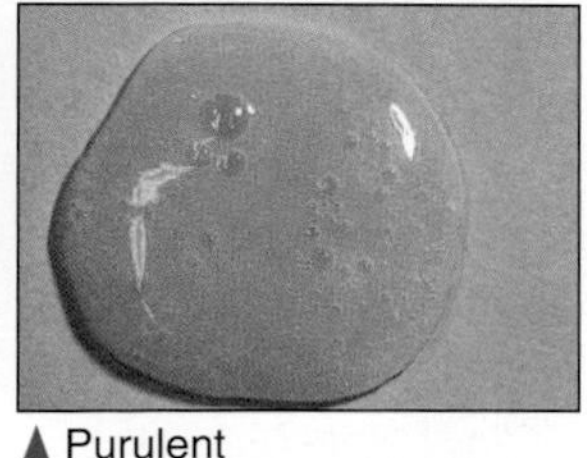
▲ Purulent
Bronchial or pneumonic infection

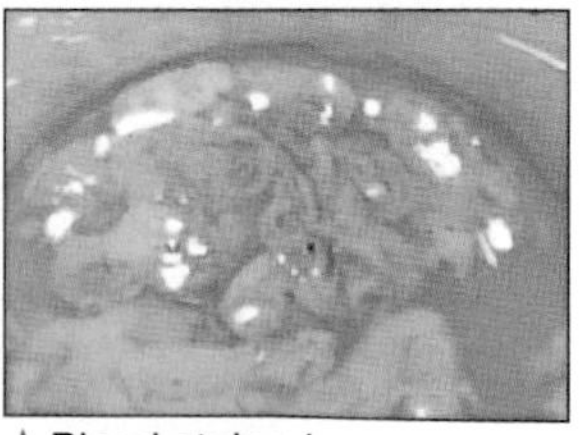
▲ Blood-stained
Cancer, tuberculosis, bronchiectasis, pulmonary embolism

Chronic obstructive pulmonary disease

Pursed lip breathing
Central cyanosis
Prolonged expiration

Reduced cricosternal distance

Use of accessory muscles

Intercostal indrawing during inspiration

Hyperinflated 'barrel' chest

Cardiac apex not palpable
Loss of cardiac dullness on percussion

Auscultation
Reduced breath sounds – wheeze

Heart sounds loudest in epigastrium

Inward movement of lower ribs on inspiration (low flat diaphragm)

Also: raised JVP, peripheral oedema if cor pulmonale

Pulmonary fibrosis

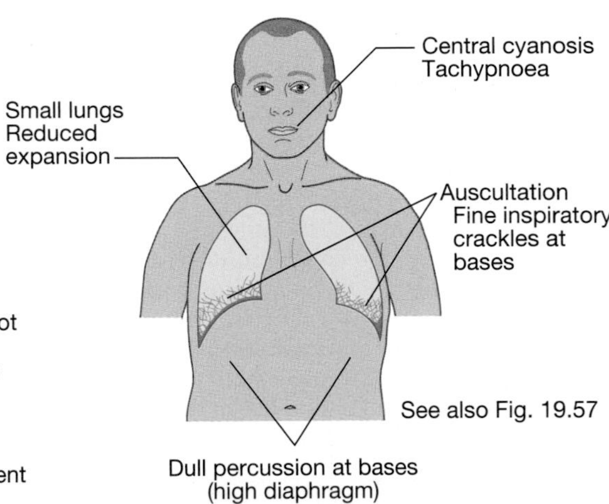

Also: finger clubbing common in idiopathic pulmonary fibrosis; raised JVP and peripheral oedema if cor pulmonale

Right middle lobe pneumonia

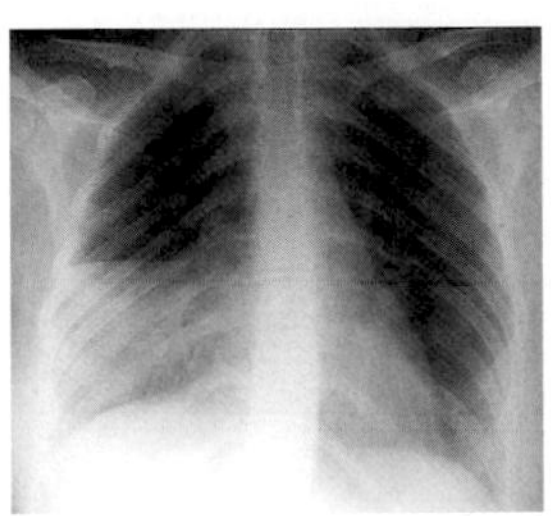

Obscures R heart border on X-ray

Inspection
- Tachypnoea
- Central cyanosis (if severe)

Palpation
- ↓Expansion on R

Percussion
- Dull R mid-zone and axilla

Auscultation
- Bronchial breath sounds and ↑vocal resonance over consolidation and whispering pectoriloquy
- Pleural rub if pleurisy

Right upper lobe collapse

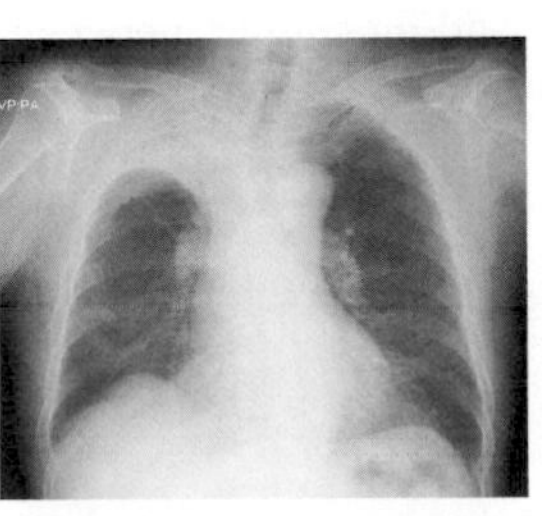

X-ray
- Deviated trachea (to R)
- Elevated horizontal fissure
- ↓Volume R hemithorax
- Central (hilar) mass may be seen

Inspection
- ↓Volume R upper zone

Palpation
- Trachea deviated to R
- ↓Expansion R upper zone

Percussion
- Dull R upper zone

Auscultation
- ↓Breath sounds with central obstruction

Right pneumothorax

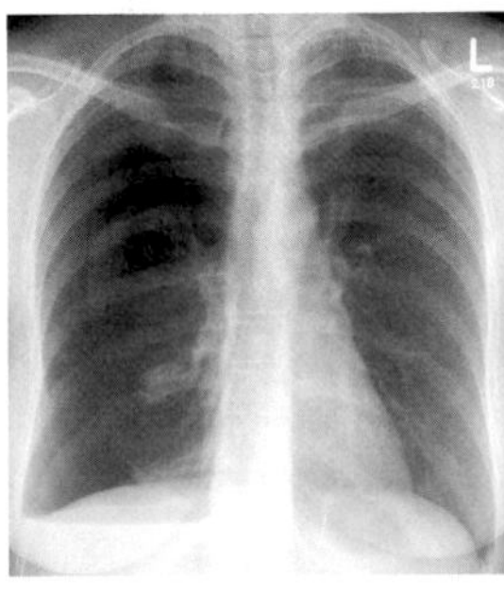

Inspection
- Tachypnoea (pain, deflation reflex)

Palpation
- ↓Expansion R side

Percussion
- Resonant or hyper-resonant on R

Auscultation
- Absent breath sounds on R

Tension pneumothorax also causes
- Deviation of trachea to opposite side
- Tachycardia and hypotension

Large right pleural effusion

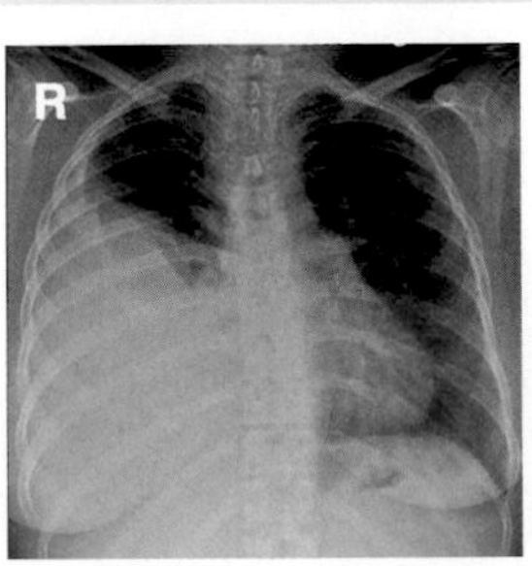

Inspection
- Tachypnoea

Palpation
- ↓Expansion on R
- Trachea and apex may be moved to L

Percussion
- Stony dull
- R mid- and lower zones

Auscultation
- Absent breath sounds and vocal resonance R base
- Bronchial breathing or crackles above effusion

Insets (Upper lobe collapse) http://3.bp.blogspot.com; *(Pneumothorax)* http://chestatlas.com; *(Pleural effusion)* www.ispub.com – see p. 731.

Respiratory disease is responsible for a major burden of morbidity and untimely death, with conditions such as tuberculosis, pandemic influenza and pneumonia the most important in world health terms. The increasing prevalence of allergy, asthma and chronic obstructive pulmonary disease (COPD) contributes to the overall burden of chronic disease in the community. By 2025, the number of cigarette smokers worldwide is anticipated to increase to 1.5 billion, ensuring a growing burden of tobacco-related respiratory conditions.

Respiratory disease covers a breadth of pathologies, including infectious, inflammatory, neoplastic and degenerative processes. The practice of respiratory medicine thus requires collaboration with a range of disciplines. Recent advances have improved the lives of many patients with obstructive lung disease, cystic fibrosis, obstructive sleep apnoea and pulmonary hypertension, but the outlook remains poor for lung and other respiratory cancers, and for some of the fibrosing lung conditions.

FUNCTIONAL ANATOMY AND PHYSIOLOGY

The lungs occupy the upper two-thirds of the bony thorax, bounded medially by the spine, the heart and the mediastinum and inferiorly by the diaphragm. During breathing, free movement of the lung surface relative to the chest wall is facilitated by sliding contact between the parietal and visceral pleura, which cover the inner surface of the chest wall and the lung respectively, and are normally in close apposition. Inspiration involves downward contraction of the dome-shaped diaphragm (innervated by the phrenic nerves originating from C3, 4 and 5) and upward, outward movement of the ribs on the costovertebral joints, caused by contraction of the external intercostal muscles (innervated by intercostal nerves originating from the thoracic spinal cord). Expiration is largely passive, driven by elastic recoil of the lungs.

The conducting airways from the nose to the alveoli connect the external environment with the extensive, thin and vulnerable alveolar surface. As air is inhaled through the upper airways, it is filtered in the nose, heated to body temperature and fully saturated with water vapour; partial recovery of this heat and moisture occurs on expiration. Total airway cross-section is smallest in the glottis and trachea, making the central airway particularly vulnerable to obstruction by foreign bodies and tumours. Normal breath sounds originate mainly from the rapid turbulent airflow in the larynx, trachea and main bronchi.

The multitude of small airways within the lung parenchyma has a very large combined cross-sectional area (over 300 cm^2 in the third-generation respiratory bronchioles), resulting in very slow flow rates. Airflow is normally silent here, and gas transport occurs largely by diffusion in the final generations. Major bronchial and pulmonary divisions are shown in Figure 19.1.

The acinus (Fig. 19.2) is the gas exchange unit of the lung and comprises branching respiratory bronchioles

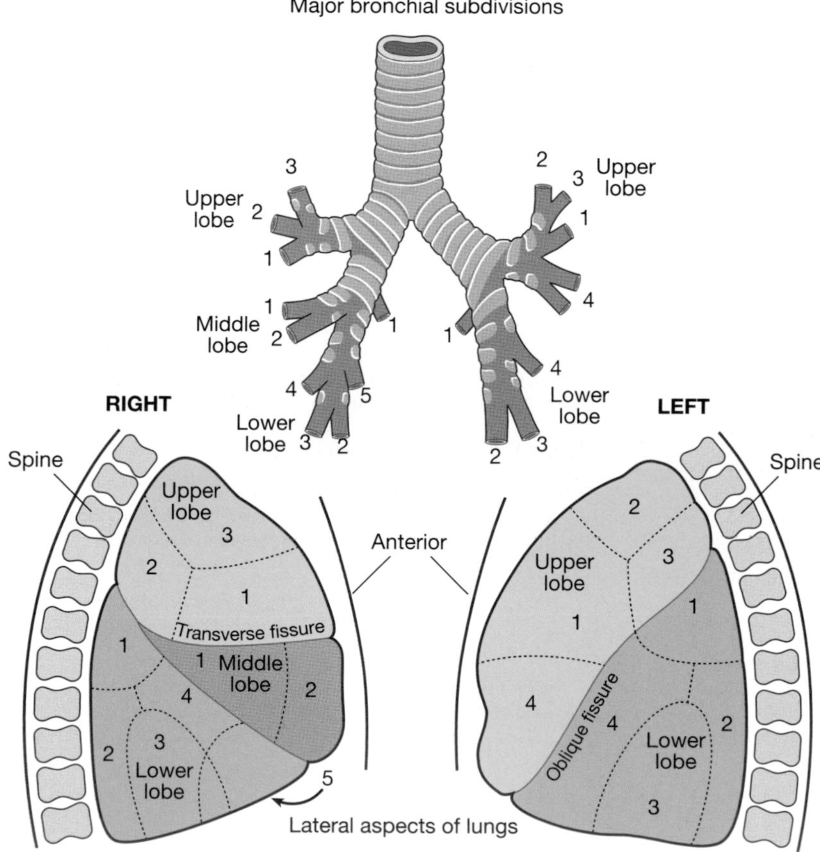

Fig. 19.1 The major bronchial divisions and the fissures, lobes and segments of the lungs. The angle of the oblique fissure means that the left upper lobe is largely anterior to the lower lobe. On the right, the transverse fissure separates the upper from the anteriorly placed middle lobe, which is matched by the lingular segment on the left side. The site of a lobe determines whether physical signs are mainly anterior or posterior. Each lobe is composed of two or more bronchopulmonary segments that are supplied by the main branches of each lobar bronchus.

Bronchopulmonary segments:
Right *Upper lobe*: (1) Anterior, (2) Posterior, (3) Apical. *Middle lobe*: (1) Lateral, (2) Medial. *Lower lobe*: (1) Apical, (2) Posterior basal, (3) Lateral basal, (4) Anterior basal, (5) Medial basal.
Left *Upper lobe*: (1) Anterior, (2) Apical, (3) Posterior, (4) Lingular. *Lower lobe*: (1) Apical, (2) Posterior basal, (3) Lateral basal, (4) Anterior basal.

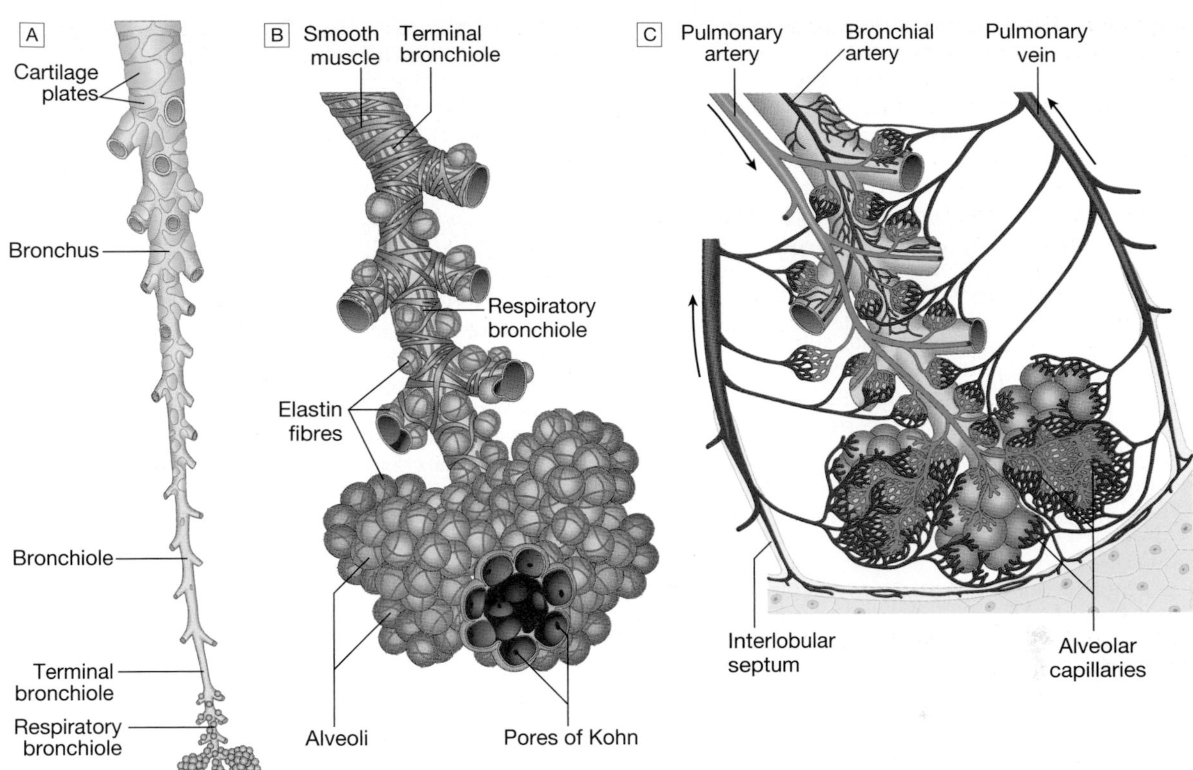

Fig. 19.2 Functional anatomy of the lung. **A** The tapering, branching bronchus is armoured against compression by plates of cartilage. The more distal bronchioles are collapsible, but held patent by surrounding elastic tissue. **B** The unit of lung supplied by a terminal bronchiole is called an acinus. The bronchiolar wall contains smooth muscle and elastin fibres. The latter also run through the alveolar walls. Gas exchange occurs in the alveoli, which are connected to each other by the pores of Kohn. **C** Vascular anatomy of an acinus. Both the pulmonary artery (carrying desaturated blood) and the bronchial artery (systemic supply to airway tissue) run along the bronchus. The venous drainage to the left atrium follows the interlobular septa. From www.Netter.com – see p. 731.

and clusters of alveoli. Here the air makes close contact with the blood in the pulmonary capillaries (gas-to-blood distance < 0.4 μm), and oxygen uptake and CO_2 excretion occur. The alveoli are lined with flattened epithelial cells (type I pneumocytes) and a few, more cuboidal, type II pneumocytes. The latter produce surfactant, which is a mixture of phospholipids that reduces surface tension and counteracts the tendency of alveoli to collapse under surface tension. Type II pneumocytes can divide to reconstitute type I pneumocytes after lung injury.

Lung mechanics

Healthy alveolar walls contain a fine network of elastin and collagen fibres (see Fig. 19.2). The volume of the lungs at the end of a tidal ('normal') breath out is called the functional residual capacity (FRC). At this volume, the inward elastic recoil of the lungs (resulting from elastin fibres and surface tension in the alveolar lining fluid) is balanced by the resistance of the chest wall to inward distortion from its resting shape, causing negative pressure in the pleural space. Elastin fibres allow the lung to be easily distended at physiological lung volumes, but collagen fibres cause increasing stiffness as full inflation is approached so that, in health, the maximum inspiratory volume is limited by the lung (rather than the chest wall). Within the lung, the weight of tissue compresses the dependent regions and distends the uppermost parts, so a greater portion of an inhaled breath passes to the basal regions, which also receive the greatest blood flow as a result of gravity. Elastin fibres in alveolar walls maintain small airway patency by radial traction on the airway walls. Even in health, however, these small airways narrow during expiration because they are surrounded by alveoli at higher pressure, but are prevented from collapsing by radial elastic traction. The volume that can be exhaled is thus limited purely by the capacity of the expiratory muscles to distort the chest wall inwards. In emphysema, loss of alveolar walls leaves the small airways unsupported, and their collapse on expiration causes air trapping and high end-expiratory volume (p. 673).

Control of breathing

The respiratory motor neurons in the posterior medulla oblongata are the origin of the respiratory cycle. Their activity is modulated by multiple external inputs in health and in disease (see Fig. 19.10, p. 657):

- Central chemoreceptors in the ventrolateral medulla sense the pH of the cerebrospinal fluid (CSF) and are indirectly stimulated by a rise in arterial PCO_2.
- The carotid bodies sense hypoxaemia but are mainly activated by arterial PO_2 values below 8 KPa (60 mmHg). They are also sensitised to hypoxia by raised arterial PCO_2.
- Muscle spindles in the respiratory muscles sense changes in mechanical load.

- Vagal sensory fibres from the lung may be stimulated by stretch, by inhaled toxins or by disease processes in the interstitium.
- Cortical (volitional) and limbic (emotional) influences can override the automatic control of breathing.

Ventilation/perfusion matching and the pulmonary circulation

To achieve optimal gas exchange within the lungs, the regional distribution of ventilation and perfusion must be matched. At segmental and subsegmental level, hypoxia constricts pulmonary arterioles and airway CO_2 dilates bronchi, helping to maintain good regional matching of ventilation and perfusion. Lung disease may create regions of relative underventilation or underperfusion, which disturb this regional matching, causing respiratory failure (p. 663). In addition to causing ventilation–perfusion mismatch, diseases that destroy capillaries or thicken the alveolar capillary membrane (e.g. emphysema or fibrosis) can impair gas diffusion directly.

The pulmonary circulation in health operates at low pressure (approximately 24/9 mmHg), and can accommodate large increases in flow with minimal rise in pressure, such as during exercise. Pulmonary hypertension occurs when vessels are destroyed by emphysema, obstructed by thrombus, involved in interstitial inflammation or thickened by pulmonary vascular disease. The right ventricle responds by hypertrophy, with right axis deviation and P pulmonale on the ECG. Pulmonary hypertension with hypoxia and hypercapnia is associated with generalised salt and water retention ('cor pulmonale'), with elevation of the jugular venous pressure (JVP) and peripheral oedema. This is thought to result mainly from a failure of the hypoxic and hypercapnic kidney to excrete sufficient salt and water.

Lung defences

Upper airway defences

Large airborne particles are trapped by nasal hairs, and smaller particles settling on the mucosa are cleared towards the oropharynx by the columnar ciliated epithelium which covers the turbinates and septum (Fig. 19.3). During cough, expiratory muscle effort against a closed glottis results in high intrathoracic pressure, which is then released explosively. The flexible posterior tracheal wall is pushed inwards by the high surrounding pressure, which reduces tracheal cross-section and thus maximises the airspeed to achieve effective expectoration. The larynx also acts as a sphincter, protecting the airway during swallowing and vomiting.

Lower airway defences

The sterility, structure and function of the lower airways are maintained by close cooperation between the innate and adaptive immune responses (pp. 72 and 76).

The innate response in the lungs is characterised by a number of non-specific defence mechanisms. Inhaled particulate matter is trapped in airway mucus and cleared by the mucociliary escalator. Cigarette smoke increases mucus secretion but reduces mucociliary clearance and predisposes towards lower respiratory tract infections, including pneumonia. Defective mucociliary transport is also a feature of several rare diseases, including Kartagener's syndrome, Young's syndrome and ciliary dysmotility syndrome, which are characterised by repeated sino-pulmonary infections and bronchiectasis.

Airway secretions contain an array of antimicrobial peptides (such as defensins, immunoglobulin A (IgA) and lysozyme), antiproteinases and antioxidants. Many assist with the opsonisation and killing of bacteria, and the regulation of the powerful proteolytic enzymes secreted by inflammatory cells. In particular, α_1-antiproteinase (A1Pi) regulates neutrophil elastase, and deficiency of this may be associated with premature emphysema.

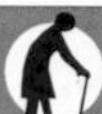

19.1 Respiratory function in old age

- **Reserve capacity**: a significant reduction in function can occur with ageing with only minimal effect on normal breathing, but the ability to combat acute disease is reduced.
- **Decline in FEV_1**: the FEV_1/FVC (forced expiratory volume/forced vital capacity, p. 652) ratio falls by around 0.2% per year from 70% at the age of 40–45 years, due to a decline in elastic recoil in the small airways with age. Smoking accelerates this decline threefold on average. Symptoms usually occur only when FEV_1 drops below 50% of predicted.
- **Increasing ventilation–perfusion mismatch**: the reduction in elastic recoil causes a tendency for the small airways to collapse during expiration, particularly in dependent areas of the lungs, thus reducing ventilation.
- **Reduced ventilatory responses to hypoxia and hypercapnia**: older people may be less tachypnoeic for any given fall in PaO_2 or rise in $PaCO_2$.
- **Impaired defences against infection**: due to reduced numbers of glandular epithelial cells, which lead to a reduction in protective mucus.
- **Decline in maximum oxygen uptake**: due to a combination of impairments in muscle, and the respiratory and cardiovascular systems. This leads to a reduction in cardiorespiratory reserve and exercise capacity.
- **Loss of chest wall compliance**: due to reduced intervertebral disc spaces and ossification of the costal cartilages; respiratory muscle strength and endurance also decline. These changes only become important in the presence of other respiratory disease.

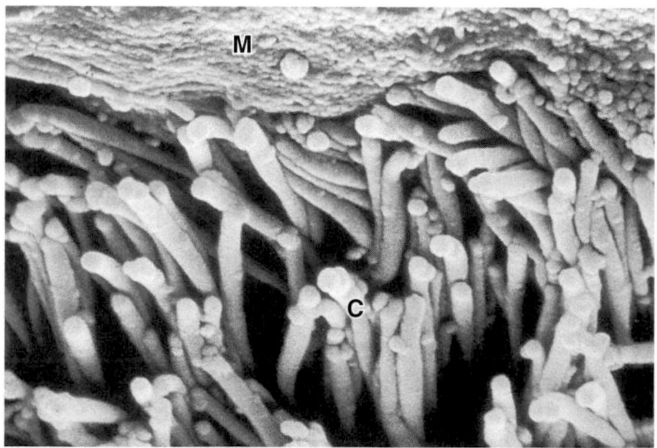

Fig. 19.3 The mucociliary escalator. Scanning electron micrograph of the respiratory epithelium showing large numbers of cilia (C) overlaid by the mucus 'raft' (M).

Macrophages engulf microbes, organic dusts and other particulate matter. They are unable to digest inorganic agents, such as asbestos or silica, which lead to their death and the release of powerful proteolytic enzymes that cause parenchymal damage. Neutrophil numbers in the airway are low, but the pulmonary circulation contains a marginated pool that may be recruited rapidly in response to bacterial infection. This may explain the prominence of lung injury in sepsis syndromes and trauma.

Adaptive immunity is characterised by the specificity of the response and the development of memory. Lung dendritic cells facilitate antigen presentation to T and B lymphocytes.

INVESTIGATION OF RESPIRATORY DISEASE

A detailed history, thorough examination and basic haematological and biochemical tests usually indicate the likely diagnosis and differential. A number of other investigations are normally required to confirm the diagnosis and/or monitor disease activity.

Imaging

The 'plain' chest X-ray

This is performed on the majority of patients suspected of having chest disease. A postero-anterior (PA) film provides information on the lung fields, heart, mediastinum, vascular structures and thoracic cage (Fig. 19.4). Additional information may be obtained from a lateral film, particularly if pathology is suspected behind the heart shadow or deep in the diaphragmatic sulci. An approach to interpreting the chest X-ray is given in Box 19.2, and common abnormalities are listed in Box 19.3.

19.2 How to interpret a chest X-ray

Name, date, orientation	Films are postero-anterior (PA) unless marked AP to denote that they are antero-posterior
Lung fields	Equal translucency? Check horizontal fissure from right hilum to sixth rib at the anterior axillary line Masses? Consolidation? Cavitation?
Lung apices	Check behind the clavicles: Masses? Consolidation? Cavitation?
Trachea	Central? (Midway between the clavicular heads) Paratracheal mass? Goitre?
Heart	Normal shape? Cardiothoracic ratio (should be < half the intrathoracic diameter) Retrocardiac mass?
Hila	Left should be higher than right Shape? (Should be concave laterally; if convex, consider mass or lymphadenopathy) Density?
Diaphragm	Right should be higher than left Hyperinflation? (No more than 10 ribs should be visible posteriorly above the diaphragm)
Costophrenic angles	Acute and well defined? (Pleural fluid or thickening, if not)
Soft tissues	Breast shadows in females Chest wall for masses or subcutaneous emphysema
Bones	Ribs, vertebrae, scapulae and clavicles Any fracture visible at bone margins or lucencies?

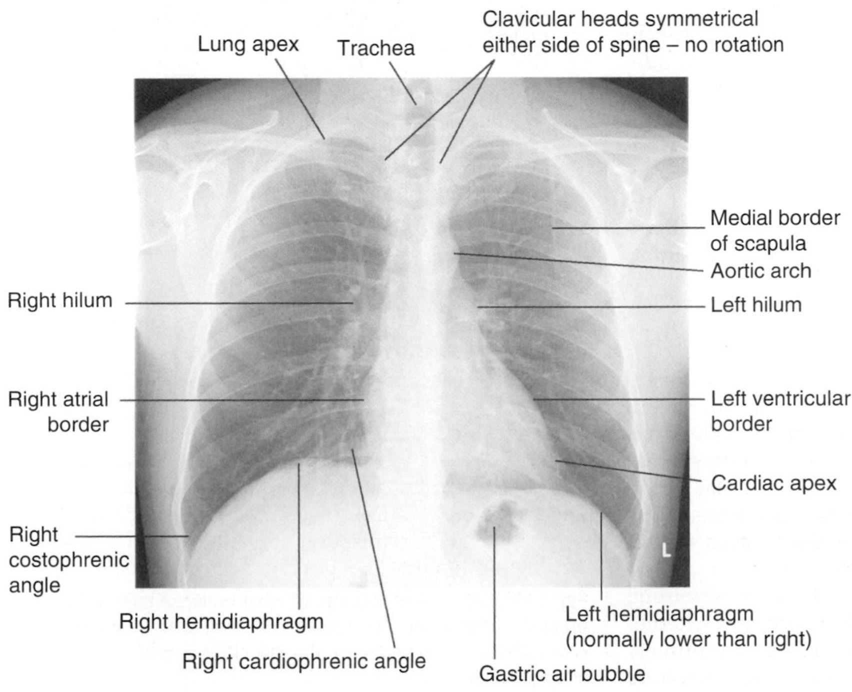

Fig. 19.4 The normal chest X-ray. The lung markings consist of branching and tapering lines radiating out from the hila. Where airways and vessels turn towards the film, they can appear as open or filled circles (see upper pole of right hilum). The scapulae may overlie the lung fields; trace the edge of bony structures to avoid mistaking them for pleural or pulmonary shadows. To check for hyperinflation, count the ribs; if more than 10 are visible posteriorly above the diaphragm, the lungs are hyperinflated. From Innes 2009 – see p. 731.

19.3 Common chest X-ray abnormalities

Pulmonary and pleural shadowing	
• **Consolidation**: infection, infarction, inflammation, and rarely bronchoalveolar cell carcinoma • **Lobar collapse**: mucus plugging, tumour, compression by lymph nodes • **Solitary nodule**: see page 660 • **Multiple nodules**: miliary tuberculosis (TB), dust inhalation, metastatic malignancy, healed varicella pneumonia, rheumatoid disease • **Ring shadows, tramlines and tubular shadows**: bronchiectasis • **Cavitating lesions**: tumour, abscess, infarct, pneumonia (*Staphylococcus/Klebsiella*), granulomatosis with polyangiitis • **Reticular, nodular and reticulonodular shadows**: diffuse parenchymal lung disease, infection • **Pleural abnormalities**: fluid, plaques, tumour	
Increased translucency	
• Bullae • Pneumothorax	• Oligaemia
Hilar abnormalities	
• **Unilateral hilar enlargement:** TB, bronchial carcinoma, lymphoma • **Bilateral hilar enlargement:** sarcoid, lymphoma, TB, silicosis	
Other abnormalities	
• Hiatus hernia	• Surgical emphysema

Increased shadowing may represent accumulation of fluid, lobar collapse or consolidation. Uncomplicated consolidation should not change the position of the mediastinum and the presence of an air bronchogram means that proximal bronchi are patent. Collapse (implying obstruction of the lobar bronchus) is accompanied by loss of volume and displacement of the mediastinum towards the affected side (Fig. 19.5).

The presence of ring shadows (thickened bronchi seen end-on), tramline shadows (thickened bronchi side-on) or tubular shadows (bronchi filled with secretions) suggests bronchiectasis, but computed tomography is a much more sensitive test than plain X-ray in bronchiectasis. The presence of pleural fluid is suggested by a dense basal shadow, which, in the erect patient, ascends towards the axilla (p. 645). In large pulmonary embolism, relative oligaemia may cause a lung field to appear abnormally dark.

Computed tomography

Computed tomography (CT) provides detailed images of the pulmonary parenchyma, mediastinum, pleura and bony structures. The displayed range of densities can be adjusted to highlight different structures, such as the lung parenchyma, the mediastinal vascular structures or bone. Sophisticated software facilitates three-dimensional reconstruction of the thorax and virtual bronchoscopy.

CT is superior to chest radiography in determining the position and size of a pulmonary lesion and whether calcification or cavitation is present. It is now routinely used in the assessment of patients with suspected lung

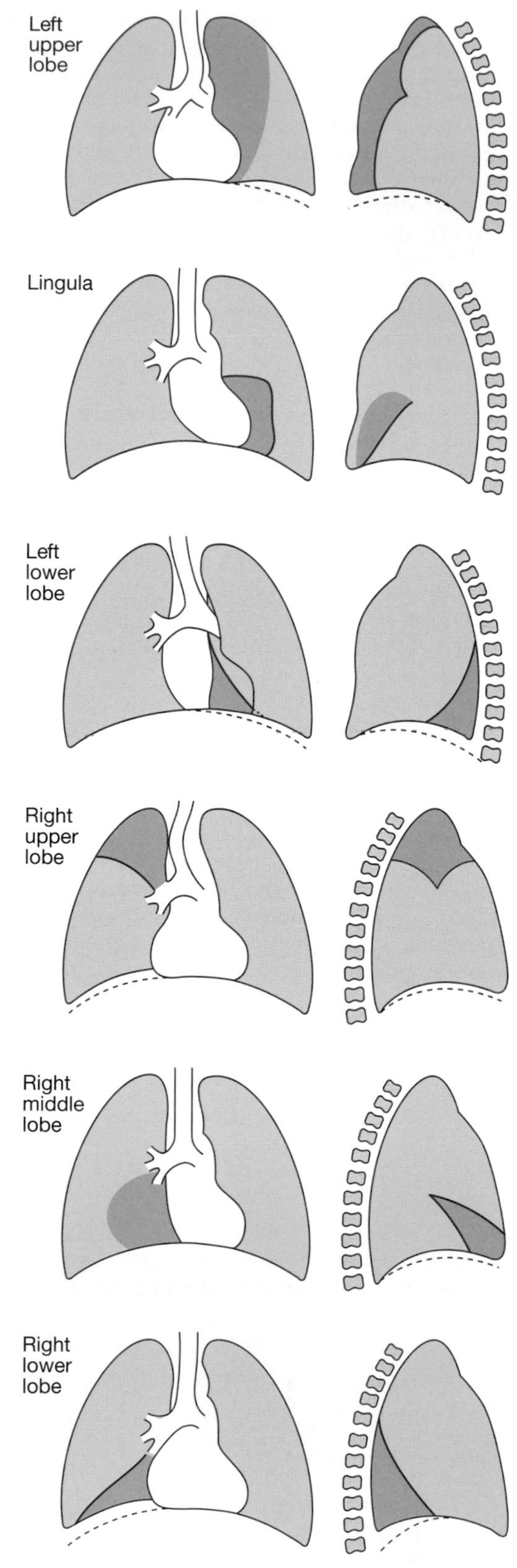

Fig. 19.5 Radiological features of lobar collapse caused by bronchial obstruction. The dotted line in the drawings represents the normal position of the diaphragm. The dark pink area represents the extent of shadowing seen on the X-ray.

cancer and facilitates guided percutaneous needle biopsy. Information on tumour stage may be gained by examining the mediastinum, liver and adrenal glands.

High-resolution CT (HRCT) uses thin sections to provide detailed images of the pulmonary parenchyma and is particularly useful in assessing diffuse parenchymal lung disease, identifying bronchiectasis (Fig. 19.30, p. 679), and assessing type and extent of emphysema.

Assessment of the pulmonary circulation

CT pulmonary angiography (CTPA) has become the investigation of choice in the diagnosis of pulmonary thromboembolism (see Fig. 19.69, p. 679), when it may either confirm the suspected embolism or highlight an alternative diagnosis. It has largely replaced the radioisotope-based ventilation–perfusion scan, although the latter continues to provide useful information in the pre-operative assessment of patients being considered for lung resection. In pulmonary hypertension, Doppler echocardiographic assessment of tricuspid regurgitant jets allows accurate non-invasive measurement of pulmonary artery pressure in most cases. Right heart catheterisation is still used in the investigation of patients with pulmonary hypertension in specialised centres, as it permits accurate measurement of response to pulmonary vasodilators.

Positron emission tomography

Positron emission tomography (PET) scanners exploit the ability of malignant tissue to absorb and metabolise glucose avidly. The radiotracer ^{18}F-fluorodeoxyglucose (FDG) is infused and rapidly taken up by malignant tissue. It is then phosphorylated but cannot be metabolised further, becoming 'trapped' in the cell. PET is useful in the investigation of pulmonary nodules, and in staging mediastinal lymph nodes and distal metastatic disease in patients with lung cancer. The negative predictive value is high; however, the positive predictive value is poor. Co-registration of PET and CT (PET-CT) enhances localisation and characterisation of metabolically active deposits (Fig. 19.6). Future advances will see the combination of PET and magnetic resonance imaging (MRI).

Ultrasound

Ultrasound is used to assess the pleural space for pleural fluid, which appears as a hypoechoic space. It also allows direct visualisation of the diaphragm and solid organs such as the liver, spleen and kidneys, thereby allowing safe pleural aspiration, biopsy and intercostal chest drain insertion. Ultrasound can also be used to guide needle biopsy of superficial lymph node or chest wall masses and provides useful information on the shape and movement of the diaphragm. Endobronchial ultrasound (EBUS) is described below.

Endoscopic examination

Laryngoscopy

The larynx may be inspected directly with a fibreoptic laryngoscope and this is useful in cases of suspected vocal cord dysfunction, when paradoxical movement of the vocal cords may mimic asthma. Left-sided lung tumours may involve the left recurrent laryngeal nerve, paralysing the left vocal cord and leading to a hoarse voice and a 'bovine' cough.

Bronchoscopy

The trachea and the first 3–4 generations of bronchi may be inspected using a flexible bronchoscope. Flexible bronchoscopy is usually performed under local anaesthesia with sedation, on an outpatient basis. Abnormal tissue in the bronchial lumen or wall can be biopsied, and bronchial brushings, washings or aspirates can be taken for cytological or bacteriological examination. Small biopsy specimens of lung tissue, taken by forceps passed through the bronchial wall (transbronchial biopsies), may be helpful in the diagnosis of bronchocentric disorders such as sarcoid, hypersensitivity pneumonitis and diffuse malignancy, but are generally too small to be of diagnostic value in other diffuse parenchymal pulmonary disease (p. 706). Transbronchial needle aspiration (TBNA) may be used to sample mediastinal lymph nodes and to stage lung cancer.

Rigid bronchoscopy requires general anaesthesia and is reserved for specific situations, such as massive haemoptysis or removal of foreign bodies (see Fig. 19.9, p. 655). Endobronchial laser therapy and endobronchial stenting may be easier with rigid bronchoscopy.

Assessment of the mediastinum

The sampling of mediastinal lymph nodes is essential in the diagnosis and staging of lung cancer and may confirm the diagnosis of non-malignant conditions, such as tuberculosis or sarcoidosis. Endobronchial

A 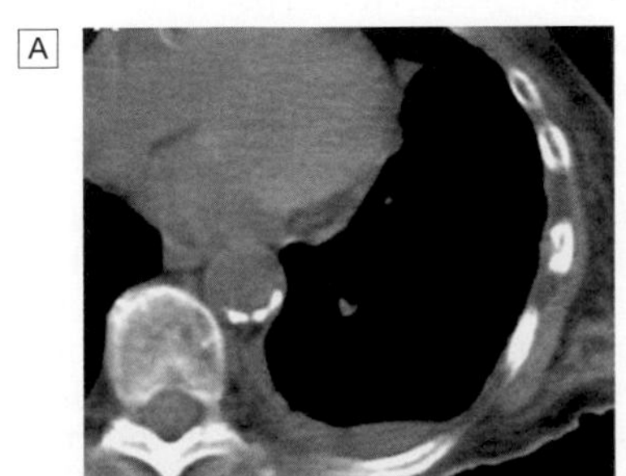

B 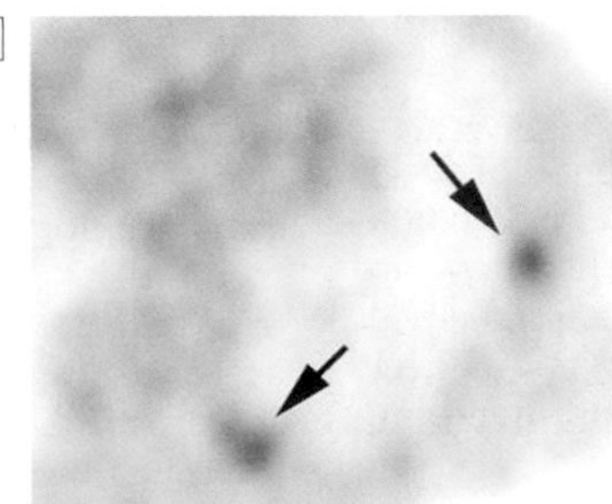

C 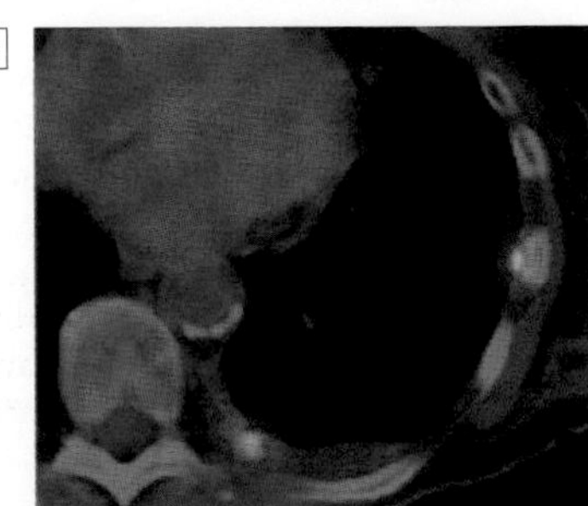

Fig. 19.6 Computed tomography and positron emission tomography combined to reveal intrathoracic metastases. **A** In a patient with lung cancer, CT shows some posterior pleural thickening. **B** PET scanning reveals FDG uptake in two pleural lesions (arrows). **C** The lesions are highlighted in yellow in the combined PET/CT image. From http://radiology.rsnajnls.org – see p. 731.

ultrasound (EBUS), using a specialised bronchoscope, allows directed needle aspiration from peribronchial nodes and is used increasingly to determine disease extent. Lymph nodes down to the main carina can also be sampled using a mediastinoscope passed through a small incision at the suprasternal notch under general anaesthetic. Lymph nodes in the lower mediastinum may be biopsied via the oesophagus using endoscopic ultrasound (EUS), an oesophageal endoscope equipped with an ultrasound transducer and biopsy needle.

Investigation of pleural disease

Core biopsy of the pleura, guided by either ultrasound or CT, has largely replaced the traditional 'blind' method of pleural biopsy using an Abram's needle. Thoracoscopy, which involves the insertion of an endoscope through the chest wall, facilitates biopsy under direct vision and is performed by many surgeons and an increasing number of physicians.

Immunological and serological tests

The presence of pneumococcal antigen (revealed by counter-immunoelectrophoresis) in sputum, blood or urine may be of diagnostic importance in pneumonia. Influenza viruses can be detected in throat swab samples by fluorescent antibody techniques. In blood, high or rising antibody titres to specific organisms (such as *Legionella*, *Mycoplasma*, *Chlamydia* or viruses) may eventually clinch a diagnosis suspected on clinical grounds but early diagnosis of *Legionella* is best done by urine antigen testing. Precipitating antibodies may indicate a reaction to fungi such as *Aspergillus* (p. 697) or to antigens involved in hypersensitivity pneumonitis (p. 719). Total levels of immunoglobulin E (IgE), and levels of IgE directed against specific antigens, can be useful in assessing the contribution of allergy to respiratory disease.

Skin tests

The tuberculin test (p. 695) may be of value in the diagnosis of tuberculosis. Skin hypersensitivity tests are useful in the investigation of allergic diseases (p. 89).

Microbiological investigations

Sputum, pleural fluid, throat swabs, blood, and bronchial washings and aspirates can be examined for bacteria, fungi and viruses. In some cases, as when *Mycobacterium tuberculosis* is isolated, the information is diagnostically conclusive but, in others, the findings must be interpreted in conjunction with the results of clinical and radiological examination.

The use of hypertonic saline to induce expectoration of sputum is useful in facilitating the collection of specimens for microbiology, particularly in patients in whom more invasive procedures, such as bronchoscopy, are not possible. The technique also allows assessment of the inflammatory cell population of the airway, which is a useful research tool in many conditions, including asthma, COPD and interstitial lung disease.

Histopathology and cytology

Histopathological examination of biopsies of pleura, lymph node or lung often allows a 'tissue diagnosis' to be made. This is particularly important in suspected malignancy or in characterising the pathological changes in interstitial lung disease. Important causative organisms, such as *M. tuberculosis*, *Pneumocystis jirovecii* or fungi, may be identified in bronchial washings, brushings or transbronchial biopsies.

Cytological examination of exfoliated cells in pleural fluid or bronchial brushings and washings, or of fine needle aspirates from lymph nodes or pulmonary lesions, can support a diagnosis of malignancy but, if this is indeterminate, a larger tissue biopsy is often necessary. Differential cell counts in bronchial lavage fluid may help to distinguish pulmonary changes due to sarcoidosis (p. 709) from those caused by idiopathic pulmonary fibrosis (p. 706) or hypersensitivity pneumonitis (p. 719).

Respiratory function testing

Respiratory function tests are used to aid diagnosis, assess functional impairment, and monitor treatment or progression of disease. Airway narrowing, lung volume and gas exchange capacity are quantified and compared with normal values adjusted for age, gender, height and ethnic origin. In diseases characterised by airway narrowing (e.g. asthma, bronchitis and emphysema), maximum expiratory flow is limited by dynamic compression of small intrathoracic airways, some of which may close completely during expiration, limiting the volume that can be expired ('obstructive' defect). Hyperinflation of the chest results, and can become extreme if elastic recoil is also lost due to parenchymal destruction, as in emphysema. In contrast, diseases that cause interstitial inflammation and/or fibrosis lead to progressive loss of lung volume ('restrictive' defect) with normal expiratory flow rates. Typical laboratory traces are illustrated in Figure 19.7.

Measurement of airway obstruction

Airway narrowing is assessed by asking patients to blow out as hard and as fast as they can into a peak flow meter or a spirometer. Peak flow meters are cheap and convenient for home monitoring of peak expiratory flow (PEF) in the detection and monitoring of asthma, but results are effort-dependent. More accurate and reproducible measures are obtained by inhaling fully, then exhaling at maximum effort into a spirometer. The forced expired volume in 1 second (FEV_1) is the volume exhaled in the first second, and the forced vital capacity (FVC) is the total volume exhaled. FEV_1 is disproportionately reduced in airflow obstruction, resulting in FEV_1/FVC ratios of less than 70%. In this situation, spirometry should be repeated following inhaled short-acting β_2-adrenoceptor agonists (e.g. salbutamol); a large improvement in FEV_1 (over 400 mL) and variability in peak flow over time are features of asthma (p. 668).

To distinguish large airway narrowing (e.g. tracheal stenosis or compression) from small airway narrowing, flow/volume loops are recorded using spirometry. These display flow in relation to lung volume (rather than time) during maximum expiration and inspiration, and the pattern of flow reveals the site of airflow obstruction (see Fig. 19.7).

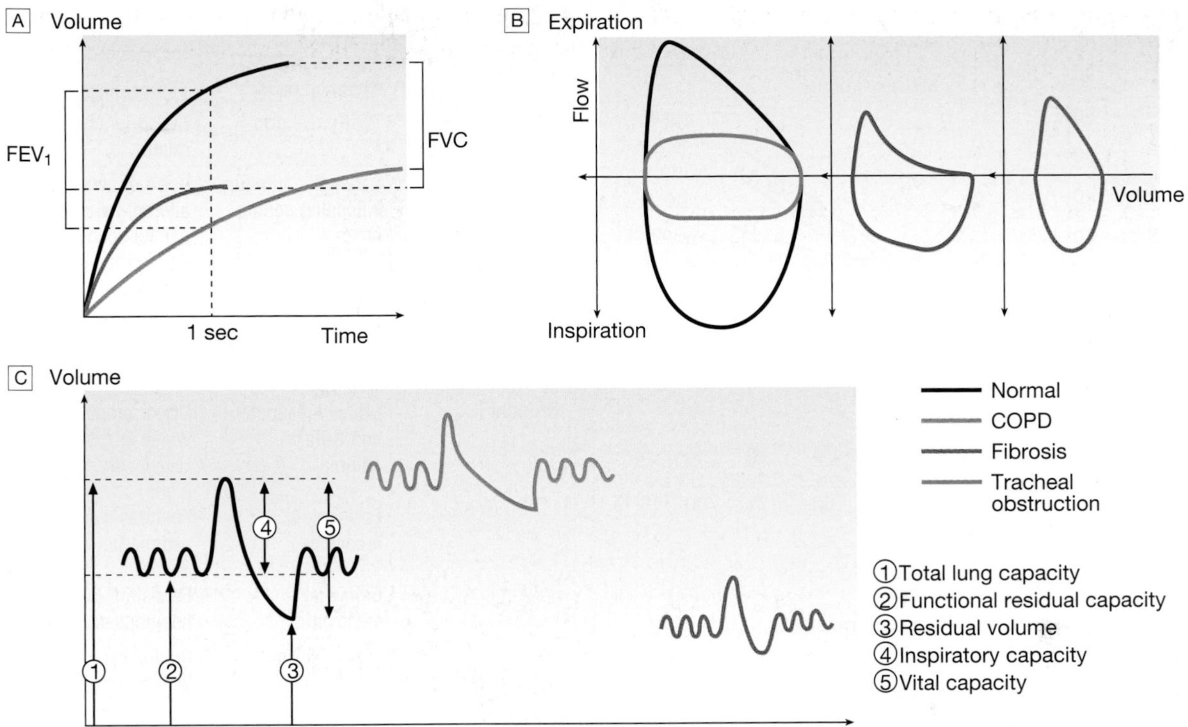

Fig. 19.7 Respiratory function tests in health and disease. **A** Volume/time traces from forced expiration in a normal subject, in COPD and in fibrosis. COPD causes slow, prolonged and limited exhalation. In fibrosis, forced expiration results in rapid expulsion of a reduced forced vital capacity (FVC). Forced expiratory volume (FEV_1) is reduced in both diseases but is disproportionately reduced, compared to FVC, in COPD. **B** The same data plotted as flow/volume loops. In COPD, collapse of intrathoracic airways limits flow, particularly during mid- and late expiration. The blue trace illustrates large airway obstruction, which particularly limits peak flow rates. **C** Lung volume measurement. Volume/time graphs during quiet breathing with a single maximal breath in and out. COPD causes hyperinflation with increased residual volume. Fibrosis causes a proportional reduction in all lung volumes.

Lung volumes

Tidal volume and vital capacity (VC – the maximum amount of air that can be expelled from the lungs after the deepest possible breath) can be measured by spirometry. Total lung capacity (TLC – the total amount of air in the lungs after taking the deepest breath possible) can be measured by asking the patient to rebreathe an inert non-absorbed gas (usually helium) and recording how much the test gas is diluted by lung gas. This measures the volume of intrathoracic gas that mixes with tidal breaths. Alternatively, lung volume may be measured by body plethysmography, which determines the pressure/volume relationship of the thorax. This method measures total intrathoracic gas volume, including poorly ventilated areas such as bullae.

Transfer factor

To measure the capacity of the lungs to exchange gas, patients inhale a test mixture of 0.3% carbon monoxide, which is taken up avidly by haemoglobin in pulmonary capillaries. After a short breath-hold, the rate of disappearance of CO into the circulation is calculated from a sample of expirate, and expressed as the TL_{CO} or carbon monoxide transfer factor. Helium is also included in the test breath to allow calculation of the volume of lung examined by the test breath. Transfer factor expressed per unit lung volume is termed K_{CO}. Common respiratory function abnormalities are summarised in Box 19.4.

19.4 How to interpret respiratory function abnormalities

	Asthma	Chronic bronchitis	Emphysema	Pulmonary fibrosis
FEV_1	↓↓	↓↓	↓↓	↓
VC	↓	↓	↓	↓↓
FEV_1/VC	↓	↓	↓	→/↑
TL_{CO}	→	→	↓↓	↓↓
K_{CO}	→/↑	→	↓	→/↓
TLC	→/↑	↑	↑↑	↓
RV	→/↑	↑	↑↑	↓

(RV = residual volume; see text for other abbreviations)

Arterial blood gases and oximetry

The measurement of hydrogen ion concentration, PaO_2 and $PaCO_2$, and derived bicarbonate concentration in an arterial blood sample is essential to assess the degree and type of respiratory failure, and for measuring acid–base status. This is discussed in detail on pages 663 and 442. Interpretation of results is made easier by blood gas diagrams (Fig. 19.8), which indicate whether any acidosis or alkalosis is due to acute or chronic respiratory derangements of $PaCO_2$, or to metabolic causes. Pulse oximeters with finger or ear probes measure the

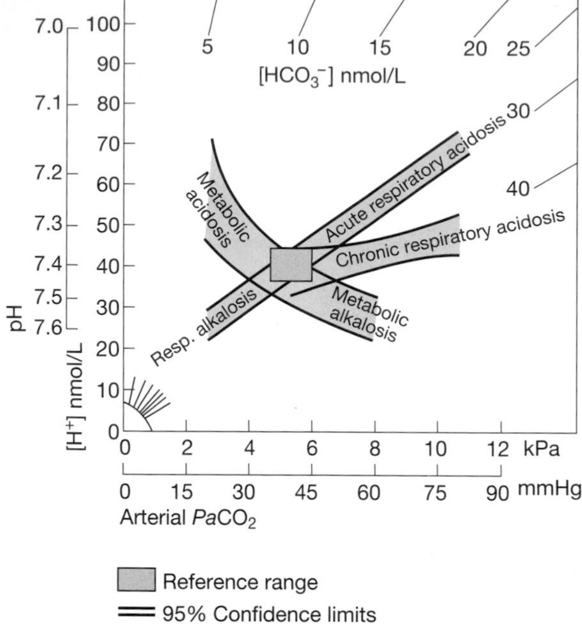

Fig. 19.8 Changes in blood [H+], PaCO₂ and plasma [HCO₃⁻] in acid–base disorders. The rectangle indicates normal limits for [H+] and $PaCO_2$. The bands represent 95% confidence limits of single disturbances in human blood. To determine the likely cause of an acid–base disorder, plot the values of [H+] and $PaCO_2$ from an arterial blood gas measurement. The diagram indicates whether any acidosis or alkalosis results primarily from a respiratory disorder of $PaCO_2$ or from a metabolic derangement. Adapted from Flenley 1971 – see p. 732.

difference in absorbance of light by oxygenated and deoxygenated blood to calculate its oxygen saturation (SaO_2). This allows non-invasive continuous assessment of oxygen saturation in patients, which is useful in assessing hypoxaemia and its response to therapy.

Exercise tests

Resting measurements may be unhelpful in early disease or in patients complaining only of exercise-induced symptoms. Exercise testing with spirometry before and after can help demonstrate exercise-induced asthma. Walk tests include the self-paced 6-minute walk and the externally paced incremental 'shuttle' test, where patients walk at increasing pace between two cones 10 m apart. These provide simple, repeatable assessments of disability and response to treatment. Cardiopulmonary bicycle exercise testing, with measurement of metabolic gas exchange, ventilation and ECG changes, is useful for quantifying exercise limitation and detecting occult cardiovascular or respiratory limitation in a breathless patient.

PRESENTING PROBLEMS IN RESPIRATORY DISEASE

Cough

Cough is the most frequent symptom of respiratory disease and is caused by stimulation of sensory nerves in the mucosa of the pharynx, larynx, trachea and bronchi. Acute sensitisation of the normal cough reflex occurs in a number of conditions, and it is typically induced by changes in air temperature or exposure to irritants, such as cigarette smoke or perfumes. The characteristics of cough originating at various levels of the respiratory tract are detailed in Box 19.5.

19.5 Cough

Origin	Common causes	Clinical features
Pharynx	Post-nasal drip	History of chronic rhinitis
Larynx	Laryngitis, tumour, whooping cough, croup	Voice or swallowing altered, harsh or painful cough Paroxysms of cough, often associated with stridor
Trachea	Tracheitis	Raw retrosternal pain with cough
Bronchi	Bronchitis (acute) and COPD	Dry or productive, worse in mornings
	Asthma	Usually dry, worse at night
	Eosinophilic bronchitis	Features similar to asthma but AHR absent
	Bronchial carcinoma	Persistent (often with haemoptysis)
Lung parenchyma	Tuberculosis	Productive (often with haemoptysis)
	Pneumonia	Dry initially, productive later
	Bronchiectasis	Productive, changes in posture induce sputum production
	Pulmonary oedema	Often at night (may be productive of pink, frothy sputum)
	Interstitial fibrosis	Dry and distressing
Drug side-effect	ACE inhibitors	Dry cough

(ACE = angiotensin-converting enzyme; AHR = airway hyper-reactivity; COPD = chronic obstructive pulmonary disease)
Based on Crompton GK. The respiratory system. In: Munro JF, Campbell IW. Macleod's clinical examination. 10th edn. Edinburgh: Churchill Livingstone; 2000 (p. 119); copyright Elsevier.

The explosive quality of a normal cough is lost in patients with respiratory muscle paralysis or vocal cord palsy. Paralysis of a single vocal cord gives rise to a prolonged, low-pitched, inefficient 'bovine' cough accompanied by hoarseness. Coexistence of an inspiratory noise (stridor) indicates partial obstruction of a major airway (e.g. laryngeal oedema, tracheal tumour, scarring, compression or inhaled foreign body) and requires urgent investigation and treatment. Sputum production is common in patients with acute or chronic cough, and its nature and appearance can provide clues to the aetiology (p. 644).

Causes of cough

Acute transient cough is most commonly caused by viral lower respiratory tract infection, post-nasal drip resulting from rhinitis or sinusitis, aspiration of a foreign

A

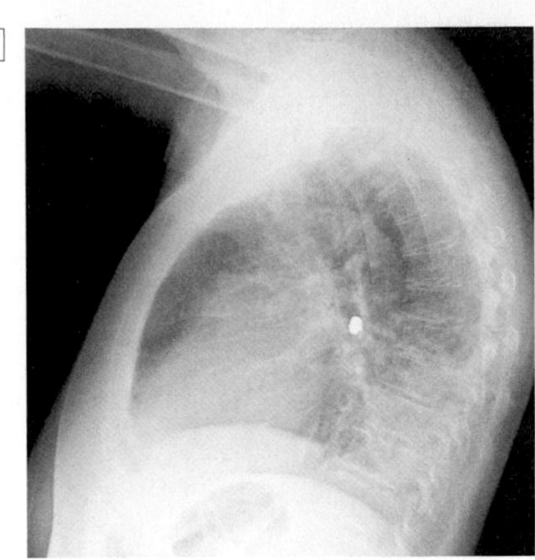

B

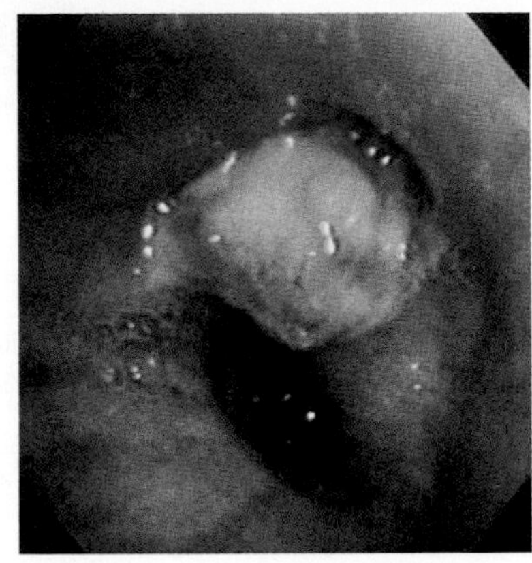

Fig. 19.9 Inhaled foreign body. **A** Chest X-ray showing a tooth lodged in a main bronchus. **B** Bronchoscopic appearance of inhaled foreign body (tooth) with a covering mucous film.

body, or throat-clearing secondary to laryngitis or pharyngitis. When cough occurs in the context of more serious diseases, such as pneumonia, aspiration, congestive heart failure or pulmonary embolism, it is usually easy to diagnose from other clinical features.

Patients with chronic cough present more of a challenge, especially when physical examination, chest X-ray and lung function studies are normal. In this context, it is most often explained by cough-variant asthma (where cough may be the principal or exclusive clinical manifestation), post-nasal drip secondary to nasal or sinus disease, or gastro-oesophageal reflux with aspiration. Diagnosis of the latter may require ambulatory oesophageal pH monitoring or a prolonged trial of anti-reflux therapy (p. 865). Between 10% and 15% of patients (particularly women) taking angiotensin-converting enzyme (ACE) inhibitors develop a drug-induced chronic cough. *Bordetella pertussis* infection in adults (p. 682) can also result in protracted cough and should be suspected in those in close contact with children. While most patients with a bronchogenic carcinoma have an abnormal chest X-ray on presentation, fibreoptic bronchoscopy or thoracic CT is advisable in most adults (especially smokers) with otherwise unexplained cough of recent onset, as this may reveal a small endobronchial tumour or unexpected foreign body (Fig. 19.9). In a small percentage of patients, dry cough may be the presenting feature of interstitial lung disease.

Breathlessness

Breathlessness or dyspnoea can be defined as the feeling of an uncomfortable need to breathe. It is unusual among sensations, as it has no defined receptors, no localised representation in the brain, and multiple causes both in health (e.g. exercise) and in diseases of the lungs, heart or muscles.

Pathophysiology

Stimuli to breathing resulting from disease processes are shown in Figure 19.10. Respiratory diseases can stimulate breathing and dyspnoea by:

- stimulating intrapulmonary sensory nerves (e.g. pneumothorax, interstitial inflammation and pulmonary embolus)
- increasing the mechanical load on the respiratory muscles (e.g. airflow obstruction or pulmonary fibrosis)
- causing hypoxia, hypercapnia or acidosis, which stimulate chemoreceptors.

In cardiac failure, pulmonary congestion reduces lung compliance and can also obstruct the small airways. Reduced cardiac output also limits oxygen supply to the skeletal muscles during exercise, causing early lactic acidaemia and further stimulating breathing via the central chemoreceptors.

Breathlessness and the effects of treatment can be quantified using a symptom scale. Patients tend to report breathlessness in proportion to the sum of the above stimuli to breathe. Individual patients differ greatly in the intensity of breathlessness reported for a given set of circumstances, but breathlessness scores during exercise within individuals are reproducible, and can be used to monitor the effects of therapy.

Differential diagnosis

Patients with breathlessness present either with chronic exertional symptoms or as an emergency with acute breathlessness, when symptoms are prominent even at rest. The causes can be classified accordingly (Box 19.6).

Chronic exertional breathlessness

The cause of breathlessness is often apparent from a careful clinical history. Key questions include:

How is your breathing at rest and overnight?

In COPD, there is a fixed, structural limit to maximum ventilation, and a tendency for progressive hyperinflation during exercise. Breathlessness is mainly apparent when walking, and patients usually report minimal symptoms at rest and overnight. In contrast, patients with significant asthma are often woken from their sleep by breathlessness with chest tightness and wheeze.

Orthopnoea, however, is common in COPD, as well as in heart disease, because airflow obstruction is made worse by cranial displacement of the diaphragm by the abdominal contents when recumbent, so many patients choose to sleep propped up. It may thus not be a useful differentiating symptom, unless there is a clear history of previous angina or infarction to suggest cardiac disease.

How much can you do on a good day?

Noting 'breathless on exertion' is not enough; the approximate distance the patient can walk on the level should be documented, along with capacity to climb

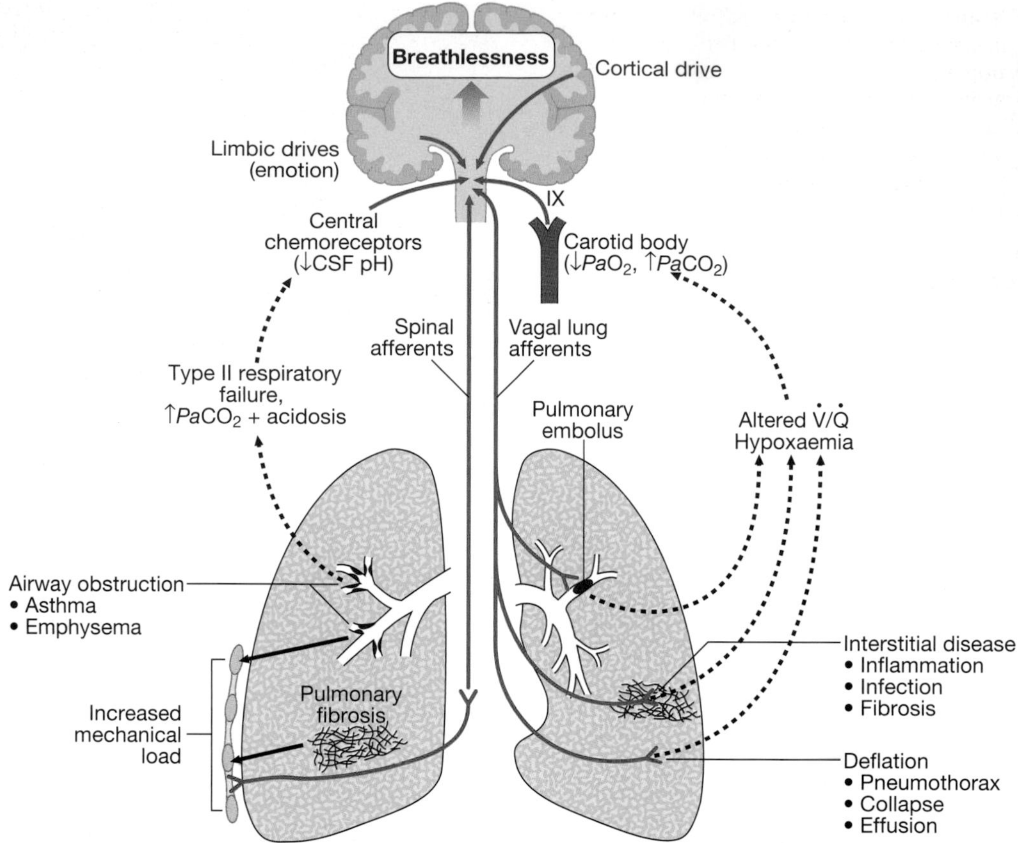

Fig. 19.10 Respiratory stimuli contributing to breathlessness. Mechanisms by which disease can stimulate the respiratory motor neurons in the medulla. Breathlessness is usually felt in proportion to the sum of these stimuli. Further explanation is given on page 543. ($\dot{V}/\dot{Q}$ = ventilation/perfusion match)

19.6 Causes of breathlessness

System	Acute dyspnoea	Chronic exertional dyspnoea
Cardiovascular	*Acute pulmonary oedema (p. 543)	Chronic heart failure (p. 543) Myocardial ischaemia (angina equivalent) (p. 544)
Respiratory	*Acute severe asthma *Acute exacerbation of COPD *Pneumothorax *Pneumonia *Pulmonary embolus ARDS Inhaled foreign body (especially in children) Lobar collapse Laryngeal oedema (e.g. anaphylaxis)	*COPD *Chronic asthma Bronchial carcinoma Interstitial lung disease (sarcoidosis, fibrosing alveolitis, extrinsic allergic alveolitis, pneumoconiosis) Chronic pulmonary thromboembolism Lymphatic carcinomatosis (may cause intolerable breathlessness) Large pleural effusion(s)
Others	Metabolic acidosis (e.g. diabetic ketoacidosis, lactic acidosis, uraemia, overdose of salicylates, ethylene glycol poisoning) Psychogenic hyperventilation (anxiety or panic-related)	Severe anaemia Obesity Deconditioning

*Denotes a common cause. (ARDS = acute respiratory distress syndrome; COPD = chronic obstructive pulmonary disease)

inclines or stairs. Variability within and between days is a hallmark of asthma; in mild asthma, the patient may be free of symptoms and signs when well. Gradual, progressive loss of exercise capacity over months and years, with consistent disability over days, is typical of COPD. When asthma is suspected, the degree of variability is best documented by home peak flow monitoring.

Relentless, progressive breathlessness that is also present at rest, often accompanied by a dry cough, suggests interstitial fibrosis. Impaired left ventricular function can also cause chronic exertional breathlessness, cough and wheeze. A history of angina, hypertension or myocardial infarction raises the possibility of a cardiac cause. This may be confirmed by a displaced apex beat, a raised JVP and cardiac murmurs (although these signs can occur in severe cor pulmonale). The chest X-ray may show cardiomegaly, and an electrocardiogram (ECG) and echocardiogram may provide evidence of left ventricular disease. Measurement of arterial blood gases may help, as, in the absence of an intracardiac shunt or pulmonary oedema, the PaO_2 in cardiac disease is normal and the $PaCO_2$ is low or normal.

Did you have breathing problems in childhood or at school?

When present, a history of childhood wheeze increases the likelihood of asthma, although this history may be absent in late-onset asthma. A history of atopic allergy also increases the likelihood of asthma.

Do you have other symptoms along with your breathlessness?

Digital or perioral paraesthesiae and a feeling that 'I cannot get a deep enough breath in' are typical features of psychogenic hyperventilation, but this cannot be diagnosed until investigations have excluded other potential causes. Additional symptoms include light-headedness, central chest discomfort or even carpopedal spasm due to acute respiratory alkalosis. These alarming symptoms may provoke further anxiety and exacerbate hyperventilation. Psychogenic breathlessness rarely disturbs sleep, frequently occurs at rest, may be provoked by stressful situations and may even be relieved by exercise. The Nijmegen questionnaire can be used to score some of the typical symptoms of hyperventilation (Box 19.7). Arterial blood gases show normal PO_2, low PCO_2 and alkalosis.

Pleuritic chest pain in a patient with chronic breathlessness, particularly if it occurs in more than one site over time, should raise suspicion of thromboembolic disease. Thromboembolism may occasionally present as chronic breathlessness with no other specific features, and should always be considered before a diagnosis of psychogenic hyperventilation is made.

Morning headache is an important symptom in patients with breathlessness, as it may signal the onset of carbon dioxide retention and respiratory failure. This is particularly significant in patients with musculoskeletal disease impairing respiratory function (e.g. kyphoscoliosis or muscular dystrophy).

Acute severe breathlessness

This is one of the most common and dramatic medical emergencies. The history and a rapid but careful examination will usually suggest a diagnosis which can be confirmed by routine investigations, including chest X-ray, ECG and arterial blood gases. Specific features that aid the diagnosis of the important causes are shown in Box 19.8.

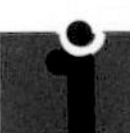

19.7 Factors suggesting psychogenic hyperventilation

- 'Inability to take a deep breath'
- Frequent sighing/erratic ventilation at rest
- Short breath-holding time in the absence of severe respiratory disease
- Difficulty in performing and/or inconsistent spirometry measures
- High score (over 26) on Nijmegen questionnaire
- Induction of symptoms during submaximal hyperventilation
- Resting end-tidal CO_2 < 4.5%
- Associated digital paraesthesiae

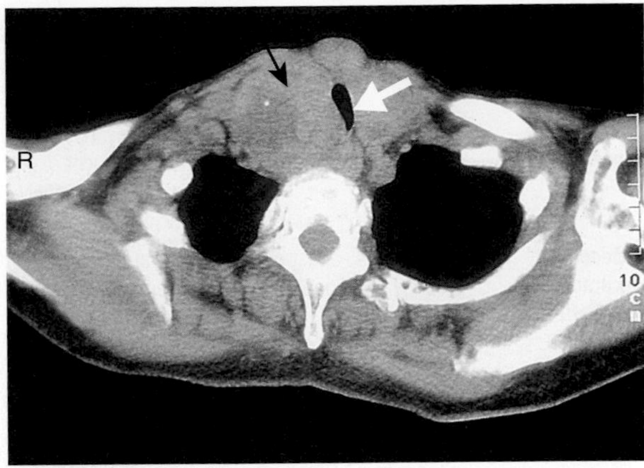

Fig. 19.11 CT showing retrosternal multinodular goitre (small arrow) causing acute severe breathlessness and stridor due to tracheal compression (large arrow).

History

It is important to establish the rate of onset and severity of the breathlessness and whether associated cardiovascular symptoms (chest pain, palpitations, sweating and nausea) or respiratory symptoms (cough, wheeze, haemoptysis, stridor – Fig. 19.11) are present. A previous history of repeated episodes of left ventricular failure, asthma or exacerbations of COPD is valuable. In the severely ill patient, it may be necessary to obtain the history from accompanying witnesses. In children, the possibility of inhalation of a foreign body (see Fig. 19.9) or acute epiglottitis should always be considered.

Clinical assessment

The following should be assessed and documented:

- level of consciousness
- degree of central cyanosis
- evidence of anaphylaxis (urticaria or angioedema)
- patency of the upper airway
- ability to speak (in single words or sentences)
- cardiovascular status (heart rate and rhythm, blood pressure and degree of peripheral perfusion).

Pulmonary oedema is suggested by pink, frothy sputum and bi-basal crackles; asthma or COPD by wheeze and prolonged expiration; pneumothorax by a silent resonant hemithorax; and pulmonary embolus by severe breathlessness with normal breath sounds. The peak expiratory flow should be measured whenever possible. Leg swelling may suggest cardiac failure or, if asymmetrical, venous thrombosis. Arterial blood gases, a chest X-ray and an ECG should be obtained to confirm the clinical diagnosis, and high concentrations of oxygen given pending results. Urgent endotracheal intubation (p. 194) may become necessary if the conscious level declines or if severe respiratory acidosis is present.

19.8 Differential diagnosis of acute breathlessness

Condition	History	Signs	CXR	ABG	ECG
Pulmonary oedema	Chest pain, palpitations, orthopnoea, cardiac history*	Central cyanosis, ↑JVP, sweating, cool extremities, basal crackles*	Cardiomegaly, oedema/pleural effusions*	↓PaO_2 ↓$PaCO_2$	Sinus tachycardia, ischaemia*, arrhythmia
Massive pulmonary embolus	Risk factors, chest pain, pleurisy, syncope*, dizziness*	Central cyanosis, ↑JVP*, absence of signs in the lung*, shock (tachycardia, hypotension)	Often normal Prominent hilar vessels, oligaemic lung fields*	↓PaO_2 ↓$PaCO_2$	Sinus tachycardia, RBBB, $S_1Q_3T_3$ pattern ↑$T(V_1–V_4)$
Acute severe asthma	History of asthma, asthma medications, wheeze*	Tachycardia, pulsus paradoxus, cyanosis (late), JVP →*, ↓peak flow, wheeze*	Hyperinflation only (unless complicated by pneumothorax)*	↓PaO_2 ↓$PaCO_2$ (↑$PaCO_2$ in extremis)	Sinus tachycardia (bradycardia in extremis)
Acute exacerbation of COPD	Previous episodes*, smoker. If in type II respiratory failure, may be drowsy	Cyanosis, hyperinflation*, signs of CO_2 retention (flapping tremor, bounding pulses)*	Hyperinflation*, bullae, complicating pneumothorax	↓ or ↓↓PaO_2 ↑$PaCO_2$ in type II failure ± ↑H^+, ↑HCO_3 in chronic type II failure	Normal, or signs of right ventricular strain
Pneumonia	Prodromal illness*, fever*, rigors*, pleurisy*	Fever, confusion, pleural rub*, consolidation*, cyanosis (if severe)	Pneumonic consolidation*	↓PaO_2 ↓$PaCO_2$ (↑ in extremis)	Tachycardia
Metabolic acidosis	Evidence of diabetes mellitus or renal disease, aspirin or ethylene glycol overdose	Fetor (ketones), hyperventilation without heart or lung signs*, dehydration*, air hunger	Normal	PaO_2 normal ↓↓$PaCO_2$, ↑H^+	
Psychogenic	Previous episodes, digital or perioral dysaesthesia	No cyanosis, no heart or lung signs, carpopedal spasm	Normal	PaO_2 normal* ↓↓$PaCO_2$, ↓H^+*	

*Valuable discriminatory feature. (ABG = arterial blood gases; RBBB = right bundle branch block)

Chest pain

Chest pain is a frequent manifestation of both cardiac (p. 539) and respiratory disease (Box 19.9). Pleurisy, a sharp chest pain aggravated by deep breathing or coughing, is a common feature of pulmonary infection or infarction; it may also occur with malignancy. On examination, rib movement may be restricted and a pleural rub may be present. Malignant involvement of the chest wall or ribs can cause gnawing, continuous local pain in the chest wall. Central chest pain suggests heart disease but also occurs with tumours affecting the mediastinum, oesophageal disease (p. 865) or disease of the thoracic aorta (p. 603). Massive pulmonary embolus may cause ischaemic cardiac pain, as well as severe breathlessness. Tracheitis produces raw upper retrosternal pain, exacerbated by the accompanying cough. Musculoskeletal chest wall pain is usually exacerbated by movement and associated with local tenderness.

Haemoptysis

Coughing up blood, irrespective of the amount, is an alarming symptom and patients nearly always seek medical advice. Care should be taken to establish that it is true haemoptysis and not haematemesis, or gum or nose bleeding. Haemoptysis must always be assumed to have a serious cause until this is excluded (Box 19.10).

Many episodes of haemoptysis remain unexplained, even after full investigation, and are likely to be due to simple bronchial infection. A history of repeated small haemoptysis, or blood-streaking of sputum, is highly suggestive of bronchial carcinoma. Fever, night sweats and weight loss suggest tuberculosis. Pneumococcal pneumonia often causes 'rusty'-coloured sputum but can cause frank haemoptysis, as can all suppurative pneumonic infections, including lung abscess (p. 687). Bronchiectasis (p. 678) and intracavitary mycetoma (p. 698) can cause catastrophic bronchial haemorrhage, and in these patients there may be a history of previous tuberculosis or pneumonia in early life. Finally, pulmonary thromboembolism is a common cause of haemoptysis and should always be considered.

Physical examination may reveal additional clues. Finger clubbing suggests bronchial carcinoma or bronchiectasis; other signs of malignancy, such as cachexia, hepatomegaly and lymphadenopathy, should also be sought. Fever, pleural rub and signs of consolidation occur in pneumonia or pulmonary infarction; a minority of patients with pulmonary infarction also have unilateral leg swelling or pain suggestive of deep venous thrombosis. Rashes, haematuria and digital infarcts

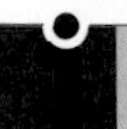

19.9 Differential diagnosis of chest pain

Central	
Cardiac	
• Myocardial ischaemia (angina) • Myocardial infarction • Myocarditis	• Pericarditis • Mitral valve prolapse syndrome
Aortic	
• Aortic dissection	• Aortic aneurysm
Oesophageal	
• Oesophagitis • Oesophageal spasm	• Mallory–Weiss syndrome
Massive pulmonary embolus	
Mediastinal	
• Tracheitis	• Malignancy
Anxiety/emotion[1]	
Peripheral	
Lungs/pleura	
• Pulmonary infarct • Pneumonia • Pneumothorax	• Malignancy • Tuberculosis • Connective tissue disorders
Musculoskeletal[2]	
• Osteoarthritis • Rib fracture/injury • Costochondritis (Tietze's syndrome)	• Intercostal muscle injury • Epidemic myalgia (Bornholm disease)
Neurological	
• Prolapsed intervertebral disc	• Herpes zoster • Thoracic outlet syndrome

[1]May also cause peripheral chest pain. [2]Can sometimes cause central chest pain.

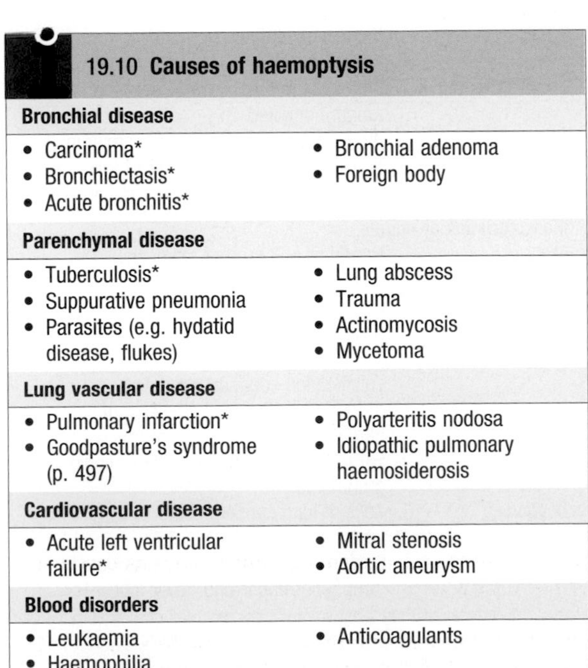

19.10 Causes of haemoptysis

Bronchial disease	
• Carcinoma* • Bronchiectasis* • Acute bronchitis*	• Bronchial adenoma • Foreign body
Parenchymal disease	
• Tuberculosis* • Suppurative pneumonia • Parasites (e.g. hydatid disease, flukes)	• Lung abscess • Trauma • Actinomycosis • Mycetoma
Lung vascular disease	
• Pulmonary infarction* • Goodpasture's syndrome (p. 497)	• Polyarteritis nodosa • Idiopathic pulmonary haemosiderosis
Cardiovascular disease	
• Acute left ventricular failure*	• Mitral stenosis • Aortic aneurysm
Blood disorders	
• Leukaemia • Haemophilia	• Anticoagulants

*More common causes.

point to an underlying systemic disease, such as a vasculitis, which may be associated with haemoptysis.

Management

In severe acute haemoptysis, the patient should be nursed upright (or on the side of the bleeding, if this is known), given high-flow oxygen and resuscitated as required. Bronchoscopy in the acute phase is difficult and often merely shows blood throughout the bronchial tree. If radiology shows an obvious central cause, then rigid bronchoscopy under general anaesthesia may allow intervention to stop bleeding; however, the source often cannot be visualised. Intubation with a divided endotracheal tube may allow protected ventilation of the unaffected lung to stabilise the patient. Bronchial arteriography and embolisation (Fig. 19.12), or even emergency surgery, can be life-saving in the acute situation.

In the vast majority of cases, however, the haemoptysis itself is not life-threatening and a logical sequence of investigations can be followed:

- chest X-ray, which may provide evidence of a localised lesion, including tumour (malignant or benign), pneumonia, mycetoma or tuberculosis
- full blood count (FBC) and clotting screen
- bronchoscopy after acute bleeding has settled, which may reveal a central bronchial carcinoma (not visible on the chest X-ray) and permit biopsy and tissue diagnosis
- CTPA, which may reveal underlying pulmonary thromboembolic disease or alternative causes not seen on the chest X-ray (e.g. pulmonary arteriovenous malformation or small or hidden tumours).

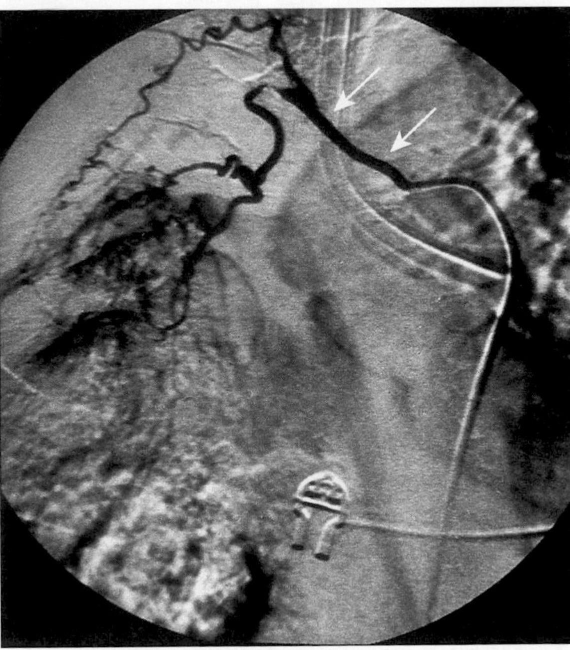

Fig. 19.12 Bronchial artery angiography. An angiography catheter has been passed via the femoral artery and aorta into an abnormally dilated right bronchial artery (arrows). Contrast is seen flowing into the lung. This patient had post-tuberculous bronchiectasis and presented with massive haemoptysis. Bronchial artery embolisation was successfully performed.

19

The incidental pulmonary nodule

The incidental finding of a pulmonary nodule (a rounded opacity measuring up to 3 cm in diameter) is common, particularly with the widespread use of thoracic CT scanning (Fig. 19.13). The differential diagnosis is extensive (Box 19.11), and whilst the majority are benign, it is important to identify a potentially treatable malignancy.

A lesion may be confidently described as benign if it appears unchanged over 2 years. If previous images are available and this can be established, no further investigation may be necessary. Otherwise, the likelihood of malignancy is assessed by considering the characteristics of the patient, including age, smoking history and any history of prior malignancy, and the appearance of the nodule in terms of its size, margin, density and location (Box 19.12). Further investigation is required in the majority of cases.

Pulmonary nodules are invariably beyond the vision of the bronchoscope and, with the notable exception of pulmonary infection (e.g. tuberculosis), bronchoscopy is usually unrewarding as the yield from blind washings is low. Endoscopic bronchoscopic ultrasound may overcome this but, for the time being, tissue is most commonly obtained using percutaneous needle biopsy under ultrasound or CT guidance. Needle biopsy may be complicated by pneumothorax in around 20% of cases and although only 3% require intercostal drainage, this technique should only be contemplated in individuals with an FEV_1 of more than 35% predicted. Haemorrhage into the lung or pleural space, air embolism and tumour seeding are rare but recognised complications.

PET scanning provides useful information about nodules of at least 1 cm in diameter, in which the presence of high metabolic activity is strongly suggestive of malignancy, while an inactive 'cold' nodule is consistent with benign disease. False-positive results may occur with some infectious or inflammatory nodules, and false-negative results with neuro-endocrine tumours and bronchiolo-alveolar cell carcinomas. Detection of neuro-endocrine tumours may be improved by the use of ^{68}Ga-Dotatoc in place of FDG.

Where tissue biopsy is contraindicated and the lesion is too small to be confidently assessed by PET, interval thoracic CT scanning may be considered. The period between scans is based upon the average tumour doubling time (Box 19.13). Changes may be difficult to assess visually and specially adapted computer programs allow more detailed topographical assessment. However, the risks of radiation exposure inherent in this approach, and the fact that further nodules are likely to be detected, need to be considered. In some circumstances, if the nodule is highly likely to be malignant and the patient is fit for surgery, the best option may be to proceed to surgical resection.

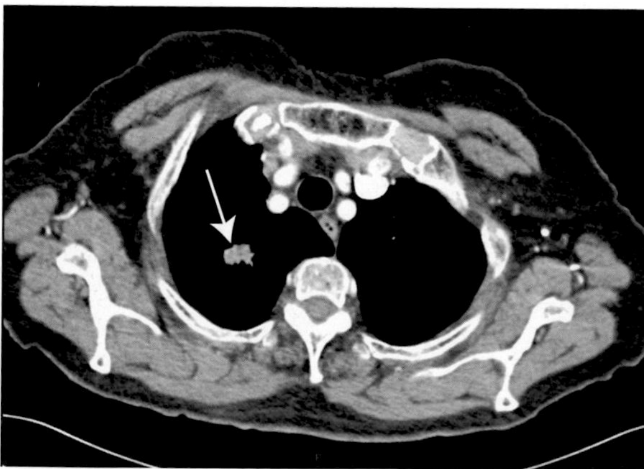

Fig. 19.13 Thoracic CT scan showing a solitary pulmonary nodule identified in the right upper lobe (arrow).

19.11 Causes of pulmonary nodules

Common causes

- Bronchial carcinoma
- Single metastasis
- Localised pneumonia
- Lung abscess
- Tuberculoma
- Pulmonary infarct

Uncommon causes

- Benign tumours
- Lymphoma
- Arteriovenous malformation
- Hydatid cyst (p. 380)
- Bronchogenic cyst
- Rheumatoid nodule
- Pulmonary sequestration
- Pulmonary haematoma
- Wegener's granuloma
- 'Pseudotumour' – fluid collection in a fissure
- Aspergilloma (usually surrounded by air 'halo')

19.12 Clinical and radiographic features distinguishing benign from malignant nodules

Feature	Risk of malignancy
Patient characteristics	
Age	Increases with age and is uncommon < age of 40
Smoking history	Increases in proportion to duration and amount smoked
Other	Increased by history of lung cancer in first-degree relative, and by exposure to asbestos, silica, uranium and radon
Characteristics of nodule	
Size	Nearly all > 3 cm but fewer than 1% < 4 mm are malignant
Margin	Usually smooth in benign lesions Spiculated suggests malignancy
Calcification or fat	Laminated or central deposition of calcification suggests granuloma 'Popcorn' pattern is suggestive of hamartoma Fat may suggest hamartoma or lipoid granuloma
Location	70% of lung cancers occur in upper lobes Benign lesions are equally distributed throughout upper and lower lobes

Note Linear or sheet-like lung opacities are unlikely to represent neoplasms and do not require follow-up. Some nodular opacities may be sufficiently typical of scarring that follow-up is not warranted.
Adapted from Fleischer Society Statement. Radiology 2005; 237:395–400.

19.13 Recommendations for follow-up of incidental nodules smaller than 8 mm[1]

Nodule size (mm) (average of length and width)	No or minimal history of smoking/ other risk factors	Smoker/other risk factors
≤ 4	No follow-up needed[2]	Follow-up CT at 12 mths; if unchanged, no further follow-up
4–6	Follow-up at 12 mths; if unchanged, no further follow-up	Initial follow-up CT at 6–12 mths, then at 18–24 mths if no change
6–8	Initial follow-up CT at 6–12 mths, then at 18–24 mths if no change	Initial follow-up CT at 3–6 mths, then at 9–12 mths if no change
> 8	Follow-up CT at around 3, 9 and 24 mths, dynamic contrast-enhanced CT, PET and/or biopsy	As for low-risk patient

[1]Excludes younger patients, and those with unexplained fever or known/ suspected malignant disease.
[2]Very low risk of malignancy (< 1%). Non-solid (ground glass) or partly solid nodules may require longer follow-up to exclude indolent adenocarcinoma.
Adapted from Radiology 2005; 237:395–400.

Pleural effusion

The accumulation of serous fluid within the pleural space is termed pleural effusion. The accumulation of frank pus is termed empyema (p. 662), that of blood is haemothorax, and that of chyle is a chylothorax. In general, pleural fluid accumulates as a result of either increased hydrostatic pressure or decreased osmotic pressure ('transudative' effusion, as seen in cardiac, liver or renal failure), or from increased microvascular pressure due to disease of the pleura or injury in the adjacent lung ('exudative' effusion). The causes of the majority of pleural effusions (Boxes 19.14 and 19.15) are identified by a thorough history, examination and relevant investigations.

Clinical assessment

Symptoms (pain on inspiration and coughing) and signs of pleurisy (a pleural rub) often precede the development of an effusion, especially in patients with underlying pneumonia, pulmonary infarction or connective tissue disease. However, when breathlessness is the only symptom, depending on the size and rate of accumulation, the onset may be insidious. The physical signs are detailed on page 645.

Investigations

Radiological investigations

The classical appearance of pleural fluid on the erect PA chest film is of a curved shadow at the lung base, blunting the costophrenic angle and ascending towards the axilla (p. 645). Fluid appears to track up the lateral chest wall. In fact, fluid surrounds the whole lung at this level, but casts a radiological shadow only where the X-ray beam passes tangentially across the fluid against the lateral chest wall. Around 200 mL of fluid is required in order for it to be detectable on a PA chest X-ray. Previous scarring or adhesions in the pleural space can cause localised effusions. Pleural fluid localised below the lower lobe ('subpulmonary effusion') simulates an elevated hemidiaphragm. Pleural fluid localised within an oblique fissure may produce a rounded opacity that may be mistaken for a tumour.

Ultrasound is more accurate than plain chest X-ray for determining the presence of fluid. A clear hypoechoic space is consistent with a transudate and the presence of moving floating densities suggests an exudate. The presence of septation suggests an evolving empyema or resolving haemothorax. CT scanning is indicated where malignant disease is suspected.

19.14 Causes of pleural effusion

Common causes

- Pneumonia ('para-pneumonic effusion')
- Tuberculosis
- Pulmonary infarction*
- Malignant disease
- Cardiac failure*
- Subdiaphragmatic disorders (subphrenic abscess, pancreatitis etc.)

Uncommon causes

- Hypoproteinaemia* (nephrotic syndrome, liver failure, malnutrition)
- Connective tissue diseases* (particularly systemic lupus erythematosus (SLE) and rheumatoid arthritis)
- Post-myocardial infarction syndrome
- Acute rheumatic fever
- Meigs' syndrome (ovarian tumour plus pleural effusion)
- Myxoedema*
- Uraemia*
- Asbestos-related benign pleural effusion

*May cause bilateral effusions.

Pleural aspiration and biopsy

In some conditions (e.g. left ventricular failure), it should not be necessary to sample fluid unless atypical features are present; appropriate treatment should be administered and the effusion re-evaluated. However, in most other circumstances, diagnostic sampling is required. Simple aspiration provides information on the colour and texture of fluid and these alone may immediately suggest an empyema or chylothorax. The presence of blood is consistent with pulmonary infarction or malignancy, but may result from a traumatic tap. Biochemical analysis allows classification into transudate and exudates (Box 19.16) and Gram stain may suggest para-pneumonic effusion. The predominant cell type provides useful information and cytological examination is essential. A low pH suggests infection but may also be seen in rheumatoid arthritis, ruptured oesophagus or advanced malignancy.

Ultrasound- or CT-guided pleural biopsy provides tissue for pathological and microbiological analysis. Where necessary, video-assisted thoracoscopy allows visualisaton of the pleura and direct guidance of a biopsy.

19.15 Pleural effusion: main causes and features

Cause	Appearance of fluid	Type of fluid	Predominant cells in fluid	Other diagnostic features
Tuberculosis	Serous, usually amber-coloured	Exudate	Lymphocytes (occasionally polymorphs)	Positive tuberculin test Isolation of *M. tuberculosis* from pleural fluid (20%) Positive pleural biopsy (80%) Raised adenosine deaminase
Malignant disease	Serous, often blood-stained	Exudate	Serosal cells and lymphocytes Often clumps of malignant cells	Positive pleural biopsy (40%) Evidence of malignancy elsewhere
Cardiac failure	Serous, straw-coloured	Transudate	Few serosal cells	Other signs of cardiac failure Response to diuretics
Pulmonary infarction	Serous or blood-stained	Exudate (rarely transudate)	Red blood cells Eosinophils	Evidence of pulmonary infarction Obvious source of embolism Factors predisposing to venous thrombosis
Rheumatoid disease	Serous Turbid if chronic	Exudate	Lymphocytes (occasionally polymorphs)	Rheumatoid arthritis: rheumatoid factor and anti-CCP antibodies Cholesterol in chronic effusion; very low glucose in pleural fluid
SLE	Serous	Exudate	Lymphocytes and serosal cells	Other signs of SLE Antinuclear factor or anti-DNA positive
Acute pancreatitis	Serous or blood-stained	Exudate	No cells predominate	Higher amylase in pleural fluid than in serum
Obstruction of thoracic duct	Milky	Chyle	None	Chylomicrons

(anti-CCP = anti-cyclic citrullinated peptide; SLE = systemic lupus erythematosus)

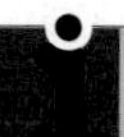

19.16 Light's criteria for distinguishing pleural transudate from exudate

Exudate is likely if one or more of the following criteria are met:

- Pleural fluid protein : serum protein ratio > 0.5
- Pleural fluid LDH : serum LDH ratio > 0.6
- Pleural fluid LDH > two-thirds of the upper limit of normal serum LDH

(LDH = lactate dehydrogenase)

Management

Therapeutic aspiration may be required to palliate breathlessness but removing more than 1.5 L at a time is associated with a small risk of re-expansion pulmonary oedema. An effusion should never be drained to dryness before establishing a diagnosis, as biopsy may be precluded until further fluid accumulates. Treatment of the underlying cause – for example, heart failure, pneumonia, pulmonary embolism or subphrenic abscess – will often be followed by resolution of the effusion. The management of pleural effusion in pneumonia, tuberculosis and malignancy is dealt with below.

Empyema

This is a collection of pus in the pleural space, which may be as thin as serous fluid or so thick that it is impossible to aspirate, even through a wide-bore needle. Microscopically, neutrophil leucocytes are present in large numbers. An empyema may involve the whole pleural space or only part of it ('loculated' or 'encysted' empyema) and is usually unilateral. It is always secondary to infection in a neighbouring structure, usually the lung, most commonly due to the bacterial pneumonias and tuberculosis. Over 40% of patients with community-acquired pneumonia develop an associated pleural effusion ('para-pneumonic' effusion) and about 15% of these become secondarily infected. Other causes are infection of a haemothorax following trauma or surgery, oesophageal rupture, and rupture of a subphrenic abscess through the diaphragm.

Both pleural surfaces are covered with a thick, shaggy, inflammatory exudate. The pus in the pleural space is often under considerable pressure, and if the condition is not adequately treated, pus may rupture into a bronchus, causing a bronchopleural fistula and pyopneumothorax, or track through the chest wall with the formation of a subcutaneous abscess or sinus, so-called empyema necessitans.

Clinical assessment

An empyema should be suspected in patients with pulmonary infection if there is severe pleuritic chest pain or persisting or recurrent pyrexia, despite appropriate antibiotic treatment. In other cases, the primary infection may be so mild that it passes unrecognised and the first definite clinical features are due to the empyema itself. Once an empyema has developed, systemic features are prominent (Box 19.17).

19.17 Clinical features of empyema

Systemic features
• Pyrexia, usually high and remittent • Rigors, sweating, malaise and weight loss • Polymorphonuclear leucocytosis, high CRP
Local features
• Pleural pain; breathlessness; cough and sputum, usually because of underlying lung disease; copious purulent sputum if empyema ruptures into a bronchus (bronchopleural fistula) • Clinical signs of pleural effusion

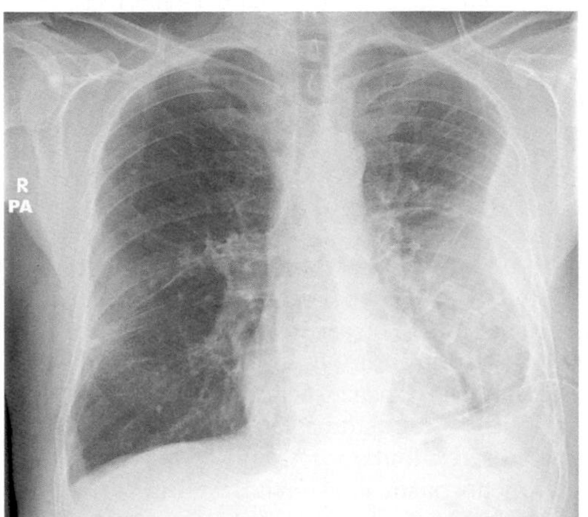

Fig. 19.14 Chest X-ray showing a 'D'-shaped shadow in the left mid-zone, consistent with an empyema. In this case, an intercostal chest drain has been inserted but the loculated collection of pus remains.

Investigations

Chest X-ray appearances may be indistinguishable from those of pleural effusion, although pleural adhesions may confine the empyema to form a 'D'-shaped shadow against the inside of the chest wall (Fig. 19.14). When air is present as well as pus (pyopneumothorax), a horizontal 'fluid level' marks the air/liquid interface. Ultrasound shows the position of the fluid, the extent of pleural thickening and whether fluid is in a single collection or multiloculated, containing fibrin and debris (Fig. 19.15). CT provides information on the pleura, underlying lung parenchyma and patency of the major bronchi.

Ultrasound or CT is used to identify the optimal site for aspiration, which is best performed using a wide-bore needle. If the fluid is thick and turbid pus, empyema is confirmed. Other features suggesting empyema are a fluid glucose of less than 3.3 mmol/L (60 mg/dL), lactate dehydrogenase (LDH) of more than 1000 U/L, or a fluid pH of less than 7.0 (H^+ over 100 nmol/L). However, pH measurement should be avoided if pus is thick, as it damages blood gas machines. The pus is frequently sterile on culture if antibiotics have already been given. The distinction between tuberculous and non-tuberculous disease can be difficult and often requires pleural biopsy, histology and culture.

Management

An empyema will only heal if infection is eradicated and the empyema space is obliterated, allowing apposition of the visceral and parietal pleural layers. This can only occur if re-expansion of the compressed lung is secured at an early stage by removal of all the pus from the pleural space. When the pus is sufficiently thin, this is most easily achieved by the insertion of a wide-bore intercostal tube into the most dependent part of the empyema space. If the initial aspirate reveals turbid fluid or frank pus, or if loculations are seen on ultrasound, the tube should be put on suction (–5 to –10 cm H_2O) and flushed regularly with 20 mL normal saline. If the organism causing the empyema can be identified, the appropriate antibiotic should be given for 2–4 weeks. Empirical antibiotic treatment (e.g. intravenous co-amoxiclav or cefuroxime with metronidazole) should be used if the organism is unknown. Intrapleural fibrinolytic therapy is of no benefit.

An empyema can often be aborted if these measures are started early, but if the intercostal tube is not providing adequate drainage - for example, when the pus is thick or loculated, surgical intervention is required to clear the empyema cavity of pus and break down any adhesions. Surgical 'decortication' of the lung may also be required if gross thickening of the visceral pleura is preventing re-expansion of the lung. Surgery is also necessary if a bronchopleural fistula develops.

Despite the widespread availability of antibiotics that are effective against pneumonia, empyema remains a significant cause of morbidity and mortality.

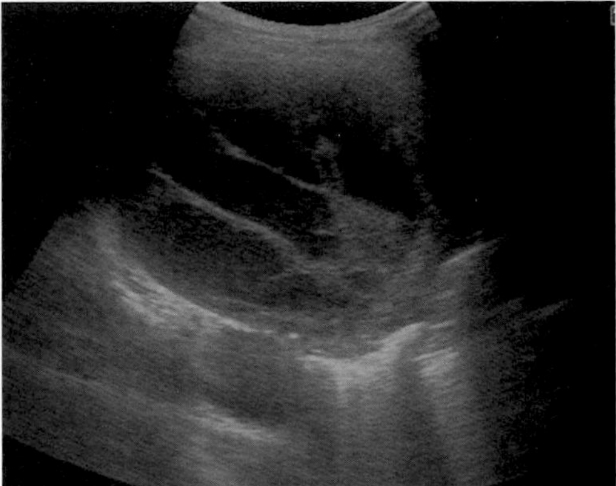

Fig. 19.15 Pleural ultrasound showing septation.

Respiratory failure

The term 'respiratory failure' is used when pulmonary gas exchange fails to maintain normal arterial oxygen and carbon dioxide levels. Its classification into types I and II is defined by the absence or presence of hypercapnia (raised $PaCO_2$).

Pathophysiology

When disease impairs ventilation of part of a lung (e.g. in asthma or pneumonia), perfusion of that region results in hypoxic and CO_2-laden blood entering the pulmonary veins. Increased ventilation of neighbouring regions of normal lung can increase CO_2 excretion, correcting arterial CO_2 to normal, but cannot augment oxygen uptake because the haemoglobin flowing through these regions is already fully saturated. Admixture of blood from the underventilated and normal regions thus results in hypoxia with normocapnia,

19

19.18 How to interpret blood gas abnormalities in respiratory failure

	Type I Hypoxia (PaO_2 < 8.0 kPa (60 mmHg)) Normal or low $PaCO_2$ (< 6.6 kPa (50 mmHg))		Type II Hypoxia (PaO_2 < 8.0 kPa (60 mmHg)) Raised $PaCO_2$ (> 6.6 kPa (50 mmHg))	
	Acute	**Chronic**	**Acute**	**Chronic**
H^+	→	→	↑	→ or ↑
Bicarbonate	→	→	→	↑
Causes	Acute asthma Pulmonary oedema Pneumonia Lobar collapse Pneumothorax Pulmonary embolus ARDS	COPD Lung fibrosis Lymphangitis carcinomatosa Right-to-left shunts	Acute severe asthma Acute exacerbation of COPD Upper airway obstruction Acute neuropathies/paralysis Narcotic drugs Primary alveolar hypoventilation Flail chest injury	COPD Sleep apnoea Kyphoscoliosis Myopathies/muscular dystrophy Ankylosing spondylitis

(ARDS = acute respiratory distress syndrome; COPD = chronic obstructive pulmonary disease)

which is called 'type I respiratory failure'. Diseases causing this include all those that impair ventilation locally with sparing of other regions (Box 19.18).

Arterial hypoxia with hypercapnia (type II respiratory failure) is seen in conditions that cause generalised, severe ventilation–perfusion mismatch, leaving insufficient normal lung to correct $PaCO_2$, or a disease that reduces total ventilation. The latter includes not just diseases of the lung but also disorders affecting any part of the neuromuscular mechanism of ventilation (see Box 19.18).

Management of acute respiratory failure

Prompt diagnosis and management of the underlying cause is crucial. In type I respiratory failure, high concentrations of oxygen (40–60% by mask) will usually relieve hypoxia by increasing the alveolar PO_2 in poorly ventilated lung units. Occasionally, however (e.g. severe pneumonia affecting several lobes), mechanical ventilation may be needed to relieve hypoxia. Patients who need high concentrations of oxygen for more than a few hours should receive humidified oxygen.

Acute type II respiratory failure is an emergency requiring immediate intervention. It is useful to distinguish between patients with high ventilatory drive (rapid respiratory rate and accessory muscle recruitment) who cannot move sufficient air, and those with reduced or inadequate respiratory effort. In the former, particularly if inspiratory stridor is present, acute upper airway obstruction from foreign body inhalation or laryngeal obstruction (angioedema, carcinoma or vocal cord paralysis) must be considered, as the Heimlich manœuvre (p. 728), immediate intubation or emergency tracheostomy may be life-saving.

More commonly, the problem is in the lungs, with severe generalised bronchial obstruction from COPD or asthma, acute respiratory distress syndrome (ARDS) arising from a variety of insults (p. 191), or occasionally tension pneumothorax (p. 728). In all such cases, high-concentration (e.g. 60%) oxygen should be administered, pending a rapid examination of the respiratory system and measurement of arterial blood gases. Patients with the trachea deviated away from a silent and resonant hemithorax are likely to have tension pneumothorax, and air should be aspirated from the pleural space and a chest drain inserted as soon as possible. Patients with generalised wheeze, scanty breath sounds bilaterally or a history of asthma or COPD should be treated with nebulised salbutamol 2.5 mg with oxygen, repeated until bronchospasm is relieved. Failure to respond to initial treatment, declining conscious level and worsening respiratory acidosis (H^+ > 50 nmol/L (pH < 7.3), $PaCO_2$ > 6.6 kPa (50 mmHg)) on blood gases are all indications that supported ventilation is required (p. 193).

A small percentage of patients with severe chronic COPD and type II respiratory failure develop abnormal tolerance to raised $PaCO_2$ and may become dependent on hypoxic drive to breathe. In these patients only, lower concentrations of oxygen (24–28% by Venturi mask) should be used to avoid precipitating worsening respiratory depression (see below). In all cases, regular monitoring of arterial blood gases is important to assess progress.

Patients with acute type II respiratory failure who have reduced drive or conscious level may be suffering from sedative poisoning, CO_2 narcosis or a primary failure of neurological drive (e.g. following intracerebral haemorrhage or head injury). History from a witness may be invaluable, and reversal of specific drugs with (for example) opiate antagonists is occasionally successful, but should not delay intubation and supported mechanical ventilation in appropriate cases.

Chronic and 'acute on chronic' type II respiratory failure

The most common cause of chronic type II respiratory failure is severe COPD. Although $PaCO_2$ may be persistently raised, there is no persisting acidaemia because the kidneys retain bicarbonate, correcting arterial pH to normal. This 'compensated' pattern, which may also occur in chronic neuromuscular disease or kyphoscoliosis, is maintained until there is a further acute illness (see Box 19.18), such as an exacerbation of COPD which precipitates an episode of 'acute on chronic' respiratory failure, with acidaemia and initial respiratory distress followed by drowsiness and eventually coma. These patients have lost their chemo-sensitivity to elevated $PaCO_2$, and so they may paradoxically depend on hypoxia for respiratory drive, and are at risk of respiratory depression if given high concentrations of oxygen – for example, during ambulance transfers or in emergency departments. Moreover, in contrast to acute severe asthma, some patients with 'acute on chronic' type II respiratory failure due to COPD may not be distressed, despite being critically ill with severe hypoxaemia, hypercapnia and acidaemia. While the physical signs of CO_2 retention (confusion, flapping tremor, bounding pulses and so on) can be helpful if present, they may not be, so arterial blood gases are mandatory in the assessment of initial severity and response to treatment.

Management

The principal aims of treatment in acute on chronic type II respiratory failure are to achieve a safe PaO_2 (> 7.0 kPa (52 mmHg)) without increasing $PaCO_2$ and acidosis, while identifying and treating the precipitating condition. In these patients, it is not necessary to achieve a normal PaO_2; even a small increase will often have a greatly beneficial effect on tissue oxygen delivery, since their PaO_2 values are often on the steep part of the oxygen saturation curve (p. 184). The risks of worsening hypercapnia and coma must be balanced against those of severe hypoxaemia, which include potentially fatal arrhythmias or severe cerebral complications.

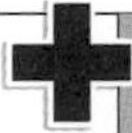

19.19 Assessment and management of 'acute on chronic' type II respiratory failure

Initial assessment

Patient may not appear distressed, despite being critically ill

- Conscious level (response to commands, ability to cough)
- CO_2 retention (warm periphery, bounding pulses, flapping tremor)
- Airways obstruction (wheeze, prolonged expiration, hyperinflation, intercostal indrawing, pursed lips)
- Cor pulmonale (peripheral oedema, raised JVP, hepatomegaly, ascites)
- Background functional status and quality of life
- Signs of precipitating cause (see Box 19.17)

Investigations

- Arterial blood gases (severity of hypoxaemia, hypercapnia, acidaemia, bicarbonate)
- Chest X-ray

Management

- Maintenance of airway
- Treatment of specific precipitating cause
- Frequent physiotherapy ± pharyngeal suction
- Nebulised bronchodilators
- Controlled oxygen therapy
  Start with 24% Venturi mask
  Aim for a PaO_2 > 7 kPa (52 mmHg) (a PaO_2 < 5 (37 mmHg) is dangerous)
- Antibiotics if evidence of infection
- Diuretics if evidence of fluid overload

Progress

- If $PaCO_2$ continues to rise or a safe PaO_2 cannot be achieved without severe hypercapnia and acidaemia, mechanical ventilatory support may be required

Immediate treatment is shown in Box 19.19. Patients who are conscious and have adequate respiratory drive may benefit from non-invasive ventilation (NIV), which has been shown to reduce the need for intubation and shorten hospital stay. Patients who are drowsy and have low respiratory drive require an urgent decision regarding intubation and ventilation, as this is likely to be the only effective treatment, even though weaning off the ventilator may be difficult in severe disease. The decision is challenging, and important factors to consider include patient and family wishes, presence of a potentially remediable precipitating condition, prior functional capacity and quality of life. The various types of non-invasive (via a face or nasal mask) or invasive (via an endotracheal tube) ventilation are detailed on pages 193–196.

Respiratory stimulant drugs, such as doxapram, tend to cause unacceptable distress due to increased dyspnoea, and have been largely superseded by intubation and mechanical ventilation in patients with CO_2 narcosis, as they provide only minor and transient improvements in arterial blood gases.

Home ventilation for chronic respiratory failure

NIV is of great value in the long-term treatment of respiratory failure due to spinal deformity, neuromuscular disease and central alveolar hypoventilation. Some patients with advanced lung disease, e.g. cystic fibrosis, also benefit from NIV for respiratory failure. In these conditions, the onset of type II respiratory failure can be very gradual. Morning headache (due to elevated $PaCO_2$) and fatigue are common symptoms but, in many cases, the diagnosis is only revealed by sleep studies or morning blood gas analysis. In the initial stages, ventilation is insufficient for metabolic needs only during sleep, when there is a physiological decline in ventilatory drive. Over time, however, CO_2 retention becomes chronic, with renal compensation of acidosis. Treatment by home-based NIV overnight is often sufficient to restore the daytime PCO_2 to normal, and to relieve fatigue and headache. In advanced disease (e.g. muscular dystrophies or cystic fibrosis), daytime NIV may also be required.

Lung transplantation

Lung transplantation is an established treatment for carefully selected patients with advanced lung disease unresponsive to medical treatment (Box 19.20).

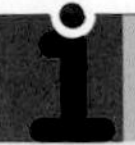

19.20 Indications for lung transplantation

Parenchymal lung disease

- Cystic fibrosis
- Emphysema
- Pulmonary fibrosis
- Obliterative bronchiolitis
- Langerhans cell histiocytosis (p. 715)
- Lymphangioleiomyomatosis (p. 715)

Pulmonary vascular disease

- Primary pulmonary hypertension
- Thromboembolic pulmonary hypertension
- Veno-occlusive disease
- Eisenmenger's syndrome (p. 631)

19

Single-lung transplantation may be used for selected patients with advanced emphysema or lung fibrosis. This is contraindicated in patients with chronic bilateral pulmonary infection, such as cystic fibrosis and bronchiectasis, because the transplanted lung is vulnerable to cross-infection in the context of post-transplant immunosuppression and for these individuals bilateral lung transplantation is the standard procedure. Combined heart–lung transplantation is still occasionally needed for patients with advanced congenital heart disease such as Eisenmenger's syndrome, and is preferred by some surgeons for the treatment of primary pulmonary hypertension unresponsive to medical therapy.

The prognosis following lung transplantation is improving steadily with modern immunosuppressive drugs: over 50% 10-year survival in some UK centres. However, chronic rejection resulting in obliterative bronchiolitis continues to afflict some recipients. Corticosteroids are used to manage acute rejection, but drugs that inhibit cell-mediated immunity specifically, such as ciclosporin, mycophenolate and tacrolimus (p. 94), are used to prevent chronic rejection. Azithromycin, statins and total lymphoid irradiation are employed to treat obliterative bronchiolitis, but late organ failure remains a significant problem.

The major factor limiting the availability of lung transplantation is the shortage of donor lungs. To improve organ availability, techniques to recondition the lungs in vitro after removal from the donor are being developed.

OBSTRUCTIVE PULMONARY DISEASES

Asthma

Asthma is a chronic inflammatory disorder of the airways, in which many cells and cellular elements play a role. The chronic inflammation is associated with airway hyper-responsiveness that leads to recurrent episodes of wheezing, breathlessness, chest tightness and coughing, particularly at night and in the early morning. These episodes are usually associated with widespread but variable airflow obstruction within the lung that is often reversible, either spontaneously or with treatment.

Epidemiology

The prevalence of asthma increased steadily over the latter part of the last century, first in the developed and then in the developing world (Fig. 19.16). Current estimates suggest that asthma affects 300 million people worldwide, with a predicted additional 100 million people affected by 2025. The socio-economic impact is enormous, as poor control leads to days lost from school or work, unscheduled health-care visits and hospital admissions.

Although the development and course of the disease, and the response to treatment, are influenced by genetic determinants, the rapid rise in prevalence implies that environmental factors are critically important in the development and expression of the disease. To date, studies have explored the potential role of indoor and outdoor allergens, microbial exposure, diet, vitamins, breastfeeding, tobacco smoke, air pollution and obesity but no clear consensus has emerged.

Pathophysiology

Airway hyper-reactivity (AHR) – the tendency for airways to narrow excessively in response to triggers that have little or no effect in normal individuals – is integral to the diagnosis of asthma and appears to be related, although not exclusively, to airway inflammation (Fig. 19.17). Other factors likely to be important in the behaviour of airway smooth muscle include the degree of airway narrowing and neurogenic mechanisms.

The relationship between atopy (the propensity to produce IgE) and asthma is well established, and in many individuals there is a clear relationship between sensitisation and allergen exposure, as demonstrated by skin prick reactivity or elevated serum specific IgE. Common examples of allergens include house dust mites, pets such as cats and dogs, pests such as cockroaches, and fungi. Inhalation of an allergen into the airway is followed by an early and late-phase bronchoconstrictor response (Fig. 19.18). Allergic mechanisms

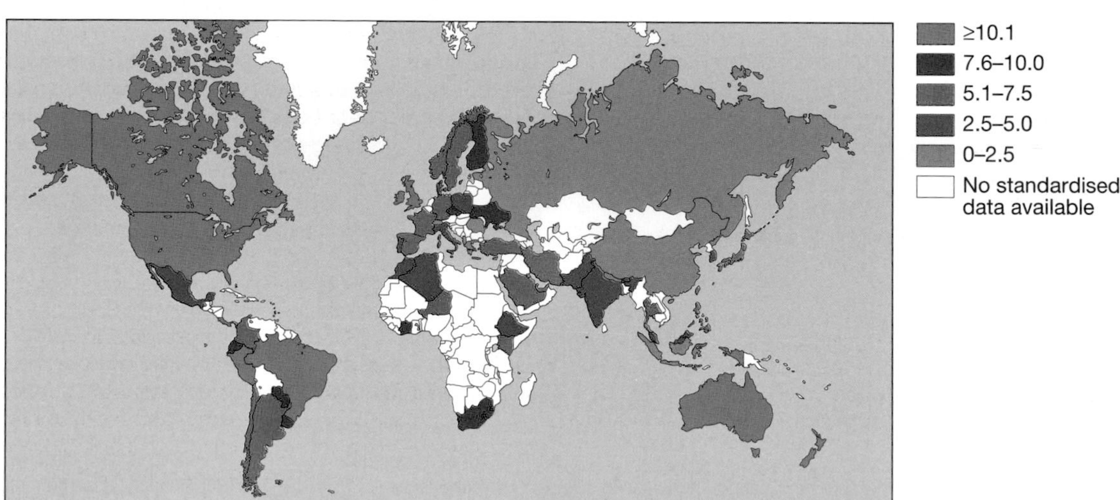

Fig. 19.16 World map showing the prevalence of clinical asthma (proportion of population (%)). From WHO – see p. 732; data drawn from the European Community Respiratory Health Study (ECRHS) and the International Study of Asthma and Allergies in Childhood (ISAAC).

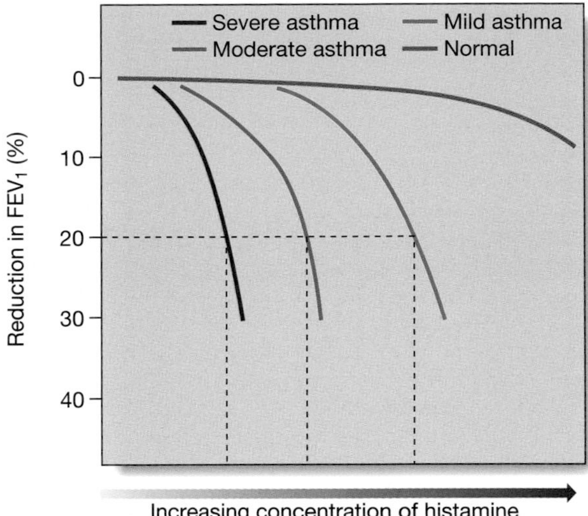

Fig. 19.17 Airway hyper-reactivity in asthma. This is demonstrated by bronchial challenge tests with sequentially increasing concentrations of either histamine, methacholine or mannitol. The reactivity of the airways is expressed as the concentration or dose of either chemical required to produce a specific decrease (usually 20%) in the FEV_1 (PC_{20} or PD_{20} respectively).

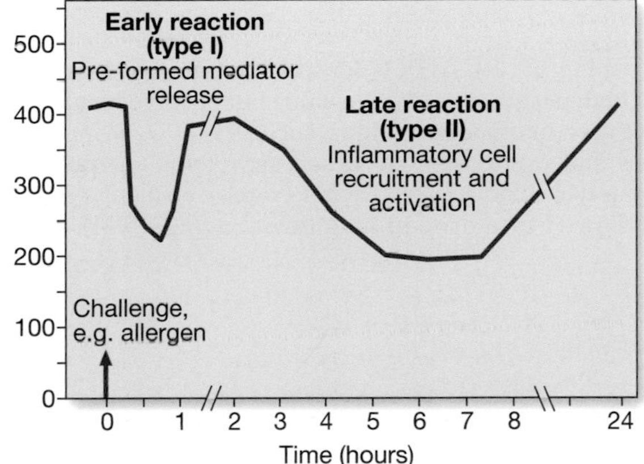

Fig. 19.18 Changes in peak flow following allergen challenge. A similar biphasic response is observed following a variety of different challenges. Occasionally, an isolated late response is seen with no early reaction.

are also implicated in some cases of occupational asthma (p. 715).

In cases of aspirin-sensitive asthma, the ingestion of salicylates results in inhibition of the cyclo-oxygenase enzymes, preferentially shunting the metabolism of arachidonic acid through the lipoxygenase pathway with resultant production of the asthmogenic cysteinyl leukotrienes. In exercise-induced asthma, hyperventilation results in water loss from the pericellular lining fluid of the respiratory mucosa, which, in turn, triggers mediator release. Heat loss from the respiratory mucosa may also be important.

In persistent asthma, a chronic and complex inflammatory response ensues, characterised by an influx of numerous inflammatory cells, the transformation and participation of airway structural cells, and the secretion of an array of cytokines, chemokines and growth factors. Examination of the inflammatory cell profile in induced sputum samples demonstrates that, although asthma is predominantly characterised by airway eosinophilia, neutrophilic inflammation predominates in some patients, while, in others, scant inflammation is observed: so-called 'pauci-granulocytic' asthma.

With increasing severity and chronicity of the disease, remodelling of the airway may occur, leading to fibrosis of the airway wall, fixed narrowing of the airway and a reduced response to bronchodilator medication.

Clinical features

Typical symptoms include recurrent episodes of wheezing, chest tightness, breathlessness and cough. Asthma is commonly mistaken for a cold or chest infection which is taking time to resolve (e.g. longer than 10 days). Classical precipitants include exercise, particularly in cold weather, exposure to airborne allergens or pollutants, and viral upper respiratory tract infections. Wheeze apart, there is often very little to find on examination. An inspection for nasal polyps and eczema should be performed. Rarely, a vasculitic rash may suggest Churg–Strauss syndrome (p. 1118).

Patients with mild intermittent asthma are usually asymptomatic between exacerbations. Individuals with persistent asthma report ongoing breathlessness and wheeze, but these are variable, with symptoms fluctuating over the course of one day, or from day to day or month to month.

Asthma characteristically displays a diurnal pattern, with symptoms and lung function being worse in the early morning. Particularly when poorly controlled, symptoms such as cough and wheeze disturb sleep and have led to the term 'nocturnal asthma'. Cough may be the dominant symptom in some patients, and the lack of wheeze or breathlessness may lead to a delay in reaching the diagnosis of so-called 'cough-variant asthma'.

Some patients with asthma have a similar inflammatory response in the upper airway. Careful enquiry should be made as to a history of sinusitis, sinus headache, a blocked or runny nose, and loss of sense of smell.

Although the aetiology of asthma is often elusive, an attempt should be made to identify any agents that may contribute to the appearance or aggravation of the condition. Particular enquiry should be made about potential allergens, such as exposure to a pet cat, guinea pig, rabbit or horse, pest infestation, exposure to moulds following water damage to a home or building, and any potential occupational agents.

In some circumstances, the appearance of asthma is triggered by medications. Beta-blockers, even when administered topically as eye drops, may induce bronchospasm, as may aspirin and other non-steroidal anti-inflammatory drugs (NSAIDs). The classical aspirin-sensitive patient is female and presents in middle age with asthma, rhinosinusitis and nasal polyps. Aspirin-sensitive patients may also report symptoms following alcohol (in particular, white wine) and foods containing salicylates. Other medications implicated include the oral contraceptive pill, cholinergic agents and prostaglandin F2α. Betel nuts contain arecoline, which is structurally similar to methacholine and can aggravate asthma. An important minority of patients develop a particularly severe form of asthma, and this appears to be more common in women. Allergic triggers are less important and airway neutrophilia predominates.

Diagnosis

The diagnosis of asthma is predominantly clinical and based on a characteristic history. Supportive evidence is provided by the demonstration of variable airflow obstruction, preferably by using spirometry (Box 19.21) to measure FEV_1 and VC. This identifies the obstructive defect, defines its severity, and provides a baseline for bronchodilator reversibility (Fig. 19.19). If spirometry is not available, a peak flow meter may be used. Patients should be instructed to record peak flow readings after rising in the morning and before retiring in the evening. A diurnal variation in PEF of more than 20% (the lowest values typically being recorded in the morning) is considered diagnostic, and the magnitude of variability provides some indication of disease severity (Fig. 19.20). A trial of corticosteroids (e.g. 30 mg daily for 2 weeks) may be useful in establishing the diagnosis, by demonstrating an improvement in either FEV_1 or PEF.

It is not uncommon for patients whose symptoms are suggestive of asthma to have normal lung function. In these circumstances, the demonstration of AHR by challenge tests may be useful to confirm the diagnosis (see Fig. 19.17). AHR is sensitive but non-specific: it has a high negative predictive value but positive results may be seen in other conditions, such as COPD, bronchiectasis and cystic fibrosis. When symptoms are predominantly related to exercise, an exercise challenge may be followed by a drop in lung function (Fig. 19.21).

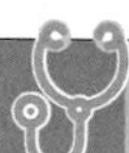

19.21 How to make a diagnosis of asthma

Compatible clinical history *plus either/or*:

- $FEV_1 \geq 15\%$* (and 200 mL) increase following administration of a bronchodilator/trial of corticosteroids
- $> 20\%$ diurnal variation on ≥ 3 days in a week for 2 weeks on PEF diary
- $FEV_1 \geq 15\%$ decrease after 6 mins of exercise

*Global Initiative for Asthma (GINA) definition accepts an increase of 12%.

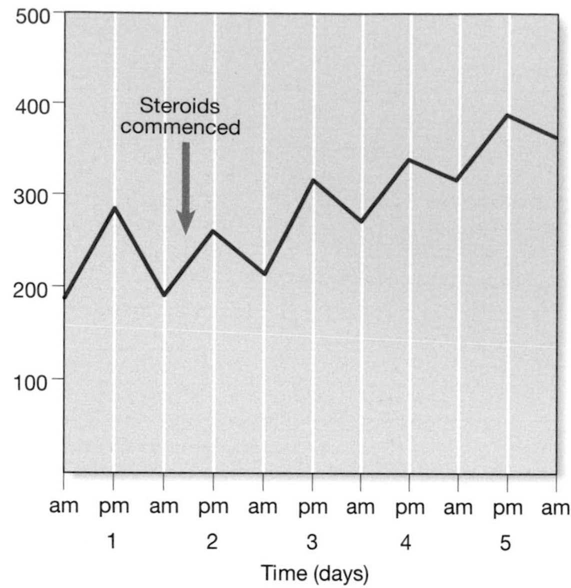

Fig. 19.20 Serial recordings of peak expiratory flow (PEF) in a patient with asthma. Note the sharp overnight fall (morning dip) and subsequent rise during the day. Following the introduction of corticosteroids, there is an improvement in PEF rate and loss of morning dipping.

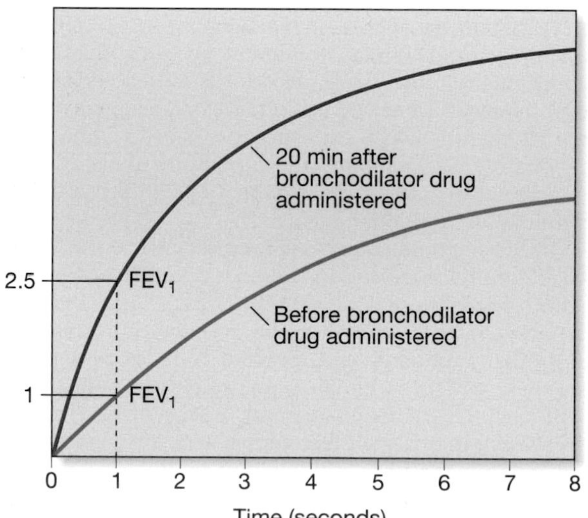

Fig. 19.19 Reversibility test. Forced expiratory manœuvres before and 20 minutes after inhalation of a β_2-adrenoceptor agonist. Note the increase in FEV_1 from 1.0 to 2.5 L.

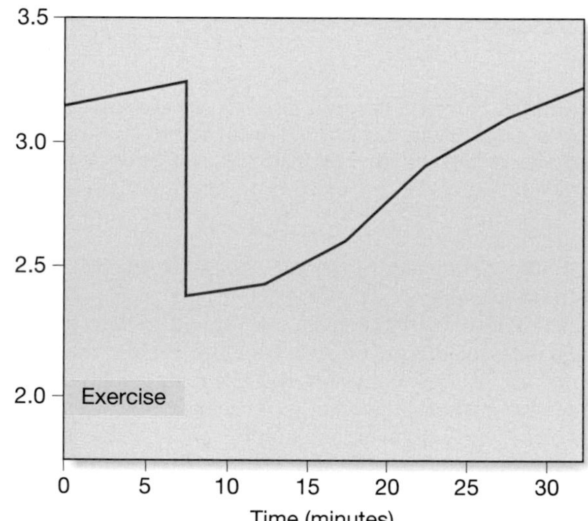

Fig. 19.21 Exercise-induced asthma. Serial recordings of FEV_1 in a patient with bronchial asthma before and after 6 minutes of strenuous exercise. Note initial rise on completion of exercise, followed by sudden fall and gradual recovery. Adequate warm-up exercise or pre-treatment with a β_2-adrenoceptor agonist, nedocromil sodium or a leukotriene antagonist can protect against exercise-induced symptoms.

Other investigations

- *Measurement of allergic status*: the presence of atopy may be demonstrated by skin prick tests. Similar information may be provided by the measurement of total and allergen-specific IgE. A full blood picture may show the peripheral blood eosinophilia.
- *Radiological examination*: chest X-ray appearances are often normal or show hyperinflation of lung fields. Lobar collapse may be seen if mucus occludes a large bronchus and, if accompanied by the presence of flitting infiltrates, may suggest that asthma has been complicated by allergic bronchopulmonary aspergillosis (p. 697). An HRCT scan may be useful to detect bronchiectasis.
- *Assessment of eosinophilic airway inflammation*: an induced sputum differential eosinophil count of greater than 2% or exhaled breath nitric oxide concentration (FE_{NO}) may support the diagnosis but is non-specific.

Management

Setting goals

Asthma is a chronic condition but may be controlled with appropriate treatment in the majority of patients. The goal of treatment should be to obtain and maintain complete control (Box 19.22), but aims may be modified according to the circumstances and the patient. Unfortunately, surveys consistently demonstrate that the majority of individuals with asthma report suboptimal control, perhaps reflecting the poor expectations of patients and their clinicians.

Whenever possible, patients should be encouraged to take responsibility for managing their own disease. A full explanation of the nature of the condition, the relationship between symptoms and inflammation, the importance of key symptoms such as nocturnal waking, the different types of medication, and, if appropriate, the use of PEF to guide management decisions, should be given. A variety of tools/questionnaires have been validated to assist in assessing asthma control. Written action plans can be helpful in developing self-management skills.

Avoidance of aggravating factors

This is particularly important in the management of occupational asthma (p. 715) but may also be relevant in atopic patients, when removing or reducing exposure to relevant antigens, such as a pet, may effect improvement. House dust mite exposure may be minimised by replacing carpets with floorboards and using mite-impermeable bedding. So far, improvements in asthma control following such measures have been difficult to demonstrate. Many patients are sensitised to several ubiquitous aeroallergens, making avoidance strategies largely impractical. Measures to reduce fungal exposure and eliminate cockroaches may be applicable in specific circumstances, and medications known to precipitate or aggravate asthma should be avoided. Smoking cessation (p. 100) is particularly important, as smoking not only encourages sensitisation, but also induces a relative corticosteroid resistance in the airway.

The stepwise approach to the management of asthma (Fig. 19.22)

Step 1: Occasional use of inhaled short-acting β_2-adrenoreceptor agonist bronchodilators

For patients with mild intermittent asthma (symptoms less than once a week for 3 months and fewer than two nocturnal episodes per month), it is usually sufficient to prescribe an inhaled short-acting β_2-agonist, such as salbutamol or terbutaline, to be used as required. However, many patients (and their physicians) underestimate the severity of asthma. A history of a severe exacerbation should lead to a step-up in treatment.

A variety of different inhaled devices are available and the choice of device should be guided by patient preference and competence in its use. The metered-dose inhaler remains the most widely prescribed (Fig. 19.23).

Step 2: Introduction of regular preventer therapy

Regular anti-inflammatory therapy (preferably inhaled corticosteroids (ICS), such as beclometasone, budesonide (BUD), fluticasone or ciclesonide) should be started in addition to inhaled β_2-agonists taken on an as-required basis for any patient who:

- has experienced an exacerbation of asthma in the last 2 years (Box 19.23)
- uses inhaled β_2-agonists three times a week or more
- reports symptoms three times a week or more
- is awakened by asthma one night per week.

For adults, a reasonable starting dose is 400 µg beclometasone dipropionate (BDP) or equivalent per day in adults, although higher doses may be required in smokers. Alternative but much less effective preventive

19.22 Levels of asthma control*

Characteristic	Controlled	Partly controlled (any present in any week)	Uncontrolled
Daytime symptoms	None (≤ twice/wk)	> twice/wk	≥ 3 features of partly controlled asthma present in any wk
Limitations of activities	None	Any	
Nocturnal symptoms/awakening	None	Any	
Need for rescue/'reliever' treatment	None (≤ twice/wk)	> twice/wk	
Lung function (PEF or FEV_1)	Normal	< 80% predicted or personal best (if known) on any day	
Exacerbation	None	≥ 1/yr	1 in any wk

*Based on GINA guidelines.

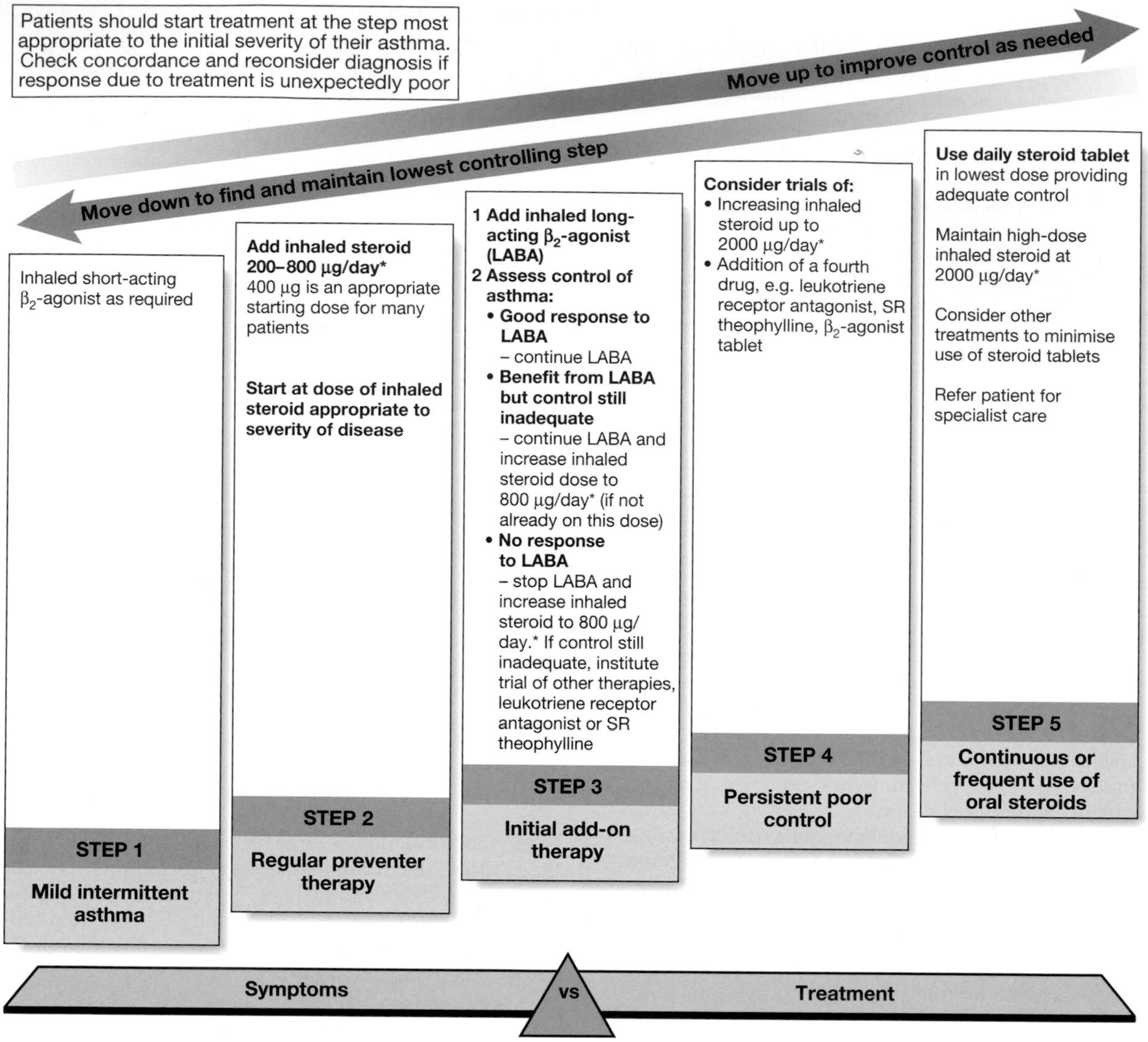

Patients should start treatment at the step most appropriate to the initial severity of their asthma. Check concordance and reconsider diagnosis if response due to treatment is unexpectedly poor

Move up to improve control as needed

Move down to find and maintain lowest controlling step

STEP 1 — Mild intermittent asthma

Inhaled short-acting β_2-agonist as required

STEP 2 — Regular preventer therapy

Add inhaled steroid 200–800 µg/day*
400 µg is an appropriate starting dose for many patients

Start at dose of inhaled steroid appropriate to severity of disease

STEP 3 — Initial add-on therapy

1 Add inhaled long-acting β_2-agonist (LABA)

2 Assess control of asthma:

- **Good response to LABA** – continue LABA
- **Benefit from LABA but control still inadequate** – continue LABA and increase inhaled steroid dose to 800 µg/day* (if not already on this dose)
- **No response to LABA** – stop LABA and increase inhaled steroid to 800 µg/day.* If control still inadequate, institute trial of other therapies, leukotriene receptor antagonist or SR theophylline

STEP 4 — Persistent poor control

Consider trials of:

- Increasing inhaled steroid up to 2000 µg/day*
- Addition of a fourth drug, e.g. leukotriene receptor antagonist, SR theophylline, β_2-agonist tablet

STEP 5 — Continuous or frequent use of oral steroids

Use daily steroid tablet in lowest dose providing adequate control

Maintain high-dose inhaled steroid at 2000 µg/day*

Consider other treatments to minimise use of steroid tablets

Refer patient for specialist care

Symptoms vs Treatment

Fig. 19.22 Management approach in adults based on asthma control. *Beclometasone dipropionate (BDP) or equivalent. From British Thoracic Society and SIGN – see p. 732.

• Remove the cap and shake the inhaler
• Breathe out gently and place the mouthpiece into the mouth
• Incline the head backwards to minimise oropharyngeal deposition
• Simultaneously, begin a slow deep inspiration, depress the canister and continue to inhale
• Hold the breath for 10 seconds

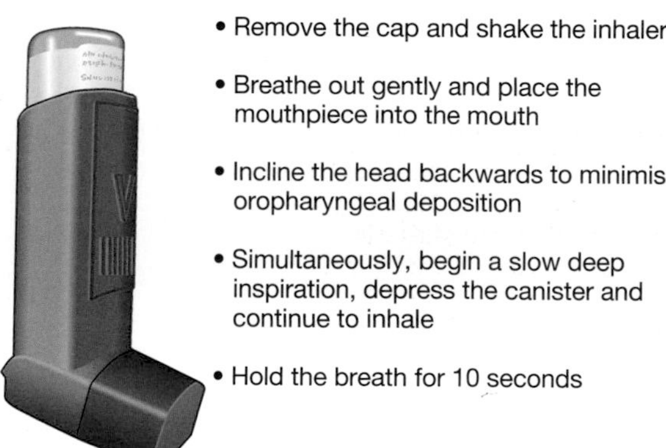

Fig. 19.23 How to use a metered-dose inhaler.

agents include chromones, leukotriene receptor antagonists, and theophyllines.

Step 3: Add-on therapy

If a patient remains poorly controlled, despite regular use of ICS, a thorough review should be undertaken of adherence, inhaler technique and ongoing exposure to modifiable aggravating factors. A further increase in the dose of ICS may benefit some patients but, in general, add-on therapy should be considered in adults taking 800 µg/day BDP (or equivalent).

Long-acting β_2-agonists (LABAs), such as salmeterol and formoterol (duration of action of at least 12 hours), represent the first choice of add-on therapy. They have consistently been demonstrated to improve asthma control and to reduce the frequency and severity of exacerbations when compared to increasing the dose of ICS alone. Fixed combination inhalers of ICS and LABAs have been developed; these are more convenient, increase compliance and prevent patients using a LABA

EBM 19.23 Inhaled corticosteroids and asthma

'Regular therapy with low-dose budesonide reduces the risk of severe exacerbations in patients with mild persistent asthma.'

- Pauwels RA, et al. Lancet 2003; 361:1066–1067.

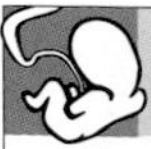

19.24 Asthma in pregnancy

- **Unpredictable clinical course**: one-third worsen, one-third remain stable and one-third improve.
- **Labour and delivery**: 90% have no symptoms.
- **Safety data**: good for β_2-agonists, inhaled steroids, theophyllines, oral prednisolone, and chromones.
- **Oral leukotriene receptor antagonists**: no evidence that these harm the fetus and they should not be stopped in women who have previously demonstrated significant improvement in asthma control prior to pregnancy.
- **Steroids**: women on maintenance prednisolone > 7.5 mg/day should receive hydrocortisone 100 mg 3–4 times daily during labour.
- **Prostaglandin F2α**: may induce bronchospasm and should be used with extreme caution.
- **Breastfeeding**: use medications as normal.
- **Uncontrolled asthma**: associated with maternal (hyperemesis, hypertension, pre-eclampsia, vaginal haemorrhage, complicated labour) and fetal (intrauterine growth restriction and low birth weight, preterm birth, increased perinatal mortality, neonatal hypoxia) complications.

as monotherapy – the latter may be accompanied by an increased risk of life-threatening attacks or asthma death. The onset of action of formoterol is similar to that of salbutamol such that, in carefully selected patients, a fixed combination of budesonide and formoterol may be used as both rescue and maintenance therapy.

Oral leukotriene receptor antagonists (e.g. montelukast 10 mg daily) are generally less effective than LABA as add-on therapy, but may facilitate a reduction in the dose of ICS and control exacerbations. Oral theophyllines may be considered in some patients but their unpredictable metabolism, propensity for drug interactions and prominent side-effects limit their widespread use.

Step 4: Poor control on moderate dose of inhaled steroid and add-on therapy: addition of a fourth drug

In adults, the dose of ICS may be increased to 2000 µg BDP/BUD (or equivalent) daily. A nasal corticosteroid preparation should be used in patients with prominent upper airway symptoms. Oral therapy with leukotriene receptor antagonists, theophyllines or a slow-release β_2-agonist may be considered. If the trial of add-on therapy is ineffective, it should be discontinued. Oral itraconazole may be contemplated in patients with allergic bronchopulmonary aspergillosis (p. 697).

Step 5: Continuous or frequent use of oral steroids

At this stage, prednisolone therapy (usually administered as a single daily dose in the morning) should be prescribed in the lowest amount necessary to control symptoms. Patients on long-term corticosteroid tablets (> 3 months) or receiving more than three or four courses per year will be at risk of systemic side-effects (p. 776). Osteoporosis can be prevented in this group by giving bisphosphonates (p. 1123). In atopic patients, omalizumab, a monoclonal antibody directed against IgE, may prove helpful in reducing symptoms and allowing a reduction in the prednisolone dose. Steroid-sparing therapies, such as methotrexate, ciclosporin or oral gold, may be considered.

Step-down therapy

Once asthma control is established, the dose of inhaled (or oral) corticosteroid should be titrated to the lowest dose at which effective control of asthma is maintained. Decreasing the dose of ICS by around 25–50% every 3 months is a reasonable strategy for most patients.

Exacerbations of asthma

The course of asthma may be punctuated by exacerbations with increased symptoms, deterioration in lung function, and an increase in airway inflammation. Exacerbations are most commonly precipitated by viral infections, but moulds (*Alternaria* and *Cladosporium*), pollens (particularly following thunderstorms) and air pollution are also implicated. Most attacks are characterised by a gradual deterioration over several hours to days but some appear to occur with little or no warning: so-called brittle asthma. An important minority of patients appear to have a blunted perception of airway narrowing and fail to appreciate the early signs of deterioration.

Management of mild to moderate exacerbations

Doubling the dose of ICS does not prevent an impending exacerbation. Short courses of 'rescue' oral corticosteroids (prednisolone 30–60 mg daily) therefore are often required to regain control. Tapering of the dose to withdraw treatment is not necessary, unless given for more than 3 weeks.

Indications for 'rescue' courses include:

- symptoms and PEF progressively worsening day by day, with a fall of PEF below 60% of the patient's personal best recording
- onset or worsening of sleep disturbance by asthma
- persistence of morning symptoms until midday
- progressively diminishing response to an inhaled bronchodilator
- symptoms sufficiently severe to require treatment with nebulised or injected bronchodilators.

Management of acute severe asthma

Box 19.25 highlights the immediate assessment requirements in acute asthma. Measurement of PEF is

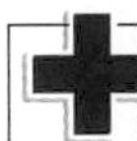

19.25 Immediate assessment of acute severe asthma

Acute severe asthma

- PEF 33–50% predicted (< 200 L/min)
- Respiratory rate ≥ 25 breaths/min
- Heart rate ≥ 110 beats/min
- Inability to complete sentences in 1 breath

Life-threatening features

- PEF < 33% predicted (< 100 L/min)
- SpO_2 < 92% or PaO_2 < 8 kPa (60 mmHg) (especially if being treated with oxygen)
- Normal or raised $PaCO_2$
- Silent chest
- Cyanosis
- Feeble respiratory effort
- Bradycardia or arrhythmias
- Hypotension
- Exhaustion
- Confusion
- Coma

Near-fatal asthma

- Raised $PaCO_2$ and/or requiring mechanical ventilation with raised inflation pressures

19

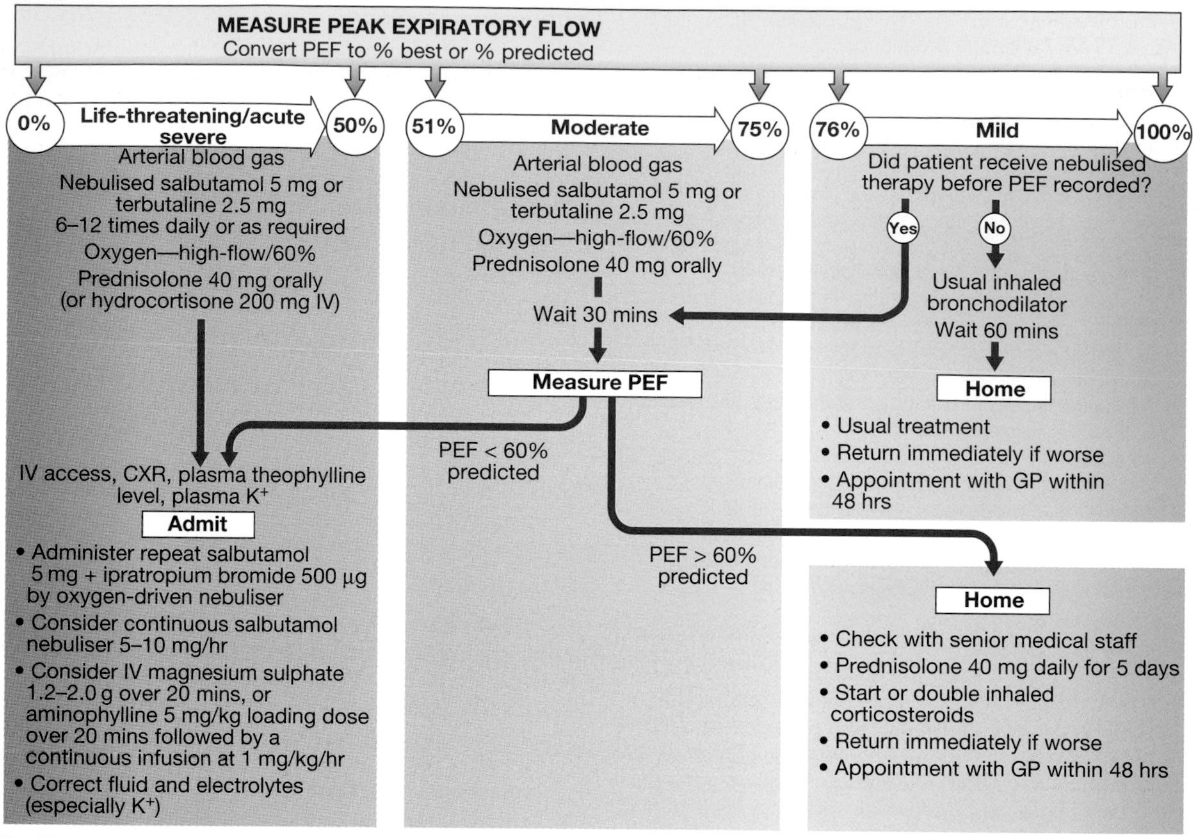

MEASURE PEAK EXPIRATORY FLOW
Convert PEF to % best or % predicted

0% — Life-threatening/acute severe — 50%

Arterial blood gas
Nebulised salbutamol 5 mg or terbutaline 2.5 mg 6–12 times daily or as required
Oxygen—high-flow/60%
Prednisolone 40 mg orally (or hydrocortisone 200 mg IV)

51% — Moderate — 75%

Arterial blood gas
Nebulised salbutamol 5 mg or terbutaline 2.5 mg
Oxygen—high-flow/60%
Prednisolone 40 mg orally

Wait 30 mins

Measure PEF

76% — Mild — 100%

Did patient receive nebulised therapy before PEF recorded?

Yes → Wait 30 mins

No → Usual inhaled bronchodilator
Wait 60 mins

Home

- Usual treatment
- Return immediately if worse
- Appointment with GP within 48 hrs

PEF < 60% predicted

IV access, CXR, plasma theophylline level, plasma K^+

Admit

- Administer repeat salbutamol 5 mg + ipratropium bromide 500 µg by oxygen-driven nebuliser
- Consider continuous salbutamol nebuliser 5–10 mg/hr
- Consider IV magnesium sulphate 1.2–2.0 g over 20 mins, or aminophylline 5 mg/kg loading dose over 20 mins followed by a continuous infusion at 1 mg/kg/hr
- Correct fluid and electrolytes (especially K^+)

PEF > 60% predicted

Home

- Check with senior medical staff
- Prednisolone 40 mg daily for 5 days
- Start or double inhaled corticosteroids
- Return immediately if worse
- Appointment with GP within 48 hrs

Fig. 19.24 Immediate treatment of patients with acute severe asthma.

mandatory, unless the patient is too ill to cooperate, and is most easily interpreted when expressed as a percentage of the predicted normal or of the previous best value obtained on optimal treatment (Fig. 19.24). Arterial blood gas analysis is essential to determine the $PaCO_2$, a normal or elevated level being particularly dangerous. A chest X-ray is not immediately necessary, unless pneumothorax is suspected.

Treatment includes the following measures:

- *Oxygen.* High concentrations (humidified if possible) should be administered to maintain the oxygen saturation above 92% in adults. The presence of a high $PaCO_2$ should not be taken as an indication to reduce oxygen concentration, but as a warning sign of a severe or life-threatening attack. Failure to achieve appropriate oxygenation is an indication for assisted ventilation.
- *High doses of inhaled bronchodilators.* Short-acting β_2-agonists are the agent of choice. In hospital, they are most conveniently given via a nebuliser driven by oxygen, but delivery of multiple doses of salbutamol via a metered-dose inhaler through a spacer device provides equivalent bronchodilatation and can be used in primary care. Ipratropium bromide provides further bronchodilator therapy and should be added to salbutamol in acute severe or life-threatening attacks.
- *Systemic corticosteroids.* These reduce the inflammatory response and hasten the resolution of an exacerbation. They should be administered to all patients with an acute severe attack. They can usually be administered orally as prednisolone, but intravenous hydrocortisone may be used in patients who are vomiting or unable to swallow.

There is no evidence base for the use of intravenous fluids but many patients are dehydrated due to high insensible water loss and will probably benefit. Potassium supplements may be necessary, as repeated doses of salbutamol can lower serum potassium.

If patients fail to improve, a number of further options may be considered. Intravenous magnesium may provide additional bronchodilatation in patients whose presenting PEF is below 30% predicted. Some patients appear to benefit from the use of intravenous aminophylline but cardiac monitoring is recommended.

PEF should be recorded every 15–30 minutes and then every 4–6 hours. Pulse oximetry should ensure that SaO_2 remains above 92%, but repeat arterial blood gases are necessary if the initial $PaCO_2$ measurements were normal or raised, the PaO_2 was below 8 kPa (60 mmHg), or the patient deteriorates. Box 19.26 lists the indications

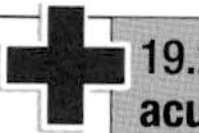

19.26 Indications for assisted ventilation in acute severe asthma

- Coma
- Respiratory arrest
- Deterioration of arterial blood gas tensions despite optimal therapy
  - PaO_2 < 8 kPa (60 mmHg) and falling
  - $PaCO_2$ > 6 kPa (45 mmHg) and rising
  - pH low and falling (H^+ high and rising)
- Exhaustion, confusion, drowsiness

for endotracheal intubation and intermittent positive pressure ventilation.

Prognosis

The outcome from acute severe asthma is generally good. Death is fortunately rare but a considerable number of deaths occur in young people and many are preventable. Failure to recognise the severity of an attack, on the part of either the assessing physician or the patient, contributes to delay in delivering appropriate therapy and to under-treatment.

Prior to discharge, patients should be stable on discharge medication (nebulised therapy should have been discontinued for at least 24 hours) and the PEF should have reached 75% of predicted or personal best. The acute attack should prompt a look for and avoidance of any trigger factors, the delivery of asthma education and the provision of a written self-management plan. The patient should be offered an appointment with a GP or asthma nurse within 2 working days of discharge, and follow-up at a specialist hospital clinic within a month.

Chronic obstructive pulmonary disease

Chronic obstructive pulmonary disease (COPD) is a preventable and treatable disease characterised by persistent airflow limitation that is usually progressive, and associated with an enhanced chronic inflammatory response in the airways and the lung to noxious particles or gases. Exacerbations and comorbidities contribute to the overall severity in individual patients. Related diagnoses include chronic bronchitis (cough and sputum on most days for at least 3 months, in each of 2 consecutive years) and emphysema (abnormal permanent enlargement of the airspaces distal to the terminal bronchioles, accompanied by destruction of their walls and without obvious fibrosis). Extra-pulmonary effects include weight loss and skeletal muscle dysfunction (Fig. 19.25). Commonly associated comorbid conditions include cardiovascular disease, cerebrovascular disease, the metabolic syndrome, osteoporosis, depression and lung cancer.

Epidemiology and aetiology

The prevalence of COPD is directly related to the prevalence of tobacco smoking and, in low- and middle-income countries, the use of biomass fuels. Current estimates suggest that 80 million people worldwide suffer from moderate to severe disease. In 2005, COPD contributed to more than 3 million deaths (5% of deaths globally), but, by 2020, it is forecast to represent the third most important cause of death worldwide. The anticipated rise in morbidity and mortality from COPD will be greatest in Asian and African countries, as a result of their increasing tobacco consumption.

Other risk factors are shown in Box 19.27. Cigarette smoking represents the most significant risk factor, and the risk of developing COPD relates to both the amount and the duration of smoking. It is unusual to develop COPD with less than 10 pack years (1 pack year = 20 cigarettes/day/year) and not all smokers develop the condition, suggesting that individual susceptibility factors are important.

Pathophysiology

COPD has both pulmonary and systemic components (see Fig. 19.25). The presence of airflow limitation,

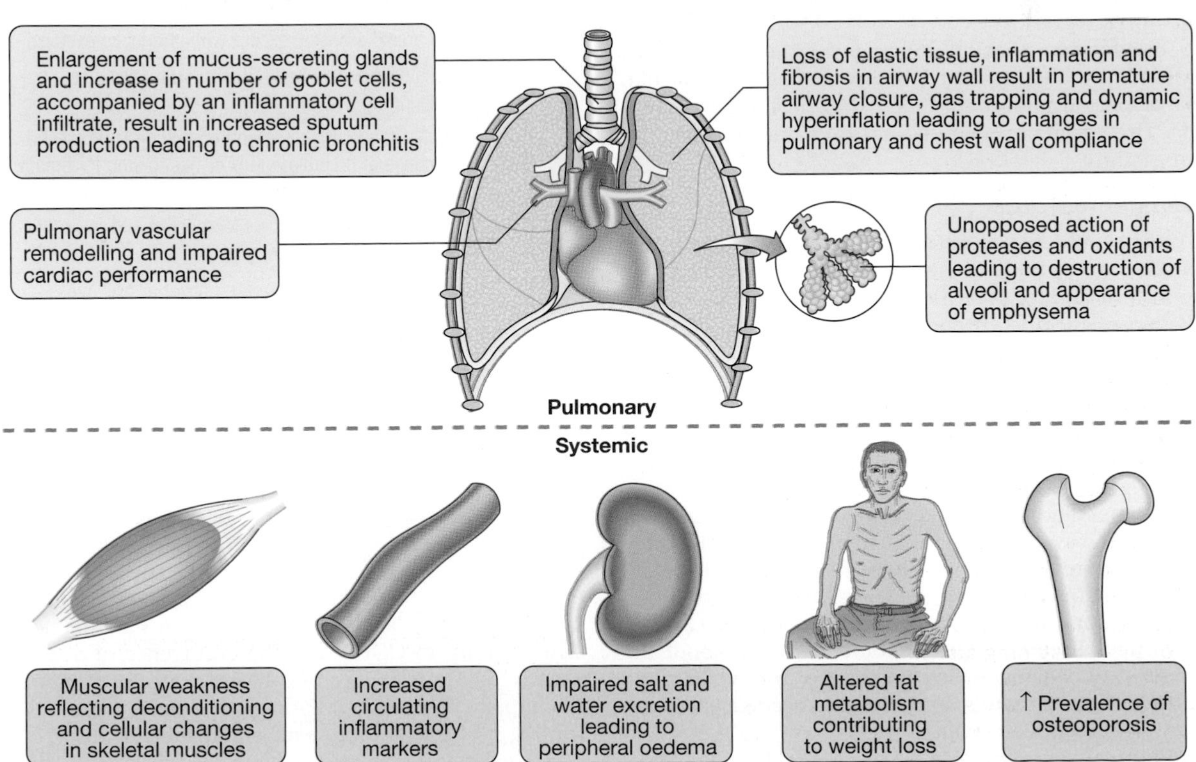

Fig. 19.25 The pulmonary and systemic features of COPD.

19.27 Risk factors for development of COPD

Environmental

- Tobacco smoke accounts for 95% of cases in UK
- Indoor air pollution; cooking with biomass fuels in confined areas in developing countries
- Occupational exposures, such as coal dust, silica and cadmium
- Low birth weight may reduce maximally attained lung function in young adult life
- Lung growth: childhood infections or maternal smoking may affect growth of lung during childhood, resulting in a lower maximally attained lung function in adult life
- Infections: recurrent infection may accelerate decline in FEV_1; persistence of adenovirus in lung tissue may alter local inflammatory response, predisposing to lung damage; HIV infection is associated with emphysema
- Low socioeconomic status
- Cannabis smoking

Host factors

- Genetic factors: α_1-antiproteinase deficiency; other COPD susceptibility genes are likely to be identified
- Airway hyper-reactivity

combined with premature airway closure, leads to gas trapping and hyperinflation, reducing pulmonary and chest wall compliance. Pulmonary hyperinflation also flattens the diaphragmatic muscles and leads to an increasingly horizontal alignment of the intercostal muscles, placing the respiratory muscles at a mechanical disadvantage. The work of breathing is therefore markedly increased, first on exercise, when the time for expiration is further shortened, but then, as the disease advances, at rest.

Emphysema (Fig. 19.26) may be classified by the pattern of the enlarged airspaces as centriacinar, panacinar or paraseptal. Bullae form in some individuals. This results in impaired gas exchange and respiratory failure.

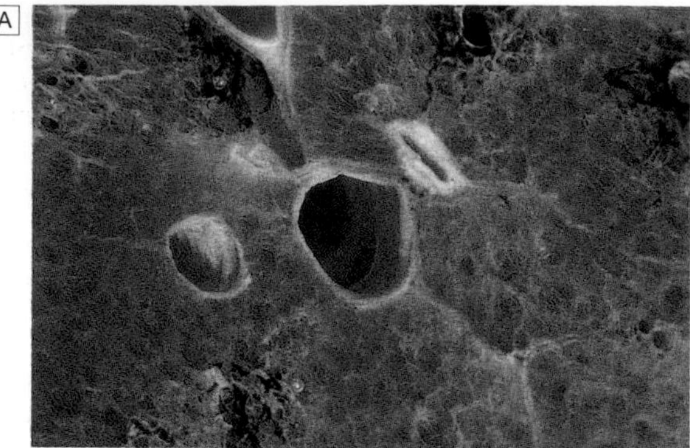

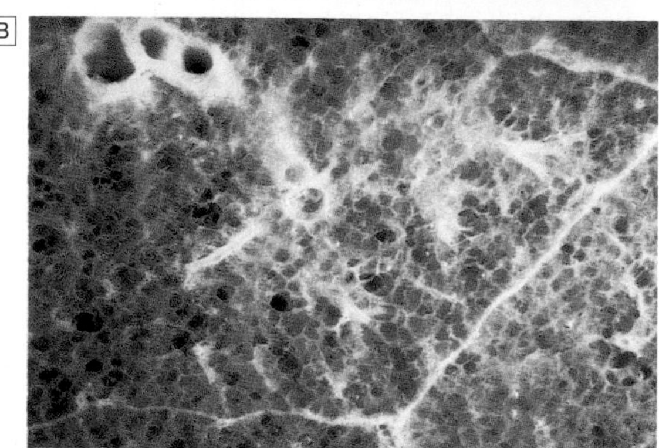

Fig. 19.26 The pathology of emphysema. **A** Normal lung. **B** Emphysematous lung showing gross loss of the normal surface area available for gas exchange.

Clinical features

COPD should be suspected in any patient over the age of 40 years who presents with symptoms of chronic bronchitis and/or breathlessness. Important differential diagnoses include chronic asthma, tuberculosis, bronchiectasis and congestive cardiac failure.

Cough and associated sputum production are usually the first symptoms, often referred to as a 'smoker's cough'. Haemoptysis may complicate exacerbations of COPD but should not be attributed to COPD without thorough investigation.

Breathlessness usually precipitates the presentation to health care. The severity should be quantified by documenting what level of exertion the patient can manage before stopping; scales such as the modified MRC dyspnoea scale may be useful (Box 19.28). In advanced disease, enquiry should be made about the presence of oedema, which may be seen for the first time during an exacerbation, and morning headaches, which may suggest hypercapnia.

Physical signs (pp. 644–645) are non-specific, correlate poorly with lung function, and are seldom obvious until the disease is advanced. Breath sounds are typically quiet. Crackles may accompany infection but, if persistent, raise the possibility of bronchiectasis. Finger clubbing is not a feature of COPD and should trigger further investigation for lung cancer or fibrosis. Pitting oedema should be sought but the frequently used term 'cor pulmonale' is actually a misnomer, as the right heart seldom 'fails' in COPD and the occurrence of oedema usually relates to failure of salt and water excretion by the hypoxic hypercapnic kidney. The body mass index (BMI – p. 114) is of prognostic significance.

Two classical phenotypes have been described: 'pink puffers' and 'blue bloaters'. The former are typically thin

19.28 Modified MRC dyspnoea scale

Grade	Degree of breathlessness related to activities
0	No breathlessness, except with strenuous exercise
1	Breathlessness when hurrying on the level or walking up a slight hill
2	Walks slower than contemporaries on level ground because of breathlessness or has to stop for breath when walking at own pace
3	Stops for breath after walking about 100 m or after a few minutes on level ground
4	Too breathless to leave the house, or breathless when dressing or undressing

(MRC = Medical Research Council)

and breathless, and maintain a normal $PaCO_2$ until the late stage of disease. The latter develop (or tolerate) hypercapnia earlier and may develop oedema and secondary polycythaemia. In practice, these phenotypes often overlap.

Investigations

Although there are no reliable radiographic signs that correlate with the severity of airflow limitation, a chest X-ray is essential to identify alternative diagnoses, such as cardiac failure, other complications of smoking such as lung cancer, and the presence of bullae. A blood count is useful to exclude anaemia or polycythaemia, and in younger patients with predominantly basal emphysema, α_1-antiproteinase should be assayed.

The diagnosis requires objective demonstration of airflow obstruction by spirometry and is established when the post-bronchodilator FEV_1/FVC is less than 70%. The severity of COPD may be defined in relation to the post-bronchodilator FEV_1 (Box 19.29). A low peak flow is consistent with COPD but is non-specific, does not discriminate between obstructive and restrictive disorders, and may underestimate the severity of airflow limitation.

Measurement of lung volumes provides an assessment of hyperinflation. This is generally performed by using the helium dilution technique (p. 653); in patients with severe COPD, and with large bullae in particular, body plethysmography is preferred because the use of helium may underestimate lung volumes. Emphysema is suggested by a low gas transfer value (p. 653). Exercise tests provide an objective assessment of exercise tolerance and a baseline for judging response to bronchodilator therapy or rehabilitation programmes; they may also be valuable when assessing prognosis. Pulse oximetry of less than 93% may indicate the need for referral for a domiciliary oxygen assessment.

The assessment of health status provides valuable clinical information. The St George's Respiratory Questionnaire (SGRQ) is a commonly used research tool but is too cumbersome for routine clinical practice. The COPD Assessment Test (CAT) employs only eight questions and the scores correlate closely with the SGRQ.

HRCT is likely to play an increasing role in the assessment of COPD, as it allows the detection, characterisation and quantification of emphysema (Fig. 19.27) and is more sensitive than a chest X-ray for detecting bullae.

19.29 Spirometric classification of COPD severity based on post-bronchodilator FEV_1

Stage	Severity	FEV_1
I	Mild*	$FEV_1/FVC < 0.70$ $FEV_1 \geq 80\%$ predicted
II	Moderate	$FEV_1/FVC < 0.70$ FEV_1 50–79% predicted
III	Severe	$FEV_1/FVC < 0.70$ FEV_1 30–49% predicted
IV	Very severe	$FEV_1/FVC < 0.70$ $FEV_1 < 30\%$ predicted or $FEV_1 < 50\%$ predicted if respiratory failure present

*Mild COPD should not be diagnosed on lung function alone if the patient is asymptomatic. Based on NICE guidelines 2010.

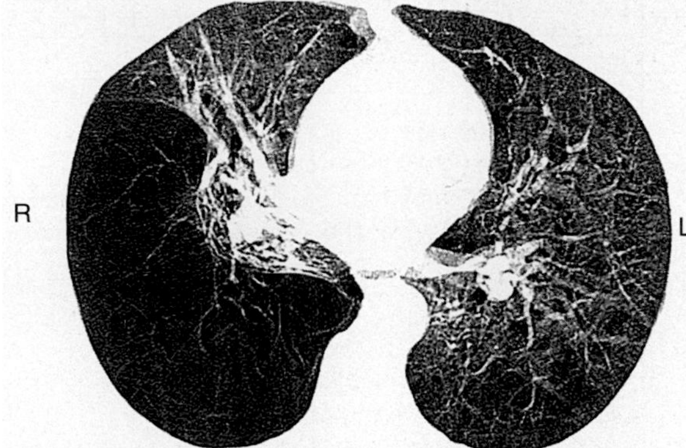

Fig. 19.27 Gross emphysema. HRCT showing emphysema, most evident in the right lower lobe.

Management

The management of COPD (Fig. 19.28) has been the subject of unjustified pessimism. It is usually possible to help breathlessness, reduce the frequency and severity of exacerbations, enhance the health status, and improve the prognosis.

Reducing exposure to noxious particles and gases

Every attempt should be made to highlight to the patient the role of smoking in the development and progression of COPD, with advice and assistance to help them stop (p. 100). Reducing the number of cigarettes smoked each day has little impact on the course and prognosis of COPD, but complete cessation is accompanied by an improvement in lung function and deceleration in the rate of FEV_1 decline (Fig. 19.29 and Box 19.30). In regions where the indoor burning of biomass fuels is important, the introduction of non-smoking cooking devices or use of alternative fuels should be encouraged.

Bronchodilators

Bronchodilator therapy is central to the management of breathlessness. The inhaled route is preferred and a number of different agents, delivered by a variety of devices, are available. Choice should be informed by patient preference and inhaler assessment. Short-acting bronchodilators, such as the β_2-agonists salbutamol and terbutaline, or the anticholinergic ipratropium bromide, may be used for patients with mild disease, but longer-acting bronchodilators, such as the β_2-agonists salmeterol, formoterol and indacaterol, or the anticholinergic tiotropium bromide, are more appropriate for patients with moderate to severe disease. Significant improvements in breathlessness may be reported, despite minimal changes in FEV_1, probably reflecting improvements in lung emptying that reduce dynamic hyperinflation and ease the work of breathing.

EBM 19.30 Smoking cessation and COPD

'Sustained smoking cessation in mild to moderate COPD is accompanied by a reduced decline in FEV_1 compared to persistent smokers.'

- Anthonisen NR, et al. Am J Respir Crit Care Med 2002; 166:675–679.

I : Mild	II : Moderate	III : Severe	IV : Very severe
• $FEV_1/FVC < 0.70$ • $FEV_1 \geq 80\%$ predicted	• $FEV_1/FVC < 0.70$ • $50\% \leq FEV_1 < 80\%$ predicted	• $FEV_1/FVC < 0.70$ • $30\% \leq FEV_1 < 50\%$ predicted	• $FEV_1/FVC < 0.70$ • $FEV_1 < 30\%$ predicted *or* $FEV_1 < 50\%$ predicted *plus* chronic respiratory failure
Active reduction of risk factor(s); influenza vaccination →	→	→	→
Add short-acting bronchodilator (when needed) →	→	→	→
	Add regular treatment with one or more long-acting bronchodilators (when needed) **Add** rehabilitation		
		Add inhaled glucocorticosteroids if repeated exacerbations	
			Add long-term oxygen if chronic respiratory failure **Consider** surgical treatments

Fig. 19.28 Global Initiative for Chronic Obstructive Lung Disease (GOLD) guidelines for treatment of COPD. Post-bronchodilator FEV_1 is recommended for the diagnosis and assessment of severity of COPD. From www.goldcopd.com – see p. 732.

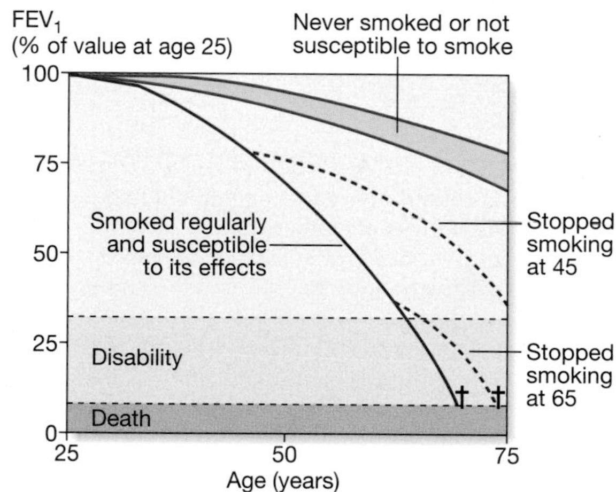

Fig. 19.29 Model of annual decline in FEV_1 with accelerated decline in susceptible smokers. When smoking is stopped, subsequent loss is similar to that in healthy non-smokers.

Oral bronchodilator therapy may be used in patients who cannot use inhaled devices efficiently. Theophylline preparations improve breathlessness and quality of life, but their use is limited by side-effects, unpredictable metabolism and drug interactions. Bambuterol, a pro-drug of terbutaline, is used on occasion. Orally active, highly selective phosphodiesterase inhibitors are currently under appraisal.

Corticosteroids

Inhaled corticosteroids (ICS) reduce the frequency and severity of exacerbations, and are currently recommended in patients with severe disease (FEV_1 < 50%) who report two or more exacerbations requiring antibiotics or oral steroids per year. Regular use is associated with a small improvement in FEV_1, but ICS do not alter the natural history of the FEV_1 decline. It is more usual to prescribe a fixed combination of an ICS and a LABA.

Oral corticosteroids are useful during exacerbations but maintenance therapy contributes to osteoporosis and impaired skeletal muscle function and should be avoided. Oral corticosteroid trials assist in the diagnosis of asthma but do not predict response to inhaled steroids in COPD.

Pulmonary rehabilitation

Exercise should be encouraged at all stages and patients reassured that breathlessness, whilst distressing, is not dangerous. Multidisciplinary programmes that incorporate physical training, disease education and nutritional counselling reduce symptoms, improve health status and enhance confidence. Most programmes include 2–3 sessions per week for 6 and 12 weeks, and are accompanied by demonstrable and sustained improvements in exercise tolerance and health status.

Oxygen therapy

Long-term domiciliary oxygen therapy (LTOT) has been shown to be of significant benefit in selected patients (Boxes 19.31 and 19.32). It is most conveniently provided

EBM 19.31 Long-term domiciliary oxygen therapy

'Long-term home oxygen therapy improves survival in selected patients with COPD complicated by severe hypoxaemia (arterial PaO_2 less than 8.0 kPa (55 mmHg)).'

- Cranston JM, et al. Domiciliary oxygen for chronic obstructive pulmonary disease. Cochrane Database of Systematic Reviews, 2005, issue 4. Art no. CD001744.

For further information: 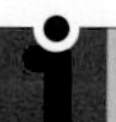 www.brit-thoracic.org.uk

19.32 Prescription of long-term oxygen therapy in COPD

Arterial blood gases measured in clinically stable patients on optimal medical therapy on at least two occasions 3 weeks apart:

- PaO_2 < 7.3 kPa (55 mmHg) irrespective of $PaCO_2$ and FEV_1 < 1.5 L
- PaO_2 7.3–8 kPa (55–60 mmHg) plus pulmonary hypertension, peripheral oedema or nocturnal hypoxaemia
- the patient has stopped smoking.

Use at least 15 hrs/day at 2–4 L/min to achieve a PaO_2 > 8 kPa (60 mmHg) without unacceptable rise in $PaCO_2$.

by an oxygen concentrator and patients should be instructed to use oxygen for a minimum of 15 hours per day; greater benefits are seen in patients who receive more than 20 hours per day. The aim of therapy is to increase the PaO_2 to at least 8 kPa (60 mmHg) or SaO_2 to at least 90%. Ambulatory oxygen therapy should be considered in patients who desaturate on exercise and show objective improvement in exercise capacity and/or dyspnoea with oxygen. Oxygen flow rates should be adjusted to maintain SaO_2 above 90%.

Surgical intervention

Patients in whom large bullae compress surrounding normal lung tissue, who otherwise have minimal airflow limitation and a lack of generalised emphysema, may be considered for bullectomy. Patients with predominantly upper lobe emphysema, with preserved gas transfer and no evidence of pulmonary hypertension, may benefit from lung volume reduction surgery (LVRS), in which peripheral emphysematous lung tissue is resected with the aim of reducing hyperinflation and decreasing the work of breathing. Both bullectomy and LVRS can be performed thoracoscopically, minimising morbidity. Lung transplantation may benefit carefully selected patients with advanced disease (p. 665).

Other measures

Patients with COPD should be offered an annual influenza vaccination and, as appropriate, pneumococcal vaccination. Obesity, poor nutrition, depression and social isolation should be addressed as far as possible. Mucolytic therapy or antioxidant agents are occasionally used but with limited evidence.

Addressing end-of-life needs is an important yet often ignored aspect of care in advanced disease. Morphine may be used for palliation of breathlessness in advanced disease and benzodiazepines in low dose may reduce anxiety. Decisions regarding resuscitation should be discussed with the patient in advance of critical illness.

Prognosis

COPD has a variable natural history but is usually progressive. The prognosis is inversely related to age and directly related to the post-bronchodilator FEV_1. Other poor prognostic indicators include weight loss and pulmonary hypertension. A composite score comprising the body mass index (B), the degree of airflow obstruction (O), a measurement of dyspnoea (D) and exercise capacity (E) may assist in predicting death from respiratory and other causes (Box 19.33). Respiratory failure, cardiac disease and lung cancer represent common modes of death.

19.33 Calculation of the BODE index

	Points on BODE index			
Variable	**0**	**1**	**2**	**3**
FEV_1	≥ 65	50–64	36–49	≤ 35
Distance walked in 6 mins (m)	≥ 350	250–349	150–249	≤ 149
MRC dyspnoea scale*	0–1	2	3	4
Body mass index	> 21	≤ 21		

A patient with a BODE score of 0–2 has a mortality rate of around 10% at 52 mths, whereas a patient with a BODE score of 7–10 has a mortality rate of around 80% at 52 mths.

*See Box 19.28.

Acute exacerbations of COPD

Acute exacerbations of COPD are characterised by an increase in symptoms and deterioration in lung function and health status. They become more frequent as the disease progresses and are usually triggered by bacteria, viruses or a change in air quality. They may be accompanied by the development of respiratory failure and/or fluid retention and are an important cause of death.

Many patients can be managed at home with the use of increased bronchodilator therapy, a short course of oral corticosteroids and, if appropriate, antibiotics. The presence of cyanosis, peripheral oedema or an alteration in consciousness indicates the need for referral to hospital. In other patients, consideration of comorbidity and social circumstances may influence decisions regarding hospital admission.

Management

In patients with an exacerbation of severe COPD, high concentrations of oxygen may cause respiratory depression and worsening acidosis (p. 665). Controlled oxygen at 24% or 28% should be used with the aim of maintaining a PaO_2 above 8 kPa (60 mmHg) (or an SaO_2 between 88% and 92%) without worsening acidosis.

Nebulised short-acting β_2-agonists, combined with an anticholinergic agent (e.g. salbutamol and ipratropium), should be administered. With careful supervision, it is usually safe to drive nebulisers with oxygen, but if

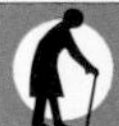

19.34 Obstructive pulmonary disease in old age

- **Asthma**: may appear de novo in old age, so airflow obstruction should not always be assumed to be due to COPD.
- **PEF recordings**: older people with poor vision have difficulty reading PEF meters.
- **Perception of bronchoconstriction**: impaired by age, so an older patient's description of symptoms may not be a reliable indicator of severity.
- **Stopping smoking**: the benefits on the rate of loss of lung function decline with age but remain valuable up to the age of 80.
- **Metered-dose inhalers**: many older people cannot use these because of difficulty coordinating and triggering the device. Even mild cognitive impairment virtually precludes their use. Frequent demonstration and re-instruction in the use of all devices are required.
- **Mortality rates for acute asthma**: higher in old age, partly because patients underestimate the severity of bronchoconstriction and also develop a lower degree of tachycardia and pulsus paradoxus for the same degree of bronchoconstriction.
- **Treatment decisions**: advanced age in itself is not a barrier to intensive care or mechanical ventilation in an acute episode of asthma or COPD, but this decision may be difficult and should be shared with the patient (if possible), the relatives and the GP.

concern exists regarding oxygen sensitivity, they may be driven by compressed air and supplemental oxygen delivered by nasal cannula.

Oral prednisolone reduces symptoms and improves lung function. Currently, doses of 30 mg for 10 days are recommended but shorter courses may be acceptable. Prophylaxis against osteoporosis should be considered in patients who receive repeated courses of steroids (p. 776).

The role of bacteria in exacerbations remains controversial and there is little evidence for the routine administration of antibiotics. They are currently recommended, however, for patients reporting an increase in sputum purulence, sputum volume or breathlessness. In most cases, simple regimens are advised, such as an aminopenicillin or a macrolide. Co-amoxiclav is only required in regions where β-lactamase-producing organisms are known to be common.

If, despite the above measures, the patient remains tachypnoeic, hypercapnic and acidotic ($PaCO_2$ > 6 kPa, $H^+ \geq 45$ (pH < 7.35)), then NIV should be commenced (p. 193). Its use is associated with reduced requirements for mechanical ventilation and reduced mortality (Box 19.35). It is not useful in patients who cannot protect their airway. Mechanical ventilation may be considered in those with a reversible cause for deterioration (e.g. pneumonia), or if there is no prior history of respiratory failure.

Exacerbations may be accompanied by the development of peripheral oedema that usually responds to diuretics. There has been a vogue for using intravenous infusions of aminophylline, but evidence for benefit is limited and there is an associated risk of inducing arrhythmias and drug interactions. The use of the respiratory stimulant doxapram has been largely superseded by the development of NIV, but it may be useful for a limited period in selected patients with a low respiratory rate.

Discharge from hospital may be planned once patients are clinically stable on their usual maintenance medication. The provision of a nurse-led 'hospital at home' team providing short-term nebuliser loan improves discharge rates and additional support for the patient.

EBM 19.35 Non-invasive ventilation in COPD exacerbations

'Non-invasive ventilation is safe and effective in patients with an acute exacerbation of COPD complicated by mild to moderate respiratory acidosis, and should be considered early in the course of respiratory failure to reduce the need for endotracheal intubation, treatment failure and mortality.'

- Lim WJ, et al. Non-invasive positive pressure ventilation for treatment of respiratory failure due to exacerbations of chronic obstructive pulmonary disease. Cochrane Database of Systematic Reviews, 2004, issue 3. Art. no. CD004104.

Bronchiectasis

Bronchiectasis means abnormal dilatation of the bronchi. Chronic suppurative airway infection with sputum production, progressive scarring and lung damage occur, whatever the cause.

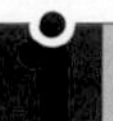

19.36 Causes of bronchiectasis

Congenital

- Cystic fibrosis
- Ciliary dysfunction syndromes
  - Primary ciliary dyskinesia (immotile cilia syndrome)
  - Kartagener's syndrome (sinusitis and transposition of the viscera)
- Primary hypogammaglobulinaemia (p. 881)

Acquired: children

- Pneumonia (complicating whooping cough or measles)
- Primary TB
- Inhaled foreign body

Acquired: adults

- Suppurative pneumonia
- Pulmonary TB
- Allergic bronchopulmonary aspergillosis complicating asthma (p. 697)
- Bronchial tumours

Aetiology and pathology

Bronchiectasis may result from a congenital defect affecting airway ion transport or ciliary function, such as cystic fibrosis (see below), or may be acquired secondary to damage to the airways by a destructive infection, inhaled toxin or foreign body. The result is chronic inflammation and infection in airways. Box 19.36 shows the common causes, of which tuberculosis is the most common worldwide.

Localised bronchiectasis may occur due to the accumulation of pus beyond an obstructing bronchial lesion, such as enlarged tuberculous hilar lymph nodes, a bronchial tumour or an inhaled foreign body (e.g. an aspirated peanut).

The bronchiectatic cavities may be lined by granulation tissue, squamous epithelium or normal ciliated epithelium. There may also be inflammatory changes in the deeper layers of the bronchial wall and hypertrophy of the bronchial arteries. Chronic inflammatory and fibrotic changes are usually found in the surrounding lung tissue, resulting in progressive destruction of the normal lung architecture in advanced cases.

Clinical features

The symptoms are shown in Box 19.37.

Physical signs in the chest may be unilateral or bilateral. If the bronchiectatic airways do not contain secretions and there is no associated lobar collapse, there are no abnormal physical signs. When there are large amounts of sputum in the bronchiectatic spaces, numerous coarse crackles may be heard over the affected areas. Collapse with retained secretions blocking a proximal bronchus may lead to locally diminished breath sounds, while advanced disease may cause scarring and overlying bronchial breathing. Acute haemoptysis is an important complication of bronchiectasis; management is described on page 659.

Investigations

In addition to common respiratory pathogens, sputum culture may reveal *Pseudomonas aeruginosa*, fungi such as *Aspergillus* and various mycobacteria. Frequent cultures

19.37 Symptoms of bronchiectasis

- **Cough**: chronic, daily, persistent
- **Sputum**: copious, continuously purulent
- **Pleuritic pain**: when infection spreads to involve pleura, or with segmental collapse due to retained secretions
- **Haemoptysis**:
  Streaks of blood common, larger volumes with exacerbations of infection
  Massive haemoptysis requiring bronchial artery embolisation sometimes occurs
- **Infective exacerbation**: increased sputum volume with fever, malaise, anorexia
- **Halitosis**: frequently accompanies purulent sputum
- **General debility**: difficulty maintaining weight, anorexia, exertional breathlessness

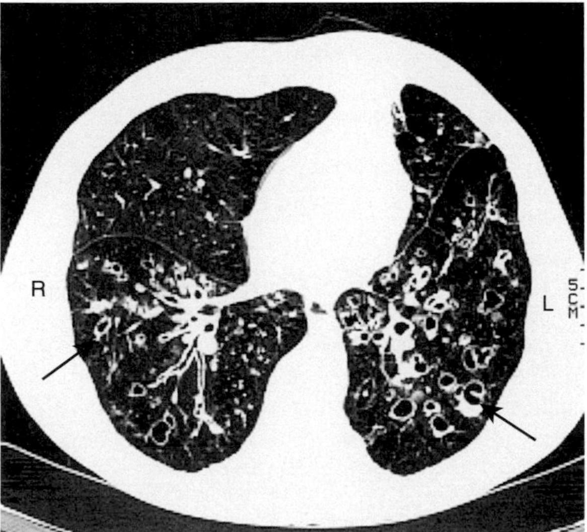

Fig. 19.30 CT of bronchiectasis. Extensive dilatation of the bronchi, with thickened walls (arrows) in both lower lobes.

are necessary to ensure appropriate treatment of resistant organisms.

Bronchiectasis, unless very gross, is not usually apparent on a chest X-ray. In advanced disease, thickened airway walls, cystic bronchiectatic spaces, and associated areas of pneumonic consolidation or collapse may be visible. CT is much more sensitive, and shows thickened, dilated airways (Fig. 19.30).

A screening test can be performed in patients suspected of having a ciliary dysfunction syndrome by measuring the time taken for a small pellet of saccharin placed in the anterior chamber of the nose to reach the pharynx, at which point the patient can taste it. This time should not exceed 20 minutes but is greatly prolonged in patients with ciliary dysfunction. Ciliary beat frequency may also be assessed from biopsies taken from the nose. Structural abnormalities of cilia can be detected by electron microscopy.

Management

In patients with airflow obstruction, inhaled bronchodilators and corticosteroids should be used to enhance airway patency.

Physiotherapy

Patients should be shown how to perform regular daily physiotherapy to assist the drainage of excess bronchial secretions. Efficiently executed, this is of great value both in reducing the amount of cough and sputum, and in preventing recurrent episodes of bronchopulmonary infection. Patients should lie in a position in which the lobe to be drained is uppermost. Deep breathing followed by forced expiratory manœuvres (the 'active cycle of breathing' technique) helps to move secretions in the dilated bronchi towards the trachea, from which they can be cleared by vigorous coughing. Devices that increase airway pressure either by a constant amount (positive expiratory pressure mask) or in an oscillatory manner (flutter valve), aid sputum clearance in some patients, and a variety of techniques should be tried to find the one that suits the individual. The optimum duration and frequency of physiotherapy depend on the amount of sputum, but 5–10 minutes twice daily is a minimum for most patients.

Antibiotic therapy

For most patients with bronchiectasis, the appropriate antibiotics are the same as those used in COPD (p. 678) but larger doses and longer courses are required, and resolution of symptoms is often incomplete. When secondary infection occurs with staphylococci and Gram-negative bacilli, in particular *Pseudomonas* species, antibiotic therapy becomes more challenging and should be guided by the microbiological sensitivities. For *Pseudomonas*, oral ciprofloxacin (500–750 mg twice daily) or ceftazidime by intravenous injection or infusion (1–2 g 3 times daily) may be required. Haemoptysis in bronchiectasis often responds to treatment of the underlying infection, although, in severe cases, percutaneous embolisation of the bronchial circulation by an interventional radiologist may be necessary.

Surgical treatment

Excision of bronchiectatic areas is only indicated in a small proportion of cases. These are usually patients in whom the bronchiectasis is confined to a single lobe or segment on CT. Unfortunately, many of the patients in whom medical treatment proves unsuccessful are also unsuitable for surgery because of either extensive bilateral bronchiectasis or coexisting severe airflow obstruction. In progressive forms of bronchiectasis, resection of destroyed areas of lung that are acting as a reservoir of infection should only be considered as a last resort.

Prognosis

The disease is progressive when associated with ciliary dysfunction and cystic fibrosis, and eventually causes respiratory failure. In other patients, the prognosis can be relatively good if physiotherapy is performed regularly and antibiotics are used aggressively.

Prevention

As bronchiectasis commonly starts in childhood following measles, whooping cough or a primary tuberculous infection, adequate prophylaxis for and treatment of these conditions are essential. The early recognition and treatment of bronchial obstruction are also important.

Cystic fibrosis

Genetics, pathogenesis and epidemiology

Cystic fibrosis (CF) is the most common fatal genetic disease in Caucasians, with autosomal recessive inheritance, a carrier rate of 1 in 25, and an incidence of about 1 in 2500 live births (pp. 48 and 53). CF is the result of mutations affecting a gene on the long arm of chromosome 7, which codes for a chloride channel known as cystic fibrosis transmembrane conductance regulator (*CFTR*); this influences salt and water movement across epithelial cell membranes. The most common *CFTR* mutation in northern European and American populations is *ΔF508*, but over a thousand mutations of this gene have now been identified. The genetic defect causes increased sodium and chloride content in sweat and increased resorption of sodium and water from respiratory epithelium (Fig. 19.31). Relative dehydration of the airway epithelium is thought to predispose to chronic bacterial infection and ciliary dysfunction, leading to bronchiectasis. The gene defect also causes disorders in the gut epithelium, pancreas, liver and reproductive tract (see below).

In the 1960s, few patients with CF survived childhood, yet with aggressive treatment of airway infection and nutritional support, life expectancy has improved dramatically, so that there are now more adults than children with CF in many developed countries. Until recently, the diagnosis was most commonly made from the clinical picture (bowel obstruction, failure to thrive, steatorrhoea and/or chest symptoms in a young child), supported by sweat electrolyte testing and genotyping. Patients with unusual phenotypes were commonly missed, however, and late diagnosis led to poorer outcomes. Neonatal screening for CF using immunoreactive trypsin and genetic testing of newborn blood samples is now routine in the UK, and should reduce delayed diagnosis and improve outcomes. Prenatal screening by amniocentesis may be offered to those known to be at high risk.

Clinical features

The lungs are macroscopically normal at birth, but bronchiolar inflammation and infections usually lead to bronchiectasis in childhood. At this stage, the lungs are most commonly infected with *Staphylococcus aureus*; however, in adulthood, many patients become colonised with *Pseudomonas aeruginosa*. Recurrent exacerbations of bronchiectasis, initially in the upper lobes but subsequently throughout both lungs, cause progressive lung damage, resulting ultimately in death from respiratory failure. Other clinical manifestations are shown in Box 19.38. Most men with CF are infertile due to failure of development of the vas deferens, but microsurgical sperm

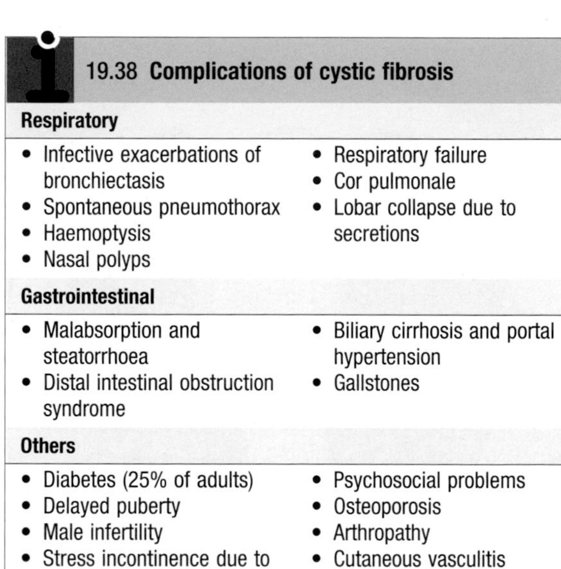

19.38 Complications of cystic fibrosis

Respiratory	
• Infective exacerbations of bronchiectasis • Spontaneous pneumothorax • Haemoptysis • Nasal polyps	• Respiratory failure • Cor pulmonale • Lobar collapse due to secretions
Gastrointestinal	
• Malabsorption and steatorrhoea • Distal intestinal obstruction syndrome	• Biliary cirrhosis and portal hypertension • Gallstones
Others	
• Diabetes (25% of adults) • Delayed puberty • Male infertility • Stress incontinence due to repeated forced cough	• Psychosocial problems • Osteoporosis • Arthropathy • Cutaneous vasculitis

A Normal

Airway lumen

Apical surface

EPITHELIAL CELL

Basal surface

① Chloride ion

② Sodium ion

cAMP

Chloride ion

Sodium ion

Water

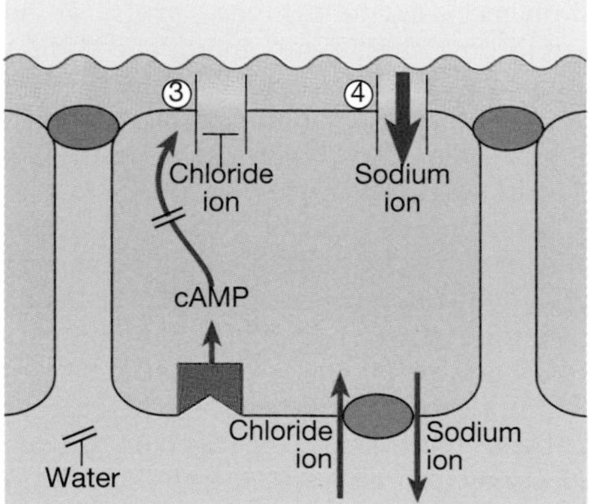

β2-adrenoceptor

Fig. 19.31 Cystic fibrosis: basic defect in the pulmonary epithelium. **A** The CF gene codes for a chloride channel (1) in the apical (luminal) membrane of epithelial cells in the conducting airways. This is normally controlled by cyclic adenosine monophosphate (cAMP) and indirectly by β-adrenoceptor stimulation, and is one of several apical ion channels which control the quantity and solute content of airway-lining fluid. Normal channels appear to inhibit the adjacent epithelial sodium channels (2). **B** In cystic fibrosis, one of many CF gene defects causes absence or defective function of this chloride channel (3). This leads to reduced chloride secretion and loss of inhibition of sodium channels, with excessive sodium resorption (4) and dehydration of the airway lining. The resulting abnormal airway-lining fluid predisposes to infection by mechanisms still to be fully explained.

aspiration and in vitro fertilisation are possible. Genotype is a poor predictor of disease severity in individuals; even siblings with matching genotypes may have different phenotypes. This suggests that other 'modifier genes', as yet unidentified, influence clinical outcome.

Management

Treatment of CF lung disease

The management of CF lung disease is that of severe bronchiectasis. All patients with CF who produce sputum should perform chest physiotherapy regularly, and more frequently during exacerbations. While infections with *Staph. aureus* can often be managed with oral antibiotics, intravenous treatment (frequently self-administered at home through an implanted subcutaneous vascular port) is usually needed for *Pseudomonas* infections. Regular nebulised antibiotic therapy (colistin or tobramycin) is used between exacerbations in an attempt to suppress chronic *Pseudomonas* infection.

Unfortunately, the bronchi of many CF patients eventually become colonised with pathogens that are resistant to most antibiotics. Resistant strains of *P. aeruginosa*, *Stenotrophomonas maltophilia* and *Burkholderia cepacia* are the main culprits, and may require prolonged treatment with unusual combinations of antibiotics. *Aspergillus* and non-tuberculous mycobacteria are also frequently found in the sputum of CF patients but, in most cases, these behave as benign 'colonisers' of the bronchiectatic airways and do not require specific therapy. Some patients have coexistent asthma, which is treated with inhaled bronchodilators and corticosteroids; allergic bronchopulmonary aspergillosis (p. 697) also occurs occasionally in CF.

Four maintenance treatments have been shown to cause modest rises in lung function and/or to reduce the frequency of chest exacerbations in CF patients (Box 19.39). Individual responses are variable and should be carefully monitored to avoid burdening patients with treatments that prove ineffective.

For advanced CF lung disease, home oxygen and NIV may be necessary to treat respiratory failure. Ultimately, lung transplantation can produce dramatic improvements but is limited by donor organ availability.

Treatment of non-respiratory manifestations of CF

There is a clear link between good nutrition and prognosis in CF. Malabsorption due to exocrine pancreatic failure is treated with oral pancreatic enzymes and vitamin supplements. The increased caloric requirements of CF patients are met by supplemental feeding, including nasogastric or gastrostomy tube feeding if required. Diabetes eventually develops in over 25% of patients and often requires insulin therapy. Osteoporosis secondary to malabsorption and chronic ill health should be sought and treated.

Novel therapies for cystic fibrosis

Small molecules designed to correct the function of particular CFTR defects are being developed, and one (ivacaftor) gives significant clinical benefits in patients with the G551D mutation. Somatic gene therapy for CF is also under development. Manufactured normal copies of the CF gene are 'packaged' in liposomes or virus vectors and administered to the airways by aerosol inhalation. Trials are under way but more efficient gene delivery methods are needed to make this practical.

19.39 Treatments that reduce chest exacerbations and/or improve lung function in cystic fibrosis

Therapy	Patients treated
Nebulised recombinant human DNase 2.5 mg daily	Age ≥ 5, FVC > 40% predicted
Nebulised tobramycin 300 mg twice daily, given in alternate mths	Patients colonised with *Pseudomonas aeruginosa*
Regular oral azithromycin 500 mg three times/wk	Patients colonised with *Pseudomonas aeruginosa*
Nebulised hypertonic saline, 4 mL 7%, twice daily	Age ≥ 6, FEV_1 > 40% predicted

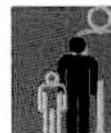

19.40 Cystic fibrosis in adolescence

- **Issues for the patient**:
  - Move to adult CF centre – loss of trusted paediatric team
  - Feelings of being different from peers due to chronic illness
  - Demanding treatments that conflict with social and school life
  - Pressure to take responsibility for self-care
  - Relationship/fertility concerns
- **Issues for the patient's parents**:
  - Loss of control over patient's treatment – feeling excluded
  - Loss of trusted paediatric team
  - Need to develop trust in adult team
  - Feelings of helplessness when adolescent rebels or will not take treatment
- **Issues for the CF team**:
  - Reluctance or refusal by patient to engage with transition
  - Management of deterioration due to non-adherence
  - Motivation of adolescents to self-care
  - Provision of adolescent-friendly health-care environment

INFECTIONS OF THE RESPIRATORY SYSTEM

Infections of the upper and lower respiratory tract are a major cause of morbidity and mortality, particularly in patients at the extremes of age, and those with pre-existing lung disease or immune suppression.

Upper respiratory tract infection

Upper respiratory tract infections (URTIs), such as coryza (the common cold), acute pharyngitis and acute tracheobronchitis, are the most common of all communicable diseases and represent the most frequent cause of short-term absenteeism from work and school. The vast majority are caused by viruses (p. 328) and, in adults, are usually short-lived and rarely serious.

Acute coryza is the most common URTI and is usually the result of rhinovirus infection. In addition to general malaise, acute coryza typically causes nasal discharge, sneezing and cough. Involvement of the pharynx results in a sore throat, that of the larynx a hoarse or lost voice.

If complicated by a tracheitis or bronchitis, chest tightness and wheeze typical of asthma occur. Specific investigation is rarely warranted and treatment with simple analgesics, antipyretics and decongestants is all that is required. Symptoms usually resolve quickly, but if repeated URTIs 'go to the chest', a more formal diagnosis of asthma ought to be considered. A variety of viruses causing URTI may also trigger exacerbations of asthma or COPD and aggravate other lung diseases.

Bordetella pertussis, the cause of whooping cough, is an important source of URTI. It is highly contagious and is notifiable in the UK. Vaccination confers protection and is usually offered in infancy, but its efficacy wanes in adult life and the infection is easily spread. Adults usually experience a mild illness similar to acute coryza, but some individuals develop paroxysms of coughing which can persist for weeks to months, earning whooping cough the designation of 'the cough of 100 days'. The diagnosis may be confirmed by bacterial culture, polymerase chain reaction (PCR) from a nasopharyngeal swab or serological testing. If the illness is recognised early in the clinical course, macrolide antibiotics may ameliorate the course.

Rhinosinusitis typically causes a combination of nasal congestion, blockage or discharge, and may be accompanied by facial pain/pressure or loss of smell. Examination usually confirms erythematous swollen nasal mucosa and pus may be evident. Nasal polyps should be sought and dental infection excluded. Treatment with topical corticosteroids, nasal decongestants and regular nasal douching are usually sufficient and, although bacterial infection is often present, antibiotics are only indicated if symptoms persist for more than 5 days. Persistent symptoms or recurrent episodes should prompt a referral to an ear, nose and throat specialist.

Influenza is discussed on page 319.

Pneumonia

Pneumonia is as an acute respiratory illness associated with recently developed radiological pulmonary shadowing, which may be segmental, lobar or multilobar. The context in which pneumonia develops is highly indicative of the likely organism(s) involved; therefore, pneumonias are usually classified as community- or hospital-acquired, or as occurring in immunocompromised hosts. 'Lobar pneumonia' is a radiological and pathological term referring to homogeneous consolidation of one or more lung lobes, often with associated pleural inflammation. 'Bronchopneumonia' refers to more patchy alveolar consolidation associated with bronchial and bronchiolar inflammation, often affecting both lower lobes.

The inflammatory response in lobar pneumonia evolves through stages of congestion, red then grey hepatisation, and finally resolution. In the first stage, the alveolar units are flooded by a proteinaceous exudate and by neutrophils and red blood cells, and numerous pneumococci may be observed. As fibrin forms on the cut surface of the affected lobe, it resembles liver and so this stage is known as 'red hepatisation'. As congestion resolves, the lung tissue becomes grey ('grey hepatisation'), and ultimately, clearance and repair mechanisms restore the normal architecture of the lung.

Community-acquired pneumonia

Figures from the UK suggest that an estimated 5–11/1000 adults suffer from community-acquired pneumonia (CAP) each year, accounting for around 5–12% of all lower respiratory tract infections. It affects all age groups but is particularly common at the extremes of age; worldwide, CAP continues to kill more children than any other illness, and its propensity to ease the passing of the frail and elderly led to pneumonia being known as the 'old man's friend'.

Most cases are spread by droplet infection and, whilst CAP may occur in previously healthy individuals, several factors may impair the effectiveness of local defences and predispose to CAP (Box 19.41). *Streptococcus pneumoniae* (Fig. 19.32) remains the most common infecting agent. The likelihood that other organisms may be involved depends on the age of the patient and the clinical context. Viral infections are important causes of CAP in children, and their contribution to adult CAP is increasingly recognised (Box 19.42).

A 'best guess' as to the likely organism may be made from the context in which pneumonia develops, but not from the clinical and radiological picture, which does not differ sufficiently from one organism to another; the term 'atypical pneumonia' has therefore been dropped. *Mycoplasma pneumoniae* is more common in young people and rare in the elderly, whereas *Haemophilus influenzae* is more common in the elderly, particularly when underlying lung disease is present. *Legionella pneumophila* occurs in local outbreaks centred on contaminated cooling towers in hotels, hospitals and other industrial buildings. *Staphylococcus aureus* is more common following an episode of influenza. Foreign travel raises the possibility of infections that might otherwise be unusual in the UK: for example, *Burkholderia pseudomallei* from South-east Asia. Travel also facilitates the spread of illnesses such as severe acute

19.41 Factors that predispose to pneumonia

- Cigarette smoking
- Upper respiratory tract infections
- Alcohol
- Corticosteroid therapy
- Old age
- Recent influenza infection
- Pre-existing lung disease
- HIV
- Indoor air pollution

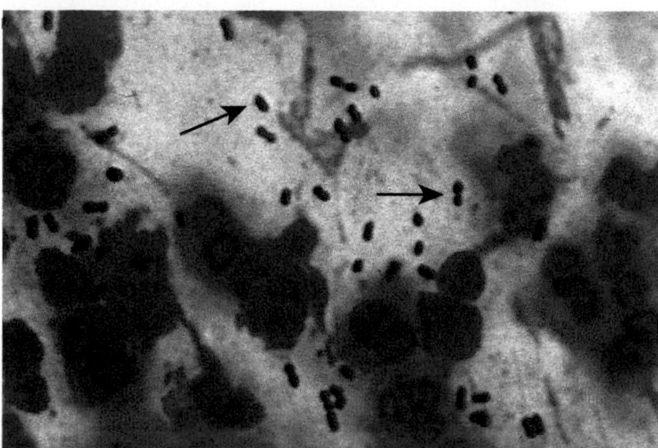

Fig. 19.32 Gram stain of sputum showing Gram-positive diplococci characteristic of *Strep. pneumoniae* (arrows).

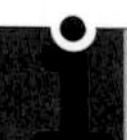

19.42 Organisms causing community-acquired pneumonia

Bacteria	
• *Streptococcus pneumoniae*	• *Chlamydia psittaci*
• *Mycoplasma pneumoniae*	• *Coxiella burnetii* (Q fever, 'querry' fever)
• *Legionella pneumophila*	• *Klebsiella pneumoniae* (Freidländer's bacillus)
• *Chlamydia pneumoniae*	• *Actinomyces israelii*
• *Haemophilus influenzae*	
• *Staphylococcus aureus*	
Viruses	
• Influenza, parainfluenza	• Cytomegalovirus (CMV)
• Measles	• Coronavirus (Urbani SARS-associated coronavirus)
• Herpes simplex	
• Varicella	
• Adenovirus	

(SARS = severe acute respiratory syndrome)

respiratory syndrome (SARS), caused by a form of coronavirus arising in the Guangdong province of China, but which spread rapidly through Hong Kong and Vietnam, and then throughout the world. Certain occupations may be associated with exposure to specific bacteria (p. 715).

Clinical features

Pneumonia, particularly lobar pneumonia, usually presents as an acute illness. Systemic features such as fever, rigors, shivering and malaise predominate and delirium may be present. The appetite is invariably lost and headache frequently reported.

Pulmonary symptoms include cough, which at first is characteristically short, painful and dry, but later accompanied by the expectoration of mucopurulent sputum. Rust-coloured sputum may be seen in patients with *Strep. pneumoniae*, and the occasional individual may report haemoptysis. Pleuritic chest pain may be a presenting feature and, on occasion, may be referred to the shoulder or anterior abdominal wall. Upper abdominal tenderness is sometimes apparent in patients with lower lobe pneumonia or if there is associated hepatitis. Less typical presentations may be seen in the very young and the elderly.

On examination, the respiratory and pulse rate may be raised and the blood pressure low, while an assessment of the mental state may reveal a delirium. These are important indicators of the severity of the illness (Fig. 19.33). Not all patients are pyrexial but this is a helpful diagnostic clue if present. Oxygen saturation on air may be low, and the patient cyanosed and distressed.

Chest signs (p. 645) vary, depending on the phase of the inflammatory response. When consolidated, the lung is typically dull to percussion and, as conduction of sound is enhanced, auscultation reveals bronchial breathing and whispering pectoriloquy; crackles are heard throughout. However, in many patients, signs are more subtle with reduced air entry only, but crackles are usually present.

An assessment of nutrition is important as, if poor, the response to treatment will be impaired, particularly in the elderly. On occasion, inferences as to the likely organism may be drawn from clinical examination. For example, the presence of herpes labialis may point to streptococcal infection, as may the finding of 'rusty' sputum. The presence of poor dental hygiene should prompt consideration of *Klebsiella* or *Actinomyces israelii*. The differential diagnosis of pneumonia is shown in Box 19.43.

19.43 Differential diagnosis of pneumonia

- Pulmonary infarction
- Pulmonary/pleural TB
- Pulmonary oedema (can be unilateral)
- Pulmonary eosinophilia (p. 713)
- Malignancy: bronchoalveolar cell carcinoma
- Rare disorders: cryptogenic organising pneumonia/bronchiolitis obliterans organising pneumonia (COP/BOOP) (p. 708)

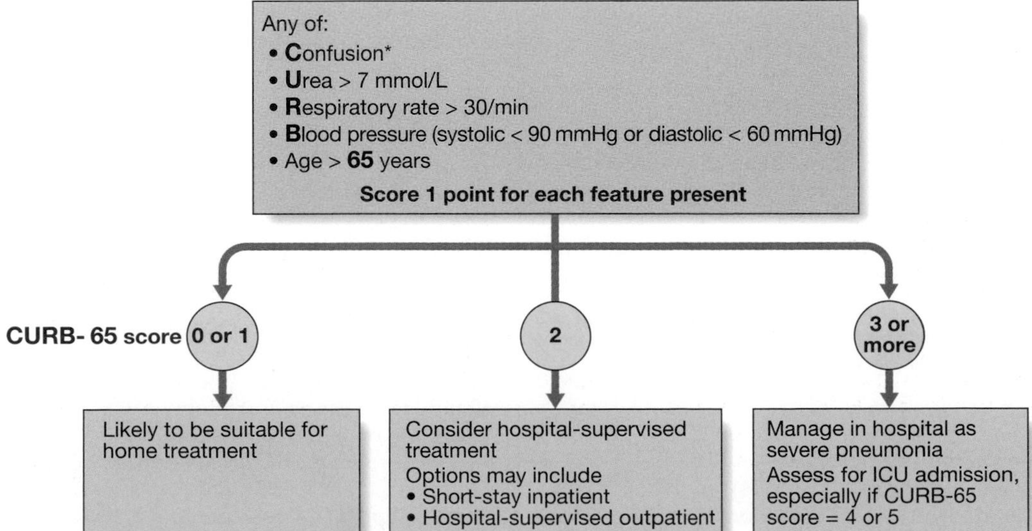

Fig. 19.33 Hospital CURB-65. *Defined as a Mental Test Score of 8 or less, or new disorientation in person, place or time. (Urea of 7 mmol/L ≅ 20 mg/dL.)

19

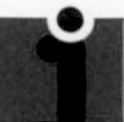

19.44 Investigations in CAP

Blood

Full blood count
- Very high (> 20×10^9/L) or low (< 4×10^9/L) white cell count: marker of severity
- Neutrophil leucocytosis > 15×10^9/L: suggests bacterial aetiology
- Haemolytic anaemia: occasional complication of *Mycoplasma*

Urea and electrolytes
- Urea > 7 mmol/L (~20 mg/dL): marker of severity
- Hyponatraemia: marker of severity

Liver function tests
- Abnormal if basal pneumonia inflames liver
- Hypoalbuminaemia: marker of severity

Erythrocyte sedimentation rate/C-reactive protein
- Non-specifically elevated

Blood culture
- Bacteraemia: marker of severity

Serology
- Acute and convalescent titres for *Mycoplasma*, *Chlamydia*, *Legionella* and viral infections

Cold agglutinins
- Positive in 50% of patients with *Mycoplasma*

Arterial blood gases
- Measure when SaO_2 < 93% or when severe clinical features to assess ventilatory failure or acidosis

Sputum

Sputum samples
- Gram stain (see Fig. 19.32), culture and antimicrobial sensitivity testing

Oropharynx swab
- PCR for *Mycoplasma pneumoniae* and other atypical pathogens

Urine
- Pneumococcal and/or *Legionella* antigen

Chest X-ray

Lobar pneumonia
- Patchy opacification evolves into homogeneous consolidation of affected lobe
- Air bronchogram (air-filled bronchi appear lucent against consolidated lung tissue) may be present (see Fig. 19.34)

Bronchopneumonia
- Typically patchy and segmental shadowing

Complications
- Para-pneumonic effusion, intrapulmonary abscess or empyema

Staph. aureus
- Suggested by multilobar shadowing, cavitation, pneumatocoeles and abscesses

Pleural fluid
- Always aspirate and culture when present in more than trivial amounts, preferably with ultrasound guidance

Investigations

The aims of investigation (Box 19.44) are to confirm the diagnosis and exclude other conditions, assess the severity and identify the development of complications. Typical chest X-ray findings in a lobar pneumonia are shown in Figure 19.34. Whilst many cases of mild to moderate CAP can be successfully managed without identification of the organism, a range of microbiological tests should be performed on patients with severe CAP.

A
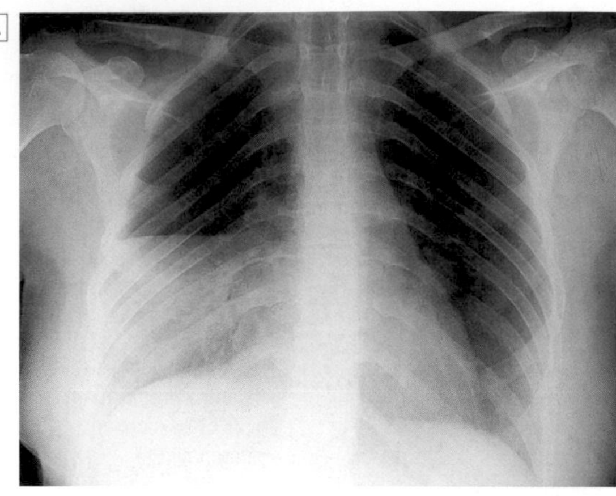

B
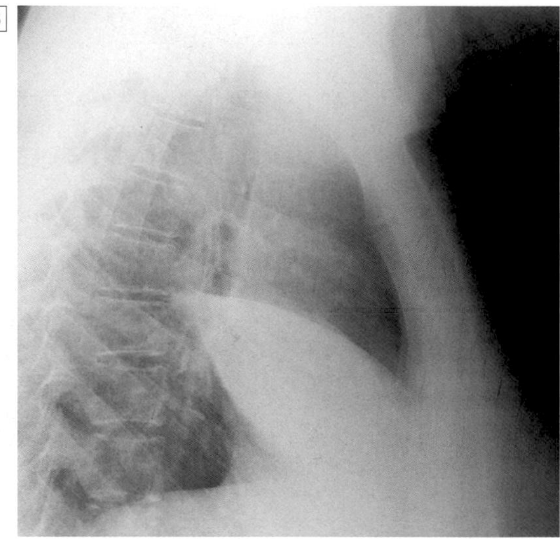

Fig. 19.34 Pneumonia of the right middle lobe. **A** PA view: consolidation in the right middle lobe with characteristic opacification beneath the horizontal fissure and loss of normal contrast between the right heart border and lung. **B** Lateral view: consolidation confined to the anteriorly situated middle lobe.

Management

The most important aspects of management are oxygenation, fluid balance and antibiotic therapy. In severe or prolonged illness, nutritional support may be required.

Oxygen

Oxygen should be administered to all patients with tachypnoea, hypoxaemia, hypotension or acidosis, with the aim of maintaining the PaO_2 at or above 8 kPa (60 mmHg) or the SaO_2 at or above 92%. High concentrations (35% or more), preferably humidified, should be used in all patients who do not have hypercapnia associated with COPD. Continuous positive airway pressure (CPAP) should be considered in those who remain hypoxic despite this, and these patients should be managed in a high-dependency or intensive care environment, where mechanical ventilation can be rapidly

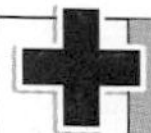

19.45 Indications for referral to ITU

- CURB score of 4–5, failing to respond rapidly to initial management
- Persisting hypoxia (PaO_2 < 8 kPa (60 mmHg)), despite high concentrations of oxygen
- Progressive hypercapnia
- Severe acidosis
- Circulatory shock
- Reduced conscious level

employed. Indications for referral to the intensive therapy unit (ITU) are summarised in Box 19.45.

Intravenous fluids

These should be considered in patients with severe illness, older patients and those who are vomiting. Otherwise, an adequate oral intake of fluid should be encouraged. Inotropic support may be required in patients with shock (p. 190).

Antibiotics

Prompt administration of antibiotics improves the outcome. The initial choice of antibiotic is guided by clinical context, severity assessment, local knowledge of antibiotic resistance patterns and any available epidemiological information. Current regimens are detailed in Box 19.46. In most patients with uncomplicated pneumonia, a 7-day course is adequate, although treatment is usually required for longer in those with *Legionella*, staphylococcal or *Klebsiella* pneumonia. Oral antibiotics are usually adequate unless the patient has a severe illness, impaired consciousness, loss of swallowing reflex, or functional or anatomical reasons for malabsorption.

It is important to relieve pleural pain, as it may prevent the patient from breathing normally and coughing efficiently. For the majority, simple analgesia with

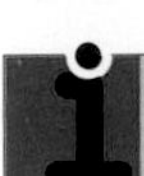

19.46 Antibiotic treatment for CAP*

Uncomplicated CAP

- Amoxicillin 500 mg 3 times daily orally

If patient is allergic to penicillin

- Clarithromycin 500 mg twice daily orally ***or*** Erythromycin 500 mg 4 times daily orally

If *Staphylococcus* is cultured or suspected

- Flucloxacillin 1–2 g 4 times daily IV ***plus***
- Clarithromycin 500 mg twice daily IV

If *Mycoplasma* or *Legionella* is suspected

- Clarithromycin 500 mg twice daily orally or IV ***or*** Erythromycin 500 mg 4 times daily orally IV ***plus***
- Rifampicin 600 mg twice daily IV in severe cases

Severe CAP

- Clarithromycin 500 mg twice daily IV ***or*** Erythromycin 500 mg 4 times daily IV ***plus***
- Co-amoxiclav 1.2 g 3 times daily IV ***or*** Ceftriaxone 1–2 g daily IV ***or*** Cefuroxime 1.5 g 3 times daily IV ***or***
- Amoxicillin 1 g 4 times daily IV ***plus*** flucloxacillin 2 g 4 times daily IV

*Adapted from British Thoracic Society Guidelines.

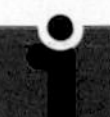

19.47 Complications of pneumonia

- Para-pneumonic effusion – common
- Empyema (p. 662)
- Retention of sputum causing lobar collapse
- Deep vein thrombosis and pulmonary embolism
- Pneumothorax, particularly with *Staph. aureus*
- Suppurative pneumonia/lung abscess
- ARDS, renal failure, multi-organ failure (p. 192)
- Ectopic abscess formation (*Staph. aureus*)
- Hepatitis, pericarditis, myocarditis, meningoencephalitis
- Pyrexia due to drug hypersensitivity

paracetamol, co-codamol or NSAIDs is sufficient. In some patients, opiates may be required but these must be used with extreme caution in patients with poor respiratory function, as they may suppress ventilation. Physiotherapy is not usually indicated in patients with CAP, but may help expectoration in those who suppress cough because of pleural pain.

Most patients respond promptly to antibiotic therapy. However, fever may persist for several days and the chest X-ray often takes several weeks or even months to resolve, especially in old age. Delayed recovery suggests either that a complication has occurred (Box 19.47), that the diagnosis is incorrect (see Box 19.43) or, alternatively, that the pneumonia may be secondary to a proximal bronchial obstruction or recurrent aspiration. The mortality rate of adults with non-severe pneumonia is very low (< 1%); hospital death rates are typically between 5 and 10% but may be as high as 50% in severe illness.

Discharge and follow-up

The decision to discharge patients depends on their home circumstances and the likelihood of complications. A chest X-ray need not be repeated before discharge in those making a satisfactory clinical recovery. Clinical review should be arranged around 6 weeks later and a chest X-ray obtained if there are persistent symptoms, physical signs or reasons to suspect underlying malignancy.

Prevention

Current smokers should be advised to stop. Influenza and pneumococcal vaccination should be considered in selected patients (p. 148). Because of the mode of spread, *Legionella pneumophila* has important public health implications and usually requires notification to the appropriate health authority. In developing countries, tackling malnourishment and indoor air pollution, and encouraging immunisation against measles, pertussis and *Haemophilus influenzae* type b are particularly important in children.

Hospital-acquired pneumonia

Hospital-acquired or nosocomial pneumonia is a new episode of pneumonia occurring at least 2 days after admission to hospital. It is the second most common hospital-acquired infection (HAI) and the leading cause of HAI-associated death. The elderly are particularly at risk, along with patients in intensive care units, especially when mechanically ventilated; in the latter case,

19.48 Factors predisposing to hospital-acquired pneumonia

Reduced host defences against bacteria
• Reduced immune defences (e.g. corticosteroid treatment, diabetes, malignancy) • Reduced cough reflex (e.g. post-operative) • Disordered mucociliary clearance (e.g. anaesthetic agents) • Bulbar or vocal cord palsy
Aspiration of nasopharyngeal or gastric secretions
• Immobility or reduced conscious level • Vomiting, dysphagia (N.B. stroke disease), achalasia or severe reflux • Nasogastric intubation
Bacteria introduced into lower respiratory tract
• Endotracheal intubation/tracheostomy • Infected ventilators/nebulisers/bronchoscopes • Dental or sinus infection
Bacteraemia
• Abdominal sepsis • IV cannula infection • Infected emboli

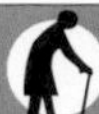

19.49 Respiratory infection in old age

- **Increased risk of and from respiratory infection**: because of reduced immune responses, increased closing volumes, reduced respiratory muscle strength and endurance, altered mucus layer, poor nutritional status and the increased prevalence of chronic lung disease.
- **Predisposing factors**: other medical conditions may predispose to infection, e.g. swallowing difficulties due to stroke increase the risk of aspiration pneumonia.
- **Atypical presentation**: older patients often present with confusion, rather than breathlessness or cough.
- **Mortality**: the vast majority of deaths from pneumonia in developed countries occur in older people.
- **Influenza**: has a much higher complication rate, morbidity and mortality. Vaccination significantly reduces morbidity and mortality in old age but uptake is poor.
- **TB**: most cases in old age represent reactivation of previous, often unrecognised disease and may be precipitated by steroid therapy, diabetes mellitus and the factors above. Cryptic miliary TB is an occasional alternative presentation. Older people more commonly suffer adverse effects from antituberculous chemotherapy and require close monitoring.

the term 'ventilator-associated pneumonia' (VAP) is used. Healthcare-associated pneumonia (HCAP) is the development of pneumonia in a person who has spent at least 2 days in hospital within the last 90 days, or has attended a haemodialysis unit, received intravenous antibiotics, or been resident in a nursing home or other long-term care facility. The factors predisposing to the development of pneumonia in a hospitalised patient are listed in Box 19.48. The organisms implicated in early-onset HAP (occurring within 4–5 days of admission) are similar to those involved in CAP. Late-onset HAP is associated with a different range of pathogens to CAP, with more Gram-negative bacteria (e.g. *Escherichia, Pseudomonas, Klebsiella* species and *Acinetobacter baumannii*), *Staph. aureus* (including the meticillin-resistant type (MRSA)) and anaerobes.

Clinical features and investigations

The diagnosis should be considered in any hospitalised or ventilated patient who develops purulent sputum (or endotracheal secretions), new radiological infiltrates, an otherwise unexplained increase in oxygen requirement, a core temperature of more than 38.3°C, and a leucocytosis or leucopenia. However, the clinical features and radiographic signs are variable and non-specific, raising a broad differential diagnosis that includes venous thromboembolism, ARDS, pulmonary oedema, pulmonary haemorrhage and drug toxicity. Therefore, in contrast to CAP, microbiological confirmation should be sought whenever possible. As in CAP, the full blood count (FBC), urea and electrolytes (U&E), erythrocyte sedimentation rate (ESR) and C-reactive protein (CRP), and arterial blood gas samples should be sent for analysis and a chest X-ray performed, but other investigations and imaging may be necessary to exclude other conditions. Adequate sputum samples may be difficult to obtain in frail elderly patients and physiotherapy should be considered to aid expectoration. In patients who are mechanically ventilated, bronchoscopy-directed protected brush specimens, bronchoalveolar lavage (BAL) or endotracheal aspirates may be obtained.

Management

The principles of management are similar to those for CAP, focusing on adequate oxygenation, appropriate fluid balance and antibiotics. However, the choice of empirical antibiotic therapy is considerably more challenging, given the diversity of pathogens and the potential for drug resistance.

In early-onset HAP, patients who have received no previous antibiotics can be treated with co-amoxiclav or cefuroxime. If the patient has received a course of recent antibiotics, then piperacillin/tazobactam or a third-generation cephalosporin should be considered.

In late-onset HAP, the choice of antibiotics must cover the Gram-negative bacteria (see above), *Staph. aureus* (including MRSA) and anaerobes. Anti-pseudomonal cover may be provided by a carbapenem (meropenem) or a third-generation cephalosporin combined with an aminoglycoside. MRSA cover may be provided by glycopeptides, such as vancomycin or linezolid. *A. baumannii* is usually sensitive to carbapenems but resistant cases may require the prolonged administration of nebulised colistin. The choice of agents is most appropriately guided by knowledge of local patterns of microbiology and antibiotic resistance. It is usual to commence broad-based cover, discontinuing less appropriate antibiotics as culture results become available. In the absence of good evidence, the duration of antibiotic therapy remains a matter for clinical judgement.

Physiotherapy is important to aid expectoration in the immobile and elderly, and nutritional support is often required.

Prevention

Despite appropriate management, the mortality from HAP is approximately 30%, so prevention is very important. Good hygiene is paramount, particularly with regard to handwashing and any equipment used. The risk of aspiration should be minimised, and the use of stress ulcer prophylaxis with proton pump inhibitors limited, as they may increase the risk of ventilator-associated pneumonia. Oral antiseptic (chlorhexidine 2%) may be used to decontaminate the upper airway, and some intensive care units employ selective decontamination of the digestive tract when the anticipated requirement for ventilation will exceed 48 hours.

Suppurative pneumonia, aspiration pneumonia and pulmonary abscess

These conditions are considered together, as their aetiology and clinical features overlap. Suppurative pneumonia is characterised by destruction of the lung parenchyma by the inflammatory process and, although microabscess formation is a characteristic histological feature, 'pulmonary abscess' is usually taken to refer to lesions in which there is a large localised collection of pus, or a cavity lined by chronic inflammatory tissue, from which pus has escaped by rupture into a bronchus.

Suppurative pneumonia and pulmonary abscess often develop after the inhalation of septic material during operations on the nose, mouth or throat under general anaesthesia, or of vomitus during anaesthesia or coma, particularly if oral hygiene is poor. Additional risk factors for aspiration pneumonia include bulbar or vocal cord palsy, stroke, achalasia or oesophageal reflux, and alcoholism. Aspiration tends to localise to dependent areas of the lung, such as the apical segment of the lower lobe in a supine patient. Suppurative pneumonia and pulmonary abscess may also complicate local bronchial obstruction from a neoplasm or foreign body.

Infections are usually due to a mixture of anaerobes and aerobes in common with the typical flora encountered in the mouth and upper respiratory tract. Isolates of *Bacteroides melaninogenicus, Fusobacterium necrophorum,* anaerobic or micro-aerophilic cocci, and *Bacteroides fragilis* may be identified. When suppurative pneumonia or a pulmonary abscess occurs in a previously healthy lung, the most likely infecting organism is *Staph. aureus* or *Klebsiella pneumoniae.*

Bacterial infection of a pulmonary infarct or a collapsed lobe may also produce a suppurative pneumonia or lung abscess. The organisms isolated from the sputum include *Strep. pneumoniae, Staph. aureus, Strep. pyogenes, H. influenzae* and, in some cases, anaerobic bacteria. In many cases, however, no pathogen can be isolated, particularly when antibiotics have been given.

Strains of community-acquired MRSA (CA-MRSA) produce the cytotoxin Panton–Valentine leukocidin. The organism is mainly responsible for suppurative skin infection but may be associated with rapidly progressive, severe, necrotising pneumonia.

Lemierre's syndrome is a rare cause of pulmonary abscesses. The usual causative agent is the anaerobe, *F. necrophorum.* The illness typically commences as a sore throat, painful swollen neck, fever, rigor, haemoptysis and dyspnoea, and spread into the jugular veins leads to thrombosis and metastatic spread of the organisms.

Injecting drug-users are at particular risk of developing haematogenous lung abscess, often in association with endocarditis affecting the pulmonary and tricuspid valves.

19.50 Clinical features of suppurative pneumonia

Symptoms

- Cough with large amounts of sputum, sometimes fetid and blood-stained
- Pleural pain common
- Sudden expectoration of copious amounts of foul sputum if abscess ruptures into a bronchus

Clinical signs

- High remittent pyrexia
- Profound systemic upset
- Digital clubbing may develop quickly (10–14 days)
- Consolidation on chest examination; signs of cavitation rarely found
- Pleural rub common
- Rapid deterioration in general health, with marked weight loss if not adequately treated

A non-infective form of aspiration pneumonia – exogenous lipid pneumonia – may follow the aspiration of animal, vegetable, or mineral oils.

The clinical features of suppurative pneumonia are summarised in Box 19.50.

Investigations and management

Radiological features of suppurative pneumonia include homogeneous lobar or segmental opacity consistent with consolidation or collapse. Abscesses are characterised by cavitation and fluid level. Occasionally, a pre-existing emphysematous bulla becomes infected and appears as a cavity containing an air–fluid level.

Aspiration pneumonia can be treated with intravenous co-amoxiclav 1.2 g 3 times daily. If an anaerobic bacterial infection is suspected (e.g. from fetor of the sputum), oral metronidazole 400 mg 3 times daily should be added. Further modification of antibiotics may be required, depending on the clinical response and the microbiological results. CA-MRSA is usually susceptible to a variety of oral non-β-lactam antibiotics, such as trimethoprim/sulfamethoxazole, clindamycin, tetracyclines and linezolid. Parenteral therapy with vancomycin or daptomycin can also be considered. *F. necrophorum* is highly susceptible to β-lactam antibiotics, and to metronidazole, clindamycin and third-generation cephalosporins. Prolonged treatment for 4–6 weeks may be required in some patients with lung abscess. Physiotherapy is of great value, especially when suppuration is present in the lower lobes or when a large abscess cavity has formed.

In most patients, there is a good response to treatment and, although residual fibrosis and bronchiectasis are common sequelae, these seldom give rise to serious morbidity. Surgery should be contemplated if no improvement occurs, despite optimal medical therapy. Removal or treatment of any obstructing endobronchial lesion is essential.

Pneumonia in the immunocompromised patient

Patients immunocompromised by drugs or disease (particularly HIV, p. 400) are at high risk of pulmonary infection. The majority of cases are caused by the same pathogens that cause pneumonia in

19.51 Causes of immune suppression-associated lung infection

	Causes	Infecting organisms
Defective phagocytic function	Acute leukaemia Cytotoxic drugs Agranulocytosis	Gram-positive bacteria, including *Staph. aureus* Gram-negative bacteria Fungi, e.g. *Candida albicans* and *Aspergillus fumigatus*
Defects in cell-mediated immunity	Immunosuppressive drugs Cytotoxic chemotherapy Lymphoma Thymic aplasia	Viruses Cytomegalovirus Herpesvirus Adenovirus Influenza Fungi *Pneumocystis jirovecii* (formerly *carinii*) *Candida albicans* *Aspergillus fumigatus*
Defects in antibody production	Multiple myeloma Chronic lymphocytic leukaemia	*Haemophilus influenzae* *Mycoplasma pneumoniae*

non-immunocompromised individuals, but in patients with more profound immunosuppression, unusual organisms or those normally considered to be of low virulence or non-pathogenic may become 'opportunistic' pathogens (Box 19.51). Therefore, the possibility of Gram-negative bacteria, especially *Pseudomonas aeruginosa*, viral agents, fungi, mycobacteria, and less common organisms such as *Nocardia asteroides* has to be considered. Infection is often due to more than one organism.

Clinical features

These typically include fever, cough and breathlessness, but are influenced by the degree of immunosuppression; symptoms are less specific in the more profoundly immunosuppressed. The speed of onset tends to be less rapid in patients with opportunistic organisms such as *Pneumocystis jirovecii* and mycobacterial infections than with bacterial infections (p. 400). In *P. jirovecii* pneumonia, symptoms of cough and breathlessness can be present for several days or weeks before the onset of systemic symptoms or the appearance of X-ray abnormalities. The clinical features of invasive pulmonary aspergillosis are described on page 698.

Diagnosis

The approach is informed by the clinical context and severity of the illness. Invasive investigations, such as bronchoscopy, BAL, transbronchial biopsy or surgical lung biopsy, are often impractical, as many patients are too ill to undergo these safely. However, 'induced sputum' (p. 652) offers a relatively safe method of obtaining microbiological samples. HRCT is useful in differentiating the likely cause:

- Focal unilateral airspace opacification favours bacterial infection, mycobacteria or *Nocardia*.
- Bilateral opacification favours *P. jirovecii* pneumonia, fungi, viruses and unusual bacteria, e.g. *Nocardia*.
- Cavitation may be seen with *N. asteroides*, mycobacteria and fungi.
- The presence of a 'halo sign' may suggest *Aspergillus* (see Fig. 19.45, p. 698).
- Pleural effusions suggest a pyogenic bacterial infection and are uncommon in *P. jirovecii* pneumonia.

Management

In theory, treatment should be based on the identified causative organism but, in practice, this is frequently unknown and broad-spectrum antibiotic therapy is required, such as a third-generation cephalosporin or a quinolone, plus an antistaphylococcal antibiotic, or an antipseudomonal penicillin plus an aminoglycoside.

Thereafter, treatment may be tailored according to the results of investigations and the clinical response. These may dictate the addition of antifungal or antiviral therapies. The management of *P. jirovecii* infection is detailed on page 400, and that of invasive aspergillosis on page 698.

Tuberculosis

Epidemiology

Tuberculosis (TB) is caused by infection with *Mycobacterium tuberculosis* (MTB), which is part of a complex of organisms including *M. bovis* (reservoir cattle) and *M. africanum* (reservoir human). Recent figures suggest a decline in the incidence of TB, but its impact on world health remains significant. In 2010, an estimated 8.8 million incident cases occurred and TB was estimated to account for nearly 1.5 million deaths, making it the second most common cause of death due to an infective disease. Furthermore, it is estimated that around one-third of the world's population has latent TB. The majority of cases occur in the world's poorest nations, who struggle to cover the costs associated with management and control programmes (Fig. 19.35). In Africa, the resurgence of TB has been largely driven by HIV disease and, in the former Soviet Union and Baltic states, by a lack of appropriate health care associated with social and political upheaval.

Pathology and pathogenesis

M. bovis infection arises from drinking non-sterilised milk from infected cows. *M. tuberculosis* is spread by the inhalation of aerosolised droplet nuclei from other infected patients. Once inhaled, the organisms lodge in the alveoli and initiate the recruitment of macrophages and lymphocytes. Macrophages undergo transformation into epithelioid and Langhans cells, which aggregate with the lymphocytes to form the classical tuberculous granuloma (Fig. 19.36). Numerous granulomas aggregate to form a primary lesion or 'Ghon focus' (a pale yellow, caseous nodule, usually a few millimetres to 1–2 cm in diameter), which is characteristically situated in the periphery of the lung. Spread of organisms to the hilar lymph nodes is followed by a similar pathological reaction, and the combination of the primary lesion and regional lymph nodes is referred to as the 'primary complex of Ranke'. Reparative processes encase the primary complex in a fibrous capsule, limiting the spread of bacilli: so-called latent TB (p. 695). If no further complications ensue, this lesion eventually

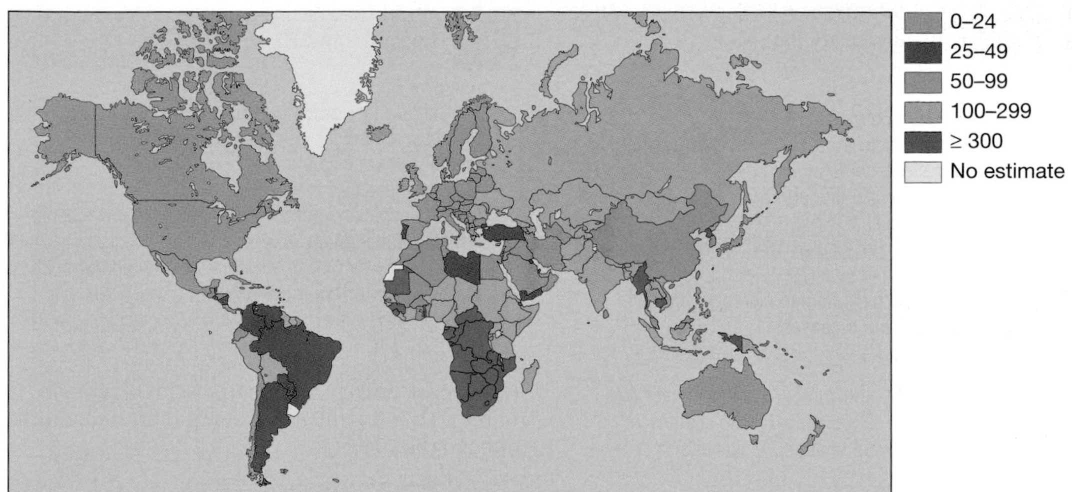

Fig. 19.35 Worldwide incidence of tuberculosis. Estimated new cases (all forms) per 100 000 population (WHO). From Maartens and Wilkinson 2007 – see p. 732.

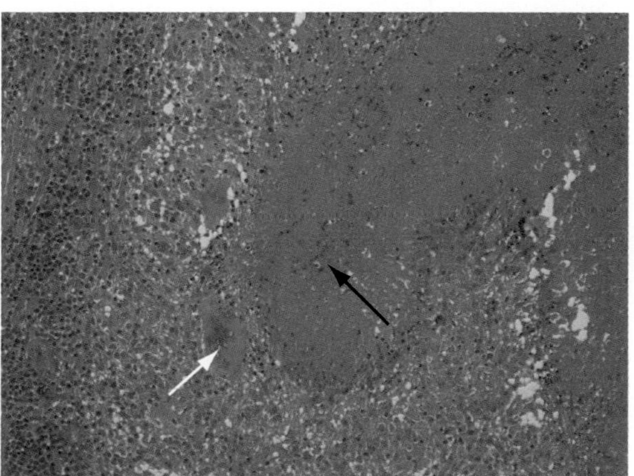

Fig. 19.36 Tuberculous granuloma. Normal lung tissue is lost and replaced by a mass of fibrous tissue with granulomatous inflammation characterised by large numbers of macrophages and multinucleate giant cells (white arrow). The central area of this focus shows caseous degeneration (black arrow).

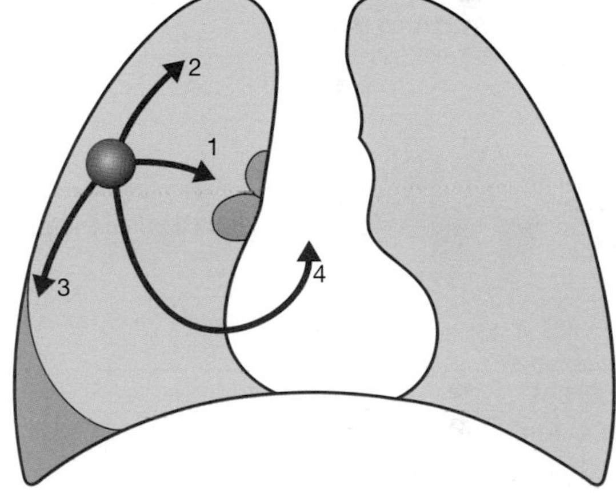

Fig. 19.37 Primary pulmonary TB. (1) Spread from the primary focus to hilar and mediastinal lymph glands to form the 'primary complex', which in most cases heals spontaneously. (2) Direct extension of the primary focus – progressive pulmonary TB. (3) Spread to the pleura – tuberculous pleurisy and pleural effusion. (4) Blood-borne spread: *few bacilli* – pulmonary, skeletal, renal, genitourinary infection, often months or years later; *massive spread* – miliary TB and meningitis.

calcifies and is clearly seen on a chest X-ray. However, lymphatic or haematogenous spread may occur before immunity is established, seeding secondary foci in other organs, including lymph nodes, serous membranes, meninges, bones, liver, kidneys and lungs, which may lie dormant for years. The only clue that infection has occurred may be the appearance of a cell-mediated, delayed-type hypersensitivity reaction to tuberculin, demonstrated by tuberculin skin testing. If these reparative processes fail, primary progressive disease ensues (Fig. 19.37). The estimated lifetime risk of developing disease after primary infection is 10%, with roughly half of this risk occurring in the first 2 years after infection. Factors predisposing to TB are summarised in Box 19.52 and the natural history of infection with TB is summarised in Box 19.53.

Clinical features: pulmonary disease

Primary pulmonary TB

Primary TB refers to the infection of a previously uninfected (tuberculin-negative) individual. A few patients develop a self-limiting febrile illness but clinical disease only occurs if there is a hypersensitivity reaction or progressive infection (Box 19.54). Progressive primary disease may appear during the course of the initial illness or after a latent period of weeks or months.

Miliary TB

Blood-borne dissemination gives rise to miliary TB, which may present acutely but more frequently is characterised by 2–3 weeks of fever, night sweats, anorexia, weight loss and a dry cough. Hepatosplenomegaly may develop and the presence of a headache may indicate coexistent tuberculous meningitis. Auscultation of the chest is frequently normal, but in more advanced disease, widespread crackles are evident. Fundoscopy may show choroidal tubercles. The classical appearances on chest X-ray are of fine 1–2 mm lesions ('millet seed') distributed throughout the lung fields, although occasionally the appearances are coarser. Anaemia and

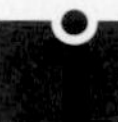

19.52 Factors increasing the risk of TB

Patient-related

- Age (children > young adults < elderly)
- First-generation immigrants from high-prevalence countries
- Close contacts of patients with smear-positive pulmonary TB
- Overcrowding (prisons, collective dormitories); homelessness (doss houses and hostels)
- Chest X-ray evidence of self-healed TB
- Primary infection < 1 yr previously
- Smoking: cigarettes and bidis (Indian cigarettes made of tobacco wrapped in temburini leaves)

Associated diseases

- Immunosuppression: HIV, anti-tumour necrosis factor (TNF) therapy, high-dose corticosteroids, cytotoxic agents
- Malignancy (especially lymphoma and leukaemia)
- Diabetes mellitus
- Chronic kidney disease
- Silicosis
- Gastrointestinal disease associated with malnutrition (gastrectomy, jejuno-ileal bypass, cancer of the pancreas, malabsorption)
- Deficiency of vitamin D or A
- Recent measles in children

19.53 Natural history of untreated primary TB

Time from infection	Manifestations
3–8 wks	Primary complex, positive tuberculin skin test
3–6 mths	Meningeal, miliary and pleural disease
Up to 3 yrs	Gastrointestinal, bone and joint, and lymph node disease
Around 8 yrs	Renal tract disease
From 3 yrs onwards	Post-primary disease due to reactivation or re-infection

Adapted from Grange JM. In: Davies PDO, ed. Clinical tuberculosis. London: Hodder Arnold; 1998.

19.54 Features of primary TB

Infection (4–8 wks)

- Influenza-like illness
- Skin test conversion
- Primary complex

Disease

- Lymphadenopathy: hilar (often unilateral), paratracheal or mediastinal
- Collapse (especially right middle lobe)
- Consolidation (especially right middle lobe)
- Obstructive emphysema
- Cavitation (rare)
- Pleural effusion
- Miliary
- Meningitis
- Pericarditis

Hypersensitivity

- Erythema nodosum
- Phlyctenular conjunctivitis
- Dactylitis

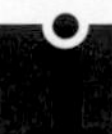

19.55 Cryptic TB

- Age over 60 yrs
- Intermittent low-grade pyrexia of unknown origin
- Unexplained weight loss, general debility (hepatosplenomegaly in 25–50%)
- Normal chest X-ray
- Blood dyscrasias; leukaemoid reaction, pancytopenia
- Negative tuberculin skin test
- Confirmation by biopsy with granulomas and/or acid-fast bacilli in liver or bone marrow

leucopenia reflect bone marrow involvement. 'Cryptic' miliary TB is an unusual presentation sometimes seen in old age (Box 19.55).

Post-primary pulmonary TB

Post-primary disease refers to exogenous ('new' infection) or endogenous (reactivation of a dormant primary lesion) infection in a person who has been sensitised by earlier exposure. It is most frequently pulmonary and characteristically occurs in the apex of an upper lobe, where the oxygen tension favours survival of the strictly aerobic organism. The onset is usually insidious, developing slowly over several weeks. Systemic symptoms include fever, night sweats, malaise, and loss of appetite and weight, and are accompanied by progressive pulmonary symptoms (Box 19.56). Very occasionally, this form of TB may present with one of the complications listed in Box 19.57. Radiological changes include ill-defined opacification in one or both of the upper lobes, and as progression occurs, consolidation, collapse and cavitation develop to varying degrees (Fig. 19.38). It is often difficult to distinguish active from quiescent disease on radiological criteria alone, but the presence of a miliary pattern or cavitation favours active disease. In extensive disease, collapse may be marked and results in significant displacement of the trachea and mediastinum. Occasionally, a caseous lymph node may drain into an adjoining bronchus, leading to tuberculous pneumonia.

Clinical features: extrapulmonary disease

Extrapulmonary tuberculosis accounts for about 20% of cases in those who are HIV-negative but is more common in HIV-positive individuals.

Lymphadenitis

Lymph nodes are the most common extrapulmonary site of disease. Cervical and mediastinal glands are affected most frequently, followed by axillary and inguinal, and more than one region may be involved. Disease may represent primary infection, spread from contiguous sites, or reactivation. Supraclavicular lymphadenopathy is often the result of spread from mediastinal disease. The nodes are usually painless and initially mobile but become matted together with time. When caseation and liquefaction occur, the swelling becomes fluctuant and may discharge through the skin with the formation of a 'collar-stud' abscess and sinus formation. Approximately half of cases fail to show any constitutional features, such as fevers or night sweats. The tuberculin test is usually strongly positive. During or after treatment, paradoxical enlargement,

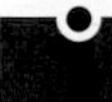

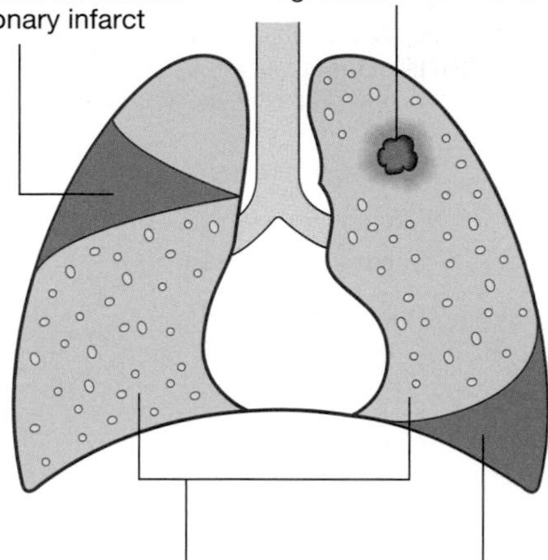
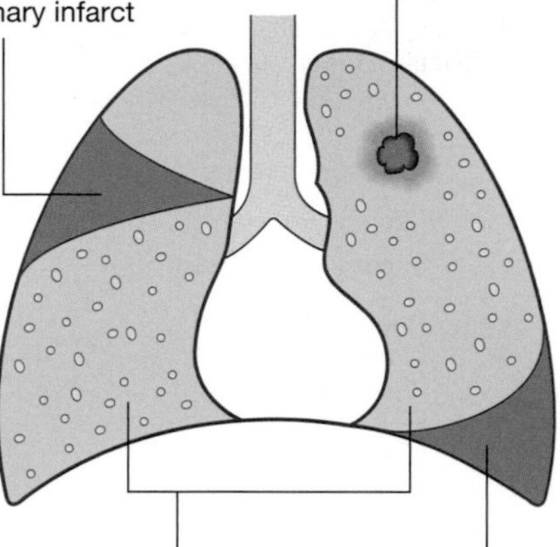

Fig. 19.38 Chest X-ray: major manifestations and differential diagnosis of pulmonary TB. Less common manifestations include pneumothorax, ARDS (p. 192), cor pulmonale and localised emphysema.

development of new nodes and suppuration may all occur but without evidence of continued infection; surgical excision is rarely necessary. In non-immigrant children in the UK, most mycobacterial lymphadenitis is caused by opportunistic mycobacteria, especially of the *M. avium* complex.

Gastrointestinal tuberculosis

TB can affect any part of the bowel and patients may present with a wide range of symptoms and signs (Fig. 19.39). Upper gastrointestinal tract involvement is rare and is usually an unexpected histological finding in an endoscopic or laparotomy specimen. Ileocaecal disease accounts for approximately half of abdominal TB cases. Fever, night sweats, anorexia and weight loss are usually prominent and a right iliac fossa mass may be palpable. Up to 30% of cases present with an acute abdomen. Ultrasound or CT may reveal thickened bowel wall, abdominal lymphadenopathy, mesenteric thickening or ascites. Barium enema and small bowel enema reveal narrowing, shortening and distortion of the bowel, with caecal involvement predominating. Diagnosis rests on obtaining histology by either colonoscopy or mini-laparotomy. The main differential diagnosis is Crohn's disease (p. 897). Tuberculous peritonitis is characterised by abdominal distension, pain and constitutional symptoms. The ascitic fluid is exudative and cellular, with a predominance of lymphocytes. Laparoscopy reveals multiple white 'tubercles' over the peritoneal and omental surfaces. Low-grade hepatic dysfunction is common in miliary disease, in which biopsy reveals

19.56 Clinical presentations of pulmonary TB

• Chronic cough, often with haemoptysis	• Asymptomatic (diagnosis on chest X-ray)
• Pyrexia of unknown origin	• Weight loss, general debility
• Unresolved pneumonia	• Spontaneous pneumothorax
• Exudative pleural effusion	

19.57 Chronic complications of pulmonary TB

Pulmonary	
• Massive haemoptysis	• Aspergilloma
• Cor pulmonale	• Lung/pleural calcification
• Fibrosis/emphysema	• Obstructive airways disease
• Atypical mycobacterial infection	• Bronchiectasis
	• Bronchopleural fistula
Non-pulmonary	
• Empyema necessitans	• Anorectal disease*
• Laryngitis	• Amyloidosis
• Enteritis*	• Poncet's polyarthritis

*From swallowed sputum.

granulomas. Occasionally, patients may be frankly icteric, with a mixed hepatic/cholestatic picture.

Pericardial disease

Disease occurs in two forms (see Fig. 19.39 and p. 639): pericardial effusion and constrictive pericarditis. Fever and night sweats are rarely prominent and the presentation is usually insidious, with breathlessness and abdominal swelling. Coexistent pulmonary disease is very rare, with the exception of pleural effusion. Pulsus paradoxus, a raised JVP, hepatomegaly, prominent ascites and peripheral oedema are common to both types. Pericardial effusion is associated with increased pericardial dullness and a globular enlarged heart on chest X-ray, and pericardial calcification occurs in around 25% of cases. Constriction is associated with an early third heart sound and, occasionally, atrial fibrillation. Diagnosis is based on the clinical, radiological and echocardiographic findings (p. 640). The effusion is frequently blood-stained. Open pericardial biopsy can be performed where there is diagnostic uncertainty. The addition of corticosteroids to anti-tuberculosis treatment has been shown to help both forms of pericardial disease.

Central nervous system disease

Meningeal disease represents the most important form of central nervous system TB. Unrecognised and untreated, it is rapidly fatal. Even when appropriate treatment is prescribed, mortality rates of 30% have been reported, whilst survivors may be left with neurological sequelae. Clinical features, investigations and management are described on page 1204.

Bone and joint disease

The spine is the most common site for bony TB (Pott's disease), which usually presents with chronic back pain and typically involves the lower thoracic and lumbar

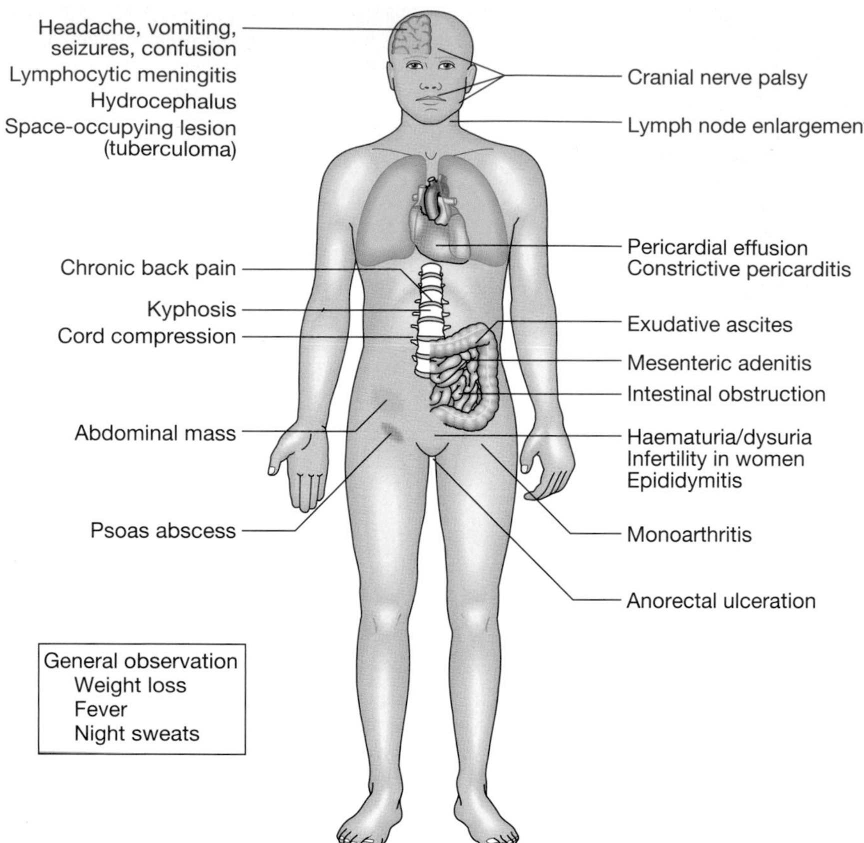

Fig. 19.39 Systemic presentations of extrapulmonary TB.

spine (see Fig. 19.39). The infection starts as a discitis and then spreads along the spinal ligaments to involve the adjacent anterior vertebral bodies, causing angulation of the vertebrae with subsequent kyphosis. Paravertebral and psoas abscess formation is common and the disease may present with a large (cold) abscess in the inguinal region. CT or MRI is valuable in gauging the extent of disease, the amount of cord compression, and the site for needle biopsy or open exploration, if required. The major differential diagnosis is malignancy, which tends to affect the vertebral body and leave the disc intact. Important complications include spinal instability or cord compression.

TB can affect any joint but most frequently involves the hip or knee. Presentation is usually insidious, with pain and swelling; fever and night sweats are uncommon. Radiological changes are often non-specific but, as disease progresses, reduction in joint space and erosions appear. Poncet's arthropathy is an immunologically mediated polyarthritis that usually resolves within 2 months of starting treatment.

Genitourinary disease

Fever and night sweats are rare with renal tract TB and patients are often only mildly symptomatic for many years. Haematuria, frequency and dysuria are often present, with sterile pyuria found on urine microscopy and culture. In women, infertility from endometritis, or pelvic pain and swelling from salpingitis or a tubo-ovarian abscess occurs occasionally. In men, genitourinary TB may present as epididymitis or prostatitis.

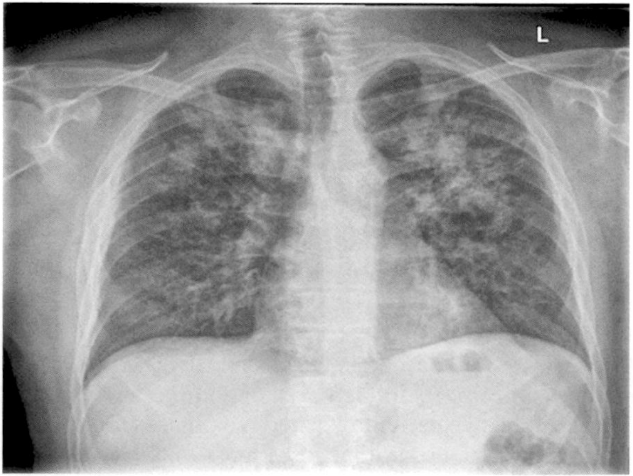

Fig. 19.40 Typical changes of tuberculosis. The chest X-ray shows bilateral upper lobe airspace shadowing with cavitation.

Diagnosis

The presence of an otherwise unexplained cough for more than 2–3 weeks, particularly in regions where TB is prevalent, or typical chest X-ray changes (Fig. 19.40), should prompt further investigation (Box 19.58). Direct microscopy of sputum remains the most important first step. The probability of detecting acid-fast bacilli is proportional to the bacillary burden in the sputum (typically positive when 5000–10 000 organisms are present). By virtue of their substantial, lipid-rich wall, tuberculous bacilli are difficult to stain. The most effective

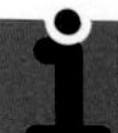

19.58 Diagnosis of TB

Specimens required

Pulmonary
- Sputum* (induced with nebulised hypertonic saline if not expectorating)
- Bronchoscopy with washings or BAL
- Gastric washing* (mainly used for children)

Extrapulmonary
- Fluid examination (cerebrospinal, ascitic, pleural, pericardial, joint): yield classically very low
- Tissue biopsy (from affected site): bone marrow/liver may be diagnostic in disseminated disease

Diagnostic tests
- Tuberculin skin test: low sensitivity/specificity; useful only in primary or deep-seated infection
- Stain
  - Ziehl–Neelsen
  - Auramine fluorescence
- Nucleic acid amplification
- Culture
  - Solid media (Löwenstein–Jensen, Middlebrook)
  - Liquid media (e.g. BACTEC or MGIT)
- Pleural fluid: adenosine deaminase
- Response to empirical antituberculous drugs (usually seen after 5–10 days)

Baseline blood tests
- FBC, CRP, ESR, U&E and LFTs

*At least 2 but preferably 3, including an early morning sample.
(BAL = bronchoalveolar lavage; MGIT = mycobacteria growth indicator tube)

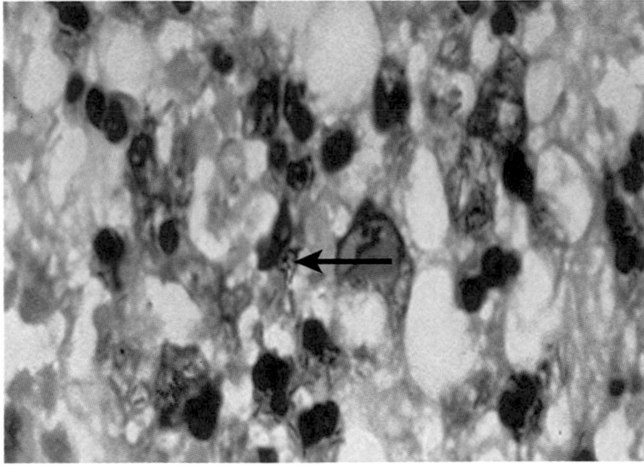

Fig. 19.41 Positive Ziehl–Neelsen stain. Mycobacteria retain the red carbol fuchsin stain, despite washing with acid and alcohol.

techniques are the Ziehl–Neelsen (Fig. 19.41) and rhodamine–auramine. The latter causes the tuberculous bacilli to fluoresce against a dark background and is easier to use when numerous specimens need to be examined; however, it is more complex and expensive, limiting use in resource-poor regions.

A positive smear is sufficient for the presumptive diagnosis of TB but definitive diagnosis requires culture. Smear-negative sputum should also be cultured, as only 10–100 viable organisms are required for sputum to be culture-positive. A diagnosis of smear-negative TB may be made in advance of culture if the chest X-ray appearances are typical of TB and there is no response to a broad-spectrum antibiotic.

MTB grows slowly and may take between 4 and 6 weeks to appear on solid medium, such as Löwenstein–Jensen or Middlebrook. Faster growth (1–3 weeks) occurs in liquid media, such as the radioactive BACTEC system or the non-radiometric mycobacteria growth indicator tube (MGIT). The BACTEC method is the most widely accepted as the reference standard in developed nations and detects mycobacterial growth by measuring the liberation of $^{14}CO_2$, following metabolism of ^{14}C-labelled substrate present in the medium.

Drug sensitivity testing is particularly important in those with a previous history of TB, treatment failure or chronic disease, and in those who are resident in or have visited an area of high prevalence of resistance, or who are HIV-positive. The detection of rifampicin resistance, using molecular tools to test for the presence of the *rpo* gene currently associated with around 95% of rifampicin-resistant cases, is important, as rifampicin forms the cornerstone of 6-month chemotherapy.

Nucleic acid amplification tests, such as the Xpert/RIF test, combine the potential to diagnose TB and detect the presence of rifampicin resistance, and may become the test of first choice in individuals with HIV or those suspected to have multi-drug-resistant tuberculosis (MDR-TB). If a cluster of cases suggests a common source, confirmation may be sought by fingerprinting of isolates with restriction-fragment length polymorphism (RFLP).

The diagnosis of extrapulmonary TB can be more challenging. There are generally fewer organisms (particularly in meningeal or pleural fluid), so culture or histopathological examination of tissue is more important. Adenosine deaminase in pleural fluid, and to a lesser extent in CSF, may assist in confirming suspected TB. In the presence of HIV, examination of sputum may still be useful, as subclinical pulmonary disease is common.

Management

Chemotherapy

The treatment of TB is based on the principle of an initial intensive phase to reduce the bacterial population rapidly, followed by a continuation phase to destroy any remaining bacteria (Box 19.59). Standard treatment involves 6 months' treatment with isoniazid and rifampicin, supplemented in the first 2 months with pyrazinamide and ethambutol. Fixed-dose tablets combining two or three drugs are preferred. Treatment should be commenced immediately in any patient who is smear-positive, or smear-negative but with typical chest X-ray changes and no response to standard antibiotics.

Six months of therapy is appropriate for all patients with new-onset pulmonary TB and most cases of extrapulmonary TB. However, 12 months of therapy is recommended for meningeal TB, including involvement of the spinal cord in cases of spinal TB; in these cases, ethambutol may be replaced by streptomycin. Pyridoxine should be prescribed in pregnant women and malnourished patients to reduce the risk of peripheral neuropathy with isoniazid. Where drug resistance is not anticipated, patients can be assumed to be non-infectious after 2 weeks of appropriate therapy.

19.59 Treatment of new TB patients (World Health Organization recommendations)

Intensive phase	Continuation phase	Comments
Standard regimen		
2 mths of HRZE	4 mths of HR	
2 mths of HRZE	4 mths of HRE	Applies only in countries with high levels of isoniazid resistance in new TB patients, and where isoniazid drug susceptibility testing in new patients is not done (or results are unavailable) before the continuation phase begins
Dosing frequency		
Daily*	Daily	Optimal
Daily*	3 times/wk	Acceptable alternative for any new patient receiving directly observed therapy
3 times/wk	3 times/wk	Acceptable alternative, provided that the patient is receiving directly observed therapy and is NOT living with HIV or living in an HIV-prevalent setting

*Daily (rather than 3 times weekly) intensive-phase dosing may help to prevent acquired drug resistance in TB patients starting treatment with isoniazid resistance. (H = isoniazid; R = rifampicin; Z = pyrazinamide; E = ethambutol) Adapted from WHO Treatment of Tuberculosis Guidelines, 4th edn.

19.60 Main adverse reactions of first-line antituberculous drugs

	Isoniazid	Rifampicin	Pyrazinamide	Streptomycin	Ethambutol
Mode of action	Cell wall synthesis	DNA transcription	Unknown	Protein synthesis	Cell wall synthesis
Major adverse reactions	Peripheral neuropathy[1] Hepatitis[2] Rash	Febrile reactions Hepatitis Rash Gastrointestinal disturbance	Hepatitis Gastrointestinal disturbance Hyperuricaemia	8th nerve damage Rash	Retrobulbar neuritis[3] Arthralgia
Less common adverse reactions	Lupoid reactions Seizures Psychoses	Interstitial nephritis Thrombocytopenia Haemolytic anaemia	Rash Photosensitisation Gout	Nephrotoxicity Agranulocytosis	Peripheral neuropathy Rash

[1]The risk may be reduced by prescribing pyridoxine. [2]More common in patients with a slow acetylator status and in alcoholics. [3]Reduced visual acuity and colour vision may be reported with higher doses and are usually reversible.

Most patients can be treated at home. Admission to a hospital unit with appropriate isolation facilities should be considered where there is uncertainty about the diagnosis, intolerance of medication, questionable treatment adherence, adverse social conditions or a significant risk of MDR-TB (culture-positive after 2 months on treatment, or contact with known MDR-TB).

Patients treated with rifampicin should be advised that their urine, tears and other secretions will develop a bright orange/red coloration, and women taking the oral contraceptive pill must be warned that its efficacy will be reduced and alternative contraception may be necessary. Ethambutol and streptomycin should be used with caution in renal failure, with appropriate dose reduction and monitoring of drug levels. Adverse drug reactions occur in about 10% of patients, but are significantly more common with HIV co-infection (Box 19.60).

Baseline liver function and regular monitoring are important for patients treated with standard therapy. Rifampicin may cause asymptomatic hyperbilirubinaemia but, along with isoniazid and pyrazinamide, may also cause hepatitis. Mild asymptomatic increases in transaminases are common but significant hepatotoxicity only occurs in 2–5%. It is appropriate to stop treatment and allow any symptoms to subside and the liver function tests (LFTs) to recover before commencing a stepwise re-introduction of the individual drugs. Less hepatotoxic regimens may be considered, including streptomycin, ethambutol and fluoroquinolone.

Corticosteroids reduce inflammation and limit tissue damage, and are currently recommended when treating pericardial or meningeal disease, and in children with endobronchial disease. They may confer benefit in TB of the ureter, pleural effusions and extensive pulmonary disease, and can suppress hypersensitivity drug reactions. Surgery should be considered in cases complicated by massive haemoptysis, loculated empyema, constrictive pericarditis, lymph node suppuration, and spinal disease with cord compression, but usually only after a full course of antituberculosis treatment.

The effectiveness of therapy for pulmonary TB is assessed by further sputum smear at 2 months and at 5 months. Treatment failure is defined as a positive sputum smear or culture at 5 months or any patient with a multidrug resistant strain, regardless of whether they are smear-positive or negative. Extrapulmonary TB must be assessed clinically or radiographically, as appropriate.

Control and prevention

The World Health Organization (WHO) is committed to reducing the incidence of TB by 2015. Supporting the development of laboratory and health-care services to improve detection and treatment of active and latent TB is an important component of this goal.

Detection of latent TB

Contact tracing is a legal requirement in many countries. It has the potential to identify the probable index case, other cases infected by the same index patient (with or without evidence of disease), and close contacts who should receive BCG vaccination (see below) or chemotherapy. Approximately 10–20% of close contacts of patients with smear-positive pulmonary TB and 2–5% of those with smear-negative, culture-positive disease have evidence of TB infection.

Cases are commonly identified using the tuberculin skin test (Box 19.61 and Fig 19.42). An otherwise asymptomatic contact with a positive tuberculin skin test but a normal chest X-ray may be treated with chemoprophylaxis to prevent infection from progressing to clinical disease. Chemoprophylaxis is also recommended for children aged less than 16 years identified during contact tracing as having a strongly positive tuberculin test, children aged less than 2 years in close contact with smear-positive pulmonary disease, those in whom recent tuberculin conversion has been confirmed, and babies of mothers with pulmonary TB. It should also be considered for HIV-infected close contacts of a patient with smear-positive disease. A course of rifampicin and isoniazid for 3 months or isoniazid for 6 months is effective.

Tuberculin skin testing may be associated with false-positive reactions in those who have had a BCG vaccination and in areas where exposure to non-tuberculous mycobacteria is high. The skin tests may also be falsely negative in the setting of immunosuppression or overwhelming infection. These limitations may be overcome by employing interferon-gamma release assays (IGRAs) (Fig. 19.43). These tests measure the release of IFN-γ from sensitised T cells in response to antigens, such as early secretory antigenic target (ESAT)-6 or culture filtrate protein (CFP)-10, that are encoded by genes specific to the MTB and are not shared with BCG or opportunistic mycobacteria. The greater specificity of these tests, combined with the logistical convenience of one blood test, as opposed to two visits for skin testing, suggests that IGRAs will replace the tuberculin skin test in low-incidence, high-income countries.

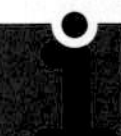

19.61 Skin testing in TB: tests using purified protein derivative (PPD)

Heaf test

- Read at 3–7 days
- Multipuncture method
  - Grade 1: 4–6 papules
  - Grade 2: Confluent papules forming ring
  - Grade 3: Central induration
  - Grade 4: > 10 mm induration

Mantoux test

- Read at 2–4 days
- 10 tuberculin units used
  - Positive when induration 5–14 mm (equivalent to Heaf grade 2) and > 15 mm (Heaf grade 3–4)

False negatives

- Severe TB (25% of cases negative)
- Newborn and elderly
- HIV (if CD4 count < 200 cells/mL)
- Malnutrition
- Recent infection (e.g. measles) or immunisation
- Immunosuppressive drugs
- Malignancy
- Sarcoidosis

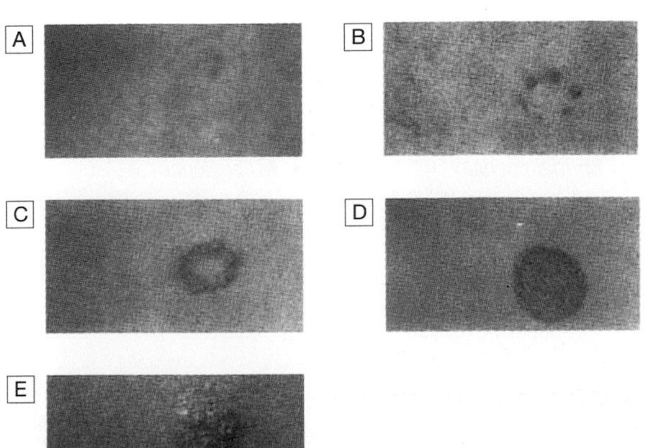

Fig. 19.42 Gradings of the Heaf test response. A Negative. B Grade 1. C Grade 2. D Grade 3. E Grade 4.

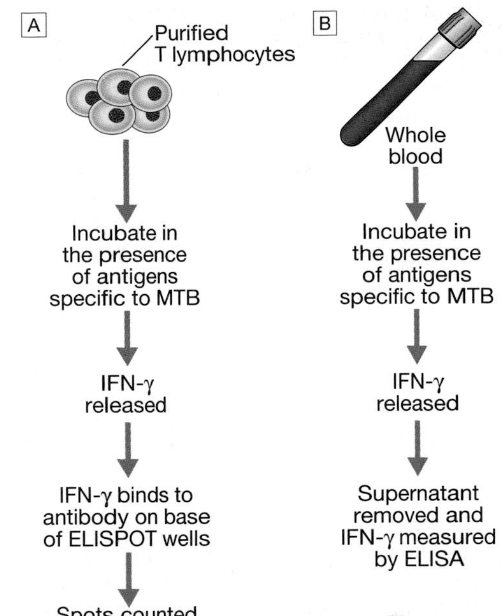

Fig. 19.43 The principles of interferon-gamma release assays. A sample of either purified T cells (T-SPOT.TB® test) or whole blood (QuantiFERON®–TB Gold test) is incubated in the presence of antigens specific to *Mycobacterium tuberculosis* (MTB). The release of interferon-gamma (IFN-γ) by the cells is measured by enzyme-lined immunosorbent assay (ELISA). (ELISPOT = enzyme-linked immunosorbent spot assay)

Directly observed therapy

Poor adherence to therapy is a major factor in prolonged illness, risk of relapse, and the emergence of drug resistance. Directly observed therapy (DOT) involves the supervised administration of therapy 3 times weekly to improve adherence. DOT has become an important control strategy in resource-poor nations. In the UK, it is currently recommended for patients thought unlikely to be adherent to therapy: homeless people and drifters, alcohol or drug users, patients with serious mental illness and those with a history of non-compliance.

TB and HIV/AIDS

The close links between HIV and TB, particularly in sub-Saharan Africa, and the potential for both diseases to overwhelm health-care funding in resource-poor nations have been recognised, with the promotion of programmes that link detection and treatment of TB with detection and treatment of HIV. It is recommended that all patients with TB should be tested for HIV disease. Mortality is high and TB is a leading cause of death in HIV patients. Full discussion of its presentation and management is given on page 400.

Drug-resistant TB

Drug-resistant TB is defined by the presence of resistance to any first-line agent. Multidrug-resistant TB (MDR-TB) is defined by resistance to at least rifampicin and isoniazid, with or without other drug resistance. Extensively drug-resistant TB (XDR-TB) is defined as resistance to at least rifampicin and isoniazid, in addition to any quinolone and at least one injectable second-line agent. The prevalence of MDR-TB is rising, particularly in the former Soviet Union, Central Asia and Africa. It is more common in those with a prior history of TB, particularly if treatment has been inadequate, and those with HIV infection. Box 19.62 lists the factors contributing to the emergence of drug-resistant TB. Diagnosis is challenging, especially in developing countries, and although cure may be possible, it requires prolonged treatment with less effective, more toxic and more expensive therapies. The mortality rate from MDR-TB is high and that from XDR-TB higher still.

Vaccines

BCG (the Calmette–Guérin bacillus), a live attenuated vaccine derived from *M. bovis*, is the most established TB vaccine. It is administered by intradermal injection and is highly immunogenic. BCG appears to be effective in preventing disseminated disease, including tuberculous meningitis, in children, but its efficacy in adults is inconsistent and new vaccines are urgently needed. Current vaccination policies vary worldwide according to incidence and health-care resources, but usually target children and other high-risk individuals. BCG is very safe, with the occasional complication of local abscess formation. It should not be administered to those who are immunocompromised (e.g. by HIV) or pregnant.

Prognosis

Following successful completion of chemotherapy, cure should be anticipated in the majority of patients. There is a small (< 5%) and unavoidable risk of relapse. Most relapses occur within 5 months and usually have the same drug susceptibility. In the absence of treatment, a patient with smear-positive TB will remain infectious for an average of 2 years; in 1 year, 25% of untreated cases will die. Death is more likely in those who are smear-positive and those who smoke. A few patients die unexpectedly soon after commencing therapy and it is possible that some have subclinical hypoadrenalism that is unmasked by a rifampicin-induced increase in steroid metabolism. HIV-positive patients have higher mortality rates and a modestly increased risk of relapse.

19.62 Factors contributing to the emergence of drug-resistant TB

- Drug shortages
- Poor-quality drugs
- Lack of appropriate supervision
- Transmission of drug-resistant strains
- Prior anti-tuberculosis treatment
- Treatment failure (smear-positive at 5 mths)

Opportunistic mycobacterial infection

Other species of environmental mycobacteria (often termed 'atypical') may cause human disease (Box 19.63). The sites commonly involved are the lungs, lymph nodes, skin and soft tissues. The most widely recognised of these mycobacteria, *M. avium* complex (MAC), is well described in severe HIV disease (CD4 count < 50 cells/mL – p. 407). However, several others (including MAC) colonise and/or infect apparently immunocompetent patients with chronic lung diseases such as COPD, bronchiectasis, pneumoconiosis, old TB, or cystic fibrosis. The clinical presentation varies from a relatively indolent course in some to an aggressive course characterised by cavitatory or nodular disease in others. Radiological appearances may be similar to classical TB, but in patients with bronchiectasis, opportunistic infection may present with lower-zone nodules. The most commonly reported organisms include *M. kansasii*, *M. malmoense*, *M. xenopi* and *M. abscessus*, but geographical variation is marked. *M. abscessus* and *M. fortuitum* grow rapidly but the majority grow slowly. More rapid diagnostic systems are under development, including DNA probes, high-performance liquid chromatography (HPLC), PCR restriction enzyme analysis (PRA) and 16S rRNA gene sequence analysis. With the exception of *M. kansasii*, drug sensitivity testing is usually unhelpful in predicting treatment response. There is usually no requirement for notification, as the organisms are not normally communicable.

19.63 Site-specific opportunistic mycobacterial disease

Pulmonary	
• *M. xenopi* • *M. kansasii*	• *M. malmoense* • MAC
Lymph node	
• MAC • *M. malmoense*	• *M. fortuitum* • *M. chelonei*
Soft tissue/skin	
• *M. leprae* • *M. ulcerans* (prevalent in Africa, northern Australia and South-east Asia)	• *M. marinum* • *M. fortuitum* • *M. chelonei*
Disseminated	
• MAC (HIV-associated) • *M. haemophilum* • *M. genavense*	• *M. fortuitum* • *M. chelonei* • BCG

(BCG = bacille Calmette–Guérin; MAC = *Mycobacterium avium* complex – *M. scrofulaceum*, *M. intracellulare* and *M. avium*)

Respiratory diseases caused by fungi

The majority of fungi encountered by humans are harmless saprophytes but in certain circumstances (Box 19.64) some species may cause disease by infecting human tissue, promoting damaging allergic reactions or producing toxins. 'Mycosis' is the term applied to disease caused by fungal infection.

Aspergillus species

Most cases of bronchopulmonary aspergillosis are caused by *Aspergillus fumigatus*, but other members of the genus (*A. clavatus*, *A. flavus*, *A. niger* and *A. terreus*) occasionally cause disease. The conditions associated with *Aspergillus* species are listed in Box 19.65.

Allergic bronchopulmonary aspergillosis

Allergic bronchopulmonary aspergillosis (ABPA) occurs as a result of a hypersensitivity reaction to germinating fungal spores in the airway wall. The condition may complicate the course of asthma and cystic fibrosis, and is a recognised cause of pulmonary eosinophilia (p. 713). The prevalence of ABPA is approximately 1–2% in asthma and 5–10% in cystic fibrosis. A variety of human leucocyte antigens (HLA) convey both an increased and a decreased risk of developing the condition, suggesting that genetic susceptibility is important.

Clinical features and investigations

Clinical features depend on the stage of the disease. Common manifestations in the early phase include fever, breathlessness, cough productive of bronchial casts, and worsening of asthmatic symptoms. The appearance of radiographic infiltrates may cause ABPA to be mistaken for pneumonia, but the diagnosis may also be suggested by segmental or lobar collapse on chest X-rays of patients whose asthma symptoms are stable. Diagnostic features are shown in Box 19.66 and the typical *Aspergillus* hyphae in Figure 19.44. If bronchiectasis develops, its symptoms and complications often overshadow those of asthma.

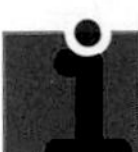

19.64 Factors predisposing to fungal disease

Systemic factors

- Diabetes mellitus
- Chronic alcoholism
- HIV
- Radiotherapy
- Corticosteroids and other immunosuppressant medication

Local factors

- Tissue damage by suppuration or necrosis
- Alteration of normal bacterial flora by antibiotic therapy

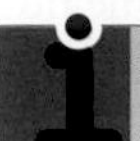

19.65 Classification of bronchopulmonary aspergillosis

- Allergic bronchopulmonary aspergillosis (asthmatic pulmonary eosinophilia)
- Extrinsic allergic alveolitis (*Aspergillus clavatus*)
- Intracavitary aspergilloma
- Invasive pulmonary aspergillosis
- Chronic and subacute pulmonary aspergillosis

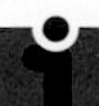

19.66 Features of allergic bronchopulmonary aspergillosis

- Asthma (in the majority of cases)
- Proximal bronchiectasis (inner two-thirds of chest CT field)
- Positive skin test to an extract of *A. fumigatus*
- Elevated total serum IgE > 417 KU/L or 1000 ng/mL
- Elevated serum IgE (*A. fumigatus*) or IgG (*A. fumigatus*)
- Peripheral blood eosinophilia > 0.5×10^9/L
- Presence or history of chest X-ray abnormalities
- Fungal hyphae of *A. fumigatus* on microscopic examination of sputum

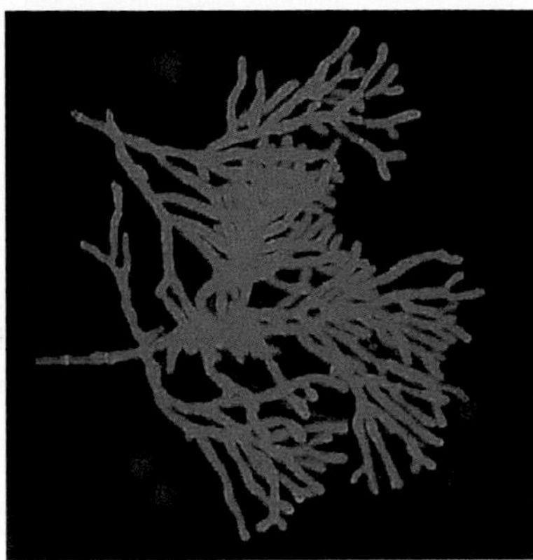

Fig. 19.44 Branching *Aspergillus* hyphae seen in ABPA. The figure shows the use of calcofluor white, a non-specific fluorochrome stain that binds to fungi and fluoresces when exposed to light of the appropriate wavelength. *Aspergillus fumigatus* was subsequently grown on culture.

Management

ABPA is generally considered an indication for regular therapy with low-dose oral corticosteroids (prednisolone 7.5–10 mg daily), with the aim of suppressing the immunopathological responses and preventing progressive tissue damage. In some patients, itraconazole (400 mg/day) facilitates a reduction in oral steroids, and a 4-month trial is usually recommended to assess its efficacy. The use of specific anti-IgE monoclonal antibodies is under consideration. Exacerbations, particularly when associated with new chest X-ray changes, should be treated promptly with prednisolone 40–60 mg daily and physiotherapy. If persistent lobar collapse occurs, bronchoscopy (usually under general anaesthetic) should be performed to remove impacted mucus and ensure prompt re-inflation.

Aspergilloma

Inhaled *Aspergillus* may lodge and germinate in areas of damaged lung tissue, forming a fungal ball or 'aspergilloma'. The upper lobes are most frequently involved and fungal balls readily form in tuberculous cavities (Fig. 19.45). Less common causes include damage from a lung abscess cavity, a bronchiectatic space, pulmonary infarct, sarcoid, ankylosing spondylitis or even a cavitated tumour. The presence of multiple aspergilloma cavities in a diseased area of lung has been termed a 'complex aspergilloma' (see below).

Clinical features and investigations

Simple aspergillomas are often asymptomatic and are identified incidentally on chest X-ray. However, they

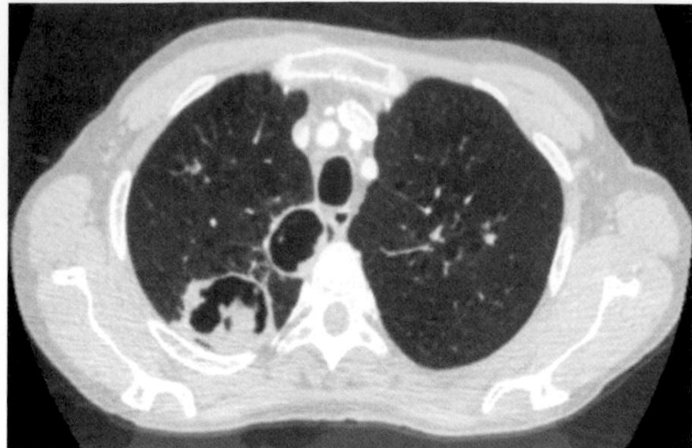

Fig. 19.45 CT of aspergilloma in the left upper lobe. The rounded fungal ball is separated from the wall of the cavity by a 'halo' of air.

may cause recurrent haemoptysis, which may be severe and life-threatening. Non-specific systemic features, such as lethargy and weight loss, may also be reported.

The fungal ball produces a tumour-like opacity on X-ray, but can be distinguished from a carcinoma by the presence of a crescent of air between the fungal ball and the upper wall of the cavity. HRCT is more sensitive (see Fig. 19.45). Elevated serum precipitins to *A. fumigatus* are found in virtually all patients. Sputum microscopy typically demonstrates scanty hyphal fragments and is usually positive on culture. Less than half exhibit skin hypersensitivity to extracts of *A. fumigatus*. Rarely, other filamentous fungi can cause intracavitary mycetoma and are identified by culture.

Management

Asymptomatic cases do not require treatment. Specific antifungal therapy is of no value and steroids may predispose to invasion. Aspergillomas complicated by haemoptysis should be excised surgically. In those unfit for surgery, palliative procedures range from local instillation of amphotericin B to bronchial artery embolisation. The latter may be used to control haemoptysis prior to definitive surgery.

Invasive pulmonary aspergillosis

Invasive pulmonary aspergillosis (IPA) is most commonly a complication of profound neutropenia caused by drugs (especially immunosuppressants) and/or disease (Box 19.67).

Clinical features and investigations

Acute IPA causes a severe necrotising pneumonia and must be considered in any immunocompromised patient who develops fever, new respiratory symptoms (particularly pleural pain or haemoptysis) or a pleural rub. Invasion of pulmonary vessels causes thrombosis and infarction, and systemic spread may occur to the brain, heart, kidneys and others organs. Tracheobronchial aspergillosis involvement is characterised by the formation of fungal plaques and ulceration.

HRCT characteristically shows macronodules (usually ≥ 1 cm), which may be surrounded by a 'halo' of low attenuation if captured early (< 5 days). Culture or histopathological evidence of *Aspergillus* in diseased tissues provides a definitive diagnosis, but the majority of patients are too ill for invasive tests such as bronchoscopy or lung biopsy. Other investigations include detection of *Aspergillus* cell wall components (galactomannan and β-1,3-glucan) in blood or BAL fluid and *Aspergillus* DNA by PCR. Diagnosis is often inferred from a combination of features (Box 19.68).

Management and prevention

IPA carries a high mortality rate, especially if treatment is delayed. The treatment of choice is voriconazole. Second-line agents include liposomal amphotericin,

19.67 Risk factors for invasive aspergillosis

- Neutropenia: risk related to duration and degree
- Solid organ or allogeneic stem cell transplantation
- Prolonged high-dose corticosteroid therapy
- Leukaemia and other haematological malignancies
- Cytotoxic chemotherapy
- Advanced HIV disease
- Severe COPD
- Critically ill patients on intensive care units
- Chronic granulomatous disease

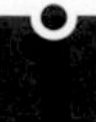

19.68 Criteria for the diagnosis of probable invasive pulmonary aspergillosis[1]

Host factors

- Recent history of neutropenia (< 0.5×10^9/L for ≥ 10 days) temporally related to the onset of fungal disease
- Recipient of allogeneic stem cell transplant
- Prolonged use of corticosteroids (average minimum 0.3 mg/kg/day prednisolone or equivalent) for > 3 wks (excludes ABPA)
- Treatment with other recognised T-cell immune suppressants, such as ciclosporin, TNF-α blockers, specific monoclonal antibodies (e.g. alemtuzumab) or nucleoside analogues during the last 90 days
- Inherited severe immune deficiency, e.g. chronic granulomatous disease or severe combined immune deficiency (p. 80)

Clinical criteria[2]

- The presence of one of the following on CT:
  1. Dense, well-circumscribed lesion(s) with or without a halo sign
  2. Air crescent sign
  3. Cavity

Tracheobronchitis

- Tracheobronchial ulceration, nodule, pseudomembrane, plaque or eschar seen on bronchoscopy

Mycological criteria

- Mould in sputum, BAL fluid or bronchial brush, indicated by one of the following:
  1. Recovery of fungal elements indicating a mould of *Aspergillus*
  2. Recovery by culture of a mould of *Aspergillus*
- Indirect tests (detection of antigen or cell wall constituents)
  1. Galactomannan antigen in plasma, serum or BAL fluid
  2. β-1,3-glucan detected in serum (detects other species of fungi, as well as *Aspergillus*)[3]

[1]Adapted from European Organisation for Research and Treatment of Cancer/Mycoses Study Group. [2]Must be consistent with the mycological findings and temporally related to current episode. [3]May be useful as a preliminary screening tool for invasive aspergillosis.

caspofungin or posaconazole. Response may be assessed clinically, radiologically and serologically (by estimation of the circulating galactomannan level). Recovery is dependent on immune reconstitution, which may be accompanied by enlargement and/or cavitation of pulmonary nodules.

Patients at risk of *Aspergillus* (and other fungal infections) should be nursed in rooms with high-efficiency particulate air (HEPA) filters and laminar airflow. In areas with high spore counts, patients are advised to wear a mask if venturing outside their hospital room. Posaconazole (200 mg 3 times daily) or itraconazole (200 mg/day) may be prescribed for primary prophylaxis, and patients with a history of definite or probable IPA should be considered for secondary prophylaxis before further immunosuppression.

Chronic and subacute pulmonary aspergillosis

Chronic pulmonary aspergillosis (CPA) is an indolent non-invasive complication of chronic lung disease, such as COPD, tuberculosis, opportunistic mycobacterial disease or fibrotic lung disease. It may be associated with malnutrition, diabetes or liver disease and co-infection with opportunistic mycobacteria. CPA may mimic tuberculosis, resulting in its delayed diagnosis. Features include cough (with or without haemoptysis), weight loss, anorexia and fatigue over months or years, with associated fever, night sweats and elevated inflammatory markers. Radiological features include thick-walled cavities (predominantly apical), pulmonary infiltrates, pleural thickening and, later, fibrosis. The terms chronic necrotising (CNPA), cavitary ('complex aspergilloma') and fibrosing pulmonary aspergillosis have been applied, depending on the predominant features. There is overlap between CNPA and 'subacute' and 'semi-invasive' aspergillosis. Subacute aspergillosis is increasingly recognised in intensive care patients, especially those with COPD. The diagnosis is made by a combination of radiological examination, histopathology, isolation of fungus from the respiratory tract and detection of *Aspergillus* IgG in serum. Treatment usually involves prolonged indefinite courses of itraconazole or voriconazole, but cure is unusual. The most frequent pattern is chronic relapse/remission with gradual deterioration. Surgical intervention is fraught with complications and should be avoided.

Other fungal infections

Mucormycosis (p. 384) may present with a pulmonary syndrome indistinguishable clinically from acute IPA. Diagnosis relies on histopathology (where available) and/or culture of the organism from diseased tissue. The principles of treatment are as for other forms of mucormycosis: correction of predisposing factors, antifungal therapy with high-dose lipid amphotericin B or posaconazole, and surgical débridement.

Histoplasmosis, coccidioidomycosis, blastomycosis and cryptococcosis are discussed on pages 384–386.

TUMOURS OF THE BRONCHUS AND LUNG

Lung cancer is the most common cause of death from cancer worldwide, causing 1.4 million deaths per year (Box 19.69). Tobacco use is the major preventable cause. Just as tobacco use and cancer rates are falling in some developed countries, both smoking and lung cancer are rising in Eastern Europe and in many developing countries. The great majority of tumours in the lung are primary bronchial carcinomas and, in contrast to many other tumours, the prognosis remains poor, with fewer than 30% of patients surviving at 1 year and 6–8% at 5 years. Carcinomas of many other organs, as well as osteogenic and other sarcomas, may cause metastatic pulmonary deposits.

19.69 The burden of lung cancer

- Strikes 900 000 men and 330 000 women each year
- Accounts for 18% of all cancer deaths
- More than a threefold increase in deaths since 1950
- Rates rising in women: female lung cancer deaths outnumber male in some Nordic countries
- Has overtaken breast cancer in several countries, making it the most common cause of cancer death in men and women

Primary tumours of the lung

Aetiology

Cigarette smoking is by far the most important cause of lung cancer. It is thought to be directly responsible for at least 90% of lung carcinomas, the risk being proportional to the amount smoked and to the tar content of cigarettes. The death rate from the disease in heavy smokers is 40 times that in non-smokers. Risk falls slowly after smoking cessation, but remains above that in non-smokers for many years. It is estimated that 1 in 2 smokers dies from a smoking-related disease, about half in middle age. The effect of 'passive' smoking is more difficult to quantify but is currently thought to be a factor in 5% of all lung cancer deaths. Exposure to naturally occurring radon is another risk. The incidence of lung cancer is slightly higher in urban than in rural dwellers, which may reflect differences in atmospheric pollution (including tobacco smoke) or occupation, since a number of industrial materials are associated with lung cancer (p. 266). In recent years, the strong link between smoking and ill health has led many Western governments to legislate against smoking in public places, and smoking prevalence and some smoking-related diseases are already declining in these countries (p. 100).

Bronchial carcinoma

The incidence of bronchial carcinoma increased dramatically during the 20th century as a direct result of the tobacco epidemic (Fig. 19.46). In women, smoking prevalence and deaths from lung cancer continue to increase, and more women now die of lung cancer than breast cancer in the USA and the UK.

Pathology

Bronchial carcinomas arise from the bronchial epithelium or mucous glands. The common cell types are listed in Box 19.70. When the tumour occurs in a large bronchus, symptoms arise early, but tumours originating in a peripheral bronchus can grow very large without

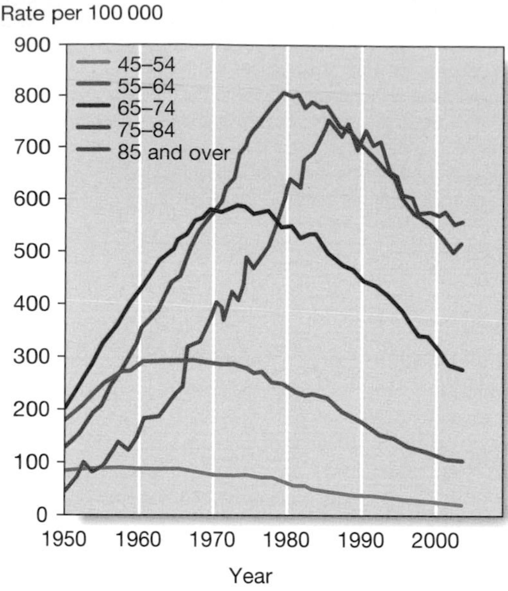

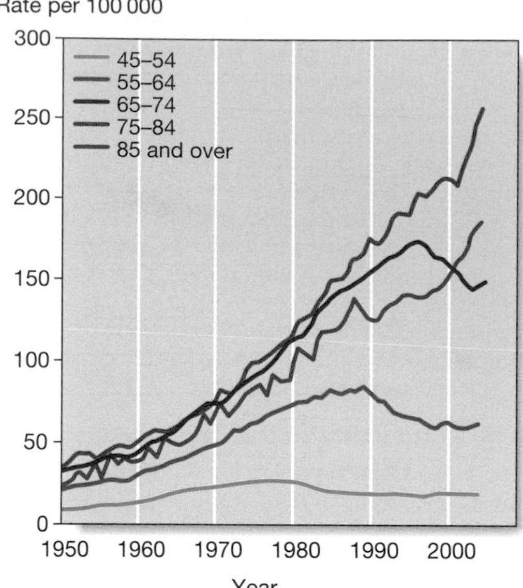

Fig. 19.46 Mortality trends from lung cancer in England and Wales, 1950–2004, by age and year of death. A Males. B Females. Note the decline in mortality from lung cancer in men towards the end of this period, reflecting a change in smoking habit.

19.70 Common cell types in bronchial carcinoma

Cell type	%
Squamous	35
Adenocarcinoma	30
Small-cell	20
Large-cell	15

producing symptoms, resulting in delayed diagnosis. Peripheral squamous tumours may undergo central necrosis and cavitation, and may resemble a lung abscess on X-ray (Fig. 19.47). Bronchial carcinoma may involve the pleura directly or by lymphatic spread, and may extend into the chest wall, invading the intercostal nerves or the brachial plexus and causing pain. Lymphatic spread to mediastinal and supraclavicular lymph nodes often occurs before diagnosis. Blood-borne metastases occur most commonly in liver, bone, brain, adrenals and skin. Even a small primary tumour may cause widespread metastatic deposits and this is a particular characteristic of small-cell lung cancers.

Clinical features

Lung cancer presents in many different ways, reflecting local, metastatic or paraneoplastic tumour effects.

- *Cough*. This is the most common early symptom. It is often dry but secondary infection may cause purulent sputum. A change in the character of a smoker's cough, particularly if associated with other new symptoms, should always raise suspicion of bronchial carcinoma.
- *Haemoptysis*. Haemoptysis is common, especially with central bronchial tumours. Although it may be caused by bronchitic infection, haemoptysis in a smoker should always be investigated to exclude a bronchial carcinoma. Occasionally, central tumours invade large vessels, causing sudden massive haemoptysis that may be fatal.
- *Bronchial obstruction*. This is another common presentation, and the clinical and radiological manifestations (Figs 19.48 and 19.5, p. 650; Box 19.71) depend on the site and extent of the obstruction, any secondary infection, and the extent of coexisting lung disease. Complete obstruction causes collapse of a lobe or lung, with breathlessness, mediastinal displacement and dullness to percussion with reduced breath sounds. Partial bronchial obstruction may cause a monophonic, unilateral wheeze that fails to clear

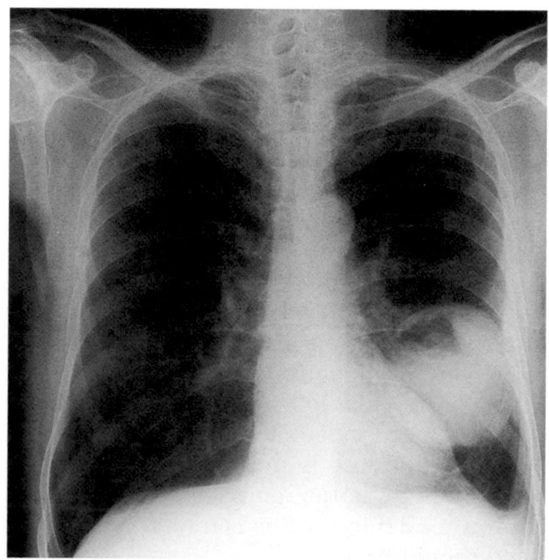

Fig. 19.47 Large cavitated bronchial carcinoma in left lower lobe.

A

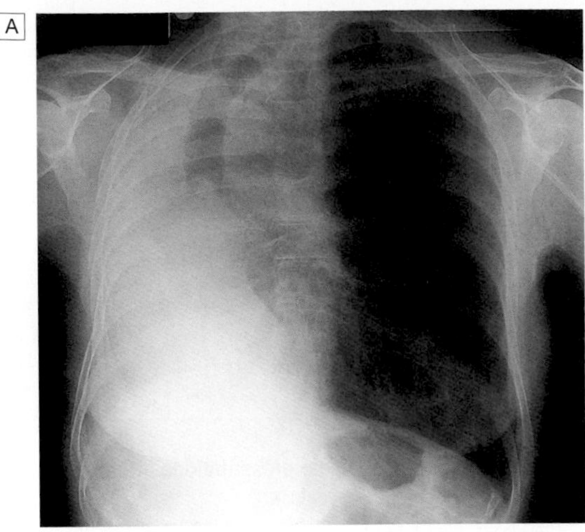

B

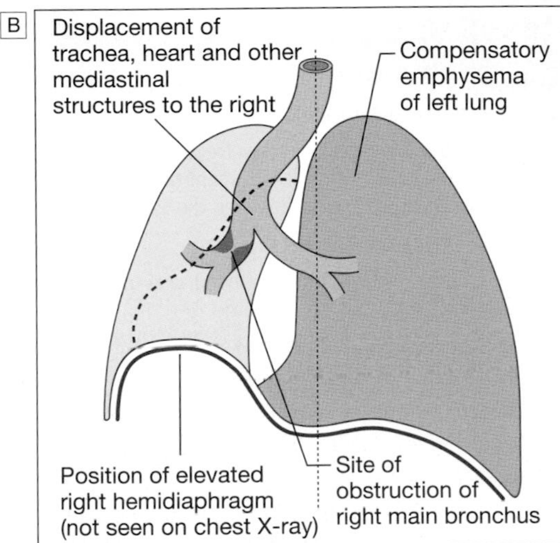

Fig. 19.48 Collapse of the right lung: effects on neighbouring structures. A Chest X-ray. B The typical abnormalities are highlighted.

19.71 Causes of large bronchus obstruction

Common

- Bronchial carcinoma or adenoma
- Enlarged tracheobronchial lymph nodes (malignant or tuberculous)
- Inhaled foreign bodies (especially right lung)
- Bronchial casts or plugs consisting of inspissated mucus or blood clot (especially asthma, cystic fibrosis, haemoptysis, debility)
- Collections of mucus or mucopus retained in the bronchi as a result of ineffective expectoration (especially postoperative following abdominal surgery)

Rare

- Aortic aneurysm
- Giant left atrium
- Pericardial effusion
- Congenital bronchial atresia
- Fibrous bronchial stricture (e.g. following tuberculosis or bronchial surgery/lung transplant)

with coughing, and may also impair the drainage of secretions to cause pneumonia or lung abscess as a presenting problem. Pneumonia that recurs at the same site or responds slowly to treatment, particularly in a smoker, should always suggest an underlying bronchial carcinoma. Stridor (a harsh inspiratory noise) occurs when the larynx, trachea or a main bronchus is narrowed by the primary tumour or by compression from malignant enlargement of the subcarinal and paratracheal lymph nodes.

- *Breathlessness.* Breathlessness may be caused by collapse or pneumonia, or by tumour causing a large pleural effusion or compressing a phrenic nerve and leading to diaphragmatic paralysis.
- *Pain and nerve entrapment.* Pleural pain usually indicates malignant pleural invasion, although it can occur with distal infection. Intercostal nerve involvement causes pain in the distribution of a thoracic dermatome. Carcinoma in the lung apex may cause Horner's syndrome (ipsilateral partial ptosis, enophthalmos, miosis and hypohidrosis of the face – p. 1172) due to involvement of the sympathetic chain at or above the stellate ganglion. Pancoast's syndrome (pain in the inner aspect of the arm, sometimes with small muscle wasting in the hand) indicates malignant destruction of the T1 and C8 roots in the lower part of the brachial plexus by an apical lung tumour.
- *Mediastinal spread.* Involvement of the oesophagus may cause dysphagia. If the pericardium is invaded, arrhythmia or pericardial effusion may occur. Superior vena cava obstruction by malignant nodes causes suffusion and swelling of the neck and face, conjunctival oedema, headache and dilated veins on the chest wall, and is most commonly due to bronchial carcinoma. Involvement of the left recurrent laryngeal nerve by tumours at the left hilum causes vocal cord paralysis, voice alteration and a 'bovine' cough (lacking the normal explosive character). Supraclavicular lymph nodes may be palpably enlarged or identified using ultrasound; if so, a needle aspirate may provide a simple means of cytological diagnosis.
- *Metastatic spread.* This may lead to focal neurological defects, epileptic seizures, personality change, jaundice, bone pain or skin nodules. Lassitude, anorexia and weight loss usually indicate metastatic spread.
- *Finger clubbing.* Overgrowth of the soft tissue of the terminal phalanx, leading to increased nail curvature and nail bed fluctuation, is often seen (p. 644).
- *Hypertrophic pulmonary osteoarthropathy (HPOA).* This is a painful periostitis of the distal tibia, fibula, radius and ulna, with local tenderness and sometimes pitting oedema over the anterior shin. X-rays reveal subperiosteal new bone formation. While most frequently associated with bronchial carcinoma, HPOA can occur with other tumours.
- *Non-metastatic extrapulmonary effects* (Box 19.72). The syndrome of inappropriate antidiuretic hormone secretion (SIADH, p. 438) and ectopic adrenocorticotrophic hormone secretion (p. 774) are usually associated with small-cell lung cancer. Hypercalcaemia may indicate malignant bone

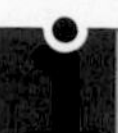

19.72 Non-metastatic extrapulmonary manifestations of bronchial carcinoma

Endocrine (Ch. 20)

- Inappropriate antidiuretic hormone secretion causing hyponatraemia
- Ectopic adrenocorticotrophic hormone secretion
- Hypercalcaemia due to secretion of parathyroid hormone-related peptides
- Carcinoid syndrome (p. 889)
- Gynaecomastia

Neurological (Ch. 26)

- Polyneuropathy
- Myelopathy
- Cerebellar degeneration
- Myasthenia (Lambert–Eaton syndrome, p. 1227)

Other

- Digital clubbing
- Hypertrophic pulmonary osteoarthropathy
- Nephrotic syndrome
- Polymyositis and dermatomyositis
- Eosinophilia

destruction or production of hormone-like peptides by a tumour. Associated neurological syndromes may occur with any type of bronchial carcinoma.

Investigations

The main aims of investigation are to confirm the diagnosis, establish the histological cell type and define the extent of the disease.

Imaging

Bronchial carcinoma produces a range of appearances on chest X-ray, from lobar collapse (see Fig. 19.5, p. 650) to mass lesions, effusion or malignant rib destruction (Fig. 19.49 and Box 19.73). CT should be performed early as it may reveal mediastinal or metastatic spread and is helpful for planning biopsy procedures: for example, in establishing whether a tumour is accessible by bronchoscopy or percutaneous CT-guided biopsy.

Biopsy and histopathology

Around three-quarters of primary lung tumours can be visualised and sampled directly by biopsy and brushing using a flexible bronchoscope. Bronchoscopy also allows an assessment of operability, from the proximity of central tumours to the main carina (Fig. 19.50).

For tumours which are too peripheral to be accessible by bronchoscope, the yield of 'blind' bronchoscopic washings and brushings from the radiologically affected area is low, and percutaneous needle biopsy under CT or ultrasound guidance is a more reliable way to obtain a histological diagnosis. There is a small risk of iatrogenic pneumothorax, which may preclude the procedure if there is extensive coexisting COPD. In patients who are unfit for invasive investigation, sputum cytology can reveal malignant cells (Fig. 19.51), although the yield is low.

In patients with pleural effusions, pleural aspiration and biopsy is the preferred investigation. Where facilities exist, thoracoscopy increases yield by allowing targeted biopsies under direct vision. In patients with metastatic disease, the diagnosis can often be confirmed

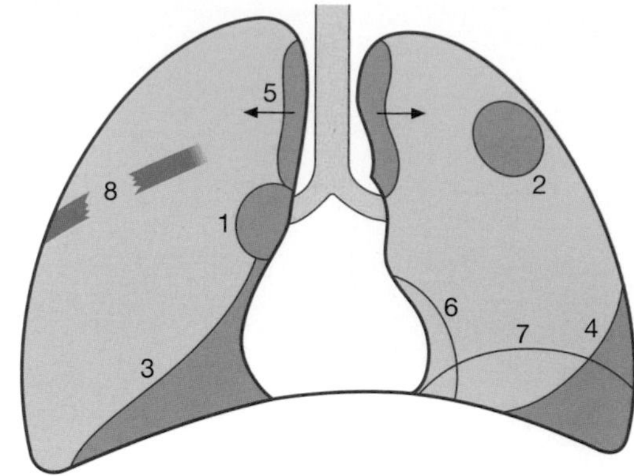

Fig. 19.49 Common radiological presentations of bronchial carcinoma. See Box 19.73 for details.

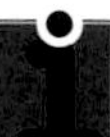

19.73 Common radiological presentations of bronchial carcinoma

1 Unilateral hilar enlargement

- Central tumour. Hilar glandular involvement. However, a peripheral tumour in the apical segment of a lower lobe can look like an enlarged hilar shadow on the PA X-ray

2 Peripheral pulmonary opacity (p. 660)

- Usually irregular but well circumscribed, and may contain irregular cavitation. Can be very large

3 Lung, lobe or segmental collapse

- Usually caused by tumour within the bronchus, leading to occlusion. Lung collapse may be due to compression of the main bronchus by enlarged lymph glands

4 Pleural effusion

- Usually indicates tumour invasion of pleural space; very rarely, a manifestation of infection in collapsed lung tissue distal to a bronchial carcinoma

5–7 Broadening of mediastinum, enlarged cardiac shadow, elevation of a hemidiaphragm

- Paratracheal lymphadenopathy may cause widening of the upper mediastinum. A malignant pericardial effusion will cause enlargement of the cardiac shadow. If a raised hemidiaphragm is caused by phrenic nerve palsy, screening will show it to move paradoxically upwards when patient sniffs

8 Rib destruction

- Direct invasion of the chest wall or blood-borne metastatic spread can cause osteolytic lesions of the ribs

by needle aspiration or biopsy of affected lymph nodes, skin lesions, liver or bone marrow.

Staging to guide treatment

The propensity of small-cell lung cancer to metastasise early dictates that patients with this are usually not suitable for surgical intervention. In patients with non-small-cell cancer, appropriate treatment and prognosis are determined by disease extent, so careful staging is required. CT scanning is used early to detect obvious local or distant spread. Enlarged upper mediastinal nodes may be sampled using a bronchoscope equipped with endobronchial ultrasound (EBUS) or by mediastinoscopy. Nodes in the lower mediastinum can be

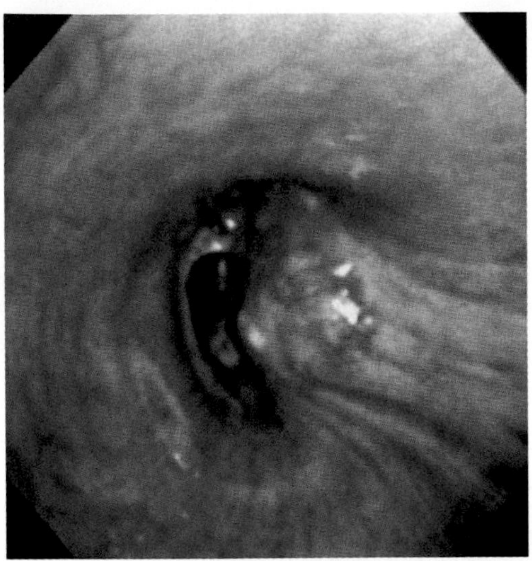

Fig. 19.50 Bronchoscopic view of a bronchogenic carcinoma. There is distortion of mucosal folds, partial occlusion of the airway lumen and abnormal tumour tissue.

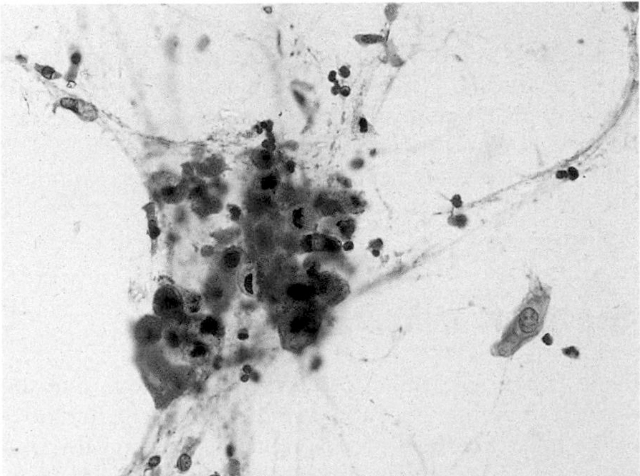

Fig. 19.51 Sputum sample showing a cluster of carcinoma cells. There is keratinisation, with orangeophilia of the cytoplasm. Non-keratinised forms are also seen. The nuclei are large and 'coal-black' in density. These features suggest squamous cell bronchogenic carcinoma.

sampled through the oesophageal wall using endoscopic ultrasound. Combined CT and PET imaging (see Fig. 19.6, p. 651) is used increasingly to detect metabolically active tumour metastases. Head CT, radionuclide bone scanning, liver ultrasound and bone marrow biopsy are generally reserved for patients with clinical, haematological or biochemical evidence of tumour spread to these sites. Information on tumour size and nodal and metastatic spread is then collated to assign the patient to one of seven staging groups that determine optimal management and prognosis (Fig. 19.52). Detailed physiological testing is required to assess whether the patient's respiratory and cardiac function is sufficient to allow aggressive treatment.

Management

Surgical resection carries the best hope of long-term survival, but some patients treated with radical radiotherapy and chemotherapy also achieve prolonged remission or cure. Unfortunately, in over 75% of cases, treatment with the aim of cure is not possible, or is inappropriate due to extensive spread or comorbidity. Such patients are offered palliative therapy and best supportive care. Radiotherapy and in some cases chemotherapy can relieve distressing symptoms.

Surgical treatment

Accurate pre-operative staging, coupled with improvements in surgical and post-operative care, now offers 5-year survival rates of over 75% in stage I disease (N0, tumour confined within visceral pleura) and 55% in stage II disease, which includes resection in patients with ipsilateral peribronchial or hilar node involvement.

Radiotherapy

While much less effective than surgery, radical radiotherapy can offer long-term survival in selected patients with localised disease in whom comorbidity precludes surgery. Radical radiotherapy is usually combined with chemotherapy when lymph nodes are involved (stage III). Highly targeted (stereotactic) radiotherapy may be given in 3–5 treatments for small lesions.

The greatest value of radiotherapy, however, is in the palliation of distressing complications, such as superior

<table>
<tr><th rowspan="2">Tumour stage</th><th colspan="4">Lymph node spread</th></tr>
<tr><th>N0
(None)</th><th>N1
(Ipsilateral hilar)</th><th>N2
(Ipsilateral mediastinal or subcarinal)</th><th>N3
(Contralateral or supraclavicular)</th></tr>
<tr><td>T1 (<3 cm)</td><td>Ia (50%)</td><td rowspan="2">IIa (36%)</td><td rowspan="3">IIIa (19%)</td><td rowspan="4">IIIb (7%)</td></tr>
<tr><td>T2a (3–5 cm)</td><td>Ib (43%)</td></tr>
<tr><td>T2b (5–7 cm)</td><td>IIa (36%)</td><td>IIb (25%)</td></tr>
<tr><td>T3 (>7 cm)</td><td>IIb (25%)</td><td colspan="2">IIIa (19%)</td></tr>
<tr><td>T4 (Invading heart, vessels, oesophagus, carina etc.)</td><td colspan="2">IIIa (19%)</td><td colspan="2">IIIb (7%)</td></tr>
<tr><td>M1 Metastases present</td><td colspan="4">IV (2%)</td></tr>
</table>

Fig. 19.52 Tumour stage and 5-year survival in non-small cell lung cancer. The figure shows the relationship between tumour extent (size, lymph node status and metastases) and average prognosis (% survival at 5 years for each clinical stage). Adapted from Detterbeck 2009 - see p. 732.

vena cava obstruction, recurrent haemoptysis, and pain caused by chest wall invasion or by skeletal metastatic deposits. Obstruction of the trachea and main bronchi can also be relieved temporarily. Radiotherapy can be used in conjunction with chemotherapy in the treatment of small-cell carcinoma, and is particularly efficient at preventing the development of brain metastases in patients who have had a complete response to chemotherapy (p. 277).

Chemotherapy

The treatment of small-cell carcinoma with combinations of cytotoxic drugs, sometimes in combination with radiotherapy, can increase the median survival from 3 months to well over a year. The use of combinations of chemotherapeutic drugs requires considerable skill and should be overseen by teams of clinical oncologists and specialist nurses. Combination chemotherapy leads to better outcomes than single-agent treatment. Regular cycles of therapy, including combinations of intravenous cyclophosphamide, doxorubicin and vincristine or intravenous cisplatin and etoposide, are commonly used. In general, chemotherapy is less effective in non-small-cell bronchial cancers. However, studies in such patients using platinum-based chemotherapy regimens have shown a 30% response rate associated with a small increase in survival. Some non-small-cell lung tumours, particularly adenocarcinomas, carry detectable mutations in the epidermal growth factor receptor (*EGFR*) gene. Patients with these mutations are particularly responsive to the tyrosine kinase inhibitors gefitinib and erlotinib.

In non-small-cell carcinoma, there is some evidence that chemotherapy given before surgery may increase survival and can effectively 'down-stage' disease with limited nodal spread. Post-operative chemotherapy is now proven to enhance survival rates when operative samples show nodal involvement by tumour.

Nausea and vomiting are common side-effects of chemotherapy and are best treated with 5-HT_3 receptor antagonists (p. 289).

Laser therapy and stenting

Palliation of symptoms caused by major airway obstruction can be achieved in selected patients using bronchoscopic laser treatment to clear tumour tissue and allow re-aeration of collapsed lung. The best results are achieved in tumours of the main bronchi. Endobronchial stents can be used to maintain airway patency in the face of extrinsic compression by malignant nodes.

General aspects of management

The best outcomes are obtained when lung cancer is managed in specialist centres by multidisciplinary teams, including oncologists, thoracic surgeons, respiratory physicians and specialist nurses. Effective communication, pain relief and attention to diet are important. Lung tumours can cause clinically significant depression and anxiety, and these may need specific therapy. The management of non-metastatic endocrine manifestations is described in Chapter 20. When a malignant pleural effusion is present, an attempt should be made to drain the pleural cavity using an intercostal drain; provided the lung fully re-expands, pleurodesis with a sclerosing agent such as talc should be performed to prevent recurrent effusion.

Prognosis

The overall prognosis in bronchial carcinoma is very poor, with around 70% of patients dying within a year of diagnosis and only 6–8% of patients surviving 5 years after diagnosis. The best prognosis is with well-differentiated squamous cell tumours that have not metastasised and are amenable to surgical resection. The clinical features and prognosis of some less common benign and malignant lung tumours are given in Box 19.74.

Secondary tumours of the lung

Blood-borne metastatic deposits in the lungs may be derived from many primary tumours, in particular those of the breast, kidney, uterus, ovary, testes and thyroid. The secondary deposits are usually multiple and bilateral. Often there are no respiratory symptoms and the diagnosis is made on radiological examination. Breathlessness may occur if a considerable amount of lung tissue has been replaced by metastatic tumour.

19.74 Rare types of lung tumour

Tumour	Status	Histology	Typical presentation	Prognosis
Adenosquamous carcinoma	Malignant	Tumours with areas of unequivocal squamous and adeno-differentiation	Peripheral or central lung mass	Stage-dependent
Neuro-endocrine (carcinoid) tumour (p. 784)	Low-grade malignant	Neuroendocrine differentiation	Bronchial obstruction, cough	95% 5-yr survival with resection
Bronchial gland adenoma	Benign	Salivary gland differentiation	Tracheobronchial irritation/obstruction	Local resection curative
Bronchial gland carcinoma	Low-grade malignant	Salivary gland differentiation	Tracheobronchial irritation/obstruction	Local recurrence occurs
Hamartoma	Benign	Mesenchymal cells, cartilage	Peripheral lung nodule	Local resection curative
Bronchoalveolar carcinoma	Malignant	Tumour cells line alveolar spaces	Alveolar shadowing, productive cough	Variable, worse if multifocal

Endobronchial deposits are uncommon but can cause haemoptysis and lobar collapse.

Lymphatic infiltration may develop in patients with carcinoma of the breast, stomach, bowel, pancreas or bronchus. 'Lymphangitic carcinomatosis' causes severe and rapidly progressive breathlessness associated with marked hypoxaemia. The chest X-ray shows diffuse pulmonary shadowing radiating from the hilar regions, often associated with septal lines, and CT demonstrates characteristic polygonal thickened interlobular septa. Palliation of breathlessness with opiates may help (p. 289).

Tumours of the mediastinum

Figure 19.53 shows the four major compartments of the mediastinum, and Box 19.75 lists likely causes of a mediastinal mass in each location.

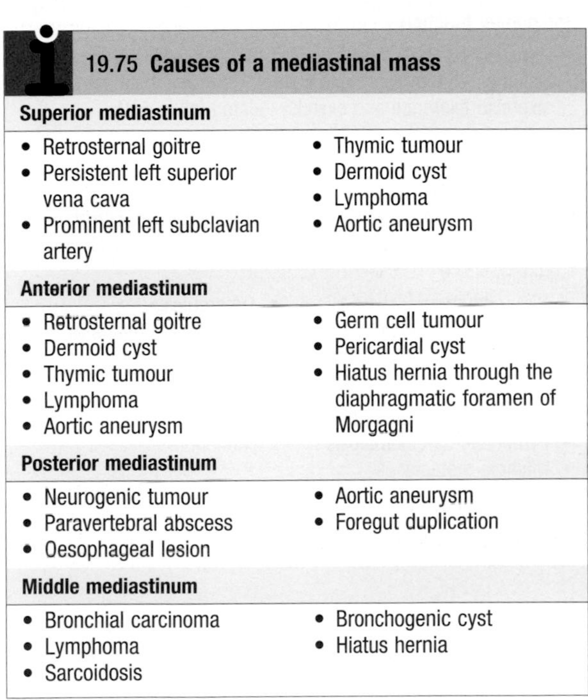

19.75 Causes of a mediastinal mass

Superior mediastinum	
• Retrosternal goitre • Persistent left superior vena cava • Prominent left subclavian artery	• Thymic tumour • Dermoid cyst • Lymphoma • Aortic aneurysm
Anterior mediastinum	
• Retrosternal goitre • Dermoid cyst • Thymic tumour • Lymphoma • Aortic aneurysm	• Germ cell tumour • Pericardial cyst • Hiatus hernia through the diaphragmatic foramen of Morgagni
Posterior mediastinum	
• Neurogenic tumour • Paravertebral abscess • Oesophageal lesion	• Aortic aneurysm • Foregut duplication
Middle mediastinum	
• Bronchial carcinoma • Lymphoma • Sarcoidosis	• Bronchogenic cyst • Hiatus hernia

Benign tumours and cysts in the mediastinum are often diagnosed when a chest X-ray is undertaken for some other reason. In general, they do not invade vital structures but may cause symptoms by compressing the trachea or the superior vena cava. A dermoid cyst may very occasionally rupture into a bronchus.

Malignant mediastinal tumours are distinguished by their power to invade as well as compress surrounding structures. As a result, even a small malignant tumour can produce symptoms, although more commonly the tumour has attained a considerable size before this happens (Box 19.76). The most common cause is mediastinal lymph node metastases from bronchogenic carcinoma, but lymphomas, leukaemia, malignant thymic tumours and germ-cell tumours can cause similar features. Aortic and innominate aneurysms have destructive features resembling those of malignant mediastinal tumours.

19.76 Clinical features of malignant mediastinal invasion

Trachea and main bronchi
• Stridor, breathlessness, cough, pulmonary collapse
Oesophagus
• Dysphagia, oesophageal displacement or obstruction on barium swallow examination
Phrenic nerve
• Diaphragmatic paralysis
Left recurrent laryngeal nerve
• Paralysis of left vocal cord with hoarseness and 'bovine' cough
Sympathetic trunk
• Horner's syndrome
Superior vena cava
• SVC obstruction: non-pulsatile distension of neck veins, subconjunctival oedema, and oedema and cyanosis of head, neck, hands and arms. Dilated anastomotic veins on chest wall
Pericardium
• Pericarditis and/or pericardial effusion

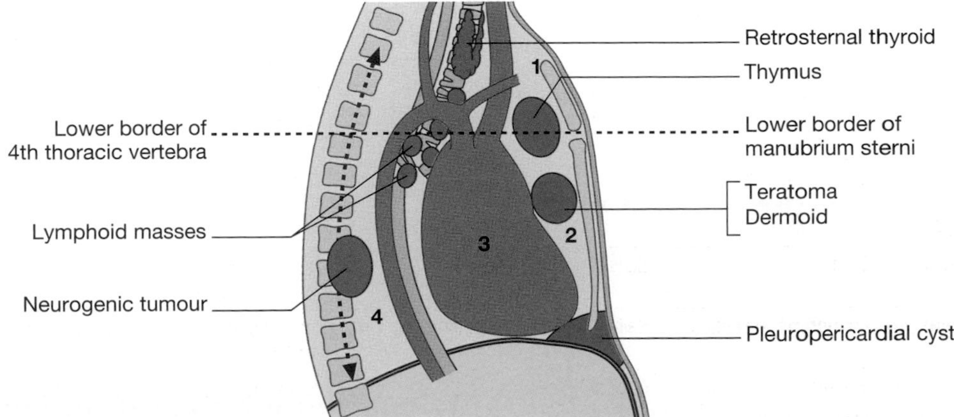

Fig. 19.53 The divisions of the mediastinum. (1) Superior mediastinum. (2) Anterior mediastinum. (3) Middle mediastinum. (4) Posterior mediastinum. Sites of the more common mediastinal tumours are also illustrated. From Johnson 1986 – see p. 732.

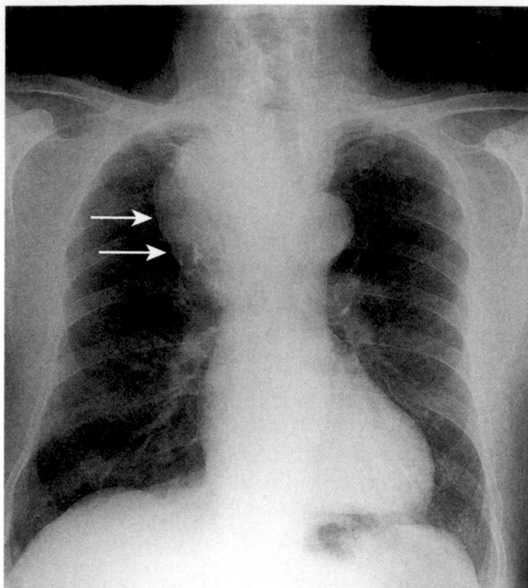

Fig. 19.54 Intrathoracic goitre (arrows) extending from right upper mediastinum.

Investigations

A benign mediastinal tumour generally appears on chest X-ray as a sharply circumscribed mediastinal opacity encroaching on one or both lung fields (Fig. 19.54). CT (or MRI) is the investigation of choice for mediastinal tumours (e.g. see Fig. 20.11B, p. 753). A malignant mediastinal tumour seldom has a clearly defined margin and often presents as a general broadening of the mediastinum.

Bronchoscopy may reveal a primary bronchial carcinoma causing mediastinal lymphadenopathy. Endobronchial ultrasound may be used to guide sampling of peribronchial masses. The posterior mediastinum can be imaged and biopsied via the oesophagus using endoscopic ultrasound (p. 651).

Mediastinoscopy under general anaesthetic can be used to visualise and biopsy masses in the superior and anterior mediastinum, but surgical exploration of the chest, with removal of part or all of the tumour, is often required to obtain a histological diagnosis.

Management

Benign mediastinal tumours should be removed surgically because most produce symptoms sooner or later. Cysts may become infected, while neural tumours have the potential to undergo malignant transformation. The operative mortality is low in the absence of coexisting cardiovascular disease, COPD or extreme age.

INTERSTITIAL AND INFILTRATIVE PULMONARY DISEASES

Diffuse parenchymal lung disease

The diffuse parenchymal lung diseases (DPLDs) are a heterogeneous group of conditions affecting the pulmonary parenchyma (interstitium) and/or alveolar lumen, which are frequently considered collectively as they share a sufficient number of clinical physiological and radiographic similarities (Box 19.77). The current classification is shown in Figure 19.55 and the potential differential diagnoses in Box 19.78. They often present with a cough that is typically dry and distressing, and breathlessness that is frequently insidious in onset but thereafter relentlessly progressive. Physical examination reveals the presence of inspiratory crackles and in many cases digital clubbing develops. Pulmonary function tests typically show a restrictive ventilatory defect in the presence of small lung volumes and reduced gas transfer. The typical radiographic findings include ground glass and reticulonodular shadowing in the earliest stages, with progression to honeycomb cysts and traction bronchiectasis. Whilst these appearances may be seen on a 'plain' chest X-ray, they are most easily appreciated on HRCT, which has assumed a central role in the evaluation of DPLD (Fig. 19.56).

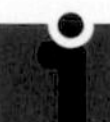

19.77 Features common to the diffuse parenchymal lung diseases

Clinical presentation

- Cough: usually dry, persistent and distressing
- Breathlessness: usually slowly progressive; insidious onset; acute in some cases

Examination findings

- Crackles: typically bilateral and basal
- Clubbing: common in idiopathic pulmonary fibrosis but also seen in other types, e.g. asbestosis
- Central cyanosis and signs of right heart failure in advanced disease

Radiology

- Chest X-ray: typically small lung volumes with reticulonodular shadowing but may be normal in early or limited disease
- HRCT: combinations of ground glass changes, reticulonodular shadowing, honeycomb cysts and traction bronchiectasis, depending on stage of disease

Pulmonary function

- Typically restrictive ventilatory defect with reduced lung volumes and impaired gas transfer; exercise tests assess exercise tolerance and exercise-related fall in SaO_2

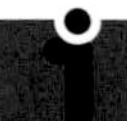

19.78 Conditions that mimic diffuse parenchymal lung disease

Infection

- Viral pneumonia
- *Pneumocystis jirovecii*
- *Mycoplasma pneumoniae*
- Tuberculosis
- Parasite, e.g. filariasis
- Fungal infection

Malignancy

- Leukaemia and lymphoma
- Lymphatic carcinomatosis
- Multiple metastases
- Bronchoalveolar carcinoma

Pulmonary oedema

Aspiration pneumonitis

Idiopathic interstitial pneumonias

The idiopathic interstitial pneumonias represent a major subgroup of DPLDs that are grouped together because

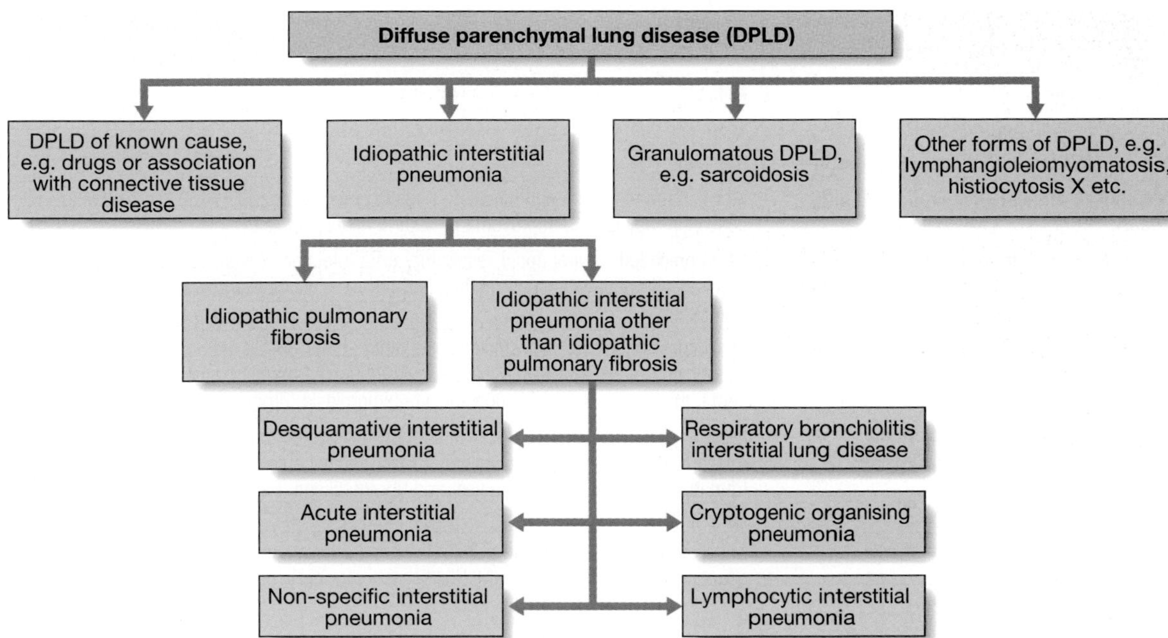

Fig. 19.55 Classification of diffuse parenchymal lung disease.

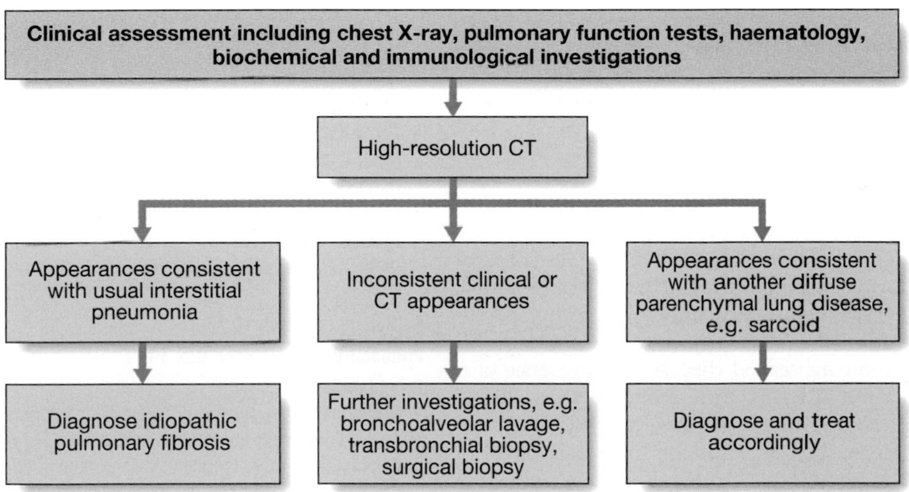

Fig. 19.56 Algorithm for the investigation of patients with interstitial lung disease following initial clinical and chest X-ray examination.

of their unknown aetiology (Box 19.79). They are often distinguished by the predominant histological pattern on tissue biopsy; hence they are frequently referred to by their pathological description – for example, usual interstitial pneumonia or non-specific interstitial pneumonia. The most important of these is idiopathic pulmonary fibrosis.

Idiopathic pulmonary fibrosis

Idiopathic pulmonary fibrosis (IPF) is defined as a progressive fibrosing interstitial pneumonia of unknown cause, occurring in adults and associated with the histological or radiological pattern of usual interstitial pneumonia (UIP). Important differentials include fibrosing diseases caused by occupational exposure, medication or connective tissue diseases, which must be excluded by careful history, examination and investigation.

The histological features of the condition are suggestive of repeated episodes of focal damage to the alveolar epithelium consistent with an autoimmune process but the aetiology remains elusive; speculation has included exposure to viruses (e.g. Epstein–Barr virus), occupational dusts (metal or wood), drugs (antidepressants) or chronic gastro-oesophageal reflux. Familial cases are rare but genetic factors that control the inflammatory and fibrotic response are likely to be important. There is a strong association with cigarette smoking.

Clinical features

IPF usually presents in the older adult and is uncommon before the age of 50 years. With the advent of

19.79 Idiopathic interstitial pneumonias

Clinical diagnosis	Notes
Usual interstitial pneumonia (UIP)	Idiopathic pulmonary fibrosis – see text
Non-specific interstitial pneumonia (NSIP)	See page 709
Respiratory bronchiolitis–interstitial lung disease	More common in men and smokers. Usually presents at age 40–60 yrs. Smoking cessation may lead to improvement. Natural history unclear
Acute interstitial pneumonia	Often preceded by viral upper respiratory tract infection. Severe exertional dyspnoea, widespread pneumonic consolidation and diffuse alveolar damage on biopsy. Prognosis often poor
Desquamative interstitial pneumonia (DIP)	More common in men and smokers. Presents at age 40–60 yrs. Insidious onset of dyspnoea. Clubbing in 50%. Biopsy shows increased macrophages in alveolar space, septal thickening and type II pneumocyte hyperplasia. Prognosis generally good
Cryptogenic organising pneumonia ('bronchiolitis obliterans organising pneumonia' – BOOP)	Presents as clinical and radiological pneumonia. Systemic features and markedly raised ESR common. Finger clubbing absent. Biopsy shows florid proliferation of immature collagen (Masson bodies) and fibrous tissue. Response to corticosteroids classically excellent
Lymphocytic interstitial pneumonia (LIP)	More common in women, slow onset over years. Investigate for associations with connective tissue disease or HIV. Unclear whether corticosteroids helpful

widespread CT scanning, it may present as an incidental finding in an otherwise asymptomatic individual but more typically presents with progressive breathlessness (which may have been insidious) and a non-productive cough. Constitutional symptoms are unusual. Clinical findings include finger clubbing and the presence of bi-basal fine late inspiratory crackles likened to the unfastening of Velcro.

Investigations

These are summarised in Box 19.80. Established IPF will be apparent on chest X-ray as bilateral lower lobe and subpleural reticular shadowing. However, the chest X-ray may be normal in individuals with early or limited disease. HRCT typically demonstrates a patchy, predominantly peripheral, subpleural and basal reticular pattern and, in more advanced disease, the presence of honeycombing cysts and traction bronchiectasis (Fig. 19.57). When these features are present, HRCT has a high positive predictive value for the diagnosis of IPF and recourse to biopsy is seldom necessary. HRCT appearances may also be sufficiently characteristic to suggest an alternative diagnosis such as hypersensitivity pneumonitis (p. 719) or sarcoidosis (p. 709). The presence of pleural plaques may suggest asbestosis (p. 718).

Pulmonary function tests classically show a restrictive defect with reduced lung volumes and gas transfer. However, lung volumes may be preserved in patients with concomitant emphysema. Dynamic tests are useful to document exercise tolerance and demonstrate exercise-induced arterial hypoxaemia, but as IPF advances, arterial hypoxaemia and hypocapnia are present at rest.

Bronchoscopy is seldom necessary unless there is a significant possibility of infection or a malignant process; lymphocytosis may suggest chronic hypersensitivity pneumonitis. The tissue samples obtained by transbronchial lung biopsy are invariably insufficient to be of value and, if tissue is required, a surgical lung biopsy should be performed. Lung biopsy should be considered in cases of diagnostic uncertainty or with atypical features. UIP is the histological pattern predominantly encountered in IPF (Fig. 19.58). However, it is also found in asbestosis, hypersensitivity pneumonitis, connective tissue diseases and drug reactions.

It is not uncommon to identify mildly positive anti-nuclear antibodies or anti-cyclic citrullinated peptide (anti-CCP), in which case repeat serological testing should be performed, as lung disease may precede the appearance of connective tissue disease.

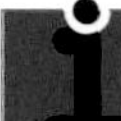

19.80 Investigations in diffuse parenchymal lung disease

Laboratory investigations
- Full blood count: lymphopenia in sarcoid; eosinophilia in pulmonary eosinophilias and drug reactions; neutrophilia in hypersensitivity pneumonitis
- Ca^{2+}: may be elevated in sarcoid
- Lactate dehydrogenase: may be elevated in active alveolitis
- Serum angiotensin-converting enzyme: non-specific indicator of disease activity in sarcoid
- ESR and CRP: non-specifically raised
- Autoimmune screen: anti-cyclic citrullinated peptide (anti-CCP) and other autoantibodies may suggest connective tissue disease

Radiology (see Box 19.77)

Pulmonary function (see Box 19.77)

Bronchoscopy
- Bronchoalveolar lavage: differential cell counts may point to sarcoid and drug-induced pneumonitis, pulmonary eosinophilias, hypersensitivity pneumonitis or cryptogenic organising pneumonia; useful to exclude infection
- Transbronchial biopsy: useful in sarcoid and differential of malignancy or infection
- Bronchial biopsy: occasionally useful in sarcoid

Video-assisted thoracoscopic lung biopsy (in selected cases)
- Allows pathological classification: presence of asbestos bodies may suggest asbestosis, silica in occupational fibrosing lung disease

Others
- Liver biopsy: may be useful in sarcoidosis
- Urinary calcium excretion: may be useful in sarcoidosis

Management and prognosis

Treatment is difficult. Although the combination of prednisolone, azathioprine and N-acetylcysteine had shown some promise, large studies suggest that it is mostly ineffective. Disappointing results have also been reported for trials of colchicine, interferon-γ 1b, bosentan and etanercept. Subject to further investigation, pirfenidone may slow the rate of decline of lung function and, by inference, improve mortality. It remains sensible to treat gastro-oesophageal reflux and to look for and treat pulmonary hypertension but, where possible, treatment with experimental agents outside clinical trials should not be tried. Where appropriate, lung transplantation should be considered. Oxygen may help breathlessness but opiates may be required to relieve severe dyspnoea. The optimum treatment for acute exacerbations is unknown but corticosteroids should probably be used.

The natural history is usually one of steady decline but some patients are prone to exacerbations, which are accompanied by an acute deterioration in breathlessness, disturbed gas exchange, and new ground glass changes or consolidation on HRCT. In advanced disease, central cyanosis is detectable and patients may develop features of right heart failure. A median survival of 3 years is widely quoted; however, the rate of disease progression varies considerably, from death within a few months to survival with minimal symptoms for many years. Serial lung function testing may provide useful prognostic information, with relative preservation of lung function suggesting longer survival, and significantly impaired gas transfer and/or desaturation on exercise heralding a poorer prognosis. The finding of high numbers of fibroblastic foci on biopsy suggests a more rapid deterioration. IPF is associated with an increased risk of carcinoma of the lung.

A

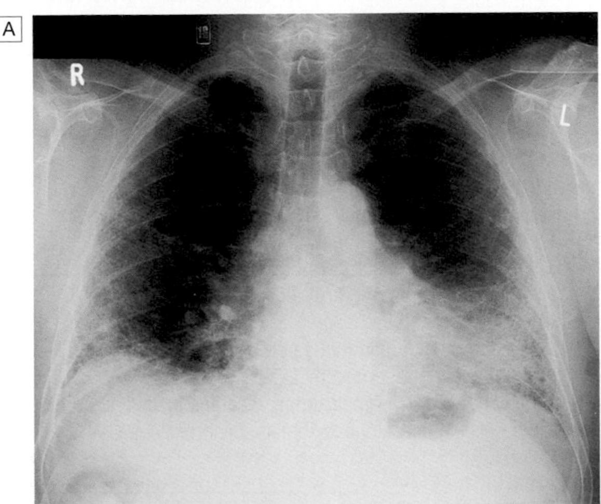

B

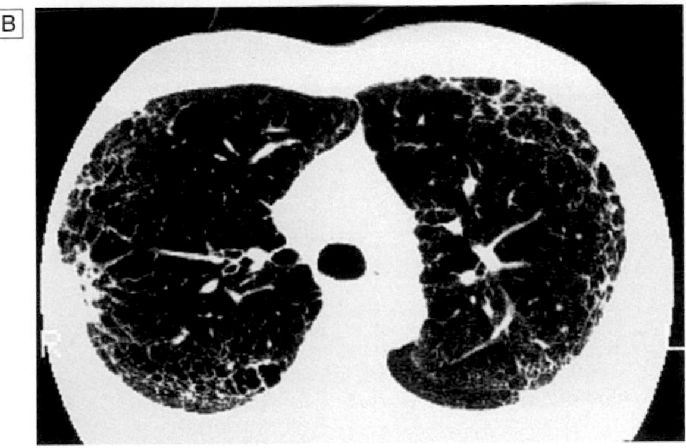

Fig. 19.57 Idiopathic pulmonary fibrosis. **A** Chest X-ray showing bilateral, predominantly lower-zone and peripheral coarse reticulonodular shadowing and small lungs. **B** The CT scan shows honeycombing and scarring which is most marked peripherally.

Non-specific interstitial pneumonia

The clinical picture of fibrotic non-specific interstitial pneumonia (NSIP) is similar to that of IPF, although patients tend to be women and younger in age. As with UIP, the condition may present as an isolated idiopathic pulmonary condition, but an NSIP pattern is often associated with connective tissue disease, certain drugs, chronic hypersensitivity pneumonitis and HIV infection; care must be taken to identify these possibilities, as the pulmonary condition may precede the appearance of connective tissue disease. HRCT findings are less specific than with IPF and lung biopsy may be required. The prognosis is significantly better than that of IPF, particularly in the cellular form of the condition, and the 5-year mortality rate is typically less than 15%.

Sarcoidosis

Sarcoidosis is a multisystem granulomatous disorder of unknown aetiology characterised by the presence of non-caseating granulomas (Fig. 19.59). It is more often described in colder parts of northern Europe. It also appears to be more common and more severe in those

A

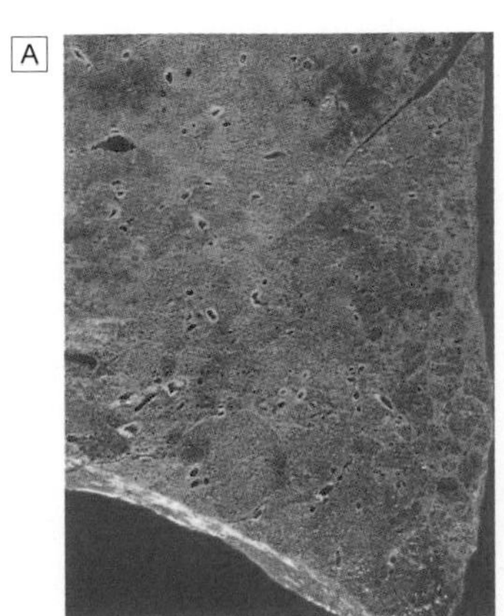

B

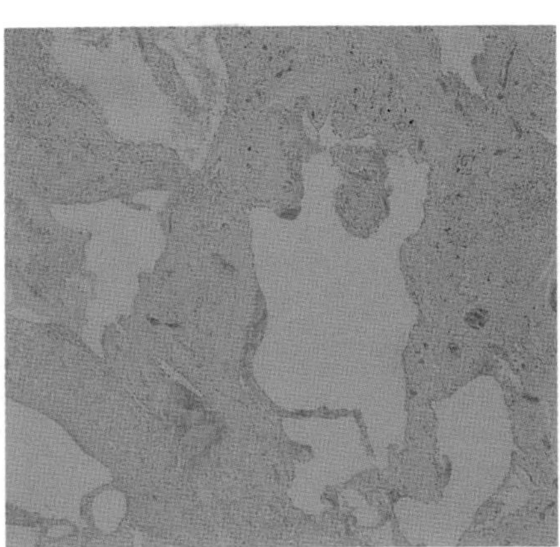

Fig. 19.58 Pathology of usual interstitial pneumonia. **A** Lung tissue showing subpleural scarring, most prominently down the posterior edge of the lower lobe. This distribution of fibrosis is typical of usual interstitial pneumonitis. The fibrosis may be associated with prominent cystic change known as 'honeycomb lung'. **B** Histology showing severe interstitial fibrosis with loss of the normal alveolar architecture and the development of 'honeycomb' cysts.

from a West Indian or Asian background, while Eskimos, Arabs and Chinese are rarely affected. The tendency for sarcoid to present in spring and summer has led to speculation about the role of infective agents, including mycobacteria, propionibacteria and viruses, but the cause remains elusive. Genetic susceptibility is supported by familial clustering; a range of class II HLA alleles confer protection from or susceptibility to the condition. Sarcoidosis occurs less frequently in smokers.

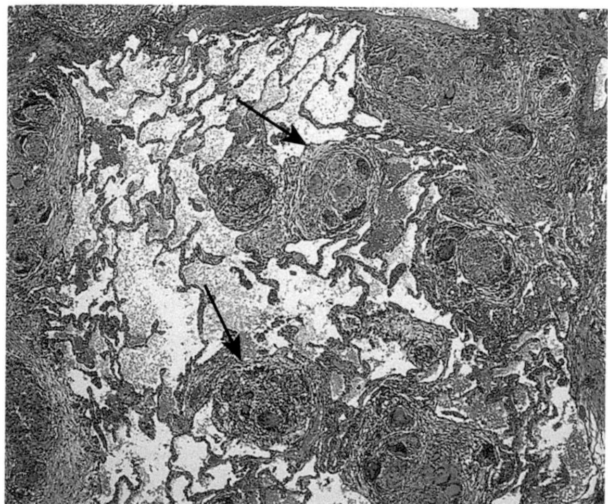

Fig. 19.59 Sarcoidosis of the lung. Histology showing non-caseating granulomas (arrows).

Clinical features

Sarcoidosis is considered with other DPLDs, as over 90% of cases affect the lungs, but the condition can involve almost any organ (Fig. 19.60 and Box 19.81). Löfgren's syndrome – an acute illness characterised by erythema nodosum, peripheral arthropathy, uveitis, bilateral hilar lymphadenopathy (BHL), lethargy and occasionally fever – is often seen in young women. Alternatively, BHL may be detected in an otherwise asymptomatic individual undergoing a chest X-ray for other purposes.

19.81 Presentation of sarcoidosis

- Asymptomatic: abnormal routine chest X-ray (~30%) or abnormal liver function tests
- Respiratory and constitutional symptoms (20–30%)
- Erythema nodosum and arthralgia (20–30%)
- Ocular symptoms (5–10%)
- Skin sarcoid (including lupus pernio) (5%)
- Superficial lymphadenopathy (5%)
- Other (1%), e.g. hypercalcaemia, diabetes insipidus, cranial nerve palsies, cardiac arrhythmias, nephrocalcinosis

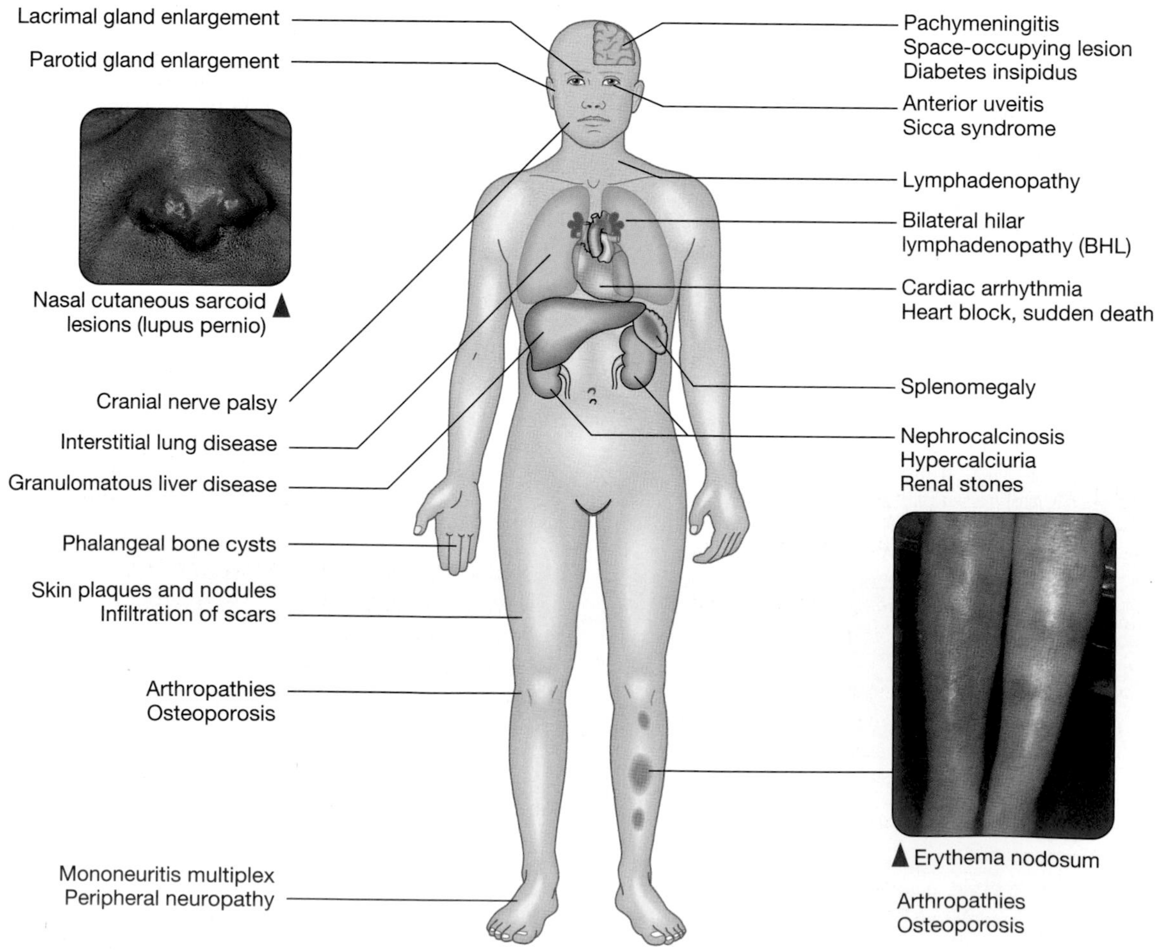

Fig. 19.60 Possible systemic involvement in sarcoidosis. *Inset (Erythema nodosum)* From Savin et al. 1997 – see p. 732.

Pulmonary disease may also present in a more insidious manner with cough, exertional breathlessness and radiographic infiltrates; chest auscultation is often unremarkable. Fibrosis occurs in 20% of cases of pulmonary sarcoidosis and may cause a silent loss of lung function. Pleural disease is uncommon and finger clubbing not a feature. Complications such as bronchiectasis, aspergilloma, pneumothorax, pulmonary hypertension and cor pulmonale have been reported but are rare.

Investigations

Lymphopenia is characteristic and liver function tests may be mildly deranged. Hypercalcaemia may be present (reflecting increased formation of calcitrol – 1,25-dihydroxyvitamin D_3 – by alveolar macrophages), particularly if the patient has been exposed to strong sunlight. Hypercalciuria may also be seen and may lead to nephrocalcinosis. Serum ACE may provide a non-specific marker of disease activity and can assist in monitoring the clinical course. Chest radiography has been used to stage sarcoid (Box 19.82). In patients with pulmonary infiltrates, pulmonary function testing may show a restrictive defect accompanied by impaired gas exchange. Exercise tests may reveal oxygen desaturation. Bronchoscopy may demonstrate a 'cobblestone' appearance of the mucosa, and bronchial and transbronchial biopsy usually shows non-caseating granulomas. The BAL fluid typically contains an increased CD4:CD8 T-cell ratio. Characteristic HRCT appearances include reticulonodular opacities that follow a perilymphatic distribution, centred on bronchovascular bundles and the subpleural areas.

The occurrence of erythema nodosum with BHL on chest X-ray is often sufficient for a confident diagnosis, without recourse to a tissue biopsy. Similarly, a typical presentation with classical HRCT features may also be accepted. Otherwise, the diagnosis should be confirmed by histological examination of the involved organ. The presence of anergy (e.g. to tuberculin skin tests) may support the diagnosis.

Management

Patients who present with acute illness and erythema nodosum are treated with NSAIDs and, if disease is severe, a short course of corticosteroids. The majority of patients enjoy spontaneous remission and so, if there is no evidence of organ damage, systemic corticosteroid therapy can be withheld for 6 months. However, prednisolone (at a starting dose of 20–40 mg/day) should be commenced immediately in the presence of hypercalcaemia, pulmonary impairment, renal impairment and uveitis (Box 19.83). Topical steroids may be useful in cases of mild uveitis, and inhaled corticosteroids have been used to shorten the duration of systemic corticosteroid use in asymptomatic parenchymal sarcoid. Patients should be warned that strong sunlight might precipitate hypercalcaemia and endanger renal function.

Features suggesting a less favourable outlook include age over 40 years, Afro-Caribbean ethnicity, persistent symptoms for more than 6 months, the involvement of more than three organs, lupus pernio and a stage III/IV chest X-ray. In patients with severe disease, methotrexate (10–20 mg/week), azathioprine (50–150 mg/day) and the use of specific tumour necrosis factor (TNF)-α inhibitors (p. 1102) have been effective. Chloroquine, hydroxychloroquine and low-dose thalidomide may be useful in cutaneous sarcoid with limited pulmonary involvement. Selected patients may be referred for consideration of single lung transplantation. The overall mortality is low (1–5%) and usually reflects cardiac involvement or pulmonary fibrosis.

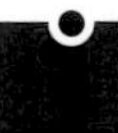

19.82 Chest X-ray changes in sarcoidosis

Stage I: BHL (usually symmetrical); paratracheal nodes often enlarged
• Often asymptomatic, but may be associated with erythema nodosum and arthralgia. The majority of cases resolve spontaneously within 1 yr
Stage II: BHL and parenchymal infiltrates
• Patients may present with breathlessness or cough. The majority of cases resolve spontaneously
Stage III: parenchymal infiltrates without BHL
• Disease less likely to resolve spontaneously
Stage IV: pulmonary fibrosis
• Can cause progression to ventilatory failure, pulmonary hypertension and cor pulmonale

(BHL = bilateral hilar lymphadenopathy)

EBM 19.83 Systemic corticosteroids in pulmonary sarcoidosis

'Oral glucocorticoids administered for 6–24 months improve chest X-ray appearances and symptoms, but there is little evidence of an improvement in lung function and there are no data from follow-up beyond 2 years.'

- Paramothayan NS, et al. Corticosteroids for pulmonary sarcoidosis. Cochrane Database of Systematic Reviews, 2005, issue 2. Art. no.: CD001114.

Lung diseases due to systemic inflammatory disease

Acute respiratory distress syndrome

See page 192.

Respiratory involvement in connective tissue disorders

Pulmonary complications of connective tissue disease are common, and affect the airways, alveoli, pulmonary vasculature, diaphragm and chest wall muscles, and chest wall itself (Box 19.84). In some instances, pulmonary disease may precede the appearance of the connective tissue disorder. Indirect associations between connective tissue disorders and respiratory complications include those due to disease in other organs, e.g. thrombocytopenia causing haemoptysis; pulmonary toxic effects of drugs used to treat the connective tissue disorder, e.g. gold and methotrexate; and secondary infection due to the disease itself, neutropenia or immunosuppressive drug regimens.

19.84 Respiratory complications of connective tissue disorders

Disorder	Airways	Parenchyma	Pleura	Diaphragm and chest wall
Rheumatoid arthritis	Bronchitis, obliterative bronchiolitis, bronchiectasis, crico-arytenoid arthritis, stridor	Pulmonary fibrosis, nodules, upper lobe fibrosis, infections	Pleurisy, effusion, pneumothorax	Poor healing of intercostal drain sites
Systemic lupus erythematosus	–	Pulmonary fibrosis, 'vasculitic' infarcts	Pleurisy, effusion	Diaphragmatic weakness (shrinking lungs)
Systemic sclerosis	Bronchiectasis	Pulmonary fibrosis, aspiration pneumonia	–	Cutaneous thoracic restriction (hidebound chest)
Dermatomyositis/ polymyositis	Bronchial carcinoma	Pulmonary fibrosis	–	Intercostal and diaphragmatic myopathy
Rheumatic fever	–	Pneumonia	Pleurisy, effusion	–

Rheumatoid disease

Pulmonary involvement in rheumatoid arthritis is important, accounting for around 10–20% of the mortality associated with the condition (p. 1096). The majority of cases occur within 5 years of the rheumatological diagnosis but pulmonary manifestations may precede joint involvement in 10–20%. Pulmonary fibrosis is the most common pulmonary manifestation. All forms of interstitial disease have been described but NSIP is probably the most frequent. A rare variant of localised upper lobe fibrosis and cavitation is occasionally seen.

Pleural effusion is common, especially in men with seropositive disease. Effusions are usually small and unilateral but can be large and bilateral. Most resolve spontaneously. Biochemical testing shows an exudate with markedly reduced glucose levels and raised LDH. Effusions that fail to resolve spontaneously may respond to a short course of oral prednisolone (30–40 mg daily) but some become chronic.

Rheumatoid pulmonary nodules are usually asymptomatic and detected incidentally on imaging. They are usually multiple and subpleural in site (Fig. 19.61). Solitary nodules can mimic primary bronchial carcinoma and, when they are multiple, the differential diagnoses include pulmonary metastatic disease. Cavitation raises the possibility of tuberculosis and predisposes to pneumothorax. The combination of rheumatoid nodules and pneumoconiosis is known as Caplan's syndrome (p. 717).

Bronchitis and bronchiectasis are both more common in rheumatoid patients. Rarely, the potentially fatal condition called obliterative bronchiolitis may develop. Bacterial lower respiratory tract infections are frequent. Treatments given for rheumatoid arthritis may also be relevant: corticosteroid therapy predisposes to infections, methotrexate may cause pulmonary fibrosis, and anti-TNF therapy has been associated with the reactivation of tuberculosis.

Systemic lupus erythematosus

Pleuropulmonary involvement is more common in lupus than in any other connective tissue disorder and may be a presenting problem, in which case it is sometimes attributed incorrectly to infection or pulmonary embolism. Up to two-thirds of patients have repeated episodes of pleurisy, with or without effusions. Effusions may be bilateral and may also involve the pericardium.

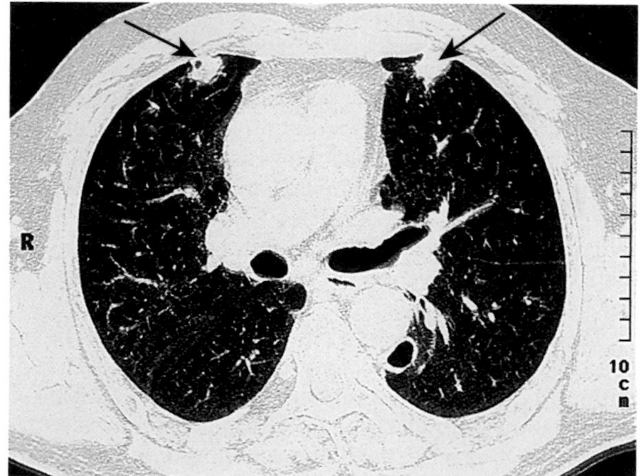

Fig. 19.61 Rheumatoid (necrobiotic) nodules. Thoracic CT just below the level of the main carina showing the typical appearance of peripheral pleural-based nodules. The nodule in the left lower lobe shows characteristic cavitation.

The most serious manifestation of lupus is an acute alveolitis, which may be associated with diffuse alveolar haemorrhage. This condition is life-threatening and requires immunosuppression.

Pulmonary fibrosis is a relatively uncommon manifestation of systemic lupus erythematosus (SLE). Some patients with SLE present with exertional dyspnoea and orthopnoea but without overt signs of pulmonary fibrosis. The chest X-ray reveals elevated diaphragms, and pulmonary function testing shows reduced lung volumes. This condition has been described as 'shrinking lungs' and has been attributed to diaphragmatic myopathy.

SLE patients with antiphospholipid antibodies are at increased risk of venous and pulmonary thromboembolism and require life-long anticoagulation.

Systemic sclerosis

Most patients with systemic sclerosis (p. 1112) eventually develop diffuse pulmonary fibrosis; at necropsy, more than 90% have evidence of lung fibrosis. In some patients, it is indolent but when progressive, as in IPF, the median survival time is around 4 years. Pulmonary fibrosis is rare in the CREST variant of progressive systemic sclerosis but isolated pulmonary hypertension may develop.

Other pulmonary complications include recurrent aspiration pneumonias secondary to oesophageal disease. Rarely, sclerosis of the skin of the chest wall may be so extensive and cicatrising as to restrict chest wall movement – this constitutes the so-called 'hidebound chest'.

Pulmonary eosinophilia and vasculitides

Pulmonary eosinophilia refers to the association of radiographic (usually pneumonic) abnormalities and peripheral blood eosinophilia. The term encompasses a group of disorders of different aetiology (Box 19.85). Eosinophils are the predominant cell recovered in sputum or BAL, and eosinophil products are likely to be the prime mediators of tissue damage.

Acute eosinophilic pneumonia

Acute eosinophilic pneumonia is an acute febrile illness (of less than 5 days' duration) characterised by diffuse pulmonary infiltrates and hypoxic respiratory failure. The pathology is usually that of diffuse alveolar damage. Diagnosis is confirmed by BAL, which characteristically demonstrates more than 25% eosinophils. The condition is usually idiopathic but drug reactions should be considered. Corticosteroids invariably induce prompt and complete resolution.

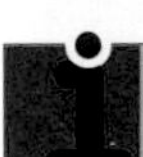

19.85 Pulmonary eosinophilia

Extrinsic (cause known)

- Helminths: e.g. *Ascaris, Toxocara, Filaria*
- Drugs: nitrofurantoin, para-aminosalicylic acid (PAS), sulfasalazine, imipramine, chlorpropamide, phenylbutazone
- Fungi: e.g. *Aspergillus fumigatus* causing allergic bronchopulmonary aspergillosis (p. 697)

Intrinsic (cause unknown)

- Cryptogenic eosinophilic pneumonia
- Churg–Strauss syndrome, diagnosed on the basis of ≥ 4 of the following features:
  - Asthma
  - Peripheral blood eosinophilia > 1.5×10^9/L (or > 10% of a total white cell count)
  - Mononeuropathy or polyneuropathy
  - Pulmonary infiltrates
  - Paranasal sinus disease
  - Eosinophilic vasculitis on biopsy of an affected site
- Hypereosinophilic syndrome
- Polyarteritis nodosa (p. 1117; rare)

Chronic eosinophilic pneumonia

Chronic eosinophilic pneumonia typically presents in an insidious manner with malaise, fever, weight loss, breathlessness and unproductive cough. The condition is more common in middle-aged females. The classical chest X-ray appearance has been likened to the photographic negative of pulmonary oedema with bilateral, peripheral and predominantly upper lobe parenchymal shadowing. The peripheral blood eosinophil count is almost always very high, and the ESR and total serum IgE are elevated. BAL reveals a high proportion of eosinophils in the lavage fluid. Response to prednisolone (20–40 mg daily) is usually dramatic. Prednisolone can usually be withdrawn after a few weeks without relapse, but long-term, low-dose therapy is occasionally necessary.

Tropical pulmonary eosinophilia

Tropical pulmonary eosinophilia occurs as a result of a mosquito-borne filarial infection caused by the tissue-dwelling human nematode *Wuchereria bancrofti* or *Brugia malayi*. The condition presents with fever, weight loss, dyspnoea and asthma-like symptoms. There is marked peripheral blood eosinophilia and elevation of total IgE. High antifilarial antibody titres are seen. The diagnosis may be confirmed by a response to treatment with diethylcarbamazine (6 mg/kg/day for 3 weeks). Tropical pulmonary eosinophilia must be distinguished from infection with *Strongyloides stercoralis* (p. 370), as corticosteroids may cause life-threatening dissemination in the latter. Ascariasis ('larva migrans') and other hookworm infestations are described in detail in Chapter 13.

Granulomatosis with polyangiitis

Granulomatosis with polyangiitis (also known as Wegener's granulomatosis) is a rare vasculitic and granulomatous condition (p. 1118). The lung is commonly involved in systemic forms of the condition but a limited pulmonary form may also occur. Respiratory symptoms include cough, haemoptysis and chest pain. Associated upper respiratory tract manifestations include nasal discharge and crusting, and otitis media. Fever, weight loss and anaemia are common. Radiological features include multiple nodules and cavitation that may resemble primary or metastatic carcinoma, or a pulmonary abscess. Tissue biopsy confirms the distinctive pattern of necrotising granulomas and necrotising vasculitis. Other respiratory complications of granulomatosis with polyangiitis include tracheal subglottic stenosis and saddle nose deformity. The differential diagnoses include mycobacterial and fungal infection and other forms of pulmonary vasculitis, including polyarteritis nodosa (pulmonary infarction), microscopic polyangiitis, Churg–Strauss syndrome (in which there is marked tissue eosinophilia and association with asthma), necrotising sarcoid, bronchocentric granulomatosis and lymphomatoid granulomatosis.

Goodpasture's syndrome

This describes the association of pulmonary haemorrhage and glomerulonephritis, in which IgG antibodies bind to the glomerular or alveolar basement membranes (see Box 17.39, p. 499). Pulmonary disease usually precedes renal involvement and includes radiographic infiltrates and hypoxia with or without haemoptysis. It occurs more commonly in men and almost exclusively in smokers.

Lung diseases due to irradiation and drugs

Radiotherapy

Targeting radiotherapy to certain tumours is inevitably accompanied by irradiation of normal lung tissue. Although delivered in divided doses, the effects are cumulative. Acute radiation pneumonitis is typically seen within 6–12 weeks and presents with cough and dyspnoea. This may resolve spontaneously but responds to corticosteroid treatment. Chronic interstitial fibrosis may present several months later with symptoms of exertional dyspnoea and cough. Changes are often confined to the area irradiated but may be bilateral. Established post-irradiation fibrosis does not usually respond to corticosteroid treatment. The pulmonary effects of radiation (p. 277) are exacerbated by treatment with cytotoxic drugs and the phenomenon of 'recall pneumonitis' describes the appearance of radiation injury in a previously irradiated area, when chemotherapy follows radiotherapy. If the patient survives, there are long-term risks of lung cancer.

Drugs

Drugs may cause a range of pulmonary conditions (Box 19.86). Pulmonary fibrosis may occur in response to a variety of drugs, but is seen most frequently with bleomycin, methotrexate, amiodarone and nitrofurantoin. Eosinophilic pulmonary reactions can also be caused by drugs. The pathogenesis may be an immune reaction similar to that in hypersensitivity pneumonitis, which specifically attracts large numbers of eosinophils into the lungs. This type of reaction is well described as a rare reaction to a variety of antineoplastic agents (e.g. bleomycin), antibiotics (e.g. sulphonamides), sulfasalazine and the anticonvulsants phenytoin and carbamazepine. Patients usually present with breathlessness, cough and fever. The chest X-ray characteristically shows patchy shadowing. Most cases resolve completely on withdrawal of the drug, but if the reaction is severe, rapid resolution can be obtained with corticosteroids.

Drugs may also cause other lung diseases, such as asthma, pulmonary haemorrhage and pleural disease. An ARDS-like syndrome of acute non-cardiogenic pulmonary oedema may present with dramatic onset of breathlessness, severe hypoxaemia and signs of alveolar oedema on the chest X-ray. This syndrome has been reported most frequently in cases of opiate overdose in drug addicts (p. 219) but also after salicylate overdose, and occasionally after therapeutic doses of drugs, including hydrochlorothiazides and some cytotoxic agents.

Rare interstitial lung diseases

See Box 19.88.

19.86 Drug-induced respiratory disease

Non-cardiogenic pulmonary oedema (ARDS)
- Hydrochlorothiazide
- Thrombolytics (streptokinase)
- IV β-adrenoceptor agonists (e.g. for premature labour)
- Aspirin and opiates (in overdose)

Non-eosinophilic alveolitis
- Amiodarone, flecainide, gold, nitrofurantoin, cytotoxic agents – especially bleomycin, busulfan, mitomycin C, methotrexate, sulfasalazine

Pulmonary eosinophilia
- Antimicrobials (nitrofurantoin, penicillin, tetracyclines, sulphonamides, nalidixic acid)
- Drugs used in joint disease (gold, aspirin, penicillamine, naproxen)
- Cytotoxic drugs (bleomycin, methotrexate, procarbazine)
- Psychotropic drugs (chlorpromazine, dosulepin, imipramine)
- Anticonvulsants (carbamazepine, phenytoin)
- Others (sulfasalazine, nadolol)

Pleural disease
- Bromocriptine, amiodarone, methotrexate, methysergide
- Induction of SLE – phenytoin, hydralazine, isoniazid

Asthma
- Pharmacological mechanisms (β-blockers, cholinergic agonists, aspirin and NSAIDs)
- Idiosyncratic reactions (tamoxifen, dipyridamole)

19.87 Interstitial lung disease in old age

- **Idiopathic pulmonary fibrosis**: the most common interstitial lung disease, with a worse prognosis.
- **Chronic aspiration pneumonitis**: must always be considered in elderly patients presenting with bilateral basal shadowing on a chest X-ray.
- **Granulomatosis with polyangiitis (Wegener's granulomatosis)**: a rare condition but more common in old age. Renal involvement is more common at presentation and upper respiratory problems are fewer.
- **Asbestosis**: symptoms may only appear in old age because of the prolonged latent period between exposure and disease.
- **Drug-induced interstitial lung disease**: more common, presumably because of the increased chance of exposure to multiple drugs.
- **Rarer interstitial disease**: sarcoidosis, idiopathic pulmonary haemosiderosis, alveolar proteinosis and eosinophilic pneumonia rarely present.
- **Increased dyspnoea**: coexistent muscle weakness, chest wall deformity (e.g. thoracic kyphosis) and deconditioning may all exacerbate dyspnoea associated with interstitial lung disease.
- **Surgical lung biopsy**: often inappropriate in the very frail. A diagnosis therefore frequently depends on clinical and HRCT findings alone.

19.88 Rare interstitial lung diseases

Disease	Presentation	Chest X-ray	Course
Idiopathic pulmonary haemosiderosis	Haemoptysis, breathlessness, anaemia	Bilateral infiltrates, often perihilar Diffuse pulmonary fibrosis	Rapidly progressive in children Slow progression or remission in adults Death from massive pulmonary haemorrhage or cor pulmonale and respiratory failure
Alveolar proteinosis	Breathlessness and cough Occasionally fever, chest pain and haemoptysis	Diffuse bilateral shadowing, often more pronounced in the hilar regions Air bronchogram	Spontaneous remission in one-third Whole-lung lavage or granulocyte macrophage–colony stimulating factor (GM–CSF) therapy may be effective
Langerhans cell histiocytosis (histiocytosis X)	Breathlessness, cough, pneumothorax	Diffuse interstitial shadowing progressing to honeycombing	Course unpredictable but may progress to respiratory failure Smoking cessation may be followed by significant improvement Poor response to immunosuppressive treatment
Neurofibromatosis	Breathlessness and cough in a patient with multiple organ involvement with neurofibromas including skin	Bilateral reticulonodular shadowing of diffuse interstitial fibrosis	Slow progression to death from respiratory failure Poor response to corticosteroid therapy
Alveolar microlithiasis	May be asymptomatic Breathlessness and cough	Diffuse calcified micronodular shadowing more pronounced in the lower zones	Slowly progressive to cor pulmonale and respiratory failure May stabilise in some
Lymphangiolelomyomatosis	Haemoptysis, breathlessness, pneumothorax and chylous effusion in females	Diffuse bilateral shadowing CT shows characteristic thin-walled cysts with well-defined walls throughout both lungs	Progressive to death within 10 yrs Oestrogen ablation and progesterone therapy of doubtful value Consider lung transplantation
Pulmonary tuberous sclerosis	Very similar to lymphangioleiomyomatosis, except occasionally occurs in men		

OCCUPATIONAL AND ENVIRONMENTAL LUNG DISEASE

The role of occupation and environmental exposure in lung disease is a particularly important area of respiratory medicine. Occupational lung disease is common and, in addition to the challenges of its diagnosis and management, often involves discussions about the workplace and, in some circumstances, lawyers. Many countries encourage the registration of cases of occupational lung disease.

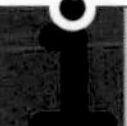

19.89 Occupational asthma

Most frequently reported causative agents

- Isocyanates
- Flour and grain dust
- Colophony and fluxes
- Latex
- Animals
- Aldehydes
- Wood dust

Workers most commonly reported to occupational asthma schemes

- Paint sprayers
- Bakers and pastry-makers
- Nurses
- Chemical workers

Occupational airway disease

Occupational asthma

Occupational asthma (OA) should be considered in any individual of working age who develops new-onset asthma, particularly if the patient reports an improvement in asthma symptoms during periods away from work, e.g. at weekends and on holiday. Workers in certain occupations appear to be at particularly high risk (Box 19.89) and the condition is more common in smokers and atopic individuals. Depending on the intensity of exposure, asthmatic symptoms usually develop within the first year of employment but are classically preceded by a latent period. Symptoms of rhinoconjunctivitis often precede the development of asthma. When OA follows exposure to high molecular weight proteins, sensitisation to the agent may be demonstrated by skin testing or measurement of specific IgE. Confirmation of OA should be sought from lung function tests, which usually involves serial recording of peak flow at work, at least 4 times per day for at least 3 weeks and, if possible, including a period away from work (Fig. 19.62). In certain circumstances, specific challenge tests are required to confirm the diagnosis.

It may be possible to remove the worker from the implicated agent but when this is not feasible,

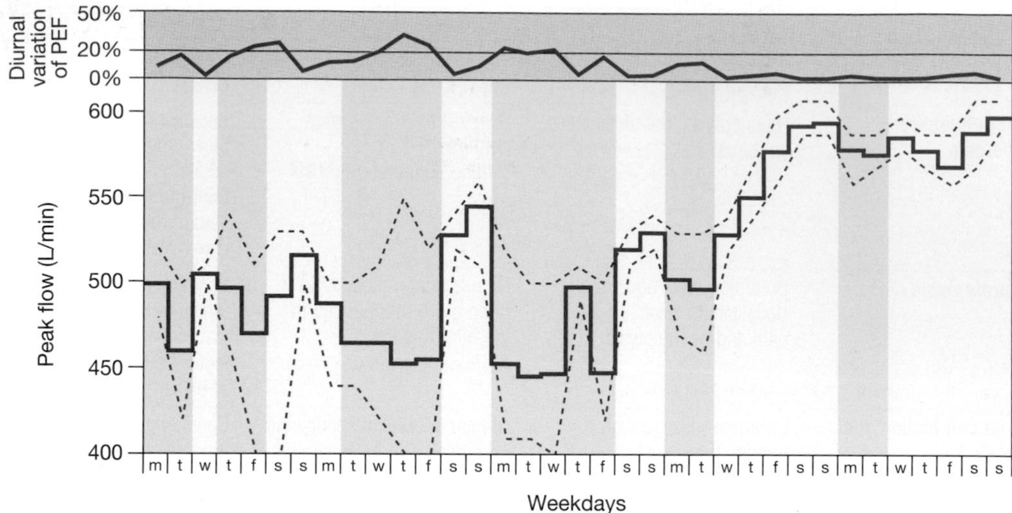

Fig. 19.62 Peak flow readings in occupational asthma. Subjects with suspected occupational asthma are asked to perform 2-hourly serial peak flows at, and away from, work. The maximum, mean and minimum values are plotted daily. Days at work are indicated by the shaded areas. The diurnal variation is displayed at the top. In this example, a period away from work is followed by a marked improvement in peak flow readings and a reduction in diurnal variation.

consideration of personal protective equipment and workplace hygiene may allow patients to retain their job and income. Specialist follow-up in such situations is highly advisable. A favourable prognosis is indicated by a short history of symptoms and normal lung function at diagnosis. Where reduction or avoidance of exposure fails to bring about resolution, the general management does not differ from that of other forms of asthma.

Reactive airways dysfunction syndrome

Reactive airways dysfunction syndrome or acute irritant-induced asthma refers to the development of a persistent asthma-like syndrome following the inhalation of an airway irritant: typically, a single specific exposure to a gas, smoke, fume or vapour in very high concentrations. Pulmonary function tests show airflow obstruction and airway hyper-reactivity, and the management is similar to that of asthma. Once developed, the condition often persists but it is common for symptoms to improve over years.

Chronic obstructive pulmonary disease

Whilst tobacco smoking remains the most important preventable cause of COPD, there is increasing recognition that other noxious particles and gases can both cause or aggravate the condition. Occupational COPD is recognised in workers exposed to coal dust, crystalline silica and cadmium. In many parts of the developing world, indoor air pollution from the burning of biomass fuels in confined spaces used for cooking contributes to the development of COPD.

Byssinosis

Byssinosis occurs in workers at cotton and flax mills who are exposed to cotton brack (dried leaf and plant debris). An acute form of the disease may occur but, more typically, byssinosis develops after 20–30 years' exposure. Typical symptoms include chest tightness or breathlessness, accompanied by a drop in lung function; classically, these are most severe on the first day of the working week ('Monday fever'), or on return to work following a period away. As the week progresses, symptoms improve and the fall in lung function becomes less dramatic. Continued exposure leads to the development of persistent symptoms and a progressive decline in FEV_1 similar to that observed in COPD.

Pneumoconiosis

Pneumoconiosis can be defined as a permanent alteration of lung structure due to the inhalation of mineral dust and the tissue reactions of the lung to its presence, excluding bronchitis and emphysema (Box 19.90). Not all dusts are pathogenic. For example, silica is highly fibrogenic, whereas iron (siderosis), tin (stannosis) and barium (baritosis) are almost inert. Beryllium causes an interstitial granulomatous disease similar to sarcoidosis. In many types of pneumoconiosis, a long period of dust exposure is required before radiological changes appear, and these may precede clinical symptoms. The most important pneumoconioses include coal worker's pneumoconiosis, silicosis and asbestosis.

Coal worker's pneumoconiosis

Coal worker's pneumoconiosis (CWP) follows prolonged inhalation of coal dust. Dust-laden alveolar macrophages aggregate to form macules in or near the centre of the secondary pulmonary lobule and a fibrotic reaction ensues, resulting in the appearance of scattered discrete fibrotic lesions. Classification is based on the size and extent of radiographic nodularity. Simple coal worker's pneumoconiosis (SCWP) refers to the appearance of small radiographic nodules in an otherwise asymptomatic individual. SCWP does not impair lung function and, once exposure ceases, will seldom progress. Progressive massive fibrosis (PMF) refers to the formation of conglomerate masses (mainly in the upper lobes), which may cavitate. The development of

19.90 Lung diseases caused by exposure to inorganic dusts

Cause	Occupation	Description	Characteristic pathological features
Coal dust	Coal mining	Coal worker's pneumoconiosis	Focal and interstitial fibrosis, centrilobular emphysema, progressive massive fibrosis
Silica	Mining, quarrying, stone dressing, metal grinding, pottery, boiler scaling	Silicosis	
Asbestos	Demolition, ship breaking, manufacture of fireproof insulating materials, pipe and boiler lagging	Asbestos-related disease	Pleural plaques, diffuse pleural thickening, acute benign pleurisy, carcinoma of lung, interstitial fibrosis, mesothelioma
Iron oxide	Arc welding	Siderosis	Mineral deposition only
Tin oxide	Tin mining	Stannosis	Tin-laden macrophages
Beryllium	Aircraft, atomic energy and electronics industries	Berylliosis	Granulomas, interstitial fibrosis

PMF is usually associated with cough, sputum that may be black (melanoptysis), and breathlessness. The chest X-ray appearances may be confused with lung cancer, tuberculosis and granulomatosis with polyangiitis. PMF may progress even after coal dust exposure ceases, and in extreme cases leads to respiratory failure and right ventricular failure.

Caplan's syndrome describes the coexistence of rheumatoid arthritis and rounded fibrotic nodules 0.5–5 cm in diameter. They show pathological features similar to a rheumatoid nodule, including central necrosis, palisading histiocytes, and a peripheral rim of lymphocytes and plasma cells. This syndrome may also occur in other types of pneumoconiosis.

Silicosis

Silicosis results from the inhalation of crystalline silica, usually in the form of quartz, by workers cutting, grinding and polishing stone. Classic silicosis is most common and usually manifests after 10–20 years of continuous silica exposure, during which time the patient remains asymptomatic. Accelerated silicosis is associated with a much shorter duration of dust exposure (typically 5–10 years), and may present as early as 1 year of exposure; as the name suggests, it follows a more aggressive course. Intense exposure to very fine crystalline silica dust can cause a more acute disease – silicoproteinosis, similar to alveolar proteinosis (see Box 19.88, p. 715).

Radiological features are similar to those of coal worker's pneumoconiosis, with multiple well-circumscribed 3–5-mm nodular opacities, predominantly in the mid- and upper zones. As the disease progresses, PMF may develop (Fig. 19.63). Enlargement of the hilar glands with an 'egg-shell' pattern of calcification is said to be characteristic but is uncommon and non-specific. Silica is highly fibrogenic and the disease is usually progressive, even when exposure ceases; hence the affected worker should always be removed from further exposure. Individuals with silicosis are at increased risk of tuberculosis (silicotuberculosis), lung cancer and COPD. Associations with renal and connective tissue disease have also been described.

Berylliosis

Exposure to beryllium is encountered in aircraft engineering and dentistry. The presence of cough, progressive breathlessness, night sweats and arthralgia in a worker exposed to dusts, fumes or vapours containing beryllium should raise suspicions of berylliosis. The radiographic appearances are similar in type and distribution to sarcoid, and biopsy shows sarcoid-like granulomas. The diagnosis may be confirmed by specialised tests of lymphocyte function.

A
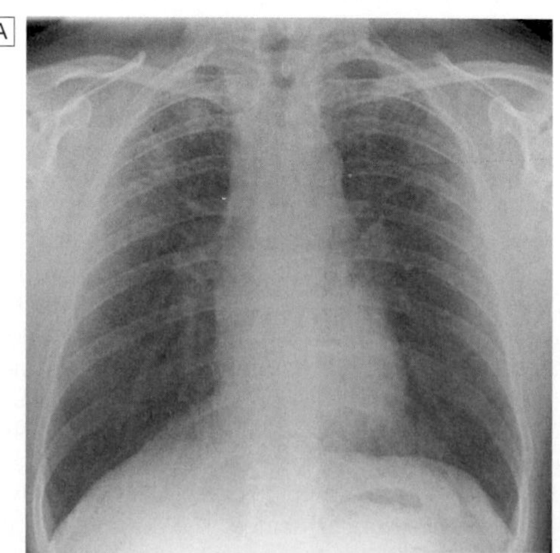

B
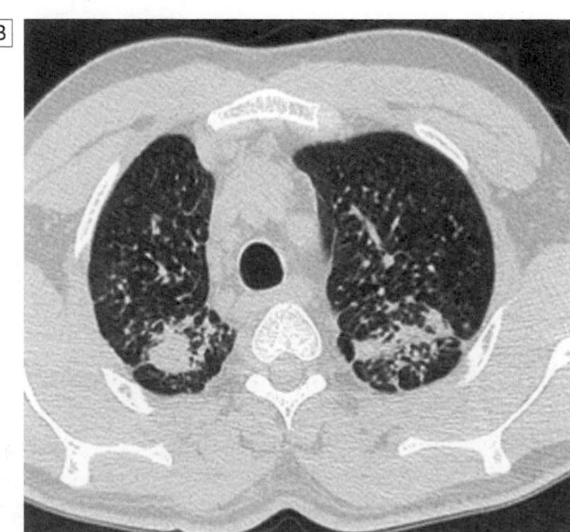

Fig. 19.63 Silicosis. A A chest X-ray from a patient with silicosis, showing the presence of small rounded nodules predominantly seen in the upper zones. B HRCT from the same patient, demonstrating conglomeration of nodules with posterior bias.

Less common pneumoconioses

Siderosis refers to the development of a benign iron oxide pneumoconiosis in welders and other iron foundry workers. Baritosis may be seen in barium process workers, and stannosis in tin refining; haematite lung occurs in iron ore miners and resembles silicosis but stains the lung red. Diamond polishers may develop hard metal disease; this condition is similar to UIP but the pathology shows a giant cell interstitial pneumonia. Popcorn worker's lung is a form of obliterative bronchiolitis following ingestion of diacetyl used in butter flavouring.

Asbestos-related lung and pleural diseases

Asbestos is a naturally occurring silicate. Its fibres may be classified as either chrysotile (white asbestos), which accounts for 90% of the world's production, or serpentine (crocidolite or blue asbestos, and amosite or brown asbestos). Its favourable thermal and chemical insulation properties led to its extensive use by the shipbuilding and construction industries throughout the latter part of the twentieth century. Exposure to asbestos may be followed by the development of both pleural and pulmonary disease, after a lengthy latent period.

Pleural plaques

Pleural plaques are the most common manifestation of past asbestos exposure, and are discrete circumscribed areas of hyaline fibrosis that may occur on the parietal pleura of the chest wall, diaphragm, pericardium or mediastinum. They are virtually always asymptomatic and are usually identified as an incidental finding on a chest X-ray (Fig. 19.64) or thoracic CT scan, particularly when partially calcified. They do not cause any impairment of lung function and are benign.

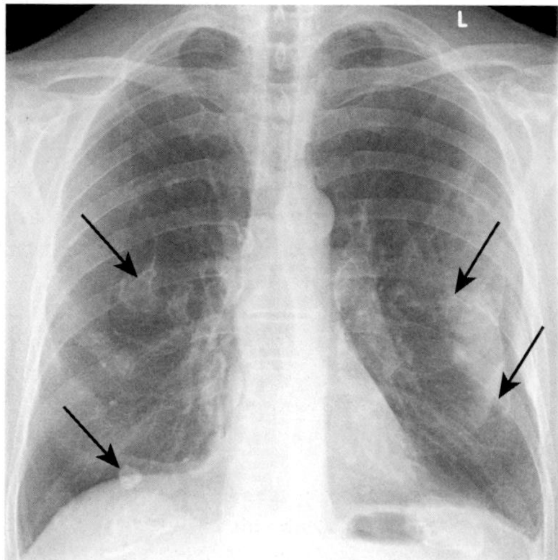

Fig. 19.64 Asbestos-related benign pleural plaques. Chest X-ray showing extensive calcified pleural plaques ('candle wax' appearance – arrows), particularly marked on the diaphragm and lateral pleural surfaces.

Acute benign asbestos pleurisy

Benign asbestos pleurisy is estimated to occur in around one-fifth of asbestos workers but many episodes are subclinical and pass unreported. When symptomatic, patients present with features of pleurisy, including mild fever and systemic disturbance. The diagnosis necessitates the exclusion of other known causes of pleurisy and pleural effusion. Repeated episodes may be followed by the development of diffuse (visceral) pleural thickening.

Diffuse pleural thickening

Diffuse pleural thickening (DPT) affects the visceral pleura and, if sufficiently extensive, may cause restrictive lung function impairment, exertional breathlessness and, occasionally, persistent chest pain. The typical appearances of DPT on chest X-ray include thickening of the pleura along the chest wall and obliteration of the costophrenic angles. Earlier manifestations of DPT, including parenchymal bands, may be detected by CT (Fig. 19.65). Occasionally, shrinkage of the visceral pleura results in the development of 'round atelectasis'. There is no treatment and the condition may progress in around one-third of individuals. In exceptionally severe cases, surgical decortication may be considered. A pleural biopsy may be required to exclude mesothelioma.

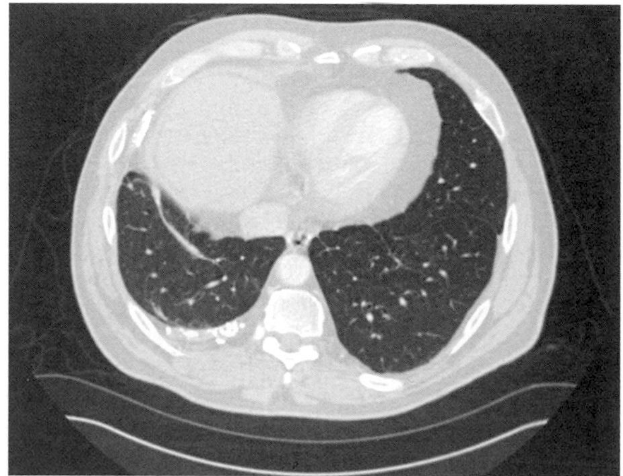

Fig. 19.65 Thoracic CT scan showing right-sided pleural thickening and an associated parenchymal band.

Asbestosis

Asbestosis is a diffuse parenchymal lung disease. Its development generally requires substantial exposure over several years, and is rare with low-level or bystander exposure. In common with other fibrosing lung diseases, asbestosis usually presents with exertional breathlessness and fine, late inspiratory crackles over the lower zones. Finger clubbing may be present. Pulmonary function tests and HRCT appearances are similar to those of UIP. These features, accompanied by a history of substantial asbestos exposure, are generally sufficient to establish the diagnosis; lung biopsy is rarely necessary. When biopsy is performed, the diagnosis is made when alveolar septal fibrosis is accompanied by an average of at least two asbestos bodies per square cm of lung tissue. In cases where there is doubt, asbestos fibre counts may be performed on lung biopsy material to establish the diagnosis.

Asbestosis is usually slowly progressive but tends to be more indolent and associated with a better prognosis than UIP; in advanced cases, however, respiratory failure and cor pulmonale may still develop. About 40% of patients (who usually smoke) develop carcinoma of the lung and 10% may develop mesothelioma.

Mesothelioma

Mesothelioma is a malignant tumour affecting the pleura or, less commonly, the peritoneum. Its occurrence almost invariably suggests past asbestos exposure, which may be low-level. There is typically a long latent interval between first exposure and the onset of clinical manifestations, such that, even though asbestos control measures have now been implemented, deaths from mesothelioma continue to increase.

Pleural mesothelioma typically presents with increasing breathlessness resulting from pleural effusion, or unremitting chest pain when there is involvement of the chest wall. As the tumour progresses, it encases the underlying lung and may invade into the parenchyma, the mediastinum and the pericardium. Metastatic disease, although often not clinically detectable in life, is a common finding on post-mortem.

Mesothelioma is almost invariably fatal. Highly selected patients may be considered for radical surgery but, in the majority, therapy is invariably directed towards palliation of symptoms. The use of chemotherapy may improve quality of life and is accompanied by a small survival benefit of around 3 months. Radiotherapy can be used to control pain and limit the risk of tumour seeding at biopsy sites. Pleural effusions are managed with drainage and pleurodesis. Typical figures for survival from onset of symptoms are around 16 months for epithelioid tumours, 10 months for sarcomatoid tumours and 15 months for biphasic tumours, with only a minority of patients surviving longer periods.

19.91 Examples of lung diseases caused by organic dusts

Disorder	Source	Antigen/agent
Farmer's lung*	Mouldy hay, straw, grain	*Micropolyspora faeni* *Aspergillus fumigatus*
Bird fancier's lung*	Avian excreta, proteins and feathers	Avian serum proteins
Malt worker's lung*	Mouldy maltings	*Aspergillus clavatus*
Cheese worker's lung*	Mouldy cheese	*Aspergillus clavatus* *Penicillium casei*
Maple bark stripper's lung*	Bark from stored maple	*Cryptostroma corticale*
Saxophone player's lung*	Reed of any wind instrument	*Fusarium* spp. *Penicillium* spp. *Cladosporium* spp.
Byssinosis	Textile industries	Cotton, flax, hemp dust
Inhalation ('humidifier') fever	Contamination of air conditioning	Thermophilic actinomycetes

*Presents as hypersensitivity pneumonitis.

Lung diseases due to organic dusts

A wide range of organic agents may cause respiratory disorders (Box 19.91). Disease results from a local immune response to animal proteins, or fungal antigens in mouldy vegetable matter. Hypersensitivity pneumonitis is the most common of these conditions.

Hypersensitivity pneumonitis

Hypersensitivity pneumonitis (HP; also called extrinsic allergic alveolitis) results from the inhalation of a wide variety of organic antigens, which give rise to a diffuse immune complex reaction in the alveoli and bronchioles. Common causes include farmer's lung and bird fancier's lung. Other examples are shown in Box 19.91. HP is not exclusively occupational or environmental, and other important causes include medications (see Box 19.86).

The pathology of hypersensitivity pneumonitis is consistent with both type III and type IV immunological mechanisms (p. 87). Precipitating IgG antibodies may be detected in the serum and a type III Arthus reaction is believed to occur in the lung, where the precipitation of immune complexes results in activation of complement and an inflammatory response in the alveolar walls, characterised by the influx of mononuclear cells and foamy histiocytes. The presence of poorly formed non-caseating granulomas in the alveolar walls suggests that type IV responses are also important. The distribution of the inflammatory infiltrate is predominantly peribronchiolar, which helps to distinguish the appearances from non-specific interstitial pneumonia and lymphocytic interstitial pneumonia. Chronic forms may be accompanied by fibrosis. For reasons that remain uncertain, there is a lower incidence of hypersensitivity pneumonitis in smokers than non-smokers.

Clinical features

The presentation of HP varies from an acute form to a more indolent pattern, depending on the antigen load. For example, the farmer exposed to mouldy hay after it was gathered and stored damp during a wet summer, or the pigeon fancier cleaning a large pigeon loft, will report influenza-like symptoms within a few hours, accompanied by cough, breathlessness and wheeze. On the other hand, the individual with low-level antigen exposure, such as to an indoor pet bird, will typically present in a more indolent fashion with slowly progressive breathlessness, and, in some cases, established fibrosis may be present by the time the disease is recognised. Chest auscultation typically reveals widespread end-inspiratory crackles and squeaks.

Investigations

In cases of acute HP, the chest X-ray typically shows ill-defined patchy airspace shadowing which, given the systemic features, may be confused with pneumonia. HRCT is more likely to show bilateral ground glass shadowing and areas of consolidation superimposed on small centrilobar nodular opacities with an upper and middle lobe predominance (Fig. 19.66). In more

A

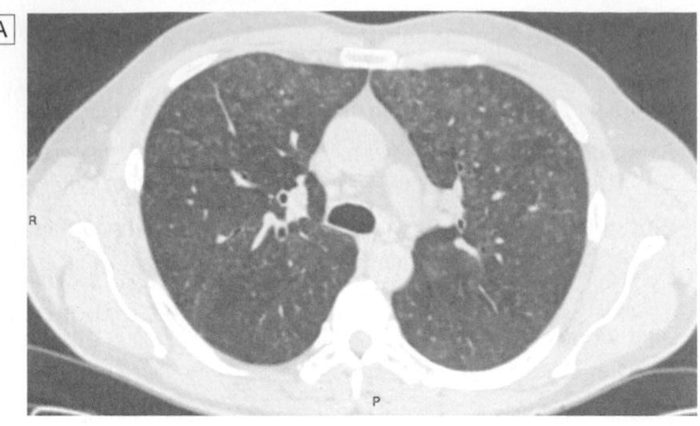

B

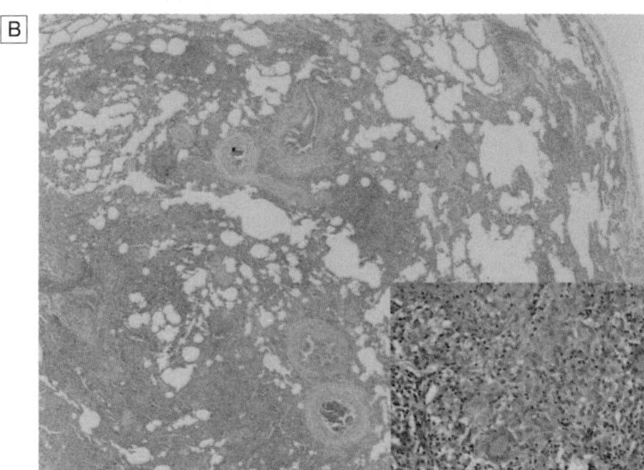

Fig. 19.66 Hypersensitivity pneumonitis. **A** HRCT showing typical patchy ground glass opacification. **B** Histology shows evidence of an interstitial inflammatory infiltrate in the lung, expanding alveolar walls, with a peribronchial distribution. Within the infiltrate, there are foci of small, poorly defined non-caseating granulomas (insert), which often lie adjacent to the airways. In this case, there is little in the way of established lung fibrosis, but this can be marked.

chronic disease, features of fibrosis, such as volume loss, linear opacities and architectural distortion, appear. In common with other fibrotic diseases, pulmonary function tests show a restrictive ventilatory defect with reduced lung volumes and impaired gas transfer, and dynamic tests may detect oxygen desaturation. In more advanced disease, type I respiratory failure is present at rest.

Diagnosis

The diagnosis of HP is usually based on the characteristic clinical and radiological features, together with the identification of a potential source of antigen in the patient's home or place of work (Box 19.92). It may be supported by a positive serum precipitin test or by more sensitive serological tests. However, the presence of precipitins without the other features does not signify a diagnosis; the great majority of farmers with positive precipitins do not have farmer's lung, and up to 15% of pigeon breeders may have positive serum precipitins yet remain healthy.

Where HP is suspected but the cause is not readily apparent, a visit to the patient's home or workplace should be made. Occasionally, if an agent previously unrecognised as causing HP is suspected, provocation testing may be necessary to prove the diagnosis; if positive, inhalation of the relevant antigen is followed after 3–6 hours by pyrexia and a reduction in VC and gas transfer factor. BAL fluid usually shows an increase in

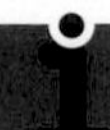

19.92 Predictive factors in the identification of hypersensitivity pneumonitis

- Exposure to a known offending antigen
- Positive precipitating antibodies to offending antigen
- Recurrent episodes of symptoms
- Inspiratory crackles on examination
- Symptoms occurring 4–8 hrs after exposure
- Weight loss

the number of CD8+ T lymphocytes, and transbronchial biopsy can occasionally provide sufficient tissue for a confident diagnosis; however, open lung biopsy may be necessary (Fig. 19.66B).

Management

If practical, the patient should cease exposure to the inciting agent. In some cases, however, this may be difficult, either because of implications for livelihood (e.g. farmers) or enthusiasm for hobbies (e.g. pigeon breeders). Dust masks with appropriate filters may minimise exposure and be combined with methods of reducing levels of antigen (e.g. drying hay before storage). In acute cases, prednisolone should be given for 3–4 weeks, starting with an oral dose of 40 mg per day. Severely hypoxaemic patients may require high-concentration oxygen therapy initially. Most patients recover completely but, if unchecked, fibrosis may progress to cause severe respiratory disability, hypoxaemia, pulmonary hypertension, cor pulmonale and eventually death.

Inhalation ('humidifier') fever

Inhalation fever shares similarities with HP. It occurs as a result of contaminated humidifiers or air-conditioning units that release a fine spray of microorganisms into the atmosphere. The illness is characterised by self-limiting fever and breathlessness; permanent sequelae are unusual. An identical syndrome can also develop after disturbing an accumulation of mouldy hay, compost or mulch. So-called 'hot tub lung' appears to be attributable to *Mycobacterium avium*. Outbreaks of HP in workers using metalworking fluids appear to be linked to *Acinetobacter* or *Ochrobactrum*.

Occupational lung cancer

Individuals exposed to substantial quantities of asbestos are at increased risk of lung cancer particularly if they smoke tobacco. Increased risks of lung cancer have also been reported in workers who develop silicosis and those exposed to radon gas, beryllium, diesel exhaust fumes, cadmium, chromium, and dust and fumes from coke plants.

Occupational pneumonia

Occupational and environmental exposures may be closely linked to the development of pneumonia. Welders appear to be at increased risk of pneumonia and pneumococcal vaccine is currently recommended for those in the trade. Farm, abattoir and hide factory workers may be exposed to *Coxiella burnetii*, the causative agent of Q fever. The organisms are excreted from milk, urine, faeces and amniotic fluid, or may be transmitted by cattle ticks or contaminated dust from the milking floor, or by drinking milk that is inadequately pasteurised. Birds (often parrots or budgerigars) infected with *Chlamydia psittaci* can cause psittacosis in humans. Sewage workers, farmers, animal handlers and veterinarians run an increased risk of contracting leptospiral pneumonia. Contact with rabbits, hares, muskrats and ground squirrels is associated with tularaemic pneumonia, caused by *Francisella tularensis* (p. 340). Anthrax (wool-sorter's disease, p. 346) may occur in workers exposed to infected hides, hair, bristle, bonemeal and animal carcases.

PULMONARY VASCULAR DISEASE

Venous thromboembolism

Deep venous thrombosis (DVT, p. 1008) and pulmonary embolism (PE) are included under this heading. The majority (80%) of pulmonary emboli arise from the propagation of lower limb DVT. Rare causes include septic emboli (from endocarditis affecting the tricuspid or pulmonary valves), tumour (especially choriocarcinoma), fat, air, amniotic fluid and placenta.

The incidence of VTE in the community is unknown; it occurs in approximately 1% of all patients admitted to hospital and accounts for around 5% of in-hospital deaths. It is a common mode of death in patients with cancer, stroke and pregnancy.

Clinical features

VTE may be difficult to diagnose. It is helpful to consider:

- Is the clinical presentation consi
- Does the patient have risk factor
- Are there any alternative diagno the patient's presentation?

Clinical presentation varies, dep size and distribution of emboli and diorespiratory reserve (Box 19.93). factor is present in 80–90% (Box 19. one or more risk factors increases the risk further still.

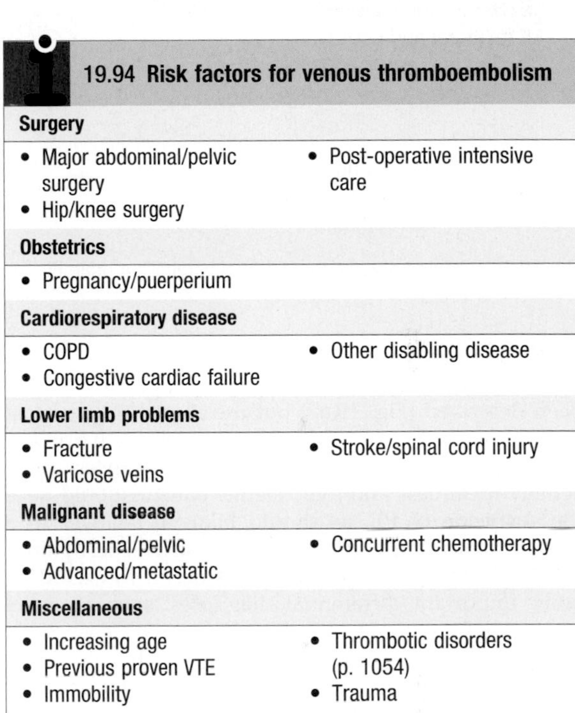

19.94 Risk factors for venous thromboembolism

Surgery	
• Major abdominal/pelvic surgery • Hip/knee surgery	• Post-operative intensive care
Obstetrics	
• Pregnancy/puerperium	
Cardiorespiratory disease	
• COPD • Congestive cardiac failure	• Other disabling disease
Lower limb problems	
• Fracture • Varicose veins	• Stroke/spinal cord injury
Malignant disease	
• Abdominal/pelvic • Advanced/metastatic	• Concurrent chemotherapy
Miscellaneous	
• Increasing age • Previous proven VTE • Immobility	• Thrombotic disorders (p. 1054) • Trauma

19.93 Features of pulmonary thromboemboli

	Acute massive PE	Acute small/medium PE	Chronic PE
Pathophysiology	Major haemodynamic effects: ↓cardiac output; acute right heart failure	Occlusion of segmental pulmonary artery → infarction ± effusion	Chronic occlusion of pulmonary microvasculature, right heart failure
Symptoms	Faintness or collapse, crushing central chest pain, apprehension, severe dyspnoea	Pleuritic chest pain, restricted breathing, haemoptysis	Exertional dyspnoea. Late symptoms of pulmonary hypertension or right heart failure
Signs	Major circulatory collapse: tachycardia, hypotension, ↑JVP, RV gallop rhythm, loud P_2, severe cyanosis, ↓urinary output	Tachycardia, pleural rub, raised hemidiaphragm, crackles, effusion (often blood-stained), low-grade fever	May be minimal early in disease. Later: RV heave, loud P_2. Terminal: signs of right heart failure
Chest X-ray	Usually normal. May be subtle oligaemia	Pleuropulmonary opacities, pleural effusion, linear shadows, raised hemidiaphragm	Enlarged pulmonary artery trunk, enlarged heart, prominent right ventricle
ECG	$S_1Q_3T_3$ anterior T-wave inversion, RBBB	Sinus tachycardia	RV hypertrophy and strain
Arterial blood gases	Markedly abnormal with ↓PaO_2 and ↓$PaCO_2$. Metabolic acidosis	May be normal or ↓PaO_2 or ↓$PaCO_2$	Exertional ↓PaO_2 or desaturation on formal exercise testing
Alternative diagnoses	Myocardial infarction, pericardial tamponade, aortic dissection	Pneumonia, pneumothorax, musculoskeletal chest pain	Other causes of pulmonary hypertension

(JVP = jugular venous pressure; PE = pulmonary embolism; RBBB = right bundle branch block; RV = ventricular)

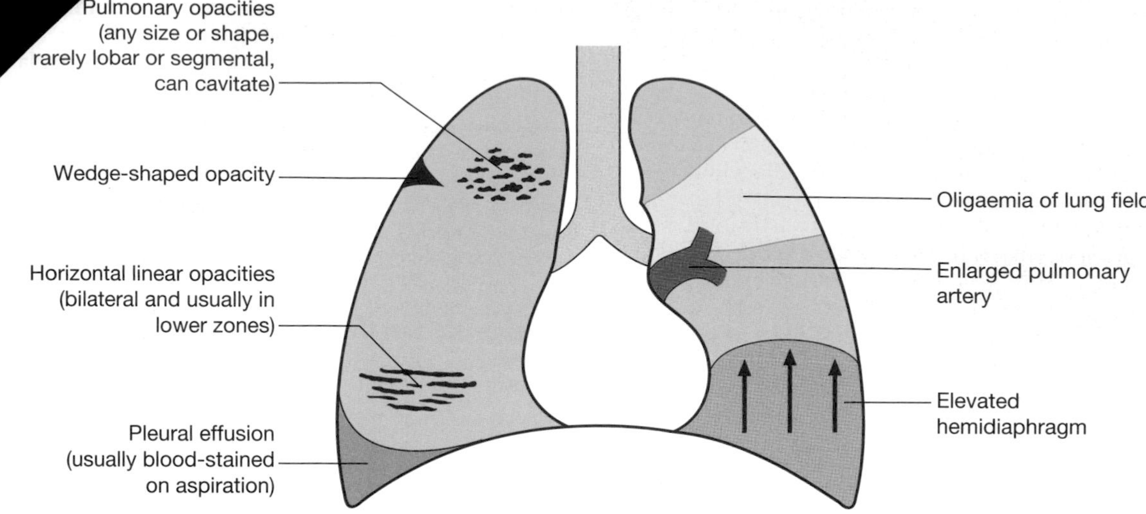

Fig. 19.67 Features of pulmonary thromboembolism/infarction on chest X-ray.

Investigations

A variety of non-specific radiographic appearances have been described (Fig. 19.67) but the chest X-ray is most useful in excluding key differential diagnoses, e.g. pneumonia or pneumothorax. Normal appearances in an acutely breathless and hypoxaemic patient should raise the suspicion of PE, as should bilateral changes in a patient presenting with unilateral pleuritic chest pain.

The ECG is often normal but is useful in excluding other important differential diagnoses, such as acute myocardial infarction and pericarditis. The most common findings in PE include sinus tachycardia and anterior T-wave inversion but these are non-specific; larger emboli may cause right heart strain revealed by an $S_1Q_3T_3$ pattern, ST-segment and T-wave changes, or the appearance of right bundle branch block.

Arterial blood gases typically show a reduced PaO_2 and a normal or low $PaCO_2$, and an increased alveolar–arterial oxygen gradient, but may be normal in a significant minority. A metabolic acidosis may be seen in acute massive PE with cardiovascular collapse.

D-dimer is a specific degradation product released into the circulation when cross-linked fibrin undergoes endogenous fibrinolysis (p. 1000). An elevated D-dimer is of limited value, as it may be raised in a variety of conditions including PE, myocardial infarction, pneumonia and sepsis. However, low levels (< 500 ng/mL, measured by ELISA), particularly where clinical risk is low, have a high negative predictive value and further investigation is usually unnecessary (Fig. 19.68). The D-dimer result should be disregarded in high-risk patients, as further investigation is mandatory even if it is normal. Other circulating markers that reflect right ventricular micro-infarction, such as troponin I and brain natriuretic peptide, are under investigation.

CT pulmonary angiography (CTPA, Fig. 19.69) is the first-line diagnostic test. It has the advantages of visualising the distribution and extent of the emboli, or highlighting an alternative diagnosis, such as consolidation, pneumothorax or aortic dissection. The sensitivity of CT scanning may be increased by simultaneous visualisation of the femoral and popliteal veins, although this is not widely practised. As the contrast media may be nephrotoxic, care should be taken in patients with renal impairment, and CTPA avoided in those with a history of allergy to iodinated contrast media.

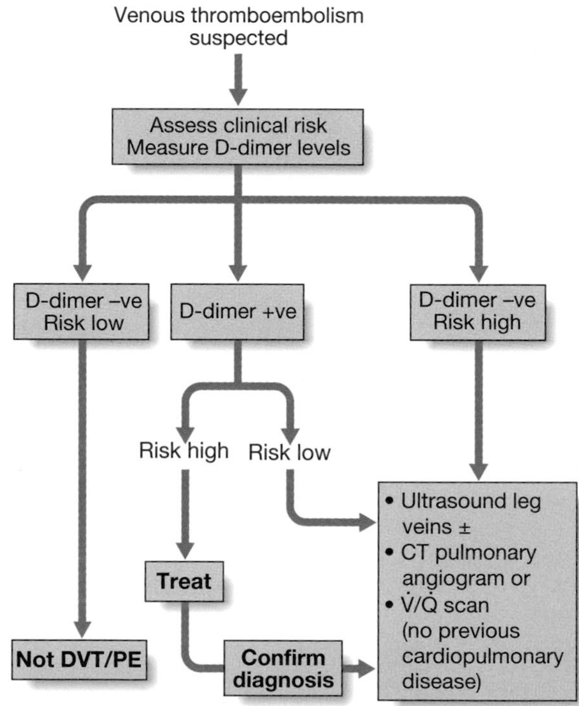

Fig. 19.68 Algorithm for the investigation of patients with suspected pulmonary thromboembolism. Clinical risk is based on the presence of risk factors for venous thromboembolism and the probability of another diagnosis.

Ventilation–perfusion scanning is seldom used nowadays, although a limited role remains in those without significant cardiopulmonary disease. Colour Doppler ultrasound of the leg veins remains the investigation of choice in patients with suspected DVT, but may also be used in patients with suspected PE, particularly if there are clinical signs in a limb, as many will have identifiable proximal thrombus in the leg veins.

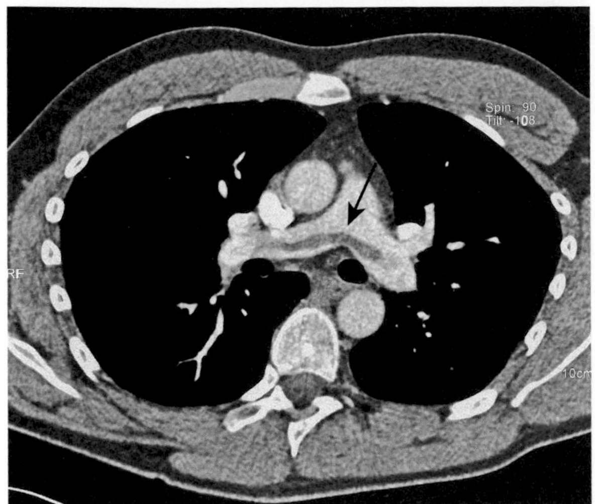

Fig. 19.69 CT pulmonary angiogram. The arrow points to a saddle embolism in the bifurcation of the pulmonary artery.

Bedside echocardiography is extremely helpful in the differential diagnosis and assessment of acute circulatory collapse (p. 544). Acute dilatation of the right heart is usually present in massive PE, and thrombus (embolism in transit) may be visible. Alternative diagnoses, including left ventricular failure, aortic dissection and pericardial tamponade, can also be identified.

Conventional pulmonary angiography has been largely superseded by CTPA but is still useful in selected settings or to deliver catheter-based therapies.

Management

General measures

Prompt recognition and treatment are potentially lifesaving. Sufficient oxygen should be given to hypoxaemic patients to maintain arterial oxygen saturation above 90%. Circulatory shock should be treated with intravenous fluids or plasma expander, but inotropic agents are of limited value as the hypoxic dilated right ventricle is already close to maximally stimulated by endogenous catecholamines. Diuretics and vasodilators should also be avoided, as they will reduce cardiac output. Opiates may be necessary to relieve pain and distress but should be used with caution in the hypotensive patient. External cardiac massage may be successful in the moribund patient by dislodging and breaking up a large central embolus.

Anticoagulation

Anticoagulation should be commenced immediately in patients with a high or intermediate probability of PE, but may be safely withheld in those with low clinical probability, pending investigation. Heparin reduces further propagation of clot and the risk of further emboli, and lowers mortality. It is most easily administered as subcutaneous low molecular weight heparin (LMWH). The dose is based on the patient's weight and there is usually no requirement to monitor tests of coagulation (p. 1018). Treatment with LMWH should continue for at least 5 days, during which time an oral anticoagulant is commenced. Fondaparinux, a synthetic pentasaccharide closely related to heparin, represents an alternative to LMWH. Warfarin – a vitamin K antagonist – remains the most commonly used oral anticoagulant. Therapy is initiated with a high loading dose, followed by a maintenance dose based on the international normalised ratio (INR). LMWH should not be discontinued until the INR is 2 or more for at least 24 hours. Due to the narrow therapeutic index of warfarin and its propensity to interact with other drugs and food, regular measurement of the INR is required throughout the duration of anticoagulation. Newer thrombin or activated factor X inhibitors offer more predictable dosing and have no requirement for coagulation monitoring; they may ultimately replace warfarin.

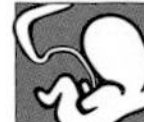

19.95 VTE and pregnancy

- **Maternal mortality**: VTE is the leading cause.
- **CTPA**: may be performed safely with fetal shielding (0.01–0.06 mGy). It is important to consider the risk of radiation to breast tissue (particularly if there is a family history of breast carcinoma) and the risk of iodinated contrast media to mother and fetus (neonatal hypothyroidism).
- **$\dot{V}/\dot{Q}$ scanning**: greater radiation dose to fetus (0.11–0.22 mGy) but less to maternal breast tissue.
- **In utero radiation exposure**: estimated incidence of childhood malignancy is about 1 in 16 000 per mGy.
- **Warfarin**: teratogenic, so VTE should be treated with LMWH during pregnancy.

Decisions regarding the duration of anticoagulation represent a balance between the risk and consequences of recurrence, and the risks of prolonged anticoagulation. In patients with an identifiable and reversible risk factor, anticoagulation may be safely discontinued following 3 months of therapy. Those with persistent prothrombotic risks or a history of previous emboli should be anticoagulated for life. In patients with cancer-associated VTE, LMWH should be continued for at least 6 months before switching to warfarin. For patients with unprovoked VTE, the appropriate duration of anticoagulation should be at least 3 months, but prolonged therapy should be considered in males (who have a higher risk of recurrent VTE than females), those in whom the D-dimer remains elevated when measured 1 month after stopping anticoagulation, those with post-thrombotic syndrome, and those in whom recurrent PE may be fatal. The disadvantages of prolonged anticoagulation range from the inconvenience of long-term INR monitoring to the more serious risk of major haemorrhage (around 3% per year). Life-threatening haemorrhage occurs in around 1% of cases per year and fatal bleeding in 0.25% cases per year.

Thrombolytic and surgical therapy

Thrombolysis is indicated in any patient presenting with acute massive PE accompanied by cardiogenic shock. In the absence of shock, the benefits are less clear but thrombolysis may be considered in those presenting with right ventricular dilatation and hypokinesis or severe hypoxaemia. Patients must be screened carefully for haemorrhagic risk, as there is a high risk of intracranial haemorrhage. Surgical pulmonary embolectomy may be considered in selected patients but carries a high mortality.

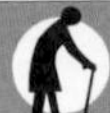

19.96 Thromboembolic disease in old age

- **Risk**: rises by a factor of 2.5 over the age of 60 yrs.
- **Prophylaxis for VTE**: should be considered in all older patients who are immobile as a result of acute illness, except when this is due to acute stroke.
- **Association with cancer**: the prevalence of cancer among those with DVT increases with age but the relative risk of malignancy with DVT falls; therefore extensive investigation is not justified if initial assessment reveals no evidence of an underlying neoplasm.
- **Warfarin**: older patients are more sensitive to the anticoagulant effects of warfarin, partly due to the concurrent use of other drugs and the presence of other pathology. Life-threatening or fatal bleeds on warfarin are significantly more common in those aged over 80 yrs.
- **Chronic immobility**: long-term anticoagulant therapy is not required as there is no associated increase in thromboembolism.

Caval filters

A patient in whom anticoagulation is contraindicated, who has suffered massive haemorrhage on anticoagulation, or recurrent VTE despite anticoagulation, should be considered for an inferior vena caval filter. Retrievable caval filters are particularly useful in patients with temporary risk factors.

Prognosis

Immediate morality is greatest in those with echocardiographic evidence of right ventricular dysfunction or cardiogenic shock. Once anticoagulation is commenced, however, the risk of mortality rapidly falls. The risk of recurrence is highest in the first 6–12 months after the initial event, and at 10 years around one-third of individuals will have suffered a further event.

Pulmonary hypertension

Pulmonary hypertension (PH) is defined as a mean pulmonary artery pressure of at least 25 mmHg at rest, as measured at right heart catheterisation. The definition may be further refined by consideration of the pulmonary wedge pressure, the cardiac output and the transpulmonary pressure gradient (mean PAP – mean PWP). The clinical classification of pulmonary hypertension is shown in Box 19.97. Further classification is based on the degree of functional disturbance, assessed using the New York Heart Association (NYHA) grades I–IV. Although respiratory failure due to intrinsic pulmonary disease is the most common cause of pulmonary hypertension, severe pulmonary hypertension may occur as a primary disorder, as a complication of connective tissue disease (e.g. systemic sclerosis), or as a result of chronic thromboembolic events.

Primary pulmonary hypertension (PPH) is a rare but important disease that affects predominantly women, aged between 20 and 30 years. Familial disease is rarer still but is known to be associated with mutations in the gene encoding type II bone morphogenetic protein receptor (*BMPR2*), a member of the TGF-β superfamily. Mutations in this gene have been identified in some patients with sporadic pulmonary hypertension.

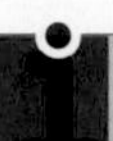

19.97 Classification of pulmonary hypertension

Pulmonary arterial hypertension

- Primary pulmonary hypertension: sporadic and familial
- Secondary to: connective tissue disease (limited cutaneous systemic sclerosis), congenital systemic to pulmonary shunts, portal hypertension, HIV infection, exposure to various drugs or toxins, and persistent pulmonary hypertension of the newborn

Pulmonary venous hypertension

- Left-sided atrial or ventricular heart disease
- Left-sided valvular heart disease
- Pulmonary veno-occlusive disease
- Pulmonary capillary haemangiomatosis

Pulmonary hypertension associated with disorders of the respiratory system and/or hypoxaemia

- COPD
- Diffuse parenchymal lung disease
- Sleep-disordered breathing
- Alveolar hypoventilation disorders
- Chronic exposure to high altitude
- Neonatal lung disease
- Alveolar capillary dysplasia
- Severe kyphoscoliosis

Pulmonary hypertension caused by chronic thromboembolic disease

- Thromboembolic obstruction of the proximal pulmonary arteries
- In situ thrombosis
- Sickle cell disease

Miscellaneous

- Inflammatory conditions
- Extrinsic compression of central pulmonary veins

Adapted from Dana Point 2008. Simonneau G, et al. Updated clinical classification of pulmonary hypertension. J Am Coll Cardiol 2009; 54:S43–S54.

Pathological features include hypertrophy of both the media and the intima of the vessel wall, and a clonal expansion of endothelial cells which take on the appearance of plexiform lesions. There is marked narrowing of the vessel lumen and this, together with the frequently observed in situ thrombosis, leads to an increase in pulmonary vascular resistance and pulmonary hypertension.

Clinical features

PH presents insidiously and is often diagnosed late. Typical symptoms include breathlessness, chest pain, fatigue, palpitation and syncope. Important signs include elevation of the jugular venous pulse (with a prominent 'a' wave if in sinus rhythm), a parasternal heave (right ventricular hypertrophy), accentuation of the pulmonary component of the second heart sound and a right ventricular third heart sound. Signs of interstitial lung disease or cardiac, liver or connective tissue disease may suggest the underlying cause.

Investigations

PH is suspected if an electrocardiograph shows a right ventricular 'strain' pattern or a chest X-ray shows enlarged pulmonary arteries, peripheral pruning and right ventricle enlargement (Fig. 19.70). Doppler assessment of the tricuspid regurgitant jet by transthoracic echocardiography provides a non-invasive estimate of

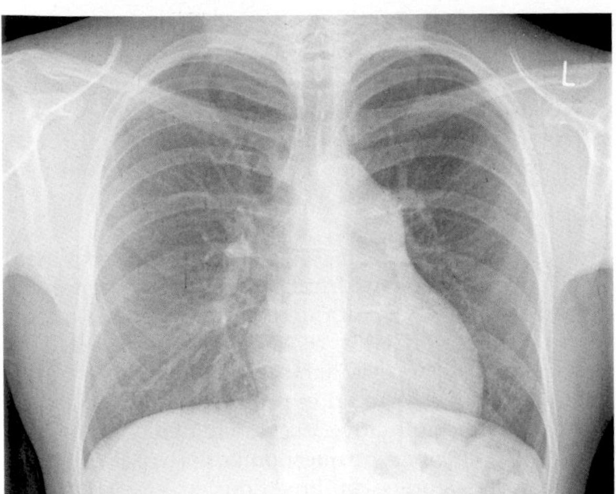

Fig. 19.70 Chest X-ray showing the typical appearance in pulmonary hypertension.

the pulmonary artery pressure, which is equal to 4 × (tricuspid regurgitation velocity)^2. Further assessment should be by right heart catheterisation to assess pulmonary haemodynamics, measure vasodilator responsiveness and thus guide further therapy.

Management

The management of PH should be guided by expert advice. General measures include diuretic therapy for right heart failure, and long-term oxygen therapy for those with chronic hypoxaemia. Unless there is an increased risk of bleeding, anticoagulation should be considered. Digoxin may be useful in patients who develop atrial tachyarrhythmias. Pregnancy carries a very high risk of death and women of child-bearing age should be counselled appropriately. Excessive physical activity that leads to distressing symptoms should be avoided but otherwise patients should be encouraged to remain active. Pneumococcal and influenza vaccination should be given.

Specific treatment options include high-dose calcium channel blockers, prostaglandins such as epoprostenol (prostacyclin) or iloprost therapy, the phosphodiesterase type 5 (PDE5) inhibitor sildenafil, and the oral endothelin antagonist bosentan. Selected patients are referred for heart–lung transplantation, and pulmonary thrombo-endarterectomy may be contemplated in those with chronic proximal pulmonary thromboembolic disease. Another alternative is atrial septostomy (the creation of a right-to-left shunt), which decompresses the right ventricle and improves haemodynamic performance.

DISEASES OF THE UPPER AIRWAY

Diseases of the nasopharynx

Allergic rhinitis

This is a disorder in which there are episodes of nasal congestion, watery nasal discharge and sneezing. It may be seasonal or perennial, and is due to an immediate hypersensitivity reaction in the nasal mucosa. Seasonal antigens include pollens from grasses, flowers, weeds or trees. Grass pollen is responsible for hay fever, the most common type of seasonal allergic rhinitis in northern Europe, which is at its peak between May and July. However this is a worldwide problem, which may be aggravated during harvest seasons.

Perennial allergic rhinitis may be a specific reaction to antigens derived from house dust, fungal spores or animal dander, but similar symptoms can be caused by physical or chemical irritants – for example, pungent odours or fumes, including strong perfumes, cold air and dry atmospheres. The phrase 'vasomotor rhinitis' is often used in this context, as the term 'allergic' is a misnomer.

Clinical features

In the seasonal type, there are frequent sudden attacks of sneezing, with profuse watery nasal discharge and nasal obstruction. These attacks last for a few hours and are often accompanied by smarting and watering of the eyes and conjunctival irritation. In perennial rhinitis, the symptoms are similar but more continuous and usually less severe. Skin hypersensitivity tests with the relevant antigen are usually positive in seasonal allergic rhinitis, but are less useful in perennial rhinitis.

Management

In those sensitised to house dust, simple measures, such as thorough dust removal from the bed area, leaving a window open and renewing old pillows, are often helpful. Avoidance of pollen and antigens from domestic pets, however desirable and beneficial, is usually impractical.

The following medications, singly or in combination, are usually effective in both seasonal and perennial allergic rhinitis:

- an antihistamine such as loratadine
- sodium cromoglicate nasal spray
- steroid nasal spray, e.g. beclometasone dipropionate, fluticasone, mometasone or budesonide.

In patients whose symptoms are very severe and seriously interfering with school, business or social activities, systemic corticosteroids are occasionally indicated, but adverse effects limit their usefulness. Vasomotor rhinitis is often difficult to treat, but may respond to ipratropium bromide, administered into each nostril 3 times daily.

Sleep-disordered breathing

A variety of respiratory disorders affect sleep or are affected by sleep. Cough and wheeze disturbing sleep are characteristic of asthma, while the hypoventilation that accompanies normal sleep can precipitate respiratory failure in patients with disordered ventilation due to kyphoscoliosis, diaphragmatic palsy or muscle disease (e.g. muscular dystrophy).

In contrast, a small but important group of disorders cause problems only during sleep. Patients with these may have normal lungs and daytime respiratory function, but during sleep have either abnormalities of ventilatory drive (central sleep apnoea) or upper airway obstruction (obstructive sleep apnoea). Of these, the obstructive sleep apnoea/hypopnoea syndrome is by far the most common and important. When this coexists with COPD, severe respiratory failure can result even if the COPD is mild.

The sleep apnoea/hypopnoea syndrome

It is now recognised that 2–4% of the middle-aged population suffer from recurrent upper airway obstruction during sleep. The resulting sleep fragmentation causes daytime sleepiness, especially in monotonous situations, resulting in a threefold increased risk of road traffic accidents and a ninefold increased risk of single-vehicle accidents.

Aetiology

Sleep apnoea results from recurrent occlusion of the pharynx during sleep, usually at the level of the soft palate. Inspiration results in negative pressure within the pharynx. During wakefulness, upper airway dilating muscles, including palatoglossus and genioglossus, contract actively during inspiration to preserve airway patency. During sleep, muscle tone declines, impairing the ability of these muscles to maintain pharyngeal patency. In a minority of people, a combination of an anatomically narrow palatopharynx and underactivity of the dilating muscles during sleep results in inspiratory airway obstruction. Incomplete obstruction causes turbulent flow, resulting in snoring (around 40% of middle-aged men and 20% of middle-aged women snore). More severe obstruction triggers increased inspiratory effort and transiently wakes the patient, allowing the dilating muscles to re-open the airway. These awakenings are so brief that patients have no recollection of them. After a series of loud deep breaths that may wake their bed partner, the patient rapidly returns to sleep, snores and becomes apnoeic once more. This cycle of apnoea and awakening may repeat itself many hundreds of times per night and results in severe sleep fragmentation and secondary variations in blood pressure, which may predispose over time to cardiovascular disease.

Predisposing factors to the sleep apnoea/hypopnoea syndrome include male gender, which doubles the risk, and obesity, which is found in about 50%, because parapharyngeal fat deposits tend to narrow the pharynx. Nasal obstruction or a recessed mandible can further exacerbate the problem. Acromegaly and hypothyroidism also predispose by causing submucosal infiltration and narrowing of the upper airway. Sleep apnoea is often familial, where the maxilla and mandible are back-set, narrowing the upper airway. Alcohol and sedatives predispose to snoring and apnoea by relaxing the upper airway dilating muscles. As a result of marked sympathetic activation during apnoea, sleep-disordered breathing is associated over time with sustained hypertension and an increased risk of coronary events and stroke. An association has also been described with insulin resistance, the metabolic syndrome and type II diabetes. Treatment of sleep apnoea reduces sympathetic drive and blood pressure, and may also improve these associated metabolic disorders.

Clinical features

Excessive daytime sleepiness is the principal symptom and snoring is virtually universal. The patient usually feels that he or she has been asleep all night but wakes unrefreshed. Bed partners report loud snoring in all body positions and often have noticed multiple breathing pauses (apnoeas). Difficulty with concentration, impaired cognitive function and work performance, depression, irritability and nocturia are other features.

Investigations

Provided that the sleepiness does not result from inadequate time in bed or from shift work, anyone who repeatedly falls asleep during the day when not in bed, who complains that his or her work is impaired by sleepiness, or who is a habitual snorer with multiple witnessed apnoeas should be referred for a sleep assessment. A more quantitative assessment of daytime sleepiness can be obtained by questionnaire (Box 19.98).

Overnight studies of breathing, oxygenation and sleep quality are diagnostic (Fig. 19.71) but the level of

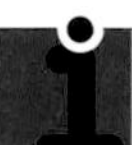

19.98 Epworth sleepiness scale

How likely are you to doze off or fall asleep in the situations described below? Choose the most appropriate number for each situation from the following scale:

0 = would never doze
1 = slight chance of dozing
2 = moderate chance of dozing
3 = high chance of dozing

- Sitting and reading
- Watching TV
- Sitting inactive in a public place (e.g. a theatre or a meeting)
- As a passenger in a car for an hour without a break
- Lying down to rest in the afternoon when circumstances permit
- Sitting and talking to someone
- Sitting quietly after a lunch without alcohol
- In a car, while stopped for a few minutes in the traffic

Normal subjects average 5.9 (SD 2.2) and patients with severe obstructive sleep apnoea average 16.0 (SD 4.4).

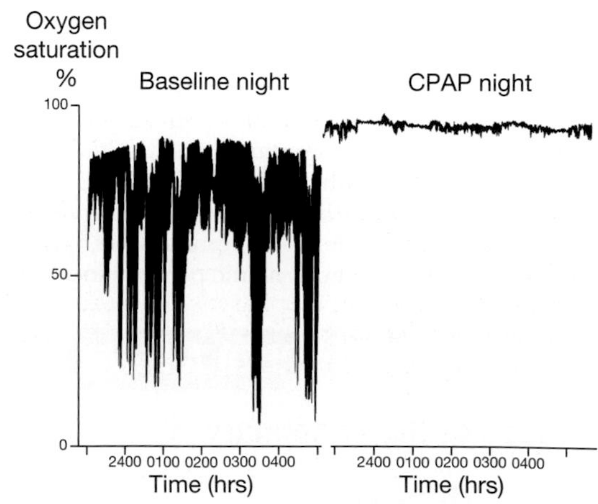

Fig. 19.71 Sleep apnoea/hypopnoea syndrome: overnight oxygen saturation trace. The left-hand panel shows the trace of a patient who had 53 apnoeas plus hypopnoeas/hour, 55 brief awakenings/hour and marked oxygen desaturation. The right-hand panel shows the effect of continuous positive airway pressure (CPAP) of 10 cm H_2O delivered through a tight-fitting nasal mask: it abolished his breathing irregularity and awakenings, and improved oxygenation.

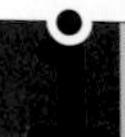

19.99 Differential diagnosis of persistent sleepiness

Lack of sleep	
• Inadequate time in bed	• Shift work
• Extraneous sleep disruption (e.g. babies/children)	• Excessive caffeine intake
	• Physical illness (e.g. pain)
Sleep disruption	
• Sleep apnoea/hypopnoea syndrome • Periodic limb movement disorder (recurrent limb movements during non-REM sleep, frequent nocturnal awakenings)	
Sleepiness with relatively normal sleep	
• Narcolepsy • Idiopathic hypersomnolence (rare) • Neurological lesions (e.g. hypothalamic or upper brainstem infarcts or tumours) • Drugs	
Psychological/psychiatric	
• Depression	

investigations depends on local resources and the probability of the diagnosis. The current threshold for diagnosing moderate sleep apnoea/hypopnoea syndrome is 15 apnoeas/hypopnoeas per hour of sleep, where an apnoea is defined as a 10-second or longer breathing pause and a hypopnoea a 10-second or longer 50% reduction in breathing.

Several other conditions can cause daytime sleepiness but can usually be excluded by a careful history (Box 19.99). Narcolepsy is a rare cause of sleepiness, occurring in 0.05% of the population (p. 1187). Idiopathic hypersomnolence occurs in younger individuals and is characterised by long nocturnal sleeps.

Management

The major hazard to patients and those around them is traffic accidents, so all drivers must be advised not to drive until treatment has relieved their sleepiness. In a minority, relief of nasal obstruction or the avoidance of alcohol may prevent obstruction. Advice to obese patients to lose weight is often unheeded, and the majority of patients need to use continuous positive airway pressure (CPAP) delivered by a nasal mask every night to splint the upper airway open. When CPAP is tolerated, the effect is often dramatic (see Fig. 19.71), with relief of somnolence and improved daytime performance, quality of life and survival. Unfortunately, 30–50% of patients do not tolerate CPAP. Mandibular advancement devices that fit over the teeth and hold the mandible forward, thus opening the pharynx, are an alternative that is effective in some patients. There is no evidence that palatal surgery is of benefit.

Laryngeal disorders

The larynx is commonly affected by acute self-limiting infections (p. 681). Other disorders include chronic laryngitis, laryngeal tuberculosis, laryngeal paralysis and laryngeal obstruction. Tumours of the larynx are relatively common, particularly in smokers. For further details, the reader should refer to an otolaryngology text.

19.100 Causes of chronic laryngitis

- Repeated attacks of acute laryngitis
- Excessive use of the voice, especially in dusty atmospheres
- Heavy tobacco smoking
- Mouth-breathing from nasal obstruction
- Chronic infection of nasal sinuses

Chronic laryngitis

The common causes are listed in Box 19.100. The chief symptoms are hoarseness or loss of voice (aphonia). There is irritation of the throat and a spasmodic cough. The disease pursues a chronic course, frequently uninfluenced by treatment, and the voice may become permanently impaired. Other causes of chronic hoarseness include use of inhaled corticosteroid treatment, tuberculosis, laryngeal paralysis or tumour.

In some patients, a chest X-ray may reveal an unsuspected bronchial carcinoma or pulmonary tuberculosis. If these are not found, laryngoscopy should be performed to exclude a local structural cause.

When no specific treatable cause is found, the voice must be rested completely. This is particularly important in public speakers and singers. Smoking should be avoided. Some benefit may be obtained from frequent inhalations of medicated steam.

Laryngeal paralysis

Interruption of the motor nerve supply of the larynx is nearly always unilateral and, because of the intrathoracic course of the left recurrent laryngeal nerve, usually left-sided. One or both recurrent laryngeal nerves may be damaged at thyroidectomy, by carcinoma of the thyroid or by anterior neck injury. Rarely, the vagal trunk itself is involved by tumour, aneurysm or trauma.

Clinical features and management

Hoarseness always accompanies laryngeal paralysis, whatever its cause. Paralysis of organic origin is seldom reversible, but when only one vocal cord is affected, hoarseness may improve or even disappear after a few weeks, as the normal cord compensates by crossing the midline to approximate with the paralysed cord on phonation.

'Bovine cough' is a characteristic feature of organic laryngeal paralysis, and lacks the explosive quality of normal coughing because the cords fail to close the glottis. Sputum clearance may also be impaired. A normal cough in patients with partial loss of voice or aphonia virtually excludes laryngeal paralysis. Stridor is occasionally present but seldom severe, except when laryngeal paralysis is bilateral.

Laryngoscopy is required to establish the diagnosis of laryngeal paralysis. The paralysed cord lies in the so-called 'cadaveric' position, midway between abduction and adduction.

The cause should be treated, if possible. In unilateral paralysis, persistent dysphonia may be improved by the injection of Teflon into the affected vocal cord. In bilateral organic paralysis, tracheal intubation, tracheostomy or plastic surgery on the larynx may be necessary.

19

Psychogenic hoarseness and aphonia

Psychogenic causes of hoarseness or aphonia may be suggested by associated symptoms in the history (p. 236). However, laryngoscopy may be necessary to exclude a physical cause. In psychogenic aphonia, only the voluntary movement of adduction of the vocal cords is seen to be impaired. Speech therapy may be helpful.

Laryngeal obstruction

Laryngeal obstruction is more liable to occur in children than in adults because of the smaller size of the glottis. Important causes are given in Box 19.101. Sudden complete laryngeal obstruction by a foreign body produces the clinical picture of acute asphyxia: violent but ineffective inspiratory efforts with indrawing of the intercostal spaces and the unsupported lower ribs, accompanied by cyanosis. Unrelieved, the condition progresses to coma and death within a few minutes. When, as in most cases, the obstruction is incomplete at first, the main clinical features are progressive breathlessness accompanied by stridor and cyanosis. Urgent treatment to prevent complete obstruction is needed.

Management

Transient laryngeal obstruction due to exudate and spasm, which may occur with acute pharyngitis in children and with whooping cough, is potentially dangerous but can usually be relieved by steam inhalation. Laryngeal obstruction from all other causes carries a high mortality and demands prompt treatment.

When a foreign body causes laryngeal obstruction in children, it can often be dislodged by turning the patient head downwards, and squeezing the chest vigorously. In adults, a sudden forceful compression of the upper abdomen (Heimlich manœuvre) may be effective. Otherwise, the cause of the obstruction should be investigated by direct laryngoscopy, which may also permit the removal of an unsuspected foreign body or the insertion of a tube past the obstruction into the trachea. Tracheostomy must be performed without delay if these procedures fail to relieve obstruction but, except in dire emergencies, this should be performed in theatre by a surgeon.

In diphtheria, antitoxin should be administered, and for other infections the appropriate antibiotic should be given. In angioedema, complete laryngeal occlusion can usually be prevented by treatment with adrenaline (epinephrine) 0.5–1 mg (0.5–1 mL of 1:1000) IM, chlorphenamine maleate (10–20 mg by slow intravenous injection) and intravenous hydrocortisone sodium succinate (200 mg).

19.101 Causes of laryngeal obstruction

- Inflammatory or allergic oedema, or exudate
- Spasm of laryngeal muscles
- Inhaled foreign body
- Inhaled blood clot or vomitus in an unconscious patient
- Tumours of the larynx
- Bilateral vocal cord paralysis
- Fixation of both cords in rheumatoid disease

Tracheal disorders

Tracheal obstruction

External compression by lymph nodes containing metastases, usually from a bronchial carcinoma, is a more frequent cause of tracheal obstruction than primary benign or malignant tumours. The trachea may also be compressed by a retrosternal goitre (see Fig. 19.11, p. 657). Rare causes include an aneurysm of the aortic arch and (in children) tuberculous mediastinal lymph nodes. Tracheal stenosis is an occasional complication of tracheostomy, prolonged intubation, granulomatosis with polyangiitis (Wegener's granulomatosis, p. 1118) or trauma.

Clinical features and management

Stridor can be detected in every patient with severe tracheal narrowing. Bronchoscopic examination of the trachea should be undertaken without delay to determine the site, degree and nature of the obstruction.

Localised tumours of the trachea can be resected, but reconstruction after resection may be technically difficult. Endobronchial laser therapy, bronchoscopically placed tracheal stents, chemotherapy and radiotherapy are alternatives to surgery. The choice of treatment depends upon the nature of the tumour and the general health of the patient. Benign tracheal strictures can sometimes be dilated but may require resection.

Tracheo-oesophageal fistula

This may be present in newborn infants as a congenital abnormality. In adults, it is usually due to malignant lesions in the mediastinum, such as carcinoma or lymphoma, eroding both the trachea and oesophagus to produce a communication between them. Swallowed liquids enter the trachea and bronchi through the fistula and provoke coughing.

Surgical closure of a congenital fistula, if undertaken promptly, is usually successful. There is usually no curative treatment for malignant fistulae, and death from overwhelming pulmonary infection rapidly supervenes.

PLEURAL DISEASE

Pleurisy, pleural effusion, empyema and asbestos-associated pleural disease have been described above.

Pneumothorax

Pneumothorax is the presence of air in the pleural space, which can either occur spontaneously, or result from iatrogenic injury or trauma to the lung or chest wall (Box 19.102). Primary spontaneous pneumothorax occurs in patients with no history of lung disease. Smoking, tall stature and the presence of apical subpleural blebs are risk factors. Secondary pneumothorax affects patients with pre-existing lung disease and is associated with higher mortality rates (Fig. 19.72).

Where the communication between the airway and the pleural space seals off as the lung deflates and does not re-open, the pneumothorax is referred to as 'closed'

(Fig. 19.73A). The mean pleural pressure remains negative, spontaneous reabsorption of air and re-expansion of the lung occur over a few days or weeks, and infection is uncommon. This contrasts with an 'open' pneumothorax, where the communication fails to seal and air continues to pass freely between the bronchial tree and pleural space (Fig. 19.73B). An example of the latter is a bronchopleural fistula, which, if large, can facilitate the transmission of infection from the airways into the pleural space, leading to empyema. An open pneumothorax is commonly seen following rupture of an emphysematous bulla, tuberculous cavity or lung abscess into the pleural space.

Occasionally, the communication between the airway and the pleural space acts as a one-way valve, allowing air to enter the pleural space during inspiration but not to escape on expiration. Large amounts of trapped air accumulate progressively in the pleural space and the intrapleural pressure rises to well above atmospheric levels. This is a tension pneumothorax. The pressure causes mediastinal displacement towards the opposite side, with compression of the opposite normal lung and impairment of systemic venous return, causing cardiovascular compromise (Fig. 19.73C).

19.102 Classification of pneumothorax

Spontaneous
Primary • No evidence of overt lung disease. Air escapes from the lung into the pleural space through rupture of a small pleural bleb, or the pulmonary end of a pleural adhesion **Secondary** • Underlying lung disease, most commonly COPD and tuberculosis; also seen in asthma, lung abscess, pulmonary infarcts, bronchogenic carcinoma, and all forms of fibrotic and cystic lung disease
Traumatic
• Iatrogenic (e.g. following thoracic surgery or biopsy) or chest wall injury

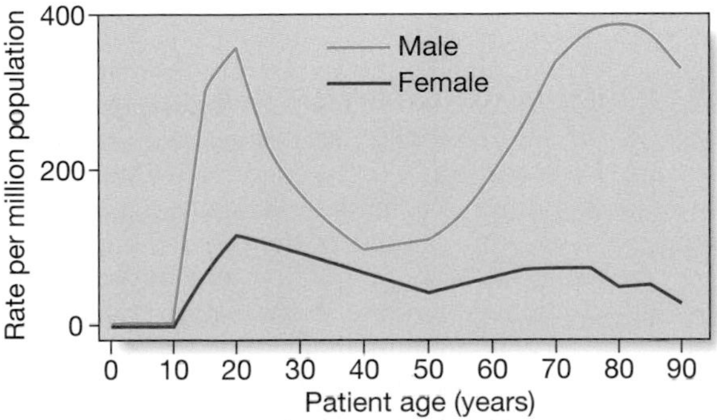

Fig. 19.72 Bimodal age distribution for hospital admissions for pneumothorax in England. The incidence of primary spontaneous pneumothorax peaks in males aged 15–30 years. Secondary spontaneous pneumothorax occurs mainly in males over 55 years.

Clinical features

The most common symptoms are sudden-onset unilateral pleuritic chest pain or breathlessness. In those individuals with underlying chest disease, breathlessness can be severe and may not resolve spontaneously. In patients with a small pneumothorax, physical examination may be normal. A larger pneumothorax (> 15% of the hemithorax) results in decreased or absent breath sounds (p. 645). The combination of absent breath sounds and resonant percussion note is diagnostic of pneumothorax.

By contrast, in tension pneumothorax there is rapidly progressive breathlessness associated with a marked tachycardia, hypotension, cyanosis and tracheal displacement away from the side of the silent hemithorax. Occasionally, tension pneumothorax may occur without mediastinal shift, if malignant disease or scarring has splinted the mediastinum.

Investigations

The chest X-ray shows the sharply defined edge of the deflated lung with complete translucency (no lung markings) between this and the chest wall (p. 645). Care must be taken to differentiate between a large pre-existing emphysematous bulla and a pneumothorax. CT is used in difficult cases to avoid misdirected attempts

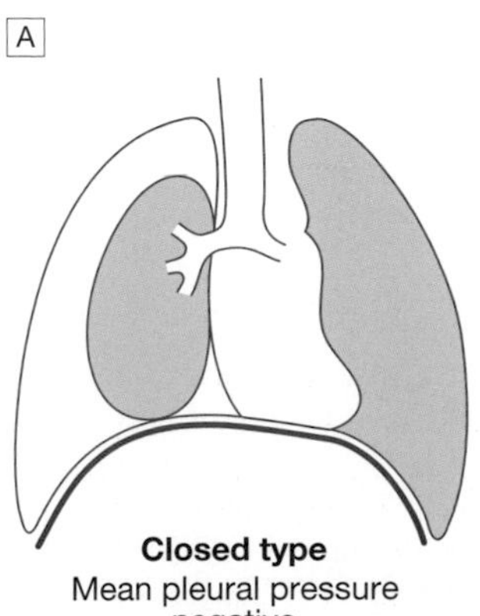

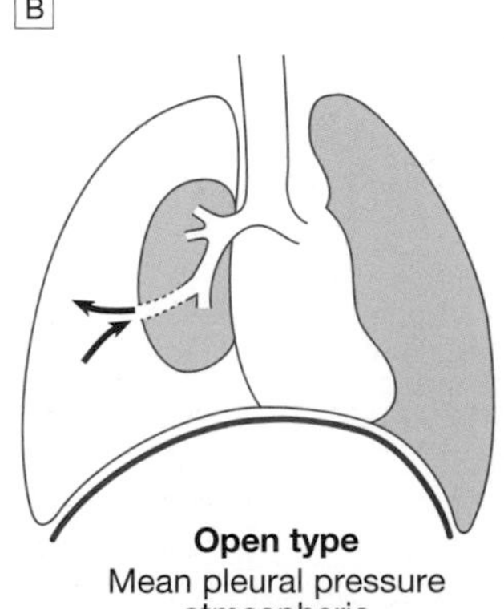

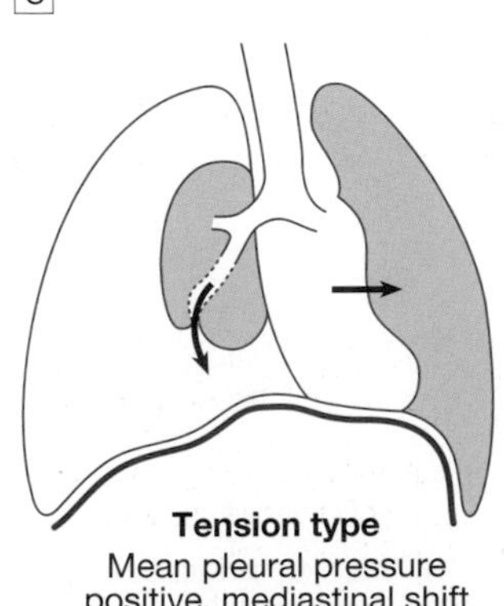

Fig. 19.73 Types of spontaneous pneumothorax. A Closed type. B Open type. C Tension (valvular) type.

at aspiration. X-rays may also show the extent of any mediastinal displacement and reveal any pleural fluid or underlying pulmonary disease.

Management

Primary pneumothorax, in which the lung edge is less than 2 cm from the chest wall and the patient is not breathless, normally resolves without intervention. In young patients presenting with a moderate or large spontaneous primary pneumothorax, percutaneous needle aspiration of air is a simple and well-tolerated alternative to intercostal tube drainage, with a 60–80% chance of avoiding the need for a chest drain (Fig. 19.74). In patients with significant underlying chronic lung disease, however, secondary pneumothorax may cause respiratory distress. In these patients, the success rate of aspiration is much lower, and intercostal tube drainage and inpatient observation are usually required, particularly in those individuals over 50 years old and those with respiratory compromise. If there is a tension pneumothorax, immediate release of the positive pressure by insertion of a blunt cannula into the pleural space may be beneficial, allowing time to prepare for chest drain insertion.

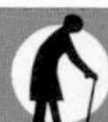

19.103 Pleural disease in old age

- **Spontaneous pneumothorax**: invariably associated with underlying lung disease in old age and has a significant mortality. Surgical or chemical pleurodesis is advised in all such patients.
- **Rib fracture**: common cause of pleural-type pain; may be spontaneous (due to coughing), traumatic or pathological. Underlying osteomalacia may contribute to poor healing, especially in the housebound with no exposure to sunlight.
- **Tuberculosis**: should always be considered and actively excluded in any elderly patient presenting with a unilateral pleural effusion.
- **Mesothelioma**: more common in older individuals than younger people due to a long latency period between asbestos exposure (often more than 20 yrs) and the development of disease.
- **Analgesia**: frail older people are particularly sensitive to the respiratory depressant effects of opiate-based analgesia and careful monitoring is required when using these agents for pleural pain.

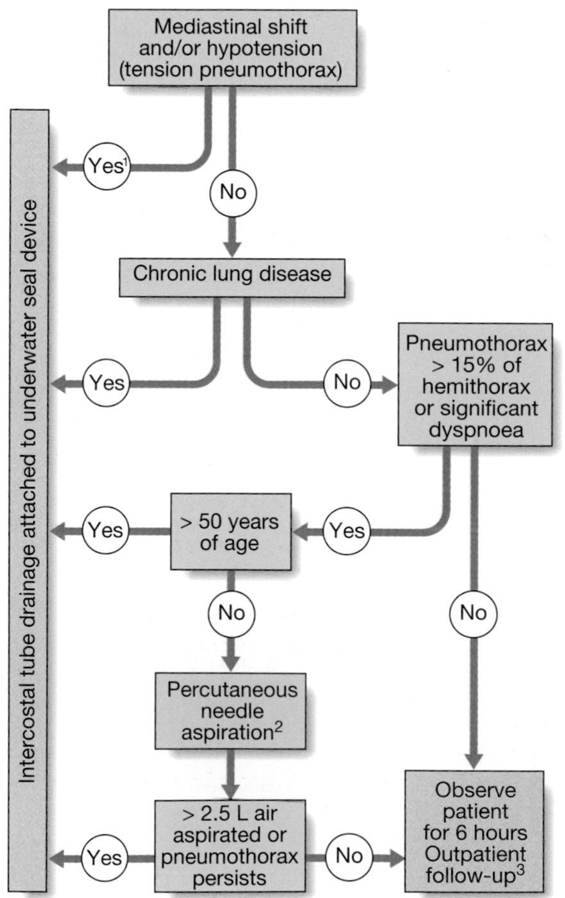

Fig. 19.74 Management of spontaneous pneumothorax.
(1) Immediate decompression prior to insertion of the intercostal drain. (2) Aspirate in the 2nd intercostal space anteriorly in the mid-clavicular line using a 16 F cannula; discontinue if resistance is felt, the patient coughs excessively, or more than 2.5 L of air are removed. (3) The post-aspiration chest X-ray is not a reliable indicator of whether a pleural leak remains, and all patients should be told to attend again immediately in the event of deterioration.

When needed, intercostal drains are inserted in the 4th, 5th or 6th intercostal space in the mid-axillary line, connected to an underwater seal or one-way Heimlich valve, and secured firmly to the chest wall. Clamping of an intercostal drain is potentially dangerous and rarely indicated. The drain should be removed the morning after the lung has fully re-inflated and bubbling has stopped. Continued bubbling after 5–7 days is an indication for surgery. If bubbling in the drainage bottle stops before full re-inflation, the tube is either blocked, kinked or displaced. Supplemental oxygen may speed resolution, as it accelerates the rate at which nitrogen is reabsorbed by the pleura.

Patients with a closed pneumothorax should be advised not to fly, as the trapped gas expands at altitude. After complete resolution, there is no clear evidence to indicate how long patients should avoid flying, although guidelines suggest that waiting 1–2 weeks, with confirmation of full inflation prior to flight, is prudent. Patients should also be advised to stop smoking and informed about the risks of a recurrent pneumothorax. Diving is potentially dangerous after pneumothorax, unless a surgical pleurodesis has sealed the lung to the chest wall.

Recurrent spontaneous pneumothorax

After primary spontaneous pneumothorax, recurrence occurs within a year of either aspiration or tube drainage in approximately 25% of patients, and should prompt definitive treatment. Surgical pleurodesis is recommended in all patients following a second pneumothorax and should be considered following the first episode of secondary pneumothorax if low respiratory reserve makes recurrence hazardous. Pleurodesis can be achieved by pleural abrasion or parietal pleurectomy at thoracotomy or thoracoscopy.

DISEASES OF THE DIAPHRAGM AND CHEST WALL

Disorders of the diaphragm

Congenital disorders

Diaphragmatic hernias

Congenital defects of the diaphragm can allow herniation of abdominal viscera. Posteriorly situated hernias through the foramen of Bochdalek are more common than anterior hernias through the foramen of Morgagni.

Eventration of the diaphragm

Abnormal elevation or bulging of one hemidiaphragm, more often the left, results from total or partial absence of muscular development of the septum transversum. Most eventrations are asymptomatic and are detected by chance on X-ray in adult life, but severe respiratory distress can be caused in infancy if the diaphragmatic muscular defect is extensive.

Acquired disorders

Elevation of a hemidiaphragm may result from paralysis or other structural causes (Box 19.104). The phrenic nerve may be damaged by bronchial carcinoma, disease of cervical vertebrae, tumours of the cervical cord, shingles, trauma (including road traffic and birth injuries), surgery, and stretching of the nerve by mediastinal masses and aortic aneurysms. Idiopathic diaphragmatic paralysis occasionally occurs in otherwise fit patients. Paralysis of one hemidiaphragm results in loss of around 20% of ventilatory capacity, but may not be noticed by otherwise healthy individuals. Ultrasound screening can be used to demonstrate paradoxical upward movement of the paralysed hemidiaphragm on sniffing. CT of the chest and neck is the best way to exclude occult disease affecting the phrenic nerve.

Bilateral diaphragmatic weakness occurs in peripheral neuropathies of any type, including Guillain–Barré syndrome (p. 1224), in disorders affecting the anterior horn cells, e.g. poliomyelitis (p. 1207), in muscular dystrophies, and in connective tissue disorders such as SLE and polymyositis (pp. 1109 and 1114).

Hiatus hernia is common (p. 865). Diaphragmatic rupture is usually caused by a crush injury and may not be detected until years later. Respiratory disorders that cause pulmonary hyperinflation, e.g. emphysema, and those that result in small stiff lungs, e.g. diffuse pulmonary fibrosis, compromise diaphragmatic function and predispose to fatigue.

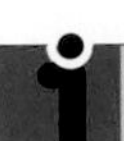

19.104 Causes of elevation of a hemidiaphragm

- Phrenic nerve paralysis
- Eventration of the diaphragm
- Decrease in volume of one lung (e.g. lobectomy, unilateral pulmonary fibrosis)
- Severe pleuritic pain
- Pulmonary infarction
- Subphrenic abscess
- Large volume of gas in the stomach or colon
- Large tumours or cysts of the liver

Deformities of the chest wall

Thoracic kyphoscoliosis

Abnormalities of alignment of the dorsal spine and their consequent effects on thoracic shape may be caused by:

- congenital abnormality
- vertebral disease, including tuberculosis, osteoporosis and ankylosing spondylitis
- trauma
- neuromuscular disease such as poliomyelitis.

Simple kyphosis (increased anteroposterior curvature) causes less pulmonary embarrassment than kyphoscoliosis (anteroposterior and lateral curvature). Kyphoscoliosis, if severe, restricts and distorts expansion of the chest wall and impairs diaphragmatic function, causing ventilation–perfusion mismatch in the lungs. Patients with severe deformity may develop type II respiratory failure (initially manifest during sleep), pulmonary hypertension and right ventricular failure. They can often be successfully treated with non-invasive ventilatory support (p. 193).

Pectus excavatum

Pectus excavatum (funnel chest) is an idiopathic condition in which the body of the sternum, usually only the lower end, is curved inwards. The heart is displaced to the left and may be compressed between the sternum and the vertebral column but only rarely is there associated disturbance of cardiac function. The deformity may restrict chest expansion and reduce vital capacity. Operative correction is rarely performed, and then only for cosmetic reasons.

Pectus carinatum

Pectus carinatum (pigeon chest) is frequently caused by severe asthma during childhood. Very occasionally, this deformity can be produced by rickets or be idiopathic.

Further information and acknowledgements

Websites

www.brit-thoracic.org.uk *Website of the British Thoracic Society with access to guidelines on a range of respiratory conditions.*

www.ersnet.org *European Respiratory Society provides information on education and research, and patient information.*

www.ginasthma.com *Global Initiative for Asthma website with a comprehensive overview of asthma.*

www.goldcopd.com *Global Initiative for Chronic Obstructive Lung Disease website containing a comprehensive overview of COPD.*

www.thoracic.org *American Thoracic Society provides information on education and research, and patient information.*

Figure acknowledgements

Page 645 insets (upper lobe collapse) http://3.bp.blogspot.com; *(pneumothorax)* http://chestatlas.com; *(pleural effusion)* www.ispub.com.

19

Fig. 19.2 www.Netter.com Illustrations 155 (bronchus, acinus) and 191 (circulation), Elsevier.

Fig. 19.4 Innes JA. Davidson's Essentials of medicine. Edinburgh: Churchill Livingstone; 2009 (Fig. 19.4, p. 791); copyright Elsevier.

Fig. 19.6A–C http://radiology.rsnajnls.org.

Fig. 19.8 Adapted from Flenley D. Lancet 1971; 1:1921.

Fig. 19.16 WHO Global surveillance, prevention and control of chronic respiratory diseases: a comprehensive approach.

Fig. 19.22 British Thoracic Society and SIGN guideline on the Management of Asthma.

Fig. 19.28 Global Initiative for Chronic Obstructive Lung Disease, www.goldcopd.com.

Fig. 19.35 Maartens G, Wilkinson RJ. Tuberculosis. Lancet 2007; 370:2030–2043.

Fig. 19.52 Adapted from Detterbeck FC, Boffa DJ, Tanoue LT. The new lung cancer staging system. Chest 2009; 136:260–271.

Fig. 19.53 Johnson N McL. Respiratory medicine. Oxford: Blackwell Science; 1986.

Fig. 19.60 inset (erythema nodosum) Savin JA, Hunter JAA, Hepburn NC. Skin signs in clinical medicine. London: Mosby–Wolfe; 1997; copyright Elsevier.

M.W.J. Strachan
J. Newell-Price

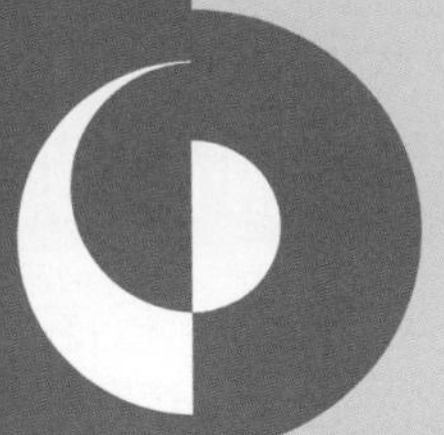

Endocrine disease 20

Clinical examination in endocrine disease 734

An overview of endocrinology 736
- Functional anatomy and physiology 736
- Endocrine pathology 736
- Investigation of endocrine disease 737
- Presenting problems in endocrine disease 737

The thyroid gland 738
- Functional anatomy, physiology and investigations 738
- Presenting problems in thyroid disease 740
  - Thyrotoxicosis 740
  - Hypothyroidism 743
  - Asymptomatic abnormal thyroid function tests 745
  - Thyroid lump or swelling 746
- Autoimmune thyroid disease 747
- Transient thyroiditis 751
- Iodine-associated thyroid disease 752
- Simple and multinodular goitre 752
- Thyroid neoplasia 754
- Congenital thyroid disease 755

The reproductive system 756
- Functional anatomy, physiology and investigations 756
- Presenting problems in reproductive disease 758
  - Delayed puberty 758
  - Amenorrhoea 759
  - Male hypogonadism 760
  - Infertility 761
  - Gynaecomastia 762
  - Hirsutism 763
- Polycystic ovarian syndrome 764
- Turner's syndrome 765
- Klinefelter's syndrome 766

The parathyroid glands 766
- Functional anatomy, physiology and investigations 766
- Presenting problems in parathyroid disease 767
  - Hypercalcaemia 767
  - Hypocalcaemia 768
- Primary hyperparathyroidism 769
- Familial hypocalciuric hypercalcaemia 770
- Hypoparathyroidism 770

The adrenal glands 771
- Functional anatomy and physiology 771
- Presenting problems in adrenal disease 773
  - Cushing's syndrome 773
  - Therapeutic use of glucocorticoids 776
  - Adrenal insufficiency 777
  - Incidental adrenal mass 779
- Primary hyperaldosteronism 780
- Phaeochromocytoma and paraganglioma 781
- Congenital adrenal hyperplasia 782

The endocrine pancreas and gastrointestinal tract 782
- Presenting problems in endocrine pancreas disease 783
  - Spontaneous hypoglycaemia 783
- Gastroenteropancreatic neuro-endocrine tumours 784

The hypothalamus and the pituitary gland 785
- Functional anatomy, physiology and investigations 786
- Presenting problems in hypothalamic and pituitary disease 787
  - Hypopituitarism 787
  - Pituitary tumour 789
  - Hyperprolactinaemia/galactorrhoea 790
- Prolactinoma 791
- Acromegaly 792
- Craniopharyngioma 793
- Diabetes insipidus 794

Disorders affecting multiple endocrine glands 795
- Multiple endocrine neoplasia 795
- Autoimmune polyendocrine syndromes 795
- Late effects of childhood cancer therapy 796

CLINICAL EXAMINATION IN ENDOCRINE DISEASE

6 Head
Eyes
- Graves' disease (see opposite)
- Diplopia
- Visual field defect (see opposite)

Hair
- Alopecia
- Frontal balding

Facial features
- Hypothyroid
- Hirsutism
- Acromegaly
- Cushing's

Mental state
- Lethargy
- Depression
- Confusion
- Libido

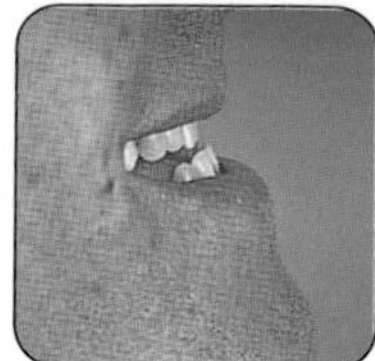

▲ Prognathism in acromegaly

5 Blood pressure
Hypertension in Cushing's and Conn's syndromes, phaeochromocytoma
Hypotension in adrenal insufficiency

4 Pulse
Atrial fibrillation
Sinus tachycardia
Bradycardia

3 Skin
Hair distribution
Dry/greasy
Pigmentation/pallor
Bruising
Vitiligo
Striae
Thickness

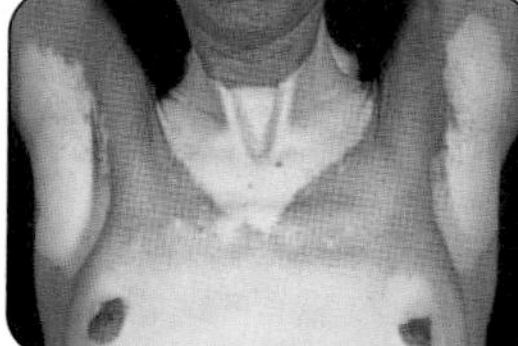

Vitiligo in organ-specific autoimmune disease ▲

2 Hands
Palmar erythema
Tremor
Acromegaly
Carpal tunnel syndrome

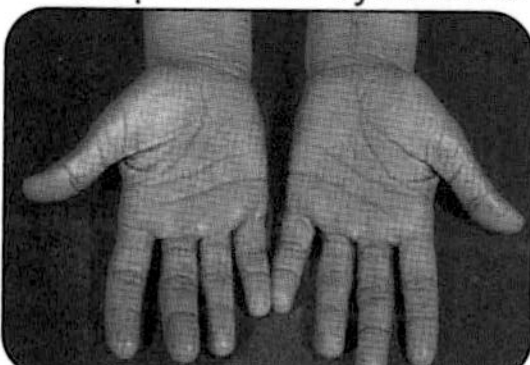

Pigmentation of creases due to high ACTH levels in Addison's disease ▲

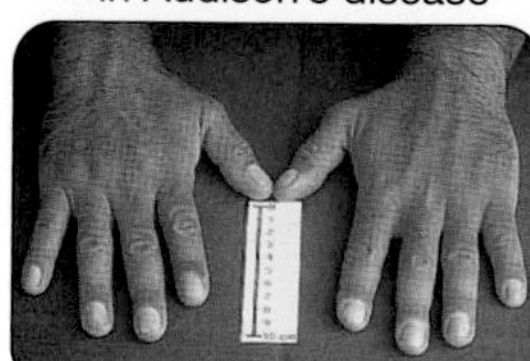

Acromegalic hands. Note soft tissue enlargement causing 'spade-like' changes ▲

1 Height and weight

Observation
- Most examination in endocrinology is by observation
- Astute observation can often yield 'spot' diagnosis of endocrine disorders
- The emphasis of examination varies depending on which gland or hormone is thought to be involved

7 Neck
Voice
- Hoarse, e.g. hypothyroid
- Virilised

Thyroid gland (see opposite)
- Goitre
- Nodules

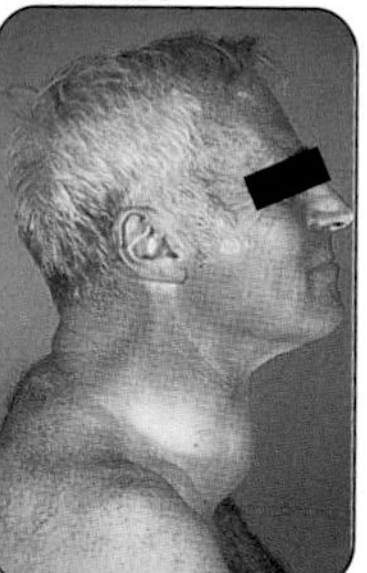

▲ Multinodular goitre

8 Breasts
Galactorrhoea
Gynaecomastia

9 Body fat
Central obesity in Cushing's syndrome and growth hormone deficiency

10 Bones
Fragility fractures (e.g. of vertebrae, neck of femur or distal radius)

11 Genitalia
Virilisation
Pubertal development
Testicular volume

12 Legs
Proximal myopathy
Myxoedema

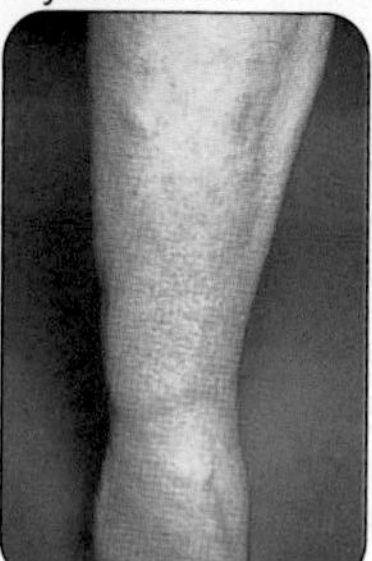

▲ Pretibial myxoedema in Graves' disease

Endocrine disease causes clinical syndromes with symptoms and signs involving many organ systems, reflecting the diverse effects of hormone deficiency and excess. The emphasis of the clinical examination depends on the gland or hormone that is thought to be abnormal.

Diabetes mellitus (described in detail in Ch. 21) and thyroid disease are the most common endocrine disorders.

6 Examination of the visual fields by confrontation

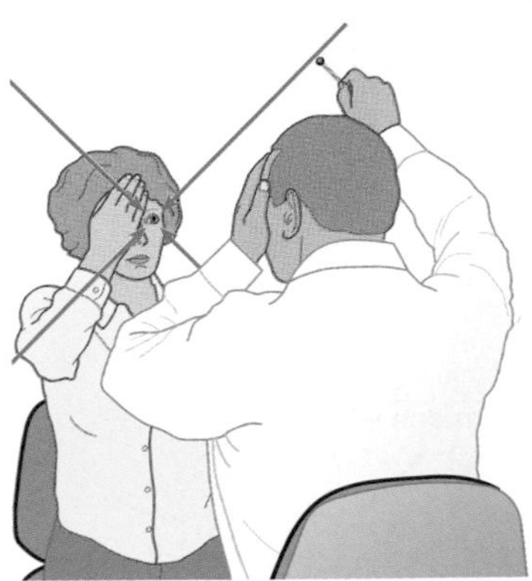

- Sit opposite patient
- You and patient cover opposite eyes
- Bring red pin (or wiggling finger) slowly into view from extreme of your vision, as shown
- Ask patient to say 'now' when it comes into view
- Continue to move pin into centre of vision and ask patient to tell you if it disappears
- Repeat in each of four quadrants
- Repeat in other eye

A bitemporal hemianopia is the classical finding in pituitary macroadenomas (p. 789)

6 Examination in Graves' ophthalmopathy

- **Inspect** from front and side
  - Periorbital oedema (Fig. 20.7)
  - Conjunctival inflammation (chemosis)
  - Corneal ulceration
  - Proptosis (exophthalmos)*
  - Lid retraction*

Normal | Proptosis | Lid retraction

- **Range of eye movements**
  - Lid lag on descending gaze*
  - Diplopia on lateral gaze

Normal | Normal descent | Lid lag descent

- **Pupillary reflexes**
  - Afferent defect (pupils constrict further on swinging light to unaffected eye, Box 26.28)
- **Vision**
  - Visual acuity impaired
  - Loss of colour vision
  - Visual field defects

Right proptosis and afferent pupillary defect

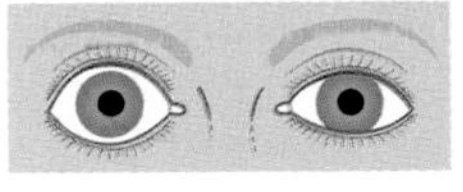

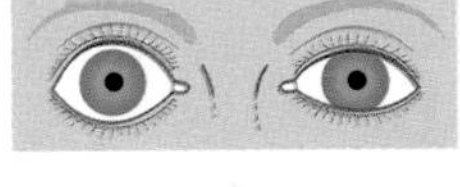

- **Ophthalmoscopy**
  - Optic disc pallor
  - Papilloedema

*Note position of eyelids relative to iris.

7 Examination of the thyroid gland

- **Inspect** from front to side
- **Palpate** from behind
  - Thyroid moves on swallowing
  - Cervical lymph nodes
  - Tracheal deviation
- **Auscultate** for bruit
  - Ask patient to hold breath
  - If present, check for radiating murmur
- **Percuss** for retrosternal thyroid
- Consider systemic signs of thyroid dysfunction (Box 20.7) incl. tremor, palmar erythema, warm peripheries, tachycardia, lid lag
- Consider signs of Graves' disease incl. ophthalmopathy, pretibial myxoedema

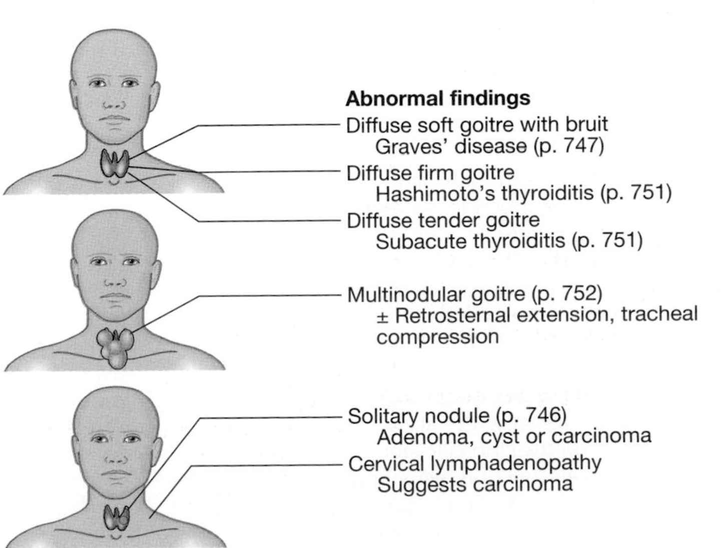

Endocrinology concerns the synthesis, secretion and action of hormones. These are chemical messengers released from endocrine glands that coordinate the activities of many different cells. Endocrine diseases can therefore affect multiple organs and systems. This chapter describes the principles of endocrinology before dealing with the function and diseases of each gland in turn.

Some endocrine disorders are common, particularly those of the thyroid, parathyroid glands, reproductive system and β cells of the pancreas (Ch. 21). For example, thyroid dysfunction occurs in more than 10% of the population in areas with iodine deficiency, such as the Himalayas, and 4% of women aged 20–50 years in the UK. Some endocrine diseases are becoming more common in association with emerging diseases; HIV infection is associated in particular with adrenal insufficiency. Less common endocrine syndromes are described later in the chapter.

Few endocrine therapies have been evaluated by randomised controlled trials, in part because hormone replacement therapy (for example, with levothyroxine) has obvious clinical benefits and placebo-controlled trials would be unethical, and in part because many endocrine diseases are rare, making trials difficult to perform. Recommendations for 'evidence-based medicine' are, therefore, relatively scarce. They relate mainly to use of therapy that is 'optional' and/or recently available, such as oestrogen replacement in post-menopausal women, androgen therapy in older men and growth hormone replacement.

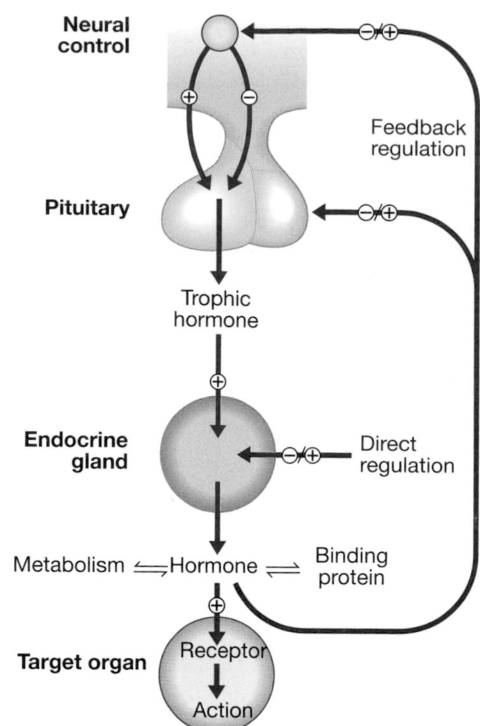

Fig. 20.1 An archetypal endocrine axis. Regulation by negative feedback and direct control is shown, along with the equilibrium between active circulating free hormone and bound or metabolised hormone.

AN OVERVIEW OF ENDOCRINOLOGY

Functional anatomy and physiology

Some endocrine glands, such as the parathyroids and pancreas, respond directly to metabolic signals, but most are controlled by hormones released from the pituitary gland. Anterior pituitary hormone secretion is controlled in turn by substances produced in the hypothalamus and released into portal blood, which drains directly down the pituitary stalk (Fig. 20.1). Posterior pituitary hormones are synthesised in the hypothalamus and transported down nerve axons, to be released from the posterior pituitary. Hormone release in the hypothalamus and pituitary is regulated by numerous stimuli and through feedback control by hormones produced by the target glands (thyroid, adrenal cortex and gonads). These integrated endocrine systems are called 'axes', and are listed in Figure 20.2.

A wide variety of molecules can act as hormones, including peptides such as insulin and growth hormone, glycoproteins such as thyroid-stimulating hormone, and amines such as noradrenaline (norepinephrine). The biological effects of hormones are mediated by binding to receptors. Many receptors are located on the cell surface. These interact with various intracellular signalling molecules on the cytosolic side of the plasma membrane to affect cell function, usually through changes in gene expression (p. 48). Some hormones, most notably steroids, triiodothyronine and vitamin D, bind to specific intracellular receptors, which directly bind to response elements on DNA to regulate gene expression (p. 42).

The classical model of endocrine function involves hormones synthesised in endocrine glands, which are released into the circulation and act at sites distant from those of secretion (as in Fig. 20.1). However, additional levels of regulation are now recognised. Many other organs secrete hormones or contribute to the peripheral metabolism and activation of pro-hormones. A notable example is the production of oestrogens from adrenal androgens in adipose tissue by the enzyme aromatase. Some hormones, such as neurotransmitters, act in a paracrine fashion to affect adjacent cells, or act in an autocrine way to affect behaviour of the cell that produces the hormone.

Endocrine pathology

For each endocrine axis or major gland, diseases can be classified as shown in Box 20.1. Pathology arising within the gland is often called 'primary' disease (for example, primary hypothyroidism in Hashimoto's thyroiditis), while abnormal stimulation of the gland is often called 'secondary' disease (for example, secondary hypothyroidism in patients with a pituitary tumour and thyroid-stimulating hormone deficiency). Some pathological processes can affect multiple endocrine glands (p. 795); these may have a genetic basis (such as organ-specific autoimmune endocrine disorders and the multiple endocrine neoplasia (MEN) syndromes) or be a consequence of therapy for another disease (for example, following treatment of childhood cancer with chemotherapy and/or radiotherapy).

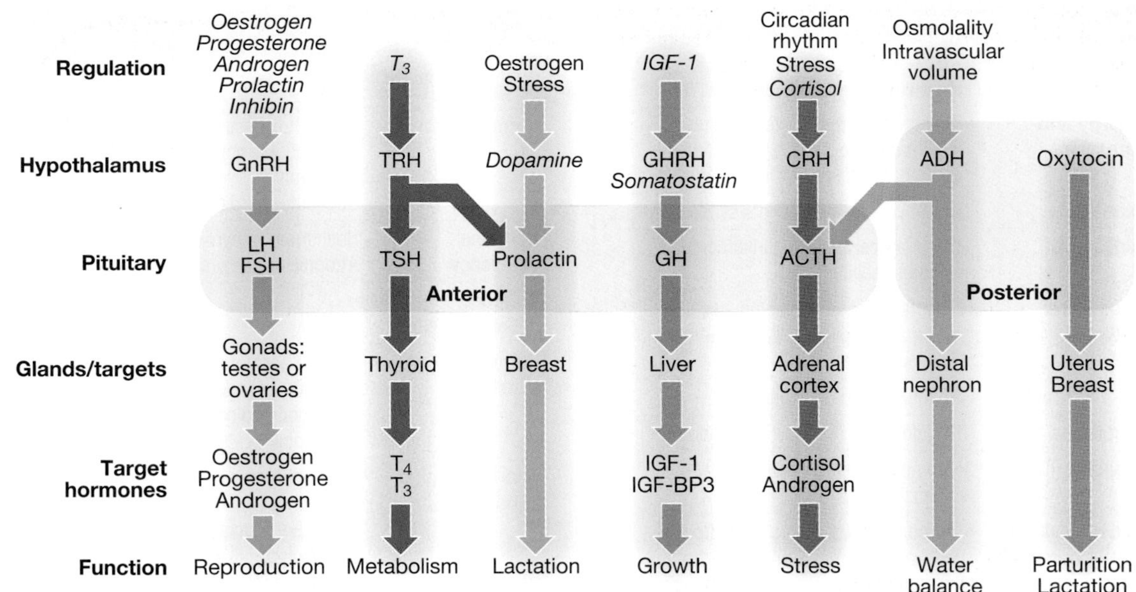

Fig. 20.2 The principal endocrine 'axes'. Some major endocrine glands are not controlled by the pituitary. These include the parathyroid glands (regulated by calcium concentrations, p. 766), the adrenal zona glomerulosa (regulated by the renin–angiotensin system, p. 771) and the endocrine pancreas (Ch. 21). Italics show negative regulation. (ACTH = adrenocorticotrophic hormone; ADH = antidiuretic hormone, arginine vasopressin; CRH = corticotrophin-releasing hormone; FSH = follicle-stimulating hormone; GH = growth hormone; GHRH = growth hormone-releasing hormone; GnRH = gonadotrophin-releasing hormone; IGF-1 = insulin-like growth factor-1; IGF-BP3 = IGF-binding protein-3; LH = luteinising hormone: T_3 = triiodothyronine; T_4 = thyroxine; TRH = thyrotrophin-releasing hormone; TSH = thyroid-stimulating hormone).

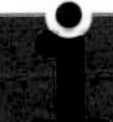

20.1 Classification of endocrine disease

Hormone excess
- Primary gland over-production
- Secondary to excess trophic substance

Hormone deficiency
- Primary gland failure
- Secondary to deficient trophic hormone

Hormone hypersensitivity
- Failure of inactivation of hormone
- Target organ over-activity/hypersensitivity

Hormone resistance
- Failure of activation of hormone
- Target organ resistance

Non-functioning tumours

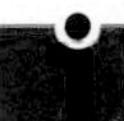

20.2 Principles of endocrine investigation

Timing of measurement
- Release of many hormones is rhythmical (pulsatile, circadian or monthly), so random measurement may be invalid and sequential or dynamic tests may be required

Choice of dynamic biochemical tests
- Abnormalities are often characterised by loss of normal regulation of hormone secretion
- If hormone deficiency is suspected, choose a stimulation test
- If hormone excess is suspected, choose a suppression test
- The more tests there are to choose from, the less likely it is that any single test is infallible, so avoid interpreting one result in isolation

Imaging
- Secretory cells also take up substrates, which can be labelled
- Most endocrine glands have a high prevalence of 'incidentalomas', so do not scan unless the biochemistry confirms endocrine dysfunction or the primary problem is a tumour

Biopsy
- Many endocrine tumours are difficult to classify histologically (e.g. adrenal carcinoma and adenoma)

Investigation of endocrine disease

Biochemical investigations play a central role in endocrinology. Most hormones can be measured in blood, but the circumstances in which the sample is taken are often crucial, especially for hormones with pulsatile secretion, such as growth hormone; those that show diurnal variation, such as cortisol; or those that demonstrate monthly variation, such as oestrogen or progesterone. Other investigations, such as imaging and biopsy, are more frequently reserved for patients who present with a tumour. The principles of investigation are shown in Box 20.2. The choice of test is often pragmatic, taking local access to reliable sampling facilities and laboratory measurements into account.

Presenting problems in endocrine disease

Endocrine diseases present in many different ways and to clinicians in many different disciplines. Classical syndromes are described in relation to individual glands in the following sections. Often, however, the

20.3 Examples of non-specific presentations of endocrine disease

Symptom	Most likely endocrine disorder(s)
Lethargy and depression	Hypothyroidism, diabetes mellitus, hyperparathyroidism, hypogonadism, adrenal insufficiency, Cushing's syndrome
Weight gain	Hypothyroidism, Cushing's syndrome
Weight loss	Thyrotoxicosis, adrenal insufficiency, diabetes mellitus
Polyuria and polydipsia	Diabetes mellitus, diabetes insipidus, hyperparathyroidism, hypokalaemia (Conn's syndrome)
Heat intolerance	Thyrotoxicosis, menopause
Palpitations	Thyrotoxicosis, phaeochromocytoma
Headache	Acromegaly, pituitary tumour, phaeochromocytoma
Muscle weakness (usually proximal)	Thyrotoxicosis, Cushing's syndrome, hypokalaemia (e.g. Conn's syndrome), hyperparathyroidism, hypogonadism
Coarsening of features	Acromegaly, hypothyroidism

presentation is with non-specific symptoms (Box 20.3) or with asymptomatic biochemical abnormalities. In addition, endocrine diseases are encountered in the differential diagnosis of common complaints discussed in other chapters of this book, including electrolyte abnormalities (Ch. 16), hypertension (Ch. 18), obesity (Ch. 5) and osteoporosis (Ch. 25). Although diseases of the adrenal glands, hypothalamus and pituitary are relatively rare, their diagnosis often relies on astute clinical observation in a patient with non-specific complaints, so it is important that clinicians are familiar with their key features.

THE THYROID GLAND

Diseases of the thyroid predominantly affect females and are common, occurring in about 5% of the population. The thyroid axis is involved in the regulation of cellular differentiation and metabolism in virtually all nucleated cells, so that disorders of thyroid function have diverse manifestations. Structural diseases of the thyroid gland, such as goitre, commonly occur in patients with normal thyroid function. Diseases of the thyroid are summarised in Box 20.4.

Functional anatomy, physiology and investigations

Thyroid physiology is illustrated in Figure 20.3. The parafollicular C cells secrete calcitonin, which is of no apparent physiological significance in humans. The follicular epithelial cells synthesise thyroid hormones by incorporating iodine into the amino acid tyrosine on the surface of thyroglobulin (Tg), a protein secreted into the colloid of the follicle. Iodide is a key substrate for thyroid hormone synthesis; a dietary intake in excess of

20.4 Classification of thyroid disease

	Primary	Secondary
Hormone excess	Graves' disease Multinodular goitre Adenoma Subacute thyroiditis	TSHoma
Hormone deficiency	Hashimoto's thyroiditis Atrophic hypothyroidism	Hypopituitarism
Hormone hypersensitivity	–	
Hormone resistance	Thyroid hormone resistance syndrome 5′-monodeiodinase deficiency	
Non-functioning tumours	Differentiated carcinoma Medullary carcinoma Lymphoma	

100 μg/day is required to maintain thyroid function in adults. The thyroid secretes predominantly thyroxine (T_4) and only a small amount of triiodothyronine (T_3); approximately 85% of T_3 in blood is produced from T_4 by a family of monodeiodinase enzymes which are active in many tissues, including liver, muscle, heart and kidney. Selenium is an integral component of these monodeiodinases. T_4 can be regarded as a pro-hormone, since it has a longer half-life in blood than T_3 (approximately 1 week compared with approximately 18 hours), and binds and activates thyroid hormone receptors less effectively than T_3. T_4 can also be converted to the inactive metabolite, reverse T_3.

T_3 and T_4 circulate in plasma almost entirely (> 99%) bound to transport proteins, mainly thyroxine-binding globulin (TBG). It is the unbound or free hormones which diffuse into tissues and exert diverse metabolic actions. Some laboratories use assays which measure total T_4 and T_3 in plasma, but it is increasingly common to measure free T_4 and free T_3. The advantage of the free hormone measurements is that they are not influenced by changes in the concentration of binding proteins; in pregnancy, for example, TBG levels are increased and total T_3 and T_4 may be raised, but free thyroid hormone levels are normal.

Production of T_3 and T_4 in the thyroid is stimulated by thyrotrophin (thyroid-stimulating hormone, TSH), a glycoprotein released from the thyrotroph cells of the anterior pituitary in response to the hypothalamic tripeptide, thyrotrophin-releasing hormone (TRH). A circadian rhythm of TSH secretion can be demonstrated with a peak at 0100 hrs and trough at 1100 hrs, but the variation is small so that thyroid function can be assessed reliably from a single blood sample taken at any time of day and does not usually require any dynamic stimulation or suppression tests. There is a negative feedback of thyroid hormones on the hypothalamus and pituitary such that in thyrotoxicosis, when plasma concentrations of T_3 and T_4 are raised, TSH secretion is suppressed. Conversely, in hypothyroidism due to disease of the thyroid gland, low T_3 and T_4 are associated with high

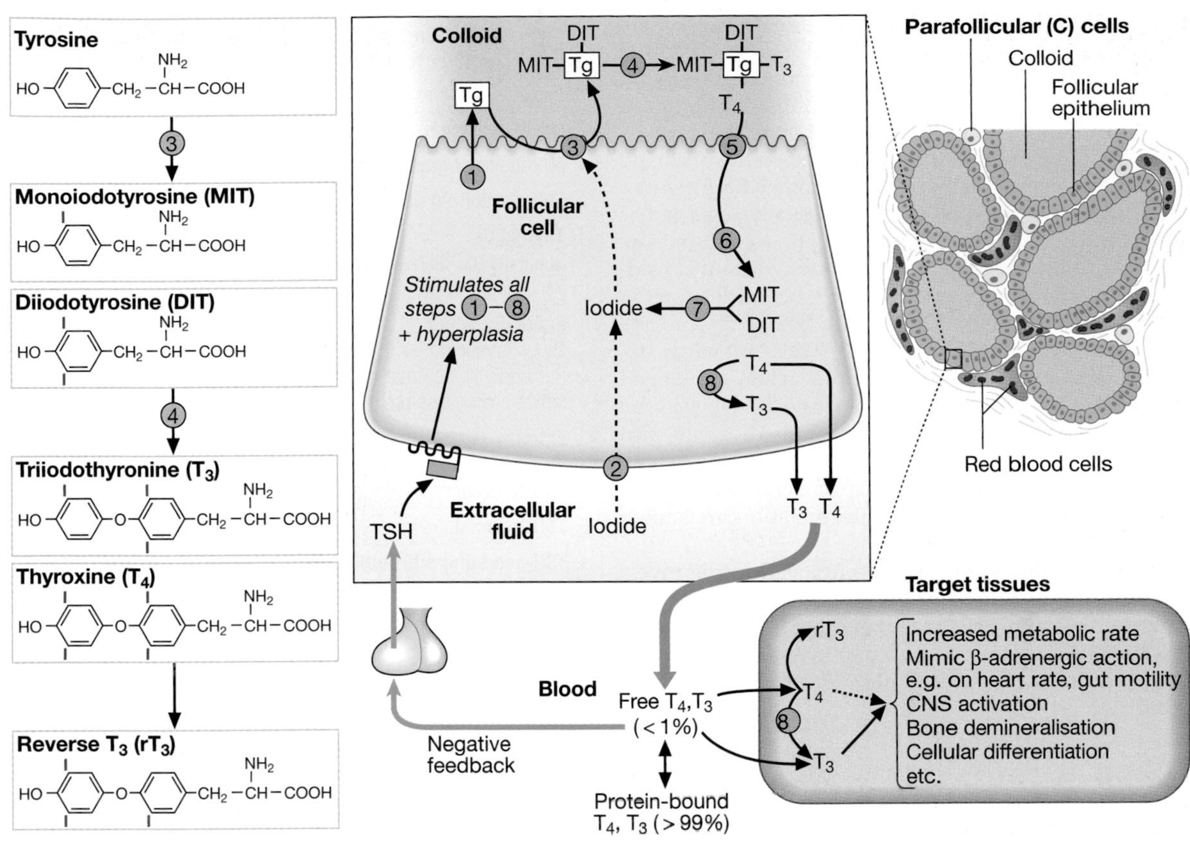

Fig. 20.3 Structure and function of the thyroid gland. (1) Thyroglobulin (Tg) is synthesised and secreted into the colloid of the follicle. (2) Inorganic iodide (I^-) is actively transported into the follicular cell ('trapping'). (3) Iodide is transported on to the colloidal surface by a transporter (pendrin, defective in Pendred's syndrome) and 'organified' by the thyroid peroxidase enzyme, which incorporates it into the amino acid tyrosine on the surface of Tg to form monoiodotyrosine (MIT) and diiodotyrosine (DIT). (4) Iodinated tyrosines couple to form T_3 and T_4. (5) Tg is endocytosed. (6) Tg is cleaved by proteolysis to free the iodinated tyrosine and thyroid hormones. (7) Iodinated tyrosine is dehalogenated to recycle the iodide. (8) T_4 is converted to T_3 by 5′-monodeiodinase.

20.5 How to interpret thyroid function test results

TSH	T_4	T_3	Most likely interpretation(s)
U.D.	Raised	Raised	Primary thyrotoxicosis
U.D.	Normal[1]	Raised	Primary T_3-toxicosis
U.D.	Normal[1]	Normal[1]	Subclinical thyrotoxicosis
U.D. or low	Raised	Low or normal	Non-thyroidal illness, amiodarone therapy
U.D.	Low	Low	Secondary hypothyroidism[4] Transient thyroiditis in evolution
Normal	Low	Low[2]	Secondary hypothyroidism[4]
Mildly elevated 5–20 mU/L	Low	Low[2]	Primary hypothyroidism Secondary hypothyroidism[4]
Elevated > 20 mU/L	Low	Low[2]	Primary hypothyroidism
Mildly elevated 5–20 mU/L	Normal[3]	Normal[2]	Subclinical hypothyroidism
Elevated 20–500 mU/L	Normal	Normal	Artefact Endogenous IgG antibodies which interfere with TSH assay
Elevated	Raised	Raised	Non-compliance with T_4 replacement – recent 'loading' dose Secondary thyrotoxicosis[4] Thyroid hormone resistance

[1]Usually upper part of reference range. [2]T_3 is not a sensitive indicator of hypothyroidism and should not be requested.
[3]Usually lower part of reference range. [4]i.e. Secondary to pituitary or hypothalamic disease. Note that TSH assays may report detectable TSH.
(U.D. = undetectable)

circulating TSH levels. The anterior pituitary is very sensitive to minor changes in thyroid hormone levels within the reference range. Although the reference range for free T_4 is 9–21 pmol/L (700–1632 pg/dL), a rise or fall of 5 pmol/L in an individual in whom the level is usually 15 pmol/L would be associated on the one hand with undetectable TSH, and on the other hand with a raised TSH. For this reason, TSH is usually regarded as the most useful investigation of thyroid function. However, interpretation of TSH values without considering thyroid hormone levels may be misleading in patients with pituitary disease (see Box 20.58, p. 787). Moreover, TSH may take several weeks to 'catch up' with T_4 and T_3 levels, for example, when prolonged suppression of TSH in thyrotoxicosis is relieved by antithyroid therapy. Heterophilic antibodies can also interfere with the TSH assay and cause a spuriously high measurement. Common patterns of abnormal thyroid function test results and their interpretation are shown in Box 20.5.

Other modalities commonly employed in the investigation of thyroid disease include measurement of antibodies against the TSH receptor or other thyroid antigens (see Box 20.8, p. 741), radioisotope imaging, fine needle aspiration biopsy and ultrasound. Their use is described below.

20.6 Causes of thyrotoxicosis and their relative frequencies

Cause	Frequency[1] (%)
Graves' disease	76
Multinodular goitre	14
Solitary thyroid adenoma	5
Thyroiditis	
Subacute (de Quervain's)[2]	3
Post-partum[2]	0.5
Iodide-induced	
Drugs (amiodarone)[2]	1
Radiographic contrast media[2]	–
Iodine prophylaxis programme[2]	–
Extrathyroidal source of thyroid hormone	
Factitious thyrotoxicosis[2]	0.2
Struma ovarii[2,3]	–
TSH-induced	
TSH-secreting pituitary adenoma	0.2
Choriocarcinoma and hydatidiform mole[4]	–
Follicular carcinoma ± metastases	0.1

[1]In a series of 2087 patients presenting to the Royal Infirmary of Edinburgh over a 10-year period.
[2]Characterised by negligible radio-isotope uptake.
[3]i.e. Ovarian teratoma containing thyroid tissue.
[4]Human chorionic gonadotrophin has thyroid-stimulating activity.

Presenting problems in thyroid disease

The most common presentations are hyperthyroidism (thyrotoxicosis), hypothyroidism and enlargement of the thyroid (goitre or thyroid nodule). Widespread availability of thyroid function tests has led to the increasingly frequent identification of patients with abnormal results who are either asymptomatic or have non-specific complaints such as tiredness and weight gain.

Thyrotoxicosis

Thyrotoxicosis describes a constellation of clinical features arising from elevated circulating levels of thyroid hormone. The most common causes are Graves' disease, multinodular goitre and autonomously functioning thyroid nodules (toxic adenoma) (Box 20.6). Thyroiditis is more common in parts of the world where relevant viral infections occur, such as North America.

Clinical assessment

The clinical manifestations of thyrotoxicosis are shown in Box 20.7 and an approach to differential diagnosis is given in Figure 20.4. The most common symptoms are weight loss with a normal or increased appetite, heat intolerance, palpitations, tremor and irritability. Tachycardia, palmar erythema and lid lag are common signs. Not all patients have a palpable goitre, but experienced clinicians can discriminate the diffuse soft goitre of Graves' disease from the irregular enlargement of a multinodular goitre. All causes of thyrotoxicosis can cause lid retraction and lid lag, due to potentiation of sympathetic innervation of the levator palpebrae muscles, but only Graves' disease causes other features of ophthalmopathy, including periorbital oedema, conjunctival irritation, exophthalmos and diplopia. Pretibial myxoedema (p. 751) and the rare thyroid acropachy (a periosteal hypertrophy, indistinguishable from finger clubbing) are also specific to Graves' disease.

Investigations

The first-line investigations are serum T_3, T_4 and TSH. If abnormal values are found, the tests should be repeated and the abnormality confirmed in view of the likely need for prolonged medical treatment or destructive therapy. In most patients, serum T_3 and T_4 are both elevated, but T_4 is in the upper part of the reference range and T_3 raised (T_3 toxicosis) in about 5%. Serum TSH is undetectable in primary thyrotoxicosis, but values can be raised in the very rare syndrome of secondary thyrotoxicosis caused by a TSH-producing pituitary adenoma. When biochemical thyrotoxicosis has been confirmed, further investigations should be undertaken to determine the underlying cause, including measurement of TSH receptor antibodies (TRAb, elevated in Graves' disease, Box 20.8) and isotope scanning, as shown in Figure 20.4. Other non-specific abnormalities are common (Box 20.9). An ECG may demonstrate sinus tachycardia or atrial fibrillation.

Radio-iodine uptake tests measure the proportion of isotope that is trapped in the whole gland, but have been largely superseded by ^{99m}technetium scintigraphy scans, which also indicate trapping, are quicker to perform with a lower dose of radioactivity, and provide a higher-resolution image. In low-uptake thyrotoxicosis, the cause is usually a transient thyroiditis (p. 751). Occasionally, patients induce 'factitious thyrotoxicosis' by consuming excessive amounts of a thyroid hormone preparation, most often levothyroxine. The exogenous thyroxine suppresses pituitary TSH secretion and hence iodine uptake, serum thyroglobulin and release of endogenous thyroid hormones. The T_4:T_3 ratio (typically

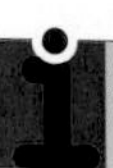

20.7 Clinical features of thyroid dysfunction

Thyrotoxicosis		Hypothyroidism	
Symptoms	**Signs**	**Symptoms**	**Signs**
Common			
Weight loss despite normal or increased appetite Heat intolerance, sweating Palpitations, tremor Dyspnoea, fatigue Irritability, emotional lability	Weight loss Tremor Palmar erythema Sinus tachycardia Lid retraction, lid lag	Weight gain Cold intolerance Fatigue, somnolence Dry skin Dry hair Menorrhagia	Weight gain
Less common			
Osteoporosis (fracture, loss of height) Diarrhoea, steatorrhoea Angina Ankle swelling Anxiety, psychosis Muscle weakness Periodic paralysis (predominantly in Chinese) Pruritus, alopecia Amenorrhoea/oligomenorrhoea Infertility, spontaneous abortion Loss of libido, impotence Excessive lacrimation	Goitre with bruit[1] Atrial fibrillation[2] Systolic hypertension/ increased pulse pressure Cardiac failure[2] Hyper-reflexia Ill-sustained clonus Proximal myopathy Bulbar myopathy[2]	Constipation Hoarseness Carpal tunnel syndrome Alopecia Aches and pains Muscle stiffness Deafness Depression Infertility	Hoarse voice Facial features: Purplish lips Malar flush Periorbital oedema Loss of lateral eyebrows Anaemia Carotenaemia Erythema ab igne Bradycardia hypertension Delayed relaxation of reflexes Dermal myxoedema
Rare			
Vomiting Apathy Anorexia Exacerbation of asthma	Gynaecomastia Spider naevi Onycholysis Pigmentation	Psychosis (myxoedema madness) Galactorrhoea Impotence	Ileus, ascites Pericardial and pleural effusions Cerebellar ataxia Myotonia

[1]In Graves' disease only. [2]Features found particularly in elderly patients.

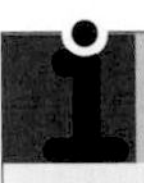

20.8 Prevalence of thyroid autoantibodies (%)

	Antibodies to:		
	Thyroid peroxidase[1]	**Thyroglobulin**	**TSH receptor[2]**
Normal population	8–27	5–20	0
Graves' disease	50–80	50–70	80–95
Autoimmune hypothyroidism	90–100	80–90	10–20
Multinodular goitre	~30–40	~30–40	0
Transient thyroiditis	~30–40	~30–40	0

[1]Thyroid peroxidase (TPO) antibodies are the principal component of what was previously measured as thyroid 'microsomal' antibodies.
[2]TSH receptor antibodies (TRAb) can be agonists (stimulatory, causing Graves' thyrotoxicosis) or antagonists ('blocking', causing hypothyroidism)

20.9 Non-specific laboratory abnormalities in thyroid dysfunction*

Thyrotoxicosis

- Serum enzymes: raised alanine aminotransferase, γ-glutamyl transferase (GGT), and alkaline phosphatase from liver and bone
- Raised bilirubin
- Mild hypercalcaemia
- Glycosuria: associated diabetes mellitus, 'lag storage' glycosuria

Hypothyroidism

- Serum enzymes: raised creatine kinase, aspartate aminotransferase, lactate dehydrogenase (LDH)
- Hypercholesterolaemia
- Anaemia: normochromic normocytic or macrocytic
- Hyponatraemia

*These abnormalities are not useful in differential diagnosis, so the tests should be avoided and any further investigation undertaken only if abnormalities persist when the patient is euthyroid.

30:1 in conventional thyrotoxicosis) is increased to above 70:1 because circulating T_3 in factitious thyrotoxicosis is derived exclusively from the peripheral monodeiodination of T_4 and not from thyroid secretion. The combination of negligible iodine uptake, high T_4:T_3 ratio and a low or undetectable thyroglobulin is diagnostic.

Management

Definitive treatment of thyrotoxicosis depends on the underlying cause and may include antithyroid drugs, radioactive iodine or surgery. A non-selective β-adrenoceptor antagonist (β-blocker), such as propranolol

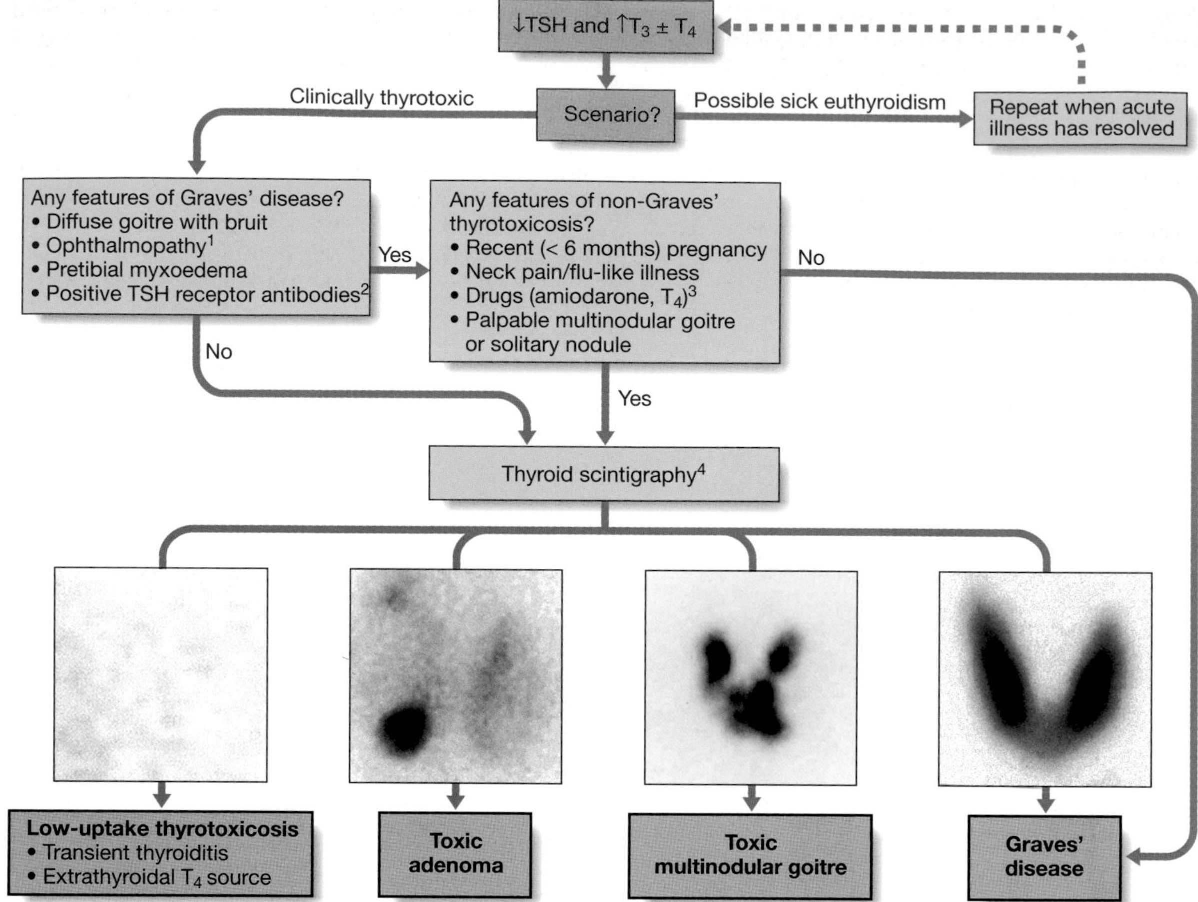

Fig. 20.4 Establishing the differential diagnosis in thyrotoxicosis. (1) Graves' ophthalmopathy refers to clinical features of exophthalmos and periorbital and conjunctival oedema, not simply the lid lag and lid retraction which can occur in all forms of thyrotoxicosis. (2) TSH receptor antibodies are very rare in patients without autoimmune thyroid disease, but only occur in 80–95% of patients with Graves' disease; a positive test is therefore confirmatory, but a negative test does not exclude Graves' disease. Other thyroid antibodies (e.g. anti-peroxidase and anti-thyroglobulin antibodies) are unhelpful in the differential diagnosis since they occur frequently in the population and are found with several of the disorders which cause thyrotoxicosis. (3) Scintigraphy is not necessary in most cases of drug-induced thyrotoxicosis. (4) ^{99m}Technetium pertechnetate scans of patients with thyrotoxicosis. In low-uptake thyrotoxicosis, most commonly due to a viral, post-partum or iodine-induced thyroiditis, there is negligible isotope detected in the region of the thyroid, although uptake is apparent in nearby salivary glands (not shown here). In a toxic adenoma there is lack of uptake of isotope by the rest of the thyroid gland due to suppression of serum TSH. In multinodular goitre there is relatively low, patchy uptake within the nodules; such an appearance is not always associated with a palpable thyroid. In Graves' disease there is diffuse uptake of isotope.

(160 mg daily) or nadolol (40–80 mg daily), will alleviate but not abolish symptoms in most patients within 24–48 hours. Beta-blockers should not be used for long-term treatment of thyrotoxicosis but are extremely useful in the short term, whilst patients are awaiting hospital consultation or following ^{131}I therapy.

Atrial fibrillation in thyrotoxicosis

Atrial fibrillation occurs in about 10% of patients with thyrotoxicosis. The incidence increases with age, so that almost half of all males with thyrotoxicosis over the age of 60 are affected. Moreover, subclinical thyrotoxicosis (p. 745) is a risk factor for atrial fibrillation. Characteristically, the ventricular rate is little influenced by digoxin, but responds to the addition of a β-blocker. Thromboembolic vascular complications are particularly common in thyrotoxic atrial fibrillation so that anticoagulation with warfarin is required, unless contraindicated. Once thyroid hormone and TSH concentrations have been returned to normal, atrial fibrillation will spontaneously revert to sinus rhythm in about 50% of patients, but cardioversion may be required in the remainder.

Thyrotoxic crisis ('thyroid storm')

This is a rare but life-threatening complication of thyrotoxicosis. The most prominent signs are fever, agitation, confusion, tachycardia or atrial fibrillation and, in the older patient, cardiac failure. It is a medical emergency, which has a mortality of 10% despite early recognition and treatment. Thyrotoxic crisis is most commonly precipitated by infection in a patient with previously unrecognised or inadequately treated thyrotoxicosis. It may also develop shortly after subtotal thyroidectomy in an ill-prepared patient or within a few days of ^{131}I therapy, when acute irradiation damage may lead to a transient rise in serum thyroid hormone levels.

Patients should be rehydrated and given propranolol, either orally (80 mg 4 times daily) or intravenously (1–5 mg 4 times daily). Sodium ipodate (500 mg per day orally) will restore serum T_3 levels to normal in

48–72 hours. This is a radiographic contrast medium which not only inhibits the release of thyroid hormones, but also reduces the conversion of T_4 to T_3 and is, therefore, more effective than potassium iodide or Lugol's solution. Dexamethasone (2 mg 4 times daily) and amiodarone have similar effects. Oral carbimazole 40–60 mg daily (p. 748) should be given to inhibit the synthesis of new thyroid hormone. If the patient is unconscious or uncooperative, carbimazole can be administered rectally with good effect, but no preparation is available for parenteral use. After 10–14 days the patient can usually be maintained on carbimazole alone.

Hypothyroidism

Hypothyroidism is a common condition with various causes (Box 20.10), but autoimmune disease (Hashimoto's thyroiditis) and thyroid failure following ^{131}I or surgical treatment of thyrotoxicosis account for over 90% of cases, except in areas where iodine deficiency is endemic. Women are affected approximately six times more frequently than men.

Clinical assessment

The clinical presentation depends on the duration and severity of the hypothyroidism. Those in whom complete thyroid failure has developed insidiously over months or years may present with many of the clinical features listed in Box 20.7. A consequence of prolonged hypothyroidism is the infiltration of many body tissues by the mucopolysaccharides, hyaluronic acid and chondroitin sulphate, resulting in a low-pitched voice, poor hearing, slurred speech due to a large tongue, and compression of the median nerve at the wrist (carpal tunnel syndrome). Infiltration of the dermis gives rise to non-pitting oedema (myxoedema), which is most marked in the skin of the hands, feet and eyelids. The resultant periorbital puffiness is often striking and may be combined with facial pallor due to vasoconstriction and anaemia, or a lemon-yellow tint to the skin caused by carotenaemia, along with purplish lips and malar flush. Most cases of hypothyroidism are not clinically obvious, however, and a high index of suspicion needs to be maintained so that the diagnosis is not overlooked in individuals complaining of non-specific symptoms such as tiredness, weight gain, depression or carpal tunnel syndrome.

The key discriminatory features in the history and examination are highlighted in Figure 20.5. Care must be taken to identify patients with transient hypothyroidism, in whom life-long levothyroxine therapy is inappropriate. This is often observed during the first 6 months after subtotal thyroidectomy or ^{131}I treatment of Graves' disease, in the post-thyrotoxic phase of subacute thyroiditis and in post-partum thyroiditis. In these conditions, levothyroxine treatment is not always necessary, as the patient may be asymptomatic during the short period of thyroid failure.

20.10 Causes of hypothyroidism

Causes	Anti-TPO antibodies[1]	Goitre[2]
Autoimmune		
Hashimoto's thyroiditis	++	±
Spontaneous atrophic hypothyroidism	–	–
Graves' disease with TSH receptor-blocking antibodies	+	±
Iatrogenic		
Radioactive iodine ablation	+	±
Thyroidectomy	+	–
Drugs		
Carbimazole, methimazole, propylthiouracil	+	±
Amiodarone	+	±
Lithium	–	±
Transient thyroiditis		
Subacute (de Quervain's) thyroiditis	+	±
Post-partum thyroiditis	+	±
Iodine deficiency, e.g. in mountainous regions	–	++
Congenital		
Dyshormonogenesis	–	++
Thyroid aplasia	–	–
Infiltrative		
Amyloidosis, Riedel's thyroiditis, sarcoidosis etc.	+	++
Secondary hypothyroidism		
TSH deficiency	–	–

[1]As shown in Box 20.8, thyroid autoantibodies are common in the healthy population, so might be present in anyone. ++ high titre; + more likely to be detected than in the healthy population; – not especially likely.
[2]Goitre: – absent; ± may be present; ++ characteristic.

Investigations

In the vast majority of cases, hypothyroidism results from an intrinsic disorder of the thyroid gland (primary hypothyroidism). In this situation, serum T_4 is low and TSH is elevated, usually in excess of 20 mU/L. Measurements of serum T_3 are unhelpful since they do not discriminate reliably between euthyroidism and hypothyroidism. Secondary hypothyroidism is rare and is caused by failure of TSH secretion in an individual with hypothalamic or anterior pituitary disease. Other non-specific abnormalities are shown in Box 20.9. In severe, prolonged hypothyroidism, the electrocardiogram (ECG) classically demonstrates sinus bradycardia with low-voltage complexes and ST segment and T-wave abnormalities. Measurement of thyroid peroxidase antibodies is helpful but further investigations are rarely required (see Fig. 20.5).

Management

Treatment is with levothyroxine replacement. It is customary to start with a low dose of 50 μg per day for 3 weeks, increasing thereafter to 100 μg per day for a further 3 weeks and finally to a maintenance dose of 100–150 μg per day. In younger patients, it is safe to initiate levothyroxine at a higher dose (for example, 100 μg per day), to allow a more rapid normalisation of thyroid hormone levels. Levothyroxine has a half-life of 7 days so it should always be taken as a single daily dose and at least 6 weeks should pass before repeating thyroid function tests and adjusting the dose, usually by 25 μg per day. Patients feel better within 2–3 weeks. Reduction in weight and periorbital puffiness occurs quickly, but the restoration of skin and hair texture and

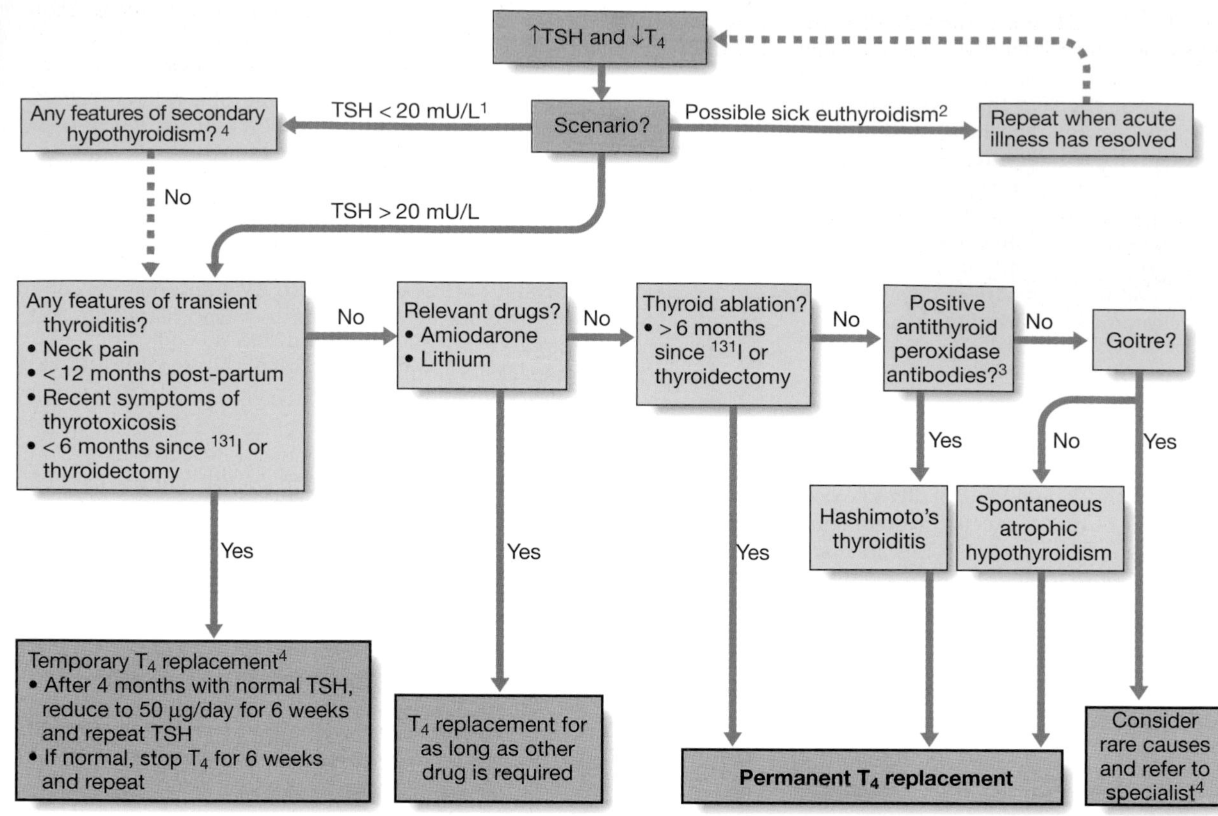

Fig. 20.5 An approach to adults with suspected primary hypothyroidism. This scheme ignores congenital causes of hypothyroidism (see Box 20.10), such as thyroid aplasia and dyshormonogenesis (associated with nerve deafness in Pendred's syndrome), which are usually diagnosed in childhood. (1) Immunoreactive TSH may be detected at normal or even modestly elevated levels in patients with pituitary failure; unless T_4 is only marginally low, TSH should be > 20 mU/L to confirm the diagnosis of primary hypothyroidism. (2) The usual abnormality in sick euthyroidism is a low TSH but any pattern can occur. (3) Thyroid peroxidase antibodies are highly sensitive but not very specific for autoimmune thyroid disease (see Boxes 20.8 and 20.10). (4) Specialist advice is most appropriate where indicated. Secondary hypothyroidism is rare, but is suggested by deficiency of pituitary hormones or by clinical features of pituitary tumour such as headache or visual field defect (p. 789). Rare causes of hypothyroidism with goitre include dyshormonogenesis and infiltration of the thyroid (see Box 20.10).

resolution of any effusions may take 3–6 months. As illustrated in Figure 20.5, most patients do not require specialist review but will require life-long levothyroxine therapy.

The dose of levothyroxine should be adjusted to maintain serum TSH within the reference range. To achieve this, serum T_4 often needs to be in the upper part of the reference range or even slightly raised, because the T_3 required for receptor activation is derived exclusively from conversion of T_4 within the target tissues, without the usual contribution from thyroid secretion. Some physicians advocate combined replacement with T_4 and T_3 or preparations of animal thyroid extract, but this approach remains controversial and is not supported by robust evidence. Some patients remain symptomatic despite normalisation of TSH and may wish to take extra levothyroxine, which suppresses TSH. However, suppressed TSH is a risk factor for osteoporosis and atrial fibrillation (p. 745; subclinical thyrotoxicosis), so this approach cannot be recommended.

It is important to measure thyroid function every 1–2 years once the dose of levothyroxine is stabilised. This encourages patient compliance with therapy and allows adjustment for variable underlying thyroid activity and other changes in levothyroxine requirements (Box 20.11). Some patients have a persistent elevation of serum TSH despite an ostensibly adequate replacement dose of levothyroxine; most commonly, this is a consequence of suboptimal compliance with therapy. There may be differences in bioavailability between the numerous generic preparations of levothyroxine and so, if an individual is experiencing marked changes in serum TSH despite optimal compliance, the prescription of a branded preparation of levothyroxine could be considered. Levothyroxine absorption is maximal when the medication is taken before bed and may be further optimised by taking a vitamin C supplement.

In some poorly compliant patients, levothyroxine is taken diligently or even in excess for a few days prior to a clinic visit, resulting in the seemingly anomalous combination of a high serum T_4 and high TSH (see Box 20.5, p. 739).

Levothyroxine replacement in ischaemic heart disease

Hypothyroidism and ischaemic heart disease are common conditions that often occur together. Although angina may remain unchanged in severity or paradoxically disappear with restoration of metabolic rate, exacerbation of myocardial ischaemia, infarction and

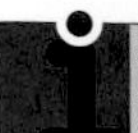

20.11 Situations in which an adjustment of the dose of levothyroxine may be necessary

Increased dose required

Use of other medication
- Increase T_4 clearance: phenobarbital, phenytoin, carbamazepine, rifampicin, sertraline*, chloroquine*
- Interfere with intestinal T_4 absorption: colestyramine, sucralfate, aluminium hydroxide, ferrous sulphate, dietary fibre supplements, calcium carbonate

Pregnancy or oestrogen therapy
- Increases concentration of serum thyroxine-binding globulin

After surgical or ^{131}I ablation of Graves' disease
- Reduces thyroidal secretion with time

Malabsorption

Decreased dose required

Ageing
- Decreases T_4 clearance

Graves' disease developing in patient with long-standing primary hypothyroidism
- Switch from production of blocking to stimulating TSH receptor antibodies

*Mechanism not fully established.

sudden death are recognised complications of levothyroxine replacement, even using doses as low as 25 μg per day. In patients with known ischaemic heart disease, thyroid hormone replacement should be introduced at low dose and increased very slowly under specialist supervision. It has been suggested that T_3 has an advantage over T_4, since T_3 has a shorter half-life and any adverse effect will reverse more quickly, but the more distinct peak in hormone levels after each dose of T_3 is a disadvantage. Coronary angioplasty or bypass surgery may be required if angina is exacerbated by levothyroxine replacement therapy.

Hypothyroidism in pregnancy

Most pregnant women with primary hypothyroidism require an increase in the dose of levothyroxine of approximately 25–50 μg daily to maintain normal TSH levels. This may reflect increased metabolism of thyroxine by the placenta and increased serum thyroxine-binding globulin during pregnancy, resulting in an increase in the total thyroid hormone pool to maintain the same free T_4 and T_3 concentrations. Inadequate maternal T_4 therapy may be associated with impaired cognitive development in an unborn child and so women are usually advised to increase their daily levothyroxine dose by 25 μg when pregnancy is confirmed. Serum TSH and free T_4 should be measured during each trimester and the dose of levothyroxine adjusted to maintain a normal TSH. See also Box 20.20 (p. 756).

Myxoedema coma

This is a very rare presentation of hypothyroidism in which there is a depressed level of consciousness, usually in an elderly patient who appears myxoedematous. Body temperature may be as low as 25°C, convulsions are not uncommon and cerebrospinal fluid (CSF) pressure and protein content are raised. The mortality rate is 50% and survival depends on early recognition and treatment of hypothyroidism and other factors contributing to the altered consciousness level, such as medication, cardiac failure, pneumonia, dilutional hyponatraemia and respiratory failure.

Myxoedema coma is a medical emergency and treatment must begin before biochemical confirmation of the diagnosis. Suspected cases should be treated with an intravenous injection of 20 μg triiodothyronine, followed by further injections of 20 μg 3 times daily until there is sustained clinical improvement. In survivors, there is a rise in body temperature within 24 hours and, after 48–72 hours, it is usually possible to switch patients to oral levothyroxine in a dose of 50 μg daily. Unless it is apparent that the patient has primary hypothyroidism, the thyroid failure should also be assumed to be secondary to hypothalamic or pituitary disease and treatment given with hydrocortisone 100 mg IM 3 times daily, pending the results of T_4, TSH and cortisol measurement (p. 787). Other measures include slow rewarming (p. 105), cautious use of intravenous fluids, broad-spectrum antibiotics and high-flow oxygen. Occasionally, assisted ventilation may be necessary.

Symptoms of hypothyroidism with normal thyroid function tests

The classic symptoms of hypothyroidism are, by their very nature, non-specific (see Box 20.3). There is a wide differential diagnosis for symptoms such as 'fatigue', 'weight gain' and 'low mood'. As has been noted, outside the context of pituitary and hypothalamic disease, serum TSH is an excellent measure of an individual's thyroid hormone status. However, some individuals believe that they have hypothyroidism despite normal serum TSH concentrations. There are a large number of websites which claim that serum TSH is not a good measure of thyroid hormone status and suggest that other factors, such as abnormalities of T_4 to T_3 conversion, may lead to low tissue levels of active thyroid hormones. Such websites often advocate a variety of tests of thyroid function of dubious scientific validity, including measurement of serum reverse T_3, 24-hour urine T_3, basal body temperature, skin iodine absorption, and levels of selenium in blood and urine. Individuals who believe they have hypothyroidism, despite normal conventional tests of thyroid function, can be difficult to manage. They require reassurance that their symptoms are being taken seriously and that organic disease has been carefully considered; if their symptoms persist, then referral to a team specialising in medically unexplained symptoms should be considered.

Asymptomatic abnormal thyroid function tests

One of the most common problems in medical practice is how to manage patients with abnormal thyroid function tests who have no obvious signs or symptoms of thyroid disease. These can be divided into three categories.

Subclinical thyrotoxicosis

Serum TSH is undetectable, and serum T_3 and T_4 are at the upper end of the reference range. This combination is most often found in older patients with multinodular goitre. These patients are at increased risk of atrial fibrillation and osteoporosis, and hence the consensus view is that they have mild thyrotoxicosis and require therapy, usually with ^{131}I. Otherwise, annual review is essential, as the conversion rate to overt thyrotoxicosis with elevated T_4 and/or T_3 concentrations is 5% each year.

Subclinical hypothyroidism

Serum TSH is raised, and serum T_3 and T_4 concentrations are at the lower end of the reference range. This may persist for many years, although there is a risk of progression to overt thyroid failure, particularly if antibodies to thyroid peroxidase are present or if the TSH rises above 10 mU/L. In patients with non-specific symptoms, a trial of levothyroxine therapy may be appropriate. In those with positive autoantibodies or TSH greater than 10 mU/L, it is better to treat the thyroid failure early rather than risk loss to follow-up and subsequent presentation with profound hypothyroidism. Levothyroxine should be given in a dose sufficient to restore the serum TSH concentration to normal.

Non-thyroidal illness ('sick euthyroidism')

This typically presents with a low serum TSH, raised T_4 and normal or low T_3, in a patient with systemic illness who does not have clinical evidence of thyroid disease. These abnormalities are caused by decreased peripheral conversion of T_4 to T_3, altered levels of binding proteins and their affinity for thyroid hormones, and often reduced secretion of TSH. During convalescence, serum TSH concentrations may increase to levels found in primary hypothyroidism. As thyroid function tests are difficult to interpret in patients with non-thyroidal illness, it is wise to avoid performing thyroid function tests unless there is clinical evidence of concomitant thyroid disease. If an abnormal result is found, treatment should only be given with specialist advice and the diagnosis should be re-evaluated after recovery.

Thyroid lump or swelling

A lump or swelling in the thyroid gland can be a source of considerable anxiety for patients. There are numerous causes but, broadly speaking, a thyroid swelling is either a solitary nodule, a multinodular goitre or a diffuse goitre (Box 20.12). Nodular thyroid disease is more common in women and occurs in approximately 30% of the adult female population. The majority of thyroid nodules are impalpable but may be identified when imaging of the neck is performed for another reason, such as during Doppler ultrasonography of the carotid arteries or computed tomographic pulmonary angiography. Increasingly, thyroid nodules are identified during staging of patients with cancer with computed tomography (CT), magnetic resonance imaging (MRI) or positron emission tomography (PET) scans. Palpable thyroid nodules occur in 4–8% of adult women and 1–2% of adult men, and classically present when the individual (or a friend or relative) notices a lump in the neck. Multinodular goitres and solitary nodules sometimes present with acute painful enlargement due to haemorrhage into a nodule.

Patients with thyroid nodules often worry that they have cancer, but the reality is that only 5–10% of thyroid nodules are malignant. A solitary nodule presenting in childhood or adolescence, particularly if there is a past history of head and neck irradiation, or one presenting in the elderly should heighten suspicion of a primary thyroid malignancy (p. 754). The presence of cervical lymphadenopathy also increases the likelihood of malignancy. Rarely, a secondary deposit from a renal, breast or lung carcinoma presents as a painful, rapidly growing, solitary thyroid nodule. Thyroid nodules identified on PET scanning have an approximately 33% chance of being malignant.

20.12 Causes of thyroid enlargement

Diffuse goitre
- Simple goitre
- Hashimoto's thyroiditis[1]
- Graves' disease
- Drugs
  Iodine, amiodarone, lithium
- Iodine deficiency (endemic goitre)[1]
- Suppurative thyroiditis[2]
- Transient thyroiditis[2]
- Dyshormonogenesis[1]
- Infiltrative
  Amyloidosis, sarcoidosis etc.
- Riedel's thyroiditis[2]

Multinodular goitre

Solitary nodule
- Colloid cyst
- Hyperplastic nodule
- Follicular adenoma
- Papillary carcinoma
- Follicular carcinoma
- Medullary cell carcinoma
- Anaplastic carcinoma
- Lymphoma
- Metastasis

[1]Goitre likely to shrink with levothyroxine therapy. [2]Usually tender.

Clinical assessment and investigations

Swellings in the anterior part of the neck most commonly originate in the thyroid and this can be confirmed by demonstrating that the swelling moves on swallowing (p. 735). It is often possible to distinguish clinically between the three main causes of thyroid swelling. There is a broad differential diagnosis of anterior neck swellings, which includes lymphadenopathy, branchial cysts, dermoid cysts and thyroglossal duct cysts (the latter are classically located in the midline and move on protrusion of the tongue). An ultrasound scan should be performed urgently, if there is any doubt as to the aetiology of an anterior neck swelling.

Serum T_3, T_4 and TSH should be measured in all patients with a goitre or solitary thyroid nodule. The finding of biochemical thyrotoxicosis or hypothyroidism (both of which may be subclinical) should lead to investigations, as already described on pages 740 and 743.

Thyroid scintigraphy

Thyroid scintigraphy with ^{99m}technetium should be performed in an individual with a low serum TSH and a nodular thyroid to confirm the presence of an autonomously functioning ('hot') nodule (see Fig. 20.4, p. 742). In such circumstances, further evaluation by fine needle aspiration is not necessary. 'Cold nodules' on scintigraphy have a much higher likelihood of malignancy, but the majority are benign and so scintigraphy is not routinely used in the evaluation of thyroid nodules when TSH is normal.

Thyroid ultrasound

If thyroid function tests are normal, an ultrasound scan will determine the nature of the thyroid swelling. Ultrasound can establish whether there is generalised or localised swelling of the thyroid. Inflammatory disorders causing a diffuse goitre, such as Graves' disease and Hashimoto's thyroiditis, demonstrate a diffuse pattern of hypoechogenicity and, in the case of Graves' disease, increased thyroid blood flow may be seen on colour flow Doppler. The presence of thyroid autoantibodies will support the diagnosis of Graves' disease or Hashimoto's thyroiditis, while their absence in a younger patient with a diffuse goitre and normal thyroid function suggests a diagnosis of 'simple goitre' (p. 752).

Ultrasound can also readily determine the size and number of nodules within the thyroid and can distinguish solid nodules from those with a cystic element. It cannot reliably distinguish benign from malignant nodules but, in experienced hands, there are some ultrasound characteristics which are associated with a higher likelihood of malignancy. These include: hypervascularity of the nodule, the presence of microcalcification and irregular, infiltrative margins. A pure cystic nodule is highly unlikely to be malignant and a 'spongiform' appearance is also highly predicative of a benign aetiology.

Fine needle aspiration

Cytological examination of a thyroid nodule, following fine needle aspiration, is recommended for most thyroid nodules over 1 cm in size. Smaller nodules should be aspirated if there is a high suspicion of malignancy on clinical or ultrasound grounds, while some clinicians will be happy to observe a nodule up to 2 cm in size with a spongiform appearance. Individuals with a multinodular goitre have the same risk of malignancy as those with a solitary nodule. Sometimes, one of the nodules in a multinodular goitre is much larger than any other (a 'dominant' nodule), but ultimately the choice of nodule to biopsy should be based on ultrasound characteristics.

Fine needle aspiration of a thyroid nodule can be performed in the outpatient clinic using a standard 21-gauge needle and a 20 mL syringe, usually making several passes through different parts of the lesion. Ultrasound-guided needle aspiration is necessary for impalpable nodules and to permit targeting of the solid component of a mixed cystic/solid nodule. Aspiration may be therapeutic in the small proportion of patients in whom the swelling is a cyst, although recurrence on more than one occasion is an indication for surgery. Cytological examination can differentiate benign (80%) from definitely malignant or indeterminate nodules (20%), of which 25–50% are confirmed as cancers at surgery. The limitations of fine needle aspiration are that it cannot differentiate between follicular adenoma and carcinoma, and that in 10–20% of cases an inadequate specimen is obtained.

Management

Solitary nodules with a solid component in which cytology either is inconclusive or shows malignant cells are treated by surgical excision. Molecular techniques may, in the future, improve the diagnostic accuracy of thyroid cytology and allow a more conservative strategy for individuals with an indeterminate biopsy (Box 20.13). Nodules in which malignancy is confirmed by formal histology are treated as described on page 754. Those which have benign cytology and a reassuring ultrasound appearance may by observed by interval ultrasound scans. In parts of the world with borderline low iodine intake, there is evidence that levothyroxine therapy, in doses that suppress serum TSH, may reduce the size of some nodules. This should not be routine practice in iodine-sufficient populations.

A diffuse or multinodular goitre may also require surgical treatment for cosmetic reasons or if there is compression of local structures (resulting in stridor or dysphagia). Levothyroxine therapy may shrink the goitre of Hashimoto's disease, particularly if serum TSH is elevated.

EBM 20.13 Molecular techniques in cytologically indeterminate thyroid nodules

'Between 60 and 70% of differentiated thyroid cancers have at least one somatic gene mutation. Using a microarray of messenger RNA transcripts from 167 genes on cytologically indeterminate thyroid nodules, the negative predictive value for lesions with a low likelihood for cancer was 94–95%. Use of this technology could, in theory, avoid unnecessary surgery.'

- Alexander EK, et al. N Engl J Med 2012; 367:705–715.

For further information: www.thyroid.org

20

Autoimmune thyroid disease

Thyroid diseases are amongst the most prevalent antibody-mediated autoimmune diseases and are associated with other organ-specific autoimmunity (Ch. 4 and p. 795). Autoantibodies may produce inflammation and destruction of thyroid tissue, resulting in hypothyroidism, goitre (in Hashimoto's thyroiditis) or sometimes even transient thyrotoxicosis ('Hashitoxicosis'), or they may stimulate the TSH receptor to cause thyrotoxicosis (in Graves' disease). There is overlap between these conditions, since some patients have multiple autoantibodies.

Graves' disease

Graves' disease can occur at any age but is unusual before puberty and most commonly affects women aged 30–50 years. The most common manifestation is thyrotoxicosis with or without a diffuse goitre. The clinical features and differential diagnosis are described on page 740. Graves' disease also causes ophthalmopathy and, rarely, pretibial myxoedema (p. 734). These extrathyroidal features usually occur in thyrotoxic patients, but can occur in the absence of thyroid dysfunction.

Graves' thyrotoxicosis

Pathophysiology

The thyrotoxicosis results from the production of IgG antibodies directed against the TSH receptor on the thyroid follicular cell, which stimulate thyroid hormone production and proliferation of follicular cells, leading to goitre in the majority of patients. These antibodies are termed thyroid-stimulating immunoglobulins or TSH receptor antibodies (TRAb) and can be detected in the serum of 80–95% of patients with Graves' disease. The concentration of TRAb in the serum is presumed to fluctuate to account for the natural history of Graves' thyrotoxicosis (Fig. 20.6). The thyroid failure seen in some patients may result from the presence of blocking antibodies against the TSH receptor, and from tissue destruction by cytotoxic antibodies and cell-mediated immunity.

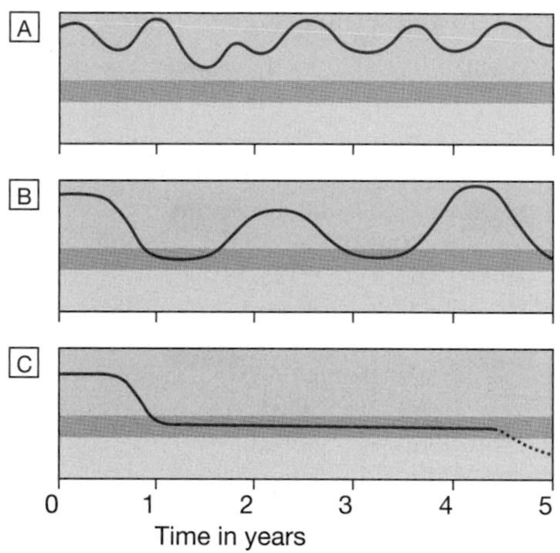

Fig. 20.6 Natural history of the thyrotoxicosis of Graves' disease. **A** and **B** The majority (60%) of patients have either prolonged periods of thyrotoxicosis of fluctuating severity, or periods of alternating relapse and remission. **C** It is the minority who experience a single short-lived episode followed by prolonged remission and, in some cases, by the eventual onset of hypothyroidism.

Graves' disease has a strong genetic component. There is 50% concordance for thyrotoxicosis between monozygotic twins but only 5% concordance between dizygotic twins. Genome-wide association studies have identified polymorphisms at the *MHC, CTLA4, PTPN22, TSHR1* and *FCRL3* loci as predisposing genetic variants. Many of these loci have been implicated in the pathogenesis of other autoimmune diseases.

A suggested trigger for the development of thyrotoxicosis in genetically susceptible individuals may be infection with viruses or bacteria. Certain strains of the gut organisms *Escherichia coli* and *Yersinia enterocolitica* possess cell membrane TSH receptors and it has been suggested that antibodies to these microbial antigens may cross-react with the TSH receptors on the host thyroid follicular cell. In regions of iodine deficiency (p. 752), iodine supplementation can precipitate thyrotoxicosis, but only in those with pre-existing subclinical Graves' disease. Smoking is weakly associated with Graves' thyrotoxicosis but strongly linked with the development of ophthalmopathy.

Management

Symptoms of thyrotoxicosis respond to β-blockade (p. 741) but definitive treatment requires control of thyroid hormone secretion. The different options are compared in Box 20.14. For patients under 40 years of age, most clinicians adopt the empirical approach of prescribing a course of carbimazole and recommending surgery if relapse occurs, while ^{131}I is employed as first- or second-line treatment in those aged over 40. A number of observational studies have linked therapeutic ^{131}I with increased incidence of some malignancies, particularly of the thyroid and gastrointestinal tract, but the results have been inconsistent; the association may be with Graves' disease rather than its therapy, and the magnitude of the effect, if any, is small. Experience from the

20.14 Comparison of treatments for the thyrotoxicosis of Graves' disease

Management	Common indications	Contraindications	Disadvantages/complications
Antithyroid drugs (carbimazole, propylthiouracil)	First episode in patients < 40 yrs	Breastfeeding (propylthiouracil suitable)	Hypersensitivity rash 2% Agranulocytosis 0.2% Hepatotoxicity (with propylthiouracil) – very rare but potentially fatal > 50% relapse rate usually within 2 yrs of stopping drug
Subtotal thyroidectomy[1]	Large goitre Poor drug compliance, especially in young patients Recurrent thyrotoxicosis after course of antithyroid drugs in young patients	Previous thyroid surgery Dependence on voice, e.g. opera singer, lecturer[2]	Hypothyroidism (~25%) Transient hypocalcaemia (10%) Permanent hypoparathyroidism (1%) Recurrent laryngeal nerve palsy[2] (1%)
Radio-iodine	Patients > 40 yrs[3] Recurrence following surgery irrespective of age Other serious comorbidity	Pregnancy or planned pregnancy within 6 mths of treatment Active Graves' ophthalmopathy[4]	Hypothyroidism, ~40% in first year, 80% after 15 yrs Most likely treatment to result in exacerbation of ophthalmopathy[4]

[1]A near-total thyroidectomy is now the favoured operation for Graves' thyrotoxicosis in many institutions and is associated with a higher risk of some complications, including hypothyroidism (nearly 100%), but a reduced risk of persistent or recurrent thyrotoxicosis.
[2]It is not only vocal cord palsy due to recurrent laryngeal nerve damage which alters the voice following thyroid surgery; the superior laryngeal nerves are frequently transected and this results in minor changes in voice quality.
[3]In many institutions, ^{131}I is used more liberally and is prescribed for much younger patients.
[4]The extent to which radio-iodine exacerbates ophthalmopathy is controversial and practice varies; some use prednisolone to reduce this risk.

Chernobyl disaster suggests that younger people are more sensitive to radiation-induced thyroid cancer. In many centres, however, ^{131}I is used extensively, even in young patients.

Antithyroid drugs. The most commonly used are carbimazole and its active metabolite, methimazole (not available in the UK). Propylthiouracil is equally effective. These drugs reduce the synthesis of new thyroid hormones by inhibiting the iodination of tyrosine (see Fig. 20.3, p. 739). Carbimazole also has an immunosuppressive action, leading to a reduction in serum TRAb concentrations, but this is not enough to influence the natural history of the thyrotoxicosis significantly.

Antithyroid drugs should be introduced at high doses (carbimazole 40–60 mg daily or propylthiouracil 400–600 mg daily). Usually, this results in subjective improvement within 10–14 days and renders the patient clinically and biochemically euthyroid at 3–4 weeks. At this point, the dose can be reduced and titrated to maintain T_4 and TSH within their reference range. In most patients, carbimazole is continued at 5–20 mg per day for 12–18 months in the hope that remission will occur. Patients with thyrotoxicosis relapse in at least 50% of cases, usually within 2 years of stopping treatment. Rarely, T_4 and TSH levels fluctuate between those of thyrotoxicosis and hypothyroidism at successive review appointments, despite good drug compliance, presumably due to rapidly changing concentrations of TRAb. In these patients, satisfactory control can be achieved by blocking thyroid hormone synthesis with carbimazole 30–40 mg daily and adding levothyroxine 100–150 μg daily as replacement therapy (a 'block and replace' regime).

Antithyroid drugs can have adverse effects. The most common is a rash. Agranulocytosis is a rare but potentially serious complication that cannot be predicted by routine measurement of white blood cell count, but which is reversible on stopping treatment. Patients should be warned to stop the drug and seek medical advice immediately, should a severe sore throat or fever develop whilst on treatment. Propylthiouracil is associated with a small but definite risk of hepatotoxicity, which, in some instances, has resulted in liver failure requiring liver transplantation, and even in death. It should, therefore, be considered second-line therapy to carbimazole and only be used during pregnancy or breastfeeding (see below), or if an adverse reaction to carbimazole has occurred.

Thyroid surgery. Patients should be rendered euthyroid with antithyroid drugs before operation. Potassium iodide, 60 mg 3 times daily orally, is often added for 2 weeks before surgery to inhibit thyroid hormone release and reduce the size and vascularity of the gland, making surgery technically easier. Traditionally, a 'subtotal' thyroidectomy is performed, in which a portion of one lobe of the thyroid is left in situ, with the aim of rendering the patient euthyroid post-operatively. While complications of surgery are rare and 80% of patients are euthyroid, 15% are permanently hypothyroid and 5% remain thyrotoxic. As a consequence, many endocrine surgeons now opt to perform a 'near-total' thyroidectomy, leaving behind only a small portion of gland adjacent to the recurrent laryngeal nerves. This strategy invariably results in permanent hypothyroidism and is probably associated with a higher risk of hypoparathyroidism, but maximises the potential for cure of thyrotoxicosis.

Radioactive iodine. ^{131}I is administered orally as a single dose, and is trapped and organified in the thyroid (see Fig. 20.3, p. 739). Although ^{131}I decays within a few weeks, it has long-lasting inhibitory effects on survival and replication of follicular cells. The variable radio-iodine uptake and radiosensitivity of the gland means that the choice of dose is empirical; in most centres, approximately 400 MBq (10 mCi) is given orally. This regimen is effective in 75% of patients within 4–12 weeks. During the lag period, symptoms can be controlled by a β-blocker or, in more severe cases, by carbimazole. However, carbimazole reduces the efficacy of ^{131}I therapy because it prevents organification of ^{131}I in the gland, and so should be avoided until 48 hours after radio-iodine administration. If thyrotoxicosis persists after 6 months, a further dose of ^{131}I can be given. The disadvantage of ^{131}I treatment is that the majority of patients eventually develop hypothyroidism. ^{131}I is usually avoided in patients with Graves' ophthalmopathy and evidence of significant active orbital inflammation. It can be administered with caution in those with mild or 'burnt-out' eye disease, when it is customary to cover the treatment with a 6-week tapering course of oral prednisolone. In women of reproductive age, pregnancy must be excluded before administration of ^{131}I and avoided for 6 months thereafter; men are also advised against fathering children for 6 months after receiving ^{131}I.

Thyrotoxicosis in pregnancy

The coexistence of pregnancy and thyrotoxicosis is unusual, as anovulatory cycles are common in thyrotoxic patients and autoimmune disease tends to remit during pregnancy, when the maternal immune response is suppressed. Thyroid function tests must be interpreted in the knowledge that thyroid-binding globulin, and hence total T_4 and T_3 levels, are increased in pregnancy and that TSH reference ranges may be lower (see Box 20.20, p. 756); a fully suppressed TSH with elevated free thyroid hormone levels indicates thyrotoxicosis. The thyrotoxicosis is almost always caused by Graves' disease. Both mother and fetus must be considered, since maternal thyroid hormones, TRAb and antithyroid drugs can all cross the placenta to some degree, exposing the fetus to the risks of thyrotoxicosis, iatrogenic hypothyroidism and goitre. Poorly controlled maternal thyrotoxicosis can result in fetal tachycardia, intra-uterine growth retardation, prematurity, stillbirth and possibly even congenital malformations.

Antithyroid drugs are the treatment of choice for thyrotoxicosis in pregnancy. Carbimazole has been associated with rare cases of embryopathy, particularly a skin defect known as aplasia cutis, and should be avoided in the first trimester. Propylthiouracil should be used in its place but, because of its potential hepatotoxicity, should be replaced with carbimazole from the beginning of the second trimester. Both drugs cross the placenta and will effectively treat thyrotoxicosis in the fetus caused by transplacental passage of TRAb. To avoid fetal hypothyroidism (which could affect brain development) and a resultant goitre, it is important to use the smallest dose of antithyroid drug (optimally, less than 150 mg propylthiouracil or 15 mg carbimazole per day) that will maintain maternal (and presumably fetal) free T_4, T_3 and TSH within their respective reference ranges. Frequent review of mother and fetus (monitoring heart rate and growth) is important. TRAb levels can be measured in the third trimester to predict the likelihood of neonatal thyrotoxicosis. When TRAb levels are not elevated, the antithyroid drug can be discontinued 4 weeks before the expected date of delivery to minimise the risk of fetal hypothyroidism at the time of maximum brain development. After delivery, if antithyroid drug is required and the patient wishes to breastfeed, then propylthiouracil is the drug of choice, as it is excreted in the milk to a much lesser extent than carbimazole. Thyroid function should be monitored periodically in the breastfed child.

If thyroid surgery is necessary because of poor drug compliance or drug hypersensitivity, it is most safely performed in the second trimester. Radioactive iodine is absolutely contraindicated, as it invariably induces fetal hypothyroidism.

Thyrotoxicosis in adolescence

Thyrotoxicosis can occasionally occur in adolescence and is almost always due to Graves' disease. The presentation may be atypical and management challenging, as summarised in Box 20.15.

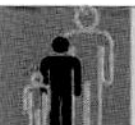

20.15 Thyrotoxicosis in adolescence

- **Presentation**: may present with a deterioration in school performance or symptoms suggestive of attention deficit hyperactivity disorder.
- **Anti-thyroid drug therapy**: prolonged courses may be required because remission rates following an 18-month course of therapy are much lower than in adults.
- **Compliance**: compliance with anti-thyroid drug therapy is often suboptimal, resulting in poor disease control which may adversely affect performance at school.
- **Radio-iodine therapy**: usually avoided in adolescents because of concerns about risk of future malignancy.

Graves' ophthalmopathy

This condition is immunologically mediated but the autoantigen has not been identified. Within the orbit (and the dermis) there is cytokine-mediated proliferation of fibroblasts which secrete hydrophilic glycosaminoglycans. The resulting increase in interstitial fluid content, combined with a chronic inflammatory cell infiltrate, causes marked swelling and ultimately fibrosis of the extraocular muscles (Fig. 20.7) and a rise in retrobulbar pressure. The eye is displaced forwards (proptosis, exophthalmos; p. 735) and in severe cases there is optic nerve compression.

Ophthalmopathy, like thyrotoxicosis (see Fig. 20.6), typically follows an episodic course and it is helpful to distinguish patients with active inflammation (periorbital oedema and conjunctival inflammation with changing orbital signs) from those in whom the inflammation has 'burnt out'. Eye disease is detectable in up to 50% of thyrotoxic patients at presentation, but active ocular inflammation may occur before or after thyrotoxic episodes (exophthalmic Graves' disease). It is more common in cigarette smokers and is exacerbated by poor

A

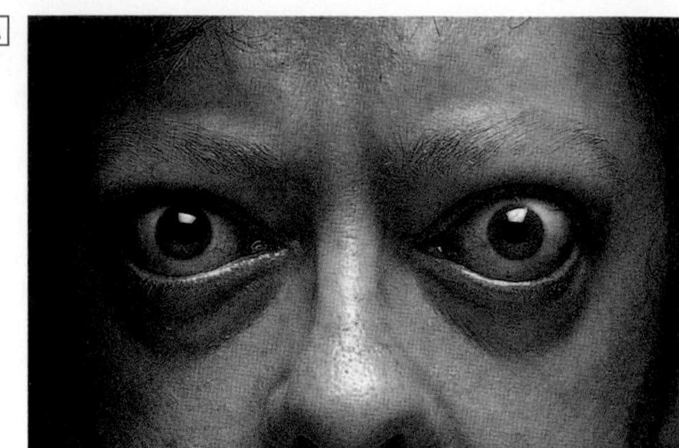

B

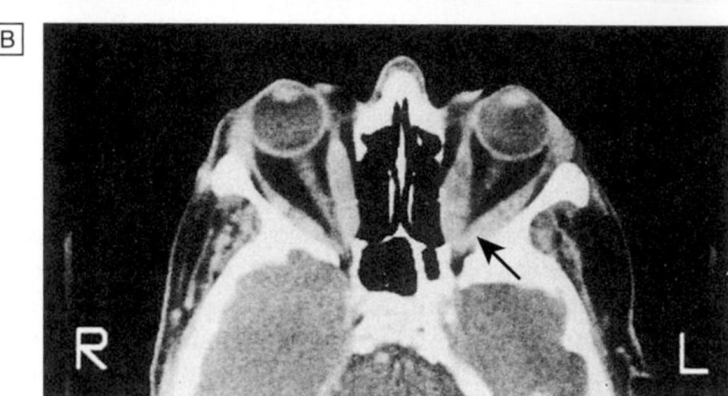

Fig. 20.7 Graves' disease. **A** Bilateral ophthalmopathy in a 42-year-old man. The main symptoms were diplopia in all directions of gaze and reduced visual acuity in the left eye. The periorbital swelling is due to retrobulbar fat prolapsing into the eyelids, and increased interstitial fluid as a result of raised intraorbital pressure. **B** Transverse CT of the orbits, showing the enlarged extraocular muscles. This is most obvious at the apex of the left orbit (arrow), where compression of the optic nerve caused reduced visual acuity.

control of thyroid function, especially hypothyroidism. The most frequent presenting symptoms are related to increased exposure of the cornea, resulting from proptosis and lid retraction. There may be excessive lacrimation made worse by wind and bright light, a 'gritty' sensation in the eye, and pain due to conjunctivitis or corneal ulceration. In addition, there may be reduction of visual acuity and/or visual fields as a consequence of corneal oedema or optic nerve compression. Other signs of optic nerve compression include reduced colour vision and a relative afferent pupillary defect (pp. 735 and 1169). If the extraocular muscles are involved and do not act in concert, diplopia results.

The majority of patients require no treatment other than reassurance. Smoking cessation should be actively encouraged. Methylcellulose eye drops and gel counter the gritty discomfort of dry eyes, and tinted glasses or side shields attached to spectacle frames reduce the excessive lacrimation triggered by sun or wind. In patients with mild Graves' ophthalmopathy, oral selenium (100 μg twice daily for 6 months) improves quality of life, reduces ocular involvement and slows progression of disease; the mechanism of action is not known but may relate to an antioxidant effect (Box 20.16). More severe inflammatory episodes are treated with glucocorticoids (e.g. daily oral prednisolone or pulsed IV methylprednisolone) and sometimes orbital radiotherapy. There is also an increasing trend to use immunosuppressant therapies, such as ciclosporin, in combination with glucocorticoids. Loss of visual acuity

EBM 20.16 Effects of selenium supplementation in mild Graves' ophthalmopathy

'Selenium therapy for 6 months was associated with improvement of both the appearance score and the visual-functioning score. The benefits persisted 6 months following cessation of therapy.'

- Marcocci C, et al. N Engl J Med 2012; 364:1920–1931.

For further information: www.thyroid.org

is an indication for urgent surgical decompression of the orbit. In 'burnt-out' disease, surgery to the eyelids and/or ocular muscles may improve conjunctival exposure, cosmetic appearance and diplopia.

Pretibial myxoedema

This infiltrative dermopathy occurs in fewer than 10% of patients with Graves' disease and has similar pathological features as occur in the orbit. It takes the form of raised pink-coloured or purplish plaques on the anterior aspect of the leg, extending on to the dorsum of the foot (p. 734). The lesions may be itchy and the skin may have a 'peau d'orange' appearance with growth of coarse hair; less commonly, the face and arms are affected. Treatment is rarely required, but in severe cases topical glucocorticoids may be helpful.

Hashimoto's thyroiditis

Hashimoto's thyroiditis is characterised by destructive lymphoid infiltration of the thyroid, ultimately leading to a varying degree of fibrosis and thyroid enlargement. There is an increased risk of thyroid lymphoma (p. 755), although this is exceedingly rare. The nomenclature of autoimmune hypothyroidism is confusing. Some authorities reserve the term 'Hashimoto's thyroiditis' for patients with positive antithyroid peroxidase autoantibodies and a firm goitre who may or may not be hypothyroid, and use the term 'spontaneous atrophic hypothyroidism' for hypothyroid patients without a goitre in whom TSH receptor-blocking antibodies may be more important than antiperoxidase antibodies. However, these syndromes can both be considered as variants of the same underlying disease process.

Hashimoto's thyroiditis increases in incidence with age and affects approximately 3.5 per 1000 women and 0.8 per 1000 men each year. Many present with a small or moderately sized diffuse goitre, which is characteristically firm or rubbery in consistency. The goitre may be soft, however, and impossible to differentiate from simple goitre (p. 752) by palpation alone. Around 25% of patients are hypothyroid at presentation. In the remainder, serum T_4 is normal and TSH normal or raised, but these patients are at risk of developing overt hypothyroidism in future years. Antithyroid peroxidase antibodies are present in the serum in more than 90% of patients with Hashimoto's thyroiditis. In those under the age of 20 years, antinuclear factor (ANF) may also be positive.

Levothyroxine therapy is indicated as treatment for hypothyroidism (p. 743), and also to shrink an associated goitre. In this context, the dose of thyroxine should be sufficient to suppress serum TSH to low but detectable levels.

Transient thyroiditis

Subacute (de Quervain's) thyroiditis

In its classical painful form, subacute thyroiditis is a transient inflammation of the thyroid gland occurring after infection with Coxsackie, mumps or adenoviruses. There is pain in the region of the thyroid that may radiate to the angle of the jaw and the ears, and is made worse by swallowing, coughing and movement of the neck. The thyroid is usually palpably enlarged and tender. Systemic upset is common. Affected patients are usually females aged 20–40 years. Painless transient thyroiditis can also occur after viral infection and in patients with underlying autoimmune disease. The condition can also be precipitated by drugs, including interferon-α and lithium.

Irrespective of the clinical presentation, inflammation in the thyroid gland occurs and is associated with release of colloid and stored thyroid hormones, but also with damage to follicular cells and impaired synthesis of new thyroid hormones. As a result, T_4 and T_3 levels are raised for 4–6 weeks until the pre-formed colloid is depleted. Thereafter, there is usually a period of hypothyroidism of variable severity before the follicular cells recover and normal thyroid function is restored within 4–6 months (Fig. 20.8). In the thyrotoxic phase, the iodine uptake is low, because the damaged follicular cells are unable to trap iodine and because TSH secretion is suppressed. Low-titre thyroid autoantibodies appear transiently in the serum, and the erythrocyte sedimentation rate (ESR) is usually raised. High-titre autoantibodies suggest an underlying autoimmune pathology and greater risk of recurrence and ultimate progression to hypothyroidism.

The pain and systemic upset usually respond to simple measures such as non-steroidal anti-inflammatory drugs (NSAIDs). Occasionally, however, it may be necessary to prescribe prednisolone 40 mg daily for 3–4 weeks. The thyrotoxicosis is mild and treatment with a β-blocker is usually adequate. Antithyroid drugs are of no benefit because thyroid hormone synthesis is impaired rather than enhanced. Careful monitoring of thyroid function and symptoms is required so that

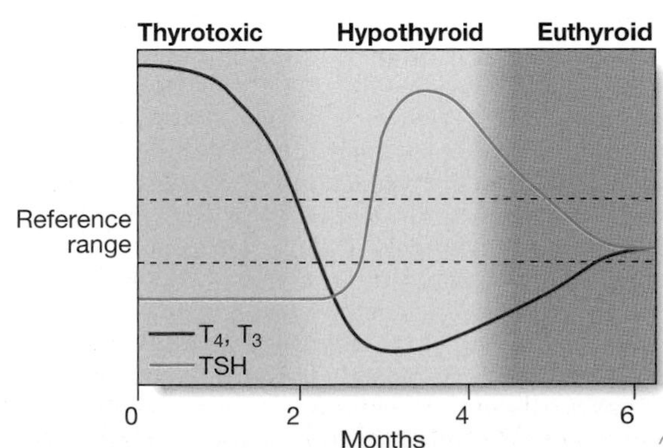

Fig. 20.8 Thyroid function tests in an episode of transient thyroiditis. This pattern might be observed in classical subacute (de Quervain's) thyroiditis, painless thyroiditis or post-partum thyroiditis. The duration of each phase varies between patients.

20

levothyroxine can be prescribed temporarily in the hypothyroid phase. Care must be taken to identify patients presenting with hypothyroidism who are in the later stages of a transient thyroiditis, since they are unlikely to require life-long levothyroxine therapy (see Fig. 20.5, p. 744).

Post-partum thyroiditis

The maternal immune response, which is modified during pregnancy to allow survival of the fetus, is enhanced after delivery and may unmask previously unrecognised subclinical autoimmune thyroid disease. Surveys have shown that transient biochemical disturbances of thyroid function occur in 5–10% of women within 6 months of delivery (see Box 20.20, p. 756). Those affected are likely to have anti-thyroid peroxidase antibodies in the serum in early pregnancy. Symptoms of thyroid dysfunction are rare and there is no association between postnatal depression and abnormal thyroid function tests. However, symptomatic thyrotoxicosis presenting for the first time within 12 months of childbirth is likely to be due to post-partum thyroiditis and the diagnosis is confirmed by a negligible radio-isotope uptake. The clinical course and treatment are similar to those of painless subacute thyroiditis (see above). Post-partum thyroiditis tends to recur after subsequent pregnancies, and eventually patients progress over a period of years to permanent hypothyroidism.

Iodine-associated thyroid disease

Iodine deficiency

Thyroid enlargement is extremely common in certain mountainous parts of the world, such as the Andes, the Himalayas and central Africa, where there is dietary iodine deficiency (endemic goitre). Most patients are euthyroid with normal or raised TSH levels, although hypothyroidism can occur with severe iodine deficiency. Iodine supplementation programmes have abolished this condition in most developed countries.

Iodine-induced thyroid dysfunction

Iodine has complex effects on thyroid function. Very high concentrations of iodine inhibit thyroid hormone release and this forms the rationale for iodine treatment of thyroid storm (p. 742) and prior to thyroid surgery for thyrotoxicosis (p. 748). Iodine administration initially enhances, but then inhibits, iodination of tyrosine and thyroid hormone synthesis (see Fig. 20.3, p. 739). The resulting effect of iodine on thyroid function varies according to whether the patient has an iodine-deficient diet or underlying thyroid disease. In iodine-deficient parts of the world, transient thyrotoxicosis may be precipitated by prophylactic iodinisation programmes. In iodine-sufficient areas, thyrotoxicosis can be precipitated by radiographic contrast medium or expectorants in individuals who have underlying thyroid disease predisposing to thyrotoxicosis, such as multinodular goitre or Graves' disease in remission. Induction of thyrotoxicosis by iodine is called the Jod–Basedow effect. Chronic excess iodine administration can, however, result in hypothyroidism. Increased iodine within the thyroid gland down-regulates iodine trapping, so that uptake is low in all circumstances.

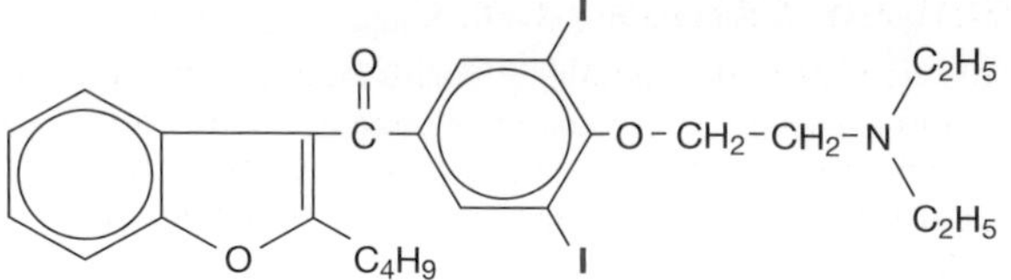

Fig. 20.9 The structure of amiodarone. Note the similarities to T_4 (see Fig. 20.3, p. 739).

Amiodarone

The anti-arrhythmic agent amiodarone has a structure that is analogous to that of T_4 (Fig. 20.9) and contains huge amounts of iodine; a 200 mg dose contains 75 mg iodine, compared with a daily dietary requirement of just 125 μg. Amiodarone also has a cytotoxic effect on thyroid follicular cells and inhibits conversion of T_4 to T_3. Most patients receiving amiodarone have normal thyroid function, but up to 20% develop hypothyroidism or thyrotoxicosis and so thyroid function should be monitored regularly. The ratio of T_4:T_3 is elevated and TSH provides the best indicator of thyroid function.

The thyrotoxicosis can be classified as either:

- type I: iodine-induced excess thyroid hormone synthesis in patients with an underlying thyroid disorder, such as nodular goitre or latent Graves' disease
- type II: thyroiditis due to a direct cytotoxic effect if amiodarone administration results in a transient thyrotoxicosis.

These patterns can overlap and can be difficult to distinguish clinically, as iodine uptake is low in both. There is no widely accepted management algorithm, although the iodine excess renders the gland resistant to radio-iodine. Antithyroid drugs may be effective in patients with the type I form, but are ineffective in type II thyrotoxicosis. Prednisolone is beneficial in the type II form. A pragmatic approach is to commence combination therapy with an antithyroid drug and glucocorticoid in patients with significant thyrotoxicosis. A rapid response (within 1–2 weeks) usually indicates a type II picture and permits withdrawal of the antithyroid therapy; a slower response suggests a type I picture, when antithyroid drugs may be continued and prednisolone withdrawn. Potassium perchlorate can also be used to inhibit iodine trapping in the thyroid. If the cardiac state allows, amiodarone should be discontinued, but it has a long half-life (50–60 days) and so its effects are long-lasting. To minimise the risk of type I thyrotoxicosis, thyroid function should be measured in all patients prior to commencement of amiodarone therapy, and amiodarone should be avoided if TSH is suppressed.

Hypothyroidism should be treated with levothyroxine, which can be given while amiodarone is continued.

Simple and multinodular goitre

These terms describe diffuse or multinodular enlargement of the thyroid, which occurs sporadically and is of unknown aetiology.

Simple diffuse goitre

This form of goitre usually presents between the ages of 15 and 25 years, often during pregnancy, and tends to be noticed by friends and relatives rather than the patient. Occasionally, there is a tight sensation in the neck, particularly when swallowing. The goitre is soft and symmetrical, and the thyroid enlarged to two or three times normal. There is no tenderness, lymphadenopathy or overlying bruit. Concentrations of T_3, T_4 and TSH are normal and no thyroid autoantibodies are detected in the serum. No treatment is necessary and the goitre usually regresses. In some, however, the unknown stimulus to thyroid enlargement persists and, as a result of recurrent episodes of hyperplasia and involution during the following 10–20 years, the gland becomes multinodular with areas of autonomous function.

Multinodular goitre

The natural history is shown in Figure 20.10. Patients with thyroid enlargement in the absence of thyroid dysfunction or positive autoantibodies (i.e. with 'simple goitre', see above) as young adults may progress to develop nodules. These nodules grow at varying rates and secrete thyroid hormone 'autonomously', thereby suppressing TSH-dependent growth and function in the rest of the gland. Ultimately, complete suppression of TSH occurs in about 25% of cases, with T_4 and T_3 levels often within the reference range (subclinical thyrotoxicosis, p. 745) but sometimes elevated (toxic multinodular goitre; see Fig. 20.4, p. 742).

Age (in years)	15–25	35–55	> 55
Goitre	Diffuse	Nodular	Nodular
Tracheal compression/ deviation	No	Minimal	Yes
T_3, T_4	Normal	Normal	Raised
TSH	Normal	Normal or undetectable	Undetectable

Fig. 20.10 Natural history of simple goitre.

Clinical features and investigations

Multinodular goitre is usually diagnosed in patients presenting with thyrotoxicosis, a large goitre with or without tracheal compression, or sudden painful swelling caused by haemorrhage into a nodule or cyst. The goitre is nodular or lobulated on palpation and may extend retrosternally; however, not all multinodular goitres causing thyrotoxicosis are easily palpable. Very large goitres may cause mediastinal compression with stridor (Fig. 20.11), dysphagia and obstruction of the superior vena cava. Hoarseness due to recurrent laryngeal nerve palsy can occur, but is far more suggestive of thyroid carcinoma.

The diagnosis can be confirmed by ultrasonography and/or thyroid scintigraphy (see Fig. 20.4, p. 742). In patients with large goitres, a flow-volume loop is a good screening test for significant tracheal compression (see Fig. 20.11). If intervention is contemplated, a CT or MRI of the thoracic inlet should be performed to quantify the degree of tracheal displacement or compression and the extent of retrosternal extension. Nodules should be evaluated for the possibility of thyroid neoplasia, as described on page 754.

Management

If the goitre is small, no treatment is necessary but annual thyroid function testing should be arranged, as the natural history is progression to a toxic multinodular goitre. Thyroid surgery is indicated for large goitres which cause mediastinal compression or which are cosmetically unattractive. ^{131}I can result in a significant reduction in thyroid size and may be of value in

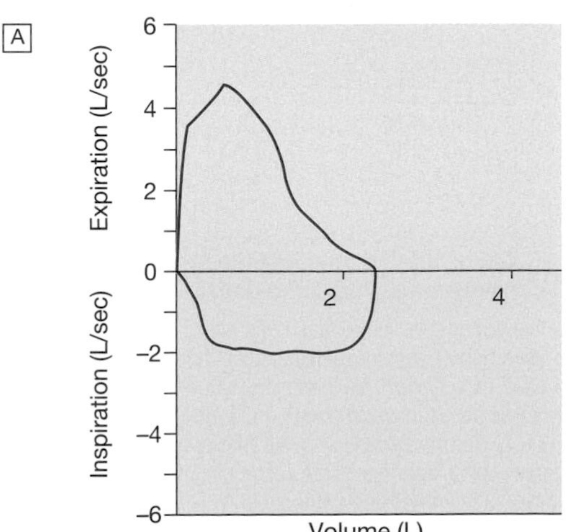

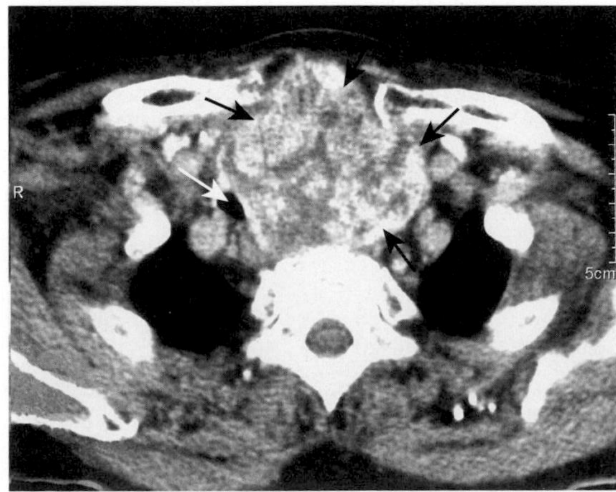

Fig. 20.11 Multinodular goitre with tracheal compression. **A** A flow-volume loop (p. 653) showing a square-shaped inspiratory curve indicating extrathoracic airflow obstruction. **B** A CT scan of the neck showing a large retrosternal goitre (black arrows) with marked deviation and compression of the trachea (white arrow).

elderly patients. Levothyroxine therapy is of no benefit in shrinking multinodular goitres in iodine-sufficient countries and may simply aggravate any associated thyrotoxicosis.

In toxic multinodular goitre, treatment is usually with ^{131}I. The iodine uptake is lower than in Graves' disease, so a higher dose may be administered (up to 800 Mbq (approximately 20 mCi)) and hypothyroidism is less common. In thyrotoxic patients with a large goitre, thyroid surgery may be indicated. Long-term treatment with antithyroid drugs is not usually employed, as relapse is invariable after drug withdrawal.

Asymptomatic patients with subclinical thyrotoxicosis (p. 745) are increasingly being treated with ^{131}I on the grounds that a suppressed TSH is a risk factor for atrial fibrillation and, particularly in post-menopausal women, osteoporosis.

Thyroid neoplasia

Patients with thyroid tumours usually present with a solitary nodule (p. 746). Most are benign and a few of these, called 'toxic adenomas', secrete excess thyroid hormones. Primary thyroid malignancy is rare, accounting for less than 1% of all carcinomas, and has an incidence of 25 per million per annum. As shown in Box 20.17, it can be classified according to the cell type of origin. With the exception of medullary carcinoma, thyroid cancer is more common in females.

Toxic adenoma

A solitary toxic nodule is the cause of less than 5% of all cases of thyrotoxicosis. The nodule is a follicular adenoma, which autonomously secretes excess thyroid hormones and inhibits endogenous TSH secretion, with subsequent atrophy of the rest of the thyroid gland. The adenoma is usually greater than 3 cm in diameter.

Most patients are female and over 40 years of age. Although many nodules are palpable, the diagnosis can be made with certainty only by thyroid scintigraphy (see Fig. 20.4, p. 742). The thyrotoxicosis is usually mild and in almost 50% of patients the plasma T_3 alone is elevated (T_3 thyrotoxicosis). ^{131}I (400–800 MBq (10–20 mCi)) is highly effective and is an ideal treatment since the atrophic cells surrounding the nodule do not take up iodine and so receive little or no radiation. For this reason, permanent hypothyroidism is unusual. A surgical hemithyroidectomy is an alternative.

20.17 Malignant thyroid tumours

Type of tumour	Frequency (%)	Age at presentation (years)	10-year survival (%)
Follicular cells			
Differentiated carcinoma			
Papillary	75–85	20–40	98
Follicular	10–20	40–60	94
Anaplastic	< 5	> 60	9
Parafollicular C cells			
Medullary carcinoma	5–8	> 40*	78
Lymphocytes			
Lymphoma	< 5	> 60	45

*Patients with medullary carcinoma as part of MEN type 2 (p. 795) may present in childhood.

Differentiated carcinoma

Papillary carcinoma

This is the most common of the malignant thyroid tumours and accounts for 90% of irradiation-induced thyroid cancer. It may be multifocal and spread is initially to regional lymph nodes. Some patients present with cervical lymphadenopathy and no apparent thyroid enlargement; in such instances, the primary lesion may be less than 10 mm in diameter.

Follicular carcinoma

This is always a single encapsulated lesion. Spread to cervical lymph nodes is rare. Metastases are blood-borne and are most often found in bone, lungs and brain.

Management

This is usually by total thyroidectomy followed by a large dose of ^{131}I (3700 MBq (approximately 100 mCi)) in order to ablate any remaining thyroid tissue, normal or malignant. Recent data indicate that a ^{131}I dose of 1100 MBq (approximately 30 mCi) may be equally as effective at thyroid ablation (Box 20.18). Thereafter, long-term treatment with levothyroxine in a dose sufficient to suppress TSH (usually 150–200 μg daily) is important, as there is evidence that growth of differentiated thyroid carcinomas is TSH-dependent. Follow-up is by measurement of serum thyroglobulin, which should be undetectable in patients whose normal thyroid has been ablated and who are taking a suppressive dose of levothyroxine. Detectable thyroglobulin is suggestive of tumour recurrence or metastases, which may be localised by ultrasound, CT, MRI or whole-body scanning with ^{131}I, and may respond to further radio-iodine therapy. Radio-iodine treatment in thyroid cancer and isotope scanning both require serum TSH concentrations to be elevated (> 20 mU/L). This may be achieved by stopping levothyroxine for 4–6 weeks, inducing symptomatic hypothyroidism, or by administering intramuscular injections of recombinant human TSH. Patients usually find the latter approach preferable but it is more expensive. Clinical

EBM 20.18 Ablative radio-iodine following thyroidectomy for differentiated thyroid cancer

'Ablative radioactive iodine has been associated with an increased risk of second malignancies. Two randomised controlled clinical trials have shown that 1100 MBq radio-iodine (30 mCi) is as effective at ablating thyroid tissue as 3700 MBq (100 mCi). Both trials also showed that preparation of patients for radio-iodine treatment with recombinant TSH was as effective as levothyroxine withdrawal.'

- Schlumberger M, et al. N Engl J Med 2012; 366:1663–1673.
- Mallick U, et al. N Engl J Med 2012; 366:1674–1685.

For further information: www.thyroid.org

trials are currently ongoing with novel anti-cancer agents, such as tyrosine kinase inhibitors, in patients with advanced papillary and follicular carcinoma that is refractive to radio-iodine.

Prognosis

Most patients with papillary and thyroid cancer will be cured with appropriate treatment. Adverse prognostic factors include older age at presentation, the presence of distant metastases, male sex and the identification of certain histological subtypes. However, radio-iodine therapy can be effective in treating even those with distant metastases, particularly small-volume disease in the lungs, and so prolonged survival is quite common.

Anaplastic carcinoma and lymphoma

These two conditions are difficult to distinguish clinically but are distinct cytologically and histologically. Patients are usually over 60 years of age and present with rapid thyroid enlargement over 2–3 months. The goitre is hard and there may be stridor due to tracheal compression and hoarseness due to recurrent laryngeal nerve palsy. There is no effective treatment for anaplastic carcinoma, although surgery and radiotherapy may be considered in some circumstances. In older patients, median survival is only 7 months.

The prognosis for lymphoma, which may arise from pre-existing Hashimoto's thyroiditis, is better (p. 1041), with a median survival of 9 years. Some 98% are non-Hodgkin's lymphomas, usually the diffuse large B-cell subtype. Treatment is with combination chemotherapy, such as the CHOP regime (p. 1045), and external beam radiotherapy.

Medullary carcinoma

This tumour arises from the parafollicular C cells of the thyroid. In addition to calcitonin, the tumour may secrete 5-hydroxytryptamine (5-HT, serotonin), various peptides of the tachykinin family, adrenocorticotrophic hormone (ACTH) and prostaglandins. As a consequence, carcinoid syndrome (p. 784) and Cushing's syndrome (p. 773) may occur.

Patients usually present in middle age with a firm thyroid mass. Cervical lymph node involvement is common but distant metastases are rare initially. Serum calcitonin levels are raised and are useful in monitoring response to treatment. Despite the very high levels of calcitonin found in some patients, hypocalcaemia is extremely rare; however, hypercalcitoninaemia can be associated with severe, watery diarrhoea.

Treatment is by total thyroidectomy with removal of regional cervical lymph nodes. Since the C cells do not concentrate iodine and are not responsive to TSH, there is no role for ^{131}I therapy or TSH suppression with levothyroxine. External beam radiotherapy may be considered in some patients at high risk of local recurrence. Vandetanib, a tyrosine kinase inhibitor, is licensed for patients with advanced medullary cancer. The prognosis is less good than for papillary and follicular carcinoma, but individuals can live for many decades with persistent disease which behaves in an indolent fashion.

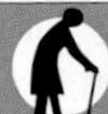

20.19 The thyroid gland in old age

Thyrotoxicosis

- **Causes**: commonly due to multinodular goitre.
- **Clinical features**: apathy, anorexia, proximal myopathy, atrial fibrillation and cardiac failure predominate.
- **Non-thyroidal illness**: thyroid function tests are performed more frequently in the elderly, but interpretation may be altered by intercurrent illness.

Hypothyroidism

- **Clinical features**: non-specific features, such as physical and mental slowing, are often attributed to increasing age and the diagnosis is delayed.
- **Myxoedema coma** (p. 745): more likely in the elderly.
- **Levothyroxine dose**: to avoid exacerbating latent or established heart disease, the starting dose should be 25 µg daily. Levothyroxine requirements fall with increasing age and few patients need more than 100 µg daily.
- **Other medication** (see Box 20.11, p. 745): may interfere with absorption or metabolism of levothyroxine, necessitating an increase in dose.

Medullary carcinoma of the thyroid may occur sporadically, or in families as part of the MEN type 2 syndrome (p. 795).

Riedel's thyroiditis

This is not a form of thyroid cancer, but the presentation is similar and the differentiation can usually only be made by thyroid biopsy. It is an exceptionally rare condition of unknown aetiology, in which there is extensive infiltration of the thyroid and surrounding structures with fibrous tissue. There may be associated mediastinal and retroperitoneal fibrosis. Presentation is with a slow-growing goitre which is irregular and stony-hard. There is usually tracheal and oesophageal compression necessitating partial thyroidectomy. Other recognised complications include recurrent laryngeal nerve palsy, hypoparathyroidism and eventually hypothyroidism.

Congenital thyroid disease

Early treatment with levothyroxine is essential to prevent irreversible brain damage in children (cretinism) with congenital hypothyroidism. Routine screening of TSH levels in heelprick blood samples obtained 5–7 days after birth (as part of the Guthrie test) has revealed an incidence of approximately 1 in 3000, resulting from thyroid agenesis, ectopic or hypoplastic glands, or dyshormonogenesis. Congenital hypothyroidism is thus six times more common than phenylketonuria. It is now possible to start thyroid replacement therapy within 2 weeks of birth. Developmental assessment of infants treated at this early stage has revealed no differences between cases and controls in most children.

Dyshormonogenesis

Several autosomal recessive defects in thyroid hormone synthesis have been described; the most common results from deficiency of the intrathyroidal peroxidase enzyme. Homozygous individuals present with congenital hypothyroidism; heterozygotes present in the first two decades of life with goitre, normal thyroid hormone levels and a raised TSH. The combination of dyshormonogenetic goitre and nerve deafness is known as Pendred's syndrome and is due to mutations in pendrin, the protein which transports iodide to the luminal surface of the follicular cell (see Fig. 20.3, p. 739).

Thyroid hormone resistance

This is a rare disorder in which the pituitary and hypothalamus are resistant to feedback suppression of TSH by T_3, sometimes due to mutations in the thyroid hormone receptor β or because of defects in monodeiodinase activity. The result is high levels of TSH, T_4 and T_3, often with a moderate goitre which may not be noted until adulthood. Thyroid hormone signalling is highly complex and involves different isozymes of both monodeiodinases and thyroid hormone receptors in different tissues. For that reason, other tissues may or may not share the resistance to thyroid hormone and there may be features of thyrotoxicosis (e.g. tachycardia). This condition can be difficult to distinguish from an equally rare TSH-producing pituitary tumour (see Box 20.5, p. 739); administration of TRH results in elevation of TSH in thyroid hormone resistance and not in TSHoma, but an MRI scan of the pituitary may be necessary to exclude a macroadenoma.

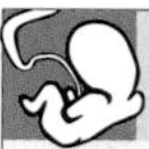

20.20 Thyroid disease in pregnancy

Normal pregnancy

- **Trimester-specific reference ranges**: should be used to interpret thyroid function test results in pregnancy. In the first trimester, TSH is lower and free T_4 and T_3 higher, in part due to thyroid stimulation by human chorionic gonadotrophin (hCG). In later pregnancy, free T_4 and T_3 are lower. Binding globulin levels are induced by oestrogen, so total T_4 and T_3 levels are invariably high.
- **Iodine requirements**: increased in pregnancy. The World Health Organization (WHO) recommends minimum intake of 200 μg/day.
- **Screening of thyroid function and autoantibodies**: not recommended for every woman, but should be performed in the first trimester in those with a personal or family history of thyroid disease, goitre, other autoimmune disease including type 1 diabetes, or when there is clinical suspicion of thyroid dysfunction.

Thyrotoxicosis

- **Hyperemesis gravidarum**: associated with thyrotoxic biochemistry, sometimes requiring antithyroid drugs.
- **Subclinical thyrotoxicosis**: not usually treated, to avoid fetal hypothyroidism.
- **Antithyroid drugs**: propylthiouracil should be used in the first trimester, with carbimazole substituted in the second and third trimesters.

Hypothyroidism

- **Preterm labour and impaired cognitive development in the offspring**: may be associated with even subclinical hypothyroidism.
- **Levothyroxine replacement therapy dose requirements**: increase by 30–50% from early in pregnancy. Monitoring to maintain TSH results within the trimester-specific reference range is recommended in early pregnancy and at least once in each trimester.

Post-partum thyroiditis

- **Screening**: not recommended for every woman, but thyroid function should be tested 4–6 weeks post-partum in those with a personal history of thyroid disease, goitre or other autoimmune disease including type 1 diabetes, those known to have positive anti-thyroid peroxidase antibodies, or when there is clinical suspicion of thyroid dysfunction.

THE REPRODUCTIVE SYSTEM

Clinical practice in reproductive medicine is shared between several specialties, including gynaecology, urology, paediatrics, psychiatry and endocrinology. The following section is focused on disorders managed by endocrinologists.

Functional anatomy, physiology and investigations

The physiology of male and female reproductive function is illustrated in Figures 20.12 and 20.13 respectively.

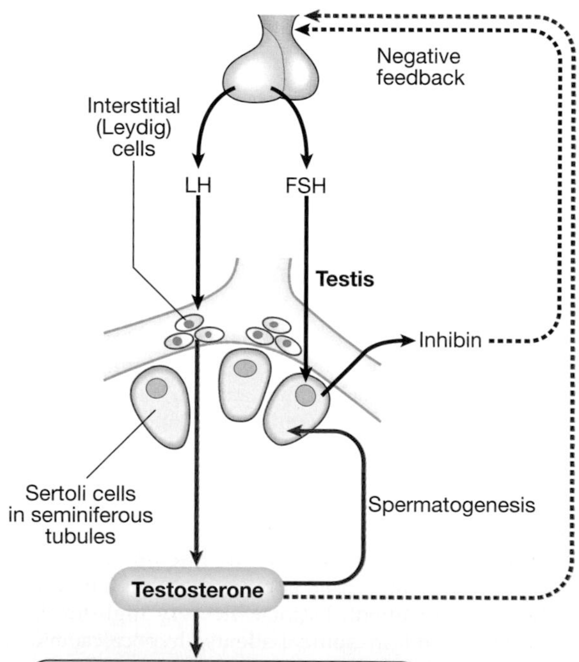

Fig. 20.12 Male reproductive physiology. (FSH = follicle-stimulating hormone; LH = luteinising hormone).

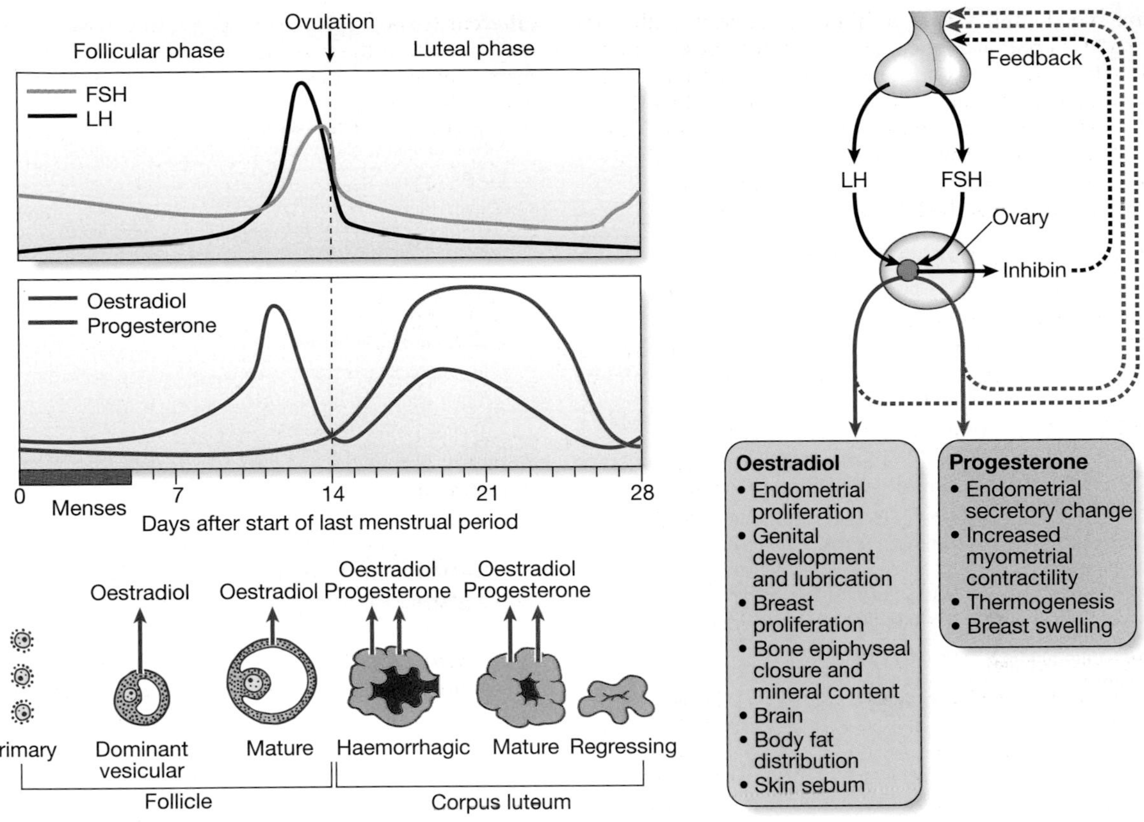

Fig. 20.13 Female reproductive physiology and the normal menstrual cycle.

20

Pathways for synthesis of sex steroids are shown in Figure 20.18 (p. 772).

The male

In the male, the testis subserves two principal functions: synthesis of testosterone by the interstitial Leydig cells under the control of luteinising hormone (LH), and spermatogenesis by Sertoli cells under the control of follicle-stimulating hormone (FSH) (but also requiring adequate testosterone). Negative feedback suppression of LH is mediated principally by testosterone, while secretion of another hormone by the testis, inhibin, suppresses FSH. The axis can be assessed easily by a random blood sample for testosterone, LH and FSH. Testosterone levels are higher in the morning and therefore, if testosterone is marginally low, sampling should be repeated in the early morning (0900 hrs). Testosterone is largely bound in plasma to sex hormone-binding globulin, and this can also be measured to calculate the 'free androgen index' or the 'bioavailable' testosterone. Testicular function can also be tested by semen analysis.

There is no equivalent of the menopause in men, although testosterone concentrations decline slowly from the fourth decade onwards.

The female

In the female, physiology varies during the normal menstrual cycle. FSH stimulates growth and development of ovarian follicles during the first 14 days after the menses. This leads to a gradual increase in oestradiol production from granulosa cells, which initially suppresses FSH secretion (negative feedback) but then, above a certain level, stimulates an increase in both the frequency and amplitude of gonadotrophin-releasing hormone (GnRH) pulses, resulting in a marked increase in LH secretion (positive feedback). The mid-cycle 'surge' of LH induces ovulation. After release of the ovum, the follicle differentiates into a corpus luteum, which secretes progesterone. Unless pregnancy occurs during the cycle, the corpus luteum regresses and the fall in progesterone levels results in menstrual bleeding. Circulating levels of oestrogen and progesterone in pre-menopausal women are, therefore, critically dependent on the time of the cycle. The most useful 'test' of ovarian function is a careful menstrual history: if menses are regular, measurement of gonadotrophins and oestrogen is not necessary. In addition, ovulation can be confirmed by measuring plasma progesterone levels during the luteal phase ('day 21 progesterone').

Cessation of menstruation (the menopause) occurs at an average age of approximately 50 years in developed countries. In the 5 years before, there is a gradual increase in the number of anovulatory cycles and this is referred to as the climacteric. Oestrogen and inhibin secretion falls and negative feedback results in increased pituitary secretion of LH and FSH (typically to levels above 30 U/L (3.3 μg/L)).

The pathophysiology of male and female reproductive dysfunction is summarised in Box 20.21.

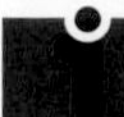

20.21 Classification of diseases of the reproductive system

	Primary	Secondary
Hormone excess	Polycystic ovarian syndrome Granulosa cell tumour Leydig cell tumour Teratoma	Pituitary gonadotrophinoma
Hormone deficiency	Menopause Hypogonadism (see Box 20.22) Turner's syndrome Klinefelter's syndrome	Hypopituitarism Kallmann's syndrome (isolated GnRH deficiency) Severe systemic illness, including anorexia nervosa
Hormone hypersensitivity	Idiopathic hirsutism	
Hormone resistance	Androgen resistance syndromes Complete ('testicular feminisation') Partial (Reifenstein's syndrome) 5α-reductase type 2 deficiency	
Non-functioning tumours	Ovarian cysts Carcinoma Teratoma Seminoma	

20.22 Causes of delayed puberty and hypogonadism

Constitutional delay

Hypogonadotrophic hypogonadism

- Structural hypothalamic/pituitary disease (see Box 20.59, p. 787)
- Functional gonadotrophin deficiency
  - Chronic systemic illness (e.g. asthma, malabsorption, coeliac disease, cystic fibrosis, renal failure)
  - Psychological stress
  - Anorexia nervosa
  - Excessive physical exercise
  - Hyperprolactinaemia
  - Other endocrine disease (e.g. Cushing's syndrome, primary hypothyroidism)
- Isolated gonadotrophin deficiency (Kallmann's syndrome)

Hypergonadotrophic hypogonadism

- Acquired gonadal damage
  - Chemotherapy/radiotherapy to gonads
  - Trauma/surgery to gonads
  - Autoimmune gonadal failure
  - Mumps orchitis
  - Tuberculosis
  - Haemochromatosis
- Developmental/congenital gonadal disorders
  - Steroid biosynthetic defects
  - Anorchidism/cryptorchidism in males
  - Klinefelter's syndrome (47XXY, male phenotype)
  - Turner's syndrome (45XO, female phenotype)

Presenting problems in reproductive disease

Delayed puberty

Puberty is considered to be delayed if the onset of the physical features of sexual maturation has not occurred by a chronological age that is 2.5 standard deviations (SD) above the national average. In the UK, this is by the age of 14 in boys and 13 in girls. Genetic factors have a major influence in determining the timing of the onset of puberty, such that the age of menarche (the onset of menstruation) is often comparable within sibling and mother–daughter pairs and within ethnic groups. However, because there is also a threshold for body weight that acts as a trigger for normal puberty, the onset of puberty can be influenced by other factors including nutritional status and chronic illness (p. 110).

Clinical assessment

The differential diagnosis is shown in Box 20.22. The key issue is to determine whether the delay in puberty is simply because the 'clock is running slow' (constitutional delay of puberty) or because there is pathology in the hypothalamus/pituitary (hypogonadotrophic hypogonadism) or the gonads (hypergonadotrophic hypogonadism). A general history and physical examination should be performed with particular reference to previous or current medical disorders, social circumstances and family history. Body proportions, sense of smell and pubertal stage should be carefully documented and, in boys, the presence or absence of testes in the scrotum noted. Current weight and height may be plotted on centile charts, along with parental heights. Previous growth measurements in childhood, which can usually be obtained from health records, are extremely useful. Healthy growth usually follows a centile. Usually, children with constitutional delay have always been small, but have maintained a normal growth velocity that is appropriate for bone age. Poor linear growth, with 'crossing of the centiles', is more likely to be associated with acquired disease. Issues that are commonly encountered in the management of adolescents with delayed puberty are summarised in Box 20.23.

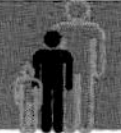

20.23 Delayed puberty

- **Aetiology**: in boys the most common cause is constitutional delay, whereas in girls there is invariably an underlying structural or functional cause.
- **Psychological effects**: whatever the underlying cause, delayed puberty is often associated with substantial psychological distress.
- **Investigations**: a karyotype should be performed in all adolescents with hypergonadotrophic hypogonadism, to exclude Turner's and Klinefelter's syndromes, unless there is an obvious precipitating cause.
- **Medical induction of puberty**: if this is being considered, it needs to be managed carefully and be carried out in a controlled fashion, to avoid premature fusion of the epiphyses.

Constitutional delay of puberty

This is the most common cause of delayed puberty. Affected children are healthy and have usually been more than 2 SD below the mean height for their age throughout childhood. There is often a history of delayed puberty in siblings or parents. Since sex steroids are essential for fusion of the epiphyses, 'bone age' can be estimated by X-rays of epiphyses, usually in the wrist and hand; in constitutional delay, bone age is lower than chronological age. Constitutional delay of puberty should be considered as a normal variant, as puberty will commence spontaneously. However, affected children can experience significant psychological distress because of their lack of physical development, particularly when compared with their peers.

Hypogonadotrophic hypogonadism

This may be due to structural, inflammatory or infiltrative disorders of the pituitary and/or hypothalamus (see Box 20.59, p. 787). In such circumstances, other pituitary hormones, such as growth hormone, are also likely to be deficient.

'Functional' gonadotrophin deficiency is caused by a variety of factors, including low body weight, chronic systemic illness (as a consequence of the disease itself or secondary malnutrition), endocrine disorders and profound psychosocial stress.

Isolated gonadotrophin deficiency is usually due to a genetic abnormality that affects the synthesis of either GnRH or gonadotrophins. The most common form is Kallmann's syndrome, in which there is primary GnRH deficiency and, in most affected individuals, agenesis or hypoplasia of the olfactory bulbs, resulting in anosmia or hyposmia. If isolated gonadotrophin deficiency is left untreated, the epiphyses fail to fuse, resulting in tall stature with disproportionately long arms and legs relative to trunk height (eunuchoid habitus).

Cryptorchidism (undescended testes) and gynaecomastia are commonly observed in all forms of hypogonadotrophic hypogonadism.

Hypergonadotrophic hypogonadism

Hypergonadotrophic hypogonadism associated with delayed puberty is usually due to Klinefelter's syndrome in boys and Turner's syndrome in girls (pp. 765 and 766). Other causes of primary gonadal failure are shown in Box 20.22.

Investigations

Key measurements are LH and FSH, testosterone (in boys) and oestradiol (in girls). Chromosome analysis should be performed if gonadotrophin concentrations are elevated. If gonadotrophin concentrations are low, then the differential diagnosis lies between constitutional delay and hypogonadotrophic hypogonadism. A plain X-ray of the wrist and hand may be compared with a set of standard films to obtain a bone age. Full blood count, renal function, liver function, thyroid function and coeliac disease autoantibodies (p. 880) should be measured, but further tests may be unnecessary if the blood tests are normal and the child has all the clinical features of constitutional delay. If hypogonadotrophic hypogonadism is suspected, neuroimaging and further investigations are required (p. 786).

Management

Puberty can be induced using low doses of oral oestrogen in girls (for example, ethinylestradiol 2 μg daily) or testosterone in boys (testosterone gel or depot testosterone esters). Higher doses carry a risk of early fusion of epiphyses. This therapy should be given in a specialist clinic where the progress of puberty and growth can be carefully monitored. In children with constitutional delay, this 'priming' therapy can be discontinued when endogenous puberty is established, usually in less than a year. In children with hypogonadism, the underlying cause should be treated and reversed if possible. If hypogonadism is permanent, sex hormone doses are gradually increased during puberty and full adult replacement doses given when development is complete.

Amenorrhoea

Primary amenorrhoea describes the condition of a female patient who has never menstruated; this usually occurs as a manifestation of delayed puberty but may also be a consequence of anatomical defects of the female reproductive system, such as endometrial hypoplasia or vaginal agenesis. Secondary amenorrhoea describes the cessation of menstruation. The causes of this common presentation are shown in Box 20.24. In non-pregnant women, secondary amenorrhoea is almost invariably a consequence of either ovarian or hypothalamic/pituitary dysfunction. Premature ovarian failure (premature menopause) is defined, arbitrarily, as occurring before 40 years of age. Rarely, endometrial adhesions (Asherman's syndrome) can form after uterine curettage, surgery or infection with tuberculosis or schistosomiasis, preventing endometrial proliferation and shedding.

Clinical assessment

The underlying cause can often be suspected from associated clinical features and the patient's age. Hypothalamic/pituitary disease and premature ovarian failure result in oestrogen deficiency, which causes a variety of symptoms usually associated with the menopause (Box 20.25). A history of galactorrhoea should be sought. Significant weight loss of any cause can cause amenorrhoea by suppression of gonadotrophins. Weight gain may suggest hypothyroidism, Cushing's syndrome or, very rarely, a hypothalamic lesion. Hirsutism, obesity and long-standing irregular periods suggest polycystic ovarian syndrome (PCOS, p. 764). The presence of other autoimmune disease raises the possibility of autoimmune premature ovarian failure.

Investigations

Pregnancy should be excluded in women of reproductive age by measuring urine or serum human chorionic

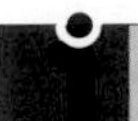

20.24 Causes of secondary amenorrhoea

Physiological
- Pregnancy
- Menopause

Hypogonadotrophic hypogonadism (see Box 20.22)

Ovarian dysfunction
- Hypergonadotrophic hypogonadism (see Box 20.22)
- Polycystic ovarian syndrome
- Androgen-secreting tumours

Uterine dysfunction
- Asherman's syndrome

20

20.25 Symptoms of oestrogen deficiency

Vasomotor effects	
• Hot flushes	• Sweating
Psychological	
• Anxiety • Irritability	• Emotional lability
Genitourinary	
• Dyspareunia • Urgency of micturition	• Vaginal infections

EBM 20.26 Hormone replacement therapy (HRT) in post-menopausal women

'Administering HRT for 5 years to 10 000 women aged 50–79 years prevents 5 hip fractures and 6 cases of colorectal cancer, while inducing 8 extra cases of breast cancer, 8 of pulmonary embolism, 7 of coronary heart disease and 8 of stroke. The risks increase with age.'

- Writing Group for the Women's Health Initiative Investigators. JAMA 2002: 288:321–333.

gonadotrophin (hCG). Serum LH, FSH, oestradiol, prolactin, testosterone, T_4 and TSH should be measured and, in the absence of a menstrual cycle, can be taken at any time. Investigation of hyperprolactinaemia is described on page 791. High concentrations of LH and FSH with low or low-normal oestradiol suggest primary ovarian failure. Ovarian autoantibodies may be positive when there is an underlying autoimmune aetiology, and a karyotype should be performed in younger women to exclude mosaic Turner's syndrome. Elevated LH, prolactin and testosterone levels with normal oestradiol are common in PCOS. Low levels of LH, FSH and oestradiol suggest hypothalamic or pituitary disease, and a pituitary MRI is indicated.

There is some overlap in gonadotrophin and oestrogen concentrations between women with hypogonadotrophic hypogonadism and PCOS. If there is doubt as to the underlying cause of secondary amenorrhoea, then the response to 5 days of treatment with an oral progestogen (e.g. medroxyprogesterone acetate 10 mg twice daily) can be assessed. In women with PCOS, the progestogen will cause maturation of the endometrium and menstruation will occur a few days after the progestogen is stopped. In women with hypogonadotrophic hypogonadism, menstruation does not occur following progestogen withdrawal because the endometrium is atrophic as a result of oestrogen deficiency. If doubt persists in distinguishing oestrogen deficiency from a uterine abnormality, the capacity for menstruation can be tested with 1 month of treatment with cyclical oestrogen and progestogen (usually administered as a combined oral contraceptive pill).

Assessment of bone mineral density by dual energy X-ray absorptiometry (DEXA, p. 1065) may be appropriate in patients with low androgen and oestrogen levels.

Management

Where possible, the underlying cause should be treated. For example, women with functional amenorrhoea due to excessive exercise and low weight should be encouraged to reduce their exercise and regain some weight. The management of structural pituitary and hypothalamic disease is described on page 790 and that of PCOS on page 764.

In oestrogen-deficient women, replacement therapy may be necessary to treat symptoms and/or to prevent osteoporosis. Women who have had a hysterectomy can be treated with oestrogen alone, but those with a uterus should be treated with combined oestrogen/progestogen therapy, since unopposed oestrogen increases the risk of endometrial cancer. Cyclical hormone replacement therapy (HRT) regimens typically involve giving oestrogen on days 1–21 and progestogen on days 14–21 of the cycle and this can be conveniently administered as the oral contraceptive pill. If oestrogenic side-effects (fluid retention, weight gain, hypertension and thrombosis) are a concern, then lower-dose oral or transdermal HRT may be more appropriate.

The timing of the discontinuation of oestrogen replacement therapy is still a matter of debate. In post-menopausal women, HRT has been shown to relieve menopausal symptoms and to prevent osteoporotic fractures but is associated with adverse effects, which are related to the duration of therapy and to the patient's age (Box 20.26). In patients with premature menopause, HRT should be continued up to the age of around 50 years, but only continued beyond this age if there are continued symptoms of oestrogen deficiency on discontinuation.

Management of infertility in oestrogen-deficient women is described on page 760.

Male hypogonadism

The clinical features of both hypo- and hypergonadotrophic hypogonadism include loss of libido, lethargy with muscle weakness, and decreased frequency of shaving. Patients may also present with gynaecomastia, infertility, delayed puberty, osteoporosis or anaemia of chronic disease. The causes of hypogonadism are listed in Box 20.22.

Investigations

Male hypogonadism is confirmed by demonstrating a low serum testosterone level. The distinction between hypo- and hypergonadotrophic hypogonadism is by measurement of random LH and FSH. Patients with hypogonadotrophic hypogonadism should be investigated as described for pituitary disease on page 786. Biochemical hypogonadism is associated with central obesity and the metabolic syndrome (p. 805); postulated mechanisms are complex and include reduction in sex hormone binding globulin by insulin resistance and reduction in GnRH and gonadotrophin secretion by cytokines or oestrogen released by adipose tissue. Testosterone levels also fall gradually with age in men (see Box 20.34, p. 766) and this is associated with gonadotrophin levels that are low or inappropriately within the 'normal' range. There is an increasing trend to measure testosterone in older men, typically as part of an assessment of erectile dysfunction. Patients with hypergonadotrophic hypogonadism should have the testes examined for cryptorchidism or atrophy,

20.27 Options for androgen replacement therapy

Route of administration	Preparation	Dose	Frequency	Comments
Intramuscular	Testosterone enantate	50–250 mg	Every 3–4 wks	Produces peaks and troughs of testosterone levels which are outside the physiological range and may be symptomatic
	Testosterone undecanoate	1000 mg	Every 3 mths	Smoother profile than testosterone enantate, less frequent injections
Subcutaneous	Testosterone pellets	600–800 mg	Every 4–6 mths	Smoother profile than testosterone enantate but implantation causes scarring and infection
Transdermal	Testosterone patch	5–10 mg	Daily	Stable testosterone levels but high incidence of skin hypersensitivity
	Testosterone gel	50–100 mg	Daily	Stable testosterone levels; transfer of gel can occur following skin-to-skin contact with another person
Oral	Testosterone undecanoate	40–120 mg	Twice daily	Very variable testosterone levels; risk of hepatotoxicity

and a karyotype performed (to identify Klinefelter's syndrome).

Management

Testosterone replacement is clearly indicated in younger men with significant hypogonadism to prevent osteoporosis and to restore muscle power and libido. Debate exists as to whether replacement therapy is of benefit in mild hypogonadism associated with ageing and central obesity, particularly in the absence of structural pituitary/hypothalamic disease or other pituitary hormone deficiency. In such instances, a therapeutic trial of testosterone therapy may be considered if symptoms are present, but the benefits of therapy must be carefully weighed against the potential for harm.

Routes of testosterone administration are shown in Box 20.27. First-pass hepatic metabolism of testosterone is highly efficient, so bioavailability of ingested preparations is poor. Doses of systemic testosterone can be titrated against symptoms; circulating testosterone levels may provide only a rough guide to dosage because they may be highly variable (see Box 20.27). Testosterone therapy can aggravate prostatic carcinoma; prostate-specific antigen (PSA) should be measured before commencing testosterone therapy in men older than 50 years and monitored annually thereafter. Haemoglobin concentration should also be monitored in older men, as androgen replacement can cause polycythaemia. Testosterone replacement inhibits spermatogenesis; treatment for fertility is described below.

Infertility

Infertility affects around 1 in 7 couples of reproductive age, often causing psychological distress. The main causes are listed in Box 20.28. In women, it may result from anovulation or abnormalities of the reproductive tract that prevent fertilisation or embryonic implantation, often damaged fallopian tubes from previous infection. In men, infertility may result from impaired sperm quality (for example, reduced motility) or reduced sperm number. Azoospermia or oligospermia is usually idiopathic, but may be a consequence of hypogonadism (see Box 20.22). Microdeletions of the Y chromosome are increasingly recognised as a cause of severely abnormal spermatogenesis. In many couples, more than one factor causing subfertility is present, and in a large proportion no cause can be identified.

20.28 Causes of infertility

Female factor (35–40%)

- Ovulatory dysfunction
  - Polycystic ovarian syndrome
  - Hypogonadotrophic hypogonadism (see Box 20.22)
  - Hypergonadotrophic hypogonadism (see Box 20.22)
- Tubular dysfunction
  - Pelvic inflammatory disease (chlamydia, gonorrhoea)
  - Endometriosis
  - Previous sterilisation
  - Previous pelvic or abdominal surgery
- Cervical and/or uterine dysfunction
  - Congenital abnormalities
  - Fibroids
  - Treatment for cervical carcinoma
  - Asherman's syndrome

Male factor (35–40%)

- Reduced sperm quality or production
  - Y chromosome microdeletions
  - Varicocoele
  - Hypergonadotrophic hypogonadism (see Box 20.22)
  - Hypogonadotrophic hypogonadism (see Box 20.22)
- Tubular dysfunction
  - Varicocoele
  - Congenital abnormality of vas deferens/epididymis
  - Previous sexually transmitted infection (chlamydia, gonorrhoea)
  - Previous vasectomy

Unexplained or mixed factor (20–35%)

Clinical assessment

A history of previous pregnancies, relevant infections and surgery is important in both men and women. A sexual history must be explored sensitively, as some couples have intercourse infrequently or only when they consider the woman to be ovulating, and psychosexual difficulties are common. Irregular and/or infrequent menstrual periods are an indicator of anovulatory cycles in the woman, in which case causes such as PCOS should be considered. In men, the testes should be examined to confirm that both are in the scrotum and to identify any structural abnormality, such as small size, absent vas deferens or the presence of a varicocoele.

Investigations

Investigations should generally be performed after a couple has failed to conceive despite unprotected intercourse for 12 months, unless there is an obvious abnormality like amenorrhoea. Both partners need to be investigated. The male partner needs a semen analysis to assess sperm count and quality. Home testing for ovulation (by commercial urine dipstick kits, temperature measurement, or assessment of cervical mucus) is not recommended, as the information is often counterbalanced by increased anxiety if interpretation is inconclusive. In women with regular periods, ovulation can be confirmed by an elevated serum progesterone concentration on day 21 of the menstrual cycle. Transvaginal ultrasound can be used to assess uterine and ovarian anatomy. Tubal patency may be examined at laparoscopy or by hysterosalpingography (HSG; a radio-opaque medium is injected into the uterus and should normally outline the fallopian tubes). In vitro assessments of sperm survival in cervical mucus may be done in cases of unexplained infertility but are rarely helpful.

Management

Couples should be advised to have regular sexual intercourse, ideally every 2–3 days throughout the menstrual cycle. It is not uncommon for 'spontaneous' pregnancies to occur in couples undergoing investigations for infertility or with identified causes of male or female subfertility.

In women with anovulatory cycles secondary to PCOS (p. 764), clomifene, which has partial anti-oestrogen action, blocks negative feedback of oestrogen on the hypothalamus/pituitary, causing gonadotrophin secretion and thus ovulation. In women with gonadotrophin deficiency or in whom anti-oestrogen therapy is unsuccessful, ovulation may be induced by direct stimulation of the ovary by daily injection of FSH and an injection of hCG to induce follicular rupture at the appropriate time. In hypothalamic disease, pulsatile GnRH therapy with a portable infusion pump can be used to stimulate pituitary gonadotrophin secretion (note that non-pulsatile administration of GnRH or its analogues paradoxically suppresses LH and FSH secretion). Whatever method of ovulation induction is employed, monitoring of response is essential to avoid multiple ovulation. For clomifene, ultrasound monitoring is recommended for at least the first cycle. During gonadotrophin therapy, closer monitoring of follicular growth by transvaginal ultrasonography and blood oestradiol levels is mandatory. 'Ovarian hyperstimulation syndrome' is characterised by grossly enlarged ovaries and capillary leak with circulatory shock, pleural effusions and ascites. Anovulatory women who fail to respond to ovulation induction or who have primary ovarian failure may wish to consider using donated eggs or embryos, surrogacy and adoption.

Surgery to restore fallopian tube patency can be effective but in vitro fertilisation (IVF) is normally recommended. IVF is widely used for many causes of infertility and in unexplained cases of prolonged (> 3 years) infertility. The success of IVF depends on age, with low success rates in women over 40 years.

Men with hypogonadotrophic hypogonadism who wish fertility are usually given injections of hCG several times a week (recombinant FSH may also be required in men with hypogonadism of pre-pubertal origin); it may take up to 2 years to achieve satisfactory sperm counts. Surgery is rarely an option in primary testicular disease but removal of a varicocoele can improve semen quality. Extraction of sperm from the epididymis for IVF, and intracytoplasmic sperm injection (ICSI, when single spermatozoa are injected into each oöcyte) are being used increasingly in men with oligospermia or poor sperm quality who have primary testicular disease. Azoospermic men may opt to use donated sperm but this may be in short supply.

Gynaecomastia

Gynaecomastia is the presence of glandular breast tissue in males. Normal breast development in women is oestrogen-dependent, while androgens oppose this effect. Gynaecomastia results from an imbalance between androgen and oestrogen activity, which may reflect androgen deficiency or oestrogen excess. Causes are listed in Box 20.29. The most common are physiological: for example, in the newborn baby (due to maternal and placental oestrogens), in pubertal boys (in whom oestradiol concentrations reach adult levels before testosterone) and in elderly men (due to decreasing testosterone concentrations). Prolactin excess alone does not cause gynaecomastia (p. 790).

Clinical assessment

A drug history is important. Gynaecomastia is often asymmetrical and palpation may allow breast tissue to be distinguished from the prominent adipose tissue around the nipple that is often observed in obesity. Features of hypogonadism should be sought (see above) and the testes examined for evidence of cryptorchidism, atrophy or a tumour.

Investigations

If a clinical distinction between gynaecomastia and adipose tissue cannot be made, then ultrasonography or mammography is required. A random blood sample

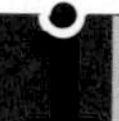

20.29 Causes of gynaecomastia

Idiopathic

Physiological

Drug-induced
- Cimetidine
- Digoxin
- Anti-androgens (cyproterone acetate, spironolactone)
- Some exogenous anabolic steroids (diethylstilbestrol)
- Cannabis

Hypogonadism (see Box 20.22)

Androgen resistance syndromes

Oestrogen excess
- Liver failure (impaired steroid metabolism)
- Oestrogen-secreting tumour (for example, of testis)
- hCG-secreting tumour (for example, of testis or lung)

should be taken for testosterone, LH, FSH, oestradiol, prolactin and hCG. Elevated oestrogen concentrations are found in testicular tumours and hCG-producing neoplasms.

Management

An adolescent with gynaecomastia who is progressing normally through puberty may be reassured that the gynaecomastia will usually resolve once development is complete. If puberty does not proceed in a harmonious manner, then there may be an underlying abnormality that requires investigation (p. 758). Gynaecomastia may cause significant psychological distress, especially in adolescent boys, and surgical excision may be justified for cosmetic reasons. Androgen replacement will usually improve gynaecomastia in hypogonadal males and any other identifiable underlying cause should be addressed if possible. The anti-oestrogen tamoxifen may also be effective in reducing the size of the breast tissue.

Hirsutism

Hirsutism refers to the excessive growth of thick terminal hair in an androgen-dependent distribution in women (upper lip, chin, chest, back, lower abdomen, thigh, forearm) and is one of the most common presentations of endocrine disease. It should be distinguished from hypertrichosis, which is generalised excessive growth of vellus hair. The aetiology of androgen excess is shown in Box 20.30.

Clinical assessment

The severity of hirsutism is subjective. Some women suffer profound embarrassment from a degree of hair growth which others would not consider remarkable. Important observations are a drug and menstrual history, calculation of body mass index, measurement of blood pressure, and examination for virilisation (clitoromegaly, deep voice, male-pattern balding, breast atrophy) and associated features, including acne vulgaris or Cushing's syndrome (p. 773). Hirsutism of recent onset associated with virilisation is suggestive of an androgen-secreting tumour but this is rare.

Investigations

A random blood sample should be taken for testosterone, prolactin, LH and FSH. If there are clinical features of Cushing's syndrome, further investigations should be performed (p. 774).

If testosterone levels are more than twice the upper limit of normal for females, idiopathic hirsutism and PCOS are less likely, especially if LH and FSH levels are low. Under these circumstances, other causes of androgen excess should be sought. Congenital adrenal hyperplasia due to 21-hydroxylase deficiency is diagnosed by a short ACTH stimulation test with measurement of 17OH-progesterone (p. 782). In patients with androgen-secreting tumours, serum testosterone does not suppress following dexamethasone (either as an overnight or a 48-hour low-dose suppression test) or oestrogen

20.30 Causes of hirsutism

Cause	Clinical features	Investigation findings	Treatment
Idiopathic	Often familial Mediterranean or Asian background	Normal	Cosmetic measures Anti-androgens
Polycystic ovarian syndrome	Obesity Oligomenorrhoea or secondary amenorrhoea Infertility	LH:FSH ratio > 2.5:1 Minor elevation of androgens* Mild hyperprolactinaemia	Weight loss Cosmetic measures Anti-androgens (Metformin, glitazones may be useful)
Congenital adrenal hyperplasia (95% 21-hydroxylase deficiency)	Pigmentation History of salt-wasting in childhood, ambiguous genitalia, or adrenal crisis when stressed Jewish background	Elevated androgens* which suppress with dexamethasone Abnormal rise in 17OH-progesterone with ACTH	Glucocorticoid replacement administered in reverse rhythm to suppress early morning ACTH
Exogenous androgen administration	Athletes Virilisation	Low LH and FSH Analysis of urinary androgens may detect drug of misuse	Stop steroid misuse
Androgen-secreting tumour of ovary or adrenal cortex	Rapid onset Virilisation: clitoromegaly, deep voice, balding, breast atrophy	High androgens* which do not suppress with dexamethasone or oestrogen Low LH and FSH CT or MRI usually demonstrates a tumour	Surgical excision
Cushing's syndrome	Clinical features of Cushing's syndrome (p. 773)	Normal or mild elevation of adrenal androgens* See investigations (p. 774)	Treat the cause (p. 775)

*e.g. Serum testosterone levels in women: < 2 nmol/L (< 58 ng/dL) is normal; 2–5 nmol/L (58–144 ng/dL) is minor elevation; > 5 nmol/L (> 144 ng/dL) is high and requires further investigation.

(30 μg daily for 7 days). The tumour should then be sought by CT or MRI of the adrenals and ovaries.

Management

This depends on the cause (see Box 20.30). Options for the treatment of PCOS and idiopathic hirsutism are similar and are described below.

Polycystic ovarian syndrome

Polycystic ovarian syndrome (PCOS) affects up to 10% of women of reproductive age. It is a heterogenous disorder (Box 20.31), often associated with obesity, for which the primary cause remains uncertain. Genetic factors probably play a role, since PCOS often affects several family members. The severity and clinical features of PCOS vary markedly between individual patients but diagnosis is usually made during the investigation of hirsutism (p. 763) or amenorrhoea/oligomenorrhoea (p. 759). Infertility may also be present (p. 761). There is no universally accepted definition, but it has been recommended that a diagnosis of PCOS requires the presence of two of the following three features:

- menstrual irregularity
- clinical or biochemical androgen excess
- multiple cysts in the ovaries (most readily detected by transvaginal ultrasound; Fig. 20.14).

Women with PCOS are at increased risk of glucose intolerance and some authorities recommend screening for type 2 diabetes and other cardiovascular risk factors associated with the metabolic syndrome (p. 805).

Management

This should be directed at the presenting complaint, but all PCOS patients who are overweight should be encouraged to lose weight, as this can improve several symptoms, including menstrual irregularity, and reduces the risk of type 2 diabetes.

20.31 Features of polycystic ovarian syndrome

Mechanisms*	Manifestations
Pituitary dysfunction	High serum LH High serum prolactin
Anovulatory menstrual cycles	Oligomenorrhoea Secondary amenorrhoea Cystic ovaries Infertility
Androgen excess	Hirsutism Acne
Obesity	Hyperglycaemia Elevated oestrogens
Insulin resistance	Dyslipidaemia Hypertension

*These mechanisms are interrelated; it is not known which, if any, is primary. PCOS probably represents the common end point of several different pathologies.

EBM 20.32 Treatment of infertility in women with PCOS

'In one randomised controlled clinical trial, 626 infertile women with PCOS were randomised to receive clomifene, metformin or combination therapy. After 6 months, the live birth rates were 22.5%, 7.2% and 26.8% respectively. Multiple births occurred in 6% of women receiving clomifene and none of those receiving metformin.'

- RS Legro, et al. New Engl J Med 2008; 356:551–566.

Menstrual irregularity and infertility

Most women with PCOS have oligomenorrhoea, with irregular, heavy menstrual periods. This may not require treatment unless fertility is desired. Metformin (p. 821), by reducing insulin resistance, may restore regular ovulatory cycles in overweight women, although it is less effective than clomifene (p. 762) at restoring fertility as measured by successful pregnancy (Box 20.32). Thiazolidinediones (p. 823) also enhance insulin sensitivity and restore menstrual regularity in PCOS, but are contraindicated in women planning pregnancy.

In women who have very few periods each year or are amenorrhoeic, the high oestrogen concentrations associated with PCOS can cause endometrial hyperplasia. Progestogens can be administered on a cyclical basis to induce regular shedding of the endometrium and a withdrawal bleed, or a progestogen-impregnated intrauterine coil can be fitted.

Hirsutism

For hirsutism, most patients will have used cosmetic measures, such as shaving, bleaching and waxing, before consulting a doctor. Electrolysis and laser treatment are effective for small areas like the upper lip and for chest hair but are expensive. Eflornithine cream inhibits ornithine decarboxylase in hair follicles and may reduce hair growth when applied daily to affected areas of the face.

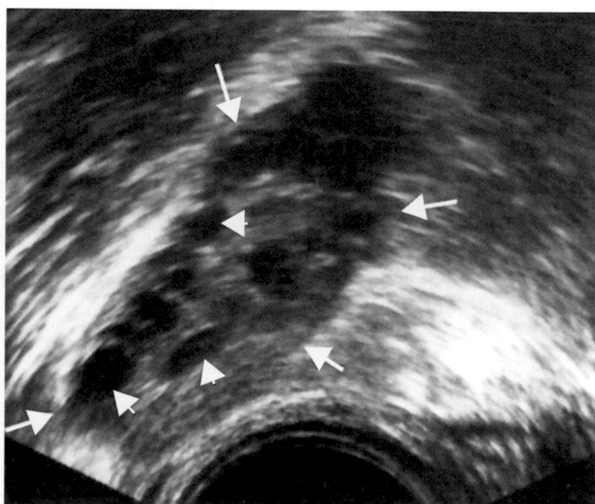

Fig. 20.14 Polycystic ovary. A transvaginal ultrasound scan showing multiple cysts (some indicated by small arrows) in the ovary (highlighted by bigger arrows) of a woman with polycystic ovarian syndrome.

20.33 Anti-androgen therapy

Mechanism of action	Drug	Dose	Hazards
Androgen receptor antagonists	Cyproterone acetate	2, 50 or 100 mg on days 1–11 of 28-day cycle with ethinylestradiol 30 μg on days 1–21	Hepatic dysfunction Feminisation of male fetus Progesterone receptor agonist Dysfunctional uterine bleeding
	Spironolactone	100–200 mg daily	Electrolyte disturbance
	Flutamide	Not recommended	Hepatic dysfunction
5α-reductase inhibitors (prevent conversion of testosterone to active dihydrotestosterone)	Finasteride	5 mg daily	Limited clinical experience; possibly less efficacious than other treatments
Suppress ovarian steroid production and elevate sex hormone-binding globulin	Oestrogen	See combination with cyproterone acetate above *or* Conventional oestrogen-containing contraceptive	Venous thromboembolism Hypertension Weight gain Dyslipidaemia Increased breast and endometrial carcinoma

If conservative measures are unsuccessful, anti-androgen therapy is given (Box 20.33). The life cycle of a hair follicle is at least 3 months and no improvement is likely before this time, when follicles have shed their hair and replacement hair growth has been suppressed. Metformin and thiazolidinediones are less effective at treating hirsutism than at restoring menstrual regularity. Unless weight is lost, hirsutism will return if therapy is discontinued. The patient should know that prolonged exposure to some agents may not be desirable and they should be stopped before pregnancy.

Turner's syndrome

Turner's syndrome affects around 1 in 2500 females. It is classically associated with a 45XO karyotype but other cytogenetic abnormalities may be responsible, including mosaic forms (e.g. 45XO/46XX or 45XO/46XY) and partial deletions of an X chromosome.

Clinical features

These are shown in Figure 20.15.

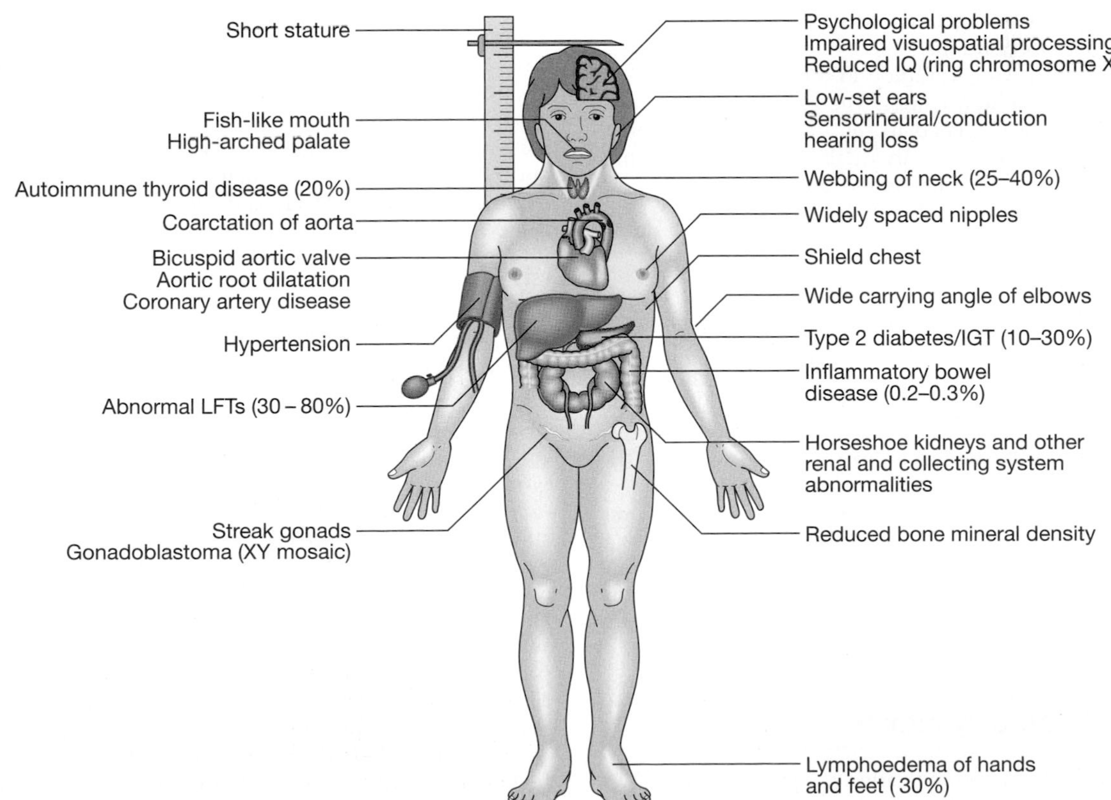

Fig. 20.15 Clinical features of Turner's syndrome (45XO). (IGT = impaired glucose tolerance).

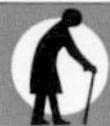

20.34 Gonadal function in old age

- **Post-menopausal osteoporosis**: a major public health issue due to the high incidence of associated fragility fractures, especially of hip.
- **Hormone replacement therapy**: should only be prescribed above the age of 50 for the short-term relief of symptoms of oestrogen deficiency.
- **Sexual activity**: many older people remain sexually active.
- **'Male menopause'**: does not occur, although testosterone concentrations do fall with age. Testosterone therapy in mildly hypogonadal men may be of benefit for body composition, muscle and bone. Large randomised trials are required to determine whether benefits outweigh potentially harmful effects on the prostate and cardiovascular system.
- **Androgens in older women**: hirsutism and balding occur. In the rare patients in whom androgen levels are elevated, this may be pathological, e.g. from an ovarian tumour.

Individuals with Turner's syndrome invariably have short stature from an early age and this is often the initial presenting symptom. It is probably due to haploinsufficiency of the *SHOX* gene, one copy of which is found on both the X and Y chromosomes, which encodes a protein that is predominantly found in bone fibroblasts.

The genital tract and external genitalia in Turner's syndrome are female in character, since this is the default developmental outcome in the absence of testes. Ovarian tissue develops normally until the third month of gestation, but thereafter there is gonadal dysgenesis with accelerated degeneration of oöcytes and increased ovarian stromal fibrosis, resulting in 'streak ovaries'. The inability of ovarian tissue to produce oestrogen results in loss of negative feedback and elevation of FSH and LH concentrations.

There is a wide variation in the spectrum of associated somatic abnormalities. The severity of the phenotype is, in part, related to the underlying cytogenetic abnormality. Mosaic individuals may have only mild short stature and may enter puberty spontaneously before developing gonadal failure.

Diagnosis and management

The diagnosis of Turner's syndrome can be confirmed by karyotype analysis. Short stature, although not directly due to growth hormone deficiency, responds to high doses of growth hormone. Prophylactic gonadectomy is recommended for individuals with 45XO/46XY mosaicism because there is an increased risk of gonadoblastoma. Pubertal development can be induced with oestrogen therapy but causes fusion of the epiphyses and cessation of growth. Therefore, the timing of pubertal induction needs to be carefully planned. Adults with Turner's syndrome require long-term oestrogen replacement therapy and should be monitored periodically for the development of aortic root dilatation, hearing loss and other somatic complications.

Klinefelter's syndrome

Klinefelter's syndrome affects approximately 1 in 1000 males and is usually associated with a 47XXY karyotype. However, other cytogenetic variants may be responsible, especially 46XY/47XXY mosaicism. The principal pathological abnormality is dysgenesis of the seminiferous tubules. This is evident from infancy (and possibly even in utero) and progresses with age. By adolescence, hyalinisation and fibrosis are present within the seminiferous tubules and Leydig cell function is impaired, resulting in hypogonadism.

Clinical features

The diagnosis is typically made in adolescents who have presented with gynaecomastia and failure to progress normally through puberty. Affected individuals usually have small, firm testes. Tall stature is apparent from early childhood, reflecting characteristically long leg length associated with 47XXY, and may be exacerbated by androgen deficiency with lack of epiphyseal closure in puberty. Other clinical features may include learning difficulties and behavioural disorders, as well as an increased risk of breast cancer and type 2 diabetes in later life. The spectrum of clinical features is wide and some individuals, especially those with 46XY/47XXY mosaicism, may pass through puberty normally and be identified only during investigation for infertility.

Diagnosis and management

Klinefelter's syndrome is suggested by the typical phenotype in a patient with hypergonadotrophic hypogonadism and can be confirmed by karyotype analysis. Individuals with clinical and biochemical evidence of androgen deficiency require androgen replacement (see Box 20.27, p. 761).

THE PARATHYROID GLANDS

Parathyroid hormone (PTH) plays a key role in the regulation of calcium and phosphate homeostasis and vitamin D metabolism, as shown in Figure 25.55 (p. 1125). The consequences of altered function of this axis in gut and renal disease are covered in Chapters 22 and 17, respectively. Other metabolic bone diseases are explored in Chapter 25. Here, the investigation of hypercalcaemia and hypocalcaemia and disorders of the parathyroid glands are discussed.

Functional anatomy, physiology and investigations

The four parathyroid glands lie behind the lobes of the thyroid and weigh between 25 and 40 mg. The parathyroid chief cells respond directly to changes in calcium concentrations via a G-protein-coupled cell surface receptor (the calcium-sensing receptor) located on the cell surface (see Fig. 25.55). When serum ionised calcium levels fall, PTH secretion rises. PTH is a single-chain polypeptide of 84 amino acids. It acts on the renal tubules to promote reabsorption of calcium and reduce reabsorption of phosphate, and on the skeleton to increase osteoclastic bone resorption and bone formation. PTH also promotes conversion of 25-hydroxycholecalciferol to the active metabolite 1,25-dihydroxycholecalciferol; the 1,25-dihydroxycholecalciferol, in turn, enhances calcium absorption from the gut.

More than 99% of total body calcium is in bone. Prolonged exposure of bone to high levels of PTH is associated with increased osteoclastic activity and new bone formation, but the net effect is to cause bone loss with mobilisation of calcium into the extracellular fluid. In contrast, pulsatile release of PTH causes net bone gain, an effect that is exploited therapeutically in the treatment of osteoporosis (p. 1124).

The differential diagnosis of disorders of calcium metabolism requires measurement of calcium phosphate, alkaline phosphatase, renal function, PTH and 25(OH)D. Although the parathyroid glands detect and respond to ionised calcium levels, most clinical laboratories only measure total serum calcium levels and about 50% of total calcium is bound to organic ions, such as citrate or phosphate, and to proteins, especially albumin. Accordingly, if the serum albumin level is reduced, total calcium concentrations should be 'corrected' by adjusting the value for calcium upwards by 0.02 mmol/L (0.4 mg/dL) for each 1 g/L reduction in albumin below 40 g/L. If albumin concentrations are significantly low, as in severe acute illness and other chronic illness such as liver cirrhosis, this correction is less accurate and measurement of ionised calcium is needed.

Calcitonin is secreted from the parafollicular C cells of the thyroid gland. Although it is a useful tumour marker in medullary carcinoma of thyroid (p. 755) and can be given therapeutically in Paget's disease of bone (p. 1129), its release from the thyroid is of no clinical relevance to calcium homeostasis in humans.

Disorders of the parathyroid glands are summarised in Box 20.35.

20.35 Classification of diseases of the parathyroid glands

	Primary	Secondary
Hormone excess	Primary hyperparathyroidism Parathyroid adenoma Parathyroid carcinoma[1] Parathyroid hyperplasia[2] Tertiary hyperparathyroidism Following prolonged secondary hyperparathyroidism	Secondary hyperparathyroidism Chronic kidney disease Malabsorption Vitamin D deficiency
Hormone deficiency	Hypoparathyroidism Post-surgical Autoimmune Inherited	
Hormone hypersensitivity	Autosomal dominant hypercalciuric hypocalcaemic (CASR-activating mutation)	
Hormone resistance	Pseudohypoparathyroidism Familial hypocalciuric hypercalcaemia	
Non-functioning tumours	Parathyroid carcinoma[1]	

[1]Parathyroid carcinomas may or may not produce PTH. [2]In multiple endocrine neoplasia (MEN) syndromes (p. 794)
(CASR = calcium-sensing receptor)

Presenting problems in parathyroid disease

Hypercalcaemia

Hypercalcaemia is one of the most common biochemical abnormalities and is often detected during routine biochemical analysis in asymptomatic patients. However, it can present with chronic symptoms, as described below, and occasionally as an acute emergency with severe hypercalcaemia and dehydration.

Causes of hypercalcaemia are listed in Box 20.36. Of these, primary hyperparathyroidism and malignant hypercalcaemia are by far the most common. Familial hypocalciuric hypercalcaemia (FHH) is a rare but important cause that needs differentiation from primary hyperparathyroidism (HPT). Lithium may cause hyperparathyroidism by reducing the sensitivity of the calcium-sensing receptor.

Clinical assessment

Symptoms and signs of hypercalcaemia include polyuria and polydipsia, renal colic, lethargy, anorexia, nausea, dyspepsia and peptic ulceration, constipation, depression, drowsiness and impaired cognition. Patients with malignant hypercalcaemia can have a rapid onset of symptoms and may have clinical features that help to localise the tumour.

The classic symptoms of primary hyperparathyroidism are described by the adage 'bones, stones and abdominal groans', but few patients present in this way nowadays and the disorder is most often picked up as an incidental finding on biochemical testing. About 50% of patients with primary hyperparathyroidism are asymptomatic while others have nonspecific symptoms such as fatigue, depression and generalised aches and pains. Some present with renal calculi and it has been estimated that 5% of first stone formers and 15% of recurrent stone formers have primary hyperparathyroidism (p. 769). Hypertension is a common feature of hyperparathyroidism. Parathyroid tumours are almost never palpable.

A family history of hypercalcaemia raises the possibility of FHH or MEN (p. 794).

20.36 Causes of hypercalcaemia

With normal or elevated PTH levels

- Primary or tertiary hyperparathyroidism
- Lithium-induced hyperparathyroidism
- Familial hypocalciuric hypercalcaemia

With low PTH levels

- Malignancy (lung, breast, myeloma, renal, lymphoma, thyroid)
- Elevated 1,25$(OH)_2$ vitamin D (vitamin D intoxication, sarcoidosis, HIV, other granulomatous disease)
- Thyrotoxicosis
- Paget's disease with immobilisation
- Milk-alkali syndrome
- Thiazide diuretics
- Glucocorticoid deficiency

Investigations

The most discriminant investigation is measurement of PTH. If PTH levels are detectable or elevated in the presence of hypercalcaemia, then primary hyperparathyroidism is the most likely diagnosis. High plasma phosphate and alkaline phosphatase accompanied by renal impairment suggest tertiary hyperparathyroidism. Hypercalcaemia may cause nephrocalcinosis and renal tubular impairment, resulting in hyperuricaemia and hyperchloraemia.

Patients with FHH can present with a similar biochemical picture to primary hyperparathyroidism but typically have low urinary calcium excretion (a ratio of urinary calcium clearance to creatinine clearance of < 0.01). The diagnosis of FHH can be confirmed by screening family members for hypercalcaemia and/or a mutation in the gene encoding the calcium-sensing receptor.

If PTH is low and no other cause is apparent, then malignancy with or without bony metastases is likely. PTH-related peptide, which is often responsible for the hypercalcaemia associated with malignancy, is not detected by PTH assays, but can be measured by a specific assay (although this is not usually necessary). Unless the source is obvious, the patient should be screened for malignancy with a chest X-ray, myeloma screen (p. 1046) and CT as appropriate.

Management

Treatment of severe hypercalcaemia and primary hyperparathyroidism is described on pages 273 and 769, respectively. FHH does not require any specific intervention.

Hypocalcaemia

Aetiology

Hypocalcaemia is much less common than hypercalcaemia. The differential diagnosis is shown in Box 20.37. The most common cause of hypocalcaemia is a low serum albumin with normal ionised calcium concentration. Conversely, ionised calcium may be low in the face of normal total serum calcium in patients with alkalosis: for example, as a result of hyperventilation.

Hypocalcaemia may also develop as a result of magnesium depletion and should be considered in patients with malabsorption, on diuretic or proton pump inhibitor therapy, and/or with a history of alcohol excess. Magnesium deficiency causes hypocalcaemia by impairing the ability of the parathyroid glands to secrete PTH (resulting in PTH concentrations that are low or inappropriately in the reference range) and may also impair the actions of PTH on bone and kidney.

Clinical assessment

Mild hypocalcaemia is often asymptomatic but, with more profound reductions in serum calcium, tetany can occur. This is characterised by muscle spasms due to increased excitability of peripheral nerves.

Children are more liable to develop tetany than adults and present with a characteristic triad of carpopedal spasm, stridor and convulsions, although one or more of these may be found independently of the others. In carpopedal spasm, the hands adopt a characteristic position with flexion of the metacarpophalangeal joints of the fingers and adduction of the thumb ('main d'accoucheur'). Pedal spasm can also occur but is less frequent. Stridor is caused by spasm of the glottis. Adults can also develop carpopedal spasm in association with tingling of the hands and feet and around the mouth, but stridor and fits are rare.

Latent tetany may be detected by eliciting Trousseau's sign; inflation of a sphygmomanometer cuff on the upper arm to more than the systolic blood pressure is followed by carpal spasm within 3 minutes. Less specific is Chvostek's sign, in which tapping over the branches of the facial nerve as they emerge from the parotid gland produces twitching of the facial muscles.

20.37 Differential diagnosis of hypocalcaemia

	Total serum calcium	Ionised serum calcium	Serum phosphate	Serum PTH	Comments
Hypoalbuminaemia	↓	↔	↔	↔	Adjust calcium upwards by 0.02 mmol/L (0.1 mg/dL) for every 1 g/L reduction in albumin below 40 g/L
Alkalosis	↔	↓	↔	↔ or ↑	Ch. 16
Vitamin D deficiency	↓	↓	↓	↑	Ch. 25
Chronic renal failure	↓	↓	↑	↑	Due to impaired vitamin D hydroxylation Serum creatinine ↑
Hypoparathyroidism	↓	↓	↑	↓	See text
Pseudohypoparathyroidism	↓	↓	↑	↑	Characteristic phenotype (see text)
Acute pancreatitis	↓	↓	↔ or ↓	↑	Usually clinically obvious Serum amylase ↑
Hypomagnesaemia	↓	↓	Variable	↓ or ↔	Treatment of hypomagnesaemia may correct hypocalcaemia

(↑ = levels increased; ↓ = levels reduced; ↔ = levels normal)

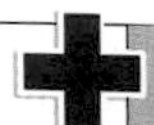

20.38 Management of severe hypocalcaemia

Immediate management
• 10–20 mL 10% calcium gluconate IV over 10–20 mins • Continuous IV infusion may be required for several hours (equivalent of 10 mL 10% calcium gluconate/hr) • Cardiac monitoring is recommended
If associated hypomagnesaemia
• 50 mmol magnesium chloride IV over 24 hours • Most parenteral magnesium will be excreted in the urine, so further doses may be required to replenish body stores

Hypocalcaemia can cause papilloedema and prolongation of the ECG QT interval, which may predispose to ventricular arrhythmias. Prolonged hypocalcaemia and hyperphosphataemia (as in hypoparathyroidism) may cause calcification of the basal ganglia, grand mal epilepsy, psychosis and cataracts. Hypocalcaemia associated with hypophosphataemia, as in vitamin D deficiency, causes rickets in children and osteomalacia in adults (p. 1125).

Management

Emergency management of hypocalcaemia associated with tetany is described in Box 20.38. Treatment of chronic hypocalcaemia is described on page 770.

Primary hyperparathyroidism

Primary hyperparathyroidism is caused by autonomous secretion of PTH, usually by a single parathyroid adenoma, which can vary in diameter from a few millimetres to several centimetres. It should be distinguished from secondary hyperparathyroidism, in which there is a physiological increase in PTH secretion to compensate for prolonged hypocalcaemia (such as in vitamin D deficiency, p. 1126), and from tertiary hyperparathyroidism, in which continuous stimulation of the parathyroids over a prolonged period of time results in adenoma formation and autonomous PTH secretion (Box 20.39). This is most commonly seen in individuals with advanced chronic kidney disease (p. 483).

The prevalence of primary hyperparathyroidism is about 1 in 800 and it is 2–3 times more common in women than men; 90% of patients are over 50 years of age. It also occurs in the familial MEN syndromes (p. 795), in which case hyperplasia or multiple adenomas of all four parathyroid glands are more likely than a solitary adenoma.

Clinical and radiological features

The clinical presentation of primary hyperparathyroidism is described on page 769. Parathyroid bone disease is now rare due to earlier diagnosis and treatment. Osteitis fibrosa results from increased bone resorption by osteoclasts with fibrous replacement in the lacunae. This may present as bone pain and tenderness, fracture and deformity. Chondrocalcinosis can occur due to deposition of calcium pyrophosphate crystals within articular cartilage. It typically affects the menisci at the knees and can result in secondary degenerative arthritis or predispose to attacks of acute pseudogout

20.39 Hyperparathyroidism

Type	Serum calcium	PTH
Primary Single adenoma (90%) Multiple adenomas (4%) Nodular hyperplasia (5%) Carcinoma (1%)	Raised	Not suppressed
Secondary Chronic renal failure Malabsorption Osteomalacia and rickets	Low	Raised
Tertiary	Raised	Not suppressed

(p. 1090). Skeletal X-rays are usually normal in mild primary hyperparathyroidism, but in patients with advanced disease characteristic changes are observed. In the early stages there is demineralisation, with subperiosteal erosions and terminal resorption in the phalanges. A 'pepper-pot' appearance may be seen on lateral X-rays of the skull. Reduced bone mineral density, resulting in either osteopenia or osteoporosis, is now the most common skeletal manifestation of hyperparathyroidism. This is usually not evident radiographically and requires assessment by DEXA (p. 1065).

In nephrocalcinosis, scattered opacities may be visible within the renal outline. There may be soft tissue calcification in arterial walls and hands and in the cornea.

Investigations

The diagnosis can be confirmed by finding a raised PTH level in the presence of hypercalcaemia, provided that FHH is excluded (p. 770). Parathyroid scanning by ^{99m}Tc-sestamibi scintigraphy (Fig. 20.16) and/or ultrasound examination can be performed prior to surgery, in an attempt to localise an adenoma and allow a targeted resection. However, negative imaging does not exclude the diagnosis.

Management

The treatment of choice for primary hyperparathyroidism is surgery, with excision of a solitary parathyroid adenoma or hyperplastic glands. Experienced surgeons will identify solitary tumours in more than 90% of cases. Patients with parathyroid bone disease run a significant risk of developing hypocalcaemia postoperatively, but the risk of this can be reduced by correcting vitamin D deficiency pre-operatively.

Surgery is usually indicated for individuals aged less than 50 years, with clear-cut symptoms or documented complications (such as peptic ulceration, renal stones, renal impairment or osteoporosis), and (in asymptomatic patients) significant hypercalcaemia (corrected serum calcium > 2.85 mmol/L (> 11.4 mg/dL)). Patients who are treated conservatively without surgery should have calcium biochemistry and renal function checked annually and bone density monitored periodically. They should be encouraged to maintain a high oral fluid intake to avoid renal stones.

Occasionally, primary hyperparathyroidism presents with severe life-threatening hypercalcaemia. This is often due to dehydration and should be managed medically with intravenous fluids and bisphosphonates, as

A

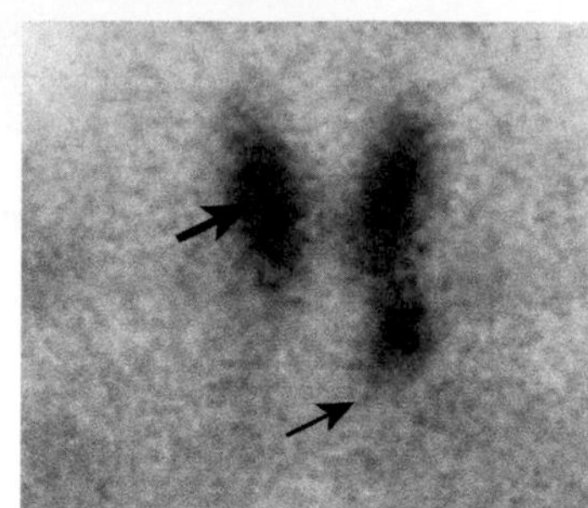

B

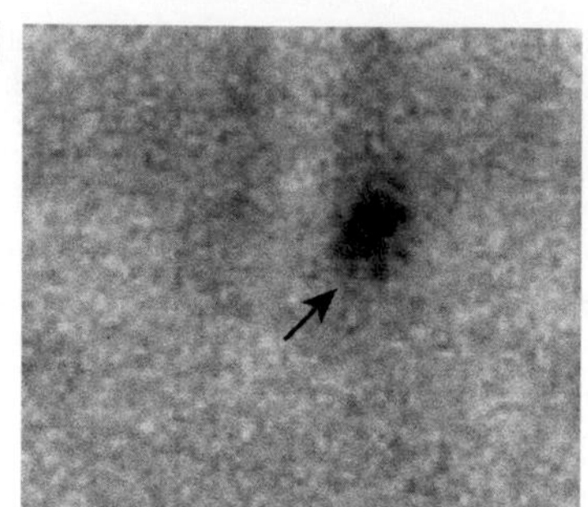

Fig. 20.16 ^{99m}Tc-sestamibi scan of a patient with primary hyperparathyroidism secondary to a parathyroid adenoma. A After 1 hour, there is uptake in the thyroid gland (thick arrow) and the enlarged left inferior parathyroid gland (thin arrow). B After 3 hours, uptake is evident only in the parathyroid.

described on page 273. If this is not effective, then urgent parathyroidectomy should be considered.

Cinacalcet is a calcimimetic which enhances the sensitivity of the calcium-sensing receptor, so reducing PTH levels, and is licensed for tertiary hyperparathyroidism and as a treatment for patients with primary hyperparathyroidism who are unwilling to have surgery or are medically unfit.

Familial hypocalciuric hypercalcaemia

This autosomal dominant disorder is caused by an inactivating mutation in one of the alleles of the calcium-sensing receptor gene, which reduces the ability of the parathyroid gland to 'sense' ionised calcium concentrations. As a result, higher than normal calcium levels are required to suppress PTH secretion. The typical presentation is with mild hypercalcaemia with PTH concentrations that are 'inappropriately' at the upper end of the reference range or are slightly elevated. Calcium-sensing receptors in the renal tubules are also affected and this leads to increased renal tubular reabsorption of calcium and hypocalciuria. The hypercalcaemia of FHH is always asymptomatic and complications do not occur. The main risk of FHH is of the patient being subjected to an unnecessary (and ineffective) parathyroidectomy if misdiagnosed as having primary hyperparathyroidism. Testing of family members for hypercalcaemia is helpful in confirming the diagnosis and it is also possible to perform genetic testing. No treatment is necessary.

Hypoparathyroidism

The most common cause of hypoparathyroidism is damage to the parathyroid glands (or their blood supply) during thyroid surgery; post-operative hypocalcaemia develops in 5.5% of patients overall but 9% of patients undergoing total thyroidectomy. Rarely, hypoparathyroidism can occur as a result of infiltration of the glands with iron in haemochromatosis (p. 972) or copper in Wilson's disease (p. 973).

There are a number of rare congenital or inherited forms of hypoparathyroidism. One form is associated with autoimmune polyendocrine syndrome type 1 (p. 795) and another with DiGeorge syndrome (p. 56). Autosomal dominant hypoparathyroidism (ADH) is the mirror image of familial hypocalciuric hypercalcaemia (see above), in that an activating mutation in the calcium-sensing receptor reduces PTH levels, resulting in hypocalcaemia and hypercalciuria.

20.40 The parathyroid glands in old age

- **Osteoporosis**: always exclude osteomalacia and hyperparathyroidism by checking vitamin D and calcium concentrations.
- **Primary hyperparathyroidism**: more common with ageing. Older people can often be observed without surgical intervention.
- **Hypercalcaemia**: may cause confusion.
- **Vitamin D deficiency**: common because of poor diet and limited exposure to the sun.

Pseudohypoparathyroidism

In this disorder, the individual is functionally hypoparathyroid but, instead of PTH deficiency, there is tissue resistance to the effects of PTH, such that PTH concentrations are markedly elevated. The PTH receptor itself is normal but the downstream signalling pathways are defective due to mutations that affect *GNAS1*, which encodes the Gsα protein, a molecule involved in signal transduction downstream of the PTH receptor and other G-protein-coupled receptors. There are several subtypes but the most common (pseudohypoparathyroidism type 1a) is characterised by hypocalcaemia and hyperphosphataemia, in association with short stature, short fourth metacarpals and metatarsals, rounded face, obesity and subcutaneous calcification; these features are collectively referred to as Albright's hereditary osteodystrophy (AHO). Type 1a pseudohypoparathyroidism occurs only when the *GNAS1* mutation is inherited on the maternal chromosome.

The term pseudopseudohypoparathyroidism is used to describe patients who have clinical features of AHO but normal serum calcium and PTH concentrations; it occurs when the *GNAS1* mutation is inherited on the paternal chromosome. The inheritance of these disorders is an example of genetic imprinting (p. 52). The difference in clinical features occurs as a result of the fact that renal cells exclusively express the maternal *GNAS1* allele, whereas both maternal and paternal alleles are expressed in other cell types; this explains why maternal inheritance is associated with hypocalcaemia and resistance to PTH (which regulates serum calcium and phosphate levels largely by an effect on the renal tubule), and why paternal inheritance is associated with skeletal and other abnormalities in the absence of hypocalcaemia and raised PTH values.

Management of hypoparathyroidism

Persistent hypoparathyroidism and pseudohypoparathyroidism are treated with oral calcium salts and vitamin D analogues, either 1α-hydroxycholecalciferol (alfacalcidol) or 1,25-dihydroxycholecalciferol (calcitriol). This therapy needs careful monitoring because of the risks of iatrogenic hypercalcaemia, hypercalciuria and nephrocalcinosis. Recombinant PTH is available as subcutaneous injection therapy for osteoporosis (p. 1120) and, although not currently licensed, has been used in hypoparathyroidism (but not in pseudohypoparathyroidism). It is much more expensive than calcium and vitamin D analogue therapy but has the advantage that it is less likely to cause hypercalciuria. There is no specific treatment for AHO other than to try to maintain calcium levels within the reference range using active vitamin D metabolites.

THE ADRENAL GLANDS

The adrenals comprise several separate endocrine glands within a single anatomical structure. The adrenal medulla is an extension of the sympathetic nervous system which secretes catecholamines into capillaries rather than synapses. Most of the adrenal cortex is made up of cells which secrete cortisol and adrenal androgens, and form part of the hypothalamic–pituitary–adrenal (HPA) axis. The small outer glomerulosa of the cortex secretes aldosterone under the control of the renin–angiotensin system. These functions are important in the integrated control of cardiovascular, metabolic and immune responses to stress.

There is increasing evidence that subtle alterations in adrenal function contribute to the pathogenesis of common diseases such as hypertension, obesity and type 2 diabetes mellitus. However, classical syndromes of adrenal hormone deficiency and excess are relatively rare.

Functional anatomy and physiology

Adrenal anatomy and function are shown in Figure 20.17. Histologically, the cortex is divided into three zones, but these function as two units (zona glomerulosa and zonae fasciculata/reticularis) which produce

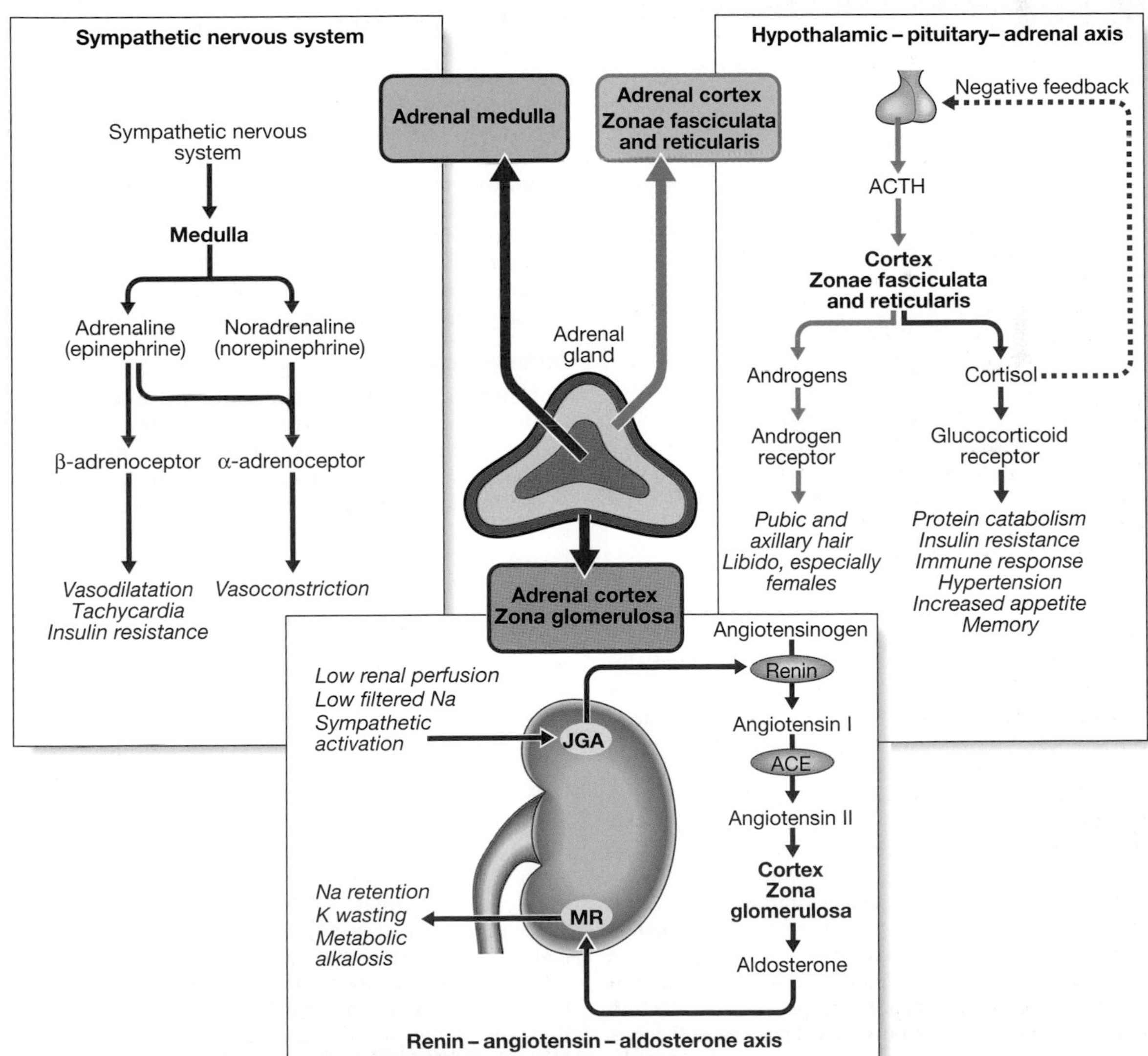

Fig. 20.17 Structure and function of the adrenal glands. (ACE = angiotensin-converting enzyme; ACTH = adrenocorticotrophic hormone; JGA = juxtaglomerular apparatus; MR = mineralocorticoid receptor).

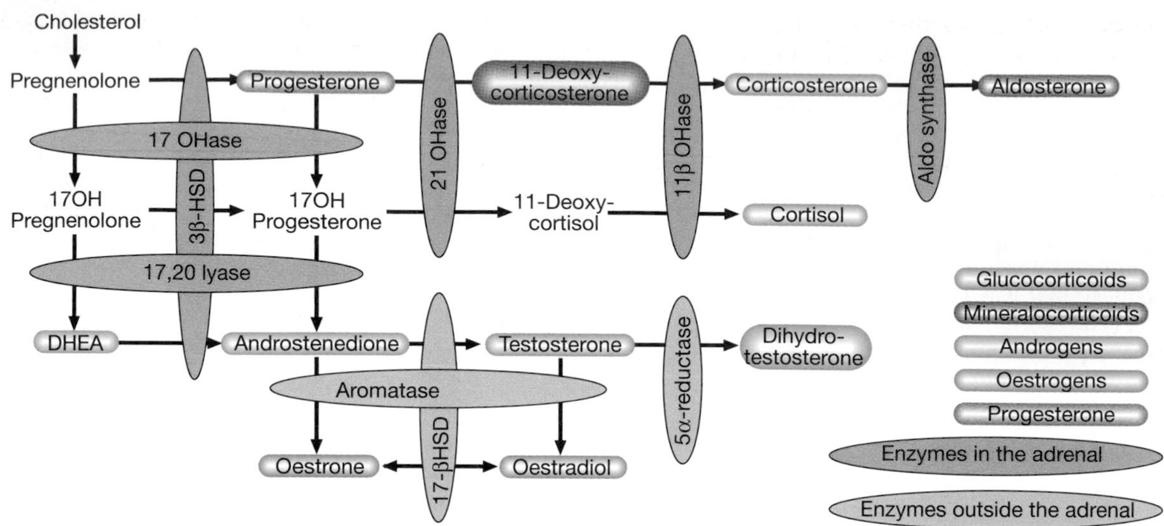

Fig. 20.18 The major pathways of synthesis of steroid hormones. (DHEA = dehydroepiandrosterone; HSD = hydroxysteroid dehydrogenase; OHase = hydroxylase)

20.41 Classification of diseases of the adrenal glands

	Primary	Secondary
Hormone excess	Non-ACTH-dependent Cushing's syndrome Primary hyperaldosteronism Phaeochromocytoma	ACTH-dependent Cushing's syndrome Secondary hyperaldosteronism
Hormone deficiency	Addison's disease Congenital adrenal hyperplasia	Hypopituitarism
Hormone hypersensitivity	11 β-hydroxysteroid dehydrogenase type 2 deficiency Liddle's syndrome	
Hormone resistance	Pseudohypoaldosteronism Glucocorticoid resistance syndrome	
Non-functioning tumours	Adenoma Carcinoma (usually functioning) Metastatic tumours	

corticosteroids in response to humoral stimuli. Pathways for the biosynthesis of corticosteroids are shown in Figure 20.18. Investigation of adrenal function is described under specific diseases below. The different types of adrenal disease are shown in Box 20.41.

Glucocorticoids

Cortisol is the major glucocorticoid in humans. Levels are highest in the morning on waking and lowest in the middle of the night. Cortisol rises dramatically during stress, including any illness. This elevation protects key metabolic functions (such as the maintenance of cerebral glucose supply during starvation) and inhibits potentially damaging inflammatory responses to infection and injury. The clinical importance of cortisol deficiency is, therefore, most obvious at times of stress.

More than 95% of circulating cortisol is bound to protein, principally cortisol-binding globulin, which is increased by oestrogens. It is the free fraction that is biologically active. Cortisol regulates cell function by binding to glucocorticoid receptors that regulate the transcription of many genes. Cortisol can also activate mineralocorticoid receptors, but it does not normally do so because most cells containing mineralocorticoid receptors also express an enzyme called 11 β-hydroxysteroid dehydrogenase type 2 (11 β-HSD2), which inactivates cortisol by converting it to cortisone. Inhibitors of 11 β-HSD2 (such as liquorice) or mutations in the gene that encodes 11 β-HSD2 cause cortisol to act as a mineralocorticoid, resulting in sodium retention and hypertension (see Box 20.50, p. 780).

Mineralocorticoids

Aldosterone is the most important mineralocorticoid. It binds to mineralocorticoid receptors in the kidney and causes sodium retention and increased excretion of potassium and protons (Ch. 16). The principal stimulus to aldosterone secretion is angiotensin II, a peptide produced by activation of the renin–angiotensin system (see Fig. 20.17). Renin activity in the juxtaglomerular apparatus of the kidney is stimulated by low perfusion pressure in the afferent arteriole, low sodium filtration leading to low sodium concentrations at the macula densa, or increased sympathetic nerve activity. As a result, renin activity is increased in hypovolaemia and renal artery stenosis, and is approximately doubled when standing up from a recumbent position.

Catecholamines

In humans, only a small proportion of circulating noradrenaline (norepinephrine) is derived from the adrenal medulla; much more is released from sympathetic nerve endings. Conversion of noradrenaline to adrenaline (epinephrine) is catalysed by catechol-o-methyltransferase (COMT), which is induced by glucocorticoids. Blood flow in the adrenal is centripetal, so that the medulla is bathed in high concentrations of cortisol and is the major source of circulating adrenaline. However, after surgical removal of the adrenal medullae, there appear to be no clinical consequences attributable to deficiency of circulating catecholamines.

Adrenal androgens

Adrenal androgens are secreted in response to ACTH and are the most abundant steroids in the blood stream. They are probably important in the initiation of puberty (adrenarche). The adrenals are also the major source of androgens in adult females and may be important in female libido.

Presenting problems in adrenal disease

Cushing's syndrome

Cushing's syndrome is caused by excessive activation of glucocorticoid receptors. It is most commonly iatrogenic, due to prolonged administration of synthetic glucocorticoids such as prednisolone. Endogenous Cushing's syndrome is uncommon but is due to chronic over-production of cortisol by the adrenal glands, either as the result of an adrenal tumour or because of excessive production of ACTH by a pituitary tumour or ectopic ACTH production by other tumours.

Aetiology

The causes are shown in Box 20.42. Amongst endogenous causes, pituitary-dependent cortisol excess (by convention, called Cushing's disease) accounts for approximately 80% of cases. Both Cushing's disease and cortisol-secreting adrenal tumours are four times more common in women than men. In contrast, ectopic ACTH syndrome (often due to a small-cell carcinoma of the bronchus) is more common in men.

Clinical assessment

The diverse manifestations of glucocorticoid excess are shown in Figure 20.19. Many of these are not specific to Cushing's syndrome and, because spontaneous Cushing's syndrome is rare, the positive predictive

20.42 Classification of endogenous Cushing's syndrome

ACTH-dependent – 80%
• Pituitary adenoma secreting ACTH (Cushing's disease) – 70% • Ectopic ACTH syndrome (bronchial carcinoid, small-cell lung carcinoma, other neuro-endocrine tumour) – 10%
Non-ACTH-dependent – 20%
• Adrenal adenoma – 15% • Adrenal carcinoma – 5% • ACTH-independent macronodular hyperplasia; primary pigmented nodular adrenal disease; McCune–Albright syndrome (together < 1%)
Hypercortisolism due to other causes (also referred to as pseudo-Cushing's syndrome)
• Alcohol excess (biochemical and clinical features) • Major depressive illness (biochemical features only, some clinical overlap) • Primary obesity (mild biochemical features, some clinical overlap)

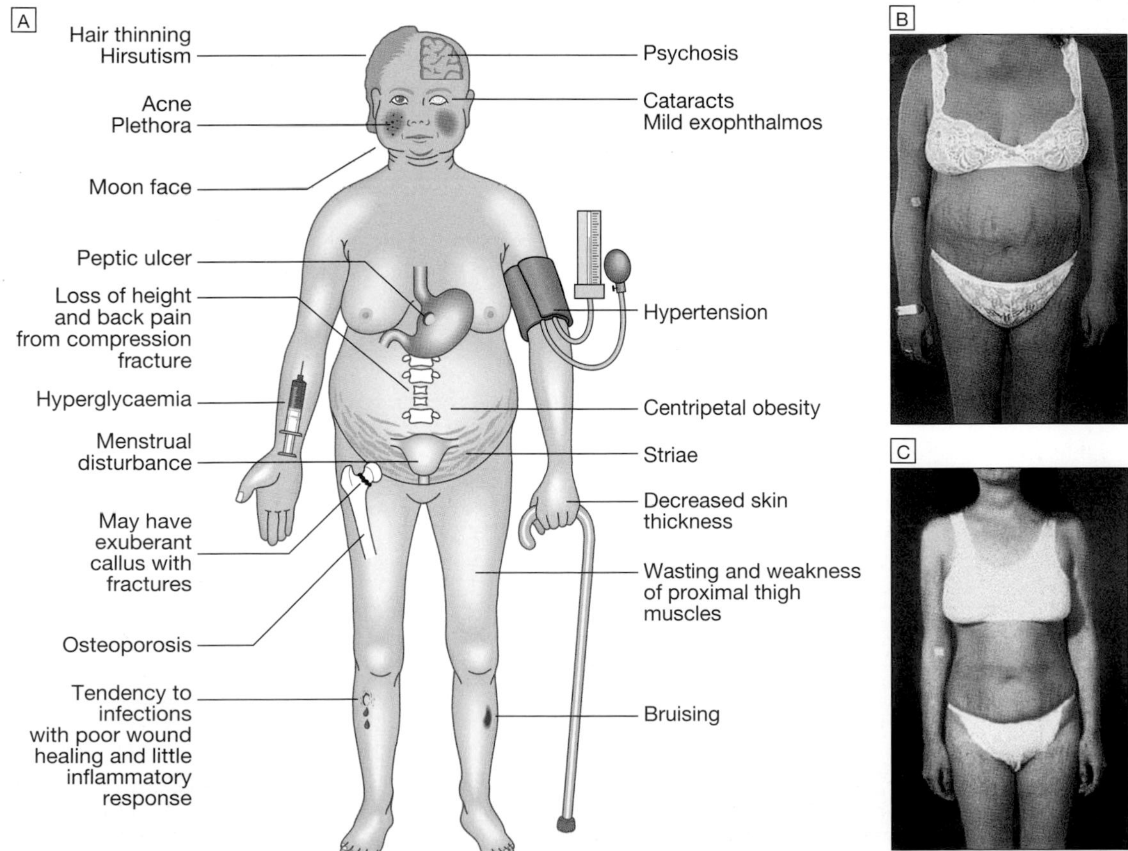

Fig. 20.19 Cushing's syndrome. **A** Clinical features common to all causes. **B** A patient with Cushing's disease before treatment. **C** The same patient 1 year after the successful removal of an ACTH-secreting pituitary microadenoma by trans-sphenoidal surgery.

value of any single clinical feature alone is low. Moreover, some common disorders can be confused with Cushing's syndrome because they are associated with alterations in cortisol secretion: for example, obesity and depression (see Box 20.42). Features which favour Cushing's syndrome in an obese patient are bruising, myopathy and thin skin. Any clinical suspicion of cortisol excess is best resolved by further investigation.

It is vital to exclude iatrogenic causes in all patients with Cushing's syndrome since even inhaled or topical glucocorticoids can induce the syndrome in susceptible individuals. A careful drug history must therefore be taken before embarking on complex investigations.

Some clinical features are more common in ectopic ACTH syndrome. Whilst ACTH-secreting pituitary tumours retain some negative feedback sensitivity to cortisol, this is absent in tumours that produce ectopic ACTH, typically resulting in higher levels of both ACTH and cortisol than are observed in pituitary-driven disease. The high ACTH levels are associated with marked pigmentation because of binding to melanocortin 1 receptors on melanocytes in the skin. The high cortisol levels also overcome the capacity of 11 β-HSD2 to inactivate cortisol in the kidney (p. 772), causing hypokalaemic alkalosis which aggravates myopathy and hyperglycaemia (by inhibiting insulin secretion). When the tumour that is secreting ACTH is malignant, then the onset is usually rapid and may be associated with cachexia. For these reasons, the classical features of Cushing's syndrome are less common in ectopic ACTH syndrome; if present, they suggest that a less aggressive tumour, such as a bronchial carcinoid, is responsible.

In Cushing's disease, the pituitary tumour is usually a microadenoma (< 10 mm in diameter); hence other features of a pituitary macroadenoma (hypopituitarism, visual failure or disconnection hyperprolactinaemia, p. 787) are rare.

Investigations

The large number of tests available for Cushing's syndrome reflects the fact that each one has limited specificity and sensitivity in isolation. Accordingly, several tests are usually combined to establish the diagnosis. Testing for Cushing's syndrome should be avoided under conditions of stress, such as an acute illness, because this activates the HPA axis, causing potentially spurious results. The diagnosis of Cushing's is a two-step process:

1. to establish whether the patient has Cushing's syndrome (Fig. 20.20)
2. to define its cause (Fig. 20.21).

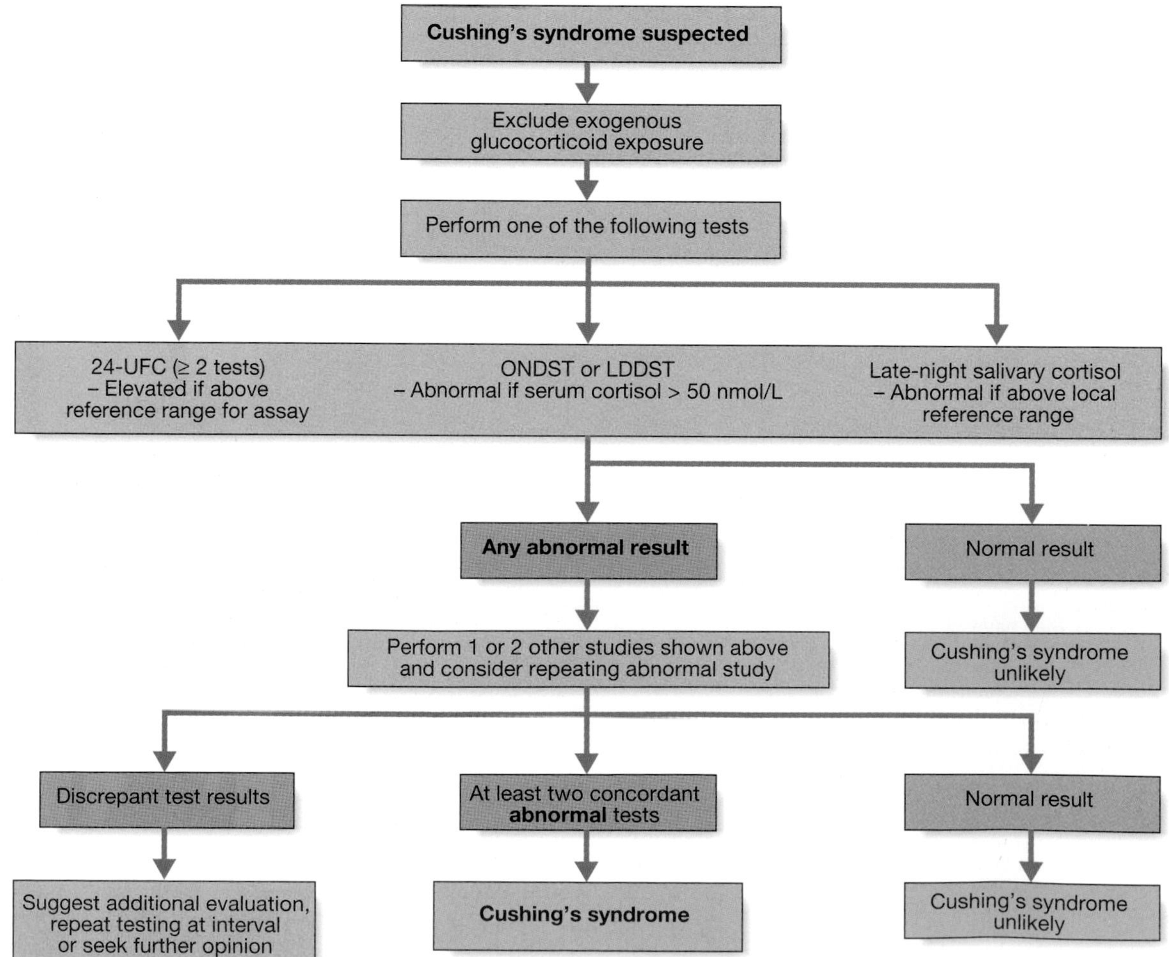

Fig. 20.20 Sequence of investigations in suspected spontaneous Cushing's syndrome. A serum cortisol of 50 nmol/L is equivalent to 1.81 μg/dL. (LDDST = low-dose dexamethasone suppression test; ONDST = overnight dexamethasone suppression test; UFC = urinary free cortisol)

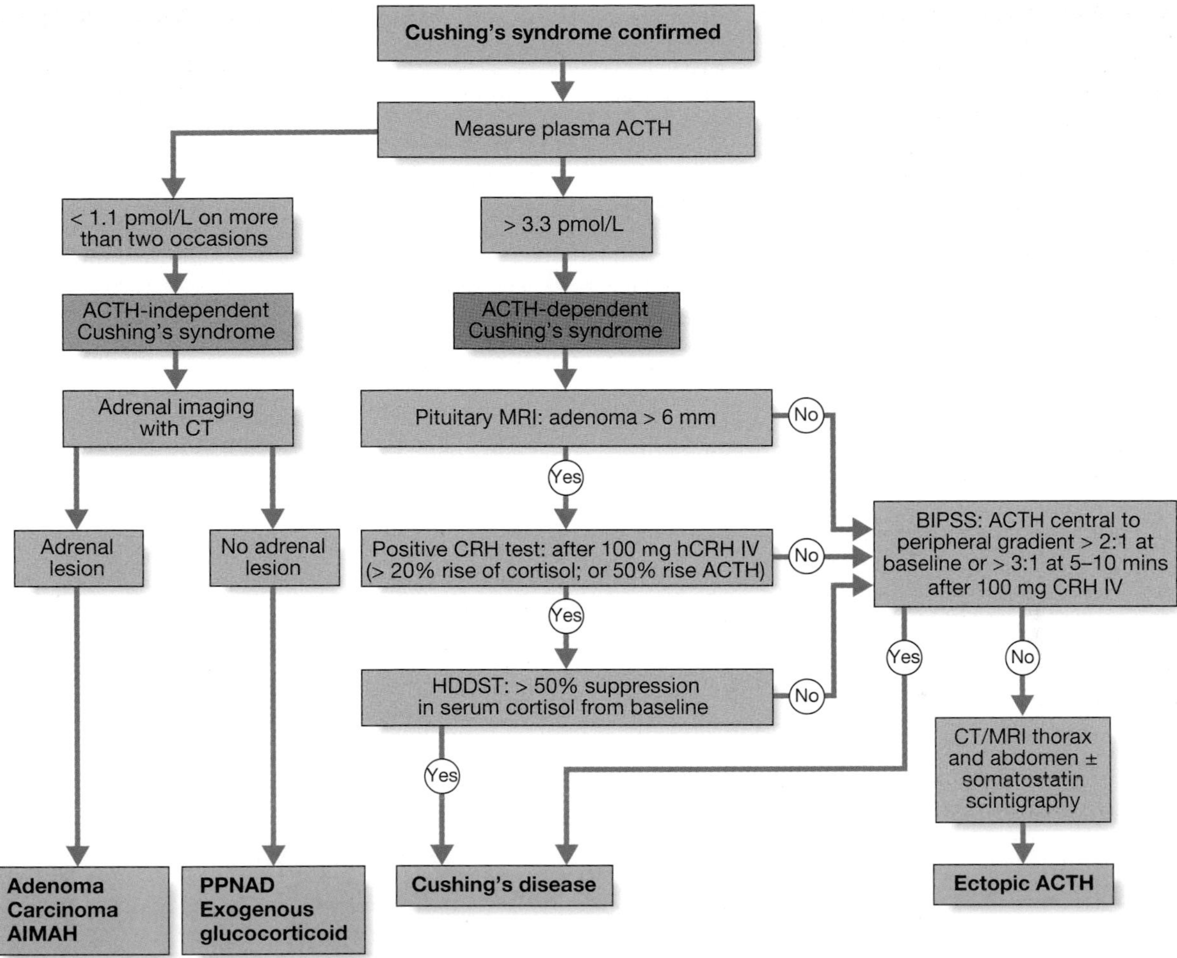

Fig. 20.21 Determining the cause of confirmed Cushing's syndrome. To convert pmol/L to ng/L, multiply by 4.541. (ACTH = adrenocorticotrophic hormone; AIMAH = ACTH-independent macronodular adrenal hyperplasia; BIPSS = bilateral inferior petrosal sinus sampling; CRH = corticotrophin-releasing hormone; HDDST = high-dose dexamethasone suppression test; PPNAD = primary pigmented nodular adrenal disease)

Some additional tests are useful in all cases of Cushing's syndrome, including plasma electrolytes, glucose, glycosylated haemoglobin and bone mineral density measurement.

Establishing the presence of Cushing's syndrome

Cushing's syndrome is confirmed by using two of three main tests:

1. failure to suppress serum cortisol with low doses of oral dexamethasone
2. loss of the normal circadian rhythm of cortisol, with inappropriately elevated late-night serum or salivary cortisol
3. increased 24-hour urine free cortisol (see Fig. 20.20).

Dexamethasone is used for suppression testing because it does not cross-react in radioimmunoassays for cortisol. An overnight dexamethasone suppression test (ONDST) involves administration of 1 mg dexamethasone at 2300 hrs and measuring serum cortisol at 0900 hrs the following day. In a low-dose dexamethasone suppression test (LDDST), serum cortisol is measured following administration of 0.5 mg dexamethasone 4 times daily for 48 hours. It is important for any oestrogens to be stopped for 6 weeks prior to investigation to allow corticosteroid-binding globulin (CBG) levels to return to normal and to avoid false-positive responses, as most cortisol assays measure total cortisol, including that bound to CBG. Cyclicity of cortisol secretion is a feature of all types of Cushing's syndrome and, if very variable, can confuse diagnosis. Use of multiple salivary cortisol samples over weeks or months can be of use in diagnosis, but an elevated salivary cortisol alone should not be taken as proof of diagnosis. In iatrogenic Cushing's syndrome, cortisol levels are low unless the patient is taking a corticosteroid (such as prednisolone) that cross-reacts in immunoassays with cortisol.

Determining the underlying cause

Once the presence of Cushing's syndrome is confirmed, measurement of plasma ACTH is the key to establishing the differential diagnosis. In the presence of excess cortisol secretion, an undetectable ACTH (below 1.1 pmol/L (5 pg/mL)) indicates an adrenal cause, while ACTH levels greater than 3.3 pmol/L (15 pg/mL) suggest a pituitary cause or ectopic ACTH. ACTH levels between these values represent a 'grey area', and further evaluation by a specialist is required. Tests to discriminate pituitary from ectopic sources of ACTH rely on the fact that pituitary tumours, but not ectopic tumours, retain some features of normal regulation of ACTH secretion. Thus, in pituitary-dependent Cushing's disease, ACTH secretion is suppressed by high-dose dexamethasone and ACTH is stimulated by corticotrophin-releasing hormone (CRH). In a high-dose dexamethasone suppression test (HDDST), serum cortisol is measured before and after administration of 2 mg of dexamethasone 4 times daily for 48 hours.

Techniques for localisation of tumours secreting ACTH or cortisol are listed in Figure 20.21. MRI detects around 60% of pituitary microadenomas secreting ACTH. If available, bilateral inferior petrosal sinus sampling (BIPSS) with measurement of ACTH is the best means of confirming Cushing's disease, unless MRI shows a tumour bigger than 6 mm. CT or MRI detects most adrenal tumours; adrenal carcinomas are usually large (> 5 cm) and have other features of malignancy (p. 779).

Management

Untreated severe Cushing's syndrome has a 50% 5-year mortality. Most patients are treated surgically, but medical therapy may be given in severe cases for a few weeks prior to operation to improve the clinical state. A number of drugs are used to inhibit corticosteroid biosynthesis, including metyrapone and ketoconazole. The dose of these agents is best titrated against serum cortisol levels or 24-hour urine free cortisol.

Cushing's disease

Trans-sphenoidal surgery carried out by an experienced surgeon with selective removal of the adenoma is the treatment of choice, with approximately 70% of patients going into immediate remission. Around 20% of patients suffer a recurrence, often years later, emphasising the need for life-long follow-up.

Laparoscopic bilateral adrenalectomy performed by an expert surgeon effectively cures ACTH-dependent Cushing's syndrome, but in patients with pituitary-dependent Cushing's syndrome, this can result in Nelson's syndrome, with an invasive pituitary macroadenoma and very high ACTH levels causing pigmentation. The risk of Nelson's syndrome may be reduced by pituitary irradiation.

Adrenal tumours

Laparoscopic adrenal surgery is the treatment of choice for adrenal adenomas. Surgery offers the only prospect of cure for adrenocortical carcinomas, but in general, prognosis is poor with high rates of recurrence, even in patients with localised disease at presentation. Radiotherapy to the tumour bed reduces the risk of local recurrence, and systemic therapy consists of the adrenolytic drug mitotane and chemotherapy, but responses are often poor.

Ectopic ACTH syndrome

Localised tumours, such as bronchial carcinoid, should be removed surgically. In patients with incurable malignancy, it is important to reduce the severity of the Cushing's syndrome using medical therapy (see above) or, if appropriate, bilateral adrenalectomy.

Therapeutic use of glucocorticoids

The remarkable anti-inflammatory properties of glucocorticoids have led to their use in a wide variety of clinical conditions but the hazards are significant. Equivalent doses of commonly used glucocorticoids are listed in Box 20.43. Topical preparations (dermal, rectal and inhaled) can also be absorbed into the systemic circulation, and although this rarely occurs to a sufficient degree to produce clinical features of Cushing's syndrome, it can result in significant suppression of endogenous ACTH and cortisol secretion. Severe Cushing's syndrome can result if there is concomitant administration of inhaled glucocorticoids and inhibitors of the liver enzyme CYP450 3A4, such as the antiretroviral drug ritonavir (p. 407).

Adverse effects of glucocorticoids

The clinical features of glucocorticoid excess are illustrated in Figure 20.19. Adverse effects are related to dose, duration of therapy, and pre-existing conditions that might be worsened by corticosteroid therapy, such as diabetes mellitus or osteoporosis. Osteoporosis is a particularly important problem because, for a given bone mineral density, the fracture risk is greater in glucocorticoid-treated patients than in post-menopausal osteoporosis. Therefore, when systemic glucocorticoids are prescribed and the anticipated duration of steroid therapy is more than 3 months, bone-protective therapy should be considered, as detailed on page 1102. Rapid changes in glucocorticoid levels can also lead to marked mood disturbances, including depression, mania and insomnia.

The anti-inflammatory effect of glucocorticoids may mask signs of disease. For example, perforation of a viscus may be masked and the patient may show no febrile response to an infection. Although there is debate about whether or not corticosteroids increase the risk of peptic ulcer when used alone, they act synergistically with NSAIDs, including aspirin, to increase the risk of serious gastrointestinal adverse effects. Latent tuberculosis may be re-activated and patients on corticosteroids should be advised to avoid contact with varicella zoster virus if they are not immune.

Management of glucocorticoid withdrawal

All glucocorticoid therapy, even if inhaled or applied topically, can suppress the HPA axis. In practice, this is only likely to result in a crisis due to adrenal insufficiency on withdrawal of treatment if glucocorticoids have been administered orally or systemically for longer than 3 weeks, if repeated courses have been prescribed within the previous year, or if the dose is higher than the equivalent of 7.5 mg prednisolone per day. In these circumstances, the drug, when it is no longer required for the underlying condition, must be withdrawn slowly at a rate dictated by the duration of treatment. If

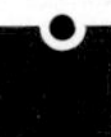

20.43 Approximate equivalent doses of glucocorticoids

- Hydrocortisone: 20 mg
- Cortisone acetate: 25 mg
- Prednisolone: 5 mg
- Dexamethasone: 0.5 mg

20.44 Advice to patients on glucocorticoid replacement therapy

Intercurrent stress
- Febrile illness: double dose of hydrocortisone

Surgery
- Minor operation: hydrocortisone 100 mg IM with pre-medication
- Major operation: hydrocortisone 100 mg 4 times daily for 24 hrs, then 50 mg IM 4 times daily until ready to take tablets

Vomiting
- Patients must have parenteral hydrocortisone if unable to take it by mouth

Steroid card
- Patient should carry this at all times; it should give information regarding diagnosis, steroid, dose and doctor

Bracelet and emergency pack
- Patients should be encouraged to buy one of these and have it engraved with the diagnosis, current treatment and a reference number for a central database
- Patients should be given a hydrocortisone emergency pack and trained in the self-administration of hydrocortisone 100 mg IM; they should be advised to take the pack on holidays/trips abroad

glucocorticoid therapy has been prolonged, then it may take many months for the HPA axis to recover. All patients must be advised to avoid sudden drug withdrawal. They should be issued with a steroid card and/or wear an engraved bracelet (Box 20.44).

Recovery of the HPA axis is aided if there is no exogenous glucocorticoid present during the nocturnal surge in ACTH secretion. This can be achieved by giving glucocorticoid in the morning. Giving ACTH to stimulate adrenal recovery is of no value, as the pituitary remains suppressed.

In patients who have received glucocorticoids for longer than a few weeks, it is often valuable to confirm that the HPA axis is recovering during glucocorticoid withdrawal. Once the dose of glucocorticoid is reduced to a minimum (e.g. 4 mg prednisolone or 0.5 mg dexamethasone per day), then measure plasma cortisol at 0900 hrs before the next dose. If this is detectable, then perform an ACTH stimulation test (see Box 20.47) to confirm that glucocorticoids can be withdrawn completely. Even once glucocorticoids have been successfully withdrawn, short-term replacement therapy is often advised during significant intercurrent illness occurring in subsequent months, as the HPA axis may not be able to respond fully to severe stress.

Adrenal insufficiency

Adrenal insufficiency results from inadequate secretion of cortisol and/or aldosterone. It is potentially fatal and notoriously variable in its presentation. A high index of suspicion is therefore required in patients with unexplained fatigue, hyponatraemia or hypotension. Causes are shown in Box 20.45. The most common is ACTH deficiency (secondary adrenocortical failure), usually because of inappropriate withdrawal of chronic glucocorticoid therapy or a pituitary tumour (p. 789).

20.45 Causes of adrenocortical insufficiency

Secondary (↓ACTH)
- Withdrawal of suppressive glucocorticoid therapy
- Hypothalamic or pituitary disease

Primary (↑ACTH)

Addison's disease

Common causes	*Rare causes*
• Autoimmune Sporadic Polyglandular syndromes (p. 795) • Tuberculosis • HIV/AIDS • Metastatic carcinoma • Bilateral adrenalectomy	• Lymphoma • Intra-adrenal haemorrhage (Waterhouse–Friedrichsen syndrome following meningococcal septicaemia) • Amyloidosis • Haemochromatosis

Corticosteroid biosynthetic enzyme defects
- Congenital adrenal hyperplasias
- Drugs
  Metyrapone, ketoconazole, etomidate

20

Congenital adrenal hyperplasias and Addison's disease (primary adrenocortical failure) are rare causes.

Clinical assessment

The clinical features of adrenal insufficiency are shown in Box 20.46. In Addison's disease, either glucocorticoid or mineralocorticoid deficiency may come first, but eventually all patients fail to secrete both classes of corticosteroid.

Patients may present with chronic features and/or in acute circulatory shock. With a chronic presentation, initial symptoms are often misdiagnosed as chronic fatigue syndrome or depression. Adrenocortical insufficiency should also be considered in patients with hyponatraemia, even in the absence of symptoms (p. 437).

Features of an acute adrenal crisis include circulatory shock with severe hypotension, hyponatraemia, hyperkalaemia and, in some instances, hypoglycaemia and hypercalcaemia. Muscle cramps, nausea, vomiting, diarrhoea and unexplained fever may be present. The crisis is often precipitated by intercurrent disease, surgery or infection.

Vitiligo occurs in 10–20% of patients with autoimmune Addison's disease (p. 734).

Investigations

Treatment should not be delayed to wait for results in patients with suspected acute adrenal crisis. Here, a random blood sample should be stored for subsequent measurement of cortisol and, if the patient's clinical condition permits, it may be appropriate to spend 30 minutes performing a short ACTH stimulation test (Box 20.47) before administering hydrocortisone. Investigations should be performed before treatment is given in patients who present with features suggestive of chronic adrenal insufficiency.

Assessment of glucocorticoids

Random plasma cortisol is usually low in patients with adrenal insufficiency but it may be within the reference

20.46 Clinical and biochemical features of adrenal insufficiency

	Glucocorticoid insufficiency	Mineralocorticoid insufficiency	ACTH excess	Adrenal androgen insufficiency
Withdrawal of exogenous glucocorticoid	+	–	–	+
Hypopituitarism	+	–	–	+
Addison's disease	+	+	+	+
Congenital adrenal hyperplasia (21 OHase deficiency)	+	+	+	–
Clinical features	Weight loss, anorexia Malaise, weakness Nausea, vomiting Diarrhoea or constipation Postural hypotension Shock Hypoglycaemia Hyponatraemia (dilutional) Hypercalcaemia	Hypotension Shock Hyponatraemia (depletional) Hyperkalaemia	Pigmentation of: Sun-exposed areas Pressure areas (e.g. elbows, knees) Palmar creases, knuckles Mucous membranes Conjunctivae Recent scars	Decreased body hair and loss of libido, especially in female

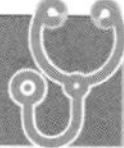

20.47 How and when to do an ACTH stimulation test

Use

- Diagnosis of primary or secondary adrenal insufficiency
- Assessment of HPA axis in patients taking suppressive glucocorticoid therapy
- Relies on ACTH-dependent adrenal atrophy in secondary adrenal insufficiency, so may not detect acute ACTH deficiency (for example, in pituitary apoplexy, p. 789)

Dose

- 250 μg $ACTH_{1-24}$ (Synacthen) by IM injection at any time of day

Blood samples

- 0 and 30 mins for plasma cortisol
- 0 mins also for ACTH (on ice) if Addison's disease is being considered (patient not known to have pituitary disease or to be taking exogenous glucocorticoids)

Results

- Normal subjects: plasma cortisol > 500 nmol/L (~18 μg/dL)* either at baseline or at 30 mins
- Incremental change in cortisol is not a criterion

*The exact cortisol concentration depends on the cortisol assay being used.

range, yet inappropriately low, for a seriously ill patient. Random measurement of plasma cortisol cannot therefore be used to confirm or refute the diagnosis, unless the value is above 500 nmol/L (> 18 μg/dL), which effectively excludes adrenal insufficiency.

More useful is the short ACTH stimulation test (also called the tetracosactrin or short Synacthen test) described in Box 20.47. Cortisol levels fail to increase in response to exogenous ACTH in patients with primary or secondary adrenal insufficiency. These can be distinguished by measurement of ACTH (which is low in ACTH deficiency and high in Addison's disease).

Assessment of mineralocorticoids

Mineralocorticoid secretion in patients with suspected Addison's disease cannot be adequately assessed by electrolyte measurements since hyponatraemia occurs in both aldosterone and cortisol deficiency (see Box 20.46 and p. 437). Hyperkalaemia is common, but not universal, in aldosterone deficiency. Plasma renin and aldosterone should be measured in the supine position. In mineralocorticoid deficiency, plasma renin activity is high, with plasma aldosterone being either low or in the lower part of the reference range.

Assessment of adrenal androgens

This is not necessary in men because testosterone from the testes is the principal androgen. In women, dehydroepiandrosterone (DHEA) and androstenedione may be measured in a random specimen of blood, though levels are highest in the morning.

Other tests to establish the cause

Patients with unexplained secondary adrenocortical insufficiency should be investigated as described on page 786. In patients with elevated ACTH, further tests are required to establish the cause of Addison's disease. Adrenal autoantibodies are frequently positive in autoimmune adrenal failure. If antibody tests are negative, imaging of the adrenal glands with CT or MRI is indicated. Tuberculosis causes adrenal calcification, visible on plain X-ray or ultrasound scan. An HIV test should be performed if risk factors for infection are present (p. 391). Adrenal metastases are a rare cause of adrenal insufficiency. Patients with evidence of autoimmune adrenal failure should be screened for other organ-specific autoimmune diseases, such as thyroid disease, pernicious anaemia and type 1 diabetes.

Management

Patients with adrenocortical insufficiency always need glucocorticoid replacement therapy and usually, but

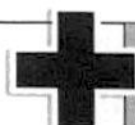

20.48 Management of adrenal crisis

Correct volume depletion

- IV saline as required to normalise blood pressure and pulse
- In severe hyponatraemia (< 125 mmol/L) avoid increases of plasma Na > 10 mmol/L/day to prevent pontine demyelination (p. 437)
- Fludrocortisone is not required during the acute phase of treatment

Replace glucocorticoids

- IV hydrocortisone succinate 100 mg stat, and 100 mg 4 times daily for first 12–24 hours
- Continue parenteral hydrocortisone (50–100 mg IM 4 times daily) until patient is well enough for reliable oral therapy

Correct other metabolic abnormalities

- Acute hypoglycaemia: IV 10% glucose
- Hyperkalaemia: should respond to volume replacement but occasionally requires specific therapy (see Box 16.17, p. 443)

Identify and treat underlying cause

- Consider acute precipitant, such as infection
- Consider adrenal or pituitary pathology (see Box 20.45)

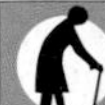

20.49 Glucocorticoids in old age

- **Adrenocortical insufficiency**: often insidious and difficult to spot.
- **Glucocorticoid therapy**: especially hazardous in older people, who are already relatively immunocompromised and susceptible to osteoporosis, diabetes, hypertension and other complications.
- **'Physiological' glucocorticoid replacement therapy**: increased risk of adrenal crisis because compliance may be poor and there is a greater incidence of intercurrent illness. Patient and carer education, with regular reinforcement of the principles described in Box 20.44, is crucial.

not always, mineralocorticoid therapy. There is some evidence that adrenal androgen replacement may also be beneficial in women. Other treatments depend on the underlying cause. The emergency management of adrenal crisis is described in Box 20.48.

Glucocorticoid replacement

Adrenal replacement therapy consists of oral hydrocortisone (cortisol) 15–20 mg daily in divided doses, typically 10 mg on waking and 5 mg at around 1500 hrs. These are physiological replacement doses which should not cause Cushingoid side-effects. The dose may need to be adjusted for the individual patient but this is subjective. Excess weight gain usually indicates over-replacement, whilst persistent lethargy or hyperpigmentation may be due to an inadequate dose or lack of absorption. Measurement of plasma cortisol levels is not usually helpful. Advice to patients dependent on glucocorticoid replacement is given in Box 20.44.

Mineralocorticoid replacement

Fludrocortisone (9α-fluoro-hydrocortisone) is administered at the usual dose of 0.05–0.15 mg daily, and adequacy of replacement may be assessed by measurement of blood pressure, plasma electrolytes and plasma renin.

Androgen replacement

Androgen replacement with DHEA (50 mg/day) is occasionally given to women with primary adrenal insufficiency who have symptoms of reduced libido and fatigue, but the evidence in support of this is not robust and treatment may be associated with side-effects such as acne and hirsutism.

Incidental adrenal mass

It is not uncommon for a mass in the adrenal gland to be identified on a CT or MRI scan of the abdomen that has been performed for another indication. Such lesions are known as adrenal 'incidentalomas'. They are present in up to 10% of adults and the prevalence increases with age.

Eighty-five per cent of adrenal incidentalomas are non-functioning adrenal adenomas. The remainder includes functional tumours of the adrenal cortex (secreting cortisol, aldosterone or androgens), phaeochromocytomas, primary and secondary carcinomas, hamartomas and other rare disorders, including granulomatous infiltrations.

Clinical assessment and investigations

There are two key questions to be resolved: is the lesion secreting hormones, and is it benign or malignant?

Patients with an adrenal incidentaloma are usually asymptomatic. However, clinical signs and symptoms of excess glucocorticoids (p. 772), mineralocorticoids (see below), catecholamines (p. 781) and, in women, androgens (p. 763) should be sought. Investigations should include a dexamethasone suppression test, urine or plasma metanephrines and, in virilised women, measurement of serum testosterone, DHEA and androstenedione. Patients with hypertension should be investigated for mineralocorticoid excess, as described below.

CT and MRI are equally effective in assessing the malignant potential of an adrenal mass, using the following parameters:

- *Size.* The larger the lesion, the greater the malignant potential. Around 90% of adrenocortical carcinomas are over 4 cm in diameter, but specificity is poor since only approximately 25% of such lesions are malignant.
- *Configuration.* Homogeneous and smooth lesions are more likely to be benign. The presence of metastatic lesions elsewhere increases the risk of malignancy, but as many as two-thirds of adrenal incidentalomas in patients with cancer are benign.
- *Presence of lipid.* Adenomas are usually lipid-rich, resulting in an attenuation of below 10 Hounsfield Units (HU) on an unenhanced CT, and in signal dropout on chemical shift MRI.
- *Enhancement.* Benign lesions demonstrate rapid washout of contrast, whereas malignant lesions tend to retain contrast.

Histology in a sample obtained by CT-guided biopsy is rarely indicated, and is not useful in distinguishing an adrenal adenoma from an adrenal carcinoma. Biopsy is occasionally helpful in confirming adrenal metastases from other cancers, but should be avoided if either phaeochromocytoma or primary adrenal cancer is suspected in order to avoid precipitation of a hypertensive crisis or seeding of tumour cells, respectively.

Management

Functional lesions and tumours of more than 4 cm in diameter should be considered for removal by adrenal surgery. In patients with radiologically benign, non-functioning lesions of less than 4 cm in diameter, surgery is only required if serial imaging suggests tumour growth. Optimal management of patients with low-grade cortisol secretion, as demonstrated by the dexamethasone suppression test, remains to be established.

Primary hyperaldosteronism

Estimates of the prevalence of primary hyperaldosteronism vary according to the screening tests employed, but it may occur in as many as 10% of people with hypertension. Indications to test for mineralocorticoid excess in hypertensive patients include hypokalaemia (including hypokalaemia induced by thiazide diuretics), poor control of blood pressure with conventional therapy, a family history of early-onset hypertension, or presentation at a young age.

Causes of excessive activation of mineralocorticoid receptors are shown in Box 20.50. It is important to differentiate primary hyperaldosteronism, caused by an intrinsic abnormality of the adrenal glands resulting in aldosterone excess, from secondary hyperaldosteronism, which is usually a consequence of enhanced activity of renin in response to inadequate renal perfusion and hypotension. Most individuals with primary hyperaldosteronism have bilateral adrenal hyperplasia (idiopathic hyperaldosteronism), while only a minority have an aldosterone-producing adenoma (APA; Conn's syndrome). Glucocorticoid-suppressible hyperaldosteronism is a rare autosomal dominant condition in which aldosterone is secreted 'ectopically' from the adrenal fasciculata/reticularis in response to ACTH. Rarely, the mineralocorticoid receptor pathway in the distal nephron is activated, even though aldosterone concentrations are low.

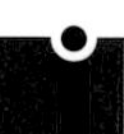

20.50 Causes of mineralocorticoid excess

With renin high and aldosterone high (secondary hyperaldosteronism)
• Inadequate renal perfusion (diuretic therapy, cardiac failure, liver failure, nephrotic syndrome, renal artery stenosis) • Renin-secreting renal tumour (very rare)
With renin low and aldosterone high (primary hyperaldosteronism)
• Adrenal adenoma secreting aldosterone (Conn's syndrome) • Idiopathic bilateral adrenal hyperplasia • Glucocorticoid-suppressible hyperaldosteronism (rare)
With renin low and aldosterone low (non-aldosterone-dependent activation of mineralocorticoid pathway)
• Ectopic ACTH syndrome • Liquorice misuse (inhibition of 11 β-HSD2) • Liddle's syndrome • 11-deoxycorticosterone-secreting adrenal tumour • Rare forms of congenital adrenal hyperplasia and 11 β-HSD2 deficiency

Clinical features

Individuals with primary hyperaldosteronism are usually asymptomatic but may have features of sodium retention or potassium loss. Sodium retention may cause oedema, while hypokalaemia may cause muscle weakness (or even paralysis, especially in Chinese), polyuria (secondary to renal tubular damage, which produces nephrogenic diabetes insipidus) and occasionally tetany (because of associated metabolic alkalosis and low ionised calcium). Blood pressure is elevated but accelerated phase hypertension is rare.

Investigations

Biochemical

Routine blood tests may show a hypokalaemic alkalosis. Sodium is usually at the upper end of the reference range in primary hyperaldosteronism, but is characteristically low in secondary hyperaldosteronism (because low plasma volume stimulates antidiuretic hormone (ADH) release and high angiotensin II levels stimulate thirst). The key measurements are plasma renin and aldosterone (see Box 20.50), and in many centres, the aldosterone : renin ratio (ARR) is employed as a screening test for primary hyperaldosteronism in hypertensive patients. Almost all antihypertensive drugs interfere with this ratio (β-blockers inhibit whilst thiazide diuretics stimulate renin secretion). Thus, individuals with an elevated ARR require further testing after stopping antihypertensive drugs for at least 2 weeks. If necessary, antihypertensive agents that have minimal effects on the renin–angiotensin system, such as calcium antagonists and α-blockers, may be substituted. Oral potassium supplementation may also be required, as hypokalaemia itself suppresses renin activity. If, on repeat testing, plasma renin is low and aldosterone concentrations are elevated, then further investigation under specialist supervision may include suppression tests (sodium loading) and/or stimulation tests (captopril or furosemide administration) to differentiate angiotensin II-dependent aldosterone secretion in idiopathic hyperplasia from autonomous aldosterone secretion typical of an APA.

Imaging and localisation

Imaging with CT or MRI will identify most APAs (Fig. 20.22), but it is important to recognise the risk of false-positives (non-functioning adrenal adenomas are common) and false-negatives (imaging may have insufficient resolution to identify adenomas with diameter of less than 0.5 cm). If the imaging is inconclusive and there is an intention to proceed with surgery on the basis of strong biochemical evidence of an APA, then adrenal vein catheterisation with measurement of aldosterone (and cortisol to confirm positioning of the catheters) is required. In some centres, this is performed even in the presence of a unilateral 'adenoma', to avoid inadvertent removal of an incidental non-functioning adenoma contralateral to the inapparent cause of aldosterone excess.

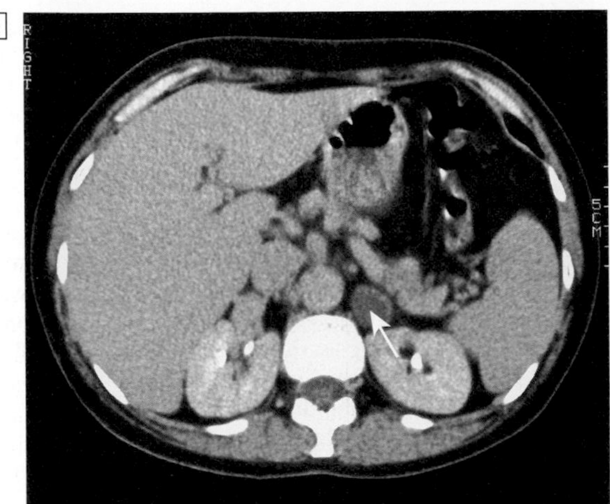

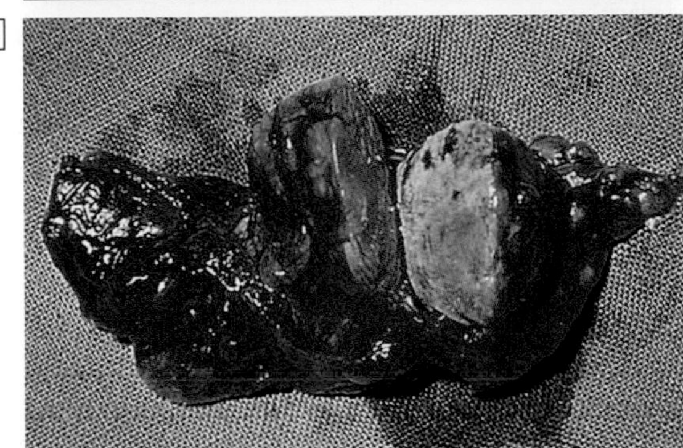

Fig. 20.22 Aldosterone-producing adenoma causing Conn's syndrome. **A** CT scan of left adrenal adenoma (arrow). **B** The tumour is 'canary yellow' because of intracellular lipid accumulation.

Management

Mineralocorticoid receptor antagonists (spironolactone and eplerenone) are valuable in treating both hypokalaemia and hypertension in all forms of mineralocorticoid excess. Up to 20% of males develop gynaecomastia on spironolactone. Amiloride (10–40 mg/day), which blocks the epithelial sodium channel regulated by aldosterone, is an alternative.

In patients with an APA, medical therapy is usually given for a few weeks to normalise whole-body electrolyte balance before unilateral adrenalectomy. Laparoscopic surgery cures the biochemical abnormality but, depending on the pre-operative duration, hypertension remains in as many as 70% of cases, probably because of irreversible damage to the systemic microcirculation.

Phaeochromocytoma and paraganglioma

These are rare neuro-endocrine tumours that may secrete catecholamines (adrenaline/epinephrine, noradrenaline/norepinephrine). Approximately 80% of these tumours occur in the adrenal medulla (phaeochromocytomas), while 20% arise elsewhere in the body in sympathetic ganglia (paragangliomas). Most are benign but approximately 15% show malignant features. Around 30% are associated with inherited disorders, including neurofibromatosis (p. 1215), von Hippel–Lindau syndrome (p. 1216) and MEN 2 (p. 795). Paragangliomas are particularly associated with mutations in the succinate dehydrogenase B, C and D genes.

20.51 Clinical features of phaeochromocytoma

- Hypertension (usually paroxysmal; often postural drop of blood pressure)
- Paroxysms of:
  - Pallor (occasionally flushing)
  - Palpitations, sweating
  - Headache
  - Anxiety (angor animi)
- Abdominal pain, vomiting
- Constipation
- Weight loss
- Glucose intolerance

Clinical features

These depend on the pattern of catecholamine secretion and are listed in Box 20.51.

Some patients present with hypertension, although it has been estimated that phaeochromocytoma accounts for less than 0.1% of cases of hypertension. The presentation may be with a complication of hypertension, such as stroke, myocardial infarction, left ventricular failure, hypertensive retinopathy or accelerated phase hypertension. The apparent paradox of postural hypotension between episodes is explained by 'pressure natriuresis' during hypertensive episodes so that intravascular volume is reduced. There may also be features of the familial syndromes associated with phaeochromocytoma. Paragangliomas are often non-functioning.

Investigations

Excessive secretion of catecholamines can be confirmed by measuring metabolites in plasma and/or urine (metanephrine and normetanephrine). There is a high 'false-positive' rate, as misleading metanephrine concentrations may be seen in stressed patients (during acute illness, following vigorous exercise or severe pain) and following ingestion of some drugs such as tricyclic antidepressants. For this reason, a repeat sample should usually be requested if elevated levels are found, although, as a rule, the higher the concentration of metanephrines, the more likely is the diagnosis of phaeochromocytoma/paraganglioma. Serum chromogranin A is often elevated and may be a useful tumour marker in patients with non-secretory tumours and/or metastatic disease. Genetic testing should be considered in individuals with other features of a genetic syndrome, with a family history of phaeochromocytoma/paraganglioma, and in those presenting under the age of 50 years.

Localisation

Phaeochromocytomas are usually identified by abdominal CT or MRI (Fig. 20.23). Localisation of paragangliomas may be more difficult. Scintigraphy using meta-iodobenzyl guanidine (MIBG) can be useful, particularly if combined with CT. ^{18}F-deoxyglucose PET is especially useful for detection of malignant disease and for confirming an imaging abnormality as a paraganglioma in an individual with underlying risk due to genetic mutation.

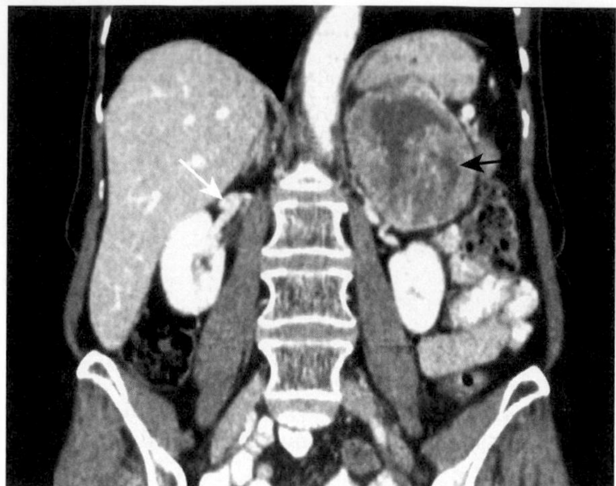

Fig. 20.23 CT scan of abdomen showing large left adrenal phaeochromocytoma. The normal right adrenal (white arrow) contrasts with the large heterogeneous phaeochromocytoma arising from the left adrenal gland (black arrow).

Management

Medical therapy is required to prepare the patient for surgery, preferably for a minimum of 6 weeks to allow restoration of normal plasma volume. The most useful drug in the face of very high circulating catecholamines is the α-blocker phenoxybenzamine (10–20 mg orally 3–4 times daily) because it is a non-competitive antagonist, unlike prazosin or doxazosin. If α-blockade produces a marked tachycardia, then a β-blocker such as propranolol can be added. On no account should a β-blocker be given before an α-blocker, as this may cause a paradoxical rise in blood pressure due to unopposed α-mediated vasoconstriction.

During surgery, sodium nitroprusside and the short-acting α-antagonist phentolamine are useful in controlling hypertensive episodes, which may result from anaesthetic induction or tumour mobilisation. Post-operative hypotension may occur and require volume expansion and, very occasionally, noradrenaline (norepinephrine) infusion, but is uncommon if the patient has been prepared with phenoxybenzamine.

Metastatic tumours may behave in an aggressive or a very indolent fashion. Management options include debulking surgery, radionuclide therapy with ^{131}I-MIBG, chemotherapy and (chemo)embolisation of hepatic metastases; some may respond to tyrosine kinase and angiogenesis inhibitors.

Congenital adrenal hyperplasia

Pathophysiology and clinical features

Inherited defects in enzymes of the cortisol biosynthetic pathway (see Fig. 20.18, p. 772) result in insufficiency of hormones downstream of the block, with impaired negative feedback and increased ACTH secretion. ACTH then stimulates the production of steroids upstream of the enzyme block. This produces adrenal hyperplasia and a combination of clinical features that depend on the severity and site of the defect in biosynthesis. All of these enzyme abnormalities are inherited as autosomal recessive traits.

The most common enzyme defect is 21-hydroxylase deficiency. This results in impaired synthesis of cortisol and aldosterone and accumulation of 17OH-progesterone, which is then diverted to form adrenal androgens. In about one-third of cases, this defect is severe and presents in infancy with features of glucocorticoid and mineralocorticoid deficiency (see Box 20.46, p. 778) and androgen excess, such as ambiguous genitalia in girls. In the other two-thirds, mineralocorticoid secretion is adequate but there may be features of cortisol insufficiency and/or ACTH and androgen excess, including precocious pseudo-puberty, which is distinguished from 'true' precocious puberty by low gonadotrophins. Sometimes the mildest enzyme defects are not apparent until adult life, when females may present with amenorrhoea and/or hirsutism (p. 763). This is called 'non-classical' or 'late-onset' congenital adrenal hyperplasia.

Defects of all the other enzymes in Figure 20.18 (p. 772) are rare. Both 17-hydroxylase and 11 β-hydroxylase deficiency may produce hypertension due to excess production of 11-deoxycorticosterone, which has mineralocorticoid activity.

Investigations

Circulating 17OH-progesterone levels are raised in 21-hydroxylase deficiency, but this may only be demonstrated after ACTH administration in late-onset cases. To avoid salt-wasting crises in infancy, 17OH-progesterone can be routinely measured in heelprick blood spot samples taken from all infants in the first week of life. Assessment is otherwise as described for adrenal insufficiency on page 778.

In siblings of affected children, antenatal genetic diagnosis can be made by amniocentesis or chorionic villus sampling. This allows prevention of virilisation of affected female fetuses by administration of dexamethasone to the mother to suppress ACTH levels.

Management

The aim is to replace deficient corticosteroids and to suppress ACTH-driven adrenal androgen production. A careful balance is required between adequate suppression of adrenal androgen excess and excessive glucocorticoid replacement resulting in features of Cushing's syndrome. In children, growth velocity is an important measurement, since either under- or over-replacement with glucocorticoids suppresses growth. In adults, there is no uniformly agreed adrenal replacement regime, and clinical features (menstrual cycle, hirsutism, weight gain, blood pressure) and biochemical profiles (plasma renin, 17OH-progesterone and testosterone levels) provide a guide.

Women with late-onset 21-hydroxylase deficiency may not require corticosteroid replacement. If hirsutism is the main problem, anti-androgen therapy may be just as effective (p. 764).

THE ENDOCRINE PANCREAS AND GASTROINTESTINAL TRACT

A series of hormones are secreted from cells distributed throughout the gastrointestinal tract and pancreas. Functional anatomy and physiology are

20.52 Classification of endocrine diseases of the pancreas and gastrointestinal tract

	Primary	Secondary
Hormone excess	Insulinoma Gastrinoma (Zollinger–Ellison syndrome) Carcinoid syndrome (secretion of 5-HT) Glucagonoma VIPoma Somatostatinoma	Hypergastrinaemia of achlorhydria Hyperinsulinaemia after bariatric surgery
Hormone deficiency	Diabetes mellitus	
Hormone resistance	Insulin resistance syndromes (e.g. type 2 diabetes mellitus, lipodystrophy, leprechaunism)	
Non-functioning tumours	Pancreatic carcinoma Pancreatic neuro-endocrine tumour	

described in Chapters 21 and 22. Diseases associated with abnormalities of these hormones are listed in Box 20.52. Most are rare, with the exception of diabetes mellitus (Ch. 21).

Presenting problems in endocrine pancreas disease

Spontaneous hypoglycaemia

Hypoglycaemia most commonly occurs as a side-effect of treatment with insulin or sulphonylurea drugs in people with diabetes mellitus. In non-diabetic individuals, symptomatic hypoglycaemia is rare, but it is not uncommon to detect venous blood glucose concentrations below 3.0 mmol/L in asymptomatic patients. For this reason, and because the symptoms of hypoglycaemia are non-specific, a hypoglycaemic disorder should only be diagnosed if all three conditions of Whipple's triad are met (Fig. 20.24). There is no specific blood glucose concentration at which spontaneous hypoglycaemia can be said to occur, although the lower the blood glucose concentration, the more likely it is to have pathological significance.

Clinical assessment

The clinical features of hypoglycaemia are described in the section on insulin-induced hypoglycaemia on page 814. Individuals with chronic spontaneous hypoglycaemia often have attenuated autonomic responses and 'hypoglycaemia unawareness', and may present with a wide variety of features of neuro-glycopenia, including odd behaviour and convulsions. The symptoms are usually episodic and relieved by consumption of carbohydrate. Symptoms occurring while fasting (such as before breakfast) or following exercise are much more likely to be representative of pathological hypoglycaemia than those which develop after food (post-prandial or 'reactive' symptoms). Hypoglycaemia should be considered in all comatose patients, even if there is an apparently obvious cause, such as hemiplegic stroke or alcohol intoxication.

Investigations

Does the patient have a hypoglycaemic disorder?

Patients who present acutely with confusion, coma or convulsions should be tested for hypoglycaemia at the bedside with a capillary blood sample and an automated meter. While this is sufficient to exclude hypoglycaemia, blood glucose meters are relatively inaccurate in the hypoglycaemic range and the diagnosis should always be confirmed by a laboratory-based glucose measurement. At the same time, a sample should be taken for later measurement, if necessary, of alcohol, insulin, C-peptide, cortisol and sulphonylurea levels. Taking these samples during an acute presentation

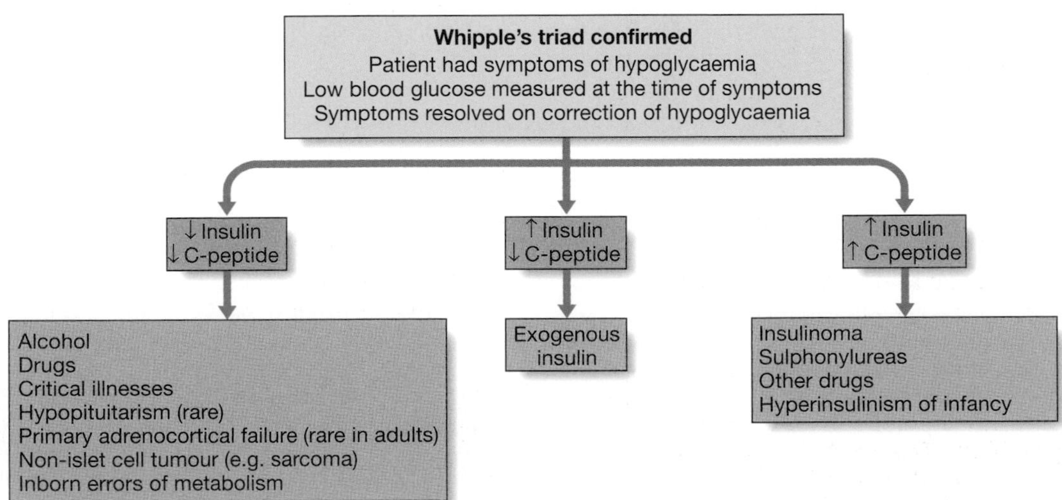

Fig. 20.24 Differential diagnosis of spontaneous hypoglycaemia. Measurement of insulin and C-peptide concentrations during an episode is helpful in determining the underlying cause.

20

prevents subsequent unnecessary dynamic tests and is of medico-legal importance in cases where poisoning is suspected.

Patients who attend the outpatient clinic with episodic symptoms suggestive of hypoglycaemia present a more challenging problem. The main diagnostic test is the prolonged (72-hour) fast. If symptoms of hypoglycaemia develop during the fast, then blood samples should be taken to confirm hypoglycaemia and for later measurement of insulin and C-peptide. Hypoglycaemia is then corrected with oral or intravenous glucose and Whipple's triad completed by confirmation of the resolution of symptoms. The absence of clinical and biochemical evidence of hypoglycaemia during a prolonged fast effectively excludes the diagnosis of a hypoglycaemic disorder.

What is the cause of the hypoglycaemia?

In the acute setting, the underlying diagnosis is often obvious. In non-diabetic individuals, alcohol excess is the most common cause of hypoglycaemia in the UK, but other drugs – for example, salicylates, quinine and pentamidine – may also be implicated. Hypoglycaemia is one of many metabolic derangements which occur in patients with hepatic failure, renal failure, sepsis or malaria.

Hypoglycaemia in the absence of insulin, or any insulin-like factor, in the blood indicates impaired gluconeogenesis and/or availability of glucose from glycogen in the liver. Hypoglycaemia associated with high insulin and low C-peptide concentrations is indicative of administration of exogenous insulin, either factitiously or feloniously. Adults with high insulin and C-peptide concentrations during an episode of hypoglycaemia are most likely to have an insulinoma, but sulphonylurea ingestion should also be considered (particularly in individuals with access to such medication, such as health-care professionals or family members of someone with type 2 diabetes). Suppressed plasma β-hydroxybutyrate helps confirm inappropriate insulin secretion during fasting. Usually, insulinomas in the pancreas are small (< 5 mm diameter) but can be identified by CT, MRI or ultrasound (endoscopic or laparoscopic). Imaging should include the liver since around 10% of insulinomas are malignant. Rarely, large non-pancreatic tumours, such as sarcomas, may cause recurrent hypoglycaemia because of their ability to produce excess pro-insulin-like growth factor-2 (pro-IGF-2).

Management

Treatment of acute hypoglycaemia should be initiated as soon as laboratory blood samples have been taken, and should *not* be deferred until formal laboratory confirmation has been obtained. Intravenous dextrose (5% or 10%) is effective in the short term in the obtunded patient, and should be followed on recovery with oral unrefined carbohydrate (starch). Continuous dextrose infusion may be necessary, especially in sulphonylurea poisoning. Intramuscular glucagon (1 mg) stimulates hepatic glucose release, but is ineffective in patients with depleted glycogen reserves, such as in alcohol excess or liver disease.

Chronic recurrent hypoglycaemia in insulin-secreting tumours can be treated by regular consumption of oral carbohydrate combined with agents that inhibit insulin secretion (diazoxide or somatostatin analogues). Insulinomas are resected when benign, providing the individual is fit enough to undergo surgery. Metastatic malignant insulinomas are incurable and are managed along the same lines as other metastatic neuro-endocrine tumours (see below).

20.53 Spontaneous hypoglycaemia in old age

- **Presentation**: may present with focal neurological abnormality. Blood glucose should be checked in all patients with acute neurological symptoms and signs, especially stroke, as these will reverse with early treatment of hypoglycaemia.

Gastroenteropancreatic neuro-endocrine tumours

Neuro-endocrine tumours (NETs) are a heterogeneous group derived from neuro-endocrine cells in many organs, including the gastrointestinal tract, lung, adrenals (phaeochromocytoma, p. 781) and thyroid (medullary carcinoma, p. 755). Most NETs occur sporadically, but a proportion are associated with genetic cancer syndromes, such as MEN 1, MEN 2 and neurofibromatosis type 1 (pp. 795 and 1215). NETs may secrete hormones into the circulation.

Gastroenteropancreatic NETs arise in organs that are derived embryologically from the gastrointestinal tract. Most commonly, they occur in the small bowel but they can also arise elsewhere in the bowel, pancreas, thymus and bronchi. The term 'carcinoid' is often used when referring to non-pancreatic gastroenteropancreatic NETs because, when initially described, they were thought to behave in an indolent fashion compared with conventional cancers. It is now recognised that there is a wide spectrum of malignant potential for all NETs; some are benign (most insulinomas and appendiceal carcinoid tumours), while others have an aggressive clinical course with widespread metastases (small-cell carcinoma of the lung). The majority of gastroenteropancreatic NETs behave in an intermediate manner, with relatively slow growth but a propensity to invade and metastasise to remote organs, especially the liver.

Clinical features

Patients with gastroenteropancreatic NETs often have a history of abdominal pain over many years prior to diagnosis and usually present with local mass effects, such as small-bowel obstruction, appendicitis, and pain from hepatic metastases. Thymic and bronchial carcinoids occasionally present with ectopic ACTH syndrome (p. 774). Pancreatic NETs can also cause hormone excess (Box 20.54) but most are non-functional. The classic 'carcinoid syndrome' (Box 20.55) occurs when vasoactive hormones reach the systemic circulation. In the case of gastrointestinal carcinoids, this invariably means that the tumour has metastasised to the liver or there are peritoneal deposits, which allow secreted hormones to gain access to the systemic circulation; hormones secreted by the primary tumour into the portal vein are metabolised and inactivated in the liver.

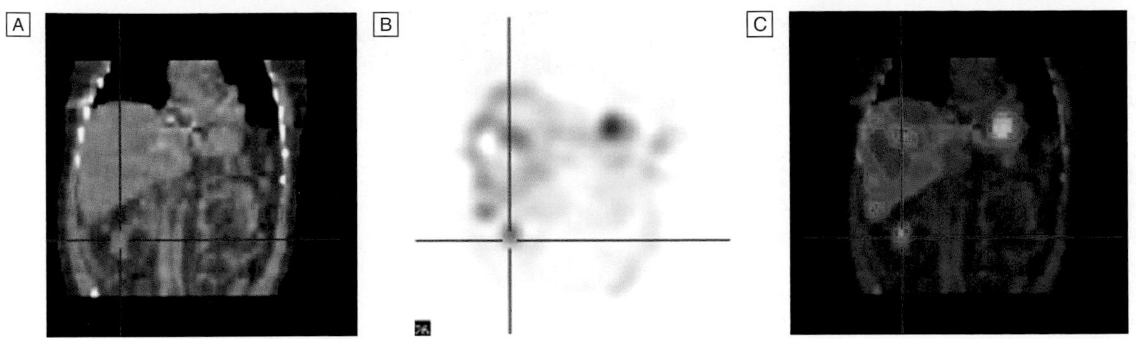

Fig. 20.25 Octreotide scintigraphy in a metastatic neuro-endocrine tumour. **A** Coronal CT scan showing hepatomegaly and a mass inferior to the liver (at the intersection of the horizontal and vertical red lines). **B** Octreotide scintogram showing patches of increased uptake in the upper abdomen. **C** When the octreotide and CT scans are superimposed, it shows that the areas of increased uptake are in hepatic metastases and in the tissue mass, which may be lymph nodes or a primary tumour.

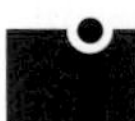

20.54 Pancreatic neuro-endocrine tumours

Tumour	Hormone	Effects
Gastrinoma	Gastrin	Peptic ulcer and steatorrhoea (Zollinger–Ellison syndrome)
Insulinoma	Insulin	Recurrent hypoglycaemia (see above)
VIPoma	Vasoactive intestinal peptide (VIP)	Watery diarrhoea and hypokalaemia
Glucagonoma	Glucagon	Diabetes mellitus, necrolytic migratory erythema
Somatostatinoma	Somatostatin	Diabetes mellitus and steatorrhoea

20.55 Clinical features of the carcinoid syndrome

- Episodic flushing, wheezing and diarrhoea
- Facial telangiectasia
- Cardiac involvement (tricuspid regurgitation, pulmonary stenosis, right ventricular endocardial plaques) leading to heart failure

Investigations

A combination of imaging with ultrasound, CT, MRI and/or radio-labelled somatostatin analogue (Fig. 20.25) will usually identify the primary tumour and allow staging, which is crucial for determining prognosis. Biopsy of the primary tumour or a metastatic deposit is required to confirm the histological type. NETs demonstrate immunohistochemical staining for the proteins chromogranin A and synaptophysin, and the histological grade may also provide prognostic information.

Carcinoid syndrome is confirmed by measuring elevated concentrations of 5-hydroxyindoleacetic acid (5-HIAA), a metabolite of serotonin, in a 24-hour urine collection. False-positives can occur, particularly if the individual has been eating certain foods, such as avocado and pineapple. Plasma chromogranin A can be measured in a fasting blood sample, along with the hormones listed in Box 20.54. All of these can be useful as tumour markers.

Management

Treatment of solitary tumours is by surgical resection. If metastatic or multifocal primary disease is present, then surgery is usually not indicated, unless there is a complication such as gastrointestinal obstruction. Diazoxide can reduce insulin secretion in insulinomas, and high doses of proton pump inhibitors suppress acid production in gastrinomas. Somatostatin analogues are effective in reducing the symptoms of carcinoid syndrome and of excess glucagon and vasoactive intestinal peptide (VIP) production. The slow-growing nature of NETs means that conventional cancer therapies, such as chemotherapy and radiotherapy, have limited efficacy. Other treatments, such as interferon, targeted radionuclide therapy with ^{131}I-MIBG and radio-labelled somatostatin analogues (which may be taken up by NET metastases), and resection/embolisation of hepatic metastases, may have a role in the palliation of symptoms but there is little evidence that they prolong life. The tyrosine kinase inhibitor sunitinib and the mammalian target of rapamycin (mTOR) inhibitor everolimus have shown benefit in progressive pancreatic NETS (Box 20.56), and should be considered as part of standard therapy.

EBM 20.56 Tyrosine kinase/mTOR inhibitors in advanced pancreatic neuro-endocrine tumours

'Two randomised controlled clinical trials showed significant improvements in progression-free survival in patients with advanced and progressive pancreatic neuro-endocrine tumours.'

- Yao JC, et al. N Engl J Med 2011; 364(6):514–523.
- Raymond E, et al. N Engl J Med 2011; 364(6):501–513.

THE HYPOTHALAMUS AND THE PITUITARY GLAND

Diseases of the hypothalamus and pituitary have an annual incidence of approximately 3:100000 and a prevalence of 30–40 per 100 000. The pituitary plays a central role in several major endocrine axes, so that investigation and treatment invariably involve several other endocrine glands.

Functional anatomy, physiology and investigations

The anatomical relationships of the pituitary are shown in Figure 20.26 and its numerous functions are shown in Figure 20.2 (p. 737). The pituitary gland is enclosed in the sella turcica and bridged over by a fold of dura mater called the diaphragma sellae, with the sphenoidal air sinuses below and the optic chiasm above. The cavernous sinuses are lateral to the pituitary fossa and contain the 3rd, 4th and 6th cranial nerves and the internal carotid arteries. The gland is composed of two lobes, anterior and posterior, and is connected to the hypothalamus by the infundibular stalk, which has portal vessels carrying blood from the median eminence of the hypothalamus to the anterior lobe and nerve fibres to the posterior lobe.

Diseases of the hypothalamus and pituitary are classified in Box 20.57. By far the most common disorder is an adenoma of the anterior pituitary gland.

A

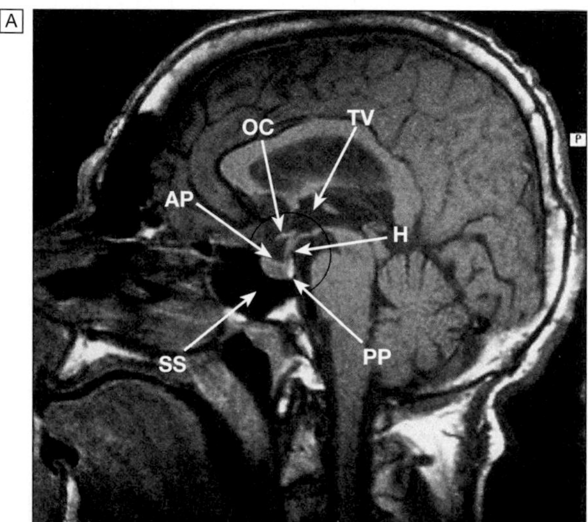

B

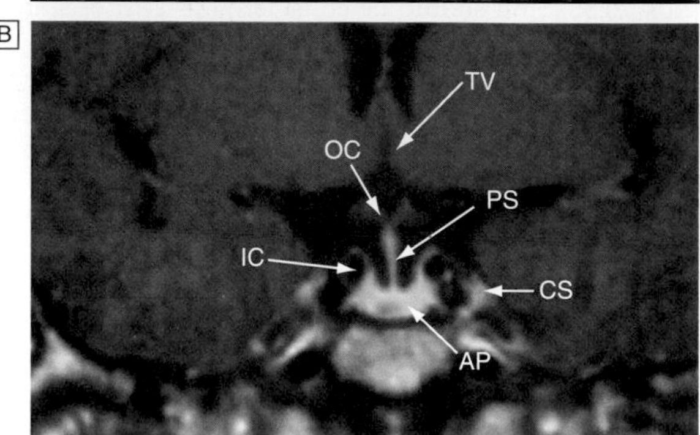

Fig. 20.26 Anatomical relationships of the normal pituitary gland and hypothalamus. See also Figure 20.2 (p. 737). A Sagittal MRI. B Coronal MRI. (AP = anterior pituitary; CS = cavernous sinus; H = hypothalamus; IC = internal carotid artery; OC = optic chiasm; PP = posterior pituitary; PS = pituitary stalk; SS = sphenoid sinus; TV = third ventricle)

20.57 Classification of diseases of the pituitary and hypothalamus

	Primary	Secondary
Non-functioning tumours	Pituitary adenoma Craniopharyngioma Metastatic tumours	
Hormone excess		
Anterior pituitary	Prolactinoma Acromegaly Cushing's disease Rare TSH-, LH-and FSH-secreting adenomas	Disconnection hyperprolactinaemia
Hypothalamus and posterior pituitary	Syndrome of inappropriate antidiuretic hormone (SIADH; p. 438)	
Hormone deficiency		
Anterior pituitary	Hypopituitarism	GnRH deficiency (Kallmann's syndrome)
Hypothalamus and posterior pituitary	Cranial diabetes insipidus	
Hormone resistance	Growth hormone resistance (Laron dwarfism) Nephrogenic diabetes insipidus	

Investigation of patients with pituitary disease

Although pituitary disease presents with diverse clinical manifestations (see below), the approach to investigation is similar in all cases (Box 20.58).

The approach to testing for hormone deficiency is outlined in Box 20.58. Details are given in the sections on individual glands elsewhere in this chapter. Tests for hormone excess vary according to the hormone in question. For example, prolactin is not secreted in pulsatile fashion, although it rises with significant psychological stress. Assuming that the patient was not distressed by venepuncture, a random measurement of serum prolactin is sufficient to diagnose hyperprolactinaemia. In contrast, growth hormone is secreted in a pulsatile fashion. A high random level does not confirm acromegaly; the diagnosis is only confirmed by failure of growth hormone to be suppressed during an oral glucose tolerance test, and a high serum insulin-like growth factor-1 (IGF-1). Similarly, in suspected ACTH-dependent Cushing's disease (p. 773), random measurement of plasma cortisol is unreliable and the diagnosis is usually made by a dexamethasone suppression test.

The most common local complication of a large pituitary tumour is compression of the optic pathway. The resulting visual field defect can be documented using a Goldman's perimetry chart.

MRI reveals 'abnormalities' of the pituitary gland in as many as 10% of 'healthy' middle-aged people. It should therefore be performed only if there is a clear biochemical abnormality or in a patient who presents with clinical features of pituitary tumour (see below). A pituitary tumour may be classified as either a macroadenoma (> 10 mm diameter) or a microadenoma (< 10 mm diameter).

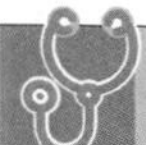

20.58 How to investigate patients with suspected pituitary hypothalamic disease

Identify pituitary hormone deficiency

ACTH deficiency
- Short ACTH stimulation test (see Box 20.47, p. 778)
- Insulin tolerance test (see Box 20.61, p. 788): only if uncertainty in interpretation of short ACTH stimulation test (e.g. acute presentation)

LH/FSH deficiency
- In the male, measure random serum testosterone, LH and FSH
- In the pre-menopausal female, ask if menses are regular
- In the post-menopausal female, measure random serum LH and FSH (which would normally be > 30 mU/L)

TSH deficiency
- Measure random serum T_4
- Note that TSH is often detectable in secondary hypothyroidism

Growth hormone deficiency
Only investigate if growth hormone replacement therapy is being contemplated; p. 789
- Measure immediately after exercise
- Consider other stimulatory tests (see Box 20.60)

Cranial diabetes insipidus
Only investigate if patient complains of polyuria/polydipsia, which may be masked by ACTH or TSH deficiency
- Exclude other causes of polyuria with blood glucose, potassium and calcium measurements
- Water deprivation test (see Box 20.66, p. 795) or 5% saline infusion test

Identify hormone excess
- Measure random serum prolactin
- Investigate for acromegaly (glucose tolerance test) or Cushing's syndrome (p. 774) if there are clinical features

Establish the anatomy and diagnosis
- Consider visual field testing
- Image the pituitary and hypothalamus by MRI or CT

Surgical biopsy is usually only performed as part of a therapeutic operation. Conventional histology identifies tumours as chromophobe (usually non-functioning), acidophil (typically prolactin- or growth hormone-secreting) or basophil (typically ACTH-secreting); immunohistochemistry may confirm their secretory capacity but is poorly predictive of growth potential of the tumour.

Presenting problems in hypothalamic and pituitary disease

The clinical features of pituitary disease are shown in Figure 20.27 overleaf. Younger women with pituitary disease most commonly present with secondary amenorrhoea (p. 759) or galactorrhoea (in hyperprolactinaemia). Post-menopausal women and men of any age are less likely to report symptoms of hypogonadism and so are more likely to present late with larger tumours causing visual field defects. Nowadays, many patients present with the incidental finding of a pituitary tumour on a CT or MRI scan.

Hypopituitarism

Hypopituitarism describes combined deficiency of any of the anterior pituitary hormones. The clinical presentation is variable and depends on the underlying lesion and the pattern of resulting hormone deficiency. The most common cause is a pituitary macroadenoma but other causes are listed in Box 20.59.

Clinical assessment

The presentation is highly variable. For example, following radiotherapy to the pituitary region, there is a characteristic sequence of loss of pituitary hormone secretion. Growth hormone secretion is often the earliest to be lost. In adults, this produces lethargy, muscle weakness and increased fat mass but these features are not obvious in isolation. Next, gonadotrophin (LH and FSH) secretion becomes impaired with, in the male, loss of libido and, in the female, oligomenorrhoea or amenorrhoea. Later, in the male there may be gynaecomastia and decreased frequency of shaving. In both sexes, axillary and pubic hair eventually become sparse or even absent and the skin becomes characteristically finer and wrinkled. Chronic anaemia may also occur. The next hormone to be lost is usually ACTH, resulting in symptoms of cortisol insufficiency (including postural hypotension and

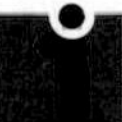

20.59 Causes of anterior pituitary hormone deficiency

Structural	
• Primary pituitary tumour Adenoma* Carcinoma (exceptionally rare) • Craniopharyngioma* • Meningioma* • Secondary tumour (including leukaemia and lymphoma)	• Chordoma • Germinoma (pinealoma) • Arachnoid cyst • Rathke's cleft cyst • Haemorrhage (apoplexy)
Inflammatory/infiltrative	
• Sarcoidosis • Infections, e.g. pituitary abscess, tuberculosis, syphilis, encephalitis	• Lymphocytic hypophysitis • Haemochromatosis • Langerhans cell histiocytosis
Congenital deficiencies	
• GnRH (Kallmann's syndrome)* – gonadotrophin-releasing hormone • GHRH* – growth hormone-releasing hormone	• TRH – thyrotrophin-releasing hormone • CRH – corticotrophin-releasing hormone
Functional*	
• Chronic systemic illness • Anorexia nervosa	• Excessive exercise
Other	
• Head injury* • (Para)sellar surgery* • (Para)sellar radiotherapy*	• Post-partum necrosis (Sheehan's syndrome) • Opiate analgesia

*The most common causes of pituitary hormone deficiency.

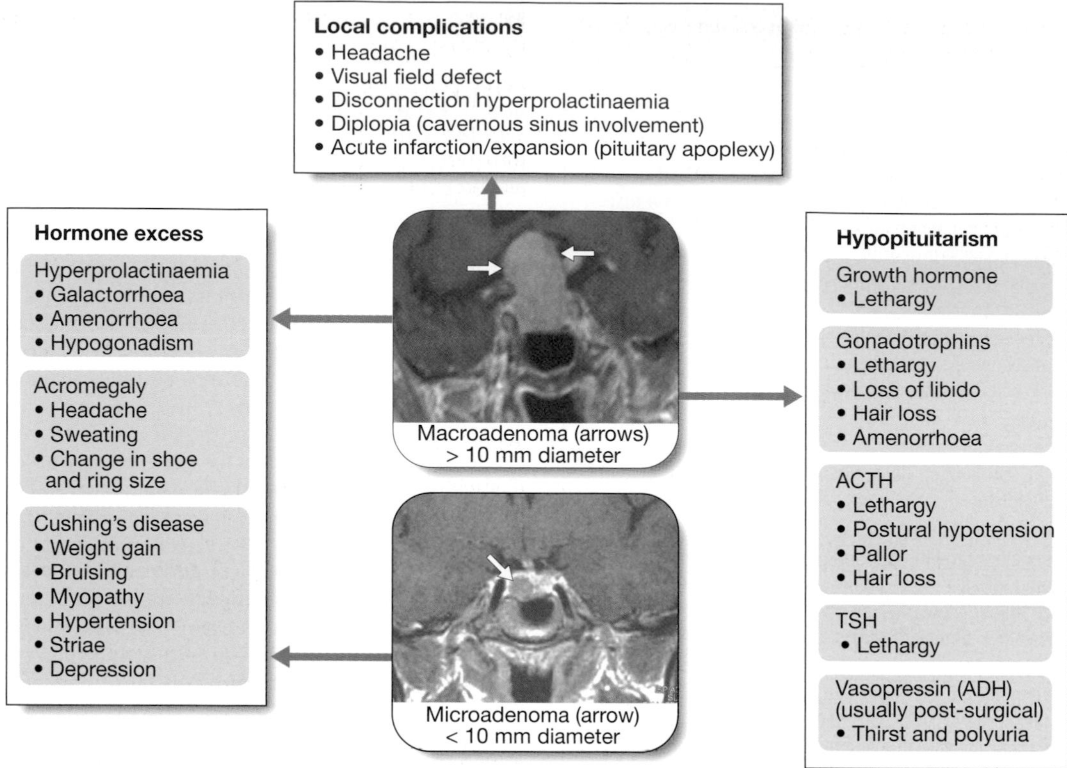

Fig. 20.27 **Common symptoms and signs to consider in a patient with suspected pituitary disease.**

a *dilutional* hyponatraemia). In contrast to primary adrenal insufficiency (p. 777), angiotensin II-dependent zona glomerulosa function is not lost and hence aldosterone secretion maintains normal plasma potassium. In contrast to the pigmentation of Addison's disease due to high levels of circulating ACTH acting on the skin melanocytes, a striking degree of pallor is usually present. Finally, TSH secretion is lost with consequent secondary hypothyroidism. This contributes further to apathy and cold intolerance. In contrast to primary hypothyroidism, frank myxoedema is rare, presumably because the thyroid retains some autonomous function. The onset of all of the above symptoms is notoriously insidious. However, patients sometimes present acutely unwell with glucocorticoid deficiency. This may be precipitated by a mild infection or injury, or may occur secondary to pituitary apoplexy (p. 789).

Other features of pituitary disease may be present (see Fig. 20.27).

Investigations

The strategy for investigation of pituitary disease is described in Box 20.58. In acutely unwell patients, the priority is to diagnose and treat cortisol deficiency (p. 776). Other tests can be undertaken later. Specific dynamic tests for diagnosing hormone deficiency are described in Boxes 20.47 (p. 778) and 20.60. More specialised biochemical tests, such as insulin tolerance tests (Box 20.61), GnRH and TRH tests, are rarely required. All patients with biochemical evidence of pituitary hormone deficiency should have an MRI or CT scan to identify pituitary or hypothalamic tumours. If a tumour is not identified, then further investigations are indicated to exclude infectious or infiltrative causes.

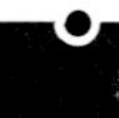

20.60 Tests of growth hormone secretion

GH levels are commonly undetectable, so a choice from the range of 'stimulation' tests is required:

- Insulin-induced hypoglycaemia
- Arginine (may be combined with GHRH)
- Glucagon
- Clonidine

Management

Treatment of acutely ill patients is similar to that described for adrenocortical insufficiency on page 778, except that sodium depletion is not an important component to correct. Chronic hormone replacement therapies are described below. Once the cause of hypopituitarism is established, specific treatment – of a pituitary macroadenoma, for example (see below) – may be required.

Cortisol replacement

Hydrocortisone should be given if there is ACTH deficiency. Suitable doses are described in the section on adrenal disease on page 779. Mineralocorticoid replacement is not required.

Thyroid hormone replacement

Levothyroxine 50–150 μg once daily should be given as described on page 743. Unlike in primary

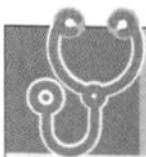

20.61 How and when to do an insulin tolerance test

Use
• Assessment of the HPA axis • Assessment of growth hormone deficiency • Indicated when there is doubt after the other tests in Box 20.58 • Usually performed in specialist centres, especially in children • IV glucose and hydrocortisone must be available for resuscitation
Contraindications
• Ischaemic heart disease • Epilepsy • Severe hypopituitarism (0800 hrs plasma cortisol < 180 nmol/L (6.6 µg/dL))
Dose
• 0.15 U/kg body weight soluble insulin IV
Aim
• To produce adequate hypoglycaemia (tachycardia and sweating with blood glucose < 2.2 mmol/L (40 mg/dL))
Blood samples
• 0, 30, 45, 60, 90, 120 mins for blood glucose, plasma cortisol and growth hormone
Results
• Normal subjects: GH > 6.7 µg/L (20 mU/L)* • Normal subjects: cortisol > 550 nmol/L (~20.2 µg/dL)*
*The precise cut-off figure for a satisfactory cortisol and GH response depends on the assay used and so varies between centres.

hypothyroidism, measuring TSH is not helpful in adjusting the replacement dose because patients with hypopituitarism often secrete glycoproteins which are measured in the TSH assays but are not bioactive. The aim is to maintain serum T_4 in the upper part of the reference range. It is dangerous to give thyroid replacement in adrenal insufficiency without first giving glucocorticoid therapy, since this may precipitate adrenal crisis.

Sex hormone replacement

This is indicated if there is gonadotrophin deficiency in women under the age of 50 and in men to restore normal sexual function and to prevent osteoporosis (p. 1120).

Growth hormone replacement

Growth hormone (GH) is administered by daily subcutaneous self-injection to children and adolescents with GH deficiency and, until recently, was discontinued once the epiphyses had fused. However, although hypopituitary adults receiving 'full' replacement with hydrocortisone, levothyroxine and sex steroids are usually much improved by these therapies, some individuals remain lethargic and unwell compared with a healthy population. Some of these patients feel better, and have objective improvements in their fat : muscle mass ratios and other metabolic parameters, if they are also given GH replacement. Treatment with GH may also help young adults to achieve a higher peak bone mineral density. The principal side-effect is sodium retention, manifest as peripheral oedema or carpal tunnel syndrome. For this reason, GH replacement should be started at a low dose, with monitoring of the response by measurement of serum IGF-1.

Pituitary tumour

Pituitary tumours produce a variety of mass effects, depending on their size and location, but also present as incidental findings on CT or MRI, or with hypopituitarism, as described above. A wide variety of disorders can present as mass lesions in or around the pituitary gland (see Box 20.59). Most intrasellar tumours are pituitary macroadenomas (most commonly non-functioning adenomas, see Fig. 20.27), whereas suprasellar masses may be craniopharyngiomas (see Fig. 20.30, p. 794). The most common cause of a parasellar mass is a meningioma.

Clinical assessment

Clinical features are shown in Figure 20.27. A common but non-specific presentation is with headache, which may be the consequence of stretching of the diaphragma sellae. Although the classical abnormalities associated with compression of the optic chiasm are bitemporal hemianopia (see Fig. 20.28) or upper quadrantanopia, any type of visual field defect can result from suprasellar extension of a tumour because it may compress the optic nerve (unilateral loss of acuity or scotoma) or the optic tract (homonymous hemianopia). Optic atrophy may be apparent on ophthalmoscopy. Lateral extension of a sellar mass into the cavernous sinus with subsequent compression of the 3rd, 4th or 6th cranial nerve may cause diplopia and strabismus, but in anterior pituitary tumours this is an unusual presentation.

Occasionally, pituitary tumours infarct or there is bleeding into cystic lesions. This is termed 'pituitary apoplexy' and may result in sudden expansion with local compression symptoms and acute-onset hypopituitarism. Non-haemorrhagic infarction can also occur in a normal pituitary gland; predisposing factors include catastrophic obstetric haemorrhage (Sheehan's syndrome), diabetes mellitus and raised intracranial pressure.

Investigations

Patients suspected of having a pituitary tumour should undergo MRI or CT. Whilst some lesions have distinctive neuro-radiological features, the definitive diagnosis is made on histology after surgery. All patients with (para)sellar space-occupying lesions should have pituitary function assessed as described in Box 20.58 (p. 787).

Management

Modalities of treatment of common pituitary and hypothalamic tumours are shown in Box 20.62. Associated hypopituitarism should be treated as described above.

Urgent treatment is required if there is evidence of pressure on visual pathways. The chances of recovery of a visual field defect are proportional to the duration of symptoms, with full recovery unlikely if the defect has been present for longer than 4 months. In the presence of a sellar mass lesion, it is crucial that serum prolactin is measured before emergency surgery is performed. If the prolactin is over 5000 mU/L, then the lesion is likely to be a macroprolactinoma and to respond

20

20.62 Therapeutic modalities for hypothalamic and pituitary tumours

	Surgery	Radiotherapy	Medical	Comment
Non-functioning pituitary macroadenoma	1st line	2nd line	–	
Prolactinoma	2nd line	2nd line	1st line Dopamine agonists	Dopamine agonists usually cause macroadenomas to shrink
Acromegaly	1st line	2nd line	2nd line Somatostatin analogues Dopamine agonists GH receptor antagonists	Medical therapy does not reliably cause macroadenomas to shrink Radiotherapy and medical therapy are used in combination for inoperable tumours
Cushing's disease	1st line	2nd line	–	Radiotherapy may be more effective in children than in adults and appears to cause less hypopituitarism in the long-term
Craniopharyngioma	1st line	2nd line	–	

to a dopamine agonist with shrinkage of the lesion, making surgery unnecessary (see Fig. 20.28).

Most operations on the pituitary are performed using the trans-sphenoidal approach via the nostrils, while transfrontal surgery via a craniotomy is reserved for suprasellar tumours. It is uncommon to be able to resect lateral extensions into the cavernous sinuses. All operations on the pituitary carry a risk of damaging normal endocrine function; this risk increases with the size of the primary lesion.

Pituitary function (see Box 20.58, p. 787) should be retested 4–6 weeks following surgery, primarily to detect the development of any new hormone deficits. Rarely, the surgical treatment of a sellar lesion can result in recovery of hormone secretion that was deficient pre-operatively.

Following surgery, usually after 3–6 months, imaging should be repeated and, if there is a significant residual mass and the histology confirms an anterior pituitary tumour, external radiotherapy may be given to reduce the risk of recurrence. Radiotherapy is not useful in patients requiring urgent therapy because it takes many months or years to be effective and there is a risk of acute swelling of the mass. Fractionated radiotherapy carries a life-long risk of hypopituitarism (50–70% in the first 10 years) and annual pituitary function tests are obligatory. There is also concern that radiotherapy might impair cognitive function, cause vascular changes and even induce primary brain tumours, but these side-effects have not been quantified reliably and are likely to be rare. Stereotactic radiosurgery, best delivered by the 'gamma knife', allows specific targeting of residual disease in a more focused fashion.

Non-functioning tumours should be followed up by repeated imaging at intervals that depend on the size of the lesion and on whether or not radiotherapy has been administered. For smaller lesions that are not causing mass effects, therapeutic surgery may not be indicated and the lesion may simply be monitored by serial neuroimaging without a clear-cut diagnosis having been established.

Hyperprolactinaemia/galactorrhoea

Hyperprolactinaemia is a common abnormality which usually presents with hypogonadism and/or galactorrhoea (lactation in the absence of breastfeeding). Since prolactin stimulates milk secretion but not breast development, galactorrhoea rarely occurs in men and only does so if gynaecomastia has been induced by hypogonadism (p. 760). The differential diagnosis of hyperprolactinaemia is shown in Box 20.63. Many drugs, especially dopamine antagonists, elevate prolactin concentrations. Pituitary tumours can cause hyperprolactinaemia by directly secreting prolactin (prolactinomas, see below), or by compressing the infundibular stalk

20.63 Causes of hyperprolactinaemia

Physiological
- Stress (e.g. post-seizure)
- Pregnancy
- Lactation
- Nipple stimulation
- Sleep
- Coitus
- Exercise
- Baby crying

Drug-induced

Dopamine antagonists
- Antipsychotics (phenothiazines and butyrophenones)
- Antidepressants
- Antiemetics (e.g. metoclopramide, domperidone)

Dopamine-depleting drugs
- Reserpine
- Methyldopa

Oestrogens
- Oral contraceptive pill

Pathological

Common
- Disconnection hyperprolactinaemia (e.g. non-functioning pituitary macroadenoma)
- Prolactinoma (usually microadenoma)
- Primary hypothyroidism
- Polycystic ovarian syndrome
- Macroprolactinaemia

Uncommon
- Pituitary tumour secreting prolactin and growth hormone
- Hypothalamic disease
- Renal failure

Rare
- Chest wall reflex (e.g. post-herpes zoster)

and thus interrupting the tonic inhibitory effect of hypothalamic dopamine on prolactin secretion ('disconnection' hyperprolactinaemia).

Prolactin usually circulates as a free (monomeric) hormone in plasma, but in some individuals prolactin becomes bound to an IgG antibody. This complex is known as macroprolactin and such patients have macroprolactinaemia (not to be confused with macro-prolactinoma, a prolactin-secreting pituitary tumour of more than 1 cm in diameter). Since macroprolactin cannot cross blood-vessel walls to reach prolactin receptors in target tissues, it is of no pathological significance. Some commercial prolactin assays do not distinguish prolactin from macroprolactin and so macroprolactinaemia is a cause of spurious hyperprolactinaemia. Identification of macroprolactin requires gel filtration chromatography or polyethylene glycol precipitation techniques, and one of these tests should be performed in all patients with hyperprolactinaemia if the prolactin assay is known to cross-react.

Clinical assessment

In women, in addition to galactorrhoea, hypogonadism associated with hyperprolactinaemia causes secondary amenorrhoea and anovulation with infertility (p. 759). Important points in the history include drug use, recent pregnancy and menstrual history. The quantity of milk produced is variable, and it may be observed only by manual expression. In men there is decreased libido, reduced shaving frequency and lethargy (p. 760). Unilateral galactorrhoea may be confused with nipple discharge, and breast examination to exclude malignancy or fibrocystic disease is important. Further assessment should address the features in Figure 20.27 (p. 788).

Investigations

Pregnancy should first be excluded before further investigations are performed in women of child-bearing potential. The upper limit of normal for many assays of serum prolactin is approximately 500 mU/L (14 ng/mL). In non-pregnant and non-lactating patients, monomeric prolactin concentrations of 500–1000 mU/L are likely to be induced by stress or drugs, and a repeat measurement is indicated. Levels between 1000 and 5000 mU/L are likely to be due to either drugs, or a microprolactinoma or 'disconnection' hyperprolactinaemia. Levels above 5000 mU/L are highly suggestive of a macroprolactinoma.

Patients with prolactin excess should have tests of gonadal function (p. 757), and T_4 and TSH should be measured to exclude primary hypothyroidism causing TRH-induced prolactin excess. Unless the prolactin falls after withdrawal of relevant drug therapy, a serum prolactin consistently above the reference range is an indication for MRI or CT scan of the hypothalamus and pituitary. Patients with a macroadenoma also need tests for hypopituitarism (see Box 20.58).

Management

If possible, the underlying cause should be corrected (for example, cessation of offending drugs and giving levothyroxine replacement in primary hypothyroidism). If dopamine antagonists are the cause, then dopamine agonist therapy is contraindicated, and if gonadal dysfunction is the primary concern, sex steroid replacement therapy may be indicated. Troublesome physiological galactorrhoea can also be treated with dopamine agonists (see Box 20.64). Management of prolactinomas is described below.

Prolactinoma

Most prolactinomas in pre-menopausal women are microadenomas because the symptoms of prolactin excess usually result in early presentation. Prolactin-secreting cells of the anterior pituitary share a common lineage with GH-secreting cells, so occasionally prolactinomas can secrete excess GH and cause acromegaly. In prolactinomas there is a relationship between prolactin concentration and tumour size: the higher the level, the bigger the tumour. Some macroprolactinomas can elevate prolactin concentrations above 100 000 mU/L. The investigation of prolactinomas is the same as for other pituitary tumours (see above).

Management

As shown in Box 20.62, several therapeutic modalities can be employed in the management of prolactinomas.

Medical

Dopamine agonist drugs are first-line therapy for the majority of patients (Box 20.64). They usually reduce

20.64 Dopamine agonist therapy: drugs used to treat prolactinomas

	Oral dose*	Advantages	Disadvantages
Bromocriptine	2.5–15 mg/day 2–3 times daily	Available for parenteral use Short half-life; useful in treating infertility Proven long-term efficacy	Ergotamine-like side-effects (nausea, headache, postural hypotension, constipation) Frequent dosing so poor compliance Rare reports of fibrotic reactions in various tissues
Cabergoline	250–1000 μg/week 2 doses/week	Long-acting, so missed doses less important Reported to have fewer ergotamine-like side-effects	Limited data on safety in pregnancy Associated with cardiac valvular fibrosis in Parkinson's disease
Quinagolide	50–150 μg/day Once daily	A non-ergot with few side-effects in patients intolerant of the above	Untested in pregnancy

*Tolerance develops for the side-effects. All of these agents, especially bromocriptine, must be introduced at low dose and increased slowly. If several doses of bromocriptine are missed, the process must start again.

A

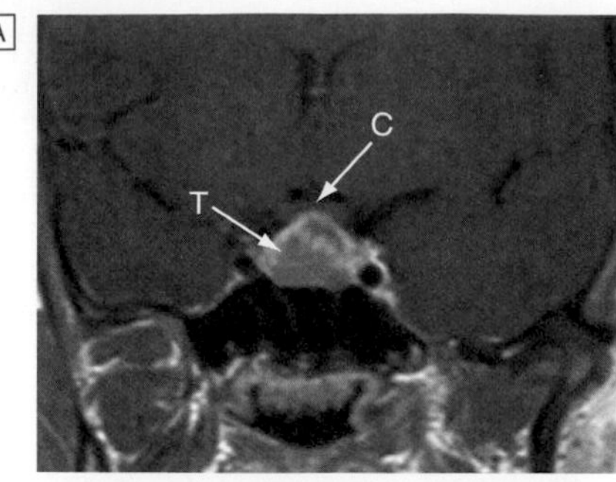

B

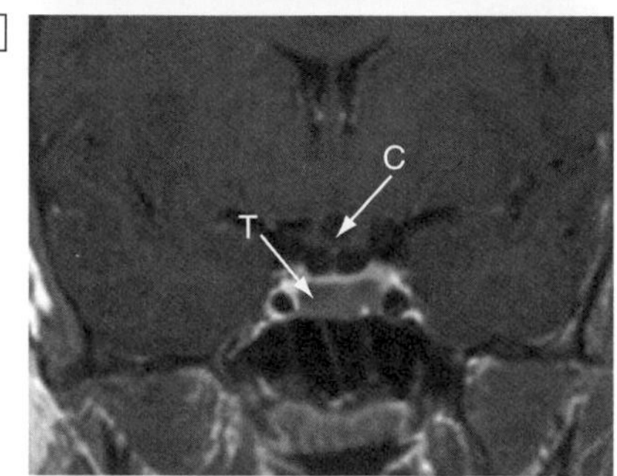

Fig. 20.28 Shrinkage of a macroprolactinoma following treatment with a dopamine agonist. **A** MRI scan showing a pituitary macroadenoma (T) compressing the optic chiasm (C). **B** MRI scan of the same tumour following treatment with a dopamine agonist. The macroadenoma, which was a prolactinoma, has decreased in size substantially and is no longer compressing the optic chiasm.

serum prolactin concentrations and cause significant tumour shrinkage after several months of therapy (Fig. 20.28), but visual field defects, if present, may improve within days of first administration. It is possible to withdraw dopamine agonist therapy without recurrence of hyperprolactinaemia after a few years of treatment in some patients with a microadenoma. Also, after the menopause, suppression of prolactin is only required in microadenomas if galactorrhoea is troublesome, since hypogonadism is then physiological and tumour growth unlikely. In patients with macroadenomas, drugs can only be withdrawn after curative surgery or radiotherapy and under close supervision.

Ergot-derived dopamine agonists (bromocriptine and cabergoline) can bind to 5-HT_{2B} receptors in the heart and elsewhere and have been associated with fibrotic reactions, particularly tricuspid valve regurgitation, when used in high doses in patients with Parkinson's disease. At the relatively low doses used in prolactinomas most data suggest that systematic screening for cardiac fibrosis is unnecessary, but if dopamine agonist therapy is prolonged, periodic screening by echocardiography or use of non-ergot agents (quinagolide) may be indicated.

Surgery and radiotherapy

Surgical decompression is usually only necessary when a macroprolactinoma has failed to shrink sufficiently with dopamine agonist therapy, and this may be because the tumour has a significant cystic component. Surgery may also be performed in patients who are intolerant of dopamine agonists. Microadenomas can be removed selectively by trans-sphenoidal surgery with a cure rate of about 80% but recurrence is not unusual; the cure rate for surgery in macroadenomas is substantially lower.

External irradiation may be required for some macroadenomas to prevent regrowth if dopamine agonists are stopped.

Pregnancy

Hyperprolactinaemia often presents with infertility, so dopamine agonist therapy may be followed by pregnancy. Patients with microadenomas should be advised to withdraw dopamine agonist therapy as soon as pregnancy is confirmed. In contrast, macroprolactinomas may enlarge rapidly under oestrogen stimulation and these patients should continue dopamine agonist therapy and need measurement of prolactin levels and visual fields during pregnancy. All patients should be advised to report headache or visual disturbance promptly.

Acromegaly

Acromegaly is caused by growth hormone (GH) secretion from a pituitary tumour, usually a macroadenoma, and carries an approximate two-fold excess mortality when untreated.

Clinical features

If GH hypersecretion occurs before puberty, then the presentation is with gigantism. More commonly, GH excess occurs in adult life and presents with acromegaly. If hypersecretion starts in adolescence and persists into adult life, then the two conditions may be combined. The clinical features are shown in Figure 20.29. The most common complaints are headache and sweating. Additional features include those of any pituitary tumour (see Fig. 20.27, p. 788).

Investigations

The clinical diagnosis must be confirmed by measuring GH levels during an oral glucose tolerance test and measuring serum IGF-1. In normal subjects, plasma GH suppresses to below 0.5 μg/L (approximately 2 mU/L). In acromegaly, GH does not suppress and in about 30% of patients there is a paradoxical rise; IGF-1 is also elevated. The rest of pituitary function should be investigated as described in Box 20.58 (p. 787). Prolactin concentrations are elevated in about 30% of patients due to co-secretion of prolactin from the tumour. Additional tests in acromegaly may include screening for colonic neoplasms with colonoscopy.

Management

The main aims are to improve symptoms and to normalise serum GH and IGF-1 to reduce morbidity and mortality. Treatment is summarised in Box 20.62.

Surgical

Trans-sphenoidal surgery is usually the first line of treatment and may result in cure of GH excess, especially in patients with microadenomas. More often, surgery serves to debulk the tumour and further second-line therapy is required, according to post-operative imaging and glucose tolerance test results.

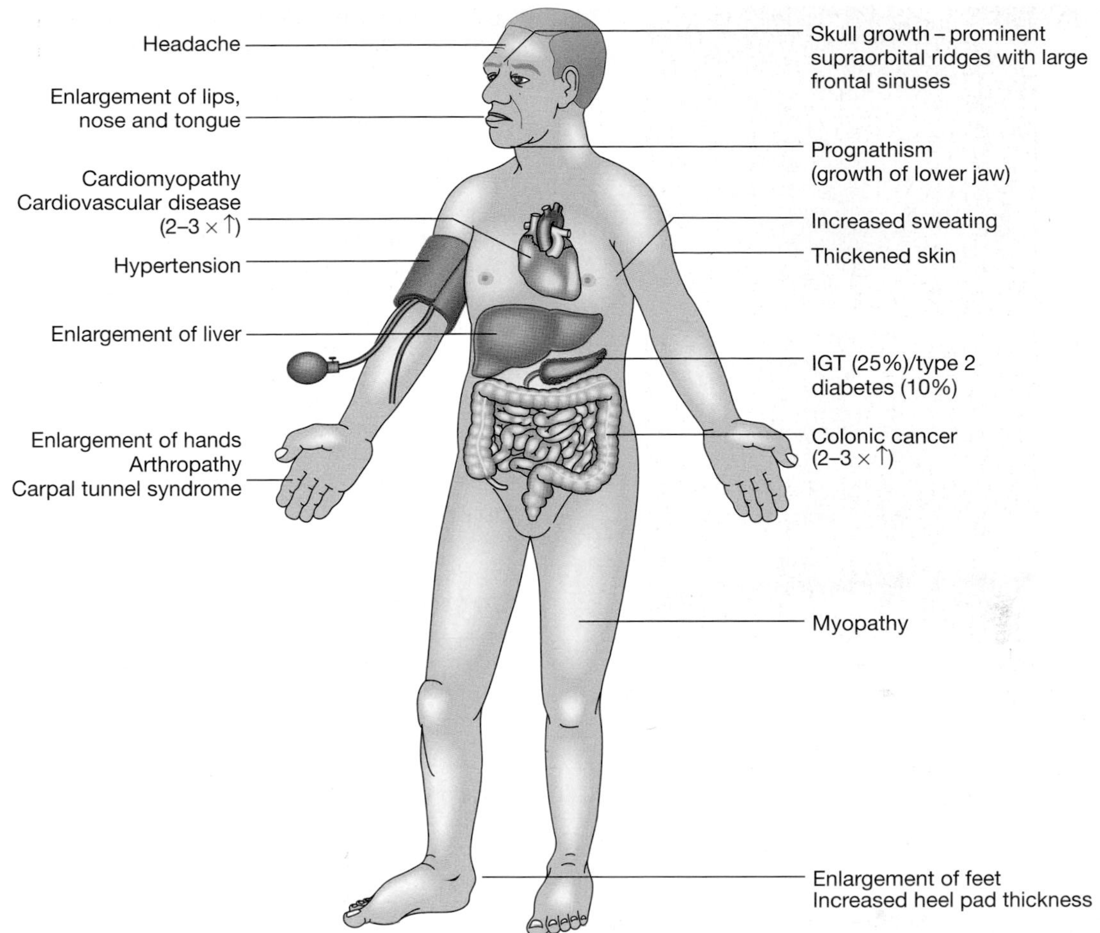

Fig. 20.29 Clinical features of acromegaly. (IGT = impaired glucose tolerance)

Radiotherapy

External radiotherapy is usually employed as second-line treatment if acromegaly persists after surgery, to stop tumour growth and lower GH levels. However, GH levels fall slowly (over many years) and there is a risk of hypopituitarism.

Medical

If acromegaly persists after surgery, medical therapy is usually employed to lower GH levels to below 1.5 μg/L (below approximately 5 mU/L) and to normalise IGF-1 concentrations. Medical therapy may be discontinued after several years in patients who have received radiotherapy. Somatostatin analogues (such as octreotide or lanreotide) can be administered as slow-release injections every few weeks. Somatostatin analogues can also be used as primary therapy for acromegaly either as an alternative or in advance of surgery, given evidence that they can induce modest tumour shrinkage in some patients. Dopamine agonists are less effective at lowering GH but may sometimes be helpful, especially with associated prolactin excess. Pegvisomant is a peptide GH receptor antagonist administered by daily self-injection and may be indicated in some patients whose GH and IGF-1 concentrations fail to suppress sufficiently following somatostatin analogue therapy.

Craniopharyngioma

Craniopharyngiomas are benign tumours that develop in cell rests of Rathke's pouch, and may be located within the sella turcica, or commonly in the suprasellar space. They are often cystic, with a solid component that may or may not be calcified (Fig. 20.30). In young people, they are diagnosed more commonly than pituitary adenomas. They may present with pressure effects on adjacent structures, hypopituitarism and/or cranial diabetes insipidus. Other clinical features directly related to hypothalamic damage may also occur. These include hyperphagia and obesity, loss of the sensation of thirst and disturbance of temperature regulation.

Craniopharyngiomas can be treated by the trans-sphenoidal route but surgery may also involve a craniotomy, with a relatively high risk of hypothalamic damage and other complications. If the tumour has a large cystic component, it may be safer to place in the cyst cavity a drain which is attached to a subcutaneous access device, rather than attempt a resection. Whatever form it takes, surgery is unlikely to be curative and radiotherapy is usually given to reduce the risk of relapse. Unfortunately, craniopharyngiomas often recur, requiring repeated surgery. They often cause considerable morbidity, usually from hypothalamic obesity, water balance problems and/or visual failure.

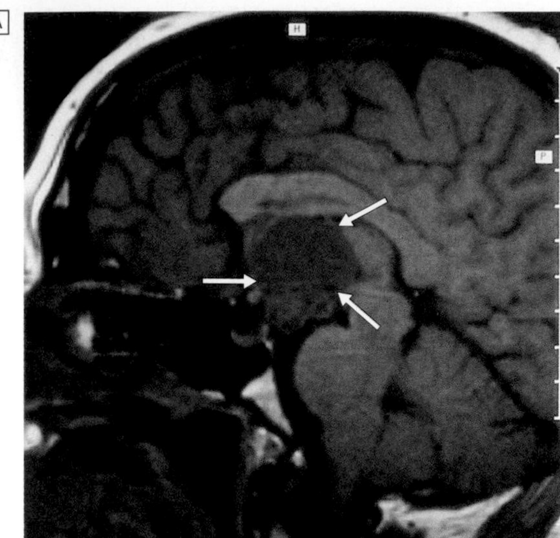

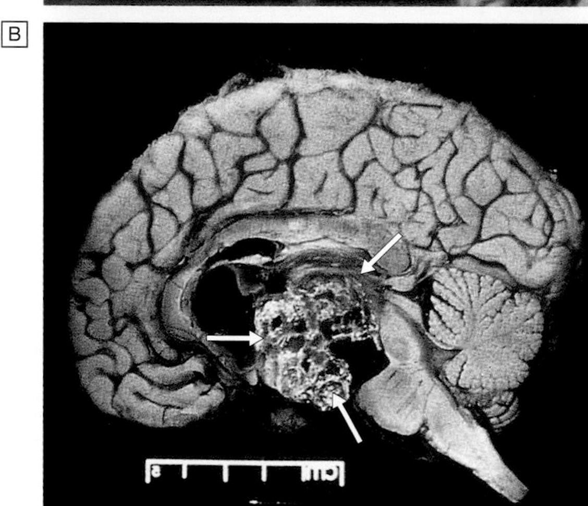

Fig. 20.30 Craniopharyngioma. **A** This developmental tumour characteristically presents in younger patients; it is often cystic and calcified, as shown in this MRI scan (arrows). **B** Pathology specimen.

Diabetes insipidus

This uncommon disorder is characterised by the persistent excretion of excessive quantities of dilute urine and by thirst. It is classified into two types:

- cranial diabetes insipidus, in which there is deficient production of ADH by the hypothalamus
- nephrogenic diabetes insipidus, in which the renal tubules are unresponsive to ADH.

The underlying causes are listed in Box 20.65.

Clinical features

The most marked symptoms are polyuria and polydipsia. The patient may pass 5–20 L or more of urine in 24 hours. This is of low specific gravity and osmolality. If the patient has an intact thirst mechanism, is conscious and has access to oral fluids, then he or she can maintain adequate fluid intake. However, in an unconscious patient or a patient with damage to the hypothalamic thirst centre, diabetes insipidus is potentially lethal. If there is associated cortisol deficiency, then diabetes insipidus may not be manifest until glucocorticoid replacement therapy is given. The most common differential diagnosis is primary polydipsia, caused by drinking excessive amounts of fluid in the absence of a defect in ADH or thirst control.

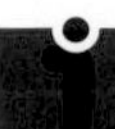

20.65 Causes of diabetes insipidus

Cranial

Structural hypothalamic or high stalk lesion
- See Box 20.59

Idiopathic

Genetic defect
- Dominant (*AVP* gene mutation)
- Recessive (DIDMOAD syndrome – association of diabetes insipidus with diabetes mellitus, optic atrophy, deafness)

Nephrogenic

Genetic defect
- V2 receptor mutation
- Aquaporin-2 mutation
- Cystinosis

Metabolic abnormality
- Hypokalaemia
- Hypercalcaemia

Drug therapy
- Lithium
- Demeclocycline

Poisoning
- Heavy metals

Chronic kidney disease
- Polycystic kidney disease
- Sickle-cell anaemia
- Infiltrative disease

Investigations

Diabetes insipidus can be confirmed if serum ADH is undetectable (although the assay for this is not widely available) or the urine is not maximally concentrated (i.e. is below 600 mOsm/kg) in the presence of increased plasma osmolality (i.e. greater than 300 mOsm/kg). Sometimes, the diagnosis can be confirmed or refuted by random simultaneous samples of blood and urine, but more often a dynamic test is required. The water deprivation test described in Box 20.66 is widely used, but an alternative is to infuse hypertonic (5%) saline and measure ADH secretion in response to increasing plasma osmolality. Thirst can also be assessed during these tests on a visual analogue scale. Anterior pituitary function and suprasellar anatomy should be assessed in patients with cranial diabetes insipidus (see Box 20.58, p. 787).

In primary polydipsia, the urine may be excessively dilute because of chronic diuresis, which 'washes out' the solute gradient across the loop of Henle, but plasma osmolality is low rather than high. DDAVP (see below) should not be administered to patients with primary polydipsia, since it will prevent excretion of water and there is a risk of severe water intoxication if the patient continues to drink fluid to excess.

In nephrogenic diabetes insipidus, appropriate further tests include plasma electrolytes, calcium and investigation of the renal tract (Chs 16 and 17).

Management

Treatment of cranial diabetes insipidus is with desamino-des-aspartate-arginine vasopressin (desmopressin, DDAVP), an analogue of ADH which has a

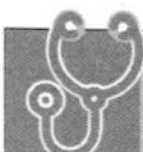

20.66 How and when to do a water deprivation test

Use

- To establish a diagnosis of diabetes insipidus and to differentiate cranial from nephrogenic causes

Protocol

- No coffee, tea or smoking on the test day
- Free fluids until 0730 hrs on the morning of the test, but discourage patients from 'stocking up' with extra fluid in anticipation of fluid deprivation
- No fluids from 0730 hrs
- Attend at 0830 hrs for body weight, plasma and urine osmolality
- Record body weight, urine volume, urine and plasma osmolality and thirst score on a visual analogue scale every 2 hrs for up to 8 hrs
- Stop the test if the patient loses 3% of body weight
- If plasma osmolality reaches > 300 mOsm/kg and urine osmolality < 600 mOsm/kg, then administer DDAVP (see text) 2 μg IM

Interpretation

- Diabetes insipidus is confirmed by a plasma osmolality > 300 mOsm/kg with a urine osmolality < 600 mOsm/kg
- Cranial diabetes insipidus is confirmed if urine osmolality rises by at least 50% after DDAVP
- Nephrogenic diabetes insipidus is confirmed if DDAVP does not concentrate the urine
- Primary polydipsia is suggested by low plasma osmolality at the start of the test

longer half-life. DDAVP is usually administered intranasally. An oral formulation is also available but bioavailability is low and rather unpredictable. In sick patients, DDAVP should be given by intramuscular injection. The dose of DDAVP should be adjusted on the basis of serum sodium concentrations and/or osmolality. The principal hazard is excessive treatment, resulting in water intoxication and hyponatraemia. Conversely, inadequate treatment results in thirst and polyuria. The ideal dose prevents nocturia but allows a degree of polyuria from time to time before the next dose (e.g. DDAVP nasal dose 5 μg in the morning and 10 μg at night).

The polyuria in nephrogenic diabetes insipidus is improved by thiazide diuretics (e.g. bendroflumethiazide 5–10 mg/day), amiloride (5–10 mg/day) and NSAIDs (e.g. indometacin 15 mg 3 times daily), although the last of these carries a risk of reducing glomerular filtration rate.

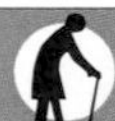

20.67 The pituitary and hypothalamus in old age

- **Late presentation**: often with large tumours causing visual disturbance, because early symptoms such as amenorrhoea and sexual dysfunction do not occur or are not recognised.
- **Coincidentally discovered pituitary tumours**: may not require surgical intervention if the visual apparatus is not involved, because of slow growth. Radiotherapy alone is sometimes employed simply to prevent further growth.
- **Hyperprolactinaemia**: less impact in post-menopausal women who are already 'physiologically' hypogonadal. Macroprolactinomas, however, require treatment because of their potential to cause mass effects.

DISORDERS AFFECTING MULTIPLE ENDOCRINE GLANDS

Multiple endocrine neoplasia

Multiple endocrine neoplasias (MEN) are rare autosomal dominant syndromes characterised by hyperplasia and formation of adenomas or malignant tumours in multiple glands. They fall into two groups, as shown in Box 20.68. Some other genetic diseases also have an increased risk of endocrine tumours; for example, phaeochromocytoma is associated with von Hippel-Lindau syndrome (p. 1216) and neurofibromatosis type 1 (p. 1215).

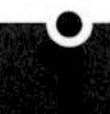

20.68 Multiple endocrine neoplasia (MEN) syndromes

MEN 1 (Wermer's syndrome)

- Primary hyperparathyroidism
- Pituitary tumours
- Pancreatic neuro-endocrine tumours (insulinoma, gastrinoma)

MEN 2 (Sipple's syndrome)

- Primary hyperparathyroidism
- Medullary carcinoma of thyroid
- Phaeochromocytoma

In addition, in MEN 2b syndrome, there are phenotypic changes (including marfanoid habitus, skeletal abnormalities, abnormal dental enamel, multiple mucosal neuromas)

The MEN syndromes should be considered in all patients with two or more endocrine tumours and in patients with solitary tumours who report other endocrine tumours in their family. Inactivating mutations in *MENIN*, a tumour suppressor gene on chromosome 11, cause MEN 1, whereas MEN 2 is caused by gain-of-function mutations in the *RET* proto-oncogene on chromosome 10. These cause constitutive activation of the membrane-associated tyrosine kinase RET, which controls the development of cells that migrate from the neural crest. In contrast, loss-of-function mutations of the RET kinase cause Hirschsprung's disease (p. 917). Genetic testing can be performed on relatives of affected individuals, after appropriate counselling (p. 67).

Individuals who carry mutations associated with MEN should be entered into a surveillance programme. In MEN 1, this typically involves annual history, examination and measurements of serum calcium, gastrointestinal hormones (see Box 20.54, p. 785) and prolactin; MRI of the pituitary and pancreas is performed at less frequent intervals. In individuals with MEN 2, annual history, examination and measurement of serum calcium and urinary catecholamine metabolites should be performed. Because the penetrance of medullary carcinoma of the thyroid is 100% in individuals with a *RET* mutation, prophylactic thyroidectomy should be performed in early childhood.

Autoimmune polyendocrine syndromes

Two distinct autoimmune polyendocrine syndromes are known: APS types 1 and 2.

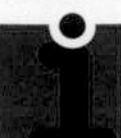

20.69 Autoimmune polyendocrine syndromes (APS)*

Type 1 (APECED)	
• Addison's disease • Hypoparathyroidism • Type 1 diabetes • Primary hypothyroidism	• Chronic mucocutaneous candidiasis • Nail dystrophy • Dental enamel hypoplasia
Type 2 (Schmidt's syndrome)	
• Addison's disease • Primary hypothyroidism • Graves' disease • Pernicious anaemia • Primary hypogonadism	• Type 1 diabetes • Vitiligo • Coeliac disease • Myasthenia gravis

*In both types of APS, the precise pattern of disease varies between affected individuals.

The most common is APS type 2 (Schmidt's syndrome), which typically presents in women between the ages of 20 and 60. It is usually defined as the occurrence in the same individual of two or more autoimmune endocrine disorders, some of which are listed in Box 20.69. The mode of inheritance is autosomal dominant with incomplete penetrance and there is a strong association with HLA-DR3 and CTLA-4.

Much less common is APS type 1, which is also termed autoimmune poly-endocrinopathy-candidiasis-ectodermal dystrophy (APECED). This is inherited in an autosomal recessive fashion and is caused by loss-of-function mutations in the autoimmune regulator gene *AIRE*, which is responsible for the presentation of self-antigens to thymocytes in utero. This is essential for the deletion of thymocyte clones that react against self-antigens and hence for the development of immune tolerance (Ch. 4). The most common clinical features are described in Box 20.69, although the pattern of presentation is variable and other autoimmune disorders are often observed.

Late effects of childhood cancer therapy

Prolonged survival is increasingly common following successful treatment of cancers in children and adolescents. The therapies used to treat these diseases, including radiotherapy and chemotherapy, may cause long-term endocrine dysfunction. In many circumstances this is predictable, such as cytotoxic chemotherapy causing future infertility and pubertal delay (especially in boys), cranial irradiation causing long-term pituitary dysfunction, and radiotherapy to the neck causing hypothyroidism and thyroid cancer. Increasing recognition of these issues has resulted in active monitoring programmes for survivors of childhood cancer, who are best seen in specialist 'late effects' multidisciplinary clinics where teams include endocrinologists, oncologists, reproductive medicine specialists, psychologists and nurse specialists.

Further information

Websites

www.british-thyroid-association.org *British Thyroid Association: provider of guidelines, e.g. for use of thyroid function tests.*

www.btf-thyroid.org *British Thyroid Foundation: a resource for patient leaflets and support for patients with thyroid disorders.*

www.endocrinology.org *British Society for Endocrinology: useful online education resources and links to patient support group.*

www.endo-society.org *American Endocrine Society: provider of clinical practice guidelines.*

www.pituitary.org.uk *Pituitary Foundation: a resource for patient and general practitioner leaflets and further information.*

www.thyroid.org *American Thyroid Association: provider of clinical practice guidelines.*

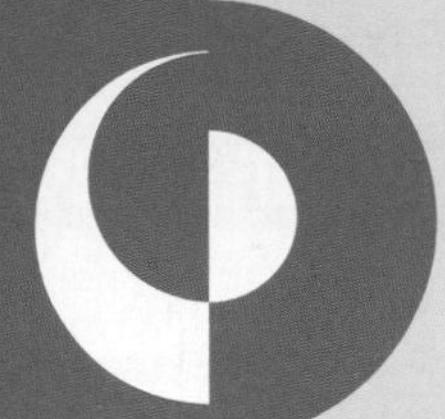

E.R. Pearson
R.J. McCrimmon

Diabetes mellitus

21

Clinical examination of the patient with diabetes 798

Functional anatomy and physiology 800
- Normal glucose and fat metabolism 800
- Aetiology and pathogenesis of diabetes 802

Investigations 807

Presenting problems in diabetes mellitus 808
- Newly discovered hyperglycaemia 808
- Long-term supervision of diabetes 811
- Diabetic ketoacidosis 811
- Hyperglycaemic hyperosmolar state 814
- Hypoglycaemia 814
- Diabetes in pregnancy 817
- Children, adolescents and young adults with diabetes 818
- Hyperglycaemia in acute myocardial infarction 818
- Surgery and diabetes 818
- Complications of diabetes 820

Management of diabetes 820
- Diet and lifestyle 820
- Drugs to reduce hyperglycaemia 821
- Insulin therapy 824
- Transplantation 826

Complications of diabetes 826
- Diabetic retinopathy 828
- Diabetic nephropathy 830
- Diabetic neuropathy 831
- The diabetic foot 833

CLINICAL EXAMINATION OF THE PATIENT WITH DIABETES

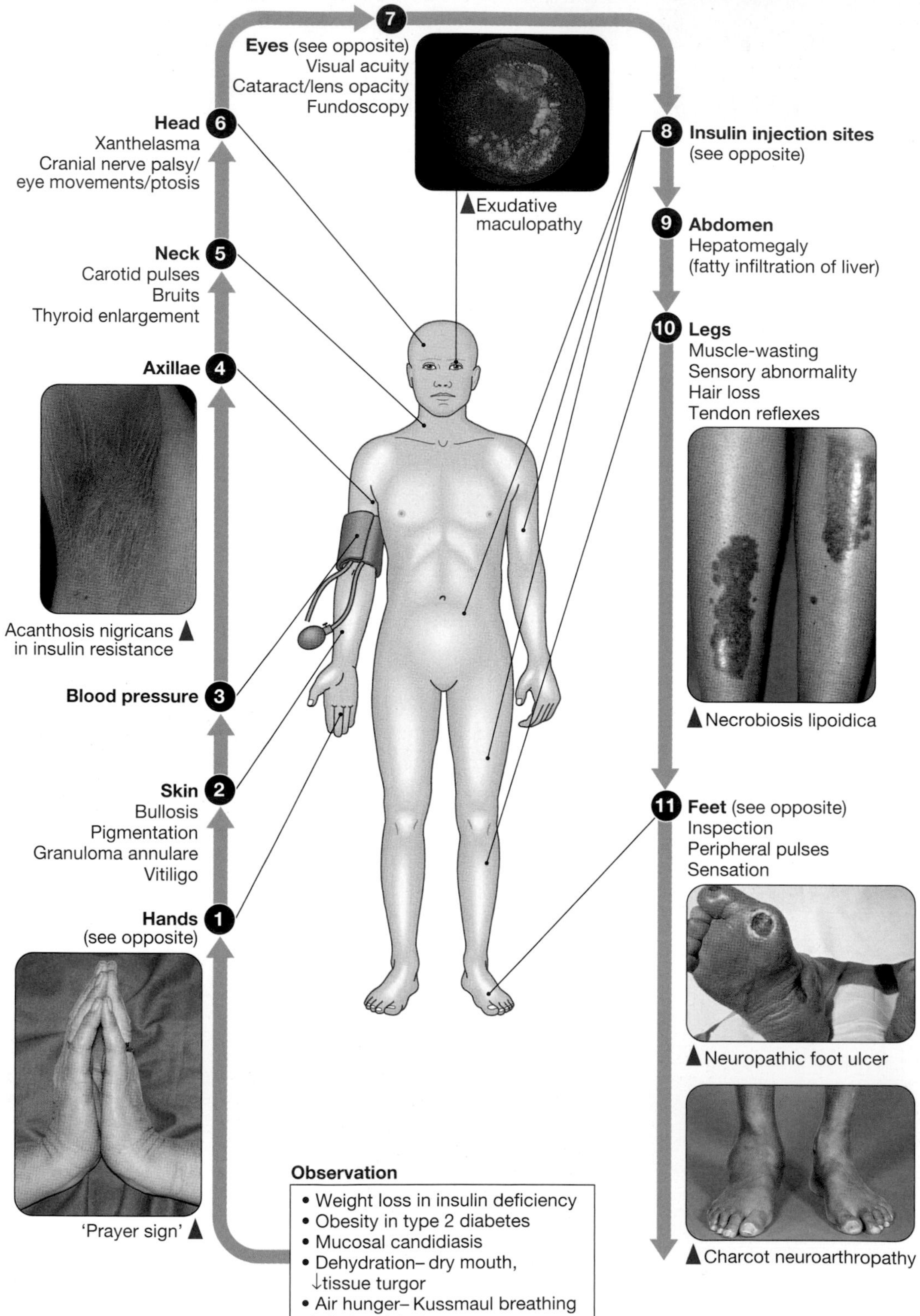

Inset (Acanthosis nigricans) From Shotliff. In: Lim 2007 – see p. 836.

Diabetes can affect every system in the body. In routine clinical practice, examination of the patient with diabetes is focused on 1 hands, 3 blood pressure, 4 and 5 axillae and neck, 7 eyes, 8 insulin injection sites and 11 feet.

7 Examination of the eyes

Visual acuity

- Distance vision using Snellen chart at 6 metres
- Near vision using standard reading chart

Visual acuity can alter reversibly with acute hyperglycaemia due to osmotic changes affecting the lens. Most patients with retinopathy do not have altered visual acuity, except after a vitreous haemorrhage or in some cases of maculopathy.

Lens opacification

- Look for the red reflex using the ophthalmoscope held 30 cm from the eye

Fundal examination

- Either use a three-field retinal camera or dilate pupils with a mydriatic (e.g. tropicamide) and examine with ophthalmoscope in a darkened room
- Note features of diabetic retinopathy (p. 828), including photocoagulation scars from previous laser treatment

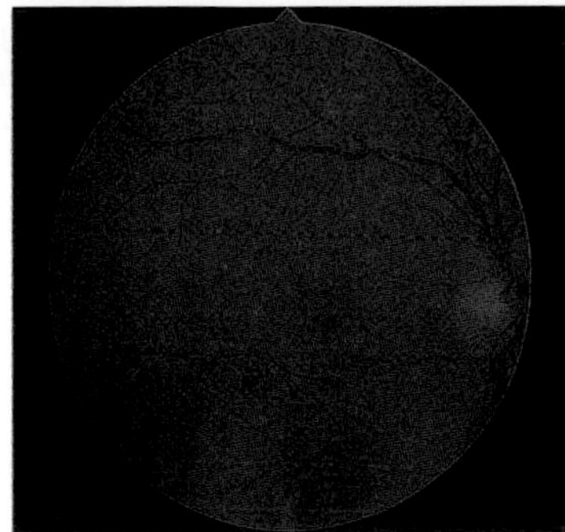

Background retinopathy.

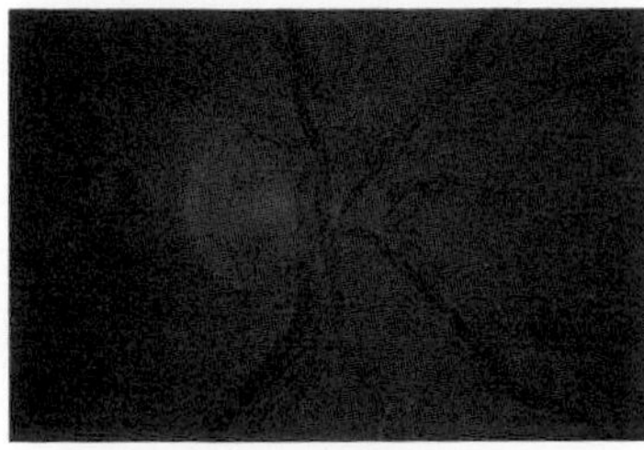

Proliferative retinopathy.

1 Examination of the hands

Several abnormalities are more common in diabetes:

- Limited joint mobility ('cheiroarthropathy') causes painless stiffness. The inability to extend (to 180°) the metacarpophalangeal or interphalangeal joints of at least one finger bilaterally can be demonstrated in the 'prayer sign'
- Dupuytren's contracture (p. 1134) causes nodules or thickening of the skin and knuckle pads
- Carpal tunnel syndrome (p. 1224) presents with wrist pain radiating into the hand
- Trigger finger (flexor tenosynovitis)
- Muscle-wasting/sensory changes may be present in peripheral sensorimotor neuropathy, although this is more common in the lower limbs

8 Insulin injection sites

Main areas used

- Anterior abdominal wall
- Upper thighs/buttocks
- Upper outer arms

Inspection

- Bruising
- Subcutaneous fat deposition (lipohypertrophy)
- Subcutaneous fat loss (lipoatrophy; associated with injection of unpurified animal insulins – now rare)
- Erythema, infection (rare)

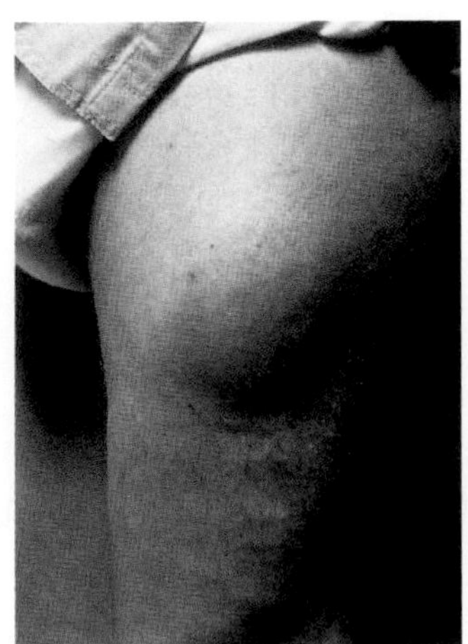

Lipohypertrophy of the upper arm.

11 Examination of the feet

Inspection

- Look for evidence of callus formation on weight-bearing areas, clawing of the toes (in neuropathy), loss of the plantar arch, discoloration of the skin (ischaemia), localised infection and ulcers
- Deformity may be present, especially in Charcot neuroarthropathy
- Fungal infection may affect skin between toes, and nails

Circulation

- Peripheral pulses, skin temperature and capillary refill may be abnormal

Sensation

- Abnormal in stocking distribution in typical peripheral sensorimotor neuropathy
- Testing light touch with monofilaments is sufficient for risk assessment; test other sensation modalities (vibration, pain, proprioception) only when neuropathy is being evaluated

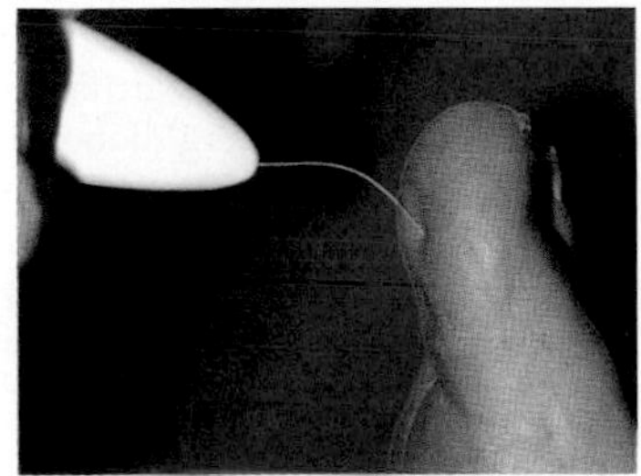

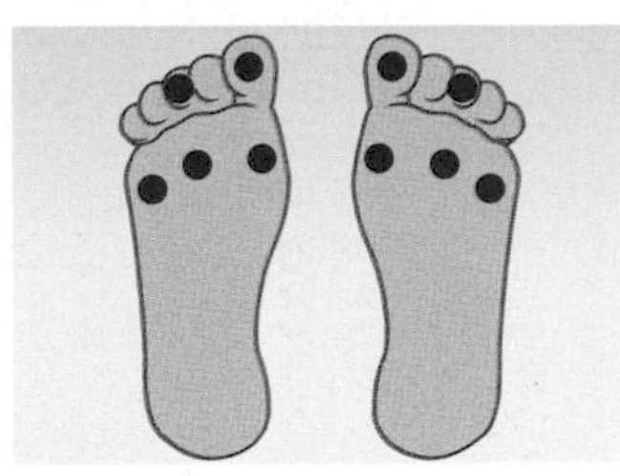

Monofilaments. The monofilament is applied gently until slightly deformed at 5 points on each foot. Callus should be avoided as sensation is reduced. If the patient feels fewer than 8 out of 10 touches, the risk of foot ulceration is increased 5–10-fold.

Reflexes

- Loss of ankle reflexes in typical sensorimotor neuropathy
- Test plantar and ankle reflexes

Diabetes mellitus is a clinical syndrome characterised by an increase in plasma blood glucose (hyperglycaemia). Diabetes has many causes (see Box 21.5, p. 807) but is most commonly due to type 1 or type 2 diabetes. Type 1 diabetes is caused by autoimmune destruction of insulin-producing cells (β cells) in the pancreas, resulting in absolute insulin deficiency, whereas type 2 diabetes is characterised by resistance to the action of insulin and an inability to produce sufficient insulin to overcome this 'insulin resistance'. Hyperglycaemia results in both acute and long-term problems. Acutely, high glucose and lack of insulin can result in marked symptoms, metabolic decompensation and hospitalisation. Chronic hyperglycaemia is responsible for diabetes-specific 'microvascular' complications affecting the eyes (retinopathy), kidneys (nephropathy) and feet (neuropathy).

There is a continuous distribution of blood glucose in the population, with no clear division between people with normal and abnormal values. The diagnostic criteria for diabetes (a fasting plasma glucose ≥ 7.0 mmol/L (126 mg/dL) or glucose 2 hours after an oral glucose challenge ≥ 11.1 mmol/L (200 mg/dL); see p. 807) have been selected to identify those who have a degree of hyperglycaemia which, if untreated, carries a significant risk of microvascular disease, and in particular diabetic retinopathy. Less severe hyperglycaemia is called 'impaired glucose tolerance'. This is not associated with a substantial risk of microvascular disease, but is connected with an increased risk of large vessel disease (e.g. atheroma leading to myocardial infarction) and with a greater risk of developing diabetes in future.

The incidence of diabetes is rising. Globally, it is estimated that 366 million people had diabetes in 2011 (approximately 8.3% of the world population, or 3 new cases every 10 seconds), and this figure is expected to reach 552 million by 2030. This global pandemic principally involves type 2 diabetes, the prevalence of which varies considerably around the world (Fig. 21.1), being associated with differences in genetic as well as environmental factors such as greater longevity, obesity, unsatisfactory diet, sedentary lifestyle, increasing urbanisation and economic development. A pronounced rise in the prevalence of type 2 diabetes occurs in migrant populations to industrialised countries, as in Asian and Afro-Caribbean immigrants to the UK or USA. Type 2 diabetes is now being observed in children and adolescents, particularly in some ethnic groups, such as Hispanics and Afro-Americans.

The incidence of type 1 diabetes is also increasing, such that between 1960 and 1996, 3% more children were diagnosed worldwide each year. Type 1 diabetes is generally more common in countries closer to the polar regions. Finland, for instance, has the highest rate of type 1 diagnosis per year at around 40 per 100 000 of the population, whereas in China the incidence is only 0.1 per 100 000 of the population. Type 1 diabetes is most common in Caucasians and more people are diagnosed in the winter months.

Diabetes is a major burden upon health-care facilities in all countries. Globally, diabetes caused 4.6 million deaths in 2011, and health-care expenditure attributed to diabetes was estimated to be at least US$465 billion, or 11% of total health-care expenditure.

FUNCTIONAL ANATOMY AND PHYSIOLOGY

Normal glucose and fat metabolism

Blood glucose is tightly regulated and maintained within a narrow range. This is essential for ensuring a continuous supply of glucose to the central nervous system. The brain has little capacity to store energy in the form of glycogen or triglyceride and the blood–brain barrier is largely impermeable to fatty acids, so the brain depends on the liver for a constant supply of glucose for oxidation and hence generation of adenosine triphosphate (ATP). Glucose homeostasis is achieved through the coordinated actions of multiple organs, but mainly reflects a balance between the entry of glucose into the circulation from the liver, supplemented by intestinal

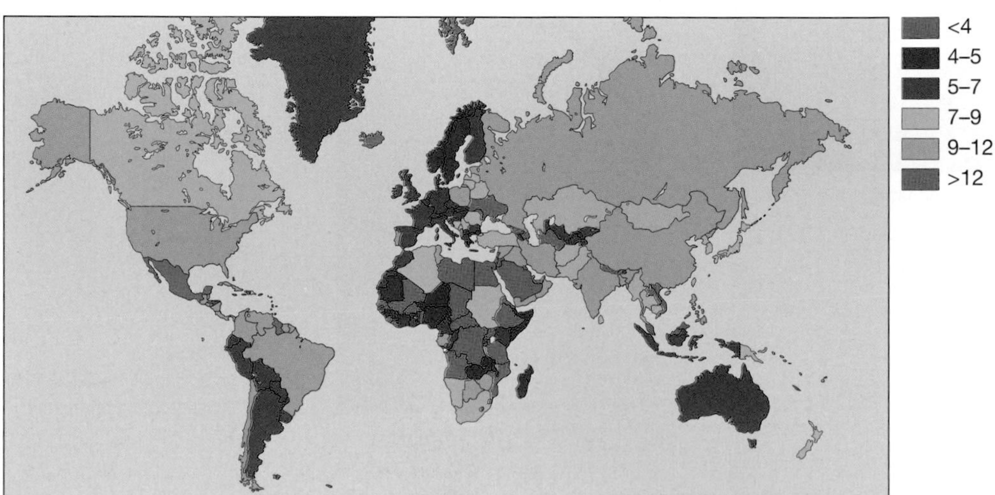

Fig. 21.1 Prevalence (%) of diabetes in those aged 20–79 years, 2011, based on estimates from the International Diabetes Federation.

absorption of glucose after meals, and the uptake of glucose by peripheral tissues, particularly skeletal muscle and brain.

After ingestion of a meal containing carbohydrate, normal blood glucose levels are maintained by:

- suppression of hepatic glucose production
- stimulation of hepatic glucose uptake
- stimulation of glucose uptake by peripheral tissues (Fig. 21.2).

Insulin, the primary regulator of glucose metabolism and storage (Box 21.1), is secreted from pancreatic β cells into the portal circulation in response to a rise in blood glucose (Fig. 21.3). A number of other factors released from the gut following food intake can augment insulin release, including amino acids and hormones such as glucagon-like peptide 1 (GLP-1) and gastrointestinal peptide (GIP). As a result, insulin release is greater when glucose is administered by mouth than when the same rise in plasma glucose is achieved by intravenous glucose infusion, a phenomenon termed the 'incretin' effect (see Fig. 21.3). The post-prandial rise in portal vein insulin and glucose, together with a fall in portal

21.1 Metabolic actions of insulin

Increase	Decrease
Carbohydrate metabolism	
Glucose transport (muscle, adipose tissue)	Gluconeogenesis
Glucose phosphorylation	Glycogenolysis
Glycogen synthesis	
Glycolysis	
Pyruvate dehydrogenase activity	
Pentose phosphate shunt	
Lipid metabolism	
Triglyceride synthesis	Lipolysis
Fatty acid synthesis (liver)	Lipoprotein lipase (muscle)
Lipoprotein lipase activity (adipose tissue)	Ketogenesis
	Fatty acid oxidation (liver)
Protein metabolism	
Amino acid transport	Protein degradation
Protein synthesis	

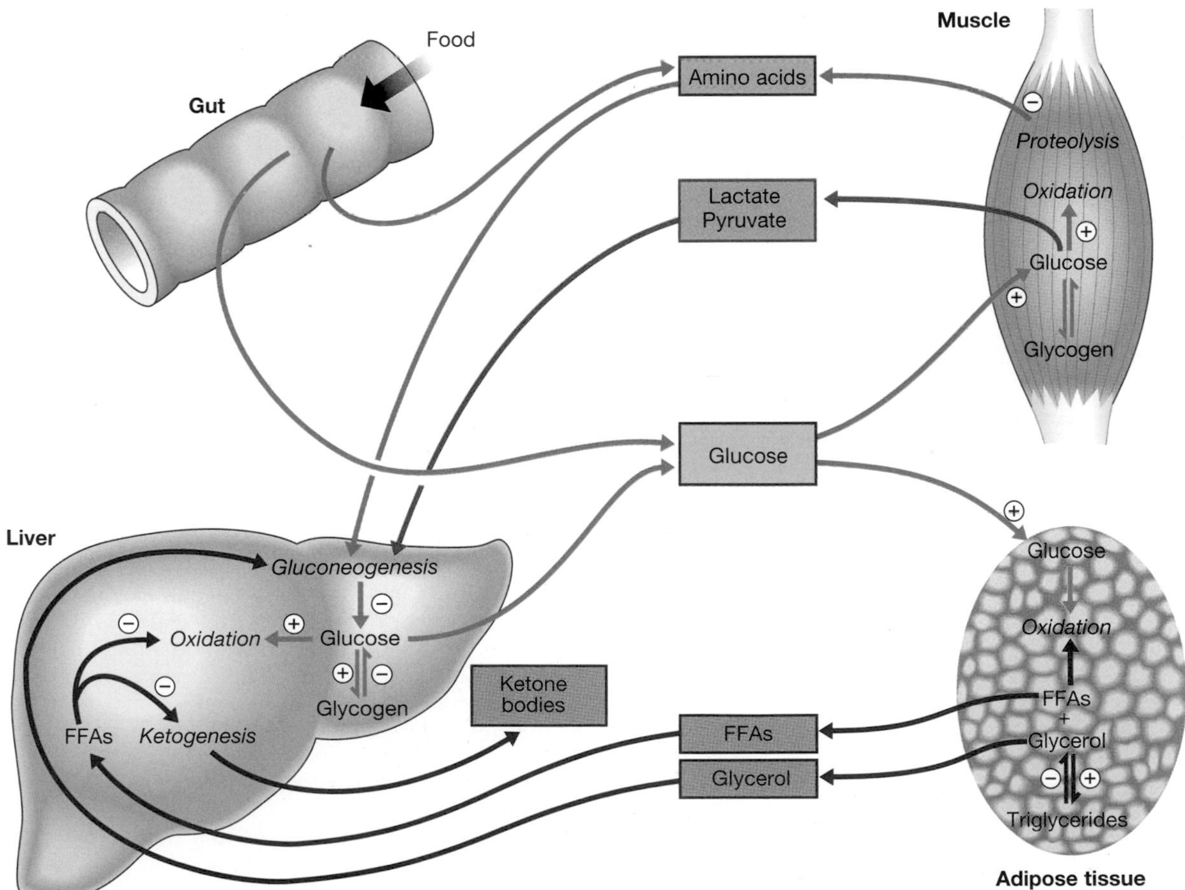

Fig. 21.2 Major metabolic pathways of fuel metabolism and the actions of insulin. ⊕ indicates stimulation and ⊖ indicates suppression by insulin. In response to a rise in blood glucose, e.g. after a meal, insulin is released, suppressing gluconeogenesis and promoting glycogen synthesis and storage. Insulin promotes the peripheral uptake of glucose, particularly in skeletal muscle, and encourages storage (as muscle glycogen). It also promotes protein synthesis and lipogenesis, and suppresses lipolysis. The release of intermediate metabolites, including amino acids (glutamine, alanine), 3-carbon intermediates in oxidation (lactate, pyruvate) and free fatty acids (FFAs), is controlled by insulin. In the absence of insulin, e.g. during fasting, these processes are reversed and favour gluconeogenesis in liver from glycogen, glycerol, amino acids and other 3-carbon precursors.

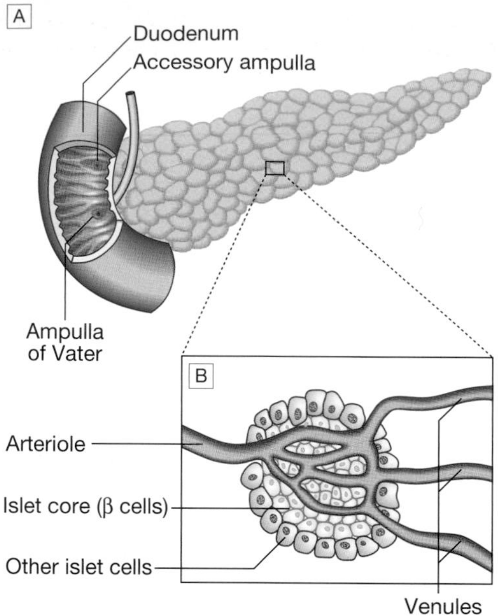

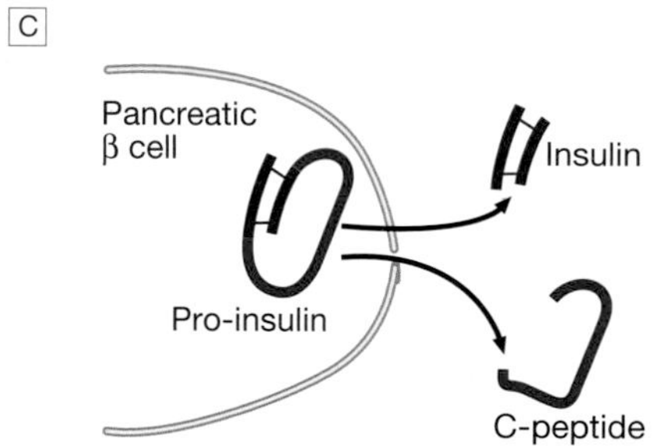

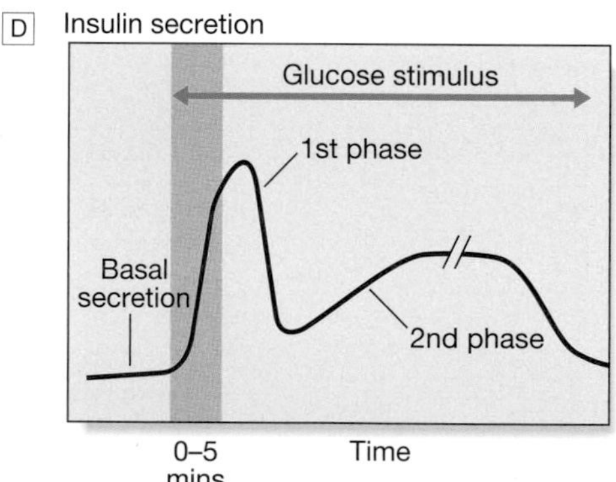

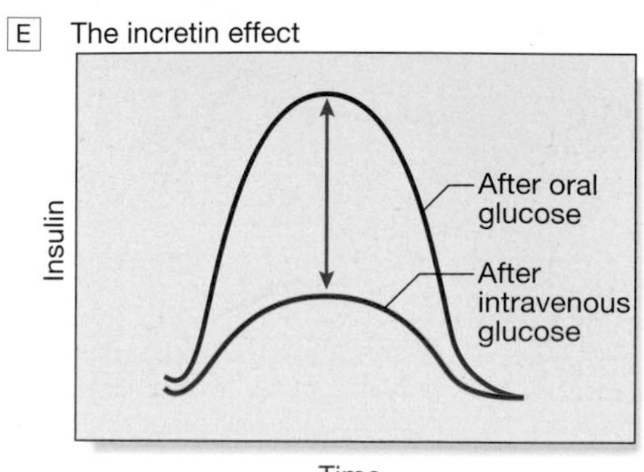

Fig. 21.3 Pancreatic structure and endocrine function. **A** The normal adult pancreas contains about 1 million islets, which are scattered throughout the exocrine parenchyma. Histology is shown in Figure 21.4. **B** The core of each islet consists of β cells that produce insulin, and is surrounded by a cortex of endocrine cells that produce other hormones, including glucagon (α cells), somatostatin (δ cells) and pancreatic polypeptide (PP cells). **C** Pro-insulin in the pancreatic β cell is cleaved to release insulin and equimolar amounts of inert C-peptide (connecting peptide). Measurement of C-peptide can be used to assess endogenous insulin secretory capacity. **D** An acute first phase of insulin secretion occurs in response to an elevated blood glucose, followed by a sustained second phase. **E** The incretin effect describes the observation that insulin secretion is greater when glucose is given by mouth than when glucose is administered intravenously to achieve the same rise in blood glucose concentrations. The additional stimulus to insulin secretion is mediated by release of peptides from the gut and these actions are exploited in incretin-based therapies (p. 823).

glucagon concentrations, suppresses hepatic glucose production and results in net hepatic glucose uptake. Depending on the size of the carbohydrate load, around one-quarter to one-third of ingested glucose is taken up in the liver. In addition, insulin stimulates glucose uptake in skeletal muscle and fat, mediated by the glucose transporter, GLUT 4.

When intestinal glucose absorption declines between meals, portal vein insulin and glucose concentrations fall while glucagon levels rise. This leads to increased hepatic glucose output via gluconeogenesis and glycogen breakdown. The liver now resumes net glucose production and glucose homeostasis is maintained. The main substrates for gluconeogenesis are glycerol and amino acids, as shown in Figure 21.2.

Adipocytes (and the liver) synthesise triglyceride from non-esterified ('free') fatty acids (FFAs) and glycerol. Insulin is the major regulator not only of glucose metabolism but also of fatty acid metabolism. High insulin levels after meals promote triglyceride accumulation. In contrast, in the fasting state, low insulin levels permit lipolysis and the release into the circulation of FFAs (and glycerol), which can be oxidised by many tissues. Their partial oxidation in the liver provides energy to drive gluconeogenesis and also produces ketone bodies (acetoacetate, which can be reduced to 3-hydroxybutyrate or decarboxylated to acetone), which are generated in hepatocyte mitochondria. Ketone bodies are organic acids which, when formed in small amounts, are oxidised and utilised as metabolic fuel. However, the rate of utilisation of ketone bodies by peripheral tissues is limited, and when the rate of production by the liver exceeds their removal, hyperketonaemia results. This occurs physiologically during starvation, when low insulin levels and high catecholamine levels increase lipolysis and delivery of FFAs to the liver.

Aetiology and pathogenesis of diabetes

In both of the common types of diabetes, environmental factors interact with genetic susceptibility to determine which people develop the clinical syndrome, and the timing of its onset. However, the underlying genes, precipitating environmental factors and pathophysiology differ substantially between type 1 and type 2 diabetes. Type 1 diabetes was previously termed 'insulin-dependent diabetes mellitus' (IDDM) and is invariably associated with profound insulin deficiency requiring replacement therapy. Type 2 diabetes was previously termed 'non-insulin-dependent diabetes mellitus' (NIDDM) because patients retain the capacity to secrete some insulin but exhibit impaired sensitivity to insulin (insulin resistance) and initially can usually be treated without insulin replacement therapy. However, 20% or more of patients with type 2 diabetes will ultimately develop profound insulin deficiency requiring replacement therapy, so that IDDM and NIDDM were misnomers.

Type 1 diabetes

Pathology

Type 1 diabetes is a T cell-mediated autoimmune disease (p. 86) involving destruction of the insulin-secreting β cells in the pancreatic islets. Progressive loss of β cell function takes place over a prolonged period (months to years), but marked hyperglycaemia, accompanied by the classical symptoms of diabetes, occurs only when 80–90% of the functional capacity of β cells has been lost.

The pathology in the pre-diabetic pancreas is characterised by 'insulitis' (Fig. 21.4), with infiltration of the islets by mononuclear cells containing activated macrophages, helper cytotoxic and suppressor T lymphocytes, natural killer cells and B lymphocytes. Initially, these lesions are patchy and, until a very late stage, lobules containing heavily infiltrated islets are seen adjacent to unaffected lobules. The destructive process is β cell-specific, the glucagon and other hormone-secreting cells in the islet remaining intact.

Islet cell antibodies are present before the clinical presentation of type 1 diabetes, and their detection can be useful in confirming a diagnosis of type 1 diabetes, but they are poorly predictive of disease progression and disappear over time (see Fig. 21.4). Type 1 diabetes is associated with other autoimmune disorders (Ch. 4), including thyroid disease (p. 738), coeliac disease (p. 880), Addison's disease (p. 777), pernicious anaemia (p. 1025) and vitiligo (p. 1295).

Genetic predisposition

Genetic factors account for about one-third of the susceptibility to type 1 diabetes, the inheritance of which is polygenic (Box 21.2). Over 20 different regions of the human genome show some linkage with type 1 diabetes but most interest has focused on the human leucocyte antigen (HLA) region within the major histocompatibility complex on the short arm of chromosome 6; this locus is designated IDDM 1. The HLA haplotypes *DR3* and/or *DR4* are associated with increased susceptibility to type 1 diabetes in Caucasians and are in 'linkage disequilibrium', i.e. they tend to be transmitted together, with the neighbouring alleles of the *HLA-DQA1* and *DQB1* genes. The latter may be the main determinants of genetic susceptibility, since these HLA class II genes code for proteins on the surface of cells which present foreign and self antigens to T lymphocytes (p. 87). Candidate gene and genome-wide association studies have also implicated other genes in type 1 diabetes, e.g. *CD25*, *PTPN22*, *IL2RA* and *IL-10*, which are involved in immune recognition of pancreatic islet antigens, T-cell development and immune regulation. The genes associated with type 1 diabetes overlap with those for other

21.2 Risk of type 1 diabetes among first-degree relatives of patients with type 1 diabetes

Relative with type 1 diabetes	% overall risk
Identical twin	35
Non-identical twin	20
HLA-identical sibling	16
Non-HLA-identical sibling	3
Father	9
Mother	3
Both parents	Up to 30

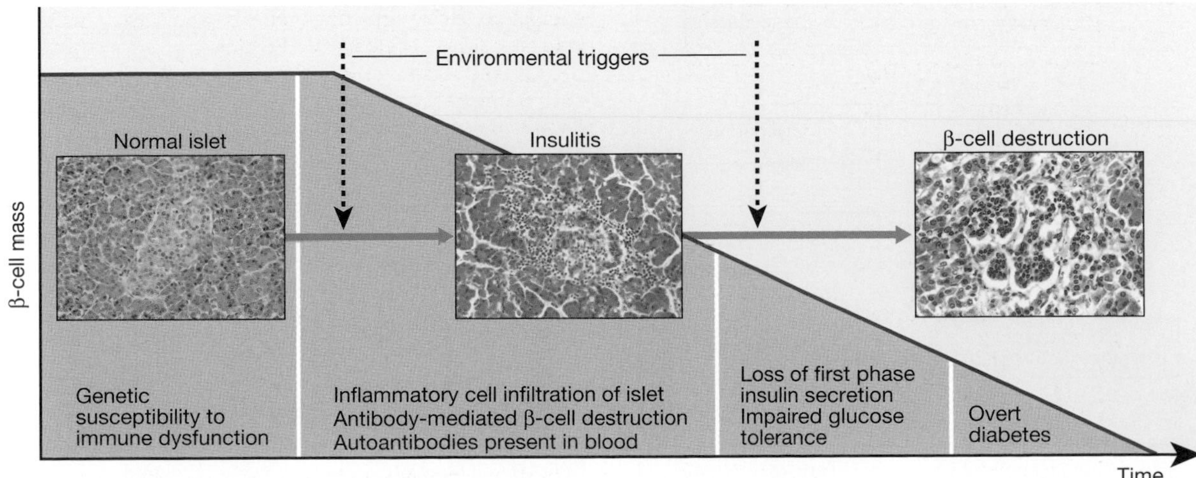

Fig. 21.4 Pathogenesis of type 1 diabetes. Proposed sequence of events in the development of type 1 diabetes. Environmental triggers are described in the text.

autoimmune disorders, such as coeliac disease and thyroid disease, consistent with clustering of these conditions in individuals or families.

Environmental predisposition

Although genetic susceptibility appears to be a prerequisite for type 1 diabetes, the concordance rate between monozygotic twins is less than 40% (see Box 21.2), and wide geographic and seasonal variations in incidence suggest that environmental factors have an important role in precipitating disease.

Although hypotheses abound, the nature of these environmental factors is uncertain. They may trigger type 1 diabetes through direct toxicity to β cells or by stimulating an autoimmune reaction directed against β cells. Potential candidates fall into three main categories: viruses, specific drugs or chemicals, and dietary constituents. Viruses implicated in the aetiology of type 1 diabetes include mumps, Coxsackie B4, retroviruses, rubella (in utero), cytomegalovirus and Epstein–Barr virus. Various dietary nitrosamines (found in smoked and cured meats) and coffee have been proposed as potentially diabetogenic toxins. Bovine serum albumin (BSA), a major constituent of cow's milk, has been implicated, since children who are given cow's milk early in infancy are more likely to develop type 1 diabetes than those who are breastfed. BSA may cross the neonatal gut and raise antibodies which cross-react with a heat-shock protein expressed by β cells. It has also been proposed that reduced exposure to microorganisms in early childhood limits maturation of the immune system and increases susceptibility to autoimmune disease (the 'hygiene hypothesis').

Metabolic disturbances in type 1 diabetes

Patients with type 1 diabetes present when progressive β-cell destruction has crossed a threshold at which adequate insulin secretion and normal blood glucose levels can no longer be sustained. Above a certain level, high glucose levels may be toxic to the remaining β cells, so that profound insulin deficiency rapidly ensues, causing the metabolic sequelae shown in Figure 21.5. Hyperglycaemia leads to glycosuria and dehydration, causing fatigue, polyuria, nocturia, thirst and polydipsia, susceptibility to urinary and genital tract infections, and later tachycardia and hypotension. Unrestrained lipolysis and proteolysis result in weight loss. Ketoacidosis occurs when generation of ketone bodies exceeds the capacity for their metabolism. Elevated blood H^+ ions drive K^+ out of the intracellular compartment, while secondary hyperaldosteronism encourages urinary loss of K^+. Thus patients usually present with a short history (typically a few weeks) of hyperglycaemic symptoms (thirst, polyuria, nocturia and fatigue), infections and weight loss, and may have developed ketoacidosis (p. 811).

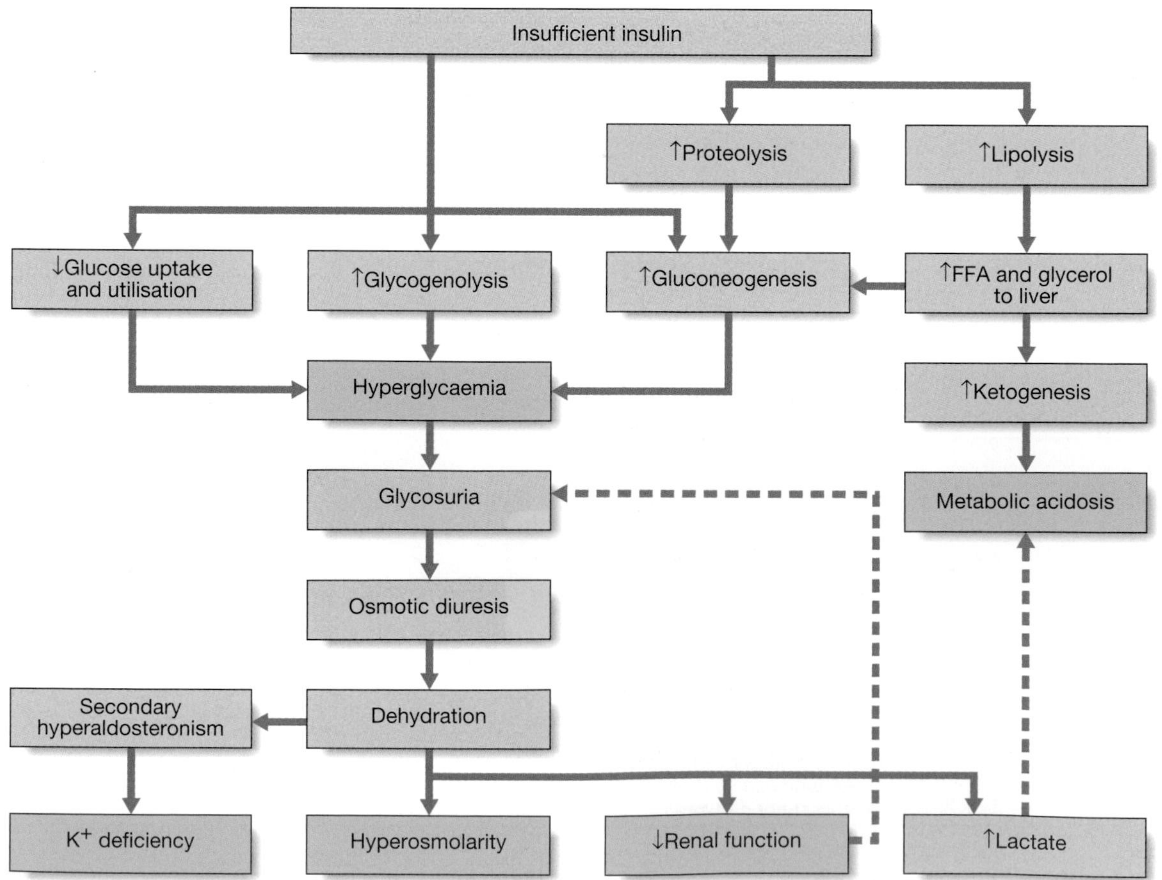

Fig. 21.5 Acute metabolic complications of insulin deficiency. (FFA = free fatty acids.)

Type 2 diabetes

Pathology

Type 2 diabetes is a diagnosis of exclusion, i.e. it is made when type 1 diabetes and other types of diabetes (see Box 21.5, p. 807) are ruled out, and is highly heterogeneous. The natural history of typical type 2 diabetes is shown in Figure 21.6. Initially, insulin resistance leads to elevated insulin secretion in order to maintain normal blood glucose levels. However, in susceptible individuals, the pancreatic β cells are unable to sustain the increased demand for insulin and a slowly progressive insulin deficiency develops. Some patients develop diabetes at a young age, usually driven by insulin resistance due to obesity and ethnicity; others, particularly the elderly, develop diabetes despite being non-obese and may have more pronounced β-cell failure. The key feature is a 'relative' insulin deficiency, such that there is insufficient insulin production to overcome the resistance to insulin action. This contrasts with type 1 diabetes, in which there is rapid loss of insulin production and an absolute deficiency, resulting in ketoacidosis and death if the insulin is not replaced.

Insulin resistance

Type 2 diabetes, or its antecedent, impaired glucose tolerance, is one of a cluster of conditions thought to be caused by resistance to insulin action. Thus, patients with type 2 diabetes often have associated disorders including hypertension, dyslipidaemia (characterised by elevated levels of small dense low-density lipoprotein (LDL) cholesterol and triglycerides, and a low level of high-density lipoprotein (HDL) cholesterol), non-alcoholic fatty liver (p. 959) and, in women, polycystic ovarian syndrome. This cluster has been termed the 'insulin resistance syndrome' or 'metabolic syndrome', and is much more common in patients who are obese.

The primary cause of insulin resistance remains unclear; it is likely that there are multiple defects in insulin signalling, affecting several tissues. One theory is centred around the adipocyte; this is particularly appealing, as obesity is a major cause of increased insulin resistance. Intra-abdominal 'central' adipose tissue is metabolically active, and releases large quantities of FFAs, which may induce insulin resistance because they compete with glucose as a fuel supply for oxidation in peripheral tissues such as muscle. In addition, adipose tissue releases a number of hormones (including a variety of peptides, called 'adipokines' because they are structurally similar to immunological 'cytokines') which act on specific receptors to influence sensitivity to insulin in other tissues. Because the venous drainage of visceral adipose tissue is into the portal vein, central obesity may have a particularly potent influence on insulin sensitivity in the liver, and thereby adversely affect gluconeogenesis and hepatic lipid metabolism.

Physical activity is another important determinant of insulin sensitivity. Inactivity is associated with down-regulation of insulin-sensitive kinases and may promote accumulation of FFAs within skeletal muscle. Sedentary people are therefore more insulin-resistant than active people with the same degree of obesity. Moreover, physical activity allows non-insulin-dependent glucose uptake into muscle, reducing the 'demand' on the pancreatic β cells to produce insulin.

Deposition of fat in the liver is a common association with central obesity and is exacerbated by insulin resistance and/or deficiency. Many patients with type 2 diabetes have evidence of fatty infiltration of the liver (non-alcoholic fatty liver disease (NAFLD)). This condition may improve with effective treatment of the diabetes and dyslipidaemia, but despite this, a few patients progress to non-alcoholic steatohepatitis (NASH, p. 959) and cirrhosis.

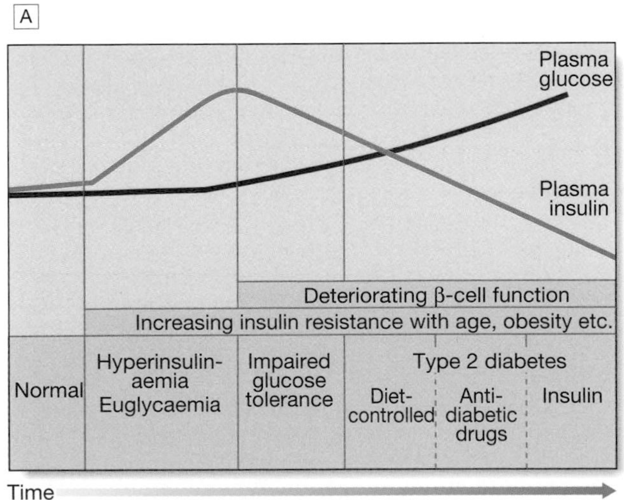

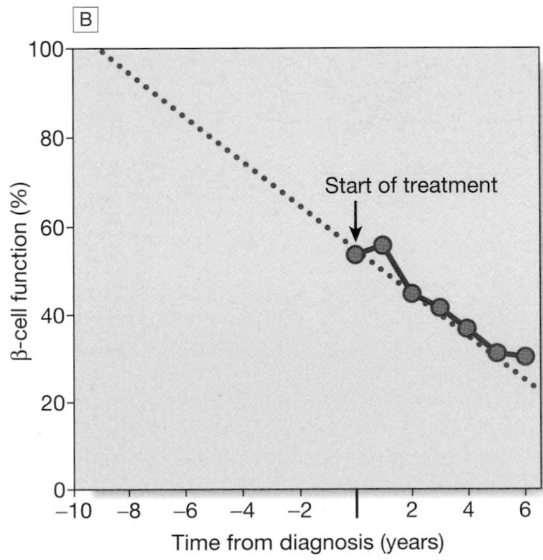

Fig. 21.6 Natural history of type 2 diabetes. **A** In the early stage of the disorder, the response to progressive insulin resistance is an increase in insulin secretion by the pancreatic cells, causing hyperinsulinaemia. Eventually, the β cells are unable to compensate adequately and blood glucose rises, producing hyperglycaemia. With further β-cell failure, glycaemic control deteriorates and treatment requirements escalate. **B** Progressive pancreatic β-cell failure in patients with type 2 diabetes in the United Kingdom Prospective Diabetes Study (UKPDS). Beta-cell function was estimated using the homeostasis model assessment (HOMA) and was already below 50% at the time of diagnosis. Thereafter, long-term incremental increases in fasting plasma glucose were accompanied by progressive β-cell dysfunction. If the slope of this progression is extrapolated, it appears that pancreatic dysfunction may have been developing for many years before diagnosis of diabetes. Part B adapted from Holman 1998 – see p. 836.

Pancreatic β-cell failure

In the early stages of type 2 diabetes, reduction in the total mass of pancreatic islet tissue is modest. At the time of diagnosis, around 50% of β-cell function has been lost and this declines progressively (see Fig. 21.6B). Some pathological changes are typical of type 2 diabetes, the most consistent of which is deposition of amyloid in the islets. In addition, elevated plasma glucose and FFAs exert toxic effects on pancreatic β cells to impair insulin secretion. However, while β-cell numbers are reduced, β-cell mass is unchanged and glucagon secretion is increased, which may contribute to hyperglycaemia.

Genetic predisposition

Genetic factors are important in type 2 diabetes, as shown by marked differences in susceptibility in different ethnic groups and by studies in monozygotic twins where concordance rates for type 2 diabetes approach 100%. However, many genes are involved and the chance of developing diabetes is also influenced very powerfully by environmental factors (Box 21.3). Genome-wide association studies have identified over 65 genes or gene regions that are associated with type 2 diabetes, each exerting a small effect. The largest effect is seen with variation in *TCF7L2*; the 10% of the population with two copies of the risk variant for this gene have a nearly twofold increase in risk of developing type 2 diabetes. Most of the genes known to contribute to risk of type 2 diabetes are involved in β-cell function or in regulation of cell cycling and turnover, suggesting that altered regulation of β-cell mass is a key factor.

21.3 Risk of developing type 2 diabetes for siblings of and individuals with type 2 diabetes

Age at onset of type 2 diabetes in proband	Age-corrected risk of type 2 diabetes for siblings (%)
25–44	53
45–54	37
55–64	38
65–80	31

Environmental and other risk factors

Diet and obesity

Epidemiological studies show that type 2 diabetes is associated with overeating, especially when combined with obesity and underactivity. Middle-aged people with diabetes eat significantly more and are fatter and less active than their non-diabetic siblings. The risk of developing type 2 diabetes increases tenfold in people with a body mass index (BMI) of more than 30 kg/m^2 (p. 115). However, although the majority of patients with type 2 diabetes are obese, only a minority of obese people develop diabetes, as the majority of obese patients are able to increase insulin secretion to compensate for the increased demand resulting from obesity and insulin resistance. Those who develop diabetes may have genetically impaired β-cell function, reduced β-cell mass, or a susceptibility of β cells to attack by toxic substances such as FFAs or inflammatory cytokines.

21.4 Diagnosis of diabetes mellitus in old age

- **Prevalence**: increases with age, affecting ~10% of people over 65 years. Half of these people are undiagnosed. Impaired β-cell function and exaggerated insulin resistance with ageing both contribute.
- **Glycosuria**: the renal threshold for glucose rises with age, so glycosuria may not develop until the blood glucose concentration is markedly raised.
- **Pancreatic carcinoma**: may present in old age with the development of diabetes, in association with weight loss and diminished appetite.

Age

Type 2 diabetes is more common in the middle-aged and elderly (Box 21.4). In the UK, it affects 10% of the population over 65, and over 70% of all cases of diabetes occur after the age of 50 years.

Metabolic disturbances in type 2 diabetes

Patients with type 2 diabetes have a slow onset of 'relative' insulin deficiency. Relatively small amounts of insulin are required to suppress lipolysis, and some glucose uptake is maintained in muscle, so that, in contrast with type 1 diabetes, lipolysis and proteolysis are not unrestrained and weight loss and ketoacidosis seldom occur. In type 2 diabetes, hyperglycaemia tends to develop slowly over months or years; because of this insidious onset many cases of type 2 diabetes are discovered coincidentally and a large number are undetected. At diagnosis, patients are often asymptomatic or give a long history (typically many months) of fatigue, with or without 'osmotic symptoms' (thirst and polyuria). In some patients with type 2 diabetes, presentation is late and pancreatic β-cell failure has reached an advanced stage of insulin deficiency (see type 1 diabetes, p. 803). These patients may present with weight loss but ketoacidosis is uncommon. However, in some ethnic groups, such as African Americans, half of those whose first presentation is with diabetic ketoacidosis have type 2 diabetes.

Intercurrent illness, e.g. with infections, increases the production of stress hormones which oppose insulin action, such as cortisol, growth hormone and catecholamines. This can precipitate an acute exacerbation of insulin resistance and insulin deficiency, and result in more severe hyperglycaemia and dehydration (see hyperglycaemic hyperosmolar state, p. 814).

Other forms of diabetes

Other causes of diabetes are shown in Box 21.5. In most cases, there is an obvious cause of destruction of pancreatic β cells. Some acquired disorders, notably other endocrine diseases such as acromegaly (p. 792) or Cushing's syndrome (p. 773), can precipitate type 2 diabetes in susceptible individuals.

A number of unusual genetic diseases are associated with diabetes. In rare families, diabetes is caused by single gene defects with autosomal dominant inheritance. These subtypes constitute less than 5% of all cases of diabetes and typically present as 'maturity-onset diabetes of the young' (MODY), i.e. non-insulin-requiring

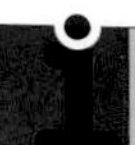

21.5 Aetiological classification of diabetes mellitus

Type 1 diabetes
- Immune-mediated
- Idiopathic

Type 2 diabetes

Other specific types
- Genetic defects of β-cell function (see Box 21.6)
- Genetic defects of insulin action (e.g. leprechaunism, lipodystrophies)
- Pancreatic disease (e.g. pancreatitis, pancreatectomy, neoplastic disease, cystic fibrosis, haemochromatosis, fibrocalculous pancreatopathy)
- Excess endogenous production of hormonal antagonists to insulin, e.g.
  Growth hormone – acromegaly
  Glucocorticoids – Cushing's syndrome
  Glucagon – glucagonoma
  Catecholamines – phaeochromocytoma
  Thyroid hormones – thyrotoxicosis
- Drug-induced (e.g. corticosteroids, thiazide diuretics, phenytoin)
- Uncommon forms of immune-mediated diabetes (e.g. IPEX (immunodysregulation polyendocrinopathy X) syndrome)
- Associated with genetic syndromes (e.g. Down's syndrome; Klinefelter's syndrome; Turner's syndrome; DIDMOAD (Wolfram's syndrome) – diabetes insipidus, diabetes mellitus, optic atrophy, nerve deafness; Friedreich's ataxia; myotonic dystrophy)

Gestational diabetes

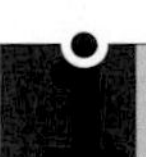

21.6 Monogenic diabetes mellitus: maturity-onset diabetes of the young (MODY)

Functional defect	Main type*	Gene mutated*
β-cell glucose sensing	MODY2	*GCK*
The set point for basal insulin release is altered, causing a high fasting glucose, but sufficient insulin is released after meals. As a result, the HbA_{1c} is often normal and microvascular complications are rare. Treatment is rarely required		
β-cell transcriptional regulation	MODY3 MODY5 MODY1	*HNF-1α* *HNF-1β* *HNF-4α*
Diabetes develops during adolescence/early adulthood and can be managed with diet and tablets for many years, but ultimately, insulin treatment is required. The HNF-1α and 4α forms respond particularly well to sulphonylurea drugs. All types are associated with microvascular complications. HNF-1β mutations also cause renal cysts and renal failure		

*Other gene mutations have been found in rare cases. For further information, see http://diabetesgenes.org.

diabetes presenting before the age of 25 years (Box 21.6). Very rarely, diabetes can develop at or soon after birth. This neonatal diabetes is usually genetic in origin, with 50% due to mutations in the K_{ATP} channel of the pancreatic β cell causing insulin deficiency and diabetic ketoacidosis. However, sulphonylurea drugs overcome the defect in potassium channel signalling, so that insulin therapy is not necessary in these cases.

INVESTIGATIONS

Urine testing

Glucose

Testing the urine for glucose with dipsticks is a common screening procedure for detecting diabetes. If possible, testing should be performed on urine passed 1–2 hours after a meal to maximise sensitivity. Glycosuria always warrants further assessment by blood testing (see below). The greatest disadvantage of urinary glucose measurement is the individual variation in renal threshold for glucose. The most frequent cause of glycosuria is a low renal threshold, which is common during pregnancy and in young people; the resulting 'renal glycosuria' is a benign condition unrelated to diabetes. Another disadvantage is that some drugs (such as β-lactam antibiotics, levodopa and salicylates) may interfere with urine glucose tests.

Ketones

Ketone bodies can be identified by the nitroprusside reaction, which measures acetoacetate, using either tablets or dipsticks. Ketonuria may be found in normal people who have been fasting or exercising strenuously for long periods, who have been vomiting repeatedly, or who have been eating a diet high in fat and low in carbohydrate. Ketonuria is therefore not pathognomonic of diabetes but, if associated with glycosuria, the diagnosis of diabetes is highly likely. In diabetic ketoacidosis (p. 811), ketones can also be detected in plasma using test sticks (see below).

Protein

Standard dipstick testing for albumin detects urinary albumin at concentrations above 300 mg/L, but smaller amounts (microalbuminuria, see Box 17.13, p. 476) can only be measured using specific albumin dipsticks or by quantitative biochemical laboratory measurement. Microalbuminuria or proteinuria, in the absence of urinary tract infection, is an important indicator of diabetic nephropathy and/or increased risk of macrovascular disease (p. 830).

Blood testing

Glucose

Laboratory glucose testing in blood relies upon an enzymatic reaction (glucose oxidase) and is cheap, usually automated and highly reliable. However, blood glucose levels depend on whether the patient has eaten recently, so it is important to consider the circumstances in which the blood sample was taken.

Blood glucose can also be measured with colorimetric or other testing sticks, which are often read with a portable electronic meter. These are used for capillary (fingerprick) testing to monitor diabetes treatment (p. 810). There is some debate as to whether self-monitoring in people with type 2 diabetes improves glycaemic control. Many countries now only offer self-monitoring to people with type 2 diabetes taking insulin therapy. To make the diagnosis of diabetes, the blood glucose concentration should be estimated using an accurate laboratory method rather than a portable technique.

21

Glucose concentrations are lower in venous than arterial or capillary (fingerprick) blood. Whole blood glucose concentrations are lower than plasma concentrations because red blood cells contain relatively little glucose. Venous plasma values are usually the most reliable for diagnostic purposes (Boxes 21.10 and 21.11).

Ketones

Blood ketone monitoring is increasingly available. Urinary ketone measurements described above are semi-quantitative, difficult to perform and retrospective (i.e. the urine has accumulated over several hours), and do not measure the major ketone in blood during diabetic ketoacidosis (DKA), beta-hydroxybutyrate (β-OHB). Whole blood ketone monitoring detects β-OHB and is useful in assisting with insulin adjustment during intercurrent illness or sustained hyperglycaemia to prevent or detect DKA. Blood ketone monitoring is also useful in monitoring resolution of DKA in hospitalised patients (Box 21.7).

21.7 Interpretation of capillary blood ketone measurements

Measurement*	Interpretation
< 0.6 mmol/L	Normal; no action required
0.6–1.5 mmol/L	Suggests metabolic control may be deteriorating; continue to monitor and seek medical advice if sustained/progressive
1.5–3.0 mmol/L	With high blood glucose (> 10 mmol/L), there is a high risk of diabetic ketoacidosis; seek medical advice
> 3.0 mmol/L	Severe ketosis; in the presence of high glucose (> 10 mmol/L) suggests presence of diabetic ketoacidosis; seek urgent medical help

*To convert to mg/dL, divide values by 0.098.

Glycated haemoglobin

Glycated haemoglobin provides an accurate and objective measure of glycaemic control integrated over a period of weeks to months.

In diabetes, the slow non-enzymatic covalent attachment of glucose to haemoglobin (glycation) increases the amount in the HbA_1 (HbA_{1c}) fraction relative to non-glycated adult haemoglobin (HbA_0). These fractions can be separated by chromatography; laboratories may report glycated haemoglobin as total glycated haemoglobin (GHb), HbA_1 or HbA_{1c}. In most countries, HbA_{1c} is the preferred measurement. The rate of formation of HbA_{1c} is directly proportional to the ambient blood glucose concentration; a rise of 1% in HbA_{1c} corresponds to an approximate average increase of 2 mmol/L (36 mg/dL) in blood glucose. Although HbA_{1c} concentration reflects the integrated blood glucose control over the lifespan of erythrocytes (120 days), HbA_{1c} is most sensitive to changes in glycaemic control occurring in the month before measurement.

Various assay methods are used to measure HbA_{1c}, but most laboratories have been reporting HbA_{1c} values (as %) aligned with the reference range that was used in the Diabetes Control and Complications Trial (DCCT).

21.8 Conversion between DCCT and IFCC units for HbA_{1c}

DCCT units (%)	IFCC units (mmol/mol)
4	20
5	31
6	42
7	53
8	64
9	75
10	86

IFCC HbA_{1c} (mmol/mol) = [DCCT HbA_{1c}(%)–2.15] × 10.929

(DCCT = Diabetes Control and Complications Trial; IFCC = International Federation of Clinical Chemistry and Laboratory Medicine)

To allow worldwide comparisons of HbA_{1c} values, the International Federation of Clinical Chemistry and Laboratory Medicine (IFCC) has developed a standard method; IFCC-standardised HbA_{1c} values are reported in mmol/mol. In 2011, many countries adopted the IFCC reference method (Box 21.8).

HbA_{1c} estimates may be erroneously diminished in anaemia or during pregnancy, and may be difficult to interpret with some assay methods in patients who have uraemia or a haemoglobinopathy.

PRESENTING PROBLEMS IN DIABETES MELLITUS

Newly discovered hyperglycaemia

Hyperglycaemia is a very common biochemical abnormality. It is frequently detected on routine biochemical analysis of asymptomatic patients, following routine dipstick testing of urine showing glycosuria, or during severe illness ('stress hyperglycaemia'). Alternatively, hyperglycaemia may present with the symptoms described in Box 21.9. Occasionally, patients present as an emergency with acute metabolic decompensation (see below). The key goals are to establish whether the patient has diabetes, and if so, what type of diabetes it is and how it should be treated.

Establishing the diagnosis of diabetes

Glycaemia can be classified into three categories: normal, impaired (pre-diabetes) and diabetes (Boxes 21.10 and 21.11). The glucose cut-off that defines diabetes is based upon the level above which there is a significant risk of microvascular complications (retinopathy, nephropathy, neuropathy). People categorised as having pre-diabetes have blood glucose levels that carry a negligible risk of microvascular complications but are at increased risk of developing diabetes. Also, because there is a continuous risk of macrovascular disease (atheroma of large conduit blood vessels) with increasing glycaemia in the population, people with pre-diabetes have increased risk of cardiovascular disease (myocardial infarction, stroke and peripheral vascular disease).

When a person has symptoms of diabetes, the diagnosis can be confirmed with either a fasting glucose

≥ 7.0 mmol/L (126 mg/dL) or a random glucose ≥ 11.1 mmol/L (200 mg/dL) (see Box 21.10). Asymptomatic individuals should have a second confirmatory test. Diabetes should not be diagnosed by capillary blood glucose results. The World Health Organization (WHO) guidelines (2011) introduced the use of HbA_{1c} for diagnosis of diabetes, with an IFCC HbA_{1c} of more than 48 mmol/mol also being diagnostic.

Pre-diabetes can be diagnosed either as 'impaired fasting glucose' (IFG), based upon a fasting plasma glucose result, or 'impaired glucose tolerance' (IGT), based upon the fasting and 2-hour oral glucose tolerance test results (OGTT; see Box 21.11). Patients with pre-diabetes should be advised of their risk of progression to diabetes, given advice about lifestyle modification to reduce this risk (as for type 2 diabetes, p. 820), and be ensured of aggressive management of cardiovascular risk factors such as hypertension and dyslipidaemia.

In some people, an abnormal blood glucose result is observed under conditions which impose a burden on the pancreatic β cells, e.g. during pregnancy, infection, myocardial infarction or other severe stress, or during treatment with diabetogenic drugs such as corticosteroids. This 'stress hyperglycaemia' usually disappears after the acute illness has resolved. However, blood glucose should be remeasured and an OGTT will often show persistence of impaired glucose tolerance.

The diagnostic criteria recommended for diabetes in pregnancy are more stringent than those for non-pregnant subjects (see Box 21.23, p. 817). Pregnant women with abnormal glucose tolerance should be referred urgently to a specialist unit for full evaluation.

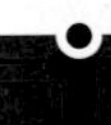

21.9 Symptoms of hyperglycaemia

- Thirst, dry mouth
- Polyuria
- Nocturia
- Tiredness, fatigue, lethargy
- Change in weight (usually weight loss)
- Blurring of vision
- Pruritus vulvae, balanitis (genital candidiasis)
- Nausea
- Headache
- Hyperphagia; predilection for sweet foods
- Mood change, irritability, difficulty in concentrating, apathy

21.10 Diagnosis of diabetes and pre-diabetes

Diabetes is confirmed by either:

- Plasma glucose in random sample or 2 hrs after a 75 g glucose load ≥ 11.1 (200 mg/dL) **or**
- Fasting plasma glucose ≥ 7.0 mmol/L (126 mg/dL)

In asymptomatic patients, two diagnostic tests are required to confirm diabetes.

'Pre-diabetes' is classified as:

- Impaired fasting glucose = fasting plasma glucose ≥ 6.0 (108 mg/dL) and < 7.0 mmol/L (126 mg/dL)
- Impaired glucose tolerance = fasting plasma glucose < 7.0 mmol/L (126 mg/dL) **and** 2-hr glucose after 75 g oral glucose drink 7.8–11.1 mmol/L (140–200 mg/dL)

When a diagnosis of diabetes is confirmed, other investigations should include plasma urea, creatinine and electrolytes, lipids, liver and thyroid function tests, and urine testing for ketones, protein or microalbuminuria.

Clinical assessment and classification

Hyperglycaemia causes a wide variety of symptoms (see Box 21.9). The classical clinical features of the two main types of diabetes are compared in Box 21.12. Symptoms of thirst, polyuria, nocturia and rapid weight loss are prominent in type 1 diabetes, but are often absent in patients with type 2 diabetes, many of whom are asymptomatic or have non-specific complaints such as chronic fatigue and malaise. Uncontrolled diabetes is associated

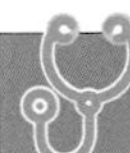

21.11 How to perform an oral glucose tolerance test (OGTT)

Which patients to test

- Fasting plasma glucose 6.1–7.0 mmol/L (110–126 mg/dL)
- Uncertainty about the diagnosis of diabetes

Preparation before the test

- Unrestricted carbohydrate diet for 3 days
- Fasted overnight for at least 8 hrs
- Rest for 30 mins
- Remain seated for the duration of the test, with no smoking

Sampling

- Measure plasma glucose before and 2 hrs after a 75 g oral glucose drink

Interpretation (venous plasma glucose)

	Fasting	2 hrs after glucose load
Impaired fasting glucose	6.1–6.9 mmol/L (110–125 mg/dL)	< 7.8 mmol/L (< 140 mg/dL)
Impaired glucose tolerance	< 7.0 mmol/L (< 126 mg/dL)	7.8–11.0 mmol/L (140–199 mg/dL)
Diabetes	≥ 7.0 mmol/L (> 126 mg/dL)	≥ 11.1 mmol/L (> 200 mg/dL)

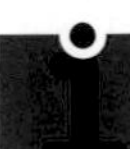

21.12 Classical features of type 1 and type 2 diabetes

	Type 1	Type 2
Typical age at onset	< 40 yrs	> 50 yrs
Duration of symptoms	Weeks	Months to years
Body weight	Normal or low	Obese
Ketonuria	Yes	No
Rapid death without treatment with insulin	Yes	No
Autoantibodies	Positive in 80–90%	Negative
Diabetic complications at diagnosis	No	25%
Family history of diabetes	Uncommon	Common
Other autoimmune disease	Common	Uncommon

with an increased susceptibility to infection and patients may present with skin sepsis (boils) or genital candidiasis, and complain of pruritus vulvae or balanitis.

While the distinction between type 1 and type 2 diabetes is usually obvious, overlap occurs, particularly in age at onset, duration of symptoms and family history. There are many patients in whom the type of diabetes is not immediately apparent. For example, patients with type 2 diabetes may present with marked and rapid weight loss and even diabetic ketoacidosis, and type 2 diabetes is increasingly diagnosed in children and young adults. Type 1 diabetes can occur at any age, not just in younger people, and may develop more insidiously; the presence of pancreatic autoantibodies confirms the diagnosis of slow-onset type 1 diabetes, termed latent autoimmune diabetes of adults (LADA). Pancreatic autoantibodies are detectable at high titre in 80–90% of patients with type 1 diabetes, so a negative result should prompt consideration of other aetiologies. Other causes of diabetes (see Box 21.5, p. 807), such as MODY, should not be forgotten, particularly in those presenting in childhood or as young adults. A history of pancreatic disease, particularly in patients with a history of alcohol excess, makes insulin deficiency more likely. Sometimes the definitive classification of the type of diabetes is only made later, once the natural history or responsiveness to different therapies becomes apparent.

Physical signs in patients with type 2 diabetes at diagnosis depend on the mode of presentation. In Western populations, more than 80% are overweight, and the obesity is often central (truncal or abdominal). Obesity is much less evident in Asians. Hypertension is present in at least 50% of patients with type 2 diabetes. Although dyslipidaemia is also common, skin lesions such as xanthelasma and eruptive xanthomas are rare. An increasing number of patients now present with NAFLD, usually identified by their elevated blood transaminase values, but they may also have non-tender hepatomegaly.

Management

The aims of management are to improve symptoms of hyperglycaemia and to minimise the risks of long-term microvascular and macrovascular complications. Treatment methods for diabetes include dietary/lifestyle modification, oral anti-diabetic drugs and injected therapies. These are described in detail on page 821. In patients with suspected type 1 diabetes, urgent treatment with insulin is required and prompt referral to a specialist is usually needed. In patients with suspected type 2 diabetes, first-line therapy involves advice about dietary and lifestyle modification. Oral anti-diabetic drugs are usually added in those who do not achieve glycaemic targets as a result, or who have severe symptomatic hyperglycaemia at diagnosis and a high HbA_{1c}. However, the guidelines in some countries are to introduce medication immediately upon diagnosis of diabetes without waiting to assess the impact of diet and lifestyle changes.

In parallel with treatment of hyperglycaemia, other risk factors for complications of diabetes need to be addressed, including treatment of hypertension (p. 609) and dyslipidaemia (p. 456), and advice on smoking cessation (p. 100).

Educating patients

It is essential that people with diabetes understand their disorder and learn to handle all aspects of their management as comprehensively and quickly as possible. Ideally, this can be achieved by a multidisciplinary team (doctor, dietitian, specialist nurse and podiatrist) in the outpatient setting. For those with newly diagnosed type 2 diabetes, structured education can be given in groups by trained educators. Those requiring insulin need to learn how to measure doses of insulin accurately with an insulin syringe or pen device, how to inject, and how to adjust the dose on the basis of blood glucose values and in relation to factors such as exercise, illness and episodic hypoglycaemia. They must therefore acquire a working knowledge of diabetes, be familiar with the symptoms of hypoglycaemia (see Box 21.19, p. 815), and have ready access to medical advice when the need arises. Information should be provided about driving (national statutory regulations and practical safety measures, Box 21.13). Providing this education is time-consuming but essential if patients are to undertake normal activities safely while maintaining good control.

Self-assessment of glycaemic control

In people with type 2 diabetes there is not usually a need for regular self-assessment of blood glucose, unless the patient is treated with insulin, or at risk of hypoglycaemia while taking sulphonylureas. Blood glucose testing can be used for self-education (i.e. demonstrating how different food and exercise regimes affect blood glucose), and may be useful in acute illness. Blood glucose targets vary according to individual circumstances, but, in general, pre-meal values between 4 and 7 mmol/L (72 and 126 mg/dL) and 2-hour post-meal values between 4 and 8 mmol/L represent optimal control.

Insulin-treated patients should be taught how to monitor their own blood glucose using capillary blood glucose meters. Immediate knowledge of blood glucose levels can be used by patients to guide their insulin dosing and to manage exercise and illness. This can be

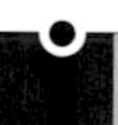

21.13 Diabetes and driving

- Licensing regulations vary considerably between countries. In the UK, diabetes requiring insulin therapy or any complication that could affect driving should be declared to the Driver and Vehicle Licensing Agency; ordinary driving licences are 'period-restricted' for insulin-treated drivers; and vocational licences (large goods vehicles and public service vehicles) may be granted but require very strict criteria to be met
- The main risk to driving performance is hypoglycaemia. Visual impairment and other complications may occasionally cause problems
- Insulin-treated diabetic drivers should:
  - Check blood glucose before driving and 2-hourly during long journeys
  - Keep an accessible supply of fast-acting carbohydrate in the vehicle
  - Take regular snacks or meals during long journeys
  - Stop driving if hypoglycaemia develops
  - Refrain from driving until at least 45 mins after treatment of hypoglycaemia (delayed recovery of cognitive function)
  - Carry identification in case of injury

supplemented with blood testing for ketones when blood glucose is high and/or during intercurrent illness.

Urine testing for glucose is not recommended because variability in renal threshold means that some patients with inadequate glycaemic control will not find glucose in their urine.

Long-term supervision of diabetes

Diabetes is a complex disorder which progresses in severity with time, so people with diabetes should be seen at regular intervals for the remainder of their lives, either at a specialist diabetic clinic or in primary care where facilities are available and staff are trained in diabetes care. A checklist for follow-up visits is given in Box 21.14. The frequency of visits is variable, ranging from weekly during pregnancy to annually in the case of patients with well-controlled type 2 diabetes.

Therapeutic goals

The target HbA_{1c} depends on the individual patient. Early on in diabetes (i.e. patients managed by diet or one or two oral agents), a target of 48 mmol/mol (6.5%) or less may be appropriate. However, a higher target of 58 mmol/mol (7.5%) may be more appropriate in older

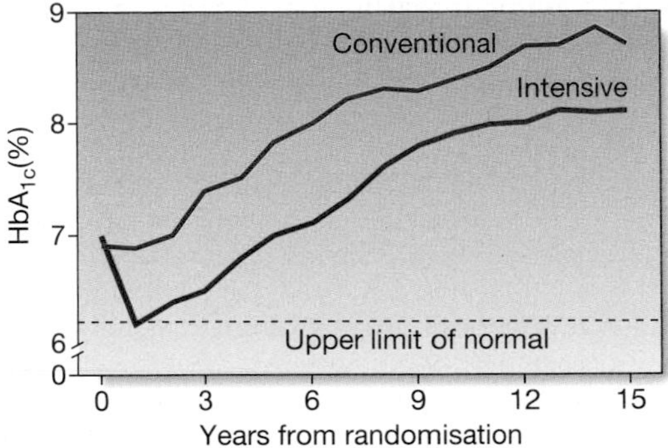

Fig. 21.7 Time course of changes in HbA_{1c} during the United Kingdom Prospective Diabetes Study (UKPDS). In the UKPDS there was loss of glycaemic control with time in patients receiving monotherapy, independently of their randomisation to conventional or intensive glycaemic control, consistent with progressive decline in β-cell function (see Fig. 21.6, p. 805). Adapted from UKPDS 1998 – see p. 836.

patients with pre-existing cardiovascular disease, or those treated with insulin and therefore at risk of hypoglycaemia. In general, the benefits of lower target HbA_{1c} (primarily a lower risk of microvascular disease) need to be weighed against any increased risks (primarily hypoglycaemia in insulin-treated patients). Type 2 diabetes is usually a progressive condition (Fig. 21.7), unless there are major diet and lifestyle changes, so that there is usually a need to increase diabetes medication over time to achieve the individualised target HbA_{1c}.

In people with type 2 diabetes, treatment of coexisting hypertension and dyslipidaemia is usually required. This can be decided by assessing absolute risk of a cardiovascular disease event (p. 581) and adjusting targets
to individual circumstances. The target for blood pre
sure is usually below 140/80 mmHg, although s
guidelines suggest 130/80 mmHg. For lipid-lo
there is a reduction in cardiovascular risk
normal cholesterol levels, but statin thera
recommended when the 10-year card
risk is at least 20%. As a general ru
anyone with type 2 diabetes wh
40 years should receive a stati
cholesterol levels. Some g
target level once the pa
others suggest a total c
(~150 mg/dL) and
2.0 mmol/L (~75
ate in type 1
data from

Di

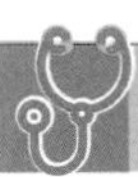

21.14 How to review a patient in the diabetes clinic

Lifestyle issues
- General health
- Work or school
- Smoking
- Alcohol intake
- Stress or depression
- Sexual health
- Exercise

Body weight and BMI

Blood pressure
- Individualised target of 130–140/70–80 mmHg, depending on risk factors and presence of nephropathy

Urinalysis
- Analyse fasting specimen for glucose, ketones, albumin (both macro- and micro-albuminuria)

Biochemistry
- Renal, liver and thyroid function
- Lipid profile and estimated 10-yr cardiovascular risk to guide need for lipid-lowering therapy (p. 581)

Glycaemic control
- Glycated haemoglobin (HbA_{1c}); individualised target between 48 and 58 mmol/mol (6.5 and 7.5%)
- Inspection of home blood glucose monitoring record (if carried out by patient)

Hypoglycaemic episodes
- Number and cause of severe (requiring assistance for treatment) events and frequency of mild (self-treated) episodes and biochemical hypoglycaemia
- Awareness of hypoglycaemia
- Driving advice

Assessment of injection sites if insulin-treated

Eye examination
- Visual acuities (near and distance)
- Ophthalmoscopy (with pupils dilated) or digital ph

Examination of lower limbs and feet
- Assessment of foot risk (p. 799)

21

comorbid conditions such as acute myocardial infarction, sepsis or pneumonia.

DKA is characteristic of type 1 diabetes (see Box 21.12) and is often the presenting problem in newly diagnosed patients. However, an increasing number of patients presenting with DKA have underlying type 2 diabetes. This appears to be particularly prevalent in African-American and Hispanic populations. In established type 1 diabetes, DKA may be precipitated by an intercurrent illness because of failure to increase insulin dose appropriately to compensate for the stress response. Sometimes, there is no evidence of a precipitating infection and DKA develops because of errors in self-management. In young patients with recurrent episodes of DKA, up to 20% may have psychological problems complicated by eating disorders.

Pathogenesis

A clear understanding of the biochemical basis and pathophysiology of DKA is essential for its efficient treatment (see Fig. 21.5, p. 804). The cardinal biochemical features are:

- hyperketonaemia (≥ 3 mmol/L) and ketonuria (more than 2+ on standard urine sticks)
- hyperglycaemia (blood glucose ≥ 11 mmol/L (~200 mg/dL))
- metabolic acidosis (venous bicarbonate < 15 mmol/L and/or venous pH < 7.3).

The hyperglycaemia causes a profound osmotic diuresis leading to dehydration and electrolyte loss, particularly of sodium and potassium. Potassium loss is exacerbated by secondary hyperaldosteronism ... result of reduc...

water, catabolism of protein and glycogen, and displacement of potassium from the intracellular compartment by H^+ ions. However, soon after treatment is started, there is likely to be a precipitous fall in the plasma potassium due to dilution of extracellular potassium by administration of intravenous fluids, the movement of potassium into cells induced by insulin, and the continuing renal loss of potassium.

The magnitude of the hyperglycaemia does not correlate with the severity of the metabolic acidosis; moderate elevation of blood glucose may be associated with life-threatening ketoacidosis. In some cases, hyperglycaemia predominates and acidosis is minimal, with patients presenting in a hyperosmolar state (p. 814).

Clinical assessment

The clinical features of ketoacidosis are listed in Box 21.16. In the fulminating case, the striking features are those of salt and water depletion, with loss of skin turgor, furred tongue and cracked lips, tachycardia, hypotension and reduced intra-ocular pressure. Breathing may be deep and sighing, the breath is usually fetid, and the sickly-sweet smell of acetone may be apparent. Mental apathy, confusion or a reduced conscious level may be present, although coma is uncommon. Indeed, a patient with dangerous ketoacidosis requiring urgent treatment may walk into the consulting room. For this reason, the term 'diabetic ketoacidosis' is to be preferred to 'diabetic coma', which implies that there is no urgency until unconsciousness supervenes. In fact, it is imperative that energetic treatment is started at the earliest ...

...ometimes a feature of DKA, par-
...nd vomiting is common. Serum
...d but rarely indicates coexisting
...l patients, pyrexia may not be
... of vasodilatation secondary to

...tant but should not delay the
... fluid and insulin replacement:
...and electrolytes, glucose and
...dosis is indicated by a
...nate < 12 mmol/L).
...*or ketones* (p. 807).

...es of diabetic ketoacidosis

- Leg cramps
- Blurred vision
- Abdominal pain

- Air hunger (Kussmaul breathing)
- Smell of acetone
- Hypothermia
- Confusion, drowsiness, coma (10%)

...es-
...some
...wering,
...even with
...py is usually
...ovascular event
...e, this means that
...o is over the age of
..., irrespective of baseline
...idelines do not suggest a
...ent is started on a statin but
...holesterol of less than 4.0 mmol/L
... an LDL cholesterol of less than
... mg/dL). Similar targets are appropri-
...diabetes, although there is a shortage of
...linical trials in this group.

...abetic ketoacidosis

Diabetic ketoacidosis (DKA) is a medical emergency and remains a serious cause of morbidity, principally in people with type 1 diabetes. Mortality is low in the UK (approximately 2%) but remains high in developing countries and among non-hospitalised patients. Mortality in DKA is most commonly caused in children and adolescents by cerebral oedema and in adults by hypokalaemia, acute respiratory distress syndrome and

...otography

- *ECG.*
- *Infection screen*: full blood count, blood and urine culture, C-reactive protein, chest X-ray. Although leucocytosis invariably occurs in DKA, this represents a stress response and does not necessarily indicate infection.

Management

DKA is a medical emergency which should be treated in hospital, preferably in a high-dependency area. If available, the diabetes specialist team should be involved. Regular clinical and biochemical review is essential, particularly during the first 24 hours of treatment. Guidelines for management of DKA are shown in Box 21.17.

Insulin

A fixed-rate intravenous insulin infusion of 0.1 U/kg body weight/hr is recommended (see Box 21.17). Exceptionally, if intravenous administration is not feasible, soluble insulin can be given by intramuscular injection (loading dose of 10–20 U, followed by 5 U hourly), or a fast-acting insulin analogue can be given hourly by subcutaneous injection (initially 0.3 U/kg body weight, then 0.1 U/kg hourly). The blood glucose concentration should fall by 3–6 mmol/L (approximately 55–110 mg/dL) per hour, or blood ketone concentrations fall by at least 0.5 mmol/L/hr. A more rapid decrease in blood glucose should be avoided, as this might precipitate hypoglycaemia and the serious complication of cerebral oedema, particularly in children. Failure of blood glucose to fall within 1 hour of commencing insulin infusion should lead to a re-assessment of insulin dose. Ketosis, dehydration, acidaemia, infection and stress combine to produce severe insulin resistance in some cases, but most will respond to a low-dose insulin regimen. When the blood glucose has fallen, 10% dextrose infusion is introduced and insulin infusion continued to encourage glucose uptake into cells and restoration of normal metabolism. In recent years, it has also become increasingly common to continue with the use of long-acting insulin analogues administered subcutaneously during the initial management of DKA; this provides background insulin for when the intravenous insulin is discontinued.

Restoration of the usual insulin regimen, by subcutaneous injection, should not be instituted until the patient is both biochemically stable and able to eat and drink normally.

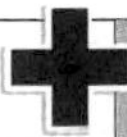

21.17 Management of diabetic ketoacidosis*

Time: 0–60 mins

1. Commence 0.9% sodium chloride
   If systolic BP > 90 mmHg, give 1 L over 60 mins
   If systolic BP < 90 mmHg, give 500 mL over 10–15 mins, then re-assess. If BP remains < 90 mmHg, seek senior review
2. Commence insulin treatment
   50 U human soluble insulin in 50 mL 0.9% sodium chloride infused intravenously at 0.1 U/kg body weight/hr
   Continue with SC basal insulin analogue if usually taken by patient
3. Perform further investigations: see text
4. Establish monitoring schedule
   Hourly capillary blood glucose and ketone testing
   Venous bicarbonate and potassium after 1 and 2 hrs, then every 2 hrs
   Plasma electrolytes every 4 hrs
   Clinical monitoring of O_2 saturation, pulse, BP, respiratory rate and urine output every hour
5. Treat any precipitating cause

Time: 60 mins to 12 hrs

- IV infusion of 0.9% sodium chloride with potassium chloride added as indicated below
  1 L over 2 hrs
  1 L over 2 hrs
  1 L over 4 hrs
  1 L over 4 hrs
  1 L over 6 hrs
- Add 10% glucose 125 mL/hr IV when glucose < 14 mmol/L
- Be more cautious with fluid replacement in elderly, young people, pregnant patients and those with renal or heart failure. If plasma sodium is > 155 mmol/L, 0.45% sodium chloride may be used.
- Adjust potassium chloride infusion

Plasma potassium (mmol/L)	Potassium replacement (mmol/L of infusion)
> 5.5	Nil
3.5–5.5	40
< 3.5	Senior review – additional potassium required

Time: 12–24 hrs

- Ketonaemia and acidosis should have resolved (blood ketones < 0.3 mmol/L, venous bicarbonate > 18 mmol/L). Request senior review if not improving
- If patient is not eating and drinking
  Continue IV insulin infusion at lower rate of 2–3 U/kg/hr
  Continue IV fluid replacement and biochemical monitoring
- If ketoacidosis has resolved and patient is able to eat and drink
  Re-initiate SC insulin with advice from diabetes team. Do not discontinue IV insulin until 30 mins after SC short-acting insulin injection

Additional procedures

- Catheterisation if no urine passed after 3 hrs
- Central venous line if cardiovascular system compromised, to allow fluid replacement to be adjusted accurately – also consider in elderly, pregnant, renal or cardiac failure, other serious comorbidities, severe DKA
- Measure arterial blood gases and repeat chest X-ray if O_2 saturation < 92%
- ECG monitoring in severe cases
- Thromboprophylaxis with low molecular weight heparin

*Adapted from Joint British Diabetes Societies guideline, NHS Diabetes (2010).

Fluid replacement

In adults, rapid fluid replacement in the first few hours is usually recommended (as in Box 21.17). Caution is recommended in children and young adults because of the risk of cerebral oedema. Most current guidelines favour correction of the extracellular fluid deficit with isotonic saline (0.9% sodium chloride). If the plasma sodium is greater than 155 mmol/L, 0.45% saline may be used initially.

Potassium

Careful monitoring of potassium is essential to the management of diabetic ketoacidosis because both hypo- and hyperkalaemia can occur and are potentially life-threatening. Potassium replacement is not usually recommended with the initial litre of fluid because prerenal failure may be present secondary to dehydration. Treatment with 0.9% sodium chloride with potassium chloride 40 mmol/L is recommended if the serum potassium is below 5.5 mmol/L and the patient is passing urine (see Box 21.17). If the potassium falls below 3.5 mmol/L, the potassium replacement regimen needs to be reviewed. Cardiac rhythm should be monitored in severe DKA because of the risk of electrolyte-induced cardiac arrhythmia.

Bicarbonate

Adequate fluid and insulin replacement should resolve the acidosis. The use of intravenous bicarbonate therapy is currently not recommended. Acidosis may reflect an adaptive response, improving oxygen delivery to the tissues, and so excessive bicarbonate may induce a paradoxical increase in cerebrospinal fluid acidosis and has been implicated in the pathogenesis of cerebral oedema in children and young adults.

Hyperglycaemic hyperosmolar state

Hyperglycaemic hyperosmolar state (HHS) is characterised by severe hyperglycaemia (> 30 mmol/L (600 mg/dL)), hyperosmolality (serum osmolality > 320 mOsm/kg), and dehydration in the absence of significant hyperketonaemia (< 3 mmol/L) or acidosis (pH > 7.3, bicarbonate > 15 mmol/L). It was previously referred to as hyperosmolar non-ketotic (HONK) coma but, as in DKA, coma is not invariable. As with DKA, there is glycosuria, leading to an osmotic diuresis, with loss of water, sodium, potassium and other electrolytes. However, in HHS, hyperglycaemia usually develops over a longer period (a few days to weeks), causing more profound hyperglycaemia and dehydration (fluid loss may be 10–22 litres in a person weighing 100 kg). The reason that patients with HHS do not develop significant ketoacidosis is unclear, although it has been speculated that insulin levels may be too low to stimulate glucose uptake in insulin-sensitive tissues, but still sufficient to prevent lipolysis and subsequent ketogenesis. A mixed picture of HHS and DKA can occur.

Although typically occurring in the elderly, HHS is increasingly seen in younger adults. Common precipitating factors include infection, myocardial infarction, cerebrovascular events or drug therapy (e.g. corticosteroids). Poor prognostic signs include hypothermia, hypotension (systolic blood pressure < 90 mmHg), tachy- or bradycardia, severe hypernatraemia (sodium > 160 mmol/L), serum osmolality > 360 mOsm/kg, and the presence of other serious comorbidities. Mortality rates are higher than in DKA – up to 20% in the USA, reflecting the age and frailty of the population and more frequent presence of comorbidities.

21.18 Principles of management of hyperglycaemic hyperosmolar state

- Measure or calculate serum osmolality frequently
- Give fluid replacement with 0.9% sodium chloride (IV). Use 0.45% sodium chloride only if osmolality is increasing, despite positive fluid balance. Target fall in plasma sodium is ≤ 10 mmol/L at 24 hrs
- Aim for positive fluid balance of 3–6 L by 12 hrs, and replacement of remaining estimated loss over next 12 hrs
- Initiate insulin IV infusion (0.05 U/kg body weight/hr) only when blood glucose is not falling with 0.9% sodium chloride alone *OR* if there is significant ketonaemia (3β-hydroxybutyrate > 1 mmol/L or urine ketones > 2+). Reduce blood glucose by no more than 5 mmol/L/hr
- Treat coexisting conditions
- Give prophylactic anticoagulation
- Assume high risk of foot ulceration

The principles of therapy are shown in Box 21.18. The aims are to normalise osmolality, replace fluid and electrolyte losses, and normalise blood glucose, at the same time preventing complications such as arterial or venous thrombosis, cerebral oedema and central pontine demyelinosis (Ch. 16). Comorbidities also need to be taken into account; for example, rapid fluid replacement may precipitate cardiac failure in patients with coronary artery disease. Historically, management of HHS has followed DKA guidelines, but increasing recognition of the differences between HHS and DKA has led to new approaches in HHS. In particular, rapid shifts in osmolality should be avoided through more measured fluid replacement regimens that are guided by serial calculations of serum osmolality. A key recommendation is that 0.9% sodium chloride solution alone is used for initial treatment, and that insulin is introduced only when the rate of fall in blood glucose has plateaued.

If osmolality cannot be measured frequently, osmolarity can be calculated as follows and used as a surrogate (based on plasma values in mmol/L):

$$\text{Plasma osmolarity} = 2[\text{Na}^+] + [\text{glucose}] + [\text{urea}]$$

The normal value is 280–290 mmol/L and consciousness is impaired when it is high (> 340 mmol/L), as commonly occurs in HHS.

Hypoglycaemia

Hypoglycaemia (blood glucose < 3.5 mmol/L (63 mg/dL)) in diabetes results in most circumstances from insulin therapy, less frequently from use of oral insulin secretagogues such as sulphonylurea drugs, and rarely with other anti-diabetic drugs. When hypoglycaemia develops in non-diabetic people, it is called 'spontaneous' hypoglycaemia, the causes and investigation of which are described on page 783. Hypoglycaemia can be a frequent occurrence in the lives of people with type 1 diabetes and has a major impact on their willingness and ability to achieve target glucose levels.

In health, a number of mechanisms are in place to ensure that glucose homeostasis is maintained. If blood glucose falls, three primary physiological defence mechanisms operate: endogenous insulin release from pancreatic β cells is suppressed; release of glucagon from pancreatic α cells is increased; and the autonomic nervous system is activated, with release of catecholamines both systemically and within the tissues. In addition, stress hormones, such as cortisol and growth hormone, are increased in the blood. These actions reduce whole-body glucose uptake and increase hepatic glucose production, maintaining a glucose supply to the brain. People with type 1 diabetes cannot regulate insulin once it is injected subcutaneously, and so it continues to act, despite developing hypoglycaemia. In addition, within 5 years of diagnosis, most patients will have lost their ability to release glucagon specifically during hypoglycaemia. This is thought to result mainly from loss of α-cell regulation by β cells. These two primary defects mean that hypoglycaemia occurs much more frequently in people with type 1 and longer-duration type 2 diabetes.

Clinical assessment

Symptoms of hypoglycaemia (Box 21.19) comprise two main groups: those related to acute activation of the autonomic nervous system and those secondary to glucose deprivation of the brain (neuroglycopenia). Symptoms of hypoglycaemia are idiosyncratic and differ with age and duration of diabetes. Hypoglycaemia also affects mood, inducing a state of increased tension and low energy. Learning to recognise the early onset of hypoglycaemia is an important aspect of the education of diabetic patients treated with insulin. The severity of hypoglycaemia is defined by the ability to self-treat; 'mild' episodes are self-treated, while 'severe' episodes require assistance for recovery.

Circumstances of hypoglycaemia

Risk factors and causes of hypoglycaemia in patients taking insulin or sulphonylurea drugs are listed in Box 21.20. Severe hypoglycaemia can have serious morbidity (e.g. convulsions, coma, focal neurological lesions) and has a mortality of up to 4% in insulin-treated patients. Rarely, sudden death during sleep occurs in otherwise healthy young patients with type 1 diabetes ('dead-in-bed syndrome') and may result from hypoglycaemia-induced cardiac arrhythmia. Severe hypoglycaemia is very disruptive and impinges on many aspects of the patient's life, including employment, driving (see Box 21.13, p. 810), travel, sport and personal relationships.

Nocturnal hypoglycaemia in patients with type 1 diabetes is common but often undetected, as hypoglycaemia does not usually waken a person from sleep. Patients may describe poor quality of sleep, morning headaches and vivid dreams or nightmares, or a partner may observe profuse sweating, restlessness, twitching or even seizures. The only reliable way to identify this problem is to measure blood glucose during the night.

Exercise-induced hypoglycaemia occurs in people with well-controlled, insulin-treated diabetes because of hyperinsulinaemia. Suppression of endogenous insulin secretion to allow increased hepatic glucose production to meet the increased metabolic demand is key to the normal physiological response to exercise. In insulin-treated diabetes, insulin levels may actually increase with exercise because of improved blood flow at the site of injection and this increases the risk of hypoglycaemia.

Awareness of hypoglycaemia

For most individuals, the glucose level (threshold) at which they first become aware of hypoglycaemia is not

21.19 Most common symptoms of hypoglycaemia

Autonomic	
• Sweating • Trembling • Pounding heart	• Hunger • Anxiety
Neuroglycopenic	
• Confusion • Drowsiness • Speech difficulty	• Inability to concentrate • Incoordination • Irritability, anger
Non-specific	
• Nausea • Tiredness	• Headache

N.B. Symptoms differ with age; children exhibit behavioural changes (such as naughtiness or irritability), while elderly people experience more prominent neurological symptoms (such as visual disturbance and ataxia).

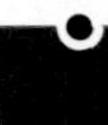

21.20 Hypoglycaemia in diabetes: common causes and risk factors

Causes of hypoglycaemia

- Missed, delayed or inadequate meal
- Unexpected or unusual exercise
- Alcohol
- Errors in oral anti-diabetic agent(s) or insulin dose/schedule/administration
- Poorly designed insulin regimen, particularly if predisposing to nocturnal hyperinsulinaemia
- Lipohypertrophy at injection sites causing variable insulin absorption
- Gastroparesis due to autonomic neuropathy causing variable carbohydrate absorption
- Malabsorption, e.g. coeliac disease
- Unrecognised other endocrine disorder, e.g. Addison's disease
- Factitious (deliberately induced)
- Breastfeeding

Risk factors for severe hypoglycaemia

- Strict glycaemic control
- Impaired awareness of hypoglycaemia
- Age (very young and elderly)
- Long duration of diabetes
- Sleep
- C-peptide negativity (indicating complete insulin deficiency)
- History of previous severe hypoglycaemia
- Renal impairment
- Genetic, e.g. angiotensin-converting enzyme (ACE) genotype

constant but varies according to the circumstances in which hypoglycaemia arises (e.g. during the night or during exercise). In addition, with longer duration of disease, and particularly in response to frequent hypoglycaemia, the threshold for generation of symptom responses to hypoglycaemia shifts to a lower glucose concentration. This cerebral adaptation has a similar effect on the counter-regulatory hormonal response to hypoglycaemia. Taken together, this means that individuals with type 1 diabetes may have reduced (impaired) awareness of hypoglycaemia. Symptoms can be experienced less intensely, or even be absent, despite blood glucose concentrations below 2.5 mmol/L (45 mg/dL). Such individuals are at an especially high risk of severe hypoglycaemia. The prevalence of impaired awareness of hypoglycaemia increases with time; overall, it affects around 20–25% of people with type 1 diabetes and under 10% with insulin-treated type 2 diabetes.

Management

Acute treatment of hypoglycaemia

Treatment of hypoglycaemia depends on its severity and on whether the patient is conscious and able to swallow (Box 21.21). Oral carbohydrate usually suffices if hypoglycaemia is recognised early. If parenteral therapy is required, then as soon as the patient is able to swallow, glucose should be given orally. Full recovery may not occur immediately and reversal of cognitive impairment may not be complete until 60 minutes after normoglycaemia is restored. When hypoglycaemia has occurred in a patient treated with a long- or intermediate-acting insulin or a long-acting sulphonylurea, such as glibenclamide, the possibility of recurrence should be anticipated; to prevent this, infusion of 10% dextrose, titrated to the patient's blood glucose, may be necessary.

If the patient fails to regain consciousness after blood glucose is restored to normal, then cerebral oedema and other causes of impaired consciousness – such as alcohol intoxication, a post-ictal state or cerebral haemorrhage – should be considered. Cerebral oedema has a high mortality and morbidity, and requires urgent treatment with mannitol and high-dose oxygen.

Following recovery, it is important to try to identify a cause and make appropriate adjustments to the patient's therapy. Unless the reason for a hypoglycaemic episode is clear, the patient should reduce the next dose of insulin by 10–20% and seek medical advice about further adjustments in dose.

The management of self-poisoning with oral anti-diabetic agents is described on page 216.

Prevention of hypoglycaemia

Patient education is fundamental to the prevention of hypoglycaemia. Risk factors for, and treatment of hypoglycaemia should be discussed. The importance of regular blood glucose monitoring and the need to have glucose (and glucagon) readily available should be stressed. A review of insulin and carbohydrate management during exercise is particularly useful. Advice for patients when travelling is summarised in Box 21.22.

Relatives and friends also need to be familiar with the symptoms and signs of hypoglycaemia and should be instructed in how to help (including how to inject glucagon).

It is important to recognise that all current insulin replacement regimens are suboptimal and do not accurately replicate normal physiological insulin profiles. Understanding the pharmacokinetics and pharmacodynamics of the insulin regimen in use by the patient will help prevent further hypoglycaemia (p. 824). For example, an individual experiencing regular nocturnal hypoglycaemia between midnight and 0200 hours may be found to be taking twice-daily soluble and intermediate-acting insulins before breakfast and before the main evening meal between 1700 and 1900 hours. In this case, the peak action of the isophane insulin will coincide with the period of maximum sensitivity to insulin – namely, 2300–0200 hours – and increase the risk of nocturnal hypoglycaemia. To address this, the evening dose of depot intermediate-acting insulin should be deferred until bedtime (after 2300 hours), shifting its peak action period to 0500–0700 hours. It is also a sensible precaution for patients to measure their blood glucose before they retire to bed and to have a carbohydrate snack if the reading is less than 6.0 mmol/L (approximately 110 mg/dL).

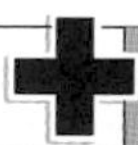

21.21 Emergency treatment of hypoglycaemia

Mild (self-treated)

- Oral fast-acting carbohydrate (10–15 g) is taken as glucose drink or tablets or confectionery
- This should be followed with a snack containing complex carbohydrate

Severe (external help required)

- If patient is semiconscious or unconscious, parenteral treatment is required:
  IV 75 mL 20% dextrose (= 15 g; give 0.2 g/kg in children)*
  Or
  IM glucagon (1 mg; 0.5 mg in children)
- If patient is conscious and able to swallow:
  Give oral refined glucose as drink or sweets (= 25 g)
  Or
  Apply glucose gel or jam or honey to buccal mucosa

*Use of 50% dextrose is no longer recommended.

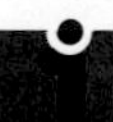

21.22 Avoidance and treatment of hypoglycaemia during travel

- Carry a supply of fast-acting carbohydrate (non-perishable, in suitable containers)
  Screwtop plastic bottles for glucose drinks
  Packets of powdered glucose (for use in hot, humid climates)
  Confectionery (foil-wrapped in hot climates)
- Companions should carry additional oral carbohydrate, and glucagon
- Perform frequent blood glucose testing (carry spare meter and/or visually read strips)
- Use fast-acting insulin analogues for long-distance air travel

Diabetes in pregnancy

During pregnancy, maternal glucose metabolism changes to optimise glucose and other nutrient delivery to the fetus. This is particularly apparent in the second half of pregnancy, when there is an increase in maternal tissue insulin resistance, such that glucose is preferentially supplied to the fetus rather than maternal tissue. This is largely driven by the maternal hormonal environment, with increased oestrogens and progestogens, and, in particular, human placental lactogen (hPL). The delivery of the placenta results in rapid decline in hPL with a rapid reversal of insulin resistance soon after birth. During pregnancy, fasting plasma glucose decreases slightly, while post-prandial blood glucose may be increased. The renal threshold for glycosuria (p. 807) is reduced in pregnancy.

In the fetus, insulin secretion is driven by fetal blood glucose levels, which are determined by the maternal glucose concentrations. Thus maternal hyperglycaemia drives fetal hyperinsulinaemia. Since insulin is a major fetal growth factor, hyperinsulinaemia in turn drives increased fetal growth, resulting in increased birth weight ('macrosomia').

Gestational diabetes

Gestational diabetes is defined as diabetes with first onset or recognition during pregnancy. This definition will include a few patients who develop type 1 diabetes during pregnancy, where prompt action and early insulin treatment will be required, and some patients who develop type 2 diabetes, or had unknown pre-existing type 2 diabetes, in whom the diabetes does not remit after pregnancy. However, the majority of gestational diabetes develops due to an inability to increase insulin secretion adequately to compensate for pregnancy-induced insulin resistance, and most women can expect to return to normal glucose tolerance immediately after pregnancy.

In contrast to non-gestational diabetes, for which the diagnostic thresholds for diabetes are based upon risk of microvascular complications, the diagnosis of gestational diabetes is based upon maternal blood glucose measures that are associated with increased fetal growth. An international consensus recommended that glucose values diagnostic of gestational diabetes should be lower than those for non-gestational diabetes (Box 21.23). Controversy remains about who should be screened, and in part the screening strategy depends on the population risk. It is widely accepted that women at high risk for gestational diabetes should have an oral glucose tolerance test at 24–28 weeks, with some guidelines recommending that all are screened by measuring HbA_{1c}, fasting blood glucose or random blood glucose at the first booking visit. With the increasing use of HbA_{1c} to diagnose diabetes, it should be noted that HbA_{1c} is unreliable after early pregnancy, when it falls due to increased red cell turnover.

Management of gestational diabetes

The aim is to normalise the maternal blood glucose and thereby reduce excessive fetal growth. The first element of management is dietary modification, in particular by reducing consumption of quick-acting refined carbohydrate. Women with gestational diabetes should undertake regular pre- and post-prandial self-monitoring of blood glucose, aiming for pre-meal blood glucose levels of less than 5.5 mmol/L (100 mg/dL) or post-meal blood glucose levels of less than 7.0 mmol/L (125 mg/dL). If treatment is necessary, metformin or glibenclamide is considered safe to use in pregnancy. Glibenclamide should be used rather than other sulphonylureas because it does not cross the placenta. Other oral therapies or injectable incretin-based therapies should not be given in pregnancy. Insulin may be required, especially in the later stages of pregnancy. If the maternal blood glucose is not well controlled prior to, and during, delivery, the resulting fetal hyperinsulinaemia leads to neonatal hyperinsulinaemia, which in turn can cause neonatal hypoglycaemia.

After delivery, maternal glucose usually rapidly returns to pre-pregnancy levels. Woman should be tested at least 6 weeks post-partum with an oral glucose tolerance test. In women with persistent mild fasting hyperglycaemia (glucose over 5.5 mmol/L (100 mg/dL)) who have a small increment (less than 3.5 mmol/L) in plasma glucose 2 hours after oral glucose, monogenic diabetes due to a mutation in GCK (encoding glucokinase) should be considered (see Box 21.6, p. 807). Those who have returned to normal glucose tolerance remain at considerable risk for developing type 2 diabetes, with a 5-year risk between 15 and 50%, depending on the population. Therefore, all women who have had gestational diabetes should be given diet and lifestyle advice to reduce their risk of developing type 2 diabetes (p. 820).

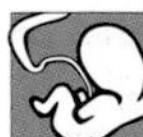

21.23 Identifying patients with gestational diabetes

Women at high risk of gestational diabetes

- BMI > 30 kg/m^2
- A previous macrosomic baby weighing ≥ 4.5 kg at birth
- Previous gestational diabetes
- A first-degree relative with diabetes
- A high-risk ethnicity – South Asian, black Caribbean or Middle Eastern

Diagnosis

- High-risk women should have a 75 g oral glucose tolerance test before 28 weeks' gestation
- Gestational diabetes is diagnosed when:
  Fasting plasma glucose ≥ 5.1 mmol/L (92 mg/dL) *or*
  1-hr plasma glucose (after glucose load) ≥ 10 mmol/L (180 mg/dL) *or*
  2-hr plasma glucose (after glucose load) ≥ 8 mmol/L (144 mg/dL)
- Consider testing high-risk women at first booking visit with an HbA_{1c} or fasting blood glucose

Pregnancy in women with established diabetes

Maternal hyperglycaemia early in pregnancy (during the first 6 weeks post-conception) can adversely affect fetal development. Consequences include cardiac, renal and skeletal malformations, of which the caudal regression syndrome is the most characteristic. The risk of fetal anomaly is about 2% for non-diabetic women, about 4% for women with well-controlled diabetes (HbA_{1c} below 53 mmol/mol (7%)), but more than 20% for those with poor glycaemic control (HbA_{1c} greater than 97 mmol/mol (11%)). Therefore, a woman with diabetes should, if possible, be helped to achieve excellent glycaemic control *before* becoming pregnant. In addition, high-dose folic acid (5 mg, rather than the usual 400 µg, daily) should be initiated before conception to reduce the risk of neural tube defects.

As for gestational diabetes, mothers should attempt to maintain near-normal blood glucose levels whilst avoiding hypoglycaemia throughout their pregnancy, as this minimises excessive fetal growth and neonatal hypoglycaemia. However, this is often difficult to achieve. Pregnancy is also associated with an increased potential for ketosis, particularly, but not exclusively, in women with type 1 diabetes. Ketoacidosis during pregnancy is dangerous for the mother and is associated with a high rate (10–35%) of fetal mortality.

Pregnancy is associated with a worsening of diabetic complications, most notably retinopathy and nephropathy, so careful monitoring of eyes and kidneys is required throughout pregnancy. If heavy proteinuria and/or renal dysfunction exist prior to pregnancy, there is a marked increase in the risk of pre-eclampsia, and renal function can deteriorate irreversibly during pregnancy. These risks need to be carefully discussed before a woman with diabetes is considering pregnancy. While the outlook for mother and child has been vastly improved over recent years, pregnancy outcomes are still not equivalent to those of non-diabetic mothers. Perinatal mortality rates remain 3–4 times those of the non-diabetic population (at around 30–40 per 1000 pregnancies) and the rate of congenital malformation is increased 5–6-fold overall.

Children, adolescents and young adults with diabetes

The management of diabetes in children and adolescents presents particular challenges, which should be addressed in specialised clinics (Box 21.24).

Hyperglycaemia in acute myocardial infarction

Hyperglycaemia is often found in patients who have sustained an acute myocardial infarction. In some, this represents stress hyperglycaemia (p. 808), some have previously undiagnosed diabetes, and many have established diabetes. Many patients with stress hyperglycaemia will have impaired glucose tolerance on a subsequent glucose tolerance test. Over and above the standard management of myocardial infarction (p. 593), hyperglycaemia should be treated with insulin rather than oral anti-diabetic agents in the peri-infarct period, aiming for near-normalisation of blood glucose. Studies have suggested that good glycaemic control using insulin therapy in hyperglycaemic patients with acute myocardial infarction may reduce their long-term mortality from coronary heart disease.

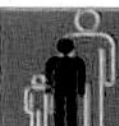

21.24 Diabetes in adolescence

- **Type of diabetes**: type 1 diabetes is predominant in children and adolescents, but type 2 diabetes is now presenting in unprecedented numbers of obese, inactive teenagers. Monogenic diabetes (MODY) should also be considered (see Box 21.6, p. 807).
- **Physiological changes**: hormonal, physical and lifestyle changes in puberty affect dietary intake, exercise patterns and sensitivity to insulin, necessitating alterations in insulin regimen.
- **Emotional changes**: adolescence is a phase of transition into independence (principally from parental care). Periods of rebellion against parental control, experimentation (e.g. with alcohol) and a more chaotic lifestyle are common, and often impact adversely on control of diabetes.
- **Glycaemic control**: a temporary deterioration in control is common, although not universal. It is sometimes more important to maintain contact and engagement with a young person than to insist on tight glycaemic control.
- **Diabetic ketoacidosis**: a few adolescents and young adults present with frequent episodes of DKA, often because of non-adherence to insulin therapy. This is more common in females. Motivating factors may include weight loss, rebellion, and manipulation of family or schooling circumstances.
- **Adolescent diabetes clinics**: these challenges are best tackled with support from a specialised multidisciplinary team, including paediatricians, physicians, nurses and psychologists. Support is required for the patient and parents.

Surgery and diabetes

Patients with diabetes are reported to have up to 50% higher peri-operative mortality than patients without diabetes. Surgery causes catabolic stress and secretion of counter-regulatory hormones (including catecholamines and cortisol) in both normal and diabetic subjects. This results in increased glycogenolysis, gluconeogenesis, lipolysis, proteolysis and insulin resistance. Starvation exacerbates this process by increasing lipolysis. In the non-diabetic person, these metabolic effects lead to a secondary increase in the secretion of insulin, which exerts a controlling influence. In diabetic patients, either there is absolute deficiency of insulin (type 1 diabetes) or insulin secretion is delayed and impaired (type 2 diabetes), so that in untreated or poorly controlled diabetes, the uptake of metabolic substrate into tissues is significantly reduced, catabolism is increased and, ultimately, metabolic decompensation in the form of diabetic ketoacidosis may develop in both types of diabetes. In addition, hyperglycaemia impairs wound healing and innate immunity, leading to increased risk of infection. Patients with diabetes are also more likely to have underlying pre-operative morbidity, especially cardiovascular disease. Finally, management errors with diabetes may cause dangerous hyperglycaemia or hypoglycaemia. Careful pre-operative assessment and peri-operative management are therefore essential, ideally with support from the diabetes specialist team.

Pre-operative assessment

Unless a surgical intervention is an emergency, patients with diabetes should be assessed well in advance of surgery so that poor glycaemic control and other risk factors can be addressed (Box 21.25). There is good evidence that higher HbA_{1c} is associated with adverse peri-operative outcome. In general, an upper limit for an acceptable HbA_{1c} should be between 64 and 75 mmol/mol (8 and 9%). However, since optimisation of care may take weeks or months to achieve, the benefits need to be weighed against the need for early surgical intervention.

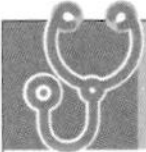

21.25 How to carry out pre-operative assessment of patients with diabetes

- Assess glycaemic control
  Consider delaying surgery and referral to the diabetes team if HbA_{1c} > 75 mmol/mol (9%). This should be weighed against the need for surgery
- Assess cardiovascular status
  Optimise blood pressure
  ECG for evidence of (possibly silent) ischaemic heart disease and to assess QTc (p. 532)
- Assess foot risk (p. 833)
  Patients with high-risk feet should have suitable pressure relief provided during post-operative nursing
- For minor/moderate operations where only one meal will be omitted, plan for the patient to be first on the list

Peri-operative management

Figure 21.8 outlines a general approach to peri-operative management of diabetes, although this may need to be adapted according to the patient, the surgical procedure and local guidelines. Patients with diabetes who are considered low-risk can attend as day cases or be admitted on the day of surgery. However, patients are often admitted the night before to ensure optimal management, and to begin intravenous insulin to optimise blood glucose, if required.

Post-operative management

Patients who need to continue fasting after surgery should be maintained on intravenous insulin and fluids until they are able to eat and drink (see Fig. 21.8). During this time, care must be taken with fluid balance and electrolyte levels. Insulin infusion necessitates dextrose infusion to maintain a supply of glucose, but this combination drives down plasma potassium (p. 440) and can result in hyponatraemia. Intravenous fluids during prolonged insulin infusion should therefore include saline and potassium supplementation. UK guidelines recommend use of dextrose/saline (0.45% saline with 5% dextrose and 0.15% potassium chloride).

Once a patient's usual treatment has been reinstated, care must be taken to continue to control the blood glucose, ideally between 4 and 10 mmol/L (70–180 mg/dL), in order to optimise wound healing and recovery.

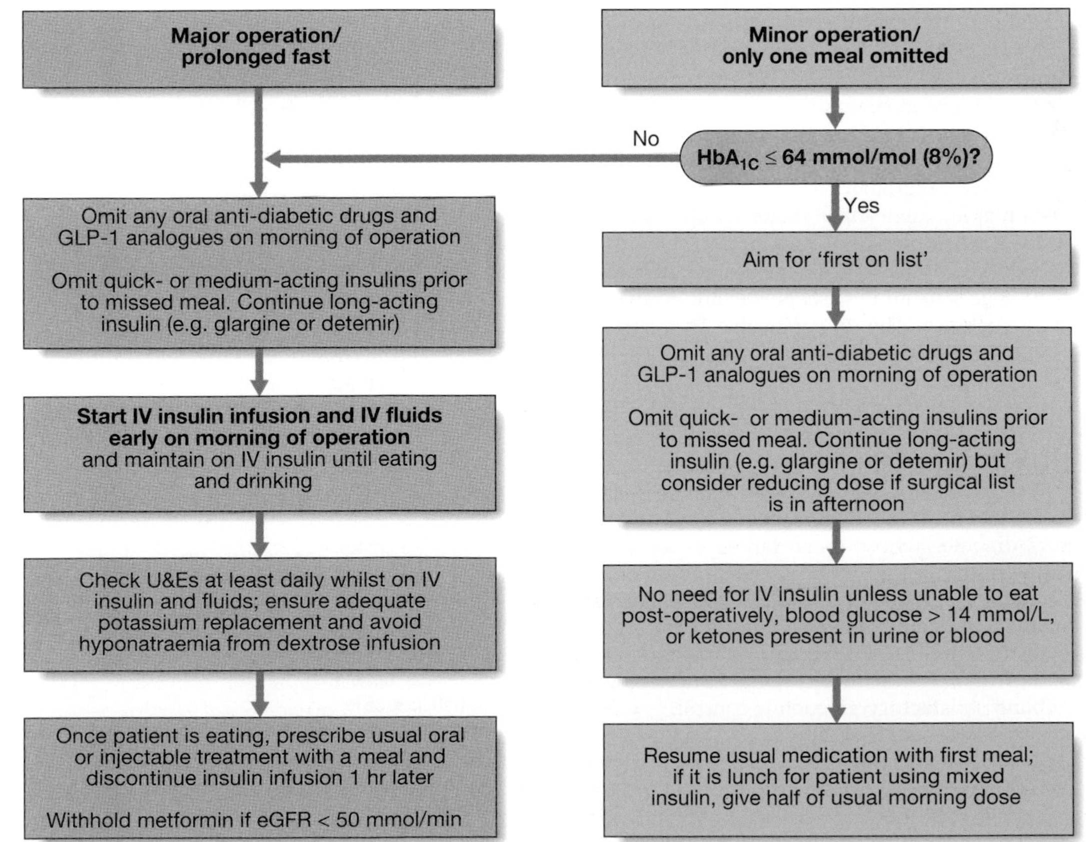

Fig. 21.8 Management of diabetic patients undergoing surgery and general anaesthesia. (Glucose > 14 mmol/L ≅ 250 mg/dL) (eGFR = estimated glomerular filtration rate; GLP-1 = glucagon-like peptide 1)

21

Patients normally controlled on tablets may require temporary subcutaneous insulin treatment until the increased 'stress' of surgery, wound healing or infection has resolved.

Complications of diabetes

Patients with long-standing diabetes are at risk of developing a variety of complications (see Box 21.31, p. 826). Moreover, as many as 25% of people with type 2 diabetes have evidence of diabetic complications at the time of initial diagnosis. Thus, diabetes may be first suspected when a patient visits an optometrist or podiatrist, or presents with hypertension or a vascular event such as an acute myocardial infarction or stroke. Blood glucose should therefore be checked in all patients presenting with such pathology. The detailed investigation and management of diabetic complications are described on pages 826–836.

MANAGEMENT OF DIABETES

In new cases of diabetes, adequate glycaemic control can be obtained by diet and lifestyle advice alone in approximately 50%, 20–30% will need oral anti-diabetic medication, and 20–30% will require insulin. Regardless of aetiology, the choice of treatment is determined by the adequacy of residual β-cell function. However, this cannot be determined easily by measurement of plasma insulin concentration because a level which is adequate in one patient may be inadequate in another, depending upon sensitivity to insulin. Consideration of the features in Box 21.12 (p. 809), and in particular the age and weight of the patient at diagnosis, usually indicate the type of treatment required. However, in each individual, the regimen adopted is effectively a therapeutic trial and should be reviewed regularly.

The ideal management for diabetes would allow the person to lead a completely normal life, to remain not only symptom-free but in good health, to achieve a normal metabolic state and to escape the long-term complications of diabetes. This is achievable to a variable degree. Setting individual goals for each patient is discussed on page 811.

Patients whose glycaemic control deteriorates after a period of satisfactory control need their therapy to be adjusted. However, this is not a homogeneous group; it includes some patients with late-onset type 1 diabetes who develop an absolute deficiency of insulin, some with type 2 diabetes whose β-cell failure is advanced, and others who are not adhering to the recommended lifestyle changes or medication. Weight loss suggests worsening β-cell function. During continuing follow-up, the majority of patients will require combinations of anti-diabetic drugs, often with additional insulin replacement, to obtain satisfactory glycaemic control.

Diet and lifestyle

The importance of lifestyle changes such as undertaking regular physical activity, observing a healthy diet and reducing alcohol consumption should not be underestimated in improving glycaemic control, but many people, particularly the middle-aged and elderly, find them difficult to sustain. Patients should also be encouraged to stop smoking.

Healthy eating

All people with diabetes need to pay special attention to their diet (Box 21.26; see also p. 110). They should have access to a dietitian at diagnosis, at review and at times of treatment change. Nutritional advice should be tailored to individuals and take account of their age and lifestyle. Many people with type 2 diabetes require dietary advice for achieving weight loss, to include caloric restriction and, in particular, reduced fat intake. Structured education programmes are available for both common types of diabetes.

Carbohydrate

Both the amount and source of carbohydrate determine post-prandial glucose (p. 112). The glycaemic index (GI) of a carbohydrate-containing food is a measure of the change in blood glucose following its ingestion relative to the rise in blood glucose observed following a liquid oral glucose tolerance test. Different foods can be ranked by their effect on post-prandial glycaemia. Consumption of foods with a low GI is encouraged because they produce a slow, gradual rise in blood glucose. Examples include starchy foods such as basmati rice, spaghetti, porridge, noodles, granary bread, and beans and lentils. However, different methods of food processing and preparation can influence the GI of foods, as can the ripeness of some foods and differences in strains of rice. In addition, while consideration of GI is useful in choosing between types of carbohydrate, it does not address the total amount consumed. Recent studies suggest short-term (6 months), very low carbohydrate diets (containing as little as 50 g carbohydrate per day – 13% of daily energy) are safe and effective means of reducing

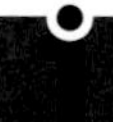

21.26 Dietary management of diabetes

Aims of dietary management

- Achieve good glycaemic control
- Reduce hyperglycaemia and avoid hypoglycaemia
- Assist with weight management:
  - Weight maintenance for type 1 diabetes and non-obese type 2 diabetes
  - Weight loss for overweight and obese type 2 diabetes
- Reduce the risk of micro- and macrovascular complications
- Ensure adequate nutritional intake
- Avoid 'atherogenic' diets or those that aggravate complications, e.g. high protein intake in nephropathy

Dietary constituents and recommended % of energy intake

- Carbohydrate: 45–60%
  - Sucrose: up to 10%
- Fat (total): < 35%
  - n-6 Polyunsaturated: < 10%
  - n-3 Polyunsaturated: eat 1 portion (140 g) oily fish once or twice weekly
  - Monounsaturated: 10–20%
  - Saturated: < 10%
- Protein: 10–15% (do not exceed 1 g/kg body weight/day)
- Fruit/vegetables: 5 portions daily

weight and improving glycaemic control. However, high dropout rates and poor adherence suggest that this type of diet is not widely applicable.

In type 1 diabetes, the development of modern insulin regimens, particularly using insulin analogues or continuous subcutaneous insulin infusion (CSII; p. 824), has allowed increased flexibility in the timing and choice of carbohydrate intake. It is now possible to match the amount of carbohydrate in a meal with a dose of short-acting insulin using methods such as Dose Adjustment for Normal Eating (DAFNE), although this is demanding and requires extensive patient education. This approach enables motivated individuals with type 1 diabetes to achieve and maintain good glycaemic control, while avoiding post-prandial hyper- and hypoglycaemia.

Fat

The intake of total fat should be restricted to less than 35% of energy intake, with less than 10% as saturated fat, and 10–20% from monounsaturated fat through consumption of oils and spreads made from olive, rapeseed or groundnut oils (see Box 21.26). The influence of dietary fats on plasma lipid profile and cardiovascular disease is discussed on page 113.

Salt

People with diabetes should follow the advice given to the general population: namely, to limit sodium intake to no more than 6 g daily.

Weight management

In patients with diabetes, weight management is important, as a high percentage of people with type 2 diabetes are overweight or obese, and many anti-diabetic drugs, including insulin, encourage weight gain. Obesity, particularly central obesity with increased waist circumference, also predicts insulin resistance and cardiovascular risk.

Management of obesity is described on page 117. Weight loss can be achieved through a reduction in energy intake and an increase in energy expenditure through physical activity. Lifestyle interventions or pharmacotherapy for obesity when associated with weight reduction have beneficial effects on HbA_{1c}, but long-term benefits in terms of glycaemic control and microvascular disease have not been adequately assessed. More recently, bariatric surgery has been shown to induce marked weight loss in obese individuals with type 2 diabetes and this is often associated with significant improvements in HbA_{1c} and withdrawal of or reduction in diabetes medications.

Exercise

All patients with diabetes should be advised to achieve a significant level of physical activity and to maintain this in the long term. This can include activities such as walking, gardening, swimming or cycling. Supervised and structured exercise programmes may be of particular benefit to people with type 2 diabetes. Various guidelines exist for physical activity in the general population. Those from the US Department of Health and Human services (2008) suggest that adults (18–64 years) should build up to achieve a weekly minimum of 2.5 hours of moderate-intensity exercise or 75 minutes of vigorous-intensity exercise, or a combination thereof. The aerobic (moderate-intensity) activity should be performed for at least 10 minutes each time and spread throughout the week, with at least 30 minutes on at least 5 days of the week. Older adults should also follow these guidelines as far as their abilities allow. Recently, it has also been suggested that a combination of both aerobic and resistance exercise may lead to greater improvements in glycaemic control.

In type 1 diabetes, exercise can increase the risk of hypoglycaemia, so patients should seek specialist advice on taking extra carbohydrate, reducing insulin doses and choosing an injection site.

Alcohol

Alcohol is recognised as having both beneficial and harmful effects on cardiovascular disease and this also appears to apply in patients with diabetes. Alcohol can therefore be taken in moderation in diabetes with the aim of keeping within national guidelines relating to recommendations for people without diabetes (e.g. in the UK, the weekly recommended maximum is 14 U for women and 21 U for men). However, alcohol can reduce hypoglycaemia awareness and, by suppressing gluconeogenesis, increase hypoglycaemia risk. In addition, all patients with diabetes should be made aware of the high calorie content of alcohol and the implications for body weight management, which are often overlooked.

Drugs to reduce hyperglycaemia

For many years, there were only a few choices of drugs available for type 2 diabetes – the biguanide metformin, the sulphonylureas and insulin. Insulin is the only treatment for type 1 diabetes. Acarbose was also available but little used in most countries. Since the late 1990s, however, several new classes of agents have been approved for use in type 2 diabetes, with more in development. Newer drugs include thiazolidinediones, dipeptidyl peptidase 4 (DPP-4) inhibitors, glucagon-like peptide 1 (GLP-1) receptor agonists, and sodium and glucose transporter 2 (SGLT2) inhibitors. The effects of these drugs are compared in Box 21.27. This makes for an exciting time in diabetes pharmacotherapy, but exactly how, when and in what order these agents should be used remains uncertain. The older drugs are cheaper and have established benefits for reducing microvascular disease; they are therefore usually recommended as first-line therapy. Use of the newer drugs is not supported by evidence for reduction in microvascular disease (because the trials have not yet been done) and they are much more expensive, so are often reserved for later therapy after failure of metformin and sulphonylureas. One guideline which follows these principles is shown in Figure 21.9. However, this does not necessarily reflect the optimum positioning of these newer drugs. As large trials, which aim to establish their cardiovascular benefit, report in the next few years, these recommendations may change dramatically.

Biguanides

Metformin is the only biguanide now available. Its long-term benefits were shown in the UK Prospective Diabetes Study (UKPDS) (p. 827), and it is now widely used

21.27 Effects of drugs used in the treatment of type 2 diabetes

	Insulin	Sulphonylureas and meglitinides	Metformin	Acarbose	Thiazolidinediones (glitazones)	DPP-4 inhibitors (gliptins)	GLP-1 receptor agonists	SGLT2 inhibitors
Fasting blood glucose	↓	↓	↓	↘	↓	↓	↓	↓
Post-prandial blood glucose	↓	↓	↓	↓	↓	↓	↓	↓
Plasma insulin	↑	↑	↓	↓	↓	↑	↑	↓
Body weight	↑	↑	→	→	↑	→	↓	↓
Risk of hypoglycaemia	++	+	–	–	–	–	–	–
Tolerability	Good	Good	Moderate	Moderate	Moderate	Good	Moderate	Limited experience

(DPP-4 = dipeptidyl peptidase 4; GLP-1 = glucagon-like peptide 1; SGLT2 = sodium and glucose transporter 2)

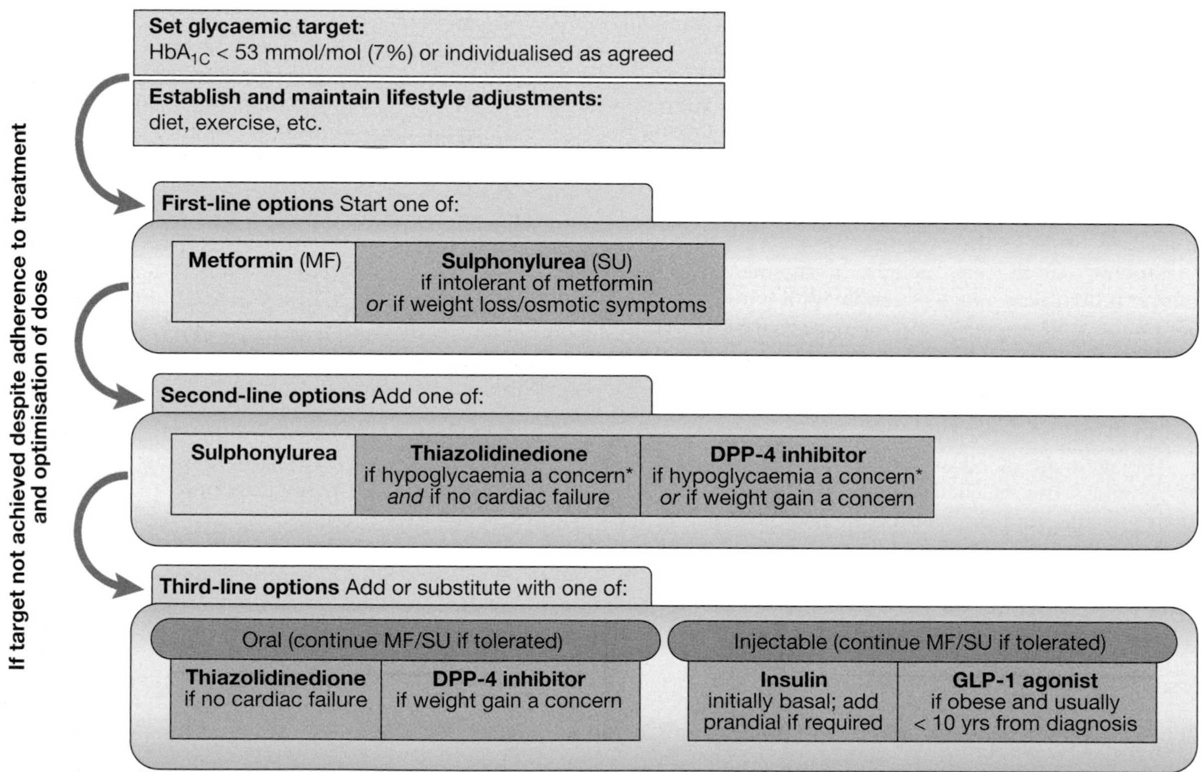

Fig. 21.9 Management of hyperglycaemia in type 2 diabetes. Purple boxes indicate the usual approach, and green boxes show alternatives which are selected according to individual circumstances. *Hypoglycaemia risk includes driving, occupational hazards and risk of falls. Note that SGLT2 inhibitors were not available when this guideline was produced. (DPP-4 = dipeptidyl peptidase 4; GLP-1 = glucagon-like peptide 1). Adapted from SIGN 116 – see p. 836.

as first-line therapy for type 2 diabetes, irrespective of body weight. Metformin is also given increasingly as an adjunct to insulin therapy in obese patients with type 1 diabetes. Approximately 25% of patients develop mild gastrointestinal side-effects with metformin, but only 5% are unable to tolerate it even at low dose. The main side-effects are diarrhoea, abdominal cramps, bloating and nausea.

Mechanism of action

The mechanism of action of metformin has not been precisely defined. Whilst classically considered an 'insulin sensitiser' because it lowers insulin levels, its main effects are on fasting glucose and are insulin-independent. Metformin reduces hepatic glucose production, may also increase insulin-mediated glucose uptake, and has effects on gut glucose uptake and utilisation. At the molecular level, metformin acts as a weak inhibitor of mitochondrial respiration, which increases intracellular adenosine monophosphate (AMP) and reduces adenosine triphosphate (ATP). This has direct effects on the flux through gluconeogenesis, and activates the intracellular energy sensor AMP-activated protein kinase (AMPK), leading to multiple beneficial metabolic effects.

Clinical use

Metformin is a potent blood glucose-lowering treatment that is weight-neutral, does not cause hypoglycaemia and has established benefits in microvascular disease. It is employed as first-line therapy in all patients who tolerate it, and its use is maintained when additional agents are added as glycaemia deteriorates (see Fig. 21.9). Metformin is usually introduced at low dose (500 mg twice daily) to minimise the risk of gastrointestinal side-effects. The usual maintenance dose is 1 g twice daily. There is a modified-release formulation of metformin which may be better tolerated by patients with gastrointestinal side-effects.

Metformin can increase susceptibility to lactic acidosis, although this is much less common than was previously thought. As metformin is cleared by the kidneys, it can accumulate in renal impairment, so the dose should be halved when estimated glomerular filtration rate (eGFR) is 30–45 mL/min, and it should not be used below an eGFR of 30 mL/min. Its use is also contraindicated in patients with impaired hepatic function and in those who drink alcohol in excess, in whom the risk of lactic acidosis is significantly increased. It should be discontinued, at least temporarily, if any other serious medical condition develops, especially one causing severe shock or hypoxia. In such circumstances, treatment with insulin should be substituted if required.

Sulphonylureas

Sulphonylureas are 'insulin secretagogues', i.e. they promote pancreatic β-cell insulin secretion. Similar to metformin, the long-term benefits of sulphonylureas in lowering microvascular complications of diabetes were established in the UK Prospective Diabetes Study (p. 827).

Mechanism of action

Sulphonylureas act by closing the pancreatic β-cell ATP-sensitive potassium (K_{ATP}) channel, decreasing K^+ efflux, which ultimately triggers insulin secretion. Meglitinides (e.g. repaglinide and nateglinide) also work in this way and, although short-acting, are essentially sulphonylurea-like drugs.

Clinical use

Sulphonylureas are an effective therapy for lowering blood glucose and are often used as an add-on to metformin, if glycaemia is inadequately controlled on metformin alone (see Fig. 21.9). The main adverse effects of sulphonylureas are weight gain and hypoglycaemia. The weight gain is not ideal in patients with diabetes who are already overweight or obese, although sulphonylureas are effective treatments in this group. Hypoglycaemia occurs because the closure of K_{ATP} channels brings about unregulated insulin secretion, even with normal or low blood glucose levels.

There are a number of sulphonylureas. In the UK, gliclazide is the most commonly used; in contrast, in the USA, glibenclamide (also known as glyburide) is widely used. Glibenclamide, however, is long-acting and prone to induce hypoglycaemia, so should be avoided in the elderly. Other sulphonylureas include glimepiride and glipizide. The dose–response of all sulphonylureas is steepest at low doses; little additional benefit is obtained when the dose is increased to maximal levels.

Alpha-glucosidase inhibitors

The α-glucosidase inhibitors delay carbohydrate absorption in the gut by inhibiting disaccharidases. Acarbose and miglitol are available and are taken with each meal. Both lower post-prandial blood glucose and modestly improve overall glycaemic control. They can be combined with a sulphonylurea. The main side-effects are flatulence, abdominal bloating and diarrhoea. They are used widely in the Far East but infrequently in the UK.

Thiazolidinediones

Mechanism of action

These drugs (also called TZDs, 'glitazones' or PPARγ agonists) bind and activate peroxisome proliferator-activated receptor-γ, a nuclear receptor present mainly in adipose tissue that regulates the expression of several genes involved in metabolism. TZDs enhance the actions of endogenous insulin, in part directly (in the adipose cells) and in part indirectly (by altering release of 'adipokines', such as adiponectin, which alter insulin sensitivity in the liver). Plasma insulin concentrations are not increased and hypoglycaemia does not occur. TZDs increase pre-adipocyte differentiation, resulting in an increase in fat mass and in body weight.

Clinical use

TZDs have been prescribed widely since the late 1990s, but recently a number of adverse effects have become apparent and their use has declined. One popular TZD, rosiglitazone, was reported to increase the risk of myocardial infarction and was withdrawn in 2010. The other TZD in common use, pioglitazone, does not appear to increase the risk of myocardial infarction but it does exacerbate cardiac failure by causing fluid retention, and recent data show that it increases the risk of bone fracture, and possibly bladder cancer. These observations have reduced the use of pioglitazone dramatically.

Pioglitazone can be very effective at lowering blood glucose in some patients and appears more effective in insulin-resistant patients. In addition, it has a beneficial effect in reducing fatty liver and NASH (p. 805). Pioglitazone is usually added to metformin with or without sulphonylurea therapy (see Fig. 21.9). It may be given with insulin therapy, when it can be very effective, but the combination of insulin and TZDs markedly increases fluid retention and risk of cardiac failure, so should be used with caution.

Incretin-based therapies: DPP-4 inhibitors and GLP-1 analogues

The incretin effect is the augmentation of insulin secretion seen when a glucose stimulus is given orally rather than intravenously, and reflects the release of incretin peptides from the gut (see Fig. 21.3, p. 802). The incretin hormones are primarily glucagon-like peptide 1 (GLP-1) and gastric inhibitory polypeptide (GIP). These are rapidly broken down by the peptidase DPP-4 (dipeptidyl peptidase 4). The incretin effect is diminished in type 2 diabetes, and this has stimulated the development of two incretin-based therapeutic approaches.

The 'gliptins', or DPP-4 inhibitors, prevent breakdown and therefore enhance concentrations of endogenous GLP-1 and GIP. The first DPP-4 inhibitor to market was sitagliptin; others now available include vildagliptin, saxagliptin and linagliptin. These drugs are very well tolerated and are weight-neutral (see Box 21.27).

The GLP-1 receptor agonists have a similar structure to GLP-1 but have been modified to resist breakdown by DPP-4. These agents are not orally active and have to be given by subcutaneous injection. However, they have a key advantage over the DPP-4 inhibitors: because the GLP-1 activity achieved is supra-physiological, it delays gastric emptying and, at the level of the hypothalamus, decreases appetite. Thus, injectable GLP-1 analogues lower blood glucose and result in weight loss – an appealing therapy, as the majority of patients with type 2 diabetes are obese. Currently available GLP-1 receptor agonists include exenatide (twice daily), exenatide MR (once weekly) and liraglutide (once daily).

Unlike sulphonylureas, both incretin-based therapies only promote insulin secretion when there is a glucose 'trigger' for insulin secretion. Thus, when the blood glucose is normal, the insulin secretion is not augmented and so these agents do not cause hypoglycaemia.

SGLT2 inhibitors

The sodium and glucose transporter 2 (SGLT2) inhibitor, dapagliflozin, was licensed for use in 2012. Glucose is filtered freely in the renal glomeruli and reabsorbed in the proximal tubules. SGLT2 is involved in reabsorption of glucose. Inhibition results in approximately 25% of the filtered glucose not being reabsorbed, with consequent glycosuria. Although this helps to lower blood glucose and results in calorie loss and subsequent weight loss, the glycosuria does result in increased urinary tract and genital fungal infections. With limited experience and evidence to date, the most appropriate position for SGLT2 inhibitors in the therapy of type 2 diabetes has yet to be established.

Insulin therapy

Manufacture and formulation

Insulin was discovered in 1921 and transformed the management of type 1 diabetes, until then a fatal disorder. Until the 1980s, insulin was obtained by extraction and purification from pancreata of cows and pigs (bovine and porcine insulins), and some patients still prefer to use animal insulins. Recombinant DNA technology enabled large-scale production of human insulin. More recently, the amino acid sequence of insulin has been altered to produce analogues of insulin, which differ in their rate of absorption from the site of injection.

The duration of action of short-acting, unmodified insulin ('soluble' or 'regular' insulin), which is a clear solution, can be extended by the addition of protamine and zinc at neutral pH (isophane or NPH insulin) or excess zinc ions (lente insulins). These modified 'depot' insulins are cloudy preparations. Pre-mixed formulations containing short-acting and isophane insulins in various proportions are available. The pharmacokinetics of these various insulins are shown in Box 21.28.

In most countries, the insulin concentration in available formulations has been standardised at 100 U/mL.

21.28 Duration of action (in hours) of insulin preparations

Insulin	Onset	Peak	Duration
Rapid-acting (insulin analogues: lispro, aspart, glulisine)	< 0.5	0.5–2.5	3–4.5
Short-acting (soluble (regular))	0.5–1	1–4	4–8
Intermediate-acting (isophane (NPH), lente)	1–3	3–8	7–14
Long-acting (bovine ultralente)	2–4	6–12	12–30
Long-acting (insulin analogues: glargine, detemir)	1–2	None	18–24

Subcutaneous multiple dose insulin therapy

In most patients, insulin is injected subcutaneously several times a day into the anterior abdominal wall, upper arms, outer thighs and buttocks (Box 21.29). Accidental intramuscular injection often occurs in children and thin adults. The rate of absorption of insulin may be influenced by many factors other than the insulin formulation, including the site, depth and volume of injection, skin temperature (warming), local massage and exercise. Absorption is delayed from areas of lipohypertrophy at injection sites (p. 799), which results from the local trophic action of insulin, so repeated injection at the same site should be avoided. Other routes of administration (intravenous and intraperitoneal) are reserved for specific circumstances.

Once absorbed into the blood, insulin has a half-life of just a few minutes. It is removed mainly by the liver and also the kidneys, so plasma insulin concentrations are elevated in patients with liver disease or renal failure. Rarely, the rate of clearance can be affected by binding to insulin antibodies (induced by use of animal insulins).

Insulin can be administered using a disposable plastic syringe with a fine needle (which can be re-used several times), but this has largely been replaced by pen

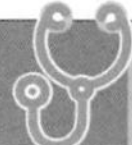

21.29 How to inject insulin subcutaneously

- Needle sited at right angle to the skin
- Subcutaneous (not intramuscular) injection
- Delivery devices: glass syringe (requires re-sterilisation), plastic syringe (disposable), pen device (reusable, some disposable), infusion pump

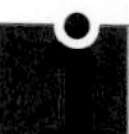

21.30 Side-effects of insulin therapy

- Hypoglycaemia
- Weight gain
- Peripheral oedema (insulin treatment causes salt and water retention in the short term)
- Insulin antibodies (with animal insulins)
- Local allergy (rare)
- Lipohypertrophy or lipoatrophy at injection sites

injectors containing insulin in cartridges sufficient for multiple dosing. These are also available as pre-loaded disposable pens.

For the most part, insulin analogues have replaced soluble and isophane insulins, especially for people with type 1 diabetes, because they allow more flexibility and convenience (see Box 21.28). Unlike soluble insulin, which should be injected 30 minutes before eating, rapid-acting insulin analogues can be administered immediately before, during or even after meals. Long-acting insulin analogues are better able than isophane insulin to maintain 'basal' insulin levels for up to 24 hours, so need only be injected once daily. Despite these pharmacokinetic benefits, the impact of insulin analogues on glycaemic control and adverse events appears to be minor.

The complications of insulin therapy are listed in Box 21.30; the most important of these is hypoglycaemia (p. 814). A common problem is fasting hyperglycaemia ('the dawn phenomenon'), which arises through a combination of the normal circadian rhythm and release of counter-regulatory hormones (growth hormone and cortisol) during the later part of the night, as well as diminishing levels of overnight isophane insulin.

Insulin dosing regimens

The choice of regimen depends on the desired degree of glycaemic control, the severity of underlying insulin deficiency, the patient's lifestyle, and his or her ability to adjust the insulin dose. The time–action profile of different insulin regimens, compared to the secretory pattern of insulin in the non-diabetic state, is shown in Figure 21.10. Most people with type 1 diabetes require two or more injections of insulin daily. In type 2 diabetes, insulin is usually initiated as a once-daily long-acting insulin, either alone or in combination with oral hypoglycaemic agents. However, in time, more frequent insulin injections are usually required.

Twice-daily administration of a short-acting and intermediate-acting insulin (usually soluble and isophane insulins), given in combination before breakfast and the evening meal, is the simplest regimen and is still used commonly in many countries. Initially, two-thirds of the total daily requirement of insulin is given in the morning in a ratio of short-acting to intermediate-acting of 1:2, and the remaining third is given in the evening. Pre-mixed formulations are available containing different proportions of soluble and isophane insulins (e.g. 30:70 and 50:50). These are useful for patients who have difficulty mixing insulins, but are inflexible as the individual components cannot be adjusted independently. They need to be resuspended by shaking the vial several times before administration. Fixed-mixture insulins also have altered pharmacodynamic profiles, such that the peak insulin action and time to peak effect are significantly reduced compared with injecting the same insulins separately.

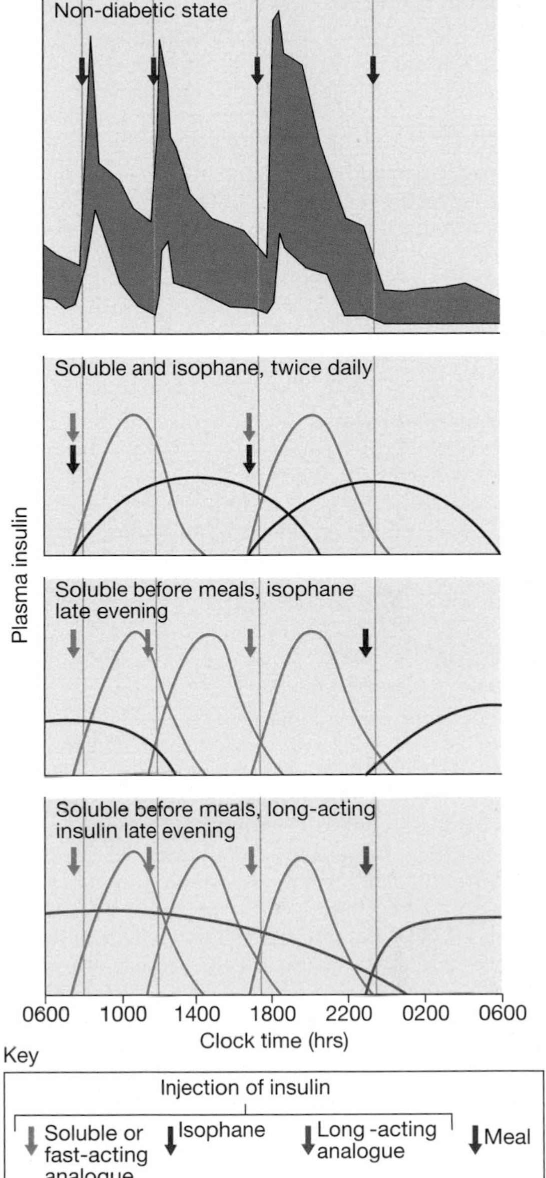

Fig. 21.10 Profiles of plasma insulin associated with different insulin regimens. The schematic profiles are compared with the insulin responses (mean ± one standard deviation) observed in non-diabetic adults shown in the top panel (shaded area). These are theoretical patterns of plasma insulin and may differ considerably in magnitude and duration of action between individuals.

Multiple injection regimens (intensive insulin therapy) are popular, with short-acting insulin being taken before each meal, and intermediate- or long-acting insulin being injected once or twice daily (basal-bolus regimen). This type of regimen allows greater freedom with regard to meal timing and more variable day-to-day physical activity.

21

Alternative insulin therapies

'Open-loop' systems are battery-powered portable pumps providing continuous subcutaneous (CSII), intraperitoneal or intravenous infusion of insulin without reference to the blood glucose concentration. The rate of insulin infusion is variable; it can be programmed to match the patient's diurnal variation in requirements and then manually boosted at mealtimes. In practice, the 'loop' is closed by the patient performing blood glucose estimations, and the use of these devices requires a high degree of patient motivation. These increasingly sophisticated systems can achieve excellent glycaemic control but widespread therapeutic use is limited by cost. The 'Artificial Pancreas' project aims to close the loop by using miniaturised glucose sensors to communicate wirelessly with the insulin pump, which would automatically adjust its rate, but this has not yet reached widespread clinical practice.

Alternative routes of insulin delivery have been investigated. Clinical trials with intrapulmonary (inhalation), transdermal and oral insulins are ongoing but as yet none has proven commercially viable.

Transplantation

Whole pancreas transplantation is carried out in a small number of patients with diabetes each year, but it presents problems relating to exocrine pancreatic secretions and long-term immunosuppression is necessary. While results are steadily improving, they remain less favourable than for renal transplantation. At present, the procedure is usually undertaken only in patients with end-stage renal failure who require a combined pancreas/kidney transplantation and in whom diabetes control is particularly difficult, e.g. because of recurrent hypoglycaemia.

Transplantation of isolated pancreatic islets (usually into the liver via the portal vein) has been achieved safely in an increasing number of centres around the world. Progress is being made towards meeting the needs of supply, purification and storage of islets, but the problems of transplant rejection, and of destruction by the patient's autoantibodies against β cells, remain. Nevertheless, the development of methods of inducing tolerance to transplanted islets and the potential use of stem cells (p. 69) means that this may still prove the most promising approach in the long term.

COMPLICATIONS OF DIABETES

Despite all the treatments now available, the outcome for patients with diabetes remains disappointing. Long-term complications of diabetes still cause significant morbidity and mortality (Boxes 21.31 and 21.32).

Excess mortality in diabetes is caused mainly by large blood vessel disease, particularly myocardial infarction and stroke. Macrovascular disease also causes substantial morbidity from myocardial infarction, stroke, angina, cardiac failure and intermittent claudication. The pathological changes of atherosclerosis in diabetic patients are similar to those in the non-diabetic population but occur earlier in life and are more extensive and severe. Diabetes amplifies the effects of the other major cardiovascular risk factors: smoking, hypertension and dyslipidaemia (Fig. 21.11). Moreover, patients with type 2 diabetes are more likely to have additional cardiovascular risk factors, which co-segregate with insulin resistance in the metabolic syndrome (p. 805).

Disease of small blood vessels is a specific complication of diabetes and is termed diabetic microangiopathy. It contributes to mortality through renal failure caused

21.31 Complications of diabetes

Microvascular/neuropathic

Retinopathy, cataract
- Impaired vision

Nephropathy
- Renal failure

Peripheral neuropathy
- Sensory loss
- Pain
- Motor weakness

Autonomic neuropathy
- Gastrointestinal problems (gastroparesis; altered bowel habit)
- Postural hypotension

Foot disease
- Ulceration
- Arthropathy

Macrovascular

Coronary circulation
- Myocardial ischaemia/infarction

Cerebral circulation
- Transient ischaemic attack
- Stroke

Peripheral circulation
- Claudication
- Ischaemia

21.32 Mortality in diabetes

Risk versus non-diabetic controls (mortality ratio)	
• Overall	2.6
• Coronary heart disease Cerebrovascular disease Peripheral vascular disease	2.8
• All other causes, including renal failure	2.7
Causes of death in diabetes (approximate proportion)	
• Cardiovascular disease	70%
• Renal failure	10%
• Cancer	10%
• Infections	6%
• Diabetic ketoacidosis	1%
• Other	3%

Risk factors for increased morbidity and mortality in diabetes
- Duration of diabetes
- Early age at onset of disease
- High glycated haemoglobin (HbA_{1c})
- Raised blood pressure
- Proteinuria; microalbuminuria
- Dyslipidaemia
- Obesity

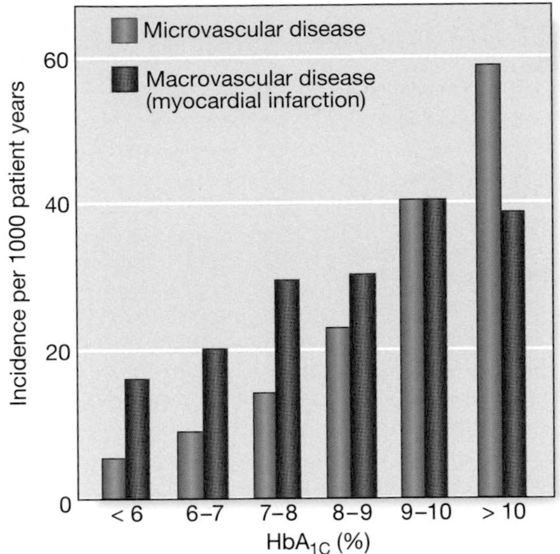

Fig. 21.11 Association between HbA_{1c} and risk of microvascular and macrovascular diabetes complications. These data were obtained amongst participants in the UK Prospective Diabetes Study and were adjusted for effects of age, sex and ethnicity; the incidences show what could be expected amongst white men aged 50–54 years at diagnosis of type 2 diabetes, followed up for 10 years. Microvascular disease included retinopathy requiring photocoagulation, vitreous haemorrhage and renal failure. Macrovascular disease included fatal and non-fatal myocardial infarction and sudden death. A 1% change in HbA_{1c} is equivalent to a reduction of 11 mmol/mol.

by diabetic nephropathy, and is responsible for substantial morbidity and disability: for example, blindness from diabetic retinopathy, difficulty in walking, chronic ulceration of the feet from peripheral neuropathy, and bowel and bladder dysfunction from autonomic neuropathy. The risk of microvascular disease is positively correlated with the duration and degree of sustained hyperglycaemia, however caused and at whatever age it develops.

Pathophysiology

The histopathological hallmark of diabetic microangiopathy is thickening of the capillary basement membrane, with associated increased vascular permeability, which occurs throughout the body. The development of the characteristic clinical syndromes of diabetic retinopathy, nephropathy, neuropathy and accelerated atherosclerosis is thought to result from the local response to generalised vascular injury. For example, in the wall of large vessels, increased permeability of arterial endothelium, particularly when combined with hyperinsulinaemia and hypertension, may increase the deposition of atherogenic lipoproteins. The mechanisms linking hyperglycaemia to these pathological changes are, however, poorly characterised.

Preventing diabetes complications

Glycaemic control

The evidence that improved glycaemic control decreases the risk of developing microvascular complications of diabetes was established by the Diabetes Control and Complications Trial (DCCT) in type 1 diabetes, and the UK Prospective Diabetes Study (UKPDS) in type 2 diabetes. The DCCT was a large study that lasted 9 years.

EBM 21.33 Glycaemic control in type 1 diabetes

'In patients with type 1 diabetes, strict glycaemic control (mean HbA_{1c} 53 mmol/mol (7%)) reduced the development of retinopathy and other microvascular complications by 76% compared with conventional therapy (mean HbA_{1c} 75 mmol/mol (9%)). On longer-term follow-up, strict glycaemic control also reduced cardiovascular events, including myocardial infarction, stroke and death from cardiovascular disease.'

- Diabetes Control and Complications Trial Research Group. N Engl J Med 1993; 329:977–986.
- Diabetes Control and Complications Trial/Epidemiology of Diabetes Interventions and Complications (DCCT/EDIC) Study Research Group. N Engl J Med 2005; 353:2643–2653.

For further information: www.diabetes.niddk.nih.gov/dm/pubs/control/

EBM 21.34 Glycaemic control in type 2 diabetes

'In patients with type 2 diabetes, intensive glycaemic control (mean HbA_{1c} 53 mmol/mol (7%)) with oral anti-diabetic drugs or insulin reduced the development of microvascular complications, particularly retinopathy, by 25% compared with conventional treatment (mean HbA_{1c} 64 mmol/mol (8%)). On longer-term follow-up, there was a significant reduction in myocardial infarction and all-cause mortality in intensively controlled patients.'

- UKPDS Group. Lancet 1998; 352:837–853, 854–865.
- Holman RR, et al. N Engl J Med 2008; 359:1577–1589.

For further information:  www.dtu.ox.ac.uk

There was a 60% overall reduction in the risk of developing diabetic complications in patients with type 1 diabetes on intensive therapy with strict glycaemic control, compared with those on conventional therapy (Box 21.33). No single factor other than glycaemic control had a significant effect on outcome. However, the group who were intensively treated to lower blood glucose had three times the rate of severe hypoglycaemia. The UKPDS showed that, in type 2 diabetes, the frequency of diabetic complications is lower and progression is slower with good glycaemic control and effective treatment of hypertension, irrespective of the type of therapy used (Box 21.34). Extrapolation from the UKPDS suggests that, for every 11 mmol/mol (1%) reduction in HbA_{1c}, there is a 21% reduction in death related to diabetes, a 14% reduction in myocardial infarction and 30–40% reduction in risk of microvascular complications (see Fig. 21.11).

These landmark trials demonstrated that diabetic complications are preventable and that the aim of treatment should be 'near-normal' glycaemia. However, more recent studies, such as the Action to Control Cardiovascular Risk in Diabetes (ACCORD), showed increased mortality in a subgroup of patients who were aggressively treated to lower HbA_{1c} to a target of less than 48 mmol/mol (6.5%). The patients in this study had poor glycaemic control at baseline, a long duration of diabetes and a high prevalence of cardiovascular disease. It appears that, whilst a low target HbA_{1c} is appropriate in younger patients with earlier diabetes who do not

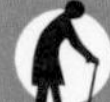

21.35 Diabetes management in old age

- **Glycaemic control**: the optimal target for glycaemic control in older people has yet to be determined. Strict glycaemic control should be avoided in frail patients with comorbidities and in older patients with long duration of diabetes.
- **Cognitive function and affect**: may benefit from improving glycaemic control.
- **Hypoglycaemia**: older people have reduced symptomatic awareness of hypoglycaemia and limited knowledge of symptoms, and are at greater risk of, and from, hypoglycaemia.
- **Mortality**: the mortality rate of older people with diabetes is more than double that of age-matched non-diabetic people, largely because of increased deaths from cardiovascular disease.

have underlying cardiovascular disease, aggressive glucose-lowering is not beneficial in older patients with long duration of diabetes and multiple comorbidities (Box 21.35).

Control of other risk factors

Randomised controlled trials have shown that aggressive management of blood pressure minimises the microvascular and macrovascular complications of diabetes. Angiotensin-converting enzyme (ACE) inhibitors are valuable in improving outcome in heart disease and in treating diabetic nephropathy (p. 830). The management of dyslipidaemia with a statin limits macrovascular disease in people with diabetes (p. 456). This often results in the necessary use of multiple medications, which exacerbates the problem of adherence to therapy by patients; it is not unusual for a patient to be taking two or more diabetes therapies, two or more blood pressure drugs and a statin.

Diabetic retinopathy

Diabetic retinopathy (DR) is one of the most common causes of blindness in adults between 30 and 65 years of age in developed countries. The prevalence of DR increases with duration of diabetes, and almost all individuals with type 1 diabetes and the majority of those with type 2 diabetes will have some degree of DR after 20 years.

Pathogenesis

Hyperglycaemia increases retinal blood flow and disrupts intracellular metabolism in retinal endothelial cells and pericytes (pericytes wrap around the outside of the capillary wall and influence blood flow and capillary permeability). This leads to impaired vascular autoregulation, increased production of vasoactive substances and endothelial cell proliferation. The resulting capillary hypoperfusion and closure cause chronic retinal ischaemia, stimulating the production of growth factors, including vascular endothelial growth factor (VEGF), which further stimulates deleterious endothelial cell growth (causing new vessel formation) and increased vascular permeability (causing retinal leakage and exudation).

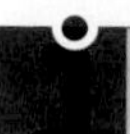

21.36 Risk factors for diabetic retinopathy

- Long duration of diabetes
- Poor glycaemic control
- Hypertension
- Hyperlipidaemia
- Pregnancy
- Nephropathy/renal disease
- Others: obesity, smoking

Clinical features

The major risk factors for DR are shown in Box 21.36. DR is a progressive condition, often classified into two stages: non-proliferative ('background') and proliferative. The earliest signs of non-proliferative DR are microaneurysms and retinal haemorrhages, sometimes inaccurately called 'dot' and 'blot' haemorrhages, respectively (Fig. 21.12A and B). As DR progresses and there is continuing capillary hypoperfusion, cotton wool spots, venous beading and intra-retinal microvascular abnormalities can be seen (Fig. 21.12C–E); this stage is referred to as pre-proliferative DR. The disease may then progress to proliferative DR, which is characterised by growth of new blood vessels on the retina or optic disc (Fig. 21.12F and G). The new vessels are abnormal and often bleed, leading to vitreous haemorrhage, subsequent fibrosis and scarring, and finally tractional retinal detachment.

In addition to proliferative and non-proliferative DR, patients may also develop clinically significant macular oedema (CSMO; see Fig. 21.12C). This can occur at any stage of DR and is characterised by increased vascular permeability and deposition of hard exudates in the central retina. CSMO is the most common cause of loss of vision in people with diabetes.

Proliferative retinopathy and severe ocular ischaemia may stimulate new vessels to grow on the anterior surface of the iris: 'rubeosis iridis'. These vessels may obstruct the drainage angle of the eye and the outflow of aqueous fluid, causing secondary glaucoma.

Loss of visual acuity

Microaneurysms, abnormalities of the veins, and small haemorrhages and exudates situated in the periphery will not interfere with vision. However, if these changes are observed near the macula, and in particular if they are accompanied by loss of visual acuity, CSMO should be suspected. Macular oedema can cause impairment of visual acuity even if this is associated with only mild peripheral non-proliferative retinopathy and no other obvious pathology. Macular oedema can only be confirmed or excluded on slit lamp retinal biomicroscopy.

Sudden visual loss occurs with vitreous haemorrhage or retinal detachment. In pre-proliferative and proliferative retinopathy, whether or not visual acuity is impaired, prompt laser treatment is important to reduce the risk of haemorrhage, fibrosis/gliosis and severe irreversible visual impairment.

Prevention

Glycaemic, blood pressure and lipid profile control

Many epidemiological studies have shown a clear relationship between glycaemic control and the incidence of DR. Large randomised controlled trials have shown convincingly that improved glycaemic control, particularly

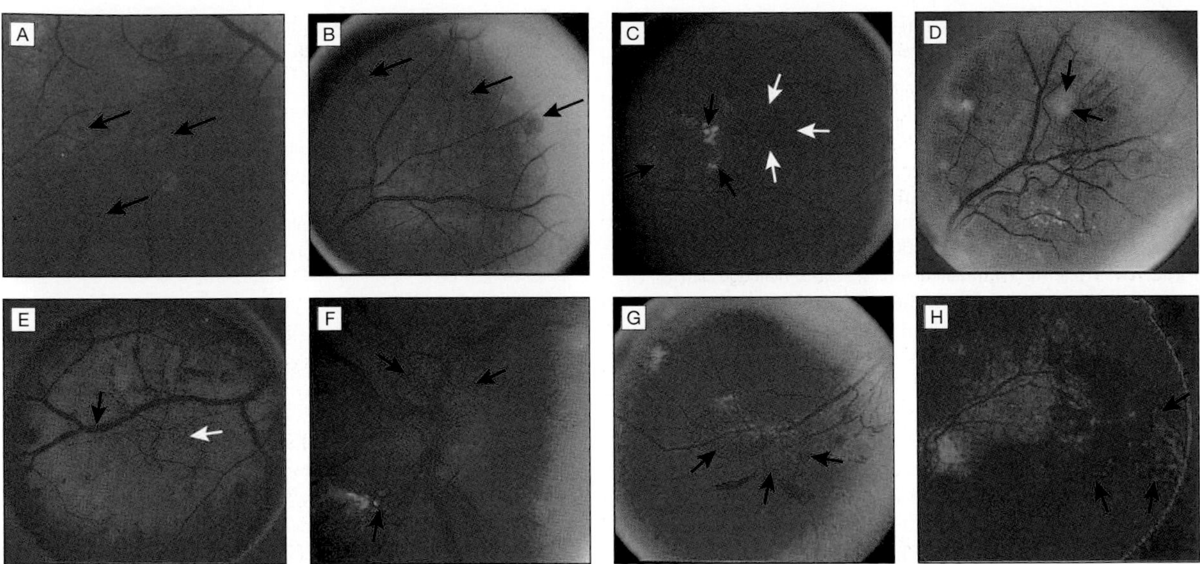

Fig. 21.12 Diabetic retinopathy. **A** *Microaneurysms.* Usually the earliest clinical abnormality, these tiny aneurysms arise mainly from the venous end of capillaries and appear as discrete, circular, dark red dots near to, but apparently separate from, the retinal vessels and no wider than a vessel at the optic disc margin (arrows). **B** *Haemorrhages.* Larger than a microaneurysm, with indistinct margins and at least as wide as a vessel at the optic disc margin, these occur in deeper layers of the retina (arrows). They result either from microaneurysms that have burst or from leaky capillaries. Superficial flame-shaped haemorrhages in the nerve fibre layer may also occur, particularly if the patient is hypertensive. **C** *Hard exudates.* These irregularly shaped lesions are formed from leaking of cholesterol, often through microaneurysms (black arrows). They can be associated with retinal oedema; if this affects the centre of the macula, it can cause clinically significant macular oedema (CSMO, white arrows), which is sight-threatening. **D** *Cotton wool spots.* These white, feathery, fluffy lesions indicate capillary infarcts within the nerve fibre layer (arrows). They are most often seen in rapidly advancing retinopathy or in association with uncontrolled hypertension. **E** *Venous beading.* In extensive retinal ischaemia, walls of veins develop saccular bulges, looking like a string of sausages (black arrow). Intra-retinal microvascular anomalies (IRMA) are spidery vessels, often with sharp corners that indicate dilatations of pre-existing capillaries (white arrow). **F** and **G** *Neovascularisation.* New vessel formation in response to widespread retinal ischaemia may arise from the venous circulation either on the optic *disc* (NVD, arrows in F) or *elsewhere* in the retina (NVE, arrows in G). Initially, fine tufts of delicate vessels form arcades on the surface of the retina; later, they may extend forwards on to the posterior surface of the vitreous. Leaking of serous products from new vessels stimulates a connective tissue reaction, with gliosis and fibrosis, that first appears as a white, cloudy haze among the network of new vessels and later extends to obliterate the area with a dense white sheet. **H** *Vitreous haemorrhage.* New vessels are fragile and liable to rupture during vitreous movement, causing a pre-retinal ('subhyaloid') or a vitreous haemorrhage (arrows), which may lead to sudden visual loss.

in the early stages of disease, reduces both the incidence and progression of DR in type 1 (see Box 21.33) and type 2 (see Box 21.34) diabetes. When blood glucose is lowered, there can be a transient deterioration of retinopathy. This relates to loss of hyperglycaemia-induced hyperperfusion in the retinal circulation and a consequent increase in ischaemia. However, this effect wears off within 18 months. Improvement in glycaemic control should therefore be effected gradually in patients with retinopathy, particularly when glycaemic control is initially poor.

Evidence from randomised controlled trials suggests that blood pressure control is also warranted to reduce the incidence and progression of DR. Early trials suggested specific benefit from angiotensin II receptor antagonists, but later studies indicate that other antihypertensive agents are similarly effective. Most guidelines recommend achieving a blood pressure of less than 130/80 mmHg. Observational studies suggest that hyperlipidaemia is a risk factor for DR, but intervention trials have not been conclusive.

Screening

Annual screening for retinopathy is essential in all diabetic patients, as the disease is asymptomatic in the early stages, when treatment is most effective. Screening is particularly important in those with risk factors. It should be undertaken by trained personnel in an organised and audited programme. The preferred method is a digital photographic system for retinal imaging, with prompt referral of patients with sight-threatening retinopathy to an ophthalmologist for examination with slit lamp biomicroscopy. If direct ophthalmoscopy is used, the pupils should be dilated for adequate examination. Unfortunately, many people with diabetes receive no regular supervision and do not attend for eye screening.

Management

Good glycaemic (HbA_{1c} around 53 mmol/mol (7%)) control and an appropriate blood pressure (< 130/80 mmHg) should be maintained to prevent onset and delay progression of diabetic eye disease. Novel agents are emerging, including ranibizumab, a monoclonal antibody fragment that binds to VEGF-A and is anti-angiogenic; it is used for diabetic macular oedema.

Retinal photocoagulation (laser treatment) is indicated in: severe proliferative or very severe non-proliferative retinopathy; new vessels elsewhere with vitreous haemorrhage; new vessels without vitreous haemorrhage in type 2 diabetes; or CSMO. Photocoagulation is used:

- to treat leaking microaneurysms and areas of retinal thickening in the macular area, and to reduce macular oedema (focal laser)

- to destroy areas of retinal ischaemia and hence lower intraocular levels of VEGF, which play a major role in the development of neovascularisation
- to reduce the risk of recurrent haemorrhage by inducing gliosis and fibrosis of new vessels (pan-retinal photocoagulation (PRP)).

Argon laser photocoagulation is the usual method. This simple procedure can be carried out under topical anaesthesia. Patients should be reviewed regularly to look for further development of new vessels and/or maculopathy. Extensive bilateral photocoagulation can cause significant visual field loss, which may interfere with driving ability and reduce night vision.

Vitrectomy is used in selected cases of advanced diabetic eye disease due to type 1 diabetes where visual loss has been caused by recurrent vitreous haemorrhage that has failed to clear or by tractional retinal detachment threatening the macula. The value of vitrectomy in type 2 diabetes is less certain. Rubeosis iridis is a severe complication requiring early and extensive PRP.

Other causes of visual loss in people with diabetes

Around 50% of visual loss in people with type 2 diabetes results from causes other than diabetic retinopathy. These include cataract, age-related macular degeneration, retinal vein occlusion, retinal arterial occlusion, non-arteritic ischaemic optic neuropathy and glaucoma. Some of these conditions are to be expected in this group, as they relate to cardiovascular risk factors (e.g. hypertension, hyperlipidaemia and smoking), all of which are prevalent in people with type 2 diabetes.

Cataract

Cataract is a permanent lens opacity and is a common cause of visual deterioration in the elderly. The lens thickens and opacifies with age; with diabetes, the increased metabolic insult to the lens causes these changes to accelerate and occur prematurely. A rare type of 'snow-flake' cataract occurs in young patients with poorly controlled diabetes. This does not usually affect vision but tends to make fundal examination difficult.

The indications for cataract extraction are similar to those for the non-diabetic population and depend on the degree of visual impairment. An additional indication in diabetes is when adequate assessment of the fundus, or laser treatment to the retina, is prevented.

Diabetic nephropathy

Diabetic nephropathy is an important cause of morbidity and mortality, and is now among the most common causes of end-stage renal failure in developed countries. About 30% of patients with type 1 diabetes have developed diabetic nephropathy 20 years after diagnosis, but the risk after this time falls to less than 1% per year, and from the outset the risk is not equal in all patients (Box 21.37). Indeed, some patients do not develop nephropathy, despite having long-standing, poorly controlled diabetes, suggesting that they are genetically protected from it. Whilst variants in a few genes have been implicated in diabetic nephropathy, the major differences in individual risk remain unexplained. Epidemiological data have indicated that the overall incidence is declining as standards of glycaemic and blood pressure control have improved.

The pattern of progression of renal abnormalities in diabetes is shown schematically in Figure 21.13. Pathologically, the first changes coincide with the onset of microalbuminuria and include thickening of the glomerular basement membrane and accumulation of matrix material in the mesangium. Subsequently, nodular deposits (Fig. 21.14) are characteristic, and glomerulosclerosis worsens as heavy proteinuria develops, until

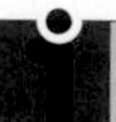

21.37 Risk factors for diabetic nephropathy

- Poor glycaemic control
- Long duration of diabetes
- Presence of other microvascular complications
- Ethnicity (e.g. Asians, Pima Indians)
- Pre-existing hypertension
- Family history of diabetic nephropathy
- Family history of hypertension

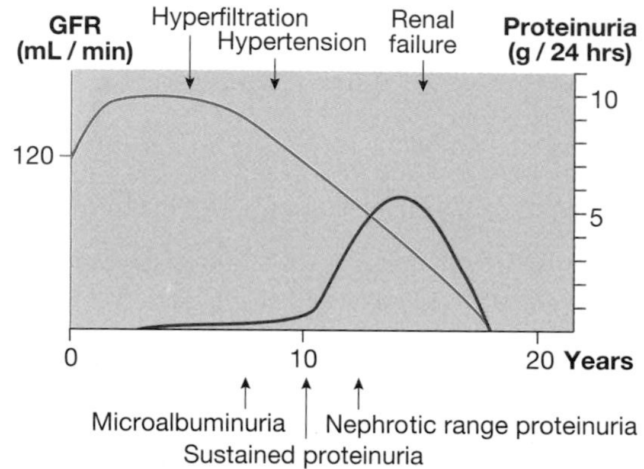

Fig. 21.13 Natural history of diabetic nephropathy. In the first few years of type 1 diabetes mellitus, there is hyperfiltration, which declines fairly steadily to return to a normal value at approximately 10 years (blue line). In susceptible patients (about 30%), after about 10 years, there is sustained proteinuria, and by approximately 14 years it has reached the nephrotic range (red line). Renal function continues to decline, with the end stage being reached at approximately 16 years.

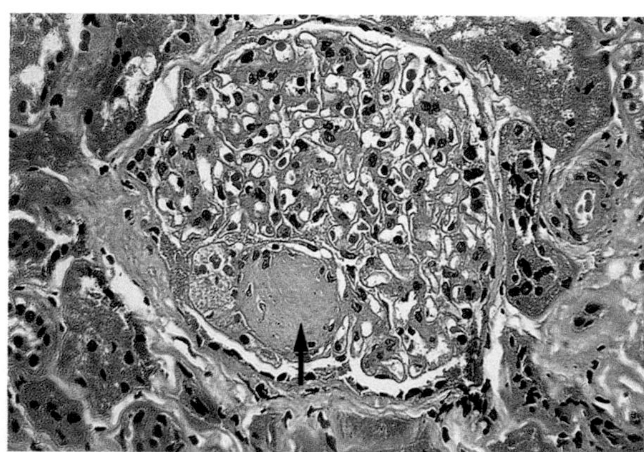

Fig. 21.14 Nodular diabetic glomerulosclerosis. There is thickening of basement membranes and mesangial expansion, and a Kimmelstiel–Wilson nodule (arrow), which is pathognomonic of diabetic kidney disease.

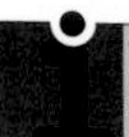

21.38 Screening for microalbuminuria

- Identifies incipient nephropathy in type 1 and type 2 diabetes; is an independent predictor of macrovascular disease in type 2 diabetes
- Risk factors include high blood pressure, poor glycaemic control, smoking
- Who to screen:
  Patients with type 1 diabetes annually from 5 yrs after diagnosis
  Patients with type 2 diabetes annually from time of diagnosis
- Early morning urine measured for albumin : creatinine ratio (ACR). Microalbuminuria present if:
  Males ACR 2.5–30 mg/mmol creatinine
  Females ACR 3.5–30 mg/mmol creatinine
- An elevated ACR should be followed by a repeat test:
  Established microalbuminuria if 2 out of 3 tests positive
  An ACR > 30 mg/mmol creatinine is consistent with overt nephropathy

glomeruli are progressively lost and renal function deteriorates.

Diagnosis and screening

Microalbuminuria (Box 21.38) is the presence in the urine of small amounts of albumin, at a concentration below that detectable using a standard urine dipstick. Overt nephropathy is defined as the presence of macroalbuminuria (albumin to creatinine ratio (ACR) > 300 mg/mmol; detectable on urine dipstick). Microalbuminuria is a good predictor of progression to nephropathy in type 1 diabetes. It is a less reliable predictor of nephropathy in older patients with type 2 diabetes, in whom it may be accounted for by other diseases (p. 476), although it is a potentially useful marker of an increased risk of macrovascular disease.

Management

The presence of established microalbuminuria or overt nephropathy should prompt vigorous efforts to reduce the risk of progression of nephropathy and of cardiovascular disease by:

- aggressive reduction of blood pressure
- aggressive cardiovascular risk factor reduction (Box 21.39).

In type 1 diabetes, ACE inhibitors have been shown to provide greater protection than equal blood pressure reduction achieved with other drugs (p. 611), and subsequent studies have shown similar benefits from angiotensin II receptor blockers (ARBs) in patients with type 2 diabetes. This benefit from blockade of the renin-angiotensin system arises from a reduction in the angiotensin II-mediated vasoconstriction of efferent arterioles in glomeruli (see Fig 17.1D, p. 465). The resulting dilatation of these vessels decreases glomeruli filtration pressure and therefore the hyperfiltration and protein leak. Both ACE inhibitors and ARBs increase risk of hyperkalaemia (p. 442) and, in the presence of renal artery stenosis (p. 494), may induce marked deterioration in renal function. Therefore, electrolytes and renal function should be checked after initiation or each dose increase. Non-dihydropyridine calcium antagonists (diltiazem, verapamil) may be suitable alternatives.

EBM 21.39 Multiple risk factor intervention in type 2 diabetes

'In type 2 patients with microalbuminuria, intensive treatment (including control of glycaemia and hypertension, with use of ACE inhibitors, statins and aspirin) reduced the risk of cardiovascular disease by 53%, of nephropathy by 61%, and of retinopathy by 58% compared with conventional treatment. On longer-term follow-up, there was a reduction in total mortality and death from cardiovascular causes.'

- Gaede P, et al. N Engl J Med 2003; 348:383–393.
- Gaede P, et al. N Engl J Med 2008; 358:580–591.

Halving the amount of albuminuria with an ACE or ARB results in a nearly 50% reduction in long-term risk of progression to end-stage renal disease. However, some patients do progress, with worsening renal function. Renal replacement therapy (p. 488) may benefit diabetic patients at an earlier stage than other patients with end-stage renal failure.

Renal transplantation dramatically improves the life of many, and any recurrence of diabetic nephropathy in the allograft is usually too slow to be a serious problem, but associated macrovascular and microvascular disease elsewhere may still progress. Pancreatic transplantation (generally carried out at the same time as renal transplantation) can produce insulin independence and delay or reverse microvascular disease, but the supply of organs is limited and this option is available to few. For further information on management, see Chapter 17.

Diabetic neuropathy

Although there is some evidence that the central nervous system is affected in long-term diabetes, the clinical impact of diabetes is mainly manifest in the peripheral nervous system. Diabetic neuropathy causes substantial morbidity and increases mortality. It is diagnosed on the basis of symptoms and signs, and after the exclusion of other causes of neuropathy (p. 1223). Depending on the criteria used for diagnosis, it affects between 50 and 90% of patients with diabetes, and of these, 15–30% will have painful diabetic neuropathy (PDN). Like retinopathy, neuropathy occurs secondary to metabolic disturbance, and prevalence is related to the duration of diabetes and the degree of metabolic control.

Pathological features can occur in any peripheral nerves. They include axonal degeneration of both myelinated and unmyelinated fibres, with thickening of the Schwann cell basal lamina, patchy segmental demyelination, and abnormal intraneural capillaries (with basement membrane thickening and microthrombi).

Various classifications of diabetic neuropathy have been proposed. One is shown in Box 21.40, but motor, sensory and autonomic nerves may be involved in varying combinations so that clinically mixed syndromes usually occur.

Clinical features

Symmetrical sensory polyneuropathy

This is frequently asymptomatic. The most common clinical signs are diminished perception of vibration

21.40 Classification of diabetic neuropathy

Somatic

- Polyneuropathy
  Symmetrical, mainly sensory and distal
  Asymmetrical, mainly motor and proximal (including amyotrophy)
- Mononeuropathy (including mononeuritis multiplex)

Visceral (autonomic)

- Cardiovascular
- Gastrointestinal
- Genitourinary
- Sudomotor
- Vasomotor
- Pupillary

sensation distally, 'glove and stocking' impairment of all other modalities of sensation (see Fig. 21.15), and loss of tendon reflexes in the lower limbs. In symptomatic patients, sensory abnormalities are predominant. Symptoms include paraesthesiae in the feet (and, rarely, in the hands), pain in the lower limbs (dull, aching and/or lancinating, worse at night, and mainly felt on the anterior aspect of the legs), burning sensations in the soles of the feet, cutaneous hyperaesthesia and an abnormal gait (commonly wide-based), often associated with a sense of numbness in the feet. Weakness and atrophy, in particular of the interosseous muscles, may develop, leading to structural changes in the foot with loss of lateral and transverse arches, clawing of the toes and exposure of the metatarsal heads. This results in increased pressure on the plantar aspects of the metatarsal heads, with the development of callus skin at these and other pressure points. Electrophysiological tests (p. 1151) demonstrate slowing of both motor and sensory conduction, and tests of vibration sensitivity and thermal thresholds are abnormal.

A diffuse small-fibre neuropathy causes altered perception of pain and temperature, and is associated with symptomatic autonomic neuropathy; characteristic features include foot ulcers and Charcot neuroarthropathy.

Asymmetrical motor diabetic neuropathy

Sometimes called diabetic amyotrophy, this presents as severe and progressive weakness and wasting of the proximal muscles of the lower (and occasionally the upper) limbs. It is commonly accompanied by severe pain, mainly felt on the anterior aspect of the leg, and hyperaesthesia and paraesthesiae. Sometimes there may also be marked loss of weight ('neuropathic cachexia'). The patient may look extremely ill and be unable to get out of bed. Tendon reflexes may be absent on the affected side(s). Sometimes there are extensor plantar responses and the cerebrospinal fluid protein is often raised. This condition is thought to involve acute infarction of the lower motor neurons of the lumbosacral plexus. Other lesions involving this plexus, such as neoplasms and lumbar disc disease, must be excluded. Although recovery usually occurs within 12 months, some deficits are permanent. Management is mainly supportive.

Mononeuropathy

Either motor or sensory function can be affected within a single peripheral or cranial nerve. Unlike the gradual progression of distal symmetrical and autonomic neuropathies, mononeuropathies are severe and of rapid onset, but they eventually recover. The nerves most commonly affected are the 3rd and 6th cranial nerves (resulting in diplopia), and the femoral and sciatic nerves. Rarely, involvement of other single nerves results in paresis and paraesthesiae in the thorax and trunk (truncal radiculopathies).

Nerve compression palsies are more common in diabetes, frequently affecting the median nerve, giving the clinical picture of carpal tunnel syndrome, and less commonly the ulnar nerve. Lateral popliteal nerve compression occasionally causes foot drop. Compression palsies may be more common because of glycosylation and thickening of connective tissue and/or because of increased susceptibility of nerves affected by diabetic microangiopathy.

Autonomic neuropathy

This is not necessarily associated with peripheral somatic neuropathy. Parasympathetic or sympathetic nerves may be predominantly affected in one or more visceral systems. The resulting symptoms and signs are listed in Box 21.41 and tests of autonomic function in Box 21.42. The development of autonomic neuropathy is less clearly related to poor metabolic control than somatic neuropathy, and improved control rarely results in improved symptoms. Within 10 years of developing overt symptoms of autonomic neuropathy, 30–50% of patients are dead, many from sudden cardiorespiratory arrest. Patients with postural hypotension (a drop in systolic pressure of 30 mmHg or more on standing from the supine position) have the highest subsequent mortality.

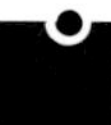

21.41 Clinical features of autonomic neuropathy

Cardiovascular

- Postural hypotension
- Resting tachycardia
- Fixed heart rate

Gastrointestinal

- Dysphagia, due to oesophageal atony
- Abdominal fullness, nausea and vomiting, unstable glycaemia, due to delayed gastric emptying ('gastroparesis')
- Nocturnal diarrhoea ± faecal incontinence
- Constipation, due to colonic atony

Genitourinary

- Difficulty in micturition, urinary incontinence, recurrent infection, due to atonic bladder
- Erectile dysfunction and retrograde ejaculation

Sudomotor

- Nocturnal sweats without hypoglycaemia
- Gustatory sweating
- Anhidrosis; fissures in the feet

Vasomotor

- Feet feel cold, due to loss of skin vasomotor responses
- Dependent oedema, due to loss of vasomotor tone and increased vascular permeability
- Bullous formation

Pupillary

- Decreased pupil size
- Resistance to mydriatics
- Delayed or absent reflexes to light

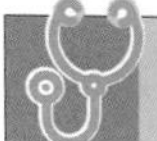

21.42 How to test cardiovascular autonomic function

Simple reflex tests

	Normal	Borderline	Abnormal
Heart rate responses			
To Valsalva manœuvre (15 secs)[1]: ratio of longest to shortest R–R interval	≥ 1.21		≤ 1.20
To deep breathing (6 breaths over 1 min): maximum–minimum heart rate	≥ 15	11–14	≤ 10
To standing after lying: ratio of R–R interval of 30th to 15th beats	≥ 1.04	1.01–1.03	≤ 1.00
Blood pressure response[2]			
To standing: systolic BP fall (mmHg)	≤ 10	11–29	≥ 30

Specialised tests

- Heart rate and blood pressure responses to sustained handgrip
- Heart rate variability using power spectral analysis of ECG monitoring
- Heart rate and blood pressure variability using time–domain analysis of ambulatory monitoring
- MIBG (met-iodobenzylguanidine) scan of the heart

[1]Omit in patients with previous laser therapy for proliferative retinopathy.
[2]Avoid arm with arteriovenous fistula in dialysed patients.

Erectile dysfunction

Erectile failure (impotence) affects 30% of diabetic males and is often multifactorial. Although neuropathy and vascular causes are common, psychological factors, including depression, anxiety and reduced libido, may be partly responsible. Alcohol and antihypertensive drugs, such as thiazide diuretics and β-adrenoceptor antagonists (β-blockers), may cause sexual dysfunction and patients have an endocrine cause such as testosterone deficiency or hyperprolactinaemia. For further information, see page 474.

Management

Management of neuropathies is outlined in Box 21.43.

21.43 Management options for peripheral sensorimotor and autonomic neuropathies

Pain and paraesthesiae from peripheral somatic neuropathies

- Intensive insulin therapy (strict glycaemic control)
- Anticonvulsants (gabapentin, pregabalin, carbamazepine, phenytoin)
- Tricyclic antidepressants (amitriptyline, imipramine)
- Other antidepressants (duloxetine)
- Substance P depleter (capsaicin – topical)
- Opiates (tramadol, oxycodone)
- Membrane stabilisers (mexiletine, IV lidocaine)
- Antioxidant (α-lipoic acid)

Postural hypotension

- Support stockings
- Fludrocortisone
- NSAIDs
- α-adrenoceptor agonist (midodrine)

Gastroparesis

- Dopamine antagonists (metoclopramide, domperidone)
- Erythromycin
- Gastric pacemaker; percutaneous enteral (jejunal) feeding (see Fig. 5.17, p. 123)

Diarrhoea (p. 857)

- Loperamide
- Broad-spectrum antibiotics
- Clonidine
- Octreotide

Constipation

- Stimulant laxatives (senna)

Atonic bladder

- Intermittent self-catheterisation (p. 1175)

Excessive sweating

- Anticholinergic drugs (propantheline, poldine, oxybutinin)
- Clonidine
- Topical antimuscarinic agent (glycopyrrolate cream)

Erectile dysfunction (p. 474)

- Phosphodiesterase type 5 inhibitors (sildenafil, vardenafil, tadalafil) – oral
- Dopamine agonist (apomorphine) – sublingual
- Prostaglandin E1 (alprostadil) – injected into corpus cavernosum or intra-urethral administration of pellets
- Vacuum tumescence devices
- Implanted penile prosthesis
- Psychological counselling; psychosexual therapy

(NSAIDs = non-steroidal anti-inflammatory drugs)

The diabetic foot

The foot is a frequent site of complications in patients with diabetes and for this reason foot care is particularly important. Tissue necrosis in the feet is a common reason for hospital admission in diabetic patients. Treatment of the foot complications of diabetes accounts for more inpatient days than any other diabetes-related complication.

Aetiology

Foot ulceration occurs as a result of trauma (often trivial) in the presence of neuropathy and/or peripheral vascular disease (see p. 600 and Fig. 21.15), with infection occurring as a secondary phenomenon following disruption of the protective epidermis. Most ulcers develop at the site of a plaque of callus skin, beneath which tissue necrosis occurs and eventually breaks through to the surface. In many cases, multiple components are involved, but sometimes neuropathy or ischaemia predominates, as illustrated in Box 21.44. Ischaemia alone accounts for a minority of foot ulcers in diabetic patients, with most being either neuropathic or neuro-ischaemic.

Charcot neuro-arthropathy is a progressive condition affecting the bones and joints of the foot; it is characterised by early inflammation and then joint dislocation, subluxation, and pathological fractures of the foot of

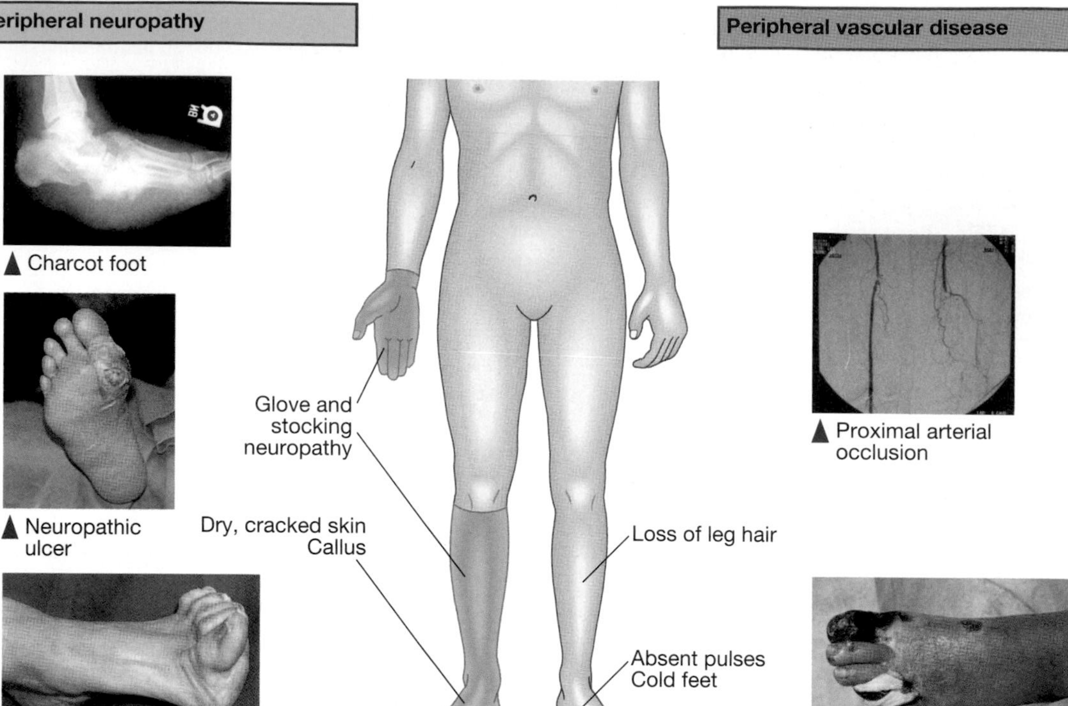

Fig. 21.15 Diabetic foot disease. Patients with diabetes can have neuropathy, peripheral vascular disease or both. Clawing of the toes is thought to be caused by intrinsic muscle atrophy and subsequent imbalance of muscle function, and causes increased pressure on the metatarsal heads and pressure on flexed toes, leading to increased callus and risk of ulceration. A Charcot foot occurs only in the presence of neuropathy, and results in bony destruction and ultimately deformity (this X-ray shows a resulting 'rocker bottom foot'). The angiogram shows disease of the superficial femoral arteries (occlusion of the left and stenosis of the right). *Insets* (*Proximal arterial occlusion*) From Medscape; (*Toe clawing*) Bowker and Pfeifer 2008; (*Neuropathic foot ulcer*) Levy and Valabhji 2008; (*Digital gangrene*) Swartz 2006 – see p. 836.

21.44 Clinical features of the diabetic foot

	Neuropathy	Ischaemia
Symptoms	None Paraesthesiae Pain Numbness	None Claudication Rest pain
Structural damage	Ulcer Sepsis Abscess Osteomyelitis Digital gangrene Charcot joint	Ulcer Sepsis Gangrene

neuropathic patients, often resulting in debilitating deformity (see Fig. 21.15 and p. 798). Charcot neuro-arthropathy can arise in any condition that causes neuropathy (including syphilis, spinal cord injury, syringomyelia and so on) but diabetes is the most common cause. The pathophysiological mechanisms remain poorly understood, but may involve unperceived trauma leading to progressive destruction (the 'neurotraumatic' theory), and/or increased blood flow resulting in a mismatch of bone destruction and synthesis (the 'neurovascular' theory). More recent evidence points to disordered inflammation mediated via the nuclear factor kappa B (NFκB)/receptor activator of NFκB ligand (RANKL) pathway, opening the way for trials of the RANKL inhibitor, denosumab (p. 1124).

Management

Management can be divided into primary prevention and treatment of an active problem. All patients should be educated in preventive measures (Box 21.45). The feet of patients with diabetes should be screened annually, following the steps listed on page 799. Two simple tests are required to grade a patient's risk: a 10 g monofilament should be used to assess sensation at five points on each foot, and foot pulses should be palpated (dorsalis pedis and/or posterior tibial). Combined with the clinical scenario, these tests guide appropriate referral and monitoring (Fig. 21.16). Removal of callus skin with a scalpel is usually best done by a podiatrist who has specialist training and experience in diabetic foot problems.

Foot ulcer

Once a foot ulcer develops, patients should ideally be referred to a multidisciplinary foot team, involving a diabetes specialist, a podiatrist, a vascular surgeon and an orthotist. Treatment involves: débridement of dead tissue; prompt, often prolonged, treatment with antibiotics if required, as infection can accelerate tissue necrosis and lead to gangrene; pressure relief using dressings; use of specialised bespoke orthotic footwear;

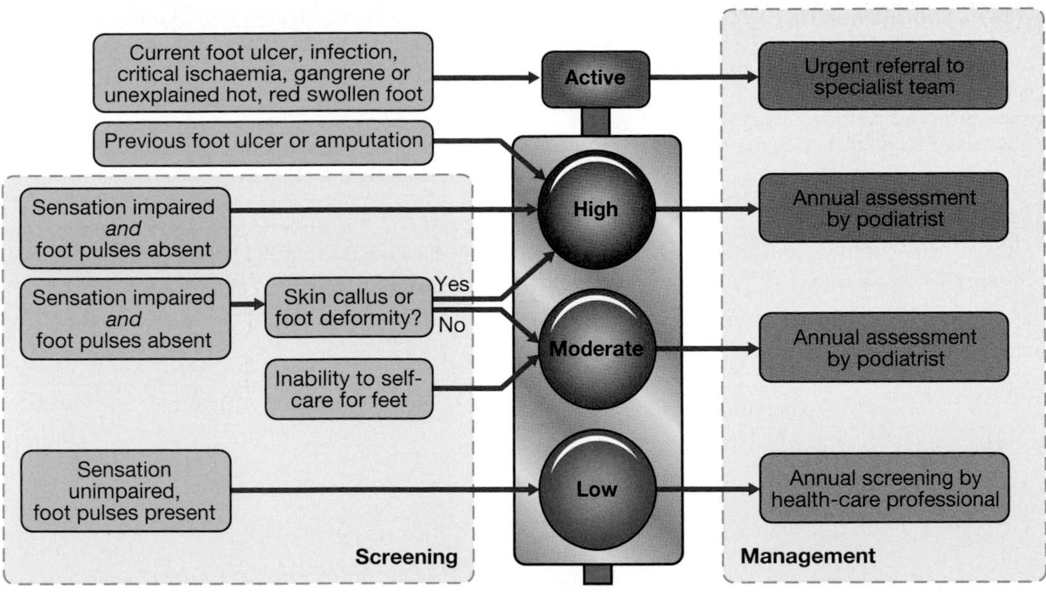

Fig. 21.16 Risk assessment and management of foot problems in diabetes. Adapted from SIGN 116 – see p. 836.

21.45 Care of the feet in patients with diabetes

- Preventive advice to all diabetic patients includes:
  - Inspect feet every day
  - Wash feet every day
  - Moisturise skin if dry
  - Cut or file toenails regularly
  - Change socks or stockings every day
  - Avoid walking barefoot
  - Check footwear for foreign bodies
  - Wear suitable, well-fitting shoes
  - Cover minor cuts with sterile dressings
  - Do not burst blisters
  - Avoid over-the-counter corn/callus remedies
- Advice to moderate- and high-risk patients is as above plus:
  - Do not attempt corn removal
  - Avoid high and low temperatures
- A podiatrist is an integral part of the diabetes team to ensure regular and effective podiatry and to educate patients in care of the feet
- Specially manufactured and fitted orthotic footwear is required to prevent recurrence of ulceration and to protect the feet of patients with Charcot neuroarthropathy

and sometimes total contact plaster cast or irremovable aircast boot. If an ulcer is neuro-ischaemic, a vascular assessment is often carried out, by ultrasound or angiography, as revascularisation by angioplasty or surgery may be required to allow the ulcer to heal. In cases of severe secondary infection or gangrene, an amputation may be required. This can be limited to the affected toe or involve more extensive limb amputation.

Charcot foot

Acute Charcot arthropathy almost always presents with signs of inflammation – a hot, red, swollen foot. Initial X-ray may show bony destruction but is often normal. As about 40% of patients with a Charcot joint also have a foot ulcer, it can be difficult to differentiate from osteomyelitis. Magnetic resonance imaging (MRI) of the foot is often helpful. The mainstay of treatment for an active Charcot foot is immobilisation and, ideally, avoidance of weight-bearing on the affected foot. The rationale is that if no pressure is applied through the foot, the destructive process involving the bones will not result in significant deformity when the acute inflammatory process subsides. Immobilisation is often achieved by a total contact plaster cast or 'aircast' boot. The acute phase often lasts 3–6 months and sometimes longer. In the post-acute phase, there is consolidation and remodelling of fracture fragments, eventually resulting in a stable foot.

Further information and acknowledgements

Websites

www.cdc.gov/diabetes/ *Diabetes Public Health Resource. Useful American site with resources for patients and health-care professionals.*

www.diabetes.org *American Diabetes Association. Includes information on research and advocacy issues.*

www.diabetes.org.uk *Diabetes UK. Includes information for patients and leaflets.*

www.idf.org *International Diabetes Federation. Useful information on international aspects of care and education.*

www.joslin.org *Joslin Diabetes Center. Well-written resource for patients and health-care professionals, and information on diabetes research.*

www.mydiabetesmyway.scot.nhs.uk/ *An interactive diabetes website for patients with diabetes and their carers.*

www.ndei.org *National Diabetes Education Initiative. Web-based education for health-care professionals, including case studies and slides.*

Figure acknowledgements

Page 798 inset (*Acanthosis nigricans*) Shotliff K. Diabetes and other metabolic diseases. In: Lim E (ed). Medicine and surgery: an integrated textbook. Elsevier; 2007, Fig. 7.11. Copyright © 2007 Edinburgh: Elsevier Ltd. All rights reserved.

Fig. 21.6B Adapted from Holman RR. Diabetes Res Clin Pract 1998; 40 (Suppl.):S21–S25.

Fig. 21.7 Adapted from UK Prospective Diabetes Study Group. UKPDS 33. Lancet 1998; 352: 837–853.

Figs 21.9 and 21.16 Adapted from Scottish Intercollegiate Guidelines Network (SIGN) guideline number 116.

Fig. 21.15 insets (*Proximal arterial occlusion*) http://emedicine.medscape.com/article/460178-overview#a0104; (*Toe clawing*) Bowker JH, Pfeifer MA. Levin and O'Neal's The diabetic foot, 7th edn. Philadelphia: Mosby; 2008; Fig. 26-9. Copyright © 2008 by Mosby, Inc., an affiliate of Elsevier; (*Neuropathic foot ulcer*) Levy MJ, Valabhji J. Vascular II: The diabetic foot. Surgery 2008; 26:25–28, Fig. 2; copyright © 2007 Elsevier Ltd; (*Digital gangrene*) Swartz MH. Textbook of physical diagnosis, 5th edn. Philadelphia: WB Saunders, 2006.

I.D. Penman
C.W. Lees

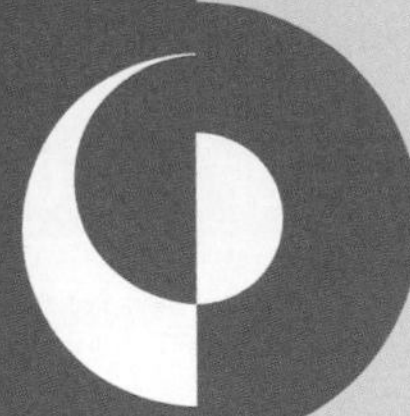

Alimentary tract and pancreatic disease 22

Clinical examination of the gastrointestinal tract 838

Functional anatomy and physiology 840
- Control of gastrointestinal function 844
- Gut hormones 845

Investigation of gastrointestinal disease 845

Presenting problems in gastrointestinal disease 851
- Dysphagia 851
- Dyspepsia 852
- Heartburn and regurgitation 852
- Vomiting 853
- Gastrointestinal bleeding 853
- Diarrhoea 857
- Malabsorption 857
- Weight loss 859
- Constipation 860
- Abdominal pain 861

Diseases of the mouth and salivary glands 863

Diseases of the oesophagus 865
- Gastro-oesophageal reflux disease 865
- Motility disorders 868
- Tumours of the oesophagus 870
- Perforation of the oesophagus 871

Diseases of the stomach and duodenum 871
- Gastritis 871
- Peptic ulcer disease 872
- Functional disorders 876
- Tumours of the stomach 877

Diseases of the small intestine 880
- Disorders causing malabsorption 880
- Motility disorders 886
- Miscellaneous disorders of the small intestine 886
- Adverse food reactions 887
- Infections of the small intestine 888
- Tumours of the small intestine 888

Diseases of the pancreas 889
- Acute pancreatitis 889
- Chronic pancreatitis 892
- Congenital abnormalities affecting the pancreas 894
- Tumours of the pancreas 895

Inflammatory bowel disease 897

Irritable bowel syndrome 907

AIDS and the gastrointestinal tract 909

Ischaemic gut injury 909

Disorders of the colon and rectum 910
- Tumours of the colon and rectum 910
- Diverticulosis 916
- Constipation and disorders of defecation 917
- Anorectal disorders 918
- Diseases of the peritoneal cavity 919
- Other disorders 919

CLINICAL EXAMINATION OF THE GASTROINTESTINAL TRACT

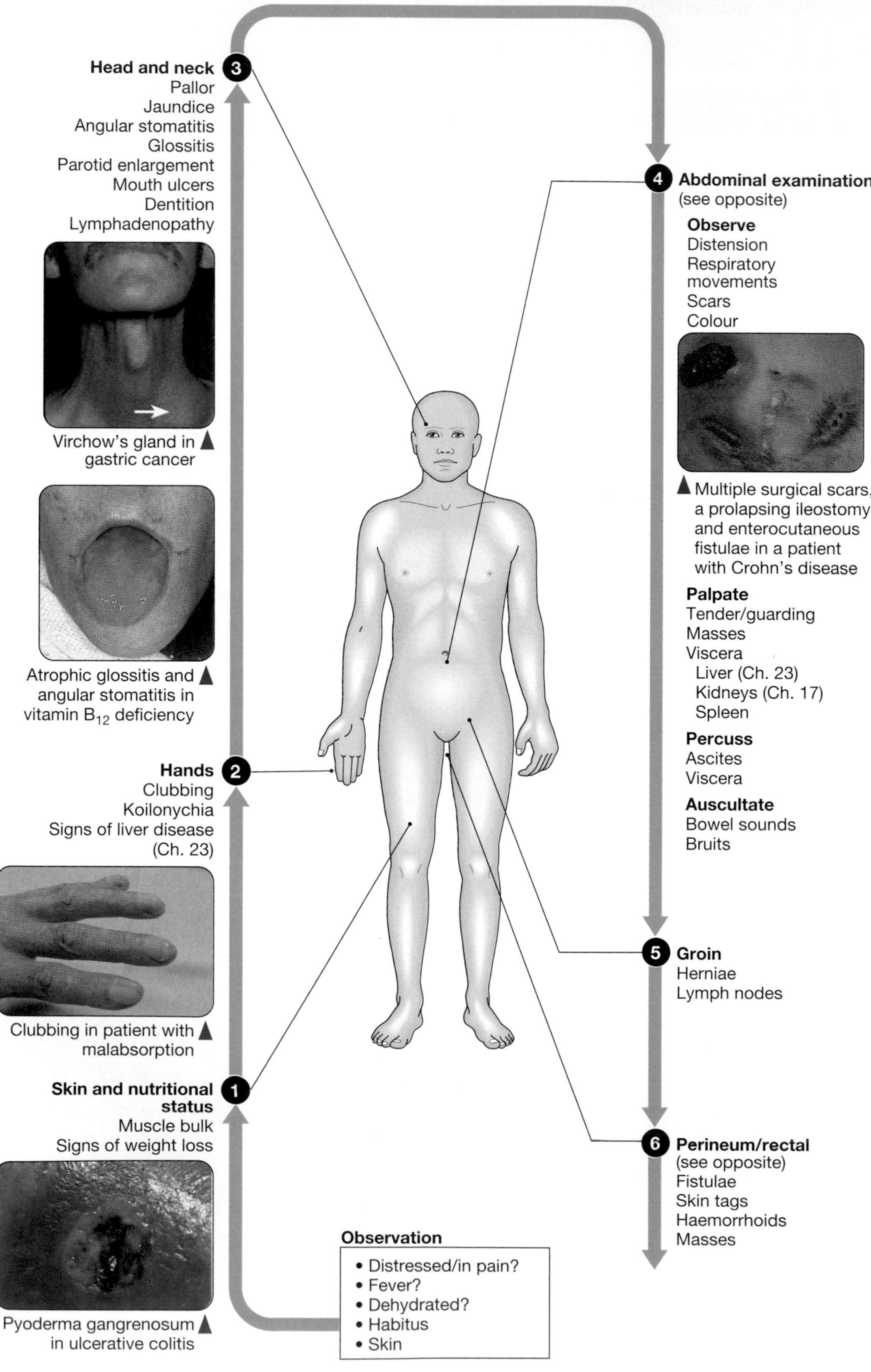

4 Abdominal examination: possible findings

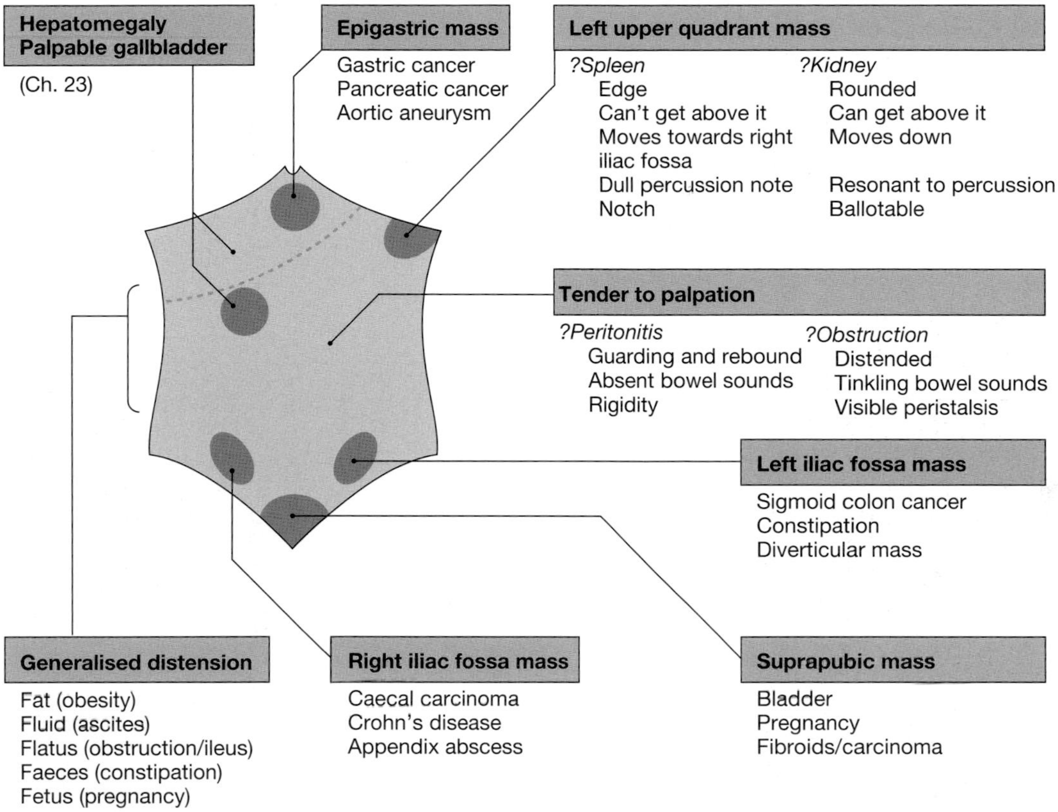

Hepatomegaly
Palpable gallbladder
(Ch. 23)
Epigastric mass
Gastric cancer
Pancreatic cancer
Aortic aneurysm
Left upper quadrant mass
?Spleen
Edge
Can't get above it
Moves towards right iliac fossa
Dull percussion note
Notch
?Kidney
Rounded
Can get above it
Moves down
Resonant to percussion
Ballotable
Tender to palpation
?Peritonitis
Guarding and rebound
Absent bowel sounds
Rigidity
?Obstruction
Distended
Tinkling bowel sounds
Visible peristalsis
Left iliac fossa mass
Sigmoid colon cancer
Constipation
Diverticular mass
Generalised distension
Fat (obesity)
Fluid (ascites)
Flatus (obstruction/ileus)
Faeces (constipation)
Fetus (pregnancy)
Right iliac fossa mass
Caecal carcinoma
Crohn's disease
Appendix abscess
Suprapubic mass
Bladder
Pregnancy
Fibroids/carcinoma

6 Rectal examination: common findings

Anal disease
Tags
Haemorrhoids
Polyps
Crohn's disease
Stool
Consistency
Colour
Steatorrhoea
Bloody/black
Faecal occult blood ⊕⊖
Tumour
Polyp
Cancer
Prolapse
Extrinsic
Tumour
Abscess
Prostate
Uterus/cervix

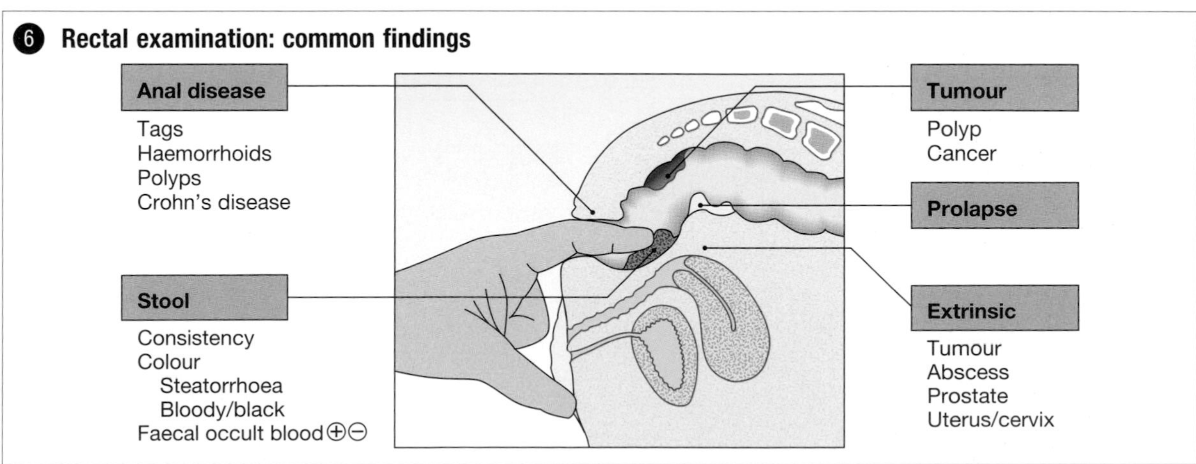

Diseases of the gastrointestinal tract are a major cause of morbidity and mortality. Approximately 10% of all general practitioner consultations in the United Kingdom are for indigestion, and 1 in 14 is for diarrhoea. Infective diarrhoea and malabsorption are responsible for much ill health and many deaths in the developing world. The gastrointestinal tract is the most common site for cancer development. Colorectal cancer is the second most common cancer in men, and population-based screening programmes exist in many countries. Functional bowel disorders affect up to 10–15% of the population and consume considerable health-care resources. The inflammatory bowel diseases, Crohn's disease and ulcerative colitis, together affect 1 in 250 people in the Western world, with substantial associated morbidity.

FUNCTIONAL ANATOMY AND PHYSIOLOGY

Oesophagus, stomach and duodenum

This muscular tube extends 25 cm from the cricoid cartilage to the cardiac orifice of the stomach. It has an upper and a lower sphincter. A peristaltic swallowing wave propels the food bolus into the stomach (Fig. 22.1).

The stomach acts as a 'hopper', retaining and grinding food, then actively propelling it into the upper small bowel (Fig. 22.2).

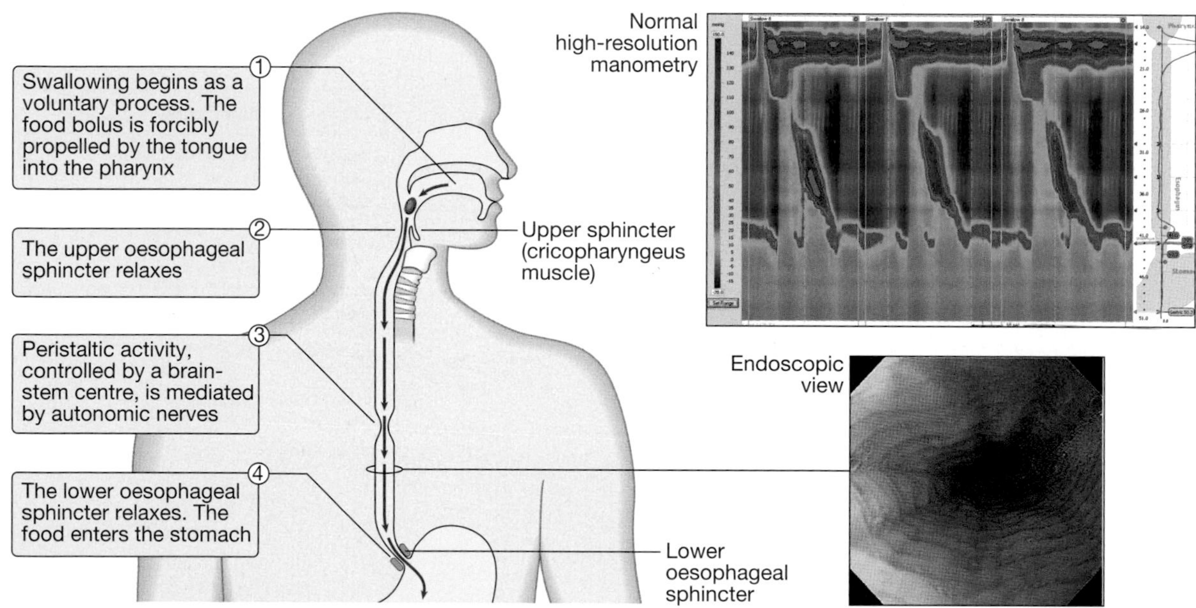

Fig. 22.1 The oesophagus: anatomy and function. The swallowing wave.

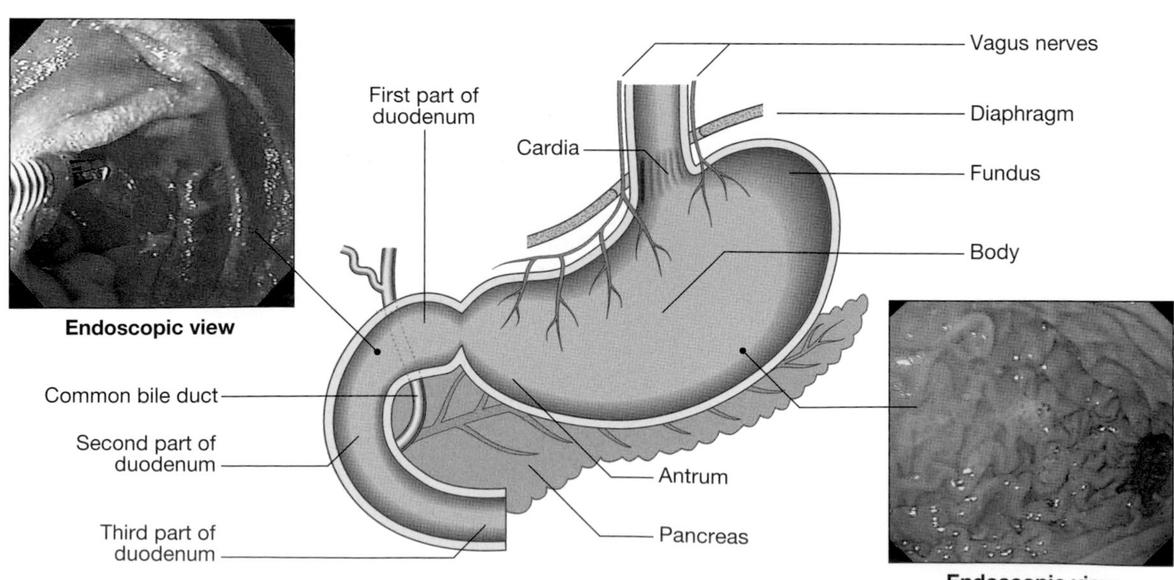

Fig. 22.2 Normal gastric and duodenal anatomy.

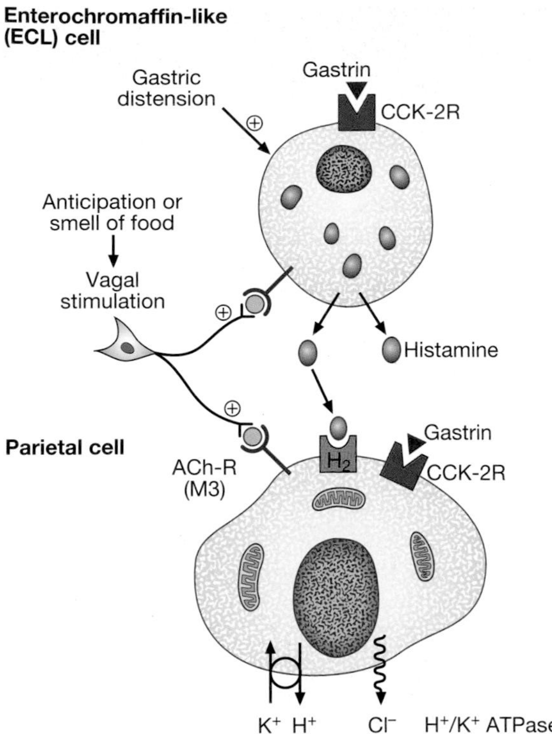

Fig. 22.3 Control of acid secretion. Gastrin released from antral G cells in response to food (protein) binds to cholecystokinin receptors (CCK-2R) on the surface of enterochromaffin-like (ECL) cells, which in turn release histamine. The histamine binds to H_2 receptors on parietal cells and this leads to secretion of hydrogen ions, in exchange for potassium ions at the apical membrane. Parietal cells also express CCK-2R and it is thought that activation of these receptors by gastrin is involved in regulatory proliferation of parietal cells. Cholinergic (vagal) activity and gastric distension also stimulate acid secretion; somatostatin, vasoactive intestinal polypeptide (VIP) and gastric inhibitory polypeptide (GIP) may inhibit it. (ACh-R = acetylcholine receptor; ATPase = adenosine triphosphatase)

Gastric secretion

Gastrin, histamine and acetylcholine are the key stimulants of acid secretion. Hydrogen and chloride ions are secreted from the apical membrane of gastric parietal cells into the lumen of the stomach by a hydrogen-potassium adenosine triphosphatase (ATPase) ('proton pump') (Fig. 22.3). The hydrochloric acid sterilises the upper gastrointestinal tract and converts pepsinogen - which is secreted by chief cells - to pepsin. The glycoprotein intrinsic factor, secreted in parallel with acid, is necessary for vitamin B_{12} absorption.

Gastrin, somatostatin and ghrelin

The hormone gastrin is produced by G cells in the antrum, whereas somatostatin is secreted from D cells throughout the stomach. Gastrin stimulates acid secretion and mucosal growth, whilst somatostatin suppresses it. Ghrelin, secreted from oxyntic glands, stimulates acid secretion but also appetite and gastric emptying.

Protective factors

Bicarbonate ions, stimulated by prostaglandins, mucins and trefoil factor family (TFF) peptides together protect the gastroduodenal mucosa from the ulcerative properties of acid and pepsin.

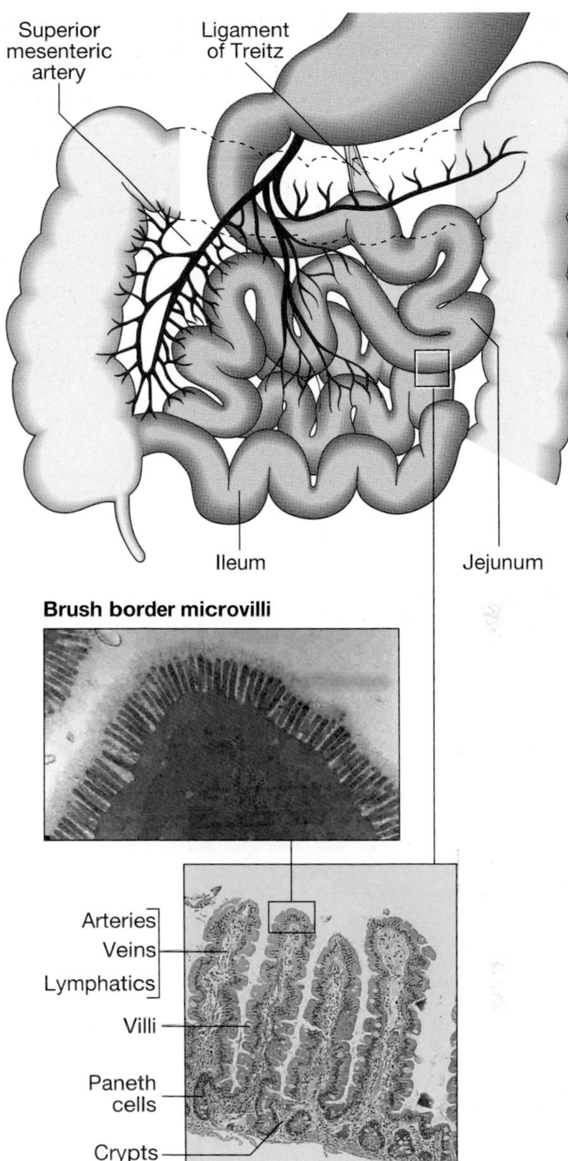

Fig. 22.4 Small intestine: anatomy. Epithelial cells are formed in crypts and differentiate as they migrate to the tip of the villi to form enterocytes (absorptive cells) and goblet cells.

Small intestine

The small bowel extends from the ligament of Treitz to the ileocaecal valve (Fig. 22.4). During fasting, a wave of peristaltic activity passes down the small bowel every 1–2 hours. Entry of food into the gastrointestinal tract stimulates small bowel peristaltic activity. Functions of the small intestine are:

- digestion (mechanical, enzymatic and peristaltic)
- absorption - the products of digestion, water, electrolytes and vitamins
- protection against ingested toxins
- immune regulation.

Digestion and absorption

Fat

Dietary lipids comprise long-chain triglycerides, cholesterol esters and lecithin. Lipids are insoluble in water

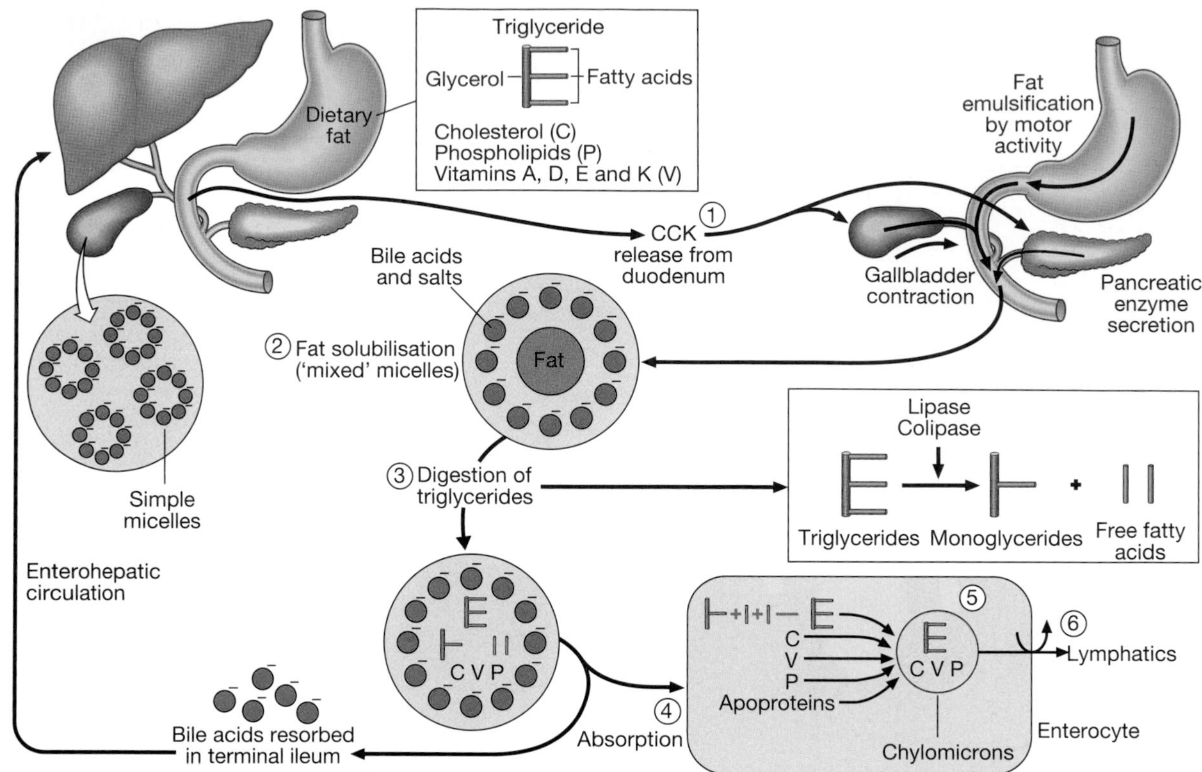

Fig. 22.5 Fat digestion. *Step 1: Luminal phase.* Fatty acids stimulate cholecystokinin (CCK) release from the duodenum and upper jejunum. The CCK stimulates release of amylase, lipase, colipase and proteases from the pancreas, causes gallbladder contraction and relaxes the sphincter of Oddi, leading bile to flow into the intestine. *Step 2: Fat solubilisation.* Bile acids and salts combine with dietary fat to form mixed micelles, which also contain cholesterol and fat-soluble vitamins. *Step 3: Digestion.* Pancreatic lipase, in the presence of its co-factor, colipase, cleaves long-chain triglycerides, yielding fatty acids and monoglycerides. *Step 4: Absorption.* Mixed micelles diffuse to the brush border of the enterocytes. Within the brush border, long-chain fatty acids bind to proteins, which transport the fatty acids into the cell, whereas cholesterol, short-chain fatty acids, phospholipids and fat-soluble vitamins enter the cell directly. The bile salts remain in the small intestinal lumen and are actively transported from the terminal ileum into the portal circulation and returned to the liver (the enterohepatic circulation). *Step 5: Re-esterification.* Within the enterocyte, fatty acids are re-esterified to form triglycerides. Triglycerides combine with cholesterol ester, fat-soluble vitamins, phospholipids and apoproteins to form chylomicrons. *Step 6: Transport.* Chylomicrons leave the enterocytes by exocytosis, enter mesenteric lymphatics, pass into the thoracic duct, and eventually reach the systemic circulation.

and undergo lipolysis and incorporation into mixed micelles before they can be absorbed into enterocytes along with the fat-soluble vitamins A, D, K and E. The lipids are processed within enterocytes and pass via lymphatics into the systemic circulation. Fat absorption and digestion can be considered as a stepwise process, as outlined in Figure 22.5.

Carbohydrates

Starch is hydrolysed by salivary and pancreatic amylases to alpha-limit dextrins containing 4–8 glucose molecules; to the disaccharide, maltose; and to the trisaccharide, maltotriose.

Disaccharides are digested by enzymes fixed to the microvillous membrane to form the monosaccharides, glucose, galactose and fructose. Glucose and galactose enter the cell by an energy-requiring process involving a carrier protein, and fructose enters by simple diffusion.

Protein

The steps involved in protein digestion are shown in Figure 22.6. Intragastric digestion by pepsin is quantitatively modest but important because the resulting polypeptides and amino acids stimulate CCK release from the mucosa of the proximal jejunum, which in turn stimulates release of pancreatic proteases, including trypsinogen, chymotrypsinogen, pro-elastases and procarboxypeptidases, from the pancreas. On exposure to brush border enterokinase, inert trypsinogen is converted to the active proteolytic enzyme trypsin, which activates the other pancreatic proenzymes. Trypsin digests proteins to produce oligopeptides, peptides and amino acids. Oligopeptides are further hydrolysed by brush border enzymes to yield dipeptides, tripeptides and amino acids. These small peptides and the amino acids are actively transported into the enterocytes, where intracellular peptidases further digest peptides to amino acids. Amino acids are then actively transported across the basal cell membrane of the enterocyte into the portal circulation and the liver.

Water and electrolytes

Absorption and secretion of electrolytes and water occur throughout the intestine. Electrolytes and water are transported by two pathways:

- *the paracellular route,* in which passive flow through tight junctions between cells is a consequence of osmotic, electrical or hydrostatic gradients
- *the transcellular route* across apical and basolateral membranes by energy-requiring specific active transport carriers (pumps).

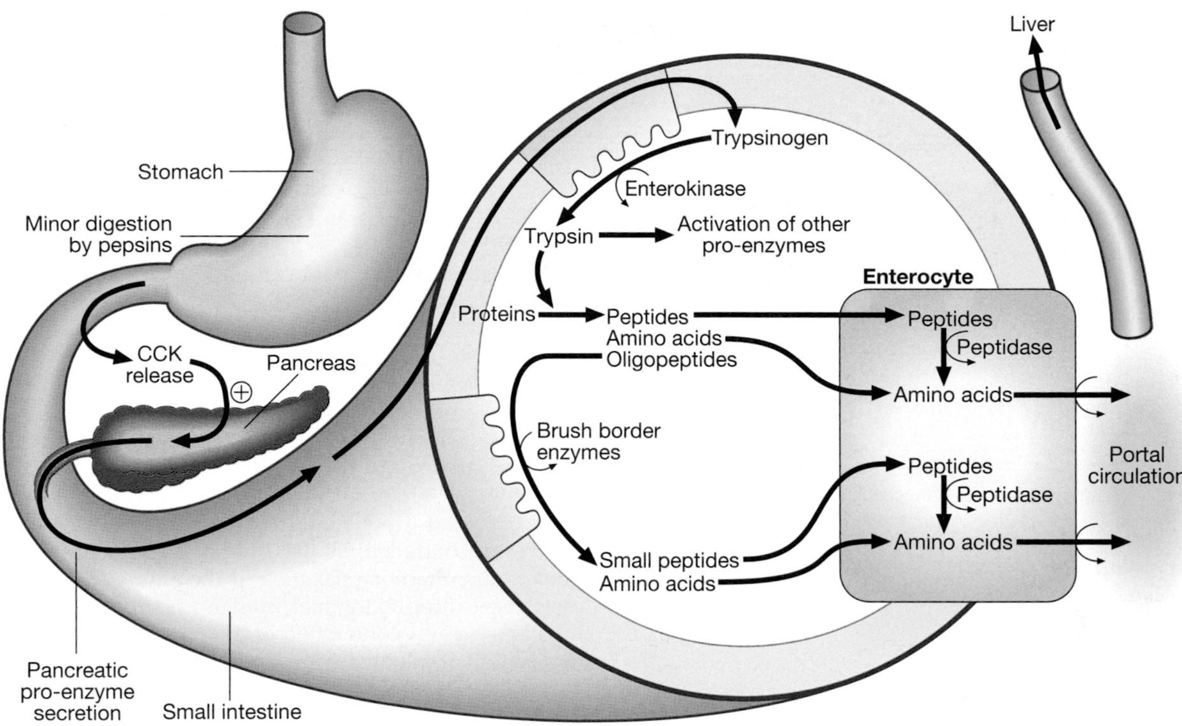

Fig. 22.6 Protein digestion.

In healthy individuals, fluid balance is tightly controlled, such that only 100 mL of the 8 litres of fluid entering the gastrointestinal tract daily is excreted in stools (Fig. 22.7).

Vitamins and trace elements

Water-soluble vitamins are absorbed throughout the intestine. The absorption of folic acid, vitamin B_{12}, calcium and iron is described on page 1024.

Protective function of the small intestine

Physical defence mechanisms

There are several levels of defence in the small bowel (Fig. 22.8). Firstly, the gut lumen contains host bacteria, mucins and secreted antibacterial products, including defensins and immunoglobulins which help combat pathogenic infections. Secondly, epithelial cells have relatively impermeable brush border membranes, and passage between cells is prevented by tight and adherens junctions. These cells can react to foreign peptides ('innate immunity') using pattern recognition receptors found on cell surfaces (Toll receptors) or intracellularly. Lastly, in the subepithelial layer, immune responses occur under control of the adaptive immune system in response to pathogenic compounds.

Immunological defence mechanisms

Gastrointestinal mucosa-associated lymphoid tissue (MALT) constitutes 25% of the total lymphatic tissue of the body and is at the heart of adaptive immunity. Within Peyer's patches, B lymphocytes differentiate to plasma cells following exposure to antigens, and these migrate to mesenteric lymph nodes, to enter the blood stream via the thoracic duct. The plasma cells return to the lamina propria of the gut through the circulation and release immunoglobulin A (IgA), which is transported

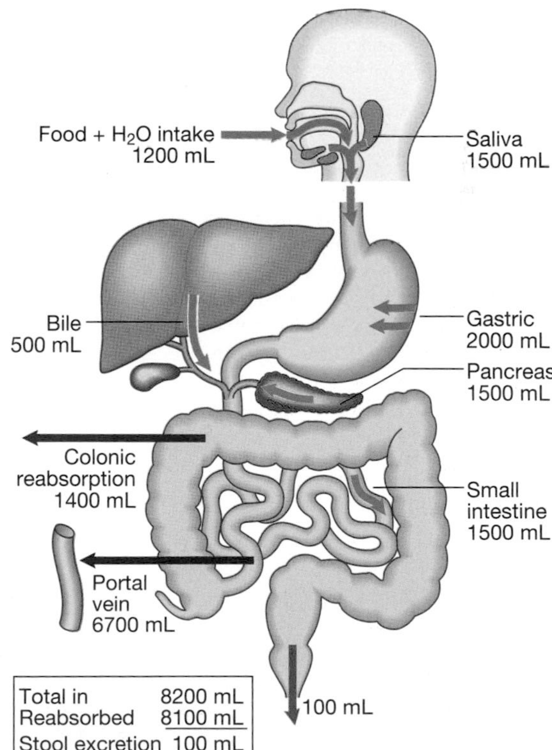

Fig. 22.7 Fluid homeostasis in the gastrointestinal tract.

into the lumen of the intestine. Intestinal T lymphocytes help localise plasma cells to the site of antigen exposure, as well as producing inflammatory mediators. Macrophages in the gut phagocytose foreign materials and secrete a range of cytokines, which mediate

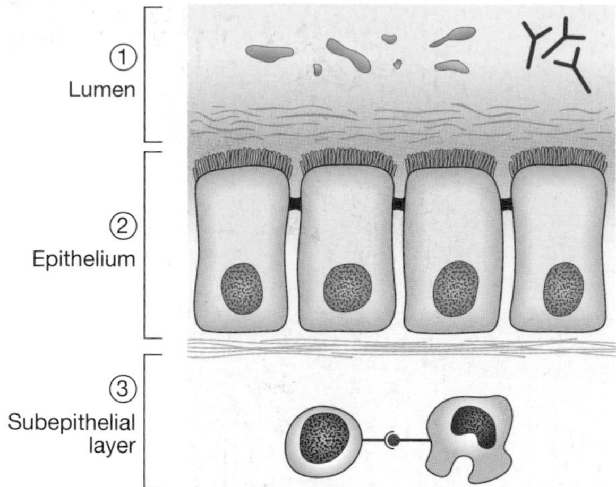

Fig. 22.8 Intestinal defence mechanisms. See text for details.

inflammation. Similarly, activation of mast-cell surface IgE receptors leads to degranulation and release of other molecules involved in inflammation.

Pancreas

The exocrine pancreas (Box 22.1) is necessary for the digestion of fat, protein and carbohydrate. Proenzymes are secreted from pancreatic acinar cells in response to circulating gastrointestinal hormones (Fig. 22.9) and are activated by trypsin. Bicarbonate-rich fluid is secreted from ductular cells to produce an optimum alkaline pH for enzyme activity.

Colon

The colon (Fig. 22.10) absorbs water and electrolytes. It also acts as a storage organ and has contractile activity. Two types of contraction occur. The first of these is segmentation (ring contraction), which leads to mixing but not propulsion; this promotes absorption of water and electrolytes. Propulsive (peristaltic contraction) waves occur several times a day and propel faeces to the rectum. All activity is stimulated after meals, probably in response to release of motilin and CCK. Faecal continence depends upon maintenance of the anorectal angle and tonic contraction of the external anal sphincters. On defecation, there is relaxation of the anorectal muscles, increased intra-abdominal pressure from the Valsalva manœuvre and contraction of abdominal muscles, and relaxation of the anal sphincters.

22.1 Pancreatic enzymes

Enzyme	Substrate	Product
Amylase	Starch and glycogen	Limit dextrans Maltose Maltriose
Lipase **Colipase**	Triglycerides	Monoglycerides and free fatty acids
Proteolytic enzymes Trypsinogen Chymotrypsinogen Pro-elastase Pro-carboxypeptidases	Proteins and polypeptides	Short polypeptides

Control of gastrointestinal function

Secretion, absorption, motor activity, growth and differentiation of the gut are all modulated by a combination of neuronal and hormonal factors.

The nervous system and gastrointestinal function

The central nervous system (CNS), the autonomic system (ANS) and the enteric nervous system (ENS) interact to regulate gut function. The ANS comprises:

- *parasympathetic pathways* (vagal and sacral efferent), which are cholinergic, and increase smooth muscle tone and promote sphincter relaxation

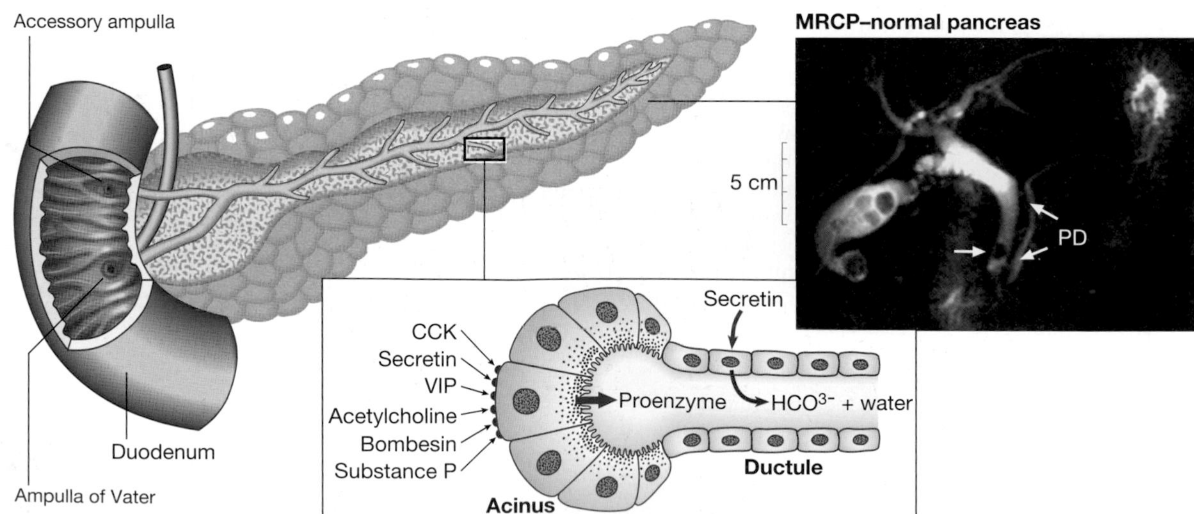

Fig. 22.9 Pancreatic structure and function. Ductular cells secrete alkaline fluid in response to secretin. Acinar cells secrete digestive enzymes from zymogen granules in response to a range of secretagogues. The photograph shows a normal pancreatic duct (PD) and side branches, as defined at magnetic resonance cholangiopancreatography (MRCP). Note the incidental calculi in the gallbladder and common bile duct (arrow). (CCK = cholecystokinin; VIP = vasoactive intestinal polypeptide)

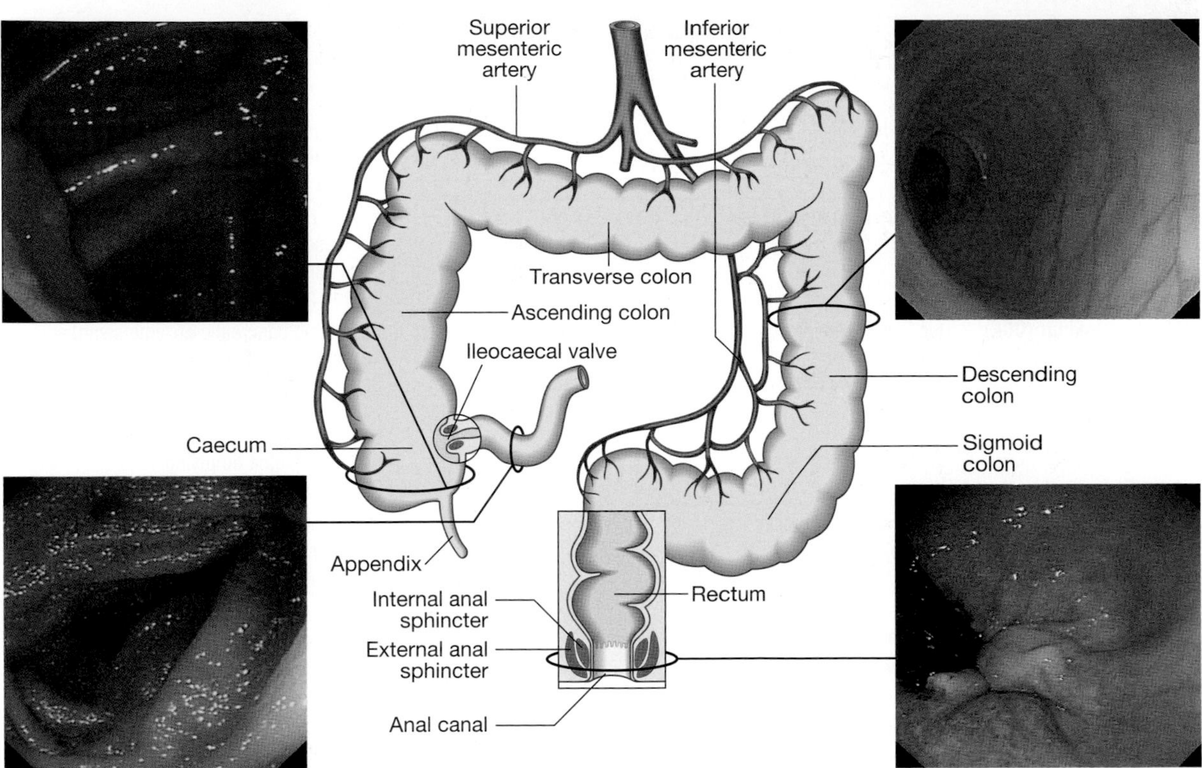

Fig. 22.10 The normal colon, rectum and anal canal.

- *sympathetic pathways*, which release noradrenaline (norepinephrine), reduce smooth muscle tone and stimulate sphincter contraction.

The enteric nervous system

In conjunction with the ANS, the ENS senses gut contents and conditions, and regulates motility, fluid exchange, secretion, blood flow and other key gut functions. It comprises two major networks intrinsic to the gut wall. The myenteric (Auerbach's) plexus in the smooth muscle layer regulates motor control; and the submucosal (Meissner's) plexus exerts secretory control over the epithelium, enteroendocrine cells and submucosal vessels. Together, these plexuses form a two-layered neuronal mesh along the length of the gut. Although connected centrally via the ANS, the ENS can function autonomously, using a variety of transmitters, including acetylcholine, noradrenaline (norepinephrine), 5-hydroxytryptamine (5-HT, serotonin), nitric oxide, substance P and calcitonin gene-related peptide (CGRP). There are local reflex loops within the ENS but also loops involving the coeliac and mesenteric ganglia and the paravertebral ganglia. The parasympathetic system generally stimulates motility and secretion, while the sympathetic system generally acts in an inhibitory manner.

Peristalsis

Peristalsis is a reflex triggered by gut wall distension, which consists of a wave of circular muscle contraction to propel contents from the oesophagus to the rectum. It can be influenced by innervation but functions independently. It results from a basic electrical rhythm originating from the interstitial cells of Cajal in the circular layer of intestinal smooth muscle. These are stellate cells of mesenchymal origin with smooth muscle features, which act as the 'pacemaker' of the gut.

Migrating motor complexes

Migrating motor complexes (MMC) are waves of contraction spreading from the stomach to the ileum, occurring at a frequency of about 5 per minute every 90 minutes or so, between meals and during fasting. They may serve to sweep intestinal contents distally in preparation for the next meal and are inhibited by eating.

Gut hormones

The origin, action and control of the major gut hormones, peptides and non-peptide signalling transmitters are summarised in Box 22.2.

INVESTIGATION OF GASTROINTESTINAL DISEASE

A wide range of tests are available for the investigation of patients with gastrointestinal symptoms. These can be classified broadly into tests of structure, tests for infection and tests of function.

Imaging

Plain X-rays

Plain X-rays of the abdomen are useful in the diagnosis of intestinal obstruction or paralytic ileus, where dilated loops of bowel and (in the erect position) fluid levels may be seen. Calcified lymph nodes, gallstones and renal stones can also be detected. Chest X-ray

22.2 Gut hormones and peptides

Hormone	Origin	Stimulus	Action
Gastrin	Stomach (G cell)	Products of protein digestion Suppressed by acid and somatostatin	Stimulates gastric acid secretion Stimulates growth of gastrointestinal mucosa
Somatostatin	Throughout GI tract (D cell)	Fat ingestion	Inhibits gastrin and insulin secretion Decreases acid secretion Decreases absorption Inhibits pancreatic secretion
Cholecystokinin (CCK)	Duodenum and jejunum (I cells); also ileal and colonic nerve endings	Products of protein digestion Fat and fatty acids Suppressed by trypsin	Stimulates pancreatic enzyme secretion Gallbladder contraction Sphincter of Oddi relaxation Satiety Decreases gastric acid secretion Reduces gastric emptying Regulates pancreatic growth
Secretin	Duodenum and jejunum (S cells)	Duodenal acid Fatty acids	Stimulates pancreatic fluid and bicarbonate secretion Decreases acid secretion Reduces gastric emptying
Motilin	Duodenum, small intestine and colon (Mo cells)	Fasting Dietary fat	Regulates peristaltic activity, including migrating motor complexes (MMC)
Gastric inhibitory polypeptide (GIP)	Duodenum (K cells) and jejunum	Glucose and fat	Stimulates insulin release (also known as glucose-dependent insulinotrophic polypeptide) Inhibits acid secretion
Vasoactive intestinal peptide (VIP)	Nerve fibres throughout GI tract	Unknown	Vasodilator Smooth muscle relaxation Water and electrolyte secretion
Ghrelin	Stomach	Fasting Inhibited by eating	Stimulates appetite, acid secretion and gastric emptying
Peptide YY	Ileum and colon	Feeding	Modulates satiety
Amylin	Pancreatic islet β-cells	Feeding	Glycaemic control

(performed with the patient in erect position) is useful in the diagnosis of suspected perforation, as it shows subdiaphragmatic free air.

Contrast studies

X-rays with contrast medium are usually performed to assess not only anatomical abnormalities but also motility. Barium sulphate provides good mucosal coating and excellent opacification but can precipitate impaction proximal to an obstructive lesion. Water-soluble contrast is used to opacify bowel prior to abdominal computed tomography and in cases of suspected perforation. The double contrast technique improves mucosal visualisation by using gas to distend the barium-coated intestinal surface. Contrast studies are useful for detecting filling defects, such as tumours, strictures, ulcers and motility disorders, but are inferior to endoscopic procedures and more sophisticated cross-sectional imaging techniques, such as computed tomography and magnetic resonance imaging. The major uses and limitations of various contrast studies are shown in Box 22.3 and Figure 22.11.

Ultrasound, computed tomography and magnetic resonance imaging

Ultrasound (US), computed tomography (CT) and magnetic resonance imaging (MRI) are key tests in the evaluation of intra-abdominal disease. They are non-invasive and offer detailed images of the abdominal contents. Their main applications are summarised in Box 22.4 and Figure 22.12.

Endoscopy

Videoendoscopes provide high-definition imaging and accessories can be passed down the endoscope to allow both diagnostic and therapeutic procedures, some of which are illustrated in Figure 22.13. Endoscopes with magnifying lenses allow almost microscopic detail to be observed, and imaging modalities, such as confocal endomicroscopy, autofluorescence and 'narrow band imaging', are increasingly used to detect subtle abnormalities not visible by standard 'white light' endoscopy.

Upper gastrointestinal endoscopy

This is performed under light intravenous benzodiazepine sedation, or using only local anaesthetic throat spray after the patient has fasted for at least 4 hours. With the patient in the left lateral position, the entire oesophagus (excluding pharynx), stomach and first two parts of duodenum can be seen. Indications, contraindications and complications are given in Box 22.5.

22.3 Contrast radiology in the investigation of gastrointestinal disease

	Barium swallow/meal	Barium follow-through	Barium enema
Indications and major uses	Motility disorders (achalasia and gastroparesis) Perforation or fistula (non-ionic contrast)	Diarrhoea and abdominal pain of small bowel origin Possible obstruction by strictures Suspected malabsorption Crohn's disease assessment	Altered bowel habit Evaluation of strictures or diverticular disease Megacolon Chronic constipation
Limitations	Risk of aspiration Poor mucosal detail Low sensitivity for early cancer Inability to biopsy	Time-consuming Radiation exposure Relative insensitivity	Difficult in frail or incontinent patients Sigmoidoscopy needed to see rectum Low sensitivity for lesions < 1 cm

A
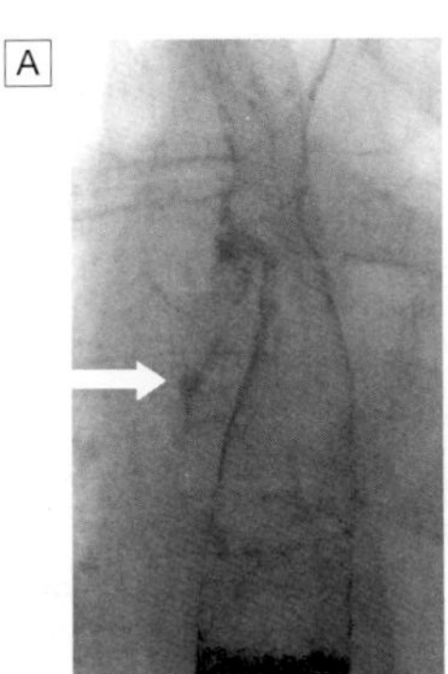
B
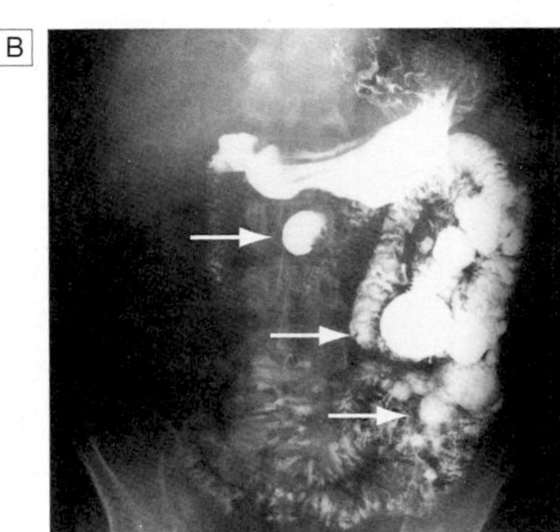
C
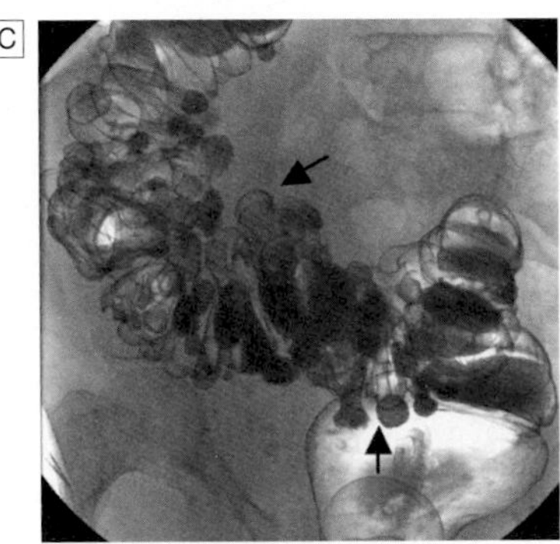

Fig. 22.11 Examples of contrast radiology. **A** Non-ionic contrast swallow shows leakage of contrast (arrow) into the mediastinum following stricture dilatation. **B** Barium follow-through. There are multiple diverticula (arrows) in this patient with jejunal diverticulosis. **C** Barium enema showing severe diverticular disease. There is tortuosity and narrowing of the sigmoid colon with multiple diverticula (arrows).

22.4 Imaging in gastroenterology

	Ultrasound	CT	MRI	CT-PET
Indications and major uses	Abdominal masses Organomegaly Ascites Biliary tract dilatation Gallstones Guided biopsy of lesions Small bowel imaging	Assess pancreatic disease Hepatic tumour deposits CT colonography ('virtual colonoscopy') Tumour staging Assess lesion vascularity Abscesses and collections	Hepatic tumour staging MRCP Pelvic/perianal disease Crohn's fistulae Small bowel visualisation	Detection of metastases not seen on ultrasound or CT Images can be fused with CT to form composite image
Limitations	Low sensitivity for small lesions Little functional information Operator-dependent Gas and obesity may obscure view	Cost Radiation dose	Claustrophobic patients Contraindicated in presence of metallic prostheses, cardiac pacemaker, cochlear implants	Signal detection depends on metabolic activity within tumour – not all are metabolically active

A
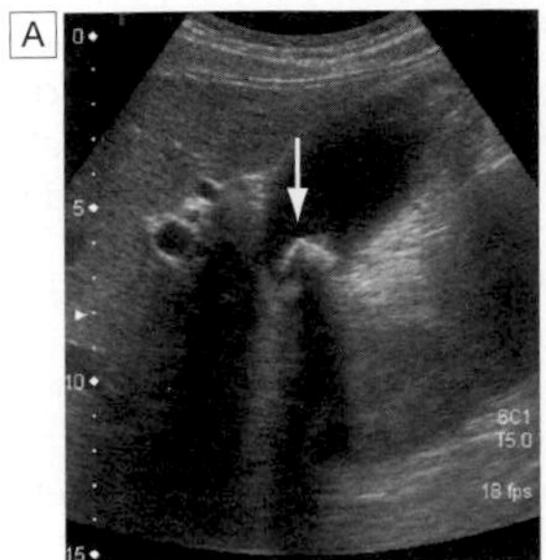
B
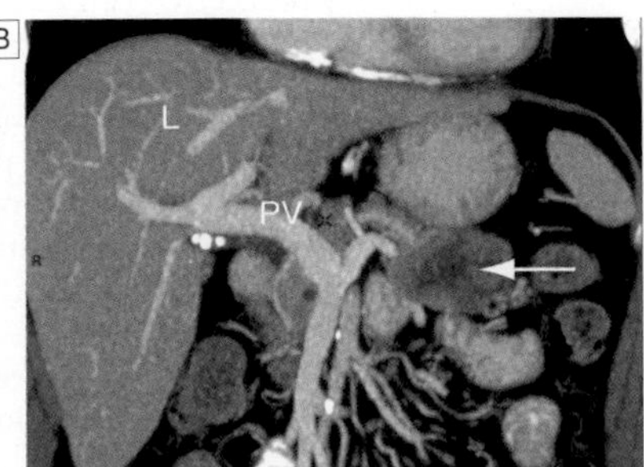

C
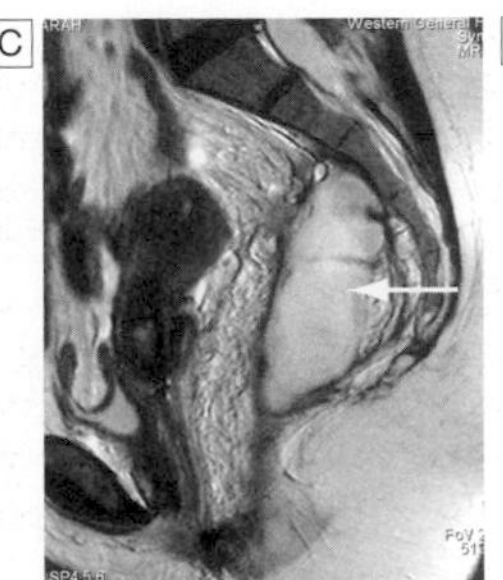
D
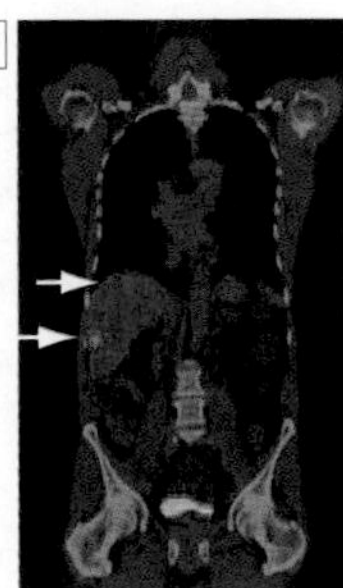

Fig. 22.12 Examples of ultrasound, CT and MRI. **A** Ultrasound showing large gallstone (arrow) with acoustic shadowing. **B** Multidetector coronal CT showing large solid and cystic malignant tumour in the pancreatic tail (arrow). (PV = portal vein; L = liver) **C** Pelvic MRI showing large pelvic abscess (arrow) posterior to the rectum in a patient with Crohn's disease. **D** Fused CT-PET image showing two liver metastases (arrows).

Control of bleeding

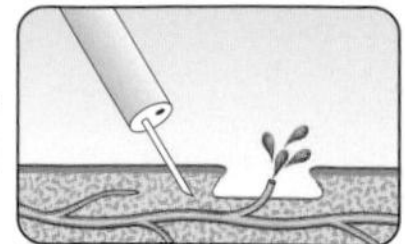
Injection sclerotherapy

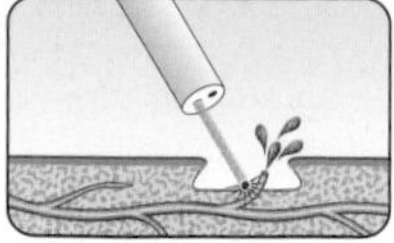
Diathermy

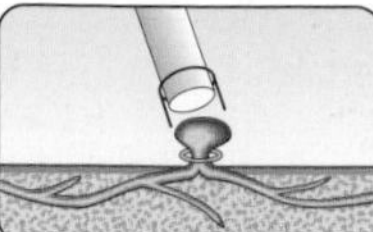
Variceal ligation

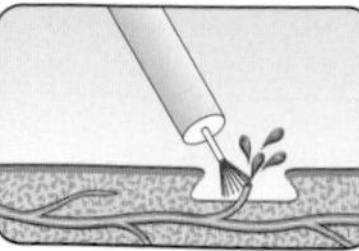
Laser therapy

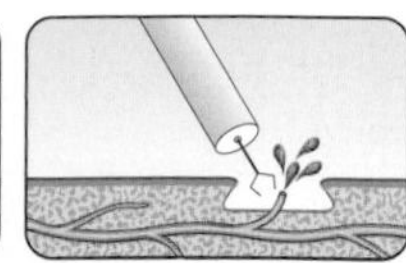
Endoscopic clipping

Treatment of tumours

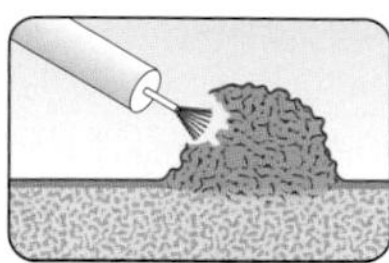
Laser therapy

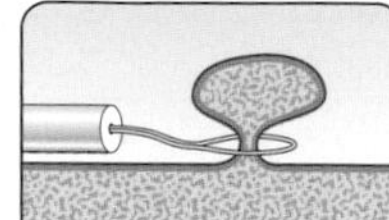
Polypectomy

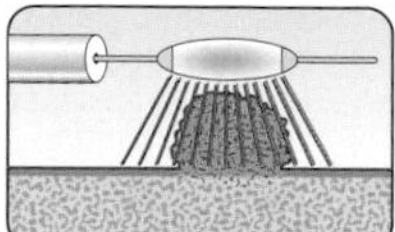
Photodynamic therapy/radiofrequency ablation

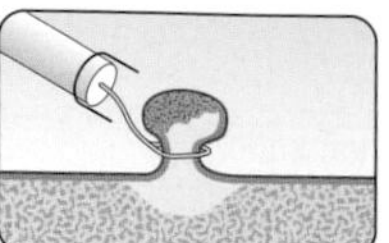
Endoscopic mucosal resection

Treatment of strictures

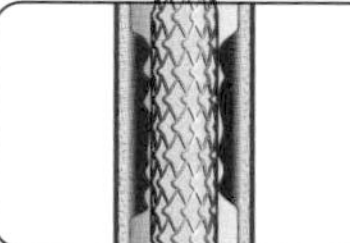
Stent insertion

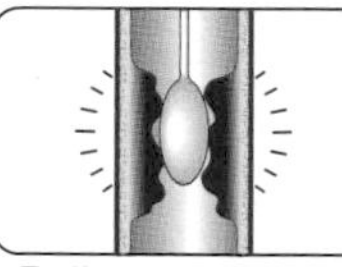
Balloon dilatation

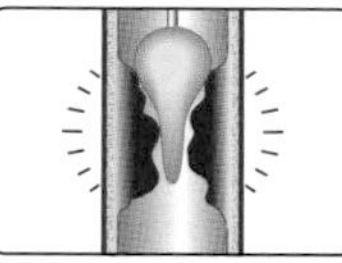
Bouginage

Management of biliary and pancreatic disease

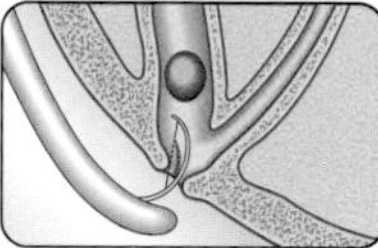
Sphincterotomy

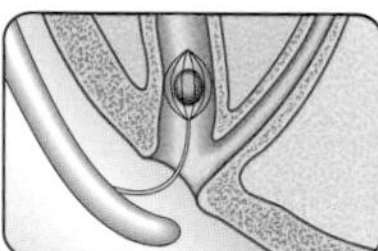
Basket retrieval

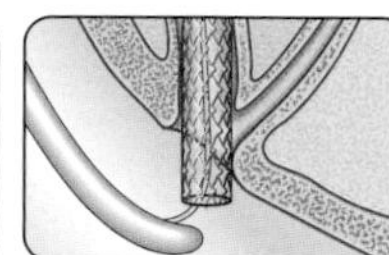
Stent insertion

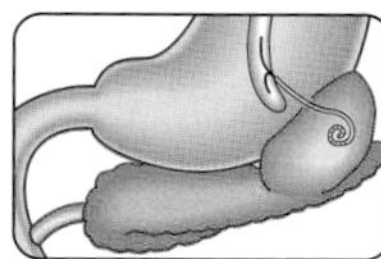
Pseudocyst drainage

Fig. 22.13 Examples of therapeutic techniques in endoscopy.

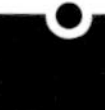

22.5 Upper gastrointestinal endoscopy

Indications

- Dyspepsia over 55 yrs of age or with alarm symptoms
- Atypical chest pain
- Dysphagia
- Vomiting
- Weight loss
- Acute or chronic gastrointestinal bleeding
- Screening for oesophageal varices in patients with chronic liver disease
- Abnormal CT scan or barium meal
- Duodenal biopsies in the investigation of malabsorption and to confirm a diagnosis of coeliac disease prior to commencement of gluten-free diet
- Therapeutic, including treatment of bleeding lesions, banding/injection of varices, dilatation of strictures, insertion of stents, placement of percutaneous gastrostomies

Contraindications

- Severe shock
- Recent myocardial infarction, unstable angina, cardiac arrhythmia*
- Severe respiratory disease*
- Atlantoaxial subluxation*
- Possible visceral perforation

Complications

- Cardiorespiratory depression due to sedation
- Aspiration pneumonia
- Perforation

*These are 'relative' contraindications; in experienced hands, endoscopy can be safely performed.

Capsule endoscopy

Capsule endoscopy (Fig. 22.14) uses a capsule containing an imaging device, battery, transmitter and antenna; as it traverses the small intestine, it transmits images to a battery-powered recorder worn on a belt round the patient's waist. After approximately 8 hours, the capsule is excreted. Images from the capsule are analysed as a video sequence and it is usually possible to localise the segment of small bowel in which lesions are seen. Abnormalities detected usually require enteroscopy for confirmation and therapy. Indications, contraindications and complications are listed in Box 22.6.

Double balloon enteroscopy

While endoscopy can reach the proximal small intestine in most patients, a newer technique called double balloon enteroscopy is also available, which uses a long endoscope with a flexible overtube. Sequential and repeated inflation and deflation of balloons on the tip of the overtube and enteroscope allow the operator to push and pull along the entire length of the small intestine to the terminal ileum, in order to diagnose or treat small bowel lesions detected by capsule endoscopy or other imaging modalities. Indications, contraindications and complications are listed in Box 22.7.

Sigmoidoscopy and colonoscopy

Sigmoidoscopy can be carried out either in the outpatient clinic using a 20 cm rigid plastic sigmoidoscope or in the endoscopy suite using a 60 cm flexible colonoscope following bowel preparation. When sigmoidoscopy is combined with proctoscopy, accurate detection of haemorrhoids, ulcerative colitis and distal colorectal neoplasia is possible. After full bowel cleansing, it is possible to examine the entire colon and the terminal ileum using a longer colonoscope. Indications, contraindications and complications of colonoscopy are listed in Box 22.8.

Magnetic resonance cholangiopancreatography

Magnetic resonance cholangiopancreatography (MRCP) has largely replaced endoscopic retrograde

A

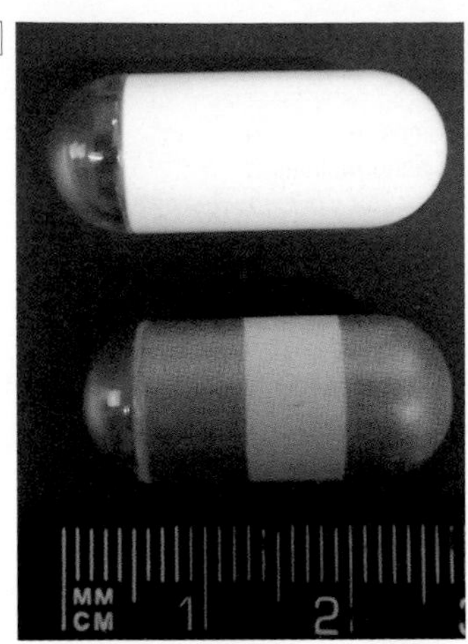

B

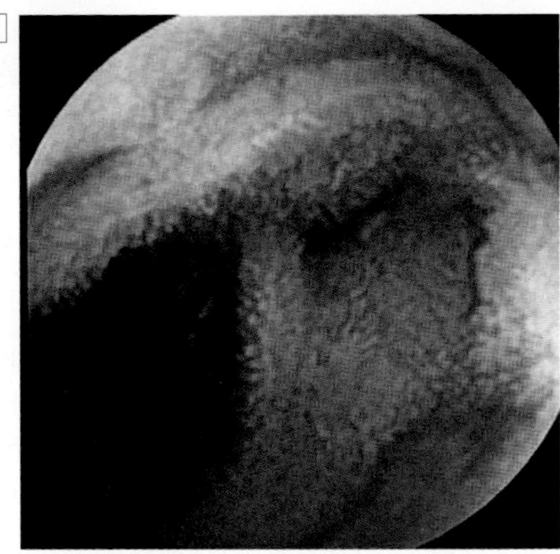

Fig. 22.14 Wireless capsule endoscopy. **A** Examples of capsules. **B** Capsule endoscopy image of bleeding jejunal vascular malformation.

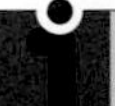

22.6 Wireless capsule endoscopy

Indications

- Obscure gastrointestinal bleeding
- Small bowel Crohn's disease
- Assessment of coeliac disease and its complications
- Screening and surveillance in familial polyposis syndromes

Contraindications

- Known or suspected small bowel stricture (risk of capsule retention)
- Caution in people with pacemakers or implantable defibrillators

Complications

- Capsule retention (< 1%)

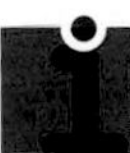

22.7 Double balloon enteroscopy

Indications

Diagnostic

- Obscure gastrointestinal bleeding
- Malabsorption or unexplained diarrhoea
- Suspicious radiological findings
- Suspected small bowel tumour
- Surveillance of polyposis syndromes

Therapeutic

- Coagulation/diathermy of bleeding lesions
- Jejunostomy placement

Contraindications

- As for upper gastrointestinal endoscopy

Complications

- As for upper gastrointestinal endoscopy
- Post-procedure abdominal pain (≤20%)
- Pancreatitis (1–3%)
- Perforation (especially after resection of large polyps)

cholangiopancreatography (ERCP) in the evaluation of obstructive jaundice since it provides comparable images of the biliary tree and pancreas, providing information that complements that obtained from CT and endoscopic ultrasound examination (EUS).

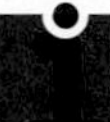

22.8 Colonoscopy

Indications*

- Suspected inflammatory bowel disease
- Chronic diarrhoea
- Altered bowel habit
- Rectal bleeding or iron deficiency anaemia
- Assessment of abnormal CT colonogram or barium enema
- Colorectal cancer screening
- Colorectal adenoma and carcinoma follow-up
- Therapeutic procedures, including endoscopic resection, dilatation of strictures, laser, stent insertion and argon plasma coagulation

Contraindications

- Acute severe ulcerative colitis (prefer unprepared flexible sigmoidoscopy)
- As for upper gastrointestinal endoscopy

Complications

- Cardiorespiratory depression due to sedation
- Perforation
- Bleeding following polypectomy

*Colonoscopy is not useful in the investigation of constipation.

Endoscopic retrograde cholangiopancreatography

Using a side-viewing duodenoscope, it is possible to cannulate the main pancreatic duct and common bile duct. Nowadays, ERCP is mainly used in the treatment of a range of biliary and pancreatic diseases that have been identified by other imaging techniques such as MRCP, EUS and CT. Indications for and risks of ERCP are listed in Box 22.9.

Histology

Biopsy material obtained during endoscopy or percutaneously can provide useful information (Box 22.11).

Tests of infection

Bacterial cultures

Stool cultures are essential in the investigation of diarrhoea, especially when it is acute or bloody, in order to identify pathogenic organisms (Ch. 13).

22.9 Endoscopic retrograde cholangiopancreatography (ERCP)

Indications

Diagnostic ERCP
- Biliary or pancreatic disease where other imaging is equivocal or is contraindicated
- Ampullary biopsy or biliary cytology

Therapeutic ERCP
- Biliary disease
  - Removal of common bile duct calculi*
  - Palliation of malignant biliary obstruction
  - Management of biliary leaks/damage complicating surgery
  - Dilatation of benign strictures
  - Primary sclerosing cholangitis
- Pancreatic disease
  - Drainage of pancreatic pseudocysts and fistulae
  - Removal of pancreatic calculi (selected cases)

Contraindications
- Severe cardiopulmonary comorbidity
- Coagulopathy

Complications
- Occur in 5–10% with a 30-day mortality of 0.5–1%

General
- As for upper endoscopy

Specific
- Biliary disease
  - Bleeding following sphincterotomy
  - Cholangitis (if biliary obstruction is not relieved by ERCP)
  - Gallstone impaction
- Pancreatic disease
  - Acute pancreatitis
  - Infection of pseudocyst

*Laparoscopic surgery is preferred in fit individuals who also require cholecystectomy.

22.10 Endoscopy in old age

- **Tolerance**: endoscopic procedures are generally well tolerated, even in very old people.
- **Side-effects from sedation**: older people are more sensitive, and respiratory depression, hypotension and prolonged recovery times are more common.
- **Bowel preparation for colonoscopy**: can be difficult in frail, immobile people. Sodium phosphate-based preparations can cause dehydration or hypotension and should be avoided in those with underlying cardiac or renal failure. Minimal preparation CT colonograms provide an excellent alternative in these individuals.
- **Antiperistaltic agents**: hyoscine should be avoided in those with glaucoma and can also cause tachyarrhythmias. Glucagon is preferred if an antiperistaltic agent is needed.

Serology

Detection of antibodies plays a limited role in the diagnosis of gastrointestinal infection caused by organisms such as *Helicobacter pylori*, *Salmonella* species and *Entamoeba histolytica*.

Breath tests

Non-invasive breath tests for *H. pylori* infection are discussed on page 873. Breath tests for suspected small intestinal bacterial overgrowth are discussed on page 882.

22.11 Reasons for biopsy or cytological examination

- Suspected malignant lesions
- Assessment of mucosal abnormalities
- Diagnosis of infection (*Candida, Helicobacter pylori, Giardia lamblia*)
- Analysis of genetic mutations

Tests of function

A number of dynamic tests can be used to investigate aspects of gut function, including digestion, absorption, inflammation and epithelial permeability. Some of the more commonly used ones are listed in Box 22.12. In the assessment of suspected malabsorption, blood tests (full blood count, erythrocyte sedimentation rate (ESR), C-reactive protein (CRP), folate, vitamin B_{12}, iron status, albumin, calcium and phosphate) are essential, and endoscopy is undertaken to obtain mucosal biopsies. Faecal calprotectin is very sensitive at detecting mucosal inflammation.

Oesophageal motility

A barium swallow can give useful information about oesophageal motility. Videofluoroscopy, with joint assessment by a speech and language therapist and a radiologist, may be necessary in difficult cases. Oesophageal manometry (see Fig. 22.1, p. 840), often in conjunction with 24-hour pH measurements, is of value in diagnosing cases of refractory gastro-oesophageal reflux, achalasia and non-cardiac chest pain. Oesophageal impedance testing is useful for detecting non-acid or gas reflux events, especially in patients with atypical symptoms or those who respond poorly to acid suppression.

Gastric emptying

This involves administering a test meal containing solids and liquids labelled with different radioisotopes and measuring the amount retained in the stomach afterwards (Box 22.13). It is useful in the investigation of suspected delayed gastric emptying (gastroparesis) when other studies are normal.

Colonic and anorectal motility

A plain abdominal X-ray taken on day 5 after ingestion of different-shaped inert plastic pellets on days 1–3 gives an estimate of whole gut transit time. The test is useful in the evaluation of chronic constipation, when the position of any retained pellets can be observed, and helps to differentiate cases of slow transit from those due to obstructed defecation. The mechanism of defecation and anorectal function can be assessed by anorectal manometry, electrophysiological tests and defecating proctography.

Radioisotope tests

Many different radioisotope tests are used (see Box 22.13). In some, structural information is obtained, such as the localisation of a Meckel's diverticulum. Others provide functional information, such as the rate of gastric emptying or ability to reabsorb bile acids. Yet

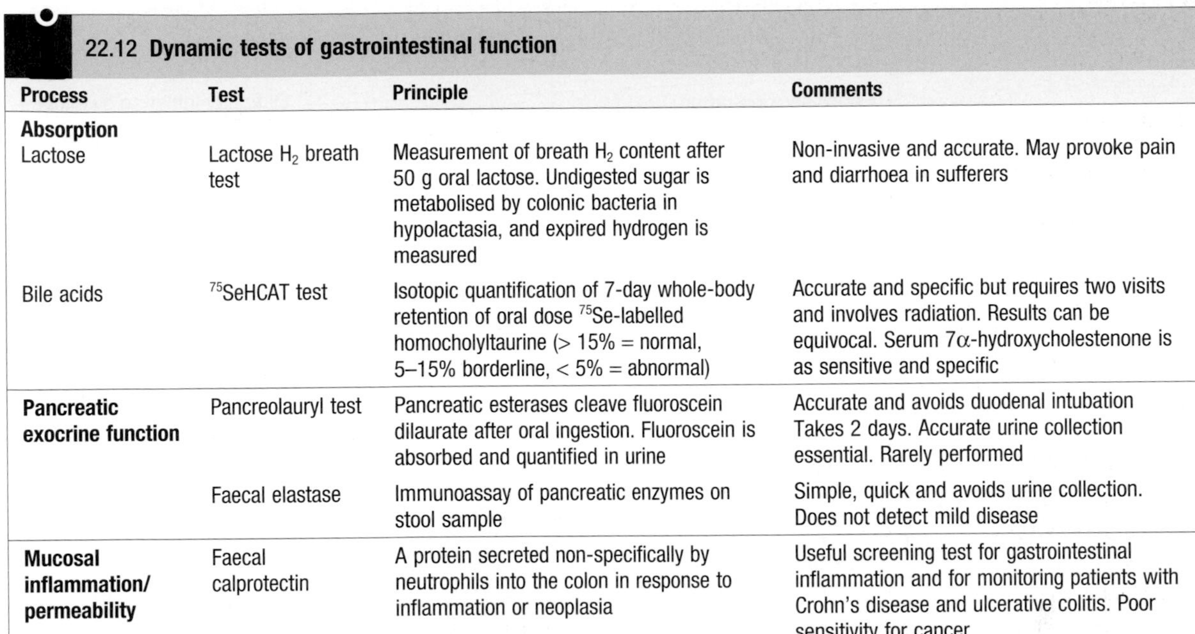

22.12 Dynamic tests of gastrointestinal function

Process	Test	Principle	Comments
Absorption Lactose	Lactose H_2 breath test	Measurement of breath H_2 content after 50 g oral lactose. Undigested sugar is metabolised by colonic bacteria in hypolactasia, and expired hydrogen is measured	Non-invasive and accurate. May provoke pain and diarrhoea in sufferers
Bile acids	^{75}SeHCAT test	Isotopic quantification of 7-day whole-body retention of oral dose ^{75}Se-labelled homocholyltaurine (> 15% = normal, 5–15% borderline, < 5% = abnormal)	Accurate and specific but requires two visits and involves radiation. Results can be equivocal. Serum 7α-hydroxycholestenone is as sensitive and specific
Pancreatic exocrine function	Pancreolauryl test	Pancreatic esterases cleave fluoroscein dilaurate after oral ingestion. Fluoroscein is absorbed and quantified in urine	Accurate and avoids duodenal intubation Takes 2 days. Accurate urine collection essential. Rarely performed
	Faecal elastase	Immunoassay of pancreatic enzymes on stool sample	Simple, quick and avoids urine collection. Does not detect mild disease
Mucosal inflammation/ permeability	Faecal calprotectin	A protein secreted non-specifically by neutrophils into the colon in response to inflammation or neoplasia	Useful screening test for gastrointestinal inflammation and for monitoring patients with Crohn's disease and ulcerative colitis. Poor sensitivity for cancer

22

22.13 Commonly used radioisotope tests in gastroenterology

Test	Isotope	Major uses and principle of test
Gastric emptying study	^{99m}Tc-sulphur ^{111}In-DTPA	Used in assessment of gastric emptying, particularly for possible gastroparesis
Urea breath test	^{13}C-urea	Used in non-invasive diagnosis of *H. pylori.* Bacterial urease enzyme splits urea to ammonia and CO_2, which is detected in expired air
Meckel's scan	^{99m}Tc-pertechnate	Diagnosis of Meckel's diverticulum in cases of obscure gastrointestinal bleeding. Isotope is injected IV and localises in ectopic parietal mucosa within diverticulum
Somatostatin receptor scan (SRS)	^{111}In-DTPA-DPheoctreotide	Labelled somatostatin analogue binds to cell surface somatostatin receptors on pancreatic neuro-endocrine tumours

others are tests of infection and rely on the presence of bacteria to hydrolyse a radio-labelled test substance followed by detection of the radioisotope in expired air, such as the urea breath test for *H. pylori.*

PRESENTING PROBLEMS IN GASTROINTESTINAL DISEASE

Dysphagia

Dysphagia is defined as difficulty in swallowing. It may coexist with heartburn or vomiting but should be distinguished from both globus sensation (in which anxious people feel a lump in the throat without organic cause) and odynophagia (pain during swallowing, usually from gastro-oesophageal reflux or candidiasis).

Dysphagia can occur due to problems in the oropharynx or oesophagus (Fig. 22.15). Oropharyngeal disorders affect the initiation of swallowing at the pharynx and upper oesophageal sphincter. The patient has difficulty initiating swallowing and complains of choking, nasal regurgitation or tracheal aspiration. Drooling, dysarthria, hoarseness and cranial nerve or other neurological signs may be present. Oesophageal disorders cause dysphagia by obstructing the lumen or by affecting motility. Patients with oesophageal disease complain of food 'sticking' after swallowing, although the level at which this is felt correlates poorly with the true site of obstruction. Swallowing of liquids is normal until strictures become extreme.

Investigations

Dysphagia should always be investigated urgently. Endoscopy is the investigation of choice because it allows biopsy and dilatation of strictures. If no abnormality is found, then barium swallow with videofluoroscopic swallowing assessment is indicated to detect major motility disorders. In some cases, oesophageal manometry is required. High-resolution manometry allows accurate classification of abnormalities. Figure 22.15 summarises a diagnostic approach to dysphagia and lists the major causes.

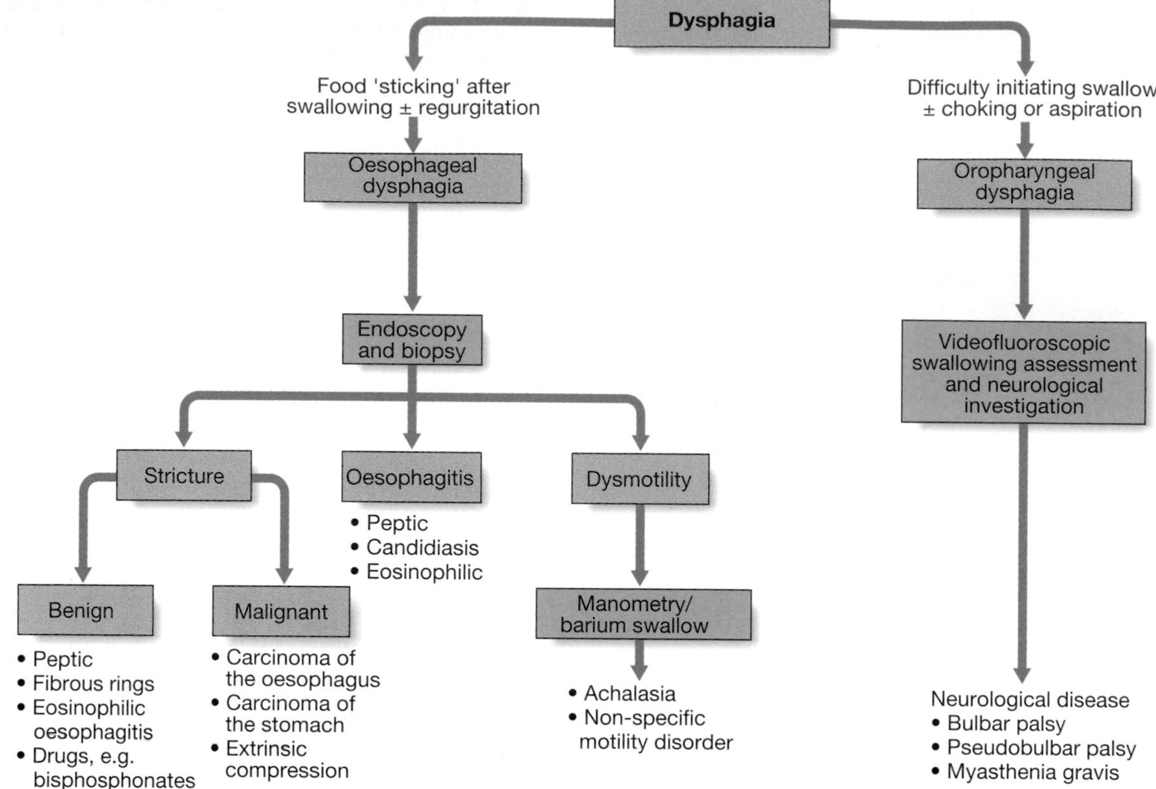

Fig. 22.15 Investigation of dysphagia.

Dyspepsia

Dyspepsia describes symptoms such as discomfort, bloating and nausea, which are thought to originate from the upper gastrointestinal tract. There are many causes (Box 22.14), including some arising outside the digestive system. Heartburn and other 'reflux' symptoms are separate entities and are considered elsewhere. Although symptoms often correlate poorly with the underlying diagnosis, a careful history is important to detect 'alarm' features requiring urgent investigation (Box 22.15) and to detect atypical symptoms which might be due to problems outside the gastrointestinal tract.

Dyspepsia affects up to 80% of the population at some time in life and most patients have no serious underlying disease. Patients who present with new dyspepsia at an age of more than 55 years and younger patients unresponsive to empirical treatment require investigation to exclude serious disease. An algorithm for the investigation of dyspepsia is outlined in Figure 22.16.

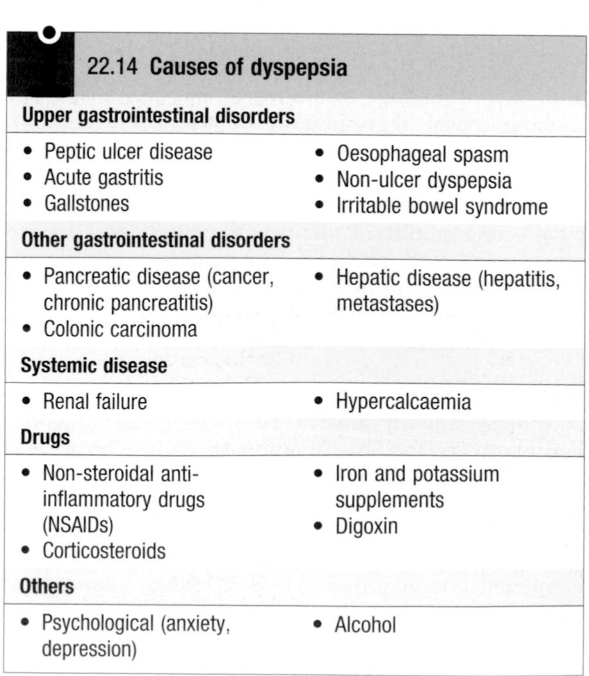

22.14 Causes of dyspepsia

Upper gastrointestinal disorders	
• Peptic ulcer disease • Acute gastritis • Gallstones	• Oesophageal spasm • Non-ulcer dyspepsia • Irritable bowel syndrome
Other gastrointestinal disorders	
• Pancreatic disease (cancer, chronic pancreatitis) • Colonic carcinoma	• Hepatic disease (hepatitis, metastases)
Systemic disease	
• Renal failure	• Hypercalcaemia
Drugs	
• Non-steroidal anti-inflammatory drugs (NSAIDs) • Corticosteroids	• Iron and potassium supplements • Digoxin
Others	
• Psychological (anxiety, depression)	• Alcohol

22.15 Alarm features in dyspepsia

• Weight loss	• Haematemesis and/or melaena
• Anaemia	• Dysphagia
• Vomiting	• Palpable abdominal mass

Heartburn and regurgitation

Heartburn describes retrosternal, burning discomfort, often rising up into the chest and sometimes accompanied by regurgitation of acidic or bitter fluid into the throat. These symptoms often occur after meals, on lying down or with bending, straining or heavy lifting. They are classical of gastro-oesophageal reflux but up to 50%

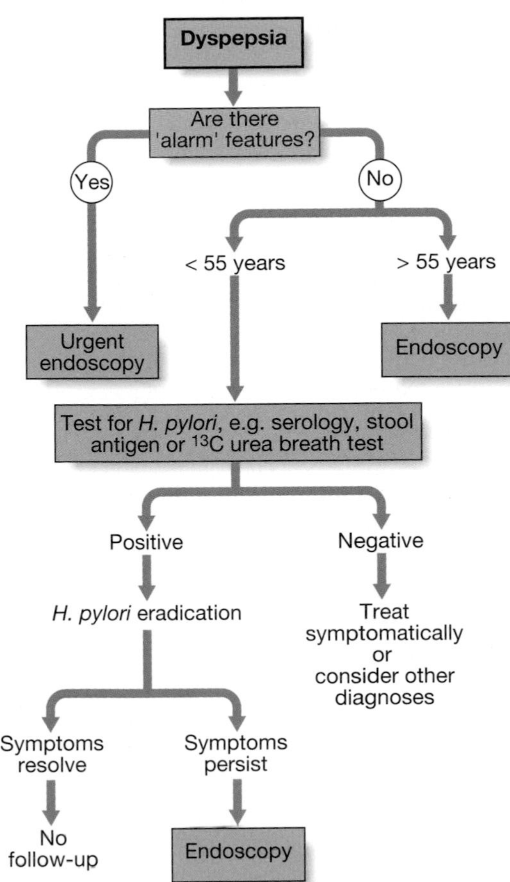

Fig. 22.16 Investigation of dyspepsia.

of patients present with other symptoms, such as chest pain, belching, halitosis, chronic cough or sore throats. In young patients with typical symptoms and a good response to dietary changes, antacids or acid suppression, investigation is not required, but in patients over 55 years of age, those with alarm symptoms or atypical features, urgent endoscopy is necessary.

Vomiting

Vomiting is a complex reflex involving both autonomic and somatic neural pathways. Synchronous contraction of the diaphragm, intercostal muscles and abdominal muscles raises intra-abdominal pressure and, combined with relaxation of the lower oesophageal sphincter, results in forcible ejection of gastric contents. It is important to distinguish true vomiting from regurgitation and to elicit whether the vomiting is acute or chronic (recurrent), as the underlying causes may differ. The major causes are shown in Figure 22.17.

Gastrointestinal bleeding

Acute upper gastrointestinal haemorrhage

This is the most common gastrointestinal emergency, accounting for 50–170 admissions to hospital per 100 000 of the population each year in the UK. The mortality of patients admitted to hospital is about 10% but there is some evidence that outcome is better when patients are treated in specialised units. Risk scoring systems have been developed to stratify risk of needing endoscopic therapy or a poor outcome (Box 22.16). The advantage

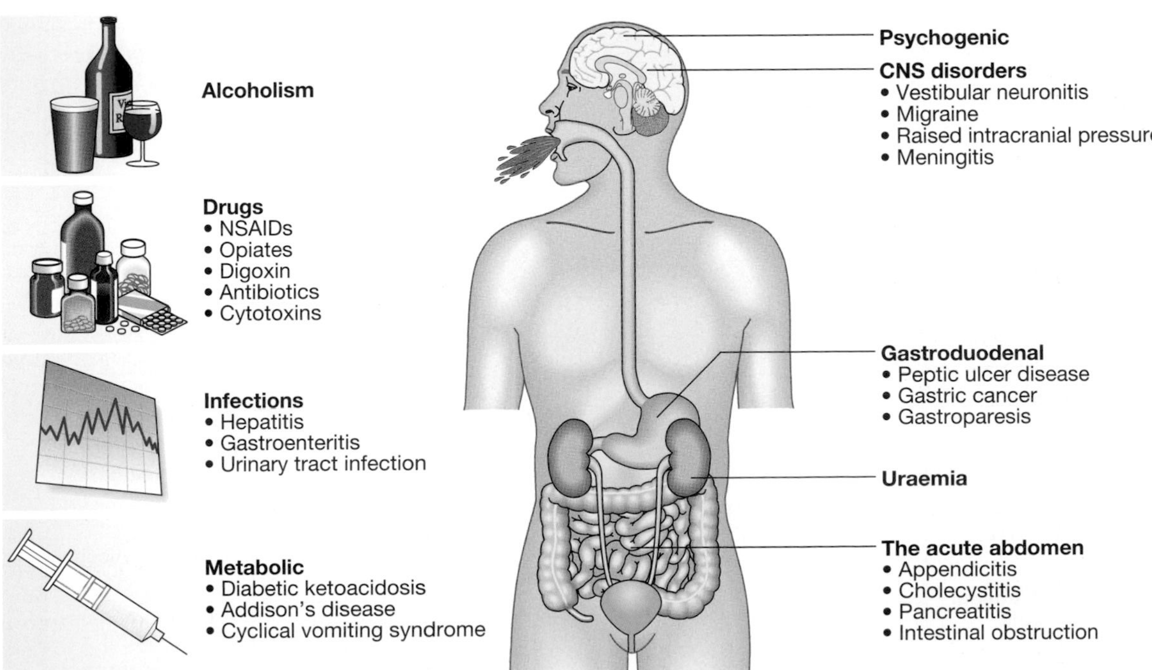

Fig. 22.17 Causes of vomiting.

22.16 Modified Blatchford score: risk stratification in acute upper GI bleeding

Admission risk marker	Score component value
Blood urea	
≥ 25 mmol/L (≥ 70 mg/dL)	6
10–25 mmol/L (28–70 mg/dL)	4
8–10 mmol/L (22.4–28 mg/dL)	3
6·5–8 mmol/L (18.2–22.4 mg/dL)	2
< 6.5 mmol/L (18.2 mg/dL)	0
Haemoglobin for men	
< 100 g/L (10 g/dL)	6
100–119 g/L (10–11.9 g/dL)	3
120–129 g/L (12–12.9 g/dL)	1
≥ 130 g/L (13 g/dL)	0
Haemoglobin for women	
< 100 g/L (10 g/dL)	6
100–119 g/L (10–11.9 g/dL)	1
≥ 120 g/L (12 g/dL)	0
Systolic blood pressure	
< 90 mmHg	3
90–99 mmHg	2
100–109 mmHg	1
> 109 mmHg	0
Other markers	
Presentation with syncope	2
Hepatic disease	2
Cardiac failure	2
Pulse ≥ 100 beats/min	1
Presentation with melaena	1
None of the above	0

of the Blatchford score is that it may be used before endoscopy to predict the need for intervention to treat bleeding. Low scores (2 or less) are associated with a very low risk of adverse outcome. The common causes are shown in Figure 22.18.

Clinical assessment

Haematemesis is red with clots when bleeding is rapid and profuse, or black ('coffee grounds') when less severe. Syncope may occur and is due to hypotension from intravascular volume depletion. Symptoms of anaemia suggest chronic bleeding. Melaena is the passage of black, tarry stools containing altered blood; it is usually caused by bleeding from the upper gastrointestinal tract, although haemorrhage from the right side of the colon is occasionally responsible. The characteristic colour and smell are the result of the action of digestive enzymes and of bacteria upon haemoglobin. Severe acute upper gastrointestinal bleeding can sometimes cause maroon or bright red stool.

Management

The principles of emergency management of non-variceal bleeding are summarised in Box 22.17 and are discussed in detail below. Management of variceal bleeding is discussed on page 946.

1. Intravenous access

The first step is to gain intravenous access using at least one large-bore cannula.

2. Initial clinical assessment

- *Define circulatory status.* Severe bleeding causes tachycardia, hypotension and oliguria. The patient is cold and sweating, and may be agitated.
- *Seek evidence of liver disease* (p. 922). Jaundice, cutaneous stigmata, hepatosplenomegaly and ascites may be present in decompensated cirrhosis.
- *Identify comorbidity.* The presence of cardiorespiratory, cerebrovascular or renal disease is important, both because these may be worsened by acute bleeding and because they increase the hazards of endoscopy and surgical operations.

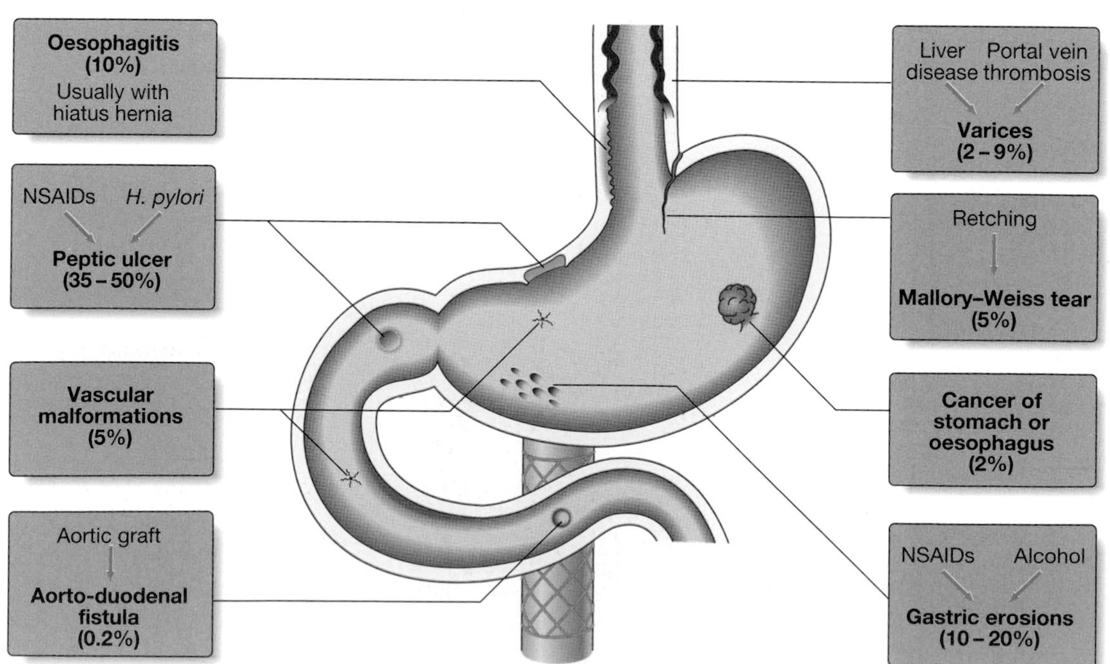

Fig. 22.18 Causes of acute upper gastrointestinal haemorrhage. (Frequency in parentheses.) (NSAIDs = non-steroidal anti-inflammatory drugs)

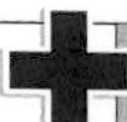

22.17 Emergency management of acute non-variceal upper gastrointestinal haemorrhage

- Gain IV access with large-bore cannula × 2
- Check full blood count, routine biochemistry and coagulation screen; cross-match blood
- Perform hourly measurements of blood pressure, pulse and urine output; consider central venous pressure monitoring in the high-dependency unit for severe bleeding
- Give IV crystalloids in patients with hypotension and tachycardia
- Transfuse with blood if blood pressure remains low and patient is actively bleeding
- Organise endoscopy for diagnosis and treatment once patient is resuscitated
- Give 72-hr proton pump inhibitor IV infusion for bleeding peptic ulcer
- Consider surgery or interventional radiological intervention (e.g. arterial embolisation) if bleeding recurs

These factors can be combined using the Blatchford score (see Box 22.16), which can be calculated at the bedside. A score of less than 3 is associated with a good prognosis, while progressively higher scores are associated with poorer outcomes.

3. Basic investigations

- *Full blood count.* Chronic or subacute bleeding leads to anaemia, but the haemoglobin concentration may be normal after sudden, major bleeding until haemodilution occurs. Thrombocytopenia may be a clue to the presence of hypersplenism in chronic liver disease.
- *Urea and electrolytes.* This test may show evidence of renal failure. The blood urea rises as the absorbed products of luminal blood are metabolised by the liver; an elevated blood urea with normal creatinine concentration implies severe bleeding.
- *Liver function tests.* These may show evidence of chronic liver disease.
- *Prothrombin time.* Check with clinical suggestion of liver disease or in anticoagulated patients.
- *Cross-matching.* At least 2 units of blood should be cross-matched.

4. Resuscitation

Intravenous crystalloid fluids should be given to raise the blood pressure, and blood should be transfused when the patient is actively bleeding with low blood pressure and tachycardia. Comorbidities should be managed as appropriate. Patients with suspected chronic liver disease should receive broad-spectrum antibiotics. Central venous pressure (CVP) monitoring may be useful in severe bleeding, particularly in patients with cardiac disease, to assist in defining the volume of fluid replacement and in identifying rebleeding.

5. Oxygen

This should be given to all patients in shock.

6. Endoscopy

This should be carried out after adequate resuscitation, ideally within 24 hours, and will yield a diagnosis in 80% of cases. Patients who are found to have major endoscopic stigmata of recent haemorrhage (Fig. 22.19) can be treated endoscopically using a thermal or mechanical modality, such as a 'heater probe' or endoscopic clips, combined with injection of dilute adrenaline (epinephrine) into the bleeding point ('dual therapy'). This may stop active bleeding and, combined with intravenous proton pump inhibitor (PPI) therapy, prevent rebleeding, thus avoiding the need for surgery (Boxes 22.18 and 22.19). Patients found to have bled from varices should be treated by band ligation (p. 946).

7. Monitoring

Patients should be closely observed, with hourly measurements of pulse, blood pressure and urine output.

EBM 22.18 Single versus dual modality endoscopic therapy in high-risk bleeding ulcers

'Adding a second procedure to adrenaline (epinephrine) injection further reduces bleeding rates from 18.5% to 10% (relative risk 0.55) and emergency surgery from 10.8% to 6.7% (relative risk 0.69). Mortality falls from 4.7% to 2.5% (relative risk 0.52; 95% confidence interval 0.38 to 1.05), without statistical significance. The risk of further bleeding decreased, regardless of which second procedure was applied (clips or thermal).'

- Vergara M, et al. Epinephrine injection versus epinephrine injection and a second endoscopic method in high risk bleeding ulcers. Cochrane Database of Systematic Reviews, 2007, issue 2. Art. no. CD005584 (updated 2009).

For further information: www.cochrane.org/cochrane-reviews

22

A
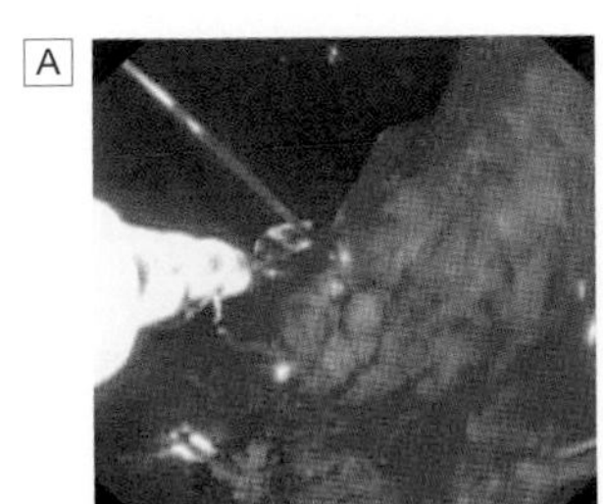
B
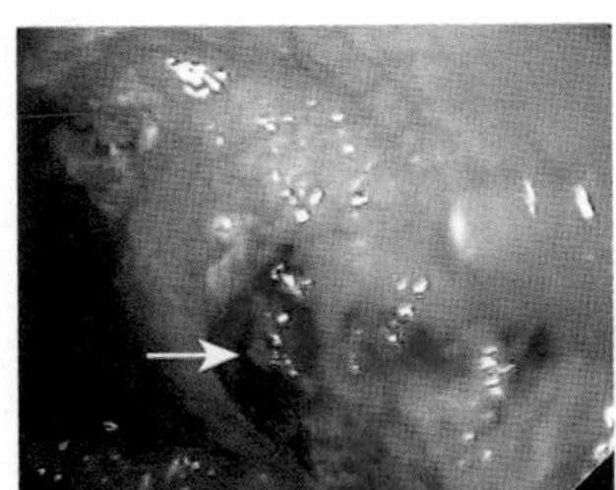
C
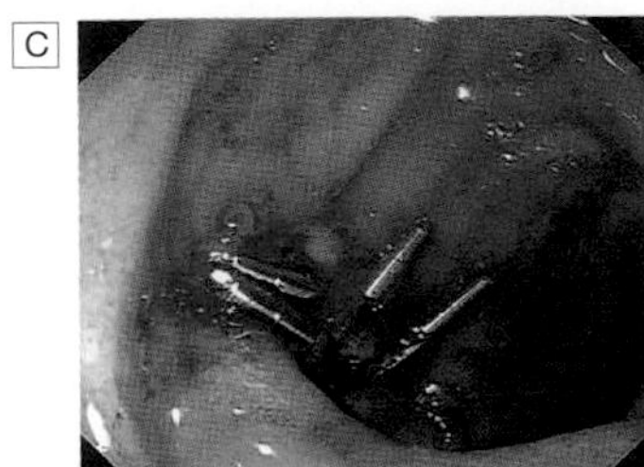

Fig. 22.19 Major stigmata of recent haemorrhage and endoscopic treatment. **A** Active arterial spurting from a gastric ulcer. An endoscopic clip is about to be placed on the bleeding vessel. When associated with shock, 80% of cases will continue to bleed or rebleed. **B** 'Visible vessel' (arrow). In reality, this is a pseudoaneurysm of the feeding artery seen here in a pre-pyloric peptic ulcer. It carries a 50% chance of rebleeding. **C** Haemostasis is achieved after endoscopic clipping of the bleeding vessel in the duodenum.

EBM 22.19 Adjunctive drug therapy for bleeding ulcers

'Intravenous proton pump inhibitor infusions reduce rebleeding ($NNT_B = 12$) and need for surgery ($NNT_B = 20$), but not mortality, in patients who have been subjected to endoscopic therapy for major peptic ulcer haemorrhage. When given prior to endoscopy, they reduce the need for endoscopic therapy and hospital stay, but not the need for surgery or mortality.'

- Leontiadis GI, et al. BMJ 2005; 330:568–575.
- Lau JY, et al. New Engl J Med 2007; 356:1631–1640.

For further information: www.sign.ac.uk

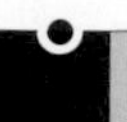

22.20 Causes of lower gastrointestinal bleeding

Severe acute	
• Diverticular disease • Angiodysplasia • Ischaemia	• Meckel's diverticulum • Inflammatory bowel disease (rarely)
Moderate, chronic/subacute	
• Fissure • Haemorrhoids • Inflammatory bowel disease • Carcinoma	• Large polyps • Angiodysplasia • Radiation enteritis • Solitary rectal ulcer

8. Surgery

Surgery is indicated when endoscopic haemostasis fails to stop active bleeding and if rebleeding occurs on one occasion in an elderly or frail patient, or twice in a younger, fitter patient. If available, angiographic embolisation is an effective alternative to surgery in frail patients.

The choice of operation depends on the site and diagnosis of the bleeding lesion. Duodenal ulcers are treated by under-running, with or without pyloroplasty. Under-running for gastric ulcers can also be carried out (a biopsy must be taken to exclude carcinoma). Local excision may be performed, but when neither is possible, partial gastrectomy is required. Following surgery for ulcer bleeding, all patients should be treated with *H. pylori* eradication therapy if they test positive for it, and should avoid NSAIDs. Successful eradication should be confirmed by urea breath or faecal antigen testing.

Lower gastrointestinal bleeding

This may be due to haemorrhage from the colon, anal canal or small bowel. It is useful to distinguish those patients who present with profuse, acute bleeding from those who present with chronic or subacute bleeding of lesser severity (Box 22.20).

Severe acute lower gastrointestinal bleeding

This presents with profuse red or maroon diarrhoea and with shock. Diverticular disease is the most common cause and is often due to erosion of an artery within the mouth of a diverticulum. Bleeding almost always stops spontaneously, but if it does not, the diseased segment of colon should be resected after confirmation of the site by angiography or colonoscopy. Angiodysplasia is a disease of the elderly, in which vascular malformations develop in the proximal colon. Bleeding can be acute and profuse; it usually stops spontaneously but commonly recurs. Diagnosis is often difficult. Colonoscopy may reveal characteristic vascular spots and, in the acute phase, visceral angiography can show bleeding into the intestinal lumen and an abnormal large, draining vein. In some patients, diagnosis is only achieved by laparotomy with on-table colonoscopy. The treatment of choice is endoscopic thermal ablation, but resection of the affected bowel may be required if bleeding continues. Bowel ischaemia due to occlusion of the inferior mesenteric artery can present with abdominal colic and rectal bleeding. It should be considered in patients (particularly the elderly) who have evidence of generalised atherosclerosis. The diagnosis is made at colonoscopy. Resection is required only in the presence of peritonitis. Meckel's diverticulum with ectopic gastric epithelium may ulcerate and erode into a major artery. The diagnosis should be considered in children or adolescents who present with profuse or recurrent lower gastrointestinal bleeding. A Meckel's ^{99m}Tc-pertechnate scan is sometimes positive but the diagnosis is commonly made only by laparotomy, at which time the diverticulum is excised.

Subacute or chronic lower gastrointestinal bleeding

This can occur at all ages and is usually due to haemorrhoids or anal fissure. Haemorrhoidal bleeding is bright red and occurs during or after defecation. Proctoscopy can be used to make the diagnosis but subjects who have altered bowel habit and those who present over the age of 40 years should undergo colonoscopy to exclude coexisting colorectal cancer. Anal fissure should be suspected when fresh rectal bleeding and anal pain occur during defecation.

Major gastrointestinal bleeding of unknown cause

In some patients who present with major gastrointestinal bleeding, upper endoscopy and colonoscopy fail to reveal a diagnosis. When severe life-threatening bleeding continues, urgent CT mesenteric angiography is indicated. This will usually identify the site if the bleeding rate exceeds 1 mL/min and then formal angiographic embolisation can often stop the bleeding. If angiography is negative or bleeding is less severe, push or double balloon enteroscopy can visualise the small intestine (Fig. 22.20) and treat the bleeding source. Wireless capsule endoscopy is often used to define a source of bleeding prior to enteroscopy. When all else fails, laparotomy with on-table endoscopy is indicated.

Chronic occult gastrointestinal bleeding

In this context, occult means that blood or its breakdown products are present in the stool but cannot be seen by the naked eye. Occult bleeding may reach 200 mL per day and cause iron deficiency anaemia. Any cause of gastrointestinal bleeding may be responsible but the most important is colorectal cancer, particularly carcinoma of the caecum, which may produce no gastrointestinal symptoms. In clinical practice, investigation of

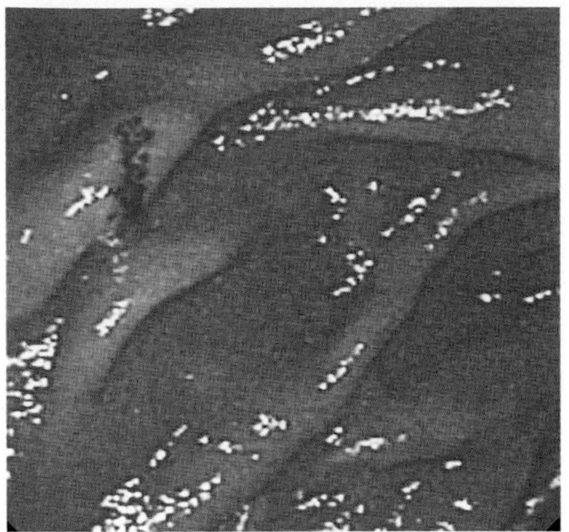

Fig. 22.20 Jejunal angiodysplastic lesion seen at enteroscopy in a patient with recurrent obscure bleeding.

the upper and lower gastrointestinal tract should be considered whenever a patient presents with unexplained iron deficiency anaemia. Testing the stool for the presence of blood is unnecessary and should not influence whether or not the gastrointestinal tract is imaged because bleeding from tumours is often intermittent and a negative faecal occult blood (FOB) test does not exclude the diagnosis. The only value of FOB testing is as a means of population screening for colonic neoplasia in asymptomatic individuals (p. 916).

Diarrhoea

Diarrhoea is defined as the passage of more than 200 g of stool daily, and measurement of stool volume is helpful in confirming this. The most severe symptom in many patients is urgency of defecation, and faecal incontinence is a common event in acute and chronic diarrhoeal illnesses.

Acute diarrhoea

This is extremely common and is usually due to faecal–oral transmission of bacteria or their toxins, viruses or parasites (Ch. 13). Infective diarrhoea is usually short-lived and patients who present with a history of diarrhoea lasting more than 10 days rarely have an infective cause. A variety of drugs, including antibiotics, cytotoxic drugs, PPIs and NSAIDs, may be responsible.

Chronic or relapsing diarrhoea

The most common cause is irritable bowel syndrome (p. 907), which can present with increased frequency of defecation and loose, watery or pellety stools. Diarrhoea rarely occurs at night and is most severe before and after breakfast. At other times, the patient is constipated and there are other characteristic symptoms of irritable bowel syndrome. The stool often contains mucus but never blood, and 24-hour stool volume is less than 200 g. Chronic diarrhoea can be categorised as being due to disease of the colon or small bowel, or to malabsorption (Box 22.21). Clinical presentation, examination of the stool, routine blood tests and imaging reveal a diagnosis in many cases. A series of negative investigations usually implies irritable bowel syndrome but some patients clearly have organic disease and need more extensive investigations.

Malabsorption

Diarrhoea and weight loss in patients with a normal diet is likely to be caused by malabsorption. The symptoms are diverse in nature and variable in severity. A few patients have apparently normal bowel habit but diarrhoea is usual and may be watery and voluminous. Bulky, pale and offensive stools which float in the toilet (steatorrhoea) signify fat malabsorption. Abdominal distension, borborygmi, cramps, weight loss and undigested food in the stool may be present. Some patients complain only of malaise and lethargy. In others,

22.21 Chronic or relapsing diarrhoea

	Colonic	Malabsorption	Small bowel
Clinical features	Blood and mucus in stool Cramping lower abdominal pain	Steatorrhoea Undigested food in the stool Weight loss and nutritional disturbances	Large-volume, watery stool Abdominal bloating Cramping mid-abdominal pain

Some causes	Inflammatory bowel disease
	Microscopic colitis
	Neoplasia
	Ischaemia
	Irritable bowel syndrome
		Pancreatic
		  Chronic pancreatitis
		  Cancer of pancreas
		  Cystic fibrosis
		Enteropathy
		  Coeliac disease
		  Tropical sprue
		  Lymphoma
		Lymphangiectasia
			Crohn's disease
			VIPoma
			Drug-induced
			  NSAIDs
			  Aminosalicylates
			  Selective serotonin re-uptake inhibitors (SSRIs)

Investigations	Faecal calprotectin Ileocolonoscopy with biopsies	Faecal elastase Ultrasound, CT and MRCP Small-bowel biopsy Barium follow-through or small-bowel MRI	Faecal calprotectin Stool volume Gut hormone profile Barium follow-through or small-bowel MRI

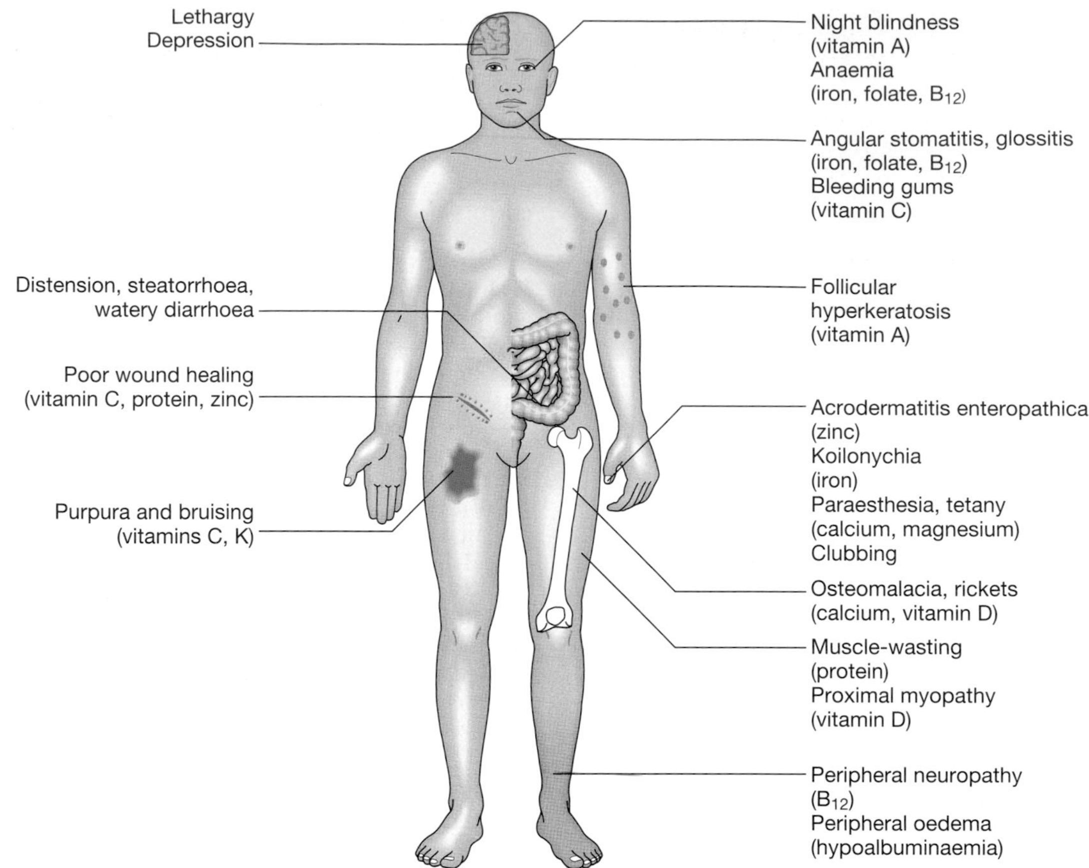

Fig. 22.21 Possible physical consequences of malabsorption.

symptoms related to deficiencies of specific vitamins, trace elements and minerals may occur (Fig. 22.21).

Pathophysiology

Malabsorption results from abnormalities of the three processes which are essential to normal digestion:

1. *Intraluminal maldigestion* occurs when deficiency of bile or pancreatic enzymes results in inadequate solubilisation and hydrolysis of nutrients. Fat and protein malabsorption results. This may also occur with small bowel bacterial overgrowth.
2. *Mucosal malabsorption* results from small bowel resection or conditions which damage the small intestinal epithelium, thereby diminishing the surface area for absorption and depleting brush border enzyme activity.
3. *'Post-mucosal' lymphatic obstruction* prevents the uptake and transport of absorbed lipids into lymphatic vessels. Increased pressure in these vessels results in leakage into the intestinal lumen, leading to protein-losing enteropathy.

Investigations

Investigations should be performed both to confirm the presence of malabsorption and to determine the underlying cause. Routine blood tests may show one or more of the abnormalities listed in Box 22.22. Tests to confirm fat and protein malabsorption should be performed, as described on page 851. An approach to the investigation of malabsorption is shown in Figure 22.22.

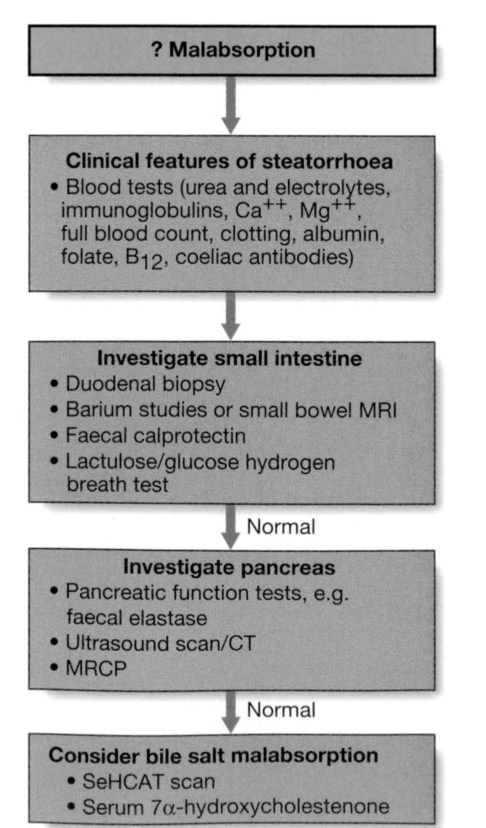

Fig. 22.22 Investigation for suspected malabsorption.

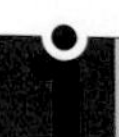

22.22 Routine blood test abnormalities in malabsorption

Haematology

- Microcytic anaemia (iron deficiency)
- Macrocytic anaemia (folate or B_{12} deficiency)
- Increased prothrombin time (vitamin K deficiency)

Biochemistry

- Hypoalbuminaemia
- Hypocalcaemia (p. 768)
- Hypomagnesaemia
- Hypophosphataemia
- Low serum zinc

Weight loss

Weight loss may be physiological, due to dieting, exercise, starvation, or the decreased nutritional intake which accompanies old age. Weight loss of more than 3 kg over 6 months is significant and often indicates the presence of an underlying disease. Hospital and general practice weight records may be valuable in confirming that weight loss has occurred, as may reweighing patients at intervals; sometimes weight is regained or stabilises in those with no obvious cause. Pathological weight loss can be due to psychiatric illness, systemic disease, gastrointestinal causes or advanced disease of many organ systems (Fig. 22.23).

Physiological

Weight loss can occur in the absence of serious disease in healthy individuals who have changes in physical activity or social circumstances. It may be difficult to be sure of this diagnosis in older patients, when the dietary history may be unreliable, and professional help from a dietitian is often valuable under these circumstances.

Psychiatric illness

Features of anorexia nervosa (p. 255), bulimia (p. 256) and affective disorders (p. 243) may only be apparent after formal psychiatric input. Alcoholic patients lose weight as a consequence of self-neglect and poor dietary intake. Depression may cause weight loss.

Systemic diseases

Chronic infections, including tuberculosis (p. 688), recurrent urinary or chest infections, and a range of parasitic and protozoan infections (Ch. 13), should be considered. A history of foreign travel, high-risk activities and specific features, such as fever, night sweats, rigors, productive cough and dysuria, must be sought. Promiscuous sexual activity and drug misuse suggest HIV-related illness (Ch. 14). Weight loss is a late feature of disseminated malignancy, but by the time the patient presents, other features of cancer are often present. Chronic inflammatory diseases, such as rheumatoid arthritis (p. 1096), and polymyalgia rheumatica (p. 1117) are often associated with weight loss.

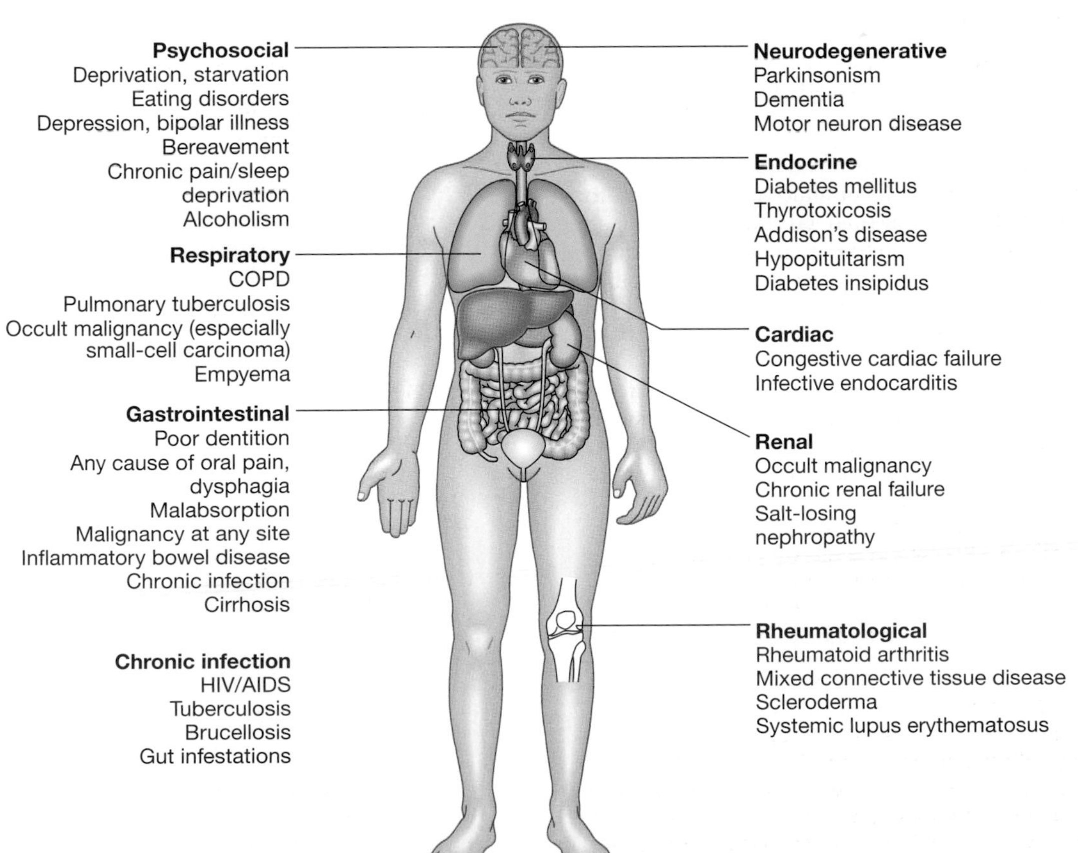

Fig. 22.23 Some important causes of weight loss.

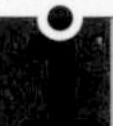

22.23 Some easily overlooked causes of unexplained weight loss

- Depression/anxiety
- Chronic pain or sleep deprivation
- Psychosocial deprivation/malnutrition in the elderly
- Existing conditions (severe chronic obstructive pulmonary disease, cardiac failure)
- Diabetes mellitus/hyperthyroidism
- Occult malignancy
- Anorexia nervosa in atypical groups
- Addison's disease/panhypopituitarism

Gastrointestinal disease

Almost any disease of the gastrointestinal tract can cause weight loss. Dysphagia and gastric outflow obstruction (pp. 851 and 875) cause weight loss by reducing food intake. Malignancy at any site may cause weight loss by mechanical obstruction, anorexia or cytokine-mediated systemic effects. Malabsorption from pancreatic diseases (p. 889) or small bowel causes may lead to profound weight loss with specific nutritional deficiencies (Ch. 5). Inflammatory diseases, such as Crohn's disease or ulcerative colitis (p. 897), cause anorexia, fear of eating and loss of protein, blood and nutrients from the gut.

Metabolic disorders and miscellaneous causes

Weight loss may occur in association with metabolic disorders, as well as end-stage respiratory and cardiac disease. Some easily overlooked causes of weight loss are listed in Box 22.23.

Investigations

In cases where the cause of weight loss is not obvious after thorough history-taking and physical examination, or where an existing condition is considered unlikely, the following investigations are indicated: urinalysis for sugar, protein and blood; blood tests, including liver function tests, random blood glucose and thyroid function tests; CRP and ESR (may be raised in unsuspected infections, such as tuberculosis, connective tissue disorders and malignancy); and faecal calprotectin. Sometimes invasive tests, such as bone marrow aspiration or liver biopsy, may be necessary to identify conditions like cryptic miliary tuberculosis (p. 689). Rarely, abdominal and pelvic imaging by CT may be necessary, but before embarking on invasive or very costly investigations, it is always worth revisiting the patient's history and reweighing at intervals.

Constipation

Constipation is defined as infrequent passage of hard stools. Patients may also complain of straining, a sensation of incomplete evacuation and either perianal or abdominal discomfort. Constipation may occur in many gastrointestinal and other medical disorders (Box 22.24).

Clinical assessment and management

The onset, duration and characteristics are important; for example, a neonatal onset suggests Hirschsprung's disease, while a recent change in bowel activity in middle age should raise the suspicion of organic disorders, such as colonic carcinoma. The presence of rectal bleeding, pain and weight loss is important, as are excessive straining, symptoms suggestive of irritable bowel syndrome, a history of childhood constipation and emotional distress.

Careful examination contributes more to the diagnosis than extensive investigation. A search should be made for general medical disorders, as well as signs of intestinal obstruction. Neurological disorders, especially spinal cord lesions, should be sought. Perineal inspection and rectal examination are essential and may reveal abnormalities of the pelvic floor (abnormal descent, impaired sensation), anal canal or rectum (masses, faecal impaction, prolapse).

It is neither possible nor appropriate to investigate every person with constipation. Most respond to increased fluid intake, dietary fibre supplementation, exercise and the judicious use of laxatives. Middle-aged or elderly patients with a short history or worrying symptoms (rectal bleeding, pain or weight loss) must be investigated promptly, by either barium enema or colonoscopy. For those with simple constipation, investigation will usually proceed along the following lines.

Initial visit

Digital rectal examination, proctoscopy and sigmoidoscopy (to detect anorectal disease), routine biochemistry, including serum calcium and thyroid function tests, and a full blood count should be carried out. If these are normal, a 1-month trial of dietary fibre and/or laxatives is justified.

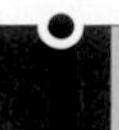

22.24 Causes of constipation

Gastrointestinal disorders	
Dietary	
• Lack of fibre and/or fluid intake	
Motility	
• Slow-transit constipation • Irritable bowel syndrome • Drugs (see below)	• Chronic intestinal pseudo-obstruction
Structural	
• Colonic carcinoma • Diverticular disease	• Hirschsprung's disease
Defecation	
• Anorectal disease (Crohn's, fissures, haemorrhoids)	• Obstructed defecation
Non-gastrointestinal disorders	
Drugs	
• Opiates • Anticholinergics • Calcium antagonists	• Iron supplements • Aluminium-containing antacids
Neurological	
• Multiple sclerosis • Spinal cord lesions	• Cerebrovascular accidents • Parkinsonism
Metabolic/endocrine	
• Diabetes mellitus • Hypercalcaemia	• Hypothyroidism • Pregnancy
Others	
• Any serious illness with immobility, especially in the elderly	• Depression

Next visit

If symptoms persist, then examination of the colon by barium enema or CT colonography is indicated to look for structural disease.

Further investigation

If no cause is found and disabling symptoms are present, then specialist referral for investigation of possible dysmotility may be necessary. The problem may be one of infrequent desire to defecate ('slow transit') or else may result from neuromuscular incoordination and excessive straining ('functional obstructive defecation', p. 913). Intestinal marker studies, anorectal manometry, electrophysiological studies and magnetic resonance proctography can all be used to define the problem.

Abdominal pain

There are four types of abdominal pain:

- *Visceral*. Gut organs are insensitive to stimuli such as burning and cutting but are sensitive to distension, contraction, twisting and stretching. Pain from unpaired structures is usually but not always felt in the midline.
- *Parietal*. The parietal peritoneum is innervated by somatic nerves, and its involvement by inflammation, infection or neoplasia causes sharp, well-localised and lateralised pain.
- *Referred pain*. (For example, gallbladder pain is referred to the back or shoulder tip.)
- *Psychogenic*. Cultural, emotional and psychosocial factors influence everyone's experience of pain. In some patients, no organic cause can be found despite investigation, and psychogenic causes (depression or somatisation disorder) may be responsible (pp. 235 and 245).

The acute abdomen

This accounts for approximately 50% of all urgent admissions to general surgical units. The acute abdomen is a consequence of one or more pathological processes (Box 22.25):

- *Inflammation*. Pain develops gradually, usually over several hours. It is initially rather diffuse until the parietal peritoneum is involved, when it becomes localised. Movement exacerbates the pain; abdominal rigidity and guarding occur.
- *Perforation*. When a viscus perforates, pain starts abruptly; it is severe and leads to generalised peritonitis.
- *Obstruction*. Pain is colicky, with spasms which cause the patient to writhe around and double up. Colicky pain which does not disappear between spasms suggests complicating inflammation.

22.25 Causes of acute abdominal pain

Inflammation	
• Appendicitis • Diverticulitis • Cholecystitis • Pelvic inflammatory disease	• Pancreatitis • Pyelonephritis • Intra-abdominal abscess
Perforation/rupture	
• Peptic ulcer • Diverticular disease	• Ovarian cyst • Aortic aneurysm
Obstruction	
• Intestinal obstruction • Biliary colic	• Ureteric colic
Other (rare)	
• See Box 22.27	

Initial clinical assessment

If there are signs of peritonitis (guarding and rebound tenderness with rigidity), the patient should be resuscitated with oxygen, intravenous fluids and antibiotics. In other circumstances, further investigations are required (Fig. 22.24).

Investigations

Patients should have a full blood count, urea and electrolytes, and amylase taken to look for evidence of dehydration, leucocytosis and pancreatitis. An erect chest X-ray may show air under the diaphragm, suggestive of perforation, and a plain abdominal film may show evidence of obstruction or ileus. An abdominal ultrasound may help if gallstones or renal stones are suspected. Ultrasonography is also useful in the detection of free fluid and any possible intra-abdominal abscess. Contrast studies, by either mouth or anus, are useful in the further evaluation of intestinal obstruction, and essential in the differentiation of pseudo-obstruction from mechanical large-bowel obstruction. Other investigations commonly used include CT (seeking evidence of pancreatitis, retroperitoneal collections or masses, including an aortic aneurysm) and angiography (mesenteric ischaemia).

Diagnostic laparotomy should be considered when the diagnosis has not been revealed by other investigations. All patients must be carefully and regularly re-assessed (every 2–4 hours) so that any change in condition that might alter both the suspected diagnosis and clinical decision can be observed and acted upon early.

Management

The general approach is to close perforations, treat inflammatory conditions with antibiotics or resection, and relieve obstructions. The speed of intervention and the necessity for surgery depend on the organ that is involved and on a number of other factors, of which the presence or absence of peritonitis is the most important. A treatment summary of some of the more common surgical conditions follows.

Acute appendicitis

This should be treated by early surgery, since there is a risk of perforation and recurrent attacks with non-operative treatment. The appendix can be removed through a conventional right iliac fossa skin crease incision or by laparoscopic techniques.

Acute cholecystitis

This can be successfully treated non-operatively but the high risk of recurrent attacks and the low morbidity of

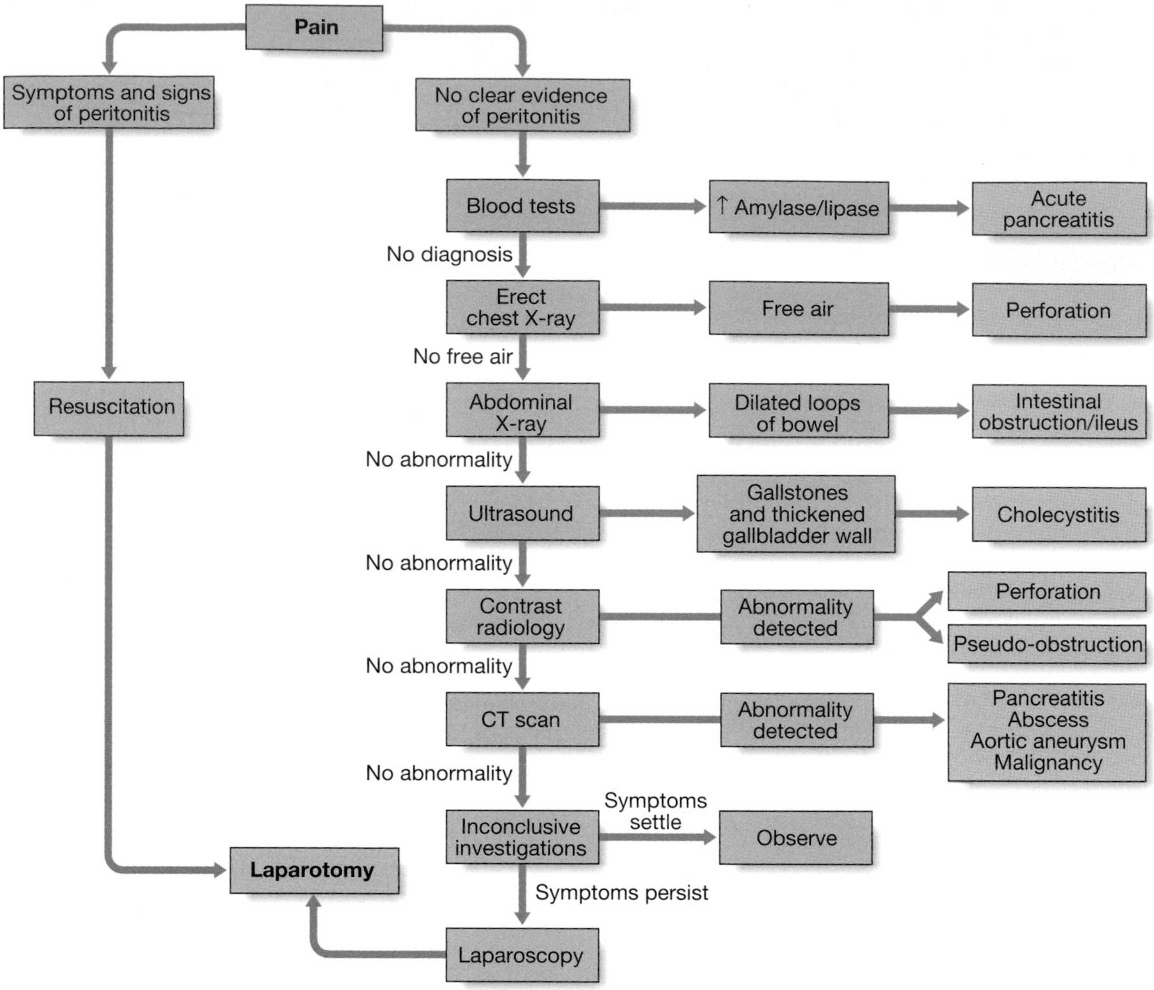

Pain
Symptoms and signs of peritonitis
No clear evidence of peritonitis
Blood tests
↑ Amylase/lipase
Acute pancreatitis
No diagnosis
Erect chest X-ray
Free air
Perforation
No free air
Resuscitation
Abdominal X-ray
Dilated loops of bowel
Intestinal obstruction/ileus
No abnormality
Ultrasound
Gallstones and thickened gallbladder wall
Cholecystitis
No abnormality
Contrast radiology
Abnormality detected
Perforation
Pseudo-obstruction
No abnormality
CT scan
Abnormality detected
Pancreatitis
Abscess
Aortic aneurysm
Malignancy
No abnormality
Inconclusive investigations
Symptoms settle
Observe
Laparotomy
Symptoms persist
Laparoscopy

Fig. 22.24 **Management of acute abdominal pain: an algorithm.**

surgery have made early laparoscopic cholecystectomy the treatment of choice.

Acute diverticulitis

Conservative therapy is standard but if perforation has occurred, resection is advisable. Depending on peritoneal contamination and the state of the patient, primary anastomosis is preferable to a Hartmann's procedure (oversew of rectal stump and end colostomy).

Small bowel obstruction

If the cause is obvious and surgery inevitable (such as with a strangulated hernia), an early operation is appropriate. If the suspected cause is adhesions from previous surgery, only those patients who do not resolve within the first 48 hours or who develop signs of strangulation (colicky pain becomes constant, peritonitis, tachycardia, fever, leucocytosis) should have surgery.

Large bowel obstruction

Pseudo-obstruction should be treated non-operatively. Some patients benefit from colonoscopic decompression, but mechanical obstruction merits resection, usually with a primary anastomosis. Differentiation between the two is made by water-soluble contrast enema.

22.26 Acute abdominal pain in old age

- **Presentation**: severity and localisation may blunt with age. Presentation may be atypical, even with perforation of a viscus.
- **Cancer**: a more common cause of acute pain in those over 70 yrs than in those under 50 yrs. Older people with vague abdominal symptoms should therefore be carefully assessed.
- **Non-specific symptoms**: intra-abdominal inflammatory conditions, such as diverticulitis, may present with non-specific symptoms, such as acute confusion or anorexia and relatively little abdominal tenderness. The reasons for this are not clear but may result from altered sensory perception.
- **Outcome of abdominal surgery**: determined by the degree of comorbid disease and whether surgery is elective or emergency, rather than by chronological age.

Perforated peptic ulcer

Surgical closure of the perforation is standard practice but some patients without generalised peritonitis can be treated non-operatively once a water-soluble contrast meal has confirmed spontaneous sealing of the perforation. Adequate and aggressive resuscitation with intravenous fluids, antibiotics and analgesia is mandatory before surgery.

For a more detailed discussion of acute abdominal pain, the reader is referred to the sister volume of this text, *Principles and Practice of Surgery*.

Chronic or recurrent abdominal pain

It is essential to take a detailed history, paying particular attention to features of the pain and any associated symptoms (Boxes 22.27 and 22.28).

Note should be made of the patient's general demeanour, mood and emotional state, signs of weight loss, fever, jaundice or anaemia. If a thorough abdominal and rectal examination is normal, a careful search should be made for evidence of disease affecting other structures, particularly the vertebral column, spinal cord, lungs and cardiovascular system.

Investigations will depend on the clinical features elicited during the history and examination:

- Endoscopy and ultrasound are indicated for epigastric pain, and for dyspepsia and symptoms suggestive of gallbladder disease
- Colonoscopy is indicated for patients with altered bowel habit, rectal bleeding or features of obstruction suggesting colonic disease.
- CT or MR angiography should be considered when pain is provoked by food in a patient with widespread atherosclerosis, since this may indicate mesenteric ischaemia.
- Persistent symptoms require exclusion of colonic or small bowel disease. However, young patients with pain relieved by defecation, bloating and alternating bowel habit are likely to have irritable bowel syndrome (p. 907). Simple investigations (blood tests, faecal calprotectin and sigmoidoscopy) are sufficient in the absence of rectal bleeding, weight loss and abnormal physical findings.
- Ultrasound, CT and faecal elastase are required for patients with upper abdominal pain radiating to the back. A history of alcohol misuse, weight loss and diarrhoea suggests chronic pancreatitis or pancreatic cancer.
- Recurrent attacks of pain in the loins radiating to the flanks with urinary symptoms should prompt investigation for renal or ureteric stones by abdominal X-ray, ultrasound and CT urography.
- A past history of psychiatric disturbance, repeated negative investigations or vague symptoms which do not fit any disease or organ pattern suggest a psychological origin for the pain (p. 236). Careful review of case notes and previous investigations, along with open and honest discussion with the patient, reduces the need for further cycles of unnecessary and invasive tests. Care must always be taken, however, not to miss rare pathology or atypical presentations of common diseases.

22.27 Extra-intestinal causes of chronic or recurrent abdominal pain

Retroperitoneal	
• Aortic aneurysm • Malignancy	• Lymphadenopathy • Abscess
Psychogenic	
• Depression • Anxiety	• Hypochondriasis • Somatisation
Locomotor	
• Vertebral compression/fracture	• Abdominal muscle strain
Metabolic/endocrine	
• Diabetes mellitus • Addison's disease	• Acute intermittent porphyria • Hypercalcaemia
Drugs/toxins	
• Corticosteroids • Azathioprine	• Lead • Alcohol
Haematological	
• Sickle-cell disease	• Haemolytic disorders
Neurological	
• Spinal cord lesions • Tabes dorsalis	• Radiculopathy

22.28 How to assess abdominal pain

- Duration
- Site and radiation
- Severity
- Precipitating and relieving factors (food, drugs, alcohol, posture, movement, defecation)
- Nature (colicky, constant, sharp or dull, wakes patient at night)
- Pattern (intermittent or continuous)
- Associated features (vomiting, dyspepsia, altered bowel habit)

Constant abdominal pain

Patients with chronic pain that is constant or nearly always present usually have features to suggest the underlying diagnosis. In a minority, no cause will be found, despite thorough investigation, leading to the diagnosis of 'chronic functional abdominal pain'. In these patients, there appears to be abnormal CNS processing of normal visceral afferent sensory input, psychosocial factors are often operative (p. 240), and the most important tasks are to provide symptom control, if not relief, and to minimise the effects of the pain on social, personal and occupational life. Patients are best managed in specialised pain clinics where, in addition to psychological support, appropriate use of drugs, including tricyclic antidepressants, gabapentin or pregabalin, ketamine and opioids, may be necessary.

DISEASES OF THE MOUTH AND SALIVARY GLANDS

Aphthous ulceration

Aphthous ulcers are superficial and painful; they occur in any part of the mouth. Recurrent ulcers afflict up to 30% of the population and are particularly common in women prior to menstruation. The cause is unknown, but in severe cases other causes of oral ulceration must be considered (Box 22.29). Occasionally, biopsy is necessary for diagnosis.

22.29 Causes of oral ulceration

Aphthous	
• Idiopathic	• Premenstrual
Infection	
• Fungal (candidiasis) • Viral (herpes simplex, HIV)	• Bacterial, including syphilis, tuberculosis
Gastrointestinal diseases	
• Crohn's disease	• Coeliac disease
Dermatological conditions	
• Lichen planus • Immunobullous disorders (p. 1292)	• Dermatitis herpetiformis • Erythema multiforme
Drugs	
• Nicorandil, NSAIDs, methotrexate, penicillamine, losartan, ACE inhibitors	• Stevens–Johnson syndrome (pp. 1264 and 1302) • Cytotoxic drugs
Systemic diseases	
• Systemic lupus erythematosus (p. 1109)	• Behçet's syndrome (p. 1119)
Neoplasia	
• Carcinoma • Leukaemia	• Kaposi's sarcoma

(ACE = angiotensin-converting enzyme; NSAIDs = non-steroidal anti-inflammatory drugs)

Management is with topical corticosteroids (such as 0.1% triamcinolone in Orabase) or choline salicylate (8.7%) gel. Symptomatic relief is achieved using local anaesthetic mouthwashes. Rarely, patients with very severe, recurrent aphthous ulcers may need oral corticosteroids.

Oral cancer

Squamous carcinoma of the oral cavity is common worldwide and the incidence has increased by 25% in the last decade in the UK. The mortality rate is around 50%, largely as a result of late diagnosis. Poor diet, alcohol excess and smoking or tobacco chewing are the traditional risk factors but high-risk, oncogenic strains of human papillomavirus (HPV-16 and HPV-18) have been identified as responsible for much of the recent increase in incidence, especially in cases affecting the base of tongue, soft palate and tonsils. In parts of Asia, the disease is common among people who chew areca nuts wrapped in leaves of the betel plant ('betel nuts').

Oral cancer may present in many ways (Box 22.30) and a high index of suspicion is required. Patients with suspicious lesions should have all possible sources of local trauma or infection treated and should be reviewed after 2 weeks, with biopsy if the lesion persists. Small cancers can be resected but extensive surgery, with neck dissection to remove involved lymph nodes, may be necessary. Some patients can be treated with radical radiotherapy alone, and sometimes radiotherapy is also given after surgery to treat microscopic residual disease. Some tumours may be amenable to photodynamic therapy (PDT), avoiding the need for surgery.

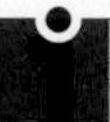

22.30 Symptoms and signs of oral cancer

- Solitary ulcer without precipitant, e.g. local trauma
- Solitary white patch ('leukoplakia') which fails to wipe off
- Solitary red patch
- Fixed lump
- Lip numbness in absence of trauma or infection
- Trismus (painful/difficult mouth opening)
- Cervical lymphadenopathy

Candidiasis

The yeast *Candida albicans* is a normal mouth commensal but it may proliferate to cause thrush. This occurs in babies, debilitated patients, patients receiving corticosteroid or antibiotic therapy, patients with diabetes and immunosuppressed patients, especially those receiving cytotoxic therapy and those with HIV infection. White patches are seen on the tongue and buccal mucosa. Odynophagia or dysphagia suggests pharyngeal and oesophageal candidiasis. A clinical diagnosis is sufficient to instigate therapy, although brushings or biopsies can be obtained for mycological examination. Oral thrush is treated using nystatin or amphotericin suspensions or lozenges. Resistant cases or immunosuppressed patients may require oral fluconazole.

Parotitis

Parotitis is due to viral or bacterial infection. Mumps causes a self-limiting acute parotitis (p. 319). Bacterial parotitis usually occurs as a complication of major surgery. It is a consequence of dehydration and poor oral hygiene, and can be avoided by good post-operative care. Patients present with painful parotid swelling and this can be complicated by abscess formation. Broad-spectrum antibiotics are required, whilst surgical drainage is necessary for abscesses. Other causes of salivary gland enlargement are listed in Box 22.31.

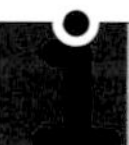

22.31 Causes of salivary gland swelling

• Infection Mumps Bacterial (post-operative) • Calculi • Sjögren's syndrome (p. 1114) • Sarcoidosis	• Tumours Benign: pleomorphic adenoma (95% of cases) Intermediate: mucoepidermoid tumour Malignant: carcinoma

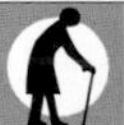

22.32 Oral health in old age

- **Dry mouth**: affects around 40% of healthy older people.
- **Gustatory and olfactory sensation**: declines and chewing power is diminished.
- **Salivation**: baseline salivary flow falls but stimulated salivation is unchanged.
- **Root caries and periodontal disease**: common partly because oral hygiene deteriorates with increasing frailty.
- **Bacteraemia and septicaemia**: may complicate Gram-negative anaerobic infection in the periodontal pockets of the very frail.

DISEASES OF THE OESOPHAGUS

Gastro-oesophageal reflux disease

Gastro-oesophageal reflux resulting in heartburn affects approximately 30% of the general population.

Pathophysiology

Occasional episodes of gastro-oesophageal reflux are common in healthy individuals. Reflux is normally followed by oesophageal peristaltic waves which efficiently clear the gullet, alkaline saliva neutralises residual acid, and symptoms do not occur. Gastro-oesophageal reflux disease develops when the oesophageal mucosa is exposed to gastroduodenal contents for prolonged periods of time, resulting in symptoms and, in a proportion of cases, oesophagitis. Several factors are known to be involved in the development of gastro-oesophageal reflux disease and these are shown in Figure 22.25.

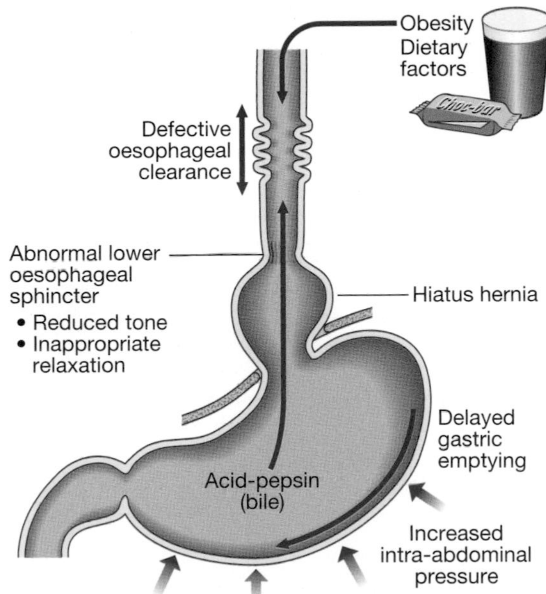

Fig. 22.25 Factors associated with the development of gastro-oesophageal reflux disease.

Abnormalities of the lower oesophageal sphincter

The lower oesophageal sphincter is tonically contracted under normal circumstances, relaxing only during swallowing (p. 840).

Some patients with gastro-oesophageal reflux disease have reduced lower oesophageal sphincter tone, permitting reflux when intra-abdominal pressure rises. In others, basal sphincter tone is normal but reflux occurs in response to frequent episodes of inappropriate sphincter relaxation.

Hiatus hernia

Hiatus hernia (Box 22.33 and Fig. 22.26) causes reflux because the pressure gradient between the abdominal and thoracic cavities, which normally pinches the hiatus, is lost. In addition, the oblique angle between the cardia and oesophagus disappears. Many patients who have large hiatus hernias develop reflux symptoms, but the relationship between the presence of a hernia and symptoms is poor. Hiatus hernia is very common in individuals who have no symptoms, and some symptomatic patients have only a very small or no hernia. Nevertheless, almost all patients who develop oesophagitis, Barrett's oesophagus or peptic strictures have a hiatus hernia.

Delayed oesophageal clearance

Defective oesophageal peristaltic activity is commonly found in patients who have oesophagitis. It is a primary abnormality, since it persists after oesophagitis has been healed by acid-suppressing drug therapy. Poor oesophageal clearance leads to increased acid exposure time.

22.33 Important features of hiatus hernia

- Herniation of the stomach through the diaphragm into the chest
- Occurs in 30% of the population over the age of 50 yrs
- Often asymptomatic
- Heartburn and regurgitation can occur
- Gastric volvulus may complicate large para-oesophageal hernias

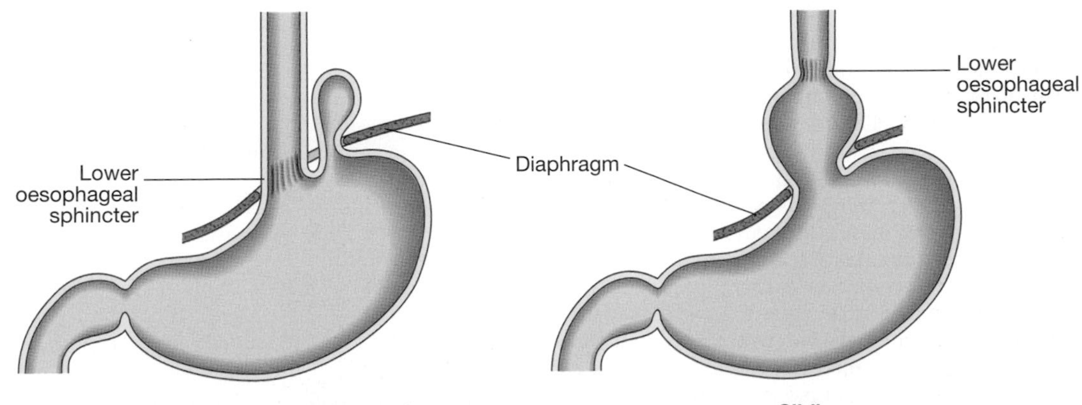

Fig. 22.26 Types of hiatus hernia.

22

Gastric contents

Gastric acid is the most important oesophageal irritant and there is a close relationship between acid exposure time and symptoms. Pepsin and bile also contribute to mucosal injury.

Defective gastric emptying

Gastric emptying is delayed in patients with gastro-oesophageal reflux disease. The reason is unknown.

Increased intra-abdominal pressure

Pregnancy and obesity are established predisposing causes. Weight loss may improve symptoms.

Dietary and environmental factors

Dietary fat, chocolate, alcohol and coffee relax the lower oesophageal sphincter and may provoke symptoms. The foods that trigger symptoms vary widely between affected individuals.

Patient factors

Visceral sensitivity and patient vigilance play a role in determining symptom severity and consulting behaviour in individual patients.

Clinical features

The major symptoms are heartburn and regurgitation, often provoked by bending, straining or lying down. 'Waterbrash', which is salivation due to reflex salivary gland stimulation as acid enters the gullet, is often present. The patient is often overweight. Some patients are woken at night by choking as refluxed fluid irritates the larynx. Others develop odynophagia or dysphagia. A variety of other features have been described, such as atypical chest pain which may be severe and can mimic angina, and may be due to reflux-induced oesophageal spasm. Others include hoarseness ('acid laryngitis'), recurrent chest infections, chronic cough and asthma (Box 22.34). The true relationship of these features to gastro-oesophageal reflux disease remains unclear.

Complications

Oesophagitis

A range of endoscopic findings, from mild redness to severe, bleeding ulceration with stricture formation, are recognised, although appearances may be completely normal (Fig. 22.27). There is a poor correlation between symptoms and histological and endoscopic findings.

Barrett's oesophagus

Barrett's oesophagus is a pre-malignant condition, in which the normal squamous lining of the lower oesophagus is replaced by columnar mucosa (columnar lined oesophagus; CLO) that may contain areas of intestinal metaplasia (Fig. 22.28). It is an adaptive response to chronic gastro-oesophageal reflux and is found in 10% of patients undergoing gastroscopy for reflux symptoms. Community-based epidemiological studies suggest that the true prevalence may be up to 1.5–5% of the population, as the condition is often asymptomatic until discovered when the patient presents with oesophageal cancer. The relative risk of oesophageal cancer is 40–120-fold increased but the absolute risk is low (0.1–0.5% per year). The epidemiology and aetiology of CLO are poorly understood. The prevalence is increasing, and it is more common in men (especially white), the obese and those over 50 years of age. It is weakly associated with smoking but not alcohol intake. The risk of cancer seems to relate to the severity and duration of reflux rather than the presence of CLO per se and it has been suggested that duodenogastro-oesophageal reflux of bile, pancreatic enzymes and pepsin, as well as gastric acid, may be important in pathogenesis. The molecular events underlying progression of CLO to dysplasia and cancer are incompletely understood but inactivation of the tumour suppression protein p16 by loss of heterozygosity or promoter hypermethylation is a key event, followed by somatic inactivation of p53, which promotes

EBM 22.34 The association between gastro-oesophageal reflux disease and asthma

'Reflux is significantly more common in asthma patients (odds ratio 5.5) and asthma is more common in patients with gastro-oesophageal reflux disease (odds ratio 2.3), compared to controls. Evidence for the direction of causality, however, is lacking.'

- Havemann BD, et al. Gut 2007; 56:1654–1664.

For further information: www.evidbasedgastro.com

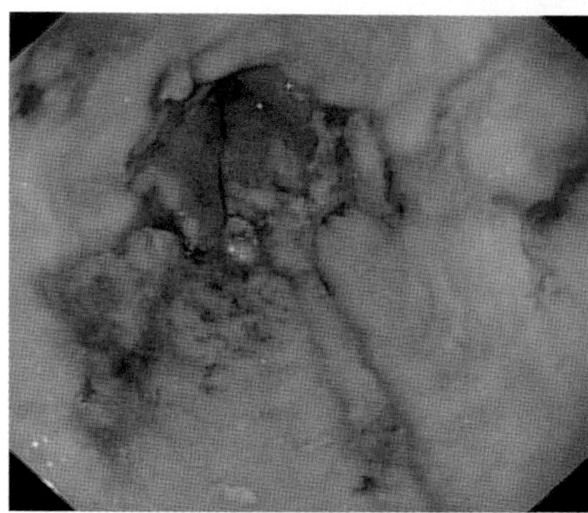

Fig. 22.27 Severe reflux oesophagitis. There is near-circumferential superficial ulceration and inflammation extending up the gullet.

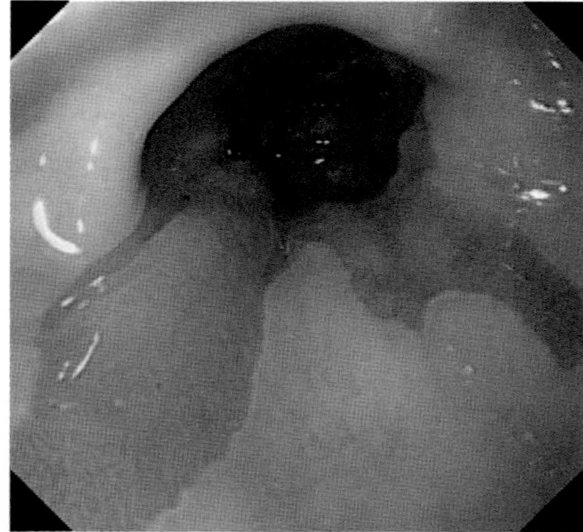

Fig. 22.28 Barrett's oesophagus. Tongues of pink columnar mucosa are seen extending upwards above the oesophago-gastric junction.

aneuploidy and tumour progression. Studies are in progress to develop biomarkers that will allow detection of those at higher cancer risk.

Diagnosis. This requires multiple systematic biopsies to maximise the chance of detecting intestinal metaplasia and/or dysplasia.

Management. Neither potent acid suppression nor anti-reflux surgery stops progression or induces regression of CLO, and treatment is only indicated for symptoms of reflux or complications, such as stricture. Endoscopic therapies, such as radiofrequency ablation or photodynamic therapy, can induce regression but, at present, are used only for those with dysplasia or intramucosal cancer. Regular endoscopic surveillance can detect dysplasia at an early stage and may improve survival but, because most CLO is undetected until cancer develops, surveillance strategies are unlikely to influence the overall mortality rate of oesophageal cancer. Surveillance is expensive and cost-effectiveness studies have been conflicting, but it is currently recommended that patients with CLO without dysplasia should undergo endoscopy at 3–5-yearly intervals and those with low-grade dysplasia at 6–12-monthly intervals.

For those with high-grade dysplasia (HGD) or intramucosal carcinoma, the treatment options are either oesophagectomy or endoscopic therapy with a combination of endoscopic resection (ER) of any visibly abnormal areas and radiofrequency ablation (RFA) of the remaining Barrett's mucosa as an 'organ-preserving' alternative to surgery. These cases should be discussed in a multidisciplinary team meeting and managed in specialist centres.

Anaemia

Iron deficiency anaemia can occur as a consequence of occult blood loss from long-standing oesophagitis. Most patients have a large hiatus hernia and bleeding can stem from subtle erosions in the neck of the sac ('Cameron lesions'). Nevertheless, hiatus hernia is very common and other causes of blood loss, particularly colorectal cancer, must be considered in anaemic patients, even when endoscopy reveals oesophagitis.

Benign oesophageal stricture

Fibrous strictures can develop as a consequence of long-standing oesophagitis, especially in the elderly and those with poor oesophageal peristaltic activity. The typical presentation is with dysphagia that is worse for solids than for liquids. Bolus obstruction following ingestion of meat causes absolute dysphagia. A history of heartburn is common but not invariable; many elderly patients presenting with strictures have no preceding heartburn.

Diagnosis is by endoscopy, when biopsies of the stricture can be taken to exclude malignancy. Endoscopic balloon dilatation or bouginage is helpful. Subsequently, long-term therapy with a PPI drug at full dose should be started to reduce the risk of recurrent oesophagitis and stricture formation. The patient should be advised to chew food thoroughly, and it is important to ensure adequate dentition.

Gastric volvulus

Occasionally, a massive intrathoracic hiatus hernia may twist upon itself, leading to a gastric volvulus. This gives rise to complete oesophageal or gastric obstruction and the patient presents with severe chest pain, vomiting and dysphagia. The diagnosis is made by chest X-ray (air bubble in the chest) and barium swallow. Most cases spontaneously resolve but recurrence is common, and surgery is usually advised after the acute episode has been treated by nasogastric decompression.

Investigations

Young patients who present with typical symptoms of gastro-oesophageal reflux, without worrying features such as dysphagia, weight loss or anaemia, can be treated empirically without investigation. Investigation is advisable if patients present over the age of 50–55 years, if symptoms are atypical or if a complication is suspected. Endoscopy is the investigation of choice. This is performed to exclude other upper gastrointestinal diseases that can mimic gastro-oesophageal reflux and to identify complications. A normal endoscopy in a patient with compatible symptoms should not preclude treatment for gastro-oesophageal reflux disease.

Twenty-four-hour pH monitoring is indicated if the diagnosis is unclear or surgical intervention is under consideration. This involves tethering a slim catheter with a terminal radiotelemetry pH-sensitive probe above the gastro-oesophageal junction. The intraluminal pH is recorded whilst the patient undergoes normal activities, and episodes of symptoms are noted and related to pH. A pH of less than 4 for more than 6–7% of the study time is diagnostic of reflux disease. In a few patients with difficult reflux, impedance testing can detect weakly acidic or alkaline reflux that is not revealed by standard pH testing.

Management

A treatment algorithm for gastro-oesophageal reflux is outlined in Figure 22.29. Lifestyle advice, including weight loss, avoidance of dietary items that the patient finds worsen symptoms, elevation of the bed head in those who experience nocturnal symptoms, avoidance of late meals and giving up smoking, should be recommended. Patients who fail to respond to these measures should be offered PPIs, which are usually effective in resolving symptoms and healing oesophagitis. Recurrence of symptoms is common when therapy is stopped and some patients require life-long treatment at the lowest acceptable dose. When dysmotility features are prominent, domperidone can be helpful. There is no evidence that *H. pylori* eradication has any therapeutic value. Proprietary antacids and alginates can also provide symptomatic benefit. H_2-receptor antagonist drugs also help symptoms without healing oesophagitis.

Long-term PPI therapy is associated with reduced absorption of iron, B_{12} and magnesium, and a small but increased risk of osteoporosis and fractures (odds ratio 1.2–1.5). The drugs also predispose to enteric infections with *Salmonella*, *Campylobacter* and possibly *Clostridium difficile*. Long-term therapy increases the risk of *Helicobacter*-associated progression of gastric mucosal atrophy (see below) and *H. pylori* eradication is advised in patients requiring PPIs for more than 1 year.

Patients who fail to respond to medical therapy, those who are unwilling to take long-term PPIs and those

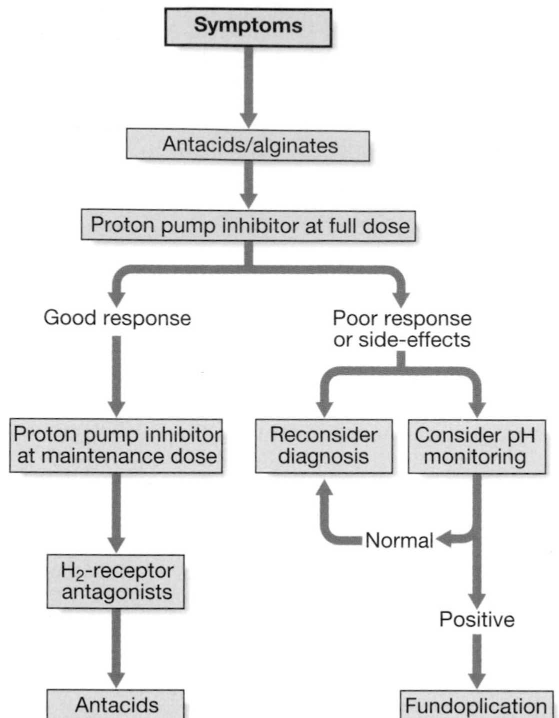

Fig. 22.29 Treatment of gastro-oesophageal reflux disease: a 'step-down' approach.

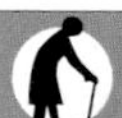

22.35 Gastro-oesophageal reflux disease in old age

- **Prevalence**: higher.
- **Severity of symptoms**: does not correlate with the degree of mucosal inflammation.
- **Complications**: late complications, such as peptic strictures or bleeding from oesophagitis, are more common.
- **Recurrent pneumonia**: consider aspiration from occult gastro-oesophageal reflux disease.

whose major symptom is severe regurgitation should be considered for laparoscopic anti-reflux surgery (see *Principles and Practice of Surgery*). Although heartburn and regurgitation are alleviated in most patients, a small minority develop complications, such as inability to vomit and abdominal bloating ('gas-bloat' syndrome').

Other causes of oesophagitis

Infection

Oesophageal candidiasis occurs in debilitated patients and those taking broad-spectrum antibiotics or cytotoxic drugs. It is a particular problem in patients with HIV-AIDS, who are also susceptible to a spectrum of other oesophageal infections (p. 399).

Corrosives

Suicide attempt by strong household bleach or battery acid is followed by painful burns of the mouth and pharynx and by extensive erosive oesophagitis. This may be complicated by oesophageal perforation with mediastinitis and by stricture formation. At the time of presentation, treatment is conservative, based upon analgesia and nutritional support; vomiting and endoscopy should be avoided because of the high risk of oesophageal perforation. After the acute phase, a barium swallow should be performed to demonstrate the extent of stricture formation. Endoscopic dilatation is usually necessary but it is difficult and hazardous because strictures are often long, tortuous and easily perforated.

Drugs

Potassium supplements and NSAIDs may cause oesophageal ulcers when the tablets are trapped above an oesophageal stricture. Liquid preparations of these drugs should be used in such patients. Bisphosphonates cause oesophageal ulceration and should be used with caution in patients with known oesophageal disorders.

Eosinophilic oesophagitis

This is more common in children but increasingly recognised in young adults. It occurs more often in atopic individuals and is characterised by eosinophilic infiltration of the oesophageal mucosa. Patients present with dysphagia or food bolus obstruction more often than heartburn, and other symptoms, such as chest pain and vomiting, may be present. Endoscopy is usually normal but mucosal rings (that sometimes need endoscopic dilatation), strictures or a narrow-calibre oesophagus can occur. Children may respond to elimination diets but these are less successful in adults, who should first be treated with PPIs. The condition can be treated with 8–12 weeks of therapy with topical corticosteroids, such as fluticasone or betamethasone. The usual approach is to prescribe a metered-dose inhaler but to tell the patient to spray this into the mouth and swallow it rather than inhale it. Refractory symptoms sometimes respond to montelukast, a leukotriene inhibitor.

Motility disorders

Pharyngeal pouch

This occurs because of incoordination of swallowing within the pharynx, which leads to herniation through the cricopharyngeus muscle and formation of a pouch. It is rare, affecting 1 in 100 000 people; it usually develops in middle life but can arise at any age. Many patients have no symptoms, but regurgitation, halitosis and dysphagia can be present. Some notice gurgling in the throat after swallowing. The investigation of choice is a barium swallow, which demonstrates the pouch and reveals incoordination of swallowing, often with pulmonary aspiration. Endoscopy may be hazardous, since the instrument may enter and perforate the pouch. Surgical myotomy ('diverticulotomy'), with or without resection of the pouch, is indicated in symptomatic patients.

Achalasia of the oesophagus

Pathophysiology

Achalasia is characterised by:

- a hypertonic lower oesophageal sphincter, which fails to relax in response to the swallowing wave
- failure of propagated oesophageal contraction, leading to progressive dilatation of the gullet.

The cause is unknown. Defective release of nitric oxide by inhibitory neurons in the lower oesophageal sphincter has been reported, and there is degeneration of ganglion cells within the sphincter and the body of the oesophagus. Loss of the dorsal vagal nuclei within the brainstem can be demonstrated in later stages. Infection with *Trypanosoma cruzi* in Chagas' disease (p. 360) causes a syndrome that is clinically indistinguishable from achalasia.

Clinical features

The presentation is with dysphagia. This develops slowly, is initially intermittent, and is worse for solids and eased by drinking liquids, and by standing and moving around after eating. Heartburn does not occur because the closed oesophageal sphincter prevents gastro-oesophageal reflux. Some patients experience episodes of chest pain due to oesophageal spasm. As the disease progresses, dysphagia worsens, the oesophagus empties poorly and nocturnal pulmonary aspiration develops. Achalasia predisposes to squamous carcinoma of the oesophagus.

Investigations

Endoscopy should always be carried out because carcinoma of the cardia can mimic the presentation and radiological and manometric features of achalasia ('pseudo-achalasia'). A barium swallow shows tapered narrowing of the lower oesophagus and, in late disease, the oesophageal body is dilated, aperistaltic and food-filled (Fig. 22.30A). Manometry confirms the high-pressure, non-relaxing lower oesophageal sphincter with poor contractility of the oesophageal body (Fig. 22.30B).

Management

Endoscopic

Forceful pneumatic dilatation using a 30–35-mm diameter fluoroscopically positioned balloon disrupts the oesophageal sphincter and improves symptoms in 80% of patients. Some patients require more than one dilatation but those needing frequent dilatation are best treated surgically. Endoscopically directed injection of botulinum toxin into the lower oesophageal sphincter induces clinical remission but relapse is common.

Surgical

Surgical myotomy (Heller's operation), performed either laparoscopically or as an open operation, is effective but is more invasive than endoscopic dilatation. Both pneumatic dilatation and myotomy may be complicated by gastro-oesophageal reflux, and this can lead to severe oesophagitis because oesophageal clearance is so poor. For this reason, Heller's myotomy is accompanied by a partial fundoplication anti-reflux procedure. PPI therapy is often necessary after surgery. Recently, a complex endoscopic technique has been developed in specialist centres (peroral endoscopic myotomy, POEM).

Other oesophageal motility disorders

Diffuse oesophageal spasm presents in late middle age with episodic chest pain that may mimic angina, but is sometimes accompanied by transient dysphagia. Some cases occur in response to gastro-oesophageal reflux. Treatment is based upon the use of PPI drugs when gastro-oesophageal reflux is present. Oral or sublingual nitrates or nifedipine may relieve attacks of pain. The results of drug therapy are often disappointing, as are the alternatives: pneumatic dilatation and surgical myotomy. 'Nutcracker' oesophagus is a condition in which extremely forceful peristaltic activity leads to episodic chest pain and dysphagia. Treatment is with nitrates or nifedipine. Some patients present with oesophageal motility disorders which do not fit into a specific disease entity. The patients are usually elderly and present with dysphagia and chest pain. Manometric abnormalities, ranging from poor peristalsis to spasm, occur. Treatment is with dilatation and/or vasodilators for chest pain.

Secondary causes of oesophageal dysmotility

In systemic sclerosis or CREST syndrome, the muscle of the oesophagus is replaced by fibrous tissue, which causes failure of peristalsis leading to heartburn and dysphagia. Oesophagitis is often severe, and benign fibrous strictures occur. These patients require

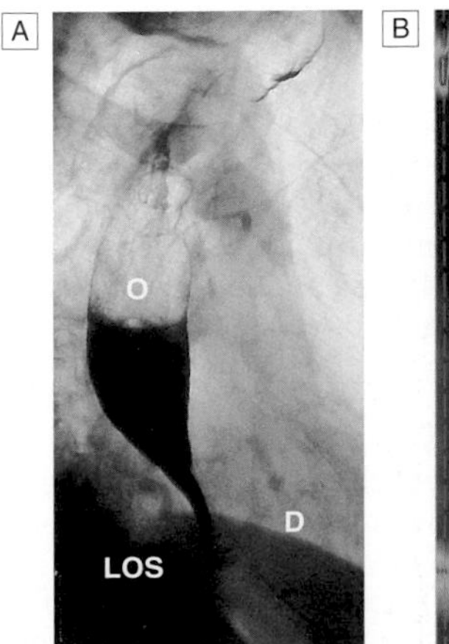

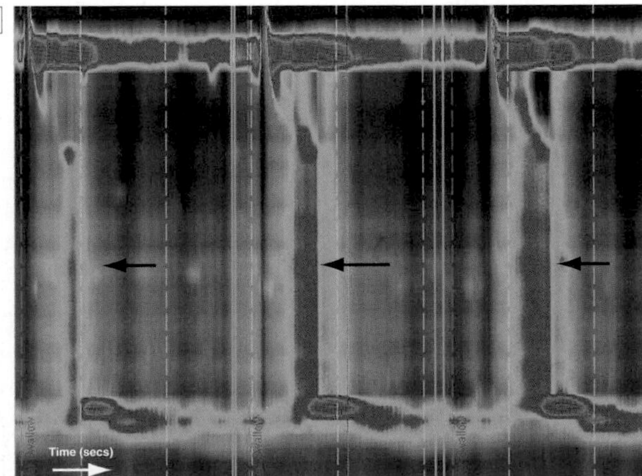

Fig. 22.30 Achalasia. **A** X-ray showing a dilated, barium-filled oesophagus (O) with fluid level and distal tapering, and a closed lower oesophageal sphincter (LOS). (D = diaphragm) **B** High-resolution manometry in achalasia showing absence of peristaltic swallowing wave in oesophageal body (black arrows) and raised LOS pressure with failure of relaxation on swallowing (white arrow). Compare with normal appearances in Figure 22.1 (p. 840).

long-term therapy with PPIs. Dermatomyositis, rheumatoid arthritis and myasthenia gravis may also cause dysphagia.

Benign oesophageal stricture

Benign oesophageal stricture is usually a consequence of gastro-oesophageal reflux disease (Box 22.36) and occurs most often in elderly patients who have poor oesophageal clearance. Rings, due to submucosal fibrosis, are found at the oesophago-gastric junction ('Schatzki ring') and cause intermittent dysphagia, often starting in middle age. A post-cricoid web is a rare complication of iron deficiency anaemia (Paterson–Kelly or Plummer–Vinson syndrome), and may be complicated by the development of squamous carcinoma. Benign strictures can be treated by endoscopic dilatation, in which wire-guided bougies or balloons are used to disrupt the fibrous tissue of the stricture.

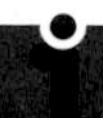

22.36 Causes of oesophageal stricture

- Gastro-oesophageal reflux disease
- Webs and rings
- Carcinoma of the oesophagus or cardia
- Eosinophilic oesophagitis
- Extrinsic compression from bronchial carcinoma
- Corrosive ingestion
- Post-operative scarring following oesophageal resection
- Post-radiotherapy
- Following long-term nasogastric intubation
- Bisphosphonates

Tumours of the oesophagus

Benign tumours

The most common is a leiomyoma. This is usually asymptomatic but may cause bleeding or dysphagia.

Carcinoma of the oesophagus

Squamous oesophageal cancer (Box 22.37) is relatively rare in Caucasians (4:100 000) but is more common in Iran, parts of Africa and China (200:100 000). Squamous cancer can occur in any part of the oesophagus, and almost all tumours in the upper oesophagus are squamous cancers. Adenocarcinomas typically arise in the lower third of the oesophagus from Barrett's oesophagus or from the cardia of the stomach. The incidence is increasing and is now approximately 5:100 000 in the UK; this is possibly because of the high prevalence of gastro-oesophageal reflux and Barrett's oesophagus in Western populations. Despite modern treatment, the overall 5-year survival of patients presenting with oesophageal cancer is only 13%.

Clinical features

Most patients have a history of progressive, painless dysphagia for solid foods. Others present acutely because of food bolus obstruction. In late stages, weight loss is often extreme; chest pain or hoarseness suggests mediastinal invasion. Fistulation between the oesophagus and the trachea or bronchial tree leads to coughing after swallowing, pneumonia and pleural effusion. Physical signs may be absent but, even at initial presentation, cachexia, cervical lymphadenopathy or other evidence of metastatic spread is common.

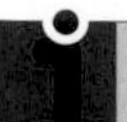

22.37 Squamous carcinoma: aetiological factors

- Smoking
- Alcohol excess
- Chewing betel nuts or tobacco
- Achalasia of the oesophagus
- Coeliac disease
- Post-cricoid web
- Post-caustic stricture
- Tylosis (familial hyperkeratosis of palms and soles)

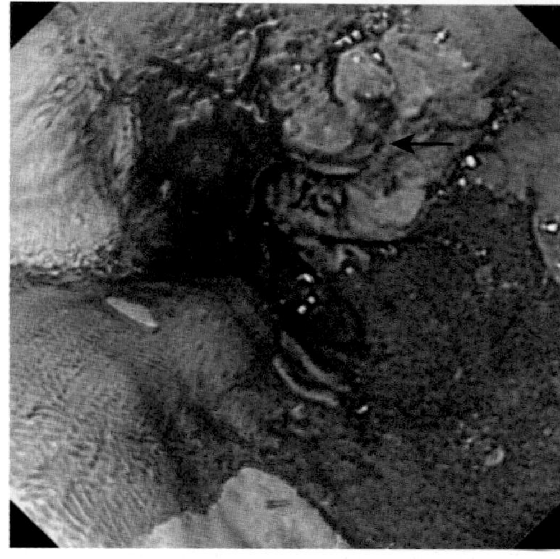

Fig. 22.31 Adenocarcinoma of the lower oesophagus. Adenocarcinoma in association with Barrett's oesophagus (arrow).

Investigations

The investigation of choice is upper gastrointestinal endoscopy (Fig. 22.31) with biopsy. A barium swallow demonstrates the site and length of the stricture but adds little useful information. Once a diagnosis has been made, investigations should be performed to stage the tumour and define operability. Thoracic and abdominal CT, often combined with positron emission tomography (CT-PET), should be carried out to identify metastatic spread and local invasion. Invasion of the aorta, major airways or coeliac axis usually precludes surgery, but patients with resectable disease on imaging should undergo EUS to determine the depth of penetration of the tumour into the oesophageal wall and to detect locoregional lymph node involvement (Fig. 22.32). These investigations will define the TNM stage of the disease (p. 268).

Management

The treatment of choice is surgery if the patient presents at a point at which resection is possible. Patients with tumours that have extended beyond the wall of the oesophagus (T3) or which have lymph node involvement (N1) have a 5-year survival of around 10%. However, this figure improves significantly if the tumour is confined to the oesophageal wall and there is no spread to lymph nodes. Overall survival following

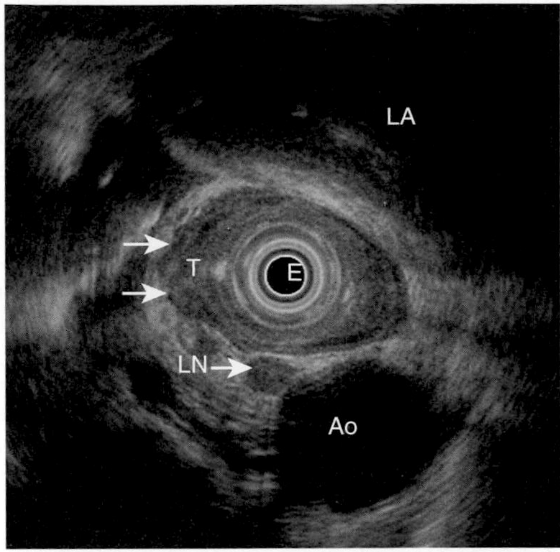

Fig. 22.32 Endoscopic ultrasound staging of oesophageal carcinoma. The tumour (T) has extended through the oesophageal wall (stage T3, arrows). A small peritumoral lymph node (LN) is also seen. (Ao = aorta; LA = left atrium; E = echoendoscope)

'potentially curative' surgery (all macroscopic tumour removed) is about 30% at 5 years, but recent studies have suggested that this can be improved by neoadjuvant chemotherapy. Although squamous carcinomas are radiosensitive, radiotherapy alone is associated with a 5-year survival of only 5%, but combined chemoradiotherapy for these tumours can achieve 5-year survival rates of 25–30%.

Approximately 70% of patients have extensive disease at presentation; in these, treatment is palliative and should focus on relief of dysphagia and pain. Endoscopic laser therapy or self-expanding metallic stents can be used to improve swallowing. Palliative radiotherapy may induce shrinkage of both squamous cancers and adenocarcinomas but symptomatic response may be slow. Quality of life can be improved by nutritional support and appropriate analgesia.

Perforation of the oesophagus

The most common cause is endoscopic perforation complicating dilatation or intubation. Malignant, corrosive or post-radiotherapy strictures are more likely to be perforated than peptic strictures. A perforated peptic stricture is managed conservatively using broad-spectrum antibiotics and parenteral nutrition; most cases heal within days. Malignant, caustic and radiotherapy stricture perforations require resection or stenting.

Spontaneous oesophageal perforation ('Boerhaave's syndrome') results from forceful vomiting and retching. Severe chest pain and shock occur as oesophago-gastric contents enter the mediastinum and thoracic cavity. Subcutaneous emphysema, pleural effusions and pneumothorax develop. The diagnosis can be made using a water-soluble contrast swallow but, in difficult cases, both CT and careful endoscopy (usually in an intubated patient) may be required. Treatment is surgical. Delay in diagnosis is a key factor in the high mortality associated with this condition.

DISEASES OF THE STOMACH AND DUODENUM

Gastritis

Gastritis is a histological diagnosis, although it can sometimes be recognised at endoscopy.

Acute gastritis

Acute gastritis is often erosive and haemorrhagic. Neutrophils are the predominant inflammatory cell in the superficial epithelium. Many cases result from aspirin or NSAID ingestion (Box 22.38). Acute gastritis often produces no symptoms but may cause dyspepsia, anorexia, nausea or vomiting, and haematemesis or melaena. Many cases resolve quickly and do not merit investigation; in others, endoscopy and biopsy may be necessary to exclude peptic ulcer or cancer. Treatment should be directed at the underlying cause. Short-term symptomatic therapy with antacids, and acid suppression using PPIs, prokinetics (domperidone) or antiemetics (metoclopramide) may be necessary.

Chronic gastritis due to *Helicobacter pylori* infection

This is the most common cause of chronic gastritis (see Box 22.38). The predominant inflammatory cells are lymphocytes and plasma cells. Correlation between symptoms and endoscopic or pathological findings is poor. Most patients are asymptomatic and do not require treatment, but patients with dyspepsia may benefit from *H. pylori* eradication.

Autoimmune chronic gastritis

This involves the body of the stomach but spares the antrum; it results from autoimmune damage to parietal

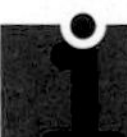

22.38 Common causes of gastritis

Acute gastritis (often erosive and haemorrhagic)
- Aspirin, NSAIDs
- *H. pylori* (initial infection)
- Alcohol
- Other drugs, e.g. iron preparations
- Severe physiological stress, e.g. burns, multi-organ failure, CNS trauma
- Bile reflux, e.g. following gastric surgery
- Viral infections, e.g. CMV, herpes simplex virus in HIV-AIDS (p. 399)

Chronic non-specific gastritis
- *H. pylori* infection
- Autoimmune (pernicious anaemia)
- Post-gastrectomy

Chronic 'specific' forms (rare)
- Infections, e.g. CMV, tuberculosis
- Gastrointestinal diseases, e.g. Crohn's disease
- Systemic diseases, e.g. sarcoidosis, graft-versus-host disease
- Idiopathic, e.g. granulomatous gastritis

(CMV = cytomegalovirus; NSAIDs = non-steroidal anti-inflammatory drugs)

22

cells. The histological features are diffuse chronic inflammation, atrophy and loss of fundic glands, intestinal metaplasia and sometimes hyperplasia of enterochromaffin-like (ECL) cells. Circulating antibodies to parietal cell and intrinsic factor may be present. In some patients, the degree of gastric atrophy is severe, and loss of intrinsic factor secretion leads to pernicious anaemia (p. 1025). The gastritis itself is usually asymptomatic. Some patients have evidence of other organ-specific autoimmunity, particularly thyroid disease. Long-term, there is a two- to threefold increase in the risk of gastric cancer (see also p. 877).

Ménétrier's disease

In this rare condition, the gastric pits are elongated and tortuous, with replacement of the parietal and chief cells by mucus-secreting cells. The cause is unknown but there is excessive production of TGF-α. As a result, the mucosal folds of the body and fundus are greatly enlarged. Most patients are hypochlorhydric. Whilst some patients have upper gastrointestinal symptoms, the majority present in middle or old age with protein-losing enteropathy (p. 886) due to exudation from the gastric mucosa. Endoscopy shows enlarged, nodular and coarse folds, although biopsies may not be deep enough to show all the histological features. Treatment with antisecretory drugs, such as PPIs with or without octreotide, may reduce protein loss and *H. pylori* eradication may be effective, but unresponsive patients require partial gastrectomy.

Peptic ulcer disease

The term 'peptic ulcer' refers to an ulcer in the lower oesophagus, stomach or duodenum, in the jejunum after surgical anastomosis to the stomach or, rarely, in the ileum adjacent to a Meckel's diverticulum. Ulcers in the stomach or duodenum may be acute or chronic; both penetrate the muscularis mucosae but the acute ulcer shows no evidence of fibrosis. Erosions do not penetrate the muscularis mucosae.

Gastric and duodenal ulcer

The prevalence of peptic ulcer (0.1–0.2%) is decreasing in many Western communities as a result of widespread use of *Helicobacter pylori* eradication therapy but it remains high in developing countries. The male-to-female ratio for duodenal ulcer varies from 5:1 to 2:1, whilst that for gastric ulcer is 2:1 or less. Chronic gastric ulcer is usually single; 90% are situated on the lesser curve within the antrum or at the junction between body and antral mucosa. Chronic duodenal ulcer usually occurs in the first part of the duodenum and 50% are on the anterior wall. Gastric and duodenal ulcers coexist in 10% of patients and more than one peptic ulcer is found in 10–15% of patients.

Pathophysiology

H. pylori

Peptic ulceration is strongly associated with *H. pylori* infection. The prevalence in developed nations rises with age, and in the UK approximately 50% of people over the age of 50 years are infected. In the developing world, infection is more common, affecting up to 90% of adults. These infections are probably acquired in childhood by person-to-person contact. The vast majority of colonised people remain healthy and asymptomatic and only a minority develop clinical disease. Around 90% of duodenal ulcer patients and 70% of gastric ulcer patients are infected with *H. pylori*. The remaining 30% of gastric ulcers are caused by NSAIDs and this proportion is increasing in Western countries as a result of *H. pylori* eradication strategies.

H. pylori is Gram-negative and spiral, and has multiple flagella at one end, which make it motile, allowing it to burrow and live beneath the mucus layer adherent to the epithelial surface. It uses an adhesin molecule (BabA) to bind to the Lewis b antigen on epithelial cells. Here the surface pH is close to neutral and any acidity is buffered by the organism's production of the enzyme urease. This produces ammonia from urea and raises the pH around the bacterium and between its two cell membrane layers. *H. pylori* exclusively colonises gastric-type epithelium and is only found in the duodenum in association with patches of gastric metaplasia. It causes chronic gastritis by provoking a local inflammatory response in the underlying epithelium (Fig. 22.33). This depends on numerous factors, notably expression of bacterial *cagA* and *vacA* genes. The cagA gene product is injected into epithelial cells, interacting with numerous cell-signalling pathways involved in cell replication and apoptosis. *H. pylori* strains expressing cagA ($cagA^+$) are more often associated with disease than $cagA^-$ strains. Most strains also secrete a large pore-forming protein called vacA, which causes increased cell permeability, efflux of micronutrients from the epithelium, induction of apoptosis and suppression of local immune cell activity. Several forms of vacA exist and pathology is most strongly associated with the s1/ml form of the toxin.

In most people, *H. pylori* causes localised antral gastritis associated with depletion of somatostatin (from D cells) and increased gastrin release from G cells. The subsequent hypergastrinaemia stimulates increased acid

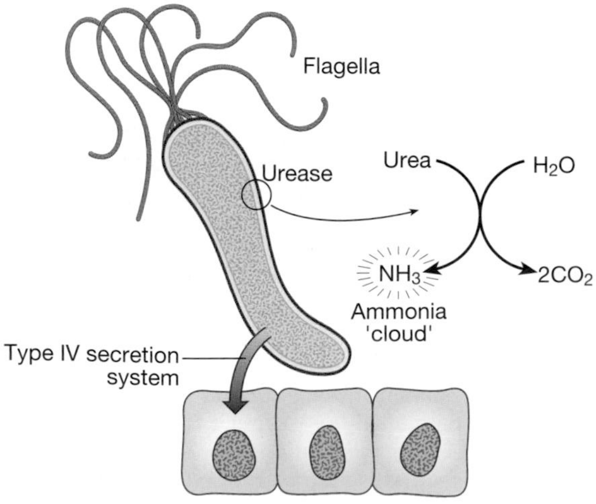

Fig. 22.33 Factors that influence the virulence of *H. pylori*.

production by parietal cells but, in the majority of cases, this has no clinical consequences. In a minority of patients, this effect is exaggerated, leading to duodenal ulceration (Fig. 22.34). In 1% of infected people, *H. pylori* causes a pangastritis, leading to gastric atrophy and hypochlorhydria. This allows other bacteria to proliferate within the stomach; these produce mutagenic nitrites from dietary nitrates, predisposing to the development of gastric cancer (Fig. 22.35). The effects of *H. pylori* are more complex in gastric ulcer patients compared to those with duodenal ulcers. The ulcer probably arises because of impaired mucosal defence resulting from a combination of *H. pylori* infection, NSAIDs and smoking, rather than excess acid.

NSAIDs

Treatment with NSAIDs is associated with peptic ulcers due to impairment of mucosal defences, as discussed on page 1078.

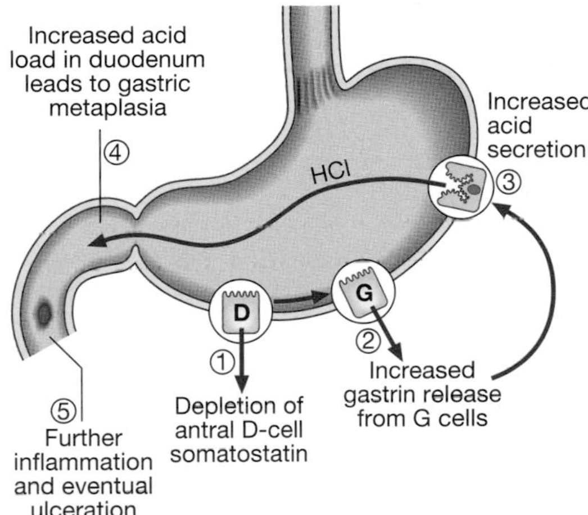

Fig. 22.34 Sequence of events in the pathophysiology of duodenal ulceration.

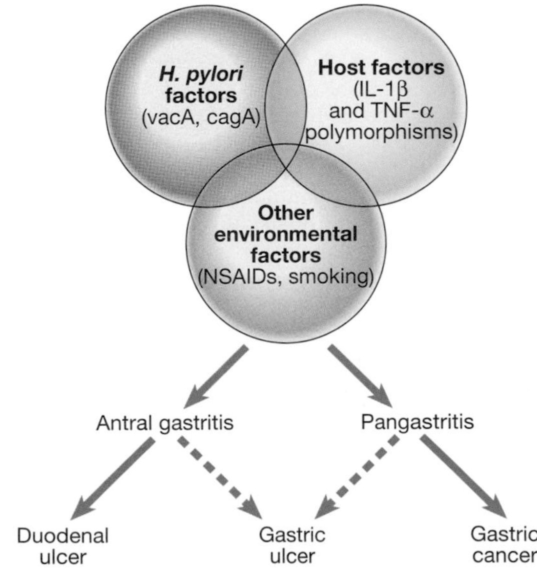

Fig. 22.35 Consequences of *H. pylori* infection.

Smoking

Smoking confers an increased risk of gastric ulcer and, to a lesser extent, duodenal ulcer. Once the ulcer has formed, it is more likely to cause complications and less likely to heal if the patient continues to smoke.

Clinical features

Peptic ulcer disease is a chronic condition with spontaneous relapses and remissions lasting for decades, if not for life. The most common presentation is with recurrent abdominal pain which has three notable characteristics: localisation to the epigastrium, relationship to food and episodic occurrence. Occasional vomiting occurs in about 40% of ulcer subjects; persistent daily vomiting suggests gastric outlet obstruction. In one-third, the history is less characteristic, especially in elderly people or those taking NSAIDs. In them, pain may be absent or so slight that it is experienced only as a vague sense of epigastric unease. Occasionally, the only symptoms are anorexia and nausea, or early satiety after meals. In some patients, the ulcer is completely 'silent', presenting for the first time with anaemia from chronic undetected blood loss, as an abrupt haematemesis or as acute perforation; in others, there is recurrent acute bleeding without ulcer pain. The diagnostic value of individual symptoms for peptic ulcer disease is poor; the history is therefore a poor predictor of the presence of an ulcer.

Investigations

Endoscopy is the preferred investigation. Gastric ulcers may occasionally be malignant and therefore must always be biopsied and followed up to ensure healing. Patients should be tested for *H. pylori* infection. The current options available are listed in Box 22.39. Some are invasive and require endoscopy; others are non-invasive. They vary in sensitivity and specificity. Breath tests or faecal antigen tests are best because of accuracy, simplicity and non-invasiveness.

22.39 Methods for the diagnosis of *Helicobacter pylori* infection

Test	Advantages	Disadvantages
Non-invasive		
Serology	Rapid office kits available Good for population studies	Lacks specificity Cannot differentiate current from past infection
^{13}C-urea breath tests	High sensitivity and specificity	Requires expensive mass spectrometer
Faecal antigen test	Cheap, specific (> 95%)	Acceptability
Invasive (antral biopsy)		
Histology	Specificity	False negatives Takes several days to process
Rapid urease tests	Cheap, quick, specific (> 95%)	Sensitivity 85%
Microbiological culture	'Gold standard' Defines antibiotic sensitivity	Slow and laborious Lacks sensitivity

Management

The aims of management are to relieve symptoms, induce healing and prevent recurrence. *H. pylori* eradication is the cornerstone of therapy for peptic ulcers, as this will successfully prevent relapse and eliminate the need for long-term therapy in the majority of patients.

H. pylori eradication

All patients with proven ulcers who are *H. pylori*-positive should be offered eradication as primary therapy. Treatment is based upon a PPI taken simultaneously with two antibiotics (from amoxicillin, clarithromycin and metronidazole) for 7 days (Box 22.40). High-dose, twice-daily PPI therapy increases efficacy of treatment, as does extending treatment to 10–14 days. Success is achieved in 80–90% of patients, although compliance, side-effects (Box 22.41) and antibiotic resistance influence this. Resistance to amoxicillin is rare but rates of metronidazole resistance reach 40% in some countries and, recently, rates of clarithromycin resistance of 20–40% have appeared. Where the latter exceed 15–20%, a quadruple therapy regimen, consisting of omeprazole (or another PPI), bismuth subcitrate, metronidazole and tetracycline (OBMT) for 10–14 days, is recommended. In areas of low clarithromycin resistance, this regimen should also be offered as second-line therapy to those who remain infected after initial therapy, once compliance has been checked. For those who are still colonised after two treatments, the choice lies between a third attempt guided by antimicrobial sensitivity testing, rescue therapy (levofloxacin, PPI and clarithromycin) or long-term acid suppression.

H. pylori and NSAIDs are independent risk factors for ulcer disease and patients requiring long-term NSAID therapy should first undergo eradication therapy to reduce ulcer risk. Subsequent co-prescription of a PPI along with the NSAID is advised but is not always necessary for patients being given low-dose aspirin, in whom the risk of ulcer complications is lower.

EBM 22.40 *H. pylori* eradication and peptic ulcer healing

'Compared to ulcer-healing drugs, *H. pylori* eradication therapy is superior for healing duodenal ulcers (RR 0.66) and affords equivalent protection against recurrence of both duodenal and gastric ulcers.'

- Ford AC, et al. Eradication therapy for peptic ulcer disease in *Helicobacter pylori* positive patients. Cochrane Database of Systematic Reviews, 2006, issue 2. Art. no. CD003840.

For further information: www.cochrane.org/cochrane-reviews

22.41 Common side-effects of *H. pylori* eradication therapy

- Diarrhoea: 30–50% of patients; usually mild but *Clostridium difficile*-associated diarrhoea can occur
- Flushing and vomiting when taken with alcohol (metronidazole)
- Nausea, vomiting
- Abdominal cramps
- Headache
- Rash

22.42 Indications for *H. pylori* eradication

Definite

- Peptic ulcer
- Extranodal marginal-zone lymphomas of MALT type
- Family history of gastric cancer
- Previous resection for gastric cancer
- *H. pylori*-positive dyspepsia
- Long-term NSAID or low-dose aspirin users
- Chronic (> 1 yr) PPI users
- Extragastric disorders:
  - Unexplained vitamin B_{12} deficiency*
  - Idiopathic thrombocytopenic purpura*
  - Iron deficiency anaemia* (see text)

Not indicated

- Gastro-oesophageal reflux disease
- Asymptomatic people without gastric cancer risk factors

*If *H. pylori*-positive on testing.

Other indications for *H. pylori* eradication are shown in Box 22.42. Eradication of the infection has proven benefits in several extragastric disorders, including unexplained B_{12} deficiency and iron deficiency anaemia, once sources of gastrointestinal bleeding have been looked for and excluded. Platelet counts improve and may normalise after eradication therapy in patients with idiopathic thrombocytopenic purpura (ITP, p. 1050); the mechanism for this is unclear.

General measures

Cigarette smoking, aspirin and NSAIDs should be avoided. Alcohol in moderation is not harmful and no special dietary advice is required.

Maintenance treatment

Continuous maintenance treatment should not be necessary after successful *H. pylori* eradication. For the minority who do require it, the lowest effective dose of PPI should be used.

Surgical treatment

Surgery is now rarely required for peptic ulcer disease but it is needed in some cases (Box 22.43).

The operation of choice for a chronic non-healing gastric ulcer is partial gastrectomy, preferably with a Billroth I anastomosis, in which the ulcer itself and the ulcer-bearing area of the stomach are resected. The reason for this is to exclude an underlying cancer. In an emergency, 'under-running' the ulcer for bleeding or 'oversewing' (patch repair) for perforation is all that is required, in addition to taking a biopsy. For giant

22.43 Indications for surgery in peptic ulcer

Emergency

- Perforation
- Haemorrhage

Elective

- Gastric outflow obstruction
- Persistent ulceration despite adequate medical therapy
- Recurrent ulcer following gastric surgery

duodenal ulcers, partial gastrectomy using a 'Polya' or Billroth II reconstruction may be required.

Complications of gastric resection or vagotomy

Up to 50% of patients who undergo gastric surgery for peptic ulcer surgery experience long-term adverse effects. In most cases, these are minor, but in 10% they significantly impair quality of life.

Dumping. Rapid gastric emptying leads to distension of the proximal small intestine as the hypertonic contents draw fluid into the lumen. This leads to abdominal discomfort and diarrhoea after eating. Autonomic reflexes release a range of gastrointestinal hormones that provoke vasomotor features, such as flushing, palpitations, sweating, tachycardia and hypotension. Patients should therefore avoid large meals with high carbohydrate content.

Chemical (bile reflux) gastropathy. Duodenogastric bile reflux leads to chronic gastropathy. Treatment with aluminium-containing antacids or sucralfate may be effective. A few patients require revisional surgery with creation of a Roux en Y loop to prevent bile reflux.

Diarrhoea and maldigestion. Diarrhoea may develop after any peptic ulcer operation and usually occurs 1–2 hours after eating. Poor mixing of food in the stomach, with rapid emptying, inadequate mixing with pancreaticobiliary secretions, rapid transit and bacterial overgrowth, may lead to malabsorption. Diarrhoea often responds to small, dry meals with a reduced intake of refined carbohydrates. Antidiarrhoeal drugs, such as codeine phosphate (15–30 mg 4–6 times daily) or loperamide (2 mg after each loose stool), are helpful.

Weight loss. Most patients lose weight shortly after surgery and 30–40% are unable to regain all the weight that is lost. The usual cause is reduced intake because of a small gastric remnant, but diarrhoea and mild steatorrhoea also contribute.

Anaemia. Anaemia is common many years after subtotal gastrectomy. Iron deficiency is the most common cause; folic acid and B_{12} deficiency are much less frequent. Inadequate dietary intake of iron and folate, lack of acid and intrinsic factor secretion, mild chronic low-grade blood loss from the gastric remnant and recurrent ulceration are responsible.

Metabolic bone disease. Both osteoporosis and osteomalacia can occur as a consequence of calcium and vitamin D malabsorption.

Gastric cancer. An increased risk of gastric cancer has been reported from several epidemiological studies. Surgery itself is an independent risk factor for late development of malignancy in the gastric remnant but the risk is higher in those with hypochlorhydria, duodenogastric reflux of bile, smoking and *H. pylori* infection. Although the relative risk is increased, the absolute risk of cancer remains low and endoscopic surveillance is not indicated following gastric surgery.

Complications of peptic ulcer disease

Perforation

When perforation occurs, the contents of the stomach escape into the peritoneal cavity, leading to peritonitis. This is more common in duodenal than in gastric ulcers, and is usually found with ulcers on the anterior wall. About one-quarter of all perforations occur in acute ulcers and NSAIDs are often incriminated. Perforation can be the first sign of ulcer, and a history of recurrent epigastric pain is uncommon. The most striking symptom is sudden, severe pain; its distribution follows the spread of the gastric contents over the peritoneum. The pain initially develops in the upper abdomen and rapidly becomes generalised; shoulder tip pain is caused by irritation of the diaphragm. The pain is accompanied by shallow respiration due to limitation of diaphragmatic movements and by shock. The abdomen is held immobile and there is generalised 'board-like' rigidity. Bowel sounds are absent and liver dullness to percussion decreases due to the presence of gas under the diaphragm. After some hours, symptoms may improve, although abdominal rigidity remains. Later, the patient's condition deteriorates as general peritonitis develops. In at least 50% of cases, an erect chest X-ray shows free air beneath the diaphragm. If not, a water-soluble contrast swallow will confirm leakage of gastroduodenal contents. After resuscitation, the acute perforation should be treated surgically, either by simple closure or by converting the perforation into a pyloroplasty if it is large. On rare occasions, a 'Polya' partial gastrectomy is required. Following surgery, *H. pylori* should be treated (if present) and NSAIDs avoided. Perforation carries a mortality of 25%, reflecting the advanced age and significant comorbidity of the population that are affected.

Gastric outlet obstruction

The causes are shown in Box 22.45. The most common is an ulcer in the region of the pylorus. The presentation is with nausea, vomiting and abdominal distension. Large quantities of gastric content are often vomited, and food eaten 24 hours or more previously may be recognised. Physical examination may show evidence of wasting and dehydration. A succussion splash may be elicited 4 hours or more after the last meal or drink.

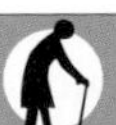

22.44 Peptic ulcer disease in old age

- **Gastroduodenal ulcers**: have a greater incidence, admission rate and mortality.
- **Causes**: high prevalence of *H. pylori*, NSAID use and impaired defence mechanisms.
- **Atypical presentations**: pain and dyspepsia are frequently absent or atypical. Older people often develop complications, such as bleeding or perforation, without a dyspeptic history.
- **Bleeding**: older patients require more intensive management (including measurement of central venous pressure) than younger because they tolerate hypovolaemic shock poorly.

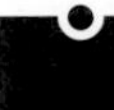

22.45 Differential diagnosis and management of gastric outlet obstruction

Cause	Management
Fibrotic stricture from duodenal ulcer (pyloric stenosis)	Balloon dilatation or surgery
Oedema from pyloric channel or duodenal ulcer	PPI therapy
Carcinoma of antrum	Surgery
Adult hypertrophic pyloric stenosis	Surgery

22

Visible gastric peristalsis is diagnostic of gastric outlet obstruction. Loss of gastric contents leads to dehydration with low serum chloride and potassium, and raised serum bicarbonate and urea concentrations. This results in enhanced renal absorption of Na^+ in exchange for H^+ and paradoxical aciduria. Endoscopy should be performed after the stomach has been emptied by a wide-bore nasogastric tube. Intravenous correction of dehydration is undertaken and, in severe cases, at least 4 L of isotonic saline and 80 mmol of potassium may be necessary during the first 24 hours. In some patients, PPI drugs heal ulcers, relieve pyloric oedema and overcome the need for surgery. Endoscopic balloon dilatation of benign stenoses may be possible in some patients, but in others partial gastrectomy is necessary, although this is best done after a 7-day period of nasogastric aspiration, which enables the stomach to return to normal size. A gastroenterostomy is an alternative operation but, unless this is accompanied by vagotomy, patients will require long-term PPI therapy to prevent stomal ulceration.

Bleeding

See page 853.

Zollinger–Ellison syndrome

This is a rare disorder characterised by the triad of severe peptic ulceration, gastric acid hypersecretion and a non-β cell islet tumour of the pancreas ('gastrinoma'). It probably accounts for about 0.1% of all cases of duodenal ulceration. The syndrome occurs in either sex at any age, although it is most common between 30 and 50 years of age.

Pathophysiology

The tumour secretes gastrin, which stimulates acid secretion to its maximal capacity and increases the parietal cell mass three- to sixfold. The acid output may be so great that it reaches the upper small intestine, reducing the luminal pH to 2 or less. Pancreatic lipase is inactivated and bile acids are precipitated. Diarrhoea and steatorrhoea result. Around 90% of tumours occur in the pancreatic head or proximal duodenal wall. At least half are multiple, and tumour size can vary from 1 mm to 20 cm. Approximately one-half to two-thirds are malignant but are often slow-growing. Adenomas of the parathyroid and pituitary glands (multiple endocrine neoplasia, MEN type 1; p. 795) are present in 20–60% of patients.

Clinical features

The presentation is with severe and often multiple peptic ulcers in unusual sites, such as the post-bulbar duodenum, jejunum or oesophagus. There is a poor response to standard ulcer therapy. The history is usually short; bleeding and perforations are common. Diarrhoea is seen in one-third or more of patients and can be the presenting feature.

Investigations

Hypersecretion of acid under basal conditions, with little increase following pentagastrin, may be confirmed by gastric aspiration. Serum gastrin levels are grossly elevated (10- to 1000-fold). Injection of the hormone secretin normally causes no change or a slight decrease in circulating gastrin concentrations, but in Zollinger–Ellison syndrome produces a paradoxical and dramatic increase in gastrin. Tumour localisation is best achieved by EUS and radio-labelled somatostatin receptor scintigraphy.

Management

Some 30% of small and single tumours can be localised and resected but many tumours are multifocal. Some patients present with metastatic disease and, in these circumstances, surgery is inappropriate. In the majority of these patients, continuous therapy with omeprazole or other PPIs can be successful in healing ulcers and alleviating diarrhoea, although double the normal dose is required. The synthetic somatostatin analogue, octreotide, given by subcutaneous injection, reduces gastrin secretion and is of value. Overall 5-year survival is 60–75% and all patients should be monitored for the later development of other manifestations of MEN 1.

Functional disorders

Functional dyspepsia

This is defined as chronic dyspepsia in the absence of organic disease. Other commonly reported symptoms include early satiety, fullness, bloating and nausea. 'Ulcer-like' and 'dysmotility-type' subgroups are often reported, but there is overlap between these and with irritable bowel syndrome.

Pathophysiology

The cause is poorly understood but probably covers a spectrum of mucosal, motility and psychiatric disorders.

Clinical features

Patients are usually young (< 40 years) and women are affected twice as commonly as men. Abdominal discomfort is associated with a combination of other 'dyspeptic' symptoms, the most common being nausea, satiety and bloating after meals. Morning symptoms are characteristic and pain or nausea may occur on waking. Direct enquiry may elicit symptoms suggestive of irritable bowel syndrome. Peptic ulcer disease must be considered, whilst in older subjects intra-abdominal malignancy is a prime concern. There are no diagnostic signs, apart perhaps from inappropriate tenderness on abdominal palpation. Symptoms may appear disproportionate to clinical well-being and there is no weight loss. Patients often appear anxious. A drug history should be taken and the possibility of a depressive illness should be considered. Pregnancy should be ruled out in young women before radiological studies are undertaken. Alcohol misuse should be suspected when early morning nausea and retching are prominent.

Investigations

The history will often suggest the diagnosis. All patients should be checked for *H. pylori* infection and patients over the age of 55 years should undergo endoscopy to exclude mucosal disease. While an ultrasound scan may detect gallstones, these are rarely responsible for dyspeptic symptoms.

Management

The most important elements are explanation and reassurance. Possible psychological factors should be explored and the concept of psychological influences on gut function should be explained. Idiosyncratic and restrictive diets are of little benefit, but smaller portions and fat restriction may help.

Up to 10% of patients benefit from *H. pylori* eradication therapy and this should be offered to infected patients. Eradication also removes a major risk factor for gastric cancer but at the cost of a small risk of side-effects and worsening symptoms of underlying gastro-oesophageal reflux disease. Drug treatment is not especially successful but merits trial. Antacids, such as hydrotalcite, are sometimes helpful. Prokinetic drugs, such as metoclopramide (10 mg 3 times daily) or domperidone (10–20 mg 3 times daily), may be given before meals if nausea, vomiting or bloating is prominent. Metoclopramide may induce extrapyramidal side-effects, including tardive dyskinesia in young subjects. H_2-receptor antagonist drugs may be tried if night pain or heartburn is troublesome. Low-dose tricyclic agents, such as amitriptyline, are of value in up to two-thirds.

Symptoms that can be associated with an identifiable cause of stress resolve with appropriate counselling. Some patients have major psychological disorders that result in persistent or recurrent symptoms and need behavioural or other formal psychotherapy (p. 240).

Functional causes of vomiting

Psychogenic retching or vomiting may arise in anxiety. It typically occurs on wakening or immediately after breakfast and only rarely later in the day. The disorder is probably a reaction to facing up to the worries of everyday life; in the young, it can be due to school phobia. Early morning vomiting also occurs in pregnancy, alcohol misuse and depression. Although functional vomiting may occur regularly over long periods, there is little or no weight loss. Children, and less often adults, sometimes suffer from acute and recurrent disabling bouts of vomiting for days at a time. The cause of this cyclical vomiting syndrome is unknown, but in some adults it is associated with cannabis use.

In all patients, it is essential to exclude other common causes (p. 853). Tranquillisers and antiemetic drugs (metoclopramide 10 mg 3 times daily, domperidone 10 mg 3 times daily, prochlorperazine 5–10 mg 3 times daily) have only a secondary place in management. Antidepressants in full dose may be effective (p. 244).

Gastroparesis

Defective gastric emptying without mechanical obstruction of the stomach or duodenum can occur as a primary event, due to inherited or acquired disorders of the gastric pacemaker, or can be secondary to disorders of autonomic nerves (particularly diabetic neuropathy) or the gastroduodenal musculature (systemic sclerosis, myotonic dystrophies and amyloidosis). Drugs such as opiates, calcium channel antagonists and those with anticholinergic activity (tricyclics, phenothiazines) can also cause gastroparesis. Early satiety and recurrent vomiting are the major symptoms; abdominal fullness and a succussion splash may be present on examination. Treatment is based upon small, frequent, low-fat meals and the use of metoclopramide and domperidone. In severe cases, nutritional failure can occur and long-term jejunostomy feeding or total parenteral nutrition is required. Surgical insertion of a gastric neurostimulator has been successful in some cases, especially those complicating diabetic autonomic neuropathy.

Tumours of the stomach

Gastric carcinoma

Gastric carcinoma is the fourth leading cause of cancer death worldwide, but there is marked geographical variation in incidence. It is most common in China, Japan, Korea (incidence 40/100 000 males), Eastern Europe and parts of South America (20/100 000). Rates in the UK are 12/100 000 for men. In most countries, the incidence is 50% lower in women. In both sexes, it rises sharply after 50 years of age. Studies of Japanese migrants to the USA have revealed a much lower incidence in second-generation migrants, confirming the importance of environmental factors. The overall prognosis is poor, with less than 30% surviving 5 years, and the best hope for improved survival lies in more efficient detection of tumours at an earlier stage.

22

Pathophysiology

Infection with *H. pylori* plays a key pathogenic role. It is associated with chronic atrophic gastritis, gastric mucosal atrophy and with gastric cancer (Fig. 22.36). It has been estimated that *H. pylori* infection may contribute to the occurrence of gastric cancer in 60–70% of cases and that acquisition of infection at an early age may be important. Although *H. pylori* infection is common in Africa, gastric cancer is uncommon and this enigma may be explained by lower life expectancy in this part of the

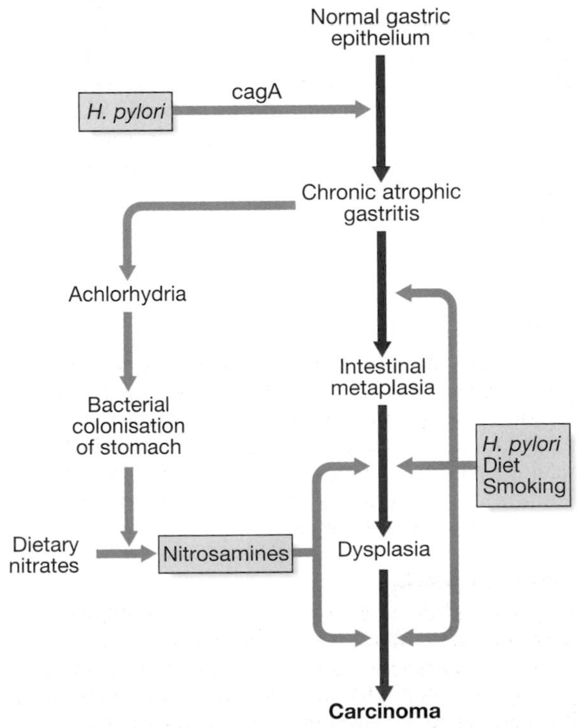

Fig. 22.36 Gastric carcinogenesis: a possible mechanism.

22.46 Risk factors for gastric cancer

- *H. pylori*
- Smoking
- Alcohol
- Dietary associations (see text)
- Autoimmune gastritis (pernicious anaemia)
- Adenomatous gastric polyps
- Previous partial gastrectomy (> 20 yrs)
- Ménétrier's disease
- Hereditary diffuse gastric cancer families (*HDC-1* mutations)
- Familial adenomatous polyposis (FAP, p. 911)

world. Although the majority of *H. pylori*-infected individuals have normal or increased acid secretion, a few become hypo- or achlorhydric and these people are thought to be at greatest risk. Chronic inflammation with generation of reactive oxygen species and depletion of the normally abundant antioxidant ascorbic acid are also important. There is strong evidence that *H. pylori* eradication, especially if achieved before irreversible pre-neoplastic changes have developed, reduces the risk of cancer development in high-risk populations and is cost-effective.

Diets rich in salted, smoked or pickled foods and the consumption of nitrites and nitrates may increase cancer risk. Carcinogenic N-nitroso-compounds are formed from nitrates by the action of nitrite-reducing bacteria which colonise the achlorhydric stomach. Diets lacking fresh fruit and vegetables, as well as vitamins C and A, may also contribute. Other risk factors are listed in Box 22.46. No predominant genetic abnormality has been identified, although cancer risk is increased two- to threefold in first-degree relatives of patients, and links with blood group A have been reported. Rarely, gastric cancer may be inherited in an autosomal dominant manner in association with mutations of the *E-cadherin* (*CDH1*) gene.

Virtually all tumours are adenocarcinomas arising from mucus-secreting cells in the base of the gastric crypts. Most develop upon a background of chronic atrophic gastritis with intestinal metaplasia and dysplasia. Cancers are either 'intestinal', arising from areas of intestinal metaplasia with histological features reminiscent of intestinal epithelium, or 'diffuse', arising from normal gastric mucosa. Intestinal carcinomas are more common and arise against a background of chronic mucosal injury. Diffuse cancers tend to be poorly differentiated and occur in younger patients. In the developing world, 50% of gastric cancers develop in the antrum; 20–30% occur in the gastric body, often on the greater curve; and 20% are found in the cardia. In Western populations, however, proximal gastric tumours are becoming more common than those arising in the body and distal stomach. This change in disease pattern may be a reflection of changes in lifestyle or the decreasing prevalence of *H. pylori* in the West. Diffuse submucosal infiltration by a scirrhous cancer (linitis plastica) is uncommon. Early gastric cancer is defined as cancer confined to the mucosa or submucosa (Fig. 22.37A). It is more often recognised in Japan, where widespread screening is practised. Some cases can be cured by endoscopic mucosal or submucosal resection (Fig. 22.37B). The majority of patients (> 80%) in the West, however, present with advanced gastric cancer.

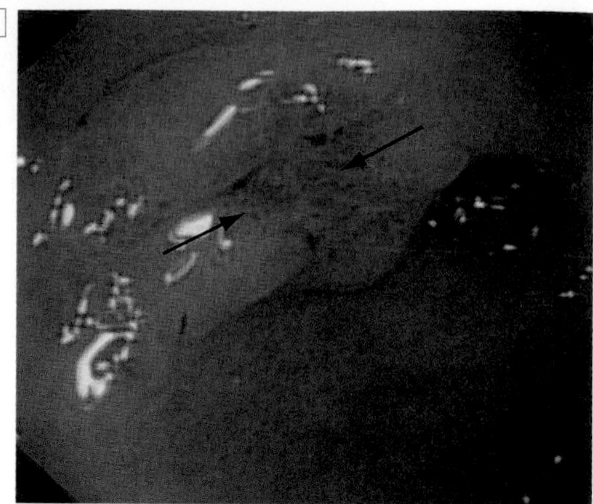

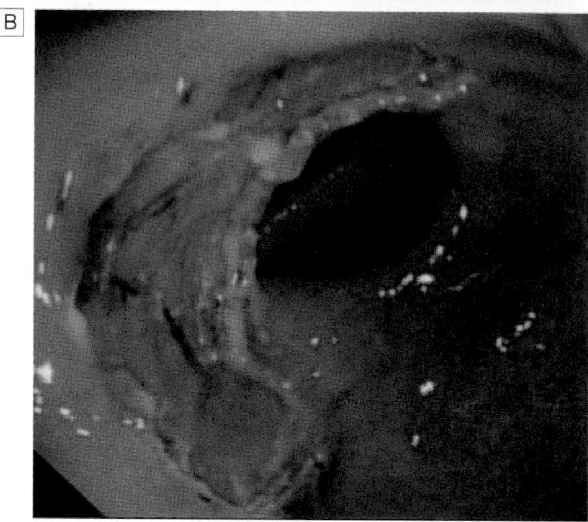

Fig. 22.37 Gastric carcinoma. **A** Endoscopic image of a small superficial pre-pyloric cancer (arrows). **B** Appearance after endoscopic mucosal resection (EMR). The tumour has been completely removed.

Clinical features

Early gastric cancer is usually asymptomatic but may be discovered during endoscopy for investigation of dyspepsia. Two-thirds of patients with advanced cancers have weight loss and 50% have ulcer-like pain. Anorexia and nausea occur in one-third, while early satiety, haematemesis, melaena and dyspepsia alone are less common. Dysphagia occurs in tumours of the gastric cardia which obstruct the gastro-oesophageal junction. Anaemia from occult bleeding is also common. Examination may reveal no abnormalities but signs of weight loss, anaemia and a palpable epigastric mass are not infrequent. Jaundice or ascites signify metastatic spread. Occasionally, tumour spread occurs to the supraclavicular lymph nodes (Troisier's sign), umbilicus (Sister Joseph's nodule) or ovaries (Krukenberg tumour). Paraneoplastic phenomena, such as acanthosis nigricans, thrombophlebitis (Trousseau's sign) and dermatomyositis, occur rarely. Metastases arise most commonly in the liver, lungs, peritoneum and bone marrow.

Investigations

Upper gastrointestinal endoscopy is the investigation of choice and should be performed promptly in any dyspeptic patient with 'alarm features' (see Box 22.15, p. 852). Multiple biopsies from the edge and base of a gastric ulcer are required. Barium meal is a poor alternative since any abnormalities must be followed by endoscopy and biopsy. Once the diagnosis is made, further imaging is necessary for staging and assessment of resectability. CT will provide evidence of intra-abdominal spread or liver metastases. Even with these techniques, laparoscopy with peritoneal washings is required to determine whether the tumour is resectable, as it is the only modality that will reliably detect peritoneal spread.

Management

Surgery

Resection offers the only hope of cure, and this can be achieved in about 90% of patients with early gastric cancer. For the majority of patients with locally advanced disease, total gastrectomy with lymphadenectomy is the operation of choice, preserving the spleen if possible. Proximal tumours involving the oesophago-gastric junction also require a distal oesophagectomy. Small, distally sited tumours can be managed by a partial gastrectomy with lymphadenectomy and either a Billroth I or a Roux en Y reconstruction. More extensive lymph node resection may increase survival rates but carries greater morbidity. Even for those who cannot be cured, palliative resection may be necessary when patients present with bleeding or gastric outflow obstruction. Following surgery, recurrence is much more likely if serosal penetration has occurred, although complete removal of all macroscopic tumour combined with lymphadenectomy will achieve a 50–60% 5-year survival. Recent evidence suggests that perioperative chemotherapy with epirubicin, cisplatin and fluorouracil (ECF) improves survival rates.

Palliative treatment

In patients with inoperable tumours, survival can be improved and palliation of symptoms achieved with chemotherapy using 5-fluorouracil and cisplatin, ECF or other platinum and taxane-based regimens. The biological agent trastuzumab may benefit some patients whose tumours over-express HER2 (see p. 268 and Box 22.47). Endoscopic laser ablation for control of dysphagia or recurrent bleeding benefits some patients. Carcinomas at the cardia or pylorus may require endoscopic dilatation or insertion of expandable metallic stents for relief of dysphagia or vomiting. A nasogastric tube may offer temporary relief of vomiting due to gastric outlet obstruction (Box 22.48).

EBM 22.47 Chemotherapy for advanced gastric cancer

'Chemotherapy significantly improves survival in comparison to best supportive care. In addition, combination chemotherapy improves survival compared to single-agent 5-fluorouracil (5-FU). All patients should be tested for their HER2 status and trastuzumab should be added to a standard 5-FU/cisplatin regimen in patients with HER2-positive tumours.'

- Wagner AD, et al. Chemotherapy for advanced gastric cancer. Cochrane Database of Systematic Reviews, 2010, issue 3. Art. no. CD004064.

For further information: www.cochrane.org/cochrane-reviews

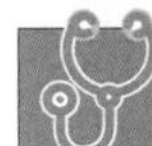

22.48 How to insert a nasogastric tube

Equipment

- 8–9F 'fine-bore' tube for feeding or 16–18F 'wide-bore' tube for drainage
- Lubricant jelly
- Cup of water and straw for sipping
- Adhesive tape
- pH (not litmus) paper
- Sickness bowl and tissues
- Catheter drainage bag and clamp (for drainage)

Technique

- A clear explanation and a calm patient are essential
- Establish a 'stop signal' for the patient to use, if needed
- Ask the patient to sit semi-upright
- Examine the nose for deformity or blockage to determine which side to use
- Measure the distance from ear to xiphoid process via the nose and mark the position on the tube
- Advance the lubricated tube tip slowly along the floor of the nasal passage to the oropharynx
- Ask the patient to sip water and advance the tube 2–3 cm with each swallow
- Stop, withdraw and retry if the patient is distressed or coughing, as the tube may have entered the larynx
- Advance until the mark on the tube reaches the tip of the nose and secure with tape
- Aspirate the contents and check pH (gastric acid confirmed if pH < 5). If in doubt, perform a chest X-ray to confirm tube position (usually necessary with feeding tubes)
- Attach the catheter drainage bag, if necessary, and clamp

Aftercare

- Flush the tube daily after feeding or drug dosing
- Check position regularly and look for signs of displacement
- Check with the pharmacist what drugs, if any, can be safely given via the tube

Gastric lymphoma

This is a rare tumour accounting for less than 5% of all gastric malignancies. The stomach is, however, the most common site for extranodal non-Hodgkin lymphoma and 60% of all primary gastrointestinal lymphomas occur at this site. Lymphoid tissue is not found in the normal stomach but lymphoid aggregates develop in the presence of *H. pylori* infection. Indeed, *H. pylori* infection is closely associated with the development of a low-grade lymphoma (classified as extranodal marginal-zone lymphomas of MALT type). EUS plays an important role in staging these lesions by accurately defining the depth of invasion into the gastric wall.

The clinical presentation is similar to that of gastric cancer, and endoscopically the tumour appears as a polypoid or ulcerating mass. While initial treatment of low-grade lesions confined to the superficial layers of the gastric wall consists of *H. pylori* eradication and close observation, 25% contain t(11:18) chromosomal translocations. In these cases, additional radiotherapy or chemotherapy is usually necessary. High-grade B-cell lymphomas should be treated by a combination of

22

rituximab, chemotherapy, surgery and radiotherapy. The choice depends on the site and extent of tumour, the presence of comorbid illnesses, and other factors, such as symptoms of bleeding and gastric outflow obstruction. The prognosis depends on the stage at diagnosis. Features predicting a favourable prognosis are stage I or II disease, small resectable tumours, tumours with low-grade histology, and age below 60 years.

Other tumours of the stomach

Gastrointestinal stromal cell tumours (GIST), arising from the interstitial cells of Cajal, are occasionally found at upper gastrointestinal endoscopy. They are differentiated from other mesenchymal tumours by expression of the *c-kit* proto-oncogene, which encodes a tyrosine kinase receptor. These tumours are usually benign and asymptomatic, but may occasionally be responsible for dyspepsia, ulceration and gastrointestinal bleeding. Small lesions (< 2 cm) are usually followed by endoscopy, while larger ones require surgical resection. Very large lesions should be treated pre-operatively with imatinib (a tyrosine kinase inhibitor) to reduce their size and make surgery easier. Imatinib can also be used for palliation of metastatic GISTs.

A variety of polyps occur. Hyperplastic polyps and fundic cystic gland polyps are common and of no consequence. Adenomatous polyps are rare but have malignant potential and should be removed endoscopically.

Occasionally, gastric carcinoid tumours are seen in the fundus and body in patients with long-standing pernicious anaemia. These benign tumours arise from ECL or other endocrine cells, and are often multiple but rarely invasive. Unlike carcinoid tumours arising elsewhere in the gastrointestinal tract, they usually run a benign and favourable course. However, large (> 2 cm) carcinoids may metastasise and should be removed. Rarely, small nodules of ectopic pancreatic exocrine tissue are found. These 'pancreatic rests' may be mistaken for gastric neoplasms and usually cause no symptoms. EUS is the most useful investigation.

DISEASES OF THE SMALL INTESTINE

Disorders causing malabsorption

Coeliac disease

Coeliac disease is an inflammatory disorder of the small bowel occurring in genetically susceptible individuals, which results from intolerance to wheat gluten and similar proteins found in rye, barley and, to a lesser extent, oats. It can result in malabsorption and responds to a gluten-free diet. The condition occurs worldwide but is more common in northern Europe. The prevalence in the UK is approximately 1%, although 50% of these people are asymptomatic. These include both undiagnosed 'silent' cases of the disease and cases of 'latent' coeliac disease – genetically susceptible people who may later develop clinical coeliac disease.

Pathophysiology

The precise mechanism of mucosal damage is unclear but immunological responses to gluten play a key role (Fig. 22.38). Tissue transglutaminase (tTG) is now recognised as the autoantigen for anti-endomysial antibodies, which are often used in serological diagnosis.

Clinical features

Coeliac disease can present at any age. In infancy, it occurs after weaning on to cereals and typically presents with diarrhoea, malabsorption and failure to thrive. In

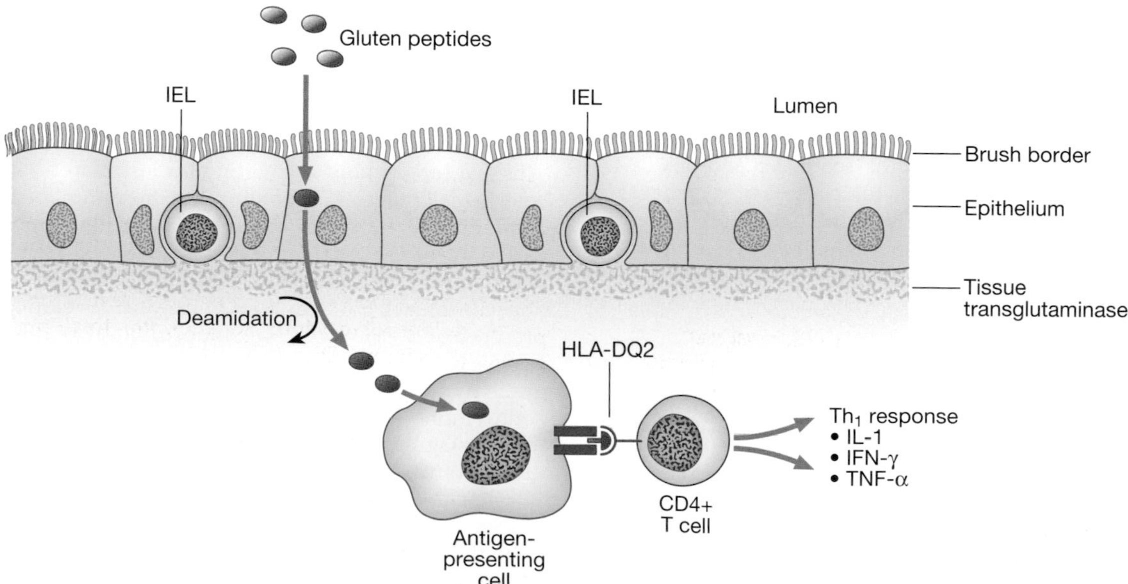

Fig. 22.38 Pathophysiology of coeliac disease. After being taken up by epithelial cells, gluten peptides are deamidated by the enzyme tissue transglutaminase in the subepithelial layer. They are then able to fit the antigen-binding motif on human leucocyte antigen (HLA)-DQ2-positive antigen-presenting cells. Recognition by CD4+ T cells triggers a Th_1 immune response with generation of pro-inflammatory cytokines – interleukin-1 (IL-1), interferon-gamma (IFN-γ) and tumour necrosis factor-alpha (TNF-α). Lymphocytes infiltrate the lamina propria, and increased intra-epithelial lymphocytes (IEL), crypt hyperplasia and villous atrophy ensue.

older children, it may present with non-specific features, such as delayed growth. Features of malnutrition are found on examination and mild abdominal distension may be present. Affected children have growth and pubertal delay, leading to short stature in adulthood.

In adults, the disease usually presents during the third or fourth decade and females are affected twice as often as males. The presentation is highly variable, depending on the severity and extent of small bowel involvement. Some have florid malabsorption, while others develop non-specific symptoms, such as tiredness, weight loss, folate deficiency or iron deficiency anaemia. Other presentations include oral ulceration, dyspepsia and bloating. Unrecognised coeliac disease is associated with mild under-nutrition and osteoporosis.

Coeliac disease is associated with other human leucocyte antigen (HLA)-linked autoimmune disorders and with certain other diseases (Box 22.49).

Investigations

These are performed to confirm the diagnosis and to look for consequences of malabsorption.

Duodenal biopsy

Endoscopic small bowel biopsy is the gold standard. The histological features are usually characteristic but other causes of villous atrophy should be considered (Box 22.50 and Fig. 22.39). Sometimes the villi appear normal but there are excess numbers of intra-epithelial lymphocytes.

Antibodies

Anti-endomysial antibodies of the IgA class are detectable by immunofluorescence in most untreated cases. They are sensitive (85–95%) and specific (approximately 99%) for the diagnosis, except in very young infants. IgG antibodies, however, must be analysed in patients with coexisting IgA deficiency. The tTG assay has replaced other blood tests in many countries, as it is easier to perform, semi-quantitative and more accurate in patients with IgA deficiency. These antibody tests constitute a valuable screening tool in patients with diarrhoea but are not a substitute for small bowel biopsy; they usually become negative with successful treatment.

A

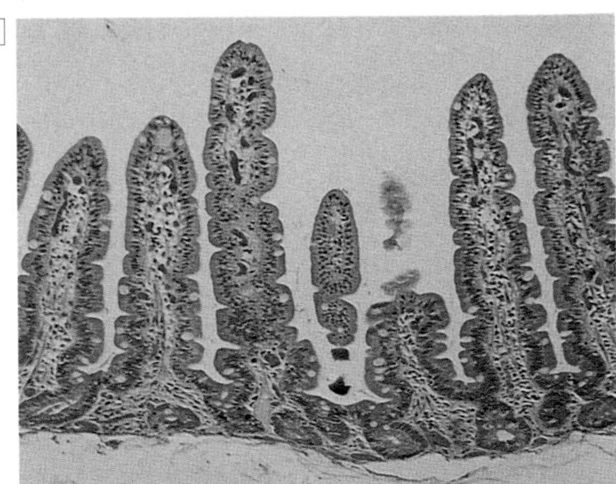

B

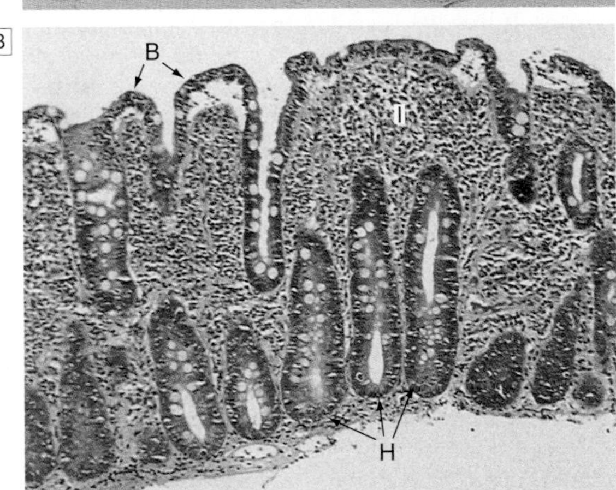

Fig. 22.39 Jejunal mucosa. **A** Normal. **B** Subtotal villous atrophy in coeliac disease. There is blunting of villi (B), crypt hyperplasia (H) and inflammatory infiltration of the lamina propria (I). From Hayes and Simpson 1995 – see p. 920.

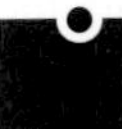

22.49 Disease associations of coeliac disease

- Insulin-dependent diabetes mellitus (2–8%)
- Thyroid disease (5%)
- Primary biliary cirrhosis (3%)
- Sjögren's syndrome (3%)
- IgA deficiency (2%)
- Pernicious anaemia
- Sarcoidosis
- Neurological complications: encephalopathy, cerebellar atrophy, peripheral neuropathy, epilepsy
- Myasthenia gravis
- Dermatitis herpetiformis
- Down's syndrome
- Enteropathy-associated T-cell lymphoma
- Small bowel carcinoma
- Squamous carcinoma of oesophagus
- Ulcerative jejunitis
- Pancreatic insufficiency
- Microscopic colitis
- Splenic atrophy

22.50 Important causes of subtotal villous atrophy

- Coeliac disease
- Tropical sprue
- Dermatitis herpetiformis
- Lymphoma
- HIV-related enteropathy
- Giardiasis
- Hypogammaglobulinaemia
- Radiation
- Whipple's disease
- Zollinger–Ellison syndrome

Haematology and biochemistry

A full blood count may show microcytic or macrocytic anaemia from iron or folate deficiency and features of hyposplenism (target cells, spherocytes and Howell–Jolly bodies). Biochemical tests may reveal reduced concentrations of calcium, magnesium, total protein, albumin or vitamin D.

Other investigations

Measurement of bone density should be considered to look for evidence of osteoporosis, especially in older patients and post-menopausal women.

Management

The aims are to correct existing deficiencies of iron, folate, calcium and/or vitamin D, and to commence a life-long gluten-free diet. This requires the exclusion of wheat, rye, barley and initially oats, although oats may be re-introduced safely in most patients after 6–12 months. Initially, frequent dietary counselling is

22

required to make sure the diet is being observed, as the most common reason for failure to improve with dietary treatment is accidental or unrecognised gluten ingestion. Mineral and vitamin supplements are also given when indicated but are seldom necessary when a strict gluten-free diet is adhered to. Booklets produced by coeliac societies in many countries, containing diet sheets and recipes for the use of gluten-free flour, are of great value. Patients should be followed up after initiation of a gluten-free diet, with assessment of symptoms, weight and nutritional status, and blood taken for measurement of tTG or anti-endomysial antibodies. Repeat small bowel biopsies are not required routinely but should be considered in patients whose symptoms fail to improve and those in whom antibody levels remain high. Dietary compliance should be carefully assessed in these circumstances. If the diet is satisfactory, then other conditions, such as pancreatic insufficiency or microscopic colitis, should be sought, as should complications of coeliac disease, such as ulcerative jejunitis or enteropathy-associated T-cell lymphoma. There remain a small number of patients who fail to respond adequately to a gluten-free diet, and these require therapy with corticosteroids or immunosuppressive drugs.

Complications

A twofold-increased risk of malignancy, particularly of enteropathy-associated T-cell lymphoma, small bowel carcinoma and squamous carcinoma of the oesophagus, has been reported.

A few patients develop ulcerative jejuno-ileitis. This may present with fever, pain, obstruction or perforation. This diagnosis can be made by barium studies or enteroscopy, but laparotomy and full-thickness biopsy may be required. Treatment is difficult. Corticosteroids are used with mixed success and some patients require surgical resection and parenteral nutrition. The course is often progressive and relentless.

Osteoporosis and osteomalacia may occur in patients with long-standing, poorly controlled coeliac disease. These complications are less common in patients who adhere strictly to a gluten-free diet.

Dermatitis herpetiformis

This is characterised by crops of intensely itchy blisters over the elbows, knees, back and buttocks (p. 1294). Immunofluorescence shows granular or linear IgA deposition at the dermo-epidermal junction. Almost all patients have partial villous atrophy on duodenal biopsy, identical to that seen in coeliac disease, even though they usually have no gastrointestinal symptoms. In contrast, fewer than 10% of coeliac patients have evidence of dermatitis herpetiformis, although both disorders are associated with the same histocompatibility antigen groups. The rash usually responds to a gluten-free diet but some patients require additional treatment with dapsone (100–150 mg daily).

Tropical sprue

Tropical sprue is defined as chronic, progressive malabsorption in a patient in or from the tropics, associated with abnormalities of small intestinal structure and function. The disease occurs mainly in the West Indies and in southern India, Malaysia and Indonesia.

Pathophysiology

The epidemiological pattern and occasional epidemics suggest that an infective agent may be involved. Although no single bacterium has been isolated, the condition often begins after an acute diarrhoeal illness. Small bowel bacterial overgrowth with *Escherichia coli*, *Enterobacter* and *Klebsiella* is frequently seen. The changes closely resemble those of coeliac disease.

Clinical features

There is diarrhoea, abdominal distension, anorexia, fatigue and weight loss. In visitors to the tropics, the onset of severe diarrhoea may be sudden and accompanied by fever. When the disorder becomes chronic, the features of megaloblastic anaemia (folic acid malabsorption) and other deficiencies, including ankle oedema, glossitis and stomatitis, are common. Remissions and relapses may occur. The differential diagnosis in the indigenous tropical population is an infective cause of diarrhoea. The important differential diagnosis in visitors to the tropics is giardiasis (p. 368).

Management

Tetracycline (250 mg 4 times daily for 28 days) is the treatment of choice and brings about long-term remission or cure. In most patients, pharmacological doses of folic acid (5 mg daily) improve symptoms and jejunal morphology. In some cases, treatment must be prolonged before improvement occurs, and occasionally patients must leave the tropics.

Small bowel bacterial overgrowth ('blind loop syndrome')

The normal duodenum and jejunum contain fewer than 10^4/mL organisms, which are usually derived from saliva. The count of coliform organisms never exceeds 10^3/mL. In bacterial overgrowth, there may be 10^8–10^{10}/mL organisms, most of which are normally found only in the colon. Disorders which impair the normal physiological mechanisms controlling bacterial proliferation in the intestine predispose to bacterial overgrowth (Box 22.51).

22.51 Causes of small bowel bacterial overgrowth

Mechanism	Examples
Hypo- or achlorhydria	Pernicious anaemia Partial gastrectomy Long-term PPI therapy
Impaired intestinal motility	Scleroderma Diabetic autonomic neuropathy Chronic intestinal pseudo-obstruction
Structural abnormalities	Gastric surgery (blind loop after Billroth II operation) Jejunal diverticulosis Enterocolic fistulae* Extensive small bowel resection Strictures*
Impaired immune function	Hypogammaglobulinaemia

*Most commonly caused by Crohn's disease.

The most important are loss of gastric acidity, impaired intestinal motility and structural abnormalities which allow colonic bacteria to gain access to the small intestine or provide a secluded haven from the peristaltic stream.

Pathophysiology

Bacterial overgrowth can occur in patients with small bowel diverticuli. Another cause is diabetic autonomic neuropathy (p. 831), which reduces small bowel motility and affects enterocyte secretion. In scleroderma, bacterial overgrowth arises because the circular and longitudinal layers of the intestinal muscle are fibrosed and motility is abnormal. In idiopathic hypogammaglobulinaemia, bacterial overgrowth occurs because the IgA and IgM levels in serum and jejunal secretions are reduced. Chronic diarrhoea and malabsorption occur because of bacterial overgrowth and recurrent gastrointestinal infections (particularly giardiasis, p. 368).

Clinical features

The patient presents with watery diarrhoea and/or steatorrhoea, with anaemia due to B_{12} deficiency. These arise because of deconjugation of bile acids, which impairs micelle formation, and because of bacterial utilisation of vitamin B_{12}. There may also be symptoms from the underlying intestinal cause.

Investigations

The diagnosis of blind loops or fistulae can often be made by barium follow-through or small bowel enema. Endoscopic duodenal biopsies are useful in excluding coeliac disease. Jejunal contents for bacteriological examination can also be aspirated at endoscopy but the laboratory analysis requires anaerobic and aerobic culture techniques. Bacterial overgrowth can also be diagnosed non-invasively using hydrogen breath tests. This simple, non-radioactive test involves serial measurement of breath samples for hydrogen after oral ingestion of 50 g glucose or lactulose; if bacteria are present within the small bowel, they rapidly metabolise the glucose, causing an early rise in exhaled hydrogen, in advance of that normally resulting from metabolism by colonic flora. Biochemical analysis may reveal low serum levels of vitamin B_{12}, with normal or elevated folate levels because the bacteria produce folic acid. Hypogammaglobulinaemia can be diagnosed by measurement of serum immunoglobulins and by intestinal biopsy, which shows reduced or absent plasma cells and nodular lymphoid hyperplasia.

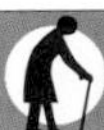

22.52 Malabsorption in old age

- **Coeliac disease**: symptoms such as dyspepsia tend to be vague; only 25% present classically with diarrhoea and weight loss. Metabolic bone disease, folate or iron deficiency, coagulopathy and small bowel lymphoma are more common.
- **Small bowel bacterial overgrowth**: more common due to atrophic gastritis, resulting in hypo- or achlorhydria; increased prevalence of jejunal diverticulosis; and long-term adverse effects of gastric surgery for ulcer disease.

Management

The underlying cause of small bowel bacterial overgrowth should be addressed, where possible. Tetracycline (250 mg 4 times daily for 7 days) is then the treatment of choice, although up to 50% of patients do not respond adequately. Metronidazole (400 mg 3 times daily) or ciprofloxacin (250 mg twice daily) is an alternative. Some patients require up to 4 weeks of treatment and, in a few, continuous rotating courses of antibiotics are necessary. Intramuscular vitamin B_{12} supplementation may be needed in chronic cases. Patients with motility disorders, such as diabetes and scleroderma, can sometimes benefit from antidiarrhoeal drugs (diphenoxylate (5 mg 3 times daily orally) or loperamide (2 mg 4–6 times daily) orally). Giardiasis should be controlled in patients with hypogammaglobulinaemia using metronidazole or tinidazole, but if symptoms fail to respond adequately, immunoglobulin infusions may be required.

Whipple's disease

This rare condition is characterised by infiltration of small intestinal mucosa by 'foamy' macrophages, which stain positive with periodic acid–Schiff (PAS) reagent. The disease is a multisystem one and almost any organ can be affected, sometimes long before gastrointestinal involvement becomes apparent (Box 22.53).

Pathophysiology

Whipple's disease is caused by infection with the Gram-positive bacillus *Tropheryma whipplei*, which becomes resident within macrophages in the bowel mucosa. Villi are widened and flattened, containing densely packed macrophages in the lamina propria, which obstruct lymphatic drainage and cause fat malabsorption.

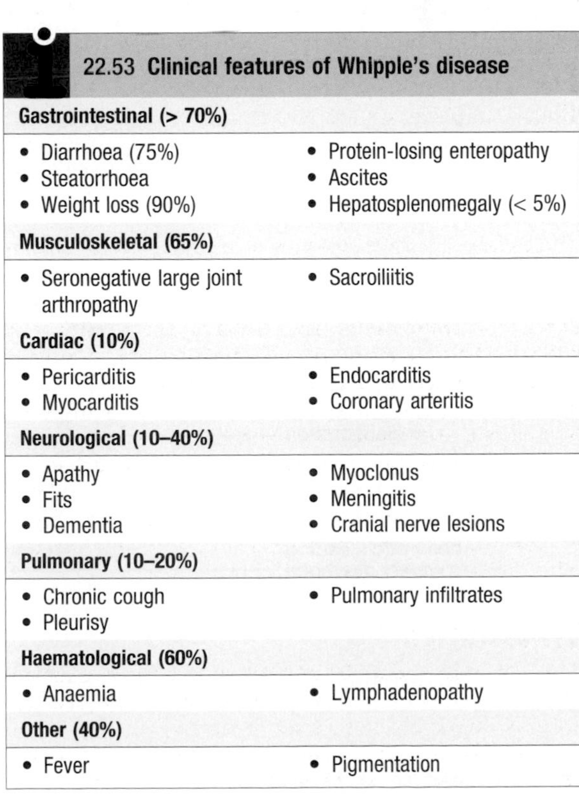

22.53 Clinical features of Whipple's disease

Gastrointestinal (> 70%)	
• Diarrhoea (75%) • Steatorrhoea • Weight loss (90%)	• Protein-losing enteropathy • Ascites • Hepatosplenomegaly (< 5%)
Musculoskeletal (65%)	
• Seronegative large joint arthropathy	• Sacroiliitis
Cardiac (10%)	
• Pericarditis • Myocarditis	• Endocarditis • Coronary arteritis
Neurological (10–40%)	
• Apathy • Fits • Dementia	• Myoclonus • Meningitis • Cranial nerve lesions
Pulmonary (10–20%)	
• Chronic cough • Pleurisy	• Pulmonary infiltrates
Haematological (60%)	
• Anaemia	• Lymphadenopathy
Other (40%)	
• Fever	• Pigmentation

22

Clinical features

Middle-aged men are most frequently affected and the presentation depends on the pattern of organ involvement. Low-grade fever is common and most patients have joint symptoms to some degree, often as the first manifestation. Occasionally, neurological manifestations may predominate.

Diagnosis

This is made by the characteristic features on small bowel biopsy, with characterisation of the bacillus by polymerase chain reaction (PCR).

Management

Whipple's disease is often fatal if untreated but responds well, at least initially, to intravenous ceftriaxone (2 g daily for 2 weeks), followed by oral co-trimoxazole for at least 1 year. Symptoms usually resolve quickly and biopsy changes revert to normal in a few weeks. Long-term follow-up is essential, as clinical relapse occurs in up to one-third of patients, often within the CNS; in this case, the same therapy is repeated or else treatment with doxycycline and hydroxychloroquine is necessary.

Ileal resection

Malabsorption can occur as a complication of small bowel resection. The most common scenario is in patients with Crohn's disease who have undergone ileal resection, leading to malabsorption of vitamin B_{12} and bile salts (Fig. 22.40). Unabsorbed bile salts pass into the colon, stimulating water and electrolyte secretion and causing diarrhoea. If hepatic synthesis of new bile salts cannot keep pace with faecal losses, fat malabsorption occurs. Another consequence is the formation of lithogenic bile, leading to gallstones. Renal calculi, rich in oxalate, develop. Normally, oxalate in the colon is bound to and precipitated by calcium. Unabsorbed bile salts preferentially bind calcium, leaving oxalate to be absorbed, with development of urinary oxalate calculi.

Patients have urgent watery diarrhoea or mild steatorrhoea. Contrast studies and tests of B_{12} and bile acid absorption (p. 850) are useful investigations. Parenteral vitamin B_{12} supplementation is necessary. Diarrhoea usually responds well to colestyramine, a resin which binds bile salts in the intestinal lumen. Aluminium hydroxide can be used as an alternative.

Short bowel syndrome

Short bowel syndrome is defined as malabsorption resulting from extensive small intestinal resection or disease. The syndrome has many causes (Box 22.54) but, in adults, it usually results from extensive surgery undertaken for Crohn's disease or mesenteric infarction. Irrespective of the underlying cause, three main types of patient are seen:

- jejunal resection with an intact ileum and colon
- jejunal and ileal resection with an intact colon (jejunum–colon)
- jejunal and ileal resection and colectomy (jejunostomy).

Pathophysiology

Patients who undergo a jejunal resection but who have an intact ileum and colon are rarely encountered and seldom require nutritional support. Those who have undergone both jejunal and ileal resection have in

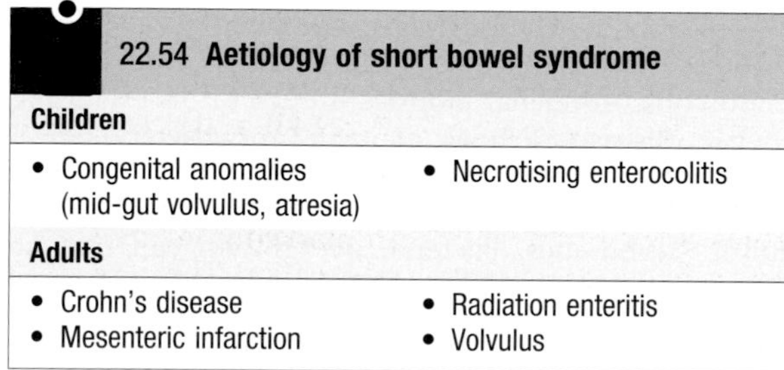

22.54 Aetiology of short bowel syndrome

Children	
• Congenital anomalies (mid-gut volvulus, atresia)	• Necrotising enterocolitis
Adults	
• Crohn's disease • Mesenteric infarction	• Radiation enteritis • Volvulus

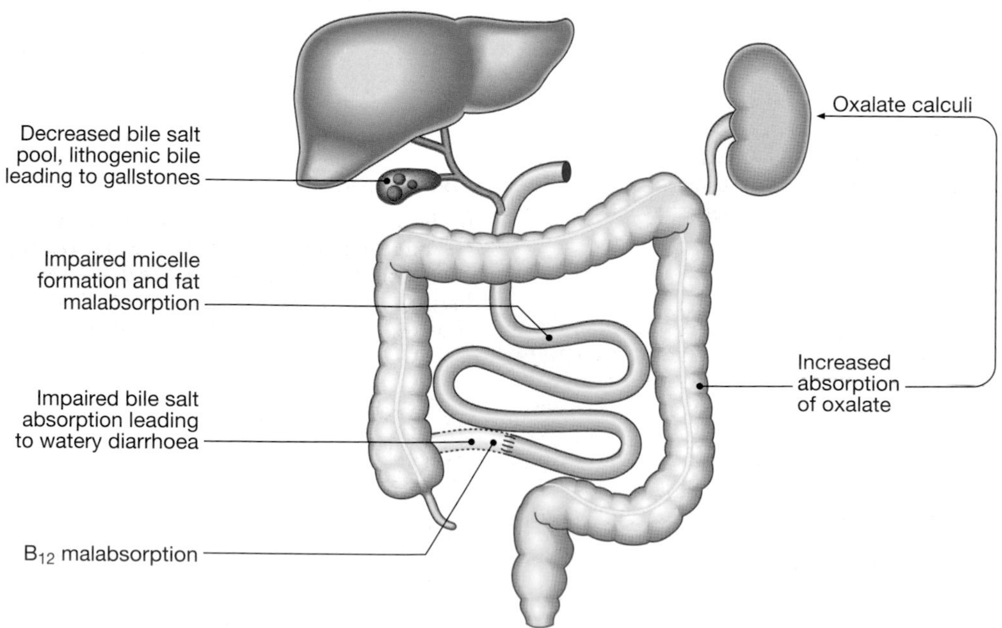

Fig. 22.40 Consequences of ileal resection.

22.55 Effects of a short bowel

	Jejunum–colon	Jejunostomy
Clinical	Gradual diarrhoea, weight loss	Rapid fluid losses
Water/electrolyte depletion	+/–	++
Malabsorption of nutrients	+	++
D-lactic acidosis	+/–	–
Oxalate renal calculi	++	–
Pigment gallstones	++	++
Gut adaptation	+	–
Impact on quality of life	Diarrhoea	High output, dehydration, parenteral nutrition

– absent; +/– can occur; + common; ++ major problem.

common the fact that they have lost a large amount of surface area for digestion and absorption, but there are important differences between jejunum–colon and jejunostomy patients (Box 22.55). Digestion and absorption are normally completed within the first 100 cm of jejunum, and enteral feeding is usually still possible if this amount of small intestine remains. The proximal small bowel normally reabsorbs most of the 8 L of fluid it receives daily (see Fig. 22.7, p. 843), and patients with a high jejunostomy are at great risk of hypovolaemia, dehydration and electrolyte losses. The presence of some or all of the colon can markedly improve these losses by increased water reabsorption. The presence of an intact ileocaecal valve ameliorates the clinical picture by slowing small intestinal transit and reducing bacterial overgrowth.

Clinical features

Severely affected patients have large volumes of jejunostomy fluid losses or, if the colon is preserved, diarrhoea and steatorrhoea. Dehydration and signs of hypovolaemia are common, as are weight loss, loss of muscle bulk and malnutrition. Some patients remain in satisfactory but precarious fluid balance until a minor intercurrent illness or intestinal upset occurs, when they can become rapidly dehydrated.

Management

In the immediate post-operative period, total parenteral nutrition (TPN) should be started and PPI therapy given to reduce gastric secretions. Enteral feeding should be cautiously introduced after 1–2 weeks under careful supervision and slowly increased as tolerated. For patients with a jejunostomy, parenteral saline is likely to be necessary if less than 100 cm of jejunum remains. If less than 75 cm of small bowel remains, TPN is also needed.

The principles of long-term management are:

- Detailed nutritional assessments at regular intervals.
- Monitoring of fluid and electrolyte balance. Patients can usually be taught how to do this for themselves. A readily available supply of oral rehydration solution is useful for intercurrent illness.
- Adequate calorie and protein intake. Fats are a good energy source and should be taken as tolerated. Medium-chain triglyceride supplements are given because they are more easily absorbed.
- Use of oral/enteral rather than parenteral nutrition whenever possible.
- Replacement of vitamin B_{12}, calcium, vitamin D, magnesium, zinc and folic acid.
- Loperamide (2–4 mg 4 times daily) or codeine phosphate (30 mg 4–6 times daily) for diarrhoea.

Octreotide (50–200 μg 2–3 times daily by subcutaneous injection) reduces gastrointestinal secretions and is useful in patients who are unable to maintain positive fluid balance. Despite these measures, some require long-term home TPN for survival and this is best managed in specialist centres. Small bowel transplantation is an option but rejection and graft-versus-host disease (p. 1017) remain significant hurdles.

Radiation enteritis and proctocolitis

Intestinal damage occurs in 10–15% of patients undergoing radiotherapy for abdominal or pelvic malignancy. The risk varies with total dose, dosing schedule and the use of concomitant chemotherapy.

Pathophysiology

The rectum, sigmoid colon and terminal ileum are most frequently involved. Radiation causes acute inflammation, shortening of villi, oedema and crypt abscess formation. These usually resolve completely but some patients develop an obliterative endarteritis affecting the endothelium of submucosal arterioles over 2–12 months. In the longer term, this can provoke a fibrotic reaction, leading to adhesions, ulceration, strictures, obstruction or fistula to adjacent organs.

Clinical features

In the acute phase, there is nausea, vomiting, cramping abdominal pain and diarrhoea. When the rectum and colon are involved, rectal mucus, bleeding and tenesmus occur. The chronic phase develops after 5–10 years in some patients and produces one or more of the problems listed in Box 22.56.

Investigations

In the acute phase, the rectal changes at sigmoidoscopy resemble ulcerative proctitis (see Fig. 22.56, p. 902). The extent of the lesion can be assessed by colonoscopy. Barium follow-through can be of diagnostic value in showing small bowel strictures, ulcers and fistulae.

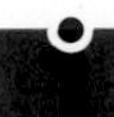

22.56 Chronic complications of intestinal irradiation

- Proctocolitis
- Bleeding from telangiectasia
- Small bowel strictures
- Fistulae: rectovaginal, colovesical, enterocolic
- Adhesions
- Malabsorption: bacterial overgrowth, bile salt malabsorption (ileal damage)

Management

Diarrhoea in the acute phase should be treated with codeine phosphate, diphenoxylate or loperamide. Local corticosteroid enemas can help proctitis, and antibiotics may be required for bacterial overgrowth. Nutritional supplements are necessary when malabsorption is present. Colestyramine (4 g as a single sachet) is useful for bile salt malabsorption. Endoscopic argon plasma coagulation therapy may reduce bleeding from proctitis. Surgery should be avoided, if possible, because the injured intestine is difficult to resect and anastomose, but may be necessary for obstruction, perforation or fistula.

Abetalipoproteinaemia

This rare autosomal recessive disorder is caused by deficiency of apolipoprotein B, which results in failure of chylomicron formation. It leads to fat malabsorption and deficiency of fat-soluble vitamins. Jejunal biopsy reveals enterocytes distended with resynthesised triglyceride and normal villous morphology. Serum cholesterol and triglyceride levels are low. A number of other abnormalities occur in this syndrome, including acanthocytosis, retinitis pigmentosa and a progressive neurological disorder with cerebellar and dorsal column signs. Symptoms may be improved by a low-fat diet supplemented with medium-chain triglycerides and vitamins A, D, E and K.

Motility disorders

Chronic intestinal pseudo-obstruction

Small intestinal motility is disordered in conditions which affect the smooth muscle or nerves of the intestine. Many cases are 'primary' (idiopathic), while others are 'secondary' to a variety of disorders or drugs (Box 22.57).

Clinical features

There are recurrent episodes of nausea, vomiting, abdominal discomfort and distension, often worse after food. Alternating constipation and diarrhoea occur and weight loss results from malabsorption (due to bacterial overgrowth) and fear of eating. There may also be symptoms of dysmotility affecting other parts of the gastrointestinal tract, such as dysphagia, and, in primary cases, features of bladder dysfunction. Some patients develop severe abdominal pain for reasons that are poorly understood and this can be difficult to manage.

Investigations

The diagnosis is often delayed and a high index of suspicion is needed. Plain X-rays show distended loops of bowel and air–fluid levels, but barium studies demonstrate no mechanical obstruction. Laparotomy is sometimes required to exclude obstruction and to obtain full-thickness biopsies of the intestine. Examination of biopsy material using specialised techniques, such as electron microscopy, and immunohistochemistry can diagnose the many rare diseases of enteric smooth muscle and nerves that can cause this syndrome.

Management

This is often difficult. Underlying causes should be addressed and further surgery avoided. Metoclopramide or domperidone may enhance motility, and antibiotics are given for bacterial overgrowth. Nutritional and psychological support is also necessary.

Miscellaneous disorders of the small intestine

Protein-losing enteropathy

This term is used when there is excessive loss of protein into the gut lumen, sufficient to cause hypoproteinaemia. Protein-losing enteropathy occurs in many gut disorders but is most common in those in which ulceration occurs (Box 22.58). In other disorders, protein loss can result from increased mucosal permeability or obstruction of intestinal lymphatic vessels. Patients present with peripheral oedema and hypoproteinaemia in the presence of normal liver function and without proteinuria. The diagnosis can be confirmed by measurement of faecal clearance of α_1-antitrypsin or ^{51}Cr-labelled albumin after intravenous injection. Other investigations should be performed to determine the underlying cause. Treatment is that of the underlying disorder, with nutritional support and measures to control peripheral oedema.

22.57 Causes of chronic intestinal pseudo-obstruction

Primary or idiopathic

- Rare familial visceral myopathies or neuropathies
- Congenital aganglionosis

Secondary

- Drugs (opiates, tricyclic antidepressants, phenothiazines)
- Smooth muscle disorders (scleroderma, amyloidosis, mitochondrial myopathies)
- Myenteric plexus disorders, e.g. paraneoplastic syndrome in small-cell lung cancer
- CNS disorders (Parkinson's disease autonomic neuropathy)
- Endocrine and metabolic disorders, (hypothyroidism, phaeochromocytoma, acute intermittent porphyria)

22.58 Causes of protein-losing enteropathy

With mucosal erosions or ulceration

- Crohn's disease
- Ulcerative colitis
- Radiation damage
- Oesophageal, gastric or colonic cancer
- Lymphoma

Without mucosal erosions or ulceration

- Ménétrier's disease
- Bacterial overgrowth
- Coeliac disease
- Tropical sprue
- Eosinophilic gastroenteritis
- Systemic lupus erythematosus

With lymphatic obstruction

- Intestinal lymphangiectasia
- Constrictive pericarditis
- Lymphoma
- Whipple's disease

Intestinal lymphangiectasia

This may be primary, resulting from congenital malunion of lymphatics, or secondary to lymphatic obstruction due to lymphoma, filariasis or constrictive pericarditis. Impaired drainage of intestinal lymphatic vessels leads to discharge of protein and fat-rich lymph into the gastrointestinal lumen. The condition presents with peripheral lymphoedema, pleural effusions or chylous ascites, and steatorrhoea. Investigations reveal hypoalbuminaemia, lymphocytopenia and reduced serum immunoglobulin concentrations. The diagnosis can be made by CT scanning and by enteroscopy and jejunal biopsy, which shows greatly dilated lacteals. Treatment consists of a low-fat diet with medium-chain triglyceride supplements.

Ulceration of the small intestine

Small bowel ulcers are uncommon and are either idiopathic or secondary to underlying intestinal disorders (Box 22.59). Ulcers are more common in the ileum, and cause bleeding, perforation, stricture formation or obstruction. Barium studies and enteroscopy confirm the diagnosis.

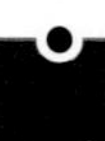

22.59 Causes of small intestinal ulcers

- Idiopathic
- Inflammatory bowel disease
- NSAIDs
- Ulcerative jejuno-ileitis
- Lymphoma and carcinoma
- Infections, (tuberculosis, typhoid, *Yersinia enterocolitica*)
- Others (radiation, vasculitis)

NSAID-associated small intestinal toxicity

These drugs cause a spectrum of small intestinal lesions ranging from erosions and ulcers to mucosal webs, strictures and, rarely, a condition known as 'diaphragm disease', in which intense submucosal fibrosis results in circumferential stricturing. The condition can present with pain, obstruction, bleeding or anaemia, and may mimic Crohn's disease, carcinoma or lymphoma. Enteroscopy or capsule endoscopy can reveal the diagnosis but sometimes this is only discovered at laparotomy.

Eosinophilic gastroenteritis

This disorder of unknown aetiology can affect any part of the gastrointestinal tract; it is characterised by eosinophil infiltration involving the gut wall, in the absence of parasitic infection or eosinophilia of other tissues. Peripheral blood eosinophilia is present in 80% of cases.

Clinical features

There are features of obstruction and inflammation, such as colicky pain, nausea and vomiting, diarrhoea and weight loss. Protein-losing enteropathy occurs and up to 50% of patients have a history of other allergic disorders. Serosal involvement may produce eosinophilic ascites.

Investigations and management

The diagnosis is made by histological assessment of multiple endoscopic biopsies, although full-thickness biopsies are occasionally required. Other investigations should be performed to exclude parasitic infection and other causes of eosinophilia. The serum IgE concentration is often raised. Dietary manipulations are rarely effective, although elimination diets, especially of milk, may benefit a few patients. Severe symptoms are treated with prednisolone (20–40 mg daily) and/or sodium cromoglicate, which stabilises mast cell membranes. The prognosis is good in the majority of patients.

Meckel's diverticulum

This is the most common congenital anomaly of the gastrointestinal tract and occurs in 0.3–3% of people, but the vast majority of affected individuals are asymptomatic throughout life. The diverticulum results from failure of closure of the vitelline duct, with persistence of a blind-ending sac arising from the anti-mesenteric border of the ileum; it usually occurs within 100 cm of the ileocaecal valve and is up to 5 cm long. Approximately 50% contain ectopic gastric mucosa; rarely, colonic, pancreatic or endometrial tissue is present. Complications most commonly occur in the first 2 years of life but are occasionally seen in young adults. Bleeding can result from ulceration of ileal mucosa adjacent to the ectopic parietal cells and presents as recurrent melaena or altered blood per rectum. The diagnosis can be made by scanning the abdomen using a gamma counter following an intravenous injection of ^{99m}Tc-pertechnate, which is concentrated by ectopic parietal cells. Other complications include intestinal obstruction, diverticulitis, intussusception and perforation. Intervention is unnecessary unless complications occur.

Adverse food reactions

Adverse food reactions are common and are subdivided into food intolerance and food allergy, the former being much more common. In food intolerance, there is an adverse reaction to food which is not immune-mediated and results from pharmacological (histamine, tyramine or monosodium glutamate), metabolic (lactase deficiency) or other mechanisms (toxins or chemical contaminants in food).

Lactose intolerance

Human milk contains around 200 mmol/L (68 g/L) of lactose, which is normally digested to glucose and galactose by the brush border enzyme lactase prior to absorption. In most populations, enterocyte lactase activity declines throughout childhood. The enzyme is deficient in up to 90% of adult Africans, Asians and South Americans, but only 5% of northern Europeans.

In cases of genetically determined (primary) lactase deficiency, jejunal morphology is normal. 'Secondary' lactase deficiency occurs as a consequence of disorders which damage the jejunal mucosa, such as coeliac disease and viral gastroenteritis. Unhydrolysed lactose enters the colon, where bacterial fermentation produces volatile short-chain fatty acids, hydrogen and carbon dioxide.

Clinical features

In most people, lactase deficiency is completely asymptomatic. However, some complain of colicky pain, abdominal distension, increased flatus, borborygmi and diarrhoea after ingesting milk or milk products. Irritable bowel syndrome may be suspected but the correct diagnosis is suggested by clinical improvement on lactose withdrawal. The lactose hydrogen breath test is a useful non-invasive confirmatory investigation.

Dietary exclusion of lactose is recommended, although most sufferers are able to tolerate small amounts of milk without symptoms. Addition of commercial lactase preparations to milk has been effective in some studies but is costly.

Intolerance of other sugars

'Osmotic' diarrhoea can be caused by sorbitol, an unabsorbable carbohydrate which is used as an artificial sweetener. Fructose contained within fruit juices may also cause diarrhoea if it is consumed in greater quantities than can be absorbed.

Food allergy

Food allergies are immune-mediated disorders, most commonly due to type I hypersensitivity reactions with production of IgE antibodies, although type IV delayed hypersensitivity reactions are also seen. Up to 20% of the population perceive themselves as suffering from food allergy but only 1–2% of adults and 5–7% of children have genuine food allergies. The most common culprits are peanuts, milk, eggs, soya and shellfish.

Clinical manifestations occur immediately on exposure and range from trivial to life-threatening or even fatal anaphylaxis. The common oral allergy syndrome results from contact with benzoic acid in certain fresh fruit juices, leading to urticaria and angioedema of the lips and oropharynx. This is not, however, an immune-mediated reaction. 'Allergic gastroenteropathy' has features similar to eosinophilic gastroenteritis, while 'gastrointestinal anaphylaxis' consists of nausea, vomiting, diarrhoea and sometimes cardiovascular and respiratory collapse. Fatal reactions to trace amounts of peanuts are well documented.

The diagnosis of food allergy is difficult to prove or refute. Skin prick tests and measurements of antigen-specific IgE antibodies in serum have limited predictive value. Double-blind placebo-controlled food challenges are the gold standard, but are laborious and are not readily available. In many cases, clinical suspicion and trials of elimination diets are used.

Treatment of proven food allergy consists of detailed patient education and awareness, strict elimination of the offending antigen, and, in some cases, antihistamines or sodium cromoglicate. Anaphylaxis should be treated as a medical emergency with resuscitation, airway support and intravenous adrenaline (epinephrine). Teachers and other carers of affected children should be trained to deal with this. Patients should wear an information bracelet and be taught to carry and use a preloaded adrenaline syringe.

Infections of the small intestine

Travellers' diarrhoea, giardiasis and amoebiasis

See pages 310, 368 and 367.

Abdominal tuberculosis

Mycobacterium tuberculosis is a rare cause of abdominal disease in Caucasians but must be considered in people in and from the developing world and in AIDS patients. Gut infection usually results from human *M. tuberculosis*, which is swallowed after coughing. Many patients have no pulmonary symptoms and a normal chest X-ray.

The area most commonly affected is the ileocaecal region. The presentation and radiological findings may be very similar to those of Crohn's disease. Abdominal pain can be acute or of several months' duration, but diarrhoea is less common in tuberculosis than in Crohn's disease. Low-grade fever is common but not invariable. Like Crohn's disease, tuberculosis can affect any part of the gastrointestinal tract, and perianal disease with fistula is recognised. Peritoneal tuberculosis may result in peritonitis with exudative ascites, associated with abdominal pain and fever. Granulomatous hepatitis occurs.

Diagnosis

Abdominal tuberculosis causes an elevated ESR; a raised serum alkaline phosphatase concentration suggests hepatic involvement. Histological confirmation should be sought by endoscopy, laparoscopy or liver biopsy. Caseation of granulomas is not always seen and acid- and alcohol-fast bacteria are often scanty. Culture may be helpful but identification of the organism may take 6 weeks and diagnosis is now possible on biopsy specimens using PCR-based techniques.

Management

When the presentation is very suggestive of abdominal tuberculosis, chemotherapy with four drugs – isoniazid, rifampicin, pyrazinamide and ethambutol (p. 691) – should be commenced, even if bacteriological or histological proof is lacking.

Cryptosporidiosis

Cryptosporidiosis and other protozoal infections, including isosporiasis (*Isospora belli*) and microsporidiosis, are dealt with on pages 369 and 399.

Tumours of the small intestine

The small intestine is rarely affected by neoplasia, and fewer than 5% of all gastrointestinal tumours occur at this site.

Benign tumours

The most common are adenomas, GIST, lipomas and hamartomas. Adenomas are most often found in the periampullary region and are usually asymptomatic, although occult bleeding or obstruction due to intussusception may occur. Transformation to adenocarcinoma is rare. Multiple adenomas are common in the duodenum of patients with familial adenomatous polyposis (FAP), who merit regular endoscopic surveillance. Hamartomatous polyps with almost no malignant potential occur in Peutz–Jeghers syndrome (p. 912).

Malignant tumours

These are rare and include, in decreasing order of frequency, adenocarcinoma, carcinoid tumour, malignant GIST and lymphoma. The majority occur in middle age or later. Kaposi's sarcoma of the small bowel may arise in patients with AIDS.

Adenocarcinomas

Adenocarcinomas occur with increased frequency in patients with FAP, coeliac disease and Peutz–Jeghers syndrome. The non-specific presentation and rarity of these lesions often lead to delay in diagnosis. Barium follow-through examination or small bowel enema studies demonstrate most lesions of this type. Enteroscopy, capsule endoscopy, mesenteric angiography and CT also play a role in investigation. Treatment is by surgical resection.

Neuro-endocrine tumours

Also known as carcinoid tumours, these are derived from enterochromaffin cells and are most common in the appendix. Localised spread and the potential for metastasis to the liver increase with primary lesions over 2 cm in diameter. They also occur in the rectum and in the appendix; those in the appendix are usually benign. Overall, these tumours are less aggressive than carcinomas and their growth is usually slow.

Symptoms depend on the location of the tumour and whether or not it is producing hormones or vasoactive peptides. The term 'carcinoid syndrome' refers to the systemic symptoms that result when secretory products of the neoplastic enterochromaffin cells reach the systemic circulation (Box 22.60). When produced by the primary tumour, they are usually metabolised in the liver and do not reach the systemic circulation. The syndrome is therefore only seen with hepatic metastases.

Management

The treatment is surgical resection. The treatment of carcinoid syndrome is palliative because hepatic metastases have already occurred, although prolonged survival is common. Surgical removal of the primary tumour and hepatic metastases may be of value, as reduction of tumour mass (cytoreductive surgery) improves symptoms. Hepatic artery embolisation is another option, since it can retard growth of hepatic deposits. Octreotide (200 μg 3 times daily by subcutaneous injection) can be used to reduce release of 5-HT, bradykinin and peptide hormones by the tumour. Cytotoxic chemotherapy with streptozotocin and 5-fluorouracil has limited benefits and is reserved as second-line therapy after other therapies have failed.

22.60 Clinical features of neuro-endocrine tumours*

- Small-bowel obstruction due to the tumour mass
- Intestinal ischaemia (due to mesenteric infiltration or vasospasm)
- Hepatic metastases causing pain, hepatomegaly and jaundice
- Flushing and wheezing
- Diarrhoea
- Cardiac involvement (tricuspid regurgitation, pulmonary stenosis, right ventricular endocardial plaques) leading to heart failure
- Facial telangiectasia

*The diagnosis is made by detecting excess levels of the 5-HT metabolite, 5-HIAA, in a 24-hr urine collection and by raised serum chromogranin A levels.

Lymphoma

Non-Hodgkin lymphoma (p. 1043) may involve the gastrointestinal tract as part of more generalised disease or may rarely arise in the gut, the small intestine being most commonly affected. Lymphomas occur with increased frequency in patients with coeliac disease, HIV-AIDS and other immunodeficiency states. Most are of B-cell origin, although lymphoma associated with coeliac disease is derived from T cells (enteropathy-associated T-cell lymphoma).

Colicky abdominal pain, obstruction and weight loss are the presenting features, and perforation is also occasionally seen. Malabsorption is a feature of diffuse bowel involvement and hepatosplenomegaly is rare.

The diagnosis is made by small bowel biopsy, radiological contrast studies and CT. Staging investigations should be performed as for lymphomas occurring elsewhere (p. 1042). Surgical resection, where possible, is the treatment of choice, with radiotherapy and combination chemotherapy reserved for those with advanced disease. The prognosis depends largely on the stage at diagnosis, cell type, patient age and the presence of 'B' symptoms (fever, weight loss, night sweats).

Immunoproliferative small intestinal disease

Immunoproliferative small intestinal disease (IPSID), also known as alpha heavy chain disease, is a rare condition occurring mainly in Mediterranean countries, the Middle East, India, Pakistan and North America. It is a variant of B-cell lymphoma of MALT type and often associated with *Campylobacter jejuni* infection. The condition varies in severity from relatively benign to frankly malignant.

The small intestinal mucosa is diffusely affected, especially proximally, by a dense lymphoplasmacytic infiltrate. Enlarged mesenteric lymph nodes are also common. Most patients are young adults, who present with malabsorption, anorexia and fever. Serum electrophoresis confirms the presence of alpha heavy chains (from the F_c portion of IgA). Prolonged remissions can be obtained with long-term antibiotic therapy, but chemotherapy is required for those who fail to respond or who have aggressive disease.

DISEASES OF THE PANCREAS

Acute pancreatitis

Acute pancreatitis accounts for 3% of all cases of abdominal pain admitted to hospital. It affects 2–28 per 100 000 of the population and is increasing in incidence. It is a potentially serious condition with an overall mortality of 10%. About 80% of all cases are mild and have a favourable outcome. About 98% of deaths from pancreatitis occur in the 20% of patients with severe disease and about one-third of these occur within the first week, usually from multi-organ failure. After this time, the majority of deaths result from sepsis, especially that

22.61 Glasgow criteria for prognosis in acute pancreatitis*

- Age > 55 yrs
- PO_2 < 8 kPa (60 mmHg)
- White blood cell count (WBC) > 15 × 10^9/L
- Albumin < 32 g/L (3.2 g/dL)
- Serum calcium < 2 mmol/L (8 mg/dL) (corrected)
- Glucose > 10 mmol/L (180 mg/dL)
- Urea > 16 mmol/L (45 mg/dL) (after rehydration)
- Alanine aminotransferase (ALT) > 200 U/L
- Lactate dehydrogenase (LDH) > 600 U/L

*Severity and prognosis worsen as the number of these factors increases. More than three implies severe disease.

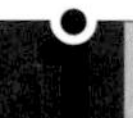

22.62 Features that predict severe pancreatitis

Initial assessment

- Clinical impression of severity
- Body mass index > 30
- Pleural effusion on chest X-ray
- APACHE II score > 8

24 hrs after admission

- Clinical impression of severity
- APACHE II score > 8
- Glasgow score > 3
- Persisting organ failure, especially if multiple
- CRP > 150 mg/L

48 hrs after admission

- Clinical impression of severity
- Glasgow score > 3
- CRP > 150 mg/L
- Persisting organ failure for 48 hrs
- Multiple or progressive organ failure

(CRP = C-reactive protein)

complicating infected necrosis. At admission, it is possible to predict patients at risk of these complications (Box 22.61). Patients who are predicted to have severe pancreatitis (Box 22.62) and those with necrosis or other complications should be managed in a specialist centre with an intensive therapy unit and multidisciplinary hepatobiliary specialists.

Pathophysiology

Acute pancreatitis occurs as a consequence of premature intracellular trypsinogen activation, releasing proteases which digest the pancreas and surrounding tissue. Triggers for this are many, including alcohol, gallstones and pancreatic duct obstruction (Fig. 22.41). There is simultaneous activation of nuclear factor kappa B (NFκB), leading to mitochondrial dysfunction, autophagy and a vigorous inflammatory response. The normal pancreas has only a poorly developed capsule, and adjacent structures, including the common bile duct, duodenum, splenic vein and transverse colon, are commonly involved in the inflammatory process. The severity of acute pancreatitis is dependent upon the balance between the activity of released proteolytic enzymes and antiproteolytic factors. The latter comprise an intracellular pancreatic trypsin inhibitor protein and circulating

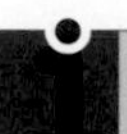

22.63 Causes of acute pancreatitis

Common (90% of cases)

- Gallstones
- Alcohol
- Idiopathic
- Post-ERCP

Rare

- Post-surgical (abdominal, cardiopulmonary bypass)
- Trauma
- Drugs (azathioprine/mercaptopurine, thiazide diuretics, sodium valproate)
- Metabolic (hypercalcaemia, hypertriglyceridaemia)
- Pancreas divisum (p. 894)
- Sphincter of Oddi dysfunction
- Infection (mumps, Coxsackie virus)
- Hereditary
- Renal failure
- Organ transplantation (kidney, liver)
- Severe hypothermia
- Petrochemical exposure

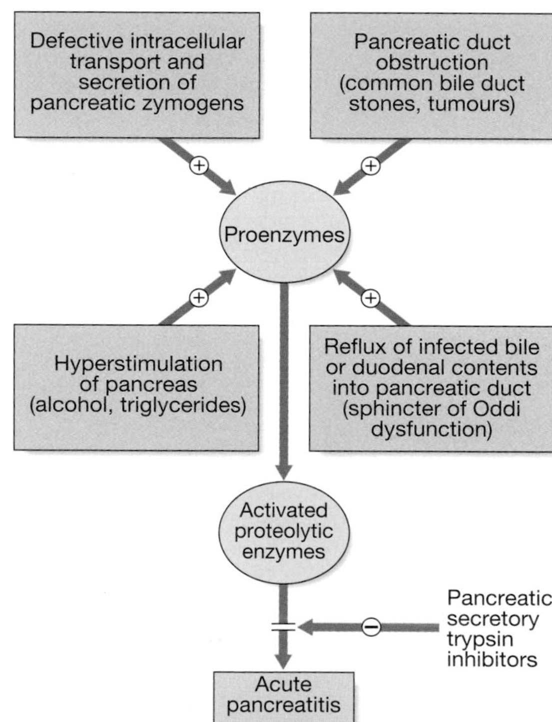

Fig. 22.41 Pathophysiology of acute pancreatitis.

β_2-macroglobulin, α_1-antitrypsin and Cl-esterase inhibitors. The causes of acute pancreatitis are listed in Box 22.63. Acute pancreatitis is often self-limiting, but in some patients with severe disease, local complications, such as necrosis, pseudocyst or abscess, occur, as well as systemic complications that lead to multi-organ failure.

Clinical features

The typical presentation is with severe, constant upper abdominal pain, of increasing intensity over 15–60 minutes, which radiates to the back. Nausea and vomiting are common. There is marked epigastric tenderness, but in the early stages (and in contrast to a perforated peptic ulcer), guarding and rebound

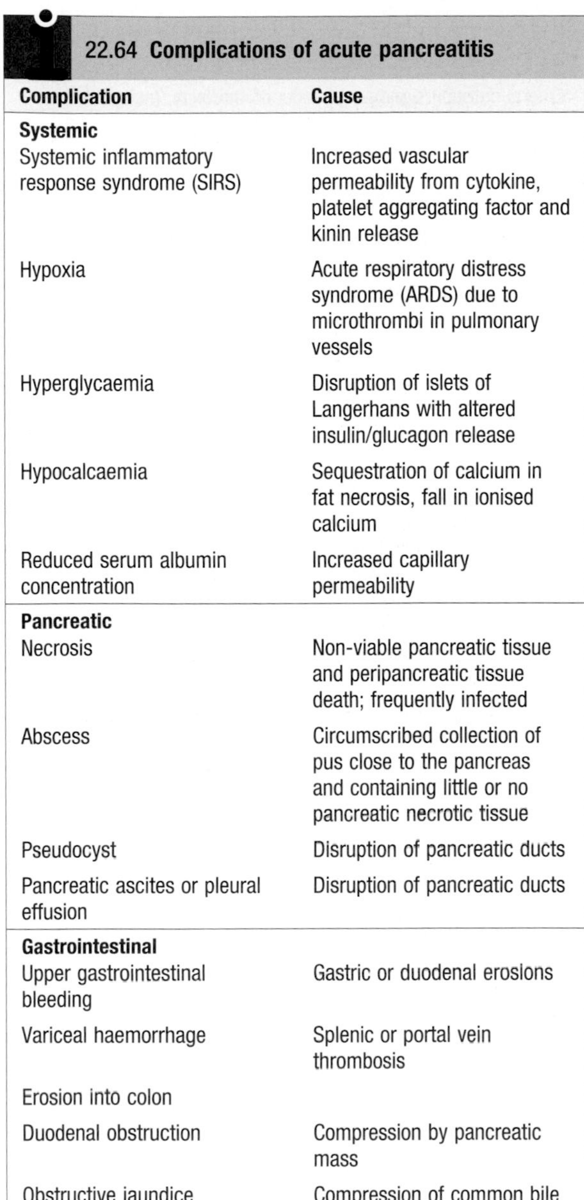

22.64 Complications of acute pancreatitis

Complication	Cause
Systemic	
Systemic inflammatory response syndrome (SIRS)	Increased vascular permeability from cytokine, platelet aggregating factor and kinin release
Hypoxia	Acute respiratory distress syndrome (ARDS) due to microthrombi in pulmonary vessels
Hyperglycaemia	Disruption of islets of Langerhans with altered insulin/glucagon release
Hypocalcaemia	Sequestration of calcium in fat necrosis, fall in ionised calcium
Reduced serum albumin concentration	Increased capillary permeability
Pancreatic	
Necrosis	Non-viable pancreatic tissue and peripancreatic tissue death; frequently infected
Abscess	Circumscribed collection of pus close to the pancreas and containing little or no pancreatic necrotic tissue
Pseudocyst	Disruption of pancreatic ducts
Pancreatic ascites or pleural effusion	Disruption of pancreatic ducts
Gastrointestinal	
Upper gastrointestinal bleeding	Gastric or duodenal erosions
Variceal haemorrhage	Splenic or portal vein thrombosis
Erosion into colon	
Duodenal obstruction	Compression by pancreatic mass
Obstructive jaundice	Compression of common bile duct

tenderness are absent because the inflammation is principally retroperitoneal. Bowel sounds become quiet or absent as paralytic ileus develops. In severe cases, the patient becomes hypoxic and develops hypovolaemic shock with oliguria. Discoloration of the flanks (Grey Turner's sign) or the periumbilical region (Cullen's sign) is a feature of severe pancreatitis with haemorrhage. The differential diagnosis includes a perforated viscus, acute cholecystitis and myocardial infarction. Various complications may occur and these are listed in Box 22.64.

A collection of fluid and debris may develop in the lesser sac, following inflammatory rupture of the pancreatic duct; this is known as a pancreatic fluid collection. It is initially contained within a poorly defined, fragile wall of granulation tissue, which matures over a 6-week period to form a fibrous capsule (Fig. 22.42). Such 'pseudocysts' are common and usually asymptomatic, resolving as the pancreatitis recovers.

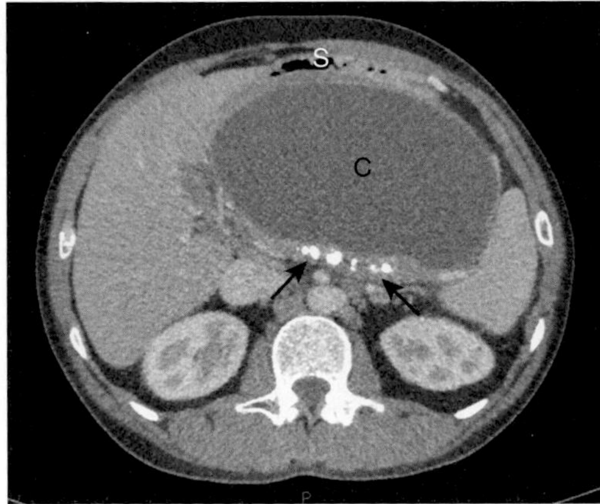

Fig. 22.42 CT showing large pancreatic pseudocyst (C) compressing the stomach (S). The pancreas is atrophic and calcified (arrows).

Pseudocysts greater than 6 cm in diameter seldom disappear spontaneously and can cause constant abdominal pain and compress or erode surrounding structures, including blood vessels, to form pseudoaneurysms. Large pseudocysts can be detected clinically as a palpable abdominal mass.

Pancreatic ascites occurs when fluid leaks from a disrupted pancreatic duct into the peritoneal cavity. Leakage into the thoracic cavity can result in a pleural effusion or a pleuro-pancreatic fistula.

Investigations

The diagnosis is based upon raised serum amylase or lipase concentrations and ultrasound or CT evidence of pancreatic swelling. Plain X-rays should be taken to exclude other diagnoses, such as perforation or obstruction, and to identify pulmonary complications. Amylase is efficiently excreted by the kidneys, and concentrations may have returned to normal if measured 24–48 hours after the onset of pancreatitis. A persistently elevated serum amylase concentration suggests pseudocyst formation. Peritoneal amylase concentrations are massively elevated in pancreatic ascites. Serum amylase concentrations are also elevated (but less so) in intestinal ischaemia, perforated peptic ulcer and ruptured ovarian cyst, whilst the salivary isoenzyme of amylase is elevated in parotitis. If available, serum lipase measurements are preferable to amylase, as they have greater diagnostic accuracy for acute pancreatitis.

Ultrasound scanning can confirm the diagnosis, although in the earlier stages the gland may not be grossly swollen. The ultrasound scan is also useful because it may show gallstones, biliary obstruction or pseudocyst formation.

Contrast-enhanced pancreatic CT 6–10 days after admission can be useful in assessing viability of the pancreas if persisting organ failure, sepsis or clinical deterioration is present, since these features may indicate that pancreatic necrosis has occurred. Necrotising pancreatitis is associated with decreased pancreatic enhancement on CT, following intravenous injection of contrast material. The presence of gas within necrotic material (Fig. 22.43) suggests infection and impending abscess formation, in which case percutaneous aspiration of material for bacterial culture should be carried out and

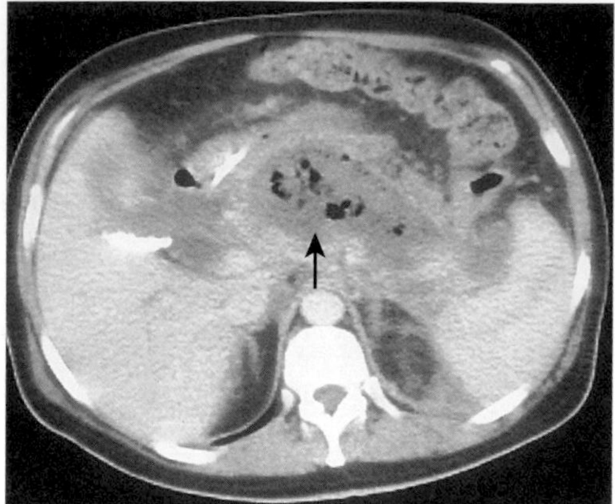

Fig. 22.43 Pancreatic necrosis. Lack of vascular enhancement of the pancreas during contrast-enhanced CT indicates necrosis (arrow). The presence of gas suggests that infection has occurred.

appropriate antibiotics prescribed. Involvement of the colon, blood vessels and other adjacent structures by the inflammatory process is best seen by CT.

Certain investigations stratify the severity of acute pancreatitis and have important prognostic value at the time of presentation (see Boxes 22.61 and 22.62). In addition, serial assessment of C-reactive protein (CRP) is a useful indicator of progress. A peak CRP > 210 mg/L in the first 4 days predicts severe acute pancreatitis with 80% accuracy. It is worth noting that the serum amylase concentration has no prognostic value.

Management

Management comprises several related steps:

- establishing the diagnosis and disease severity
- early resuscitation, according to whether the disease is mild or severe
- detection and treatment of complications
- treating the underlying cause.

Opiate analgesics should be given to treat pain and hypovolaemia should be corrected using normal saline or other crystalloids. All severe cases should be managed in a high-dependency or intensive care unit. A central venous line and urinary catheter should be established to monitor patients with shock. Oxygen should be given to hypoxic patients, and those who develop systemic inflammatory response syndrome (SIRS) may require ventilatory support. Hyperglycaemia should be corrected using insulin, but it is not usually necessary to correct hypocalcaemia by intravenous calcium injection, unless tetany occurs.

Nasogastric aspiration is only required if paralytic ileus is present. Enteral feeding, if tolerated, should be started at an early stage in patients with severe pancreatitis because they are in a severely catabolic state and need nutritional support (Box 22.65). Enteral feeding decreases endotoxaemia and so may reduce systemic complications. Nasogastric feeding is just as effective as the nasojejunal route. Prophylaxis of thromboembolism with subcutaneous low-molecular-weight heparin is also advisable. The use of prophylactic, broad-spectrum intravenous antibiotics, such as imipenem or cefuroxime, to prevent infection of pancreatic necrosis is of unproven benefit but they are often given empirically.

EBM 22.65 Enteral versus total parenteral nutritional (TPN) support in acute pancreatitis

'Enteral nutrition significantly reduced mortality, multiple organ failure, systemic infections and the need for operative interventions, compared to TPN. Enteral nutrition should be considered the standard of care for patients with acute pancreatitis requiring nutritional support.'

- Al-Omran M, et al. Cochrane Database of Systematic Reviews, 2010, issue 1. Art. no. CD002837.

For further information: www.cochrane.org/cochrane-reviews

Patients who present with cholangitis or jaundice in association with severe acute pancreatitis should undergo urgent ERCP to diagnose and treat choledocholithiasis. In less severe cases of gallstone pancreatitis, biliary imaging (using MRCP or EUS) can be carried out after the acute phase has resolved. If the liver function tests return to normal and ultrasound has not demonstrated a dilated biliary tree, laparoscopic cholecystectomy with an on-table cholangiogram is appropriate because any common bile duct stones have probably passed. When the operative cholangiogram detects residual common bile duct stones, these should be removed by laparoscopic exploration of the duct or by post-operative ERCP. Cholecystectomy should be undertaken within 2 weeks of resolution of pancreatitis – and preferably during the same admission – to prevent further potentially fatal attacks of pancreatitis. Patients with necrotising pancreatitis or pancreatic abscess require urgent endoscopic or minimally invasive retroperitoneal pancreatic (MIRP) necrosectomy to debride all cavities of necrotic material. Pancreatic pseudocysts can be treated by drainage into the stomach, duodenum or jejunum. This is usually performed after an interval of at least 6 weeks, once a pseudocapsule has matured, by surgical or endoscopic cystogastrostomy.

Chronic pancreatitis

Chronic pancreatitis is a chronic inflammatory disease characterised by fibrosis and destruction of exocrine pancreatic tissue. Diabetes mellitus occurs in advanced cases because the islets of Langerhans are involved.

Pathophysiology

Around 80% of cases in Western countries result from alcohol misuse. In southern India, severe chronic calcific pancreatitis occurs in non-alcoholics, possibly as a result of malnutrition and cassava consumption. Other causes are listed in Box 22.66. The pathophysiology of chronic pancreatitis is shown in Figure 22.44.

Clinical features

Chronic pancreatitis predominantly affects middle-aged alcoholic men. Almost all present with abdominal pain. In 50%, this occurs as episodes of 'acute pancreatitis', although each attack results in a degree of permanent pancreatic damage. Relentless, slowly progressive chronic pain without acute exacerbations affects 35% of patients, whilst the remainder have no pain but present with diarrhoea. Pain is due to a combination of increased pressure within the pancreatic ducts and

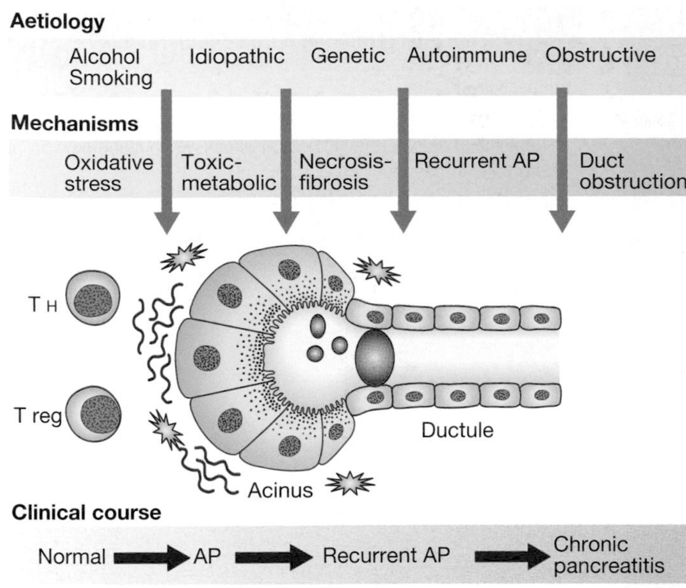

Fig. 22.44 Pathophysiology of chronic pancreatitis. Alcohol and other risk factors may trigger acute pancreatitis (AP) through multiple mechanisms. The first (or 'sentinel') episode of acute pancreatitis initiates an inflammatory response involving T-helper cells. Ongoing exposure to alcohol drives further inflammation but this is modified by regulatory T cells with subsequent fibrosis, via activation of pancreatic stellate cells. A cycle of inflammation and fibrosis ensues, with development of chronic pancreatitis. Alcohol is the most relevant risk factor, as it is involved at multiple steps.

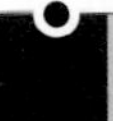

22.66 Causes of chronic pancreatitis*

Toxic–metabolic	
• Alcohol • Tobacco	• Hypercalcaemia • Chronic renal failure
Idiopathic	
• Tropical	• Early-/late-onset types
Genetic	
• Hereditary pancreatitis (cationic trypsinogen mutation)	• *SPINK-1* mutation • Cystic fibrosis
Autoimmune	
• Isolated or as part of multi-organ problem	
Recurrent and severe acute pancreatitis	
• Recurrent acute pancreatitis	• Post-necrotic
Obstructive	
• Ductal adenocarcinoma • Intraductal papillary mucinous neoplasia	• Pancreas divisum • Sphincter of Oddi stenosis

*These can be memorised by the mnemonic 'TIGARO'. Gallstones do not cause chronic pancreatitis but may be observed as an incidental finding.

direct involvement of peripancreatic nerves by the inflammatory process. Pain may be relieved by leaning forwards or by drinking alcohol. Approximately one-fifth of patients chronically consume opiate analgesics. Weight loss is common and results from a combination of anorexia, avoidance of food because of post-prandial pain, malabsorption and/or diabetes. Steatorrhoea occurs when more than 90% of the exocrine tissue has been destroyed; protein malabsorption only develops in the most advanced cases. Overall, 30% of patients are diabetic, but this figure rises to 70% in those with chronic calcific pancreatitis. Physical examination reveals a thin, malnourished patient with epigastric tenderness. Skin pigmentation over the abdomen and back is common and results from chronic use of a hot water bottle (*erythema ab igne*). Many patients have features of other alcohol- and smoking-related diseases. Complications are listed in Box 22.67.

22.67 Complications of chronic pancreatitis

- Pseudocysts and pancreatic ascites, which occur in both acute and chronic pancreatitis
- Obstructive jaundice due to benign stricture of the common bile duct as it passes through the diseased pancreas
- Duodenal stenosis
- Portal or splenic vein thrombosis leading to segmental portal hypertension and gastric varices
- Peptic ulcer

22.68 Investigations in chronic pancreatitis

Tests to establish the diagnosis

- Ultrasound
- CT (may show atrophy, calcification or ductal dilatation)
- Abdominal X-ray (may show calcification)
- MRCP
- Endoscopic ultrasound

Tests of pancreatic function

- Collection of pure pancreatic juice after secretin injection (gold standard but invasive and seldom used)
- Pancreolauryl test (see Box 22.12, p. 851)
- Faecal pancreatic elastase

Tests of anatomy prior to surgery

- MRCP

Investigations

Investigations (Box 22.68 and Fig. 22.45) are carried out to:

- make a diagnosis of chronic pancreatitis
- define pancreatic function
- demonstrate anatomical abnormalities prior to surgical intervention.

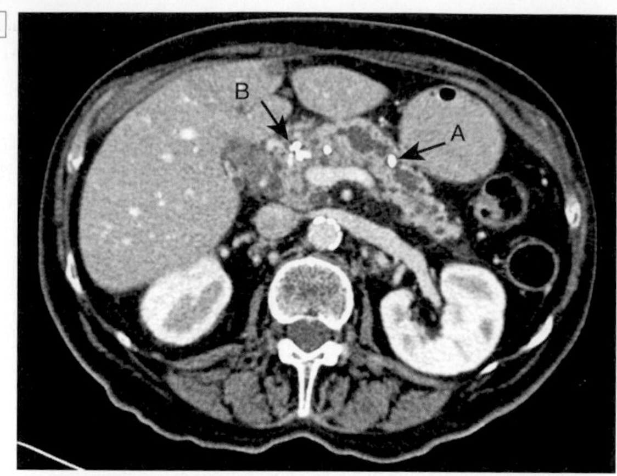

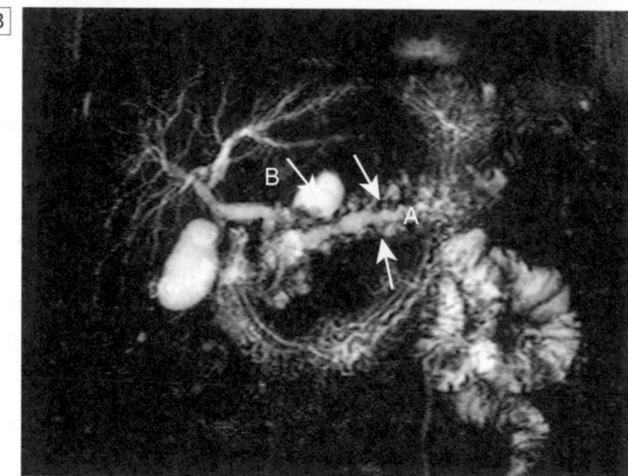

Fig. 22.45 Imaging in chronic pancreatitis. **A** CT scan showing a grossly dilated and irregular duct with a calcified stone (arrow A). Note the calcification in the head of the gland (arrow B). **B** MRCP of the same patient showing marked ductal dilatation with abnormal dilated side branches (arrows A). A small cyst is also present (arrow B).

Management

Alcohol misuse

Alcohol avoidance is crucial in halting progression of the disease and reducing pain.

Pain relief

A range of analgesic drugs, particularly NSAIDs, are valuable, but the severe and unremitting nature of the pain often leads to opiate use with the risk of addiction. Oral pancreatic enzyme supplements suppress pancreatic secretion and their regular use reduces analgesic consumption in some patients. Patients who are abstinent from alcohol and who have severe chronic pain which is resistant to conservative measures should be considered for surgical or endoscopic pancreatic therapy (Box 22.69). Coeliac plexus neurolysis sometimes produces long-lasting pain relief, although relapse occurs in the majority of cases. In some patients, MRCP does not show a surgically or endoscopically correctable abnormality and, in these patients, the only surgical approach is total pancreatectomy. Unfortunately, even after this operation, some patients continue to experience pain. Moreover, the procedure causes diabetes, which may be difficult to control, with a high risk of hypoglycaemia (since both insulin and glucagon release are absent), and significant morbidity and mortality.

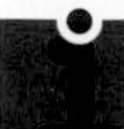

22.69 Intervention in chronic pancreatitis
Endoscopic therapy
• Dilatation or stenting of pancreatic duct strictures • Removal of calculi (mechanical or shock-wave lithotripsy) • Drainage of pseudocysts
Surgical methods
• Partial pancreatic resection, preserving the duodenum • Pancreatico-jejunostomy

Malabsorption

This is treated by dietary fat restriction (with supplementary medium-chain triglyceride therapy in malnourished patients) and oral pancreatic enzyme supplements. A PPI is added to optimise duodenal pH for pancreatic enzyme activity.

Management of complications

Surgical or endoscopic therapy may be necessary for the management of pseudocysts, pancreatic ascites, common bile duct or duodenal stricture and the consequences of portal hypertension. Many patients with chronic pancreatitis also require treatment for other alcohol- and smoking-related diseases and for the consequences of self-neglect and malnutrition.

Autoimmune pancreatitis

Autoimmune pancreatitis (AIP) is a form of chronic pancreatitis that can mimic cancer but which responds to corticosteroids. It is characterised by abdominal pain, weight loss or obstructive jaundice, without acute attacks of pancreatitis. Blood tests reveal increased serum IgG or IgG4, and the presence of other autoantibodies. Imaging shows a diffusely enlarged pancreas, narrowing of the pancreatic duct and stricturing of the lower bile duct. AIP may occur alone or with other autoimmune disorders, such as Sjögren's syndrome, primary sclerosing cholangitis (PSC) or inflammatory bowel disease. The response to steroids is usually excellent but some patients require azathioprine.

Congenital abnormalities affecting the pancreas

Pancreas divisum

This is due to failure of the primitive dorsal and ventral ducts to fuse during embryonic development of the pancreas. As a consequence, most of the pancreatic drainage occurs through the smaller accessory ampulla rather than through the major ampulla. The condition occurs in 7–10% of the normal population and is usually asymptomatic, but some patients develop acute pancreatitis, chronic pancreatitis or atypical abdominal pain.

Annular pancreas

In this congenital anomaly, the pancreas encircles the second/third part of the duodenum, leading to gastric outlet obstruction. Annular pancreas is associated with malrotation of the intestine, atresias and cardiac anomalies.

Cystic fibrosis

This disease is considered in detail on page 680. The major gastrointestinal manifestations are pancreatic insufficiency and meconium ileus. Peptic ulcer and hepatobiliary disease may also occur. In cystic fibrosis, pancreatic secretions are protein- and mucus-rich. The resultant viscous juice forms plugs which obstruct the pancreatic ductules, leading to progressive destruction of acinar cells. Steatorrhoea is universal and the large-volume bulky stools predispose to rectal prolapse. Malnutrition is compounded by the metabolic demands of respiratory failure and by diabetes, which develops in 40% of patients by adolescence.

Most patients now survive well into adulthood and heart/lung transplantation can further prolong life. Optimal treatment depends upon an assiduous team approach to respiratory, nutritional and hepatobiliary complications. Nutritional counselling and supervision are important to ensure intake of high-energy foods, providing 120–150% of the recommended intake for normal subjects. Fats are an important calorie source and, despite the presence of steatorrhoea, fat intake should not be restricted. Supplementary fat-soluble vitamins are also necessary. High-dose oral pancreatic enzymes are required, in doses sufficient to control steatorrhoea and stool frequency. A PPI aids fat digestion by producing an optimal duodenal pH. Diabetic patients usually require insulin injections rather than oral hypoglycaemic agents.

Meconium ileus

Mucus-rich plugs within intestinal contents can obstruct the small or large intestine. Meconium ileus is treated by the mucolytic agent N-acetylcysteine, given orally, by Gastrografin enema or by gut lavage using polyethylene glycol. In resistant cases of meconium ileus, surgical resection may be necessary.

Tumours of the pancreas

Pancreatic carcinoma affects 10–15 per 100 000 in Western populations, rising to 100 per 100 000 in those over the age of 70. Men are affected twice as often as women. The disease is associated with increasing age, smoking and chronic pancreatitis. Between 5 and 10% of patients have a genetic predisposition (hereditary pancreatitis, MEN, hereditary non-polyposis colon cancer (HNPCC) and familial atypical mole multiple melanoma syndrome (FAMMM). Overall survival is only 3–5%, with median survival of 6–10 months for those with locally advanced disease and 3–5 months if metastases are present.

Pathophysiology

Some 90% of pancreatic neoplasms are adenocarcinomas which arise from the pancreatic ducts. These tumours involve local structures and metastasise to regional lymph nodes at an early stage. Most patients have advanced disease at the time of presentation.

Clinical features

Many patients are asymptomatic until an advanced stage, when they present with central abdominal pain, weight loss and obstructive jaundice (Fig. 22.46). The pain results from invasion of the coeliac plexus and is characteristically incessant and gnawing. It often radiates from the upper abdomen through to the back and may be eased a little by bending forwards. Almost all patients lose weight and many are cachectic. Around 60% of tumours arise from the head of the pancreas, and involvement of the common bile duct results in the development of obstructive jaundice, often with severe pruritus. A few patients present with diarrhoea, vomiting from duodenal obstruction, diabetes mellitus, recurrent venous thrombosis, acute pancreatitis or depression. Physical examination reveals clear evidence of weight loss. An abdominal mass due to the tumour itself, a palpable gallbladder or hepatic metastasis is commonly found. A palpable gallbladder in a jaundiced patient is usually the consequence of distal biliary obstruction by a pancreatic cancer (Courvoisier's sign).

Investigations

The diagnosis is usually made by ultrasound and contrast-enhanced CT (Fig. 22.47). Diagnosis in non-jaundiced patients is often delayed because presenting symptoms are relatively non-specific. Fit patients with small localised tumours should undergo staging to define operability. EUS or laparoscopy with laparoscopic ultrasound will define tumour size, involvement of blood vessels and metastatic spread. In patients unsuitable for surgery because of advanced disease, frailty or comorbidity, EUS or CT-guided cytology or biopsy can be used to confirm the diagnosis. MRCP and ERCP are sensitive methods of diagnosing pancreatic cancer and are valuable when the diagnosis is in doubt, although differentiation between cancer and localised chronic pancreatitis can be difficult. The main role of ERCP is to insert a stent into the common bile duct to relieve obstructive jaundice in inoperable patients.

Management

Surgical resection is the only method of effecting cure, and 5-year survival in patients undergoing a complete resection is around 12%. Recent trials have demonstrated improved survival (21–29%) with adjuvant chemotherapy using gemcitabine. Unfortunately, only 10–15% of tumours are resectable for cure, since most are locally advanced at the time of diagnosis. For the great majority of patients, treatment is palliative. Chemotherapy with FOLFIRINOX (5-fluorouracil, leucovorin, irinotecan and oxaliplatin) improves median survival to 11 months. Pain relief can be achieved using analgesics but, in some patients, coeliac plexus neurolysis may be required. Jaundice can be relieved by choledochojejunostomy in fit patients, whereas percutaneous or endoscopic stenting is preferable in the elderly and those with very advanced disease. Ampullary or periampullary adenocarcinomas are rare neoplasms which arise from the ampulla of Vater or adjacent duodenum. They are often polypoid and may ulcerate; they frequently infiltrate the duodenum but behave less aggressively than pancreatic adenocarcinoma. Around 25% of patients undergoing resection of ampullary or periampullary tumours survive for 5 years, in contrast to patients with pancreatic ductal cancer.

Cystic neoplasms of the pancreas are increasingly being seen with widespread use of CT. These are a heterogeneous group; serous cystadenomas rarely, if ever, become malignant and do not require surgery.

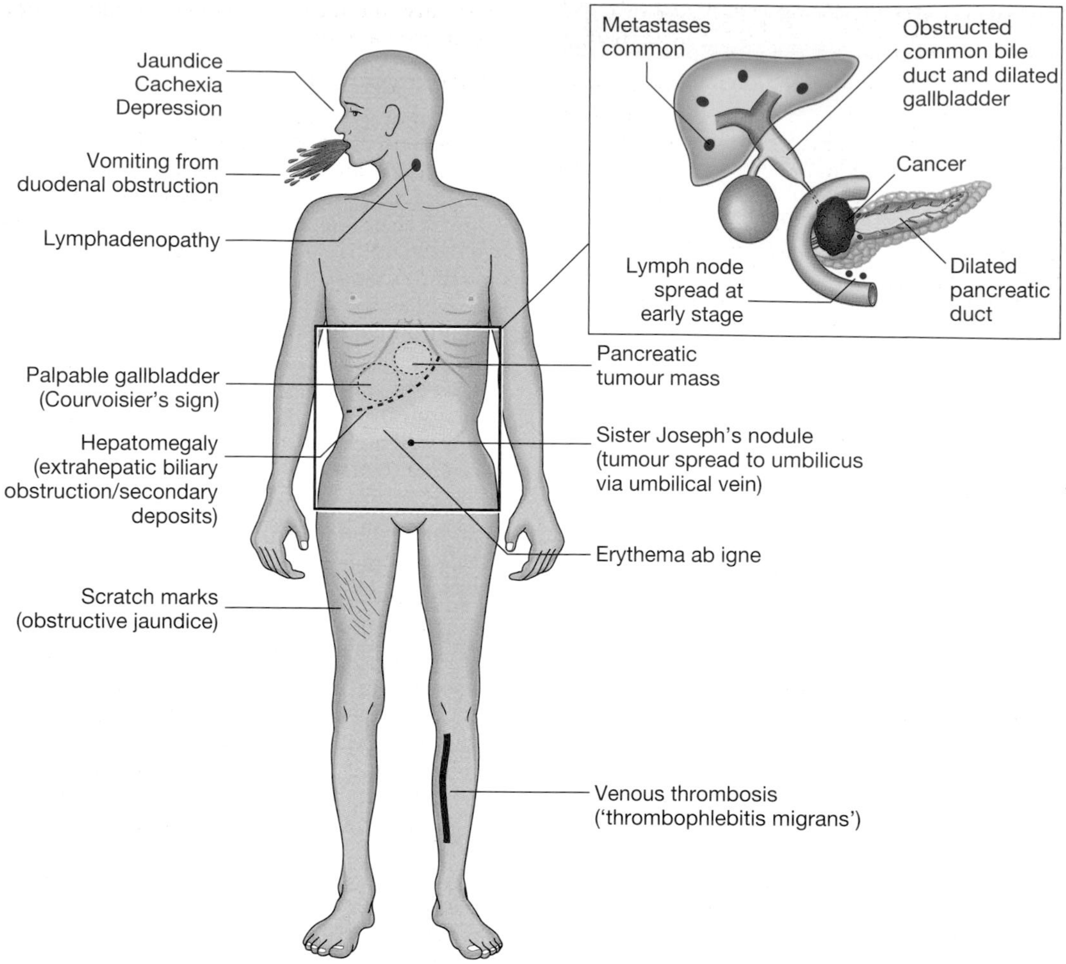

Jaundice
Cachexia
Depression

Vomiting from duodenal obstruction

Lymphadenopathy

Palpable gallbladder (Courvoisier's sign)

Hepatomegaly (extrahepatic biliary obstruction/secondary deposits)

Scratch marks (obstructive jaundice)

Metastases common

Obstructed common bile duct and dilated gallbladder

Cancer

Lymph node spread at early stage

Dilated pancreatic duct

Pancreatic tumour mass

Sister Joseph's nodule (tumour spread to umbilicus via umbilical vein)

Erythema ab igne

Venous thrombosis ('thrombophlebitis migrans')

Fig. 22.46 Features of pancreatic cancer.

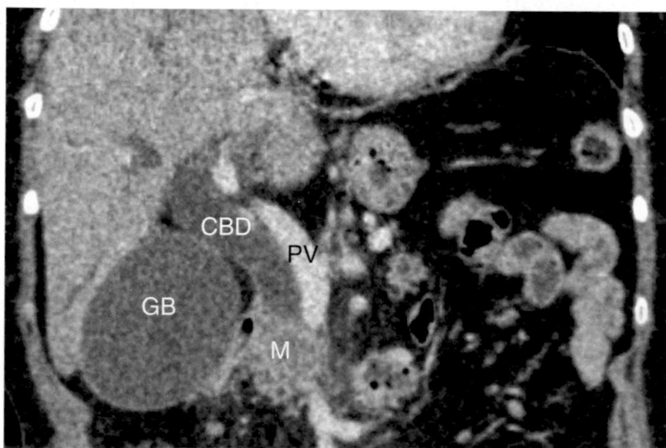

Fig. 22.47 Carcinoma of the pancreatic head. A large mass (M) in the head of pancreas involves the portal vein (PV) and obstructs the common bile duct (CBD). The gallbladder (GB) is distended.

Mucinous cysts occur more often in women, are usually in the pancreatic tail and display a spectrum of behaviour from benign to frankly malignant. Aspiration of the cyst contents for cytology and measurement of carcino-embryonic antigen (CEA) and amylase concentrations in fluid obtained at EUS can help determine whether a lesion is mucinous or not. In fit patients, all mucinous lesions should be resected. A variant, called intraductal papillary mucinous neoplasia (IPMN), is often discovered coincidentally on CT, frequently in elderly men. This may affect the main pancreatic duct with marked dilatation and plugs of mucus, or may affect a side branch. The histology varies from villous adenomatous change to dysplasia or carcinoma. Since IPMN is a pre-malignant but indolent condition, the decision to resect or to monitor depends on age and fitness of the patient and location, size and evolution of lesions.

Pancreatic neuro-endocrine tumours

These can occur in association with parathyroid and pituitary adenomas (MEN 1, p. 795). The majority of endocrine tumours are non-secretory and, although malignant, grow slowly and metastasise late. Other tumours secrete hormones and present because of their endocrine effects (see Box 20.54, p. 784). Neuro-endocrine pancreatic tumours may be single, but are frequently multifocal and arise from other clusters of neuro-endocrine cells derived from neural crest tissues. They are localised by CT and endoscopic ultrasound. ^{111}In-labelled DTPA is very sensitive in the diagnosis of glucagonoma.

INFLAMMATORY BOWEL DISEASE

Ulcerative colitis and Crohn's disease are chronic inflammatory bowel diseases which pursue a protracted relapsing and remitting course, usually extending over years. The diseases have many similarities and it is sometimes impossible to differentiate between them. A crucial distinction is that ulcerative colitis only involves the colon, while Crohn's disease can involve any part of the gastrointestinal tract from mouth to anus. A summary of the main features of ulcerative colitis and Crohn's disease is provided in Box 22.70.

The incidence of inflammatory bowel disease (IBD) varies widely between populations. There was a dramatic increase in the incidence of Crohn's disease in the Western world, starting in the second half of the last century and coinciding with the introduction of a more 'hygienic' environment with the advent of domestic refrigeration and the widespread use of antibiotics. The developing world has seen similar patterns, as these countries adopt an increasingly Westernised lifestyle.

In the West, the incidence of ulcerative colitis is stable at 10–20 per 100000, with a prevalence of 100–200 per 100000, while the incidence of Crohn's disease is increasing and is now 5–10 per 100000, with a prevalence of 50–100 per 100000. Both diseases most commonly start in the second and third decades of life, with a second smaller incidence peak in the seventh decade. Approximately 240000 people are affected by IBD in the UK (approximately 1.4 million in the USA), equating to a prevalence of about 1 in 250. Life expectancy in patients with IBD is similar to that of the general population. Although many patients require surgery and admission to hospital for other reasons, with substantial associated morbidity, the majority have an excellent work record and pursue a normal life.

Pathophysiology

Inflammatory bowel disease has both environmental and genetic components, and evidence from genome-wide association studies suggests that genetic variants that predispose to Crohn's disease may have undergone positive selection by protecting against infectious diseases, including tuberculosis (Box 22.71). It is thought that IBD develops because these genetically susceptible individuals mount an abnormal inflammatory response to environmental triggers, such as intestinal bacteria. This leads to inflammation of the intestine with release of inflammatory mediators, including TNF, IL-12 and IL-23, which cause tissue damage (Fig. 22.48). In both diseases, the intestinal wall is infiltrated with acute and chronic inflammatory cells but there are important differences between the conditions in the distribution of lesions and in histological features (Fig. 22.49).

Ulcerative colitis

Inflammation invariably involves the rectum (proctitis) and spreads proximally in a continuous manner to involve the entire colon in some cases (pancolitis). In long-standing pancolitis, the bowel can become shortened and post-inflammatory 'pseudopolyps' develop; these are normal or hypertrophied residual mucosa within areas of atrophy. The inflammatory process is limited to the mucosa and spares the deeper layers of the bowel wall (Fig. 22.50). Both acute and chronic inflammatory cells infiltrate the lamina propria and the crypts ('cryptitis'). Crypt abscesses are typical. Goblet cells lose their mucus and, in long-standing cases, glands become distorted. Dysplasia, characterised by heaping

22.70 Comparison of ulcerative colitis and Crohn's disease

	Ulcerative colitis	Crohn's disease
Age group	Any	Any
Gender	M = F	Slight female preponderance
Incidence	Stable	Increasing
Ethnic group	Any	Any; more common in Ashkenazi Jews
Genetic factors	*HLA-DR*103*; colonic epithelial barrier function (*HNF4a, LAMB1, CDH1*)	Defective innate immunity and autophagy (*NOD2, ATG16L1, IRGM*)
Risk factors	More common in non-/ex-smokers Appendicectomy protects	More common in smokers
Anatomical distribution	Colon only; begins at anorectal margin with variable proximal extension	Any part of gastrointestinal tract; perianal disease common; patchy distribution, skip lesions
Extra-intestinal manifestations	Common	Common
Presentation	Bloody diarrhoea	Variable; pain, diarrhoea, weight loss all common
Histology	Inflammation limited to mucosa; crypt distortion, cryptitis, crypt abscesses, loss of goblet cells	Submucosal or transmural inflammation common; deep fissuring ulcers, fistulae; patchy changes; granulomas
Management	5-ASA; corticosteroids; azathioprine; biological therapy (anti-TNF); colectomy is curative	Corticosteroids; azathioprine; methotrexate; biological therapy (anti-TNF); nutritional therapy; surgery for complications is not curative; 5-ASA not effective

(5-ASA = 5-aminosalicylic acid; TNF = tumour necrosis factor)

22

of cells within crypts, nuclear atypia and increased mitotic rate, may herald development of colon cancer.

Crohn's disease

The sites most commonly involved are, in order of frequency, the terminal ileum and right side of colon, colon alone, terminal ileum alone, ileum and jejunum. The entire wall of the bowel is oedematous and thickened, and there are deep ulcers which often appear as linear fissures; thus the mucosa between them is described as 'cobblestone'. These may penetrate through the bowel wall to initiate abscesses or fistulae involving the bowel, bladder, uterus, vagina and skin of the perineum. The

22.71 Factors associated with the development of inflammatory bowel disease

Genetic

- Both CD and UC common in Ashkenazi Jews
- 10% have first-degree relative/≥1 close relative with IBD
- High concordance in identical twins (40–50% CD; 20–25% UC)
- 163 susceptibility loci identified at genome-wide levels of significance; most confer susceptibility to both CD and UC; many are also susceptibility loci for other inflammatory conditions (esp. ankylosing spondylosis and psoriasis)
- UC and CD both associated with genetic variants at HLA locus, and with multiple genes involved with immune signalling (esp. IL-23 and IL-10 pathways)
- CD associated with genetic defects in innate immunity and autophagy (*NOD2, ATG16L1* and *IRGM* genes)
- UC associated with genetic defects in barrier function
- *NOD2* associated with ileal and stricturing disease, and hence need for resectional surgery
- *HLA-DR*103* associated with severe UC

Environmental

- UC more common in non-smokers and ex-smokers
- CD more common in smokers (relative risk = 3)
- CD associated with low-residue, high-refined-sugar diet
- Commensal gut microbiota altered (dysbiosis) in CD and UC
- Appendicectomy protects against UC

(CD = Crohn's disease; HLA = human leucocyte antigen; IL = interleukin; IBD = inflammatory bowel disease; UC = ulcerative colitis)

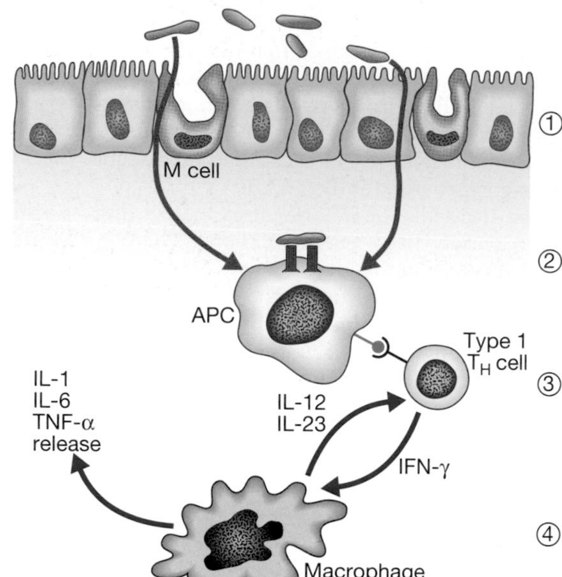

Fig. 22.48 Pathogenesis of inflammatory bowel disease. (1) Bacterial antigens are taken up by specialised M cells, pass between leaky epithelial cells or enter the lamina propria through ulcerated mucosa. (2) After processing, they are presented to type 1 T-helper cells by antigen-presenting cells (APC) in the lamina propria. (3) T-cell activation and differentiation results in a Th_1 T cell-mediated cytokine response (4) with secretion of cytokines, including interferon-gamma (IFN-γ). Further amplification of T cells perpetuates the inflammatory process with activation of non-immune cells and release of other important cytokines, including interleukin (IL)-12, IL-23, IL-1 IL-6 and tumour necrosis factor (TNF). These pathways occur in all normal individuals exposed to an inflammatory insult and this is self-limiting in healthy subjects. In genetically predisposed persons, dysregulation of innate immunity may trigger inflammatory bowel disease.

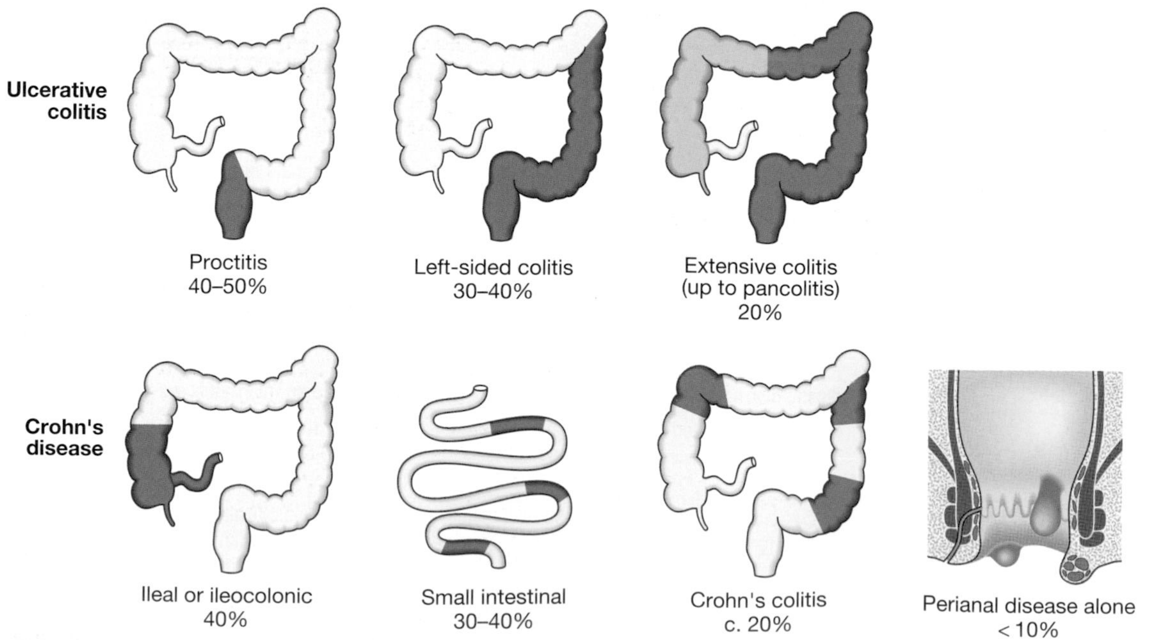

Fig. 22.49 Common patterns of disease distribution in inflammatory bowel disease.

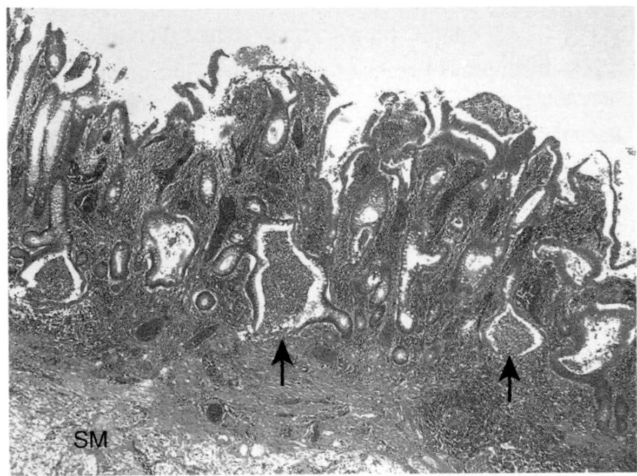

Fig. 22.50 Histology of ulcerative colitis. There is surface ulceration and inflammation is confined to the mucosa with excess inflammatory cells in the lamina propria, loss of goblet cells, and crypt abscesses (arrows). (SM = submucosa)

A

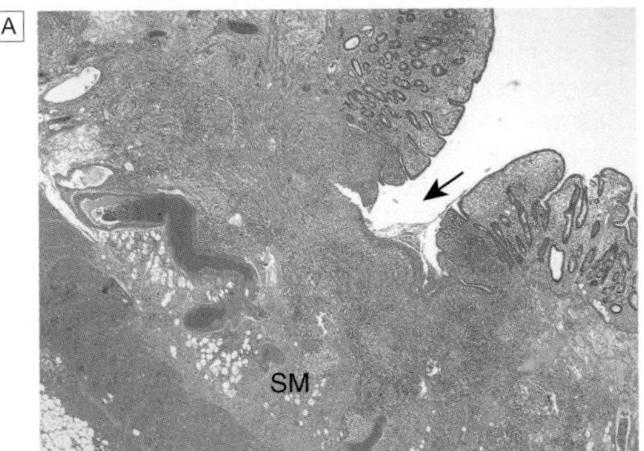

B

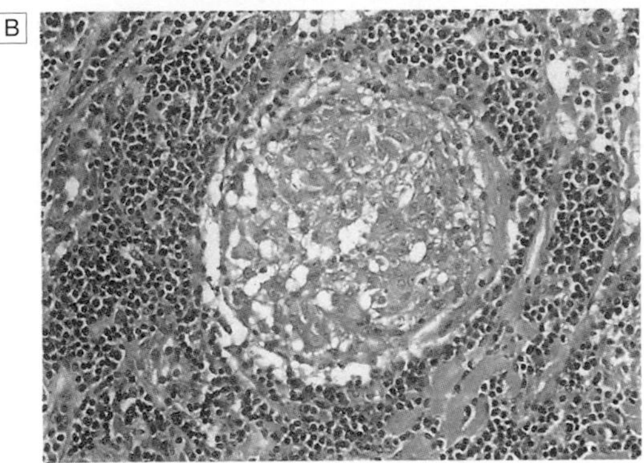

Fig. 22.51 Histology of Crohn's disease. **A** Inflammation is 'transmural'; there is fissuring ulceration (arrow), with inflammation extending into the submucosa (SM). **B** At higher power, a characteristic non-caseating granuloma is seen.

mesenteric lymph nodes are enlarged and the mesentery is thickened. Crohn's disease has a patchy distribution and the inflammatory process is interrupted by islands of normal mucosa. On histological examination, the bowel wall is thickened with a chronic inflammatory infiltrate throughout all layers (Fig. 22.51).

Clinical features

Ulcerative colitis

The cardinal symptoms are rectal bleeding with passage of mucus and bloody diarrhoea. The presentation varies, depending on the site and severity of the disease (see Fig. 22.49), as well as the presence of extra-intestinal manifestations. The first attack is usually the most severe and is followed by relapses and remissions. Emotional stress, intercurrent infection, gastroenteritis, antibiotics or NSAID therapy may all provoke a relapse. Proctitis causes rectal bleeding and mucus discharge, accompanied by tenesmus. Some patients pass frequent, small-volume fluid stools, while others pass pellety stools due to constipation upstream of the inflamed rectum. Constitutional symptoms do not occur. Left-sided and extensive colitis causes bloody diarrhoea with mucus, often with abdominal cramps. In severe cases, anorexia, malaise, weight loss and abdominal pain occur, and the patient is toxic, with fever, tachycardia and signs of peritoneal inflammation (Box 22.72).

22.72 Assessment of disease severity in ulcerative colitis

	Mild	Severe
Daily bowel frequency	< 4	≥ 6*
Blood in stools	+/–	+++
Stool volume	< 200 g/24 hrs	> 400 g/24 hrs
Pulse	< 90 beats/min	≥ 90 beats/min*
Temperature	Normal	≥ 37.8°C*
Haemoglobin	Normal	< 100 g/L (< 10 g/dL)*
Erythrocyte sedimentation rate	Normal	> 30 mm/hr* (or equivalent C-reactive protein)
Serum albumin	> 35 g/L (> 3.5 g/dL)	< 30 g/L (< 3 g/dL)
Abdominal X-ray	Normal	Dilated bowel and/or mucosal islands
Sigmoidoscopy	Normal or granular mucosa	Blood in lumen

*The Truelove–Witts criteria for acute severe ulcerative colitis are ≥ 6 bloody stools/24 hrs plus one or more of anaemia, fever, tachycardia and high inflammatory markers.

Crohn's disease

The major symptoms are abdominal pain, diarrhoea and weight loss. Ileal Crohn's disease (Figs 22.52 and 22.53) may cause subacute or even acute intestinal obstruction. The pain is often associated with diarrhoea, which is usually watery and does not contain blood or mucus. Almost all patients lose weight because they avoid food, since eating provokes pain. Weight loss may also be due to malabsorption, and some patients present with features of fat, protein or vitamin deficiencies. Crohn's colitis presents in an identical manner to ulcerative colitis, but rectal sparing and the presence of perianal disease are features which favour a diagnosis of Crohn's disease. Many patients present with symptoms of both small bowel and colonic disease. A few patients present with isolated perianal disease, vomiting from jejunal strictures or severe oral ulceration.

Physical examination often reveals evidence of weight loss, anaemia with glossitis and angular

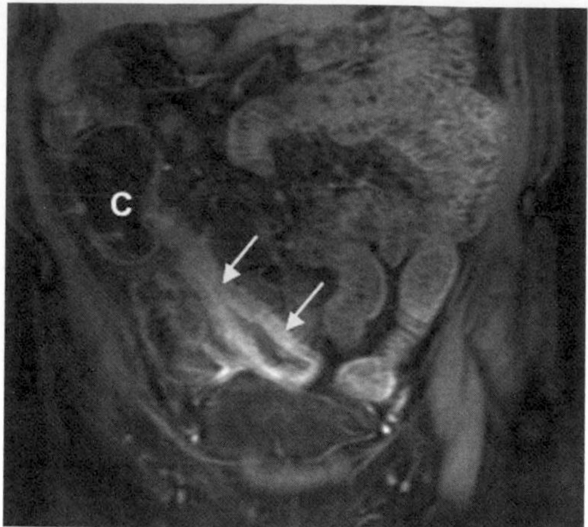

Fig. 22.52 Ileal Crohn's disease. MRI scan showing a thickened narrowed loop of ileum with enhancement after MR contrast (arrows), consistent with active Crohn's disease. Normal small bowel can be seen at the top right of the image. (C = caecum)

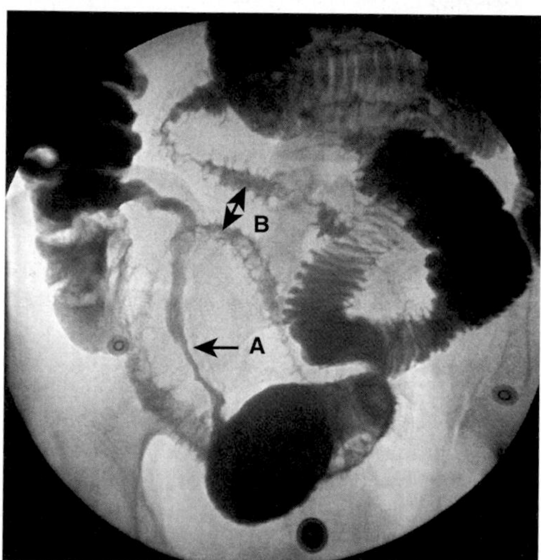

Fig. 22.53 Barium follow-through showing terminal ileal Crohn's disease. A long stricture is present (arrow A), and more proximally there is ulceration with characteristic 'rose thorn' ulcers (arrow B).

stomatitis. There is abdominal tenderness, most marked over the inflamed area. An abdominal mass may be palpable and is due to matted loops of thickened bowel or an intra-abdominal abscess. Perianal skin tags, fissures or fistulae are found in at least 50% of patients.

Differential diagnosis

The differential diagnosis is summarised in Box 22.73. The most important issue is to distinguish the first attack of acute colitis from infection. In general, diarrhoea lasting longer than 10 days in Western countries is unlikely to be the result of infection, whereas a history of foreign travel, antibiotic exposure (pseudomembranous colitis) or homosexual contact increases the possibility of infection, which should be excluded by the appropriate investigations (see below). The diagnosis of Crohn's disease is usually more straightforward and is made on the basis of imaging and clinical presentation, but in atypical cases, biopsy or surgical resection is necessary to exclude other diseases (Box 22.74).

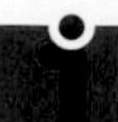

22.73 Conditions which can mimic ulcerative or Crohn's colitis

Infective

Bacterial

- *Salmonella*
- *Shigella*
- *Campylobacter jejuni*
- *E. coli* 0157
- Gonococcal proctitis
- Pseudomembranous colitis
- *Chlamydia* proctitis

Viral

- Herpes simplex proctitis
- Cytomegalovirus

Protozoal

- Amoebiasis

Non-infective

- Ischaemic colitis
- Collagenous colitis
- NSAIDs
- Diverticulitis
- Radiation proctitis
- Behçet's disease
- Colonic carcinoma

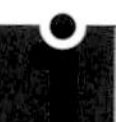

22.74 Differential diagnosis of small bowel Crohn's disease

- Other causes of right iliac fossa mass
  - Caecal carcinoma*
  - Appendix abscess*
- Infection (tuberculosis, *Yersinia*, actinomycosis)
- Mesenteric adenitis
- Pelvic inflammatory disease
- Lymphoma

*Common; other causes are rare.

Complications

Life-threatening colonic inflammation

This can occur in both ulcerative colitis and Crohn's colitis. In the most extreme cases, the colon dilates (toxic megacolon) and bacterial toxins pass freely across the diseased mucosa into the portal and then systemic circulation. This complication arises most commonly during the first attack of colitis and is recognised by the features described in Box 22.72. An abdominal X-ray should be taken daily because, when the transverse colon is dilated to more than 6 cm (Fig. 22.54), there is a high risk of colonic perforation, although this complication can also occur in the absence of toxic megacolon.

Haemorrhage

Haemorrhage due to erosion of a major artery is rare but can occur in both conditions.

Fistulae

These are specific to Crohn's disease. Enteroenteric fistulae can cause diarrhoea and malabsorption due to blind loop syndrome. Enterovesical fistulation causes recurrent urinary infections and pneumaturia. An enterovaginal fistula causes a faeculent vaginal discharge. Fistulation from the bowel may also cause perianal or ischiorectal abscesses, fissures and fistulae.

Cancer

The risk of dysplasia and cancer increases with the duration and extent of uncontrolled colonic inflammation. Thus patients who have long-standing, extensive colitis are at highest risk. Oral mesalazine therapy reduces the

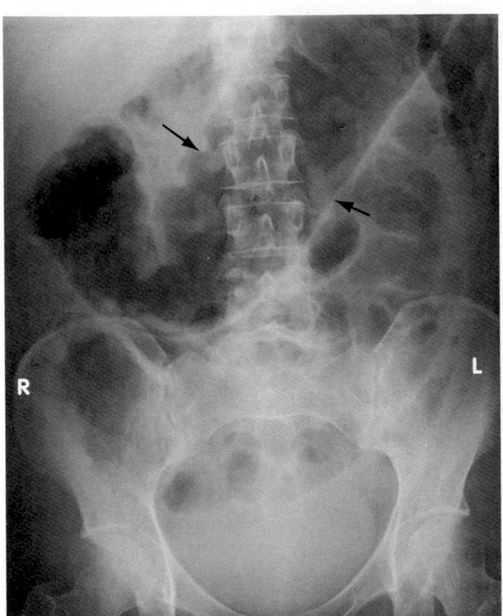

Fig. 22.54 Plain abdominal X-ray showing a grossly dilated colon due to severe ulcerative colitis. There is also marked mucosal oedema and 'thumb-printing' (arrows).

risk of dysplasia and neoplasia in ulcerative colitis. Azathioprine also seems to reduce the risk of colorectal cancer in ulcerative colitis and Crohn's colitis. This protective effect probably extends to any medical treatment that results in sustained healing of the colonic mucosa. The cumulative risk for dysplasia in ulcerative colitis may be as high as 20% after 30 years but is probably lower for Crohn's colitis. The risk is particularly high in patients who have concomitant primary sclerosing cholangitis for unknown reasons. Tumours develop in areas of dysplasia and may be multiple. Patients with long-standing colitis are therefore entered into surveillance programmes beginning 10 years after diagnosis. Targeted biopsies of areas that show abnormalities on staining with indigo carmine or methylene blue increase the chance of detecting dysplasia and this technique (termed pancolonic chromo-endoscopy) has replaced colonoscopy with random biopsies taken every 10 cm in screening for malignancy. The procedure allows patients to be stratified into high-, medium- or low-risk groups to determine the interval between surveillance procedures. If high-grade dysplasia is found, panproctocolectomy is usually recommended because of the high risk of colon cancer.

Extra-intestinal complications

Extra-intestinal complications are common in IBD and may dominate the clinical picture. Some of these occur during relapse of intestinal disease; others appear unrelated to intestinal disease activity (Fig. 22.55).

Investigations

Investigations are necessary to confirm the diagnosis, define disease distribution and activity, and identify complications. Full blood count may show anaemia resulting from bleeding or malabsorption of iron, folic acid or vitamin B_{12}. Serum albumin concentration falls as a consequence of protein-losing enteropathy, inflammatory disease or poor nutrition. The ESR and CRP are elevated in exacerbations and in response to abscess formation. Faecal calproctectin has a high sensitivity for detecting gastrointestinal inflammation and may be elevated, even when the CRP is normal. It is particularly useful in distinguishing inflammatory bowel disease from irritable bowel syndrome at diagnosis, and for subsequent monitoring of disease activity.

Bacteriology

At initial presentation, stool microscopy, culture and examination for *Clostridium difficile* toxin or for ova and cysts, blood cultures and serological tests should be performed. These investigations may need to be repeated in established disease to exclude superimposed enteric infection in patients who present with exacerbations of IBD. During acute flares necessitating hospital admission, three separate stool samples should be sent for bacteriology to maximise sensitivity.

Endoscopy

Patients who present with diarrhoea plus raised inflammatory markers or alarm features, such as weight loss, rectal bleeding and anaemia, should undergo ileocolonoscopy. Flexible sigmoidoscopy is occasionally performed to make a diagnosis, especially during acute severe presentations when ileocolonoscopy may confer an unacceptable risk; ileocolonoscopy should still be performed at a later date, however, in order to evaluate disease extent. In ulcerative colitis, there is loss of vascular pattern, granularity, friability and contact bleeding, with or without ulceration (Fig. 22.56). In Crohn's disease, patchy inflammation, with discrete, deep ulcers, strictures and perianal disease (fissures, fistulae and skin tags), is typically observed, often with rectal sparing. In established disease, colonoscopy may show active inflammation with pseudopolyps or a complicating carcinoma. Biopsies should be taken from each anatomical segment (terminal ileum, right colon, transverse colon, left colon and rectum) to confirm the diagnosis and define disease extent, and also to seek dysplasia in patients with long-standing colitis. In Crohn's disease, wireless capsule endoscopy is useful in the identification of small bowel inflammation but should be avoided in the presence of strictures. Enteroscopy may be required to make a histological diagnosis of small bowel Crohn's disease, when the inflamed segment is out of reach of standard endoscopes. All children and most adults with Crohn's disease should have upper gastrointestinal endoscopy and biopsy to complete their staging. Not only is upper gastrointestinal Crohn's disease relatively common in this group, but it may help to make a definitive diagnosis in patients who otherwise appear to have non-specific colonic inflammation.

Radiology

Barium enema is a less sensitive investigation than colonoscopy in patients with colitis and, where colonoscopy is incomplete, a CT colonogram is preferred. Small bowel imaging is essential to complete staging of Crohn's disease. Traditional contrast imaging by barium follow-through demonstrates affected areas of the bowel as narrowed and ulcerated, often with multiple strictures (see Fig. 22.53). This has now largely been replaced by MRI enterography, which does not involve exposure to radiation and is a sensitive way of detecting extra-intestinal manifestations and of assessing pelvic and

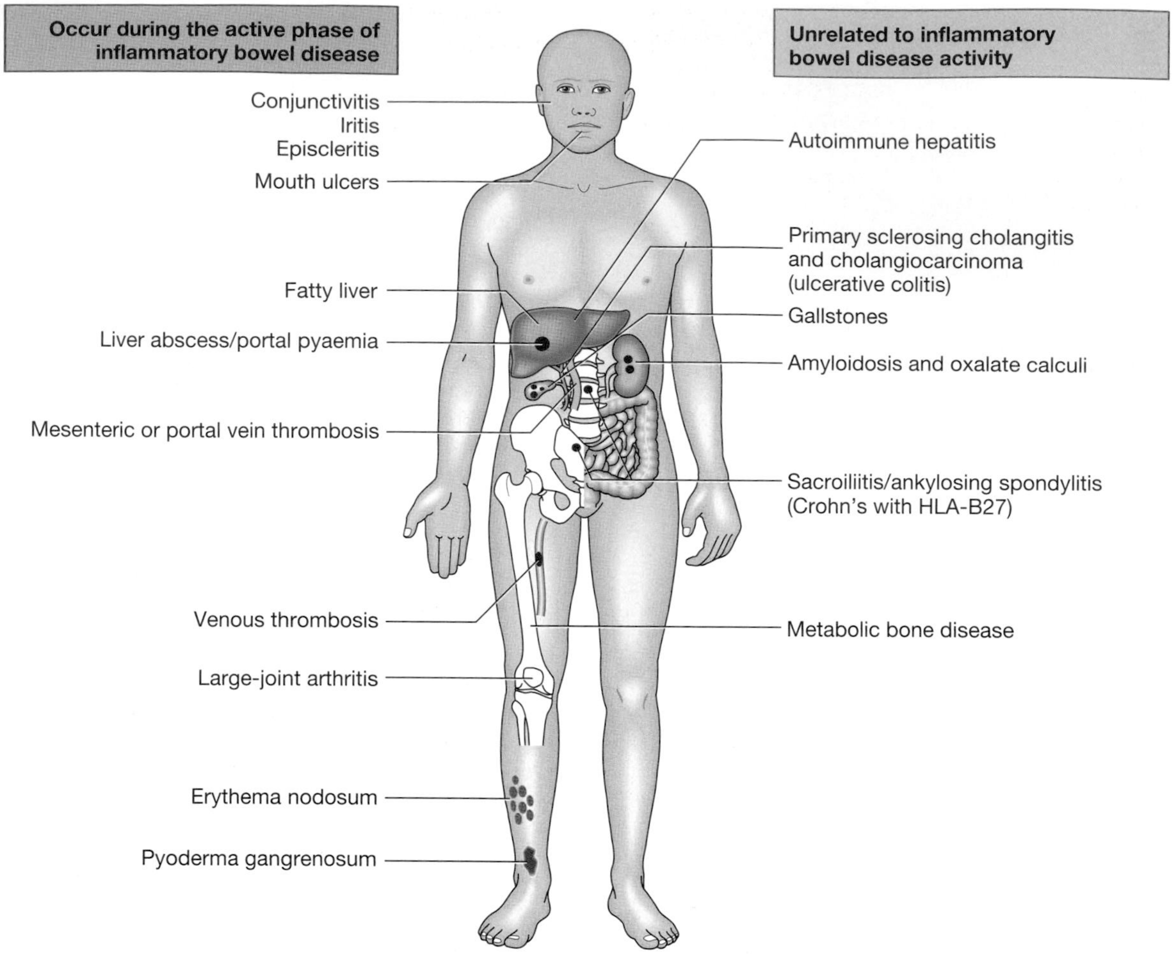

Occur during the active phase of inflammatory bowel disease

Conjunctivitis
Iritis
Episcleritis
Mouth ulcers
Fatty liver
Liver abscess/portal pyaemia
Mesenteric or portal vein thrombosis
Venous thrombosis
Large-joint arthritis
Erythema nodosum
Pyoderma gangrenosum

Unrelated to inflammatory bowel disease activity

Autoimmune hepatitis
Primary sclerosing cholangitis and cholangiocarcinoma (ulcerative colitis)
Gallstones
Amyloidosis and oxalate calculi
Sacroiliitis/ankylosing spondylitis (Crohn's with HLA-B27)
Metabolic bone disease

Fig. 22.55 Systemic complications of inflammatory bowel disease. (See also Chs 19 and 20.)

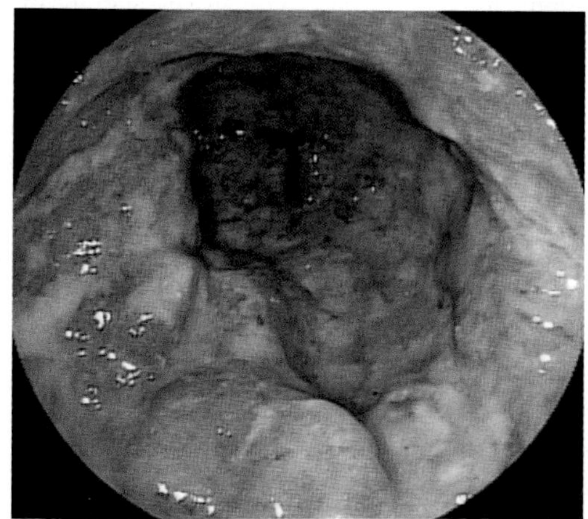

Fig. 22.56 Sigmoidoscopic view of moderately active ulcerative colitis. Mucosa is erythematous and friable with contact bleeding. Submucosal blood vessels are no longer visible.

perineal involvement. These studies use an orally administered small bowel-distending agent and intravenous contrast to provide transmural imaging that can usefully distinguish between predominantly inflammatory strictures (that should respond to anti-inflammatory medical strategies) and fibrotic strictures (that require a mechanical solution, such as surgical resection, stricturoplasty or endoscopic balloon dilatation). A plain abdominal X-ray is essential in the management of patients who present with severe active disease. Dilatation of the colon (see Fig. 22.54), mucosal oedema (thumb-printing) or evidence of perforation may be found. In small bowel Crohn's disease, there may be evidence of intestinal obstruction or displacement of bowel loops by a mass. Ultrasound is a very powerful tool to detect small bowel inflammation and stricture formation, but it is rather operator-dependent. The role of CT is limited to screening for complications, such as perforation or abscess formation, in the acutely unwell.

Management

Drugs that are used in the treatment of IBD are listed in Box 22.75. Although medical therapy plays an important role, optimal management depends on establishing a multidisciplinary team-based approach involving physicians, surgeons, radiologists, nurse specialists and dietitians. Both ulcerative colitis and Crohn's disease are life-long conditions and have important psychosocial implications; specialist nurses, counsellors and patient support groups have key roles in education, reassurance and coping. The key aims of medical therapy are to:

- treat acute attacks (induce remission)
- prevent relapses (maintain remission)

22.75 Drugs used in the treatment of inflammatory bowel disease

Class	Mechanism of action	Notes
Aminosalicylates (mesalazine (Asacol, Salofalk, Pentasa, Mezavant), olsalazine, sulfasalazine, balsalazide)	Modulate cytokine release from mucosa Delivered to colon by one of three mechanisms: 1. pH-dependent (Asacol, Salofalk) 2. time-dependent (Pentasa) 3. bacterial breakdown by colonic bacteria from a carrier molecule (sulfasalazine, balsalazide)	No proven value in CD Available as oral or topical (enema/suppository) Sulfasalazine causes side-effects in 10–45%: headache, nausea, diarrhoea, blood dyscrasias Other aminosalicylates better tolerated; diarrhoea, headache in 2–5% Rarely, renal impairment (check urea and electrolytes 6-monthly)
Corticosteroids (prednisolone, hydrocortisone, budesonide)	Anti-inflammatory Budesonide is a potent corticosteroid efficiently cleared from circulation by liver, thereby minimising adrenocortical suppression and steroid side-effects	Topical, oral or IV, according to disease severity Budesonide considered for active ileitis and ileocolitis High vigilance for complications Never used for maintenance therapy Calcium/vitamin D supplements
Thiopurines (azathioprine, mercaptopurine)	Immunomodulation by inducing T-cell apoptosis Azathioprine is metabolised in liver to mercaptopurine, then by thiopurine methyltransferase (TPMT) to thioguanine nucleotides	Effective after 12 wks of starting therapy Complications leading to drug withdrawal in ~20%. Flu-like syndrome with myalgia, nausea and vomiting Leucopenia in 3%, particularly in inherited TPMT deficiency (TPMT levels checked prior to therapy) Hepatotoxicity; pancreatitis 60% of those intolerant of azathioprine will tolerate mercaptopurine Increase in lymphoma (approximately 2–3-fold) and non-melanoma skin cancer (life-long sun protection advised) Metabolite levels can be measured to tailor therapy
Methotrexate	Anti-inflammatory	Intolerance in 10–18%. Maximal efficacy when given by SC injection once weekly. Nausea, stomatitis, diarrhoea, hepatotoxicity and pneumonitis. Co-prescription of folic acid and antiemetics. Teratogenic; robust contraception required for females of child-bearing age
Ciclosporin	Inhibits T-cell activation	Rescue therapy to prevent surgery in UC responding poorly to corticosteroids. No value in CD Major side-effects in 0–17%: nephrotoxicity, infections, neurotoxicity (including fits) Minor complications in up to 50%: tremor, paraesthesiae, abnormal liver function tests, hirsutism
Anti-TNF antibodies (infliximab and adalimumab)	Suppress inflammation and induce apoptosis of inflammatory cells	Moderately to severely active CD, including fistulating disease Moderate–severe UC and acute severe UC as rescue therapy Acute (anaphylactic) and delayed (serum sickness) infusion reactions after multiple infusions; anti-drug antibody titres and drug levels can be measured Contraindicated in the presence of infections; reactivation of latent tuberculosis Increased risk of infections and possibly of malignancy
Antibiotics	Antibacterial	Useful in perianal CD and pouchitis Major concern is peripheral neuropathy with long-term metronidazole
Antidiarrhoeal agents (loperamide, co-phenoxylate)	Reduce gut motility and small bowel secretion Loperamide improves anal function	Avoided in acute flare-ups of disease May precipitate colonic dilatation

- prevent bowel damage
- detect dysplasia and prevent carcinoma
- select appropriate patients for surgery.

Ulcerative colitis

Active proctitis. Most patients with ulcerative proctitis respond to a 1 g mesalazine suppository but some will additionally require oral 5-aminosalicylate (5-ASA) therapy. Topical corticosteroids are less effective and are reserved for patients who are intolerant of topical mesalazine. Patients with resistant disease may require treatment with systemic corticosteroids and immunosuppressants.

Active left-sided or extensive ulcerative colitis. In mild to moderately active cases, the combination of a once-daily oral and a topical 5-ASA preparation ('top and tail approach') is usually effective. The topical preparation (1 g foam or liquid enema) is typically withdrawn after 1 month. The oral 5-ASA is continued long-term to prevent relapse and minimise the risk of dysplasia. In patients who do not respond to this approach within 2–4 weeks, oral prednisolone (40 mg daily, tapered by 5 mg/week over an 8-week total course) is indicated. Corticosteroids should never be used for maintenance therapy. At the first signs of corticosteroid resistance (lack of efficacy) or in patients who require high corticosteroid doses to maintain control, immunosuppressive therapy with a thiopurine should be introduced.

Severe ulcerative colitis. Patients who fail to respond to maximal oral therapy and those who present with acute severe colitis (meeting the Truelove–Witts criteria; see Box 22.72) are best managed in hospital and should be monitored jointly by a physician and surgeon:

- clinically: for the presence of abdominal pain, temperature, pulse rate, stool blood and frequency
- by laboratory testing: haemoglobin, white cell count, albumin, electrolytes, ESR and CRP
- radiologically: for colonic dilatation on plain abdominal X-rays.

All patients should be given supportive treatment with intravenous fluids to correct dehydration, and enteral nutritional support should be provided for malnourished patients (Box 22.76). Intravenous corticosteroids (methylprednisolone 60 mg or hydrocortisone 400 mg/day) should be given by intravenous infusion or bolus injection. Topical and oral aminosalicylates have no role to play in the acute severe attack. Response to therapy is judged over the first 3 days. Patients who do not respond promptly to corticosteroids should be considered for medical rescue therapy with ciclosporin (intravenous infusion or oral) or infliximab (5 mg/kg), which, in approximately 60% of cases, can avoid the need for urgent colectomy.

Patients who develop colonic dilatation (> 6 cm), those whose clinical and laboratory measurements deteriorate and those who do not respond after 7–10 days' maximal medical treatment usually require urgent colectomy. Subtotal colectomy can also be performed laparoscopically, given sufficient local expertise.

Maintenance of remission. Life-long maintenance therapy is recommended for all patients with left-sided or extensive disease but is not necessary in those with proctitis (although 20% of these patients will develop proximal 'extension' over the lifetime of their disease). Once-daily oral 5-aminosalicylates are the preferred first-line agents. Sulfasalazine has a higher incidence of side-effects but is equally effective and can be considered in patients with coexistent arthropathy. Patients who frequently relapse despite aminosalicylate drugs should be treated with thiopurines.

Crohn's disease

Principles of treatment. Crohn's disease is a progressive condition which may result in stricture or fistula formation if suboptimally treated. It is therefore important to agree long-term treatment goals with the patient; these are to induce remission and then maintain corticosteroid-free remission with a normal quality of life. Treatment should focus on monitoring the patient carefully for evidence of disease activity and complications (Box 22.77), and ensuring that mucosal healing is achieved.

Induction of remission. Corticosteroids remain the mainstay of treatment for active Crohn's disease. The drug of first choice in patents with ileal disease is budesonide, since it undergoes 90% first-pass metabolism in the liver and has very little systemic toxicity. A typical regimen is 9 mg once daily for 6 weeks, with a gradual reduction in dose over the subsequent 2 weeks when therapy is stopped. If there is no response to budesonide within 2 weeks, the patient should be switched to prednisolone, which has greater potency. This is typically given in a dose of 40 mg daily, reducing by 5 mg/week over 8 weeks, at which point treatment is stopped. Oral prednisolone in the above dose regimen is the treatment of choice for inducing remission in colonic Crohn's disease. Calcium and vitamin D supplements should be co-prescribed in patients who are on corticosteroids, to try to compensate for their inhibitory effect on intestinal calcium absorption.

As an alternative to corticosteroid therapy, enteral nutrition with either an elemental (constituent amino acids) or polymeric (liquid protein) diet may induce remission. Both types of diet are equally effective but the polymeric one is more palatable when taken by mouth. It is particularly effective in children, in whom equal efficacy to corticosteroids has been demonstrated, and in extensive ileal disease in adults. As well as resting the gut and providing excellent nutritional support, it also

22.76 Medical management of fulminant ulcerative colitis

- Admit to hospital for intensive therapy and monitoring
- Intravenous fluids and correction of electrolyte imbalance
- Transfusion if haemoglobin < 100 g/L (< 10 g/dL)
- IV methylprednisolone (60 mg daily) or hydrocortisone (400 mg daily)
- Antibiotics until enteric infection excluded
- Nutritional support
- Subcutaneous low-molecular-weight heparin for prophylaxis of venous thromboembolism
- Avoidance of opiates and antidiarrhoeal agents
- Consider infliximab (5 mg/kg) or ciclosporin (2 mg/kg) in stable patients not responding to 3–5 days of corticosteroids

22.77 Monitoring of inflammatory bowel disease

- Assess symptoms, including extra-intestinal manifestations
- Examine for abdominal mass or perianal disease
- Perform full blood count, urea and electrolytes, liver function tests, albumin, CRP
- Check haematinics (B_{12}, folate, iron studies) at least annually
- Check faecal calprotectin (to monitor each disease flare/change in therapy and assess response)
- Stool cultures (at each flare to exclude infection)
- Assess mucosal healing: surrogate markers (CRP/calprotectin), ileocolonoscopy and/or small bowel MRI
- Enrol patient in a dedicated IBD clinic (can be nurse-led or phone clinic for stable, uncomplicated patients)
- Arrange IBD multidisciplinary meeting for acutely ill or complex patients
- Check vaccinations are up to date; ensure surveillance colonoscopy scheduled where appropriate

has a direct anti-inflammatory effect. It is an effective bridge to urgent staging investigations at first presentation and can be given by mouth or by nasogastric tube. With sufficient explanation, encouragement and motivation, most patients will tolerate it well.

Some patients with severe colonic disease require admission to hospital for intravenous corticosteroids. In severe ileal or panenteric disease, induction therapy with an anti-TNF agent is appropriate, provided that acute perforating complications, such as abscess, have not occurred. Both infliximab and adalimumab are licensed for use in the UK. Randomised trials have demonstrated that combination therapy with an anti-TNF antibody and a thiopurine is the most effective strategy for inducing and maintaining remission in luminal Crohn's patients. This strategy is more effective than anti-TNF monotherapy, which, in turn, is more effective than thiopurine monotherapy. Following induction of remission, a substantial proportion of patients (20–30%) remain well without the requirement for maintenance therapy. Patients with evidence of persistently active disease require further treatment (see below).

Maintenance therapy. Immunosuppressive treatment with thiopurines (azathioprine and mercaptopurine) forms the core of maintenance therapy, but methotrexate is also effective and can be given once weekly, either orally or by subcutaneous injection. Women of child-bearing potential who are prescribed methotrexate must use a robust contraceptive method, since it is teratogenic. Combination therapy with an immunosuppressant and an anti-TNF antibody is the most effective strategy but costs are high and there is an increased risk of serious adverse effects. In the UK, the use of anti-TNF therapy is limited to specific patient subgroups with severe disease (Boxes 22.78 and 22.79). Careful monitoring of disease activity (see Box 22.77) is the key to maintaining sustained remission and preventing the accumulation of bowel damage in Crohn's disease. Cigarette smokers should be strongly counselled to stop smoking at every possible opportunity. Those that do not manage to stop smoking fare much worse, with increased rates of relapse and surgical intervention.

Fistulae and perianal disease. Fistulae may develop in relation to active Crohn's disease and are often associated with sepsis. The first step is to define the site by imaging (usually MRI of the pelvis). Surgical exploration by an examination under anaesthetic is usually then required, to delineate the anatomy and drain abscesses. Seton sutures can be inserted through fistula tracts to ensure adequate drainage and to prevent future sepsis. Corticosteroids are ineffective. For simple perianal disease, metronidazole and/or ciprofloxacin are first-line therapies. Thiopurines can be used in chronic disease but do not usually result in fistula healing. Infliximab and adalimumab can heal fistulae and perianal disease in many patients and are indicated when the measures described above have been ineffective.

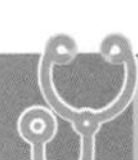

22.78 How to give anti-TNF therapy in inflammatory bowel disease

- Infliximab (5 mg/kg IV infusion) is given as 3 loading doses (at 0, 2 and 6 wks), with 8-weekly maintenance thereafter
- Adalimumab is given as SC injections, which patients can be trained to give themselves. Loading dose is 160 mg, followed by 80 mg 2 wks later and 40 mg every second wk thereafter; some patients require dose escalation to 40 mg once weekly
- Concomitant immunosuppression with a thiopurine or methotrexate may be more efficacious than monotherapy but has more side-effects
- Anti-TNF therapy is contraindicated in the presence of active infection and latent tuberculosis without appropriate prophylaxis; it carries an increased risk of opportunistic infections and possible increased risk of malignancy; and, rarely, multiple sclerosis may be unmasked in susceptible individuals. Counselling about the risk–benefit for each patient is important
- Prior to therapy, latent tuberculosis must be excluded
- Certolizumab is effective for luminal Crohn's disease but is not licensed in Europe
- Etanercept is not effective in Crohn's disease

EBM 22.79 Biological therapy in the management of inflammatory bowel disease

'Infliximab or adalimumab is recommended for patients with severely active Crohn's disease not responding to conventional immunosuppressive therapy, including corticosteroids, or where such therapies are contraindicated. Infliximab is also licensed for use in children and for fistulating Crohn's disease, and is an effective rescue therapy for patients with acute severe ulcerative colitis not responding to intravenous corticosteroids. Infliximab and adalimumab are also both effective for moderately active ulcerative colitis.'

- Crohn's disease – management in adults, children and young people. NICE guideline, Oct 2012.

For further information: http://guidance.nice.org.uk/CG152

Surgical treatment

Ulcerative colitis

Up to 60% of patients with extensive ulcerative colitis eventually require surgery. The indications are listed in Box 22.80. Impaired quality of life, with impact upon occupation and on social and family life, is the most important of these. Surgery involves removal of the entire colon and rectum, and cures the patient. One-third of those with pancolitis undergo colectomy within 5 years of diagnosis. Before surgery, patients must be counselled by doctors, stoma nurses and patients who have undergone similar surgery. The choice of procedure is either panproctocolectomy with ileostomy, or proctocolectomy with ileal–anal pouch anastomosis. The

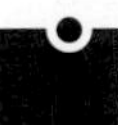

22.80 Indications for surgery in ulcerative colitis

Impaired quality of life
- Loss of occupation or education
- Disruption of family life

Failure of medical therapy
- Dependence on oral corticosteroids
- Complications of drug therapy

Fulminant colitis

Disease complications unresponsive to medical therapy
- Arthritis
- Pyoderma gangrenosum

Colon cancer or severe dysplasia

22

sister surgical text to this book, *Principles and Practice of Surgery*, should be consulted for further details.

Crohn's disease

The indications for surgery are similar to those for ulcerative colitis. Operations are often necessary to deal with fistulae, abscesses and perianal disease, and may also be required to relieve small or large bowel obstruction. In contrast to ulcerative colitis, surgery is not curative and disease recurrence is the rule. The only method that has consistently been shown to reduce post-operative recurrence is smoking cessation. Antibiotics are effective in the short term only. It is common to undertake colonoscopy 6 months after surgery to inspect and biopsy the anastomosis and neo-terminal ileum. Patients with endoscopic recurrence are then prescribed thiopurines.

Surgery should be as conservative as possible in order to minimise loss of viable intestine and to avoid creation of a short bowel syndrome. Obstructing or fistulating small bowel disease may require resection of affected tissue. Patients who have localised segments of Crohn's colitis may be managed by segmental resection and/or multiple stricturoplasties, in which the stricture is not resected but instead incised in its longitudinal axis and sutured transversely. Others who have extensive colitis require total colectomy but ileal–anal pouch formation should be avoided because of the high risk of recurrence within the pouch and subsequent fistulae, abscess formation and pouch failure.

Historical datasets show that around 80% of Crohn's patients undergo surgery at some stage, and 70% of these require more than one operation during their lifetime. Clinical recurrence following resectional surgery is present in 50% of all cases at 10 years. Emerging data demonstrate that aggressive medical therapy, coupled with intense monitoring, probably reduces the requirement for surgery substantially.

IBD in special circumstances

Childhood

Chronic ill health in childhood or adolescent IBD may result in growth failure, metabolic bone disease and delayed puberty. Loss of schooling and social contact, as well as frequent hospitalisation, can have important psychosocial consequences. Treatment is similar to that described for adults and may require corticosteroids, immunosuppressive drugs, biological agents and surgery. Monitoring of height, weight and sexual development is crucial. Children with IBD should be managed by specialised paediatric gastroenterologists and transitioned to adult care in dedicated clinics (Box 22.81).

Pregnancy

A women's ability to become pregnant is adversely affected by active IBD. Pre-conceptual counselling should focus on optimising disease control. During pregnancy, the rule of thirds applies - roughly one-third of women improve, one-third get worse and one third remain stable with active disease. In the post-partum period, these changes sometimes reverse spontaneously. Drug therapy, including aminosalicylates, corticosteroids and azathioprine, can be safely continued throughout pregnancy but methotrexate must be avoided, both during pregnancy and if the patient is trying to conceive (Box 22.82). Anti-TNF agents are transmitted through

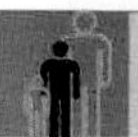

22.81 Inflammatory bowel disease in adolescence

- **Delayed growth and pubertal development**: chronic active inflammation, malabsorption, malnutrition and long-term corticosteroids contribute to short stature and delayed development, with physical and psychological consequences.
- **Metabolic bone disease**: more common with chronic disease beginning in childhood, resulting from chronic inflammation, dietary deficiency and malabsorption of calcium and vitamin D.
- **Drug side-effects and compliance issues**: young people are more likely to require azathioprine or biological therapy than adults. Poor compliance with therapy is more common than with adults, as younger patients may feel well, lack self-motivation to adhere and believe that drugs are ineffective or cause side-effects.
- **Loss of time from education**: physical illness, surgery, fatigue in chronic IBD, privacy and dignity issues, and social isolation may all contribute.
- **Emotional difficulties**: may result from difficulties coping with illness, problems forming interpersonal relationships, and issues relating to body image or sexual function.

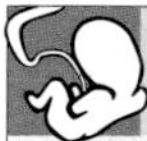

22.82 Pregnancy and inflammatory bowel disease

Pre-conception

- Outcomes are best when pregnancy is carefully planned and disease is in remission
- Methotrexate must be stopped; other IBD drugs should be continued until discussed with a specialist
- Aminosalicylates and azathioprine are safe in pregnancy
- Corticosteroids are probably safe
- Safety of biological therapy in pregnancy is unclear; use only when absolutely necessary
- Daily folic acid supplements are recommended

Pregnancy

- Two-thirds of patients in remission will remain so in pregnancy
- Active disease is likely to remain active
- Severe active disease carries an increased risk of premature delivery and low birth weight
- Gentle flexible sigmoidoscopy is safe after the first trimester
- X-rays should be avoided
- Colonoscopy can be performed safely if the potential benefits outweigh the risks

Labour

- Needs careful discussion between patient, gastroenterologist and obstetrician
- Normal labour and vaginal delivery are possible for most
- Caesarean section may be preferred for patients with perianal Crohn's or an ileo-anal pouch to reduce risks of pelvic floor damage, fistulation and late incontinence

Breastfeeding

- Safe and does not exacerbate IBD
- Data on the risk to babies from drugs excreted in breast milk are limited; most are probably safe
- Patients should discuss breastfeeding and drug therapy carefully with their doctor

the placenta (but not breast milk) and are usually omitted during the last trimester.

Metabolic bone disease

Patients with IBD are prone to developing osteoporosis due to effects of chronic inflammation, corticosteroids, weight loss, malnutrition and malabsorption. Osteomalacia can also occur in Crohn's disease that is complicated by malabsorption, but is less common than osteoporosis. The risk of osteoporosis increases with age and with the dose and duration of corticosteroid therapy.

Microscopic colitis

Microscopic colitis, which comprises two related conditions, lymphocytic colitis and collagenous colitis, has no known cause. The presentation is with watery diarrhoea. The colonoscopic appearances are normal but histological examination of biopsies shows a range of abnormalities. It is therefore recommended that biopsies of the right and left colon plus terminal ileum should be undertaken in all patients undergoing colonoscopy for diarrhoea. Collagenous colitis is characterised by the presence of a submucosal band of collagen, often with a chronic inflammatory infiltrate. The disease is more common in women and may be associated with rheumatoid arthritis, diabetes, coeliac disease and some drug therapies, such as NSAIDs or PPIs. Treatment with budesonide is usually effective but the condition will recur in some patients on discontinuation of therapy.

IRRITABLE BOWEL SYNDROME

Irritable bowel syndrome (IBS) is characterised by recurrent abdominal pain in association with abnormal defecation in the absence of a structural abnormality of the gut. About 10–15% of the population are affected at some time but only 10% of these consult their doctors because of symptoms. Nevertheless, IBS is the most common cause of gastrointestinal referral and accounts for frequent absenteeism from work and impaired quality of life. Young women are affected 2–3 times more often than men. Coexisting conditions, such as non-ulcer dyspepsia, chronic fatigue syndrome, dysmenorrhoea and fibromyalgia, are common. Between 5 and 10% of patients have a history of physical or sexual abuse.

Pathophysiology

The cause of IBS is incompletely understood but biopsychosocial factors are thought to play an important role, along with luminal factors, such as diet and the gut microbiota, as discussed below.

Behavioural and psychosocial factors

Most patients seen in general practice do not have psychological problems but about 50% of patients referred to hospital have a psychiatric illness, such as anxiety, depression, somatisation and neurosis. Panic attacks are also common. Acute psychological stress and overt psychiatric disease are known to alter visceral perception and gastrointestinal motility. There is an increased prevalence of abnormal illness behaviour, with frequent consultations for minor symptoms and reduced coping ability (p. 236). These factors contribute to but do not cause IBS.

Physiological factors

There is some evidence that IBS may be a serotoninergic (5-HT) disorder, as evidenced by relatively excessive release of 5-HT in diarrhoea-predominant IBS (D-IBS) and relative deficiency with constipation-predominant IBS (C-IBS). Accordingly, 5-HT_3 receptor antagonists are effective in D-IBS, while 5-HT_4 agonists improve bowel function in C-IBS. There is some evidence that IBS may represent a state of low-grade gut inflammation or immune activation, not detectable by tests, with raised numbers of mucosal mast cells, which sensitise enteric neurons by releasing histamine and tryptase. Some patients respond positively to mast cell stabilisers, such as ketotifen, which supports a pathogenic role of mast cells in at least some patients. Immune activation may be associated with altered CNS processing of visceral pain signals. This is more common in women and in D-IBS, and may be triggered by a prior episode of gastroenteritis with *Salmonella* or *Campylobacter* species.

Luminal factors

Both quantitative and qualitative alterations in intestinal bacterial contents (the gut microbiota) have been reported. Small intestinal bacterial overgrowth (SIBO) may be present in some patients and lead to symptoms. This 'gut dysbiosis' may explain the response to probiotics or the non-absorbable antibiotic rifaximin that has been reported in trials.

Dietary factors are also important. Some patients have chemical food intolerances (not allergy) to poorly absorbed, short-chain carbohydrates (lactose, fructose and sorbitol, among others), collectively known as FODMAPs (fermentable oligo-, di- and monosaccharides, and polyols). Their fermentation in the colon leads to bloating, pain, wind and altered bowel habit. Non-coeliac gluten sensitivity (negative coeliac serology and normal duodenal biopsies) seems to be present in some IBS patients, while others may be intolerant of chemicals such as salicylates or benzoates, found in certain foods.

Clinical features

The most common presentation is that of recurrent abdominal discomfort (Box 22.83). This is usually colicky or cramping in nature, felt in the lower abdomen and relieved by defecation. Abdominal bloating worsens throughout the day; the cause is unknown but it is not due to excessive intestinal gas. The bowel habit is variable. Most patients alternate between episodes of diarrhoea and constipation, but it is useful to classify patients as having predominantly constipation or predominantly diarrhoea. Those with constipation tend to pass infrequent pellety stools, usually in association with abdominal pain or proctalgia. Those with diarrhoea have frequent defecation but produce low-volume stools and rarely have nocturnal symptoms. Passage of mucus is

22.83 Rome III criteria for diagnosis of irritable bowel syndrome

Recurrent abdominal pain or discomfort at least 3 days/mth in the last 3 months, associated with *two or more* of the following:

- Improvement with defecation
- Onset associated with a change in frequency of stool
- Onset associated with a change in form (appearance) of stool

common but rectal bleeding does not occur. Patients do not lose weight and are constitutionally well. Physical examination is generally unremarkable, with the exception of variable tenderness to palpation.

Diagnosis

The diagnosis is clinical in nature and can be made confidently in most patients using the Rome criteria combined with the absence of alarm symptoms, without resorting to complicated tests (Box 22.84). Full blood count and faecal calprotectin, with or without sigmoidoscopy, are usually done and are normal in IBS. Colonoscopy should be undertaken in older patients (over 40 years of age) to exclude colorectal cancer. Endoscopic examination is also required in patients who report rectal bleeding to exclude colon cancer and IBD. Those who present atypically require investigations to exclude other gastrointestinal diseases. Diarrhoea-predominant patients justify investigations to exclude coeliac disease (p. 880), microscopic colitis (p. 907), lactose intolerance (p. 887), bile acid malabsorption (p. 851), thyrotoxicosis (p. 740) and, in developing countries, parasitic infection.

Management

The most important steps are to make a positive diagnosis and reassure the patient. Many patients are concerned that they have developed cancer, and a cycle of anxiety leading to colonic symptoms, which further heighten anxiety, can be broken by explanation that

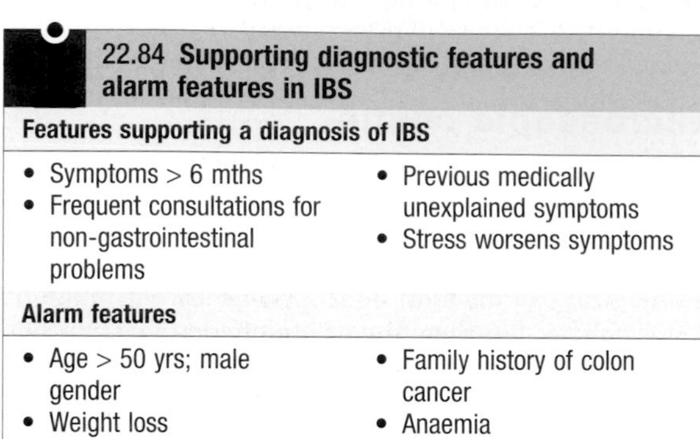

22.84 Supporting diagnostic features and alarm features in IBS

Features supporting a diagnosis of IBS	
• Symptoms > 6 mths • Frequent consultations for non-gastrointestinal problems	• Previous medically unexplained symptoms • Stress worsens symptoms
Alarm features	
• Age > 50 yrs; male gender • Weight loss • Nocturnal symptoms	• Family history of colon cancer • Anaemia • Rectal bleeding

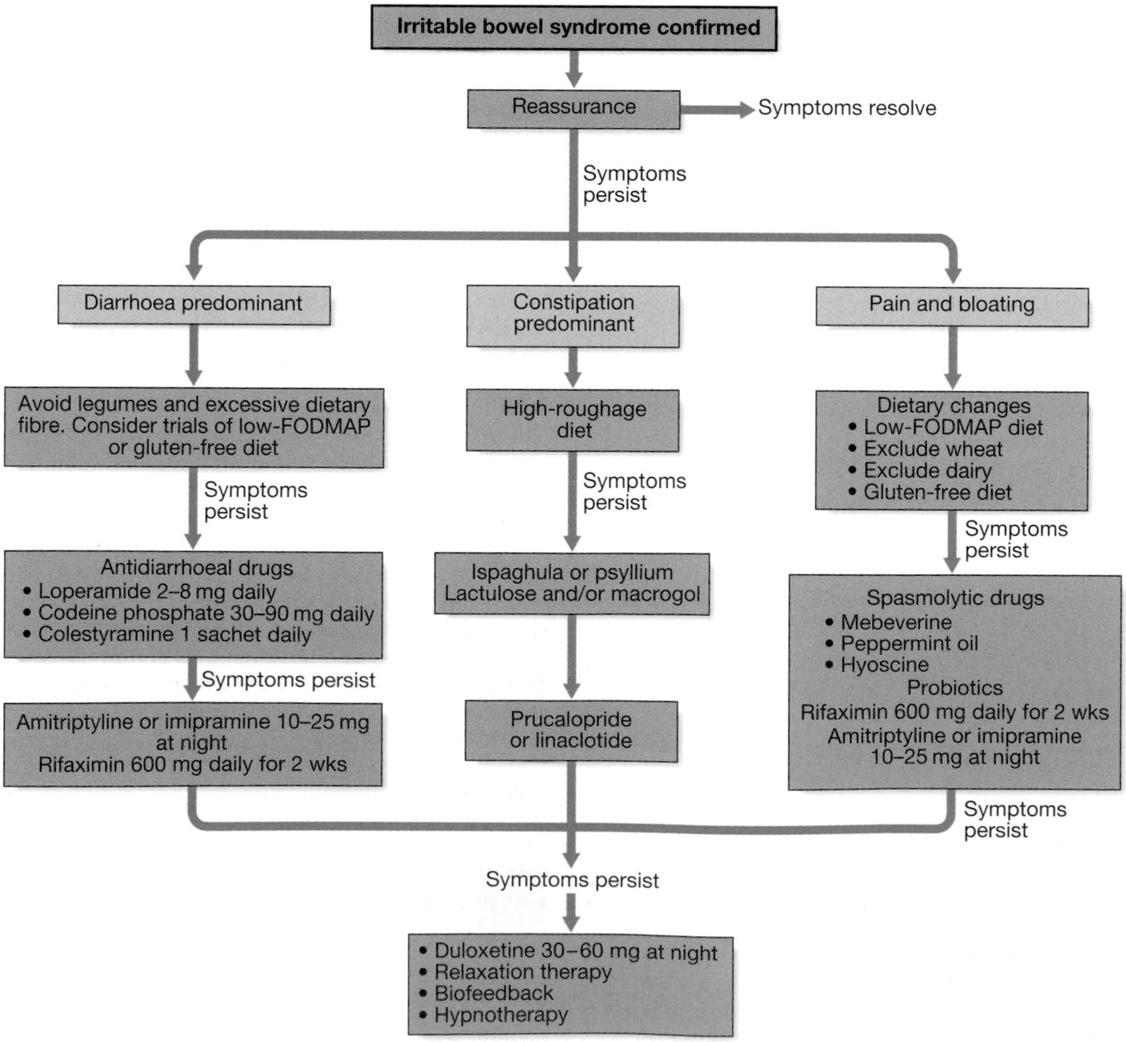

Irritable bowel syndrome confirmed
Reassurance
Symptoms resolve
Symptoms persist
Diarrhoea predominant
Constipation predominant
Pain and bloating
Avoid legumes and excessive dietary fibre. Consider trials of low-FODMAP or gluten-free diet
Symptoms persist
Antidiarrhoeal drugs
• Loperamide 2–8 mg daily
• Codeine phosphate 30–90 mg daily
• Colestyramine 1 sachet daily
Symptoms persist
Amitriptyline or imipramine 10–25 mg at night
Rifaximin 600 mg daily for 2 wks
High-roughage diet
Symptoms persist
Ispaghula or psyllium
Lactulose and/or macrogol
Prucalopride or linaclotide
Dietary changes
• Low-FODMAP diet
• Exclude wheat
• Exclude dairy
• Gluten-free diet
Symptoms persist
Spasmolytic drugs
• Mebeverine
• Peppermint oil
• Hyoscine
Probiotics
Rifaximin 600 mg daily for 2 wks
Amitriptyline or imipramine 10–25 mg at night
Symptoms persist
Symptoms persist
• Duloxetine 30–60 mg at night
• Relaxation therapy
• Biofeedback
• Hypnotherapy

Fig. 22.57 Management of irritable bowel syndrome. (FODMAP = fermentable oligo-, di- and monosaccharides, and polyols)

symptoms are not due to a serious underlying disease but instead are the result of behavioural, psychosocial, physiological and luminal factors described above. In patients who fail to respond to reassurance, treatment is traditionally tailored to the predominant symptoms (Fig. 22.57). Up to 20% may benefit from a wheat-free diet, some may respond to lactose exclusion, and excess intake of caffeine or artificial sweeteners, such as sorbitol, should be addressed. A more restrictive, 'low-FODMAP' diet, supervised by a dietitian, with gradual re-introduction of different food groups, may help some patients, as may a trial of a gluten-free diet. Probiotics, in capsule form, can be effective if taken for several months, although the optimum combination of bacterial strains and dose have yet to be clarified.

Patients with intractable symptoms sometimes benefit from several months of therapy with a tricyclic antidepressant, such as amitriptyline or imipramine (10–25 mg orally at night). Side-effects include dry mouth and drowsiness but these are usually mild and the drug is generally well tolerated, although patients with features of somatisation tolerate the drug poorly and lower doses should be used. It may act by reducing visceral sensation and by altering gastrointestinal motility. Anxiety and affective disorders may also require specific treatment (pp. 242 and 243). The 5-HT_4 agonist prucalopride, the guanylate cyclase-C receptor agonist linaclotide, and chloride channel activators, such as lubiprostone, can be effective in constipation-predominant IBS.

Trials of anti-inflammatory agents, such as ketotifen or mesalazine, and the antibiotic rifaximin may be considered in some patients with difficult symptoms but are best prescribed only after specialist referral.

Psychological interventions, such as cognitive behavioural therapy, relaxation and gut-directed hypnotherapy, should be reserved for the most difficult cases. A range of complementary and alternative therapies exist; most lack a good evidence base but are popular and help some patients (Box 22.85).

Most patients have a relapsing and remitting course. Exacerbations often follow stressful life events, occupational dissatisfaction and difficulties with interpersonal relationships.

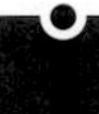

22.85 Complementary and alternative therapies for IBS

Manipulative and body-based
• Massage, chiropractic
Mind–body interventions
• Meditation, hypnosis*, cognitive therapy
Biologically based
• Herbal products*, dietary additives, probiotics*
Energy healing
• Biofield therapies (reiki), bio-electromagnetic field therapies
Alternative medical systems
• Ayurvedic, homeopathy, traditional Chinese medicine

*Some evidence for benefit exists.
From Hussain Z, et al. Aliment Pharmacol Ther 2006; 23:465–471.

AIDS AND THE GASTROINTESTINAL TRACT

Patients with HIV-AIDS may develop several symptoms referable to the gastrointestinal tract, as discussed in detail on page 399. Consider HIV testing in all patients with atypical or unexplained gastrointestinal symptoms and those resident in areas of high prevalence.

ISCHAEMIC GUT INJURY

Ischaemic gut injury is usually the result of arterial occlusion. Severe hypotension and venous insufficiency are less frequent causes (p. 198). The presentation is variable, depending on the different vessels involved and the acuteness of the event. Diagnosis is often difficult.

Acute small bowel ischaemia

An embolus from the heart or aorta to the superior mesenteric artery is responsible for 40–50% of cases, thrombosis of underlying atheromatous disease for approximately 25%, and non-occlusive ischaemia due to hypotension complicating myocardial infarction, heart failure, arrhythmias or sudden blood loss for approximately 25%. Vasculitis and venous occlusion are rare causes. The clinical spectrum ranges from transient alteration of bowel function to transmural haemorrhagic necrosis and gangrene. Patients usually have evidence of cardiac disease and arrhythmia. Almost all develop abdominal pain that is more impressive than the physical findings. In the early stages, the only physical signs may be a silent, distended abdomen or diminished bowel sounds, peritonitis only developing later.

Leucocytosis, metabolic acidosis, hyperphosphataemia and hyperamylasaemia are typical. Plain abdominal X-rays show 'thumb-printing' due to mucosal oedema. Mesenteric or CT angiography reveals an occluded or narrowed major artery with spasm of arterial arcades, although most patients undergo laparotomy on the basis of a clinical diagnosis without angiography. Resuscitation, management of cardiac disease and intravenous antibiotic therapy, followed by laparotomy, are key steps. If treatment is instituted early, embolectomy and vascular reconstruction may salvage some small bowel. In these rare cases, a 'second look' laparotomy should be undertaken 24 hours later and further necrotic bowel resected. In patients at high surgical risk, thrombolysis may sometimes be effective. The results of therapy depend on early intervention; patients treated late have a 75% mortality rate. Survivors often have nutritional failure from short bowel syndrome (p. 884) and require intensive nutritional support, including home parenteral nutrition and anticoagulation. Small bowel transplantation is promising in selected patients. Patients with mesenteric venous thrombosis also require surgery if there are signs of peritonitis but are otherwise treated with anticoagulation. Investigations for underlying prothrombotic disorders should be performed (p. 1054).

Acute colonic ischaemia

The splenic flexure and descending colon have little collateral circulation and lie in 'watershed' areas of arterial supply. The spectrum of injury ranges from reversible colopathy to transient colitis, colonic stricture, gangrene and fulminant pancolitis. Arterial thromboembolism is usually responsible but colonic ischaemia can also follow severe hypotension, colonic volvulus, strangulated hernia, systemic vasculitis or hypercoagulable states. Ischaemia of the descending and sigmoid colon is also a complication of abdominal aortic aneurysm surgery (where the inferior mesenteric artery is ligated). The patient is usually elderly and presents with sudden onset of cramping, left-sided, lower abdominal pain and rectal bleeding. Symptoms usually resolve spontaneously over 24–48 hours and healing occurs in 2 weeks. Some may develop a fibrous stricture or segment of colitis. A minority develop gangrene and peritonitis. The diagnosis is established by colonoscopy within 48 hours of presentation; otherwise, mucosal ulceration may have resolved. Resection is required for peritonitis.

Chronic mesenteric ischaemia

This results from atherosclerotic stenosis of the coeliac axis, superior mesenteric artery and inferior mesenteric artery. At least two of the three vessels must be affected for symptoms to develop. The typical presentation is with dull but severe mid- or upper abdominal pain developing about 30 minutes after eating. Weight loss is common because the patient is reluctant to eat, and some experience diarrhoea. Physical examination shows evidence of generalised arterial disease. An abdominal bruit is sometimes audible but is non-specific. The diagnosis is made by mesenteric angiography. Treatment is by vascular reconstruction or percutaneous angioplasty, if the patient's clinical condition permits. The condition is frequently complicated by intestinal infarction, if left untreated.

DISORDERS OF THE COLON AND RECTUM

Tumours of the colon and rectum

Polyps and polyposis syndromes

Polyps may be neoplastic or non-neoplastic. The latter include hamartomas, metaplastic ('hyperplastic') polyps and inflammatory polyps. These have no malignant potential. Polyps may be single or multiple and vary from a few millimetres to several centimetres in size.

Colorectal adenomas are extremely common in the Western world and the prevalence rises with age; 50% of people over 60 years of age have adenomas, and in half of these the polyps are multiple. They are more common in the rectum and distal colon and are either pedunculated or sessile. Histologically, they are classified as either tubular, villous or tubulovillous, according to the glandular architecture. Nearly all forms of colorectal carcinoma develop from adenomatous polyps, although not all polyps carry the same degree of risk. Features associated with a higher risk of subsequent malignancy are listed in Box 22.86.

Adenomas are usually asymptomatic and discovered incidentally. Occasionally, they cause bleeding and anaemia. Villous adenomas can secrete large amounts of mucus, causing diarrhoea and hypokalaemia.

22.86 Risk factors for malignant change in colonic polyps

- Large size (> 2 cm)
- Multiple polyps
- Villous architecture
- Dysplasia

A

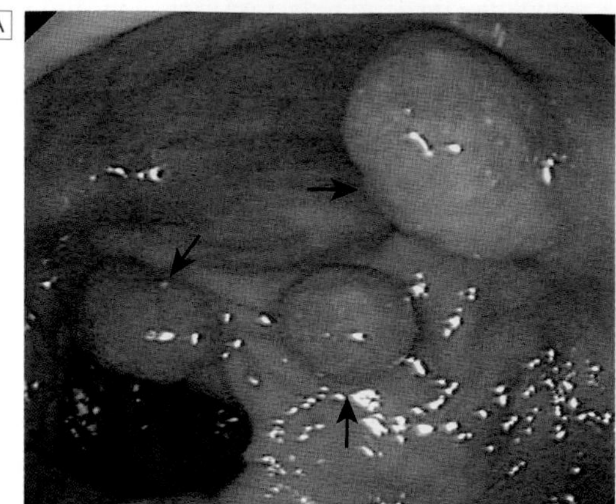

B

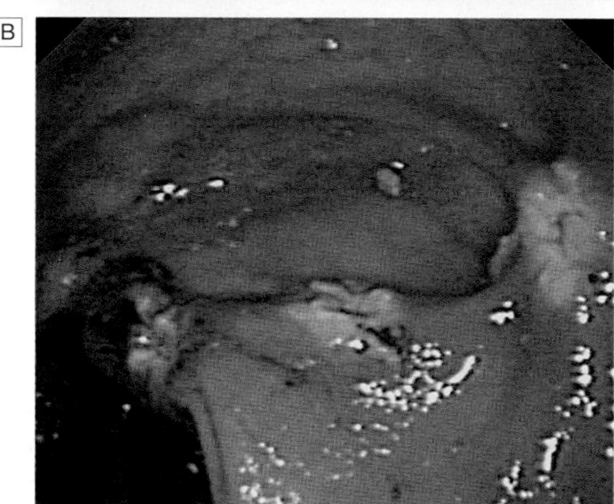

Fig. 22.58 Adenomatous colonic polyps. **A** Before colonoscopic polypectomy (arrows show polyps). **B** After polypectomy.

Discovery of a polyp at sigmoidoscopy is an indication for colonoscopy because proximal polyps are present in 40–50% of such patients. Colonoscopic polypectomy should be carried out wherever possible, as this considerably reduces subsequent colorectal cancer risk (Fig. 22.58). Very large or sessile polyps can sometimes be removed safely by endoscopic mucosal resection (EMR) but many require surgery. Once all polyps have been removed, surveillance colonoscopy should be undertaken at 3–5-year intervals, as new polyps develop in 50% of patients. Patients over 75 years of age do not require repeated colonoscopies, as their subsequent lifetime cancer risk is low.

Between 10 and 20% of polyps show histological evidence of malignancy. When cancer cells are found within 2 mm of the resection margin of the polyp, when the polyp cancer is poorly differentiated or when lymphatic invasion is present, segmental colonic resection is recommended because residual tumour or lymphatic spread (in up to 10%) may be present. Malignant polyps without these features can be followed up by surveillance colonoscopy.

Polyposis syndromes are classified by histopathology (Box 22.87). It should be noted that, while the

22.87 Gastrointestinal polyposis syndromes

	Neoplastic	Non-neoplastic*			
	Familial adenomatous polyposis	Peutz–Jeghers syndrome	Juvenile polyposis	Cronkhite–Canada syndrome	Cowden's disease
Inheritance	Autosomal dominant	Autosomal dominant	Autosomal dominant in 1/3	None	Autosomal dominant
Oesophageal polyps	–	–	–	+	+
Gastric polyps	+	+	+	+++	+++
Small bowel polyps	++	+++	++	++	++
Colonic polyps	+++	++	++	+++	+
Other features	Colorectal cancer, bleeding, extra-intestinal features (Box 22.88)	Pigmentation, bleeding, intussusception, bowel and other cancers	Colorectal cancer	Hair loss, pigmentation, nail dystrophy, malabsorption	Many congenital anomalies, oral and cutaneous hamartomas, thyroid and breast tumours

– absent; + may occur; ++ common; +++ very common. *The polyps themselves are not neoplastic but cancer risk is increased in several syndromes.

hamartomatous polyps in Peutz–Jeghers syndrome and juvenile polyposis are not themselves neoplastic, these disorders are associated with an increased risk of malignancy of the breast, colon, ovary and thyroid.

Familial adenomatous polyposis

Familial adenomatous polyposis (FAP) is an uncommon autosomal dominant disorder affecting 1 in 13 000 of the population and accounting for 1% of all colorectal cancers. It results from germline mutation of the tumour suppressor *APC* gene, followed by acquired mutation of the remaining allele (Ch. 3). The *APC* gene is large and over 1400 different mutations have been reported, but most are loss-of-function mutations resulting in a truncated APC protein. This protein normally binds to and sequesters β-catenin but is unable to do so when mutated, allowing β-catenin to translocate to the nucleus, where it up-regulates the expression of many genes.

Around 20% of cases arise as new mutations and have no family history. Hundreds to thousands of adenomatous colonic polyps develop in 80% of patients by age 15 (Fig. 22.59), with symptoms such as rectal bleeding beginning a few years later. In those affected, cancer will develop within 10–15 years of the appearance of adenomas and 90% of patients will develop colorectal cancer by the age of 50 years. Despite surveillance, approximately 1 in 4 patients with FAP have cancer by the time they undergo colectomy.

A second gene involved in base excision repair (MutY homolog, *MUTYH*) has been identified which may give rise to colonic polyposis. *MUTYH* displays autosomal recessive inheritance and leads to tens to hundreds of polyps and proximal colon cancer. This variant is referred to as *MUTYH*-associated polyposis (MAP).

Non-neoplastic cystic fundic gland polyps occur in the stomach but adenomatous polyps also occur uncommonly. Duodenal adenomas occur in over 90% and are most common around the ampulla of Vater. Malignant transformation to adenocarcinoma occurs in 10% and is the leading cause of death in those who have had prophylactic colectomy. Many extra-intestinal features are also seen in FAP (Box 22.88).

Desmoid tumours occur in up to one-third of patients and usually arise in the mesentery or abdominal wall. Although benign, they may become very large, causing compression of adjacent organs, intestinal obstruction or vascular compromise, and are difficult to remove. They

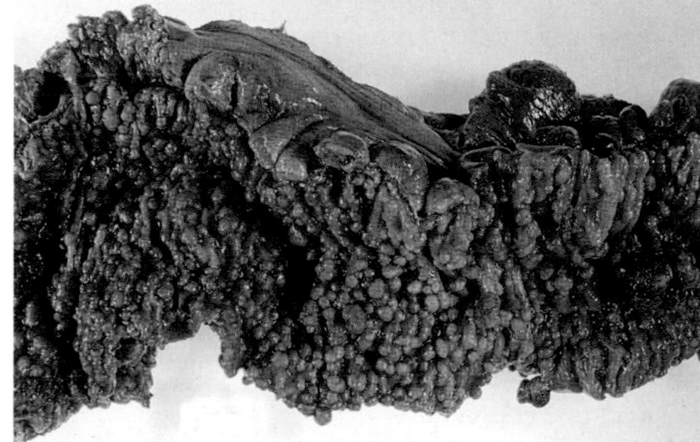

Fig. 22.59 Familial adenomatous polyposis. There are hundreds of adenomatous polyps throughout the colon.

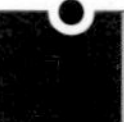

22.88 Extra-intestinal features of familial adenomatous polyposis

- Congenital hypertrophy of the retinal pigment epithelium (CHRPE, 70–80%)
- Epidermoid cysts (extremities, face, scalp)* (50%)
- Benign osteomas, especially skull and angle of mandible* (50–90%)
- Dental abnormalities (15–25%)*
- Desmoid tumours (10–15%)
- Other malignancies (brain, thyroid, liver, 1–3%)

*Gardner's syndrome.

sometimes respond to hormonal therapy with tamoxifen, and the NSAID sulindac may lead to regression in some, by unknown mechanisms. Congenital hypertrophy of the retinal pigment epithelium (CHRPE) occurs in some and is seen as dark, round, pigmented retinal lesions. When present in an at-risk individual, they are 100% predictive of the presence of FAP. A variant, Turcot's syndrome, is characterised by FAP with primary CNS tumours (astrocytoma or medulloblastoma).

Early identification of affected individuals before symptoms develop is essential. The diagnosis can be excluded if sigmoidoscopy is normal. In newly diagnosed cases, genetic testing should be carried out to confirm the diagnosis and identify the causal mutation. Subsequently, all first-degree relatives should also undergo testing (p. 60). In families with known FAP, family members should undergo mutation testing at 13–14 years of age and patients who are found to have the mutation should be offered colectomy after school or college education has been completed. The operation of choice is total proctocolectomy with ileal pouch–anal anastomosis. Periodic upper gastrointestinal endoscopy every 1–3 years is recommended to detect and monitor duodenal and periampullary adenomas. If large, these may be amenable to endoscopic resection.

Peutz–Jeghers syndrome

Multiple hamartomatous polyps occur in the small intestine and colon, as well as melanin pigmentation of the lips, mouth and digits (Fig. 22.60). Most cases are asymptomatic, although chronic bleeding, anaemia or intussusception can occur. There is a significant risk of small bowel or colonic adenocarcinoma and of cancer of the pancreas, lung, ovary, breast and endometrium. It is an autosomal dominantly inherited disorder, most commonly resulting from truncating mutations in a serine–threonine kinase gene on chromosome 19p (*STK11*). Diagnosis requires two of the three following features:

- small bowel polyposis
- mucocutaneous pigmentation
- a family history suggesting autosomal dominant inheritance.

The diagnosis can be made by genetic testing but this may be inconclusive, since mutations in genes other than *STK11* can cause the disorder. Affected people should undergo regular upper endoscopy, colonoscopy, and small bowel and pancreatic imaging. Polyps greater than 1 cm in size should be removed. Testicular examination is essential for men, while women should undergo pelvic examination, cervical smears and regular mammography. Asymptomatic relatives of affected patients should also undergo screening.

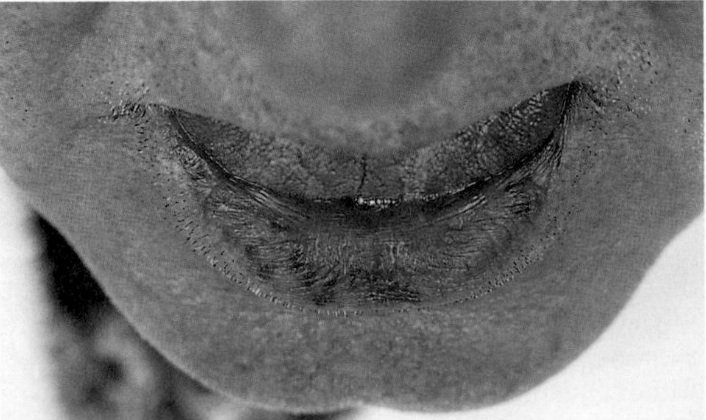

Fig. 22.60 Peutz–Jeghers syndrome. Typical lip pigmentation.

Juvenile polyposis

In juvenile polyposis (JPS), tens to hundreds of mucus-filled hamartomatous polyps are found in the colorectum. One-third of cases are inherited in an autosomal dominant manner and up to 20% develop colorectal cancer before the age of 40. The criteria for diagnosis are:

- ten or more colonic juvenile polyps
- juvenile polyps elsewhere in the gut, *or*
- any polyps in those with a family history.

Germline mutations in the *SMAD4* gene are often found, as are *PTEN* mutations. Colonoscopy with polypectomy should be performed every 1–3 years and colectomy considered for extensive involvement.

Colorectal cancer

Although relatively rare in the developing world, colorectal cancer is the second most common internal malignancy and the second leading cause of cancer deaths in Western countries. In the UK, the incidence is 50–60 per 100 000, equating to 30 000 cases per year. The condition becomes increasingly common over the age of 50 years.

Pathophysiology

Both environmental and genetic factors are important in colorectal carcinogenesis (Fig. 22.61). Environmental factors account for 70% of all 'sporadic' colorectal cancers. This figure is based on the wide geographical variation in incidence and the decrease in risk seen in migrants who move from high- to low-risk countries. Dietary factors are most important and these are summarised in Box 22.89; other recognised risk factors are listed in Box 22.90.

Colorectal cancer development results from the accumulation of multiple genetic mutations arising from two major pathways: chromosomal instability and microsatellite instability (Fig. 22.62).

- *Chromosomal instability.* Mutations or deletions of portions of chromosomes arise, with loss of heterozygosity (LOH) and inactivation of specific tumour suppressor genes. In LOH, one allele of a gene is deleted but gene inactivation only occurs when a subsequent unrelated mutation affects the other allele.
- *Microsatellite instability.* This involves germline mutations in one of six genes encoding enzymes involved in repairing errors that occur normally during DNA replication (DNA mismatch repair); these genes are designated *hMSH2, hMSH6, hMLH1, hMLH3, hPMS1* and *hPMS2*. Replication errors accumulate and can be detected in 'microsatellites' of repetitive DNA sequences. They also occur in important regulatory genes, resulting in a genetically unstable phenotype and accumulation of multiple somatic mutations throughout the genome that eventually lead to cancer. A few sporadic cancers develop this way, as do most cases of hereditary non-polyposis colon cancer (HNPCC).

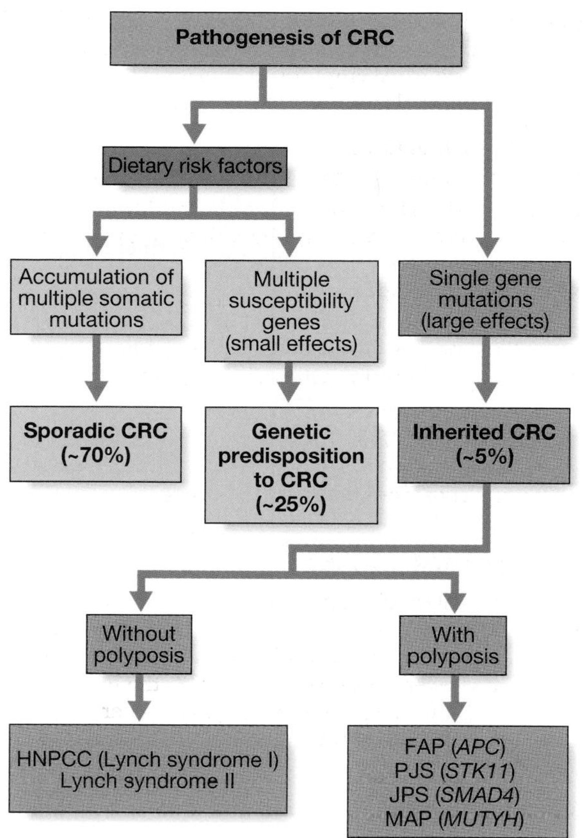

Fig. 22.61 Pathogenesis of colorectal cancer (CRC). (FAP = familial adenomatous polyposis; HNPCC = hereditary non-polyposis colon cancer; JPS = juvenile polyposis syndrome; MAP = *MUTYH*-associated polyposis; PJS = Peutz–Jeghers syndrome)

22.89 Dietary risk factors for colorectal cancer

Risk factor	Comments
Increased risk	
Red meat*	High saturated fat and protein content Carcinogenic amines formed during cooking
Saturated animal fat*	High faecal bile acid and fatty acid levels May affect colonic prostaglandin turnover
Decreased risk	
Dietary fibre*	Effects vary with fibre type; shortened transit time, binding of bile acids and effects on bacterial flora proposed
Fruit and vegetables	Green vegetables contain anticarcinogens, such as flavonoids Little evidence for protection from vitamins A, C, E
Calcium	Binds and precipitates faecal bile acids
Folic acid	Reverses DNA hypomethylation
Omega-3 fatty acids	May be of modest benefit

*Evidence is inconsistent and a clear relationship is unproven.

22.90 Non-dietary risk factors for colorectal cancer

Medical conditions

- Colorectal adenomas (p. 910)
- Long-standing extensive ulcerative colitis or Crohn's colitis (p. 897), especially if associated with primary sclerosing cholangitis (PSC)
- Ureterosigmoidostomy
- Acromegaly
- Pelvic radiotherapy

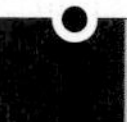

Others

- Obesity and sedentary lifestyle – may be related to diet
- Smoking (relative risk 1.5–3.0)
- Alcohol (weak association)
- Cholecystectomy (effect of bile acids in right colon)
- Type 2 diabetes (hyperinsulinaemia)
- Use of aspirin or NSAIDs (COX-2 inhibition) and perhaps statins associated with *reduced* risk

22.91 Modified Amsterdam criteria* for hereditary non-polyposis colon cancer

- Three or more relatives with colon cancer (at least one first-degree)
- Colorectal cancer in two or more generations
- At least one member affected under 50 yrs of age
- FAP excluded

*These criteria are strict and may miss some families with mutations. HNPCC should also be considered in individuals with colorectal or endometrial cancer under 45 yrs of age.

About 5–10% of colon cancers are caused by HNPCC. Pedigrees with this disorder have an autosomal dominant mode of inheritance and a positive family history of colon cancer occurring at a young age. The lifetime risk in affected individuals is 80%, with a mean age at cancer development of 45 years. In contrast to sporadic colon cancer, two-thirds of tumours occur proximally. The diagnostic criteria are listed in Box 22.91. In a subset of patients, there is also an increased incidence of cancers of the endometrium, ovary, urinary tract, stomach, pancreas, small intestine and CNS, related to inheritance of different mismatch repair gene mutations. Those who fulfil the criteria for HNPCC should be referred for pedigree assessment, genetic testing (see above) and colonoscopy. These should begin around 25 years of age or 5–10 years earlier than the youngest case of cancer in the family. Colonoscopy needs to be repeated every 1–2 years but, even then, interval cancers can still occur.

A family history of colorectal cancer can be obtained in 20% of patients who do not fulfil the criteria for HNPCC. In these families, the lifetime risk of developing colon cancer is 1 in 12 and 1 in 6, respectively, when one or two first-degree relatives are affected. The risk is even higher if relatives were affected at an early age. The genes responsible for these cases are unknown, however. Most tumours arise from malignant transformation of a benign adenomatous polyp. Over 65% occur in the rectosigmoid and a further 15% recur in the caecum or ascending colon. Synchronous tumours are present in 2–5% of patients. Spread occurs through the bowel wall. Rectal cancers may invade the pelvic viscera and side walls. Lymphatic invasion is common at presentation, as

	Normal	Early adenoma	Intermediate adenoma	Late adenoma	Carcinoma
Key gene(s)		*APC* (adenomatous polyposis coli)	*K-ras*	*DCC* (deleted in colon cancer) *SMAD4*	*p53*
Chromosome		5q	12p	18q	17p
Normal function		Inhibits translocation of β-catenin to nucleus and suppresses cell growth	Transmembrane GTP-binding protein mediating mitogenic signals (p21)	*DCC* regulates apoptosis and has a tumour suppressor function *SMAD4* regulates cell growth	Upregulated during cell damage to arrest cell cycle and allow DNA repair or apoptosis to occur
Alteration		Truncating mutations	Gain-of-function mutations	Allelic deletion or silencing (*DCC*) Gain-of-function mutations (*SMAD4*)	Allelic deletion; gain-of-function mutations
Effect		Progression to early adenoma development	Cell proliferation	Enhanced tumour growth, invasion and metastasis	Cell proliferation; impaired apoptosis

Further mutations
- Anchorage independence
- Protease synthesis
- Telomerase synthesis
- Multidrug resistance
- Evasion of immune system

Fig. 22.62 The multistep origin of cancer: molecular events implicated in colorectal carcinogenesis. (GTP = guanine triphosphate)

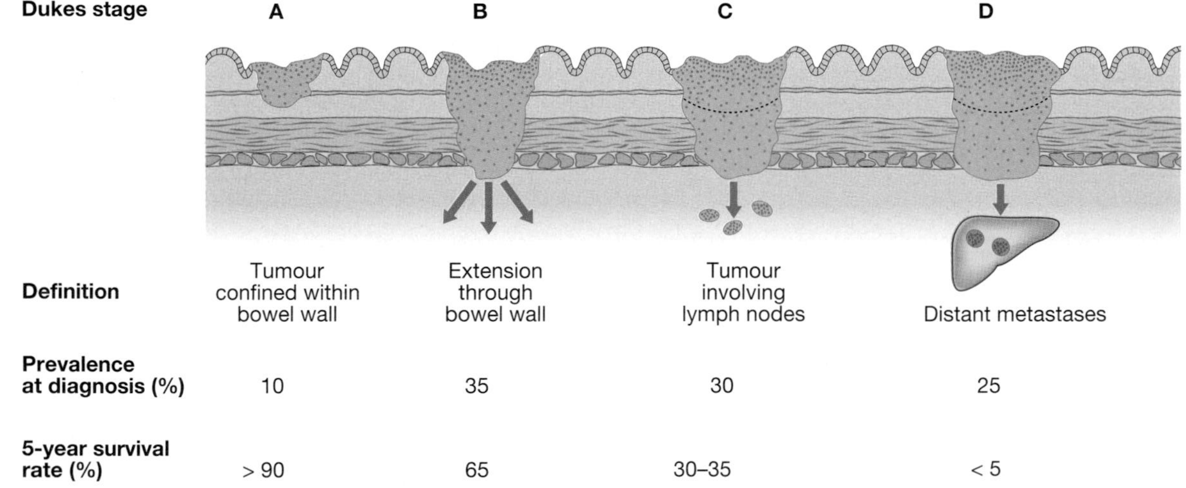

Fig. 22.63 Modified Dukes classification and survival in colorectal cancer.

is spread through both portal and systemic circulations to reach the liver and, less commonly, the lungs. Tumour stage at diagnosis is the most important determinant of prognosis (Fig. 22.63).

Clinical features

Symptoms vary depending on the site of the carcinoma. In tumours of the left colon, fresh rectal bleeding is common and obstruction occurs early. Tumours of the right colon present with anaemia from occult bleeding or with altered bowel habit, but obstruction is a late feature. Colicky lower abdominal pain is present in two-thirds of patients and rectal bleeding occurs in 50%. A minority present with features of either obstruction or perforation, leading to peritonitis, localised abscess or fistula formation. Carcinoma of the rectum usually causes early bleeding, mucus discharge or a feeling of incomplete emptying. Between 10 and 20% of patients present with iron deficiency anaemia or weight loss. On examination, there may be a palpable mass, signs of anaemia or hepatomegaly from metastases. Low rectal tumours may be palpable on digital examination.

Investigations

Colonoscopy is the investigation of choice because it is more sensitive and specific than barium enema. Furthermore, lesions can be biopsied and polyps removed. Patients in whom colonoscopy is incomplete and those who are at high risk of complications can be investigated by CT colonography (virtual colonoscopy). This is a sensitive and non-invasive technique for diagnosing tumours and polyps of more than 6 mm diameter. When the diagnosis of colon cancer has been made, CT of chest, abdomen and pelvis should be performed as a staging investigation, particularly to detect hepatic metastases. Pelvic MRI or endoanal ultrasound should be used for local staging of rectal cancer. Measurement of serum carcinoembryonic antigen (CEA) levels are of limited value in diagnosis, since values are normal in many patients, but CEA testing can be helpful during follow-up to monitor for the prescience of recurrence.

Management

Surgery

All patients should be discussed at a multidisciplinary team meeting. Those with locally advanced rectal cancer should be offered neoadjuvant radiotherapy or chemoradiotherapy to increase the subsequent chance of a complete (R0) surgical resection. A 1-week course of radiotherapy just prior to surgery reduces the risk of local recurrence in operable rectal cancer. The tumour should be removed, along with adequate resection margins and pericolic lymph nodes. Continuity should be restored by direct anastomosis, wherever possible. Carcinomas within 2 cm of the anal verge may require abdominoperineal resection and formation of a colostomy. All patients should be counselled pre-operatively about the possible need for a stoma. Total mesorectal excision (TME) reduces recurrence rates and increases survival in rectal cancer. Metastatic disease confined to liver or lung should be considered for resection, as this can be potentially curative if there is truly no disease at other sites. Post-operatively, patients should undergo colonoscopy after 6–12 months and then at 5 years to search for local recurrence or development of new lesions, which occur in 6% of cases.

Adjuvant therapy

About 30–40% of patients have lymph node involvement at presentation (see Fig. 22.63) and are, therefore, at risk of recurrence. Most recurrences are within 3 years of diagnosis and affect the liver, lung, distant lymph nodes and peritoneum. Adjuvant chemotherapy with 5-fluorouracil/folinic acid or capecitabine, preferably in combination with oxaliplatin, can reduce the risk of recurrence in patients with Dukes stage C cancers and some high-risk Dukes B cancers. Post-operative radiotherapy reduces the risk of local recurrence in rectal cancer if operative resection margins are involved.

Palliation of advanced disease

Surgical resection of the primary tumour is appropriate for some patients with metastases to treat obstruction, bleeding or pain. Palliative chemotherapy with 5-fluorouracil/folinic acid, capecitabine, oxaliplatin or irinotecan improves survival. Patients with advanced metastatic disease may be treated with monoclonal antibodies using bevacizumab or cetuximab, either alone or together with chemotherapy. Pelvic radiotherapy is sometimes useful for distressing rectal symptoms such as pain, bleeding or severe tenesmus. Endoscopic laser therapy or insertion of an expandable metal stent can be used to relieve obstruction (Fig. 22.64).

A

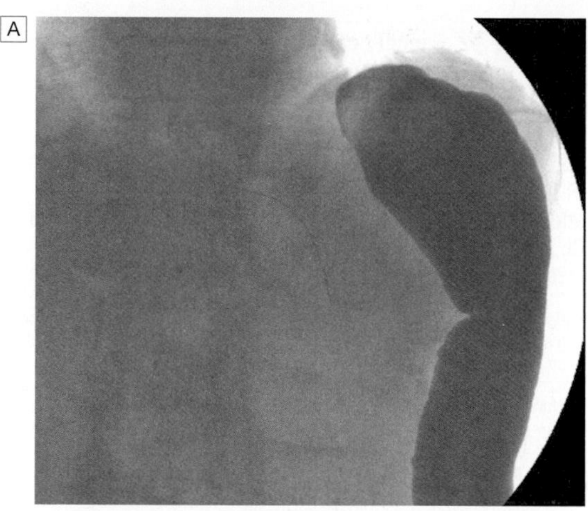

B

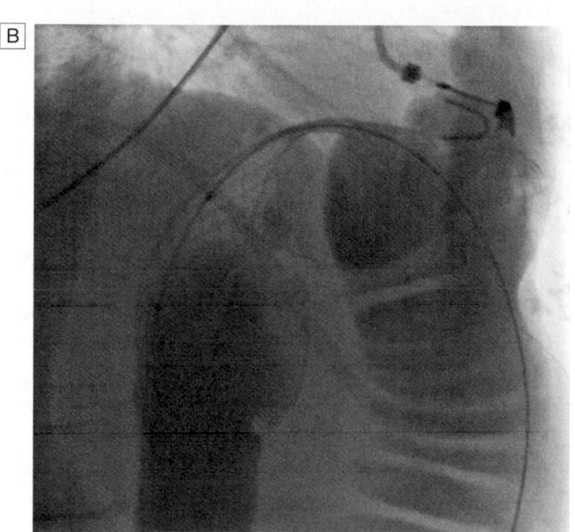

C

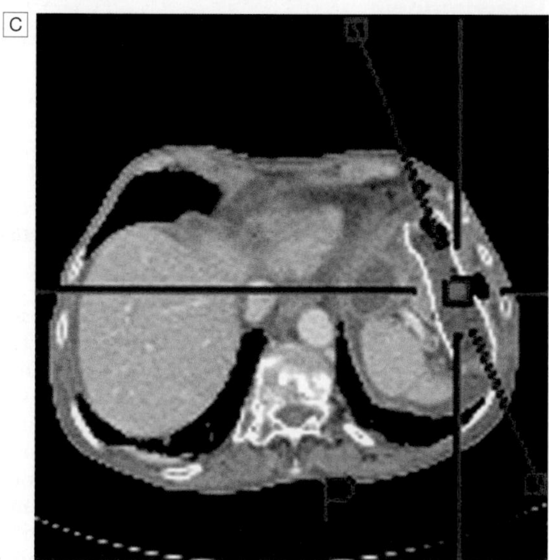

Fig. 22.64 Placement of a colonic stent for an inoperable cancer with impending obstruction. [A] The contrast study demonstrates an obstruction. [B] The stent is deployed across the tumour. [C] A satisfactory position is demonstrated on subsequent CT scanning.

EBM 22.92 Faecal occult blood (FOB) testing and colon cancer mortality

'Combined results from four randomised controlled trials show that participants allocated to screening by FOB testing had a 16% reduction in the relative risk of colorectal cancer mortality (RR 0.84, CI: 0.78–0.90). When adjusted for screening attendance, there was a 25% relative risk reduction (RR 0.75, CI: 0.66–0.84) for those attending at least one round of FOB screening.'

- Hewitson P, et al. Screening for colorectal cancer using the faecal occult blood test, Hemoccult. Cochrane Database of Systematic Reviews, 2007, issue 1. Art. no. CD001216; CD001216.pub2 (up to date 2010).

For further information: www.cochrane.org/cochrane-reviews

Prevention and screening

Secondary prevention aims to detect and remove lesions at an early or pre-malignant stage. Several potential methods exist:

- Population-based screening of people over the age of 50 years by regular *faecal occult blood (FOB) testing* reduces colorectal cancer mortality (Box 22.92) and increases the proportion of early cancers detected. The sensitivity and specificity of these tests need to be improved.
- *Colonoscopy* remains the gold standard but is expensive and carries risks; many countries lack the resources to offer this form of screening.
- *Flexible sigmoidoscopy* is an alternative option and has been shown to reduce overall colorectal cancer mortality by approximately 35% (70% for cases arising in the rectosigmoid). It is recommended in the USA every 5 years in all persons over the age of 50.
- Screening for high-risk patients by *molecular genetic analysis* is an exciting prospect but is not yet available.

Diverticulosis

Diverticula are acquired and are most common in the sigmoid and descending colon of middle-aged people. Asymptomatic diverticula (diverticulosis) are present in over 50% of people above the age of 70 years. Symptomatic diverticular disease supervenes in 10–25% of cases, while complicated diverticulosis (acute diverticulitis, pericolic abscess, bleeding, perforation or stricture) is uncommon.

Pathophysiology

A life-long refined diet with a relative deficiency of fibre is widely thought to be responsible and the condition is rare in populations with a high dietary fibre intake, such as in Asia, where it more often affects the right side of the colon. It is postulated that small-volume stools require high intracolonic pressures for propulsion and this leads to herniation of mucosa between the taeniae coli (Fig. 22.65). Diverticula consist of protrusions of mucosa covered by peritoneum. There is commonly hypertrophy of the circular muscle coat. Inflammation is thought to result from impaction of diverticula with faecoliths. This may resolve spontaneously or progress to cause haemorrhage, perforation, local abscess

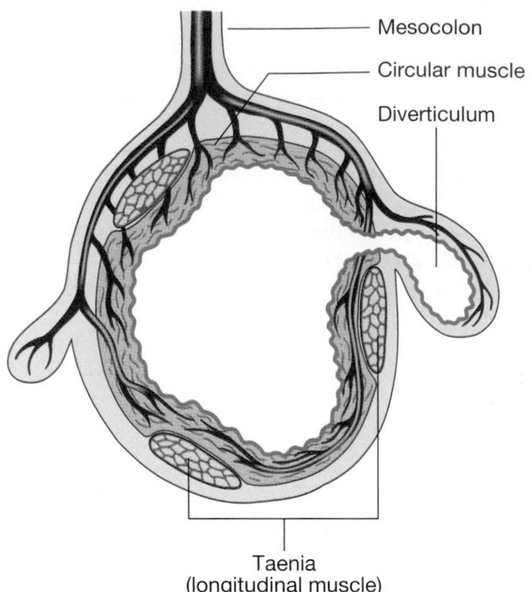

Fig. 22.65 The human colon in diverticulosis. The colonic wall is weak between the taeniae. The blood vessels that supply the colon pierce the circular muscle and weaken it further by forming tunnels. Diverticula usually emerge through these points of least resistance.

formation, fistula and peritonitis. Repeated attacks of inflammation lead to thickening of the bowel wall, narrowing of the lumen and eventual obstruction.

Clinical features

Symptoms are usually the result of associated constipation or spasm. Colicky pain is suprapubic or felt in the left iliac fossa. The sigmoid colon may be palpable and, in attacks of diverticulitis, there is local tenderness, guarding, rigidity ('left-sided appendicitis') and sometimes a palpable mass. During these episodes, there may be diarrhoea, rectal bleeding or fever. The differential diagnosis includes colorectal cancer, ischaemic colitis, inflammatory bowel disease and infection. Diverticular disease may be complicated by perforation, pericolic abscess, fistula formation (usually colovesical) or acute rectal bleeding. These complications are more common in patients who take NSAIDs or aspirin. After one attack of diverticulitis, the recurrence rate is around 3% per year. Over 10–30 years, perforation, obstruction or bleeding may occur, each affecting 5% of patients.

Investigations

Investigations are usually performed to exclude colorectal neoplasia. Barium enema can be used to confirm the presence of diverticula (see Fig. 22.11C, p. 847), strictures and fistulae. If barium studies are performed, flexible sigmoidoscopy is also necessary to exclude a coexisting neoplasm, which is easily missed radiologically. In severe diverticulosis, colonoscopy requires expertise and carries a risk of perforation. CT is used to assess complications, such as perforation or pericolic abscess.

Management

Diverticular disease that is asymptomatic and discovered coincidentally requires no treatment. Constipation can be relieved by a high-fibre diet, with or without a bulking laxative (ispaghula husk, 1–2 sachets daily), taken with plenty of fluids. Stimulant laxatives (see Box 22.93 below) should be avoided. Antispasmodics may sometimes help. Acute attacks of diverticulitis should be treated with 7 days of metronidazole (400 mg 3 times daily orally), along with co-amoxiclav (500/125 mg 4 times daily). Severe cases require intravenous fluids, intravenous antibiotics, analgesia and nasogastric suction, but randomised trials show no benefit from acute resection compared to conservative management, and emergency surgery is reserved for severe haemorrhage or perforation. Percutaneous drainage of acute paracolic abscesses can be effective and avoids the need for emergency surgery. Patients who have repeated attacks of obstruction should undergo elective surgery once the acute episode has settled, in order to resect the affected segment of bowel with restoration of continuity by primary anastomosis.

Constipation and disorders of defecation

The clinical approach to patients with constipation and its aetiology have been described on page 860.

Simple constipation

Simple constipation is extremely common and does not signify underlying organic disease. It usually responds to increased dietary fibre or the use of bulking agents; an adequate fluid intake is also essential. Many types of laxative are available, and these are listed in Box 22.93.

Severe idiopathic constipation

This occurs almost exclusively in young women and often begins in childhood or adolescence. The cause is unknown but some have 'slow transit' with reduced motor activity in the colon. Others have 'obstructed defecation', resulting from inappropriate contraction of the external anal sphincter and puborectalis muscle (anismus). The condition is often resistant to treatment. Bulking agents may exacerbate symptoms but prokinetic agents or balanced solutions of polyethylene glycol '3350' benefit some patients with slow transit. Glycerol suppositories and biofeedback techniques are used for those with obstructed defecation. Others benefit from agents such as prucalopride or linaclotide. Rarely, subtotal colectomy may be necessary as a last resort.

22.93 Laxatives

Class	Examples
Bulk-forming	Ispaghula husk, methylcellulose
Stimulants	Bisacodyl, dantron (only for terminally ill patients), docusate, senna
Faecal softeners	Docusate, arachis oil enema
Osmotic laxatives	Lactulose, lactitol, magnesium salts
Others	Polyethylene glycol (PEG)*, phosphate enema*

*Used mainly for bowel preparation prior to investigation or surgery.

Faecal impaction

In faecal impaction, a large, hard mass of stool fills the rectum. This tends to occur in disabled, immobile or institutionalised patients, especially the frail elderly or those with dementia. Constipating drugs, autonomic neuropathy and painful anal conditions also contribute. Megacolon, intestinal obstruction and urinary tract infections may supervene. Perforation and bleeding from pressure-induced ulceration are occasionally seen. Treatment involves adequate hydration and careful digital disimpaction after softening the impacted stool with arachis oil enemas. Stimulants should be avoided.

Melanosis coli and laxative misuse syndromes

Long-term consumption of stimulant laxatives leads to accumulation of lipofuscin pigment in macrophages in the lamina propria. This imparts a brown discoloration to the colonic mucosa, often described as resembling 'tiger skin'. The condition is benign and resolves when the laxatives are stopped. Prolonged laxative use may rarely result in megacolon or 'cathartic colon', in which barium enema demonstrates a featureless mucosa, loss of haustra and shortening of the bowel. Surreptitious laxative misuse is a psychiatric condition seen in young women, some of whom have a history of bulimia or anorexia nervosa (pp. 255 and 256). They complain of refractory watery diarrhoea. Laxative use is usually denied and may continue, even when patients are undergoing investigation. Screening of urine for laxatives may reveal the diagnosis.

Hirschsprung's disease

This disease is characterised by constipation and colonic dilatation (megacolon) due to congenital absence of ganglion cells in the large intestine. The incidence is approximately 1:5000. About one-third of patients have a positive family history and, in these families, the disease is inherited in an autosomal dominant manner with incomplete penetrance. About 50% of familial cases and 15% of sporadic cases have mutations affecting the *RET* proto-oncogene, which is also implicated in multiple endocrine neoplasia type 2 (MEN 2) (p. 795). Unlike MEN 2, which is caused by activating *RET* mutations, Hirschprung's disease is caused by loss-of-function mutations. Although *RET* is the most important susceptibility gene, some patients with *RET* mutations do not develop clinical disease, and mutations in other genes have been identified which interact to cause the disease. All of the genes are implicated in Hirschprung's disease are involved in the regulation of enteric neurogenesis, and the mutations cause failure of migration of neuroblasts into the gut wall during embryogenesis. Ganglion cells are absent from nerve plexuses, most commonly in a short segment of the rectum and/or sigmoid colon. As a result, the internal anal sphincter fails to relax. Constipation, abdominal distension and vomiting usually develop immediately after birth but a few cases do not present until childhood or adolescence. The rectum is empty on digital examination.

Barium enema shows a small rectum and colonic dilatation above the narrowed segment. Full-thickness biopsies are required to demonstrate nerve plexuses and confirm the absence of ganglion cells. Histochemical stains for acetylcholinesterase are also used. Anorectal manometry demonstrates failure of the rectum to relax with balloon distension. Treatment involves resection of the affected segment.

Acquired megacolon

This may develop in childhood as a result of voluntary withholding of stool during toilet training. In such cases, it presents after the first year of life and is distinguished from Hirschsprung's disease by the urge to defecate and the presence of stool in the rectum. It usually responds to osmotic laxatives.

In adults, acquired megacolon has several causes. It is seen in depressed or demented patients, either as part of the condition or as a side-effect of antidepressant drugs. Prolonged misuse of stimulant laxatives may cause degeneration of the myenteric plexus, while interruption of sensory or motor innervation may be responsible in a number of neurological disorders. Patients taking large doses of opioid analgesics can develop a megacolon: so-called 'narcotic bowel syndrome'. Scleroderma and hypothyroidism are other recognised causes.

Most patients can be managed conservatively by treatment of the underlying cause, high-residue diets, laxatives and the judicious use of enemas. Prokinetics are helpful in a minority of patients. Subtotal colectomy is a last resort for the most severely affected patients.

Acute colonic pseudo-obstruction

Acute colonic pseudo-obstruction (Ogilvie's syndrome) has many causes (Box 22.95) and is characterised by sudden onset of painless, massive enlargement of the proximal colon; there are no features of mechanical obstruction. Bowel sounds are normal or high-pitched, rather than absent. Left untreated, it may progress to perforation, peritonitis and death.

Abdominal X-rays show colonic dilatation with air extending to the rectum. Caecal diameter greater than 10 cm is associated with a high risk of perforation. Single-contrast or water-soluble barium enemas demonstrate the absence of mechanical obstruction.

Management consists of treating the underlying disorder and correcting any biochemical abnormalities. The anticholinesterase, neostigmine, is effective in enhancing parasympathetic activity and gut motility. Decompression, either with a rectal tube or by colonoscopy, may be effective but needs to be repeated until the condition resolves. In severe cases, surgical or fluoroscopic defunctioning caecostomy is necessary.

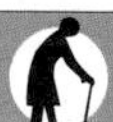

22.94 Constipation in old age

- **Evaluation**: particular attention should be paid to immobility, dietary fluid and fibre intake, drugs and depression.
- **Immobility**: predisposes to constipation by increasing the colonic transit time; the longer this is, the greater the fluid absorption and the harder the stool.
- **Bulking agents**: can make matters worse in patients with slow transit times and should be avoided.
- **Overflow diarrhoea**: if faecal impaction develops, paradoxical overflow diarrhoea may occur. If antidiarrhoeal agents are given, the underlying impaction may worsen and result in serious complications, such as stercoral ulceration and bleeding.

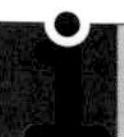

22.95 Causes of acute colonic pseudo-obstruction

- Trauma, burns
- Recent surgery
- Drugs (opiates, phenothiazines)
- Respiratory failure
- Electrolyte and acid–base disorders
- Diabetes mellitus
- Uraemia

Anorectal disorders

Faecal incontinence

The normal control of anal continence is described on page 844. Common causes of incontinence are listed in Box 22.96. High-risk patients include frail older people, women after childbirth and those with severe neurological/spinal disorders, learning difficulties or cognitive impairment.

Patients are often embarrassed to admit incontinence and may complain only of 'diarrhoea'. A careful history and examination, especially of the anorectum and perineum, may help to establish the underlying cause. Endoanal ultrasound is valuable for defining the integrity of the anal sphincters, while anorectal physiology and MR proctography are also useful investigations.

Management

This is often very difficult. Underlying disorders should be treated and diarrhoea managed with loperamide, diphenoxylate or codeine phosphate. Attention must be paid to a proper diet and adequate fluid intake. Pelvic floor exercises, biofeedback and bowel retraining techniques help some patients, and those with confirmed anal sphincter defects may benefit from sphincter repair operations. Where sphincter repair is not appropriate, a trial of sacral nerve stimulation is undertaken with a view to insertion of a permanent stimulator but, if unsuccessful, creation of a neo-sphincter may be possible, by graciloplasty or by an artificial anal sphincter.

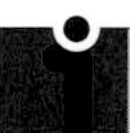

22.96 Causes of faecal incontinence

- Obstetric trauma: childbirth, hysterectomy
- Severe diarrhoea
- Faecal impaction
- Congenital anorectal anomalies
- Anorectal disease: haemorrhoids, rectal prolapse, Crohn's disease
- Neurological disorders: spinal cord or cauda equina lesions, dementia

Haemorrhoids

Haemorrhoids (commonly known as piles) arise from congestion of the internal and/or external venous plexuses around the anal canal. They are extremely common in adults. The aetiology is unknown, although they are associated with constipation and straining, and may develop for the first time during pregnancy. First-degree piles bleed, while second-degree piles prolapse but retract spontaneously. Third-degree piles are those which require manual replacement after prolapsing. Bright red rectal bleeding occurs after defecation. Other symptoms include pain, pruritus ani and mucus discharge. Treatment involves measures to prevent constipation and straining. Band ligation is effective for many, but a minority of patients require haemorrhoidectomy, which is usually curative. Recently, haemorrhoidal artery ligation operation (HALO) procedures have been developed and may replace surgery. HALO involves using Doppler ultrasound to identify all the arteries feeding the haemorrhoids and ligating them.

Pruritus ani

This is common and can stem from many causes (Box 22.97), most of which result in contamination of the perianal skin with faecal contents.

Itching may be severe and results in an itch–scratch–itch cycle which exacerbates the problem. When no underlying cause is found, all local barrier ointments and creams must be stopped. Good personal hygiene is essential, with careful washing after defecation. The perineal area must be kept dry and clean. Bulk-forming laxatives may reduce faecal soiling.

22.97 Causes of pruritus ani

Local anorectal conditions	
• Haemorrhoids • Fistula, fissures	• Poor hygiene
Infections	
• Threadworms	• Candidiasis
Skin disorders	
• Contact dermatitis • Psoriasis	• Lichen planus
Other	
• Diarrhoea or incontinence of any cause	• Irritable bowel syndrome • Anxiety

Solitary rectal ulcer syndrome

This is most common in young adults and occurs on the anterior rectal wall. It is thought to result from localised chronic trauma and/or ischaemia associated with disordered puborectalis function and mucosal prolapse. The ulcer is seen at sigmoidoscopy and biopsies show a characteristic accumulation of collagen.

Symptoms include minor bleeding and mucus per rectum, tenesmus and perineal pain. Treatment is often difficult but avoidance of straining at defecation is important and treatment of constipation may help. Marked mucosal prolapse is treated surgically.

Anal fissure

In this common problem, traumatic or ischaemic damage to the anal mucosa results in a superficial mucosal tear, most commonly in the midline posteriorly. Spasm of the internal anal sphincter exacerbates the condition. Severe pain occurs on defecation and there may be minor bleeding, mucus discharge and pruritus. The skin may be indurated and an oedematous skin tag, or 'sentinel pile', adjacent to the fissure is common.

Avoidance of constipation with bulk-forming laxatives and increased fluid intake is important. Relaxation of the internal sphincter is normally mediated by nitric oxide, and 0.2% glyceryl trinitrate, which donates nitric oxide and improves mucosal blood flow, is effective in 60–80% of patients. Diltiazem cream (2%) can be used as an alternative. Resistant cases may respond to injection of botulinum toxin into the internal anal sphincter to induce relaxation. Manual dilatation under anaesthesia leads to long-term incontinence and should not be considered. The majority of cases can be treated without surgery, but where these measures fail, healing can be achieved surgically by lateral internal anal sphincterotomy or advancement anoplasty.

Anorectal abscesses and fistulae

Perianal abscesses develop between the internal and external anal sphincters and may point at the perianal skin. Ischiorectal abscesses occur lateral to the sphincters in the ischiorectal fossa. They usually result from infection of anal glands by normal intestinal bacteria. Crohn's disease (p. 897) is sometimes responsible.

Patients complain of extreme perianal pain, fever and/or discharge of pus. Spontaneous rupture may lead to the development of fistulae. These may be superficial or track through the anal sphincters to reach the rectum. Abscesses are drained surgically and superficial fistulae are laid open with care to avoid sphincter damage.

Diseases of the peritoneal cavity

Peritonitis

Surgical peritonitis occurs as the result of a ruptured viscus (for details see this book's companion text, *Principles and Practice of Surgery*). Peritonitis may also complicate ascites in chronic liver disease (spontaneous bacterial peritonitis, p. 941) or may occur in children in the absence of ascites, due to infection with *Streptococcus pneumoniae* or β-haemolytic streptococci (p. 331).

Chlamydial peritonitis is a complication of pelvic inflammatory disease (p. 422). The patient presents with right upper quadrant pain, pyrexia and a hepatic rub (the Fitz-Hugh–Curtis syndrome). Tuberculosis may cause peritonitis and ascites (p. 688).

Tumours

The most common is secondary adenocarcinoma from the ovary or gastrointestinal tract. Mesothelioma is a rare tumour complicating asbestos exposure. It presents as a diffuse abdominal mass, due to omental infiltration, and with ascites. The prognosis is extremely poor.

Other disorders

Endometriosis

Ectopic endometrial tissue can become embedded on the serosal aspect of the intestine, most frequently in the sigmoid and rectum. The overlying mucosa is usually intact. Cyclical engorgement and inflammation result in pain, bleeding, diarrhoea, constipation, and adhesions or obstruction. Low backache is frequent. The onset is usually between 20 and 45 years and is more common in nulliparous women. Bimanual examination may reveal tender nodules in the pouch of Douglas. Endoscopic studies only reveal the diagnosis if carried out during menstruation, when a bluish mass with intact overlying mucosa is apparent. In some patients, laparoscopy is required. Treatment options include laparoscopic diathermy and hormonal therapy with progestogens (e.g. norethisterone), gonadotrophin-releasing hormone analogues or danazol.

Pneumatosis cystoides intestinalis

In this rare condition, multiple gas-filled submucosal cysts line the colonic and small bowel walls. The cause is unknown, but the condition may be seen in patients with chronic cardiac or pulmonary disease, pyloric obstruction, scleroderma or dermatomyositis. Most patients are asymptomatic, although there may be abdominal cramp, diarrhoea, tenesmus, rectal bleeding and mucus discharge. The cysts are recognised on sigmoidoscopy, plain abdominal X-rays or barium enema. Therapies reported to be effective include prolonged high-flow oxygen, elemental diets and antibiotics.

Further information and acknowledgements

Books and journal articles

Canard JM, Letard J-C, Palazzo L, Penman I, Lennon AM. Gastrointestinal endoscopy in practice. Edinburgh: Churchill Livingstone; 2011.

Feldman M, Friedman LS, Brandt LJ. Sleisenger and Fordtran's gastrointestinal and liver disease. 9th edn. Philadelphia: Saunders; 2010.

Websites

www.bsg.org.uk *British Society of Gastroenterology.*

www.coeliac.org.uk *Coeliac UK.*

www.ecco-ibd.eu *European Crohn's and Colitis Organisation.*

www.gastro.org *American Gastroenterological Association and American Digestive Health Foundation.*

www.isg.org.in *Indian Society of Gastroenterology.*

www.nacc.org.uk *Crohn's and Colitis UK.*

Figure acknowledgement

Fig. 22.39AB Hayes P, Simpson K. Gastroenterology and liver disease. Edinburgh: Churchill Livingstone; 1995; copyright Elsevier.

Q.M. Anstee
D.E.J. Jones

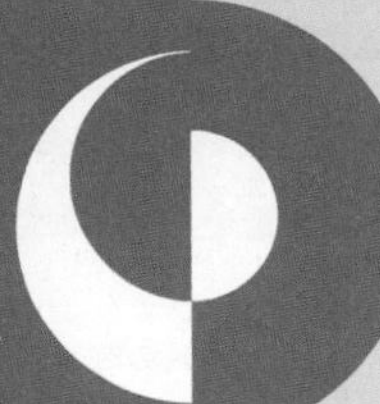

Liver and biliary tract disease 23

Clinical examination of the abdomen for liver and biliary disease 922

Functional anatomy and physiology 924
- Applied anatomy 924
- Hepatic function 926

Investigation of liver and hepatobiliary disease 928
- Liver blood biochemistry 928
- Haematological tests 929
- Immunological tests 929
- Imaging 930
- Histological examination 931
- Non-invasive markers of hepatic fibrosis 932

Presenting problems in liver disease 932
- Acute liver failure 932
- Abnormal liver function tests 935
- Jaundice 936
- Hepatomegaly 938
- Ascites 938
- Hepatic encephalopathy 941
- Variceal bleeding 942

Cirrhosis 942

Portal hypertension 945

Infections and the liver 948
- Viral hepatitis 948
- HIV infection and the liver 955
- Liver abscess 956

Alcoholic liver disease 957

Non-alcoholic fatty liver disease 959

Autoimmune liver and biliary disease 961
- Autoimmune hepatitis 962
- Primary biliary cirrhosis 963
- Primary sclerosing cholangitis 965
- IgG4-associated cholangitis 966

Liver tumours and other focal liver lesions 966
- Primary malignant tumours 967
- Secondary malignant tumours 969
- Benign tumours 970

Drugs and the liver 970
- Drug-induced liver injury 970

Inherited liver diseases 972
- Haemochromatosis 972
- Wilson's disease 973
- Alpha$_1$-antitrypsin deficiency 974
- Gilbert's syndrome 974

Vascular liver disease 975
- Hepatic arterial disease 975
- Portal venous disease 975
- Hepatic venous disease 976
- Nodular regenerative hyperplasia of the liver 977

Pregnancy and the liver 977
- Intercurrent and pre-existing liver disease 977
- Pregnancy-associated liver disease 977

Liver transplantation 978
- Indications and contraindications 978
- Complications 979
- Prognosis 979

Cholestatic and biliary disease 980
- Chemical cholestasis 980
- Benign recurrent intrahepatic cholestasis 980
- Intrahepatic biliary disease 980
- Extrahepatic biliary disease 981
- Secondary biliary cirrhosis 981
- Gallstones 981
- Cholecystitis 983
- Choledocholithiasis 984
- Tumours of the gallbladder and bile duct 985
- Miscellaneous biliary disorders 986

CLINICAL EXAMINATION OF THE ABDOMEN FOR LIVER AND BILIARY DISEASE

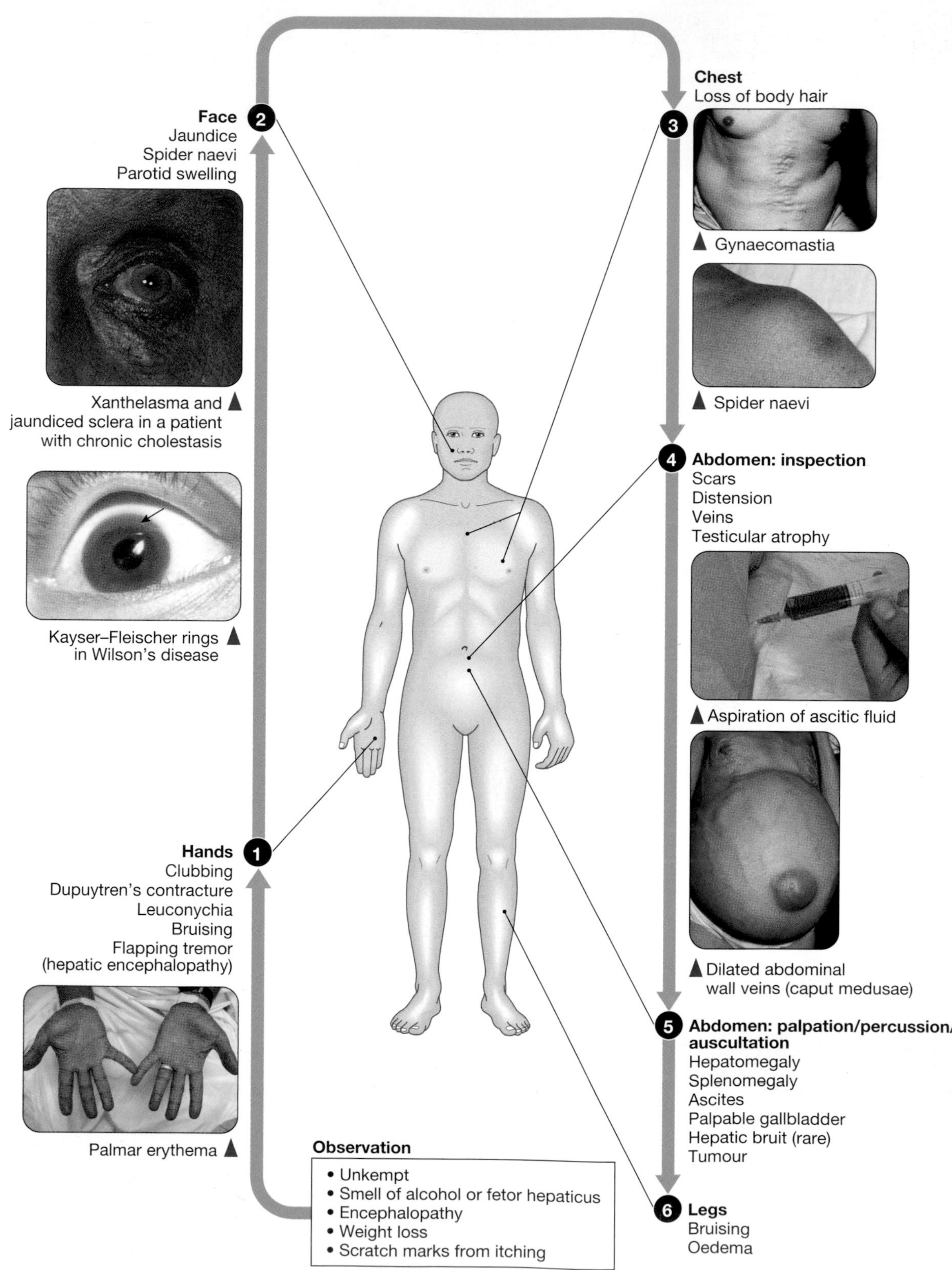

Insets (*Spider naevi*) From Hayes and Simpson 1995; (*Aspiration*) Strachan 2008; (*Palmar erythema*) Martin 2011 – see p. 988.

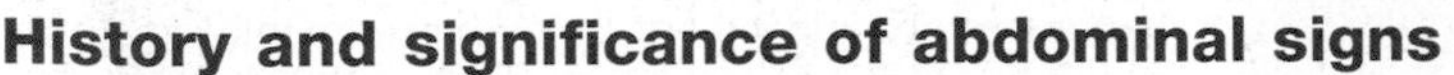

History and significance of abdominal signs

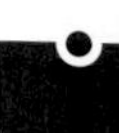

Presenting clinical features of liver disease

Presenting features of liver disease represent combined effects of:

Impairment of liver function and metabolic sequelae of this

- Jaundice (failure of bilirubin clearance)
- Encephalopathy (failure of clearance of by-products of metabolism)
- Bleeding (impaired liver synthesis of clotting factors)
- Hypoglycaemia

Ongoing presence of aetiological factors (e.g. alcohol)

- Effects of aetiological agent, e.g. intoxication, withdrawal, cognitive impairment *versus*
- Effects of liver injury from agent, e.g. encephalopathy

Effects of chronic liver injury (> 6 mths)

Catabolic status (± poor nutrition)
- Skin thinning ('paper-money skin')
- Loss of muscle bulk
- Leuconychia

Impaired albumin synthesis
- Reduced oncotic pressure (contributes to ascites)

Reduced aldosterone clearance
- Na^+ retention (contributes to ascites)

Reduced oestrogen clearance
- Mild feminisation of males (loss of body hair, gynaecomastia)

5 Assessment of liver size

Clinical assessment of hepatomegaly is important in diagnosing liver disease.

- Start in the right iliac fossa.
- Progress up the abdomen 2 cm with each breath (through open mouth).
- Confirm the lower border of the liver by percussion.
- Detect if smooth or irregular, tender or non-tender; ascertain shape.
- Identify the upper border by percussion.

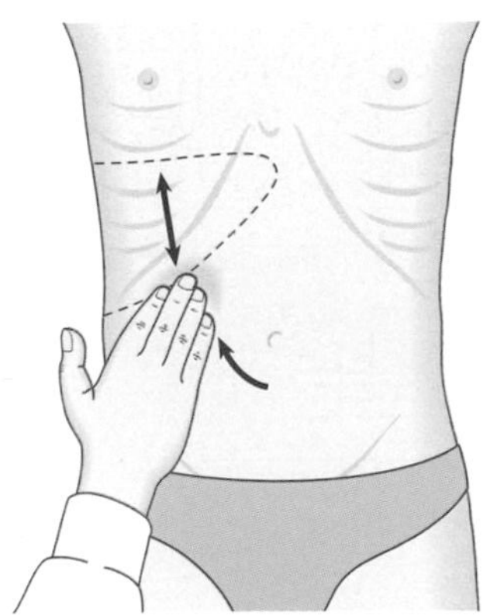

Ascites

Causes	Associated clinical findings
Exudative (high protein)	
Carcinoma	Weight loss ± hepatomegaly
Tuberculosis	Weight loss + fever
Transudative (low protein)	
Cirrhosis	Hepatomegaly Splenomegaly Spider naevi
Renal failure (including nephrotic syndrome)	Generalised oedema
Congestive heart failure	Peripheral oedema Elevated jugular venous pressure (JVP)

1 Assessment of encephalopathy

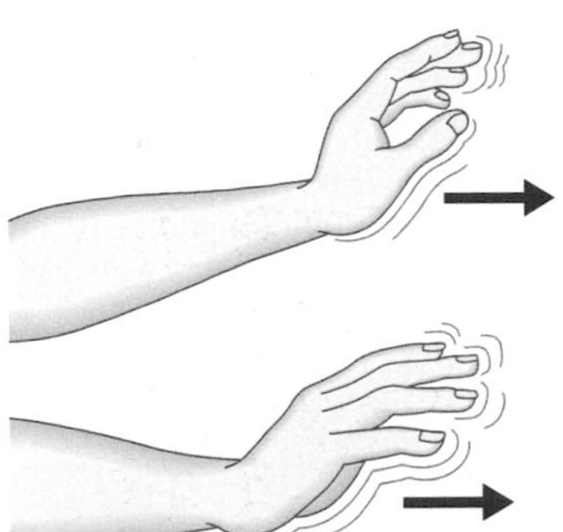

Flapping tremor. Jerky forward movements every 5–10 seconds when arms are outstretched and hands are dorsiflexed suggest hepatic encephalopathy. The movements are coarser than those seen in tremor.

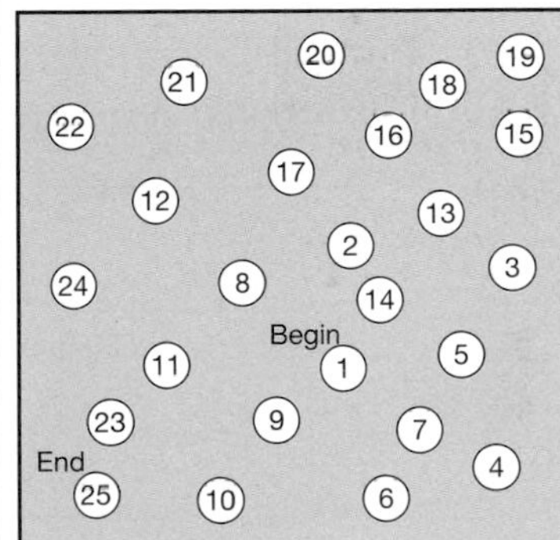

Number connection test. These 25 numbered circles can normally be joined together within 30 seconds. Serial observations may provide useful information as long as the position of the numbers is varied to avoid the patient learning their pattern.

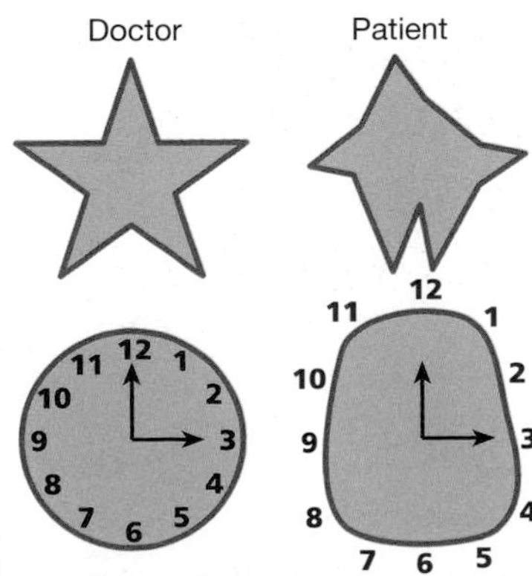

Constructional apraxia. Drawing stars and clocks may reveal marked abnormality.

FUNCTIONAL ANATOMY AND PHYSIOLOGY

Applied anatomy

Normal liver structure and blood supply

The liver weighs 1.2–1.5 kg and has multiple functions, including key roles in metabolism, control of infection, elimination of toxins and by-products of metabolism. It is classically divided into left and right lobes by the falciform ligament, but a more useful functional division is into the right and left hemilivers, based on blood supply (Fig. 23.1). These are further divided into eight segments according to subdivisions of the hepatic and portal veins. Each segment has its own branch of the hepatic artery and biliary tree. The segmental anatomy of the liver has an important influence on imaging and treatment of liver tumours, given the increasing use of surgical resection. A liver segment is made up of multiple smaller units known as lobules, comprised of a central vein, radiating sinusoids separated from each other by single liver cell (hepatocyte) plates, and peripheral portal tracts. The functional unit of the liver is the hepatic acinus (Fig. 23.2).

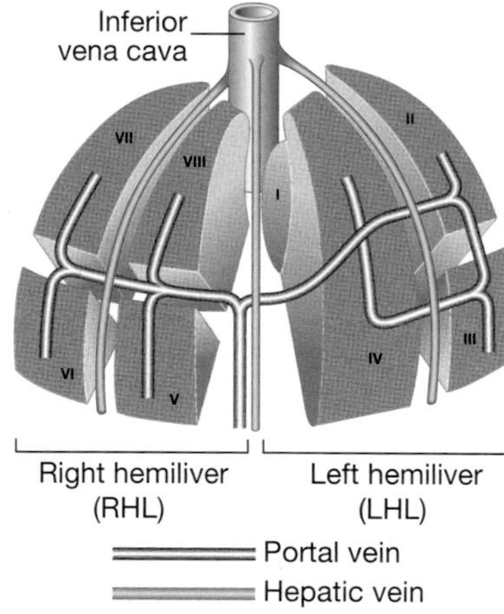

Fig. 23.1 Liver blood supply.

Blood flows into the acinus via a single branch of the portal vein and hepatic artery situated centrally in the portal tracts. Blood flows outwards along the hepatic sinusoids into one of several tributaries of the hepatic vein at the periphery of the acinus. Bile, formed by active and passive excretion by hepatocytes into channels called cholangioles which lie between them, flows in the opposite direction from the periphery of the acinus. The cholangioles converge in interlobular bile ducts in the portal tracts. The hepatocytes in each acinus lie in three zones, depending on their position relative to the portal tract. Those in zone 1 are closest to the terminal branches of the portal vein and hepatic artery, and are richly supplied with oxygenated blood, and blood containing the highest concentration of nutrients and toxins. Conversely, hepatocytes in zone 3 are furthest from the portal tracts and closest to the hepatic veins, and are therefore relatively hypoxic and exposed to lower concentrations of nutrients and toxins compared to zone 1. The different perfusion and toxin exposure patterns, and thus vulnerability, of hepatocytes in the different zones contribute to the often-patchy nature of liver injury.

Liver cells

Hepatocytes comprise 80% of liver cells. The remaining 20% are the endothelial cells lining the sinusoids,

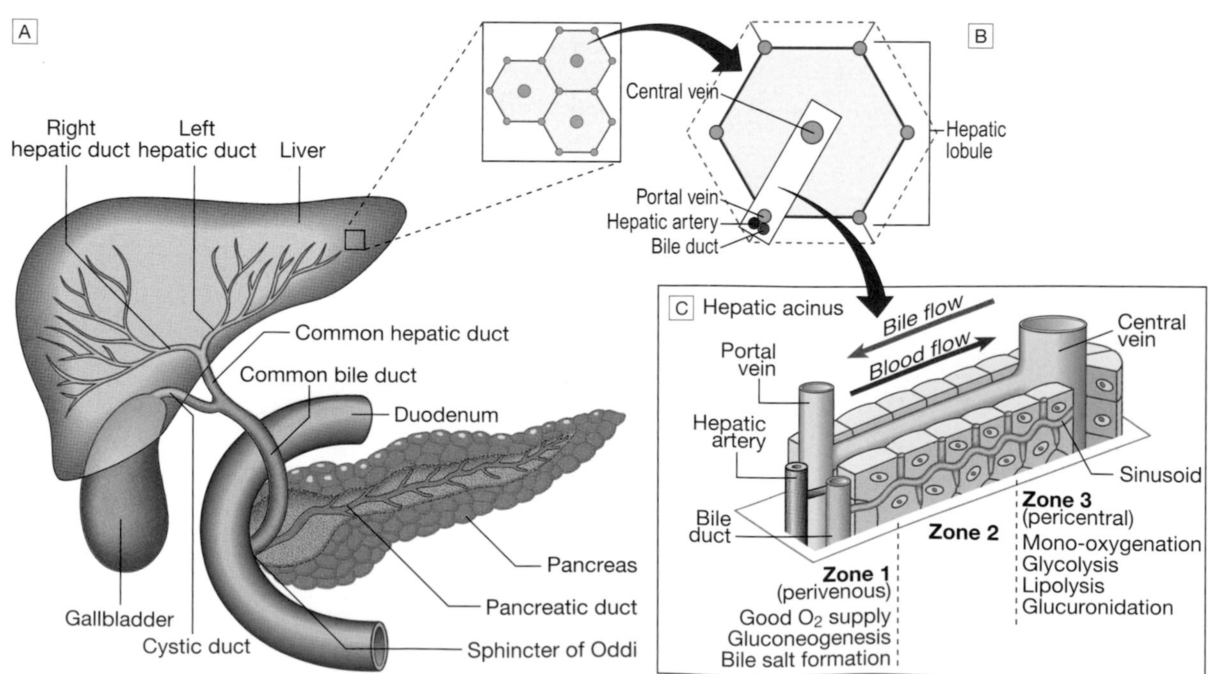

Fig. 23.2 Liver structure and microstructure. **A** Liver anatomy showing relationship with pancreas, bile duct and duodenum. **B** Hepatic lobule. **C** Hepatic acinus.

epithelial cells lining the intrahepatic bile ducts, cells of the immune system (including macrophages (Kupffer cells) and unique populations of atypical lymphocytes), and a key population of non-parenchymal cells called stellate or Ito cells.

Endothelial cells line the sinusoids (Fig. 23.3), a network of capillary vessels that differ from other capillary beds in the body in that there is no basement membrane. The endothelial cells have gaps between them (fenestrae) of about 0.1 micron in diameter, allowing free flow of fluid and particulate matter to the hepatocytes. Individual hepatocytes are separated from the leaky sinusoids by the space of Disse, which contains stellate cells that store vitamin A and play an important part in regulating liver blood flow. They may also be immunologically active and play a role in the liver's contribution to defence against pathogens. The key role of stellate cells in terms of pathology is in the development of hepatic fibrosis, the precursor of cirrhosis. They undergo activation in response to cytokines produced following liver injury, differentiating into myofibroblasts, which are the major producers of the collagen-rich matrix that forms fibrous tissue (Fig. 23.4).

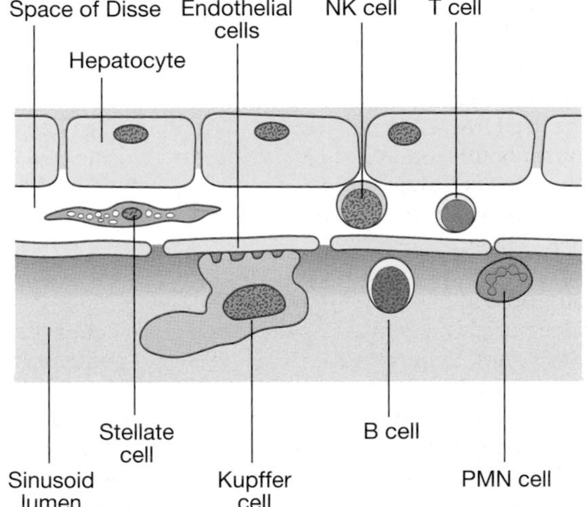

Fig. 23.3 Non-parenchymal liver cells. (B = B lymphocytes; NK = natural killer cells; PMN = polymorphonuclear leucocytes; T = T lymphocytes).

Blood supply

The liver is unique as an organ as it has dual perfusion, receiving a majority of its supply via the portal vein, which drains blood from the gut via the splanchnic circulation and is the principal route for nutrient trafficking to the liver, and a minority from the hepatic artery. The portal venous contribution is 50–90%. The dual perfusion system, and the variable contribution from portal vein and hepatic artery, can have important effects on the clinical expression of liver ischaemia (which typically exhibits a less dramatic pattern than

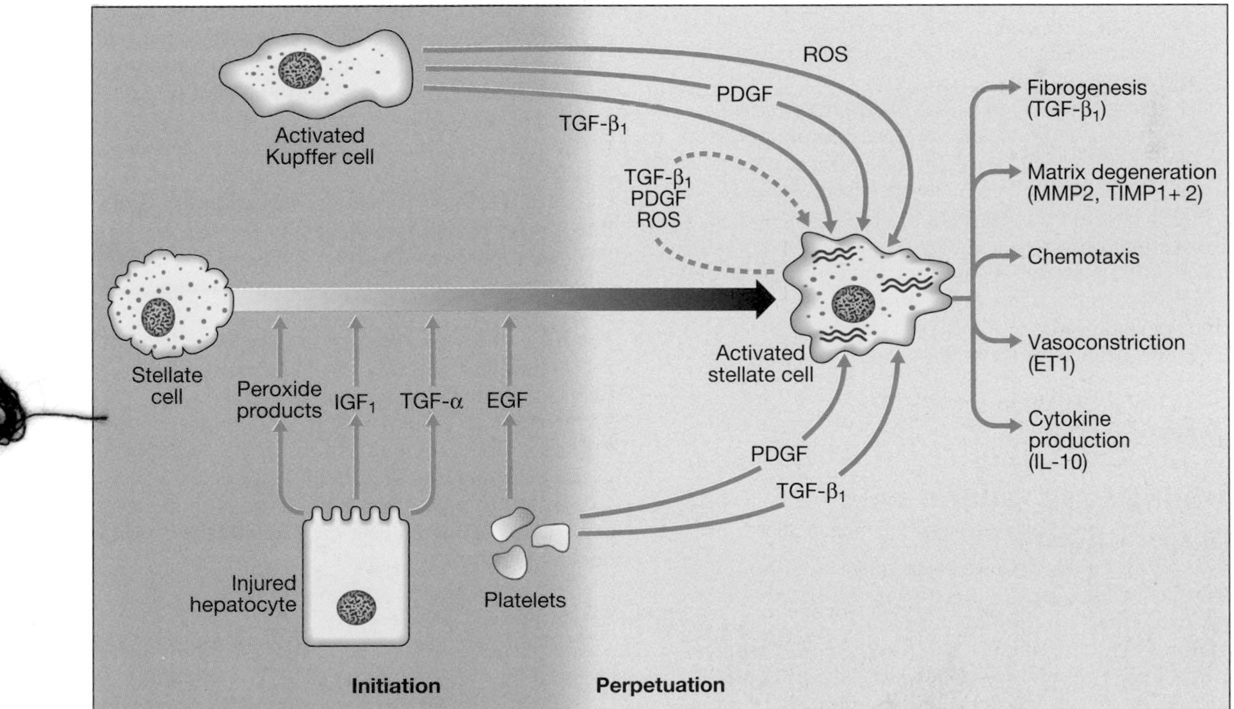

Fig. 23.4 Pathogenic mechanisms in hepatic fibrosis. Stellate cell activation occurs under the influence of cytokines released by other cell types in the liver, including hepatocytes, Kupffer cells (tissue macrophages), platelets and lymphocytes. Once stellate cells become activated, they can perpetuate their own activation by synthesis of transforming growth factor-beta (TGF-β_1,) and platelet-derived growth factor (PDGF) through autocrine loops. Activated stellate cells produce TGF-β_1, stimulating the production of collagen matrix, as well as inhibitors of collagen breakdown. The inhibitors of collagen breakdown, matrix metalloproteinase 2 and 9 (MMP2 and MMP9), are inactivated in turn by tissue inhibitors TIMP1 and TIMP2, which are increased in fibrosis. Inflammation also contributes to fibrosis, with the cytokine profile produced by Th2 lymphocytes, such as interleukin-6 and 13 (IL-6 and IL-13). Activated stellate cells also produce endothelin 1 (ET1), which may contribute to portal hypertension. (EGF = epidermal growth factor; IGF_1 = insulin-like growth factor 1; ROS = reactive oxygen species).

ischaemia in other organs, a fact that can sometimes lead to it being missed clinically), and can raise practical challenges in liver transplant surgery.

Biliary system and gallbladder

Hepatocytes provide the driving force for bile flow by creating osmotic gradients of bile acids, which form micelles in bile (bile acid-dependent bile flow), and of sodium (bile acid-independent bile flow). Bile is secreted by hepatocytes and flows from cholangioles to the biliary canaliculi. The canaliculi join to form larger intrahepatic bile ducts, which in turn merge to form the right and left hepatic ducts. These ducts join as they emerge from the liver to form the common hepatic duct, which becomes the common bile duct after joining the cystic duct (see Fig. 23.2). The common bile duct is approximately 5 cm long and 4–6 mm wide. The distal portion of the duct passes through the head of the pancreas and usually joins the pancreatic duct before entering the duodenum through the ampullary sphincter (sphincter of Oddi). It should be noted, though, that the anatomy of the lower common bile duct can vary widely. Common bile duct pressure is maintained by rhythmic contraction and relaxation of the sphincter of Oddi; this pressure exceeds gallbladder pressure in the fasting state, so that bile normally flows into the gallbladder, where it is concentrated tenfold by resorption of water and electrolytes.

The gallbladder is a pear-shaped sac typically lying under the right hemiliver, with its fundus located anteriorly behind the tip of the 9th costal cartilage. Anatomical variation is common and should be considered when assessing patients clinically and radiologically. The function of the gallbladder is to concentrate, and provide a reservoir for, bile. Gallbladder tone is maintained by vagal activity, and cholecystokinin released from the duodenal mucosa during feeding causes gallbladder contraction and reduces sphincter pressure, so that bile flows into the duodenum. The body and neck of the gallbladder pass postero-medially towards the porta hepatis, and the cystic duct then joins it to the common hepatic duct. The cystic duct mucosa has prominent crescentic folds (valves of Heister), giving it a beaded appearance on cholangiography.

Hepatic function

Carbohydrate, amino acid and lipid metabolism

The liver plays a central role in carbohydrate, lipid and amino acid metabolism, and is also involved in metabolising drugs and environmental toxins (Fig. 23.5). An important and increasingly recognised role for the liver is in the integration of metabolic pathways, regulating the response of the body to feeding and starvation. Abnormality in metabolic pathways and their regulation can play an important role both in liver disease (e.g. non-alcoholic fatty liver disease (NAFLD)) and in diseases that are not conventionally regarded as diseases of the liver (such as type II diabetes mellitus and inborn errors of metabolism). Hepatocytes have specific pathways to handle each of the nutrients absorbed from the gut and carried to the liver via the portal vein.

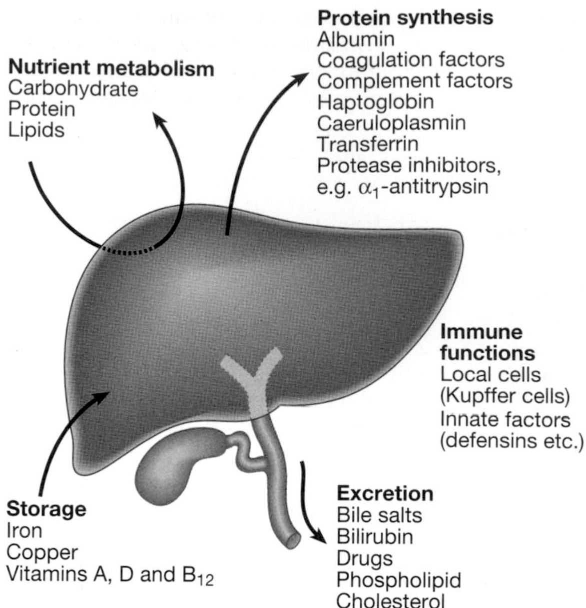

Fig. 23.5 Important liver functions.

- Amino acids from dietary proteins are used for synthesis of plasma proteins, including albumin. The liver produces 8–14 g of albumin per day, and this plays a critical role in maintaining oncotic pressure in the vascular space and in the transport of small molecules like bilirubin, hormones and drugs throughout the body. Amino acids that are not required for the production of new proteins are broken down, with the amino group being converted ultimately to urea.
- Following a meal, more than half of the glucose absorbed is taken up by the liver and stored as glycogen or converted to glycerol and fatty acids, thus preventing hyperglycaemia. During fasting, glycogen is broken down to release glucose (gluconeogenesis), thereby preventing hypoglycaemia (p. 800).
- The liver plays a central role in lipid metabolism, producing very low-density lipoproteins and further metabolising low- and high-density lipoproteins (see Fig. 16.14, p. 452). Dysregulation of lipid metabolism is thought to have a critical role in the pathogenesis of NAFLD. Lipids are now recognised to play a key part in the pathogenesis of hepatitis C, facilitating viral entry into hepatocytes.

Clotting factors

The liver produces key proteins that are involved in the coagulation cascade. Many of these coagulation factors (II, VII, IX and X) are post-translationally modified by vitamin K-dependent enzymes, and their synthesis is impaired in vitamin K deficiency (p. 997). Reduced clotting factor synthesis is an important and easily accessible biomarker of liver function in the setting of liver injury. Prothrombin time (PT; or the International Normalised Ratio, INR) is therefore one of the most important clinical tools available for the assessment of hepatocyte function. Note that the deranged PT or INR seen in liver disease may not directly equate to increased bleeding risk, as these tests do not capture the concurrent reduced synthesis of *anticoagulant* factors, including protein C and protein S. In general, therefore, correction of PT using blood products before minor invasive procedures should be guided by clinical risk rather than the absolute value of the PT.

Bilirubin metabolism and bile

The liver plays a central role in the metabolism of bilirubin and is responsible for the production of bile (Fig. 23.6). Between 425 and 510 mmol (250–300 mg) of unconjugated bilirubin is produced from the catabolism of haem daily. Bilirubin in the blood is normally almost all unconjugated and, because it is not water-soluble, is bound to albumin and does not pass into the urine. Unconjugated bilirubin is taken up by hepatocytes at the sinusoidal membrane, where it is conjugated in the endoplasmic reticulum by UDP-glucuronyl transferase, producing bilirubin mono- and diglucuronide. Impaired conjugation by this enzyme is a cause of inherited hyperbilirubinaemias (see Box 23.17, p. 937). These bilirubin conjugates are water-soluble and are exported into the bile canaliculi by specific carriers on the hepatocyte membranes. The conjugated bilirubin is excreted in the bile and passes into the duodenal lumen.

Once in the intestine, conjugated bilirubin is metabolised by colonic bacteria to form stercobilinogen, which may be further oxidised to stercobilin. Both stercobilinogen and stercobilin are then excreted in the stool, contributing to its brown colour. Biliary obstruction results in reduced stercobilinogen in the stool, and the stools become pale. A small amount of stercobilinogen (4 mg/day) is absorbed from the bowel, passes through the liver, and is excreted in the urine, where it is known as urobilinogen or, following further oxidisation, urobilin. The liver secretes 1–2 L of bile daily. Bile contains bile acids (formed from cholesterol), phospholipids, bilirubin and cholesterol. Several biliary transporter proteins have been identified (Fig. 23.7). Mutations in genes encoding these proteins have been identified in inherited intrahepatic biliary diseases presenting in childhood, and in adult-onset disease such as intrahepatic cholestasis of pregnancy and gallstone formation.

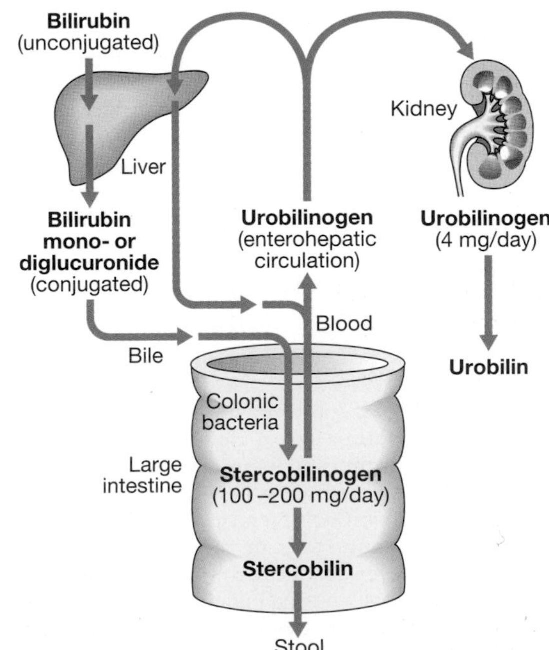

Fig. 23.6 Pathway of bilirubin excretion.

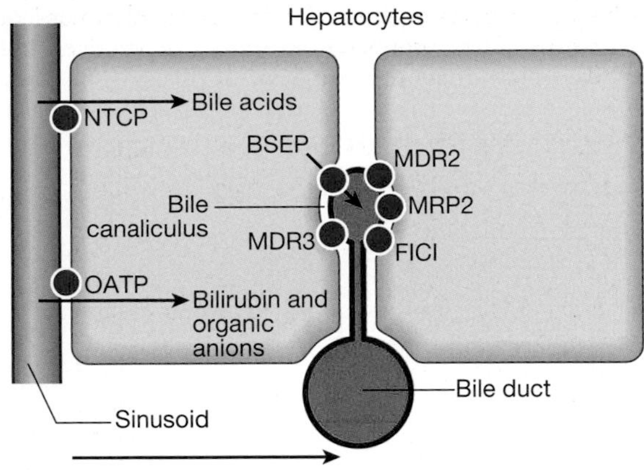

Fig. 23.7 Biliary transporter proteins. On the hepatocyte basolateral membrane, NTCP (sodium taurocholate co-transporting polypeptide) mediates uptake of conjugated bile acids from portal blood. At the canalicular membrane, these bile acids are secreted via BSEP (bile salt export pump) into bile. MDR3 (multidrug resistance protein 3), also situated on the canalicular membrane, transports phospholipid to the outer side of the membrane. This solubilises bile acids, forming micelles and protecting bile duct membranes from bile salt damage. FIC1 (familial intrahepatic cholestasis 1) moves phosphatidylserine from the inside to the outside of the canalicular membrane; mutations result in familial cholestasis syndrome in childhood. MDR2 (multidrug resistance 2) regulates transport of glutathione. MRP2 (multidrug resistance protein 2) transports bilirubin and is induced by rifampicin. OATP (organic anion transporter protein) transports bilirubin and organic anions.

Storage of vitamins and minerals

Vitamins A, D and B_{12} are stored by the liver in large amounts, while others, such as vitamin K and folate, are stored in smaller amounts and disappear rapidly if dietary intake is reduced. The liver is also able to metabolise vitamins to more active compounds, e.g. 7-dehydrocholesterol to 25(OH) vitamin D. Vitamin K is a fat-soluble vitamin and so the inability to absorb fat-soluble vitamins, as occurs in biliary obstruction, results in a coagulopathy. The liver also stores minerals such as iron, in ferritin and haemosiderin, and copper, which is excreted in bile.

Immune regulation

Approximately 9% of the normal liver is composed of immune cells (see Fig. 23.3). Cells of the innate immune system include Kupffer cells derived from blood monocytes, the liver macrophages and natural killer (NK) cells, as well as 'classical' B and T cells of the adaptive immune response (p. 76). An additional type of atypical lymphocyte, with phenotypic features of both T cells and NK cells is thought to play an important role in host defence, through linking of innate and adaptive immunity. The enrichment of such cells in the liver reflects the unique importance of the liver in preventing microorganisms from the gut entering the systemic circulation.

Kupffer cells constitute the largest single mass of tissue-resident macrophages in the body and account for 80% of the phagocytic capacity of this system. They remove aged and damaged red blood cells, bacteria, viruses, antigen–antibody complexes and endotoxin. They also produce a wide variety of inflammatory mediators that can act locally or may be released into the systemic circulation.

The immunological environment of the liver is unique in that antigens presented within it tend to induce immunological tolerance. This is of importance in liver transplantation, where classical major histocompatibility (MHC) barriers may be crossed, and also in chronic viral infections, when immune responses may be attenuated. The mechanisms that underlie this phenomenon have not been fully defined.

INVESTIGATION OF LIVER AND HEPATOBILIARY DISEASE

Investigations play an important role in the management of liver disease in three settings:

- identification of the presence of liver disease
- establishing the aetiology
- understanding disease severity (in particular, identification of cirrhosis with its complications).

When planning investigations it is important to be clear as to which of these goals is being addressed.

Suspicion of the presence of liver disease is normally based on blood biochemistry abnormality ('liver function tests', or 'LFTs'), undertaken either as a result of clinical suspicion or, increasingly, in the setting of health screening. Less commonly, suspicion arises after a structural abnormality is identified on imaging.

Aetiology is typically established through a combination of history, specific blood tests and, where appropriate, imaging and liver biopsy.

Staging of disease (in essence, the identification of cirrhosis) is largely histological, although there is increasing interest in non-invasive approaches, including novel imaging modalities, serum markers of fibrosis and the use of predictive scoring systems.

The aims of investigation in patients with suspected liver disease are shown in Box 23.1.

Liver blood biochemistry

Liver blood biochemistry (LFTs) includes the measurement of serum bilirubin, aminotransferases, alkaline phosphatase, gamma-glutamyl transferase and albumin. Most analytes measured by LFTs are not truly 'function' tests but, given that they are released by injured hepatocytes, instead provide biochemical evidence of liver cell damage. Liver function per se is best assessed by the serum albumin, PT and bilirubin because of the role played by the liver in synthesis of albumin and clotting factors and in clearance of bilirubin. Although LFT abnormalities are often non-specific, the patterns are frequently helpful in directing further investigations. Also, levels of bilirubin and albumin and the PT are related to clinical outcome in patients with severe liver disease, reflected by their use in several prognostic scores: the Child–Pugh and MELD scores in cirrhosis (see Boxes 23.30 and 23.32, p. 944), the Glasgow score in alcoholic hepatitis (see Box 23.54, p. 959) and the King's College Hospital criteria for liver transplantation in acute liver failure (see Box 23.11, p. 934).

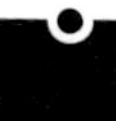

23.1 Aims of investigations in patients with suspected liver disease

- Detect hepatic abnormality
- Measure the severity of liver damage
- Detect the pattern of liver function test abnormality: hepatitic or obstructive/cholestatic
- Identify the specific cause
- Investigate possible complications

Bilirubin and albumin

The degree of elevation of bilirubin can reflect the degree of liver damage. A raised bilirubin often occurs earlier in the natural history of biliary disease (e.g. primary biliary cirrhosis) than in disease of the liver parenchyma (e.g. cirrhosis) where the hepatocytes are primarily involved. Swelling of the liver within its capsule in inflammation can, however, sometimes impair bile flow and cause an elevation of bilirubin level that is disproportionate to the degree of liver injury. Caution is therefore needed in interpreting the level of liver injury purely on the basis of bilirubin elevation.

Serum albumin levels are often low in patients with liver disease. This is due to a change in the volume of distribution of albumin, and reduced synthesis. Since the plasma half-life of albumin is about 2 weeks, albumin levels may be normal in acute liver failure but are almost always reduced in chronic liver failure.

Alanine aminotransferase and aspartate aminotransferase

Alanine aminotransferase (ALT) and aspartate aminotransferase (AST) are located in the cytoplasm of the hepatocyte; AST is also located in the hepatocyte mitochondria. Although both transaminase enzymes are widely distributed, expression of ALT outside the liver is relatively low and this enzyme is therefore considered more specific for hepatocellular damage. Large increases of aminotransferase activity favour hepatocellular damage, and this pattern of LFT abnormality is known as 'hepatitic'.

Alkaline phosphatase and gamma-glutamyl transferase

Alkaline phosphatase (ALP) is the collective name given to several different enzymes that hydrolyse phosphate esters at alkaline pH. These enzymes are widely distributed in the body, but the main sites of production are the liver, gastrointestinal tract, bone, placenta and kidney. ALPs are post-translationally modified, resulting in the production of several different isoenzymes, which differ in abundance in different tissues. ALP enzymes in the liver are located in cell membranes of the hepatic sinusoids and the biliary canaliculi. Accordingly, levels rise with intrahepatic and extrahepatic biliary obstruction and with sinusoidal obstruction, as occurs in infiltrative liver disease.

23.2 'Hepatitic' and 'cholestatic'/'obstructive' liver function tests

Pattern	AST/ALT	GGT	ALP
Biliary obstruction	↑	↑↑	↑↑↑
Hepatitis	↑↑↑	↑	↑
Alcohol/enzyme-inducing drugs	N/↑	↑↑	N

N = normal; ↑ mild elevation (< twice normal); ↑↑ moderate elevation (2–5 times normal); ↑↑↑ marked elevation (> 5 times normal).
(ALT = alanine aminotransferase; ALP = alkaline phosphatase; AST = aspartate aminotransferase; GGT = gamma-glutamyltransferase)

23.3 Drugs that increase levels of gamma-glutamyltransferase

- Barbiturates
- Carbamazepine
- Ethanol
- Griseofulvin
- Isoniazid
- Rifampicin
- Phenytoin

Gamma-glutamyl transferase (GGT) is a microsomal enzyme found in many cells and tissues of the body. The highest concentrations are located in the liver, where it is produced by hepatocytes and by the epithelium lining small bile ducts. The function of GGT is to transfer glutamyl groups from gamma-glutamyl peptides to other peptides and amino acids.

The pattern of a modest increase in aminotransferase activity and large increases in ALP and GGT activity favours biliary obstruction and is commonly described as 'cholestatic' or 'obstructive' (Box 23.2). Isolated elevation of the serum GGT is relatively common, and may occur during ingestion of microsomal enzyme-inducing drugs, including alcohol (Box 23.3), but also in NAFLD.

Other biochemical tests

Other widely available biochemical tests may become altered in patients with liver disease:

- Hyponatraemia occurs in severe liver disease due to increased production of antidiuretic hormone (ADH; Fig. 16.5, p. 435).
- Serum urea may be reduced in hepatic failure, whereas levels of urea may be increased following gastrointestinal haemorrhage.
- When high levels of urea are accompanied by raised bilirubin, high serum creatinine and low urinary sodium, this suggests hepatorenal failure, which carries a grave prognosis.
- Significantly elevated ferritin suggests haemochromatosis. Modest elevations can be seen in inflammatory disease and alcohol excess.

Haematological tests

Blood count

The peripheral blood count is often abnormal and can give a clue to the underlying diagnosis:

- *A normochromic normocytic anaemia* may reflect recent gastrointestinal haemorrhage, whereas chronic blood loss is characterised by a hypochromic microcytic anaemia secondary to iron deficiency. A high erythrocyte mean cell volume (macrocytosis) is associated with alcohol misuse, but target cells in any jaundiced patient also result in a macrocytosis. Macrocytosis can persist for a long period of time after alcohol cessation, making it a poor marker of ongoing consumption.
- *Leucopenia* may complicate portal hypertension and hypersplenism, whereas leucocytosis may occur with cholangitis, alcoholic hepatitis and hepatic abscesses. Atypical lymphocytes are seen in infectious mononucleosis, which may be complicated by an acute hepatitis.
- *Thrombocytopenia* is common in cirrhosis and is due to reduced platelet production, and increased breakdown because of hypersplenism. Thrombopoietin, required for platelet production, is produced in the liver and levels fall with worsening liver function. Thus platelet levels are usually more depressed than white cells and haemoglobin in the presence of hypersplenism in patients with cirrhosis. A low platelet count is often an indicator of chronic liver disease, particularly in the context of hepatomegaly. Thrombocytosis is unusual in patients with liver disease but may occur in those with active gastrointestinal haemorrhage and, rarely, in hepatocellular carcinoma.

Coagulation tests

These are often abnormal in patients with liver disease. The normal half-lives of the vitamin K-dependent coagulation factors in the blood are short (5–72 hours) and so changes in the prothrombin time occur relatively quickly following liver damage; these changes provide valuable prognostic information in patients with both acute and chronic liver failure. An increased PT is evidence of severe liver damage in chronic liver disease. Vitamin K does not reverse this deficiency if it is due to liver disease, but will correct the PT if the cause is vitamin K deficiency, as may occur with biliary obstruction due to non-absorption of fat-soluble vitamins.

Immunological tests

A variety of tests are available to evaluate the aetiology of hepatic disease (Boxes 23.4 and 23.5). The presence of liver-related autoantibodies can be suggestive of the presence of autoimmune liver disease (although false-positive results can occur in non-autoimmune inflammatory disease such as NAFLD). Elevation in overall

23.4 Chronic liver disease screen

- Hepatitis B surface antigen
- Hepatitis C antibody
- Liver autoantibodies (antinuclear antibody, smooth muscle antibody, antimitochondrial antibody)
- Immunoglobulins
- Ferritin
- α_1-antitrypsin
- Caeruloplasmin

23

23.5 How to identify the cause of LFT abnormality

Diagnosis	Clinical clue	Initial test	Additional tests
Alcoholic liver disease	History	LFTs AST > ALT; high MCV	Random blood alcohol
Non-alcoholic fatty liver disease (NAFLD)	Metabolic syndrome (central obesity, diabetes, hypertension)	LFTs	Liver biopsy
Chronic hepatitis B **Chronic hepatitis C**	Injection drug use; blood transfusion	HBsAg HCV antibody	HBeAg, HBeAb HBV-DNA HCV-RNA
Primary biliary cirrhosis	Itching; raised ALP	AMA	Liver biopsy
Primary sclerosing cholangitis	Inflammatory bowel disease	MRCP	ANCA
Autoimmune hepatitis	Other autoimmune diseases	ASMA, ANA, LKM, immunoglobulin	Liver biopsy
Haemochromatosis	Diabetes/joint pain	Transferrin saturation, ferritin	HFE gene test
Wilson's disease	Neurological signs; haemolysis	Caeruloplasmin	24-hr urinary copper
α_1-antitrypsin	Lung disease	α_1-antitrypsin level	α_1-antitrypsin genotype
Drug-induced liver disease	Drug/herbal remedy history	LFTs	Liver biopsy
Coeliac disease	Malabsorption	Endomysial antibody	Small bowel biopsy

(ALP = alkaline phosphatase; ALT = alanine aminotransferase; AMA = antimitochondrial antibody; ANA = antinuclear antibody; ANCA = antineutrophil cytoplasmic antibodies; ASMA = anti-smooth muscle antibody; AST = aspartate aminotransferase; HBeAb = antibody to hepatitis B e antigen; HBeAg = hepatitis B e antigen; HBsAg = hepatitis B surface antigen; HBV = hepatitis B virus; HCV = hepatitis C virus; HFE = haemochromatosis (high iron/Fe); LKM = liver-kidney microsomal antibody; MCV = mean cell volume; MRCP = magnetic resonance cholangiopancreatography)

serum immunoglobulin levels can also be suggestive of autoimmunity (immunoglobulin (Ig)G and IgM). Elevated serum IgA can be seen, often in more advanced alcoholic liver disease and NAFLD, although the association is not specific.

Imaging

Several imaging techniques can be used to determine the site and general nature of structural lesions in the liver and biliary tree. In general, however, imaging techniques are unable to identify hepatic inflammation and have poor sensitivity for liver fibrosis unless advanced cirrhosis with portal hypertension is present.

Ultrasound

Ultrasound is non-invasive and most commonly used as a 'first-line' test to identify gallstones, biliary obstruction (Fig. 23.8) or thrombosis in the hepatic vasculature. Ultrasound is good for the identification of splenomegaly and abnormalities in liver texture, but is less effective at identifying diffuse parenchymal disease. Focal lesions, such as tumours, may not be detected if they are below 2 cm in diameter and have echogenic characteristics similar to normal liver tissue. Bubble-based contrast media are now routinely used and can enhance discriminant capability. Doppler ultrasound allows blood flow in the hepatic artery, portal vein and hepatic veins to be investigated. Endoscopic ultrasound provides high-resolution images of the pancreas, biliary tree and liver (see Fig. 23.45, p. 985).

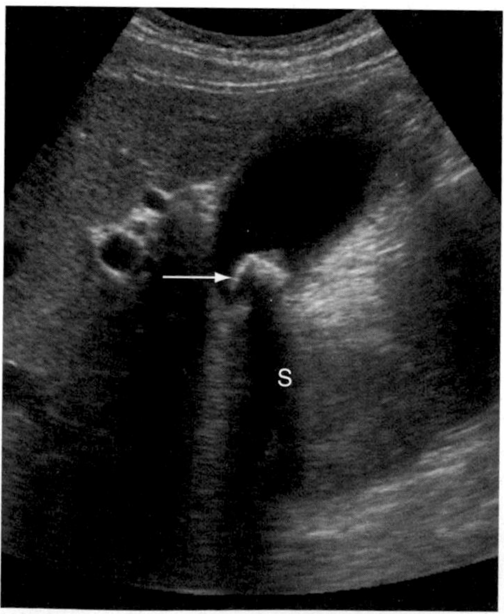

Fig. 23.8 Ultrasound showing a stone in the gallbladder. Stone (arrow) with acoustic shadow (S).

Computed tomography and magnetic resonance imaging

Computed tomography (CT) detects smaller focal lesions in the liver, especially when combined with contrast injection (Fig. 23.9). Magnetic resonance imaging (MRI) can also be used to localise and confirm the aetiology of focal liver lesions, particularly primary and secondary tumours.

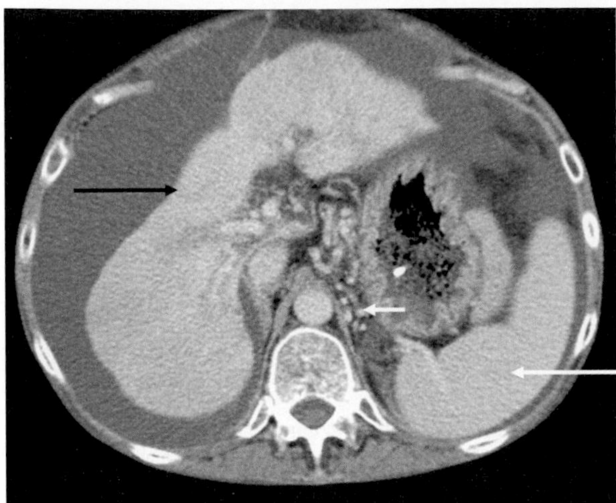

Fig. 23.9 CT scan in a patient with cirrhosis. The liver is small and has an irregular outline (black arrow), the spleen is enlarged (long white arrow), fluid (ascites) is seen around the liver, and collateral vessels are present around the proximal stomach (short white arrow).

Hepatic angiography is seldom used nowadays as a diagnostic tool, since CT and MRI are both able to provide images of hepatic vasculature, but it still has a therapeutic role in the embolisation of vascular tumours such as hepatocellular carcinoma. Hepatic venography is now rarely performed.

Cholangiography

Cholangiography can be undertaken by magnetic resonance cholangiopancreatography (MRCP, Fig. 23.10), endoscopy (endoscopic retrograde cholangiopancreatography, ERCP, Fig. 23.11) or the percutaneous approach (percutaneous transhepatic cholangiography, PTC). The latter does not allow the ampulla of Vater or pancreatic duct to be visualised. MRCP is as good as ERCP at providing images of the biliary tree but has fewer complications and is the diagnostic test of choice.

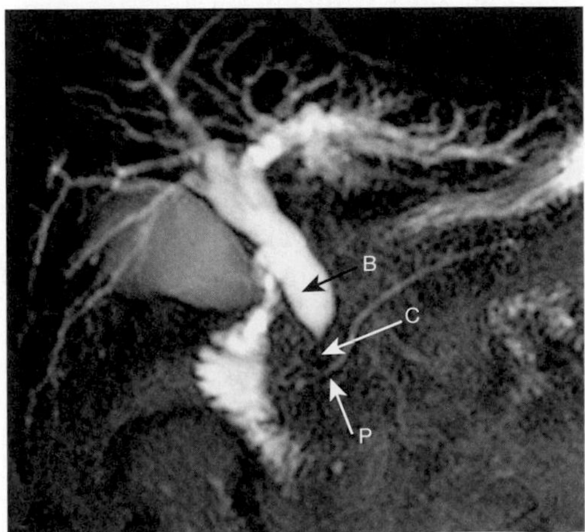

Fig. 23.10 MRCP showing a biliary stricture due to cholangiocarcinoma in the distal common bile duct (C). The proximal common bile duct (B) is dilated but the pancreatic duct (P) is normal.

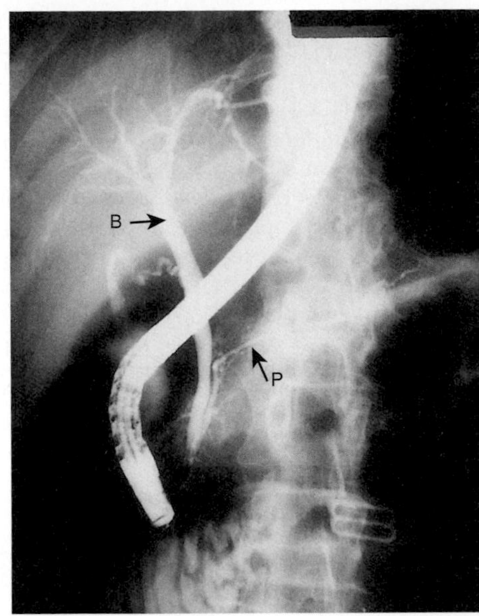

Fig. 23.11 ERCP showing the normal biliary (B) and pancreatic (P) duct system.

23

Both endoscopic and percutaneous approaches allow therapeutic interventions, such as the insertion of biliary stents across malignant bile duct strictures. The percutaneous approach is only used if it is not possible to access the bile duct endoscopically.

Histological examination

An ultrasound-guided liver biopsy can confirm the severity of liver damage and provide aetiological information. It is performed percutaneously with a Trucut or Menghini needle, usually through an intercostal space under local anaesthesia, or radiologically using a transjugular approach.

Percutaneous liver biopsy is a relatively safe procedure if the conditions detailed in Box 23.6 are met, but carries a mortality of about 0.01%. The main complications are abdominal and/or shoulder pain, bleeding and biliary peritonitis. Biliary peritonitis is rare and usually occurs when a biopsy is performed in a patient with obstruction of a large bile duct. Liver biopsies can be carried out in patients with defective haemostasis if:

- the defect is corrected with fresh frozen plasma and platelet transfusion
- the biopsy is obtained by the transjugular route, *or*

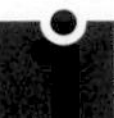

23.6 Conditions required for safe percutaneous liver biopsy

- Cooperative patient
- Prothrombin time < 4 secs prolonged
- Platelet count > 80 × 10^9/L
- Exclusion of bile duct obstruction, localised skin infection, advanced chronic obstructive pulmonary disease, marked ascites and severe anaemia

- the procedure is conducted percutaneously under ultrasound control and the needle track is then plugged with procoagulant material.

In patients with potentially resectable malignancy, biopsy should be avoided due to the potential risk of tumour dissemination. Operative or laparoscopic liver biopsy may sometimes be valuable.

Although the pathological features of liver disease are complex, with several features occurring together, liver disorders can be broadly classified histologically into fatty liver (steatosis), hepatitis (inflammation, 'grade') and cirrhosis (fibrosis, 'stage'). The use of special histological stains can help in determining aetiology. The clinical features and prognosis of these changes are dependent on the underlying aetiology, and are discussed in the relevant sections below.

Non-invasive markers of hepatic fibrosis

Non-invasive markers of liver fibrosis have been developed and can reduce the need for liver biopsy to assess the extent of fibrosis in some settings.

Serological markers of hepatic fibrosis, such as α_2-macroglobulin, haptoglobin and routine clinical biochemistry tests, are used in the Fibrotest®. The ELF® (Enhanced Liver Fibrosis) serological assay uses a combination of hyaluronic acid, procollagen peptide III (PIIINP) and tissue inhibitor of metalloproteinase 1 (TIMP1). These tests are good at differentiating severe fibrosis from mild scarring, but are limited in their ability to detect subtle changes. A number of non-commercial scores based on standard biochemical and anthropometric indices have also been described that provide similar levels of sensitivity and specificity (e.g. the FIB4 Score).

An alternative to serological markers is transient elastography in which ultrasound-based shock waves are sent through the liver to measure liver stiffness as a surrogate for hepatic fibrosis. Once again, this test is good at differentiating severe fibrosis from mild scarring, but is limited in its ability to detect subtle changes, and validity may be affected by obesity.

PRESENTING PROBLEMS IN LIVER DISEASE

Liver injury may be either acute or chronic. The main causes are listed in Figure 23.12 and discussed in detail later in the chapter.

- *Acute liver injury* may present with non-specific symptoms of fatigue and abnormal LFTs, or with jaundice and acute liver failure.
- *Chronic liver injury* is defined as hepatic injury, inflammation and/or fibrosis occurring in the liver for more than 6 months. In the early stages, patients can be asymptomatic with fluctuating abnormal LFTs. With more severe liver damage, however, the presentation can be with jaundice, portal hypertension or other signs of cirrhosis and hepatic decompensation (Box 23.7).

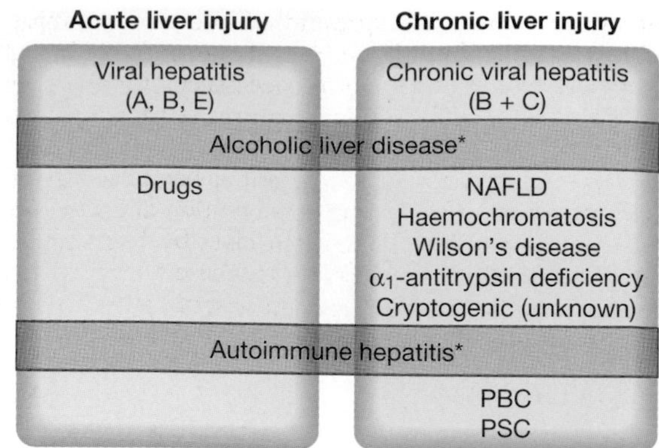

Fig. 23.12 Causes of acute and chronic liver injury. *Although there is often evidence of chronic liver disease at presentation, may present acutely with jaundice. In alcoholic liver disease this is due to superimposed alcoholic hepatitis. (NAFLD = non-alcoholic fatty liver disease; PBC = primary biliary cirrhosis; PSC = primary sclerosing cholangitis).

23.7 Presentation of liver disease

Severity	Acute liver injury	Chronic liver injury
Mild/moderate	Abnormal LFTs	Abnormal LFTs
Severe	Jaundice	Signs of cirrhosis ± portal hypertension
Very severe	Acute liver failure	Chronic liver failure* Jaundice Ascites Hepatic encephalopathy Portal hypertension with variceal bleeding

*May not occur until several years after cirrhosis has presented.

Acute liver failure

Acute liver failure is an uncommon but serious condition. The presentation is with progressive deterioration in liver function and mental changes progressing from confusion to coma. The syndrome was originally defined further as occurring within 8 weeks of onset of the precipitating illness, in the absence of evidence of pre-existing liver disease. This distinguishes it from instances in which hepatic encephalopathy represents a deterioration in chronic liver disease.

Liver failure occurs when there is insufficient metabolic and synthetic function for the needs of the patient. Although the direct cause is usually acute loss of functional hepatocytes, this can occur in different settings, which have implications for outcome and treatment. In a patient whose liver was previously normal (fulminant liver failure), the level of injury needed to cause liver failure, and thus the patient risk, is very high. In a patient with pre-existing chronic liver disease, the additional acute insult needed to precipitate liver failure is much less. It is critical, therefore, to understand whether liver failure is a true acute event or an acute deterioration on a background of pre-existing injury (which may itself not have been diagnosed). Although ultimately liver biopsy may be necessary, it is the presence or absence of the clinical features suggesting chronicity that guides the clinician.

More recently, newer classifications have been developed to reflect differences in presentation and outcome of acute liver failure. One such classification divides acute liver failure into hyperacute, acute and subacute, according to the interval between onset of jaundice and encephalopathy (Box 23.8).

Pathophysiology

Any cause of liver damage can produce acute liver failure, provided it is sufficiently severe (Fig. 23.13). Acute viral hepatitis is the most common cause worldwide, whereas paracetamol toxicity (p. 212) is the most frequent cause in the UK. Acute liver failure occurs occasionally with other drugs, or from *Amanita phalloides* (mushroom) poisoning, in pregnancy, in Wilson's disease, following shock (p. 190) and, rarely, in extensive malignant disease of the liver. In 10% of cases the cause of acute liver failure remains unknown and these patients are often labelled as having 'non-A–E viral hepatitis' or 'cryptogenic' acute liver failure.

23.8 Classification of acute liver failure

Type	Time: jaundice to encephalopathy	Cerebral oedema	Common causes
Hyperacute	< 7 days	Common	Viral, paracetamol
Acute	8–28 days	Common	Cryptogenic, drugs
Subacute	29 days–12 weeks	Uncommon	Cryptogenic, drugs

Clinical assessment

Cerebral disturbance (hepatic encephalopathy and/or cerebral oedema) is the cardinal manifestation of acute liver failure, but in the early stages this can be mild and episodic and so its absence does not exclude a significant acute liver injury. The initial clinical features are often subtle and include reduced alertness and poor concentration, progressing through behavioural abnormalities such as restlessness and aggressive outbursts, to drowsiness and coma (Box 23.9). Cerebral oedema may occur due to increased intracranial pressure, causing unequal or abnormally reacting pupils, fixed pupils, hypertensive episodes, bradycardia, hyperventilation, profuse sweating, local or general myoclonus, focal fits or decerebrate posturing. Papilloedema occurs rarely and is a late sign. More general symptoms include weakness, nausea and vomiting. Right hypochondrial discomfort is an occasional feature.

The patient may be jaundiced; however, this may not be present at the outset (e.g. in paracetamol overdose) and there are a number of exceptions, including Reye's syndrome, in which jaundice is rare. Occasionally, death may occur in fulminant cases of acute liver failure before

23.9 How to assess clinical grade of hepatic encephalopathy

Clinical grade	Clinical signs
Grade 1	Poor concentration, slurred speech, slow mentation, disordered sleep rhythm
Grade 2	Drowsy but easily rousable, occasional aggressive behaviour, lethargic
Grade 3	Marked confusion, drowsy, sleepy but responds to pain and voice, gross disorientation
Grade 4	Unresponsive to voice, may or may not respond to painful stimuli, unconscious

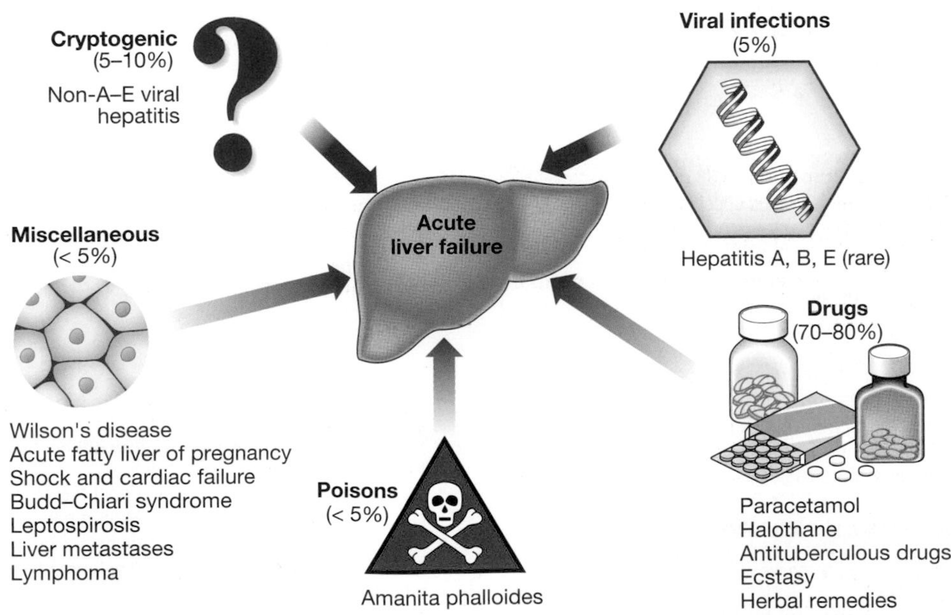

Fig. 23.13 Causes of acute liver failure in the UK. The relative frequency of the different causes varies according to geographical area.

jaundice develops. Fetor hepaticus can be present. The liver is usually of normal size but later becomes smaller. Hepatomegaly is unusual and, in the presence of a sudden onset of ascites, suggests venous outflow obstruction as the cause (Budd–Chiari syndrome, p. 976). Splenomegaly is uncommon and never prominent. Ascites and oedema are late developments and may be a consequence of fluid therapy. Other features are related to the development of complications (see below).

Investigations

The patient should be investigated to determine the cause of the liver failure and the prognosis (Boxes 23.10 and 23.11). Hepatitis B core IgM antibody is the best screening test for acute hepatitis B infection, as liver damage is due to the immunological response to the virus, which has often been eliminated, and the test for HBsAg may be negative. The PT rapidly becomes prolonged as coagulation factor synthesis fails; this is the laboratory test of greatest prognostic value and should be carried out at least twice daily. Its prognostic importance emphasises the necessity of avoiding the use of fresh frozen plasma to correct raised PT in acute liver failure, except in the setting of frank bleeding. Factor V levels can be used instead of the PT to assess the degree of liver impairment. The plasma bilirubin reflects the degree of jaundice. Plasma aminotransferase activity is particularly high after paracetamol overdose, reaching 100–500 times normal, but falls as liver damage progresses and is not helpful in determining prognosis. Plasma albumin remains normal unless the course is prolonged. Percutaneous liver biopsy is contraindicated because of the severe coagulopathy, but biopsy can be undertaken using the transjugular route if appropriate.

Management

Patients with acute liver failure should be treated in a high-dependency or intensive care unit as soon as progressive prolongation of the PT occurs or hepatic encephalopathy is identified (Box 23.12), so that prompt treatment of complications can be initiated (Box 23.13). Conservative treatment aims to maintain life in the hope that hepatic regeneration will occur, but early transfer to a specialised transplant unit should always be considered. *N*-acetylcysteine therapy may improve

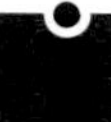

23.10 Investigations to determine the cause of acute liver failure

- Toxicology screen of blood and urine
- HBsAg, IgM anti-HBc
- IgM anti-HAV
- Anti-HEV, HCV, cytomegalovirus, herpes simplex, Epstein–Barr virus
- Caeruloplasmin, serum copper, urinary copper, slit-lamp eye examination
- Autoantibodies: ANA, ASMA, LKM, SLA
- Immunoglobulins
- Ultrasound of liver and Doppler of hepatic veins

(ANA = antinuclear antibody; ASMA = anti-smooth muscle antibody; LKM = liver-kidney microsomal antibody; SLA = soluble liver antigen)

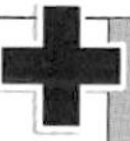

23.11 Adverse prognostic criteria in acute liver failure*

- $H^+ > 50$ nmol/L (pH < 7.3) at or beyond 24 hrs following the overdose

Or

- Serum creatinine > 300 μmol/L (≅ 3.38 mg/dL) *plus* prothrombin time > 100 secs *plus* encephalopathy grade 3 or 4

Non-paracetamol cases

- Prothrombin time > 100 secs

Or

- Any three of the following:
  - Jaundice to encephalopathy time > 7 days
  - Age < 10 or > 40 yrs
  - Indeterminate or drug-induced causes
  - Bilirubin > 300 μmol/L (≅ 17.6 mg/dL)
  - Prothrombin time > 50 secs

Or

- Factor V level < 15% and encephalopathy grade 3 or 4

*Predict a mortality rate of ≥ 90% and are an indication for referral for possible liver transplantation.

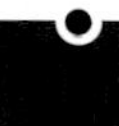

23.12 Monitoring in acute liver failure

Cardiorespiratory

- Pulse
- Blood pressure
- Central venous pressure
- Respiratory rate

Neurological

- Intracranial pressure monitoring (specialist units, p. 198)
- Conscious level

Fluid balance

- Hourly output (urine, vomiting, diarrhoea)
- Input: oral, intravenous

Blood analyses

- Arterial blood gases
- Peripheral blood count (including platelets)
- Sodium, potassium, HCO^{3-}, calcium, magnesium
- Creatinine, urea
- Glucose (2-hourly in acute phase)
- Prothrombin time

Infection surveillance

- Cultures: blood, urine, throat, sputum, cannula sites
- Chest X-ray
- Temperature

23.13 Complications of acute liver failure

- Encephalopathy and cerebral oedema
- Hypoglycaemia
- Metabolic acidosis
- Infection (bacterial, fungal)
- Renal failure
- Multi-organ failure (hypotension and respiratory failure)

outcome, particularly in patients with acute liver failure due to paracetamol poisoning. Liver transplantation is an increasingly important treatment option for acute liver failure, and criteria have been developed to identify patients unlikely to survive without a transplant (see Box 23.11). Patients should, wherever possible, be transferred to a transplant centre before these criteria are met to allow time for assessment and to maximise the time for a donor liver to become available. Survival following liver transplantation for acute liver failure is improving, and 1-year survival rates of about 60% can be expected.

Abnormal liver function tests

Frequently, LFTs are requested in patients who have no symptoms or signs of liver disease, as part of routine health checks, insurance medicals and drug monitoring. When abnormal results are found, it is important for the clinician to be able to interpret them and to investigate patients appropriately. Many patients with chronic liver disease are asymptomatic or have vague, non-specific symptoms. Apparently asymptomatic abnormal LFTs are therefore a common occurrence. When LFTs are measured routinely prior to elective surgery, 3.5% of patients are discovered to have mildly elevated transaminases. The prevalence of abnormal LFTs has been reported to be as high as 10% in some studies. The most common abnormalities are alcoholic (p. 957) or non-alcoholic fatty liver disease (p. 959). Since effective medical treatments are now available for many types of chronic liver disease, further evaluation is usually warranted to make sure the patient does not have a treatable condition. Although transient mild abnormalities in LFTs may not be clinically significant, the majority of patients with persistently abnormal LFTs do have significant liver disease. Biochemical abnormalities in chronic liver disease often fluctuate over time, and therefore even mild abnormalities can indicate significant underlying disease and so warrant follow-up and investigation.

When abnormal LFTs are detected, a thorough history should be compiled to determine the patient's alcohol consumption, drug use (prescribed drugs or otherwise), risk factors for viral hepatitis (e.g. blood transfusion, injecting drug use, tattoos), the presence of autoimmune diseases, family history, neurological symptoms, and the presence of features of the metabolic syndrome (p. 805), including diabetes and/or obesity (see Box 23.5, p. 930, and Box 5.18, p. 115). The presence or absence of stigmata of chronic liver disease does not reliably identify those individuals with significant disease, and investigations are indicated, even in the absence of these signs.

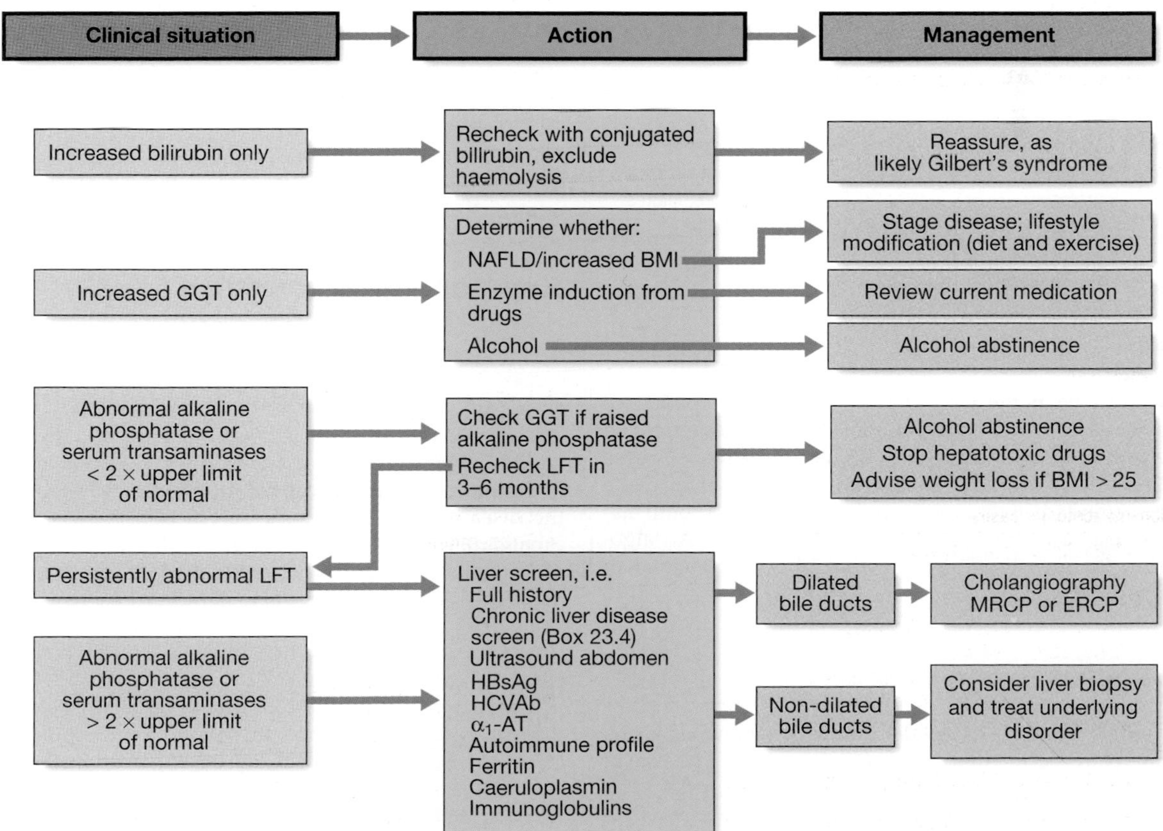

Fig. 23.14 Suggested management of abnormal LFTs in asymptomatic patients. *No further investigation needed.

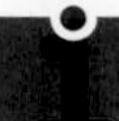

23.14 Common causes of elevated serum transaminases

Minor elevation (< 100 U/L*)	
• Chronic hepatitis C • Chronic hepatitis B	• Haemochromatosis • Fatty liver disease
Moderate elevation (100–300 U/L*)	
As above plus: • Alcoholic hepatitis • Non-alcoholic steatohepatitis	• Autoimmune hepatitis • Wilson's disease
Major elevation (> 300 U/L*)	
• Drugs (e.g. paracetamol) • Acute viral hepatitis • Autoimmune liver disease • Ischaemic liver	• Toxins (e.g. *Amanita phalloides* poisoning) • Flare of chronic hepatitis B

*Note: These ranges are indicative but do not rigidly discriminate between different aetiologies

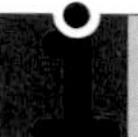

23.15 Causes of cholestatic jaundice

Intrahepatic	
• Primary biliary cirrhosis • Primary sclerosing cholangitis • Alcohol • Drugs • Hepatic infiltrations (lymphoma, granuloma, amyloid, metastases)	• Cystic fibrosis • Severe bacterial infections • Pregnancy (p. 977) • Inherited cholestatic liver disease, e.g. benign recurrent intrahepatic cholestasis • Chronic right heart failure
Extrahepatic	
• Carcinoma Ampullary Pancreatic Bile duct (cholangiocarcinoma) Liver metastases	• Choledocholithiasis • Parasitic infection • Traumatic biliary strictures • Chronic pancreatitis

Both the pattern of LFT abnormality, hepatitic or obstructive, and the degree of elevation are helpful in determining the cause of underlying liver disease (Boxes 23.14 and 23.15). The investigations that make up a standard liver screen and additional or confirmatory tests are shown in Boxes 23.4 and 23.5. An algorithm for investigating abnormal LFTs is provided in Figure 23.14.

Jaundice

Jaundice is usually detectable clinically when the plasma bilirubin exceeds 40 μmol/L (~2.5 mg/dL). The causes of jaundice overlap with the causes of abnormal LFTs discussed above. In a patient with jaundice it is useful to consider whether the cause might be pre-hepatic, hepatic or post-hepatic and there are often important clues in the history (Box 23.16).

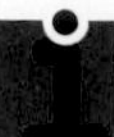

23.16 Key history points in patients with jaundice

Symptoms*
- Itching preceding jaundice
- Abdominal pain (suggests stones)
- Weight loss (chronic liver disease and malignancy)
- Dark urine and pale stools
- Fever ± rigors
- Dry eyes/dry mouth
- Fatigue

Recent drug history

Other
- Exposure to intravenous drug or blood transfusions
- Travel history and country of birth
- Metabolic syndrome (increased body mass index ± type 2 diabetes/hypertension)
- Autoimmune disease history
- Alcohol history
- Inflammatory bowel disease
- Family history of liver disease, autoimmune disease or the metabolic syndrome

*Symptoms may be absent and abnormal LFTs detected incidentally.

Pre-hepatic jaundice

This is caused either by haemolysis or by congenital hyperbilirubinaemia, and is characterised by an isolated raised bilirubin level.

In haemolysis, destruction of red blood cells or their marrow precursors causes increased bilirubin production. Jaundice due to haemolysis is usually mild because a healthy liver can excrete a bilirubin load six times greater than normal before unconjugated bilirubin accumulates in the plasma. This does not apply to newborns, who have less capacity to metabolise bilirubin.

The most common form of non-haemolytic hyperbilirubinaemia is Gilbert's syndrome, an inherited disorder of bilirubin metabolism (Box 23.17). Other inherited disorders of bilirubin metabolism are very rare.

Hepatocellular jaundice

Hepatocellular jaundice results from an inability of the liver to transport bilirubin into the bile, occurring as a consequence of parenchymal disease. Bilirubin transport across the hepatocytes may be impaired at any point between uptake of unconjugated bilirubin into the cells and transport of conjugated bilirubin into the canaliculi. In addition, swelling of cells and oedema resulting from the disease itself may cause obstruction of the biliary canaliculi. In hepatocellular jaundice the concentrations of both unconjugated and conjugated bilirubin in the blood increase. Hepatocellular jaundice can be due to acute or chronic injury (see Fig. 23.12), and clinical features of acute or chronic liver disease may be detected clinically (see Box 23.7, p. 932).

Characteristically, jaundice due to parenchymal liver disease is associated with increases in transaminases (AST, ALT), but increases in other LFTs, including cholestatic enzymes (GGT, ALP) may occur, and suggest specific aetiologies (see below). Acute jaundice in the presence of an ALT of greater than 1000 U/L is highly suggestive of an infectious cause (e.g. hepatitis A, B), drugs (e.g. paracetamol) or hepatic ischaemia.

23.17 Congenital non-haemolytic hyperbilirubinaemia

Syndrome	Inheritance	Abnormality	Clinical features	Treatment
Unconjugated hyperbilirubinaemia				
Gilbert's	Autosomal dominant	↓ Glucuronyl transferase ↓ Bilirubin uptake	Mild jaundice, especially with fasting	No treatment necessary
Crigler–Najjar				
Type I	Autosomal recessive	Absent glucuronyl transferase	Rapid death in neonate (kernicterus)	
Type II	Autosomal dominant	↓↓ Glucuronyl transferase	Presents in neonate	Phenobarbital, ultraviolet light or liver transplant
Conjugated hyperbilirubinaemia				
Dubin–Johnson	Autosomal recessive	↓ Canalicular excretion of organic anions, including bilirubin	Mild	No treatment necessary
Rotor's	Autosomal recessive	↓ Bilirubin uptake ↓ Intrahepatic binding	Mild	No treatment necessary

Imaging is essential, in particular to identify features suggestive of cirrhosis, to define the patency of the hepatic vasculature, and to obtain evidence of portal hypertension. Liver biopsy has an important role in defining the aetiology of hepatocellular jaundice and the extent of liver injury.

Obstructive (cholestatic) jaundice

Cholestatic jaundice may be caused by:

- failure of hepatocytes to initiate bile flow
- obstruction of the bile ducts or portal tracts
- obstruction of bile flow in the extrahepatic bile ducts between the porta hepatis and the papilla of Vater.

In the absence of treatment, cholestatic jaundice tends to become progressively more severe because conjugated bilirubin is unable to enter the bile canaliculi and passes back into the blood, and also because there is a failure of clearance of unconjugated bilirubin arriving at the liver cells. The causes of cholestatic jaundice are listed in Box 23.15. Cholestasis may result from defects at more than one of these levels. Those confined to the extrahepatic bile ducts may be amenable to surgical or endoscopic correction.

Clinical features (Box 23.18) comprise those due to cholestasis itself, those due to secondary infection (cholangitis) and those of the underlying condition (Box 23.19). Obstruction of the bile duct drainage due to blockage of the extrahepatic biliary tree is characteristically associated with pale stools and dark urine. Pruritus may be a dominant feature and can be accompanied by skin excoriations. Peripheral stigmata of chronic liver disease are absent. If the gallbladder is palpable, the jaundice is unlikely to be caused by biliary obstruction due to gallstones, probably because a chronically

23.18 Clinical features and complications of cholestatic jaundice

Cholestasis

Early features

- Jaundice
- Dark urine
- Pale stools
- Pruritus

Late features

- Malabsorption (vitamins A, D, E and K): weight loss, steatorrhoea, osteomalacia, bleeding tendency
- Xanthelasma and xanthomas

Cholangitis

- Fever
- Rigors
- Pain (if gallstones present)

23.19 Clinical features suggesting an underlying cause of cholestatic jaundice*

Clinical feature	Causes
Jaundice	
Static or increasing	Carcinoma Primary biliary cirrhosis Primary sclerosing cholangitis
Fluctuating	Choledocholithiasis Stricture Pancreatitis Choledochal cyst Primary sclerosing cholangitis
Abdominal pain	Choledocholithiasis Pancreatitis Choledochal cyst
Cholangitis	Stone Stricture Choledochal cyst
Abdominal scar	Stone Stricture
Irregular hepatomegaly	Hepatic carcinoma
Palpable gallbladder	Carcinoma below cystic duct (usually pancreas)
Abdominal mass	Carcinoma Pancreatitis (cyst) Choledochal cyst
Occult blood in stools	Ampullary tumour

*Each of the diseases listed here can give rise to almost any of the clinical features shown, but the box indicates the most likely cause of the clinical features listed.

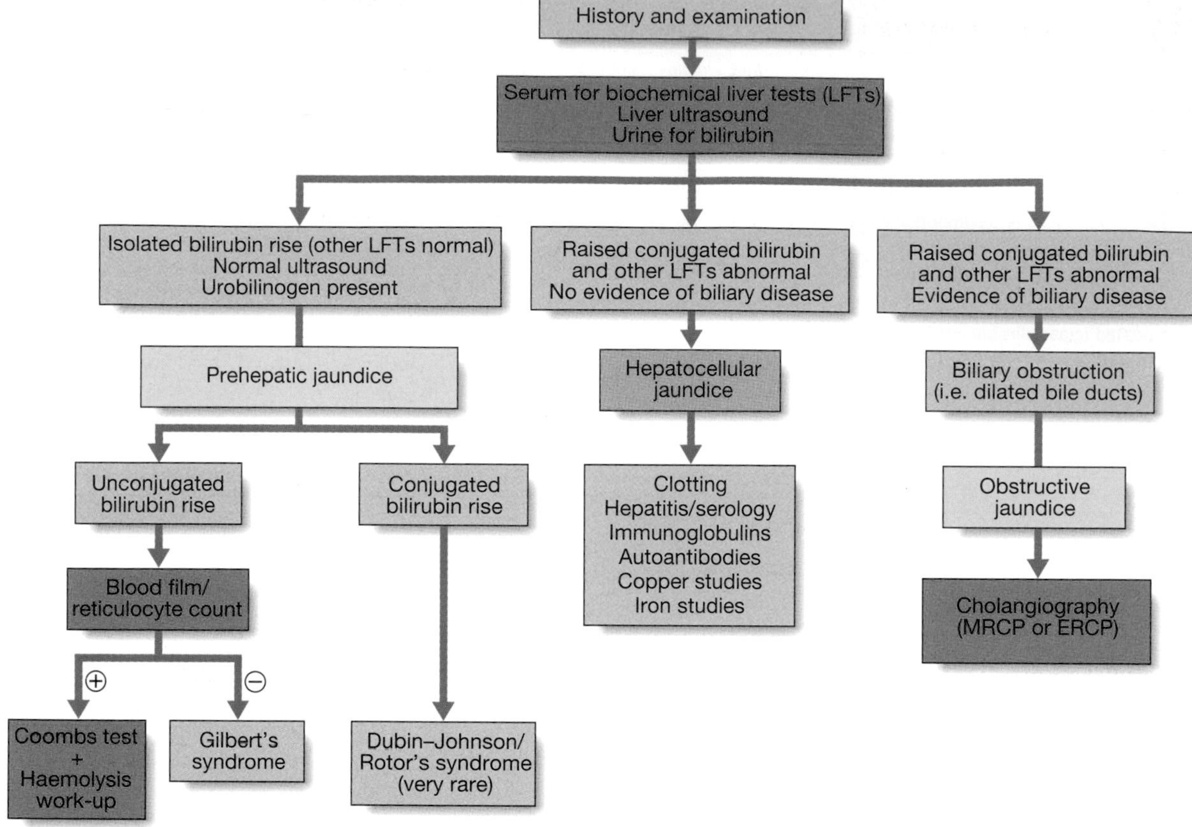

Fig. 23.15 Investigation of jaundice.

inflamed stone-containing gallbladder cannot readily dilate. This is Courvoisier's Law, and suggests that jaundice is due to a malignant biliary obstruction (e.g. pancreatic cancer). Cholangitis is characterised by 'Charcot's triad' of jaundice, right upper quadrant pain and fever. Cholestatic jaundice is characterised by a relatively greater elevation of ALP and GGT than the aminotransferases.

Ultrasound is indicated to determine whether there is evidence of mechanical obstruction and dilatation of the biliary tree (Fig. 23.15). Management of cholestatic jaundice depends on the underlying cause and is discussed in the relevant sections below.

Hepatomegaly

Hepatomegaly may occur as the result of a general enlargement of the liver or because of primary or secondary liver tumour (Box 23.20). The most common liver tumour in Western countries is liver metastasis, whereas primary liver cancer complicating chronic viral hepatitis is more common in the Far East. Unlike metastases, neuro-endocrine tumours typically cause massive hepatomegaly but without significant weight loss. Cirrhosis can be associated with either hepatomegaly or reduced liver size in advanced disease. Although all causes of cirrhosis can involve hepatomegaly, it is much more common in alcoholic liver disease and haemochromatosis. Hepatomegaly may resolve in patients with alcoholic cirrhosis when they stop drinking.

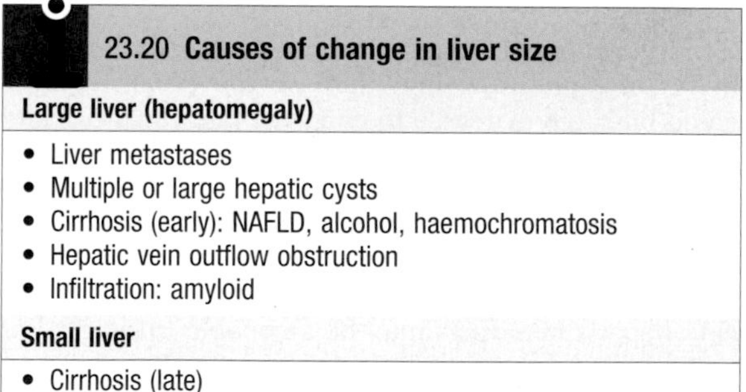

23.20 Causes of change in liver size

Large liver (hepatomegaly)
• Liver metastases • Multiple or large hepatic cysts • Cirrhosis (early): NAFLD, alcohol, haemochromatosis • Hepatic vein outflow obstruction • Infiltration: amyloid
Small liver
• Cirrhosis (late)

Ascites

Ascites is present when there is accumulation of free fluid in the peritoneal cavity. Small amounts of ascites are asymptomatic, but with larger accumulations of fluid (> 1 L) there is abdominal distension, fullness in the flanks, shifting dullness on percussion and, when the ascites is marked, a fluid thrill. Other features include eversion of the umbilicus, herniae, abdominal striae, divarication of the recti and scrotal oedema. Dilated superficial abdominal veins may be seen if the ascites is due to portal hypertension.

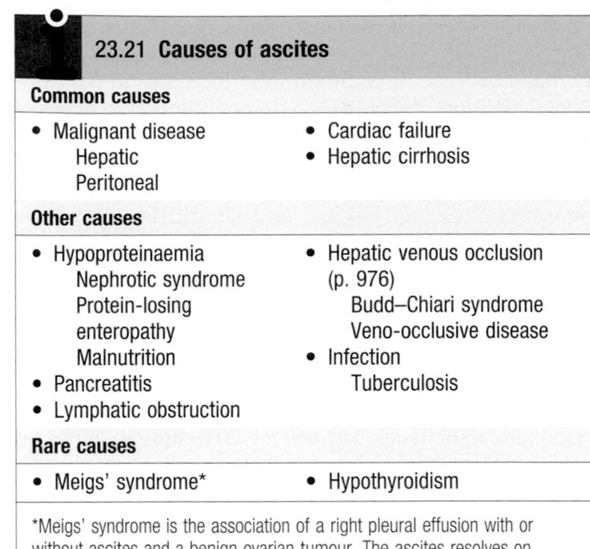

23.21 Causes of ascites

Common causes	
• Malignant disease Hepatic Peritoneal	• Cardiac failure • Hepatic cirrhosis
Other causes	
• Hypoproteinaemia Nephrotic syndrome Protein-losing enteropathy Malnutrition • Pancreatitis • Lymphatic obstruction	• Hepatic venous occlusion (p. 976) Budd–Chiari syndrome Veno-occlusive disease • Infection Tuberculosis
Rare causes	
• Meigs' syndrome*	• Hypothyroidism

*Meigs' syndrome is the association of a right pleural effusion with or without ascites and a benign ovarian tumour. The ascites resolves on removal of the tumour.

Pathophysiology

Ascites has numerous causes, the most common of which are malignant disease, cirrhosis and heart failure. Many primary disorders of the peritoneum and visceral organs can also cause ascites, and these need to be considered even in a patient with chronic liver disease (Box 23.21). Splanchnic vasodilatation is thought to be the main factor leading to ascites in cirrhosis. This is mediated by vasodilators (mainly nitric oxide) that are released when portal hypertension causes shunting of blood into the systemic circulation. Systemic arterial pressure falls due to pronounced splanchnic vasodilatation as cirrhosis advances. This leads to activation of the renin–angiotensin system with secondary aldosteronism, increased sympathetic nervous activity, increased atrial natriuretic hormone secretion and altered activity of the kallikrein–kinin system (Fig. 23.16). These systems tend to normalise arterial pressure but produce salt and water retention. In this setting the combination of splanchnic arterial vasodilatation and portal hypertension alters intestinal capillary permeability, promoting accumulation of fluid within the peritoneum.

Investigations

Ultrasonography is the best means of detecting ascites, particularly in the obese and those with small volumes of fluid. Paracentesis (if necessary under ultrasonic guidance) can be used to obtain ascitic fluid for analysis. The appearance of ascitic fluid may point to the underlying cause (Box 23.22). Pleural effusions are found in about 10% of patients, usually on the right side (hepatic hydrothorax); most are small and only identified on chest X-ray, but occasionally a massive hydrothorax occurs. Pleural effusions, particularly those on the left side, should not be assumed to be due to the ascites.

Measurement of the protein concentration and the serum–ascites albumin gradient (SAAG) are used to distinguish a transudate from an exudate. Cirrhotic patients typically develop a transudate with a total protein concentration below 25 g/L and relatively few cells. However, in up to 30% of patients, the total protein concentration is more than 30 g/L. In these cases, it is useful to calculate the SAAG by subtracting the concentration of the ascites fluid albumin from the serum albumin. A gradient of more than 11 g/L is 96% predictive that ascites is due to portal hypertension. Venous outflow obstruction due to cardiac failure or hepatic venous outflow obstruction can also cause a transudative ascites, as indicated by an albumin gradient above 11 g/L but, unlike in cirrhosis, the total protein content is usually above 25 g/L.

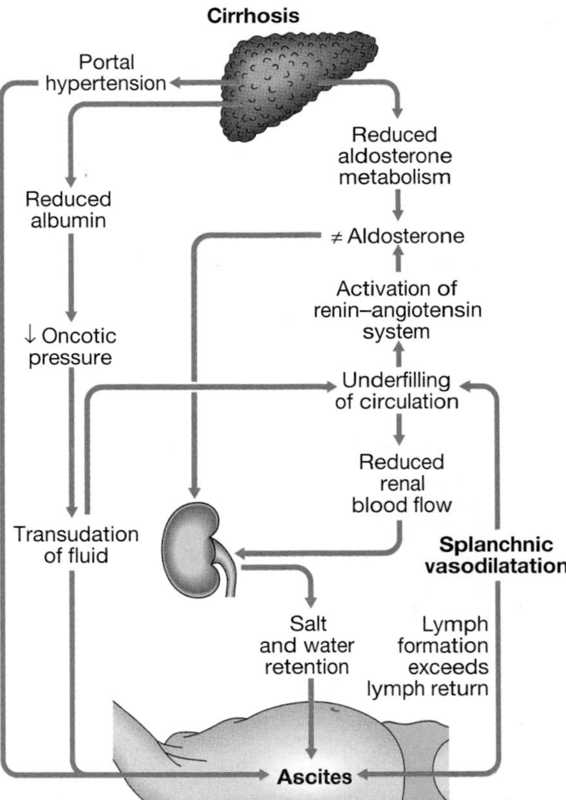

Fig. 23.16 Pathogenesis of ascites.

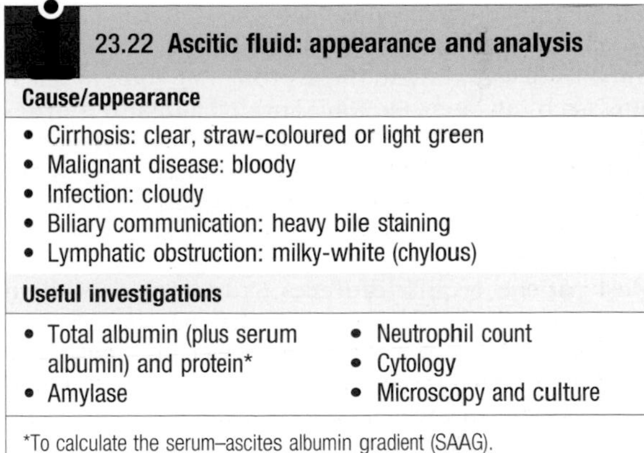

23.22 Ascitic fluid: appearance and analysis

Cause/appearance	
• Cirrhosis: clear, straw-coloured or light green • Malignant disease: bloody • Infection: cloudy • Biliary communication: heavy bile staining • Lymphatic obstruction: milky-white (chylous)	
Useful investigations	
• Total albumin (plus serum albumin) and protein* • Amylase	• Neutrophil count • Cytology • Microscopy and culture

*To calculate the serum–ascites albumin gradient (SAAG).

Exudative ascites (ascites protein concentration > 25 g/L or a SAAG < 11 g/L) raises the possibility of infection (especially tuberculosis), malignancy, hepatic venous obstruction, pancreatic ascites or, rarely, hypothyroidism. Ascites amylase activity above 1000 U/L identifies pancreatic ascites, and low ascites glucose concentrations suggest malignant disease or tuberculosis. Cytological examination may reveal malignant cells (one-third of cirrhotic patients with a bloody tap have a hepatocellular carcinoma). Polymorphonuclear leucocyte counts above 250×10^6/L strongly suggest infection (spontaneous bacterial peritonitis, see below). Laparoscopy can be valuable in detecting peritoneal disease.

Management

Successful treatment relieves discomfort but does not prolong life; if over-vigorous, it can produce serious disorders of fluid and electrolyte balance and precipitate hepatic encephalopathy (p. 941). Treatment of transudative ascites is based on restricting sodium and water intake, promoting urine output with diuretics and, if necessary, removing ascites directly by paracentesis. Exudative ascites due to malignancy is treated with paracentesis, but fluid replacement is generally not required. During management of ascites, the patient should be weighed regularly. Diuretics should be titrated to remove no more than 1 L of fluid daily, so body weight should not fall by more than 1 kg daily to avoid excessive fluid depletion.

Sodium and water restriction

Restriction of dietary sodium intake is essential to achieve negative sodium balance, and a few patients can be managed satisfactorily by this alone. Restriction of sodium intake to 100 mmol/day ('no added salt diet') is usually adequate. Drugs containing relatively large amounts of sodium, and those promoting sodium retention such as non-steroidal anti-inflammatory drugs (NSAIDs), must be avoided (Box 23.23). Restriction of water intake to 1.0–1.5 L/day is necessary only if the plasma sodium falls below 125 mmol/L.

Diuretics

Most patients require diuretics in addition to sodium restriction. Spironolactone (100–400 mg/day) is the first-line drug because it is a powerful aldosterone antagonist; it can cause painful gynaecomastia and hyperkalaemia, in which case amiloride (5–10 mg/day) can be substituted. Some patients also require loop diuretics, such as furosemide, but these can cause fluid and electrolyte imbalance and renal dysfunction. Diuresis may be improved if patients are rested in bed, perhaps because renal blood flow increases in the horizontal position. Patients who do not respond to doses of 400 mg spironolactone and 160 mg furosemide, or who are unable to tolerate these doses due to hyponatraemia or renal impairment, are considered to have refractory or diuretic-resistant ascites and should be treated by other measures.

23.23 Some drugs containing relatively large amounts of sodium or causing sodium retention

High sodium content	
• Alginates • Antacids • Antibiotics • Phenytoin	• Sodium valproate • Effervescent preparations (e.g. aspirin, calcium, paracetamol)
Sodium retention	
• Carbenoxolone • Corticosteroids • Metoclopramide	• NSAIDs • Oestrogens

Paracentesis

First-line treatment of refractory ascites is large-volume paracentesis. Paracentesis to dryness is safe, provided the circulation is supported with an intravenous colloid such as human albumin (6–8 g per litre of ascites removed, usually as 100 mL of 20% human albumin solution (HAS) for every 1.5–2 L of ascites drained) or another plasma expander. Paracentesis can be used as an initial therapy or when other treatments fail.

Transjugular intrahepatic portosystemic stent shunt

A transjugular intrahepatic portosystemic stent shunt (TIPSS) (p. 947) can relieve resistant ascites but does not prolong life; it may be an option where the only alternative is frequent, large-volume paracentesis. It can be used in patients awaiting liver transplantation or in those with reasonable liver function, but can aggravate encephalopathy in those with poor function.

Peritoneo-venous shunt

The peritoneo-venous shunt is a long tube with a non-return valve running subcutaneously from the peritoneum to the internal jugular vein in the neck; it allows ascitic fluid to pass directly into the systemic circulation. Complications, including infection, superior vena caval thrombosis, pulmonary oedema, bleeding from oesophageal varices and disseminated intravascular coagulopathy, limit its use and insertion of these shunts is now rare.

Complications

Renal failure

Renal failure can occur in patients with ascites. It can be pre-renal due to vasodilatation from sepsis and/or diuretic therapy, or due to hepatorenal syndrome.

Hepatorenal syndrome

This occurs in 10% of patients with advanced cirrhosis complicated by ascites. There are two clinical types; both are mediated by renal vasoconstriction due to underfilling of the arterial circulation.

- *Type 1 hepatorenal syndrome* is characterised by progressive oliguria, a rapid rise of the serum creatinine and a very poor prognosis (without treatment, median survival is less than 1 month). There is usually no proteinuria, a urine sodium excretion of less than 10 mmol/day and a urine/plasma osmolarity ratio of more than 1.5. Other non-functional causes of renal failure must be excluded before the diagnosis is made. Treatment consists of albumin infusions in combination with terlipressin and is effective in about two-thirds of patients. Haemodialysis should not be used routinely because it does not improve the outcome.

Patients who survive should be considered for liver transplantation.

- *Type 2 hepatorenal syndrome* usually occurs in patients with refractory ascites, is characterised by a moderate and stable increase in serum creatinine, and has a better prognosis.

Spontaneous bacterial peritonitis

Spontaneous bacterial peritonitis (SBP) may present with abdominal pain, rebound tenderness, absent bowel sounds and fever in a patient with obvious features of cirrhosis and ascites. Abdominal signs are mild or absent in about one-third of patients, and in these patients hepatic encephalopathy and fever are the main features. Diagnostic paracentesis may show cloudy fluid, and an ascites neutrophil count above 250×10^6/L almost invariably indicates infection. The source of infection cannot usually be determined, but most organisms isolated are of enteric origin and *Escherichia coli* is most frequently found. Ascitic culture in blood culture bottles gives the highest yield of organisms. SBP needs to be differentiated from other intra-abdominal emergencies, and the finding of multiple organisms on culture should arouse suspicion of a perforated viscus.

Treatment should be started immediately with broad-spectrum antibiotics, such as cefotaxime or piperacillin/tazobactam). Recurrence of SBP is common but may be reduced with prophylactic quinolones such as norfloxacin or ciprofloxacin (Box 23.24).

EBM 23.24 Antibiotics and spontaneous bacterial peritonitis (SBP)

'In patients with a previous episode of SBP and continued ascites, norfloxacin 400 mg/day prevents recurrence (NNT_B 4.5).'

'In patients with cirrhosis who have had a gastrointestinal haemorrhage, prophylactic antibiotics reduce the risk of bacterial peritonitis (NNT_B 12.5) and improve survival (NNT_B 11).'

- Gines P, et al. Hepatology 1990; 12:716.
- Bernard B, et al. Hepatology 1999; 29:1655–1661.

For further information: www.easl.eu/_clinical-practice-guideline/

Prognosis

Only 10–20% of patients survive 5 years from the first appearance of ascites due to cirrhosis. The outlook is not universally poor, however, and is best in those with well-maintained liver function and a good response to therapy. The prognosis is also better when a treatable cause for the underlying cirrhosis is present or when a precipitating cause for ascites, such as excess salt intake, is found. The mortality at 1 year is 50% following the first episode of bacterial peritonitis.

Hepatic encephalopathy

Hepatic encephalopathy is a neuropsychiatric syndrome caused by liver disease. As it progresses, confusion is followed by coma. Confusion needs to be differentiated from delirium tremens and Wernicke's encephalopathy, and coma from subdural haematoma, which can occur in alcoholics after a fall (Box 23.25). Features include changes of intellect, personality, emotions and consciousness, with or without neurological signs. The degree of encephalopathy can be graded from 1 to 4, depending on these features, and this is useful in assessing response to therapy (see Box 23.9, p. 933). When an episode develops acutely, a precipitating factor may be found (Box 23.26). The earliest features are very mild and easily overlooked but, as the condition becomes more severe, apathy, inability to concentrate, confusion, disorientation, drowsiness, slurring of speech and eventually coma develop. Convulsions sometimes occur. Examination usually shows a flapping tremor (asterixis), inability to perform simple mental arithmetic tasks or to draw objects such as a star (constructional apraxia; p. 923), and, as the condition progresses, hyper-reflexia and bilateral extensor plantar responses. Hepatic encephalopathy rarely causes focal neurological signs; if these are present, other causes must be sought. Fetor hepaticus, a sweet musty odour to the breath, is usually present but is more a sign of liver failure and portosystemic shunting than of hepatic encephalopathy. Rarely, chronic hepatic encephalopathy (hepatocerebral degeneration) gives rise to variable combinations of cerebellar dysfunction, Parkinsonian syndromes, spastic paraplegia and dementia.

23.25 Differential diagnosis of hepatic encephalopathy

- Intracranial bleed (subdural, extradural haematoma, p. 1218)
- Drug or alcohol intoxication (pp. 252 and 254)
- Delirium tremens/alcohol withdrawal (p. 253)
- Wernicke's encephalopathy (p. 253)
- Primary psychiatric disorders (p. 242)
- Hypoglycaemia (p. 814)
- Neurological Wilson's disease (p. 1198)
- Post-ictal state

23.26 Factors precipitating hepatic encephalopathy

- Drugs (especially sedatives, antidepressants)
- Dehydration (including diuretics, paracentesis)
- Portosystemic shunting
- Infection
- Hypokalaemia
- Constipation
- ↑Protein load (including GI bleeding)

Pathophysiology

Hepatic encephalopathy is thought to be due to a disturbance of brain function provoked by circulating neurotoxins that are normally metabolised by the liver. Accordingly, most affected patients have evidence of liver failure and portosystemic shunting of blood, but the balance between these varies from individual to individual. Some degree of liver failure is a key factor, as portosystemic shunting of blood alone hardly ever causes encephalopathy. The 'neurotoxins' causing encephalopathy are unknown, but they are thought to be mainly nitrogenous substances produced in the gut, at least in part by bacterial action. These substances are normally metabolised by the healthy liver and excluded from the systemic circulation. Ammonia has traditionally been considered an important factor. Recent interest has focused on γ-aminobutyric acid (GABA) as a mediator, along with octopamine, amino acids, mercaptans and fatty acids that can act as neurotransmitters. The brain in cirrhosis may also be sensitised to other factors such as drugs that can precipitate hepatic encephalopathy (see Box 23.26). Disruption of the function of the blood–brain barrier is a feature of acute hepatic failure and may lead to cerebral oedema.

Investigations

The diagnosis can usually be made clinically, but when doubt exists, an electroencephalogram (EEG) shows diffuse slowing of the normal alpha waves with eventual development of delta waves. The arterial ammonia is usually increased in patients with hepatic encephalopathy. However, increased concentrations can occur in the absence of clinical encephalopathy, rendering this investigation of little diagnostic value.

Management

The principles are to treat or remove precipitating causes (see Box 23.26) and to suppress the production of neurotoxins by bacteria in the bowel. Dietary protein restriction is rarely needed and is no longer recommended as first-line treatment because it is unpalatable and can lead to a worsening nutritional state in already malnourished patients. Lactulose (15–30 mL 3 times daily) is increased gradually until the bowels are moving twice daily. It produces an osmotic laxative effect, reduces the pH of the colonic content, thereby limiting colonic ammonia absorption, and promotes the incorporation of nitrogen into bacteria. Rifaximin (400 mg 3 times daily) is a well-tolerated, non-absorbed antibiotic that acts by reducing the bacterial content of the bowel and has been shown to be effective. It can be used in addition, or as an alternative, to lactulose if diarrhoea becomes troublesome. Chronic or refractory encephalopathy is one of the main indications for liver transplantation.

Variceal bleeding

Acute upper gastrointestinal haemorrhage from gastro-oesophageal varices (Fig. 23.17) is common in chronic liver disease. Investigation and management are discussed on page 853 and the specific management of variceal bleeding on page 946.

CIRRHOSIS

Cirrhosis is characterised by diffuse hepatic fibrosis and nodule formation. It can occur at any age, has significant morbidity and is an important cause of premature death. Worldwide, the most common causes are chronic viral hepatitis, prolonged excessive alcohol consumption and NAFLD. Cirrhosis is the most common cause of portal hypertension and its complications.

The causes of cirrhosis are listed in Box 23.27; any condition leading to persistent or recurrent hepatocyte death, such as chronic hepatitis C infection, alcoholic liver disease (ALD) or NAFLD may lead to cirrhosis. It may also occur in prolonged biliary damage or obstruction, as is found in primary biliary cirrhosis (PBC), primary sclerosing cholangitis and post-surgical biliary strictures. Persistent blockage of venous return from the liver, such as occurs in veno-occlusive disease and Budd–Chiari syndrome, can also result in cirrhosis.

Pathophysiology

Following liver injury, stellate cells in the space of Disse (see Fig. 23.3, p. 925) are activated by cytokines produced by Kupffer cells and hepatocytes. This transforms the stellate cell into a myofibroblast-like cell, capable of producing collagen, pro-inflammatory cytokines and

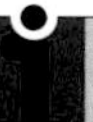

23.27 Causes of cirrhosis

- Alcohol
- Chronic viral hepatitis (B or C)
- Non-alcoholic fatty liver disease
- Immune
  - Primary sclerosing cholangitis
  - Autoimmune liver disease
- Biliary
  - Primary biliary cirrhosis
  - Secondary biliary cirrhosis
  - Cystic fibrosis
- Genetic
  - Haemochromatosis
  - Wilson's disease
  - α_1-antitrypsin deficiency
- Cryptogenic (unknown – 15%)
- Chronic venous outflow obstruction
- Any chronic liver disease

A
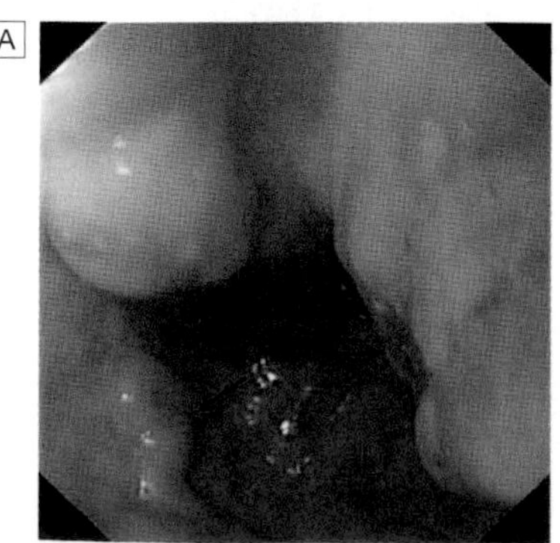

B
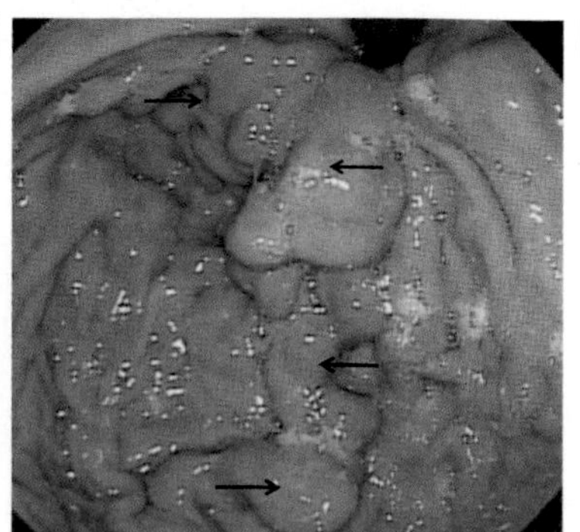

C
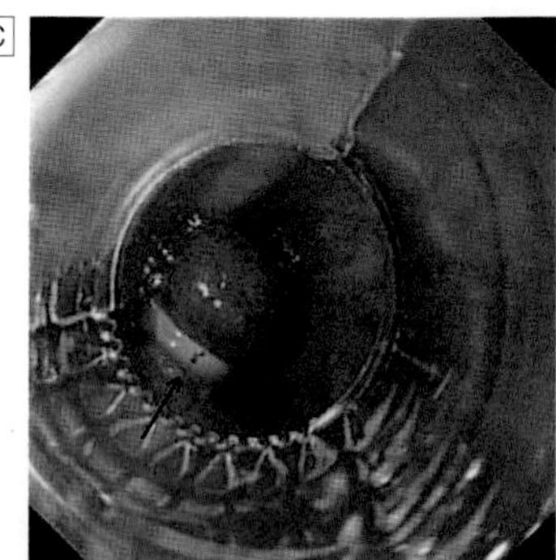

Fig. 23.17 Varices: endoscopic views. **A** Oesophageal varices (arrows) at the lower end of the oesophagus. **B** Gastric varices (arrows). **C** Appearance of oesophageal varices following application of strangulating bands (band ligation, arrow).

A

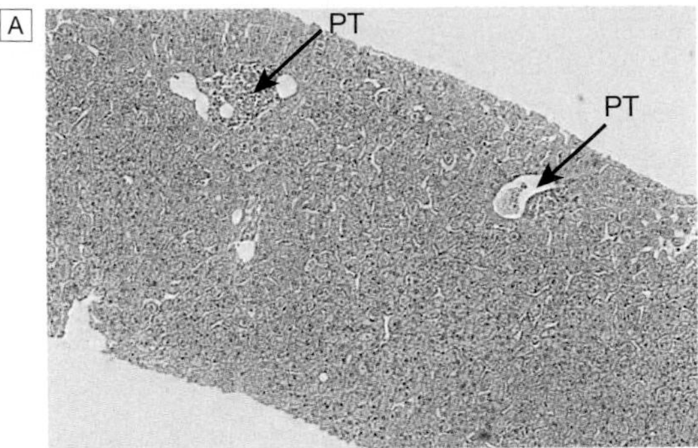

B

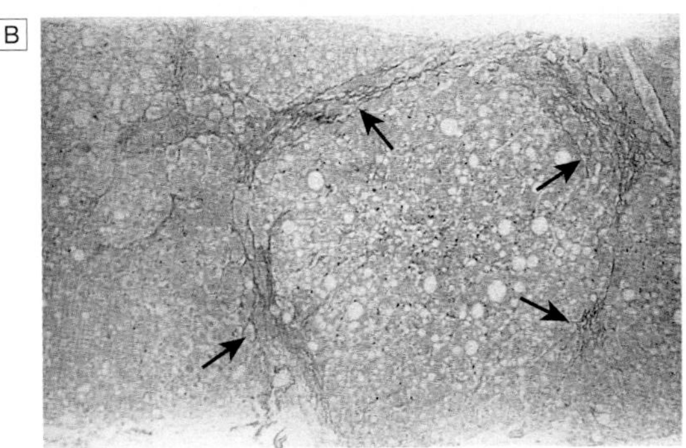

C

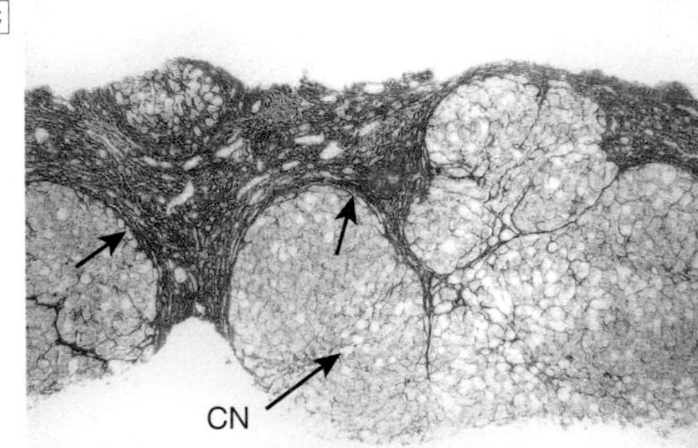

Fig. 23.18 Histological features in normal liver, hepatic fibrosis and cirrhosis. **A** Normal liver. Columns of hepatocytes 1–2 cells thick radiate from the portal tracts (PT) to the central veins. The portal tract contains a normal intralobular bile duct branch of the hepatic artery and portal venous radical. **B** Bridging fibrosis (stained pink, arrows) spreading out around the hepatic vein and single liver cells (pericellular) and linking adjacent portal tracts and hepatic veins. **C** A cirrhotic liver. The liver architecture is disrupted. The normal arrangement of portal tracts and hepatic veins is now lost and nodules of proliferating hepatocytes are broken up by strands of pink/orange-staining fibrous tissue (arrows) forming cirrhotic nodules (CN).

other mediators that promote hepatocyte damage and tissue fibrosis (see Fig. 23.4, p. 925).

Cirrhosis is a histological diagnosis (Fig. 23.18). It evolves over years as progressive fibrosis and widespread hepatocyte loss lead to distortion of the normal liver architecture that disrupts the hepatic vasculature, causing portosystemic shunts. These changes usually affect the whole liver, but in biliary cirrhosis (e.g. PBC) they can be patchy. Cirrhosis can be classified histologically into:

- *Micronodular cirrhosis*, characterised by small nodules about 1 mm in diameter and typically seen in alcoholic cirrhosis.
- *Macronodular cirrhosis*, characterised by larger nodules of various sizes. Areas of previous collapse of the liver architecture are evidenced by large fibrous scars.

Clinical features

The clinical presentation is highly variable. Some patients are asymptomatic and the diagnosis is made incidentally at ultrasound or at surgery. Others present with isolated hepatomegaly, splenomegaly, signs of portal hypertension (p. 945) or hepatic insufficiency. When symptoms are present, they are often non-specific and include weakness, fatigue, muscle cramps, weight loss, anorexia, nausea, vomiting and upper abdominal discomfort (Box 23.28). Cirrhosis will occasionally present because of shortness of breath due to a large right pleural effusion, or with hepatopulmonary syndrome (p. 975).

Hepatomegaly is common when the cirrhosis is due to ALD or haemochromatosis. Progressive hepatocyte destruction and fibrosis gradually reduce liver size as the disease progresses in other causes of cirrhosis. A reduction in liver size is especially common if the cause is viral hepatitis or autoimmune liver disease. The liver is often hard, irregular and non-tender. Jaundice is mild when it first appears and is due primarily to a failure to excrete bilirubin. Palmar erythema can be seen early in the disease, but is of limited diagnostic value, as it occurs in many other conditions associated with a hyperdynamic circulation, including normal pregnancy, as well as being found in some healthy people. Spider telangiectasias occur and comprise a central arteriole (which occasionally raises the skin surface), from which small vessels radiate. They vary in size from 1 to 2 mm in diameter, and are usually found only above the nipples. One or two small spider telangiectasias may be present in about 2% of healthy people and may occur transiently in greater numbers in the third trimester of pregnancy, but otherwise they are a strong indicator of liver disease. Florid spider telangiectasia, gynaecomastia and parotid enlargement are most common in alcoholic cirrhosis. Pigmentation is most striking in haemochromatosis and in any cirrhosis associated with prolonged cholestasis. Pulmonary arteriovenous shunts also develop, leading to hypoxaemia and eventually to central cyanosis, but this is a late feature.

Endocrine changes are noticed more readily in men, who show loss of male hair distribution and testicular

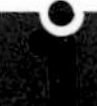

23.28 Clinical features of hepatic cirrhosis

- Hepatomegaly (although liver may also be small)
- Jaundice
- Ascites
- Circulatory changes: spider telangiectasia, palmar erythema, cyanosis
- Endocrine changes: loss of libido, hair loss
  Men: gynaecomastia, testicular atrophy, impotence
  Women: breast atrophy, irregular menses, amenorrhoea
- Haemorrhagic tendency: bruises, purpura, epistaxis
- Portal hypertension: splenomegaly, collateral vessels, variceal bleeding
- Hepatic (portosystemic) encephalopathy
- Other features: pigmentation, digital clubbing, Dupuytren's contracture

23.29 Features of chronic liver failure

- Worsening synthetic liver function
  - Prolonged PT
  - Low albumin
- Jaundice
- Portal hypertension
- Variceal bleeding
- Hepatic encephalopathy
- Ascites
  - Spontaneous bacterial peritonitis
  - Hepatorenal failure

atrophy. Gynaecomastia is common and can be due to drugs such as spironolactone. Easy bruising becomes more frequent as cirrhosis advances.

Splenomegaly and collateral vessel formation are features of portal hypertension, which occurs in more advanced disease (see below). Ascites also signifies advanced disease. Evidence of hepatic encephalopathy also becomes common with disease progression. Non-specific features of chronic liver disease include clubbing of the fingers and toes. Dupuytren's contracture is traditionally regarded as a complication of cirrhosis, but the evidence for this is weak. Chronic liver failure develops when the metabolic capacity of the liver is exceeded. It is characterised by the presence of encephalopathy and/or ascites. The term 'hepatic decompensation' or 'decompensated liver disease' is often used when chronic liver failure occurs.

Other clinical and laboratory features may be present (Box 23.29); these include peripheral oedema, renal failure, jaundice, and hypoalbuminaemia and coagulation abnormalities due to defective protein synthesis.

Management

This includes treatment of the underlying cause, maintenance of nutrition and treatment of complications, including ascites, hepatic encephalopathy, portal hypertension and varices. Once the diagnosis of cirrhosis is made, endoscopy should be performed to screen for oesophageal varices (p. 946) and repeated every 2 years. As cirrhosis is associated with an increased risk of hepatocellular carcinoma (HCC), patients should be placed under regular surveillance for it (p. 967).

Chronic liver failure due to cirrhosis can also be treated by liver transplantation. This currently accounts for about three-quarters of all liver transplants (p. 978).

Prognosis

The overall prognosis in cirrhosis is poor. Many patients present with advanced disease and/or serious complications that carry a high mortality. Overall, only 25% of patients survive 5 years from diagnosis but, where liver function is good, 50% survive for 5 years and 25% for up to 10 years. The prognosis is more favourable when the underlying cause of the cirrhosis can be corrected, as in alcohol misuse, haemochromatosis or Wilson's disease.

Laboratory tests give only a rough guide to prognosis in individual patients. Deteriorating liver function, as evidenced by jaundice, ascites or encephalopathy, indicates a poor prognosis unless a treatable cause such as infection is found. Increasing bilirubin, falling albumin (or an albumin concentration < 30 g/L), marked hyponatraemia (< 120 mmol/L) not due to diuretic therapy, and a prolonged PT are all bad prognostic features (Boxes 23.30 and 23.31). The Child–Pugh score and, more recently, the MELD (Model for End-stage Liver Disease) score can be used to assess prognosis. The MELD is more difficult to calculate at the bedside but, unlike the Child–Pugh score, includes renal function; if this is impaired, it is known to be a poor prognostic feature in end-stage disease (Box 23.32). Although

23.30 Child–Pugh classification of prognosis in cirrhosis

Score	1	2	3
Encephalopathy	None	Mild	Marked
Bilirubin (μmol/L)*			
PBC/sclerosing cholangitis	< 68	68–170	> 170
Other causes of cirrhosis	< 34	34–50	> 50
Albumin (g/L)	> 35	28–35	< 28
PT (seconds prolonged)	< 4	4–6	> 6
Ascites	None	Mild	Marked

Add the individual scores: < 7 = Child's A, 7–9 = Child's B, > 9 = Child's C

*To convert bilirubin in μmol/L to mg/dL, divide by 17.

23.31 Survival in cirrhosis

Child–Pugh grade	Survival (%) 1 year	5 years	10 years	Hepatic deaths (%)
A	82	45	25	43
B	62	20	7	72
C	42	20	0	85

Based on Powell LW, Mortimer R, Harris OD. Cirrhosis of the liver: a comparative study of the four major aetiological groups. Med J Aust 1971; 1:941–950.

23.32 One-year survival rate depending on MELD score

MELD score	One-year survival (%) No complications	Complications*
< 9	97	90
10–19	90	85
20–29	70	65
30–39	70	50

MELD from SI units

$10 \times (0.378$ [ln serum bilirubin (μmol/L) + 1.12 [ln INR] + 0.957 [ln serum creatinine (μmol/L)] + 0.643)

MELD from non-SI units

3.8 [ln serum bilirubin (mg/dL)] + 11.2 [ln INR] + 9.3 [ln serum creatinine (mg/dL)] + 6.4

ln = natural log. To calculate online, go to http://optn.transplant.hrsa.gov/resources/MeldPeldCalculator.asp?index=98.

*'Complications' means the presence of ascites, encephalopathy or variceal bleeding.

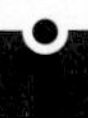

these scores give a guide to prognosis, the course of cirrhosis can be unpredictable, as complications such as variceal bleeding may occur.

PORTAL HYPERTENSION

This frequently complicates cirrhosis but has other causes. The normal hepatic venous pressure gradient (difference between the wedged hepatic venous pressure and free hepatic venous pressure, see below) is 5–6 mm Hg. Clinically significant portal hypertension is present when the gradient exceeds 10 mm Hg and risk of variceal bleeding increases beyond a gradient of 12 mm Hg. Increased vascular resistance is common. Causes are classified in accordance with the main sites of obstruction to blood flow in the portal venous system (Fig. 23.19). Extrahepatic portal vein obstruction is the usual source of portal hypertension in childhood and adolescence, while cirrhosis causes at least 90% of cases of portal hypertension in adults in developed countries. Schistosomiasis is the most common cause of portal hypertension worldwide but is infrequent outside endemic areas (e.g. Egypt; p. 376).

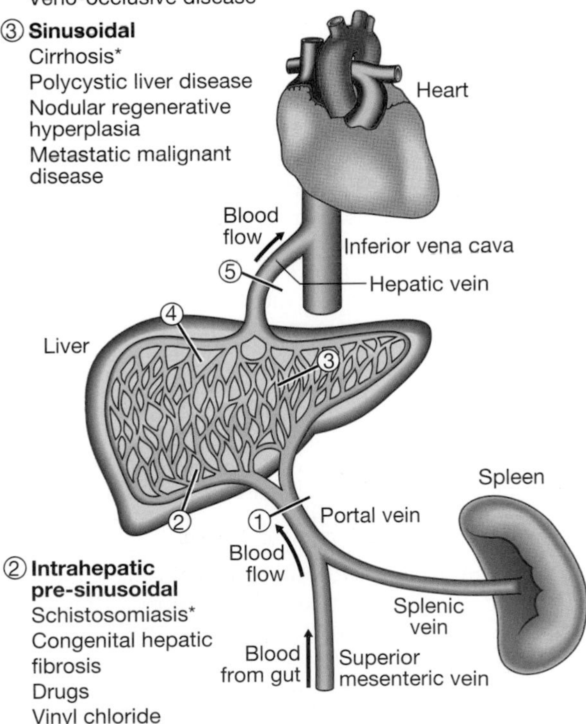

Fig. 23.19 Classification of portal hypertension according to site of vascular obstruction. *Most common cause. Note that splenic vein occlusion can also follow pancreatitis, leading to gastric varices.

23.33 Complications of portal hypertension

- Variceal bleeding: oesophageal, gastric, other (rare)
- Congestive gastropathy
- Hypersplenism
- Ascites
- Iron deficiency anaemia
- Renal failure
- Hepatic encephalopathy

Clinical features

The clinical features result principally from portal venous congestion and collateral vessel formation (Box 23.33). Splenomegaly is a cardinal finding, and a diagnosis of portal hypertension is unusual when splenomegaly cannot be detected clinically or by ultrasonography. The spleen is rarely enlarged more than 5 cm below the left costal margin in adults, but more marked splenomegaly can occur in childhood and adolescence. Collateral vessels may be visible on the anterior abdominal wall and occasionally several radiate from the umbilicus to form a caput medusae. Rarely, a large umbilical collateral vessel has a blood flow sufficient to give a venous hum on auscultation (Cruveilhier–Baumgarten syndrome). The most important collateral vessel formation occurs in the oesophagus and stomach, and this can be a source of severe bleeding. Rectal varices also cause bleeding and are often mistaken for haemorrhoids (which are no more common in portal hypertension than in the general population). Fetor hepaticus results from portosystemic shunting of blood, which allows mercaptans to pass directly to the lungs.

Ascites occurs as a result of renal sodium retention and portal hypertension that may be due, for example, to post-hepatic portal hypertension (hepatic outflow obstruction, p. 939) or cirrhosis.

The most important consequence of portal hypertension is variceal bleeding, which commonly arises from oesophageal varices located within 3–5 cm of the gastro-oesophageal junction, or from gastric varices. The size of the varices, endoscopic variceal features such as red spots and stripes, high portal pressure and liver failure are all general factors that predispose to bleeding. Drugs capable of causing mucosal erosion, such as salicylates and NSAIDs, can also precipitate bleeding. Variceal bleeding is often severe, and recurrent if preventative treatment is not given.

Pathophysiology

Increased portal vascular resistance leads to a gradual reduction in the flow of portal blood to the liver and simultaneously to the development of collateral vessels, allowing portal blood to bypass the liver and enter the systemic circulation directly. Portosystemic shunting occurs, particularly in the gastrointestinal tract and especially the distal oesophagus, stomach and rectum, in the anterior abdominal wall, and in the renal, lumbar, ovarian and testicular vasculature. Stomal varices can also occur at the site of an ileostomy. As collateral vessel formation progresses, more than half of the portal blood flow may be shunted directly to the systemic circulation. Increased portal flow contributes to portal hypertension but is not the dominant factor.

Investigations

The diagnosis is often made clinically. Portal venous pressure measurements are rarely needed for clinical assessment or routine management, but can be used to confirm portal hypertension and to differentiate sinusoidal and pre-sinusoidal forms. Pressure measurements are made by using a balloon catheter inserted using the transjugular route (via the inferior vena cava into a hepatic vein and then hepatic venule) to measure the wedged hepatic venous pressure (WHVP). This is an indirect measurement of portal vein pressure. Thrombocytopenia is common due to hypersplenism, and platelet counts are usually in the region of $100 \times 10^9/L$; values below $50 \times 10^9/L$ are uncommon. Leucopenia occurs occasionally but anaemia is seldom attributed directly to hypersplenism; if anaemia is found, a source of bleeding should be sought.

The most useful investigation is endoscopy to determine whether gastro-oesophageal varices are present (see Fig. 23.17, p. 942). Once the diagnosis of cirrhosis is made, endoscopy should be performed to screen for oesophageal varices (and repeated every 2 years). Ultrasonography often shows features of portal hypertension, such as splenomegaly and collateral vessels, and can sometimes indicate the cause, such as liver disease or portal vein thrombosis. CT and MRI angiography can identify the extent of portal vein clot and are used to identify hepatic vein patency.

Management

Acute upper gastrointestinal haemorrhage from gastro-oesophageal varices is a common manifestation of chronic liver disease. In the presence of portal hypertension, the risk of a variceal bleed occurring within 2 years varies from 7% for small varices up to 30% for large varices. The mortality following a variceal bleed has improved to around 15% overall but is still about 45% in those with poor liver function (i.e. Child–Pugh C).

The management of portal hypertension is largely focused on the prevention and/or control of variceal haemorrhage. However, it should be remembered that bleeding can also result from peptic ulceration, which is more common in patients with liver disease than in the general population. The investigation and management of gastrointestinal bleeding are dealt with in more detail on page 853.

Primary prevention of variceal bleeding

If non-bleeding varices are identified at endoscopy, β-adrenoceptor antagonist (β-blocker) therapy with propranolol (80–160 mg/day) or nadolol is effective in reducing portal venous pressure. Administration of these drugs at doses that reduce the heart rate by 25% has been shown to be effective in the primary prevention of variceal bleeding (Box 23.34). The efficacy of β-blockers in primary prevention is similar to that of prophylactic banding, which may also be considered, particularly in patients that are unable to tolerate β-blocker therapy. Carvedilol, a non-cardioselective vasodilating β-blocker, is also effective.

Management of acute variceal bleeding

The priority in acute bleeding is to restore the circulation with blood and plasma, not least because shock reduces liver blood flow and causes further deterioration of liver function. The source of bleeding should always be confirmed by endoscopy, because about 20% of patients are bleeding from non-variceal lesions. Management of acute variceal bleeding is described in Box 23.35 and illustrated in Figure 23.20. All patients with cirrhosis and gastrointestinal bleeding should receive prophylactic broad-spectrum antibiotics, such as oral ciprofloxacin or intravenous cephalosporin, because sepsis is common and treatment with antibiotics has been shown to improve outcomes. The measures used to control acute variceal bleeding include vasoactive medications (e.g. terlipressin), endoscopic therapy (banding or sclerotherapy), balloon tamponade, transjugular intrahepatic portosystemic stent shunting (TIPSS) and, rarely, oesophageal transection.

Pharmacological reduction of portal venous pressure. Terlipressin is a synthetic vasopressin analogue that, in contrast to vasopressin, can be given by intermittent injection rather than continuous infusion. It reduces portal blood flow and/or intrahepatic resistance and hence reduces portal pressure. It reduces mortality in the setting of acute variceal bleeding. The dose is 2 mg IV 4 times daily until bleeding stops, and then 1 mg 4 times daily for up to 72 hours. Caution is needed in patients with severe ischaemic heart disease or peripheral vascular disease because of the drug's vasoconstrictor properties.

Banding ligation and sclerotherapy. This is the most widely used initial treatment and is undertaken if possible at the time of diagnostic endoscopy (see Fig. 23.17C, p. 942). It stops variceal bleeding in 80% of patients and can be repeated if bleeding recurs. Band ligation involves

EBM 23.34 Primary prevention of variceal bleeding

'In patients with cirrhosis, treatment with propranolol reduces variceal bleeding by 47% (NNT_B 10), death from bleeding by 45% (NNT_B 25) and overall mortality by 22% (NNT_B 16).'

- Hayes PC, et al. Lancet 1990; 336:153–156.

For further information: www.bsg.org.uk

23.35 Emergency management of bleeding

Management	Reason
IV fluids (colloid)	Extracellular volume replacement
Vasopressor (terlipressin)	Reduces portal pressure, acute bleeding and risk of early rebleeding
Prophylactic antibiotics (cephalosporin IV)	Reduces incidence of SBP
Emergency endoscopy	Confirms variceal rather than ulcer bleed
Variceal band ligation	To stop bleeding
Proton pump inhibitor	To prevent peptic ulcers
Phosphate enema and/or lactulose	To prevent hepatic encephalopathy

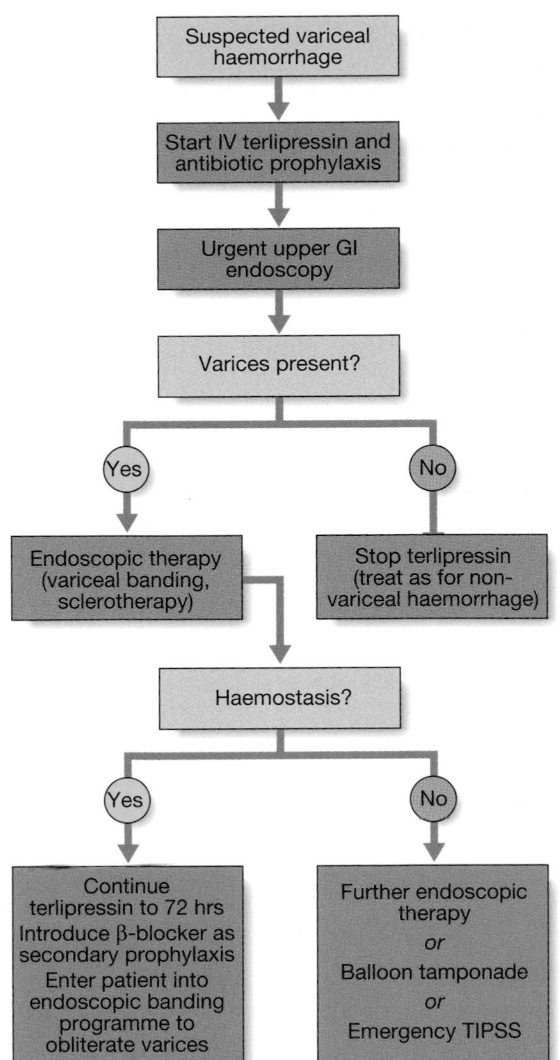

Fig. 23.20 Management of acute bleeding from oesophageal varices. (TIPSS = transjugular intrahepatic portosystemic stent shunt).

the varices being sucked into a cap placed on the end of the endoscope, allowing them to be occluded with a tight rubber band. The occluded varix subsequently sloughs with variceal obliteration. Banding is repeated every 4–6 weeks until the varices are obliterated. Regular follow-up endoscopy is required to identify and treat any recurrence of varices. Band ligation has fewer side-effects than, and has largely replaced, sclerotherapy, a technique in which varices are injected with a sclerosing agent. Banding is associated with a lower risk of oesophageal perforation or stricturing than sclerotherapy. Prophylactic acid suppression with proton pump inhibitors reduces the risk of secondary bleeding from banding-induced ulceration.

Active bleeding may make endoscopic therapy difficult. Protection of the patient's airway with endotracheal intubation may aid the endoscopist, facilitating endoscopic therapy, and significantly reduce the risk of pulmonary aspiration.

Balloon tamponade. This technique employs a Sengstaken–Blakemore tube possessing two balloons that exert pressure in the fundus of the stomach and in

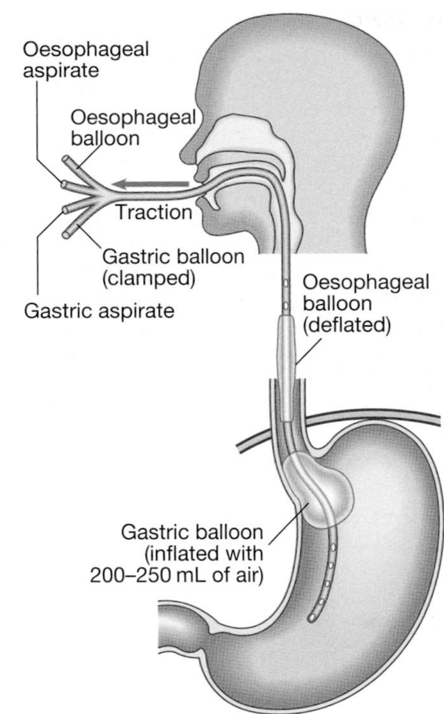

Fig. 23.21 Sengstaken–Blakemore tube.

the lower oesophagus respectively (Fig. 23.21). Additional lumens allow material to be aspirated from the stomach and from the oesophagus above the oesophageal balloon. This technique may be used in the event of life-threatening haemorrhage if early endoscopic therapy is not available or is unsuccessful.

Endotracheal intubation prior to tube insertion reduces the risk of pulmonary aspiration. The tube should be passed through the mouth and its presence in the stomach should be checked by auscultating the upper abdomen while injecting air and by radiology. The safest technique is to inflate the balloon in the stomach under direct endoscopic vision. Gentle traction is essential to maintain pressure on the varices. Initially, only the gastric balloon should be inflated, with 200–250 mL of air, as this will usually control bleeding. Inflation of the gastric balloon must be stopped if the patient experiences pain because inadvertent inflation in the oesophagus can cause oesophageal rupture. If the oesophageal balloon needs to be used because of continued bleeding, it should be deflated for about 10 minutes every 3 hours to avoid oesophageal mucosal damage. Pressure in the oesophageal balloon should be monitored with a sphygmomanometer, and should not exceed 40 mm Hg. Balloon tamponade will almost always stop oesophageal and gastric fundal variceal bleeding, but is only a bridge to more definitive therapy. Self-expanding removable oesophageal stents are a new alternative in patients with bleeding oesophageal, but not gastric, varices.

TIPSS. This technique uses a stent placed between the portal vein and the hepatic vein within the liver to provide a portosystemic shunt and therefore reduce portal pressure (Fig. 23.22). It is carried out under radiological control via the internal jugular vein; prior patency of the portal vein must be determined angiographically,

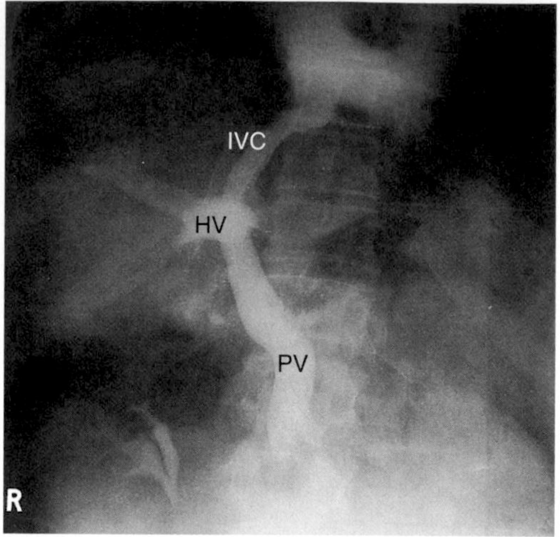

Fig. 23.22 Transjugular intrahepatic portosystemic stent shunt (TIPSS). X-ray showing placement of TIPSS within the portal vein (PV), allowing blood to flow from the portal vein into the hepatic vein (HV) and then the inferior vena cava (IVC).

EBM 23.36 Secondary prevention of variceal bleeding in patients with cirrhosis

'While TIPSS is more effective than endoscopic treatment in reducing variceal rebleeding, it does not improve survival and is associated with more encephalopathy.'

- Jalan R, et al. Gut 2000; 6:1–15.
- Laine L. Hepatology 1995; 22:663–665.

For further information: www.bsg.org.uk

coagulation deficiencies may require correction with fresh frozen plasma, and antibiotic cover is provided. Successful shunt placement stops and prevents variceal bleeding. Further bleeding necessitates investigation and treatment (e.g. angioplasty) because it is usually associated with shunt narrowing or occlusion. Hepatic encephalopathy may occur following TIPSS and is managed by reducing the shunt diameter. Although TIPSS is associated with less rebleeding than endoscopic therapy, survival is not improved (Box 23.36).

Portosystemic shunt surgery. Surgery prevents recurrent bleeding, but carries a high mortality and often leads to encephalopathy. In practice, portosystemic shunts are now reserved for patients in whom other treatments have not been successful and are offered only to those with good liver function.

Oesophageal transection. Rarely, surgical transection of the varices may be performed as a last resort when bleeding cannot be controlled by other means, but operative mortality is high.

Secondary prevention of variceal bleeding

Beta-blockers are used as a secondary measure to prevent recurrent variceal bleeding. Following successful treatment by endoscopic therapy, patients should be entered into an oesophageal banding programme with repeated sessions of therapy at 1- to 2-week intervals until the varices are obliterated. In selected individuals, TIPSS may also be considered in this setting.

Congestive gastropathy

Long-standing portal hypertension causes chronic gastric congestion recognisable at endoscopy as multiple areas of punctate erythema ('snake skin gastropathy'). Rarely, similar lesions occur more distally in the gastrointestinal tract. These areas may become eroded, causing bleeding from multiple sites. Acute bleeding can occur but repeated minor bleeding causing iron-deficiency anaemia is more common. Anaemia may be prevented by oral iron supplements but repeated blood transfusions can become necessary. Reduction of the portal pressure using propranolol (80–160 mg/day) is the best initial treatment. If this is ineffective, a TIPSS procedure can be undertaken.

INFECTIONS AND THE LIVER

The liver may be subject to a number of different infections. These include hepatotropic viral infections, and bacterial and protozoal infections. Each has specific clinical features and requires targeted therapies.

Viral hepatitis

This must be considered in anyone presenting with hepatitic liver blood tests (high transaminases). The causes are listed in Box 23.37.

All these viruses cause illnesses with similar clinical and pathological features and which are frequently anicteric or even asymptomatic. They differ in their tendency to cause acute and chronic infections. The features of the major hepatitis viruses are shown in Box 23.38.

Clinical features of acute infection

A non-specific prodromal illness characterised by headache, myalgia, arthralgia, nausea and anorexia usually precedes the development of jaundice by a few days to 2 weeks. Vomiting and diarrhoea may follow, and abdominal discomfort is common. Dark urine and pale stools may precede jaundice. There are usually few physical signs. The liver is often tender but only minimally enlarged. Occasionally, mild splenomegaly and cervical lymphadenopathy are seen. These are more frequent in children or those with Epstein–Barr virus (EBV) infection. Symptoms rarely last longer than 3–6 weeks. Complications may occur (Box 23.39) but are rare.

Investigations

A hepatitic pattern of LFTs develops, with serum transaminases typically between 200 and 2000 U/L in an

23.37 Causes of viral hepatitis

Common	
• Hepatitis A • Hepatitis B ± hepatitis D	• Hepatitis C • Hepatitis E
Less common	
• Cytomegalovirus	• Epstein–Barr virus
Rare	
• Herpes simplex	• Yellow fever

23.38 Features of the main hepatitis viruses

	Hepatitis A	Hepatitis B	Hepatitis C	Hepatitis D	Hepatitis E
Virus					
Group	Enterovirus	Hepadna virus	Flavivirus	Incomplete virus	Calicivirus
Nucleic acid	RNA	DNA	RNA	RNA	RNA
Size (diameter)	27 nm	42 nm	30–38 nm	35 nm	27 nm
Incubation (wks)	2–4	4–20	2–26	6–9	3–8
Spread					
Faeces	Yes	No	No	No	Yes
Blood	Uncommon	Yes	Yes	Yes	No
Saliva	Yes	Yes	Yes	Unknown	Unknown
Sexual	Uncommon	Yes	Uncommon	Yes	Unknown
Vertical	No	Yes	Uncommon	Yes	No
Chronic infection	No	Yes	Yes	Yes	No (rarely in immune-compromised)
Prevention					
Active	Vaccine	Vaccine	No	Prevented by hepatitis B vaccination	No
Passive	Immune serum globulin	Hyperimmune serum globulin	No		No

Note All body fluids are potentially infectious, although some (e.g. urine) are less infectious than others.

23.39 Complications of acute viral hepatitis

- Acute liver failure
- Cholestatic hepatitis (hepatitis A)
- Aplastic anaemia
- Chronic liver disease and cirrhosis (hepatitis B and C)
- Relapsing hepatitis

acute infection (usually lower and fluctuating in chronic infections). The plasma bilirubin reflects the degree of liver damage. The ALP rarely exceeds twice the upper limit of normal. Prolongation of the PT indicates the severity of the hepatitis but rarely exceeds 25 seconds, except in rare cases of acute liver failure. The white cell count is usually normal with a relative lymphocytosis. Serological tests confirm the aetiology of the infection.

Management

Most individuals do not need hospital care. Drugs such as sedatives and narcotics, which are metabolised in the liver, should be avoided. No specific dietary modifications are needed. Alcohol should be avoided during the acute illness. Elective surgery should be avoided in cases of acute viral hepatitis, as there is a risk of post-operative liver failure.

Liver transplantation is very rarely indicated for acute viral hepatitis complicated by liver failure, but is commonly performed for complications of cirrhosis resulting from chronic hepatitis B and C infection.

Hepatitis A

The hepatitis A virus (HAV) belongs to the picornavirus group of enteroviruses. HAV is highly infectious and is spread by the faecal–oral route. Infected individuals, who may be asymptomatic, excrete the virus in faeces for about 2–3 weeks before the onset of symptoms and then for a further 2 weeks or so. Infection is common in children but often asymptomatic, and so up to 30% of adults will have serological evidence of past infection but give no history of jaundice. Infection is also more common in areas of overcrowding and poor sanitation. In occasional outbreaks, water and shellfish have been the vehicles of transmission. In contrast to hepatitis B, a chronic carrier state does not occur.

Investigations

Only one HAV antigen has been found and infected people make an antibody to this antigen (anti-HAV). Anti-HAV is important in diagnosis, as HAV is only present in the blood transiently during the incubation period. Excretion in the stools occurs for only 7–14 days after the onset of the clinical illness and the virus cannot be grown readily. Anti-HAV of the IgM type, indicating a primary immune response, is already present in the blood at the onset of the clinical illness and is diagnostic of an acute HAV infection. Titres of this antibody fall to low levels within about 3 months of recovery. Anti-HAV of the IgG type is of no diagnostic value, as HAV infection is common and this antibody persists for years after infection, but it can be used as a marker of previous HAV infection. Its presence indicates immunity to HAV.

Management

Infection in the community is best prevented by improving social conditions, especially overcrowding and poor sanitation. Individuals can be given substantial protection from infection by active immunisation with an inactivated virus vaccine.

Immunisation should be considered for individuals with chronic hepatitis B or C infections. Immediate protection can be provided by immune serum globulin if this is given soon after exposure to the virus. The protective effect of immune serum globulin is attributed to its anti-HAV content. Immunisation should be considered for those at particular risk, such as close contacts of HAV-infected patients, the elderly, those with other major disease and perhaps pregnant women.

Immune serum globulin can be effective in an outbreak of hepatitis, in a school or nursery, as injection of those at risk prevents secondary spread to families. People travelling to endemic areas are best protected by vaccination.

Acute liver failure is rare in hepatitis A (0.1%) and chronic infection does not occur. However, HAV infection in patients with chronic liver disease may cause serious or life-threatening disease. In adults, a cholestatic phase with elevated ALP levels may complicate infection. There is no role for antiviral drugs in the therapy of HAV infection.

Hepatitis B

The hepatitis B virus consists of a core containing DNA and a DNA polymerase enzyme needed for virus replication. The core of the virus is surrounded by surface protein (Fig. 23.23). The virus, also called a Dane particle, and an excess of its surface protein (known as hepatitis B surface antigen) circulate in the blood. Humans are the only source of infection.

Hepatitis B is one of the most common causes of chronic liver disease and hepatocellular carcinoma worldwide. Approximately one-third of the world's population have serological evidence of past or current infection with hepatitis B and approximately 350–400 million people are chronic HBsAg carriers.

Hepatitis B may cause an acute viral hepatitis; however, acute infection is often asymptomatic, particularly when acquired at birth. Many individuals with chronic hepatitis B are also asymptomatic.

The risk of progression to chronic liver disease depends on the source and timing of infection (Box 23.40). Vertical transmission from mother to child in the perinatal period is the most common cause of infection worldwide and carries the highest risk of ongoing chronic infection. In this setting, adaptive immune responses to HBV may be absent initially, with apparent immunological tolerance. Several mechanisms contribute towards this.

- Firstly, the introduction of antigen in the neonatal period is tolerogenic.
- Secondly, the presentation of such antigen within the liver, as described above, promotes tolerance; this is particularly evident in the absence of a significant innate or inflammatory response.
- Finally, very high loads of antigen may lead to so-called 'exhaustion' of cellular immune responses. However, the state of tolerance is not permanent and may be reversed as a result of therapy, or through spontaneous changes in innate responses such as interferon-alpha and NK cells, accompanied by host-mediated immunopathology.

Chronic hepatitis can lead to cirrhosis or HCC, usually after decades of infection (Fig. 23.24). Chronic HBV infection is a dynamic process that can be divided into five phases (Box 23.41); however, these are not necessarily sequential and not all patients will go through all phases. It should be remembered that the virus is not directly cytotoxic to cells; rather it is an immune response to viral antigens displayed on infected hepatocytes that initiates liver injury. This explains why there may be very high levels of viral replication but little hepatocellular damage during the 'immune tolerant' phase.

23.40 Source of hepatitis B infection and risk of chronic infection

Horizontal transmission (10%)
• Injection drug use • Infected unscreened blood products • Tattoos/acupuncture needles • Sexual (homosexual and heterosexual) • Close living quarters/playground play as a toddler (may contribute to high rate of horizontal transmission in Africa)
Vertical transmission (90%)
• HBsAg-positive mother

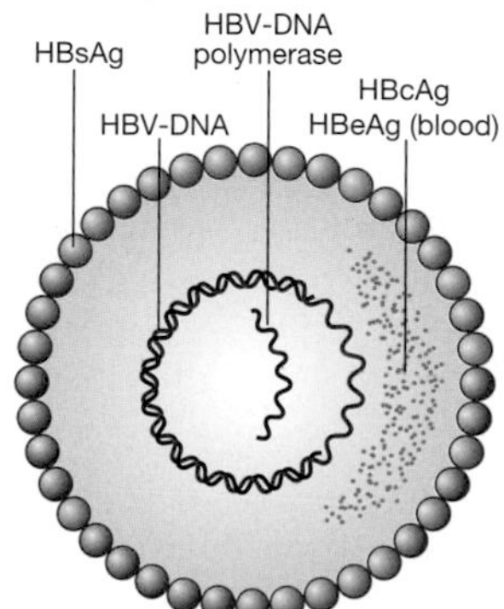

Fig. 23.23 Schematic diagram of hepatitis B virus. Hepatitis B surface antigen (HBsAg) is a protein that makes up part of the viral envelope. Hepatitis B core antigen (HBcAg) is a protein that makes up the capsid or core part of the virus (found in the liver but not in blood). Hepatitis B e antigen (HBeAg) is part of the HBcAg that can be found in the blood and indicates infectivity.

Investigations

Serology

HBV contains several antigens to which infected persons can make immune responses (Fig. 23.25); these antigens and their antibodies are important in identifying HBV infection (Boxes 23.41 and 23.42), although the widespread availability of polymerase chain reaction (PCR) techniques to measure viral DNA levels in peripheral blood means that longitudinal monitoring is now also frequently guided by direct assessment of viral load.

Hepatitis B surface antigen (HBsAg). HBsAg is an indicator of active infection, and a negative test for HBsAg makes HBV infection very unlikely. In acute liver failure from hepatitis B, the liver damage is mediated by viral clearance and so HBsAg is negative, with evidence of recent infection shown by the presence of hepatitis B core IgM. HBsAg appears in the blood late in the incubation period, but before the prodromal phase of acute type B hepatitis; it may be present for a few days only, disappearing even before jaundice has developed, but usually lasts for 3–4 weeks and can

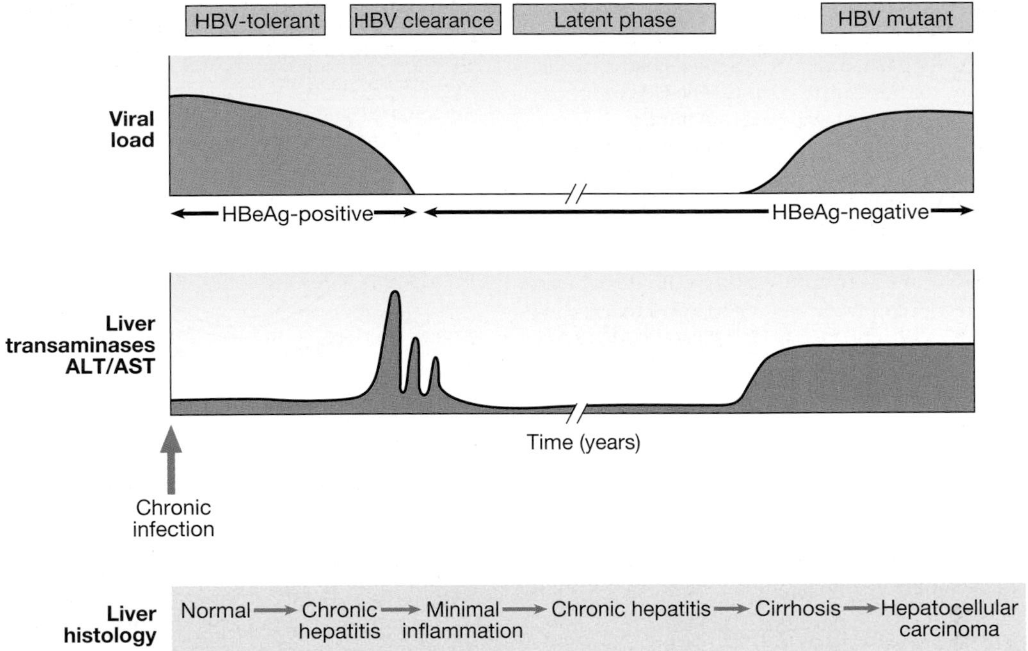

Fig. 23.24 Natural history of chronic hepatitis B infection. There is an initial immunotolerant phase with high levels of virus and normal liver biochemistry. An immunological response to the virus then occurs, with elevation in serum transaminases, which causes liver damage: chronic hepatitis. If this response is sustained over many years and viral clearance does not occur promptly, chronic hepatitis may result in cirrhosis. In individuals with a successful immunological response, viral load falls, HBe antibody develops and there is no further liver damage. Some individuals may subsequently develop HBV-DNA mutants that escape from immune regulation, and viral load again rises with further chronic hepatitis. Mutations in the core protein result in the virus's inability to secrete HBe antigen despite high levels of viral replication; such individuals have HBeAg-negative chronic hepatitis. (ALT = alanine aminotransferase; AST = aspartate aminotransferase)

23.41 The five phases of chronic hepatitis B virus infection

Phase	HBsAg	HBeAg	Anti-HBe Ab	Viral load	ALT	Histology	Notes
'Immune tolerant' phase	+	+	–	+++	Normal/ Low	Normal/minimal necroinflammation	Prolonged in perinatally infected individuals; may be short or absent if infected as an adult. High viral load and so very infectious
'Immune reactive' HBeAg-positive chronic hepatitis phase	+	+	–	++	Raised	Moderate/severe necroinflammation	May last weeks or years. High risk of cirrhosis or HCC if prolonged. Increased chance of spontaneous loss of HBeAg with seroconversion to anti-HBe Ab-positive state
'Inactive carrier' phase	+	–	+	–/+	Normal	Normal/minimal necroinflammation	Low risk of cirrhosis or HCC in majority
HBeAg-negative chronic hepatitis phase	+	–	+	Fluctuating +/++	Raised/ Fluctuating	Moderate/severe necroinflammation	May represent late immune reactivation or presence of 'pre-core mutant' HBV. High risk of cirrhosis or HCC
HBsAg-negative phase	–	–	+	–/±	Normal	Normal	Ultrasensitive techniques may detect low-level HBV even after HBsAg loss

persist for up to 5 months. The persistence of HBsAg for longer than 6 months indicates chronic infection. Antibody to HBsAg (anti-HBs) usually appears after about 3–6 months and persists for many years or perhaps permanently. Anti-HBs implies either a previous infection, in which case anti-HBc (see below) is usually also present, or previous vaccination, in which case anti-HBc is not present.

Hepatitis B core antigen (HBcAg). HBcAg is not found in the blood, but antibody to it (anti-HBc) appears early

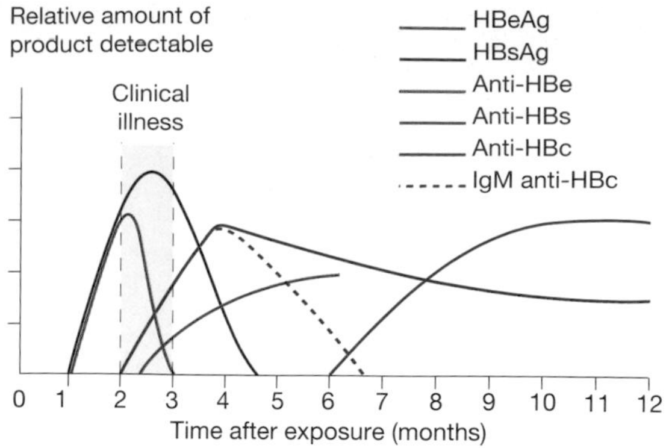

Fig. 23.25 Serological responses to hepatitis B virus infection. (HBeAg = hepatitis B e antigen; anti-HBe = antibody to HBeAg; HBsAg = hepatitis B surface antigen; anti-HBs = antibody to HBsAg; anti-HBc = antibody to hepatitis B core antigen)

23.42 How to interpret the serological tests of acute hepatitis B virus infection

Interpretation	HBsAg	Anti-HBc IgM	Anti-HBc IgG	Anti-HBs
Incubation period	+	+	–	–
Acute hepatitis				
Early	+	+	–	–
Established	+	+	+	–
Established (occasional)	–	+	+	–
Convalescence				
(3–6 months)	–	±	+	±
(6–9 months)	–	–	+	+
Post-infection	–	–	+	±
Immunisation without infection	–	–	–	+

+ Positive; – negative; ± present at low titre or absent.

in the illness and rapidly reaches a high titre, which subsides gradually but then persists. Anti-HBc is initially of IgM type, with IgG antibody appearing later. Anti-HBc (IgM) can sometimes reveal an acute HBV infection when the HBsAg has disappeared and before anti-HBs has developed (see Fig. 23.25 and Box 23.42).

Hepatitis B e antigen (HBeAg). HBeAg is an indicator of viral replication. In acute hepatitis B it may appear only transiently at the outset of the illness; its appearance is followed by the production of antibody (anti-HBe). The HBeAg reflects active replication of the virus in the liver.

Chronic HBV infection (see below) is marked by the presence of HBsAg and anti-HBc (IgG) in the blood. Usually, HBeAg or anti-HBe is also present; HBeAg indicates continued active replication of the virus in the liver. The absence of HBeAg usually implies low viral replication; the exception is HBeAg-negative chronic hepatitis B (also called 'pre-core mutant' infection, discussed below), in which high levels of viral replication, serum HBV-DNA and hepatic necroinflammation are seen, despite negative HBeAg.

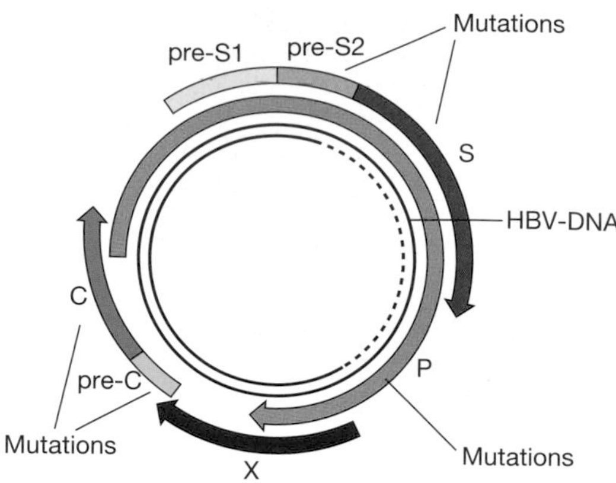

Fig. 23.26 The site of HBV-DNA mutations. HBV-DNA encodes four proteins: a DNA polymerase needed for viral replication (P), a surface protein (S), a core protein (C) and an X protein. The pre-C and C regions encode a core protein and an e antigen. Although mutations in the hepatitis B virus are frequent, certain mutations have important clinical consequences. Pre-C encodes a signal sequence needed for the C protein to be secreted from the liver cell into serum as e antigen. A mutation in the pre-core region leads to a failure of secretion of e antigen into serum, and so individuals have high levels of viral production but no detectable e antigen in the serum. Mutations can also occur in the surface protein and may lead to the failure of vaccination to prevent infection since surface antibodies are produced against the native S protein. Mutations also occur in the DNA polymerase during antiviral treatment with lamivudine.

Viral load and genotype

HBV-DNA can be measured by PCR in the blood. Viral loads are usually in excess of 10^5 copies/mL in the presence of active viral replication, as indicated by the presence of e antigen. In contrast, in those with low viral replication, HBsAg- and anti-HBe-positive, viral loads are less than 10^5 copies/mL. The exception is in patients who have a mutation in the pre-core protein, which means they cannot secrete e antigen into serum (Fig. 23.26). Such individuals will be anti-HBe-positive but have a high viral load and often evidence of chronic hepatitis. These mutations are common in the Far East, and those patients affected are classified as having e antigen-negative chronic hepatitis. They respond differently to antiviral drugs from those with classical e antigen-positive chronic hepatitis.

Measurement of viral load is important in monitoring antiviral therapy and identifying patients with pre-core mutants. Specific HBV genotypes (A–H) can also be identified using PCR. In some settings these may be useful in guiding therapy, as genotype A tends to respond better to pegylated interferon alfa, compared to genotypes C and D.

Management of acute hepatitis B

Treatment is supportive, with monitoring for acute liver failure, which occurs in less than 1% of cases. There is no definitive evidence that antiviral therapy reduces the severity or duration of acute hepatitis B.

Full recovery occurs in 90–95% of adults following acute HBV infection. The remaining 5–10% develop a chronic hepatitis B infection that usually continues for life, although later recovery occasionally occurs. Infection passing from mother to child at birth leads to chronic infection in the child in 90% of cases and recovery is rare. Chronic infection is also common in immunodeficient individuals, such as those with Down's syndrome or human immunodeficiency virus (HIV) infection. Fulminant liver failure due to acute hepatitis B occurs in less than 1% of cases.

Recovery from acute HBV infection occurs within 6 months and is characterised by the appearance of antibody to viral antigens. Persistence of HBeAg beyond this time indicates chronic infection. Combined HBV and HDV infection causes more aggressive disease.

Management of chronic hepatitis B

Treatments are still limited, as no drug is consistently able to eradicate hepatitis B infection completely (i.e. render the patient HBsAg-negative). The goals of treatment are HBeAg seroconversion, reduction in HBV-DNA and normalisation of the LFTs. The indication for treatment is a high viral load in the presence of active hepatitis, as demonstrated by elevated serum transaminases and/or histological evidence of inflammation and fibrosis. The oral antiviral agents are more effective in reducing viral loads in patients with e antigen-negative chronic hepatitis B than in those with e antigen-positive chronic hepatitis B, as the pre-treatment viral loads are lower.

Most patients with chronic hepatitis B are asymptomatic and develop complications such as cirrhosis and hepatocellular carcinoma only after many years (see Fig. 23.24). Cirrhosis develops in 15–20% of patients with chronic HBV over 5–20 years. This proportion is higher in those who are e antigen-positive.

Two different types of drug are used to treat hepatitis B: direct-acting nucleoside/nucleotide analogues and pegylated interferon-alfa.

Direct-acting nucleoside/nucleotide antiviral agents

Orally administered nucleoside/nucleotide antiviral agents are the mainstay of therapy. These act by inhibiting the reverse transcription of pre-genomic RNA to HBV-DNA by HBV-DNA polymerase but do not directly affect the cccDNA (covalently closed circular DNA) template for viral replication, and so relapse is common if treatment is withdrawn. One major concern is the selection of antiviral-resistant mutations with long-term treatment. This is particularly important with some of the older agents, such as lamivudine, as mutations induced by previous antiviral exposure may also induce resistance to newer agents. Entecavir and tenofovir (see below) are potent antivirals with a high barrier to genetic resistance, and so are the most appropriate first-line agents.

Lamivudine. Although effective, long-term therapy is often complicated by the development of HBV-DNA polymerase mutants (e.g. the 'YMDD variant'), which may occur after 9 months and are characterised by a rise in viral load during treatment. Telbivudine is more potent but is also susceptible to viral resistance. Adefovir is associated with development of HBV-DNA mutants at a lower rate than with lamivudine; 2% are identified after 2 years of treatment but this figure increases to 18% after 3 years.

Entecavir and tenofovir. Monotherapy with entecavir or tenofovir is more effective than either lamivudine or adefovir in reducing viral load in HBeAg-positive and HBeAg-negative chronic hepatitis (Boxes 23.43 and 23.44). Antiviral resistance mutations occur in only 1–2% after 3 years of entecavir drug exposure. Both drugs have anti-HIV action and so their use as monotherapy is contraindicated in HIV-positive patients, as it may lead to HIV antiviral drug resistance. Current European guidelines advise that the other nucleoside/nucleotide antivirals should not be used as first-line monotherapy due to the induction of viral mutations, unless more potent drugs with a high barrier to resistance are not available or appropriate.

EBM 23.43 Entecavir and telbivudine in chronic hepatitis B infection

'In HBeAg-positive patients, 48 weeks of treatment with entecavir suppresses HBV-DNA levels in 67%, compared to 36% with lamivudine and 60% with telbivudine. Anti-HBe seroconversion occurs in 21% following a year of entecavir, lamivudine or telbivudine. In HBeAg-negative chronic hepatitis, HBV-DNA negativity is achieved in 90% with entecavir, compared to 72% with lamivudine and 88% with telbivudine at 1 year. Treatment also improves histology and liver biochemistry.'

- Chang T-T. N Engl J Med 2006; 354:1001–1010.
- Lai C-L. N Engl J Med 2007; 357:2576–2588.
- Lai C-L. N Engl J Med 2006; 354:1011–1020.

For further information: www.easl.eu/_clinical-practice-guideline/

EBM 23.44 Tenofovir for chronic hepatitis B

'Among patients with chronic HBV infection, tenofovir at a daily dose of 300 mg had superior antiviral efficacy with a similar safety profile as compared with adefovir 10 mg daily. In HBeAg-positive patients, tenofovir suppressed HBV-DNA to < 400 copies/mL in 76% of patients, compared with 13% of those given adefovir ($p < 0.001$).'

- Marcellin P, et al. NEJM 2008; 359:2442–2445.

Interferon-alfa

This is most effective in patients with a low viral load and serum transaminases greater than twice the upper limit of normal, in whom it acts by augmenting a native immune response. In HBeAg-positive chronic hepatitis, 33% lose e antigen after 4–6 months of treatment, compared to 12% of controls. Response rates are lower in HBeAg-negative chronic hepatitis, even when patients are given longer courses of treatment. Interferon is contraindicated in the presence of cirrhosis, as it may cause a rise in serum transaminases and precipitate liver failure. Longer-acting pegylated interferons that can be given once weekly have been evaluated in both HBeAg-positive and HBeAg-negative chronic hepatitis (Box 23.45). Side-effects are common and include fatigue, depression, irritability, bone marrow suppression and the triggering of autoimmune thyroid disease.

Liver transplantation

Historically, liver transplantation was contraindicated in hepatitis B because infection often recurred in the graft. However, the use of post-liver transplant prophylaxis with direct-acting antiviral agents and hepatitis B immunoglobulins has reduced the re-infection rate to 10% and increased 5-year survival to 80%, making transplantation an acceptable treatment option.

EBM 23.45 Pegylated interferons in chronic hepatitis B infection

'In HBeAg-positive chronic hepatitis, treatment with pegylated interferon for 6 months eliminates HBeAg in 35% of patients, and normalises liver biochemistry in 25%. In HBeAg-negative chronic hepatitis, treatment with pegylated interferon for 12 months leads to normal liver biochemistry in 60% of patients, and sustained suppression of hepatitis B virus load below 400 copies/mL in 20%.'

- Cooksley WG, et al. J Viral Hep 2003; 10:298–302.
- Marcellin P. N Engl J Med 2004; 351:1206–1217.

For further information: www.easl.eu/_clinical-practice-guideline

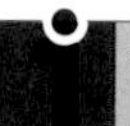

23.46 At-risk groups meriting hepatitis B vaccination in low-endemic areas

- Parenteral drug users
- Men who have sex with men
- Close contacts of infected individuals
  - Newborn of infected mothers
  - Regular sexual partners
- Patients on chronic haemodialysis
- Patients with chronic liver disease
- Medical, nursing and laboratory personnel

Prevention

Individuals are most infectious when markers of continuing viral replication, such as HBeAg, and high levels of HBV-DNA are present in the blood. HBV-DNA can be found in saliva, urine, semen and vaginal secretions. The virus is about ten times more infectious than hepatitis C, which in turn is about ten times more infectious than HIV.

A recombinant hepatitis B vaccine containing HBsAg is available (Engerix) and is capable of producing active immunisation in 95% of normal individuals. The vaccine should be offered to those at special risk of infection who are not already immune, as evidenced by anti-HBs in the blood (Box 23.46). The vaccine is ineffective in those already infected by HBV. Infection can also be prevented or minimised by the intramuscular injection of hyperimmune serum globulin prepared from blood containing anti-HBs. This should be given within 24 hours, or at most a week, of exposure to infected blood in circumstances likely to cause infection (e.g. needlestick injury, contamination of cuts or mucous membranes). Vaccine can be given together with hyperimmune globulin (active–passive immunisation).

Neonates born to hepatitis B-infected mothers should be immunised at birth and given immunoglobulin. Hepatitis B serology should then be checked at 12 months of age.

Hepatitis D (Delta virus)

The hepatitis D virus (HDV) is an RNA-defective virus that has no independent existence; it requires HBV for replication and has the same sources and modes of spread. It can infect individuals simultaneously with HBV, or can superinfect those who are already chronic carriers of HBV. Simultaneous infections give rise to acute hepatitis, which is often severe but is limited by recovery from the HBV infection. Infections in individuals who are chronic carriers of HBV can cause acute hepatitis with spontaneous recovery, and occasionally simultaneous cessation of the chronic HBV infection occurs. Chronic infection with HBV and HDV can also occur, and this frequently causes rapidly progressive chronic hepatitis and eventually cirrhosis.

HDV has a worldwide distribution. It is endemic in parts of the Mediterranean basin, Africa and South America, where transmission is mainly by close personal contact and occasionally by vertical transmission from mothers who also carry HBV. In non-endemic areas, transmission is mainly a consequence of parenteral drug misuse.

Investigations

HDV contains a single antigen to which infected individuals make an antibody (anti-HDV). Delta antigen appears in the blood only transiently, and in practice diagnosis depends on detecting anti-HDV. Simultaneous infection with HBV and HDV followed by full recovery is associated with the appearance of low titres of anti-HDV of IgM type within a few days of the onset of the illness. This antibody generally disappears within 2 months but persists in a few patients. Superinfection of patients with chronic HBV infection leads to the production of high titres of anti-HDV, initially IgM and later IgG. Such patients may then develop chronic infection with both viruses, in which case anti-HDV titres plateau at high levels.

Management

Effective management of hepatitis B prevents hepatitis D.

Hepatitis C

This is caused by an RNA flavivirus. Acute symptomatic infection with hepatitis C is rare. Most individuals are unaware of when they became infected and are only identified when they develop chronic liver disease. Eighty per cent of individuals exposed to the virus become chronically infected and late spontaneous viral clearance is rare.

Hepatitis C is the cause of what used to be known as 'non-A, non-B hepatitis'.

Hepatitis C infection is usually identified in asymptomatic individuals screened because they have risk factors for infection, such as previous injecting drug use (Box 23.47), or have incidentally been found to have abnormal liver blood tests. Although most individuals remain asymptomatic until progression to cirrhosis occurs, fatigue can complicate chronic infection and is unrelated to the degree of liver damage.

Investigations

Serology and virology

The HCV protein contains several antigens that give rise to antibodies in an infected person and these are used in diagnosis. It may take 6–12 weeks for antibodies to appear in the blood following acute infection such as a needlestick injury. In these cases, hepatitis C RNA can be identified in the blood as early as 2–4 weeks after infection. Active infection is confirmed by the presence of serum hepatitis C RNA in anyone who is antibody-positive. Anti-HCV antibodies persist in serum even after viral clearance, whether spontaneous or post-treatment.

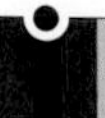

23.47 Risk factors for the acquisition of chronic hepatitis C infection

- Intravenous drug misuse (95% of new cases in the UK)
- Unscreened blood products
- Vertical transmission (3% risk)
- Needlestick injury (3% risk)
- Iatrogenic parenteral transmission (i.e. contaminated vaccination needles)
- Sharing toothbrushes/razors

EBM 23.48 Treatment of hepatitis C

'The addition of ribavirin to pegylated interferon-alfa therapy improves the overall sustained virological response from 33% to 55%.'

- Manns MP, et al. Lancet 2001; 358:958–965.
- Hadziyannis SJ, et al. Ann Intern Med 2004; 140:346–553.

For further information: www.easl.eu/_clinical-practice-guideline/

Molecular analysis

There are six common viral genotypes, the distribution of which varies worldwide. Genotype has no effect on progression of liver disease but does affect response to treatment. Genotype 1 is most common in northern Europe and is less easy to eradicate than genotypes 2 and 3 with traditional pegylated interferon alfa/ribavirin-based treatments.

Liver function tests

LFTs may be normal or show fluctuating serum transaminases between 50 and 200 U/L. Jaundice is rare and only usually appears in end-stage cirrhosis.

Liver histology

Serum transaminase levels in hepatitis C are a poor predictor of the degree of liver fibrosis and so a liver biopsy is often required to stage the degree of liver damage. The degree of inflammation and fibrosis can be scored histologically. The most common scoring system used in hepatitis C is the Metavir system, which scores fibrosis from 1 to 4, the latter equating to cirrhosis.

Management

The aim of treatment is to eradicate infection. Until recently, the treatment of choice was dual therapy with pegylated interferon-alfa given as a weekly subcutaneous injection, together with oral ribavirin, a synthetic nucleotide analogue (Box 23.48). The main side-effects of ribavirin are haemolytic anaemia and teratogenicity. Side-effects of interferon are significant and include flu-like symptoms, irritability and depression, all of which can affect quality of life. Virological relapse can occur in the first 3 months after stopping treatment, and cure is defined as loss of virus from serum 6 months after completing therapy (sustained virological response, or SVR). The length of treatment and efficacy depend on viral genotype (12 months' treatment for genotype 1 results in a 40% SVR, whereas 6 months' treatment for genotype 2 or 3 leads to an SVR in > 70%). Response to treatment is better in patients who have an early virological response, as defined by negativity of HCV-RNA in serum 1 month after starting therapy, and it may be possible to shorten the duration of therapy in this patient group.

The recent availability of triple therapy with the addition of protease inhibitors such as telaprevir and boceprevir to standard pegylated interferon/ribavirin has provided a significant advance in therapy, with SVR rates for genotype 1 individuals comparable to those previously only achieved in genotypes 2 and 3.

Liver transplantation should be considered when complications of cirrhosis occur, such as diuretic-resistant ascites. Unfortunately, hepatitis C almost always recurs in the transplanted liver and up to 15% of patients will develop cirrhosis in the liver graft within 5 years of transplantation.

There is no active or passive protection against HCV. Progression from chronic hepatitis to cirrhosis occurs over 20–40 years. Risk factors for progression include male gender, immunosuppression (such as co-infection with HIV), prothrombotic states and heavy alcohol misuse. Not everyone with hepatitis C infection will necessarily develop cirrhosis but approximately 20% do so within 20 years. Once cirrhosis has developed, the 5- and 10-year survival rates are 95% and 81% respectively. One-quarter of people with cirrhosis will develop complications within 10 years and, once complications like ascites have arisen, the 5-year survival is around 50%. Once cirrhosis is present, 2–5% per year will develop primary hepatocellular carcinoma.

Hepatitis E

Hepatitis E is caused by an RNA virus that is endemic in India and the Middle East. An increase in prevalence has recently been noted in northern Europe and infection is no longer seen only in travellers from an endemic area.

The clinical presentation and management of hepatitis E are similar to that of hepatitis A. Disease is spread via the faecal–oral route; in most cases, it presents as a self-limiting acute hepatitis and does not usually cause chronic liver disease, although some cases have been described, usually in immunocompromised patients.

Hepatitis E differs from hepatitis A in that infection during pregnancy is associated with the development of acute liver failure, which has a high mortality. In acute infection, IgM antibodies to HEV are positive.

Other forms of viral hepatitis

Non-A, non-B, non-C (NANBNC) or non-A–E hepatitis is the term used to describe hepatitis thought to be due to a virus that is not HAV, HBV, HCV or HEV. Other viruses that affect the liver probably exist, but the viruses described above now account for the majority of hepatitis virus infections. Cytomegalovirus and EBV infection cause abnormal LFTs in most patients, and occasionally jaundice occurs. Herpes simplex is a rare cause of hepatitis in adults, and most of these patients are immunocompromised. Abnormal LFTs are also common in chickenpox, measles, rubella and acute HIV infection.

HIV infection and the liver

Several causes of abnormal LFTs occur in HIV infection, as shown in Box 23.49. This topic is discussed in more detail on page 400.

23.49 Causes of abnormal liver blood tests in HIV infection

Hepatitic blood tests	
• Chronic hepatitis C • Chronic hepatitis B	• Antiretroviral drugs • Cytomegalovirus
Cholestatic blood tests	
• Tuberculosis • Atypical mycobacterium	• Sclerosing cholangitis due to cryptosporidia

23.50 Causes of pyogenic liver abscesses

- Biliary obstruction (cholangitis)
- Haematogenous
  Portal vein (mesenteric infections)
  Hepatic artery (bacteraemia)
- Direct extension
- Trauma
  Penetrating or non-penetrating
- Infection of liver tumour or cyst

Liver abscess

Liver abscesses are classified as pyogenic, hydatid or amoebic.

Pyogenic liver abscess

Pyogenic liver abscesses are uncommon but important because they are potentially curable, carry significant morbidity and mortality if untreated, and are easily overlooked. The mortality of liver abscesses is 20–40%; failure to make the diagnosis is the most common cause of death. Older patients and those with multiple abscesses also have a higher mortality.

Pathophysiology

Infection can reach the liver in several ways (Box 23.50). Pyogenic abscesses are most common in older patients and usually result from ascending infection due to biliary obstruction (cholangitis) or contiguous spread from an empyema of the gallbladder. They can also complicate dental sepsis. Abscesses complicating suppurative appendicitis used to be common in young adults but are now rare. Immunocompromised patients are particularly likely to develop liver abscesses. Single lesions are more common in the right liver; multiple abscesses are usually due to infection secondary to biliary obstruction. *E. coli* and various streptococci, particularly *Strep. milleri*, are the most common organisms; anaerobes, including streptococci and *Bacteroides*, can often be found when infection has been transmitted from large bowel pathology via the portal vein, and multiple organisms are present in one-third of patients.

Clinical features

Patients are generally ill with fever, and sometimes rigors and weight loss. Abdominal pain is the most common symptom and is usually in the right upper quadrant, sometimes with radiation to the right shoulder. The pain may be pleuritic in nature. Tender hepatomegaly is found in more than 50% of patients. Mild jaundice may be present, becoming severe if large abscesses cause biliary obstruction. Atypical presentations are common and explain the frequency with which the diagnosis is made only at postmortem. This is a particular problem in patients with gradually developing illnesses or pyrexia of unknown origin without localising features. Necrotic colorectal metastases can be misdiagnosed as hepatic abscess.

Investigations

Liver imaging is the most revealing investigation and shows 90% or more of symptomatic abscesses. Needle aspiration under ultrasound guidance confirms the diagnosis and provides pus for culture. A leucocytosis is frequently found, plasma ALP activity is usually increased, and the serum albumin is often low. The chest X-ray may show a raised right diaphragm and lung collapse, or an effusion at the base of the right lung. Blood cultures are positive in 50–80%. Abscesses caused by gut-derived organisms require active exclusion of significant colonic pathology, such as a colonoscopy to exclude colorectal carcinoma.

Management

This includes prolonged antibiotic therapy and drainage of the abscess. Associated biliary obstruction and cholangitis require biliary drainage (preferably endoscopically). Pending the results of culture of blood and pus from the abscess, treatment should be commenced with a combination of antibiotics such as ampicillin, gentamicin and metronidazole. Aspiration or drainage with a catheter placed in the abscess under ultrasound guidance is required if the abscess is large or if it does not respond to antibiotics. Surgical drainage is rarely undertaken, although hepatic resection may be indicated for a chronic persistent abscess or 'pseudotumour'.

Hydatid cysts

Hydatid cysts are caused by *Echinococcus granulosus* infection (p. 380). They have an outer layer derived from the host, an intermediate laminated layer and an inner germinal layer. They can be single (Fig. 23.27) or multiple. Chronic cysts become calcified. The cysts may

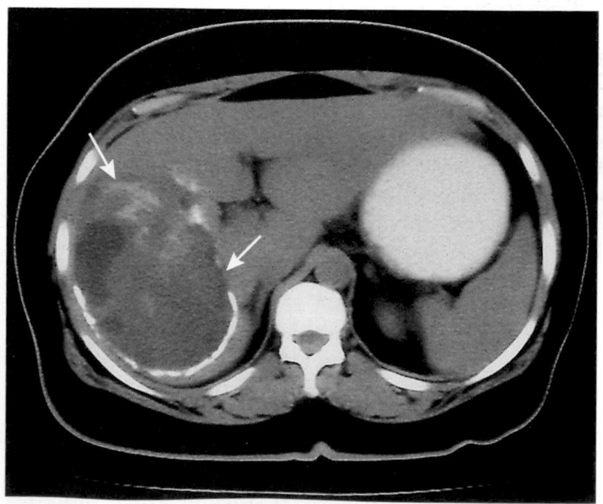

Fig. 23.27 Hydatid cyst of the liver on CT (arrows).

be asymptomatic but may present with abdominal pain or a mass. Peripheral blood eosinophilia is present in 20% of cases, whilst X-rays may show calcification of the rim of the abscess. CT reliably shows the cyst(s), and *Echinococcus* enzyme-linked immunosorbent assay (ELISA) has 90% sensitivity for hepatic hydatid cysts. Rupture or secondary infection of cysts can occur, and a communication with the intrahepatic biliary tree can then result, with associated biliary obstruction.

All patients should be treated medically with albendazole or mebendazole prior to definitive therapy. In the absence of communications with the biliary tree, treatment consists of percutaneous aspiration of the cyst followed by the injection of 100% ethanol into the cysts and then re-aspiration of the cyst contents (PAIR). Where there is communication between the cyst and biliary system, surgical removal of the intact cyst is the preferred treatment.

Amoebic liver abscesses

Amoebic liver abscesses are caused by *Entamoeba histolytica* infection (p. 367). Up to 50% of cases do not have a previous history of intestinal disease. Although amoebic liver abscesses are most often found in endemic areas, patients can present with no history of travel to these places. Abscesses are usually large, single and located in the right lobe; multiple abscesses may occur in advanced disease. Fever and abdominal pain or swelling are the most common symptoms. Diagnosis may depend on cyst aspiration revealing the classic anchovy sauce appearance of the cyst fluid. Analysis of serum for *Entamoeba* antibodies by immunoassay carries 99% sensitivity and over 90% specificity, and is more accurate than stool analysis in amoebic liver disease. Treatment is described on page 368.

ALCOHOLIC LIVER DISEASE

Alcohol is one of the most common causes of chronic liver disease worldwide, with consumption continuing to increase in many countries. Patients with alcoholic liver disease (ALD) may also have risk factors for other liver diseases (e.g. coexisting NAFLD or chronic viral hepatitis infection), and these may interact to increase disease severity.

In the UK, a unit of alcohol contains 8 g of ethanol (Box 23.51). A threshold of 14 units/week in women and 21 units/week in men is generally considered safe. The risk threshold for developing ALD is variable but begins at 30 g/day of ethanol. However, there is no clear linear relationship between dose and liver damage. For many, consumption of more than 80 g/day, for more than 5 years, is required to confer significant risk of advanced liver disease. The average alcohol consumption of a man with cirrhosis is 160 g/day for over 8 years. Some of the risk factors for ALD are:

- *Drinking pattern*. ALD and alcohol dependence are not synonymous; many of those who develop ALD are not alcohol-dependent and most dependent drinkers have normal liver function. Liver damage is more likely to occur in continuous rather than intermittent or 'binge' drinkers, as this pattern gives the liver a chance to recover. It is therefore recommended that people should have at least two alcohol-free days each week. The type of beverage does not affect risk.
- *Gender*. The incidence of alcoholic liver disease is increasing in women, who have higher blood ethanol levels than men after consuming the same amount of alcohol. This may be related to the reduced volume of distribution of alcohol.
- *Genetics*. Alcoholism is more concordant in monozygotic than dizygotic twins. Whilst polymorphisms in the genes involved in alcohol metabolism, such as aldehyde dehydrogenase, may alter drinking behaviour, they have not been linked to ALD. Recently, the patatin-like phospholipase domain-containing 3 (*PNPLA3*) gene, also known as adiponutrin, has been implicated in the pathogenesis of both ALD and NAFLD (p. 959).
- *Nutrition*. Obesity increases the incidence of liver-related mortality by over fivefold in heavy drinkers. Ethanol itself produces 7 kcal/g (29.3 kJ/g) and many alcoholic drinks also contain sugar, which further increases the calorific value and may contribute to weight gain. Excess alcohol consumption is frequently associated with nutritional deficiencies that contribute to morbidity.

23.51 Amount of alcohol in an average drink

Alcohol type	% alcohol by volume	Amount	Units*
Beer	3.5	440 mL (1 pint)	2
	9	440 mL (1 pint)	4
Wine	10	125 mL	1
	12	750 mL	9
'Alcopops'	6	330 mL	2
Sherry	17.5	750 mL	13
Vodka/rum/gin	37.5	25 mL	1
Whisky/brandy	40	700 mL	28

*1 unit = 8 g.

Pathophysiology

Alcohol reaches peak blood concentrations after about 20 minutes, although this may be influenced by stomach contents. It is metabolised almost exclusively by the liver via one of two pathways (Fig. 23.28).

Approximately 80% of alcohol is metabolised to acetaldehyde by the mitochondrial enzyme, alcohol dehydrogenase (ADH). Acetaldehyde is then metabolised to acetyl-CoA and acetate by aldehyde dehydrogenase. This generates NADH from NAD (nicotinamide adenine dinucleotide), which changes the redox potential of the cell. Acetaldehyde forms adducts with cellular proteins in hepatocytes that activate the immune system, contributing to cell injury.

The remaining 20% of alcohol is metabolised by the microsomal ethanol-oxidising system (MEOS) pathway. Cytochrome CYP2E1 is an enzyme that oxidises ethanol to acetate. It is induced by alcohol, and during metabolism of ethanol it releases oxygen free radicals, leading to lipid peroxidation and mitochondrial damage. The CYP2E1 enzyme also metabolises acetaminophen, and

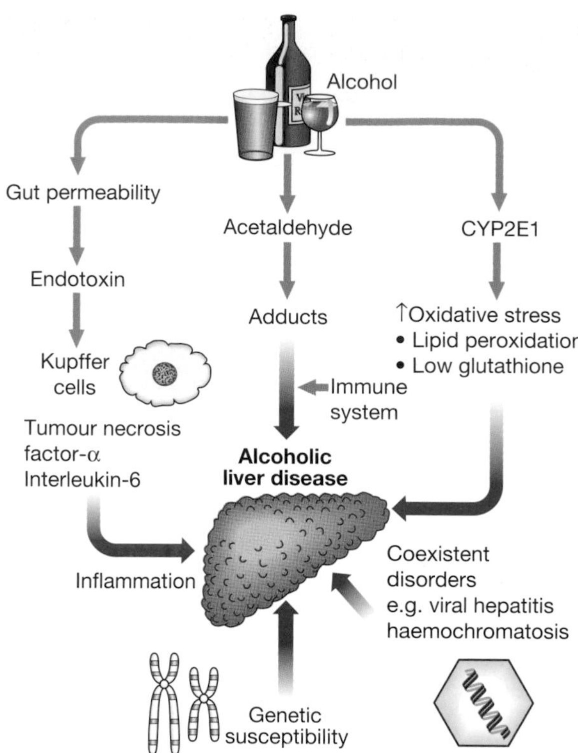

Fig. 23.28 Factors involved in the pathogenesis of alcoholic liver disease.

23.52 Pathological features of alcoholic liver disease

- Alcoholic hepatitis
  Lipogranuloma
  Neutrophil infiltration
  Mallory's hyaline
  Pericellular fibrosis
- Macrovesicular steatosis
- Fibrosis and cirrhosis
- Central hyaline sclerosis

hence chronic alcoholics are more susceptible to hepatotoxicity from low doses of paracetamol.

It is thought that pro-inflammatory cytokines may also be involved in inducing hepatic damage in alcoholic hepatitis, since endotoxin is released into the blood because of increased gut permeability, leading to release of tumour necrosis factor alpha (TNF-α), interleukin (IL)-1, IL-2 and IL-8 from immune cells. All of these cytokines have been implicated in the pathogenesis of liver fibrosis (see Fig. 23.4, p. 925).

The pathological features of alcoholic liver disease are shown in Box 23.52. In about 80% of patients with severe alcoholic hepatitis, cirrhosis will coexist at presentation. Iron deposition is common and does not necessarily indicate haemochromatosis. Figure 23.30 (p. 960) shows the histological features of alcoholic liver disease, which are identical to those of non-alcoholic steatohepatitis.

Clinical features

ALD has a wide clinical spectrum ranging from mild abnormalities of LFTs on biochemical testing to advanced cirrhosis. The liver is often enlarged in ALD, even in the presence of cirrhosis. Stigmata of chronic liver disease, such as palmar erythema, are more common in alcoholic cirrhosis than in cirrhosis of other aetiologies. Alcohol misuse may also cause damage of other organs and this should be specifically looked for (see Box 10.35, p. 253). Three types of ALD are recognised (Box 23.53) but these overlap considerably, as do the pathological changes seen in the liver.

23.53 Clinical syndromes of alcoholic liver disease

Fatty liver

- Asymptomatic abnormal liver biochemistry
- Normal/large liver

Alcoholic hepatitis

- Jaundice
- Malnutrition
- Hepatomegaly
- Features of portal hypertension (e.g. ascites, encephalopathy)

Cirrhosis

- Stigmata of chronic liver disease
- Ascites/varices/encephalopathy
- Large, normal or small liver
- Hepatocellular carcinoma

Alcoholic fatty liver disease

Alcoholic fatty liver disease (AFLD) usually presents with elevated transaminases in the absence of hepatomegaly. It has a good prognosis and steatosis usually disappears after 3 months of abstinence.

Alcoholic hepatitis

This presents with jaundice and hepatomegaly; complications of portal hypertension may also be present. It has a significantly worse prognosis than AFLD. About one-third of patients die in the acute episode, particularly those with hepatic encephalopathy or a prolonged PT. Cirrhosis often coexists; if not present, it is the likely outcome if drinking continues. Patients with acute alcoholic hepatitis often deteriorate during the first 1–3 weeks in hospital. Even if they abstain, it may take up to 6 months for jaundice to resolve. In patients presenting with jaundice who subsequently abstain, the 3- and 5-year survival is 70%. In contrast, those who continue to drink have 3- and 5-year survival rates of 60% and 34% respectively.

Alcoholic cirrhosis

Alcoholic cirrhosis often presents with a serious complication, such as variceal haemorrhage or ascites, and only half of such patients will survive 5 years from presentation. However, most who survive the initial illness and who become abstinent will survive beyond 5 years.

Investigations

Investigations aim to establish alcohol misuse, to exclude alternative or additional coexistent causes of liver disease and to assess the severity of liver damage. The clinical history from patient, relatives and friends is important to establish alcohol misuse duration and severity. Biological markers, particularly macrocytosis in the absence of anaemia, may suggest and support a history of alcohol misuse. A raised GGT is not specific for alcohol misuse and may also be elevated in the

23.54 How to assess prognosis using the Glasgow alcoholic hepatitis score

Score	1	2	3
Age	< 50	> 50	
WCC (× 10^9/L)	< 15	> 15	
Urea (mmol/L)	< 5	> 5	
PT ratio	< 1.5	1.5–2.0	> 2.0
Bilirubin (μmol/L)	< 125	125–250	> 250
A score ≥ 9 is associated with a 40% 28-day survival, compared to 80% for patients with a score < 9.			

(PT = prothrombin time; WCC = white cell count)

presence of other conditions, including NAFLD. The level may not therefore return to normal with abstinence if chronic liver disease is present, and GGT should not be relied on as an indicator of ongoing alcohol consumption. The presence of jaundice may suggest alcoholic hepatitis. Determining the extent of liver damage often requires a liver biopsy.

In alcoholic hepatitis, PT and bilirubin are used to calculate a 'discriminant function' (DF), also known as the Maddrey score, which enables the clinician to assess prognosis (PT = prothrombin time; serum bilirubin in μmol/L is divided by 17 to convert to mg/dL):

$$\mathbf{DF = [4.6 \times Increase\ in\ PT\ (sec)] + Bilirubin\ (mg/dL)}$$

A value over 32 implies severe liver disease with a poor prognosis and is used to guide treatment decisions (see below). A second scoring system, the Glasgow score, uses the age, white cell count and renal function, in addition to PT and bilirubin, to assess prognosis with a cutoff of 9 (Box 23.54).

Management

Cessation of alcohol consumption is the single most important treatment and prognostic factor. Life-long abstinence is the best advice. General health and life expectancy are improved when this occurs, irrespective of the stage of liver disease. Abstinence is even effective at preventing progression, hepatic decompensation and death once cirrhosis is present. Treatment of alcohol dependency is discussed on page 253. In the acute presentation of ALD it is important to identify and anticipate alcohol withdrawal and Wernicke's encephalopathy, which need treating in parallel with the liver disease and any complications of cirrhosis.

Nutrition

Good nutrition is very important, and enteral feeding via a fine-bore nasogastric tube may be needed in severely ill patients.

Corticosteroids

These are of value in patients with severe alcoholic hepatitis (Maddrey's discriminative score > 32) and increase survival (Box 23.55). A similar improvement in 28-day survival from 52% to 78% is seen when steroids are given to those with a Glasgow score of more than 9. Sepsis is the main side-effect of steroids, and existing sepsis and variceal haemorrhage are the main contraindications to their use. If the bilirubin has not fallen 7 days after starting steroids, the drugs are unlikely to reduce mortality and should be stopped.

EBM 23.55 Corticosteroids in alcoholic hepatitis

'In severe alcoholic hepatitis, corticosteroids improve survival at 28 days from 65% to 85% (NNT_B 5).'

- Mathurin R, et al. J Hepatol 2002; 36:480–487.

For further information: EASL Guidelines: http://www.easl.eu/_clinical-practice-guideline/issue-9-june-2012-clinical-practice-guidelines-on-the-management-of-alcoholic-liver-disease

EBM 23.56 Pentoxifylline in alcoholic hepatitis

'In severe alcoholic hepatitis, oral pentoxifylline reduces inpatient mortality, particularly from hepatorenal failure, from 46% to 25% (NNT_B 5).'

- Akriviadis E, et al. Gastroenterology 2000; 119:1637–1648.

For further information: www.easl.eu/_clinical-practice-guideline/

Pentoxifylline

Pentoxifylline, which has a weak anti-TNF action, may be beneficial in severe alcoholic hepatitis. It reduces the incidence of hepatorenal failure and its use is not complicated by sepsis (Box 23.56). It is not known whether corticosteroids, pentoxifylline or a combination is superior in the treatment of alcoholic hepatitis.

Liver transplantation

The role of liver transplantation in the management of ALD remains controversial. In many centres, ALD is a common indication for liver transplantation. The challenge is to identify patients with an unacceptable risk of returning to harmful alcohol consumption. Many programmes require a 6-month period of abstinence from alcohol before a patient is considered for transplantation. Although this relates poorly to the incidence of alcohol relapse after transplantation, liver function may improve to the extent that transplantation is no longer necessary. The outcome of transplantation for ALD is good and, if the patient remains abstinent, there is no risk of disease recurrence. Transplantation for alcoholic hepatitis has a poorer outcome and is seldom performed.

NON-ALCOHOLIC FATTY LIVER DISEASE

Non-alcoholic fatty liver disease (NAFLD) represents a spectrum of liver disease encompassing simple fatty infiltration (steatosis), fat and inflammation (non-alcoholic steatohepatitis, NASH) and cirrhosis, in the absence of excessive alcohol consumption (typically a threshold of < 20 g/day for women and < 30 g/day for men is adopted) (Fig. 23.29). While simple steatosis has not been associated with liver-related morbidity, NASH is linked with progressive liver fibrosis, cirrhosis and liver cancer, as well as increased cardiovascular risk. The true extent of associated morbidity is not well defined;

however, in one study NASH was associated with a greater than tenfold increased risk of liver-related death (2.8% vs 0.2%) and a doubling of cardiovascular risk over a mean follow-up of 13.7 years.

NAFLD is strongly associated with obesity, dyslipidaemia, insulin resistance and type 2 (non-insulin dependent) diabetes mellitus, and so may be considered to be the hepatic manifestation of the 'metabolic syndrome' (p. 805). Increasingly sedentary lifestyles and changing dietary patterns mean that the prevalence of obesity and insulin resistance has increased, making NAFLD the leading cause of liver dysfunction in the non-alcoholic, viral hepatitis-negative population in Europe and North America. Estimates vary between populations; however, one large European study found NAFLD to be present in 94% of obese patients (body mass index (BMI) > 30 kg/m^2), 67% of overweight patients (BMI > 25 kg/m^2) and 25% of normal-weight patients. The overall prevalence of NAFLD in patients with type 2 diabetes ranges from 40% to 70%. Histological NASH was found in 3–16% of apparently healthy potential living liver-donors in Europe and 6–15% in USA.

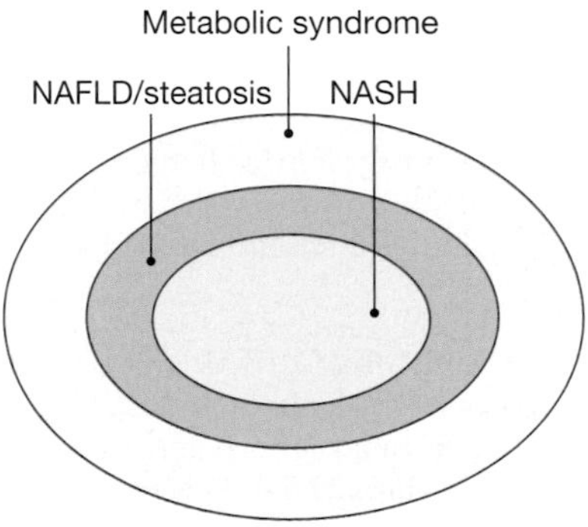

Fig. 23.29 The spectrum of non-alcoholic fatty liver disease.

Pathophysiology

Whilst the majority of patients with the metabolic syndrome develop steatosis, only a minority exhibit NASH or fibrosis. The initiating events in NAFLD are based on the development of obesity and insulin resistance, leading to increased hepatic free fatty acid flux. This imbalance between the rate of import/synthesis and the rate of export/catabolism of fatty acids in the liver leads to the development of steatosis. This may be an adaptive response through which hepatocytes store potentially toxic lipids as relatively inert triglyceride. A 'two-hit' hypothesis has been proposed to describe the pathogenesis of NAFLD, the 'first hit' causing steatosis that then progresses to steatohepatitis if a 'second hit' occurs. In reality, progression probably follows hepatocellular injury caused by a combination of several different 'hits', including:

- oxidative stress due to free radicals produced during fatty acid oxidation
- direct lipotoxicity
- gut-derived endotoxin
- cytokine release (TNF-α etc.)
- endoplasmic reticulum stress.

Cellular damage triggers a mixture of immune-mediated hepatocellular injury and cell death, which leads to stellate cell activation and hepatic fibrosis (Fig. 23.30).

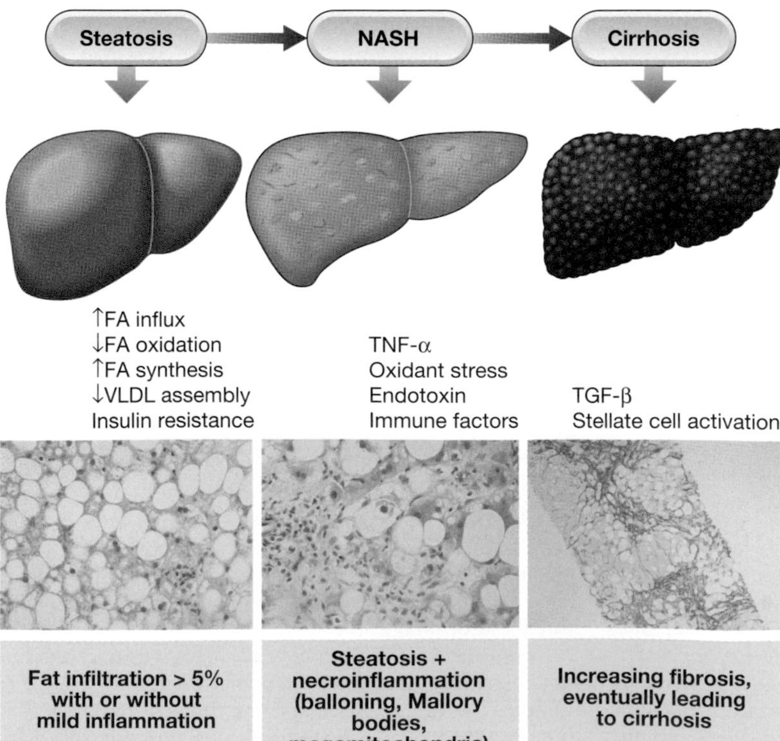

Fig. 23.30 Features of non-alcoholic fatty liver disease and non-alcoholic steatohepatitis. Rate of progression is determined by environmental (dietary) and genetic factors. (FA = fatty acids; TGF-β = transforming growth factor beta; TNF-α = tumour necrosis factor alpha; VLDL = very low-density lipoproteins)

As with many other liver diseases, subtle inter-patient genetic variations and environmental factors interact to determine disease progression. *PNPLA3* and its product, adiponutrin, may influence disease severity.

Clinical features

NAFLD is frequently asymptomatic, although it may be associated with fatigue and mild right upper quadrant discomfort. It is commonly identified as an incidental biochemical abnormality during routine blood tests. Alternatively, patients with progressive NASH may present late in the natural history of the disease with complications of cirrhosis and portal hypertension, such as variceal haemorrhage, or HCC.

The average age of NASH patients is 40–50 years (50–60 years for NASH–cirrhosis); however, the emerging epidemic of childhood obesity means that NASH is present in increasing numbers of younger patients. Most patients with NAFLD have insulin resistance and exhibit features of the metabolic syndrome (p. 805). Recognised independent risk factors for disease progression are age over 45 years, presence of diabetes (or severity of insulin resistance), obesity (BMI > 30 kg/m^2) and hypertension. These factors help with identification of 'high-risk' patient groups. NAFLD is also associated with polycystic ovary syndrome, obstructive sleep apnoea and small-bowel bacterial overgrowth.

Investigations

Investigation of patients with suspected NAFLD should be directed first towards exclusion of excess alcohol consumption and other liver diseases (including viral, autoimmune and other metabolic causes), and then at confirming the presence of NAFLD, discriminating simple steatosis from NASH and determining the extent of any hepatic fibrosis that is present.

Biochemical tests

There is no single diagnostic blood test for NAFLD. Elevations of serum ALT and AST are modest, and usually less than twice the upper limit of normal. ALT levels fall as hepatic fibrosis increases and the characteristic AST : ALT ratio of less than 1 seen in NASH reverses (AST : ALT > 1) as disease progresses towards cirrhosis, meaning that steatohepatitis with advanced disease may be present even in those with normal-range ALT levels. Other laboratory abnormalities that may be present include non-specific elevations of GGT, low-titre ANA in 20–30% of patients and elevated ferritin levels.

Imaging

Ultrasound is most often used and provides a qualitative assessment of hepatic fat content, as the liver appears 'bright' due to increased echogenicity; however, sensitivity is limited when fewer than 33% of hepatocytes are steatotic. Alternatives include CT, MRI or MR spectroscopy, which offer greater sensitivity for detecting lesser degrees of steatosis, but these are resource-intensive and not widely used in routine practice. Currently, no routine imaging modality can distinguish simple steatosis from steatohepatitis or accurately quantify hepatic fibrosis short of cirrhosis.

Liver biopsy

Liver biopsy remains the 'gold standard' investigation for diagnosis and assessment of degree of inflammation and extent of liver fibrosis. The histological definition of NASH is based on a combination of three lesions (steatosis, hepatocellular injury and inflammation; see Fig. 23.30) with a mainly centrilobular, acinar zone 3, distribution. Specific features include hepatocyte ballooning degeneration with or without acidophil bodies or spotty necrosis and a mild, mixed inflammatory infiltrate. These may be accompanied by Mallory–Denk bodies. Perisinusoidal fibrosis is a characteristic feature of NASH. Histological scoring systems are widely used to assess disease severity semi-quantitatively.

It is important to note that hepatic fat content tends to diminish as cirrhosis develops and so NASH is likely to be under-diagnosed in the setting of advanced liver disease, where it is thought to be the underlying cause of 30–75% of cases in which no specific aetiology is readily identified (so-called 'cryptogenic cirrhosis').

Management

As a marker of the metabolic syndrome, identification of NAFLD should prompt screening for and treatment of cardiovascular risk factors in all patients. However, in recognition of the greater morbidity associated with NASH as opposed to simple steatosis, liver-targeted treatment should be focused particularly on those patients with NASH.

Non-pharmacological treatment

Current treatment comprises lifestyle interventions to promote weight loss and improve insulin sensitivity through dietary changes and physical exercise. Sustained weight reduction of 7–10% is associated with significant improvement in histological and biochemical NASH severity.

Pharmacological treatment

No pharmacological agents are currently licensed specifically for NASH therapy. Treatment directed at coexisting metabolic disorders, such as dyslipidaemia and hypertension, should be given. Although use of HMG-CoA reductase inhibitors (statins) does not ameliorate NAFLD, there does not appear to be any increased risk of hepatotoxicity or other side-effects from these agents, and so they may be used to treat dyslipidaemia. Specific insulin-sensitising agents, in particular glitazones, may help selected patients, while positive results with high-dose vitamin E (800 U/day) have been tempered by evidence that high doses may be associated with an increased risk of prostate cancer and all-cause mortality, which has limited its use.

AUTOIMMUNE LIVER AND BILIARY DISEASE

The liver is an important target for autoimmune injury. The clinical picture is dictated by the nature of the autoimmune process and, in particular, the target cell for immune injury. The disease patterns are quite distinctive for primary hepatocellular injury (in the context of autoimmune hepatitis) and biliary epithelial cell injury (primary biliary cirrhosis and primary sclerosing cholangitis).

Autoimmune hepatitis

Autoimmune hepatitis is a disease of immune-mediated liver injury characterised by the presence of serum antibodies and peripheral blood T lymphocytes reactive with self-proteins, a strong association with other autoimmune diseases (Box 23.57), and high levels of serum immunoglobulins – in particular, elevation of IgG. Although most commonly seen in women, particularly in the second and third decades of life, it can develop in either sex at any age. The reasons for the breakdown in immune tolerance in autoimmune hepatitis remain unclear, although cross-reactivity with viruses such as HAV and EBV in immunogenetically susceptible individuals (typically those with human leucocyte antigen (HLA)-DR3 and DR4, particularly HLA-DRB3*0101 and HLA-DRB1*0401) has been suggested as a mechanism.

Pathophysiology

Several subtypes of this disorder have been proposed that have differing immunological markers. Although the different patterns can be associated with variation in disease aspects such as response to immunosuppressive therapy, histological patterns are similar in the different settings and the basic approach to treatment (complete control of liver injury using immunosuppressive drugs and maintained with appropriate therapy) is the same. The formal classification into disease types has fallen out of favour in recent years.

The most frequently seen autoantibody pattern is high titre of antinuclear and anti-smooth muscle antibodies, typically associated with IgG hyperglobulinaemia (type I autoimmune hepatitis in the old classification), frequently seen in young adult females. Disease characterised by the presence of anti-LKM (liver–kidney microsomal) antibodies, recognising cytochrome P450-IID6 expressed on the hepatocyte membrane, is typically seen in paediatric populations and can be more resistant to treatment than ANA-positive disease. Adult onset of anti-LKM can be seen in chronic HCV infection. This was classified as type II disease in the old system. More recently, a pattern of antibody reactivity with anti-soluble liver antigen has been described in typically adult patients, often with aggressive disease and usually lacking autoantibodies of other specificities.

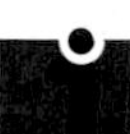

23.57 Conditions associated with autoimmune hepatitis

- Migrating polyarthritis
- Urticarial rashes
- Lymphadenopathy
- Hashimoto's thyroiditis
- Thyrotoxicosis
- Myxoedema
- Pleurisy
- Coombs-positive haemolytic anaemia
- Transient pulmonary infiltrates
- Ulcerative colitis
- Glomerulonephritis
- Nephrotic syndrome

Clinical features

The onset is usually insidious, with fatigue, anorexia and jaundice. In about one-quarter of patients, the onset is acute, resembling viral hepatitis, but resolution does not occur. This acute presentation can lead to extensive liver necrosis and liver failure. Other features include fever, arthralgia, vitiligo and epistaxis. Amenorrhoea can occur. Jaundice is mild to moderate or occasionally absent, but signs of chronic liver disease, especially spider naevi and hepatosplenomegaly, can be present. Associated autoimmune disease, such as Hashimoto's thyroiditis or rheumatoid arthritis, is often present and can modulate the clinical presentation.

Investigations

Serological tests for autoantibodies are often positive (Box 23.58), but low titres of these antibodies occur in some healthy people and in patients with other inflammatory liver diseases. ANA also occur in connective tissue diseases and other autoimmune diseases (with an identical pattern of homogenous nuclear staining) while anti-smooth muscle antibody has been reported in infectious mononucleosis and a variety of malignant diseases. Anti-microsomal antibodies (anti-LKM) occur particularly in children and adolescents. Elevated serum IgG levels are an important diagnostic and treatment response feature if present, but the diagnosis is still possible in the presence of normal IgG levels. If the diagnosis of autoimmune hepatitis is suspected, liver biopsy should be performed. It typically shows interface hepatitis, with or without cirrhosis.

Management

Treatment with corticosteroids is life-saving in autoimmune hepatitis, particularly during exacerbations of active and symptomatic disease. Initially, prednisolone 40 mg/day is given orally; the dose is then gradually reduced as the patient and LFTs improve. Maintenance therapy should only be instituted once LFTs are normal (as well as IgG if elevated). Approaches to maintenance include reduced-dose prednisolone (ideally below 5–10 mg/day), usually in the context of azathioprine 1.0–1.5 mg/kg/day (Box 23.59). Azathioprine can also be used as the sole maintenance immunosuppressive

23.58 Frequency of autoantibodies in chronic non-viral liver diseases and in healthy people

Disease	Antinuclear antibody (%)	Anti-smooth muscle antibody (%)	Antimitochondrial antibody*
Healthy controls	5	1.5	0.01
Autoimmune hepatitis	80	70	15
Primary biliary cirrhosis	25	35	95
Cryptogenic cirrhosis	40	30	15

*Patients with antimitochondrial antibody frequently have cholestatic LFTs and may have primary biliary cirrhosis (see text).

EBM 23.59 Immunosuppression in autoimmune hepatitis

'In autoimmune hepatitis, treatment with prednisolone ± azathioprine improves serum biochemistry and hepatic histology. It also improves survival at 10 years from 27% to 63% (NNT_B 2.7).'

'In patients who have been in remission for more than 1 year, increasing the dose of azathioprine (from 1 to 2 mg/kg) and withdrawing prednisolone reduces steroid side-effects and does not increase the risk of relapse.'

- Kirk AP, et al. Gut 1980; 21:78–83.
- Johnson PJ, et al. N Engl J Med 1995; 333:958–963.

agent in patients with low-activity disease. Newer agents such as mycophenolate mofetil (MMF) are increasingly being used but formal evidence to inform practice in this area is lacking. Patients should be monitored for acute exacerbations (LFT and IgG screening with patients alerted to the possible symptoms) and such exacerbations should be treated with corticosteroids. Although treatment can significantly reduce the rate of progression to cirrhosis, end-stage disease can be seen in patients despite treatment.

Primary biliary cirrhosis

Primary biliary cirrhosis (PBC) is a chronic, progressive cholestatic liver disease that predominantly affects middle-aged women. It is strongly associated with the presence of antimitochondrial antibodies (AMA), which are diagnostic, and is characterised by a granulomatous inflammation of the portal tracts, leading to progressive damage and eventually loss of the small and middle-sized bile ducts. This in turn leads to fibrosis and cirrhosis of the liver. The condition typically presents with an insidious onset of itching and/or tiredness; it may also be found incidentally as the result of routine blood tests.

Epidemiology

The prevalence of PBC varies across the world. It is relatively common in northern Europe and North America but is rare in Africa and Asia. There is a strong female-to-male predominance of 9:1; it is also more common amongst cigarette smokers. Clustering of cases has been reported, suggesting an environmental trigger in susceptible individuals.

Pathophysiology

Immune mechanisms are clearly involved. The condition is closely associated with other autoimmune non-hepatic diseases, such as thyroid disease, and there is a genetic association with HLA-DR8, together with polymorphisms in a number of other genes regulating the nature of the immune response (e.g. IL-12 and its receptor). AMA are directed at pyruvate dehydrogenase complex, a mitochondrial enzyme complex that plays a key role in cellular energy generation. PBC-specific ANA (such as those directed at the nuclear pore antigen gp210) have a characteristic staining pattern in immunofluorescence assays (selectively binding to the nuclear rim or nuclear dots), which means that they should

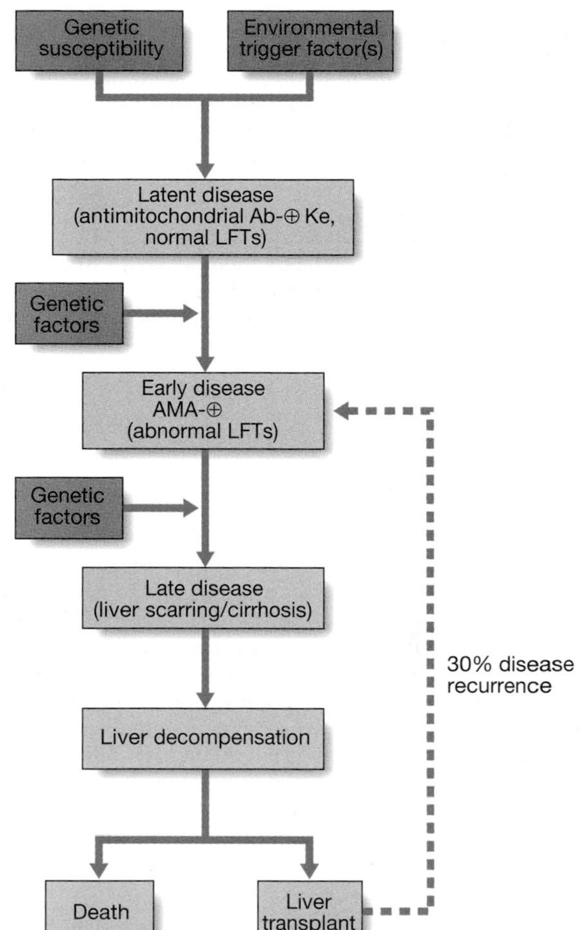

Fig. 23.31 Natural history of primary biliary cirrhosis.

not be mistaken for the homogenously staining ANA seen in autoimmune hepatitis. Elevations in serum immunoglobulin levels are frequent but, unlike in autoimmune hepatitis, elevation is typically of IgM.

Pathologically, chronic granulomatous inflammation destroys the interlobular bile ducts; progressive lymphocyte-mediated inflammatory damage causes fibrosis, which spreads from the portal tracts to the liver parenchyma and eventually leads to cirrhosis. A model of the natural history of the disease process is shown in Figure 23.31.

Clinical features

Systemic symptoms such as fatigue are common and may precede diagnosis for years. Pruritus, which can be a feature of any cholestatic disease, is a common presenting complaint and may precede jaundice by months or years. Jaundice is rarely a presenting feature. The itching is usually worse on the limbs. Although there may be right upper abdominal discomfort, fever and rigors do not occur. Bone pain or fractures can rarely result from osteomalacia (fat-soluble vitamin malabsorption) or, more commonly, from osteoporosis (hepatic osteodystrophy).

Initially, patients are well nourished but weight loss can occur as the disease progresses. Scratch marks may be found in patients with severe pruritus.

Jaundice is only prominent late in the disease and can become intense. Xanthomatous deposits occur in a minority, especially around the eyes. Mild hepatomegaly is common and splenomegaly becomes increasingly common as portal hypertension develops. Liver failure may supervene.

Associated diseases

Autoimmune and connective tissue diseases occur with increased frequency in PBC, particularly the sicca syndrome (p. 1114), systemic sclerosis, coeliac disease (p. 879) and thyroid diseases. Hypothyroidism should always be considered in patients with fatigue.

Diagnosis and investigations

The LFTs show a pattern of cholestasis (see Box 23.2, p. 929). Hypercholesterolaemia is common and worsens as disease progresses; however, it is of no diagnostic value. AMA is present in over 95% of patients, and when it is absent the diagnosis should not be made without obtaining histological evidence and considering cholangiography (MRCP or ERCP) to exclude other biliary disease. ANA and anti-smooth muscle antibodies are present in around 15% of patients (see Box 23.58); autoantibodies found in associated diseases may also be present. Ultrasound examination shows no sign of biliary obstruction. Liver biopsy is only necessary if there is diagnostic uncertainty. The histological features of PBC correlate poorly with the clinical features; portal hypertension can develop before the histological onset of cirrhosis.

Management

The hydrophilic bile acid, ursodeoxycholic acid (UDCA), at a dose of 13–15 mg/kg/day improves bile flow, replaces toxic hydrophobic bile acids in the bile acid pool, and reduces apoptosis of the biliary epithelium. Clinically, UDCA improves LFTs, may slow down histological progression and has few side-effects (Box 23.60); it is therefore widely used in the treatment of PBC and should be regarded as the optimal first-line treatment. A significant minority of patients either fail to normalise their LFTs with UDCA or show an inadequate response, and such patients have an increased risk of developing end-stage liver disease compared to patients showing a full response. There is currently no consensus as to how to treat such patients. Immunosuppressants, such as corticosteroids, azathioprine, penicillamine and ciclosporin, have all been trialled in PBC. None shows overall benefit when given to unselected patients. Whether they offer benefit to the specific subgroup of UDCA non-responding patients requiring second-line approaches to treatment is not clear.

Liver transplantation should be considered once liver failure has developed and may be indicated in patients with intractable pruritus. Serum bilirubin remains the most reliable marker of declining liver function. Transplantation is associated with an excellent 5-year survival of over 80%, although the disease will recur in over one-third of patients at 10 years.

Pruritus

This is the main symptom requiring treatment. The cause is unknown but up-regulation of opioid receptors and increased levels of endogenous opioids may play a role. First-line treatment is with the anion-binding resin colestyramine, which probably acts by binding potential pruritogens in the intestine and increasing their excretion in the stool. A dose of 4–16 g/day orally is used. The powder is mixed in orange juice and the main dose (8 g) taken before and after breakfast, when maximal duodenal bile acid concentrations occur. Colestyramine may bind other drugs in the gut (most obviously UDCA), and adequate spacing should be used between drugs. Colestyramine is sometimes ineffective, especially in complete biliary obstruction, and can be difficult for some patients to tolerate. Alternative treatments include rifampicin (150 mg/day, titrated up to a maximum of 600 mg/day as required and contingent on there being no deterioration in LFTs), naltrexone (an opioid antagonist; 25 mg/day initially, increasing up to 300 mg/day), plasmapheresis and a liver support device (e.g. a molecular adsorbent recirculating system (MARS)).

Fatigue

Fatigue affects about one-third of patients with PBC. The cause is unknown but it may reflect intracerebral changes due to cholestasis. Unfortunately, once depression, hypothyroidism and coeliac disease have been excluded, there is currently no specific treatment. The impact on patients' lives can be substantial.

Malabsorption

Prolonged cholestasis is associated with steatorrhoea and malabsorption of fat-soluble vitamins, which should be replaced as necessary. Coeliac disease should be excluded since its incidence is increased in PBC.

Bone disease

Osteopenia and osteoporosis are common, and normal post-menopausal bone loss is accelerated. Baseline bone density should be measured (p. 1122) and treatment started with replacement calcium and vitamin D_3. Bisphosphonates should be used if there is evidence of osteoporosis. Osteomalacia is rare.

EBM 23.60 Ursodeoxycholic acid (UDCA) in primary biliary cirrhosis

'In primary biliary cirrhosis, UDCA therapy (13–15 mg/kg/day) improves biochemical markers of cholestasis and jaundice. Some randomised trials have shown that UDCA treatment significantly slows disease progression, but whether it affects mortality or transplantation rates remains controversial.'

- Poupon RE, et al. Gastroenterology 1997; 113:884–890.
- Corpechot C, et al. Hepatology 2000; 32:1196–1199.
- Goulis J, et al. Lancet 1999; 354:1053–1060.

For further information: www.easl.eu/_clinical-practice-guideline/

Overlap syndromes

AMA-negative PBC ('autoimmune cholangitis')

A few patients demonstrate the clinical, biochemical and histological features of PBC but do not have detectable AMA in the serum. Serum transaminases, serum Ig levels and titres of ANA tend to be higher than in AMA-positive PBC. However, the clinical course mirrors classical PBC and these patients should be considered to have a variant of PBC.

PBC/autoimmune hepatitis overlap

A few patients with AMA and cholestatic LFTs have elevated transaminases, high serum immunoglobulins and interface hepatitis on liver histology; in such individuals a trial of corticosteroid therapy may be beneficial.

Primary sclerosing cholangitis

Primary sclerosing cholangitis (PSC) is a cholestatic liver disease caused by diffuse inflammation and fibrosis; it can involve the entire biliary tree and leads to the gradual obliteration of intrahepatic and extrahepatic bile ducts, and ultimately biliary cirrhosis, portal hypertension and hepatic failure. Although considered as an autoimmune disease, evidence for an autoimmune pathophysiology is weaker than is the case for PBC and autoimmune hepatitis. The incidence is about 6.3/100 000 in Caucasians. Cholangiocarcinoma develops in about 10–30% of patients during the course of the disease.

PSC is twice as common in young men. Most patients present at age 25–40 years, although the condition may be diagnosed at any age and is an important cause of chronic liver disease in children. The generally accepted diagnostic criteria are:

- generalised beading and stenosis of the biliary system on cholangiography (Fig. 23.32)
- absence of choledocholithiasis (or history of bile duct surgery)
- exclusion of bile duct cancer, by prolonged follow-up.

The term 'secondary sclerosing cholangitis' is used to describe the typical bile duct changes described above when a clear predisposing factor for duct fibrosis can be identified. The causes of secondary sclerosing cholangitis are shown in Box 23.61.

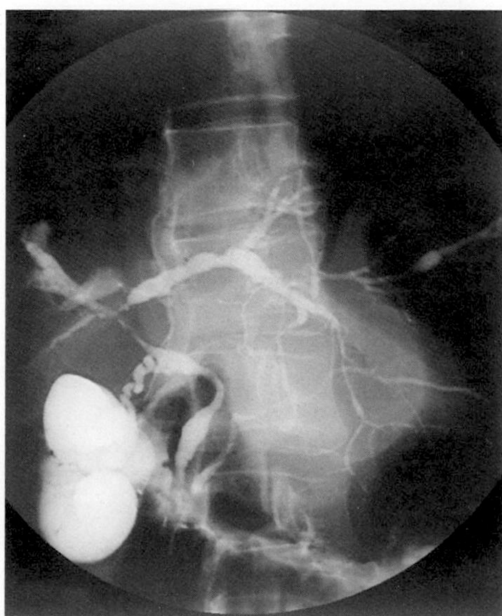

Fig. 23.32 A percutaneous cholangiogram in sclerosing cholangitis, showing characteristic irregularity of the biliary tree.

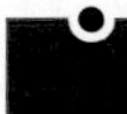

23.61 Causes of secondary sclerosing cholangitis

- Previous bile duct surgery with stricturing and cholangitis
- Bile duct stones causing cholangitis
- Intrahepatic infusion of 5-fluorodeoxyuridine
- Insertion of formalin into hepatic hydatid cysts
- Insertion of alcohol into hepatic tumours
- Parasitic infections (e.g. *Clonorchis*)
- Autoimmune pancreatitis/IgG4-associated cholangitis
- Acquired immunodeficiency syndrome (AIDS; probably infective as a result of cytomegalovirus or *Cryptosporidium*)

23.62 Diseases associated with primary sclerosing cholangitis

- Ulcerative colitis
- Crohn's colitis
- Chronic pancreatitis
- Retroperitoneal fibrosis
- Riedel's thyroiditis
- Retro-orbital tumours
- Immune deficiency states
- Sjögren's syndrome
- Angio-immunoplastic lymphadenopathy
- Histiocytosis X
- Autoimmune haemolytic anaemia
- Autoimmune pancreatitis/ IgG4-associated cholangitis

23

Pathophysiology

The cause of PSC is unknown but there is a close association with inflammatory bowel disease, particularly ulcerative colitis (Box 23.62). About two-thirds of patients have coexisting ulcerative colitis, and PSC is the most common form of chronic liver disease in ulcerative colitis. Between 3% and 10% of patients with ulcerative colitis develop PSC, particularly those with extensive colitis or pancolitis. The prevalence of primary sclerosing cholangitis is lower in patients with Crohn's colitis (about 1%). Patients with PSC and ulcerative colitis are at greater risk of colorectal neoplasia than those with ulcerative colitis alone, and those who develop colorectal neoplasia are at greater risk of cholangiocarcinoma.

It is currently believed that PSC is an immunologically mediated disease, triggered in genetically susceptible individuals by toxic or infectious agents, which may gain access to the biliary tract through a leaky, diseased colon. A close link with HLA haplotype A1 B8 DR3 DRW52A has been identified. This haplotype is commonly found in association with other organ-specific autoimmune diseases (e.g. autoimmune hepatitis).

The importance of immunological factors has been emphasised by reports showing humoral and cellular abnormalities in PSC. Perinuclear antineutrophil cytoplasmic antibodies (ANCA) have been detected in the sera of 60–80% of patients with PSC with or without ulcerative colitis, and in 30–40% of patients with ulcerative colitis alone. The antibody is not specific for PSC and is found in other chronic liver diseases (e.g. 50% of patients with autoimmune hepatitis).

Clinical features

The diagnosis is often made incidentally when persistently raised serum ALP is discovered in an individual with ulcerative colitis. Common symptoms include fatigue, intermittent jaundice, weight loss, right upper quadrant abdominal pain and pruritus. Attacks of acute cholangitis are uncommon and usually follow biliary instrumentation. Physical examination is abnormal in about 50% of symptomatic patients; the most common findings are jaundice and hepatomegaly/splenomegaly. The condition may be associated with many other diseases (see Box 23.62).

Investigations

Biochemical screening usually reveals a cholestatic pattern of LFTs but ALP and bilirubin levels may vary widely in individual patients during the course of the disease. For example, ALP and bilirubin values increase during acute cholangitis, decrease after therapy, and sometimes fluctuate for no apparent reason. Modest elevations in serum transaminases are usually seen, whereas hypoalbuminaemia and clotting abnormalities are found only at a late stage. In addition to ANCA, low titres of serum ANA and anti-smooth muscle antibodies may be found in PSC but have no diagnostic significance; serum AMA is absent.

The key investigation is now MRCP, which is usually diagnostic, revealing multiple irregular stricturing and dilatation (see Fig. 23.32). ERCP should be reserved for patients in whom therapeutic intervention is likely to be necessary and should follow MRCP.

On liver biopsy the characteristic early features of PSC are periductal 'onion-skin' fibrosis and inflammation, with portal oedema and bile ductular proliferation resulting in expansion of the portal tracts (Fig. 23.33). Later, fibrosis spreads, progressing inevitably to biliary cirrhosis; obliterative cholangitis leads to the so-called 'vanishing bile duct syndrome'.

Management

There is no cure for PSC, but management of cholestasis and its complications and specific treatment of the disease process are indicated. UDCA is widely used, although the evidence to support this is limited. UDCA may have benefit in terms of reducing colon carcinoma risk.

The course of PSC is variable. In symptomatic patients, median survival from presentation to death or liver transplantation is about 12 years. About 75% of asymptomatic patients survive 15 years or more. Most patients die from liver failure, about 30% die from bile duct carcinoma, and the remainder die from colonic cancer or complications of colitis. Immunosuppressive agents, including prednisolone, azathioprine, methotrexate and ciclosporin, have been tried; generally, results have been disappointing.

Symptomatic patients often have pruritus. Management is as for PBC. Fatigue appears to be less prominent than in PBC, although it is still present in some patients.

Management of complications

Broad-spectrum antibiotics (e.g. ciprofloxacin) should be given for acute attacks of cholangitis but have no proven value in preventing attacks. If cholangiography shows a well-defined obstruction to the extrahepatic bile ducts ('dominant stricture'), mechanical relief can be obtained by placement of a plastic stent or by balloon dilatation performed at ERCP. It is important, in this situation, actively to consider the possibility of cholangiocarcinoma (the differential diagnosis for dominant extrahepatic stricture). Fat-soluble vitamin replacement is necessary in jaundiced patients. Metabolic bone disease (usually osteoporosis) is a common complication that requires treatment (p. 1120).

Surgical treatment

Surgical resection of the extrahepatic bile duct and biliary reconstruction have a limited role in the management of non-cirrhotic patients with dominant extrahepatic disease. Orthotopic transplantation is the only surgical option in patients with advanced liver disease; 5-year survival is 80–90% in most centres. Unfortunately, the condition may recur in the graft and there are no identified therapies able to prevent this. Cholangiocarcinoma is a contraindication to transplantation. Colon carcinoma risk can be increased in patients following transplant because of the effects of immune suppression and enhanced surveillance should be instituted.

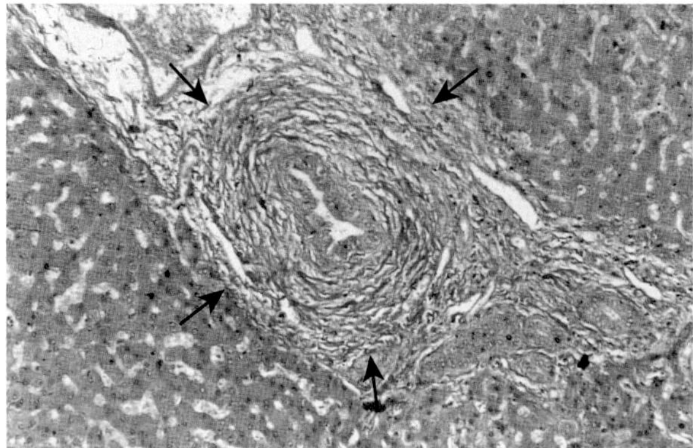

Fig. 23.33 Primary sclerosing cholangitis. Note onion-skin scarring (arrows) surrounding a bile duct.

IgG4-associated cholangitis

This recently reported disease (as well as its nomenclature) is closely related to autoimmune pancreatitis (which is present in more than 90% of the patients; p. 894). IgG4-associated cholangitis (IAC) often presents with obstructive jaundice (due to either hilar stricturing/ intrahepatic sclerosing cholangitis or a low bile duct stricture), and cholangiographic appearances suggest PSC with or without hilar cholangiocarcinoma. The serum IgG4 is often raised and liver biopsy shows a lymphoplasmacytic infiltrate, with IgG4-positive plasma cells. An important observation is that, compared to PSC, IAC appears to respond well to steroid therapy.

LIVER TUMOURS AND OTHER FOCAL LIVER LESIONS

Identification of a hepatic mass lesion is common, both in patients with known pre-existing liver disease and as a primary presentation. Although primary and secondary malignant tumours are important potential diagnoses, benign disease is frequent. The finding of a liver mass, with its association in the minds of patients with metastatic malignant disease, creates a high level of anxiety, a factor that should always be borne in mind. The critical steps to be taken in diagnosing hepatic mass lesions are:

- determining the presence, nature and severity of any underlying chronic liver disease, as the differential diagnosis is very different in patients with and without chronic liver disease
- use of optimal (usually multiple) imaging modalities.

Primary malignant tumours

Hepatocellular carcinoma

Hepatocellular carcinoma (HCC) is the most common primary liver tumour, and the sixth most common cause of cancer worldwide. Cirrhosis is present in 75–90% of individuals with HCC and is an important risk factor for the disease. The risk is between 1% and 5% in cirrhosis caused by hepatitis B and C. There is also an increased risk in cirrhosis due to haemochromatosis, alcohol, NASH and α_1-antitrypsin deficiency. In northern Europe, 90% of those with HCC have underlying cirrhosis, compared with 30% in Taiwan, where hepatitis B is the main risk factor. The age-adjusted incidence rates vary from 28 per 100 000 in South-east Asia (reflecting the prevalence of hepatitis B) to 10 per 100 000 in southern Europe and 5 per 100 000 in northern Europe. Chronic hepatitis B infection increases the risk of HCC 100-fold and is the major risk factor worldwide. The risk of HCC is 0.4% per year in the absence of cirrhosis and 2–6% in cirrhosis. The risk is four times higher in HBeAg-positive individuals than in those who are HBeAg-negative. Hepatitis B vaccination has led to a fall in HCC in countries with a high prevalence of hepatitis B. The incidence in Europe and North America has risen recently, probably related to the increased prevalence of hepatitis C and NASH cirrhosis. The risk is higher in men and rises with age.

Macroscopically, the tumour usually appears as a single mass in the absence of cirrhosis, or as a single nodule or multiple nodules in the presence of cirrhosis. It takes its blood supply from the hepatic artery and tends to spread by invasion into the portal vein and its radicals. Lymph node metastases are common, while lung and bone metastases are rare. Well-differentiated tumours can resemble normal hepatocytes and can be difficult to distinguish from normal liver.

Clinical features

Patients typically present with HCC in one of two ways. Commonly, those with underlying cirrhosis develop a deterioration in their liver function, with worsening ascites and/or jaundice or variceal haemorrhage. Other characteristic symptoms can include weight loss, anorexia and abdominal pain. This often-rapid deterioration can, however, be the event that leads to previously occult cirrhosis becoming clinically apparent, meaning that absence of an established diagnosis of cirrhosis does not preclude a diagnosis of HCC complicating cirrhosis. Examination may reveal hepatomegaly or a right hypochondrial mass. Tumour vascularity can lead to an abdominal bruit, and hepatic rupture with intra-abdominal bleeding may occur. The advanced nature of the disease that presents in this way makes curative therapy unlikely.

The second presentation is through screening of patients at risk of HCC. The disease is typically detected much earlier in its natural history, significantly increasing the treatment options.

Investigations

Serum markers

Alpha-fetoprotein (AFP) is produced by 60% of HCCs. Levels increase with the size of the tumour and are often normal or only minimally elevated in small tumours detected by ultrasound screening. Serum AFP can also rise in the presence of active hepatitis B and C viral replication; very high levels are seen in acute hepatic necrosis, such as that following paracetamol toxicity. AFP is used in conjunction with ultrasound in screening but, in view of low sensitivity and specificity, levels need to be interpreted with caution. Nevertheless, in the absence of a marked hepatic flare of disease, a progressively rising AFP, or AFP over 400 ng/mL (normal is < 10 ng/mL), warrants an aggressive search for HCC. In HCC patients with elevated AFP levels, serial measurements can be a useful biomarker of disease progression/response to treatment.

Imaging

Ultrasound will detect focal liver lesions as small as 2–3 cm. The use of ultrasound contrast agents has increased sensitivity and specificity, but is highly user-dependent. Ultrasound may also show evidence of portal vein involvement and features of coexistent cirrhosis. Multidetector row CT, following intravenous contrast, identifies HCC by its classical hypervascular appearance (Fig. 23.34). Small lesions of less than 2 cm can be difficult to differentiate from hyperplastic nodules in cirrhosis. MRI can be used instead of CT. Angiography is now seldom performed and has been superseded by the above techniques. Combination of imaging modalities more accurately diagnoses and stages the extent of disease, and using at least two modalities

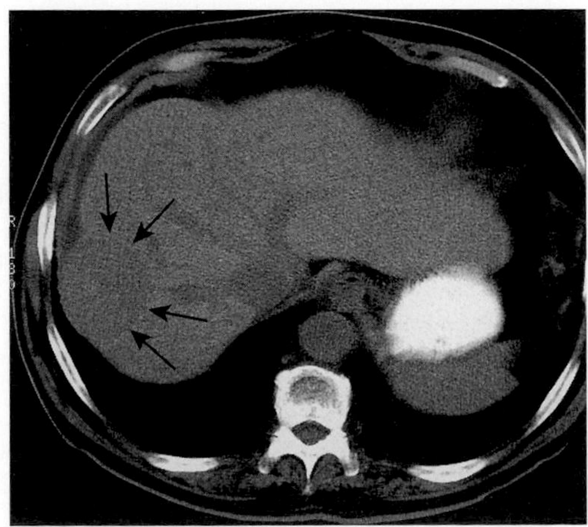

Fig. 23.34 CT showing a large hepatocellular carcinoma (arrows).

(typically, CT or MRI following initial screening ultrasound identification of a mass lesion) is recommended.

Liver biopsy

Histological confirmation is advisable in patients with large tumours who do not have cirrhosis or hepatitis B, in order to confirm the diagnosis and exclude metastatic tumour. Biopsy should be avoided in patients who may be eligible for transplantation or surgical resection because there is a small (< 2%) risk of tumour seeding along the needle tract. In all cases of potential HCC where biopsy is being considered, the impact that a confirmed diagnosis will have on therapy must be weighed against the risks of bleeding. If biopsy will not change management, then its appropriateness should be considered carefully.

Role of screening

Screening for HCC, by ultrasound scanning and AFP measurements at 6-month intervals, is indicated in high-risk patients, such as those with cirrhosis due to hepatitis B and C, haemochromatosis, alcohol, NASH and α_1-antitrypsin deficiency. It may also be indicated in individuals with chronic hepatitis B (who carry an increased risk of HCC, even in the absence of cirrhosis). Although no randomised controlled studies of outcome have been undertaken, screening identifies smaller tumours, often less than 3 cm in size, which are more likely to be cured by surgical resection, local ablative therapy or transplantation (Box 23.63). The role of screening in other forms of chronic liver disease, such as autoimmune hepatitis and PBC, is unclear. This is compounded by the fact that disease staging by biopsy is no longer standard practice in conditions such as PBC, so formal documentation of the presence of cirrhosis, which might be the trigger for commencement of HCC screening, rarely takes place.

Management

This is different for patients with cirrhosis and those without (see Box 23.63). In the presence of cirrhosis, tumour size, multicentricity, extent of liver disease (Child–Pugh score) and performance status dictate appropriate therapy. An algorithm for managing those with cirrhosis is shown in Figure 23.35.

Prognosis depends on tumour size, the presence of vascular invasion, and liver function in those with cirrhosis. Screening has improved the outlook through early detection.

EBM 23.63 Guidelines for screening and management of hepatocellular carcinoma

'Cirrhotic patients who would be suitable for curative therapy if diagnosed with hepatocellular carcinoma should be offered screening with 6-monthly ultrasound and AFP testing.'

'Curative therapies for hepatocellular carcinoma include liver transplantation, hepatic resection and ablative therapy. Treatment depends on the presence/absence of cirrhosis, underlying liver function, tumour size and tumour multicentricity.'

- European Association for the Study of the Liver Clinical Guidelines. J Hepatol 2012; 56:908–943.

For further information: www.aasld.org/practiceguidelines/

Hepatic resection

This is the treatment of choice for non-cirrhotic patients. The 5-year survival in this group is about 50%. However, there is a 50% recurrence rate at 5 years; this may be due to a second de novo tumour or recurrence of the original tumour. Few patients with cirrhosis are suitable for hepatic resection because of the high risk of hepatic failure; nevertheless, surgery is offered, particularly in the Far East, to some cirrhotic patients with small tumours and good liver function (Child–Pugh A with no portal hypertension).

Liver transplantation

Transplantation has the benefit of curing underlying cirrhosis and removing the risk of a second, de novo tumour in an at-risk patient. The requirement for immunosuppression creates its own risks of reactivation, however, if residual or metastatic disease is present, and assessment of patients for suitability for liver transplantation focuses on the exclusion of extrahepatic and vascular-invading disease. The 5-year survival following liver transplantation is 75% for patients with single tumours less than 5 cm in size or three tumours smaller than 3 cm (the Milan criteria). Unfortunately, the underlying liver disease, in particular hepatitis C, may recur in the transplanted liver and can result in recurrent cirrhosis giving rise to de novo HCC risk, now complicated by the presence of immunosuppression.

Percutaneous therapy

Percutaneous ethanol injection into the tumour under ultrasound guidance is efficacious (80% cure rate) for tumours of 3 cm or smaller. Recurrence rates (50% at 3 years) are similar to those following surgical resection. Radiofrequency ablation, using a single electrode inserted into the tumour under radiological guidance, is an alternative that takes longer to perform but may cause more complete tumour necrosis. Improvements in percutaneous therapy, with the combination of low patient impact, relative efficacy and capacity for repeat treatment, are making these approaches attractive, particularly in patients in whom major surgery would be inappropriate. Their role in primary therapy as an alternative to curative resection or transplantation remains to be established.

Trans-arterial chemo-embolisation

Hepatocellular cancers are not radiosensitive and the response rate to chemotherapy with drugs such as doxorubicin is only around 30%. In contrast, hepatic artery embolisation with Gelfoam and doxorubicin is more effective, with survival rates of 60% in cirrhotic patients with unresectable HCC and good liver function (compared with 20% in untreated patients) at 2 years. Unfortunately, any survival benefit is lost at 4 years. Trans-arterial chemo-embolisation (TACE) is contraindicated in decompensated cirrhosis and multifocal HCC. TACE is now most frequently used as a holding first intervention whilst the tumour is being assessed and the definitive management plan is being developed.

Chemotherapy

Sorafenib improves survival from 7.9 to 10.7 months in cirrhotic patients. The drug is a multikinase inhibitor with activity against Raf, vascular endothelial growth

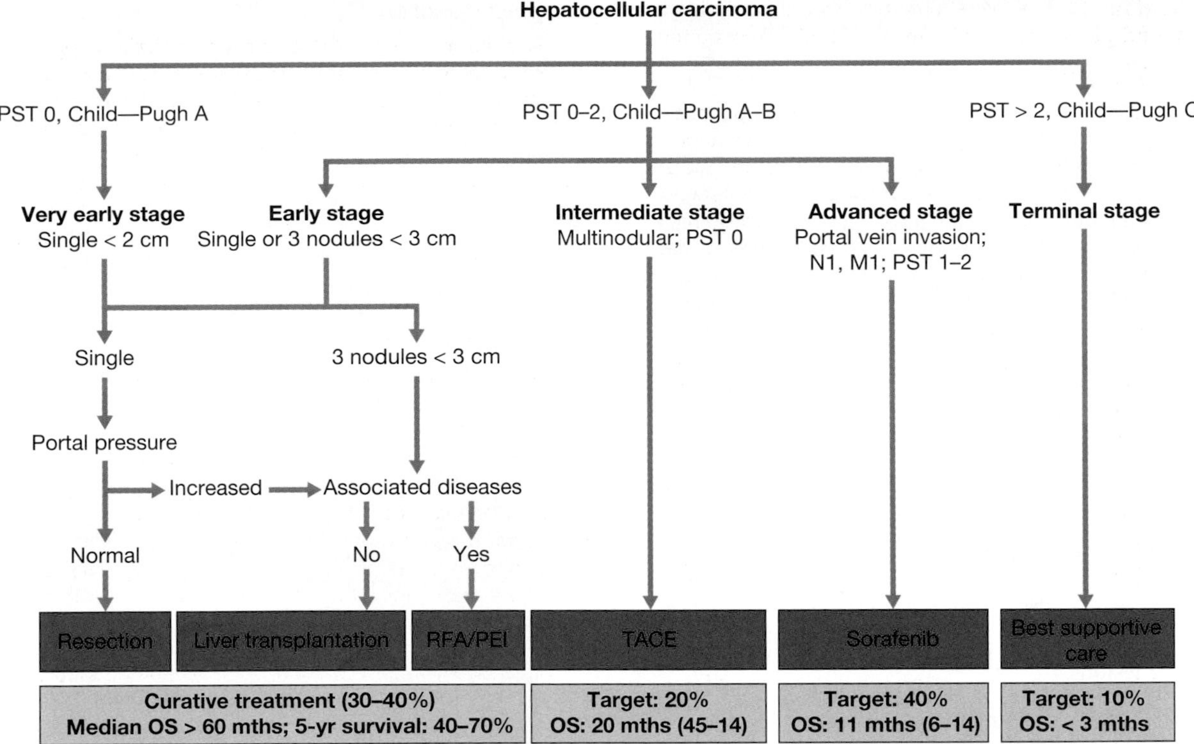

Fig. 23.35 Management of hepatocellular carcinoma complicating cirrhosis. Performance status (PST; see Box 11.3, p. 268): 0 = fully active, no symptoms; > 2 = limited self-care, confined to bed or chair for 50% of waking hours. Child–Pugh score: see Box 23.30, p. 944. N1, M1: lymph node involvement and metastases (for TNM classification, see Box 11.4, p. 268) (OS = overall survival; PEI = percutaneous ethanol injection; RFA = radiofrequency ablation; TACE = trans-arterial chemo-embolisation). Based on EASL–EORTC Clinical Practice Guidelines 2012 – see p. 988.

factor (VEGF) and platelet-derived growth factor (PDGF) signalling, and is the first systemic therapy to prolong survival in HCC. The ultimate role of sorafenib in HCC – in particular, when and how best to use it – remains to be established.

Fibrolamellar hepatocellular carcinoma

This rare variant differs from HCC in that it occurs in young adults, equally in males and females, in the absence of hepatitis B infection and cirrhosis. The tumours are often large at presentation and the AFP is usually normal. Histology of the tumour reveals malignant hepatocytes surrounded by a dense fibrous stroma. The treatment of choice is surgical resection. This variant of HCC has a better prognosis following surgery than an equivalent-sized HCC, two-thirds of patients surviving beyond 5 years.

Other primary malignant tumours

These are rare but include haemangio-endothelial sarcomas. Cholangiocarcinoma (bile duct cancer) typically presents with bile duct obstruction rather than as a hepatic mass lesion, although the latter occasionally occurs.

Secondary malignant tumours

These are common and usually originate from carcinomas in the lung, breast, abdomen or pelvis. They may be single or multiple. Peritoneal dissemination frequently results in ascites.

Clinical features

The primary neoplasm is asymptomatic in 50% of patients, being detected on either radiological, endoscopic or blood biochemistry screening. There is liver enlargement and weight loss; jaundice may be present.

Investigations

A raised ALP activity is the most common biochemical abnormality but LFTs may be normal. Ascitic fluid, if present, has a high protein content and may be blood-stained; cytology sometimes reveals malignant cells. Imaging shows filling defects (Fig. 23.36); laparoscopy may reveal the tumour and facilitates liver biopsy.

Management

Hepatic resection can improve survival for slow-growing tumours such as colonic carcinomas, and is an approach that should be actively explored in patients who are fit for liver resection, have had the primary tumour resected and in whom extrahepatic disease has been excluded. Patients with neuro-endocrine tumours, such as gastrinomas, insulinomas and glucagonomas, and those with lymphomas may benefit from surgery, hormonal treatment or chemotherapy. Unfortunately, palliative treatment to relieve pain is all that is available for most patients; this may include arterial embolisation of the tumour masses.

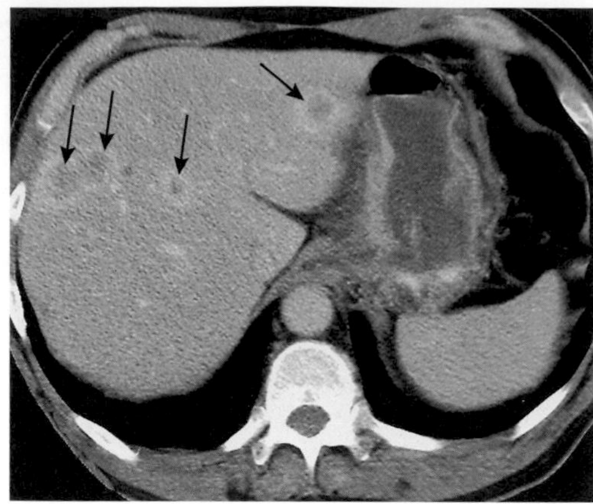

Fig. 23.36 CT showing multiple liver metastases (arrows).

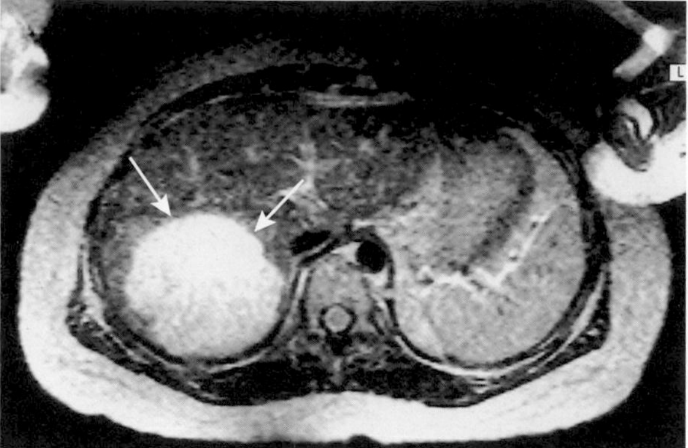

Fig. 23.37 MRI showing a haemangioma (arrows) in the liver.

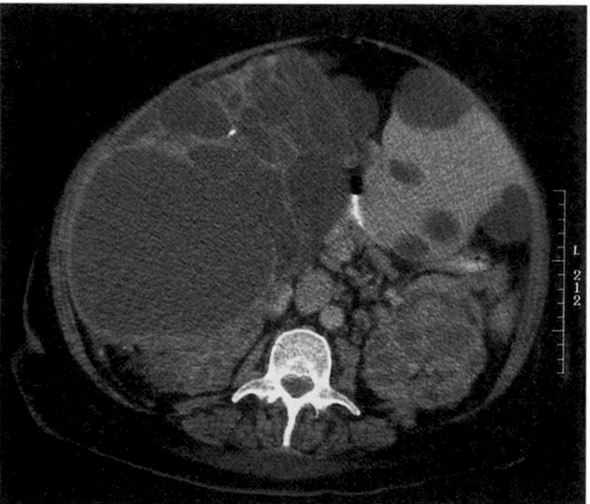

Fig. 23.38 CT showing multiple cysts in the liver and kidneys in polycystic disease.

Benign tumours

The increasing use of ultrasound scanning has led to more frequent identification of incidental benign focal liver lesions.

Hepatic adenomas

These are rare vascular tumours that may present as an abdominal mass, or with abdominal pain or intraperitoneal bleeding. They are more common in women and may be caused by oral contraceptives, androgens and anabolic steroids. Resection is indicated for the relief of symptoms. Hepatic adenomas can increase in size during pregnancy. Large or rapidly growing adenomas can, rarely, rupture, causing intraperitoneal bleeding.

Haemangiomas

These are the most common benign liver tumours and are present in 1–20% of the population. Most are smaller than 5 cm and rarely cause symptoms (Fig. 23.37). The diagnosis is usually made by ultrasound, but CT may show a low-density lesion with delayed arterial filling. Surgery is only needed for very large symptomatic lesions or where the diagnosis is in doubt.

Focal nodular hyperplasia

Focal nodular hyperplasia (FNH) is common in women under the age of 40. The lesions are usually asymptomatic but can be up to 10 cm in diameter; they can be differentiated from adenoma because of a focal central scar seen on CT or MRI. Histologically, they consist of nodular regeneration of hepatocytes but without fibrosis. They may be multiple but only rarely need resection.

Cystic liver disease and liver abscess

Isolated or multiple simple cysts are common in the liver and are a relatively frequent finding on ultrasound screening. They can be associated with polycystic renal disease (Fig. 23.38). They are intrinsically benign and require no therapy, other than in rare cases where the mass effect of very large or multiple cysts causes abdominal discomfort. In such cases, percutaneous or surgical debulking can be attempted but recurrence is typical. Liver abscesses are discussed on page 956.

DRUGS AND THE LIVER

The liver is the primary site of drug metabolism and an important target for drug-induced injury. Pre-existing liver disease may affect the capacity of the liver to metabolise drugs, and unexpected toxicity may occur when patients with liver disease are given drugs in normal doses. Box 23.64 also shows drugs that should be avoided in patients with cirrhosis, as they can exacerbate known complications of cirrhosis. The possibility of undiagnosed underlying liver injury should always be considered in patients exhibiting unexpected effects following drug exposure.

Drug-induced liver injury

Drug toxicity should always be considered in the differential diagnosis of patients presenting with acute liver failure, jaundice or abnormal liver biochemistry. Some typical patterns of drug toxicity are listed in Box 23.65; the most common picture is of a mixed cholestatic hepatitis. The presence of jaundice indicates more severe liver damage. Although acute liver failure can occur, most drug reactions are self-limiting and chronic liver damage is rare. Abnormal LFTs often take weeks to

23.64 Drugs to be avoided in cirrhosis

Drug	Problem	Toxicity
NSAIDs	Reduced renal blood flow Mucosal ulceration	Hepatorenal failure Bleeding varices
ACE inhibitors	Reduced renal blood flow	Hepatorenal failure
Codeine	Constipation	Hepatic encephalopathy
Narcotics	Constipation, drug accumulation	Hepatic encephalopathy
Anxiolytics	Drug accumulation	Hepatic encephalopathy

(ACE = angiotensin-converting enzyme)

23.65 Examples of common causes of drug-induced hepatotoxicity

Pattern	Drug
Cholestasis	Chlorpromazine High-dose oestrogens
Cholestatic hepatitis	NSAIDs Co-amoxiclav Statins
Acute hepatitis	Rifampicin Isoniazid
Non-alcoholic steatohepatitis	Amiodarone
Venous outflow obstruction	Busulfan Azathioprine
Fibrosis	Methotrexate

normalise following a drug-induced hepatitis, and it may take months for them to normalise following a cholestatic hepatitis. Occasionally, permanent bile duct loss (ductopenia) follows a cholestatic drug reaction, such as that due to co-amoxiclav, resulting in chronic cholestasis with persistent symptoms such as itching.

The key to diagnosing acute drug-induced liver disease is to take a detailed drug history (Box 23.66), looking for temporal relationships between drug exposure and onset of liver abnormality (bearing in mind the fact that liver injury can frequently take weeks or even months to develop following exposure). A liver biopsy should be considered if there is suspicion of pre-existing liver disease or if blood tests fail to improve when the suspect drug is withdrawn.

Where drug-induced liver injury is suspected or cannot be excluded, the potential culprit drug should be discontinued unless it is impossible to do so safely.

Types of liver injury

Different histological patterns of liver injury may occur with drug injury.

Cholestasis

Pure cholestasis (selective interference with bile flow in the absence of liver injury) can occur with oestrogens; this was common when high concentrations of

23.66 The diagnosis of acute drug-induced liver disease

- Tabulate the drugs taken
  - Prescribed
  - Self-administered
- Establish whether hepatotoxicity is reported in the literature
- Relate the time at which the drugs were taken to the onset of illness
  - 4 days to 8 weeks (usual)
- Establish the effect of stopping the drugs on normalisation of liver biochemistry
  - Hepatitic LFTs (2 months)
  - Cholestatic/mixed LFTs (6 months)
- Exclude other causes
  - Viral hepatitis
  - Biliary disease
- Consider liver biopsy

N.B. Challenge tests with drugs should be avoided.

oestrogens (50 μg/day) were used as contraceptives. Both the current oral contraceptive pill and hormone replacement therapy can be safely used in chronic liver disease.

Chlorpromazine and antibiotics such as flucloxacillin are examples of drugs that cause cholestatic hepatitis, which is characterised by inflammation and canalicular injury. Co-amoxiclav is the most common antibiotic to cause abnormal LFTs but, unlike other antibiotics, it may not produce symptoms until 10–42 days after it is stopped. Anabolic steroids used by body-builders may also cause a cholestatic hepatitis. In some cases (e.g. NSAIDs and cyclo-oxygenase (COX)-2 inhibitors) there is overlap with acute hepatocellular injury.

Hepatocyte necrosis

Many drugs cause an acute hepatocellular necrosis with high serum transaminase concentrations; paracetamol is the best known. Inflammation is not always present but does accompany necrosis in liver injury due to diclofenac (an NSAID) and isoniazid (an anti-tuberculous drug). Granulomas may be seen in liver injury following the use of allopurinol. Acute hepatocellular necrosis has also been described following the use of several herbal remedies, including germander, comfrey and jin bu huan. Recreational drugs, including cocaine and ecstasy, can also cause severe acute hepatitis.

Steatosis

Microvesicular hepatocyte fat deposition, due to direct effects on mitochondrial beta-oxidation, can follow exposure to tetracyclines and sodium valproate (see Box 23.69, p. 978). Macrovesicular hepatocyte fat deposition has been described with tamoxifen, and amiodarone toxicity can produce a similar histological picture to NASH.

Vascular/sinusoidal lesions

Drugs such as the alkylating agents used in oncology can damage the vascular endothelium and lead to hepatic venous outflow obstruction. Chronic overdose of vitamin A can damage the sinusoids and trigger local fibrosis that can result in portal hypertension.

Hepatic fibrosis

Most drugs cause reversible liver injury and hepatic fibrosis is very uncommon. Methotrexate, however, as well as causing acute liver injury when it is started, can lead to cirrhosis when used in high doses over a long period of time. Risk factors for drug-induced hepatic fibrosis include pre-existing liver disease and a high alcohol intake.

INHERITED LIVER DISEASES

The inherited diseases are an important and probably under-diagnosed group of liver diseases. In addition to the 'classical' conditions such as haemochromatosis and Wilson's disease, the important role played by the liver in the expression of the inborn errors of metabolism should be remembered, as should the potential for genetic underpinning for intrahepatic cholestasis.

Haemochromatosis

Haemochromatosis is a condition in which the amount of total body iron is increased; the excess iron is deposited in, and causes damage to, several organs, including the liver. It may be primary or secondary to other diseases (Box 23.67).

Hereditary haemochromatosis

In hereditary haemochromatosis (HHC), iron is deposited throughout the body and total body iron may reach 20–60 g (normally 4 g). The important organs involved are the liver, pancreatic islets, endocrine glands and heart. In the liver, iron deposition occurs first in the periportal hepatocytes, extending later to all hepatocytes. The gradual development of fibrous septa leads to the formation of irregular nodules, and finally regeneration results in macronodular cirrhosis. An excess of liver iron can occur in alcoholic cirrhosis but this is mild by comparison with haemochromatosis.

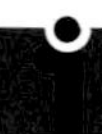

23.67 Causes of haemochromatosis

Primary haemochromatosis

- Hereditary haemochromatosis
- Congenital acaeruloplasminaemia
- Congenital atransferrinaemia

Secondary iron overload

- Parenteral iron-loading (e.g. repeated blood transfusion)
- Iron-loading anaemia (thalassaemia, sideroblastic anaemia, pyruvate kinase deficiency)
- Liver disease

Complex iron overload

- Juvenile haemochromatosis
- Neonatal haemochromatosis
- Alcoholic liver disease
- Porphyria cutanea tarda
- African iron overload (Bantu siderosis)

Pathophysiology

The disease is caused by increased absorption of dietary iron and is inherited as an autosomal recessive trait. Approximately 90% of patients are homozygous for a single-point mutation resulting in a cysteine to tyrosine substitution at position 282 (C282Y) in the HFE protein, which has structural and functional similarity to the HLA proteins. The mechanisms by which HFE regulates iron absorption are unclear. However, it is believed that HFE normally interacts with the transferrin receptor in the basolateral membrane of intestinal epithelial cells. In HHC, it is thought that the lack of functional HFE causes a defect in uptake of transferrin-associated iron, leading to up-regulation of enterocyte iron-specific divalent metal transporters and excessive iron absorption. A histidine to aspartic acid mutation at position 63 (H63D) in HFE causes a less severe form of haemochromatosis that is most commonly found in patients who are compound heterozygotes also carrying a C282Y mutated allele. Fewer than 50% of C282Y homozygotes will develop clinical features of haemochromatosis; therefore other factors must also be important. HHC may promote accelerated liver disease in patients with alcohol excess or hepatitis C infection. Iron loss in menstruation and pregnancy can delay the onset of HHC in females.

Clinical features

Symptomatic disease usually presents in men over 40 years with features of liver disease (often with hepatomegaly), diabetes mellitus or heart failure. Fatigue and arthropathy are early symptoms but are frequently absent. Leaden-grey skin pigmentation due to excess melanin occurs, especially in exposed parts, axillae, groins and genitalia: hence the term 'bronzed diabetes'. Once again, absence of this feature does not preclude the diagnosis. Impotence, loss of libido, testicular atrophy and arthritis with chondrocalcinosis secondary to calcium pyrophosphate deposition are also common. Cardiac failure or cardiac dysrhythmia may occur due to iron deposition in the heart.

Investigations

Serum iron studies show a greatly increased ferritin, a raised plasma iron and saturated plasma iron-binding capacity. Transferrin saturation of more than 45% is suggestive of iron overload. Significant liver disease is unusual in patients with ferritin lower than 1000 μg/L. The differential diagnoses for elevated ferritin are inflammatory disease or excess ethanol consumption for modest elevations (< 1000 μg/L). Very significant ferritin elevation can be seen in adult Still's disease. In terms of imaging techniques, MRI has high specificity for iron overload, but poor sensitivity. Liver biopsy allows assessment of fibrosis and distribution of iron (hepatocyte iron characteristic of haemochromatosis). The Hepatic Iron Index (HII) provides quantification of liver iron (μmol of iron per g dry weight of liver/age in years). HII of more than 1.9 suggests genetic haemochromatosis (Fig. 23.39). Both the C282Y and the H63D mutations can be identified by genetic testing, which is now in routine clinical use.

Management

Treatment consists of weekly venesection of 500 mL blood (250 mg iron) until the serum iron is normal;

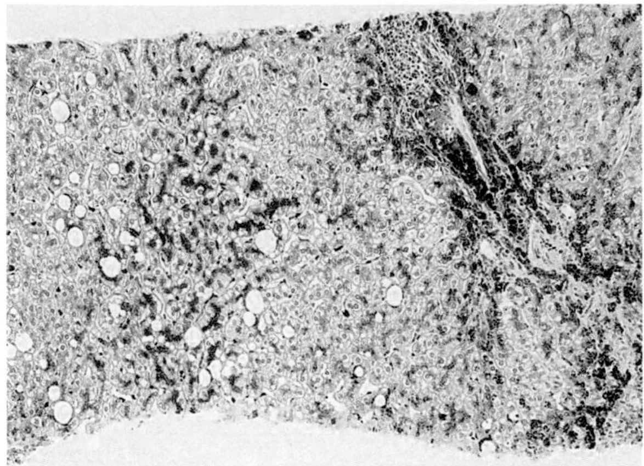

Fig. 23.39 Liver histology: haemochromatosis. This Perls stain shows accumulating iron within hepatocytes, which is stained blue. There is also accumulation of large fat globules in some hepatocytes (macrovesicular steatosis). Iron also accumulates in Kupffer cells and biliary epithelial cells.

this may take 2 years or more. The aim is to reduce ferritin to under 50 μg/L. Thereafter, venesection is continued as required to keep the serum ferritin normal. Liver and cardiac problems improve after iron removal, but joint pain is less predictable and can improve or worsen after iron removal. Diabetes mellitus does not resolve after venesection. Other therapy includes that for cirrhosis and diabetes mellitus. First-degree family members should be investigated, preferably by genetic screening and also by checking the plasma ferritin and iron-binding saturation. Liver biopsy is only indicated in asymptomatic relatives if the LFTs are abnormal and/or the serum ferritin is greater than 1000 μg/L because these features are associated with significant fibrosis or cirrhosis. Asymptomatic disease should also be treated by venesection until the serum ferritin is normal.

Pre-cirrhotic patients with HHC have a normal life expectancy, and even cirrhotic patients have a good prognosis compared with other forms of cirrhosis (three-quarters of patients are alive 5 years after diagnosis). This is probably because liver function is well preserved at diagnosis and improves with therapy. Screening for hepatocellular carcinoma (p. 967) is mandatory because this is the main cause of death, affecting one-third of patients with cirrhosis irrespective of therapy. Venesection reduces but does not abolish the risk of hepatocellular carcinoma in the presence of cirrhosis.

Secondary haemochromatosis

Many conditions, including chronic haemolytic disorders, sideroblastic anaemia, other conditions requiring multiple blood transfusion (generally over 50 L), porphyria cutanea tarda, dietary iron overload and occasionally alcoholic cirrhosis, are associated with widespread secondary siderosis. The features are similar to primary haemochromatosis, but the history and clinical findings point to the true diagnosis. Some patients are heterozygotes for the *HFE* gene and this may contribute to the development of iron overload.

Wilson's disease

Wilson's disease (hepatolenticular degeneration) is a rare but important autosomal recessive disorder of copper metabolism caused by a variety of mutations in the *ATP7B* gene on chromosome 13. Total body copper is increased, with excess copper deposited in, and causing damage to, several organs.

Pathophysiology

Normally, dietary copper is absorbed from the stomach and proximal small intestine, and is rapidly taken into the liver, where it is stored and incorporated into caeruloplasmin, which is secreted into the blood. The accumulation of excessive copper in the body is ultimately prevented by its excretion, the most important route being via bile. In Wilson's disease, there is almost always a failure of synthesis of caeruloplasmin; however, some 5% of patients have a normal circulating caeruloplasmin concentration and this is not the primary pathogenic defect. The amount of copper in the body at birth is normal, but thereafter it increases steadily; the organs most affected are the liver, basal ganglia of the brain, eyes, kidneys and skeleton.

The *ATP7B* gene encodes a member of the copper-transporting P-type adenosine triphosphatase family, which functions to export copper from various cell types. At least 200 different mutations have been described. Most cases are compound heterozygotes with two different mutations in *ATP7B*. Attempts to correlate the genotype with the mode of presentation and clinical course have not shown any consistent patterns. The large number of culprit mutations means that, in contrast to haemochromatosis, genetic diagnosis is not routine in Wilson's disease, although it may have a role in screening families following identification of the genotype in an index patient.

Clinical features

Symptoms usually arise between the ages of 5 and 45 years. Hepatic disease occurs predominantly in childhood and early adolescence, although it can present in adults in their fifties. Neurological damage causes basal ganglion syndromes and dementia, which tends to present in later adolescence. These features can occur alone or simultaneously. Other manifestations include renal tubular damage and osteoporosis, but these are rarely presenting features.

Liver disease

Episodes of acute hepatitis, sometimes recurrent, can occur, especially in children, and may progress to fulminant liver failure. The latter is characterised by the liberation of free copper into the blood stream, causing massive haemolysis and renal tubulopathy. Chronic hepatitis can also develop insidiously and eventually present with established cirrhosis; liver failure and portal hypertension may supervene. The possibility of Wilson's disease should be considered in any patient under the age of 40 presenting with recurrent acute hepatitis or chronic liver disease of unknown cause, especially when accompanied by haemolysis.

Neurological disease

Clinical features include a variety of extrapyramidal features, particularly tremor, choreoathetosis, dystonia, parkinsonism and dementia (Ch. 26). Unusual clumsiness for age may be an early symptom. Neurological disease typically develops after the onset of liver disease and can be prevented by effective treatment started following diagnosis in the liver disease phase. This increases the importance of diagnosis in the liver phase beyond just allowing effective management of liver disease.

Kayser–Fleischer rings

These constitute the most important single clinical clue to the diagnosis and can be seen in 60% of adults with Wilson's disease (less often in children but almost always in neurological Wilson's disease), albeit sometimes only by slit-lamp examination. Kayser–Fleischer rings are characterised by greenish-brown discoloration of the corneal margin appearing first at the upper periphery (see p. 922). They disappear with treatment.

Investigations

A low serum caeruloplasmin is the best single laboratory clue to the diagnosis. However, advanced liver failure from any cause can reduce the serum caeruloplasmin, and occasionally it is normal in Wilson's disease. Other features of disordered copper metabolism should therefore be sought; these include a high free serum copper concentration, a high urine copper excretion of greater than 0.6 μmol/24 hrs (38 μg/24 hrs) and a very high hepatic copper content. Measuring 24-hour urinary copper excretion whilst giving D-penicillamine is a useful confirmatory test; more than 25 μmol/24 hrs is considered diagnostic of Wilson's disease.

Management

The copper-binding agent, penicillamine, is the drug of choice. The dose given must be sufficient to produce cupriuresis and most patients require 1.5 g/day (range 1–4 g). The dose can be reduced once the disease is in remission but treatment must continue for life, even through pregnancy. Care must be taken to ensure that re-accumulation of copper does not occur. Abrupt discontinuation of treatment must be avoided because this may precipitate acute liver failure. Toxic effects occur in one-third of patients and include rashes, protein-losing nephropathy, lupus-like syndrome and bone marrow depression. If these do occur, trientine dihydrochloride (1.2–2.4 g/day) and zinc (50 mg 3 times daily) are potential alternatives.

Liver transplantation is indicated for fulminant liver failure or for advanced cirrhosis with liver failure. The value of liver transplantation in severe neurological Wilson's disease is unclear. Prognosis is excellent, provided treatment is started before there is irreversible damage. Siblings and children of patients with Wilson's disease must be investigated and treatment should be given to all affected individuals, even if they are asymptomatic.

Alpha$_1$-antitrypsin deficiency

Alpha$_1$-antitrypsin (α_1-AT) is a serine protease inhibitor (Pi) produced by the liver. The mutated form of α_1-AT (PiZ) cannot be secreted into the blood by liver cells because it is retained within the endoplasmic reticulum of the hepatocyte. Homozygous individuals (PiZZ) have low plasma α_1-AT concentrations, although globules containing α_1-AT are found in the liver, and these people may develop hepatic and pulmonary disease. Liver manifestations include cholestatic jaundice in the neonatal period (neonatal hepatitis), which can resolve spontaneously, chronic hepatitis and cirrhosis in adults, and, in the long term, HCC. Alpha$_1$-AT deficiency is a not uncommon exacerbating factor for liver disease of other aetiologies, and the possibility of dual pathology should be considered in patients in whom severity of disease, such as ALD, appears disproportionate to the level of underlying insult.

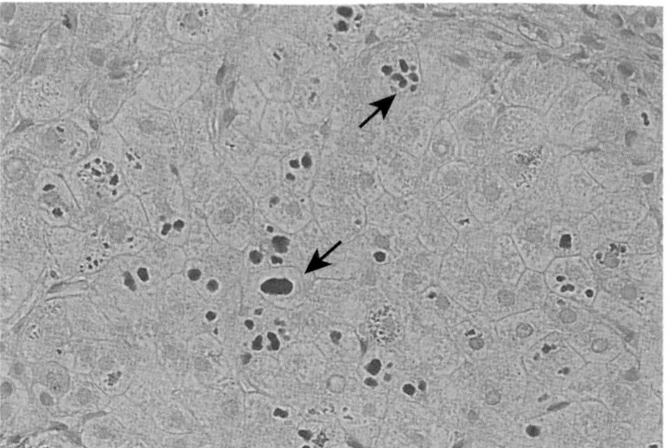

Fig. 23.40 Liver histology in α_1-antitrypsin deficiency. Accumulation of periodic acid–Schiff-positive granules (arrows) within individual hepatocytes is shown in this section from a patient with α_1-AT deficiency.

There are no clinical features distinguishing liver disease due to α_1-AT deficiency from liver disease due to other causes, and the diagnosis is made from the low plasma α_1-AT concentration and genotyping for the presence of the mutation. Alpha$_1$-AT-containing globules can be demonstrated in the liver (Fig. 23.40) but this is not necessary to make the diagnosis. Occasionally, patients with liver disease and minor reductions of plasma α_1-AT concentrations have α_1-AT variants other than PiZZ, but the relationship of these to liver disease is uncertain.

There is no specific treatment; the risk of severe and early-onset emphysema means that all patients should be advised to stop smoking.

Gilbert's syndrome

Gilbert's syndrome is by far the most common inherited disorder of bilirubin metabolism (see Box 23.17, p. 937). It is an autosomal dominant trait caused by a mutation in the promoter region of the UDP-glucuronyl transferase enzyme, which leads to reduced enzyme expression. This results in decreased conjugation of bilirubin, which accumulates as unconjugated bilirubin in the blood. The levels of unconjugated bilirubin increase during fasting, as fasting reduces levels of UDP-glucuronyl transferase.

Clinical features

The typical presentation is with isolated elevation of bilirubin, typically, although not exclusively, in the setting of physical stress or illness. There are no stigmata of chronic liver disease other than jaundice. Increased excretion of bilirubin and hence stercobilinogen leads to normal-coloured or dark stools, and increased urobilinogen excretion causes the urine to turn dark on standing as urobilin is formed. In the presence of haemolysis, pallor due to anaemia and splenomegaly due to excessive reticulo-endothelial activity are usually present.

Investigations

The plasma bilirubin is usually less than 100 μmol/L (~6 mg/dL) and the LFTs are otherwise normal. There is no bilirubinuria because the hyperbilirubinaemia is predominantly unconjugated. Hepatic histology is normal and liver biopsy is not recommended for the investigation of patients with possible Gilbert's syndrome. The condition is not associated with liver injury and thus has an excellent prognosis, needs no treatment, and is clinically important only because it may be mistaken for more serious liver disease.

VASCULAR LIVER DISEASE

Metabolically, the liver is highly active and has large oxygen requirements. This places it at risk of ischaemic injury in settings of impaired perfusion. The risk is mitigated, however, by the dual perfusion of the liver (via portal vein as well as hepatic artery), with the former representing a low-pressure perfusion system that offers protection against the potential effects of arterial hypotension. The single outflow through the hepatic vein and the low-pressure perfusion system of the portal vein make the liver vulnerable to venous thrombotic ischaemia in the context of Budd–Chiari syndrome and portal vein thrombosis, respectively.

Hepatic arterial disease

Liver ischaemia

Liver ischaemic injury is relatively common during hypotensive or hypoxic events and is under-diagnosed. The characteristic pattern is one of rising transaminase values in the days following such an event (e.g. prolonged seizures). Liver synthetic dysfunction and encephalopathy are uncommon but can occur. Liver failure is very rare. Diagnosis typically rests on clinical suspicion and exclusion of other potential aetiologies. Treatment is aimed at optimising liver perfusion and oxygen delivery. Outcome is dictated by the morbidity and mortality associated with the underlying disease, given that liver ischaemia frequently occurs in the context of other organ ischaemia in high-risk patients.

Liver arterial disease

Hepatic arterial disease is rare outside the setting of liver transplantation and is difficult to diagnose. It can cause significant liver damage. Hepatic artery occlusion may result from inadvertent injury during biliary surgery or may be caused by emboli, neoplasms, polyarteritis nodosa, blunt trauma or radiation. It usually causes severe upper abdominal pain with or without signs of circulatory shock. LFTs show raised transaminases (AST or ALT usually > 1000 U/L), as in other causes of acute liver damage. Patients usually survive if the liver and portal blood supply are otherwise normal.

Hepatic artery aneurysms are extrahepatic in three-quarters of cases and intrahepatic in one-quarter. Atheroma, vasculitis, bacterial endocarditis and surgical or biopsy trauma are the main causes. They usually lead to bleeding into the biliary tree, peritoneum or intestine, and are best diagnosed by angiography. Treatment is radiological or surgical. Any of the vasculitides can affect the hepatic artery but this rarely causes symptoms.

Hepatic artery thrombosis is a recognised complication of liver transplantation and typically occurs in the early post-transplant period. Clinical features are often related to bile duct rather than liver ischaemia because of the dominant role of the hepatic artery in extrahepatic bile duct perfusion. Manifestations can include bile duct anastomotic failure with bile leak or the development of late bile duct strictures. Diagnosis and initial intervention are radiological in the first instance, with ERCP and biliary stenting being the principal approaches to the treatment of bile duct injury.

Portal venous disease

Portal hypertension

See page 945.

Portal vein thrombosis

Portal venous thrombosis as a primary event is rare, but can occur in any condition predisposing to thrombosis. It may also complicate intra-abdominal inflammatory or neoplastic disease, and is a recognised cause of portal hypertension. Acute portal venous thrombosis causes abdominal pain and diarrhoea, and may rarely lead to bowel infarction, requiring surgery. Treatment is otherwise based on anticoagulation, although there are no randomised data on efficacy. An underlying thrombophilia needs to be excluded. Subacute thrombosis can be asymptomatic but may subsequently lead to extrahepatic portal hypertension (p. 945). Ascites is unusual in non-cirrhotic portal hypertension, unless the albumin is particularly low.

Portal vein thrombosis can arise as a secondary event in patients with cirrhosis and portal hypertension, and is a recognised cause of decompensation in patients with previously stable cirrhosis. In patients showing such decompensation, portal vein patency should be assessed by ultrasound with Doppler flow studies.

Hepatopulmonary syndrome

This condition is characterised by resistant hypoxaemia (PaO_2 < 9.3 kPa or 70 mm Hg), intrapulmonary vascular dilatation in patients with cirrhosis, and portal hypertension. Clinical features include finger clubbing, cyanosis, spider naevi and a characteristic reduction in arterial oxygen saturation on standing. The hypoxia is due to intrapulmonary shunting through direct arteriovenous communications. Nitric oxide (NO) overproduction may be important in pathogenesis. The hepatopulmonary syndrome can be treated by liver transplantation but, if severe (PaO_2 < 6.7 kPa or 50 mm Hg), is associated with an increased operative risk.

Portopulmonary hypertension

This unusual complication of portal hypertension is similar to 'primary pulmonary hypertension' (p. 724). It is defined as pulmonary hypertension with increased pulmonary vascular resistance and a normal pulmonary artery wedge pressure in a patient with portal hypertension. The condition is caused by vasoconstriction and obliteration of the pulmonary arterial system, and leads to breathlessness and fatigue.

Hepatic venous disease

Obstruction to hepatic venous blood flow can occur in the small central hepatic veins, the large hepatic veins, the inferior vena cava or the heart (see Fig. 23.19, p. 945). The clinical features depend on the cause and on the speed with which obstruction develops, and can mimic many other forms of chronic liver disease, sometimes leading to delayed diagnosis. Congestive hepatomegaly and ascites are, however, the most consistent features. The possibility of hepatic venous obstruction should always be considered in patients with an atypical liver presentation.

Budd–Chiari syndrome

This uncommon condition is caused by thrombosis of the larger hepatic veins and sometimes the inferior vena cava. Many patients have haematological disorders such as myelofibrosis, primary proliferative polycythaemia, paroxysmal nocturnal haemoglobinuria, or antithrombin III, protein C or protein S deficiencies (Ch. 24). Pregnancy and oral contraceptive use, obstruction due to tumours (particularly carcinomas of the liver, kidneys or adrenals), congenital venous webs and occasionally inferior vena caval stenosis are the other main causes. The underlying cause cannot be found in about 50% of patients, although this percentage is falling as molecular diagnostic tools (such as the JAK2 mutation in myelofibrosis) increase our capacity to diagnose underlying haematological disorders. Hepatic congestion affecting the centrilobular areas is followed by centrilobular fibrosis, and eventually cirrhosis supervenes in those who survive long enough.

Clinical features

Acute venous occlusion causes rapid development of upper abdominal pain, marked ascites and occasionally acute liver failure. More gradual occlusion causes gross ascites and, often, upper abdominal discomfort. Hepatomegaly, frequently with tenderness over the liver, is almost always present. Peripheral oedema occurs only when there is inferior vena cava obstruction. Features of cirrhosis and portal hypertension develop in those who survive the acute event.

Investigations

The LFTs vary considerably, depending on the presentation, and can show the features of acute hepatitis. Ascitic fluid analysis shows a protein concentration above 25 g/L (exudate) in the early stages; however, this often falls later in the disease. Doppler ultrasound may reveal obliteration of the hepatic veins and reversed flow or associated thrombosis in the portal vein. CT may show enlargement of the caudate lobe, as it often has a separate venous drainage system that is not involved in the disease. CT and MRI may also demonstrate occlusion of the hepatic veins and inferior vena cava. Liver biopsy demonstrates centrilobular congestion with fibrosis, depending on the duration of the illness. Venography is only needed if CT and MRI are unable to demonstrate the hepatic venous anatomy clearly.

Management

Predisposing causes should be treated as far as possible; where recent thrombosis is suspected, thrombolysis with streptokinase, followed by heparin and oral anticoagulation, should be considered. Ascites is initially treated medically but often with only limited success. Short hepatic venous strictures can be treated with angioplasty. In the case of more extensive hepatic vein occlusion, many patients can be managed successfully by insertion of a covered TIPSS, followed by anticoagulation. Surgical shunts, such as portacaval shunts, are less commonly performed now that TIPSS is available. Occasionally, a web can be resected or an inferior vena caval stenosis dilated. Progressive liver failure is an indication for liver transplantation and life-long anticoagulation.

Prognosis without transplantation or shunting is poor, particularly following an acute presentation with liver failure. A 3-year survival of 50% is reported in those who survive the initial event. The 1- and 10-year survival following liver transplantation is 85% and 69% respectively, and this compares with a 5- and 10-year survival of 87% and 37% following surgical shunting.

Veno-occlusive disease

Veno-occlusive disease (VOD) is a rare condition characterised by widespread occlusion of the small central hepatic veins. Pyrrolizidine alkaloids in *Senecio* and *Heliotropium* plants used to make teas, as well as cytotoxic drugs and hepatic irradiation, are all recognised causes. VOD may develop in 10–20% of patients following haematopoietic stem cell transplantation (usually within the first 20 days), and carries a 90% mortality in severe cases. Pathogenesis involves obliteration and fibrosis of terminal hepatic venules due to deposition of red cells, haemosiderin-laden macrophages and coagulation factors. In this setting, VOD is thought to relate to preconditioning therapy with irradiation and cytotoxic chemotherapy. The clinical features are similar to those of the Budd–Chiari syndrome (see above). Investigations show evidence of venous outflow obstruction histologically but, in contrast to Budd–Chiari, the large hepatic veins appear patent radiologically. Transjugular liver biopsy (with portal pressure measurements) may make the diagnosis. Traditionally, treatment has been supportive, but defibrotide shows promise (the drug binds to vascular endothelial cells, promoting fibrinolysis and suppressing coagulation).

Cardiac disease

Hepatic damage, due primarily to congestion, may develop in all forms of right heart failure (p. 548);

usually, the clinical features are predominantly cardiac. Very rarely, long-standing cardiac failure and hepatic congestion give rise to cardiac cirrhosis. Cardiac causes of acute and chronic liver disease are under-diagnosed. Treatment is that of the underlying heart disease.

Nodular regenerative hyperplasia of the liver

This is the most common cause of non-cirrhotic portal hypertension in developed countries; it is characterised by small hepatocyte nodules throughout the liver without fibrosis, which can result in sinusoidal compression. It is believed to be due to damage to small hepatic arterioles and portal venules. It occurs in older people and is associated with many conditions, including connective tissue disease, haematological diseases and immunosuppressive drugs, such as azathioprine. The condition is usually asymptomatic, but occasionally presents with portal hypertension or with an abdominal mass. The diagnosis is made by liver biopsy, which, in contrast to cirrhosis, shows nodule formation in the absence of fibrous septa. Liver function is good and the prognosis is very favourable. Management is based on treatment of the portal hypertension.

PREGNANCY AND THE LIVER

The inter-relationship between liver disease and pregnancy can be a complex one and a source of real anxiety for both patient and clinicians. Three possibilities need to be borne in mind when faced with a pregnant woman with a liver abnormality:

- that this represents a worsening of pre-existing chronic liver or biliary disease (although pregnancy may be the first time a woman's liver biochemistry has been tested, so this may not have previously been diagnosed)
- that this represents a genuine first presentation of liver disease that is not intrinsically related to pregnancy
- that this represents a genuine pregnancy-associated liver injury process.

It is critical to obtain information relating to liver disease risk factors and pre-pregnancy liver status to establish whether any abnormality was present before pregnancy. In general, the earlier in pregnancy that liver abnormality presents, the more likely it is to represent either pre-existing liver disease or non-pregnancy-related acute liver disease. Equally, the best outcome for both mother and baby results from optimising the physical condition of the mother, and in situations of deteriorating liver function (which can be steep in late pregnancy) consideration should always be given to early delivery if the fetus is viable. Joint management between hepatologists and obstetricians is essential.

Intercurrent and pre-existing liver disease

Acute hepatitis A can occur during pregnancy but has no effect on the fetus. Chronic hepatitis B requires identification in pregnancy because of long-term health implications for the mother and the effectiveness of perinatal vaccination (with or without pre-delivery maternal antiviral therapy) in reducing neonatal acquisition of chronic hepatitis B. Maternal transmission of hepatitis C occurs in 1% of cases, and there is no convincing evidence that the mode of delivery affects this. Hepatitis E is reported to progress to acute liver failure much more commonly in pregnancy, with a 20% maternal mortality. Pregnancy may be associated with either worsening or improvement of autoimmune hepatitis, although improvement during pregnancy and rebound post-partum is the most common pattern seen. Complications of portal hypertension may be a particular issue in the second and third trimesters.

Gallstones (p. 981) are more common during pregnancy, and may present with cholecystitis or biliary obstruction. The diagnosis can usually be made with ultrasound. In biliary obstruction due to gallstones, therapeutic ERCP can be safely performed, but lead protection for the fetus is essential and X-ray screening must be kept to a minimum.

Pregnancy-associated liver disease

The following conditions occur only during pregnancy, may recur in subsequent pregnancies and resolve after delivery of the baby. The causes of abnormal LFTs in pregnancy, which include pregnancy-associated liver disease, are shown in Box 23.68.

Acute cholestasis of pregnancy

This accounts for 20% of cases of jaundice in pregnancy; it usually occurs in the third trimester of pregnancy but can arise earlier. It may be linked with intrauterine growth retardation and premature birth, but is most

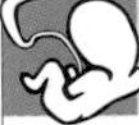

23.68 Abnormal liver function tests in pregnancy

- **Liver function tests**: ALT levels and albumin normally fall in pregnancy. ALP levels can rise due to the contribution of placental ALP.
- **Pre-existing liver disease**: pregnancy is uncommon in cirrhosis because cirrhosis causes relative infertility. Variceal bleeding can occur if varices present prior to conception, and ascites or polyhydramnios should be treated with amiloride rather than spironolactone. Penicillamine for Wilson's disease and azathioprine for autoimmune liver disease should be continued during pregnancy. Autoimmune liver disease can flare up post-partum.
- **Unrelated liver disease**: viral- and drug-induced hepatitis must be excluded in the presence of an elevated ALT. Immunoglobulin/vaccination given to the fetus at birth prevents transmission of hepatitis B to the fetus if the mother is infected. Gallstones are more common in pregnancy and post-partum, and are a cause of a raised ALP level. Biliary imaging with ultrasound and MRCP is safe. ERCP to remove stones can be performed safely with shielding of the fetus from radiation.
- **Pregnancy-related liver diseases**: occur predominantly in the third trimester and resolve post-partum. Maternal and fetal mortality and morbidity are prevented by early delivery.

characteristically associated with intrauterine fetal death if the pregnancy goes beyond 36 weeks of gestation. The condition characteristically presents with itching and cholestatic LFTs. A normal bilirubin and hepatitic LFTs do not, however, preclude the diagnosis. Bile salts are elevated in the serum and this represents a useful clinical test. Delivery leads to resolution and should be considered from 36 weeks onwards. Pregnancy should not be allowed to continue beyond term because of a steep rise in the risk of intrauterine death. UDCA (15 mg/kg daily) effectively controls itching and probably prevents premature birth. The major issue with UDCA in acute cholestasis of pregnancy is the relatively long time required to achieve effective levels within the bile pool, which renders it of little use in patients presenting in the very end stages of pregnancy. Cholestasis recurs in 60% of future pregnancies and the opportunities available for screening based on previous risk make UDCA a much more viable therapy in this setting.

Acute fatty liver of pregnancy

This is more common in twin and first pregnancies, and may arise more frequently when the fetus is male. It occurs in 1 in 14 000 pregnancies in the USA. It typically presents between 31 and 38 weeks of pregnancy with vomiting and abdominal pain followed by jaundice. In severe cases, this may be followed by lactic acidosis, coagulopathy, encephalopathy and renal failure. Hypoglycaemia can also occur. The features are characteristic of a defect in beta-oxidation of fatty acids in the mitochondria that leads to the formation of small fat droplets in liver cells (known as microvesicular fatty liver). Some women are heterozygous for loss-of-function mutations in the long-chain 3-hydroxyacyl-CoA dehydrogenase (*LCHAD*) gene. Other causes of microvesicular steatosis that have a similar clinical presentation outside pregnancy are shown in Box 23.69. Differentiation from toxaemia of pregnancy (which is more common) can be achieved by the finding of high serum uric acid levels and the absence of haemolysis. Overlap between acute fatty liver of pregnancy, HELLP (see below) and toxaemia of pregnancy can occur. Early diagnosis, specialist care and delivery of the fetus have led to a fall in maternal and perinatal mortality to 1% and 7% respectively.

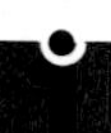

23.69 Hepatic mitochondrial cytopathies

- Acute fatty liver of pregnancy
- Drugs: sodium valproate, tetracyclines
- Reye's syndrome (aspirin toxicity in childhood)
- Toxins: *Bacillus cereus*

Toxaemia of pregnancy and HELLP

The HELLP syndrome (haemolysis, elevated liver enzymes and low platelets) is a variant of pre-eclampsia that tends to affect multiparous women. It usually presents at 27–36 weeks of pregnancy with hypertension, proteinuria and fluid retention, although, as with all liver diseases of pregnancy, the presentation can be highly variable and all potential diagnoses should be considered in all patients. Jaundice only occurs in 5% of cases. Blood tests may show low haemoglobin, with fragmented red cells, markedly elevated serum transaminases and raised D-dimers. The condition can be complicated by hepatic infarction and rupture. Maternal complications also include disseminated intravascular coagulation and placental abruption. Maternal mortality is 1% and perinatal mortality can be up to 30%. Delivery usually leads to prompt resolution, and disease recurs in fewer than 5% of subsequent pregnancies.

LIVER TRANSPLANTATION

The outcome following liver transplantation has improved significantly over the last decade so that elective transplantation in low-risk individuals now has a 1-year survival rate of more than 90% and is an effective treatment for end-stage liver disease. The number of procedures is limited by cadaveric donor availability, and in many parts of the world this has led to living donor transplant programmes. Despite this, 10% of those listed for liver transplantation will die while awaiting a donor liver. The main complications of liver transplantation relate to rejection, complications of long-term immunosuppression and disease recurrence in the liver graft.

Indications and contraindications

Currently, around 9500 liver transplants are undertaken in Europe and the USA annually. About 10% are performed for acute liver failure, 6% for metabolic diseases, 71% for cirrhosis and 11% for hepatocellular carcinoma. Most patients are under 60 years of age, and only 10% are aged between 60 and 70 years. Indications for elective transplant assessment are listed in Box 23.70. In North America the most common indication is hepatitis C cirrhosis, about 10–20% of transplants being for alcoholic cirrhosis (Fig. 23.41). Patients with alcoholic liver disease need to show a capacity for abstinence.

The main contraindications to transplantation are sepsis, extrahepatic malignancy, active alcohol or other substance misuse, and marked cardiorespiratory dysfunction.

Patients are matched for ABO blood group and size, but do not require HLA-matching with donors, as the

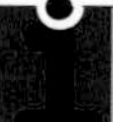

23.70 Indications for liver transplant assessment for cirrhosis

Complications

- First episode of bacterial peritonitis
- Diuretic-resistant ascites
- Recurrent variceal haemorrhage
- Hepatocellular carcinoma < 5 cm
- Persistent hepatic encephalopathy

Poor liver function

- Bilirubin > 100 μmol/L (5.8 mg/dL) in primary biliary cirrhosis
- MELD score > 12
- Child–Pugh grade C

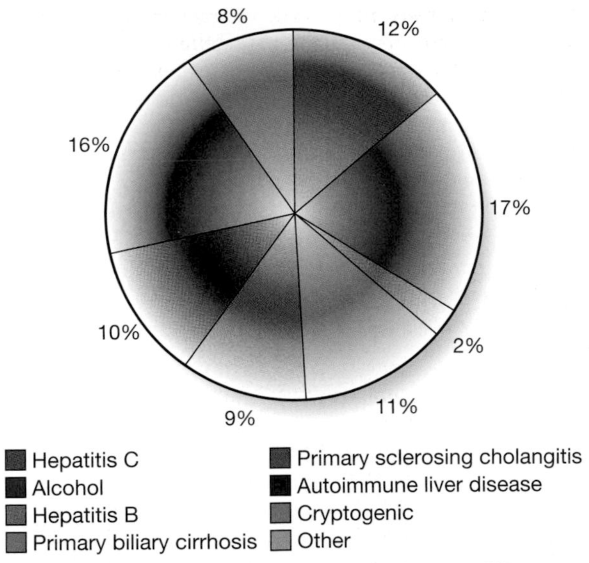

Fig. 23.41 Indications for liver transplantation in the UK between 2001 and 2005.

liver is a relatively immune-privileged organ compared with heart or kidney.

In many parts of the world, the MELD score (see Box 23.32, p. 944) is used to identify and prioritise patients for transplantation. In the UK, a similar score that also incorporates serum sodium, the United Kingdom End-Stage Liver Disease score (UKELD), is used to guide recipient selection. To be listed for elective (non-super-urgent) transplantation in the UK, patients must have a greater than 50% projected post-transplant 5-year survival and fall into one of three categories:

- *Category 1*: estimated 1-year mortality without transplantation of more than 9% (equivalent to a UKELD score of more than 49 points)
- *Category 2*: HCC diagnosed radiologically by two concordant modalities; based on CT, a single lesion of less than 5 cm maximum diameter or fewer than three lesions each less than 3 cm in diameter without macrovascular invasion or metastases.
- *Category 3*: 'variant syndromes', including diuretic-resistant ascites, hepatopulmonary syndrome, chronic hepatic encephalopathy, intractable pruritus, familial amyloidosis, primary hyperlipidaemia, polycystic liver disease and recurrent cholangitis.

Super-urgent listing is reserved for patients with acute liver failure according to specific criteria.

Two types of transplant are increasingly used because of insufficient cadaveric donors:

- *Split liver transplantation.* A cadaveric donor liver can be split into two, with the larger right lobe used in an adult and the smaller left lobe used in a child. This practice has led to an increase in procedures despite a shortage of donor organs.
- *Living donor transplantation.* This is normally performed using the left lateral segment or the right lobe. The donor mortality is significant at 0.5–1%. Pre-operative assessment includes looking at donor liver size and psychological status.

Complications

Early complications

Primary graft non-function

This is a state of hepatocellular dysfunction arising as a consequence of liver paresis that results from ischaemia following removal from the donor and prior to reperfusion in the recipient. Factors that increase the likelihood of primary non-function include increasing donor age, degree of steatosis in the liver, and the length of ischaemia. Treatment is supportive until recovery of function. Occasionally, recovery is not seen and re-transplant is necessary.

Technical complications

These include hepatic artery thrombosis, which may necessitate re-transplantation. Anastomotic biliary strictures can also occur; these may respond to endoscopic balloon dilatation and stenting, or require surgical reconstruction. Portal vein thrombosis is rare.

Rejection

Less immunosuppression is needed following liver transplantation than with kidney or heart/lung grafting. Initial immunosuppression is usually with tacrolimus or ciclosporin, prednisolone and azathioprine or mycophenolate. Some patients can eventually be maintained on a single agent. Acute cellular rejection occurs in 60–80% of patients, commonly at 5–10 days post transplant and usually within the first 6 weeks, but can arise at any point. This normally responds to 3 days of high-dose intravenous methylprednisolone.

Infections

Bacterial infections, such as pneumonia and wound infections, can occur in the first few weeks after transplantation. Cytomegalovirus (primary infection or reactivation) is a common infection in the 3 months after transplantation and can cause hepatitis. Patients who have never had cytomegalovirus infection but who receive a liver from a donor who has been exposed are at greatest risk of infection, and are usually given prophylactic antiviral therapy such as valganciclovir. Herpes simplex virus reactivation or, rarely, primary infection may occur. Prophylaxis is given to recipients who have had previous exposure to tuberculosis for the first 6 months after transplantation to prevent reactivation.

Late complications

These include recurrence of the initial disease in the graft and complications due to the immunosuppressive therapy, such as renal impairment from ciclosporin. Metabolic syndrome is common, being described in about 50% of transplant recipients within 6 months in the USA. Chronic vascular rejection is rare, occurring in only 5% of cases.

Prognosis

The outcome following transplantation for acute liver failure is worse than for chronic liver disease because

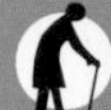

23.71 Liver disease in old age

- **Alcoholic liver disease**: 10% of cases present over the age of 70 years, when disease is more likely to be severe and has a worse prognosis.
- **Hepatitis A**: causes more severe illness and runs a more protracted course.
- **Primary biliary cirrhosis**: one-third of cases are over 65 years.
- **Liver abscess**: more than 50% of all cases in the UK are over 60 years.
- **Hepatocellular carcinoma**: approximately 50% of cases present over the age of 65 years in the UK.
- **Surgery**: older people are less likely to survive liver surgery (including transplantation) because comorbidity is more prevalent.

most patients have multi-organ failure at the time of transplantation. The 1-year survival is 65% and falls only a little to 59% at 5 years. The 1-year survival for patients with cirrhosis is over 90%, falling to 70–75% at 5 years.

CHOLESTATIC AND BILIARY DISEASE

The concepts of biliary and cholestatic disease, and the important distinctions between them, can be a source of confusion. 'Cholestasis' relates to a biochemical abnormality (typically elevation of ALP and, if the process is significant, elevation in serum bile acid levels and bilirubin) resulting from an abnormality in bile flow. The cause can range from inherited or acquired dysfunction of transporter molecules responsible for the production of canalicular bile to physical obstruction of the extrahepatic bile duct. 'Biliary disease' relates to pathology at any level from the small intrahepatic bile ducts to the sphincter of Oddi. Although there is very significant overlap between cholestatic and biliary disease, there are scenarios where cholestasis can exist without biliary disease (transporter disease or pure drug-induced cholestasis) and where biliary disease can exist without cholestasis (when disease of the bile duct does not impact on bile flow). These anomalies should always be borne in mind, and cholestasis and biliary disease always effectively distinguished.

Chemical cholestasis

Pure cholestasis can occur as an inherited condition (see p. 972), as a consequence of cholestatic drug reactions (p. 971) or as acute cholestasis of pregnancy (p. 977). A more frequent, but less recognised, acquired biochemical cholestasis occurs in sepsis ('cholangitis lente'). This biochemical phenomenon is one of the causes of LFT abnormality in sepsis, does not require specific treatment, and has a prognostic significance conferred by the underlying septic process.

Mutations in the biliary transporter proteins on the hepatocyte canalicular membrane (familial intrahepatic cholestasis 1, FIC1), illustrated in Figure 23.7 (p. 927), have been shown to cause an inherited intrahepatic biliary disease in childhood, characterised by raised ALP levels and progression to a biliary cirrhosis. It is also becoming increasingly clear that these proteins contribute to intrahepatic biliary disease in adulthood.

Benign recurrent intrahepatic cholestasis

This rare condition usually presents in adolescence and is characterised by recurrent episodes of cholestasis, lasting 1–6 months. It is now known to be mediated by mutations in the *ATP8B1* gene, which lies on chromosome 18 and encodes FIC1.

Episodes start with pruritus, while painless jaundice develops later. LFTs show a cholestatic pattern. Liver biopsy shows cholestasis during an episode but is normal between episodes. Treatment is required to relieve the symptoms of cholestasis, such as pruritus, and the long-term prognosis is good.

Intrahepatic biliary disease

Inflammatory and immune disease

The small intrahepatic bile ducts appear to be specifically vulnerable to immune injury, and ductopenic injury ('vanishing bile duct syndrome') can be a feature of a number of chronic conditions, including graft-versus-host disease (GVHD), sarcoidosis and, in the setting of liver transplantation, ductopenic rejection. Intrahepatic small bile duct injury occurs most frequently in PBC, an autoimmune cholestatic disease, and less frequently in PSC (Box 23.72).

Caroli's disease

This is very rare and is characterised by segmental saccular dilatations of the intrahepatic biliary tree. The

23.72 Comparison of primary biliary cirrhosis and primary sclerosing cholangitis

	PBC	PSC
Gender (F:M)	10:1	1:3
Age	Older: median age 50–55 yrs	Younger: median age 20–40 yrs
Disease associations	Non-organ-specific autoimmune disease (e.g. Sjögren's syndrome) and autoimmune thyroid disease	Ulcerative colitis
Autoantibody profile	90% AMA +ve	65–85% pANCA +ve (but this is non-specific and not diagnostic)
Predominant bile-duct injury	Intrahepatic	Extrahepatic > intrahepatic

(AMA = antimitochondrial antibodies; pANCA = perinuclear antineutrophil cytoplasmic antibodies)

whole liver is usually affected, and extrahepatic biliary dilatation occurs in about one-quarter of patients. Recurrent attacks of cholangitis (see Box 23.18, p. 937) may cause hepatic abscesses. Complications include biliary stones and cholangiocarcinoma. Antibiotics are required for episodes of cholangitis. Occasionally, localised disease can be treated by segmental liver resection, and liver transplantation may sometimes be required.

Congenital hepatic fibrosis

This is characterised by broad bands of fibrous tissue linking the portal tracts in the liver, abnormalities of the interlobular bile ducts, and sometimes a lack of portal venules. The renal tubules may show cystic dilatation (medullary sponge kidney, p. 506), and eventually renal cysts may develop. The condition can be inherited as an autosomal recessive trait. Liver involvement causes portal hypertension with splenomegaly and bleeding from oesophageal varices that usually presents in adolescence or in early adult life. The prognosis is good because liver function is preserved. Treatment may be required for variceal bleeding and occasionally cholangitis. Patients can present during childhood with renal failure if the kidneys are severely affected.

Cystic fibrosis

Cystic fibrosis (p. 680) is associated with a biliary cirrhosis in about 5% of individuals. Splenomegaly and an elevated ALP are characteristic. Complications do not normally arise until late adolescence or early adulthood, when bleeding due to variceal haemorrhage may occur. UDCA improves liver blood tests but it is not known whether the drug can prevent progression of liver disease. Deficiency of fat-soluble vitamins (A, D, E and K) may need to be treated in view of both biliary and pancreatic disease.

Extrahepatic biliary disease

Diseases of the extrahepatic biliary tree typically present with the clinical features of impaired bile flow (obstructive jaundice and fat malabsorption). Obstructive disease is frequently a consequence of stricturing following gallstone passage and associated infection and inflammation or post-surgical intervention. PSC frequently involves the extrahepatic biliary tree, and its differential, IgG4 disease, is an important and potentially treatable cause of disease (p. 966). Malignant diseases (cholangiocarcinoma or carcinoma of the head of pancreas should be considered in all patients with extrahepatic biliary obstruction.

Choledochal cysts

This term applies to cysts anywhere in the biliary tree (Fig. 23.42). The great majority cause diffuse dilatation of the common bile duct (type I), but others take the form of biliary diverticula (type II), dilatation of the intraduodenal bile duct (type III) and multiple biliary cysts (type IV). The last type merges with Caroli's disease (see above). In the neonate, they may present with jaundice or biliary peritonitis. Recurrent jaundice, abdominal pain and cholangitis may arise in the adult.

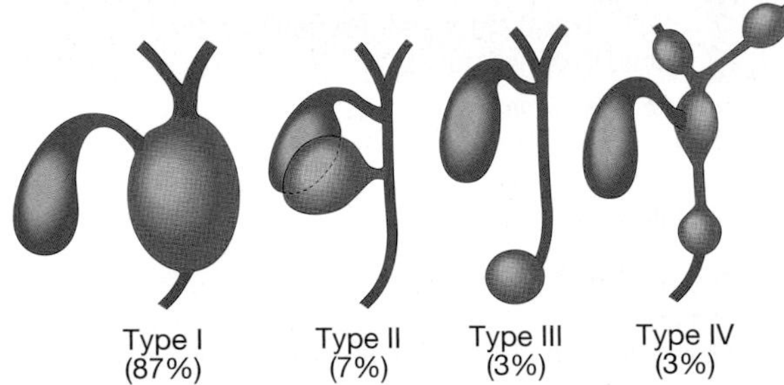

Fig. 23.42 Classification and frequency of choledochal cysts. From Shearman and Finlayson 1989 – see p. 988.

Liver abscess and biliary cirrhosis may develop, and there is an increased incidence of cholangiocarcinoma. Excision of the cyst with hepatico-jejunostomy is the treatment of choice.

Secondary biliary cirrhosis

Secondary biliary cirrhosis develops after prolonged large duct biliary obstruction due to gallstones, benign bile duct strictures or sclerosing cholangitis (see below). Carcinomas rarely cause secondary biliary cirrhosis because few patients survive long enough. The clinical features are those of chronic cholestasis with episodes of ascending cholangitis or even liver abscess (p. 956). Cirrhosis, ascites and portal hypertension are late features. Relief of biliary obstruction may require endoscopic or surgical intervention. Cholangitis requires treatment with antibiotics, which can be given continuously if attacks recur frequently.

Gallstones

Gallstone formation is the most common disorder of the biliary tree and it is unusual for the gallbladder to be diseased in the absence of gallstones. In developed countries, gallstones occur in 7% of males and 15% of females aged 18–65 years, with an overall prevalence of 11%. In individuals under 40 years there is a 3:1 female preponderance, whereas in the elderly the sex ratio is about equal. In developed countries, the incidence of symptomatic gallstones appears to be increasing and they occur at an earlier age. Gallstones are less frequent in India, the Far East and Africa. There has been much debate over the role of diet in cholesterol gallstone disease; an increase in dietary cholesterol, fat, total calories and refined carbohydrate or lack of dietary fibre has been implicated. At present, the best data support an association between simple refined sugar in the diet and gallstones.

Pathophysiology

Gallstones are conveniently classified into cholesterol or pigment stones, although the majority are of mixed composition. Cholesterol stones are most common in developed countries, whereas pigment stones are more frequent in developing countries. Gallstones contain varying quantities of calcium salts, including calcium bilirubinate, carbonate, phosphate and palmitate, which

23.73 Risk factors and mechanisms for cholesterol gallstones

↑ Cholesterol secretion

- Old age
- Female gender
- Pregnancy
- Obesity
- Rapid weight loss

Impaired gallbladder emptying

- Pregnancy
- Gallbladder stasis
- Fasting
- Total parenteral nutrition
- Spinal cord injury

↓ Bile salt secretion

- Pregnancy

23.74 Composition of and risk factors for pigment stones

	Black	Brown
Composition	Polymerised calcium bilirubinates* Mucin glycoprotein Calcium phosphate Calcium carbonate Cholesterol	Calcium bilirubinate crystals* Mucin glycoprotein Cholesterol Calcium palmitate/ stearate
Risk factors	Haemolysis Age Hepatic cirrhosis Ileal resection/disease	Infected bile Stasis

*Major component.

23.75 Pathogenic factors leading to the production of lithogenic bile

- Defective bile salt synthesis
- Excessive intestinal loss of bile salts
- Over-sensitive bile salt feedback
- Excessive cholesterol secretion
- Abnormal gallbladder function

are radio-opaque. Gallstone formation is multifactorial, and the factors involved are related to the type of gallstone (Boxes 23.73 and 23.74).

Cholesterol gallstones

Cholesterol is held in solution in bile by its association with bile acids and phospholipids in the form of micelles and vesicles. Biliary lipoproteins may also have a role in solubilising cholesterol. In gallstone disease the liver produces bile that contains an excess of cholesterol, because there is either a relative deficiency of bile salts or a relative excess of cholesterol ('lithogenic' bile). Disorders with the potential to induce lithogenic bile are shown in Box 23.75. Factors initiating crystallisation of cholesterol in lithogenic bile (nucleation factors) are also important in determining the rate at which crystals form from saturated bile. Factors favouring nucleation (mucus, calcium, fatty acids, other proteins) and antinucleating factors (apolipoproteins) have been described.

Pigment stones

Brown crumbly pigment stones are almost always the consequence of bacterial or parasitic biliary infection. They are common in the Far East, where infection allows bacterial β-glucuronidase to hydrolyse conjugated bilirubin to its free form, which then precipitates as calcium bilirubinate. The mechanism of black pigment gallstone formation in developed countries is not satisfactorily explained. Haemolysis is important, as these stones occur in chronic haemolytic disease.

Biliary sludge

This describes gelatinous bile that contains numerous microspheroliths of calcium bilirubinate granules and cholesterol crystals, as well as glycoproteins; it is an important precursor to the formation of gallstones in the majority of patients. Biliary sludge is frequently formed under normal conditions, but then either dissolves or is cleared by the gallbladder; only in about 15% of patients does it persist to form cholesterol stones. Fasting, parenteral nutrition and pregnancy are also associated with sludge formation.

Clinical features

Only 10% of individuals with gallstones develop clinical evidence of gallstone disease. Symptomatic stones within the gallbladder (Box 23.76) manifest as either biliary pain ('biliary colic') or cholecystitis (see below). If a gallstone becomes acutely impacted in the cystic duct, the patient will experience pain. The term 'biliary colic' is a misnomer because the pain does not rhythmically increase and decrease in intensity like other forms of colic. Typically, the pain occurs suddenly and persists for about 2 hours; if it continues for more than 6 hours, a complication such as cholecystitis or pancreatitis may be present. Pain is usually felt in the epigastrium (70% of patients) or right upper quadrant (20%), and radiates to the interscapular region or the tip of the right scapula, but other sites include the left upper quadrant and the lower chest. The pain can mimic intrathoracic disease, oesophagitis, myocardial infarction or dissecting aneurysm.

Combinations of fatty food intolerance, dyspepsia and flatulence not attributable to other causes have been referred to as 'gallstone dyspepsia'. These symptoms are not now recognised as being caused by

23.76 Clinical features and complications of gallstones

Clinical features

- Asymptomatic (80%)
- Biliary colic
- Acute cholecystitis
- Chronic cholecystitis

Complications

- Empyema of the gallbladder
- Porcelain gallbladder
- Choledocholithiasis
- Acute pancreatitis
- Fistulae from gallbladder to duodenum/colon
- Pressure on/inflammation of the common bile duct by a gallstone in the cystic duct (Mirizzi's syndrome)
- Gallstone ileus
- Cancer of the gallbladder

gallstones and are best regarded as functional dyspepsia (p. 852).

Acute and chronic cholecystitis is described below.

A mucocele may develop if there is slow distension of the gallbladder from continuous secretion of mucus; if this material becomes infected, an empyema supervenes. Calcium may be secreted into the lumen of the hydropic gallbladder, causing 'limey' bile, and if calcium salts are precipitated in the gallbladder wall, the radiological appearance of 'porcelain' gallbladder results.

Gallstones in the gallbladder (cholecystolithiasis) migrate to the common bile duct (choledocholithiasis, p. 984) in approximately 15% of patients and cause biliary colic. Rarely, fistulae develop between the gallbladder and the duodenum, colon or stomach. If this occurs, air will be seen in the biliary tree on plain abdominal X-rays. If a stone larger than 2.5 cm in diameter has migrated into the gut, it may impact either at the terminal ileum or occasionally in the duodenum or sigmoid colon. The resultant intestinal obstruction may be followed by 'gallstone ileus'. Gallstones impacted in the cystic duct may cause stricturing of the common hepatic duct and the clinical picture of extrahepatic biliary diseases (with its important differential of malignant bile duct stricture). The more common cause of jaundice due to gallstones is a stone passing from the cystic duct into the common bile duct (choledocholithiasis), which may also result in cholangitis or acute pancreatitis. It is usually very small stones that precipitate acute pancreatitis, due (it is thought) to oedema at the ampulla as the stone passes into the duodenum (no stone is seen within the bile duct in 80% of cases of presumed gallstone pancreatitis, suggesting stone passage). Previous stone passage is also the likely cause of most cases of benign papillary fibrosis, which is most commonly seen in patients with previous or present gallstone disease (it may present with jaundice, obstructive LFTs with biliary dilatation, post-cholecystectomy pain or acute pancreatitis).

Cancer of the gallbladder is uncommon (p. 985) but in over 95% of cases is associated with gallstones. The diagnosis is usually made as an incidental histological finding following cholecystectomy for gallstone disease.

Investigations

Ultrasound is the investigation of choice for diagnosing gallstones. Most stones are diagnosed by transabdominal ultrasound, which has a greater than 92% sensitivity and 99% specificity for gallbladder stones (see Fig. 23.8, p. 930). CT (Fig. 23.43) and MRCP are excellent modalities for detecting complications of gallstones (distal bile duct stone or gallbladder empyema), but are inferior to ultrasound in defining their presence in the gallbladder. When recurrent attacks of otherwise unexplained acute pancreatitis occur, this may result from 'microlithiasis' in the gallbladder or common bile duct, and this is best assessed by endoscopic ultrasound (EUS).

Management

Asymptomatic gallstones found incidentally should not be treated because the majority will never cause symptoms. Symptomatic gallstones are best treated surgically by laparoscopic cholecystectomy, with the severity of symptoms being balanced against the individual patient surgical risk in deciding whether surgery is warranted.

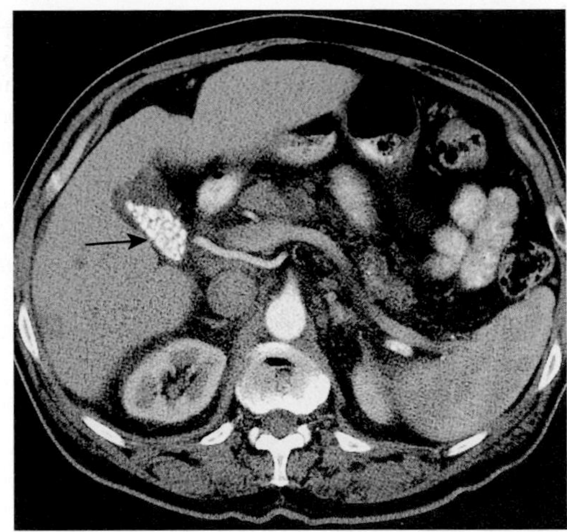

Fig. 23.43 CT showing gallstones within the gallbladder (arrow).

23.77 Treatment of gallstones

Gallbladder stones

- Cholecystectomy: open or laparoscopic
- Oral bile acids: chenodeoxycholic or ursodeoxycholic (low rate of stone dissolution)

Bile duct stones

- Lithotripsy (endoscopic or extracorporeal shock wave, ESWL)
- Endoscopic sphincterotomy and balloon trawl
- Surgical bile duct exploration

Various techniques can be used to treat common bile duct stones (Box 23.77).

Cholecystitis

Acute cholecystitis

Pathophysiology

Acute cholecystitis is almost always associated with obstruction of the gallbladder neck or cystic duct by a gallstone. Occasionally, obstruction may be by mucus, parasitic worms or a bile tumour, or may follow endoscopic bile duct stenting. The pathogenesis is unclear but the initial inflammation is possibly chemically induced. This leads to gallbladder mucosal damage, which releases phospholipase, converting biliary lecithin to lysolecithin, a recognised mucosal toxin. At the time of surgery, approximately 50% of cultures of the gallbladder contents are sterile. Infection occurs eventually, and in elderly patients or those with diabetes mellitus a severe infection with gas-forming organisms can cause emphysematous cholecystitis. Acalculous cholecystitis can occur in the intensive care setting and in association with parenteral nutrition, sickle cell disease and diabetes mellitus.

Clinical features

The cardinal feature is pain in the right upper quadrant but also in the epigastrium, the right shoulder tip or the interscapular region. Differentiation between biliary colic (p. 982) and acute cholecystitis may be difficult;

features suggesting cholecystitis include severe and prolonged pain, fever and leucocytosis.

Examination shows right hypochondrial tenderness, rigidity worse on inspiration (Murphy's sign) and occasionally a gallbladder mass (30% of cases). Fever is present but rigors are unusual. Jaundice occurs in less than 10% of patients and is usually due to passage of stones into the common bile duct, or compression or even stricturing of the common bile duct following stone impaction in the cystic duct (Mirizzi's syndrome). Gallbladder perforation occurs in 10–15% of cases, and gallbladder empyema may arise.

Investigations

Peripheral blood leucocytosis is common, except in the elderly patient, in whom the signs of inflammation may be minimal. Minor increases of transaminases and amylase may be encountered. Amylase should be measured to detect acute pancreatitis (p. 889), which may be a potentially serious complication of gallstones. Only when the amylase is higher than 1000 U/L can pain be confidently attributed to acute pancreatitis, since moderately elevated levels of amylase can occur in many other causes of abdominal pain. Plain X-rays of the abdomen and chest may show radio-opaque gallstones, and rarely intrabiliary gas due to fistulation of a gallstone into the intestine; they are important in excluding lower lobe pneumonia and a perforated viscus. Ultrasonography detects gallstones and gallbladder thickening due to cholecystitis, but gallbladder empyema or perforation is best assessed by CT.

Management

Medical

This consists of bed rest, pain relief, antibiotics and intravenous fluids. Moderate pain can be treated with NSAIDs but more severe pain should be managed with opiates. A cephalosporin (such as cefuroxime) or piperacillin/tazobactam is the usual antibiotic of choice, but metronidazole is normally added in severely ill patients and local prescribing practice may vary. Nasogastric aspiration is only needed for persistent vomiting. Cholecystitis usually resolves with medical treatment, but the inflammation may progress to an empyema or perforation and peritonitis.

Surgical

Urgent surgery is the optimal treatment when cholecystitis progresses in spite of medical therapy and when complications such as empyema or perforation develop. Operation should be carried out within 5 days of the onset of symptoms. Delayed surgery after 2–3 months is no longer favoured. When cholecystectomy may be difficult due to extensive inflammatory change, percutaneous gallbladder drainage can be performed, with subsequent cholecystectomy 4–6 weeks later. Recurrent biliary colic or cholecystitis is frequent if the gallbladder is not removed.

Chronic cholecystitis

Chronic inflammation of the gallbladder is almost invariably associated with gallstones. The usual symptoms are those of recurrent attacks of upper abdominal pain, often at night and following a heavy meal. The clinical features are similar to those of acute calculous cholecystitis but milder. The patient may recover spontaneously or following analgesia and antibiotics. Patients are usually advised to undergo elective laparoscopic cholecystectomy.

Acute cholangitis

Acute cholangitis is caused by bacterial infection of bile ducts and occurs in patients with other biliary problems, such as choledocholithiasis (see below), biliary strictures or tumours, or after ERCP. Jaundice, fever (with or without rigors) and right upper quadrant pain are the main presenting features ('Charcot's triad'). Treatment is with antibiotics, relief of biliary obstruction and removal (if possible) of the underlying cause.

Choledocholithiasis

Stones in the common bile duct (choledocholithiasis) occur in 10–15% of patients with gallstones (Fig. 23.44), which have usually migrated from the gallbladder. Primary bile duct stones are rare but can develop within the common bile duct many years after a cholecystectomy, and are sometimes related to biliary sludge arising from dysfunction of the sphincter of Oddi. In Far Eastern countries, primary common bile duct stones are thought to follow bacterial infection secondary to parasitic infections with *Clonorchis sinensis*, *Ascaris lumbricoides* or *Fasciola hepatica* (pp. 377, 371 and 379). Common bile duct stones can cause bile duct obstruction and may be complicated by cholangitis due to secondary bacterial infection, septicaemia, liver abscess and biliary stricture.

Clinical features

Choledocholithiasis may be asymptomatic, may be found incidentally by operative cholangiography at

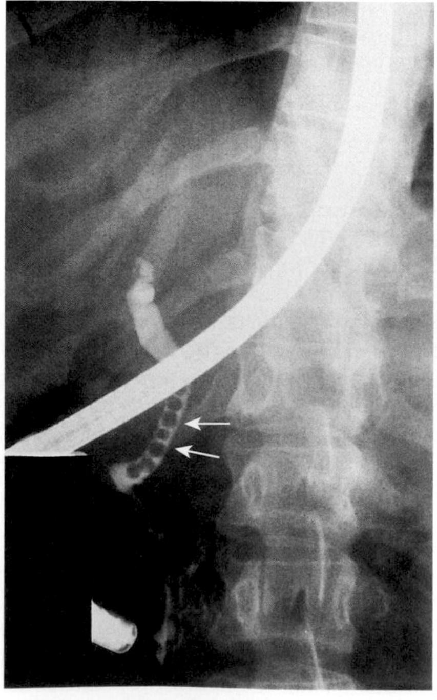

Fig. 23.44 ERCP showing common duct stones (arrows).

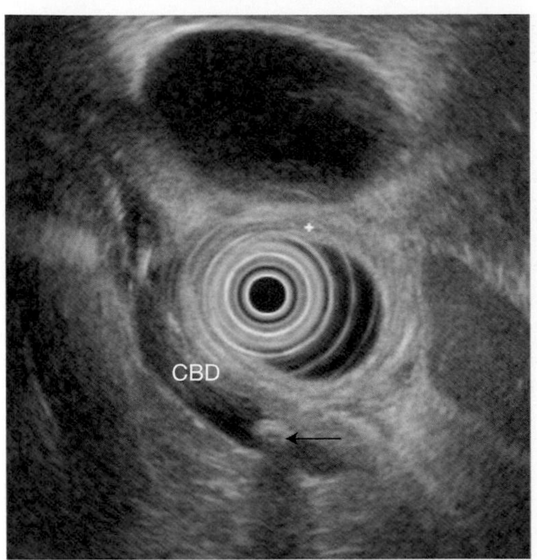

Fig. 23.45 Endoscopic ultrasound (EUS) image in a patient with cholangitis. The dilated common bile duct (CBD) contains a small stone (arrow), which causes acoustic shadowing.

cholecystectomy, or may manifest as recurrent abdominal pain with or without jaundice. The pain is usually in the right upper quadrant, and fever, pruritus and dark urine may be present. Rigors may be a feature; jaundice is common and usually associated with pain. Physical examination may show the scar of a previous cholecystectomy; if the gallbladder is present, it is usually small, fibrotic and impalpable.

Investigations

The LFTs show a cholestatic pattern and there is bilirubinuria. If cholangitis is present, the patient usually has a leucocytosis. The most convenient method of demonstrating obstruction to the common bile duct is by transabdominal ultrasound. This shows dilated extrahepatic and intrahepatic bile ducts, together with gallbladder stones (Fig. 23.45), but does not always reveal the cause of the obstruction in the common bile duct; 50% of bile duct stones are missed on ultrasound, particularly those in the distal common bile duct. EUS is extremely accurate at identifying bile duct stones. MRCP is non-invasive, and is indicated when intervention is not necessarily mandatory (e.g. the patient with possible bile duct stones but no jaundice or sepsis).

Management

Cholangitis should be treated with analgesia, intravenous fluids and broad-spectrum antibiotics, such as cefuroxime and metronidazole (local prescribing practice may vary). Blood cultures should be taken before the antibiotics are administered. Patients also require urgent decompression of the biliary tree and stone removal. ERCP with biliary sphincterotomy and stone extraction is the treatment of choice and is successful in about 90% of patients. If ERCP fails, other approaches include percutaneous transhepatic drainage and combined ('rendezvous') endoscopic procedures, extracorporeal shock wave lithotripsy (ESWL) and surgery.

Surgical treatment of choledocholithiasis is performed less frequently than ERCP because it carries higher morbidity and mortality. Before the common bile duct is explored, the diagnosis of choledocholithiasis should be confirmed by intraoperative cholangiography. If gallstones are found, the bile duct is explored, all stones are removed, stone clearance is checked by cholangiography or choledochoscopy, and a T-tube is inserted into the common bile duct. It is now possible to achieve these goals laparoscopically in specialist centres.

Recurrent pyogenic cholangitis

This disease occurs predominantly in South-east Asia. Biliary sludge, calcium bilirubinate concretions and stones accumulate in the intrahepatic bile ducts, with secondary bacterial infection. Patients present with recurrent attacks of upper abdominal pain, fever and cholestatic jaundice. Investigation of the biliary tree demonstrates that both the intrahepatic and the extrahepatic portions are filled with soft biliary mud. Eventually, the liver becomes scarred and liver abscesses and secondary biliary cirrhosis develop. The condition is difficult to manage, and requires drainage of the biliary tract with extraction of stones, antibiotics and, in certain patients, partial resection of damaged areas of the liver.

Tumours of the gallbladder and bile duct

Carcinoma of the gallbladder

This is an uncommon tumour, occurring more often in females and usually in those over the age of 70 years. More than 90% are adenocarcinomas; the remainder are anaplastic or, rarely, squamous tumours. Gallstones are present in 70–80% of cases and are thought to be important in the aetiology of the tumour. Individuals with a calcified gallbladder ('porcelain gallbladder', p. 983) are at high risk of malignant change, and gallbladder polyps over 1 cm in size are associated with increased risk of malignancy; preventative cholecystectomy should be considered in such patients. Chronic infection with *Salmonella*, especially in areas where typhoid is endemic, is also a risk factor.

Carcinoma of the gallbladder may be diagnosed incidentally and is found in 1–3% of gallbladders removed at cholecystectomy for gallstone disease. It may manifest as repeated attacks of biliary pain and later persistent jaundice and weight loss. A gallbladder mass may be palpable in the right hypochondrium. LFTs show cholestasis, and porcelain gallbladder may be found on X-ray. The tumour can be diagnosed by ultrasonography and staged by CT. The treatment is surgical excision, but local extension of the tumour beyond the wall of the gallbladder into the liver, lymph nodes and surrounding tissues is invariable and palliative management is usually all that can be offered. Survival is generally short, death typically occurring within 1 year in patients presenting with symptoms.

Cholangiocarcinoma

Cholangiocarcinoma (CCA) is an uncommon tumour that can arise anywhere in the biliary tree, from the intrahepatic bile ducts (20–25% of cases) and the confluence of the right and left hepatic ducts at the liver

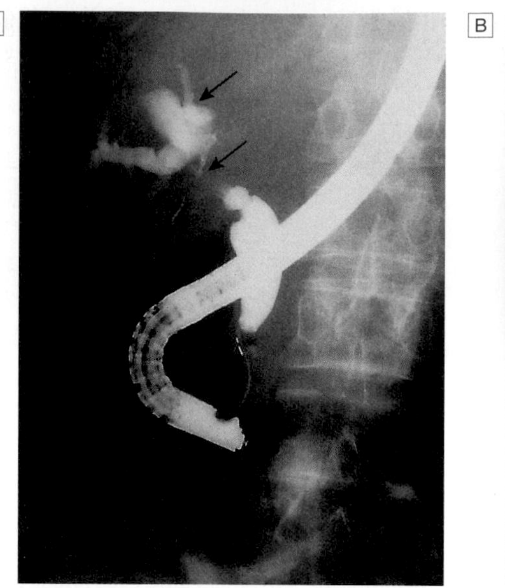

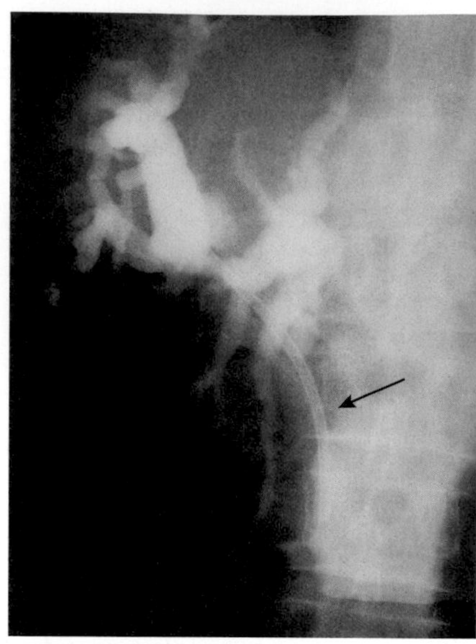

Fig. 23.46 Cholangiocarcinoma. **A** ERCP showing malignant biliary stricture (bottom arrow) and dilated intrahepatic bile ducts above (top arrow). **B** Post-ERCP stenting showing plastic endobiliary stent (arrow), which will drain bile from the dilated ducts above the stricture into the duodenum.

hilum (50–60%) to the distal common bile duct (20%). It accounts for only 1.5% of all cancers but the incidence is increasing. The cause is unknown but the tumour is associated with gallstones, primary and secondary sclerosing cholangitis, Caroli's disease and choledochal cysts (see Fig. 23.42, p. 981). In the Far East, particularly northern Thailand, chronic liver fluke infection (*Clonorchis sinensis*) is a major risk factor for the development of CCA in men. Primary sclerosing cholangitis carries a lifetime risk of CCA of approximately 20%, although only 5% of CCAs relate to primary sclerosing cholangitis. Chronic biliary inflammation appears to be a common factor in the development of biliary dysplasia and cancer that is shared by all the predisposing causes.

Tumours typically invade the lymphatics and adjacent vessels, with a predilection for spread within perineural sheaths. The presentation is usually with obstructive jaundice. About 50% of patients also have upper abdominal pain and weight loss. The diagnosis is made by a combination of CT and MRI but can be difficult to confirm in patients with sclerosing cholangitis. Serum levels of the tumour marker CA19-9 are elevated in up to 80% of cases, although this may occur in biliary obstruction of any cause. In the setting of biliary obstruction, ERCP may result in positive biliary cytology. Endoscopic ultrasound-fine needle aspiration (EUS-FNA) of bile duct masses is sometimes possible, and in specialist centres single-operator cholangioscopy with biopsy is now established. CCAs can be treated surgically in about 20% of patients, which improves 5-year survival from less than 5% to 20–40%. Surgery involves excision of the extrahepatic biliary tree with or without a liver resection and a Roux loop reconstruction. However, most patients are treated by stent insertion across the malignant biliary stricture, using endoscopic or transhepatic techniques (Fig. 23.46). Combination chemotherapy is increasingly used and palliation with endoscopic photodynamic therapy has provided encouraging results.

Carcinoma at the ampulla of Vater

Nearly 40% of all adenocarcinomas of the small intestine arise in relationship to the ampulla of Vater, and present with pain, anaemia, vomiting and weight loss. Jaundice may be intermittent or persistent. The diagnosis is made by duodenal endoscopy and biopsy of the tumour, but staging by CT/MRI is essential. Ampullary carcinoma must be differentiated from carcinoma of the head of the pancreas and a cholangiocarcinoma because these latter conditions both have a worse prognosis. Imaging may show a 'double duct sign' with stricturing of both the common bile duct and pancreatic duct at the ampulla and upstream dilatation of the ducts. EUS is the most sensitive method of assessing and staging ampullary or periampullary tumours.

Curative surgical treatment can be undertaken by pancreaticoduodenectomy, and the 5-year survival may be as high as 50%. If resection is impossible, palliative surgical bypass or stenting may be necessary.

Benign gallbladder tumours

These are uncommon, often asymptomatic and usually found incidentally at operation or postmortem. Cholesterol polyps, sometimes associated with cholesterolosis, papillomas and adenomas, are the main types.

Miscellaneous biliary disorders

Post-cholecystectomy syndrome

Dyspeptic symptoms following cholecystectomy (post-cholecystectomy syndrome) occur in about 30% of patients, depending on how the condition is defined, how actively symptoms are sought and the original indication for cholecystectomy. The syndrome occurs most frequently in women, in patients who have had symptoms for more than 5 years before cholecystectomy, and when the operation was undertaken for non-calculous

23.78 Causes of post-cholecystectomy symptoms

Immediate post-surgical	
• Bleeding • Biliary peritonitis • Abscess	• Bile duct trauma/transection • Fistula
Biliary	
• Common bile duct stones • Benign stricture • Tumour • Cystic duct stump syndrome	• Disorders of the ampulla of Vater (e.g. benign papillary fibrosis; sphincter of Oddi dysfunction)
Extrabiliary	
• Non-ulcer dyspepsia • Peptic ulcer • Pancreatic disease	• Gastro-oesophageal reflux • Irritable bowel syndrome • Functional abdominal pain

gallbladder disease. An increase in bowel habit resulting from bile acid diarrhoea occurs in about 5–10% of patients after cholecystectomy, and often responds to colestyramine 4–8 g daily. Severe post-cholecystectomy syndrome occurs in only 2–5% of patients. The main causes are listed in Box 23.78.

The usual symptoms include right upper quadrant pain, flatulence, fatty food intolerance, and occasionally jaundice and cholangitis. The LFTs may be abnormal and sometimes show cholestasis. Ultrasonography is used to detect biliary obstruction, and EUS or MRCP is used to seek common bile duct stones. If retained bile duct stones are excluded, sphincter of Oddi dysfunction should be considered (see below). Other investigations that may be required include upper gastrointestinal endoscopy, small bowel radiology and pancreatic function tests. The possibility of a functional illness should also be considered.

Sphincter of Oddi dysfunction

The sphincter of Oddi is a small smooth muscle sphincter situated at the junction of the bile duct and pancreatic duct in the duodenum. Sphincter of Oddi dysfunction (SOD) is characterised by an increase in contractility that produces a benign non-calculous obstruction to the flow of bile or pancreatic juice. This may cause pancreaticobiliary pain, deranged LFTs or recurrent pancreatitis. A clinical classification system, based on clinical history, laboratory results and ERCP findings, is widely used (Boxes 23.79 and 23.80).

Clinical features

Patients with SOD, who are predominantly female, present with symptoms and signs suggestive of either biliary or pancreatic disease.

- *Patients with biliary-type SOD* experience recurrent, episodic biliary-type pain. They have often had a cholecystectomy but the gallbladder may be intact.
- *Patients with pancreatic SOD* usually present with unexplained recurrent attacks of pancreatitis.

Investigations

The diagnosis is established by excluding gallstones, including microlithiasis, and demonstrating a dilated or

23.79 Classification of biliary sphincter of Oddi dysfunction

Biliary type I
• Biliary-type pain • Abnormal liver enzymes (ALT/AST > twice normal on two or more occasions) • Dilated common bile duct (> 12 mm diameter) • Delayed drainage of ERCP contrast beyond 45 mins
Biliary type II
• Biliary-type pain with one or two of the above criteria
Biliary type III
• Biliary-type pain with no other abnormalities

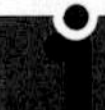

23.80 Classification of pancreatic sphincter of Oddi dysfunction

Pancreatic type I
• Pancreatic-type pain • Twice normal amylase or lipase • Pancreatic duct > 6 mm in the head or 5 mm in the body
Pancreatic type II
• Pancreatic-type pain with only one of the above criteria
Pancreatic type III
• Pancreatic-type pain with no other abnormalities

slowly draining bile duct. The gold standard for diagnosis is sphincter of Oddi manometry. This is not, however, widely available and is associated with a high rate of procedure-related pancreatitis.

Management

All biliary SOD patients with type I disease are treated with endoscopic sphincterotomy. The results are good but patients should be warned that there is a high risk of complications, particularly acute pancreatitis. Manometry should ideally be performed in all suspected SOD type II and III patients, and 'speculative' sphincterotomy should be avoided. In type III patients without documented evidence of sphincter hypertension, medical therapy with nifedipine and/or low-dose amitriptyline may be tried. The role of botulinum toxin ('botox') injection into the sphincter to improve sphincter function remains unclear.

Pancreatic SOD can be treated with pancreatic stenting followed by pancreatic sphincterotomy, carried out in specialised units. Emerging evidence suggests that all patients being investigated by ERCP for suspected SOD should also undergo prophylactic pancreatic duct stenting, because this significantly reduces the rate of procedure-related acute pancreatitis.

Cholesterolosis of the gallbladder

In this condition, lipid deposits in the submucosa and epithelium appear as multiple yellow spots on the pink mucosa, giving rise to the description 'strawberry gallbladder'. Cholesterolosis of the gallbladder is usually asymptomatic but may occasionally present with right upper quadrant pain. Small, fixed filling defects may be visible on ultrasonography; the radiologist can usually differentiate between gallstones and cholesterolosis.

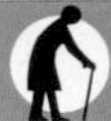

23.81 **Gallbladder disease in old age**

- **Gallstones**: by the age of 70 years, prevalence is around 30% in women and 19% in men.
- **Acute cholecystitis**: tends to be severe, may have few localising signs, and is associated with a high frequency of empyema and perforation. If such complications supervene, mortality may reach 20%.
- **Cholecystectomy**: mortality after urgent cholecystectomy for acute uncomplicated cholecystitis is not significantly higher than in younger patients.
- **Endoscopic sphincterotomy and removal of common duct stones**: well tolerated by older patients, with lower mortality than surgical common bile duct exploration.
- **Cancer of the gallbladder**: a disease of old age, with a 1-year survival of 10%.

The condition is usually diagnosed at cholecystectomy; if the diagnosis is made radiologically, cholecystectomy may be indicated, depending on symptoms.

Adenomyomatosis of the gallbladder

In this condition, there is hyperplasia of the muscle and mucosa of the gallbladder. The projection of pouches of mucous membrane through weak points in the muscle coat produces Rokitansky–Aschoff sinuses. There is much disagreement over whether adenomyomatosis is a cause of right upper quadrant pain or other gastrointestinal symptoms. It may be diagnosed by oral cholecystography, when a halo or ring of opacified diverticula can be seen around the gallbladder. Other appearances include deformity of the body of the gallbladder or marked irregularity of the outline. Localised adenomyomatosis in the region of the gallbladder fundus causes the appearance of a 'Phrygian cap'. Most patients are treated by cholecystectomy but only after excluding other diseases in the upper gastrointestinal tract.

IgG4-associated cholangitis

This recently reported disease often presents with obstructive jaundice and is discussed fully on page 966.

Further information and acknowledgements

Books and journal articles

Day CP. Non-alcoholic fatty liver disease: current concepts and management strategies. Clin Med 2008; 6:19–25.

Neuberger J, Gimson A, Davies M, et al. Selection of patients for liver transplantation and allocation of donated livers in the UK. Gut 2008; 57:252–257.

Ratziu V, Bellentani S, Cortez-Pinto H, et al. A position statement on NAFLD/NASH based on the EASL 2009 special conference. J Hepatol 2010; 53:372–384.

Websites

www.aasld.org *American Association for the Study of Liver Diseases (guidelines available).*

www.bsg.org.uk *British Society of Gastroenterology (guidelines available).*

www.easl.ch *European Association for the Study of the Liver (guidelines available).*

www.eltr.org *European Liver Transplant Registry.*

www.unos.org *United Network for Organ Sharing: US transplant register.*

Figure acknowledgements

Page 922 insets (*Spider naevi*) Hayes P, Simpson K. Gastroenterology and liver disease. Edinburgh: Churchill Livingstone; 1995; copyright Elsevier; (*Aspiration*) Strachan M. Davidson's clinical cases. Edinburgh: Churchill Livingstone; 2008 (Fig. 65.1); (*Palmar erythema*) Martin P. Approach to the patient with liver disease. In: Goldman's Cecil Medicine, Goldman L and Schafter AI. 24th edn. Philadelphia: WB Saunders; 2012; Fig. 1148-2, p. 954.

Fig. 23.35 Based on EASL–EORTC Clinical Practice Guidelines, Management of hepatocellular carcinoma. Journal of Hepatology 2012, 56:908–943.

Fig. 23.42 Shearman DC, Finlayson NDC. Diseases of the gastrointestinal tract and liver. 2nd edn. Edinburgh: Churchill Livingstone; 1989; copyright Elsevier.

H.G. Watson
J.I.O. Craig
L.M. Manson

Blood disease 24

Clinical examination in blood disease 990

Functional anatomy and physiology 992
- Haematopoiesis 992
- Blood cells and their functions 994
- Haemostasis 996

Investigation of diseases of the blood 998
- The full blood count 998
- Blood film examination 998
- Bone marrow examination 998
- Investigation of coagulation 999

Presenting problems in blood disease 1001
- Anaemia 1001
- High haemoglobin 1003
- Leucopenia (low white cell count) 1004
- Leucocytosis (high white cell count) 1005
- Lymphadenopathy 1005
- Splenomegaly 1006
- Bleeding 1006
- Thrombocytopenia (low platelet count) 1007
- Thrombocytosis (high platelet count) 1008
- Pancytopenia 1008
- Infection 1008
- Venous thrombosis 1008

Blood products and transfusion 1011
- Blood products 1011
- Adverse effects of transfusion 1012
- Safe transfusion procedures 1015

Haematopoietic stem cell transplantation 1017

Anticoagulant and antithrombotic therapy 1018
- Heparins 1018
- Coumarins 1019
- Prophylaxis of venous thrombosis 1020

Anaemias 1021
- Iron deficiency anaemia 1021
- Anaemia of chronic disease 1023
- Megaloblastic anaemia 1024
- Haemolytic anaemia 1026
- Haemoglobinopathies 1031

Haematological malignancies 1035
- Leukaemias 1035
- Lymphomas 1041
- Paraproteinaemias 1045

Aplastic anaemia 1048
- Primary idiopathic acquired aplastic anaemia 1048
- Secondary aplastic anaemia 1048

Myeloproliferative neoplasms 1048

Bleeding disorders 1049
- Disorders of primary haemostasis 1049
- Coagulation disorders 1050

Thrombotic disorders 1054

CLINICAL EXAMINATION IN BLOOD DISEASE

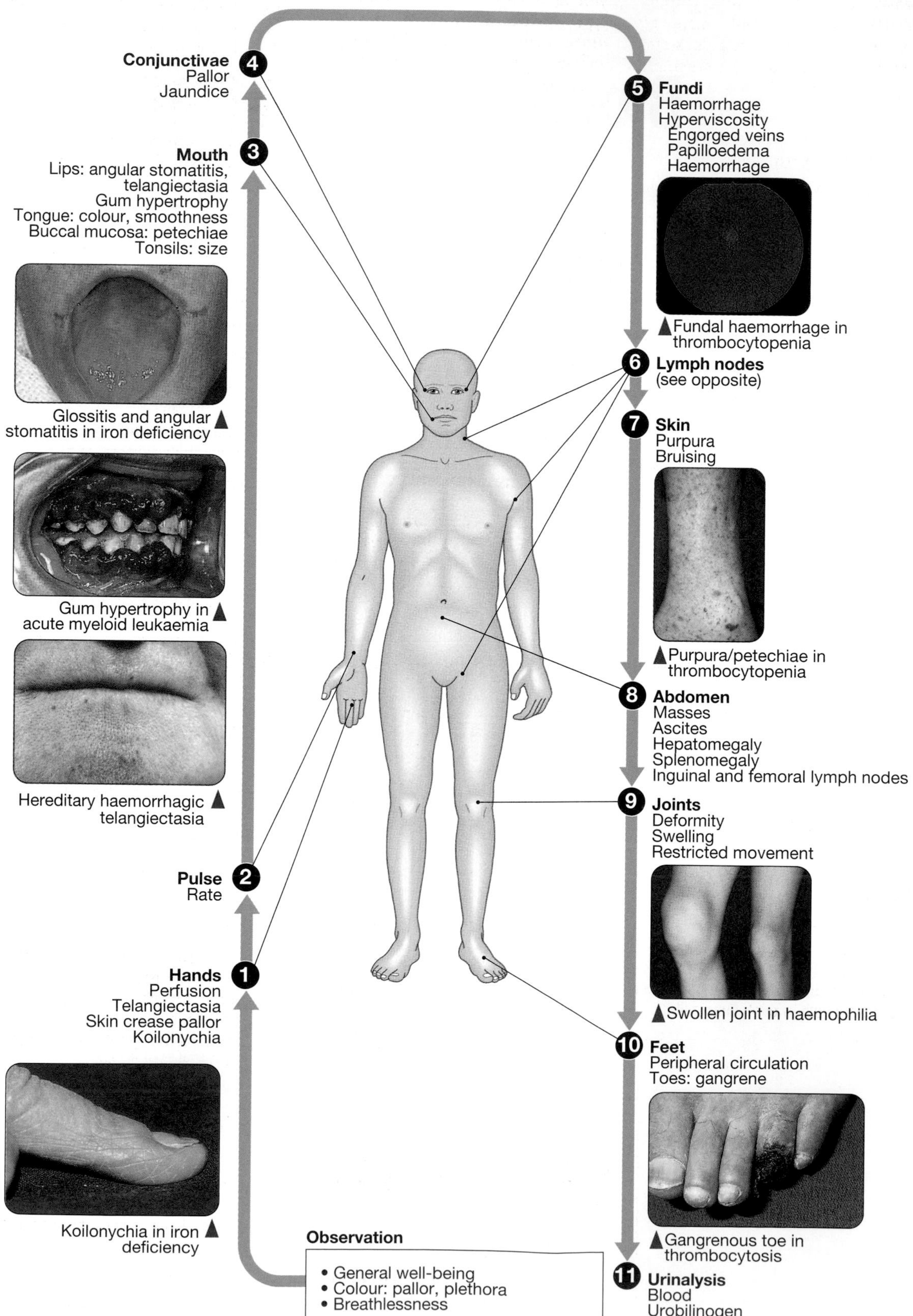

Insets (*Glossitis*) From Hoffbrand, et al. 2010; (*Petechiae*) Young, et al. 2006 – see p. 1056.

Abnormalities detected in the blood are caused not only by primary diseases of the blood and lymphoreticular systems, but also by diseases affecting other systems of the body. The clinical assessment of patients with haematological abnormalities must include a general history and examination, as well as a search for symptoms and signs of abnormalities of red cells, white cells, platelets, haemostatic systems, lymph nodes and lymphoreticular tissues.

6 Lymphadenopathy

Lymphadenopathy can be caused by benign or malignant disease. The clinical points to clarify are shown in the box.

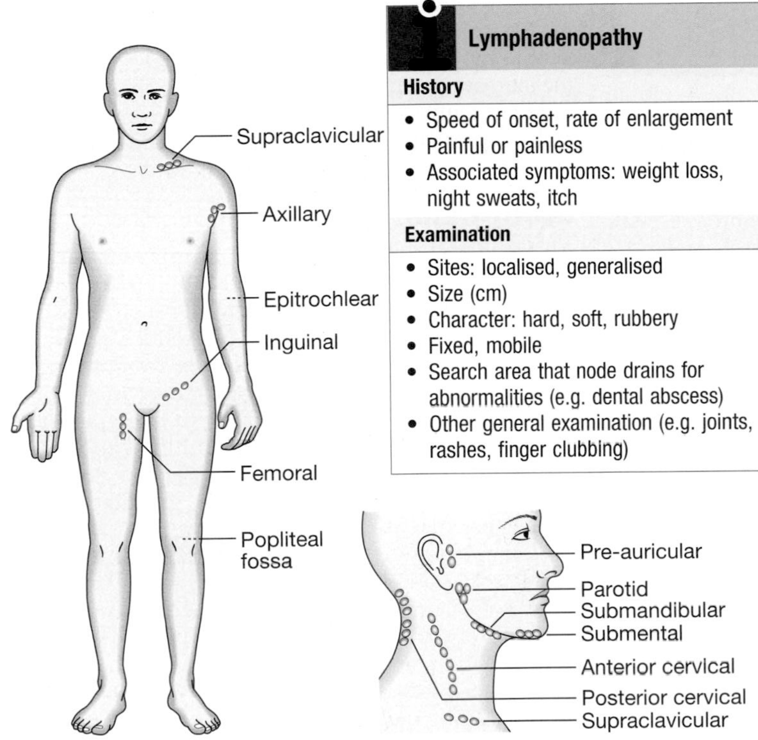

Lymphadenopathy

History

- Speed of onset, rate of enlargement
- Painful or painless
- Associated symptoms: weight loss, night sweats, itch

Examination

- Sites: localised, generalised
- Size (cm)
- Character: hard, soft, rubbery
- Fixed, mobile
- Search area that node drains for abnormalities (e.g. dental abscess)
- Other general examination (e.g. joints, rashes, finger clubbing)

8 Examination of the spleen

- Move hand up from right iliac fossa, towards left upper quadrant on expiration.
- Keep hand still and ask patient to take a deep breath through the mouth to feel spleen edge being displaced downwards.
- Place your left hand around patient's lower ribs and approach costal margin to pull spleen forwards.
- To help palpate small spleens, roll the patient on to the right side and examine as before.

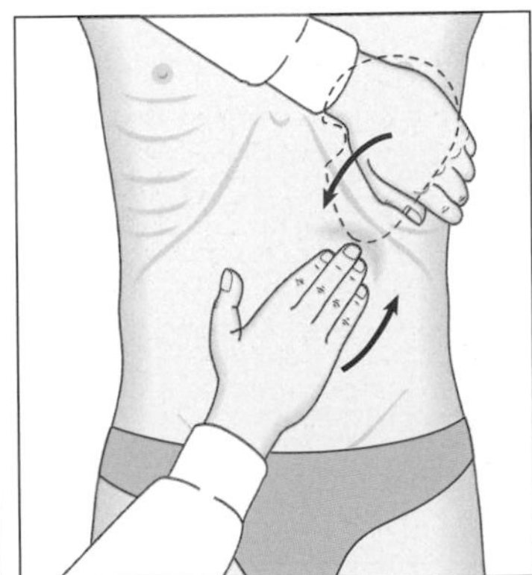

Characteristics of the spleen

- Notch
- Superficial
- Dull to percussion
- Cannot get examining hand between ribs and spleen
- Moves well with respiration

Anaemia

Symptoms and signs help to indicate the clinical severity of anaemia. A full history and examination is needed to identify the underlying cause.

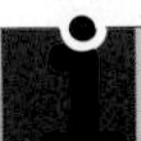

Anaemia

Non-specific symptoms

- Tiredness
- Lightheadedness
- Breathlessness
- Development/worsening of ischaemic symptoms, e.g. angina or claudication

Non-specific signs

- Mucous membrane pallor
- Tachypnoea
- Raised jugular venous pressure
- Tachycardia
- Flow murmurs
- Ankle oedema
- Postural hypotension

Bleeding

Bleeding can be due to congenital or acquired abnormalities in the clotting system. History and examination help to clarify the severity and underlying cause of the bleeding.

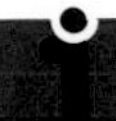

Bleeding

History

- Site of bleed
- Duration of bleed
- Precipitating causes, including previous surgery or trauma
- Family history
- Drug history
- Age at presentation
- Other medical conditions, e.g. liver disease

Examination

There are two main patterns of bleeding:

1. **Mucosal bleeding**
   Reduced number or function of platelets (e.g. bone marrow failure or aspirin) or von Willebrand factor (e.g. von Willebrand disease)
   - Skin: petechiae, bruises
   - Gum and mucous membrane bleeding
   - Fundal haemorrhage
   - Post-surgical bleeding
2. **Coagulation factor deficiency**
   (e.g. haemophilia or warfarin)
   - Bleeding into joints (haemarthrosis) or muscles
   - Bleeding into soft tissues
   - Retroperitoneal haemorrhage
   - Intracranial haemorrhage
   - Post-surgical bleeding

Disorders of the blood cover a wide spectrum of illnesses, ranging from some of the most common disorders affecting mankind (anaemias) to relatively rare conditions such as leukaemias and congenital coagulation disorders. Although the latter are uncommon, advances in cellular and molecular biology have had major impacts on their diagnosis, treatment and prognosis. Haematological changes occur as a consequence of diseases affecting any system and give important information in the diagnosis and monitoring of many conditions.

FUNCTIONAL ANATOMY AND PHYSIOLOGY

Blood flows throughout the body in the vascular system, and consists of:

- red cells, which transport oxygen from the lungs to the tissues
- white cells, which defend against infection
- platelets, which interact with blood vessels and clotting factors to maintain vascular integrity and prevent bleeding
- plasma, which contains proteins with many functions, including antibodies and coagulation factors.

Haematopoiesis

Haematopoiesis describes the formation of blood cells, an active process that must maintain normal numbers of circulating cells and be able to respond rapidly to increased demands such as bleeding or infection. During development, haematopoiesis occurs in the liver and spleen, and subsequently in red bone marrow in the medullary cavity of all bones. In childhood, red marrow is progressively replaced by fat (yellow marrow), so that, in adults, normal haematopoiesis is restricted to the vertebrae, pelvis, sternum, ribs, clavicles, skull, upper humeri and proximal femora. However, red marrow can expand in response to increased demands for blood cells.

Bone marrow contains a range of immature haematopoietic precursor cells and a storage pool of mature cells for release at times of increased demand. Haematopoietic cells interact closely with surrounding connective tissue stroma, made up of reticular cells, macrophages, fat cells, blood vessels and nerve fibres (Fig. 24.1). In normal marrow, nests of red cell precursors cluster around a central macrophage, which provides iron and also phagocytoses nuclei from red cells prior to their release into the circulation. Megakaryocytes are large cells which produce and release platelets into vascular sinuses. White cell precursors are clustered next to the bone trabeculae; maturing cells migrate into the marrow spaces towards the vascular sinuses. Plasma cells are antibody-secreting mature B cells which normally represent less than 5% of the marrow population and are scattered throughout the intertrabecular spaces.

Stem cells

All blood cells are derived from pluripotent haematopoietic stem cells. These comprise only 0.01% of the total marrow cells, but they can self-renew (i.e. make more stem cells) or differentiate to produce a hierarchy of lineage-committed stem cells. The resulting primitive progenitor cells cannot be identified morphologically, so they are named according to the types of cell (or colony) they form during cell culture experiments. CFU–GM (colony-forming unit - granulocyte, monocyte) are stem cells that produce granulocytic and monocytic lines, CFU–E produce erythroid cells, and CFU–Meg produce megakaryocytes and ultimately platelets (Fig. 24.2).

Growth factors, produced in bone marrow stromal cells and elsewhere, control the survival, proliferation, differentiation and function of stem cells and their progeny. Some, such as interleukin-3 (IL-3), stem cell factor (SCF) and granulocyte, macrophage-colony-stimulating factor (GM–CSF), act on a wide number of cell types at various stages of differentiation. Others,

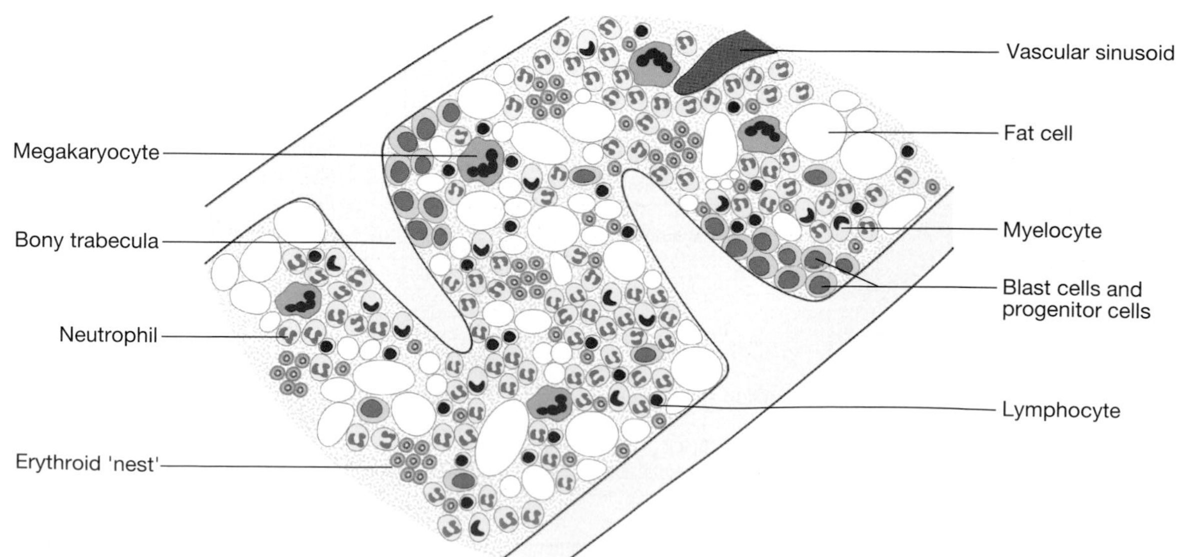

Fig. 24.1 Structural organisation of normal bone marrow.

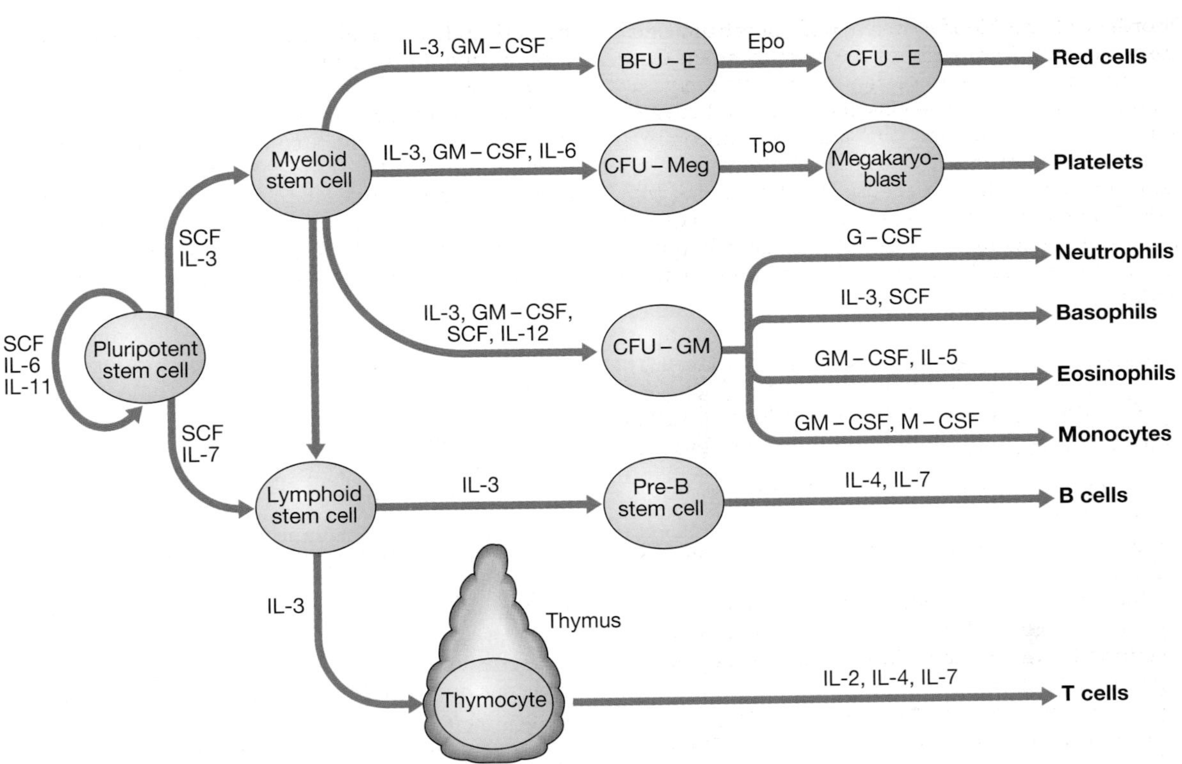

Fig. 24.2 Stem cells and growth factors in haematopoietic cell development. (BFU-E = burst-forming unit – erythroid; CFU–E = colony-forming unit – erythroid; CFU–GM = colony-forming unit – granulocyte, monocyte; CFU–Meg = colony-forming unit – megakaryocyte; Epo = erythropoietin; G–CSF = granulocyte–colony-stimulating factor; GM–CSF = granulocyte, macrophage–colony-stimulating factor; IL = interleukin; M–CSF = macrophage–colony-stimulating factor; SCF = stem cell factor; Tpo = thrombopoietin)

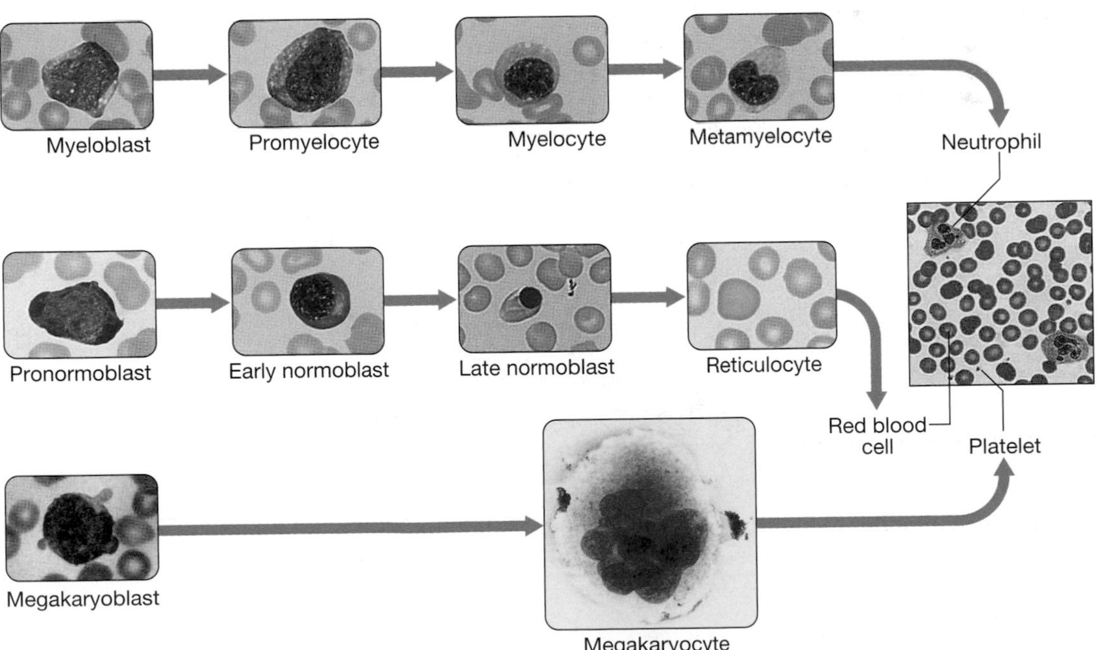

Fig. 24.3 Maturation pathway of red cells, granulocytes and platelets. The image on the right is normal blood film.

such as erythropoietin (Epo), granulocyte-colony-stimulating factor (G-CSF) and thrombopoietin (Tpo), are lineage-specific. Many of these growth factors are now synthesised by recombinant DNA technology and used as treatments: for example, Epo to correct renal anaemia and G-CSF to hasten neutrophil recovery after chemotherapy.

The bone marrow also contains stem cells which can differentiate into non-haematological cells, such as nerve, skeletal muscle, cardiac muscle, liver and blood vessel endothelium. This is termed stem-cell plasticity and may have exciting clinical applications in the future (Ch. 3).

Blood cells and their functions

Red cells

Red cell precursors formed in the bone marrow from the erythroid (CFU–E) progenitor cells are called erythroblasts or normoblasts (Fig. 24.3). These divide and acquire haemoglobin, which turns the cytoplasm pink; the nucleus condenses and is extruded from the cell. The first non-nucleated red cell is a reticulocyte, which still contains ribosomal material in the cytoplasm, giving these large cells a faint blue tinge ('polychromasia'). Reticulocytes lose their ribosomal material and mature over 3 days, during which time they are released into the circulation. Increased numbers of circulating reticulocytes (reticulocytosis) reflect increased erythropoiesis. Proliferation and differentiation of red cell precursors is stimulated by erythropoietin, a polypeptide hormone produced by renal interstitial peritubular cells in response to hypoxia. Failure of erythropoietin production in patients with renal failure (p. 478) causes anaemia, which can be treated with exogenous recombinant erythropoietin.

Normal mature red cells circulate for about 120 days. They are 8 μm biconcave discs lacking a nucleus but filled with haemoglobin, which delivers oxygen to the tissues. In order to pass through the smallest capillaries, the red cell membrane is deformable, with a lipid bilayer to which a 'skeleton' of filamentous proteins is attached via special linkage proteins (Fig. 24.4). Inherited abnormalities of any of these proteins result in loss of membrane as cells pass through the spleen, and the formation of abnormally shaped red cells called spherocytes or elliptocytes (see Fig. 24.8D, p. 999). Red cells are exposed to osmotic stress in the pulmonary and renal circulation; in order to maintain homeostasis, the membrane contains ion pumps, which control intracellular levels of sodium, potassium, chloride and bicarbonate. In the absence of mitochondria, the energy for these functions is provided by anaerobic glycolysis and the pentose phosphate pathway in the cytosol. Membrane glycoproteins inserted into the lipid bilayer also form the antigens recognised by blood grouping (see Fig. 24.4). The ABO and Rhesus systems are the most commonly recognised (p. 1012), but over 400 blood group antigens have been described.

Haemoglobin

Haemoglobin is a protein specially adapted for oxygen transport. It is composed of four globin chains, each surrounding an iron-containing porphyrin pigment molecule termed haem. Globin chains are a combination of two alpha and two non-alpha chains; haemoglobin A ($\alpha\alpha/\beta\beta$) represents over 90% of adult haemoglobin, whereas haemoglobin F ($\alpha\alpha/\gamma\gamma$) is the predominant type in the fetus. Each haem molecule contains a ferrous ion (Fe^{2+}), to which oxygen reversibly binds; the affinity for oxygen increases as successive oxygen molecules bind. When oxygen is bound, the beta chains 'swing' closer together; they move apart as oxygen is lost. In the 'open' deoxygenated state, 2,3 diphosphoglycerate (DPG), a product of red cell metabolism, binds to the haemoglobin molecule and lowers its oxygen affinity. These complex interactions produce the sigmoid shape of the oxygen dissociation curve (Fig. 24.5). The position of this curve depends upon the concentrations of 2,3 DPG, H^+ ions and CO_2; increased levels shift the curve to the right and cause oxygen to be released more readily, e.g. when

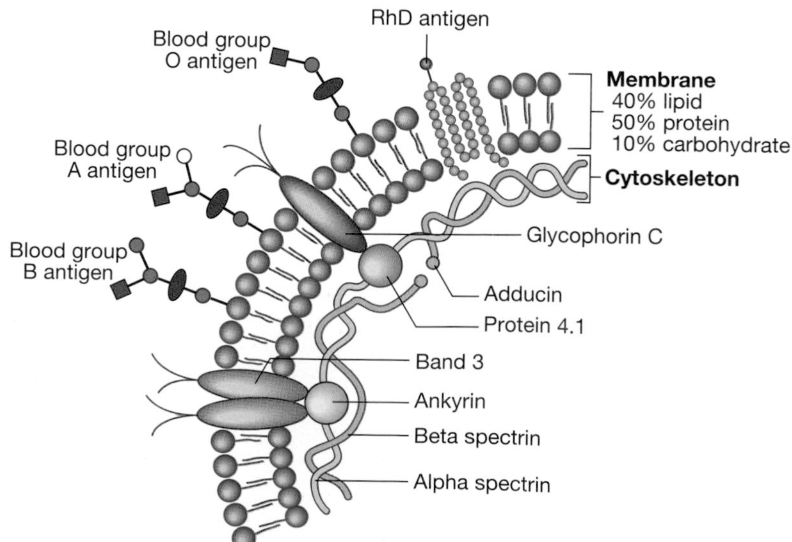

Fig. 24.4 Normal structure of red cell membrane. Red cell membrane flexibility is conferred by attachment of cytoskeletal proteins. Important transmembrane proteins include band 3 (an ion transport channel) and glycophorin (involved in cytoskeletal attachment and gas exchange, and a receptor for *Plasmodium falciparum* in malaria). Antigens on the red blood cell determine an individual's blood group. There are about 22 blood group systems (groups of carbohydrate or protein antigens controlled by a single gene or by multiple closely linked loci); the most important clinically are the ABO and Rhesus (Rh) systems (p. 1012). The ABO genetic locus has three main allelic forms: A, B and O. The A and B alleles encode glycosyltransferases that introduce N-acetylgalactosamine (open circle) and D-galactose (blue circle), respectively, on to antigenic carbohydrate molecules on the membrane surface. People with the O allele produce an O antigen, which lacks either of these added sugar groups. Rh antigens are transmembrane proteins.

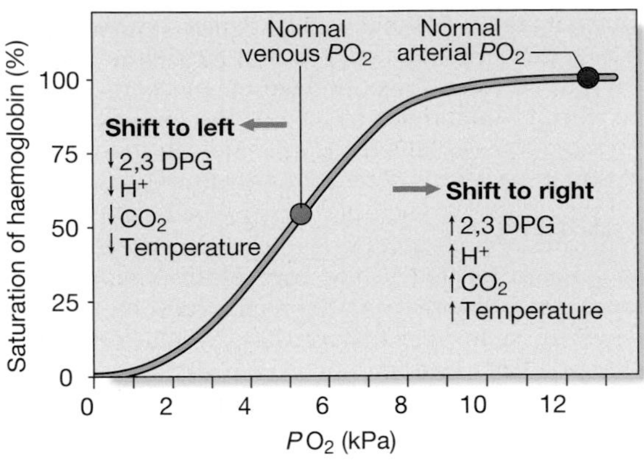

Fig. 24.5 The haemoglobin oxygen dissociation curve. Factors are listed which shift the curve to the right (more oxygen released from blood) and to the left (less oxygen released) at given PO_2. (To convert kPa to mmHg, multiply by 7.5.)

red cells reach hypoxic tissues. Haemoglobin F is unable to bind 2,3 DPG and has a left-shifted oxygen dissociation curve, which, together with the low pH of fetal blood, ensures fetal oxygenation.

Genetic mutations affecting the haem-binding pockets of globin chains or the 'hinge' interactions between globin chains result in haemoglobinopathies or unstable haemoglobins. Alpha globin chains are produced by two genes on chromosome 16, and beta globin chains by a single gene on chromosome 11; imbalance in the production of globin chains results in the thalassaemias (p. 1034). Defects in haem synthesis cause the porphyrias (p. 458).

Destruction

Red cells at the end of their lifespan of approximately 120 days are phagocytosed by the reticulo-endothelial system. Amino acids from globin chains are recycled and iron is removed from haem for re-use in haemoglobin synthesis. The remnant haem structure is degraded to bilirubin and conjugated with glucuronic acid before being excreted in bile. In the small bowel, bilirubin is converted to stercobilin; most of this is excreted, but a small amount is reabsorbed and excreted by the kidney as urobilinogen. Increased red cell destruction due to haemolysis or ineffective haematopoiesis results in jaundice and increased urinary urobilinogen. Free intravascular haemoglobin is toxic and is normally bound by haptoglobins, which are plasma proteins produced by the liver.

White cells

White cells or leucocytes in the blood consist of granulocytes (neutrophils, eosinophils and basophils), monocytes and lymphocytes (see Fig. 24.12, p. 1004). Granulocytes and monocytes are formed from bone marrow CFU-GM progenitor cells during myelopoiesis. The first recognisable granulocyte in the marrow is the myeloblast, a large cell with a small amount of basophilic cytoplasm and a primitive nucleus with open chromatin and nucleoli. As the cells divide and mature, the nucleus segments and the cytoplasm acquires specific neutrophilic, eosinophilic or basophilic granules (see Fig. 24.3). This takes about 14 days. The cytokines G-CSF, GM-CSF and M-CSF are involved in the production of myeloid cells, and G-CSF can be used clinically to hasten recovery of blood neutrophil counts after chemotherapy.

Myelocytes or metamyelocytes are normally found only in the marrow but may appear in the circulation in infection or toxic states. The appearance of more primitive myeloid precursors in the blood is often associated with the presence of nucleated red cells and is termed a 'leucoerythroblastic' picture; this indicates a serious disturbance of marrow function.

Neutrophils

Neutrophils, the most common white blood cells in the blood of adults, are 10–14 μm in diameter, with a multilobular nucleus containing 2–5 segments and granules in their cytoplasm. Their main function is to recognise, ingest and destroy foreign particles and microorganisms (p. 72). A large storage pool of mature neutrophils exists in the bone marrow. Every day, some 10^{11} neutrophils enter the circulation, where cells may be circulating freely or attached to endothelium in the marginating pool. These two pools are equal in size; factors such as exercise or catecholamines increase the number of cells flowing in the blood. Neutrophils spend 6–10 hours in the circulation before being removed, principally by the spleen. Alternatively, they pass into the tissues and either are consumed in the inflammatory process or undergo apoptotic cell death and phagocytosis by macrophages.

Eosinophils

Eosinophils represent 1–6% of the circulating white cells. They are a similar size to neutrophils but have a bilobed nucleus and prominent orange granules on Romanowsky staining. Eosinophils are phagocytic and their granules contain a peroxidase capable of generating reactive oxygen species and proteins involved in the intracellular killing of protozoa and helminths (p. 311). They are also involved in allergic reactions (e.g. atopic asthma, p. 666; see also p. 89).

Basophils

These cells are less common than eosinophils, representing less than 1% of circulating white cells. They contain dense black granules which obscure the nucleus. Mast cells resemble basophils but are found only in the tissues. These cells are involved in hypersensitivity reactions (p. 75).

Monocytes

Monocytes are the largest of the white cells, with a diameter of 12–20 μm and an irregular nucleus in abundant pale blue cytoplasm containing occasional cytoplasmic vacuoles. These cells circulate for a few hours and then migrate into tissue, where they become macrophages, Kupffer cells or antigen-presenting dendritic cells. The former phagocytose debris, apoptotic cells and microorganisms (see Box 4.1, p. 74).

Lymphocytes

Lymphocytes are derived from pluripotent haematopoietic stem cells in the bone marrow. There are two main types: T cells (which mediate cellular immunity) and B cells (which mediate humoral immunity) (p. 77). Lymphoid cells that migrate to the thymus develop into T cells, whereas B cells develop in the bone marrow.

The majority (about 80%) of lymphocytes in the circulation are T cells. Lymphocytes are heterogeneous, the smallest being the size of red cells and the largest the size of neutrophils. Small lymphocytes are circular with scanty cytoplasm but larger cells are more irregular with abundant blue cytoplasm. Lymphocyte subpopulations have specific functions and lifespan can vary from a few days to many years. Cell surface antigens ('cluster of differentiation' (CD) antigens), which appear at different points of lymphocyte maturation, are used to classify lymphomas and lymphoid leukaemias.

Haemostasis

Blood must be maintained in a fluid state in order to function as a transport system, but must be able to solidify to form a clot following vascular injury in order to prevent excessive bleeding, a process known as haemostasis. Successful haemostasis is localised to the area of tissue damage and is followed by removal of the clot and tissue repair. This is achieved by complex interactions between the vascular endothelium, platelets, coagulation factors, natural anticoagulants and fibrinolytic enzymes (Fig. 24.6). Dysfunction of any of these components may result in haemorrhage or thrombosis.

Platelets

Platelets are formed in the bone marrow from megakaryocytes. Megakaryocytic stem cells (CFU–Meg) divide to form megakaryoblasts, which undergo a process called 'endomitotic reduplication', in which there is division of the nucleus but not the cell. This creates mature megakaryocytes, large cells with several nuclei and cytoplasm containing platelet granules. Large numbers of platelets then fragment off from each megakaryocyte into the circulation. The formation and maturation of megakaryocytes are stimulated by thrombopoietin produced in the liver. Platelets circulate for 8–10 days before they are destroyed in the

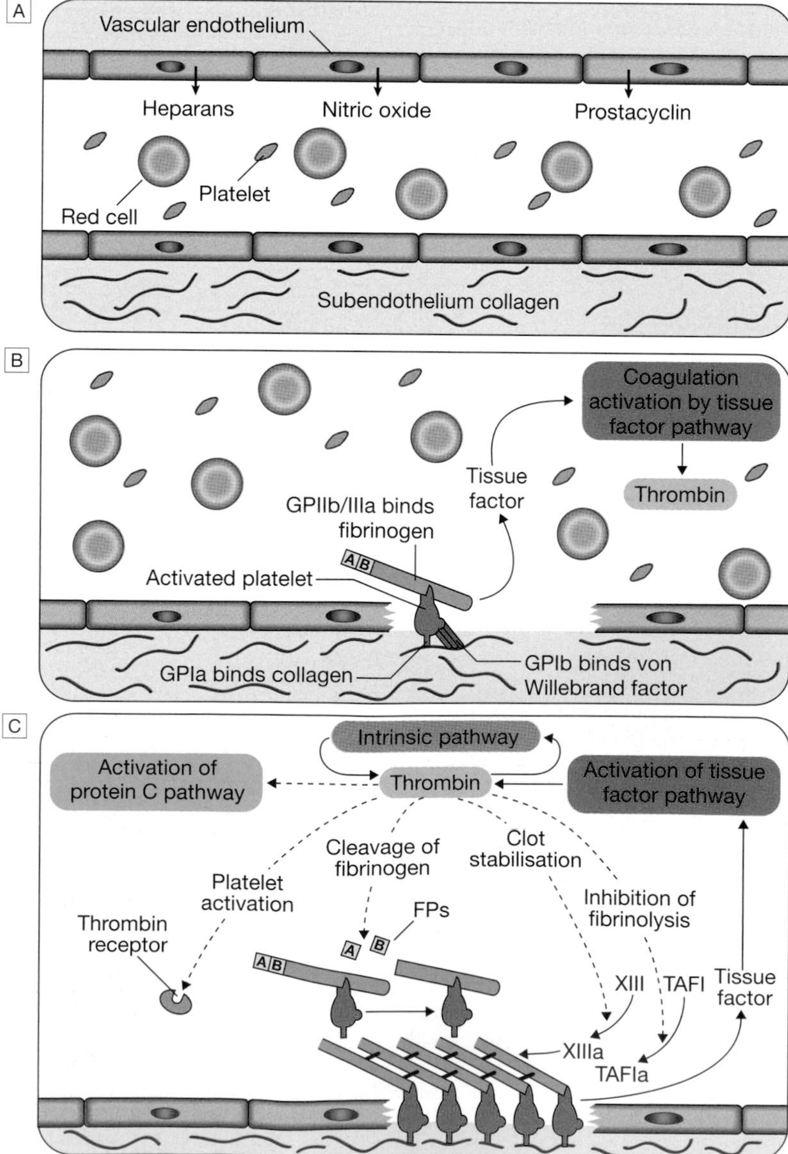

Fig. 24.6 The stages of normal haemostasis.

A *Stage 1 Pre-injury conditions encourage flow* The vascular endothelium produces substances (including nitric oxide, prostacyclin and heparans) to prevent adhesion of platelets and white cells to the vessel wall. Platelets and coagulation factors circulate in a non-activated state.

B *Stage 2 Early haemostatic response: platelets adhere; coagulation is activated.* At the site of injury, the endothelium is breached, exposing subendothelial collagen. Small amounts of tissue factor (TF) are released. Platelets bind to collagen via a specific receptor, glycoprotein Ia (GPIa), causing a change in platelet shape and its adhesion to the area of damage by the binding of other receptors (GPIb and GPIIb/IIIa) to von Willebrand factor and fibrinogen, respectively. Coagulation is activated by the tissue factor (extrinsic) pathway, generating small amounts of thrombin.

C *Stage 3 Fibrin clot formation: platelets become activated and aggregate; fibrin formation is supported by the platelet membrane; stable fibrin clot forms.* The adherent platelets are activated by many pathways, including binding of adenosine diphosphate (ADP), collagen, thrombin and adrenaline (epinephrine) to surface receptors. The cyclo-oxygenase pathway converts arachidonic acid from the platelet membrane into thromboxane A_2, which causes aggregation of platelets. Activation of the platelets results in release of the platelet granule contents, enhancing coagulation further (see Fig. 24.7). Thrombin plays a key role in the control of coagulation: the small amount generated via the TF pathway massively amplifies its own production; the 'intrinsic' pathway becomes reticulo-endothelial system. Some 30% of peripheral platelets are normally pooled in the spleen and do not circulate.

Under normal conditions platelets are discoid, with a diameter of 2–4 μm (Fig. 24.7). The surface membrane invaginates to form a tubular network, the canalicular system, which provides a conduit for the discharge of the granule content following platelet activation. Drugs which inhibit platelet function and thrombosis include aspirin (cyclo-oxygenase inhibitor), clopidogrel (adenosine diphosphate (ADP)-mediated activation inhibitor), dipyridamole (phosphodiesterase inhibitor), and the IIb/IIIa inhibitors abciximab, tirofiban and eptifibatide (which prevent fibrinogen binding; p. 594).

Clotting factors

The coagulation system consists of a cascade of soluble inactive zymogen proteins designated by Roman numerals. When proteolytically cleaved and activated, each is capable of activating one or more components of the cascade. Activated factors are designated by the suffix 'a'. Some of these reactions require phospholipid and calcium. Coagulation occurs by two pathways: it is initiated by the extrinsic (or tissue factor) pathway and amplified by the 'intrinsic pathway' (see Fig. 24.6).

Clotting factors are synthesised by the liver, although factor V is also produced by platelets and endothelial cells. Factors II, VII, IX and X require post-translational carboxylation to allow them to participate in coagulation. The carboxylase enzyme responsible for this in the liver is vitamin K-dependent. Vitamin K is converted to an epoxide in this reaction and must be reduced to its active form by a reductase enzyme. This reductase is inhibited by warfarin, and this is the basis of the anticoagulant effect of coumarins (p. 1019). Congenital (e.g. haemophilia) and acquired (e.g. liver failure) causes of coagulation factor deficiency are associated with bleeding.

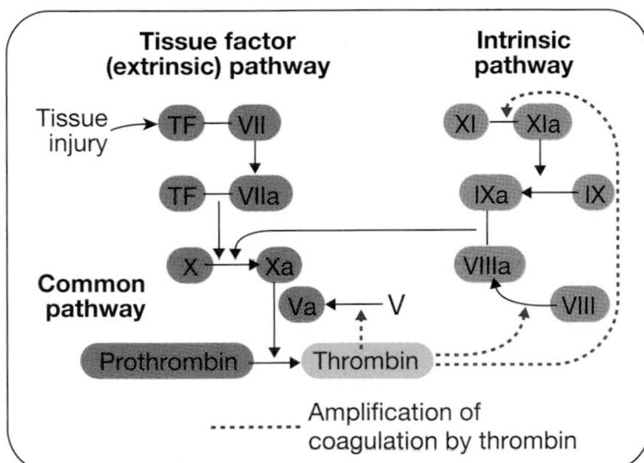

activated and large amounts of thrombin are generated. Thrombin directly causes clot formation by cleaving fibrinopeptides (FP) from fibrinogen to produce fibrin. Fibrin monomers are cross-linked by factor XIII, which is also activated by thrombin. Having had a key role in clot formation and stabilisation, thrombin then starts to regulate clot formation in two main ways: (a) activation of the protein C (PC) pathway (a natural anticoagulant), which reduces further coagulation; (b) activation of thrombin-activatable fibrinolysis inhibitor (TAFI), which inhibits fibrinolysis (see D and E).

D

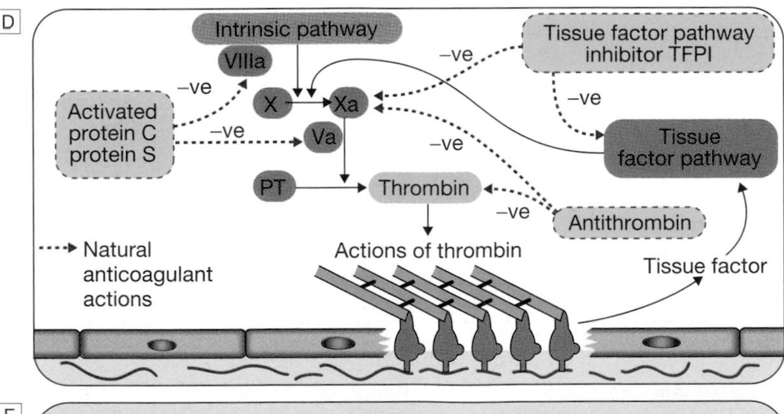

D *Stage 4 Limiting clot formation: natural anticoagulants reverse activation of coagulation factors.* Once haemostasis has been secured, the propagation of clot is curtailed by anticoagulants. Antithrombin is a serine protease inhibitor synthesised by the liver, which destroys activated factors such as XIa, Xa and thrombin (IIa). Its major activity against thrombin and Xa is enhanced by heparin and fondaparinux, explaining their anticoagulant effect. Tissue factor pathway inhibitor (TFPI) binds to and inactivates VIIa and Xa. Activation of PC occurs following binding of thrombin to membrane-bound thrombomodulin; activated protein C (aPC) binds to its co-factor protein S (PS), and cleaves Va and VIIIa. PC and PS are vitamin K-dependent and are depleted by coumarin anticoagulants such as warfarin.

E

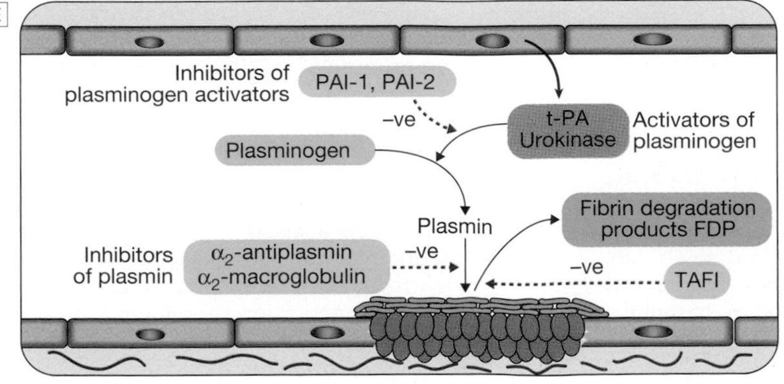

E *Stage 5 Fibrinolysis: plasmin degrades fibrin to allow vessel recanalisation and tissue repair.* The insoluble clot needs to be broken down for vessel recanalisation. Plasmin, the main fibrinolytic enzyme, is produced when plasminogen is activated, e.g. by tissue plasminogen activator (t-PA) or urokinase in the clot. Plasmin hydrolyses the fibrin clot, producing fibrin degradation products, including the D-dimer. This process is highly regulated; the plasminogen activators are controlled by an inhibitor called plasminogen activator inhibitor (PAI), the activity of plasmin is inhibited by α_2-antiplasmin and α_2-macroglobulin, and fibrinolysis is further inhibited by the thrombin-activated TAFI.

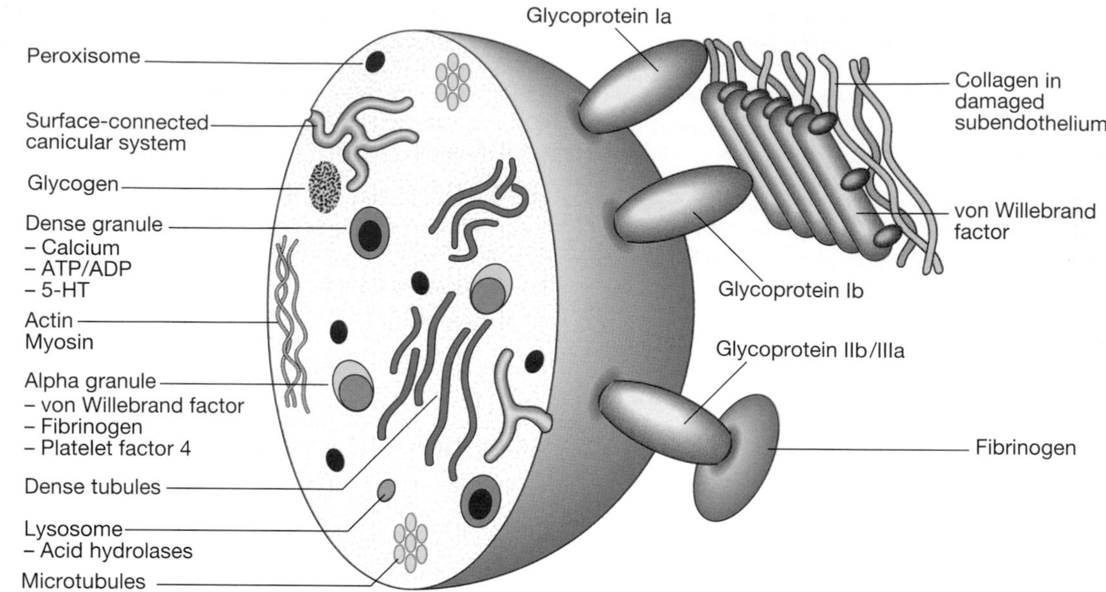

Fig. 24.7 Normal platelet structure. (5-HT = 5-hydroxytryptamine, serotonin; ADP = adenosine diphosphate; ATP = adenosine triphosphate)

INVESTIGATION OF DISEASES OF THE BLOOD

The full blood count

To obtain a full blood count (FBC), anticoagulated blood is processed through automated blood analysers which use a variety of technologies (particle-sizing, radio-frequency and laser instrumentation) to measure the haematological parameters. These include numbers of circulating cells, the proportion of whole blood volume occupied by red cells (the haematocrit, Hct), and the red cell indices which give information about the size of red cells (mean cell volume, MCV) and the amount of haemoglobin present in the red cells (mean cell haemoglobin, MCH). Blood analysers can differentiate types of white blood cell and give automated counts of neutrophils, lymphocytes, monocytes, eosinophils and basophils. It is important to appreciate, however, that a number of conditions can lead to spurious results (Box 24.1). The reference ranges for a number of common haematological parameters in adults are given in Chapter 29.

24.1 Spurious FBC results from autoanalysers

Result	Explanation
Increased haemoglobin	Lipaemia, jaundice, very high white cell count
Reduced haemoglobin	Improper sample mixing, blood taken from vein into which an infusion is flowing
Increased red cell volume (MCV)	Cold agglutinins, non-ketotic hyperosmolarity
Increased white cell count	Nucleated red cells present
Reduced platelet count	Clot in sample, platelet clumping

Blood film examination

Although technical advances in full blood count analysers have resulted in fewer blood samples requiring manual examination, scrutiny of blood components prepared on a microscope slide (the 'blood film') can often yield valuable information (Box 24.2 and Fig. 24.8). Analysers cannot identify abnormalities of red cell shape and content (e.g. Howell–Jolly bodies, basophilic stippling, malaria parasites) or fully define abnormal white cells such as blasts.

Bone marrow examination

In adults, bone marrow for examination is usually obtained from the posterior iliac crest. After a local anaesthetic, marrow can be sucked out from the medullary space, stained and examined under the microscope (bone marrow aspirate). In addition, a core of bone may be removed (trephine biopsy), fixed and decalcified before sections are cut for staining (Fig. 24.9). A bone marrow aspirate is used to assess the composition and morphology of haematopoietic cells or abnormal infiltrates. Further investigations may be performed, such as cell surface marker analysis (immunophenotyping), chromosome and molecular studies to assess malignant disease, or marrow culture for suspected tuberculosis. A trephine biopsy is superior for assessing marrow cellularity, marrow fibrosis, and infiltration by abnormal cells such as metastatic carcinoma.

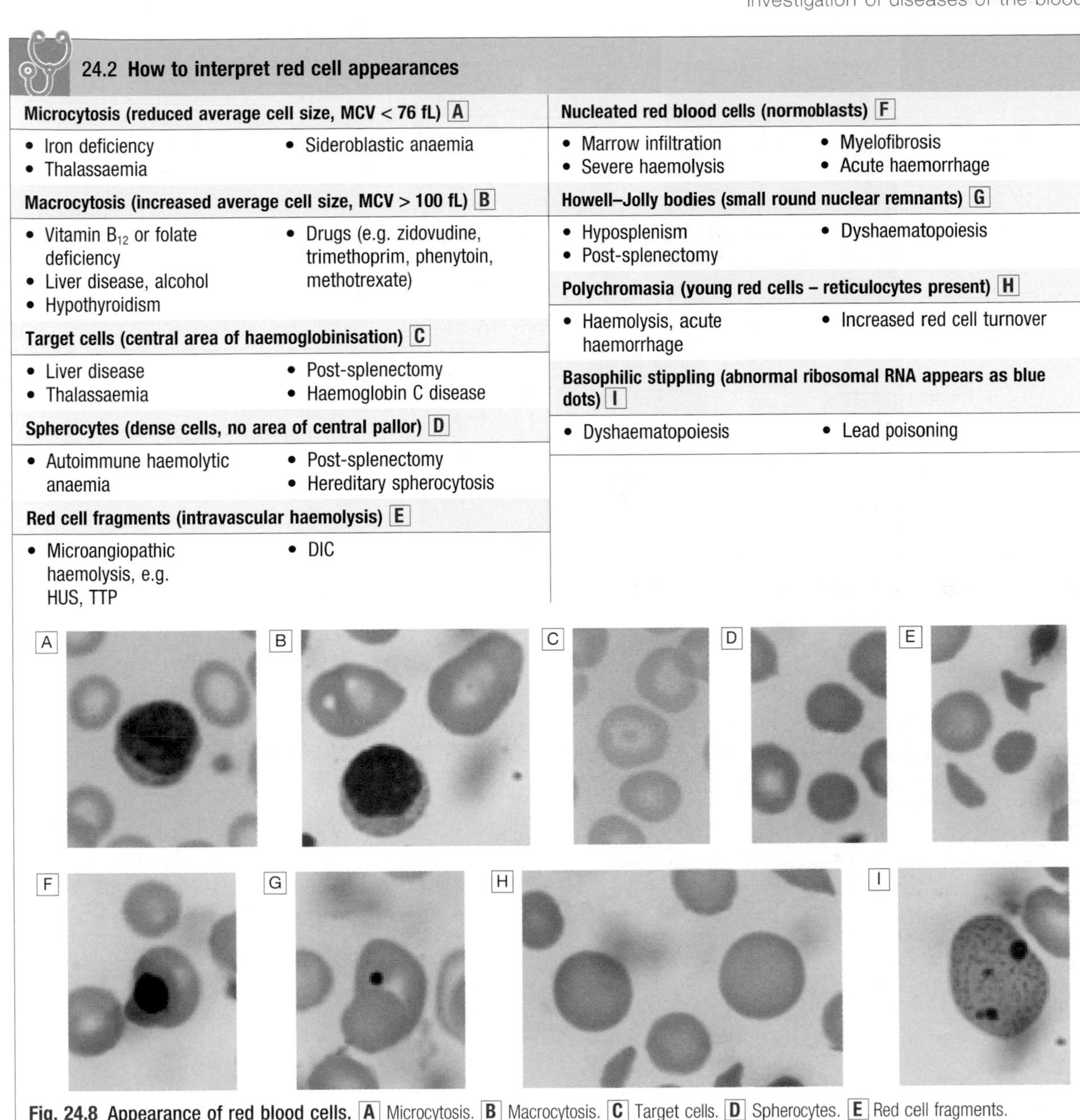

24.2 How to interpret red cell appearances

Microcytosis (reduced average cell size, MCV < 76 fL) A	**Nucleated red blood cells (normoblasts) F**
• Iron deficiency • Thalassaemia • Sideroblastic anaemia	• Marrow infiltration • Severe haemolysis • Myelofibrosis • Acute haemorrhage
Macrocytosis (increased average cell size, MCV > 100 fL) B	**Howell–Jolly bodies (small round nuclear remnants) G**
• Vitamin B_{12} or folate deficiency • Liver disease, alcohol • Hypothyroidism • Drugs (e.g. zidovudine, trimethoprim, phenytoin, methotrexate)	• Hyposplenism • Post-splenectomy • Dyshaematopoiesis
Target cells (central area of haemoglobinisation) C	**Polychromasia (young red cells – reticulocytes present) H**
• Liver disease • Thalassaemia • Post-splenectomy • Haemoglobin C disease	• Haemolysis, acute haemorrhage • Increased red cell turnover
Spherocytes (dense cells, no area of central pallor) D	**Basophilic stippling (abnormal ribosomal RNA appears as blue dots) I**
• Autoimmune haemolytic anaemia • Post-splenectomy • Hereditary spherocytosis	• Dyshaematopoiesis • Lead poisoning
Red cell fragments (intravascular haemolysis) E	
• Microangiopathic haemolysis, e.g. HUS, TTP • DIC	

Fig. 24.8 Appearance of red blood cells. A Microcytosis. B Macrocytosis. C Target cells. D Spherocytes. E Red cell fragments. F Nucleated red blood cells. G Howell–Jolly bodies. H Polychromasia. I Basophilic stippling.

(DIC = disseminated intravascular coagulation; HUS = haemolytic uraemic syndrome; MCV = mean cell volume; TTP = thrombotic thrombocytopenic purpura)

Investigation of coagulation

Bleeding disorders

In patients with clinical evidence of a bleeding disorder (p. 991), there are recommended screening tests (Box 24.3).

Coagulation tests measure the time to clot formation in vitro in a plasma sample after the clotting process is initiated by activators and calcium. The result of the test sample is compared with normal controls. The tissue factor ('extrinsic') pathway (see Fig 24.6) is assessed by the prothrombin time (PT), and the 'intrinsic' pathway by the activated partial thromboplastin time (APTT), sometimes known as the partial thromboplastin time with kaolin (PTTK). Coagulation is delayed by deficiencies of coagulation factors and by the presence of inhibitors of coagulation, such as heparin. The approximate reference ranges and causes of abnormalities are shown in Box 24.3. If both the PT and APTT are prolonged, this indicates either deficiency or inhibition of the final common pathway (which includes factors X, V, prothrombin and fibrinogen) or global coagulation factor deficiency involving more than one factor, as occurs in disseminated intravascular coagulation (DIC, pp. 201 and 1055). Further specific tests may be performed based on interpretation of the clinical scenario and results of these screening tests. A mixing test with normal plasma

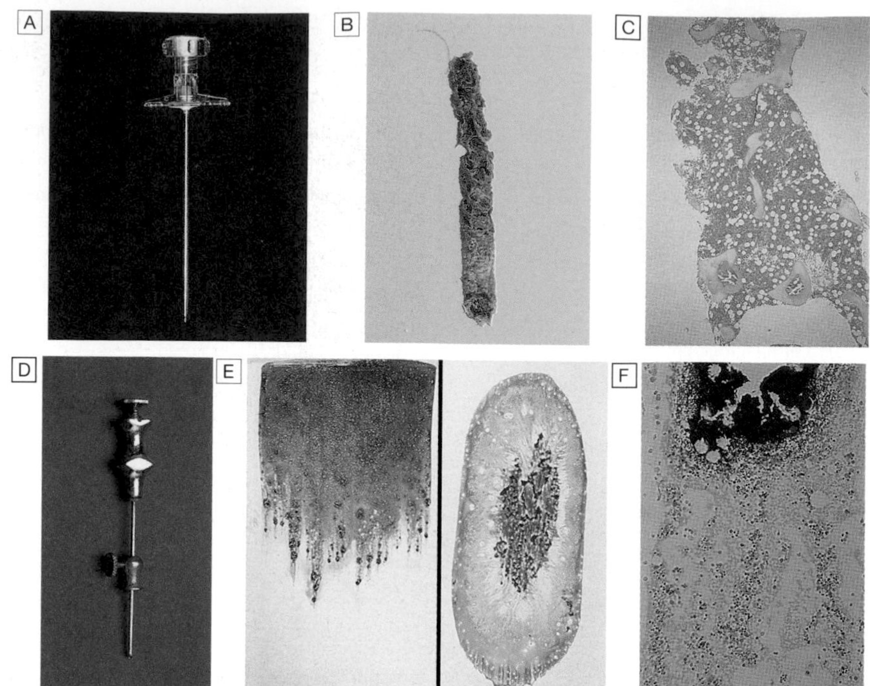

Fig. 24.9 Bone marrow aspirate and trephine. **A** Trephine biopsy needle. **B** Macroscopic appearance of a trephine biopsy. **C** Microscopic appearance of stained section of trephine. **D** Bone marrow aspirate needle. **E** Stained macroscopic appearance of marrow aspirate: smear (left) and squash (right). **F** Microscopic appearance of stained marrow particles and trails of haematopoietic cells.

24.3 Coagulation screening tests

Investigation	Reference range*	Situations in which tests may be abnormal
Platelet count	150–400 × 10^9/L	Thrombocytopenia
Prothrombin time (PT)	9–12 secs	Deficiencies of factors II, V, VII or X Severe fibrinogen deficiency
Activated partial thromboplastin time (APTT)	26–36 secs	Deficiencies of factors II, V, VIII, IX, X, XI, XII Severe fibrinogen deficiency Unfractionated heparin therapy Antibodies against clotting factors Lupus anticoagulant
Fibrinogen concentration	1.5–4.0 g/L	Hypofibrinogenaemia, e.g. liver failure, DIC

N.B. International normalised ratio (INR) is used only to monitor coumarin therapy and is not a coagulation screening test.
*Ranges are approximate and may vary between laboratories.
(DIC = disseminated intravascular coagulation)

allows differentiation between a coagulation factor deficiency (the prolonged time corrects) and the presence of an inhibitor of coagulation (the prolonged time does not correct); the latter may be chemical (heparins) or an antibody (most often a lupus anticoagulant but occasionally a specific inhibitor of one of the coagulation factors, typically factor VIII). Von Willebrand disease may present with a normal APTT; further investigation of suspected cases is detailed on page 1053.

Platelet function has historically been assessed by the bleeding time, measured as the time to stop bleeding after a standardised incision. However, most centres have abandoned the use of this test. Platelet function can be assessed in vitro by measuring aggregation in response to various agonists, such as adrenaline (epinephrine), collagen, thrombin and ADP, or by measuring the constituents of the intracellular granules, e.g. adenosine triphosphate (ATP)/ADP.

Coagulation screening tests are also performed in patients with suspected DIC, when clotting factors and platelets are consumed, resulting in thrombocytopenia and prolonged PT and APTT. In addition, there is evidence of active coagulation with consumption of fibrinogen and generation of fibrin degradation products (D-dimers). Note, however, that fibrinogen is an acute phase protein which may also be elevated in inflammatory disease (p. 82).

Monitoring anticoagulant therapy

The international normalised ratio (INR) is validated only to assess the therapeutic effect of coumarin anticoagulants, including warfarin. INR is the ratio of the patient's PT to that of a normal control, raised to the power of the international sensitivity index of the thromboplastin used in the test (ISI, derived by comparison with an international reference standard material).

Monitoring of heparin therapy is, on the whole, only required with unfractionated heparins. Therapeutic anticoagulation prolongs the APTT relative to a control sample by a ratio of approximately 1.5–2.5. Low molecular weight heparins have such a predictable dose response that monitoring of the anticoagulant effect is not required, except in patients with renal impairment (glomerular filtration rate less than 30 mL/min). When monitoring is indicated, an anti-Xa activity assay rather than APTT should be used.

Thrombotic disorders

Measurement of plasma levels of D-dimers derived from fibrin degradation is useful in excluding the diagnosis of active venous thrombosis in some patients (see Fig. 24.15, p. 1010).

A variety of tests exist which may help to explain an underlying propensity to thrombosis, especially venous thromboembolism (thrombophilia) (Box 24.4). Examples of possible indications for testing are given in Box 24.5. In most patients, the results do not affect clinical management (p. 1054) but they may influence the duration of anticoagulation (e.g. antiphospholipid antibodies, p. 1055), justify family screening in inherited thrombophilias (p. 1054), or suggest additional management strategies to reduce thrombosis risk (e.g. in myeloproliferative disease and paroxysmal nocturnal haemoglobinuria; p. 1031). Anticoagulants can interfere with some of these assays; for example, warfarin reduces protein C and S levels and affects measurement of lupus anticoagulant, while heparin interferes with antithrombin and lupus anticoagulant assays. Therefore these tests, when required, should be performed when the patient is not taking anticoagulants.

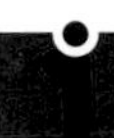

24.4 Investigation of possible thrombophilia

Full blood count

Plasma levels
- Antithrombin
- Protein C
- Protein S (free)
- Antiphospholipid antibodies/lupus anticoagulant and anticardiolipin antibody

Thrombin/reptilase time (for dysfibrinogenaemia)

Genetic testing
- Factor V Leiden
- Prothrombin G20210A
- *JAK-2* mutation

Flow cytometry
- Screen for glycerol phosphatidyl inositol (GPI)-linked cell surface proteins (CD14, 16, 55, 59), deficient in paroxysmal nocturnal haemoglobinuria

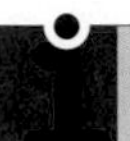

24.5 Indications for thrombophilia testing*

- Venous thrombosis < 45 yrs
- Recurrent venous thrombosis
- Family history of unprovoked or recurrent thrombosis
- Combined arterial and venous thrombosis
- Venous thrombosis at an unusual site
  - Cerebral venous thrombosis
  - Hepatic vein (Budd–Chiari syndrome)
  - Portal vein, mesenteric vein

*Antiphospholipid antibodies should be sought where clinical criteria for antiphospholipid syndrome (APS) are fulfilled (p. 1055). Thrombophilia testing may explain the diagnosis without necessarily affecting management.

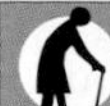

24.6 Haematological investigations in old age

- **Blood cell counts and film components**: not altered in general by ageing alone, although haemoglobin concentrations fall with increasing age.
- **Ratio of bone marrow cells to marrow fat**: falls.
- **Neutrophils**: maintained throughout life, although leucocytes may be less readily mobilised by bacterial invasion in old age.
- **Lymphocytes**: functionally compromised by age due to a T cell-related defect in cell-mediated immunity.
- **Clotting factors**: no major changes, although mild congenital deficiencies may be first noticed in old age.
- **Erythrocyte sedimentation rate (ESR)**: raised above the reference range, but usually in association with chronic or subacute disease. In truly healthy older people, the ESR range is very similar to that in younger people.

PRESENTING PROBLEMS IN BLOOD DISEASE

Anaemia

Anaemia refers to a state in which the level of haemoglobin in the blood is below the reference range appropriate for age and sex. Other factors, including pregnancy and altitude, also affect haemoglobin levels and must be taken into account when considering whether an individual is anaemic. The clinical features of anaemia reflect diminished oxygen supply to the tissues (p. 991). A rapid onset of anaemia (e.g. due to blood loss) causes more profound symptoms than a gradually developing anaemia. Individuals with cardiorespiratory disease are more susceptible to symptoms of anaemia.

The clinical assessment and investigation of anaemia should gauge its severity and define the underlying cause (Box 24.7).

Clinical assessment

- *Iron deficiency anaemia* (p. 1021) is the most common type of anaemia worldwide. A thorough gastrointestinal history is important, looking in particular for symptoms of blood loss. Menorrhagia

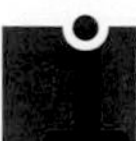

24.7 Causes of anaemia

Decreased or ineffective marrow production
- Lack of iron, vitamin B_{12} or folate
- Hypoplasia/myelodysplasia
- Invasion by malignant cells
- Renal failure
- Anaemia of chronic disease

Normal marrow production but increased removal of cells
- Blood loss
- Haemolysis
- Hypersplenism

24

is a common cause of anaemia in pre-menopausal females, so women should always be asked about their periods.

- *A dietary history* should assess the intake of iron and folate, which may become deficient in comparison to needs (e.g. in pregnancy or during periods of rapid growth; pp. 1025 and 125).
- *Past medical history* may reveal a disease which is known to be associated with anaemia, such as rheumatoid arthritis (anaemia of chronic disease), or previous surgery (e.g. resection of the stomach or small bowel, which may lead to malabsorption of iron and/or vitamin B_{12}).
- *Family history and ethnic background* may raise suspicion of haemolytic anaemias, such as the haemoglobinopathies and hereditary spherocytosis. Pernicious anaemia may also be familial.
- *A drug history* may reveal the ingestion of drugs which cause blood loss (e.g. aspirin and anti-inflammatory drugs), haemolysis (e.g. sulphonamides) or aplasia (e.g. chloramphenicol).

On examination, as well as the general physical findings of anaemia shown on page 991, there may be specific findings related to the aetiology of the anaemia; for example, a patient may be found to have a right iliac fossa mass due to an underlying caecal carcinoma. Haemolytic anaemias can cause jaundice. Vitamin B_{12} deficiency may be associated with neurological signs, including peripheral neuropathy, dementia and signs of subacute combined degeneration of the cord (p. 1025). Sickle-cell anaemia (p. 1032) may result in leg ulcers, stroke or features of pulmonary hypertension. Anaemia may be multifactorial and the lack of specific symptoms and signs does not rule out silent pathology.

Investigations

Schemes for the investigation of anaemias are often based on the size of the red cells, which is most accurately indicated by the MCV in the FBC. Commonly, in the presence of anaemia:

- A normal MCV (normocytic anaemia) suggests either acute blood loss or the anaemia of chronic disease (ACD) (Fig. 24.10).
- A low MCV (microcytic anaemia) suggests iron deficiency or thalassaemia (see Fig. 24.10).
- A high MCV (macrocytic anaemia) suggests vitamin B_{12} or folate deficiency or myelodysplasia (Fig. 24.11).

Specific types of anaemia and their management are described later in this chapter (p. 1021).

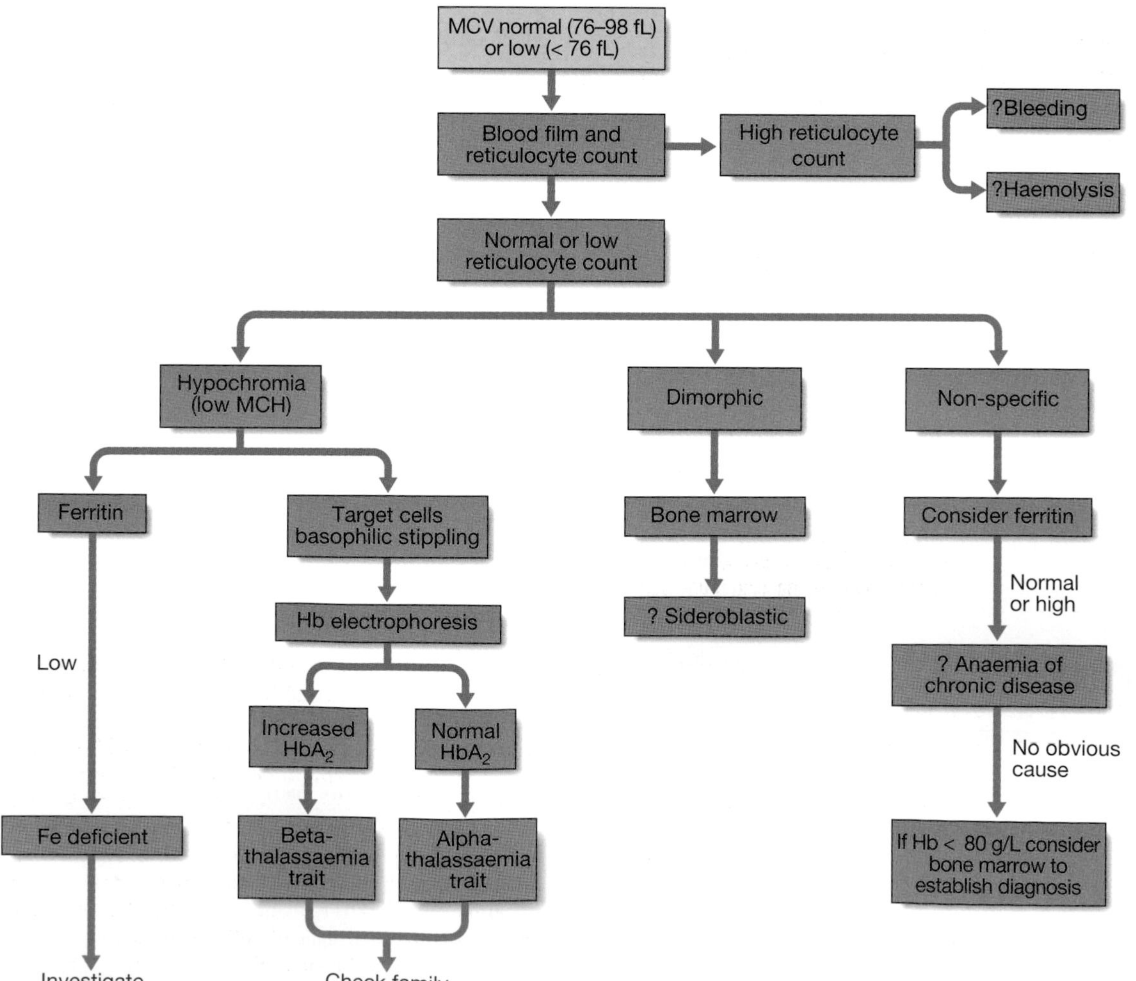

Fig. 24.10 Investigation of anaemia with normal or low MCV.

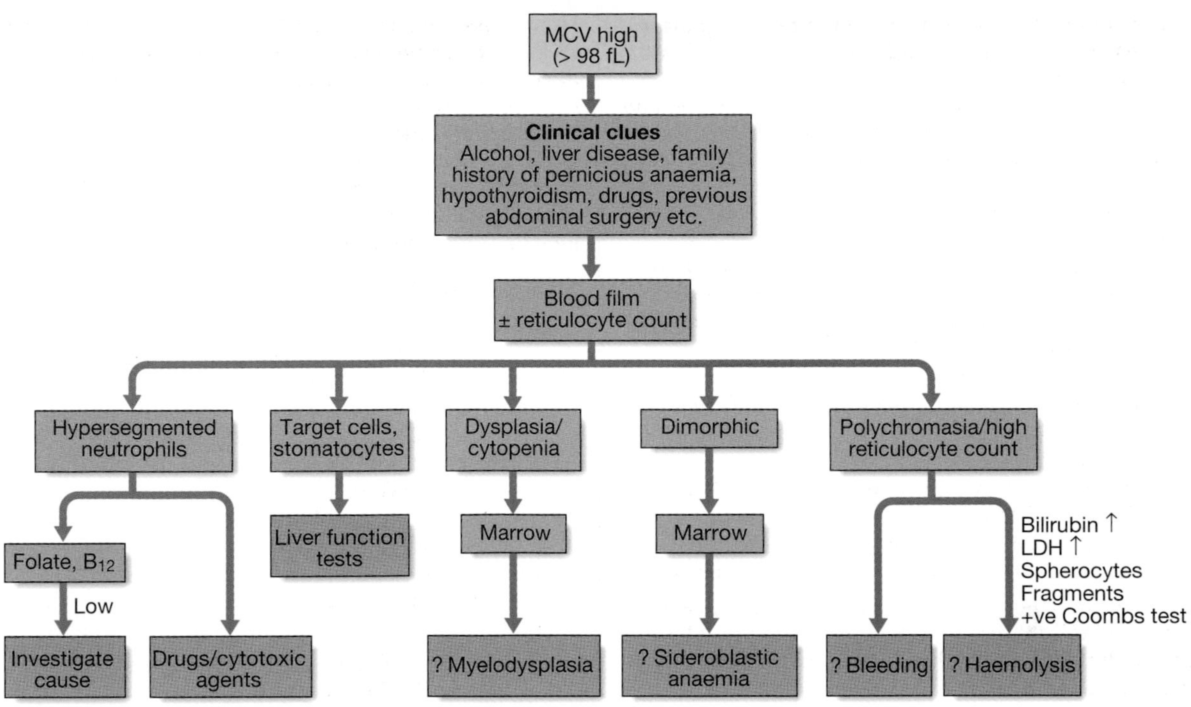

Fig. 24.11 Investigation of anaemia with high MCV. (LDH = lactate dehydrogenase)

24.8 Classification and causes of erythrocytosis

	Absolute erythrocytosis	Relative (low-volume) erythrocytosis
Haematocrit	High	High
Red cell mass	High	Normal
Plasma volume	Normal	Low
Causes	*Primary* Myeloproliferative disorder Polycythaemia rubra vera (primary proliferative polycythaemia) *Secondary* High erythropoietin due to tissue hypoxia High altitude Cardiorespiratory disease High-affinity haemoglobins Inappropriately increased erythropoietin Renal disease (hydronephrosis, cysts, carcinoma) Other tumours (hepatoma, bronchogenic carcinoma, uterine fibroids, phaeochromocytoma, cerebellar haemangioblastoma) Exogenous erythropoietin administration Performance-enhancing drug-taking in athletes	Diuretics Smoking Obesity Alcohol excess Gaisbock's syndrome

High haemoglobin

Patients with a persistently raised haematocrit (Hct) (> 0.52 males, > 0.48 females) for more than 2 months should be investigated. 'True' polycythaemia (or absolute erythrocytosis) indicates an excess of red cells, while 'relative' (or 'low-volume') polycythaemia is due to a decreased plasma volume. Causes are shown in Box 24.8.

Clinical assessment and investigations

Males and females with Hct values of over 0.60 and over 0.56, respectively, can be assumed to have an absolute erythrocytosis. A clinical history and examination will identify most patients with polycythaemia secondary to hypoxia. The presence of hypertension, smoking, excess alcohol consumption and/or diuretic use is consistent with low-volume polycythaemia (Gaisbock's syndrome). In polycythaemia rubra vera (PRV), a mutation in a kinase, *JAK-2 V617F*, is found in over 90% of cases (p. 1049). Patients with PRV have an increased risk of arterial thromboses, particularly stroke, and venous thromboembolism. They may also have aquagenic pruritus (worse after a hot bath), hepatosplenomegaly and gout (due to high red cell turnover).

If the *JAK-2* mutation is absent and there is no obvious secondary cause, a measurement of red cell mass is required to confirm an absolute erythrocytosis, followed by further investigations to exclude hypoxia, and causes of inappropriate erythropoietin secretion. Red cell mass measurement is performed by radiolabelling an aliquot of the patient's red cells, re-injecting them and measuring the dilution of the isotope.

Leucopenia (low white cell count)

A reduction in the total numbers of circulating white cells is called leucopenia. This may be due to a reduction in all types of white cell or in individual cell types (usually neutrophils or lymphocytes). Leucopenia may occur in isolation or as part of a reduction in all three haematological lineages (pancytopenia; p. 1008).

Neutropenia

A reduction in neutrophil count (usually less than 1.5×10^9/L, but dependent on age and race) is called neutropenia. The main causes are listed in Box 24.9. Drug-induced neutropenia is not uncommon (Box 24.10). Clinical manifestations range from no symptoms to overwhelming sepsis. The risk of bacterial infection is related to the degree of neutropenia, with counts lower than 0.5×10^9/L considered to be critically low. Fever is the first and often only manifestation of infection. A sore throat, perianal pain or skin inflammation may be present. The lack of neutrophils allows the patient to become septicaemic and shocked within hours if immediate antibiotic therapy is not commenced. Management is discussed on page 302.

Lymphopenia

This is an absolute lymphocyte count of less than 1×10^9/L. The causes are shown in Box 24.9. Although minor reductions may be asymptomatic, deficiencies in cell-mediated immunity may result in infections (with organisms such as fungi, viruses and mycobacteria) and a propensity to lymphoid and other malignancies (particularly those associated with viral infections such as

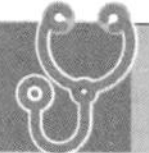

24.9 How to interpret white blood cell results

Neutrophils A

Neutrophilia
- Infection: bacterial, fungal
- Trauma: surgery, burns
- Infarction: myocardial infarct, pulmonary embolus, sickle-cell crisis
- Inflammation: gout, rheumatoid arthritis, ulcerative colitis, Crohn's disease
- Malignancy: solid tumours, Hodgkin lymphoma
- Myeloproliferative disease: polycythaemia, chronic myeloid leukaemia
- Physiological: exercise, pregnancy

Neutropenia
- Infection: viral, bacterial (e.g. *Salmonella*), protozoal (e.g. malaria)
- Drugs: see Box 24.10
- Autoimmune: connective tissue disease
- Alcohol
- Bone marrow infiltration: leukaemia, myelodysplasia
- Congenital: Kostmann's syndrome
- Constitutional: Afro-Caribbean and Middle Eastern descent

Eosinophils B

Eosinophilia
- Allergy: hay fever, asthma, eczema
- Infection: parasitic
- Drug hypersensitivity: e.g. gold, sulphonamides
- Vasculitis, e.g. Churg–Strauss syndrome, granulomatosis with polyangiitis (Wegener's granulomatosis)
- Connective tissue disease: polyarteritis nodosa
- Malignancy: solid tumours, lymphomas
- Primary bone marrow disorders: myeloproliferative disorders, hypereosinophilic syndrome (HES), acute myeloid leukaemia

Basophils C

Basophilia
- Myeloproliferative disease: polycythaemia, chronic myeloid leukaemia
- Inflammation: acute hypersensitivity, ulcerative colitis, Crohn's disease
- Iron deficiency

Monocytes D

Monocytosis
- Infection: bacterial (e.g. tuberculosis)
- Inflammation: connective tissue disease, ulcerative colitis, Crohn's disease
- Malignancy: solid tumours, chronic myelomonocytic leukaemia

Lymphocytes E

Lymphocytosis
- Infection: viral, bacterial (e.g. *Bordetella pertussis*)
- Lymphoproliferative disease: chronic lymphocytic leukaemia, lymphoma
- Post-splenectomy

Lymphopenia
- Inflammation: connective tissue disease
- Lymphoma
- Renal failure
- Sarcoidosis
- Drugs: corticosteroids, cytotoxics
- Congenital: severe combined immunodeficiency
- HIV infection

A 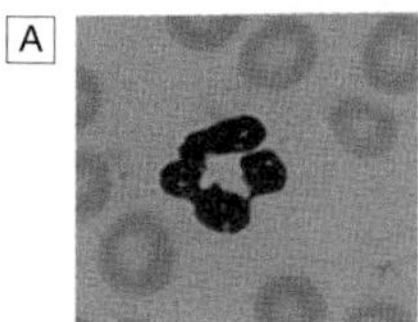
B 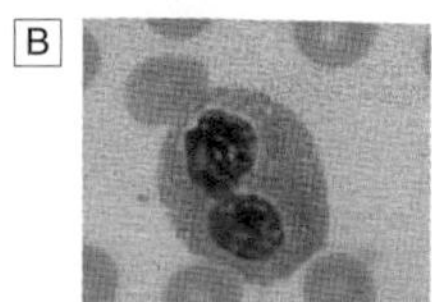
C 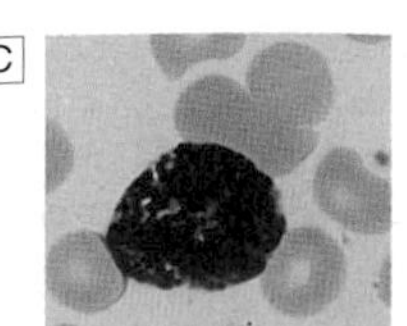
D 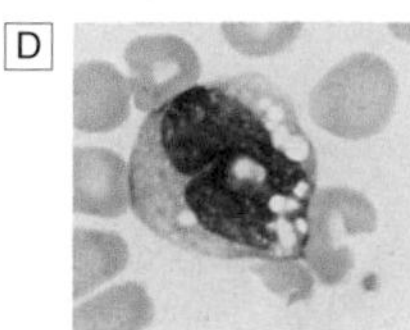
E 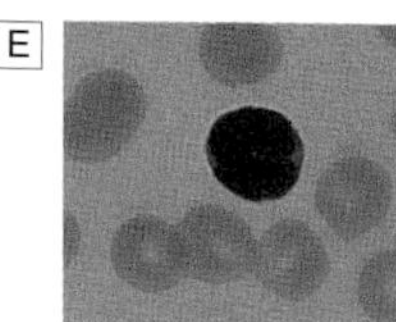

Fig. 24.12 Appearance of white blood cells. A Neutrophil. B Eosinophil. C Basophil. D Monocyte. E Lymphocyte.

24.10 Drugs that can induce neutropenia

Group	Examples
Analgesics/anti-inflammatory agents	Gold, penicillamine, naproxen
Antithyroid drugs	Carbimazole, propylthiouracil
Anti-arrhythmics	Quinidine, procainamide
Antihypertensives	Captopril, enalapril, nifedipine
Antidepressants/ psychotropics	Amitriptyline, dosulepin, mianserin
Antimalarials	Pyrimethamine, dapsone, sulfadoxine, chloroquine
Anticonvulsants	Phenytoin, sodium valproate, carbamazepine
Antibiotics	Sulphonamides, penicillins, cephalosporins
Miscellaneous	Cimetidine, ranitidine, chlorpropamide, zidovudine

Epstein–Barr virus (EBV), human papillomavirus (HPV) and human herpesvirus 8 (HHV-8)).

Leucocytosis (high white cell count)

An increase in the total numbers of circulating white cells is called leucocytosis. This is usually due to an increase in a specific type of cell (see Box 24.9). It is important to realise that an increase in a single type of white cell (e.g. eosinophils or monocytes) may not increase the total white cell count (WCC) above the upper limit of normal and will only be apparent if the 'differential' of the white count is examined.

Neutrophilia

An increase in the number of circulating neutrophils is called a neutrophilia or a neutrophil leucocytosis. It can result from an increased production of cells from the bone marrow or redistribution from the marginated pool. The normal neutrophil count depends upon age, race and certain physiological parameters. During pregnancy, not only is there an increase in neutrophils but also earlier forms such as metamyelocytes can be found in the blood. The causes of a neutrophilia are shown in Box 24.9.

Eosinophilia

A high eosinophil count of more than $0.5 \times 10^9/L$ is usually secondary to infection (especially parasites; p. 311), allergy (e.g. eczema, asthma, reactions to drugs; p. 89), immunological disorders (e.g. polyarteritis, sarcoidosis) or malignancy (e.g. lymphomas) (see Box 24.9). Usually, such eosinophilia is short-lived.

In the rarer primary disorders, there is a persistently raised, often clonal, eosinophilia: for example, in myeloproliferative disorders, subtypes of acute myeloid leukaemia and idiopathic hypereosinophilic syndrome (HES). Recently, specific mutations in receptor tyrosine kinase genes have been found in some primary eosinophilias (e.g. causing re-arrangements of platelet-derived growth factor receptors α and β or c-kit), which allow diagnosis and, in some cases, specific therapy with tyrosine kinase inhibitors such as imatinib.

Eosinophil infiltration can damage many organs (e.g. heart, lungs, gastrointestinal tract, skin, musculoskeletal system); therefore evaluation of eosinophilia includes not only the identification of any underlying cause and its appropriate treatment, but also assessment of any related organ damage.

Lymphocytosis

A lymphocytosis is an increase in circulating lymphocytes above that expected for the patient's age. In adults, this is greater than $3.5 \times 10^9/L$. Infants and children have higher counts; age-related reference ranges should be consulted. Causes are shown in Box 24.9; the most common is viral infection.

Lymphadenopathy

Enlarged lymph glands may be an important indicator of haematological disease but they are not uncommon in reaction to infection or inflammation (Box 24.11). The sites of lymph node groups, and symptoms and signs that may help elucidate the underlying cause are shown on page 991. Nodes which enlarge in response to local infection or inflammation ('reactive nodes') usually expand rapidly and are painful, whereas those due to haematological disease are more frequently painless. Localised lymphadenopathy should elicit a search for a source of inflammation in the appropriate drainage area:

- the scalp, ear, mouth, face or teeth for neck nodes
- the breast for axillary nodes
- the perineum or external genitalia for inguinal nodes.

Generalised lymphadenopathy may be secondary to infection, connective tissue disease or extensive skin disease, but is more likely to signify underlying haematological malignancy. Weight loss and drenching night sweats that may require a change of night clothes are associated with haematological malignancies, particularly lymphoma.

Initial investigations in lymphadenopathy include an FBC (to detect neutrophilia in infection or evidence of haematological disease), an ESR and a chest X-ray (to detect mediastinal lymphadenopathy). If the findings suggest malignancy, a formal cutting needle or excision

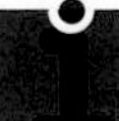

24.11 Causes of lymphadenopathy

Infective
- Bacterial: streptococcal, tuberculosis, brucellosis
- Viral: Epstein–Barr virus (EBV), human immunodeficiency virus (HIV)
- Protozoal: toxoplasmosis
- Fungal: histoplasmosis, coccidioidomycosis

Neoplastic
- Primary: lymphomas, leukaemias
- Secondary: lung, breast, thyroid, stomach

Connective tissue disorders
- Rheumatoid arthritis
- Systemic lupus erythematosus (SLE)

Sarcoidosis

Amyloidosis

Drugs
- Phenytoin

biopsy of a representative node is indicated to obtain a histological diagnosis.

Splenomegaly

The spleen may be enlarged due to involvement by lymphoproliferative disease, the resumption of extramedullary haematopoiesis in myeloproliferative disease, enhanced reticulo-endothelial activity in autoimmune haemolysis, expansion of the lymphoid tissue in response to infections, or vascular congestion as a result of portal hypertension (Box 24.12). Hepatosplenomegaly is suggestive of lympho- or myeloproliferative disease, liver disease or infiltration (e.g. with amyloid). Associated lymphadenopathy is suggestive of lymphoproliferative disease. An enlarged spleen may cause abdominal discomfort, accompanied by back pain and abdominal bloating due to stomach compression. Splenic infarction produces severe abdominal pain radiating to the left shoulder tip, associated with a splenic rub on auscultation. Rarely, spontaneous or traumatic rupture and bleeding may occur.

Investigation should focus on the suspected cause. Imaging of the spleen by ultrasound or computed tomography (CT) will detect variations in density in the spleen, which may be a feature of lymphoproliferative disease; it also allows imaging of the liver and abdominal lymph nodes. Biopsy of enlarged abdominal or superficial lymph nodes may provide the diagnosis. A chest X-ray or CT of the thorax will detect mediastinal lymphadenopathy. An FBC may show pancytopenia secondary to hypersplenism, when the enlarged spleen has become overactive, destroying blood cells prematurely. If other abnormalities are present, such as abnormal lymphocytes or a leuco-erythroblastic blood film, a bone marrow examination is indicated. Screening for infectious or liver disease (p. 928) may be appropriate. If all investigations are unhelpful, splenectomy may be diagnostic but is rarely carried out in these circumstances.

24.12 Causes of splenomegaly

Congestive	
Portal hypertension	
• Cirrhosis • Hepatic vein occlusion • Portal vein thrombosis	• Stenosis or malformation of portal or splenic vein
Cardiac	
• Chronic congestive cardiac failure	• Constrictive pericarditis
Infective	
Bacterial	
• Endocarditis • Septicaemia • Tuberculosis	• Brucellosis • Salmonella
Viral	
• Hepatitis • Epstein–Barr	• Cytomegalovirus
Protozoal	
• Malaria* • Leishmaniasis (kala-azar)*	• Trypanosomiasis
Fungal	
• Histoplasmosis	
Inflammatory/granulomatous disorders	
• Felty's syndrome in rheumatoid arthritis • Sarcoidosis	• Systemic lupus erythematosus
Haematological	
Red cell disorders	
• Megaloblastic anaemia • Haemoglobinopathies	• Hereditary spherocytosis
Autoimmune haemolytic anaemias	
Myeloproliferative disorders	
• Chronic myeloid leukaemia* • Myelofibrosis*	• Polycythaemia rubra vera • Essential thrombocythaemia
Neoplastic	
• Leukaemias, including chronic myeloid leukaemia*	• Lymphomas
Other malignancies	
• Metastatic cancer – rare	
Lysosomal storage diseases	
• Gaucher's disease	• Niemann–Pick disease
Miscellaneous	
• Cysts, amyloid, thyrotoxicosis	

*Causes of massive splenomegaly.

Bleeding

Normal bleeding is seen following surgery and trauma. Pathological bleeding occurs when structurally abnormal vessels rupture or when a vessel is breached in the presence of a defect in haemostasis. This may be due to a deficiency or dysfunction of platelets, to the coagulation factors, or occasionally to excessive fibrinolysis, which is most commonly observed following therapeutic thrombolysis (p. 596).

Clinical assessment

'Screening' blood tests (see Box 24.3, p. 1000) do not reliably detect all causes of pathological bleeding (e.g. von Willebrand disease, scurvy, certain anticoagulant drugs and the causes of purpura listed in Box 24.13) and should not be used indiscriminately. A careful clinical evaluation is the key to diagnosis of bleeding disorders (p. 1049). It is important to consider the following:

- *Site of bleeding.* Bleeding into muscle and joints, along with retroperitoneal and intracranial haemorrhage, indicates a likely defect in coagulation factors. Purpura, prolonged bleeding from superficial cuts, epistaxis, gastrointestinal haemorrhage or menorrhagia is more likely to be due to thrombocytopenia, a platelet function disorder or von Willebrand disease. Recurrent bleeds at a single site suggest a local structural abnormality.
- *Duration of history.* It may be possible to assess whether the disorder is congenital or acquired.
- *Precipitating causes.* Bleeding arising spontaneously indicates a more severe defect than bleeding that occurs only after trauma.
- *Surgery.* Ask about operations. Dental extractions, tonsillectomy and circumcision are stressful tests of

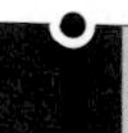

24.13 Causes of non-thrombocytopenic purpura

- Senile purpura
- Factitious purpura
- Henoch–Schönlein purpura (pp. 501 and 1119)
- Vasculitis (p. 1115)
- Paraproteinaemias
- Purpura fulminans, e.g. in DIC secondary to sepsis

the haemostatic system. Immediate post-surgical bleeding suggests defective platelet plug formation and primary haemostasis; delayed haemorrhage is more suggestive of a coagulation defect. In post-surgical patients, persistent bleeding from a single site is more likely to indicate surgical bleeding than a bleeding disorder.

- *Family history.* While a positive family history may be present in patients with inherited disorders, the absence of affected relatives does not exclude a hereditary bleeding diathesis; about one-third of cases of haemophilia arise in individuals without a family history, and deficiencies of factor VII, X and XIII are recessively inherited. Recessive disorders are more common in cultures where there is consanguineous marriage.
- *Drugs.* Use of antithrombotic, anticoagulant and fibrinolytic drugs must be elicited. Drug interactions with warfarin and drug-induced thrombocytopenia should be considered. Some 'herbal' remedies may result in a bleeding diathesis.

Clinical examination may reveal different patterns of skin bleeding. Petechial purpura is minor bleeding into the dermis that is flat and non-blanching (Fig. 24.13). Petechiae are typically found in patients with thrombocytopenia or platelet dysfunction. Palpable purpura occurs in vasculitis. Ecchymosis, or bruising, is more extensive bleeding into deeper layers of the skin. The lesions are initially dark red or purple but become yellow as haemoglobin is degraded. Retroperitoneal bleeding presents with a flank haematoma. Telangiectasia of lips and tongue points to hereditary haemorrhagic telangiectasia (p. 1049). Joints should be examined for evidence of haemarthroses. A full examination is important, as it may give clues to an underlying associated systemic illness such as a haematological or other malignancy, liver disease, renal failure, connective tissue disease and possible causes of splenomegaly.

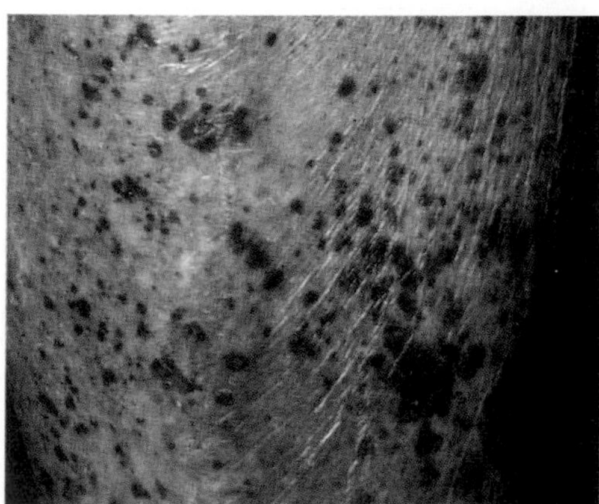

Fig. 24.13 Petechial purpura.

Investigations

Screening investigations and their interpretation are described on page 999. If the patient has a history that is strongly suggestive of a bleeding disorder and all the preliminary screening tests give normal results, further investigations, such as measurement of von Willebrand factor and assessment of platelet function, should be performed (p. 1053).

Thrombocytopenia (low platelet count)

A reduced platelet count may arise by one of two mechanisms:

- decreased or abnormal production (bone marrow failure and hereditary thrombocytopathies)

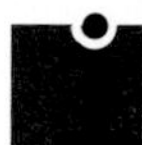

24.14 Causes of thrombocytopenia

Decreased production

Marrow hypoplasia
- Childhood bone marrow failure syndromes, e.g. Fanconi's anaemia, dyskeratosis congenita, amegakaryocytic thrombocytopenia
- Idiopathic aplastic anaemia
- Drug-induced: cytotoxics, antimetabolites
- Transfusion-associated graft-versus-host disease

Marrow infiltration
- Leukaemia
- Myeloma
- Carcinoma (rare)
- Myelofibrosis
- Osteopetrosis
- Lysosomal storage disorders, e.g. Gaucher's disease

Haematinic deficiency
- Vitamin B_{12} and/or folate deficiency

Familial (macro-)thrombocytopathies
- Myosin heavy chain abnormalities, e.g. Alport's syndrome, Fechner's syndrome
- Bernard Soulier disease
- Montreal platelet syndrome
- Wiskott–Aldrich syndrome (small platelets)

Increased consumption

Immune mechanisms
- Idiopathic thrombocytopenic purpura*
- Neonatal alloimmune thrombocytopenia
- Post-transfusion purpura
- Drug-associated, especially quinine and vancomycin

Coagulation activation
- Disseminated intravascular coagulation (see Box 24.70, p. 1056)

Mechanical pooling
- Hypersplenism

Thrombotic microangiopathies
- Haemolytic uraemic syndrome
- Liver disease
- Thrombotic thrombocytopenic purpura
- Pre-eclampsia

Others
- Gestational thrombocytopenia
- Type 2B von Willebrand disease

*Associated conditions include collagen vascular diseases (particularly SLE), B cell malignancy, HIV infection and antiphospholipid syndrome.

- increased consumption following release into the circulation (immune-mediated, DIC or sequestration).

Spontaneous bleeding does not usually occur until the platelet count falls below 20×10^9/L, unless their function is also compromised. Purpura and spontaneous bruising are characteristic but there may also be oral, nasal, gastrointestinal or genitourinary bleeding. Severe thrombocytopenia (< 10×10^9/L) may result in retinal haemorrhage and potentially fatal intracranial bleeding, but this is rare.

Investigations are directed at the possible causes listed in Box 24.14. A blood film is the single most useful initial investigation. Examination of the bone marrow may reveal increased megakaryocytes in consumptive causes of thrombocytopenia, or the underlying cause of bone marrow failure in leukaemia, hypoplastic anaemia or myelodysplasia.

Treatment (if required) depends on the underlying cause. Platelet transfusion is rarely required and is usually confined to patients with bone marrow failure and platelet counts below 10×10^9/L, or to clinical situations with actual or predicted serious haemorrhage.

Thrombocytosis (high platelet count)

The most common reason for a raised platelet count is that it is reactive to another process such as infection, connective tissue disease, malignancy, iron deficiency, acute haemolysis or gastrointestinal bleeding (Box 24.15). The presenting clinical features are usually those of the underlying disorder and haemostasis is rarely affected. Reactive thrombocytosis is distinguished from the myeloproliferative disorders by the presence of uniform small platelets, lack of splenomegaly, and the presence of an associated disorder. The key to diagnosis is the clinical history and examination, combined with observation of the platelet count over time (reactive thrombocytosis gets better with resolution of the underlying cause).

The platelets are a product of an abnormally expanding clone of cells in the myeloproliferative disorders, chronic myeloid leukaemia and some forms of myelodysplasia. Patients with PRV, essential thrombocythaemia and occasionally myelofibrosis may present with thrombosis or, rarely, bleeding. Stroke and transient ischaemic attacks, amaurosis fugax, and digital ischaemia or gangrene are also features. In addition, patients with myeloproliferative disorders present with features such as itching after exposure to water (aquagenic pruritus), splenomegaly and systemic upset.

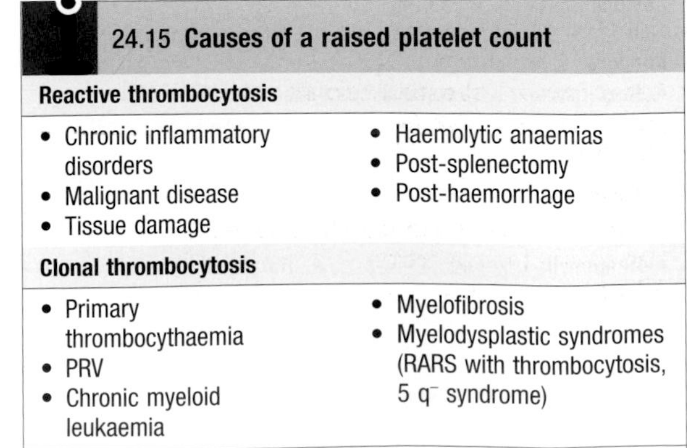

24.15 Causes of a raised platelet count

Reactive thrombocytosis	
• Chronic inflammatory disorders • Malignant disease • Tissue damage	• Haemolytic anaemias • Post-splenectomy • Post-haemorrhage
Clonal thrombocytosis	
• Primary thrombocythaemia • PRV • Chronic myeloid leukaemia	• Myelofibrosis • Myelodysplastic syndromes (RARS with thrombocytosis, 5 q⁻ syndrome)

(PRV = polycythaemia rubra vera; RARS = refractory anaemia with sideroblasts)

Pancytopenia

Pancytopenia refers to the combination of anaemia, leucopenia and thrombocytopenia. It may be due to reduced production of blood cells as a consequence of bone marrow suppression or infiltration, or there may be peripheral destruction or splenic pooling of mature cells. Causes are shown in Box 24.16. A bone marrow aspirate and trephine are usually required to establish the diagnosis.

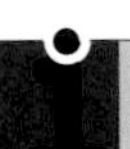

24.16 Causes of pancytopenia

Bone marrow failure	
• Hypoplastic/aplastic anaemia (p. 1048): inherited, idiopathic, viral, drugs	
Bone marrow infiltration	
• Acute leukaemia • Myeloma • Lymphoma • Carcinoma	• Haemophagocytic syndrome • Myelodysplastic syndromes
Ineffective haematopoiesis	
• Megaloblastic anaemia • Acquired immunodeficiency syndrome (AIDS)	
Peripheral pooling/destruction	
• Hypersplenism: portal hypertension, Felty's syndrome, malaria, myelofibrosis • Systemic lupus erythematosus (SLE)	

Infection

Infection is a major complication of haematological disorders. It relates to the immunological deficit caused by the disease itself, or its treatment with chemotherapy and/or immunotherapy (pp. 1004 and 302).

Venous thrombosis

While the most common presentation of venous thromboembolic disease (VTE) is with deep vein thrombosis (DVT) of the leg and/or pulmonary embolism (PE; see also p. 721), similar principles apply to rarer manifestations such as jugular vein thrombosis, upper limb DVT, cerebral sinus thrombosis (p. 1247) and intra-abdominal venous thrombosis (e.g. Budd–Chiari syndrome; p. 976).

DVT has an annual incidence of approximately 1:1000 in Western populations and the case mortality is 1–3%. It is increasingly common with ageing, and many of the deaths are related to coexisting medical conditions, such as active cancer. Risk factors for DVT and PE are often present (Box 24.17). Figure 24.14 illustrates some of the causes and consequences of VTE disease.

Clinical assessment

Lower limb DVT characteristically starts in the distal veins, causing pain, swelling, an increase in temperature

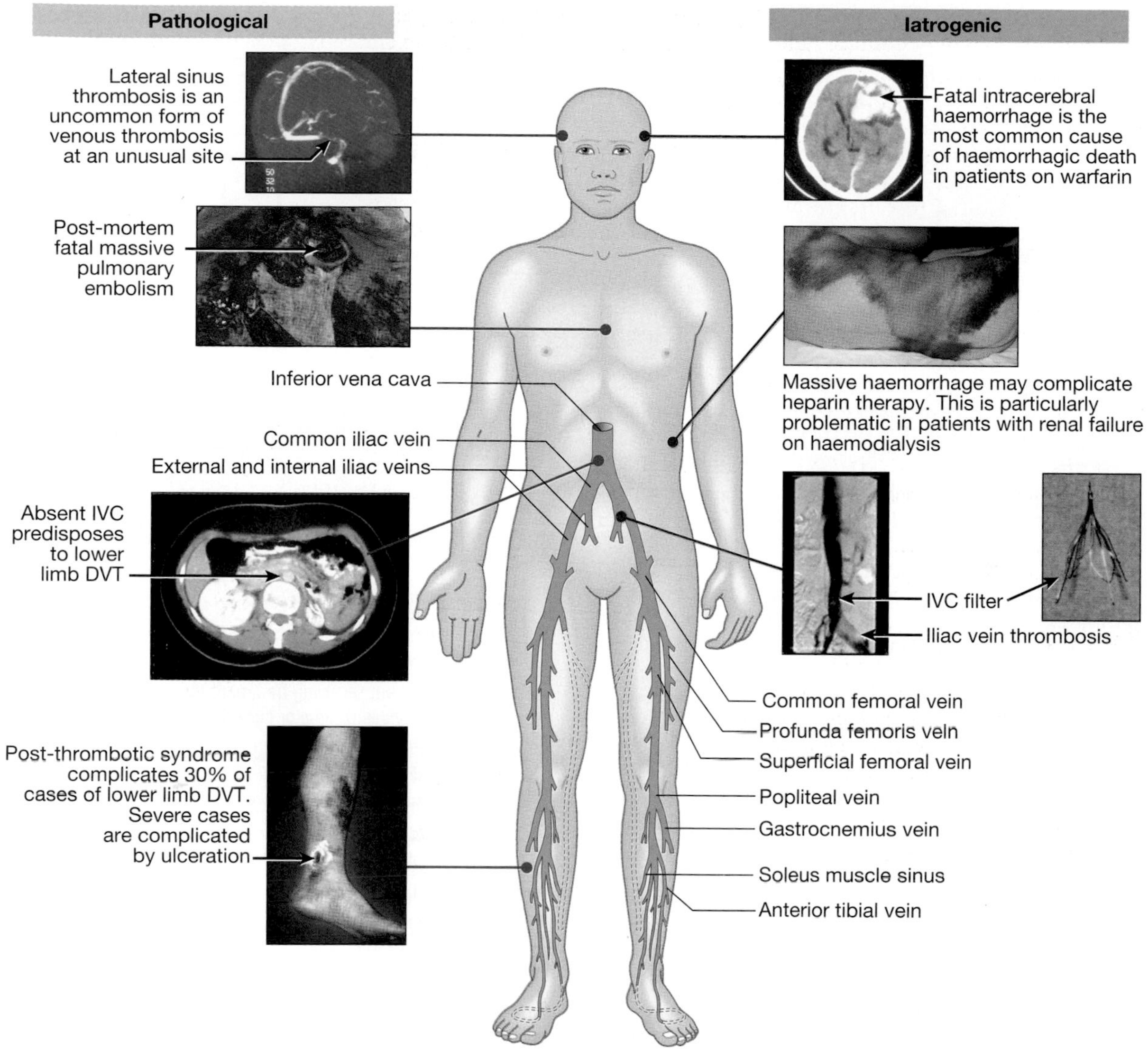

Pathological

Lateral sinus thrombosis is an uncommon form of venous thrombosis at an unusual site

Post-mortem fatal massive pulmonary embolism

Inferior vena cava

Common iliac vein

External and internal iliac veins

Absent IVC predisposes to lower limb DVT

Post-thrombotic syndrome complicates 30% of cases of lower limb DVT. Severe cases are complicated by ulceration

Iatrogenic

Fatal intracerebral haemorrhage is the most common cause of haemorrhagic death in patients on warfarin

Massive haemorrhage may complicate heparin therapy. This is particularly problematic in patients with renal failure on haemodialysis

IVC filter

Iliac vein thrombosis

Common femoral vein

Profunda femoris vein

Superficial femoral vein

Popliteal vein

Gastrocnemius vein

Soleus muscle sinus

Anterior tibial vein

Fig. 24.14 Causes and consequences of venous thromboembolic disease and its treatment. (IVC = inferior vena cava)

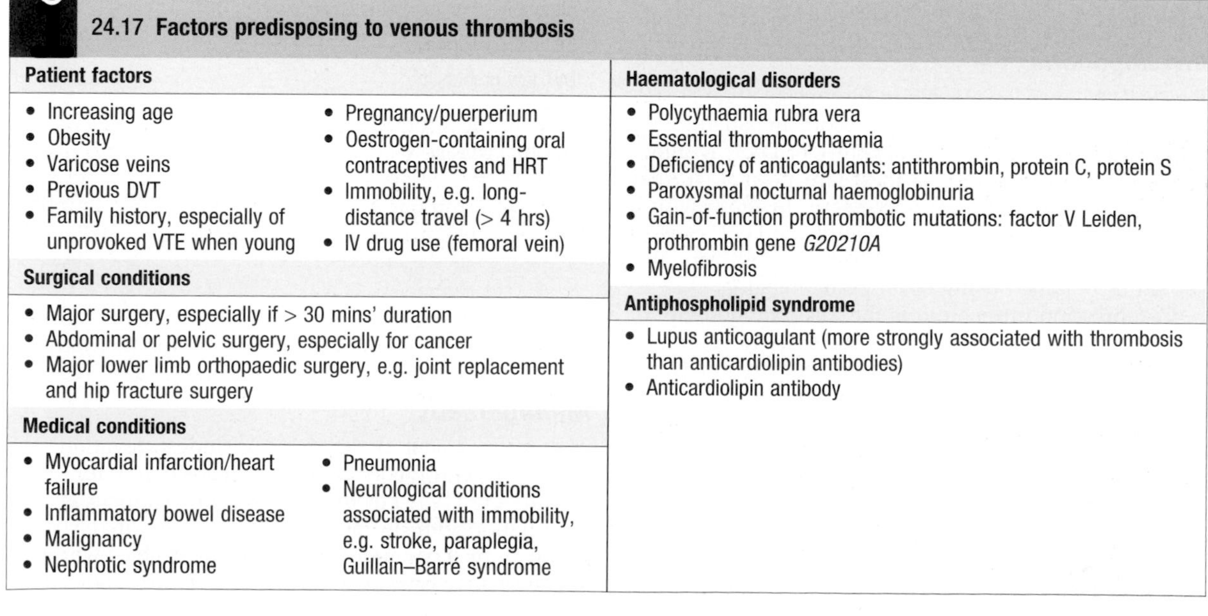

24.17 Factors predisposing to venous thrombosis

Patient factors

- Increasing age
- Obesity
- Varicose veins
- Previous DVT
- Family history, especially of unprovoked VTE when young
- Pregnancy/puerperium
- Oestrogen-containing oral contraceptives and HRT
- Immobility, e.g. long-distance travel (> 4 hrs)
- IV drug use (femoral vein)

Surgical conditions

- Major surgery, especially if > 30 mins' duration
- Abdominal or pelvic surgery, especially for cancer
- Major lower limb orthopaedic surgery, e.g. joint replacement and hip fracture surgery

Medical conditions

- Myocardial infarction/heart failure
- Inflammatory bowel disease
- Malignancy
- Nephrotic syndrome
- Pneumonia
- Neurological conditions associated with immobility, e.g. stroke, paraplegia, Guillain–Barré syndrome

Haematological disorders

- Polycythaemia rubra vera
- Essential thrombocythaemia
- Deficiency of anticoagulants: antithrombin, protein C, protein S
- Paroxysmal nocturnal haemoglobinuria
- Gain-of-function prothrombotic mutations: factor V Leiden, prothrombin gene *G20210A*
- Myelofibrosis

Antiphospholipid syndrome

- Lupus anticoagulant (more strongly associated with thrombosis than anticardiolipin antibodies)
- Anticardiolipin antibody

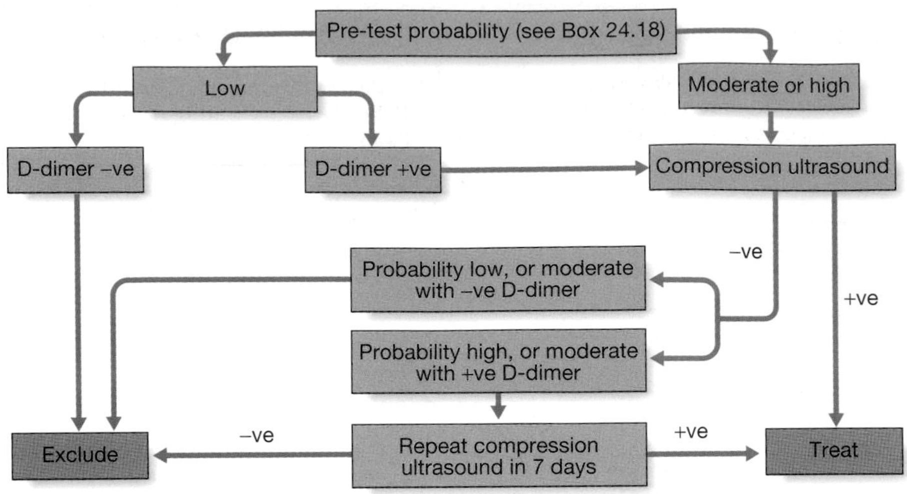

Fig. 24.15 Investigation of suspected deep vein thrombosis. Pre-test probability is calculated in Box 24.18.

and dilatation of the superficial veins. Often, however, symptoms and signs are minimal. It is typically unilateral but may be bilateral, and clot may extend proximally into the inferior vena cava. Bilateral DVT is more commonly seen with underlying malignancy or anomalies of the inferior vena cava. The differential diagnosis of unilateral leg swelling includes a spontaneous or traumatic calf muscle tear or a ruptured Baker's cyst, both characterised by sudden onset and localised tenderness. Infective cellulitis is usually distinguished by marked skin erythema and heat localised within a well-demarcated area of the leg and may be associated with an obvious source of entry of infection (e.g. insect bite, leg ulcer).

Risk factors for DVT should be considered (see Box 24.17), and examination should include assessment for malignancy. Symptoms and signs of PE should be sought (p. 721), particularly in those with proximal thrombosis; asymptomatic PE is thought to be present in approximately 30% of patients with lower limb DVT.

Clinical criteria can be used to rank patients according to their likelihood of DVT or PE: for example, by using scoring systems such as the Wells score (Box 24.18).

Investigations

Figure 24.15 gives an algorithm for investigation of suspected DVT based on initial Wells score. In patients with a low ('unlikely') pre-test probability of DVT, D-dimer levels can be measured; if these are normal, further investigation for DVT is unnecessary. In those with a moderate or high ('likely') probability of DVT or with elevated D-dimer levels, objective diagnosis of DVT should be obtained using appropriate imaging.

Compression ultrasound is the imaging modality of choice in most centres. It has a sensitivity for proximal DVT (clot involving the popliteal vein or above) of 99.5%. Sensitivity and specificity are lower for diagnosing calf vein thrombosis. Contrast venography is an alternative that is now rarely used. In patients with proven DVT, further imaging to diagnose PE is not required unless massive PE is clinically suspected or there is otherwise unexplained breathlessness (p. 722).

Predisposing factors, particularly pelvic malignancy and those listed in Box 24.17, should be considered and investigation pursued. In occasional patients, further investigation for an underlying thrombophilic condition may be considered (see Boxes 24.4 and 24.5, p. 1001).

24.18 Predicting the pre-test probability of deep vein thrombosis using the Wells score*

Clinical characteristic	Score
Active cancer (patient receiving treatment for cancer within previous 6 mths or currently receiving palliative treatment)	1
Paralysis, paresis or recent plaster immobilisation of lower extremities	1
Recently bedridden for ≥ 3 days, or major surgery within previous 4 wks	1
Localised tenderness along distribution of deep venous system	1
Entire leg swollen	1
Calf swelling at least 3 cm larger than that on asymptomatic side (measured 10 cm below tibial tuberosity)	1
Pitting oedema confined to symptomatic leg	1
Collateral superficial veins (non-varicose)	1
Alternative diagnosis at least as likely as DVT	–2
Clinical probability	**Total score**
DVT low probability	≤ 1
DVT moderate probability	1–2
DVT high probability	≥ 2

*A dichotomised revised Wells score, which classifies patients as 'unlikely' or 'likely', may also be used. From Wells PS. New Engl J Med 2003; 349:1227; copyright © 2003 Massachusetts Medical Society.

Management

The management of leg DVT includes elevation and analgesia. Thrombolysis may be considered for limb-threatening DVT, but the mainstay of treatment is anticoagulation with low molecular weight heparin (LMWH), followed by a coumarin anticoagulant, such as warfarin. An alternative is the oral Xa inhibitor, rivaroxaban, which

EBM 24.19 Treatment of venous thromboembolism

'In patients with active cancer, treatment of deep vein thrombosis with low molecular weight heparin (LMWH) for 6 months is superior in preventing recurrence of thrombosis to short-period LMWH followed by warfarin.'

- Lee AY, et al. N Engl J Med 2003; 349(2):146–153.

has a rapid onset of action and can be used immediately from diagnosis without the need for LMWH. Treatment of acute VTE with LMWH should continue for at least 5 days. If a coumarin is being introduced, the heparin should continue until the INR has been in the target range (2–3; pp. 1000 and 1018) for 2 days. Patients who have had a DVT and have a strong contraindication to anticoagulation, and those who, despite therapeutic anticoagulation, continue to have new pulmonary emboli, should have an inferior vena cava filter inserted to prevent life-threatening PE.

The optimal initial duration of anticoagulation is between 6 weeks and 6 months. Patients who have thrombosis in the presence of a temporary risk factor, which is then removed, can usually be treated for shorter periods (e.g. 3 months) than those who sustain unprovoked thrombosis. In patients with active cancer and VTE, there is evidence that LMWH should be continued for 6 months rather than being replaced by a coumarin (Box 24.19). Evidence indicates that periods of anticoagulation of more than 6 months do not alter the rate of recurrence following discontinuation of therapy.

Recurrence of DVT is about 2–3% per annum in patients who have a medical temporary risk factor at presentation and about 8% per annum in those with apparently unprovoked DVT. Recurrence plateaus at around 30–40% at 5 years. Post-thrombotic syndrome is due to damage of venous valves by the thrombus. It results in persistent leg swelling, heaviness and discoloration. The most severe complication of this syndrome is ulceration around the medial malleolus.

BLOOD PRODUCTS AND TRANSFUSION

Blood transfusion from an unrelated donor to a recipient inevitably carries some risk, including adverse immunological interactions between the host and infused blood (p. 94) and transmission of infectious agents. Although there are many compelling clinical indications for blood component transfusion, there are also many clinical circumstances in which transfusion is conventional but the evidence for its effectiveness is limited. In these settings, allogeneic transfusion may be avoided by following protocols that recommend use of low haemoglobin thresholds for red cell transfusion (Box 24.20), perioperative blood salvage and antifibrinolytic drugs.

Blood products

Blood components are prepared from whole blood collected from individual donors and include red cells, platelets, plasma and cryoprecipitate (Box 24.22).

Plasma derivatives are licensed pharmaceutical products produced on a factory scale from large volumes of

EBM 24.20 Red cell transfusion in critically ill patients

'A restrictive strategy of red cell transfusion is at least as effective as, and possibly superior to, a liberal transfusion strategy in critically ill patients. A restrictive strategy allows transfusion when Hb is below 70 g/L and maintains Hb at 70–90 g/L, whereas a liberal strategy allows transfusion when Hb is below 100 g/L and maintains Hb at 100–120 g/L.'

- Hébert PC, et al. N Eng J Med 1999; 340(6):409–417.

For further information: www.transfusionguidelines.org.uk
www.learnbloodtransfusion.org.uk

EBM 24.21 Fluid resuscitation in critically ill patients

'In patients with trauma, burns or following surgery, there is no evidence that resuscitation with albumin or other colloid solutions reduces the risk of death compared to resuscitation with crystalloid solutions.'

- Perel P, Roberts I. Colloids versus crystalloids for fluid resuscitation in critically ill patients. Cochrane Database of Systematic Reviews, 2011, issue 3. Art. no. CD000567.

human plasma obtained from many people and treated to remove transmissible infection. Examples include:

- *Coagulation factors.* Concentrates of factors VIII and IX are used for the treatment of conditions such as haemophilia A, haemophilia B and von Willebrand disease. Coagulation factors made by recombinant DNA technology are now preferred due to perceived lack of infection risk but plasma-derived products are still used in many countries.
- *Immunoglobulins.* Intravenous immunoglobulin (IVIgG) is administered as regular replacement therapy to reduce infective complications in patients with immunodeficiency. A short, high-dose course of IVIgG may also be effective in some immunological disorders, including immune thrombocytopenia (p. 1049) and Guillain–Barré syndrome (p. 1224). IVIgG can cause acute reactions and must be infused strictly according to the manufacturer's product information. There is a risk of renal dysfunction in susceptible patients and, in these circumstances, immunoglobulin products containing low or no sucrose are preferred. Anti-zoster immunoglobulin has a role in the prophylaxis of varicella zoster (p. 317). Anti-Rhesus D immunoglobulin is used in pregnancy to prevent haemolytic disease of the newborn (see Box 24.24 below).
- *Human albumin.* This is available in two strengths. The 5% solution can be used as a colloid resuscitation fluid, but it is no more effective and is more expensive than crystalloid solutions (Box 24.21). Human albumin 20% solution is used in the management of hypoproteinaemic oedema in nephrotic syndrome (p. 476), and ascites in chronic liver disease (p. 938). It is hyperoncotic and expands plasma volume by more than the amount infused.

Blood donation

A safe supply of blood components depends on a well-organised system with regular donation by healthy individuals who have no excess risk of infections transmissible in blood (Fig. 24.16). Blood donations are obtained by

24.22 Blood components and their use

Component	Major haemorrhage	Other indications
Red cell concentrate[1] Most of the plasma is removed and replaced with a solution of glucose and adenine in saline to maintain viability of red cells ABO compatibility with recipient is essential	Replace acute blood loss: increase circulating red cell mass to relieve clinical features caused by insufficient oxygen delivery	*Severe anaemia* If no cardiovascular disease, transfuse to maintain Hb at 70 g/L If known or likely to have cardiovascular disease, maintain Hb at 90 g/L
Platelet concentrate One adult dose is made from four donations of whole blood, or from a single platelet apheresis donation ABO compatibility with recipient is preferable	Maintain platelet count > 50×10^9/L, or in multiple or CNS trauma > 100×10^9/L Each adult dose has a minimum of 2.4×10^{11} platelets, which raises platelet count by 40×10^9/L unless there is consumptive coagulopathy, e.g. DIC	*Thrombocytopenia*, e.g. in acute leukaemia Maintain platelet count > 10×10^9/L if not bleeding Maintain platelet count > 20×10^9/L if minor bleeding or at risk (sepsis, concurrent use of antibiotics, abnormal clotting) Increase platelet count > 50×10^9/L for minor invasive procedure (e.g. lumbar puncture, gastroscopy and biopsy, insertion of indwelling lines, liver biopsy, laparotomy) or if acute, major blood loss Increase platelet count > 100×10^9/L for operations in critical sites such as brain or eyes
Fresh frozen plasma[2] 150–300 mL plasma from one donation of whole blood ABO compatibility with recipient is recommended	Dilutional coagulopathy with a PT prolonged > 50% is likely after replacement of 1–1.5 blood volumes with red cell concentrate Initial dose of FFP 15 mL/kg Further doses only if bleeding continues and guided by PT and APTT	*Replacement of coagulation factor deficiency* If no virally inactivated or recombinant product is available *TTP* Plasma exchange (using virus-inactivated plasma if available) is frequently effective
Cryoprecipitate[2] Fibrinogen and coagulation factor concentrated from plasma by controlled thawing 10–20 mL pack contains fibrinogen 150–300 mg, factor VIII 80–120 U, von Willebrand factor 80–120 U In UK, supplied as pools of 5 U	May be indicated if fibrinogen < 0.8 g/L due to dilution and DIC Pooled units (of 10 donations) containing 3 g fibrinogen in 300 mL raise fibrinogen by 1 g/L	*von Willebrand disease and haemophilia* If virus-inactivated or recombinant products are not available

[1]**Whole blood** is an alternative to red cell concentrate. ABO compatibility with recipient is essential.
[2]Pooled plasma can be treated with solvent and detergent or single units treated with methylene blue as an additional viral inactivation step. Virus-inactivated plasma is indicated for large-volume exposure, as in treatment of thrombotic thrombocytopenic purpura, and for treatment of children in the UK born after 1995.
(APTT = activated partial thromboplastin time; CNS = central nervous system; DIC = disseminated intravascular coagulation; FFP = fresh frozen plasma; PT = prothrombin time; TTP = thrombotic thrombocytopenic purpura)

either venesection of a unit of whole blood or collection of a specific component, such as platelets, by apheresis. During apheresis, the donor's blood is drawn via a closed system into a machine which separates the components by centrifugation and collects the desired fraction into a bag, returning the rest of the blood to the donor. Each donation must be tested for hepatitis B (HBV), hepatitis C (HCV), HIV and human T cell lymphotropic (HTLV) virus nucleic acid and/or antibodies. Platelet concentrates may be tested for bacterial contamination. The need for other microbiological tests depends on local epidemiology. For example, testing for *Trypanosoma cruzi* (Chagas' disease; p. 360) is necessary in areas of South America and the USA where infection is prevalent; tests for West Nile virus have been required in the USA since this agent became prevalent; plasma donated in the UK is not used at present for producing pooled plasma derivatives in view of concerns about transmission of variant Creutzfeldt–Jakob disease (vCJD; p. 1211).

Adverse effects of transfusion

Death directly attributable to transfusion is rare, at less than 0.3 per 100 000 transfusions. However, relatively minor symptoms of transfusion reactions (fever, itch or urticaria) occur in up to 3% of transfusions, usually in patients who have had repeated transfusions. Any symptoms or signs that arise during a transfusion must be taken seriously, as they may be the first warnings of a serious reaction. Figure 24.18 (p. 1016) outlines the symptoms and signs, management and investigation of acute reactions to blood components.

Red cell incompatibility

Red blood cell membranes contain numerous cell surface molecules which are potentially antigenic (see Fig. 24.4, p. 994). The ABO and Rh(D) antigens are the most important in routine transfusion and antenatal practice.

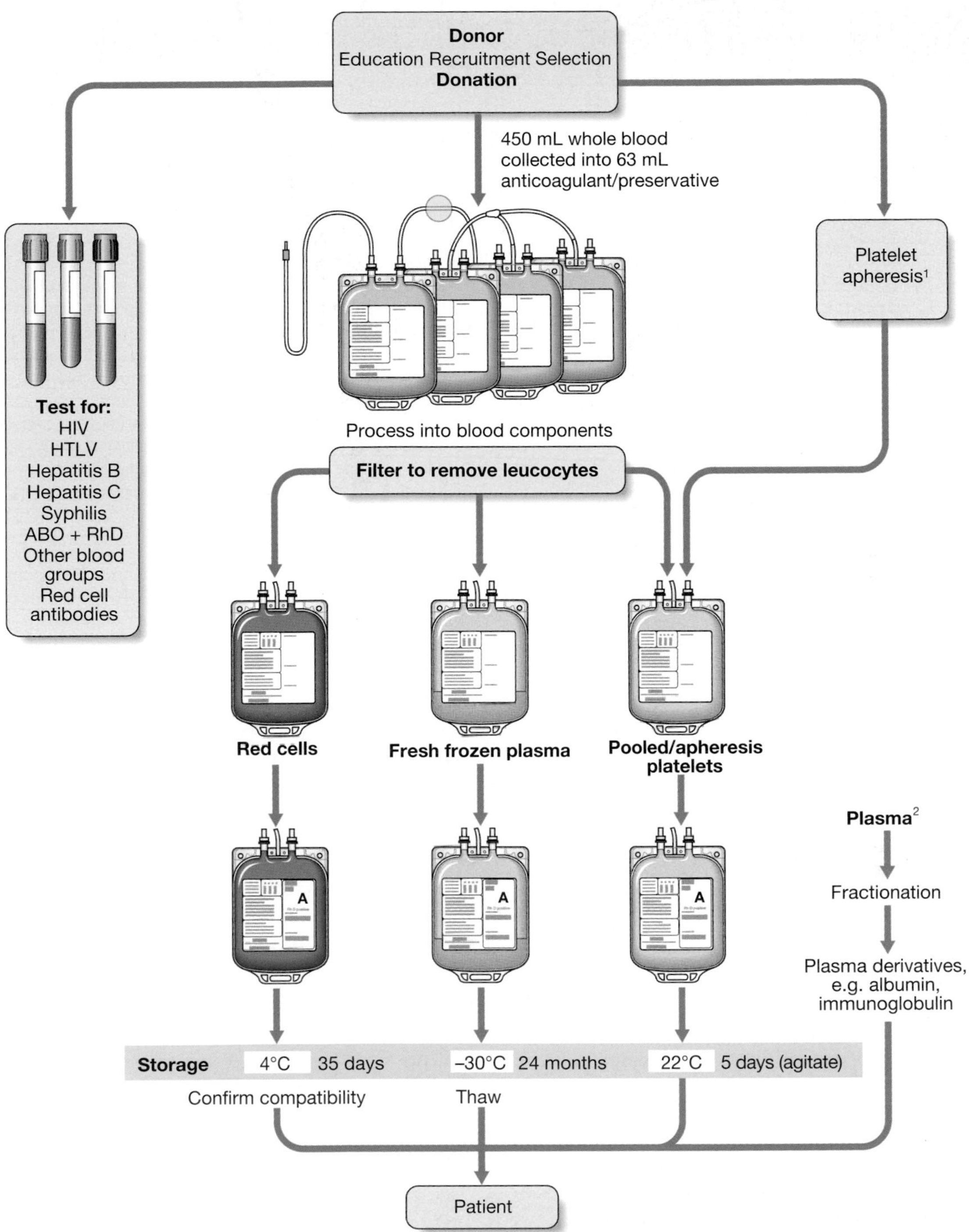

Fig. 24.16 Blood donation, processing and storage. [1]Platelet apheresis involves circulating the donor's blood through a cell separator to remove platelets before returning other blood components to the donor. [2]In the UK, plasma for fractionation is imported as a precautionary measure against variant Creutzfeldt–Jakob disease. (HIV = human immunodeficiency virus; HTLV = human T cell lymphotropic virus)

ABO blood groups

The frequency of the ABO antigens varies among different populations. The ABO blood group antigens are oligosaccharide chains that project from the red cell surface. These chains are attached to proteins and lipids that lie in the red cell membrane. The ABO gene encodes a glycosyltransferase that catalyses the final step in the synthesis of the chain which has three common alleles: A, B and O. The O allele encodes an inactive enzyme, leaving the ABO antigen precursor (called the H antigen) unmodified. The A and B alleles encode enzymes that differ by four amino acids and hence attach different sugars to the end of the chain. Individuals are tolerant to their own ABO antigens, but do not suppress B cell clones producing antibodies against ABO antigens that they do not carry themselves (Box 24.23). They are therefore capable of mounting a humoral immune response to these 'foreign' antigens.

24.23 ABO blood group antigens and antibodies

ABO blood group	Red cell A or B antigens	Antibodies in plasma	UK frequency (%)
O	None	Anti-A and anti-B	46
A	A	Anti-B	42
B	B	Anti-A	9
AB	A and B	None	3

ABO-incompatible red cell transfusion

If red cells of an incompatible ABO group are transfused (especially if a group O recipient is transfused with group A, B or AB red cells), the *recipient's* IgM anti-A, anti-B or anti-AB binds to the *transfused* red cells. This activates the full complement pathway (p. 75), creating pores in the red cell membrane and destroying the transfused red cells in the circulation (intravascular haemolysis). The anaphylatoxins C3a and C5a, released by complement activation, liberate cytokines such as tumour necrosis factor (TNF), interleukin 1 (IL-1) and IL-8, and stimulate degranulation of mast cells with release of vasoactive mediators. All these substances may lead to inflammation, increased vascular permeability and hypotension, which may, in turn, cause shock and renal failure. Inflammatory mediators can also cause platelet aggregation, lung peribronchial oedema and smooth muscle contraction. About 20–30% of ABO-incompatible transfusions cause some degree of morbidity, and 5–10% cause or contribute to a patient's death. The main reason for this relatively low morbidity is the lack of potency of ABO antibodies in group A or B subjects; even if the recipient is group O, those who are very young or very old usually have weaker antibodies that do not lead to the activation of large amounts of complement.

The Rhesus D blood group and haemolytic disease of the newborn

About 15% of Caucasians are Rhesus-negative; that is, they lack the Rhesus D (RhD) red cell surface antigen (see Fig. 24.4, p. 994). In other populations (e.g. in Chinese and Bengalis), only 1–5% are Rhesus-negative. RhD-negative individuals do not normally produce substantial amounts of anti-RhD antibodies. However, if RhD-positive red cells enter the circulation of an RhD-negative individual, IgG antibodies are produced. This can occur during pregnancy if the mother is exposed to fetal cells via fetomaternal haemorrhage, or following transfusion. If a woman is so sensitised, during a subsequent pregnancy anti-RhD antibodies can cross the placenta; if the fetus is RhD-positive, haemolysis with severe fetal anaemia and hyperbilirubinaemia can result. This can cause severe neurological damage or death due to haemolytic disease of the newborn (HDN). Therefore, an RhD-negative female who may subsequently become pregnant should never be transfused with RhD-positive blood.

In RhD-negative women, administration of anti-RhD immunoglobulin (anti-D) perinatally can block the immune response to RhD antigen on fetal cells and is the only effective product for preventing the development of Rhesus antibodies (Box 24.24).

HDN can also be caused by other alloantibodies against red cell antigens, usually after previous pregnancies or transfusions. These antigens include Rhc,

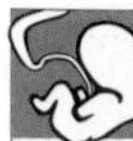

24.24 Rhesus D blood groups in pregnancy

- **Haemolytic disease of the newborn (HDN)**: occurs when the mother has anti-red cell IgG antibodies that cross the placenta and haemolyse fetal red cells.
- **Screening for HDN in pregnancy**: at the time of booking (12–16 wks) and again at 28–34 wks gestation, every pregnant woman should have a blood sample sent for determination of ABO and RhD group and testing for red cell alloantibodies that may be directed against paternal blood group antigens present in fetal red cells.
- **Anti-D immunoglobulin prophylaxis in a pregnant woman who is RhD-negative**: antenatal anti-D prophylaxis is offered at 28–34 wks to RhD-negative pregnant women who have no evidence of immune anti-D. This prevents the formation of antibodies that could cause HDN. Following delivery of an RhD-positive baby, the mother is given further anti-D within 72 hrs; a maternal sample is checked for remaining fetal red cells and additional anti-D is given if indicated. Additional anti-D is also given after potential sensitising events antenatally (e.g. early bleeding). Doses vary according to national recommendations.

RhC, RhE, Rhe, and the Kell, Kidd and Duffy antigen systems. HDN can also occur if there is fetomaternal ABO incompatibility, most commonly seen in a group O mother with a group A fetus. The fetus is generally less severely affected by ABO incompatibility than by RhD, Rhc or Kell antigen mismatch.

Other immunological complications of transfusion

Rare but serious complications include transfusion-associated lung injury (TRALI) and transfusion-associated graft-versus-host disease (TA GVHD). The latter occurs when there is sharing of a human leucocyte antigen (HLA) haplotype between donor and recipient, which allows transfused lymphocytes to engraft, proliferate and recognise the recipient as foreign, resulting in acute GVHD (p. 1017). Prevention is by gamma- or X-ray irradiation of blood components before their administration to prevent lymphocyte proliferation. Those at risk of TA GVHD who must receive irradiated blood components include: patients with congenital T cell immunodeficiencies or Hodgkin lymphoma; patients with aplastic anaemia receiving immunosuppressive therapy with anti-thymocyte globulin; recipients of haematopoietic stem cell transplants or of blood from a family member; neonates who have received an intrauterine transfusion; and patients taking T lymphocyte-suppressing drugs, such as fludarabine and other purine analogues.

Transfusion-transmitted infection

Over the past 30 years, HBV, HIV-1 and HCV have been identified and effective tests introduced to detect and exclude infected donations. Where blood is from 'safe' donors and correctly tested, the current risk of a donated unit being infectious is very small. By 2010 in the UK, the estimated chance that a unit of blood from a 'safe' donor might transmit one of the viruses for which blood is tested was 1 in 6.4 million units for HIV-1, 1 in 100 million for HCV and 1 in 1.4 million for HBV. However, some patients who received transfusions before these tests were available suffered serious consequences from infection; this serves as a reminder to avoid non-essential transfusion, since it is impossible to exclude the emergence of new or currently unrecognised transfusion-transmissible infection. Licensed plasma derivatives that have been virus-inactivated do not transmit HIV, HTLV, HBV, HCV, cytomegalovirus or other lipid-enveloped viruses.

vCJD is a human prion disease linked to bovine spongiform encephalitis (BSE; p. 1211). The risk of a recipient acquiring the agent of vCJD from a transfusion is uncertain, but of 16 recipients of blood from donors who later developed the disease, 3 have died with clinical vCJD and 1 other had postmortem pathological features of infection.

Bacterial contamination of a blood component – usually platelets – is extremely rare (e.g. no reports in the UK in either 2010 or 2011) but can result in severe bacteraemia/septicaemia in the recipient.

Safe transfusion procedures

The proposed transfusion and any alternatives should be discussed with the patient or, if that is not possible, with a relative, and this should be documented. Some patients, e.g. Jehovah's Witnesses, may refuse transfusion and require specialised management to survive profound anaemia following blood loss.

Pre-transfusion testing

To ensure that red cells supplied for transfusion are compatible with the intended recipient, the transfusion laboratory will perform either a 'group and screen' procedure or a 'cross-match'. In the group and screen procedure, the red cells from the patient's blood sample are tested to determine the ABO and RhD type, and the patient's serum is also tested against an array of red cells expressing the most important antigens to detect any red cell antibodies. Any antibody detected can be identified by further testing, so that red cell units that lack the corresponding antigen can be selected. The patient's sample can be held in the laboratory for up to a week, so that the hospital blood bank can quickly prepare compatible blood without the need for a further patient sample. Conventional cross-matching consists of the group and antibody screen, followed by direct confirmation of the compatibility of individual units of red cells with the patient's serum. Full cross-matching takes about 45 minutes if no red cell antibodies are present, but may require hours if a patient has multiple antibodies.

Blood can be supplied by 'electronic issue', without the need for compatibility cross-matching, if the laboratory's computer system shows that the patient's ABO and RhD groups have been identified and confirmed on two separate occasions and their antibody screen is negative.

Bedside procedures for safe transfusion

Errors leading to patients receiving the wrong blood are an important avoidable cause of mortality and morbidity. Most incompatible transfusions result from failure to adhere to standard procedures for taking correctly labelled blood samples from the patient and ensuring that the correct pack of blood component is transfused into the intended patient. In the UK in 2011, there were 247 reports of transfusion of an incorrect blood component (8 per 100 000 units transfused). Every hospital where blood is transfused should have a written transfusion policy used by all staff who order, check or administer blood products (Fig. 24.17). Management of suspected transfusion reactions is shown in Figure 24.18.

Taking blood for pre-transfusion testing

- Positively identify the patient at the bedside
- Label the sample tube and complete the request form clearly and accurately after identifying the patient
- Do not write forms and labels in advance

Administering blood

- Positively identify the patient at the bedside
- Ensure that the identification of each blood pack matches the patient's identification
- Check that the ABO and RhD groups of each pack are compatible with the patient's
- Check each pack for evidence of damage
- If in doubt, do not use and return to the blood bank
- Complete the forms that document the transfusion of each pack

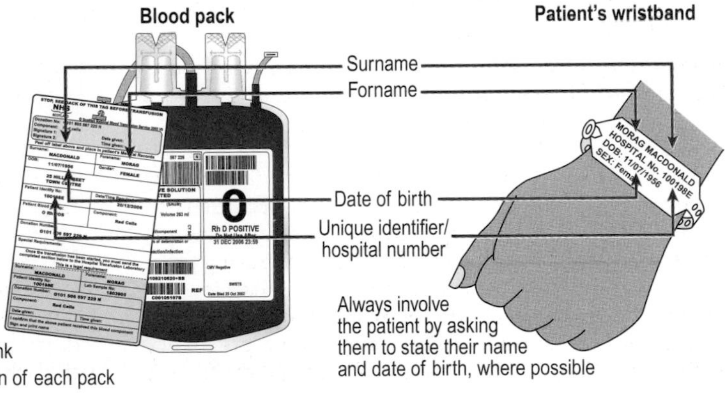

Record-keeping

- Record in the patient's notes the reason for transfusion, the product given, dose, any adverse effects and the clinical response

Observations

- Transfusions should only be given when the patient can be observed
- Blood pressure, pulse and temperature should be monitored before and 15 minutes after starting each pack
- In concious patients, further observations are only needed if the patient has symptoms or signs of a reaction
- In unconscious patients, check pulse and temperature at intervals during transfusion
- Signs of abnormal bleeding during the transfusion could be due to disseminated intravascular coagulation resulting from an acute haemolytic reaction

Fig. 24.17 Bedside procedures for safe blood transfusion. The patient's safety depends on adherence to standard procedures for taking samples for compatibility testing, administering blood, record-keeping and observations.

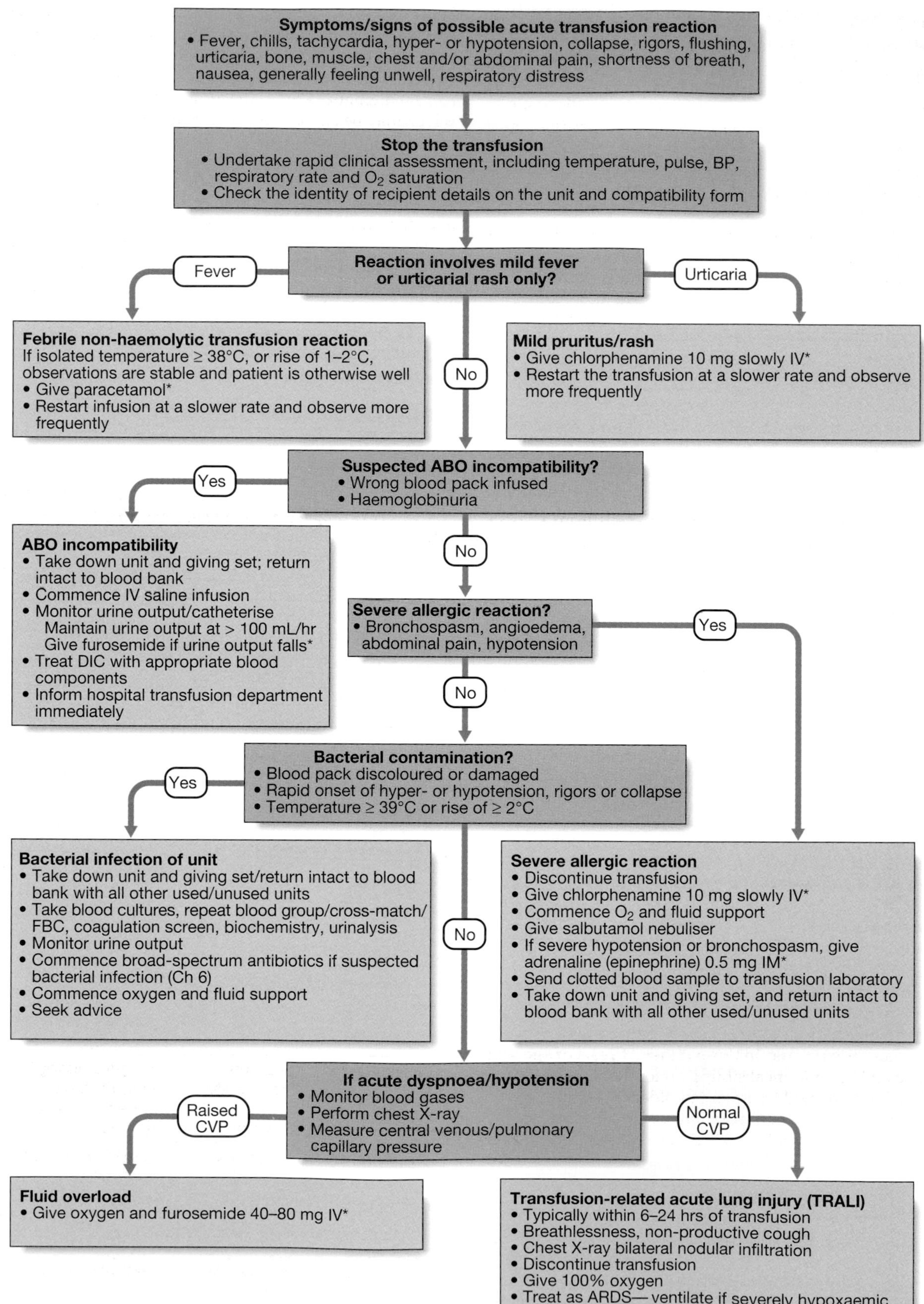

Fig. 24.18 Investigation and management of acute transfusion reactions. *Use size-appropriate dose in children. (ARDS = acute respiratory distress syndrome; DIC = disseminated intravascular coagulation; FBC = full blood count)

HAEMATOPOIETIC STEM CELL TRANSPLANTATION

Transplantation of haematopoietic stem cells (HSCT) has offered the only hope of 'cure' in a variety of haematological and non-haematological disorders (Box 24.25). As standard treatment improves, the indications for HSCT are being refined and extended, although its use remains most common in haematological malignancies. The type of HSCT is defined according to the donor and source of stem cells:

- In *allogeneic* HSCT, the stem cells come from a *donor* – either related (usually an HLA-identical sibling) or a closely HLA-matched volunteer unrelated donor (VUD).
- In an *autologous* transplant, the stem cells are harvested from the *patient* and stored in the vapour phase of liquid nitrogen until required. Stem cells can be harvested from the bone marrow or from the blood.

Allogeneic HSCT

Healthy bone marrow or blood stem cells from a donor are infused intravenously into the recipient, who has been suitably 'conditioned'. The conditioning treatment (chemotherapy with or without radiotherapy) destroys malignant cells and immunosuppresses the recipient, as well as ablating the recipient's haematopoietic tissues (myeloablation). The infused donor cells 'home' to the marrow, engraft and produce enough erythrocytes, granulocytes and platelets for the patient's needs after about 3–4 weeks. During this period of aplasia, patients are at risk of infection and bleeding, and require intensive supportive care as described on page 1038. It may take several years to regain normal immunological function and patients remain at risk from opportunistic infections, in particular in the first year.

An advantage of receiving allogeneic donor stem cells is that the donor's immune system can recognise residual recipient malignant cells and destroy them. This immunological 'graft versus disease' effect is a powerful tool against many haematological tumours and can be boosted post transplantation by the infusion of T cells taken from the donor, so-called donor lymphocyte infusion (DLI).

Considerable morbidity and mortality are associated with HSCT. The best results are obtained with minimal residual disease, and in those under 20 years of age who have an HLA-identical sibling donor. Reduced-intensity HSCT has enabled treatment of older or less fit patients. In this form of transplantation, rather than using very intensive conditioning which causes morbidity from organ damage, relatively low doses of drugs, such as fludarabine and cyclophosphamide, are used to immunosuppress the recipient and allow donor stem cells to engraft. The emerging donor immune system then eliminates malignant cells via the 'graft versus disease' effect, which may be boosted by the elective use of donor T cell infusions post transplant.

Complications

These are outlined in Boxes 24.26 and 24.27. The risks and outcomes of transplantation depend upon several patient- and disease-related factors. In general, 25% die from procedure-related complications, such as infection and GVHD, and there remains a significant risk of relapse of the haematological malignancy. The long-term survival for patients undergoing allogeneic HSCT in acute leukaemia is around 50%.

Graft-versus-host disease

Graft-versus-host disease (GVHD) is caused by the cytotoxic activity of donor T lymphocytes which become

24.25 Indications for allogeneic HSCT

- Neoplastic disorders affecting stem cell compartments (e.g. leukaemias)
- Failure of haematopoiesis (e.g. aplastic anaemia)
- Major inherited defects in blood cell production (e.g. thalassaemia, immunodeficiency diseases)
- Inborn errors of metabolism with missing enzymes or cell lines

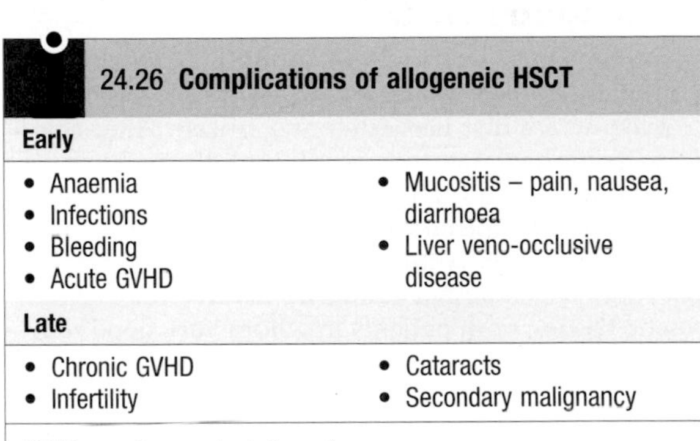

24.26 Complications of allogeneic HSCT

Early	
• Anaemia • Infections • Bleeding • Acute GVHD	• Mucositis – pain, nausea, diarrhoea • Liver veno-occlusive disease
Late	
• Chronic GVHD • Infertility	• Cataracts • Secondary malignancy

(GVHD = graft-versus-host disease)

24.27 Infections during recovery from HSCT

Infection	Time after HSCT	Management
Herpes simplex (p. 325)	0–4 wks (aplastic phase)	Aciclovir prophylaxis and therapy
Bacterial, fungal	0–4 wks (aplastic phase)	As for acute leukaemia (p. 1036) – antibiotic and antifungal prophylaxis and therapy
Cytomegalovirus (p. 321)	5–21 wks (cell-mediated immune deficiency)	Antigen screening in blood (PCR) and pre-emptive therapy (e.g. ganciclovir)
Varicella zoster (p. 316)	After 13 wks	Aciclovir prophylaxis and therapy
Pneumocystis jirovecii (p. 400)	8–26 wks	Co-trimoxazole
Encapsulated bacteria	8 wks to years (immunoglobulin deficiency, prolonged with GVHD)	Prophylaxis and revaccination

(GVHD = graft-versus-host disease; PCR = polymerase chain reaction)

24

sensitised to their new host, regarding it as foreign. This may cause either an acute or a chronic form of GVHD.

Acute GVHD occurs in the first 100 days after transplant in about one-third of patients. It can affect the skin, causing rashes, the liver, causing jaundice, and the gut, causing diarrhoea, and may vary from mild to lethal. Prevention includes HLA-matching of the donor, immunosuppressant drugs, including methotrexate, ciclosporin, alemtuzumab or antithymocyte globulin. Severe presentations are very difficult to control and, despite high-dose corticosteroids, may result in death.

Chronic GVHD may follow acute GVHD or arise independently; it occurs later than acute GVHD. It often resembles a connective tissue disorder, and carries an increased risk of infection, although in mild cases a rash may be the only manifestation. Chronic GVHD is usually treated with corticosteroids and prolonged immunosuppression with, for example, ciclosporin. However, associated with chronic GVHD are the graft-versus-leukaemia effect and a lower relapse rate of the underlying malignancy.

Autologous HSCT

This procedure can also be used in haematological malignancies. The patient's own stem cells from blood or marrow are first harvested and frozen. After conditioning myeloablative therapy, the autologous stem cells are reinfused into the blood stream in order to rescue the patient from the marrow damage and aplasia caused by chemotherapy. Autologous HSCT may be used for disorders which do not primarily involve the haematopoietic tissues, or in patients in whom very good remissions have been achieved. The preferred source of stem cells for autologous transplants is peripheral blood. These stem cells engraft more quickly, marrow recovery occurring within 2–3 weeks. There is no risk of GVHD and no immunosuppression is required. Thus autologous stem cell transplantation carries a lower procedure-related mortality rate than allogeneic HSCT at around 5%, but there is a higher rate of recurrence of malignancy. Whether the stem cells should be treated (purged) in an attempt to remove any residual malignant cells remains controversial.

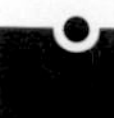

24.28 Indications for anticoagulation

Indication	INR
Heparin/LMWH	
• Prevention and treatment of VTE	
• Percutaneous coronary intervention	
• Post-thrombolysis for MI	
• Unstable angina pectoris	
• Non-Q wave MI	
• Acute peripheral arterial occlusion	
• Cardiopulmonary bypass	
• Haemodialysis and haemofiltration	
Coumarins (warfarin etc.)	
• Prevention and treatment of VTE	Therapeutic INR 2.5
• Arterial embolism	Therapeutic INR 2.5
• Atrial fibrillation with specific stroke risk factors (p. 562)	Therapeutic INR 2.5
• Mobile mural thrombus post-MI	Therapeutic INR 2.5
• Extensive anterior MI	Therapeutic INR 2.5
• Dilated cardiomyopathy	Therapeutic INR 2.5
• Cardioversion	Therapeutic INR 2.5
• Ischaemic stroke in antiphospholipid syndrome	Therapeutic INR 2.5
• Mitral stenosis and mitral regurgitation with atrial fibrillation	Therapeutic INR 2.5
• Recurrent venous thrombosis whilst on warfarin	INR 3.5
• Mechanical prosthetic cardiac valves	INR 3.5
Rivaroxaban	
• Prevention and treatment of VTE	
• Atrial fibrillation with risk factor for stroke	
Dabigatran etexilate	
• Prevention of VTE	
• Atrial fibrillation with risk factors for stroke	
Apixaban	
• Prevention of VTE	

(INR = international normalised ratio; LMWH = low molecular weight heparin; MI = myocardial infarction; VTE = venous thromboembolism)

ANTICOAGULANT AND ANTITHROMBOTIC THERAPY

There are numerous indications for anticoagulant and antithrombotic medications (Box 24.28). The guiding principles are outlined here, but management in specific indications is discussed elsewhere in the book. Broadly speaking, antiplatelet medications are of greater efficacy in the prevention of arterial thrombosis and of less value in the prevention of VTE. Thus, antiplatelet agents, such as aspirin and clopidogrel, are the drugs of choice in acute coronary events and in ischaemic cerebrovascular disease, while warfarin and other anticoagulants are favoured in VTE. In some extremely prothrombotic situations, such as coronary artery stenting, a combination of anticoagulant and antiplatelet drugs is used.

A range of anticoagulant and antithrombotic drugs is used in clinical practice (Box 24.29). Newer agents allow predictable anticoagulation without the need for frequent monitoring and dose titration. Although warfarin remains the mainstay for oral anticoagulation, newer oral anticoagulants (dabigatran, rivaroxaban and apixaban), which can be given at fixed doses with predictable effects and no need for monitoring, have now been approved for the prevention of perioperative VTE, the treatment of established VTE and the prevention of cardioembolic stroke in patients with atrial fibrillation.

Heparins

Unfractionated heparin (UFH) and low molecular weight heparins (LMWH) both act by binding via a specific pentasaccharide to antithrombin which potentiates its natural anticoagulant activity (see Fig. 24.6, p. 996). Increased cleavage of activated proteases, particularly factor Xa and thrombin (IIa), accounts for the anticoagulant effect. LMWHs preferentially augment antithrombin activity against factor Xa. For the licensed indications, LMWHs are at least as efficacious as UFH but have several advantages:

- LMWHs are nearly 100% bioavailable and therefore produce reliable dose-dependent anticoagulation.

24.29 Modes of action of anticoagulant and antithrombotic drugs

Mode of action	Drug
Antiplatelet drugs	
Cyclo-oxygenase (COX) inhibition	Aspirin
Adenosine diphosphate (ADP) receptor inhibition	Clopidogrel Prasugrel Ticagrelor
Glycoprotein IIb/IIIa inhibition	Abciximab Tirofiban Eptifibatide
Phosphodiesterase inhibition	Dipyridamole
Oral anticoagulants	
Vitamin K antagonism	Warfarin/coumarins
Direct thrombin inhibition	Dabigatran
Direct Xa inhibition	Rivaroxaban Apixaban
Injectable anticoagulants	
Antithrombin-dependent inhibition of thrombin and Xa	Heparin
Antithrombin-dependent inhibition of Xa	Fondaparinux Idraparinux
Direct thrombin inhibition	Lepirudin Argatroban Bivalirudin

- LMWHs do not require monitoring of their anticoagulant effect (except possibly in patients with very low body weight and with a glomerular filtration rate below 30 mL/min).
- LMWHs have a half-life of around 4 hours when given subcutaneously, compared with 1 hour for UFH. This permits once-daily dosing by the subcutaneous route, rather than the therapeutic continuous intravenous infusion or prophylactic twice-daily subcutaneous administration required for UFH.
- While rates of bleeding are similar between products, the risk of osteoporosis and heparin-induced thrombocytopenia is much lower for LMWH.
- However, UFH is more completely reversed by protamine sulphate in the event of bleeding and at the end of cardiopulmonary bypass, for which UFH remains the drug of choice.

LMWHs are widely used for the prevention and treatment of VTE, the management of acute coronary syndromes and for most other scenarios listed in Box 24.28. In some situations, UFH is still favoured by some clinicians, though there is little evidence that it is advantageous, except when rapid reversibility is required. UFH is useful in patients with a high risk of bleeding: for example, those who have peptic ulceration or may require surgery. It is also favoured in the treatment of life-threatening thromboembolism: for example, major PE with significant hypoxaemia, hypotension and right-sided heart strain. In this situation, UFH is started with a loading intravenous dose of 80 U/kg., followed by a continuous infusion of 18 U/kg/hr initially. The level of anticoagulation should be assessed by the APTT after 6 hours and, if satisfactory, twice daily thereafter. It is usual to aim for a patient APTT which is 1.5–2.5 times the control time of the test.

Heparin-induced thrombocytopenia

Heparin-induced thrombocytopenia (HIT) is a rare complication of heparin therapy, caused by induction of anti-heparin/PF4 antibodies which bind to and activate platelets via an Fc receptor. This results in platelet activation and a prothrombotic state, with a paradoxical thrombocytopenia. HIT is more common in surgical than medical patients (especially cardiac and orthopaedic patients), with use of UFH rather than LMWH, and with higher doses of heparin.

Clinical features

Patients present, typically 5–14 days after starting heparin treatment, with a fall in platelet count of more than 30% from baseline. The count may still be in the reference range. They may be asymptomatic, or develop venous or arterial thrombosis and skin lesions, including overt skin necrosis. Affected patients may complain of pain or itch at injection sites and of systemic symptoms, such as shivering, following heparin injections. Patients who have received heparin in the preceding 100 days and who have preformed antibodies may develop acute systemic symptoms and an abrupt fall in platelet count in the first 24 hours after re-exposure.

Investigations

The pre-test probability of the diagnosis is assessed using the 4Ts scoring system. This assigns a score based on:

- the thrombocytopenia
- the timing of the fall in platelet count
- the presence of new thrombosis
- the likelihood of another cause for the thrombocytopenia.

Individuals at low risk need no further test; those with intermediate and high likelihood scores should have the diagnosis confirmed or refuted using an anti-PF4 enzyme-linked immunosorbent assay (ELISA).

Management

Heparin should be discontinued as soon as HIT is diagnosed and an alternative anticoagulant which does not cross-react with the antibody substituted. Argatroban (a direct thrombin inhibitor) and danaparoid (a heparin analogue) are licensed for use in the UK. In asymptomatic patients with HIT who do not receive an alternative anticoagulant, around 50% will sustain a thrombosis in the subsequent 30 days. Patients with established thrombosis have a poor prognosis.

Coumarins

Although several coumarin anticoagulants are used around the world, warfarin is the most common.

Coumarins inhibit the vitamin K-dependent post-translational carboxylation of factors II, VII, IX and X in the liver. This results in anticoagulation due to an effective deficiency of these factors. This is monitored by the INR, a standardised test based on measurement of the prothrombin time (p. 1000). Recommended target INR values for specific indications are given in Box 24.28.

Warfarin anticoagulation typically takes 3–5 days to become established, even using initial loading doses. Patients who require rapid initiation of therapy may receive higher initiation doses of warfarin. A typical regime in this situation is to give 10 mg warfarin on the first and second days, with 5 mg on the third day; subsequent doses are titrated against the INR. Patients without an urgent need for anticoagulation (e.g. atrial fibrillation) can have warfarin introduced slowly using lower doses. Low-dose regimens are associated with a lower risk of the patient developing a supratherapeutic INR, and hence a lower bleeding risk. The duration of warfarin therapy depends on the clinical indication, and while treatment of DVT or preparation for cardioversion requires a limited duration, anticoagulation to prevent cardioembolic stroke in atrial fibrillation or from heart valve disease is long-term.

The major problems with warfarin are:

- a narrow therapeutic window
- metabolism that is affected by many factors
- numerous drug interactions.

Drug interactions are common through protein binding and metabolism by the cytochrome P450 system. Inter-individual differences in warfarin doses required to achieve a therapeutic INR are mostly accounted for by naturally occurring polymorphisms in the *CYP2C9* and the *VKORC1* genes and dietary intake of vitamin K.

Major bleeding is the most common serious side-effect of warfarin and occurs in 1–2% of patients each year. Fatal haemorrhage, most commonly intracranial, occurs in about 0.25% per annum. There are scoring systems which predict the annual bleeding risk and these can be used to help compare the risks and benefits of warfarin for an individual patient (Box 24.30). There are also some specific contraindications to anticoagulation (see Box 24.30). Management of warfarin includes strategies for over-anticoagulation and for bleeding:

- If the INR is above the therapeutic level, warfarin should be withheld or the dose reduced. If the patient is not bleeding, it may be appropriate to give a small dose of vitamin K either orally or IV (1–2.5 mg), especially if the INR is greater than 8.
- In the event of bleeding, withhold further warfarin. Minor bleeding can be treated with 1–2.5 mg of vitamin K IV. Major haemorrhage should be treated as an emergency with vitamin K 5–10 mg slowly IV, combined with coagulation factor replacement. This should optimally be a prothrombin complex concentrate (30–50 U/kg) which contains factors II, VII, IX and X; if that is not available, fresh frozen plasma (15–30 mL/kg) should be given.

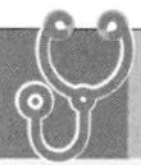

24.30 How to assess risks of anticoagulation

Contraindications

- Recent surgery, especially to eye or CNS
- Pre-existing haemorrhage state, e.g. liver disease, haemophilia, thrombocytopenia
- Pre-existing structural lesions, e.g. peptic ulcer
- Recent cerebral or gastrointestinal haemorrhage
- Uncontrolled hypertension
- Cognitive impairment
- Frequent falls

Bleeding risk score*

- Age > 65 yrs (1 point)
- Previous gastrointestinal bleed (1 point)
- Previous stroke (1 point)
- Medical illness (1 point)
  Recent myocardial infarction
  Renal failure
  Anaemia
  Diabetes mellitus

Score: annual rate of major haemorrhage

0 = 3%
1–2 = 12%
3–4 = 30–48%

*Other bleeding risk scores have been applied to different clinical circumstances, e.g. HAS-BLED score in atrial fibrillation.

Prophylaxis of venous thrombosis

All patients admitted to hospital should be assessed for their risk of developing VTE and appropriate prophylactic measures put in place. Both medical and surgical patients are at increased risk. A summary of the risk categories is given in Box 24.31. Early mobilisation of patients is important to prevent DVT. Patients at medium

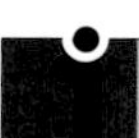

24.31 Antithrombotic prophylaxis

Indications

Patients in the following categories should be considered for specific antithrombotic prophylaxis:

Moderate risk of DVT

Major surgery

- In patients > 40 yrs or with other risk factor for VTE

Major medical illness, e.g.

- Heart failure
- MI with complications
- Sepsis
- Inflammatory conditions, including inflammatory bowel disease
- Active malignancy
- Nephrotic syndrome
- Stroke and other conditions leading to lower limb paralysis

High risk of DVT

- Major abdominal or pelvic surgery for malignancy or with history of DVT or known thrombophilia (see Box 24.4, p. 1001)
- Major hip or knee surgery
- Neurosurgery

Methods of VTE prophylaxis

Mechanical

- Intermittent pneumatic compression
- Mechanical foot pumps
- Graduated compression stockings

Pharmacological

- LMWHs
- Unfractionated heparin
- Fondaparinux
- Dabigatran
- Rivaroxaban
- Apixaban
- Warfarin

(DVT = deep vein thrombosis; MI = myocardial infarction; VTE = venous thromboembolism)

or high risk require additional antithrombotic measures; these may be pharmacological or mechanical. There is increasing evidence in high-risk groups, such as patients who have had major lower limb orthopaedic surgery and abdominal or pelvic cancer surgery, for protracted thromboprophylaxis for as long as 30 days after the procedure. Particular care should be taken with the use of pharmacological prophylaxis in patients with a high risk of bleeding or with specific risks of haemorrhage related to the site of surgery or the use of spinal or epidural anaesthesia.

ANAEMIAS

Around 30% of the total world population is anaemic and half of these, some 600 million people, have iron deficiency. The classification of anaemia by the size of the red cells (MCV) indicates the likely cause (see Figs 24.10 and 24.11, pp. 1002 and 1003).

Red cells in the bone marrow must acquire a minimum level of haemoglobin before being released into the blood stream (Fig. 24.19). Whilst in the marrow compartment, red cell precursors undergo cell division, driven by erythropoietin. If red cells cannot acquire haemoglobin at a normal rate, they will undergo more divisions than normal and will have a low MCV when finally released into the blood. The MCV is low because component parts of the haemoglobin molecule are not fully available: that is, iron in iron deficiency, globin chains in thalassaemia, haem ring in congenital sideroblastic anaemia and, occasionally, poor iron utilisation in the anaemia of chronic disease.

In megaloblastic anaemia, the biochemical consequence of vitamin B_{12} or folate deficiency is an inability to synthesise new bases to make DNA. A similar defect of cell division is seen in the presence of cytotoxic drugs or haematological disease in the marrow, such as myelodysplasia. In these states, cells haemoglobinise normally but undergo fewer cell divisions, resulting in circulating red cells with a raised MCV. The red cell membrane is composed of a lipid bilayer which will freely exchange with the plasma pool of lipid. Conditions such as liver disease, hypothyroidism, hyperlipidaemia and pregnancy are associated with raised lipids and may also cause a raised MCV. Reticulocytes are larger than mature red cells, so when the reticulocyte count is raised – for example, in haemolysis – this may also increase the MCV.

Iron deficiency anaemia

This occurs when iron losses or physiological requirements exceed absorption.

Blood loss

The most common explanation in men and post-menopausal women is gastrointestinal blood loss (p. 853). This may result from occult gastric or colorectal malignancy, gastritis, peptic ulceration, inflammatory bowel disease, diverticulitis, polyps and angiodysplastic lesions. Worldwide, hookworm and schistosomiasis are the most common causes of gut blood loss (pp. 369 and 376). Gastrointestinal blood loss may be exacerbated by the chronic use of aspirin or non-steroidal anti-inflammatory drugs (NSAIDs), which cause intestinal

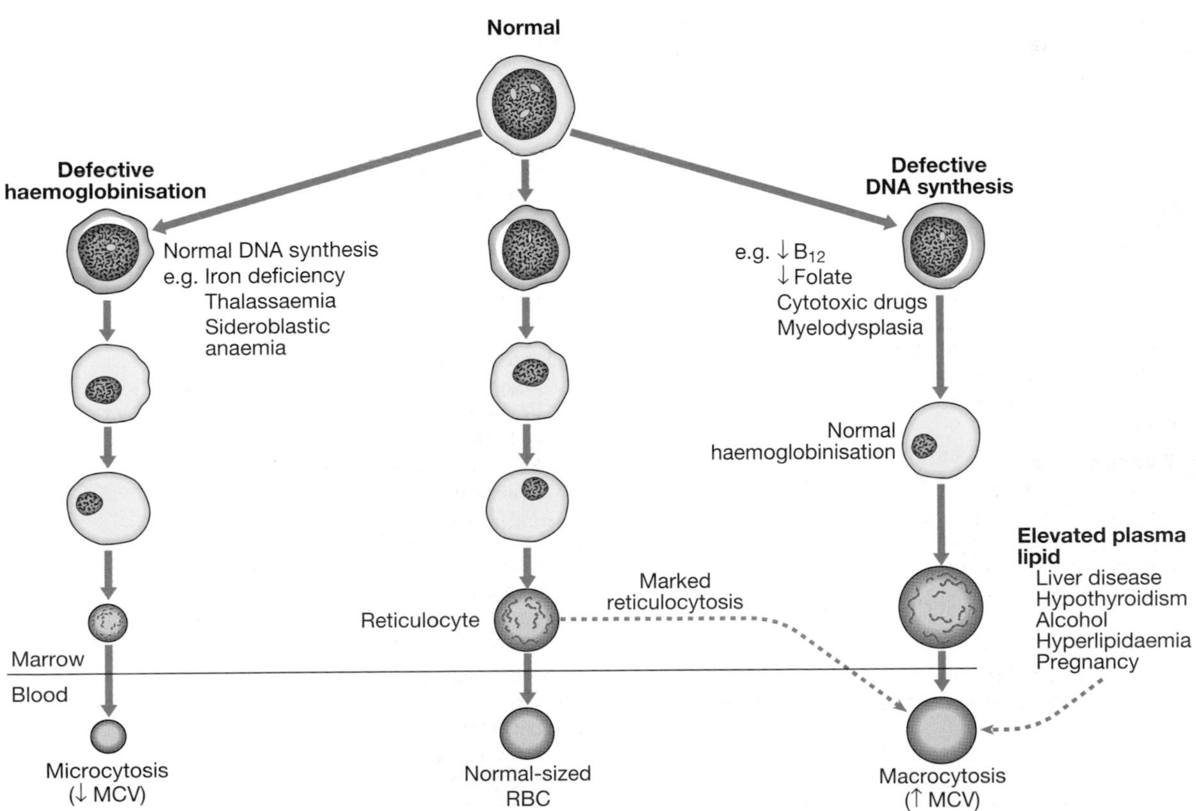

Fig. 24.19 Factors which influence the size of red cells in anaemia. In microcytosis, the MCV is < 76 fL. In macrocytosis, the MCV is > 100 fL. (MCV = mean cell volume; RBC = red blood cell)

24

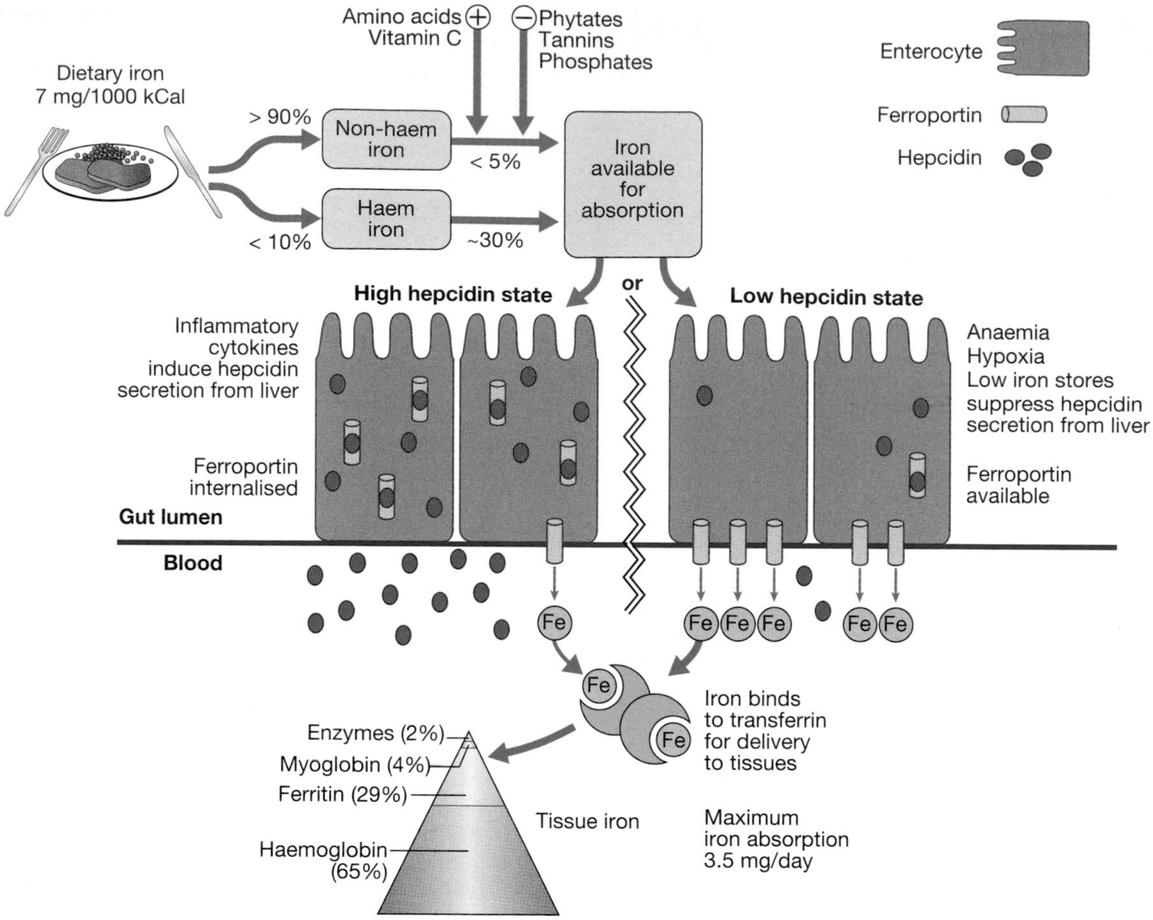

Amino acids ⊕
Vitamin C
⊖ Phytates
Tannins
Phosphates
Enterocyte
Ferroportin
Hepcidin
Dietary iron
7 mg/1000 kCal
> 90%
Non-haem iron
< 5%
< 10%
Haem iron
~30%
Iron available for absorption
High hepcidin state
or
Low hepcidin state
Inflammatory cytokines induce hepcidin secretion from liver
Ferroportin internalised
Gut lumen
Blood
Anaemia
Hypoxia
Low iron stores suppress hepcidin secretion from liver
Ferroportin available
Fe
Iron binds to transferrin for delivery to tissues
Enzymes (2%)
Myoglobin (4%)
Ferritin (29%)
Haemoglobin (65%)
Tissue iron
Maximum iron absorption 3.5 mg/day

Fig. 24.20 The regulation of iron absorption, uptake and distribution in the body. The transport of iron is regulated in a similar fashion to enterocytes in other iron-transporting cells such as macrophages.

erosions and impair platelet function. In women of child-bearing age, menstrual blood loss, pregnancy and breastfeeding contribute to iron deficiency by depleting iron stores; in developed countries, one-third of pre-menopausal women have low iron stores but only 3% display iron-deficient haematopoiesis. Very rarely, chronic haemoptysis or haematuria may cause iron deficiency.

Malabsorption

A dietary assessment should be made in all patients to ascertain their iron intake (p. 130). Gastric acid is required to release iron from food and helps to keep iron in the soluble ferrous state (Fig. 24.20). Achlorhydria in the elderly or that due to drugs such as proton pump inhibitors may contribute to the lack of iron availability from the diet, as may previous gastric surgery. Iron is absorbed actively in the upper small intestine and hence can be affected by coeliac disease (p. 880).

Physiological demands

At times of rapid growth, such as infancy and puberty, iron requirements increase and may outstrip absorption. In pregnancy, iron is diverted to the fetus, the placenta and the increased maternal red cell mass, and is lost with bleeding at parturition (Box 24.32).

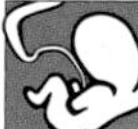

24.32 Haematological physiology in pregnancy

- **Full blood count**: increased plasma volume (40%) lowers normal Hb (reference range reduced to > 105 g/L at 28 wks). The MCV may increase by 5 fL. A progressive neutrophilia occurs. Gestational thrombocytopenia (rarely $< 60 \times 10^9$/L) is a benign phenomenon.
- **Depletion of iron stores**: iron deficiency is a common cause of anaemia in pregnancy and, if present, should be treated with oral iron supplement.
- **Vitamin B_{12}**: serum levels are physiologically low in pregnancy but deficiency is uncommon.
- **Folate**: tissue stores may become depleted, and folate supplementation is recommended in all pregnancies (see Box 5.32, p. 125).
- **Coagulation factors**: from the second trimester, procoagulant factors increase approximately threefold, particularly fibrinogen, von Willebrand factor and factor VIII. This causes activated protein C resistance and a shortened activated partial thromboplastin time (APTT), and contributes to a prothrombotic state.
- **Anticoagulants**: levels of protein C increase from the second trimester, while levels of free protein S fall as C4b binding protein increases.

24.33 Investigations to differentiate anaemia of chronic disease from iron deficiency anaemia

	Ferritin	Iron	TIBC	Transferrin saturation	Soluble transferrin receptor
Iron deficiency anaemia	↓	↓	↑	↓	↑
Anaemia of chronic disease	↑/Normal	↓	↓	↓	↓/Normal

(TIBC = total iron binding capacity)

Investigations

Confirmation of iron deficiency

Plasma ferritin is a measure of iron stores in tissues and is the best single test to confirm iron deficiency (Box 24.33). It is a very specific test; a subnormal level is due to iron deficiency or, very rarely, hypothyroidism or vitamin C deficiency. Ferritin levels can be raised in liver disease and in the acute phase response; in these conditions, a ferritin level of up to 100 μg/L may still be compatible with low bone marrow iron stores.

Plasma iron and total iron binding capacity (TIBC) are measures of iron availability; hence they are affected by many factors besides iron stores. Plasma iron has a marked diurnal and day-to-day variation and becomes very low during an acute phase response but is raised in liver disease and haemolysis. Levels of transferrin, the binding protein for iron, are lowered by malnutrition, liver disease, the acute phase response and nephrotic syndrome, but raised by pregnancy and the oral contraceptive pill. A transferrin saturation (i.e. iron/TIBC × 100) of less than 16% is consistent with iron deficiency but is less specific than a ferritin measurement.

All proliferating cells express membrane transferrin receptors to acquire iron; a small amount of this receptor is shed into blood, where it can be detected in a free soluble form. At times of poor iron stores, cells up-regulate transferrin receptor expression and the levels of soluble plasma transferrin receptor increase. This can now be measured by immunoassay and used to distinguish storage iron depletion in the presence of an acute phase response or liver disease, when a raised level indicates iron deficiency. In difficult cases, it may still be necessary to examine a bone marrow aspirate for iron stores.

Investigation of the cause

This will depend upon the age and sex of the patient, as well as the history and clinical findings. In men and in post-menopausal women with a normal diet, the upper and lower gastrointestinal tract should be investigated by endoscopy or radiological studies. Serum anti-endomysial or anti-transglutaminase antibodies and possibly a duodenal biopsy are indicated (p. 881) to detect coeliac disease. In the tropics, stool and urine should be examined for parasites (p. 311).

Management

Unless the patient has angina, heart failure or evidence of cerebral hypoxia, transfusion is not necessary and oral iron replacement is appropriate. Ferrous sulphate 200 mg 3 times daily (195 mg of elemental iron per day) is adequate and should be continued for 3–6 months to replete iron stores. Many patients suffer gastrointestinal side-effects with ferrous sulphate, including dyspepsia and altered bowel habit. When this occurs, reduction in dose to 200 mg twice daily or a switch to ferrous gluconate 300 mg twice daily (70 mg of elemental iron per day) should be tried. Delayed-release preparations are not useful, since they release iron beyond the upper small intestine, where it cannot be absorbed.

The haemoglobin should rise by around 10 g/L every 7–10 days and a reticulocyte response will be evident within a week. A failure to respond adequately may be due to non-compliance, continued blood loss, malabsorption or an incorrect diagnosis. Patients with malabsorption or chronic gut disease may need parenteral iron therapy. Previously, iron dextran or iron sucrose was used, but new preparations of iron isomaltose and iron carboxymaltose have fewer allergic effects and are preferred. Doses required can be calculated based on the patient's starting haemoglobin and body weight. Observation for anaphylaxis following an initial test dose is recommended.

Anaemia of chronic disease

Anaemia of chronic disease (ACD) is a common type of anaemia, particularly in hospital populations. It occurs in the setting of chronic infection, chronic inflammation or neoplasia. The anaemia is not related to bleeding, haemolysis or marrow infiltration, is mild, with haemoglobin in the range of 85–115 g/L, and is usually associated with a normal MCV (normocytic, normochromic), though this may be reduced in long-standing inflammation. The serum iron is low but iron stores are normal or increased, as indicated by the ferritin or stainable marrow iron.

Pathogenesis

It has recently become clear that the key regulatory protein that accounts for the findings characteristic of ACD is hepcidin, which is produced by the liver (see Fig. 24.20). Hepcidin production is induced by pro-inflammatory cytokines, especially IL-6. Hepcidin binds to ferroportin on the membrane of iron-exporting cells, such as small intestinal enterocytes and macrophages, internalising the ferroportin and thereby inhibiting the export of iron from these cells into the blood. The iron remains trapped inside the cells in the form of ferritin, levels of which are therefore normal or high in the face of significant anaemia. Inhibition or blockade of hepcidin is a potential target for treatment of this form of anaemia.

Diagnosis and management

It is often difficult to distinguish ACD associated with a low MCV from iron deficiency. Box 24.33 summarises the investigations and results. Examination of the marrow may ultimately be required to assess iron stores directly. A trial of oral iron can be given in difficult situations. A positive response occurs in true iron deficiency but not in ACD. Measures which reduce the severity of the underlying disorder generally help to improve the ACD.

Megaloblastic anaemia

This results from a deficiency of vitamin B_{12} or folic acid, or from disturbances in folic acid metabolism. Folate is an important substrate of, and vitamin B_{12} a co-factor for, the generation of the essential amino acid methionine from homocysteine. This reaction produces tetrahydrofolate, which is converted to thymidine monophosphate for incorporation into DNA. Deficiency of either vitamin B_{12} or folate will therefore produce high plasma levels of homocysteine and impaired DNA synthesis.

The end result is cells with arrested nuclear maturation but normal cytoplasmic development: so-called nucleocytoplasmic asynchrony. All proliferating cells will exhibit megaloblastosis; hence changes are evident in the buccal mucosa, tongue, small intestine, cervix, vagina and uterus. The high proliferation rate of bone marrow results in striking changes in the haematopoietic system in megaloblastic anaemia. Cells become arrested in development and die within the marrow; this ineffective erythropoiesis results in an expanded hypercellular marrow. The megaloblastic changes are most evident in the early nucleated red cell precursors, and haemolysis within the marrow results in a raised bilirubin and lactate dehydrogenase (LDH), but without the reticulocytosis characteristic of other forms of haemolysis (p. 1026). Iron stores are usually raised. The mature red cells are large and oval, and sometimes contain nuclear remnants. Nuclear changes are seen in the immature granulocyte precursors and a characteristic appearance is that of 'giant' metamyelocytes with a large 'sausage-shaped' nucleus. The mature neutrophils show hypersegmentation of their nuclei, with cells having six or more nuclear lobes. If severe, a pancytopenia may be present in the peripheral blood.

Vitamin B_{12} deficiency, but not folate deficiency, is associated with neurological disease in up to 40% of cases, although advanced neurological disease due to B_{12} deficiency is now uncommon in the developed world. The main pathological finding is focal demyelination affecting the spinal cord, peripheral nerves, optic nerves and cerebrum. The most common manifestations are sensory, with peripheral paraesthesiae and ataxia of gait. The clinical and diagnostic features of megaloblastic anaemia are summarised in Boxes 24.34 and 24.35, and the neurological features of B_{12} deficiency in Box 24.36.

24.34 Clinical features of megaloblastic anaemia

Symptoms

- Malaise (90%)
- Breathlessness (50%)
- Paraesthesiae (80%)
- Sore mouth (20%)
- Weight loss
- Altered skin pigmentation
- Impotence
- Poor memory
- Depression
- Personality change
- Hallucinations
- Visual disturbance

Signs

- Smooth tongue
- Angular cheilosis
- Vitiligo
- Skin pigmentation
- Heart failure
- Pyrexia

24.35 Investigations in megaloblastic anaemia

Investigation	Result
Haemoglobin	Often reduced, may be very low
MCV	Usually raised, commonly > 120 fL
Erythrocyte count	Low for degree of anaemia
Blood film	Oval macrocytosis, poikilocytosis, red cell fragmentation, neutrophil hypersegmentation
Reticulocyte count	Low for degree of anaemia
Leucocyte count	Low or normal
Platelet count	Low or normal
Bone marrow	Increased cellularity, megaloblastic changes in erythroid series, giant metamyelocytes, dysplastic megakaryocytes, increased iron in stores, pathological non-ring sideroblasts
Serum ferritin	Elevated
Plasma lactate dehydrogenase (LDH)	Elevated, often markedly

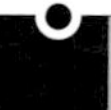

24.36 Neurological findings in B_{12} deficiency

Peripheral nerves

- Glove and stocking paraesthesiae
- Loss of ankle reflexes

Spinal cord

- Subacute combined degeneration of the cord
  - Posterior columns – diminished vibration sensation and proprioception
  - Corticospinal tracts – upper motor neuron signs

Cerebrum

- Dementia
- Optic atrophy

Autonomic neuropathy

Vitamin B_{12}

Vitamin B_{12} absorption

The average daily diet contains 5–30 μg of vitamin B_{12}, mainly in meat, fish, eggs and milk – well in excess of the 1 μg daily requirement. In the stomach, gastric enzymes release vitamin B_{12} from food and at gastric pH it binds to a carrier protein termed R protein. The gastric parietal cells produce intrinsic factor, a vitamin B_{12}-binding protein which optimally binds vitamin B_{12} at pH 8. As gastric emptying occurs, pancreatic secretion raises the pH and vitamin B_{12} released from the diet switches from the R protein to intrinsic factor. Bile also contains vitamin B_{12} which is available for reabsorption in the intestine. The vitamin B_{12}–intrinsic factor complex binds to specific receptors in the terminal ileum, and vitamin B_{12} is actively transported by the enterocytes to plasma, where it binds to transcobalamin II, a transport protein produced by the liver, which carries it to the tissues for utilisation. The liver stores enough vitamin B_{12} for 3 years and this, together with the enterohepatic circulation, means that vitamin B_{12} deficiency takes years to become manifest, even if all dietary intake is stopped or severe B_{12} malabsorption supervenes.

Blood levels of vitamin B_{12} provide a reasonable indication of tissue stores and are usually diagnostic of deficiency. Levels of cobalamins fall in normal pregnancy. Reference ranges vary between laboratories but levels below 150 ng/L are common and, in the last trimester, 5–10% of women have levels below 100 ng/L. Spuriously low B_{12} values occur in women using the oral contraceptive pill and in patients with myeloma, in whom paraproteins can interfere with vitamin B_{12} assays.

Causes of vitamin B_{12} deficiency

Dietary deficiency

This only occurs in strict vegans but the onset of clinical features can occur at any age between 10 and 80 years. Less strict vegetarians often have slightly low vitamin B_{12} levels but are not tissue vitamin B_{12}-deficient.

Gastric pathology

Release of vitamin B_{12} from the food requires normal gastric acid and enzyme secretion, and this is impaired by hypochlorhydria in elderly patients or following gastric surgery. Total gastrectomy invariably results in vitamin B_{12} deficiency within 5 years, often combined with iron deficiency; these patients need life-long 3-monthly vitamin B_{12} injections. After partial gastrectomy, vitamin B_{12} deficiency only develops in 10–20% of patients by 5 years; an annual injection of vitamin B_{12} should prevent deficiency in this group.

Pernicious anaemia

This is an organ-specific autoimmune disorder in which the gastric mucosa is atrophic, with loss of parietal cells causing intrinsic factor deficiency. In the absence of intrinsic factor, less than 1% of dietary vitamin B_{12} is absorbed. Pernicious anaemia has an incidence of 25/100 000 population over the age of 40 years in developed countries, but an average age of onset of 60 years. It is more common in individuals with other autoimmune disease (Hashimoto's thyroiditis, Graves' disease, vitiligo, hypoparathyroidism or Addison's disease; Ch. 20) or a family history of these or pernicious anaemia. The finding of anti-intrinsic factor antibodies in the context of B_{12} deficiency is diagnostic of pernicious anaemia without further investigation. Antiparietal cell antibodies are present in over 90% of cases but are also present in 20% of normal females over the age of 60 years; a negative result makes pernicious anaemia less likely but a positive result is not diagnostic. The Schilling test, involving measurement of absorption of radio-labelled B_{12} after oral administration before and after replacement of intrinsic factor, has fallen out of favour with the availability of autoantibody tests, greater caution in the use of radioactive tracers, and limited availability of intrinsic factor.

Small bowel pathology

One-third of patients with pancreatic exocrine insufficiency fail to transfer dietary vitamin B_{12} from R protein to intrinsic factor. This usually results in slightly low vitamin B_{12} values but no tissue evidence of vitamin B_{12} deficiency.

Motility disorders or hypogammaglobulinaemia can result in bacterial overgrowth, and the ensuing competition for free vitamin B_{12} can lead to deficiency. This is corrected to some extent by appropriate antibiotics.

A small number of people heavily infected with the fish tapeworm (p. 378) develop vitamin B_{12} deficiency.

Inflammatory disease of the terminal ileum, such as Crohn's disease, may impair the absorption of vitamin B_{12}–intrinsic factor complex, as may surgery on that part of the bowel.

Folate

Folate absorption

Folates are produced by plants and bacteria; hence dietary leafy vegetables (spinach, broccoli, lettuce), fruits (bananas, melons) and animal protein (liver, kidney) are a rich source. An average Western diet contains more than the minimum daily intake of 50 µg but excess cooking destroys folates. Most dietary folate is present as polyglutamates; these are converted to monoglutamate in the upper small bowel and actively transported into plasma. Plasma folate is loosely bound to plasma proteins such as albumin and there is an enterohepatic circulation. Total body stores of folate are small and deficiency can occur in a matter of weeks.

Folate deficiency

The causes and diagnostic features of folate deficiency are shown in Boxes 24.37 and 24.38. The edentulous elderly or psychiatric patient is particularly susceptible to dietary deficiency and this is exacerbated in the presence of gut disease or malignancy. Pregnancy-induced folate deficiency is the most common cause of megaloblastosis worldwide and is more likely in the context of twin pregnancies, multiparity and hyperemesis

24.37 Causes of folate deficiency

Diet
• Poor intake of vegetables
Malabsorption
• e.g. Coeliac disease
Increased demand
• Cell proliferation, e.g. haemolysis • Pregnancy
Drugs*
• Certain anticonvulsants (e.g. phenytoin) • Contraceptive pill • Certain cytotoxic drugs (e.g. methotrexate)

*Usually only a problem in patients deficient in folate from another cause.

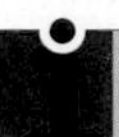

24.38 Investigation of folic acid deficiency

Diagnostic findings
• Serum folate levels may be low but are difficult to interpret • Low red cell folate levels indicate prolonged folate deficiency and are probably the most relevant measure
Corroborative findings
• Macrocytic dysplastic blood picture • Megaloblastic marrow

gravidarum. Serum folate is very sensitive to dietary intake; a single folate-rich meal can normalise it in a patient with true folate deficiency, whereas anorexia, alcohol and anticonvulsant therapy can reduce it in the absence of megaloblastosis. For this reason, red cell folate levels are a more accurate indicator of folate stores and tissue folate deficiency.

Management of megaloblastic anaemia

If a patient with a severe megaloblastic anaemia is very ill and treatment must be started before vitamin B_{12} and red cell folate results are available, that treatment should always include both folic acid and vitamin B_{12}. The use of folic acid alone in the presence of vitamin B_{12} deficiency may result in worsening of neurological deficits.

Rarely, if severe angina or heart failure is present, transfusion can be used in megaloblastic anaemia. The cardiovascular system is adapted to the chronic anaemia present in megaloblastosis, and the volume load imposed by transfusion may result in decompensation and severe cardiac failure. In such circumstances, exchange transfusion or slow administration of 1 U of red cells with diuretic cover may be given cautiously.

Vitamin B_{12} deficiency

Vitamin B_{12} deficiency is treated with hydroxycobalamin 1000 μg IM for 6 doses 2 or 3 days apart, followed by maintenance therapy of 1000 μg every 3 months for life. The reticulocyte count will peak by the 5th–10th day after starting replacement therapy. The haemoglobin will rise by 10 g/L every week until normalised. The response of the marrow is associated with a fall in plasma potassium levels and rapid depletion of iron stores. If an initial response is not maintained and the blood film is dimorphic (i.e. shows a mixture of microcytic and macrocytic cells), the patient may need additional iron therapy. A sensory neuropathy may take 6–12 months to correct; long-standing neurological damage may not improve.

Folate deficiency

Oral folic acid 5 mg daily for 3 weeks will treat acute deficiency and 5 mg once weekly is adequate maintenance therapy. Prophylactic folic acid in pregnancy prevents megaloblastosis in women at risk, and reduces the risk of fetal neural tube defects (p. 125). Prophylactic supplementation is also given in chronic haematological disease associated with reduced red cell lifespan (e.g. haemolytic anaemias). There is some evidence that supraphysiological supplementation (400 μg/day) can reduce the risk of coronary and cerebrovascular disease by lowering plasma homocysteine levels. This has led the US Food and Drug Administration to introduce fortification of bread, flour and rice with folic acid.

Haemolytic anaemia

Haemolysis indicates that there is shortening of the normal red cell lifespan of 120 days. There are many causes, as shown in Figure 24.21. To compensate, the bone marrow may increase its output of red cells six- to eightfold by increasing the proportion of red cells produced, expanding the volume of active marrow, and releasing reticulocytes prematurely. Anaemia only occurs if the rate of destruction exceeds this increased production rate.

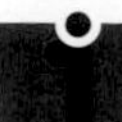

24.39 Investigation results indicating active haemolysis

Hallmarks of haemolysis	
• ↓Haemoglobin	• ↑Reticulocytes
• ↑Unconjugated bilirubin	• ↑Urinary urobilinogen
• ↑Lactate dehydrogenase	
Additional features of intravascular haemolysis	
• ↓Haptoglobin	• Positive urinary haemosiderin
• ↑Methaemalbumin	• Haemoglobinuria

Results of investigations which establish the presence of haemolysis are shown in Box 24.39. Red cell destruction overloads pathways for haemoglobin breakdown in the liver (p. 927), causing a modest rise in unconjugated bilirubin in the blood and mild jaundice. Increased reabsorption of urobilinogen from the gut results in an increase in urinary urobilinogen (pp. 936 and 994). Red cell destruction releases LDH into the serum. The bone marrow compensation results in a reticulocytosis, and sometimes nucleated red cell precursors appear in the blood. Increased proliferation of the bone marrow can result in a thrombocytosis, neutrophilia and, if marked, immature granulocytes in the blood, producing a leucoerythroblastic blood film. The appearances of the red cells may give an indication of the likely cause of the haemolysis:

- Spherocytes are small, dark red cells which suggest autoimmune haemolysis or hereditary spherocytosis.
- Sickle cells suggest sickle-cell disease.
- Red cell fragments indicate microangiopathic haemolysis.

The compensatory erythroid hyperplasia may give rise to folate deficiency, with megaloblastic blood features.

The differential diagnosis of haemolysis is determined by the clinical scenario in combination with the results of blood film examination and Coombs testing for antibodies directed against red cells (see below and Fig. 24.21).

Extravascular haemolysis

Physiological red cell destruction occurs in the reticulo-endothelial cells in the liver or spleen, so avoiding free haemoglobin in the plasma. In most haemolytic states, haemolysis is predominantly extravascular.

To confirm the haemolysis, patients' red cells can be labelled with ^{51}chromium. When re-injected, they can be used to determine red cell survival; when combined with body surface radioactivity counting, this test may indicate whether the liver or the spleen is the main source of red cell destruction. However, it is seldom performed in clinical practice.

Intravascular haemolysis

Less commonly, red cell lysis occurs within the blood stream due to membrane damage by complement (ABO transfusion reactions, paroxysmal nocturnal haemoglobinuria), infections (malaria, *Clostridium perfringens*),

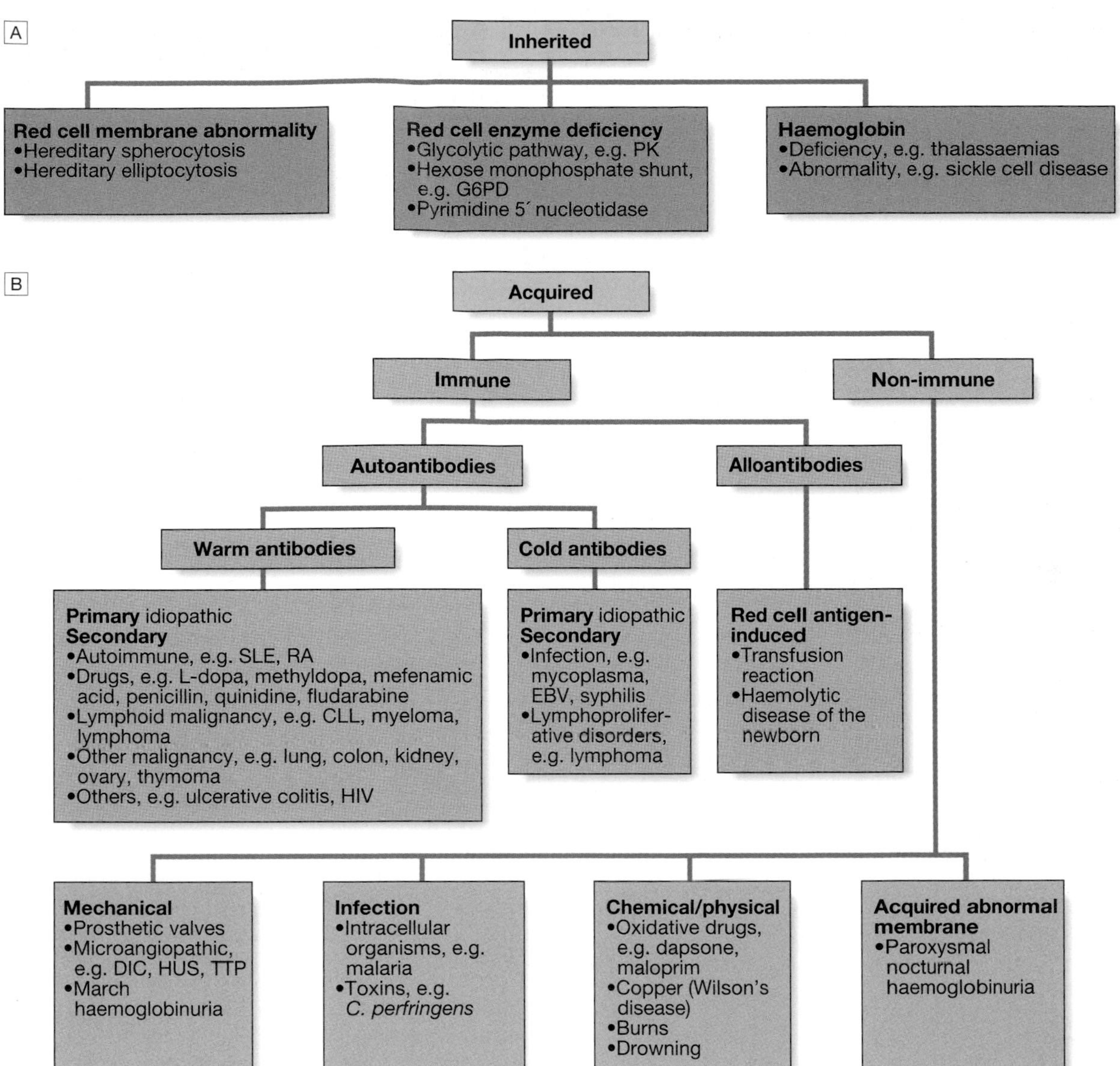

Fig. 24.21 Causes of haemolysis. A Inherited causes. B Acquired causes. (CLL = chronic lymphatic leukaemia; DIC = disseminated intravascular coagulation; EBV = Epstein–Barr virus; G6PD = glucose-6-phosphate dehydrogenase; HUS = haemolytic uraemic syndrome; PK = pyruvate kinase; RA = rheumatoid arthritis; SLE = systemic lupus erythematosus; TTP = thrombotic thrombocytopenic purpura)

mechanical trauma (heart valves, DIC) or oxidative damage (e.g. drugs such as dapsone and maloprim). When intravascular red cell destruction occurs, free haemoglobin is released into the plasma. Free haemoglobin is toxic to cells and binding proteins have evolved to minimise this risk. Haptoglobin is an α_2-globulin produced by the liver, which binds free haemoglobin, resulting in a fall in its levels during active haemolysis. Once haptoglobins are saturated, free haemoglobin is oxidised to form methaemoglobin, which binds to albumin, in turn forming methaemalbumin, which can be detected spectrophotometrically in the Schumm's test. Methaemoglobin is degraded and any free haem is bound to a second binding protein called haemopexin. If all the protective mechanisms are saturated, free haemoglobin may appear in the urine (haemoglobinuria). When fulminant, this gives rise to black urine, as in severe *falciparum* malaria infection (p. 353). In smaller amounts, renal tubular cells absorb the haemoglobin, degrade it and store the iron as haemosiderin. When the tubular cells are subsequently sloughed into the urine, they give rise to haemosiderinuria, which is always indicative of intravascular haemolysis.

Red cell membrane defects

The structure of the red cell membrane is shown in Figure 24.4 (p. 994). The basic structure is a cytoskeleton 'stapled' on to the lipid bilayer by special protein complexes. This structure ensures great deformability and elasticity; the red cell diameter is 8 μm but the narrowest capillaries in the circulation are in the spleen, measuring just 2 μm in diameter. When the normal red cell structure is disturbed, usually by a quantitative or functional deficiency of one or more proteins in the cytoskeleton, cells lose their elasticity. Each time such cells pass through the spleen, they lose membrane relative to their cell volume. This results in an increase in mean cell haemoglobin concentration (MCHC), abnormal cell shape (see Box 24.2, p. 999) and reduced red cell survival due to extravascular haemolysis.

Hereditary spherocytosis

This is usually inherited as an autosomal dominant condition, although 25% of cases have no family history and represent new mutations. The incidence is approximately 1:5000 in developed countries but this may be an underestimate, since the disease may present de novo in patients aged over 65 years and is often discovered as a chance finding on a blood count. The most common abnormalities are deficiencies of beta spectrin or ankyrin (see Fig. 24.4, p. 994). The severity of spontaneous haemolysis varies. Most cases are associated with an asymptomatic compensated chronic haemolytic state with spherocytes present on the blood film, a reticulocytosis and mild hyperbilirubinaemia. Pigment gallstones are present in up to 50% of patients and may cause symptomatic cholecystitis. Occasional cases are associated with more severe haemolysis; these may be due to coincidental polymorphisms in alpha spectrin or co-inheritance of a second defect involving a different protein.

The clinical course may be complicated by crises:

- *A haemolytic crisis* occurs when the severity of haemolysis increases; this is rare, and usually associated with infection.
- *A megaloblastic crisis* follows the development of folate deficiency; this may occur as a first presentation of the disease in pregnancy.
- *An aplastic crisis* occurs in association with parvovirus B19 infection (p. 315). Parvovirus causes a common exanthem in children, but if individuals with chronic haemolysis become infected, the virus directly invades red cell precursors and temporarily switches off red cell production. Patients present with severe anaemia and a low reticulocyte count.

Investigations

The patient and other family members should be screened for features of compensated haemolysis (see Box 24.39). This may be all that is required to confirm the diagnosis. Haemoglobin levels are variable, depending on the degree of compensation. The blood film will show spherocytes but the direct Coombs test (see Fig. 24.22) is negative, excluding immune haemolysis. An osmotic fragility test may show increased sensitivity to lysis in hypotonic saline solutions but is limited by lack of sensitivity and specificity. More specific flow cytometric tests, detecting binding of eosin-5-maleimide to red cells, are recommended in borderline cases.

Management

Folic acid prophylaxis, 5 mg daily, should be given for life. Consideration may be given to splenectomy, which improves but does not normalise red cell survival. Potential indications include moderate to severe haemolysis with complications (anaemia and gallstones), although splenectomy should be delayed until after 6 years of age in view of the risk of sepsis. Guidelines for the management of patients after splenectomy are presented in Box 24.40.

Acute, severe haemolytic crises require transfusion support, but blood must be cross-matched carefully and transfused slowly as haemolytic transfusion reactions may occur (p. 1016).

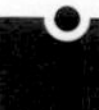

24.40 Management of the splenectomised patient

- Vaccinate with pneumococcal, *Haemophilus influenzae* type B, meningococcal group C and influenza vaccines at least 2–3 wks before elective splenectomy. Vaccination should be given after emergency surgery but may be less effective
- Pneumococcal re-immunisation should be given at least 5-yearly and influenza annually. Vaccination status must be documented
- Life-long prophylactic penicillin V 500 mg twice daily is recommended. In penicillin-allergic patients, consider a macrolide
- Patients should be educated regarding the risks of infection and methods of prophylaxis
- A card or bracelet should be carried to alert health professionals to the risk of overwhelming sepsis
- In septicaemia, patients should be resuscitated and given IV antibiotics to cover pneumococcus, *Haemophilus* and meningococcus, according to local resistance patterns
- The risk of cerebral malaria is increased in the event of infection
- Animal bites should be promptly treated with local disinfection and antibiotics, to prevent serious soft tissue infection and septicaemia

Hereditary elliptocytosis

This term refers to a heterogeneous group of disorders that produce an increase in elliptocytic red cells on the blood film and a variable degree of haemolysis. This is due to a functional abnormality of one or more anchor proteins in the red cell membrane, e.g. alpha spectrin or protein 4.1. Inheritance may be autosomal dominant or recessive. Hereditary elliptocytosis is less common than hereditary spherocytosis in Western countries, with an incidence of 1/10 000, but is more common in equatorial Africa and parts of South-east Asia. The clinical course is variable and depends upon the degree of membrane dysfunction caused by the inherited molecular defect(s); most cases present as an asymptomatic blood film abnormality, but occasional cases result in neonatal haemolysis or a chronic compensated haemolytic state. Management of the latter is the same as for hereditary spherocytosis.

A characteristic variant of hereditary elliptocytosis occurs in South-east Asia, particularly Malaysia and Papua New Guinea, with stomatocytes and ovalocytes in the blood. This has a prevalence of up to 30% in some communities because it offers relative protection from malaria and thus has sustained a high gene frequency. The blood film is often very abnormal and immediate differential diagnosis is broad.

Red cell enzymopathies

The mature red cell must produce energy via ATP to maintain a normal internal environment and cell volume whilst protecting itself from the oxidative stress presented by oxygen carriage. Anaerobic glycolysis via the Embden–Meyerhof pathway generates ATP, and the hexose monophosphate shunt produces nicotinamide adenine dinucleotide phosphate (NADPH) and glutathione to protect against oxidative stress. The impact of functional or quantitative defects in the enzymes in these pathways depends upon the importance of the steps affected and the presence of alternative pathways. In general, defects in the hexose monophosphate shunt pathway result in periodic haemolysis precipitated by episodic oxidative stress, whilst those in the Embden–Meyerhof pathway result in shortened red cell survival and chronic haemolysis.

Glucose-6-phosphate dehydrogenase deficiency

The enzyme glucose-6-phosphate dehydrogenase (G6PD) is pivotal in the hexose monophosphate shunt pathway. Deficiencies result in the most common human enzymopathy, affecting 10% of the world's population, with a geographical distribution which parallels the malaria belt because heterozygotes are protected from malarial parasitisation. The enzyme is a heteromeric structure made of catalytic subunits which are encoded by a gene on the X chromosome. The deficiency therefore affects males and rare homozygous females (p. 53), but it is carried by females. Carrier heterozygous females are usually only affected in the neonatal period or in the presence of extreme lyonisation, producing selective inactivation of the non-affected X chromosome.

Over 400 subtypes of G6PD are described. The most common types associated with normal activity are the B^+ enzyme present in most Caucasians and 70% of Afro-Caribbeans, and the A^+ variant present in 20% of Afro-Caribbeans. The two common variants associated with reduced activity are the A^- variety in approximately 10% of Afro-Caribbeans, and the Mediterranean or B^- variety in Caucasians. In East and West Africa, up to 20% of males and 4% of females (homozygotes) are affected and have enzyme levels of about 15% of normal. The deficiency in Caucasian and Oriental populations is more severe, with enzyme levels as low as 1%.

Clinical features and investigation findings are shown in Box 24.41.

Management aims to stop any precipitant drugs and treat any underlying infection. Acute transfusion support may be life-saving.

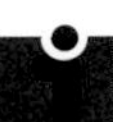

24.41 Glucose-6-phosphate dehydrogenase deficiency

Clinical features

- Acute drug-induced haemolysis to (e.g.):
  - Analgesics: aspirin, phenacetin
  - Antimalarials: primaquine, quinine, chloroquine, pyrimethamine
  - Antibiotics: sulphonamides, nitrofurantoin, ciprofloxacin
  - Miscellaneous: quinidine, probenecid, vitamin K, dapsone
- Chronic compensated haemolysis
- Infection or acute illness
- Neonatal jaundice: may be a feature of the B^- enzyme
- Favism, i.e. acute haemolysis after ingestion of broad beans (*Vicia faba*)

Laboratory features

Non-spherocytic intravascular haemolysis during an attack
The blood film will show:
- Bite cells (red cells with a 'bite' of membrane missing)
- Blister cells (red cells with surface blistering of the membrane)
- Irregularly shaped small cells
- Polychromasia reflecting the reticulocytosis
- Denatured haemoglobin visible as Heinz bodies within the red cell cytoplasm with a supravital stain such as methyl violet

G6PD level
- Can be indirectly assessed by screening methods which usually depend upon the decreased ability to reduce dyes
- Direct assessment of G6PD is made in those with low screening values
- Care must be taken close to an acute haemolytic episode because reticulocytes may have higher enzyme levels and give rise to a false normal result

Pyruvate kinase deficiency

This is the second most common red cell enzyme defect. It results in deficiency of ATP production and a chronic haemolytic anaemia. It is inherited as an autosomal recessive trait. The extent of anaemia is variable; the blood film shows characteristic 'prickle cells' which resemble holly leaves. Enzyme activity is only 5–20% of normal. Transfusion support may be necessary.

Pyrimidine 5′ nucleotidase deficiency

The pyrimidine 5′ nucleotidase enzyme catalyses the dephosphorylation of nucleoside monophosphates and is important during the degradation of RNA in reticulocytes. It is inherited as an autosomal recessive trait and is as common as pyruvate kinase deficiency in Mediterranean, African and Jewish populations. The accumulation of excess ribonucleoprotein results in coarse basophilic stippling (see Box 24.2, p. 999), associated with a chronic haemolytic state. The enzyme is very sensitive to inhibition by lead and this is the reason why basophilic stippling is a feature of lead poisoning.

Autoimmune haemolytic anaemia

This results from increased red cell destruction due to red cell autoantibodies. The antibodies may be IgG or M, or more rarely IgE or A. If an antibody avidly fixes complement, it will cause intravascular haemolysis, but if complement activation is weak, the haemolysis will be extravascular. Antibody-coated red cells lose membrane to macrophages in the spleen and hence spherocytes are present in the blood. The optimum temperature at which the antibody is active (thermal specificity) is used to classify immune haemolysis:

- *Warm antibodies* bind best at 37°C and account for 80% of cases. The majority are IgG and often react against Rhesus antigens.
- *Cold antibodies* bind best at 4°C but can bind up to 37°C in some cases. They are usually IgM and bind complement. To be clinically relevant, they must act within the range of normal body temperatures. They account for the other 20% of cases.

Warm autoimmune haemolysis

The incidence of warm autoimmune haemolysis is approximately 1/100 000 population per annum; it occurs at all ages but is more common in middle age and in females. No underlying cause is identified in up to 50% of cases. The remainder are secondary to a wide variety of other conditions (see Fig. 24.21B).

Investigations

There is evidence of haemolysis and spherocytes on the blood film. The diagnosis is confirmed by the direct

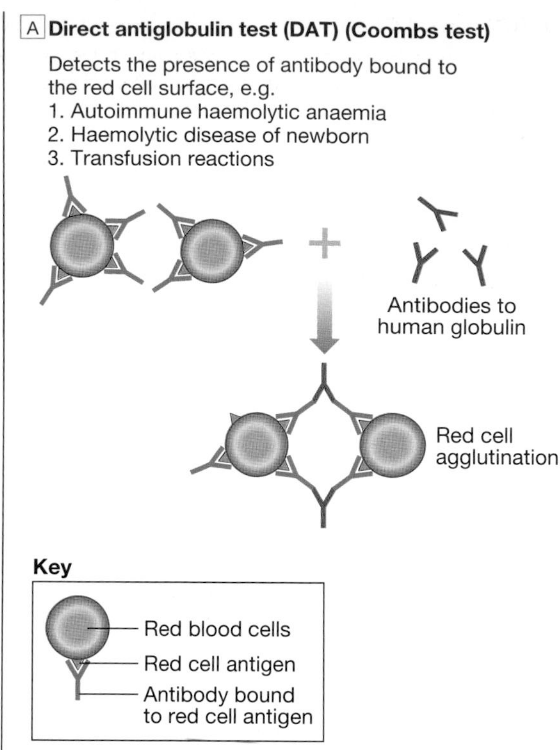

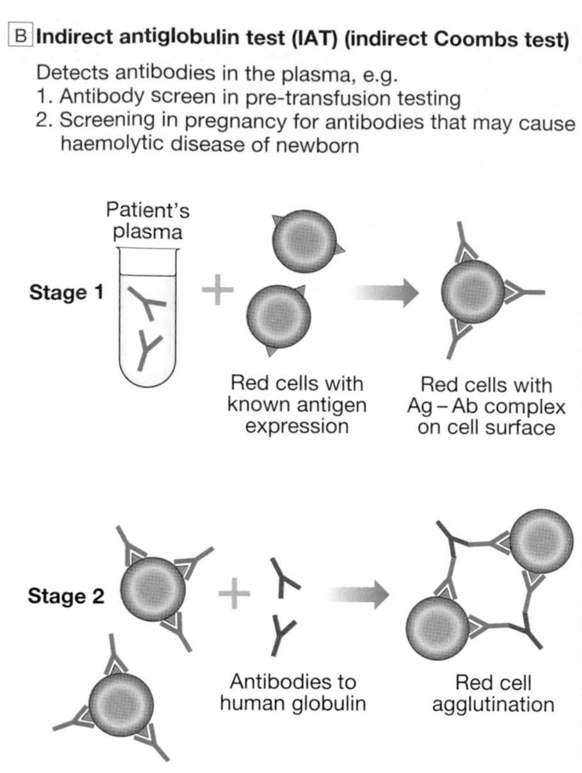

Fig. 24.22 Direct and indirect antiglobulin tests.

Coombs or antiglobulin test (Fig. 24.22). The patient's red cells are mixed with Coombs reagent, which contains antibodies against human IgG/M/complement. If the red cells have been coated by antibody in vivo, the Coombs reagent will induce their agglutination and this can be detected visually. The relevant antibody can be eluted from the red cell surface and tested against a panel of typed red cells to determine against which red cell antigen it is directed. The most common specificity is Rhesus and most often anti-e; this is helpful when choosing blood to cross-match. The direct Coombs test can be negative in the presence of brisk haemolysis. A positive test requires about 200 antibody molecules to attach to each red cell; with a very avid complement-fixing antibody, haemolysis may occur at lower levels of antibody-binding. The standard Coombs reagent will miss IgA or IgE antibodies. Around 10% of all warm autoimmune haemolytic anaemias are Coombs test-negative.

Management

If the haemolysis is secondary to an underlying cause, this must be treated and any implicated drugs stopped.

It is usual to treat patients initially with prednisolone 1 mg/kg orally. A response is seen in 70–80% of cases but may take up to 3 weeks; a rise in haemoglobin will be matched by a fall in bilirubin, LDH and reticulocyte levels. Once the haemoglobin has normalised and the reticulocytosis resolved, the corticosteroid dose can be reduced slowly over about 10 weeks. Corticosteroids work by decreasing macrophage destruction of antibody-coated red cells and reducing antibody production.

Transfusion support may be required for life-threatening problems, such as the development of heart failure or rapid unabated falls in haemoglobin. The least incompatible blood should be used but this may still give rise to transfusion reactions or the development of alloantibodies.

If the haemolysis fails to respond to corticosteroids or can only be stabilised by large doses, then splenectomy should be considered. This removes a main site of red cell destruction and antibody production, with a good response in 50–60% of cases. The operation can be performed laparoscopically with reduced morbidity. If splenectomy is not appropriate, alternative immunosuppressive therapy with azathioprine or cyclophosphamide may be considered. This is least suitable for young patients, in whom long-term immunosuppression carries a risk of secondary neoplasms. The anti-CD20 (B cell) monoclonal antibody, rituximab, has shown some success in difficult cases.

Cold agglutinin disease

This is due to antibodies, usually IgM, which bind to the red cells at low temperatures and cause them to agglutinate. It may cause intravascular haemolysis if complement fixation occurs. This can be chronic when the antibody is monoclonal, or acute or transient when the antibody is polyclonal.

Chronic cold agglutinin disease

This affects elderly patients and may be associated with an underlying low-grade B cell lymphoma. It causes a low-grade intravascular haemolysis with cold, painful and often blue fingers, toes, ears or nose (so-called acrocyanosis). The latter is due to red cell agglutination in the small vessels in these colder exposed areas. The blood film shows red cell agglutination and the MCV may be spuriously high because the automated analysers detect aggregates as single cells. Monoclonal IgM usually has anti-I or, less often, anti-i specificity. Treatment is directed at any underlying lymphoma but if the disease is idiopathic, then patients must keep extremities warm, especially in winter. Some patients respond to corticosteroid therapy and blood transfusion may be considered, but the cross-match sample must be placed in a transport flask at a temperature of 37°C and blood administered via a blood-warmer. All patients should receive folic acid supplementation.

Other causes of cold agglutination

Cold agglutination can occur in association with *Mycoplasma pneumoniae* or with infectious mononucleosis. Paroxysmal cold haemoglobinuria is a very rare cause seen in children, in association with viral or bacterial infection. An IgG antibody binds to red cells in the peripheral circulation but lysis occurs in the central circulation when complement fixation takes place. This antibody is termed the Donath–Landsteiner antibody and has specificity against the P antigen on the red cells.

Alloimmune haemolytic anaemia

Alloimmune haemolytic anaemia is caused by antibodies against non-self red cells, and occurs after unmatched transfusion (p. 1016), or after maternal sensitisation to paternal antigens on fetal cells (haemolytic disease of the newborn, p. 1014).

Non-immune haemolytic anaemia

Physical trauma

Physical disruption of red cells may occur in a number of conditions and is characterised by the presence of red cell fragments on the blood film and markers of intravascular haemolysis:

- *Mechanical heart valves.* High flow through incompetent valves or periprosthetic leaks through the suture ring holding a valve in place result in shear stress damage.
- *March haemoglobinuria.* Vigorous exercise, such as prolonged marching or marathon running, can cause red cell damage in the capillaries in the feet.
- *Thermal injury.* Severe burns cause thermal damage to red cells, characterised by fragmentation and the presence of microspherocytes in the blood.
- *Microangiopathic haemolytic anaemia.* Fibrin deposition in capillaries can cause severe red cell disruption. It may occur in a wide variety of conditions: disseminated carcinomatosis, malignant or pregnancy-induced hypertension, haemolytic uraemic syndrome (p. 495), thrombotic thrombocytopenic purpura (p. 1056) and disseminated intravascular coagulation (p. 1055).

Infection

Plasmodium falciparum malaria (p. 353) may be associated with intravascular haemolysis; when severe, this is termed blackwater fever because of the associated haemoglobinuria. *Clostridium perfringens* septicaemia (p. 305), usually in the context of ascending cholangitis, may cause severe intravascular haemolysis with marked spherocytosis due to bacterial production of a lecithinase which destroys the red cell membrane.

Chemicals or drugs

Dapsone and sulfasalazine cause haemolysis by oxidative denaturation of haemoglobin. Denatured haemoglobin forms Heinz bodies in the red cells, visible on supravital staining with brilliant cresyl blue. Arsenic gas, copper, chlorates, nitrites and nitrobenzene derivatives may all cause haemolysis.

Paroxysmal nocturnal haemoglobinuria

Paroxysmal nocturnal haemoglobinuria (PNH) is a rare acquired, non-malignant clonal expansion of haematopoietic stem cells deficient in GPI-anchor protein; it results in intravascular haemolysis and anaemia because of increased sensitivity of red cells to lysis by complement. Episodes of intravascular haemolysis result in haemoglobinuria, most noticeable in early morning urine, which has a characteristic red–brown colour. The disease is associated with an increased risk of venous thrombosis in unusual sites, such as the liver or abdomen. PNH is also associated with hypoplastic bone marrow failure, aplastic anaemia and myelodysplastic syndrome (pp. 1048 and 1041). Management is supportive with transfusion and treatment of thrombosis. Recently, the anti-complement C5 monoclonal antibody eculizumab was shown to be effective in reducing haemolysis.

Haemoglobinopathies

These diseases are caused by mutations affecting the genes encoding the globin chains of the haemoglobin molecule. Normal haemoglobin is comprised of two alpha and two non-alpha globin chains. Alpha globin chains are produced throughout life, including in the fetus, so severe mutations may cause intrauterine death. Production of non-alpha chains varies with age; fetal haemoglobin (HbF-$\alpha\alpha/\gamma\gamma$) has two gamma chains, while the predominant adult haemoglobin (HbA-$\alpha\alpha/\beta\beta$) has two beta chains. Thus, disorders affecting the beta chains do not present until after 6 months of age. A constant small amount of haemoglobin A_2 (HbA_2-$\alpha\alpha/\delta\delta$, usually less than 2%) is made from birth.

The geographical distribution of the common haemoglobinopathies is shown in Figure 24.23. The haemoglobinopathies can be classified into qualitative or quantitative abnormalities.

Qualitative abnormalities – abnormal haemoglobins

In qualitative abnormalities (called the abnormal haemoglobins), there is a functionally important alteration in the amino acid structure of the polypeptide chains of the globin chains. Several hundred such variants are known; they were originally designated by letters of the alphabet, e.g. S, C, D or E, but are now described by names usually taken from the town or district in which they were first described. The best-known example is haemoglobin S, found in sickle-cell anaemia. Mutations around the haem-binding pocket cause the haem ring to fall out of the structure and produce an unstable haemoglobin. These substitutions often change the charge of the globin chains, producing different electrophoretic mobility, and this forms the basis for the

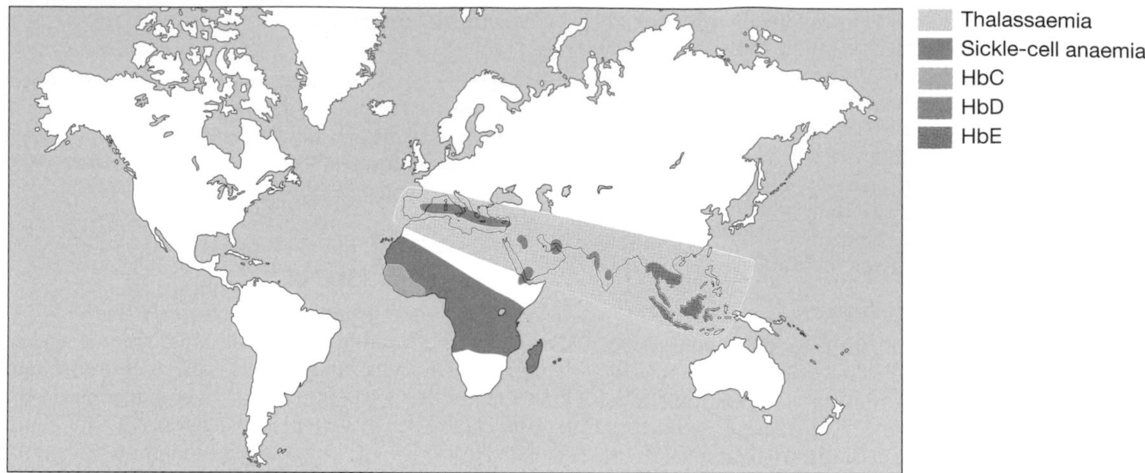

Fig. 24.23 The geographical distribution of the haemoglobinopathies. From Hoffbrand and Pettit 1992 – see p. 1056.

diagnostic use of haemoglobin electrophoresis to identify haemoglobinopathies.

Quantitative abnormalities – thalassaemias

In quantitative abnormalities (the thalassaemias), there are mutations causing a reduced rate of production of one or other of the globin chains, altering the ratio of alpha to non-alpha chains. In alpha-thalassaemia excess beta chains are present, whilst in beta-thalassaemia excess alpha chains are present. The excess chains precipitate, causing red cell membrane damage and reduced red cell survival.

Sickle-cell anaemia

Sickle-cell disease results from a single glutamic acid to valine substitution at position 6 of the beta globin polypeptide chain. It is inherited as an autosomal recessive trait (p. 53). Homozygotes only produce abnormal beta chains that make haemoglobin S (HbS, termed SS), and this results in the clinical syndrome of sickle-cell disease. Heterozygotes produce a mixture of normal and abnormal beta chains that make normal HbA and HbS (termed AS), and this results in the clinically asymptomatic sickle-cell trait.

Epidemiology

The heterozygote frequency is over 20% in tropical Africa (see Fig. 24.23). In black American populations, sickle-cell trait has a frequency of 8%. Individuals with sickle-cell trait are relatively resistant to the lethal effects of *falciparum* malaria in early childhood; the high prevalence in equatorial Africa can be explained by the survival advantage it confers in areas where *falciparum* malaria is endemic. However, homozygous patients with sickle-cell anaemia do not have correspondingly greater resistance to *falciparum* malaria.

Pathogenesis

When haemoglobin S is deoxygenated, the molecules of haemoglobin polymerise to form pseudocrystalline structures known as 'tactoids'. These distort the red cell membrane and produce characteristic sickle-shaped cells (Fig. 24.24). The polymerisation is reversible when re-oxygenation occurs. The distortion of the red cell membrane, however, may become permanent and the red cell 'irreversibly sickled'. The greater the concentration of sickle-cell haemoglobin in the individual cell, the more easily tactoids are formed, but this process may be enhanced or retarded by the presence of other haemoglobins. Thus, the abnormal haemoglobin C variant participates in the polymerisation more readily than haemoglobin A, whereas haemoglobin F strongly inhibits polymerisation.

Clinical features

Sickling is precipitated by hypoxia, acidosis, dehydration and infection. Irreversibly sickled cells have a shortened survival and plug vessels in the microcirculation. This results in a number of acute syndromes, termed 'crises', and chronic organ damage (Fig. 24.24):

- Painful *vaso-occlusive crisis*. Plugging of small vessels in the bone produces acute severe bone pain. This affects areas of active marrow: the hands and feet in children (so-called dactylitis) or the femora, humeri, ribs, pelvis and vertebrae in adults. Patients usually have a systemic response with tachycardia, sweating and a fever. This is the most common crisis.
- *Sickle chest syndrome*. This may follow a vaso-occlusive crisis and is the most common cause of death in adult sickle disease. Bone marrow infarction results in fat emboli to the lungs, which cause further sickling and infarction, leading to ventilatory failure if not treated.
- *Sequestration crisis*. Thrombosis of the venous outflow from an organ causes loss of function and acute painful enlargement. In children, the spleen is the most common site. Massive splenic enlargement may result in severe anaemia, circulatory collapse and death. Recurrent sickling in the spleen in childhood results in infarction and adults may have no functional spleen. In adults, the liver may undergo sequestration with severe pain due to capsular stretching. Priapism is a complication seen in affected men.
- *Aplastic crisis*. Infection with human parvovirus B19 results in a severe but self-limiting red cell aplasia. This produces a very low haemoglobin, which may cause heart failure. Unlike in all other sickle crises, the reticulocyte count is low.

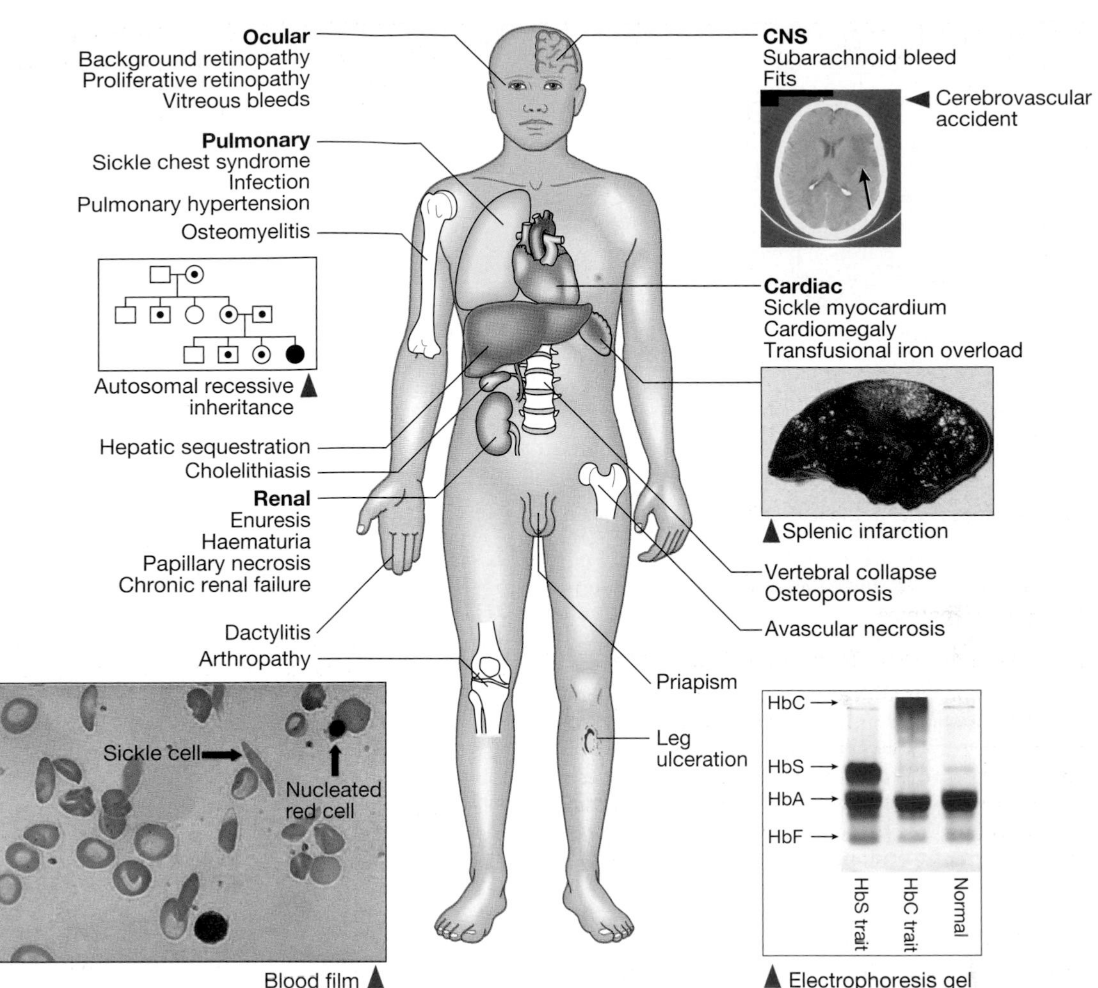

Fig. 24.24 Clinical and laboratory features of sickle-cell disease.

Investigations

Patients with sickle-cell disease have a compensated anaemia, usually around 60–80 g/L. The blood film shows sickle cells, target cells and features of hyposplenism. A reticulocytosis is present. The presence of HbS can be demonstrated by exposing red cells to a reducing agent such as sodium dithionite; HbA gives a clear solution, whereas HbS polymerises to produce a turbid solution. This forms the basis of emergency screening tests before surgery in appropriate ethnic groups but cannot distinguish between sickle-cell trait and disease. The definitive diagnosis requires haemoglobin electrophoresis to demonstrate the absence of HbA, 2–20% HbF and the predominance of HbS. Both parents of the affected individual will have sickle-cell trait.

Management

All patients with sickle-cell disease should receive prophylaxis with daily folic acid, and penicillin V to protect against pneumococcal infection, which may be lethal in the presence of hyposplenism. These patients should be vaccinated against pneumococcus, meningococcus, *Haemophilus influenzae* B, hepatitis B and seasonal influenza.

Vaso-occlusive crises are managed by aggressive rehydration, oxygen therapy, adequate analgesia (which often requires opiates) and antibiotics. Transfusion should be with fully genotyped blood wherever possible. Simple top-up transfusion may be used in a sequestration or aplastic crisis. A regular transfusion programme to suppress HbS production and maintain the HbS level below 30% may be indicated in patients with recurrent severe complications, such as cerebrovascular accidents in children or chest syndromes in adults. Exchange transfusion, in which a patient is simultaneously venesected and transfused to replace HbS with HbA, may be used in life-threatening crises or to prepare patients for surgery.

A high HbF level inhibits polymerisation of HbS and reduces sickling. Patients with sickle-cell disease and high HbF levels have a mild clinical course with few crises. Some agents are able to increase synthesis of HbF and this has been used to reduce the frequency of severe crises. The oral cytotoxic agent hydroxycarbamide has been shown to have clinical benefit with acceptable side-effects in children and adults who have recurrent severe crises.

Relatively few allogeneic stem cell transplants from HLA-matched siblings have been performed but this procedure appears to be potentially curative (p. 1017).

Prognosis

In Africa, few children with sickle-cell anaemia survive to adult life without medical attention. Even with standard medical care, approximately 15% die by the age of 20 years and 50% by the age of 40 years.

Other abnormal haemoglobins

Another beta chain haemoglobinopathy, haemoglobin C (HbC) disease, is clinically silent but associated with microcytosis and target cells on the blood film. Compound heterozygotes inheriting one HbS gene and one HbC gene from their parents have haemoglobin SC disease, which behaves like a mild form of sickle-cell disease. SC disease is associated with a reduced frequency of crises but is not uncommonly linked with complications in pregnancy and retinopathy.

The thalassaemias

Thalassaemia is an inherited impairment of haemoglobin production, in which there is partial or complete failure to synthesise a specific type of globin chain. In alpha-thalassaemia, disruption of one or both alleles on chromosome 16 may occur, with production of some or no alpha globin chains. In beta-thalassaemia, defective production usually results from disabling point mutations causing no (β^0) or reduced (β^-) beta chain production.

Beta-thalassaemia

Failure to synthesise beta chains (beta-thalassaemia) is the most common type of thalassaemia, most prevalent in the Mediterranean area. Heterozygotes have thalassaemia minor, a condition in which there is usually mild anaemia and little or no clinical disability, which may be detected only when iron therapy for a mild microcytic anaemia fails. Homozygotes (thalassaemia major) either are unable to synthesise haemoglobin A or, at best, produce very little; after the first 4–6 months of life, they develop profound hypochromic anaemia. The diagnostic features are summarised in Box 24.42. Intermediate grades of severity occur.

Management and prevention

See Box 24.43. Cure is now a possibility for selected children, with allogeneic haematopoietic stem cell transplantation (p. 1017).

It is possible to identify a fetus with homozygous beta-thalassaemia by obtaining chorionic villous material for DNA analysis sufficiently early in pregnancy to allow termination. This examination is only appropriate if both parents are known to be carriers (beta-thalassaemia minor) and will accept a termination.

Alpha-thalassaemia

Reduced or absent alpha chain synthesis is common in Southeast Asia. There are two alpha gene loci on chromosome 16 and therefore each individual carries four alpha gene alleles.

- If one is deleted, there is no clinical effect.
- If two are deleted, there may be a mild hypochromic anaemia.
- If three are deleted, the patient has haemoglobin H disease.
- If all four are deleted, the baby is stillborn (hydrops fetalis).

Haemoglobin H is a beta-chain tetramer, formed from the excess of beta chains, which is functionally useless, so that patients rely on their low levels of HbA for oxygen transport. Treatment of haemoglobin H

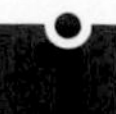

24.42 Diagnostic features of beta-thalassaemia

Beta-thalassaemia major (homozygotes)

- Profound hypochromic anaemia
- Evidence of severe red cell dysplasia
- Erythroblastosis
- Absence or gross reduction of the amount of haemoglobin A
- Raised levels of haemoglobin F
- Evidence that both parents have thalassaemia minor

Beta-thalassaemia minor (heterozygotes)

- Mild anaemia
- Microcytic hypochromic erythrocytes (not iron-deficient)
- Some target cells
- Punctate basophilia
- Raised haemoglobin A_2 fraction

24.43 Treatment of beta-thalassaemia major

Problem	Management
Erythropoietic failure	Allogeneic HSCT from HLA-compatible sibling Transfusion to maintain Hb > 100 g/L Folic acid 5 mg daily
Iron overload	Iron therapy contraindicated Iron chelation therapy
Splenomegaly causing mechanical problems, excessive transfusion needs	Splenectomy; see Box 24.40

(Hb = haemoglobin; HLA = human leucocyte antigen; HSCT = haematopoietic stem cell transplantation)

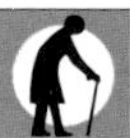

24.44 Anaemia in old age

- **Mean haemoglobin**: falls with age in both sexes but remains well within the reference range. When a low haemoglobin does occur, it is generally due to disease.
- **Anaemia can never be considered 'normal' in old age.**
- **Symptoms**: may be subtle and insidious. Cardiovascular features such as dyspnoea and oedema, and cerebral features such as dizziness and apathy, tend to predominate.
- **Ferritin**: if lower than 45 μg/L in older people, is highly predictive of iron deficiency.
- **Serum iron and transferrin**: fall with age because of the prevalence of other disorders, and are not reliable indicators of deficiency.
- **Most common cause of iron deficiency**: gastrointestinal blood loss.
- **Most common cause of vitamin B_{12} deficiency**: pernicious anaemia, as the prevalence of chronic atrophic gastritis rises in old age.
- **Neuropsychiatric symptoms associated with vitamin B_{12} deficiency**: well-established association but a causal relationship has not been clearly shown. Dementia associated with vitamin B_{12} deficiency in the absence of haematological abnormalities is rare.
- **Anaemia of chronic disease**: frequent in old age because of the rising prevalence of diseases that inhibit iron transport.

disease is similar to that of beta-thalassaemia of intermediate severity, involving folic acid supplementation, transfusion if required and avoidance of iron therapy.

HAEMATOLOGICAL MALIGNANCIES

Haematological malignancies arise when the processes controlling proliferation or apoptosis are corrupted in blood cells. If mature differentiated cells are involved, the cells will have a low growth fraction and produce indolent neoplasms, such as the low-grade lymphomas or chronic leukaemias, when patients have an expected survival of many years. In contrast, if more primitive stem cells are involved, the cells can have the highest growth fractions of all human neoplasms, producing rapidly progressive, life-threatening illnesses such as the acute leukaemias or high-grade lymphomas. Involvement of pluripotent stem cells produces the most aggressive acute leukaemias. In general, haematological neoplasms are diseases of elderly patients, the exceptions being acute lymphoblastic leukaemia, which predominantly affects children, and Hodgkin lymphoma, which affects people aged 20–40 years. Management of young patients with haematological malignancy is particularly challenging (Box 24.45).

Leukaemias

Leukaemias are malignant disorders of the haematopoietic stem cell compartment, characteristically associated with increased numbers of white cells in the bone marrow and/or peripheral blood. The course of leukaemia may vary from a few days or weeks to many years, depending on the type.

Epidemiology and aetiology

The incidence of leukaemia of all types in the population is approximately 10/100 000 per annum, of which just under half are cases of acute leukaemia. Males are affected more frequently than females, the ratio being about 3:2 in acute leukaemia, 2:1 in chronic lymphocytic leukaemia and 1.3:1 in chronic myeloid leukaemia.

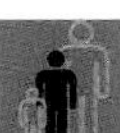

24.45 Consequences of haematological malignancy in adolescence

- **Tailored management protocols**: the most effective treatment schedules for leukaemia and lymphoma differ between children and adults. Adolescent patients may be most appropriately managed in specialist centres.
- **Psychosocial effects**: adolescents undergoing treatment for haematological malignancy may suffer significant consequences for their schooling and social development, and require support from a multidisciplinary team.
- **'Late effects'**: adolescents who have been treated with chemotherapy and/or radiotherapy in childhood may be at risk of a wide range of complications, depending on the region irradiated, radiation dose and the drugs used. Particularly relevant complications in this age group include short stature, growth hormone deficiency, delayed puberty, and cognitive dysfunction affecting schooling (after cranial irradiation). Life-long follow-up is often undertaken to detect and manage these late effects and to deal with consequences such as infertility and secondary malignancy.

24.46 Risk factors for leukaemia

Ionising radiation

- After atomic bombing of Japanese cities (myeloid leukaemia)
- Radiotherapy for ankylosing spondylitis
- Diagnostic X-rays of the fetus in pregnancy

Cytotoxic drugs

- Especially alkylating agents (myeloid leukaemia, usually after a latent period of several years)
- Industrial exposure to benzene

Retroviruses

- One rare form of T-cell leukaemia/lymphoma appears to be associated with a retrovirus similar to the viruses causing leukaemia in cats and cattle

Genetic

- Identical twin of patients with leukaemia
- Down's syndrome and certain other genetic disorders

Immunological

- Immune deficiency states (e.g. hypogammaglobulinaemia)

Geographical variation in incidence does occur, the most striking being the rarity of chronic lymphocytic leukaemia in the Chinese and related races. Acute leukaemia occurs at all ages. Acute lymphoblastic leukaemia shows a peak of incidence in children aged 1–5 years. All forms of acute myeloid leukaemia have their lowest incidence in young adult life and there is a striking rise over the age of 50. Chronic leukaemias occur mainly in middle and old age.

The cause of the leukaemia is unknown in the majority of patients. Several risk factors, however, have been identified (Box 24.46).

Terminology and classification

Leukaemias are traditionally classified into four main groups:

- acute lymphoblastic leukaemia (ALL)
- acute myeloid leukaemia (AML)
- chronic lymphocytic leukaemia (CLL)
- chronic myeloid leukaemia (CML).

In acute leukaemia, there is proliferation of primitive stem cells, leading to an accumulation of blasts, predominantly in the bone marrow, which causes bone marrow failure. In chronic leukaemia, the malignant clone is able to differentiate, resulting in an accumulation of more mature cells. Lymphocytic and lymphoblastic cells are those derived from the lymphoid stem cell (B cells and T cells). Myeloid refers to the other lineages: that is, precursors of red cells, granulocytes, monocytes and platelets (see Fig. 24.2, p. 993).

The diagnosis of leukaemia is usually suspected from an abnormal blood count, often a raised white count, and is confirmed by examination of the bone marrow. This includes the morphology of the abnormal cells, analysis of cell surface markers (immunophenotyping), clone-specific chromosome abnormalities and molecular changes. These results are incorporated in the World Health Organization (WHO) classification of tumours of haematopoietic and lymphoid tissues; the subclassification of acute leukaemias is shown in Box 24.47. The features in the bone marrow not only provide an

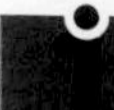

24.47 WHO classification of acute leukaemia

Acute myeloid leukaemia (AML) with recurrent genetic abnormalities
- AML with t(8;21), gene product AML-ETO
- AML with eosinophilia inv(16) or t(16;16), gene product CBFβ-MYH11
- Acute promyelocytic leukaemia t(15;17), gene product PML-RARA
- AML with t(9;11)(p22;q23), gene product MLLT3-MLL
- AML with t(6;9)(p23;q34), gene product DEK-NUP214
- AML with inv(3)(q21q26.2) or t(3;3)(q21;q26.2), gene product RPN1-EVI1

Acute myeloid leukaemia with myelodysplasia-related changes
- e.g. Following a myelodysplastic syndrome

Therapy-related myeloid neoplasms
- e.g. Alkylating agent or topoisomerase II inhibitor

Myeloid sarcoma

Myeloid proliferations related to Down's syndrome

Acute myeloid leukaemia not otherwise specified
- e.g. AML with or without differentiation, acute myelomonocytic leukaemia, erythroleukaemia, megakaryoblastic leukaemia, myeloid sarcoma

Acute lymphoblastic leukaemia (ALL)
- Precursor B ALL
- Precursor T ALL

accurate diagnosis but also give valuable prognostic information, allowing therapy to be tailored to the patient's disease.

Acute leukaemia

There is a failure of cell maturation in acute leukaemia. Proliferation of cells which do not mature leads to an accumulation of primitive cells which take up more and more marrow space at the expense of the normal haematopoietic elements. Eventually, this proliferation spills into the blood. Acute myeloid leukaemia (AML) is about four times more common than acute lymphoblastic leukaemia (ALL) in adults. In children, the proportions are reversed, the lymphoblastic variety being more common. The clinical features are usually those of bone marrow failure (anaemia, bleeding or infection – pp. 1001, 1006 and 1008).

Investigations

Blood examination usually shows anaemia with a normal or raised MCV. The leucocyte count may vary from as low as $1 \times 10^9/L$ to as high as $500 \times 10^9/L$ or more. In the majority of patients, the count is below $100 \times 10^9/L$. Severe thrombocytopenia is usual but not invariable. Frequently, blast cells are seen in the blood film but sometimes blast cells may be infrequent or absent. A bone marrow examination will confirm the diagnosis. The bone marrow is usually hypercellular, with replacement of normal elements by leukaemic blast cells in varying degrees (but more than 20% of the cells) (Fig. 24.25). The presence of Auer rods in the cytoplasm of blast cells indicates a myeloblastic type of leukaemia. Classification and prognosis are determined by immunophenotyping, chromosome and molecular analysis, as shown in Figure 24.26.

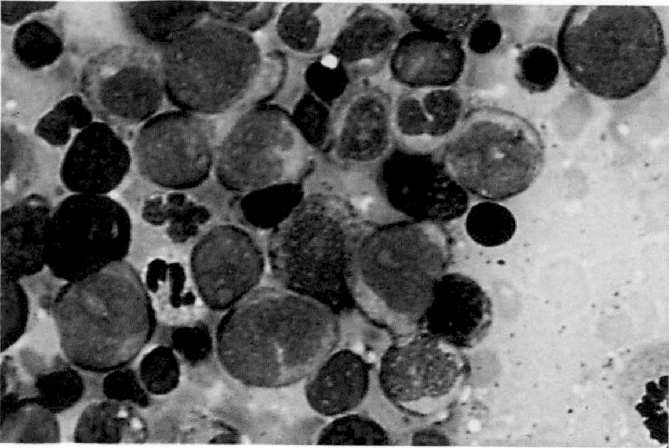

Fig. 24.25 Acute myeloid leukaemia. Bone marrow aspirate showing infiltration with large blast cells which display nuclear folding and prominent nucleoli.

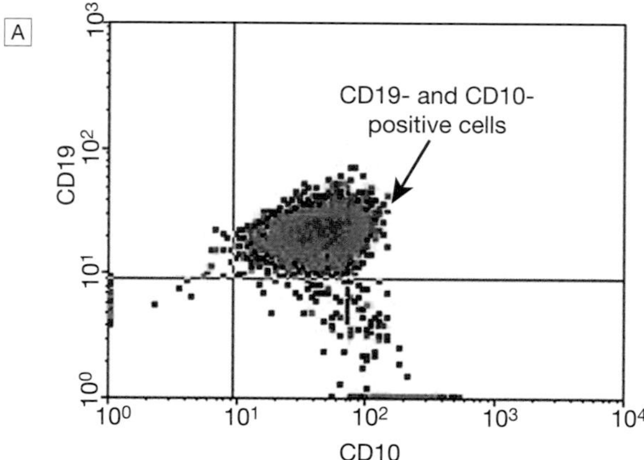

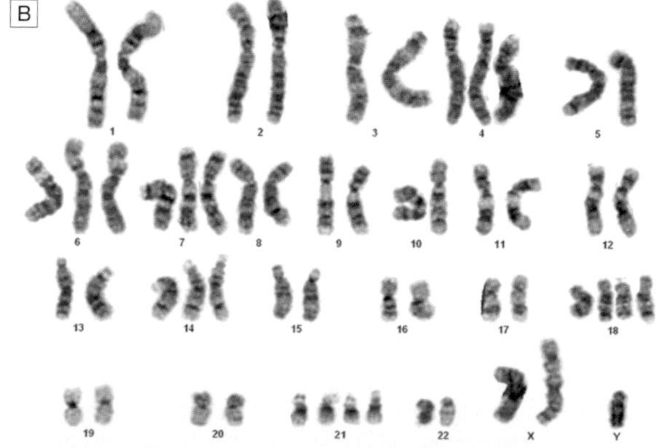

Fig. 24.26 Investigation of acute lymphoblastic leukaemia (ALL). **A** Flow cytometric analysis of blasts labelled with the fluorescent antibodies anti-CD19 (y axis) and anti-CD10 (x axis). ALL blasts are positive for both CD19 and CD10 (arrow). **B** Chromosome analysis (karyotype) of blasts showing additional chromosomes X, 4, 6, 7, 14, 18 and 21.

Management

The general strategy for acute leukaemia is shown in Figure 24.27. The first decision must be whether or not to give specific treatment. This is generally aggressive, has numerous side-effects, and may not be appropriate for the very elderly or patients with serious comorbidities (Chs 7 and 11). In these patients, supportive

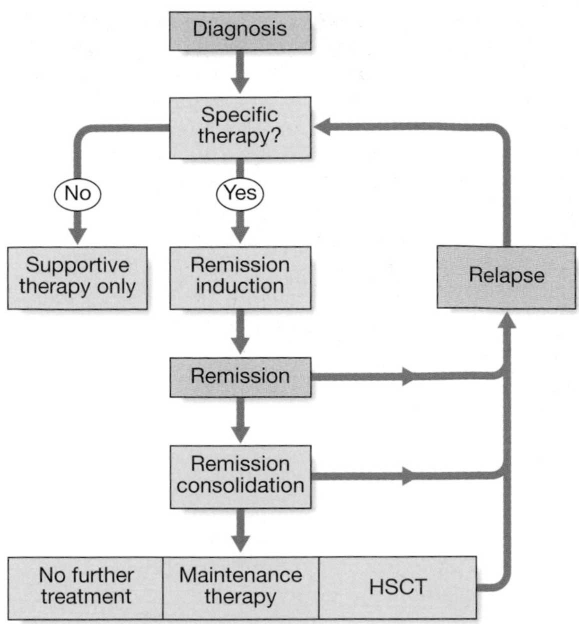

Fig. 24.27 Treatment strategy in acute leukaemia. (HSCT = haematopoietic stem cell transplantation)

treatment can effect considerable improvement in well-being.

Specific therapy

If a decision to embark on specific therapy has been taken, the patient should be prepared as recommended in Box 24.48. It is unwise to attempt aggressive management of acute leukaemia unless adequate services are available for the provision of supportive therapy.

The aim of treatment is to destroy the leukaemic clone of cells without destroying the residual normal stem cell compartment from which repopulation of the haematopoietic tissues will occur. There are three phases:

- *Remission induction.* In this phase, the bulk of the tumour is destroyed by combination chemotherapy. The patient goes through a period of severe bone marrow hypoplasia, requiring intensive support and inpatient care from a specially trained multidisciplinary team.
- *Remission consolidation.* If remission has been achieved, residual disease is attacked by therapy during the consolidation phase. This consists of a number of courses of chemotherapy, again resulting in periods of marrow hypoplasia. In poor-prognosis leukaemia, this may include haematopoietic stem cell transplantation.
- *Remission maintenance.* If the patient is still in remission after the consolidation phase for ALL, a period of maintenance therapy is given, with the individual as an outpatient and treatment consisting of a repeating cycle of drug administration. This may extend for up to 3 years if relapse does not occur.

In patients with ALL, it is necessary to give prophylactic treatment to the central nervous system, as this is a sanctuary site where standard therapy does not penetrate. This usually consists of a combination of cranial irradiation, intrathecal chemotherapy and high-dose methotrexate, which crosses the blood–brain barrier.

Thereafter, specific therapy is discontinued and the patient observed.

The detail of the schedules for these treatments can be found in specialist texts. The drugs most commonly employed are listed in Box 24.49. Generally, if a patient fails to go into remission with induction treatment, alternative drug combinations may be tried, but the outlook is poor unless remission can be achieved. Disease which relapses during treatment or soon after the end of treatment carries a poor prognosis and is difficult to treat. The longer after the end of treatment that relapse occurs, the more likely it is that further treatment will be effective.

In some patients, alternative palliative chemotherapy, not designed to achieve remission, may be used to curb excessive leucocyte proliferation. Drugs used for this purpose include hydroxycarbamide and

24.48 Preparation for specific therapy in acute leukaemia

- Existing infections identified and treated (e.g. urinary tract infection, oral candidiasis, dental, gingival and skin infections)
- Anaemia corrected by red cell concentrate transfusion
- Thrombocytopenic bleeding controlled by platelet transfusions
- If possible, central venous catheter (e.g. Hickman line) inserted to facilitate access to the circulation for delivery of chemotherapy, fluids, blood products and other supportive drugs
- Tumour lysis risk assessed and prevention started: fluids with allopurinol or rasburicase
- Therapeutic regimen carefully explained to the patient and informed consent obtained
- Consideration of entry into clinical trial

24.49 Drugs commonly used in the treatment of acute leukaemia

Phase	ALL	AML
Induction	Vincristine (IV) Prednisolone (oral) L-asparaginase (IM) Daunorubicin (IV) Methotrexate (intrathecal) Imatinib (oral)*	Daunorubicin (IV) Cytarabine (IV) Etoposide (IV and oral)
Consolidation	Daunorubicin (IV) Cytarabine (IV) Etoposide (IV) Methotrexate (IV) Imatinib (oral)*	Cytarabine (IV) Amsacrine (IV) Mitoxantrone (IV)
Maintenance	Prednisolone (oral) Vincristine (IV) Mercaptopurine (oral) Methotrexate (oral) Imatinib (oral)*	

*If Philadelphia chromosome-positive.

24

mercaptopurine. The aim is to reduce the blast count without inducing bone marrow failure.

Supportive therapy

Aggressive and potentially curative therapy, which involves periods of severe bone marrow failure, would not be possible without appropriate supportive care. The following problems commonly arise.

Anaemia. Anaemia is treated with red cell concentrate transfusions.

Bleeding. Thrombocytopenic bleeding requires platelet transfusions, unless the bleeding is trivial. Prophylactic platelet transfusion should be given to maintain the platelet count above 10×10^9/L. Coagulation abnormalities occur and need accurate diagnosis and treatment (p. 1050).

Infection. Fever (> 38°C) lasting over 1 hour in a neutropenic patient indicates possible septicaemia (see also p. 296). Parenteral broad-spectrum antibiotic therapy is essential. Empirical therapy is given according to local bacteriological resistance patterns: for example, with a combination of an aminoglycoside (e.g. gentamicin) and a broad-spectrum penicillin (e.g. piperacillin/tazobactam) or a single-agent beta-lactam (e.g. meropenem). The organisms most commonly associated with severe neutropenic sepsis are Gram-positive bacteria, such as *Staphylococcus aureus* and *Staph. epidermidis*, which are present on the skin and gain entry via cannulae and central lines. Gram-negative infections often originate from the gastrointestinal tract, which is affected by chemotherapy-induced mucositis; organisms such as *Escherichia coli*, *Pseudomonas* and *Klebsiella* spp. are likely to cause rapid clinical deterioration and must be covered with the initial empirical antibiotic therapy. Gram-positive infection may require vancomycin therapy. If fever has not resolved after 3–5 days, empirical antifungal therapy (e.g. a liposomal amphotericin B preparation, voriconazole or caspofungin) is added.

Patients with ALL are susceptible to infection with *Pneumocystis jirovecii* (p. 400), which causes a severe pneumonia. Prophylaxis with co-trimoxazole is given during chemotherapy. Diagnosis may require either bronchoalveolar lavage or open lung biopsy. Treatment is with high-dose co-trimoxazole, initially intravenously, changing to oral treatment as soon as possible.

Oral and pharyngeal candida infection is common. Fluconazole is effective for the treatment of established local infection and for prophylaxis against systemic candidaemia. Prophylaxis against other systemic fungal infections, including *Aspergillus*, using itraconazole or posaconazole, for example, is usual practice during high-risk intensive chemotherapy. This is often used along with sensitive markers of early fungal infection to guide treatment initiation (a 'pre-emptive approach').

For systemic fungal infection with *Candida* or aspergillosis, intravenous liposomal amphotericin or voriconazole is required.

Reactivation of herpes simplex infection (p. 325) occurs frequently around the lips and nose during ablative therapy for acute leukaemia, and is treated with aciclovir. This may also be prescribed prophylactically to patients with a history of cold sores or elevated antibody titres to herpes simplex. Herpes zoster manifesting as chickenpox or, after reactivation, as shingles (p. 318) should be treated in the early stage with high-dose aciclovir, as it can be fatal in immunocompromised patients.

The value of isolation facilities, such as laminar flow rooms, is debatable but may contribute to staff awareness of careful reverse barrier nursing practice. The isolation can be psychologically stressful for the patient.

Metabolic problems. Frequent monitoring of fluid balance and renal, hepatic and haemostatic function is necessary. Patients are often severely anorexic and diarrhoea is common as a consequence of the side-effects of therapy; they may find drinking difficult and hence require intravenous fluids and electrolytes. Renal toxicity occurs with some antibiotics (e.g. aminoglycosides) and antifungal agents (amphotericin). Cellular breakdown during induction therapy (tumour lysis syndrome) releases intracellular ions and nucleic acid breakdown products, causing hyperkalaemia, hyperuricaemia, hyperphosphataemia and hypocalcaemia. This may cause renal failure. Allopurinol and intravenous hydration are given to try to prevent this. In patients at high risk of tumour lysis syndrome, prophylactic rasburicase (a recombinant urate oxidase enzyme) can be used. Occasionally, dialysis may be required.

Psychological problems. Psychological support is a key aspect of care. Patients should be kept informed, and their questions answered and fears allayed as far as possible. A multidisciplinary approach to patient care involves input from many services, including psychology. Key members of the team include haematology specialist nurses, who are often the central point of contact for patients and families throughout the illness.

Haematopoietic stem cell transplantation

This is described on page 1017. In patients with high-risk acute leukaemia, allogeneic HSCT can improve 5-year survival from 20% to around 50%.

Prognosis

Without treatment, the median survival of patients with acute leukaemia is about 5 weeks. This may be extended to a number of months with supportive treatment.

24.50 Outcome in adult acute leukaemia

Disease/risk	Risk factors	5-yr overall survival
Acute myeloid leukaemia		
Good risk	Promyelocytic leukaemia t(15;17) t(8;21) inv 16 or t(16;16)	76%
Poor risk	Cytogenetic abnormalities −5, −7, del 5q, abn(3q), complex (> 5)	21%
Intermediate risk	AML with none of the above	48%
Acute lymphoblastic leukaemia		
Poor risk	Philadelphia chromosome High white count > 100×10^9/L Abnormal short arm of chromosome 11 t(1;19)	20%
Standard	ALL with none of the above	37%

Patients who achieve remission with specific therapy have a better outlook. Around 80% of adult patients under 60 years of age with ALL or AML achieve remission, although remission rates are lower for older patients. However, the relapse rate continues to be high. Box 24.50 shows the survival in ALL and AML, and the influence of prognostic features.

Advances in treatment have led to steady improvement in survival from leukaemia. Advances include the introduction of drugs such as ATRA (all transretinoic acid) in acute promyelocytic leukaemia, which has greatly reduced induction deaths from bleeding in this good-risk leukaemia. Current trials aim to improve survival, especially in standard and poor-risk disease, with strategies that include allogeneic HSCT and targeted therapies such as anti-CD33 monoclonal antibodies and FLT3 inhibitors.

Chronic myeloid leukaemia

Chronic myeloid leukaemia (CML) is a myeloproliferative stem cell disorder resulting in proliferation of all haematopoietic lineages but manifesting predominantly in the granulocytic series. Maturation of cells proceeds fairly normally. The disease occurs chiefly between the ages of 30 and 80 years, with a peak incidence at 55 years. It is rare, with an annual incidence in the UK of 1.8/100 000, and accounts for 20% of all leukaemias. It is found in all races.

The defining characteristic of CML is the chromosome abnormality known as the Philadelphia (Ph) chromosome. This is a shortened chromosome 22 resulting from a reciprocal translocation of material with chromosome 9. The break on chromosome 22 occurs in the breakpoint cluster region (BCR). The fragment from chromosome 9 that joins the BCR carries the *abl* oncogene, which forms a fusion gene with the remains of the BCR. This *BCR ABL* fusion gene codes for a 210 kDa protein with tyrosine kinase activity, which plays a causative role in the disease as an oncogene (p. 59), influencing cellular proliferation, differentiation and survival. In some patients in whom conventional chromosomal analysis does not detect a Ph chromosome, the BCR ABL gene product is detectable by molecular techniques.

Natural history

The disease has three phases:

- *A chronic phase,* in which the disease is responsive to treatment and is easily controlled, which used to last 3–5 years. With the introduction of imatinib therapy, this phase has been prolonged to longer than 8 years in many patients.
- *An accelerated phase* (not always seen), in which disease control becomes more difficult.
- *Blast crisis,* in which the disease transforms into an acute leukaemia, either myeloid (70%) or lymphoblastic (30%), which is relatively refractory to treatment. This is the cause of death in the majority of patients; therefore survival is dictated by the timing of blast crisis, which cannot be predicted. Prior to imatinib therapy (see below), approximately 10% of patients per year would transform. In those treated with imatinib for up to 5 years, only between 0.5 and 2.5% have transformed each year.

Clinical features

Symptoms at presentation may include lethargy, weight loss, abdominal discomfort and sweating, but about 25% of patients are asymptomatic at diagnosis. Splenomegaly is present in 90%; in about 10%, the enlargement is massive, extending to over 15 cm below the costal margin. A friction rub may be heard in cases of splenic infarction. Hepatomegaly occurs in about 50%. Lymphadenopathy is unusual.

Investigations

FBC results are variable between patients. There is usually a normocytic, normochromic anaemia. The leucocyte count can vary from 10 to 600 × 10^9/L. In about one-third of patients, there is a very high platelet count, sometimes as high as 2000 × 10^9/L. In the blood film, the full range of granulocyte precursors, from myeloblasts to mature neutrophils, is seen but the predominant cells are neutrophils and myelocytes (see Fig. 24.3, p. 993). Myeloblasts usually constitute less than 10% of all white cells. There is often an absolute increase in eosinophils and basophils, and nucleated red cells are common. If the disease progresses through an accelerated phase, the percentage of more primitive cells increases. Blast transformation is characterised by a dramatic increase in the number of circulating blasts. In patients with thrombocytosis, very high platelet counts may persist during treatment, in both chronic and accelerated phases, but usually drop dramatically at blast transformation. Basophilia tends to increase as the disease progresses.

Bone marrow should be obtained to confirm the diagnosis and phase of disease by morphology, chromosome analysis to demonstrate the presence of the Ph chromosome, and RNA analysis to demonstrate the presence of the BCR ABL gene product. Blood LDH levels are elevated and the uric acid level may be high due to increased cell breakdown.

Management

Chronic phase

Imatinib, dasatinib and nilotinib specifically inhibit BCR ABL tyrosine kinase activity and reduce the uncontrolled proliferation of white cells. They are recommended as first-line therapy in chronic-phase CML, producing complete cytogenetic response (disappearance of the Ph chromosome) in 76% at 18 months of therapy (Box 24.51). Patients are monitored by repeated bone marrow examination until there is a complete cytogenetic response, and then by 3-monthly real-time quantitative polymerase chain reaction (PCR) for BCR ABL mRNA transcripts in blood. For those failing to respond or progress on imatinib, options include second-generation tyrosine kinase inhibitors, such as dasatinib or nilotinib, allogeneic HSCT (p. 1017), or

EBM 24.51 Tyrosine kinase inhibition in chronic myeloid leukaemia

'As first-line therapy in CML, imatinib is better tolerated and induces a cytogenetic response in ~87% of cases at 18 months, compared with ~35% response to interferon plus cytarabine.'

- O'Brien SG for the IRIS Investigators. N Engl J Med 2003; 348:994–1004.

24

classical cytotoxic drugs such as hydroxycarbamide (hydroxyurea) or interferon. Hydroxycarbamide was previously used widely for initial control of disease, and is still useful in this context or in palliative situations. It does not diminish the frequency of the Ph chromosome or affect the onset of blast cell transformation. Interferon-alfa was considered first-line treatment before imatinib was developed. It was given alone or with the chemotherapy agent Ara-C, and controlled CML chronic phase in about 70% of patients.

Accelerated phase and blast crisis

Management is more difficult. For patients presenting in accelerated phase, imatinib is indicated if the patient has not already received it. Hydroxycarbamide can be an effective single agent and low-dose cytarabine can also be tried. When blast transformation occurs, the type of blast cell should be determined. Response to appropriate acute leukaemia treatment (see Box 24.49) is better if disease is lymphoblastic than if it is myeloblastic. Given the very poor response in myeloblastic transformation, there is a strong case for supportive therapy only, particularly in older patients.

Patients progressing to advanced-phase disease on imatinib may respond to a second-generation tyrosine kinase inhibitor and may be considered for allogeneic HSCT (p. 1017).

Chronic lymphocytic leukaemia

Chronic lymphocytic leukaemia (CLL) is the most common variety of leukaemia, accounting for 30% of cases. The male to female ratio is 2:1 and the median age at presentation is 65–70 years. In this disease, B lymphocytes, which would normally respond to antigens by transformation and antibody formation, fail to do so. An ever-increasing mass of immuno-incompetent cells accumulates, to the detriment of immune function and normal bone marrow haematopoiesis.

Clinical features

The onset is usually insidious. Indeed, in around 70% of patients, the diagnosis is made incidentally on a routine FBC. Presenting problems may be anaemia, infections, painless lymphadenopathy, and systemic symptoms such as night sweats or weight loss. However, these more often occur later in the course of the disease.

Investigations

The diagnosis is based on the peripheral blood findings of a mature lymphocytosis ($> 5 \times 10^9/L$) with characteristic morphology and cell surface markers. Immunophenotyping reveals the lymphocytes to be monoclonal B cells expressing the B cell antigens CD19 and CD23, with either kappa or lambda immunoglobulin light chains and, characteristically, an aberrant T cell antigen, CD5.

Other useful investigations in CLL include a reticulocyte count and a direct Coombs test, as autoimmune haemolytic anaemia may occur (p. 1029). Serum immunoglobulin levels should be estimated to establish the degree of immunosuppression, which is common and progressive. Bone marrow examination by aspirate and trephine is not essential for the diagnosis of CLL, but may be helpful in difficult cases, for prognosis (patients with diffuse marrow involvement have a poorer prognosis) and to monitor response to therapy. The main prognostic factor is stage of disease (Box 24.52); however, malignant cell characteristics, such as CD38 expression, abnormalities of chromosome 11 or 17, and absence of mutations of IgV_H genes, also indicate a poorer prognosis.

24.52 Staging of chronic lymphocytic leukaemia

Clinical stage A (60% patients)
• No anaemia or thrombocytopenia and fewer than three areas of lymphoid enlargement
Clinical stage B (30% patients)
• No anaemia or thrombocytopenia, with three or more involved areas of lymphoid enlargement
Clinical stage C (10% patients)
• Anaemia and/or thrombocytopenia, regardless of the number of areas of lymphoid enlargement

Management

No specific treatment is required for most clinical stage A patients, unless progression occurs. Life expectancy is usually normal in older patients. The patient should be offered clear information about CLL, and be reassured about the indolent nature of the disease, as the diagnosis of leukaemia inevitably causes anxiety.

Treatment is only required if there is evidence of bone marrow failure, massive or progressive lymphadenopathy or splenomegaly, systemic symptoms such as weight loss or night sweats, a rapidly increasing lymphocyte count or autoimmune haemolytic anaemia or thrombocytopenia. Initial therapy for those requiring treatment (stages B and C) may consist of oral chemotherapy with the alkylating agent chlorambucil. This will reduce the abnormal lymphocyte mass and produce symptomatic improvement in most patients. More recently, the purine analogue fludarabine, in combination with the alkylating agent cyclophosphamide and the anti-CD20 monoclonal antibody rituximab, has increased remission rates and disease-free survival, although there are increased risks of infection and secondary malignancies. Bone marrow failure or autoimmune cytopenias may respond to corticosteroids.

Supportive care is increasingly required in progressive disease, e.g. transfusions for symptomatic anaemia or thrombocytopenia, prompt treatment of infections and, for some patients with hypogammaglobulinaemia, immunoglobulin replacement. Radiotherapy may be used for lymphadenopathy which is causing discomfort or local obstruction, and for symptomatic splenomegaly. Splenectomy may be required to improve low blood counts due to autoimmune destruction or to hypersplenism, and can relieve massive splenomegaly.

Prognosis

The majority of clinical stage A patients have a normal life expectancy but patients with advanced CLL are more likely to die from their disease or infectious complications. Survival is influenced by prognostic features of the leukaemia and whether patients can tolerate intensive treatment. In those treated with chemotherapy and rituximab, 90% are alive 4 years later (Box 24.53).

EBM 24.53 Chemotherapy plus anti-CD20 monoclonal antibody therapy in CLL

'The addition of rituximab (R) to first-line chemotherapy (with fludarabine and cyclophosphamide, RFC) improves median progression free survival (51.8 compared with 32.8 months) and overall survival in CLL. The time to 25% of patients dying was 62.5 months with RFC and 46.8 months with chemotherapy alone.'

- Hallek M, et al. Lancet 2010; 376:21 164–21 174.

Rarely, CLL transforms to an aggressive high-grade lymphoma, called Richter's transformation.

Prolymphocytic leukaemia

This is a variant of chronic lymphocytic leukaemia found mainly in males over the age of 60 years; 25% of cases are of the T cell variety. There is typically massive splenomegaly with little lymphadenopathy and a very high leucocyte count, often in excess of $400 \times 10^9/L$; the characteristic cell is a large lymphocyte with a prominent nucleolus. Treatment is generally unsuccessful and the prognosis very poor. Leukapheresis, splenectomy and chemotherapy may be tried.

Hairy cell leukaemia

This is a rare chronic B-cell lymphoproliferative disorder. The male to female ratio is 6:1 and the median age at diagnosis is 50 years. Presenting symptoms are those of general ill health and recurrent infections. Splenomegaly occurs in 90% but lymph node enlargement is unusual.

Severe neutropenia, monocytopenia and the characteristic hairy cells in the blood and bone marrow are typical. These cells usually have a B lymphocyte immunotype but they also characteristically express CD25 and CD103. Recently, all patients with hairy cell leukaemia have been found to have a mutation in the *BRAF* gene.

Over recent years, a number of treatments, including cladribine and deoxycoformycin, have been shown to produce long-lasting remissions.

Myelodysplastic syndrome

Myelodysplastic syndrome (MDS) consists of a group of clonal haematopoietic disorders which represent steps in the progression to the development of leukaemia. MDS presents with consequences of bone marrow failure (anaemia, recurrent infections or bleeding), usually in older people (median age at diagnosis is 69 years). The overall incidence is 4/100 000 in the population, rising to more than 30/100 000 in the over-seventies. The blood film is characterised by cytopenias and abnormal-looking (dysplastic) blood cells, including macrocytic red cells and hypogranular neutrophils with nuclear hyper- or hyposegmentation. The bone marrow is hypercellular, with dysplastic changes in all three cell lines. Blast cells may be increased but do not reach the 20% level that indicates acute leukaemia. Chromosome analysis frequently reveals abnormalities, particularly of chromosome 5 or 7. The WHO classification of MDS is shown in Box 24.54.

24.54 WHO classification of myelodysplastic syndromes

Disease	Bone marrow findings
Refractory anaemia (RA)	Blasts < 5% Erythroid dysplasia only
Refractory anaemia with sideroblasts (RARS)	Blasts < 5% Ringed sideroblasts > 15%
Refractory cytopenias with multilineage dysplasia (RCMD)	Blasts < 5% 2–3 lineage dysplasia
Refractory anaemia with excess blasts (RAEB)	Blasts 5–20% 2–3 lineage dysplasia
Myelodysplastic syndrome with 5q–	Myelodysplastic syndrome associated with a del (5q) cytogenetic abnormality Blasts < 5% Often normal or increased blood platelet count
Myelodysplastic syndrome unclassified	None of the above or inadequate material

Inevitably, MDS progresses to AML, although the time to progression varies (from months to years) with the subtype of MDS, being slowest in refractory anaemia and most rapid in refractory anaemia with excess of blasts. An international prognostic scoring system (IPSS) predicts clinical outcome based upon karyotype and cytopenias in blood, as well as percentage of bone marrow blasts. In low-risk patients, median survival is 5.7 years and time for 25% of patients to develop AML is 9.4 years; equivalent figures in high-risk patients are 0.4 and 0.2 years, respectively.

Management

For the vast majority of patients who are elderly, the disease is incurable, and supportive care with red cell and platelet transfusions is the mainstay of treatment. A trial of erythropoietin and granulocyte-colony-stimulating factor (G-CSF) is recommended in some patients with early disease to improve haemoglobin and white cell counts. For younger patients with higher-risk disease, allogeneic HSCT may afford a cure. Transplantation should be preceded by intensive chemotherapy in those with more advanced disease. More recently, the hypomethylating agent azacytidine has improved survival by a median of 9 months for high-risk patients, and in the UK is recommended for those not eligible for transplantation.

Lymphomas

These neoplasms arise from lymphoid tissues, and are diagnosed from the pathological findings on biopsy as Hodgkin or non-Hodgkin lymphoma. The majority are of B cell origin. Non-Hodgkin lymphomas are classified as low- or high-grade tumours on the basis of their proliferation rate.

- *High-grade tumours* divide rapidly, are typically present for a matter of weeks before diagnosis, and may be life-threatening.
- *Low-grade tumours* divide slowly, may be present for many months before diagnosis, and typically behave in an indolent fashion.

Hodgkin lymphoma

The histological hallmark of Hodgkin lymphoma (HL) is the presence of Reed–Sternberg cells, large malignant lymphoid cells of B cell origin (Fig. 24.28). They are often only present in small numbers but are surrounded by large numbers of reactive non-malignant T cells, plasma cells and eosinophils.

The epidemiology of HL is shown in Box 24.55 and its histological WHO classification in Box 24.56.

Nodular lymphocyte-predominant HL is slow-growing, localised and rarely fatal. Classical HL is divided into four histological subtypes from the appearance of the Reed–Sternberg cells and surrounding reactive cells. The nodular sclerosing type is more common in young patients and in women. Mixed cellularity is more common in the elderly. Lymphocyte-rich HL usually presents in men. Lymphocyte-depleted HL is rare and probably represents large-cell or anaplastic non-Hodgkin lymphoma.

Clinical features

There is painless, rubbery lymphadenopathy, usually in the neck or supraclavicular fossae; the lymph nodes may fluctuate in size. Young patients with nodular sclerosing disease may have large mediastinal masses which are surprisingly asymptomatic but may cause dry cough and some breathlessness. Isolated subdiaphragmatic nodes occur in fewer than 10% at diagnosis. Hepatosplenomegaly may be present but does not always indicate disease in those organs. Spread is contiguous from one node to the next and extranodal disease, such as bone, brain or skin involvement, is rare.

Investigations

Treatment of HL depends upon the stage at presentation; therefore investigations aim not only to diagnose lymphoma but also to determine the extent of disease (Box 24.57).

- *FBC* may be normal. If a normochromic, normocytic anaemia or lymphopenia is present, this is a poor prognostic factor. An eosinophilia or a neutrophilia may be present.
- *ESR* may be raised.
- *Renal function tests* are required to ensure function is normal prior to treatment.
- *Liver function* may be abnormal in the absence of disease or may reflect hepatic infiltration. An obstructive pattern may be caused by nodes at the porta hepatis.

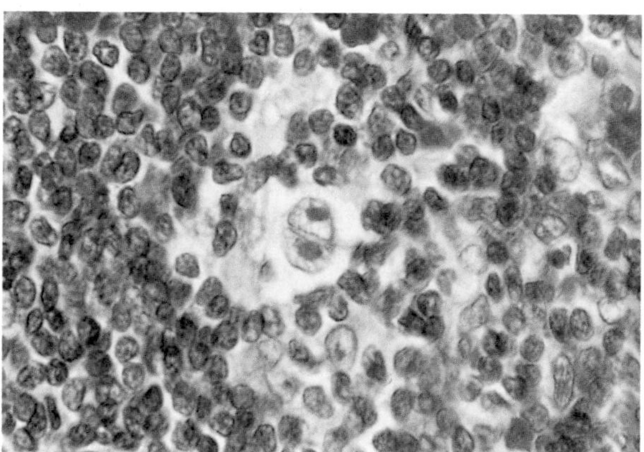

Fig. 24.28 Hodgkin lymphoma. In the centre of this lymph node biopsy is a large typical Reed–Sternberg cell with two nuclei containing a prominent eosinophilic nucleolus.

24.55 Epidemiology and aetiology of Hodgkin lymphoma

Incidence
- ~4 new cases/100 000 population/yr

Sex ratio
- Slight male excess (1.5 : 1)

Age
- Median age 31 yrs; first peak at 20–35 yrs and second at 50–70 yrs

Aetiology
- Unknown
- More common in patients from well-educated backgrounds and small families
- Three times more likely with a past history of infectious mononucleosis but no definitive causal link to Epstein–Barr virus infection is proven

24.56 WHO pathological classification of Hodgkin lymphoma

Type	Histology classification	Proportion of HL
Nodular lymphocyte-predominant HL		5%
Classical HL	Nodular sclerosing	70%
	Mixed cellularity	20%
	Lymphocyte-rich	5%
	Lymphocyte-depleted	Rare

24.57 Clinical stages of Hodgkin lymphoma (Ann Arbor classification)

Stage	Definition
I	Involvement of a single lymph node region (I) or extralymphatic* site (I_E)
II	Involvement of two or more lymph node regions (II) or an extralymphatic site and lymph node regions on the same side of (above or below) the diaphragm (II_E)
III	Involvement of lymph node regions on both sides of the diaphragm with (III_E) or without (III) localised extralymphatic involvement or involvement of the spleen (III_S), or both (III_{SE})
IV	Diffuse involvement of one or more extralymphatic tissues, e.g. liver or bone marrow

Each stage is subclassified:
- **A** No systemic symptoms
- **B** Weight loss > 10%, drenching sweats, fever

*The lymphatic structures are defined as the lymph nodes, spleen, thymus, Waldeyer's ring, appendix and Peyer's patches.

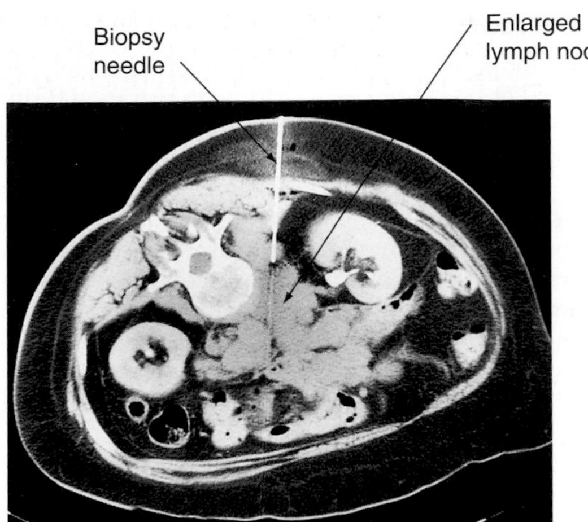

Fig. 24.29 CT-guided percutaneous needle biopsy of retroperitoneal nodes involved by lymphoma.

- *LDH measurements* showing raised levels are an adverse prognostic factor.
- *Chest X-ray* may show a mediastinal mass.
- *CT scan* of chest, abdomen and pelvis permits staging. Bulky disease (> 10 cm in a single node mass) is an adverse prognostic feature.
- *Lymph node biopsy* may be undertaken surgically or by percutaneous needle biopsy under radiological guidance (Fig. 24.29).

Management

Historically, radiotherapy to lymph nodes alone has been used to treat localised stage IA or stage IIA disease effectively, with no adverse prognostic features. Careful planning of radiotherapy is required to limit the doses delivered to normal tissues. Fertility is usually preserved after radiotherapy. Young women receiving breast irradiation during the treatment of chest disease have an increased risk of breast cancer and should participate in a screening programme. Patients continuing to smoke after lung irradiation are at particular risk of lung cancer.

Clinical trials have shown that patients with early-stage disease have better outcomes if chemotherapy is included in their treatment. The majority of HL patients are now treated with chemotherapy and adjunctive radiotherapy. The ABVD regimen (doxorubicin, vinblastine, bleomycin and dacarbazine) is widely used in the UK. Standard therapy of early-stage patients usually includes additional treatment with radiotherapy to the involved lymph nodes after four courses of ABVD. Treatment response is assessed clinically and by repeat CT and newer scanning modalities such as positron emission tomography (PET). ABVD chemotherapy can cause cardiac and pulmonary toxicity, due to doxorubicin and bleomycin, respectively. The incidence of infertility and secondary myelodysplasia/AML is low with this regime.

Patients with advanced-stage disease are most commonly managed with chemotherapy alone. Standard treatment in the UK is 6–8 cycles of ABVD, followed by an assessment of response. As with early disease, achieving PET-negative remission predicts a better long-term remission rate. Overall, the long-term disease control/cure rates are lower with advanced disease.

24.58 The Hasenclever prognostic index for advanced Hodgkin lymphoma

Score 1 for each of the following risk factors present at diagnosis:

- Age > 45 yrs
- Male gender
- Serum albumin < 40 g/L
- Haemoglobin < 105 g/L
- Stage IV disease
- White blood count > 15 × 10^9/L
- Lymphopenia < 0.6 × 10^9/L

Score	5-yr rate of freedom from progression (%)	5-yr rate of overall survival (%)
0–1	79	90
> 2	60	74
> 3	55	70
> 4	47	59

Patients with disease which is resistant to therapy may be considered for autologous HSCT (p. 1018).

Prognosis

Over 90% of patients with early-stage HL achieve complete remission when treated with chemotherapy followed by involved field radiotherapy, and the great majority are cured. The major challenge is how to reduce treatment intensity, and hence long-term toxicity, without reducing the excellent cure rates in this group.

Between 50 and 70% of those with advanced-stage HL can be cured. The Hasenclever index (Box 24.58) can be helpful in assigning approximate chances of cure when discussing treatment plans with patients. Patients who fail to respond to initial chemotherapy or relapse within a year have a poor prognosis but some may achieve long-term survival after autologous HSCT. Patients relapsing after 1 year may obtain long-term survival with further chemotherapy alone.

Non-Hodgkin lymphoma

Non-Hodgkin lymphoma (NHL) represents a monoclonal proliferation of lymphoid cells of B cell (70%) or T cell (30%) origin. The incidence of these tumours increases with age, to 62.8/million population per annum at age 75 years, and the overall rate is increasing at about 3% per year.

The epidemiology of NHL is shown in Box 24.59. Previous classifications were based principally on histological appearances. The current WHO classification stratifies according to cell lineage (T or B cells) and incorporates clinical features, histology, chromosomal abnormalities and cell surface markers of the malignant cells. Clinically, the most important factor is grade, which is a reflection of proliferation rate. High-grade NHL has high proliferation rates, rapidly produces symptoms, is fatal if untreated, but is potentially curable. Low-grade NHL has low proliferation rates, may be asymptomatic for many months before presentation, runs an indolent course, but is not curable by conventional therapy. Of all cases of NHL in the developed world, over two-thirds are either diffuse large B-cell NHL (high-grade) or follicular NHL (low-grade) (Fig. 24.30). Other forms of NHL, including Burkitt lymphoma, mantle cell lymphoma, MALT lymphomas and T-cell lymphomas, are less common.

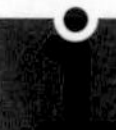

24.59 Epidemiology and aetiology of non-Hodgkin lymphoma

Incidence
- 12 new cases/100 000 people/year

Sex ratio
- Slight male excess

Age
- Median age 65–70 yrs

Aetiology
- No single causative abnormality described
- Lymphoma is a late manifestation of HIV infection (p. 405)
- Specific lymphoma types are associated with viruses: e.g. Epstein–Barr virus (EBV) with post-transplant NHL, human herpesvirus 8 (HHV8) with a primary effusion lymphoma, and human T-cell lymphotropic virus (HTLV) with adult T-cell leukaemia lymphoma
- Gastric lymphoma can be associated with *Helicobacter pylori* infection
- Some lymphomas are associated with specific chromosomal translocations; the t(14;18) in follicular lymphoma results in the dysregulated expression of the BCL-2 gene product, which inhibits apoptotic cell death. The t(8;14) found in Burkitt lymphoma and the t(11;14) in mantle cell lymphoma alter function of c-myc and cyclin D1, respectively, resulting in malignant proliferation
- Lymphoma occurs in congenital immunodeficiency states and in immunosuppressed patients after organ transplantation

A

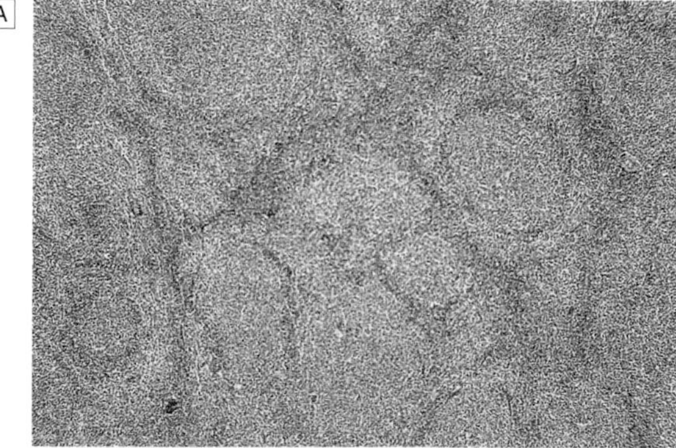

B

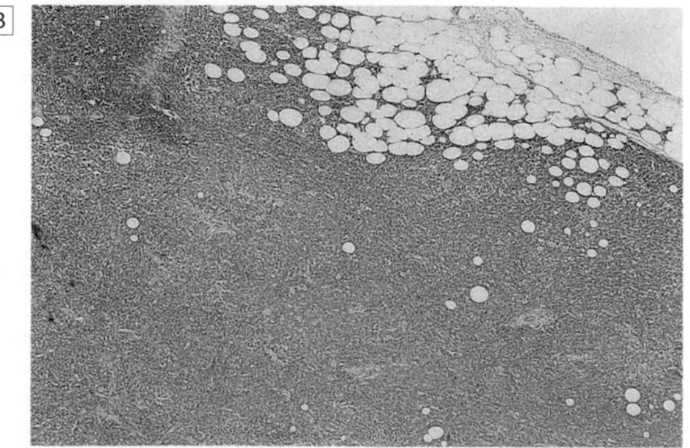

Fig. 24.30 Histology of non-Hodgkin lymphoma. **A** (Low-grade) follicular or nodular pattern. **B** (High-grade) diffuse pattern.

Clinical features

Unlike Hodgkin lymphoma, NHL is often widely disseminated at presentation, including in extranodal sites. Patients present with lymph node enlargement, which may be associated with systemic upset: weight loss, sweats, fever and itching. Hepatosplenomegaly may be present. Sites of extranodal involvement include the bone marrow, gut, thyroid, lung, skin, testis, brain and, more rarely, bone. Bone marrow involvement is more common in low-grade (50–60%) than high-grade (10%) disease. Compression syndromes may occur, including gut obstruction, ascites, superior vena cava obstruction and spinal cord compression.

The same staging system (see Box 24.57) is used for both HL and NHL, but NHL is more likely to be stage III or IV at presentation.

Investigations

These are as for HL, but in addition the following should be performed:

- *Bone marrow aspiration and trephine.*
- *Immunophenotyping of surface antigens to distinguish T from B cell tumours.* This may be done on blood, marrow or nodal material.
- *Cytogenetic analysis to detect chromosomal translocations* and molecular testing for T cell receptor or immunoglobulin gene rearrangements, if available.
- *Immunoglobulin determination.* Some lymphomas are associated with IgG or IgM paraproteins, which serve as markers for treatment response.
- *Measurement of uric acid levels.* Some very aggressive high-grade NHLs are associated with very high urate levels, which can precipitate renal failure when treatment is started.
- *HIV testing.* This may be appropriate if risk factors are present (p. 392).

Management

Low-grade NHL

Asymptomatic patients may not require therapy. Indications for treatment include marked systemic symptoms, lymphadenopathy causing discomfort or disfigurement, bone marrow failure or compression syndromes. In follicular lymphoma, the options are:

- *Radiotherapy.* This can be used for localised stage I disease, which is rare.
- *Chemotherapy.* Most patients will respond to oral therapy with chlorambucil, which is well tolerated but not curative. More intensive intravenous chemotherapy in younger patients produces better quality of life but no survival benefit. Humanised monoclonal antibodies ('biological' therapy; see p. 1102) can be used to target surface antigens on tumour cells, and induce tumour cell apoptosis directly. The anti-CD20 antibody rituximab has been shown to induce durable clinical responses in up to 60% of patients when given alone, and acts synergistically when given with chemotherapy. Rituximab (R) in combination with cyclophosphamide, vincristine and prednisolone (R-CVP) is commonly used as first-line therapy.
- *Transplantation.* Particular interest centres on the role of high-dose chemotherapy and HSCT in

EBM 24.60 Chemotherapy plus anti-CD20 therapy in high-grade non-Hodgkin lymphoma

'The addition of rituximab to CHOP chemotherapy in diffuse large B-cell NHL improved the 10-year overall survival from 27.6% to 43.5%.'

- Coiffier B, et al. Blood 2010; 116:2040–2045.

patients with relapsed disease. Such high-dose therapy improves disease-free survival but longer follow-up is awaited before conclusions can be drawn about cure.

High-grade NHL

Patients with diffuse large B-cell NHL need treatment at initial presentation:

- *Chemotherapy.* The majority (> 90%) are treated with intravenous combination chemotherapy, typically with the CHOP regimen (cyclophosphamide, doxorubicin, vincristine and prednisolone). When combined with CHOP chemotherapy, the biological therapy rituximab (R) increases the complete response rates and improves overall survival. R-CHOP is currently recommended as first-line therapy for those with stage II or greater diffuse large B-cell lymphoma (Box 24.60).
- *Radiotherapy.* A few stage I patients without bulky disease may be suitable for radiotherapy. Radiotherapy is also indicated for a residual localised site of bulk disease after chemotherapy, and for spinal cord and other compression syndromes.
- *HSCT.* Autologous HSCT (p. 1018) benefits patients with relapsed chemosensitive disease.

Prognosis

Low-grade NHL runs an indolent remitting and relapsing course, with an overall median survival of 10 years. Transformation to a high-grade NHL occurs in 3% per annum and is associated with poor survival.

In diffuse large B-cell high-grade NHL treated with R-CHOP, some 75% of patients overall respond initially to therapy and 50% will have disease-free survival at 5 years. The prognosis for patients with NHL is further refined according to the international prognostic index (IPI). For high-grade NHL, 5-year survival ranges from 75% in those with low-risk scores (age < 60 years, stage I or II, one or fewer extranodal sites, normal LDH and good performance status) to 25% in those with high-risk scores (increasing age, advanced stage, concomitant disease and a raised LDH).

Relapse is associated with a poor response to further chemotherapy (< 10% 5-year survival), but in patients under 65 years, HSCT improves survival.

Paraproteinaemias

A gammopathy refers to over-production of one or more classes of immunoglobulin. It may be polyclonal in association with acute or chronic inflammation, such as infection, sarcoidosis, autoimmune disorders or some malignancies. Alternatively, a monoclonal increase in a single immunoglobulin class may occur in association with normal or reduced levels of the other immunoglobulins. Such monoclonal proteins (also called M-proteins, paraproteins or monoclonal gammopathies) occur as a feature of myeloma, lymphoma and amyloidosis, in connective tissue disease such as rheumatoid arthritis or polymyalgia rheumatica, in infection such as HIV, and in solid tumours. In addition, they may be present with no underlying disease. Gammopathies are detected by plasma immunoelectrophoresis.

Monoclonal gammopathy of uncertain significance

In monoclonal gammopathy of uncertain significance (MGUS, also known as benign monoclonal gammopathy), a paraprotein is present in the blood but with no other features of myeloma, Waldenström macroglobulinaemia (see below), lymphoma or related disease. It is a common finding associated with increasing age; a paraprotein can be found in 1% of the population aged over 50 years, increasing to 5% over 80 years.

Clinical features and investigations

Patients are usually asymptomatic, and the paraprotein is found on blood testing for other reasons. The routine blood count and biochemistry are normal, the paraprotein is usually present in small amounts with no associated immune paresis, and there are no lytic bone lesions. The bone marrow may have increased plasma cells but these usually constitute less than 10% of nucleated cells.

Prognosis

After follow-up of 20 years, only one-quarter of cases will progress to myeloma or a related disorder (i.e. around 1% per annum). Patients with low-level IgG paraproteins without reductions in IgM and IgA levels and with normal serum free light chain level are highly unlikely to progress at any time.

Waldenström macroglobulinaemia

This is a low-grade lymphoplasmacytoid lymphoma associated with an IgM paraprotein, causing clinical features of hyperviscosity syndrome. It is a rare tumour occurring in the elderly and affects males more commonly.

Patients classically present with features of hyperviscosity, such as nosebleeds, bruising, confusion and visual disturbance. However, presentation may be with anaemia, systemic symptoms, splenomegaly or lymphadenopathy. Patients are found on investigation to have an IgM paraprotein associated with a raised plasma viscosity. The bone marrow has a characteristic appearance, with infiltration of lymphoid cells and prominent mast cells.

Management

If patients show symptoms of hyperviscosity and anaemia, plasmapheresis is required to remove IgM and make blood transfusion possible. Chemotherapy with alkylating agents, such as chlorambucil, has been the mainstay of treatment, controlling disease in over 50%. Fludarabine may be more effective but has more side-effects. Rituximab can also be effective. The median survival is 5 years.

Multiple myeloma

This is a malignant proliferation of plasma cells. Normal plasma cells are derived from B cells and produce immunoglobulins which contain heavy and light chains. Normal immunoglobulins are polyclonal, which means that a variety of heavy chains are produced and each may be of kappa or lambda light chain type (p. 77). In myeloma, plasma cells produce immunoglobulin of a single heavy and light chain, a monoclonal protein commonly referred to as a paraprotein. In some cases, only light chain is produced and this appears in the urine as Bence Jones proteinuria. The frequency of different isotypes of monoclonal protein in myeloma is shown in Box 24.61.

Although a small number of malignant plasma cells are present in the circulation, the majority are present in the bone marrow. The malignant plasma cells produce cytokines, which stimulate osteoclasts and result in net bone reabsorption. The resulting lytic lesions cause bone pain, fractures and hypercalcaemia. Marrow involvement can result in anaemia or pancytopenia.

24.61 Classification of multiple myeloma

Type of monoclonal (M)-protein	Relative frequency (%)
IgG	55
IgA	21
Light chain only	22
Others (D, E, non-secretory)	2

Clinical features and investigations

The incidence of myeloma is 4/100 000 new cases per annum, with a male to female ratio of 2:1. The median age at diagnosis is 60–70 years and the disease is more common in Afro-Caribbeans. The clinical features are demonstrated in Figure 24.31.

Diagnosis of myeloma requires two of the following criteria:

- increased malignant plasma cells in the bone marrow
- serum and/or urinary M-protein
- skeletal lytic lesions.

Bone marrow aspiration, plasma and urinary electrophoresis, and a skeletal survey are thus required. Other investigations are listed in Box 24.62. Normal immunoglobulin levels, i.e. the absence of immunoparesis, should cast doubt on the diagnosis. Paraproteinaemia can cause an elevated ESR (p. 85) but this is a non-specific test; only approximately 5% of patients with a persistently elevated ESR above 100 mm/hr have underlying myeloma.

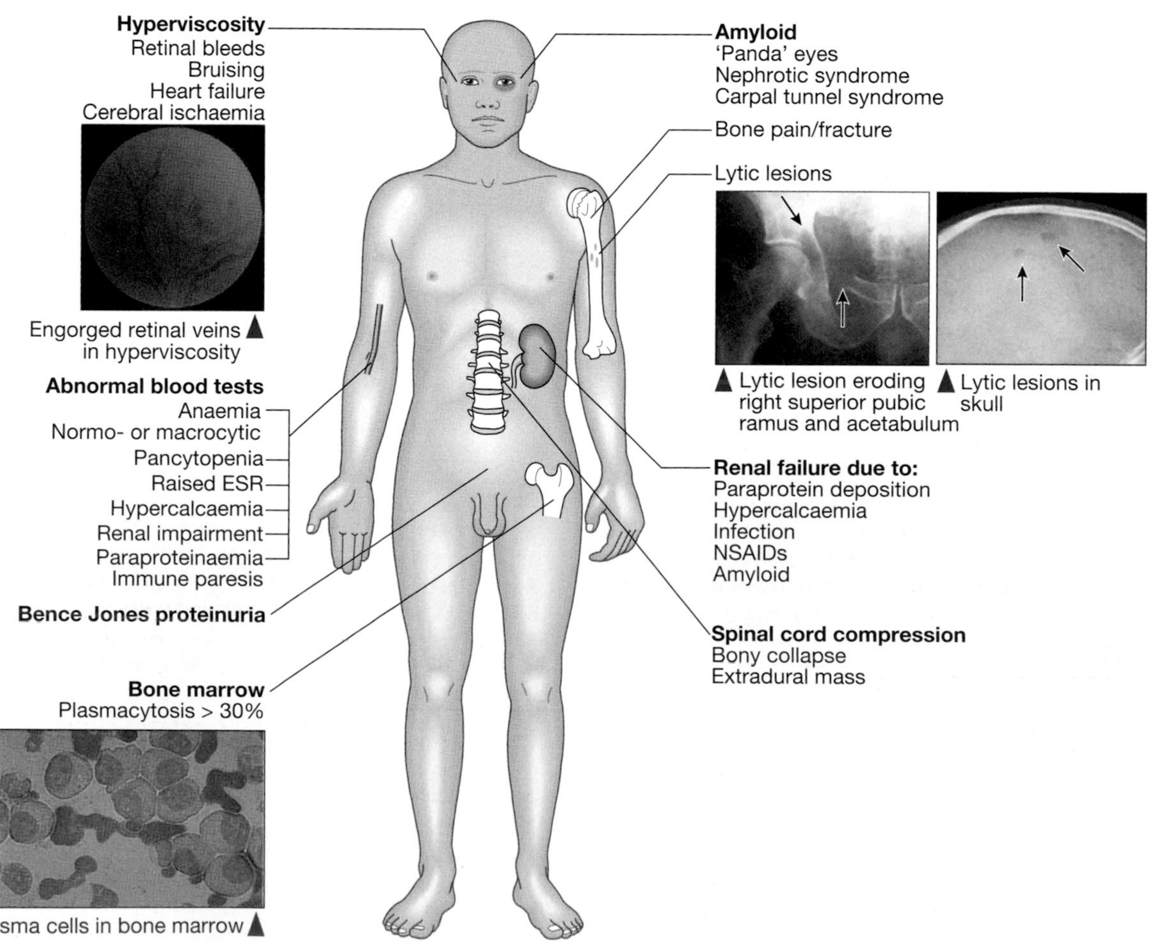

Fig. 24.31 Clinical and laboratory features of multiple myeloma.

24.62 Rationale for investigations in multiple myeloma

Question	Investigations
Presence of lytic lesions, bone fractures?	X-rays (skeletal survey)[1] Alkaline phosphatase[1]
Spinal cord compression?	MRI spine[2]
Presence of urine or plasma M-protein?	Blood and urine protein electrophoresis
Type of M-protein?	Blood and urine immunoelectrophoresis
Amount of M-protein?	Quantification of M-protein
Degree of immune paresis?	Plasma immunoglobulins
Presence of plasma cells in bone marrow?	Bone marrow aspiration and trephine
Degree of bone marrow failure?	Full blood count
Renal function?	Urea and electrolytes, creatinine, urate
Presence of hypercalcaemia?	Blood calcium and albumin
Poor prognostic factors at diagnosis?	β_2 microglobulin > 5.5 mg/L, albumin < 35 g/L

[1]In the absence of fractures, the plasma alkaline phosphatase and isotope bone scan will be normal despite the lytic lesions.
[2]All investigations shown above are routine in myeloma, except MRI of the spine, which is reserved for those with clinical indications.

EBM 24.63 Autologous haematopoietic stem cell transplantation in multiple myeloma

'The addition of autologous HSCT to conventional intravenous chemotherapy improves survival from 42 to 54 months.'

- Child JA, et al. N Engl J Med 2003; 348:1875–1883.

For further information: www.ukmf.org.uk

24.64 Haematological malignancy in old age

- **Median age**: approximately 70 yrs for most haematological malignancies.
- **Poor-risk biological features**: adverse cytogenetics or the presence of a multidrug resistance phenotype are more frequent.
- **Prognosis**: increasing age is an independent adverse variable in acute leukaemia and aggressive lymphoma.
- **Chemotherapy**: may be less well tolerated. Older people are more likely to have antecedent cardiac, pulmonary or metabolic problems, tolerate systemic infection less well and metabolise cytotoxic drugs differently.
- **Cure rates**: similar to those in younger patients, in those who do tolerate treatment.
- **Decision to treat**: should be based on the individual's biological status, the level of social support available, and the patient's wishes and those of the immediate family, but not on chronological age alone.

Management

If patients are asymptomatic with no evidence of end organ damage (e.g. to kidneys, bone marrow or bone), treatment may not be required.

Immediate support

- High fluid intake to treat renal impairment and hypercalcaemia (p. 767).
- Analgesia for bone pain.
- Bisphosphonates for hypercalcaemia and to delay other skeletal related events (p. 1123).
- Allopurinol to prevent urate nephropathy.
- Plasmapheresis, if necessary, for hyperviscosity.

Chemotherapy with or without HSCT

Myeloma therapy has improved with the addition of novel agents, initially thalidomide and more recently the proteasome inhibitor bortezomib, to first-line treatments. In older patients, thalidomide combined with the alkylating agent melphalan and prednisolone has increased the median overall survival to more than 4 years. Thalidomide has both anti-angiogenic effects against tumour blood vessels and immunomodulatory effects. It can cause somnolence, constipation, peripheral neuropathy and thrombosis. It is vital that females of child-bearing age use adequate contraception, as thalidomide is teratogenic. Treatment is administered until paraprotein levels have stopped falling. This is termed 'plateau phase' and can last for weeks or years.

In younger, fitter patients, standard treatment includes first-line chemotherapy to maximum response and then an autologous HSCT, which improves quality of life and prolongs survival (Box 24.63) but does not cure myeloma. The role of allogeneic transplantation (p. 1017) and of reduced-intensity allografting after autologous transplantation in younger patients is under evaluation.

When myeloma progresses, treatment is given to induce a further plateau phase. In the UK at present, bortezomib is recommended, followed by lenalidomide if there is subsequent progression.

Radiotherapy

This is effective for localised bone pain not responding to simple analgesia and for pathological fractures. It is also useful for the emergency treatment of spinal cord compression complicating extradural plasmacytomas.

Bisphosphonates

Long-term bisphosphonate therapy reduces bone pain and skeletal events. These drugs protect bone (p. 1123) and may cause apoptosis of malignant plasma cells. There is evidence that intravenous zoledronate in combination with anti-myeloma therapy confers a survival advantage over oral bisphosphonates. Osteonecrosis of the jaw may be associated with long-term use; therefore regular dental review is advisable.

Prognosis

The international staging system (ISS) identifies poor prognostic features, including a high β_2-microglobulin and low albumin at diagnosis (ISS stage 3, median survival 29 months). Those with a normal albumin and a low β_2-microglobulin (ISS stage 1) have a median survival of 62 months. Use of autologous HSCT and advances in drug therapy have increased survival, with over one-third of patients now surviving for 5 years, compared with only one-quarter 10 years ago. The outlook may improve further with new drugs and combinations of treatments.

APLASTIC ANAEMIA

Primary idiopathic acquired aplastic anaemia

This is a rare disorder in Europe and North America, with 2–4 new cases per million population per annum. The disease is much more common in certain other parts of the world: for example, east Asia. The basic problem is failure of the pluripotent stem cells, producing hypoplasia of the bone marrow with a pancytopenia in the blood. The diagnosis rests on exclusion of other causes of secondary aplastic anaemia (see below) and rare congenital causes, such as Fanconi's anaemia.

Clinical features and investigations

Patients present with symptoms of bone marrow failure, usually anaemia or bleeding, and less commonly, infections. An FBC demonstrates pancytopenia, low reticulocytes and often macrocytosis. Bone marrow aspiration and trephine reveal hypocellularity.

Management

All patients will require blood product support and aggressive management of infection. The prognosis of severe aplastic anaemia managed with supportive therapy only is poor and more than 50% of patients die, usually in the first year. The curative treatment for patients under 30 years of age with severe idiopathic aplastic anaemia is allogeneic HSCT if there is an available donor (p. 1017). Those with a compatible sibling donor should proceed to transplantation as soon as possible; they have a 75–90% chance of long-term cure. In older patients, immunosuppressive therapy with ciclosporin and antithymocyte globulin gives 5-year survival rates of 75%. Such patients may relapse or other clonal disorders of haematopoiesis may evolve, such as paroxysmal nocturnal haemoglobinuria (p. 1031), myelodysplastic syndrome (p. 1041) and acute myeloid leukaemia (p. 1036). They must be followed up long-term.

Secondary aplastic anaemia

Causes of this condition are listed in Box 24.65. It is not practical to list all the drugs which have been suspected of causing aplasia. It is important to check the reported side-effects of all drugs taken over the preceding months. In some instances, the cytopenia is more selective and affects only one cell line, most often the neutrophils. Frequently, this is an incidental finding, with no ill health. It probably has an immune basis but this is difficult to prove.

The clinical features and methods of diagnosis are the same as for primary idiopathic aplastic anaemia. An underlying cause should be treated or removed but otherwise management is as for the idiopathic form.

24.65 Causes of secondary aplastic anaemia

- Drugs
  - Cytotoxic drugs
  - Antibiotics – chloramphenicol, sulphonamides
  - Antirheumatic agents – penicillamine, gold, phenylbutazone, indometacin
  - Antithyroid drugs
  - Anticonvulsants
  - Immunosuppressants – azathioprine
- Chemicals
  - Benzene toluene solvent misuse – glue-sniffing
  - Insecticides – chlorinated hydrocarbons (DDT), organophosphates and carbamates (pp. 220 and 222)
- Radiation
- Viral hepatitis
- Pregnancy
- Paroxysmal nocturnal haemoglobinuria

MYELOPROLIFERATIVE NEOPLASMS

These make up a group of chronic conditions characterised by clonal proliferation of marrow precursor cells, and include polycythaemia rubra vera (PRV), essential thrombocythaemia, myelofibrosis, and chronic myeloid leukaemia (p. 1039). Although the majority of patients are classifiable as having one of these disorders, some have overlapping features and there is often progression from one to another, e.g. PRV to myelofibrosis. The recent discovery of the molecular basis of these disorders will lead to changes in classification and treatment; a mutation in the gene on chromosome 9 encoding the signal transduction molecule *JAK-2* has been found in more than 90% of PRV cases and 50% of those with essential thrombocythaemia and myelofibrosis.

Myelofibrosis

In myelofibrosis, the marrow is initially hypercellular, with an excess of abnormal megakaryocytes which release growth factors, e.g. platelet-derived growth factor, to the marrow microenvironment, resulting in a reactive proliferation of fibroblasts. As the disease progresses, the marrow becomes fibrosed.

Most patients present over the age of 50 years, with lassitude, weight loss and night sweats. The spleen can be massively enlarged due to extramedullary haematopoiesis (blood cell formation outside the bone marrow), and painful splenic infarcts may occur.

The characteristic blood picture is leucoerythroblastic anaemia, with circulating immature red blood cells (increased reticulocytes and nucleated red blood cells) and granulocyte precursors (myelocytes). The red cells are shaped like teardrops (teardrop poikilocytes), and giant platelets may be seen in the blood. The white count varies from low to moderately high, and the platelet count may be high, normal or low. Urate levels may be high due to increased cell breakdown, and folate deficiency is common. The marrow is often difficult to aspirate and a trephine biopsy shows an excess of megakaryocytes, increased reticulin and fibrous tissue replacement. The presence of a *JAK-2* mutation supports the diagnosis.

Management and prognosis

Median survival is 4 years from diagnosis, but ranges from 1 year to over 20 years. Treatment is directed at control of symptoms, e.g. red cell transfusions for anaemia. Folic acid should be given to prevent deficiency. Cytotoxic therapy with hydroxycarbamide may help control spleen size, the white cell count or systemic symptoms. Splenectomy may be required for a grossly enlarged spleen or symptomatic pancytopenia secondary to splenic pooling of cells and hypersplenism. HSCT may be considered for younger patients. Ruxolitinib, an inhibitor of *JAK-2*, has recently been licensed for use.

Essential thrombocythaemia

Increased proliferation of megakaryocytes results in a raised level of circulating platelets that are often dysfunctional. Prior to making a diagnosis of essential thrombocythaemia (ET), reactive causes of thrombocytosis must be excluded (p. 1008). The presence of a *JAK-2* mutation supports the diagnosis but is not universal. Patients present at a median age of 60 years with vascular occlusion or bleeding, or with an asymptomatic isolated raised platelet count. A small percentage transform to acute leukaemia and others to myelofibrosis.

It is likely that most patients with ET benefit from low-dose aspirin to reduce the risk of occlusive vascular events. Low-risk patients (age < 40 years, platelet count < 1000×10^9/L and no bleeding or thrombosis) may not require treatment to reduce the platelet count. For those with a platelet count above 1000×10^9/L, with symptoms, or with other risk factors for thrombosis such as diabetes or hypertension, treatment to control platelet counts should be given. Agents include oral hydroxycarbamide or anagrelide, an inhibitor of megakaryocyte maturation. Intravenous radioactive phosphorus (^{32}P) may be useful in old age.

Polycythaemia rubra vera

Polycythaemia rubra vera (PRV) occurs mainly in patients over the age of 40 years and presents either as an incidental finding of a high haemoglobin, or with symptoms of hyperviscosity, such as lassitude, loss of concentration, headaches, dizziness, blackouts, pruritus and epistaxis. Some patients present with manifestations of peripheral arterial disease or a cerebrovascular accident. Venous thromboembolism may also occur. Peptic ulceration is common, sometimes complicated by bleeding. Patients are often plethoric and many have a palpable spleen at diagnosis.

Investigation of polycythaemia is discussed on page 1002. The diagnosis of PRV now rests upon the demonstration of a high haematocrit and the presence of the *JAK-2* mutation. In the occasional *JAK-2*-negative cases, a raised red cell mass and absence of causes of a secondary erythrocytosis must be established. The spleen is enlarged, neutrophil and platelet counts are frequently raised, an abnormal karyotype may be found in the marrow, and in vitro culture of the marrow can be used to demonstrate autonomous growth in the absence of added growth factors.

Management and prognosis

Aspirin reduces the risk of thrombosis. Venesection gives prompt relief of hyperviscosity symptoms. Between 400 and 500 mL of blood (less if the patient is elderly) are removed and the venesection is repeated every 5–7 days until the haematocrit is reduced to below 45%. Less frequent but regular venesection will maintain this level until the haemoglobin remains reduced because of iron deficiency.

Suppression of marrow proliferation with hydroxycarbamide or interferon-alfa may reduce the risk of vascular occlusion, control spleen size and reduce transformation to myelofibrosis. Radioactive phosphorus (5 mCi of ^{32}P IV) is reserved for older patients, as it increases the risk of transformation to acute leukaemia by 6- to 10-fold.

Median survival after diagnosis in treated patients exceeds 10 years. Some patients survive more than 20 years; however, cerebrovascular or coronary events occur in up to 60% of patients. The disease may convert to another myeloproliferative disorder, with about 25% developing acute leukaemia or myelofibrosis.

BLEEDING DISORDERS

Disorders of primary haemostasis

The initial formation of the platelet plug (see Fig. 24.6A, p. 996; also known as 'primary haemostasis') may fail in thrombocytopenia (p. 1007), von Willebrand disease (p. 1053), and also in platelet function disorders and diseases affecting the vessel wall.

Vessel wall abnormalities

Vessel wall abnormalities may be:

- congenital, such as hereditary haemorrhagic telangiectasia
- acquired, as in a vasculitis (p. 1115) or scurvy.

Hereditary haemorrhagic telangiectasia

Hereditary haemorrhagic telangiectasia (HHT) is a dominantly inherited condition caused by mutations in the genes encoding endoglin and activin receptor-like kinase, which are endothelial cell receptors for transforming growth factor-beta (TGF-β), a potent angiogenic cytokine. Telangiectasia and small aneurysms are found on the fingertips, face and tongue, and in the nasal passages, lung and gastrointestinal tract. A significant proportion of these patients develop larger pulmonary arteriovenous malformations (PAVMs) that cause arterial hypoxaemia due to a right-to-left shunt. These predispose to paradoxical embolism, resulting in stroke or cerebral abscess. All patients with HHT should be screened for PAVMs; if these are found, ablation by percutaneous embolisation should be considered.

Patients present either with recurrent bleeds, particularly epistaxis, or with iron deficiency due to occult gastrointestinal bleeding. Treatment can be difficult because of the multiple bleeding points but regular iron therapy often allows the marrow to compensate for blood loss. Local cautery or laser therapy may prevent single lesions from bleeding. A variety of medical therapies have been tried but none has been found to be universally effective.

Ehlers–Danlos disease

Vascular Ehlers–Danlos syndrome (type 4) is a rare autosomal dominant disorder (1/100 000) caused by a defect in type 3 collagen which results in fragile blood vessels and organ membranes, leading to bleeding and organ rupture. Classical joint hypermobility (p. 1134) is often limited in this form of the disease but skin changes and facial appearance are typical. The diagnosis should be considered when there is a history of bleeding but normal laboratory tests.

Scurvy

Vitamin C deficiency affects the normal synthesis of collagen and results in a bleeding disorder characterised by perifollicular and petechial haemorrhage, bruising and subperiosteal bleeding. The key to diagnosis is the dietary history (p. 129).

Platelet function disorders

Bleeding may result from thrombocytopenia (see Box 24.14, p. 1007) or from congenital or acquired abnormalities of platelet function. The most common acquired disorders are iatrogenic, resulting from the use of aspirin, clopidogrel, dipyridamole and the IIb/IIIa inhibitors to prevent arterial thrombosis (see Box 24.29, p. 1019). Inherited platelet function abnormalities are relatively rare. Congenital abnormalities may be due to deficiency of the membrane glycoproteins, e.g. Glanzmann's thrombasthenia (IIb/IIIa) or Bernard–Soulier disease (Ib), or due to the presence of defective platelet granules, e.g. a deficiency of dense (delta) granules (see Fig. 24.7, p. 998) giving rise to storage pool disorders. The congenital macrothrombocytopathies that are due to mutations in the myosin heavy chain gene *MYH-9* are characterised by large platelets, inclusion bodies in the neutrophils (Döhle bodies) and a variety of other features, including sensorineural deafness and renal abnormalities.

Apart from Glanzmann's thrombasthenia, these conditions are mild disorders, with bleeding typically occurring after trauma or surgery but rarely spontaneously. Glanzmann's is an autosomal recessive condition associated with a variable but often severe bleeding disorder. These conditions are usually managed by local mechanical measures, but antifibrinolytics, such as tranexamic acid, may be useful and, in severe bleeding, platelet transfusion may be required. Recombinant VIIa is licensed for the treatment of resistant bleeding in Glanzmann's thrombasthenia.

Thrombocytopenia

Thrombocytopenia occurs in many disease processes, as listed in Box 24.14 (p. 1007), many of which are discussed elsewhere in this chapter.

Idiopathic thrombocytopenic purpura

Idiopathic thrombocytopenic purpura (ITP) is mediated by autoantibodies, most often directed against the platelet membrane glycoprotein IIb/IIIa, which sensitise the platelet, resulting in premature removal from the circulation by cells of the reticulo-endothelial system. It is not a single disorder; some cases occur in isolation while others are associated with underlying immune dysregulation in conditions such as connective tissue diseases, HIV infection, B cell malignancies, pregnancy and certain drug therapies. However, the clinical presentation and pathogenesis are similar, whatever the cause of ITP.

Clinical features and investigations

The presentation depends on the degree of thrombocytopenia. Spontaneous bleeding typically occurs only when the platelet count is below 20×10^9/L. At higher counts, the patient may complain of easy bruising or sometimes epistaxis or menorrhagia. Many cases with counts of more than 50×10^9/L are discovered by chance.

In adults, ITP more commonly affects females and may have an insidious onset. Unlike ITP in children, it is unusual for there to be a history of a preceding viral infection. Symptoms or signs of a connective tissue disease may be apparent at presentation or emerge several years later. Patients aged over 65 years should have a bone marrow examination to look for an accompanying B cell malignancy and appropriate autoantibody testing performed if a diagnosis of connective tissue disease is likely. HIV testing should be considered. The peripheral blood film is normal, apart from a greatly reduced platelet number, whilst the bone marrow reveals an obvious increase in megakaryocytes.

Management

Many patients with stable compensated ITP and a platelet count of more than 30×10^9/L do not require treatment to raise the platelet count, except at times of increased bleeding risk, such as surgery and biopsy. First-line therapy for patients with spontaneous bleeding is with prednisolone 1 mg/kg daily to suppress antibody production and inhibit phagocytosis of sensitised platelets by reticuloendothelial cells. Administration of intravenous immunoglobulin (IVIg) can raise the platelet count by blocking antibody receptors on reticuloendothelial cells, and is combined with corticosteroid therapy if there is severe haemostatic failure or a slow response to steroids alone. Persistent or potentially life-threatening bleeding should be treated with platelet transfusion in addition to the other therapies.

The condition may become chronic, with remissions and relapses. Relapses should be treated by re-introducing corticosteroids. If a patient has two relapses, or primary refractory disease, splenectomy is considered, with the precautions shown in Box 24.40 (p. 1028). Splenectomy produces complete remission in about 70% of patients and improvement in a further 20–25%, so that, following splenectomy, only 5–10% of patients require further medical therapy. If severe thrombocytopenia with or without significant bleeding persists despite splenectomy, second-line therapy with the thrombopoietin analogue romiplostim or the thrombopoietin receptor agonist eltrombopag should be considered. Low-dose corticosteroid therapy, immunosuppressants such as rituximab, ciclosporin and tacrolimus should be considered in cases where the approaches above are ineffective.

Coagulation disorders

Normal coagulation is explained in Figure 24.6 (p. 996). Coagulation factor deficiency may be congenital or acquired, and may affect one or several of the coagulation factors (Box 24.66). Inherited disorders are almost uniformly related to decreased synthesis, as a result of

24.66 Causes of coagulopathy

Congenital

X-linked
- Haemophilia A and B

Autosomal
- Von Willebrand disease
- Factor II, V, VII, X, XI and XIII deficiencies
- Combined II, VII, IX and X deficiency
- Combined V and VIII deficiency
- Hypofibrinogenaemia
- Dysfibrinogenaemia

Acquired

Under-production
- Liver failure

Increased consumption
- Coagulation activation
  Disseminated intravascular coagulation (DIC)
- Immune-mediated
  Acquired haemophilia and von Willebrand syndrome
- Others
  Acquired factor X deficiency (in amyloid)
  Acquired von Willebrand syndrome in Wilms tumour

Drug-induced

Inhibition of function
- Heparins
- Argatroban
- Fondaparinux
- Rivaroxaban
- Apixaban
- Dabigatran

Inhibition of synthesis
- Warfarin

mutation in the gene encoding a key protein in coagulation. Von Willebrand disease is the most common inherited bleeding disorder. Haemophilia A and B are the most common single coagulation factor deficiencies, but inherited deficiencies of all the other coagulation factors are seen. Acquired disorders may be due to under-production (e.g. in liver failure), increased consumption (e.g. in disseminated intravascular coagulation) or inhibition of function (such as heparin therapy or immune inhibitors of coagulation, e.g. acquired haemophilia A).

Haemophilia A

Factor VIII deficiency resulting in haemophilia A affects 1/10 000 individuals. It is the most common congenital coagulation factor deficiency. Factor VIII is primarily synthesised by the liver and endothelial cells, and has a half-life of about 12 hours. It is protected from proteolysis in the circulation by binding to von Willebrand factor (vWF).

Genetics

The factor VIII gene is located on the X chromosome. Severe haemophilia is associated with large deletions, while single-base changes more often result in moderate or mild disease (Box 24.67). As the gene is on the X chromosome, haemophilia A is a sex-linked disorder (p. 53). Thus all daughters of haemophiliacs are obligate carriers and they, in turn, have a 1 in 4 chance of each pregnancy resulting in the birth of an affected male

24.67 Severity of haemophilia (ISTH criteria)

Severity	Factor VIII or IX level	Clinical presentation
Severe	< 0.01 U/mL	Spontaneous haemarthroses and muscle haematomas
Moderate	0.01–0.05 U/mL	Mild trauma or surgery causes bleeding
Mild	> 0.05 to 0.4 U/mL	Major injury or surgery results in excess bleeding

(ISTH = International Society on Thrombosis and Haemostasis)

baby, a normal male baby, a carrier female or a normal female. Antenatal diagnosis by chorionic villous sampling is possible in families with a known mutation.

Haemophilia 'breeds true' within a family; all members have the same factor VIII gene mutation and a similarly severe or mild phenotype. Female carriers of haemophilia may have reduced factor VIII levels because of random inactivation of their normal X chromosome in the developing fetus (lyonisation). This can result in a mild bleeding disorder; thus all known or suspected carriers of haemophilia should have their factor VIII level measured.

Clinical features

The extent and patterns of bleeding are closely related to residual factor VIII levels. Patients with severe haemophilia (< 1% of normal factor VIII levels) present with spontaneous bleeding into skin, muscle and joints. Retroperitoneal and intracranial bleeding is also a feature. Babies with severe haemophilia have an increased risk of intracranial haemorrhage and, although there is insufficient evidence to recommend routine caesarean section for these births, it is appropriate to avoid head trauma and to perform imaging of the newborn within the first 24 hours of life. Individuals with moderate and mild haemophilia (factor VIII levels 1–40%) present with the same pattern of bleeding, but usually after trauma or surgery, when bleeding is greater than would be expected from the severity of the insult.

The major morbidity of recurrent bleeding in severe haemophilia is musculoskeletal. Bleeding is typically into large joints, especially knees, elbows, ankles and hips. Muscle haematomas are also characteristic, most commonly in the calf and psoas muscles. If early treatment is not given to arrest bleeding, a hot, swollen and very painful joint or muscle haematoma develops. Recurrent bleeding into joints leads to synovial hypertrophy, destruction of the cartilage and secondary osteoarthrosis (Fig. 24.32). Complications of muscle haematomas depend on their location. A large psoas bleed may extend to compress the femoral nerve; calf haematomas may increase pressure within the inflexible fascial sheath, causing a compartment syndrome with ischaemia, necrosis, fibrosis, and subsequent contraction and shortening of the Achilles tendon.

Management

In severe haemophilia A, bleeding episodes should be treated by raising the factor VIII level, usually by

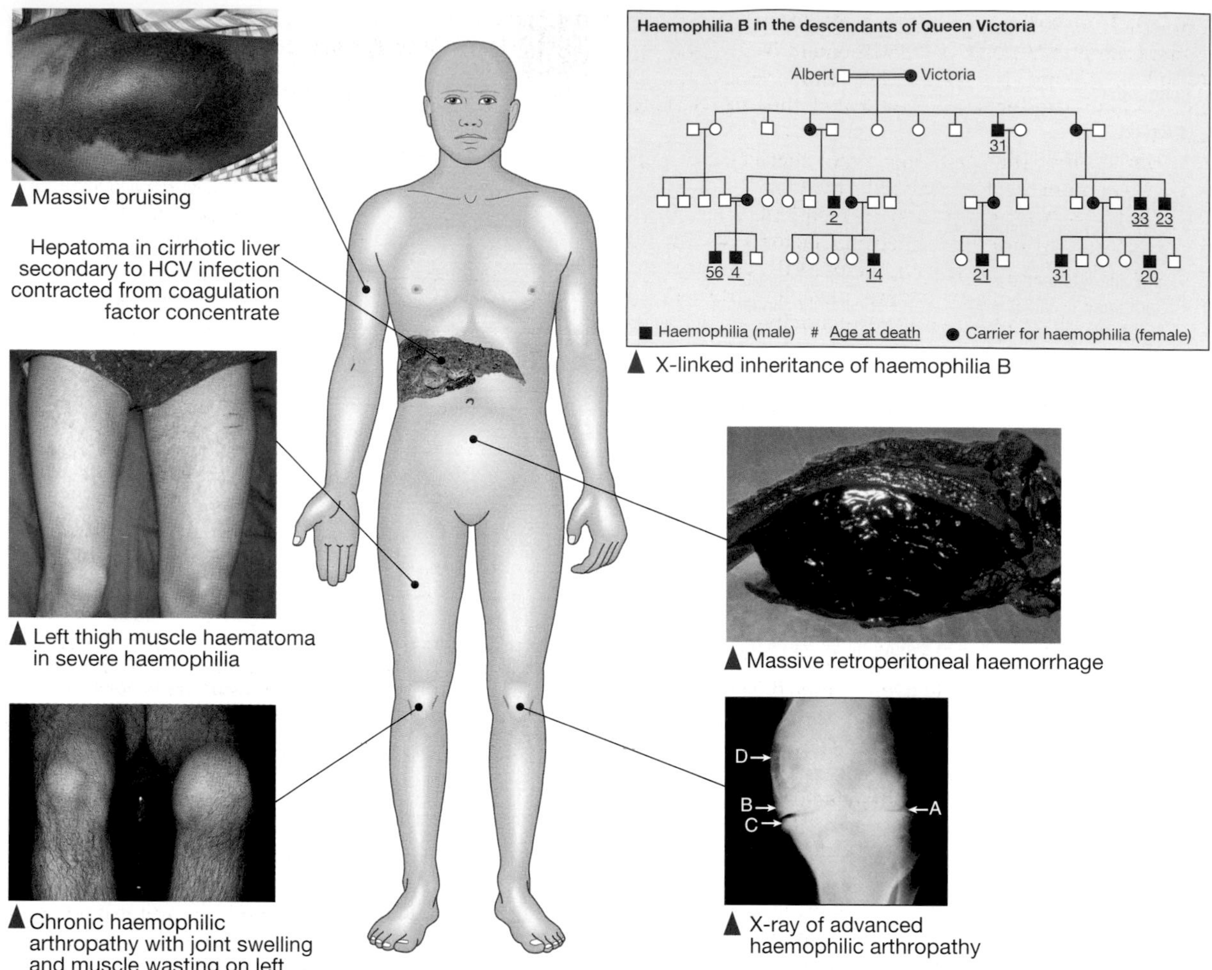

Fig. 24.32 Clinical manifestations of haemophilia. On the knee X-ray, repeated bleeds have led to broadening of the femoral epicondyles, and there is no cartilage present, as evidenced by the close proximity of the femur and tibia (A); sclerosis (B), osteophyte (C) and bony cysts (D) are present. (HCV = hepatitis C virus). *Inset (Massive bruising)* From Hoffbrand 2000 – see p. 1056.

intravenous infusion of factor VIII concentrate. Factor VIII concentrates are freeze-dried and stable at 4°C and can therefore be stored in domestic refrigerators, allowing patients to treat themselves at home at the earliest indication of bleeding. Factor VIII concentrate prepared from blood donor plasma is now screened for HBV, HCV and HIV, and undergoes two separate virus inactivation processes during manufacture; these preparations have a good safety record. However, factor VIII concentrates prepared by recombinant technology are now widely available and, although more expensive, are perceived as being safer than those derived from human plasma. In addition to raising factor VIII concentrations, resting of the bleeding site by either bed rest or a splint reduces continuing haemorrhage. Once bleeding has settled, the patient should be mobilised and physiotherapy used to restore strength to the surrounding muscles. All non-immune potential recipients of pooled blood products should be offered hepatitis A and B immunisation.

The vasopressin receptor agonist DDAVP (p. 794) raises the vWF and factor VIII levels by 3–4-fold, which is useful in arresting bleeding in patients with mild or moderate haemophilia A. The dose required for this purpose is higher than that used in diabetes insipidus, usually 0.3 μg/kg given intravenously or subcutaneously. Alternatively, the same effect can be achieved by intranasal administration of 300 μg. Following repeated administration of DDAVP, patients need to be monitored for evidence of water retention, which can result in significant hyponatraemia. DDAVP is contraindicated in patients with a history of severe arterial disease because of a propensity to provoke a thrombotic event.

In addition to treatment 'on demand' for bleeding, factor VIII can be administered 2 or 3 times per week as 'prophylaxis' to prevent bleeding in severe haemophilia. This is most appropriate in children, but its widespread use is limited by the high cost of factor VIII preparations. New concentrates of factor VIII (and factor IX) will soon add to the treatment options for these conditions.

Complications of coagulation factor therapy

Before 1986, coagulation factor concentrates from human plasma were not virally inactivated with heat or chemicals, and many patients became infected with HIV and hepatitis viruses HBV and HCV. In exposed patients with severe haemophilia, infection with HCV is almost universal, 80–90% have evidence of HBV exposure, and 60% became HIV-positive. Management is described in Chapters 23 and 14. Since 1989, viral inactivation of these blood products has eradicated the risk of viral infection.

Concern that the infectious agent that causes vCJD (p. 1211) might be transmissible by blood and blood products has been confirmed in recipients of red cell transfusion, and in one recipient of factor VIII. Pooled plasma products, including factor VIII concentrate, are now manufactured from plasma collected in countries with a low incidence of bovine spongiform encephalopathy.

Another serious complication of factor VIII infusion is the development of anti-factor VIII antibodies, which arise in about 20% of severe haemophiliacs. Such antibodies rapidly neutralise therapeutic infusions, making treatment relatively ineffective. Infusions of activated clotting factors, e.g. VIIa or factor VIII inhibitor bypass activity (FEIBA), may stop bleeding.

Haemophilia B (Christmas disease)

Aberrations of the factor IX gene, which is also present on the X chromosome, result in a reduction of the plasma factor IX level, giving rise to haemophilia B. This disorder is clinically indistinguishable from haemophilia A but is less common. The frequency of bleeding episodes is related to the severity of the deficiency of the plasma factor IX level. Treatment is with a factor IX concentrate, used in much the same way as factor VIII for haemophilia A. Although factor IX concentrates shared the problems of virus transmission seen with factor VIII, they do not commonly induce inhibitor antibodies (< 1% patients); when this does occur, however, it may be heralded by the development of a severe allergic-type reaction.

Von Willebrand disease

Von Willebrand disease is a common but usually mild bleeding disorder caused by a quantitative (types 1 and 3) or qualitative (type 2) deficiency of von Willebrand factor (vWF), a protein synthesised by endothelial cells and megakaryocytes, which is involved in both platelet function and coagulation. It normally forms a multimeric structure which is essential for its interaction with subendothelial collagen and platelets (see Fig. 24.7, p. 998). vWF acts as a carrier protein for factor VIII, to which it is non-covalently bound; deficiency of vWF lowers the plasma factor VIII level. vWF also forms bridges between platelets and subendothelial components (e.g. collagen; see Fig. 24.6, p. 996), allowing platelets to adhere to damaged vessel walls; deficiency of vWF therefore leads to impaired platelet plug formation. Blood group antigens (A and B) are expressed on vWF, reducing its susceptibility to proteolysis; as a result, people with blood group O have lower circulating vWF levels than individuals with non-O groups. This needs to be borne in mind when making a diagnosis of von Willebrand disease.

Most patients with von Willebrand disease have a type 1 disorder, characterised by a quantitative decrease in a normal functional protein. Patients with type 2 disorders inherit vWF molecules that are functionally abnormal. The type of abnormality depends on the site of the mutation in the *vWD* gene. Patients with mutations in platelet binding have type 2A disease, those with mutations in the platelet glycoprotein Ib binding site have type 2B, those with mutations in the factor VIII binding site have type 2N disease, and those with other abnormalities in platelet binding have type 2M. The patterns of laboratory abnormality accompanying these types are described in Box 24.68. The gene for vWF is located on chromosome 12 and the disease is usually inherited as an autosomal dominant, except in cases of type 2N and type 3, when it is recessive.

24.68 Classification of von Willebrand disease

Type	Defect	Inheritance	Investigations
1	Partial quantitative	AD	Parallel decrease in vWF: Ag and VIII:c
2A	Qualitative	AD	Absent HWM of vWF Ratio of vWF activity to antigen < 0.7
2B	Qualitative	AD	Reduced HWM of vWF Enhanced platelet agglutination (RIPA)
2M	Qualitative	AD	Normal multimers of vWF Abnormal platelets Interactions
2N	Qualitative	AR	Defective binding of vWF to VIII Low VIII
3	Severe quantitative	AR or CH	Very low vWF activity and VIII:c Absent multimers

(AD = autosomal dominant; AR = autosomal recessive; CH = compound heterozygote; HWM = high-weight multimers of vWF; RIPA = ristocetin-induced platelet agglutination; VIII:c = coagulation factor VIII activity in functional assay; vWF = von Willebrand factor; vWF:Ag = vWF antigen measured by ELISA)

Clinical features

Patients present with haemorrhagic manifestations similar to those in individuals with reduced platelet function. Superficial bruising, epistaxis, menorrhagia and gastrointestinal haemorrhage are common. Bleeding episodes are usually much less common than in severe haemophilia and excessive haemorrhage may only be observed after trauma or surgery. Within a single family, the disease has variable penetrance, so that some members may have quite severe and frequent bleeds, whereas others are relatively asymptomatic.

Investigations

The disorder is characterised by reduced activity of vWF and factor VIII. The disease can be classified using a combination of assays which include functional and antigenic measures of vWF, multimeric analysis of the protein, and specific tests of function to determine binding to platelet glycoprotein Ib (RIPA) and factor VIII (see Box 24.68). In addition, analysis for mutations in the *vWF* gene is informative in most cases.

Management

Many episodes of mild haemorrhage can be successfully treated by local means or with DDAVP, which raises the vWF level, resulting in a secondary increase in factor VIII.

Tranexamic acid may be useful in mucosal bleeding. For more serious or persistent bleeds, haemostasis can be achieved with selected factor VIII concentrates which contain considerable quantities of vWF in addition to factor VIII. Young children and patients with severe arterial disease should not receive DDAVP, and patients with type 2B disease develop thrombocytopenia which may be troublesome following DDAVP. Bleeding in type 3 patients responds to nothing apart from concentrate.

Rare inherited bleeding disorders

Severe deficiencies of factor VII, X and XIII occur as autosomal recessive disorders. They are rare but are associated with severe bleeding. Typical features include haemorrhage from the umbilical stump and intracranial haemorrhage. Factor XIII deficiency is typically associated with female infertility.

Factor XI deficiency may occur in heterozygous or homozygous individuals. Bleeding is very variable and is not accurately predicted by coagulation factor levels. In general, severe bleeding is confined to patients with levels below 15% of normal.

Acquired bleeding disorders

Disseminated intravascular coagulation (DIC) is an important cause of bleeding which begins with exaggerated and inappropriate intravascular coagulation. It is discussed under thrombotic disease on page 1055.

Liver disease

In severe parenchymal liver disease (Ch. 23), bleeding may arise from many different causes. Pathological sources of potential major bleeding, such as oesophageal varices or peptic ulcer, are more likely. There is reduced hepatic synthesis: for example, of factors V, VII, VIII, IX, X, XI, prothrombin and fibrinogen. Clearance of plasminogen activator is reduced. Thrombocytopenia may occur secondary to hypersplenism in portal hypertension. In cholestatic jaundice, there is reduced vitamin K absorption, leading to deficiency of factors II, VII, IX and X. Treatment with plasma products or platelet transfusion should be reserved for acute bleeds or to cover interventional procedures such as liver biopsy. Vitamin K deficiency can be readily corrected with parenteral administration of vitamin K.

Renal failure

The severity of the haemorrhagic state in renal failure is proportional to the plasma urea concentration (p. 478). Bleeding manifestations are those of platelet dysfunction, with gastrointestinal haemorrhage being particularly common. The causes are multifactorial, including anaemia, mild thrombocytopenia and the accumulation of low molecular weight waste products, normally excreted by the kidney, which inhibit platelet function. Treatment is by dialysis to reduce the urea concentration. Rarely, in severe or persistent bleeding, platelet concentrate infusions and red cell transfusions are indicated. Increasing the concentration of vWF, either by cryoprecipitate or by DDAVP, may promote haemostasis.

THROMBOTIC DISORDERS

Venous thromboembolic disease (VTE) and its treatment have many clinical manifestations. The approach to patients with the most common presentation, deep venous thrombosis of the leg, is described on page 1008.

Pulmonary embolism is discussed on page 721. Anticoagulant therapy is discussed on page 1010. Predisposing factors for VTE are listed in Box 24.17 (p. 1009). In a small proportion of cases, there is an underlying haematological disorder predisposing to venous thrombosis, detected using the tests described in Boxes 24.4 and 24.5 (p. 1001). These disorders include myeloproliferative disorders and paroxysmal nocturnal haemoglobinuria, which are discussed above (pp. 1048 and 1031). They also include inherited and acquired conditions, described below.

Inherited abnormalities of coagulation

Several inherited conditions predispose to VTE, and have several points in common that are worth noting:

- None of them is strongly associated with arterial thrombosis.
- All are associated with a slightly increased incidence of adverse outcome of pregnancy, including recurrent early fetal loss, but there are no data to indicate that any specific intervention changes that outcome.
- Apart from in antithrombin deficiency and homozygous factor V Leiden, most carriers of these genes will never have an episode of VTE; if they do, it will be associated with the presence of an additional temporary risk factor.
- There is little evidence that detection of these abnormalities predicts recurrence of VTE.
- None of these conditions per se requires treatment with anticoagulants. Patients with thrombosis should receive anticoagulation, as discussed on page 1009. Patients who are deemed to be at high risk of thrombosis, e.g. those with antithrombin deficiency in pregnancy, should receive treatment or prophylactic doses of heparin to cover the period of risk only.

Antithrombin deficiency

Antithrombin (AT) is a serine protease inhibitor (SERPIN) which inactivates the activated coagulation factors IIa, IXa, Xa and XIa. Heparins, fondaparinux and idraparinux achieve their therapeutic effect by potentiating the activity of AT. Familial deficiency of AT is inherited as an autosomal dominant; homozygosity for mutant alleles is not compatible with life. Around 70% of affected individuals will have an episode of VTE before the age of 60 years and the relative risk for thrombosis compared with the background population is 10–20. Pregnancy is a high-risk period for VTE and this requires fairly aggressive management with doses of LMWH which are greater than the usual prophylactic doses (≥ 100 U/kg/day). AT concentrate (either plasma-derived or recombinant) is available; this is required for cardiopulmonary bypass and may be used as an adjunct to heparin in surgical prophylaxis.

Protein C and S deficiencies

Protein C and S are vitamin K-dependent natural anticoagulants involved in switching off coagulation factor activation (factors Va and VIIIa) and thrombin generation (see Fig. 24.6E, p. 997). Inherited deficiency of either protein C or S results in a prothrombotic state with a fivefold relative risk of VTE compared with the background population.

Factor V Leiden

Factor V Leiden results from a gain-of-function, single-base pair mutation which prevents the cleavage and hence inactivation of activated factor V. This results in a relative risk of venous thrombosis of 5 in heterozygotes and 50 or more in rare homozygotes. The mutation is found in about 5% of Northern Europeans, 2% of Hispanics, 1.2% of African-Americans, 0.5% of Asian-Americans and 1.25% of Native Americans, and is rare in Chinese and Malay people.

Prothrombin G20210A

This gain-of-function mutation in the non-coding 3′ end of the prothrombin gene is associated with an increased plasma level of prothrombin. It is present in about 2% of Northern Europeans but is rare in native populations of Korea, China, India and Africa. In the heterozygous state, it is associated with a 2–3-fold increase in risk of VTE compared with the background population.

Antiphospholipid syndrome

Antiphospholipid syndrome (APS) is a clinicopathological entity in which a constellation of clinical conditions, alone or in combination, is found in association with a persistently positive test for an antiphospholipid antibody. The antiphospholipid antibodies are heterogeneous and typically are directed against proteins which bind to phospholipids (Box 24.69). Although causal roles for these antibodies have been proposed, the mechanisms underlying the clinical features of APS are not clear. In clinical practice, two types of test are used, which detect:

- antibodies which bind to negatively charged phospholipid on an ELISA plate (called an anticardiolipin antibody test)
- those which interfere with phospholipid-dependent coagulation tests like the APTT or the dilute Russell viper venom time (DRVVT; called a lupus anticoagulant test).

The term antiphospholipid antibody encompasses both a lupus anticoagulant and an anticardiolipin antibody; individuals may be positive for one or both of these activities.

Clinical features and management

APS may present in isolation (primary APS) or in association with one of the conditions shown in Box 24.69, most typically systemic lupus erythematosus (secondary APS). Most patients present with a single manifestation and APS is now most frequently diagnosed in women with adverse outcomes of pregnancy. It is extremely important to make the diagnosis in patients with APS, whatever the manifestation, because it affects the prognosis and management of arterial thrombosis, VTE and pregnancy.

Arterial thrombosis, typically stroke, associated with APS should be treated with warfarin, as opposed to aspirin. APS-associated VTE is one of the situations in which the predicted recurrence rate is high enough to indicate long-term anticoagulation after a first event. In women with APS, it is likely that intervention with heparin and possibly aspirin increases the chance of a successful pregnancy outcome.

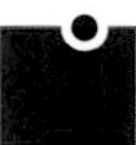

24.69 Antiphospholipid syndrome

Clinical manifestations

- Adverse pregnancy outcome
    - Recurrent first trimester abortion (≥ 3)
    - Unexplained death of morphologically normal fetus after 10 wks' gestation
    - Severe early pre-eclampsia
- Venous thromboembolism
- Arterial thromboembolism
- Livedo reticularis, catastrophic APS, transverse myelitis, skin necrosis, chorea

Conditions associated with secondary APS

- Systemic lupus erythematosus
- Rheumatoid arthritis
- Systemic sclerosis
- Behçet's syndrome
- Temporal arteritis
- Sjögren's syndrome

Targets for antiphospholipid antibodies

- β_2-glycoprotein 1
- Protein C
- Annexin V
- Prothrombin (may result in haemorrhagic presentation)

Disseminated intravascular coagulation

Disseminated intravascular coagulation (DIC) may complicate a range of illnesses (Box 24.70). It is characterised by systemic activation of the pathways involved in coagulation and its regulation. This may result in the generation of intravascular fibrin clots causing multi-organ failure, with simultaneous coagulation factor and platelet consumption causing bleeding. The systemic coagulation activation is induced either through cytokine pathways, which are activated as part of a systemic inflammatory response, or by the release of procoagulant substances such as tissue factor. In addition, sub-optimal function of the natural anticoagulant pathways and dysregulated fibrinolysis contribute to DIC. There is consumption of platelets, coagulation factors (notably factors V and VIII) and fibrinogen. The lysis of fibrin clot results in production of fibrin degradation products (FDPs), including D-dimers.

Investigations

DIC should be suspected when any of the conditions listed in Box 24.70 are met. Measurement of coagulation times (APTT and PT; p. 1000), along with fibrinogen, platelet count and FDPs, helps in the assessment of prognosis and aids clinical decision-making with regard to both bleeding and thrombotic complications.

Management

Therapy is primarily aimed at the underlying cause. These patients will often require intensive care to deal with concomitant issues, such as acidosis, dehydration, renal failure and hypoxia. Blood component therapy, such as fresh frozen plasma, cryoprecipitate and platelets, should be given if the patient is bleeding or to cover interventions with high bleeding risk, but should not be

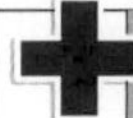

24.70 Disseminated intravascular coagulation

Underlying conditions

- Infection/sepsis
- Trauma
- Obstetric, e.g. amniotic fluid embolism, placental abruption, pre-eclampsia
- Severe liver failure
- Malignancy, e.g. solid tumours and leukaemias
- Tissue destruction, e.g. pancreatitis, burns
- Vascular abnormalities, e.g. vascular aneurysms, liver haemangiomas
- Toxic/immunological, e.g. ABO incompatibility, snake bites, recreational drugs

ISTH scoring system for diagnosis of DIC

Presence of an associated disorder	Essential
Platelets	> 100 = 0 < 100 = 1 < 50 = 2
Elevated fibrin degradation products	No increase = 0 Moderate = 2 Strong = 3
Prolonged prothrombin time	< 3 sec = 0 > 3 sec but < 6 sec = 1 > 6 sec = 2
Fibrinogen	> 1 g/L = 0 < 1 g/L = 1

Total score
≥ 5 = Compatible with overt DIC
< 5 = Repeat monitoring over 1–2 days

(ISTH = International Society for Thrombosis and Haemostasis)

prescribed routinely based on coagulation tests and platelet counts alone. Prophylactic doses of heparin should be given, unless there is a clear contraindication. Established thrombosis should be treated cautiously with therapeutic doses of unfractionated heparin, unless clearly contraindicated. Patients with DIC should not, in general, be treated with antifibrinolytic therapy, e.g. tranexamic acid.

Thrombotic thrombocytopenic purpura

Like DIC and also heparin-induced thrombocytopenia (p. 1018), thrombotic thrombocytopenic purpura (TTP) is a disorder in which thrombosis is accompanied by paradoxical thrombocytopenia. TTP is characterised by a pentad of findings, although few patients have all five components:

- thrombocytopenia
- microangiopathic haemolytic anaemia
- neurological sequelae
- fever
- renal impairment.

24.71 Haemostasis and thrombosis in old age

- **Thrombocytopenia**: not uncommon because of the rising prevalence of disorders in which it may be a secondary feature, and also because of the greater use of drugs that can cause it.
- **'Senile' purpura**: presumed to be due to an age-associated loss of subcutaneous fat and the collagenous support of small blood vessels, making them more prone to damage from minor trauma.
- **Thrombosis**: more frequent in old age. This may be due to stasis, to which older people are prone; some studies show increased platelet aggregation with age, and others age-associated hyperactivity of the haemostatic system which could create a prothrombotic state.

It is an acute autoimmune disorder mediated by antibodies against ADAMTS-13 (a disintegrin and metalloproteinase with a thrombospondin type-1 motif).

This enzyme normally cleaves vWF multimers to produce normal functional units, and its deficiency results in large vWF multimers which cross-link platelets. The features are of microvascular occlusion by platelet thrombi affecting key organs, principally brain and kidneys. It is a rare disorder (1 in 750 000 per annum), which may occur alone or in association with drugs (ticlopidine, ciclosporin), HIV, shiga toxins and malignancy. It should be treated by emergency plasma exchange. Corticosteroids, aspirin and rituximab also have a role in management. Untreated mortality rates are 90% in the first 10 days, and even with appropriate therapy, the mortality rate is 20–30% at 6 months.

Further information and acknowledgements

Websites

www.bcshguidelines.com *British Committee for Standards in Haematology guidelines.*

www.cibmtr.org *International Bone Marrow Transplant Registry.*

www.transfusionguidelines.org.uk *Contains the UK Transfusion Services' Handbook of Transfusion Medicine and links to other relevant sites.*

www.ukhcdo.org *UK Haemophilia Centre Doctors' Organisation.*

Figure acknowledgements

Page 990 insets (Glossitis) Hoffbrand VA, John E, Pettit JE, Vyas P. Hypochromic anemias. In: Color atlas of clinical hematology. 4th edn. Philadelphia: Mosby; 2010; Fig. 5.12; *(Petechiae)* Young NS, Gerson SL, High KA (eds). Clinical hematology. St Louis: Mosby; 2006.

Fig. 24.23 Hoffbrand AV, Pettit JE. Essential haematology. 3rd edn. Edinburgh: Blackwell Science; 1992.

Fig. 24.32 inset (Massive bruising) Hoffbrand VA. Color atlas of clinical hematology. 3rd edn. Philadelphia: Mosby; 2000; pp. 281–283.

S.H. Ralston
I.B. McInnes

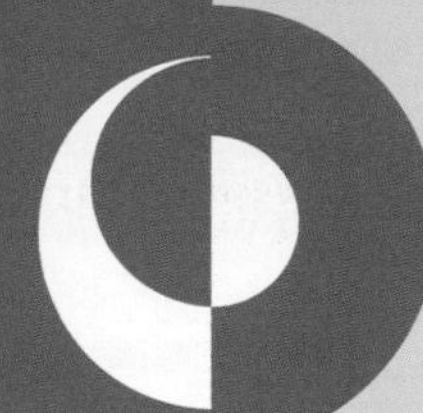

Rheumatology and bone disease 25

Clinical examination of the musculoskeletal system 1058

Functional anatomy and physiology 1060

Investigation of musculoskeletal disease 1064
- Joint aspiration 1064
- Imaging 1064
- Blood tests 1066
- Tissue biopsy 1068
- Electromyography 1068

Presenting problems in musculoskeletal disease 1069
- Acute monoarthritis 1069
- Polyarthritis 1069
- Fracture 1071
- Generalised musculoskeletal pain 1071
- Back pain 1072
- Regional musculoskeletal pain 1074
  - Neck pain 1074
  - Shoulder pain 1074
  - Elbow pain 1075
  - Hand and wrist pain 1075
  - Hip pain 1075
  - Knee pain 1075
  - Ankle and foot pain 1076
- Muscle pain and weakness 1076

Principles of management of musculoskeletal disorders 1077
- Education and lifestyle interventions 1077
- Pharmacological treatment 1078
- Non-pharmacological interventions 1080

Osteoarthritis 1081

Crystal-induced arthritis 1086
- Gout 1087
- Calcium pyrophosphate dihydrate crystal deposition disease 1090
- Basic calcium phosphate deposition disease 1091

Fibromyalgia 1092

Bone and joint infection 1094
- Septic arthritis 1094
- Viral arthritis 1095
- Osteomyelitis 1095
- Tuberculosis 1096

Rheumatoid arthritis 1096
- Pathophysiology 1096
- Clinical features 1097
- Investigations 1100
- Management 1100

Juvenile idiopathic arthritis 1103

Seronegative spondyloarthropathies 1104
- Ankylosing spondylitis 1105
- Reactive arthritis 1107
- Psoriatic arthritis 1108
- Enteropathic arthritis 1109

Connective tissue diseases 1109
- Systemic lupus erythematosus 1109
- Systemic sclerosis 1112
- Mixed connective tissue disease 1113
- Sjögren's syndrome 1114
- Polymyositis and dermatomyositis 1114
- Inclusion body myositis 1115

Vasculitis 1115
- Takayasu's disease 1116
- Kawasaki disease 1116
- Polyarteritis nodosa 1117
- Giant cell arteritis and polymyalgia rheumatica 1117
- Antineutrophil cytoplasmic antibody-associated vasculitis 1118
- Churg–Strauss syndrome 1118
- Henoch–Schönlein purpura 1119
- Cryoglobulinaemic vasculitis 1119
- Behçet's syndrome 1119
- Relapsing polychondritis 1119

Diseases of bone 1120
- Osteoporosis 1120
- Osteomalacia and rickets 1125
- Paget's disease of bone 1128
- Other bone diseases 1130
  - Reflex sympathetic dystrophy syndrome 1130
  - Osteonecrosis 1130
  - Scheuermann's osteochondritis 1130
  - Polyostotic fibrous dysplasia 1131
  - Osteogenesis imperfecta 1131
  - Osteopetrosis 1131
  - Sclerosing bone dysplasias 1131

Bone and joint tumours 1131
- Osteosarcoma 1132
- Metastatic bone disease 1132

Rheumatological involvement in other diseases 1132
- Malignant disease 1132
- Endocrine disease 1132
- Haematological disease 1133
- Neurological disease 1133

Miscellaneous conditions 1133
- Spondylolisis and spondylolisthesis 1133
- Diffuse idiopathic skeletal hyperostosis 1133
- Pigmented villonodular synovitis 1134
- Joint hypermobility 1134
- Dupuytren's contracture 1134
- Carpal tunnel syndrome 1134
- Trigger finger 1134
- Periodic fever syndromes 1135
- Anterior tibial compartment syndrome 1135
- Synovitis–acne–pustulosis–hyperostosis–osteitis syndrome 1135

CLINICAL EXAMINATION OF THE MUSCULOSKELETAL SYSTEM

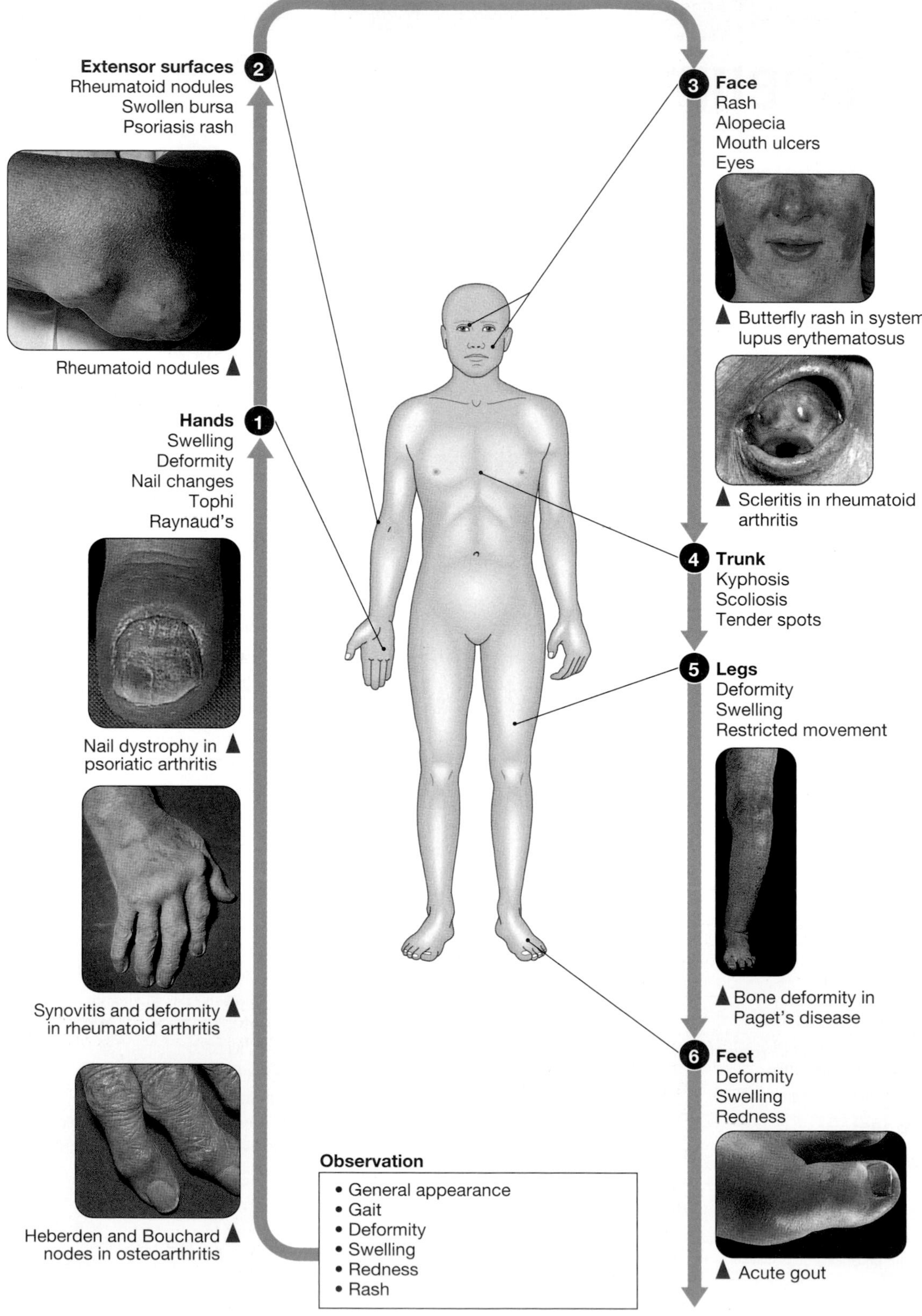

General Assessment of Locomotor System (GALS)

1 Gait

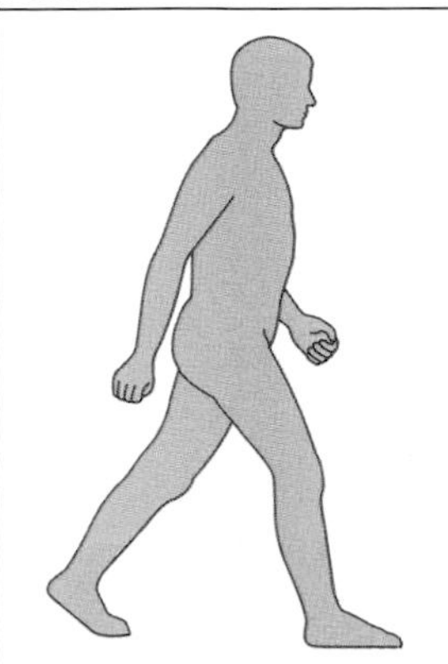

Ask patient to walk for a few steps, then come back. Look for pain or limp

2 Arms

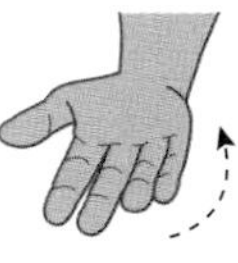

Inspect hands for swelling or deformity

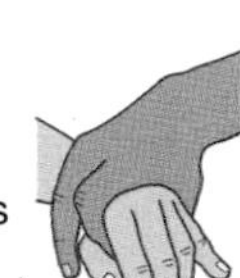

Ask patient to make a fist and open and close fingers (tests hand function)

Squeeze metacarpals (tests for inflammation)

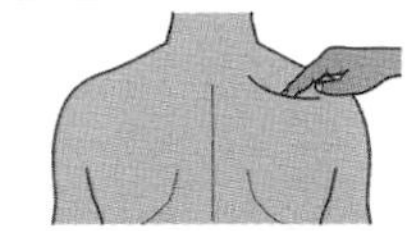

Press over supraspinatus (tests for hyperalgesia)

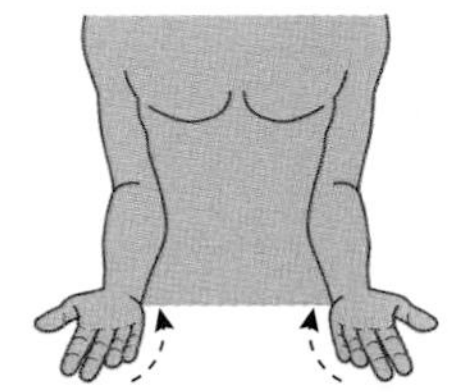

Patient turns palms up and down with elbows at side (tests supination and pronation of wrists and elbow)

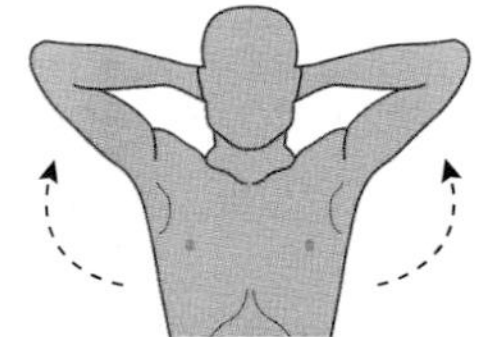

Ask patient to put hands behind head (tests shoulder movements)

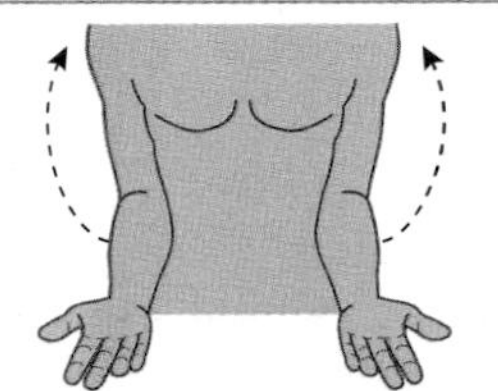

Patient flexes elbows to touch shoulder (tests elbow flexion)

3 Legs

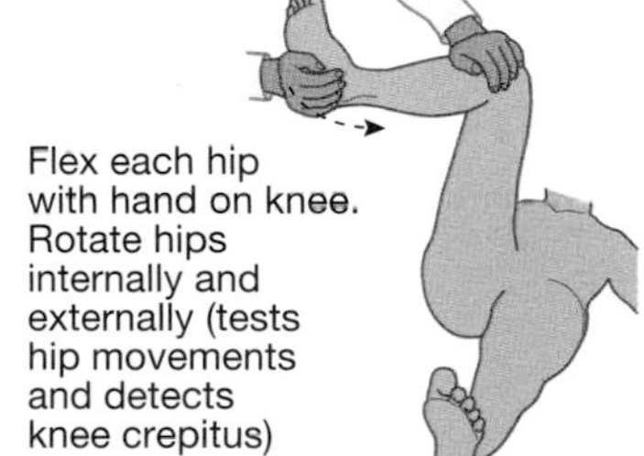

Flex each hip with hand on knee. Rotate hips internally and externally (tests hip movements and detects knee crepitus)

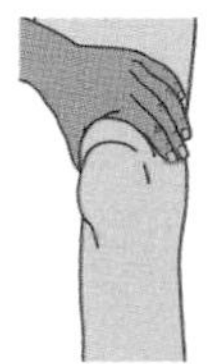

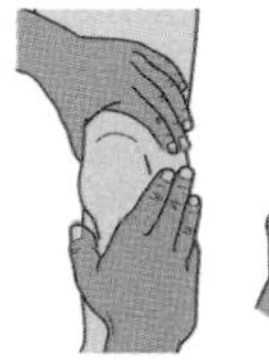

Palpate each knee for warmth and swelling (tests for synovitis and effusion)

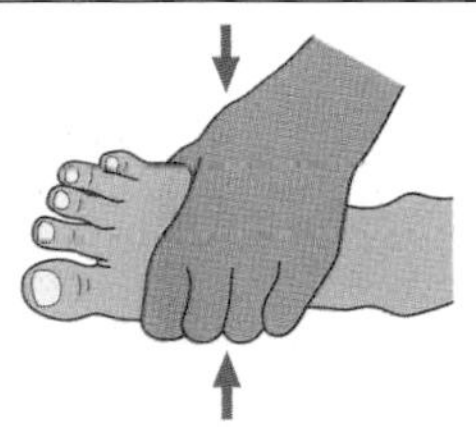

Inspect ankles and feet. Squeeze forefoot (tests for metatarsophalangeal synovitis)

4 Spine

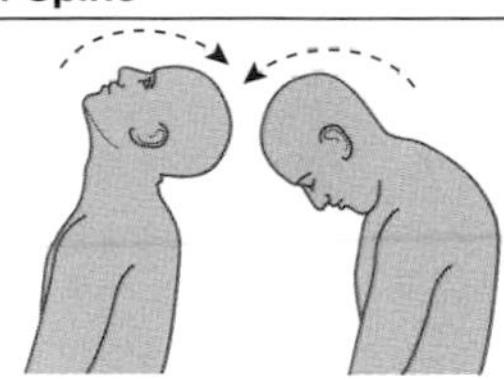

Patient looks at ceiling and then puts chin on chest (tests flexion and extension cervical spine)

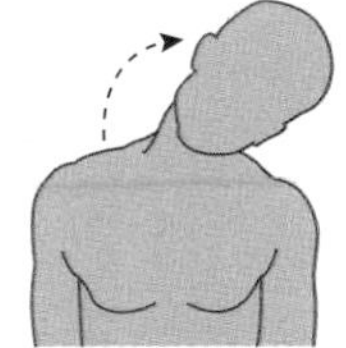

Ask patient to try to put ear on shoulder (tests lateral flexion cervical spine)

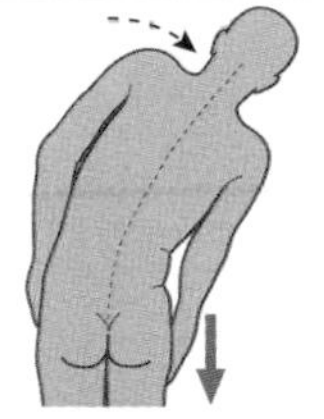

Patient slides hand down leg to knee (tests lateral spine flexion)

Inspect spine from behind and side, looking for scoliosis, kyphosis or localised deformity. Ask patient to touch toes

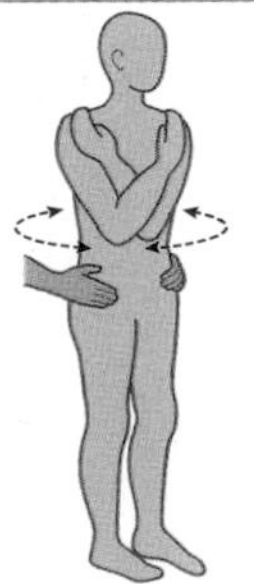

Stand behind patient and hold their pelvis. Ask them to turn from side to side without moving their feet (tests thoracolumbar rotation)

5 Record results

A normal screen

G✓	A	M
A	✓	✓
L	✓	✓
S	✓	✓

G = gait
A = arms
L = legs
S = spine
A = appearance
M = movement

Example of an abnormal screen

G✗	A	M
A	✓	✓
L	✗	✗
S	✓	✓

Antalgic gait
Right knee
Varus
↓Flexion
Crepitus^{++}
Effusion
Diagnosis: osteoarthritis right knee

Disorders of the musculoskeletal system affect all ages and ethnic groups. In the UK, about 25% of new consultations in general practice are for musculoskeletal symptoms. Musculoskeletal diseases may arise from processes affecting bones, joints, muscles, or connective tissues such as skin and tendon. The principal manifestations are pain and impairment of locomotor function.

25.1 Relative prevalence of musculoskeletal disorders

	Prevalence	Gender ratio	Age association
'Non-inflammatory' conditions			
Neck and back pain	20%	F = M	–
Osteoarthritis			
Knee	10%	F > M	++
Hip	4%	F = M	+
Osteoporosis	15%	F > M	++
Regional 'soft tissue' pain	10%	F > M	++
Fibromyalgia	3%	F > M	++
'Inflammatory' conditions			
Rheumatoid arthritis	1%	F > M	+
Gout	1.5%	M > F	–
Seronegative spondyloarthritis	0.8%	F = M	–
Polymyalgia rheumatica	0.04%	F > M	++
Connective tissue diseases (mainly lupus)	0.02%	F > M	–

Diseases of the musculoskeletal system tend to be more common in women and most increase in frequency with increasing age. The two most common disorders are osteoarthritis and osteoporosis (Box 25.1). Osteoarthritis is the most common type of arthritis and affects up to 80% of people over the age of 75. Osteoporosis is the most common bone disease and affects 50% of women and 20% of men by their eighth decade. Diseases of the musculoskeletal system are the most common cause of physical disability in older people and account for one-third of physical disability at all ages.

FUNCTIONAL ANATOMY AND PHYSIOLOGY

The musculoskeletal system is responsible for movement of the body, provides a structural framework to protect internal organs, and acts as a reservoir for storage of calcium and phosphate in the regulation of mineral homeostasis. The main components of the musculoskeletal system are depicted in Figure 25.1.

Bone

Bones fall into two main types based on their embryonic development. Flat bones, such as the skull, develop by intramembranous ossification, in which embryonic fibroblasts differentiate directly into bone within

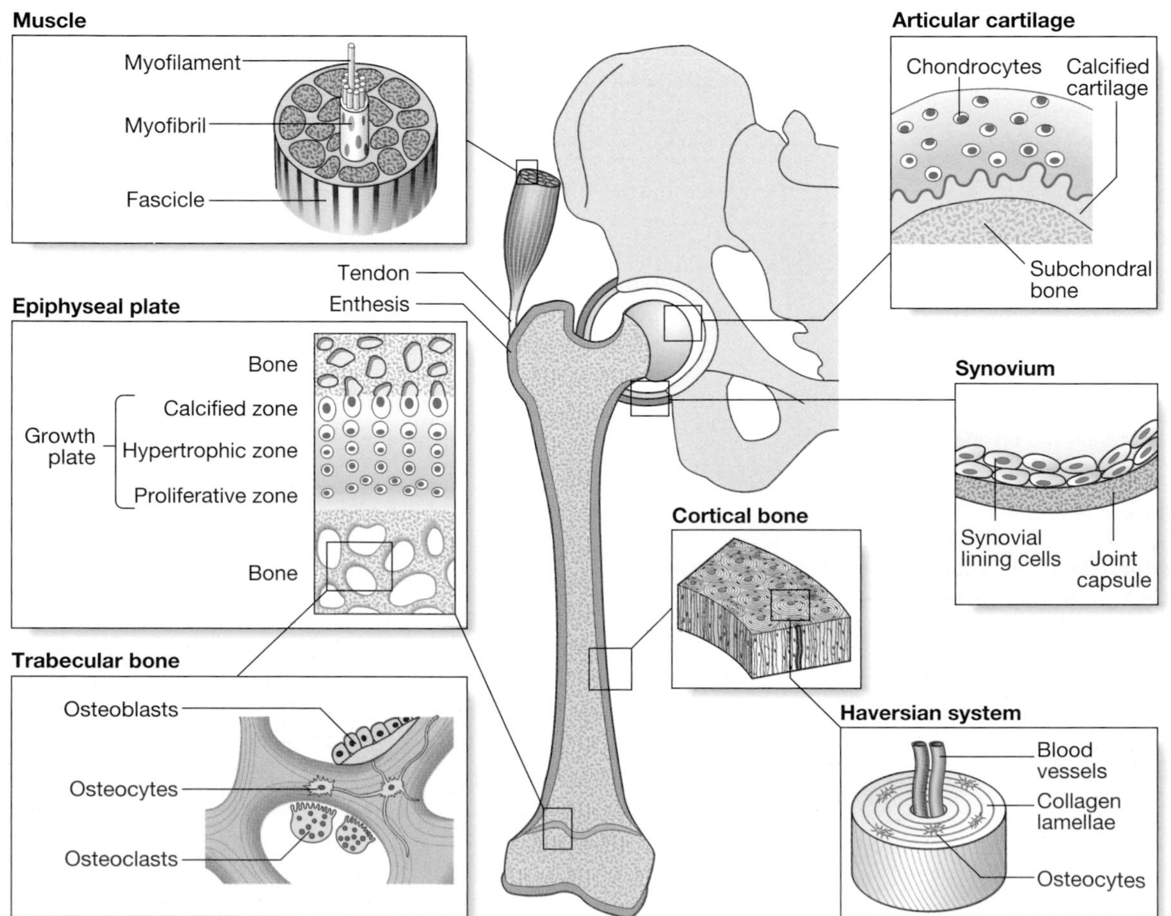

Fig. 25.1 Structure of the major musculoskeletal tissues.

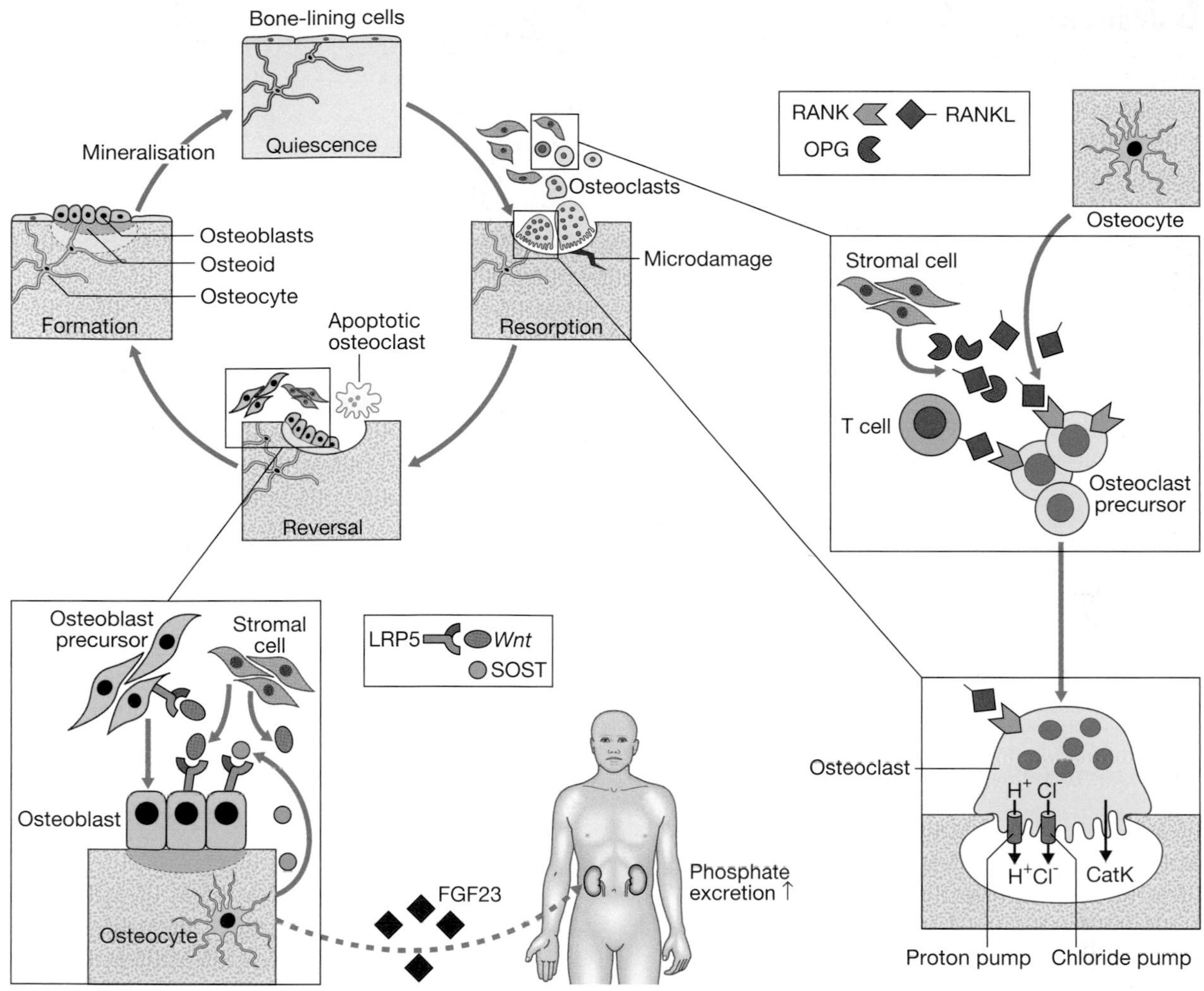

Fig. 25.2 Regulation of bone remodelling. Bone is renewed and repaired during the bone remodelling cycle, in which old and damaged bone is removed by osteoclasts and replaced by osteoblasts. Osteocytes play a central role in bone remodelling by secreting RANKL, which promotes osteoclast differentiation and activity by binding to RANK. Osteocytes regulate bone formation by producing SOST, which binds to the LRP5 receptor and prevents its activation by members of the Wnt family. Osteocytes also regulate phosphate homeostasis by producing fibroblast growth factor 23 (FGF23), which is a circulating hormone that acts on the kidney to promote phosphate excretion. (CatK = cathepsin K; LRP5 = lipoprotein receptor protein 5; OPG = osteoprotegerin; RANK = receptor activator of nuclear factor kappa B; RANKL = RANK ligand; SOST = sclerostin)

condensations of mesenchymal tissue during early fetal life. Long bones, such as the femur and radius, develop by endochondral ossification from a cartilage template. During development, the cartilage is invaded by vascular tissue containing osteoprogenitor cells and is gradually replaced by bone from centres of ossification situated in the middle and at the ends of the bone. A thin remnant of cartilage called the growth plate or epiphysis remains at each end of long bones, and chondrocyte proliferation here is responsible for skeletal growth during childhood and adolescence. During puberty, the rise in levels of sex hormones halts cell division in the growth plate. The cartilage remnant then disappears as the epiphysis fuses and longitudinal bone growth ceases.

The normal skeleton has two forms of bone tissue (see Fig. 25.1). Cortical bone is formed from Haversian systems, comprising concentric lamellae of bone tissue surrounding a central canal that contains blood vessels. Cortical bone is dense and forms a hard envelope around the long bones. Trabecular or cancellous bone fills the centre of the bone and consists of an interconnecting meshwork of trabeculae, separated by spaces filled with bone marrow.

There are three main cell types in bone:

- *Osteoclasts:* multinucleated cells of haematopoietic origin, responsible for bone resorption.
- *Osteoblasts:* mononuclear cells of mesenchymal origin, responsible for bone formation.
- *Osteocytes:* these differentiate from osteoblasts during bone formation and become embedded in bone matrix. Osteocytes are responsible for sensing and responding to mechanical loading of the skeleton and play a critical role in regulating bone formation and bone resorption, by producing receptor activator of nuclear factor kappa B ligand (RANKL) and sclerostin (SOST). They also play a central role in regulating phosphate metabolism by producing the hormone fibroblast growth factor 23 (FGF23), which acts on the kidney to promote phosphate excretion (Fig. 25.2).

Bone matrix and mineral

The most abundant protein of bone is type I collagen, which is formed from two α1 peptide chains and one α2 chain wound together in a triple helix. Type I collagen is proteolytically processed inside the cell before being laid down in the extracellular space, releasing propeptide fragments that can be used as biochemical markers of bone formation (p. 1066). Subsequently, the collagen fibrils become 'cross-linked' to one another by pyridinium molecules, a process that enhances bone strength. When bone is broken down by osteoclasts, the cross-links are released, providing biochemical markers of bone resorption. Bone is normally laid down in an orderly fashion, but when bone turnover is high, as in Paget's disease or severe hyperparathyroidism, it is laid down in a chaotic pattern, giving rise to 'woven bone', which is mechanically weak. Bone matrix also contains growth factors, other structural proteins and proteoglycans, thought to be involved in helping bone cells attach to bone matrix and in regulating bone cell activity. The other major component of bone is mineral, comprised of calcium and phosphate crystals deposited between the collagen fibrils in the form of hydroxyapatite [$Ca_{10}(PO_4)_6(OH)_2$]. Mineralisation is essential for bone's rigidity and strength, but over-mineralisation can increase brittleness, which contributes to bone fragility in diseases like osteogenesis imperfecta (p. 1131).

Bone remodelling

Bone remodelling is required for renewal and repair of the skeleton throughout life (see Fig. 25.2). It starts with the attraction of osteoclast precursors in peripheral blood to the target site, probably by local release of chemotactic factors from areas of microdamage. The osteoclast precursors differentiate into mature osteoclasts in response to RANKL, which is produced by osteocytes, activated T cells and bone marrow stromal cells. RANKL activates the RANK receptor, which is expressed on osteoclasts and precursors. This is blocked by osteoprotegerin (OPG), a decoy receptor for RANKL that inhibits osteoclast formation. Mature osteoclasts attach to the bone surface by a tight sealing zone, and secrete hydrochloric acid and proteolytic enzymes such as cathepsin K into the space underneath. The acid dissolves the mineral and cathepsin K degrades collagen. When resorption is complete, osteoclasts undergo programmed cell death, and bone formation begins with the attraction of osteoblast precursors to the resorption site. These differentiate into mature osteoblasts, which deposit new bone matrix in the resorption lacuna, until the hole is filled. Some osteoblasts become trapped in bone matrix and differentiate into osteocytes. These act as biomechanical sensors and produce several molecules that influence bone remodelling and phosphate metabolism. Bone formation is stimulated by Wnt proteins, which bind to and activate lipoprotein-related receptor protein 5 (LRP5), expressed on osteoblasts. This process is inhibited by SOST, which is produced by osteocytes (see Fig. 25.2). Initially, the newly formed bone matrix (osteoid) is uncalcified but subsequently becomes mineralised to form mature bone. Alkaline phosphatase (ALP), produced by osteoblasts, plays an important role in bone mineralisation by degrading pyrophosphate, an inhibitor of mineralisation. Bone remodelling is regulated by circulating hormones such as parathyroid hormone (PTH) and oestrogen, and locally produced factors such as cytokines (Box 25.2). Many systemic hormones exert effects on bone turnover by affecting local expression of RANK, RANKL, OPG, SOST and molecules in the Wnt/LRP5 pathway (Fig. 25.2, Box 25.2).

25.2 Regulators of bone remodelling

Factor	Bone resorption	Bone formation
Parathyroid hormone (PTH)	↑	↑
Receptor activator of nuclear factor kappa B ligand (RANKL)	↑	↔
Osteoprotegerin (OPG)	↓	↔
Sclerostin (SOST)	↔	↓
Interleukin-1 (IL-1)	↑	↓
Tumour necrosis factor-α (TNF-α)	↑	↓
Thyroid hormone	↑	↑
Glucocorticoids	↑	↓↓
Oestrogen/testosterone	↓	↑
Mechanical loading	↓	↑

Joints

Bones are linked by joints. There are three main subtypes: fibrous, fibrocartilaginous and synovial (Box 25.3).

Fibrous and fibrocartilaginous joints

These comprise a simple bridge of fibrous or fibrocartilaginous tissue joining two bones together where there is little requirement for movement. The intervertebral disc is a special type of fibrocartilaginous joint in which an amorphous area, called the nucleus pulposus, lies in the centre of the fibrocartilaginous bridge. The nucleus has a high water content and acts as a cushion to improve the disc's shock-absorbing properties.

Synovial joints

Complex structures containing several cell types, these are found where a wide range of movement is needed (Fig. 25.3).

Articular cartilage

This avascular tissue covers the bone ends in synovial joints. Cartilage cells (chondrocytes) are responsible for synthesis and turnover of cartilage, which consists of a mesh of type II collagen fibrils that extend through a hydrated 'gel' of proteoglycan molecules. The most

25.3 Types of joint

Type	Range of movement	Examples
Fibrous	Minimal	Skull sutures
Fibrocartilaginous	Limited	Symphysis pubis Costochondral junctions Intervertebral discs Sacroiliac joints
Synovial	Large	Most limb joints Temporomandibular Costovertebral

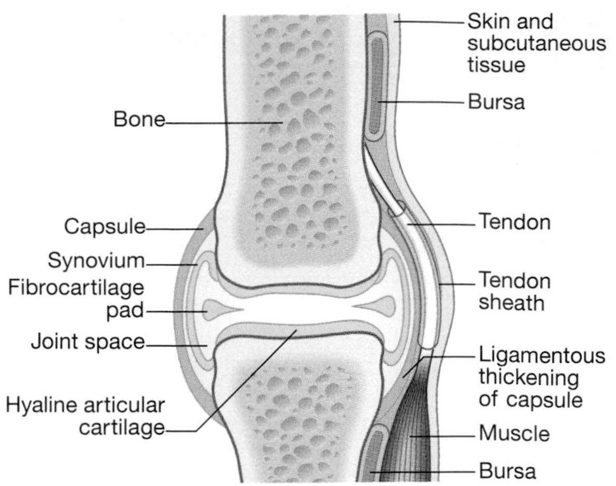

Fig. 25.3 Structure of a synovial joint.

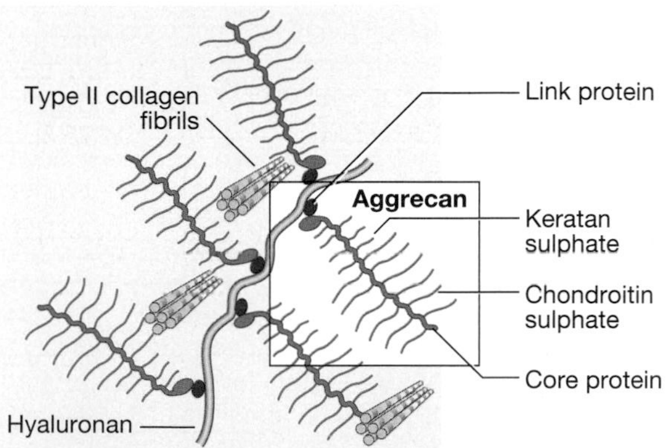

Fig. 25.4 Ultrastructure of articular cartilage.

important proteoglycan is aggrecan, which consists of a core protein to which several glycosaminoglycan (GAG) side-chains are attached (Fig. 25.4). The GAGs are polysaccharides that consist of long chains of disaccharide repeats comprising one normal sugar and an amino sugar. The most abundant GAGs in aggrecan are chondroitin sulphate and keratan sulphate. Hyaluronan is another important GAG that binds to aggrecan molecules to form very large complexes with a total molecular weight of more than 100 million. Aggrecan has a strong negative charge and avidly binds water molecules to assume a shape that occupies the maximum possible volume available. The expansive force of the hydrated aggrecan, combined with the restrictive strength of the collagen mesh, gives articular cartilage excellent shock-absorbing properties.

With ageing, the concentration of chondroitin sulphate decreases, whereas that of keratan sulphate increases, resulting in reduced water content and shock-absorbing properties. These changes differ from those found in osteoarthritis (p. 1081), where there is abnormal chondrocyte division, loss of proteoglycan from matrix and an increase in water content. Cartilage matrix is constantly turning over and in health there is a perfect balance between synthesis and degradation. Degradation of cartilage matrix is carried out by aggrecanases and matrix metalloproteinases, responsible for the breakdown of proteins and proteoglycans, and by glycosidases, responsible for the breakdown of GAGs. Pro-inflammatory cytokines, such as interleukin-1 (IL-1) and tumour necrosis factor (TNF), stimulate production of aggrecanase and metalloproteinases, which contribute to cartilage degradation in inflammatory arthritis.

Synovial fluid

The surfaces of articular cartilage are separated by a space filled with synovial fluid, a viscous liquid that lubricates the joint. It is an ultrafiltrate of plasma, into which synovial cells secrete hyaluronan and proteoglycans.

Intra-articular discs

Some joints contain fibrocartilaginous discs within the joint space that act as shock absorbers. The most clinically important are the menisci of the knee. These are avascular structures that remain viable by diffusion of oxygen and nutrients from the synovial fluid.

The synovial membrane, joint capsule and bursae

The bones of synovial joints are connected by the joint capsule, a fibrous structure richly supplied with blood vessels, nerves and lymphatics, which encases the joint. Ligaments are discrete, regional thickenings of the capsule that act to stabilise joints (see Fig. 25.3). The inner surface of the joint capsule is the synovial membrane, comprising an outer layer of blood vessels and loose connective tissue that is rich in type I collagen, and an inner layer 1–4 cells thick consisting of two main cell types. Type A synoviocytes are phagocytic cells derived from the monocyte/macrophage lineage and are responsible for removing particulate matter from the joint cavity; type B synoviocytes are fibroblast-like cells that secrete synovial fluid. Most inflammatory and degenerative joint diseases associate with thickening of the synovial membrane and infiltration by lymphocytes, polymorphs and macrophages.

Bursae are hollow sacs lined with synovium and contain a small amount of synovial fluid. They help tendons and muscles move smoothly in relation to bones and other articular structures.

Skeletal muscle

Skeletal muscles are responsible for body movements and respiration. Muscle consists of bundles of cells (myocytes) embedded in fine connective tissue containing nerves and blood vessels. Myocytes are large, elongated, multinucleated cells formed by fusion of mononuclear precursors (myoblasts) in early embryonic life. The nuclei lie peripherally and the centre of the cell contains actin and myosin molecules, which interdigitate with one another to form the myofibrils that are responsible for muscle contraction. The molecular mechanisms of skeletal muscle contraction are the same as for cardiac muscle (p. 531). Myocytes contain many mitochondria that provide the large amounts of adenosine triphosphate (ATP) necessary for muscle contraction, and are rich in the protein myoglobin, which acts as a reservoir for oxygen during contraction.

Individual myofibrils are organised into bundles (fasciculi) that are bound together by a thin layer of connective tissue (the perimysium). The surface of the muscle is surrounded by a thicker layer of connective tissue, the epimysium, which merges with the perimysium to form the muscle tendon. Tendons are tough, fibrous structures that attach muscles to a point of insertion on the bone surface called the enthesis.

INVESTIGATION OF MUSCULOSKELETAL DISEASE

Clinical history and examination usually provide sufficient information for the diagnosis and management of most musculoskeletal diseases. Investigations are helpful in confirming the diagnosis, assessing disease activity and indicating prognosis.

Joint aspiration

Joint aspiration with examination of synovial fluid (SF) is pivotal in patients suspected of having septic arthritis, crystal arthritis or intra-articular bleeding. It should be done in all patients with acute monoarthritis, and samples sent for microbiology and clinical chemistry.

It is possible to obtain SF by aspiration from most peripheral joints, and only a small volume is required for diagnostic purposes. Normal SF is present in small volume, and is clear and either colourless or pale yellow with a high viscosity. It contains few cells. With joint inflammation, the volume increases, the cell count and the proportion of neutrophils rise (causing turbidity), and the viscosity reduces (due to enzymatic degradation of hyaluronan and aggrecan). Turbid fluid with a high neutrophil count occurs in sepsis, crystal arthritis and reactive arthritis. High concentrations of urate crystals or cholesterol can make SF appear white. Non-uniform blood-staining usually reflects needle trauma to the synovium. Uniform blood-staining is most commonly due to a bleeding diathesis, trauma or pigmented villonodular synovitis (p. 1134), but can occur in severe inflammatory synovitis. A lipid layer floating above blood-stained fluid is diagnostic of intra-articular fracture and is caused by release of bone marrow fat into the joint.

Crystals can be identified by compensated polarised light microscopy of fresh SF (to avoid crystal dissolution and post-aspiration crystallisation). Urate crystals are long and needle-shaped, and show a strong light intensity and negative birefringence (Fig. 25.5A). Calcium pyrophosphate crystals are smaller, rhomboid in shape and usually less numerous than urate, and have weak intensity and positive birefringence (Fig. 25.5B).

A

B

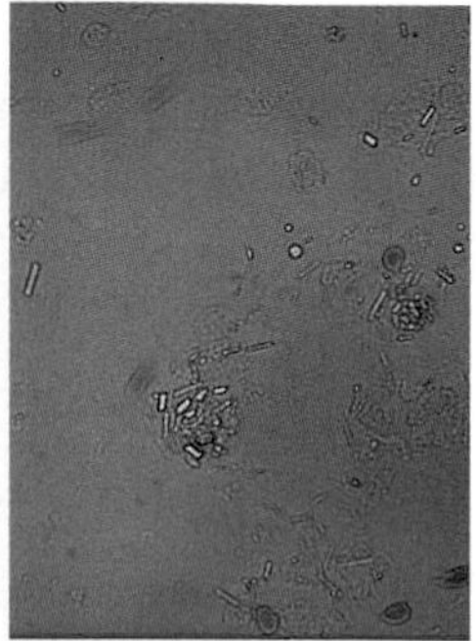

Fig. 25.5 Compensated polarised light microscopy of synovial fluids (× 400). **A** Monosodium urate crystals showing bright negative birefringence under polarised light and needle-shaped morphology. **B** Calcium pyrophosphate crystals showing weak positive birefringence under polarised light and are few in number. They are more difficult to detect than urate crystals.

Imaging

Plain radiography

Radiographs show anatomical changes that are of value in the differential diagnosis of many bone and joint diseases (Box 25.4). The bones and joints to be X-rayed are usually selected on the basis of symptoms or patterns of involvement identified at clinical assessment.

Radiographs are of diagnostic value in osteoarthritis (OA), where they demonstrate joint space narrowing that tends to be focal rather than widespread, as in inflammatory arthritis. Other features of OA detected on X-ray include osteophytes, subchondral sclerosis, bone cysts and calcified loose bodies within the synovium (see Fig. 25.20, p. 1084). Radiographs may show erosions and sclerosis of the sacroiliac joints and syndesmophytes in the spine in patients with seronegative spondyloarthritis (see Fig. 25.36, p. 1106). In peripheral joints, so-called proliferative erosions, associated with new bone formation and a periosteal reaction, may be observed. In tophaceous gout, well-defined punched-out erosions may occur (see Fig. 25.26, p. 1089). Calcification of cartilage, tendons and soft tissues or muscle may occur in chondrocalcinosis (see Fig. 25.27, p. 1090), calcific periarthritis and connective tissue diseases.

Radiographs are of limited value in the diagnosis of rheumatoid arthritis (RA) since features such as erosions, joint space narrowing and periarticular osteoporosis may only be detectable after several months or even years. The main indication for radiographs in RA is in the assessment of advanced disease, when structural damage of the joints is suspected and arthroplasty is being considered. Early evidence of articular damage in RA is more usually obtained using magnetic resonance imaging or ultrasonography.

25.4 X-ray abnormalities in selected rheumatic diseases

Rheumatoid arthritis	
• Periarticular osteoporosis • Bone erosions	• Joint space narrowing
Osteoporosis	
• Osteopenia • Vertebral fractures	• Non-vertebral fractures
Paget's disease	
• Bone expansion • Abnormal trabecular pattern • Osteolysis	• Osteosclerosis • Pseudofractures
Spondyloarthritis	
• Sacroiliitis • Syndesmophytes	• Ligament calcification • Squaring of vertebral bodies
Osteoarthritis	
• Joint space narrowing • Osteophytes • Subchondral sclerosis	• Peaking of tibial spines • Subchondral cysts

Radionuclide bone scan

This is useful in patients suspected of having metastatic bone disease and Paget's disease. It involves gamma-camera imaging following an intravenous injection of ^{99m}Tc-bisphosphonate. Early post-injection images reflect vascularity and can show increased perfusion of inflamed synovium, Pagetic bone, or primary or secondary bone tumours. Delayed images taken a few hours later reflect bone remodelling as the bisphosphonate localises to sites of active bone turnover. Scintigraphy has a high sensitivity for detecting important bone and joint pathology that is not apparent on plain X-rays (Box 25.5). Single photon emission computed tomography (SPECT) combines radionuclide imaging with computed tomography. It can provide accurate anatomical localisation of abnormal tracer uptake within the bone and is of particular value in the assessment of patients with chronic low back pain of unknown cause.

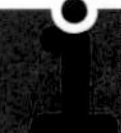

25.5 Conditions detected by isotope bone scanning

- Paget's disease of bone
- Bone metastases
- Stress fractures
- Reflex sympathetic dystrophy (algodystrophy, p. 1130)
- Hypertrophic pulmonary osteoarthropathy (p. 1132)

Magnetic resonance imaging

Magnetic resonance imaging (MRI) gives detailed information on anatomy, allowing three-dimensional visualisation of bone and soft tissues that cannot be adequately assessed by plain X-rays. The technique is valuable in the assessment and diagnosis of many musculoskeletal diseases (Box 25.6). T1-weighted sequences are useful for defining anatomy, whereas T2-weighted sequences are useful for assessing tissue water content, which is often increased in synovitis and other inflammatory disorders (Fig. 25.6). Contrast agents, such as gadolinium, can be administered to increase sensitivity in detecting erosions and synovitis.

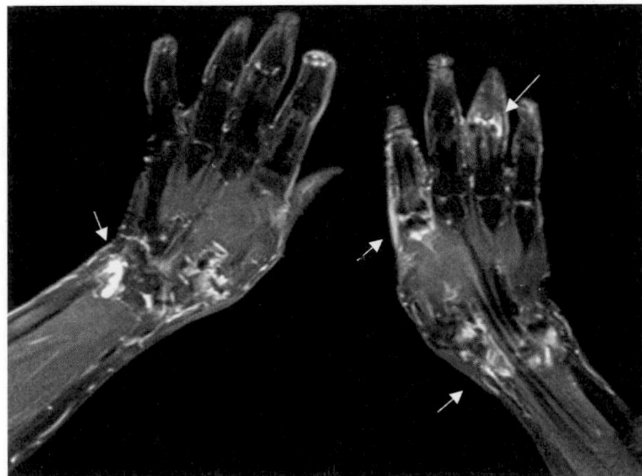

Fig. 25.6 Magnetic resonance image showing synovitis. Coronal fat-saturated post-contrast T1-weighted image shows extensive enhancement consistent with synovitis (white areas, arrowed) in both wrists and at the second metacarpophalangeal joint and proximal interphalangeal joints of the right hand.

25.6 Conditions detected by magnetic resonance imaging

- Osteonecrosis
- Intervertebral disc disease
- Nerve root entrapment
- Spinal cord compression
- Spinal stenosis
- Sepsis
- Reflex sympathetic dystrophy syndrome
- Malignancy
- Fractures
- Meniscal disease
- Synovitis
- Sacroiliitis and enthesitis
- Inflammatory myositis
- Rotator cuff tears, bursitis and tenosynovitis

Ultrasonography

Ultrasonography is a useful investigation for confirmation of small joint synovitis and erosion, for anatomical confirmation of periarticular lesions, and for guided aspiration and injection of joints and bursae. Ultrasound is more sensitive than clinical examination for the detection of early synovitis and is used increasingly in the diagnosis and assessment of patients with suspected inflammatory arthritis. In addition to locating synovial thickening and effusions, ultrasound can detect increased blood flow within synovium using power Doppler imaging, an option that is available on most modern ultrasound machines (Fig. 25.7).

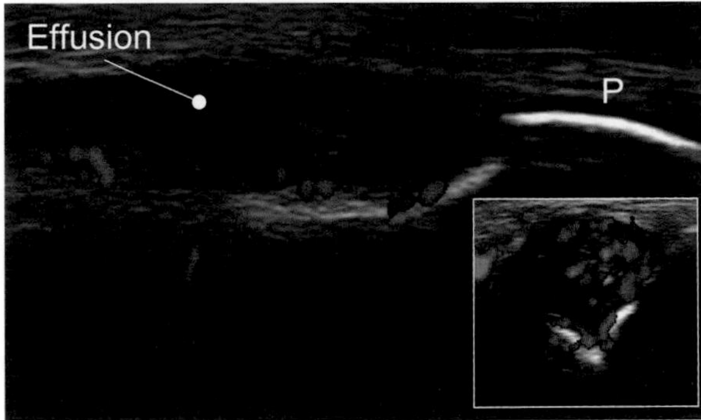

Fig. 25.7 Ultrasound image showing synovitis. Lateral image of a metacarpophalangeal joint in inflammatory arthritis. The periosteum (P) of the phalanx shows as a white line. The dark, hypo-echoic area indicates an effusion. The coloured areas demonstrated by power Doppler indicate increased vascularity. The inset shows a transverse image of the same joint.

Computed tomography

Computed tomography (CT) can be used in the assessment of patients with bone and joint disease but has largely been superseded by MRI, which gives better visualisation of soft tissue structures. CT may be used when MRI is contraindicated, or for evaluation of articular regions in which an adjacent joint replacement creates image artefacts on MRI.

Bone mineral density

Bone mineral density (BMD) measurements play a key role in the diagnosis and management of osteoporosis. The technique of choice is dual energy X-ray absorptiometry (DEXA), which is usually performed at the lumbar spine and hip, and provides images of the region studied. This technique works on the principle that calcium in bone attenuates passage of X-ray beams through the tissue in proportion to the amount of mineral present. The greater the amount of bone mineral present, the higher the BMD value. Most DEXA scanners give a BMD readout expressed as grams of hydroxyapatite/cm^2, and as a T-score and Z-score value. The T-score is a measure of the number of standard deviations by which the patient's BMD value differs from that in a young healthy control, whereas the BMD Z-score is a measure of the number of standard deviations by which the BMD deviates from that of age-matched controls (Fig. 25.8). Osteoporosis is defined by a T-score value of 2.5 or below (shaded red in the figure), whereas osteopenia is diagnosed when the T-score lies between −1.0 and −2.5 (shaded pink). Many healthy people, especially above the age of 50, have BMD values in the osteopenic range. Values of BMD above −1.0 and below +2.5 are considered normal, whereas values above +2.5 can be found in osteosclerotic diseases and OA. Results need to be interpreted carefully. It is possible for BMD values to lie in the normal or osteopenic range in patients who have osteoporosis, due to coexisting conditions such as aortic calcification, vertebral compression fractures, degenerative disc disease and OA. These can sometimes be suspected on the basis of antero-posterior or lateral DEXA images, but abnormal appearances should be confirmed by X-ray or other imaging as appropriate.

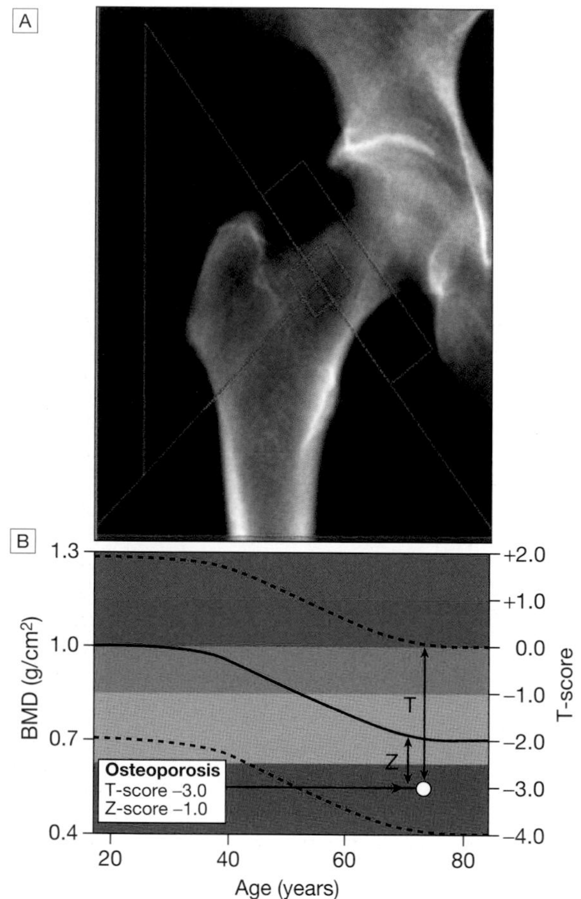

Fig. 25.8 Typical output from a dual energy X-ray absorptiometry (DEXA) scanner. **A** DEXA scan of the hip. **B** Bone mineral density (BMD) values plotted in g/cm^2 (left axis) and as the T-score values (right axis). The solid line represents the population average plotted against age, and the interrupted lines are ± 2 standard deviations from the average. The patient shown, aged 72, has an osteoporotic T-score of −3.0 but a Z-score of −1.0, which is within the 'normal range' for that age, reflecting the fact that bone is lost with age.

Blood tests

Haematology

Abnormalities in the full blood count (FBC) often occur in inflammatory rheumatic diseases but changes are usually non-specific. Examples include neutrophilia in vasculitis, acute gout and sepsis; neutropenia in lupus; and a raised erythrocyte sedimentation rate (ESR) in many inflammatory diseases. Reduced levels of haemoglobin are a common and important finding in a range of rheumatological disorders. Many disease-modifying antirheumatic drugs (DMARDs) cause marrow toxicity and require regular monitoring of the FBC.

Biochemistry

Routine biochemistry is useful for assessing metabolic bone disease, muscle diseases and gout. Several bone diseases, including Paget's disease, renal bone disease and osteomalacia, give a characteristic pattern that can be helpful diagnostically (Box 25.7). Serum levels of uric acid are usually raised in gout but a normal level does not exclude it, especially during an acute attack, when urate levels temporarily fall. Equally, an elevated serum uric acid does not confirm the diagnosis, since most hyperuricaemic people never develop gout. Levels of C-reactive protein (CRP) are a useful marker of infection and inflammation, and are more specific than the ESR. An exception is in connective tissue diseases such as systemic lupus erythematosus (SLE) and systemic sclerosis, where CRP may be normal but ESR raised in active

25.7 Biochemical abnormalities in bone disease

	Serum calcium	Serum phosphate	Serum ALP	Serum PTH	Serum 25(OH)D
Osteoporosis	N	N	N	N	N or ↓
Paget's disease	N	N	↑↑	N or ↑	N
Renal osteodystrophy	↓	↑↑	↑	↑↑	N
Vitamin D-deficient osteomalacia	N or ↓	N or ↓	↑↑	↑↑	↓
Hypophosphataemic rickets	N	↓↓	↑	N or ↑	N

(ALP = alkaline phosphatase; N = normal; PTH = parathyroid hormone; single arrow = increased or decreased; double arrow = greatly increased or decreased)

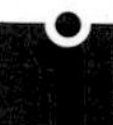

25.8 Causes of an elevated serum creatine kinase

- Inflammatory myositis ± vasculitis
- Muscular dystrophy
- Motor neuron disease
- Alcohol, drugs (N.B. statins)
- Trauma, strenuous exercise, long lie after a fall
- Myocardial infarction*
- Hypothyroidism, metabolic myopathy
- Viral myositis

*The CK-MB cardiac-specific isoform is disproportionately elevated compared with total CK.

inflammatory disease. Accordingly, an elevated CRP in a patient with lupus or scleroderma suggests an intercurrent illness such as sepsis rather than active disease. More detail on the interpretation of CRP and ESR changes is given on page 84. Serum creatine kinase (CK) levels are useful in the diagnosis of myopathy or myositis, but specificity and sensitivity are poor and raised levels may occur in some conditions (Box 25.8). Biochemical monitoring of renal and hepatic function is important in ongoing care of patients on DMARD therapy.

Autoantibodies

Autoantibody tests are widely used in the diagnosis of rheumatic diseases. False-positive results are common but high antibody titres or concentrations are generally of greater clinical significance. Whatever test is used, the results must be interpreted in light of the clinical picture and the different detection and assay systems used in different hospitals.

Rheumatoid factor

Rheumatoid factor (RF) is an antibody directed against the Fc fragment of human immunoglobulin. In routine clinical practice, IgM rheumatoid factor is usually measured, although different methodologies allow measurement of IgG and IgA RFs too. Positive RF occurs in a wide variety of diseases and some normal adults (Box 25.9), particularly with increasing age. Although the specificity is poor, about 70% of patients with RA test positive. High RF titres are associated with more severe disease and extra-articular disease.

Anti-citrullinated peptide antibodies

Anti-citrullinated peptide antibodies (ACPA) recognise peptides in which the amino acid arginine has been converted to citrulline by peptidylarginine deiminase, an enzyme abundant in inflamed synovium and in a variety of mucosal structures. ACPA have similar sensitivity to RF for RA (70%) but much higher specificity (> 95%), and are increasingly being used in preference to RF in the diagnosis of RA. ACPA are associated with more severe disease progression, and can be detected in asymptomatic patients several years before the development of RA. Their pathological role is still debated but it is likely that they amplify the synovial response at an inflammatory stimulus.

Antinuclear antibodies

Antinuclear antibodies (ANA) are directed against one or more components of the cell nucleus, including nucleic acids themselves, and the proteins concerned with processing of DNA or RNA. They occur in many inflammatory rheumatic diseases but are also found at low titre in normal individuals and in other diseases (Box 25.10). High titres of ANA are of greater diagnostic significance but circulating levels are not associated with disease severity or activity. The most common indication for ANA testing is in patients suspected of having SLE or connective tissue diseases. ANA has high sensitivity for SLE (virtually 100%) but low specificity (10–40%). A negative ANA virtually excludes SLE but a positive result does not confirm it.

Anti-DNA antibodies bind to double-stranded DNA and are highly specific for SLE (95%) but sensitivity is poor (30%). They can be useful in disease monitoring since very high titres are associated with more severe disease, including renal or central nervous system (CNS) involvement, and an increase in antibody titre may precede relapse.

Antibodies to extractable nuclear antigens (ENA) act as markers for certain connective tissue diseases and some complications of SLE, but sensitivity and specificity are poor (Box 25.11). For example, antibodies to Sm are found in a minority of patients with SLE but are associated with renal involvement. Antibodies to Ro occur in SLE and in Sjögren's syndrome (in association with anti-La antibodies), and are associated with a

25.9 Conditions associated with a positive rheumatoid factor

Disease	Frequency (%)
Rheumatoid arthritis with nodules and extra-articular manifestations	100
Rheumatoid arthritis (overall)	70
Sjögren's syndrome	90
Mixed essential cryoglobulinaemia	90
Primary biliary cirrhosis	50
Infective endocarditis	40
Systemic lupus erythematosus	30
Tuberculosis	15
Age > 65 yrs	20

Normal healthy people can be positive for rheumatoid factor.

25.10 Conditions associated with a positive antinuclear antibody

Condition	Approximate frequency
Diseases where ANA is useful in diagnosis	
Systemic lupus erythematosus	100%
Systemic sclerosis	60–80%
Sjögren's syndrome	40–70%
Dermatomyositis or polymyositis	30–80%
Mixed connective tissue disease	100%
Autoimmune hepatitis	100%
Diseases where ANA is not useful in diagnosis	
Rheumatoid arthritis	30–50%
Autoimmune thyroid disease	30–50%
Malignancy	Varies widely
Infectious diseases	Varies widely

N.B. 5% of healthy individuals have an ANA titre > 1:80.

25

25.11 Conditions associated with antibodies to extractable nuclear antigens

Antibody (target/other name)	Disease association
Anti-centromere antibody	CREST variant of systemic sclerosis (sensitivity 60%, specificity 98%) Occasionally found in primary Raynaud's syndrome
Anti-histone antibody	Drug-induced lupus (80%)
Anti-Jo-1 (anti-histidyl-tRNA synthetase)	Polymyositis, dermatomyositis or polymyositis–systemic sclerosis overlap (20–30%). Particularly associated with interstitial lung disease
Anti-La antibody (anti-SS-B)	Sjögren's syndrome (60%) SLE (20–60%)
Anti-ribonucleoprotein antibody (anti-RNP)	Mixed connective tissue disease (100%) SLE (25–50%), usually in conjunction with anti-Sm antibodies
Anti-Ro antibody (anti-SS-A)	SLE (35–60%): associated with photosensitivity, thrombocytopenia and subacute cutaneous lupus Maternal anti-Ro antibodies associated with neonatal lupus and congenital heart block Sjögren's syndrome (40–80%)
Anti-RNA polymerase	Diffuse systemic sclerosis (15%)
Anti Sm (anti-Smith antibody)	SLE (15–30%); associated with renal disease
Anti-Scl-70 (anti-topoisomerase I antibody)	Diffuse systemic sclerosis (15%); associated with more severe organ involvement, including pulmonary fibrosis

(CREST = calcinosis, Raynaud's, oesophageal dysmotility, sclerodactyly, telangiectasia)

photosensitive rash and congenital heart block. Antibodies to ribonuclear protein (RNP) occur in SLE and also in mixed connective tissue disease, where features of lupus, myositis and systemic sclerosis coexist. Anti-topoisomerase 1 (also termed Scl-70) antibodies occur in diffuse systemic sclerosis, whereas anti-centromere antibodies are more specific for limited systemic sclerosis.

Antiphospholipid antibodies

Antiphospholipid antibodies bind to a number of phospholipid binding proteins, but the most clinically relevant are those that target beta$_2$-glycoprotein 1 (β_2GP1). They may be detected in SLE and other connective tissue diseases or can be present in isolation or in the antiphospholipid antibody syndrome (p. 1055).

Antineutrophil cytoplasmic antibodies

Antineutrophil cytoplasmic antibodies (ANCA) are IgG antibodies directed against the cytoplasmic constituents of granulocytes and are useful in the diagnosis and monitoring of systemic vasculitis. Two common patterns are described by immunofluorescence: cytoplasmic fluorescence (c-ANCA), which is caused by antibodies to proteinase-3 (PR3); and perinuclear fluorescence (p-ANCA), which is caused by antibodies to myeloperoxidase (MPO) and other proteins such as lactoferrin and elastase. These antibodies are not specific for vasculitis and positive results may be found in autoimmune liver disease, malignancy, infection (bacterial and human immunodeficiency virus, HIV), inflammatory bowel disease, rheumatoid arthritis, SLE and pulmonary fibrosis.

Tissue biopsy

Tissue biopsy is useful in confirming the diagnosis in certain musculoskeletal diseases.

Synovial biopsy can be useful in selected patients with chronic inflammatory monoarthritis or tenosynovitis to rule out chronic infectious causes, especially mycobacterial infections. Characteristic changes on MRI can obviate the need for biopsy in many cases of suspected tumour. Whatever the indication, synovial biopsy can be obtained arthroscopically (by conventional means or via use of needle arthroscope) or using ultrasound guidance under local anaesthetic.

Temporal artery biopsy can be of value in patients suspected of having temporal arteritis, especially when the presentation is atypical, but a negative result does not exclude the diagnosis. Biopsies of affected tissues, such as skin, lung, nasopharynx, gut, kidney and muscle, can be of value in the diagnosis of systemic vasculitis and granulomatosis with polyangiitis (also known as Wegener's granulomatosis).

Muscle biopsy plays an important role in the investigation of myopathy and inflammatory myositis. It is usually taken from the quadriceps or deltoid through a small skin incision under local anaesthetic. Since myositis can be patchy in nature, MRI is sometimes used to localise the best site for biopsy. Immunohistochemical staining, together with plain histology, gives information on primary and secondary muscle and neuromuscular disease. Repeat biopsies are sometimes used to monitor the response to treatment.

Bone biopsy is occasionally required where non-invasive tests give inconclusive results and in the diagnosis of infiltrative disorders, chronic infections and malignancy. If a systemic disorder of mineralisation, such as osteomalacia, is suspected, the biopsy can be taken from the iliac crest using a large-diameter (8-mm) trephine needle under local anaesthetic, and processed without demineralisation. For focal lesions, the biopsy should be taken under X-ray guidance or at open surgery, from an affected site.

Electromyography

Electromyography (p. 1152) is of value in the investigation of suspected myopathy and inflammatory myositis, when it shows the diagnostic triad of:

- spontaneous fibrillation
- short-duration action potentials in a polyphasic disorganised outline
- repetitive bouts of high-voltage oscillations on needle contact with diseased muscle.

PRESENTING PROBLEMS IN MUSCULOSKELETAL DISEASE

Acute monoarthritis

This term is used to describe sudden pain and swelling in a single joint. The most important causes are crystal arthritis, sepsis and reactive arthritis. Other potential causes are shown in Box 25.12.

Clinical assessment

The clinical history, pattern of joint involvement, speed of onset, and age and gender of the patient all give clues to the most likely diagnosis. Reactive arthritis (p. 1107) is the most common cause in young men, gout in middle-aged men and pseudogout in older women. Gout classically affects the first metatarsophalangeal (MTP) joint, whereas the wrist and shoulder are typical sites for pseudogout. A very rapid onset (6–12 hours) is suggestive of gout or pseudogout; joint sepsis develops more slowly and continues to progress until treated. Haemarthrosis typically causes a large effusion, in the absence of periarticular swelling or skin change, in a patient who has suffered an injury. Pigmented villonodular synovitis (p. 1134) also presents with synovial swelling and a large effusion, although the onset is gradual. A previous diarrhoeal illness or recent sexual contact suggests reactive arthritis, whereas intercurrent illness, dehydration or surgery may act as a trigger for crystal-induced arthritis. Rheumatoid arthritis seldom presents with monoarthritis and a sudden increase in pain and swelling involving a single joint in a patient with pre-existing RA is strongly suggestive of sepsis. Osteoarthritis can present with pain and stiffness affecting a single joint, but the onset is gradual and there is seldom evidence of significant joint swelling.

Investigations

Aspiration of the affected joint is mandatory. The fluid should be sent for culture and Gram stain to seek the presence of organisms, and should be checked by microscopy for crystals. Blood cultures should also be taken in patients suspected of having septic arthritis. CRP levels and ESR are raised in sepsis, crystal arthritis and reactive arthritis, and this can be useful in assessing the response to treatment. Serum uric acid measurements may be raised in gout but a normal level does not exclude the diagnosis.

Management

If there is any suspicion of sepsis, intravenous antibiotics (Box 25.52, p. 1095) should be given promptly, pending the results of cultures. Otherwise, management should be directed towards the underlying cause.

25.12 Causes of acute monoarthritis

Common

- Septic arthritis
- Gout
- Pseudogout
- Reactive arthritis
- Trauma
- Haemarthrosis
- Seronegative spondyloarthritis
  - Psoriatic arthritis
  - Ankylosing spondylitis
  - Enteropathic arthritis

Less common

- Erythema nodosum
- Rheumatoid arthritis
- Juvenile idiopathic arthritis
- Pigmented villonodular synovitis
- Foreign body reaction
- Other infection
  - Gonococcal
  - Tuberculosis
- Leukaemia*
- Osteomyelitis*

*In children, both leukaemia and osteomyelitis may present with monoarthritis.

Polyarthritis

This term is used to describe pain and swelling affecting five or more joints or joint groups. The possible causes are listed in Box 25.13.

25.13 Causes of polyarthritis

Cause	Characteristics
Common	
Rheumatoid arthritis	Symmetrical, small and large joints, upper and lower limbs
Viral arthritis	Symmetrical, small joints; may be associated with rash and prodromal illness; self-limiting
Osteoarthritis	Symmetrical, targets PIP, DIP and first CMC joints in hands, knees, hips, back and neck; associated with Heberden's and Bouchard's nodes
Psoriatic arthritis	Asymmetrical, targets PIP and DIP joints of hands and feet (sausage appearance on examination), nail pitting, large joints also affected
Ankylosing spondylitis and enteropathic arthritis	Tends to affect large joints, lower more than upper limbs, possible history of inflammatory back pain
SLE	Symmetrical, typically affecting small joints, clinical evidence of synovitis unusual
Less common	
Juvenile idiopathic arthritis	Symmetrical, small and large joints, upper and lower limbs
Chronic gout	Affects distal more than proximal joints, history of acute attacks
Chronic sarcoidosis (p. 709)	Symmetrical, small and large joints
Polymyalgia rheumatica	Symmetrical, small and large joints
Rare	
Systemic sclerosis and polymyositis	Small and large joints
Hypertrophic osteoarthropathy	Small joints, clubbing
Haemochromatosis (p. 972)	Small and large joints
Acromegaly (p. 792)	Mainly large joints and spine

(CMC = carpometacarpal; DIP = distal interphalangeal; PIP = proximal interphalangeal)

25

Clinical assessment

The hallmarks of inflammatory arthritis are early morning stiffness and worsening of symptoms with inactivity, along with synovial swelling and tenderness on examination. Clinical features in other systems can be helpful in determining the underlying cause (Box 25.14). The most important diagnosis to consider is rheumatoid arthritis, which is characterised by symmetrical involvement of the small joints of the hands and feet, often in association with other joints. Viral arthritis should also be considered. This presents with an acute symmetrical inflammatory polyarthritis affecting small and large joints of upper and lower limbs, often with a rash.

The pattern of involvement can be helpful in reaching a diagnosis (Fig. 25.9). Asymmetry, lower limb predominance and greater involvement of large joints are characteristic of seronegative spondyloarthritis. Other extra-articular features may also be present, giving a clue to the diagnosis. In psoriatic arthritis, the small joints of the hand and feet are often affected, but with involvement of the proximal and distal interphalangeal (PIP and DIP) joints, as opposed to the metacarpophalangeal (MCP) and PIP joints in RA. The pattern of involvement also tends to be asymmetrical in psoriatic arthritis, and other clues such as nail pitting and a rash may be present. SLE can be associated with polyarthritis but more usually causes polyarthralgia and tenosynovitis (p. 1110).

Investigations

Blood samples should be taken for routine haematology, biochemistry, ESR, CRP, viral serology and an immunological screen, including ANA, RF and ACPA. Ultrasound examination or MRI may be required to confirm the presence of synovitis if this is not obvious clinically.

25.14 Extra-articular features of inflammatory arthritis

Clinical feature	Disease association
Skin, nails and mucous membranes	
Psoriasis, nail pitting and dystrophy	Psoriatic arthritis
Raynaud's phenomenon	SLE, systemic sclerosis
Photosensitivity	SLE
Livedo reticularis	SLE
Splinter haemorrhages, nail-fold infarcts	Vasculitis
Oral ulcers	SLE, reactive arthritis, Behçet's syndrome
Large nodules (mainly extensor surfaces)	RA, gout
Clubbing	Enteropathic arthritis, metastatic lung cancer, endocarditis
Eyes	
Uveitis	Seronegative spondyloarthritis
Conjunctivitis	Reactive arthritis
Episcleritis, scleritis	RA, vasculitis
Heart, lungs	
Pleuro-pericarditis	SLE, RA
Fibrosing alveolitis	RA, SLE, other connective tissue disease
Abdominal organs	
Hepatosplenomegaly	RA, SLE
Haematuria, proteinuria	SLE, vasculitis, systemic sclerosis
Urethritis	Reactive arthritis
Fever, lymphadenopathy	Infection, systemic juvenile idiopathic arthritis

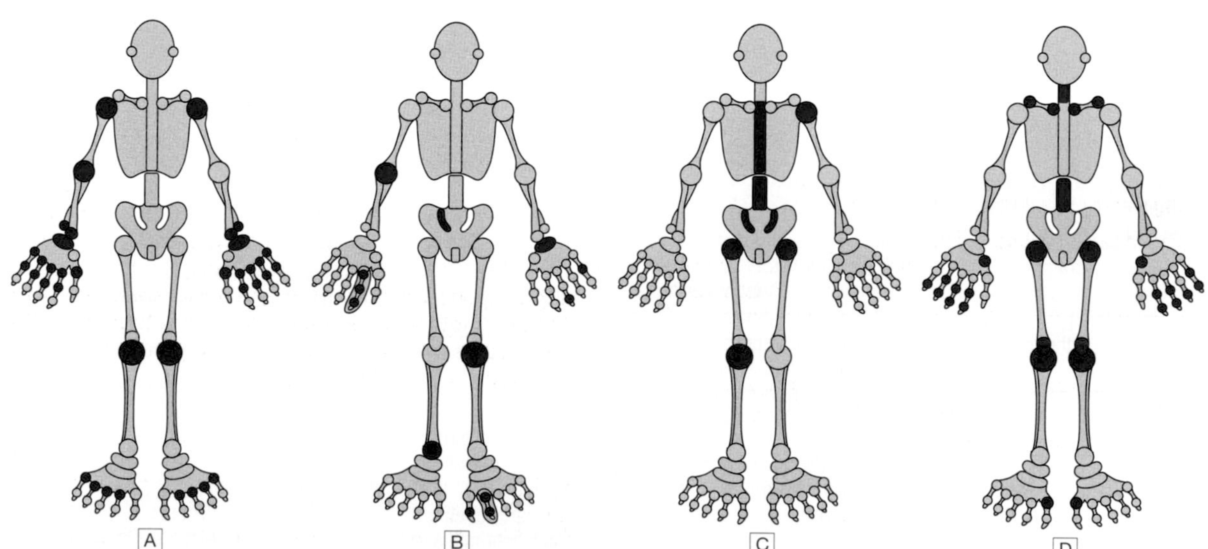

Fig. 25.9 Patterns of joint involvement in different forms of polyarthritis. **A** Rheumatoid arthritis typically targets the metacarpophalangeal and proximal interphalangeal joints of the hands and metatarsophalangeal joints of the feet, as well as other joints, in a symmetrical pattern. **B** Psoriatic arthritis targets proximal and distal interphalangeal joints of the hands and larger joints in an asymmetrical pattern. Sacroiliitis (often asymmetrical) may occur. **C** Ankylosing spondylitis targets the spine, sacroiliac joints and large peripheral joints in an asymmetrical pattern. **D** Osteoarthritis targets the proximal and distal interphalangeal joints of the hands, first carpometacarpal joint at the base of the thumb, knees, hips, lumbar and cervical spine.

Management

Management should be directed at the underlying condition, but treatment with non-steroidal anti-inflammatory drugs (NSAIDs) and analgesics may be required for symptom control until a diagnosis has been made.

Fracture

Fractures are a common presenting symptom of osteoporosis, but they also occur in other bone diseases, in osteopenia and in some patients with normal bone.

Clinical assessment

The presentation is with localised bone pain, which is worsened by movement of the affected limb or region. There is usually a history of trauma but spontaneous fractures can occur in the absence of trauma in those with severe osteoporosis. Fractures can be divided into several subtypes, based on the precipitating event and presence or absence of an underlying disease (Box 25.15). The main differential diagnosis is soft tissue injury, but fracture should be suspected when there is marked pain and swelling, abnormal movement of the affected limb, crepitus or deformity. Femoral neck fractures typically produce a shortened, externally rotated leg that is painful to move.

Investigations

Radiographs of the affected site should be taken in at least two planes and examined for discontinuity of the cortical outline (Box 25.16). In addition to demonstrating the fracture, X-rays may also show evidence of an underlying disorder, such as osteoporosis, Paget's disease or osteomalacia. If the X-ray fails to show evidence of a fracture but clinical suspicion remains high, MRI should be performed, since this can demonstrate fractures that are radiographically occult. Patients who are over the age of 50 and present with fragility fractures should be screened for the presence of osteoporosis by DEXA.

Management

Management of fracture in the acute stage requires adequate pain relief, with opiates if necessary, reduction of the fracture to restore normal anatomy, and immobilisation of the affected limb to promote healing. This can be achieved either by the use of an external cast or splint or by internal fixation. Femoral neck fractures present a special management problem since non-union and avascular necrosis are common. This is especially true with intracapsular hip fractures, which should be treated by joint replacement surgery. Following the fracture, rehabilitation is required with physiotherapy and a supervised exercise programme (this is especially important in older patients to prevent muscle-wasting and loss of mobility). Elderly patients with hip fracture also benefit from nutritional supplementation. Patients with high-energy and fatigue fractures generally require no further investigation or treatment once the fracture has healed. If the DEXA examination or other investigation shows evidence of osteoporosis or other metabolic bone disease, this should be treated appropriately (p. 172).

25.15 Characteristics of different fracture types

Fracture type	Precipitation factor	Disease
Fragility fracture	Fall from standing height or less	Osteoporosis Osteopenia
Vertebral fracture	Bending, lifting, falling	Osteoporosis
Stress fracture	Running, excessive training	Normal
High-energy fracture	Major trauma	Normal
Pathological fracture	Spontaneous, minimal trauma	Malignancy Paget's disease Osteomalacia

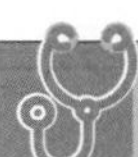

25.16 How to investigate a suspected fracture

- Order X-rays in two projections at right angles to one another
- Include the whole bone and the joints at either end (this may reveal an additional unsuspected fracture)
- Check for evidence of displacement
- Check for a break in the cortex
- In suspected vertebral fracture, check for depression of the end plate
- If clinical suspicion is high but no fracture is seen, request MRI

Generalised musculoskeletal pain

Clinical assessment

Clinical history and examination can often indicate the underlying cause (Box 25.17). Relentlessly progressive pain occurring in association with weight loss suggests malignant disease with bone metastases. Generalised bone pain may also occur in Paget's disease if the disease is widespread, but Pagetic pain is usually more focal and localised to the site of involvement (p. 1128). Widespread pain can occur in OA but this also tends to be localised to sites of involvement, such as the lumbar spine, hips, knees and hands. Signs of OA may be apparent on clinical examination. Osteomalacia (p. 1125) can cause generalised bone pain that is associated with bone tenderness and limb girdle weakness. Fibromyalgia can present with generalised pain particularly affecting the trunk, back and neck. Accompanying features include fatigue, poor concentration and focal areas of hyperalgesia. Another potential cause is joint hypermobility, the features of which should be apparent on clinical examination (p. 1134).

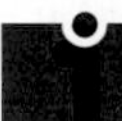

25.17 Causes of generalised pain

- Metastatic bone disease
- Fibromyalgia (p. 1092)
- Joint hypermobility
- Osteomalacia (p. 1125)
- Osteoarthritis
- Paget's disease
- Polymyalgia rheumatica (p. 1117)
- Myositis (p. 1114)

Investigations

Radionuclide bone scanning is of value in patients suspected of having bone metastases and Paget's disease, along with further imaging as appropriate. Myeloma (p. 1046) should be excluded by plasma and urinary protein electrophoresis. If these results are positive, a radiological skeletal survey should be performed, since the isotope bone scan may be normal in myeloma. Routine biochemistry, vitamin D levels and PTH measurement should be performed if osteomalacia is suspected. In Paget's disease, ALP may be elevated but can be normal in localised disease. Laboratory investigations are normal in patients with fibromyalgia and benign hypermobility.

Management

Management should be directed towards the underlying cause. Chronic pain of unknown cause and that associated with fibromyalgia responds poorly to analgesics and NSAID, but may respond partially to antineuropathic agents such as amitriptyline, duloxetine, gabapentin and pregabalin.

Back pain

Back pain is a common symptom that affects 60–80% of people at some time in their lives. Although the prevalence has not increased, reported disability from back pain has risen significantly in the last 30 years. In Western countries, back pain is the most common cause of sickness-related work absence. In the UK, 7% of adults consult their GP each year with back pain. The most important causes are summarised in Box 25.18.

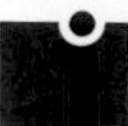

25.18 Causes of low back pain

- Mechanical back pain
- Prolapsed intervertebral disc
- Osteoarthritis
- Vertebral fracture (p. 1071)
- Spinal stenosis
- Paget's disease
- Spondylolysis (p. 1133)
- Bone metastases
- Spondylolisthesis (p. 1133)
- Arachnoiditis
- Scheuermann's disease (p. 1130)

Clinical assessment

The main purpose of clinical assessment is to differentiate the self-limiting disorder of acute mechanical back pain from serious spinal pathology, as summarised in Figure 25.10. Mechanical back pain is the most common cause of acute back pain in people aged 20–55. This accounts for more than 90% of episodes, and is usually acute and associated with lifting or bending. It is exacerbated by activity and is generally relieved by rest (Box 25.19). It is usually confined to the lumbar–sacral region, buttock or thigh, is asymmetrical, and does not radiate beyond the knee (which would imply nerve root irritation). On examination, there may be asymmetric local paraspinal muscle spasm and tenderness, and painful restriction of some but not all movements. Low back pain is more common in manual workers, particularly those in occupations that involve heavy lifting and twisting. The prognosis is generally good. After 2 days,

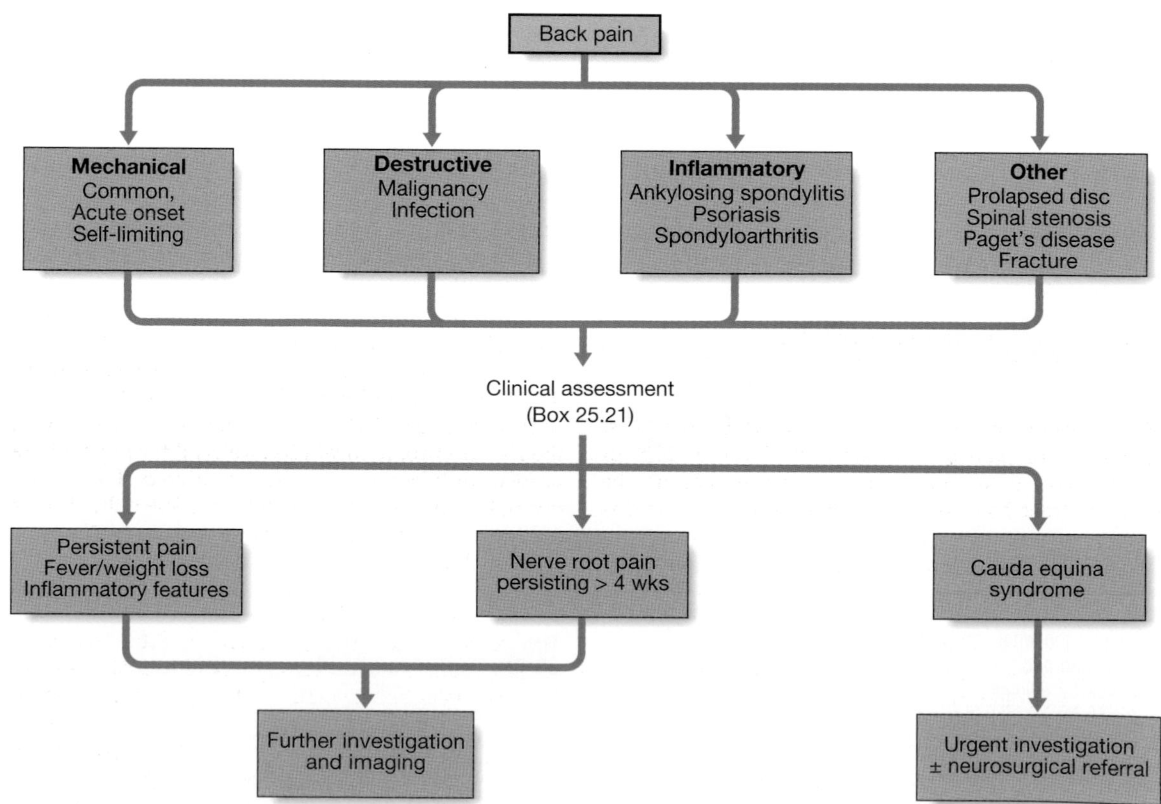

Fig. 25.10 Initial triage assessment of back pain.

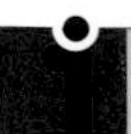

25.19 Features of mechanical low back pain

- Pain varies with physical activity (improved with rest)
- Sudden onset, precipitated by lifting or bending
- Recurrent episodes
- Pain limited to back or upper leg
- No clear-cut nerve root distribution
- No systemic features
- Prognosis good (90% recovery at 6 wks)

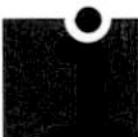

25.20 Red flags for possible spinal pathology

History

- Age: presentation < 20 yrs or > 55 yrs
- Character: constant, progressive pain unrelieved by rest
- Location: thoracic pain
- Past medical history: carcinoma, tuberculosis, HIV, systemic corticosteroid use, osteoporosis
- Constitutional: systemic upset, sweats, weight loss
- Major trauma

Examination

- Painful spinal deformity
- Severe/symmetrical spinal deformity
- Saddle anaesthesia
- Progressive neurological signs/muscle-wasting
- Multiple levels of root signs

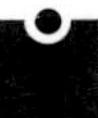

25.21 Clinical features of radicular pain

Nerve root pain

- Unilateral leg pain worse than low back pain
- Pain radiates beyond knee
- Paraesthesia in same distribution
- Nerve irritation signs (reduced straight leg raising that reproduces leg pain)
- Motor, sensory or reflex signs (limited to one nerve root)
- Prognosis reasonable (50% recovery at 6 wks)

Cauda equina syndrome

- Difficulty with micturition
- Loss of anal sphincter tone or faecal incontinence
- Saddle anaesthesia
- Gait disturbance
- Pain, numbness or weakness affecting one or both legs

30% are better and 90% have recovered by 6 weeks. Recurrences of pain may occur and about 10–15% of patients go on to develop chronic back pain that may be difficult to treat. Psychological elements, such as job dissatisfaction, depression and anxiety, are important risk factors for the transition to chronic pain and disability.

Back pain secondary to serious spinal pathology has different characteristics (Box 25.20). If there is clinical evidence of spinal cord or nerve root compression, or a cauda equina lesion (Box 25.21), urgent investigation is needed. Spinal stenosis presents with leg discomfort on walking that is relieved by rest (pseudoclaudication). Bending forwards or walking uphill may also relieve the pain. Common causes include Paget's disease, in which enlargement of the vertebrae may encroach on the spinal canal, and osteoarthritis of the spine, in which osteophytes can have the same effect. Patients may adopt a characteristic simian posture, with a forward stoop and slight flexion at hips and knees.

Degenerative disc disease is a common cause of chronic low back pain. Prolapse of an intervertebral disc presents with nerve root pain, which can be accompanied by a sensory deficit, motor weakness, and asymmetrical reflexes. Examination may reveal a positive sciatic or femoral stretch test. About 70% of patients improve by 4 weeks. Inflammatory back pain due to seronegative spondyloarthritis has a gradual onset and almost always occurs before the age of 40. It is associated with morning stiffness and improves with movement. Spondylolisthesis (p. 1133) may cause back pain that is typically aggravated by standing and walking. Occasionally, diffuse idiopathic skeletal hyperostosis (DISH; p. 1133) can cause back pain but it is usually asymptomatic. Arachnoiditis is a rare cause of chronic severe low back pain. It is due to chronic inflammation of the nerve root sheaths in the spinal canal and can complicate meningitis, spinal surgery, or myelography with oil-based contrast agents.

Investigations

Investigations are not required in patients with acute mechanical back pain. Those with persistent pain (> 6 weeks) or red flags (see Box 25.20) should undergo further investigation. MRI is the investigation of choice since it can demonstrate spinal stenosis, cord compression or nerve root compression, as well as inflammatory changes in spondyloarthropathy, and infectious causes such as spinal abscess. Plain radiographs can be of value in patients suspected of having vertebral compression fractures, OA and degenerative disc disease. If metastatic disease is suspected, radionuclide bone scan or SPECT should be considered. Additional investigations that may be required include routine biochemistry and haematology with measurement of ESR and CRP (to screen for sepsis and inflammatory disease), protein and urinary electrophoresis (for myeloma) and prostate specific antigen (for prostate carcinoma).

Management

Education is important in patients with mechanical back pain. It should emphasise the self-limiting nature of the condition and the fact that exercise is helpful rather than damaging. Regular analgesia and/or NSAIDs may be required to improve mobility and facilitate exercise. Return to work and normal activity should take place as soon as possible. Bed rest is not helpful and may increase the risk of chronic disability. Referral for physiotherapy or manipulation should be considered if a return to normal activities has not been achieved by 6 weeks. Low-dose tricyclic antidepressant drugs may help pain, sleep and mood.

Other treatment modalities that are occasionally used include epidural and facet joint injection, traction and lumbar supports, though there is little evidence to support their use (Box 25.22). Malignant disease, osteoporosis, Paget's disease and spondyloarthropathies require specific treatment of the underlying condition.

Surgery is required in less than 1% of patients with low back pain but may be needed in spinal stenosis, in spinal cord compression and in some patients with nerve root compression.

EBM 25.22 Management of low back pain

- Reassure patients (favourable prognosis)
- Advise patients to stay active
- Prescribe medication if necessary (preferably at fixed time intervals)
- Paracetamol
- NSAID
- Consider opioids, muscle relaxants
- Discourage bed rest
- Consider spinal manipulation for pain relief
- Do not advise lumbar supports, back-specific exercises, traction, acupuncture, epidural or facet injections.

- Koes BW. BMJ 2006; 332:1430–1434.

Regional musculoskeletal pain

Regional musculoskeletal pain is a common presenting complaint, usually occurring as the result of age-related degenerative disease of tendons and ligaments, OA and repetitive strain injuries due to overuse.

Neck pain

Neck pain is a common symptom that can occur following injury (for example, whiplash), after falling asleep in an awkward position, as a result of stress, or in association with OA of the spine. The causes are shown in Box 25.23. Most cases resolve spontaneously or with a short course of NSAID or analgesics, and a soft collar. Patients with persistent pain that follows a nerve root distribution and those with neurological signs and symptoms should be investigated by MRI scan, and if necessary referred for a neurosurgical opinion.

25.23 Causes of neck pain

Mechanical	
• Postural • Whiplash injury	• Disc prolapse • Cervical spondylosis
Inflammatory	
• Infections • Spondylitis • Juvenile idiopathic arthritis	• RA • Polymyalgia rheumatica
Metabolic	
• Osteoporosis • Osteomalacia	• Paget's disease
Neoplasia	
• Metastases • Myeloma	• Lymphoma • Intrathecal tumours
Other	
• Fibromyalgia	• Torticollis
Referred pain	
• Pharynx • Cervical lymph nodes • Teeth • Angina pectoris	• Aortic aneurysm • Pancoast tumour • Diaphragm

Shoulder pain

Shoulder pain is a common complaint in both genders over the age of 40, and is most often due to degenerative disease of tendons in the rotator cuff (Box 25.24). Varying pain patterns associated with common lesions are shown in Figure 25.11. Management is symptomatic, with analgesics, NSAID, local corticosteroid injections and physiotherapy aimed at restoring normal movement and function. Surgery may be required in patients who have debilitating symptoms in association with rotator cuff tears. Adhesive capsulitis (frozen shoulder) presents with upper arm pain that can progress over 4–10 weeks before subsiding over a similar time course. Restriction of glenohumeral movement is characteristic. In the early phase, there is marked anterior joint/capsular tenderness and stress pain in a capsular pattern; later there is painless restriction, often of all movements. Frozen shoulder is more common in diabetes mellitus, but may also be triggered by a rotator cuff tear, local trauma, myocardial infarction or hemiplegia. Treatment in the early stage is with analgesia, intra- and extracapsular steroid injection, and regular 'pendulum' exercises of the arm to prevent the capsule from over-tightening. Mobilising and strengthening exercises are the sole treatment in the painless 'frozen' stage. The natural

25.24 Clinical findings in shoulder pain

Rotator cuff lesion

- Pain reproduced by resisted active movement:
  Abduction: supraspinatus
  External rotation: infraspinatus, teres minor
  Internal rotation: subscapularis

Subacromial bursitis

- Pain on full abduction but no pain on resisted active abduction

Bicipital (long head) tendinitis

- Tender over bicipital groove
- Pain reproduced by resisted active wrist supination or elbow flexion

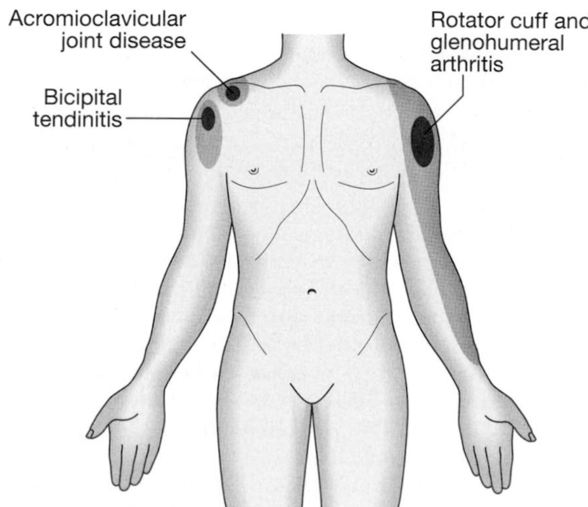

Fig. 25.11 Pain patterns around the shoulder. The dark shading indicates sites of maximum pain.

history is for slow but complete recovery, sometimes taking up to 2 years.

Elbow pain

The most common causes are repetitive strain injury affecting the lateral epicondyle (tennis elbow) and medial epicondyle (golfer's elbow) (Box 25.25). Management is by rest, analgesics and topical or systemic NSAID. Symptoms may also respond to local application of glyceryl trinitrate patches. Local corticosteroid injections may be required in resistant cases. Olecranon bursitis can also follow local repetitive trauma but other causes include infections, gout and RA.

25.25 Local causes of elbow pain

Lesion	Pain	Examination findings
Tennis elbow	Lateral epicondyle Radiation to extensor forearm	Tender over epicondyle Pain reproduced by resisted active wrist extension
Golfer's elbow	Medial epicondyle Radiation to flexor forearm	Tender over epicondyle Pain reproduced by resisted active wrist flexion
Olecranon bursitis	Olecranon	Fluctuant tender swelling over olecranon

Hand and wrist pain

Pain from hand or wrist joints is well localised to the affected joint, except for pain from the first metacarpal joint, commonly targeted by OA; although maximal at the thumb base, the pain often radiates down the thumb and to the radial aspect of the wrist. Non-articular causes of hand pain include:

- Tenosynovitis: flexor or extensor (pain and swelling, with or without fine crepitus on volar or extensor aspect). De Quervain's tenosynovitis involves the tendon sheaths of abductor pollicis longus and extensor pollicis brevis, and produces pain maximal over the radial aspect of the distal forearm and wrist. It usually occurs as the result of a repetitive strain injury. There is tenderness (with or without warmth, linear swelling and fine crepitus) over the distal radius and marked pain on forced ulnar deviation of the wrist with the thumb held across the patient's palm (Finkelstein's sign).
- Raynaud's phenomenon (p. 602).
- C8/T1 radiculopathy.
- Reflex sympathetic dystrophy (p. 1130).

Hip pain

Pain from the hip joint is usually maximal deep in the anterior groin, with variable radiation to the buttock, anterolateral thigh, knee or shin (Fig. 25.12). Trochanteric bursitis is a common cause (Box 25.26), typically affecting obese women, and occurring in isolation or secondary to an abnormal gait, such as in hip or knee OA. Pain in the hip region may also be referred from the back. Root entrapment can cause pain in the lateral thigh (T12–L1) or the inguinal region and lateral thigh (L2–4), but is worsened by coughing and straining more than by movement and is often accompanied by sensory disturbance. Other less common causes include psoas abscess, retroperitoneal haemorrhage or pelvic inflammation, which can cause inguinal and lateral thigh pain that is aggravated by resisted hip flexion.

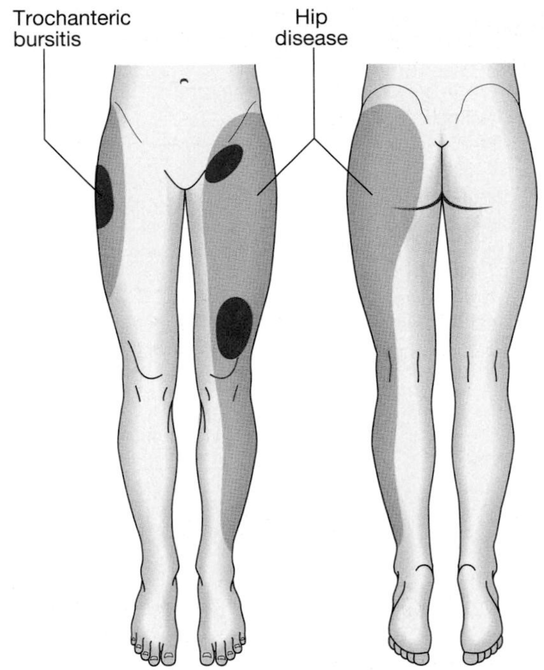

Fig. 25.12 Pain patterns of hip disease and trochanteric bursitis. The dark shading indicates sites of maximum pain.

25.26 Local causes of hip pain

Lesion	Pain	Examination findings
Trochanteric bursitis	Upper lateral thigh, worse on lying on that side at night	Tender over greater trochanter
Gluteal enthesopathy	Upper lateral thigh, worse on lying on that side at night	Tender over greater trochanter Pain reproduced by resisted active hip abduction
Adductor tendinitis	Upper inner thigh Usually clearly sports-related	Tender over adductor origin/tendon/muscle Pain reproduced by resisted active hip adduction
Ischiogluteal bursitis	Buttock, worse on sitting	Tender over ischial prominence
Iliopectineal bursitis	Anterior groin	Tender (± fluctuant swelling) lateral to femoral pulse, not worsened by internal rotation of hip (cf. hip pain)

Knee pain

The most common cause of knee pain is OA, the features of which are described on page 1082. Pain that is associated with locking of the knee (sudden painful inability to extend fully) is usually due to a meniscal tear or osteochondritis dissecans. Referred pain from the hip

25.27 Local causes of knee pain

Lesion	Pain	Examination findings
Pre-patellar bursitis	Anterior patella	Tender fluctuant swelling in front of patella
Superficial and deep infrapatellar bursitis	Anterior knee, inferior to patella	Tender fluctuant swelling in front of (superficial) or behind (deep) patella tendon
Anserine bursitis	Upper medial tibia	Tenderness (± warmth, swelling) over upper medial tibia
Inferior medial collateral ligament enthesopathy	Upper medial tibia	Localised tenderness of upper medial tibia Pain reproduced by valgus stress on partly flexed knee
Popliteal cyst (Baker's cyst)	Popliteal fossa	Tender swelling of popliteal fossa, usually reducible by massage with knee in mid-flexion
Patella tendon enthesopathy	Anterior upper tibia	Tenderness and firm swelling of tibial tubercle
Osteochondritis (Osgood–Schlatter disease)	Anterior upper tibia	Affects adolescents Pain on resisted active knee extension

may present at the knee and is reproduced by hip not knee movement. Pain from periarticular lesions is well localised to the involved structure (Box 25.27). Anterior knee pain may be due to bursitis occurring as the result of repetitive occupational kneeling, as well as infection and gout. Anterior knee pain, aggravated by sports, may occur in adolescent girls but is usually self-limiting. Rarely, anterior knee pain may be the result of chondromalacia patellae, in which degenerative changes of the articular cartilage occur.

Ankle and foot pain

Pain from the mortice joint of the ankle (the tibiofibular–talar joint) is felt between the malleoli and is worse on weight-bearing. Pain from the subtalar joint is also worse on weight-bearing on uneven surfaces. The mortice joint is commonly affected by OA, whereas RA tends to affect the subtalar joint. Pain under the heel can arise from plantar fasciitis or subcalcaneal bursitis. Pain affecting the back of the heel may be due to Achilles tendinitis or bursitis. Patients with seronegative spondyloarthritis may develop enthesopathy affecting this region, resulting in plantar fasciitis, which presents with pain and tenderness under the heel, or as Achilles enthesitis, which presents with pain at the tendon insertion into the calcaneus. The MTP joints of the feet are commonly involved in RA. The presentation is with pain on walking below the metatarsal heads, often described as 'walking on marbles'. Patients with active inflammation of the MTP joints have pain when the forefoot is squeezed (p. 1059). Involvement of the first MTP joint is common in OA and is associated with a valgus deformity (hallux valgus). This joint is also a classical target in acute gout. Claw foot (pes cavus) can be associated with anterior foot pain and is characterised by a high arch and clawing of the toes. It may be an isolated phenomenon or secondary to neurological disorders such as Friedreich's ataxia (p. 1199) or spina bifida (p. 1222). Management should follow the general principles outlined on page 1077. Bursitis and enthesitis resistant to standard measures may respond to local steroid injections. Morton's neuroma is the name given to an entrapment neuropathy of the interdigital nerves of the feet, which presents with shooting pain that is usually located between the third and fourth metatarsal heads. Women are most commonly affected. Local sensory loss and a palpable tender swelling between the metatarsal heads may be detected. Footwear adjustment, with or without a local corticosteroid injection, often helps but surgical decompression may be required if symptoms persist.

Muscle pain and weakness

Muscle pain and weakness can arise from a variety of causes. It is important to distinguish between a subjective feeling of generalised weakness or fatigue, and an objective weakness with loss of muscle power and function. The former is a non-specific manifestation of many diseases, including depression, whereas the latter is often a sign of primary muscle disease.

Clinical assessment

Proximal muscle weakness suggests the presence of a myopathy or myositis, which typically causes difficulty with standing from a seated position, squatting and lifting overhead. The causes are shown in Box 25.28. Worsening of symptoms on exercise and post-exertional cramps suggest a metabolic myopathy, such as glycogen storage disease (p. 450). A strong family history and onset in childhood or early adulthood suggests muscular dystrophy (p. 1228). Alcohol excess can cause an inflammatory myositis and atrophy of type 2 muscle fibres. Proximal myopathy may be a complication of corticosteroid therapy and of osteomalacia. Myopathy and myositis can also occur in association with statin use and viral infections, including HIV infection, when it may be due to HIV itself or treatment with zidovudine. Clinical examination should document the presence, pattern and severity of muscle weakness, and the latter should be assessed using the Medical Research Council (MRC) scale, in which muscle strength is graded on a six-point scale ranging from no power (0) to full power (5).

Investigations

Investigations should include routine biochemistry and haematology, ESR, and measurement of CRP and CK. Serum 25(OH) vitamin D levels and PTH should be checked in suspected osteomalacia. Raised CK levels suggest muscle pathology but do not establish the cause. The ESR and CRP may be raised in inflammatory myositis. Muscle biopsy and electromyography (EMG) are usually required to make the diagnosis, but MRI can be used to identify focal areas of muscle abnormality and increase the diagnostic yield from muscle biopsies.

Management

Management is determined by the cause but all patients with muscle disease may benefit from physiotherapy and graded exercises to maximise muscle function.

25.28 Causes of proximal muscle pain or weakness

Inflammatory	
• Polymyositis • Dermatomyositis	• Inclusion body myositis • Polymyalgia rheumatica
Endocrine (Ch. 20)	
• Hypothyroidism • Hyperthyroidism	• Cushing's syndrome • Addison's disease
Metabolic (Ch. 16)	
• Myophosphorylase deficiency • Phosphofructokinase deficiency • Hypokalaemia	• Carnitine deficiency • Myoadenylate deaminase deficiency • Osteomalacia (p. 1125)
Drugs/toxins	
• Alcohol • Cocaine • Fibrates	• Statins • Penicillamine • Zidovudine
Infections (Ch. 13)	
• Viral (HIV, cytomegalovirus, rubella, Epstein–Barr, echo) • Parasitic (schistosomiasis, cysticercosis, toxoplasmosis)	• Bacterial (*Clostridium perfringens*, staphylococci, tuberculosis, *Mycoplasma*)

PRINCIPLES OF MANAGEMENT OF MUSCULOSKELETAL DISORDERS

Although management of musculoskeletal disease depends on the underlying diagnosis, certain aspects of management are common to many disorders. The general aims of management are to:

- educate the patient
- control pain
- optimise function
- modify the disease process where this is possible
- identify and treat related comorbidity.

These aims are interrelated and success in one area often benefits others. Successful management requires careful assessment of the person as a whole, as well as his or her musculoskeletal system. The management plan should be individualised and patient-centred, should involve all necessary members of the multidisciplinary team, and should be agreed and understood by both the patient and involved practitioners. It must also take into account:

- the person's daily activity requirements, and work and recreational aspirations
- risk factors and associations of the musculoskeletal condition (obesity, muscle weakness, non-restorative sleep)
- the person's perceptions and knowledge of the condition
- medications and coping strategies already tried by the patient
- comorbid disease and its therapy
- the availability, costs and logistics of appropriate evidence-based interventions.

25.29 Core interventions for patients with rheumatic diseases

Core	

• Education
• Exercise
  Aerobic conditioning
  Strengthening
• Simple analgesia
	• Reduction of adverse mechanical factors
	  Pacing of activities
	  Appropriate footwear
	• Weight reduction if obese

Other options	

• Other analgesic drugs
  Oral NSAIDs
  Topical agents
  Opioid analgesics
  Amitriptyline
  Gabapentin/pregabalin
• Disease-modifying therapy
	• Local corticosteroid injections
	• Physical treatments
	  Heat, cold, aids, appliances
	• Surgery
	• Coping strategies

Simple and safe interventions should be tried first. Symptoms and signs will change with time, so the plan requires regular review and re-adjustment. Effective management may require the expertise of a variety of health professionals, with a coordinated multidisciplinary team approach.

Core interventions that should be considered for everyone with a painful musculoskeletal condition are listed in Box 25.29. There are also other non-pharmacological and drug options, the choice depending largely on the nature and severity of the diagnosis.

Education and lifestyle interventions

Education

Patients must always be informed about the nature of their condition and its investigation, treatment and prognosis, as education can improve outcome. Information and therapist contact can reduce pain and disability, improve self-efficacy and reduce the health-care costs of many musculoskeletal conditions, including OA and RA. The mechanisms are unclear but in part may result from improved adherence. Benefits are modest but potentially long-lasting, safe and cost-effective (Box 25.30). Education can be provided through one-to-one discussion, written literature, patient-led group education classes and interactive computer programs. Inclusion of the patient's partner or carer is often appropriate; this is essential for childhood conditions but also helps in many chronic adult conditions, such as RA or fibromyalgia.

Exercise

Two types of exercise should be prescribed (Box 25.30):

- Aerobic fitness training can produce long-term reduction in pain and disability. It improves well-being, encourages restorative sleep and benefits common comorbidity such as obesity, diabetes, chronic heart failure and hypertension.
- Local strengthening exercise for muscles that act over compromised joints also reduces pain and disability, with improvements in the reduced muscle strength, proprioception, coordination and

EBM 25.30 Education and exercise in the management of arthritis

'Both patient education and exercise regimens have a modest, yet clinically important influence on patients' well-being.'

'Both aerobic walking and home-based quadriceps-strengthening exercises reduce pain and disability from knee osteoarthritis.'

- Devos-Combey L, et al. J Rheumatol 2006; 33:744–756.
- Roddy E, et al. Ann Rheum Dis 2005; 64:544–548.

balance that associate with chronic arthritis. 'Small amounts often' of strengthening exercise are better than protracted sessions performed infrequently.

Joint protection

Excessive impact-loading and adverse repetitive use of a compromised joint or periarticular tissue can often be reduced: for example, cessation of contact sports, or altered use of machinery or tools at the workplace. Simple 'pacing' of activities - dividing physically onerous tasks into shorter segments with brief breaks in between - is helpful. Use of shock-absorbing footwear with thick soft soles can reduce impact-loading through feet, knees, hips and back, and improve symptoms at these sites. A walking stick held on the contralateral side takes the weight off a painful hip, knee or foot.

Weight loss

Obesity aggravates pain at most sites of the body through increased mechanical strain and is a risk factor for more rapid progression of joint damage in patients with arthritis. This should be explained to obese patients and strategies offered on how to lose and then maintain an appropriate weight (p. 117).

Pharmacological treatment

Analgesics

Paracetamol (1 g up to 4 times daily) is the oral analgesic of first choice and, if successful, the preferred long-term oral analgesic. It inhibits prostaglandin synthesis in the brain but has less effect on peripheral prostaglandin production. It is generally well tolerated and has few adverse effects and drug interactions. There is a possible increased risk of both gastrointestinal events and cardiovascular disease with chronic usage, but it is uncertain whether this is due to the underlying disease or the drug itself. If paracetamol fails to achieve an adequate response, it can be used in combination with opioids such as codeine and dihydrocodeine in compound analgesic preparations like co-codamol (codeine and paracetamol) or co-dydramol (dihydrocodeine and paracetamol). Although these are more effective than paracetamol, side-effects include constipation, headache and confusion, especially in the elderly. The centrally acting analgesics tramadol and meptazinol may be useful for temporary control of severe pain unresponsive to other measures. Both may cause nausea, bowel upset, dizziness and somnolence, and withdrawal symptoms after chronic use. The non-opioid analgesic nefopam (30–90 mg 3 times daily) can help moderate pain, though side-effects (nausea, anxiety, dry mouth) often limit its use. Patients with severe or intractable pain may require stronger opioid analgesics such as oxycodon and morphine.

Non-steroidal anti-inflammatory drugs

These are among the most widely prescribed drugs, but their use has declined over recent years because of concerns about an increased risk of cardiovascular disease. Oral NSAIDs are particularly useful in the management of pain that has an inflammatory component, and a long-acting NSAID taken in the evening may help reduce early morning stiffness. There is marked variability in individual tolerance and response; patients who do not respond to one NSAID may still gain relief from another. The mechanism of NSAID action is through inhibition of prostaglandin H synthase and cyclo-oxygenase (COX) enzymes. Arachidonic acid, derived from membrane phospholipids, is metabolised to produce prostaglandins and leukotrienes by the COX and 5-lipoxygenase pathways respectively (Fig. 25.13). There are two isoforms of COX, encoded by different genes. COX-1 is constitutively expressed and fulfils a 'housekeeping' function in the gastric mucosa, platelets and kidneys. The COX-2 enzyme is largely induced at sites of inflammation, producing prostaglandins that cause local pain and inflammation, but COX-2 is also up-regulated in the CNS, where it plays a role in the central mediation of pain and fever. Traditional NSAIDs, such as ibuprofen, diclofenac and naproxen, inhibit both COX enzymes, whereas newer NSAIDs, such as celecoxib and etoricoxib, selectively inhibit COX-2. Whilst NSAIDs have anti-inflammatory activity, they are not thought to have a disease-modifying effect in either OA or inflammatory rheumatic diseases.

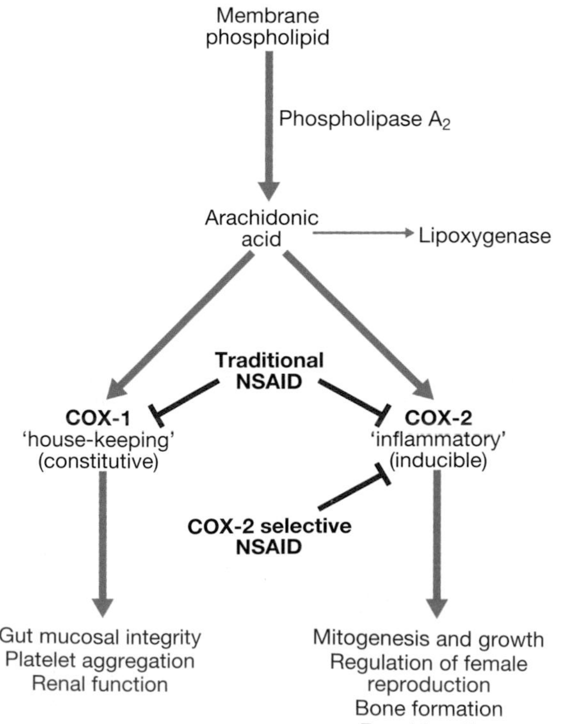

Fig. 25.13 COX-1 and COX-2 pathways.

25.31 Commonly used NSAIDs and their relative risk of gastrointestinal bleeding and perforation

Drug	Daily adult dose	Doses/ day	Idiosyncratic side-effects, comments
Very low risk			
Celecoxib	100–200 mg	1–2	Selective COX-2 inhibitor
Etoricoxib	60–120 mg	1	Selective COX-2 inhibitor
Low risk			
Ibuprofen	600–1600 mg	3–4	Weak anti-inflammatory effect at this dose
Etodolac	600 mg	1	Partially selective COX-2 inhibitor
Meloxicam	7.5–15 mg	1	Partially selective COX-2 inhibitor
Nabumetone	1–2 g	1–2	Partially selective COX-2 inhibitor
Medium risk			
Ibuprofen	1600–2400 mg	3–4	
Naproxen	500–1000 mg	1–2	
Diclofenac	75–150 mg	2–3	Abnormal liver function tests
High risk			
Indometacin	50–200 mg	3–4	High incidence of dyspepsia and CNS side-effects (headache, dizziness, confusion)
Ketoprofen	100–200 mg	2–4	
Highest risk			
Piroxicam	20–30 mg	1–2	Restricted use in those > 60 yrs
Azapropazone	600–200 mg	2–4	Uricosuric action. Restricted use in those > 60 yrs

Non-selective NSAIDs can damage the gastric and duodenal mucosal barrier and are associated with an increased risk of upper gastrointestinal ulceration, bleeding and perforation. The adjusted increased risk (odds ratio) of bleeding or perforation from all NSAIDs is 4–5, though differences exist between NSAIDs (Box 25.31). Dyspepsia is a poor guide to the presence of NSAID-associated ulceration and bleeding, and the principal risk factors are shown in Box 25.32. Co-prescription of omeprazole (20 mg daily) or misoprostol (200 µg twice or 3 times daily) reduces but does not eliminate NSAID-induced ulceration and bleeding, but H_2-antagonists in standard doses are ineffective. The COX-2 selective NSAIDs celecoxib and etoricoxib are much less likely to cause gastrointestinal toxicity but benefit is attenuated in patients on low-dose aspirin. In the UK, National Institute for Health and Clinical Excellence (NICE) guidelines advise that a proton pump inhibitor (PPI) should be co-prescribed

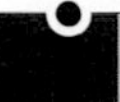

25.32 Risk factors for NSAID-induced ulcers

- Age > 60 yrs*
- Past history of peptic ulcer*
- Past history of adverse event with NSAID
- Concomitant corticosteroid use
- High-dose or multiple NSAID
- High-risk NSAID (see Box 25.31)

*The most important risk factors.

25.33 Recommendations for the use of NSAID

- Use with caution in patients with cardiovascular disease
- Use the lowest dose for the shortest time possible to control symptoms
- Avoid NSAID in patients on warfarin
- Allow 2–3 weeks to assess efficacy. If response is inadequate, consider trial of another NSAID
- Never prescribe more than one NSAID at a time
- Co-prescribe proton pump inhibitor for patients with risk factors for gastrointestinal adverse effects (see Box 25.32)

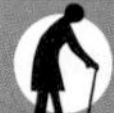

25.34 Use of oral NSAID in old age

- **Gastrointestinal complications**: age is a strong risk factor for bleeding and perforation and peptic ulceration. Elderly patients are more likely to die if they suffer NSAID-associated bleeding or perforation.
- **Cardiovascular disease**: use NSAID with caution in patients with cardiovascular disease. Therapy with NSAID may exacerbate hypertension and heart failure.
- **Renal disease**: use of NSAID may cause renal impairment.

with all NSAIDs, including COX-2 selective NSAIDs, even though the risk of gastrointestinal events with these is low. Since chronic PPI therapy is associated with an increased risk of hip fracture, the merits of giving PPI therapy with a COX-2 selective drug need to be weighed up carefully.

Other side-effects of NSAID include fluid retention and renal impairment due to inhibition of renal prostaglandin production, non-ulcer-associated dyspepsia, abdominal pain and altered bowel habit, and rashes. Interstitial nephritis, asthma and anaphylaxis can also occur but are rare. Recommendations for NSAID prescribing are summarised in Box 25.33. Because of the risk of adverse effects, NSAIDs should be used with great care in the elderly (Box 25.34).

Topical agents

Topical NSAID creams and gels and capsaicin (chilli extract; 0.025%) cream can help in the treatment of OA and superficial periarticular lesions affecting hands, elbows and knees. They may be used as monotherapy or as an adjunct to oral analgesics. Topical NSAIDs can penetrate superficial tissues and even reach the joint capsule, though intrasynovial levels mainly reflect blood-borne drug delivery. Capsaicin selectively binds to the protein transient receptor potential vanilloid type 1 (TRPV1), which is a heat-activated calcium channel on the surface of peripheral type C nociceptor fibres. Initial application causes a burning sensation but continued use depletes presynaptic substance P, with subsequent pain reduction that is optimal after 1–2 weeks.

Non-pharmacological interventions

Physical and occupational therapy

Local heat, ice packs, wax baths and other local external applications can induce muscle relaxation and temporary relief of symptoms in a range of rheumatic diseases.

Hydrotherapy induces muscle relaxation and facilitates enhanced movement in a warm, pain-relieving environment without the restraints of gravity and normal load-bearing. Various manipulative techniques may also help improve restricted movement. The combination of these with education and therapist contact enhances their benefits.

Splints can give temporary rest and support for painful joints and periarticular tissues, and prevent harmful involuntary postures during sleep. Prolonged rest, however, must be avoided.

Orthoses are more permanent appliances used to reduce instability and excessive abnormal movement. They include working wrist splints, knee orthoses, and iron and T-straps to control ankle instability. Orthoses are particularly suited to severely disabled patients in whom a surgical option is inappropriate, and often need to be custom-made for the individual.

Aids and appliances can provide dignity and independence to patients with respect to activities of daily living. Common examples are a raised toilet seat, raised chair height, extended handles on taps, a shower instead of a bath, thick-handled cutlery, and extended 'hands' to pull on tights and socks. Full assessment and advice from an occupational therapist maximise the benefits of these.

Surgery

A variety of surgical interventions can relieve pain and conserve or restore function in patients with bone, joint and periarticular disease (Box 25.35). Soft tissue release and tenosynovectomy may reduce inflammatory symptoms, improve function and prevent or retard tendon damage for variable periods, sometimes indefinitely. Synovectomy of joints does not prevent disease progression but may be indicated for pain relief when drugs, physical therapy and intra-articular injections have provided insufficient relief. The main approaches for damaged joints are osteotomy (cutting bone to alter joint mechanics and load transmission), excision arthroplasty (removing part or all of the joint), joint replacement (insertion of prosthesis in place of the excised joint) and arthrodesis (joint fusion). Surgical fixation of fractures is frequently required in patients with osteoporosis and other bone diseases.

The main aims of surgery are to provide pain relief and improve function and quality of life. If surgery is to be successful, the aims and consequences of each operation should be considered as part of an integrated programme of management and rehabilitation, by multidisciplinary teams of surgeons, allied health professionals and physicians, and carefully explained to the patient. Assessment of motivation, social support and environment is no less important than careful consideration of patients' general health, their risks for major surgery, the extent of disease in other joints, and their ability to mobilise following surgery. For some severely compromised people, pain relief and functional independence are better served by provision of a suitable wheelchair, home adjustments and social services than by surgery that is technically successful but following which the patient cannot mobilise.

25.35 Surgical procedures in rheumatology and bone disease

Procedure	Indication
Soft tissue release	
Carpal tunnel	Median nerve compression
Tarsal tunnel	Posterior tibial nerve entrapment
Flexor tenosynovectomy	Relief of 'trigger' fingers
Ulnar nerve transposition	Ulnar nerve entrapment at elbow
Fasciotomy	Severe Dupuytren's contracture
Tendon repairs and transfers	
Hand extensor tendons	Extensor tendon rupture
Thumb and finger flexor tendons	Flexor tendon rupture
Synovectomy	
Wrist and extensor tendon sheath (+ excision of radial head)	Pain relief and prevention of extensor tendon rupture in RA, resistant inflammatory synovitis
Knee synovectomy	Resistant inflammatory synovitis
Osteotomy	
Femoral osteotomy	Early OA of hip
Tibial osteotomy	Unicompartmental knee OA Deformed tibia in OA or Paget's disease
Excision arthroplasty	
First metatarsophalangeal joint (Keller's procedure)	Painful hallux valgus
Radial head	Painful distal radio-ulnar joint
Lateral end of clavicle	Painful acromioclavicular joint
Metatarsal head	Painful subluxed metatarsophalangeal joints
Joint replacement arthroplasty	
Knee, hip, shoulder, elbow	Painful damaged joints in OA and RA
Arthrodesis	
Wrist	Damaged joint: pain relief, improvement of grip
Ankle/subtalar joints	Damaged joint: pain relief, stabilisation of hindfoot
Fracture repair	
Hip arthroplasty	Fractured neck of femur
External fixation	Multiple fractures, open fractures
Intramedullary nailing	Tibial and femur fractures
Screw, plating and wiring	Wrist and other fractures
Other procedures	
Nerve root decompression	Spinal stenosis, nerve entrapment
Kyphoplasty	Painful vertebral fracture
Vertebroplasty	Painful vertebral fracture

Self-help and coping strategies

These help patients to cope better with, and adjust to, chronic pain and disability. They may be useful at any

25.36 Self-help and coping strategies

- Yoga and relaxation techniques to reduce stress
- Avoiding negative situations or activities that produce stress, and increasing pleasant activities that give satisfaction
- Information and discussion to alter beliefs about and perspectives on disease
- Reducing or avoiding catastrophising and maladaptive pain behaviour
- Imagery and distraction techniques for pain
- Expanding social contact and better use of social services

stage but are particularly so for patients with incurable problems, who have tried all available treatment options. The aim is to increase self-management through self-assessment and problem-solving, so that patients can recognise negative but potentially remediable aspects of their mood (stress, frustration, anger or low self-esteem) and their situation (physical, social, financial). These may then be addressed by changes in attitude and behaviour, as shown in Box 25.36.

Involvement of the spouse or partner in mutual goal-setting can improve partnership adjustment. Such approaches are often an element of group education classes and pain clinics, but may require more formal clinical psychological input.

OSTEOARTHRITIS

Osteoarthritis (OA) is by far the most common form of arthritis. It is strongly associated with ageing and is a major cause of pain and disability in older people. Osteoarthritis is characterised by focal loss of articular cartilage, subchondral osteosclerosis, osteophyte formation at the joint margin, and remodelling of joint contour with enlargement of affected joints. Inflammation can occur but is not a prominent feature. Joint involvement in OA follows a characteristic distribution, mainly targeting the hips, knees, PIP and DIP joints of the hands, neck and lumbar spine (see Fig. 25.9). The prevalence of OA rises progressively with age and it has been estimated that 45% of all people develop knee OA and 25% hip OA at some point during life. Although some of these patients are asymptomatic, the lifetime risk of having a total hip or knee replacement for OA in someone aged 50 is about 11% in women and 8% in men. Symptoms attributable to OA are more prevalent in women, except at the hip, where men are equally affected.

Pathophysiology

OA is a complex disorder with both genetic and environmental components (Fig. 25.14). Repetitive adverse loading of joints during occupation or competitive sports is also an important predisposing factor in farmers (hip OA), miners (knee OA) and elite or professional athletes (knee OA). For most people, however, participation in recreational sport does not appear to increase the risk of OA, unless there has been significant joint trauma. Congenital abnormalities of the joint, such as slipped femoral epiphysis, are also associated with a high risk of OA, presumably due to abnormal load distribution within the joint, and this is also thought to be the explanation for the increased risk of OA in Paget's disease of bone. Obesity is another strong risk factor. Although this is likely to be due in part to increased mechanical loading of the joints, it has been speculated that cytokines released from adipose tissue may also play a role. The increased incidence of OA in women has led to speculation that sex hormones may play a causal role. While there is no evidence to suggest that circulating sex hormone levels or reproductive history predispose to OA, some studies have shown a lower prevalence of OA in women who use hormone replacement therapy (HRT), as compared with non-users. Genetic factors play a key role in the pathogenesis of OA, and family-based studies have estimated that the heritability of OA ranges between about 43% at the knee to between 60% and 65% at the hip and hand, respectively. Recent genome-wide association studies have identified several loci that predispose to OA, but many others remain to be discovered.

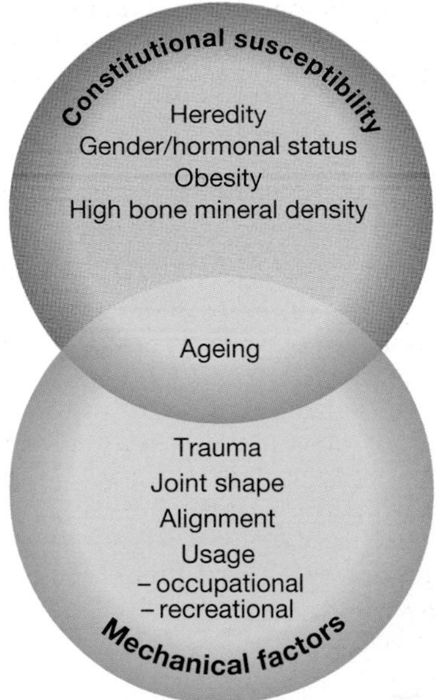

Fig. 25.14 Risk factors for the development of osteoarthritis.

Major alterations in cartilage structure are characteristic of OA. Chondrocytes divide to produce nests of metabolically active cells (Fig. 25.15A). Initially, matrix components are produced at an increased rate, but at the same time there is increased degradation of the major structural components of cartilage, including aggrecan and type II collagen (see Fig. 25.4, p. 1063). Eventually, the concentration of aggrecan in matrix falls and makes the cartilage vulnerable to load-bearing injury. Fissuring of the cartilage surface ('fibrillation') then occurs, leading to the development of deep vertical clefts (Fig. 25.15B), localised chondrocyte death and decreased cartilage thickness; this is focal rather than generalised in nature and mainly affects the maximum load-bearing part of the joint, although, eventually, large parts of the cartilage surface can be damaged. Calcium pyrophosphate and basic calcium phosphate crystals often become deposited in the abnormal cartilage.

The subchondral bone is also abnormal, with osteosclerosis and subchondral cyst formation (Fig. 25.15C).

A 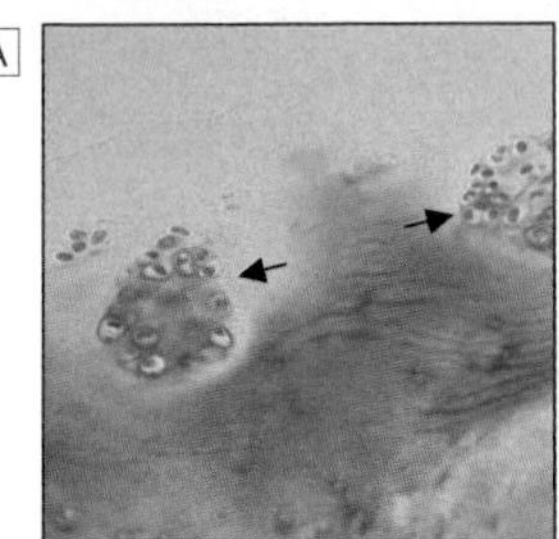

B 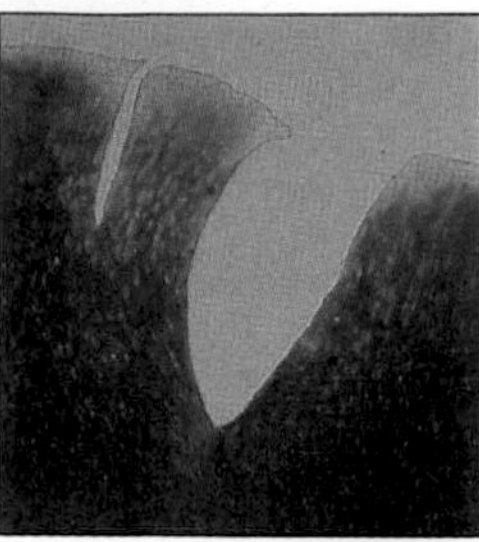

C 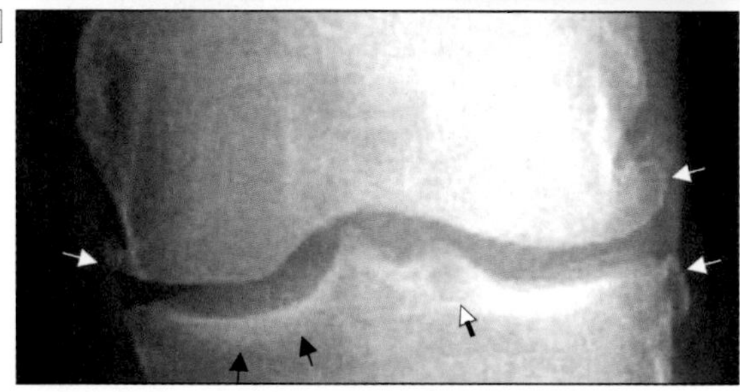

Fig. 25.15 Pathological changes in osteoarthritis. **A** Abnormal nests of proliferating chondrocytes (arrows) interspersed with matrix devoid of normal chondrocytes. **B** Fibrillation of cartilage in OA. **C** Radiograph of knee joint affected by OA, showing osteophytes at joint margin (white arrows), subchondral sclerosis (black arrows) and subchondral cyst (open arrow).

Fibrocartilage is produced at the joint margin, which undergoes endochondral ossification to form osteophytes. Bone remodelling and cartilage thinning slowly alter the shape of the OA joint, increasing its surface area. Patients with OA also have higher BMD values at sites distant from the joint, and this is particularly related to osteophyte formation. The reason for this is not completely understood but it may reflect the fact that common signalling pathways are involved in the regulation of bone and cartilage metabolism.

The synovium undergoes variable degrees of hyperplasia, and inflammatory changes may sometimes be observed, although to a much lesser extent than in RA and other inflammatory arthropathies. Osteochondral bodies commonly occur within the synovium, reflecting chondroid metaplasia or secondary uptake and growth of damaged cartilage fragments. The outer capsule also thickens and contracts, usually retaining the stability of the remodelling joint. The muscles surrounding affected joints commonly show evidence of wasting and non-specific type II fibre atrophy.

Clinical features

The main presenting symptoms are pain and functional restriction in a patient over the age of 45, but more often over 60 years. The causes of pain in OA are not completely understood but may relate to increased pressure in subchondral bone (mainly causing night pain), trabecular microfractures, capsular distension and low-grade synovitis, or may result from bursitis and enthesopathy secondary to altered joint mechanics. Typical OA pain has the characteristics listed in Box 25.37. For many people, functional restriction of the hands, knees or hips is an equal, if not greater, problem than pain. The clinical findings vary according to severity but are principally those of joint damage.

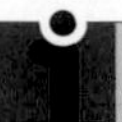

25.37 Symptoms and signs of osteoarthritis

Pain

- Insidious onset over months or years
- Variable or intermittent over time ('good days, bad days')
- Mainly related to movement and weight-bearing, relieved by rest
- Only brief (< 15 mins) morning stiffness and brief (< 5 mins) 'gelling' after rest
- Usually only one or a few joints painful

Clinical signs

- Restricted movement due to capsular thickening, or blocking by osteophyte
- Palpable, sometimes audible, coarse crepitus due to rough articular surfaces
- Bony swelling around joint margins
- Deformity, usually without instability
- Joint-line or periarticular tenderness
- Muscle weakness and wasting
- Synovitis mild or absent

The correlation between the presence of structural change, pain and disability varies markedly according to site. It is stronger at the hip than the knee, and poor at most small joints. Risk factors for pain and disability may differ from those for structural change. At the knee, for example, reduced quadriceps muscle strength and adverse psychosocial factors (anxiety, depression) correlate more strongly with pain and disability than the degree of radiographic change.

Radiological evidence of OA is very common in middle-aged and older people, and the disease may coexist with other conditions, so it is important to remember that pain in a patient with OA may be due to another cause. Generalised OA, knee OA, hip OA and spine OA (spondylosis) will be considered individually.

Generalised nodal OA

Characteristics of this common form of OA are shown in Box 25.38. Some patients are asymptomatic whereas others develop pain, stiffness and swelling of one or more PIP joints of the hands from the age of about 40 years onward. Gradually, these develop posterolateral swellings on each side of the extensor tendon that slowly enlarge and harden to become Heberden's (DIP) and Bouchard's (PIP) nodes (Fig. 25.16). Typically, each joint goes through a phase of episodic symptoms (1–5 years) while the node evolves and OA develops. Once OA is fully established, symptoms may subside and hand function often remains good. Affected joints are enlarged as the result of osteophyte formation and

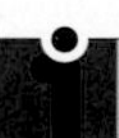

25.38 Characteristics of generalised nodal osteoarthritis

- Polyarticular finger interphalangeal joint OA
- Heberden's (± Bouchard's) nodes
- Marked female preponderance
- Peak onset in middle age
- Good functional outcome for hands
- Predisposition to OA at other joints, especially knees
- Strong genetic predisposition

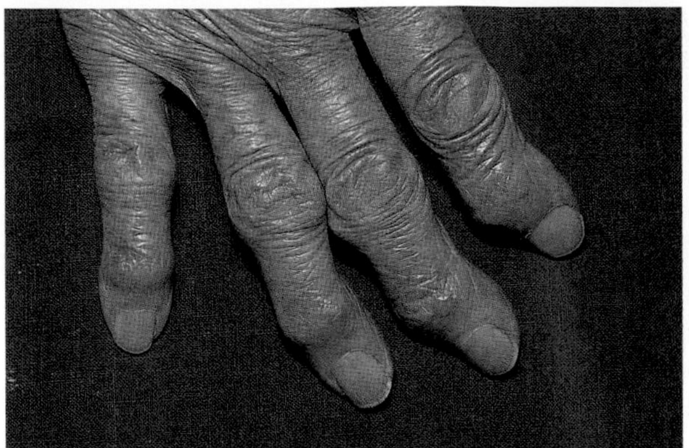

Fig. 25.16 Nodal osteoarthritis. Heberden's nodes and lateral (radial/ulnar) deviation of distal interphalangeal joints, with mild Bouchard's nodes at the proximal interphalangeal joints.

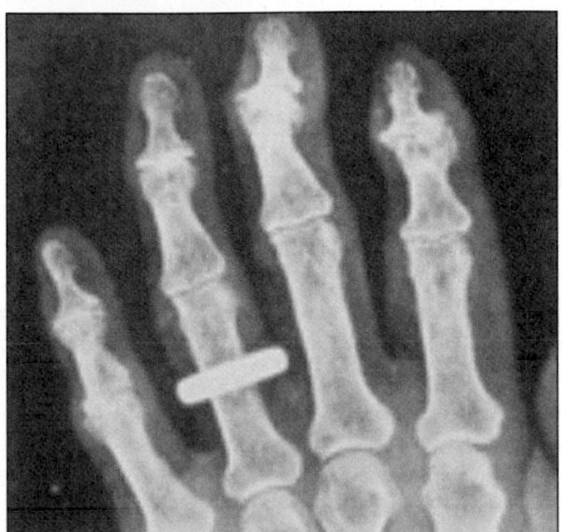

Fig. 25.17 X-ray appearances in hand osteoarthritis. There is marked loss of joint space at all of the distal interphalangeal joints, with osteophyte formation most marked at the first and second DIP joints. The fifth proximal interphalangeal joint also shows loss of joint space with osteophyte formation.

often show characteristic lateral deviation, reflecting the asymmetric focal cartilage loss of OA (Fig. 25.17). Involvement of the first carpometacarpal joint (CMC) is also common, leading to pain on trying to open bottles and jars and functional impairment. Clinically, it may be detected by the presence of crepitus on joint movement, and squaring of the thumb base.

Generalised nodal OA has a very strong genetic component: the daughter of an affected mother has a 1 in 3 chance of developing nodal OA herself. People with nodal OA are at increased risk of OA at other sites, especially the knee.

Knee OA

OA principally targets the patello-femoral and medial tibio-femoral compartments at this site but eventually spreads to affect the whole of the joint (Fig. 25.18). It may be isolated or occur as part of generalised nodal OA. Most patients, particularly women, have bilateral and symmetrical involvement. With men, trauma is a more important risk factor and may result in unilateral OA.

The pain is usually localised to the anterior or medial aspect of the knee and upper tibia. Patello-femoral pain is usually worse going up and down stairs or inclines.

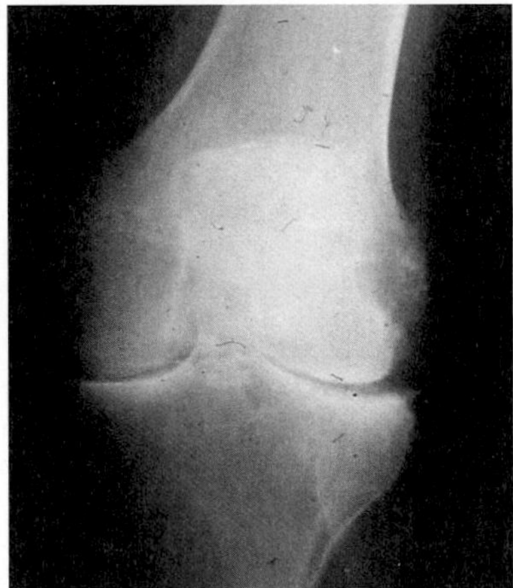

Fig. 25.18 X-ray appearances in knee osteoarthritis. There is almost complete loss of joint space affecting both compartments, and sclerosis of subchondral bone.

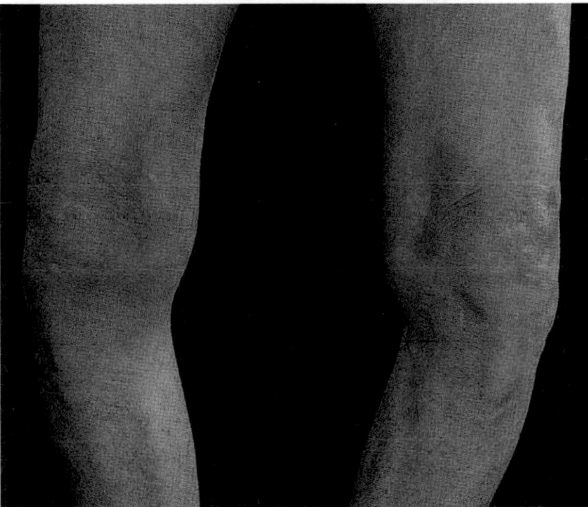

Fig. 25.19 Typical varus deformity resulting from marked medial tibio-femoral osteoarthritis.

Posterior knee pain suggests the presence of a complicating popliteal cyst (Baker's cyst). Prolonged walking, rising from a chair, getting in or out of a car, or bending to put on shoes and socks may be difficult. Local examination findings may include:

- a jerky, asymmetric (antalgic) gait with less time weight-bearing on the painful side
- a varus (Fig. 25.19), less commonly valgus, and/or fixed flexion deformity
- joint-line and/or periarticular tenderness (secondary anserine bursitis and medial ligament enthesopathy (see Box 25.27, p. 1076), causing tenderness of the upper medial tibia)
- weakness and wasting of the quadriceps muscle
- restricted flexion/extension with coarse crepitus
- bony swelling around the joint line.

Calcium pyrophosphate dihydrate (CPPD) crystal deposition in association with OA is most common at the knee. This may result in a more overt inflammatory component (stiffness, effusions) and super-added acute attacks of synovitis ('pseudogout', p. 1090), which may predict more rapid radiographic and clinical progression.

Hip OA

Hip OA most commonly targets the superior aspect of the joint (Fig. 25.20). This is often unilateral at presentation, frequently progresses with superolateral migration of the femoral head, and has a poor prognosis. The less common central (medial) OA shows more central cartilage loss and is largely confined to women. It is often bilateral at presentation and may associate with generalised nodal OA. It has a better prognosis than superior hip OA and progression to axial migration of the femoral head is uncommon.

The hip shows the best correlation between symptoms and radiographic change. Hip pain is usually maximal deep in the anterior groin, with variable radiation to the buttock, anterolateral thigh, knee or shin. Lateral hip pain, worse on lying on that side with tenderness over the greater trochanter, suggests secondary trochanteric bursitis. Common functional difficulties are the same as for knee OA; in addition, restricted hip abduction in women may cause pain on intercourse. Examination may reveal:

- an antalgic gait
- weakness and wasting of quadriceps and gluteal muscles
- pain and restriction of internal rotation with the hip flexed – the earliest and most sensitive sign of hip OA; other movements may subsequently be restricted and painful
- anterior groin tenderness just lateral to the femoral pulse
- fixed flexion, external rotation deformity of the hip
- ipsilateral leg shortening with severe joint attrition and superior femoral migration.

Although obesity is not a major risk factor for development of hip OA, it is associated with more rapid progression.

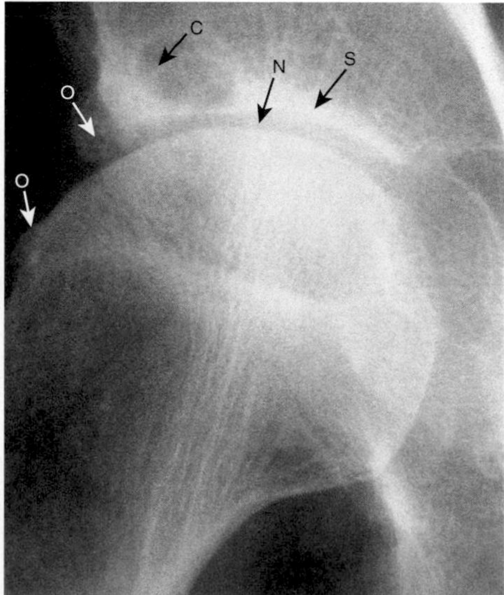

Fig. 25.20 X-ray of hip showing changes of osteoarthritis. Note the superior joint space narrowing (N), subchondral sclerosis (S), marginal osteophytes (white arrows) and cysts (C).

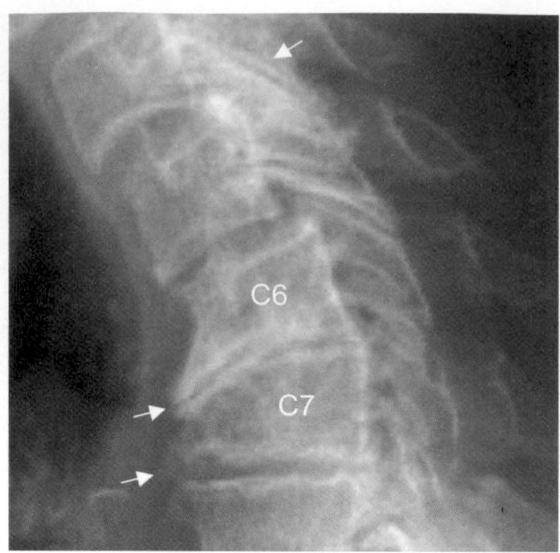

Fig. 25.21 X-ray of spine showing typical changes of osteoarthritis. Cervical spondylosis showing disc space narrowing between C6 and C7, osteophytes at the anterior vertebral body margins (arrows) and osteosclerosis at the apophyseal joints.

Spine OA

The cervical and lumbar spine are predominantly targeted by OA, then referred to as cervical spondylosis and lumbar spondylosis, respectively (Fig. 25.21). Spine OA may occur in isolation or as part of generalised OA. The typical presentation is with pain localised to the low back region or the neck, although radiation of pain to the arms, buttocks and legs may also occur due to nerve root compression. The pain is typically relieved by rest and worse on movement. On physical examination, the range of movement may be limited and loss of lumbar lordosis is typical. The straight leg-raising test or femoral stretch test may be positive and neurological signs may be seen in the legs where there is complicating spinal stenosis or nerve root compression.

Early-onset OA

Unusually, typical symptoms and signs of OA may present before the age of 45. In most cases, a single joint is affected and there is a clear history of previous trauma. However, specific causes of OA need to be considered in people with early-onset disease affecting several joints, especially those not normally targeted by OA, rare causes need to be considered (Box 25.39). Kashin–Beck disease is a rare form of OA that occurs in children, typically between the ages of 7 and 13, in some regions

25.39 Causes of early-onset osteoarthritis
Monoarticular
• Previous trauma, localised instability
Pauciarticular or polyarticular

• Juvenile idiopathic arthritis (p. 1103)
• Metabolic or endocrine disease
  Haemochromatosis (p. 972)
  Ochronosis
  Acromegaly (p. 792)
• Spondylo-epiphyseal dysplasia
• Late avascular necrosis
• Neuropathic joint
• Kashin–Beck disease

of China. The cause is unknown but suggested predisposing factors are selenium deficiency and contamination of cereals with mycotoxin-producing fungi.

Erosive OA

This term is used to describe rare patients with hand OA who have a more prolonged symptom phase, more overt inflammation, more disability and worse outcome than those with nodal OA. Distinguishing features include preferential targeting of PIP joints, subchondral erosions on X-rays, occasional ankylosis of affected joints and lack of association with OA elsewhere. It is unclear whether erosive OA is part of the spectrum of hand OA or a discrete subset.

Investigations

A plain X-ray of the affected joint should be performed and often this will show one or more of the typical features of OA (see Figs 25.17–25.21). In addition to providing diagnostic information, X-rays are used to assess the severity of structural change, which is useful if joint replacement surgery is being considered. Non-weight-bearing postero-anterior views of the pelvis are adequate for assessing hip OA. Patients with suspected knee OA should have standing antero-posterior radiographs taken to assess tibio-femoral cartilage loss, and a flexed skyline view to assess patello-femoral involvement. Spine OA can often be diagnosed on plain X-ray, which typically shows evidence of disc space narrowing and osteophytes. If nerve root compression or spinal stenosis is suspected, MRI should be performed.

Routine biochemistry, haematology and autoantibody tests are usually normal. Synovial fluid aspirated from an affected joint is viscous with a low cell count. Radioisotope bone scans performed for other reasons often show, as an incidental finding, discrete increased uptake in OA joints due to increased bone remodelling.

Unexplained early-onset OA requires additional investigation, guided by the suspected underlying condition. X-rays may show typical features of dysplasia or avascular necrosis, widening of joint spaces in acromegaly, multiple cysts and chondrocalcinosis in haemochromatosis (p. 972), or disorganised architecture in neuropathic joints.

Management

Treatment follows the principles outlined on pages 1077–1081 and in Box 25.40. Measures that are pertinent in older people are summarised in Box 25.41.

Education and other general measures

It is important to explain the nature of the condition fully, outlining the role of relevant risk factors (obesity, heredity, trauma) and the fact that established structural changes are permanent but that pain and function can improve. The prognosis should also be discussed (good for nodal hand OA, more optimistic for knee than hip OA), as should how appropriate action can improve the prognosis of large-joint OA. Exercise has beneficial effects in OA, including both strengthening and aerobic exercise, preferably with reinforcement by

EBM 25.40 Management of osteoarthritis

'The following measures have been shown to be effective:
- weight loss (if overweight)
- quadriceps strengthening exercises (knee OA)
- paracetamol and/or topical NSAID
- oral NSAID
- joint replacement surgery for disabling symptoms.'

For further information 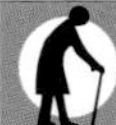 www.nice.org.uk/CG59

25.41 Osteoarthritis in old age

- **Pain and disability**: OA is the principal cause in old age.
- **Calcium phosphate deposition disease**: may cause acute attacks of synovitis (pseudogout) on a background of chronic OA.
- **Falls**: reduced muscle strength and pain associated with lower limb OA increase the risk.
- **Muscle strengthening exercises**: safely reduce the pain and disability of knee OA with accompanying improvements in balance and reduced tendency to fall.
- **Oral paracetamol and topical NSAID**: safe in older people, with no important drug interactions or contraindications.
- **Intra-articular injection of corticosteroid**: a very safe and often effective treatment, particularly useful for tiding a patient over a special event.
- **Total joint replacement**: an excellent cost-effective treatment for severe disabling knee or hip OA in older people. There is no age limit for joint replacement surgery.

a physiotherapist (see Box 25.30, p. 1078). Quadriceps strengthening exercises are particularly beneficial in knee OA. Weight loss can have a substantial beneficial effect on symptoms if the patient is obese and is probably one of the most effective treatments for reducing pain, particularly in OA of the lower limbs. Shock-absorbing footwear, pacing of activities, use of a walking stick for painful knee or hip OA, or provision of built-up shoes to equalise leg lengths can all improve symptoms.

Analgesics and anti-inflammatory drugs

If symptoms do not respond to non-pharmacological measures, paracetamol should be given. Addition of a topical NSAID, and then capsaicin, for knee and hand OA can also be helpful. Oral NSAID should be considered in patients who remain symptomatic. These drugs are significantly more effective than paracetamol and can be successfully combined with paracetamol or compound analgesics such as co-codamol if the pain is severe. Opiates may occasionally be required. For temporary benefit of moderate to severe pain, intra-articular injection of corticosteroids can be helpful (see below). Local physical therapies such as heat or cold can sometimes give temporary relief. Acupuncture and transcutaneous electrical nerve stimulation (TENS) have also been shown to be effective in knee OA. Antineuropathic drugs, such as amitriptyline, gabapentin and pregabalin, are sometimes used in patients with symptoms that are difficult to control, but the evidence base for their use is poor.

Corticosteroid injections

Intra-articular corticosteroid injections are effective in the treatment of knee OA and are also used for symptomatic relief in the treatment of OA at the first CMC joint. The duration of effect is usually short but trials of serial corticosteroid injections every 3 months in knee OA have shown efficacy for up to 1 year.

Chondroitin and glucosamine

Chondroitin sulphate and glucosamine sulphate have been used alone and in combination for the treatment of knee OA. There is evidence from randomised controlled trials that these agents can improve knee pain to a small extent (3–5%), as compared with placebo. Although NICE did not consider these differences to be clinically significant, the beneficial effects of paracetamol in knee OA are equally small.

Hyaluronan injections

In knee OA, intra-articular injection of one of several forms of hyaluronan (polymers of hyaluronate), usually given as a course of weekly injections for 3–5 weeks, may give modest pain relief for several months. However, evidence for efficacy is heterogeneous and the expense of this treatment and the common requirement for serial injection mean that hyaluronan injections are not recommended for OA by NICE.

Disease-modifying therapies

There are no licensed drugs that can halt the progression of OA. Glucosamine sulphate was shown in one study to slow the rate of radiological progression in knee OA and to reduce the number of subjects who progressed to joint replacement but the study has been criticised on methodological grounds. A recent randomised controlled trial suggested that strontium ranelate might also be effective in reducing the rate of progression of knee OA but it is not licensed for this indication.

Surgery

Surgery should be considered for patients with OA whose pain, stiffness and reduced function impact significantly on their quality of life and are refractory to other treatments. Osteotomy can prolong the life of malaligned joints and relieve pain by reducing intraosseous pressure, but is performed infrequently. Total joint replacement surgery is by far the most common surgical procedure for patients with OA. It can transform the quality of life for people with severe knee or hip OA and is indicated when there is significant structural damage on X-ray, and pain and functional impairment are limiting quality of life despite the use of medical therapy. Although surgery should not be undertaken at an early stage during the development of OA, it is important to consider it before functional limitation has become advanced since this may compromise the surgical outcome. Patient-specific factors, such as age, gender, smoking and presence of obesity, should not be barriers to referral for joint replacement.

Only a small proportion of patients with OA progress to the extent that total joint replacement is required, but OA is by far the most frequent indication for a total joint replacement. Over 95% of joint replacements continue to function well into the second decade after surgery and most provide life-long, pain-free function. However, some 20% of patients are not satisfied with the outcome, and a few experience little or no improvement in pain.

CRYSTAL-INDUCED ARTHRITIS

A variety of crystals can deposit in and around joints and cause an acute inflammatory arthritis, as well as a

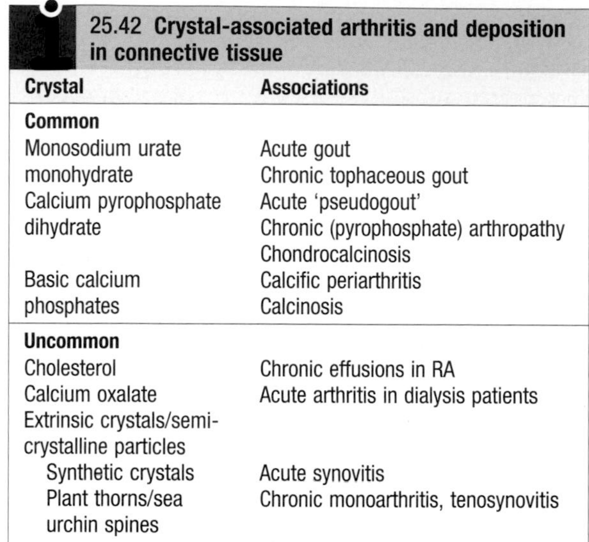

25.42 Crystal-associated arthritis and deposition in connective tissue

Crystal	Associations
Common	
Monosodium urate monohydrate	Acute gout Chronic tophaceous gout
Calcium pyrophosphate dihydrate	Acute 'pseudogout' Chronic (pyrophosphate) arthropathy Chondrocalcinosis
Basic calcium phosphates	Calcific periarthritis Calcinosis
Uncommon	
Cholesterol	Chronic effusions in RA
Calcium oxalate	Acute arthritis in dialysis patients
Extrinsic crystals/semi-crystalline particles	
Synthetic crystals	Acute synovitis
Plant thorns/sea urchin spines	Chronic monoarthritis, tenosynovitis

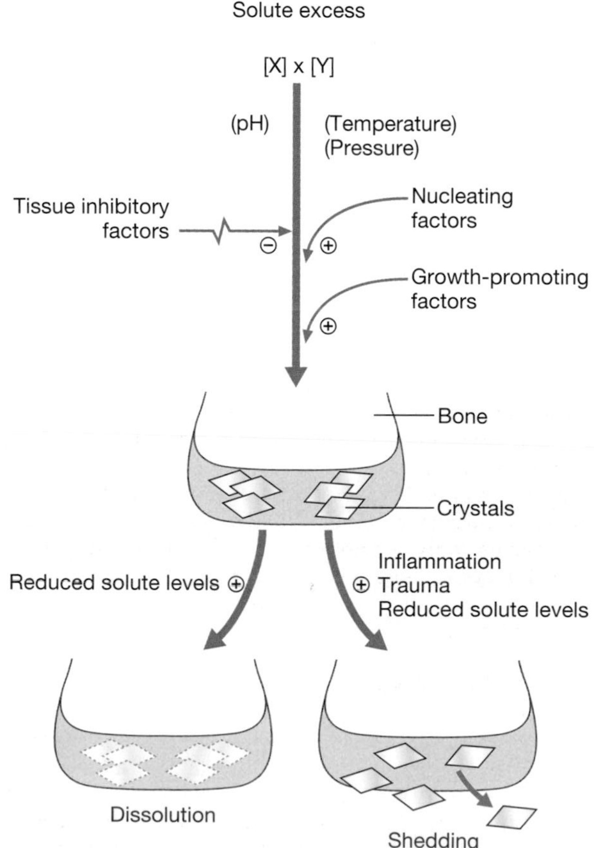

Fig. 25.22 Factors affecting the balance of crystal formation and tissue concentration.

more chronic arthritis associated with progressive joint damage (Box 25.42). Crystals can be the primary pathogenic agent, as in gout, or an accessory factor, as in calcium pyrophosphate deposition disease, in which crystals are deposited in joints that are already abnormal. Several factors influence crystal formation (Fig. 25.22). There must be sufficient concentration of the chemical components (ionic product), but whether a crystal then forms depends on the balance of tissue factors that promote and inhibit crystal nucleation and growth. Many tissues are supersaturated for the various products but depend on natural inhibitors to prevent crystallisation. The inflammatory potential of crystals resides in their physical irregularity and high negative surface charge, which can induce inflammation and damage cell membranes. Crystals may also cause mechanical damage to tissues and act as wear particles at the joint surface. Crystals can paradoxically reside in cartilage or tendon for years without causing inflammation or symptoms, and it is only when they are released that they trigger inflammation. This may occur spontaneously but can also result from local trauma, changes in the concentration of the components that form crystals, or be part of an acute phase response due to intercurrent illness or surgery.

Gout

Gout is an inflammatory disease caused by deposition of monosodium urate monohydrate crystals in and around synovial joints.

Epidemiology

The prevalence of gout varies between populations but is approximately 1–2%, with a greater than 5:1 male preponderance. It is the most common inflammatory arthritis in men and in older women. The risk of developing gout increases with age and with serum uric acid (SUA) levels, which are normally distributed in the general population. Levels are higher in men, increase with age and are associated with body weight. Levels are higher in some ethnic groups (such as Maoris and Pacific islanders). Hyperuricaemia is defined as an SUA level greater than 2 standard deviations above the mean for the population. Gout has become more common over recent years in parallel with increased longevity and the higher prevalence of metabolic syndrome, of which hyperuricaemia is an integral component. Although hyperuricaemia is an independent risk factor for hypertension, vascular disease, renal disease and cardiovascular events, only a minority of hyperuricaemic people develop gout. There is currently no evidence to support the use of urate-lowering therapy in patients with asymptomatic hyperuricaemia.

Pathophysiology

About one-third of the body uric acid pool is derived from dietary sources and two-thirds from endogenous purine metabolism (Fig. 25.23). The concentration of uric acid in body fluids depends on the balance between endogenous synthesis, and elimination by the kidneys (two-thirds) and gut (one-third). Purine nucleotide synthesis and degradation are regulated by a network of enzyme pathways. Xanthine oxidase catalyses the end conversion of hypoxanthine to xanthine and then xanthine to uric acid.

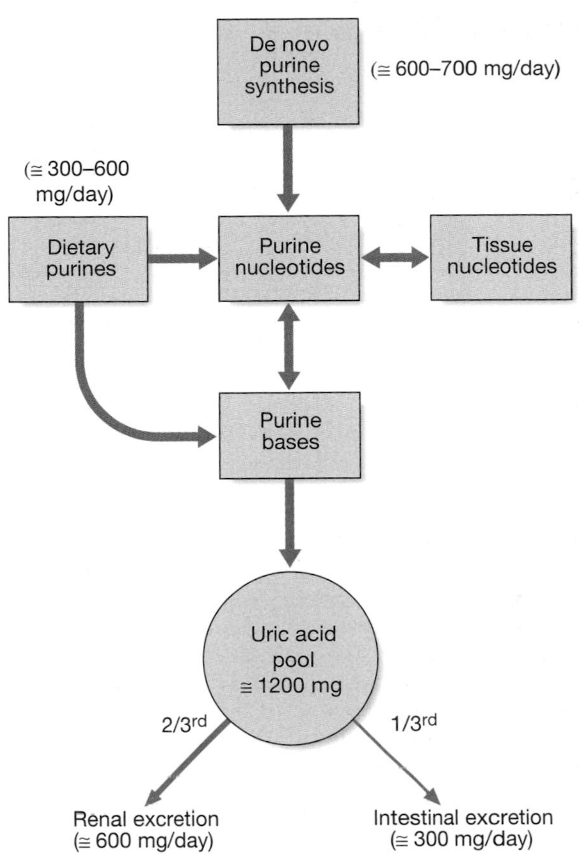

Fig. 25.23 The uric acid pool. Origins and disposal of uric acid.

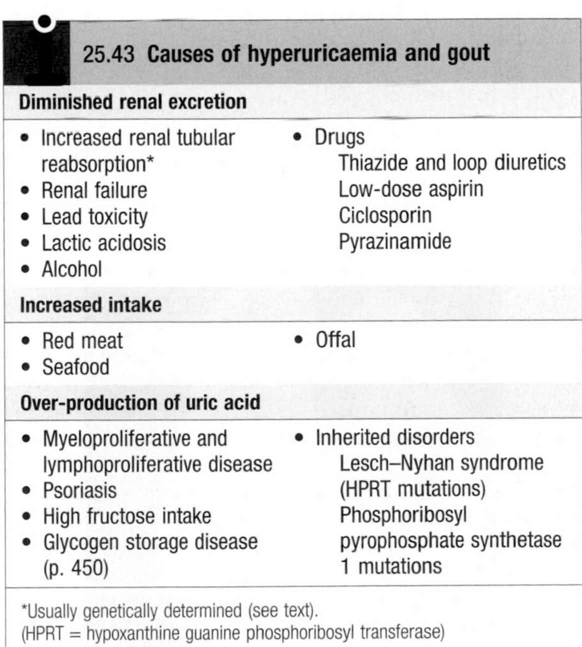

25.43 Causes of hyperuricaemia and gout

Diminished renal excretion	
• Increased renal tubular reabsorption* • Renal failure • Lead toxicity • Lactic acidosis • Alcohol	• Drugs Thiazide and loop diuretics Low-dose aspirin Ciclosporin Pyrazinamide
Increased intake	
• Red meat • Seafood	• Offal
Over-production of uric acid	
• Myeloproliferative and lymphoproliferative disease • Psoriasis • High fructose intake • Glycogen storage disease (p. 450)	• Inherited disorders Lesch–Nyhan syndrome (HPRT mutations) Phosphoribosyl pyrophosphate synthetase 1 mutations

*Usually genetically determined (see text).
(HPRT = hypoxanthine guanine phosphoribosyl transferase)

The causes of hyperuricaemia are shown in Box 25.43. In over 90% of patients, the main abnormality is reduced uric acid excretion by the renal tubules, which impairs the body's ability to respond to a purine load. In many cases, this is genetically determined and recent studies

25

have identified polymorphisms in several genes that are associated with gout, the most important of which is *SLC2A9*, which regulates urate excretion by the kidney. Impaired renal excretion of urate also accounts for the occurrence of hyperuricaemia in chronic renal failure, and for the association between hyperuricaemia and treatment with thiazide diuretics.

Other risk factors for gout include metabolic syndrome (p. 805), high alcohol intake (predominantly beer, which contains guanosine), generalised osteoarthritis, a diet relatively high in red meat or fructose or relatively low in vitamin C or coffee, and lead poisoning (saturnine gout). The association between OA and gout is thought to be due to reduction in levels of proteoglycan and other inhibitors of crystal formation in osteoarthritic cartilage, predisposing to crystal formation.

Some patients develop gout because they overproduce uric acid. The mechanisms are poorly understood, except in the case of a few rare disorders, in which gout is inherited in a Mendelian manner as the result of mutations in genes responsible for purine synthesis (see Box 25.43). Lesch–Nyhan syndrome for example, is an X-linked recessive form of gout that is also associated with mental retardation, self-mutilation and choreoathetosis. Such conditions should be suspected if other clinical features are present or there is an early age at onset with a positive family history. Severe hyperuricaemia can also occur in patients with leukaemia undergoing chemotherapy due to increased purine turnover.

Clinical features

The classical presentation is with an acute monoarthritis, which in over 50% of cases affects the first MTP joint (Fig. 25.24). Other common sites are the ankle, midfoot, knee, small joints of hands, wrist and elbow. The axial skeleton and large proximal joints are rarely involved. Typical features include:

- rapid onset, reaching maximum severity in 2–6 hours, and often waking the patient in the early morning
- severe pain, often described as the 'worst pain ever'
- extreme tenderness, such that the patient is unable to wear a sock or to let bedding rest on the joint
- marked swelling with overlying red, shiny skin
- self-limiting over 5–14 days, with complete resolution.

During the attack, the joint shows signs of marked synovitis, swelling and erythema. There may be accompanying fever, malaise and even confusion, especially if a large joint such as the knee is involved. As the attack subsides, pruritus and desquamation of overlying skin are common. The main differential diagnosis is septic arthritis, infective cellulitis or reactive arthritis. Acute attacks may also manifest as bursitis, tenosynovitis or cellulitis, which have the same clinical characteristics. Many patients describe milder episodes lasting just a few days. Some have attacks in more than one joint. Others have further attacks in other joints a few days later (cluster attacks), the first possibly acting as a trigger. Simultaneous polyarticular attacks are unusual.

Some people never have a second episode after an acute attack. In others, several years may elapse before the next attack. In many, however, a second attack occurs within 1 year and may progress to chronic gout, with chronic pain and joint damage, and occasionally severe deformity and functional impairment. Patients with uncontrolled hyperuricaemia who suffer multiple attacks of acute gout may also progress to chronic gout.

Crystals may be deposited in the joints and soft tissues to produce irregular firm nodules called tophi. These have a predilection for the extensor surfaces of fingers, hands, forearm, elbows, Achilles tendons and sometimes the helix of the ear. Tophi have a white colour, differentiating them from rheumatoid nodules (Fig. 25.25). Tophi can ulcerate, discharging white gritty material, become infected or induce a local inflammatory response, with erythema and pus in the absence of secondary infection. They are usually a feature of long-standing gout but can sometimes develop within

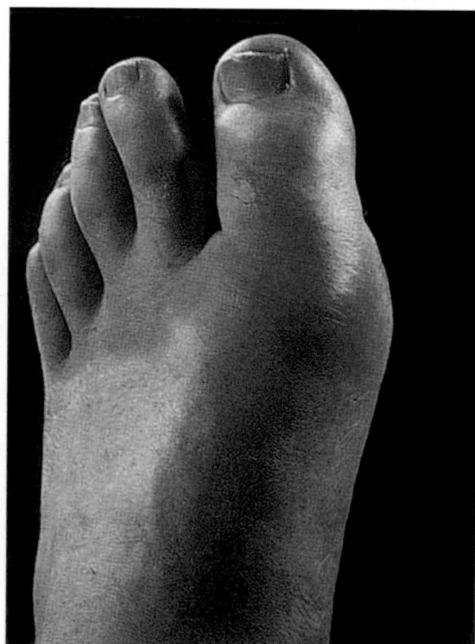

Fig. 25.24 Podagra. Acute gout causing swelling, erythema and extreme pain and tenderness of the first metatarsophalangeal joint.

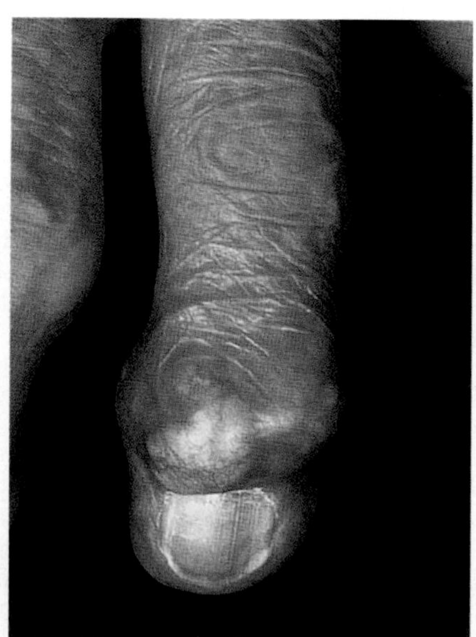

Fig. 25.25 Tophus with white monosodium urate monohydrate crystals visible beneath the skin. Diuretic-induced gout in a patient with pre-existing nodal OA.

12 months in patients with chronic renal failure. Occasionally, tophi may develop in the absence of previous acute attacks, especially in patients on thiazide therapy who have coexisting OA.

In addition to causing musculoskeletal disease, chronic hyperuricaemia may be complicated by renal stone formation (p. 507) and, if severe, renal impairment due to the development of interstitial nephritis as the result of urate deposition in the kidney. This is particularly common in patients with chronic tophaceous gout who are on diuretic therapy.

Investigations

The diagnosis of gout can be confirmed by the identification of urate crystals in the aspirate from a joint, bursa or tophus (see Fig. 25.5A, p. 1064). In acute gout, synovial fluid shows increased turbidity due to the greatly elevated cell count (> 90% neutrophils). In chronic gout, the appearance is more variable but occasionally the fluid appears white due to the high crystal load. Between attacks, aspiration of an asymptomatic first MTP joint or knee may still reveal crystals.

A biochemical screen, including renal function, uric acid, glucose and lipid profile, should be performed because of the association with metabolic syndrome. Although hyperuricaemia is usually present, this does not confirm the diagnosis. Conversely, normal uric acid levels during an attack do not exclude gout, as serum urate falls during the acute phase response. Elevated ESR and CRP and a neutrophilia are typical of acute gout, and they return to normal as the attack subsides. Tophaceous gout may be accompanied by a modest but chronic elevation in ESR and CRP.

Radiographs are usually normal in acute gout but well-demarcated erosions may be seen in patients with chronic or tophaceous gout (Fig. 25.26). Tophi may also be visible on X-rays as soft tissue swellings. In late disease, destructive changes may occur similar to those in other forms of advanced inflammatory arthritis.

Management

Oral NSAIDs are effective for pain relief in the acute attack and are the standard treatment, but have to be prescribed with caution in old age. Local ice packs can also be used for symptomatic relief. Patients with recurrent episodes can keep a supply of an NSAID and take it as soon as the first symptoms occur, continuing until the attack resolves. Oral colchicine, which works by inhibiting microtubule assembly in neutrophils, is also very effective. It is usually given in doses of 0.5 mg twice or 3 times daily. The most common adverse effects are nausea, vomiting and diarrhoea. Joint aspiration can give pain relief, and may be combined with an intra-articular steroid injection if the diagnosis is clear and infection can be excluded. A short course of oral or intramuscular corticosteroids can also be highly effective in treating acute attacks.

Patients who have more than one acute attack within 12 months and those with complications should be offered urate-lowering therapy (Box 25.44). The long-term therapeutic aim is to prevent attacks occurring by bringing uric acid levels below the level at which monosodium urate monohydrate crystals form. A therapeutic target of 360 μmol/L (6 mg/dL) is recommended in the British Society of Rheumatology guidelines, whereas the European League Against Rheumatism guidelines recommend a threshold of 300 μmol/L (5 mg/dL).

Allopurinol is the drug of first choice. It is a xanthine oxidase inhibitor, which reduces the conversion of hypoxanthine and xanthine to uric acid. The recommended starting dose is 100 mg daily, or 50 mg in older patients and in renal impairment. The dose of allopurinol should be increased by 100 mg every 4 weeks (50 mg in the elderly and those with renal impairment) until the target uric acid level is achieved, side-effects occur or the maximum recommended dose is reached (900 mg/day). Acute flares of gout often occur following initiation of urate-lowering therapy. The patient should be warned about this and told to continue therapy, even if an attack occurs. The risk of flares can be reduced by administration of oral colchicine (0.5 mg twice daily) or NSAID therapy for the first few months. In the longer term, annual monitoring of uric acid levels is recommended. In most patients, urate-lowering therapy needs to be continued indefinitely.

Febuxostat is a xanthine oxidase inhibitor that is useful in patients who fail to respond adequately to allopurinol, and those in whom it is contraindicated or has been poorly tolerated. It undergoes hepatic metabolism and so no dose adjustment is required for renal impairment. It is more effective than allopurinol at reducing uric acid levels and, as a result, commonly provokes attacks at the recommended starting dose (80 mg daily). In view of this, treatment with colchicine or NSAID should be considered for the initial 6 months.

Uricosuric drugs, such as probenecid or sulfinpyrazone, can be effective but require several doses each day and maintenance of a high urine flow to avoid uric

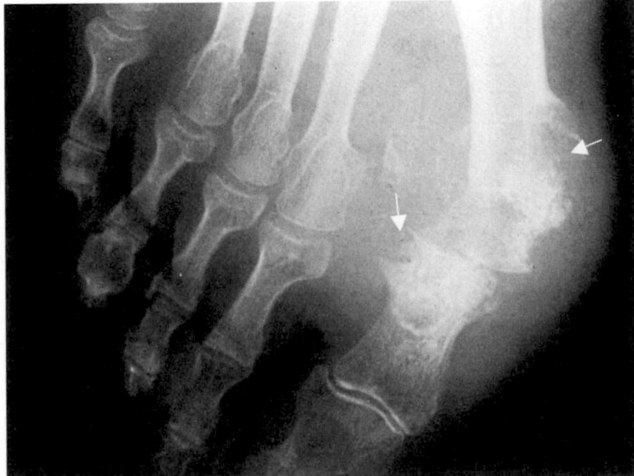

Fig. 25.26 Erosive arthritis in chronic gout. Punched-out erosions are visible (arrows), in association with a destructive arthritis affecting the first metatarsophalangeal joint.

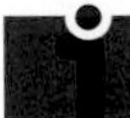

25.44 Indications for urate-lowering drugs

- Recurrent attacks of acute gout
- Tophi
- Evidence of bone or joint damage
- Renal impairment
- Nephrolithiasis
- Very high levels of serum uric acid

25

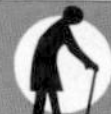

25.45 Gout in old age

- **Aetiology**: a higher proportion of older patients have gout secondary to diuretic use and chronic kidney disease. Gout is often associated with OA.
- **Presentation**: may be atypical, with painful tophi and chronic symptoms, rather than acute attacks. Joints of the upper limbs are more frequently affected.
- **Management**: acute attacks are best treated by aspiration and intra-articular injection of corticosteroids, followed by early mobilisation. NSAID and colchicine should be used with caution because of increased risk of toxicity. Low doses of allopurinol (50 mg/day) should be given, and increased gradually to avoid toxicity.

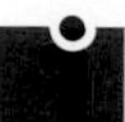

25.46 Risk factors for chondrocalcinosis

Common

- Age
- Osteoarthritis*
- Primary hyperparathyroidism

Rare

- Familial*
- Haemochromatosis*
- Hypophosphatasia
- Hypomagnesaemia
- Wilson's disease

*May be associated with structural damage to affected joints.

acid crystallisation in renal tubules. Salicylates antagonise the uricosuric action of these drugs and should be avoided. Uricosurics are contraindicated in over-producers, those with renal impairment and in urolithiasis (they increase stone formation). The uricosuric benzbromarone can be very effective and safe in mild to moderate renal impairment, but can cause hepatotoxicity. It is not licensed in the UK for the treatment of hyperuricaemia.

Pegloticase is a biological treatment in which the enzyme uricase has been conjugated to monomethoxy-polyethylene glycol. It is indicated for the treatment of tophaceous gout resistant to standard therapy and is administered as an intravenous infusion every 2 weeks for up to 6 months. It is highly effective at controlling hyperuricaemia and causes regression of tophi. The main adverse effects are infusion reactions (which can be treated with antihistamines or steroids) and flares of gout during the first 3 months of therapy. A limiting factor for longer-term treatment is the development of antibodies to pegloticase, which occur in a high proportion of cases and are associated with an impaired therapeutic response.

In addition to drug treatment, predisposing factors should be corrected if possible. Patients should be advised to lose weight where appropriate and to reduce excessive alcohol intake, especially beer. Thiazide diuretics should be stopped if possible and substituted with angiotensin-converting enzyme (ACE) inhibitors, as these have a uricosuric effect. Patients should be advised to avoid large amounts of seafood and offal, which have a high purine content, but a highly restrictive diet is not necessary.

Calcium pyrophosphate dihydrate crystal deposition disease

This condition is associated with deposition of calcium pyrophosphate dihydrate (CPPD) crystals within articular and hyaline cartilage and is sometimes known as 'pseudogout'. It is rare under the age of 55, but occurs in 10–15% of people between the ages of 65 and 75 years and in 30–60% of those over 85. The knee (hyaline cartilage and menisci) is by far the most common site, followed by the wrist (triangular fibrocartilage) and pelvis (symphysis pubis). Risk factors are shown in Box 25.46. In many patients, chondrocalcinosis is asymptomatic

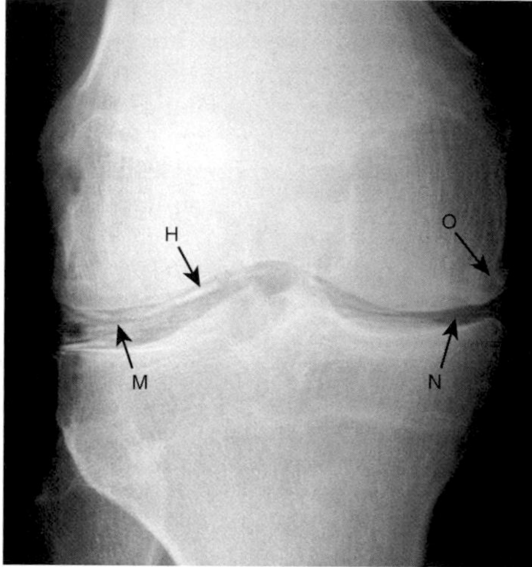

Fig. 25.27 Chondrocalcinosis of the knee. The X-ray shows calcification of the fibrocartilaginous menisci (M) and articular hyaline cartilage (H). There is also narrowing (N) and osteophyte (O) of the medial tibio-femoral compartment.

and an incidental finding on X-ray examination, but others present with an acute inflammatory arthritis (pseudogout) or a chronic inflammatory arthropathy superimposed on a background of OA, especially at the knee (Fig. 25.27), associated with joint damage and functional limitation.

Pathophysiology

The underlying mechanisms of crystal deposition are poorly understood. Clinical studies have shown that pyrophosphate levels are raised in patients with CPPD crystal deposition disease, possibly due to over-production, but why this occurs is unclear. In hypophosphatasia, the predisposing factor is thought to be impaired degradation of pyrophosphate due to mutations in the genes that encode ALP. OA is thought to predispose to CPPD crystal deposition disease because of a reduction in the amounts of proteoglycan and other natural inhibitors of crystal formation in the abnormal cartilage.

Clinical features

A common presentation is with an acute inflammatory arthritis that resembles acute gout, sometimes termed 'pseudogout'. Examination reveals a warm, tender erythematous joint with signs of a large effusion. Fever is common and the patient may appear confused and ill. The knee is most commonly affected, followed by the wrist, shoulder, ankle and elbow. Trigger factors include trauma, intercurrent illness and surgery. Sepsis and gout are the main differential diagnoses.

Chronic arthropathy may also occur in association with CPPD crystal deposition disease, affecting the same joints that are involved in acute pseudogout. The presentation is with chronic pain, early morning stiffness, inactivity gelling and functional impairment. Acute attacks of pseudogout may be superimposed. Affected joints usually show features of OA, with varying degrees of synovitis. Effusion and synovial thickening are usually most apparent at knees and wrists; wrist involvement may result in carpal tunnel syndrome. Inflammatory features may be sufficiently pronounced to suggest RA, but tenosynovitis and extra-articular involvement are absent, and large and medium rather than small joints are targeted. Severe damage and instability of knees or shoulders may occasionally lead to consideration of a neuropathic joint, but no neurological abnormalities will be found.

Investigations

Examination of synovial fluid using compensated polarised microscopy will demonstrate CPPD crystals (see Fig. 25.5B, p. 1064) and permit distinction from gout. The aspirated fluid is often turbid and may be uniformly blood-stained, reflecting the severity of inflammation. Since sepsis and pseudogout can coexist, Gram stain and culture of the fluid should be performed to exclude sepsis, even if CPPD crystals are identified in synovial fluid.

X-rays of the affected joint may show evidence of calcification in hyaline cartilage and/or fibrocartilage, although absence of calcification does not exclude the diagnosis. Signs of OA are frequently present. Screening for secondary causes (see Box 25.46) should be undertaken, especially in patients who present under the age of 25 and those with polyarticular disease.

Management

Joint aspiration can often provide symptomatic relief in pseudogout and sometimes no further treatment is required. Patients with persistent symptoms can be treated with intra-articular corticosteroids, colchicine or NSAID. Since most patients with pseudogout are elderly, NSAID must be used with caution. Early active mobilisation is also important. Chronic pyrophosphate-induced arthropathy should be managed as for OA (p. 1085).

Basic calcium phosphate deposition disease

Basic calcium phosphate (BCP) deposition disease is caused by the deposition of hydroxyapatite or apatite crystals and other basic calcium phosphate salts (octacalcium phosphate, tricalcium phosphate) in soft tissues. The main affected sites are tendons, ligaments and hyaline cartilage in patients with degenerative disease, and skeletal muscle and subcutaneous tissues in connective tissue diseases.

25.47 Rheumatic diseases associated with basic calcium phosphate deposition

Disease	Site of calcification
Calcific periarthritis	Tendons and ligaments
Dermatomyositis and polymyositis	Subcutaneous tissue
Systemic sclerosis and CREST syndrome	Subcutaneous tissue
Mixed connective tissue disease	Subcutaneous tissue
Paget's disease of bone	Blood vessels
Ankylosing spondylitis	Ligaments
Fibrodysplasia ossificans progressiva	Subcutaneous tissues and muscle
Milwaukee shoulder syndrome	Tendons and ligaments
Albright's hereditary osteodystrophy	Muscle

(CREST = calcinosis, Raynaud's, oesophageal dysmotility, sclerodactyly, telangiectasia)

Pathophysiology

Under normal circumstances, inhibitors of mineralisation, such as pyrophosphate and proteoglycans, inhibit calcification of soft tissues. When these protective mechanisms break down, abnormal calcification occurs. There are many causes (Box 25.47). In most situations, calcification is of no consequence, but when the crystals are released, an inflammatory reaction may be initiated, causing local pain and inflammation.

Calcific periarthritis

Deposition of BCP in tendons may result in an acute inflammatory response. The most commonly affected site is the supraspinatus tendon (Fig. 25.28) but other sites may also be affected, including the tendons around the hip, feet and hands. The presentation is with acute pain, swelling and local tenderness that develops rapidly

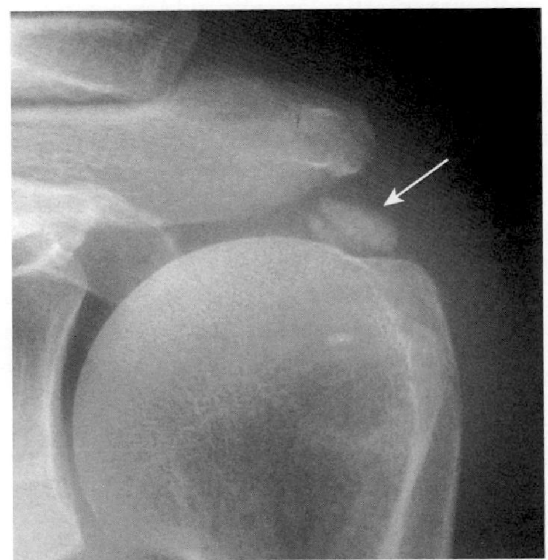

Fig. 25.28 Shoulder X-ray showing supraspinatus tendon calcification (arrow).

25

over 4–6 hours. The overlying skin may be hot and red, raising the possibility of infection. Attacks sometimes occur spontaneously but can also be triggered by trauma. Modest systemic upset and fever are common. X-rays show tendon calcification. If the affected joint or bursa is aspirated, inflammatory fluid containing many calcium-staining (alizarin red S) aggregates may be obtained. During an acute attack, there may be a neutrophilia with an elevation in ESR and CRP. Routine biochemistry is normal. Treatment is with analgesics and NSAID. Attacks may also respond to a local injection of corticosteroid. The condition usually resolves spontaneously over 1–3 weeks and this is often accompanied by dispersal and disappearance of small to medium-sized BCP deposits on X-ray. Large deposits sometimes accumulate, causing limitation of joint movement, and may require surgical removal.

Acute inflammatory arthritis

Deposition of BCP occurs commonly in OA, both alone and in combination with CPPD crystals, when it is referred to as mixed crystal deposition disease. It may present with pseudogout or be an incidental finding.

Milwaukee shoulder syndrome

This is a rare syndrome, in which extensive deposition of BCP crystals in large joints is associated with progressive joint destruction. It is more common in women than in men. The onset is gradual with joint pain, sometimes precipitated by injury or overuse. The disease progresses over a few months to cause severe pain and disability, associated with joint destruction. X-rays show joint space narrowing, osteophytes and calcification. Aspiration yields large volumes of relatively non-inflammatory fluid containing abundant BCP aggregates and often cartilage fragments. The differential diagnosis is end-stage avascular necrosis, chronic sepsis or neuropathic joint. There is no acute phase response and synovial fluid cultures are negative.

Treatment is with analgesics, intra-articular injection of corticosteroids, local physical treatments and physiotherapy. The clinical outcome is poor, however, and most patients require joint replacement. The cause is incompletely understood but it has been speculated that deposition of BCP crystals activates collagenase and other proteases in articular cells, which are responsible for the tissue damage.

Connective tissue disease

Deposition of BCP may occur in the subcutaneous tissues and muscle of patients with scleroderma and other connective tissue disease. Usually, the deposits are asymptomatic but can be associated with pain and local ulceration. There is no specific treatment.

FIBROMYALGIA

This is a common cause of generalised regional pain and disability, and is frequently associated with medically unexplained symptoms in other systems (p. 236). The prevalence in the UK and US is about 2–3%. Although fibromyalgia can occur at any age, including adolescence, it increases in prevalence with age, to reach a peak of 7% in women aged over 70. There is a strong female predominance of around 10:1. Risk factors include life events that cause psychosocial distress, such as marital disharmony, alcoholism in the family, injury or assault, low income and self-reported childhood abuse (Box 25.48). It occurs in a wide variety of races and cultures.

EBM 25.48 Predisposing factors for fibromyalgia

'Epidemiological studies show that widespread body pain, fatigue, psychological distress and multiple hyperalgesic tender sites cluster together and associate with stressful life events.'

- Wolfe F, et al. Arthritis Rheum 1995; 38:19–28.
- Croft P, et al. BMJ 1994; 309:696–699.

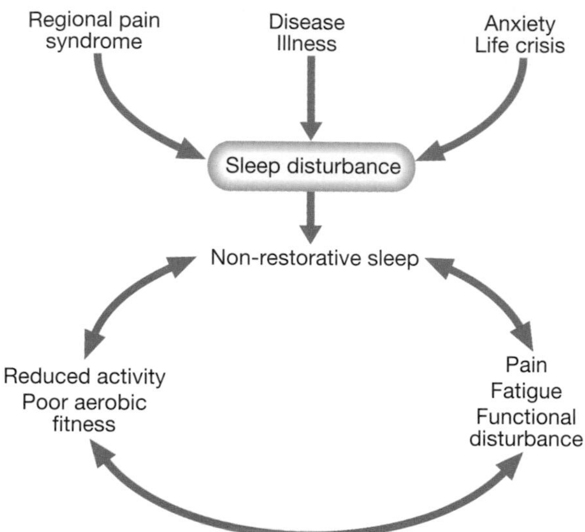

Fig. 25.29 Possible causative mechanisms in fibromyalgia.

Pathophysiology

The cause of fibromyalgia is poorly understood but two abnormalities that may be interrelated (Fig. 25.29) have been consistently reported in affected patients.

Sleep abnormality

Delta waves are characteristic of deep stages of non-rapid eye movement (non-REM) sleep, usually occurring in the first few hours and thought to have an important restorative function. People with fibromyalgia have reduced delta sleep in a pattern distinct from that seen with depression. Furthermore, deprivation of delta but not REM sleep in normal volunteers produces the symptoms and signs of fibromyalgia, supporting it as a non-restorative sleep disorder.

Abnormal peripheral and central pain processing

A reduced threshold of pain perception and tolerance at characteristic sites throughout the body is characteristic of fibromyalgia. Affected people have peripheral sensitisation and spinal cord 'wind-up' (pain amplification), with an exaggerated skin flare response to topically applied capsaicin, and frequent occurrence of dermatographism and allodynia (normally non-noxious stimuli become painful). Abnormal central pain processing is suggested by altered cerebrospinal fluid levels of substance P (increased) and serotonin (reduced); reduced basal levels of regional cerebral blood flow in the caudate and thalamus with an augmented processing response on functional MRI; low basal free cortisol and reduction in evening trough; and altered descending inhibition via the hypothalamic–pituitary–adrenal and growth hormone somatomedin axes.

Clinical features

The main presenting feature is widespread pain, which is often worst in the neck and back (Box 25.49). The pain is characteristically diffuse and unresponsive to analgesics and NSAID. Physiotherapy often makes it worse. Fatiguability, most prominent in the morning, is another major problem and disability is often marked. Although people can usually dress, feed and groom themselves, they may be unable to perform tasks such as shopping or housework. They may have experienced major difficulties at work or even retire because of pain and fatigue.

Examination is unremarkable, apart from the presence of hyperalgesia on moderate digital pressure in multiple sites (Fig. 25.30). The tenderness can be quantitated using metered dolorimeters but moderate digital pressure, enough just to whiten the nail, is sufficient for clinical diagnosis. Patients with other musculoskeletal diseases can develop fibromyalgia and it is important to determine to what extent symptoms are related to fibromyalgia or a coexisting disease.

25.49 Clinical features in fibromyalgia

Usual symptoms

- Multiple regional pain
- Marked fatigability
- Marked disability
- Broken, non-restorative sleep
- Low affect, irritability, weepiness
- Poor concentration, forgetfulness

Variable locomotor symptoms

- Early morning stiffness
- Swelling of hands, fingers
- Numbness, tingling of all fingers

Additional, variable, non-locomotor symptoms

- Non-throbbing bifrontal headache (tension headache)
- Colicky abdominal pain, bloating, variable bowel habit (irritable bowel syndrome)
- Bladder fullness, nocturnal frequency (irritable bladder)
- Hyperacusis, dyspareunia, discomfort when touched (allodynia)
- Frequent side-effects with drugs (chemical sensitivity)

Investigations and management

There are no abnormalities on routine blood tests or imaging, but it is important to screen for other conditions that could contribute to some of the patient's symptoms (Box 25.50).

The aims of management are to educate the patient about the condition, achieve pain control and improve sleep. Wherever possible, education should include the

25.50 Minimum investigation screen in fibromyalgia

Test	Condition screened
Full blood count	Anaemia, lymphopenia of SLE
Erythrocyte sedimentation rate, C-reactive protein	Inflammatory disease
Thyroid function	Hypothyroidism
Calcium, alkaline phosphatase	Hyperparathyroidism, osteomalacia
Antinuclear antibodies	SLE

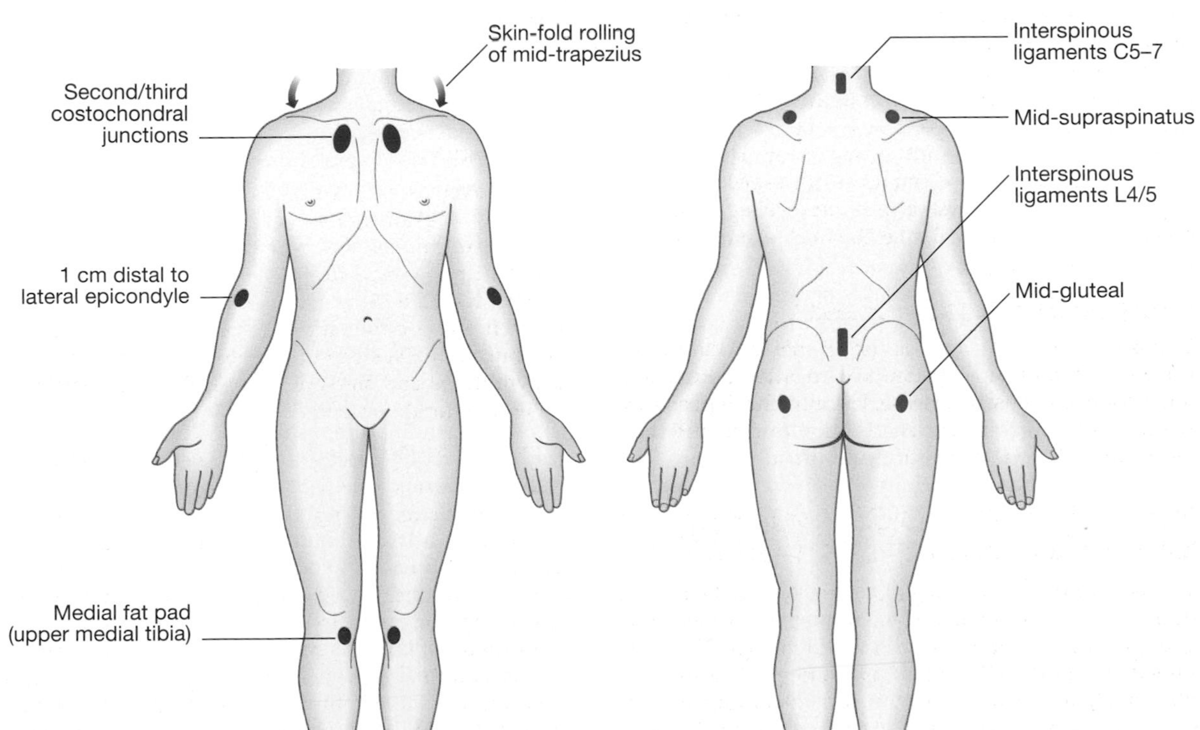

Fig. 25.30 Typical tender spots in fibromyalgia.

spouse, family or carer. It should be acknowledged that the cause of fibromyalgia is not fully understood but the widespread pain does not reflect inflammation, tissue damage or disease. The model of a self-perpetuating cycle of poor sleep and pain (see Fig. 25.29) is a useful framework for problem-based management. Understanding the diagnosis can often help the patient come to terms with the symptoms. Repeat or drawn-out investigation may reinforce beliefs in occult serious pathology and should be avoided.

Low-dose amitriptyline (10–75 mg at night), with or without fluoxetine, may help by encouraging delta sleep and reducing spinal cord wind-up. Many people with fibromyalgia, however, are intolerant of even small doses of amitriptyline. There is limited evidence for the use of tramadol, serotonin–noradrenaline (norepinephrine) re-uptake inhibitors (SNRIs) such as duloxetine, and the anticonvulsants pregabalin and gabapentin. A graded increase in aerobic exercise can improve well-being and sleep quality. The use of self-help strategies and a cognitive behavioural approach with relaxation techniques should be encouraged. Sublimated anxiety relating to distressing life events should be specifically explored with appropriate counselling. There are patient organisations that provide additional information and support.

The prognosis for hospital-diagnosed fibromyalgia is poor. Although treatment may improve quality of life and ability to cope, most people do not lose their symptoms over 5 years. Subjects diagnosed in primary care, or who have sublimated anxiety that can be successfully addressed, may fare better.

BONE AND JOINT INFECTION

Septic arthritis

Septic arthritis is the most rapid and destructive joint disease, and is associated with significant morbidity and a mortality of 10%. This has not improved over the last 20 years, despite advances in antimicrobial therapy. The incidence is 2–10 per 100 000 in the general population, and 30–70 per 100 000 in those with pre-existing joint disease or joint replacement.

Septic arthritis is usually due to haematogenous spread from either skin or upper respiratory tract; infection from direct puncture wounds or secondary to joint aspiration is uncommon. Risk factors include increasing age, pre-existing joint disease (principally RA), diabetes mellitus, immunosuppression (by drugs or disease) and intravenous drug misuse. In RA, the skin is a frequent portal of entry because of maceration of skin between the toes due to joint deformity and difficulties with foot hygiene due to hand deformity. Box 25.51 describes the particular considerations in old age.

Clinical features

The usual presentation is with acute or subacute monoarthritis and fever. The joint is usually swollen, hot and red, with pain at rest and on movement. Although any joint can be affected, lower limb joints, such as the knee and hip, are commonly targeted. Patients with pre-existing arthritis may present with multiple joint involvement.

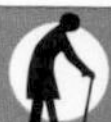

25.51 Joint and bone infection in old age

- **Vertebral infection**: more common. Recognition may be delayed, as symptoms may be attributed to compression fractures caused by osteoporosis.
- **Peripheral vascular disease**: leads to more frequent involvement of the bones of the feet, and diabetic foot ulcers are also commonly complicated by osteomyelitis.
- **Prosthetic joint infections**: now more common because of the increased frequency of prosthetic joint insertion in older people.
- **Gram-negative bacilli**: more frequent pathogens than in younger people.

In adults, the most likely organism is *Staphylococcus aureus*, particularly in patients with RA and diabetes. In young, sexually active adults, disseminated gonococcal infection occurs in up to 3% of untreated gonorrhoea, usually presenting with migratory arthralgia, low-grade fever and tenosynovitis, which may precede the development of oligo- or monoarthritis. Painful pustular skin lesions may also be present. Amongst the elderly and intravenous drug users, Gram-negative bacilli or group B, C and G streptococci are important causes. Group A streptococci, pneumococci, meningococci and *Haemophilus influenzae* are occasionally isolated.

Investigations

The pivotal investigation is joint aspiration but blood cultures should also be taken. The synovial fluid is usually turbid or blood-stained but may appear normal. If the joint is not readily accessible, aspiration should be performed under imaging guidance or in theatre. Prosthetic joints should only be aspirated in theatre.

Synovial fluid should be sent for Gram stain and culture; cultures are positive in around 90% of cases, but the Gram stain is positive in only 50%. In contrast, synovial fluid culture is positive in only 30% of gonococcal infections, making it important to obtain concurrent cultures from the genital tract (positive in 70–90% of cases). There is a leucocytosis with raised ESR and CRP in most patients, but these features may be absent in elderly or immunocompromised patients, or early in the disease course. Serial measurements of CRP and ESR are useful in following the response to treatment.

Management

The principles of management are summarised in Box 25.52. The patient should be admitted to hospital for pain relief and administration of parenteral antibiotics. Flucloxacillin (2 g IV 4 times daily) is the antibiotic of first choice pending the results of cultures, since it will cover most staphylococcal and streptococcal infections. If there is reason to suspect a Gram-negative infection, then a cephalosporin or gentamicin should be added. Microbiology advice should be sought in complicated situations such as intravenous drug users, patients in intensive care and those who might be colonised by resistant organisms. It is traditional to continue intravenous antibiotics for 2 weeks and to follow this with oral treatment for another 4 weeks, but there is no evidence to support the optimal duration of treatment. Joint aspiration should be performed using a large-bore needle once or twice daily. If this is not possible,

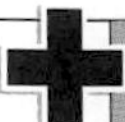

25.52 Emergency management of suspected septic arthritis

Admit patient to hospital
Perform urgent investigations • Aspirate joint Send synovial fluid for Gram stain and culture Use imaging guidance if required (e.g. for hip) • Send blood for culture, routine biochemistry and haematology, including ESR and CRP • Consider sending other samples (sputum, urine, wound swab) for culture, depending on patient history, to determine primary source of infection
Commence intravenous antibiotic
• Flucloxacillin 2 g 4 times daily • If penicillin-allergic, give clindamycin 450–600 mg 4 times daily • If at high risk of Gram-negative sepsis (elderly, frail, recurrent urinary tract infection), add a cephalosporin (cefuroxime 1.5 g 3 times daily)
Relieve pain
• Oral and/or intravenous analgesics • Consider local ice-packs
Aspirate joint
• Perform serial needle aspiration to dryness (1–3 times/day or as required) • Consider arthroscopic drainage if needle aspiration difficult
Arrange physiotherapy
• Early regular passive movement, progressing to active movements once pain controlled and effusion not re-accumulating

arthroscopic or open surgical drainage may need to be undertaken. Regular passive movement should be undertaken from the outset, and active movements encouraged once the condition has stabilised. Infected prosthetic joints require management by the orthopaedic team, but often prolonged antibiotic treatment on its own is ineffective and removal of the prosthesis is required for eradication of the infection.

Arthritis may be a feature of Lyme disease caused by members of the *Borrelia* species of microorganisms. It is generally a late manifestation, which usually affects large joints. Brucellosis presents with an acute febrile illness, followed in some cases by the development of localised infection, which can result in arthritis, bursitis, osteomyelitis, sacroiliitis and paravertebral or psoas abscesses. These conditions are discussed on pages 332 and 333.

Viral arthritis

The usual presentation is with acute polyarthritis, following a febrile illness, which may be accompanied by a rash. Most cases of viral arthritis are self-limiting and settle down within 4–6 weeks. Human parvovirus (mainly B19, p. 315) arthropathy is the most common in Europe; adults may not have the characteristic 'slapped cheek' facial rash seen in children. The diagnosis can be confirmed by a rise in specific IgM. Polyarthritis may also occur rarely with hepatitis B and C, rubella (including rubella vaccination) and HIV infection. A variety of

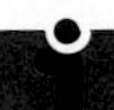

25.53 Musculoskeletal manifestations of HIV

Manifestation	Comment
• Non-specific arthralgia	Most common; intermittent and polyarticular
• Reactive arthritis • Psoriatic arthritis • Idiopathic lower limb inflammatory oligoarthritis	Especially in men who have sex with men
• Osteonecrosis • Myositis • Vasculitis • Sjögren's-like disease	Unclear if related to HIV or its treatment, or intercurrent disease

mosquito-borne viruses may cause epidemics of acute polyarthritis, including Ross River (Australia, Pacific), Chikungunya and O'nyongnyong (Asia, Africa), and Mayaro viruses (South America). A wide variety of articular symptoms have been associated with HIV, mainly in the later stages of infection (Box 25.53). Management is symptomatic, with NSAID and analgesics.

Osteomyelitis

In osteomyelitis, the primary site of infection is bone and bone marrow. Any part of a bone may be involved but there is preferential targeting of the juxta-epiphyseal regions of long bones adjacent to joints. The usual source is through haematogenous spread, although directly introduced infection may complicate trauma or orthopaedic surgery. The organisms most frequently implicated are staphylococci, *Pseudomonas* and *Mycobacterium tuberculosis*. Osteomyelitis occurs most commonly in childhood and adolescence. Risk factors include diabetes mellitus (especially involving the foot), compromised immunity (including AIDS) and sickle cell disease, which particularly increases the risk of *Salmonella* infection. The infection often results in a florid inflammatory response, with a greatly increased intraosseous pressure. If untreated, the condition may cause localised areas of osteonecrosis, leading to the development of a fragment of necrotic bone that is called a sequestrum. Eventual perforation of the cortex by pus stimulates local new bone formation (involucrum) in the periosteum, often leading to the development of sinuses that discharge through the skin.

Clinical features and investigations

The presentation is with localised bone pain and tenderness, often accompanied by malaise, night sweats and pyrexia. The adjacent joint may be painful to move and may develop a sterile effusion or secondary septic arthritis. X-rays may show evidence of osteopenia, localised osteolysis and osteonecrosis, but the imaging modality of choice is MRI, which is much more sensitive for detecting early changes. Cultures should be performed, where possible, by open or imaging-guided biopsy. Blood cultures should be taken, which may also reveal the causative organism.

Management

Early recognition and management is critical; once osteomyelitis becomes established and chronic, it may prove very hard to eradicate the infection with antibiotics alone. The principles are those followed for septic arthritis, with parenteral antibiotics for at least 2 weeks, followed by oral antibiotics for at least 4 weeks. Resection of the infected bone and subsequent reconstruction are often required. Complications of chronic osteomyelitis include secondary amyloidosis (p. 86) and skin malignancy at the margin of a discharging sinus (Marjolin's ulcer).

Tuberculosis

Tuberculosis can affect the musculoskeletal system, usually targeting the spine (Pott's disease) or large joints such as the hip, knee or ankle. The presentation is with pain, swelling and fever. The X-ray changes are non-specific and mycobacteria are seldom identified in the synovial fluid, so tissue biopsy is required for a definite diagnosis. Medical management is described on page 693. In some cases, surgical débridement may be required for extensive joint disease, and spinal involvement may require surgical stabilisation and decompression.

RHEUMATOID ARTHRITIS

Rheumatoid arthritis (RA) is the most common persistent inflammatory arthritis, occurring throughout the world and in all ethnic groups. The prevalence is lowest in black Africans and Chinese, and highest in Pima Indians. In Caucasians, approximately 0.8–1.0% are affected, with a female to male ratio of 3:1. The clinical course is prolonged, with intermittent exacerbations and remissions. Patients with RA have an increased mortality when compared with age-matched controls, primarily due to an increased risk of cardiovascular disease. This is most marked in those with severe disease, with a reduction in expected lifespan by 8–15 years. Around 40% of RA patients are registered as disabled within 3 years of onset, and around 80% are moderately to severely disabled within 20 years. Functional capacity decreases most rapidly at the beginning of disease and the functional status of patients within their first year of RA is often predictive of long-term outcome. Factors that associate with a poorer prognosis are disability at presentation, female gender, involvement of MTP joints, radiographic damage at presentation, smoking and a positive RF or ACPA. It is likely that the prognosis of RA will improve as more effective treatment regimens are introduced in patients with early disease. In former years, around 25% of patients required a large joint replacement but rates are now falling, probably reflecting more aggressive and effective medical therapy.

Pathophysiology

Genetic, epigenetic and environmental factors are implicated in the pathogenesis of RA. The concordance rate of RA is higher in monozygotic (12–15%) than in dizygotic twins (3%), and there is an increased frequency of disease in first-degree relatives of patients. Genome-wide association studies have detected more than 30 loci that are associated with the risk of developing RA or with severity of disease once it is established. Many of the risk genes are involved in the function of the immune system, and include major histocompatibility complex (MHC) class II, *PTPN22*, *CD40L* and *CTLA4*. The MHC class II gene, *HLA-DR4*, is the major susceptibility haplotype in most ethnic groups, occurring in 50–75% of Caucasian patients with RA, compared to 20–25% of the normal population. However, *DR1* is more important in Indians and Israelis, and *DW15* in Japanese. It has long been thought that RA may be triggered by an infectious agent in a genetically susceptible host, but a specific pathogen has not been identified. Periodontal disease and oral pathogens have been implicated, as have gastrointestinal organisms, and viruses such as Epstein–Barr and cytomegalovirus. Cigarette smoking is a strong risk factor for developing RA, especially in people with *HLA-DR4*, and is also associated with greater disease severity and reduced responsiveness to DMARD and biological treatment. Susceptibility is increased post-partum and by breastfeeding, indicating that hormone/immune interactions may be important.

The clinical onset of RA is characterised by infiltration of the synovial membrane with lymphocytes, plasma cells, dendritic cells and macrophages. $CD4^+$ T lymphocytes, including Th1 cells (interferon-gamma (IFN-γ) producers) and Th17 cells (IL-17A, IL-17F and IL-22 producers), play a central role by interacting with other cells in the synovium. Lymphoid follicles form within the synovial membrane in which T cell–B cell interactions lead B cells to produce cytokines and autoantibodies, including RF and ACPA. Synovial macrophages are activated by immune complexes and local damage-associated molecules acting via Toll-like receptors, to produce pro-inflammatory cytokines, including TNF, IL-1, IL-6 and IL-15. These act on synovial fibroblasts, to promote swelling of the synovial membrane and damage to soft tissues and cartilage. Fibroblasts, in particular, form a rich source of inflammatory cytokines, chemokines, leukotrienes and matrix metalloproteinases that drive local tissue damage and remodelling. Similarly, activation of osteoclasts by RANKL and chondrocytes by cytokines such as IL-1 and TNF drives destruction of bone and cartilage respectively (Fig. 25.31). The RA joint is hypoxic and this promotes new blood vessel formation (neoangiogenesis). Thus the inflamed synovium becomes vascularised, with highly activated endothelial cells supporting the recruitment of yet more leucocytes to perpetuate the inflammatory process. Amongst the range of inflammatory mediators present in the RA joint, TNF plays an important role by regulating production of other cytokines, whose actions are shown in Figure 25.31, and by activating the endothelium. IL-6 similarly plays a critical inflammatory role within the joint and also in regulating the systemic effects of RA by inducing the acute phase response, anaemia of chronic disease, fatigue and reduced cognitive function.

The inflammatory granulation tissue (pannus) formed by the above sequence of events spreads over and under the articular cartilage, which is progressively eroded and destroyed. Maturation of osteoclasts in the synovial membrane and in adjacent bone combine to erode bony structures. Later, fibrous or bony ankylosis may occur. Muscles adjacent to inflamed joints atrophy and may be infiltrated with lymphocytes. This leads to progressive biomechanical dysfunction and may further amplify destruction.

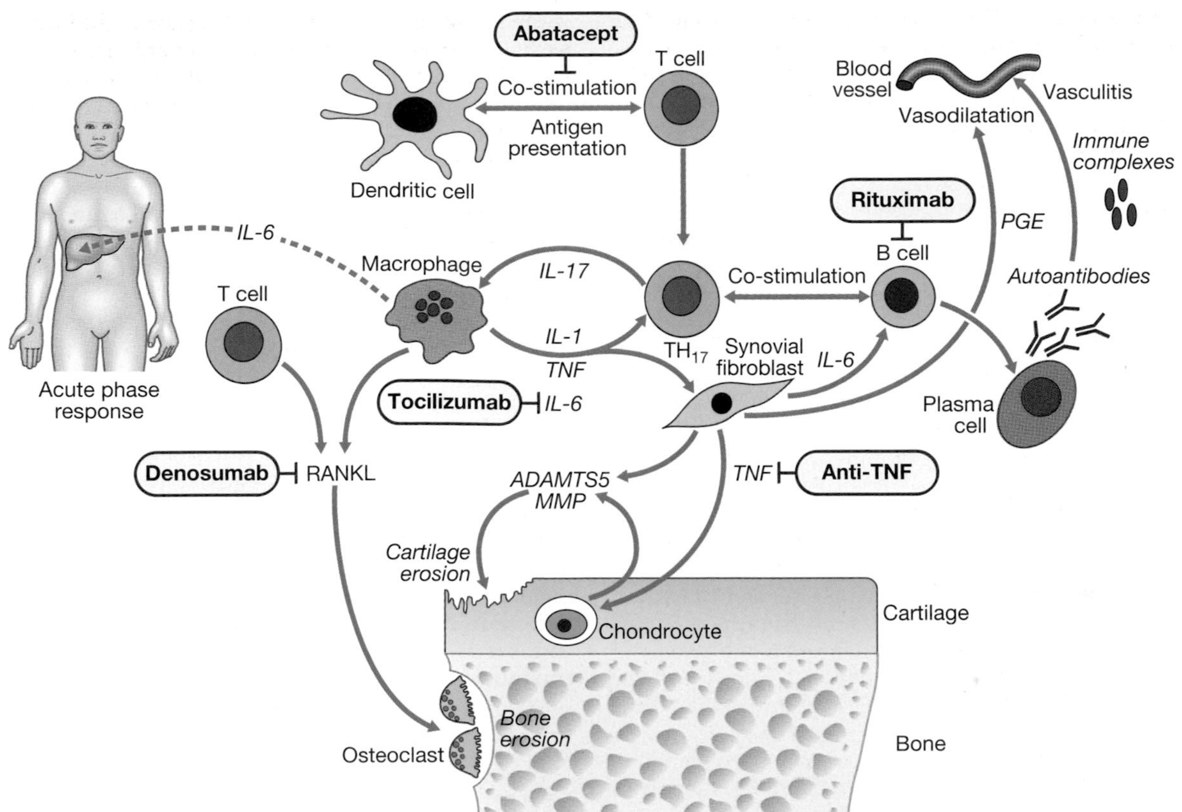

Fig. 25.31 Pathophysiology of rheumatoid arthritis. Some of the cytokines and cellular interactions believed to be important in RA are shown, along with the targets for currently available biological drugs. (ADAMTS5 = aggrecanase; IL = interleukin; MMP = matrix metalloproteinases; PGE = prostaglandin E; TNF = tumour necrosis factor; RANKL = RANK ligand)

Rheumatoid nodules consist of a central area of fibrinoid material surrounded by a palisade of proliferating mononuclear cells. Similar granulomatous lesions may occur in the pleura, lung, pericardium and sclera. Lymph nodes in RA are often hyperplastic, showing many lymphoid follicles with large germinal centres and numerous plasma cells in the sinuses and medullary cords. Immunofluorescence confirms RF and ACPA synthesis by plasma cells in synovium and lymph nodes. The bone marrow in RA is similarly hyperplastic, with evidence of lymphocyte activation and proliferation and local cytokine production. The bone marrow forms a selective survival niche for plasma cells that, in turn, produce autoantibodies. Importantly, these plasma cells are CD20-negative and, as such, escape therapies that target CD20, such as rituximab (see below).

Clinical features

The typical presentation is with pain, joint swelling and stiffness affecting the small joints of the hands, feet and wrists. Large joint involvement, systemic symptoms and extra-articular features may also occur. Clinical criteria for the diagnosis of RA are shown in Box 25.54.

Sometimes RA has a very acute onset, with florid morning stiffness, polyarthritis and pitting oedema. This occurs more commonly in old age. Other patients may present with proximal muscle stiffness mimicking

25.54 Criteria for diagnosis of rheumatoid arthritis*

Criterion	Score
Joints affected	
1 large joint	0
2–10 large joints	1
1–3 small joints	2
4–10 small joints	5
Serology	
Negative RF and ACPA	0
Low positive RF or ACPA	2
High positive RF or ACPA	3
Duration of symptoms	
$<$ 6 wks	0
$>$ 6 wks	1
Acute phase reactants	
Normal CRP and ESR	0
Abnormal CRP or ESR	1
Patients with a score $\geq$ 6 are considered to have definite RA.	

*European League Against Rheumatism/American College of Rheumatology 2010 Criteria.
(ACPA = anti-citrullinated peptide antibodies; CRP = C-reactive protein; ESR = erythrocyte sedimentation rate; RF = rheumatoid factor)

25

polymyalgia rheumatica (p. 1117). Occasionally, the onset is palindromic, with relapsing and remitting episodes of pain, stiffness and swelling that last for only a few hours or days.

Examination reveals typical features of symmetrical swelling of the MCP and PIP joints. These and other joints are tender on pressure when actively inflamed and have stress pain on passive movement. Erythema is unusual and its presence suggests coexistent sepsis. Characteristic deformities may develop with long-standing uncontrolled disease, including 'swan neck' deformity, the boutonnière or 'button hole' deformity, and a Z deformity of the thumb (Fig. 25.32B). Dorsal subluxation of the ulna at the distal radio-ulnar joint is common and may contribute to rupture of the fourth and fifth extensor tendons. Triggering of fingers may occur because of nodules in the flexor tendon sheaths. Deformities of the hand are less common now, as a result of more aggressive treatment.

In the foot, dorsal subluxation of the MTP joints may result in 'cock-up' toe deformities. This causes pain on weight-bearing on the exposed MTP heads and development of secondary adventitious bursae and callosities. In the hindfoot, calcaneovalgus (eversion) is the most common deformity, reflecting damage to the ankle and subtalar joint. This is often associated with loss of the longitudinal arch (flat foot) due to rupture of the tibialis posterior tendon.

Popliteal ('Baker's') cysts may occur in combination with knee synovitis, where synovial fluid communicates with the cyst but is prevented from returning to the joint by a valve-like mechanism. Rupture, often induced by knee flexion in the presence of a large effusion, leads to calf pain and swelling that may mimic a deep venous thrombosis (DVT).

A

B

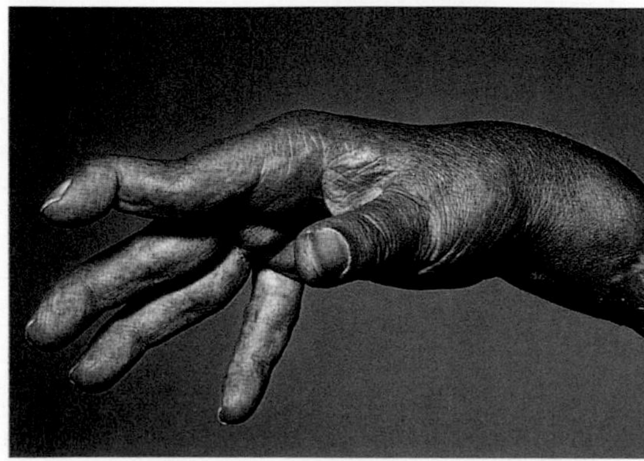

Fig. 25.32 The hand in rheumatoid arthritis. A Ulnar deviation of the fingers with wasting of the small muscles of the hands and synovial swelling at the wrists, the extensor tendon sheaths, the metacarpophalangeal and proximal interphalangeal joints. B 'Swan neck' deformity of the fingers.

Extra-articular features

Anorexia, weight loss and fatigue are common and may occur throughout the disease course. Generalised osteoporosis and muscle-wasting result from systemic inflammation. Extra-articular features are most common in patients with long-standing seropositive erosive disease but may occasionally occur at presentation, especially in men. Most are due to serositis, granuloma and nodule formation or vasculitis (Box 25.55).

Cutaneous and vascular features

Rheumatoid nodules occur almost exclusively in seropositive patients, usually at sites of pressure or friction, such as the extensor surfaces of the forearm (Fig. 25.33), sacrum, Achilles tendon and toes. They may be complicated by ulceration and secondary infection. Rheumatoid vasculitis may occur in older seropositive patients and is indicated by systemic symptoms (fatigue, fever) and multiple extra-articular features. Vasculitis can vary

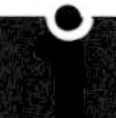

25.55 Extra-articular manifestations of rheumatoid disease

Systemic	
• Fever	• Fatigue
• Weight loss	• Susceptibility to infection
Musculoskeletal	
• Muscle-wasting	• Bursitis
• Tenosynovitis	• Osteoporosis
Haematological	
• Anaemia	• Eosinophilia
• Thrombocytosis	
Lymphatic	
• Felty's syndrome (see Box 25.56)	• Splenomegaly
Nodules	
• Sinuses	• Fistulae
Ocular	
• Episcleritis	• Scleromalacia
• Scleritis	• Keratoconjunctivitis sicca
Vasculitis	
• Digital arteritis	• Mononeuritis multiplex
• Ulcers	• Visceral arteritis
• Pyoderma gangrenosum	
Cardiac	
• Pericarditis	• Conduction defects
• Myocarditis	• Coronary vasculitis
• Endocarditis	• Granulomatous aortitis
Pulmonary	
• Nodules	• Bronchiolitis
• Pleural effusions	• Caplan's syndrome
• Fibrosing alveolitis	
Neurological	
• Cervical cord compression	• Peripheral neuropathy
• Compression neuropathies	• Mononeuritis multiplex
Amyloidosis (p. 86)	

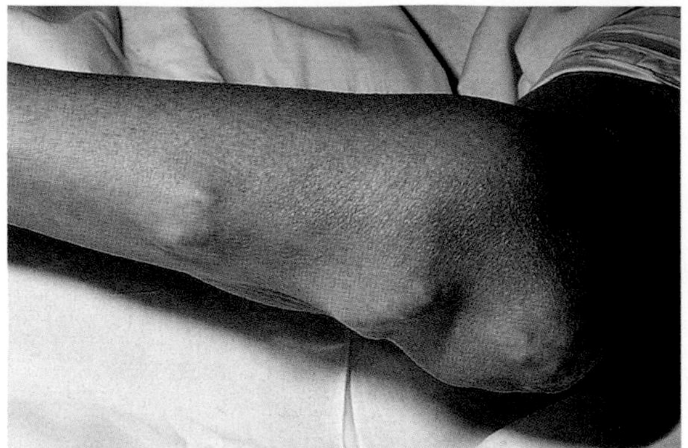

Fig. 25.33 Rheumatoid nodules and olecranon bursitis. Nodules were palpable within as well as outside the bursa.

from relatively benign nail-fold infarcts to widespread cutaneous ulceration and skin necrosis. Rarely, involvement of medium-sized arteries can lead to mesenteric, renal or coronary artery occlusion.

Ocular involvement

The most common symptom is dry eyes (keratoconjunctivitis sicca) due to secondary Sjögren's syndrome (p. 1114). Painless episcleritis frequently accompanies nodular seropositive disease; it may cause intense redness of superficial vessels but sight is unimpaired. Scleritis is more serious and potentially sight-threatening; the eye is red and painful, vision is impaired, and the sclera shows a deep red blush beneath the individual red superficial vessels (p. 1058). Scleromalacia is painless bilateral thinning of the sclera, with the affected area appearing blue or grey (the colour of the underlying choroid). Corneal melting is a rare but devastating manifestation. It occurs in long-standing disease and is associated with systemic vasculitis. It causes pain, redness and blurred vision with corneal thinning. If it is untreated, progression to perforation is common, so urgent high-dose steroid and immunosuppressive therapy is indicated.

Cardiac and pulmonary involvement

Cardiac involvement occurs in up to 30% of patients with seropositive RA but is usually asymptomatic. Symptomatic pericardial effusions and constrictive pericarditis are rare. Occasionally, granulomatous lesions can cause heart block, cardiomyopathy, coronary artery occlusion or aortic regurgitation. Serositis is commonly asymptomatic but may present as pleurisy or breathlessness. Pulmonary fibrosis can occur in advanced RA and may cause dyspnoea (p. 712). In addition to the above manifestations, which are due to the direct effects of the inflammatory process, the risk of atheroma and cardiovascular disease is increased in RA. This is caused by a combination of conventional risk factors, such as high cholesterol, smoking, hypertension and reduced physical activity, and the effects of inflammatory factors, such as immune complexes, cytokines and chemokines, on the endothelium and adipose tissue. The risk of cardiovascular disease may be increased by NSAID and corticosteroids, whereas there is some evidence that DMARD and biological medicines are protective.

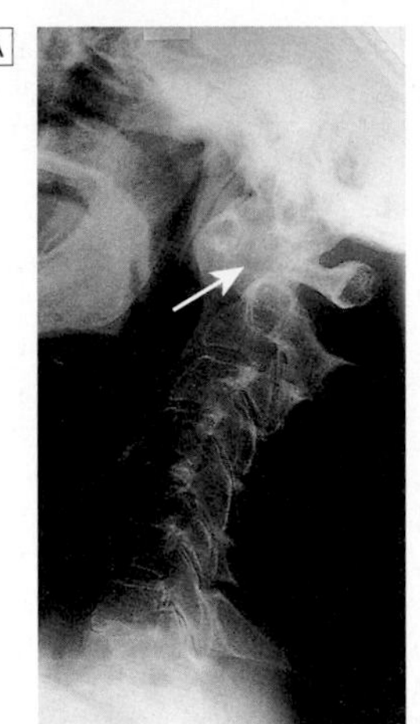

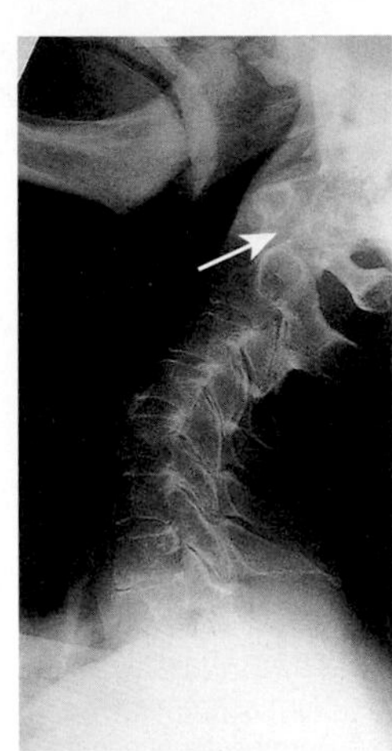

Fig. 25.34 Subluxation of cervical spine. **A** Flexion, showing widening of the space (arrow) between the odontoid peg of the axis (behind) and the anterior arch of the atlas (in front). **B** Extension, showing reduction in this space.

Neurological complications

Peripheral entrapment neuropathies may result from compression by hypertrophied synovium or by joint subluxation. Median nerve compression in the carpal tunnel is most common and bilateral compression can occur as an early presenting feature of RA. Other syndromes include ulnar nerve compression at the elbow or wrist, compression of the lateral popliteal nerve at the head of the fibula, and tarsal tunnel syndrome (entrapment of the posterior tibial nerve in the flexor retinaculum), which causes burning, tingling and numbness in the distal sole and toes. Diffuse symmetrical peripheral neuropathy and mononeuritis multiplex may occur in patients with rheumatoid vasculitis.

Cervical cord compression can result from subluxation of the cervical spine at the atlanto-axial joint or at a subaxial level (Fig. 25.34). Atlanto-axial subluxation is a common finding in long-standing RA and is due to erosion of the transverse ligament posterior to the odontoid peg. If unrecognised, it can lead to cord compression or sudden death following minor trauma or manipulation. Atlanto-axial subluxation should be suspected in any RA patient who describes new onset of occipital headache, particularly if symptoms of paraesthesia or electric shock are present in the arms. The onset is often insidious, with subtle loss of function that is initially attributed to active disease. Reflexes and power can be very difficult to assess in the presence of marked joint damage and therefore sensory or upper motor signs are most important. Patients with spinal cord compression may require operative stabilisation and fixation, though the outcome is poor if the patient already has tetraparesis.

Other complications

Amyloidosis is a rare complication of prolonged active disease and usually presents with nephrotic syndrome. Microcytic anaemia can occur due to iron deficiency resulting from NSAID-induced gastrointestinal blood loss, and normochromic, normocytic anaemia with thrombocytosis is present in active disease. Felty's syndrome is the association of splenomegaly and

25.56 Felty's syndrome

Risk factors

- Age of onset 50–70 yrs
- Female > male
- Caucasians > blacks
- Long-standing RA
- Deforming but inactive disease
- Seropositive for RF

Common clinical features

- Splenomegaly
- Lymphadenopathy
- Weight loss
- Skin pigmentation
- Keratoconjunctivitis sicca
- Vasculitis, leg ulcers
- Recurrent infections
- Nodules

Laboratory findings

- Normochromic, normocytic anaemia
- Neutropenia
- Abnormal liver function
- Thrombocytopenia
- Impaired T- and B-cell immunity

neutropenia with RA (Box 25.56). Generalised and local lymphadenopathy affecting nodes draining actively inflamed joints may both occur. Patients with persistent lymphadenopathy should be biopsied since there is an increased risk of lymphoma in patients with long-standing RA.

Investigations

The diagnosis of RA is based on clinical grounds but investigations are useful in confirming the diagnosis and assessing disease activity (Box 25.57). The ESR and CRP are usually raised but normal results do not exclude the diagnosis. ACPA are positive in about 70% of cases and are highly specific for RA, occurring in many patients before clinical onset of the disease. Similarly RF is positive in about 70% of cases, many of whom also test positive for ACPA. Low titres of RF are found in about 10% of the normal population and in other diseases (p. 1067).

Ultrasound examination and MRI are not routinely required in patients with obvious clinical signs. Their main value is in patients with symptoms suggestive of an inflammatory arthritis, where there is uncertainty about the presence of synovitis. They are also a sensitive means of detecting early erosions. Plain X-rays of the hands, wrist and feet are of limited value in early RA but certain changes are characteristic, including peri-articular osteoporosis and marginal joint erosions. The main indication for X-ray is in the assessment of patients with problem joints to determine if significant structural damage has occurred. Patients who are suspected of having atlanto-axial disease should have lateral X-rays taken in flexion and extension, and the degree of cord compression should be established with MRI. In patients with Baker's cyst, ultrasound may be required to establish the diagnosis, since DVT and Baker's cyst may coexist.

The DAS28 score is widely used to assess disease activity, the response to treatment and the need for biological therapy. It involves counting the number of swollen and tender joints in the upper limbs and knees, and combining this with the ESR and the patient's assessment of his/her general health on a visual analogue scale, to generate a numerical score. The higher the value, the more active the disease (Box 25.58).

25.57 Investigations and monitoring of rheumatoid arthritis

To establish diagnosis

- Clinical criteria
- ESR and CRP
- Ultrasound or MRI
- Rheumatoid factor and anti-citrullinated peptide antibodies

To monitor disease activity and drug efficacy

- Pain (visual analogue scale)
- Early morning stiffness (minutes)
- Joint tenderness
- Joint swelling
- DAS28 score
- ESR and CRP
- Ultrasound

To monitor disease damage

- X-rays
- Functional assessment

To monitor drug safety

- Urinalysis
- Full blood count
- Urea, creatinine and liver function tests

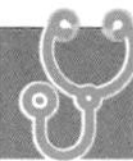

25.58 How to calculate the DAS28 score

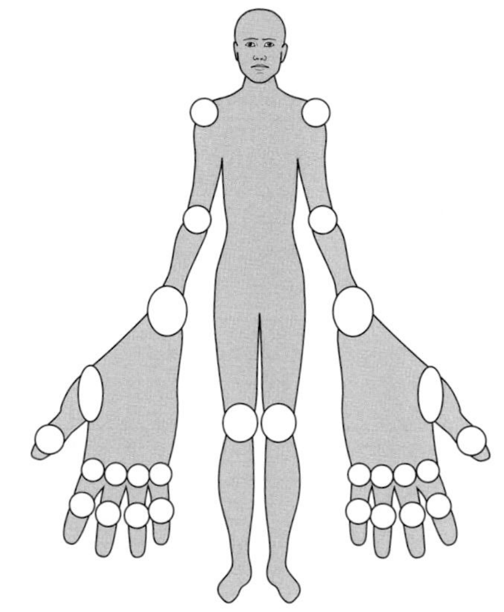

- Count the number of tender joints
- Count the number of swollen joints
- Measure the ESR
- Ask the patient to rate global activity of arthritis during the past week from 0 (no symptoms) to 100 (very severe)
- Enter data into an online calculator[1] or work out using a formula[2]

[1]www.4s-dawn.com/DAS28.
[2]DAS28 = 0.56 × square root (tender joints) + 0.28 × square root (swollen joints) + 0.70 × $\log_e$(ESR) + 0.014 (global activity score)

Management

The mainstay of treatment in RA comprises the early use of small-molecule disease-modifying antirheumatic drugs (DMARDs), and corticosteroids for induction of remission. There is evidence that early use of DMARD therapy improves clinical outcome in RA. Partial or non-response to DMARD therapy should prompt escalation of the dose or use of an additional DMARD, with progression to biological drugs if necessary (Fig. 25.35). Regular monitoring of DMARD therapy is essential because of the risk of liver and haematological toxicity. Some DMARDs are contraindicated in pregnancy, especially during the first trimester (Box 25.59). Patients who wish to become pregnant should be counselled to stop DMARD treatment while they try to conceive. Since RA almost always undergoes remission during pregnancy, it is usually possible to manage the condition without DMARD therapy over this period. Details of the dose regimens, toxicity and monitoring requirements are shown in Box 25.60.

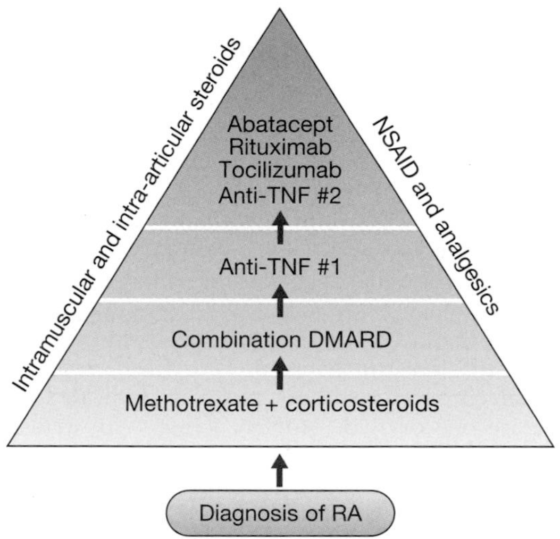

Fig. 25.35 Management of early rheumatoid arthritis. See text for details of each drug. (DMARD = disease-modifying antirheumatic drug; NSAID = non-steroidal anti-inflammatory drug; TNF = tumour necrosis factor)

25.59 Rheumatoid arthritis in pregnancy

- **Immunological changes in pregnancy**: most patients with RA go into remission during pregnancy.
- **Conception**: methotrexate and leflunomide should be discontinued for at least 3 months before trying to conceive.
- **Paracetamol**: the oral analgesic of choice during pregnancy.
- **Oral NSAIDs and selective COX-2 inhibitors**: can be used after implantation up until the last trimester.
- **Corticosteroids**: may be used to control disease flares; the main maternal risks are hypertension, glucose intolerance and osteoporosis.
- **DMARDs that may be used**: sulfasalazine, hydroxychloroquine, azathioprine or ciclosporin if required to control inflammation.
- **DMARDs that must be avoided**: methotrexate, leflunomide, cyclophosphamide, gold and penicillamine.
- **Biological therapies**: safety during pregnancy is currently unclear.
- **Breastfeeding**: methotrexate, leflunomide, cyclophosphamide, ciclosporin, azathioprine, sulfasalazine and hydroxychloroquine are contraindicated.

25.60 Commonly used small-molecule disease-modifying antirheumatic drugs in rheumatoid arthritis

Drug	Mechanism of action	Usual maintenance dose	Principal side-effects	Monitoring requirement	Monitoring frequency
Methotrexate	Inhibits DNA synthesis and cell division	5–25 mg/wk	GI upset, stomatitis, rash, alopecia, hepatotoxicity, acute pneumonitis	FBC, LFTs	Initially monthly, then every 3 mths
Sulfasalazine	Unknown	2–4 g/day	Nausea, GI upset, rash, hepatitis, neutropenia, pancytopenia (rare)	FBC, LFTs	Monthly for 3 mths, then 3-monthly
Hydroxychloroquine	Unknown	200–400 mg/day	Rash, nausea, diarrhoea, headache, corneal deposits, retinopathy (rare)	Visual acuity, fundoscopy	12-monthly
Leflunomide	Blocks T-cell division	10–20 mg/day	Nausea, GI upset, rash, alopecia, hepatitis, hypertension	FBC, LFTs, BP	2–4-weekly
D-Penicillamine	Unknown	250–750 mg/day	Rash, stomatitis, metallic taste, proteinuria, thrombocytopenia	FBC, urine (for protein)	Initially 1–2-weekly; 4–6-weekly for maintenance
Gold	Unknown	50 mg/mth by IM injection	Rash, stomatitis, alopecia, proteinuria, thrombocytopenia, myelosuppression	FBC, urine (protein)	Each injection
Ciclosporin	Blocks T-cell activation	150–300 mg/day	Nausea, GI upset, renal impairment, hypertension	FBC, LFTs, U&E, BP	2–4-weekly

(BP = blood pressure; FBC = full blood count; LFT = liver function tests; U&E = urea and electrolytes)

Disease-modifying antirheumatic drugs

Methotrexate

Methotrexate is the anchor DMARD in RA. It is usually given as a starting weekly oral dose of 7.5–10 mg and this is increased in 2.5 mg increments every 2–4 weeks until benefit occurs or toxicity is limiting. The maximum recommended dose is 25 mg. The benefits of methotrexate usually start to appear within 1–2 months but a 6-month course should be given before concluding that it has been ineffective. The most common adverse effects are nausea, vomiting and malaise within 24–48 hours of administration. Patients who experience these can sometimes be successfully treated with subcutaneous methotrexate. Folic acid (5 mg/week) reduces the incidence of adverse effects without reducing efficacy. Patients should be warned of drug interaction with sulphonamides and to avoid excess alcohol, which enhances methotrexate hepatotoxicity. Acute pulmonary toxicity (pneumonitis) is rare but can occur at any time during treatment. Patients should therefore be warned to seek early advice if they develop any new respiratory symptoms. Methotrexate should be stopped immediately if pneumonitis is suspected and high-dose steroids should be given.

Sulfasalazine

Sulfasalazine (SSZ) is widely used, both alone and in combination with methotrexate and other drugs. The mechanism of action is incompletely understood. Nausea and gastrointestinal intolerance are the main adverse effects. The usual starting dose is 500 mg daily, building up gradually to a maintenance dose of 2–4 g/day. The patient should be warned of possible orange staining of urine and contact lenses. Monitoring should be performed for liver and haematological toxicity.

Hydroxychloroquine

Hydroxycholoroquine is given in a dose of 400 mg daily, usually in combination with other DMARDs. Ocular toxicity can occur with long-term use due to retinal damage. It is usual to check visual acuity before starting treatment and to repeat this periodically whilst treatment is continued.

Leflunomide

Leflunomide can be used alone or in combination with other drugs. It works by inhibiting lymphocyte proliferation and activation. It is usually well tolerated and has low marrow toxicity, but may cause liver dysfunction. The usual maintenance dose is 10–20 mg/day. It is possible to give a loading dose of 100 mg on 3 consecutive days at the start of treatment, but this is seldom used in routine clinical practice. Monitoring should be performed for liver and haematological toxicity.

Gold, penicillamine and ciclosporin A

These are only occasionally used due to the availability of drugs with a better risk–benefit profile. Gold (sodium aurothiomalate) is given by deep intramuscular injection of 50 mg after an initial 10 mg test dose. Treatment is continued weekly for up to 6 months until benefit occurs, when the frequency is reduced to fortnightly and then monthly. Penicillamine is given in a starting dose of 125–250 mg daily on an empty stomach, and increased in 125-mg increments every 6 weeks until benefit occurs or adverse effects develop. Ciclosporin A inhibits lymphocyte division and activation. It is given in a dose of 150–300 mg/day with monitoring of blood pressure and renal function.

Corticosteroids

Systemic corticosteroids have disease-modifying activity, but their primary role is in the induction of remission in patients with early RA who are starting synthetic DMARD treatment. Various regimens have been used but there is little evidence to suggest that one is superior to another. One strategy is to give a high dose of oral prednisolone initially (60 mg daily) and to reduce and stop this gradually over a period of 3 months as the DMARD starts to take effect. Another is to employ low-dose prednisolone (5–10 mg daily for 6–24 months) or to give intramuscular injections of methylprednisolone or triamcinolone every 6–8 weeks. Intramuscular steroids are often used to treat flares of disease activity in patients who are established on DMARD therapy. Intra-articular corticosteroids are primarily indicated when there are one or two 'problem joints' with persistent synovitis despite good general control of the disease. Although corticosteroids are very useful, they also have significant adverse effects (p. 776). In the context of RA, osteoporosis is probably the most important since this is a known complication of RA, even in the absence of corticosteroid therapy. Accordingly DEXA scanning followed by bone protection should be considered in any patient with RA who is expected to be on more than 7.5 mg prednisolone daily for more than 3 months.

Biological therapies

The use of biological agents (often abbreviated to 'biologics') is reserved for the treatment of patients who have high disease activity despite having had an adequate trial of traditional DMARDs. These agents are targeted towards specific cytokines and other cell-surface molecules regulating the immune response. Although generally well tolerated, biological therapies increase the risk of serious infections due to suppression of the immune response. Although biological treatment is more effective than standard DMARD therapy, treatment costs are significantly greater. Because of this, many countries have set guidelines restricting their use. Current UK recommendations are that biological therapy should be initiated only in active RA (DAS28 > 5.1; p. 1100) when an adequate trial of at least two other DMARDs (including methotrexate) has failed. Details of the individual agents, their mechanisms of action and their toxicity are shown in Box 25.61.

Anti-TNF therapy

Anti-TNF therapy is the first-line biological drug in RA. Several agents are available, as summarised in Box 25.61. With the exception of infliximab, which must be prescribed with methotrexate to reduce the risk of neutralising antibodies developing, these agents can be used as monotherapy. In clinical practice, however, most are co-prescribed with methotrexate, as this is more efficacious. The main adverse effects are serious infections

25.61 Commonly used biological drugs in rheumatoid arthritis

Drug	Usual maintenance dose	Comment	NICE[1]
Anti-TNF-α			
Etanercept	50 mg every wk SC	Decoy receptor for TNF-α	Yes
Infliximab	3 mg/kg every 8 wks IV	Antibodies to TNF. Infliximab must be given in combination with methotrexate	Yes
Adalimumab	40 mg every 2 wks SC		Yes
Certolizumab	200 mg every 2 wks SC		Yes
Golimumab	50 mg every 4 wks SC		Yes
Anti-B-cell therapy			
Rituximab	1000 mg IV; repeat after 2 wks	Pre-medication with methylprednisolone 100 mg IV, chlorphenamine 10 mg IV and paracetamol given 30 min prior to each infusion	Yes[2]
Inhibitor of T-cell activation			
Abatacept	125 mg SC once a week	Favourable safety profile	Yes[2]
Anti-IL6			
Tocilizumab	8 mg/kg every 4 wks IV	More effective than anti-TNF in methotrexate-intolerant patients	Yes
Anti IL-1			
Anakinra	100 mg daily, SC	Less effective than other biological drugs	No

[1]Recommended for use by the National Institute of Clinical Excellence in the UK.
[2]Second-line, if patient has failed to respond to at least one TNF inhibitor.

and reactivation of latent tuberculosis. There is evidence that TNF blockade can increase the risk of some malignancies, particularly basal cell carcinoma of the skin, and that it can accelerate progression of cancer in patients with prior malignant disease. In contrast, the risk of vascular disease in RA patients seems to be reduced by anti-TNF therapy.

Rituximab

Rituximab is an antibody directed against the CD20 receptor, which is expressed on B lymphocytes and immature plasma cells. It is given by two intravenous infusions, 2 weeks apart, usually in combination with intravenous corticosteroid. It causes depletion of peripheral and synovial B cells, which is sustained for several months after administration. The treatment is repeated usually when signs of improvement are wearing off (anything from 6 months to 1 year). It is mostly used in the treatment of patients with resistant RA who have failed to respond to TNF blockade.

Abatacept

Abatacept is an agent in which the Fc domain of IgG is fused to the extracellular domain of CTLA4. It blocks the interaction between CD28 and CD80/86 that is required for full activation of T cells following antigen presentation by dendritic cells or macrophages. Abatacept has a good safety profile and is as efficacious as anti-TNF therapy in biological-naïve patients who fail to respond to conventional DMARD therapy.

Tocilizumab

This agent is an antibody directed against the IL-6 receptor, and is licensed for the treatment of rheumatoid arthritis. It prevents IL-6 activating its receptor within the synovial membrane and in other tissues such as liver and muscle. It has similar efficacy to anti-TNF therapy and is licensed for use as monotherapy or in combination with methotrexate. Adverse effects include leucopenia, hypercholesterolaemia and an increased risk of infections. It is generally used as second-line treatment in patients who have failed to respond to anti-TNF therapy, except in those who are intolerant of methotrexate, in which case it is used as a first-line treatment.

Anakinra

Anakinra is a decoy receptor for IL-1. It has some activity in RA but is seldom used since it appears to be less effective than other biological drugs.

Other treatments

Surgery

Synovectomy of the wrist or finger tendon sheaths of the hands may be required for pain relief or to prevent tendon rupture when medical interventions have failed. In later stages when joint damage has occurred, osteotomy, arthrodesis or arthroplasty may be required (see Box 25.35, p. 1080).

General measures

The general principles outlined on page 1077 should be followed. Physical rest, analgesics and NSAID may be required to control symptoms. Passive exercises and joint protection measures should be encouraged with the aim of conserving function in affected joints. During treatment, periodic assessment of disease activity, progression and disability is essential. In the vast majority, management is outpatient- or day patient-based, but hospital admission can be helpful in patients with very active disease for a period of bed rest, multiple joint injections, splinting, regular hydrotherapy, physiotherapy and education.

JUVENILE IDIOPATHIC ARTHRITIS

Inflammatory arthritis occurs rarely in children. Several distinct subtypes are recognised (Box 25.62). Systemic juvenile idiopathic arthritis (JIA; formerly known as

25.62 Clinical features of juvenile idiopathic arthritis

Subtype	Frequency	Clinical features	Immunology
Systemic JIA	5%	Fever, rash, arthralgia, hepatosplenomegaly	Autoantibody-negative
Oligoarthritis (≤ 4 joints)	60%	Large-joint arthritis, uveitis	ANA-positive
Polyarthritis (≥ 5 joints)	20%	Polyarthritis. May be extended form of oligoarthritis	ANA-positive
Enthesis-related	5%	Sacroiliitis, enthesopathy	HLA-B27-positive
Rheumatoid factor-positive	5%	Polyarthritis, similar to RA	RF-positive, ACPA-positive
Psoriatic arthritis	5%	Same as adult disease (p. 1108)	Autoantibody-negative
(ACPA = anti-citrullinated peptide antibodies; ANA = antinuclear antibody; HLA = human leucocyte antigen; RF = rheumatoid factor)			

25.63 Juvenile idiopathic arthritis in adolescence

- **Uveitis**: may be clinically silent and persist into adulthood, necessitating routine screening for eye involvement.
- **Persistence into adulthood**: persists in 50% of cases, especially in systemic disease, necessitating long-term follow-up.
- **Reduced peak bone mass**: common in polyarthritis and systemic JIA but little data on fracture risk, and evidence base for treatment is poor
- **Biological drugs**: effective in JIA but long-term safety remains unclear.

Still's disease) is a systemic disorder characterised by fever, rash, arthritis, hepatosplenomegaly and serositis in association with a raised ESR and CRP. Autoantibody tests are negative.

Oligoarthritis is the most common form, accounting for about 60% of cases. Two subtypes are recognised, depending on the extent of involvement, but they probably form part of a single disease spectrum. Oligoarticular JIA is more common in females and tends to affect large joints in an asymmetrical pattern. There is an association with uveitis and many patients are ANA-positive. Rheumatoid factor-negative polyarthritis is a heterogeneous form. Some patients are ANA-positive and these probably represent a subtype of oligoarticular JIA with more extensive joint involvement. Other patients present with polyarticular disease that is similar to adult seronegative RA. Juvenile forms of ankylosing spondylitis and psoriatic arthritis also occur.

Patients with JIA should be referred to a paediatric rheumatologist. The principles of management are similar to those in adult inflammatory disease, and corticosteroids and methotrexate are required for systemic JIA. Recent trials indicate that TNF blockers, IL-1 inhibitors and tocilizumab may also be effective. Steroids and methotrexate are also indicated for oligoarticular and polyarticular JIA, with progression to anti-TNF therapy in poor responders.

The prognosis of oligoarthritis is good and in many patients the condition resolves at puberty. Polyarticular and systemic JIA have a poorer prognosis, however, and in about 50% of cases the disease remains active into adulthood, requiring extended follow-up by adult rheumatology services. Common issues encountered during transition of paediatric patients into adulthood are shown in Box 25.63.

Adult-onset Still's disease

This is a rare systemic inflammatory disorder of unknown cause, similar to juvenile idiopathic arthritis, which presents with intermittent fever, rash and arthralgia. Splenomegaly, hepatomegaly and lymphadenopathy may be present. Investigations typically show evidence of an acute phase response, with a markedly elevated serum ferritin. Tests for RF and ANA are negative. Most patients respond to corticosteroids but DMARDs may also be required as steroid-sparing agents. Anecdotal reports indicate that anakinra (p. 1103), anti-TNF therapy and tocilizumab may be helpful in patients with resistant disease, but none of these has been tested in a randomised trial.

SERONEGATIVE SPONDYLOARTHROPATHIES

These comprise a group of related inflammatory joint diseases, which show considerable overlap in their clinical features and a shared immunogenetic association with the HLA-B27 antigen (Box 25.64). They include:

- ankylosing spondylitis
- axial spondyloarthritis
- reactive arthritis, including Reiter's syndrome
- psoriatic arthritis
- arthropathy associated with inflammatory bowel disease.

The synovitis is non-specific and is often indistinguishable from RA. However, the distinctive feature of this group of diseases is the marked degree of extrasynovial inflammation, especially of the enthesis but also of the joint capsule, periosteum, cartilage and subchondral bone. There is a striking association with carriage of the HLA-B27 allele, particularly for ankylosing spondylitis (> 95%) and reactive arthritis (90%), and especially associated with sacroiliitis, uveitis or balanitis. Understanding of the cause is incomplete but an aberrant response to infection is thought to be involved in genetically predisposed individuals. In some situations, a triggering organism can be identified, as in reactive arthritis following bacterial dysentery or chlamydial urethritis, but in others the environmental trigger remains obscure. Familial clustering not only is common to the specific condition occurring in the proband, but also may extend to other diseases in the seronegative spondyloarthopathy group.

25.64 Clinical features common to seronegative spondyloarthritis

- Asymmetrical inflammatory oligoarthritis (lower > upper limb)
- Sacroiliitis and inflammatory spondylitis
- Inflammatory enthesitis
- Tendency for familial aggregation
- RF and ACPA negative
- Absence of nodules and other extra-articular features of RA
- Typical overlapping extra-articular features:
  - Mucosal inflammation: conjunctivitis, buccal ulceration, urethritis, prostatitis, bowel ulceration
  - Pustular skin lesions and nail dystrophy
  - Anterior uveitis
  - Aortic root fibrosis (aortic incompetence, conduction defects)
  - Erythema nodosum

Ankylosing spondylitis

Ankylosing spondylitis (AS) is characterised by a chronic inflammatory arthritis predominantly affecting the sacroiliac joints and spine, which can progress to bony fusion of the spine. The onset is typically between the ages of 20 and 30, with a male preponderance of about 3:1. In Europe, more than 90% of those affected are HLA-B27-positive. The overall prevalence is less than 0.5% in most populations. Over 75% of patients are able to remain in employment and enjoy a good quality of life. Even if severe ankylosis develops, functional limitation may not be marked as long as the spine is fused in an erect posture.

Pathophysiology

Ankylosing spondylitis is thought to arise from an as yet ill-defined interaction between environmental pathogens and the host immune system in genetically susceptible individuals. Increased faecal carriage of *Klebsiella aerogenes* occurs in patients with established AS and may relate to exacerbation of both joint and eye disease. Wider alterations in the human gut microbial environment are increasingly implicated, which could lead to increased levels of circulating cytokines such as IL-23 that can activate enthesial or synovial T cells. The HLA-B27 molecule itself is implicated through its antigen-presenting function (it is a class I MHC molecule) or because of its propensity to form homodimers that activate leucocytes. HLA-B27 molecules may also misfold, causing increased endoplasmic reticulum stress. This could lead to inflammatory cytokine release by macrophages and dendritic cells, thus triggering inflammatory disease.

Clinical features

The cardinal feature is low back pain and early morning stiffness with radiation to the buttocks or posterior thighs. Symptoms are exacerbated by inactivity and relieved by movement. The disease tends to ascend slowly, ultimately involving the whole spine, although some patients present with symptoms of the thoracic or cervical spine. As the disease progresses, the spine becomes increasingly rigid as ankylosis occurs. Secondary osteoporosis of the vertebral bodies

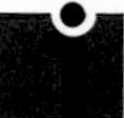

25.65 Extra-articular features of ankylosing spondylitis

- Anterior uveitis (25%) and conjunctivitis (20%)
- Prostatitis (80% men): usually asymptomatic
- Cardiovascular disease
  - Aortic incompetence
  - Mitral incompetence
  - Cardiac conduction defects
  - Pericarditis
- Amyloidosis
- Atypical upper lobe pulmonary fibrosis

frequently occurs, leading to an increased risk of vertebral fracture.

Early physical signs include a reduced range of lumbar spine movements in all directions and pain on sacroiliac stressing. As the disease progresses, stiffness increases throughout the spine and chest expansion becomes restricted. Spinal fusion varies in its extent and in most cases does not cause a gross flexion deformity, but a few patients develop marked kyphosis of the dorsal and cervical spine that may interfere with forward vision. This may prove incapacitating, especially when associated with fixed flexion contractures of hips or knees. Pleuritic chest pain aggravated by breathing is common and results from costovertebral joint involvement. Plantar fasciitis, Achilles tendinitis and tenderness over bony prominences such as the iliac crest and greater trochanter may all occur, reflecting inflammation at the sites of tendon insertions (enthesitis).

Up to 40% of patients also have peripheral arthritis. This is usually asymmetrical, affecting large joints such as the hips, knees, ankles and shoulders. In about 10% of cases, involvement of a peripheral joint may antedate spinal symptoms, and in a further 10%, symptoms begin in childhood, as in the syndrome of oligoarticular juvenile idiopathic arthritis.

Fatigue is a major complaint and may result from both chronic interruption of sleep due to pain, and chronic systemic inflammation with direct effects of inflammatory cytokines on the brain. Acute anterior uveitis is the most common extra-articular feature, which occasionally precedes joint disease. Other extra-articular features are occasionally observed but are rare (Box 25.65). Disease activity in AS can be assessed by the Bath Ankylosing Spondylitis Disease Activity Index (BASDAI), a questionnaire in which patients and their physician rate severity of various symptoms (Box 25.66). This is important in assessing eligibility for biological treatment. The criteria for the diagnosis of classical AS and axial spondyloarthropathy (SpA) are shown in Box 25.67. The criteria for axial SpA were developed to take account of the fact that X-rays may be normal in patients with early AS.

Investigations

In established AS, radiographs of the sacroiliac joint show irregularity and loss of cortical margins, widening of the joint space and subsequently sclerosis, joint space narrowing and fusion. Lateral thoracolumbar spine X-rays may show anterior 'squaring' of vertebrae due to erosion and sclerosis of the anterior corners and periostitis of the waist. Bridging syndesmophytes may also be

25

seen. These are areas of calcification that follow the outermost fibres of the annulus (Fig. 25.36). In advanced disease, ossification of the anterior longitudinal ligament and facet joint fusion may also be visible. The combination of these features may result in the typical 'bamboo' spine (Fig. 25.37). Erosive changes may be seen in the symphysis pubis, the ischial tuberosities and peripheral joints. Osteoporosis and atlanto-axial dislocation can occur as late features. Patients with early disease can have normal X-rays, and if clinical suspicion is high, MRI should be performed. This is much more sensitive for detection of early sacroiliitis than X-ray (Fig. 25.38) and can also detect inflammatory changes in the lumbar spine.

25.66 Bath Ankylosing Spondylitis Disease Activity Index

Question	Score
1. How would you describe the overall level of fatigue or tiredness you have experienced?	1–10
2. How would you describe the overall level of neck, back or hip pain you have had?	1–10
3. How would you describe the overall level of pain and swelling you have had in joints other than the neck, back or hip?	1–10
4. How would you describe the overall level of discomfort you have had from any areas tender to touch or pressure?	1–10
5. How would you describe the overall level of discomfort you have had from the time you wake up?	1–10
6. How long does your morning stiffness last from the time you wake up?	0 hr to 2+ hrs

The patient is asked to complete each question. The score is calculated by taking the average of all 6 questions, where duration of morning stiffness in minutes is coded in 12-minute increments from none (1) to 120 (10). Online calculators are also available at http://basdai.com

25.67 Diagnostic criteria for ankylosing spondylitis and axial spondyloarthritis

Axial spondyloarthritis	Ankylosing spondylitis
Imaging	
Sacroiliitis on MRI only	Bilateral sacroiliitis on X-ray, even if changes are mild Unilateral sacroiliitis on X-ray if changes are definite
History	
Back pain > 3 mths which has four of the following characteristics: 1. improved by exercise 2. not relieved by rest 3. insidious onset 4. night pain 5. age at onset < 40 Good response of back pain to NSAID Family history of spondyloarthritis History of inflammatory bowel disease	Back pain > 3 mths improved by exercise and not relieved by rest
Clinical examination	
Arthritis Enthesitis Uveitis Dactylitis Psoriasis	Limitation of lumbar spine movement in sagittal and frontal planes Chest expansion reduced
Investigations	
HLA-B27-positive Elevated CRP	

Axial spondyloarthritis is diagnosed when there is sacroiliitis on MRI plus one other feature on history, clinical examination or investigation. The diagnosis can also be made in patients who are HLA-B27-positive with two or more clinical features in the absence of sacroiliitis
Ankylosing spondylitis can be diagnosed when X-ray evidence of sacroiliitis occurs with one other feature on history or clinical examination

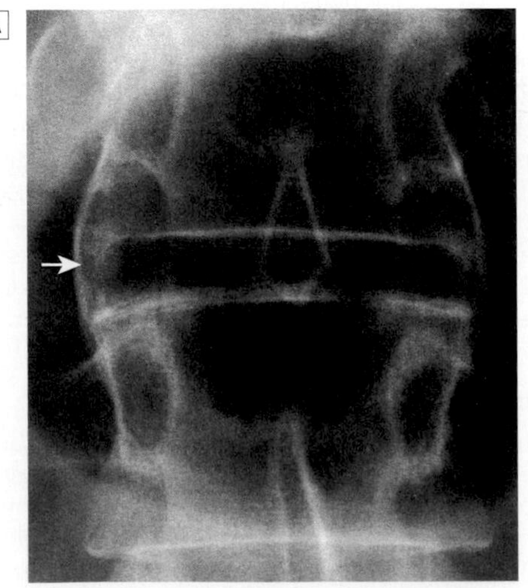

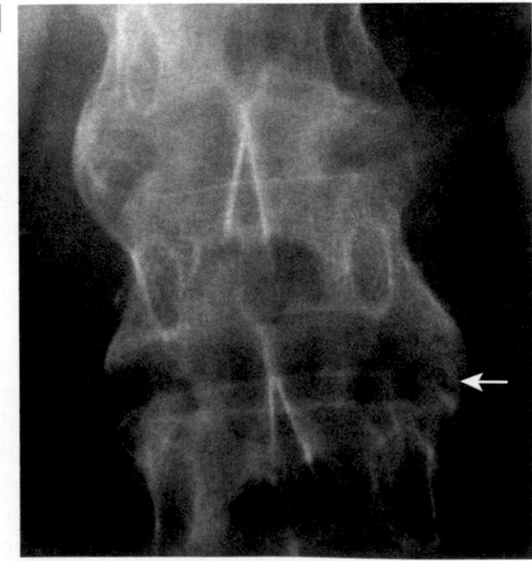

Fig. 25.36 X-ray changes in spondyloarthropathies. **A** Fine symmetrical marginal syndesmophytes typical of ankylosing spondylitis (arrow). **B** Coarse, asymmetrical non-marginal syndesmophytes typical of psoriatic/Reiter's spondylitis (arrow).

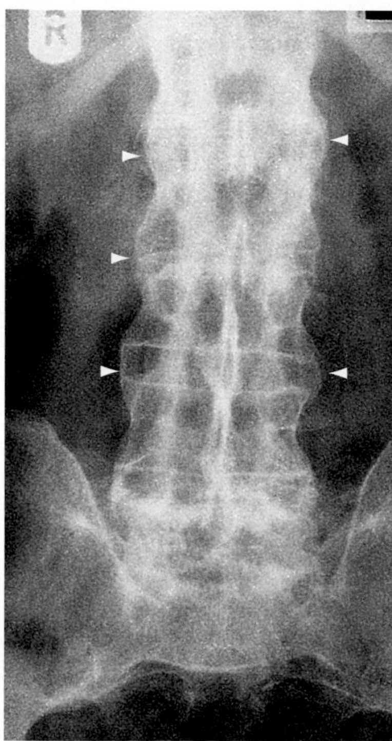

Fig. 25.37 'Bamboo' spine of severe late ankylosing spondylitis. Note the symmetrical marginal syndesmophytes (arrows), sacroiliac joint fusion and generalised osteopenia.

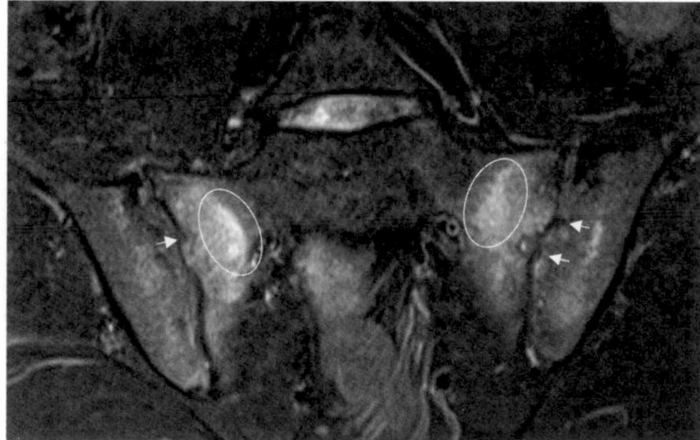

Fig. 25.38 MRI appearances in sacroiliitis. Coronal MRI short T1 inversion recovery (STIR) sequence showing bilateral sacroiliitis in early ankylosing spondylitis. Bone marrow oedema (circles) is present around both sacroiliac joints, which show irregularities due to erosions (arrows).

The ESR and CRP are usually raised in active disease but may be normal. Testing for HLA-B27 can be helpful, especially in patients with back pain suggestive of an inflammatory cause, when other investigations have yielded equivocal results. Autoantibodies such as RF, ACPA and ANA are negative.

Management

The aims of management are to relieve pain and stiffness, maintain a maximal range of skeletal mobility and avoid the development of deformities. Education and appropriate physical activity are the cornerstones of management. Early in the disease, patients should be taught to perform daily back extension exercises, including a morning 'warm-up' routine, and to punctuate prolonged periods of inactivity with regular breaks. Swimming is ideal exercise. Poor posture must be avoided. NSAIDs and analgesics are often effective in relieving symptoms and may alter the underlying course of the disease. A long-acting NSAID at night is helpful for alleviation of morning stiffness. Peripheral arthritis can be treated with methotrexate or sulfasalazine, but these drugs have no effect on axial disease. Anti-TNF therapy should be considered in patients who are inadequately controlled on standard therapy with a BASDAI score of ≥ 4.0 and a spinal pain score of ≥ 4.0. Anti-TNF therapy frequently improves symptoms but has not been shown to prevent ankylosis or alter natural history of the disease. Other biological interventions using agents developed for RA have been disappointing, suggesting fundamental differences in disease pathogenesis.

Local corticosteroid injections can be useful for persistent plantar fasciitis, other enthesopathies and peripheral arthritis. Oral corticosteroids may be required for acute uveitis but do not help spinal disease. Severe hip, knee or shoulder restriction may require surgery. Total hip arthroplasty has largely removed the need for difficult spinal surgery in those with advanced deformity.

Reactive arthritis

Reactive arthritis (previously known as Reiter's disease) is predominantly a disease of young men, with a male preponderance of 15:1. It is the most common cause of inflammatory arthritis in men aged 16–35 but may occur at any age. Between 1 and 2% of patients with non-specific urethritis seen at genitourinary medicine clinics have reactive arthritis (p. 415). Following an epidemic of *Shigella* dysentery, 20% of HLA-B27-positive men developed reactive arthritis. Reactive arthritis may present with the triad described in Box 25.68 but many patients present with arthritis only.

Clinical features

The onset is typically acute, with an inflammatory oligoarthritis that is asymmetrical and targets lower limb joints, such as the knees, ankles, midtarsal and MTP joints. It occasionally presents with single joint

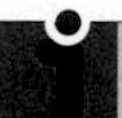

25.68 Reiter's disease

Classic triad*	
• Non-specific urethritis • Conjunctivitis (~50%)	• Reactive arthritis
Additional extra-articular features	
• Circinate balanitis (20–50%) • Keratoderma blennorrhagica (15%)	• Nail dystrophy • Buccal erosions (10%)
Precipitated by	
• Bacterial dysentery, mainly *Salmonella, Shigella, Campylobacter* or *Yersinia* • Sexually acquired infection with *Chlamydia*	

*Incomplete forms with just one or two of the classic triad are more frequent than the full syndrome.

25

involvement and no clear history of an infectious trigger. There may be considerable systemic disturbance, with fever and weight loss. Achilles tendinitis or plantar fasciitis may also be present. The first attack of arthritis is usually self-limiting, but recurrent or chronic arthritis develops in more than 60% of patients, and about 10% still have active disease 20 years after the initial presentation. Low back pain and stiffness are common and 15–20% of patients develop sacroiliitis. Spondylitis, chronic erosive arthritis, recurrent acute arthritis and uveitis are the major causes of long-term morbidity.

Several extra-articular features may occur (see Box 25.68). Circinate balanitis starts as vesicles on the coronal margin of the prepuce and glans penis, later rupturing to form superficial erosions with minimal surrounding erythema, some coalescing to give a circular pattern. Lesions are often painless and may escape notice. Keratoderma blennorrhagica begins as discrete waxy, yellow-brown vesico-papules with desquamating margins, occasionally coalescing to form large crusty plaques. The palms and soles are particularly affected but spread may occur to the scrotum, scalp and trunk. These lesions are indistinguishable from pustular psoriasis. Nail dystrophy with subungual hyperkeratosis is common and indistinguishable from psoriatic nail dystrophy. Mouth ulcers manifest as shallow red painless patches on tongue, palate, buccal mucosa and lips, lasting only a few days. Conjunctivitis may accompany the first acute episode. Uveitis is rare with the first attack but occurs in 30% of patients with recurring or chronic arthritis.

Other complications are rare but include aortic incompetence, conduction defects, pleuro-pericarditis, peripheral neuropathy, seizures and meningoencephalitis.

Investigations

The diagnosis is usually made clinically but joint aspiration may be required to exclude crystal arthritis and articular infection. Synovial fluid is leucocyte-rich and may contain multinucleated macrophages (Reiter's cells). ESR and CRP are raised during an acute attack. Urethritis may be confirmed in the 'two-glass test' by demonstration of mucoid threads in the first-void specimen that clear in the second. High vaginal swabs may reveal *Chlamydia* on culture. Except for post-*Salmonella* arthritis, stool cultures are usually negative by the time the arthritis presents, but serum agglutinin tests may help confirm previous dysentery. RF, ACPA and ANA are negative.

In chronic or recurrent disease, X-rays show periarticular osteoporosis, joint space narrowing and proliferative erosions. Another characteristic feature is periostitis, especially of metatarsals, phalanges and pelvis, and large, 'fluffy' calcaneal spurs. In contrast to AS, radiographic sacroiliitis is often asymmetrical and sometimes unilateral, and syndesmophytes are predominantly coarse and asymmetrical, often extending beyond the contours of the annulus ('non-marginal') (see Fig. 25.36B). X-ray changes in the peripheral joints and spine are identical to those in psoriasis.

Management

The acute attack should be treated with rest, oral NSAIDs and analgesics. Intra-articular steroids may be required in patients with severe synovitis. Non-specific chlamydial urethritis is usually treated with a short course of doxycycline or a single dose of azithromycin, and this may reduce the frequency of arthritis in sexually acquired cases. Treatment with DMARDs should be considered for patients with persistent marked symptoms, recurrent arthritis or severe keratoderma blennorrhagica. Anterior uveitis is a medical emergency requiring topical, subconjunctival or systemic corticosteroids.

Psoriatic arthritis

Psoriatic arthritis (PsA) occurs in 7–20% of patients with psoriasis and in up to 0.6% of the general population. The onset is usually between 25 and 40 years of age. Most patients (70%) have pre-existing psoriasis but in 20% the arthritis predates the occurrence of skin disease. Occasionally, the arthritis and psoriasis develop synchronously.

Clinical features

The presentation is with pain and swelling affecting the joints and entheses. Several patterns of joint involvement are recognised but the course is generally one of intermittent exacerbation followed by varying periods of complete or near-complete remission. Destructive arthritis and disability are uncommon, except in the case of arthritis mutilans.

- *Asymmetrical inflammatory oligoarthritis* affects about 40% of patients and often presents abruptly with a combination of synovitis and adjacent periarticular inflammation. This occurs most characteristically in the hands and feet, when synovitis of a finger or toe is coupled with tenosynovitis, enthesitis and inflammation of intervening tissue to give a 'sausage digit' or dactylitis (Fig. 25.39A). Large joints, such as the knee and ankle, may also be involved, sometimes with very large effusions.
- *Symmetrical polyarthritis* occurs in about 25% of cases. It predominates in women and may strongly resemble RA, with symmetrical involvement of small and large joints in both upper and lower limbs. Nodules and other extra-articular features of RA are absent and arthritis is generally less extensive and more benign. Much of the hand deformity often results from tenosynovitis and soft tissue contractures.
- *Distal IPJ arthritis* is an uncommon but characteristic pattern affecting men more often than women. It targets finger DIP joints and surrounding periarticular tissues, almost invariably with accompanying nail dystrophy (Fig. 25.39B).
- *Psoriatic spondylitis* presents a similar clinical picture to AS but with less severe involvement. It may occur alone or with any of the other clinical patterns described above and is typically unilateral or asymmetric in severity.
- *Arthritis mutilans* is a deforming erosive arthritis targeting the fingers and toes that occurs in 5% of cases of PsA. Prominent cartilage and bone destruction results in marked instability. The encasing skin appears invaginated and 'telescoped' ('main en lorgnette') and the finger can be pulled back to its original length.

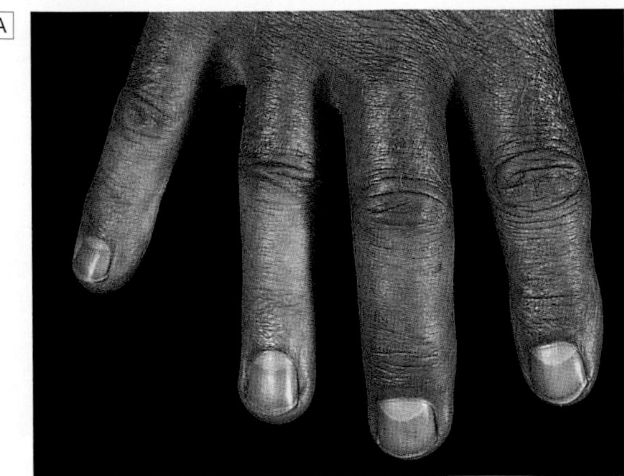

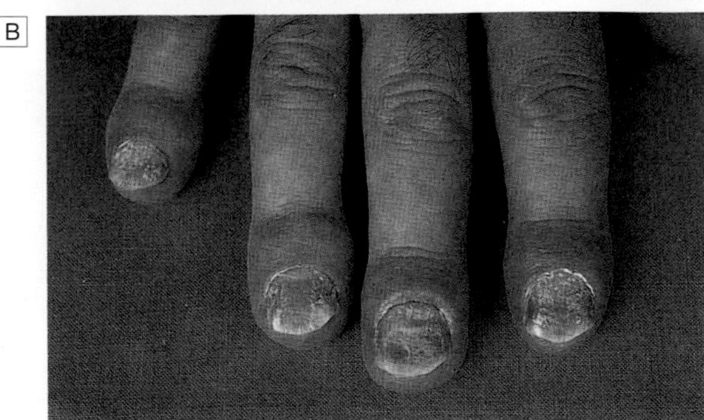

Fig. 25.39 Psoriatic arthropathy. **A** 'Sausage' middle finger of a patient with psoriatic arthritis. **B** Typical distal interphalangeal joint pattern with accompanying nail dystrophy (pitting and onycholysis).

Nail changes include pitting, onycholysis, subungual hyperkeratosis and horizontal ridging. They are found in 85% of those with PsA and only 30% of those with uncomplicated psoriasis, and can occur in the absence of skin disease. The characteristic rash of psoriasis (p. 1286) may be widespread, or confined to the scalp, natal cleft and umbilicus, where it is easily overlooked. Conjunctivitis can occur, whereas uveitis is mainly confined to HLA-B27-positive individuals with sacroiliitis and spondylitis.

Investigations

The diagnosis is made on clinical grounds. Autoantibodies are generally negative and acute phase reactants, such as ESR and CRP, are raised in only a proportion of patients with active disease. X-rays may be normal or show erosive change with joint space narrowing. Features that favour PsA over RA include the characteristic distribution (see Fig 25.9, p. 1070) of proliferative erosions with marked new bone formation, absence of periarticular osteoporosis and osteosclerosis. Imaging of the axial skeleton often reveals features similar to those in chronic reactive arthritis, with coarse, asymmetrical, non-marginal syndesmophytes and asymmetrical sacroiliitis. MRI and ultrasound with power Doppler are increasingly employed to detect synovial inflammation and inflammation at the entheses.

Management

Therapy with NSAID and analgesics may be sufficient to control symptoms in mild disease. Intra-articular steroid injections can control synovitis in problem joints. Splints and prolonged rest should be avoided because of the tendency to fibrous and bony ankylosis. Patients with spondylitis should be prescribed the same exercise and posture regime as in AS.

Therapy with DMARDs should be considered for persistent synovitis unresponsive to conservative treatment. Methotrexate is the drug of first choice since it may also help skin psoriasis, but other DMARDs may also be effective, including sulfasalazine, ciclosporin and leflunomide. DMARD monitoring should take place with particular attention to liver function since abnormalities are common in PsA. Hydroxychloroquine is generally avoided, as it can cause exfoliative skin reactions. Anti-TNF treatment should be considered for patients with active synovitis who respond inadequately to standard DMARDs. This is effective for both PsA and psoriasis. Other biological treatments, such as ustekinumab, are emerging, which target the IL-12/23 receptor. Ustekinumab is highly effective in the treatment of psoriatic skin disease and is often effectve in PsA.

The retinoid acitretin (p. 1267) is effective for skin lesions and, anecdotally, may also help arthritis, but it is teratogenic so must be avoided in young women. It also causes mucocutaneous side-effects, hyperlipidaemia, myalgias and extraspinal calcification. Photochemotherapy with methoxypsoralen and long-wave ultraviolet light (psoralen + UVA, PUVA) is primarily used for skin disease, but can also help those with synchronous exacerbations of inflammatory arthritis.

Enteropathic arthritis

An acute inflammatory oligoarthritis occurs in around 10% of patients with ulcerative colitis and 20% of those with Crohn's disease. It predominantly affects the large lower limb joints (knees, ankles, hips) but wrists and small joints of the hands and feet can also be involved. The arthritis usually coincides with exacerbations of the underlying bowel disease, and sometimes is accompanied by aphthous mouth ulcers, iritis and erythema nodosum. It improves with effective treatment of the bowel disease, and can be cured by total colectomy in patients with ulcerative colitis. Patients with inflammatory bowel disease may also develop sacroiliitis (16%) and AS (6%), which are clinically and radiologically identical to classic AS. These can predate or follow the onset of bowel disease and there is no correlation between activity of the spondylitis and bowel disease. The arthritis often remits with treatment of the bowel disease but DMARD and biological treatment is occasionally required.

CONNECTIVE TISSUE DISEASES

These share overlapping clinical features, characterised by dysregulation of immune responses, autoantibody production often directed at components of the cell nucleus, and widespread tissue damage.

Systemic lupus erythematosus

Systemic lupus erythematosus (SLE) is a rare disease with a prevalence that ranges from about 0.03% in

Caucasians to 0.2% in Afro-Caribbeans. Some 90% of affected patients are female and the peak age at onset is between 20 and 30 years. Lupus is associated with considerable morbidity and a five-fold increase in mortality compared to age- and gender-matched controls, mainly because of an increased risk of premature cardiovascular disease.

Pathophysiology

The cause of SLE is incompletely understood but genetic factors play an important role. There is a higher concordance in monozygotic twins and the disease is strongly associated with polymorphic variants at the HLA locus. In a few instances, SLE is associated with inherited mutations in complement components C1q, C2 and C4, in the immunoglobulin receptor FcγRIIIb or in the DNA exonuclease *TREX1*. Genome-wide association studies have identified common polymorphisms near several other genes that predispose to SLE, most of which are involved in regulating immune cell function. From an immunological standpoint, the characteristic feature of SLE is autoantibody production. These autoantibodies have specificity for a wide range of targets but many are directed against antigens present within the cell or within the nucleus. This has led to the hypothesis that SLE may occur because of defects in apoptosis or in the clearance of apoptotic cells, which causes inappropriate exposure of intracellular antigens on the cell surface, leading to polyclonal B- and T-cell activation and autoantibody production. This is supported by the fact that environmental factors that cause flares of lupus, such as UV light and infections, increase oxidative stress and cause cell damage. Whatever the underlying cause of the autoantibody production, immune complex formation is thought to be an important mechanism of tissue damage in active SLE, leading to vasculitis and organ damage.

Clinical features

Symptoms such as fever, weight loss and mild lymphadenopathy may occur during flares of disease activity, whereas others such as fatigue, malaise and fibromyalgia-like symptoms can be constant and not particularly associated with active inflammatory disease.

Arthritis

Arthralgia is a common symptom, occurring in 90% of patients, and is often associated with early morning stiffness. Tenosynovitis may also occur but clinically apparent synovitis with joint swelling is rare. Joint deformities may occur (Jaccoud's arthropathy) as the result of tendon damage, but joint erosions do not occur.

Raynaud's phenomenon

Raynaud's syndrome (p. 602) is common and may antedate other symptoms by months or years. A common presentation is Raynaud's in combination with arthralgia or arthritis (Fig. 25.40). Raynaud's associated with SLE and other connective tissue disease needs to be differentiated from primary Raynaud's, which is common in healthy young women. Features in favour of secondary Raynaud's include age at onset of over 25 years, absence of a family history of Raynaud's, and occurrence in a male. Examination of capillary nail-fold loops using an ophthalmoscope (and oil placed on the skin) may help distinguish primary from secondary Raynaud's. Loss of the normal loop pattern, with capillary 'fallout' and dilatation and branching of loops, supports connective tissue disease.

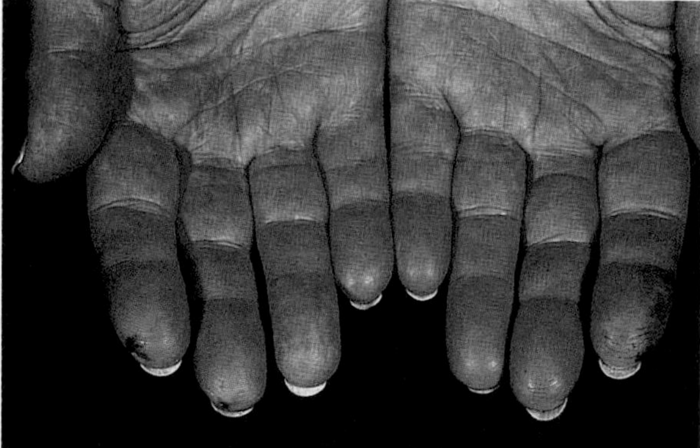

Fig. 25.40 Severe secondary Raynaud's phenomenon leading to digital ulceration.

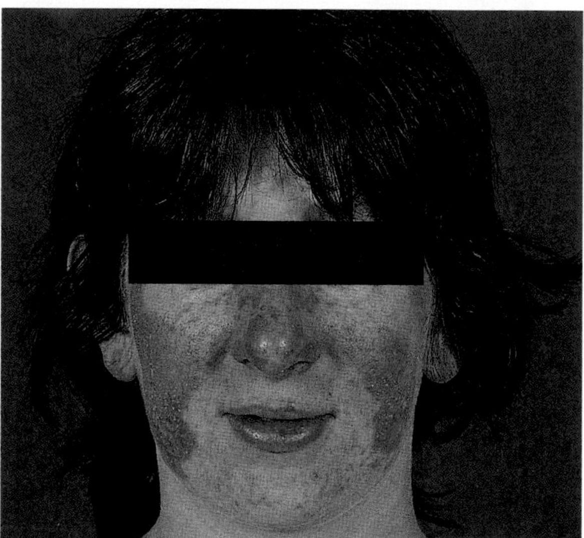

Fig. 25.41 Butterfly (malar) rash of systemic lupus erythematosus, sparing the nasolabial folds.

Skin

Rash is common in SLE and is classically precipitated by exposure to UV light. Three distinct types occur:

- The classic butterfly facial rash (up to 20% of patients). This is erythematous, raised and painful or itchy, and occurs over the cheeks with sparing of the nasolabial folds (Fig. 25.41).
- The subacute cutaneous lupus erythematosus (SCLE) rash, which is migratory, non-scarring and either annular or psoriaform.
- The discoid lupus rash characterised by hyperkeratosis and follicular plugging, with scarring alopecia if it occurs on the scalp.

Diffuse, usually non-scarring alopecia may also occur with active disease. Other skin manifestations include periungual erythema (reflecting dilated capillary loops), vasculitis and livedo reticularis (Fig. 25.42), which is also a common feature of the antiphospholipid syndrome (p. 1055).

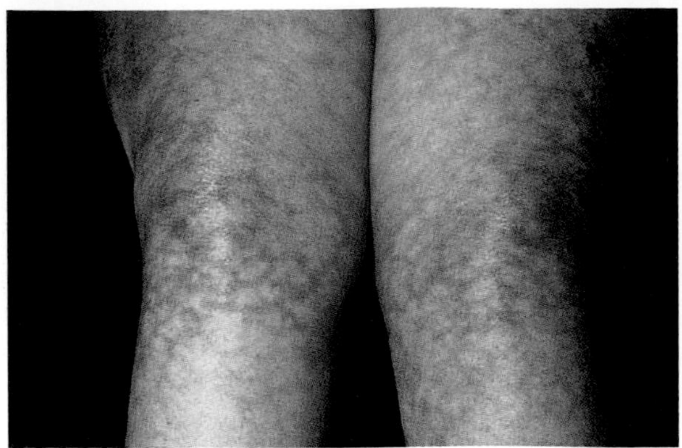

Fig. 25.42 Livedo reticularis in systemic lupus erythematosus.

Kidney

Renal involvement is one of the main determinants of prognosis, and regular monitoring of urinalysis and blood pressure is essential. The typical renal lesion is a proliferative glomerulonephritis (p. 498), characterised by heavy haematuria, proteinuria and casts on urine microscopy.

Cardiovascular

The most common manifestation is pericarditis. Myocarditis and Libman–Sacks endocarditis can also occur. The endocarditis is due to accumulation on the heart valves of sterile fibrin containing vegetations, which is thought to be a manifestation of hypercoagulability associated with antiphospholipid antibodies. The risk of atherosclerosis is greatly increased, as is the risk of stroke and myocardial infarction. This is thought to be multifactorial due to the adverse effects of inflammation on the endothelium, chronic steroid therapy and the procoagulant effects of antiphospholipid antibodies.

Lung

Lung involvement is common and most frequently manifests as pleurisy or pleural effusion. Other features include pneumonitis, atelectasis, reduced lung volume and pulmonary fibrosis that leads to breathlessness. The risk of thromboembolism is increased, especially in patients with antiphospholipid antibodies.

Neurological

Fatigue, headache and poor concentration are common, and often occur in the absence of laboratory evidence of active disease. More specific features of cerebral lupus include visual hallucinations, chorea, organic psychosis, transverse myelitis and lymphocytic meningitis.

Haematological

Neutropenia, lymphopenia, thrombocytopenia or haemolytic anaemia may occur, due to antibody-mediated destruction of peripheral blood cells. The degree of lymphopenia is a good guide to disease activity.

Gastrointestinal

Mouth ulcers may occur and may or may not be painful. Mesenteric vasculitis is a serious complication, which can present with abdominal pain, bowel infarction or perforation.

25.69 Revised American Rheumatism Association criteria for systemic lupus erythematosus

Features	Characteristics
Malar rash	Fixed erythema, flat or raised, sparing the nasolabial folds
Discoid rash	Erythematous raised patches with adherent keratotic scarring and follicular plugging
Photosensitivity	Rash due to unusual reaction to sunlight
Oral ulcers	Oral or nasopharyngeal ulceration, which may be painless
Arthritis	Non-erosive, involving two or more peripheral joints
Serositis	Pleuritis (history of pleuritic pain or rub, or pleural effusion) *or* pericarditis (rub, ECG evidence or effusion)
Renal disorder	Persistent proteinuria > 0.5 g/day *or* cellular casts (red cell, granular or tubular)
Neurological disorder	Seizures or psychosis, in the absence of provoking drugs or metabolic derangement
Haematological disorder	Haemolytic anaemia *or* leucopenia* ($< 4 \times 10^9$/L) *or* lymphopenia* ($< 1 \times 10^9$/L) *or* thrombocytopenia* ($< 100 \times 10^9$/L) in the absence of offending drugs
Immunological disorder	Anti-DNA antibodies in abnormal titre *or* presence of antibody to Sm antigen *or* positive antiphospholipid antibodies
ANA disorder	Abnormal titre of ANA by immunofluorescence
A person has SLE if any 4 out of these 11 features are present serially or simultaneously.	

*On two separate occasions.

Investigations

The diagnosis is based on a combination of clinical features and laboratory abnormalities. To fulfil the classification criteria for SLE, at least 4 of the 11 factors shown in Box 25.69 must be present or have occurred in the past. Patients should be screened for ANA and antibodies to extractable nuclear antigens, and have complement levels checked along with routine haematology and biochemistry. Patients with active SLE almost always test positive for ANA, but ANA-negative SLE can very rarely occur in the presence of antibodies to the Ro antigen. Anti-dsDNA antibodies are characteristic of severe active SLE but only occur in around 30% of cases. Similarly, patients with active disease tend to have low levels of C3 and C4, but this may be the result of inherited complement deficiency that predisposes to SLE. Studies of other family members can help to differentiate inherited deficiency from complement consumption. A raised ESR, leucopenia and lymphopenia are typical of active SLE, along with anaemia, haemolytic anaemia and thrombocytopenia. CRP is often normal in active SLE, except in the presence of serositis, and an elevated CRP suggests coexisting infection.

Management

The therapeutic goals are to educate the patient about the nature of the illness, to control symptoms and to prevent organ damage. Patients should be advised to avoid sun and UV light exposure and to employ sun blocks (factor 25–50).

Mild to moderate disease

Patients with mild disease restricted to skin and joints can sometimes be managed with analgesics, NSAID and hydroxychloroquine (200–400 mg daily). Frequently, however, corticosteroids are also necessary (prednisolone 5–20 mg/day), often in combination with immunosuppressants such as methotrexate, azathioprine or mycophenolate mofetil (MMF). Increased doses of steroids may be required for flares in activity or complications such as pleurisy or pericarditis. The monoclonal antibody belimumab, which targets the β-cell growth factor BLyS, has recently been shown to be effective in patients with active SLE who have responded inadequately to standard therapy.

Life-threatening disease

High-dose corticosteroids and immunosuppressants are required for the treatment of renal, CNS and cardiac involvement. A commonly used regimen is pulse methylprednisolone (10 mg/kg IV), coupled with cyclophosphamide (15 mg/kg IV), repeated at 2–3-weekly intervals for six cycles. Cyclophosphamide may cause haemorrhagic cystitis, but the risk can be minimised by good hydration and co-prescription of mesna, which binds its urotoxic metabolites. Because of the risk of azoospermia and anovulation (which may be permanent), pre-treatment sperm or ova collection and storage need to be considered prior to treatment with cyclophosphamide.

Mycophenolate mofetil has been used successfully in combination with high-dose steroids for renal involvement in SLE, with results equivalent to those of pulse cyclophosphamide but fewer adverse effects. The role of belimumab in life-threatening SLE remains to be established since clinical trials of this agent excluded patients with renal and cerebral lupus.

Maintenance therapy

Following control of the acute episode, the patient should be switched to oral immunosuppressive medication. A typical regimen is to start oral prednisolone in a dose of 40–60 mg daily on cessation of pulse therapy, gradually reducing to reach a target of 10–15 mg/day or less by 3 months. Azathioprine (2–2.5 mg/kg/day), methotrexate (10–25 mg/week) or MMF (2–3 g/day) should also be prescribed. The long-term aim is to continue the lowest dose of corticosteroids and immunosuppressant that will maintain remission. Cardiovascular risk factors, such as hypertension and hyperlipidaemia, should be controlled and patients advised to stop smoking.

Lupus patients with the antiphospholipid antibody syndrome (p. 1055) who have had previous thrombosis require life-long warfarin therapy.

Systemic sclerosis

Systemic sclerosis, or scleroderma, is a generalised disorder of connective tissue affecting the skin, internal organs and vasculature. It is characterised by sclerodactyly in combination with Raynaud's and digital

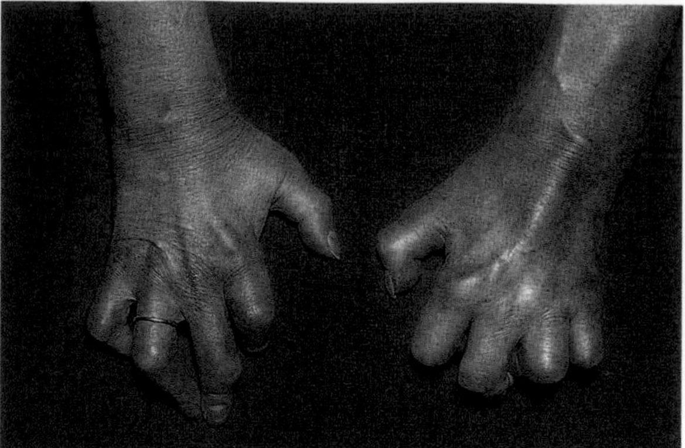

Fig. 25.43 Systemic sclerosis. Hands showing tight, shiny skin, sclerodactyly, flexion contractures of the fingers and thickening of the left middle finger extensor tendon sheath.

ischaemia (Fig. 25.43). The peak age of onset is in the fourth and fifth decades, and overall prevalence is 10–20 per 100 000, with a 4 : 1 female preponderance. It is subdivided into diffuse cutaneous systemic sclerosis (DCSS: 30% of cases) and limited cutaneous systemic sclerosis (LCSS: 70% of cases). Many patients with LCSS have features that are phenotypically grouped into the 'CREST' syndrome (**C**alcinosis, **R**aynaud's, o**E**sophageal involvement, **S**clerodactyly and **T**elangiectasia). The prognosis in DCSS is poor, with a 5-year survival of approximately 70%. Features that associate with a poor prognosis include older age, diffuse skin disease, proteinuria, high ESR, a low TLCO (gas transfer factor for carbon monoxide) and pulmonary hypertension.

Pathophysiology

The cause of systemic sclerosis is poorly understood. There is evidence for a genetic component, and associations with alleles at the HLA locus have been found. The disease occurs in all ethnic groups, and race may influence severity, since DCSS is significantly more common in black women than white. Isolated cases have been reported in which a systemic sclerosis-like disease has been triggered by exposure to silica dust, vinyl chloride, hypoxyresins and trichloroethylene. There is clear evidence of immunological dysfunction: T lymphocytes, especially those of the Th17 subtype, infiltrate the skin and there is abnormal fibroblast activation, leading to increased production of extracellular matrix in the dermis, primarily type I collagen. This results in symmetrical thickening, tightening and induration of the skin (sclerodactyly). Arterial and arteriolar narrowing occurs due to intimal proliferation and vessel wall inflammation. Endothelial injury causes release of vasoconstrictors and platelet activation, resulting in further ischaemia, which is thought to exacerbate the fibrotic process.

Clinical features

Skin

Initially, there is non-pitting oedema of fingers and flexor tendon sheaths. Subsequently, the skin becomes shiny and taut, and distal skin creases disappear. This is accompanied by erythema and tortuous dilatation of capillary loops in the nail-fold bed, readily visible with

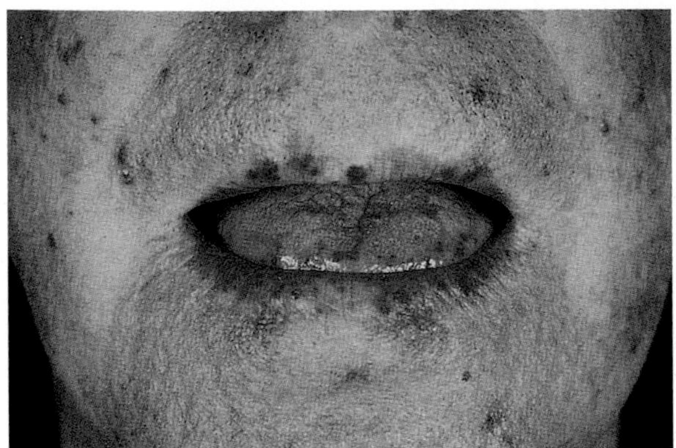

Fig. 25.44 Typical facial appearance in the CREST syndrome.

an ophthalmoscope or dissecting microscope (and oil placed on the skin). The face and neck are usually involved next, with thinning of the lips and radial furrowing. In some patients, skin thickening stops at this stage. Skin involvement restricted to sites distal to the elbow or knee (apart from the face) is classified as 'limited disease' or CREST syndrome (Fig. 25.44). Involvement proximal to the knee and elbow and on the trunk is classified as 'diffuse disease'.

Raynaud's phenomenon

This is a universal feature and can precede other features by many years. Involvement of small blood vessels in the extremities may cause critical tissue ischaemia, leading to skin ulceration over pressure areas, localised areas of infarction and pulp atrophy at the fingertips.

Musculoskeletal features

Arthralgia, morning stiffness and flexor tenosynovitis are common. Restricted hand function is due to skin rather than joint disease and erosive arthropathy is uncommon. Muscle weakness and wasting can occur due to myositis.

Gastrointestinal involvement

Smooth muscle atrophy and fibrosis in the lower two-thirds of the oesophagus lead to reflux with erosive oesophagitis. Dysphagia and odynophagia may also occur. Involvement of the stomach causes early satiety and occasionally outlet obstruction. Recurrent occult upper gastrointestinal bleeding may indicate a 'watermelon' stomach (antral vascular ectasia), which occurs in up to 20% of patients. Small intestine involvement may lead to malabsorption due to bacterial overgrowth and intermittent bloating, pain or constipation. Dilatation of large or small bowel due to autonomic neuropathy may cause pseudo-obstruction with nausea, vomiting, abdominal discomfort and distension, often worse after food.

Pulmonary involvement

This is a major cause of morbidity and mortality. Pulmonary hypertension complicates long-standing disease and is six times more prevalent in LCSS than in DCSS. It presents with rapidly progressive dyspnoea (more rapid than interstitial lung disease), right heart failure and angina, often in association with severe digital ischaemia. Fibrosing alveolitis mainly affects patients with DCSS who have topoisomerase 1 antibodies.

Renal involvement

One of the main causes of death is hypertensive renal crisis, characterised by rapidly developing malignant hypertension and renal failure. Hypertensive renal crisis is much more likely to occur in DCSS than in LCSS, and in patients with topoisomerase 1 antibodies.

Investigations

Scleroderma is primarily a clinical diagnosis but various laboratory abnormalities are characteristic. The ESR is usually elevated and raised levels of IgG are common, but CRP values tend to be normal unless there is severe organ involvement or coexisting infection. ANA is positive in about 70%, and approximately 30% of patients with DCSS have antibodies to topoisomerase 1 (Scl-70). About 60% of patients with CREST syndrome have anticentromere antibodies (p. 1068).

Management

No treatments are available that halt or reverse the fibrotic changes that underlie the disease. The focus of management, therefore, is to ameliorate the effects of the disease on target organs.

- *Raynaud's syndrome and digital ulcers.* Raynaud's should be treated by avoidance of cold exposure and use of mittens (heated mittens are available), supplemented if necessary with calcium antagonists. Intermittent infusions of prostacyclin may benefit severe digital ischaemia. The endothelin 1 antagonist bosentan can be of value in promoting healing of digital ulcers. If these become infected, antibiotics may be required, but as these penetrate tissues poorly in scleroderma, they need to be given at higher doses for a longer duration than usual.
- *Oesophageal reflux* should be treated with proton pump inhibitors and anti-reflux agents. Antibiotics may be required for bacterial overgrowth syndromes, and metoclopramide or domperidone may help patients with symptoms of pseudo-obstruction.
- *Hypertension* should be treated aggressively with ACE inhibitors, even if renal impairment is present.
- *Joint involvement* may be treated with analgesics and/or NSAID. If synovitis is present, immunosuppressants such as methotrexate can also be of value.
- *Pulmonary hypertension* may be treated with bosentan. In selected patients, heart–lung transplantation may be considered. Corticosteroids and cytotoxic drugs are indicated in patients who have coexisting myositis or fibrosing alveolitis.

Mixed connective tissue disease

Mixed connective tissue disease (MCTD) is a condition in which the clinical features of SLE, systemic sclerosis and myositis may all occur in the same patient. It most commonly presents with synovitis and oedema of the hands, in combination with Raynaud's phenomenon and muscle pain or weakness. Most patients have anti-ribonucleoprotein (RNP) antibodies, but these can occur in SLE without overlap features. Management focuses on treating the individual components of the syndrome.

Sjögren's syndrome

This is an autoimmune disorder of unknown cause, characterised by lymphocytic infiltration of salivary and lachrymal glands, leading to glandular fibrosis and exocrine failure. The typical age of onset is between 40 and 50, with a 9:1 female preponderance. The disease may occur in isolation (primary Sjögren's syndrome) or in patients with other autoimmune diseases (secondary Sjögren's syndrome).

Clinical features

The eye symptoms, termed keratoconjunctivitis sicca, are due to a lack of lubricating tears, which, in turn, reflects inflammatory infiltration of the lacrimal glands. Conjunctivitis and blepharitis are frequent, and may lead to filamentary keratitis due to tenacious mucous filaments binding to the cornea and conjunctiva. Oral involvement manifests as a dry mouth and typically the patient needs to sip water to swallow food. There is a high incidence of dental caries. Other sites of extraglandular involvement are listed in Box 25.70. The disease is associated with a 40-fold increased lifetime risk of lymphoma.

Investigations

The diagnosis can be established by the Schirmer tear test, which measures tear flow over 5 minutes using absorbent paper strips placed on the lower eyelid; a normal result is more than 6 mm of wetting. Staining with rose Bengal may show punctate epithelial abnormalities over the area not covered by the open eyelid. If the diagnosis remains in doubt, it can be confirmed by lip biopsy, which shows focal lymphocytic infiltrate of the minor salivary glands. Most patients have an elevated ESR and hypergammaglobulinaemia, and one or more autoantibodies, including ANA and RF. Anti-Ro and anti-La antibodies are commonly present (see Box 25.11, p. 1068).

Management

No treatments that have disease-modifying effects have yet been identified and management is symptomatic. Lachrymal substitutes, such as hypromellose, should be used during the day in combination with more viscous lubricating ointment at night. Soft contact lenses can be useful for corneal protection in patients with filamentary keratitis, and occlusion of the lachrymal ducts is occasionally needed. Artificial saliva and oral gels can be tried for xerostomia but are often not effective. Stimulation of saliva flow by sugar-free chewing gum or lozenges may be helpful. Adequate post-prandial oral hygiene and prompt treatment of oral candidiasis are essential. Vaginal dryness is treated with lubricants such as K-Y jelly. Extraglandular and musculoskeletal manifestations may respond to steroids, and if so, immunosuppressive drugs can be added for their steroid-sparing effect. Fatigue is difficult to treat; this is usually due to non-restorative sleep (often because of xerostomia) and is unresponsive to steroids. Immunosuppression does not improve sicca symptoms. If lymphadenopathy or salivary gland enlargement develops, biopsy should be performed to exclude malignancy.

25.70 Features of Sjögren's syndrome

Risk factors	
• Age of onset 40–60 • Female > male	• HLA-B8/DR3
Common clinical features	
• Keratoconjunctivitis sicca • Xerostomia • Salivary gland enlargement	• Non-erosive arthritis • Raynaud's phenomenon • Fatigue
Less common features	
• Low-grade fever • Interstitial lung disease • Anaemia, leucopenia • Thrombocytopenia • Cryoglobulinaemia • Vasculitis	• Peripheral neuropathy • Lymphadenopathy • Lymphoreticular lymphoma • Glomerulonephritis • Renal tubular acidosis
Autoantibodies frequently detected	
• RF • ANA • SS-A (anti-Ro)	• SS-B (anti-La) • Gastric parietal cell • Thyroid
Associated autoimmune disorders	
• SLE • Progressive systemic sclerosis	• Primary biliary cirrhosis • Chronic active hepatitis • Myasthenia gravis

Polymyositis and dermatomyositis

Polymyositis and dermatomyositis are related disorders that are characterised by an inflammatory process affecting skeletal muscle. In dermatomyositis, characteristic skin changes also occur. Both diseases are rare, with an incidence of 2–10 cases per million/year. They can occur in isolation or in association with other autoimmune diseases, such as SLE, systemic sclerosis and Sjögren's syndrome. The cause is unknown, although there is evidence for a genetic contribution.

Clinical features

The typical presentation of polymyositis is with symmetrical proximal muscle weakness, usually affecting the lower limbs more than the upper. The onset is usually between 40 and 60 years of age and is typically gradual, over a few weeks. Myositis is usually widespread but focal disease can also occur. Affected patients report difficulty rising from a chair, climbing stairs and lifting, sometimes in combination with muscle pain. Systemic features of fever, weight loss and fatigue are common. Respiratory or pharyngeal muscle involvement can lead to ventilatory failure or aspiration that requires urgent treatment. Interstitial lung disease occurs in up to 30% of patients and is strongly associated with the presence of antisynthetase (Jo-1) antibodies.

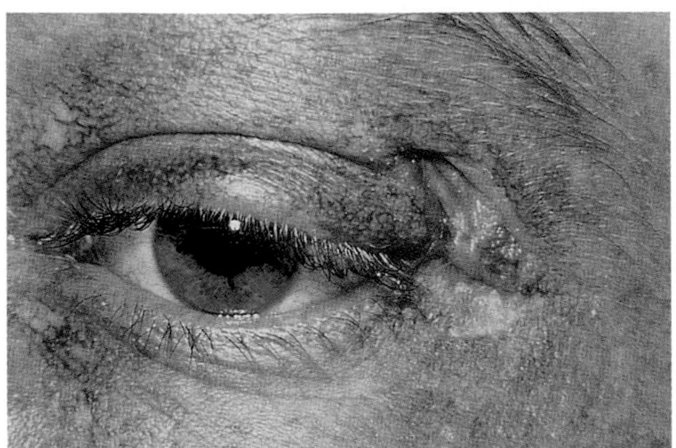

Fig. 25.45 Typical eyelid appearance in dermatomyositis. Note the oedema and telangiectasia.

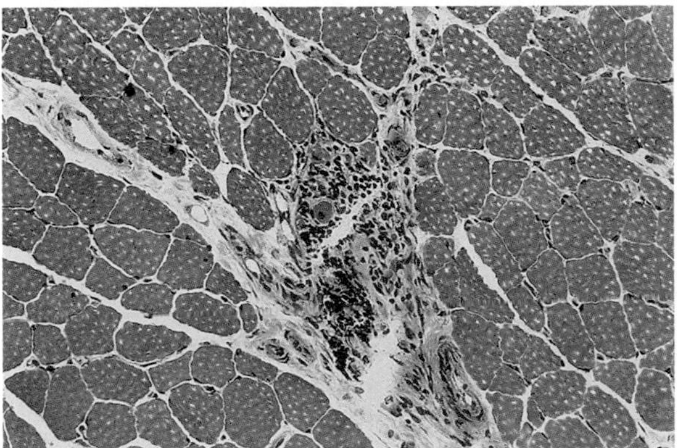

Fig. 25.46 Muscle biopsy from a patient with inflammatory myositis. The sample shows an intense inflammatory cell infiltrate in an area of degenerating and regenerating muscle fibres.

Dermatomyositis presents similarly but in combination with characteristic skin lesions. These include Gottron's papules, which are scaly, erythematous or violaceous, psoriaform plaques occurring over the extensor surfaces of PIP and DIP joints, and a heliotrope rash that is a violaceous discoloration of the eyelid in combination with periorbital oedema (Fig. 25.45). Similar rashes occur on the upper back, chest and shoulders ('shawl' distribution). Periungual nail-fold capillaries are often enlarged and tortuous. There is about a threefold increased risk of malignancy in patients with dermatomyositis and polymyositis. This may be apparent at the time of presentation, but the risk remains increased for at least 5 years following diagnosis.

Investigations

Muscle biopsy is the pivotal investigation and shows the typical features of fibre necrosis, regeneration and inflammatory cell infiltrate (Fig. 25.46). Occasionally, however, a biopsy may be normal, particularly if myositis is patchy. In such cases, MRI is used to identify areas of abnormal muscle for biopsy. Serum levels of CK are usually raised and are a useful measure of disease activity, although a normal CK does not exclude the diagnosis, particularly in juvenile myositis. EMG can confirm the presence of myopathy and exclude neuropathy. Screening for underlying malignancy should be undertaken routinely, and should include CT of chest/abdomen/pelvis, upper and lower gastrointestinal endoscopy, and mammography in women.

Management

Oral corticosteroids (prednisolone 1 mg/kg daily) are the mainstay of initial treatment, but high-dose intravenous methylprednisolone (1 g/day for 3 days) may be required in patients with respiratory or pharyngeal weakness. If there is a good response, steroids should be reduced by approximately 25% per month to a maintenance dose of 5–7.5 mg. Although most patients respond well to corticosteroids, many need additional immunosuppressive therapy. Azathioprine and methotrexate are the agents of first choice, but ciclosporin, cyclophosphamide, tacrolimus or MMF can be used as alternatives. Intravenous immunoglobulin may be effective in refractory cases. Relapses may occur in association with a rising CK, and indicate the need for additional therapy. If the patient relapses or fails to respond to treatment, this may be due to steroid-induced myopathy. A further biopsy should be performed and may show type 2 fibre atrophy in steroid-induced myopathy, as opposed to necrosis and regeneration in active myositis.

Inclusion body myositis

This is an inflammatory disease of muscle of unknown cause with a genetic component, which is associated with the accumulation of abnormal protein aggregates in affected tissue. It presents with muscle weakness in those over the age of 40 and is more common in men. Although proximal weakness does occur, distal involvement is more usual and may be asymmetrical. Investigation is the same as for polymyositis (p. 1115) and typically reveals a slightly elevated CK and both myopathic and neurogenic changes on EMG. Muscle biopsy shows abnormal fibres containing rimmed vacuoles and filamentous inclusions in the nucleus and cytoplasm. Treatment can be tried with high-dose corticosteroids, immunosuppressants and immunoglobulin, as described for polymyositis, but the therapeutic response is often poor.

VASCULITIS

These are a heterogeneous group of diseases characterised by inflammation and necrosis of blood-vessel walls, with associated damage to skin, kidney, lung, heart, brain and gastrointestinal tract. There is a wide spectrum of involvement and disease severity, ranging from mild and transient disease affecting only the skin, to life-threatening fulminant disease with multiple organ failure. Principal sites of involvement for the main types of vasculitis are summarised in Figure 25.47. The clinical features result from a combination of local tissue ischaemia (due to vessel inflammation and narrowing) and the systemic effects of widespread inflammation. Systemic vasculitis should be considered in any patient with fever, weight loss, fatigue, evidence of multisystem involvement, rashes, raised inflammatory markers and abnormal urinalysis (Box 25.71).

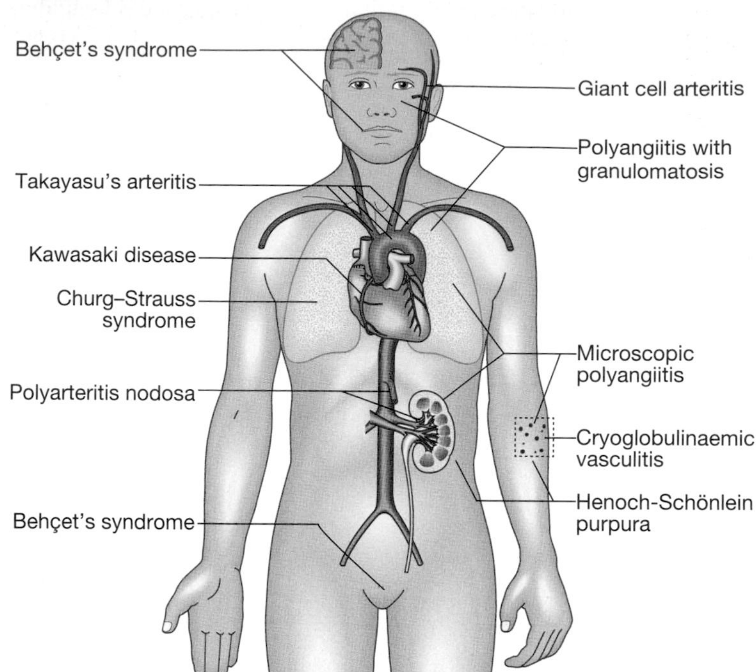

Fig. 25.47 Types of vasculitis. The anatomical targets of different forms of vasculitis are shown.

25.71 Clinical features of systemic vasculitis

Systemic	
• Malaise • Fever • Night sweats	• Weight loss with arthralgia and myalgia
Rashes	
• Palpable purpura • Pulp infarcts	• Ulceration • Livedo reticularis
Ear, nose and throat	
• Epistaxis • Recurrent sinusitis	• Deafness
Respiratory	
• Haemoptysis • Cough	• Poorly controlled asthma
Gastrointestinal	
• Abdominal pain (due to mucosal inflammation or enteric ischaemia)	• Mouth ulcers • Diarrhoea
Neurological	
• Sensory or motor neuropathy	

Takayasu's disease

Takayasu's disease predominantly affects the aorta, its major branches and occasionally the pulmonary arteries. The typical age at onset is between 25 and 30 years, with an 8:1 female preponderance. It has a worldwide distribution but is most common in Asia. Takayasu's is characterised by granulomatous inflammation of the vessel wall, leading to vessel occlusion or weakening of the vessel wall. It presents with claudication, fever, arthralgia and weight loss. The vessels most commonly affected are the aorta and carotid, ulnar, brachial, radial and axillary arteries. Clinical examination may reveal loss of pulses, bruits, hypertension and aortic incompetence. Investigation will identify an acute phase response and normocytic, normochromic anaemia, but the diagnosis is based on angiography, which reveals coarctation, occlusion and aneurysmal dilatation. The distribution of involvement is classified into four types:

- type 1: localised to the aorta and its branches
- type 2: localised to the descending thoracic and abdominal aorta
- type 3: combines features of 1 and 2
- type 4: involves the pulmonary artery.

Treatment is with high-dose steroids and immunosuppressants, as described for SLE. With appropriate treatment, the 5-year survival is 83%.

Kawasaki disease

Kawasaki disease is a vasculitis that mostly affects the coronary vessels. It presents as an acute systemic disorder, usually affecting children under 5 years. It occurs mainly in Japan and other Asian countries, such as China and Korea, but other ethnic groups may also be affected. Presentation is with fever, generalised rash, including palms and soles, inflamed oral mucosa and conjunctival injection resembling a viral exanthem. The cause is unknown but is thought to be the result of an abnormal immune response to an infectious trigger. Cardiovascular complications include coronary arteritis, leading to myocardial infarction, transient coronary dilatation, myocarditis, pericarditis, peripheral vascular insufficiency and gangrene. Treatment is with aspirin (5 mg/kg daily for 14 days) and intravenous gammaglobulin (400 mg/kg daily for 4 days).

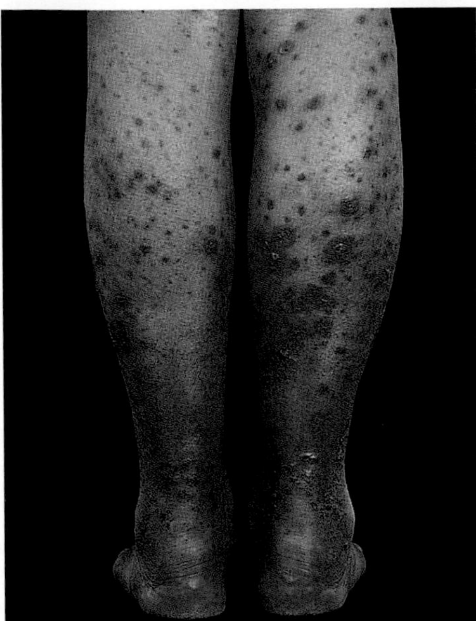

Fig. 25.48 Rash of systemic vasculitis (palpable purpura).

Polyarteritis nodosa

Polyarteritis nodosa has a peak incidence between the ages of 40 and 50, with a male preponderance of 2:1. The annual incidence is around 2/1 000000. Hepatitis B is an important risk factor, and the incidence is 10 times higher in the Inuit of Alaska, in whom hepatitis B infection is endemic. Presentation is with fever, myalgia, arthralgia and weight loss, in combination with manifestations of multisystem disease. The most common skin lesions are palpable purpura (Fig. 25.48), ulceration, infarction and livedo reticularis (see Fig. 25.42, p. 1111). Pathological changes comprise necrotising inflammation and vessel occlusion, and in 70% of patients, arteritis of the vasa nervorum leads to neuropathy, which is typically symmetrical and affects both sensory and motor function. Severe hypertension and/or renal impairment may occur due to multiple renal infarctions, but glomerulonephritis is rare (in contrast to microscopic polyangiitis). The diagnosis is confirmed by angiography, which shows multiple aneurysms and smooth narrowing of mesenteric, hepatic or renal systems, or by muscle or sural nerve biopsy, which reveals the histological changes above. Treatment is with high-dose steroids and immunosuppressants, as described for SLE.

Giant cell arteritis and polymyalgia rheumatica

Giant cell arteritis (GCA) is a granulomatous arteritis that predominantly affects medium-sized arteries in the head and neck. It is commonly associated with polymyalgia rheumatica (PMR), which presents with symmetrical muscle pain and stiffness affecting the shoulder and pelvic girdles. Since many patients with GCA have symptoms of PMR, and many patients with PMR go on to develop GCA if untreated, many rheumatologists consider them to be different manifestations of the same

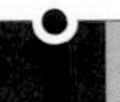

25.72 Conditions that can mimic polymyalgia rheumatica

- Fibromyalgia
- Hypothyroidism
- Cervical spondylosis
- RA
- Systemic vasculitis
- Inflammatory myopathy (particularly inclusion body myositis, p. 1115)
- Malignancy

underlying disorder. Both diseases are rare under the age of 60 years. The average age at onset is 70, with a female preponderance of about 3:1. The overall prevalence is about 20 per 100000 in those over the age of 50 years.

Clinical features

The cardinal symptom of GCA is headache, which is often localised to the temporal or occipital region and may be accompanied by scalp tenderness. Jaw pain develops in some patients, brought on by chewing or talking, due to ischaemia of the masseter muscles. Visual disturbance can occur and a catastrophic presentation is with blindness in one eye due to occlusion of the posterior ciliary artery. On fundoscopy, the optic disc may appear pale and swollen with haemorrhages, but these changes may take 24–36 hours to develop and the fundi may initially appear normal. Other visual symptoms include loss of visual acuity, reduced colour perception and papillary defects. Rarely, neurological involvement may occur, with transient ischaemic attacks, brainstem infarcts and hemiparesis.

The cardinal features of PMR are symmetrical muscle pain and stiffness affecting the shoulder and pelvic girdles. Constitutional symptoms, such as weight loss, fatigue, malaise and night sweats, are common. The onset of symptoms is usually fairly sudden over a few days, but may be more insidious. On examination, there may be stiffness and painful restriction of active shoulder movement but passive movements are preserved. Muscles may be tender to palpation but weakness and muscle-wasting are absent. Other conditions that mimic PMR are shown in Box 25.72.

Investigations

The typical laboratory abnormality is an elevated ESR, often with a normochromic, normocytic anaemia. CRP may also be elevated and in some cases this precedes elevation of the ESR. Rarely, PMR and GCA can present with a normal ESR. The diagnosis is usually based on a combination of the typical clinical features, raised ESR and prompt response to steroid. However, if there is doubt concerning the diagnosis of GCA, a temporal artery biopsy may be undertaken. Characteristic biopsy findings are fragmentation of the internal elastic lamina with necrosis of the media in combination with a mixed inflammatory cell infiltrate. Whilst a positive biopsy is helpful, a negative biopsy does not exclude the diagnosis because the lesions are focal. Ultrasound or arteriography may be used to help guide the biopsy.

Management

Corticosteroids are the treatment of choice and should be commenced urgently in suspected GCA because of the risk of visual loss (Box 25.73). Response to treatment

25.73 Emergency management of giant cell arteritis

- Take blood for ESR and CRP
- Commence prednisolone 40–60 mg daily
- Review patient in 3–4 days
- Continue steroids in patients whose symptoms have resolved, with gradual reduction in dose
- Organise temporal artery biopsy in patients with poor or equivocal response

is dramatic, such that symptoms will have completely resolved within 48–72 hours of starting corticosteroid therapy in virtually all patients. It is customary to use higher doses in GCA (60–80 mg prednisolone) than in PMR (15–30 mg), although the evidence base for this is weak. In both conditions the steroid dose should be progressively reduced, guided by symptoms and ESR, with the aim of reaching a dose of 10–15 mg by about 8 weeks. Thereafter, the rate of reduction should be slower – by 1 mg per month – until an acceptable dose is achieved (5–7.5 mg daily). If symptoms recur, the dose should be increased to that which previously controlled the symptoms, and reduction attempted again in another few weeks. Most patients need steroids for an average of 12–24 months. Some patients also require steroid-sparing agents, such as methotrexate or azathioprine, if they require a maintenance dose of prednisolone of more than 7.5 mg daily. Prophylaxis against osteoporosis should be given in patients with low BMD.

Antineutrophil cytoplasmic antibody-associated vasculitis

Antineutrophil cytoplasmic antibody (ANCA)-associated vasculitis is a life-threatening disorder characterised by inflammatory infiltration of small blood vessels, fibrinoid necrosis and the presence of circulating antibodies to ANCA. The combined incidence is about 10–15/1 000 000. Two subtypes are recognised. Microscopic polyangiitis (MPA) is a necrotising small-vessel vasculitis found with rapidly progressive glomerulonephritis, often in association with alveolar haemorrhage. Cutaneous and gastrointestinal involvement is common and other features include neuropathy (15%) and pleural effusions (15%). Patients are usually myeloperoxidase (MPO) antibody-positive. In granulomatosis with polyangiitis (also known as Wegener's granulomatosis (WG)), the vasculitis is characterised by granuloma formation, mainly affecting the nasal passages, airways and kidney. A minority of patients present with glomerulonephritis. The most common presentation of WG is with epistaxis, nasal crusting and sinusitis, but haemoptysis and mucosal ulceration may also occur. Deafness may be a feature due to inner ear involvement, and proptosis may occur because of inflammation of the retro-orbital tissue (Fig. 25.49). This causes diplopia due to entrapment of the extra-ocular muscles, or loss of vision due to optic nerve compression. Disturbance of colour vision is an early feature of optic nerve compression. Untreated nasal disease ultimately leads to destruction of bone and cartilage. Migratory pulmonary infiltrates and nodules

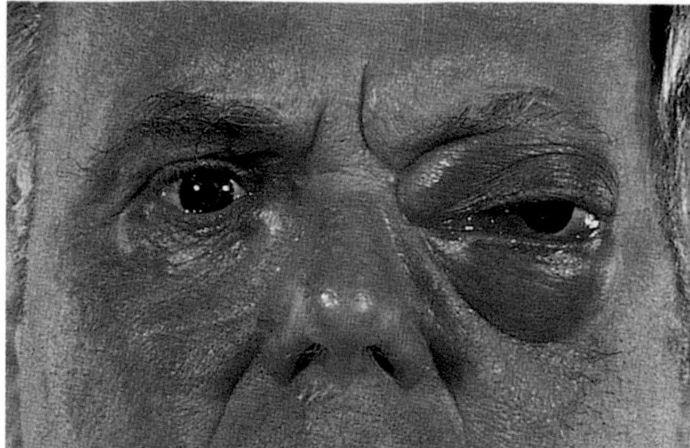

Fig. 25.49 Eye involvement in granulomatosis with polyangiitis.

occur in 50% of patients. Patients with WG are usually proteinase-3 (PR3) antibody-positive.

Patients with active disease usually have a leucocytosis with an elevated CRP and ESR, in association with raised ANCA levels. Complement levels are usually normal or slightly elevated. Imaging of the upper airways or chest with MRI can be useful in localising abnormalities but, where possible, the diagnosis should be confirmed by biopsy of the kidney or lesions in the sinuses and upper airways.

Management is with high-dose steroids and cyclophosphamide, as described for SLE, followed by maintenance therapy with lower-dose steroids and azathioprine, methotrexate or mycophenolate mofetil (MMF). Rituximab in combination with high-dose steroids is equally effective as oral cyclophosphamide at inducing remission in ANCA-associated vasculitis. Both MPA and WG have a tendency to relapse, and patients must be followed on a regular and long-term basis to check for clinical signs of recurrence. Measurements of ESR, CRP and levels of ANCA antibodies are useful in monitoring disease activity.

Churg–Strauss syndrome

Churg–Strauss syndrome (CSS) is a small-vessel vasculitis with an incidence of about 1–3 per 1 000 000; it is associated with eosinophilia. Some patients have a prodromal period for many years, characterised by allergic rhinitis, nasal polyposis and late-onset asthma that is often difficult to control. The typical acute presentation is with a triad of skin lesions (purpura or nodules), asymmetric mononeuritis multiplex and eosinophilia. Pulmonary infiltrates and pleural or pericardial effusions due to serositis may be present. Up to 50% of patients have abdominal symptoms provoked by mesenteric vasculitis. Patients with active disease have raised levels of ESR and CRP and an eosinophilia. Although antibodies to MPO or PR3 can be detected in up to 60% of cases, CSS is considered to be a distinct disorder from the other ANCA-associated vasculitides. Biopsy of an affected site reveals a small-vessel vasculitis with eosinophilic infiltration of the vessel wall. Management is with high-dose steroids and cyclophosphamide, followed by maintenance therapy with low-dose steroids and azathioprine, methotrexate or MMF.

Henoch–Schönlein purpura

Henoch–Schönlein purpura (HSP) is a small-vessel vasculitis caused by immune complex deposition following an infectious trigger. It is predominantly a disease of children and young adults. The usual presentation is with purpura over the buttocks and lower legs, accompanied by abdominal pain, gastrointestinal bleeding and arthralgia. Nephritis can also occur and may present up to 4 weeks after the onset of other symptoms. Biopsy of affected tissue shows a vasculitis with IgA deposits in the vessel wall. HSP is usually a self-limiting disorder that settles spontaneously without specific treatment. Corticosteroids and immunosuppressive therapy may be required in patients with more severe disease, particularly in the presence of nephritis.

Cryoglobulinaemic vasculitis

This is a small-vessel vasculitis that can develop in some patients with circulating cryoglobulins, which are immunoglobulins that precipitate out in the cold. Cryoglobulins are classified into three types (see Box 4.14, p. 88), and types II and III are associated with vasculitis. The typical presentation is with a vasculitic rash over the lower limbs, arthralgia, Raynaud's phenomenon and neuropathy. Some cases are secondary to hepatitis infection and others are secondary to other autoimmune diseases. Affected patients should be screened for evidence of hepatitis B and C infection, and if the results are positive, these should be treated appropriately (pp. 952 and 955). There is no consensus as to how best to treat cryoglobulinaemic vasculitis in the absence of an obvious trigger. Corticosteroids and immunosuppressive therapy are often used empirically but their efficacy is uncertain.

Behçet's syndrome

This is a vasculitis of unknown aetiology that characteristically targets small arteries and venules. It is rare in Western Europe but more common in 'Silk Route' countries around the Mediterranean and Japan, where there is a strong association with HLA-B51.

Oral ulcers are universal (Fig. 25.50). Unlike aphthous ulcers, they are usually deep and multiple, and last for 10–30 days. Genital ulcers are also a common problem, occurring in 60–80% of cases. The usual skin lesions are erythema nodosum or acneiform lesions, but migratory thrombophlebitis and vasculitis also occur. Ocular involvement is common and may include anterior or posterior uveitis or retinal vasculitis. Neurological involvement occurs in 5% and mainly involves the brainstem, although the meninges, hemispheres and cord can also be affected, causing pyramidal signs, cranial nerve lesions, brainstem symptoms or hemiparesis. Recurrent thromboses also occur. Renal involvement is extremely rare.

The diagnosis is primarily made on clinical grounds (Box 25.74) but one characteristic feature that can be of diagnostic value is the pathergy test, which involves pricking the skin with a needle and looking for evidence of pustule development within 48 hours.

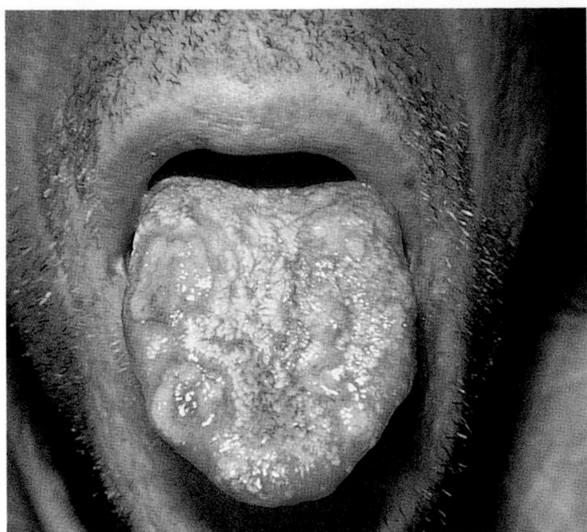

Fig. 25.50 Oral ulceration in Behçet's syndrome.

25.74 Criteria for the diagnosis of Behçet's syndrome

- Recurrent oral ulceration: minor aphthous, major aphthous or herpetiform ulceration at least three times in 12 mths

Plus two of the following:

- Recurrent genital ulceration
- Eye lesions: anterior uveitis, posterior uveitis, cells in vitreous on slit-lamp examination, retinal vasculitis
- Skin lesions: erythema nodosum, pseudofolliculitis, papulopustular lesions, acneiform nodules
- Positive pathergy test

Oral ulceration can be managed with topical steroid preparations (soluble prednisolone mouthwashes, steroid pastes). Colchicine can be effective for erythema nodosum and arthralgia. Thalidomide (100–300 mg per day for 28 days initially) is very effective for resistant oral and genital ulceration but is teratogenic and neurotoxic. Steroids and immunosuppressants are indicated for uveitis and neurological disease.

Relapsing polychondritis

Relapsing polychondritis is a rare inflammatory disease of cartilage that classically presents with acute pain and swelling of one or both ear pinnae, sparing the lower, non-cartilaginous portion. Around 30% of patients have coexisting autoimmune or connective tissue disease. Involvement of tracheobronchial cartilage leads to hoarse voice, cough, stridor or expiratory wheeze. Other manifestations include collapse of the bridge of the nose, scleritis, hearing loss and cardiac valve dysfunction. Cartilage biopsy shows an inflammatory infiltrate in the perichondrium. Both ESR and CRP are raised in active disease. Pulmonary function tests, including flow volume loops, should be performed to assess the degree of laryngotracheal disease, since this is an important cause of mortality. Mild disease usually responds to low-dose steroids or NSAID, whereas major tracheobronchial involvement requires high-dose steroids and immunosuppressants, as described for SLE.

DISEASES OF BONE

Osteoporosis

Osteoporosis is the most common bone disease and affects millions of people worldwide. Fractures related to osteoporosis are estimated to affect around 30% of women and 12% of men in developed countries, and are a major public health problem. In the UK alone, fractures are sustained by over 250 000 individuals annually, with treatment costs of about £1.75 billion. Osteoporotic fractures can affect any bone, but the most common sites are the forearm (Colles fracture), spine (vertebral fracture) and hip (Fig. 25.51). Of these, hip fractures are the most serious. Their immediate mortality is about 12% and there is a continued increase in mortality of about 20% when compared with age-matched controls. Treatment of hip fracture accounts for the majority of the healthcare costs associated with osteoporosis.

The defining feature of osteoporosis is reduced bone density, which causes a micro-architectural deterioration of bone tissue and leads to an increased risk of fracture. The prevalence of osteoporosis increases with age, reflecting the fact that bone density declines with age, especially in women (Fig. 25.52). The age-related decline in bone mass is accompanied by an increased risk of fractures (Fig. 25.53). This is due in part to the fall in bone density, but more importantly, to the increased risk of falling, which increases with age (p. 172).

Pathophysiology

Osteoporosis occurs because of a defect in attaining peak bone mass and/or because of accelerated bone loss. In normal individuals, bone mass increases during skeletal growth to reach a peak between the ages of 20 and 40 years but falls thereafter (see Fig. 25.52). In women there is an accelerated phase of bone loss after the menopause due to oestrogen deficiency, which causes uncoupling of bone resorption and bone formation, such that the amount of bone removed by osteoclasts exceeds the rate of new bone formation by osteoblasts. Age-related bone loss is a distinct process that accounts for the gradual bone loss that occurs with advancing age in both genders. Bone resorption is not particularly increased but bone formation is reduced and fails to keep pace with bone resorption. Accumulation of fat in the bone marrow space also occurs because of an age-related decline in the ability of bone marrow stem cells to differentiate into osteoblasts and an increase in their ability to differentiate into adipocytes.

Peak bone mass and bone loss are regulated by both genetic and environmental factors. Genetic factors account for up to 80% of the population variance in peak bone mass and other determinants of fracture risk, such as bone turnover and bone size. Polymorphisms have been identified in several genes that contribute to the pathogenesis of osteoporosis and many of these are in the RANK and Wnt signalling pathways, which play a critical role in regulating bone turnover (see Fig. 25.2, p. 1061). However, these account for only a small proportion of the genetic contribution to osteoporosis and many additional genetic variants remain to be discovered.

Environmental factors, such as exercise and calcium intake during growth and adolescence, are important in maximising peak bone mass and in regulating rates of post-menopausal bone loss. Smoking has a detrimental effect on bone mineral density (BMD) and is associated with an increased fracture risk, partly because female smokers have an earlier menopause than non-smokers. Heavy alcohol intake is a recognised cause of osteoporosis and fractures, but moderate intake does not substantially alter risk.

Post-menopausal osteoporosis

This is the most common cause of osteoporosis because of the effects of oestrogen deficiency, as described above. Early menopause (below the age of 45 years) is a particularly important risk factor.

Male osteoporosis

Osteoporosis is less common in men and a secondary cause can be identified in about 50% of cases. The most common are hypogonadism, corticosteroid use (see below) and alcoholism. In hypogonadism, the pathogenesis is as described for post-menopausal osteoporosis, as testosterone deficiency results in an increase in bone turnover and uncoupling of bone resorption from bone formation. Genetic factors are probably important in the 50% of cases with no identifiable cause.

Corticosteroid-induced osteoporosis

This is an important cause of osteoporosis that relates to dose and duration of corticosteroid therapy. Although there is no 'safe' dose of corticosteroid, the risk increases when the dose of prednisolone exceeds 7.5 mg daily and is continued for more than 3 months. Corticosteroids have adverse effects on calcium metabolism and bone cell function. A key abnormality is reduced bone

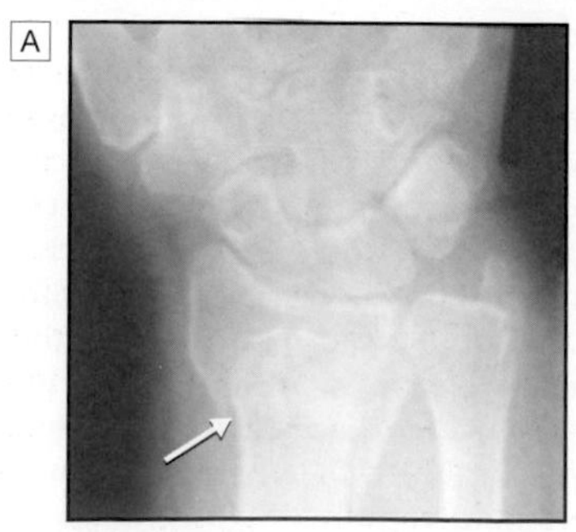

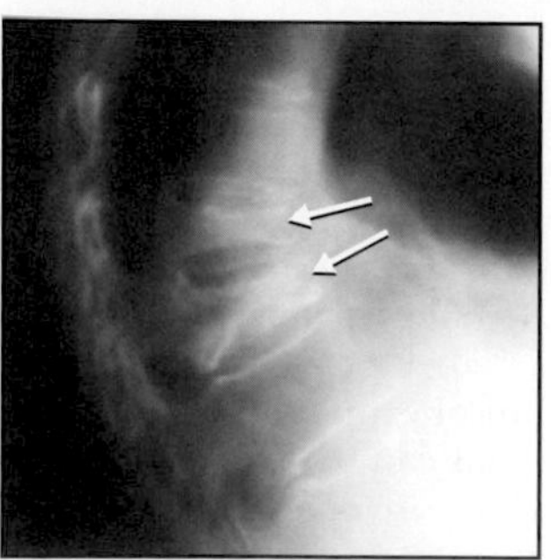

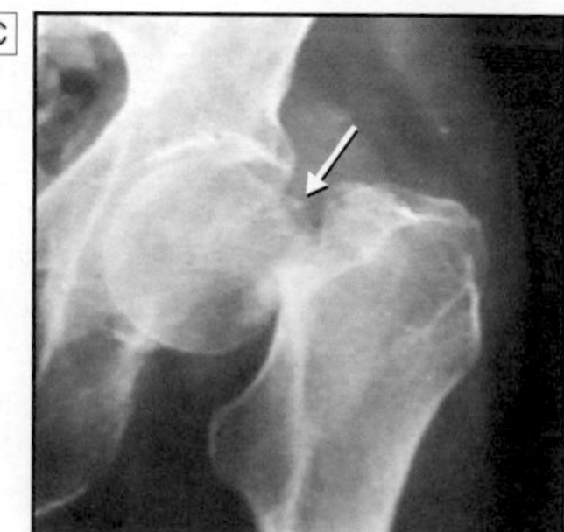

Fig. 25.51 Osteoporotic fractures: X-rays. A Wrist (Colles fracture). B Spine. C Hip.

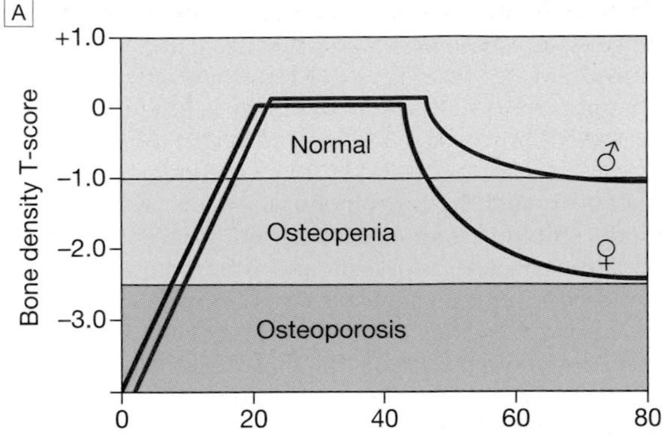

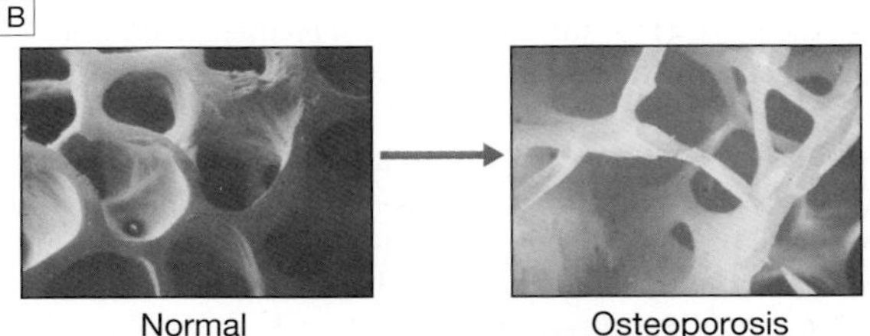

Fig. 25.52 Changes in bone mass and microstructure with age. A Changes in bone mass with age in men (blue line) and women (red line). B Scanning electron micrographs of normal bone (left) and osteoporotic bone (right).

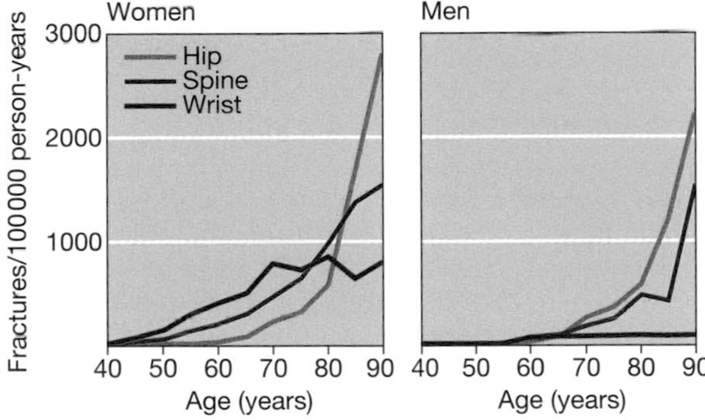

Fig. 25.53 Relationship between age and the incidence of osteoporotic fractures. Changes in the incidence of wrist fractures, vertebral fractures and hip fractures with age.

formation due to a direct inhibitory effect on osteoblast function and steroid-induced osteoblast and osteocyte apoptosis. Corticosteroids also inhibit intestinal calcium absorption and cause a renal leak of calcium, and this tends to reduce serum calcium, leading to secondary hyperparathyroidism with increased osteoclastic bone resorption. Hypogonadism may also occur with high-dose steroids.

Pregnancy-associated osteoporosis

This is a rare condition that typically presents with back pain and multiple vertebral fractures during the second or third trimester. The cause is unknown but may relate to an exaggeration of the bone loss that normally occurs during pregnancy, in patients with pre-existing low bone mass.

Other causes

Osteoporosis can occur as a complication of many diseases and drug treatments (Box 25.75). Primary hyperparathyroidism causes bone loss because sustained elevation in PTH increases bone turnover, and bone formation cannot keep pace with resorption. A similar mechanism operates in thyrotoxicosis, driven by raised levels of thyroid hormones. Cushing's disease is a rare cause, identical in mechanism to corticosteroid-induced osteoporosis. Anorexia nervosa causes osteoporosis through calcium deficiency, low body weight and hypogonadism, whereas malabsorption predisposes to it through malnutrition, calcium and vitamin D deficiency and consequent secondary hyperparathyroidism. Chronic HIV infection predisposes to osteoporosis because of low body weight, chronic immune activation and antiretroviral therapy. Inflammatory diseases increase bone resorption and suppress bone formation through release of pro-inflammatory cytokines such as IL-1 and TNF, and increased expression of RANK by lymphocytes. Similar mechanisms operate in certain cancers, which release a variety of bone-resorbing factors, including TNF, lymphotoxin and parathyroid hormone-related protein (PTHrP). Gaucher's disease (p. 451) and systemic mastocytosis also cause release of bone resorbing factors. Thiazolidinediones such as rosiglitazone inhibit osteoblast differentiation and promote adipocyte differentiation in the bone marrow, leading to reduced bone formation and bone loss. Aromatase inhibitors cause osteoporosis by reducing peripheral conversion of adrenal androgens to oestrogen, whereas gonadotrophin-releasing hormone agonists do so by causing hypogonadism.

25.75 Secondary causes of osteoporosis and osteoporotic fractures

Endocrine disease	
• Hypogonadism • Hyperthyroidism	• Hyperparathyroidism • Cushing's syndrome
Inflammatory disease	
• Inflammatory bowel disease • Ankylosing spondylitis	• RA
Drugs	
• Corticosteroids • Gonadotrophin-releasing hormone (GnRH) agonists • Aromatase inhibitors • Thyroxine over-replacement	• Thiazolidinediones • Sedatives • Anticonvulsants • Alcohol intake > 3 U/day • Heparin
Gastrointestinal disease	
• Malabsorption	• Chronic liver disease
Lung disease	
• Chronic obstructive pulmonary disease	• Cystic fibrosis
Miscellaneous	
• Myeloma • Homocystinuria • Anorexia nervosa* • Highly trained athletes* • HIV infection • Gaucher's disease	• Systemic mastocytosis • Immobilisation • Body mass index < 18 • Heavy smokers • Autoantibodies to osteoprotegerin (OPG)

*Hypogonadism also plays a role in osteoporosis associated with these conditions.

25

Clinical features

Patients with osteoporosis are asymptomatic until a fracture occurs. Osteoporotic spinal fracture may present with acute back pain or gradual onset of height loss and kyphosis with chronic pain. The pain of acute vertebral fracture can occasionally radiate to the anterior chest or abdominal wall and be mistaken for a myocardial infarction or intra-abdominal pathology, but worsening of pain by movement and local tenderness both suggest vertebral fracture. Peripheral osteoporotic fractures present with local pain, tenderness and deformity, often after an episode of minimal trauma. In patients with hip fracture, the affected leg is shortened and externally rotated. Many patients present with incidental osteopenia on an X-ray performed for other reasons.

Investigations

The pivotal investigation is dual energy X-ray absorptiometry (DEXA) at the lumbar spine and hip (see Fig. 25.8, p. 1066). This should be considered in patients with clinical risk factors for osteoporosis (Box 25.76), and those with an elevated 10-year fracture risk as defined by a fracture risk assessment tool (websites listed on p. 1135). Figure 25.54 provides an algorithm for the investigation of patients with suspected osteoporosis based on clinical risk factors, fracture risk assessment and DEXA.

A history should be taken to identify any predisposing causes, such as early menopause, excessive alcohol intake, smoking and corticosteroid therapy. Signs of endocrine disease, neoplasia and inflammatory disease should be sought on clinical examination. A falls history should be taken and a 'get up and go' test performed, especially in older patients (p. 167). Renal function, liver function, thyroid function, immunoglobulins and ESR, with screening for coeliac disease (anti-tissue transglutaminase (tTG) antibodies), should be performed. Serum 25(OH) vitamin D and PTH measurements are useful to exclude vitamin D deficiency and secondary hyperparathyroidism. Primary hyperparathyroidism should be suspected if hypercalcaemia is present (p. 769). Levels of sex hormones and gonadotrophins should be measured in men with osteoporosis and women under the age of 50. Transiliac bone biopsy is sometimes required in early-onset osteoporosis of unknown cause or when coexisting osteomalacia is suspected.

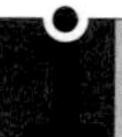

25.76 Indications for bone densitometry

- Low trauma fracture age > 50 years*
- Clinical features of osteoporosis (height loss, kyphosis)
- Osteopenia on plain X-ray
- Corticosteroid therapy (> 7.5 mg prednisolone daily for > 3 mths)
- Family history of hip fracture
- Low body weight (BMI < 18)
- Early menopause (< 45 yrs)
- Diseases associated with osteoporosis
- Increased fracture risk on risk factor analysis (FRAX or QFracture)
- Assessing response of osteoporosis to treatment

*Defined as a fracture that occurs as the result of a fall from standing height or less.

Management

The aim of treatment is to reduce the risk of fracture and this can be achieved by a combination of non-pharmacological and pharmacological approaches.

Non-pharmacological interventions

Advice on smoking cessation, moderation of alcohol intake, adequate dietary calcium intake and exercise should be given. Those with recurrent falls or unsteadiness on a 'get up and go' test should be referred to a multidisciplinary falls prevention team (p. 172). Hip protectors can reduce the risk of hip fracture in selected patients but adherence is often poor.

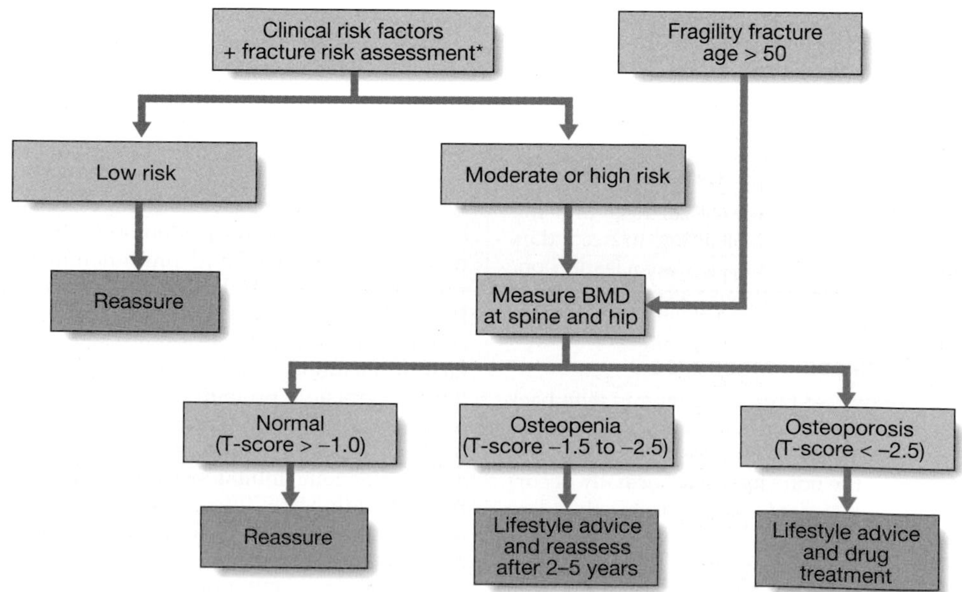

Fig. 25.54 Algorithm for the investigation of patients with suspected osteoporosis. *Using FRAX® or QFracture (see Further information, p. 1135). (BMD = bone mineral density)

Drug treatment

Several drugs have been shown to reduce the risk of osteoporotic fractures in randomised controlled trials. Their effects on vertebral and non-vertebral fracture are also summarised in Box 25.77.

Drug treatment should be considered in patients with BMD T-score values below −2.5 or below −1.5 in corticosteroid-induced osteoporosis, because there is evidence that fractures occur at a higher BMD value in steroid users and that drugs prevent fracture in patients with T-scores at this level. Treatment should also be considered in patients with vertebral fractures, irrespective of BMD, unless they resulted from significant trauma.

Bisphosphonates

Bisphosphonates inhibit bone resorption by binding to hydroxyapatite crystals on the bone surface. When osteoclasts attempt to resorb bone that contains bisphosphonate, the drug is released within the cell, where it inhibits key signalling pathways that are essential for osteoclast function. Although bisphosphonates primarily target the osteoclast, bone formation is also suppressed because of coupling between bone formation and bone resorption and an inhibitory effect on osteoblasts. However, the balance of effect on bone turnover is favourable, resulting in a gain in bone density due partly to increased mineralisation of bone. Bisphosphonate treatment typically leads to an increase in spine BMD of about 5–8% and in hip BMD of 2–4% during the first 3 years of treatment and plateaus thereafter.

Alendronic acid is the bisphosphonate used most frequently. It reduces risk of vertebral fractures by 40% and non-vertebral fractures by about 25% in postmenopausal women with osteoporosis. Risedronate is an alternative with similar efficacy, but may be better tolerated in patients with a history of gastrointestinal upset. Both drugs are effective in the treatment of corticosteroid-induced osteoporosis. They can also be used to treat male osteoporosis but neither has been shown to prevent non-vertebral fractures in men. Ibandronate is sometimes used but the evidence for prevention of non-vertebral fractures is less robust. Zoledronic acid is effective in the treatment of post-menopausal osteoporosis, corticosteroid-induced osteoporosis and osteoporosis in men. It reduces the risk of vertebral fracture by about 75% with similar effects to alendronic acid on non-vertebral fractures. It is especially useful for secondary prevention of fractures in elderly patients with hip fracture and reduces mortality in this group, being the only treatment that has been shown to modify this. Etidronate reduces the risk of vertebral fracture but the effects on non-vertebral fracture are less robust than those of other bisphosphonates. It is now seldom used.

Oral bisphosphonates are poorly absorbed from the gastrointestinal tract and should be taken on an empty stomach with plain water; no food should be eaten for 30–45 minutes after administration. Upper gastrointestinal upset occurs in about 5% so oral bisphosphonates should be used with caution in patients with existing gastro-oesophageal reflux disease. They should be avoided in patients with oesophageal stricture or achalasia, since tablets may stick in the oesophagus, causing ulceration and perforation. The most common adverse effect with intravenous bisphosphonates is a transient influenza-like illness characterised by fever, malaise, anorexia and generalised aches, which occurs 24–48 hours after administration. This is self-limiting but can be treated with paracetamol or NSAID if necessary. It predominantly occurs after the first exposure and tolerance develops thereafter. Other adverse effects are shown in Box 25.78. Osteonecrosis of the jaw (ONJ) is characterised by the presence of necrotic bone in the mandible or maxilla, typically occurring after tooth extraction when the socket fails to heal. Most ONJ cases have occurred in cancer patients with coexisting morbidity, such as infection and diabetes, who have received high doses of intravenous bisphosphonates; this complication is very rare in patients who are treated with the

25.77 Effects of drugs on the risk of osteoporotic fractures

Drug	Regimen	Vertebral fracture	Non-vertebral fracture	Hip fracture
Alendronic acid	70 mg/wk orally	+	+	+
Risedronate	35 mg/wk orally	+	+	+
Ibandronate	150 mg/mth orally 3 mg 3-monthly IV	+	+/–	–
Zoledronic acid	5 mg annually IV	+	+	+
Denosumab	60 mg 6-monthly SC	+	+	+
Strontium ranelate	2 g daily orally	+	+	+/–
Hormone replacement therapy	Various preparations	+	+	+
PTH 1-34	20 μg/day SC	+	+	–
PTH 1-84	100 μg/day SC	+	–	–
Raloxifene	60 mg/day orally	+	–	–
Tibolone	1.25 mg/day orally	+	+	–
Calcium/vitamin D	500 mg calcium and 800 U vitamin D orally	–	+/–	–

(+ effective, – not effective; +/– equivocal results, or efficacy based on post-hoc subgroup analysis of clinical trials.)

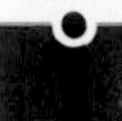

25.78 Adverse effects of bisphosphonates

Common
• Upper gastrointestinal intolerance (oral) • Acute phase response (intravenous)
Less common
• Atrial fibrillation (intravenous zoledronic acid) • Renal impairment (intravenous zoledronic acid) • Atypical subtrochanteric fractures
Rare
• Uveitis • Osteonecrosis of the jaw

dose regimes used in osteoporosis. None the less, all patients receiving bisphosphonates for any reason should be advised to pay attention to good oral hygiene. There is no evidence that temporarily stopping medication in patients undergoing tooth extraction is necessary or alters the occurrence of ONJ. Atypical subtrochanteric fractures have been described in patients who have received long-term bisphosphonates, and may be the result of over-suppression of normal bone remodelling. In the vast majority, the benefits of bisphosphonate therapy far outweigh the risks, but it is important that treatment is targeted to patients with low BMD who are most likely to benefit.

Denosumab

Denosumab is a monoclonal antibody that neutralises the effects of RANKL (see Figure 25.2, p. 1061); it is administered by subcutaneous injection every 6 months in the treatment of osteoporosis. It is a powerful inhibitor of bone resorption and reduces the risk of hip fractures by 40%, vertebral fractures by 70% and other non-vertebral fractures by 20%. It has few adverse effects but there are isolated reports of ONJ with long-term use. Unlike bisphosphonates, its duration of action is short and it must be administered on a long-term basis to maintain its effect on bone mass and bone turnover.

Calcium and vitamin D

Calcium and vitamin D have limited efficacy in the prevention of osteoporotic fractures when given in isolation but are widely used as an adjunct to other treatments, most often as combination preparations containing 500 mg calcium and 800 U vitamin D. They are of greatest value in preventing fragility fractures in elderly or institutionalised patients who are at high risk of calcium and vitamin D deficiency (Box 25.79).

Strontium ranelate

Strontium ranelate reduces vertebral fracture risk by about 50% after 3 years and non-vertebral fracture risk by 12%. The mechanism of action is poorly understood. It has a weak inhibitory effect on bone resorption, stimulates biochemical markers of bone formation and is incorporated within hydroxyapatite crystals in place of calcium. Large changes in BMD (12%) occur, although this is partly an artefact due to substitution of strontium for calcium in bone mineral. The most common adverse effect is diarrhoea. Strontium is contraindicated in patients with cardiovascular disease due to an increased

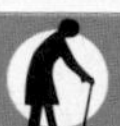

25.79 Osteoporosis in old age

- **Bone loss**: due to increased bone turnover, with an age-related defect switch in differentiation of bone marrow stromal cells to form adipocytes as opposed to osteoblasts.
- **Fractures due to osteoporosis**: common cause of morbidity and mortality, although fracture healing is not delayed by age.
- **Recurrent fractures**: those who suffer a fragility fracture are at increased risk of further fracture, so should be investigated for osteoporosis and treated if this is confirmed.
- **Falls**: risk factors for falls (such as visual and neuromuscular impairments) are independent risk factors for hip fracture in elderly women, so intervention to prevent falls is as important as treatment of osteoporosis (p. 172).
- **Intravenous zoledronic acid**: reduces mortality and subsequent fracture in elderly patients with hip fractures.
- **Calcium and vitamin D**: reduce the risk of fractures in those who are housebound or living in care homes.

risk of myocardial infarction. There is also an increased risk of venous thrombosis. Rarely, a severe rash occurs, and this is an indication to stop treatment.

Parathyroid hormone

PTH is an anabolic agent that works by stimulating new bone formation. The most widely used preparation is the 1-34 fragment of PTH (teriparatide) given by single daily subcutaneous injection of 20 μg. Teriparatide increases BMD by 10% or more in osteoporotic subjects and reduces risk of vertebral fractures by about 65% and non-vertebral fractures by 50%. It is also effective in corticosteroid-induced osteoporosis and appears superior to alendronate in terms of BMD gain and vertebral fracture reduction. It is also effective in male osteoporosis. PTH is expensive and is usually reserved for patients with severe osteoporosis (BMD T-score of –3.5 to –4.0 or below) and those who have failed to respond adequately to other treatments. The recommended duration of treatment is 24 months, after which patients should receive an antiresorptive drug, such as a bisphosphonate, to maintain the increase in BMD. Teriparatide should not be administered at the same time as bisphosphonates, as this blunts the anabolic effect. In patients who are being treated with teriparatide because of failure to respond, existing treatments should be stopped. The 1-84 fragment of PTH acts in a similar way to teriparatide but the evidence for prevention of non-vertebral fracture is less robust.

Hormone replacement therapy, raloxifene and tibolone

Cyclical HRT with oestrogen and progestogen prevents post-menopausal bone loss and reduces the risk of vertebral and non-vertebral fractures in post-menopausal women. It is primarily indicated for the prevention of osteoporosis in women with an early menopause (p. 760) and for treatment of women with osteoporosis in their early fifties who have troublesome menopausal symptoms. HRT should be avoided in older women with established osteoporosis because it significantly increases the risk of breast cancer and cardiovascular disease. Raloxifene acts as a partial agonist at oestrogen receptors in bone and liver but as an antagonist in breast and endometrium, and is classified as a selective oestrogen receptor modulator (SERM). It results in a modest increase in BMD (2%) and a 40% reduction in vertebral fractures, but does not influence the risk of non-vertebral fracture and can provoke muscle cramps and worsen hot flushes. It increases the risk of VTE to a similar extent as HRT but reduces the risk of breast cancer; it does not influence the risk of cardiovascular disease. Bazedoxifene is a related SERM that has similar effects to raloxifene. Tibolone is a steroid that has partial agonist activity at oestrogen, progestogen and androgen receptors. It has similar effects on BMD to raloxifene and has been found to prevent vertebral and non-vertebral fractures in post-menopausal osteoporosis. Treatment is associated with a slightly increased risk of stroke but a reduced risk of breast cancer.

Other drugs

Calcitonin is an osteoclast inhibitor that has weak anti-fracture efficacy but is no longer used in the treatment of osteoporosis because of concerns about an increased risk of cancer with long-term use. It is occasionally used (unlicensed) in the short-term treatment of patients with acute vertebral fracture, when it is given by subcutaneous or intramuscular injection (100–200 U daily). Calcitriol (1,25$(OH)_2D_3$), the active metabolite of vitamin D, is licensed for treatment of osteoporosis, but it is seldom used since the data on fracture prevention are less robust than for other agents.

Duration of therapy and monitoring response

Oral bisphosphonates are usually given on a long-term basis for osteoporosis with periodic review of the continued need for therapy at 5-yearly intervals. The evidence base on duration of treatment is limited. Alendronate and risedronate appear to be safe and effective for up to 10 years in most patients, although one randomised trial with alendronate showed that overall fracture rates were similar in those given 5 years' therapy as opposed to 10. Studies with intravenous zoledronic acid have shown that 3 years' treatment give equal protection from fractures as 6 years' treatment. Other drug treatments, such as HRT, raloxifene and denosumab, need to be given continuously for a beneficial effect. The optimal duration of treatment for strontium has not been established. For anabolic drugs such as PTH, a 2-year course of treatment is given and followed by long-term anti-resorptive therapy.

The response to drug treatment can be assessed by repeating BMD measurements after 2–3 years. However, changes in BMD do not predict anti-fracture efficacy well and there is little evidence that monitoring by BMD or markers improves adherence. It may, however, reassure the patient that the treatment is working. Since the precision of spine BMD (approximately 1%) is better than hip (approximately 2.5%), spine BMD is best for monitoring. To be sure that a change has occurred, about twice the precision (about 2% for spine, 5% for hip) is required. This means that, under normal circumstances, at least 2 years should have elapsed before a repeat scan is performed. Biochemical markers of bone turnover, such as N-telopeptide (NTX), respond more quickly than BMD and can be used to assess adherence, but the correlation with anti-fracture efficacy is modest. Treatment response can also be established by measuring change in patient height (to assess progression of vertebral osteoporosis) and documenting the occurrence of clinical fractures.

Surgery

Orthopaedic surgery is frequently required to reduce and stabilise osteoporotic fractures. Patients with intracapsular fracture of the femoral neck generally require hemi-arthroplasty or total hip replacement in view of the high risk of avascular necrosis.

Vertebroplasty and kyphoplasty

Vertebroplasty (VP) is sometimes used in the treatment of painful vertebral compression fractures. It involves injecting methyl methacrylate (MMA) into the affected vertebral body. Although VP has been found to give better pain relief than medical therapy in the short term, recent randomised controlled trials that compared VP with a sham procedure showed no benefit (Box 25.80), indicating that the reduction in pain may be a placebo response. Kyphoplasty (KP) is used under similar circumstances but in this case a needle is introduced into the affected vertebral body and a balloon is inflated, which is then filled with MMA. This procedure is more effective than medical treatment at relieving pain in the short term, with results similar to VP. The effects of KP have not so far been compared with a sham procedure. Both procedures are generally safe but serious adverse effects include spinal cord compression, and fat embolus may occur.

EBM 25.80 Vertebroplasty in painful vertebral fractures

'Meta-analysis of individual patient data from two placebo controlled trials of vertebroplasty showed no advantage of active treatment over a sham procedure.'

- Staples MP, et al BMJ 2011; 343:d3952.

Management of recurrent fracture

Since the treatments for osteoporosis are incompletely effective at preventing fracture, it is not uncommon to encounter patients who suffer recurrent fractures whilst on treatment. In these circumstances it is useful to perform DEXA to determine whether BMD has increased, provided that sufficient time has elapsed to assess this (see above). If BMD has increased, then treatment should be continued. If there has been no BMD response or significant bone loss has occurred, the patient should be questioned about adherence and asked if the treatment is being taken correctly. This is particularly important with oral bisphosphonates, where absorption is poor and is inhibited by food. If the patient appears to be taking the medication correctly and significant bone loss has occurred, then a different treatment should be considered.

Osteomalacia and rickets

These conditions are characterised by defective mineralisation of bone due to vitamin D deficiency, resistance to the effects of vitamin D or hypophosphataemia. Osteomalacia describes a syndrome in adults of defective bone mineralisation, bone pain, increased bone

25.81 Causes of osteomalacia and rickets

Cause	Predisposing factor	Mechanism
Vitamin D deficiency		
Classical	Lack of sunlight exposure and poor diet	Reduced cholecalciferol synthesis in the skin/low levels of vitamin D in diet
Gastrointestinal disease	Malabsorption	Malabsorption of dietary vitamin D and calcium
Failure of 1,25 vitamin D synthesis		
Chronic renal failure	Hyperphosphataemia and kidney damage	Impaired conversion of $25(OH)D_3$ to $1,25(OH)_2D_3$
Vitamin D-resistant rickets type I (autosomal recessive)	Loss-of-function mutations in renal 25(OH)D 1α-hydroxylase enzyme	Impaired conversion of $25(OH)D_3$ to $1,25(OH)_2D_3$
Vitamin D receptor defects		
Vitamin D-resistant rickets type II (autosomal recessive)	Loss-of-function mutations in vitamin D receptor	Impaired response to $1,25(OH)_2D_3$
Defects in phosphate and pyrophosphate metabolism		
Hypophosphataemic rickets (X-linked dominant)	Mutations in *PHEX*	Increased FGF23 production (mechanism unclear)
Autosomal dominant hypophosphataemic rickets	Mutation in *FGF23*	Mutant FGF23 is resistant to degradation
Autosomal recessive hypophosphataemic rickets	*DMP1* mutation	Increased production of FGF23 Local deficiency of DMP1 inhibits mineralisation
Tumour-induced hypophosphataemic osteomalacia	Ectopic production of FGF23 by tumour	Over-production of FGF23
Hypophosphatasia	Mutations in bone-specific alkaline phosphatase	Inhibition of bone mineralisation due to accumulation of pyrophosphate in bone
Iatrogenic and other		
Bisphosphonate therapy	High-dose etidronate/pamidronate	Drug-induced impairment of mineralisation
Aluminium	Use of aluminium-containing phosphate binders or aluminium in dialysis fluid	Aluminium-induced impairment of mineralisation
Fluoride	High fluoride in water	Fluoride inhibits mineralisation

fragility and fractures. Rickets is the equivalent syndrome in children and is characterised by enlargement of the growth plate and bone deformity. The disease remains prevalent in frail older people who have a poor diet and limited sunlight exposure, and in some Muslim women who live in northern latitudes. There are four main causes of osteomalacia and rickets (Box 25.81).

Vitamin D deficiency

The most common cause of osteomalacia and rickets is vitamin D deficiency, which can result from either lack of sunlight exposure, from which the majority of vitamin D is derived; dietary deficiency (Fig. 25.55); or malabsorption of vitamin D in patients with gastrointestinal disease.

Pathophysiology

The source of vitamin D and pathways involved in regulating its metabolism are shown in Figure 25.55. In normal individuals, vitamin D (also known as cholecalciferol) comes from two sources: about 70% is made in the skin from 7-dehydrocholesterol under the influence of ultraviolet light, whereas the remaining 30% is derived from the diet. On entering the circulation, vitamin D is hydroxylated in the liver to form 25(OH) vitamin D and this is further hydroxylated in the kidney to form $1,25(OH)_2D$, the biologically active metabolite. The $1,25(OH)_2D$ primarily acts on the gut to increase intestinal calcium absorption but also acts on the skeleton to stimulate bone remodelling. Synthesis of $1,25(OH)_2D$ is regulated by a negative feedback loop orchestrated by the parathyroid glands. When vitamin D levels fall – for example, as the result of reduced sunlight exposure or dietary lack – 25(OH)D and $1,25(OH)_2D$ levels also fall, resulting in a reduction in calcium absorption from the gut. This causes serum calcium levels to fall, and this is detected by calcium-sensing receptors on the parathyroid chief cells, which respond by secreting parathyroid hormone (PTH). The raised levels of PTH restore calcium levels to normal by stimulating production of $1,25(OH)_2D$, reducing renal calcium excretion and increasing bone resorption. Renal phosphate excretion also increases, lowering serum phosphate levels. Initially, these changes are effective in maintaining normal levels of serum calcium but, with prolonged vitamin D deficiency, reserves of 25(OH)D become progressively depleted (through increased conversion of 25(OH)D to $1,25(OH)_2D$), leading to hypocalcaemia and hypocalcaemia with progressive demineralisation of the skeleton and the clinical syndromes of osteomalacia and rickets.

Clinical features

Vitamin D deficiency in children causes delayed development, muscle hypotonia, craniotabes (small unossified areas in membranous bones of the skull that yield to finger pressure with a cracking feeling), bossing of the frontal and parietal bones and delayed anterior fontanelle closure, enlargement of epiphyses at the lower end of the radius, and swelling of the rib costochondral junctions ('rickety rosary'). Osteomalacia in adults presents insidiously. Mild osteomalacia can be asymptomatic or

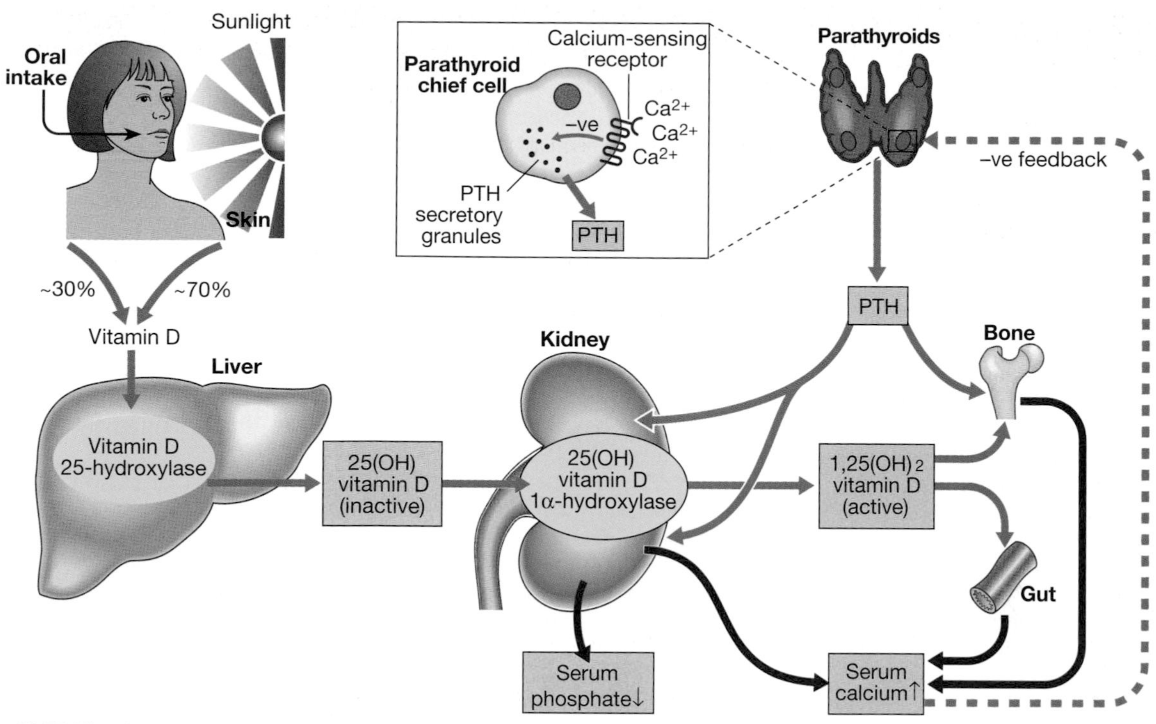

Fig. 25.55 Vitamin D metabolism. There is close interaction between vitamin D, serum calcium and parathyroid hormone (PTH). See text for details.

present with fractures and mimic osteoporosis. More severe osteomalacia presents with muscle and bone pain, general malaise and fragility fractures. Proximal muscle weakness is prominent and the patient may walk with a waddling gait and struggle to climb stairs or get out of a chair. There may be bone and muscle tenderness on pressure and focal bone pain can occur due to fissure fractures of the ribs and pelvis.

Investigations

The diagnosis can usually be made on a biochemical screen with measurement of serum 25(OH)D and PTH. Typically, serum ALP levels are raised, 25(OH)D levels are low or undetectable, and PTH is elevated. Serum calcium and phosphate levels may also be low but normal values do not exclude the diagnosis. X-rays are normal until advanced disease, when focal radiolucent areas (pseudofractures or Looser's zones) may be seen in ribs, pelvis and long bones (Fig. 25.56A). Radiographic osteopenia is common and the presence of vertebral crush fractures may cause confusion with osteoporosis. In children, there is thickening and widening of the epiphyseal plate. Radionuclide bone scan can show multiple hot spots in the ribs and pelvis at the site of fractures and the appearance may be mistaken for metastases. Where there is doubt, the diagnosis can be confirmed by bone biopsy, which shows the pathognomonic features of increased thickness and extent of osteoid seams (Fig. 25.56B).

Management

Osteomalacia and rickets respond promptly to treatment with vitamin D (250–1000 μg daily), with rapid clinical improvement, an elevation in serum 25(OH)D and a reduction in PTH. Serum ALP levels sometimes rise initially as mineralisation of bone increases, but eventually fall to within the reference range as the bone disease heals. After 3–4 months, treatment can generally be stopped or the dose of vitamin D reduced to a maintenance level of 10–20 μg of cholecalciferol daily, except in patients with underlying disease such as malabsorption, in whom higher doses may be required.

A

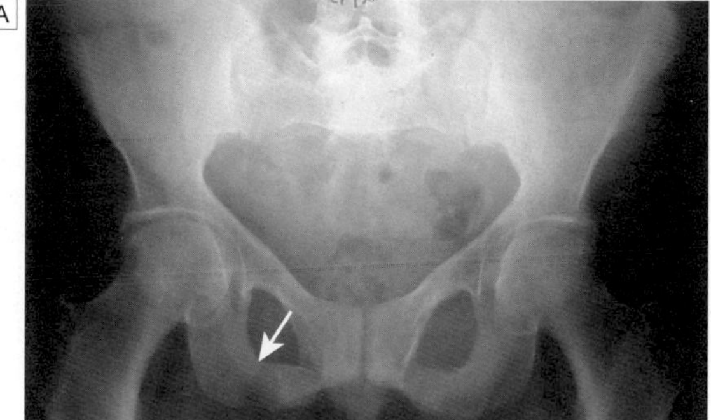

B

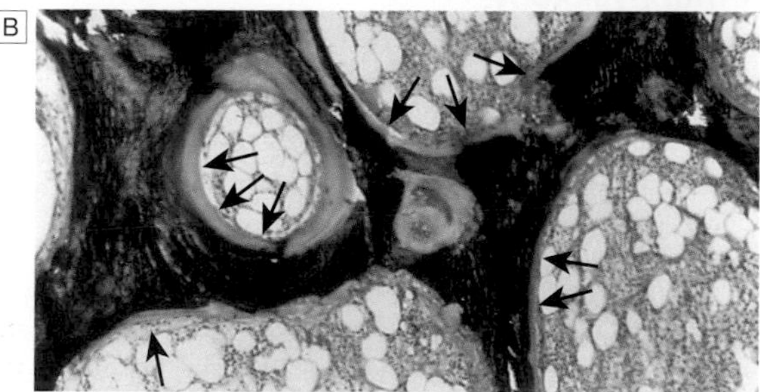

Fig. 25.56 Osteomalacia. **A** X-ray of the pelvis showing Looser's zones (arrow). **B** Photomicrograph of bone biopsy from osteomalacic patient showing thick osteoid seams (stained light blue) that cover almost all of the bone surface. Calcified bone is stained dark blue.

Vitamin D-resistant rickets

The term vitamin D-resistant rickets (VDRR) describes osteomalacia and rickets caused by:

- inactivating mutations in the 25-hydroxyvitamin D 1α-hydroxylase (CYP27B1) enzyme, which converts 25(OH)D to the active metabolite $1,25(OH)_2D_3$ (type I VDRR)
- inactivating mutations in the vitamin D receptor, which impair its ability to activate transcription (type II VDRR).

Clinical features are similar to those of infantile rickets and the diagnosis is usually first suspected when the patient fails to respond to vitamin D supplementation. Since both are recessive disorders, consanguinity is common but there may or may not be a positive family history. Biochemical features of type I disease are similar to vitamin D deficiency, except that levels of 25(OH)D are normal. In type II disease, 25(OH)D is normal but PTH and $1,25(OH)_2D_3$ values are raised. Type I can be treated with the active vitamin D metabolites, 1α-hydroxyvitamin D (1–2 μg daily, orally) or 1,25 dihydroxyvitamin D (0.25–1.5 μg daily, orally), with or without calcium supplements, depending upon the patient's diet. Type II VDRR is extremely difficult to treat but sometimes responds partially to very high doses of active vitamin D metabolites and calcium and phosphate supplements.

Renal rickets and osteomalacia

Osteomalacia and rickets occur in patients with chronic renal failure due to defects in synthesis of renal $1,25(OH)_2D_3$ or due to over-aggressive treatment with oral phosphate binders. Pathogenesis and management are discussed on page 486.

Hypophosphataemic rickets and osteomalacia

Rickets and osteomalacia can occur as the result of inherited or acquired defects in renal tubular phosphate reabsorption, and rarely in patients with tumours that secrete phosphaturic substances (see Box 25.81).

Pathophysiology

Circulating levels of FGF23 play a critical role in regulating serum phosphate by modulating expression of sodium-dependent phosphate transporters in the kidney, which are responsible for renal tubular phosphate reabsorption. Osteocytes are the main source of FGF23 and levels of expression are regulated by the proteins DMP1 and PHEX, which are also produced by osteocytes (see Fig. 25.2, p. 1061). Inherited mutations affecting these proteins are summarised in Box 25.81 and account for most cases of hypophosphataemic rickets. Acquired hypophosphataemic rickets is mostly caused by over-production of FGF23 by tumours.

Clinical features and diagnosis

The hereditary disorders usually present in childhood with rickets. The diagnosis is made on the basis of the early age at onset and the presence of hypophosphataemia with renal phosphate wasting, in the absence of vitamin D deficiency. Molecular diagnosis can define the causal mutation. Tumour-induced hypophosphataemic osteomalacia presents with severe, rapidly progressive symptoms in patients with no obvious predisposing factor for osteomalacia. Strenuous efforts should be made to identify the underlying, usually occult tumour with whole-body MRI or CT.

Management

Treatment is with phosphate supplements (1–4 g daily) and active metabolites of vitamin D (1α-hydroxyvitamin D, 1–2 μg daily, or 1,25 dihydroxyvitamin D, 0.25–1.5 μg daily) to promote intestinal calcium and phosphate absorption. The aim is to ameliorate symptoms, restore normal growth, maintain serum phosphate levels within the reference range and normalise ALP levels. Levels of calcium, phosphate, ALP and renal function should be monitored. Tumour-induced osteomalacia can be managed in the same way but ideally should be treated with surgical excision of the tumour since this is curative.

Hypophosphatasia

Hypophosphatasia is an autosomal recessive disorder caused by inactivating mutations in the *TNALP* gene that impair ALP function, resulting in accumulation of pyrophosphate and inhibition of bone mineralisation. Chondrocalcinosis may also occur. The diagnosis should be suspected in osteomalacic patients with low or undetectable levels of serum ALP but normal levels of calcium, phosphate, PTH and vitamin D metabolites. Medical treatment with injections of recombinant ALP has recently been introduced with promising results.

Other causes of osteomalacia

These are summarised in Box 25.81. Aluminium intoxication is now rare due to reduced use of aluminium-containing phosphate binders and removal of aluminium from the water supplies used in dialysis. If aluminium intoxication is suspected, the diagnosis can be confirmed by demonstration of aluminium at the calcification front in a bone biopsy. Osteomalacia due to bisphosphonates has mostly been described in patients with Paget's disease receiving etidronate and high-dose pamidronate. It is usually asymptomatic and healing occurs when treatment is stopped. Excessive fluoride intake causes osteomalacia due to direct inhibition of mineralisation and is common in parts of the world where there is a high fluoride content in drinking water. The condition reverses when fluoride intake is reduced.

Paget's disease of bone

Paget's disease of bone (PDB) is a common condition characterised by focal areas of increased and disorganised bone remodelling. It mostly affects the axial skeleton, and bones that are commonly involved include the pelvis, femur, tibia, lumbar spine, skull and scapula. It is seldom diagnosed before the age of 40, but gradually increases in incidence thereafter to affect up to 8% of the UK population by the age of 85. The disease is common in Caucasians from north-west and southern Europe but is rare in Scandinavians, Asians, Chinese and Japanese. These ethnic differences persist after migration, supporting the importance of genetic factors in the aetiology, but the incidence of PDB has fallen in some countries over the past 25 years, suggesting that environmental triggers also play a role.

Pathophysiology

The primary abnormality is increased osteoclastic bone resorption, accompanied by marrow fibrosis, increased vascularity of bone and increased osteoblast activity. Bone in PDB is architecturally abnormal and has reduced mechanical strength. Osteoclasts in PDB are increased in number, are unusually large and contain characteristic nuclear inclusion bodies. Genetic factors are important and mutations in the *SQSTM1* gene are a common cause of classical PDB. The presence of nuclear inclusion bodies in osteoclasts has fuelled speculation that PDB might be caused by a slow virus infection with measles or distemper but the evidence is conflicting. Biomechanical factors may help determine the pattern of involvement, since PDB often starts at sites of muscle insertions into bone and, in some cases, localises to bones or limbs that have been subjected to repetitive trauma or overuse. Involvement of subchondral bone can compromise the joint and predispose to OA ('Pagetic arthropathy').

Clinical features

The classic presentation is with bone pain, deformity, deafness and pathological fractures, but many patients are asymptomatic and diagnosed from an abnormal X-ray or blood test performed for another reason. Clinical signs include bone deformity and expansion, increased warmth over affected bones, and pathological fracture. Bone deformity is most evident in weight-bearing bones such as the femur and tibia, but when the skull is affected the patient may complain that hats no longer fit due to cranial enlargement. Neurological problems, such as deafness, cranial nerve defects, nerve root pain, spinal cord compression and spinal stenosis, are recognised complications due to enlargement of affected bones and encroachment upon the spinal cord and nerve foraminae. Surprisingly, deafness seldom results from compression of the auditory nerve, but is conductive due to osteosclerosis of the temporal bone. The increased vascularity of Pagetic bone makes operative procedures difficult and, in extreme cases, can precipitate high-output cardiac failure in elderly patients with limited cardiac reserve. Osteosarcoma is a rare but serious complication that presents with subacute onset of increasing pain and swelling of an affected site.

Investigations

The characteristic features are an elevated serum ALP and bone expansion on X-ray, with alternating areas of radiolucency and osteosclerosis (Fig. 25.57B). ALP is normal in about 5% of cases, usually because of monostotic involvement. Radionuclide bone scanning is useful to define the presence and extent of disease (Fig. 25.57A). If the bone scan is positive, X-rays should be taken of an affected bone to confirm the diagnosis. Bone biopsy is not usually required but may help to exclude osteosclerotic metastases in cases of diagnostic uncertainty.

Management

The main indication for treatment with inhibitors of bone resorption is bone pain thought to be due to increased metabolic activity (Box 25.82). It is often difficult to differentiate this from pain due to complications such as bone deformity, nerve compression symptoms and OA. If there is doubt, it can be worthwhile giving a therapeutic trial of antiresorptive therapy to determine whether the symptoms improve. A positive response indicates that the pain was due to increased metabolic activity. The aminobisphosphonates pamidronate, zoledronate and risedronate are more effective than simple bisphosphonates such as etidronate and tiludronate at suppressing bone turnover in PDB, but their effects on pain are similar. Although bisphosphonates suppress bone turnover in PDB, there is no evidence to show that they alter the natural history or prevent complications. Calcitonin can be used as an alternative but is less convenient to administer and more expensive. Repeated courses of bisphosphonates or calcitonin can be given if symptoms recur. If symptoms do not respond to antiresorptive therapy, it is likely that the pain is due to a complication of the disease and this should be managed according to the principles described on page 1085.

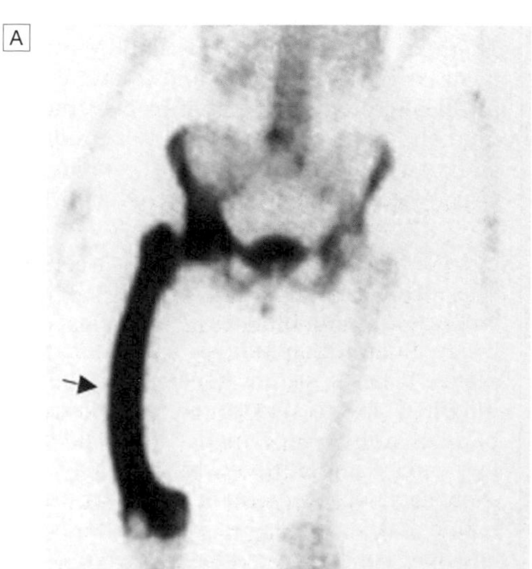

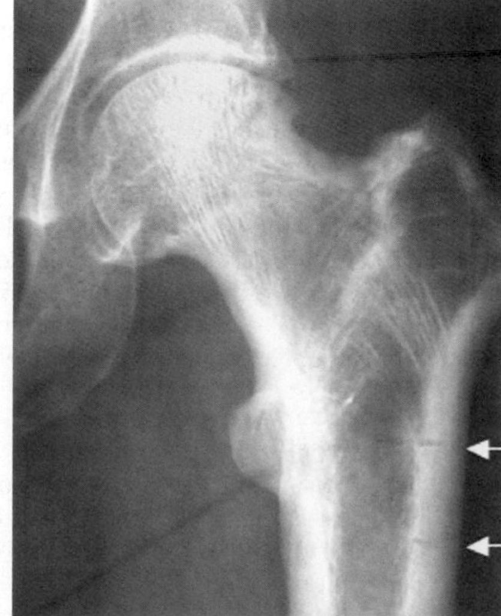

Fig. 25.57 Paget's disease. **A** Isotope bone scan from a patient with Paget's disease, illustrating the intense tracer uptake and deformity of the affected femur. **B** The typical radiographic features with expansion of the femur, alternating areas of osteosclerosis and radiolucency of the trochanter, and pseudofractures breaching the bone cortex (arrows).

25

25.82 Medical management of Paget's disease

Drug	Route of administration	Dose	Inhibitory effect on bone turnover
Etidronate	Oral	400 mg daily for 3–6 mths	+
Tiludronate	Oral	400 mg daily for 3–6 mths	+
Risedronate	Oral	30 mg daily for 2 mths	++
Pamidronate	IV	1–3 × 60 mg	++
Zoledronic acid	IV	1 × 5 mg	+++
Calcitonin	SC	100–200 U 3 times weekly for 2–3 mths	+

+ moderately effective; ++ effective; +++ highly effective.

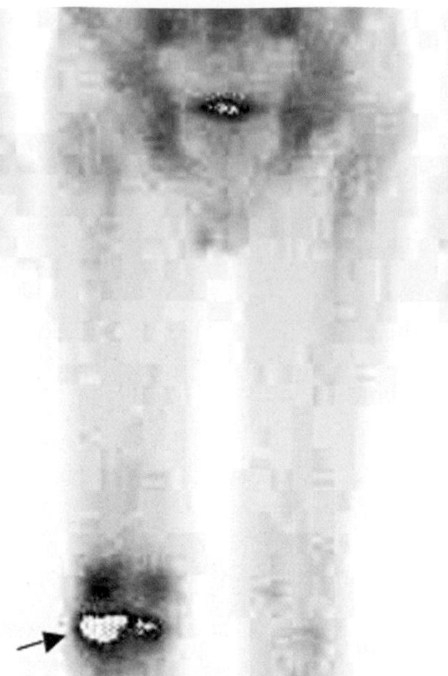

Fig. 25.58 Reflex sympathetic dystrophy. Isotope bone scan showing increased uptake in femoral condyle.

Other bone diseases

Reflex sympathetic dystrophy syndrome

Reflex sympathetic dystrophy syndrome (RSDS), or algodystrophy, presents with gradual onset of severe pain, swelling and local tenderness, usually affecting a limb extremity. It is characterised by localised osteoporosis of the affected limb and evidence of regional autonomic dysfunction, such as abnormal sweating, colour and temperature change. It is commonly triggered by fracture, occurring in up to 25% of patients with Colles fracture. It can also associate with soft tissue injury, pregnancy and intercurrent illness, or can develop spontaneously. The cause is unknown but overactivity of the sympathetic nervous system is thought to be responsible for many of its features.

The diagnosis is clinical but supported by patchy osteoporosis of the affected bone on X-ray, by a local increase in isotope uptake on bone scanning (Fig. 25.58), or by marrow oedema on MRI. The differential diagnosis includes infection and malignancy. Usually, the diagnosis of RSD is clear on clinical grounds and by the absence of an acute phase response or other systemic features of malignancy, but a biopsy of the affected site can be undertaken if necessary and typically shows local osteopenia only.

The aims of treatment are to control pain and encourage mobilisation. Analgesics, NSAID, antineuropathic agents, calcitonin, corticosteroids, β-adrenoceptor antagonists (β-blockers), sympathectomy and bisphosphonates have all been tried, but none is particularly effective. Although some cases resolve with time, many have persistent symptoms and fail to regain normal function.

Osteonecrosis

Osteonecrosis describes death of bone due to impairment of its blood supply. The most commonly affected sites are the femoral head, humeral head and femoral condyles. In some cases, the condition occurs as the result of direct trauma that interrupts the blood supply to the affected bone. This is the reason for osteonecrosis of the femoral head in patients with subtrochanteric fractures of the femoral neck, and patients with thrombophilia and haemoglobinopathies such as sickle cell disease. Other important predisposing factors include high-dose corticosteroid treatment, alcohol excess, SLE and radiotherapy, but in many of these conditions, the pathophysiology is poorly understood. The presentation is with pain localised to the affected site, which is exacerbated by weight-bearing. The diagnosis can be confirmed by MRI, which shows evidence of subchondral necrotic bone and bone marrow oedema. X-rays are normal in the early stages but later may show evidence of osteosclerosis and deformity of the affected bone. There is no specific treatment. Management should focus on controlling pain and encouraging mobilisation (p. 1085). Symptoms often improve spontaneously with time but joint replacement may be required in patients who have persisting pain in association with significant structural damage to the affected joint.

Scheuermann's osteochondritis

This disorder predominantly affects adolescent boys, who develop a dorsal kyphosis in association with irregular radiographic ossification of the vertebral end plates. It has a strong genetic component and may be inherited in an autosomal dominant manner. Most patients are asymptomatic but back pain, aggravated by exercise and relieved by rest, may occur. Excessive exercise and heavy manual labour before epiphyseal fusion has occurred may aggravate symptoms. Management consists of advice to avoid excessive activity, and protective postural exercises. Rarely, corrective surgery may be required if there is severe deformity. During adulthood, Scheuermann's osteochondritis can sometimes be complicated by the development of secondary OA, which may cause back pain. Occasionally, the vertebral deformity and kyphosis can be mistaken for osteoporotic vertebral fractures during adult life, but this can be excluded by DEXA examination, which typically shows normal or raised BMD values in Scheuermann's disease.

Polyostotic fibrous dysplasia

This is an acquired disorder caused by mutations in the *GNAS1* gene, characterised by focal or multifocal bone pain, bone deformity and expansion, and pathological fractures. Associated features include endocrine dysfunction, especially precocious puberty, and café-au-lait skin pigmentation (McCune–Albright syndrome). The diagnosis is made by imaging, which shows focal, predominantly osteolytic lesions and bone expansion on X-ray, and focal increased uptake on bone scan. The condition can resemble Paget's disease of bone but the earlier age of onset and pattern of involvement are usually distinctive. Management is symptomatic. Surgery is sometimes required for treatment of fracture and deformity. Very rarely, malignant change can occur and should be suspected if there is a sudden increase in pain and swelling. There is limited evidence that intravenous pamidronate may help bone pain and promote healing of lytic lesions.

Osteogenesis imperfecta

Osteogenesis imperfecta (OI) is the name given to a group of disorders characterised by severe osteoporosis and multiple fractures in infancy and childhood. Most cases are caused by mutations in the *COL1A1* and *COL1A2* genes, which encode the proteins that make up type I collagen. This results either in reduced collagen production (in mild OI) or in formation of abnormal collagen chains that are rapidly degraded (in severe OI). Most patients have dominant inheritance but recessive forms have been described, caused by mutations in the *CRTAP* and *LEPRE* genes, which are involved in post-translational modification of collagen. Many patients have no family history and are presumed to have new mutations. Severity varies from neonatal lethal (type II), through very severe with multiple fractures in infancy and childhood (types III and IV), to mild (type I), in which affected patients typically have blue sclerae. The diagnosis of OI is usually obvious clinically. In childhood, the disease can be mistaken for non-accidental injury and in adulthood for osteoporosis. In such cases, genetic testing can be of diagnostic value. Treatment is multidisciplinary, involving surgical reduction and fixation of fractures and correction of limb deformities, and physiotherapy and occupational therapy for rehabilitation of patients with bone deformity. Bisphosphonates are widely used in the treatment of OI, especially intravenous pamidronate in children, but there is limited evidence that this prevents fractures or deformity.

Osteopetrosis

Osteopetrosis is a rare group of inherited diseases caused by failure of osteoclast function. Presentation is highly variable, ranging from a lethal disorder that presents with bone marrow failure in infancy to a milder and sometimes asymptomatic form that presents in adulthood. Severe osteopetrosis is inherited in an autosomal recessive manner and presents with failure to thrive, delayed dentition, cranial nerve palsies (due to absent cranial foramina), blindness, anaemia and recurrent infections due to bone marrow failure. The adult-onset type (Albers–Schönberg disease) shows autosomal dominant inheritance and presents with bone pain, cranial nerve palsies, osteomyelitis, OA or fracture, or is sometimes detected as an incidental radiographic finding. The responsible mutations either affect the genes that regulate osteoclast differentiation (*RANK*, *RANKL*), causing 'osteoclast-poor' osteopetrosis, or affect the genes involved in bone resorption, causing 'osteoclast-rich' osteopetrosis. These include mutations in the *TCIRG1* gene, which encodes a component of the osteoclast proton pump, and mutations in the *CLCN7* gene, which encodes the osteoclast chloride pump. Management is difficult. IFN-γ treatment can improve blood counts and reduce frequency of infections, but in severe cases haematopoietic stem cell transplantation is required to provide a source of osteoclasts that resorb bone normally.

Sclerosing bone dysplasias

These are rare diseases characterised by osteosclerosis and increased bone formation. Van Buchem's disease and sclerosteosis are recessive disorders caused by loss-of-function mutations in the *SOST* gene (see Fig. 25.2, p. 1061). The resulting lack of sclerostin causes increased bone formation and bone overgrowth, leading to enlargement of the cranium and jaw, tall stature and cranial nerve palsies. There is no effective treatment. High bone mass syndrome is a benign disorder characterised by unusually high bone density. Most patients are asymptomatic but bone overgrowth in the palate can occur. Treatment is not usually required. Camurati–Engelmann disease is an autosomal dominant condition caused by gain of function in the *TGFB1* gene. It presents with bone pain, muscle weakness and osteosclerosis mainly affecting the diaphysis of long bones. Corticosteroids can help the bone pain, although analgesics are also usually required.

BONE AND JOINT TUMOURS

Primary tumours of bones and joints are rare, have a peak incidence in childhood and adolescence, and can be benign or malignant (Box 25.83). Paget's disease of

25.83 Primary tumours of the musculoskeletal system

Cell type	Benign	Malignant
Osteoblast	Osteoid osteoma	Osteosarcoma
Chondrocyte	Chondroma Osteochondroma	Chondrosarcoma
Fibroblast	Fibroma	Fibrosarcoma
Bone marrow cell	Eosinophilic granuloma	Ewing's sarcoma
Endothelial cell	Haemangioma	Angiosarcoma
Osteoclast precursor	Giant cell tumour	Malignant giant cell tumour

bone (p. 1128) accounts for most cases of osteosarcoma occurring above the age of 40.

Osteosarcoma

Osteosarcoma presents with local pain, swelling and tenderness. X-rays may show expansion of the bone with a surrounding soft tissue mass, often containing islands of calcification, but further evaluation by MRI or CT is necessary to determine the extent of tumour. The diagnosis can be confirmed by biopsy but this should be done after referral to a specialist team. Treatment depends on histological type but generally involves surgical removal of the tumour, followed by chemotherapy and radiotherapy. The prognosis is excellent with benign tumours and also generally good in cases that present in childhood and adolescence. The prognosis is poor in elderly patients with osteosarcoma related to Paget's disease of bone.

Metastatic bone disease

Metastatic bone disease may present in a variety of ways: with localised or generalised progressive bone pain, generalised regional pain, symptoms of spinal cord compression, or acute pain due to pathological fracture. Systemic features, such as weight loss and anorexia, and symptoms referable to the primary tumour are often present. The tumours that most commonly metastasise to bone are myeloma and those of bronchus, breast, prostate, kidney and thyroid. Management is discussed in Chapter 11.

RHEUMATOLOGICAL INVOLVEMENT IN OTHER DISEASES

Many systemic diseases can affect the locomotor system, and many drugs may cause adverse locomotor effects (Box 25.84). The most common examples are described here. Bone disease in sarcoidosis is described on page 710, haemophilia on page 1051 and sickle cell anaemia on page 1032.

Malignant disease

Malignant disease can cause a variety of non-metastatic musculoskeletal problems (Box 25.85). One of the most striking is hypertrophic pulmonary osteoarthropathy, characterised by clubbing and painful swelling of the limbs, periosteal new bone formation and arthralgia/arthritis. The most common causes are bronchial carcinoma and mesothelioma (pp. 699 and 719), but the condition can be inherited when it is caused by inactivating mutations in the *HPGD* gene, which is responsible for degradation of PGE_2, suggesting that over-production of prostaglandins may generally play a causal role in clubbing. Bone scans show increased periosteal uptake before new bone is apparent on X-ray. The course follows that of the underlying malignancy and resolves if this is cured.

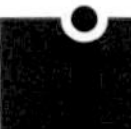

25.85 Rheumatological manifestations of malignancy

- Polyarthritis
- Dermatomyositis and polymyositis
- Hypophosphataemic osteomalacia
- Hypertrophic osteoarthropathy
- Vasculitis, connective tissue disease
- Raynaud's syndrome
- Polymyalgia rheumatica-like syndrome

Endocrine disease

Hypothyroidism (p. 743) may present with carpal tunnel syndrome, or rarely with very painful, symmetrical proximal myopathy with muscle hypertrophy. Both resolve with thyroxine replacement. Hyperparathyroidism (p. 769) predisposes to calcium pyrophosphate dihydrate deposition disease and to calcific periarthritis, especially in patients with renal disease.

25.84 Drug-induced effects on the musculoskeletal system

Musculoskeletal problem	Principal drug
Secondary gout	Thiazides, furosemide, alcohol
Osteoporosis	Corticosteroids, heparin, glitazones, aromatase inhibitors, GnRH agonists
Osteomalacia	Anticonvulsants, etidronate and pamidronate (high-dose)
Osteonecrosis	Corticosteroids, alcohol
Drug-induced lupus syndrome	Procainamide, hydralazine, isoniazid, chlorpromazine
Arthralgias or arthritis	Corticosteroid withdrawal, glibenclamide, methyldopa, ciclosporin, isoniazid, barbiturates
Myalgia	Corticosteroid withdrawal, L-tryptophan, fibrates, statins
Myopathy	Corticosteroids, chloroquine
Myositis, myasthenia	Penicillamine, statins
Cramps	Corticosteroids, ACTH, diuretics, carbenoxolone
Vasculitis	Amphetamines, thiazides

(ACTH = adrenocorticotrophic hormone; GnRH = gonadotrophin-releasing hormone)

Diabetes mellitus (Ch. 21) commonly causes diabetic cheiroarthropathy characterised by tightening of skin and periarticular structures, causing flexion deformities of the fingers that may be painful. Diabetic osteopathy presents as forefoot pain with radiographic progression from osteopenia to complete osteolysis of the phalanges and metatarsals. Diabetes also predisposes to adhesive capsulitis, Dupuytren's contracture, septic arthritis and Charcot's joints.

Acromegaly (p. 792) can be associated with mechanical back pain, with normal or excessive (not restricted) movement; carpal tunnel syndrome; Raynaud's syndrome; and an arthropathy (50%). The arthropathy mainly affects the large joints and has clinical similarities to OA but with normal or an increased range of movement. X-rays may show widening of joint spaces, squaring of bone ends, generalised osteopenia and tufting of terminal phalanges. It does not improve with treatment of the acromegaly.

Haematological disease

Haemochromatosis (p. 972) is complicated by an arthropathy in about 50% of cases. It typically presents between the ages of 40 and 50, and may predate other features of the disease. The small joints of the hands and wrists are typically affected but the hips, shoulders and knees may also be involved. The X-ray changes resemble OA but cysts are often multiple and prominent, with little osteophyte formation. Involvement of the radiocarpal and MCP joints may occur, which is unusual in primary OA, and about 30% have calcium pyrophosphate dihydrate deposition disease and/or pseudogout. Treatment of the haemochromatosis does not influence the arthropathy, and management of the arthropathy is as described for OA. Haemophilia (p. 1051) can be complicated by haemarthrosis, which, if recurrent, can result in the development of secondary osteoarthritis. Sickle-cell disease (p. 1032) may be complicated by bone pain, osteonecrosis and osteomyelitis. Thalassaemia (p. 1033) may be complicated by bone deformity, especially affecting the craniofacial bones, and by osteoporosis.

Neurological disease

Neurological disease may result in rapidly destructive arthritis of joints, first described by Charcot in association with syphilis. The cause is incompletely understood but may involve repetitive trauma as the result of sensory loss and altered blood flow secondary to impaired sympathetic nervous system control. The main predisposing diseases and sites of involvement are:

- diabetic neuropathy (hindfoot)
- syringomyelia (shoulder, elbow, wrist)
- leprosy (hands, feet)
- tabes dorsalis (knees, spine).

The presentation is with subacute or chronic monoarthritis. Pain can occur, especially at the onset, but once the joint is severely deranged, pain is often minimal and signs become disproportionately greater than symptoms. The joint is often grossly swollen, with effusion, crepitus, marked instability and deformity, but usually no increased warmth. X-rays show disorganisation of normal joint architecture and often multiple loose bodies (Fig. 25.59), and either no (atrophic) or gross (hypertrophic) new bone formation. Management principally involves orthoses and occasionally arthrodesis.

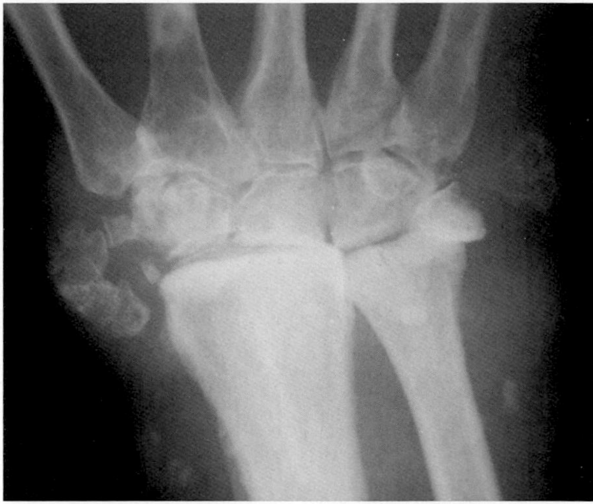

Fig. 25.59 Wrist X-ray showing a neuropathic (Charcot) joint in a patient with syringomyelia. Note the disorganised architecture with complete loss of the proximal carpal row, bony fragments and soft tissue swelling.

MISCELLANEOUS CONDITIONS

Spondylolysis and spondylolisthesis

Spondylolysis describes a break in the integrity of the neural arch. The principal cause is an acquired defect in pars interarticularis due to a fracture, mainly seen in gymnasts, dancers and runners, in whom it is an important cause of back pain. Spondylolisthesis describes the condition where a defect causes slippage of a vertebra on the one below. This may be congenital, post-traumatic or degenerative. Rarely, it can result from metastatic destruction of the posterior elements. Uncomplicated spondylolysis does not cause symptoms but spondylolisthesis can cause low back pain aggravated by standing and walking. Occasionally, symptoms of nerve root or spinal compression may occur. The diagnosis can be made on lateral X-rays of the lumbar spine but MRI may be required if there is neurological involvement. Advice on posture and muscle-strengthening exercises is required in mild cases. Surgical fusion is indicated for severe and recurrent low back pain. Surgical decompression is mandatory prior to fusion in patients with significant lumbar stenosis or symptoms of cauda equina compression.

Diffuse idiopathic skeletal hyperostosis

Diffuse idiopathic skeletal hyperostosis (DISH) is a common disorder, affecting 10% of men and 8% of women over the age of 65, and associated with obesity,

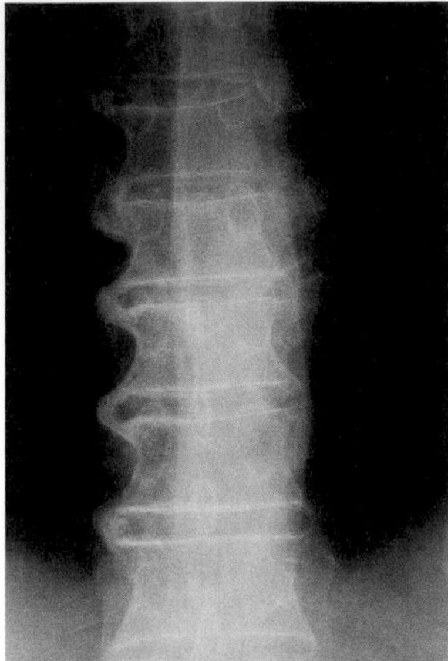

Fig. 25.60 Diffuse idiopathic skeletal hyperostosis (DISH). Antero-posterior X-ray of thoracic spine showing right-sided, flowing new bone joining more than four contiguous vertebrae. The disc spaces are preserved.

hypertension and type 2 diabetes mellitus. It is characterised by florid new bone formation along the anterolateral aspect of at least four contiguous vertebral bodies (Fig. 25.60). DISH is distinguished from lumbar spondylosis by the absence of disc space narrowing and marginal vertebral body sclerosis, and from ankylosing spondylitis by the absence of sacroiliitis or apophyseal joint fusion. It is usually an asymptomatic radiographic finding but can cause back pain or pain at peripheral sites, such as the heel in association with calcaneal spur formation.

Pigmented villonodular synovitis

Pigmented villonodular synovitis is an uncommon proliferative disorder of synovium, which typically affects young adults. It is caused by a somatic chromosomal translocation in synovial cells that places the *CSF1* gene downstream of the *COL6A3* gene promoter. The result is local over-production of macrophage colony-stimulating factor (M-CSF), which causes accumulation of macrophages in the joint. The presentation is with joint swelling, limitation of movement and local discomfort. The diagnosis can be confirmed by MRI or synovial biopsy. Treatment is by surgical or radiation synovectomy.

Joint hypermobility

Hypermobility is a relatively uncommon disorder associated with joint laxity. It may be primary or secondary to inherited diseases, such as Marfan's syndrome (p. 603), Ehlers–Danlos syndrome (p. 1050) and osteogenesis imperfecta (p. 1131). Benign joint hypermobility syndrome is diagnosed clinically when the modified Beighton score is 4 or above in the presence of arthralgia in four or more joints (Box 25.86). There is no specific treatment, apart from the general principles listed on page 1077.

25.86 Modified Beighton score for joint hypermobility

Clinical test	Score
Extend little finger > 90°	(1 point each side)
Bring thumb back parallel to/touching forearm	(1 point each side)
Extend elbow > 10°	(1 point each side)
Extend knee > 10°	(1 point each side)
Touch floor with flat of hands, legs straight	(1 point)

Hypermobile = a score of 6 or more points out of a possible 9 for epidemiological studies, or 4 or more points (with arthralgia in four or more joints) for a clinical diagnosis of the benign joint hypermobility syndrome.

Dupuytren's contracture

Dupuytren's contracture results from fibrosis and contracture of the superficial palmar fascia of the hands. The patient is unable to extend the fingers fully and there is puckering of the skin with palpable nodules. The ring and little fingers are usually the first and worst affected. It is usually painless, but causes problems due to limitation of hand function and snagging of the curled fingers in pockets. It is age-related, usually bilateral and more common in men. There is a strong genetic component and sometimes may be familial, with dominant inheritance. It can be associated with plantar fibromatosis, Peyronie's disease, alcohol misuse and chronic vibration injury. It is very slowly progressive. Often no treatment is required, but it can be treated medically by local injections of collagenase or surgically by fasciotomy if symptoms are troublesome.

Carpal tunnel syndrome

This is a common nerve entrapment syndrome caused by compression of the median nerve at the wrist. It presents with numbness, tingling and pain in a median nerve distribution (p. 1224). The most common causes are hypothyroidism, diabetes mellitus, RA, obesity and pregnancy, especially in the third trimester. In some patients no underlying cause may be identified. Carpal tunnel syndrome often responds to treatment of the underlying condition, but other options include local steroid injections and surgical decompression.

Trigger finger

This occurs as the result of stenosing tenosynovitis in the flexor tendon sheath, with intermittent locking of the finger in flexion. It can arise spontaneously or in association with inflammatory diseases like RA. Symptoms usually respond to local steroid injections but surgical decompression is occasionally required.

Periodic fever syndromes

These are a group of rare inherited disorders that present with intermittent attacks of fever, rash, arthralgia and myalgia. They usually occur in childhood but may present for the first time in adulthood. They are discussed in more detail on page 85.

Anterior tibial compartment syndrome

This is characterised by severe pain in the front of the lower leg, aggravated by exercise and relieved by rest. Symptoms result from fascial compression of the muscles in the anterior tibial compartment and may be associated with foot drop. Treatment is by surgical decompression.

Synovitis–acne–pustulosis–hyperostosis–osteitis syndrome

The synovitis–acne–pustulosis–hyperostosis–osteitis (SAPHO) syndrome is an uncommon disorder characterised by bone pain and swelling due to a sterile osteomyelitis and hyperostosis predominantly targeting the clavicles and bones of the anterior chest wall. Other features include a pustulotic rash affecting the palms and soles of the feet, sacroiliitis and synovitis of peripheral joints. It most commonly presents in children and young or middle-aged adults. Various treatments have been used, including corticosteroids, DMARDs, bisphosphonates and TNF blockers, with varying degrees of success. The cause is unknown but has been suggested to be an autoimmune process triggered by a bacterial or viral pathogen.

Further information

Journal articles

Ralston SH. Paget's disease of bone. N Engl J Med 2013; 368:644–650.

Rudwaleit M. New approaches to diagnosis and classification of axial and peripheral spondyloarthropathies. Curr Opin Rheum 2010; 22:275–280.

Sambrook P, Cooper C. Osteoporosis. Lancet 2006; 367:2010–2018.

Scott DL, Woolf F, Huizinga TW. Rheumatoid arthritis. Lancet 2010; 376:1094–1108.

Zhang W, Doherty M, et al. EULAR recommendations for gout. Part 2: Management. Ann Rheum Dis 2006; 65:1312–1324.

Websites

www.4s-dawn.com/DAS28

www.basdai.com/BASDAI.php *BASDAI calculator.*

www.nice.org.uk/CG59 *Osteoarthritis.*

www.nice.org.uk/TA161 and www.nice.org.uk/TA160 *Osteoporosis.*

www.omim.org *Online Mendelian Inheritance in Man (OMIM): genetic diseases.*

www.shef.ac.uk/FRAX/ and www.qfracture.org/ *Fracture risk assessment tools.*

J.P. Leach
R.J. Davenport

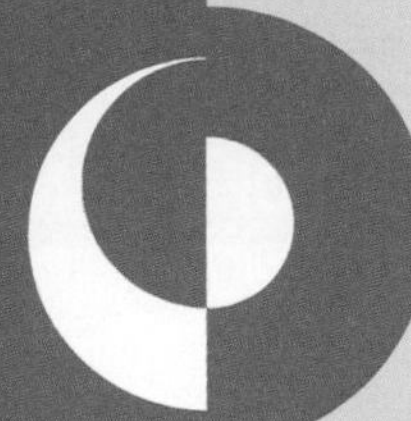

Neurological disease 26

Clinical examination of the nervous system 1138

Functional anatomy and physiology 1140

Functional anatomy of the nervous system 1141
Localising lesions in the brainstem 1148

Investigation of neurological disease 1149

Neuroimaging 1149
Neurophysiological testing 1151

Presenting problems in neurological disease 1155

Headache and facial pain 1156
Dizziness, blackouts and 'funny turns' 1157
Status epilepticus 1159
Coma 1159
Delirium 1161
Amnesia 1161
Weakness 1162
Sensory disturbance 1164
Abnormal movements 1165
Abnormal perception 1167
Altered balance and vertigo 1167
Abnormal gait 1168
Abnormal speech and language 1168
Disturbance of smell 1169
Visual disturbance and ocular abnormalities 1169
Hearing disturbance 1173
Bulbar symptoms – dysphagia and dysarthria 1173
Bladder, bowel and sexual disturbance 1174
Personality change 1175
Sleep disturbance 1175
Psychiatric disorders 1175

Functional symptoms 1175

Headache syndromes 1176

Epilepsy 1178

Vestibular disorders 1186

Disorders of sleep 1187

Excessive daytime sleepiness (hypersomnolence) 1187
Parasomnias 1187

Neuro-inflammatory diseases 1188

Multiple sclerosis 1188
Acute disseminated encephalomyelitis 1192
Transverse myelitis 1193
Neuromyelitis optica 1193

Paraneoplastic neurological disorders 1193

Neurodegenerative diseases 1194

Movement disorders 1194
Ataxias 1198
Tremor disorders 1199
Dystonia 1200
Hemifacial spasm 1200
Motor neuron disease 1200
Spinal muscular atrophy 1201

Infections of the nervous system 1201

Meningitis 1201
Parenchymal viral infections 1205
Parenchymal bacterial infections 1208
Diseases caused by bacterial toxins 1209
Transmissible spongiform encephalopathies 1211

Intracranial mass lesions and raised intracranial pressure 1211

Raised intracranial pressure 1212
Brain tumours 1213
Paraneoplastic neurological disease 1216
Hydrocephalus 1216
Idiopathic intracranial hypertension 1217
Head injury 1218

Disorders of cerebellar function 1218

Disorders of the spine and spinal cord 1218

Cervical spondylosis 1218
Lumbar spondylosis 1219
Spinal cord compression 1220
Intrinsic diseases of the spinal cord 1222

Diseases of peripheral nerves 1223

Entrapment neuropathy 1224
Multifocal neuropathy 1224
Polyneuropathy 1224
Guillain–Barré syndrome 1224
Chronic polyneuropathy 1225
Brachial plexopathy 1225
Lumbosacral plexopathy 1226
Spinal root lesions 1226

Diseases of the neuromuscular junction 1226

Myasthenia gravis 1226
Other myasthenic syndromes 1227

Diseases of muscle 1228

CLINICAL EXAMINATION OF THE NERVOUS SYSTEM

Observation

- General appearance
- Mood (e.g. anxious, depressed)
- Facial expression (or lack thereof)
- Handedness
- Nutritional status
- Blood pressure

1 Stance and gait
Posture
Romberg's test
Arm swing
Pattern of gait
Tandem (heel-toe) gait

2 Back
Scoliosis
Operative scars
Evidence of spina bifida occulta
Winging of scapula

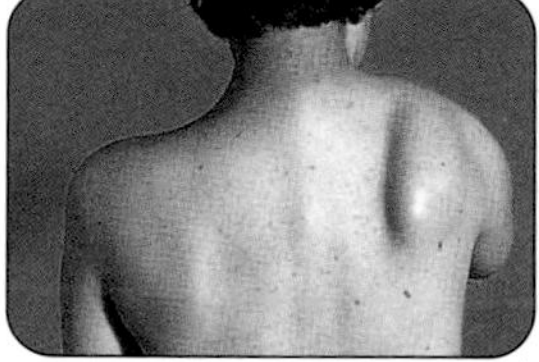

Winging of right scapula (muscular dystrophy)

3 Neck and skull
Skull size and shape
Neck stiffness and Kernig's test
Carotid bruit

4 Cranial nerves

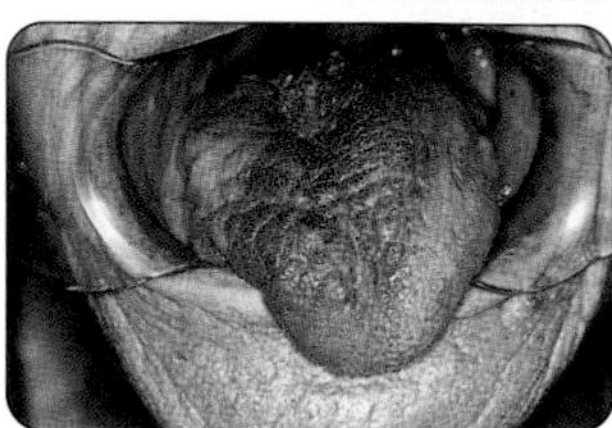

Right 12th nerve palsy: wasting of right side of tongue

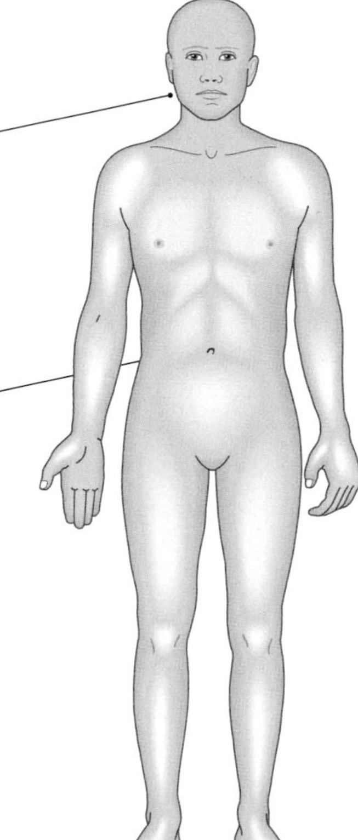

5 Optic fundi
Papilloedema
Optic atrophy
Cupping of disc (glaucoma)
Hypertensive changes
Signs of diabetes

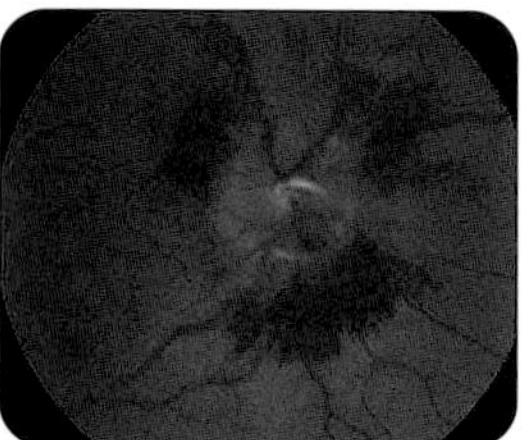

Haemorrhagic papilloedema

6 Motor
Wasting, fasciculation
Abnormal posture
Abnormal movements
Tone (including clonus)
Strength
Coordination
Tendon reflexes
Abdominal reflexes
Plantar reflexes

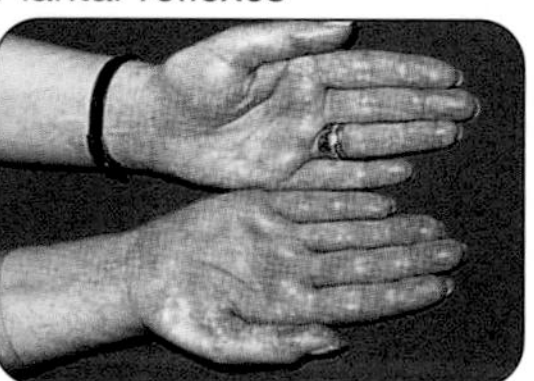

Wasting of right thenar eminence due to cervical rib

7 Sensory
Pin-prick, temperature
Joint position, vibration
Two-point discrimination

8 Higher cerebral function
Orientation
Memory
Speech and language
Localised cortical functions

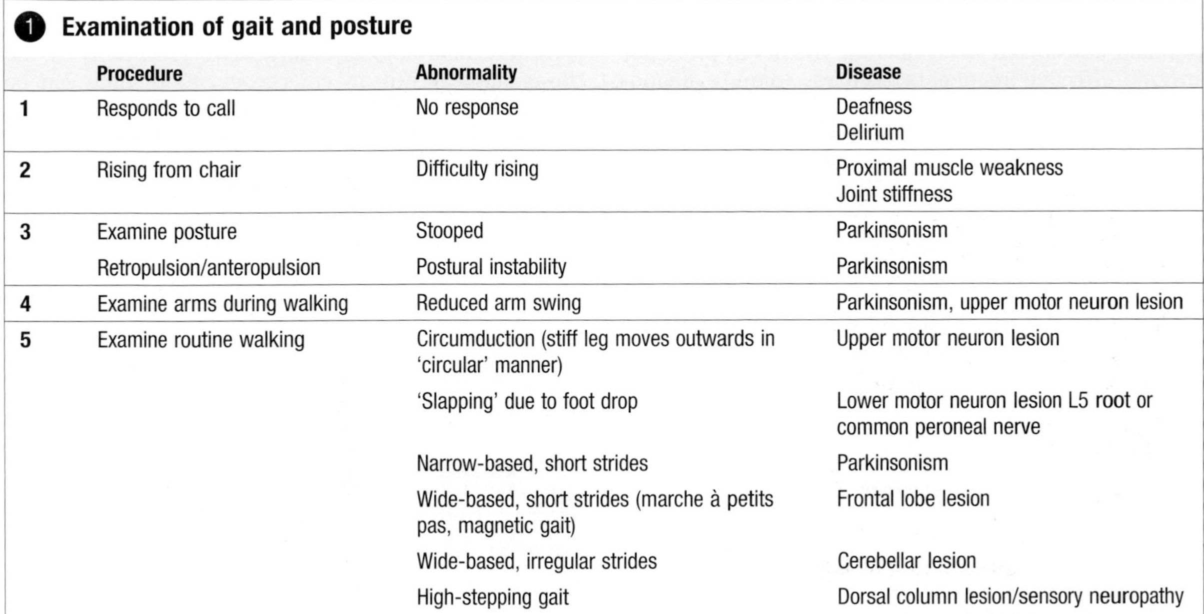

1 Examination of gait and posture

	Procedure	Abnormality	Disease
1	Responds to call	No response	Deafness Delirium
2	Rising from chair	Difficulty rising	Proximal muscle weakness Joint stiffness
3	Examine posture	Stooped	Parkinsonism
	Retropulsion/anteropulsion	Postural instability	Parkinsonism
4	Examine arms during walking	Reduced arm swing	Parkinsonism, upper motor neuron lesion
5	Examine routine walking	Circumduction (stiff leg moves outwards in 'circular' manner)	Upper motor neuron lesion
		'Slapping' due to foot drop	Lower motor neuron lesion L5 root or common peroneal nerve
		Narrow-based, short strides	Parkinsonism
		Wide-based, short strides (marche à petits pas, magnetic gait)	Frontal lobe lesion
		Wide-based, irregular strides	Cerebellar lesion
		High-stepping gait	Dorsal column lesion/sensory neuropathy

4 Examination of cranial nerves

Nerve	Name	Tests
I	Olfactory	Ask patient about sense of smell (only examine if reported change)
II	Optic	Visual acuity Visual fields 'Swinging' torch test for relative afferent pupillary defect Ophthalmoscopy
III	Oculomotor	Eye movements (nystagmus) Eyelid movement Pupil size, symmetry, reactions
IV	Trochlear	Eye movements
V	Trigeminal	Facial sensation Corneal reflex Ask patient about taste
VI	Abducens	Eye movements
VII	Facial	Facial symmetry and movements Ask patient about taste
VIII	Vestibulocochlear	Hearing (rub fingertips next to each ear) Tuning fork tests (Rinne and Weber) Hallpike test for benign positional vertigo
IX	Glossopharyngeal	Gag reflex (sensory)
X	Vagus	Palatal elevation (uvula deviates to side opposite lesion) Gag reflex (motor) Cough (bovine)
XI	Accessory	Look for wasting of trapezius/sternocleidomastoid Elevation of shoulders Turning head to right and left
XII	Hypoglossal	Look for wasting/fasciculation Tongue protrusion (deviates to side of lesion)

6 Root values of tendon reflexes

Reflex	Root value
Upper limb	
Biceps jerk	C5/C6
Supinator jerk	C5/C6
Triceps jerk	C7
Finger jerk	C8
Lower limb	
Knee jerk	L3/L4
Ankle jerk	S1

Neurological examination in old age

- **Pupils**: tend to be smaller, which makes fundoscopy more difficult.
- **Limb tone**: difficult to assess because of poor relaxation and concomitant joint disease.
- **Ankle reflexes**: may be bilaterally absent.
- **Gait assessment**: more difficult because of concurrent musculoskeletal disease and pre-existing neurological deficits.
- **Sensory testing**: especially difficult when there is cognitive impairment.
- **Vibration sense**: may be reduced in the lower legs.

Neurology has long been misperceived as a specialty in which intricate clinical examination and numerous investigations are required to diagnose obscure and untreatable conditions. In fact, it requires careful history-taking with a lesser contribution from targeted examination and considered investigation. The development of specific, effective treatments has made accurate diagnosis essential.

The brain, spinal cord and peripheral nerves combine to allow us to perceive and react to the external world, while maintaining a stable internal environment. The brain provides a platform for processing information and forming a response and, in doing so, both forms and is affected by our personality and mental state. Nervous system disorders are common, accounting for around 10% of the UK's general practice consultations, 20% of acute medical admissions, and most chronic physical disability. While pathological and anatomical localisation is important, skill is required to identify those neurological symptoms *not* associated with neurological disease, to differentiate patients requiring investigation and treatment from those who need reassurance.

Initially, it is important to exclude conditions that constitute neurological emergencies (Box 26.1). If the presentation is not an emergency, more time can be taken to reach a diagnosis. The history should provide a hypothesis for the site and nature of the potential pathology, which a focused examination may refine and inform what further investigation would be useful. A discussion with the patient about possible interventions and rehabilitation may then take place.

As Stroke has become a specific subspecialty in many centres, it is described in a separate chapter, although it is clearly a neurological condition. This chapter should be read with it, to help clarify how the presentation, diagnosis and management of stroke differ from other conditions.

26.1 Neurological emergencies

- Status epilepticus (p. 1159)
- Stroke (if thrombolysis available) (p. 1237)
- Guillain–Barré syndrome (p. 1224)
- Myasthenia gravis (if bulbar and/or respiratory) (p. 1226)
- Spinal cord compression (p. 1220)
- Subarachnoid haemorrhage (p. 1246)
- Neuroleptic malignant syndrome (p. 249)

FUNCTIONAL ANATOMY AND PHYSIOLOGY

Cells of the nervous system

The nervous system comprises billions of connections between billions of specialised cells, supplied by a complex network of specialised blood vessels. In addition to neurons, there are three types of glial cells. Astrocytes

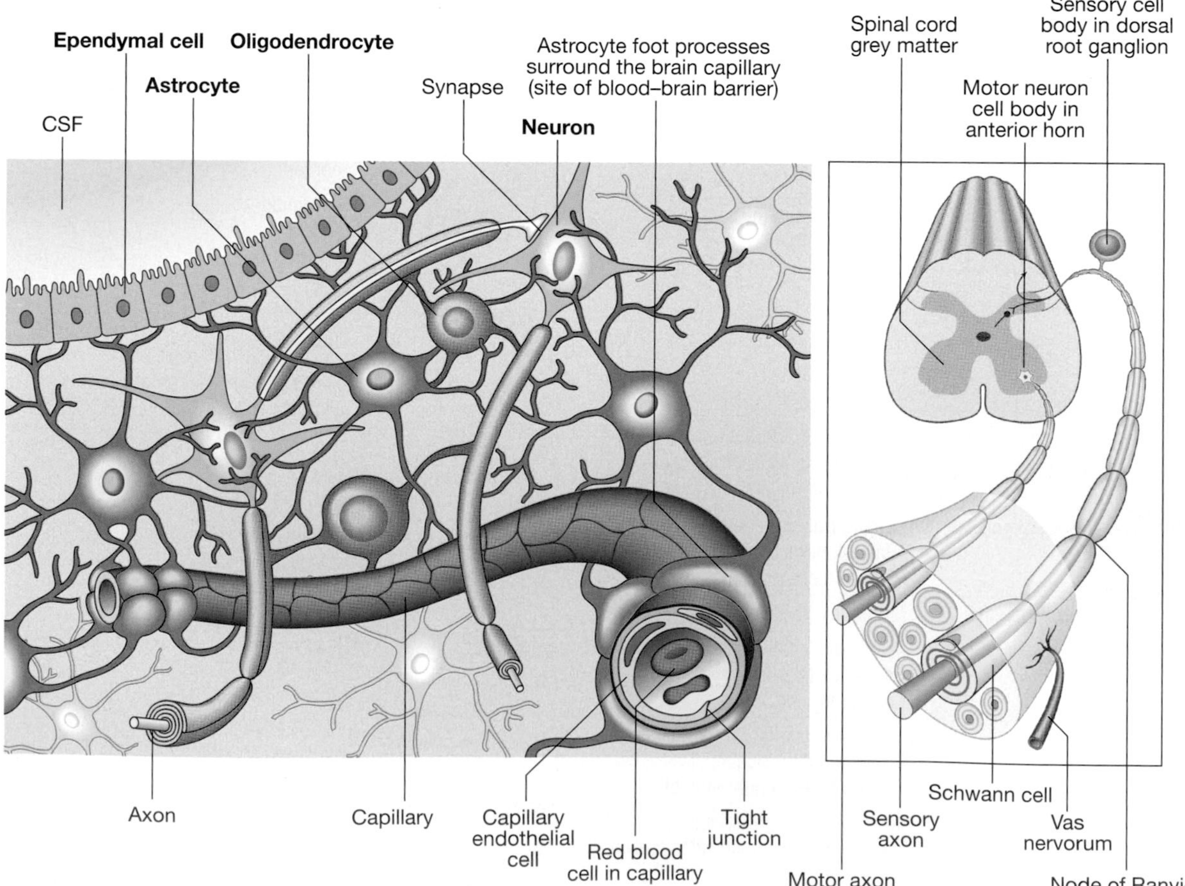

Fig. 26.1 Cells of the nervous system. (CSF = cerebrospinal fluid)

form the structural framework for neurons and control their biochemical environment. Astrocyte foot processes are intimately associated with blood vessels, forming the blood–brain barrier (Fig. 26.1). Oligodendrocytes are responsible for the formation and maintenance of the myelin sheath, which surrounds axons and is essential for the rapid transmission of action potentials by saltatory conduction. Microglial cells derive from monocytes/macrophages and play a role in fighting infection and removing damaged cells. Peripheral neurons have axons invested in myelin made by Schwann cells. Ependymal cells line the cerebral ventricles.

Generation and transmission of the nervous impulse

The role of the central nervous system (CNS) is to generate outputs in response to external stimuli and changes in internal conditions. Each neuron receives input by synaptic transmission from dendrites (branched projections of other neurons), which may sum to produce output in the form of an action potential. This is conducted down axons, with synaptic transmission to other neurons or, in the motor system, to muscle cells. These processes require the maintenance of an electrochemical gradient across neuron cell membranes by specialised membrane ion channels. Synaptic transmission involves the release of neurotransmitters that modulate the function of the target cell by interacting with structures on the cell surface, including ion channels and other cell surface receptors (Fig. 26.2). At least 20 different neurotransmitters are known to act at different sites in the nervous system, and all are potentially amenable to pharmacological manipulation.

The neuronal cell bodies may receive synaptic input from thousands of other neurons. The synapsing neuron terminals are also subject to feedback regulation via receptor sites on the pre-synaptic membrane, modifying the release of transmitter across the synaptic cleft. In addition to such acute effects, some neurotransmitters produce long-term modulation of metabolic function or gene expression. This effect probably underlies more complex processes in, for example, long-term memory.

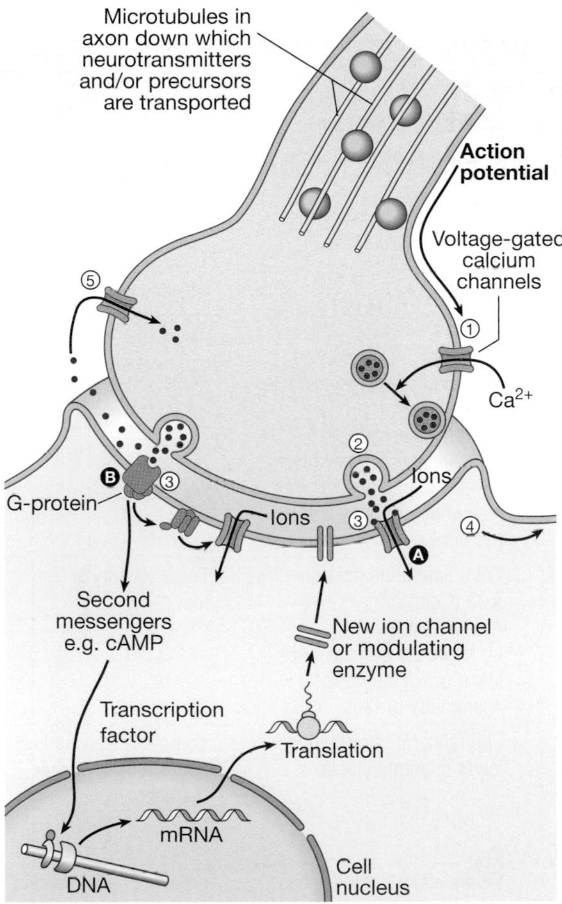

Fig. 26.2 Neurotransmission and neurotransmitters. (1) An action potential arriving at the nerve terminal depolarises the membrane and this opens voltage-gated calcium channels. (2) Entry of calcium causes the fusion of synaptic vesicles containing neurotransmitters with the pre-synaptic membrane and release of the neurotransmitter across the synaptic cleft. (3) The neurotransmitter binds to receptors on the post-synaptic membrane either (A) to open ligand-gated ion channels which, by allowing ion entry, depolarise the membrane and initiate an action potential (4), or (B) to bind to metabotrophic receptors that activate an effector enzyme (e.g. adenylyl cyclase) and thus modulate gene transcription via the intracellular second messenger system, leading to changes in synthesis of ion channels or modulating enzymes. (5) Neurotransmitters are taken up at the pre-synaptic membrane and/or metabolised. (cAMP = cyclic adenosine monophosphate; DNA = deoxyribonucleic acid; mRNA = messenger ribonucleic acid)

Functional anatomy of the nervous system

Major components of the nervous system and their interrelationships are depicted in Figure 26.3.

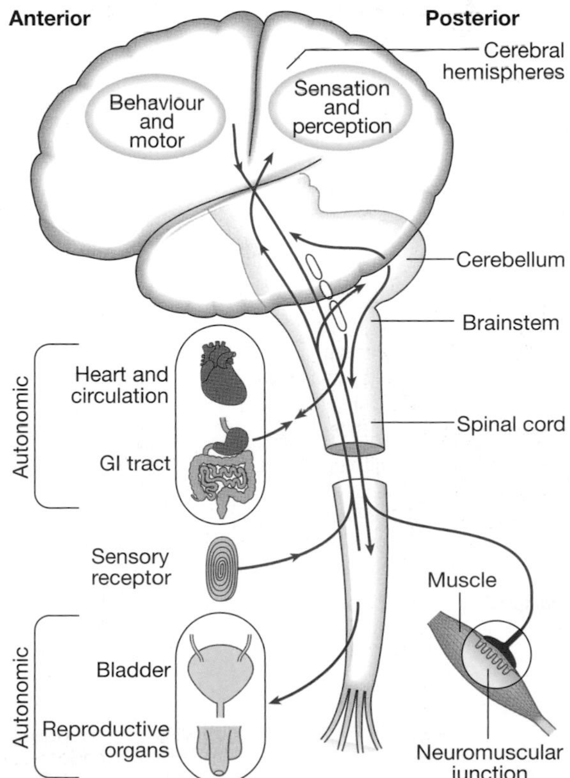

Fig. 26.3 The major anatomical components of the nervous system.

Cerebral hemispheres

The cerebral hemispheres coordinate the highest level of nervous function, the anterior half dealing with executive ('doing') functions and the posterior half constructing a perception of the environment. Each cerebral hemisphere has four functionally specialised lobes (Fig. 26.4 and Box 26.2), but some functions are lateralised, and this depends on cerebral dominance (i.e. the hemisphere in which language is represented). Cerebral dominance aligns limb dominance with language function: in right-handed individuals the left hemisphere is almost always dominant, while around half of left-handers have a dominant right hemisphere.

The frontal lobes are concerned with executive function, movement, behaviour and planning. In addition to the primary and supplementary motor cortex, there are specialised areas for the control of eye movements, speech (Broca's area) and micturition.

The parietal lobes integrate sensory perception. The primary sensory cortex lies in the post-central gyrus of the parietal lobe. Much of the remainder is devoted to 'association' cortex, which processes and interprets input from the various sensory modalities. The supramarginal and angular gyri of the dominant parietal lobe form part of the language area (p. 1169). Close to these are regions dealing with numerical function. The non-dominant parietal lobe is concerned with spatial awareness and orientation.

The temporal lobes contain the primary auditory cortex and primary vestibular cortex. On the inner medial sides lie the olfactory cortex and the parahippocampal cortex, which is involved in memory function. The temporal lobes also contain much of the limbic system, including the hippocampus and the amygdala, which are involved in memory and emotional processing. The dominant temporal lobe also participates in language functions, particularly verbal

26.2 Cortical lobar functions

		Effects of damage		
Lobe	**Function**	**Cognitive/behavioural**	**Associated physical signs**	**Positive phenomena**
Frontal	Personality Emotional control Social behaviour Contralateral motor control Language Micturition	Disinhibition Lack of initiation Antisocial behaviour Impaired memory Expressive dysphasia Incontinence	Impaired smell Contralateral hemiparesis Frontal release signs[1]	Seizures – often nocturnal with motor activity Versive head movements
Parietal: dominant	Language Calculation	Dysphasia Acalculia Dyslexia Apraxia[3] Agnosia[5]	Contralateral hemisensory loss Astereognosis[2] Agraphaesthesia[4] Contralateral homonymous lower quadrantanopia Asymmetry of optokinetic nystagmus (OKN)	Focal sensory seizures
Parietal: non-dominant	Spatial orientation Constructional skills	Neglect of contralateral side Spatial disorientation Constructional apraxia Dressing apraxia	Contralateral hemisensory loss Astereognosis[2] Agraphaesthesia[4] Contralateral homonymous lower quadrantanopia Asymmetry of OKN	Focal sensory seizures
Temporal: dominant	Auditory perception Language Verbal memory Smell Balance	Receptive aphasia Dyslexia Impaired verbal memory	Contralateral homonymous lower quadrantanopia	Complex hallucinations (smell, sound, vision, memory)
Temporal: non-dominant	Auditory perception Melody/pitch perception Non-verbal memory Smell Balance	Impaired non-verbal memory Impaired musical skills (tonal perception)	Contralateral homonymous upper quadrantanopia	Complex hallucinations (smell, sound, vision, memory)
Occipital	Visual processing	Visual inattention Visual loss Visual agnosia	Homonymous hemianopia (macular sparing)	Simple visual hallucinations (e.g. phosphenes, zigzag lines)

[1]Grasp reflex, palmomental response, pout response.
[2]Inability to determine three-dimensional shape by touch.
[3]Inability to perform complex movements in the presence of normal motor, sensory and cerebellar function.
[4]Inability to 'read' numbers or letters drawn on hand, with the eyes shut.
[5]Inability to recognise familiar objects, e.g. faces.

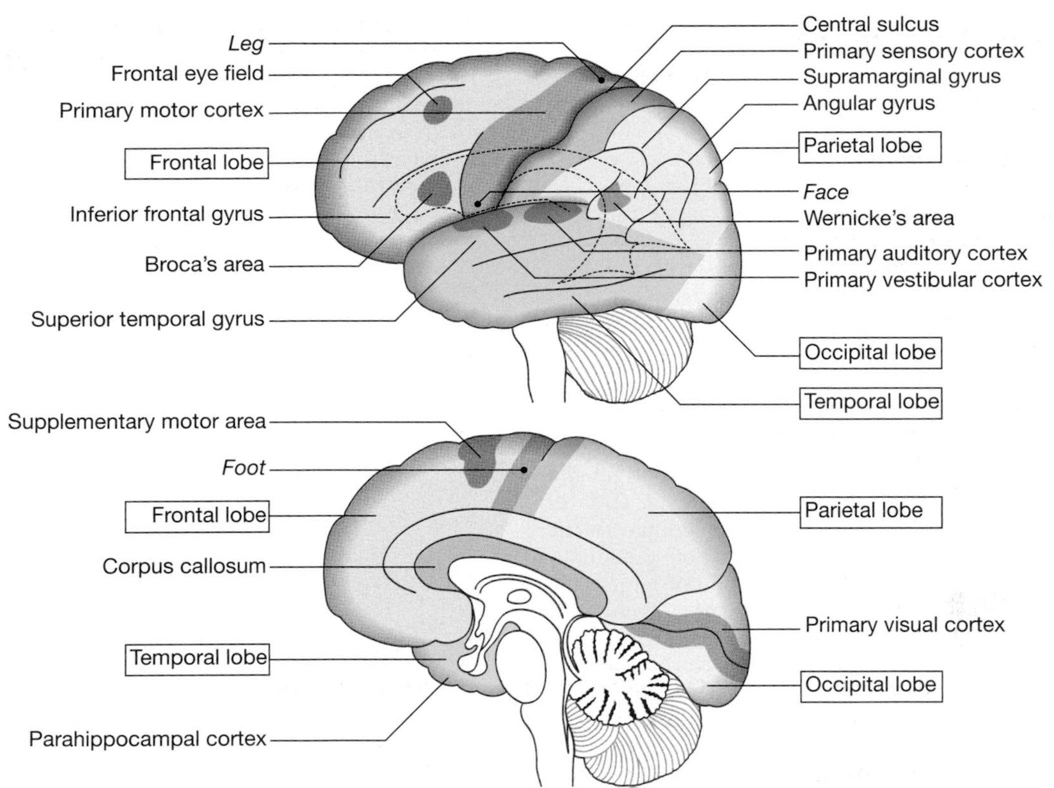

Fig. 26.4 The anatomy of the cerebral cortex.

comprehension (Wernicke's area). Musical processing occurs across both temporal lobes, rhythm on the dominant side and melody/pitch on the non-dominant.

The occipital lobes are responsible for visual interpretation. The contralateral visual hemifield is represented in each primary visual cortex, with surrounding areas processing specific visual submodalities such as colour, movement or depth, and the analysis of more complex visual patterns such as faces.

Deep to the grey matter in the cortices, and the white matter (composed of neuronal axons), are collections of cells known as the basal ganglia that are concerned with motor control; the thalamus, which is responsible for the level of attention to sensory perception; the limbic system, concerned with emotion and memory; and the hypothalamus, responsible for homeostasis, such as temperature and appetite control. The cerebral ventricles contain cerebrospinal fluid (CSF), which cushions the brain during cranial movement.

CSF is formed in the lateral ventricles and protects and nourishes the CNS. The CSF flows from third to fourth ventricles and through foramina in the brainstem to dissipate over the surface of the CNS, eventually being reabsorbed into the cerebral venous system (see Fig. 26.41, p. 1217).

The brainstem

In addition to containing all the sensory and motor pathways entering and leaving the hemispheres, the brainstem houses the nuclei and projections of the cranial nerves, as well as other important collections of neurons in the reticular formation (Fig. 26.5). Cranial nerve nuclei provide motor control to muscles of the head (including

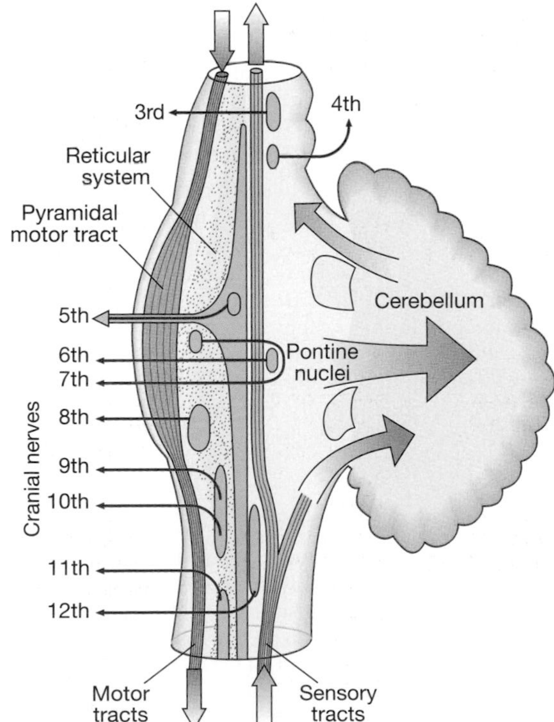

Fig. 26.5 Anatomy of the brainstem.

the face and eyes) and coordinate sensory input from the special sense organs and the face, nose, mouth, larynx and pharynx. They also relay autonomic messages, including pupillary, salivary and lacrimal functions. The reticular formation is predominantly involved in the control of conjugate eye movements, the maintenance of balance, cardiorespiratory control and the maintenance of arousal.

The spinal cord

The spinal cord is the route for virtually all communication between the extracranial structures and the CNS. Afferent and efferent fibres are grouped in discrete bundles but collections of cells in the grey matter are responsible for lower-order motor reflexes and the primary processing of sensory information, including pain.

Sensory peripheral nervous system

The sensory cell bodies of peripheral nerves are situated just outside the spinal cord, in the dorsal root ganglia in the spinal exit foramina, whilst the distal ends of their neurons utilise various specialised endings for the conversion of external stimuli into action potentials. Sensory nerves consist of a combination of large, fast, myelinated axons (which carry information about joint position sense and commands to muscles) and smaller, slower, unmyelinated axons (which carry information about pain and temperature, as well as autonomic function).

Motor peripheral nervous system

The anterior horns of the spinal cord comprise lower motor cell bodies. To increase conduction speed, peripheral motor nerve axons are wrapped in myelin produced by Schwann cells. Motor neurons release acetylcholine across the neuromuscular junction, which changes the muscle end-plate potential and initiates muscle contraction.

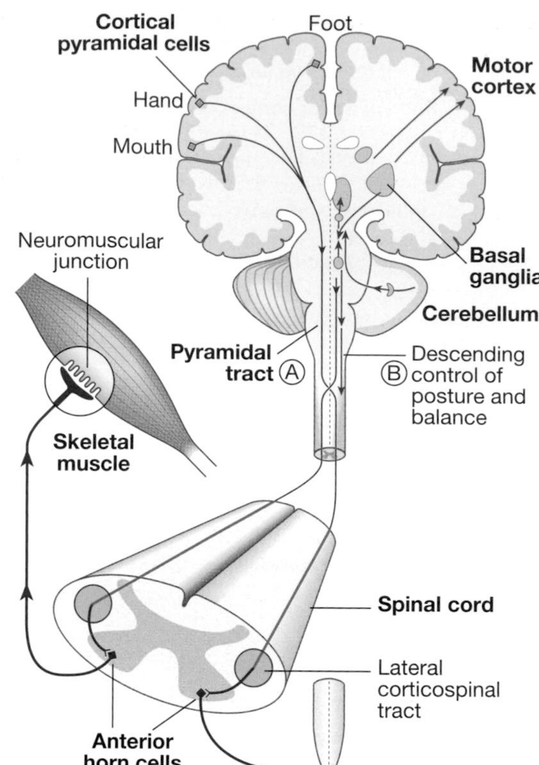

Fig. 26.6 The motor system. Neurons from the motor cortex descend as the pyramidal tract in the internal capsule and cerebral peduncle to the ventral brainstem, where most cross low in the medulla (A). In the spinal cord the upper motor neurons form the corticospinal tract in the lateral column before synapsing with the lower motor neurons in the anterior horns. The activity in the motor cortex is modulated by influences from the basal ganglia and cerebellum. Pathways descending from these structures control posture and balance (B).

The autonomic system

The autonomic system regulates the cardiovascular and respiratory systems, the smooth muscle of the gastrointestinal tract, and many exocrine and endocrine glands throughout the body. The autonomic system is controlled centrally by diffuse modulatory systems in the brainstem, limbic system, hypothalamus and frontal lobes, which are concerned with arousal and background behavioural responses to threat. Autonomic output divides functionally and pharmacologically into two divisions: the parasympathetic and sympathetic systems.

The motor system

A programme of movement formulated by the premotor cortex is converted into a series of signals in the motor cortex that are transmitted to the spinal cord in the pyramidal tract (Fig. 26.6). This passes through the internal capsule and the ventral brainstem before decussating in the medulla to enter the lateral columns of the spinal cord. The pyramidal tract 'upper motor neurons' synapse with the anterior horn cells of the spinal cord grey matter, which form the lower motor neurons.

Any movement necessitates changes in posture and muscle tone, sometimes in quite separate muscle groups to those involved in the actual movement. The motor system consists of a hierarchy of controls that maintain body posture and muscle tone, on which any movement is superimposed. In the grey matter of the spinal cord, the lowest order of the motor hierarchy controls reflex responses to stretch. Muscle spindles sense lengthening of the muscle; they provide the afferent side of the stretch reflex and initiate a monosynaptic reflex leading to protective or reactive muscle contraction. Inputs from the brainstem are largely inhibitory. Polysynaptic connections in the spinal cord grey matter control more complex reflex actions of flexion and extension of the limbs that form the basic building blocks of coordinated actions, but complete control requires input from the extrapyramidal system and the cerebellum.

Lower motor neurons

Lower motor neurons in the anterior horn of the spinal cord innervate a group of muscle fibres termed a 'motor unit'. Loss of lower motor neurons causes loss of contraction within this unit, resulting in weakness and reduced muscle tone. Subsequently, denervated muscle fibres atrophy, causing muscle wasting, and depolarise spontaneously, causing 'fibrillations'. Except in the tongue, these are usually only perceptible on electromyelography (EMG; p. 1152). With the passage of time, neighbouring intact neurons sprout to provide re-innervation, but the neuromuscular junctions of the enlarged motor units are unstable and depolarise spontaneously, causing fasciculations (which are large enough to be visible to the naked eye). Fasciculations therefore imply chronic partial denervation with re-innervation.

Upper motor neurons

Upper motor neurons have both inhibitory and excitatory influence on the function of anterior horn motor neurons. Lesions affecting the upper motor neuron result in increased tone, most evident in the strongest muscle groups (i.e. the extensors of the lower limbs and the flexors of the upper limbs). The weakness of upper motor neuron lesions is conversely more pronounced in the opposing muscle groups. Loss of inhibition will also lead to brisk reflexes and enhanced reflex patterns of movement, such as flexion withdrawal to noxious stimuli and spasms of extension. The increased tone is more apparent during rapid stretching ('spastic catch'), but may suddenly give way with sustained tension (the 'clasp-knife' phenomenon). More primitive reflexes are also released, manifest as extensor plantar responses. Spasticity may not be present until some weeks after the onset of an upper motor neuron lesion. Chronic spasticity in a patient with a spinal cord lesion may also be exacerbated by increased sensory input – for example, from a pressure sore or urinary tract infection.

The extrapyramidal system

Circuits between the basal ganglia and the motor cortex constitute the extrapyramidal system, which controls muscle tone, body posture and the initiation of movement (see Fig. 26.6). Lesions of the extrapyramidal system produce an increase in tone that, unlike spasticity, is continuous throughout the range of movement at any speed of stretch ('lead pipe' rigidity). Involuntary movements are also a feature of extrapyramidal lesions (p. 1165), and tremor in combination with rigidity produces typical 'cogwheel' rigidity. Extrapyramidal lesions also cause slowed and clumsy movements (bradykinesia), which characteristically reduce in size with repetition, as well as postural instability, which can precipitate falls.

The cerebellum

The cerebellum fine-tunes and coordinates movements initiated by the motor cortex. It also participates in the planning and learning of skilled movements through reciprocal connections with the thalamus and cortex, and in articulation of speech. A lesion in a cerebellar hemisphere causes lack of coordination on the same side of the body. Cerebellar dysfunction impairs the smoothness of eye movements, causing nystagmus and renders speech dysarthric. In the limbs, the initial movement is normal, but as the target is approached, the accuracy of the movement deteriorates, producing an 'intention tremor'. The distances of targets are misjudged (dysmetria), resulting in 'past-pointing'. The ability to produce rapid, accurate, regularly alternating movements is also impaired (dysdiadochokinesis). The central vermis of the cerebellum is concerned with the coordination of gait and posture. Disorders of this therefore produce a characteristic ataxic gait (see below).

Vision

The neurological organisation of visual pathways is shown in Figure 26.7. Fibres from ganglion cells in the retina pass to the optic disc and then backwards through the lamina cribrosa to the optic nerve. Nasal optic nerve fibres (subserving the temporal visual field) cross at the chiasm, but temporal fibres do not. Hence, fibres in each optic tract and further posteriorly carry representation of contralateral visual space. From the lateral geniculate nucleus, lower fibres pass through the temporal lobes on their way to the primary visual area in the occipital cortex, while the upper fibres pass through the parietal lobe.

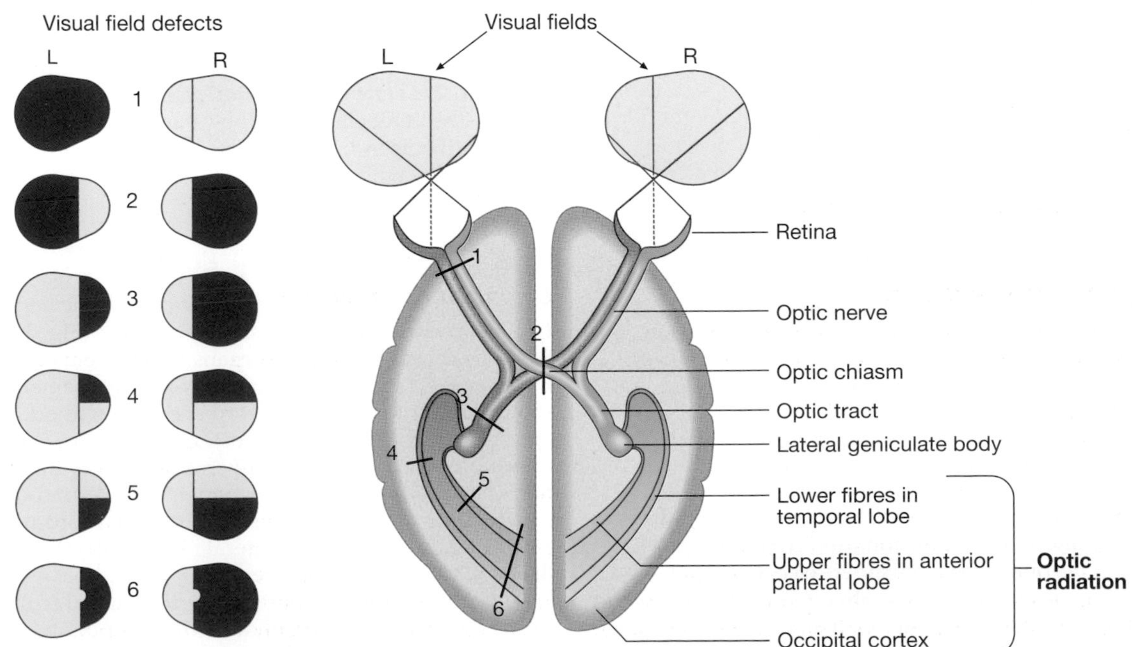

Fig. 26.7 Visual pathways and visual field defects. Schematic representation of eyes and brain in transverse section.

26

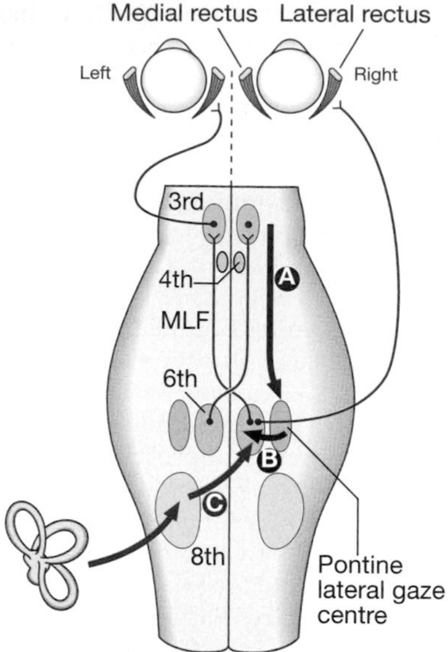

Fig. 26.8 Control of conjugate eye movements. Downward projections pass from the cortex to the pontine lateral gaze centre (A). The pontine gaze centre projects to the 6th cranial nerve nucleus (B), which innervates the ipsilateral lateral rectus and projects to the contralateral 3rd nerve nucleus (and hence medial rectus) via the medial longitudinal fasciculus (MLF). Tonic inputs from the vestibular apparatus (C) project to the contralateral 6th nerve nucleus via the vestibular nuclei.

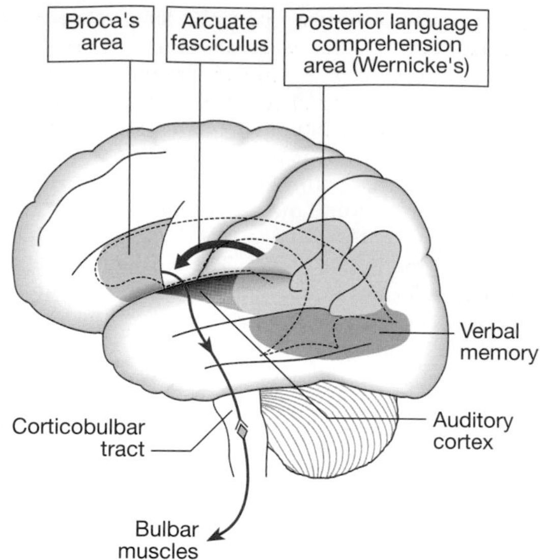

Fig. 26.9 Areas of the cerebral cortex involved in the generation of spoken language.

Normally, the eyes move conjugately (in unison), though horizontal convergence allows visual fusion of objects at different distances. The control of eye movements begins in the cerebral hemispheres, particularly within the frontal eye fields, and the pathway then descends to the brainstem with input from the visual cortex, superior colliculus and cerebellum. Horizontal and vertical gaze centres in the pons and mid-brain, respectively, coordinate output to the ocular motor nerve nuclei (3, 4 and 6), which are connected to each other by the medial longitudinal fasciculus (MLF) (Fig. 26.8). The MLF is particularly important in coordinating horizontal movements of the eyes. The extraocular muscles are then supplied by the oculomotor (3rd), trochlear (4th) and abducens (6th) cranial nerves.

The pupillary response to light is due to a combination of parasympathetic and sympathetic activity. Parasympathetic fibres originate in the Edinger–Westphal subnucleus of the 3rd nerve, and pass with the 3rd nerve to synapse in the ciliary ganglion before supplying the constrictor pupillae of the iris. Sympathetic fibres originate in the hypothalamus, pass down the brainstem and cervical spinal cord to emerge at T1, return up to the eye in association with the internal carotid artery, and supply the dilator pupillae.

Speech

Much of the cerebral cortex is involved in the process of forming and interpreting communicating sounds, especially in the dominant hemisphere (see Box 26.2, p. 1142). Decoding of speech sounds (phonemes) is carried out in the upper part of the posterior temporal lobe. The attribution of meaning, as well as the formulation of the language required for the expression of ideas and concepts, occurs predominantly in the lower parts of the anterior parietal lobe (the angular and supramarginal gyri). The temporal speech comprehension region is referred to as Wernicke's area (Fig. 26.9). Other parts of the temporal lobe contribute to verbal memory, where lexicons of meaningful words are 'stored'. Parts of the non-dominant parietal lobe appear to contribute to non-verbal aspects of language in recognising meaningful intonation patterns (prosody).

The frontal language area is in the posterior end of the dominant inferior frontal gyrus known as Broca's area. This receives input from the temporal and parietal lobes via the arcuate fasciculus. The motor commands generated in Broca's area pass to the cranial nerve nuclei in the pons and medulla, as well as to the anterior horn cells in the spinal cord. Nerve impulses to the lips, tongue, palate, pharynx, larynx and respiratory muscles result in the series of ordered sounds recognised as speech. The cerebellum also plays an important role in coordinating speech, and lesions of the cerebellum lead to dysarthria, where the problem lies in motor articulation of speech.

The somatosensory system

Sensory information from the limbs ascends the nervous system in two anatomically discrete systems (Fig. 26.10). Fibres from proprioceptive organs and those mediating well-localised touch (including vibration) enter the spinal cord at the posterior horn and pass without synapsing into the ipsilateral posterior columns. Neural fibres conveying pain and temperature sensory information (nociceptive neurons) synapse with second-order neurons that cross the midline in the spinal cord before ascending in the contralateral anterolateral spinothalamic tract to the brainstem.

The second-order neurons of the dorsal column sensory system cross the midline in the upper medulla to ascend through the brainstem. Here they lie just medial to the (already crossed) spinothalamic pathway.

Brainstem lesions can therefore cause sensory loss affecting all modalities of the contralateral side of the body. Sensory loss on the face due to brainstem lesions is dependent on the anatomy of the trigeminal fibres within the brainstem. Fibres from the back of the face (near the ears) descend within the brainstem to the upper part of the spinal cord before synapsing, the second-order neurons crossing the midline and then ascending with the spinothalamic fibres. Fibres conveying sensation from progressively more forward areas of the face descend a shorter distance in the brainstem. Thus, sensory loss in the face from low brainstem lesions is in a 'balaclava helmet' distribution, as the longer descending trigeminal fibres are affected. Both the dorsal column and spinothalamic tracts end in the thalamus, relaying from there to the parietal cortex.

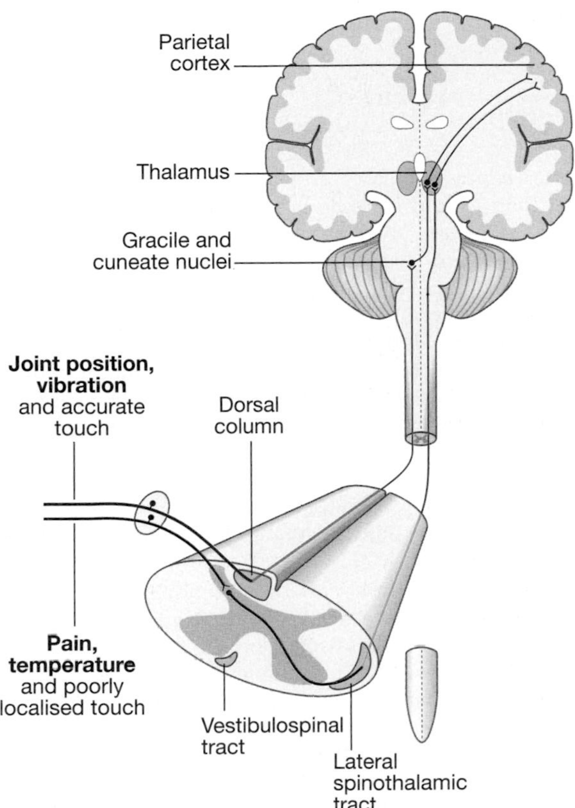

Fig. 26.10 The main somatic sensory pathways.

Pain

Pain is a complex percept that is only partly related to activity in nociceptor neurons (Fig. 26.11). In the posterior horn of the spinal cord, the second-order neuron of the spinothalamic tract is affected by a number of influences in addition to its synapse with the fibres from nociceptors. Branches from the larger mechanoceptor fibres destined for the posterior column also synapse with the second-order spinothalamic neurons and with interneurons of the grey matter of the posterior horn. The nociceptor neurons release neurotransmitters (such as substance P), in addition to excitatory transmitters, which influence the excitability of the spinothalamic neurons. Activity in the posterior horn neurons is modulated by fibres descending from the peri-aqueductal grey matter of the mid-brain and raphe nuclei of the medulla. Neurons of this 'descending analgesia system' are activated by endogenous opiate (endorphin) peptides. The spinal cord's posterior horn is therefore much more than a relay station in pain transmission; its complexity allows it to 'gate' and modulate painful sensation before it ascends in the spinothalamic tract. In the diencephalon, the perception of pain is further influenced by the rich interconnections of the thalamus with the limbic system.

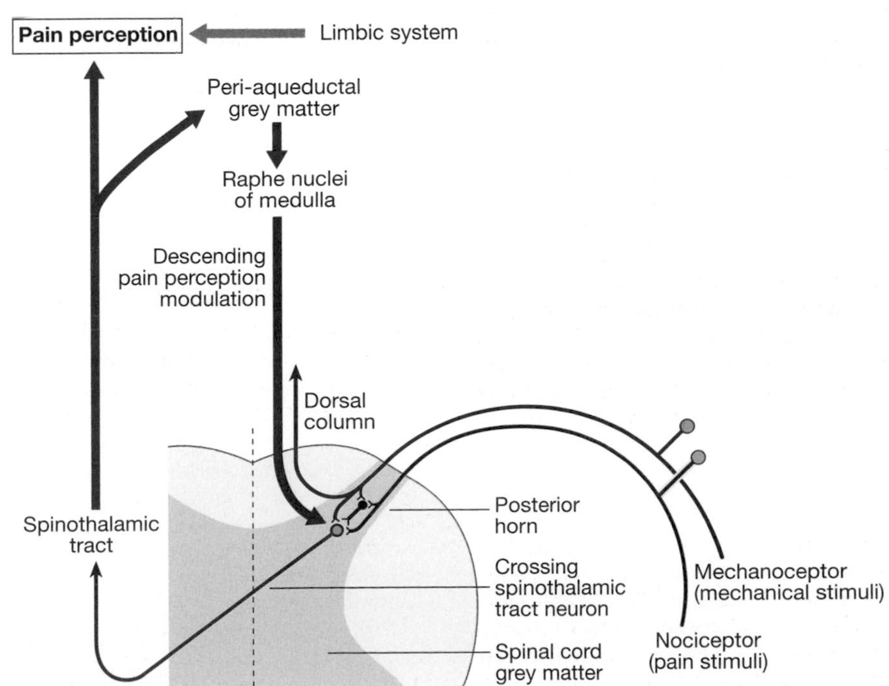

Fig. 26.11 The pain perception system.

Sphincter control

The sympathetic supply to the bladder leaves from T11–L2 to synapse in the inferior hypogastric plexus, while the parasympathetic supply leaves from S2–4. In addition, a somatic supply to the external (voluntary) sphincter arises from S2–4, travelling via the pudendal nerves.

Storage of urine is maintained by inhibiting parasympathetic activity and thus relaxing the detrusor muscle of the bladder wall. Continence is maintained by simultaneous sympathetic and somatic (via the pudendal nerve) mediated tonic contraction of the urethral sphincters. Voiding is usually under conscious control, and triggered by relaxation of tonic inhibition on the pontine micturition centre from higher centres, leading to relaxation of the pelvic floor muscles and external and internal urethral sphincters, along with parasympathetic-mediated detrusor contraction.

Personality and mood

The physiology and pathology of mood disorders are discussed elsewhere (Ch. 10) but it is important to remember that any process affecting brain function will have some effect on mood and affect. Conversely, mood disorder will have a significant effect on perception and function. It can be difficult to disentangle whether psychological and psychiatric changes are the cause or the effect of any neurological symptoms.

Sleep

The function of sleep is unknown but it is required for good health. Sleep is controlled by the reticular activating system in the upper brainstem and diencephalon. It is composed of different stages that can be visualised on electroencephalography (EEG). As drowsiness occurs, normal EEG background alpha rhythm disappears and activity becomes dominated by deepening slow-wave activity. As sleep deepens and dreaming begins, the limbs become flaccid, movements are 'blocked' and EEG signs of rapid eye movements (REM) are superimposed on the slow wave. REM sleep persists for a short spell before another slow-wave spell starts, the cycle repeating several times throughout the night. REM periods become longer as the sleep period progresses. REM sleep seems to be the most important part of the sleep cycle for refreshing cognitive processes, and REM sleep deprivation causes tiredness, irritability and impaired judgement.

Localising lesions in the brainstem

After taking a history and examining the patient, the clinician should have an idea of the nature and site of any pathology. Given the density of tracts and nuclei in the brainstem (see Fig. 26.5), detailed localisation may be possible on the basis of history and examination alone, to be confirmed or refuted by investigation.

Brainstem lesions typically present with symptoms due to cranial nerve, cerebellar and upper motor neuron dysfunction and are most commonly caused by vascular disease. Since the anatomy of the brainstem is very precisely organised, it is usually possible to localise the site of a lesion on the basis of careful history and examination in order to determine exactly which tracts/nuclei are affected, usually invoking the fewest number of lesions.

For example, in a patient presenting with sudden onset of upper motor neuron features affecting the right face, arm and leg in association with a left 3rd nerve palsy, the lesion will be in the left cerebral peduncle in the brainstem and the pathology is likely to have been a small stroke, as the onset was sudden. This combination of signs is known as Weber's syndrome, and is one of several well-described brainstem syndromes, which are listed in Box 26.3. The effects of individual cranial nerve deficits are discussed in the sections on eye movements (p. 1169) and on facial weakness, sensory loss in brainstem lesions, dysphonia and dysarthria, and bulbar symptoms (pp. 1163, 1165, 1168 and 1173).

26.3 Major focal brainstem syndromes

Name of syndrome	Site of lesions	Clinical features
Weber	Anterior cerebral peduncle (mid-brain)	Ipsilateral 3rd palsy Contralateral upper motor neuron 7th palsy Contralateral hemiplegia
Claude	Cerebral peduncle Involving red nucleus	Ipsilateral 3rd palsy Contralateral cerebellar signs
Parinaud	Dorsal mid-brain (tectum)	Vertical gaze palsy Convergence disorders Convergence retraction nystagmus Pupillary and lid disorders
Millard–Gubler	Ponto-medullary junction	Ipsilateral 6th palsy Ipsilateral lower motor neuron 7th palsy Contralateral hemiplegia
Wallenberg	Lateral medulla	Ipsilateral 5th, 9th, 10th, 11th palsy Ipsilateral Horner's syndrome Ipsilateral cerebellar signs Contralateral spinothalamic sensory loss Vestibular disturbance

INVESTIGATION OF NEUROLOGICAL DISEASE

Experienced clinicians will make around 90% of neurological diagnoses on history alone, with a lesser contribution from examination and investigation. As investigations become more complex and more easily available, it is tempting to adopt a 'scan first, think later' approach to neurology. The frequency of 'false-positive' results, the wide range of normality and the unnecessary expense, inconvenience and worry caused to patients should encourage a more thoughtful approach. Investigation may include assessment of structure (imaging) and function (neurophysiology). Neurophysiological testing has become so complex that in many countries it constitutes a separate specialty focusing on electroencephalography, evoked potentials, nerve conduction studies and electromyography.

Neuroimaging

Neurological imaging has traditionally allowed assessment of structure only. Various techniques are available, including X-rays (plain X-rays, computed tomography (CT), CT angiography, myelography and angiography), magnetic resonance (MR imaging (MRI), MR angiography (MRA)) and ultrasound (Doppler imaging of blood vessels). The uses and limitations of each of these are shown in Box 26.4.

It is now possible to use imaging techniques to assess CNS function. Single photon emission clinical tomography (SPECT) scanning can use the lipid-soluble properties of radioactive tracers to mark cerebral blood flow at the time of injection. This can be useful in investigating dementia or epilepsy. SPECT can also be used in the diagnosis of movement disorders: for example, by examining dopamine activity to assess the function of the basal ganglia in patients with possible parkinsonism.

Functional MRI (fMRI) can be used to assess blood flow during specific tasks (e.g. speaking, remembering, calculation), which can provide 'maps' of cortical function that are accurate enough to help plan lesionectomy and epilepsy surgery. Similarly, MR spectroscopy is being developed to identify the chemical composition of specific regions, providing clues as to whether lesions are ischaemic, neoplastic or inflammatory.

Head and orbit

Plain skull X-rays are now largely restricted to the diagnosis of fractures and sinus disease. CT or MRI is needed for intracranial imaging. CT will show bone and calcification well, and will easily image collections of blood. It will also detect abnormalities of the brain and ventricles, such as atrophy, tumours, cysts, abscesses, vascular lesions and hydrocephalus. Diagnostic yield is often improved by the use of intravenous contrast and thinner slicing using spiral CT. Surrounding bone structures render posterior fossa CT images less useful, and CT is less sensitive to white matter changes than MRI.

MRI resolution is unaffected by bone and so is more useful in the investigation of posterior fossa disease. Its sensitivity to cortical and white matter changes makes it effective in picking up inflammatory conditions such as multiple sclerosis, and in investigating epilepsy.

26.4 Imaging techniques for the nervous system

Technique	Applications	Advantages	Disadvantages	Comments
X-ray/CT	Plain X-rays, CT, CTA Radiculography Myelography Intra-arterial angiography	Widely available Relatively cheap Relatively quick	Ionising radiation Contrast reactions Invasive (myelography and angiography)	X-rays: used for fractures or foreign bodies CT: first line for stroke Intra-arterial angiography: gold standard for vascular lesions
MRI	Structural imaging MRA Functional MRI MR spectroscopy	High-quality soft tissue images, useful for posterior fossa and temporal lobes No ionising radiation Non-invasive	Expensive Less widely available MRA images blood flow, not vessel anatomy Claustrophobic Pacemakers contraindicate MRI Contrast (gadolinium) reactions	Functional MR and spectroscopy: mainly research tools
Ultrasound	Doppler Duplex scans	Cheap Quick Non-invasive	Operator-dependent Poor anatomical definition	Screening tool to assess need for carotid endarterectomy
Radio-isotope	Isotope brain scan SPECT PET	In vivo imaging of functional anatomy (ligand binding, blood flow)	Poor spatial resolution Ionising radiation Expensive Not widely available	Isotope scans obsolete. SPECT: useful in movement disorders, epilepsy and dementias PET: mainly research tool

(CT = computed tomography; CTA = computed tomographic angiography; MRA = magnetic resonance angiography; MRI = magnetic resonance imaging; PET = positron emission tomography; SPECT = single photon emission clinical tomography)

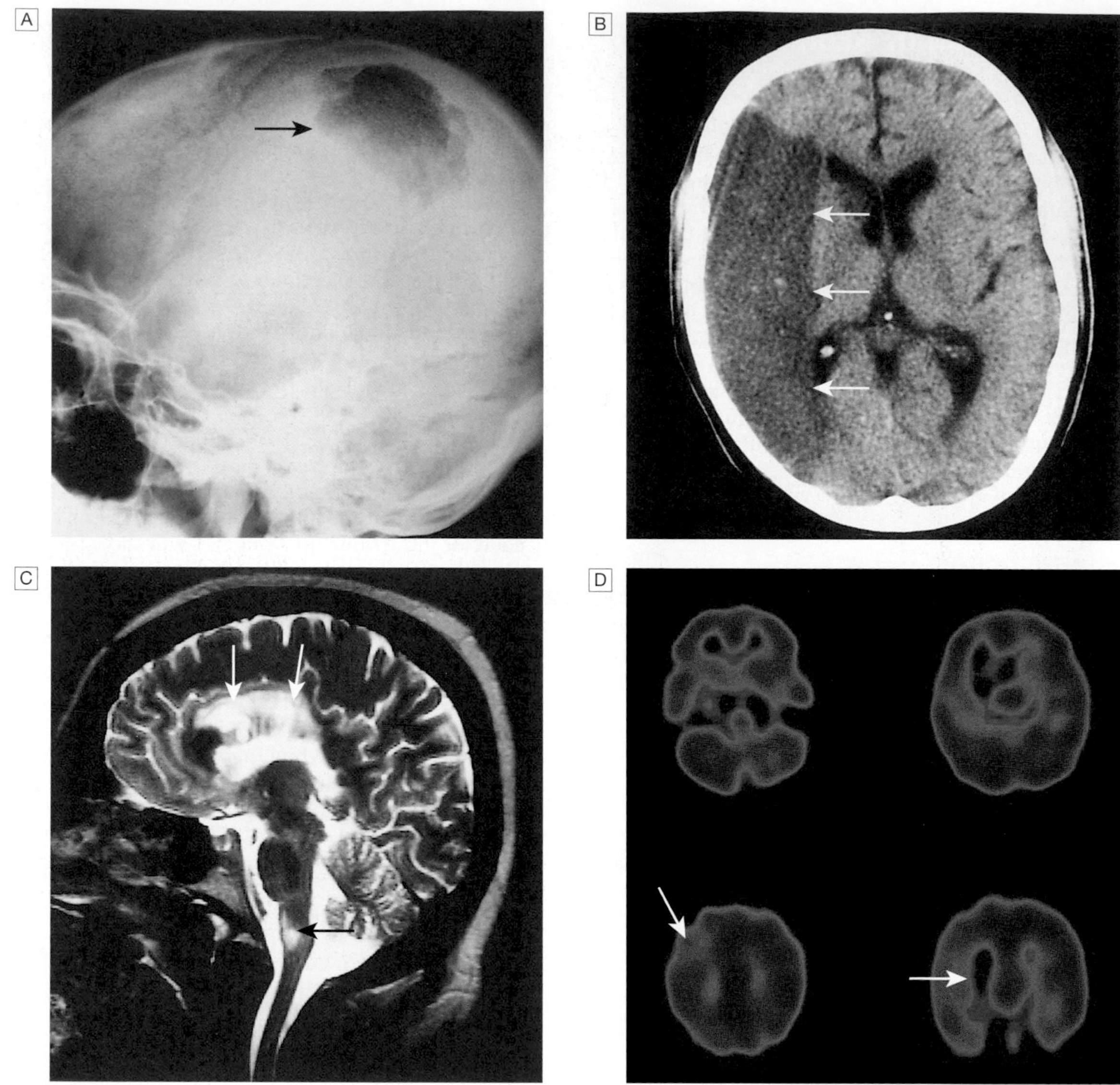

Fig. 26.12 Different techniques of imaging the head and brain. **A** Skull X-ray showing lytic skull lesion (eosinophilic granuloma – arrow). **B** CT showing complete middle cerebral artery infarct (arrows). **C** MRI showing widespread areas of high signal in multiple sclerosis (arrows). **D** SPECT after caudate infarct showing relative hypoperfusion of overlying right cerebral cortex (arrows).

Different MRI techniques will increase sensitivity to acute ischaemic stroke and may allow detection of abnormalities by filtering signals from other tissues (e.g. adipose tissues in the orbits).

Examples of brain imaged by the various techniques are shown in Figure 26.12.

Cervical, thoracic and lumbar spine

Plain X-rays are useful in the investigation of trauma to vertebrae, but their value in providing information about non-bony tissues is limited, which makes them far less helpful in the assessment of inflammatory and degenerative conditions of the spine. MRI has transformed the investigation of these areas, since it can give information not only about the vertebrae and intervertebral discs, but also about their effects on the spinal cord and nerve roots. Myelography is an invasive technique involving injection of contrast into the lumbar theca. While the outline of the nerve roots and spinal cord provides information about abnormal structure, the accuracy and wide availability of MRI have reduced the need for this. Myelography may still be used for technical reasons or where MRI is unavailable, contraindicated, or precluded by the patient's claustrophobia. Examples of the cervical spine imaged by plain X-rays, myelography and MRI are shown in Figure 26.13.

Blood vessels

Imaging of the extra- and intracranial blood vessels and disturbance of arterial or venous blood flow is described in Chapter 27.

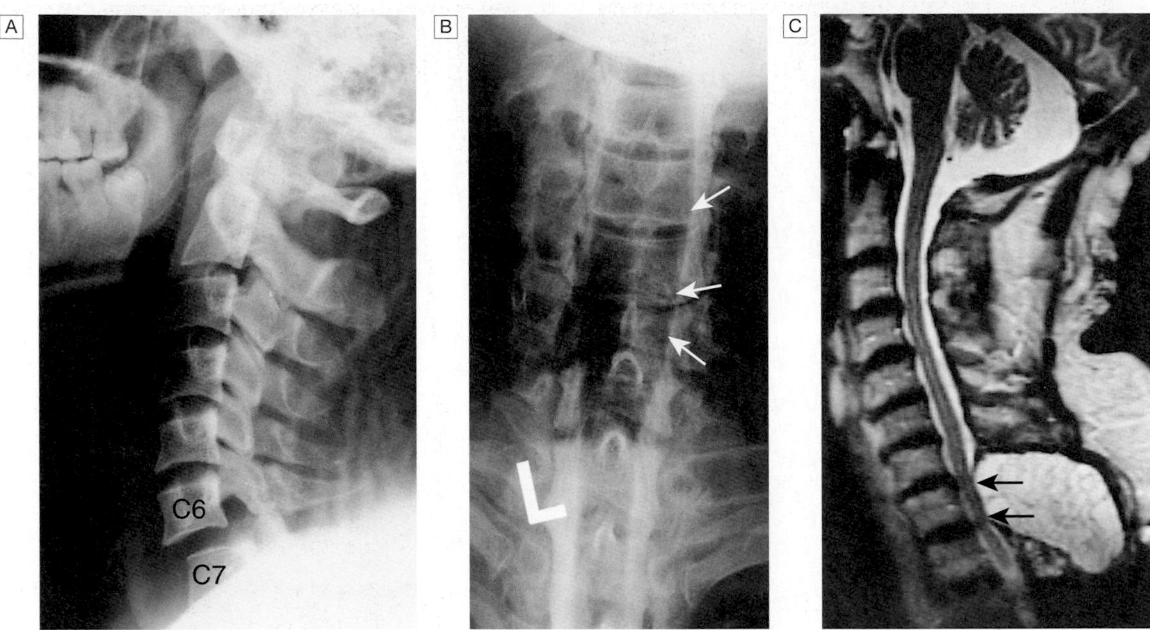

Fig. 26.13 Different techniques of imaging the cervical spine. **A** Lateral X-ray showing bilateral C6/7 facet dislocation. **B** Myelogram showing widening of cervical cord due to astrocytoma (arrows). **C** MRI showing posterior epidural compression from adenocarcinomatous metastasis to the posterior arch of T1 (arrows).

Neurophysiological testing

Electroencephalography

The electroencephalogram (EEG) is used to detect electrical activity arising in the cerebral cortex. The EEG involves placing electrodes on the scalp to record the amplitude and frequency of the resulting waveforms. With closed eyes, the normal background activity is 8–13 Hz (known as alpha rhythm), most prominent occipitally and suppressed on eye opening. Other frequency bands seen over different parts of the brain in different circumstances are beta (faster than 13/s), theta (4–8/s) and delta (slower than 4/s). Normal EEG changes evolve with age and with alertness; lower frequencies predominate in the very young and during sleep.

In recent years, digital technology has allowed longer, cleaner EEG recordings that can be analysed in a number of ways and recorded alongside contemporaneous video of any clinical 'event'. Meanwhile, the development of intracranial recording allows more sensitive monitoring via surgically placed electrodes in and around lesions to help increase the efficacy and improve the safety of epilepsy surgery.

Abnormalities in the EEG result from a number of conditions. Examples include an increase in fast frequencies (beta) seen with sedating drugs such as benzodiazepines, or marked focal slowing noted over a structural lesion such as a tumour or an infarct. Improved quality and accessibility of imaging have made EEG redundant in lesion localisation, except in the specialist investigation of epilepsy (p. 1182). EEG remains useful in progressive and continuous disorders such as reduced consciousness (p. 1159), in encephalitis (p. 1205), and in certain dementias such as Creutzfeldt–Jakob disease (p. 1211).

Since sleep induces marked changes in cerebral activity, EEG can be useful in characterising those conditions where sleep patterns are disturbed. In paroxysmal disorders such as epilepsy, EEG is at its most useful when it captures activity during one of the events in question. Up to 5% of some normal populations may demonstrate epileptiform discharges on EEG which prevent its use as a screening test for epilepsy. Over 50% of patients with proven epilepsy will have a normal 'routine' EEG, and, conversely, the presence of epileptiform features does not of itself make a diagnosis (most notably in younger patients with a family history of epilepsy). In view of this, the EEG should not be used where epilepsy is merely 'suspected'.

The EEG in epilepsy is predominantly used in its classification and prognosis, and in some patients to localise the seat of epileptiform discharges when surgery is being considered. During an epileptic seizure, high-voltage disturbances of background activity ('discharges') will often be noted. These may be generalised, as in the 3-Hz 'spike and wave' of childhood absence epilepsy, or more focal, as in localisation-related epilepsies (Fig. 26.14). Techniques such as hyperventilation or photic stimulation can be used to increase the yield of epileptiform changes, particularly in the generalised epilepsy syndromes. While some argue that it is possible to detect 'spikes' and 'sharp waves' to lend support to a clinical diagnosis, these are non-specific and therefore not diagnostic.

Nerve conduction studies

Electrical stimulation of a nerve causes an impulse to travel both efferently and afferently along the

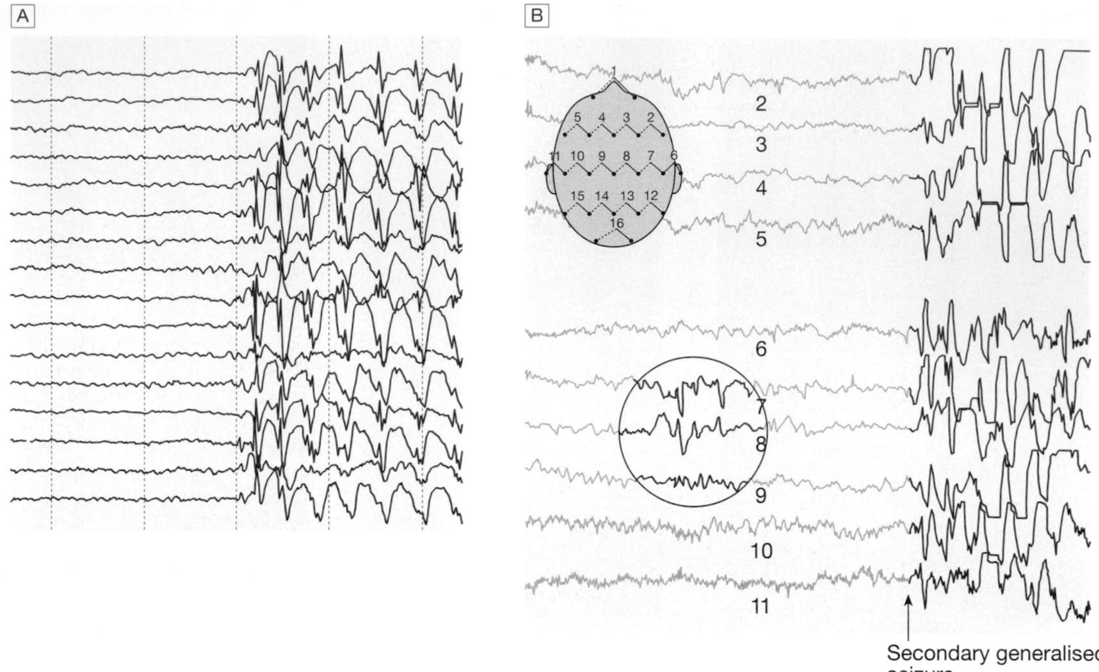

Fig. 26.14 EEGs in epilepsy. **A** Generalised epileptic discharge, as seen in epilepsy syndromes such as childhood absence or juvenile myoclonic epilepsy. **B** Focal sharp waves over the right parietal region (circled), with spread of discharge to cause a generalised tonic–clonic seizure.

underlying axons. Nerve conduction studies (NCS) make use of this, recording action potentials as they pass along peripheral nerves and (with motor nerves) as they pass into the muscle belly. Digital recording has enhanced sensitivity and reproducibility of these tiny potentials. By measuring the time taken to traverse a known distance, it is possible to calculate nerve conduction velocities (NCVs). Healthy nerves at room temperature will conduct at a speed of 40–50 m/s. If the recorded potential is smaller than expected, this provides evidence of a reduction in the overall number of functioning axons. Significant slowing of conduction velocity, in contrast, suggests impaired saltatory conduction due to peripheral nerve demyelination. Such changes in NCS may be diffuse (as in a hereditary demyelinating peripheral neuropathy, p. 1223), focal (as in pressure palsies, p. 1224) or multifocal (e.g. Guillain–Barré syndrome, p. 1224; mononeuritis multiplex, p. 1224). The information gained can allow the disease responsible for peripheral nerve dysfunction to be better deduced (see Box 26.99, p. 1223).

Stimulation of motor nerves allows for the recording of compound muscle action potentials (CMAPs) over muscles (Fig. 26.15). These are around 500 times larger than sensory nerve potentials, typically around 1–20 millivolts. Since a proportion of stimulated impulses in motor nerves will 'reflect' back to the anterior horn cell body (forming the 'F' wave), it is also possible to obtain some information about the condition of nerve roots.

Repetitive nerve stimulation (RNS) at 3–15/s provides consistent CMAPs in healthy muscle. In myasthenia gravis (p. 1226), where there is partial blockage of acetylcholine receptors, however, there is a diagnostic fall (decrement) in CMAP amplitude. In contrast, an increasing CMAP with high-frequency RNS is seen in Lambert–Eaton myasthenic syndrome (p. 1227).

Electromyography

Electromyography (EMG) is usually performed with NCS, and involves needle recording of muscle electrical potential during rest and contraction. At rest, muscle is electrically silent but loss of nerve supply causes muscle membrane to become unstable, manifest as fibrillations, positive sharp waves ('spontaneous activity') or fasciculations. During muscle contraction, motor unit action potentials are recorded. Axonal loss or destruction will result in fewer motor units. Resultant sprouting of remaining units will lead to increasing size of each individual unit on EMG. Myopathy, in contrast, will cause muscle fibre splitting, which will result in a large number of smaller units on EMG. Other abnormal activity, such as myotonic discharges, may signify abnormal ion channel conduction, as in myotonic dystrophy or myotonia congenita.

Specialised single fibre EMG (SFEMG) can be used to investigate neuromuscular junction transmission. Measuring 'jitter' and 'blocking' can identify the effect of antibodies in reducing the action of acetylcholine on the receptor.

Evoked potentials

The cortical response to visual, auditory or electrical stimulation can be measured on an EEG as an evoked potential (EP). If a stimulus is provided – for example, to the eye – the tiny EEG response can be discerned when averaging 100–1000 repeated stimuli. Assessing the latency (the time delay) and amplitude can give information about the integrity of the relevant pathway.

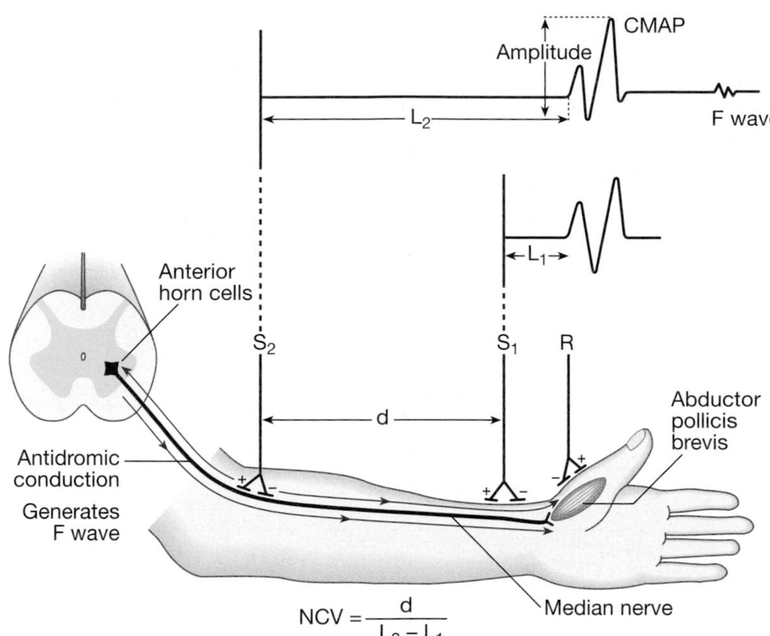

Fig. 26.15 Motor nerve conduction tests. Electrodes (R) on the muscle (abductor pollicis here) record the compound muscle action potential (CMAP) after stimulation at the median nerve at the wrist (S_1) and from the elbow (S_2). The velocity from elbow to wrist can be determined if the distance between the two stimulating electrodes (d) is known. A prolonged L_1 (L = latency) would be caused by dysfunction distally in the median nerve (e.g. in carpal tunnel syndrome). A prolonged L_2 is caused by slow nerve conduction (as in demyelinating neuropathy). The F wave is a small delayed response that appears when the electrical signal travels backwards to the anterior horn cell, sparking a second action potential in a minority of fibres (see text). (NCV = nerve conduction velocity)

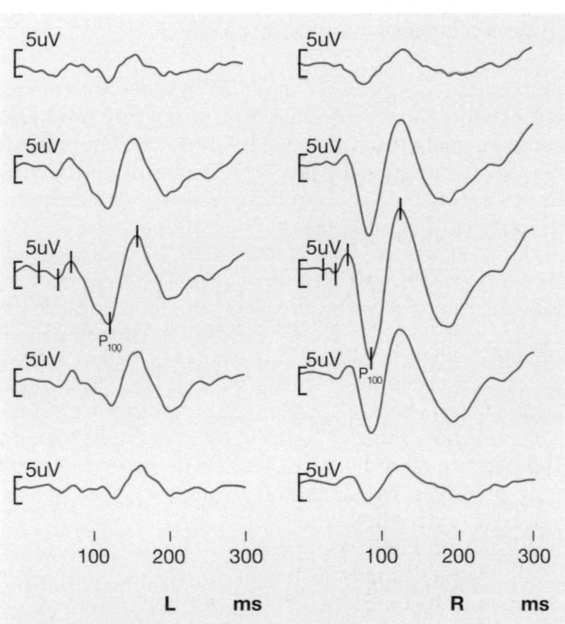

Fig. 26.16 Visual evoked responses (VER) recording. The abnormality is in the left hemisphere, with delay in latency and a reduction in signal of the P_{100}.

MRI now provides more information about CNS pathways, thus reducing reliance on EPs. In practice, visual evoked potentials (VEPs) are most commonly used to help differentiate CNS demyelination from small-vessel white-matter changes (Fig. 26.16).

Magnetic stimulation

Central conduction times can also be measured using electromagnetic induction of action potentials in the cortex or spinal cord by the local application of specialised coils. Again, MRI has made this largely redundant, other than for research.

Routine blood tests

Many systemic conditions that can affect the nervous system can be identified by simple blood tests. Nutritional deficiencies, metabolic disturbances, inflammatory conditions, or infections may all present or be associated with neurological symptoms, and basic blood tests (full blood count, erythrocyte sedimentation rate, C-reactive protein, biochemical screening) may provide clues. Specific blood tests will be highlighted in the relevant subsections of this chapter.

Immunological tests

Recent developments have seen a host of new immune-mediated conditions emerge in clinical neurology, with effects ranging from muscle and neuromuscular junction disturbance (causing weakness and muscle pain) to specific neuronal ion channels (causing cognitive decline, epilepsy and psychiatric changes). The last decade has seen the identification of many causative antibodies (see Boxes 26.62 and 26.63, p. 1194), and it is likely that further conditions will turn out to have an immune basis.

Genetic testing

An increasing number of inherited neurological conditions can now be diagnosed by DNA analysis (p. 60). These include diseases caused by increased numbers of trinucleotide repeats, such as Huntington's disease (p. 1198), myotonic dystrophy (p. 1228) and some types of spinocerebellar ataxia (p. 1199). Mitochondrial DNA can also be sequenced to diagnose relevant disorders (p. 60).

Lumbar puncture

Lumbar puncture (LP) is the technique used to obtain a CSF sample and provides an indirect measure of intracranial pressure. After local anaesthetic injection, a needle is inserted between lumbar spinous processes

26.5 How to interpret CSF results

	Normal	Subarachnoid haemorrhage	Acute bacterial meningitis	Viral meningitis	Tuberculous meningitis	Multiple sclerosis
Pressure	50–250 mm of water	Increased	Normal/ increased	Normal	Normal/increased	Normal
Colour	Clear	Blood-stained Xanthochromic	Cloudy	Clear	Clear/cloudy	Clear
Red cell count ($\times 10^6$/L)	0–4	Raised	Normal	Normal	Normal	Normal
White cell count ($\times 10^6$/L)	0–4	Normal/slightly raised	1000–5000 polymorphs	10–2000 lymphocytes	50–5000 lymphocytes	0–50 lymphocytes
Glucose	> 50–60% of blood level	Normal	Decreased	Normal	Decreased	Normal
Protein	< 0.45 g/L	Increased	Increased	Normal/ increased	Increased	Normal/ increased
Microbiology	Sterile	Sterile	Organisms on Gram stain and/or culture	Sterile/virus detected	Ziehl–Nielson/auramine stain or tuberculosis culture positive	Sterile
Oligoclonal bands	Negative	Negative	Can be positive	Can be positive	Can be positive	Often positive

(usually between L3 and L4) through the dura and into the spinal canal. Intracranial pressure can be deduced (if patients are lying on their side) and CSF removed for analysis. CSF pressure measurement is important in the diagnosis and monitoring of idiopathic intracranial hypertension (p. 1217). In this condition, the LP itself is therapeutic.

CSF is normally clear and colourless, and the tests that are usually performed include a naked eye examination of the CSF and centrifugation to determine the colour of the supernatant (yellow, or xanthochromic, some hours after subarachnoid haemorrhage (p. 1246). Routine analysis will involve a cell count, as well as assay of glucose and protein.

CSF assessment is important in investigating infections (meningitis or encephalitis), subarachnoid haemorrhage and inflammatory conditions (multiple sclerosis, sarcoidosis and cerebral lupus). Normal values and abnormalities found in specific conditions are shown in Box 26.5.

More sophisticated analysis allows measurement of antibody formation solely within the CNS (oligoclonal bands), genetic analysis (e.g. polymerase chain reaction (PCR) for herpes simplex or tuberculosis), immunological tests (paraneoplastic antibodies) and cytology (to detect malignant cells).

If there is a cranial space-occupying lesion causing raised intracranial pressure, LP presents a theoretical risk of downward shift of intracerebral contents, a potentially fatal process known as coning (p. 1212). Consequently, LP is contraindicated if there is any clinical suggestion of raised intracranial pressure (papilloedema), depressed level of consciousness, or focal neurological signs suggesting a cerebral lesion, until imaging (by CT or MRI) has excluded a space-occupying lesion or hydrocephalus. When there is a risk of local haemorrhage (thrombocytopenia, disseminated intravascular coagulation or anticoagulant treatment), then caution should be exercised or specific measures should be taken. LP can be safely performed in patients on antiplatelet drugs or low-dose heparin, but may be unsafe in patients who are fully anticoagulated due to the increased risk of epidural haematoma.

About 30% of LPs are followed by a postural headache, due to reduced CSF pressure. The frequency of headache can be reduced by using smaller or atraumatic needles. Other rarer complications involve transient radicular pain, and pain over the lumbar region during the procedure. Aseptic technique renders secondary infections such as meningitis extremely rare.

Biopsy

Biopsies of nervous tissue (peripheral nerve, muscle, meninges or brain) are occasionally required for diagnosis.

Nerve biopsy can help in the investigation of peripheral neuropathy. Usually, a distal sensory nerve (sural or radial) is targeted. Histological examination can help identify underlying causes, such as vasculitides or infiltrative disorders like amyloid. Nerve biopsy should not be undertaken lightly since there is an appreciable morbidity; it should be reserved for cases where the diagnosis is in doubt after routine investigations and where it will influence management.

Muscle biopsy is performed more frequently and is indicated for the differentiation of myositis and myopathies. These conditions can usually be distinguished by histological examination, and enzyme histochemistry can be useful when mitochondrial diseases and storage diseases are suspected. The quadriceps muscle is most commonly biopsied but other muscles may also be sampled if they are involved clinically. Although pain and infection can follow the procedure, these are less of a problem than after nerve biopsy.

Brain biopsy is required when imaging fails to clarify the nature of intracerebral lesions: for example, in unexplained degenerative diseases such as unusual cases of dementia and in patients with brain tumour. Most biopsies are performed stereotactically through a burr-hole in the skull, which lowers complication rates. Nevertheless, haemorrhage, infection and death still occur and brain biopsy should only be considered if a diagnosis is otherwise elusive.

PRESENTING PROBLEMS IN NEUROLOGICAL DISEASE

While history is important in all medical specialties, it is especially key in neurology, where many neurological diagnoses have no confirmatory test. History-taking allows doctor and patient to get to know one another – many neurological diseases follow chronic paths, and this may be the first of many such consultations. It also allows the clinician to obtain information about the patient's affect, cognition and psychiatric state.

History-taking is a highly active process and, whilst there are generic templates (Box 26.6), each individual story will follow its own course, and diagnostic considerations during the history will guide further questioning.

It is important to be clear about what patients mean by certain words. Patients may find it difficult to describe symptoms – for instance, weakness may be called 'numbness', while there are many possible interpretations of 'dizziness'. These must be clarified; even in emergency situations, a clear, accurate history is the foundation of any management plan. While the story should come primarily from the patient, input from eye-witnesses and family members is crucial if the patient is unable to provide details or if there has been loss of consciousness. This need for corroboration and clarification means the telephone is as important as any investigation.

The aim of the history is to answer two key issues: where is the lesion and what is the lesion (Box 26.7)? These should remain uppermost in the doctor's mind whilst eliciting the history. Some common combinations of symptoms may suggest particular locations for a lesion (Box 26.8). Enquiry about handedness is important; lateralisation of the dominant hand helps designate the dominant hemisphere, which in turn may help to localise any pathologies, or to plan rehabilitation or treatment strategies in asymmetrical disorders such as stroke or Parkinson's disease.

Epidemiology must be borne in mind; how likely is it that this particular patient has any specific condition under consideration? For example, a 20-year-old with right-sided headache and tenderness will not have temporal arteritis, but this is an important possibility if such symptoms present in a 78-year-old female.

Determining the evolution and speed of onset and progression of a disease is important (Box 26.9). For example, if right-hand weakness occurred overnight, it would suggest a stroke in an older person or an acute entrapment neuropathy in a younger one. Evolution over several days, however, might make demyelination (multiple sclerosis) a possible diagnosis, or perhaps a subdural haematoma if the weakness was preceded by a head injury in an older person taking warfarin. Progression over weeks might bring an intracranial mass lesion or motor neuron disease into the differential. Slow progression over a year or so, with difficulty in using the hand, could suggest a degenerative process such as Parkinson's disease. The impact on day-to-day activities, such as walking, climbing stairs and carrying out fine hand movements, should also be established in order to gauge the level of associated disability.

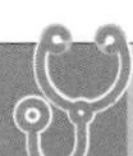

26.6 How to take a neurological history

Introduction

- Age and sex
- Handedness

Presenting complaint

- Symptoms (clarify: see text)
- Overall pattern: intermittent or persistent?
  - If intermittent, how often do symptoms occur and how long do they last?
- Speed of onset: seconds, minutes, hours, days, weeks, months, years, decades?
- Better, worse or the same over time?
- Associated symptoms (including non-neurological)
- Disability caused by symptoms
  - Change in walking
  - Difficulty with fine hand movements, e.g. writing, fastening buttons, using cutlery
- Effect on work, family life and leisure

Background

- Previous neurological symptoms and whether similar to current symptoms
- Previous medical history
- Domestic situation
- Driving licence status
- Medications (current and at time of symptom onset)
- Alcohol/smoking habits
- Recreational drug and other toxin exposure
- Family history and developmental history
- What are patient's thoughts/fears/concerns?

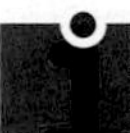

26.7 The key diagnostic questions

Where is the lesion?

- Is it neurological?
- If so, to which part of the nervous system does it localise?
  - Central versus peripheral
  - Sensory versus motor versus both

What is the lesion?

- Hereditary or congenital
- Acquired
  - Traumatic
  - Infective
  - Neoplastic
  - Degenerative
  - Inflammatory or immune-mediated
  - Vascular
  - Functional

26.8 How to 'localise' neurological disease

Combination of symptoms/signs	Probable site	Possible pathology	Other important information
Painless loss of hemilateral function	Cerebral cortex	Usually vascular, inflammatory or neoplastic	Associated systemic symptoms Tempo of evolution
Pyramidal weakness of all four limbs or both legs, bladder signs, sensory loss	Spinal cord	Usually vascular, inflammatory or neoplastic	Associated systemic symptoms Tempo of evolution
Cranial nerve lesions, with limb pyramidal signs or sensory loss ± sphincter disturbance	Brainstem Mid-brain Pons Medulla	Usually vascular or inflammatory Rarely neoplastic	Associated systemic symptoms Tempo of evolution
Visual loss + pyramidal signs and/or cerebellar signs	Widespread cerebral lesions	Usually inflammatory Less commonly vasculitic	Tempo of evolution
Weakness and/or sensory loss in a combination of individual peripheral nerves	Several peripheral nerves ('mononeuritis multiplex')	Usually inflammatory or diabetic	Associated systemic symptoms
Widespread LMN and UMN signs	Upper and lower motor neurons	Motor neuron disease Cervical myeloradiculopathy	Associated localised cervical symptoms
Distal loss of sensation and/or weakness	Generalised peripheral nerves	See causes of neuropathy (p. 1223)	Associated systemic symptoms

(LMN/UMN = lower/upper motor neuron)

26.9 The evolution of symptoms

Onset	Evolution	Possible causes
Sudden (minutes to hours)	Stable/improvement	Vascular (stroke/transient ischaemic attack (TIA)) Nerve entrapment syndromes Functional
Gradual	Progressive over days	Demyelination Infection
Gradual	Progressive over weeks to months	Neoplastic/paraneoplastic
Gradual	Progressive over months to years	Genetic Degenerative

Estimates of the frequency and duration of specific events are essential when taking details of a paroxysmal disorder such as migraine and epilepsy. Vague terms such as 'a lot' or 'sometimes' are unhelpful, and it can assist the patient if choices are given to estimate numbers, such as once a day, week or month.

Many neurological symptoms are not explained by disease. Describing these as 'functional' is less pejorative and more acceptable to patients than 'psychogenic' or 'hysterical'. Functional symptoms require considerable experience in diagnosis, and are frequently missed (p. 1175).

Headache and facial pain

Headache is common and causes considerable worry, but rarely represents sinister disease. The causes may be divided into primary (benign) or secondary, and most patients, whether presenting in clinic or as emergencies, have primary syndromes (Box 26.10). The tempo of evolution of headache is critical; sudden-onset headache, maximal immediately, is always a 'red flag' (Box 26.11) and should prompt rapid assessment in hospital for possible subarachnoid hemorrhage or other sinister causes, even though only 10–25% of patients harbour serious pathology. Clues to other possible causes (e.g. rash in meningitis) should be sought (p. 1201). Headache that evolves over hours to days is much less likely to be sinister.

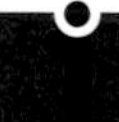

26.10 Primary and secondary headache syndromes

Primary headache syndromes

- Migraine (with or without aura)
- Tension-type headache
- Trigeminal autonomic cephalalgia (including cluster headache)
- Primary stabbing/coughing/exertional/sex-related headache
- Thunderclap headache
- New daily persistent headache syndrome

Secondary causes of headache

- Medication overuse headache (chronic daily headache)
- Intracerebral bleeding (subdural haematoma, subarachnoid or intracerebral haemorrhage)
- Raised intracranial pressure (brain tumour, idiopathic intracranial hypertension)
- Infection (meningitis, encephalitis, brain abscess)
- Inflammatory disease (temporal arteritis, other vasculitis, arthritis)
- Referred pain from other structures (orbit, temporomandibular joint, neck)

For full diagnostic listings see www.ihs-classification.org/en/

26.11 'Red flag' symptoms in headache

Symptom	Possible explanation
Sudden onset (maximal immediately or within minutes)	Subarachnoid haemorrhage Cerebral venous sinus thrombosis Pituitary apoplexy Meningitis
Focal neurological symptoms (other than for typically migrainous)	Intracranial mass lesion Vascular Neoplastic Infection
Constitutional symptoms Weight loss General malaise Pyrexia Meningism Rash	Meningoencephalitis Neoplastic (lymphoma or metastases) Inflammatory (vasculitic)
Raised intracranial pressure (worse on wakening/lying down, associated vomiting)	Intracranial mass lesion
New onset aged > 60 yrs	Temporal arteritis

It is important to establish whether the headache comes and goes, with periods of no headache in between (usually migraine), or whether it is present all or almost all the time. Associated symptoms, such as preceding visual symptoms, nausea/vomiting or photophobia/phonophobia, may support a diagnosis of migraine, but others, such as progressive focal symptoms or constitutional upset like weight loss or fever, may suggest a more sinister cause (e.g. cancer or meningitis). The behaviour of the patient during headache is often instructive; migraine patients typically retire to bed to sleep in a dark room, whereas cluster headache often induces agitated and restless behaviour.

Headache duration may indicate a diagnosis; headaches that have been present for months or years are almost never sinister (although paradoxically worry patients), whereas new-onset headache, especially in the elderly, is more of a concern. In a patient over 60 years with head pain localised to one or both temples, temporal arteritis (p. 1117) should be considered, especially if temporal pulses are absent and/or the arteries are enlarged and tender. Most outpatients with headache will have migraine (intermittent, lasting a few hours, associated with migrainous symptoms) or chronic daily headache syndrome (often present for months to years, without associated symptoms and refractory to analgesia). These are easy to recognise but patients are often very worried about their symptoms, so it is important to elicit such concerns and to explain why sinister disease is unlikely and investigation is rarely required. Sinusitis, 'eye strain', food allergies and uncomplicated hypertension are almost never the explanation for persistent headache.

Ocular pain

Assuming ocular disease (such as acute glaucoma) has been excluded, ocular pain may be due to trigeminal autonomic cephalalgias (TACs) or, rarely, inflammatory or infiltrative lesions at the apex of the orbit or the cavernous sinus, when 3rd, 4th, 5th or 6th cranial nerve involvement is usually evident.

Facial pain

Pain in the face can be due to dental or temporomandibular joint problems. Acute sinusitis is usually apparent from other features of sinus congestion/infection and may cause localised pain over the affected sinus, but is almost never the explanation for persistent facial pain or headache.

Facial pain is not uncommon in migraine but some syndromes can present solely with facial pain. The most common neurological causes of facial pain are trigeminal neuralgia, herpes zoster (shingles) and post-herpetic neuralgia, all characterised by their extreme severity. In trigeminal neuralgia, the patient describes bouts of brief (seconds), lancinating pain ('electric shocks'), most frequently felt in the second and third divisions of the nerve and often triggered by talking or chewing. Facial shingles most commonly affects the first (ophthalmic) division of the trigeminal nerve, and pain usually precedes the rash. Post-herpetic neuralgia may follow, typically a continuous burning pain throughout the affected territory, with marked sensitivity to light touch (allodynia) and resistance to treatment. Destructive lesions of the trigeminal nerve usually cause numbness rather than pain.

Persistent idiopathic facial pain is most frequently seen in middle-aged women, who report persistent pain, with no abnormal signs or investigations, and is similar to other forms of idiopathic chronic pain.

Dizziness, blackouts and 'funny turns'

Episodic lost or altered consciousness is a frequent symptom in primary care and hospital practice. The terms used for such spells vary so much among patients that they should not be taken for granted. Some patients use 'blackout' to describe a purely visual symptom, rather than loss of consciousness. Some individuals may understand 'dizziness' to mean an abnormal perception of movement (vertigo), but others will mean a feeling of faintness, and yet others unsteadiness (Box 26.12). The clinician thus needs to elucidate the exact nature of the symptoms that the patient experiences (Fig. 26.17).

The history should always be supplemented by a direct eye-witness account if available. Often a history of 'shaking' as described to the first aider will become 'fitting' when described to the ambulance crew, which then is reported as 'definite seizure' in the emergency room. Careful history with corroboration will usually establish whether there has been full consciousness, altered consciousness, vertigo, transient amnesia or something else. Vertigo is caused by an alteration in function of the peripheral vestibular organs or the central control mechanisms of balance and posture, and will be discussed elsewhere (p. 1167).

Loss of consciousness

Consciousness may be defined as an awareness of the environment and ability to respond to it. Loss of consciousness (LOC), other than in sleep, suggests a global dysfunction of the brain. This most commonly occurs

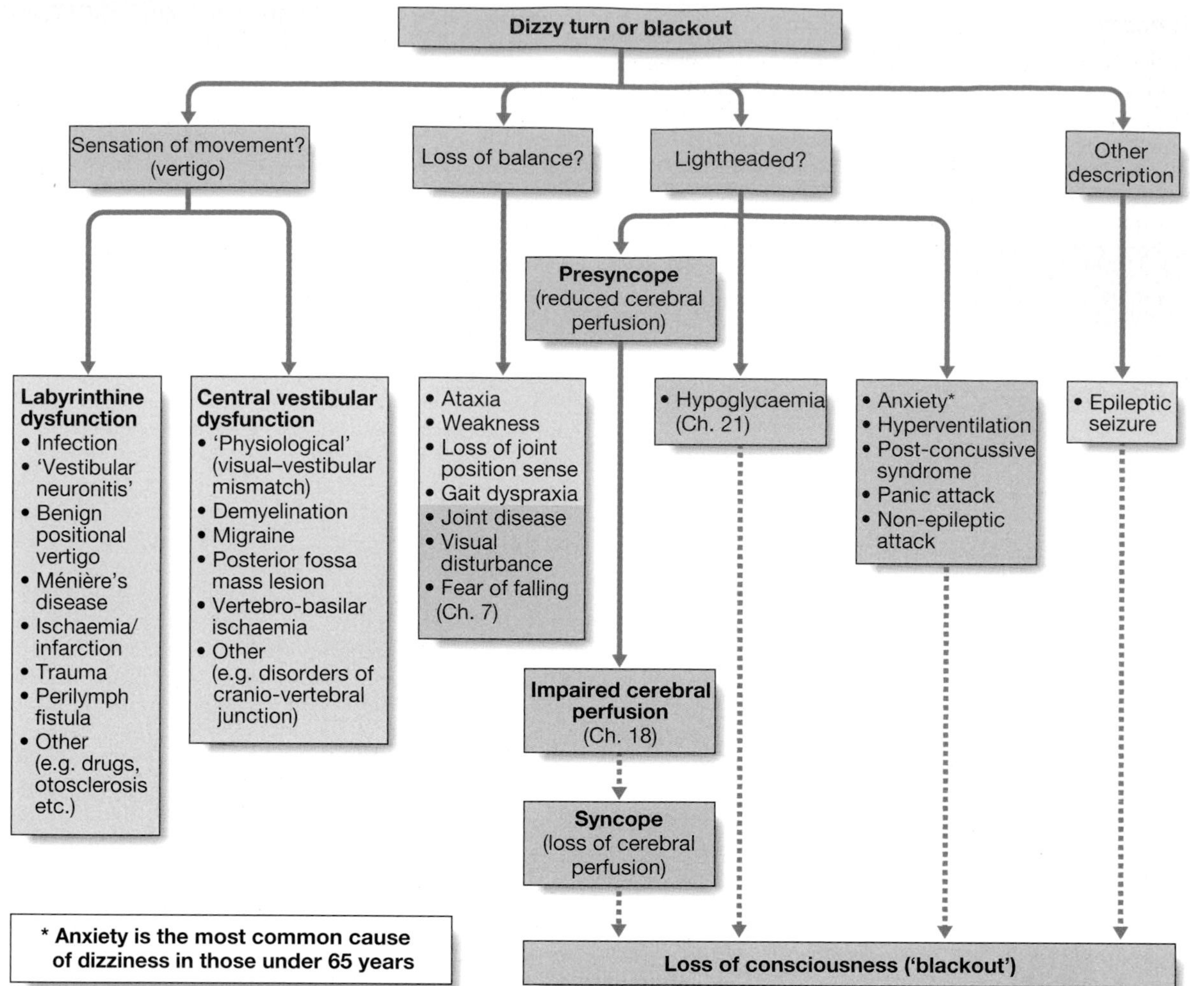

Fig. 26.17 A diagnostic approach to the patient with dizziness, funny turns or blackouts. (Neurological causes are shown in green.)

26.12 Dizziness in old age

- **Prevalence**: common, affecting up to 30% of people aged > 65 yrs.
- **Symptoms**: most frequently described as a combination of unsteadiness and lightheadedness.
- **Most common causes**: postural hypotension, cardiovascular disease, cervical spondylosis. Many patients have more than one underlying cause.
- **Arrhythmia**: can present with lightheadedness either at rest or on activity.
- **Anxiety**: frequently associated with dizziness but rarely the only cause.
- **Falls**: multidisciplinary workup is required if dizziness is associated with falls.

26.13 How to differentiate seizures from syncope

	Seizure	Syncope
Aura (e.g. olfactory)	+	–
Cyanosis	+	–
Tongue-biting	+	–/+
Post-ictal confusion	+	–
Post-ictal amnesia	+	–
Post-ictal headache	+	–
Rapid recovery	–	+

because of temporary loss of blood supply to the whole brain (syncope or faint). Alternatively, LOC can occur due to a sudden electrical dysfunction of the brain, as occurs during a seizure. Whilst most episodes of transient LOC are due to syncope or seizure, psychogenic blackouts (also known as non-epileptic seizure or pseudoseizure) need to be considered in the differential diagnosis.

No amount of investigation can replace a clear history in these circumstances. The subjective experience is important, but objective description from an eye-witness (even if only by telephone) is equally helpful. Features in the history useful in distinguishing a seizure from syncope are shown in Box 26.13.

Syncope

Typically, syncope is preceded by a brief feeling of light-headedness. Neurocardiogenic syncope (p. 555) is more likely on standing, and may be provoked by pain or emotion. There may be darkening of vision, ringing in the ears, symptoms of hyperventilation, distal tingling, feelings of nausea, clamminess or sweating. The LOC is gradual and brief, and the patient recovers quickly without confusion as long as he or she has assumed a horizontal position. There is often some brief stiffening and limb twitching, which requires differentiation from seizure-like movements. It is rare for syncope to cause injury or to cause amnesia after regaining awareness. During a syncopal attack, incontinence of urine can occur. Tongue-biting is less common in syncope and, if present, usually involves little trauma.

Cardiac syncope (p. 555), caused by a sudden drop in cardiac output, may be provoked by exertion in those with severe aortic stenosis, ischaemia or hypertrophic obstructive cardiomyopathy, or without warning in patients with cardiac arrhythmia.

Seizures

The diagnosis of generalised tonic–clonic seizures, in which there is loss of consciousness, falling to the ground and clonic movements (p. 1180), is easy but lack of eye-witness accounts can leave uncertainty. Less dramatic seizures, such as absences (p. 1181) or some focal seizures (p. 1180), which cause alteration of consciousness without the patient falling to the ground, may merely be experienced as 'lost time'. Since epileptic seizures are the result of specific processes that vary from patient to patient, their manifestation tends to be intermittent and stereotyped and often clusters in time, for reasons incompletely understood.

Non-epileptic attack disorder, psychogenic seizures, pseudoseizures, psychogenic non-epileptic seizures

This disorder is recognised in all cultures but nomenclature has yet to be standardised. Around 10% of patients referred to a first seizure clinic will have LOC resulting from psychological reactions to circumstances or traumatic life events. Clinical pointers to the diagnosis include specific emotional triggers, partially retained awareness, dramatic movements or vocalisation, very prolonged duration (up to hours), rapid recovery or subsequent emotional distress. Diagnosis is important, as such patients are at significant risk of being harmed by inappropriate treatment if they are assumed to have epilepsy. Conversely, a hasty diagnosis may lead to treatment being withheld in atypical or prolonged seizures. Specialist help is necessary to plan management.

Status epilepticus

Status epilepticus is seizure activity not resolving spontaneously, or recurrent seizure with no recovery of consciousness in between. Persisting seizure activity has a recognised mortality and is a medical emergency.

Diagnosis is usually clinical and can be made on the basis of the description of prolonged rigidity and/or clonic movements with loss of awareness. As seizure activity becomes prolonged, movements may become more subtle. Cyanosis, pyrexia, acidosis and sweating may occur, and complications include aspiration, hypotension, cardiac arrhythmias and renal or hepatic failure.

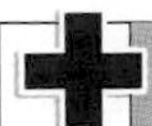

26.14 Management of status epilepticus

Initial

- Ensure airway is patent; give oxygen to prevent cerebral hypoxia
- Check pulse, blood pressure, BM stix® and respiratory rate
- Secure intravenous access
- Send blood for:
  - Glucose, urea and electrolytes, calcium and magnesium, liver function, anti-epileptic drug levels
  - Full blood count and clotting screen
  - Storing a sample for future analysis (e.g. drug misuse)
- If seizures continue for > 5 mins: give diazepam 10 mg IV (or rectally) *or* lorazepam 4 mg IV; repeat *once only* after 15 mins
- Correct any metabolic trigger, e.g. hypoglycaemia

Ongoing

If seizures continue after 30 mins

- IV infusion (with cardiac monitoring) with one of:
  - Phenytoin: 15 mg/kg at 50 mg/min
  - Fosphenytoin: 15 mg/kg at 100 mg/min
  - Phenobarbital: 10 mg/kg at 100 mg/min
- Cardiac monitor and pulse oximetry
  - Monitor neurological condition, blood pressure, respiration; check blood gases

If seizures still continue after 30–60 mins

- Transfer to intensive care
  - Start treatment for refractory status with intubation, ventilation and general anaesthesia using propofol or thiopental
  - EEG monitor

Once status controlled

- Commence longer-term anticonvulsant medication with one of:
  - Sodium valproate 10 mg/kg IV over 3–5 mins, then 800–2000 mg/day
  - Phenytoin: give loading dose (if not already used as above) of 15 mg/kg, infuse at < 50 mg/min, then 300 mg/day
  - Carbamazepine 400 mg by nasogastric tube, then 400–1200 mg/day
- Investigate cause

In patients with pre-existing epilepsy, the most likely cause is a fall in anti-epileptic drug levels. In de novo status epilepticus, it is essential to exclude precipitants such as infection (meningitis, encephalitis), neoplasia and metabolic derangement (hypoglycaemia, hyponatraemia, hypocalcaemia). Treatment and investigation are outlined in Box 26.14.

Coma

Conscious level should be measured using the Glasgow Coma Scale (GCS, Box 26.15). Although developed for use in head injury, GCS is widely used in medical coma, but disorders that affect language or limb function (e.g. left hemisphere stroke, locked-in syndrome) may reduce its usefulness. Nevertheless, it provides useful prognostic information, and serial recordings can plot improvement or deterioration. It is important to record the three components of the scale, rather than just the sum score. Thus, a description of eye-opening (E2) and withdrawing (M4) to pain and making sounds only (V2) provides a much more useful picture than GCS 8.

Persisting loss of consciousness or coma (defined as GCS ≤ 8) occurs if the arousal mechanisms in the brainstem and diencephalon are disturbed, and localises to either the brainstem or both cerebral hemispheres. There are many causes of coma (Box 26.16), including neurological (structural or non-structural brain disease) or non-neurological (e.g. type II respiratory failure). The mode of onset of coma and any precipitating event is crucial to establishing the cause, and should be obtained from family or other witnesses (by telephone if

26.15 Glasgow Coma Scale

Eye-opening (E)	
• Spontaneous	4
• To speech	3
• To pain	2
• Nil	1
Best motor response (M)	
• Obeys commands	6
• Localises	5
• Withdraws	4
• Abnormal flexion	3
• Extensor response	2
• Nil	1
Verbal response (V)	
• Orientated	5
• Confused conversation	4
• Inappropriate words	3
• Incomprehensible sounds	2
• Nil	1
Coma score = E + M + V	
Always present GCS as breakdown, not a sum score (unless 3 or 15)	
• Minimum sum	3
• Maximum sum	15

26.16 Causes of coma

Metabolic disturbance	
• Drug overdose • Diabetes mellitus Hypoglycaemia Ketoacidosis Hyperosmolar coma • Hyponatraemia	• Uraemia • Hepatic failure • Respiratory failure • Hypothermia • Hypothyroidism • Thiamin deficiency
Trauma	
• Cerebral contusion • Extradural haematoma • Subdural haematoma	• Global axonal injury (deceleration)
Vascular disease	
• Subarachnoid haemorrhage • Brainstem infarction/ haemorrhage	• Intracerebral haemorrhage • Cerebral venous sinus thrombosis
Infections	
• Meningitis • Encephalitis	• Cerebral abscess • Systemic sepsis
Others	
• Epilepsy • Brain tumour	• Functional ('pseudo-coma')

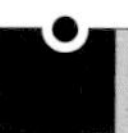

26.17 UK criteria for the diagnosis of brain death

Preconditions for considering a diagnosis of brain death

- The patient is deeply comatose
  - (a) There must be no suspicion that coma is due to depressant drugs, such as narcotics, hypnotics, tranquillisers
  - (b) Hypothermia has been excluded – rectal temperature must exceed 35°C
  - (c) There is no profound abnormality of serum electrolytes, acid–base balance or blood glucose concentrations, and any metabolic or endocrine cause of coma has been excluded
- The patient is maintained on a ventilator because spontaneous respiration has been inadequate or has ceased. Drugs, including neuromuscular blocking agents, must have been excluded as a cause of the respiratory failure
- The diagnosis of the disorder leading to brain death has been firmly established. There must be no doubt that the patient is suffering from irremediable structural brain damage

Tests for confirming brain death

- All brainstem reflexes are absent
  - (a) The pupils are fixed and unreactive to light
  - (b) The corneal reflexes are absent
  - (c) The vestibulo-ocular reflexes are absent – there is no eye movement following the injection of 20 mL of ice-cold water into each external auditory meatus in turn
  - (d) There are no motor responses to adequate stimulation within the cranial nerve distribution
  - (e) There is no gag reflex and no reflex response to a suction catheter in the trachea
- No respiratory movement occurs when the patient is disconnected from the ventilator long enough to allow the carbon dioxide tension to rise above the threshold for stimulating respiration ($PaCO_2$ must reach 6.7 kPa (50 mmHg))

The diagnosis of brain death should be made by two experienced doctors, one of whom should be a consultant and the other a consultant or specialist registrar. The tests are usually repeated after an interval of 24 hours, depending on the clinical circumstances, before brain death is finally confirmed.

necessary). Failure to obtain an adequate history for patients in coma is a common cause of diagnostic delay. Once the patient is stable from a cardiorespiratory perspective, examination should include accurate assessment of conscious level (see below) and thorough general medical examination, looking for clues such as needle tracks indicating drug abuse, rashes, fever and focal signs of infection, including neck stiffness or evidence of head injury. Focal neurological signs may suggest a structural explanation (stroke or tumour) or may be falsely localising (p. 1212).

Brain death and minimally conscious states

Coma is loss of consciousness related to loss of brain function. Brain death is a state in which cortical and brainstem function is irreversibly lost. Diagnostic criteria for brain death vary between countries (Box 26.17); if satisfied, these criteria allow support to be withdrawn and natural death to occur. Diagnosing brain death is complex and should only be done by a clinician with appropriate expertise, as clinical differentiation from reduced consciousness can be challenging (Box 26.18). The 'locked-in' syndrome, in which the patient is paralysed except for eye movements, requires preserved hemisphere function (and thus consciousness), but a strategically placed lesion in the ventral pons (usually infarction) causes complete paralysis. The vegetative state implies some retention of brainstem function and minimal cortical function, with loss of awareness of the environment. Minimally conscious states imply retention of awareness and intact brainstem function. Confident distinction between these states is important and requires careful assessment, often over a period of time. Brain death is, by definition, irreversible, but other states may offer hope for improvement. Difficult ethical issues regarding management often arise.

Delirium

Delirium is a common result of cortical impairment and is more common in old age. It manifests as a disturbance of arousal with global impairment of mental function causing drowsiness with disorientation, perceptual errors and muddled thinking. Fluctuation is typical and confusion is often worse at night. Emotional disturbance (anxiety, irritability or depression) and psychomotor changes (agitation, restlessness or retardation) are common. The assessment and management of this condition are covered in more detail on page 173.

Amnesia

Memory disturbance is a common symptom. In the absence of significant functional impairment (e.g. inability to work, dyspraxias, loss of daily function), many patients will prove to have benign memory dysfunction related to age, mood or psychiatric disorders. Investigation and treatment of the dementias are discussed elsewhere (p. 250).

Temporary loss of memory may be due to a transient toxic confusional state, the post-ictal period after seizure, or transient global amnesia. These are usually distinguished on the basis of the history.

Transient global amnesia

This predominantly affects middle-aged patients with an abrupt, discrete loss of anterograde memory function lasting up to a few hours. During the episode, patients are unable to record new memories, and this results in repetitive questioning, the hallmark of this condition. Consciousness is preserved and patients may perform even complex motor acts normally. During the attack there is retrograde amnesia for the events of the past

26.18 Classification of brain death and reduced conscious states

Diagnosis	Features	Investigation	Prognosis
Brain death	See Box 26.17	Cranial imaging for primary cause EEG – no electrical activity Cranial Doppler – no cortical blood flow	Invariably fatal
Vegetative state (VS) 'Persistent VS' > 1 mth 'Permanent VS' > 1 yr	No reaction to verbal stimuli Some reaction to noxious stimuli Sleep–wake cycles (periods of eye opening) Maintained respiratory drive Intact brainstem reflexes Occasional automatic movements (yawning, swallowing)	Cranial imaging for primary cause Maintained cortical blood flow	Prognosis better post trauma
Minimally conscious state	Some reaction to verbal stimuli Some reaction to noxious stimuli Spontaneous movements Intact brainstem reflexes	EEG demonstrates reactivity	
Locked-in syndrome	Some retained cranial nerve reflexes Some response to verbal stimuli (e.g. eye movements to communicate) No limb movement to noxious stimuli	Imaging for primary cause	Depends on cause – recovery unlikely to progress beyond 6 mths

few days, weeks or years. After 4–6 hours, memory function and behaviour return to normal but the patient has persistent, complete amnesia for the duration of the attack itself. There are no seizure markers and, unlike epileptic amnesia, transient global amnesia recurs in around 10–20% only. A vascular aetiology is unlikely and amnesia may be due to a benign process similar to migraine, occurring in the hippocampus. The patient has no physical signs and, if imaging is normal and no seizure markers are present, then the patient can be reassured.

Persistent amnesia

Patients with persistent memory disturbance must have serious neurological disease excluded. Symptoms corroborated by relatives or colleagues are likely to be more significant than those noted by the patient only. Where poor concentration is at the heart of cognitive deterioration, it is more likely to be due to an underlying mood disorder.

It is important to assess the timing of onset and to establish which aspects of memory are affected. Complaints of getting lost or of losing complex abilities are more pathological than word-finding difficulties. Disturbance of episodic or working memory (previously called 'short-term memory') must be distinguished from semantic memory (memory for concept-based knowledge unrelated to specific experiences). Episodic memory is selectively impaired in Korsakoff's syndrome (often secondary to alcohol) or bilateral temporal lobe damage. It can also be seen in conjunction with other types of dementia. Progressive deterioration over months suggests an underlying dementia, but it is important to perform a full medical assessment to detect any underlying medical problem.

It is important to identify and treat depression (p. 243) in patients with memory loss. Depression may present as a 'pseudo-dementia', with concentration and memory impairment as dominant features, and this is often reversible with antidepressant medication. However, any patient with dementia (particularly of the Alzheimer's type) may develop depression in the early stages of their illness. Specific causes of progressive dementia, with their treatment and investigation, are listed elsewhere (p. 250).

Weakness

The assessment of weakness requires the application of basic anatomy, physiology and some pathology to the interpretation of the history and clinical findings. Points to consider are shown in Boxes 26.19 and 26.20, and in Figure 26.18. The pattern and evolution of weakness and the clinical signs provide clues to the site and nature of the lesion.

26.19 Distinguishing signs in upper versus lower motor neuron syndromes

	Upper motor neuron lesion	Lower motor neuron lesion
Inspection	Normal (may be wasting in chronic lesions)	Wasting, fasciculation
Tone	Increased with clonus	Normal or decreased, no clonus
Pattern of weakness	Preferentially affects extensors in arms, flexors in leg Hemiparesis, paraparesis or tetraparesis	Typically focal, in distribution of nerve root or peripheral nerve, with associated sensory changes
Deep tendon reflexes	Increased	Decreased/absent
Plantar response	Extensor (Babinski sign)	Flexor

26.20 How to assess weakness

Clinical finding	Likely level of lesion/diagnosis
Pattern and distribution	
Isolated muscles	Radiculopathy or mononeuropathy
Both limbs on one side (hemiparesis)	Cerebral hemisphere, less likely cord or brainstem
One limb	Neuronopathy, plexopathy, cord/brain
Both lower limbs (paraparesis)	Spinal cord; look for a sensory level
Fatigability	Mysasthenia gravis
Bizarre, fluctuating, not following anatomical rules	Functional
Signs	
Upper motor neuron	Brain/spinal cord
Lower motor neuron	Peripheral nervous system
Evolution of the weakness	
Sudden and improving	Stroke/mononeuropathy
Evolving over months or years	Meningioma, cervical spondylotic myelopathy
Gradually worsening over days or weeks	Cerebral mass, demyelination
Associated symptoms	
Absence of sensory involvement	Motor neuron disease, myopathy, myasthenia

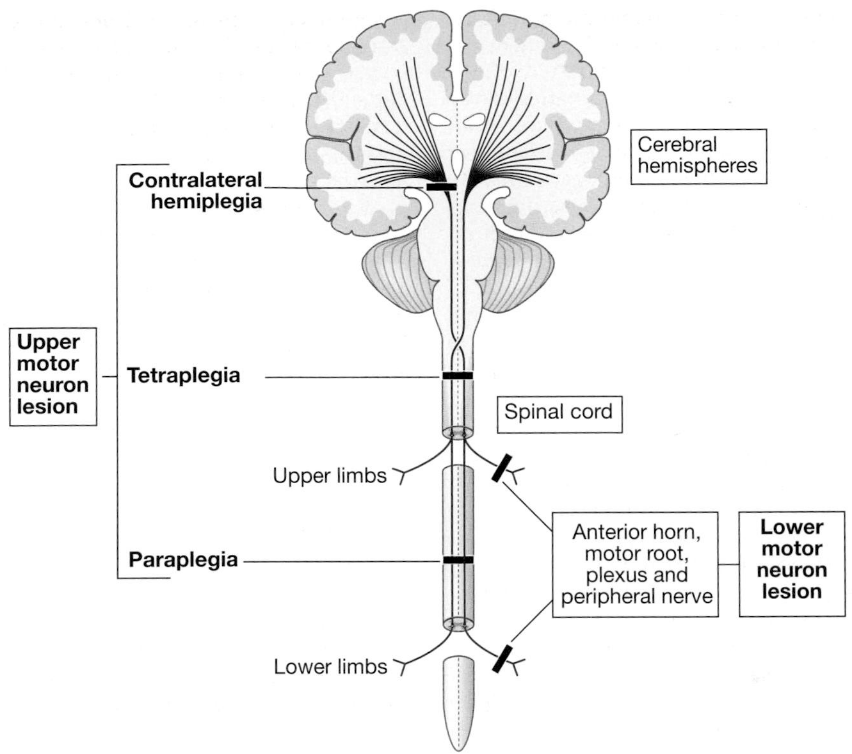

Fig. 26.18 Patterns of motor loss according to the anatomical site of the lesion.

It is important to establish whether the patient has loss of power rather than reduced sensation or generalised fatigue. Pain may restrict movement and thus mimic weakness. Paradoxically, sensory neglect (p. 1164) may leave patients unaware of even severe weakness.

Patients with parkinsonism may complain of weakness; extrapyramidal signs of rigidity (cogwheel or lead pipe) and bradykinesia should be evident, and a resting tremor, usually asymmetrical, may provide a further clue (p. 1194). Observation is as important as formal strength testing. Movement restricted by pain should be apparent, and other features (contractures, wasting, fasciculations, abnormal movements/postures) all provide diagnostic clues. Simple observation of the patient walking into the consulting room may be diagnostic.

Weakness is a common functional symptom. Functional weakness does not conform to typical organic patterns, and the signs in Box 26.19 are absent. On examination, the signs are often variable (e.g. the patient can walk but appears to have no leg movement when assessed on the couch), and strength may appear to 'give way', with the patient able to achieve full power for brief bursts. This does not occur in disease. Hoover's sign is useful to confirm functional weakness, and relies on the normal phenomenon of simultaneous hip extension when the contralateral hip flexes. In functional weakness, one may see hip extension weakness (rare in organic disease), which then returns to full strength on testing contralateral hip flexion. This sign may be demonstrated to the patient in a non-confrontational manner, to show that the potential limb power is intact.

Facial weakness

Facial nerve palsy (Bell's palsy)

One of the most common causes of facial weakness is Bell's palsy, a lower motor neuron lesion of the 7th (facial) nerve, affecting all ages and both sexes.

The lesion is within the facial canal. Symptoms usually develop subacutely over a few hours, with pain around the ear preceding the unilateral facial weakness. Patients often describe the face as 'numb', but there is no objective sensory loss (except to taste if the chorda tympani is involved). Hyperacusis may occur if the nerve to stapedius is involved, and there may be diminished salivation and tear secretion. Examination reveals an ipsilateral lower motor neuron facial nerve palsy. Vesicles in the ear or on the palate may indicate primary herpes zoster infection (p. 318).

Steroids improve recovery rates if started within 72 hours of onset but antiviral drugs are not effective. Taping the eye shut overnight helps prevent exposure keratitis and corneal abrasion. About 80% of patients recover spontaneously within 12 weeks. Plastic surgery may be considered for the minority left with facial disfigurement after 12 months. Recurrence is unusual and should prompt further investigation. Aberrant re-innervation may occur during recovery, producing unwanted facial movements, such as eye closure when the mouth is moved (synkinesis), or 'crocodile tears' (tearing during salivation).

Unlike Bell's palsy, lesions with an upper motor neuron origin partly spare the upper face. Cortical lesions may cause a facial weakness either in isolation or with associated hemiparesis and speech difficulties.

Sensory disturbance

Sensory symptoms are common and are frequently benign. Patients often find sensory symptoms difficult to describe, and sensory examination is difficult for both doctor and patient. While neurological disease can cause sensory symptoms, systemic disorders can also be responsible. Tingling in both hands and around the mouth can occur as the result of hyperventilation (p. 657) or hypocalcaemia (p. 768). When there is dysfunction of the relevant cerebral cortex, the patient's perception of the wholeness or actual presence of the relevant part of the body may be distorted.

Numbness and paraesthesia

The history may give the best clues to localisation and pathology. Certain common patterns are recognised: in migraine, the aura may consist of spreading tingling or paraesthesia, followed by numbness evolving over 20–30 minutes over one half of the body, often splitting the tongue. Sensory loss caused by a stroke or transient ischaemic attack (TIA) occurs much more rapidly and is typically negative (numbness) rather than positive (tingling). Rarely, unpleasant paraesthesia of sensory epilepsy spreads within seconds. The sensory alteration of inflammatory spinal cord lesions often ascends from one or both lower limbs to a distinct level on the trunk over hours to days. Psychogenic sensory change can occur as a manifestation of anxiety or as part of a conversion disorder (p. 246). In such cases, the distribution usually does not conform to a known anatomical pattern nor fit with any organic disease. Care must be taken in diagnosing non-organic sensory problems; a careful history and examination will ensure there is no other objective neurological deficit.

Sensory neurological examination needs to be undertaken and interpreted with care since the findings depend, by definition, on subjective reports. However, the reported distribution of sensory loss can be useful when combined with the coexisting deficits of motor and/or cranial nerve function (Fig. 26.19).

Sensory loss in peripheral nerve lesions

Here the symptoms are usually of sensory loss and paraesthesia. Single nerve lesions cause disturbance in the sensory distribution of the nerve, whereas in diffuse neuropathies the longest neurons are affected first, giving a characteristic 'glove and stocking' distribution. If smaller nerve fibres are preferentially affected (e.g. in diabetic neuropathy), temperature and pin-prick (pain) are reduced, whilst vibration sense and proprioception (modalities served by the larger, well-myelinated, sensory nerves) may be spared. In contrast, vibration and proprioception are particularly affected if the neuropathy is demyelinating in character (p. 1224), producing symptoms of tightness and swelling with impairment of proprioception and vibration sensation.

Sensory loss in nerve root lesions

These typically present with pain as a prominent feature, either within the spine or in the limb plexuses. It is often felt in the myotome rather than the dermatome. The

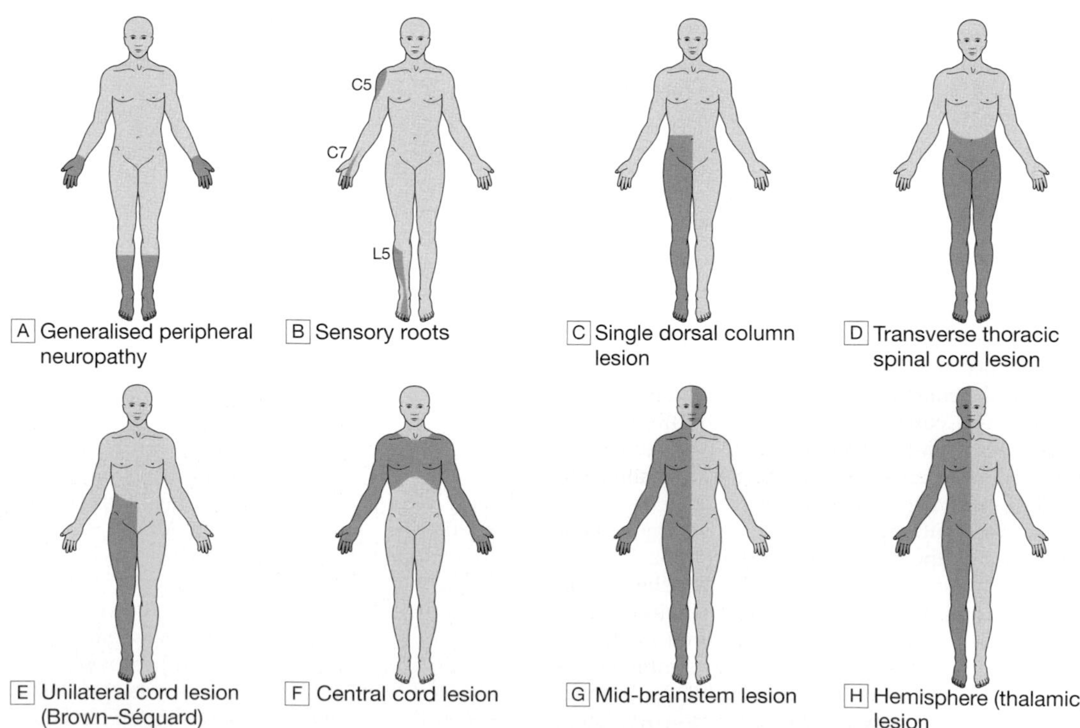

Fig. 26.19 Patterns of sensory loss. **A** Generalised peripheral neuropathy. **B** Sensory roots: some common examples. **C** Single dorsal column lesion (proprioception and some touch loss). **D** Transverse thoracic spinal cord lesion. **E** Unilateral cord lesion (Brown–Séquard): ipsilateral dorsal column (and motor) deficit and contralateral spinothalamic deficit. **F** Central cord lesion: 'cape' distribution of spinothalamic loss. **G** Mid-brainstem lesion: ipsilateral facial sensory loss and contralateral loss on body below the vertex. **H** Hemisphere (thalamic) lesion: contralateral loss on one side of face and body.

nerve root involved may be deduced from the dermatomal pattern of sensory loss, although overlap may lead to this being smaller than expected.

Sensory loss in spinal cord lesions

Transverse lesions of the spinal cord produce loss of all sensory modalities below that segmental level, although the clinical level may only be manifest 2–3 segments lower than the anatomical site of the lesion. Very often, there is a band of paraesthesia or hyperaesthesia at the top of the area of sensory loss. Clinical examination may reveal dissociated sensory loss, i.e. different patterns in the spinothalamic and dorsal columnar pathways. If the transverse lesion is vascular due to anterior spinal artery thrombosis, the spinothalamic pathways may be affected while the posterior one-third of the spinal cord (the dorsal column modalities) may be spared.

Lesions damaging one side of the spinal cord will produce loss of spinothalamic modalities (pain and temperature) on the opposite side, and of dorsal column modalities (joint position and vibration sense) on the same side of the body – the Brown–Séquard syndrome (p. 1221).

Lesions in the centre of the spinal cord (such as syringomyelia: see Box 26.98 and Fig. 26.46, p. 1222) spare the dorsal columns but involve the spinothalamic fibres crossing the cord from both sides over the length of the lesion. There is no sensory loss in segments above and below the lesion; this is described as 'suspended' sensory loss. There is sometimes reflex loss at the level of the lesion if afferent fibres of the reflex arc are affected.

An isolated lesion of the dorsal columns is not uncommon in multiple sclerosis. This produces a characteristic unpleasant, tight feeling over the limb(s) involved and, while there is no loss of pin-prick or temperature sensation, the associated loss of proprioception may severely limit function of the affected limb(s).

Sensory loss in brainstem lesions

Lesions in the brainstem can be associated with sensory loss, but the distribution depends on the site of the lesion. A lesion limited to the trigeminal nucleus or its sensory projections will cause ipsilateral facial sensory disturbance. For example, pain resembling trigeminal neuralgia can be seen in patients with multiple sclerosis. The anatomy of the trigeminal connections means that lesions in the medulla or spinal cord can give rise to 'balaclava' patterns of sensory loss (p. 1147). Sensory pathways running up from the spinal cord can also be damaged in the brainstem, resulting in simultaneous sensory loss in arm(s) and/or leg(s).

Sensory loss in hemispheric lesions

The temporal, parietal and occipital lobes receive sensory information regarding the various modalities of touch, vision, hearing and balance (see Box 26.2, p. 1142). The initial points of entry into the cortex are the respective primary cortical areas (see Fig. 26.4, p. 1143). Damage to any of these primary areas will result in reduction or loss of the ability to perceive that particular modality: 'negative' symptomatology. Abnormal excitation of these areas can result in a false perception ('positive' symptoms), the most common of which is migrainous visual aura (flashing lights or teichopsiae).

Cortical lesions are more likely to cause a mixed motor and sensory loss. Substantial lesions of the parietal cortex (as in large strokes) can cause severe loss of proprioception and may even abolish conscious awareness of the existence of the affected limb(s). The resulting loss of function in the limb may be impossible to distinguish from paralysis. Pathways are so tightly packed in the thalamus that even small lacunar strokes can cause isolated contralateral hemisensory loss.

Neuropathic pain

Neuropathic pain is a positive neurological symptom caused by dysfunction of the pain perception apparatus, in contrast to nociceptive pain, which is secondary to pathological processes such as inflammation. Neuropathic pain has distinctive features and typically provokes a very unpleasant, persistent, burning sensation. There is often increased sensitivity to touch, so that light brushing of the affected area causes exquisite pain (allodynia). Painful stimuli are felt as though they arise from a larger area than that touched, and spontaneous bursts of pain may also occur. Pain may be elicited by other modalities (allodynia) and is considerably affected by emotional influences. The most common causes of neuropathic pain are diabetic neuropathies, trigeminal and post-herpetic neuralgias, and trauma to a peripheral nerve. Treatment of these syndromes can be difficult. Drugs that modulate various parts of the nociceptive system, such as gabapentin, carbamazepine or tricyclic antidepressants, may help. Localised treatment (topical treatment or nerve blocks) sometimes succeeds but may increase the sensory deficit and worsen the situation. Electrical stimulation has occasionally proved successful. For further information, see Chapter 12.

Abnormal movements

Disorders of movement lead to either extra, unwanted movement (hyperkinetic disorders) or too little movement (hypokinetic disorders) (Box 26.21). In either case, the lesion often localises to the basal ganglia, although some tremors are related to cerebellar or brainstem disturbance. Functional movement disorders are common, and may mimic all of the organic syndromes below. The most important hypokinetic disorder is Parkinson's disease (p. 1194). Parkinsonism is a clinical description of a collection of symptoms, including tremor, bradykinesia and rigidity. Whilst the history is always important, observation is clearly vital; much of the skill in diagnosing movement disorders lies in pattern recognition. Once it is established whether the problem is hypo- or hyperkinetic, the next task is to categorise the movements further, accepting that there is often overlap. Videoing the movements (with the patient's permission), so that they can be shown to a movement disorder expert, may provide a quick diagnosis in cases of uncertainty.

Tremor

Tremor is caused by alternating agonist/antagonist muscle contractions and produces a rhythmical oscillation of the body part affected. In the assessment of tremor, the position, body part affected, frequency and

26.21 Movement disorders

Description	Features	Examples
Hypokinetic disorders		
Parkinsonism	Akinesia Rigidity Tremor Loss of postural reflexes Other features depending on cause	Idiopathic Parkinson's disease Other degenerative syndromes Drug-induced (See Box 26.64)
Catatonia	Mutism Sustained posturing and waxy flexibility	Usually psychiatric; if neurological, is most commonly of vascular origin
Hyperkinetic disorders		
Tremor	Rhythmical oscillation of body part (see Box 26.22)	Essential tremor Parkinson's disease Drug-induced
Chorea	Jerky, brief, involuntary movements	Huntington's disease Drug-induced
Tics	Stereotyped, repetitive movements, briefly suppressible	Tourette's syndrome
Myoclonus	Shock-like muscle jerks	Epilepsy Hypnic jerks (p. 1187) Focal cortical disease
Dystonia	Sustained muscle contraction causing abnormal postures ± tremor	Genetic Generalised dystonic syndromes Focal dystonias in adults (e.g. torticollis)
Others	Various	Paroxysmal hyperkinetic dyskinesias Hemifacial spasm Tardive syndromes

26.22 Causes and characteristics of tremors

	Body part affected	Position	Frequency	Amplitude	Character
Physiological	Both arms > legs	Posture, movement	High	Small (fine)	Enhanced by anxiety, emotion, drugs, toxins
Parkinsonism	Unilateral or asymmetrical Arm > leg, chin, never head	Rest Postural and re-emergent may occur	Low (3–4 Hz)	Moderate	Typically pill-rolling, thumb and index finger, other features of parkinsonism
Essential tremor	Bilateral arms, head	Movement	High (8–10 Hz)	Low to moderate	Family history; 50% respond to alcohol
Dystonic	Head, arms, legs	Posture	Variable	Variable	Other features of dystonia, often jerky tremors
Functional	Any	Any	Variable	Variable	Distractible

amplitude should be considered, as these provide diagnostic clues (Box 26.22).

Other hyperkinetic syndromes

Non-rhythmic involuntary movements include chorea, athetosis, ballism, dystonia, myoclonus and tics. They are categorised by clinical appearance, and coexistence and overlap are common, such as in choreoathetosis.

- *Chorea*: jerky, brief, purposeless involuntary movements, appearing as fidgety movements affecting different areas; they suggest disease in the caudate nucleus (as in Huntington's disease, p. 1198) and are a common complication of prolonged levodopa treatment for Parkinson's disease. Other causes are shown in Box 26.23.
- *Athetosis*: slower, writhing movement of the limbs, often combined with chorea and having similar causes.
- *Ballism*: a more dramatic form of chorea, causing often-violent flinging movements of one limb (monoballism) or one side of the body (hemiballism). The lesion localises to the contralateral subthalamic nucleus and the most common cause is stroke.
- *Dystonia*: sustained involuntary muscle contraction that causes abnormal postures or movement. It may

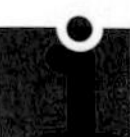

26.23 Causes of chorea

Hereditary
- Huntington's disease (HD) and HD-like syndromes
- Wilson's disease
- Neuroacanthocytosis
- Dentato-rubro-pallidoluysian atrophy
- Benign hereditary chorea
- Paroxysmal dyskinesias

Cerebral birth injury (including kernicterus)

Cerebral trauma

Drugs
- Levodopa
- Antipsychotics
- Anticonvulsants
- Oral contraceptive

Metabolic
- Disorders affecting thyroid, parathyroid, glucose, sodium, calcium and magnesium balance
- Pregnancy

Autoimmune
- Post-streptococcal (Sydenham's chorea)
- Antiphospholipid antibody syndrome
- Systemic lupus erythematosus (SLE)

Structural lesions of basal ganglia (usually caudate)
- Vascular
- Demyelination
- Brain tumour

be generalised (usually in childhood-onset genetic syndromes) or, more commonly, focal/segmental (such as in torticollis, when the head is twisted repeatedly to one side). Some dystonias only occur with specific tasks, such as writer's cramp or other occupational 'cramps'. Dystonic tremor is associated, and is asymmetrical and of large amplitude.

- *Myoclonus*: brief, isolated, random jerks of muscle groups. This is physiological at the onset of sleep (hypnic jerks). Similarly, a myoclonic jerk is a component of the normal startle response, which may be exaggerated in some rare (mostly genetic) disorders. Myoclonus may occur in disorders of the cerebral cortex, such as some forms of epilepsy. Alternatively, myoclonus can arise from subcortical structures or, more rarely, from segments of the spinal cord.
- *Tics*: stereotyped repetitive movements, such as blinking, winking, head shaking or shoulder shrugging. Unlike dyskinesias, the patient may be able to suppress them, although only for a short time. Isolated tics are common in childhood and usually disappear. Tourette's syndrome is defined by the presence of multiple motor and vocal tics that may evolve over time; it is frequently associated with psychiatric disease, including obsessive compulsions, depression, self-harm or attention deficit disorder. Tics may also occur in Huntington's and Wilson's diseases, or after streptococcal infection.

Abnormal perception

The parietal lobes are involved in the higher processing and integration of the primary sensory information. This takes place in areas referred to as 'association' cortex, damage to which gives rise to sensory (including visual) inattention, disorders of spatial perception, and disruption of spatially orientated behaviour, leading to apraxia. Apraxia is the inability to perform complex, organised activity in the presence of normal basic motor, sensory and cerebellar function (after weakness, numbness and ataxia have been excluded as causes). Examples of complex motor activities include dressing, using cutlery and geographical orientation. Other abnormalities that can result from damage to the association cortex involve difficulty reading (dyslexia) or writing (dysgraphia), or the inability to recognise familiar objects (agnosia). The results of damage to particular lobes of the brain are given in Box 26.2 (p. 1142).

Altered balance and vertigo

Balance is a complicated dynamic process that requires ongoing modification of both axial and limb muscles to compensate for the effects of gravity and alterations in body position and load (and hence centre of gravity) in order to prevent a person from falling. This requires input from a variety of sensory modalities (visual, vestibular and proprioceptive), processing by the cerebellum and brainstem, and output via a number of descending pathways (e.g. vestibulospinal, rubrospinal and reticulospinal tracts).

Disorders of balance can therefore arise from any part of this process. Disordered input (loss of vision, vestibular disorders or lack of joint position sense), processing (damage to vestibular nuclei or cerebellum) or motor function (spinal cord lesions, leg weakness of any cause) can all impair balance. The patient may complain of different symptoms, depending on the location of the lesion. For example, loss of joint position sense or cerebellar function may result in a sensation of unsteadiness, while damage to the vestibular nuclei or labyrinth may result in an illusion of movement such as vertigo (see below). A careful history is vital. Since vision can often compensate for lack of joint position sense, patients with peripheral neuropathies or dorsal column loss will often find their problem more noticeable in the dark.

Examination of such patients may yield physical signs that again depend on the site of the lesion. Sensory abnormalities may be manifest as altered visual acuities or visual fields, possibly with abnormalities on fundoscopy, altered eye movements (including nystagmus, p. 1171), impaired vestibular function (p. 1186) or lack of joint position sense. Disturbance of cerebellar function may be manifest as nystagmus, dysarthria or ataxia, or difficulty with gait (unsteadiness or inability to perform tandem gait, p. 1168). Leg weakness, if present, will be detectable on examination of the limbs.

Vertigo

Vertigo is defined as an abnormal perception of movement of the environment or self, and occurs because of conflicting visual, proprioceptive and vestibular information about a person's position in space. Vertigo commonly arises from imbalance of vestibular input and is within the experience of most people, since this is the 'dizziness' that occurs after someone has spun round vigorously and then stops. Bilateral labyrinthine dysfunction often causes some unsteadiness. Labyrinthine vertigo usually lasts days at a time, though it may recur, whilst vertigo arising from central (brainstem) disorders is often persistent and accompanied by other brainstem signs. Benign paroxysmal positional vertigo (p. 1186) lasts a few seconds on head movement. A careful history will reveal the likely cause in most patients.

Abnormal gait

Many neurological disorders can affect gait. Observing patients as they walk into the consulting room can be very informative, although formal examination is also important. Neurogenic gait disorders need to be distinguished from those due to skeletal abnormalities, usually characterised by pain producing an antalgic gait, or limp. Gait alteration incompatible with any anatomical or physiological deficit may be due to functional disorders.

Pyramidal gait

Upper motor neuron lesions cause characteristic extension of the affected leg. The resultant tendency for the toes to strike the ground on walking requires the leg to swing outwards at the hip (circumduction). Nevertheless, a shoe on the affected side worn down at the toes may provide evidence of this type of gait. In hemiplegia, the asymmetry between affected and normal sides is obvious on walking, but in paraparesis both lower limbs swing slowly from the hips in extension and are dragged stiffly over the ground - described as 'walking in mud'.

Foot drop

In normal walking, the heel is the first part of the foot to hit the ground. A lower motor neuron lesion affecting the leg will cause weakness of ankle dorsiflexion, resulting in a less controlled descent of the foot, which makes a slapping noise as it hits the ground. In severe cases, the foot will have to be lifted higher at the knee to allow room for the inadequately dorsiflexed foot to swing through, resulting in a high-stepping gait.

Myopathic gait

During walking, alternating transfer of the body's weight through each leg requires adequate hip abduction. In proximal muscle weakness, usually caused by muscle disease, the hips are not properly fixed by these muscles and trunk movements are exaggerated, producing a rolling or waddling gait.

Ataxic gait

An ataxic gait can result from lesions in the cerebellum, vestibular apparatus or peripheral nerves. Patients with lesions of the central portion of the cerebellum (the vermis) walk with a characteristic broad-based gait 'as if drunk' (cerebellar function is particularly sensitive to alcohol). Patients with acute vestibular disturbances walk similarly but the accompanying vertigo is characteristic. Inability to walk heel to toe may be the only sign of less severe cerebellar dysfunction.

Proprioceptive defects can also cause an ataxic gait. The impairment of joint position sense makes walking unreliable, especially in poor light. The feet tend to be placed on the ground with greater emphasis, presumably to enhance proprioceptive input, resulting in a 'stamping' gait.

Apraxic gait

In an apraxic gait, power, cerebellar function and proprioception are normal on examination of the legs. The patient may be able to carry out complex motor tasks (e.g. bicycling motion) while recumbent and yet cannot formulate the motor act of walking. In this higher cerebral dysfunction, the feet appear stuck to the floor and the patient cannot walk. Gait apraxia is a sign of diffuse bilateral hemisphere disease (such as normal pressure hydrocephalus) or diffuse frontal lobe disease.

Marche à petits pas

This gait is characterised by small, slow steps and marked instability. It differs from the festination found in Parkinson's disease (see below) in that it lacks increasing pace and freezing. The usual cause is small-vessel cerebrovascular disease, and there are accompanying bilateral upper motor neuron signs.

Extrapyramidal gait

The rigidity and bradykinesia of basal ganglia dysfunction (p. 1194) lead to a stooped posture and characteristic gait difficulties, with problems initiating walking and controlling the pace of the gait. Patients may become stuck whilst trying to start walking or when walking through doorways ('freezing'). The centre of gravity will be moved forwards to aid propulsion, which, with poor axial control, can lead to an accelerating pace of shuffling and difficulty stopping. This produces the festinant gait: initial stuttering steps that quickly increase in frequency while decreasing in length.

Abnormal speech and language

Speech disturbance may be isolated to disruption of sound output (dysarthria) or may involve language disturbance (dysphasia). Dysphonia (reduction in the sound/volume) is usually due to mechanical laryngeal disruption, whereas dysarthria is more typically neurological in origin. Dysphasia is always neurological and localises to the dominant cerebral hemisphere (usually left, regardless of handedness). Combinations of speech and swallowing problems are explained below (p. 1173).

Dysphonia

Dysphonia describes hoarse or whispered speech. The most common cause is laryngitis, but dysphonia can also result from a lesion of the 10th cranial nerve or disease of the vocal cords, including laryngeal dystonia. Parkinsonism may cause hypophonia with marked reduction in speech volume, often in association with dysarthria, making speech difficult to understand.

Dysarthria

Dysarthria is characterised by poorly articulated or slurred speech and can occur in association with lesions of the cerebellum, brainstem and lower cranial nerves, as well as in myasthenia or myopathic disease. Language function is not affected. The quality of the speech tends to differ depending on the cause, but it can be very

26.24 Causes of dysarthria

Type	Site	Characteristics	Associated features
Myopathic	Muscles of speech	Indistinct, poor articulation	Weakness of face, tongue and neck
Myasthenic	Motor end plate	Indistinct with fatigue and dysphonia Fluctuating severity	Ptosis, diplopia, facial and neck weakness
Bulbar	Brainstem	Indistinct, slurred, often nasal	Dysphagia, diplopia, ataxia
'Scanning'	Cerebellum	Slurred, impaired timing and cadence, 'sing-song'	Ataxia of limbs and gait, tremor of head/limbs Nystagmus
Spastic ('pseudo-bulbar')	Pyramidal tracts	Indistinct, breathy, mumbling	Poor rapid tongue movements, increased reflexes and jaw jerk
Parkinsonian	Basal ganglia	Indistinct, rapid, stammering, quiet	Tremor, rigidity, slow shuffling gait
Dystonic	Basal ganglia	Strained, slow, high-pitched	Dystonia, athetosis

difficult to distinguish the different types clinically (Box 26.24). Dysarthria is discussed further in the section on bulbar symptoms (p. 1173).

Dysphasia

Dysphasia (or aphasia) is a disorder of the language content of speech. It can occur with lesions over a wide area of the dominant hemisphere (Fig. 26.20). Dysphasia may be categorised according to whether the speech output is fluent or non-fluent. Fluent aphasias, also called receptive aphasias, are impairments related mostly to the input or reception of language, with difficulties either in auditory verbal comprehension or in the repetition of words, phrases or sentences spoken by others. Speech is easy and fluent, but there are difficulties related to the output of language as well, such as paraphasia (either substitution of similar-sounding non-words, or incorrect words) and neologisms (non-existent words). Examples include Wernicke's aphasia (which localises to the superior posterior temporal lobe), transcortical sensory aphasia, conduction aphasia and anomic aphasia.

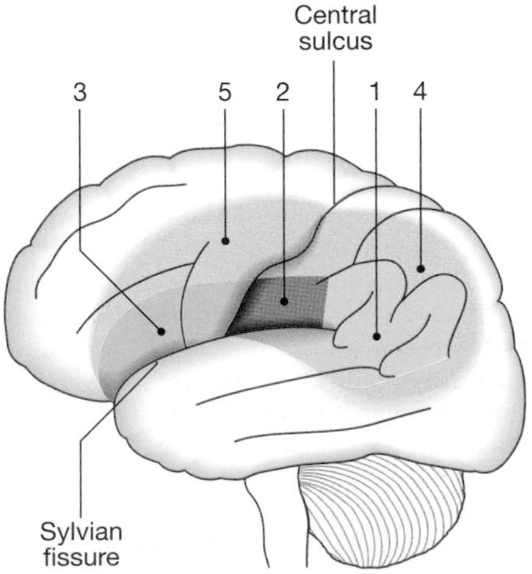

Non-fluent aphasias, also called expressive aphasias, are difficulties in articulating, but in most cases there is relatively good auditory verbal comprehension. Examples include Broca's aphasia (associated with pathologies in the inferior frontal region), transcortical motor aphasia and global aphasia.

'Pure' aphasias are selective impairments in reading, writing or the recognition of words. These disorders may be quite selective. For example, a person is able to read but not write, or is able to write but not read. Examples include pure alexia, agraphia and pure word deafness.

Dysphasia (a focal symptom) is frequently misinterpreted as confusion (which is non-focal). Dysphasia can be misheard/misspelt as dysphagia, and for this reason some prefer to use 'aphasia' to avoid confusion.

Fig. 26.20 Classification of cortical speech problems. (1) Wernicke's aphasia: fluent dysphasia with poor comprehension and poor repetition. (2) Conduction aphasia: fluent aphasia with good comprehension and poor repetition. (3) Broca's aphasia: non-fluent aphasia with good comprehension and poor repetition. (4) Transcortical sensory aphasia: fluent aphasia with poor comprehension and good repetition. (5) Transcortical motor aphasia: non-fluent aphasia with good comprehension and good repetition. Large lesions affecting all of regions 1–5 cause global aphasia.

Disturbance of smell

Symptomatic olfactory loss almost always is due to local causes (nasal obstruction), follows head injury or is idiopathic. Hyposmia may occur early in Parkinson's disease. Frontal lobe lesions are a rare cause. Positive olfactory symptoms may arise from Alzheimer's disease or epilepsy.

Visual disturbance and ocular abnormalities

Disturbances of vision may be due to primary ocular disease or to disorders of the central connections and visual cortex. Visual symptoms are usually negative (loss of vision) but sometimes are positive, most commonly in migraine. Eye movements may be disturbed, giving rise to double vision (diplopia) or blurred vision.

Visual loss

Visual loss can occur as the result of lesions in any areas between the retina and the visual cortex. Patterns of

26.25 Clinical manifestations of visual field loss

Site of lesion	Common causes	Complaint	Visual field loss	Associated physical signs
Retina/optic disc	Vascular disease (including vasculitis) Glaucoma Inflammation	Partial/complete visual loss depending on site, involving one or both eyes	Altitudinal field defect Arcuate scotoma	Reduced acuity Visual distortion (macula) Abnormal retinal appearance
Optic nerve	Optic neuritis Sarcoidosis Tumour Leber's hereditary optic neuropathy	Partial/complete loss of vision in one eye Often painful Central vision particularly affected	Central or paracentral scotoma Monocular blindness	Reduced acuity Reduced colour vision Relative afferent pupillary defect Optic atrophy (late)
Optic chiasm	Pituitary tumour Craniopharyngioma Sarcoidosis	May be none Rarely diplopia ('hemifield slide')	Bitemporal hemianopia	Pituitary function abnormalities
Optic tract	Tumour Inflammatory disease	Disturbed vision to one side of midline	Incongruous contralateral homonymous hemianopia	
Temporal lobe	Stroke Tumour Inflammatory disease	Disturbed vision to one side of midline	Contralateral homonymous upper quadrantanopia	Memory/language disorders
Parietal lobe	Stroke Tumour Inflammatory disease	Disturbed vision to one side of midline Bumping into things	Contralateral homonymous lower quadrantanopia	Contralateral sensory disturbance Asymmetry of optokinetic nystagmus
Occipital lobe	Stroke Tumour Inflammatory disease	Disturbed vision to one side of midline Difficulty reading Bumping into things	Homonymous hemianopia (may be macula-sparing)	Damage to other structures supplied by posterior cerebral circulation

visual field loss are explained by the anatomy of the visual pathways (see Fig. 26.7, p. 1145). Associated clinical manifestations are described in Box 26.25. Visual symptoms affecting one eye only are liable to be due to lesions anterior to the optic chiasm.

Transient visual loss is quite common and sudden-onset visual loss lasting less than 15 minutes is likely to have a vascular origin. It may be difficult to know whether the visual loss was monocular (carotid circulation) or binocular (vertebrobasilar circulation), and it can help to ask if the patient tried closing each eye in turn to see whether the symptom affected one eye or both. Visual field testing is an important part of the examination, either at the bedside or formally with perimetry. Field defects become more symmetrical (congruous), the closer the lesion comes to the visual cortex.

Migrainous visual symptoms are very common and, when associated with typical headache and other migraine features, rarely pose a diagnostic challenge. However, they may occur in isolation, making distinction from TIA difficult, but TIAs typically cause negative (transient blindness) symptoms, whereas migraine causes positive phenomena (see below). TIAs often last for a shorter time (a few minutes), compared to the 10–60-minute duration of migraine aura, and will have an abrupt onset and end, unlike the gradual evolution of a migraine aura.

Positive visual phenomena

The most common cause is migraine; patients may describe silvery zigzag lines (fortification spectra) or flashing coloured lights (teichopsia), usually preceding the headache. Simple flashes of light (phosphenes) may indicate damage to the retina (e.g. detachment) or to the primary visual cortex. Formed visual hallucinations may be caused by drugs, or may be due to epilepsy or 'release phenomena' in a blind visual field (Charles Bonnet's syndrome).

Double vision

Subtle double vision (diplopia) may be reported as blurred rather than double vision and most commonly arises from misalignment of the eyes. Monocular diplopia is rare and indicates ocular disease, while binocular diplopia suggests a probable neurological cause. Closing either eye in turn will abort binocular diplopia. Once the presence of binocular diplopia is confirmed, it should be established whether the diplopia is maximal in any particular direction of gaze, whether the images are separated horizontally or vertically, and whether there are any associated symptoms or signs, such as ptosis or pupillary disturbance.

Binocular diplopia occurs when eye movement is impaired, so that the image is not projected to the same points on the two retinae. It may result from central disorders or from disturbance of the ocular motor nerves, muscles or the neuromuscular junction (see Fig. 26.8, p. 1146). The pattern of double vision, along with any associated features, usually allows inference of which nerves/muscles are affected, whilst the mode of onset and other features (e.g. fatigability in myasthenia) provide further clues about the cause.

The causes of ocular motor nerve palsies are listed in Box 26.26.

26.26 Common causes of damage to cranial nerves 3, 4 and 6

Site	Common pathology	Nerve(s) involved	Associated features
Brainstem	Infarction Haemorrhage Demyelination Intrinsic tumour	3 (mid-brain) 6 (ponto-medullary junction)	Contralateral pyramidal signs Ipsilateral lower motor neuron facial palsy Other brainstem/cerebellar signs
Intrameningeal	Meningitis (infective/malignant)	3, 4 and/or 6	Meningism, features of primary disease course
	Raised intracranial pressure	6 3 (uncal herniation)	Papilloedema Features of space-occupying lesion
	Aneurysms	3 (posterior communicating artery) 6 (basilar artery)	Pain Features of subarachnoid haemorrhage
	Cerebello-pontine angle tumour	6	8, 7, 5 nerve lesions (order of likelihood) Ipsilateral cerebellar signs
	Trauma	3, 4 and/or 6	Other features of trauma
Cavernous sinus	Infection/thrombosis Carotid artery aneurysm Caroticocavernous fistula	3, 4 and/or 6	May be 5 nerve involvement also Pupil may be fixed, mid-position (sympathetic plexus on carotid may also be affected)
Superior orbital fissure	Tumour (e.g. sphenoid wing meningioma) Granuloma	3, 4 and/or 6	May be proptosis, chemosis
Orbit	Vascular (e.g. diabetes, vasculitis) Infections Tumour Granuloma Trauma	3, 4 and/or 6	Pain Pupil often spared in vascular 3rd nerve palsy

Nystagmus

Nystagmus describes a repetitive to-and-fro movement of the eyes. Usually slow drifts are the primary abnormal movement, each followed by fast (corrective) phases. Nystagmus occurs because the control systems of the eyes are defective, causing them to drift off target; corrections then become necessary to return fixation to the object of interest, causing nystagmus. The direction of the fast phase is usually designated as the direction of the nystagmus because it is easier to see. Nystagmus may be horizontal, vertical or torsional, and usually involves both eyes synchronously. It may be a physiological phenomenon in response to sustained vestibular stimulation or movement of the visual world (optokinetic nystagmus). There are many causes of pathological nystagmus, the most common sites of lesions being the vestibular system, brainstem and cerebellum.

In vestibular lesions, damage to one of the horizontal canals or its connections will allow the tonic output from the healthy, contralateral side to cause the eyes to drift towards the side of the lesion. This elicits recurrent compensatory fast movements away from the side of the lesion, manifest as unidirectional horizontal nystagmus. Vertical and torsional components can be seen with damage to other parts of the vestibular apparatus. The nystagmus of peripheral labyrinthine lesions is accompanied by vertigo and usually by nausea, vomiting and unsteadiness, but as the CNS habituates, the nystagmus disappears (fatigues) quite quickly. Central vestibular nystagmus is more persistent.

The brainstem and the cerebellum are involved in maintaining eccentric positions of gaze. Lesions will therefore allow the eyes to drift back in towards primary position, producing nystagmus with fast component beats in the direction of gaze (gaze-evoked nystagmus). This is the most common type of 'central' nystagmus; it is most commonly bidirectional and not usually accompanied by vertigo. Other signs of brainstem dysfunction may be evident. Brainstem disease may also cause vertical nystagmus.

Unilateral cerebellar lesions may result in gaze-evoked nystagmus when looking in the direction of the lesion, where the fast phases are directed towards the side of the lesion. Cerebellar hemisphere lesions also cause 'ocular dysmetria', an overshoot of target-directed, fast eye movements (saccades) resembling 'past-pointing' in limbs.

Nystagmus also occurs as a consequence of drug toxicity and nutritional deficiency (e.g. thiamin). The severity is variable, and it may or may not result in visual degradation, though it may be associated with a sensation of movement of the visual world (oscillopsia). Nystagmus may occur as a congenital phenomenon, in which case both phases are equal and 'pendular' rather than having alternating fast and slow components.

Ptosis

Various disorders may cause drooping of the eyelids (ptosis) and these are listed in Box 26.27.

26.27 Common causes of ptosis

Mechanism	Causes	Associated clinical features
3rd nerve palsy	Isolated palsy (see Box 26.26) Central/supranuclear lesion	Ptosis is usually complete Extraocular muscle palsy (eye 'down and out') Depending on site of lesion, other cranial nerve palsies (e.g. 4, 5 and 6) or contralateral upper motor neuron signs
Sympathetic lesion (Horner's syndrome: see Fig. 26.21**)**	Central (hypothalamus/brainstem) Peripheral (lung apex, carotid artery pathology) Idiopathic	Ptosis is partial Lack of sweating on affected side Depending on site of lesion, brainstem signs, signs of apical lung/brachial plexus disease, or ipsilateral carotid artery stroke
Myopathic	Myasthenia gravis Dystrophia myotonica	Extraocular muscle palsies More widespread muscle weakness, with fatigability in myasthenia Progressive external ophthalmoplegia Other characteristic features of individual causes
Other	Pseudo-ptosis (e.g. blepharospasm) Local orbital/lid disease Age-related levator dehiscence	Eyebrows depressed rather than raised May be local orbital abnormality

26.28 Pupillary disorders

Disorder	Cause	Ophthalmological features	Associated features
3rd nerve palsy	See Box 26.27	Dilated pupil Extraocular muscle palsy (eye is typically 'down and out') Complete ptosis	Other features of 3rd nerve palsy (see Box 26.27)
Horner's syndrome (see Fig. 26.21)	Lesion to sympathetic supply	Small pupil Partial ptosis Iris heterochromia (if congenital)	Ipsilateral failure of sweating (anhidrosis)
Holmes–Adie syndrome (tonic pupil)	Lesion of ciliary ganglion (usually idiopathic)	Dilated pupil Light-near dissociation (accommodate but do not react to light) Vermiform movement of iris during contraction Disturbance of accommodation	Generalised areflexia
Argyll Robertson pupil	Dorsal mid-brain lesion (syphilis or diabetes)	Small, irregular pupils Light-near dissociation	Other features of tabes dorsalis (p. 1209)
Local pupillary damage	Trauma/inflammatory disease	Irregular pupils, often with adhesions to lens (synechiae) Variable degree of reactivity	Other features of trauma/underlying inflammatory disease (e.g. cataract, blindness etc.)
Relative afferent pupillary defect (Marcus Gunn pupil)	Damage to optic nerve	Pupils symmetrical but degree of dilatation depends on which eye stimulated	Decreased visual acuity/colour vision Central scotoma Papilloedema/optic disc pallor

Abnormal pupillary responses

Abnormal pupillary responses may arise from lesions at several points between the retina and brainstem. Lesions of the oculomotor nerve, ciliary ganglion and sympathetic supply produce characteristic ipsilateral disorders of pupillary function. 'Afferent' defects result from damage to an optic nerve, impairing the direct response of a pupil to light, although leaving the consensual response from stimulation of the normal eye intact. Structural damage to the iris itself can also result in pupillary abnormalities. Causes are given in Box 26.28. An example is shown in Figure 26.21.

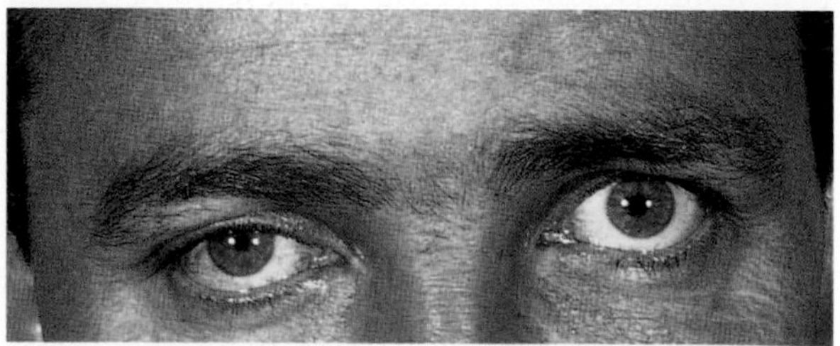

Fig. 26.21 Right-sided Horner's syndrome due to paravertebral metastasis at T1. There is ipsilateral partial ptosis and a small pupil.

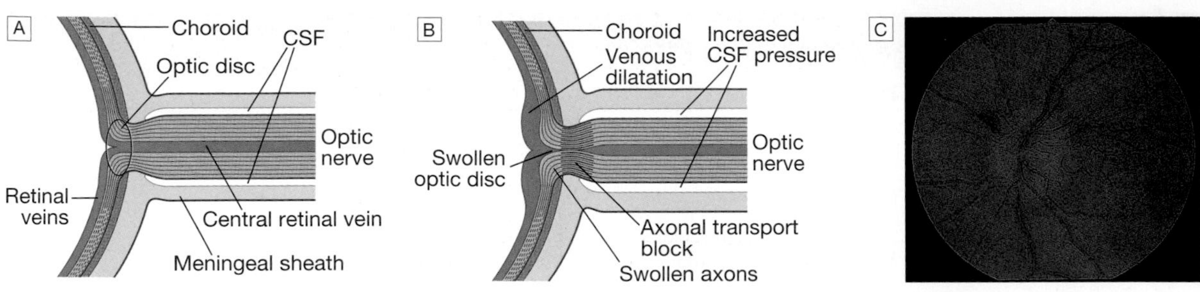

Fig. 26.22 Mechanism of optic disc oedema (papilloedema). A Normal. B Disc oedema (e.g. due to cerebral tumour). C Fundus photograph of the left eye showing optic disc oedema with a small haemorrhage on the nasal side of the disc.

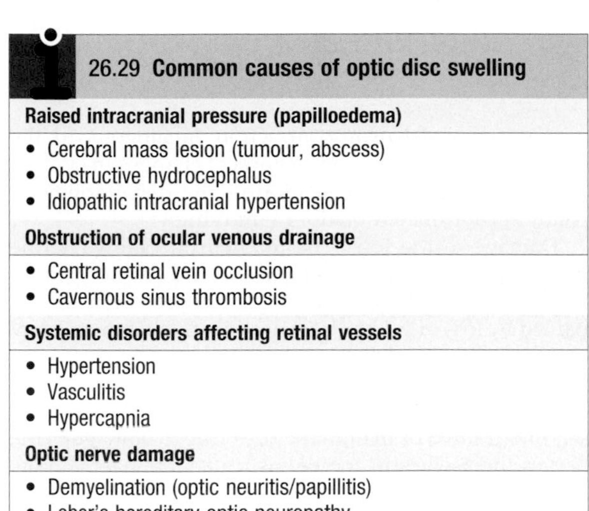

26.29 Common causes of optic disc swelling

Raised intracranial pressure (papilloedema)

- Cerebral mass lesion (tumour, abscess)
- Obstructive hydrocephalus
- Idiopathic intracranial hypertension

Obstruction of ocular venous drainage

- Central retinal vein occlusion
- Cavernous sinus thrombosis

Systemic disorders affecting retinal vessels

- Hypertension
- Vasculitis
- Hypercapnia

Optic nerve damage

- Demyelination (optic neuritis/papillitis)
- Leber's hereditary optic neuropathy
- Anterior ischaemic optic neuropathy
- Toxins (e.g. methanol)
- Infiltration of optic disc
- Sarcoidosis
- Glioma
- Lymphoma

Papilloedema

There are several causes of swelling of the optic disc, but the term 'papilloedema' is reserved for swelling secondary to raised intracranial pressure, when obstructed axoplasmic flow from retinal ganglion cells results in swollen nerve fibres, which in turn cause capillary and venous congestion, producing papilloedema. The earliest sign is the cessation of venous pulsation seen at the disc, progression causing the disc margins to become red (hyperaemic). Disc margins become indistinct and haemorrhages may occur in the retina (Fig. 26.22). Lack of papilloedema never excludes raised intracranial pressure. Other causes of optic disc swelling are listed in Box 26.29. Some normal variations of disc appearance (e.g. optic nerve drusen) can mimic disc swelling.

Optic atrophy

Loss of nerve fibres causes the optic disc to appear pale, as the choroid becomes visible (Fig. 26.23). A pale disc (optic atrophy) follows optic nerve damage, and causes include previous optic neuritis or ischaemic damage, long-standing papilloedema, optic nerve compression,

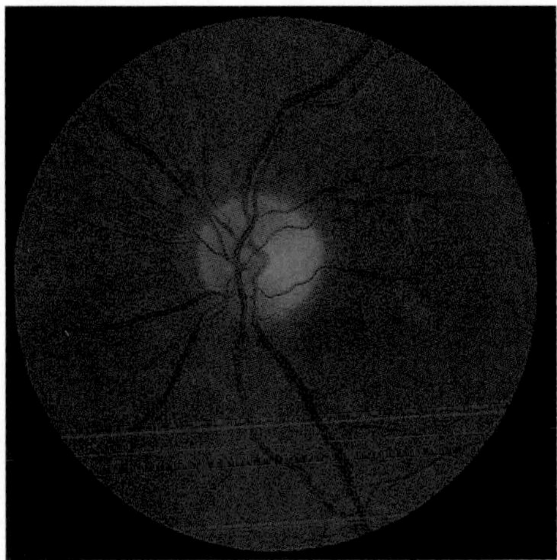

Fig. 26.23 Fundus photograph of the left eye of a patient with familial optic atrophy. Note marked pallor of optic disc.

trauma and degenerative conditions (e.g. Friedreich's ataxia, p. 1199).

Hearing disturbance

Each cochlear organ has bilateral cortical representation, so unilateral hearing loss is a result of peripheral organ damage. Bilateral hearing dysfunction is usual, and is most commonly due to age-related degeneration or noise damage, although infection and drugs (particularly diuretics and aminoglycoside antibiotics) can be a primary cause. Prominent deafness may suggest a mitochondrial disorder (see Box 26.109, p. 1229).

Bulbar symptoms – dysphagia and dysarthria

Swallowing is a complex activity involving the coordinated action of lips, tongue, soft palate, pharynx and larynx, which are innervated by cranial nerves 7, 9, 10, 11 and 12. Structural causes of dysphagia are considered on page 851. Neurological mechanisms are vulnerable to damage at different points, resulting in dysphagia that is usually accompanied by dysarthria. Tempo is again crucial: acute onset of dysphagia may occur as a result of brainstem stroke or a rapidly developing neuropathy,

26.30 Causes of pseudobulbar and bulbar palsy

	Pseudobulbar	Bulbar
Genetic	–	Kennedy's disease (X-linked bulbospinal neuronopathy)
Vascular	Bilateral hemisphere (lacunar) infarction	Medullary infarction (see Box 26.3, p. 1148)
Degenerative	Motor neuron disease (p. 1200)	Motor neuron disease Syringobulbia
Inflammatory/infective	Multiple sclerosis (p. 1188) Cerebral vasculitis	Myasthenia (p. 1226) Guillain–Barré syndrome (p. 1224) Poliomyelitis (p. 1207) Lyme disease (p. 334) Vasculitis
Neoplastic	High brainstem tumours	Brainstem glioma Malignant meningitis

such as Guillain–Barré syndrome or diphtheria. Intermittent fatigable muscle weakness (including dysphagia) would suggest myasthenia gravis. Dysphagia developing over weeks or months may be seen in motor neuron disease, polymyositis, basal meningitis and inflammatory brainstem disease. More slowly developing dysphagia suggests a myopathy or possibly a brainstem or skull-base tumour.

Pathologies affecting lower cranial nerves (9, 10, 11 and 12) frequently manifest bilaterally, producing dysphagia and dysarthria. The term 'bulbar palsy' is used to describe lower motor neuron lesions, either within the medulla or outside the brainstem. The tongue is wasted and fasciculating, and palatal movement is reduced.

Upper motor neuron innervation of swallowing is bilateral, so persistent dysphagia is unusual with a unilateral upper motor lesion (the exception being in the acute stages of, for example, a hemispheric stroke). Widespread lesions above the medulla will cause upper motor neuron bulbar paralysis, known as 'pseudobulbar palsy'. Here the tongue is small and contracted, and moves slowly; the jaw jerk is brisk. Causes of bulbar and pseudobulbar palsies are shown in Box 26.30.

Bladder, bowel and sexual disturbance

Whilst isolated disturbances of bladder, bowel and sexual function are rarely the sole presenting features of neurological disease, they are common complications of many chronic disorders such as multiple sclerosis, stroke and dementia, and are frequently found post head injury. Abnormalities in these functions considerably reduce quality of life for patients. Incontinence and its management are discussed elsewhere (pp. 472, 918 and 175).

Bladder dysfunction

The anatomy and physiology involved in controlling bladder functions are discussed on page 466 but it is worth emphasising the role of the pontine micturition centre, which is itself under higher control via inputs from the pre-frontal cortex, mid-brain and hypothalamus.

In the absence of conscious control (e.g. in coma or dementia), distension of the bladder to near-capacity evokes reflex detrusor contraction (analogous to the muscle stretch reflex), and reciprocal changes in sympathetic activation and relaxation of the distal sphincter result in coordinated bladder emptying.

Damage to the lower motor neuron pathways (the pelvic and pudendal nerves) produces a flaccid bladder and sphincter with overflow incontinence, often accompanied by loss of pudendal sensation. Such damage may be due to disease of the conus medullaris or sacral nerve roots, either within the dura (as in inflammatory or carcinomatous meningitis) or as they pass through the sacrum (trauma or malignancy), or due to damage to the nerves themselves in the pelvis (infection, haematoma, trauma or malignancy).

Damage to the pons or spinal cord results in an 'upper motor neuron' pattern of bladder dysfunction due to uncontrolled over-activity of the parasympathetic supply. The bladder is small and highly sensitive to being stretched. This results in frequency, urgency and urge incontinence. Loss of the coordinating control of the pontine micturition centre will also result in the phenomenon of detrusor–sphincter dyssynergia, in which detrusor contraction and sphincter relaxation are not coordinated; the spastic bladder will often try to empty against a closed sphincter. This manifests as both urgency and an inability to pass urine, which is distressing and painful. The resultant incomplete bladder emptying predisposes to urinary infection, and the prolonged high bladder pressure may result in renal failure; post-micturition bladder ultrasound may confirm incomplete bladder emptying. More severe lesions of the spinal cord, as in spinal cord compression or trauma, can result in painless urinary retention, as bladder sensation, normally carried in the lateral spinothalamic tracts, will be cut off.

Damage to the frontal lobes gives rise to loss of awareness of bladder fullness and consequent incontinence. Coexisting cognitive impairment may result in inappropriate micturition. These features are seen typically in hydrocephalus, frontal tumours, dementia and bifrontal subdural haematomas.

When a patient presents with bladder symptoms, it is important to try to localise the lesion on the basis of history and examination, remembering that most bladder problems are not neurological unless there are overt neurological signs. Clinical features and management are summarised in Box 26.31.

26.31 Neurogenic bladder: clinical features and treatment

	Site of lesion	Result	Treatment
Atonic (lower motor neuron)	Lesions of sacral segments of cord (conus medullaris) Lesions of sacral roots and nerves	Loss of detrusor contraction Difficulty initiating micturition Bladder distension with overflow	Intermittent self-catheterisation In-dwelling catheterisation
Hypertonic (upper motor neuron)	Pyramidal tract lesion in spinal cord or brainstem	Urgency with urge incontinence Bladder sphincter incoordination (dyssynergia) Incomplete bladder emptying	Anticholinergics: Solifenacin Tolterodine Imipramine Intermittent self-catheterisation
Cortical	Post-central Pre-central Frontal	Loss of awareness of bladder fullness Difficulty initiating micturition Inappropriate micturition Loss of social control	Intermittent or in-dwelling catheterisation

Rectal dysfunction

The rectum has an excitatory cholinergic input from the parasympathetic sacral outflow, and inhibitory sympathetic supply similar to the bladder. Continence depends largely on skeletal muscle contraction in the puborectalis and pelvic floor muscles supplied by the pudendal nerves, as well as the internal and external anal sphincters. Damage to the autonomic components usually causes constipation (a common early symptom in Parkinson's disease) but diabetic neuropathy can be associated with diarrhoea. Lesions affecting the conus medullaris, the somatic S2–4 roots and the pudendal nerves may cause faecal incontinence.

Erectile failure and ejaculatory failure

These related functions are under autonomic control via the pelvic nerves (parasympathetic, S2–4) and hypogastric nerves (sympathetic, L1–2). Descending influences from the cerebrum are important for erection, but it can occur as a reflex phenomenon in response to genital stimulation. Erection is largely parasympathetic, and may be impaired by a number of drugs, including anticholinergic, antihypertensive and antidepressant agents. Sympathetic activity is important for ejaculation, and may be inhibited by α-adrenoceptor antagonists (α-blockers). For further information on erectile failure, see page 474.

Personality change

While this is often due to psychiatric illness, neurological conditions that alter the function of the frontal lobes can cause personality change and mood disorder (see Box 26.2, p. 1142). Personality change due to a frontal lobe disorder may occur as the result of structural damage due to stroke, trauma, tumour or hydrocephalus. The nature of any change may help localise the lesion.

Patients with mesial frontal lesions become increasingly withdrawn, unresponsive and mute (abulic), often in association with urinary incontinence, gait apraxia and an increase in tone known as gegenhalten, in which the patient varies the resistance to movement in proportion to the force exerted by the examiner.

Patients with lesions of the dorsolateral pre-frontal cortex develop a dysexecutive syndrome, which involves difficulties with speech, motor planning and organisation. Those with orbitofrontal lesions of the frontal lobes, in contrast, become disinhibited, displaying grandiosity or irresponsible behaviour. Memory is substantially intact but frontal release signs may emerge, such as a grasp reflex, palmomental response or pout. Proximity to the olfactory bulb and tracts means that inferior frontal lobe tumours may be associated with anosmia.

Disturbance to the cortical areas responsible for speech or memory can result in changes that may be interpreted as changes in personality.

Sleep disturbance

Disturbances of sleep are common and are not usually due to neurological disease. Patients may complain of insomnia (difficulty sleeping), excessive daytime sleepiness, disturbed behaviour during night-time sleep, parasomnia (sleep walking and talking, or night terrors) or disturbing subjective experiences during sleep and/or its onset (nightmares, hypnagogic hallucinations, sleep paralysis). A careful history (from the bed-partner as well as the patient) usually allows specific causes of sleep disturbance to be identified and these are discussed in more detail on page 1187.

Psychiatric disorders

Psychiatric disorders are described in Chapter 10 but may cause or result from neurological problems. Care is needed in their identification, as effective management will help the underlying neurological illness.

FUNCTIONAL SYMPTOMS

Many patients presenting with neurological symptoms do not have a defined neurological disease and are best described as having functional symptoms (p. 236). Some

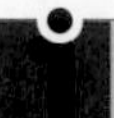

26.32 Clinical features suggestive of functional disorder

- Situational provocation
- Associated psychological disorders
  - Anxiety
  - Depression
- Lack of anatomical coherence to neurological symptoms
- Florid or bizarre descriptions of individual symptoms
- History of other medically unexplained symptoms
- Hoover's sign (p. 1163)
- Predisposing history of childhood neglect or abuse

of these are psychogenic (or conversion) disorders. Such patients often have unexplained symptoms affecting multiple systems and a long list of consultations and negative tests from other medical specialties when they present. Considering the possibility of a functional origin may save the patient further unnecessary, invasive and inconvenient investigation and anxiety.

Weakness and sensory symptoms predominate among functional symptoms, but pain or loss of consciousness can occur. Associated symptoms, such as tiredness, lethargy, poor concentration, bowel upset (irritable bowel syndrome) and gynaecological complaints, are common. A functional origin of neurological problems should always be considered, as it can allow for more rapid diagnosis and avoid unnecessarily painful or hazardous investigation. Some clinical features may hint at a functional origin for symptoms (Box 26.32). It is the clinician's job to elicit the context of the patient's symptoms in a sensitive and non-judgemental way. Whatever the illness, it is important to acknowledge that mood and sleep disturbance will exacerbate neurological symptoms, thus increasing disability resulting from neurological disorders. The best practitioners have the skill to carry the patient with them when describing the patterns of behaviour contributing to symptoms.

Assessment to detect an underlying or exacerbating mood disorder is vital in all patients, ensuring that depression and anxiety are managed to minimise their secondary effects on neurological symptoms.

HEADACHE SYNDROMES

Headaches may be classified as primary or secondary, depending on the underlying cause (see Box 26.10, p. 1156). Secondary headache may be due to structural, infective, inflammatory or vascular conditions, which are discussed later in this chapter. The primary headache syndromes are described here.

Tension-type headache

This is the most common type of headache and is experienced to some degree by the majority of the population.

Pathophysiology

Tension headache is incompletely understood. Emotions and anxiety are common precipitants and there is sometimes an associated depressive illness. Anxiety about the headache itself may lead to continuation of symptoms, and patients often become convinced of a serious underlying condition. Muscular spasms may worsen this in some patients.

Clinical features

The pain of tension headache is usually characterised as 'dull', 'tight' or like a 'pressure', and there may be a sensation of a band round the head or pressure at the vertex. It is of constant character and generalised, but often radiates forwards from the occipital region. In contrast to migraine, the pain can remain unabated for weeks or months without interruption, although the severity may vary, and there is no associated vomiting or photophobia. Activities are usually continued throughout, and the pain may be less noticeable when the patient is occupied. The pain is usually less severe in the early part of the day, becoming more troublesome as the day goes on. Tenderness may be present over the skull vault or in the occiput but is easily distinguished from the triggered pains of trigeminal neuralgia and the exquisite tenderness of temporal arteritis. Analgesics may be taken with chronic regularity despite little effect, and may serve to perpetuate the symptoms (see 'Medication overuse headache' below).

Management

Most benefit is given by providing a careful assessment, followed by discussion of likely precipitants and reassurance that the prognosis is good. Excessive use of analgesia, particularly those containing codeine, may maintain and exacerbate the headache (analgesic headache). Physiotherapy (with muscle relaxation and stress management) may help and low-dose amitriptyline can provide benefit. There is evidence that patients benefit from a perception that their problem has been taken seriously and rigorously assessed. Investigation may contribute to such reassurance, especially if concerns about an underlying lesion are strong, but patients should understand the purpose and likely outcome of such imaging.

Migraine

Migraine usually appears before middle age; it affects about 20% of females and 6% of males at some point in life. Some patients assume that migraine is a term encompassing any severe headache but it has a characteristic presentation, discussed below.

Pathophysiology

The cause of migraine is unknown but there is increasing evidence that the aura (see below) is due to dysfunction of ion channels causing a spreading front of cortical depolarisation (excitation) followed by hyperpolarisation (depression of activity). This process (the 'spreading depression of Leão') spreads over the cortex at a rate of about 3 mm/minute, corresponding to the aura's symptomatic spread. The headache phase is associated with vasodilatation of extracranial vessels and may be relayed by hypothalamic activity. Activation of the trigeminovascular system is probably important. A genetic contribution is implied by frequently positive family history, and similar phenomena occurring in disorders such as CADASIL (p. 1242). The female preponderance and the frequency of migraine attacks at certain points in the menstrual cycle also suggest hormonal influences. Oestrogen-containing oral contraception sometimes exacerbates migraine, and increases the small risk of stroke in patients who suffer from migraine with aura. Doctors and patients often over-estimate the role of dietary precipitants such as cheese, chocolate or red wine. When psychological factors contribute, the migraine attack often occurs after a period of stress, being more likely on Friday evening at the end of the working week or at the beginning of a holiday.

Clinical features

Some patients report a prodrome of malaise, irritability or behavioural change for some hours or days. Around 20% of patients experience an aura, and are said to have migraine with aura (previously known as classical migraine). The aura is most often visual, consisting of fortification spectra, which are shimmering, silvery zigzag lines that march across the visual fields for up to 40 minutes, sometimes leaving a trail of temporary visual field loss (scotoma). In some there is a sensory aura of tingling followed by numbness, spreading over 20–30 minutes, from one part of the body to another. Dominant hemisphere involvement may also cause transient speech disturbance. The 80% of patients with characteristic headache but no 'aura' are said to have migraine without aura (previously called 'common' migraine).

Migraine headache is usually severe and throbbing, with photophobia, phonophobia and vomiting lasting from 4 to 72 hours. Movement makes the pain worse, and patients prefer to lie in a quiet, dark room.

Caution should be taken in ascribing the cause of an individual's limb weakness or isolated aura without headache to migraine. In such cases, other structural disorders of the brain, or even focal epilepsy, need to be considered.

In a smaller number of patients, the symptoms of the aura do not resolve, leaving more permanent neurological disturbance. This persistent migrainous aura may occur with or without evidence of brain infarction.

Management

Avoidance of identified triggers or exacerbating factors (such as the combined contraceptive pill) may prevent attacks. Treatment of an acute attack consists of simple analgesia with aspirin, paracetamol or non-steroidal anti-inflammatory agents. Nausea may require an antiemetic such as metoclopramide or domperidone. Severe attacks can be aborted by one of the increasing number of 'triptans' (e.g. sumatriptan), which are potent 5-hydroxytryptamine (5-HT) agonists. These can be administered orally, by subcutaneous injection or by nasal spray. Care should be taken to avoid accelerating use. Caution is needed with ergotamine preparations since they may lead to dependence. Overuse of any analgesia, including triptans, may contribute to associated medication overuse headache.

If attacks are frequent (more than 3–4 per month), prophylaxis should be considered. Many drugs can be used, but the most frequently used are vasoactive drugs (calcium channel blockers and β-adrenoceptor antagonists (β-blockers)), antidepressants (amitriptyline, dosulepin) and anti-epileptic drugs (valproate, topiramate). Women with aura should avoid oestrogen treatment for either oral contraception or hormone replacement, although the increased risk of ischaemic stroke is minimal.

Medication overuse headache

With increasing availability of over-the-counter medication, headache syndromes perpetuated by analgesia intake are becoming much more common. Medication overuse headache (MOH) can complicate any other headache syndrome, but is especially associated with migraine and tension headache. The medications that are the most common culprits are compound analgesia (particularly codeine and other opiate-containing preparations) and triptans, and MOH is usually associated with use on more than 10–15 days per month.

Management is by withdrawal of the responsible analgesics; patients should be warned that the initial effect will be to exacerbate the headache. Migraine prophylactics may be helpful in reducing the rebound headaches. In severe cases, hospital admission with or without a course of corticosteroids may be helpful.

Cluster headache

Cluster headaches (also known as migrainous neuralgia) are much less common than migraine. There is a 5:1 male predominance and onset is usually in the third decade.

Pathophysiology

The cause is unknown, but this type of headache differs from migraine in its character, lack of genetic predisposition, lack of provoking dietary factors, opposing gender imbalance and different drug effect. Functional imaging studies have suggested abnormal hypothalamic activity. Patients are more often smokers with a higher than average alcohol consumption.

Clinical features

Cluster headache is strikingly periodic, featuring runs of identical headaches beginning at the same hour for weeks at a time (the eponymous 'cluster'). Patients may experience either one or several attacks within a 24-hour period. Cluster headache causes severe, unilateral periorbital pain with autonomic features, such as unilateral lacrimation, nasal congestion and conjunctival injection (occasionally with the other features of Horner's syndrome). The pain, though severe, is characteristically brief (30–90 minutes). In contrast to the behaviour of those with migraine, patients are often highly agitated during the headache phase. The cluster period is typically a few weeks, followed by remission for months to years, but a small proportion do not experience remission.

Management

Acute attacks can usually be halted by subcutaneous injections of sumatriptan or by inhalation of 100% oxygen. The brevity of the attack probably prevents other migraine therapies from being effective. Migraine prophylaxis is often ineffective too but attacks can be prevented in some patients by sodium valproate, verapamil, methysergide or short courses of oral corticosteroids. Patients with severe debilitating clusters can be helped with lithium therapy, although this requires monitoring (p. 245).

26.33 Benign paroxysmal headaches

	Character of pain	Duration	Location	Comment
Ice pick	Stabbing	Very brief (split-second)	Variable, usually temporoparietal	Benign, more common in migraine
Ice cream	Sharp, severe	30–120 secs	Bitemporal/occipital	Obvious trigger by cold stimuli
Exertional/ coital	Bursting, thunderclap	Severe for mins then less severe for hrs	Generalised	Subarachnoid haemorrhage needs to be excluded
Cough	Bursting	Secs to mins	Occipital or generalised	Intracranial pathology needs to be excluded (especially craniocervical junction)
Cluster headache (migrainous neuralgia)	Severe unilateral, with ptosis, tearing, conjunctival injection, unilateral nasal congestion	30–90 mins 1–3 times per day	Periorbital	Usually in men, occurring in clusters over weeks/ months
Chronic paroxysmal hemicrania	Severe unilateral with cluster headache-like autonomic features (see above)	5–20 mins, frequently through day	Periorbital/temporal	Usually in women, responds to indometacin
SUNCT*	Severe, sharp, triggered by touch or neck movements	15–120 secs, repetitive through day	Periorbital	May respond to carbamazepine

*Short-lasting, Unilateral, Neuralgiform headache with Conjunctival injection, Tearing, rhinorrhoea and forehead sweating.

Trigeminal neuralgia

This is characterised by unilateral lancinating facial pain, most commonly involving the second and/or third divisions of the trigeminal nerve territory, usually in patients over the age of 50 years.

Pathophysiology

Trigeminal neuralgia is thought to be caused by an irritative lesion involving the trigeminal root zone, in some cases an aberrant loop of artery. Other compressive lesions, usually benign, are occasionally found. Trigeminal neuralgia associated with multiple sclerosis may result from a plaque of demyelination in the brainstem.

Clinical features

The pain is repetitive, severe and very brief. It may be triggered by touch, a cold wind or eating. Physical signs are usually absent, although the spasms may make the patient wince and sit silently (tic douloureux). Similar symptoms may occur in multiple sclerosis or with other brainstem lesions, in which case there may be associated sensory changes in the trigeminal nerve territory or elsewhere. There is a tendency for the condition to remit and relapse over many years.

Management

The pain usually responds at least partially to carbamazepine. It is wise to start with a low dose and increase gradually, according to effect. In patients who cannot tolerate carbamazepine, gabapentin, pregabalin, amitriptyline or steroids may be effective. The possibility of surgical treatment should be entertained, especially where response is incomplete in younger patients. Decompression of the vascular loop encroaching on the trigeminal root is said to have a 90% success rate. Otherwise, localised injection of alcohol or phenol into a peripheral branch of the nerve may be effective.

Headaches associated with specific activities

These usually affect men in their thirties and forties. Patients develop a sudden, severe headache with exertion, including sexual activity. There is usually no vomiting and no neck stiffness, and the headache lasts less than 10–15 minutes, though a less severe dullness may persist for some hours. Subarachnoid haemorrhage needs to be excluded by CT and/or CSF examination (see Fig. 27.12, p. 1246) after a first event. The pathogenesis of these headaches is unknown. Although frightening, attacks are usually brief and patients may only need reassurance and simple analgesia for the residual headache. The syndrome may recur, and prevention may be necessary with propranolol or indometacin.

Other headache syndromes

A number of rare headache syndromes produce pains about the eye similar to cluster headaches (Box 26.33). These include chronic paroxysmal hemicrania and SUNCT (short-lasting unilateral neuralgiform headaches with conjunctival injection and tearing). The recognition of these syndromes is useful since they often respond to specific treatments such as indometacin.

EPILEPSY

A seizure can be defined as the occurrence of signs and/or symptoms due to abnormal, excessive or synchronous

26.34 Classification of seizures (2010 ILAE Classification)

Generalised seizures

- Tonic–clonic (in any combination)
- Absence
  - Typical
  - Atypical
  - Absence with special features
- Myoclonic absence
- Eyelid myoclonia
- Myoclonic
  - Myoclonic
  - Myoclonic atonic
  - Myoclonic tonic
- Clonic
- Tonic
- Atonic

Focal seizures

- Without impairment of consciousness or awareness (was 'simple partial')
  - Focal motor
  - Focal sensory
- With impairment of consciousness or awareness (was 'complex partial')
- Evolving to a bilateral, convulsive seizure (was 'secondarily generalised seizure')
  - Tonic
  - Clonic
  - Tonic–clonic

Unknown

- Epileptic spasms

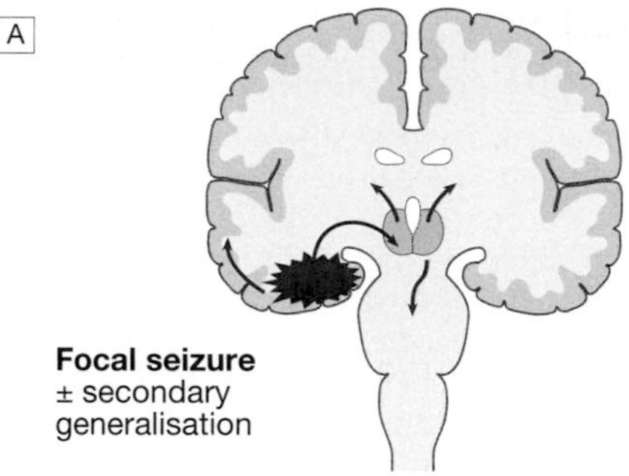

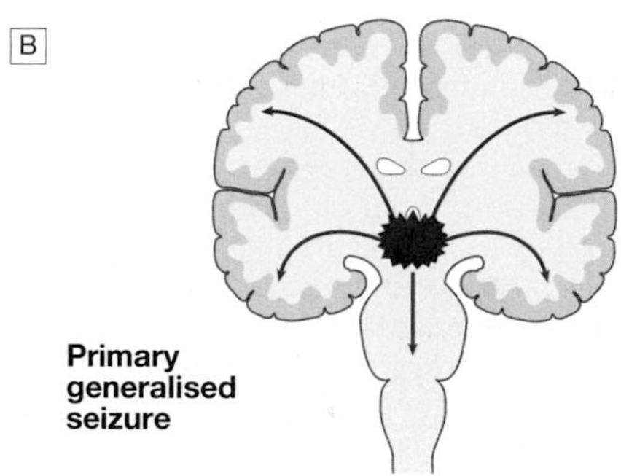

Fig. 26.24 The pathophysiological classification of seizures. **A** A focal seizure originates from a paroxysmal discharge in a focal area of the cerebral cortex (often the temporal lobe); the seizure may subsequently spread to the rest of the brain (secondary generalisation) via diencephalic activating pathways. **B** In primary generalised seizures the abnormal electrical discharges originate from the diencephalic activating system and spread simultaneously to all areas of the cortex.

neuronal activity in the brain. 'Epilepsy' is the tendency to have unprovoked seizures. The lifetime risk of seizure is about 5%, although incidence is highest at the extremes of age. Whilst the prevalence of active epilepsy in European countries is about 0.5%, the figure in developing countries may be higher because of parasitic illnesses such as cysticercosis (p. 380).

Historical terms such as 'grand mal' (implying tonic-clonic seizures) and 'petit mal' (intended by its originators to mean 'absence seizures' but commonly used to describe 'anything other than grand mal') have been superseded. Subsequent revisions, including terms such as 'complex partial' and 'simple partial', have been imprecise and confusing, carrying little information about underlying pathology, treatment or prognosis. The modern equivalents for these terms will be given below, but it is preferable to adhere to the 2010 iteration of the International League Against Epilepsy's classification (Box 26.34).

Pathophysiology

To function normally, the brain must achieve an ongoing balance between excitation and inhibition, in order to remain responsive to the environment without continued unrestrained spontaneous activity. The inhibitory transmitter gamma-aminobutyric acid (GABA) is particularly important, acting on ion channels to enhance chloride inflow and reduce the chances of action potential formation. Excitatory amino acids (glutamate and aspartate) allow influx of sodium and calcium, producing the opposite effect. It is likely that many seizures result from an imbalance between this excitation and inhibition. Intracellular recordings during seizures demonstrate a paroxysmal depolarisation shift in neuronal membrane potential, predisposing to recurrent action potentials. In vivo, epileptic cortex shows repetitive discharges involving large groups of neurons.

Seizures may be related to a localised disturbance in the cortex, becoming manifest in the first instance as focal seizures. Any disturbance of cortical architecture and function can precipitate this, whether focal infection, tumour, hamartoma or trauma-related scarring. If focal seizures remain localised, the symptoms experienced depend on which cortical area is affected. If areas in the temporal lobes become involved, then awareness of the environment becomes impaired but without associated tonic–clonic movements. When both hemispheres are involved, either at onset or after spread, the seizure becomes generalised (Fig. 26.24).

In seizures that are generalised at onset, the abnormal activity probably originates in the central mechanisms controlling cortical activation (see Fig. 26.24) and spreads rapidly. Such epilepsies constitute around 30% of all epilepsy, and are likely to reflect widespread disturbance of structure or function. Animal models have revealed mutations in genes for ion channels and receptors that cause seizures. In humans, many generalised epilepsies will have a genetic basis, and these almost always become apparent before the age of 35.

Seizure activity is usually apparent on EEG as spike and wave discharges (see Fig. 26.14, p. 1152). Other generalised seizure activity may involve merely brief loss of awareness (absence seizures), single jerks (myoclonus) or loss of tone (atonic seizures), as detailed in Box 26.34.

Clinical features

Seizure type and epilepsy type

To classify seizure type, the clinician should ask first whether there is a focal onset, and second whether the seizures conform to one of the recognised patterns (see Box 26.34). Epilepsy that starts in patients beyond their mid-thirties will almost invariably reflect a focal cerebral event. Where activity remains focal, this will be obvious. Even when generalised tonic–clonic seizures occur, seizures beginning in one cortical area will cause positive neurological symptoms and signs corresponding to the normal function of that area. Occipital onset will cause visual changes (lights and blobs of colour), temporal lobe onset will cause false recognition (déjà vu), sensory strip involvement will cause sensory alteration (burning, tingling), and motor strip involvement will cause jerking.

Patients can experience more than one type of seizure attack, and it is important to document each attack type and the patient's age at its onset, along with its frequency, duration and typical features. Any triggers should be identified (Box 26.35). The type of seizure, other clinical features and investigations can then be used to determine the epilepsy syndrome, as discussed below. Where there is doubt about the type, this is best stated and a full classification should be deferred until the evolution of the clinical features clarifies the picture.

Some patients will give a history of a previous local cortical insult, and it can be reasonably (but not invariably) inferred that this is the seat of epileptogenesis.

Focal seizures

The classification of focal seizures is shown in Box 26.34. They are caused by localised cortical activity with retained awareness. The localisation of such symptoms is described above. A spreading pattern of seizure may occur, the abnormal sensation spreading much faster (in seconds) than a migrainous focal sensory attack.

Awareness may become impaired if spread occurs to the temporal lobes (previously 'complex partial seizure'). Patients stop and stare blankly, often blinking repetitively, making smacking movements of their lips or displaying other automatisms, such as picking at their clothes. After a few minutes, consciousness returns but the patient may be muddled and feel drowsy for a period of up to an hour. The age of onset, preceding aura, longer duration and post-ictal symptoms usually make these easy to differentiate from childhood absence seizures (see below).

26.35 Trigger factors for seizures

- Sleep deprivation
- Missed doses of anti-epileptic drugs in treated patients
- Alcohol (particularly withdrawal)
- Recreational drug misuse
- Physical and mental exhaustion
- Flickering lights, including TV and computer screens (generalised epilepsy syndromes only)
- Intercurrent infections and metabolic disturbances
- Uncommon: loud noises, music, reading, hot baths

26.36 Causes of focal seizures

Idiopathic

- Benign Rolandic epilepsy of childhood
- Benign occipital epilepsy of childhood

Focal structural lesions

Genetic

- Tuberous sclerosis (p. 1302)
- Autosomal dominant frontal lobe epilepsy
- Autosomal dominant partial epilepsy with auditory features (ADPEAF)
- von Hippel–Lindau disease (p. 1216)
- Neurofibromatosis (p. 1215)
- Cerebral migration abnormalities

Infantile hemiplegia

Dysembryonic

- Cortical dysgenesis
- Sturge–Weber syndrome

Mesial temporal sclerosis (associated with febrile convulsions)

Cerebrovascular disease (Ch. 27)

- Intracerebral haemorrhage
- Cerebral infarction
- Arteriovenous malformation
- Cavernous haemangioma

Tumours (primary and secondary) (p. 1213)

Trauma (including neurosurgery)

Infective (p. 1201)

- Cerebral abscess (pyogenic)
- Toxoplasmosis
- Cysticercosis
- Tuberculoma
- Subdural empyema
- Encephalitis
- Human immunodeficiency virus (HIV)

Inflammatory

- Sarcoidosis
- Vasculitis

Seizures arising from the anterior parts of the frontal lobe may produce bizarre behaviour patterns, including limb posturing, sleep walking, or even frenetic ill-directed motor activity with incoherent screaming. Video EEG may be necessary to differentiate these from psychogenic attacks (which are more common), but abruptness of onset, stereotyped nature, relative brevity and nocturnal preponderance may indicate the frontal onset. Causes of focal seizures are given in Box 26.36.

Generalised seizures

Tonic–clonic seizures. An initial 'aura' may be experienced by the patient, depending on the cortical area from which the seizure originates (as above). The patient then becomes rigid (tonic) and unconscious, falling heavily if standing ('like a log') and risking facial injury. During this phase, breathing stops and central cyanosis may occur. As cortical discharges reduce in frequency, the limbs produce jerking (clonic) movements for a variable time. Afterwards, there is a flaccid state of deep coma, which can persist for some minutes. The patient may be confused, disorientated and/or amnesic after regaining consciousness. During the attack, urinary incontinence and tongue-biting may occur. A severely bitten, bleeding tongue after an attack of loss of consciousness is pathognomonic of a generalised seizure. Subsequently, the patient usually feels unwell and sleepy, with headache and myalgia.

26.37 Causes of generalised tonic–clonic seizures

Generalisation from focal seizures
- See Box 26.36

Genetic
- Inborn errors of metabolism (p. 64)
- Storage diseases (p. 450)
- Phakomatoses (e.g. tuberous sclerosis, p. 1302)

Cerebral birth injury

Hydrocephalus

Cerebral anoxia

Drugs
- Antibiotics: penicillin, isoniazid, metronidazole
- Antimalarials: chloroquine, mefloquine
- Ciclosporin
- Cardiac anti-arrhythmics: lidocaine, disopyramide
- Psychotropic agents: phenothiazines, tricyclic antidepressants, lithium
- Amphetamines (withdrawal)

Alcohol (especially withdrawal)

Toxins
- Organophosphates (sarin)
- Heavy metals (lead, tin)

Metabolic disease
- Hypocalcaemia
- Hyponatraemia
- Hypomagnesaemia
- Hypoglycaemia
- Renal failure
- Liver failure

Infective
- Post-infectious encephalopathy
- Meningitis (p. 1201)

Inflammatory
- Multiple sclerosis (uncommon) (p. 1188)
- SLE (p. 1109)

Diffuse degenerative diseases
- Alzheimer's disease (uncommonly) (p. 251)
- Creutzfeldt–Jakob disease (rarely) (p. 1211)

Witnesses are usually frightened by the event, often believe the person to be dying, and may struggle to give a clear account of the episode. Some may not describe the tonic or clonic phase, and may not mention cyanosis or tongue-biting. In less typical episodes, post-ictal confusion, or sequelae such as headache or myalgia, may be the main pointers to the diagnosis. Causes of generalised tonic–clonic seizures are listed in Box 26.37.

Absence seizures. Absence seizures (previously 'petit mal') always start in childhood. The attacks are rarely mistaken for focal seizures because of their brevity. They can occur so frequently (20–30 times a day) that they are mistaken for daydreaming or poor concentration in school.

Myoclonic seizures. These are typically brief, jerking movements, predominating in the arms. In epilepsy, they are more marked in the morning or on awakening from sleep, and tend to be provoked by fatigue, alcohol or sleep deprivation.

Atonic seizures. These are seizures involving brief loss of muscle tone, usually resulting in heavy falls with or without loss of consciousness. They only occur in the context of epilepsy syndromes that involve other forms of seizure.

Tonic seizures. These are associated with a generalised increase in tone and an associated loss of awareness. They are usually seen as part of an epilepsy syndrome and are unlikely to be isolated.

Clonic seizures. Clonic seizures are similar to tonic-clonic seizures. The clinical manifestations are similar but without a preceding tonic phase.

Seizures of uncertain generalised or focal nature

Epileptic spasms. While these are highlighted in the classification system, they are unusual in adult practice and occur mainly in infancy. They signify widespread cortical disturbance and take the form of marked contractions of the axial musculature, lasting a fraction of a second but recurring in clusters of 5–50, often on awakening.

Epilepsy syndromes

Many patients with epilepsy fall into specific patterns, depending on seizure type(s), age of onset and treatment responsiveness: the so-called electroclinical syndromes (Box 26.38). It is anticipated that genetic testing will ultimately demonstrate similarities in molecular pathophysiology.

Box 26.39 highlights the more common epilepsy syndromes, which are largely of early onset and are sensitive to sleep deprivation, hyperventilation, alcohol and

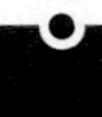

26.38 Electroclinical epilepsy syndromes

Adolescence to adulthood
- Juvenile absence epilepsy (JAE)
- Juvenile myoclonic epilepsy (JME)
- Epilepsy with generalised tonic–clonic seizures alone
- Progressive myoclonus epilepsies (PME)
- Autosomal dominant epilepsy with auditory features (ADEAF)
- Other familial temporal lobe epilepsies

Less specific age relationship
- Familial focal epilepsy with variable foci (childhood to adult)
- Reflex epilepsies

Distinctive constellations
- Mesial temporal lobe epilepsy with hippocampal sclerosis (MTLE with HS)
- Rasmussen's syndrome
- Gelastic (from the Greek word for laughter) seizures with hypothalamic hamartoma
- Hemiconvulsion–hemiplegia–epilepsy

Epilepsies with structural–metabolic causes
- Malformations of cortical development (hemimegalencephaly, heterotopias etc.)
- Neurocutaneous syndromes (tuberous sclerosis complex, Sturge–Weber etc.)
- Tumour
- Infection
- Trauma
- Angioma
- Perinatal insults
- Stroke etc.

Epilepsies of unknown cause

Conditions with epileptic seizures traditionally not diagnosed
- Benign neonatal seizures (BNS)
- Febrile seizures (FS)

26.39 Common epilepsy syndromes

	Age of onset	Type of seizure	EEG features	Treatment	Prognosis
Childhood absence epilepsy	4–8 yrs	Frequent brief absences	3/sec spike and wave	Ethosuximide Sodium valproate Levetiracetam	40% develop GTCS, 80% remit in adulthood
Juvenile absence epilepsy	10–15 yrs	Less frequent absences than childhood absence	Poly-spike and wave	Sodium valproate Levetiracetam	80% develop GTCS, 80% seizure-free in adulthood
Juvenile myoclonic epilepsy	15–20 yrs	GTCS, absences, morning myoclonus	Poly-spike and wave, photosensitivity	Sodium valproate Levetiracetam	90% remit with AEDs but relapse if AED withdrawn
GTCS on awakening	10–25 yrs	GTCS, sometimes myoclonus	Spike and wave on waking and sleep onset	Sodium valproate Levetiracetam	65% controlled with AEDs but relapse off treatment

(AED = anti-epileptic drug; GTCS = generalised tonic–clonic seizures)

photic stimulation. Epilepsies that do not fit into any of these diagnostic categories can be delineated first on the basis of the presence or absence of a known structural or metabolic condition (presumed cause), and then on the basis of the primary mode of seizure onset (generalised versus focal).

Investigations

Single seizure

All patients with transient loss of consciousness should have a 12-lead ECG. Where seizure is suspected or definite, patients should have imaging with either CT or MRI, although the yield is low unless focal signs are present. EEG may help to assess prognosis once a firm diagnosis has been made. The recurrence rate after a first seizure is approximately 40%, and most recurrent attacks occur within a month or two of the first. Further seizures are less likely if an identified trigger can be avoided (see Box 26.35).

Other investigations for infective, toxic and metabolic causes (Box 26.40) may be appropriate. An EEG performed immediately after a seizure may be more helpful in showing focal features than if performed after a delay.

Epilepsy

The same investigations are required in a patient with suspected epilepsy (Box 26.40). Where more than one seizure has occurred, an EEG may help to establish the type of epilepsy and guide therapy. As imaging becomes more sensitive, focal changes are picked up more often. Investigations should be revisited if the epilepsy is intractable to treatment.

Inter-ictal EEG is abnormal in only about 50% of patients with recurrent seizures, so it cannot be used to exclude epilepsy. The sensitivity can be increased to about 85% by prolonging recording time and including a period of natural or drug-induced sleep, but this does not replace a well-taken history. Ambulatory EEG recording or video EEG monitoring may help with differentiation of epilepsy from other attack disorders if these are sufficiently frequent.

Indications for imaging are summarised in Box 26.41. Imaging cannot establish a diagnosis of epilepsy but identifies any structural cause. It is not required if a confident diagnosis of a recognised epilepsy syndrome (e.g. juvenile myoclonic epilepsy) can be made. While CT will exclude a major structural cause of epilepsy, MRI is required to demonstrate subtle changes such as hippocampal sclerosis, which may direct or inform surgical intervention.

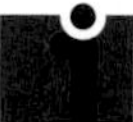

26.40 Investigation of epilepsy

From where is the epilepsy arising?
- Standard EEG
- Sleep EEG
- EEG with special electrodes (foramen ovale, subdural)

What is the cause of the epilepsy?

Structural lesion?
- CT
- MRI

Metabolic disorder?
- Urea and electrolytes
- Liver function tests
- Blood glucose
- Serum calcium, magnesium

Inflammatory or infective disorder?
- Full blood count, erythrocyte sedimentation rate, C-reactive protein
- Chest X-ray
- Serology for syphilis, HIV, collagen disease
- CSF examination

Are the attacks truly epileptic?
- Ambulatory EEG
- Videotelemetry

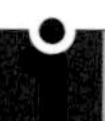

26.41 Indications for brain imaging in epilepsy

- Epilepsy starting after the age of 16 yrs
- Seizures having focal features clinically
- EEG showing a focal seizure source
- Control of seizures difficult or deteriorating

Management

It is important to explain the nature and cause of seizures to patients and their relatives, and to instruct relatives in the first aid management of seizures (Box 26.42).

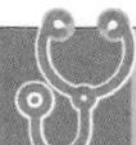

26.42 How to administer first aid for seizures

- Move person away from danger (fire, water, machinery, furniture)
- After convulsions cease, turn person into 'recovery' position (semi-prone)
- Ensure airway is clear but do **NOT** insert anything in mouth (tongue-biting occurs at seizure onset and cannot be prevented by observers)
- If convulsions continue for more than 5 mins or recur without person regaining consciousness, summon urgent medical attention
- Do not leave person alone until fully recovered (drowsiness and confusion can persist for up to 1 hr)

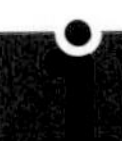

26.43 Epilepsy: outcome after 20 years

- 50% are seizure-free, without drugs, for the previous 5 yrs
- 20% are seizure-free for the previous 5 yrs but continue to take medication
- 30% continue to have seizures in spite of anti-epileptic therapy

Many people with epilepsy feel stigmatised and may become unnecessarily isolated from work and social life. It should be emphasised that epilepsy is a common disorder that affects 0.5–1% of the population, and that full control of seizures can be expected in approximately 70% of patients (Box 26.43).

Immediate care

Little can or needs to be done for a person during a major seizure except for first aid and common-sense manœuvres to limit damage or secondary complications (see Box 26.42). Advice should be given that on no account should anything be inserted into the patient's mouth. The management of status epilepticus is described on page 1159.

Lifestyle advice

Patients should be advised to avoid activities where they might place themselves or others at risk if they have a seizure. This applies at work, at home and at leisure. At home, only shallow baths (or showers) should be taken. Prolonged cycle journeys should be discouraged until reasonable freedom from seizures has been achieved. Activities requiring prolonged proximity to water (swimming, fishing or boating) should always be carried out in the company of someone who is aware of the risks and the potential need for rescue measures. Driving regulations vary between countries, and the patient should be made aware of these (Box 26.44). Certain occupations, such as firefighter or airline pilot, are not open to anyone who has a previous or active diagnosis of epilepsy; further information is available from epilepsy support organisations.

The recognised mortality of epilepsy should be discussed at around the time of diagnosis. This should be done with care and sensitivity, and with the aim of motivating the patient to adapt habits and lifestyle to optimise epilepsy control.

26.44 UK driving regulations

Private use

Single seizure

- Cease driving until at least 6 mths have passed without recurrence. Driver and Vehicle Licensing Authority (DVLA) may restore a full licence sooner if recurrence risk is low

Epilepsy (i.e. more than one seizure over the age of 5 yrs)

- Cease driving immediately
- Licence restored when patient is free from all types of seizure for 1 yr *or* seizures have occurred *exclusively* during sleep for a period of at least 3 yrs
- Licence will require renewal every 3 yrs thereafter until patient is seizure-free for 10 yrs

Withdrawal of anticonvulsants

- Cease driving during withdrawal period and for 6 mths thereafter

Vocational drivers (heavy goods and public service vehicles)

- No licence permitted if any seizure has occurred after the age of 5 yrs until patient is off medication and seizure-free for more than 10 yrs, and has no potentially epileptogenic brain lesion

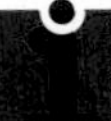

26.45 Guidelines for anticonvulsant therapy

- Start with one first-line drug (see Box 26.46)
- Start at a low dose; gradually increase dose until effective control of seizures is achieved or side-effects develop (drug levels may be helpful)
- Optimise compliance (use minimum number of doses per day)
- If first drug fails (seizures continue or side-effects develop), start second first-line drug, followed if possible by gradual withdrawal of first
- If second drug fails (seizures continue or side-effects develop), start second-line drug in combination with preferred first-line drug at maximum tolerated dose (beware interactions)
- If this combination fails (seizures continue or side-effects develop), replace second-line drug with alternative second-line drug
- If this combination fails, check compliance and reconsider diagnosis (Are events seizures? Occult lesion? Treatment compliance/alcohol/drugs confounding response?)
- Consider alternative, non-drug treatments (e.g. epilepsy surgery, vagal nerve stimulation)
- Use minimum number of drugs in combination at any one time

Anticonvulsant therapy

Anticonvulsant drug treatment (anti-epileptic drugs, or AEDs) should be considered after more than one unprovoked seizure. The decision to start treatment should be shared with the patient, to enhance compliance. A wide range of drugs is available. These agents either increase inhibitory neurotransmission in the brain or alter neuronal sodium channels to prevent abnormally rapid transmission of impulses. In the majority of patients, full control is achieved with a single drug. Dose regimens should be kept as simple as possible. Guidelines are listed in Box 26.45. For seizures of focal onset, one large

26.46 Guidelines for choice of anti-epileptic drug

Epilepsy type	First-line	Second-line	Third-line
Focal onset and/or secondary GTCS	Lamotrigine	Carbamazepine Levetiracetam Sodium valproate Topiramate Zonisamide Lacosamide	Clobazam Gabapentin Oxcarbazepine Phenobarbital Phenytoin Pregabalin Primidone Tiagabine
GTCS	Sodium valproate Levetiracetam	Lamotrigine Topiramate Zonisamide	Carbamazepine Phenytoin Primidone Phenobarbital Acetazolamide
Absence	Ethosuximide	Sodium valproate	Lamotrigine Clonazepam
Myoclonic	Sodium valproate	Levetiracetam Clonazepam	Lamotrigine Phenobarbital

N.B. Use as few drugs as possible at the lowest possible dose.

study suggests that lamotrigine is the best-tolerated monotherapy, which, alongside its favourable side-effect profile and relative lack of pharmacokinetic interactions, makes it a good first-line drug, although caution must be exercised with oral contraceptive use. Unclassified or specific syndromes respond best to valproate. Problems in pregnancy mean that sodium valproate should not be used in women of reproductive age unless the benefits outweigh the risks. The first choice should be an established first-line drug (Box 26.46), with more recently introduced drugs as second choice.

Monitoring therapy

Some practitioners confuse epilepsy care with serum level monitoring. The newer drugs have much more predictable pharmacokinetics than the older ones, and the only indication for measuring serum levels is if there is doubt that the patient is taking the medication. Blood levels need to be interpreted carefully, and dose changes made to treat the patient rather than to bring a serum level into the 'therapeutic range'. Some centres advocate serum level monitoring during pregnancy (notably with lamotrigine) but the evidence of benefit for this is not strong.

Epilepsy surgery

Some patients with drug-resistant epilepsy benefit from surgical resection of epileptogenic brain tissue. Less invasive treatments, including vagal nerve stimulation or deep brain stimulation, may also be helpful in some patients. All those who continue to experience seizures despite appropriate drug treatment should be considered for surgical treatment. Planning such interventions will require intensive specialist assessment and investigation to identify the site of seizure onset and the dispensability of any targets for resection, i.e. whether the area of brain involved is necessary for a critical function such as vision or motor function.

Withdrawing anticonvulsant therapy

Withdrawal of medication may be considered after a patient has been seizure-free for more than 2 years. Childhood-onset epilepsy, particularly classical absence seizures, carries the best prognosis for successful drug withdrawal. Other epilepsy syndromes, such as juvenile myoclonic epilepsy, have a marked tendency to recur after drug withdrawal.

Seizures that begin in adult life, particularly those with partial features, are also likely to recur, especially if there is an identified structural lesion. Overall, the recurrence rate after drug withdrawal depends on the individual's epilepsy history. An individualised estimate may be gained from the SIGN guideline tables (see 'Further information', p. 1230).

Patients should be advised of the risks of recurrence, to allow them to decide whether or not they wish to withdraw. If undertaken, withdrawal should be done slowly, reducing the drug dose gradually over weeks or months. Withdrawal may necessitate precautions around driving or occupation (see Box 26.44).

Contraception

Some AEDs induce hepatic enzymes that metabolise synthetic hormones, increasing the risk of contraceptive failure. This is most marked with carbamazepine, phenytoin and barbiturates, but clinically significant effects can be seen with lamotrigine and topiramate. If the AED cannot be changed, this can be overcome by giving higher-dose preparations of the oral contraceptive. Sodium valproate and levetiracetam have no interaction with hormonal contraception.

Pregnancy and reproduction

Epilepsy presents specific management problems during pregnancy (Box 26.47). There is usually great concern about teratogenesis associated with AEDs. It is important to recognise that the background risk of severe fetal

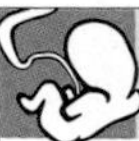

26.47 Epilepsy in pregnancy

- **Provision of pre-conception counselling is best practice**: start folic acid 5 mg daily for 2 mths before conception to reduce the risk of fetal malformations.
- **Fetal malformation**: risk is minimised if a single drug is used.
  Carbamazepine and lamotrigine have the lowest incidence of major fetal malformations.
  The risk with sodium valproate is higher but should be carefully balanced against its benefits.
  Levetiracetam may be safe, but avoid other newer drugs if possible.
- **Learning difficulties in children**: IQ may be lower when children are exposed to valproate in utero, so its use should always be considered carefully.
- **Haemorrhagic disease of the newborn**: anticonvulsants increase risk. Give oral vitamin K 20 mg daily to the mother during the last month of pregnancy and give IM vitamin K 1 mg to the infant at birth.
- **Increased frequency of seizures**: where breakthrough seizures occur, monitor anticonvulsant levels and adjust the dose regimen accordingly.
- **Pharmacokinetic effects of pregnancy**: carbamazepine levels may fall in the third trimester. Lamotrigine and levetiracetam levels may fall early in pregnancy. Some advocate monitoring of levels.

malformation in the population is around 2–3%. The modern AED most associated with teratogenesis is sodium valproate, which, at high dose, increases the risk to around 6–7%. Long-term observational studies show that most of the commonly used AEDs can be given safely in pregnancy.

Pre-conception treatment with folic acid (5 mg daily), along with use of the smallest effective doses of as few AEDs as possible, may reduce the risk of fetal abnormalities. The risks of abrupt AED withdrawal to the mother should be stressed.

Seizures may become more frequent during pregnancy, particularly if pharmacokinetic changes decrease serum levels of AEDs (see Box 26.47).

Menstrual irregularities and reduced fertility are more common in women with epilepsy, and are also increased by sodium valproate. Patients with epilepsy are at greater risk of osteoporosis, almost independently of the drug used. Some centres advocate vitamin D supplementation in any patient with epilepsy, but the higher female risk of osteoporosis makes this most important in women.

Prognosis

The outcome of newly diagnosed epilepsy is generally good. Overall, generalised seizures are more readily controlled than focal seizures. The presence of a structural lesion reduces the chances of freedom from seizures. The overall prognosis for epilepsy is shown in Box 26.43.

Status epilepticus

Presentation and management are described on page 1159. While generalised status epilepticus is most easily recognised, non-convulsive status may be less dramatic and less easily diagnosed. It may cause only altered

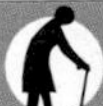

26.48 Epilepsy in old age

- **Incidence and prevalence**: late-onset epilepsy is very common and the annual incidence in those over 60 yrs is rising.
- **Fits and faints**: the features that usually differentiate these may be less definitive than in younger patients.
- **Non-convulsive status epilepticus**: can present as confusion in the elderly.
- **Cerebrovascular disease**: the underlying cause of seizures in 30–50% of patients over the age of 50 yrs. A seizure may occur with an overt stroke or with occult vascular disease.
- **AED regimens**: keep as simple as possible and take care to avoid interactions with other drugs being prescribed.
- **Carbamazepine-induced hyponatraemia**: increases significantly with age; particularly important in patients on diuretics or those with heart failure.
- **Withdrawal of anticonvulsant therapy**: late-onset epilepsy often recurs when drug treatment is stopped, so drug withdrawal should not be attempted where it was commenced appropriately.

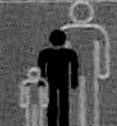

26.49 Epilepsy in adolescence

- **Effect on school/education**: seizures, AEDs and psychological complications of epilepsy may hamper education. Fear may make some educational institutions unduly restrictive.
- **Effect on family relationships**: parents may adopt a protective role, which can lead to epilepsy (and AEDs) becoming a point of assertion and rebellion.
- **Effect on career choice**: epilepsy may exclude or restrict employment in the emergency services and armed forces.
- **Alcohol**: may affect sleep pattern; excess may be associated with poor AED compliance.
- **Illicit drugs**: may affect seizure threshold and be associated with poor AED compliance.
- **Sleep disturbance**: may be worsened by social activities and computer games.
- **Oral contraception**: interactions with AED can occur. Use may not always be disclosed to parents.

awareness, confusion or wandering with automatisms. In an intensive care unit setting, EEG monitoring is essential to ensure that diagnosis and treatment are optimised.

Non-epileptic attack disorder

The difficulty with nomenclature is discussed on page 1179. Patients may present with attacks that resemble epileptic seizures but which are caused by psychological phenomena and have no abnormal epileptic discharges. Such attacks may be very prolonged, sometimes mimicking status epilepticus. Epileptic and non-epileptic attacks may coexist, and time and effort are needed to clarify the relative contribution of each, allowing more accurate and comprehensive treatment.

Non-epileptic attack disorder (NEAD) may be accompanied by dramatic flailing of the limbs and arching of the back, with side-to-side head movements and vocalising. Cyanosis and severe biting of the tongue are rare, but urinary incontinence can occur. Distress and crying are common following non-epileptic attacks. The distinction between epileptic attacks originating in the frontal lobes and non-epileptic attacks may be especially difficult, and may require videotelemetry with prolonged EEG recordings. Non-epileptic attacks are three times more common in women than in men and have been linked with a history of past or ongoing life trauma. They are not necessarily associated with formal psychiatric illness. Patients and carers may need reassurance that hospital admission is not required for every attack. Prevention requires psychotherapeutic interventions rather than drug therapy (p. 246).

VESTIBULAR DISORDERS

Vertigo is the typical symptom caused by vestibular dysfunction, and most patients with vertigo have acute vestibular failure, benign paroxysmal positional vertigo or Ménière's disease. Central (brain) causes of vertigo are rare by comparison, with the exception of migraine (p. 1176).

Acute vestibular failure

Although commonly called 'labyrinthitis' or 'vestibular neuronitis', acute vestibular failure is a more accurate term, as most cases are idiopathic. It usually presents as isolated severe vertigo with vomiting and unsteadiness. It begins abruptly, often on waking, and many patients are initially bed-bound. The vertigo settles within a few days, though head movement may continue to provoke transient symptoms (positional vertigo) for some time. During the acute attack, nystagmus (p. 1171) will be present for a few days.

Cinnarizine, prochlorperazine or betahistine provides symptomatic relief but should not be used long-term as this may delay recovery. A small proportion of patients fail to recover fully, and complain of ongoing imbalance and dysequilibrium rather than vertigo; vestibular rehabilitation by a physiotherapist may help.

Benign paroxysmal positional vertigo

Benign paroxysmal positional vertigo (BPPV) is due to the presence of otolithic debris from the saccule or utricle affecting the free flow of endolymph in the semicircular canals (cupulolithiasis). It may follow minor head injury but typically is spontaneous. The history is diagnostic, with transient (seconds) vertigo precipitated by movement (typically, rolling over in bed or getting into or out of bed). Although benign, and usually self-limiting after a few weeks or months, patients are often very alarmed by the symptoms. The diagnosis can be confirmed by the 'Hallpike manœuvre' to demonstrate positional nystagmus (Fig. 26.25). Treatment comprises explanation and reassurance, along with positioning procedures designed to return otolithic debris from the semicircular canal to saccule or utricle (such as the Epley manœuvre) and/or to re-educate the brain to cope with the inappropriate signals from the labyrinth (such as Cawthorne–Cooksey exercises: see 'Further information').

Ménière's disease

This is due to an abnormality of the endolymph that causes episodes of vertigo accompanied by tinnitus and fullness in the ear, each attack typically lasting a few hours. Over the years, patients may develop progressive deafness (typically low-tone on audiometry). Examination is typically normal in between attacks. The diagnosis is clinical, supported by abnormal audiometry. Ménière's disease is idiopathic, but a similar syndrome may be caused by middle ear trauma or infection. Management includes a low-salt diet, vestibular sedatives for acute attacks, and occasionally surgery.

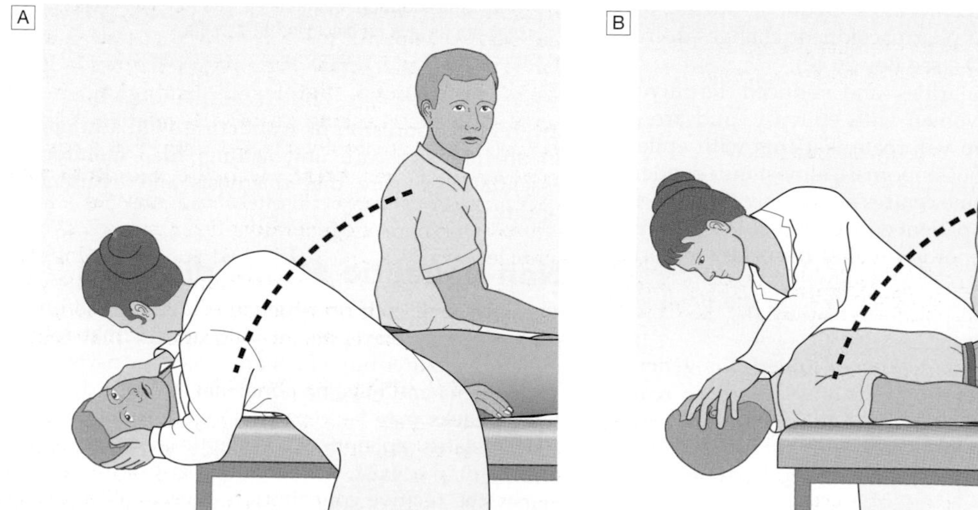

Fig. 26.25 The Hallpike manœuvre for diagnosis of benign paroxysmal positional vertigo (BPPV). Patients are asked to keep their eyes open and look at the examiner as their head is swung briskly backwards through 120° to overhang the edge of the couch. **A** Perform first with the right ear down. **B** Perform next with the left ear down. The examiner looks for nystagmus (usually accompanied by vertigo). In BPPV, the nystagmus typically occurs in A or B only and is torsional, the fast phase beating towards the lower ear. Its onset is usually delayed a few seconds, and it lasts 10–20 seconds. As the patient is returned to the upright position, transient nystagmus may occur in the opposite direction. Both nystagmus and vertigo typically decrease (fatigue) on repeat testing.

DISORDERS OF SLEEP

Sleep disturbances include too much sleep (hypersomnolence or excessive daytime sleepiness), insufficient or poor-quality sleep (insomnia), and abnormal behaviour during sleep (parasomnias). Insomnia is usually caused by psychological or psychiatric disorders, shift work and other environmental causes, pain and so on, and will not be discussed further. Many symptoms and disorders may affect sleep and sleep quality (e.g. pain, depression/anxiety, parkinsonism).

Excessive daytime sleepiness (hypersomnolence)

There are primary and secondary causes (Box 26.50). The most common causes are impaired sleep due to lifestyle issues or sleep-disordered breathing (p. 725). Sleepiness may be measured using the Epworth Sleepiness Score (see Box 19.98, p. 726). Most causes will be identified by a detailed history from the patient and their bed partner, and a 2-week sleep diary.

Narcolepsy

This has a prevalence of about 1 in 2000, with peak onset in adolescence and early middle age. The key symptom is sudden, irresistible 'sleep attacks', often in inappropriate circumstances such as whilst eating or talking. Other characteristic features help distinguish this from excessive daytime sleepiness (Box 26.51). Symptoms may be due to loss of hypocretin-secreting hypothalamic neurons. Diagnosis requires sleep study with sleep latency testing (demonstrating rapid onset of REM sleep). Treatment is with sodium oxybate, modafinil, dexamfetamine or methylphenidate. Cataplexy may respond to sodium oxybate, clomipramine or venlafaxine.

26.50 Causes of hypersomnolence

Primary causes

- Narcolepsy
- Idiopathic hypersomnolence
- Brain injury

Secondary causes (due to poor-quality sleep)

- Obstructive sleep apnoea
- Pain
- Restless legs/periodic limb movements of sleep
- Parkinsonism and other neurodegenerative diseases
- Depression/anxiety
- Medication
- Environmental factors (noise, temperature etc.)

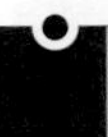

26.51 Narcolepsy symptoms

Sleep attacks

- Brief, frequent and unlike normal somnolence

Cataplexy

- Sudden loss of muscle tone triggered by surprise, laughter, strong emotion etc.

Hypnagogic or hypnapompic hallucinations

- Frightening hallucinations experienced during sleep onset or waking due to intrusion of REM sleep during wakefulness (can occur in normal people)

Sleep paralysis

- Brief paralysis on waking (can occur in normal people)

Parasomnias

Parasomnias are abnormal motor behaviours that occur around sleep. They may arise in either REM or non-REM sleep, with characteristic features and timing. Non-REM parasomnias tend to occur early in sleep. Parasomnias should be distinguished from other motor disturbances (such as periodic limb movements, hypnic jerks or sleep talking) and sleep-onset epileptic seizures (p. 1182). History from a sleeping partner or other witness is essential.

Non-REM parasomnias

These are due to incomplete arousal from non-REM sleep, and manifest as night terrors, sleep walking and confusional arousals (sleep drunkenness). They typically occur within an hour or two of sleep onset, are common in children, and usually of no pathological significance. Rarely, they persist into adulthood and may become increasingly complex, including dressing, moving objects, eating, drinking or even acts of violence. Patients have little or no recollection of the episodes, even though they appear 'awake'. They may be triggered by alcohol or unfamiliar sleeping situations, and can be familial. Treatment is usually not required, but clonazepam can be used.

REM sleep behaviour disorder

In REM sleep behaviour disorder (RBD), patients 'act out' their dreams during REM sleep, due to failure of the usual muscle atonia. Sleep partners provide typical histories of patients 'fighting' or 'struggling' in their sleep, sometimes causing injury to themselves or to their partner. They are easily roused from this state, with recollection of their dream, unlike in non-REM states. RBD is more common in men, and may be an early symptom of neurodegenerative diseases such as alpha synucleinopathies (p. 1195), perhaps preceding more typical symptoms of these conditions by years. Polysomnography will confirm absence of atonia during REM sleep. Clonazepam is the most successful treatment.

Restless legs syndrome

Restless legs syndrome (RLS) is common, with a prevalence of up to 10%, but many patients never seek medical attention. It is characterised by unpleasant leg (and sometimes arm) sensations that are eased by movement (motor restlessness); the diagnosis is clinical (Box 26.52). It has a strong familial tendency and can present with daytime somnolence due to poor sleep. It is usually idiopathic, but may be associated with haematinic deficiency, pregnancy, peripheral neuropathy, Parkinson's disease or uraemia. It should be distinguished from

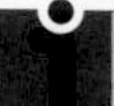

26.52 Diagnostic criteria for restless legs syndrome

A need to move the legs, usually accompanied or caused by uncomfortable, unpleasant sensations in the legs, with the following features:

- only present or worse during periods of rest or inactivity such as lying or sitting
- partially or totally relieved by movement such as walking or stretching, at least as long as the activity continues
- generally worse or occurs only in the evening or night.

akathisia, the daytime motor restlessness that is an adverse effect of anti-psychotic drugs. Treatment, if required, is with dopaminergic drugs (dopamine agonists or levodopa, p. 1196) or benzodiazepines.

Periodic limb movements in sleep

Unlike RLS, period limb movements in sleep (PLMS) only occurs during sleep and causes repetitive flexion movements of the limbs, usually in the early (non-REM) stages of sleep. Although patients are unaware of the symptoms, they may disturb sleep quality and often disturb partners. The pathological significance of PLMS is uncertain and it often occurs in normal health. There is an overlap with RLS. Treatment is most successful with clonazepam or dopaminergic drugs.

NEURO-INFLAMMATORY DISEASES

Multiple sclerosis

Multiple sclerosis (MS) is an important cause of long-term disability in adults, especially in the UK, where the prevalence is about 120 per 100 000. The annual incidence is around 7 per 100 000, while the lifetime risk of developing MS is about 1 in 400. The incidence of MS is higher in Northern Europeans, and the disease is about twice as common in females.

Pathophysiology

There is evidence that both genetic and environmental factors play a causative role. The prevalence of MS is low near the equator and increases in the temperate zones of both hemispheres. Most importantly, people retain the risk of developing the disease in the zone in which they grew up, indicating that environmental exposures during growth and development are important. Prevalence also correlates with environmental factors, such as sunlight exposure, vitamin D and exposure to Epstein–Barr virus (EBV), although causative mechanisms remain unclear. Genetic factors are also relevant; the risk of familial recurrence in MS is 15%, with highest risk in first-degree relatives (age-adjusted risk: 4–5% for siblings and 2–3% for parents or offspring). Monozygotic twins have a concordance rate of 30%. The genes that predispose to MS are incompletely defined but inheritance appears to be polygenic, with influences from genes for human leucocyte antigen (HLA) typing, interleukin receptors, *CLEC16A* (C-type lectin domain family 16 member A) and *CD226* genes. An immune hypothesis is supported by increased levels of activated T lymphocytes in the CSF and increased immunoglobulin synthesis within the CNS.

Initial CNS inflammation in MS involves entry of activated T lymphocytes across the blood–brain barrier.

A

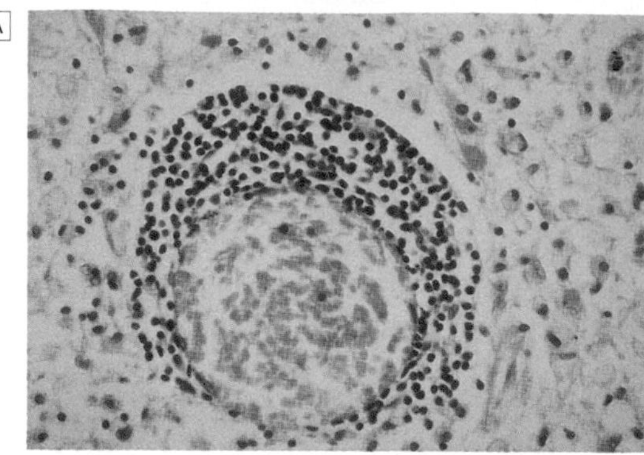

B

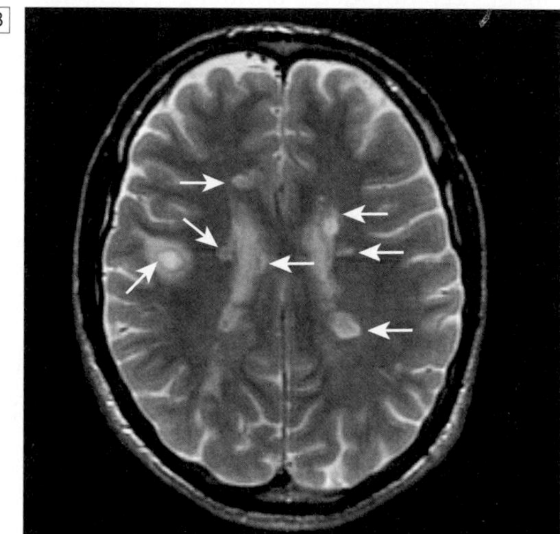

C

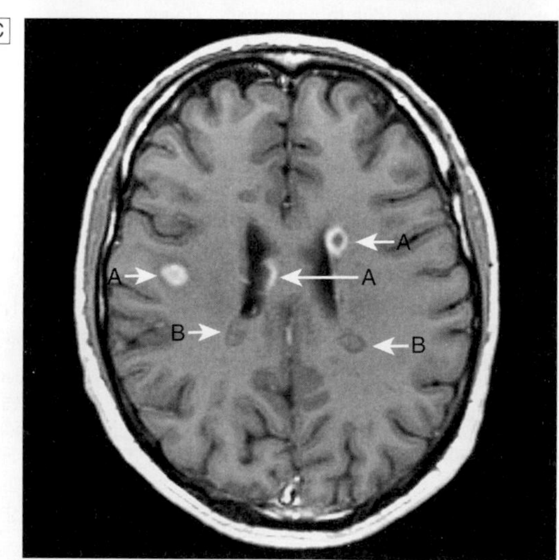

Fig. 26.26 Multiple sclerosis. **A** Photomicrograph from demyelinating plaque, showing perivascular cuffing of blood vessel by lymphocytes. **B** Brain MRI in multiple sclerosis. Multiple high-signal lesions (arrows) seen particularly in the paraventricular region on T2 image. **C** In T1 image with gadolinium enhancement, recent lesions (A arrows) show enhancement, suggesting active inflammation (enhancement persists for 4 weeks); older lesions (B arrows) show no enhancement but low signal, suggesting gliosis.

These recognise myelin-derived antigens on the surface of the nervous system's antigen-presenting cells, the microglia, and undergo clonal proliferation. The resulting inflammatory cascade releases cytokines and initiates destruction of the oligodendrocyte–myelin unit by macrophages. Histologically, the resultant lesion is a plaque of inflammatory demyelination, most commonly in the periventricular regions of the brain, the optic nerves, and the subpial regions of the spinal cord (Fig. 26.26). This begins as a circumscribed area of disintegration of the myelin sheath, accompanied by infiltration by activated lymphocytes and macrophages, often with conspicuous perivascular inflammation. After the acute attack, gliosis follows, leaving a shrunken grey scar.

Much of the initial acute clinical deficit is caused by the effect of inflammatory cytokines on transmission of the nervous impulse rather than structural disruption of the myelin, and may explain the rapid recovery of some deficits and probably the acute benefit from corticosteroids. In the long term, accumulating myelin loss reduces the efficiency of impulse propagation or causes complete conduction block, contributing to sustained impairment of CNS functions. Inflammatory mediators released during the acute attack (particularly nitric oxide) probably also initiate axonal damage, which is a feature of the latter stages of the disease. In established MS there is progressive axonal loss, probably due to the successive damage from acute attacks and the subsequent loss of neurotrophic factors from oligodendrocytes. This axonal loss may account for the phase of the disease characterised by progressive and persistent disability (Fig. 26.27).

Clinical features

A diagnosis of MS requires the demonstration of otherwise unexplained CNS lesions separated in time and space (Box 26.53). The peak age of onset of MS is the

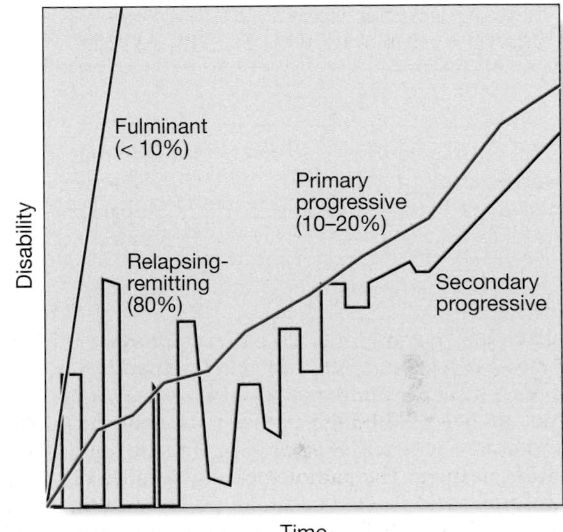

Fig. 26.27 The progression of disability in fulminant, relapsing–remitting and progressive multiple sclerosis.

26.53 The Macdonald criteria for the diagnosis of multiple sclerosis (2011)[1]

Clinical presentation[2]	Additional evidence required for diagnosis of MS
Two or more attacks with either Objective clinical evidence of at least 2 lesions *or* Objective clinical evidence of 1 attack with reasonable evidence (on clinical history) of at least 1 prior attack	None
Two or more attacks with objective clinical evidence of 1 lesion	Dissemination in 'space' demonstrated by MRI ≥ 1 lesion in at least 2 of the MS-typical regions[3] (multiple lesions in different sites) *or* Await further clinical attack at different anatomical site
One attack with objective clinical evidence of ≥ 2 lesions	Dissemination in 'time' demonstrated by Evolving MRI showing combined enhancing (new) and non-enhancing (old) lesions *or* New T2 or enhancing lesion on repeat MRI *or* Await further (second) clinical attack at different anatomical site
One attack with clinical evidence of only 1 lesion (clinically isolated syndrome)	Dissemination in 'space' demonstrated by ≥ 1 T2 lesion in at least 2 MS-typical regions *or* Dissemination in 'time', demonstrated by simultaneous enhancing and non-enhancing lesions *or* New T2 or enhancing lesions on repeat MRI *or* Await further (second) clinical attack
Insidious neurological progression suggestive of MS	1 yr of progression plus 2 of the following: Evidence for dissemination in space with ≥ 1 T2 lesions in MS-typical regions Evidence for dissemination in space based on ≥ 2 lesions in the spinal cord Positive CSF (evidence of oligoclonal band and/or elevated immunoglobulin (Ig) G index)

[1]Published by the International Panel on MS Diagnosis (Ann Neurol 2011; 69:292–302). If the clinical presentation in the left-hand column is associated with the features in the right-hand column, the diagnosis is MS. If there is incomplete association, the diagnosis is 'possible MS'.
[2]Assumes other possible causes for CNS inflammation (e.g. sarcoidosis, SLE) have been excluded.
[3]MS-typical regions = periventricular, juxtacortical, infratentorial, spinal cord.

fourth decade; onset before puberty or after the age of 60 years is rare. Where there is widespread inflammation, this usually leads to widespread symptoms and/or signs. Symptoms and signs of MS usually come on over days or weeks, resolving over weeks or months. Rarely, a more rapid stroke-like presentation may occur. Around 80% of patients have a relapsing and remitting clinical course of episodic dysfunction of the CNS with variable intervening recovery. Of the remaining 20%, most follow a slowly progressive clinical course, while a tiny minority have a fulminant variety leading to early death (see Fig. 26.27). Frequent relapses with incomplete recovery indicate a poor prognosis for the patient. Some milder cases have an interval of years or even decades between attacks, while in others (particularly if optic neuritis is the initial manifestation) there is no recurrence of disease. In some individuals, a phase of secondary progression, caused by secondary axonal degeneration, supersedes the phase of relapse and remission.

There are a number of clinical symptoms and syndromes suggestive of MS, occurring either at presentation or during the course of the illness (Box 26.54). The physical signs observed in MS are determined by the anatomical site of demyelination. Combined spinal cord and brainstem signs are common, although evidence of previous optic neuritis may be found in the form of an afferent pupillary deficit. Significant intellectual impairment only supervenes late in the disease, when loss of frontal functions and impairment of memory are common.

The prognosis for patients with MS is difficult to predict with confidence, especially early in the disease. About 15% of patients have a single attack of demyelination and do not suffer further events, whilst those with relapsing and remitting MS experience, on average, 1–2 events every 2 years. Approximately 5% of patients die within 5 years of disease onset, whilst others have a benign outcome. Prognosis is good for patients with optic neuritis and only sensory relapses. Overall, about one-third of patients are disabled to the point of needing help with walking after 10 years, and this proportion rises to about one-half after 15 years. It would appear likely (though this is as yet unproven) that disease-modifying drugs will have an effect on future prognostication.

Investigations

There is no single diagnostic test that is definitive for MS, and the results of investigation need to be combined with the clinical picture in order to make a diagnosis (Box 26.55). Other conditions should be excluded, and investigations should provide support for the diagnosis, with evidence for a chronic widespread inflammatory condition. Following the first clinical event, investigations may help prognosis by confirming the disseminated nature of the disease. MRI is the most sensitive technique for imaging lesions in brain and spinal cord (Fig. 26.28) and in excluding other causes that have provoked the neurological deficit. However, the MRI appearances in MS may be confused with those of small-vessel disease or cerebral vasculitis, and these diagnoses should be considered and excluded. Visual evoked potentials (p. 1152) can detect clinically silent lesions in up to 70% of patients, but auditory and somatosensory evoked potentials are seldom of diagnostic value.

The CSF may show a lymphocytic pleocytosis in the acute phase and oligoclonal bands of IgG in 70–90% of patients between attacks. Oligoclonal bands are not specific for MS and only denote intrathecal inflammation. These can appear in other disorders, which should be excluded by examination and other investigations. It is important to exclude other potentially treatable conditions, such as infection, vitamin B_{12} deficiency and spinal cord compression.

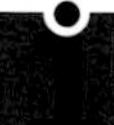

26.54 Clinical features of multiple sclerosis

Common presentations of multiple sclerosis

- Optic neuritis
- Relapsing/remitting sensory symptoms
- Subacute painless spinal cord lesion
- Acute brainstem syndrome
- Subacute loss of function of upper limb (dorsal column deficit)
- 6th cranial nerve palsy

Other symptoms and syndromes suggestive of CNS demyelination

- Afferent pupillary defect and optic atrophy (previous optic neuritis)
- Lhermitte's symptom (tingling in spine or limbs on neck flexion)
- Progressive non-compressive paraparesis
- Partial Brown–Séquard syndrome (p. 1221)
- Internuclear ophthalmoplegia with ataxia
- Postural ('rubral', 'Holmes') tremor
- Trigeminal neuralgia (p. 1178) under the age of 50
- Recurrent facial palsy

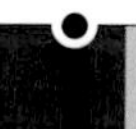

26.55 Investigations in a patient suspected of having multiple sclerosis

Exclude other structural disease and identify plaques of demyelination

- Image area of clinical involvement (MRI, myelography)

Demonstrate other sites of involvement

- Imaging (MRI)
- Visual evoked potentials
- Other evoked potentials

Demonstrate inflammatory nature of lesion(s)

- CSF examination
  - Cell count
  - Protein electrophoresis (oligoclonal bands)

Exclude other conditions

- Chest X-ray
- Serum angiotensin-converting enzyme (ACE) – sarcoidosis
- Serum B_{12}
- Antinuclear antibodies – SLE
- Antiphospholipid antibodies

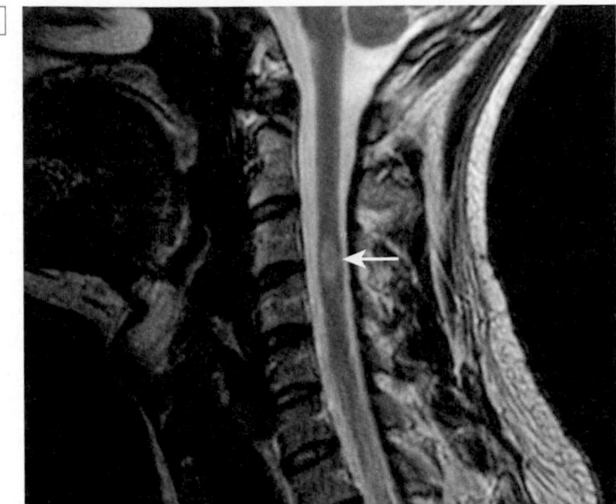

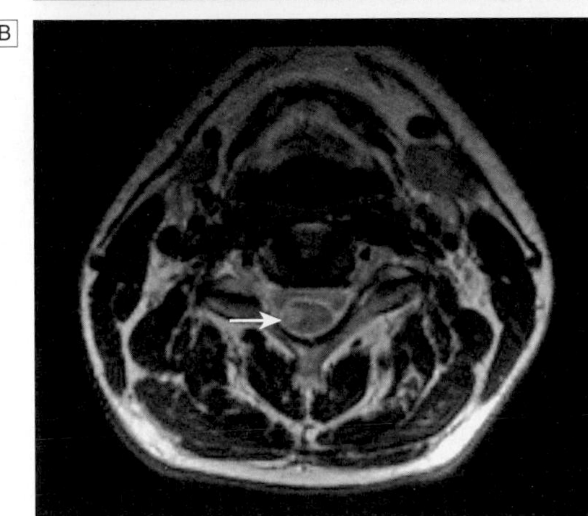

Fig. 26.28 Multiple sclerosis: demyelinating lesion in cervical spinal cord, high-signal T2 images (arrow). **A** Sagittal plane. **B** Axial plane.

EBM 26.56 Corticosteroids in multiple sclerosis

'There is evidence favouring corticosteroids (methylprednisolone) for acute exacerbations of multiple sclerosis, but there are insufficient data to estimate reliably the effect of corticosteroids on prevention of new exacerbations and reduction of long-term disability.'

'There is currently no evidence that long-term corticosteroid treatment delays progression of long-term disability in multiple sclerosis.'

- Filippini G, et al. Corticosteroids or ACTH for acute exacerbations in multiple sclerosis. Cochrane Database of Systematic Reviews, 2000, issue 4. Art. no.: CD001331.
- Ciccone A, et al. Corticosteroids for long term treatment in multiple sclerosis. Cochrane Database of Systematic Reviews, 2008, issue 1. Art. no.: CD006264.

For further information: www.cochrane.org/cochrane-reviews

EBM 26.57 Disease-modifying therapies in multiple sclerosis

'Beta-interferons have a modest effect on exacerbations and disease progression in relapsing–remitting MS but do not prevent the development of permanent physical disability on slowly progressive multiple sclerosis.'

'Natalizumab reduces relapses and disability at 2 years in relapsing–remitting multiple sclerosis.'

- Rice GP, et al. Interferon in relapsing remitting multiple sclerosis. Cochrane Database of Systematic Reviews, 2001, issue 4. Art. no.: CD002002.
- La Mantia L, et al. Interferon beta for secondary progressive multiple sclerosis. Cochrane Database of Systematic Reviews, 2011, issue 1. Art. no.: CD005181.
- Pucci E, et al. Natalizumab for relapsing remitting multiple sclerosis. Cochrane Database of Systematic Reviews, 2011, issue 10. Art. no.: CD007621.

For further information: www.cochrane.org/cochrane-reviews

Management

The management of MS involves four different strands: treatment of the acute episode, prevention of future relapses, treatment of complications and management of the patient's disability.

The acute episode

In a function-threatening exacerbation of MS, pulses of high-dose steroid, given either intravenously or orally over 3–5 days, will shorten the duration of the acute episode (Box 26.56). Prolonged administration of steroids does not alter the long-term outcome and causes severe adverse effects and should therefore be avoided. Pulses of steroids can be given up to three times in a year but use should be restricted to those individuals with significant function-threatening deficits. Prophylaxis to prevent the occurrence of steroid-induced osteoporosis (p. 1120) should be considered in patients requiring multiple courses of corticosteroids.

Disease-modifying treatment

Despite its immune basis, the administration of long-term steroids, standard chemotherapies and immunoglobulin is not practical or helpful in established MS. This motivated the search for innovative immuno-active treatments.

In relapsing and remitting MS, an increasing number of beta-interferons have been used to reduce relapse rates and improve long-term outlook. Their pharmacological properties tend to vary, but there has been no good trial evidence clinically separating the licensed compounds. Subcutaneous or intramuscular interferon-beta reduces the number of relapses by some 30%, with a small effect on long-term disability (Box 26.57). Long-term effects are usually local and development of antibodies should be sought; their development should preclude further long-term treatment. Other treatments are shown in Box 26.58.

Glatiramer acetate is a parenterally administered oligopeptide that may act as a competitor antigen, but in addition it increases numbers of regulatory CD4 T cells in relapsing–remitting MS, thereby helping to reduce relapse rates. Unlike other immunomodulatory treatments used for MS, glatiramer antibodies do not block function and actually appear to enhance efficacy.

Mitoxantrone was initially developed as a chemotherapeutic agent and has been shown to decrease the relapse rate in MS, as well as lowering the number of MRI lesions and reducing disability with long-term use. Its similarity to doxorubicin is reflected in its adverse effects, the most notable of which is cardiotoxicity.

26.58 Disease-modifying treatments in multiple sclerosis

Treatment	Mode of action	Comment
Interferon-beta	Immune modulation	In widespread use for reducing relapse rate (RCT evidence)
Glatiramer acetate	Immune modulation	Similar efficacy to interferon-beta (RCT evidence)
Fingolimod	Immune modulation	Superior efficacy to interferon-beta in RCTs
Monoclonal antibody to alpha4-integrin (natalizumab)	Immune modulation (blocks lymphocyte entry into CNS)	Recently introduced. Possibly more effective than interferon-beta and glatiramer acetate (RCT evidence)
Mitoxantrone	Immune suppression (cytotoxic)	Trials favour early use in aggressive disease

(RCT = randomised controlled clinical trial)

Natalizumab is a monoclonal antibody to an antigen expressed on activated T cells and monocytes, and has been associated with a dramatic fall in the number of lesions evident on MRI, with a corresponding decrease in the number of relapses and reduction in axonal damage. Rarely, neutralising antibodies block its efficacy and indicate that the drug should be withdrawn. Progressive multifocal leucoencephalopathy (PML) has been seen in some natalizumab-treated patients. Occasional cases of CNS lymphoma and toxoplasmosis may be related to drug use.

Other newer immunomodulatory treatments have been developed, including fingolimod, which is derived from the ascomycete metabolite ISP-1 (myriocin) and can be given orally. Further studies are needed to predict which immune treatment should be tried in which patients.

Special diets, including a gluten-free diet or linoleic acid supplements, and hyperbaric oxygen therapy are popular with patients but their efficacy has not yet been proven.

Treatment of symptoms, complications and disability

Treatments for the complications of MS are summarised in Box 26.59. It is important to provide patients with a careful explanation of the nature of the disease and its outcome. When and if disability occurs, patients and their relatives need appropriate support. Specialist nurses working in a multidisciplinary team of health-care professionals are of great value in managing the chronic phase of the disease. Periods of physiotherapy and occupational therapy may improve functional capacity in those patients who become disabled, and guidance can be provided on the provision of aids at home, reducing handicap. Care of the bladder is particularly important. Urgency and frequency can be treated pharmacologically (see Box 26.31, p. 1175), but this may lead to a degree of retention with an attendant risk of infection. Retention can be managed initially by intermittent urinary catheterisation (performed by the patient, if possible), but an in-dwelling catheter may become necessary. Sexual dysfunction is a frequent source of distress. Sildenafil or tadalafil helps impotence in men, and skilled counselling and prosthetic aids are often beneficial.

26.59 Treatment of complications in multiple sclerosis

Spasticity

- Physiotherapy
- Baclofen (usually oral)
- Dantrolene
- Gabapentin
- Sativex®
- Tizanidine
- Intrathecal baclofen
- Local (IM) injection of botulinum toxin
- Chemical neuronectomy

Ataxia

- Isoniazid
- Clonazepam

Dysaesthesia

- Carbamazepine
- Gabapentin
- Phenytoin
- Amitriptyline

Bladder symptoms

- See Box 26.31, p. 1175

Fatigue

- Amantadine
- Modafinil
- Amitriptyline

Impotence

- Sildenafil 50–100 mg/24 hrs
- Tadalafil

26.60 Multiple sclerosis in pregnancy

- **Counselling**: provision of pre-conception counselling is best practice.
- **Relapse risk**: endocrine effects on the immune system ensure that relapse risk drops during pregnancy.
- **Disease-modifying drugs**: risk of teratogenicity means that all disease-modifying drugs should ideally be stopped 6–8 wks before conception and recommenced after breastfeeding has stopped.
- **Post-partum relapse rate**: rebound of immune system activity means that the highest risk of relapse is in the first year after delivery.

Acute disseminated encephalomyelitis

This is an acute monophasic demyelinating condition in which there are areas of perivenous demyelination widely disseminated throughout the brain and spinal cord. The illness may apparently arise spontaneously but often occurs a week or so after a viral infection, especially measles and chickenpox, or following vaccination, suggesting that it is immunologically mediated.

Clinical features

Headache, vomiting, pyrexia, confusion and meningism may be presenting features, often with focal or multifocal brain and spinal cord signs. Seizures or coma may occur. A minority of patients who recover have further episodes.

Investigations

MRI shows multiple high-signal areas in a pattern similar to that of MS, although often with large confluent areas of abnormality. The CSF may be normal or show an increase in protein and lymphocytes (occasionally over 100×10^6 cells/L); oligoclonal bands may be found in the acute episode but, unlike in MS, will not persist beyond clinical recovery. The clinical picture may be very similar to a first relapse of MS.

Management

The disease may be fatal in the acute stages but is otherwise self-limiting. Treatment with high-dose intravenous methylprednisolone, using the same regimen as for a relapse of MS, is recommended.

Transverse myelitis

Transverse myelitis is an acute, usually monophasic, demyelinating disorder affecting the spinal cord. It is usually thought to be post-infectious in origin. It occurs at any age and presents with a subacute paraparesis with a sensory level, accompanied by severe pain in the neck or back at the onset. MRI should distinguish this from an external lesion affecting the spinal cord. CSF examination shows cellular pleocytosis, often with polymorphs at the onset. Oligoclonal bands are usually absent. Treatment is with high-dose intravenous methylprednisolone. The outcome is variable: one-third have static deficit, one-third go on to develop MS and one-third recover with no subsequent relapse. Some clinical features may predict the development of MS after transverse myelitis (Box 26.61).

26.61 Prognostic features predicting multiple sclerosis after transverse myelitis

Increased risk	
• Severe weakness • Catastrophic onset • Initial lancinating pain • Sensory disturbance at cervical level	• Spinal shock • Incontinence • Presence of 14-3-3 protein in CSF
Decreased risk	
• Subacute onset over days • Young onset • Retained posterior column function	• Retained tendon reflexes • Early recovery

Neuromyelitis optica

Neuromyelitis optica (also known as Devic's disease) is the occurrence of transverse myelitis and bilateral optic neuritis. The disease has been recognised for many years, particularly in Asia. The majority of cases are associated with an antibody to a neuronal membrane channel, aquaporin 4. If changes are seen on brain MRI (this is variable), they are typically high-signal lesions restricted to periventricular regions. Spinal MRI scans show lesions that are typically longer than three spinal segments (unlike the shorter lesions of MS). Clinical deficits tend to recover less well than in MS, and the disease may be more aggressive with more frequent relapses. Treatment with older immunosuppressive agents, such as steroids, azathioprine or cyclophosphamide, and/or plasmapheresis seems to be more effective than in MS.

PARANEOPLASTIC NEUROLOGICAL DISORDERS

Neurological disease may occur with systemic malignant tumours in the absence of cerebral metastases. It is now recognised that, in the majority of these cases, antigen production in the body of the tumour leads to development of antibodies to parts of the CNS. Paraneoplastic conditions are increasingly recognised, and the number of antibodies identified is also increasing (Boxes 26.62 and 26.63). These syndromes are particularly associated with small-cell carcinoma of lung, ovarian tumours, and lymphomas. Autoantibodies are found in the serum and/or CSF, and biopsy will show a lymphocytic infiltrate of the neural tissue affected.

Clinical presentations

These are summarised in Boxes 26.62 and 26.63. In most instances, the neurological condition progresses quite rapidly over a few months, preceding the malignant disease in around half of cases. The range of clinical patterns is so wide that paraneoplastic disease should be considered in the diagnosis of any unusual progressive neurological syndrome. The paraneoplastic disorders of the peripheral nervous system particularly affect the synaptic cleft (p. 1141).

Investigations and management

The presence of characteristic autoantibodies in the context of a suspicious clinical picture may be diagnostic. The causative tumour may be very small and therefore CT of the chest or abdomen or PET scanning may be necessary to find it. These investigations should only be pursued when paraneoplastic disease has been proven, rather than when it is suspected. The CSF often shows an increased protein and lymphocyte count with oligoclonal bands.

Treatment is directed at the primary tumour. Occasionally, successful therapy of the tumour is associated with improvement of the paraneoplastic syndrome. Some improvement may occur following administration of intravenous immunoglobulin.

26.62 Paraneoplastic disorders of the central nervous system

Clinical presentation	Associated tumour	Antibodies demonstrated
Limbic encephalitis	SCLC	Anti-Hu, anti-CV2, PCA-2, anti-VGKC, anti-Ma1, anti-amphiphysin, anti-Ri, ANNA-3, anti-VGCC, anti-Zic4, anti-GluR1/2, anti-GABAR
	Testicular, breast	Anti-Ma2, anti-GluR1/2
	Thymoma	Anti-VGKC, anti-CV2, anti-GluR1/2
	Ovarian/testicular teratoma	Anti-NMDAR
Myelopathy	SCLC, thymoma, others	Anti-CV2, anti-amphiphysin, anti-aquaporin
Motor neuron disease	SCLC, others	Anti-Hu
Stiff-person syndrome	Breast, SCLC, thymoma, others	Anti-amphiphysin, anti-Ri, anti-GAD, anti-GlyR
Cerebellar degeneration	Breast, ovarian, others	Anti-Yo, anti-Ma1, anti-Ri
	SCLC, others	Anti-Hu, anti-CV2, PCA-2, ANNA-3, anti-amphiphysin, anti-VGCC, anti-Ri, anti-Zic4, anti-GAD
	Lymphoma	Anti-Tr, anti-mGluR1
Multifocal encephalomyelitis	SCLC, thymoma	Anti-Hu, anti-CV2, anti-VGKC, anti-Ma1, anti-amphiphysin, anti-Ri, ANNA-3
Opsoclonus–myoclonus	Breast, ovarian	Anti-Ri, anti-Yo, anti-amphiphysin
	SCLC	Anti Hu, anti-Ri, anti-CV2, anti-amphiphysin, anti-VGCC
	Neuroblastoma	Anti-Hu
	Testicular	Anti-Ma1/2, anti-CV2
Extrapyramidal encephalitis	SCLC, thymoma, testicular	Anti-CV2, anti-Hu, anti-VGKC, anti-Ma
Optic neuritis	SCLC	Anti-CV2, anti-aquaporin
Retinal degeneration	SCLC	Anti-recoverin

(ANNA = anti-neuronal nucleolar antibody; GABAR = GABA receptor; GAD = glutamic acid decarboxylase; GluR = glutamate receptor; PCA = Purkinje cell antibody; SCLC = small-cell lung cancer; VGCC = voltage-gated calcium channel; VGKC = voltage-gated potassium channel)

26.63 Paraneoplastic disorders of the peripheral nervous system

Clinical presentation	Associated tumour	Antibodies demonstrated
Neuromyotonia	Thymoma, SCLC, others	Anti-VGKC
Myasthenia gravis	Thymoma	Anti-Achr, anti-MuSK
Sensorimotor polyneuropathy	Lymphoma, SCLC, others	Anti-HU, anti-CV2, ANNA-3, anti-Ma1, anti-amphiphysin
Lambert–Eaton syndrome	SCLC	Anti-VGCC
Motor neuropathy	Lymphoma, SCLC, others	Anti-Hu, anti-Yo, anti-CV2
Sensory neuropathy	Lymphoma, SCLC, others	Anti-Hu, anti-Yo, anti-CV2
Polymyositis/dermatomyositis	Lung, breast	Anti-Jo1

(MuSK = muscle-specific kinase; for other abbreviations, see Box 26.62)

NEURODEGENERATIVE DISEASES

Whilst MS is the most common cause of disability in young people in the UK, vascular and neurodegenerative diseases are increasingly important in later life. The neurodegenerative diseases are united in having a pathological process that leads to specific neuronal death, causing relentlessly progressive symptoms that increase in incidence in older age. The precise causes are not yet known. Alzheimer's disease (p. 251) and Parkinson's disease are the most common.

Movement disorders

Movement disorders present with a wide range of symptoms. They may be genetic or acquired, and the most important is Parkinson's disease. Most movement disorders are categorised clinically, with few confirmatory investigations available other than for those with a known gene abnormality.

Idiopathic Parkinson's disease

Parkinsonism is a clinical syndrome characterised primarily by bradykinesia (p. 1165), with associated increased

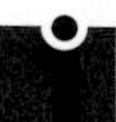

26.64 Causes of parkinsonism

Idiopathic Parkinson's disease (at least 80% of parkinsonism)

Cerebrovascular disease

Drugs and toxins
- Antipsychotic drugs (older and 'atypical')
- Metoclopramide, prochlorperazine
- Tetrabenazine
- Sodium valproate
- Lithium
- Manganese
- MPTP

Other degenerative diseases
- Dementia with Lewy bodies
- Progressive supranuclear palsy
- Multiple system atrophy
- Corticobasal degeneration
- Alzheimer's disease

Genetic
- Huntington's disease
- Fragile X tremor ataxia syndrome
- Dopa-responsive dystonia
- Spinocerebellar ataxias (particularly SCA 3)
- Wilson's disease

Anoxic brain injury

(MPTP = methyl-phenyl-tetrahydropyridine)

tone (rigidity), tremor and loss of postural reflexes. There are many causes (Box 26.64) but the most common is Parkinson's disease (PD). PD has an annual incidence of about 18/100 000 in the UK and a prevalence of about 180/100 000. Age has a critical influence on incidence and prevalence, the latter rising to 300–500/100 000 after 80 years of age. Average age of onset is about 60 years, and fewer than 5% of patients present under the age of 40. Genetic factors are increasingly recognised and several single genes causing parkinsonism have been identified, although they only account for a very small proportion of cases overall. Having a first-degree relative with PD confers a 2–3 times increased risk of developing PD. It is a progressive and incurable condition, with a variable prognosis. Whilst motor symptoms are the most common presenting features, non-motor symptoms (particularly cognitive impairment, depression and anxiety) become increasingly common as the disease progresses, and significantly reduce quality of life.

Pathophysiology

Although mutations in several genes have been identified in a few cases, in most patients the cause remains unknown. The discovery that methyl-phenyl-tetrahydropyridine (MPTP) caused severe parkinsonism in young drug users suggested that PD might be due to an environmental toxin but none has been convincingly identified. The pathological hallmarks of PD are depletion of the pigmented dopaminergic neurons in the substantia nigra and the presence of α-synuclein and other protein inclusions in nigral cells (Lewy bodies – Fig. 26.29). It is thought that environmental or genetic factors alter the α-synuclein protein, rendering it toxic and leading to Lewy body formation within the nigral cells. Lewy bodies are also found in the basal ganglia, brainstem and cortex, and increase with disease progression. PD is recognised as a synucleinopathy alongside multiple system atrophy and dementia with Lewy bodies. The loss of dopaminergic neurotransmission is responsible for many of the clinical features.

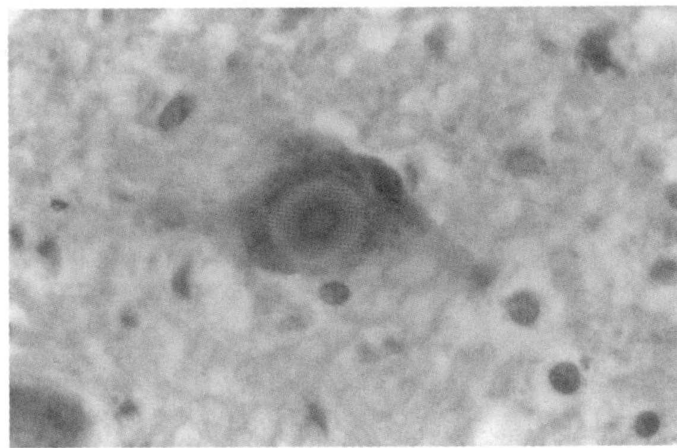

Fig. 26.29 Parkinson's disease. High power (× 400) of substantia nigra of a patient with Parkinson's disease showing classical Lewy body (haematoxylin and eosin).

Clinical features

Non-motor symptoms, including reduction in sense of smell (hyposmia), constipation and REM sleep behavioural disturbance (RBD), may precede the development of typical motor features by many years, but patients rarely present at this stage. The motor symptoms are almost always initially asymmetrical. The hallmark is bradykinesia, leading to classic symptoms such as increasingly small handwriting, difficulty with tying shoelaces or buttoning, and difficulty rolling over in bed. Tremor is an early feature but may not be apparent in at least 20% of people with PD. It is typically a unilateral rest tremor (p. 1165) affecting limbs, jaw and chin, but not the head. In some patients, tremor remains the dominant symptom for many years. Rigidity causes stiffness and a flexed posture. Although postural righting reflexes are impaired early on in the disease, falls tend not to occur until later. As the disease advances, speech becomes softer and indistinct. There are a number of abnormalities on neurological examination (Box 26.65).

Although the features are initially unilateral, gradual bilateral involvement evolves with time. Cognition is spared in early disease; if impaired, it should trigger consideration of alternative diagnoses, such as dementia with Lewy bodies.

Non-motor symptoms

Some non-motor symptoms (NMS) precede the onset of more typical symptoms by many years (see above). Depression or anxiety may also be presenting features of PD. For most patients, however, NMS become increasingly common and disabling as PD progresses. Cognitive impairment, including dementia, is the symptom most likely to impair quality of life for patients and their carers. Estimates of dementia frequency range from 30 to 80%, depending on definitions and length of follow-up. Other distressing NMS include other neuropsychiatric features (anxiety, depression, apathy, hallucinosis/psychosis), sleep disturbance and hypersomnolence, fatigue, pain, sphincter disturbance and constipation, sexual problems (erectile failure, loss of libido or hypersexuality) and drooling.

Investigations

The diagnosis is clinical. Structural imaging (CT or MRI) is usually normal for age and thus rarely helpful,

26.65 Physical signs in Parkinson's disease

General

- Expressionless face (hypomimia)
- Soft, rapid, indistinct speech (dysphonia)
- Flexed (stooped) posture
- Impaired postural reflexes

Gait

- Slow to start walking (failure of gait ignition)
- Rapid, short stride length, tendency to shorten (festination)
- Reduction of arm swing
- Impaired balance on turning

Tremor

Resting (3–4 Hz, moderate amplitude): most common
- Asymmetric, usually first in arm/hand ('pill rolling')
- May affect legs, jaw and chin, but not head
- Intermittent, present at rest, often briefly abolished by movement of the limb, exacerbated by walking

Postural (6–8 Hz, moderate amplitude)
- Present immediately on stretching out arms

Re-emergent tremor (3–4 Hz, moderate amplitude)
- Initially no tremor on stretching arms out, rest tremor re-emerges after a few seconds

Rigidity

- Cogwheel type, mostly upper limbs (due to tremor superimposed upon rigidity)
- Lead pipe type

Akinesia (fundamental feature)

- Slowness of movement
- Fatiguing and decrease in size of repetitive movements

Normal findings (if abnormal, consider other causes)

- Power, deep tendon reflexes, plantar responses
- Eye movements
- Sensory and cerebellar examination

although it may support a suspected vascular cause. Functional dopaminergic imaging (SPECT or PET) is abnormal, even at early stages (Fig. 26.30), but does not differentiate between the different forms of degenerative parkinsonism (see Box 26.64) and so is not specific for PD. In younger patients, specific investigations may be appropriate (e.g. exclusion of Huntington's and Wilson's diseases). Some patients with family histories may wish to consider genetic testing, although the role of genetic counselling is uncertain at present.

Management

Drug therapy

Drug treatment for PD remains symptomatic rather than curative, and there is no evidence that any of the currently available drugs are neuroprotective. Levodopa (LD) remains the most effective treatment available, but other agents include dopamine agonists, anticholinergics, inhibitors of monoamine oxidase (MAOI)-B and catechol-O-methyl-transferase (COMT), and amantadine. Debate continues about when to start treatment, and with which drug. In general, most specialists recommend initiating treatment when symptoms are impacting on everyday life; whether it is best to start with LD, a dopamine agonist or MAOI-B remains unclear, but most accept that the most effective, best-tolerated and cheapest drug is LD. Many motor symptoms, such as tremor, freezing, falling, head-drop and abnormal flexion, are quite resistant to treatment. Some NMS, such as anxiety or depression, may respond to drug or non-drug treatments. In the UK, rivastigmine is licensed for use in PD-associated dementia, although its effect is modest at best. Many other NMS are resistant to treatment. Evidence-based statements regarding diagnosis and drug management of PD are listed in Box 26.66.

Levodopa. LD is the precursor to dopamine. When administered orally, more than 90% is decarboxylated to dopamine peripherally in the gastrointestinal tract and blood vessels, and only a small proportion reaches the brain. This peripheral conversion is responsible for the high frequency of adverse effects, and to avoid this, LD is combined with a dopa decarboxylase inhibitor (DDI); the inhibitor does not cross the blood–brain barrier, thus avoiding unwanted decarboxylation-blocking in the brain. Two DDIs, carbidopa and benserazide, are available as combination preparations with LD, as Sinemet® and Madopar®, respectively.

LD is most effective at relieving the akinesia and rigidity; tremor response is often less satisfactory, and it has no effect on many motor (posture, freezing) and non-motor symptoms. Failure of akinesia/rigidity to respond to LD 1000 mg/day should prompt reconsideration of the diagnosis. Although controlled-release versions of LD exist, these are usually best reserved for use overnight, as their variable bioavailability makes them difficult to use throughout the day. Madopar® is also available as a dispersible tablet for more rapid-onset effect.

Adverse effects include postural hypotension, nausea and vomiting, which may be offset by domperidone. LD may exacerbate or trigger hallucinations, and abnormal LD-seeking behaviour may occur uncommonly

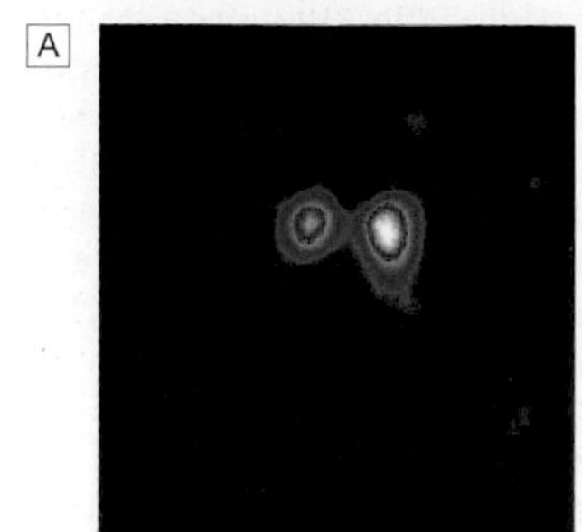

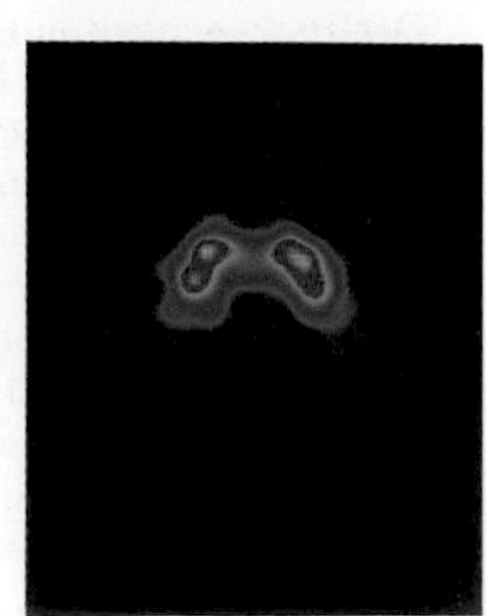

Fig. 26.30 Imaging in Parkinson's disease. **A** SPECT scan in Parkinson's disease showing reduced dopamine activity in the basal ganglia. **B** Normal.

EBM 26.66 Management of Parkinson's disease

Early treatment

'Patients with early PD may be considered for treatment with:
- levodopa plus dopa decarboxylase inhibitor *or*
- oral or transdermal dopamine agonists *or*
- monoamine oxidase B inhibitors.'

'Ergot-derived dopamine agonists should not be used as first-line treatment.'

'Anticholinergic drugs should not be used as first-line treatment.'

Motor fluctuations

'Motor fluctuations may be treated with either monoamine oxidase B inhibitors or dopamine agonists.'

'Dopamine agonists may be used to manage motor complications in patients with advanced PD. The non-ergot agonists are preferable to the ergot agonists.'

'Intermittent or infusions of subcutaneous apomorphine may be used to manage advanced PD.'

'Catechol-O-methyl-transferase (COMT) inhibitors may be used to reduce off-time in patients with advanced PD.'

- SIGN 113. Diagnosis and pharmacological management of Parkinson's disease, 2010.

For further information: www.sign.ac.uk

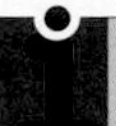

26.67 Dopamine agonists*

Ergot-derived
- Bromocriptine
- Lisuride
- Pergolide
- Cabergoline

Non-ergot-derived
- Ropinirole
- Pramipexole
- Rotigotine (transdermal patch)
- Apomorphine (subcutaneous)

*Oral unless otherwise stated.

(dopamine dysregulation syndrome) in which the patient takes excessive doses of LD.

As PD progresses, the response to LD becomes less predictable in many patients, leading to motor fluctuations. This end-of-dose deterioration is due to progressive loss of dopamine storage capacity by dwindling numbers of striatonigral neurons. LD-induced involuntary movements (dyskinesia) may occur as a peak-dose phenomenon or as a biphasic phenomenon (occurring during both the build-up and wearing-off phases). More complex fluctuations present as sudden, unpredictable changes in response, in which periods of parkinsonism ('off' phases) alternate with improved mobility but with dyskinesias ('on' phases). Motor complication management is difficult; wearing-off effects may respond to increased dose or frequency of LD or the addition of a COMT inhibitor (see below). More complex fluctuations may be improved by the addition of dopamine agonists (including continuous infusion of apomorphine), use of intrajejunal LD via a percutaneous endoscopic jejunostomy, or deep brain stimulator implantation.

Dopamine receptor agonists. Originally introduced in the hope of delaying the initiation of LD, and thus delaying motor complications, several dopamine agonists are available, and may be delivered orally, transdermally or subcutaneously (Box 26.67).

The ergot-derived agonists are no longer recommended because of rare but serious fibrotic effects. With the exception of apomorphine, all the agonists are considerably less powerful than LD in relieving parkinsonism, have more adverse effects (nausea, vomiting, confusion and hallucinations, impulse control disorders) and are more expensive. Their role in the management of PD (monotherapy or adjunctive) remains uncertain, and evidence is accruing to suggest that their usefulness as initial monotherapy is short-lasting.

MAOI-B inhibitors. Monoamine oxidase type B facilitates breakdown of excess dopamine in the synapse. Two inhibitors are used in PD: selegiline and rasagiline. The effects of both are modest, although usually well tolerated. Neither is neuroprotective, despite initial hopes.

COMT inhibitors. Catechol-O-methyl-transferase (along with dopa decarboxylase) is involved in peripheral breakdown of LD. Two inhibitors are available: entacapone and tolcapone (which also inhibits central COMT). Entacapone has a modest effect and is most useful for early wearing-off. It is available either as a single tablet taken with each LD/DDI dose, or as a combination tablet with LD and DDI. The more potent tolcapone is less used because of rare but serious hepatotoxicity.

Amantadine. This has a mild, usually short-lived effect on bradykinesia and is rarely used unless patients are unable to tolerate other drugs. It is more commonly employed as a treatment for LD-induced dyskinesias, although again benefit is modest and short-lived. Adverse effects include livedo reticularis, peripheral oedema, confusion and other anticholinergic effects.

Anticholinergic drugs. These were the main treatment for PD prior to the introduction of LD. Their role now is limited by lack of efficacy (apart from an effect on tremor sometimes) and adverse effects, including dry mouth, blurred vision, constipation, urinary retention, confusion and hallucinosis. Several anticholinergics are available, including trihexyphenidyl (benzhexol) and orphenadrine.

Surgery

Destructive neurosurgery was commonly used before the introduction of LD. In the last 20 years, stereotactic surgery has emerged and most commonly involves deep brain stimulation (DBS), rather than the destructive approach of previous eras. Various targets have been identified, including the thalamus (though this is only effective for tremor), globus pallidus and subthalamic nucleus. DBS is usually reserved for patients with medically refractory tremor or motor fluctuations, and careful patient selection is vital to success. Intracranial delivery of fetal grafts or specific growth factors remains experimental.

Physiotherapy, occupational therapy and speech therapy

Patients at all stages of PD benefit from physiotherapy, which helps reduce rigidity and corrects abnormal posture. Occupational therapists can provide equipment to help overcome functional limitations, such as rails for stairs and the toilet, and bathing equipment. Speech therapy can help where dysarthria and dysphonia interfere with communication, and advice may also be provided to those with dysphagia on the use of altered-texture diets. As with many complex neurological disorders, patients with PD should ideally be managed by a multidisciplinary team, including PD specialist nurses.

Other parkinsonian syndromes

Cerebrovascular disease and drug-induced parkinsonism are the most common alternative causes of parkinsonism (see Box 26.64). There are several degenerative conditions that cause parkinsonism, including multiple system atrophy, progressive supranuclear palsy and corticobasal degeneration. They typically have a more rapid progression than PD and tend to be resistant to treatment with LD. They are defined pathologically and identification during life is difficult. There are other conditions that may rarely manifest as parkinsonism, including Huntington's and Wilson's diseases.

Multiple system atrophy

Multiple system atrophy (MSA) is characterised by parkinsonism, autonomic failure and cerebellar symptoms, with either parkinsonism (MSA-P) or cerebellar features (MSA-C) predominating. It is much less common than PD, with a prevalence of about 4/100000. Although early distinction between PD and MSA-P may be difficult, early falls, postural instability and lack of response to LD are clues. The pathological hallmark is α-synuclein-containing glial cytoplasmic inclusions found in the basal ganglia, cerebellum and motor cortex. Management is symptomatic and the prognosis is less good than for PD, with mean survival from symptom onset of fewer than 10 years, and early disability. Cognition is preserved.

Progressive supranuclear palsy

Progressive supranuclear palsy (PSP) presents with symmetrical parkinsonism, cognitive impairment, early falls and bulbar symptoms. The characteristic eye movement disorder, with slowed vertical saccades leading to impairment of up and down gaze, may take years to emerge. PSP has different pathological features, being associated with abnormal accumulation of tau (τ) proteins and degeneration of the substantia nigra, subthalamic nucleus and mid-brain. It is therefore a tauopathy rather than synucleinopathy. The prevalence is about 5/100000, with average survival similar to that in MSA. There is no treatment, and the parkinsonism usually does not respond to LD.

Corticobasal degeneration

Corticobasal degeneration (CBD) is less common than MSA or PSP, and the clinical manifestations are variable, including parkinsonism, dystonia, myoclonus and 'alien limb' phenomenon, whereby a limb (usually upper) moves about or interferes with the other limb without apparent conscious control. Cortical symptoms, especially apraxia, are common and may be the only features in some cases, including dementia. A number of other diseases may present with a corticobasal syndrome, including other dementias. CBD is a tauopathy with widespread deposition throughout the brain, and has similar survival rates to MSA and PSP.

Wilson's disease

This is an autosomal recessive disorder causing a defect of copper metabolism (p. 973). It is a treatable cause of various movement disorders, including tremor, dystonia, parkinsonism and ataxia; psychiatric symptoms may also occur. Wilson's should always be excluded in younger patients presenting with any movement disorder.

Huntington's disease

Huntington's disease (HD) is an autosomal dominant disorder, usually presenting in adults but occasionally children. It is due to expansion of a trinucleotide CAG repeat in the *Huntingtin* gene on chromosome 4 (p. 65). The disease frequently demonstrates the phenomenon of anticipation, in which there is a younger age at onset as the disease is passed through generations, due to progressive expansion of the repeat. The prevalence is about 4–8/100000.

Clinical features

HD typically presents with a progressive behavioural disturbance, abnormal movements (usually chorea), and cognitive impairment leading to dementia. Onset under 18 years is rare, but patients may then present with parkinsonism rather than chorea (the 'Westphal variant'). There is always a family history, although this may be concealed.

Investigations and management

The diagnosis is confirmed by genetic testing; presymptomatic testing for other family members is available but must be preceded by appropriate counselling (p. 67). Brain imaging may show caudate atrophy but is not a reliable test. There are a number of HD mimics.

Management is symptomatic. The chorea may respond to neuroleptics such as risperidone or sulpiride, or other drugs such as tetrabenazine. Depression and anxiety are common, and may be helped by medication.

Ataxias

The ataxias are a heterogeneous group of inherited and acquired disorders, presenting either with pure ataxia or in association with other neurological and non-neurological features. The differential is wide (Boxes 26.68 and 26.69), and diagnosis is guided by age of onset, evolution and clinical features. A significant proportion of cases remain idiopathic despite investigation.

The hereditary ataxias are a group of inherited disorders in which degenerative changes occur to varying

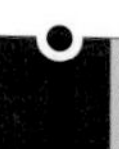

26.68 Causes of acquired ataxia

Structural lesions	
• Brain tumour	• Brain abscess
Toxic	
• Drugs: lithium, phenytoin, amiodarone, toluene, 5-fluorouracil, cytosine arabinoside • Alcohol • Heavy metals/chemicals: mercury, lead, thallium	
Infection/post-infectious	
• HIV • Varicella zoster • Whipple's disease	• Miller Fisher syndrome (p. 1224)
Degenerative	
• Multiple system atrophy • Sporadic Creutzfeldt–Jakob disease	• Idiopathic (or sporadic) late-onset cerebellar ataxia
Inflammatory/immune-mediated	
• Multiple sclerosis • Gluten ataxia (coeliac disease)	• Paraneoplastic ataxia • Hashimoto encephalopathy
Metabolic	
• Vitamin B_1 or E deficiency • Hypothyroidism	• Hypoparathyroidism
Vascular	
• Stroke (ischaemic or haemorrhagic)	• Vascular malformations • Superficial siderosis

extents in the cerebellum, brainstem, pyramidal tracts, spinocerebellar tracts, and optic and peripheral nerves, and which influence the clinical manifestations. Onset ranges from infancy to adulthood, with recessive, sex-linked or dominant inheritance (see Box 26.69). Whilst the genetic abnormality has been identified for some, allowing diagnostic testing, this is not currently the case for many of the hereditary ataxias.

Tremor disorders

Tremor (p. 1165) is a feature of many disorders, but the most important clinical syndromes are PD, essential tremor, drug-induced tremors (Box 26.70) and functional (psychogenic) tremors.

Essential tremor

This has a prevalence of about 300/100 000 and may display a dominant pattern of inheritance, although no genes have thus far been identified. It may present at any age with a bilateral arm tremor (8–10 Hz), rarely at rest but typical with movement. The head and voice may be involved. The tremor improves in about 50% of patients with small amounts of alcohol. There are no specific tests, and it should be distinguished from other tremor syndromes, including dystonic tremor. Beta-blockers and primidone are sometimes helpful, and DBS of the thalamus is an effective treatment for severe cases.

26.69 Inherited ataxias

Inheritance pattern	Age of onset	Clinical features
Autosomal dominant		
Episodic ataxias	Childhood and early adulthood	Brief episodes of ataxia, sometimes induced by stress or startle. May develop progressive ataxia
Spinocerebellar ataxias (SCA)	Childhood to middle age	Over 30 subtypes identified thus far. Progressive ataxia, sometimes associated with other features, including retinitis pigmentosa, pyramidal tract abnormalities, peripheral neuropathy and cognitive deficits
Dentato-rubro-pallidoluysian atrophy (DRPLA)	Childhood to middle age	Children present with myoclonic epilepsy and progressive ataxia. Adults have progressive ataxia with psychiatric features, dementia and choreoathetosis
Autosomal recessive		
Friedreich's ataxia	Childhood/adolescence (late onset possible)	Ataxia, nystagmus, dysarthria, spasticity, areflexia, proprioceptive impairment, diabetes mellitus, optic atrophy, cardiac abnormalities. Usually chair-bound
Ataxia telangiectasia	Childhood	Progressive ataxia, athetosis, telangiectasia on conjunctivae, impaired DNA repair, immune deficiency, tendency to malignancies
Abetalipoproteinaemia	Childhood	Steatorrhoea, sensorimotor neuropathy, retinitis pigmentosa, malabsorption of vitamins A, D, E, K
Hereditary ataxia with vitamin E deficiency	< 20 yrs	Similar to Friedreich's ataxia, visual loss or retinitis pigmentosa, chorea
Others	Usually young onset	Numerous, with genes only identified in some
X-linked		
Fragile X tremor ataxia syndrome	> 50 yrs	Tremor, ataxia, parkinsonism, autonomic failure, cognitive impairment and dementia
Adrenoleucodystrophy	Childhood to adult	Impaired adrenal and cognitive function, sometimes spastic paraparesis
Mitochondrial disease	Various	Ataxia features in several mitochondrial diseases, including Kearns–Sayre syndrome, MELAS, MERRF, Leigh's syndrome (p. 46)

(MELAS = mitochondrial myopathy, encephalopathy, lactic acidosis and stroke-like episodes; MERRF = myoclonic epilepsy with ragged red fibres)

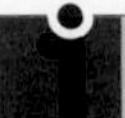

26.70 Drug-induced tremor (usually postural)*

- β-agonists (e.g. salbutamol)
- Theophylline
- Sodium valproate
- Thyroxine
- Lithium
- Tricyclic antidepressants
- Recreational drugs (e.g. amphetamines)
- Alcohol
- Caffeine

*Drugs causing parkinsonism and associated tremor are listed in Box 26.64.

Dystonia

Dystonia is characterised by a focal increase in tone affecting muscles in the limbs or trunk. It may be a feature of a number of neurological conditions (PD, Wilson's disease), or occur secondary to brain damage (trauma, stroke) or drugs (tardive syndromes). Dystonia also occurs as a primary disorder. In childhood onset, the cause is usually genetic and dystonia is generalised but adult onset is usually focal; examples include a twisted neck (torticollis), repetitive blinking (blepharospasm) or tremor. Task-specific symptoms (e.g. writer's cramp, musician's dystonia) are often dystonic. Treatment is difficult but botulinum toxin injections or DBS may be useful.

Hemifacial spasm

This usually presents after middle age with intermittent twitching around one eye, spreading ipsilaterally to other facial muscles. The spasms are exacerbated by talking, eating and stress. Hemifacial spasm is usually idiopathic (similarly to trigeminal neuralgia, it has been suggested that it is due to an aberrant arterial loop irritating the 7th nerve just outside the pons), but may be symptomatic and secondary to structural lesions or MS. Drug treatment is not effective but injections of botulinum toxin into affected muscles help, although these usually have to be repeated every 3 months or so. In refractory cases, microvascular decompression may be considered.

Motor neuron disease

Motor neuron disease (MND) is a neurodegenerative condition caused by loss of upper and lower motor neurons in the spinal cord, cranial nerve nuclei and motor cortex. Annual incidence is about 2/100 000, with a prevalence of about 7/100 000. Most cases are sporadic but between 5 and 10% of cases are familial. Abnormalities in the superoxide dismutase (*SOD1*) gene account for about 20% of such cases, and recently an expanded repeat sequence in the *C9ORF72* gene on chromosome 9 has been associated with MND and frontotemporal dementia. The most common form of MND is amyotrophic sclerosis (ALS), and many use the terms MND and ALS interchangeably. ALS is characterised by a combination of upper and lower motor neuron signs; there are rarer, pure lower (progressive muscular atrophy) or upper (progressive lateral sclerosis) motor neuron variants of MND. The average age of onset is 65, with 10% presenting before 45 years.

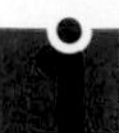

26.71 Clinical features of motor neuron disease

Onset

- Usually after the age of 50 yrs
- Very uncommon before the age of 30 yrs
- Affects males more commonly than females

Symptoms

- Limb muscle weakness, cramps, occasionally fasciculation
- Disturbance of speech/swallowing (dysarthria/dysphagia)

Signs

- Wasting and fasciculation of muscles
- Weakness of muscles of limbs, tongue, face and palate
- Pyramidal tract involvement, causing spasticity, exaggerated tendon reflexes, extensor plantar responses
- External ocular muscles and sphincters usually remain intact
- No objective sensory deficit

Course

- Symptoms often begin focally in one part and spread gradually but relentlessly to become widespread

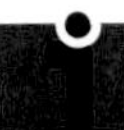

26.72 Patterns of involvement in motor neuron disease

Progressive muscular atrophy

- Predominantly spinal motor neurons affected
- Weakness and wasting of distal limb muscles at first
- Fasciculation in muscles
- Tendon reflexes may be absent

Progressive bulbar palsy

- Early involvement of tongue, palate and pharyngeal muscles
- Dysarthria/dysphagia
- Wasting and fasciculation of tongue
- Pyramidal signs may also be present

Amyotrophic lateral sclerosis (ALS)

- Combination of distal and proximal muscle-wasting and weakness, fasciculation
- Spasticity, exaggerated reflexes, extensor plantars
- Bulbar and pseudobulbar palsy follow eventually
- Pyramidal tract features may predominate

Clinical features

MND typically presents focally, either with limb onset (e.g. foot drop) or with bulbar symptoms; respiratory onset is rare but respiratory failure is a common terminal event. Sensory, autonomic and visual symptoms do not occur, although cramp is common (Box 26.71). Examination reveals a combination of lower and upper motor neuron signs (e.g. brisk reflexes in wasted, fasciculating muscles) without sensory involvement (Box 26.72). Cognitive impairment is under-recognised in MND: up to 50% will have a mainly executive impairment on formal testing, and around 10% develop a frontotemporal dementia (FTD). About 10% of patients presenting with FTD will develop ALS within a few years of dementia onset. MND is relentlessly progressive and up to 50% die within 2 years of diagnosis.

Investigations

Clinical features are often typical but alternative diagnoses should be excluded. Exclusion of treatable causes, such as immune-mediated multifocal motor neuropathy with conduction block (p. 1224) and cervical myelo-radiculopathy, is essential. Blood tests are usually normal, other than a mildly raised creatine kinase. Sensory and motor nerve conduction studies are normal but there may be reduction in amplitude of motor action potentials due to axonal loss. Electromyography will usually confirm the typical features of widespread denervation and re-innervation. Spinal fluid analysis is not usually necessary. DNA testing may become more important as genetic factors become clearer.

Management

Patients should be managed within a multidisciplinary service, including physiotherapists, speech and occupational therapists, dietitians, ventilatory and feeding support, and palliative care teams, with neurological and respiratory input. Riluzole is licensed for ALS but has only a modest effect (Box 26.73). Non-invasive ventilatory support and/or feeding by percutaneous gastrostomy may improve quality of life in selected patients. Rapid access to palliative care teams is essential for patients as they enter the terminal stages of MND.

EBM 26.73 Effective treatments for amyotrophic lateral sclerosis/motor neuron disease

'Riluzole 100 mg daily is reasonably safe and may prolong median survival by about 2–3 months in patients with ALS.'

'Non-invasive ventilation significantly prolongs survival and improves or maintains quality of life in people with ALS. Survival and some measures of quality of life were significantly improved in the subgroup of people with better bulbar function, but not in those with severe bulbar impairment.'

- Radunovic A, et al. Mechanical ventilation for amyotrophic lateral sclerosis/motor neuron disease. Cochrane Database of Systematic Reviews, 2009, issue 4. Art. no.: CD004427.
- Miller RG, et al. Riluzole for amyotrophic lateral sclerosis (ALS)/motor neuron disease (MND). Cochrane Database of Systematic Reviews, 2012, issue 3. Art. no.: CD001447.

For further information: www.cochrane.org/cochrane-reviews

Spinal muscular atrophy

This is a group of genetically determined disorders affecting spinal and cranial lower motor neurons, characterised by proximal and distal wasting, fasciculation and weakness of muscles. Involvement is usually symmetrical but occasional localised forms occur. With the exception of the infantile form, progression is slow and the prognosis better than for MND.

INFECTIONS OF THE NERVOUS SYSTEM

The clinical features of nervous system infections depend on the location of the infection (the meninges or the parenchyma of the brain and spinal cord), the causative organism (virus, bacterium, fungus or parasite), and whether the infection is acute or chronic.

26.74 Infections of the nervous system

Bacterial infections	
• Meningitis • Suppurative encephalitis • Brain abscess • Paravertebral (epidural) abscess • Tuberculosis (Ch. 19)	• Neurosyphilis • Leprosy (peripheral nerves)* • Diphtheria (peripheral nerves)* • Tetanus (motor cells)
Viral infections	
• Meningitis • Encephalitis • Transverse myelitis • Progressive multifocal leucoencephalopathy • Poliomyelitis	• Subacute sclerosing panencephalitis (late sequel) • Rabies • HIV infection (Ch. 14)
Prion diseases	
• Creutzfeldt–Jakob disease	• Kuru
Protozoal infections	
• Malaria* • Toxoplasmosis (in immune-suppressed)*	• Trypanosomiasis* • Amoebic abscess*
Helminthic infections	
• Schistosomiasis (spinal cord)* • Cysticercosis*	• Hydatid disease* • Strongyloidiasis*
Fungal infections	
• *Candida* meningitis or brain abscess	• Cryptococcal meningitis

*These infections are discussed in Chapter 13.

The major infections of the nervous system are listed in Box 26.74. The frequency of these varies geographically. Helminthic infections, such as cysticercosis and hydatid disease, and protozoal infections are described in Chapter 13.

Meningitis

Acute infection of the meninges presents with a characteristic combination of pyrexia, headache and meningism. Meningism consists of headache, photophobia and stiffness of the neck, often accompanied by other signs of meningeal irritation, including Kernig's sign (extension at the knee with the hip joint flexed causes spasm in the hamstring muscles) and Brudzinski's sign (passive flexion of the neck causes flexion of the hips and knees). Meningism is not specific to meningitis and can occur in patients with subarachnoid haemorrhage. The severity of clinical features varies with the causative organism, as does the presence of other features such as a rash. Abnormalities in the CSF (see Box 26.5, p. 1154) are important in distinguishing the cause of meningitis. Causes of meningitis are listed in Box 26.75.

Viral meningitis

Viruses are the most common cause of meningitis, usually resulting in a benign and self-limiting illness requiring no specific therapy. It is much less serious

26

26.75 Causes of meningitis

Infective	
Bacteria (see Box 26.76)	
Viruses	
• Enteroviruses (echo, Coxsackie, polio)	• Epstein–Barr
• Mumps	• HIV
• Influenza	• Lymphocytic choriomeningitis
• Herpes simplex	• Mollaret's meningitis (herpes simplex virus type 2)
• Varicella zoster	
Protozoa and parasites	
• Cysticerci	• Amoeba
Fungi	
• *Cryptococcus neoformans*	• *Blastomyces*
• *Candida*	• *Coccidioides*
• *Histoplasma*	• *Sporothrix*
Non-infective ('sterile')	
Malignant disease	
• Breast cancer	• Leukaemia
• Bronchial cancer	• Lymphoma
Inflammatory disease (may be recurrent)	
• Sarcoidosis	• Behçet's disease
• SLE	

than bacterial meningitis unless there is associated encephalitis (which is rare). A number of viruses can cause meningitis (see Box 26.75), the most common being enteroviruses. Where specific immunisation is not employed, the mumps virus is a common cause.

Clinical features

Viral meningitis occurs mainly in children or young adults, with acute onset of headache and irritability and the rapid development of meningism. The headache is usually the most severe feature. There may be a high pyrexia but focal neurological signs are rare.

Investigations

The diagnosis is made by lumbar puncture. The CSF usually contains an excess of lymphocytes but glucose and protein levels are commonly normal; the protein level may be raised. It is extremely important to verify that the patient has not received antibiotics (for whatever cause) prior to the lumbar puncture, as this picture can also be found in partially treated bacterial meningitis.

Management

There is no specific treatment and the condition is usually benign and self-limiting. The patient should be treated symptomatically in a quiet environment. Recovery usually occurs within days, although a lymphocytic pleocytosis may persist in the CSF. Meningitis may also occur as a complication of a systemic viral infection such as mumps, measles, infectious mononucleosis, herpes zoster and hepatitis. Whatever the virus, complete recovery without specific therapy is the rule.

Bacterial meningitis

Many bacteria can cause meningitis but geographical patterns vary, as does age-related sensitivity (Box 26.76).

26.76 Bacterial causes of meningitis

Age of onset	Common	Less common
Neonate	Gram-negative bacilli (*Escherichia coli*, *Proteus*) Group B streptococci	*Listeria monocytogenes*
Pre-school child	*Haemophilus influenzae* *Neisseria meningitidis* *Streptococcus pneumoniae*	*Mycobacterium tuberculosis*
Older child and adult	*Neisseria meningitidis* *Streptococcus pneumoniae*	*Listeria monocytogenes* *Mycobacterium tuberculosis* *Staphylococcus aureus* (skull fracture) *Haemophilus influenzae*

Bacterial meningitis is usually part of a bacteraemic illness, although direct spread from an adjacent focus of infection in the ear, skull fracture or sinus can be causative. Antibiotics have rendered this less common but mortality and morbidity remain significant. An important factor in determining prognosis is early diagnosis and the prompt initiation of appropriate therapy. The meningococcus and other common causes of meningitis are normal commensals of the upper respiratory tract. New and potentially pathogenic strains are acquired by the air-borne route but close contact is necessary. Epidemics of meningococcal meningitis occur particularly in cramped living conditions or where the climate is hot and dry. The organism invades through the nasopharynx, producing septicaemia and leading to meningitis.

Pathophysiology

The meningococcus (*Neisseria meningitidis*) is now the most common cause of bacterial meningitis in Western Europe after *Streptococcus pneumoniae*, whilst in the USA *Haemophilus influenzae* remains common. In India, *H. influenzae* B and *Strep. pneumoniae* are probably the most common causes of bacterial meningitis, especially in children. *Strep. suis* is a rare zoonotic cause of meningitis associated with contact with pigs. The infection stimulates an immune response, causing the pia–arachnoid membrane to become congested and infiltrated with inflammatory cells. Pus then forms in layers, which may later organise to form adhesions. These may obstruct the free flow of CSF, leading to hydrocephalus, or they may damage the cranial nerves at the base of the brain. Hearing loss is a frequent complication. The CSF pressure rises rapidly, the protein content increases, and there is a cellular reaction that varies in type and severity according to the nature of the inflammation and the causative organism. An obliterative endarteritis of the leptomeningeal arteries passing through the meningeal exudate may produce secondary cerebral infarction. Pneumococcal meningitis is often associated with a very purulent CSF and a high mortality, especially in older adults.

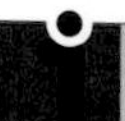

26.77 Complications of meningococcal septicaemia

- Meningitis
- Rash (morbilliform, petechial or purpuric)
- Shock
- Intravascular coagulation
- Renal failure
- Peripheral gangrene
- Arthritis (septic or reactive)
- Pericarditis (septic or reactive)

Clinical features

Headache, drowsiness, fever and neck stiffness are the usual presenting features. In severe bacterial meningitis the patient may be comatose and later there may be focal neurological signs. Ninety percent of patients with meningococcal meningitis will have two of the following: fever, neck stiffness, altered consciousness and rash. When accompanied by septicaemia, it may present very rapidly, with abrupt onset of obtundation due to cerebral oedema. Complications of meningococcal septicaemia are listed in Box 26.77. Chronic meningococcaemia is a rare condition in which the patient can be unwell for weeks or even months with recurrent fever, sweating, joint pains and transient rash. It usually occurs in the middle-aged and elderly, and in those who have previously had a splenectomy. In pneumococcal and *Haemophilus* infections there may be an associated otitis media. Pneumococcal meningitis may be associated with pneumonia and occurs especially in older patients and alcoholics, as well as those without functioning spleens. *Listeria monocytogenes* is an increasing cause of meningitis and rhombencephalitis (brainstem encephalitis) in the immunosuppressed, people with diabetes, alcoholics and pregnant women (p. 339). It can also cause meningitis in neonates.

Investigations

Lumbar puncture is mandatory unless there are contraindications (p. 1154). If the patient is drowsy and has focal neurological signs or seizures, is immunosuppressed, has undergone recent neurosurgery or has suffered a head injury, it is wise to obtain a CT to exclude a mass lesion (such as a cerebral abscess) before lumbar puncture because of the risk of coning. This should not, however, delay treatment of a presumptive meningitis. If lumbar puncture is deferred or omitted, it is essential to take blood cultures and to start empirical treatment (Fig. 26.31). Lumbar puncture will help differentiate the causative organism: in bacterial meningitis the CSF is cloudy (turbid) due to the presence of many neutrophils (often $> 1000 \times 10^6$ cells/L), the protein content is significantly elevated and the glucose reduced. Gram film and culture may allow identification of the organism. Blood cultures may be positive. PCR techniques can be used on both blood and CSF to identify bacterial DNA. These methods are useful in detecting meningococcal infection and in typing the organism.

Management

There is an untreated mortality rate of around 80%, so action must be swift. If bacterial meningitis is suspected, the patient should be given parenteral benzylpenicillin immediately (intravenous is preferable) and prompt hospital admission should be arranged. The only contraindication is a history of penicillin anaphylaxis.

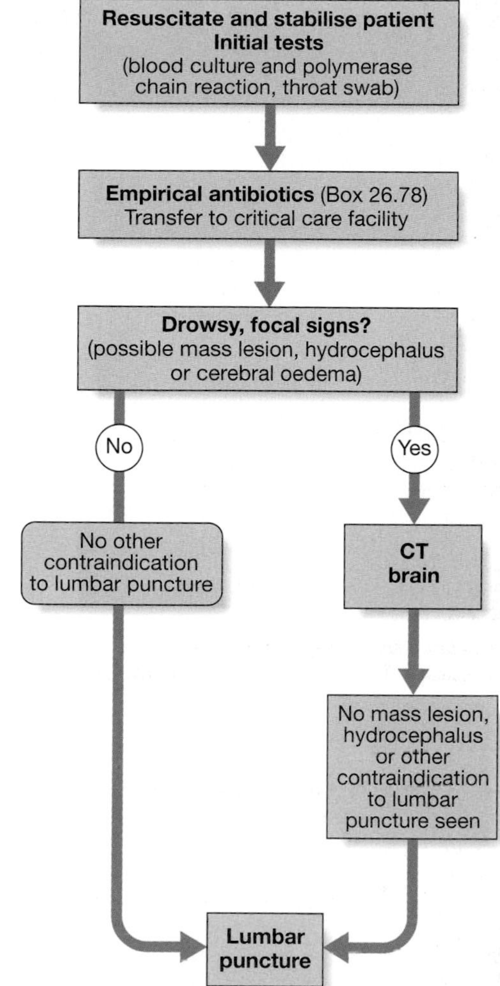

Fig. 26.31 The investigation of meningitis.

Recommended empirical therapy before the cause of meningitis is known is given in Box 26.78, and the preferred antibiotic when the organism is known after CSF examination is stipulated in Box 26.79. Adjunctive corticosteroid therapy is useful in both children and adults (Box 26.80) in developed countries where the incidence of penicillin resistance is low, but its role in settings where there are high rates of resistance or in under-developed countries where there are high rates of untreated HIV is unclear.

In meningococcal disease, mortality is doubled if the patient presents with features of septicaemia rather than meningitis. Individuals likely to require intensive care facilities and expertise include those with cardiac, respiratory or renal involvement, and those with CNS depression prejudicing the airway. Early endotracheal intubation and mechanical ventilation protect the airway and may prevent the development of the acute respiratory distress syndrome (ARDS, p. 192). Adverse prognostic features include hypotensive shock, a rapidly developing rash, a haemorrhagic diathesis, multisystem failure and age over 60 years.

Prevention of meningococcal infection

Close contacts of patients with meningococcal infection (Box 26.81) should be given 2 days of oral rifampicin. In

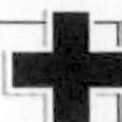

26.78 Treatment of pyogenic meningitis of unknown cause

1. Adults aged 18–50 yrs with or without a typical meningococcal rash

- Cefotaxime 2 g IV 4 times daily *or*
- Ceftriaxone 2 g IV twice daily

2. Patients in whom penicillin-resistant pneumococcal infection is suspected, or in areas with a significant incidence of penicillin resistance in the community

As for (1) but add:

- Vancomycin 1 g IV twice daily *or*
- Rifampicin 600 mg IV twice daily

3. Adults aged > 50 yrs and those in whom *Listeria monocytogenes* infection is suspected (brainstem signs, immunosuppression, diabetic, alcoholic)

As for (1) but add:

- Ampicillin 2 g IV 6 times daily *or*
- Co-trimoxazole 50 mg/kg IV daily in two divided doses

4. Patients with a clear history of anaphylaxis to β-lactams

- Chloramphenicol 25 mg/kg IV 4 times daily *plus*
- Vancomycin 1 g IV twice daily

5. Adjunctive treatment (see text)

- Dexamethasone 0.15 mg/kg 4 times daily for 2–4 days

26.79 Chemotherapy of bacterial meningitis when the cause is known

Pathogen	Regimen of choice	Alternative agents
N. meningitidis	Benzylpenicillin 2.4 g IV 6 times daily for 5–7 days	Cefuroxime, ampicillin Chloramphenicol*
Strep. pneumoniae (sensitive to β-lactams, MIC < 1 mg/L)	Cefotaxime 2 g IV 4 times daily *or* ceftriaxone 2 g IV twice daily for 10–14 days	Chloramphenicol*
Strep. pneumoniae (resistant to β-lactams)	As for sensitive strains but add vancomycin 1 g IV twice daily *or* rifampicin 600 mg IV twice daily	Vancomycin *plus* rifampicin* Moxifloxacin Gatifloxacin
H. influenzae	Cefotaxime 2 g IV 4 times daily *or* ceftriaxone 2 g IV twice daily for 10–14 days	Chloramphenicol*
L. monocytogenes	Ampicillin 2 g IV 6 times daily *plus* gentamicin 5 mg/kg IV daily	Ampicillin 2 g IV 4-hourly *plus* co-trimoxazole 50 mg/kg daily in two divided doses
Strep. suis	Cefotaxime 2 g IV 4 times daily *or* ceftriaxone 2 g IV twice daily for 10–14 days	Chloramphenicol*

*For patients with a history of anaphylaxis to β-lactam antibiotics.
(MIC = minimum inhibitory concentration)

EBM 26.80 Adjunctive dexamethasone for bacterial meningitis

Corticosteroids significantly reduce hearing loss and neurological sequelae, but do not reduce overall mortality.

- Brouwer MC, et al. Corticosteroids for acute bacterial meningitis. Cochrane Database of Systematic Reviews, 2010, issue 9. Art. no.: CD004405.

For further information: 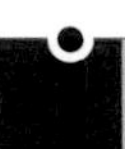 www.cochrane.org/cochrane-reviews

26.81 Chemoprophylaxis following meningococcal exposure

Close contacts warranting chemoprophylaxis

- Household contacts (including persons who ate or slept in the same dwelling as the patient during the 7 days prior to disease onset)
- Child-care and nursery-school contacts
- Persons having contact with patient's oral secretions during the 7 days prior to disease onset
  - Kissing
  - Sharing of toothbrushes
  - Sharing of eating utensils
  - Mouth-to-mouth resuscitation
  - Unprotected contact during endotracheal intubation
- Aircraft contacts for persons seated next to the patient for > 8 hrs

Persons at low risk in whom chemoprophylaxis is not recommended

- Casual contact (e.g. at school or work) without direct exposure to patient's oral secretions
- Indirect contact only (contact with a high-risk contact and not a case)
- Health-care worker without direct exposure to patient's oral secretions

adults, a single dose of ciprofloxacin is an alternative. If not treated with ceftriaxone, the index case should be given similar treatment to clear infection from the nasopharynx before hospital discharge. Vaccines are available for most meningococcal subgroups but not group B, which is among the most common serogroup isolated in many countries.

Tuberculous meningitis

Tuberculous meningitis is now uncommon in developed countries in previously healthy individuals, although it is still seen in those born in endemic areas and in the immunocompromised. It remains common in developing countries and is seen more frequently as a secondary infection in patients with the acquired immunodeficiency syndrome (AIDS).

Pathophysiology

Tuberculous meningitis most commonly occurs shortly after a primary infection in childhood or as part of miliary tuberculosis (p. 689). The usual local source of infection is a caseous focus in the meninges or brain substance adjacent to the CSF pathway. The brain is covered by a greenish, gelatinous exudate, especially around the base, and numerous scattered tubercles are found on the meninges.

26.82 Clinical features and staging of tuberculous meningitis

Symptoms	
• Headache	• Depression
• Vomiting	• Confusion
• Low-grade fever	• Behaviour changes
• Lassitude	
Signs	
• Meningism (may be absent)	• Depression of conscious level
• Oculomotor palsies	• Focal hemisphere signs
• Papilloedema	
Staging of severity	
• Stage I (early): non-specific symptoms and signs without alteration of consciousness	
• Stage II (intermediate): altered consciousness without coma or delirium + minor focal neurological signs	
• Stage III (advanced): stupor or coma, severe neurological deficits, seizures or abnormal movements	

Clinical features

The clinical features and staging criteria are listed in Box 26.82. Onset is much slower than in other bacterial meningitis – over 2–8 weeks. If untreated, it is fatal in a few weeks but complete recovery is usual if treatment is started at stage I (see Box 26.82). When treatment is initiated later, the rate of death or serious neurological deficit may be as high as 30%.

Investigations

Lumbar puncture should be performed if the diagnosis is suspected. The CSF is under increased pressure. It is usually clear but, when allowed to stand, a fine clot ('spider web') may form. The fluid contains up to 500×10^6 cells/L, predominantly lymphocytes, but can contain neutrophils. There is a rise in protein and a marked fall in glucose. The tubercle bacillus may be detected in a smear of the centrifuged deposit from the CSF but a negative result does not exclude the diagnosis. The CSF should be cultured but, as this result will not be known for up to 6 weeks, treatment must be started without waiting for confirmation. Brain imaging may show hydrocephalus, brisk meningeal enhancement on enhanced CT or MRI, and/or an intracranial tuberculoma.

Management

As soon as the diagnosis is made or strongly suspected, chemotherapy should be started using one of the regimens that include pyrazinamide, described on page 693. The use of corticosteroids in addition to anti-tuberculous therapy has been controversial. Recent evidence suggests that it improves mortality, especially if given early, but not focal neurological damage. Surgical ventricular drainage may be needed if obstructive hydrocephalus develops. Skilled nursing is essential during the acute phase of the illness, and adequate hydration and nutrition must be maintained.

Other forms of meningitis

Fungal meningitis (especially cryptococcosis – p. 384) usually occurs in patients who are immunosuppressed and is a recognised complication of HIV infection (p. 401). The CSF findings are similar to those of tuberculous meningitis, but the diagnosis can be confirmed by microscopy or specific serological tests.

In some areas, meningitis may be caused by spirochaetes (leptospirosis, Lyme disease and syphilis – pp. 336, 334 and 419), rickettsiae (typhus fever – p. 350) or protozoa (amoebiasis – p. 367).

Meningitis can also be due to non-infective pathologies. This is seen in recurrent aseptic meningitis due to SLE, Behçet's disease or sarcoidosis, as well as a condition of previously unknown origin known as Mollaret's syndrome, in which the recurrent meningitis is associated with epithelioid cells in the spinal fluid ('Mollaret' cells). Recent evidence suggests that this condition may be due to human herpes virus type 2, and is therefore infective after all. Meningitis can also be seen due to direct invasion of the meninges by neoplastic cells ('malignant meningitis' – see Box 26.75, p. 1202).

Parenchymal viral infections

Infection of the substance of the nervous system will produce symptoms of focal dysfunction (deficits and/or seizures) with general signs of infection, depending on the acuteness of the infection and the type of organism.

Viral encephalitis

A range of viruses can cause encephalitis but only a minority of patients have a history of recent viral infection. In Europe, the most serious cause of viral encephalitis is herpes simplex (p. 325), which probably reaches the brain via the olfactory nerves. Varicella zoster is also an important cause. The development of effective therapy for some forms of encephalitis has increased the importance of clinical diagnosis and virological examination of the CSF. In some parts of the world, viruses transmitted by mosquitoes and ticks (arboviruses) are an important cause of encephalitis. The epidemiology of some of these infections is changing. Japanese encephalitis (p. 328) has spread relentlessly across Asia to Australia, and there have been outbreaks of West Nile encephalitis in Romania, Israel and New York. HIV may cause encephalitis with a subacute or chronic presentation, but occasionally has an acute presentation with seroconversion.

Pathophysiology

The infection provokes an inflammatory response that involves the cortex, white matter, basal ganglia and brainstem. The distribution of lesions varies with the type of virus. For example, in herpes simplex encephalitis, the temporal lobes are usually primarily affected, whereas cytomegalovirus can involve the areas adjacent to the ventricles (ventriculitis). Inclusion bodies may be present in the neurons and glial cells and there is an infiltration of polymorphonuclear cells in the perivascular space. There is neuronal degeneration and diffuse glial proliferation, often associated with cerebral oedema.

Clinical features

Viral encephalitis presents with acute onset of headache, fever, focal neurological signs (aphasia and/or hemiplegia, visual field defects) and seizures. Disturbance of consciousness ranging from drowsiness to deep coma supervenes early and may advance dramatically. Meningism occurs in many patients. Rabies presents a distinct clinical picture and is described below.

Investigations

Imaging by CT scan may show low-density lesions in the temporal lobes but MRI is more sensitive in detecting early abnormalities. Lumbar puncture should be performed once imaging has excluded a mass lesion. The CSF usually contains excess lymphocytes but polymorphonuclear cells may predominate in the early stages. The CSF may be normal in up to 10% of cases. Some viruses, including the West Nile virus, may cause a sustained neutrophilic CSF. The protein content may be elevated but the glucose is normal. The EEG is usually abnormal in the early stages, especially in herpes simplex encephalitis, with characteristic periodic slow-wave activity in the temporal lobes. Virological investigations of the CSF, including PCR for viral DNA, may reveal the causative organism but treatment initiation should not await this.

Management

Optimum treatment for herpes simplex encephalitis (aciclovir 10 mg/kg IV 3 times daily for 2–3 weeks) has reduced mortality from 70% to around 10%. This should be given early to all patients suspected of suffering from viral encephalitis.

Some survivors will have residual epilepsy or cognitive impairment. For details of post-infectious encephalomyelitis, see page 1192. Anticonvulsant treatment may be needed (p. 1183) and raised intracranial pressure may indicate the need for dexamethasone.

Brainstem encephalitis

This presents with ataxia, dysarthria, diplopia or other cranial nerve palsies. The CSF is lymphocytic, with a normal glucose. The causative agent is presumed to be viral. However, *Listeria monocytogenes* may cause a similar syndrome with meningitis (and often a polymorphonuclear CSF pleocytosis) and requires specific treatment with ampicillin 500 mg 4 times daily (see Box 26.79).

Rabies

Rabies is caused by a rhabdovirus that infects the central nervous tissue and salivary glands of a wide range of mammals, and is usually conveyed by saliva through bites or licks on abrasions or on intact mucous membranes. Humans are most frequently infected from dogs and bats. In Europe, the maintenance host is the fox. The incubation period varies in humans from a minimum of 9 days to many months but is usually between 4 and 8 weeks. Severe bites, especially if on the head or neck, are associated with shorter incubation periods. Human rabies is a rare disease, even in endemic areas. However, because it is usually fatal, major efforts are directed at limiting its spread and preventing its importation into uninfected countries, such as the UK.

Clinical features

At the onset there may be fever, and paraesthesia at the site of the bite. A prodromal period of 1–10 days, during which the patient becomes increasingly anxious, leads to the characteristic 'hydrophobia'. Although the patient is thirsty, attempts at drinking provoke violent contractions of the diaphragm and other inspiratory muscles. Delusions and hallucinations may develop, accompanied by spitting, biting and mania, with lucid intervals in which the patient is markedly anxious. Cranial nerve lesions develop and terminal hyperpyrexia is common. Death ensues, usually within a week of the onset of symptoms.

Investigations

During life, the diagnosis is usually made on clinical grounds but rapid immunofluorescent techniques can detect antigen in corneal impression smears or skin biopsies.

Management

Established disease

Only a few patients with established rabies have survived. All received some post-exposure prophylaxis (see below) and needed intensive care facilities to control cardiac and respiratory failure. Otherwise, only palliative treatment is possible once symptoms have appeared. The patient should be heavily sedated with diazepam, supplemented by chlorpromazine if needed. Nutrition and fluids should be given intravenously or through a gastrostomy.

Pre-exposure prophylaxis

Pre-exposure prophylaxis is required by those who handle potentially infected animals professionally, those who work with rabies virus in laboratories and those who live at special risk in rabies-endemic areas. Protection is afforded by intradermal injections of human diploid cell strain vaccine, or two intramuscular injections given 4 weeks apart, followed by yearly boosters.

Post-exposure prophylaxis

The wounds should be thoroughly cleaned, preferably with a quaternary ammonium detergent or soap; damaged tissues should be excised and the wound left unsutured. Rabies can usually be prevented if treatment is started within a day or two of biting. Delayed treatment may still be of value. For maximum protection, hyperimmune serum and vaccine are required.

The safest antirabies antiserum is human rabies immunoglobulin. The dose is 20 U/kg body weight; half is infiltrated around the bite and half is given intramuscularly at a different site from the vaccine. Hyperimmune animal serum may be used but hypersensitivity reactions, including anaphylaxis, are common.

The safest vaccine, free of complications, is human diploid cell strain vaccine; 1.0 mL is given intramuscularly on days 0, 3, 7, 14, 30 and 90. In developing countries, where human rabies globulin may not be obtainable, 0.1 mL of vaccine may be given intradermally into eight sites on day 1, with single boosters on days 7 and 28. Where human products are not available and when risk of rabies is slight (licks on the skin, or minor bites of covered arms or legs), it may be justifiable to delay starting treatment while observing the biting animal or awaiting examination of its brain, rather than use the older vaccine.

Poliomyelitis

Pathophysiology

Disease is caused by one of three polioviruses, which constitutes a subgroup of the enteroviruses. Poliomyelitis has become much less common in developed countries following the widespread use of oral vaccines but is still a problem in the developing world, especially parts of Africa. Infection usually occurs through the nasopharynx.

The virus causes a lymphocytic meningitis and infects the grey matter of the spinal cord, brainstem and cortex. There is a particular propensity to damage anterior horn cells, especially in the lumbar segments.

Clinical features

The incubation period is 7–14 days. Figure 26.32 illustrates the various features of the infection. Many patients recover fully after the initial phase of a few days of mild fever and headache. In other individuals, after a week of well-being, there is a recurrence of pyrexia, headache and meningism. Weakness may start later in one muscle group and can progress to widespread paresis. Respiratory failure may supervene if intercostal muscles are paralysed or the medullary motor nuclei are involved. Epidemics vary widely in terms of the incidence of non-paralytic cases and in mortality rate. Death occurs from respiratory paralysis. Muscle weakness is maximal at the end of the first week and gradual recovery may then take place over several months. Muscles showing no signs of recovery after a month will probably not regain useful function. Second attacks are very rare but occasionally patients show late deterioration in muscle bulk and power many years after the initial infection (this is termed the 'post-polio syndrome').

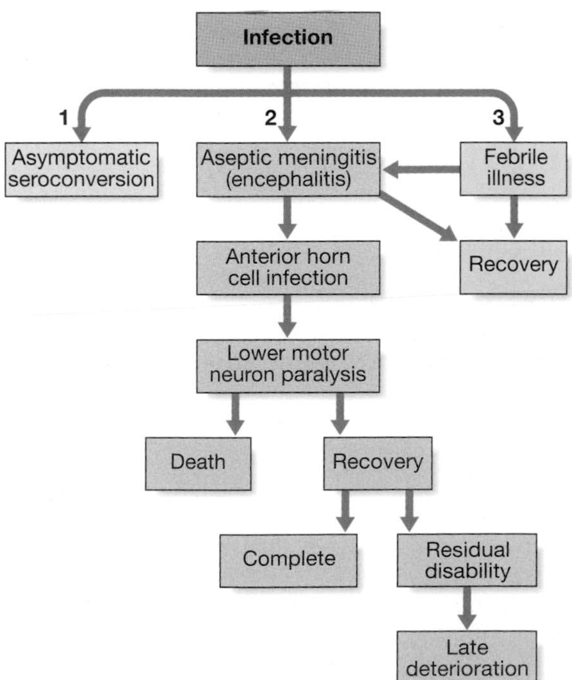

Fig. 26.32 Poliomyelitis. Possible consequences of infection.

Investigations

The CSF shows a lymphocytic pleocytosis, a rise in protein and a normal sugar content. Poliomyelitis virus may be cultured from CSF and stool.

Management

Established disease

In the early stages, bed rest is imperative because exercise appears to worsen the paralysis or precipitate it. At the onset of respiratory difficulties, a tracheostomy and ventilation are required. Subsequent treatment is by physiotherapy and orthopaedic measures.

Prophylaxis

Prevention of poliomyelitis is by immunisation with live (Sabin) vaccine. In developed countries where polio is now very rare, the live vaccine has been replaced by the killed vaccine in childhood immunisation schedules.

Herpes zoster (shingles)

Herpes zoster is the result of reactivation of the varicella zoster virus that has lain dormant in a nerve root ganglion following chickenpox earlier in life. Reactivation may be spontaneous (as usually occurs in the middle-aged or elderly) or due to immunosuppression (as in patients with diabetes, malignant disease or AIDS). Full details are given on page 318.

Subacute sclerosing panencephalitis

This is a rare, chronic, progressive and eventually fatal complication of measles, presumably a result of an inability of the nervous system to eradicate the virus. It occurs in children and adolescents, usually many years after the primary virus infection. There is generalised neurological deterioration and onset is insidious, with intellectual deterioration, apathy and clumsiness, followed by myoclonic jerks, rigidity and dementia.

The CSF may show a mild lymphocytic pleocytosis and the EEG demonstrates characteristic periodic bursts of triphasic waves. Although there is persistent measles-specific IgG in serum and CSF, antiviral therapy is ineffective and death ensues within a few years.

Progressive multifocal leucoencephalopathy

This was originally described as a rare complication of lymphoma, leukaemia or carcinomatosis, but has become more frequent as a feature of AIDS (p. 402). It is an infection of oligodendrocytes by human polyomavirus JC, which causes widespread demyelination of the white matter of the cerebral hemispheres. Clinical signs include dementia, hemiparesis and aphasia, which progress rapidly, usually leading to death within weeks or months. Areas of low density in the white matter are seen on CT but MRI is more sensitive, showing diffuse high signal in the cerebral white matter on T2-weighted images. The only treatment available is to restore the immune response (by treating AIDS or any other cause of immunosuppression).

Parenchymal bacterial infections

Cerebral abscess

Bacteria may enter the cerebral substance through penetrating injury, by direct spread from paranasal sinuses or the middle ear, or secondary to septicaemia. The site of abscess formation and the likely causative organism are both related to the source of infection (Box 26.83). Initial infection leads to local suppuration followed by loculation of pus within a surrounding wall of gliosis, which in a chronic abscess may form a tough capsule. Haematogenous spread may lead to multiple abscesses.

Clinical features

A cerebral abscess may present acutely with fever, headache, meningism and drowsiness, but more commonly presents over days or weeks as a cerebral mass lesion with little or no evidence of infection. Seizures, raised intracranial pressure and focal hemisphere signs occur alone or in combination. Distinction from a cerebral tumour may be impossible on clinical grounds.

Investigations

Lumbar puncture is potentially hazardous in the presence of raised intracranial pressure and CT should always precede it. CT reveals single or multiple low-density areas, which show ring enhancement with contrast and surrounding cerebral oedema (Fig. 26.33). There may be an elevated white blood cell count and ESR in patients with active local infection. The possibility of cerebral toxoplasmosis or tuberculous disease secondary to HIV infection (p. 402) should always be considered.

Management and prognosis

Antimicrobial therapy is indicated once the diagnosis is made. The likely source of infection should guide the choice of antibiotic (see Box 26.83). In neurosurgical patients, the addition of vancomycin should be considered. Surgical drainage by burr-hole aspiration or excision may be necessary, especially where the presence of a capsule may lead to a persistent focus of infection.

A

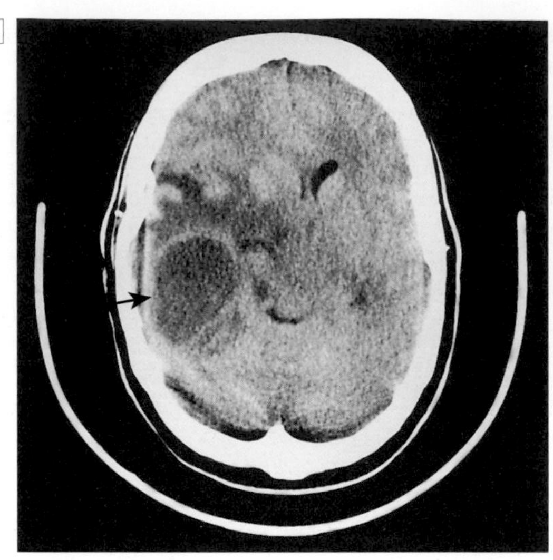

B

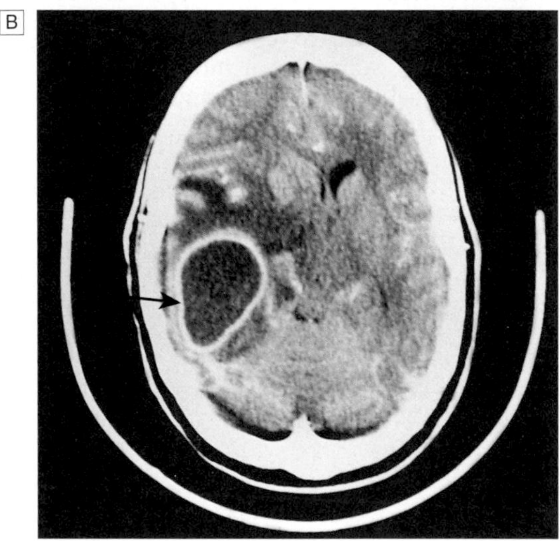

Fig. 26.33 Right temporal cerebral abscess (arrows), with surrounding oedema and midline shift to the left. **A** Unenhanced CT image. **B** Contrast-enhanced CT image.

26.83 Aetiology and treatment of bacterial cerebral abscess

Site of abscess	Source of infection	Likely organisms	Recommended treatment
Frontal lobe	Paranasal sinuses Teeth	Streptococci Anaerobes	Cefotaxime 2–3 g IV 4 times daily *plus* Metronidazole 500 mg IV 3 times daily
Temporal lobe **Cerebellum**	Middle ear Sphenoid sinus Mastoid/middle ear	Streptococci Enterobacteriaceae *Pseudomonas* spp. Anaerobes	Ampicillin 2–3 g IV 3 times daily *plus* Metronidazole 500 mg IV 3 times daily *plus either* Ceftazidime 2 g IV 3 times daily *or* Gentamicin* 5 mg/kg IV daily
Any site	Penetrating trauma	Staphylococci	Flucloxacillin 2–3 g IV 4 times daily *or* Cefuroxime 1.5 g IV 3 times daily
Multiple	Metastatic and cryptogenic	Streptococci Anaerobes	Benzylpenicillin 1.8–2.4 g IV 4 times daily if endocarditis or cyanotic heart disease Otherwise cefotaxime 2–3 g IV 4 times daily *plus* Metronidazole 500 mg IV 3 times daily

*Monitor gentamicin levels.

Epilepsy frequently develops and is often resistant to treatment.

Despite advances in therapy, the mortality rate remains at 10–20% and this may partly relate to delay in diagnosis and initiation of treatment.

Subdural empyema

This is a rare complication of frontal sinusitis, osteomyelitis of the skull vault or middle ear disease. A collection of pus in the subdural space spreads over the surface of the hemisphere, causing underlying cortical oedema or thrombophlebitis. Patients present with severe pain in the face or head and pyrexia, often with a history of preceding paranasal sinus or ear infection. The patient then becomes drowsy, with seizures and focal signs such as a progressive hemiparesis.

The diagnosis rests on a strong clinical suspicion in patients with a local focus of infection. Careful assessment with contrast-enhanced CT or MRI may show a subdural collection with underlying cerebral oedema. Management requires aspiration of pus via a burr-hole and appropriate parenteral antibiotics. Any local source of infection must be treated to prevent re-infection.

Spinal epidural abscess

The characteristic clinical features are pain in a root distribution and progressive transverse spinal cord syndrome with paraparesis, sensory impairment and sphincter dysfunction. Features of the primary focus of infection may be less obvious and thus can be overlooked. The resurgence of resistant staphylococcal infection and intravenous drug misuse has contributed to a recent marked rise in incidence.

X-ray changes occur late if present, so MRI or myelography should precede urgent neurosurgical intervention. Decompressive laminectomy with draining of the abscess relieves the pressure on the dura. Organisms may be grown from the pus or blood. Surgery, together with appropriate antibiotics, may prevent complete and irreversible paraplegia.

Lyme disease

This can cause numerous neurological problems, including polyradiculopathy, meningitis, encephalitis and mononeuritis multiplex (p. 334).

Neurosyphilis

Neurosyphilis may present as an acute or chronic process and may involve the meninges, blood vessels and/or parenchyma of the brain and spinal cord. The decade to 2008 saw a ten-fold increase in the incidence of syphilis, mostly as a result of misguided relaxation of safe sex measures with the advent of effective antiretroviral treatments for AIDS. Parallel increases in neurosyphilis are inevitable. The clinical manifestations are diverse and early diagnosis and treatment remain important.

Clinical features

The clinical and pathological features of the three most common presentations are summarised in Box 26.84. Neurological examination reveals signs indicative of the anatomical localisation of lesions. Delusions of grandeur suggest general paresis of the insane, but more commonly there is simply progressive dementia. Small and irregular pupils that react to convergence but not light, as described by Argyll Robertson (see Box 26.28, p. 1172), may accompany any neurosyphilitic syndrome, but most commonly tabes dorsalis.

26.84 Clinical and pathological features of neurosyphilis

Type	Pathology	Clinical features
Meningovascular (5 yrs)*	Endarteritis obliterans Meningeal exudate Granuloma (gumma)	Stroke Cranial nerve palsies Seizures/mass lesion
General paralysis of the insane (5–15 yrs)*	Degeneration in cerebral cortex/ cerebral atrophy Thickened meninges	Dementia Tremor Bilateral upper motor signs
Tabes dorsalis (5–20 yrs)*	Degeneration of sensory neurons Wasting of dorsal columns Optic atrophy	Lightning pains Sensory ataxia Visual failure Abdominal crises Incontinence Trophic changes
Any of the above		Argyll Robertson pupils (p. 1172)

*Interval from primary infection.

Investigations

Routine screening for syphilis is warranted in many neurological patients. Serological tests (p. 420) are positive in the serum in most patients, but CSF examination is essential if neurological involvement is suspected. Active disease is suggested by an elevated cell count, usually lymphocytic, and the protein content may be elevated to 0.5–1.0 g/L with an increased gamma globulin fraction. Serological tests in the CSF are usually positive, but progressive disease can occur with negative CSF serology.

Management

The injection of procaine benzylpenicillin (procaine penicillin) and probenecid for 17 days is essential in the treatment of neurosyphilis of all types (p. 421). Further courses of penicillin must be given if symptoms are not relieved, if the condition continues to advance or if the CSF continues to show signs of active disease. The cell count returns to normal within 3 months of completion of treatment, but the elevated protein takes longer to subside and some serological tests may never revert to normal. Evidence of clinical progression at any time is an indication for renewed treatment.

Diseases caused by bacterial toxins

Tetanus

This disease results from infection with *Clostridium tetani*, a commensal in the gut of humans and domestic animals that is found in soil. Infection enters the body through wounds, which may be trivial. It is rare in the

UK, occurring mostly in gardeners and farmers, but a recent increase has been seen in intravenous drug misusers. By contrast, the disease is common in many developing countries, where dust contains spores derived from animal and human excreta. Unhygienic practices soon after birth may lead to infection of the umbilical stump or site of circumcision, causing tetanus neonatorum. Tetanus is still one of the major killers of adults, children and neonates in developing countries, where the mortality rate can be nearly 100% in the newborn and around 40% in others.

In circumstances unfavourable to the growth of the organism, spores are formed and these may remain dormant for years in the soil. Spores germinate and bacilli multiply only in the anaerobic conditions that occur in areas of tissue necrosis or if the oxygen tension is lowered by the presence of other organisms, particularly if aerobic. The bacilli remain localised but produce an exotoxin with an affinity for motor nerve endings and motor nerve cells.

The anterior horn cells are affected after the exotoxin has passed into the blood stream and their involvement results in rigidity and convulsions. Symptoms first appear from 2 days to several weeks after injury – the shorter the incubation period, the more severe the attack and the worse the prognosis.

Clinical features

By far the most important early symptom is trismus – spasm of the masseter muscles, which causes difficulty in opening the mouth and in masticating; hence the name 'lockjaw'. Lockjaw in tetanus is painless, unlike the spasm of the masseters due to dental abscess, septic throat or other causes. Conditions that can mimic tetanus include hysteria and phenothiazine overdosage, or overdose in intravenous drug misusers.

In tetanus, the tonic rigidity spreads to involve the muscles of the face, neck and trunk. Contraction of the frontalis and the muscles at the angles of the mouth leads to the so-called 'risus sardonicus'. There is rigidity of the muscles at the neck and trunk of varying degree. The back is usually slightly arched ('opisthotonus') and there is a board-like abdominal wall.

In the more severe cases, violent spasms lasting for a few seconds to 3–4 minutes occur spontaneously, or may be induced by stimuli such as movement or noise. These convulsions are painful, exhausting and of very serious significance, especially if they appear soon after the onset of symptoms. They gradually increase in frequency and severity for about 1 week and the patient may die from exhaustion, asphyxia or aspiration pneumonia. In less severe illness, convulsions may not commence until a week or so after the first sign of rigidity, and in very mild infections they may never appear. Autonomic involvement may cause cardiovascular complications, such as hypertension. Rarely, the only manifestation of the disease may be 'local tetanus' – stiffness or spasm of the muscles near the infected wound – and the prognosis is good if treatment is commenced at this stage.

Investigations

The diagnosis is made on clinical grounds. It is rarely possible to isolate the infecting organism from the original locus of entry.

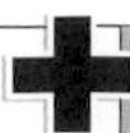

26.85 Treatment of tetanus

Neutralise absorbed toxin
- IV injection of 3000 U of human tetanus antitoxin

Prevent further toxin production
- Débridement of wound
- Benzylpenicillin 600 mg IV 4 times daily (metronidazole if patient is allergic to penicillin)

Control spasms
- Nurse in a quiet room
- Avoid unnecessary stimuli
- IV diazepam
- If spasms continue, paralyse patient and ventilate

General measures
- Maintain hydration and nutrition
- Treat secondary infections

Management

Established disease

Management of established disease should begin as soon as possible, as shown in Box 26.85.

Prevention

Tetanus can be prevented by immunisation and prompt treatment of contaminated wounds by débridement and antibiotics. In patients with a contaminated wound, the immediate danger of tetanus can be greatly reduced by the injection of 1200 mg of penicillin followed by a 7-day course of oral penicillin. For those allergic to penicillin, erythromycin should be used. When the risk of tetanus is judged to be present, an intramuscular injection of 250 U of human tetanus antitoxin should be given, along with toxoid which should be repeated 1 month and 6 months later. For those already immunised, only a booster dose of toxoid is required.

Botulism

Botulism is caused by the neurotoxins of *Clostridium botulinum*, which are extremely potent and cause disease after ingestion of even picogram amounts. Its classical form is an acute onset of bilateral cranial neuropathies associated with symmetric descending weakness.

Anaerobic conditions are necessary for the organism's growth. It may contaminate and thrive in many foodstuffs, where sealing and preserving provide the requisite conditions. Contaminated honey has been implicated in infant botulism, in which the organism colonises the gastrointestinal tract. Wound botulism is a growing problem in injection drug-users.

The toxin causes predominantly bulbar and ocular palsies (difficulty in swallowing, blurred or double vision, ptosis), progressing to limb weakness and respiratory paralysis. Criteria for the clinical diagnosis are shown in Box 26.86.

Management includes assisted ventilation and general supportive measures until the toxin eventually dissociates from nerve endings 6–8 weeks following ingestion. A polyvalent antitoxin is available for post-exposure prophylaxis and for the treatment of suspected botulism. It specifically neutralises toxin types A, B and E and is not effective against infantile botulism (in which

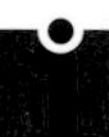

26.86 The US Centers for Disease Control (CDC) definition of botulism

Three main syndromes
1. Infantile 2. Food-borne 3. Wound infection
Clinical features
• Absence of fever • Symmetrical neurological deficits • Patient remains responsive • Normal or slow heart rate and normal blood pressure • No sensory deficits with the exception of blurred vision

active growth of the organism allows continued toxin production).

Transmissible spongiform encephalopathies

Transmissible spongiform encephalopathies (TSEs) include a number of veterinary and medical conditions that are characterised by the histopathological triad of cortical spongiform change, neuronal cell loss and gliosis. Associated with these changes, there is deposition of amyloid made up of an altered form of a normally occurring protein, the prion protein.

The precise nature of the infective agent is not yet clear but almost certainly involves the cascade formation of an abnormal prion protein. TSEs may also occur spontaneously or as an inherited disorder. Diseases affecting animals include bovine and feline spongiform encephalopathies (BSE and FSE). These diseases achieved media prominence in the 1990s, when a form of Creutzfeldt–Jakob disease emerged that was associated with prion protein ingestion.

Creutzfeldt–Jakob disease

Creutzfeldt–Jakob disease (CJD) is the best-characterised human TSE. Some 10% of cases arise due to a mutation in the gene coding for the prion protein. The sporadic form is the most common, occurring in middle-aged to elderly patients. Clinical features usually involve a rapidly progressive dementia, with myoclonus and a characteristic EEG pattern (repetitive slow-wave complexes), although a number of other features, such as visual disturbance or ataxia, may also be seen. These are particularly common in CJD transmitted by inoculation (e.g. by infected dura mater grafts). Death occurs after a mean of 4–6 months. There is no effective treatment.

Variant Creutzfeldt–Jakob disease

A variant of CJD (vCJD) emerged in the late 1990s, affecting a small number of patients in the UK. The causative agent appears to be identical to that causing BSE in cows, and the disease may have been a result of the epidemic of BSE in the UK a decade earlier. Patients affected by vCJD are typically younger than those with sporadic CJD and present with neuropsychiatric changes and sensory symptoms in the limbs, followed by ataxia, dementia and death. Progression is slightly slower than in patients with sporadic CJD (mean time to death is over a year). Characteristic EEG changes are not present, but MRI brain scans show characteristic high-signal changes in the pulvinar in a high proportion of cases (Fig. 26.34). Brain histology is distinct, with very florid plaques containing the prion proteins. Abnormal prion protein has been identified in tonsil specimens from sufferers of vCJD, leading to the suggestion that the disease could be transmitted by reticulo-endothelial tissue (like TSEs in animals but unlike sporadic CJD in humans). This has caused great concern in the UK, leading to precautionary measures such as leucodepletion of all blood used for transfusion, and the mandatory use of disposable surgical instruments wherever possible for tonsillectomy, appendicectomy and ophthalmological procedures. The incidence of vCJD has now declined dramatically but surveillance and research continue.

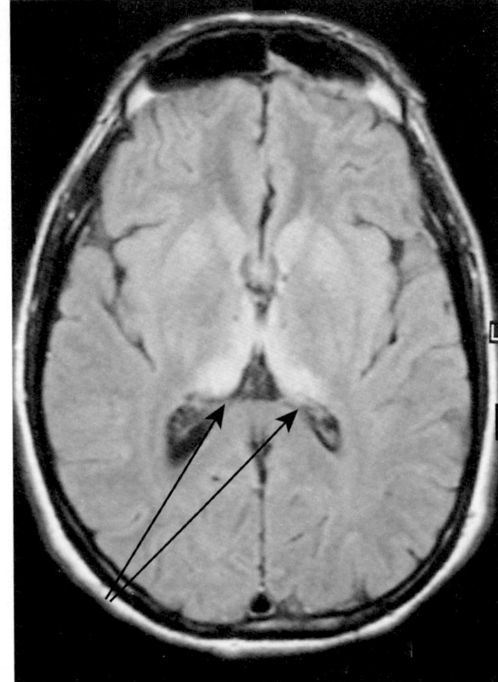

Fig. 26.34 MRI in variant Creutzfeldt–Jakob disease. Arrows indicate bilateral pulvinar hyperintensity.

Other TSE syndromes

Other extremely rare, inherited human TSEs include Gerstmann–Sträussler–Scheinker disease, fatal familial insomnia and kuru. Kuru occurred only in members of a cannibalistic New Guinea tribe and was probably transmitted by people eating the brains of dead tribal members. Clinical features include progressive ataxia and dementia.

INTRACRANIAL MASS LESIONS AND RAISED INTRACRANIAL PRESSURE

Many different types of mass lesion may arise within the intracranial cavity (Box 26.87). In developing countries, tuberculoma and other infections are frequent causes, but in the West, intracranial haemorrhage and brain

26.87 Common causes of raised intracranial pressure

Mass lesions
• Intracranial haemorrhage (traumatic or spontaneous) Extradural haematoma Subdural haematoma Intracerebral haemorrhage • Cerebral tumour (particularly posterior fossa lesions or high-grade gliomas: see Box 26.89) • Infective Cerebral abscess Tuberculoma Cysticercosis (p. 380) Hydatid cyst (p. 380) • Colloid cyst (in ventricles)
Disturbance of CSF circulation
• Obstructive (non-communicating) hydrocephalus: obstruction within ventricular system • Communicating hydrocephalus: site of obstruction outside ventricular system
Obstruction to venous sinuses
• Cerebral venous thrombosis • Trauma (depressed fractures overlying sinuses)
Diffuse brain oedema or swelling
• Meningo-encephalitis • Trauma (diffuse head injury, near-drowning) • Subarachnoid haemorrhage • Metabolic (e.g. water intoxication) • Idiopathic intracranial hypertension

26.88 Clinical features of intracranial mass lesions

Presentation	Features
Seizures	Focal onset ± generalised spread
Focal symptoms	Progressive loss of function Weakness Numbness Dysphasia Cranial neuropathy
False localising signs	Unilateral/bilateral 6th nerve palsies Contralateral 3rd nerve (usually pupil first)
Raised intracranial pressure (usually aggressive tumours causing vasogenic oedema or obstructive hydrocephalus)	Headache worse on lying/straining Vomiting Diplopia (6th nerve involvement) Papilloedema Bradycardia, raised blood pressure Impaired conscious level
Stroke/TIA-like symptoms	Acute haemorrhage into tumour Paroxysmal 'tumour attacks'
Cognitive/behavioural change	Usually frontal mass lesions
Endocrine abnormalities	Pituitary tumours
Incidental finding	Asymptomatic but identified on imaging (meningiomas commonly)

(TIA = transient ischaemic attack)

tumours are more common. The clinical features depend on the site of the mass, its nature and its rate of expansion. Symptoms and signs (see Box 26.88) are produced by a number of mechanisms.

Raised intracranial pressure

Raised intracranial pressure (RIP) may be caused by mass lesions, cerebral oedema, obstruction to CSF circulation causing hydrocephalus, impaired CSF absorption and cerebral venous obstruction (see Box 26.87).

Clinical features

In adults, intracranial pressure is less than 10–15 mmHg. The features of RIP are listed in Box 26.88. The speed of pressure increase influences presentation. If slow, compensatory mechanisms may occur, including alteration in the volume of fluid in CSF spaces and venous sinuses, which minimise symptoms. Rapid pressure increase (as in aggressive tumours) does not permit these compensatory mechanisms to occur, leading to early symptoms, including sudden death. Papilloedema is not always present, either because the pressure rise has been too rapid or because of anatomical anomalies of the meningeal sheath of the optic nerve.

A false localising sign is one in which the pathology is remote from the site of the expected lesion; in RIP, the 6th cranial nerve (unilateral or bilateral) is most commonly affected, but the 3rd, 5th and 7th nerves may also be involved. Sixth nerve palsies are thought to be due either to stretching of the long slender nerve or to compression against the petrous temporal bone ridge.

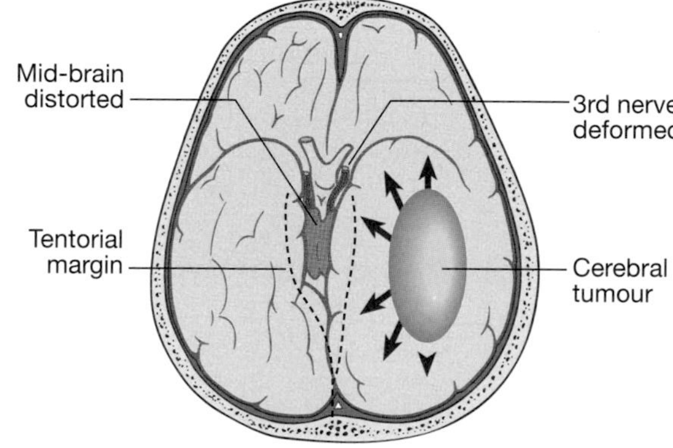

Fig. 26.35 Cerebral tumour displacing medial temporal lobe and causing pressure on the mid-brain and 3rd cranial nerve.

Trans-tentorial herniation of the uncus may compress the ipsilateral 3rd nerve and usually involves the pupillary fibres first, causing a dilated pupil; however, a false localising contralateral 3rd nerve palsy may also occur, perhaps due to extrinsic compression by the tentorial margin. Vomiting, coma, bradycardia and arterial hypertension are later features of RIP.

The rise in intracranial pressure from a mass lesion may cause displacement of the brain. Downward displacement of the medial temporal lobe (uncus) through the tentorium due to a large hemisphere mass may cause 'temporal coning' (Fig. 26.35). This may stretch the 3rd and/or 6th cranial nerves, or cause pressure on the contralateral cerebral peduncle (causing ipsilateral upper motor neuron signs), and is usually accompanied by progressive coma. Downward movement of the

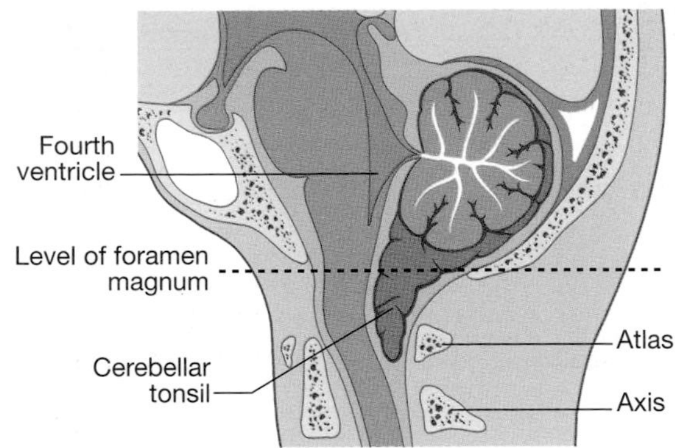

Fig. 26.36 Tonsillar cone. Downward displacement of the cerebellar tonsils below the level of the foramen magnum.

cerebellar tonsils through the foramen magnum may compress the medulla – 'tonsillar coning' (Fig. 26.36). This may result in brainstem haemorrhage and/or acute obstruction of the CSF pathways. As coning progresses, coma and death occur unless the condition is rapidly treated.

Management

Primary management of RIP should be targeted at relieving the cause (e.g. surgical decompression of mass lesion, steroids to reduce vasogenic oedema or shunt procedure to relieve hydrocephalus). Supportive treatment includes maintenance of fluid balance, blood pressure control, head elevation, and use of diuretics such as mannitol. Intensive care support may be needed (p. 199).

Brain tumours

Primary brain tumours are a heterogeneous collection of neoplasms arising from the brain tissue or meninges, and vary from benign to highly malignant. Primary malignant brain tumours (Box 26.89) are rare, accounting for 1% of all adult tumours but a higher proportion in children. The most common benign brain tumour is a meningioma. Primary brain tumours do not metastasise due to the absence of lymphatic drainage in the brain. There are rare pathological subtypes, however, such as medulloblastoma, which do have a propensity to metastasise; the reasons for this are not clear. Most cerebral tumours are sporadic but may be associated with genetic syndromes such as neurofibromatosis or tuberous sclerosis. Brain tumours are not classified by the usual TNM system but by the WHO grading I–IV; this is based on histology (e.g. nuclear pleomorphism, presence of mitoses and presence of necrosis), with grade I being the most benign and grade IV the most malignant. Gliomas account for 60% of brain tumours, with the aggressive glioblastoma multiforme (WHO grade IV) being the most common glioma, followed by meningiomas (20%) and pituitary tumours (10%). Although the lower-grade gliomas (I and II) may be very indolent, with prognosis measured in terms of many years, these tumours may transform to higher-grade disease at any time, with a resultant sharp decline in life expectancy.

Most malignant brain tumours are due to metastases, with intracranial metastases complicating about 20% of extracranial malignancies. The rate is higher with primaries in the bronchus, breast and gastrointestinal tract (Fig. 26.37). Metastases usually occur in the white matter of the cerebral or cerebellar hemispheres, but there are diffuse leptomeningeal types.

26.89 Primary brain tumours

Histological type	Common site	Age
Malignant		
Glioma (astrocytoma)	Cerebral hemisphere	Adulthood
		Childhood/adulthood
	Cerebellum	Childhood/young adulthood
	Brainstem	
Oligodendroglioma	Cerebral hemisphere	Adulthood
Medulloblastoma	Posterior fossa	Childhood
Ependymoma	Posterior fossa	Childhood/ adolescence
Cerebral lymphoma	Cerebral hemisphere	Adulthood
Benign		
Meningioma	Cortical dura Parasagittal Sphenoid ridge Suprasellar Olfactory groove	Adulthood (often incidental finding)
Neurofibroma	Acoustic neuroma	Adulthood
Craniopharyngioma	Suprasellar	Childhood/ adolescence
Pituitary adenoma	Pituitary fossa	Adulthood
Colloid cyst	Third ventricle	Any age
Pineal tumours	Quadrigeminal cistern	Childhood (teratomas) Young adulthood (germ cell)

Clinical features

The presentation is variable and usually influenced by the rate of growth. High-grade disease (WHO grade III and IV) tends to present with a short 4–6-week history of mass effect (headache, nausea secondary to RIP), while more indolent tumours can present with slowly progressive focal neurological deficits, depending on their location (see Box 26.88); generalised or focal seizures are common. Headache, if present, is usually accompanied by focal deficits or seizures, and isolated stable headache is almost never due to intracranial tumour.

The size of the primary tumour is of far less prognostic significance than its location within the brain. Tumours within the brainstem will result in early neurological deficits, while those in the frontal region may be quite large before symptoms occur.

Investigations

Diagnosis is by neuroimaging (Figs 26.38 and 26.39) and pathological grading following biopsy or resection where this is possible. The more malignant tumours are more likely to demonstrate contrast enhancement on imaging. If the tumour appears to be metastatic, further investigation to find the primary will be required.

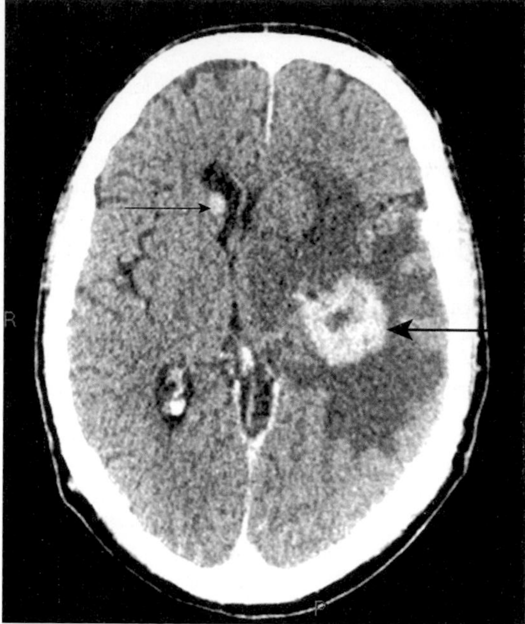

Fig. 26.37 Contrast-enhanced CT head showing a large metastasis within the left hemisphere (large arrow). There is surrounding cerebral oedema, and a smaller metastasis (small arrow) within the wall of the right lateral ventricle. The primary lesion was a lung carcinoma.

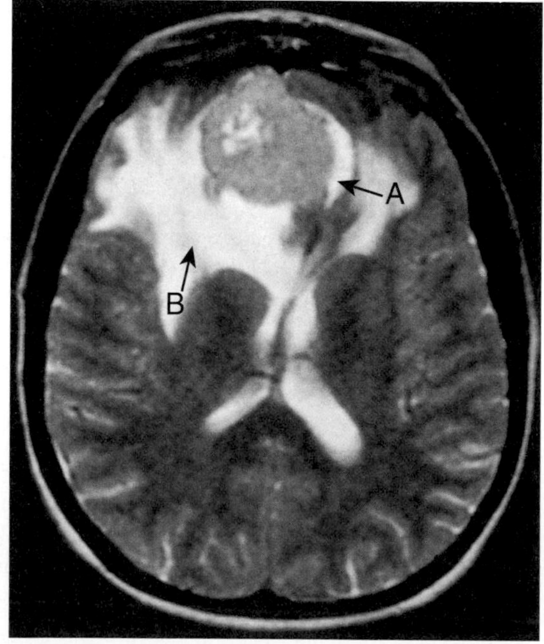

Fig. 26.38 MRI showing a meningioma in the frontal lobe (arrow A) with associated oedema (arrow B).

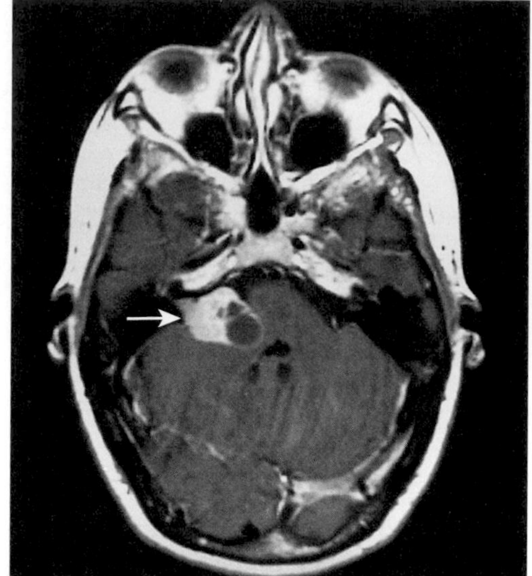

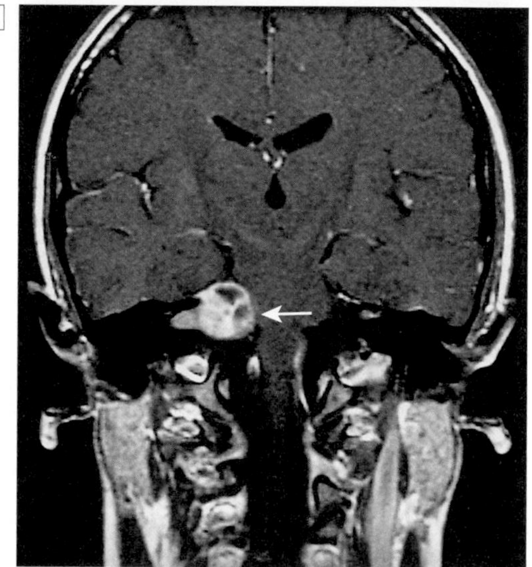

Fig. 26.39 MRI of an acoustic neuroma (arrows) in the posterior fossa compressing the brainstem. **A** Axial image. **B** Coronal image.

Management

Brain tumours are treated with a combination of surgery, radiotherapy and chemotherapy, depending on the type of tumour and the patient. Advancing age is the most powerful negative prognostic factor in CNS tumours, so best supportive care (including steroid therapy) may be most appropriate in older patients with metastases or high-grade disease. Treatment may not always be indicated in indolent (low-grade, WHO I or II) disease, and watchful waiting after surgery is often appropriate in such situations.

Dexamethasone given orally (or intravenously where RIP is acutely or severely raised) may reduce the vasogenic oedema typically associated with metastases and high-grade gliomas.

Prolactin- or growth hormone-secreting pituitary adenomas (p. 789) may respond well to treatment with dopamine agonists (such as bromocriptine, cabergoline or quinagolide); in this situation, imaging and hormone levels may be all that is required to establish a formal diagnosis, precluding the need for surgery.

Surgical

The mainstay of primary treatment is surgery, either resective (full or partial debulking) or biopsy, depending on the site and likely radiological diagnosis. Clearly, if a tumour occurs in an area of brain that is highly important for normal function (e.g. motor strip), then biopsy may be the only safe surgical intervention but, in general, maximal safe resection is the optimal surgical management. Meningiomas and acoustic neuromas offer the best prospects for complete removal and thus cure. Some meningiomas can recur, however, particularly those of the sphenoid ridge when partial excision is often all that is possible. Thereafter, post-operative surveillance may be required, as radiotherapy is effective at preventing further growth of residual tumour. Pituitary adenomas may be removed by a trans-sphenoidal route, avoiding the need for a craniotomy. Unfortunately, gliomas, which account for the majority of brain tumours, cannot be completely excised, since infiltration spreads well beyond the apparent radiological boundaries of the intracranial mass. Recurrence is therefore the rule, even if the mass of the tumour is apparently removed completely; partial excision ('debulking') may be useful in alleviating symptoms caused by RIP, but although there is increasing evidence that the degree of surgical excision may have a positive influence on survival, this has not yet been demonstrated in a randomised study.

Radiotherapy and chemotherapy

In the majority of primary CNS tumours, radiation and chemotherapy are used to control disease and extend survival rather than for cure. Meningioma and pituitary adenoma offer the best chance of life-long remission. The gliomas are incurable; high-grade, WHO IV disease still carries a median survival of just over a year. In this situation, patient and family should always be involved in decisions regarding treatment. The diagnosis, and often the symptoms, are devastating, and support from palliative care and social work is crucial at an early stage. In WHO grade III disease, prognosis is a little better (2–4 years) and in rarer, more indolent tumours, very prolonged survival is possible.

Advances have been made recently in terms of therapeutic outcome. Standard care for WHO grade IV glioblastoma multiforme is now combination radiotherapy with oral temozolomide chemotherapy; although this improves median survival of the population from only 12 to 14.5 months, up to 25% of patients survive for more than 2 years (compared to approximately 10% with radiotherapy alone). Ten percent will survive more than 5 years with temozolomide (virtually unheard of with radiotherapy alone). Benefits are more likely in well-debulked patients who are younger and fitter. Implantation of chemotherapy gives a small survival benefit.

Understanding of the molecular biology of brain tumours has allowed the use of biomarkers to guide therapy and prognostic discussions. In patients with methylation of the promoter region of the *MGMT* (methyl guanine methyl transferase) gene (about 30% of the population), 2-year survival is almost 50%. MGMT reduces the cytotoxicity of temozolomide, and this mutation also reduces the enzyme's activity, rendering the tumour more sensitive to chemotherapy. In grade II and III gliomas, the presence of the loss of heterozygocity (LOH) 1p19q chromosomal abnormality confers chemosensitivity and thus improves prognosis. The presence of a rare mutation in the *IDH-1* (isocitrate dehydrogenase) gene confers a very favourable prognosis in patients with glioblastoma.

There is a small group of highly malignant grade IV tumours that can be cured with aggressive therapy. Patients with medulloblastomas have a good chance of long-term survival with maximal surgery followed by irradiation of the whole brain and spine; younger patients may also benefit from concomitant and adjuvant chemotherapy. Older patients do not tolerate this, however.

Once tumours relapse, chemotherapy response rates are low and survival is short in high-grade disease. In the more uncommon low-grade tumours, repeated courses of chemotherapy can result in much more prolonged survival.

In metastatic disease, radiotherapy offers a modest improvement in survival but with costs in terms of quality of life; treatment therefore needs careful discussion with the patient. Benefits may be superior in breast cancer but there is little to separate other pathologies. Occasional chemosensitive cancers, such as small-cell lung cancer, may benefit from systemic chemotherapy, but intracerebral metastases represent a late stage of disease and have a short prognosis.

Prognosis

The WHO histological grading system is a powerful predictor of prognosis in primary CNS tumours, though it does not yet take account of individual biomarkers. For each tumour type and grade, advancing age and deteriorating functional status are the next most important negative prognostic features. The overall 5-year survival rate of about 14% in adults masks a wide variation that depends on tumour type.

Acoustic neuroma

This is a benign tumour of Schwann cells of the 8th cranial nerve, which may arise in isolation or as part of neurofibromatosis type 2 (see below). When sporadic, acoustic neuroma occurs after the third decade and is more frequent in females. The tumour commonly arises near the nerve's entry point into the medulla or in the internal auditory meatus, usually on the vestibular division. Acoustic neuromas account for 80–90% of tumours at the cerebellopontine angle.

Clinical features

Acoustic neuroma typically presents with unilateral progressive hearing loss, sometimes with tinnitus. Vertigo is an unusual symptom, as slow growth allows compensatory brainstem mechanisms to develop. In some cases, progressive enlargement leads to distortion of the brainstem and/or cerebellar peduncle, causing ataxia and/or cerebellar signs in the limbs. Distortion of the fourth ventricle and cerebral aqueduct may cause hydrocephalus (see below), which may be the presenting feature. Facial weakness is unusual at presentation but facial palsy may follow surgical removal of the tumour. The tumour may be identified incidentally on cranial imaging.

Investigations

MRI is the investigation of choice (see Fig. 26.39).

Management

Surgery is the treatment of choice. If the tumour can be completely removed, the prognosis is excellent, although deafness is a common complication of surgery. Stereotactic radiosurgery (radiotherapy) may be appropriate for some lesions.

Neurofibromatosis

Neurofibromatosis encompasses two clinically and genetically separate conditions, with an autosomal dominant pattern of inheritance. The more common neurofibromatosis type 1 (NF1) is caused by mutations in the *NF1* gene on chromosome 17, half of which are new mutations. NF1 is characterised by neurofibromas (benign peripheral nerve sheath tumours) and skin involvement (Fig. 26.40), and may affect numerous systems (Box 26.90). Neurofibromatosis type 2 (NF2) is caused by mutations of the *NF2* gene on chromosome 22, and is characterised by schwannomas (benign peripheral nerve sheath tumours comprising Schwann cells only), with little skin involvement; the clinical manifestations are more restricted to the eye and nervous system (see Box 26.90). Malignant change may occur in NF1 neurofibromas but is rare in NF2 schwannomas. The prevalence of NF1 and NF 2 is about 20–50 per 100 000 and 1.5 per 100 000 respectively.

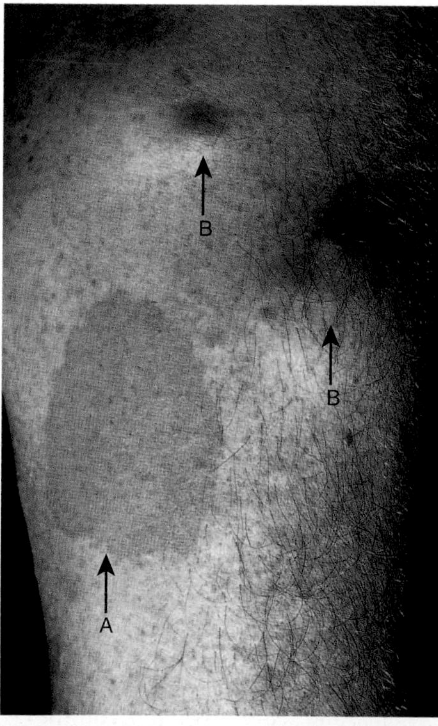

Fig. 26.40 A café au lait spot (arrow A) and subcutaneous nodules (arrows B) on the forearm of a patient with neurofibromatosis type 1.

Von Hippel–Lindau disease

This rare autosomal dominant disease is caused by mutations of the *VHL* tumour suppressor gene on chromosome 3. It promotes development of tumours affecting the kidney, adrenal gland, CNS, eye, inner ear, epididymis and pancreas, which may undergo malignant change. Benign haemangiomas and haemangioblastomas affect about 80% of patients, mostly in the cerebellum and retina.

26.90 Neurofibromatosis types 1 and 2: clinical features

Neurofibromatosis 1	Neurofibromatosis 2
Skin	
Cutaneous/subcutaneous neurofibromas Angiomas Café au lait patches (> 6) Axillary/groin freckling Hypopigmented patches	Much less commonly affected than NF1 Café au lait patches (usually < 6) Cutaneous schwannomas: plaque lesions Subcutaneous schwannomas
Eyes	
Lisch nodules (iris fibromas) Glaucoma Congenital ptosis	Cataracts Retinal hamartoma Optic nerve meningioma
Nervous system	
Plexiform neurofibromas Malignant peripheral nerve sheath tumours Aqueduct stenosis Slight tonsillar descent Cognitive impairment Epilepsy	Vestibular schwannomas Cranial nerve schwannomas (not 1 and 2) Spinal schwannomas Peripheral nerve schwannomas Cranial meningiomas Spinal meningiomas Spinal/brainstem ependymomas Spinal/cranial astrocytoma
Bone	
Scoliosis Osteoporosis Pseudoarthrosis	
Cardiorespiratory systems	
Pulmonary stenosis Hypertension Renal artery stenosis Compression from neurofibroma causing restrictive lung defect	
Gastrointestinal system	
Gastrointestinal stromal tumour Dysplasia Duodenal carcinoid tumour	

Paraneoplastic neurological disease

Paraneoplastic neurological syndromes often present before the underlying tumour declares itself and cause considerable disability. They are discussed in full on page 1193.

Hydrocephalus

Hydrocephalus is the excessive accumulation of CSF within the brain, and may be caused either by increased CSF production, by reduced CSF absorption, or by obstruction of the circulation (Fig. 26.41). Symptoms range from none to sudden death, depending upon the speed at which and degree to which hydrocephalus develops. The causes are listed in Box 26.91. The terms

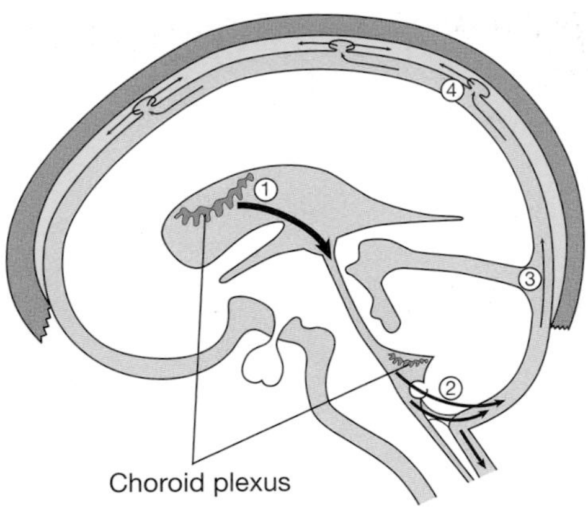

Fig. 26.41 The circulation of cerebrospinal fluid. (1) CSF is synthesised in the choroid plexus of the ventricles, and flows from the lateral and third ventricles through the aqueduct to the fourth ventricle. (2) At the foramina of Luschka and Magendie it exits the brain, flowing over the hemispheres (3) and down around the spinal cord and roots in the subarachnoid space. (4) It is then absorbed into the dural venous sinuses via the arachnoid villi.

26.91 Causes of hydrocephalus

Congenital malformations	
• Aqueduct stenosis • Chiari malformations • Dandy–Walker syndrome • Benign intracranial cysts	• Vein of Galen aneurysms • Congenital CNS infections • Craniofacial anomalies
Acquired causes	
• Mass lesions (especially those in the posterior fossa) Tumour Colloid cyst of third ventricle Abscess Haematoma	• Absorption blockages due to: Inflammation (e.g. meningitis, sarcoidosis) Intracranial haemorrhage

'communicating' and 'non-communicating' (also known as obstructive) hydrocephalus refer to blockage either outside or within the ventricular system respectively (Fig. 26.42).

Normal pressure hydrocephalus

Normal pressure hydrocephalus (NPH) is a controversial entity, said to involve intermittent rises in CSF pressure, particularly at night. It is described in old age as being associated with a triad of gait apraxia, dementia and urinary incontinence.

Management

Diversion of the CSF by means of a shunt placed between the ventricular system and the peritoneal cavity or right atrium may result in rapid relief of symptoms in obstructive hydrocephalus. The outcome of shunting in NPH is much less predictable and, until a good response can be predicted, the management of individual cases will remain uncertain.

A

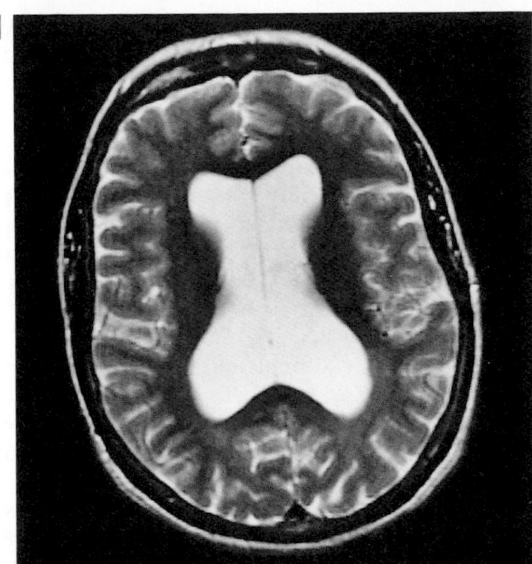

B

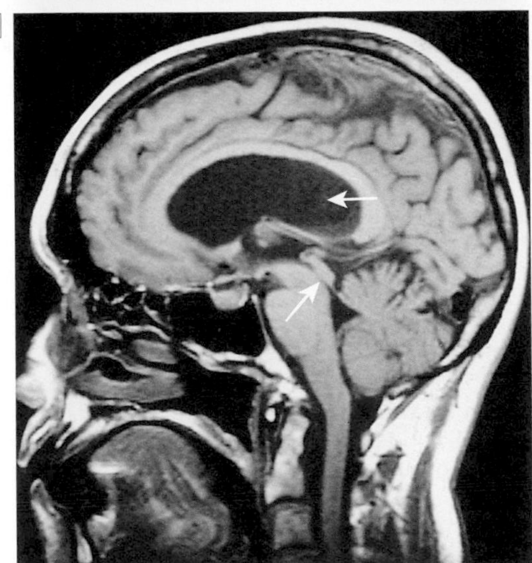

Fig. 26.42 MRI of hydrocephalus due to aqueduct stenosis. **A** Axial T2-weighted image (CSF appears white): note the dilated lateral ventricles. **B** Sagittal T2-weighted image (CSF appears black): note the dilated ventricles (top arrow) and narrowed aqueduct (bottom arrow).

Idiopathic intracranial hypertension

This usually occurs in obese young women. The annual incidence is about 3 per 100 000. RIP occurs in the absence of a structural lesion, hydrocephalus or other identifiable cause. The aetiology is uncertain but there may be a defect of CSF reabsorption by the arachnoid villi. It may be associated with a number of drugs, including tetracycline, and with vitamin A and its derivatives.

Clinical features

The usual presentation is with headache, sometimes accompanied by diplopia and visual disturbance (most commonly transient obscurations of vision associated with changes in posture). Clinical examination reveals papilloedema but little else. False localising cranial nerve palsies (usually of the 6th nerve) may be present.

It is important to record visual fields accurately for future monitoring.

Investigations

Brain imaging is required to exclude a structural or other (e.g. cerebral venous sinus thrombosis, p. 1247) cause. The ventricles are typically normal in size or small ('slit' ventricles). The diagnosis may be confirmed by lumbar puncture, which shows raised CSF pressure (usually > 30 cm CSF) but normal CSF constituents.

Management

Management can be difficult and there is no evidence to support any specific treatment. Weight loss in overweight patients may be helpful but is difficult to achieve. Acetazolamide or topiramate may help to lower intracranial pressure, the latter perhaps aiding weight loss in some patients. Repeated lumbar puncture is an effective treatment for headache, but may be technically difficult in obese patients and is often poorly tolerated. Patients failing to respond, in whom chronic papilloedema threatens vision, may require optic nerve sheath fenestration or a lumbo-peritoneal shunt.

Head injury

Diagnosis of head trauma is usually clear – either from the history or from signs of external trauma to the head. Brain injury is more likely with skull fracture but can occur without. Individual cranial nerves may be damaged in fractures of the facial bones or skull base. Intracranial effects can be substantial and take several forms: extradural haematoma (collection of blood between the skull and dura); subdural haematoma (collection of blood between the dura and the surface of the brain); and intracerebral haematoma or diffuse axonal injury.

Whatever pathology occurs, the resultant RIP may lead to coning (see Figs 26.35 and 26.36). Haematomas are identified by CT and management is by surgical drainage, usually via a burr-hole. Penetrating skull fractures lead to increased infection risk. Long-term sequelae include headache, cognitive decline and depression, all contributing to significant social, work, personality and family difficulties.

Subdural haematoma may occur spontaneously, particularly in patients on anticoagulants, in old age, and with alcohol misuse. There may or may not be a history of trauma. Patients present with subacute impairment of brain function, both globally (obtundation and coma) and focally (hemiparesis, seizures). Headache may not be present. The diagnosis should always be considered in those who present with reduced conscious level.

DISORDERS OF CEREBELLAR FUNCTION

Cerebellar dysfunction can manifest as incoordination of limb function, gait ataxia (p. 1168), speech or eye movements. Acute dysfunction may be caused by alcohol or prescription drugs (especially the sodium channel-blocking anti-epileptic drugs, phenytoin and carbamazepine).

Inflammatory changes in the cerebellum may cause symptoms in the aftermath of some infections (especially herpes zoster) or as a paraneoplastic phenomenon. The hereditary spinocerebellar ataxias are described on page 1198; they manifest as progressive ataxias in middle and old age, often with other neurological features that aid specific diagnosis.

DISORDERS OF THE SPINE AND SPINAL CORD

The spinal cord and spinal roots may be affected by intrinsic disease or by disorders of the surrounding meninges and bones. The clinical presentation of these conditions depends on the anatomical level at which the cord or roots are affected, as well as the nature of the pathological process involved. It is important to recognise when the spinal cord is at risk of compression (p. 1220) so that urgent action can be taken.

Cervical spondylosis

Cervical spondylosis is the result of osteoarthritis in the cervical spine. It is characterised by degeneration of the intervertebral discs and osteophyte formation. Such 'wear and tear' is extremely common and radiological changes are frequently found in asymptomatic individuals over the age of 50. Spondylosis may be associated with neurological dysfunction. In order of frequency, the C5/6, C6/7 and C4/5 vertebral levels affect C6, C7 and C5 roots, respectively (Fig. 26.43).

Cervical radiculopathy

Acute onset of compression of a nerve root occurs when a disc prolapses laterally. More gradual onset may be due to osteophytic encroachment of the intervertebral foramina.

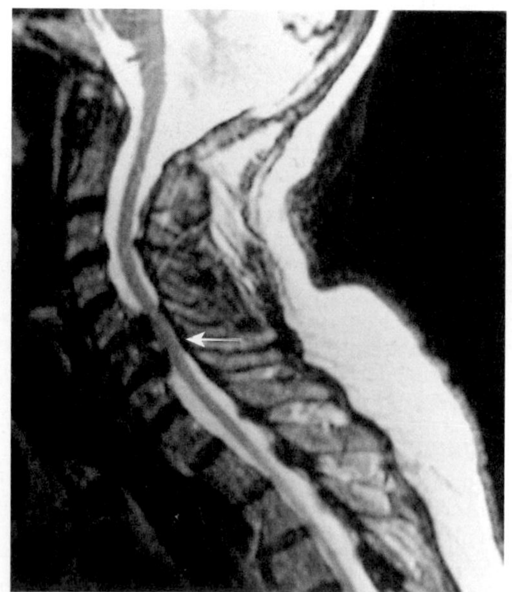

Fig. 26.43 MRI showing cervical cord compression (arrow) in cervical spondylosis.

26.92 Physical signs in cervical root compression

Root	Muscle weakness	Sensory loss	Reflex loss
C5	Biceps, deltoid, spinati	Upper lateral arm	Biceps
C6	Brachioradialis	Lower lateral arm, thumb, index finger	Supinator
C7	Triceps, finger and wrist extensors	Middle finger	Triceps

Clinical features

The patient complains of pain in the neck that may radiate in the distribution of the affected nerve root. The neck is held rigidly and neck movements may exacerbate pain. Paraesthesia and sensory loss may be found in the affected segment and there may be lower motor neuron signs, including weakness, wasting and reflex impairment (Box 26.92).

Investigations

Where there is no trauma, imaging should not be carried out for isolated cervical pain. X-rays offer limited benefit, except in excluding destructive lesions. MRI is the investigation of choice in those with radicular symptoms. Electrophysiological studies rarely add to clinical examination and have become less important with the emergence of MRI.

Management

Conservative treatment with analgesics and physiotherapy results in resolution of symptoms in the great majority of patients, but a few require surgery in the form of discectomy or radicular decompression.

Cervical myelopathy

Dorsomedial herniation of a disc and the development of transverse bony bars or posterior osteophytes may result in pressure on the spinal cord or the anterior spinal artery, which supplies the anterior two-thirds of the cord (see Fig. 26.43).

Clinical features

The onset is usually insidious and painless, but acute deterioration may occur after trauma, especially hyperextension injury. Upper motor neuron signs develop in the limbs, with spasticity of the legs usually appearing before the arms are involved. Sensory loss in the upper limbs is common, producing tingling, numbness and proprioception loss in the hands, with progressive clumsiness. Sensory manifestations in the legs are much less common. Neurological deficit usually progresses gradually and disturbance of micturition is a very late feature.

Investigations

MRI (see Fig. 26.43) (or rarely myelography) will direct surgical intervention. MRI also provides information on the state of the spinal cord at the level of compression.

Management

Surgical procedures, including laminectomy and anterior discectomy, may arrest progression of disability but neurological improvement is not the rule. The decision as to whether surgery should be undertaken may be difficult. Manual manipulation of the cervical spine is of no proven benefit and may precipitate acute neurological deterioration.

Prognosis

The prognosis of cervical myelopathy is variable. In many patients, the condition stabilises or even improves without intervention. If progression results in sphincter dysfunction or pyramidal signs, surgical decompression should be considered.

Lumbar spondylosis

This term covers degenerative disc disease and osteoarthritic change in the lumbar spine. Pain in the distribution of the lumbar or sacral roots ('sciatica') is almost always due to disc protrusion but can be a feature of other rare but important disorders, including spinal tumour, malignant disease in the pelvis and tuberculosis of the vertebral bodies.

Lumbar disc herniation

While acute lumbar disc herniation is often precipitated by trauma (usually lifting heavy weights while the spine is flexed), genetic factors may also be important. The nucleus pulposus may bulge or rupture through the annulus fibrosus, giving rise to pressure on nerve endings in the spinal ligaments, changes in the vertebral joints or pressure on nerve roots.

Pathophysiology

The altered mechanics of the lumbar spine result in loss of lumbar lordosis and there may be spasm of the paraspinal musculature. Root pressure is suggested by limitation of flexion of the hip on the affected side if the straight leg is raised (Lasègue's sign). If the third or fourth lumbar root is involved, Lasègue's sign may be negative, but pain in the back may be induced by hyperextension of the hip (femoral nerve stretch test). The roots most frequently affected are S1, L5 and L4; the signs of root pressure at these levels are summarised in Box 26.93.

26.93 Physical signs in lumbar root compression

Disc level	Root	Sensory loss	Weakness	Reflex loss
L3/L4	L4	Inner calf	Inversion of foot	Knee
L4/L5	L5	Outer calf and dorsum of foot	Dorsiflexion of hallux/toes	
L5/S1	S1	Sole and lateral foot	Plantar flexion	Ankle

Clinical features

The onset may be sudden or gradual. Alternatively, repeated episodes of low back pain may precede sciatica by months or years. Constant aching pain is felt in the lumbar region and may radiate to the buttock, thigh, calf and foot. Pain is exacerbated by coughing or straining but may be relieved by lying flat.

Investigations

Plain X-rays of the lumbar spine are of little value in the diagnosis of lumbar disc disease, although they may show other conditions such as malignant infiltration of a vertebral body. While CT can provide helpful images of the disc protrusion and/or narrowing of the exit foramina, MRI is the investigation of choice if available, since soft tissues are well imaged.

Management

Some 90% of patients with sciatica recover following conservative treatment with analgesia and early mobilisation; bed rest does not help recovery. The patient should be instructed in back-strengthening exercises and advised to avoid physical manœuvres likely to strain the lumbar spine. Injections of local anaesthetic or corticosteroids may be useful adjunctive treatment if symptoms are due to ligamentous injury or joint dysfunction. Surgery may have to be considered if there is no response to conservative treatment or if progressive neurological deficits develop. Central disc prolapse with bilateral symptoms and signs and disturbance of sphincter function requires urgent surgical decompression.

Lumbar canal stenosis

This occurs with a congenitally narrowed lumbar spinal canal, exacerbated by the degenerative changes that commonly occur with age.

Pathophysiology

The symptoms of spinal stenosis are thought to be due to local vascular compromise secondary to the canal stenosis, rendering the nerve roots ischaemic and intolerant of the increased demand that occurs on exercise.

Clinical features

Patients, who are usually elderly, develop exercise-induced weakness and paraesthesia in the legs ('spinal claudication'). These symptoms progress with continued exertion, often to the point that the patient can no longer walk, but are quickly relieved by a short period of rest. Physical examination at rest shows preservation of peripheral pulses with absent ankle reflexes. Weakness or sensory loss may only be apparent if the patient is examined immediately after exercise.

Investigations

The investigation of first choice is MRI, but contraindications (body habitus, metallic implants) may make CT or myelography necessary.

Management

Lumbar laminectomy may provide relief of symptoms and recovery of normal exercise tolerance.

Spinal cord compression

Spinal cord compression is one of the more common neurological emergencies encountered in clinical practice and the usual causes are listed in Box 26.94. A space-occupying lesion within the spinal canal may damage nerve tissue either directly by pressure or indirectly by interfering with blood supply. Oedema from venous obstruction impairs neuronal function, and ischaemia from arterial obstruction may lead to necrosis of the spinal cord. The early stages of damage are reversible but severely damaged neurons do not recover; hence the importance of early diagnosis and treatment.

Clinical features

The onset of symptoms of spinal cord compression is usually slow (over weeks) but can be acute as a result of trauma or metastases, especially if there is associated arterial occlusion. The symptoms are shown in Box 26.95.

Pain and sensory symptoms occur early, while weakness and sphincter dysfunction are usually late manifestations. The signs vary according to the level of the cord compression and the structures involved. There may be

26.94 Causes of spinal cord compression

Site	Frequency	Causes
Vertebral	80%	Trauma (extradural) Intervertebral disc prolapse Metastatic carcinoma (e.g. breast, prostate, bronchus) Myeloma Tuberculosis
Meninges (intradural, extramedullary)	15%	Tumours (e.g. meningioma, neurofibroma, ependymoma, metastasis, lymphoma, leukaemia) Epidural abscess
Spinal cord (intradural, intramedullary)	5%	Tumours (e.g. glioma, ependymoma, metastasis)

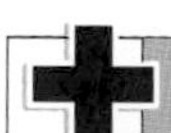

26.95 Symptoms of spinal cord compression

Pain

- Localised over the spine or in a root distribution, which may be aggravated by coughing, sneezing or straining

Sensory

- Paraesthesia, numbness or cold sensations, especially in the lower limbs, which spread proximally, often to a level on the trunk

Motor

- Weakness, heaviness or stiffness of the limbs, most commonly the legs

Sphincters

- Urgency or hesitancy of micturition, leading eventually to urinary retention

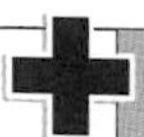

26.96 Signs of spinal cord compression

Cervical, above C5

- Upper motor neuron signs and sensory loss in all four limbs
- Diaphragm weakness (phrenic nerve)

Cervical, C5–T1

- Lower motor neuron signs and segmental sensory loss in the arms; upper motor neuron signs in the legs
- Respiratory (intercostal) muscle weakness

Thoracic cord

- Spastic paraplegia with a sensory level on the trunk
- Weakness of legs, sacral loss of sensation and extensor plantar responses

Cauda equina

- Spinal cord ends approximately at the T12/L1 spinal level and spinal lesions below this level can only cause lower motor neuron signs by affecting the cauda equina

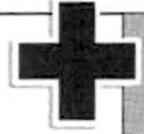

26.97 Investigation of acute spinal cord syndrome

- MRI of spine or myelography
- Plain X-rays of spine
- Chest X-ray
- CSF
- Serum B_{12}

tenderness to percussion over the spine if there is vertebral disease and this may be associated with a local kyphosis. Involvement of the roots at the level of the compression may cause dermatomal sensory impairment and corresponding lower motor signs. Interruption of fibres in the spinal cord causes sensory loss (p. 1164) and upper motor neuron signs below the level of the lesion, and there is often disturbance of sphincter function. The distribution of these signs varies with the level of the lesion (Box 26.96).

The Brown–Séquard syndrome (see Fig. 26.19E, p. 1164) results if damage is confined to one side of the cord; the findings are explained by the anatomy of the sensory tracts (see Fig. 26.10, p. 1147). With compressive lesions, there is usually a band of pain at the level of the lesion in the distribution of the nerve roots subject to compression.

Investigations

Patients with a history of acute or subacute spinal cord syndrome should be investigated urgently, as listed in Box 26.97. The investigation of choice is MRI (Fig. 26.44), as it can define the extent of compression and associated soft-tissue abnormality (Fig. 26.45). Plain X-rays may show bony destruction and soft-tissue abnormalities. Routine investigations, including chest X-ray, may provide evidence of systemic disease. If myelography is performed, CSF should be taken for analysis; in cases of complete spinal block, this shows a normal cell count with a very elevated protein causing yellow discoloration of the fluid (Froin's syndrome). The risk of acute deterioration after myelography in spinal cord compression means that the neurosurgeons should be alerted before it is undertaken. Where a secondary tumour is causing the compression, needle biopsy may be required to establish a tissue diagnosis.

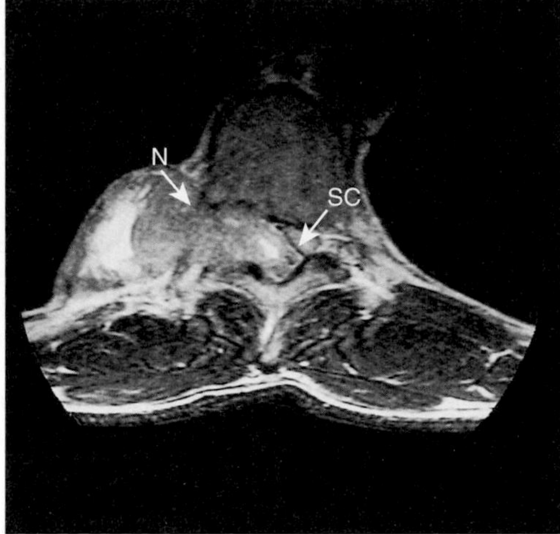

Fig. 26.44 Axial MRI of thoracic spine. A neurofibroma (N) is compressing the spinal cord (SC) and emerging in a 'dumbbell' fashion through the vertebral foramen into the paraspinal space.

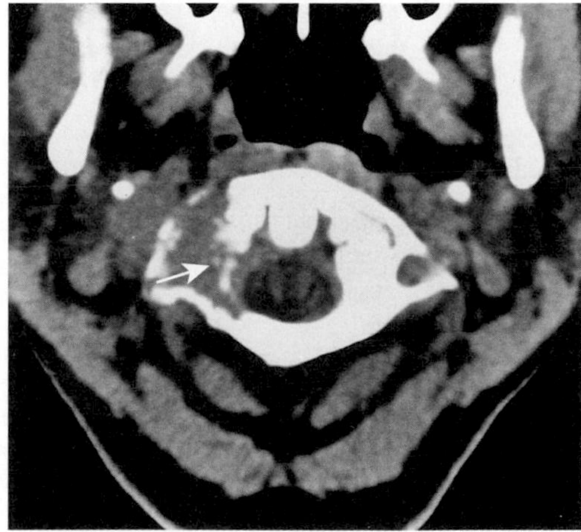

Fig. 26.45 CT myelogram of cervical spine at the level of C2 showing bony erosion of vertebra by a metastasis (arrow).

Management

Treatment and prognosis depend on the nature of the underlying lesion. Benign tumours should be surgically excised, and a good functional recovery can be expected unless a marked neurological deficit has developed before diagnosis. Extradural compression due to malignancy is the most common cause of spinal cord compression in developed countries and has a poor prognosis. Useful function can be regained if treatment, such as radiotherapy, is initiated within 24 hours of the onset of severe weakness or sphincter dysfunction; management should involve close cooperation with both oncologists and neurosurgeons.

Spinal cord compression due to tuberculosis is common in some areas of the world, and may require surgical treatment. This should be followed by appropriate antituberculous chemotherapy (p. 693) for an extended period. Traumatic lesions of the vertebral column require specialised neurosurgical treatment.

Intrinsic diseases of the spinal cord

There are many disorders that interfere with spinal cord function due to non-compressive involvement of the spinal cord itself. A list of these disorders is given in Box 26.98. The symptoms and signs are generally similar to those that would occur with extrinsic compression (see Boxes 26.95 and 26.96), although a suspended sensory loss (see Fig. 26.19F, p. 1164) can only occur with intrinsic disease such as syringomyelia. Urinary symptoms usually occur earlier in the course of an intrinsic cord disorder than with compressive disorders.

Investigation of intrinsic disease starts with imaging to exclude a compressive lesion. MRI provides most information about structural lesions such as diastematomyelia, syringomyelia (Fig. 26.46) or intrinsic tumours. Non-specific signal change may be seen in the spinal cord in inflammatory (see Fig. 26.28, p. 1191) or infective conditions and other disorders such as vitamin B_{12} deficiency. Lumbar puncture or blood tests may be required to make a specific diagnosis.

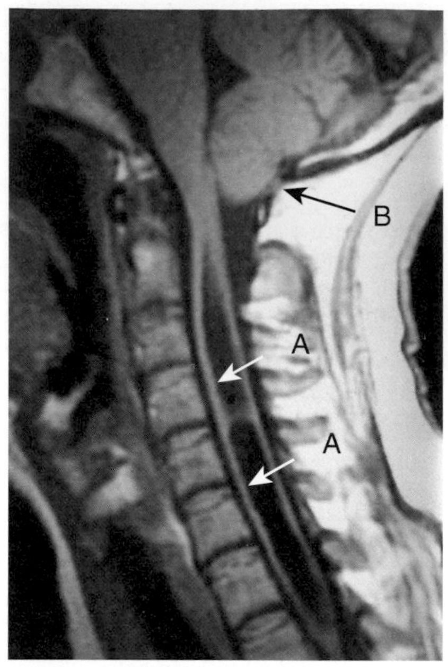

Fig. 26.46 MRI scan showing syrinx (arrows A), with herniation of cerebellar tonsils (arrow B).

26.98 Intrinsic diseases of the spinal cord

Type of disorder	Condition	Clinical features
Congenital	Diastematomyelia (spina bifida)	Features variably present at birth and deteriorate thereafter LMN features, deformity and sensory loss of legs Impaired sphincter function Hairy patch or pit over low back Incidence reduced by increased maternal intake of folic acid during pregnancy
	Hereditary spastic paraplegia	Onset usually in adult life Autosomal dominant inheritance usual Slowly progressive UMN features affecting legs > arms Little or no sensory loss
Infective/ inflammatory	Transverse myelitis due to viruses (HZV), schistosomiasis, HIV, MS, sarcoidosis	Weakness and sensory loss, often with pain, developing over hours to days UMN features below lesion Impaired sphincter function
Vascular	Anterior spinal artery infarct Intervertebral disc embolus	Abrupt onset Anterior horn cell loss (LMN) at level of lesion UMN features below it Spinothalamic sensory loss below lesion but dorsal column sensation spared
	Spinal AVM/dural fistula	Onset variable (acute to slowly progressive) Variable LMN, UMN, sensory and sphincter disturbance Symptoms and signs often not well localised to site of AVM
Neoplastic	Glioma, ependymoma	Weakness and sensory loss often with pain, developing over months to years UMN features below lesion in cord; additional LMN features in conus Impaired sphincter function
Metabolic	Vitamin B_{12} deficiency (subacute combined degeneration)	Progressive spastic paraparesis with proprioception loss Absent reflexes due to peripheral neuropathy ± Optic nerve and cerebral involvement (p. 129)
Degenerative	Motor neuron disease	Relentlessly progressive LMN and UMN features, associated bulbar weakness No sensory involvement (p. 1200)
	Syringomyelia	Gradual onset over months or years, pain in cervical segments Anterior horn cell loss (LMN) at level of lesion, UMN features below it Suspended spinothalamic sensory loss at level of lesion, dorsal columns preserved. See Figures 26.19F (p. 1164) and 26.46

(AVM = arteriovenous malformation; HIV = human immunodeficiency virus; HZV = herpes zoster virus; LMN = lower motor neuron; MS = multiple sclerosis; UMN = upper motor neuron)

DISEASES OF PERIPHERAL NERVES

Disorders of the peripheral nervous system are common and may affect the motor, sensory or autonomic components, either in isolation or combination. The site of pathology may be nerve root (radiculopathy), nerve plexus (plexopathy) or nerve (neuropathy). Neuropathies may present as mononeuropathy (single nerve affected), multiple mononeuropathies ('mononeuritis multiplex') or a symmetrical polyneuropathy (Box 26.99). Cranial nerves 3–12 share the same tissue characteristics as peripheral nerves elsewhere and are subject to the same range of diseases.

Pathophysiology

Damage may occur to the nerve cell body (axon) or the myelin sheath (Schwann cell), leading to axonal or demyelinating neuropathies. The distinction is important, as only demyelinating neuropathies are usually susceptible to treatment; making the distinction requires neurophysiology (nerve conduction studies and electromyography, pp. 1151 and 1152). Neuropathies can occur in association with many systemic diseases, toxins and drugs (Box 26.100).

Clinical features

Motor nerve involvement produces features of a lower motor neuron lesion (p. 1162). Symptoms and signs of sensory nerve involvement depend on the type of sensory nerve involved (p. 1164); small-fibre neuropathies are often painful. Autonomic involvement may cause postural hypotension, disturbance of sweating, cardiac rhythm, and gastrointestinal, bladder and sexual functions; isolated autonomic neuropathies are rare, and more commonly complicate other neuropathies.

Investigations

The investigations required reflect the wide spectrum of causes (Box 26.101). Neurophysiological tests are key in discriminating between demyelinating and axonal neuropathies, and in identifying entrapment neuropathies. Most neuropathies are of the chronic axonal type.

26.99 Causes of polyneuropathy	
Genetic	
• Charcot–Marie–Tooth disease (CMT) • Hereditary neuropathy with liability to pressure palsies (HNPP) • Hereditary sensory ± autonomic neuropathies (HSN, HSAN) • Familial amyloid polyneuropathy • Hereditary neuralgic amyotrophy	
Drugs	
• Amiodarone • Antibiotics (dapsone, isoniazid, metronidazole, ethambutol) • Antiretrovirals • Chemotherapy (cisplatin, vincristine, thalidomide) • Phenytoin	
Toxins	
• Alcohol • Nitrous oxide (recreational use) • Rarely: lead, arsenic, mercury, organophosphates, solvents	
Vitamin deficiencies	
• Thiamin • Pyridoxine	• Vitamin B_{12} • Vitamin E
Infections	
• HIV • Leprosy	• Brucellosis
Inflammatory	
• Guillain–Barré syndrome • Chronic inflammatory demyelinating polyradiculoneuropathy • Vasculitis (polyarteritis nodosa, granulomatosis with polyangiitis (also known as Wegener's granulomatosis), rheumatoid arthritis, SLE) • Paraneoplastic (antibody-mediated)	
Systemic medical conditions	
• Diabetes • Renal failure	• Sarcoidosis
Malignant disease	
• Infiltration	
Others	
• Paraproteinaemias • Amyloidosis	• Critical illness polyneuropathy/myopathy

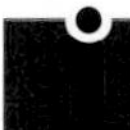

26.100 Common causes of axonal and demyelinating chronic polyneuropathies	
Axonal	
• Diabetes mellitus • Alcohol • Uraemia • Cirrhosis • Amyloid • Myxoedema • Acromegaly • Paraneoplastic	• Drugs and toxins (see Box 26.99) • Deficiency states (see Box 26.99) • Hereditary • Infection (see Box 26.99) • Idiopathic
Demyelinating	
• Chronic inflammatory demyelinating polyradiculoneuropathy • Multifocal motor neuropathy • Paraprotein-associated demyelinating neuropathy • Charcot–Marie–Tooth disease type I and type X	

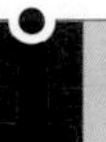

26.101 Investigation of peripheral neuropathy	
Initial tests	
• Glucose (fasting) • Erythrocyte sedimentation rate, C-reactive protein • Full blood count • Urea and electrolytes • Liver function tests	• Serum protein electrophoresis • Vitamin B_{12}, folate • ANA, ANCA • Chest X-ray • HIV testing
If initial tests are negative	
• Nerve conduction studies • Vitamins E and A • Genetic testing (see Box 26.99)	• Lyme serology (p. 335) • Serum ACE • Serum amyloid
(ACE = angiotensin-converting enzyme; ANCA = antineutrophil cytoplasmic antibody; ANA = antineutrophil antibody)	

26.102 Symptoms and signs in common entrapment neuropathies

Nerve	Symptoms	Muscle weakness/ muscle-wasting	Area of sensory loss
Median (at wrist) (carpal tunnel syndrome)	Pain and paraesthesia on palmar aspect of hands and fingers, waking the patient from sleep. Pain may extend to arm and shoulder	Abductor pollicis brevis	Lateral palm and thumb, index, middle and lateral half 4th finger
Ulnar (at elbow)	Paraesthesia on medial border of hand, wasting and weakness of hand muscles	All small hand muscles, excluding abductor pollicis brevis	Medial palm and little finger, and medial half 4th finger
Radial	Weakness of extension of wrist and fingers, often precipitated by sleeping in abnormal posture, e.g. arm over back of chair	Wrist and finger extensors, supinator	Dorsum of thumb
Common peroneal	Foot drop, trauma to head of fibula	Dorsiflexion and eversion of foot	Nil or dorsum of foot
Lateral cutaneous nerve of the thigh (meralgia paraesthetica)	Tingling and dysaesthesia on lateral border of thigh	Nil	Lateral border of thigh

Entrapment neuropathy

Focal compression or entrapment is the usual cause of a mononeuropathy. Symptoms and signs of entrapment neuropathy are listed in Box 26.102. Entrapment neuropathies may affect anyone, but diabetes, excess alcohol or toxins, or genetic syndromes may be predisposing causes. Unless axonal loss has occurred, entrapment neuropathies will recover, provided the primary cause is removed, either by avoiding the precipitation of activity or by surgical decompression.

Multifocal neuropathy

Multifocal neuropathy (mononeuritis multiplex) is characterised by lesions of multiple nerve roots, peripheral nerves or cranial nerves (Box 26.103). Vasculitis is a common cause, either as part of a systemic disease or isolated to the nerves, or it may arise on a background of a polyneuropathy (e.g. diabetes). Multifocal motor neuropathy (MMN) with conduction block is a rare pure motor neuropathy, typically affecting the arms; it is associated with anti-GM1 antibodies in about 50%, and responds to intravenous immunoglobulin.

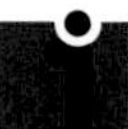

26.103 Causes of multifocal mononeuropathy

Axonal (defined on nerve conduction studies)

- Vasculitis (systemic or non-systemic)
- Diabetes mellitus
- Sarcoidosis
- Infection (HIV, hepatitis C, Lyme disease, leprosy, diphtheria)

Focal demyelination with/without conduction block

- Multifocal motor neuropathy
- Multiple compression neuropathies (usually in association with underlying disease, such as diabetes or alcoholism)
- Multifocal acquired demyelinating sensory and motor neuropathy (MADSAM)
- Hereditary neuropathy with a predisposition to pressure palsy (autosomal dominant, peripheral myelin protein 22 gene)
- Lymphoma

Polyneuropathy

A polyneuropathy is typically associated with a 'length-dependent' pattern, occurring in the longest peripheral nerves first and affecting the distal lower limbs before the upper limbs. Sensory symptoms and signs develop in an ascending 'glove and stocking' distribution (p. 1164). In inflammatory demyelinating neuropathies, the pathology may be more patchy, affecting the upper rather than lower limbs.

Guillain–Barré syndrome

Guillain–Barré syndrome (GBS) is a heterogeneous group of immune-mediated conditions with an incidence of 1–2/100 000/year. In Europe and North America, the most common variant is an acute inflammatory demyelinating polyneuropathy (AIDP). Axonal variants, either motor (acute motor axonal neuropathy, AMAN) or sensorimotor (acute motor and sensory axonal neuropathy, AMSAN), are more common in China and Japan, and account for 10% of GBS in Western countries (often associated with *Campylobacter jejuni*). The hallmark is an acute paralysis evolving over days or weeks with loss of tendon reflexes. About two-thirds of those with AIDP have a prior history of infection, and an autoimmune response triggered by the preceding infection causes demyelination. A number of GBS variants have been described, associated with specific anti-ganglioside antibodies; the best-recognised is Miller Fisher syndrome, which involves anti-GQ1b antibodies.

Clinical features

Distal paraesthesia and pain precede muscle weakness that ascends rapidly from lower to upper limbs, and is more marked proximally than distally. Facial and bulbar weakness commonly develops, and respiratory weakness requiring ventilatory support occurs in 20% of cases. Weakness progresses over a maximum of 4 weeks (usually less). Rapid deterioration to respiratory failure can develop within hours. Examination shows diffuse weakness with loss of reflexes. Miller Fisher syndrome presents with internal and external ophthalmoplegia, ataxia and areflexia.

Investigations

The CSF protein is raised, but may be normal in the first 10 days. There is usually no increase in CSF white cell count (> 10×10^6 cells/L suggests an alternative diagnosis). Electrophysiological changes may emerge after a week or so, with conduction block and multifocal motor slowing, sometimes most evident proximally as delayed F waves (p. 1152). Antibodies to the ganglioside GM1 are found in about 25%, usually the motor axonal form. Other causes of an acute neuromuscular paralysis should be excluded (e.g. poliomyelitis, botulism, diphtheria, spinal cord syndromes or myasthenia), via the history and examination rather than investigations.

Management

Supportive measures to prevent pressure sores and deep venous thrombosis are essential. Regular monitoring of respiratory function (vital capacity) is needed in the acute phase, as respiratory failure may develop with little warning. Active treatment with plasma exchange or intravenous immunoglobulin therapy shortens the duration of ventilation and improves prognosis (Box 26.104). Overall, 80% of patients recover completely within 3–6 months, 4% die and the remainder suffer residual neurological disability, which can be severe. Adverse prognostic features include older age, rapid deterioration to ventilation and evidence of axonal loss on EMG.

EBM 26.104 Intravenous immunoglobulin and plasma exchange in Guillain–Barré syndrome

'In severe Guillain–Barré syndrome (GBS), intravenous immunoglobulin (IVIg) started within 2 weeks of onset hastens recovery as much as plasma exchange (PE). Adverse events are not significantly more frequent with either treatment, but IVIg is significantly much more likely to be completed than PE.'

'In mild GBS, 2 sessions of PE are significantly superior to none; in moderate disease, 4 sessions are significantly superior to 2; and in severe disease, 6 sessions are not significantly better than 4. PE is more beneficial when started within 7 days of disease onset rather than later, but is still beneficial in patients treated up to 30 days after disease onset.'

- Hughes RAC, et al. Intravenous immunoglobulin for Guillain–Barré syndrome. Cochrane Database of Systematic Reviews, 2012, issue 7. Art. no.: CD002063.
- Raphaël JC, et al. Plasma exchange for Guillain–Barré syndrome. Cochrane Database of Systematic Reviews, 2012, issue 7. Art. no.: CD001798.

For further information: www.cochrane.org/cochrane-reviews

Chronic polyneuropathy

The most common axonal and demyelinating causes of polyneuropathy are shown in Box 26.100. A chronic symmetrical axonal polyneuropathy, evolving over months or years, is the most common form of chronic neuropathy. Diabetes mellitus is the most common cause but in about 25–50% no cause can be found.

Hereditary neuropathy

Charcot–Marie–Tooth disease (CMT) is an umbrella term for the inherited neuropathies. This group of syndromes has different clinical and genetic features. The most common CMT is the autosomal dominantly inherited CMT type 1, usually caused by duplication of the *PMP-22* gene on chromosome 17. Common signs are distal wasting ('inverted champagne bottle' legs), often with pes cavus, and predominantly motor involvement. X-linked and recessively inherited forms of CMT, causing demyelinating or axonal neuropathies, also occur.

Chronic demyelinating polyneuropathy

The acquired chronic demyelinating neuropathies include chronic inflammatory demyelinating peripheral neuropathy (CIDP), multifocal motor neuropathy (see above) and paraprotein-associated demyelinating neuropathy. CIDP typically presents with relapsing or progressive motor and sensory changes, evolving over more than 8 weeks (in distinction to the more acute GBS). It is important to recognise, as it usually responds to corticosteroids, plasma exchange or intravenous immunoglobulin.

Some 10% of patients with acquired demyelinating polyneuropathy have an abnormal serum paraprotein, sometimes associated with a lymphoproliferative malignancy. They may also demonstrate positive antibodies to myelin-associated glycoprotein (anti-MAG antibodies).

Brachial plexopathy

Trauma usually damages either the upper or the lower parts of the brachial plexus, according to the mechanics of the injury. The clinical features depend on the anatomical site of the damage (Box 26.105). Lower parts of the brachial plexus are vulnerable to infiltration from breast or apical lung tumours (Pancoast tumour, p. 701)

26.105 Physical signs in brachial plexus lesions

Site	Affected muscles	Sensory loss
Upper plexus (Erb–Duchenne)	Biceps, deltoid, spinati, rhomboids, brachioradialis (triceps, serratus anterior)	Patch over deltoid
Lower plexus (Déjerine–Klumpke)	All small hand muscles, claw hand (ulnar wrist flexors)	Ulnar border of hand/forearm
Thoracic outlet syndrome	Small hand muscles, ulnar forearm	Ulnar border of hand/forearm/upper arm

26

or damage by therapeutic irradiation; they may also be compressed by a cervical rib or fibrous band between C7 and the first rib at the thoracic outlet.

An acute brachial plexopathy of probable inflammatory origin may present with 'neuralgic amyotrophy'. Severe shoulder pain precedes the appearance of a patchy upper brachial plexus lesion, with motor and/or sensory involvement. There is no specific treatment and recovery is often incomplete; it may recur in about 25%, and there is a rare autosomal dominant hereditary form. The appearance of vesicles should indicate the alternative diagnosis of motor zoster.

Lumbosacral plexopathy

Lumbosacral plexus lesions may be caused by neoplastic infiltration or compression by retroperitoneal haematomas. A small-vessel vasculopathy can produce a unilateral or bilateral lumbar plexopathy in association with type 2 diabetes mellitus ('diabetic amyotrophy') or an idiopathic form in non-diabetic patients. This presents with painful wasting of the quadriceps with weakness of knee extension and an absent knee reflex.

Spinal root lesions

Spinal root lesions (radiculopathy) are described above. Clinical features include muscle weakness and wasting and dermatomal sensory and reflex loss, which reflect the pattern of the roots involved. Pain in the muscles innervated by the affected roots may be prominent.

DISEASES OF THE NEUROMUSCULAR JUNCTION

Myasthenia gravis

This is the most common cause of acutely evolving, fatigable weakness and preferentially affects ocular, facial and bulbar muscles.

Pathophysiology

Myasthenia gravis is an autoimmune disease, most commonly caused by antibodies to acetylcholine receptors in the post-junctional membrane of the neuromuscular junction, which are found in around 80% of affected patients. The resultant blockage of neuromuscular transmission and complement-mediated inflammatory response reduces the number of acetylcholine receptors and damages the end plate (Fig. 26.47). Other antibodies can produce a similar clinical picture, most notably autoantibodies to muscle-specific kinase (MuSK), which is involved in the regulation and maintenance of acetylcholine receptors.

About 15% of patients (mainly those with late onset) have a thymoma, most of the remainder displaying thymic follicular hyperplasia. Myasthenic patients are at greater risk of associated organ-specific autoimmune diseases. As with other autoimmune processes, triggers are not always evident, but some drugs (e.g. penicillamine) can trigger an antibody-mediated myasthenic syndrome that may persist after drug withdrawal. Other drugs, especially aminoglycosides and quinolones, may exacerbate the neuromuscular blockade and should be avoided in patients with myasthenia.

Clinical features

Myasthenia gravis usually presents between the ages of 15 and 50 years and there is a female preponderance in younger patients. In older patients, males are more commonly affected. It tends to run a relapsing and remitting course.

The most evident symptom is fatigable muscle weakness; movement is initially strong but rapidly weakens as muscle use continues. Worsening of symptoms towards the end of the day or following exercise is characteristic. There are no sensory signs or signs of involvement of the CNS, although weakness of the oculomotor muscles may mimic a central eye movement disorder. The first symptoms are usually intermittent ptosis or diplopia, but weakness of chewing, swallowing, speaking or limb movement also occurs. Any limb muscle may be affected, most commonly those of the shoulder girdle; the patient is unable to undertake tasks above shoulder level, such as combing the hair, without frequent rests. Respiratory muscles may be involved and respiratory failure is an avoidable cause of death. Aspiration may occur if the cough is ineffectual. Ventilatory support is required where weakness is severe or of abrupt onset.

Investigations

Intravenous injection of the short-acting anticholinesterase, edrophonium bromide (the Tensilon® test), is less widely used than before. Improvement in muscle function occurs within 30 seconds and usually persists for 2–3 minutes, but the test is not universally specific or sensitive. Cover with intravenous atropine is necessary to avoid bradycardia. Planning the assessment beforehand (e.g. speech or limb movements) allows some objectivity in gauging the effect.

Repetitive stimulation during nerve conduction studies may show a characteristic decremental response (p. 1151) if the muscle has been clinically affected. Anti-MuSK antibodies are more common in acetylcholine receptor antibody-negative patients with prominent bulbar involvement. All patients should have a thoracic CT to exclude thymoma, especially those without anti-acetylcholine receptor antibodies. Screening for associated autoimmune disorders, particularly thyroid disease, is important.

Management

The goals of treatment are to maximise the activity of acetylcholine at remaining receptors in the neuromuscular junctions and to limit or abolish the immunological attack on motor end plates.

The duration of action of acetylcholine is prolonged by inhibiting acetylcholinesterase. The most commonly used anticholinesterase drug is pyridostigmine. Muscarinic side-effects, including diarrhoea and colic, may be controlled by propantheline. Overdosage of anticholinesterase drugs may cause a 'cholinergic crisis' due to depolarisation block of motor end plates, with muscle fasciculation, paralysis, pallor, sweating, excessive salivation and small pupils. This may be

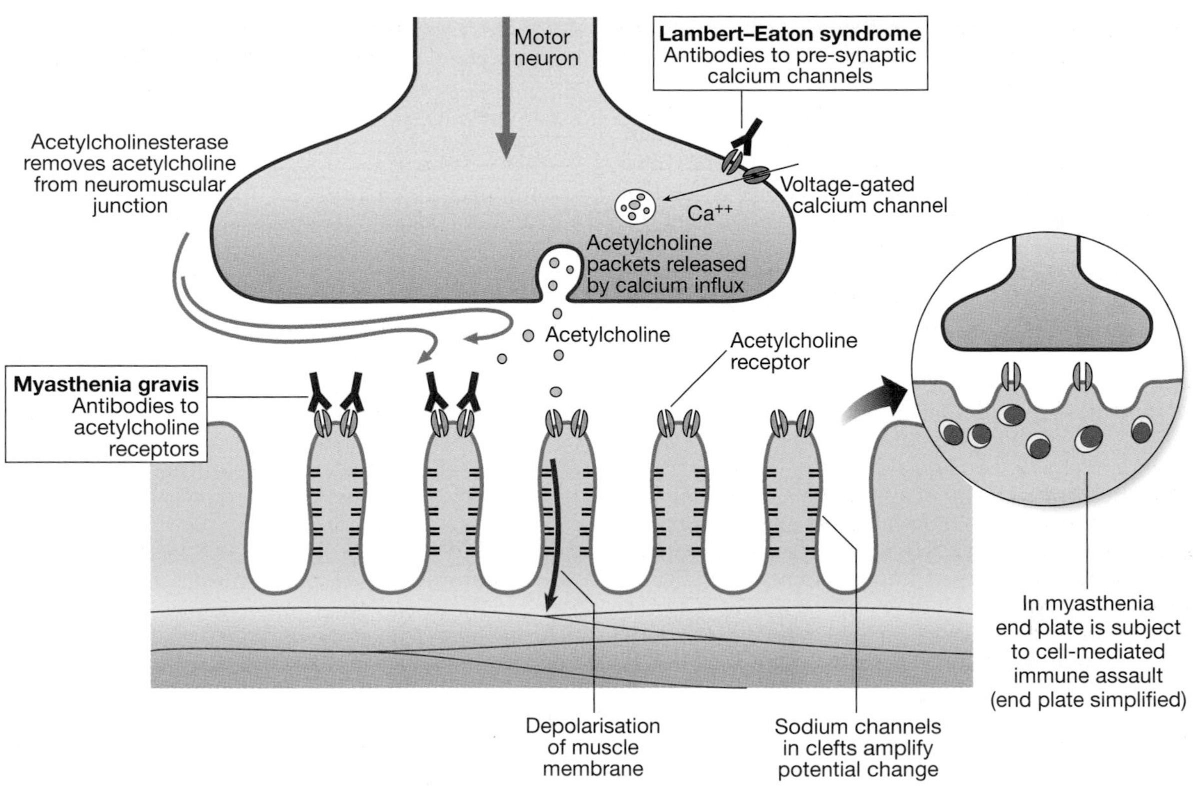

Fig. 26.47 Myasthenia gravis and Lambert–Eaton myasthenic syndrome (LEMS). In myasthenia there are antibodies to the acetylcholine receptors on the post-synaptic membrane, which block conduction across the neuromuscular junction (NMJ). Myasthenic symptoms can be transiently improved by inhibition of acetylcholinesterase (e.g. with Tensilon® – edrophonium bromide), which normally removes the acetylcholine. A cell-mediated immune response produces simplification of the post-synaptic membrane, further impairing the 'safety factor' of neuromuscular conduction. In LEMS, antibodies to the pre-synaptic voltage calcium channels impair release of acetylcholine from the motor nerve ending; calcium is required for the acetylcholine-containing vesicle to fuse with the pre-synaptic membrane for release into the NMJ.

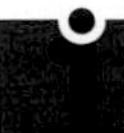

26.106 Immunological treatment of myasthenia

Acute treatments

Intravenous immunoglobulin
- Reduces production of antibodies and rapidly reduces weakness

Plasma exchange
- Removing antibody from the blood may produce marked improvement; this is usually brief, so is normally reserved for myasthenic crisis or for pre-operative preparation

Long-term treatments

Corticosteroid treatment
- Improvement is commonly preceded by marked exacerbation of myasthenic symptoms, so treatment should be initiated in hospital
- Usually necessary to continue treatment for months or years, risking adverse effects

Pharmacological immunosuppression treatment
- Azathioprine 2.5 mg/kg daily reduces the necessary dosage of steroids and may allow their withdrawal. Effect on clinical features may be delayed for months
- Mycophenolate: less commonly used

Thymectomy
- Should be considered in any antibody-positive patient under 45 yrs with symptoms not confined to extraocular muscles, unless the disease has been established for more than 7 yrs
- May be required for thymoma

distinguished from severe weakness due to exacerbation of myasthenia ('myasthenic crisis') by the clinical features and, if necessary, by the injection of a small dose of edrophonium.

The immunological treatment of myasthenia is outlined in Box 26.106. Thymectomy may improve overall prognosis but awaits clinical trial confirmation. Prognosis is variable and remissions may occur spontaneously. When myasthenia is entirely ocular, prognosis is excellent and disability slight. Young female patients with generalised disease may benefit from thymectomy, whilst older patients are less likely to have a remission despite treatment. Rapid progression of the disease more than 5 years after onset is uncommon.

Other myasthenic syndromes

Other rarer conditions can present with muscle weakness due to impaired transmission across the neuromuscular junction. The most common of these is the Lambert–Eaton myasthenic syndrome (LEMS), which can occur as an inflammatory or paraneoplastic phenomenon. Antibodies to pre-synaptic voltage-gated calcium channels (see Fig. 26.47) impair transmitter release. Patients may have autonomic dysfunction (e.g. dry mouth) in addition to muscle weakness, but the cardinal clinical sign is absence of tendon reflexes, which return after sustained contraction of the relevant muscle. The condition is associated with underlying malignancy in a high percentage of cases and investigation must be directed towards identifying any neoplasm. The condition is diagnosed electrophysiologically by the presence of post-tetanic potentiation of motor response to nerve stimulation at a frequency of 20–50/s. Treatment is with 3,4-diaminopyridine, or pyridostigmine and immunosuppression.

DISEASES OF MUSCLE

Muscle disease, either hereditary or acquired, is rare. Most typically, it presents with a proximal symmetrical weakness. Diagnosis is dependent on recognition of clinical clues, such as cardiorespiratory involvement, evolution, family history, exposure to drugs, the presence of contractures, myotonia and other systemic features, and on investigation findings, most importantly EMG and muscle biopsy. Hereditary syndromes include the muscular dystrophies, muscle channelopathies, metabolic myopathies (including mitochondrial diseases) and congenital myopathies.

Muscular dystrophies

These are inherited disorders with progressive muscle destruction, and may be associated with cardiac and/or respiratory involvement and sometimes non-myopathic features (Box 26.107). Myotonic dystrophy is the most common, with a prevalence of about 12/100 000.

Clinical features

The pattern of the clinical features is defined by the specific syndromes. Onset is often in childhood, although some patients, especially those with myotonic dystrophy, may present as adults. Wasting and weakness are usually symmetrical, without fasciculation or sensory loss, and tendon reflexes are usually preserved until a late stage. Weakness is usually proximal, except in myotonic dystrophy type 1, when it is distal.

Investigations

The diagnosis can be confirmed by specific molecular genetic testing, supplemented with EMG and muscle biopsy if necessary. Creatine kinase is markedly elevated in the dystrophinopathies (Duchenne and Becker) but is normal or moderately elevated in the other dystrophies. Screening for an associated cardiac abnormality (cardiomyopathy or dysrhythmia) is important.

Management

There is no specific therapy for most of these conditions but physiotherapy and occupational therapy help patients cope with their disability. Steroids are used in Duchenne muscular dystrophy. Treatment of associated cardiac failure or arrhythmia (with pacemaker insertion if necessary) may be required; similarly, management of respiratory complications (including nocturnal hypoventilation) can improve quality of life. Improvements in non-invasive ventilation have led to significant improvements in survival for patients with

26.107 The muscular dystrophies

Type	Genetics	Age of onset	Muscles affected	Other features
Myotonic dystrophy (DM1)	Autosomal dominant; expanded triplet repeat chromosome 19q	Any	Face (including ptosis), sternomastoids, distal limb, generalised later	Myotonia, cognitive impairment, cardiac conduction abnormalities, lens opacities, frontal balding, hypogonadism
Proximal myotonic myopathy (PROMM; DM2)	Autosomal dominant; quadruplet repeat expansion in *Zn finger protein 9* gene chromosome 3q	8–50	Proximal, especially thigh, sometimes muscle hypertrophy	As for DM1 but cognition not affected Muscle pain
Duchenne	X-linked; deletions in *dystrophin* gene Xp21	< 5 yrs	Proximal and limb girdle	Cardiomyopathy and respiratory failure
Becker	X-linked; deletions in *dystrophin* gene Xp21	Childhood/ early adult	Proximal and limb girdle	Cardiomyopathy, respiratory failure uncommon
Limb girdle	Many mutations on different chromosomes	Childhood/ early adult	Limb girdle	Very variable depending on genetic subtype, some involve cardiac and respiratory systems
Facioscapulohumeral (FSH)	Autosomal dominant; tandem repeat deletion chromosome 4q35	7–30 yrs	Face and upper limb girdle, distal lower limb weakness	Pain in shoulder girdle common, deafness Cardiorespiratory involvement rare
Oculopharyngeal	Autosomal dominant and recessive; triplet repeat expansion in *PABP2* gene chromosome 14q	30–60 yrs	Ptosis, external ophthalmoplegia, dysphagia, tongue weakness	Mild lower limb weakness
Emery–Dreifuss	X-linked recessive; mutations in *emerin* gene	4–5 yrs	Humero-peroneal, proximal limb girdle later	Contractures develop early Cardiac involvement leads to sudden death

Duchenne muscular dystrophy. Genetic counselling is important.

Inherited metabolic myopathies

There are a large number of rare inherited disorders that interfere with the biochemical pathways that maintain the energy supply (adenosine triphosphate, ATP) to muscles. These are mostly recessively inherited deficiencies in the enzymes necessary for glycogen or fatty acid (β-oxidation) metabolism (Box 26.108). They typically present with muscle weakness and pain.

Mitochondrial disorders

Mitochondrial diseases are discussed on page 65. Mitochondria are present in all tissues and dysfunction causes widespread effects, on vision (optic atrophy, retinitis pigmentosa, cataracts), hearing (sensorineural deafness), and the endocrine, cardiovascular, gastrointestinal and renal systems. Any combination of these should raise the suspicion of a mitochondrial disorder, especially if there is evidence of maternal transmission.

Mitochondrial dysfunction can be caused by alterations in either mitochondrial DNA or genes encoding for oxidative processes. Genetic abnormalities or mutations in mitochondrial DNA may affect single individuals and single tissues (most commonly muscle). Thus, patients with exercise intolerance, myalgia and sometimes recurrent myoglobinuria may have isolated pathogenic mutations in genes encoding for oxidation pathways.

Inherited disorders of the oxidative pathways of the respiratory chain in mitochondria cause a group of disorders, either restricted to the muscle or associated with non-myopathic features (Box 26.109). Many of these mitochondrial disorders are inherited via the mitochondrial genome, down the maternal line (p. 53). Diagnosis is based on clinical appearances, supported by muscle biopsy appearance (usually with 'ragged red' and/or cytochrome oxidase negative fibres), and specific mutations either on blood or, more reliably, muscle testing. Mutations may be due either to point mutations or to deletions of mitochondrial DNA.

A disorder called Leber hereditary optic neuropathy (LHON) is characterised by acute or subacute loss of vision, most frequently in males, due to bilateral optic atrophy. Three point mutations account for more than 90% of LHON cases.

Channelopathies

Inherited abnormalities of the sodium, calcium and chloride ion channels in striated muscle produce various syndromes of familial periodic paralysis, myotonia and malignant hyperthermia, which may be recognised by

26.108 Inherited disorders of muscle metabolism

	Disease	Clinical features	Diagnosis
Carbohydrate (glycogen) metabolism	Myophosphorylase deficiency (McArdle's disease): autosomal recessive	Exercise-induced myalgia, stiffness, weakness (with 'second wind' phenomenon), myoglobinuria	Creatine kinase (CK) elevated Muscle biopsy Enzyme assay
	Acid maltase deficiency (Pompe's disease): autosomal recessive	Infantile form: death within 2 yrs Childhood: death in 20–30s Adult: progressive proximal myopathy with respiratory failure	CK elevated Blood lymphocyte analysis for glycogen granules Muscle biopsy Enzyme assay
Lipid metabolism (β-oxidation)	Carnitine-palmitoyl transferase (CPT) deficiency	Myalgia *after* exercise, myoglobinuria, weakness	CK normal between attacks Urinary organic acids Enzyme assays Muscle biopsy

26.109 Mitochondrial syndromes

Syndrome	Clinical features
Myoclonic epilepsy with ragged red fibres (MERRF)	Myoclonic epilepsy, cerebellar ataxia, dementia, sensorineural deafness ± peripheral neuropathy, optic atrophy and multiple lipomas
Mitochondrial myopathy, encephalopathy, lactic acidosis and stroke-like episodes (MELAS)	Episodic encephalopathy, stroke-like episodes often preceded by migraine-like headache, nausea and vomiting
Chronic progressive external ophthalmoplegia (CPEO)	Progressive ptosis and external oculomotor palsy, proximal myopathy ± deafness, ataxia and cardiac conduction defects
Kearns–Sayre syndrome	Like CPEO but early age of onset (< 20 yrs), heart block, pigmentary retinopathy
Mitochondrial neurogastrointestinal encephalomyopathy (MNGIE)	Progressive ptosis, external oculomotor palsy, gastrointestinal dysmotility (often pseudo-obstruction), diffuse leucoencephalopathy, thin body habitus, peripheral neuropathy and myopathy
Neuropathy, ataxia and retinitis pigmentosa (NARP)	Weakness, ataxia and progressive loss of vision, along with dementia, seizures and proximal weakness

26.110 Muscle channelopathies

Channel	Muscle disease	Gene and inheritance	Clinical features
Sodium	Paramyotonia congenita	*SCN4A* (17q35) Autosomal dominant	Cold-evoked myotonia with episodic weakness provoked by exercise and cold
	Potassium-aggravated myotonia	*SCN4A*	Pure myotonia without weakness provoked by potassium
	Hyperkalaemic periodic paralysis	*SCN4A* Autosomal dominant	Brief (mins to hrs), frequent episodes of weakness provoked by rest, cold, potassium, fasting, pregnancy, stress Less common than hypokalaemic periodic paralysis
	Hypokalaemic periodic paralysis	*SCN4A* Autosomal dominant (one-third new mutations)	Longer (hrs to days) episodic weakness triggered by rest, carbohydrate loading, cold
Chloride	Myotonia congenita		
	Thomsen's disease	*CLCN1* Autosomal dominant	Myotonia usually mild, little weakness
	Becker's disease	*CLCN1* Autosomal recessive	Myotonia often severe, transient weakness
Calcium	Hypokalaemic periodic paralysis	*CACNA1S* Autosomal dominant	Episodic weakness triggered by carbohydrate meal
	Malignant hyperthermia	*CACNA1S*, *CACNL2A* Autosomal dominant	Hyperpyrexia due to excess muscle activity, precipitated by drugs, usually anaesthetic agents; most common cause of death during general anaesthetic
Potassium	Andersen–Tawil syndrome	*KCNJ2* Autosomal dominant	Similar to hypokalaemic periodic paralysis, associated with cardiac and non-myopathic features (skeletal and facial)
Ryanodine receptor	Malignant hyperthermia	*RYR1* (19q13)	As malignant hyperthermia above
	Central core and multicore disease	*RYR1* Mostly autosomal dominant	Present in infancy with mild progressive weakness

26.111 Causes of acquired proximal myopathy

Inflammatory (p. 1114)

- Polymyositis
- Dermatomyositis
- Inclusion body myositis (additional distal effects)

Endocrine and metabolic

- Hypothyroidism
- Hyperthyroidism
- Acromegaly
- Cushing's syndrome (including iatrogenic)
- Addison's disease
- Conn's syndrome
- Osteomalacia
- Hypokalaemia (liquorice, diuretic and purgative abuse)
- Hypercalcaemia (disseminated bony metastases)

Toxic

- Alcohol (chronic and acute syndromes)
- Amphetamines/cocaine/heroin
- Vitamin E
- Organophosphates
- Snake venoms

Drugs

- Corticosteroids
- Statins
- Amiodarone
- Beta-blockers
- Opiates
- Chloroquine
- Ciclosporin
- Vincristine
- Clofibrate
- Zidovudine

Paraneoplastic

- Carcinomatous neuromyopathy
- Dermatomyositis

their clinical characteristics and potassium abnormalities (Box 26.110). Genetic testing is available.

Acquired myopathies

These include the inflammatory myopathies, or myopathy associated with a range of metabolic and endocrine disorders, or drug and toxin exposure (Box 26.111).

Further information

Websites

www.aneuroa.org/ *American Neurological Association.*

www.dizziness-and-balance.com/disorders/bppv/bppv.html *and* www.brainandspine.org.uk/about_us/index.html *Diagnosing benign paroxysmal positional vertigo.*

www.ihs-classification.org/en/ *International Headache Society; full access to 2nd edition of International Classification of Headache Disorders.*

www.ninds.nih.gov *National Institute of Neurological Disorders and Stroke.*

www.sign.ac.uk *Relevant SIGN guidelines – all available for free download:*

SIGN 70 Diagnosis and management of epilepsy in adults

SIGN 107 Diagnosis and management of headache

SIGN 113 Diagnosis and management of Parkinson's disease.

www.wfneurology.org *World Federation of Neurology.*

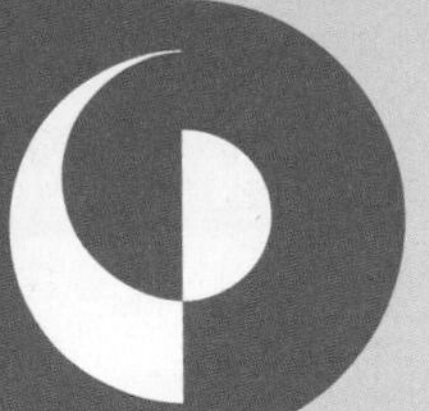

P. Langhorne

Stroke disease 27

Clinical examination in stroke disease 1232

Functional anatomy and physiology 1234

Investigations 1235

Presenting problems 1236

- Weakness 1236
- Speech disturbance 1236
- Visual deficit 1237
- Visuo-spatial dysfunction 1237
- Ataxia 1237
- Headache 1237
- Seizure 1237
- Coma 1237

Stroke 1237

- Pathophysiology 1237
- Clinical features 1239
- Investigations 1240
- Management 1242

Subarachnoid haemorrhage 1246

- Clinical features 1246
- Investigations 1246
- Management 1246

Cerebral venous disease 1247

- Clinical features 1247
- Investigations and management 1247

CLINICAL EXAMINATION IN STROKE DISEASE

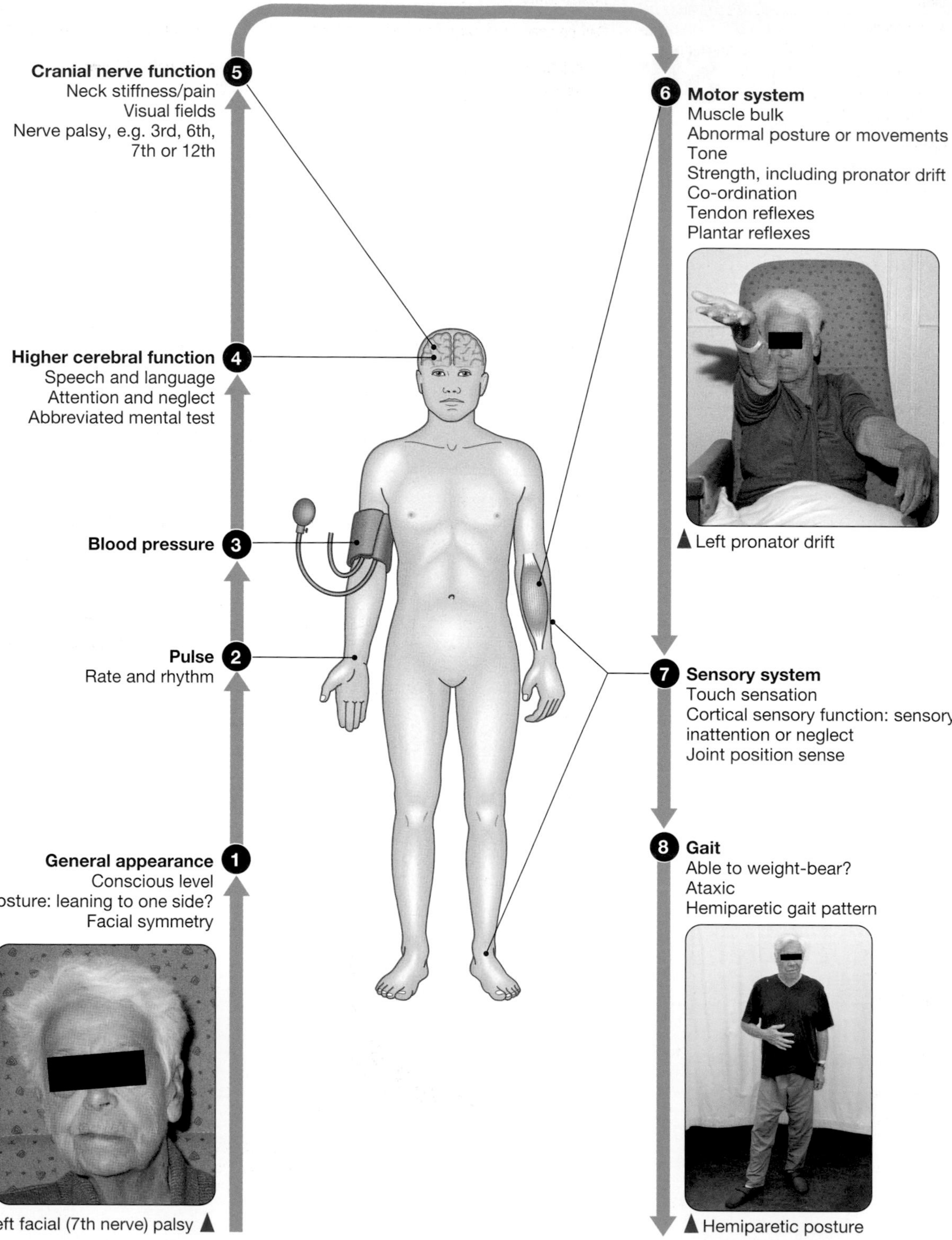

Left facial (7th nerve) palsy ▲

▲ Left pronator drift

▲ Hemiparetic posture

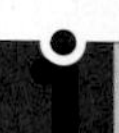

General examination

Skin
• Xanthelasma • Rash (arteritis, splinter haemorrhages) • Colour change (limb ischaemia, deep vein thrombosis) • Pressure injury
Eyes
• Arcus senilis • Diabetic retinopathy • Hypertensive retinopathy • Retinal emboli
Cardiovascular system
• Heart rhythm (?atrial fibrillation) • Blood pressure (high or low) • Carotid bruit • Jugular venous pulse (raised if heart failure, low in hypovolaemia) • Murmurs (source of embolism) • Peripheral pulses and bruits (?generalised arteriopathy)
Respiratory system
• Signs of pulmonary oedema or infection • Oxygen saturation
Abdomen
• Palpable bladder (urinary retention)
Locomotor
• Injuries sustained during collapse • Comorbidities that influence recovery e.g. osteoarthritis

Rapid assessment of suspected stroke

Rosier scale

Can be used by emergency staff to indicate probability of a stroke in acute presentations:

Unilateral facial weakness	+1	Loss of consciousness	–1
Unilateral grip weakness	+1	Seizure	–1
Unilateral arm weakness	+1		
Unilateral leg weakness	+1		
Speech loss	+1		
Visual field defect	+1		

Total (–2 to +6); score of > 0 indicates stroke is possible cause

Exclude hypoglycaemia

- Bedside blood glucose testing with BMstix

Language deficit

- The history and examination may indicate a language deficit
- Check comprehension ('lift your arms, close your eyes') to identify a receptive dysphasia
- Ask patient to name people/objects (e.g. nurse, watch, pen) to identify a nominal dysphasia
- Check articulation (ask patient to repeat phrases after you) for dysarthria

Motor deficit

Subtle pyramidal signs

- Check for pronator drift: ask patient to hold out arms and maintain their position with eyes closed (see opposite)
- Check for clumsiness of fine finger movements

Sensory and visual inattention

- Establish that sensation/visual field is intact on testing one side at a time
- Retest sensation/visual fields on simultaneous testing of both sides; the affected side will no longer be felt/seen
- Perform clock drawing test (see below)

Truncal ataxia

- Check if patient can sit up or stand without support

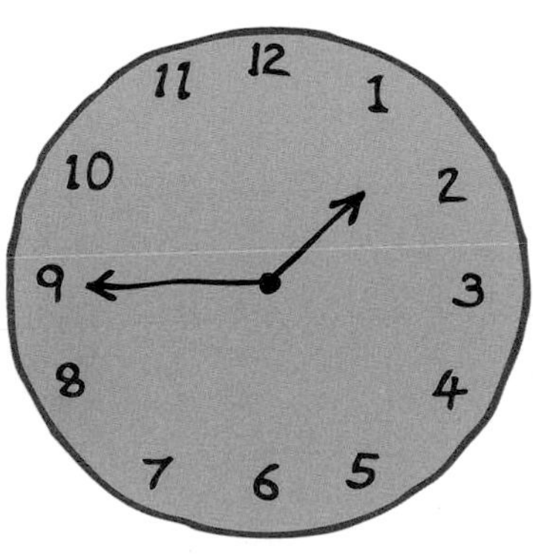

A

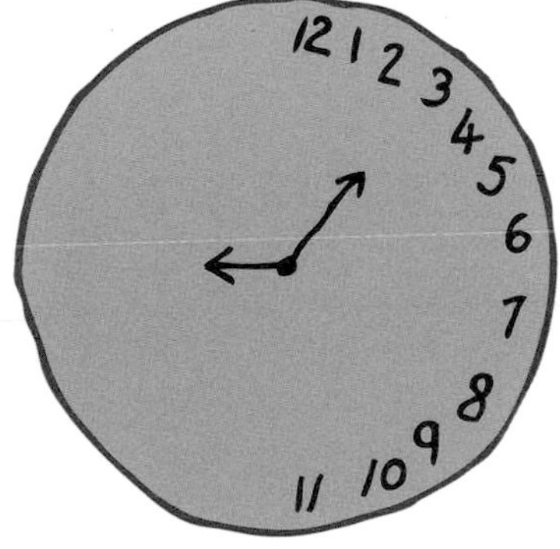

B

Clock drawing test A Image drawn by doctor. B Image drawn by patient with left-sided neglect.

Cerebrovascular disease is the third most common cause of death in high-income countries after cancers and ischaemic heart disease, and the most common cause of severe physical disability. It includes a range of disorders of the central nervous system (Fig. 27.1). Stroke is the most common clinical manifestation of cerebrovascular disease, and results in episodes of brain dysfunction due to focal ischaemia or haemorrhage. Subarachnoid haemorrhage (SAH) and cerebral venous thrombosis (CVT) will be discussed separately, since their pathophysiology, clinical manifestations and management are distinct from those of stroke. Vascular dementia is described in Chapters 10 and 26.

FUNCTIONAL ANATOMY AND PHYSIOLOGY

The main arterial supply of the brain comes from the internal carotid arteries, which supply the anterior brain, and the vertebral and basilar arteries (vertebrobasilar

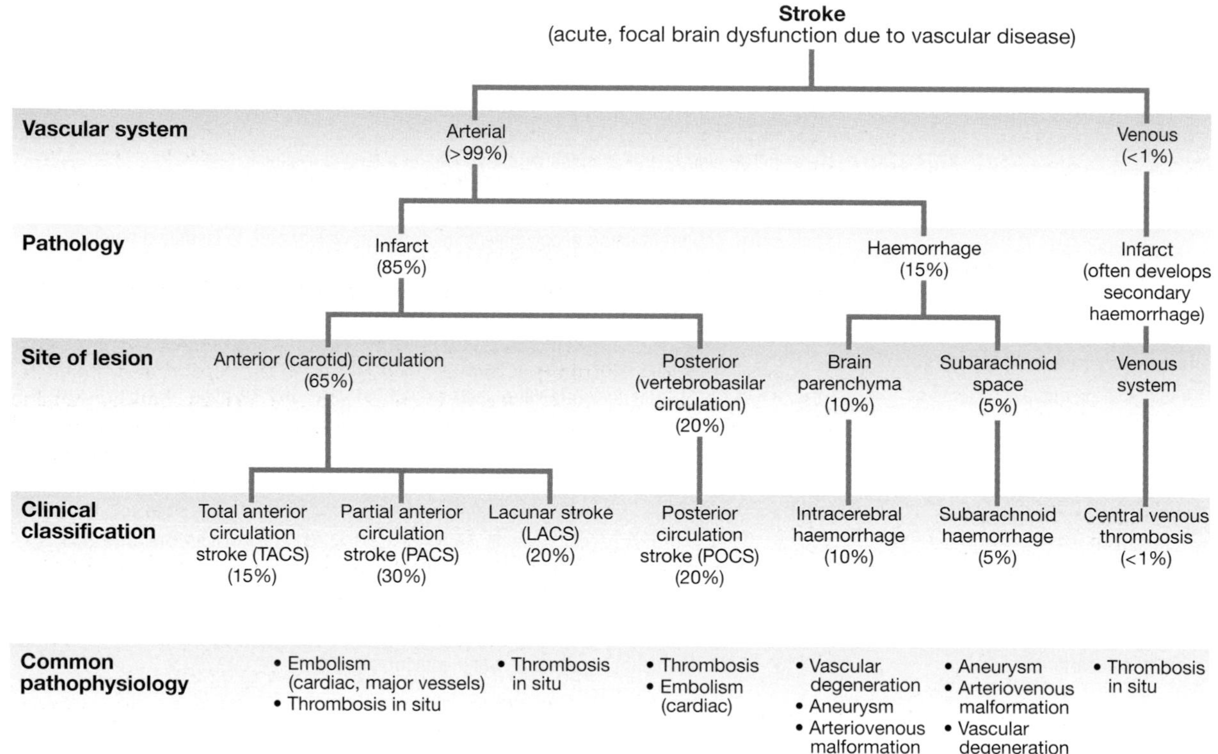

Fig. 27.1 **A classification of stroke disease.**

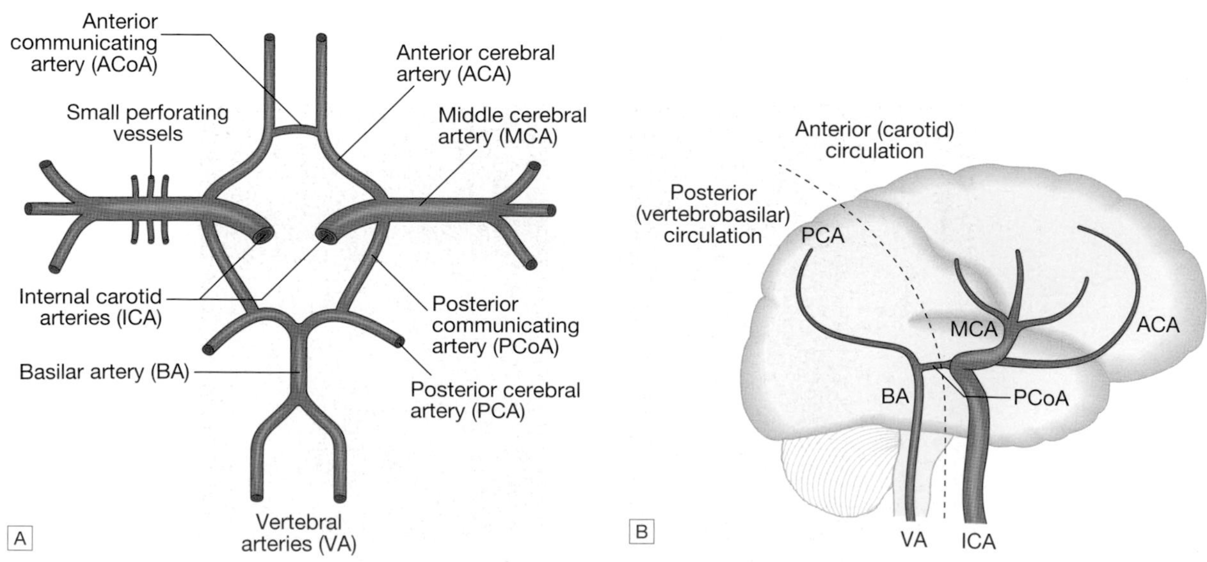

Fig. 27.2 **Arterial circulation of the brain.** **A** Horizontal view. **B** Lateral view.

system), which provide the posterior circulation. The anterior and middle cerebral arteries supply the frontal and parietal lobes, while the posterior cerebral artery supplies the occipital lobe. The vertebral and basilar arteries perfuse the brain stem, mid-brain and cerebellum (Fig. 27.2). The functions of each of these areas of the brain are described on page 1141. Communicating arteries provide connections between the anterior and posterior circulations and between left and right hemispheres, creating protective anastomotic connections that form the circle of Willis. In health, regulatory mechanisms maintain a constant cerebral blood flow across a wide range of arterial blood pressures to meet the high resting metabolic activity of brain tissue; cerebral blood vessels dilate when systemic blood pressure is lowered and constrict when it is raised. This autoregulatory mechanism can be disrupted after stroke. The venous collecting system is formed by a collection of sinuses over the surface of the brain, which drain into the jugular veins (Fig. 27.3).

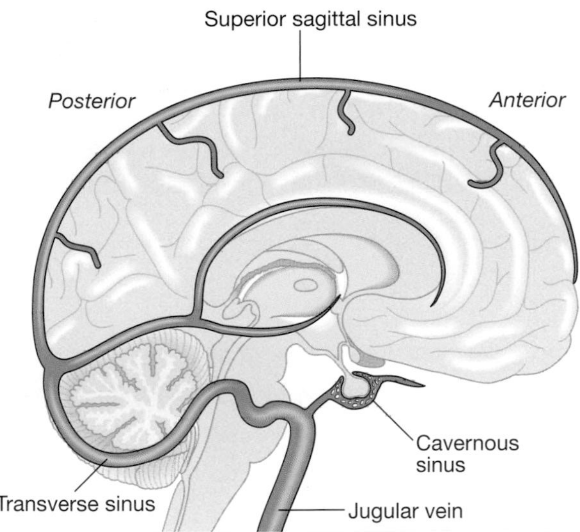

Fig. 27.3 Venous circulation of the brain.

INVESTIGATIONS

A range of investigations may be required to answer specific questions about brain structure and function and about the function of the vascular system.

Neuroimaging

Computed tomography (CT) scanning is the mainstay of stroke imaging. It allows the rapid identification of intracerebral bleeding and stroke 'mimics' (i.e. pathologies other than stroke that have similar presentations), such as tumours. Magnetic resonance imaging (MRI) is used when there is diagnostic uncertainty or delayed presentation, and when more information on brain structure and function is required (Fig. 27.4). Contraindications to MRI include cardiac pacemakers and claustrophobia on entering the scanner. These techniques are described on page 1149.

Vascular imaging

Various techniques are used to obtain images of extracranial and intracranial blood vessels (Fig. 27.5). The least invasive is ultrasound (Doppler or duplex scanning), which is used to image the carotid and the vertebral arteries in the neck. In skilled hands, reliable information can be provided about the degree of arterial stenosis and the presence of ulcerated plaques. Blood flow in the intracerebral vessels can be examined using transcranial Doppler. While the anatomical resolution is limited, it is improving and many centres no longer require formal angiography before proceeding to carotid endarterectomy (see below). Blood flow can also be detected by specialised sequences in MR angiography (MRA) but the anatomical resolution is still not comparable to that of intra-arterial angiography, which outlines blood vessels by the injection of radio-opaque contrast intravenously or intra-arterially. The X-ray images obtained can be enhanced by the use of computer-assisted digital subtraction or spiral CT. Because of the significant risk of complications, intra-arterial contrast angiography is reserved for patients in whom

27

A
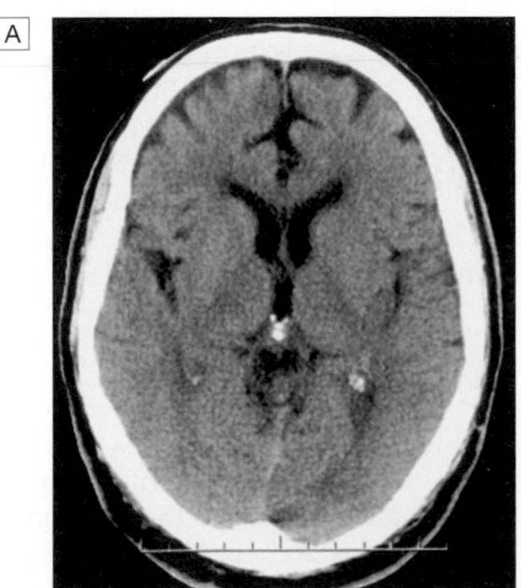

B
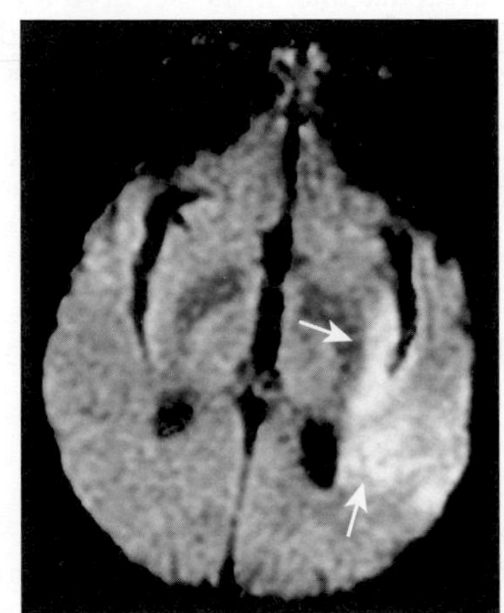

Fig. 27.4 Acute stroke seen on CT scan with corresponding MRI appearance. A CT may show no evidence of early infarction. B Corresponding image seen on MRI diffusion weighted imaging (DWI) with changes of infarction in middle cerebral artery (MCA) territory (arrows).

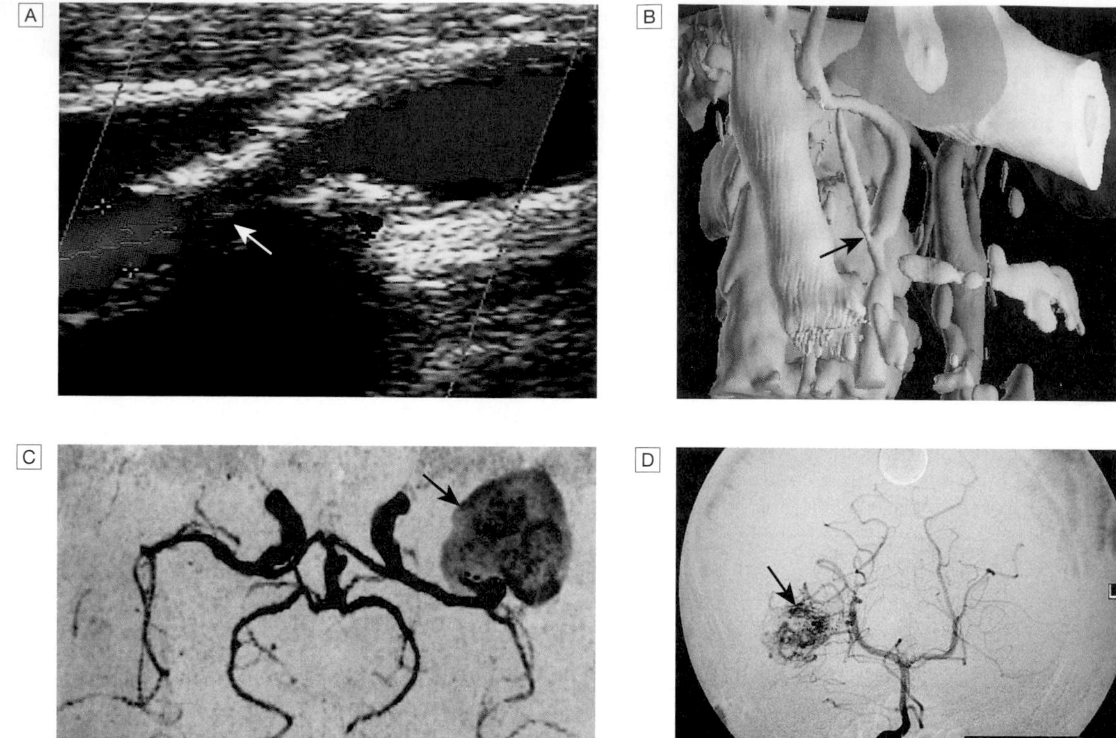

Fig. 27.5 Different techniques of imaging blood vessels. **A** Doppler scan showing 80% stenosis of the internal carotid artery (arrow). **B** Three-dimensional reconstruction of CT angiogram showing stenosis at the carotid bifurcation (arrow). **C** MR angiogram showing giant aneurysm at the middle cerebral artery bifurcation (arrow). **D** Intra-arterial angiography showing arteriovenous malformation (arrow).

non-invasive methods have provided a contradictory picture or incomplete information, or in whom it is necessary to image the intracranial circulation in detail: for example, to delineate a saccular aneurysm, an arteriovenous malformation or vasculitis.

Blood tests

These help identify underlying causes of cerebrovascular disease: for example, blood glucose (diabetes mellitus), triglycerides and cholesterol (hyperlipidaemia) or full blood count (polycythaemia) in stroke. Erythrocyte sedimentation rate (ESR) and immunological tests, such as measurement of antineutrophil cytoplasmic antibodies (ANCA) (p. 1068), may be required when vasculitis is suspected. Genetic testing for rarer inherited conditions, such as CADASIL (cerebral autosomal dominant arteriopathy with subcortical infarcts and leucoencephalopathy), may be indicated.

Lumbar puncture

Lumbar puncture (p. 1153) is largely reserved for the investigation of SAH.

Cardiovascular investigations

Electrocardiography (ECG; p. 532) and echocardiography (p. 537) may reveal abnormalities that may cause cardiac embolism in stroke.

PRESENTING PROBLEMS

Most vascular lesions develop suddenly within a matter of minutes or hours, and so should be considered in the differential diagnosis of patients with any acute neurological presentation.

Weakness

Unilateral weakness is the classical presentation of stroke and, much more rarely, of cerebral venous thrombosis. The weakness is sudden, progresses rapidly and follows a hemiplegic pattern (see Fig. 26.18, p. 1163). There is rarely any associated abnormal movement. Reflexes are initially reduced but then become increased with a spastic pattern of increased tone (see Box 26.20, p. 1162). Upper motor neuron weakness of the face (7th cranial nerve) is often present.

Speech disturbance

Dysphasia and dysarthria are the most common presentations of disturbed speech in stroke (p. 1168). Dysphasia indicates damage to the dominant frontal or parietal lobe (see Box 26.2, p. 1142), while dysarthria is a non-localising feature reflecting weakness or incoordination of the face, pharynx, lips, tongue or palate.

Visual deficit

Visual loss in stroke can be due to unilateral optic ischaemia (called amaurosis fugax if transient), caused by disturbance of blood flow in the internal carotid artery and ophthalmic artery, which leads to monocular blindness. Ischaemic damage to the occipital cortex or post-chiasmic nerve tracts results in a contralateral hemianopia (p. 1169).

Visuo-spatial dysfunction

Damage to the non-dominant cortex often results in contralateral visuo-spatial dysfunction, such as sensory or visual neglect and apraxia (inability to perform complex tasks despite normal motor, sensory and cerebellar function; p. 1167). This is sometimes misdiagnosed as acute confusion.

Ataxia

Stroke causing damage to the cerebellum and its connections can present as an acute ataxia (p. 1168) and there may be associated brainstem features such as diplopia (p. 1170) and vertigo (p. 1167). The differential diagnosis includes vestibular disorders (p. 1186).

Headache

Sudden severe headache is the cardinal symptom of SAH but also occurs in intracerebral haemorrhage. Although some degree of headache is common in acute ischaemic stroke, it is rarely a dominant feature (p. 1156). Headache also occurs in cerebral venous disease.

Seizure

Seizure is unusual in acute stroke but may be generalised or focal in cerebral venous disease.

Coma

Coma is an uncommon feature of stroke, though it may occur with a brainstem event. If it is present in the first 24 hours, it usually indicates a subarachnoid or intracerebral haemorrhage (see Box 26.16, p. 1160).

STROKE

Stroke is a common medical emergency. The incidence rises steeply with age, and in many lower- and middle-income countries it is rising in association with less healthy lifestyles. About one-fifth of patients with an acute stroke die within a month of the event and at least half of those who survive are left with physical disability.

Pathophysiology

Of the 180–300 patients per 100 000 population presenting annually with a stroke, 85% sustain a cerebral infarction due to inadequate blood flow to part of the brain, and most of the remainder have an intracerebral haemorrhage (see Fig. 27.1).

Cerebral infarction

Cerebral infarction is mostly caused by thromboembolic disease secondary to atherosclerosis in the major extracranial arteries (carotid artery and aortic arch). About 20% of infarctions are due to embolism from the heart, and a further 20% are due to thrombosis in situ caused by intrinsic disease of small perforating vessels (lenticulostriate arteries), producing so-called lacunar infarctions. The risk factors for ischaemic stroke reflect the risk factors for the underlying vascular disease (Box 27.1). About 5% are due to rare causes, including vasculitis (p. 1115), endocarditis (p. 625) and cerebral venous disease (see below). Cerebral infarction takes some hours to complete, even though the patient's deficit may be maximal shortly after the vascular occlusion. After the occlusion of a cerebral artery, infarction may be forestalled by the opening of anastomotic channels from other arterial territories that restore perfusion to its territory. Similarly, reduction in perfusion pressure leads to compensatory homeostatic changes to maintain tissue oxygenation (Fig. 27.6). These compensatory changes can sometimes prevent occlusion of even a carotid artery from having any clinically apparent effect.

However, if and when these homeostatic mechanisms fail, the process of ischaemia starts, and ultimately leads to infarction unless the vascular supply is restored. As the cerebral blood flow declines, different neuronal functions fail at various thresholds (Fig. 27.7). Once blood flow falls below the threshold for the maintenance of electrical activity, neurological deficit develops. At this level of blood flow, the neurons are still viable; if

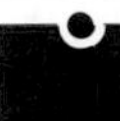

27.1 Risk factors for stroke

Fixed risk factors

- Age
- Gender (male > female except at extremes of age)
- Race (Afro-Caribbean > Asian > European)
- Previous vascular event
    - Myocardial infarction
    - Stroke
    - Peripheral vascular disease
- Heredity
- High fibrinogen

Modifiable risk factors

- Blood pressure
- Cigarette smoking
- Hyperlipidaemia
- Heart disease
    - Atrial fibrillation
    - Congestive cardiac failure
    - Infective endocarditis
- Diabetes mellitus
- Excessive alcohol intake
- Oestrogen-containing drugs
    - Oral contraceptive pill
    - Hormone replacement therapy
- Polycythaemia

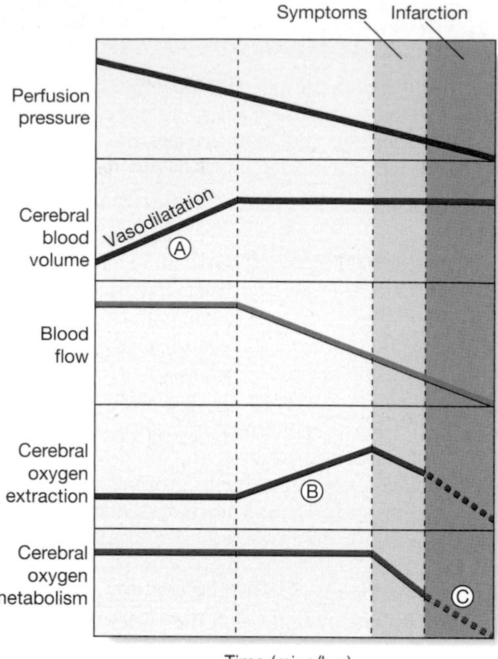

Fig. 27.6 Homeostatic responses to falling perfusion pressure in the brain following arterial occlusion. Vasodilatation initially maintains cerebral blood flow (A), but after maximal vasodilatation further falls in perfusion pressure lead to a decline in blood flow. An increase in tissue oxygen extraction, however, maintains the cerebral metabolic rate for oxygen (B). Still further falls in perfusion, and therefore blood flow, cannot be compensated; cerebral oxygen availability falls and symptoms appear, then infarction (C).

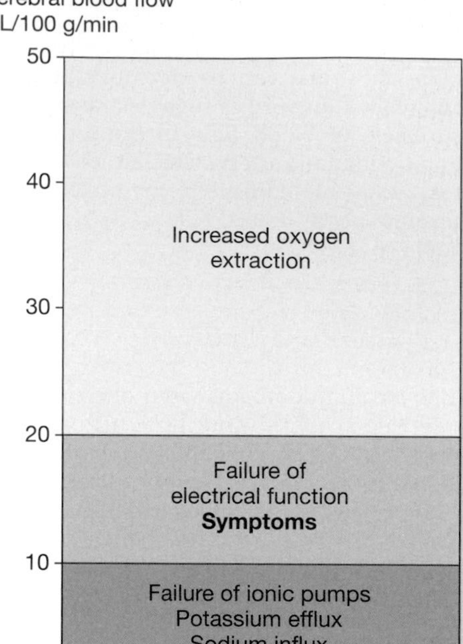

Fig. 27.7 Thresholds of cerebral ischaemia. Symptoms of cerebral ischaemia appear when the blood flow has fallen to less than half of normal and energy supply is insufficient to sustain neuronal electrical function. Full recovery can occur if this level of flow is returned to normal but not if it is sustained. Further blood flow reduction below the next threshold causes failure of cell ionic pumps and starts the ischaemic cascade, leading to cell death.

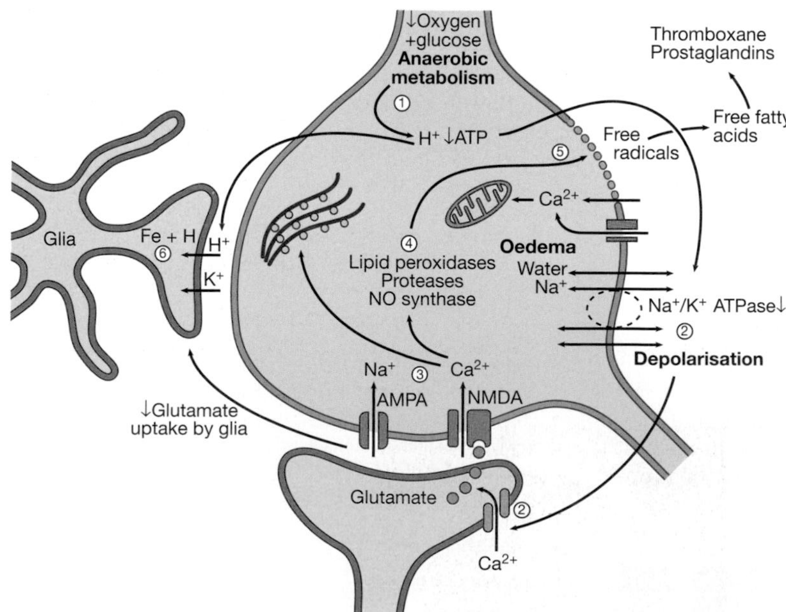

Fig. 27.8 The process of neuronal ischaemia and infarction. (1) Reduction of blood flow reduces supply of oxygen and hence ATP. H^+ is produced by anaerobic metabolism of available glucose. (2) Energy-dependent membrane ionic pumps fail, leading to cytotoxic oedema and membrane depolarisation, allowing calcium entry and releasing glutamate. (3) Calcium enters cells via glutamate-gated channels and (4) activates destructive intracellular enzymes (5), destroying intracellular organelles and cell membrane, with release of free radicals. Free fatty acid release activates pro-coagulant pathways that exacerbate local ischaemia. (6) Glial cells take up H^+, can no longer take up extracellular glutamate and also suffer cell death, leading to liquefactive necrosis of whole arterial territory.

the blood flow increases again, function returns and the patient will have had a transient ischaemic attack (TIA). However, if the blood flow falls further, a level is reached at which irreversible cell death starts. Hypoxia leads to an inadequate supply of adenosine triphosphate (ATP), which leads to failure of membrane pumps, thereby allowing influx of sodium and water into the cell (cytotoxic oedema) and the release of the excitatory neurotransmitter glutamate into the extracellular fluid. Glutamate opens membrane channels, allowing the influx of calcium and more sodium into the neurons. Calcium entering the neurons activates intracellular enzymes that complete the destructive process. The release of inflammatory mediators by microglia and astrocytes causes death of all cell types in the area of maximum ischaemia. The infarction process is worsened by the anaerobic production of lactic acid (Fig. 27.8) and consequent fall in tissue pH. There have been attempts to develop neuroprotective drugs to slow down the processes leading to irreversible cell death but so far these have proved disappointing.

The final outcome of the occlusion of a cerebral blood vessel therefore depends upon the competence of the circulatory homeostatic mechanisms, the metabolic demand, and the severity and duration of the reduction in blood flow. Higher brain temperature, as occurs in fever, and higher blood sugar have both been associated with a greater volume of infarction for a given reduction in cerebral blood flow. Subsequent restoration of blood flow may cause haemorrhage into the infarcted area ('haemorrhagic transformation'). This is particularly likely in patients given antithrombotic or thrombolytic drugs, and in patients with larger infarcts.

Radiologically, a cerebral infarct can be seen as a lesion that comprises a mixture of dead brain tissue that is already undergoing autolysis, and tissue that is ischaemic and swollen but recoverable (the 'ischaemic penumbra'). The infarct swells with time and is at its maximal size a couple of days after stroke onset. At this stage, it may be big enough to exert mass effect both clinically and radiologically; sometimes, decompressive craniectomy is required (see below). After a few weeks, the oedema subsides and the infarcted area is replaced by a sharply defined fluid-filled cavity.

Intracerebral haemorrhage

Intracerebral haemorrhage causes about 10% of acute stroke events but is more common in low-income countries. It usually results from rupture of a blood vessel within the brain parenchyma but may also occur in a patient with an SAH (see below) if the artery ruptures into the brain substance as well as into the subarachnoid space. Haemorrhage frequently occurs into an area of brain infarction and, if the volume of haemorrhage is large, it may be difficult to distinguish from primary intracerebral haemorrhage both clinically and radiologically (Fig. 27.9). The risk factors and underlying causes of intracerebral haemorrhage are listed in Box 27.2. The explosive entry of blood into the brain parenchyma causes immediate cessation of function in that area as neurons are structurally disrupted and white-matter fibre tracts are split apart. The haemorrhage itself may expand over the first minutes or hours, or it may be associated with a rim of cerebral oedema, which, along with the haematoma, acts like a mass lesion to cause progression of the neurological deficit. If big enough, this can cause shift of the intracranial contents, producing transtentorial coning and sometimes rapid death (p. 1212). If the patient survives, the haematoma is gradually absorbed, leaving a haemosiderin-lined slit in the brain parenchyma.

27.2 Causes of intracerebral haemorrhage and associated risk factors

Disease	Risk factors
Complex small-vessel disease with disruption of vessel wall	Age Hypertension High cholesterol
Amyloid angiopathy	Familial (rare) Age
Impaired blood clotting	Anticoagulant therapy Blood dyscrasia Thrombolytic therapy
Vascular anomaly	Arteriovenous malformation Cavernous haemangioma
Substance misuse	Alcohol Amphetamines Cocaine

Clinical features

Acute stroke and TIA are characterised by a rapid-onset, focal deficit of brain function. The typical presentation occurs over minutes, affects an identifiable area of the brain and is 'negative' in character (i.e. abrupt loss of function without positive features such as abnormal movement). Provided that there is a clear history of this, the chance of a brain lesion being anything other than vascular is 5% or less (Box 27.3). If symptoms progress over hours or days, other diagnoses must be excluded. Confusion and memory or balance disturbance are more often due to stroke mimics. Transient symptoms, such as syncope, amnesia, confusion and dizziness, do not reflect focal cerebral dysfunction, but are often

A

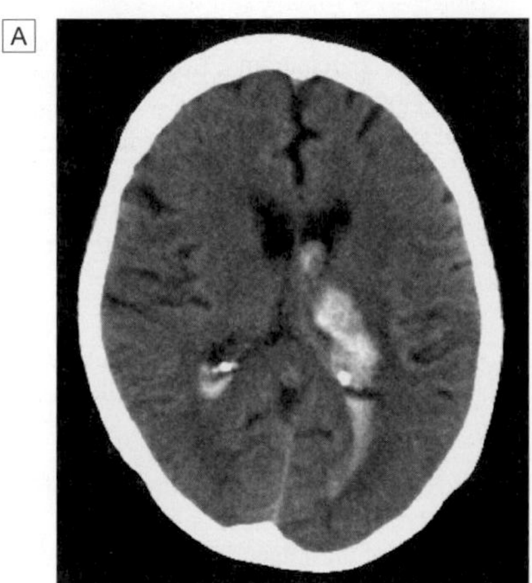

B

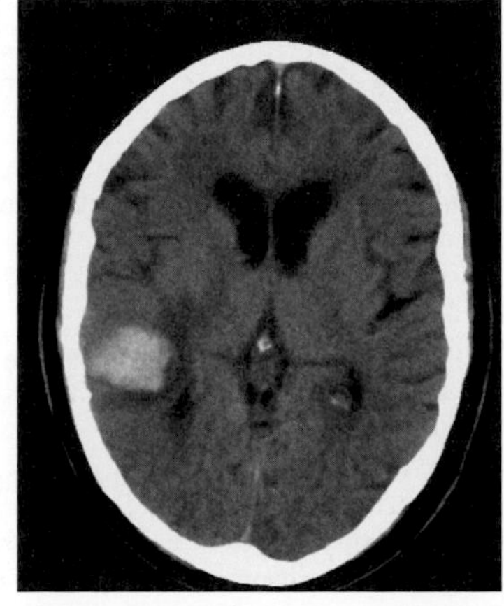

Fig. 27.9 CT scans showing intracerebral haemorrhage. **A** Basal ganglia haemorrhage with intraventricular extension. **B** Small cortical haemorrhage.

27

27.3 Differential diagnosis of stroke and TIA

'Structural' stroke mimics	
• Primary cerebral tumours • Metastatic cerebral tumours • Subdural haematoma	• Cerebral abscess • Peripheral nerve lesions (vascular or compressive) • Demyelination
'Functional' stroke mimics	
• Todd's paresis (after epileptic seizure) • Hypoglycaemia • Migrainous aura (with or without headache)	• Focal seizures • Ménière's disease or other vestibular disorder • Conversion disorder (p. 246) • Encephalitis

27.4 Characteristic features of stroke and non-stroke syndromes ('stroke mimics')

Feature	Stroke	Stroke mimics
Symptom onset	Sudden (minutes)	Often slower onset
Symptom progression	Rapidly reaches maximum severity	Often gradual onset
Severity of deficit	Unequivocal	May be variable/ uncertain
Pattern of deficit	Hemispheric pattern	May be non-specific with confusion, memory loss, balance disturbance
Loss of consciousness	Uncommon	More common

mistakenly attributed to TIA (see Fig. 26.17, p. 1158, and Box 27.4). Public health campaigns to raise awareness of the emergency nature of stroke exploit the fact that weakness of the face or arm, or disturbance of speech is the commonest presentation.

The clinical presentation of stroke depends upon which arterial territory is involved and the size of the lesion (see Fig. 27.1). These will both have a bearing on management, such as suitability for carotid endarterectomy. The neurological deficit can be identified from the patient's history and (if it is persistent) the neurological examination. The presence of a unilateral motor deficit, a higher cerebral function deficit such as aphasia or neglect, or a visual field defect usually places the lesion in the cerebral hemisphere. Ataxia, diplopia, vertigo and/or bilateral weakness usually indicate a lesion in the brainstem or cerebellum. Different combinations of these deficits define several stroke syndromes (Fig. 27.10), which reflect the site and size of the lesion and may provide clues to underlying pathology.

Reduced conscious level usually indicates a large-volume lesion in the cerebral hemisphere but may result from a lesion in the brainstem or complications such as obstructive hydrocephalus, hypoxia or severe systemic infection. The combination of severe headache and vomiting at the onset of the focal deficit is suggestive of intracerebral haemorrhage.

General examination may provide clues to the cause, and identify important comorbidities and complications.

Several terms have been used to classify strokes, often based on the duration and evolution of symptoms.

- *Transient ischaemic attack (TIA)* describes a stroke in which symptoms resolve within 24 hours – an arbitrary cutoff that has little value in practice, apart from perhaps indicating that underlying cerebral haemorrhage or extensive cerebral infarction is extremely unlikely. The term TIA traditionally also includes patients with amaurosis fugax, usually due to a vascular occlusion in the retina.
- *Stroke* describes those events in which symptoms last more than 24 hours. The differential diagnosis of patients with symptoms lasting a few minutes or hours is similar to those with persisting symptoms (see Box 27.3).
- *Progressing stroke (or stroke in evolution)* describes a stroke in which the focal neurological deficit worsens after the patient first presents. Such worsening may be due to increasing volume of infarction, haemorrhagic transformation or increasing cerebral oedema.
- *Completed stroke* describes a stroke in which the focal deficit persists and is not progressing.

When assessing a patient within hours of symptom onset, it is not possible to distinguish stroke from TIA unless symptoms have already resolved. In clinical practice, it is important to distinguish those patients with strokes who have persisting focal neurological symptoms when seen from those whose symptoms have resolved.

Investigations

Investigation of acute stroke aims to confirm the vascular nature of the lesion, distinguish cerebral infarction from haemorrhage and identify the underlying vascular disease and risk factors (Box 27.5).

27.5 Investigation of a patient with an acute stroke

Diagnostic question	Investigation
Is it a vascular lesion?	CT/MRI
Is it ischaemic or haemorrhagic?	CT/MRI
Is it a subarachnoid haemorrhage?	CT/lumbar puncture
Is there any cardiac source of embolism?	Electrocardiogram (ECG) 24-hour ECG Echocardiogram
What is the underlying vascular disease?	Duplex ultrasound of carotids Magnetic resonance angiography (MRA) CT angiography (CTA) Contrast angiography
What are the risk factors?	Full blood count Cholesterol Blood glucose
Is there an unusual cause?	Erythrocyte sedimentation rate (ESR) Serum protein electrophoresis Clotting/thrombophilia screen

Clinical syndrome	Common symptoms	Common cause	CT scan features
Total anterior circulation syndrome (TACS) 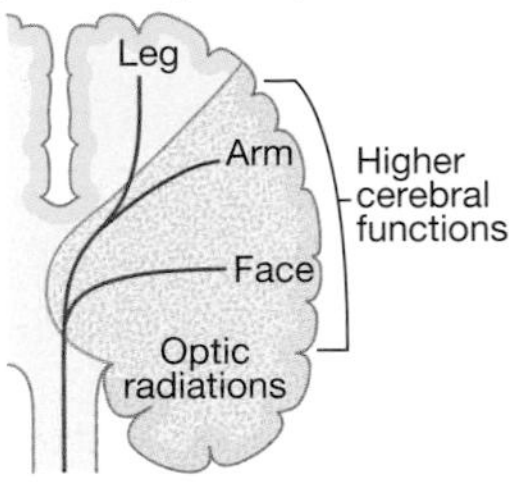	Combination of: Hemiparesis Higher cerebral dysfunction (e.g. aphasia) Hemisensory loss Homonymous hemianopia (damage to optic radiations)	Middle cerebral artery occlusion (Embolism from heart or major vessels)	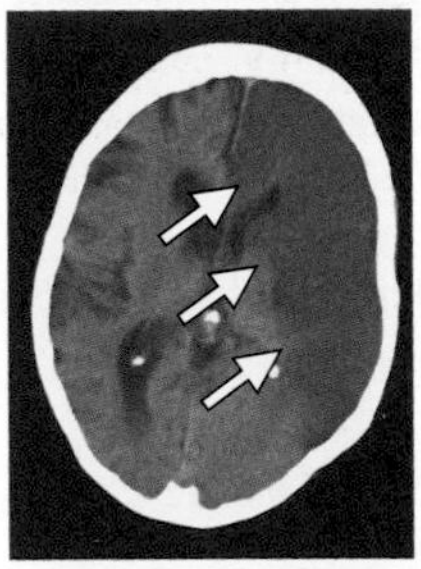
Partial anterior circulation syndrome (PACS) 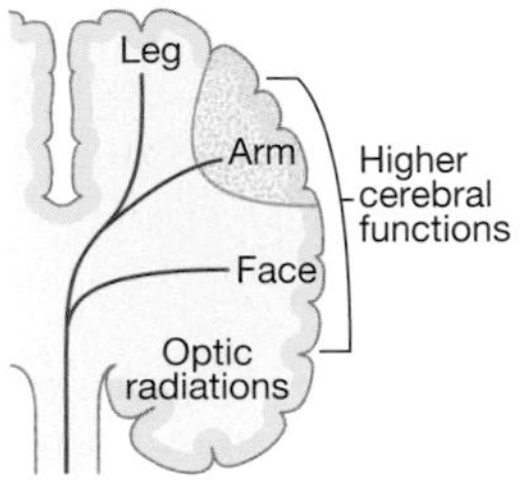	Isolated motor loss (e.g. leg only, arm only, face) Isolated higher cerebral dysfunction (e.g. aphasia, neglect) Mixture of higher cerebral dysfunction and motor loss (e.g. aphasia with right hemiparesis)	Occlusion of a branch of the middle cerebral artery or anterior cerebral artery (Embolism from heart or major vessels)	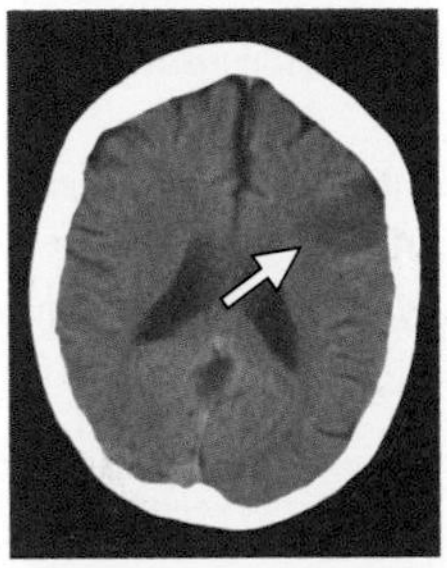
Lacunar syndrome (LACS) 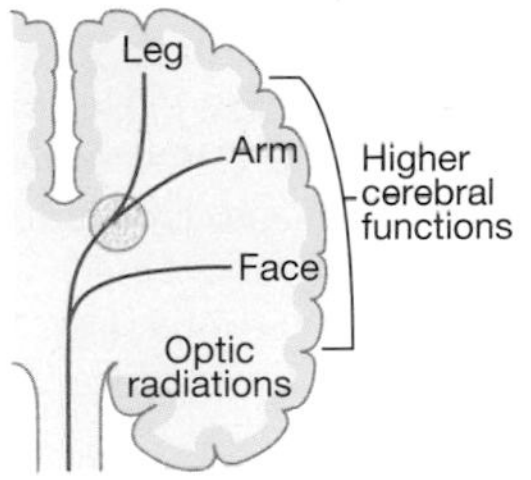	Pure motor stroke – affects two limbs Pure sensory stroke Sensory-motor stroke No higher cerebral dysfunction or hemianopia	Thrombotic occlusion of small perforating arteries (Thrombosis in situ)	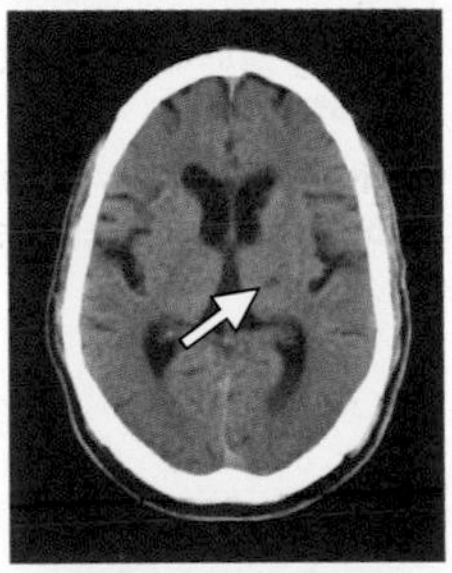
Posterior circulation stroke (POCS) (lateral view) 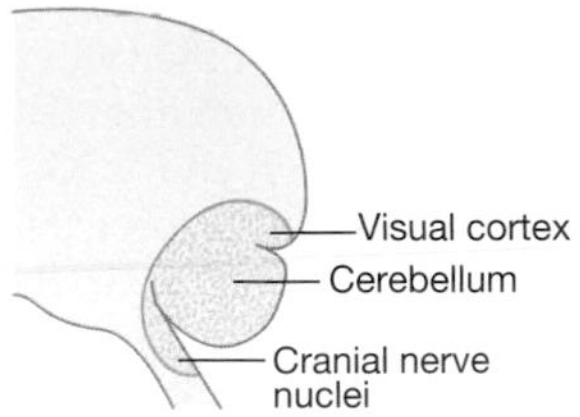	Homonymous hemianopia (damage to visual cortex) Cerebellar syndrome Cranial nerve syndromes	Occlusion in vertebral, basilar or posterior cerbral artery territory (Cardiac embolism or thrombosis in situ)	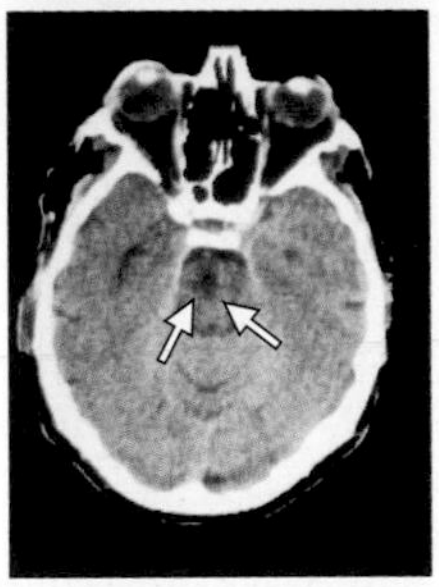

Fig. 27.10 Clinical and radiological features of the stroke syndromes. The top three diagrams show coronal sections of the brain, and the bottom one shows a sagittal section. The anatomical locations of cerebral functions are shown with the nerve tracts in green. A motor (or sensory) deficit (shown by the red shaded areas) can occur with damage to the relevant cortex (PACS), nerve tracts (LACS) or both (TACS). The corresponding CT scans show horizontal slices at the level of the lesion, highlighted by the arrows.

Risk factor analysis

Initial investigation includes a range of simple blood tests to detect common vascular risk factors and markers of rarer causes, an ECG and brain imaging. Where there is uncertainty about the nature of the stroke, further investigations are indicated. This especially applies to younger patients, who are less likely to have atherosclerotic disease (Box 27.6).

Neuroimaging

Brain imaging with either CT or MRI should be performed in all patients with acute stroke. Exceptions are where results would not influence management, such as in the advanced stage of a terminal illness. CT remains the most practical and widely available method of imaging the brain. It will usually exclude non-stroke lesions, including subdural haematomas and brain tumours, and will demonstrate intracerebral haemorrhage within minutes of stroke onset (see Fig. 27.9). However, especially within the first few hours after symptom onset, CT changes in cerebral infarction may be completely absent or only very subtle. Changes often develop over time (see Fig. 27.11, p. 1245), but small cerebral infarcts may never show up on CT scans. For most purposes, a CT scan performed within 24 hours is

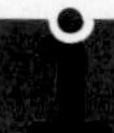

27.6 Causes and investigation of acute stroke in young patients

Cause	Investigation
Cerebral infarct	
Cardiac embolism	Echocardiography (including transoesophageal)
Premature atherosclerosis	Serum lipids
Arterial dissection	MRI Angiography
Thrombophilia	Protein C, protein S Antithrombin III Factor V Leiden, prothrombin
Homocystinuria (p. 449)	Urinary amino acids Methionine loading test
Antiphospholipid antibody syndrome (p. 1055)	Anticardiolipin antibodies/ lupus anticoagulant
Systemic lupus erythematosus	Antinuclear antibodies
Vasculitis	ESR C-reactive protein Antineutrophil cytoplasmic antibody (ANCA)
CADASIL (cerebral autosomal dominant arteriopathy with subcortical infarcts and leucoencephalopathy)	MRI brain Genetic analysis Skin biopsy
Mitochondrial cytopathy	Serum lactate White cell mitochondrial DNA Muscle biopsy Mitochondrial molecular genetics
Fabry's disease	Alpha-galactosidase levels
Neurovascular syphilis	Syphilis serology
Primary intracerebral haemorrhage	
Arteriovenous malformation (AVM)	MRI/angiography
Drug misuse	Drug screen (amphetamine, cocaine)
Coagulopathy	Prothrombin time (PT) and activated partial thromboplastin time (APTT) Platelet count
Subarachnoid haemorrhage	
Saccular ('berry') aneurysm	MRI/angiography
AVM	MRI/angiography
Vertebral dissection	MRI/angiography

adequate but there are certain circumstances in which an immediate CT scan is essential (Box 27.7). Even in the absence of changes suggesting infarction, abnormal perfusion of brain tissue can be imaged with CT after injection of contrast media (i.e. perfusion scanning). This can be useful in guiding immediate treatment of ischaemic stroke.

MRI is not as widely available as CT and scanning times are longer. However, MRI diffusion weighted imaging (DWI) can detect ischaemia earlier than CT, and other MRI sequences can also be used to demonstrate abnormal perfusion (see Fig. 27.4). MRI is more sensitive than CT in detecting strokes affecting the brainstem and

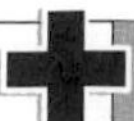

27.7 Indications for emergency CT/MRI in acute stroke

- Patient on anticoagulants or with abnormal coagulation
- Consideration of thrombolysis or immediate anticoagulation
- Deteriorating conscious level or rapidly progressing deficits
- Suspected cerebellar haematoma, to exclude hydrocephalus

cerebellum, and unlike CT, can reliably distinguish haemorrhagic from ischaemic stroke even several weeks after the onset. CT and MRI may reveal clues as to the nature of the arterial lesion. For example, there may be a small, deep lacunar infarct indicating small-vessel disease, or a more peripheral infarct suggesting an extracranial source of embolism (see Fig. 27.10). In a haemorrhagic lesion, the location might indicate the presence of an underlying vascular malformation, saccular aneurysm or amyloid angiopathy.

Vascular imaging

Many ischaemic strokes are caused by atherosclerotic thromboembolic disease of the major extracranial vessels. Detection of extracranial vascular disease can help establish why the patient has had an ischaemic stroke and, in highly selected patients, may lead on to specific treatments, including carotid endarterectomy to reduce the risk of further stroke (see below). The presence or absence of a carotid bruit is not a reliable indicator of the degree of carotid stenosis. Extracranial arterial disease can be non-invasively identified with duplex ultrasound, MRA or CT angiography (see Fig. 27.5), or occasionally intra-arterial contrast radiography as above.

Cardiac investigations

Approximately 20% of ischaemic strokes are due to embolism from the heart. The most common causes are atrial fibrillation, prosthetic heart valves, other valvular abnormalities and recent myocardial infarction. These may be identified by clinical examination and ECG, but a transthoracic or transoesophageal echocardiogram is also required to confirm the presence of a clinically apparent cardiac source or to identify an unsuspected source such as endocarditis, atrial myxoma, intracardiac thrombus or patent foramen ovale. Such findings may lead on to specific cardiac treatment.

Management

Management is aimed at minimising the volume of brain that is irreversibly damaged, preventing complications (Box 27.8), reducing the patient's disability and handicap through rehabilitation, and reducing the risk of recurrent stroke or other vascular events. With TIA there is no brain damage and disability, so the priority is to reduce the risk of further vascular events.

Supportive care

Early admission of patients to a specialised stroke unit facilitates coordinated care from a specialised multidisciplinary team (Box 27.9), and has been shown to reduce both mortality and residual disability amongst survivors. Consideration of a patient's rehabilitation needs

27.8 Complications of acute stroke

Complication	Prevention	Treatment
Chest infection	Nurse semi-erect Avoid aspiration (nil by mouth, nasogastric tube, possible gastrostomy)	Antibiotics Physiotherapy
Epileptic seizures	Maintain cerebral oxygenation Avoid metabolic disturbance	Anticonvulsants
Deep venous thrombosis/ pulmonary embolism	Maintain hydration Early mobilisation Anti-embolism stockings Heparin (for high-risk patients only)	Anticoagulation (exclude haemorrhagic stroke first)
Painful shoulder	Avoid traction injury Shoulder/arm supports Physiotherapy	Physiotherapy Local corticosteroid injections
Pressure sores	Frequent turning Monitor pressure areas Avoid urinary damage to skin	Nursing care Pressure-relieving mattress
Urinary infection	Avoid catheterisation if possible Use penile sheath	Antibiotics
Constipation	Appropriate aperients and diet	Appropriate aperients
Depression and anxiety	Maintain positive attitude and provide information	Antidepressants

EBM 27.9 Specialist stroke units

'Admitting 1000 patients to a stroke unit prevents about 50 patients from being dead or dependent at 6 months.'

- Stroke Unit Trialists' Collaboration. Cochrane Database of Systematic Reviews 2007, issue 4. Art. no.: CD000197.

For further information: www.cochrane.org/cochrane-reviews

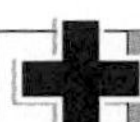

27.10 Management of acute stroke

Airway

- Perform bedside swallow screen and keep patient nil by mouth if swallowing unsafe or aspiration occurs

Breathing

- Check respiratory rate and oxygen saturation and give oxygen if saturation < 95%

Circulation

- Check peripheral perfusion, pulse and blood pressure and treat abnormalities with fluid replacement, anti-arrhythmics and inotropic drugs as appropriate

Hydration

- If signs of dehydration, give fluids parenterally or by nasogastric tube

Nutrition

- Assess nutritional status and provide nutritional supplements if necessary
- If dysphagia persists for > 48 hrs, start feeding via a nasogastric tube

Medication

- If patient is dysphagic, consider alternative routes for essential medications

Blood pressure

- Unless there is heart or renal failure, evidence of hypertensive encephalopathy or aortic dissection, do not lower blood pressure in first week as it may reduce cerebral perfusion. Blood pressure often returns towards patient's normal level within first few days

Blood glucose

- Check blood glucose and treat when levels are ≥ 11.1 mmol/L (200 mg/dL) (by insulin infusion or glucose/ potassium/insulin (GKI)
- Monitor closely to avoid hypoglycaemia

Temperature

- If pyrexic, investigate and treat underlying cause
- Control with antipyretics, as raised brain temperature may increase infarct volume

Pressure areas

- Reduce risk of skin breakdown:
  - Treat infection
  - Maintain nutrition
  - Provide pressure-relieving mattress
  - Turn immobile patients regularly

Incontinence

- Check for constipation and urinary retention; treat appropriately
- Avoid urinary catheterisation unless patient is in acute urinary retention or incontinence is threatening pressure areas

Mobilisation

- Avoid bed rest

should commence at the same time as acute medical management. Dysphagia is common and can be detected by an early bedside test of swallowing. This allows hydration, feeding and medication to be given safely, if necessary by nasogastric tube or intravenously. In the acute phase, a checklist may be useful (Box 27.10) to ensure that all the factors that might influence outcome have been addressed.

The patient's neurological deficits may worsen during the first few hours or days after their onset. This is most common in those with lacunar infarcts but may occur in other patients, due to extension of the area of infarction, haemorrhage transformation, or the development of oedema with consequent mass effect. It is important to distinguish these patients from those who are deteriorating as a result of complications such as hypoxia, sepsis, epileptic seizures or metabolic abnormalities that may be reversed more easily. Patients with cerebellar haematomas or infarcts with mass effect may develop obstructive hydrocephalus and some will benefit from insertion of a ventricular drain and/or decompressive

EBM 27.11 Role of treatments in acute stroke

Treatment	Target group	Approximate proportion of patients eligible for treatment	NNT to prevent 1 death or disability in those treated
Aspirin[1]	Acute ischaemic stroke	90%	80
Thrombolysis with rt-PA[2]	Acute ischaemic stroke		
	Treated within 3 hrs of onset	10%	9
	Treated within 3–4.5 hrs of onset	10%	20
Decompressive hemicraniectomy[3]	Large cerebral infarction	< 1%	2
Stroke unit care[4]	Acute stroke	80%	20

- [1]Sandercock P, et al. Cochrane Database of Systematic Reviews 2008, issue 3. Art. no.: CD000029.
- [2]Lees KR, et al. Lancet 2010; 375:1695–1703.
- [3]Vahedi K, et al. Lancet Neurol 2007; 6(3):215–222.
- [4]Stroke Unit Trialists' Collaboration. Cochrane Database of Systematic Reviews 2007, issue 4. Art. no.: CD000197.

For further information: www.cochrane.org/cochrane-reviews

(NNT = number needed to treat; rtPA = tissue plasminogen activator)

surgery (Box 27.11). Some patients with large haematomas or infarction with massive oedema in the cerebral hemispheres may benefit from anti-oedema agents, such as mannitol or artificial ventilation. Surgical decompression to reduce intracranial pressure should be considered in appropriate patients.

Thrombolysis

Intravenous thrombolysis with recombinant tissue plasminogen activator (rt-PA) increases the risk of haemorrhagic transformation of the cerebral infarct with potentially fatal results. However, if it is given within 4.5 hours of symptom onset to carefully selected patients, the haemorrhagic risk is offset by an improvement in overall outcome (see Box 27.11). The earlier treatment is given, the greater the benefit.

Aspirin

In the absence of contraindications, aspirin (300 mg daily) should be started immediately after an ischaemic stroke unless rt-PA has been given, in which case it should be withheld for at least 24 hours. Aspirin reduces the risk of early recurrence and has a small but clinically worthwhile effect on long-term outcome (see Box 27.11); it may be given by rectal suppository or by nasogastric tube in dysphagic patients.

Heparin

Anticoagulation with heparin has been widely used to treat acute ischaemic stroke in the past. Whilst it reduces the risk of early ischaemic recurrence and venous thromboembolism, it increases the risk of both intracranial and extracranial haemorrhage. Furthermore, routine use of heparin does not result in better long-term outcomes, and therefore it should not be used in the routine management of acute stroke. It is unclear whether heparin might provide benefit in selected patients, such as those with recent myocardial infarction, arterial dissection or progressing strokes. Intracranial haemorrhage must be excluded on brain imaging before considering anticoagulation.

Coagulation abnormalities

In those with intracerebral haemorrhage, coagulation abnormalities should be reversed as quickly as possible to reduce the likelihood of the haematoma enlarging. This most commonly arises in those on warfarin therapy. There is no evidence that clotting factors are useful in the absence of a clotting defect.

Management of risk factors

The approaches used are summarised in Figure 27.11. The average risk of a further stroke is 5–10% within the first week of a stroke or TIA, perhaps 15% in the first year and 5% per year thereafter. The risks are not substantially different for intracerebral haemorrhage. Patients with ischaemic events should be put on long-term antiplatelet drugs and statins to lower cholesterol. For patients in atrial fibrillation, the risk can be reduced by about 60% by using oral anticoagulation to achieve an INR of 2–3. The role of newer oral anticoagulants (such as dabigatran) is currently being investigated. The risk of recurrence after both ischaemic and haemorrhagic strokes can be reduced by blood pressure reduction, even for those with relatively normal blood pressures (Box 27.12).

Carotid endarterectomy and angioplasty

A small proportion of patients with a carotid territory ischaemic stroke or TIA will have a greater than 50% stenosis of the carotid artery on the side of the brain lesion. Such patients have a greater than average risk of stroke recurrence. For those without major residual disability, removal of the stenosis has been shown to reduce the overall risk of recurrence, although the operation itself carries about a 5% risk of stroke (see Box 27.12). Surgery is most effective in patients with more severe stenoses (70–99%) and in those in whom it is performed within the first couple of weeks after the TIA or ischaemic stroke. Carotid angioplasty and stenting are technically feasible but have not been shown to be as effective as endarterectomy for the

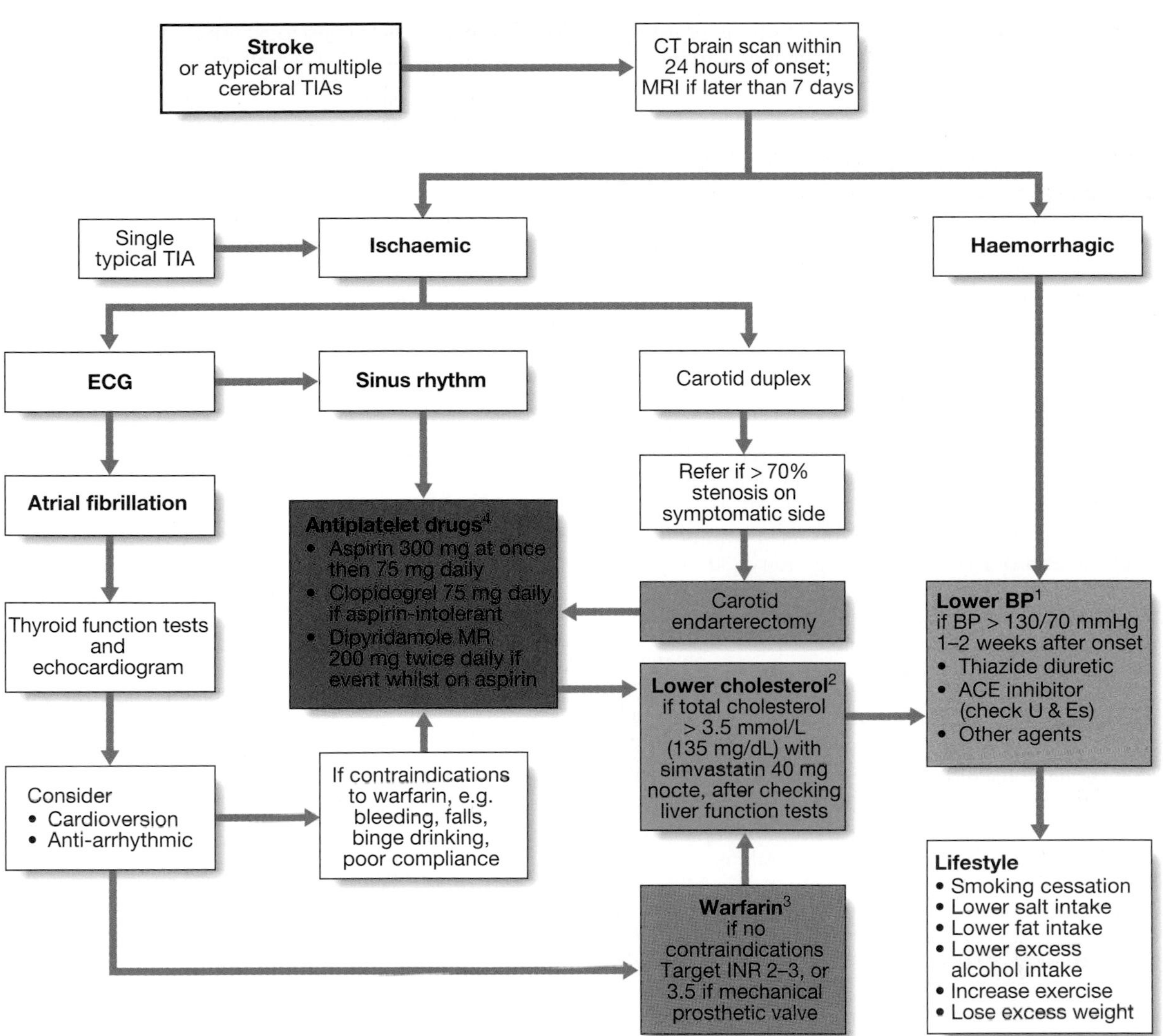

Fig. 27.11 Strategies for secondary prevention of stroke. (1) Lower BP with caution in patients with postural hypotension, renal impairment or bilateral carotid stenosis. (2) Pravastatin 40 mg can be used as an alternative to simvastatin in patients on warfarin or digoxin. (3) Warfarin and aspirin can be used in combination in patients with prosthetic heart valves. (4) The combination of aspirin and clopidogrel is only indicated in patients with unstable angina who demonstrate ECG or enzyme changes.

EBM 27.12 Strategies for secondary prevention

Treatment	Target group	Approximate proportion of patients eligible for treatment	NNT to prevent 1 recurrent stroke
Antiplatelet drugs (clopidogrel, aspirin/dipyridamole[1]	Ischaemic stroke or TIA (in sinus rhythm)	90%	100
Statins[2]	Ischaemic stroke or TIA	80%	60
Blood pressure-lowering[3]	All stroke (ischaemic or haemorrhagic) with blood pressure > 130/80 mmHg	60%	50
Anticoagulation with warfarin (or newer oral anticoagulant)[4]	Ischaemic stroke patients in atrial fibrillation	20%	15
Carotid endarterectomy[5]	Ischaemic stroke or TIA Recently symptomatic severe carotid stenosis	< 10%	15

- [1]Antithrombotic Trialists' Collaboration. BMJ 2002; 324:71–86.
- [2]Heart Protection Study Collaborative Group. Lancet 2002; 360:7–22 and SPARCL investigators. N Engl J Med 2006; 355:549–559.
- [3]PROGRESS Collaborative Group. Lancet 2001; 358:1033–1041.
- [4]Lip GYH, et al. Lancet 2012; 379:648–661.
- [5]Rothwell PM, et al. Lancet 2003; 361:107–116.

For further information: www.cochrane.org/cochrane-reviews

majority of eligible patients. Endarterectomy of asymptomatic carotid stenosis has been shown to reduce the subsequent risk of stroke, but the small absolute benefit does not justify its routine use.

SUBARACHNOID HAEMORRHAGE

Subarachnoid haemorrhage (SAH) is less common than ischaemic stroke or intracerebral haemorrhage (see Fig. 27.1) and affects about 6/100000 of the population. Women are affected more commonly than men and the condition usually presents before the age of 65. The immediate mortality of aneurysmal SAH is about 30%; survivors have a recurrence (or rebleed) rate of about 40% in the first 4 weeks and 3% annually thereafter.

Eighty-five percent of SAH are caused by saccular or 'berry' aneurysms arising from the bifurcation of cerebral arteries (see Fig. 27.2), particularly in the region of the circle of Willis. The most common sites are in the anterior communicating artery (30%), posterior communicating artery (25%) or middle cerebral artery (20%). There is an increased risk in first-degree relatives of those with saccular aneurysms, and in patients with polycystic kidney disease (p. 505) and congenital connective tissue defects such as Ehlers–Danlos syndrome (p. 1045). In about 10% of cases, SAH are non-aneurysmal haemorrhages (so-called perimesencephalic haemorrhages), which have a very characteristic appearance on CT and a benign outcome in terms of mortality and recurrence. Five percent of SAH are due to arteriovenous malformations and vertebral artery dissection.

Clinical features

SAH typically presents with a sudden, severe, 'thunderclap' headache (often occipital), which lasts for hours or even days, often accompanied by vomiting, raised blood pressure and neck stiffness or pain. It commonly occurs on physical exertion, straining and sexual excitement. There may be loss of consciousness at the onset, so SAH should be considered if a patient is found comatose. About 1 patient in 8 with a sudden severe headache has SAH and, in view of this, all who present in this way require investigation to exclude it (Fig. 27.12).

On examination, the patient is usually distressed and irritable, with photophobia. There may be neck stiffness due to subarachnoid blood but this may take some hours to develop. Focal hemisphere signs, such as hemiparesis or aphasia, may be present at onset if there is an associated intracerebral haematoma. A third nerve palsy may be present due to local pressure from an aneurysm of the posterior communicating artery, but this is rare. Fundoscopy may reveal a subhyaloid haemorrhage, which represents blood tracking along the subarachnoid space around the optic nerve.

Investigations

CT brain scanning and lumbar puncture are required. The diagnosis of SAH can be made by CT, but a negative result does not exclude it, since small amounts of blood in the subarachnoid space cannot be detected by CT (see Fig. 27.12). Lumbar puncture should be performed 12 hours after symptom onset if possible, to allow detection of xanthochromia (p. 1153). If either of these tests is positive, cerebral angiography (see Fig. 27.5) is required to determine the optimal approach to prevent recurrent bleeding.

Management

Nimodipine (30–60 mg IV for 5–14 days, followed by 360 mg orally for a further 7 days) is usually given to prevent delayed ischaemia in the acute phase. Insertion of platinum coils into an aneurysm (via an endovascular procedure) or surgical clipping of the aneurysm neck reduces the risk of both early and late recurrence. Coiling is associated with fewer perioperative complications and better outcomes than surgery; where

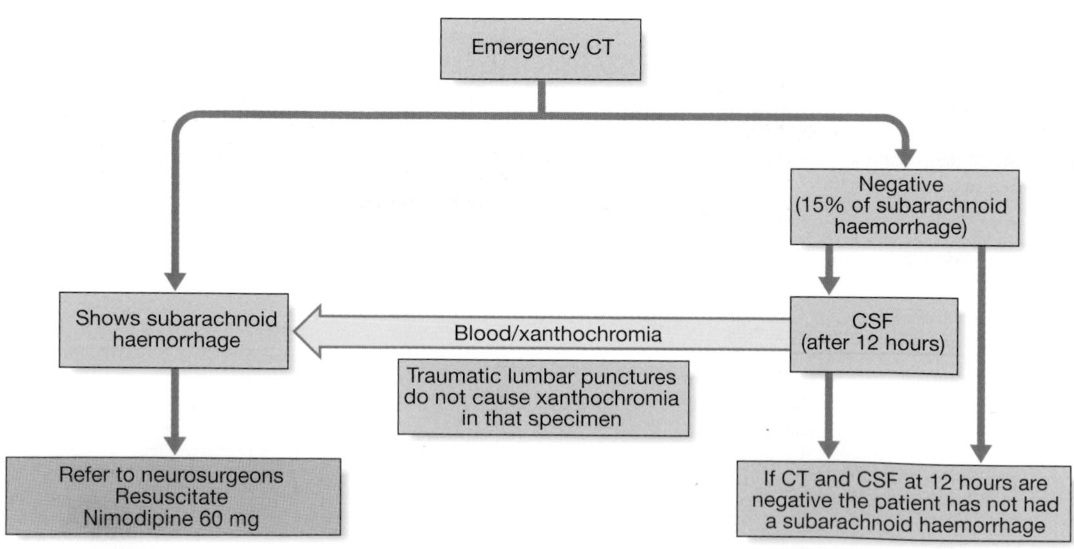

Fig. 27.12 Investigation of subarachnoid haemorrhage.

feasible, it is now the procedure of first choice. Arteriovenous malformations can be managed either by surgical removal, by ligation of the blood vessels that feed or drain the lesion, or by injection of material to occlude the fistula or draining veins. Treatment may also be required for complications of SAH, which include obstructive hydrocephalus (that may require drainage via a shunt), delayed cerebral ischaemia due to vasospasm (which may be treated with vasodilators), hyponatraemia (best managed by fluid restriction) and systemic complications associated with immobility, such as chest infection and venous thrombosis.

CEREBRAL VENOUS DISEASE

Thrombosis of the cerebral veins and venous sinuses (cerebral venous thrombosis) is much less common than arterial thrombosis. However, it has been recognised with increasing frequency in recent years, as access to non-invasive imaging of the venous sinuses using MR venography has increased. The main causes are listed in Box 27.13.

Clinical features

Cerebral venous sinus thrombosis usually presents with symptoms of raised intracranial pressure, seizures and focal neurological symptoms. The clinical features vary according to the sinus involved (Box 27.14 and see Fig. 27.3, p. 1235). Cortical vein thrombosis presents with focal cortical deficits such as aphasia and hemiparesis (depending on the area affected), and epilepsy (focal or generalised). The deficit can increase if spreading thrombophlebitis occurs.

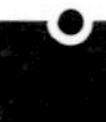

27.13 Causes of cerebral venous thrombosis

Predisposing systemic causes	
• Dehydration	• Thrombophilia (p. 1001)
• Pregnancy	• Hypotension
• Behçet's disease (p. 1119)	• Oral contraceptive use
Local causes	
• Paranasal sinusitis	• Facial skin infection
• Meningitis, subdural empyema	• Otitis media, mastoiditis
• Penetrating head and eye wounds	• Skull fracture

27.14 Clinical features of cerebral venous thrombosis

Cavernous sinus thrombosis
• Proptosis, ptosis, headache, external and internal ophthalmoplegia, papilloedema, reduced sensation in trigeminal first division • Often bilateral, patient ill and febrile
Superior sagittal sinus thrombosis
• Headache, papilloedema, seizures • Clinical features may resemble idiopathic intracranial hypertension (p. 1217) • May involve veins of both hemispheres, causing advancing motor and sensory focal deficits
Transverse sinus thrombosis
• Hemiparesis, seizures, papilloedema • May spread to jugular foramen and involve cranial nerves 9, 10 and 11

Investigations and management

MR venography demonstrates a filling defect in the affected vessel.

Anticoagulation, initially with heparin followed by warfarin, is usually beneficial, even in the presence of venous haemorrhage. In selected patients, the use of endovascular thrombolysis has been advocated. Management of underlying causes and complications, such as persistently raised intracranial pressure, is also important.

About 10% of cerebral venous sinus thrombosis, particularly cavernous sinus thrombosis, is associated with infection (most commonly *Staphylococcus aureus*), which necessitates antibiotic treatment. Otherwise, the treatment of choice is anticoagulation.

Further information

Websites

www.eso-stroke.org/pdf/ESO%20Guidelines_update_Jan_2009.pdf *European Stroke Organisation guidelines.*

www.nhs.uk/actfast/pages/stroke.aspx *Details of the FAST (face, arms, speech, time) campaign to raise public awareness of the emergency nature of stroke.*

www.rcplondon.ac.uk/resources/stroke-guidelines *Royal College of Physicians of London stroke guideline.*

www.stroketraining.org *Stroke training awareness and resources website.*

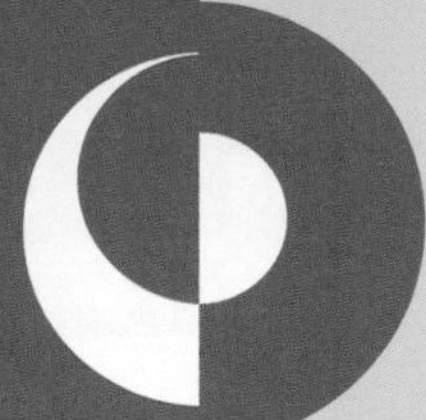

S.H. Ibbotson
R.S. Dawe

Skin disease 28

Clinical examination in skin disease 1250

Functional anatomy and physiology 1252

Investigations 1254

Presenting problems in skin disease 1256

- Lumps – new or changing lesions 1256
- Rashes – papulosquamous eruptions 1257
- Blisters 1258
- Itch (pruritus) 1258
- Photosensitivity 1260
- Leg ulcers 1262
- Abnormal skin colour 1263
- Hair and nail abnormalities 1264
- Acute skin failure 1264

Therapeutics 1264

- Topical treatment of skin disease 1264
- Phototherapy and photochemotherapy 1266
- Systemic therapies 1267
- Dermatological surgery 1268
- Other physical therapies 1268

Skin tumours 1269

- Pathogenesis of skin malignancy 1269
- Malignant tumours 1270
- Benign lesions that may be confused with skin cancers 1274

Common skin infections and infestations 1275

- Bacterial infections 1275
- Viral infections 1278
- Fungal infections 1279
- Scabies 1280
- Lice 1281

Acne and rosacea 1281

Eczemas 1283

Psoriasis and other erythematous scaly eruptions 1286

Lichen planus and lichenoid eruptions 1289

Urticaria 1290

Bullous diseases 1291

- Toxic epidermal necrolysis 1292
- Immunobullous diseases 1292

Pigmentation disorders 1295

- Decreased pigmentation 1295
- Increased pigmentation 1296

Hair disorders 1296

Nail disorders 1297

- Common nail changes and disorders 1297
- Nail changes in systemic disease 1298
- The nail in congenital disease 1299

Skin disease in general medicine 1299

- Conditions involving cutaneous vasculature 1299
- Connective tissue disease 1300
- Granulomatous disease 1301
- Metabolic disease 1301
- Abnormal deposition disorders 1302
- Genetic disorders 1302
- Reactive disorders 1302
- Drug eruptions 1303

CLINICAL EXAMINATION IN SKIN DISEASE

Observation

The patient must be undressed, with make-up and dressings removed, and examined in good lighting. Consider the following:
- Age
- General health
- Distress
- Scratching

1 Distribution of rash
Symmetrical vs asymmetrical
Proximal vs distal vs facial
Localised vs widespread

2 If symmetrical
Extensor, e.g. psoriasis
Flexor, e.g. eczema

3 Involvement of hands, including nail folds and finger webs

4 Nail involvement

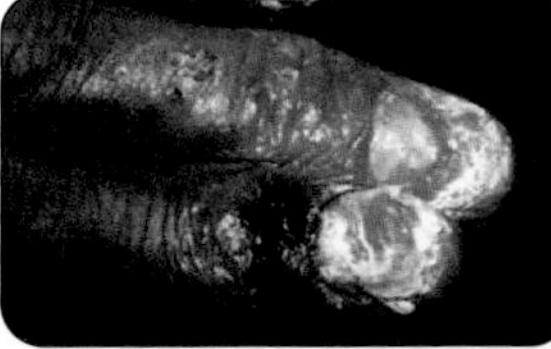

▲ Psoriatic changes in nails and peri-ungual involvement

5 Involvement of axillae/groin
e.g. hidradenitis suppurativa

6 Morphology of rash
Monomorphic or polymorphic

7 Individual lesions
Discrete, grouped, confluent, reticulate (lace-like), linear

8 Morphology of individual lesions
Use a hand lens in good lighting to assist
Use correct terminology, e.g. macules, papules, pustules

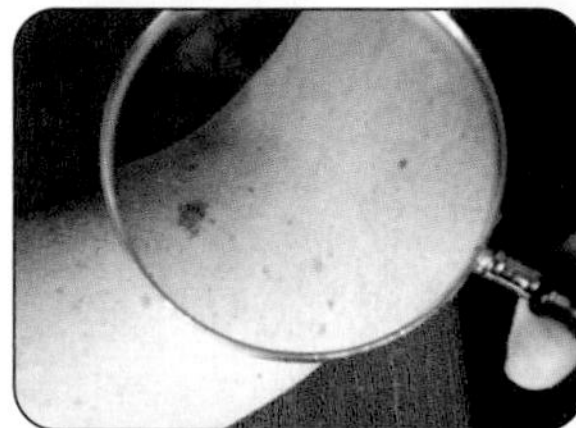

Hand lens ▲

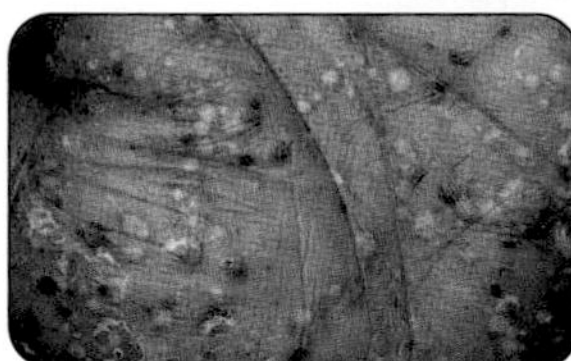

Palmoplantar pustulosis ▲

9 Examination of scalp
Hair loss
Scalp changes

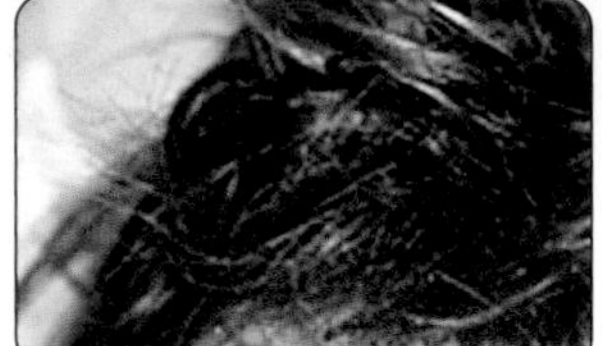

▲ Heavy infestation with head lice

10 Involvement of face
Central
Hairline
Cheeks and nasal bridge: 'butterfly' distribution
Sparing of light-protected sites, e.g. behind ears, under chin

11 Eye involvement
e.g. Conjunctivitis/blepharitis in rosacea or eyelash loss in alopecia areata

12 Oral and genital involvement

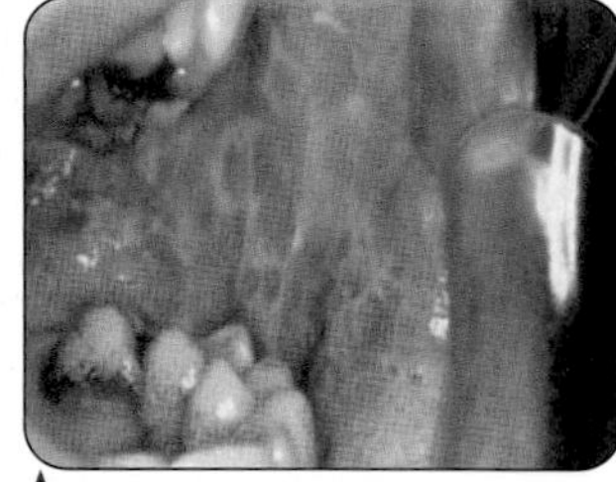

▲ Reticulate (lacy) network on buccal mucosa in lichen planus. May also be genital involvement

13 Joint involvement
e.g. Psoriatic arthritis

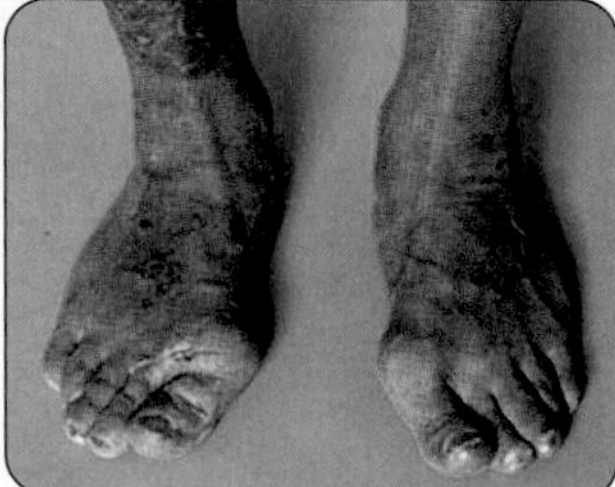

▲ Arthritis, plaque psoriasis and psoriatic nail dystrophy

14 General medical examination
Including lymph nodes and other systems as indicated

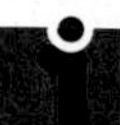

Key points in the history and examination in skin disease

It may be tempting to examine the skin before anything else. This is a mistake; take a history first, and then examine the skin and the rest of the patient.

History

History-taking should follow general principles:
- What was the onset of the condition and what is its course (coming and going, fluctuating severity, persistent, progressing)?
- Are there any excerbating or relieving factors?
- Is there a past history of skin disease, atopy or autoimmune disease?
- What is the patient's medication and allergy history? This is important, as drug-induced eruptions are common
- What is the social history? Several factors, including occupation, might be relevant both in making a diagnosis and in deciding on the best treatment approach
- How does this condition affect my patient? A widespread eruption may have little effect on one individual's quality of life, whereas another person might be severely troubled by what appears to be a minor problem to an outside observer

Examination

- Assessment requires particular emphasis on examination of the skin, hair, nails, mucous membranes and peripheral lymph nodes

Terminology

- Correct use of terminology for examination findings (see below) helps in making a differential diagnosis and allows you to describe the findings so that colleagues can visualise the process

Assessment of disease severity

- Tools for objective assessment of disease severity, such as the Psoriasis Area and Severity Index (PASI) score, can be useful in determining treatment responses (p. 1288)
- Skin disease can have major psychological effects, and the impact on patients can be gauged by dermatology health-related life quality indices, e.g. the Dermatology Life Quality Index (DLQI)

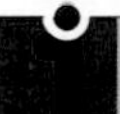

Terms used to describe skin lesions

Lesion types

- **Macule**: a circumscribed flat area of skin of ≤ 1 cm diameter that appears different from the skin surrounding it, usually because of different colour
- **Patch**: the same as a macule but larger (see Fig. 28.38, p. 1295)
- **Papule**: a discrete elevation of skin of ≤ 1 cm diameter (see Fig. 28.23, p. 1279)
- **Nodule**: similar to a papule but having significant depth (into dermis or even subcutaneous layer) and usually > 1 cm in diameter (see Fig. 28.9, p. 1270)
- **Plaque**: a raised area of skin with a flat top, > 1 cm in diameter (see Fig. 28.32A, p. 1287)
- **Vesicle and bulla**: a small (≤ 1 cm) and a larger (> 1 cm in diameter) fluid-filled blister, respectively (see Fig. 28.37A, p. 1294)
- **Pustule**: a visible accumulation of pus in a blister (see opposite)

Other terms

- **Abscess**: a localised collection of pus in a cavity
- **Atrophy**: an area of thin, translucent skin caused by loss of epidermis, dermis or subcutaneous fat, e.g. secondary to excess topical corticosteroids (see Fig. 28.8, p. 1265)
- **Burrow**: a linear or curvilinear papule, caused by a burrowing scabies mite (see Fig. 28.25A, p. 1280)
- **Comedone**: a plug of keratin and sebum in a dilated pilosebaceous orifice
- **Crust**: dried exudate of blood or serous fluid (see Fig. 28.17, p. 1275)
- **Erosion**: an area of skin denuded by complete or partial loss of the epidermis
- **Excoriation**: a linear ulcer or erosion resulting from scratching
- **Fissure**: a slit-shaped deep ulcer, e.g. in irritant dermatitis of the hands
- **Petechiae, purpura and ecchymosis**: petechiae are pinhead-sized, flat macules of extravascular blood in the dermis; purpura are larger and may be palpable; ecchymosis ('bruise') is the term used to describe bleeding that involves deeper structures
- **Scale**: a flake arising from the stratum corneum. Any condition with a thickened stratum corneum, i.e. hyperkeratosis, can cause scaling. An immature thickened and cohesive stratum corneum, e.g. as in psoriasis or Bowen's disease, gives characteristic optical and physical properties that cause a different scale from that due to a thickened, but otherwise normal, stratum corneum (see Fig. 28.11, p. 1271)
- **Scar**: replacement of normal structures by fibrous tissue at the site of an injury
- **Sinus**: a cavity or channel that permits the escape of pus or fluid
- **Stria**: a linear, atrophic, pink, purple or white band caused by connective tissue changes (see Fig. 28.8, p. 1265)
- **Telangiectasia**: visible dilatation of small cutaneous blood vessels (see Fig. 28.9A, p. 1270)
- **Ulcer**: an area from which the epidermis and at least the upper part of the dermis have been lost (see Fig. 28.7, p. 1263)
- **Weal**: an evanescent discrete area of dermal oedema, often centrally white due to masking of local blood supply by fluid; weals can be papules, macules, patches and plaques, and are the hallmark of urticaria (see Fig. 28.34, p. 1291)

Disease affecting the human skin is common, and is important because the absence of normal skin function, as well as sometimes being life-threatening, can severely impair quality of life. This may be exacerbated by the fact that people with skin disease may suffer the effects of stigma, on occasion stemming from others' belief that skin changes are the result of contagious disease.

Skin diseases affect all ages and number more than two thousand. Assessment of the skin is valuable in the management of anyone presenting with any medical problem and, conversely, assessment of the other body systems is important when managing primarily skin disease. This chapter concentrates on those skin diseases seen most frequently and those that are important as components of general medical conditions affecting other organ systems along with the skin. Skin infections, including those related to the human immunodeficiency virus (HIV), are also discussed in Chapters 13, 14 and 15.

FUNCTIONAL ANATOMY AND PHYSIOLOGY

The skin covers just under 2 m^2 in the average adult. The outer layer is the epidermis, a stratified squamous epithelium consisting mainly of keratinocytes. The epidermis is attached to, but separated from, the underlying dermis by the basement membrane. The dermis is less cellular and supports blood vessels, nerves and epidermal-derived appendages (hair follicles and sweat glands). Below it is the subcutis, consisting of adipose tissue.

Epidermis

On most sites, the epidermis is only 0.1–0.2 mm thick, except on the palms or soles where it can extend to several millimetres. Keratinocytes make up approximately 90% of epidermal cells (Fig. 28.1). The main proliferative compartment is the basal layer. Keratinocytes synthesise a range of structural proteins, such as keratins, loricrin and filaggrin (filament aggregating protein), that play key roles in maintaining normal cutaneous physiology. There are more than 50 types of keratin and their expression varies by body site, site within the epidermis and disease state. Mutations of certain keratin genes can result in blistering disorders (p. 1291) and ichthyosis (characterised by scale without major inflammation). As keratinocytes migrate from the basal layer, they differentiate, producing a variety of protein and lipid products. Keratinocytes undergo apoptosis in the granular layer before losing their nuclei and becoming the flattened corneocytes of the stratum corneum (keratin layer). The epidermis is a site of lipid production, and the ability of the stratum corneum to act as a hydrophobic barrier is the result of its 'bricks and mortar' design; dead corneocytes with highly cross-linked protein membranes ('bricks') lie within a metabolically active lipid layer synthesised by keratinocytes ('mortar'). Terminal differentiation of keratinocytes relies on the keratin filaments being aggregated and this is, in part, mediated by filaggrin. Mutations of the filaggrin gene are found in icthyosis vulgaris, and occur in some patients with atopic eczema (p. 1283).

The skin is a barrier against physical stresses. Cell-to-cell attachments must be able to transmit and dissipate stress, a function performed by desmosomes. Diseases that affect desmosomes, such as pemphigus (p. 1294), result in blistering due to keratinocyte separation.

The remaining 10% of epidermal cells are:

- *Langerhans' cells*: dendritic, bone marrow-derived cells that circulate between the epidermis and local lymph nodes. Their prime function is antigen presentation to lymphocytes. Other dermal antigen-presenting dendritic cells are also present.
- *Melanocytes*: predominantly in the basal layer and of neural crest origin. They synthesise the pigment melanin from tyrosine, package it in melanosomes and transfer it to surrounding keratinocytes via their dendritic processes.
- *Merkel cells*: occur in the basal layer and are thought to play a role in signal transduction of fine touch. Their embryological derivation is unclear.

Basement membrane

The basement membrane (see Fig. 28.1) is an anchor for the epidermis and allows movement of cells and nutrients between dermis and epidermis. The cell membrane of the epidermal basal cell is attached to the basement membrane via hemi-desmosomes. The lamina lucida lies immediately below the basal cell membrane and is composed predominantly of laminin. Anchoring filaments extend through the lamina lucida to attach to the lamina densa. This electron-dense layer consists mostly of type IV collagen; from it extend loops of type VII collagen, forming anchoring fibrils that fasten the basement membrane to the dermis.

Dermis

The dermis is vascular and supports the epidermis structurally and nutritionally. It varies in thickness from just over 1 mm on the inner forearm to 4 mm on the back. Fibroblasts are the predominant cells; others include mast cells, mononuclear phagocytes, T lymphocytes, dendritic cells, neurons and endothelial cells. The acellular part of the dermis consists mainly of fibres, including collagen I and III, elastin and reticulin, synthesised by fibroblasts. Support is provided by an amorphous ground substance (mostly glycosaminoglycans, hyaluronic acid and dermatan sulphate), whose production and catabolism are altered by hormonal changes and ultraviolet radiation (UVR). Based on the pattern of collagen fibrils, the superficial dermis is termed the 'papillary dermis', and the deeper, coarser part is the 'reticular dermis'.

Epidermal appendages

Hair follicles

There are 3–5 million hair follicles, epidermal invaginations that develop during the second trimester. They occur throughout the skin, with the exception of palms, soles and parts of the genitalia (glabrous skin). The highest density of hair follicles is on the scalp (500–1000/cm^2). Newborns are covered with fine 'lanugo' hairs, which are usually non-pigmented and lack a central medulla; these are subsequently replaced by vellus hair, which is similar but more likely to be

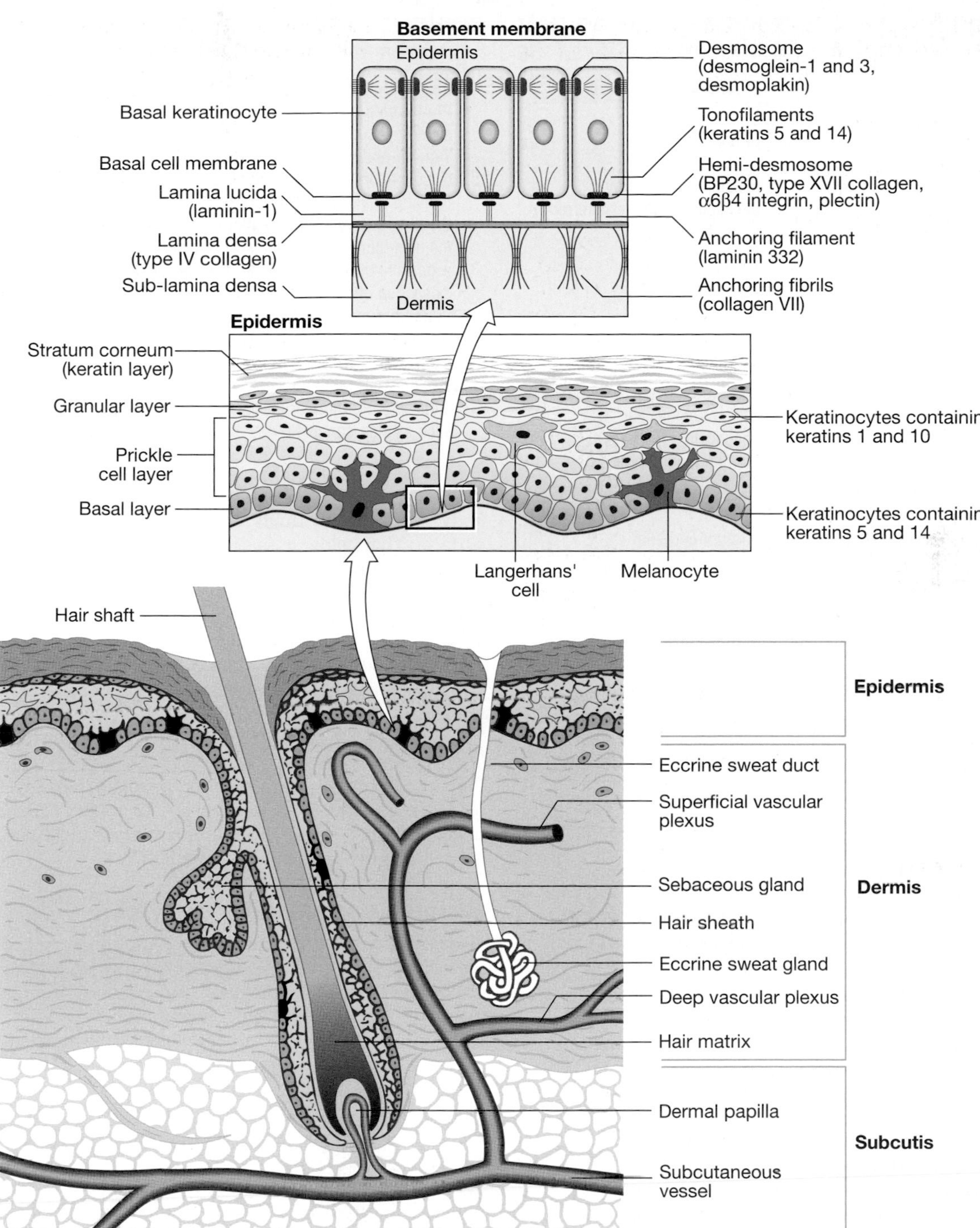

Fig. 28.1 Structure of normal skin.

pigmented. By contrast, scalp hair becomes terminal hair, which is thicker with a central medulla, is usually pigmented and grows longer. At puberty, vellus hairs in hormonally sensitive regions, such as the axillary and genital areas, become terminal.

Human hairs grow in a cycle with three phases: anagen (active hair growth), catagen (transitional phase) and telogen (resting phase). The duration of each phase varies by site. On the scalp, anagen lasts several years, catagen a few days and telogen around 3 months. The length of hair at different sites reflects the differing lengths of anagen.

Sebaceous glands

Sebaceous glands are epidermal downgrowths, usually associated with hair follicles and comprised of modified keratinocytes. The cells of the sebaceous gland (sebocytes) produce a range of lipids, discharging the contents into the duct around the hair follicle. Sebum excretion is under hormonal control, with androgens

28.1 Functions of the skin

Function	Structure/cell involved
Protection against:	
Chemicals, particles, desiccation	Stratum corneum
Ultraviolet radiation (UVR)	Melanin produced by melanocytes and transferred to keratinocytes Stratum corneum hyperproliferation
Antigens, haptens	Langerhans' cells, lymphocytes, mononuclear phagocytes, mast cells, dermal dendritic cells
Microorganisms	Stratum corneum, Langerhans' cells, mononuclear phagocytes, mast cells, dermal dendritic cells
Maintenance of fluid balance	
Prevents loss of water, electrolytes and macromolecules	Stratum corneum
Shock absorber	
Strong, elastic and compliant covering	Dermis and subcutaneous fat
Sensation	Specialised nerve endings mediating pain and withdrawal Itch leading to scratch and (e.g.) removal of a parasite
Vitamin D synthesis	Keratinocytes
Metabolism e.g. Detoxification of xenobiotics, retinoid metabolism, isomerisation of urocanic acid	Predominantly keratinocytes
Temperature regulation	Eccrine sweat glands and blood vessels
Protection, and fine manipulation of small objects	Nails
Hormonal	
Steroidogenesis, testosterone synthesis and conversion to other androgenic steroids	Hair follicles, sebaceous glands
Conversion of thyroxine (T4) to triiodothyronine (T3)	Keratinocytes
Pheromonal	
(Importance unknown in humans)	Apocrine sweat glands, possibly sebaceous glands
Psychosocial, grooming and sexual behaviour	Appearance, tactile quality of skin, hair, nails

increasing it (as do progesterones, to a lesser degree) and oestrogens reducing it. In animals, sebum is important for hair waterproofing but its role in humans is unclear.

Sweat glands

Eccrine sweat glands develop in the second trimester and are also epidermal invaginations found all over the body. Their coiled ducts open directly on to the skin surface. They play a major role in thermoregulation and, unusually, are innervated by cholinergic fibres of the sympathetic nervous system. Eccrine glands of the palms and soles are innervated differently and are activated in the 'fight or flight' response. Apocrine sweat glands are restricted to the axillae and the mammary and genital areas, are connected to hair follicles and are not involved in thermoregulation.

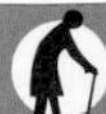

28.2 Skin changes in old age

- **Chronological ageing**: due to the intrinsic ageing process.
- **Photoageing**: due to cumulative UVR exposure and superimposed on intrinsic ageing.
- **Typical changes include**: atrophy, laxity, yellow discoloration, wrinkling, dryness, irregular pigmentation, and thinning and greying of hair.
- **Causes**: age-related alterations in structure and function of the skin, cumulative effects of environmental insults, especially UVR and smoking, cutaneous consequences of disease in other organ systems.
- **Consequences**: reduction in immune and inflammatory responses, reduction in absorption and clearance of topical medications, reduced healing, increased susceptibility to irritants, dermatitis, adverse drug effects (including topical corticosteroid-induced atrophy and purpura) and diseases such as skin cancer.

Nails

Fingernail growth commences at approximately 8 weeks of gestation and is complete by 32 weeks. Toenails develop slightly later. The anatomy of the nail apparatus is covered later in the chapter (p. 1297).

Blood vessels and nerves

Human skin has a plentiful blood supply, arranged in superficial and deep plexuses consisting of arterioles, arterial and venous capillaries, and venules. The upper plexus in the papillary dermis communicates with the lower plexus at the junction between the dermis and the subcutis. Capillary loops arise from terminal arterioles in the horizontal papillary plexus. Blood vessels are supplied by sympathetic and parasympathetic nerves, with the relative contributions of the pathways differing by site. Sympathetic signals are important in mediating autonomic-induced vasoconstriction. The blood supply of skin is far greater than that required for normal skin physiology and reflects the importance of skin in thermoregulation.

Functions of the skin

The skin has many functions, all of which can be affected by disease (Box 28.1). Skin changes associated with ageing are shown in Box 28.2.

INVESTIGATIONS

Magnifying glass

A hand lens used under good lighting conditions (ideally daylight) is valuable in examination of the skin.

Wood's light

Wood's light is a long-wavelength ultraviolet A/short-wavelength visible (violet) light source that can be used in various ways. In hypopigmentation, such as in vitiligo, it can help in appreciating the extent of disease. In pigmented conditions, such as melasma, it can determine whether pigmentation is mainly epidermal (sharp cut-off under Wood's lamp) or mixed epidermal and dermal (ill-defined cut-off). Wood's lamp can also be used to help with the diagnosis of some fungal infections because of their characteristic fluorescence.

Dermatoscopy and diascopy

Dermatoscopy (also known as dermoscopy and epiluminescence microscopy) is increasingly performed with hand-held dermatoscopes. What makes dermatoscopy unique is the fact that it allows visualisation through contact of a glass plate on the instrument with a liquid film applied to the skin, or through special optics to allow non-contact dermatoscopy, enabling deeper structures to be seen without interference by reflection and refraction of light in the epidermis.

Diascopy is simply pressing on the lesion with a glass slide. This provides some of the effect of dermatoscopy, but is mainly used to remove blood from vascular lesions to make the appearance of the lesion clearer.

Histopathology

Histopathological examination of skin biopsies is especially useful for tumour diagnosis. When a dermatologist or pathologist with dermatopathology expertise is involved, it can also assist in the diagnosis of inflammatory skin diseases. It is rare for histopathology of a previously undiagnosed inflammatory skin disease to provide a diagnosis on its own; clinico-pathological correlation is key. Most biopsies are stained with haematoxylin and eosin, but other stains may be useful in special situations, such as for fungal hyphae, iron or mucin. Direct immunofluorescence can also be undertaken on a fresh skin biopsy, allowing antigen visualisation using fluorescein-labelled antibodies; this is especially important in the diagnosis of autoimmune bullous disorders.

Microbiology

Bacteriology

Bacterial swabs may identify a causative infective agent. However, organisms identified from the skin surface may not be implicated in the underlying disease but reflect colonisation of skin damaged by a primary disease. Potential pathogens grown from the skin surface are not always the cause. For example, cellulitis is nearly always caused by pyogenic streptococci, whereas a surface skin swab will often show *Staphylococcus aureus*, which may not be the cause of the cellulitis.

Virology

A number of techniques, including immunofluorescence and polymerase chain reaction (PCR), are available to diagnose herpes simplex or herpes zoster viruses from vesicle fluid (p. 139).

Mycology

Scale, nail clippings (or scrapings of crumbly subungual hyperkeratosis) and plucked hairs can be examined by light microscopy. If potassium hydroxide and a simple light microscope are available, this can be performed in any outpatient clinic. Microbiology laboratories will also examine samples and can culture for fungi and yeasts.

Patch testing

Patch testing investigates delayed, cell-mediated, type IV hypersensitivity, which manifests as dermatitis. It is a provocation test with potential allergens (see Box 28.26, p. 1285) applied, at concentrations and in vehicles to minimise false positive and false negative reactions, under occlusion to the back for 48 hours before examination. When interpreting patch test readings, it is important to determine the clinical relevance of any allergic reactions before giving avoidance advice.

Photopatch testing is similar to patch testing, but investigates delayed hypersensitivity to an agent (usually a sunscreen or a non-steroidal anti-inflammatory (NSAID)) after the absorption of UVR. It involves applying substances in duplicate and irradiating one set with UVR (typically UVA, 5 J/cm^2), with readings then conducted in a similar manner to patch testing.

Prick tests and specific immunoglobulin E testing

Prick tests are used to investigate cutaneous type I (immediate) hypersensitivity to various antigens such as pollen, house dust mite or dander. Skin is pricked with commercially available stylets through a dilution of the appropriate antigen solution (p. 90). Alternatively, specific immunoglobulin E (IgE) levels to antigens can be measured in serum, and occasionally challenge tests are undertaken (p. 90).

Phototesting

Phototesting is important for assessing suspected photosensitivity. The mainstay investigation is monochromator phototesting, which involves exposing the patient's back to increasing doses of irradiation using narrow wavebands across the solar spectrum and then assessing responses, using the minimal erythema dose (MED) at each waveband. This is the dose required to cause just perceptible skin reddening and is compared with values for the normal population. If a patient has reduced MEDs (i.e. develops erythema at lower doses than healthy subjects), this indicates abnormal photosensitivity. Thus, monochromator phototesting can be used to determine whether a patient is abnormally photosensitive, which wavebands are involved and how sensitive the patient is (p. 1260). Provocation testing can be performed with a broadband (usually UVA) source to induce rash at a test site (most useful for polymorphic light eruption) and can be helpful for diagnosis.

Patients who are referred for phototherapy will also usually undergo an MED test, in which they are exposed to a series of test doses of the light source that will be used therapeutically (often narrowband UVB), and the MED is determined 24 hours later (or 72–96 hours for the psoralen–ultraviolet A (PUVA) minimal phototoxic dose) (p. 1266). This allows treatment regimens to be individualised, based on a patient's erythemal responses, and may detect abnormal photosensitivity.

PRESENTING PROBLEMS IN SKIN DISEASE

The major presentations in dermatology are outlined below. Detail about the underlying disorders is mostly provided in the disease-specific sections later on.

Lumps – new or changing lesions

A 'new or changed lesion' is one of the key dermatology presentations. The challenge is to distinguish between benign and malignant disease (p. 1269). Detailed history-taking and examination are essential:

- *Lesion*: Is this new or has a pre-existing lesion changed? What is the nature of the change - is it in size, colour, shape or surface? Has change been rapid or slow? Are there other features - pain, itch, inflammation, bleeding or ulceration?
- *Patient*: What is the patient's age? Are they fair-skinned and freckled? Has there been much sun exposure? Have they used sunbeds or lived in sunny climates? Have they used photoprotection?
- *Site*: Is it sun-exposed or covered? The scalp, face, upper limbs and back in men, and face, hands and lower legs in women, are the most chronically sun-exposed sites.
- *Are there other similar lesions?* These might include actinic keratoses (see Fig. 28.11, p. 1271) or basal cell papillomas (see Fig. 28.15, p. 1274).
- *Morphology of the lesion*: Tenderness, size, symmetry, regularity of border, colour, surface characteristics and the presence of features such as crust, scale and ulceration must be assessed. Stretching the skin and using a magnifying lens can be helpful, e.g. in detecting the raised, pearled edge of a basal cell carcinoma (p. 1270).
- *Dermatoscopy*: This can be used to detect the presence of abnormal vessels, such as in basal cell carcinoma or the characteristic keratin cysts in basal cell papillomas. It is invaluable for assessing pigmented and vascular lesions (Fig. 28.2).

Is it a melanocytic naevus or a malignant melanoma?

This is a common differential and one that it is critical to resolve correctly.

- The precise nature of the change should be determined (as above). Listen to the patient and pay attention to subtle changes, as patients know their skin well.

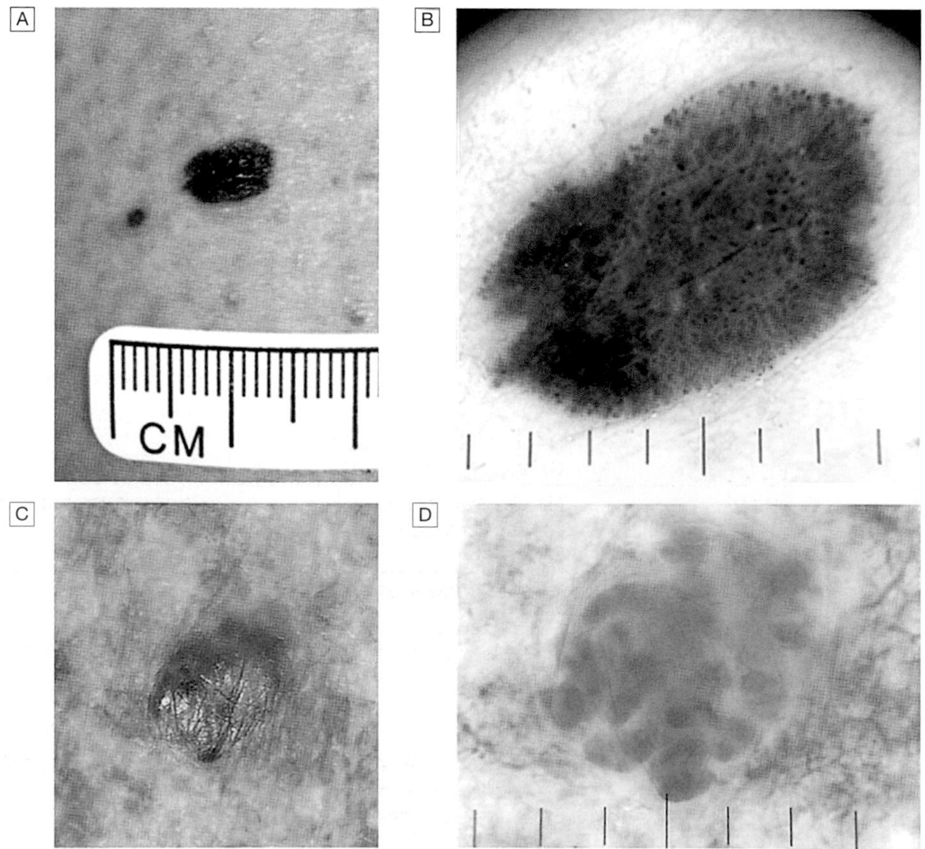

Fig. 28.2 Dermatoscopy. **A** A changing lesion. **B** Dermatoscopy highlights the abnormal pigment network and other features suggestive of melanoma. Excision biopsy confirmed the diagnosis of superficial spreading malignant melanoma (Breslow thickness 0.8 mm). **C** Another changing lesion. **D** Dermatoscopy highlights the vascular lacunae of this benign angioma and the patient was reassured.

- If the patient has other pigmented lesions, then these should be examined too, as they may be informative. For example, if the presenting lesion looks different from the others, then suspicion is needed; conversely, if the patient has multiple basal cell papillomas, this may be reassuring - although do not be falsely reassured.
- Is there a positive family history of melanoma? A suspicious naevus in a patient with a first-degree relative with melanoma probably warrants excision.

The ABCDE 'rule' is a guide to the characteristic features of melanoma (Box 28.3 and see Fig. 28.2), although, ideally, melanomas should be diagnosed before the diameter is greater than 0.5 cm. Loss of normal skin markings in a pigmented lesion may be suggestive of melanoma. Conversely, normal skin markings and fine hairs dispersed evenly over a lesion are reassuring but do not exclude melanoma. The Glasgow seven-point checklist is another useful guide:

- major features: change in size, shape and colour
- minor features: diameter over 0.5 cm, inflammation, oozing or bleeding, and itch or altered sensation.

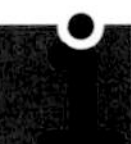

28.3 ABCDE features of malignant melanoma

- **A**symmetry
- **B**order irregular
- **C**olour irregular
- **D**iameter > 0.5 cm
- **E**levation irregular

(+ Loss of skin markings)

Rashes – papulosquamous eruptions

A rash is the other common presentation in dermatology. The main categories of scaly rashes are listed in Box 28.4. Diagnosis can often be made on clinical grounds, although a biopsy may be required. Important aspects of the history are:

- *Age at onset and duration of rash?* For example, atopic eczema often starts in early childhood and psoriasis between 15 and 40 years, and both may be chronic. Infective or drug-induced rashes are more likely to be of short duration and the latter occur in relation to drug ingestion. Duration of individual lesions is also important, as, for example, in urticaria.
- *Body site at onset and distribution?* For example, flexural sites are involved in atopic eczema and extensor surfaces and scalp in psoriasis. Symmetry is often indicative of an endogenous disease, such as psoriasis, whereas asymmetry is more common with exogenous causes, such as contact dermatitis or infections like herpes zoster.
- *Is it itchy?* For example, eczema is usually extremely itchy and psoriasis less so.
- *Was there a preceding illness or were systemic symptoms present?* Examples include guttate psoriasis precipitated by a β-haemolytic streptococcal throat infection; almost all patients with infectious mononucleosis (p. 320) treated with amoxicillin will develop an erythematous maculopapular eruption; the rash of secondary syphilis follows a history

28.4 Causes and clinical features of common scaly rashes

Diagnosis	Distribution	Morphology	Associated signs
Atopic eczema (p. 1283)	Face and flexures	Poorly defined erythema, scaling Vesicles Lichenification if chronic	Shiny nails Infra-orbital crease 'Dirty neck' (grey-brown discoloration)
Psoriasis (p. 1286)	Extensor surfaces Lower back	Well-defined Erythematous plaques Silvery scale	Nail pitting, onycholysis Scalp involvement Axillae and genital areas often affected Joint involvement Köbner phenomenon
Pityriasis rosea (p. 1289)	'Fir tree' pattern on trunk	Well-defined Small, erythematous plaques Collarette of scale	Herald patch
Drug eruption (p. 1303)	Widespread	Macules and papules Erythema and scale Exfoliation	Possible mucosal involvement or erythroderma
Pityriasis versicolor (p. 1280)	Upper trunk and shoulders	Hypo- and hyper-pigmented scaly patches	
Lichen planus (p. 1289)	Distal limbs Flexural aspect of wrists Lower back	Shiny, flat-topped, violaceous papules Wickham's striae	White lacy network on buccal mucosa Nail changes Scarring alopecia Köbner phenomenon
Tinea corporis (p. 1279)	Asymmetrical Often isolated lesions	Erythematous, often annular plaques Peripheral scale (sometimes pustules) Expansion with central clearing	Possible associated nail, scalp, groin involvement
Secondary syphilis (p. 419)	Trunk and proximal limbs Palms and soles	Red macules and papules, which become 'gun-metal' grey	History of chancre Systemic symptoms, e.g. malaise and fever

of chancre at the site of inoculation; malaise and arthralgia are common in drug eruptions and vasculitis.

The morphology of the rash and the characteristics of individual lesions are important (see Box 28.4).

Blisters

There are a limited number of conditions that present with blisters (Box 28.5). Blistering occurs due to loss of cell adhesion within the epidermis or sub-epidermal region (see Fig. 28.1, p. 1253), and the clinical presentation depends on the site or level of blistering within the skin, which in turn reflects the underlying pathogenesis (p. 1291):

- Intact blisters are not often seen if the split is high in the epidermis (below the stratum corneum), as the blister roof is so fragile that it ruptures easily, leaving erosions (e.g. pemphigus foliaceus, staphylococcal scalded skin syndrome (see Fig. 28.18, p. 1276) and bullous impetigo).
- If the split is lower in the epidermis, then intact flaccid blisters and erosions may be seen (e.g. pemphigus vulgaris and toxic epidermal necrolysis (see Fig. 28.36, p. 1292)).
- If the split is sub-epidermal, then tense-roofed blisters occur (e.g. bullous pemphigoid (see Fig. 28.37, p. 1294), epidermolysis bullosa acquisita and porphyria cutanea tarda (see Fig. 28.47, p. 1302)).
- If there are foci of separation at different levels of the epidermis, as in a dermatitis (p. 1283), multilocular bullae (made up of coalescing vesicles) occur.

A history of onset, progression, mucosal involvement, drugs and systemic symptoms should be taken. Clinical assessment of the distribution, extent and morphology of the rash should then be made. The Nikolsky sign is useful: sliding pressure from a finger on normal-looking epidermis can dislodge the epidermis in conditions with intra-epidermal defects, such as pemphigus and toxic epidermal necrolysis.

28.5 Causes of acquired blisters

	Localised	Generalised
Vesicular	Herpes simplex Herpes zoster Impetigo Pompholyx	Eczema herpeticum* Dermatitis herpetiformis Acute eczema
Bullous	Impetigo Cellulitis Stasis oedema Acute eczema Insect bites Fixed drug eruption	Toxic epidermal necrolysis* Erythema multiforme Stevens–Johnson syndrome* Bullous pemphigoid Pemphigus* Epidermolysis bullosa acquisita Lupus erythematosus Porphyria cutanea tarda/ pseudoporphyria Drug eruptions

*Usually also mucosal involvement.

A systematic approach to diagnosis is required:

1. *Exclude infection*: e.g. herpes simplex, varicella zoster or *Staph. aureus*.
2. *Consider common skin disorders in which blistering* uncommonly *occurs*: e.g. severe peripheral oedema, cellulitis, allergic contact dermatitis and eczema.
3. *Remember that bullae may develop in drug eruptions*: e.g. fixed drug eruption (p. 1303), erythema multiforme (p. 1302) and vasculitis (p. 1115). Toxic epidermal necrolysis (TEN) is a medical emergency (p. 1292).
4. *Consider immunobullous disease* (p. 1292): the age of the patient may be informative (see Box 28.35, p. 1293).

Investigations and management are guided by the clinical presentation and differential diagnosis, and are described in this chapter under the specific diseases.

Itch (pruritus)

Itch is an unpleasant sensation that leads to scratching or rubbing. The terms 'itch' and 'pruritus' are synonymous; however, 'pruritus' is often used when itch is generalised. Itch can arise from primary cutaneous disease or from systemic disease, which may cause itch by central or peripheral mechanisms. Even when the mechanism is peripheral, there are not always signs of primary skin disease.

The nerve endings that signal itch are in the epidermis or near the dermo–epidermal junction. Transmission is by unmyelinated slow-conducting C fibres through the spinothalamic tract to the thalamus and then the cortex. There is an inhibitory relationship between pain and itch. Scratching either causes inhibition of itch receptors by stimulating ascending sensory pathways that inhibit itch at the spinal cord (Wall's 'gate' mechanism), or interferes directly with cutaneous itch fibres by direct damage.

The mechanisms of itch in most systemic diseases remain unclear. The itch of kidney disease, for example, may be mediated by circulating endogenous opioids. The clinical observation that peritoneal dialysis helps reduce itch more frequently than haemodialysis is consistent with this, smaller molecules generally being dialysed more readily if the peritoneal membrane is used rather than a dialysis machine membrane.

Clinical assessment

Diagnosis is important and full assessment, through history, examination and, sometimes, investigations, is necessary. When a patient presents with generalised

28.6 Primary skin diseases causing pruritus

Generalised pruritus

- Scabies
- Eczemas
- Pre-bullous pemphigoid
- Urticarias
- Xeroderma of old age
- Psoriasis

Localised pruritus

- Eczemas
- Lichen planus
- Dermatitis herpetiformis
- Pediculosis
- Tinea infections

28.7 Secondary causes of pruritus

Medical condition	Cause of pruritus	Treatment*
Liver disease	Central opioid effect Elevation in bile salts may contribute	Naltrexone Colestyramine Rifampicin Sedative antihistamines UVB
Renal failure	Unknown; uraemia contributes	UVB Oral activated charcoal
Haematological disease		
Anaemia	Iron deficiency	Iron replacement
Polycythaemia rubra vera	Unknown (often aquagenic pruritus)	
Lymphoma Leukaemia Myeloma	Unknown	
Endocrine disease		
Diabetes mellitus	Increased infection risk, e.g. candidiasis, tinea	Treatment of infection
Thyrotoxicosis	Unknown	Emollients
Hypothyroidism	Unknown	Emollients
Carcinoid syndrome (p. 782)	5HT-mediated	
HIV infection	Infection, infestation, e.g. *Candida*	Treatment of infection
	Eosinophilic folliculitis	Local corticosteroids, UVB
	Seborrhoeic dermatitis	Anti-pityrosporal treatment
	Unknown	UVB
Malignancy	Unknown	
Psychogenic	Unknown	Psychotherapy, anxiolytics, antidepressants

*In addition to specific treatment of the primary condition. (5-HT = 5-hydroxytryptamine, serotonin).

28.8 Causes of pruritus in pregnancy

Diagnosis	Pregnancy, gestation and features	Treatment
Polymorphic eruption of pregnancy (pruritic urticarial papules and plaques, PUPP)	Typically first pregnancy and uncommonly recurs 3rd trimester, after delivery Polymorphic urticated papules and plaques, start in striae	Chlorphenamine, emollients Topical steroids
Acute cholestasis of pregnancy (p. 977)	3rd trimester and commonly recurs in subsequent pregnancies Abnormal liver function tests Increased fetal and maternal risk	Emollients Chlorphenamine Colestyramine UVB Early delivery
Pemphigoid gestationis	Any stage, often 2nd trimester and commonly recurs in subsequent pregnancies Urticated erythema, blistering initially periumbilical Characteristic histology and immunofluorescence	Topical or oral corticosteroids
Prurigo gestationis	2nd trimester Excoriated papules	Emollients Topical corticosteroids Chlorphenamine UVB
Pruritic folliculitis	3rd trimester Sterile pustules on trunk	Topical corticosteroids UVB

itch, it is important to determine whether skin changes are primary (a process in the skin causing itch) or secondary (skin changes caused by rubbing and scratching because of itch). Many common primary skin disorders are associated with itch (Box 28.6). If itch is not connected with primary skin disease, many causes should be considered (Box 28.7); these include liver diseases (mainly cholestatic diseases, such as primary biliary cirrhosis), malignancies (e.g. generalised itch may be the presenting feature of lymphoma), haematological conditions (e.g. generalised itch in chronic iron deficiency or water contact-provoked (aquagenic) intense itch in polycythaemia), endocrine diseases (including hypo- and hyperthyroidism), chronic kidney disease (in which severity of itch is not always clearly associated with plasma creatinine concentration) and psychogenic causes (such as in 'delusions of infestation'). Pruritus is common in pregnancy and may be due to one of the pregnancy-specific dermatoses. Diagnosis is particularly important in pregnancy, as some disorders can be associated with increased fetal risk (Box 28.8).

Management

There are no consistently effective therapies to suppress itch, regardless of its cause but establishing the diagnosis is the first step. If a clear-cut diagnosis is not apparent, various non-specific approaches can be used for symptom control. It is important to re-assess the patient intermittently in order to avoid missing the diagnosis.

Approaches to symptomatic relief include sedation, often with H_1 antagonist antihistamines; emollients; and counter-irritants (such as topical menthol-containing preparations). UVB phototherapy is useful in itch stemming from a variety of causes, although the only randomised controlled study evidence of its efficacy in generalised itch not caused by a skin disease is for the itch of chronic kidney disease. Other treatments include tricyclic antidepressants (probably through similar mechanisms to those involved when these drugs are used for chronic pain) and opiate antagonists. Itch can be severe and its effects on quality of life are not always appreciated.

Photosensitivity

Cutaneous photosensitivity is an abnormal response of the skin to ultraviolet (UVR) or visible radiation. The sun is the natural source but patients may also be exposed to artificial sources of UVR through the use of sunbeds and/or phototherapy (p. 1266). Chronic UVR exposure increases skin cancer risk and photoageing (p. 1254). Acute exposure can induce erythema (redness) as a normal response (Fig. 28.3). However, abnormal photosensitivity occurs when a patient reacts to lower doses than would normally cause a response, either with a heightened erythemal reaction or the development of a rash. Photoaggravated skin diseases are exacerbated by sunlight but not caused by it. The main photosensitive and photoaggravated diseases are listed in Box 28.9.

Sunlight consists mainly of visible light, and the UVR component is divided into three wavebands (Fig. 28.4):

- *UVC* (280–300 nm), which is absorbed by ozone and does not reach the earth's surface.
- *UVB* (300–320 nm), which constitutes less than 10% of UVR exposure but is around 1000-fold more biologically effective than UVA and so accounts for the erythemal 'sunburning' effects of sunlight.
- *UVA* (320–400 nm), which is the most abundant UVR component reaching the earth's surface.

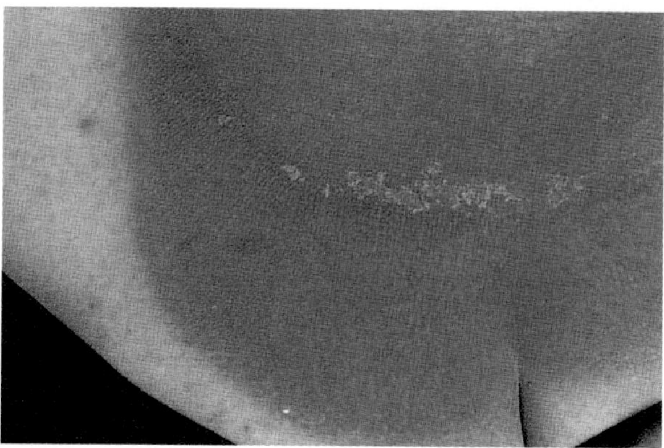

Fig. 28.3 Sunburn. Acute exposure to ultraviolet radiation results in an erythemal response which peaks 12–24 hours later. Sensitivity depends on the individual's constitutive skin phototype.

28.9 The photosensitivity and photoaggravated diseases

Cause	Condition	Clinical features
Idiopathic	Polymorphic light eruption (PLE)	Itchy, papulovesicular rash on photo-exposed sites; face and back of hands often spared. Often hours of UVR exposure needed to provoke; lasts a few days; affects 20% in Northern Europe, more common in young women
	Chronic actinic dermatitis (CAD)	Chronic dermatitis on sun-exposed sites. Most common in elderly males. UVB, UVA and often visible light photosensitivity. Most also have contact allergies
	Solar urticaria	Immediate-onset urticaria on photo-exposed sites, usually UVA and visible light photosensitivity. Can occur at any age
	Actinic prurigo	Uncommon, presents in childhood. Often familial. Some similarities to PLE, although scarring occurs
	Hydroa vacciniforme	Rare childhood photodermatosis. Varioliform scarring
Drugs	Variety of mechanisms	Usually UVA (and visible) light photosensitivity
	Phototoxicity	Most common. Exaggerated sunburn and exfoliation. Many drugs such as thiazides, tetracyclines, fluoroquinolones, quinine, NSAIDs
	Pseudoporphyria	e.g. NSAIDs, retinoids, tetracyclines, furosemide
	Photoallergy	Usually to topical agents, such as sunscreens and NSAIDs
Metabolic	Porphyrias	Mainly porphyria cutanea tarda and erythropoietic protoporphyria (p. 458).
	Pellagra	Photoexposed site dermatitis due to tryptophan deficiency (see Fig. 16.17, p. 459)
Photogenodermatoses	Xeroderma pigmentosum	Rare. Defect in DNA excision repair, abnormal photosensitivity, photoageing and skin cancer. May be neurological features
Photo-aggravation of pre-existing conditions	e.g. Lupus erythematosus	Can also be drug-induced, e.g. by thiazides (see Box 28.44, p. 1304)
	Erythema multiforme	p. 1302
	Rosacea	p. 1283

(NSAID = non-steroidal anti-inflammatory drug)

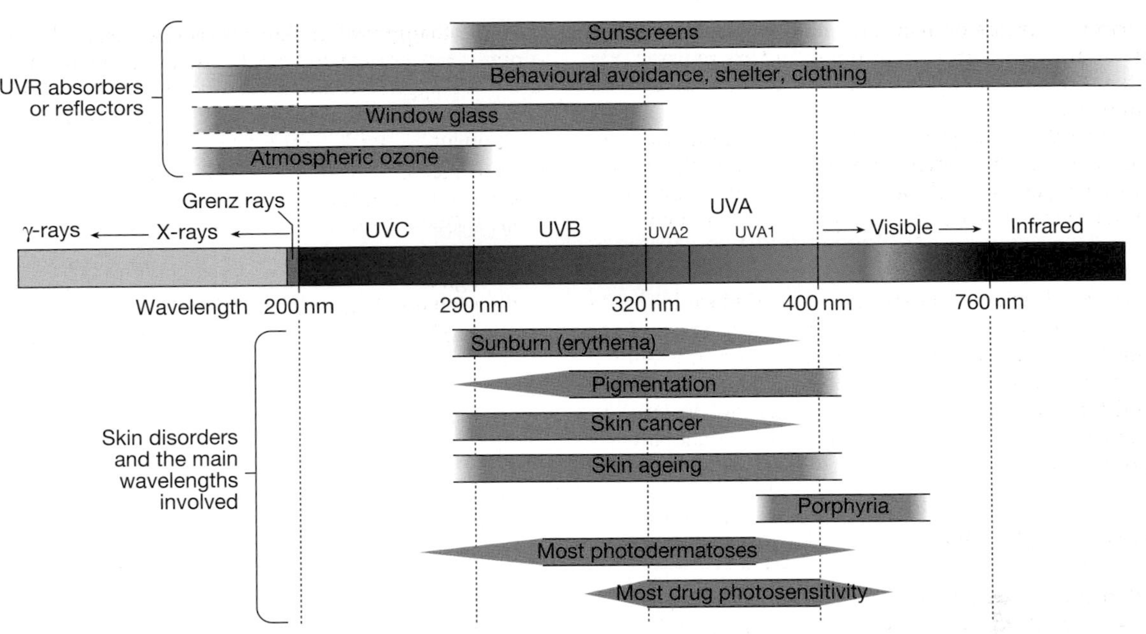

Fig. 28.4 The electromagnetic spectrum. The action spectrum is not well defined for many conditions and, for some, is approximate and may vary between patients. The action spectrum for non-melanoma skin cancer mirrors that for erythema. The action spectrum for melanoma is not known but includes UVB. Photoprotection measures vary, depending on condition, although the mainstay always includes behavioural modification and clothing cover.

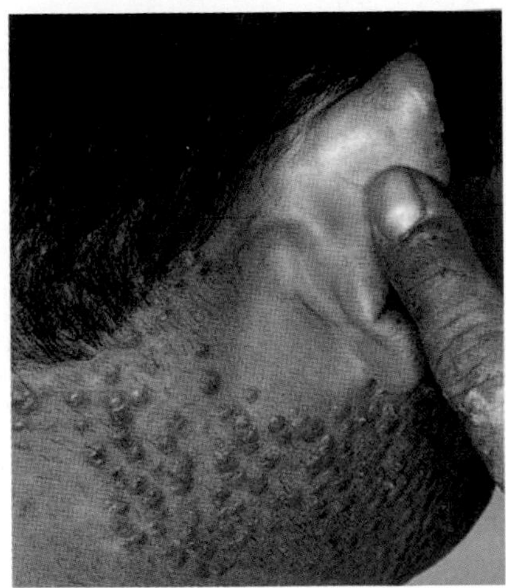

Fig. 28.5 Chronic actinic dermatitis. Note the sharp cut-off and sparing behind the ear in the shadow cast by the earlobe (Wilkinson's triangle).

Patients with photosensitivity diseases can be abnormally sensitive to UVB, UVA, visible light (over 400 nm) or, commonly, a combination of wavebands. UVB is absorbed by window glass, whereas UVA and visible light are transmitted through glass.

Clinical assessment

History-taking is essential, as the patient may not have the rash when assessed. Seasonal pattern and distribution of rash are important. Key sites are the face (particularly nose, cheeks and forehead), top of ears, neck (Fig. 28.5), bald scalp, back of hands and forearms. Sparing is often seen under the chin and nose, behind the ears, on the upper eyelids and the distal digits – as we normally walk about with our eyes open and fingers flexed! It can be misleading if there is covered site involvement (patients who are sensitive to UVA and visible light may be affected through clothing, and some photosensitive conditions, such as actinic prurigo, typically also involve covered sites), or if habitually exposed sites, such as the face, are not involved (this 'hardening' phenomenon is commonly seen in polymorphic light eruption (PLE)). Furthermore, if patients have UVA and/or visible light photosensitivity, they will commonly experience perennial symptoms and may not be aware of the association with daylight exposure. Although some conditions, such as solar urticaria, develop rapidly after sunlight exposure, others, such as cutaneous lupus, can take several days to evolve.

Investigations and management

If photosensitivity is suspected, the patient should be referred to a specialist centre for monochromator phototesting (p. 1255), if feasible. Other investigations will often include provocation, patch or photopatch testing, and screening for lupus and the porphyrias (p. 1301).

Management depends on the diagnosis. If there is a phototoxic drug or chemical cause, this must be addressed: for instance, by stopping the drug or treating the porphyria. Counselling regarding sun avoidance is essential: keeping out of direct sun in the middle of the day, covering up with clothing, wearing hats with a wide brim and careful use of high-factor sunscreens. Paradoxically, in some conditions, particularly PLE and solar urticaria, phototherapy can be used to induce 'hardening'; the mechanism is uncertain. Other approaches may be necessary, depending on disease and severity, and may include antihistamines (useful in two-thirds of patients with solar urticaria) and systemic immunosuppression (sometimes required in the idiopathic photodermatoses). Patients with photosensitivity are at risk of vitamin D deficiency, as UVB-induced cutaneous photosynthesis of vitamin D is an important source (p. 126). Patients should optimise dietary vitamin D intake and take supplements if levels are low (p. 1127).

Sunscreens

Sunscreen agents can be divided into two categories: chemical sunscreens, which absorb specific wavelengths of UVR, and physical sunscreens, which reflect UVR and the shorter visible wavelengths (see Fig. 28.4). Current sunscreen products are highly refined and most contain several sunscreen agents, offering protection against UVB and most UVA wavelengths. If a patient has photosensitivity to the longer wavelengths of UVA and the visible part of the spectrum, then conventional sunscreens that offer maximal protection in the UVB region will not be beneficial and specific reflectant sunscreens will be required. Historically, due to visible light reflection, these agents were less cosmetically acceptable, although current formulations, some of which are tinted, have reduced this problem.

Sunscreen protection levels are described by sun protection factor (SPF). This is the ratio of the dose of UVR required to produce skin erythema in the presence and absence of the sunscreen. Thus, a sunscreen of SPF20 theoretically means that it would take 20 times as long for a person to develop sunburn in the presence of the sunscreen, as compared to not using it. Therefore, SPF is really a sunburn protection factor and is not a good guide to how well a sunscreen will perform in protecting against other reactions (such as skin pain in erythropoietic protoporphyria). SPF values are determined under experimental conditions and, in practice, people use 25–33% of the amount of sunscreen required to achieve the stated SPF – thus, a sunscreen of SPF30 will, in practice, offer an SPF10 at best, and patients need to be counselled regarding application. There is also no such thing as a 'sunblock', as all sunscreens offer, at best, only partial protection and are no substitute for modifying behaviour and covering up.

Leg ulcers

Ulceration of the skin is defined as complete epidermal loss, thus exposing dermal (or deeper) layers. 'Leg ulcer' is not a diagnosis. Making a comprehensive diagnosis is the key to management. Ulcers on the lower leg are frequently caused by vascular disease, particularly, at least in part, venous hypertension. For each cause of leg ulceration there are several different underlying pathologies that have to be considered (Box 28.10).

Clinical assessment

A detailed history of the onset and course of leg ulceration and predisposing conditions should be taken. The site and surrounding skin should be assessed. Varicose veins are often present, although not inevitably. The site of ulceration may help indicate the cause (Fig. 28.6).

Appropriate investigations include:

- *Urinalysis* for glycosuria.
- *Full blood count* to detect anaemia and blood dyscrasias.

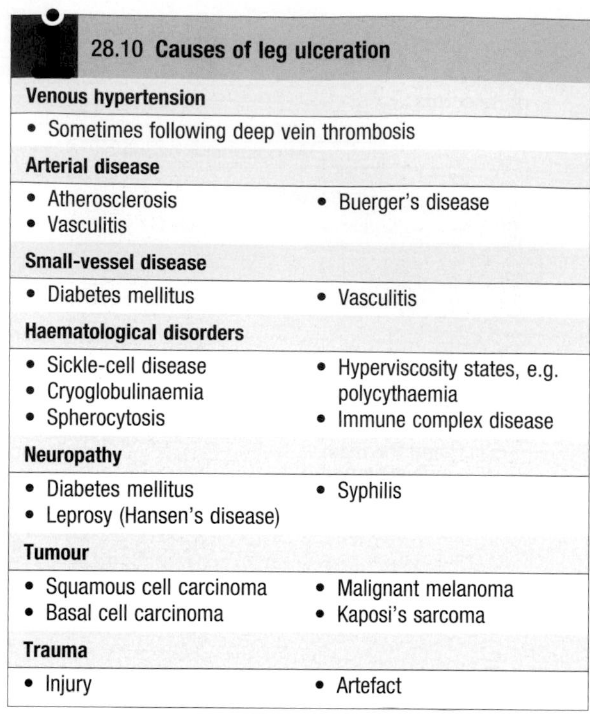

28.10 Causes of leg ulceration

Venous hypertension	
• Sometimes following deep vein thrombosis	
Arterial disease	
• Atherosclerosis • Vasculitis	• Buerger's disease
Small-vessel disease	
• Diabetes mellitus	• Vasculitis
Haematological disorders	
• Sickle-cell disease • Cryoglobulinaemia • Spherocytosis	• Hyperviscosity states, e.g. polycythaemia • Immune complex disease
Neuropathy	
• Diabetes mellitus • Leprosy (Hansen's disease)	• Syphilis
Tumour	
• Squamous cell carcinoma • Basal cell carcinoma	• Malignant melanoma • Kaposi's sarcoma
Trauma	
• Injury	• Artefact

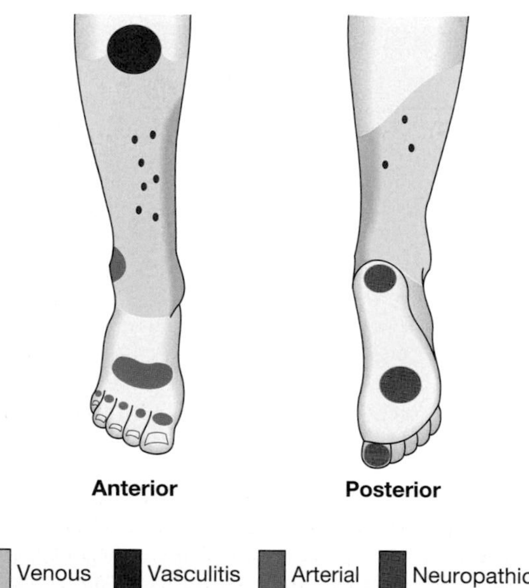

Fig. 28.6 Causes of lower limb ulceration. The main types of leg ulcer tend to affect particular sites.

- *Bacterial swab* if there is a purulent discharge, rapid extension, cellulitis, lymphangitis or septicaemia. This can guide antibiotic therapy for secondary infection but pathogenic bacteria are not always the same as those identified from the ulcer surface.
- *Doppler ultrasound* to assess arterial circulation. The normal ratio of ankle systolic pressure to brachial systolic pressure (ABPI) is 1.1 or more; if it is below 0.8, this suggests significant arterial disease. However, arterial calcification, such as in diabetes, can produce a spuriously high ABPI.

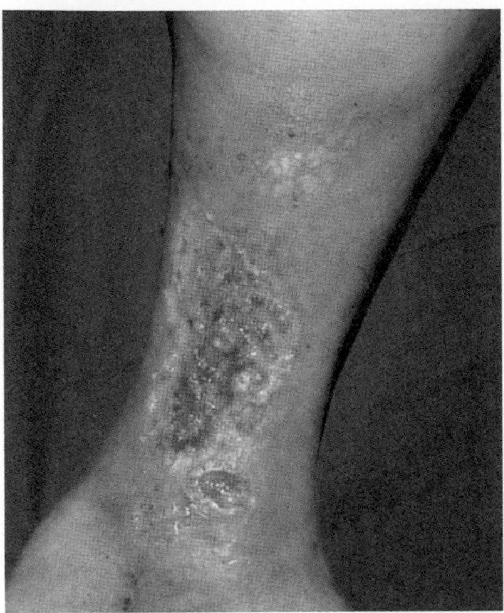

Fig. 28.7 A chronic venous ulcer on the medial lower leg, with surrounding lipodermatosclerosis.

Leg ulceration due to venous disease

Varicose veins, a history of deep venous thrombosis and obesity are predisposing factors. Incompetent valves in the deep and perforating veins of the lower leg result in retrograde flow of blood to the superficial system, and a rise in capillary pressure ('venous hypertension'). Pericapillary fibrin cuffing occurs, leading to impairment of local tissue oxygenation and homeostasis.

The first symptom in venous ulceration is often heaviness of the legs, followed by oedema. Haemosiderin pigmentation, pallor and firmness of surrounding skin, and sometimes venous/gravitational eczema (p. 1285) subsequently develop. This progresses to lipodermatosclerosis – firm induration due to fibrosis of the dermis and subcutis, which may produce the well-known 'inverted champagne bottle' appearance. Ulceration, often precipitated by trauma or infection, follows. Venous ulcers typically occur on the medial lower leg (Fig. 28.7).

Complications of venous leg ulceration include bacterial colonisation and infection, and contact allergic dermatitis to topical medicaments, dressings and bandages. Lipodermatosclerosis may cause lymphoedema and hyperkeratosis, and, rarely, a squamous cell carcinoma (SCC) may develop in a long-standing venous ulcer (Marjolin's ulcer).

Leg ulceration due to arterial disease

Deep, painful, punched-out ulcers on the lower leg, especially the shin and foot and in the context of intermittent claudication, are likely to be due to arterial disease. Risk factors include smoking, hypertension, diabetes and hyperlipidaemia. The foot is cold and dusky and the skin atrophic and hairless. Peripheral pulses are absent or reduced. If the ABPI is below 0.8, a vascular surgical assessment should be sought (p. 601).

Leg ulceration due to vasculitis

Vasculitis can cause leg ulceration directly through epidermal necrosis due to damage to the underlying vasculature or indirectly due to neuropathy (e.g. in systemic polyarteritis nodosa, p. 1117).

Leg ulceration due to neuropathy

The most common causes of neuropathic ulcers are diabetes and Hansen's disease (leprosy). Microangiopathy also contributes to ulceration in diabetes (p. 833). The ulcers occur over weight-bearing areas, such as the heel. In the presence of neuropathy, protection of skin from trauma is essential to prevent ulceration.

Management

Making a diagnosis is the first step. General advice on exercise, weight loss and smoking cessation is important. Underlying factors, such as diabetes or anaemia, must be treated. Oedema must be reduced by leg elevation and, if there is no arterial compromise, graduated compression bandaging from toes to knees to enhance venous return and improve healing. Compression bandaging is effective for individuals with an ABPI of more than 0.8 but should be avoided if the ABPI is less than 0.8.

If the ulcer is purulent, weak potassium permanganate soaks may help, and exudate and slough can be removed with normal saline or clean water. Dressings do not themselves heal leg ulcers, but can reduce discomfort and odour and, by reducing colonisation by potential pathogens, may reduce the frequency of secondary infection. A variety of dressings may be used, including non-adherent and absorbent (alginates, hydrogels, hydrocolloids) types. The frequency of dressing changes will vary: heavily exudative ulcers may need daily dressings, whereas changes once weekly may suffice.

Surrounding eczema should be suppressed with a topical corticosteroid. Commonly, this is venous eczema, but there should be a low threshold for referral for patch testing, as contact allergy to topical applications is common (p. 1255). Systemic antibiotics are only indicated if there is evidence of infection, as opposed to colonisation. Various techniques of split thickness grafting (such as pinch and mince grafts) may hasten healing of clean ulcers but do not reduce recurrence risk. Leg ulcers can be very persistent. Symptomatic relief, including oral analgesics, and sometimes chronic pain treatments (such as tricyclic antidepressants) are important. Once the ulcer has healed, ongoing use of compression hosiery may limit the risk of recurrence.

Abnormal skin colour

Loss of skin pigmentation (depigmentation), reduction in pigmentation (hypopigmentation) and increased pigment (hyperpigmentation) are features of a variety of disorders. Detailed history-taking and examination, including use of a Wood's light, are required to establish the diagnosis. Investigations will depend on the presentation. For example, microscopy of skin scrapings should be undertaken if hypopigmentation is associated with inflammation and scaling; screening for autoimmune disease may be required if vitiligo is suspected; and investigation for endocrine disease or the porphyrias may be appropriate in hyperpigmentation. Further details of the specific conditions are included later (p. 1295).

Hair and nail abnormalities

Many conditions affect the skin appendages, particularly hair and nails. Conditions causing hair loss (alopecia) are listed in Box 28.39 (p. 1296). Nail changes may be a marker for systemic disease (e.g. iron deficiency) or a feature of certain skin conditions (e.g. psoriasis).

Acute skin failure

Acute skin failure is a medical emergency. Several conditions can cause widespread and acute failure of many skin functions (see Box 28.1, p. 1254), including thermoregulation, fluid balance control and barrier to infection. A lot of these conditions involve widespread dilatation of the dermal vasculature and can provoke high-output cardiac failure; they are also associated with increased protein loss from the skin and often from the gut. Many lead to acute skin failure by causing erythroderma (erythema affecting at least 80% of the body surface area), although severe autoimmune blistering diseases and the spectrum of Stevens–Johnson syndrome–toxic epidermal necrolysis (TEN) disease can produce acute skin failure without erythroderma.

Eczema, psoriasis, drug eruptions and cutaneous T-cell lymphoma (Sézary syndrome, p. 1272) are amongst the diseases which can either present with, or progress to, erythroderma. Other causes include the psoriasis-like condition, pityriasis rubra pilaris, and rare types of ichthyosis. Erythroderma may occur at any age and is associated with severe morbidity and significant mortality (see Fig. 28.32D, p. 1287). Older people are at greatest risk, especially if they have comorbidities. It may appear suddenly or evolve slowly. In dark skin, the presence of pigmentation may mask erythema, giving a purplish hue.

Erythrodermic patients are usually systemically unwell with shivering and hypothermia, secondary to excess heat loss. They may also be pyrexial, however, and unable to lose heat due to damage to sweat gland function and sweat duct occlusion. Tachycardia and hypotension may be present because of volume depletion. Peripheral oedema is common in erythroderma, owing to low albumin and high-output cardiac failure. Lymph nodes may be enlarged, either as a reaction to skin inflammation or, rarely, due to lymphomatous infiltration.

Management of erythroderma

Regardless of the cause, important aspects of the management of erythroderma include supportive measures to ensure adequate hydration, maintenance of core temperature and adequate nutrition. Insensible fluid loss can be many litres above what is normal. Protein may be lost directly from the skin and because of the protein-losing enteropathy that often accompanies conditions such as erythrodermic psoriasis. To reduce the risks of infection, any intravenous cannulae should be sited in peripheral veins, if possible. In the initial management of acute erythroderma, urinary catheterisation is often required (for patient comfort and accurate fluid balance monitoring) but such catheters should be removed as soon as possible. Frequent application of a simple ointment emollient (such as white soft paraffin/liquid paraffin mix) is usually appropriate.

THERAPEUTICS

Topical treatment of skin disease

Many skin diseases are treated effectively by topical therapies alone. Selection of the appropriate active drug/ingredient and vehicle is essential. Ointments are preferred for dry skin conditions, such as chronic eczemas, as they are more hydrating and contain fewer excipients than creams, and so allergy risk is reduced. In contrast, creams are not as hydrating and have greater allergic potential due to a higher content of excipients, although patients find creams easier to apply and so compliance may be better. Gels and lotions can be easier to use on hair-bearing sites. The molecular weight and lipid–water coefficient of a drug determine its skin penetration, with larger, water-soluble, polar molecules penetrating poorly. In skin disease, if the stratum corneum is impaired - as in eczema - increased drug absorption occurs. Occlusion under dressings also increases absorption. Drugs can be used in different potencies or concentrations, or in combination with other active ingredients, and many are available in more than one formulation. The properties of different vehicles are listed in Box 28.11. Overall, compliance with topical treatments can be problematic, so it is essential for patients to know exactly what is required of them and for regimens to be kept as simple as possible.

Emollients

These are mainstays in the treatment of eczema, psoriasis and many other conditions, and are used to moisturise, lubricate, protect and 'soften' skin. They are essentially vehicles without active drug and are available in many formulations: creams, ointments, gels, and bath, shower and soap substitutes. White soft paraffin is the most effective and is widely used.

Topical corticosteroids

Glucocorticoids are available in a variety of formulations, although most commonly as creams and ointments. Corticosteroids are available in different potencies and strengths (Box 28.12) and selection of the correct product will depend on the patient, the condition being treated, body site and duration of expected use. Mild topical corticosteroids are used in delicate areas, such as the face or genitals, and close supervision of corticosteroid use at these sites is required. In contrast, very potent corticosteroids may be required under occlusion for chronic resistant disease such as nodular prurigo.

Although the adverse cutaneous effects of chronic corticosteroid use are well known and include atrophy, striae (Fig. 28.8), purpura and telangiectasiae, infection risk and systemic absorption (causing suppression of the hypothalamic–pituitary–adrenal axis and Cushingoid features), under-treatment is more common in practice. Patients should use the lowest potency of steroid for the shortest period to gain control of their disease, but this will vary between individuals and diseases. Initial use of a more potent corticosteroid, with reduction in potency or frequency of application as control is gained, is a sensible approach. Tolerance ('tachyphylaxis') can develop with chronic use, so intermittent courses of

28.11 Characteristics of vehicles used in topical treatments

Vehicle	Definition	Use	Site	Cosmetic acceptability	Risk of contact sensitisation
Creams	Emulsions of oil and water, e.g. aqueous cream	Acute presentations Cooling, soothing Well absorbed Mild emollients	All sites, including mucous membranes and flexures, but not hair-bearing areas	Very good Helps compliance	Significant, due to preservatives, antimicrobials and often lanolin
Ointments	Greasy preparations Insoluble in water, e.g. white soft paraffin Soluble, e.g. emulsifying ointment	Chronic dry skin conditions Occlusive and emollient Hydrating Mildly anti-inflammatory	Avoid hair-bearing areas and flexures	Moderate	Low
Lotions	Water-based Liquid formulations	Cooling effect Used to clean the skin and remove exudates Often antiseptic and astringent (e.g. potassium permanganate)	Large areas of the skin and the scalp	Good, but can sting if in an alcoholic base	Rarely
Gels	Thickened lotions Hydrophilic and hydrophobic bases	For specific sites	Hair-bearing areas and the face	Good	Low
Pastes	Semi-solid preparations consisting of finely powdered solids suspended in an ointment	Occlusive, protective Hydrating Used for circumscribed skin lesions, e.g. psoriasis, lichen simplex chronicus	Any area of skin Often used in medicated bandages	Moderate	Moderate

28.12 Potencies and strengths of commonly used topical corticosteroid preparations*

Mild
- Hydrocortisone 0.5%, 1%, 2.5%
- Hydrocortisone 1% and fusidic acid 2% (Fucidin H)

Moderate
- Clobetasone butyrate 0.05% (Eumovate)
- Betamethasone valerate 0.025% (Betnovate RD)
- Fluocinolone acetonide 0.00625% (Synalar 1 : 4)

Potent
- Betamethasone valerate 0.1% (Betnovate)
- Betamethasone valerate 0.1% and clioquinol 3% (Betnovate-C)
- Fluocinolone acetonide 0.025% (Synalar)
- Hydrocortisone butyrate 0.1% (Locoid)
- Mometasone furoate 0.1% (Elocon)

Very potent
- Clobetasol propionate 0.05% (Dermovate)

*UK trade names are given in brackets.

treatment are advised. Caution is required with corticosteroid use in psoriasis, as rebound, unstable or pustular psoriasis can occur with sudden cessation of use. Nevertheless, corticosteroids are invaluable for many sites, particularly the flexures. Topical corticosteroids are often formulated in combination with antiseptics, antibiotics or antifungals, and their controlled use may be appropriate, e.g. in infected eczema or flexural psoriasis. Intralesional injections of corticosteroids can be used in a variety of indications, including nodular prurigo, keloid scar, acne cysts and alopecia areata.

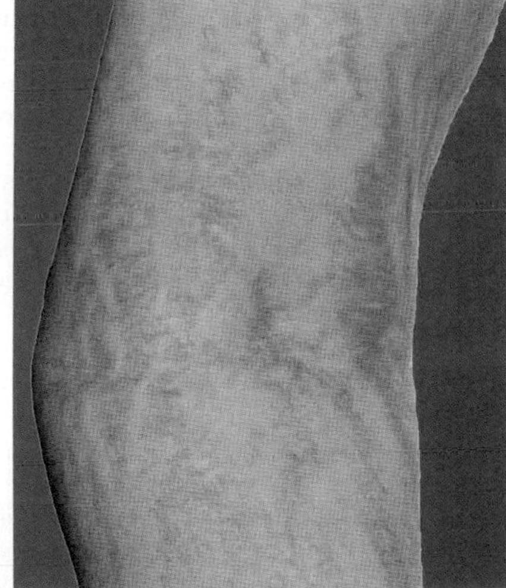

Fig. 28.8 Striae induced by excess prolonged potent topical corticosteroid use.

Dithranol and coal tar

These treatments are used mainly for psoriasis; they increase cellular differentiation and inhibit proliferation. Although often effective, they are messy and time-consuming. Modified versions of Goeckerman's regimen (the combination of coal tar and UVB) are still in use. Short-contact dithranol therapy using higher concentrations applied for 15–30 minutes can be used. Dithranol is highly irritant and causes brown staining of skin and purple discoloration of light hair. In recent years, efforts have been made to improve the tolerance of tar and dithranol preparations, but at reduced efficacy. Overall, the use of tar and dithranol has reduced in recent years.

Calcipotriol

Calcipotriol is a vitamin D agonist and is mainly used in psoriasis. It increases differentiation and reduces proliferation, and therefore lowers plaque scale and thickness. It is applied once to twice daily and, if less than 100 g of ointment is used each week, does not cause hypercalcaemia. Patient compliance is improved, as calcipotriol is odourless and does not stain. Irritancy is the main side-effect, although often temporary. Calcipotriol is a mainstay of primary care management of psoriasis.

Calcineurin inhibitors

Topical tacrolimus and, in children, pimecrolimus can be used to treat eczema and a variety of other conditions. They are calcineurin inhibitors and cause local cutaneous immunosuppression. They have an important role as steroid-sparing agents, e.g. in eczema. Initial burning and stinging may limit use but are usually transient. Caution should be employed with sun exposure and these agents should not be used in combination with phototherapy because of their immunosuppressive effects.

Anti-infective agents

Before antibiotics are used, antiseptics should be considered, as they cover a wide range of organisms and help reduce the risk of antibiotic resistance. Antiseptics can be extremely important in the treatment of patients with eczema and are often employed in combination formulations: for example, with emollients. Antibiotics can be used either for their anti-infective properties – for example, topical fusidic acid for impetigo, or for their anti-inflammatory properties – such as topical erythromycin or clindamycin for mild inflammatory acne vulgaris, or topical metronidazole for rosacea.

Anti-comedogenic agents

Benzoyl peroxide is widely used in mild comedonal acne and has both anti-comedogenic and antiseptic effects. It is an irritant, which may contribute to the therapeutic response, but this can be minimised by adjusting treatment regimes. Azelaic acid has both antimicrobial and anti-comedogenic action in acne vulgaris. Topical retinoids, in particular *all-trans* retinoic acid and adapalene, are widely employed for mild to moderate comedonal acne vulgaris. Again, irritancy is an adverse effect but dose adjustments reduce this.

Other anti-infective agents

These can be used topically for mild viral disease, such as aciclovir for prophylaxis or treatment of herpes simplex virus (cold sore) infection. Topical imidazoles are widely employed for superficial fungal and yeast infections, such as clotrimazole for candidal infections and ketoconazole for pityriasis versicolor or seborrhoeic folliculitis. Terbinafine is commonly applied topically for superficial dermatophyte infections, such as tinea pedis. Scabies and lice infections can be treated with topical permethrin or malathion.

Topical treatment for dysplasia and non-melanoma skin cancer

Medical treatment for non-melanoma skin cancer and dysplasia is a developing area and facilitates treatment of field carcinogenesis. The anti-metabolite, 5-fluorouracil (p. 1271), is used topically, mainly for actinic keratosis. Subclinical disease can be treated, highlighting the advantages of these field-directed approaches. Diclofenac in a hyaluronic acid gel base can also be employed topically for low-grade actinic keratosis; the rationale for its use is the over-expression of cyclo-oxygenase (COX)-2 in actinic keratosis. Ingenol mebutate is also now in use for actinic keratosis.

Immune response modifiers

Imiquimod was introduced for the treatment of anogenital warts but can be used for actinic keratosis, Bowen's disease, basal cell carcinoma and lentigo maligna. Its mechanism of action is via stimulation of endogenous Th2 immune responses and release of cytokines, including interferon-gamma. It can cause significant inflammation, requiring dose adjustments, but can treat subclinical disease.

Dressings

A 'wound' covering is called a dressing. Box 28.13 shows the indications for their use. The active agent, vehicle and 'wound' type should be considered. Wet lesions should be treated with wet dressings, e.g. acute eczema with potassium permanganate soaks, emollients and topical corticosteroids under wet wraps. A topical corticosteroid in a cream formulation and a paste bandage is used to soothe and cool inflamed skin. Chronic eczema may be treated with a potent topical corticosteroid in an ointment formulation and occlusion with paste bandage to ease itching and scratching. Dressings for venous leg ulcers are described on page 1263.

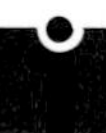

28.13 Indications for dressings

- Protection
- Symptomatic relief from pain or itch
- Maintenance of direct application of topical treatment
- Possible improvement in healing time
- Reduction of exudate
- Reduction of odour

Phototherapy and photochemotherapy

Ultraviolet radiation (UVR) treatments (most commonly, narrowband ultraviolet B and psoralen-ultraviolet A (PUVA)) are used in the management of many different diseases. The best study evidence for their efficacy is in psoriasis, atopic eczema, vitiligo and chronic urticaria, although there is some controlled study evidence for other phototherapy use, such as UVB to treat the generalised itch of kidney disease.

Psoralens are natural photosensitisers found in a number of plants. Psoralen molecules intercalate between the two strands of DNA and, upon excitation with UVA, photons cross-link the DNA strands. It is thus a pro-drug that is distributed throughout the body after oral administration, but only activated in skin that is exposed to UVA. Alternatively, psoralens can be applied in a bath before irradiation with UVA ('bath PUVA'). PUVA is a more complex treatment than UVB and has greater adverse effects; in particular, cumulative exposure to high PUVA treatment numbers increases the risk of skin cancer, particularly squamous cell carcinoma. Therefore, PUVA is generally used for poor responders to UVB, or in a few diseases for which it is the first-line phototherapy choice, such as plaque-stage cutaneous T-cell lymphoma.

Longer-wavelength UVA1 (340–400 nm) is also being investigated for use in several conditions, particularly the fibrosing skin diseases, such as morphoea, although is not widely available at present.

Systemic therapies

General information is provided here, with disease-specific details given later on.

Antibiotics

Antibiotics are generally used for their anti-infective properties, particularly for staphylococcal and streptococcal skin infections. In these indications, the correct antibiotic should be selected, based on bacterial sensitivity and patient factors. As examples, oral flucloxacillin may be indicated for infected eczema, intravenous benzyl penicillin and flucloxacillin for cellulitis, and erythromycin for a patient with a staphylococcal carbuncle who is penicillin-allergic. Optimal therapeutic doses and courses must be chosen. Several antibiotics, such as tetracyclines, erythromycin and trimethoprim, can be used for their anti-inflammatory effects in indications like acne vulgaris, bullous pemphigoid and pyoderma gangrenosum. Oxytetracycline is commonly given for acne but must be taken on an empty stomach, in a dose of up to 1.5 g a day. It has a good safety profile, even with long-term use. Lymecycline is an alternative and is taken once daily, with or without food, thereby improving compliance. Doxycycline is another option but commonly causes photosensitivity. Minocycline may be given, but with caution, as it can cause hyperpigmentation, autoimmune hepatitis and drug-induced lupus, and monitoring is required.

Hormonal treatments

In women with acne, oestrogen-containing oral contraceptives can be a useful adjunct, as they are associated with a small reduction in sebum production. Combined oestrogen and anti-androgen (such as cyproterone acetate) contraceptives can also be effective, particularly in women with acne and hirsutism, as seen in polycystic ovary syndrome (p. 764).

Antifungals

The azoles (ketoconazole, miconazole), triazoles (itraconazole, fluconazole) and triallylamines (terbinafine) are used most widely in fungal skin disease. Topical or systemic use is based on clinical presentation. For example, dermatophyte nail infection requires prolonged oral terbinafine, whereas an isolated patch of tinea corporis will respond rapidly to topical treatment.

Antivirals

Systemic antivirals are indicated for significant viral skin disease. For example, systemic aciclovir is given for eczema herpeticum (see Fig. 13.13C, p. 326).

Antihistamines

A range of H_1 and H_2 antagonists are used in dermatology. For diseases in which histamine in the skin is relevant (such as urticaria), non-sedating antihistamines should be given: for example, fexofenadine or cetirizine. For pruritic conditions such as eczema, the sedating effect of antihistamines like hydroxyzine is important. Leukotriene receptor antagonists, such as montelukast, may be added to antihistamine regimes.

Retinoids

Oral retinoids are widely used in a range of conditions, including acne, psoriasis and other keratinisation disorders. They have several functions, including promotion of differentiation, reduction in hyperkeratosis, sebum production and *Propionibacterium acnes*, and anti-inflammatory effects. Isotretinoin (13-*cis*-retinoic acid) is commonly given for moderate or severe acne, at a dose of 0.5–1 mg/kg over 4 months. Low-dose continuous isotretinoin may also be used for longer periods. Acitretin can be effective in psoriasis and other keratinisation disorders, such as ichthyosis, as can alitretinoin (9-*cis*-retinoic acid) in hand and foot eczema, and bexarotene in cutaneous T-cell lymphoma.

Retinoid side-effects include drying of the skin and mucous membranes, abnormalities in liver function or hepatitis, and increase in serum triglycerides (levels should be checked before and during therapy). Depression and suicide have been reported in association with isotretinoin, although a causal role has not been established. However, pre-drug screening for depressive symptoms should be undertaken. Alitretinoin and bexarotene can cause hypothyroidism. Systemic retinoids are teratogenic; females must have a negative pregnancy test before, during and after therapy. Pregnancy must be avoided for 2 months after isotretinoin, but for 2 years after acitretin, due to differences in drug disposition.

Immunosuppressant and immunomodulatory drugs

Systemic corticosteroids

Corticosteroids, particularly prednisolone, are widely used in inflammatory and immune-based skin diseases, such as eczema, immunobullous disease and connective tissue disorders. The usual steroid side-effects occur (pp. 776 and 1102), and often other immunosuppressants are added in as steroid-sparing agents (see below).

Methotrexate

Methotrexate can be highly effective for psoriasis, eczema and several other skin diseases. In dermatology, it is used once weekly. It is an immunosuppressant (p. 1102), which is important therapeutically but also increases susceptibility to infection. It causes myelosuppression and has adverse interactions with other commonly used drugs, such as NSAIDs. Methotrexate is hepatotoxic and long-term use can be associated with hepatic fibrosis/cirrhosis; regular monitoring of liver function tests and a full blood count is required.

Hydroxycarbamide

This is an alternative immunosuppressant to methotrexate, although it appears to be less effective for psoriasis and the risk of myelosuppression is greater.

Ciclosporin

Ciclosporin (p. 1102) is an immunosuppressant with rapid onset of action and is effective in inducing clearance of psoriasis and eczema. Caution and monitoring are required, as, in addition to immunosuppression, hypertension and nephrotoxicity are important adverse effects. Furthermore, ciclosporin should be used only with caution after phototherapy, particularly PUVA, because of the increased risk of skin cancer. Chronic use of ciclosporin is not advised.

Azathioprine

This is an anti-metabolite that is converted to 6-mercaptopurine; it inhibits DNA and RNA synthesis. Azathioprine is mutagenic and detoxified via the enzyme thiopurine methyl transferase (TPMT), now routinely measured prior to drug commencement to allow individualised and safer treatment. Side-effects include myelosuppression and gastrointestinal upset.

Mycophenolate mofetil

This immunosuppressant may be effective in diseases such as psoriasis but caution is needed, as myelosuppression can occur.

Dapsone

Dapsone is an immunomodulator and may be used in diseases where neutrophils are implicated, such as dermatitis herpetiformis (p. 1294). Haemolysis, methaemoglobinaemia and hypersensitivity can occur, and monitoring is required (pp. 158 and 350).

Antimalarials

The antimalarials, such as hydroxychloroquine, have multiple anti-inflammatory actions but are of particular use in cutaneous lupus (pp. 1102 and 1112).

Fumarates

The active component of fumaric acid ester therapy is dimethyl fumarate, and efficacy in psoriasis has been confirmed. Common adverse effects are flushing and diarrhoea. Lymphopenia is expected at effective doses.

Biological therapies

An increasing variety of monoclonal antibodies, fusion proteins and cytokines has been shown to be effective for psoriasis, and these agents are sometimes used in other recalcitrant skin diseases. The anti-tumour necrosis factor-alpha (TNF-α) therapies have the longest track record (p. 1102). These include etanercept (a human recombinant TNF-α receptor fusion protein), and infliximab and adalimumab (both anti-TNF-α monoclonal antibodies). Potential side-effects include reactivation of latent tuberculosis and development of other opportunistic infections. The long-term risks of skin and other cancers are not yet well quantified. Other biological therapies (often abbreviated to 'biologics') include B cell-targeted treatments, such as rituximab, which may be used in pemphigus vulgaris, lupus erythematosus, dermatomyositis and other immune-based diseases (p. 1102), and omalizumab (an IgE monoclonal). While introduced to treat allergic asthma, the latter may also prove useful in non-allergic diseases such as chronic urticaria (pp. 91 and 671). Intravenous immunoglobulin, pooled from donor plasma, is often used in immune complex disease, such as dermatomyositis (p. 81).

Dermatological surgery

The choice of procedure is critical; for example, basal cell papillomas should be treated by cryotherapy or curettage, and melanomas widely excised. Most dermatological surgical procedures are performed under local anaesthetic. Knowledge of local anatomy is essential, particularly the locations of vessels and nerves. In certain sites, local cutaneous nerve blocks are useful (e.g. fingers, sole of foot and nose). Some sites are associated with particular risks, such as keloidal scarring on the upper trunk of young patients, unsightly scars over the scapulae, and poor healing and risk of ulceration following procedures on the lower legs.

Excisional biopsy

The lesion is removed and sent for histology. The most common indication is suspicion of malignancy. The lesion and line of excision should be marked out. Basal cell carcinoma (BCC) is usually excised with a 4 mm margin, whereas initial excision of suspicious pigmented lesions is usually with a 2 mm margin with further excision arranged if melanoma is confirmed (p. 1273). It is important to excise down to the appropriate anatomical plane. Depending on body site, a range of procedures can minimise the resulting defect. Healing by secondary intention can also achieve good cosmetic results.

Mohs' micrographic surgery

Mohs' micrographic surgery is employed to ensure adequate tumour excision margins, while conserving unaffected tissue. It is most commonly used for BCC. The method involves processing to allow examination of all margins and is done in stages (usually on the same day) until all of the tumour is removed. The procedure is time-consuming (so can be arduous for elderly, frail patients) and requires particular surgical and pathology skills. It should be considered for recurrent and for morphoeic and ill-defined BCC, and at sites where tissue conservation is particularly important, such as eyelid skin.

Curettage

Curettage involves using a small, spoon-shaped implement (curette), not only as a definitive treatment but also to obtain histology. The latter may, however, be compromised, as tissue architecture is not well preserved and it may be difficult to distinguish between dysplasia and invasive malignancy. Curettage may be effective for basal cell papillomas, actinic keratoses, intra-epidermal carcinoma and superficial BCC.

Other physical therapies

Cryotherapy

Cryotherapy is a destructive treatment that uses liquid nitrogen. The freezing and thawing process causes cell wall and membrane destruction and cell death. Liquid nitrogen can be applied either with a cotton bud or, more effectively, with a spray gun. A wide variety of conditions can be treated but it is essential for the correct diagnosis to be made first, if necessary by diagnostic biopsy. Cryotherapy should not be employed to treat melanocytic naevi. Benign lesions, such as viral warts and basal cell papillomas, respond well, and cryotherapy can also be effective for actinic keratoses, Bowen's disease or superficial non-melanoma skin cancer. Malignant indications require more vigorous treatment, usually with two freeze–thaw cycles, and this is normally carried out in secondary care. Considerable inflammation, blistering and pigmentary change, particularly hypopigmentation, can occur.

Laser therapy

Laser therapy involves treatment with monochromatic light. Skin components, such as haemoglobin and melanin, absorb specific wavelengths of electromagnetic radiation, and these wavelengths can therefore be used to destroy these targets selectively and to treat certain skin disorders. Lasers targeting haemoglobin are employed for vascular abnormalities, such as spider naevi, telangiectasiae and port wine stains, and lasers targeting melanin can treat benign pigmentary disorders or pigment in tattoos or from drug (e.g. minocycline) deposition; the latter can also be used for hair removal if the hair is pigmented. Light delivery in short pulses restricts damage to the treated site.

The carbon dioxide laser emits infrared light that is absorbed by water in tissues and can therefore be used for destructive purposes. The depth of effect can be controlled, such that the carbon dioxide laser is widely employed for resurfacing in photorejuvenation or acne scarring. Significant morbidity is associated with this destructive laser and general anaesthesia is required.

Photodynamic therapy

Photodynamic therapy (PDT) is widely used in dermatology, predominantly for actinic keratoses, Bowen's disease and superficial BCC. Topical 'porphyrin' PDT is the most common type; it involves the application of a porphyrin pro-drug to the lesion, which is taken up and converted by the cell's haem cycle to a photosensitiser, protoporphyrin IX. This is then photochemically activated by visible (usually red) light in the presence of oxygen, which causes the production of reactive oxygen species, inflammation and destruction of treated tissue. The photosensitiser is taken up relatively selectively in diseased skin, and so inflammation and adverse effects in normal skin are minimised. PDT is as effective for superficial non-melanoma skin cancer and dysplasia as other treatments like cryotherapy and 5-fluorouracil, but may be preferred for sites of poor healing, such as the lower leg, or where cosmetic outcome is important, due to the selectivity of treatment. Pain during irradiation occurs during PDT, although adjustments to the irradiation regime can reduce discomfort.

Radiotherapy and grenz (Bucky) ray therapy

Radiotherapy can be employed for several skin conditions, including non-melanoma skin cancer or lentigo maligna that is not suitable for surgical treatment, but its use in dermatology has declined. Scarring and poikiloderma can occur at treated sites, although these are minimised if fractionated regimens are chosen. Superficial radiotherapy is now rarely employed to treat benign dermatoses. Even more superficial ionising radiation (grenz, or Bucky, rays) can be useful for localised dermatoses that are having severe effects on quality of life, if conventional treatments have been inadequate; for example, it may avoid exposure to the risks of systemic therapy for a patient with severe and hitherto unresponsive scalp psoriasis.

SKIN TUMOURS

Pathogenesis of skin malignancy

Skin cancer is the most common malignancy in fair-skinned populations. It is categorised as non-melanoma skin cancer (NMSC) and melanoma. NMSC is further subdivided into basal cell carcinoma (BCC), the most common skin cancer, and squamous cell carcinoma (SCC). The latter has precursor non-invasive states of intra-epithelial carcinoma (Bowen's disease; BD) and dysplasia (actinic keratosis; AK). Melanoma is much less common than NMSC, but because of its metastatic risk it is the cause of most skin cancer deaths.

UVR is a complete carcinogen and is the main environmental risk factor for skin cancer, which is much more common in countries with high ambient sun exposure, such as Australia. Skin cancer risk also increases if an individual migrates to such a country at a young age, particularly less than 10 years. Epidemiological evidence supports a close link between chronic UVR exposure and risk of SCC and AK, and a modest link between sun exposure and BCC risk. Melanoma usually arises on sites that are intermittently exposed to UVR, and episodes of sunburn have been implicated as a risk factor for melanoma. Sunbed exposure is also a risk for both melanoma and NMSC (Box 28.14). Strategies to reduce sun exposure are therefore important for skin cancer prevention (Box 28.15).

There may also be identifiable genetic predispositions for skin cancer, such as in xeroderma pigmentosum, an autosomal recessive condition caused by an inherited defect in DNA excision repair (pp. 267 and 67), or basal cell naevus (Gorlin's) syndrome, an autosomal dominant disorder in which the *PTCH* tumour suppressor gene on chromosome 9 is defective (p. 267). Cutaneous immune surveillance is also critical and immunosuppressed organ transplant recipients have a greatly increased risk of skin cancer, particularly SCC. Interestingly, patients who have received high numbers of

EBM 28.14 Sunbeds and skin cancer

'Recent meta-analyses have confirmed that there is an association between sunbed use and both melanoma and non-melanoma skin cancer, particularly when exposure commences in early life.'

- Boniol M, et al. Br Med J 2012; 345:14.
- Wehner MR, et al. Br Med J 2012; 345:15.

28

EBM 28.15 Sunscreens and skin cancer

'Sunscreen use attenuates the development of new naevi on intermittently sun-exposed sites in white-skinned (particularly freckled) schoolchildren living in areas of high ambient sun exposure. There is good evidence that regular sunscreen use in adults reduces the development of actinic keratosis and squamous cell carcinoma. There is also evidence to support a preventative role for regular sunscreen use in melanoma and, to a lesser extent, basal cell carcinoma.'

- Green AC, et al. J Clin Oncol 2011; 29:257–263.
- Ulrich C, et al. Br J Dermatol 2009; 161 (suppl. 3):78–84.

PUVA treatments (more than 150), which are immunosuppressive, are also at increased risk of skin cancer, particularly SCC. Despite UVB being a complete carcinogen, there is no evidence that UVB phototherapy markedly increases skin cancer risk, although ongoing vigilance is required. Ionising radiation, notably radiotherapy, thermal radiation and chemical carcinogens, such as arsenic or coal tar, can increase NMSC risk, particularly SCC. A role for oncogenic human papillomaviruses in NMSC development is also implicated, particularly in immunosuppressed patients with NMSC; viral DNA is detected in more than 80% of this group. Chronic inflammation is also a risk factor for SCC, which may arise in chronic skin ulcers, in skin inflammation, as in lupus, or in patients with the scarring genetic skin disease, dystrophic epidermolysis bullosa (see Box 28.32, p. 1292), in which up to 50% of patients develop SCC.

Malignant tumours

Basal cell carcinoma

The incidence of NMSC has increased dramatically over the last 30 years and basal cell carcinoma (BCC) accounts for more than 70% of cases. In Europe, the ratio of BCC to SCC is 4–5:1 in immunocompetent patients. BCC is a malignant tumour that rarely metastasises; it is thought to derive from immature pluripotent epidermal cells and is composed of cells with similarities to basal layer epidermis and appendages. Lesions typically occur at sites of moderate sun exposure, particularly the face, and are slow-growing. Incidence increases with age and males are more commonly affected. Lesions may ulcerate and invade locally; hence the term 'rodent ulcer'. Mutations in the *PTCH* tumour suppressor gene have been identified and an aberrant hedgehog signalling pathway is implicated in pathogenesis.

Clinical features

Early BCCs usually present as pale, translucent papules or nodules, with overlying superficial telangiectatic vessels (nodular BCC). If untreated, they will increase in size and ulcerate, to form a crater with a rolled, pearled edge and ectatic vessels (Fig. 28.9). There may be some pigmentation or a cystic component. A superficial multifocal type can occur, often on the trunk, and may be large (up to 10 cm in diameter); there may be multiple lesions. Superficial BCC usually presents as a red/brown plaque or patch with a raised, thread-like edge, which is often best seen by stretching the skin; this helps to distinguish it from Bowen's disease. Less commonly, a morphoeic, infiltrative BCC presents as an ill-defined, slowly enlarging, sclerotic yellow/grey plaque.

A

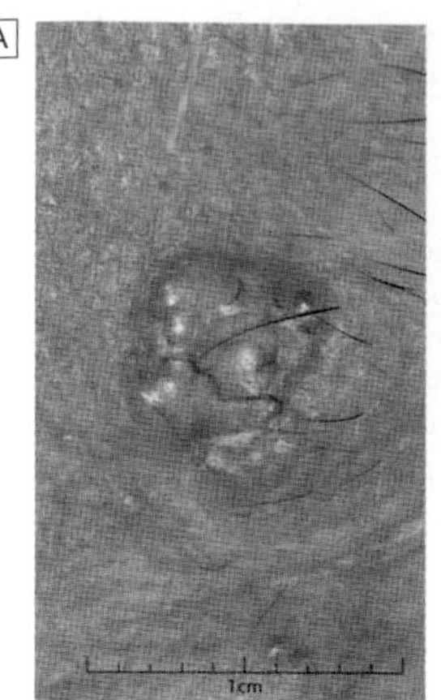

B

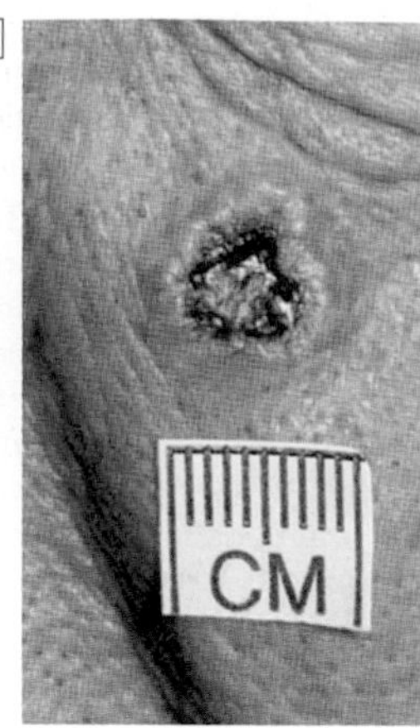

Fig. 28.9 Basal cell carcinoma. **A** A nodular BCC showing the translucent nature of the tumour and the abnormal arborising vessels. **B** An ulcerated BCC showing the raised rolled edge.

Management

Management involves early diagnosis and establishment of the correct treatment approach, taking into account patient and lesion factors (Box 28.16). Surgery is often the treatment of choice, although, increasingly, the place of non-surgical therapies is being recognised for low-risk BCC in patients in whom surgery is not appropriate. For example, an early nodular BCC in a fit patient is best excised surgically, whereas large, multiple, superficial BCCs on the trunk of a frail elderly patient with comorbidities may be best treated by a non-surgical approach, such as PDT or the immunomodulator

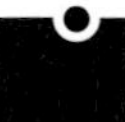

28.16 Management of non-melanoma skin cancer and pre-cancer

Basal cell carcinoma

- Excision results in the lowest recurrence rates
- Mohs' micrographic surgery is effective for high-risk BCC
- Medical treatments are often appropriate for low-risk superficial tumours in patients with comorbidities
- Cryotherapy and topical 5-fluorouracil can be used for superficial BCC
- Topical photodynamic therapy and topical imiquimod are both effective in superficial BCC
- BCC in patients with Gorlin's syndrome should not be treated with radiotherapy
- Hedgehog pathway inhibitors are being investigated for advanced inoperable BCC

Squamous cell carcinoma (and precursors actinic keratosis and Bowen's disease)

- Excision is the treatment of choice for invasive SCC
- Most recurrences or metastases occur within 5 years
- Medical management is not usually considered for invasive SCC
- There have been many advances in the medical management of field-change carcinogenesis, actinic keratoses and Bowen's disease, e.g. photodynamic therapy, imiquimod and other immunomodulators, new formulations of 5-fluorouracil, diclofenac in hyaluronic acid gel and ingenol mebutate

imiquimod (p. 426). Cryotherapy can be effective for BCC but can cause blistering and scarring, so is best suited to small, superficial lesions at low-risk sites. Curettage and cautery may also be effective for selected lesions. Management of infiltrative morphoeic BCC and/or lesions at difficult sites, such as around the eye, may require more complex surgical excision with margin control (Mohs'). If the primary tumour is not completely excised, re-excision or follow-up may be advised, as not all tumours that are incompletely excised recur. However, this is not recommended for tumours at high-risk sites or with infiltrative morphoeic BCC, where complete excision is advisable. Radiotherapy is less commonly used because of the risk of scarring, but can be invaluable for large lesions in frail patients. Clearance of more than 90% of tumours should be achieved. Non-surgical approaches are associated with higher recurrence rates than surgery (often up to 25% over 5 years) but may be most appropriate in some circumstances.

Squamous cell carcinoma

Squamous cell carcinoma (SCC) is a malignancy that arises from epidermal keratinocytes and is the second most common skin cancer, occurring more frequently in elderly males and smokers.

Clinical features

SCC usually occurs on chronically sun-exposed sites, such as bald scalp, tops of ears, face and back of hands. The clinical presentation may be diverse, ranging from rapid development of a painful keratotic nodule in a pre-existing area of dysplasia (Fig. 28.10) to the de novo presentation of an erythematous, infiltrated, often-warty nodule or plaque that may ulcerate. The clinical appearance depends on histological grading; well-differentiated tumours more often present as defined keratotic nodules (see Fig. 28.10), whereas poorly differentiated tumours tend to be ill-defined and infiltrative, and may ulcerate. SCC has metastatic potential; some tumours, such as those on lip and ears and in immunosuppressed patients, behave more aggressively and are more likely to metastasise to draining lymph nodes.

Management

Early diagnosis is important and complete surgical excision is the usual treatment of choice. Other options include curettage and cautery for small, low-risk lesions and radiotherapy if surgery is not feasible (see Box 28.16). Excision with a 3–4 mm margin has a cure rate of approximately 90–95% for most SCC. High-risk SCC, such as those with poorly differentiated histology or at high-risk sites, and metastatic disease require management via a multidisciplinary team. In patients who are at high risk for further SCC, systemic retinoids may have a role in reducing the rate of SCC development, but rapid appearance of tumours occurs on drug cessation.

Actinic keratosis

Actinic keratoses (AK) are hyperkeratotic erythematous lesions arising on chronically sun-exposed sites. Histology shows dysplasia, although the diagnosis of typical AK is usually made on clinical grounds (Fig. 28.11). They are very common in fair-skinned people who have had significant sun exposure, are often multiple and increase with age. Prevalence is much higher in Australia than in the UK and some surveys have shown a prevalence of more than 50% in those over 40 years old. The rate of progression to SCC is less than 0.1% and spontaneous resolution is possible. However, SCC can also arise de novo and without progression from AK. Increase in size, ulceration, bleeding, pain or tenderness can be indicative of transformation into SCC.

Management

A range of treatment options are available for AK (see Box 28.16). Emollients and photoprotection, including high-factor sunscreens, may suffice for mild disease. Single or low numbers of lesions of AK can be effectively treated with cryotherapy. Multiple lesions require field-directed therapy, such as 5-fluorouracil, imiquimod, diclofenac in hyaluronic acid, PDT or ingenol mebutate. Hyperkeratotic lesions may require curettage and cautery.

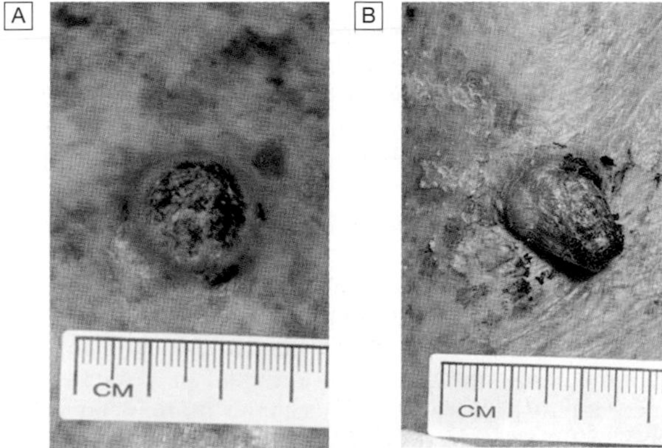

Fig. 28.10 Squamous cell carcinoma. **A** A centrally keratinous, symmetrical, well-differentiated SCC. Clinically, this could be confused with keratoacanthoma. **B** An SCC arising from an area of epidermal dysplasia.

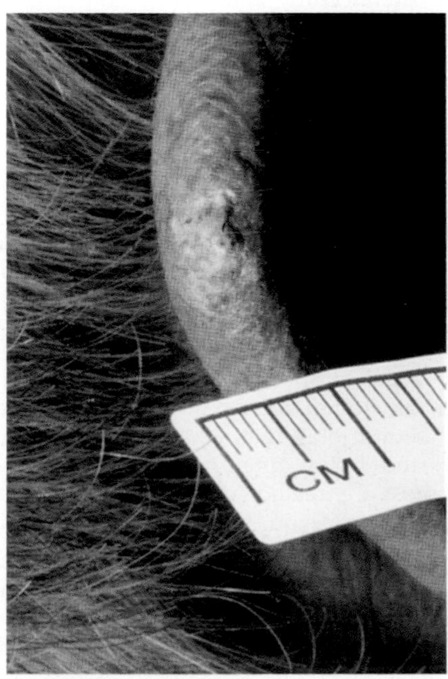

Fig. 28.11 Actinic keratosis. Close-up of a hyperkeratotic AK on the ear.

28

Intra-epidermal carcinoma (Bowen's disease)

Clinical features

Bowen's disease (BD) usually presents as a slowly enlarging, erythematous, scaly plaque on the lower legs of fair-skinned elderly women but may occur at other sites (Fig. 28.12). It can be confused with eczema or psoriasis, but is usually asymptomatic and does not respond to topical steroids. It may also be hard to distinguish from superficial BCC. Diagnostic biopsy shows intra-epidermal carcinoma but no invasion through the basement membrane. Transformation into SCC occurs in 3% or less.

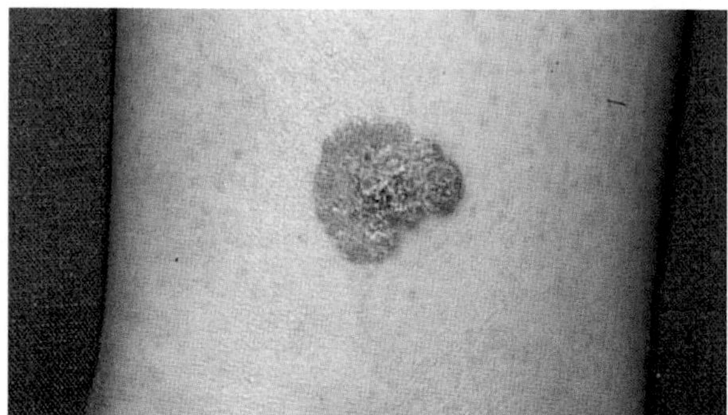

Fig. 28.12 Intra-epidermal carcinoma (Bowen's disease). The lower leg is a common site and lesions are often treated non-surgically.

Management

Incisional biopsy is usually undertaken to confirm the diagnosis, although histology may be obtained by curettage. The latter also serves to treat the lesion but does not allow distinction from SCC to be made, due to loss of tissue architecture and orientation. Non-surgical therapies are commonly preferred (see Box 28.16), especially on the lower legs, as they are associated with improved healing and reduced risk of ulceration at this site.

Keratoacanthoma

Although benign, this squamous tumour is often difficult to distinguish from SCC and is thus included in this section. It has a striking clinical presentation of rapid growth over weeks to months and subsequent spontaneous resolution. It is thought to be associated with chronic sun exposure and most commonly occurs on the central face. The classical appearance is of an isolated dome-shaped nodule often of 5 cm or more in diameter, with a central keratin plug (Fig. 28.13). Clinically and histologically, the lesion often resembles SCC (see Fig. 28.10A); most are treated surgically, either by curettage and cautery or excision, to rule out SCC and to avoid the unsightly scar after spontaneous resolution.

Cutaneous lymphomas

The most common form of cutaneous T-cell lymphoma is mycosis fungoides (MF). This can persist for years in patch and plaque stages, often resembling eczema or psoriasis. Only sometimes does it progress through

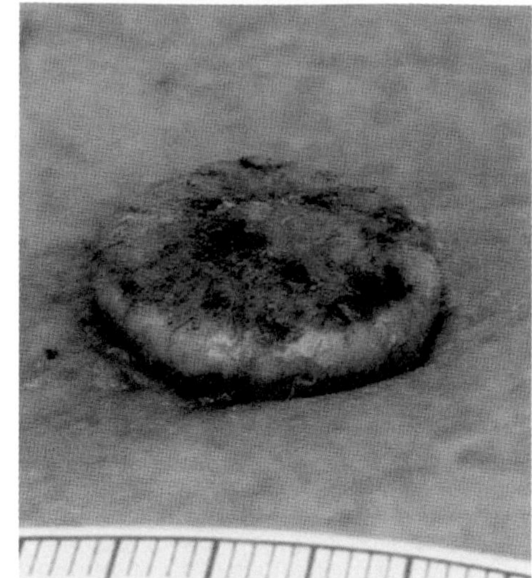

Fig. 28.13 Keratoacanthoma.

to nodules and finally a systemic stage. B-cell lymphomas, on the other hand, usually present as nodules or plaque-like tumours. The diagnosis of cutaneous T-cell lymphoma requires a high index of suspicion, particularly in patients thought to have unusual recalcitrant forms of eczema or psoriasis.

Treatment is symptomatic and there is no evidence that it alters prognosis. In the early stages of cutaneous T-cell lymphoma, systemic or local corticosteroids may be indicated; alternatively, PUVA (for plaque stage MF) or narrowband UVB phototherapy (for patch stage MF) may be used. Once lesions have moved beyond plaque stage, localised radiotherapy, electron beam radiation or systemic anti-lymphoma regimens may be needed. Management often requires collaboration between dermatologists, pathologists and haematological oncologists.

Melanoma

Melanoma is a malignant tumour of epidermal melanocytes and has metastatic potential. There has been a steady rise in melanoma incidence in fair-skinned populations over recent decades, with the highest figures in Australasia. Primary prevention and early detection are essential, as, despite advances, therapy for advanced and metastatic disease is unsatisfactory. Most melanomas are sporadic and risk factors are genetic and environmental: fair skin, freckles, red hair, number of naevi and sunlight exposure. Thus, patients with multiple atypical naevi (dysplastic naevus syndrome) and fair-skinned subjects, often with variant alleles in the melanocortin-1 gene, are at increased risk of melanoma. The type of sunlight exposure is under debate but intermittent exposure, sunburn and sunbed use are implicated. Any family history of melanoma increases individual risk but a strong family history is rare. In familial cases, an autosomal dominant inheritance with incomplete penetrance can occur. Mutations in genes coding for the p16 (*CDKN2A*) tumour suppressor gene or its binding site are implicated and, in these patients, the lifetime risk of melanoma increases to more than 50%. Advances in molecular technology have identified other susceptibility genes and potential genetic targets for therapeutic intervention in advanced disease.

Clinical features

Melanoma can occur at any age and site and in either sex, but typically affects the leg in females and back in males. It is rare before puberty. The classification of invasive malignant melanoma is shown in Box 28.17. Early lesions may be in situ and pre-invasive before becoming an invasive SSM.

Any change in naevi or development of new lesions should be assessed to exclude malignancy and, for this, the dermatoscope is invaluable (see Fig. 28.2, p. 1256). Real-time non-invasive imaging techniques are being investigated as tools to assist in diagnosis but are largely experimental. If in doubt, excision is advised.

Superficial spreading melanoma

Superficial spreading melanoma (SSM) is the most common type in Caucasians. It usually presents as a slowly enlarging, macular, pigmented lesion, with increasing irregularity in shape and pigment; this superficial, radial growth phase can last for approximately 2 years. Subsequently, the lesion becomes palpable and this is indicative of the development of vertical growth phase invasive disease in the dermis; this now has the potential to invade lymphatics and vessels and become metastatic (Fig. 28.14). Approximately 50% of melanomas arise from a pre-existing naevus.

Nodular melanoma

Nodular melanoma is most common in the fifth and sixth decades, particularly in men and on the trunk (see Fig. 28.14). This may account in part for the increased mortality rates from melanoma in men, as these are tumours with greater metastatic risk. They often present as a rapidly growing nodule that may bleed and ulcerate. Nodular melanomas may be heavily pigmented, or relatively amelanotic and erythematous, and be confused with benign vascular lesions. A rim of pigmentation may, however, be seen under the dermatoscope. Lesions may develop de novo or from a pre-existing naevus or SSM.

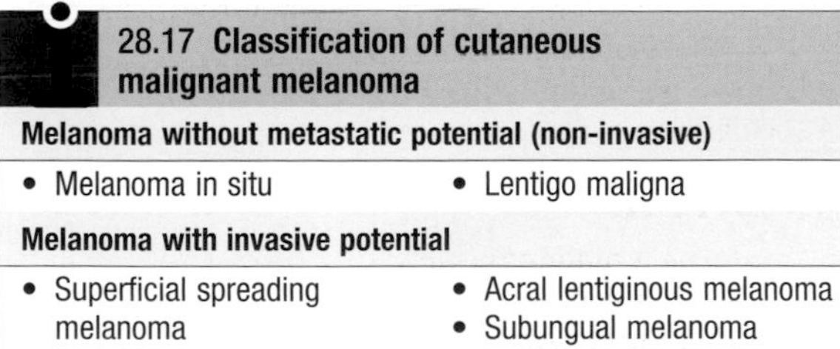

28.17 Classification of cutaneous malignant melanoma

Melanoma without metastatic potential (non-invasive)	
• Melanoma in situ	• Lentigo maligna
Melanoma with invasive potential	
• Superficial spreading melanoma • Nodular melanoma	• Acral lentiginous melanoma • Subungual melanoma • Lentigo maligna melanoma

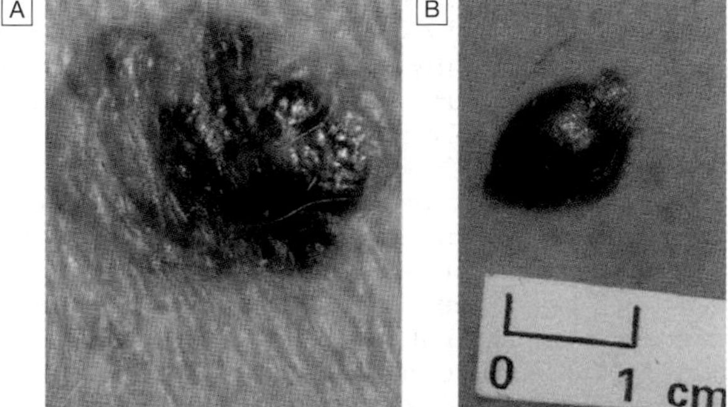

Fig. 28.14 Superficial spreading melanoma. **A** A superficial spreading malignant melanoma with a palpable area indicative of vertical growth phase (Breslow thickness 1.3 mm). **B** A nodular malignant melanoma arising de novo and with Breslow thickness 3.5 mm.

Lentigo maligna melanoma

This is biologically distinct and arises from a prolonged pre-invasive phase, lentigo maligna. It occurs as a very slowly expanding, pigmented, macular lesion, usually on photo-exposed head and neck sites of elderly patients; histology shows in situ changes only. This phase may last for several years before a nodule of invasive melanoma develops in a proportion of cases (lentigo maligna melanoma).

Acral lentiginous or palmoplantar melanoma

This accounts for only approximately 10% of melanoma in fair-skinned races but is more common in dark-skinned people, accounting for 50% of cases and indicating that UVR exposure may not be implicated in acral melanoma risk.

Subungual melanoma

This form of melanoma is rare. It may present as a painless, proximally expanding streak of pigmentation arising from the nail matrix, and progresses to nail dystrophy and involvement of the adjacent nail fold (Hutchinson's sign).

Management

Initial excision of a suspicious lesion should be performed with a 2 mm margin, where possible. Surgical excision is usually required, although radiotherapy or imiquimod may be used for lentigo maligna, if surgery is not feasible. The Breslow thickness of tumour (i.e. the maximal depth from granular cell layer to deepest tumour cells) is critical for management and prognosis. The clinical staging of extent of melanoma is essential, in order to establish whether disease is primary and localised, or if there is nodal or metastatic spread.

Wide excision of melanoma with a low risk of metastasis (i.e. stage 1 disease, Breslow thickness less than 1 mm) with a 1 cm clear margin is accepted practice. The margin of excision for more advanced disease is controversial, although a 2–3 cm margin for thicker tumours is common practice as an attempt to reduce risk of local recurrence (Box 28.18). The majority of tumours can be excised without the need for grafting. For tumours with a Breslow thickness of 1 mm or more, a sentinel lymph node biopsy may be offered. This is usually performed at the time of wider excision and involves injection of radio-labelled blue dye at the site of the primary melanoma, allowing identification of the draining 'sentinel' node by radioscintigraphy; this sentinel node is then removed and examined in detail by histology, immunohistochemistry and/or PCR of melanocyte gene products to look for tumour deposits. If the biopsy is positive, local lymphadenectomy is usually offered. This procedure may provide additional prognostic information but there is no evidence of improved survival rates in patients who have undergone this procedure. Local recurrence of disease and

EBM 28.18 Margin of excision of melanoma

'There is no evidence that radical surgery (4–6 cm excision margins) reduces the risk of local recurrence or survival compared with more conservative surgery.

Recommended surgical excision margins:

- Breslow thickness < 1 mm: 1 cm margin
- Breslow thickness 1.01–2 mm: 1–2 cm margin
- Breslow thickness 2.1–4 mm: 2–3 cm margin
- Breslow thickness > 4 mm: 3 cm margin.'

- Marsden JR, et al., British Association of Dermatologists. Br J Dermatol 2010; 163:238–256.

For further information: www.cochrane.org/cochrane-reviews

palpable local node involvement should be treated surgically.

Prognosis for metastatic disease is poor and chemotherapy is palliative. Melanoma is immunogenic and immunotherapy may be used in patients with advanced disease, although there is no evidence of improved overall survival. Other biological and gene therapies and vaccines are being investigated. Genetic advances have facilitated the introduction of tumour-targeted treatments for late-stage disease, such as *B-Raf* and *c-Kit* inhibitors for patients expressing these gene mutations, and this approach is under further investigation.

Prognosis

The Breslow thickness of the primary tumour is the most important prognostic factor in stage I disease, although other indices, including mitotic rate and presence/absence of ulceration, are also important. Patients with a primary tumour of less than 1 mm have more than a 95% chance of disease-free survival at 10 years, but this figure drops to approximately 50% for a tumour of greater than 3.5 mm thickness. Survival rates fall to less than 10% for those with advanced nodal or metastatic disease. In general, the prognosis is better in females and for tumours at certain sites, such as the leg.

Benign lesions that may be confused with skin cancers

In practice, it is often difficult to distinguish between skin cancer and a benign lesion on clinical grounds. Benign melanocytic naevi and basal cell papillomas can often be mistaken for melanoma, even by dermatologists. If there is any doubt, histology is required.

Freckle (ephelis)

Histologically, a freckle consists of normal numbers of melanocytes, but with focal increases in melanin in keratinocytes. They are most common on sun-exposed sites in fair-skinned individuals, particularly children and in those with red hair, and on the face. There is a familial tendency. Clinically, freckles are brown macules, which darken following UVR exposure.

Lentigines

A lentigo consists of increased numbers of melanocytes along the basement membrane, but without formation of the nests that occur in melanocytic naevi. These lesions usually occur at sites of chronic sun exposure (see the background skin changes in Fig. 28.10A), become more common with age, and are often referred to as 'liver spots' or 'age spots'. They can vary in colour from light to very dark brown. Distinction from melanoma is essential and histology may be required.

Haemangiomas

Benign vascular tumours or hamartomas are common and include Campbell de Morgan spots, which present as pink/red papules on the upper half of the body. They can sometimes be difficult to distinguish from melanocytic lesions, particularly if they are thrombosed or occur on particular sites, such as the lip or genitalia. The dermatoscope is helpful for this (see Fig. 28.2, p. 1256).

Basal cell papilloma (seborrhoeic wart)

Basal cell papillomas (seborrhoeic warts or keratoses) are common, benign epidermal tumours (Fig. 28.15). The name is misleading, as they do not involve sebaceous glands. They can be confused with melanoma and may be cosmetically troublesome. They may be flat, raised, pedunculated or warty-surfaced, and can appear to be 'stuck on'. They occur in both sexes and with increasing age, and are most common on the face and trunk. The colour may vary from yellow to almost black and the surface may seem 'greasy', with pinpoint keratin plugs visible, particularly with a magnifying lens. If there is no diagnostic doubt, they can be left alone or treated by cryotherapy or curettage. If the differential diagnosis includes melanoma, excision biopsy should be undertaken.

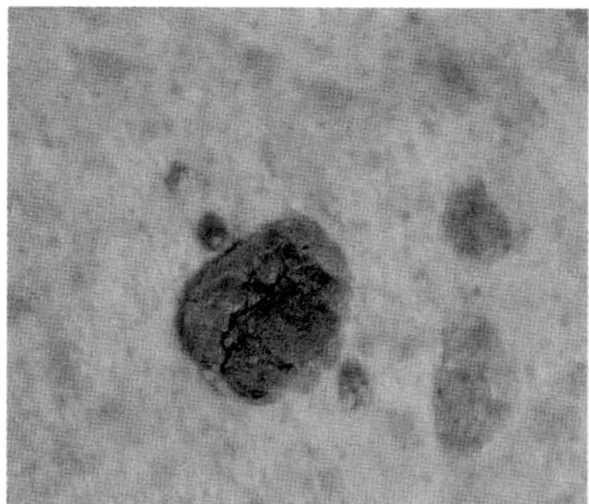

Fig. 28.15 A typical basal cell papilloma. Note the neighbouring basal cell papillomas and the coincidental benign angiomas (Campbell de Morgan spots).

Melanocytic naevi

Melanocytic naevi (moles) are localised benign clonal proliferations of melanocytes. Their cause is unknown but may relate to abnormalities of the normal migratory pattern of melanocytes during development. It is quite normal to have 20–50, although, interestingly, individuals with red hair have fewer. Genetic and environmental factors are implicated. Monozygotic twins have higher concordance in naevi numbers than dizygotic twins. Individuals who have had greater sun exposure have higher numbers of naevi. Most melanocytic naevi appear in childhood and early adult life, or during pregnancy

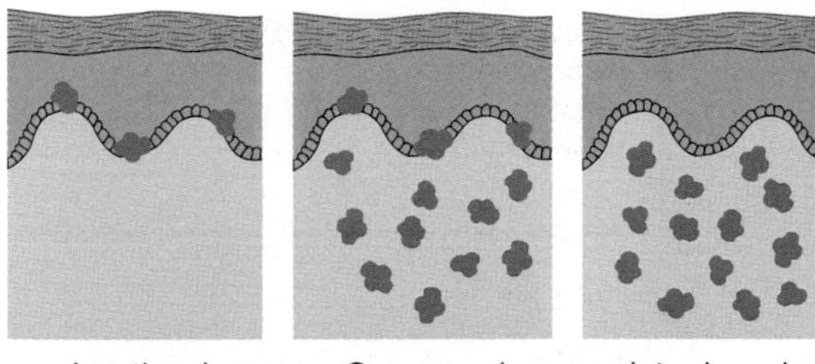

Fig. 28.16 Classification of melanocytic naevi. Classification is based on microscopic location of the nests of naevus cells.

or oestrogen therapy. The onset of a new mole is less common after the age of 25 years. Congenital melanocytic naevi occur at or shortly after birth.

Clinical features

Acquired melanocytic naevi are classified according to the microscopic location of the melanocyte nests (Fig. 28.16). Junctional naevi are usually macular, circular or oval, and mid- to dark brown. Compound and intradermal naevi are nodules, because of the dermal component, and may be hair-bearing. Intradermal naevi are usually less pigmented than compound naevi. Their surface may be smooth, cerebriform, hyperkeratotic or papillomatous.

Some individuals have large numbers of naevi, often at unusual sites, such as the scalp, palms or soles, and these may often appear 'atypical' in terms of variability in pigmentation, size and shape. Some may be very dark or pink and may show a depigmented or inflamed halo. If these naevi are removed, then 'dysplastic changes' are often seen. Such naevi are known to occur in some rare families with an inherited melanoma predisposition. However, the significance of such changes in non-familial cases is unclear and there is no consensus on management and follow-up.

Although approximately 50% of melanomas arise in pre-existing naevi, most naevi do not become malignant; although a changing naevus must be taken seriously, most will not be melanomas. Malignant change is most likely in large congenital melanocytic naevi (risk may correlate with the size of the lesion) and possibly in families who have been diagnosed as showing large numbers of atypical naevi with a history of melanoma.

Management

Melanocytic naevi are normal and do not require excision, unless malignancy is suspected or they become repeatedly inflamed or traumatised. Advice on photoprotection is important for fair-skinned individuals with multiple naevi.

Blue naevi

These are melanocytic naevi in which there is a proliferation of spindled melanocytes relatively deep within the dermis. Light scattering means that the pigment appears blue rather than brown. They may be difficult to distinguish from nodular melanoma and are therefore often excised.

Dermatofibroma

A dermatofibroma is a characteristically firm, often pigmented, raised lesion, most commonly found on the lower legs. Its aetiology is unclear, although a reactive process secondary to insect bites or trauma is one hypothesis. There is frequently a ring of pigment around the lesion and dimpling when the skin is pinched, reflecting epidermal tethering.

Acrochordon (skin tag)

Acrochordons are benign pedunculated lesions, most common in skin flexures. They may be confused with melanocytic naevi.

Lipoma

Lipomas are benign tumours of adipocytes, which are characteristically soft and lie more deeply in the skin than epidermal tumours. A variant, angiolipoma, is typically painful.

COMMON SKIN INFECTIONS AND INFESTATIONS

Bacterial infections

Impetigo

Impetigo is a common and highly contagious superficial bacterial skin infection. There are two main presentations: bullous impetigo, caused by a staphylococcal epidermolytic toxin, and non-bullous impetigo (Fig. 28.17), which can be caused by either *Staphylococcus aureus* or streptococcus, or both together. Staphylococcus is the most common agent in temperate climates, whereas streptococcal impetigo is more often seen in hot, humid areas. All ages can contract the infection but non-bullous disease particularly affects young children, often in late summer. It can be sporadic, although outbreaks can arise in conditions of overcrowding and poor hygiene or in institutions. A widespread form can occur in neonates. Predisposing factors are minor skin abrasions and the existence of other skin conditions, such as infestations or eczema.

In non-bullous impetigo, a thin-walled vesicle develops; it rapidly ruptures and is rarely seen intact. Dried

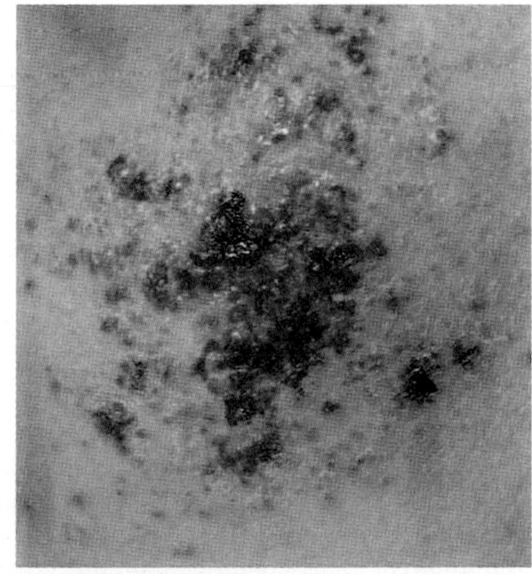

Fig. 28.17 Non-bullous impetigo.

exudate, forming golden crusting, arises on an erythematous base. In bullous disease, the toxins cleave desmoglein-1, causing a superficial epidermal split and the occurrence of intact blisters with clear to cloudy fluid, which last for 2–3 days. The face, scalp and limbs are commonly affected but other sites can also be involved, particularly if there are predisposing factors such as eczema. Lesions may be single or multiple and coalesce. Constitutional symptoms are uncommon. A bacterial swab should be taken from blister fluid or active lesion before treatment commences. Around one-third of the population are nasal carriers of *Staphylococcus*, so swabs from the nostrils should also be obtained.

In mild, localised disease, topical treatment with mupirocin or fusidic acid usually suffices and limits the spread of infection. The use of topical antiseptics and soap and water to remove infected crusts is also helpful. Staphylococcal carriage should be treated, with mupirocin topically to the nostrils if swabs are positive. In severe cases, an oral antibiotic, such as flucloxacillin or erythromycin, is indicated. If a nephritogenic streptococcus is suspected, then systemic antibiotics should be given, as post-streptococcal glomerulonephritis can occur (p. 498). Underlying disease, such as infestations, must be treated and cross-infection minimised. Scarring does not occur but there may be temporary dyspigmentation.

Staphylococcal scalded skin syndrome

Staphylococcal scalded skin syndrome (SSSS) is a potentially serious exfoliating condition occurring predominantly in children, particularly neonates (Fig. 28.18). It is caused by systemic circulation of epidermolytic toxins from a *Staph. aureus* infection. The same toxins are implicated in bullous impetigo, which is a localised form of SSSS. The focus of infection may be minor skin trauma, the umbilicus, urinary tract or nasopharynx. The child presents with fever, irritability and skin tenderness. Erythema usually begins in the groin, axillae and around the mouth. Blisters and superficial erosions develop over 1–2 days and can rapidly involve large areas, with severe systemic upset. Bacterial swabs should be obtained from possible primary sites of infection. A skin snip should also be taken for urgent histology. This is a sample of the superficial peeling skin removed by 'snipping with scissors', without the need for local anaesthetic. It shows a split beneath the stratum corneum, and differentiates SSSS from toxic epidermal necrolysis, in which the whole epidermis is affected (see Fig. 28.36, p. 1292). Systemic antibiotics (e.g. flucloxacillin) and intensive supportive measures should be commenced immediately. Bacterial swabs from nostrils, axillae and groins should be taken from family members to exclude staphylococcal carriage. Although the acute presentation of SSSS is often severe, rapid recovery and absence of scarring are usual, as the epidermal split is superficial.

Toxic shock syndrome

This condition is characterised by fever, desquamating rash, circulatory collapse and multi-organ involvement (p. 331). It is caused by staphylococcal toxins and early cases were thought to arise with tampon use. Intensive supportive care and systemic antibiotics are required.

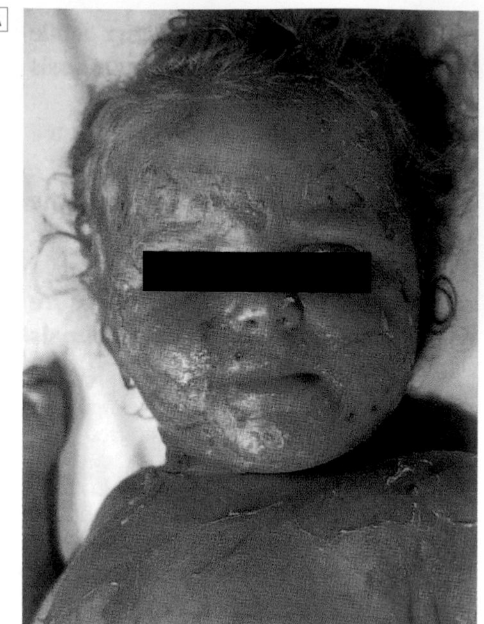

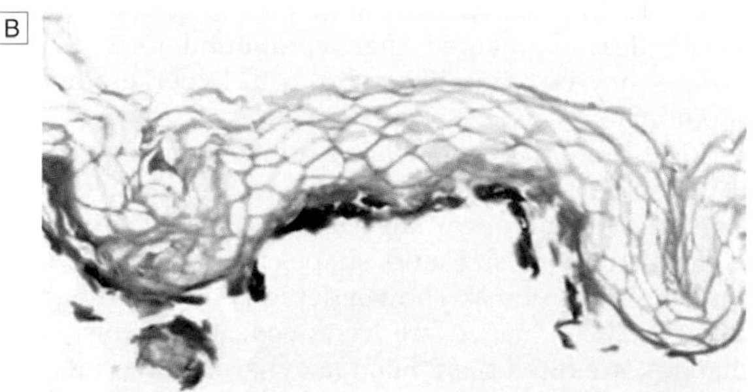

Fig. 28.18 Staphylococcal scalded skin syndrome. **A** Extensive erythema and superficial peeling of the skin. From Savin, et al. 2002 – see p. 1305. **B** The condition was rapidly diagnosed by examination of a frozen section of skin snip.

Ecthyma

Ecthyma is caused by either staphylococcus or streptococcus, or both together and is characterised by adherent crusts overlying ulceration. It occurs worldwide but is more common in the tropics. In Europe, it occurs more frequently in children. Predisposing factors include poor hygiene, malnutrition and underlying skin disease, such as scabies. It is commonly seen in drug abusers, and minor trauma can predispose to lesion development.

Folliculitis, furuncles and carbuncles

Hair follicle inflammation can be superficial, involving just the ostium of the follicle (folliculitis) or deep (furuncles and carbuncles).

Superficial folliculitis

This is very common, usually minor and subacute or chronic. Primary lesions are follicular pustules and erythema. It is often infective, caused by *Staph. aureus*, but can also be sterile and caused by physical (e.g. traumatic epilation) or chemical (e.g. mineral oil) injury. Staphylococcal folliculitis is most common in children and often

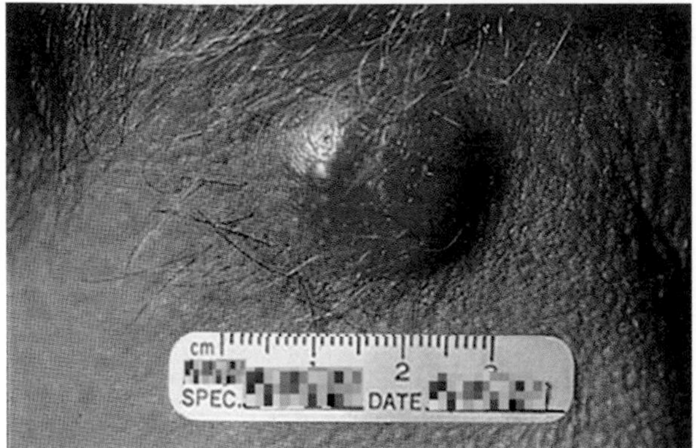

Fig. 28.19 Staphylococcal carbuncle.

occurs on the scalp or limbs. Pustules usually resolve without scarring in 7–10 days but can become chronic. In older children and adults, they may progress to a deeper form of folliculitis. The condition is often self-limiting and may respond to irritant removal and antiseptics. More severe cases may require topical or systemic antibiotics and treatment of *Staph. aureus* carrier sites.

Deep folliculitis (furuncles and carbuncles)

A furuncle (boil) is an acute *Staph. aureus* infection of the hair follicle, usually with necrosis. It is most common in young adults and males. It is usually sporadic but epidemics occasionally occur. Malnutrition, diabetes and HIV predispose, although most cases arise in healthy subjects. Any body site can be involved but neck, buttocks and anogenital areas are common. Infection is often associated with chronic *Staph. aureus* carriage in the nostrils and perineum, and may be due to resistant strains, such as meticillin-resistant organisms (MRSA). Friction caused by tight clothing may be contributory. Initially, an inflammatory follicular nodule develops and becomes pustular, fluctuant and tender. Crops of lesions sometimes occur. There may be fever and mild constitutional upset. Lesions rupture over days to weeks, discharge pus, become necrotic and leave a scar.

If a deep *Staph. aureus* infection of a group of contiguous hair follicles occurs, this is termed a carbuncle and is associated with intense deep inflammation (Fig. 28.19). This usually occurs in middle-aged men, often with predisposing conditions such as diabetes or immunosuppression. A carbuncle is an exquisitely tender nodule, usually on the neck, shoulders or hips, associated with severe constitutional symptoms. Discharge, necrosis and scarring are usual. Bacterial swabs must be taken and treatment is with anti-staphylococcal antibiotics, e.g. flucloxacillin, and sometimes incision and drainage.

Other staphylococcal toxins may also be pathogenic. For example, Panton–Valentine leukocidin-producing *Staph. aureus* can cause recurrent abscesses and may be difficult to eradicate.

Cellulitis and erysipelas

Cellulitis is inflammation of subcutaneous tissue, due to bacterial infection (Fig. 28.20). In contrast, erysipelas is bacterial infection of the dermis and upper subcutaneous tissue (Fig. 28.21), although in practice it may be difficult to distinguish between them. These conditions are most commonly caused by group A streptococcus. However, culture of swabs from affected sites is often negative. There is frequently a source of organism entry, such as an ear infection, varicose eczema/ulcer or tinea pedis, and swabs should also be taken from these sites. Diabetes and immunosuppression are predisposing factors. The patient usually has malaise, fever and leucocytosis, and streptococcal serology will often be positive. The face (erysipelas) and legs (cellulitis) are most often affected and the site is hot, painful, erythematous and oedematous. Blistering often occurs and may be haemorrhagic. Regional lymphadenopathy is common. Erysipelas typically has a well-defined edge due to its more superficial level of involvement, whereas cellulitis is typically ill-defined. Treatment is usually with intravenous anti-streptococcal antibiotics, such as benzylpenicillin, with erythromycin or ciprofloxacin as an alternative for penicillin-allergic patients. Milder cases may be treated with oral antibiotics. If cases are untreated, sequelae include lymphoedema, cavernous sinus thrombosis, septicaemia and glomerulonephritis.

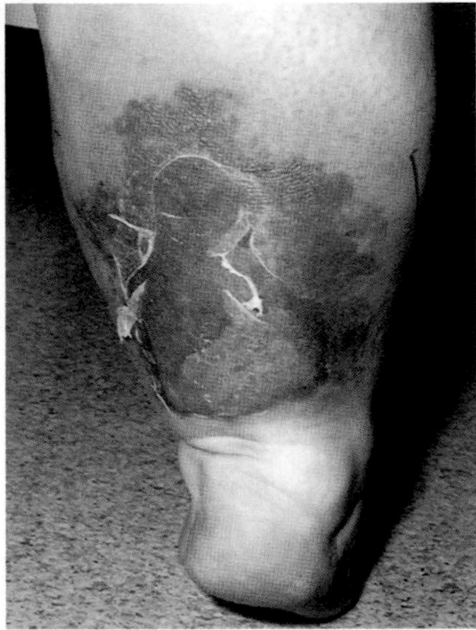

Fig. 28.20 Acute cellulitis of the leg. Note the chronic lymphoedema and the haemorrhagic blistering. Blister fluid was positive for group G streptococci.

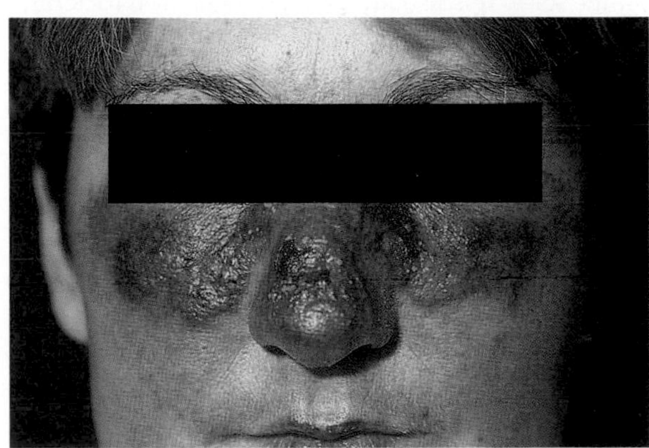

Fig. 28.21 Erysipelas. Note the blistering and the crusted rash with raised, erythematous edge. The yellow discoloration is due to topical iodine treatment.

Necrotising soft tissue infections and anthrax

See pages 305 and 347, respectively.

Erythrasma

Erythrasma is a mild, chronic, localised, superficial skin infection caused by *Corynebacterium minutissimum*, which is part of the normal skin flora. Warmth and humidity predispose to this infection, which usually occurs in flexures and toe clefts. It is asymptomatic or mildly itchy and lesions are well defined, red/brown and scaly. *C. minutissimum* has characteristic coral-pink fluorescence under Wood's light. Microscopy and culture of skin scrapings can confirm the diagnosis but are not usually needed if Wood's light examination is positive. A topical azole (clotrimazole or miconazole) or fusidic acid is usually effective. Oral erythromycin can be used for extensive or resistant disease. Antiseptics can be used to prevent disease recurrence.

Pitted keratolysis

This is another superficial skin infection with *Corynebacterium*, producing characteristic circular erosions ('pits') on the soles. It is usually asymptomatic. The bacterium can be identified in skin scrapings and typically occurs in association with hyperhidrosis, which must be treated to prevent recurrence. Treatment is as for erythrasma.

Other skin infections

Syphilis and the non-venereal treponematoses are described on pages 419 and 332. Lyme disease is described on page 334.

Viral infections

Herpesvirus infections

The cutaneous manifestations of the human herpesviruses are described on page 325.

Papillomaviruses and viral warts

Viral warts are extremely common and are caused by the DNA human papillomavirus (HPV). There are over 90 subtypes, based on DNA sequence analysis, causing different clinical presentations. Transmission is by direct virus contact, in living or shed skin, and is encouraged by trauma and moisture (e.g. swimming pools). Genital warts are spread by sexual activity and show a clear relationship with cervical and intra-epithelial cancers of the genital area. HPV-16 and 18 appear to inactivate tumour suppressor gene pathways and lead to squamous cell carcinoma of the cervix or intra-epithelial carcinoma of the genital skin (p. 425). Vaccinations are now available against HPV-16 and 18 and are recommended for adolescent females before they become sexually active. The relationship between skin HPV and skin cancer is unclear. Individuals who are systemically immunosuppressed, e.g. after organ transplantation, have greatly increased risks of skin cancer and HPV infection, but a causal link is not certain.

Clinical features

Common warts are initially smooth, skin-coloured papules, which become hyperkeratotic and 'warty'. They are most common on the hands (Fig. 28.22) but can occur on the face, genitalia and limbs, and are often multiple. Plantar warts (verrucae) have a slightly protruding rough surface and horny rim and are often painful on walking. Paring reveals capillary loops that distinguish plantar warts from corns.

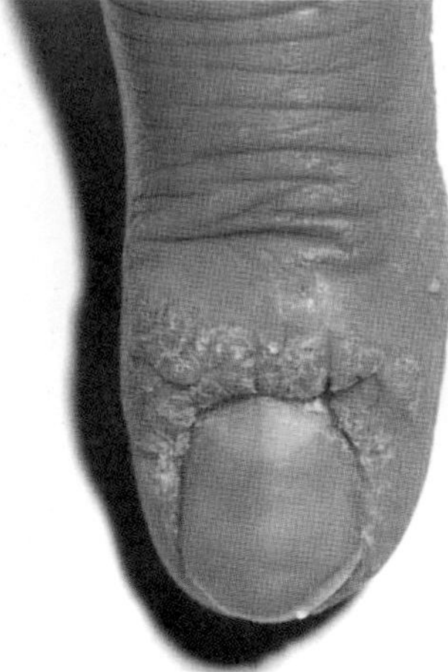

Fig. 28.22 Viral wart on the finger. The capillary loops are evident within the warty hyperkeratosis. Periungual sites are common and more difficult to treat.

Other varieties of wart include:

- *mosaic warts*: mosaic-like sheets of warts
- *plane warts*: smooth, flat-topped papules, usually on the face and backs of hands; they may be pigmented and therefore misdiagnosed
- *facial warts*: often filiform
- *genital warts*: may be papillomatous and exuberant.

Management

Most viral warts resolve spontaneously, although this may take years and active treatment is therefore often sought. However, asymptomatic warts generally should not be treated. Viral warts are particularly problematic and more recalcitrant to treatment in immunosuppressed patients following organ transplantation.

Treatments are destructive. Salicylic acid or salicylic/lactic acid combinations and regular wart paring for several months is the first approach (Box 28.19). Cryotherapy is usually the next step and is repeated 2–4-weekly. However, caution is required, particularly on the hands, as over-vigorous cryotherapy can lead to scarring, nail dystrophy and even tendon rupture. Periungual and subungual warts can be problematic, and nail cutting and electrodessication may help. Several other therapies have been used for recalcitrant warts,

EBM 28.19 Treatment of viral skin warts

'Salicylic acid is the most consistently effective treatment. For certain types (such as filiform warts on the face), cryotherapy is generally the treatment of choice but, for common hand and foot warts, a salicylic acid wart paint should be used first.'

- Kwok CS, et al. Topical treatments for cutaneous warts. Cochrane Database of Systematic Reviews, 2012, issue 9. Art. no.: CD001781.

For further information: www.cochrane.org/cochrane-reviews

including systemic retinoids, intralesional bleomycin or interferon injections, and contact sensitisation with, for example, diphencyprone. Imiquimod and PDT may also be beneficial, particularly for multiple warts in immunosuppressed patients.

Molluscum contagiosum

Molluscum contagiosum is caused by a DNA poxvirus skin infection. It is most common in children over the age of 1 year, particularly those with atopic dermatitis. It also frequently occurs in immunosuppressed patients, including those with HIV (p. 388). Lesions are dome-shaped, 'umbilicated', skin-coloured papules with central punctum (Fig. 28.23). They are often multiple and found at sites of apposition, such as the side of the chest and the inner arm. Spontaneous resolution occurs but can take months. Prior to resolution, they often become inflamed and may leave small, atrophic scars. Destructive therapies may be painful and risk scarring, and the decision not to treat is often sensible. Gentle squeezing with forceps after bathing can hasten resolution. Topical salicylic acid, podophyllin, trichloroacetic acid, cryotherapy or curettage is an alternative. Efficacy with imiquimod has recently been reported.

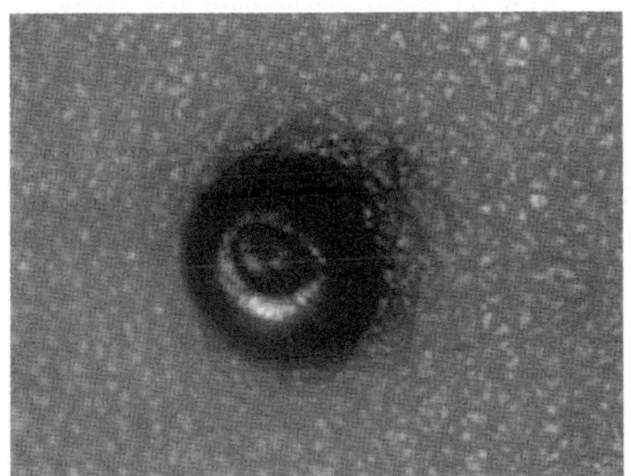

Fig. 28.23 Molluscum contagiosum. Note the central umbilication.

Orf

Orf is a parapoxvirus skin infection and is an occupational risk for those who work with sheep and goats. Inoculation of virus, usually into finger skin, causes significant inflammation and necrosis, which typically resolves within 2–6 weeks. No specific treatment is required, unless there is secondary infection. Erythema multiforme (p. 1302) can be provoked by orf.

Other viral exanthems

See page 313.

Fungal infections

Fungal skin infections can be superficial (dermatophytes and yeasts) or, less commonly, deep (chromomycosis or sporotrichosis); the latter are more often seen in tropical climates or in the immunocompromised. Dermatophyte infections (ringworm) are extremely common and usually caused by fungi of the *Microsporum*, *Trichophyton* and *Epidermophyton* species. The fungi can originate from soil (geophilic) or animals (zoophilic), or be confined to human skin (anthropophilic). Dermatophyte infections usually present with skin (tinea corporis), scalp (tinea capitis), groin (tinea cruris), foot (tinea pedis) and/or nail (onychomycosis) involvement (Fig. 28.24).

Tinea corporis

Tinea corporis should feature in the differential diagnosis of a red, scaly rash (p. 1257). Typically, lesions are erythematous, annular and scaly, with well-defined edge and central clearing. There may also be pustules at the active edge. Lesions are usually asymmetrical and may be single or multiple. The degree of inflammation is dependent on the organism involved and the host immune response. *Microsporum canis* (from dogs) and *Trichophyton verrucosum* (from cats) are common culprits. Ill-advised use of topical steroids can modify the clinical presentation and increase disease extension (tinea incognito).

Tinea cruris

This is extremely common worldwide and is usually caused by *Trichophyton rubrum*. Itchy, erythematous plaques develop in the groins and extend on to the thighs, with a raised active edge (Fig. 28.24A).

Tinea pedis (athlete's foot)

This is the most common fungal infection in the UK and USA, and is usually caused by anthropophilic fungi, such as *T. rubrum*, *T. interdigitale* and *Epidermophyton*

A

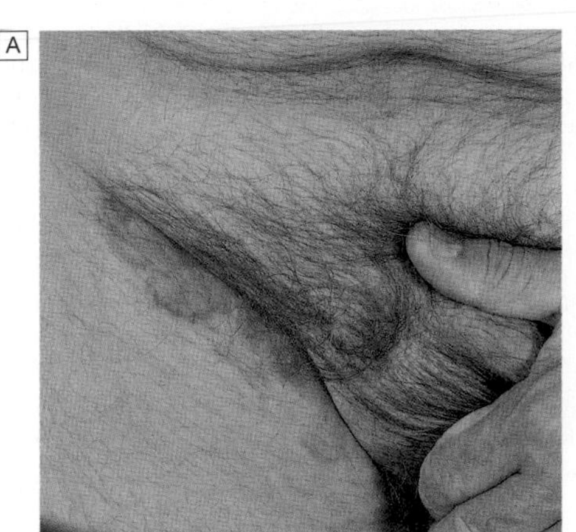

B

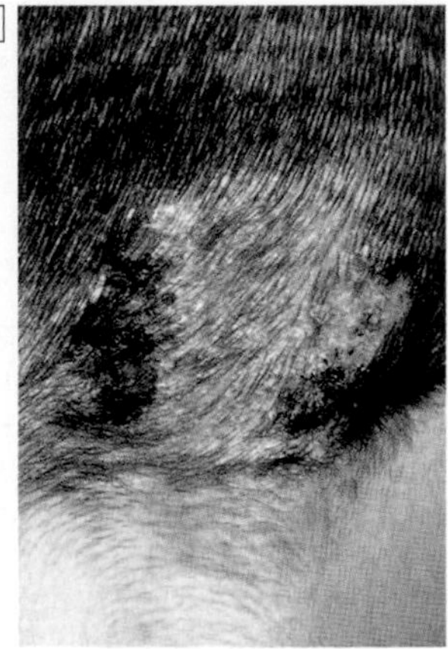

Fig. 28.24 Dermatophyte infections. **A** *Trichophyton rubrum* infection of the groin (tinea cruris). **B** *Microsporum canis* infection of the scalp (tinea capitis).

28

floccosum. It typically presents as an itchy rash between the toes, with peeling, fissuring and maceration. Involvement of one sole or palm (tinea manuum) with fine scaling is characteristic of *T. rubrum* infection. Vesiculation or blistering is more often seen with *T. mentagrophytes*.

Tinea capitis

This is a dermatophyte infection of scalp hair shafts and is most common in children (Fig. 28.24B). It typically presents as an area of scalp inflammation and scaling, often with pustules and partial hair loss. Infection may be within the shaft (endothrix, e.g. *T. tonsurans*), causing patchy hair loss, with broken hairs at the surface ('black dot'), little inflammation and no fluorescence with Wood's light. Infection outside the hair shaft (ectothrix, e.g. *Microsporum audouinii* (anthropophilic)) shows minimal inflammation; *M. canis* (from dogs and cats) infections are more inflammatory and can be identified by green fluorescence with Wood's light. Kerion is a boggy, inflammatory area of tinea capitis, usually caused by zoophilic fungi (e.g. cattle ringworm; *T. verrucosum*).

Onychomycosis

This is a fungal infection of the nail plate and the species involved are generally those that cause tinea capitis or tinea pedis. Onychomycosis usually presents with yellow/brown nail discoloration, crumbling, thickening and subungual hyperkeratosis. Usually, some nails are spared, there is asymmetry and toenails are more commonly involved.

Diagnosis and management

Skin scrapings, hair pluckings or nail clippings must be taken from areas of disease activity, typically the advancing lesion edge, in order to confirm the diagnosis by microscopy and culture (p. 1255). Topical antifungals (e.g. terbinafine or miconazole) may suffice, although systemic treatment (terbinafine, griseofulvin or itraconazole) may be required for stubborn or extensive disease and scalp or nail involvement. In addition to systemic antifungals, a short course of systemic corticosteroid may be required for kerion to limit hair loss.

Candidiasis

This is a superficial skin or mucosal infection caused by a yeast-like fungus, *Candida albicans* (p. 381). Infections are usually not serious, unless the patient is immunocompromised, when deeper tissues can be involved (p. 389). The organism has a predilection for warm, moist environments and typical presentations are napkin candidiasis in babies, genital and perineal candidiasis, intertrigo and oral candidiasis. Diagnosis can be confirmed by microscopy and culture of skin swabs, and treatment is with topical or systemic antifungals, such as azoles.

Pityriasis versicolor

Pityriasis versicolor is a persistent, superficial skin condition caused by a common commensal yeast, *Malassezia furfur*. It occurs in men and women and in different races. It is found more frequently in warmer, humid climates, and is usually more severe and persistent in the immunocompromised. It is characterised by scaly, oval macules on the upper trunk, usually hypopigmented but occasionally hyperpigmented. Hypopigmentation is more obvious after sun exposure and tanning. The diagnosis can be confirmed by microscopy of skin scrapings, showing 'spaghetti and meatballs' hyphae. Treatment with selenium sulphide or ketoconazole shampoos, and topical or systemic azole antifungal agents is usually effective, although, because these yeasts are skin commensals, recurrence is common and maintenance topical therapy may be required. Altered pigmentation can persist for months after treatment.

Scabies

Scabies is caused by the mite, *Sarcoptes scabiei*. It can lead to secondary infection, sometimes with complications, such as glomerulonephritis due to nephritogenic streptococci. It spreads in households and environments where there is intimate personal contact. The diagnosis is made by identifying the scabietic burrow (p. 312 and Fig. 28.25) and visualising the mite (by extracting with a needle or using a dermatoscope). In small children, the palms and soles can be involved, with pustules. Pruritus is prominent. The clinical features include secondary eczematisation elsewhere on the body; the face and scalp are rarely affected, except in infants. Involvement of the genitals in males and of the nipples commonly occurs. Even after successful treatment, itch can continue and occasionally nodular lesions persist.

Topical treatment of the affected individual and all asymptomatic family members/physical contacts is required to ensure eradication. Two applications 1 week apart of an aqueous solution of permethrin or malathion

A

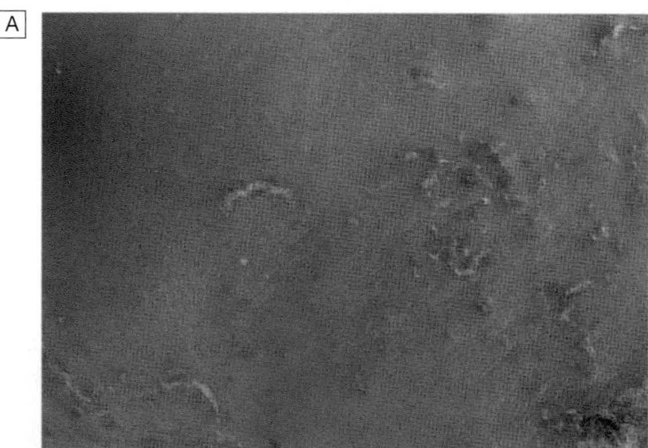

B

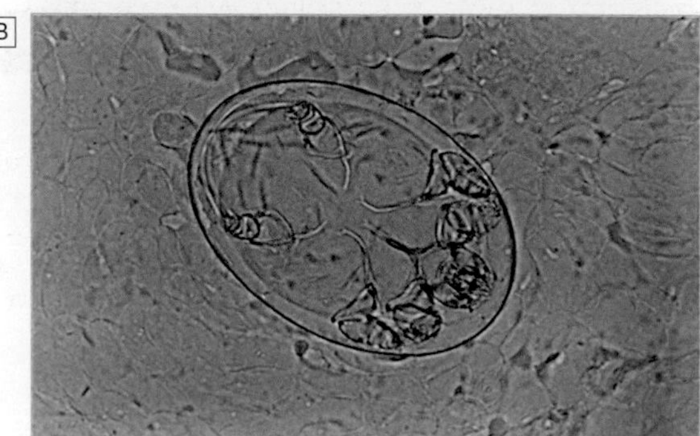

Fig. 28.25 Scabies. **A** Burrows evident on the palm of the hand. **B** A mite still in its egg, seen on light microscopy of scrapings over a burrow. Note that the mite has only six legs, unlike adult mites, which have eight.

to the whole body, excluding the head, are usually successful. If there is poor compliance, immunosuppression or heavy infestation (crusted 'Norwegian' scabies), systemic treatment with a single dose of ivermectin is sometimes appropriate.

Lice

Head lice

Infestation with the head louse, *Pediculus humanus capitis*, is common. It is highly contagious and spread by direct head-to-head contact. Scalp itch leads to scratching, secondary infection and cervical lymphadenopathy. The diagnosis is confirmed by identifying the living louse or nymph on the scalp or on a black sheet of paper after careful fine-toothed combing of wet hair following conditioner application. The empty egg cases ('nits') are easily seen on the hair shaft (p. 1250) and are hard to dislodge.

Treatment is recommended for the affected individual and any infected household/school contacts. Eradication in school populations is difficult because of poor compliance and treatment resistance. Malathion, permethrin or carbaryl, in lotion or aqueous formulations, should be applied twice at an interval of 7–10 days. Rotational treatments within a community may avoid resistance. Regular 'wet-combing' (physical removal of live lice by regular combing of conditioned wet hair) may be less effective than pharmacological treatments. Vaseline should be applied to eyelashes/brows twice daily for at least a fortnight.

Body lice

These are similar to head lice but live on clothing, particularly in seams, and feed on the skin. Poor hygiene and overcrowded conditions predispose. Itch, excoriation and secondary infection occur. Dry cleaning and high-temperature washing or insecticide treatment of clothes are required.

Pubic (crab) lice

Usually, these are sexually acquired and very itchy. Malathion or carbaryl in an aqueous base is the treatment of choice, applied on two occasions to the whole body, as body hair can also be infested. Contacts should also be treated.

ACNE AND ROSACEA

Acne vulgaris

Acne is chronic inflammation of the pilosebaceous units. The condition is extremely common; it generally starts after puberty and there are reports of it affecting over 90% of adolescents. It is usually most severe in the late teenage years but can persist into the thirties and forties, particularly in females (Box 28.20).

Aetiology

The key components are increased sebum production; colonisation of pilosebaceous ducts by *Propionibacterium acnes*, which in turn causes inflammation; and hypercornification and occlusion of pilosebaceous ducts (Fig. 28.26). Severity of acne is associated with sebum excretion rate, which increases at puberty. Both androgens and progestogens increase sebum excretion and oestrogens reduce it, although the hormonal effects may also reflect end-organ sensitivity, as most patients have normal hormone profiles. There may be a positive family history; there is high concordance in monozygotic twins and it is likely that genetic factors are important in some families, but candidate genes have not been confirmed.

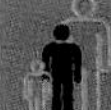

28.20 Acne in adolescence

- **Epidemiology**: acne vulgaris is most common between the ages of 12 and 20. It often begins around 10–13 years of age, lasts 5–10 years and usually resolves by age 20–25.
- **Emotional effects**: at all ages acne can have negative effects on self-esteem, but it is especially important to assess how it affects an adolescent. The consequences (whether acne is objectively severe or not) can be devastating, leading to embarrassment, school avoidance, life-long effects on ability to form friendships, attract partners, and acquire and keep employment.
- **Treatment**: effective treatments aim to improve the condition and prevent worsening (including later scarring), and to restore emotional well-being and self-esteem.

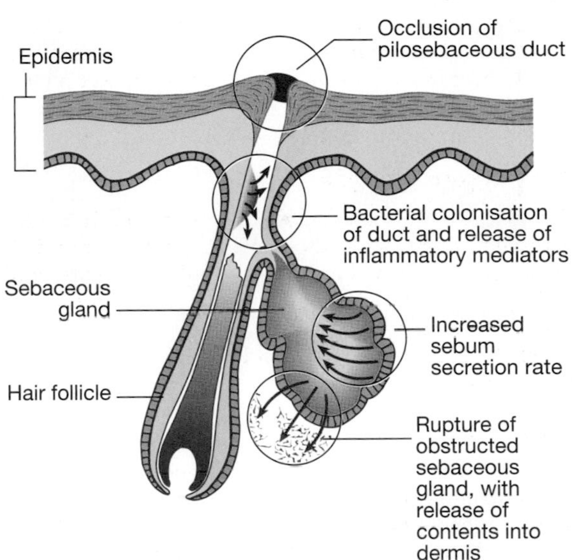

Fig. 28.26 Pathogenesis of acne.

Clinical features

Acne usually affects the face and often the trunk. Greasiness of the skin may be obvious (seborrhoea). The hallmark is the comedone: open comedones (blackheads) are dilated keratin-filled follicles, which appear as black papules due to the keratin debris; closed comedones (whiteheads) usually have no visible follicular opening and are caused by accumulation of sebum and keratin deeper in the pilosebaceous ducts. Inflammatory papules, nodules and cysts occur and may arise from comedones (Fig. 28.27). Scarring may follow deep-seated or superficial acne and may be keloidal.

There are distinct clinical variants:

- *Acne conglobata*: characterised by comedones, nodules, abscesses, sinuses and cysts, usually with

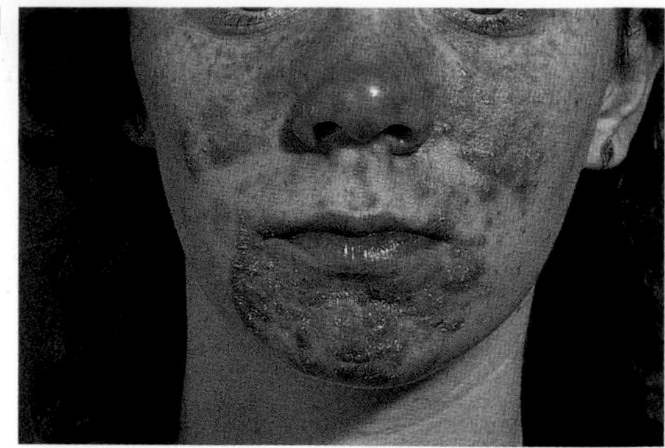

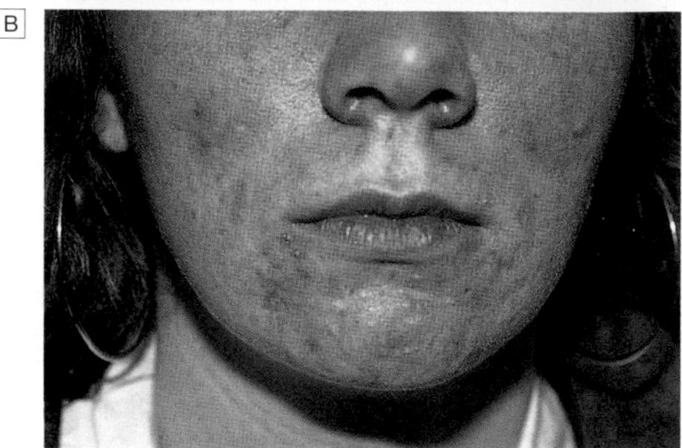

Fig. 28.27 Cystic acne in a teenager. **A** Before treatment. **B** After prolonged systemic antibiotic treatment.

marked scarring. It is rare, usually affecting adult males, and most commonly occurs on trunk and upper limbs. It may be associated with hidradenitis suppurativa (a chronic, inflammatory disorder of apocrine glands, predominantly affecting axillae and groins), scalp folliculitis and pilonidal sinus.

- *Acne fulminans*: a rare but severe presentation of acne, associated with fever, arthralgias and systemic inflammation, with raised neutrophil count and plasma viscosity. It is usually found on the trunk in adolescent males. Costochondritis can occur.
- *Acne excoriée*: describes self-inflicted excoriations due to compulsive picking of pre-existing or imagined acne lesions. It usually affects teenage girls and underlying psychological problems are common.
- *Secondary acne*: comedonal acne can be caused by greasy cosmetics or occupational exposure to oils, tars or chlorinated aromatic hydrocarbons. Predominantly pustular acne can occur in patients using systemic or topical corticosteroids, oral contraceptives, anticonvulsants, lithium or antineoplastic drugs, such as the epidermal growth factor receptor (EGFR) inhibitor, cetuximab. Most patients with acne do not have an underlying endocrine disorder. However, acne is a common feature of polycystic ovary syndrome (p. 764), which should be suspected if acne is moderate to severe and associated with hirsutism and menstrual irregularities. Virilisation should also raise suspicion of an androgen-secreting tumour.

Investigations

Investigations are not required in typical acne vulgaris. Secondary causes and suspected underlying endocrine disease or virilisation should be investigated (p. 763).

Management

Mild to moderate disease

Mild disease is usually managed with topical therapy (p. 1264). If comedones predominate, then topical benzoyl peroxide or retinoids should be used. Treatment should initially be applied at low concentrations for short duration and increased as tolerated. Azelaic acid may also be useful for mild acne. Patients with mild inflammatory acne should respond to topical antibiotics, such as erythromycin or clindamycin, which can be used in combination with other treatments.

For moderate inflammatory acne, a systemic tetracycline, such as oxytetracycline or lymecycline, should be used at adequate dose for 3–6 months in the first instance (p. 1267; Fig. 28.27B). If the case fails to respond, then alternatives include erythromycin or trimethoprim.

Oestrogen-containing oral contraceptives or a combined oestrogen/anti-androgen (such as cyproterone acetate) contraceptive may provide additional benefit in women. Patients should be referred for consideration of isotretinoin (13 *cis*-retinoic acid) if there is a failure to respond adequately to 6 months of therapy with these combined systemic and topical approaches (p. 1267).

Moderate to severe disease

Isotretinoin has revolutionised the treatment of moderate to severe acne that has not responded adequately to other therapies. It has a multifactorial mechanism of action, with reduction in sebum excretion by over 90%, follicular hypercornification and *P. acnes* colonisation. A typical course lasts for 4 months. Sebum excretion usually returns to baseline over the space of a year after treatment is stopped, although clinical benefit is usually longer-lasting. Many patients will not require further treatment, although a second or third course of isotretinoin may be required. A low-dose continuous or intermittent-dose regimen may be considered for a longer duration, in patients who relapse after a higher-dose regimen. Combination with systemic steroid may be required in the short term for severe acne, in order to minimise the risk of disease flare early in the treatment course. Thorough screening and monitoring are required, given the side-effect profile of isotretinoin (p. 1267).

Other treatments and physical measures

Intralesional injections of triamcinolone acetonide may be required for inflamed acne nodules or cysts, which can also be incised and drained, or excised under local anaesthetic. Scarring may be prevented by adequate treatment of active acne. Keloid scars may respond to intralesional steroid and/or silicone dressings. Carbon dioxide laser, microdermabrasion, chemical peeling or localised excision can also be considered for scarring. UVB phototherapy or PDT can occasionally be used in patients with inflammatory acne who are unable to use conventional therapy, such as isotretinoin. There is no convincing evidence to support a causal association between diet and acne. The psychological impact of acne must not be underestimated and should be considered in management decisions (see Box 28.20).

Rosacea

This chronic inflammatory condition affects the central face and consists of flushing, erythema, papules, pustules and telangiectasiae. The cause is unknown. Rosacea is distinct from acne vulgaris; sebum excretion is normal and comedones are absent. The relative contribution of *Demodex* mite and cutaneous vasomotor instability to the pathogenesis of rosacea remains poorly defined.

Clinical features and diagnosis

Rosacea most commonly affects fair-skinned, middle-aged females and can be exacerbated by heat, sunlight and alcohol. The convexities of nose, forehead, cheeks and chin are typically involved (Fig. 28.28). The condition is heterogeneous and, in some, intermittent flushing, followed by fixed erythema and telangiectasiae, predominate; in others, papules and pustules are prominent. Sebaceous gland hyperplasia and soft tissue overgrowth of the nose (rhinophyma) can occur, particularly in males. Conjunctivitis and blepharitis may also occur. Facial lymphoedema can be an added complication. Usually, no investigations are required and the diagnosis is obvious clinically. However, it must be distinguished from acne vulgaris, systemic lupus erythematosus, photosensitivity disorders and seborrhoeic dermatitis (the latter may coexist with rosacea).

Management

Mild disease may respond to topical antimicrobials, such as metronidazole or azelaic acid. Tetracycline or erythromycin for 3–6 months is usually effective in inflammatory pustular disease resistant to topical therapy (p. 1264). Relapse may require intermittent or chronic antibiotic use. Erythema and telangiectasiae do not respond well to antibiotics but laser therapy can be effective. Systemic isotretinoin may be helpful in severe resistant disease and rhinophyma may need laser therapy or surgery.

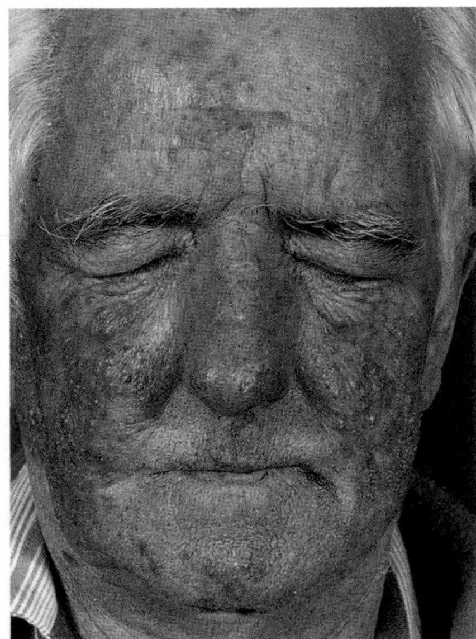

Fig. 28.28 Rosacea. Typical erythematous papulopustular rosacea affecting the mid-face.

ECZEMAS

The terms 'eczema' and 'dermatitis' are synonymous. Eczema can be acute or chronic and there are several causes. Acutely, epidermal oedema (spongiosis) and intra-epidermal vesiculation (producing multilocular blisters) predominate, whereas with chronicity there is more epidermal thickening (acanthosis). Vasodilatation and T-cell lymphocytic infiltration of the upper dermis also occur.

Clinical features

There are several patterns of eczema (Box 28.21) and environmental causes may be identifiable. The clinical features are similar, irrespective of the cause (Box 28.22).

Atopic eczema

Generalised, prolonged hypersensitivity to common environmental antigens, such as pollen and house dust mite, is the hallmark of atopy, in which there is a genetic predisposition to produce excess IgE. Atopic individuals manifest one or more of a group of diseases that includes asthma, hay fever, food and other allergies, and atopic eczema. There are strong familial associations with atopic diseases. The diagnosis of atopic eczema is made using clinical criteria (Box 28.23). Its prevalence has increased 2–5-fold since the early 1980s, and the disease now affects 1 in 10 schoolchildren.

Aetiology

Genetic factors are important. Epidermal barrier impairment is a major, and perhaps primary, factor in this form of eczema. Mutations in the filaggrin gene have been identified as important in some. Environmental factors, such as exposure to allergens in utero or during childhood, may also have an aetiological role and 60–80% of

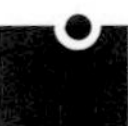

28.21 Classification of eczema
Endogenous
• Atopic, seborrhoeic
Exogenous
• Irritant, allergic, photoallergic, chronic actinic dermatitis
Characteristic patterns and morphology
• Asteatotic, discoid, gravitational, lichen simplex, pompholyx

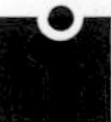

28.22 The clinical morphology of eczema
Acute
• Erythema, oedema, usually typically ill-defined • Papules, vesicles and occasionally bullae • Exudation, fissuring • Scaling
Chronic
• May be as above but less oedema, vesiculation and exudate • Lichenification: skin thickening with pronounced skin markings, secondary to chronic rubbing and scratching • Fissures, excoriations • Dyspigmentation: hyper- and hypopigmentation can occur

28.23 Diagnostic criteria for atopic eczema

Pruritus and at least three of the following are required:

- History of itch in skin creases (or cheeks if < 4 yrs)
- History of asthma/hay fever (or in a first-degree relative if < 4 yrs)
- Dry skin (xeroderma)
- Visible flexural eczema (cheeks, forehead, outer limbs if < 4 yrs)
- Onset in first 2 yrs of life

individuals are genetically susceptible to the induction of IgE-mediated sensitisation to environmental allergens such as food and animal hair. Decreased skin barrier function may also allow greater penetration of allergens through the epidermis, and thus cause immune stimulation and subsequent inflammation.

Clinical features

Atopic eczema is extremely itchy and scratching accounts for many of the signs (Fig. 28.29). Widespread cutaneous dryness (roughness) is another feature. The distribution and character of the rash vary with age (Box 28.24). Complications are listed in Box 28.25.

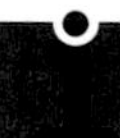

28.24 Atopic eczema: distribution and character of rash

Babies and infants

- Often acute and facial involvement prominent
- Trunk involved but nappy area usually spared

Children

- Flexures: behind knees, antecubital fossae, wrists and ankles

Adults

- Face and trunk usually involved, limb involvement not restricted to flexures
- Lichenification common

A

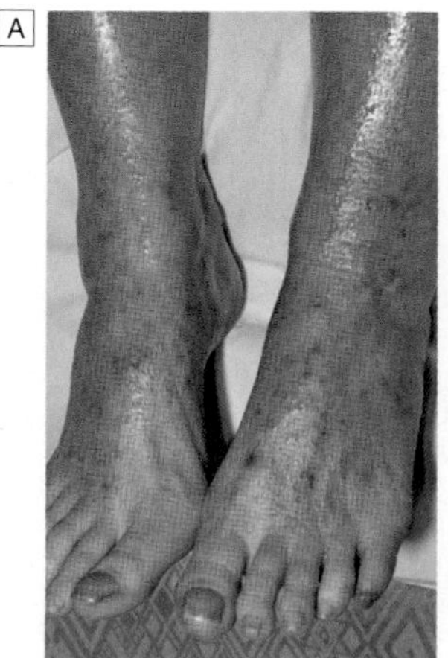

B

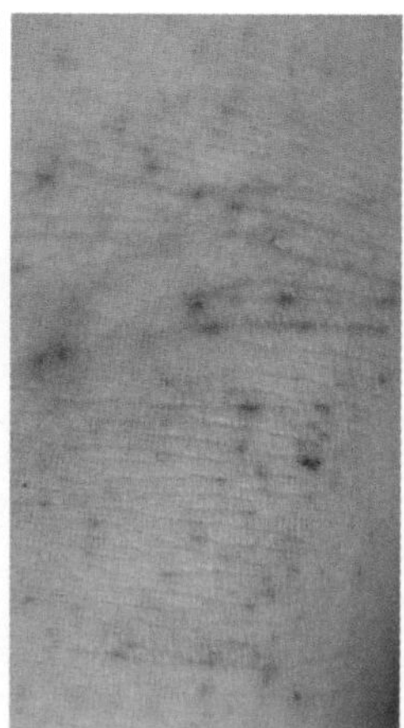

Fig. 28.29 Atopic eczema. A This patient had life-long chronic atopic eczema and experienced a generalised flare of disease triggered by infection. B Lichenification of chronic flexural eczema secondary to rubbing and scratching.

28.25 Complications of atopic eczema

Secondary infection

Bacterial

- *Staph. aureus* most common

Viral

- Herpes simplex virus can cause a widespread severe eruption – eczema herpeticum
- Papillomavirus and molluscum contagiosum are more common in atopic eczema, especially if treated with topical corticosteroids

Increased susceptibility to irritants

- Defective barrier function

Increased susceptibility to allergy

- Food allergy – mainly relevant in infants. Eggs, cow's milk, protein, fish, wheat and soya may cause an immediate urticarial eruption rather than exacerbation of eczema
- Increased risk of sensitisation to type IV allergens because of impaired barrier function

Impact on life and health

- Poor sleep, loss of schooling, behavioural difficulties, failure to thrive in children
- Impact on sleep, work, relationships, hobbies, psychology and quality of life in adults

Seborrhoeic eczema

This is an erythematous scaly rash affecting the scalp (dandruff), central face, nasolabial folds, eyebrows, central chest and upper back. It is associated with, and may be due to, overgrowth of *Pityrosporum* yeasts. When severe, it may resemble psoriasis. Severe or recalcitrant seborrhoeic eczema can be a marker of immunodeficiency, including HIV infection (p. 397).

Discoid eczema

This is common and characteristically consists of discrete coin-shaped eczematous lesions, which are often impetiginised and most commonly occur on the limbs of men. It is an eczema type that can be due to any chronic itchy condition, whether primarily of skin (e.g. atopic eczema) or another system (e.g. renal failure).

Irritant eczema

Detergents, alkalis, acids, solvents and abrasives are common irritants. Strong irritants have acute effects, whereas weaker irritants commonly cause chronic eczema, especially of the hands, after prolonged exposure. Individual susceptibility varies and the elderly, atopic and fair-skinned are predisposed. Irritant eczema accounts for most occupational cases of eczema and is a significant cause of time off work.

Allergic contact eczema

This occurs due to a delayed hypersensitivity reaction following contact with antigens or haptens. Previous allergen exposure is required for sensitisation and the reaction is specific to the allergen or closely related chemicals. Common allergens are listed in Box 28.26.

Allergy persists indefinitely and eczema occurs at sites of allergen contact and can secondarily spread

28.26 Common type IV delayed hypersensitivity allergens

Allergen	Source
Nickel	Jewellery, jean studs, bra clips, watches
Dichromate	Cement, leather, matches
Rubber chemicals	Clothing, shoes, rubber gloves, tyres
Colophony	Sticking plaster, collodion, nail varnish
Paraphenylenediamine	Hair dye, clothing, tattoos
Balsam of Peru	Perfumes, citrus fruits, shower/bath products
Neomycin, benzocaine	Topical medications
Parabens	Preservative in cosmetics and creams
Wool alcohols	Lanolin, cosmetics, creams
Epoxy resin	Resin adhesives, glues

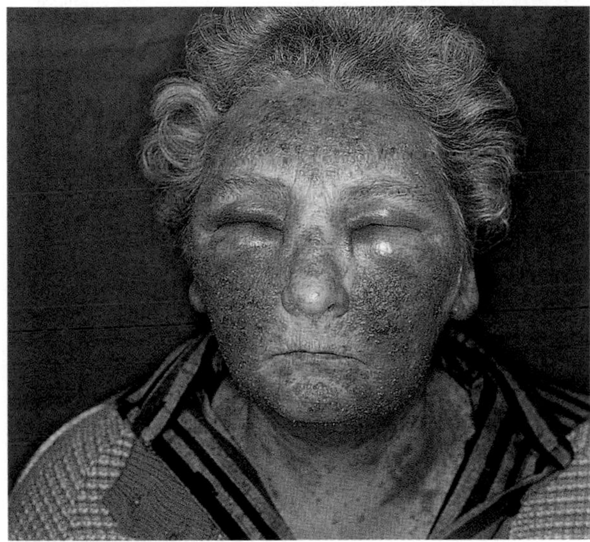

Fig. 28.30 Allergic contact eczema. This was caused by the application of an antihistamine cream. The acute eczematous reaction and bilateral periorbital oedema are typical.

beyond this. There are many recognisable patterns, e.g. eczema of the earlobes, wrists and umbilicus due to contact with nickel in earrings, watches and jeans studs, or eczema of the hands and wrists due to rubber gloves. Oedema may also be a feature (Fig. 28.30).

Asteatotic eczema

This occurs in dry skin and is common in the elderly. Low humidity caused by central heating, over-washing, diuretics and cholesterol-lowering drugs predispose. The most common site is the lower legs and a 'crazy paving' pattern of fine fissuring on an erythematous background is seen.

Gravitational (stasis) eczema

This occurs on the lower legs and is often associated with signs of venous insufficiency: oedema, loss of hair, induration, lipodermatosclerosis and ulceration.

Lichen simplex

Lichenification of eczema occurs secondary to chronic rubbing and scratching, and lichen simplex is a localised form. Common sites include the neck, lower legs and the anogenital region.

Pompholyx

Intensely itchy vesicles and bullae occur on the palms, palmar surface and sides of the fingers and soles. Pompholyx may have several causes, which include atopic eczema, irritant and contact allergic dermatitis and fungal infection.

Investigation of eczema

Patch tests are performed if contact allergic dermatitis is suspected (see Box 28.26). IgE and specific IgE tests are not routinely undertaken in atopic eczema and, similarly, prick tests are not usually helpful. Bacterial and viral swabs for microscopy and culture are useful in suspected secondary infection. Individuals with atopic eczema have an increased susceptibility to herpes simplex virus (HSV), and are at risk of developing a widespread infection, eczema herpeticum. The presence of small, punched-out lesions on a background of worsening eczema suggests the possibility of secondary HSV infection. Skin scrapings to rule out secondary fungal infection should be considered. Skin biopsy is not usually required unless there is diagnostic doubt, e.g. of a drug adverse effect or cutaneous lymphoma.

General management of eczema

Regular use of emollients (e.g. emulsifying ointment) is the mainstay treatment in all eczema types, as they limit water loss and help reduce the amount of topical corticosteroid used. Emollients are used as bath additives and soap substitutes, and directly on to the skin, and are often combined with antiseptics. Sedative antihistamines are useful if sleep is interrupted, but non-sedating antihistamines are ineffective (Box 28.27).

Topical corticosteroids

Topical corticosteroid ointments are preferred for chronic eczema, whereas cream or lotion-based treatment may be more appropriate for acute eczema. Treatment is once to twice daily (p. 1264). Hydrocortisone (1%) or clobetasone butyrate is generally used on the face, with potent or very potent corticosteroid use restricted to trunk and limbs. It is preferable to use a more potent intensive regime initially and taper according to response. As a rough guide, 200 g of a mildly

EBM 28.27 Antihistamines and itch in atopic eczema

'There is currently no high-level evidence to support or refute the efficacy or safety of oral H_1 antihistamines used as monotherapy for eczema. As for various causes of itch not mediated primarily by histamine in the skin, however, sedative (but not non-sedating) antihistamines may offer symptomatic relief.'

Apfelbacher CJ, et al. Cochrane Database of Systematic Reviews, 2013, issue 2. Art. no.: CD007770.

For further information: www.cochrane.org/cochrane-reviews

potent, 50 g of a moderately potent or 30 g of a potent corticosteroid per week would be appropriate (see Box 28.11). Very potent topical corticosteroids should not be used long-term. The side-effects of topical corticosteroid therapy need to be considered when patients are using them for a long period of time, although 'steroid phobia' and under-treatment of eczema are often more of a problem. Particular care should be taken on certain sites, such as the face and flexures, and in children and the elderly (see Box 28.2 and Fig. 28.8, p. 1265). The least potent corticosteroid that is effective should be used for the shortest possible time. The topical calcineurin inhibitors, tacrolimus and pimecrolimus, may be useful steroid-sparing agents, particularly on the face.

Atopic eczema

The impact of atopic eczema on the quality of life of the patient and parents must not be under-estimated. Information and ongoing support from health-care systems and patient support groups, such as the National Eczema Society in the UK, are essential. Mainstays of treatment are emollients and topical steroids, and tar and ichthammol paste bandages may be required. Secondary infection should be treated. Identification and avoidance of allergens are important. Phototherapy, usually with narrowband UVB, is generally the next step, if topical therapies are insufficient. PUVA or UVA1 is sometimes used. Topical calcineurin inhibitors may be applied, and systemic immunosuppression with intermittent ciclosporin, oral corticosteroids, azathioprine or methotrexate may be needed.

Seborrhoeic eczema

Topical azoles, such as ketoconazole shampoo and cream, often combined with mild corticosteroid, are mainstays. Treatment often needs to be repeated.

Irritant eczema

Irritant avoidance, including protective clothing (e.g. gloves), is essential. Emollients and topical corticosteroids are indicated.

Contact allergic eczema

Allergen avoidance is key and may involve a change of occupation or hobbies. Treatment with emollients and topical corticosteroids helps.

Gravitational eczema

Topical corticosteroids should be applied to eczematous areas but not ulcers. There is a high risk of sensitisation to topical preservatives (e.g. chlorocresol), antibiotics (e.g. neomycin) and bandages (e.g. rubber additives). Oedema and ulceration are treated by leg elevation and compression bandages (p. 1263).

PSORIASIS AND OTHER ERYTHEMATOUS SCALY ERUPTIONS

Psoriasis

Psoriasis is a chronic inflammatory, hyperproliferative skin disease. It is characterised by well-defined, erythematous scaly plaques, particularly affecting extensor surfaces and scalp, and usually follows a relapsing and remitting course. Psoriasis affects approximately 1.5–3% of Caucasians and is less common in Asian, South American and African populations. It occurs equally in both sexes and at any age; although it is uncommon under the age of 5 years, more than 50% present before the age of 30 years. The age of onset follows a bimodal distribution, with an early-onset type in the teenage or early adult years, often with a family history of psoriasis and more severe disease course. The later-onset type is typically seen between 50 and 60 years, usually without a family history and a less severe disease course.

Aetiology and pathogenesis

The pathogenesis of psoriasis is multifactorial and genetic and environmental factors are important. The genetic component is complex and polygenic. Twin studies indicate concordance rates of 60–75% and 15–20% for psoriasis arising in monozygotic and dizygotic twins, respectively, with similarities in age of onset, nature and severity of disease in familial cases. If one parent has psoriasis, the chance of a child being affected is about 15–20%; if both parents have the disease, this rises to 50% and the risk is increased further if a sibling has the disease. Advances in molecular biology have facilitated the identification of several genes with significant linkage to psoriasis. The most replicated gene is *PSORS1*, located within the major histocompatibility complex (MHC) on chromosome 6 (human leucocyte antigen (HLA) Cw6) and encoding an epidermal protein, corneodesmosin. It is thought that this gene accounts for almost half of the heritability of psoriasis.

There are several environmental triggers for psoriasis becoming manifest in a genetically predisposed subject (Box 28.28). Although the theory is controversial, stress

28.28 Exacerbating factors in psoriasis

Trauma

- Psoriatic lesions can appear at sites of skin trauma, such as scratches or surgical wounds (Köbner isomorphic phenomenon)

Infection

- β-haemolytic streptococcal throat infections often precede guttate psoriasis (see Fig. 28.32B)
- Severe psoriasis may be the initial presentation of HIV infection

Sunlight

- A minority of patients experience exacerbation of psoriasis after sun exposure, mainly due to Köbnerisation at sites of sunburn or polymorphic light eruption

Drugs

- Antimalarials, β-adrenoceptor antagonists (β-blockers), lithium, NSAIDs and anti-TNF-α drugs, such as infliximab, are examples of drugs that can exacerbate psoriasis
- 'Rebound' flare of psoriasis may occur after withdrawal of systemic corticosteroids or potent topical corticosteroids. Rebound psoriasis is often unstable and may be pustular

Psychological factors

- Anxiety and stress may exacerbate psoriasis in predisposed individuals

(NSAID = non-steroidal anti-inflammatory drug; TNF-α = tumour necrosis factor alpha)

may exacerbate psoriasis in susceptible individuals and psoriasis is itself a cause of psychological stress. Likewise, there is a higher incidence of smoking and heavy alcohol consumption in patients with psoriasis but it is unclear whether this is cause or effect.

The histological changes of psoriasis are shown in Figure 28.31. The main features are:

- keratinocyte hyperproliferation and abnormal differentiation, leading to retention of nuclei in the stratum corneum
- inflammation, with a T-cell lymphocytic infiltrate and release of cytokines and adhesion molecules, such as interleukins, TNF-α and intercellular adhesion molecule (ICAM)-1
- vascular changes, with tortuosity of dermal capillary loop vessels and release of mediators, such as vascular endothelial growth factor (VEGF).

The initiating event is unknown; whilst hyperproliferation was considered the primary step, this has not been confirmed and may, in fact, be secondary to inflammation or vascular changes.

Disordered cell proliferation is reflected by an increase in the mitotic index and in keratinocyte and T-lymphocyte apoptosis in psoriatic plaques. The transit time for keratinocyte migration, from basal layer to shedding from stratum corneum, is shortened from approximately 28 to 5 days, so that immature cells reach the stratum corneum prematurely. Proliferation rate is also less markedly increased in non-lesional skin. Similarly, even the clinically unaffected nails of patients with psoriasis grow more quickly than those of controls.

Interestingly, the HLA association, efficacy of immunosuppressants and development of psoriasis in haematopoietic stem cell transplant recipients from donors with psoriasis support an immune pathogenesis, but the mechanisms and sequence of events are unclear.

Clinical features

Psoriasis has several different presentations (Fig. 28.32).

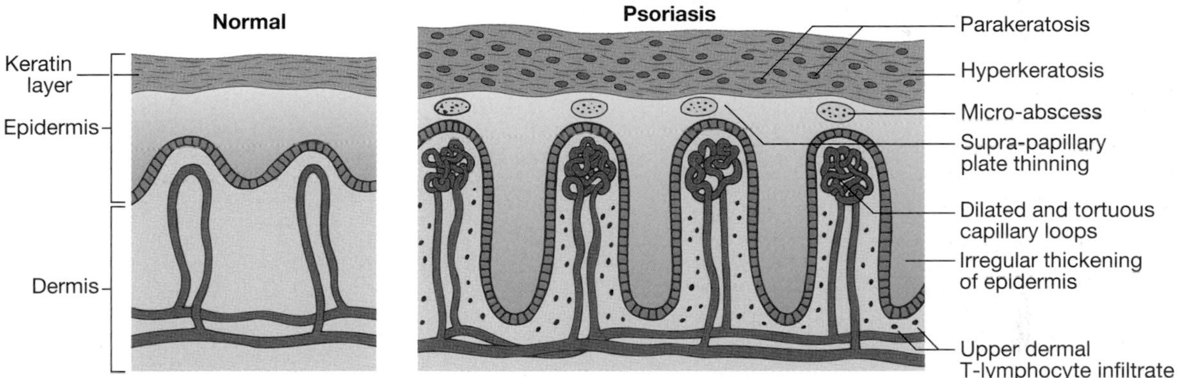

Fig. 28.31 The histology of psoriasis.

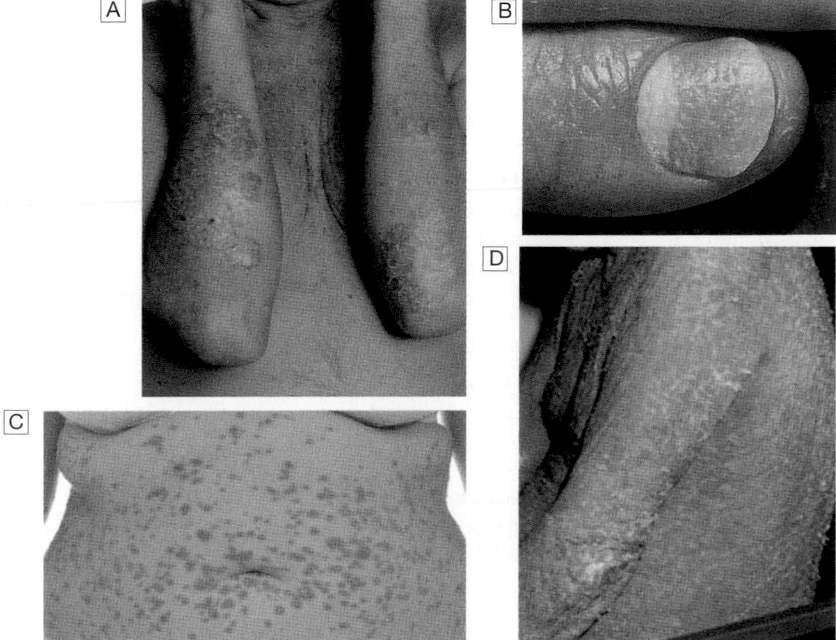

Fig. 28.32 Psoriasis. **A** Chronic plaque psoriasis, most prominent on extensor surfaces. **B** Nail involvement, with coarse pitting and separation from the nail plate (onycholysis). **C** Guttate psoriasis following a streptococcal throat infection. **D** Erythrodermic psoriasis.

Plaque psoriasis

This is the most common presentation and usually represents more stable disease. The typical lesion is a raised, well-demarcated erythematous plaque of variable size (Fig. 28.32A). In untreated disease, silver/white scale is evident and more obvious on scraping the surface. The most common sites are the extensor surfaces, notably elbows and knees, and the lower back. Others include:

- *Scalp*: involvement is seen in approximately 60% of patients. Typically, easily palpable, erythematous scaly plaques are evident within hair-bearing scalp and there is clear demarcation at or beyond the hair margin. Occipital involvement is common and difficult to treat. Less often, fine diffuse scaling may be present and difficult to distinguish from seborrhoeic dermatitis. Involvement of other 'seborrhoeic sites', such as eyebrows, nasolabial folds and the pre-sternal area, is not uncommon and again may be confused with seborrhoeic dermatitis. Temporary hair loss can occur but permanent loss is unusual.
- *Nails*: involvement is common, with 'thimble pitting', onycholysis (separation of the nail from the nail bed, Fig. 28.32B), subungual hyperkeratosis and periungual involvement (p. 1250).
- *Flexures*: psoriasis of the natal cleft and submammary and axillary folds is usually symmetrical, erythematous and smooth, without scale.
- *Palms*: psoriasis of the palms can be difficult to distinguish from eczema.

Guttate psoriasis

This is most common in children and adolescents and is often the initial presentation (Fig. 28.32C). It is commonly associated with HLA Cw6. It may present shortly after a streptococcal throat infection and rapidly evolves. Individual lesions are droplet-shaped, small (usually less than 1 cm in diameter), erythematous, scaly and numerous. An episode of guttate psoriasis may clear spontaneously or with topical treatment within a few months, but UVB phototherapy is often required and is highly effective. Guttate psoriasis often heralds the onset of plaque psoriasis in adulthood.

Erythrodermic psoriasis

Generalised erythrodermic psoriasis is a medical emergency (Fig. 28.32D).

Pustular psoriasis

Pustular psoriasis may be generalised or localised. Generalised pustular psoriasis is uncommon, unstable and life-threatening. It will often emerge in the context of plaque disease and the onset is usually sudden, with large numbers of small sterile pustules on an erythematous background, often merging into sheets, with waves of new pustules in subsequent days. The patient is usually febrile and systemically unwell, and this must be dealt with as a medical emergency (p. 1264). Localised pustular psoriasis of the palms and soles (palmoplantar pustulosis) is more common, chronic and closely associated with smoking; small, sterile pustules and erythema develop and resolve with pigmentation and scaling (p. 1250). A localised form of sterile pustulosis of a few digits (acropustulosis) can also occur. It is unclear whether these localised forms of pustulosis are truly psoriatic.

Arthropathy

Between 5% and 10% of individuals with psoriasis develop an inflammatory arthropathy, which can take on a number of patterns (pp. 1250 and 1109).

Assessment and investigations

Biopsy is not required in typical cases but may be performed if there is diagnostic doubt. An infection screen, particularly throat swab for streptococcus, may be informative in guttate psoriasis. Assessment of impact on life (e.g. using the Dermatology Life Quality Index, or DLQI) and psoriasis severity (e.g. using the Psoriasis Area and Severity Index, or PASI) (p. 1251) is essential. Rheumatology assessment should be performed if the patient has joint symptoms or signs. Due to the association of psoriasis with insulin resistance, cardiovascular risk factors should be assessed (p. 805). HIV testing should be considered in severe or recalcitrant psoriasis.

Management

Patient counselling about diagnosis and management is paramount. Psoriasis can have a major impact on all aspects of life (work, school, leisure, personal relationships and self-esteem) and this must not be underestimated. Reassurance is also needed, as the condition is generally not life-threatening. Advice regarding reduction in risk factors for cardiovascular disease should be given (smoking cessation, reduction of alcohol intake, adequate exercise and a normal body mass index). Patients need to be involved in their own management, as the disease is usually chronic and the benefit/risk profile of treatments needs to be discussed and tailored to individuals. The end-point for treatment also needs to be discussed because complete disease clearance may not be practical or appropriate and patients vary considerably in their treatment requirements. Extent of disease and impact on quality of life must be taken into account. Patient compliance with topical and systemic therapies is essential and dependent on the treatment practicalities.

The treatment approach generally follows a stepwise progression, as summarised in Box 28.29. Treatment categories are outlined in Box 28.30. If topical treatment is insufficient, then UVB phototherapy or PUVA should usually be the next step. If the patient continues to have active disease or early recurrence, then the addition of systemic retinoid (usually acitretin) or use of immunosuppressants, such as methotrexate as first choice, then

EBM 28.29 Assessment and management of psoriasis

- 'Access to appropriate information and services must be facilitated for patients with psoriasis.
- Disease severity and impact must be assessed.
- Associated arthritis must be assessed and managed.
- Comorbidities, such as cardiovascular risk, must be addressed.
- Topical therapies are first-line, followed by second- and third-line treatments (see below).
- Topical corticosteroids must be used safely.'

For further information: 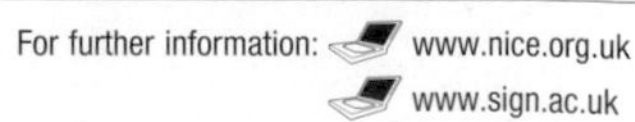
www.nice.org.uk
www.sign.ac.uk

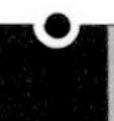

28.30 Treatment categories in psoriasis

Topical agents
• Emollients, tars, dithranol, vitamin D agonists, retinoids, corticosteroids
Photo(chemo)therapies
• UVB, PUVA, (excimer laser)
Systemic agents
• Retinoids • Immunosuppressants, e.g. methotrexate, ciclosporin, mycophenolate, hydroxycarbamide • Immunomodulators, e.g. fumaric acid esters • Biological immunosuppressants, e.g. infliximab, etanercept, adalimumab
Intensive inpatient or day-patient care
• Topical agents and photo(chemo)therapies under medical supervision

ciclosporin, mycophenolate mofetil or hydroxycarbamide, may be considered. In severe, unresponsive disease, fumaric acid esters or biological therapies, such as TNF-α, interleukin (IL)-12 or IL-23 antagonists, may be required (p. 1102).

Individualised management is essential. For example, a patient with localised plaque psoriasis on elbows, knees and sacrum should respond to topical treatment only, whereas a patient with guttate psoriasis is likely to need phototherapy as a first-line approach because of difficulties in topical drug application in extensive disease. A patient with extensive chronic plaque psoriasis and significant arthropathy would be better suited to a systemic drug, such as methotrexate, than phototherapy, which would be unlikely to improve joint symptoms.

Pityriasis rosea

This is an acute, self-limiting exanthem that particularly affects young adults and occurs worldwide, with a slight female predominance. It usually occurs in spring and summer, although no infective agent has been identified and its aetiology is unknown.

Clinical features and management

Pityriasis rosea is characterised by the appearance of a 'herald patch', an oval lesion (1–2 cm) with a central pinkish (salmon-coloured) centre, a darker periphery and a characteristic collarette of scale. It is followed 1–2 weeks later by a widespread papulosquamous eruption, which is typically arranged in a symmetrical 'Christmas tree' pattern on the trunk. Individual lesions also have a collarette of scale. An inverse variant with flexural involvement can occur. Mucosal involvement is rare. There is a small risk of recurrence. Symptomatic relief can be achieved with emollients and mild topical steroids. Post-inflammatory hyperpigmentation can supervene, particularly in darker skin types.

Other causes of an erythematous papulosquamous rash

Secondary syphilis (p. 419), pityriasis versicolor (p. 1280) and fungal infection with *Tinea corporis* (p. 1279) can all cause an erythematous papulosquamous rash and must be considered in the differential diagnosis.

Pityriasis lichenoides chronica

This is rare but typically presents within the first three decades of life. The aetiology is unclear but the condition is part of a spectrum and remits spontaneously. The more acute variety (pityriasis lichenoides et varioliformis acuta, PLEVA) presents as crops of papules that rapidly evolve with central necrosis, each attack lasting up to 3 months. The more chronic variety presents as a persistent, widespread, scaly eruption. Characteristically, lesions are brown papules with a mica-like scale ('cornflake'). The condition fluctuates but can persist for months or years. Emollients, topical steroids and long-term oral erythromycin can occasionally be helpful. UVB phototherapy or PUVA is usually effective, although recurrences are high.

Drug eruptions

It is essential to consider a drug cause in anyone presenting with an erythematous maculopapular or papulosquamous eruption, and a careful drug history is critical (p. 1303). Exfoliation ('peeling') and post-inflammatory hyper- or, less commonly, hypopigmentation, can occur.

LICHEN PLANUS AND LICHENOID ERUPTIONS

Lichen planus

Lichen planus occurs worldwide; it typically presents as a pruritic rash and the mucosae, hair and nails may be involved.

Aetiology and pathology

The cause is unknown; a viral trigger was considered but has not been substantiated. An autoimmune pathogenesis is suspected, as there is an association with inflammatory bowel disease, primary biliary cirrhosis, autoimmune hepatitis, hepatitis B and C, alopecia areata, myasthenia gravis (p. 1226) and thymoma, and there are similarities with graft-versus-host disease (GVHD, p. 1017). An immune reaction to unknown antigen is plausible. Lichen planus can occasionally occur in families and possible HLA associations have been proposed, although there is no clear inheritance pattern. There are characteristic histological changes, with hyperkeratosis, basal cell degeneration and a heavy, band-like T-lymphocyte infiltrate in the papillary dermis, with affinity for the epidermis (epidermotropism). The dermo-epidermal junction has a 'sawtooth' appearance.

Clinical features

Lichen planus occurs in both sexes and at any age, although usually between 30 and 60 years. It generally presents on the distal limbs, most commonly on the flexural aspects of the wrists and forearms (Fig. 28.33), and on the lower back. It is intensely itchy and lesions are violaceous, shiny, flat-topped, polygonal papules, with a characteristic fine lacy, white network on the surface (Wickham's striae). New lesions may appear at sites of skin trauma (Köbner phenomenon) and the

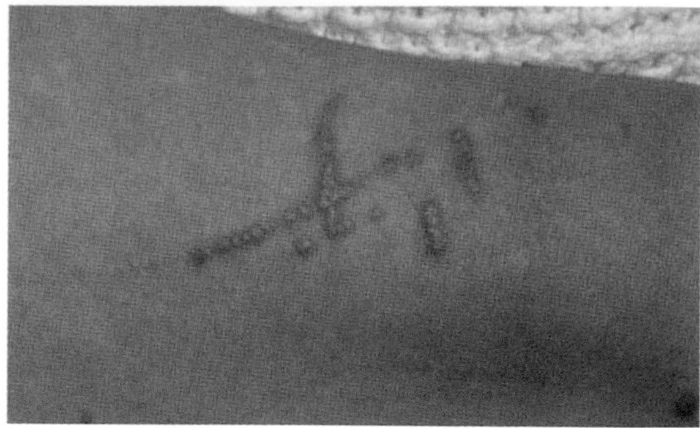

Fig. 28.33 Lichen planus. Violaceous papules on the flexural aspect of forearm, arising at a site of minor linear trauma (Köbner phenomenon).

rash may become generalised. Individual lesions may last for many months and can become hypertrophic and modified by scratching, particularly on the lower legs. The eruption usually remits over months, but can become chronic, particularly with hypertrophic disease. Post-inflammatory pigmentary change is common, particularly in darker skin types. Mucous membrane involvement occurs in 30–70% of patients, usually as a network of white, lacy striae on the buccal mucosae (p. 1250) and tongue. These oral changes are often asymptomatic and should be sought on examination. Genital and other mucosal surfaces can also be affected (pp. 416 and 418). Nail involvement occurs in about 10% and can range from longitudinal ridging to a destructive nail dystrophy, scarring (pterygium) and nail loss (p. 1298). Scalp involvement usually presents as an inflammatory scarring alopecia, often with tufting of residual hairs. The classical presentation of lichen planus is unmistakable but less common, atypical variants, which include annular, atrophic, actinic, linear, bullous, follicular, pigmented and ulcerative types, can be a diagnostic challenge.

Diagnosis

A skin biopsy should be performed if there is diagnostic doubt. A careful drug history must be taken as, although the classical presentation of lichen planus is usually 'idiopathic', the main differential is a drug-induced lichenoid reaction (see below). Other differential diagnoses include psoriasis, pityriasis rosea, pityriasis lichenoides chronica and secondary syphilis. Screening for underlying disease, such as hepatitis, must be considered.

Management

The condition is usually self-limiting, although rarely, particularly with oral lichen planus, it may persist for years. Treatment is symptomatic and potent local corticosteroids (topical, with occlusion or by injection for hypertrophic disease, or as oral rinse for oral involvement) may help the intense itch; short courses of systemic corticosteroids are sometimes required for extensive disease. UVB, PUVA or UVA1 can be beneficial and, for recalcitrant disease, retinoids or immunosuppressants such as ciclosporin may be needed. A low but significant risk of malignant transformation exists with persistent oral and genital disease, so active treatment, surveillance and smoking cessation are important.

Lichenoid eruptions

Drug-induced lichenoid reactions that are clinically and histologically difficult to distinguish from idiopathic lichen planus are important to identify. The culprits are gold, quinine, proton pump inhibitors, sulphonamides, penicillamine, antimalarials, antituberculous drugs, thiazide diuretics, β-blockers, angiotensin-converting enzyme (ACE) inhibitors, NSAIDs, sulphonylureas, lithium and dyes in colour developers (Box 28.44, p. 1304).

Graft-versus-host disease

In the acute stage of graft-versus-host disease (GVHD, p. 1017), there is a distinctive dermatitis associated with hepatitis. After about 3 months, chronic GVHD can present with a lichenoid eruption on the palms, soles, face and upper trunk. Progressive sclerodermatous skin thickening may lead to contractures and limited mobility.

URTICARIA

Urticaria ('hives') is caused by localised dermal oedema secondary to a temporary increase in capillary permeability. If oedema involves subcutaneous or submucosal layers, the term angioedema is used. Acute urticaria may be associated with angioedema of the lips, face, tongue, throat and, rarely, wheezing, abdominal pain, headaches and even anaphylaxis (p. 91).

Urticaria present for less than 6 weeks is considered to be acute, and chronic if it continues for more than 6 weeks. Individual weals last for less than 24 hours; if they persist, urticarial vasculitis needs to be considered. Clarification of duration can be achieved by drawing around the weal and re-assessing 24 hours later.

History-taking should probe for possible causes (Box 28.31). Physical triggers can also be assessed in challenge testing, such as eliciting dermographism or pressure testing. Enquiry about family history is important in angioedema. Examination may be unremarkable or weals may be evident (Fig. 28.34).

Mast cell degranulation and release of histamine and other vasoactive mediators is the basis of urticaria (Fig. 28.35). Chronic spontaneous urticaria (previously called 'chronic idiopathic' or 'chronic ordinary'

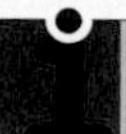

28.31 Causes of urticaria

Acute and chronic urticaria

- Autoimmune: due to antibodies that cross-link the IgE receptor on mast cells
- Allergens: in foods, medications and inhalants
- Drugs: (see Box 28.44, p. 1304)
- Contact: e.g. latex, animal saliva
- Physical: e.g. heat, cold, pressure, sun, sweat, water
- Infection: e.g. intestinal parasites
- Others: e.g. systemic lupus erythematosus (SLE), pregnancy
- Idiopathic: Chronic spontaneous urticaria and angioedema

Urticarial vasculitis

- Hepatitis B
- SLE
- Idiopathic

urticaria) is the most common chronic urticaria and has an autoimmune pathogenesis in some cases.

Investigations

Investigations should be guided by the history and possible causes but are often negative, particularly in acute urticaria. Some or all of the following may be appropriate:

- *full blood count*: eosinophilia in parasitic infection or drug cause
- *erythrocyte sedimentation rate (ESR) or plasma viscosity*: elevated in vasculitis
- *urea and electrolytes, thyroid and liver function tests, iron studies*: may reveal an underlying systemic disorder
- *total IgE and specific IgE to possible allergens*: e.g. shellfish, peanut, house dust mite
- *antinuclear factor*: positive in systemic lupus erythematosus (SLE) and often positive in urticarial vasculitis
- *complement C_3 and C_4 levels*: if these are low due to complement consumption, *C_1 esterase inhibitor* activity should be measured
- *skin biopsy*: if urticarial vasculitis is suspected
- *challenge tests*: to confirm physical urticarias.

Fig. 28.34 Urticaria. Erythema, reflecting dilated dermal vessels, and oedema (with upper dermal oedema obscuring the erythema centrally) are evident. Note the absence of epidermal changes.

Management

Removal or treatment of any trigger is essential, although this may not be identified in the majority of cases. Urticaria may be precipitated by aspirin, NSAIDs, codeine and opioids, and it is advisable to suggest alternatives such as paracetamol. In chronic urticaria, non-sedating antihistamines, such as fexofenadine, loratadine or cetirizine, are usually beneficial. If, after 2 weeks, there is lack of response, an alternative non-sedating antihistamine should be used and an H_2-blocker, such as cimetidine or ranitidine, is often added. Mast cell stabilisers or leukotriene receptor antagonists, such as montelukast, may be added for more recalcitrant disease. For chronic urticaria, narrowband UVB phototherapy is valuable. Systemic corticosteroids are widely prescribed for urticaria, but often need to be used at high doses and are only appropriate for occasional short courses. Patients with a history of life-threatening anaphylaxis, as in peanut or wasp sting allergy, should carry a self-administered adrenaline (epinephrine) injection kit. The management of anaphylaxis and hereditary angioedema is discussed on pages 92 and 94.

BULLOUS DISEASES

Blistering can occur at any level in the skin and, as such, there are a variety of different presentations, depending on the underlying defect and level of involvement. Our knowledge of the molecular basis of many blistering disorders has considerably advanced as we come to understand the processes of cutaneous cell

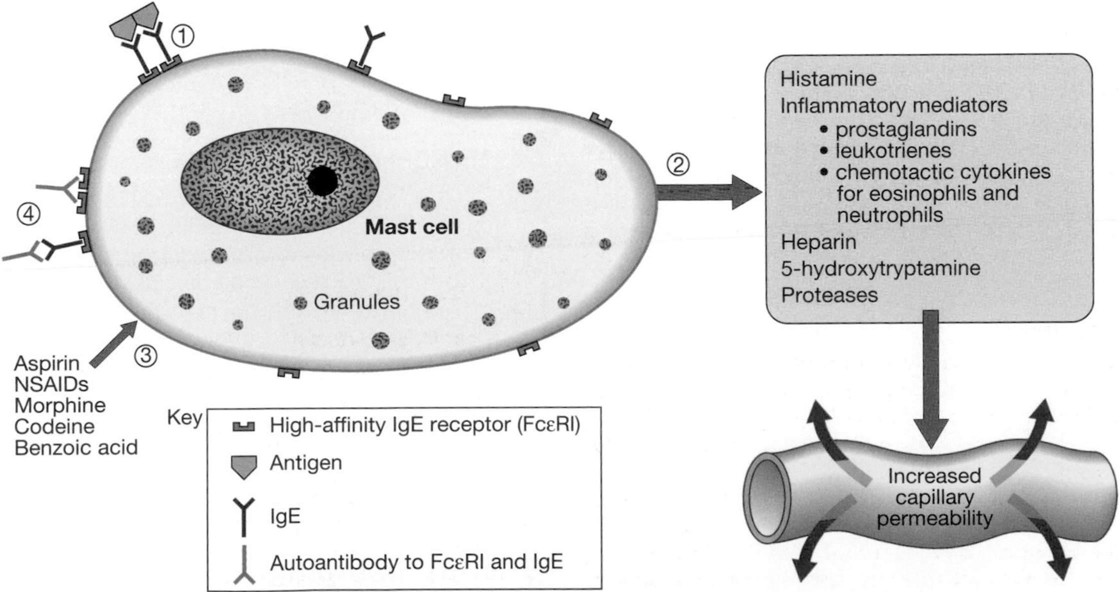

Fig. 28.35 Pathogenesis of urticaria. Mast cell degranulation occurs in a variety of ways. (1) Type I hypersensitivity causes degranulation. (2) Spontaneous mast cell degranulation in chronic urticaria. (3) Chemical mast cell degranulation. (4) Autoimmunity, with IgE antibodies directed against IgE receptors or IgE itself. Histamine and the leukotrienes are especially relevant mediators in urticaria. Heparin release is probably not a major factor in urticaria, but plays a role in the osteoporosis frequent in the mastocytoses (conditions of excess mast cells).

28.32 Classification of epidermolysis bullosa

Type	Mode of inheritance	Level of blister*	Abnormality
Simple	Autosomal dominant	Epidermal basal cell	Keratins 5 and 14
Junctional	Autosomal recessive	Lamina lucida	Laminin-5 and $\alpha_6\ \beta_4$ integrin
Dystrophic	Autosomal dominant and recessive	Dermis below lamina densa	Collagen VII

*See Fig. 28.1, p. 1253.

adhesion. Studies of the rare genetic blistering disorders, particularly epidermolysis bullosa, which present at birth (Box 28.32) have facilitated this. This section concentrates on primary blistering skin diseases.

Toxic epidermal necrolysis

Toxic epidermal necrolysis (TEN) is a medical emergency, as the extensive mucocutaneous blistering is associated with a high mortality rate. It is usually drug-induced (see Box 28.44, p. 1304), particularly by anticonvulsants, sulphonamides, sulphonylureas, NSAIDs, allopurinol and antiretroviral therapy. Usually 1–4 weeks after drug commencement, the patient becomes systemically unwell and often pyrexial, and erythema and blistering develop, initially on the trunk but rapidly involving all skin. Sheets of blisters coalesce and denude, and the underlying skin is painful and erythematous (Fig. 28.36). Mucous membrane involvement and blistering are usual. A disease severity score (Box 28.33) is used to predict outcome. The main differential diagnosis is SSSS (p. 1276), although the diagnosis is usually obvious in an adult patient with a culprit drug. Skin snip allows early diagnosis and is preferred to full-thickness skin biopsy in the acute stage.

Identification and discontinuation of the causative drug are essential. Intensive care in a dedicated dermatology ward or intensive care or burns unit is of paramount importance. Treatment is supportive, with regular sterile dressings and emollients, careful attention to fluid balance and monitoring for infection. Urethral and ocular involvement is common and must be looked for and treated symptomatically, as ocular and urethral scarring in survivors can be problematic. Sepsis and multi-organ failure are major risks. Systemic corticosteroids are contraindicated, as they are associated with increased mortality. Intravenous immunoglobulins have been studied but there is no good evidence for improved outcomes (Box 28.34).

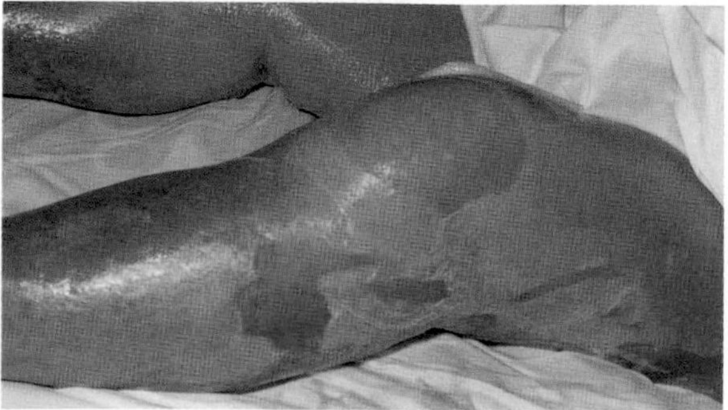

Fig. 28.36 Toxic epidermolytic necrolysis. Note the extensive erythema, oedema and epidermal loss secondary to carbamazepine.

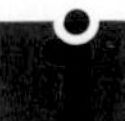

28.33 Disease severity score for toxic epidermal necrolysis (TEN): SCORTEN

Factor

- Age > 40 yrs
- Heart rate > 120 beats/min
- Cancer or haematological malignancy
- Involved body surface area > 10%
- Blood urea > 10 mmol/L (28 mg/dL)
- Serum bicarbonate < 20 mmol/L (20 meq/L)
- Blood glucose ≥ 14 mmol/L (252 mg/dL)

Mortality rates

- 0–1 factor present = 3%
- 2 factors = 12%
- 3 factors = 35%
- 4 factors = 58%
- ≥ 5 factors = 90%

Bastuji-Garin S, et al. J Invest Dermatol 2000; 115:149–153.

EBM 28.34 Intravenous immunoglobulin (IVIg) for toxic epidermal necrolysis

'The treatment of TEN involves stopping likely drug causes and supportive management. Although it is sometimes used, there is no good evidence of benefit from IVIg. Randomised studies of such interventions are needed.'

- Huang YC, et al. Br J Dermatol 2012; 167:424–432.

For further information: www.cochrane.org/cochrane-reviews

Immunobullous diseases

The age of the patient may be informative in suspected immunobullous disease (Box 28.35). The key investigation is an elliptical biopsy taken from the edge of a recent blister (Box 28.36). The sample is halved and one half put in formalin for subsequent histology, whilst the other is sent fresh for direct immunofluorescence. Serum should also be sent for indirect immunofluorescence in suspected immunobullous disease (p. 1255). Several of these blistering disorders are associated with underlying diseases, which should be considered. Many patients will require immunosuppression. Blister fluid should always be sent for culture to exclude viral or bacterial infection.

Bullous pemphigoid

Bullous pemphigoid (BP) is the most common immunobullous disease and occurs worldwide. It is a disease of the elderly, with an average age of onset of 65 years; males and females are equally affected. A range of autoantibodies develop, the best characterised being antibodies BP-230 and BP-180, directed against the hemi-desmosomal BP antigens, BPAg-1 (intracellular) and BPAg-2 (transmembranous type XVII collagen), respectively. Antibody–antigen binding initiates complement activation and inflammation, hemi-desmosomal damage and consequent subepidermal blistering.

28.35 Age of onset in immunobullous skin disorders

Disease	Age
Pemphigus vulgaris	40–60 yrs
Pemphigus foliaceus	Any age (endemic form, e.g. in parts of Brazil and South Africa, from teenage years on)
Bullous pemphigoid	60s and over
Dermatitis herpetiformis	Young, associated with coeliac disease
Linear IgA disease	Any age
Pemphigoid gestationis	Pregnant females
Epidermolysis bullosa acquisita	Any age
Bullous lupus erythematosus	Young black female

Clinical features and diagnosis

There is often a lengthy prodrome of an itchy, urticated, erythematous rash prior to the development of tense bullae (Fig. 28.37A). Milia may develop due to basement membrane disruption. Mucosal involvement is uncommon. Histology shows subepidermal blistering with an eosinophil-rich inflammatory infiltrate. Direct immunofluorescence demonstrates the presence of IgG and C3 at the basement membrane (Fig. 28.37B). Indirect immunofluorescence may show positive titres of circulating anti-epidermal antibodies. Distinction from epidermolysis bullosa acquisita requires immunofluorescence studies using the patient's serum on salt-split skin. In BP, the immunoreactants localise to the epidermal side (hemi-desmosome) of split skin, whereas in epidermolysis bullosa acquisita they localise to the base of the split (type VII collagen/anchoring fibrils).

Management

Very potent topical steroids to all sites may be sufficient in frail elderly patients (Box 28.37). Tetracyclines, such as doxycycline, have an important role and may limit the use of systemic corticosteroids. However, most require systemic corticosteroids, often combined with azathioprine. There is evidence to support the use of intravenous immunoglobulin as a steroid-sparing therapy in BP. The condition often burns out over a few years.

28

28.36 Clinical and investigation findings in the immunobullous disorders

Disease	Site of blisters	Nature of blisters	Mucous membrane involvement	Antigen	Circulating antibody (indirect IF)	Fixed antibody (direct IF)
Pemphigus vulgaris	Trunk, head	Flaccid, fragile, many erosions	100%	Desmoglein-1 and 3 (120 kD)	IgG	IgG, C_3 intercellular (epidermal)
Pemphigus foliaceus	Trunk	Often not present, multiple erosions, may mimic dermatitis	No	Desmoglein-1	IgG	IgG, C_3 intercellular (epidermal)
Bullous pemphigoid	Trunk, flexures and limbs	Tense, milia as resolve	Occasional	BP-230 and 180	IgG (70%)	IgG, C_3 at BMZ
Dermatitis herpetiformis	Elbows, lower back, buttocks	Excoriated and often not present	No	Unknown	Anti-endomysial and tissue transglutaminase	Granular IgA in papillary dermis
Linear IgA disease	Widespread	Tense, often annular configuration, 'string of beads'	Frequent	Unknown	50% have low titres of circulating antibody	Linear IgA at BMZ
Pemphigoid gestationis	Periumbilical and limbs	Tense, milia as resolve	Rare	Collagen XVII (part of hemi-desmosome, BP-180)	Circulating antibodies to BP-180 (type XVII collagen) (and BP-230)	C_3 at BMZ
Epidermolysis bullosa acquisita	Widespread	Tense, scarring, milia	Common (50%)	Type VII collagen	IgG (anti-type VII collagen)	IgG at BMZ
Bullous lupus erythematosus	Widespread	Tense	Rare	Type VII collagen	Anti-type VII collagen	IgG, IgA, IgM at BMZ

(BMZ = basement membrane zone; IF = immunofluorescence)

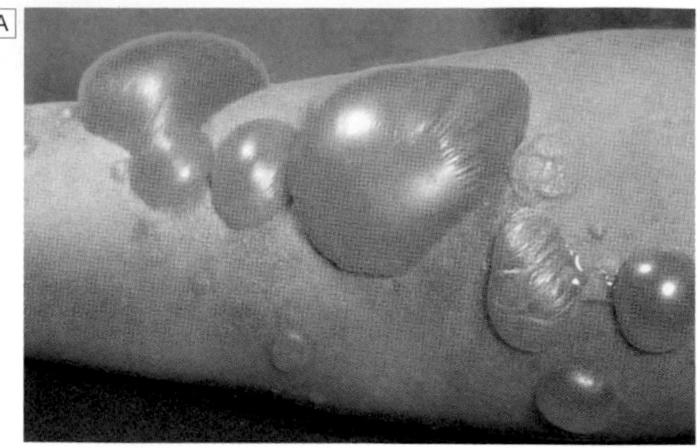

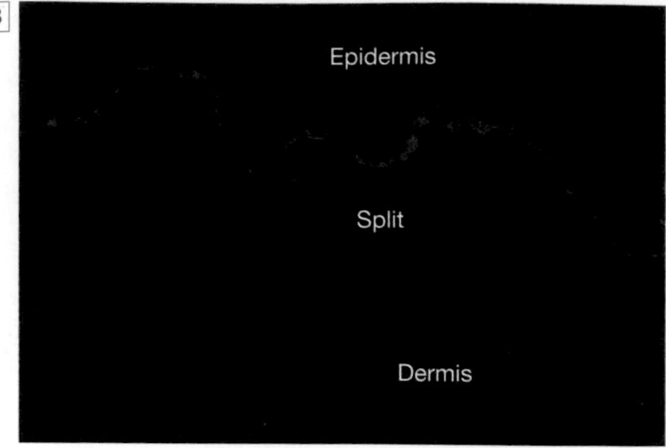

Fig. 28.37 Bullous pemphigoid. **A** Large, tense, unilocular blisters. **B** Immunofluorescence on salt-split skin, showing a subepidermal blister and linear IgG and C3 deposition at the basement membrane zone.

EBM 28.37 Treatment of bullous pemphigoid

'Very potent topical corticosteroids are effective. However, in extensive disease, applications by patients or carers may be difficult. If systemic corticosteroids are needed, there is generally no advantage in using doses greater than 0.75 mg/kg/day of prednisolone.'

- Kirtschig G, et al. Interventions for bullous pemphigoid. Cochrane Database of Systematic Reviews, 2010, issue 10. Art. no.: CD002292.

Pemphigus

Pemphigus is less common than BP and patients are usually younger. Typically, IgG1 and IgG4 autoantibodies, directed against desmogleins-1 and 3, develop, resulting in intra-epidermal blistering. Secondary causes are drugs (e.g. penicillamine or captopril) and underlying malignancy ('paraneoplastic pemphigus'). Pemphigus foliaceus is a very superficial form, in which antibodies are directed against desmoglein-1 only and affect just the most superficial epidermis.

Clinical features and diagnosis

Skin and mucosae are usually involved, although disease may be restricted to mucosae only, which may be severely affected. Due to the higher level of split within the epidermis, the blisters are flaccid, easily ruptured and often not seen intact. Erosions are common and the Nikolsky sign is positive. The trunk is usually affected. The condition is associated with significant morbidity and mortality. Histology shows intra-epidermal blistering and acantholysis, with positive direct immunofluorescence. The titres of circulating epidermal autoantibodies can also be used to monitor disease activity. Investigations should screen for associated autoimmune disease or malignancy if paraneoplastic pemphigus is suspected.

Management

Pemphigus is more difficult to control than BP and high-dose systemic corticosteroids are usually required. Azathioprine, cyclophosphamide and intravenous immunoglobulins may be used as steroid-sparing agents. Often, long-term treatment is required to prevent relapse.

Dermatitis herpetiformis

Dermatitis herpetiformis (DH) is an autoimmune blistering disorder that is strongly associated with gluten intolerance. Fewer than 10% of individuals with coeliac disease develop DH, although almost all patients with DH have evidence of partial villous atrophy on investigation, even if asymptomatic (p. 881). The pathogenesis is unknown.

Intact vesicles or blisters are often not seen, as the condition is so pruritic that excoriations on extensor surfaces of arms, knees, buttocks, shoulders and scalp may be the only signs.

Subepidermal vesiculation in the dermal papillae and a neutrophil- and eosinophil-rich infiltrate is seen histologically. Direct immunofluorescence shows granular IgA in the papillary dermis. Anti-endomysial antibodies and tissue transglutaminase should be assessed, and jejunal biopsy undertaken if indicated. A gluten-free diet may suffice but, if not, the condition is usually highly responsive to dapsone.

Linear IgA disease

This occurs in children (chronic bullous disease of childhood) and adults, and is usually self-limiting, although it can be active for a few years. Drugs, notably vancomycin, are a secondary cause. Blisters can arise on erythematous, urticated or otherwise normal-looking skin and often form an annular configuration at the edge of the lesion: 'clusters of jewels' (herpetiform) and 'string of beads' (annular/polycyclic). Mucosal involvement is common and ophthalmology input important, as long-term scarring is a risk. Linear IgA is seen at the basement membrane on direct immunofluorescence and localises to either roof or floor of salt-split skin. Dapsone, sulfapyridine, prednisolone, colchicine or intravenous immunoglobulin may be effective.

Epidermolysis bullosa acquisita

This chronic blistering disease affects skin and mucosae, and may be difficult to distinguish from other immunobullous blistering diseases. It is caused by an IgG antibody to type VII collagen, which provokes subepidermal blistering and a mixed inflammatory infiltrate. Blisters often follow trauma, and milia develop. The condition may be associated with inflammatory bowel disease, rheumatoid arthritis, multiple myeloma and lymphoma. It is difficult to treat, as it often does not respond to immunosuppressants.

Porphyria cutanea tarda and pseudoporphyria

These conditions may also cause blistering (see Boxes 28.9 and 28.44, pp. 1260 and 1304).

PIGMENTATION DISORDERS

Decreased pigmentation

Disorders causing hypopigmentation and/or depigmentation include:

- vitiligo
- albinism
- pityriasis alba: depigmented areas on the face, particularly in children, with or without scale and usually considered to be eczematous
- pityriasis versicolor (p. 1280): hypopigmentation or, less commonly, hyperpigmentation can occur
- idiopathic guttate hypomelanosis: multiple small areas of depigmentation arising in chronically sun-exposed skin
- rarely, phenylketonuria (p. 449) and hypopituitarism.

Vitiligo

Vitiligo is an acquired condition affecting 1% of the population worldwide. Focal loss of melanocytes results in the development of patches of hypopigmentation. A positive family history of vitiligo is relatively common in those with extensive disease, and this type is also associated with other autoimmune diseases. Trauma and sunburn may (through the Köbner phenomenon) precipitate the appearance of vitiligo. The pathogenesis is unclear and, whilst melanocytes may be the target of a cell-mediated autoimmune attack, it is not known why only focal areas are affected.

Clinical features

Generalised vitiligo is often symmetrical and involves hands, wrists, knees and neck, as well as areas around body orifices (Fig. 28.38). The hair of the scalp, beard, eyebrows and lashes may also depigment. Segmental vitiligo is restricted to one part of the body but not necessarily a dermatome. The patches of depigmentation are sharply defined, and in Caucasians may be surrounded by hyperpigmentation. Spotty perifollicular pigment may be seen within the depigmentation and is often the first sign of repigmentation. Sensation in the depigmented patches is normal (unlike in tuberculoid leprosy, p. 347). Wood's light examination enhances the contrast between pigmented and non-pigmented skin. The course is unpredictable but most patches remain static or enlarge; a few repigment spontaneously.

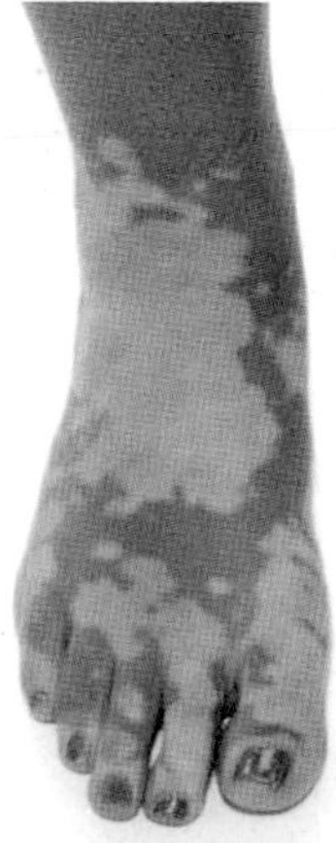
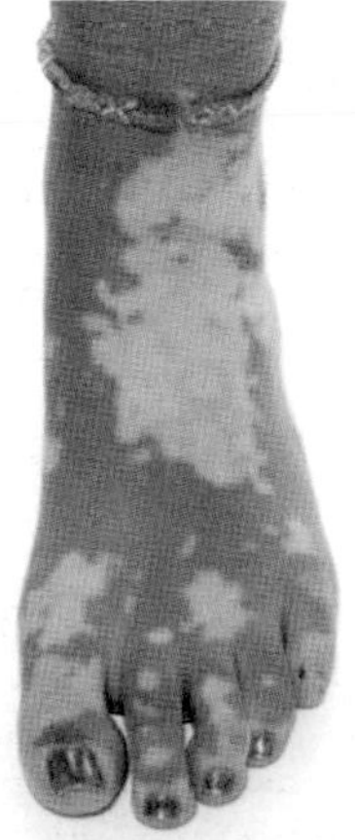

Fig. 28.38 Vitiligo. Symmetrical localised patches of depigmented skin.

Management

Protecting the patches from excessive sun exposure with clothing or sunscreen may be helpful to avoid sunburn. Camouflage cosmetics may be beneficial, particularly in those with dark skin, as can potent topical corticosteroids. Phototherapy with narrowband UVB or PUVA can be used. Narrowband UVB is the most effective repigmentary treatment available for generalised vitiligo, but even very prolonged courses often do not produce a satisfactory outcome. The absence of leucotrichia (white hairs in the area of vitiligo) and a trichrome pattern (three colours - normal skin colour, hypopigmentation and depigmentation) are good prognostic features. Vitiligo on the face, trunk and proximal limbs is more likely to respond than that on hands and feet. Autologous melanocyte transfer, using a range of techniques including split-skin grafts and blister roof grafts, is sometimes used on dermabraded recipient skin.

The impact of vitiligo differs markedly between populations. In the Indian subcontinent, the effects are more readily discernible than in pale-skinned individuals in northern Europe. Depigmentation is also seen in Hansen's disease (leprosy), which means that individuals with vitiligo are often stigmatised.

Oculocutaneous albinism

Albinism results from a range of genetic abnormalities that lead to reduced melanin biosynthesis in the skin and eyes; the number of melanocytes is normal (in contrast to vitiligo). Albinism is usually inherited as an autosomal recessive trait and there are several different types and presentations.

Type 1 albinism is due to a defect in the tyrosinase gene, whose product is rate-limiting in the production of melanin. Affected individuals have an almost complete absence of pigment in the skin and hair at birth, with consequent pale skin and white hair, and failure of melanin production in the iris and retina. Patients have photophobia, poor vision not correctable with refraction, rotatory nystagmus, and an alternating strabismus associated with abnormalities in the decussation of nerve fibres in the optic tract.

A second form of albinism is due to a defect in the *P* gene, which encodes an ion channel protein in the melanosome. Patients may have gross reduction of melanin in the skin and in the eyes, but may be more mildly affected than type 1 albinos. Establishing the subtype of albinism requires genetic analysis, as there is considerable phenotypic heterogeneity.

Oculocutaneous albinos are at grossly increased risk of sunburn and skin cancer. In equatorial regions, many die from SCC or, more rarely, melanoma in early adult life. Interestingly, they may develop pigmented melanocytic naevi and freckle in response to sun exposure.

Management

Strict photoprotection (p. 1261), with sun avoidance (including occupational exposure), clothing, hats and sunscreens, is important. Early diagnosis and treatment of skin tumours is essential.

Increased pigmentation

- *Diffuse hyperpigmentation*: most commonly due to hypermelanosis but other pigments may be deposited in the skin, e.g. orange discoloration with carotenaemia and bronze with haemochromatosis (p. 972).
- *Endocrine pigmentation*: may occur in several conditions. Melasma (chloasma) describes discrete patches of facial pigmentation that occur in pregnancy and in some women taking oral contraceptives. The mechanism for this localised increased hormonal sensitivity is unknown. Diffuse pigmentation, sometimes worse in the skin creases, may be a feature of Addison's disease (p. 777), Cushing's syndrome (p. 773), Nelson's syndrome (p. 776) and chronic renal failure due to increased levels of pituitary melanotrophic peptides, including adrenocorticotrophic hormone (ACTH, p. 776).
- *Photoexposed site hyperpigmentation*: occurs in some of the porphyrias and can be drug-induced.
- *Drug-induced pigmentation* (Box 28.38): may be diffuse or localised. It is not always due to hypermelanosis but sometimes is caused by deposition of the drug or a metabolite.
- *Focal hypermelanosis*: seen in lesions such as freckles and lentigines, characterised by focal areas of increased pigmentation.

Establishing the cause is important. Photoprotection may minimise the risk of increasing pigmentation. Topical hydroquinone preparations can be used for skin lightening in some types of hyperpigmentation, although caution is required, particularly in darker skin types.

28.38 Drug-induced pigmentation

Drug	Appearance
Amiodarone	Photo-exposed sites, slate-grey
Arsenic	Diffuse bronze pigmentation Raindrop depigmentation
Bleomycin	Usually flexural, brown
Busulfan	Diffuse brown
Chloroquine	Photo-exposed sites, blue-grey
Clofazimine	Red
Mepacrine	Yellow
Minocycline	Temples, shins, gingiva, sclera, scar sites, slate-grey
Phenothiazines	Photo-exposed sites, slate-grey
Psoralens	Photo-exposed sites, brown

HAIR DISORDERS

These can be subdivided into loss of hair (alopecia, Box 28.39) or excess hair (hirsutism or hypertrichosis), and alopecia into localised/diffuse and scarring/non-scarring. Common examples are described below. Examples of inflammatory scarring (lichen planus, discoid lupus) and non-scarring (tinea capitis, psoriasis, seborrhoeic eczema) alopecia are mentioned elsewhere.

Alopecia areata

The usual presentation of this common autoimmune disorder is as well-defined, localised, non-inflammatory, non-scarring patches of alopecia, usually on the scalp (Fig. 28.39). Pathognomonic 'exclamation mark' hairs are seen (broken hairs, tapering towards the scalp) during active hair loss. A diffuse pattern can uncommonly occur on the scalp. Eyebrows, eyelashes, beard and body hair can be affected. Alopecia totalis describes complete loss of scalp hair, and alopecia universalis is complete loss of all hair. Nail pitting may occur (p. 1298). Spontaneous regrowth is usual for small patches of alopecia but the prognosis is less good for larger patches, more extensive involvement, early onset and an association with atopy. In addition to atopy, alopecia areata is associated with other autoimmune diseases, particularly thyroid disease, and with Down's syndrome.

Androgenetic alopecia

Male-pattern baldness is physiological in men over 20 years old, although it can also occur in teenagers. It is also found in women, particularly post-menopause. Characteristically, this involves bitemporal recession initially and subsequent involvement of the crown ('male pattern'), although it is often diffuse in women.

28.39 Classification and causes of alopecia

Localised	Diffuse
Non-scarring	
Tinea capitis Alopecia areata Androgenetic alopecia Traumatic (trichotillomania, traction, cosmetic) Syphilis	Androgenetic alopecia Telogen effluvium Hypothyroidism Hyperthyroidism Hypopituitarism Diabetes mellitus HIV disease Nutritional (especially iron) deficiency Liver disease Post-partum Alopecia areata Syphilis Drug-induced, e.g. chemotherapy, retinoids
Scarring	
Idiopathic Developmental defects Discoid lupus erythematosus Herpes zoster Pseudopelade Tinea capitis/kerion Morphoea (en coup de sabre)	Discoid lupus erythematosus Radiotherapy Folliculitis decalvans Lichen planopilaris

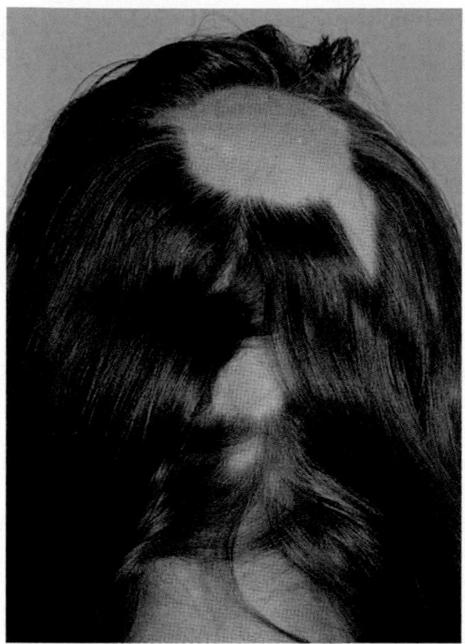

Fig. 28.39 Alopecia areata.

Investigations and management

Important investigations include full blood count, renal and liver function tests, iron studies, thyroid function, autoantibody screen and syphilis serology, as several systemic diseases, particularly iron deficiency and hypothyroidism, can cause diffuse non-scarring alopecia. Hair pull tests may help to establish the ratio of anagen to telogen hairs but require expertise for interpretation. Scrapings and pluckings are sent for mycology if there is localised inflammation. Scalp biopsy and direct immunofluorescence of a scarring alopecia may confirm a diagnosis of lichen planus or discoid lupus erythematosus, but expert interpretation is needed.

The impact of alopecia on quality of life must not be underestimated, and psychological support is required as treatment is difficult. It is important to establish realistic expectations. Underlying conditions must be treated. Alopecia areata may respond to topical or intralesional corticosteroids. Some males with androgenetic alopecia may be helped by systemic finasteride. Topical minoxidil can be used in males and females with androgenetic alopecia but, if an effect is obtained, treatment must be continued and is expensive. In females, anti-androgen therapy, such as cyproterone acetate, can be used. Wigs are often appropriate for extensive alopecia. Scalp surgery and autologous hair transplants are expensive but can be used for androgenetic alopecia.

Hypertrichosis

Hypertrichosis is a generalised or localised increase in hair and may be congenital or acquired. It can be primary or secondary: for example, to drugs such as ciclosporin, minoxidil or diazoxide, malignancy or eating disorders. Laser therapy or eflornithine, which inhibits ornithine decarboxylase and arrests hair growth whilst it is being used, may be helpful. When the hypertrichosis follows a male pattern, it is called hirsutism.

Hirsutism

Hirsutism is the growth of terminal hair in a male pattern in a female (p. 763). The cause of most cases is unknown and, while it may occur in hyperandrogenism, Cushing's syndrome and polycystic ovary syndrome, only a small minority of patients have a demonstrable hormonal abnormality. Psychological distress is often significant and oral contraceptives containing an anti-androgen (e.g. cyproterone acetate), laser therapy or topical eflornithine may be beneficial.

NAIL DISORDERS

The nails can be affected by both local and systemic disease. The nail apparatus consists of the nail matrix and the nail plate, which arises from the matrix and lies on the nail bed (Fig. 28.40). The cells of the matrix and, to a lesser extent the bed, produce the keratinous plate.

Important information may be obtained from nail fold examination, including dilated capillaries and ragged cuticles in connective tissue disease (Fig. 28.41) and the boggy inflammation of paronychia. The latter commonly occurs chronically in individuals undertaking wet work, in those with diabetes or poor peripheral circulation, and subsequent to increased cosmetic nail procedures and vigorous manicuring.

Common nail changes and disorders

Normal variants

Longitudinal ridging and beading of the nail plate occur with age. White transverse patches (striate leuconychia) are often caused by airspaces within the plate.

Effects of trauma

- *Nail biting/picking* is a very common habit. Repetitive proximal nail fold trauma (often thumb nail) results in transverse ridging and central furrowing of the nail.
- *Chronic trauma* from poorly-fitting shoes and sport can cause thickening and disordered growth of the nail (onychogryphosis) and subsequent ingrowing toenails.

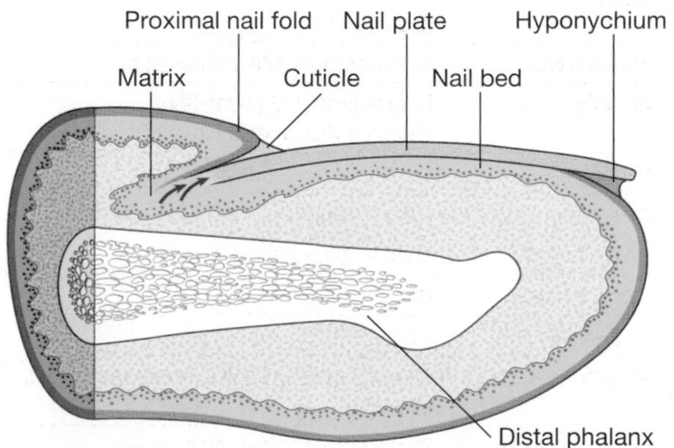

Fig. 28.40 The nail plate and bed. Arrows indicate the direction of nail growth.

- *Splinter haemorrhages* are fine, linear, dark brown longitudinal streaks in the plate (see Fig. 18.93, p. 627). They are usually subsequent to trauma, especially if distal. Uncommonly, they can occur in nail psoriasis and are a hallmark of infective endocarditis (p. 625).
- *Subungual haematoma* is red, purple or grey–brown discoloration of the nail plate, usually of the big toe (Fig. 28.42). These haematomas are usually due to trauma, although a history of this may not be clear. The main differential is subungual melanoma, although rapid onset, lack of nail-fold involvement and proximal clearing as the nail grows are clues to the diagnosis of haematoma. If there is diagnostic doubt, a biopsy may be needed.

A

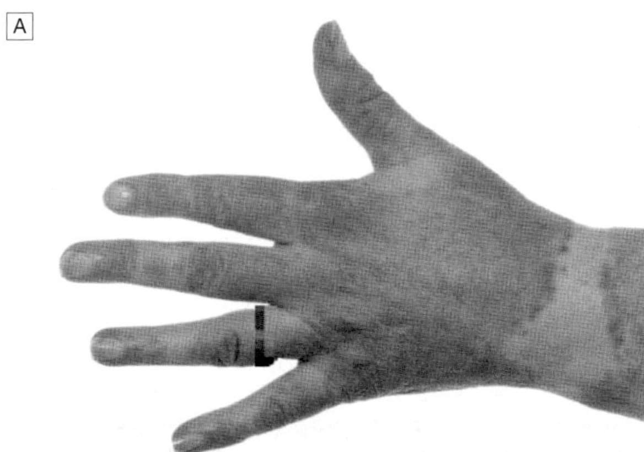

B

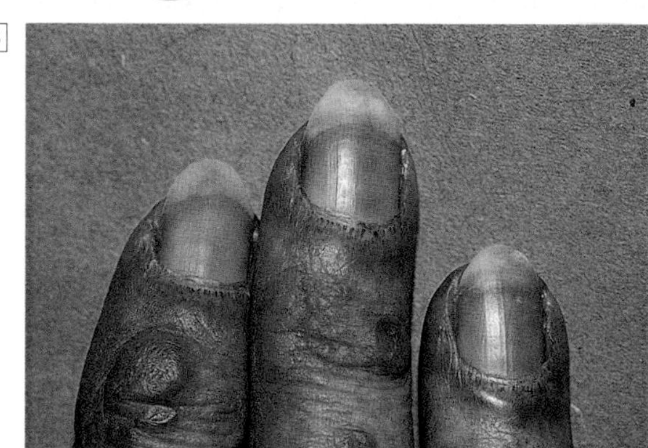

Fig. 28.41 Dermatomyositis. A Photoaggravation. B Note the prominent periungual involvement. Erythema, dilated and tortuous capillaries in the proximal nail fold, and ragged cuticles are features of connective tissue disease.

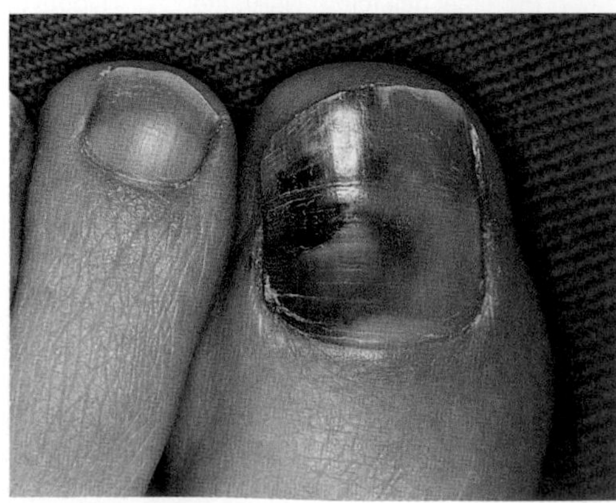

Fig. 28.42 Subungual haematoma.

The nails in common skin diseases

- *Dermatophyte infection/onychomycosis*: this is described on page 1280.
- *Psoriasis*: nail involvement is common (see Fig. 28.32B, p. 1287).
- *Eczema*: nails may be shiny due to rubbing skin. Fine pitting can occur. If there is periungual eczema, the nail may become dystrophic, with thickening and transverse ridging. Paronychia is common.
- *Lichen planus*: there may be longitudinal ridging and thinning of the nail, giving a sandpaper texture (trachyonychia), erythematous streaks (erythronychia), subungual hyperkeratosis, pigmentation and, in severe cases, pterygium and a destructive nail dystrophy.
- *Alopecia areata*: nail plate pitting and trachyonychia can occur.

Nail changes in systemic disease

The nails may be affected in many systemic diseases and important examples are detailed below:

- *Beau's lines*: horizontal ridges/indentations in nail plate occur simultaneously in all nails (Fig. 28.43B). They typically follow a systemic illness and are thought to be due to temporary growth arrest of cells in the nail matrix; they subsequently migrate out as the nail grows. Normal nail growth is approximately 0.1 mm/day for fingers and 0.05 mm/day for toes, so the timing of the systemic upset can usually be estimated by the position of the Beau's lines.
- *Koilonychia*: this concave or spoon-shaped nail plate deformity is due to iron deficiency (Fig. 28.43C).
- *Clubbing*: in the early stages, the angle between the proximal nail and nail fold is lost. In its more established form, there may be swelling of the distal digits (Figs 28.43D and E) or toe. Causes include bronchogenic carcinoma, asbestosis (especially with mesothelioma), suppurative or fibrosing lung disease, cyanotic congenital heart disease, infective endocarditis, inflammatory bowel disease, biliary cirrhosis and thyrotoxicosis; rarely, clubbing can be familial or idiopathic.
- *Nail discoloration:* whitening may occur in hypoalbuminaemia. 'Half-and-half' nails (white proximally and red/brown distally) may be found in renal failure. Drugs (e.g. antimalarials) occasionally discolour nails.

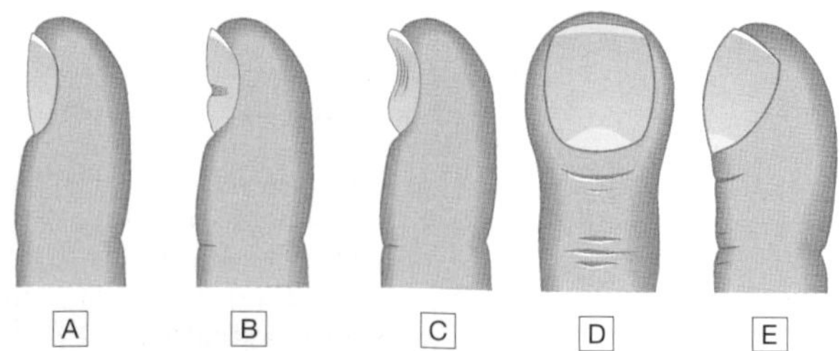

Fig. 28.43 The nail in systemic disease. A Normal nail. B Beau's line. C Koilonychia. D and E Digital clubbing.

The nail in congenital disease

Nails can be affected in congenital diseases, such as pachyonychia congenita, a rare, usually autosomal dominant, condition caused by mutations in differentiation-specific keratin genes 6A, 6B, 16 and 17. This results in palmoplantar keratoderma and gross nail discoloration and thickening, due to subungual hyperkeratosis, from birth.

SKIN DISEASE IN GENERAL MEDICINE

Many skin conditions present to other medical specialties. These are listed in Box 28.40 and the most common of those not discussed elsewhere are detailed below.

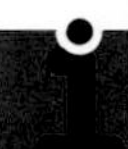

28.40 Skin problems in general medicine

Primary skin problems	
• Cellulitis • Vasculitis	• Leg ulcers • Pressure sores
Skin involvement in multisystem disease	
• Genetic (e.g. neurofibromatosis and tuberous sclerosis) • Xanthomas • Amyloidosis	• Porphyria • Sarcoidosis • SLE • Systemic sclerosis
Non-specific and variable skin reactions to systemic disease	
• Urticaria • Erythema multiforme • Annular erythemas • Erythema nodosum	• Pyoderma gangrenosum • Sweet's syndrome • Generalised pruritus
Skin conditions associated with malignancy	
• Dermatomyositis • Generalised pruritus	• Acanthosis nigricans • Superficial thrombophlebitis
Skin problems associated with specific medical disorders	
• Liver: generalised pruritus, pigmentation, spider naevi, palmar erythema, nail clubbing • Kidney: generalised pruritus, uraemic frost, pigmentation • Diabetes mellitus: necrobiosis lipoidica, diabetic dermopathy • Cutaneous Crohn's disease	
Skin problems secondary to treatment of systemic disease	
• Drug eruptions	
Miscellaneous	
• Granuloma annulare	• Morphoea

Conditions involving cutaneous vasculature

Vasculitis

Vasculitis usually presents as palpable purpura (see Fig. 25.42 and p. 1115). Causes include drugs, infection, connective tissue disease, malignancy and Henoch–Schönlein purpura. The diagnosis is confirmed by skin biopsy, with histology and immunofluorescence examination. Investigation should seek systemic involvement (particularly renal). Identification and removal or treatment of the cause is important but often difficult.

Neutrophilic dermatoses

These include pyoderma gangrenosum, Sweet's acute febrile neutrophilic dermatosis and the neutrophilic dermatosis of rheumatoid disease, and are characterised by intense inflammation, mainly consisting of neutrophils, around dermal blood vessels. There can be damage to vessels ('vasculopathy') but usually no frank vasculitis.

Pyoderma gangrenosum

The initial lesion of pyoderma gangrenosum (PG) is usually a painful, tender, inflamed nodule or pustule, which breaks down centrally and rapidly progresses to an ulcer with an indurated, undermined purplish or pustular edge (Fig. 28.44). Lesions may be single or multiple and are classified as ulcerative, pustular, bullous or vegetative. PG usually occurs in adults and, although it may occur in isolation, is usually associated with underlying disease, particularly inflammatory bowel disease, inflammatory arthritis, blood dyscrasias, immunodeficiencies and HIV infection. Investigation should be made with these associations in mind. The diagnosis is largely clinical, as histology is not specific. Analgesia, treatment of secondary bacterial infection and supportive dressings are important. Very potent topical corticosteroids or calcineurin inhibitors may be beneficial. Systemic treatment with tetracyclines, systemic steroids, dapsone, ciclosporin or other immunosuppressants is often required. Once healing has taken place, recurrences are typically only intermittent.

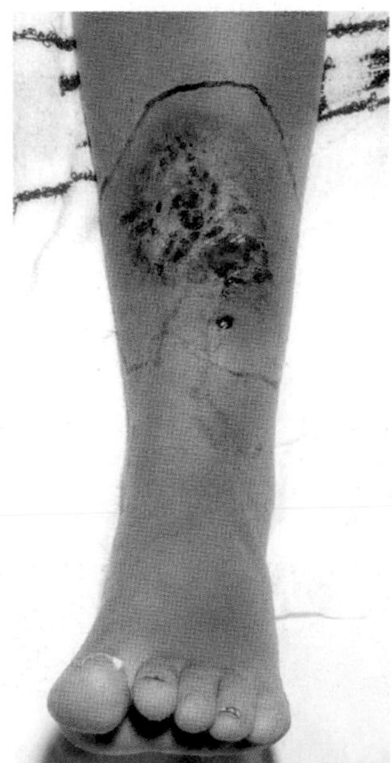

Fig. 28.44 Pyoderma gangrenosum. This young patient had Crohn's disease. Note the cribriform pattern of re-epithelialisation, which is characteristic of this condition.

Pressure sores

Localised, prolonged, pressure-induced ischaemia can lead to the development of pressure sores, which can occur in up to 30% of the hospitalised elderly. They are associated with considerable morbidity, mortality and expense to health services. The main risk factors are immobility, poor nutrition, local tissue hypoxia – for example, with anaemia, peripheral vascular disease, diabetes, sepsis and skin atrophy – or barrier impairment, such as in eczema.

A localised area of erythema develops at sites of bony prominences (particularly sacrum, greater trochanter, ischial and calcaneal tuberosities, and lateral malleolus). This progresses to a blister and then erosion, which will develop into a deep necrotic ulcer, usually colonised by *Pseudomonas aeruginosa* if pressure is not alleviated.

Prevention is key and involves identification of at-risk patients and regular repositioning and use of pressure-relieving mattresses. Predisposing factors, such as anaemia and poor nutrition, should be corrected. Once established, significant infection must be treated and necrotic tissue debrided. Dressings encourage granulation and surgical intervention may be needed.

Connective tissue disease

Lupus erythematosus

The autoimmune disorder lupus erythematosus (p. 1109) can be subdivided into systemic lupus erythematosus (SLE) and cutaneous lupus, which includes discoid lupus (DLE) and subacute cutaneous lupus erythematosus (SCLE). DLE typically presents as scaly red plaques, with follicular plugging, usually on photo-exposed sites of the face, head and neck, which resolve with scarring and pigmentary change. If the scalp is involved, scarring alopecia occurs (Fig. 28.45). Most patients with DLE do not develop SLE. Patients with SCLE may have extensive cutaneous involvement, usually aggravated by sun exposure, with an annular, polycyclic or papulosquamous eruption. Systemic involvement is uncommon and the prognosis usually good. There is a strong association with antibodies to Ro/SS-A antigen. A diagnosis of cutaneous lupus is confirmed by histopathology and direct immunofluorescence. SLE is a serious multisystem disorder and cutaneous manifestations include photosensitivity with malar (butterfly) rash, Raynaud's phenomenon, chilblains, livedo reticularis and vasculitis. Investigations and management of SLE are outlined elsewhere on page 1111. The possibility of drug-induced lupus should always be considered (see Boxes 25.84, p. 1113; 28.43, p. 1303; and 28.44, p. 1304). Cutaneous lupus may respond to topical corticosteroids or immunosuppressants. Antimalarials and photoprotection are important in the management of cutaneous lupus, and systemic immunosuppression may be required for resistant disease. Paradoxically, low-dose UVA1 phototherapy can sometimes be effective for lupus.

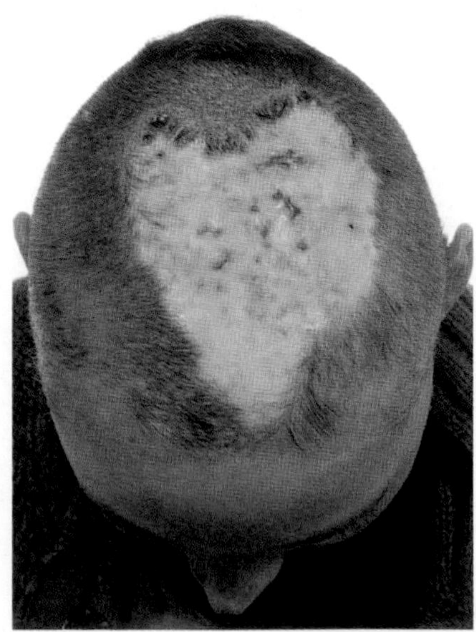

Fig. 28.45 Scarring inflammatory alopecia. This patient had systemic lupus erythematosus and additional cutaneous features of scarring inflammatory discoid lupus erythematosus.

Systemic sclerosis

Systemic sclerosis is an autoimmune multisystem disease that usually presents in middle age and is characterised by progressive cutaneous and connective tissue sclerosis, vascular abnormalities and associated autoantibodies (p. 1112). The earliest feature is usually Raynaud's phenomenon, followed by progressive skin tightening and oedema. Constricted mouth opening and perioral radial furrows, with matted telangiectasiae and pigmentary change, are common. Fixed flexion deformities of the hands, ulceration, calcification, scarring and gangrene of digits may develop. Dilated nail-fold capillaries and ragged cuticles are the norm. Investigation and management are described on page 1113.

Morphoea

Morphoea is a localised cutaneous form of scleroderma that can affect any site at any age. It usually presents as a thickened violaceous plaque, which may become hyper- or hypopigmented. Plaques can become generalised. Linear forms exist and, if in the scalp, there will be scarring hair loss (en coup de sabre). There is no systemic involvement. Topical corticosteroids or immunosuppressants or phototherapy, particularly PUVA or UVA1, can be effective, and systemic immunosuppression may be used for resistant extensive disease.

Dermatomyositis

This is a rare multisystem disease, predominantly affecting skin, muscles and blood vessels (p. 1114). The cause is unknown. There may be an autoimmune mechanism in childhood cases, whereas in adults there is often an underlying malignancy. Dermatomyositis typically presents between 40 and 60 years and is more common in females. In juvenile patients, calcinosis often occurs. The typical cutaneous features are of a violaceous 'heliotrope' erythema periorbitally and involving the upper eyelids. There may be more extensive involvement, with violaceous erythema on the upper trunk and limbs, linear erythematous streaks on the back of hands and fingers, and papules over the knuckles (Gottron's papules). Tortuous dilated nail-fold capillaries, often best seen with a dermatoscope, and ragged cuticles are usually evident. Photoaggravation of the cutaneous features is often prominent (see Fig. 28.41, p. 1298). Tenderness and proximal muscle weakness are indicative of an inflammatory proximal myopathy. Other systems, such as the respiratory tract, may be involved. Investigations include creatine kinase levels and searching for an underlying malignancy (p. 1115). Treatment usually requires high-dose corticosteroids and/or other immunosuppressants.

Granulomatous disease

Granuloma annulare

This is common and may be reactive, although a trigger is usually not apparent. The hallmark is the presence of dermal granulomas, which are usually palisading and associated with alteration of dermal collagen (necrobiosis). The condition is generally asymptomatic and may present as an isolated dermal lesion with a raised papular annular edge or be more generalised. An association between generalised disease and diabetes has been proposed but not confirmed. Lesions often resolve spontaneously. Intralesional steroids or cryotherapy can be used for localised disease, and UVB or UVA1 phototherapy or PUVA for generalised disease.

Necrobiosis lipoidica

This condition has some histological features in common with granuloma annulare, although necrobiosis predominates. The lesion has a characteristic yellow, waxy, atrophic appearance, often with violaceous edge (Fig. 28.46). Underlying blood vessels are easily seen because of tissue atrophy. Necrobiosis lipoidica typically appears on the shins and is prone to ulceration after trauma. There is a strong association with diabetes: most patients with necrobiosis lipoidica have or develop diabetes, although less than 1% of diabetic patients develop necrobiosis lipoidica. Treatment is difficult and includes potent topical or intralesional steroids, PUVA or UVA1 phototherapy and systemic immunosuppression.

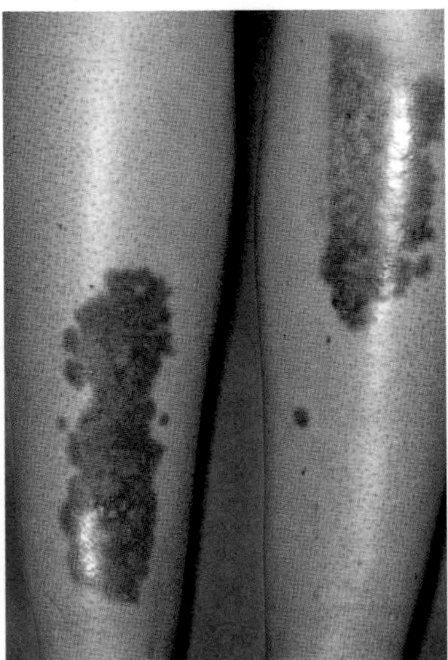

Fig. 28.46 Necrobiosis lipoidica. Atrophic yellow plaques with violaceous edges, on the shins of a patient with diabetes mellitus.

Sarcoidosis

This condition is characterised by the presence of non-caseating granulomas. The cause is unknown, although infectious and genetic factors have been proposed. It is usually a multisystem disease (p. 709), with skin lesions in about one-third of patients. Cutaneous features can occur in isolation and include violaceous infiltrated dermal plaques and nodules, which can affect any site but particularly digits and nose (lupus pernio), more generalised hyper-/hypopigmented or annular papules and plaques, infiltrative changes in scars and erythema nodosum (see Fig. 19.60. p. 710). It is more common and often more severe in black Africans and African-Americans. Investigation and management are described on page 711. Cutaneous disease may respond to topical or intralesional steroids, cryotherapy, UVA1, laser or PDT (p. 1269). Systemic disease usually requires systemic corticosteroids and/or other immunosuppressants. Responses to anti-TNF biological therapies are reported.

Cutaneous Crohn's disease

Cutaneous Crohn's disease (p. 897) is rare but may present as perianal and peristomal infiltrative plaques, lymphoedema, sinuses or fistulae, and oral granulomatous disease. These changes are termed 'metastatic' Crohn's and histology shows non-caseating granulomas. Reactive skin changes can also occur (e.g. erythema nodosum and pyoderma gangrenosum, pp. 1299 and 1303). Treatment is of the underlying disease (p. 902).

Metabolic disease

Porphyrias

The porphyrias (described on p. 458) are a diverse group of diseases, each due to insufficient activity of an enzyme in the porphyrin–haem biosynthetic pathway. Those that cause skin features do so because porphyrins in the skin absorb visible light. The most common skin presentations are photoexposed site blistering and fragility, and pain on daylight exposure.

Photoexposed site blistering and fragility

Acquired porphyria cutanea tarda (PCT) is the most common porphyria to cause these symptoms (and, in most parts of the world, the most common of all the porphyrias). PCT is due to a chronic liver disease (e.g. alcohol, hepatitis C), in combination with liver iron overload. Recognition is important, as the underlying liver disease is usually only diagnosed on investigation of the skin presentation. Typical features are increased skin fragility, blistering erosions, hypertrichosis and milia occurring on light-exposed areas, such as the backs of the hands (Fig. 28.47). Other features may include facial hypertrichosis, hyperpigmentation and morphoea-like changes. Other porphyrias that can cause similar skin features include variegate porphyria and hereditary coproporphyria. It is important not to miss these, as acute neurovisceral attacks (which never occur in PCT) are possible, often triggered by drugs (p. 1303). Pseudoporphyria usually presents like PCT but is most frequently caused by a drug (commonly naproxen; see Box 28.44, p. 1304) or by sunbed use. 'Uraemic porphyria' in renal failure presents like PCT but is caused by raised porphyrins due to impaired elimination rather than an enzyme defect.

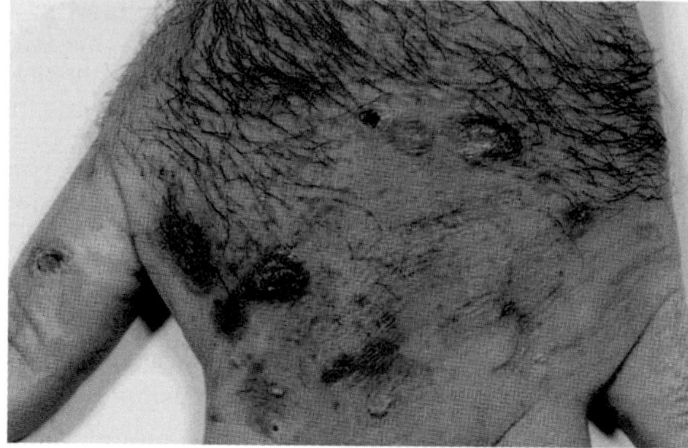

Fig. 28.47 Porphyria cutanea tarda. Skin fragility, blistering, scarring, milia and hypertrichosis on the back of hands and fingers in a patient with hepatitis C.

Pain on daylight exposure

Erythropoietic protoporphyria is a rare inherited porphyria but is important to consider. The presentation is usually in early childhood, although the diagnosis is often delayed, in part because physical signs are often minimal despite the prominence of symptoms on sunlight exposure. Erythropoietic protoporphyria is due to ferrochelatase deficiency, which leads to accumulation of lipid-soluble protoporphyrins in the skin. Multiple pigment gallstones, anaemia (usually only problematic if it is misdiagnosed as being caused by iron deficiency) and, rarely, severe liver disease can occur.

Abnormal deposition disorders

Xanthomas

Deposits of fatty material in the skin, subcutaneous fat and tendons may be the first clue to primary or secondary hyperlipidaemia (see p. 453 and Fig. 16.15).

Amyloidosis

Cutaneous amyloid may present as periocular plaques in primary systemic amyloidosis (p. 86) and amyloid associated with multiple myeloma, but is uncommon in systemic amyloidosis secondary to rheumatoid arthritis or other chronic inflammatory diseases. Amyloid infiltration of blood vessels may manifest as 'pinch purpura' following skin trauma. Macular amyloid is more common in darker skin types and appears as pruritic grey/brown macules or patches, usually on the back. Potent topical steroids can be beneficial, although it is often treatment-resistant.

Genetic disorders

Neurofibromatosis

This is described in detail on page 1215.

Tuberous sclerosis

This is an autosomal dominant condition, with two genetic loci identified: *TSC-1* (chromosome 9), encoding hamartin, and *TSC-2* (chromosome 16), encoding tuberin. The hallmark is of hamartomas in many systems. The classic triad of clinical features comprises learning disability, epilepsy and skin lesions but there is marked heterogeneity in clinical features. Skin changes include pale oval (ash leaf) macules that occur in early childhood; yellowish/pink papules in the mid-face (angiofibromas, 'adenoma sebaceum'), occurring in adolescence; periungual and subungual fibromas; and connective tissue naevi (shagreen patches, often on lower back). Gum hyperplasia, retinal phakomas (fibrous overgrowths), renal, lung and heart tumours, cerebral gliomas and calcified basal ganglia may also occur.

Reactive disorders

Erythema multiforme

Erythema multiforme has characteristic clinical and histological features and can be triggered by a variety of factors (Box 28.41); a cause is not always identified. The disease is a reaction pattern and likely to have an immunological basis. Lesions are multiple, erythematous, annular, targetoid 'bull's eyes' (Fig. 28.48) and may blister. Stevens–Johnson syndrome (pp. 1264 and 1302) is a severe form of erythema multiforme with marked

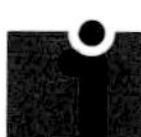

28.41 Provoking factors in erythema multiforme
Infections
• Viral, e.g. herpes simplex, orf, infectious mononucleosis, hepatitis B, HIV • *Mycoplasma* and other bacterial infections
Drugs
• e.g. Sulphonamides, penicillins, barbiturates and carbamazepine
Systemic disease
• Sarcoidosis, malignancy, SLE
Other
• Radiotherapy, pregnancy

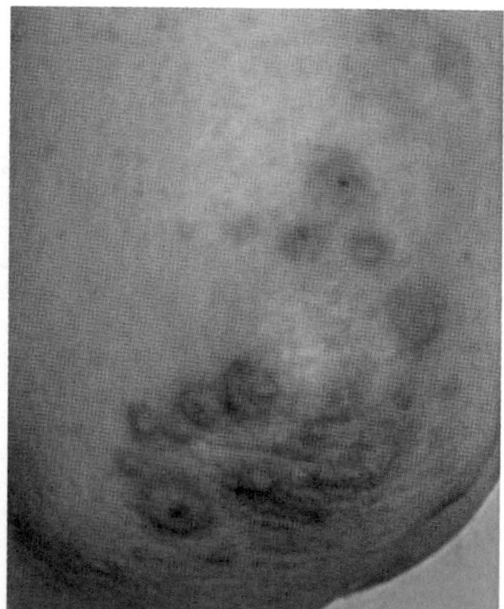

Fig. 28.48 Erythema multiforme in a young woman. Herpes simplex virus infection was the trigger.

blistering, mucosal involvement (mouth, eyes and genitals) and systemic upset.

Identification and removal/treatment of any trigger are essential. Analgesia and topical steroids may provide symptomatic relief. Supportive care is required in Stevens–Johnson syndrome, including ophthalmology input. Systemic corticosteroids may increase risk of infection and a role for intravenous immunoglobulins is controversial.

Erythema nodosum

This is characterised histologically by a septal panniculitis of subcutaneous fat (see Fig. 19.60, p. 710). An identified trigger is often present (Box 28.42). Lesions are typically painful, indurated violaceous nodules on the shins and lower legs. Systemic upset, arthralgias and fever are common. Spontaneous resolution occurs over a month or so, leaving bruise-like marks. Any underlying cause should be identified and removed or treated. Bed rest, leg elevation and oral NSAIDs may offer symptomatic relief. Systemic corticosteroids are uncommonly required and must be avoided in infection. Dapsone and potassium iodide have been effective for stubborn disease.

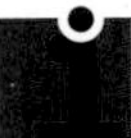

28.42 Provoking factors in erythema nodosum

Infections
• Bacteria, e.g. streptococci, mycobacteria, *Brucella*, *Mycoplasma*, *Rickettsia*, *Chlamydia* • Viruses, e.g. hepatitis B and infectious mononucleosis • Fungi
Drugs
• e.g. Sulphonamides, sulphonylureas, oral contraceptives
Systemic disease
• e.g. Sarcoidosis, inflammatory bowel disease, malignancy

Acquired reactive perforating dermatosis

The hallmark of this condition is transepidermal elimination of dermal material, particularly collagen and elastic tissue. It presents as keratotic papules, particularly in patients with diabetes and chronic renal disease. Treatment with topical steroids, retinoids, PUVA or UVA1 therapy may help. There are other related perforating dermopathies, with characteristic histology.

Annular erythemas

This group of chronic, poorly defined, annular, erythematous and often scaly eruptions can be further subdivided and may be secondary to an identifiable cause. Erythema chronicum migrans can be associated with Lyme disease (*Borrelia burgdorferi*) (p. 334). Erythema marginatum can occur in rheumatic fever (p. 614) or Still's disease (p. 1104). Erythema gyratum repens typically presents as concentric circles of erythema and scale with an advancing edge and is usually associated with underlying malignancy. Erythema annulare centrifugum presents with expanding, scaly, erythematous rings, with central fading. A trigger may not be apparent but possible associations include fungal infection, drugs, autoimmune or endocrine diseases, such as lupus or thyroid disease, and malignancy, particularly haematological. An underlying trigger must be sought and removed/treated. Topical steroids or phototherapy may be helpful for chronic disease.

Acanthosis nigricans

Hyperkeratosis and pigmentation are typical and affected sites have a velvety texture. The flexures, especially axillae and, in dark-skinned people, sides of neck, are involved (pp. 271, 272, 798). There are several types, all associated with insulin resistance. Most often, acanthosis nigricans is found in conjunction with obesity and regresses with weight loss. It can be associated with malignancy, usually adenocarcinoma (particularly gastric), when it is usually more extensive and pruritic, and can involve mucous membranes.

Drug eruptions

Virtually all drugs may have cutaneous adverse effects (Fig. 28.49) and this should be considered in the

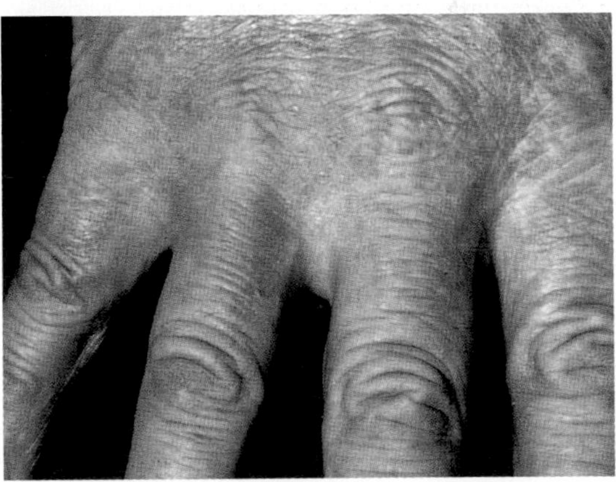

Fig. 28.49 Drug eruption. Always think about possible drug causes of any rash. This was doxycycline-induced photosensitivity in a farmer.

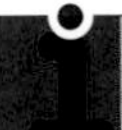

28.43 Types of drug eruption

Non-immunological (non-allergic)
All are predictable. • Striae due to corticosteroids (see Fig. 28.8, p. 1265) • Asteatosis with statins • Candidal infections with antibiotics • Worsening of psoriasis with lithium, β-blockers, antimalarials, NSAIDs • Urticaria with aspirin due to mast cell degranulation • Bradykinin-mediated angioedema due to ACE inhibitors • Doxycycline photosensitivity • Dapsone haemolysis
Immunological (allergic)
• Immediate IgE-mediated hypersensitivity (type I): penicillin-induced urticaria and anaphylaxis • Antibody-mediated (type II): penicillin-induced haemolysis • Immune complex-mediated (type III): drug-induced serum sickness or vasculitis • Delayed hypersensitivity (type IV): drug-induced erythema multiforme, lichenoid or pemphigus-like reaction; drug-induced lupus, e.g. thiazide

28.44 Clinical patterns of drug eruptions

Reaction pattern	Clinical features	Examples of causative drugs
Exanthematous	Erythema, maculopapular	Antibiotics (especially ampicillin), anticonvulsants, gold, penicillamine, NSAIDs, carbimazole, biological therapies, e.g. adalimumab
Urticaria and angioedema	Sometimes accompanied by angioedema Angioedema alone	Salicylates, opiates, NSAIDs, antibiotics, dextran ACE inhibitors
Lichenoid	Violaceous, lichen planus-like, dyspigmentation	Gold, penicillamine, antimalarials, thiazides, NSAIDs, β-blockers, ACE inhibitors, sulphonamides, lithium, sulphonylurea, proton pump inhibitors, quinine, antituberculous, dyes in colour developers
Purpura and vasculitis	Palpable purpura and necrosis	Allopurinol, antibiotics, ACE inhibitors, NSAIDs, aspirin, anticonvulsants, diuretics, oral contraceptives
Erythema multiforme	Target-like lesions and bullae on extensor aspects of limbs	See Box 28.41, p. 1302
Erythema nodosum	Tender, painful, dusky, erythematous nodules on shins	See Box 28.42, p. 1303
Exfoliative dermatitis	May be erythroderma	Allopurinol, carbamazepine, barbiturates, penicillins, PAS, isoniazid, gold, lithium, penicillamine, ACE inhibitors
Toxic epidermal necrolysis	Rapid evolution, extensive blistering, erythema, necrolysis, mucosal involvement	Anticonvulsants, antibiotics, especially sulphonamides, NSAIDs, terbinafine, sulphonylureas, antiretrovirals, allopurinol
Photosensitivity (p. 1260)	Photo-exposed site rash, may be sunburn-like, exfoliation, lichenoid	Thiazides, amiodarone, quinine, NSAIDs, tetracyclines, fluoroquinolones, phenothiazines, sulphonamides, retinoids, psoralens
Drug-induced lupus	Photosensitivity, discoid lesions, urticarial or erythema multiforme-like. May have positive lupus serology and anti-histone antibodies	Allopurinol, thiazides, ACE inhibitors, PAS, anticonvulsants, β-blockers, gold, hydralazine, minocycline, penicillamine, lithium
Psoriasiform rash	Rash like psoriasis	See Box 28.28 (p. 1286)
DRESS	Facial oedema, fever, extensive rash, lymphadenopathy, eosinophilia and systemic involvement, e.g. hepatitis	Anticonvulsants, trimethoprim, minocycline, allopurinol, dapsone, terbinafine
AGEP/toxic pustuloderma	Rapid onset of sterile, non-follicular pustules on erythematous base	Ampicillin/amoxicillin, erythromycin, quinolones, sulphonamides, terbinafine, diltiazem, hydroxychloroquine
Acneiform eruptions	Rash resembles acne	Lithium, anticonvulsants, oral contraceptives, androgenic or glucocorticoid steroids, antituberculous drugs, EGFR-antagonists, e.g. cetuximab
Pigmentation		See Box 28.38 (p. 1296)
Bullous eruptions	Often at pressure sites and may be other features, e.g. purpura, milia	Barbiturates, penicillamine
Pseudoporphyria	May be indistinguishable from porphyria cutanea tarda clinically	NSAIDS, tetracyclines, retinoids, furosemide, nalidixic acid
Exacerbation of acute hepatic porphyrias		See page 1301 Always check all drugs for safety of use in porphyrias against standard guidelines
Drug-induced immunobullous disease	May be like pemphigoid, pemphigus, dermatomyositis, scleroderma, epidermolysis bullosa acquisita	Penicillamine, ACE inhibitors, vancomycin
Fixed drug eruptions	Round/oval, erythema, oedema ± bullae Same site every time drug is given Pigmentation on resolution	Tetracyclines, sulphonamides, penicillins, quinine, NSAIDs, barbiturates, anticonvulsants
Hair loss	Diffuse	Cytotoxic agents, oral retinoids, anticoagulants, anticonvulsants, antithyroid drugs, lithium, oral contraceptives, infliximab
Hypertrichosis	Excessive hair growth in non-androgenic distribution	Diazoxide, minoxidil, ciclosporin

(ACE = angiotensin-converting enzyme; AGEP = acute generalised exanthematous pustulosis; DRESS = drug rash with eosinophilia and systemic symptoms; EGFR = epidermal growth factor receptor; NSAID = non-steroidal anti-inflammatory drug; PAS = para-aminosalicylic acid)

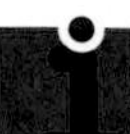

28.45 Diagnostic clues to drug eruptions

- Past history of reaction to suspected drug
- Introduction of suspected drug a few days to weeks before onset of rash
- Recent prescription of a drug commonly associated with rashes (e.g. penicillin, sulphonamide, thiazide, allopurinol)
- Symmetrical eruption that fits with a well-recognised pattern, caused by a current drug
- Resolution of rash following drug cessation

differential diagnosis of most presentations of skin disease. Drugs can exert their adverse effects via several mechanisms, which can be broadly subdivided into non-immunological and immunological (Box 28.43).

Clinical features

Cutaneous drug reactions typically present in specific patterns (Box 28.44). Non-immunologically mediated reactions can theoretically occur in anyone given sufficient exposure to drug, although idiosyncratic factors, such as genetic predisposition, may render some more susceptible. There is limited information on genetic determinants of drug responses and adverse effects, although advances have been made, e.g. with azathioprine (p. 1268). Immunologically mediated cutaneous drug eruptions typically commence within days to weeks of starting the drug. Detailed history-taking relating to prescribed and non-prescribed medications is essential and there may be other clues (Box 28.45).

Investigations and management

The suspected drug must be stopped. If drug-induced photosensitivity is considered, the patient should be phototested whilst on the drug to confirm the diagnosis; testing should be repeated after drug withdrawal to confirm resolution of photosensitivity (p. 1255). An eosinophilia and abnormalities in liver function tests may occur in adverse drug reactions and, for example, specific IgE to penicillin may be raised in penicillin-induced rash but, otherwise, specific investigations are not available. Rechallenge with drug is not usually undertaken unless the reaction is mild, as this can be risky. Drug withdrawal may not be straightforward and substitute drugs may be required. Antihistamines and/or topical or systemic corticosteroids may provide supportive management, depending on the type of cutaneous reaction. The management of anaphylaxis is described on page 92.

Further information and acknowledgements

Books and journal articles

Burns T, Breachnach S, Cox N, Griffiths C (eds). Rook's textbook of dermatology, 8th edn. Oxford: Wiley-Blackwell; 2010.

Goldsmith LA, Fitzpatrick TB. Fitzpatrick's dermatology in general medicine, 8th edn. New York: McGraw-Hill Professional; 2012.

Websites

www.bad.org.uk *Guidelines and patient information for many skin diseases.*

www.nice.org.uk *Guidelines for skin malignancy, atopic eczema, psoriasis and photodynamic therapy.*

www.sign.ac.uk *No. 72: Cutaneous melanoma (Feb 2004; review report 2012). No. 120: Management of chronic venous leg ulcers (Aug 2010). No. 121: Diagnosis and management of psoriasis and psoriatic arthritis in adults (Oct 2010). No. 125: Management of atopic eczema in primary care (Mar 2011).*

Figure acknowledgements

Fig. 28.18A Savin JA, Dahl M, Hunter JAA. Clinical dermatology. 3rd edn. Oxford: Blackwell; 2002.

28

S.W. Walker

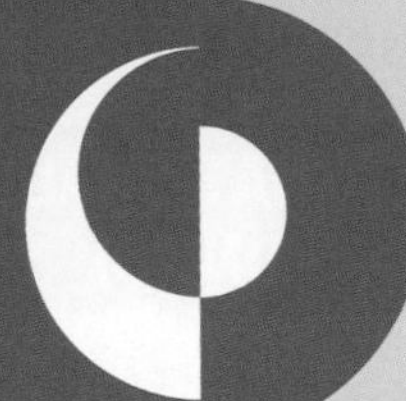

29 Laboratory reference ranges

Notes on the International System of Units (SI units) 1308

Laboratory reference ranges in adults 1308

Urea and electrolytes in venous blood 1308
Analytes in arterial blood 1308
Hormones in venous blood 1309
Other common analytes in venous blood 1310
Common analytes in urine 1311
Analytes in cerebrospinal fluid 1311
Analytes in faeces 1311
Haematological values 1312

NOTES ON THE INTERNATIONAL SYSTEM OF UNITS (SI UNITS)

Système International (SI) units are a specific subset of the metre–kilogram–second system of units and were agreed upon as the everyday currency for commercial and scientific work in 1960, following a series of international conferences organised by the International Bureau of Weights and Measures. SI units have been adopted widely in clinical laboratories but non-SI units are still used in many countries. For that reason, values in both units are given for common measurements throughout this textbook and commonly used non-SI units are shown in this chapter. However, the SI unit system is recommended.

Examples of basic SI units

Length	metre (m)
Mass	kilogram (kg)
Amount of substance	mole (mol)
Energy	joule (J)
Pressure	pascal (Pa)
Volume	The basic SI unit of volume is the cubic metre (1000 litres). For convenience, however, the litre (L) is used as the unit of volume in laboratory work.

Examples of decimal multiples and submultiples of SI units

Factor	*Name*	*Prefix*
10^{6}	mega-	M
10^{3}	kilo-	k
10^{-1}	deci-	d
10^{-2}	centi-	c
10^{-3}	milli-	m
10^{-6}	micro-	μ
10^{-9}	nano-	n
10^{-12}	pico-	p
10^{-15}	femto-	f

Exceptions to the use of SI units

By convention, blood pressure is excluded from the SI unit system and is measured in mmHg (millimetres of mercury) rather than pascals.

Mass concentrations (e.g. g/L, μg/L) are used in preference to molar concentrations for all protein measurements and for substances which do not have a sufficiently well-defined composition.

Some enzymes and hormones are measured by 'bioassay', in which the activity in the sample is compared with the activity (rather than the mass) of a standard sample that is provided from a central source. For these assays, results are given in standardised 'units', or 'international units', which depend upon the activity in the standard sample and may not be readily converted to mass units.

LABORATORY REFERENCE RANGES IN ADULTS

Reference ranges are largely those used in the Departments of Clinical Biochemistry and Haematology, Lothian Health University Hospitals Division, Edinburgh, UK. Values are shown in both SI units and, where appropriate, non-SI units. Many reference ranges vary between laboratories, depending on the assay method used and on other factors; this is especially the case for enzyme assays. The origin of reference ranges and the interpretation of 'abnormal' results are discussed on pages 4–6. No details are given here of the collection requirements, which may be critical to obtaining a meaningful result. Unless otherwise stated, reference ranges shown apply to adults; values in children may be different.

Many analytes can be measured in either serum (the supernatant of clotted blood) or plasma (the supernatant of anticoagulated blood). A specific requirement for one or the other may depend on a kit manufacturer's recommendations. In other instances, the distinction is critical (e.g. plasma is required for measurement of fibrinogen, since it is largely absent from serum; serum is required for electrophoresis to detect paraproteins because fibrinogen migrates as a discrete band in the zone of interest).

29.1 Urea and electrolytes in venous blood

	Reference range	
Analysis	**SI units**	**Non-SI units**
Sodium	135–145 mmol/L	135–145 meq/L
Potassium*	3.6–5.0 mmol/L	3.6–5.0 meq/L
Chloride	95–107 mmol/L	95–107 meq/L
Urea	2.5–6.6 mmol/L	15–40 mg/dL
Creatinine	60–120 μmol/L	0.68–1.36 mg/dL

*Serum values are, on average, 0.3 mmol/L higher than plasma.

29.2 Analytes in arterial blood

	Reference range	
Analysis	**SI units**	**Non-SI units**
Bicarbonate	21–29 mmol/L	21–29 meq/L
Hydrogen ion	37–45 nmol/L	pH 7.35–7.43
$PaCO_2$	4.5–6.0 kPa	34–45 mmHg
PaO_2	12–15 kPa	90–113 mmHg
Oxygen saturation	> 97%	

29.3 Hormones in venous blood

Hormone	Reference range: SI units	Non-SI units
Adrenocorticotrophic hormone (ACTH) (plasma)	1.5–11.2 pmol/L (0700–1000 hrs)	7–51 ng/L
Aldosterone		
Supine (at least 30 mins)	30–440 pmol/L	1.09–15.9 ng/dL
Erect (at least 1 hr)	110–860 pmol/L	3.97–31.0 ng/dL
Cortisol	Dynamic tests are required – see Ch. 20	
Follicle-stimulating hormone (FSH)		
Male	1.0–10.0 U/L	0.2–2.2 ng/mL
Female	3.0–10.0 U/L (early follicular)	0.7–2.2 ng/mL
	> 30 U/L (post-menopausal)	> 6.7 ng/mL
Gastrin (plasma, fasting)	< 120 ng/L	< 120 pg/mL
Growth hormone (GH)	Dynamic tests are usually required – see Ch. 20 < 0.5 μg/L excludes acromegaly (if IGF1 in reference range) > 6 μg/L excludes GH deficiency	–
Insulin	Highly variable and interpretable only in relation to plasma glucose and body habitus	
Luteinising hormone (LH)		
Male	1.0–9.0 U/L	0.11–1.0 μg/L
Female	2.0–9.0 U/L (early follicular)	0.2–1.0 μg/L
	> 20 U/L (post-menopausal)	> 2.2 μg/L
17β-Oestradiol		
Male	< 160 pmol/L	< 43 pg/mL
Female: early follicular	75–140 pmol/L	20–38 pg/mL
post-menopausal	< 150 pmol/L	< 41 pg/mL
Parathyroid hormone (PTH)	1.6–7.5 pmol/L	16–75 pg/mL
Progesterone (in luteal phase in women)		
Consistent with ovulation	> 30 nmol/L	> 9.3 ng/mL
Probable ovulatory cycle	15–30 nmol/L	4.7–9.3 ng/mL
Anovulatory cycle	< 10 nmol/L	< 3 ng/mL
Prolactin (PRL)	25–630 mU/L	–
Renin concentration		
Supine (at least 30 mins)	5–40 mU/L	–
Sitting (at least 15 mins)	5–45 mU/L	–
Erect (at least 1 hr)	16–63 mU/L	–
Testosterone		
Male	10–30 nmol/L	2.9–8.6 ng/mL
Female	0.3–1.9 nmol/L	0.1–0.9 ng/mL
Thyroid-stimulating hormone (TSH)	0.2–4.5 mU/L	–
Thyroxine (free), (free T_4)	9–21 pmol/L	700–1632 pg/dL
Triiodothyronine (free), (free T_3)	2.6–6.2 pmol/L	160–400 pg/dL

Notes

1. A number of hormones are unstable and collection details are critical to obtaining a meaningful result. Refer to local laboratory handbook.
2. Values in the table are only a guideline; hormone levels can often only be meaningfully understood in relation to factors such as sex (e.g. testosterone), age (e.g. FSH in women), pregnancy (e.g. thyroid function tests, prolactin), time of day (e.g. cortisol) or regulatory factors (e.g. insulin and glucose, PTH and [Ca^{2+}]).
3. Reference ranges may be critically method-dependent.

(IGF1 = insulin-like growth factor 1)

29

29.4 Other common analytes in venous blood

Analyte	Reference range: SI units	Reference range: Non-SI units
α_1-antitrypsin	1.1–2.1 g/L	110–210 mg/dL
Alanine aminotransferase (ALT)	10–50 U/L	–
Albumin	35–50 g/L	3.5–5.0 g/dL
Alkaline phosphatase	40–125 U/L	–
Amylase	< 100 U/L	–
Aspartate aminotransferase (AST)	10–45 U/L	–
Bilirubin (total)	3–16 µmol/L	0.18–0.94 mg/dL
Calcium (total)	2.1–2.6 mmol/L	4.2–5.2 meq/L or 8.5–10.5 mg/dL
Carboxy-haemoglobin	0.1–3.0%	–
Caeruloplasmin	0.16–0.47 g/L	16–47 mg/dL
Cholesterol (total)	Ideal level varies according to cardiovascular risk (see cardiovascular risk chart, p. 582), so reference ranges can be misleading. The following values were described by the European Atherosclerosis Society:	
Mild increase	5.2–6.5 mmol/L	200–250 mg/dL
Moderate increase	6.5–7.8 mmol/L	250–300 mg/dL
Severe increase	> 7.8 mmol/L	> 300 mg/dL
HDL-cholesterol	Ideal level varies according to cardiovascular risk, so reference ranges can be misleading. According to the National Cholesterol Education Programme Adult Treatment Panel III (ATPIII), a low HDL-cholesterol is:	
Low	< 1.0 mmol/L	< 40 mg/dL
Complement		
C3	0.73–1.4 g/L	–
C4	0.12–0.3 g/L	–
Total haemolytic complement	0.086–0.410 g/L	–
Copper	10–22 µmol/L	64–140 µg/dL
C-reactive protein (CRP)	< 5 mg/L Highly sensitive CRP assays also exist which measure lower values and may be useful in estimating cardiovascular risk	
Creatine kinase (CK; total)		
Male	55–170 U/L	–
Female	30–135 U/L	–
Creatine kinase MB isoenzyme	< 6% of total CK	–
Ethanol	Not normally detectable	
Marked intoxication	65–87 mmol/L	300–400 mg/dL
Stupor	87–109 mmol/L	400–500 mg/dL
Coma	> 109 mmol/L	> 500 mg/dL
Gamma-glutamyl transferase (GGT)	Male 10–55 U/L Female 5–35 U/L	–
Glucose (fasting)	3.6–5.8 mmol/L See p. 808 for definitions of impaired glucose tolerance and diabetes mellitus, and p. 783 for definition of hypoglycaemia	65–104 mg/dL
Glycated haemoglobin (HbA_{1c})	4.0–6.0% 20–42 mmol/mol Hb See p. 808 for diagnosis of diabetes mellitus	–
Immunoglobulins (Ig)		
IgA	0.8–4.5 g/L	–
IgE	0–250 kU/L	–
IgG	6.0–15.0 g/L	–
IgM	0.35–2.90 g/L	–
Lactate	0.6–2.4 mmol/L	5.40–21.6 mg/dL
Lactate dehydrogenase (LDH; total)	125–220 U/L	–
Lead	< 0.5 µmol/L	< 10 µg/dL
Magnesium	0.75–1.0 mmol/L	1.5–2.0 meq/L or 1.82–2.43 mg/dL
Osmolality	280–296 mmol/kg	–
Osmolarity	280–296 mosm/L	–
Phosphate (fasting)	0.8–1.4 mmol/L	2.48–4.34 mg/dL
Protein (total)	60–80 g/L	6–8 g/dL
Triglycerides (fasting)	0.6–1.7 mmol/L	53–150 mg/dL
Troponins	Values consistent with myocardial infarction are crucially dependent upon which troponin is measured (I or T) and on the method employed. Interpret in context of clinical presentation. See p. 535	
Tryptase	0–135 mg/L	–
Urate		
Male	0.12–0.42 mmol/L	2.0–7.0 mg/dL
Female	0.12–0.36 mmol/L	2.0–6.0 mg/dL
Vitamin D, 25(OH)D		
Normal	> 50 nmol/L	> 20 ng/mL
Deficiency	< 14 nmol/L	< 5.6 ng/mL
Inadequate stores	< 25 nmol/L	< 10 ng/mL
Zinc	10–18 µmol/L	65–118 µg/dL

29.5 Common analytes in urine

Analyte	Reference range: SI units	Reference range: Non-SI units
Albumin	Definitions of microalbuminuria are given on p. 476 Proteinuria is defined below	
Calcium (normal diet)	Up to 7.5 mmol/24 hrs	Up to 15 meq/24 hrs or 300 mg/24 hrs
Copper	< 0.6 μmol/24 hrs	< 38 μg/24 hrs
Cortisol	20–180 nmol/24 hrs	7.2–65 μg/24 hrs
Creatinine		
Male	6.3–23 mmol/24 hrs	712–2600 mg/24 hrs
Female	4.1–15 mmol/24 hrs	463–1695 mg/24 hrs
5-hydroxyindole-3-acetic acid (5-HIAA)	10–42 μmol/24 hrs	1.9–8.1 mg/24 hrs
Metadrenalines		
Normetadrenaline	0.4–3.4 μmol/24 hrs	73–620 μg/24 hrs
Metadrenaline	0.3–1.7 μmol/24 hrs	59–335 μg/24 hrs
Oxalate	0.04–0.49 mmol/24 hrs	3.6–44 mg/24 hrs
Phosphate	15–50 mmol/24 hrs	465–1548 mg/24 hrs
Potassium*	25–100 mmol/24 hrs	25–100 meq/24 hrs
Protein	< 0.3 g/L	< 0.03 g/dL
Sodium*	100–200 mmol/24 hrs	100–200 meq/24 hrs
Urate	1.2–3.0 mmol/24 hrs	202–504 mg/24 hrs
Urea	170–600 mmol/24 hrs	10.2–36.0 g/24 hrs
Zinc	3–21 μmol/24 hrs	195–1365 μg/24 hrs

*The urinary output of electrolytes such as sodium and potassium is normally a reflection of dietary intake. This can vary widely. The values quoted are appropriate to a 'Western' diet.

29.6 Analytes in cerebrospinal fluid

Analysis	Reference range: SI units	Reference range: Non-SI units
Cells	$< 5 \times 10^6$ cells/L (all mononuclear)	< 5 cells/mm^3
Glucose[1]	2.3–4.5 mmol/L	41–81 mg/dL
IgG index[2]	< 0.65	–
Total protein	0.14–0.45 g/L	0.014–0.045 g/dL

[1]Interpret in relation to plasma glucose. Values in CSF are typically approximately two-thirds of plasma levels.
[2]A crude index of increase in IgG attributable to intrathecal synthesis.

29.7 Analytes in faeces

Analyte	Reference range: SI units	Reference range: Non-SI units
Calprotectin	< 50 μg/g	–
Elastase	> 200 μg/g	–

29

29.8 Haematological values

Analysis	Reference range: SI units	Reference range: Non-SI units
Bleeding time (Ivy)	< 8 mins	–
Blood volume		
Male	65–85 mL/kg	–
Female	60–80 mL/kg	–
Coagulation screen		
Prothrombin time (PT)	10.5–13.5 secs	–
Activated partial thromboplastin time (APTT)	26–36 secs	–
D-dimers		
Interpret in relation to clinical presentation	< 230 ng/mL	–
Erythrocyte sedimentation rate (ESR)	Higher values in older patients are not necessarily abnormal	
Adult male	0–10 mm/hr	–
Adult female	3–15 mm/hr	–
Ferritin		
Male (and post-menopausal female)	20–300 μg/L	20–300 ng/mL
Female (pre-menopausal)	15–200 μg/L	15–200 ng/mL
Fibrinogen	1.5–4.0 g/L	0.15–0.4 g/dL
Folate		
Serum	2.8–20 μg/L	2.8–20 ng/mL
Red cell	120–500 μg/L	120–500 ng/mL
Haemoglobin		
Male	130–180 g/L	13–18 g/dL
Female	115–165 g/L	11.5–16.5 g/dL
Haptoglobin	0.4–2.4 g/L	0.04–0.24 g/dL
Iron		
Male	14–32 μmol/L	78–178 μg/dL
Female	10–28 μmol/L	56–157 μg/dL
Leucocytes (adults)	$4.0–11.0 \times 10^9$/L	$4.0–11.0 \times 10^3$/mm^3
Differential white cell count		
Neutrophil granulocytes	$2.0–7.5 \times 10^9$/L	$2.0–7.5 \times 10^3$/mm^3
Lymphocytes	$1.5–4.0 \times 10^9$/L	$1.5–4.0 \times 10^3$/mm^3
Monocytes	$0.2–0.8 \times 10^9$/L	$0.2–0.8 \times 10^3$/mm^3
Eosinophil granulocytes	$0.04–0.4 \times 10^9$/L	$0.04–0.4 \times 10^3$/mm^3
Basophil granulocytes	$0.01–0.1 \times 10^9$/L	$0.01–0.1 \times 10^3$/mm^3
Mean cell haemoglobin (MCH)	27–32 pg	–
Mean cell volume (MCV)	78–98 fl	–
Packed cell volume (PCV) or haematocrit		
Male	0.40–0.54	–
Female	0.37–0.47	–
Platelets	$150–350 \times 10^9$/L	$150–350 \times 10^3$/mm^3
Red cell count		
Male	$4.5–6.5 \times 10^{12}$/L	$4.5–6.5 \times 10^6$/mm^3
Female	$3.8–5.8 \times 10^{12}$/L	$3.8–5.8 \times 10^6$/mm^3
Red cell lifespan		
Mean	120 days	–
Half-life (^{51}Cr)	25–35 days	–
Reticulocytes (adults)	$25–85 \times 10^9$/L	$25–85 \times 10^3$/mm^3
Transferrin	2.0–4.0 g/L	0.2–0.4 g/dL
Transferrin saturation		
Male	25–56%	–
Female	14–51%	–
Vitamin B_{12}		
Normal	> 210 ng/L	–
Intermediate	180–200 ng/L	–
Low	< 180 ng/L	–

Index

Page numbers followed by an 'f' indicate index entries that relate to a figure; numbers followed by a 'b' indicate entries that relate to a box.

A

AAA *see* Abdominal aortic aneurysms
Abacavir, 407b
  adverse reactions, 409
  pharmacodynamics, 25b
Abatacept, 1103, 1103b
Abbey pain scale, 285
Abciximab
  myocardial infarction, 594
  platelet inhibition, 594, 997
Abdomen
  examination
    blood disorders, 990f
    cancer, 261b
    cardiovascular disease, 526f
    gastrointestinal disease, 838f
    liver and biliary disease, 923
    renal/urinary tract disease, 462f–463f
  palpation, 839b
  percussion, 839b
  swelling *see* Ascites
Abdominal aortic aneurysms (AAA), 604–605, 605b
Abdominal examination, 839b
Abdominal pain, 285b, 861–863
  acute, 861–863, 861b, 862f
  assessment, 863b
  chronic/recurrent, 863, 863b
  constant, 863
  diabetic ketoacidosis, 812, 812b
  irritable bowel syndrome, 907–908
  liver abscess, 956–957, 970
  lower abdomen, 418
  management, 861–863
  older people, 862b
  pancreatitis
    acute, 890–891
    chronic, 892–893
  peptic ulcer, perforated, 862–863
Abdominal tuberculosis, 691, 888
Abducens (6th cranial) nerve
  damage to, 1171b
  tests, 1139b
Abetalipoproteinaemia, 886, 1199b
Abnormal perception, 234, 1167
ABO blood groups, 1013–1014, 1014b
ABPA *see* Allergic bronchopulmonary aspergillosis
ABPI *see* Ankle:brachial pressure index
Abscess
  anorectal, 919
  cerebral, 1208–1209, 1208f
  collar-stud, 690–691
  definition, 1251b
  infective endocarditis, 625–629
  intra-abdominal, 200b
  liver, 956–957, 970
    amoebic, 368, 957
    pyogenic, 956, 956b
  lung, 109f, 297f
  pancreatic, 297f
  perinephric, 512
  pulmonary, 687
  spinal epidural, 1209
Absence seizures, 1181
Absidia, 384
Absorption, 21–22
  gastrointestinal tract, 21, 841–843
  interactions, 28
  parenteral, 21
  tests, 851b
  topical, 21–22
  see also Malabsorption
ABVD regimen, Hodgkin's disease, 1043
Acamprosate, 254
Acanthocytes, 463b
Acanthosis, 1283
Acanthosis nigricans, 271b, 272, 799b, 1303
Acarbose, 822b, 823
Accessory (11th cranial) nerve, tests, 1139b
Acclimatisation
  to altitude, 107
  to heat, 106
Accommodation, sheltered, 249
ACCORD trial, 827–828
ACD *see* Anaemia, of chronic disease
ACE (angiotensin-converting enzyme), 432
ACE inhibitors
  adverse reactions, 26b, 176b
    angioedema, 93b
    cough, 611–612
    hyperkalaemia, 440
    skin reactions
  aortic regurgitation
  atherosclerosis prevention, 583b
  chronic renal failure, 487–488
  contraindication, cirrhosis, 971b
  diabetic cardiovascular disease, 828
  diabetic nephropathy, 828
  drug interactions, 28b
  effect on renal function, 36b, 502, 522, 522b
  heart failure, 551, 551b
    dosages, 552b
    site of action, 552f
  hypertension, 611, 613b
  microalbuminuria in type 1 diabetes, 831
  mitral regurgitation, 619–620
  myocardial infarction, 599
  pregnancy, 37b
Acetaldehyde metabolism, 957
Acetazolamide, 434–435
  altitude illness, 107
  epilepsy, 1184b
  idiopathic intracranial hypertension, 1218
Acetyl-CoA, 957
Acetylcholine, 841
Acetylcholinesterase (AChE), 1227f
  poisoning, 209b
Acetylcysteine, 212, 709
Achalasia of oesophagus, 868–869, 869f
AChE *see* Acetylcholinesterase
Achilles tendinitis, 1107–1108
Achilles tendon xanthoma, 454f
Achlorhydria, 877f, 882b
Achondroplasia, 58
  inheritance, 59
Aciclovir
  herpesvirus infections, 161–162, 161b, 318b, 326
    bone marrow transplant patients, 1017b
    chickenpox/shingles, 317b
    genital, 424–425
    HIV/AIDS, 397
    oral hairy leukoplakia, 398
    viral encephalitis, 1206
  nephrotoxicity, 522b
  in pregnancy, 154b
Acid-base balance, 443–444, 444f
  critically ill patients, 187
  disorders, 443–447, 660b
    mixed, 447
    presenting problems, 444–447, 445b
  renal control, 444
Acidosis
  lactic, 445
    diabetics, 823
    poisoning, 209b
  metabolic, 445–446, 445b
    acute kidney injury, 482
    chronic renal failure, 485
    critically ill patients, 180f–181f, 187
    diabetic ketoacidosis, 812
    differential diagnosis, 658b
    hypothermia, 104–105
    malaria, 357b
    near-drowning, 108
    poisoning, 209b
  renal tubular, 446, 446b
  respiratory, 445b, 447
Acids, poisoning, 210, 210b
Acinetobacter spp., 136f
Acinus, 646, 647f, 924f
Acitretin
  psoriasis, 1267
  psoriatic arthritis, 1109
Acne, 1281–1283, 1281b, 1281f
  conglobata, 1281–1282
  cystic, 1282f
  excoriée, 1282
  fulminans, 1282
  secondary, 1282
  vulgaris, 1281–1283
Acneiform eruptions, 1304b
Acoustic neuroma, 1215–1216
Acrochordon, 1275
Acrocyanosis, 88b, 1030–1031
Acrodermatitis chronica atrophica, 335
Acrodermatitis enteropathica, 131–132
Acromegaly, 790b, 792–793, 793f
  musculoskeletal manifestations, 1133
ACTH *see* Adrenocorticotrophic hormone
Actin, 48
Actinic dermatitis, chronic, 1261f
Actinic keratosis, 1266, 1271, 1271f
Actinobacillus actinomycetemcomitans, 626
Actinomadura, 382
Actinomyces spp., 137f
Actinomyces israelii, 341
Actinomycetes, 135, 341
Actinomycetoma, 341
Action potential, 1141
Activated partial thromboplastin time (APTT), 999–1000, 1000b
  reference values, 1312b
Activated protein C (APC), 185
Activities of daily living (ADL), 167
  Barthel Index, 177, 177b
Acupuncture, pain management, 288, 288f
Acute abdomen, 861–863, 862f
Acute confusional states, older people, 473b
Acute coronary syndrome, 589–600
  chest pain, 543
  complications, 596–598
  management, 542f
  see also Angina, unstable; Myocardial infarction
Acute intermittent porphyria, 460b
Acute interstitial nephritis (AIN), 502–503, 502b
Acute interstitial pneumonia (AIP), 708b
Acute kidney injury (AKI), 197–198, 197b, 478–483
  causes, 479f
  clinical features, 479–481, 480b–481b
  criteria, 481b
  differential diagnosis, 481b
  interstitial, 502–503, 502b
  investigations, 480b
  malaria, 357b
  management, 482, 482b
  non-oliguric, 502–503
  older people, 483b
  pathophysiology, 479–483
  post-renal, 481
  pre-renal, 479
  pregnancy, 521
  recovery, 483

renal, 479–481
renal replacement therapy, 483, 491
screening tests, 468
Acute limb ischaemia, 603, 603b
Acute lung injury (ALI), 192
Acute mountain sickness (AMS), 107
Acute phase proteins, 82
Acute phase response, 138
ferritin levels in, 1023
musculoskeletal disease, 1092
retroperitoneal fibrosis, 511
rheumatic disease, 1089
Acute Physiology Assessment and Chronic Health Evaluation (APACHE II), 204
Acute renal failure (ARF) *see* Acute kidney injury
Acute respiratory distress syndrome (ARDS), 192, 192b
definition, 193b
drug-induced, 714b
mechanical ventilation, 196b
near-drowning victims, 108
Acute tubular necrosis (ATN), 185
drug-induced, 522b
Adalimumab
inflammatory bowel disease, 903b, 905b
rheumatoid arthritis, 1103b
skin reactions, 1268
Adams-Stokes attacks, 572
Adapalene, 1266
Adaptive immunity, 76–78
ADCC *see* Antibody-dependent cellular cytotoxicity
Addenbrooke's Cognitive Examination-Revised (ACE-R), 234
Addison's disease, 777b
Adefovir, hepatitis B, 953
Adefovir dipivoxil, 161b, 162
Adenine, 42, 43f
Adenocarcinoma
ampullary/periampullary, 895
bronchial, 700b
oesophagus, 870f–871f
pancreatic, 895
prostate, 517
renal, 515–516, 516f
small intestine, 889
of unknown origin, 282
Adenoma
adrenal, 772b
Conn's syndrome, 781f
Cushing's syndrome, 773b, 774
bronchial, 701b, 704b
colorectal, 849b, 910
familial adenomatous polyposis, 911–912
hepatic, 970
parathyroid, 769
periampullary, 888
pituitary, 790b
sebaceum, 1302
small intestine, 888
toxic, thyroid, 754
Adenomatosis of gallbladder, 988
Adenosine, 568, 575b–576b, 576
Adenosine diphosphate *see* ADP
Adenosine monophosphate, cyclic (cAMP), 47f
Adenosine triphosphate *see* ATP
Adenosquamous carcinoma of lung, 704b
Adenoviruses
diarrhoea, 328
respiratory infection, 674b, 688b
ADH *see* Antidiuretic hormone
Adhesion factors, 185
Adhesion molecules, 79
ADHR *see* Autosomal dominant hypophosphataemic rickets
Adipocytes, 802
Adipokines, 115–116, 805
Adiponectin, 115–116, 823
Adjustment disorders, 232, 242
depressive, 235
prevalence, 232b
ADL *see* Activities of daily living
Adolescents
allergy, 93b
congenital heart disease, 635b
cystic fibrosis, 681b
diabetes mellitus, 818, 818b
haematological malignancy, 1035b
infections, 313, 313b
inflammatory bowel disease, 906b
juvenile idiopathic arthritis, 1104b
renal disease, 521, 521b
ADP (adenosine diphosphate), 45f
ADP receptor inhibitors, 1019b
Adrenal crisis, 779b
Adrenal glands, 771–782
diseases
classification, 772b
presenting problems, 773–780
functional anatomy and physiology, 771–773, 771f
incidental mass (incidentaloma), 779–780
older people, 779b
Adrenal hyperplasia, congenital, 763b, 782
Adrenal insufficiency, 777–779, 777b–778b
Adrenal tumours
Cushing's syndrome, 776
see also Phaeochromocytoma
Adrenalectomy, 781
Cushing's syndrome/disease, 776
Adrenaline
anaphylaxis, 91–92, 92b
angioedema, 92b
circulatory effects, 191b
urticaria, 1290
Adrenarche, 773
Adrenocorticotrophic hormone (ACTH)
Cushing's syndrome, 271b
deficiency, hypopituitarism, 777b, 787b
ectopic ACTH syndrome, 776
ectopic production, 271b
excess, 777b–778b
reference values, venous blood, 1309b
stimulation test (tetracosactide test; short Synacthen test), 778b
Adrenoleucodystrophy, 1199b
Adriamycin *see* Doxorubicin
Adult polycystic kidney disease (PKD), 505–507, 506b, 506f
Advance directives, 171, 291
Advanced life support (ALS), 558–559, 559f
Adverse drug reactions, 24–28, 26b
classification, 25–27, 27b
older people, 175–176, 176b
pharmacovigilance, 27–28
prevalence, 24–27
risk factors, 26b
TREND analysis, 27b
see also individual drugs
Aedes spp.
Chikungunya virus, 329
dengue, 322
yellow fever, 323
AEDs (antiepilepsy drugs) *see* Anticonvulsants
AF *see* Atrial fibrillation
Affective (mood) disorders
bipolar, 243–245
organic, 235b
Affinity, 18
Affluence, health consequences, 101–102, 101b
AFP (α-fetoprotein)
hepatocellular carcinoma, 967
as tumour marker, 78, 270b
African tick bite fever, 350, 351b
African trypanosomiasis (sleeping sickness), 309b, 358–360, 359f
Afterload, 183
heart failure, 550–551
reduction, 191
Age/ageing, 165–177
atherosclerosis and, 602b
biological, 167
biology, 168–169
chronological, 167
diabetes and, 806b, 828b
physiological changes, 169–170, 169f
syndrome of premature ageing see Werner's syndrome
see also Older people
Agglutination, cold, 1030–1031
Agglutination test, 142
leishmaniasis, 363–364
leptospirosis, 338
microscopic, 338
sporotrichosis, 383
trypanosomiasis, 359
tularaemia, 340
Aggrecan, 1062–1063
Aggressive behaviour, 237–238, 237f
Agitation, terminal, 290
Agnosia, 1167
Agonists, 18
Agoraphobia, 243
Agranulocytosis, 694b, 749
AHR *see* Airway hyper-reactivity
AIDS *see* HIV infection/AIDS
Aids and appliances, musculoskeletal disease, 1080
AIN *see* Acute interstitial nephritis
AIP *see* Acute interstitial pneumonia
Air travel, 107–108
Airflow obstruction, 653f
assessment in COPD, 675
Airway hyper-reactivity (AHR), 667f
Airways, 646f
asthma, 667f
assessment, 669
defences, 648–649, 648f
maintenance, critically ill patients, 188–189
obstruction, 270b
reactive dysfunction syndrome, 716
sleep apnoea, 726–727
stroke patients, 1243b
upper airway disease, 725–728
Akathisia, 248, 1187–1188
AKI *see* Acute kidney injury
Akinesia, 1196b
Alanine aminotransferase (ALT), 928, 1310b
Albendazole
cysticercosis, 380
helminthic infections, 162, 370–372, 375
filariases, 373
hydatid disease, 381
microsporidiosis, 399b
Albers-Schöberg disease, 1131
Albinism
inheritance, 1295
oculocutaneous, 1295–1296
Albright's hereditary osteodystrophy, 1091b
Albumin, 1011
AKI, 480b
plasma, liver function test, 928
reference values
urine, 1311b
venous blood, 1310b
urinary, 1311b
see also Hypoalbuminaemia
Albumin solutions, 482b
ascites, 940
Albuminuria, diabetes mellitus, 831, 831b
Alcohol, 100
abstinence from, 20b
amount in average drink, 957b
atherosclerotic vascular disease and, 581
cardiomyopathy and
dependence, 252–254, 252b
diabetics, 821
dietary, energy provided by, 110
drug interactions, 28b
heart muscle disease and
liver disease and, 957–959
mortality, 100f
pharmacokinetics and, 24b
poisoning, 209b
thiamin deficiency and, 124–126
see also Ethanol
Alcohol misuse, 100, 100f, 240, 252–254
aetiology, 252–254
diagnosis, 253
effects, 253, 253b
liver disease *see* Alcoholic liver disease
management, 253–254
maternal, 253b
pancreatitis, 892–893
prevalence, 232b
prognosis, 253–254
Alcohol withdrawal, 20b, 253b
management, 253–254
Alcoholic fatty liver disease (AFLD), 931–932
Alcoholic liver disease, 957–959
clinical features, 958, 958b
liver function tests, 930b
older people, 980b
pathophysiology, 957–959, 958b, 958f
Aldosterone, 772
deficiency, 442
plasma potassium and, 435, 439–440
reference range, 1309b
resistance, 442
see also Hyperaldosteronism
Alendronate
dosage regimen, 35b
osteoporosis, 1123, 1123b
Alfacalcidol (1,25-hydroxycholecalciferol), 770–771
Alfentanil, 287
Alginates, 867
Algodystrophy, 1130
ALI *see* Acute lung injury
Alimentary tract, 837–920
see also Gastrointestinal tract
Alkaline phosphatase
liver function test, 928–929
placental, as tumour marker, 268, 270b
reference values, venous blood, 1310b
sclerosing cholangitis, 966
serum
Paget's disease, 1129
rickets/osteomalacia, 1127
Alkalis, poisoning, 210b
Alkalosis, 768b
hypokalemic, Cushing's syndrome
metabolic, 445b, 446–447, 447f
respiratory, 445b, 447
Alkaptonuria, 475b
Alkylating agents, 746
Alleles, 51–53
Allelic heterogeneity, 59
Allergens, 90
asthma, 667f
contact eczema, 1283–1284

Allergic alveolitis, extrinsic *see* Hypersensitivity pneumonitis
Allergic bronchopulmonary aspergillosis (ABPA), 697, 697b
Allergic contact eczema, 1284–1285, 1285f
Allergic rhinitis, 725
Allergy, 89–94, 90b
clinical assessment, 90
food, 888
hygiene hypothesis, 89
investigations, 90
challenge test, 90
patch tests, 1255, 1285
skin prick tests, 90
management, 90–91
pathology, 89
in pregnancy, 94b
presenting problems, 90–93
spiders, 225b
susceptibility to, 89
Allodynia, 1092–1093
fibromyalgia, 1092–1093
Allopurinol
acute leukaemia patients, 1037b, 1038
drug interactions, 28b
gout, 1089
hepatotoxicity, 36b, 971
pharmacodynamics, 25b
renal stone prevention, 509–510, 509b
skin reactions, 1292
Alopecia, 1296b
androgenetic, 1296
drug-induced, 1304b
scarring inflammatory, 1300f
Alopecia areata, 1296–1297, 1297f
nails in, 1297f, 1298
Alpha heavy chain disease, 889
Alpha particles, 102b
Alpha-blockers
benign prostatic hypertrophy, 613b
hypertension, 612, 613b
phaeochromocytoma, 782
α-fetoprotein (AFP)
hepatocellular carcinoma, 967
as tumour marker, 268, 270b
α-glucosidase inhibitors, 822b, 823
α-thalassaemia, 1034–1035
α-tocopherol *see* Vitamin E
α_1-antichymotrypsin, 82
α_1-antitrypsin, 82
faecal clearance, 886
liver disease, 930b
reference values, venous blood, 1310b
α_1-antitrypsin deficiency, 974, 974f
inheritance, 58b
Alport's syndrome, 502, 502f
ALS *see* Advanced life support
ALT *see* Alanine aminotransferase
Alteplase, 595
Alternaria, 671
Alternative medicine, 15
Altitude, effects/illness, 106–108, 106f
Aluminium
osteomalacia, 1126b
poisoning, 223
Aluminium hydroxide
diarrhoea, 884
phosphorus deficiency, 130
renal osteodystrophy, 488
Alveolar macrophages, 385, 711
Alveolar microlithiasis, 715b
Alveolar proteinosis, 715b
Alveolitis, 338, 712
extrinsic *see* Hypersensitivity pneumonitis
fibrosing, 543b, 1070b
cryptogenic *see* Pulmonary fibrosis, idiopathic systemic sclerosis
non-eosinophilic, drug-induced, 714b
Alzheimer's disease, 250b, 251–252, 251f
familial, 251–252
see also Dementia
Amanita phalloides poisoning, 308
Amantadine, 161b, 162
multiple sclerosis, 1192b
Parkinson's disease, 1197
Amastigotes, leishmaniasis, 363f
Amaurosis fugax, 1008
AmBisome, 364
Amelanotic melanoma, 269
Amenorrhoea, secondary, 759–760, 759b
American Psychiatric Association (DSM-IV) (4th ed), 232
American trypanosomiasis (Chagas disease), 309b, 360–361
Amikacin
actinomycetoma, 341
nocardiosis, 341
Amiloride, 435, 940
diabetes insipidus, 795
mineralocorticoid excess, 781
Amino acids, 114b
essential, 114b
metabolism, 926
disorders of, 449
Aminoglycosides, 151b, 156–157
adverse reactions, 157
brucellosis, 333
dosages, 157, 157f
effect of renal insufficiency
mechanism of action, 150b
nephrotoxicity, 36b
pharmacokinetics, 156–157
in pregnancy, 154b
Aminopenicillins, 154b, 155
Aminophylline
asthma, 672, 672f
COPD, 678
Aminosalicylates, inflammatory bowel disease, 860, 903b
Aminotransferases (transaminases), 928
acute liver failure, 934
hypothermia, 104–105
non-alcoholic fatty liver disease, 961
plasma
liver function test, 928
reference range, 1310b
viral hepatitis, 951f
Amiodarone
adverse reactions
hyperpigmentation, 1296b
pulmonary fibrosis, 714
arrhythmias, 575b, 576
atrial fibrillation, 565–566
atrial flutter, 564
tachyarrhythmias, 570
causing thyroid dysfunction, 742–743
heart failure, 553
hepatotoxicity, 971b
structure, 745b
thyrotoxicosis, 742–743, 752
Amitriptyline, 244b
fibromyalgia, 1094
headache, 1176
herpes zoster, 319, 397
irritable bowel syndrome, 909
migraine prevention, 1177
multiple sclerosis, 1192b
musculoskeletal pain, 1072
neuropathic pain, 285b, 288b, 833b
non-ulcer dyspepsia, 877
pain management, 288b
post-herpetic neuralgia, 397
psychiatric disorder, 244b
sphincter of Oddi dysfunction
Amlodipine
angina, 587b
unstable, 594
hypertension, 612
Ammonia, 464
hepatic encephalopathy, 942
Ammonium chloride, 446
Amnesia, 1161–1162
persistent, 1162
post-ictal, 1158b
transient global, 1161–1162
Amniocentesis, 63b
Amodiaquine, malaria, 356
Amoebiasis, 367–368, 368f
incubation period, 145b, 310b
Amoebic liver abscess, 368, 957
Amoeboma, 368, 368f
Amoxicillin, 154b
diphtheria, 346
gonorrhoea, 422b
Helicobacter pylori eradication, 874
listeriosis, 339
Lyme disease, 335
pneumonia, 685b
skin reactions, infectious mononucleosis, 321, 321f
urinary tract infection, 513b
Amphetamines, misuse, 218
Amphotericin/amphotericin B, 160, 160b
aspergillosis, 698–699
blastomycosis, 386
candidiasis, 383
coccidioidomycosis, 386
cryptococcal infections, HIV-related, 403
fusariosis, 384
histoplasmosis, 385–386
leishmaniasis, 364–365, 367
lipid formulations, 160
mucormycosis, 699
mycetoma, 382
nephrotoxicity, 446b, 522b
neutropenic sepsis, 274
P. marneffei infection, 385
sporotrichosis, 383
systemic fungal infections, 698
Ampicillin, 151b, 154b
cerebral abscess, 1208b
drug interactions, 155
enteric fever, 340
infective endocarditis, 628b
listeriosis, 339
liver abscess, 956
meningitis, 1204b
skin reactions, 321, 1304b
infectious mononucleosis, 321, 321f
Ampulla of Vater, carcinoma, 986
AMS *see* Acute mountain sickness
Amsacrine, acute leukaemia, 1037b
Amygdala, 1142–1143
Amylase, 842f, 844b
pancreatic, 112–113
reference values, venous blood, 1310b
salivary, 72
serum
hypothermia, 104–105
pancreatitis, 239b, 891
Amylin, 846b
Amyloid A, serum, 82
Amyloid angiopathy, 250b, 1239b
Amyloid deposition, type 2 diabetes, 806
Amyloid in plaques, Alzheimer's disease, 251–252
Amyloidosis, 86, 86b
heart disease, 86
rheumatoid arthritis, 1099–1100
skin lesions, 1302
Amylose, 112–113
Amyotrophic lateral sclerosis, 1200b–1201b
Amyotrophy
diabetic, 832
neuralgic, 1223b, 1226
ANA *see* Antinuclear antibody
Anabolic steroids, 970
Anaemia(s), 991–992, 1001–1011, 1021–1035, 1021f
after gastric resection, 845–846
ancylostomiasis, 310
aplastic, 1028, 1032, 1048, 1048b
causes, 1001b
of chronic disease (ACD), 1023, 1023b
clinical assessment, 1001–1002
haemolytic, 1026–1031, 1026b, 1027f
alloimmune, 1031
autoimmune, 1029–1031
microangiopathic, 1031
non-immune, 1031
HIV infection/AIDS, 404–405
investigation, 1002, 1002f–1003f
iron deficiency, 1001–1002, 1021–1023
alimentary tract disorders, 867
ancylostomiasis, 310
leucoerythroblastic, 1048–1049
leukaemia patients, 1038
macrocytic, 1002
malaria, 357b
megaloblastic, 1024–1026
microcytic, 1002
normocytic, normochromic, 929
older people, 1034b
pernicious, 1025
refractory, 1041b
renal failure
acute
chronic, 485b, 488
rheumatoid arthritis, 1099–1100
sickle-cell, 1032–1034, 1033f
sideroblastic
signs and symptoms, 991b
Anaesthesia
diabetics, 819f
leprosy, 348
Anagrelide, 1049
Anakinra, 1103, 1103b
Anal canal, 845f
Anal cancer, HIV-related, 405
Anal fissure, 919
Analgesia
bone metastases, 275
cholecystitis, 984
critically ill patients, 202–203
low back pain, 1073
musculoskeletal disorders, 1078–1080
myocardial infarction, 593–594
osteoarthritis, 1085
palliative care, 286–288
pancreatic cancer, 895
pancreatitis, 894
pleural pain, 685
post-herpetic neuralgia, 397
renal colic, 509
Analgesic headache, 1176
Analgesic ladder (WHO), 286–287, 287f
Analgesics
adjuvant, 288, 288b
poisoning, 212–213
see also specific drugs
Anaphylactic shock, 190
urticaria, 1290
Anaphylactoid reactions, 92, 92b
antivenom, 230
Anaphylaxis, 87, 421
causes, 92b
clinical signs, 91–92, 91f
gastrointestinal, 888
horse serum, 346
iatrogenic, 27b, 92b
management, 92, 92b
Anaplasma phagocytophila, 334

ANCAs (antineutrophil cytoplasmic antibodies), 1068, 1118
Ancylostoma caninum, 375–376
Ancylostoma duodenale, 312b, 369, 370f
  life cycle, 370f
Ancylostomiasis (hookworm), 369–370, 370f
Andersen-Tawil syndrome, 1230b
Andersen's disease, 450b
Androgen receptor antagonists, 765b
Androgen replacement therapy, 761b, 763b, 779
  polycystic ovarian syndrome, 764b
Androgens
  adrenal, 773, 778
    excess, 763b
    insufficiency, 778b
  excess, hirsutism, 763b
  exogenous, 763b
  older women, 766b
  tumours secreting, 763–764
Anergy, 86–87
Aneuploidy, 62, 849
Aneurysms
  aortic, 603–605, 604f
    abdominal, 604–605, 605b
    pain, 604
    syphilitic, 604
    thoracic, 604
  saccular (berry), 506, 632
  ventricular, 597–598
  see also Microaneurysms
Angelman's syndrome, 46, 54b, 56b
Angina
  aortic stenosis, 620
  at rest, 596–597
  crescendo, 589
    pain, 540
  decubitus, 540
  nocturnal, 586
  older people, 595b
  pain, 583–584
  post-infarct, 597
  precipitating factors, 584b
  Prinzmetal's, 589
  stable, 583–589
    clinical features, 583–589, 583b
    invasive treatment, 587–589
    investigations, 541–543, 541f
    management, 585, 585b, 586f
    with normal coronary arteries, 589
    prognosis, 589
    risk stratification, 584b
  unstable, 589–600
    clinical features, 583b, 590–593, 590b
    pain, 590
    risk stratification, 591, 591f
    treatment, 594
  variant, 589
  warm-up, 583–584
Angina equivalent, 544
Angiodysplasia, 856
Angioedema, 93, 93f
  ACE-inhibitor associated, 93b
  drug-induced, 1304b
  hereditary, 93b, 93f, 94
  idiopathic, 93b
  laryngeal obstruction, 93
  types of, 93b
  urticaria, 1290
Angiogenesis, 264, 264f–265f
Angiography
  arteriovenous malformation, 1242b
  bronchial artery, 659f
  coronary, 218, 538–539, 538f
  CT, 469, 537, 537f
  digital subtraction, 601–602
  hepatobiliary disease, 931, 967–968
  intra-arterial, 1236f
  magnetic resonance, 946
  mesenteric, 856, 861, 889, 910
  nervous system, 1149, 1149b
  pulmonary, 723
    CT, pulmonary embolism, 651, 722
  renal, 610b
  visceral, 856
Angiomatosis, bacillary, 349, 352b
Angioplasty
  angina, 744–745
  coronary, 587f, 595b, 595f
  renal artery stenosis, 495
  stroke, 1244–1246
Angiosarcoma, 1131b
Angiostrongylus cantonensis, 309b
Angiotensin II, 772
Angiotensin II receptor antagonists
  effect on renal function, 487b
  heart failure, 551–552, 552b
  hypertension, 611–612, 613b
  microalbuminuria in diabetes, 831
  renal failure, 487–488
Angiotensin-converting enzyme *see* ACE
Angiotensin-converting enzyme inhibitors *see* ACE inhibitors
Angular cheilitis, HIV/AIDS, 398
Angular stomatitis, 128, 838f, 899–900
Anhedonia, 234
Anidulafungin, 160b
Anion gap
  acidosis, 445, 445b
  poisoning, 209b
Anismus, 917
Ankle:brachial pressure index (ABPI), 1262
Ankle pain, 1076
Ankylosing spondylitis, 1091b, 1105–1107
  clinical features, 1105, 1105b
  HLA associations, 1105
  inflammatory bowel disease and, 902f
Annulus fibrosus, 529–530
Anogenital warts, 425–426
Anophthalmia, 59
Anorectal disorders, 918–919
Anorectal motility tests, 850
Anorexia
  cancer patients, 271b
  rheumatoid arthritis, 1095
Anorexia nervosa, 255–256, 256b
  osteoporosis, 1121
Anosmia, 759
Anosognosia, 252
ANP *see* Atrial natriuretic peptide
Anserine bursitis, 1076b
Antacids
  bile reflux, 851
  drug interactions, 28
  sodium content, 940b
Antagonists, 18–19
Antalgic gait, 172b
Anterior tibial compartment syndrome, 1135
Anthracyclines, 280b
Anthrax, 309b, 346–347
  bioterrorism, 145
  cutaneous, 346
  gastrointestinal, 346
  immunisation, 149b
  incubation period, 145b, 310b
  inhalational, 347
Anthropometry, 114–115
Anti-androgen therapy, 765b
Anti-anxiety drugs, 241b
Anti-arrhythmic drugs, 573–577
  adverse reactions, 575b, 1005b
  classification, 573–577, 574b
    by site of action, 574f
  dosages, 575b
  principles of use, 575b–576b
  see also individual drugs
Anti-B-cell therapy, 1103b
Anti-cancer drugs *see* Chemotherapy
Anti-CCP antibodies, 239b, 708
Anti-centromere antibodies, 1068b
Anti-comedogenic agents, 1266
Anti-cyclic citrullinated peptide antibodies (ACPA), 1067
Anti-D, 1014
Anti-DNA antibodies, 1067
Anti-epilepsy drugs (AEDs) *see* Anticonvulsants
Anti-herpesvirus agents, 161–162, 161b
Anti-histone antibodies, 1062–1063
Anti-IL1 therapy, 1103b
Anti-IL6 therapy, 1103b
Anti-inflammatory drugs
  asthma, 667–668
  osteoarthritis, 1085
  see also individual drugs
Anti-Jo-1 antibodies, 1068b
Anti-La antibodies, 1068b
Anti-LKM antibodies, 962
Anti-oestrogens, 129–130, 278
Anti-ribonucleoprotein antibody, 1068b
Anti-RNA polymerase, 1068b
Anti-Ro antibody, 1068b
Anti-Smith antibody, 1068b
Anti-smooth muscle antibodies, 962b
Anti-T-cell induction agents, 96b
Anti-thymocyte globulin (ATG), 96b
Anti-TNF therapy
  ankylosing spondylitis, 1107
  inflammatory bowel disease, 903b, 905b
  rheumatoid arthritis, 1102–1103, 1103b
Anti-topoisomerase I antibody, 1068b
Antibiotic therapy
  acne, 1282
  acute leukaemia, 1038
  adverse reactions, 26b
  cerebral abscess, 1208–1209
  cholecystitis, 984
  choledocholithiasis, 985
  cystic fibrosis, 681
  diabetic foot ulcers, 834–835
  diarrhoea associated with, 138b, 308
  gastroenteritis/acute diarrhoea, 307–308
  Helicobacter pylori eradication, 874
  hepatotoxicity, 971b
  infective endocarditis, 628, 628b
  inflammatory bowel disease, 902–905, 903b
  meningitis, 1204b
  osteomyelitis, 1095–1096
  pneumonia
    community-acquired, 685
    hospital-acquired, 686
    suppurative/aspirational, 687
  prophylactic
    infective endocarditis
    pancreatitis, 892
    spontaneous bacterial peritonitis, 941
  respiratory tract infections
    bronchiectasis, 679
    COPD, 677
    cystic fibrosis, 681
    pneumonia *see* pneumonia, above
  sepsis, 201, 201b
  septic arthritis, 1094–1095, 1095b
  skin disorders in systemic sclerosis, 1113
  staphylococcal infections *see individual infections*
  travellers' diarrhoea, 311b
  urinary tract infection, 513b
  vesico-ureteric reflux, 505b
Antibiotics
  adverse reactions, 1005b
  aminoglycosides, 151b, 156–157
  beta-lactam, 154–156, 154b, 155f
  drug interactions, 26b
  folate antagonists, 158
  glycopeptides, 157–158
  ketolides, 156
  lincosamides, 156
  macrolides, 151b, 156
  nitroimidazoles, 158
  prophylactic *see individual conditions*
  quinolones, 157, 157b
  skin reactions, 321, 321f
  sodium content, 940b
Antibody-dependent cellular cytotoxicity (ADCC), 75
Antibody/antibodies, 77b
  deficiencies, 78b, 80–82, 81b, 81f
  detection, 141–142, 141f
  see also Autoantibodies
Anticardiolipin antibodies, 1055, 1242b
Anticholinergics
  adverse reactions, 176b
  bladder dysfunction, 1175b
  COPD, 677–678
  Parkinson's disease, 1197
  poisoning, 213b
Anticholinesterases
  Alzheimer's disease, 251
  myasthenia gravis, 1226–1227
  neurotoxic envenoming, 230
α_1-Antichymotrypsin, 82
Anticoagulants/anticoagulation, 1018–1021
  adverse reactions, 26b
  angina, unstable, 594, 594b
  atrial fibrillation, stroke prevention, 567b
  coagulation screening, 1000b, 1312b
  drug interactions, 1020
  indications, 1018b
  mechanism of action, 1019b
  monitoring, 1000–1001
  myocardial infarction, 594, 594b
  obliterative cardiomyopathy
  older people, 724b
  oral, in renal/hepatic disease, 36b
  poisoning, 224b
  pregnancy, 1022b
  prosthetic heart valves and, 629b
  pulmonary embolism, 723
  risk assessment, 1020b
  rodenticides, 224b
  stroke patients, 1245b
  valvular heart disease, 620b
  venous thromboembolism, 723, 1010–1011
  see also specific anticoagulants
Anticodons, 44–45
Anticonvulsants
  epilepsy, 1183–1184
    choice of drug, 1183b–1184b
    withdrawal, 1184
  pain management, 288b
  poisoning, 224b
  skin reactions, 1304b
  use in pregnancy, 66
Antidepressants, 241b, 244, 244b
  adverse reactions, 176b, 1005b
  alcohol withdrawal, 254
  anxiety disorder, 243
  dosage regimen, 35b
  irritable bowel syndrome, 909
  medically unexplained somatic symptoms, 247b
  older people, 36b, 176b
  poisoning, 213–214
  tricyclic, 241b, 244, 244b
    irritable bowel syndrome, 909
    neuropathic pain, 288b
    poisoning, 209b, 213–214
    sphincter of Oddi dysfunction

Antidiabetic drugs, oral *see* Oral hypoglycaemics
Antidiarrhoeal drugs, 308
  inflammatory bowel disease, 903b
  irritable bowel syndrome, 908f
Antidiuretic hormone (ADH; arginine vasopressin; vasopressin), 432, 438
  diabetes insipidus, 794–795
  ectopic production, 271b
  inappropriate secretion, 438b
    cancer patients, 271b
Antiemetics
  chemotherapy, 277
  myocardial infarction, 546
  palliative care, 290b
  receptor site activity, 290b
  staphylococcal food poisoning, 341
Antifreeze poisoning, 222–223
Antifungal agents, 159–160, 160b, 1267
Antigen processing and presentation, 78
Antiglobulin (Coombs) test, 1030f
Antihistamines, 90, 1267
  allergic rhinitis, 725
  eczema, 1285b
  food allergy, 888
  labyrinthitis, 1186
  pruritus, 1260
  urticaria, 1291
Antihypertensive drugs, 611–612
  adverse reactions, 1005b
  benefit, 610b
  choice, 612
    influence of comorbidity, 613b
  chronic renal failure, 487, 488b
  combinations, 612f
  dosage regimen, 35b
  effect of old age, 36b, 610b
  renal artery stenosis, 495
  stroke prevention, 1246f
Antimalarials, 163, 356–357, 1268
  adverse reactions, 1005b
  poisoning, 215
  prophylactic, 153b
  see also individual drugs
Antimetabolites, 263f
Antimicrobial agents
  combination therapy, 150–151
  development of refined and new agents
  mechanisms of action, 150–154, 150b
  pharmacokinetics/pharmacodynamics, 152–154, 153f
  in pregnancy, 154b
  resistance to, 151–152, 152f
  selection, 151b
  susceptibility testing, 143, 143f
  therapeutic drug monitoring, 154
  see also Antibiotics
Antimicrobial therapy, 151b
  duration of, 152, 153b
  in old age, 154b
  principles, 149–154, 150f
  prophylactic, 152, 153b
  see also Antibiotic therapy
Antimitochondrial antibodies, 962b, 963
Antimonials, leishmaniasis, 364
Antimotility agents, 308
Antineutrophil cytoplasmic antibodies (ANCAs), 520, 1068, 1118
Antinuclear antibody (ANA)
  liver disease, 962b
  musculoskeletal disease, 1067–1068, 1067b
  renal disease, 468
Antioxidants, 82, 648
Antiparasitic agents, 162–164
Antiphospholipid antibodies, 1068
Antiphospholipid (antibody) syndrome, 1055, 1055b
Antiplatelet therapy, 1019b
  angina, 585
    unstable, 594, 594b
  myocardial infarction, 594, 594b
  obliterative cardiomyopathy, 638
  peri-operative, 600
  pre-eclampsia, 521
  stroke prevention, 1245b
Antiproteinases, 648
Antipsychotics (neuroleptics), 241b
  adverse reactions, 26b, 249b
  poisoning, 216
  schizophrenia, 249b
  terminal agitation, 290
Antiretroviral therapy, 161b, 407–410, 407b
  choice of regimen, 407–408
  complications, 408–409
  criteria for starting, 408, 408b
  monitoring efficacy, 408
  pregnancy, 314b
  resistance, 408
  see also individual drugs
Antirheumatic drugs
  rheumatoid arthritis, 1100–1103
  slow-acting (DMARDs) *see* Disease-modifying antirheumatic drugs
Antisecretory agents, 308
Antiseptics, 1266
Antisocial (psychopathic) personality disorder, 255
Antithrombin, 185
  deficiency, 1054
Antithymocyte globulin
  aplastic anaemia, 1048
  graft versus host disease, 1018
Antithyroid drugs
  adverse reactions, 749, 1005b
  Graves' disease, 748b, 749
    in pregnancy, 748b, 749–750
  skin reactions, 749
Antitoxin, diphtheria, 346
Antitrypsin
  liver function tests, 930b
  reference values, venous blood, 1310b
Antituberculous drugs, 693–694
  adverse reactions, 694b
  HIV/AIDS patients, 406–407
Antivenins
  scorpion, 230
  snake, 230
  spider, 230
Antivenom, 230
Antiviral agents, 161, 161b, 1267
  see also Antiretroviral drugs
Anuria, 471–472
Anxiety/anxiety disorders, 242–243
  alcohol and, 253
  classification, 243b
  differential diagnosis, 235b
  generalised, 243
  hyperventilation
  management, 243
  in palliative care patients, 290
  panic disorder, 243
  phobic, 243
  presyncope *see* Presyncope
  prevalence, 232b
  stroke patients, 1243b
  symptoms, 234–235, 235b
Aorta
  ascending
    dilatation, 535f
    syphilis, 420
  coarctation, incidence, 630b
  diseases, 603–607, 604f
Aortic aneurysms, 603–605, 604f
  abdominal, 604–605, 605b
  pain, 604
  syphilitic, 604
  thoracic, 604
Aortic dissection, 604f, 605–607, 605b, 606f
  pain, 541, 606
Aortic regurgitation, 527b, 623–624, 623b, 623f
  clinical features, 623–624, 623b
  investigations, 624, 624b
    chest X-ray, 535f
Aortic stenosis, 527b, 620–623, 621f
  congenital, 620
  Doppler echocardiography, 536f
  heart murmurs, 562b, 621
  incidence, 630b
  investigations, 621, 621b
  older people, 622b
Aortic valve
  balloon valvuloplasty, 621–623
  disease, 620–624
  replacement, 621–624
Aortitis, 604
  syphilis, 604
APACHE II, 204
Apatite crystals, deposition, 1091
APD *see* Automated peritoneal dialysis
APECED *see* Autoimmune polyendocrinopathy-candidiasis-ectodermal dystrophy
Aphasia *see* Dysphasia
Aphonia, 728
Aphthous ulceration, 863–864, 864b
Apixaban, indications, 1018b
Aplasia cutis, 749–750
Aplastic anaemia, 1048, 1048b
  secondary, 1048
Aplastic crisis, 1028, 1032
Apnoea, sleep, 726–727
Apo A1 deficiency, 455–456, 456b
Apo A1 Milano, 455–456, 456b
Apocrine glands, 1254
Apolipoproteins, 450, 451f
Apomorphine, Parkinson's disease, 1197b
Apoptosis, 50, 262
Apoptotic bodies, 50
Appendicitis, acute, 861
Apraxia, 1167
  constructional, 923f
  gait, 172b, 1168
Apronectomy, 120
APS *see* Autoimmune polyendocrine syndromes
APTT *see* Activated partial thromboplastin time
Aquaporins, 48
Ara-C *see* Cytarabine
Arachidonic acid, 138, 667
Arachis oil enemas, 917, 917b
Arachnoiditis, 1073
Arboviruses, 309b, 1205
ARDS *see* Acute respiratory distress syndrome
ARF (acute renal failure) *see* Renal failure, acute
Argentinian haemorrhagic fever, 325b
Arginine, 114b
Arginine vasopressin *see* Antidiuretic hormone
Argyll Robertson pupils, 1172b
Arms, claudication, 602
Aromatase inhibitors
  cancer treatment, 280
  osteoporosis and, 1132b
Arrhythmias, 562–579, 583b
  breathlessness, 544
  during dialysis, 492b
  electrophysiology, 539
  heart failure, 546b, 549
  hypertrophic cardiomyopathy, 637–638
  hypothermia, 104f
  mitral valve prolapse, 618
  myocardial infarction, 596, 596b, 598
  palpitation, 243, 556–557, 556b, 556f
  (pre-)syncope, 555
  sudden death, 557–560, 557b, 583b
  treatment
    drugs, 573–577
    non-drug therapy, 577–579
  see also specific arrhythmias
Arsenic
  hyperpigmentation from, 1296b
  poisoning, 223, 223b
Artemether, malaria, 356
Artemisinin, 163, 354
Arterial blood gases, 653–654, 654f
  analysis, 1308b
  asthma, 671–672
  critically ill patients, 187–188
  pneumonia, 684b
  pulmonary embolism, 721b, 722
  respiratory failure, 192b, 664b
  venous thromboembolism
Arterial disease
  hepatic, 975
  leg ulceration, 1263
  limbs
    lower, 1263
    upper, 602
  peripheral, 600–603, 600b
Arterial gas embolism, 109
Arterial pressure waveform, 187
Arterial pulse
  distinction from venous pulse, 527b
  examination, 527b
Arterialisation, 491
Arteries, great, transposition, 630b, 635b
Arteriography
  coronary, 585
  renal, 470
Arteritis
  giant cell, 1117–1118
  Takayasu's, 1116
Artesunate, malaria, 356
Arthritis
  chronic ('pyrophosphate'), 1086b
  crico-arytenoid, 712b
  crystal-induced, 1086–1092
  drug-induced, 1132b
  enteropathic, 1109
  HIV-related, 404
  juvenile idiopathic, 1103–1104, 1104b
  Lyme disease, 334–336, 1209
  monoarthritis
    acute, 1069, 1069b
    chronic inflammatory, 1068
  mutilans, 1108
  oligoarthritis, 1104, 1104b
  osteoarthritis, 1081–1086
    for detailed entry see Osteoarthritis
  polyarthritis *see* Polyarthritis
  psoriatic, 1104b, 1108–1109, 1109f
    erosions, 1109
  reactive, 1107–1108, 1107b
  rheumatic fever, 615
  rheumatoid, 1096–1103
    for detailed entry see Rheumatoid arthritis
  septic, 1094–1095
    synovial fluid analysis, 1094
  SLE, 1110
  viral, 1095
Arthrodesis, 1080b
Arthropathy
  haemophilic
  psoriasis, 1288
  reactive, sexually acquired, 423
Arthroplasty
  excision, 1080b
  joint replacement, 1080b
Asbestos-related disease, 714b, 717b, 718–719
  diffuse pleural thickening, 718, 718f
  pleural plaques, 714b, 718, 718f
  pleurisy, 718

Asbestosis, 718–719
Ascariasis, 312b
Ascaris lumbricoides (roundworm), 312b, 371, 984
Aschoff nodules, 614
Ascites, 270b, 923b, 938–941
appearance, 939b
Budd-Chiari syndrome, 976
causes, 939–941, 939b, 939f
cirrhosis, 944
heart failure, 549f
oedema, 478
pancreatic, 891, 891b
portal hypertension, 945
renal failure, 940
serum-ascites albumin gradient (SAAG), 939
Ascorbic acid *see* Vitamin C
Ash leaf macules, 1302f
Asherman's syndrome, 759
L-Asparaginase, acute leukaemia, 1037b
Aspartate, 114b
Aspartate aminotransferase (AST), 928
myocardial infarction, 593f
Aspergilloma, 697–698, 698f
Aspergillosis, 383
acute leukaemia patients, 1038
bronchopulmonary, 697–699
allergic, 697, 697b
chronic/subacute, 699
classification, 697b
invasive, 698–699, 698b
chemoprophylaxis, 153b
Aspergillus spp., 78b, 79, 382f
cystic fibrosis, 681
endocarditis, 626
immunocompromised patients, 302
Aspergillus clavatus, 697
Aspergillus flavus, 266b, 697
Aspergillus fumigatus
immunocompromised patient, 688b
respiratory infections, 697, 697f, 719b
Aspergillus niger, 697
Aspergillus terreus, 697
Asphyxia/asphyxiation
laryngeal obstruction, 728, 728b
self-harm, 238–239
Aspiration pneumonia, 687
malaria, 357b
Aspirin
adverse reactions, 26b
angina, 585
unstable, 594b
arthritis, rheumatic fever, 615
asthma association, 667
atherosclerotic vascular disease prevention, 583b
atrial fibrillation, stroke prevention, 567
coronary artery bypass grafting, 588
coronary heart disease, myocardial infarction, 594
dosage regimen, 35b
drug interactions, 28b
hypertension, 613
Kawasaki disease, 1116
microalbuminuria in diabetes, 831b
myeloproliferative disorders, 1049
myocardial infarction, 599
pericarditis, 597
peripheral vascular disease
platelet inhibition, 1050
poisoning, 212–213
pre-eclampsia prevention
rheumatic fever, 615
stroke patients, 1244
AST *see* Aspartate aminotransferase
Asteatotic eczema, 1285
Asterixis (flapping tremor), 923b
Asthma, 666–673
acute severe, 658b, 671b
management, 671–673, 672b, 672f
prognosis, 673
atopic, 669
brittle, 671
clinical features, 667–668
cough-variant, 667
diagnosis, 668–669, 668b–669b
drug-induced, 667–668, 714b
epidemiology, 666–673
exacerbations, 671–673
exercise-induced, 668f
and gastro-oesophageal reflux disease, 866b
investigations, 669
management, 669, 669b, 670f
nocturnal, 667, 669b
occupational, 666–667, 669, 715–716, 715b
management, 669
peak flow readings, 716f
older people, 677b
pathophysiology, 666–667
pregnancy, 671b
prevalence, 666f
respiratory function abnormalities, 653b
Astrocytes, 1140–1141
Astrocytoma, 911–912, 1151f
Astroviruses, 327
Asystole, 558
Ataxia telangiectasia, 267b, 1199b
gene test, 267
Ataxia(s), 1198–1199
acquired, 1199b
cerebellar, 272, 1229b
episodic, 1199b
Friedreich's, 1199b
genetics/inheritance, 56b
hereditary, 1198–1199, 1199b
sensory, 1209b
spinocerebellar, 1199b
stroke, 1237
Ataxic gait, 172b, 1168
Atazanavir, 407b
Atenolol, 575b
angina, 594
drug interactions, 28b
hypertension, 612
Atheroembolic renal disease, 469b, 496
Atheroembolism, 469b, 496f, 602
Atherosclerosis, 452–453, 579–583
chronic renal failure
diabetics, 826–827
heart transplant recipients
older people, 602b
pathophysiology, 579–583
prevention, 581–583, 582b–583b
renal artery stenosis and, 494
risk factors, 581, 582f
stages, 580f
Athetosis, 1166
Athletes, sudden death, 638
Athlete's foot, 1279–1280
Atlantoaxial subluxation, rheumatoid arthritis, 1099
Atmospheric pollution, 102
ATN *see* Acute tubular necrosis
Atomic absorption, 428b
Atopic asthma, 669
Atopic eczema, 1283–1284, 1284f
complications, 1284b
diagnosis, 1284b
management, 1286
pruritus, 1284
rash, 1257b, 1284b
Atopy, 90, 666–667
see also Allergy
Atorvastatin, 598
Atovaquone
malaria, 163, 356
ATP (adenosine triphosphate)
myocardial contraction, 530
serum, bone disease, 1066b
ATP synthase, 46b
Atria, 528, 528f
Atrial ectopic beats, 564, 564f
Atrial fibrillation (AF), 564–567, 565f
causes, 565b
hypertension, 609
lone, 565
management, 565–567
mechanisms, 565f
mitral valve disease, 616
myocardial infarction, 596
older people, 566b
paroxysmal, 565–566
permanent, 566
persistent, 566
pre-excited, 568
stroke risk, 567b
thromboembolism prevention, 566–567
thyrotoxicosis, 742
Wolff-Parkinson-White syndrome, 568–569, 568f
Atrial filling pressure, 182
Atrial flutter, 564, 564f
Atrial myxoma, 639
Atrial natriuretic peptide (ANP), 432
Atrial septal defect, 632–633, 633f
closure devices, 633f
incidence, 630b
Atrial tachyarrhythmias, 564–567
Atrial tachycardia, 564
Atrioventricular (AV) block, 571–573, 571f–572f, 572b
chronic, 573
myocardial infarction, 572–573
Atrioventricular (AV) dissociation, 570f
Atrioventricular (AV) node, 529–530, 529f
re-entry tachycardia, 567–569, 568f
Atrophy, skin, definition, 1251b
Atropine
acute cholinergic syndrome, 221
arrhythmias, 575b, 576–577
AV block, 572
carbamate poisoning, 222
cardiotoxic drug poisoning, 214–215
organophosphorus poisoning, 221
Attributable fraction, 99b
Audit *see* Clinical audit
Auerbach's plexus, 845
Aura, 1158b
migraine, 1156b
seizures/epilepsy, 1158b
Auscultation
heart, 527b
heart murmurs, 560–562, 561b
respiratory disease, 261b, 683
Austin Flint murmur, 623–624
Australian tick typhus, 351b
Autoantibodies, 88
chronic liver disease, 962b
musculoskeletal disease, 1067–1068
primary biliary cirrhosis, 963
thyroid, 741b
Autoimmune disease, 86–88, 87b
classification, 87, 88b
gastritis, 871–872
haemolytic anaemia, 1029–1031
investigations, 88
liver, 961–966
physiology and pathology, 86–87
polyendocrine syndrome, 770
predisposing factors, 87, 87b
pregnancy, 94b, 521
thyroid, 747–751
Autoimmune hepatitis, 962–963, 962b
immunosuppression in, 963b
immunosuppressive therapy, 962–963
liver function tests, 930b
Autoimmune lymphoproliferative syndrome, 80
Autoimmune polyendocrine syndromes (APS), 795–796, 796b
Autoimmune polyendocrinopathy-candidiasis-ectodermal dystrophy (APECED), 796, 796b
Automated peritoneal dialysis (APD), 492
Autonomic dysfunction, somatoform, 232b, 246
Autonomic nervous system, 844–845, 1144
diabetics, 832, 832b–833b
tests of cardiovascular autonomic function, 833b
Autonomy, respect for, 10–11
Autophagy, 46–47, 262
Autosomal dominant hypophosphataemic rickets (ADHR), 1126b
Autosomal dominant inheritance, 51–53
Autosomal dominant polycystic kidney disease (PKD), 62b
Autosomal recessive inheritance, 53
Autosomes, 42
AV *see* Atrioventricular
Avian influenza, 320
Axial spondyloarthritis, 1106b
Axons
neuropathy, 1224
peripheral nerve, 1140–1141
Azapropazone, 1079b
Azathioprine, 96b, 1268
adverse reactions, 1268
autoimmune haemolysis, 1030
autoimmune hepatitis, 962–963
biliary cirrhosis, 964
drug interactions, 28b
eczema, 1286
hepatotoxicity, 971b
inflammatory bowel disease, 903b
interstitial lung disease, 709
myasthenia gravis, 1227b
myositis, 1115
organ transplant patients, 96b, 553
rheumatic disease, 1101b
SLE, 1112
Azelaic acid, 1266, 1283
Azithromycin, 151b
bacillary angiomatosis, HIV/AIDS patients, 398
cystic fibrosis, 681b
enteric fever, 340
Mycobacterium avium complex, 407
STIs
chlamydial infection, 353, 423b
syphilis, 421
trachoma, 353
Azoles, 159–160
Aztreonam, 151b, 154b, 155f

B

B lymphocytes (B cells), 77
combined B/T lymphocyte deficiencies, 80, 81f
gastrointestinal system, 843–844
leukaemia
chronic lymphocytic, 1040
hairy cell, 1041
lymphoma, 879–880, 1272
and primary antibody deficiencies, 81f
Babesia microti, 304b
Babesiosis, 309b, 358

Bacillary angiomatosis, 349, 352b
Bacillary dysentery, 345
Bacille Calmette-Guérin *see* BCG
Bacillus spp., 136f
Bacillus anthracis, 346
Bacillus cereus, food poisoning, 306, 341, 341f
Back, examination, cardiovascular disease, 526f
Back pain, 1072–1073
 ankylosing spondylitis, 1105
 prevalence, 1060b
 red flags, 1073b
 triage, 1072f
 see also Low back pain
Baclofen, multiple sclerosis, 1192b
Bactec system, tuberculosis diagnosis, 693
Bacteraemia, 303
 definition, 184b
 homeless people, 352
Bacteria, 135, 136f
 endogenous commensal, 72
 identification, 136b
 toxins, diseases caused by, 138b, 1209–1211
Bacterial infections, 329–353
 and cancer, 266b
 gastrointestinal, 341–345
 HIV/AIDS patients, 398–399, 400b, 401
 immune deficiency and, 78b
 nervous system, 347, 1202–1204, 1202b
 respiratory, 345–347
 sexually transmitted, 419–423
 skin, soft tissue and bone, 329–333, 1275–1278
 systemic, 333–341
 see also specific infections
Bacteriophages, 134–135
Bacteriuria
 asymptomatic, 513
 catheter-related, 513
 treatment in pregnancy, 520b
Bacteroides spp., 136f–137f, 151b
Bacteroides fragilis, 687
Bacteroides melaninogenicus, 687
Bad news, giving, 4
Baker's (popliteal) cyst, 1076b, 1098
 rupture, 1098
Balance
 disorders of, 1167–1168
 see also Dizziness; Vertigo
Balanitis, 415
 anaerobic, 416b
 circinate, 416b, 1108
 plasma cell (of Zoon), 416b
Balanoposthitis, 415
Balkan nephropathy, 503–504
Ballism, 1166
Balloon dilatation, 510–511, 587f
Balloon tamponade, variceal bleeding, 928, 947f
Balloon valvuloplasty
 aortic valve, 621–623
 mitral valve, 618, 618b
Balsalazide, 903b
Balsam of Peru, 1285b
Bamboo spine, 1105–1106, 1107f
Bambuterol, COPD, 675
Bandages, compression, leg ulcers, 1263
Banding, variceal bleeding, 928
Barbiturates, 217b
 misuse, 254
 skin reactions, 1304b
 withdrawal symptoms, 20b
Bardet-Biedl syndrome, 49
Bare lymphocyte syndrome, 80
Bariatric surgery, 119–120, 119b, 120f
Baritosis, 718
Barium studies
 constipation, 861
 diverticulosis, 916
 gastrointestinal disease, 847b
 gastrointestinal tuberculosis, 691
 inflammatory bowel disease, 901–902
 oesophageal disorders, 705b, 850, 869f
 pharyngeal pouch, 868
Barotrauma, 109
Barrett's (columnar lined) oesophagus, 866–867
 carcinoma and, 866–867
Barthel Index of Activities of Daily Living, 177, 177b
Bartonella henselae, 352, 398
Bartonella quintana, 352, 398
Bartonellosis, 352–353, 352b
Bartter's syndrome, 441, 510
Basal cell carcinoma, 1270–1271, 1270b, 1270f
Basal cell papilloma, 1274, 1274f
Basal ganglia, 1143
Basal metabolic rate (BMR), 110, 111f
 in overnutrition, 112
Basement membrane, skin, 1252, 1253f
Basic calcium phosphate (BCP) crystal deposition, 1091–1092, 1091b
Basic life support (BLS), 558, 558f
Basophilia, 1004b
Basophilic stippling, 999f
Basophils, 75, 995, 1004f
 count, 1312b
Bath Ankylosing Spondylitis Disease Activity Index, 1105, 1106b
Batten's disease, 46–47
Battery acid poisoning, 868
Bayes' theorem, 6b
BCG (bacille Calmette-Guérin)
 intravesical, bladder cancer, 517
 leprosy, 350
 tuberculosis, 696
BCP *see* Basic calcium phosphate
BCR *see* Breakpoint cluster region
Beau's lines, 1298, 1298f
Becker muscular dystrophy, 1228b
Becker's disease, 1230b
Beckwith-Wiederman syndrome, 54b
Beclometasone, 21–22, 670f
Behaviour
 assessment in psychiatric disorders, 233
 disturbed and aggressive, 237–238, 237f
  older people, 238b
Behaviour therapy, 241
Behavioural rating scale for pain, 285
Behçet's syndrome, 1119, 1119b
Beighton score, modified, 1134b
Bejel, 333, 333b
Beliefs, abnormal, 234
Bell's palsy, 1163
Bence Jones protein, 477–478
Bence Jones proteinuria, 477–478, 1046
Bendroflumethiazide, 795
Beneficence, 11
Benign paroxysmal positional vertigo, 1186, 1186f
Benign prostatic hyperplasia (BPH), 472, 514–515
 incontinence and, 473
Benserazide, 1196
Benzamides, substituted, 249b
Benzathine penicillin
 prophylactic, 615–616
 syphilis, 421
Benzbromarone, 1071
Benzene, 266b, 1035b
Benzisoxazole, 249b
Benznidazole, trypanosomiasis, 163, 360–361
Benzocaine, allergy, 1285b
Benzodiazepines, 241b
 adverse reactions, 26b, 176b
 alcohol withdrawal, 253–254
 anxiety disorder, 241b, 243
 delirium, 174–175
 drug interactions, 28b
 misuse, 217
 overdose, 217
 palliative care, 289
 respiratory depression, 237–238
 stress reactions, 242
 terminal agitation, 677
 withdrawal symptoms, 20b, 254b
Benzoyl peroxide, 1266
Benzylpenicillin, 154b, 155f
 anthrax, 347
 cerebral abscess, 1208b
 infective endocarditis, 628, 628b
 meningitis, 1204b
 neurosyphilis, 1209
 procaine *see* Procaine penicillin
 rheumatic fever, 615
 soft tissue infections, 1267
 streptococcal infection, 331
 tetanus, 1210b
Bereavement, 233
Beri-beri, 128
Bernard-Soulier syndrome, 1050
Bernoulli equation, modified, 536–537
Berry aneurysms, 506, 632
Berylliosis, 717, 717b
Beta particles, 102–103, 102b
Beta-adrenoceptor agonists, 241b
 anaphylaxis, 92b
 asthma, 669–671
 COPD, 675
Beta-blockers (beta-adrenoceptor antagonists)
 adverse reactions, 26b, 176b
 angina, 586
  unstable, 594
 anxiety disorders, 243
 arrhythmias, 574–576
  atrial fibrillation, 565–566
  atrial flutter, 564
  tachyarrhythmias, 570
  ventricular tachycardia, 570
 asthma association, 667–668
 atherosclerosis prevention, 583
 cardiomyopathy, 638
 essential tremor, 1199
 heart failure, 552, 552b
  site of action, 552f
 hypertension, 612, 613b
 Marfan's syndrome, 604
 mitral stenosis, 618
 myocardial infarction, 599, 599b
 phaeochromocytoma, 782
 poisoning, 214
 skin reactions, 1304b
 thyrotoxicosis, 741–742
 variceal bleeding, 946
β-carotene, porphyria management, 460
Beta-lactam antibiotics, 154–156, 154b, 155f
 adverse reactions, 154–155
 drug interactions, 155
 mechanism of action, 150b
 pharmacokinetics, 154–155
β-oxidation, 971
β-thalassaemia, 1034, 1034b
Betamethasone, 1265b
Bevacizumab, 279
Bezold-Jarisch reflex, 555–556
Bi-level positive airway pressure (BIPAP), 194, 195f
Bicarbonate
 acid-base balance, 187
 acid-base disorders, 430b, 660b
  diabetic ketoacidosis, 814
 arterial blood, 1308b
 see also Sodium bicarbonate
Biguanides, 216, 821–823
Bile, 927
 lithogenic, 982b
 reflux, 875
Bile acid sequestering resins, 434
Bile acid tests, 851b
Bile ducts
 dilatation, 360
 flukes, 378
 stones, 983b
  pancreatitis, 890
 vanishing bile duct syndrome
Bile salts, 842f
 malabsorption, 884
Bilevel positive airway pressure *see* BIPAP
Bilharziasis *see* Schistosomiasis
Biliary cirrhosis
 investigations, 964
 primary, 963–965, 963f
  AMA-negative, 964–965
  liver function tests, 930b
  older people, 980b
  overlap syndromes, 964–965
 secondary, 981
Biliary colic, 982
Biliary disease, 980–988
 autoimmune, 961–966
 clinical examination, 922f
 extrahepatic, 981
 intrahepatic, 980–981
 investigation, 928–932
 see also Liver disease
Biliary sludge, 982
Biliary system, functional anatomy, 926
Biliary tract diseases, HIV-related, 400
Biliary transport proteins, 927f
Bilirubin
 alcoholic liver disease, 959
 excretion, 927f
 liver function test, 928
 metabolism, 927
 plasma
  acute liver failure, 934b
  jaundice, 936
 reference values, venous blood, 1310b
 viral hepatitis, 948–949
 see also Hyperbilirubinemia
Bilirubinuria, 475b
Bioavailability, 21
Biochemical investigations, 428–429, 428b
 bone disease, 1066–1067
 liver disease, 928–929
Biochemical markers
 cancer, 269, 270b
 myocardial damage, 593, 593f
Biofeedback, faecal incontinence, 918
Biological therapies, 15
 cancer, 278–279
 psoriasis, 1289b
 psychiatric disorders, 240–241
 rheumatoid arthritis, 1102–1103
 skin disease, 1268
Biomarkers
 cardiac, 593, 593f
 tumours, 269, 270b
Biopsy
 bone, 1068, 1127
 bone marrow, 1000f
 brain, 1155
 cancer diagnosis, 276
 gastrointestinal tract, 850b
  inflammatory bowel disease, 900
  small bowel biopsy, coeliac disease, 881
 kidney, 471, 471b, 503f
 liver, 931–932, 931b, 961
 lung
  bronchial carcinoma, 702
  interstitial disease, 706–707

lymph node, 1042f
muscle, 1068, 1115f, 1154
neurological disease, 1154–1155
pleural, 661
tuberculosis, 401
prostate, 518
pyrexia of unknown origin, 299b
sentinel lymph node, 1274
skin, 1255, 1268
synovial, 1068
temporal artery, 1068
transbronchial, 688
trephine, 1000f
Bioterrorism, 145
Biotin, 129
deficiency, 129
dietary sources, 125b
RNI, 125b
BIPAP/BiPAP *see* Bi-level positive airway pressure
Biphosphonates *see* Bisphosphonates
Bipolar disorder, 243–245
Birch oral allergy syndrome, 94
Bird fancier's lung, 719b
Bisacodyl, 917b
Bismuth, 308, 874
Bisoprolol, 575b
angina, 586
arrhythmias, 576
hypertension, 612
Bisphosphonates
adverse reactions, 1124b
biliary cirrhosis, 964
bone metastases, 275, 275b
hypercalcaemia, 273, 769–770
multiple myeloma, 1047
osteomalacia and, 1126b
osteoporosis, 1123–1124
Paget's disease, 1129
Bites
snake, 225b
spider, 225b
Bithionol, 162
Bitot's spots, 127
Black urine, 1026–1027
Blackheads *see* Comedones
Blackouts, 1157–1159, 1158f
alcoholic, 253
older people, 172
Blackwater fever, 356f, 1031
Bladder, 466
atonic, 1175b
dysfunction, 1174
flaccid, 1174
hypertonic, 1175b
incomplete emptying, 514–515
multiple sclerosis, 1192
overactive (spastic), 1174
stones, 507
tumours, 516–517, 517f
incidence, 262f
ultrasound, 468–469
Bladder neck
dyssynergia, 1174
obstruction, 377, 472
incontinence and, 473
Blalock-Taussig shunt, 635
Blast cells, 992f
Blast crisis, 1039–1040
Blastomyces dermatitidis, 386
Blastomycosis, 386
Blatchford score, 854b
Bleach, poisoning, 224b
Bleeding, 991–992, 1006–1007
chronic renal failure, 485
examination/investigation, 991b
gastrointestinal, 853–857
endoscopic therapy, 852b, 855
iron deficiency, 1021–1023
NSAIDs and, 1021–1022
spontaneous, malaria, 357b
variceal see Variceal bleeding
see also Haemorrhage
Bleeding disorders, 1049–1054
acquired, 1054
congenital, 1054
investigation, 999–1000
Bleeding time, 1000, 1312b
Bleomycin
Hodgkin's disease, 1043
hyperpigmentation from, 1296b
Blind loop syndrome, 882–883, 882b
Blindness
leprosy, 348–349
night, 127
river blindness, 374–375
vitamin A deficiency
see also Vision, loss
Blistering, 1301
Blisters, 1258, 1258b
at birth, 1291–1292
definition, 1251b
Blocks and gaps, 11
Blood, 992–997
arterial
analysis, 1308b
asthma, 671–672
respiratory failure, 664b
venous thromboembolism
components, 1012b
culture, 140f, 141, 303–304, 303b
donation/processing/storage, 1011–1012, 1013f
oxygenation, 182–183
Blood cells, 994–996
formation, 992–994, 992f–993f
see also Platelets; Red cells; White cells
Blood count, 998, 998b
AKI, 480b
gastrointestinal bleeding, 855
hepatobiliary disease, 929
multiple myeloma, 1047b
musculoskeletal disease, 1066
pregnancy, 1022b
see also Platelets; Red cells; White cells
Blood diseases/disorders, 989–1056
clinical examination, 990f, 991b
genetic, 995, 1051
HIV infection/AIDS, 404–405
investigation, 998–1001
malignancies, 1035–1048
older people, 1047b
presenting problems, 1001–1011
pruritus, 1259b
rheumatoid arthritis, 1099–1100
SLE, 1111
see also individual disorders
Blood film examination, 998, 999b, 999f
Blood flow
cardiovascular system, 528f, 530–531
Doppler echocardiography, 536–537, 536f
resistance to, 530
liver, 924f, 925–926
Blood gases *see* Arterial blood gases
Blood group antigens, 994, 1013
Blood groups
ABO, 1013–1014, 1014b
rhesus D, 1014, 1014b
Blood pool imaging, ventricular function assessment, 539
Blood pressure
cardiovascular disease and chronic renal failure, 488b
control
chronic renal failure
diabetes, 811
critically ill patients, 185
endocrine disease, 734f
measurement, 608, 608b
ambulatory, 608
home, 608
respiration effects, 532b
stroke patients, 1243b
target levels, 611b
see also Hypertension
Blood products, 1011–1012, 1012b
virus transmission
Blood tests, 1006, 1153, 1312b
abdominal pain, 861
diabetes mellitus, 807–808
gastrointestinal haemorrhage, 855
hepatobiliary disease, 929
inflammatory bowel disease, 901
malabsorption, 858
musculoskeletal disease, 1066–1068
neurological disease, 1153
older people, 1001b
pneumonia, 579
renal disease, 468
stroke, 1236
see also Haematological values
Blood transfusion
adverse reactions, 1012–1015
acute reactions, 1016f
infection transmission, 1014–1015
bedside procedures, 1015, 1015f
exchange
malaria, 357
megaloblastic anaemia, 1026
sickle-cell disease, 1033
gastrointestinal haemorrhage
haemolytic anaemia, 1026–1027
hereditary spherocytosis, 1028
immunological complications, 1014
see also Blood groups
Jehovah's Witnesses, 11
megaloblastic anaemia, 1026
pre-transfusion testing/ cross-matching, 1015
red cell incompatibility, 1012–1014
safe procedures, 1015
sickle-cell disease, 1033
Blood vessels
effects of hypertension, 608
imaging
cerebrovascular disease, 1149–1150, 1235–1236
nervous disease, 1235–1236
see also Vascular
Blood volume, reference values, 1312b
Blood-brain barrier, 1140–1141
Blood-stream infection, 300, 303
see also Bacteraemia
Bloom's syndrome, 267b
BLS *see* Basic life support
'Blue bloaters', 674–675
Blue finger syndrome, 602
Blue naevus, 1275
BMD *see* Bone mineral density
BMI *see* Body mass index
BMR *see* Basal metabolic rate
BNP *see* Brain natriuretic peptide
Bocavirus, 328
Boceprevir, 161b, 162, 955
Body dysmorphic disorder, 246
Body lice, 1281
Body mass index (BMI), 114–115
and cardiovascular disease risk, 116f
and diabetes risk, 116f
and obesity, 117, 117b
older people, 166f
and pancreatitis, 890b
undernutrition, 120b
Body packers/stuffers, 219, 219f
Body weight, pharmacokinetics and, 24b
Body-based therapy, 15
Boerhaave's syndrome, 871
Bohr effect, 183
Boils, 809
Bolam test, 14
Bolivian haemorrhagic fever, 325b
Bone
age-related changes, 1121f
anatomy, 1060–1064
biopsy, 1068, 1127
cortical, 1060f
erosion, 1097f
fractures *see* Fractures
infection, 1094–1096
older people, 1094b
loss of mass, 1121f
see also Osteopenia
matrix, 1062
mineralisation, 1062
in osteoarthritis, 1081–1086
pain, 270b
remodelling, 1061f, 1062, 1062b
resorption, 1061, 1061f
primary biliary cirrhosis, 963
trabecular (cancellous), 1060f
woven, 1062
Bone age, 758
Bone densitometry
indications for, 1122b
osteoporosis, 1122b
Bone diseases, 1120–1131
biochemical abnormalities, 1066b
diabetes, 833–834
metabolic
after gastric resection, 875
chronic renal failure, 486–488
coeliac disease, 881
inflammatory bowel disease, 907
metastatic, 275
radionuclide scan, 275, 1065
scintigraphy, 1065
tuberculosis, 691–692
tumours
metastatic, 275, 275b, 1132
primary, 1131–1132, 1131b
see also individual conditions
Bone marrow
aplastic anaemia, 1048
biopsy, 1000f
pyrexia of unknown origin, 298–299
examination, 998
fibrosis, 998
leukaemia, 1040
myelodysplastic syndrome, 1041
myelofibrosis, 1048
structure and function, 992f
tumours, 1131b
Bone marrow transplantation *see* Haematopoietic stem cell transplantation
Bone mineral density (BMD), 1065–1066
hyperparathyroidism, 769
measurements, 760
osteoporosis, 1122b
secondary amenorrhoea, 760
Bone pain, 285b
BOOP *see* Bronchiolitis obliterans organising pneumonia
Bordetella pertussis infection, 682
Bornholm's disease, 541
Borrelia spp., 335b
infections, 334–336
relapsing fever, 336
Borrelia afzelii, 334, 335b
Borrelia burgdorferi, 334, 335b, 1303
Borrelia garinii, 334, 335b
Bortezomib, 1047
Bosentan, 1113
Botfly, 313f
Botulinum toxin, 1210
achalasia, 869
anal fissure, 919
biliary sphincter dysfunction, 900
dystonia, 1200
hemifacial spasm, 1200
Botulism, 138b, 1210–1211, 1211b
wound, 1210
Bouchard's nodes, 1058f, 1069b, 1082–1083
Bouginage, 848f, 867
Boutonneuse fever, 350, 351b

Boutonnière deformity of fingers, 1098
Bovine serum albumin (BSA), 804
Bovine spongiform encephalopathy (BSE), 1015
Bowel
  disturbance, 1174–1175
  whole bowel irrigation, 210, 210b
  see also Colon; Small intestine
Bowen's disease, 1270b, 1272, 1272f
BPH *see* Benign prostatic hyperplasia
Brachial plexopathy, 1225–1226
Brachial plexus lesions, 1225–1226, 1225b
Brachytherapy, 277–278
Bradford Hill criteria, 99
Bradycardia
  sinus, 563, 563b
    myocardial infarction, 596
Bradykinesia, 1145
  Parkinson's disease, 1163
Brain
  arterial circulation, 1234f
  biopsy, 1155
  cerebral hemispheres, 1142–1143
  effects of alcohol, 253
  imaging, 1149–1150, 1150f
    epilepsy, 1155
    stroke, 1235–1236, 1235f–1236f, 1241–1242
  ischaemia, 199b, 572, 1046f
  schizophrenia, 247–249
  structure and function, psychiatric disorders, 233
  tumours, 1213–1216, 1213b, 1214f
    dementia, 250b
    incidence, 262f
    metastatic, 274, 274b
  venous circulation, 1235f
  see also specific regions, and entries under cerebral
Brain death, 1160b, 1161
Brain injury, 1218
Brain natriuretic peptide (BNP), 432, 535
  heart failure, 549
Brainstem, 1143–1144, 1143f
  death, 203
  encephalitis, 1206
  lesions, 1148, 1148b, 1165
Breakpoint cluster region (BCR)
  abl oncogene, 1039
  Philadelphia chromosome, 1039
Breast cancer, 279–280
  clinical features, 280
  epidemiology, 267b
  familial, 67
  incidence, 262f
  investigations, 280
  older people, 271b
  pathogenesis, 279–280
  screening, 271b, 279, 762–763, 912
  sites of metastasis, 280
  staging, 279b
  survival rates, 279b
  treatment, 280, 280b
    hormonal, 280
    local disease, 280
    metastatic disease, 280
    post-operative, 280
Breastfeeding
  drugs and, 36–37, 37b
  HIV/AIDS patients, 409–410
Breath tests, gastroenterology, 850
Breathing
  control of, 647–648
  divers, 109
  ketoacidosis, 812, 812b
  management, critically ill patients, 188–189
  rescue (mouth-to-mouth), 558
  sleep-disordered, 725–727
  stroke patients, 1243b
  see also Respiration
Breathlessness (dyspnoea)
  acute, 656b
    at rest, 655
    severe, 657
  bronchial carcinoma, 701
  causes, 543b, 656b
  and chest pain, 543–544, 657
  chronic exertional, 655–657, 656b
  COPD, 655
  differential diagnosis, 655, 658b
  heart disease, valvular, 616
  modified MRC scale, 674b
  palliative care, 289, 289b
  paroxysmal nocturnal, 544
  pathophysiology, 655, 656f
  psychogenic, 657b–658b
  respiratory disease, 655–657
Briquet's syndrome, 236b, 245
British National Formulary, 33
Broca's aphasia, 1169f
Broca's area, 1146
Bromocriptine
  neuroleptic malignant syndrome, 249
  Parkinson's disease, 1197b
  pituitary adenoma, 1214
  prolactinoma, 791b, 792
Bronchi
  obstruction, 704–705
    clinical and radiological manifestations, 650
  see also Bronchial carcinoma
Bronchial artery, 647f
  angiography, 659f
  embolisation, 698
Bronchial carcinoma, 699–704
  cell types, 700b
  clinical features, 700–702, 700f, 701b
  extrapulmonary manifestations, 702b
  investigations, 702–703, 703f
  large-cell, 700b
  management, 703–704
  metastases, 701
  pathology, 699–700
  prognosis, 704
  radiological presentations, 702–703, 702b, 702f
  small-cell, 700b
    management, 704
  squamous cell, 703f
  staging, 702–703
Bronchial gland
  adenoma, 704b
  carcinoma, 704b
Bronchiectasis, 678–679, 679f
  aspergillosis, 697
  causes, 678b
  connective tissue disorders, 712
  cystic fibrosis, 680–681
  symptoms, 679b
Bronchiolitis, 328
  obliterative, 666
    connective tissue disorders, 712
  respiratory bronchiolitis-interstitial lung disease (RB-ILD), 708b
Bronchiolitis obliterans organising pneumonia (BOOP), 708b
Bronchitis
  acute, 654b, 659b
  chronic, 653b, 673
    see also Chronic obstructive pulmonary disease
  connective tissue disorders, 712
  respiratory function abnormalities, 653b
Bronchoalveolar carcinoma, 704b
Bronchoalveolar lavage, 711
Bronchoconstriction, 677b
Bronchodilator therapy
  asthma, 669–672
  COPD, 675–676
Bronchopleural fistula, 728–729
Bronchopneumonia, 682
Bronchopulmonary segments, 646f
Bronchoscopy, 651–652
  bronchial carcinoma, 702
  cough, 655
  haemoptysis, 659
  interstitial lung disease, 708
  management of ventilated/intubated patient
  mediastinal tumours, 706
Bronchospasm, pain, 541
Bronzed diabetes, 972
Brown-Séquard syndrome, 1165, 1221
Bruce protocol for exercise tolerance testing, 534b
Brucella abortus, 333
Brucella canis, 333
Brucella melitensis, 333
Brucella suis, 333
Brucellosis, 309b, 333–334, 334f
  incubation period, 145b, 310b
  in pregnancy, 314b
  treatment, 334b
Brudzinski's sign, 1201
Brugada syndrome, 571
Brugia malayi, 312b, 372b, 372f, 713
Bruise, definition, 1251b
BSA *see* Bovine serum albumin
BSE *see* Bovine spongiform encephalopathy
Bubonic plague, 338
Buccal administration, 21
Budd-Chiari syndrome, 933–934, 976
Budesonide (BUD), 903b
Buerger's disease, 603–605
Buerger's sign, 601b
Bulbar palsy, 1174, 1174b
  motor neuron disease, 1174, 1200b
Bulimia nervosa, 256, 256b
Bullae
  definition, 1251b
  pulmonary, 650b, 674
Bullous impetigo, 1258b, 1276
Bullous pemphigoid, 1292–1293, 1293b, 1294f
Bumetanide
  hypertension, 611
  oedema, 478
Bundle branch blocks, 573, 573b
  left, 573f
  right, 573f
Bundle of His, 529–530, 529f
Bupropion, 101b, 213b
Burkholderia cenocepacia, 79
Burkholderia pseudomallei, 304b, 309b, 340, 682–683
Burkitt's lymphoma, 266b, 320
Burns
  haemolysis and, 1031
  sunburn, 1260f
Burrow, definition, 1251b
Bursae, 1063
Bursitis
  hip, 1075b, 1075f
  illopectineal, 1075b
  ischiogluteal, 1075b
  knee, 1076b
  olecranon, 1075b, 1099f
  subacromial, 1074b
  subcalcaneal, 1076
  trochanteric, 1075b, 1075f
Buruli ulcer, 333
Buschke-Loewenstein tumour, 425
Buspirone, 213b
Busulfan (busulphan)
  hepatotoxicity, 971b
  hyperpigmentation from, 1296b
Butterfly (malar) rash, 1110f
Button hole deformity of fingers, 1098
Butyrophenones, 241b
  schizophrenia, 249b
Byssinosis, 716, 719b

C

C-peptide, 783–784, 783f
C-reactive protein (CRP), 72, 84–85, 84b
  AKI, 480b
  pancreatitis, 892
  reference values, venous blood, 1310b
C1 inhibitor deficiency (hereditary angioedema), 94
  acquired, 94
C4d staining, 95
Cabergoline
  nephrotoxicity, 522b
  Parkinson's disease, 1197b
  pituitary tumours, 1214
  prolactinoma, 791b
CABG *see* Coronary artery bypass grafting
Cachexia, 124
  cancer, 122f, 290
  cardiac, 549
  neuropathic, 832
CADASIL, 1176–1177
Cadherin-1, 265
Cadmium
  lung disease and, 716
  poisoning, 308
Caecum, carcinoma, 913–914
Caeruloplasmin, 1310b
  Wilson's disease, 974
Café au lait macules, 1216f
Caffeine, 129
cagA *see* Cytotoxin-associated gene
Calabar swelling, 373
Calcific periarthritis, 1091–1092, 1091b, 1091f
Calcification
  arterial, 537, 602b
  ectopic, 486–487
  metastatic, 449
  musculoskeletal disease, 1064
  renal, 507f
Calcimimetics, 488
Calcineurin inhibitors, 96b, 1266
Calcinosis
  CREST syndrome, 1091b, 1112, 1113f
  nephrocalcinosis, 507, 522b
Calcipotriol, 1266
Calcitonin, 767
  hypercalcaemia, 273
  osteoporosis, 1125
  Paget's disease, 1129, 1130b
  as tumour marker, 270b
Calcitonin-gene-related peptide (CGRP), 845
Calcitriol (1,25-dihydroxycholecalciferol), hypoparathyroidism, 766, 770–771
Calcium, 130
  absorption, 129
  AKI, 480b
  channelopathies, 1230b
  deficiency, 130
  dietary sources, 131b
  excess, 130
  homeostasis, PTH/vitamin D and, 49b
  hyperparathyroidism, 769b
  myocardial contraction, 530
  osteomalacia, 1125–1128
  osteoporosis, 1123b, 1124
  reference values
    urine, 1311b
    venous blood, 1310b
  RNI, 131b
  serum, bone disease, 1066b
  see also Hypercalcaemia; Hypocalcaemia
Calcium antagonists (channel blockers)
  adverse reactions, 26b
  angina, 586–587
    unstable, 594

arrhythmias, 536–537
hypertension, 612, 613b
hypertrophic cardiomyopathy, 638
mitral stenosis, 618
non-dihydropyridine, microalbuminuria in diabetes, 831
poisoning, 214–215
pulmonary hypertension, 725
Raynaud's symptoms, 1113
Calcium carbonate, 488
Calcium gluconate
cardiotoxic drug poisoning, 214–215
drug interactions, 28b
hypermagnesaemia, 448
Calcium oxalate
crystals, 222–223
stones, 507b
Calcium phosphate, stones, 507b
Calcium pyrophosphate crystals, 769
Calcium pyrophosphate dihydrate (CPPD) deposition, 1086–1087, 1090–1091
Calcium therapy
hypoparathyroidism, 770–771
osteoporosis, 1124
rickets/osteomalacia, 1128
tetany, 768
Calcium and vitamin D supplements, 1124
Calculi (stones)
bile duct, 984–985
pancreatitis, 890
gallbladder *see* Gallstones
renal, 507–510, 507b
staghorn, 493b, 507
urinary tract, 507–510
see also Gallstones
Calicivirus, 949b
Calprotectin, faecal, 851b, 1311b
Cameron lesions, 867
cAMP (cyclic adenosine monophosphate), 47f
Campbell de Morgan spots, 1274
Campomelic dysplasia, 59
Campylobacter
diarrhoea, 306, 399
food poisoning, 306
Guillain-Barré syndrome, 342
Campylobacter jejuni, 342
Camurati-Engelmann disease, 1131
Cancer, 259–282, 266b
aetiology, 266–267
environmental, 266–267, 266b
genetic, 267
biochemical markers, 269, 270b
clinical assessment, 260f, 261b
dementia, 250b
emergency situations, 272–274, 273b
familial, 59, 66–67
hallmarks of, 262–266
angiogenesis, 264, 264f–265f
evasion of growth suppressors, 264
evasion of immune destruction, 266
genome instability/mutation, 262–266
invasion and metastasis, 265, 265f
replicative immortality, 264
reprogramming of energy metabolism, 265
resistance to cell death, 262
sustained proliferative signalling, 263
tumour-promoting inflammation, 265–266
histology, 268–269
cytogenetic analysis, 269
electron microscopy, 269
immunohistochemistry, 268
light microscopy, 268
HIV-related, 405, 405b
imaging, 269
incidence, 262f
inheritance, 267b
investigations, 268–269
local features, 270b
metastases, 265, 274–276
of unknown origin, 282
musculoskeletal manifestations, 1132, 1132b
neurological paraneoplastic syndromes, 271–272, 272b, 1193, 1194b, 1216
obesity and, 115b
older people, 271b
pain management, 275
predisposition syndromes, 267b
presenting problems, 269–272, 270b–271b, 1259b
renal effects, 519, 519b
screening
breast cancer, 271b, 279, 762–763, 912
cervical cancer, 281
prostate cancer, 518
staging, TNM classification, 268b
treatment/management, 276–279
adjuvant, 276
biological, 278–279
chemoprevention, 276
chemotherapy, 276–277
hormonal, 278
immunotherapy, 278
late effects, 796
neoadjuvant, 276
older people
palliative, 276
radiotherapy, 277–278
surgical, 276
see also Chemotherapy; *and specific cancers*
Cancer antigen 19.9 (CA-19.9), 270b
Cancer antigen 125 (CA-125), 270b
Cancer cachexia syndrome, 122f, 290
Candesartan
heart failure, 552b
myocardial infarction, 599
Candida spp., 134, 137f, 304b, 381, 383
acute leukaemia patients
endocarditis, 626
Candida albicans, 383, 1280
immunocompromised patients, 398
Candida dubliniensis, 383
Candida glabrata, 383
Candida krusei, 383
Candida parapsilosis, 383
Candida tropicalis, 383
Candidiasis, 381, 416b, 1280
acute disseminated, 383
genital, 417b–418b
hepatosplenic (chronic disseminated), 383
HIV/AIDS patients, 398–399, 399f
oesophageal, 868
HIV/AIDS, 399, 399f
oral, 864
HIV/AIDS, 398
pseudomembranous, 398
systemic, 383
Cannabis, 216–217
Cannula-related infection, 330, 330b
Capacity, lack of, 11
CAPD *see* Continuous ambulatory peritoneal dialysis
Capecitabine, 276, 915
Capillary leak syndrome, 323–324
Caplan's syndrome, 712, 717
Capnocytophaga canimorsus, 304b
Capnography, 188, 188f
Capsaicin
herpes zoster, 319, 397
osteoarthritis, 1079–1080, 1085
topical, 397
Capsule endoscopy, 848, 849f
Capsulitis (frozen shoulder), 1074–1075
Caput medusae, 945
Carbamate insecticides, 222
Carbamazepine
bipolar disorder
epilepsy, 1184b
hyponatraemia, 1185b
multiple sclerosis, 1192b
pain management, 285b, 1165
pharmacodynamics, 25b
pharmacokinetics, 25b
poisoning, 224b
status epilepticus, 1159b
trigeminal neuralgia, 1178
Carbapenems, 154b, 156
Carbaryl, 1281
Carbenoxolone, 441
Carbidopa, 1196
Carbimazole, 742–743, 748b, 749
pregnancy, 749–750
Carbohydrates, 112–113
diabetic diet, 820–821
dietary, 113b
energy provided by, 110
recommended intake, 114b
digestion, 842
effects of insulin
metabolism, 926
disorders of, 449–450, 1229b
see also Diabetes mellitus
Carbon dioxide (CO_2)
arterial blood ($PaCO_2$), 188, 660b, 1308b
emissions, 102
Carbon monoxide poisoning, 209b, 219–220
Carbonic acid/bicarbonate buffer system, 430–431, 444
Carbonic anhydrase, 131
Carbonic anhydrase inhibitors, 434–435
Carboplatin, 280–281
Carboxyhaemoglobin (COHb)
levels in carbon monoxide poisoning, 209b
reference range, 1310b
Carboxypenicillins, 154b, 155
Carbuncles, 1277, 1277f
Carcinoembryonic antigen (CEA), 268, 270b
Carcinogenesis, multistep
Carcinoid syndrome, 784, 785b, 889
pellagra, 128
valvular heart disease, 624
Carcinoid tumours
gastric, 880
lung, 704b
small intestine, 889, 889b
Carcinoma
ampulla of Vater, 986
anaplastic, thyroid, 755
basal cell, 270b, 1102–1103, 1256
follicular, thyroid, 754
gallbladder, 985
gastric, 877–879, 878f
hepatocellular, 967–969
medullary, thyroid, 755
oesophagus, 870–871, 870b, 871f
papillary, thyroid, 754
squamous cell
oesophagus, 870b
skin, 1271, 1271f
see also sites of carcinoma
Card agglutination trypanosomiasis test (CATT), 359
Cardiac arrest, 557–560
aetiology, 557–560
management, 558–559
survivors, 559–560
Cardiac asthma, 543
Cardiac biomarkers, 535
Cardiac cachexia, 549
Cardiac catheterisation, 538–539
aortic regurgitation, 624b
aortic stenosis, 621b
mitral valve disease, 617, 619b
Cardiac glycosides *see* Digoxin
Cardiac output, 530
factors influencing, 547
heart failure, 546
measurement, 186–187
optimization of, 191
Cardiac pacemakers
code, 578b
permanent, 564, 578–579
rate-responsive, 578–579
sinoatrial disease, 564
temporary, 578, 578f
Cardiac (pericardial) tamponade, 191, 532
see also Heart
Cardiac resynchronisation therapy (CRT), 579, 579b
Cardiac tamponade, 532, 545–546, 545b, 640
Cardiobacterium hominis, 626
Cardiogenic shock, 190, 544–546, 544f–545f
Cardiomegaly, 535
Cardiomyopathy, 636–638
arrhythmogenic right ventricular, 638
dilated, 636–637
HIV-related, 405
hypertrophic, 637–638, 638b
obliterative, 638
restrictive, 638
types, 637f
Cardiopulmonary disorders, SLE, 1111
Cardiopulmonary resuscitation (CPR), 204b
see also Basic life support
Cardiothoracic ratio, 535
Cardiovascular disorders, 525–641
chronic renal failure, 486
dyspnoea *see* Dyspnoea
genetic, 629–636, 629b–630b
hypertension *see* Hypertension
investigation, 532–539
lipids and *see* Atherosclerosis
New York Heart Association functional classification, 539b
presenting problems, 539–562
rheumatoid arthritis, 1099
risk factors, 581
obesity, 116f
syphilis, 420
therapeutic procedures, 577–579
Cardiovascular heart disease, risk prediction chart, 582f
Cardiovascular reflex tests, diabetes mellitus, 833b
Cardiovascular system, clinical examination, 526f
Cardioversion, 577
atrial fibrillation, 566
direct current (DC), arrhythmias, 564
tachyarrhythmias, 570
Carditis, 614–615
Care *see* Health care
Carey Coombs murmur, 614–615
Carnitine-palmityl transferase (CPT) deficiency, 1229b
Caroli's syndrome, 980–981
Carotene, 126
Carotid endarterectomy, 1244–1246, 1246f
Carotid pulse, 104, 189
Carotid sinus hypersensitivity, 554f, 556
Carotid sinus massage, 723
Carotid sinus syndrome, 556
Carpal tunnel syndrome, 1134
diabetes, 832
rheumatoid arthritis, 1099

Carrion's disease, 352, 352b
Cartilage
  articular, 1062–1063, 1063f
  calcification, 1064
  erosion, 1064
  osteoarthritis, 1084
Carvedilol, 946
  arrhythmias, 574–576
  hypertension, 612
Casal's necklace, 128, 128f
Caspases, 50
Caspofungin, 160, 160b
  acute leukaemia patients, 1001
  aspergillosis, 698–699
Cassava, 892
Castleman's disease, 298b, 326
Cat scratch disease, 352
Catalase, 47
Cataplexy, 1187
Cataract
  diabetics, 830
  'snow-flake', 830
Catatonia, 1166b
Catechol-O-methyl-transferase (COMT) inhibitors, Parkinson's disease, 1197
Catecholamines, 772
  drug interactions, 28b
Cathepsin K (CatK), 1061f
Catheter ablation therapy
  arrhythmias, 577–578
    tachyarrhythmias, 568–569
Catheters/catheterisation
  bacteriuria, 513
  bladder dysfunction, 1175b
  cardiac, 538–539, 538f
    aortic regurgitation, 624b
    aortic stenosis, 621b
    mitral valve disease, 617b, 619b
    therapeutic procedures, 534
  peripherally inserted central catheter, 124
  pulmonary artery, critically ill patients, 185–186, 186f
  therapeutic procedures, 577–579
  urinary retention, 515
Cathinones, 218
CatK *see* Cathepsin K
CATT *see* Card agglutination trypanosomiasis test
Cauda equina claudication, 1221b
Cauda equina syndrome, 1073b
Caval filters, 724
Cawthorne-Cooksey exercises, 1186
CBT *see* Cognitive behaviour therapy
CCK *see* Cholecystokinin
CD4 cells, 74b, 78
  HIV infection/AIDS, 392, 395b
CD8 cells, 78, 392
CDKs *see* Cyclin-dependent kinases
CEA *see* Carcinoembryonic antigen
Cefaclor, 156b
Cefalexin, 156b
  urinary tract infection, 513b
Cefazolin, 156b
Cefepime, 151b, 156b
Cefixime, 156b
  gonorrhoea, 422b
Cefotaxime, 151b, 156b
  cerebral abscess, 1208b
  meningitis, 1204b
  spontaneous bacterial peritonitis, 941
Cefoxitin, 156b
Cefradine, 156b
Ceftaroline, 156b
Ceftazidime, 151b, 155f, 156b
  bronchiectasis, 679
  melioidosis, 340
Ceftobiprole, 156b
Ceftriaxone, 151b, 156b
  leptospirosis, 338
  meningitis, 1204b
  nocardiosis, 341
  pneumonia, 401
    pyogenic meningitis, 1204b
  STIs
    congenital syphilis, 421
    gonorrhoea, 422b
  Whipple's disease, 884
Cefuroxime, 151b, 155f, 156b
  brucellosis, 335
  cerebral abscess, 1208b
  cholangitis, 985
  cholecystitis, 984
  empyema, 663
  meningitis, 1204b
  pancreatitis, 892
  pneumonia, 685b, 686
  prophylactic, 153b
  septic arthritis, 1095b
  urinary tract infection
Cefuroxime axetil, 335
Celecoxib, 1079b
Cell, 47f
  cerebrospinal fluid analysis, 1153–1154, 1154b, 1311b
  death, 50
    programmed (apoptosis), 50, 262
  division, 49–50
  functional anatomy, 42–50
  nervous system, 1140f
  senescence, 50
Cell adhesion molecules, 264f, 531–532
Cell biology, 42–50
Cell cycle, 263, 263f
  checkpoints, 49
  regulation, 263
  stimulation, 263
Cell differentiation, 49–50
Cell migration, 49–50
Cell (plasma) membrane, 47–48
  receptors, 48–49
  transport across, 48
Cellular immunity, 78
Cellular signalling, 48–49, 49b
Cellulitis, 1277, 1277f
  anaerobic, 305, 305b
Central core disease, 1230b
Central nervous system
  effects of hypertension, 609
  HIV infection/AIDS, 402–404
  SLE, 1111
  tuberculosis, 691
  tumours, 1213–1216, 1213b, 1214f
Central venous catheter infections, 303–304
Central venous pressure (CVP)
  gastrointestinal haemorrhage, 855
  monitoring, 182b, 185
    factors influencing, 183f, 186b
Cephalosporins, 151b, 155–156, 156b
  cholecystitis, 984
  Clostridium difficile infection, 344
  effect of renal insufficiency, 36b
  pneumonia, 687
  in pregnancy, 154b
Cephamycins, 155–156
Cerebellar ataxia, 272, 1229b
Cerebellar degeneration, 1194b
  cancer-related, 271b, 272
Cerebellar dysfunction, 1218
Cerebellum, 1145
Cerebral abscess, 1208–1209, 1208b, 1208f
Cerebral cortex
  anatomy, 1143f
  lobar functions, 1142b
    effects of damage, 1142b
Cerebral hemispheres, 1142–1143, 1143f
  lesions, 1165
Cerebral infarction, 1237–1239, 1238f
Cerebral ischaemia, 199b, 572, 1046f
Cerebral oedema
  acute liver failure, 933b
  high-altitude, 107
  hypoglycaemia, 813
  stroke patients, 1239–1240
Cerebral perfusion pressure, 199
Cerebral tumours *see* Brain, tumours
Cerebral venous disease, 1247
  causes, 1247b
  clinical features, 1247, 1247b
  investigations and management, 1247
Cerebrospinal fluid (CSF), 1143
  analysis, 1153–1154, 1154b, 1311b
  circulation, 1217f
  encephalomyelitis, 1193
  Guillain-Barré syndrome, 1225
  meningitis, 1202–1203, 1205
  multiple sclerosis, 1190
  subacute sclerosing panencephalitis, 1207
  syphilis, 421
  viral encephalitis, 1206
  see also Lumbar puncture
Cerebrotendinous xanthomatosis, 456b
Cerebrovascular disease *see specific conditions*
Certolizumab, 1103b
Cervical cancer, 281
  HIV-related, 405
  incidence, 262f
  screening, 281
  treatment, 281
Cervical cord compression, 1221f
  cervical spondylosis, 1218f
  rheumatoid arthritis, 1099
Cervical spine
  spondylosis, 1218–1219
  spondylotic myelopathy, 1219
  spondylotic radiculopathy, 1218–1219
  subluxation, rheumatoid arthritis, 1099, 1099f
Cervicitis
  chlamydial, 353b
  gonococcal, 418
Cestodes (tapeworms), 312b, 378–381
Cetirizine, 1267
Cetuximab, 282, 915, 1282
CF *see* Cystic fibrosis
CFTR *see* Cystic fibrosis transmembrane conductance regulator
CFU-E (colony-forming unit-erythroid), 992, 994
CFU-GM (colony-forming unit-granulocyte, monocyte), 992
CFU-Meg (colony-forming unit-megakaryocyte), 992, 996–997
CGRP (calcitonin-gene-related peptide)
Chagas disease, 309b, 360–361
  transfusion-transmitted, 1011–1012
Chain of infection, 134f
Chain of survival, cardiac arrest, 558, 558f
Chancre, 415–416
  trypanosomal, 359
Chancroid, 424b
Channelopathies, 1229–1230, 1230b
Charcoal, activated, 210, 210b
  antidiabetic overdose, 216
  antimalarial overdose, 215
  benzodiazepine overdose, 217
  digoxin/oleander poisoning, 215
  gammahydroxybutyrate poisoning, 218
  NSAID overdose, 213
  salicylate poisoning, 213
  tricyclic antidepressant poisoning, 213
Charcot joints, 1133, 1133f
Charcot neuro-arthropathy, 833–835
Charcot-Marie-Tooth disease, 48, 1225
Charcot's triad, 937–938
Charles Bonnet's syndrome, 1170
CHART *see* Continuous hyper-fractionated accelerated radiotherapy
CHD *see* Coronary heart disease
Cheese worker's lung, 719b
Cheiroarthropathy, 1133
Chelating agents, 103
Chemical cholestasis, 980
Chemical mutagens, 266b
Chemical poisoning, 219–223
Chemoembolisation, hepatocellular carcinoma, 968
Chemokine receptor inhibitors, 407b
Chemoprophylaxis, 152, 153b
  malaria, 153b, 357–358
Chemotherapy, 276–277
  adjuvant, 276
    breast cancer, 280, 280b
    bronchial carcinoma, 704
    colorectal cancer, 915
    pancreatic cancer, 895
  administration, 276–277
  adverse reactions, 277, 277f
  brain tumours, 1215
  bronchial carcinoma, 703–704
  combination, 276
  gastric cancer, 879b
  Hodgkin's disease, 1043
  leukaemia
    acute, 1037b
    chronic lymphocytic, 1040
    chronic myeloid, 1039–1040
  malignant melanoma
  myeloma, 1047
  neoadjuvant, 276
  non-Hodgkin's lymphoma, 1044
  palliative, 276
  platinum-based, 280–281, 704
  prostate cancer, 518, 518b
  tuberculosis, 693–694
    HIV/AIDS patients, 406–407
Chernobyl nuclear power explosion, 102
Chest pain, 539–543
  ankylosing spondylitis, 1105
  cardiac disease
    aortic dissection, 541, 606
    differential diagnosis, 659b
    ischaemic, 539f–540f
  causes, 541b
    gastrointestinal, 540
    musculoskeletal, 541
    psychological, 540
    respiratory, 657–658
  characteristics, 539–543
  differential diagnosis, 540–541, 659b
  evaluation, 541–543
Chest radiography/X-ray, 649–650, 649f
  abnormalities, 650b
  AKI, 480b
  bronchiectasis, 679
  cardiovascular disorders
    aortic regurgitation, 535f
    chronic constrictive pericarditis, 641f
    congenital, 629
    heart failure, 550, 550f
    mitral valve, 535f
    myocardial infarction, 593
  cardiovascular system, 535–536
  COPD, 675
  empyema, 663f
  pacemaker/defibrillator, 553f
  pleural effusion, 661, 662b
  respiratory disease, 649–650, 650f
    abnormalities, 650b
    ARDS, 193f
    aspergillosis, 697
    asthma, 669
    bronchial carcinoma, 700f

bronchial obstruction/lung collapse, 701f
bronchiectasis, 679
COPD, 675
empyema, 663f
haemoptysis, 659
HIV-related pulmonary disease, 397b, 400b, 401f
inhaled foreign body, 655f
interpretation, 649b
interstitial, 707f, 709f
lobar collapse, 650f
mediastinal tumours, 706f
pleural effusion, 661
pleural plaques, 718f
Pneumocystis jirovecii pneumonia, 401f
pneumonia, 684
pneumothorax, 729–730
pulmonary embolism, 721b, 722f
pulmonary hypertension, 725f
pulmonary oedema, 482f
sarcoidosis, 711b
silicosis, 717f
tuberculosis, 401f, 691f–692f
Chest wall deformities, 731
Cheyne-Stokes respiration, 544
Chickenpox, 316–318, 317f
immunisation, 318
incubation period, 145b
period of infectivity, 144b
pneumonia, 317
prophylaxis, 317–318
rash, 317
varicella zoster immunoglobulin, 318b
Chiclero's ulcer, 366
Chief cells, 766
Chikungunya virus, 309b, 329, 1095
Chilblains, 105
Child-Pugh classification, cirrhosis prognosis, 944b
Childbirth, associated psychiatric disorders, 257
Childhood absence epilepsy, 1182b
Children
genetic testing, 63
inflammatory bowel disease, 906
STIs, 414–415
Chiropractic, 16, 909b
Chlamydia spp., 353, 353b
Chlamydia pneumoniae, 353b
Chlamydia psittaci, 353b
Chlamydia trachomatis, 135, 151b, 353, 353b, 417
in pregnancy, 314b, 414b
Chlamydial infection, 353, 423
men, 417, 423
treatment, 423b
urethritis, 415, 1104, 1108
women, 423
Chloasma, 1296
Chlorambucil
chronic lymphocytic leukaemia, 1040
non-Hodgkin's lymphoma, 1044
Waldenström's macroglobulinaemia, 1045
Chloramphenicol, 151b, 159
contraindication
pregnancy, 154b
renal insufficiency, 36b
enteric fever, 340
mechanism of action, 150b
meningitis, 1204b
plague, 338–339
in pregnancy, 154b
pyogenic meningitis, 1204b
in renal/hepatic disease, 36b
rickettsial fevers, 352
Chloride, 132
channelopathies, 1230b
disorders of, 430b
reference values, venous blood, 1308b
Chloroquine
adverse reactions, 26
hyperpigmentation, 1296b
leprosy reactions, 350
malaria, 163, 358b
prevention, 357
myopathy, 1132b, 1230b
poisoning, 215
resistance to, 353, 356
Chlorphenamine, 38b
anaphylaxis, 92b
diphtheria, 728
pruritus, 1016f
Chlorpromazine, 249b
alcohol withdrawal syndrome, 254
diarrhoea, 308
hepatotoxicity, 971, 971b
long QT syndrome, 571b
and lupus syndrome, 1132b
poisoning, 216
rabies, 1206
schizophrenia, 249b
Chlorpropamide, 216
neutropenia, 1005b
Cholangiocarcinoma, 969, 985–986, 986f
Cholangiography
biliary cirrhosis, 964
percutaneous transhepatic (PTC)
sclerosing cholangitis, 945b
Cholangiopancreatography
endoscopic retrograde *see* ERCP
magnetic resonance *see* MRCP
Cholangiopathy, HIV-related, 400
Cholangitis
acute, 937–938
autoimmune, 964–965
and biliary cirrhosis, 980b
IgG4-associated, 966, 988
liver flukes, 378, 379b
primary sclerosing, 965–966, 980b
recurrent pyogenic, 985
sclerosing, 902f, 930b, 965–966
stone disease, 937b
Cholecalciferol *see* Vitamin D
Cholecystectomy
pancreatitis, 892
post-cholecystectomy syndrome, 987b
Cholecystitis, 983–984
acute, 861–862, 983–984
chronic, 984
gallstones, 982
Cholecystography, oral, 988
Cholecystokinin (CCK), 846b
Cholecystolithiasis, 983
Choledochal cysts, 981, 981f
Choledochojejunostomy, 895
Choledocholithiasis, 983–985
Choledochoscopy, 985
Cholera, 138b, 309b, 344–345
fluid loss, 344
immunisation, 345
incubation period, 145b, 310b
Cholera sicca, 344
Cholestasis, 980–988
benign recurrent intrahepatic, 980
biliary cirrhosis, 964
chemical, 980
drug-induced, 971, 971b
obstetric (of pregnancy), 977–978, 1259b
pruritus, 1259b
sclerosing cholangitis, 966
Cholestatic jaundice, 936b–937b, 937–938
Cholesterol, 450
absorption, 113
atheroembolism, 469b, 496
and cardiovascular disease, 452–453
dietary, 113, 114b, 451
gallstones, 982
low-density lipoprotein, 48, 451
lowering, 456–457
atherosclerosis prevention, 583b
coronary heart disease, 582
myocardial infarction, 598
peripheral vascular disease, 601b
metabolism, 85
plasma
measurement, 453
target levels, 811
reference values, venous blood, 5, 1310b
reverse transport, 452, 452f
see also Hypercholesterolaemia
Cholesterol absorption inhibitors, 434
Cholesterol ester transfer protein, 452
Cholesterolosis of gallbladder, 986–988
Choline salicylate, 864
Cholinergic syndrome, organophosphate poisoning, 220–222, 221b
Chondrocalcinosis, 1090b, 1090f
Chondrocytes
osteoarthritis, 1081
tumours, 1131b
Chondroitin sulphate, 1062–1063, 1086
Chondroma, 1131b
Chondromalacia patellae, 1075–1076
Chondrosarcoma, 1131b
CHOP regimen, non-Hodgkin's lymphoma, 1045
Chorea, 1166, 1166b
causes, 1167b
Huntington's disease, 65, 1198
Chorionic villus sampling (CVS), 63b
Choroid plexus, 1217f
Christmas disease (haemophilia B), 1053
Chromatin, 42
Chromatography, 428b
Chromium, 132
deficiency, 132
Chromoblastomycosis, 381–382
Chromogranin A, 785
Chromomycosis (chromoblastomycosis), 381–382
Chromosomal disorders, 56b, 57f, 66
see also specific conditions
Chromosomes, 42
abnormalities *see* Mutation(s)
analysis, 57f
leukaemia, 1039
myelodysplastic syndrome, 1041
deletions, 55, 56b
duplications, 55–56, 57f
sex, 42
abnormalities, 50–51
see also X chromosome; Y chromosome
translocations, 57f, 879–880, 1044
Chronic bronchitis, 653b, 673
Chronic fatigue syndrome, 246
Chronic interstitial nephritis (CIN), 503–504
drug induced, 504b
Chronic obstructive pulmonary disease *see* COPD
Chronic relapsing syndrome, 321
Chronic renal failure (CRF) *see* Renal failure, chronic
CHRPE *see* Congenital hypertrophy of retinal pigment epithelium
Chrysops, loiasis, 373
Churg-Strauss syndrome (CSS), 1118
Chvostek's sign, 447, 768
Chylomicrons, 113
Chylothorax, 661
Chyluria, lymphatic filariasis, 372
Chymotrypsinogen, 844b
Ciclesonide, 669
Ciclosporin, 96b
adverse reactions
chronic interstititial nephritis, 504b, 522b
musculoskeletal, 1132b
proximal myopathy, 1230b
aplastic anaemia, 1048
asthma, 671
drug interactions, 28b
eczema, 1268
heart transplant patients, 553
HSCT, 1018
immunosuppression, 96b, 493
inflammatory bowel disease, 903b, 904
lichen planus, 1290
liver transplant patients, 979
lung transplant patients, 666
myositis, 1115
nephrotoxicity, 979
psoriasis, 1268, 1289b
pyoderma gangrenosum, 1299
renal transplantation patients
rheumatic disease, 1101b, 1102
skin reactions, 1304b
Cidofovir
adverse reactions
CMV, 322
herpesvirus infection, 161b, 162
Ciguatera poisoning, 308
Ciguatoxin, 308
Cilia, 49
Ciliary dysfunction syndrome, 678b, 679
Ciliary dysmotility syndrome, 648
Cilostazol, 601
Cimetidine
drug interactions, 28–29
effect of renal insufficiency, 466b
neutropenia, 1005b
urticaria, 1291
CIN *see* Chronic interstitial nephritis
Cinacalcet, 770
Ciprofloxacin, 151b, 157b
anthrax, 347
bacillary dysentery, 345
bronchiectasis, 679
brucellosis, 334b
cellulitis, 1278
cholangitis, 966
cholera, 345
drug interactions, 28
inflammatory bowel disease, 860
intestinal bacterial overgrowth, 883
meningococcal infection, 1203–1204
plague, 338–339
prophylactic, 153b
spontaneous bacterial peritonitis, 941
Q fever, 352
STIs
chancroid, 424b
gonorrhoea, 422b
urinary tract infection, 513b
variceal bleeding, 946
Circulation
changes at birth, 630f
coronary, 530
critically ill patients
management, 189
monitoring, 185–187
effects of vasoactive drug infusions, 191b
enterohepatic, 22
fetal, 630f
portal, 464
stroke patients, 1243b
Circulatory failure (shock), 190–191
acute, 190, 544–546, 544f–545f
management, 190–191, 191b

  myocardial infarction, 597
  prognosis, 191
  for detailed entry see Shock
Circumduction, 1168
Circumflex artery (CX)
  coronary circulation, 529f
  occlusion, 538f
Cirrhosis, 942–945, 943f
  alcoholic, 958, 958b
  ascites, 944
  biliary, 963–965
    investigations, 964
    older people, 980b
    secondary, 981
  cardiac, 976–977
  causes, 942b
  Child-Pugh classification, 944b
  clinical features, 943–944, 943b
  cryptogenic, 961
  drugs to avoid, 971b
  haemochromatosis and, 943, 972–973
  hepatic encephalopathy, 923b, 941–942, 941b
  hepatocellular carcinoma, 967, 969f
  non-alcoholic fatty liver disease, 926, 944b, 959–961, 960f
  prognosis, 944–945, 944b
  viral hepatitis, 949b
Cisplatin
  bronchial carcinoma, 704
  endometrial cancer, 281
  gastric cancer, 879b
  head and neck tumours, 282
  and hypomagnesaemia, 448b
  nephrotoxicity, 479–481, 522b
  and peripheral neuropathy, 1223b
Citalopram, 244b, 290
Citric acid (Krebs) cycle, 128
Citrobacter spp., 151b
Citrobacter freundii, 303–304
CJD *see* Creutzfeld-Jakob disease
CK *see* Creatine kinase
Cladophialophora bantiana, 382–383
Cladophialophora carrionii, 381
Cladosporium spp., 671
Cladribine, 1041
Clarithromycin
  drug interactions, 28b
  Helicobacter pylori eradication, 874
  leprosy, 350
  Mycobacterium avium complex, 406b
  pneumonia, 685b
  in pregnancy, 154b
Clasp-knife phenomenon, 1145
Clathrin-coated pits, 48
Claude's syndrome, 1148b
Claudication
  arm, 602
  cauda equina, 1221b
  intermittent, 601
Claw foot, 1076
Clearance, 22–23, 23f
CLI (critical limb ischaemia)
Climacteric, 757
Climate change, 102
Clindamycin, 151b
  acne vulgaris, 1282
  babesiosis, 358
  bacterial vaginosis, 417b
  gas gangrene, 305
  malaria, 356
  MRSA, 331
  necrotising fasciitis, 305
  in pregnancy, 154b
  septic arthritis, 1095b
  soft tissue infections, 305
Clinical audit, 15, 15b, 15f
Clinical decision making, 7–9
  conflict of opinion, 12
  end of life, 291–292
  ethical analysis, 12–13, 13b
  ethical issues, 11–12, 12f
  heuristics, 8b
  informed consent, 10–11
  lack of capacity for, 11
Clinical endpoints, 39
Clinical ethics, 10–11
  scenario, 13
  see also Ethics
Clinical governance, 14b
Clinical pharmacology, 18–24
Clinical psychologist, 2b
Clinical trials, 32, 32f
CLM *see* Cutaneous larva migrans
CLO *see* Columnar lined (Barrett's) oesophagus
Clobazam, 1184b
Clobetasol, 416b, 418b, 1265b
Clobetasone butyrate, 1265b
  eczema, 1285–1286
Clock drawing test, 1233f
Clofazimine
  hyperpigmentation from, 1296b
  leprosy, 349b, 350
Clomethiazole, effect of old age, 36b
Clomifene, 762, 764
Clomipramine, 244b
  narcolepsy, 1187
Clonazepam
  epilepsy, 1184b
  multiple sclerosis, 1192b
  periodic limb movement syndrome, 1188
  sleep disorders, 1187
Clonidine
  delirium, 203
  diarrhoea, 833b
  opiate withdrawal, 255
Clonorchiasis, 379b
Clonorchis spp., 163
Clonorchis sinensis, 312b, 378, 379b, 984–986
Clopidogrel
  acute coronary syndrome, 594b
  angina, 585
    unstable, 594b
  myocardial infarction, 594b, 599
  peripheral arterial disease, 601b
  pharmacokinetics, 25b
  platelet inhibition, 1050
  prophylactic, 599, 1245b, 1245f
  stroke prevention, 1245b, 1245f
Clostridia, soft tissue infections, 305b
Clostridium spp., 136f–137f
Clostridium botulinum, 138b, 139, 1210
Clostridium difficile, 137f, 138b, 151b, 304b, 343–344, 344f
  diarrhoea, 399
Clostridium novyi, injecting drug users, 299–300
Clostridium perfringens, 308
  food poisoning, 342
  intravascular haemolysis, 1031
  septicaemia, 305
Clostridium tetani, 138b
Clotrimazole, 160b
  erythrasma, 1278
  genital candidiasis, 417b
Clotting *see* Coagulation
Clozapine
  drug interactions, 28b
  schizophrenia, 249b
Clubbing, digital, 1298, 1298f
  congenital heart disease, 631
  lung cancer, 271
Clue cells, 417f
Cluster headache, 1177, 1178b
CMAPs *see* Compound motor action potentials
CMV *see* Controlled mandatory ventilation
CMV (cytomegalovirus) *see* Cytomegalovirus infection
CNS *see* Central nervous system
Co-amoxiclav, 151b
  diverticulosis, 916–917
  empyema, 663
  hepatotoxicity, 971, 971b
  prophylactic, 153b
  respiratory tract infection
    pneumonia, 685b, 687
    upper, 678
  urinary tract infection, 513b
Co-artemether, 356
Co-proxamol, 219
Co-trimoxazole, 151b, 158
  adverse reactions
  brucellosis, 334b
  cyclosporiasis, 369
  isosporiasis, 399b, 406b
  listeriosis, 339
  melioidosis, 340
  meningitis, 1204b
  mycetoma, 341
  nocardiosis, 341
  P. jirovecii pneumonia, 400, 406b
    bone marrow transplants, 1017b
    leukaemia patients, 1038
  prophylactic, 153b
  prophylaxis, 406
  toxoplasmosis, HIV/AIDS patients, 402, 406b
  Whipple's disease, 884
Coagulation, disseminated intravascular, 201, 1000
Coagulation cascade, 996f–997f
Coagulation disorders, 1050–1054, 1051b
  acquired, 1051b, 1054
  congenital, 1051b, 1054–1056
  genetic testing, 62b
  investigation, 999–1001
  malaria, 357b
  stroke, 1244
Coagulation factors, 926–927, 997
  complications of therapy, 1052–1053
  concentrates, 1011
  older people, 1001b
  pregnancy, 1022b
  see also specific factors
Coagulation screen, 1000b, 1312b
  hepatobiliary disease, 929
Coagulation system inhibitors *see* Anticoagulants
Coal dust, lung disease and, 602–603, 674b
Coal tar, 1265–1266
Coal worker's pneumoconiosis, 716–717
Coarctation of aorta, 632, 632f
  incidence, 630b
  radiofemoral delay, 630f
Cobalamin *see* Vitamin B_{12}
Cobalt, 132
Cocaine misuse, 218
Coccidioides immitis, 386
Coccidioides posadasii, 386
Coccidioidomycosis, 386
Cock-up toe deformities, 1098
Codeine, 286
  contraindication, cirrhosis, 971b
  diarrhoea, 918
    inflammatory bowel disease, 903b
    irritable bowel syndrome, 908f
  effect of hepatic impairment, 971b
  headache, 1176
  malignant disease, 286
  pharmacokinetics, 25b
Codons, 43
Coeliac disease, 880–882
  anaemia, 1025b
  and dermatitis herpetiformis, 1293b, 1294
  disease associations, 881b
  investigations, 881, 881f
  liver function tests, 930b
  older people, 883b
  pathophysiology, 880, 880f
  small intestine tumours, 888–889
Coeliac plexus neurolysis, 894
Coffee, 129–130
  diabetogenic effect, 804
Cog wheel rigidity, 1145
Cognitive behaviour therapy (CBT), 241
  eating disorders, 256
  hypochondriasis, 245
  medically unexplained somatic symptoms, 247b
  obsessive-compulsive disorder, 243
  schizophrenia, 249
  somatoform disorders, 247b
Cognitive decline, general *see* Dementia
Cognitive function, assessment, 234
Cognitive impairment, 234
  HIV-related, 402
Cognitive therapy (CT), 241
COHb *see* Carboxyhaemoglobin
Coitus, headache and, 1178b
Colchicine
  arthralgia, 1119
  erythema nodosum, 1119
  familial Mediterranean fever, 85
  gout, 1089
Cold agglutinin disease, 1030–1031
Cold injury, 105, 105f
  see also Hypothermia
Cold sore, 326, 326f
Cold treatment
  musculoskeletal disorders
  see also Cryotherapy
Colectomy, 904–906
  prophylactic, 912
Colesevalam, 434
Colestipol, 434
Colestyramine, 434
  bile salt malabsorption, 886
  dyslipidaemia, 457
  ileal resection, 884
  irritable bowel syndrome, 908f
  post-cholecystectomy syndrome, 986–987
  primary biliary cirrhosis, 964
  pruritus, 1259b
  radiation enteritis, 886
Colic
  biliary, 982
  renal, 507–510
  ureteral, 507–508
Colipase, 844b
Colistin, 151b
Colitis
  collagenous, 900b, 907
  cytomegalovirus, HIV/AIDS patients, 399
  microscopic (lymphocytic), 907
  pseudomembranous, 138b
  ulcerative *see* Ulcerative colitis
Collagen, 1253f
  osteoarthritis, 1081
Collagenase, 72–73, 82–83
Collar-stud abscess, 690–691
Colles fracture, 1120
Colloid cyst, 1212b–1213b
Colloids, 482b
Colon, 844, 845f
  acute pseudo-obstruction, 918, 918b
  cancer *see* Colorectal cancer
  disorders of, 910–920
  diverticulosis, 916–917, 916f
  ischaemia, 909–910
  motility tests, 850
  obstruction, 862
  polyps/polyposis, 910–912, 911b
    adenomatous, 910f, 911–912
    see also Familial adenomatous polyposis
  structure and function, 844
  tumours, 910–916
    see also Colorectal cancer

Colonoscopy, 848, 849b
abdominal pain, 863
acute colonic pseudo-obstruction, 918
colorectal cancer, 913, 916
constipation, 861
gastrointestinal haemorrhage, 856
inflammatory bowel disease, 904b, 908
older people, 850b
polyps, 910, 912
radiation enteritis, 885
virtual, 914–915
Colony-forming unit-erythroid *see* CFU-E
Colony-forming unit-granulocyte monocyte *see* CFU-GM
Colony-forming unit-megakaryocyte *see* CFU-Meg
Colophony, 1285b
Colorectal cancer, 912–916
clinical features, 914
colonic polyps and, 910
development, 914f
diagnosis, 913b
Dukes staging, 914f
familial adenomatous polyposis coli, 67, 267b, 910f–911f, 911–912, 911b
genetics, 54b
hereditary non-polyposis, 895, 913b, 913f
incidence, 262f
inflammatory bowel disease, 900–901
investigations, 914–915
management, 915
palliative therapy, 915, 915f
pathophysiology, 912–914, 913f
prevention/screening, 916
risk factors, 913b
staging, 914f
Colorimetric chemical reaction, 428b
Columnar lined (Barrett's) oesophagus (CLO), 866–867
Coma, 198–200, 1159–1161
causes, 199b, 1160b
diabetics *see* Diabetic ketoacidosis
malaria, 357b
myxoedema, 745
poisoning, 211b
respiratory failure, 664–665
stroke patients, 1237
Comedones
acne, 1281–1282
definition, 1251b
Common cold, 681–682
Common peroneal nerve entrapment, 1224b
Communication, 4
doctor-patient, 4b
medical interview, 4b
of risk, 7, 7f
Comorbidities in older people, 170
Compartment syndrome, 301, 1051
anterior tibial, 1135
injecting drug users, 299–300
Complement, 74–75
activation, 75f
measurement, 88
deficiencies, 78b, 79
low, glomerulonephritis associated with, 501b
total haemolytic, 1310b
Complement fixation test (CFT), 142
Complement membrane attack complex, 75f
Complementary and alternative medicine (CAM), 15–16
evidence, 16
integrated health care, 16
pain management, 288
regulation, 16
safety, 16
Compound motor action potentials (CMAPs), 1152
Compressed air, physics of breathing, 109b
Compression bandages, leg ulcers, 1263
Computed tomography *see* CT (computed tomography)
COMT *see* Catechol-O-methyl-transferase inhibitors
Concentration, assessment, 234
Conduction, heart, 562–579
Condyloma, giant, 425
Condylomata lata, 419–420
Confidentiality, 11
Conflict resolution, 12
Confusion Assessment Method (CAM), 174b
Confusion/confusional states, 238
cerebral oedema, 107
older people, 24, 168
post-ictal, 1158b
terminal illness, 290
Congenital abnormalities
diaphragm
heart, 629–636, 629b–630b
adult patients, 635–636, 635b
maternal diabetes and, 818
pancreas, 894–895
rubella and, 315b
urinary tract, 510–511
Congenital adrenal hyperplasia, 763b, 782
Congenital hypertrophy of retinal pigment epithelium (CHRPE), 911–912, 911b
Congestive gastropathy, 948
Coning, 1154
Conjunctivitis
gonococcal, 422
psoriatic arthritis, 1108–1109
reactive arthritis, 1108
Connective tissue, crystal deposition, 1086–1087, 1086f
Connective tissue diseases, 1109–1115, 1300–1301
inherited, 65
management, DMARDs
mixed, 1091b, 1092, 1113–1114
prevalence, 1060b
respiratory involvement, 711–713, 712b
Conn's syndrome, 441, 781f
Consciousness
episodic loss/alteration, 1157–1159
AV block, 572
epilepsy *see* Epilepsy
seizures, 1159
see also Coma; Syncope
minimally conscious states, 1161, 1161b
Consent
artificial nutritional support, 124b
discontinuation of dialysis, 490
informed, 10–11
to organ donation, 203
Consequentialism, 10
Constipation, 860–861, 917–918
causes, 860b
clinical assessment, 860–861
diabetic neuropathy, 832b–833b
diverticulosis, 916–917
irritable bowel syndrome, 907–908
older people, 918b
stroke patients, 1243b
Consultation, communication in, 2
Contact allergic eczema, 1286
Contact inhibition, 264
Continence
faecal, 844
see also Incontinence
Continuous ambulatory peritoneal dialysis (CAPD), 492
problems, 493b
Continuous hyperfractionated accelerated radiotherapy (CHART), 703
Continuous positive airway pressure (CPAP), 191b, 193–194, 193f
drowning victims, 108
sleep apnoea, 727
Continuous professional development (CPD), 14
Contraception
epilepsy, 1184
oral *see* Oral contraception/contraceptives
Contrast media, nephrotoxicity, 469b
Controlled mandatory ventilation (CMV), 195f
Conus medullaris, spinal cord compression, 272b
Conversion (dissociative) disorder, 246, 246b
Coombs test, 1030f
COP *see* Cryptogenic organising pneumonia
COPD, 644f, 673–678
BODE index, 677b
classification, 675b
clinical features, 673f, 674–675, 675f
exertional dyspnoea, 655, 674b
epidemiology, 673–677
exacerbations, 674–675
acute, 658b, 677–678
investigations, 675
management, 675–677, 675b, 676f
occupational, 716
older people, 677b
palliative care, 284
pathophysiology, 673–674, 674f
prognosis, 677
respiratory failure, 663–666
risk factors, 674b
Coping strategies
fibromyalgia, 1093–1094
musculoskeletal disease, 1080–1081, 1081b
Copper
deficiency, 119b
dietary sources, 131b
excess, Wilson's disease, 132, 973
refeeding diet, 122b
reference values
urine, 1311b
venous blood, 1310b
RNI, 131b
Coproporphyria, hereditary, 460b
Copy number variants, 55–56
polymorphic, 56–57
Cor pulmonale, 548
Cordocentesis, 63b
Cordylobia anthropophaga, 381
Cori disease, 450b
Corneal arcus, hyperlipidaemia, 454f
Corneal melting, 1099
Corneocytes, 102
Coronary angiography, 538f, 599
Coronary angioplasty, 587f, 595b, 595f
Coronary arteries, 529–530, 529f
angiography, 526f
calcification, 537, 602b
occlusion, 1099
spasm, 589
stenosis, 538f
stenting, 1018
Coronary arteriography, 585
Coronary artery bypass grafting (CABG), 585
angina, 588–589, 588f, 589b
vs. PCI, 589b
Coronary artery disease (CAD), 583–600
clinical manifestations, 583b
diabetics, 818
hyperlipidaemia and, 581
hypertension and, 581
obesity and, 115b
pathology, 583b
prognosis, 589
risk factors, 581
Coronary artery spasm, 589
Coronary blood flow, resistance to
Coronary circulation, 530
Coronary syndromes, acute *see* Acute coronary syndrome
Coronaviruses, 145b, 328, 683b
Corrosives
oesophagitis, 868
poisoning, 224b
Corticobasal degeneration, 1198
Corticosteroids
acute lung injury, 196
adverse reactions, 26, 1265f
osteoporosis, 1120–1121
allergy, 90, 92b
biliary cirrhosis, 964
blood disorders
autoimmune haemolysis, 1030
chronic lymphocytic leukaemia, 1040
cluster headache, 1177
congenital adrenal hyperplasia, 782
critically ill patients, 196, 201
giant cell arteritis, 1117–1118
hepatitis
alcoholic, 959, 959b
autoimmune, 962–963
inflammatory bowel disease, 860, 903b
inhaled, asthma, 669–670, 670b
leprosy reactions, 349b
medication overuse headache, 1177
musculoskeletal disorders
ankylosing spondylitis, 1107
myositis, 1073
osteoarthritis, 1086
SLE, 1112
vasculitis, 1117–1118
neurological disorders
meningitis, 1204b
multiple sclerosis, 1191b
myasthenia gravis, 1227b
sciatica, 1220
pain management, 288b
palliative care, 285b, 288b
pericarditis, 597
pre-eclampsia, 521
pregnancy, 37b
pruritus, 1259b
renal disease
acute interstitial nephritis, 503
glomerulonephritis, 499b–500b, 500
respiratory disease
allergic rhinitis, 725
aspergillosis, 698
asthma, 669–670, 670b
COPD, 676
interstitial lung disease, 708b, 709
sarcoidosis, 711b
tuberculosis, 694
rheumatic disease, 1102
rheumatic fever, 615
skin disorders, 1267
adverse reactions, 1303b
alopecia areata, 1297
atopic eczema, 1285–1286
bullous pemphigoid, 1294b
lichen planus, 1290
photosensitivity, 1295
psoriasis, 1289b
topical, 1264–1265, 1265b
urticaria, 1291
vitiligo, 1295
systemic, 1267
topical, 1264–1265, 1285–1286
transplantation reactions, 96b

trichinosis, 375
weight gain, 117b
withdrawal symptoms, 20b
see also Cortisol; Glucorticoids; Hydrocortisone; Mineralocorticoids; Prednisolone
Corticotrophin-releasing hormone (CRH), 737f, 774f, 775–776
Corticotrophin-releasing hormone test, 774f
Cortisol, 772
deficiency, 794
hypopituitarism, 788
levels
adrenal insufficiency, 777, 779
Cushing's syndrome, 775–776
reference values
urine, 1311b
venous blood, 1309b
see also Hydrocortisone
Cortisone acetate, equivalent dose, 776b
Corynebacterium spp., 136f–137f
Corynebacterium diphtheriae, 138b, 345
Corynebacterium minutissimum, 1278
Coryza, acute, 681–682
Costs *see* Economics
Cotton wool spots
diabetic retinopathy, 828
hypertension, 609
Cough, 654–655, 654b
asthma, 667
at high altitude, 107
bovine, 701, 727
bronchial carcinoma, 700
COPD, 674
and headache, 1178, 1178b
laryngeal nerve paralysis, 651
palliative care, 289
pneumonia, 683
upper respiratory tract infections, 648, 681–682
Cough reflex, 654
Coumarins *see* Warfarin
Councilman bodies, 324
Counselling
dietary
coeliac disease, 881–882
COPD, 676
hyperlipidaemia, 456
genetic, 67–68
HIV diagnosis, 393b
post-traumatic stress disorder, 242
Coupled enzymatic reaction, 428b
Courvoisier's Law, 937
Cowden's syndrome, 267b, 911b
Cowpox, 327
COX *see* Cyclo-oxygenase
Coxibs *see* NSAIDs; and individual drugs
Coxiella burnetii, 135, 352
endocarditis, 626
pneumonia, 720–721
Coxsackie viruses, 319, 326–327
myocarditis, 639b
CPAP *see* Continuous positive airway pressure
CPD *see* Continuous professional development
CPPD *see* Calcium pyrophosphate dihydrate
CPR *see* Cardiopulmonary resuscitation
CPT deficiency *see* Carnitine-palmityl transferase deficiency
Crab lice, 416b
Crack cocaine, 218
Cramps
abdominal *see* Abdominal pain
drug-induced, 1132b
heat, 106
occupational, 1200
Cranial nerves
examination, 1140f
lesions/diseases, 1171b
nuclei, 1143–1144
see also specific nerves by name
Craniopharyngioma, 790b, 793, 794f
Creams, 1265b
Creatine kinase (CK)
acute coronary syndromes, 593f
elevated, 1067b
hypothermia, 104–105
muscular dystrophies, 1228
musculoskeletal disease, 1067b
myocardial infarction, 593f
myopathy, 1066–1067
myositis, 1066–1067
reference values, venous blood, 1310b
Creatinine, 430b
AKI, 197b
chronic renal failure, 484f, 487b
clearance, 508b
older people, 483b
diabetes mellitus, 484f
hepatorenal syndrome, 940–941
microalbuminuria, 831b
reference values
urine, 1311b
venous blood, 1308b
serum levels, 467f
AKI, 480b
diabetes mellitus, 484f
CREST syndrome, 1091b, 1112, 1113f
Cretinism, 131
Creutzfeld-Jakob disease (CJD), 329b, 1211
variant (vCJD), 1211, 1211f
transmission in blood products, 1015
CRF (chronic renal failure) *see* Renal failure, chronic
CRH *see* Corticotrophin-releasing hormone
Crico-arytenoid arthritis, 712b
Crigler-Najjar syndrome, 937b
Crimean-Congo haemorrhagic fever, 309b, 324, 325b
Critical care/critically ill patient, 179–204
admission guidelines, 183
assessment, 188–189
circulatory support, 189
clinical decision-making, 189–190, 189b
clinical examination/assessment, 180f–181f
discharge, 203, 203b
fluid resuscitation, 1011b
gastrointestinal support, 198
hepatic support, 198
infection sites, 200b
management
on admission, 201b
daily, 202
monitoring, 185–188
circulation, 185–187
respiratory function, 187–188
mortality, 204b
neurological support, 198–200
nutrition, 198
older people, 204b
outcome, 204
outreach, 203
oxygen delivery, 182–184
physiology, 182–185
presenting problems, 190–201
recognition, 180f–181f, 181b, 188–190
red cell transfusion, 1011b
referral, 189–190
renal support, 197–198, 197b
respiratory support, 191–197
scoring systems, 181b, 204, 204b
transport of patient, 324
withdrawal of care, 203
Critical illness polyneuropathy, 200
Critical limb ischaemia (CLI), 601–602, 601f
Crohn's disease
arthritis, 1109
childhood, 906
clinical features, 899–900, 900f
comparison with ulcerative colitis, 897b
complications, 900–901, 901f–902f
cutaneous, 1301
differential diagnosis, 900b
investigations, 901–902
management, 904–906
metastatic, 1301
pathophysiology, 898–899, 899f
perianal, 860, 919
pregnancy, 906b
prognosis, 906
pyoderma gangrenosum, 1299f
sclerosing cholangitis and, 965
small bowel, 1025
Cronkhite-Canada syndrome, 911b
Cross-infection, 134
see also Health care-acquired infections
Croup, 328, 654b
Crouzon syndrome, 49
CRP *see* C-reactive protein
CRT *see* Cardiac resynchronisation therapy
Crust, skin, definition, 1251b
Cruveilhier-Baumgarten syndrome, 945
Cryoglobulinaemic vasculitis, 1119
Cryoglobulins/cryoglobulinaemia, 88, 88b
Cryoprecipitate, 1012b
Cryosurgery, chromoblastomycosis, 381–382
Cryotherapy, 1268–1269
anogenital warts, 426
basal cell papilloma, 1274
granuloma annulare, 1301
leishmaniasis, 367
molluscum contagiosum, 426, 1279
sarcoidosis, 1301
skin cancer, 1270b, 1271
warts, 426
Cryptitis, 897–898, 897b
Cryptococcus gattii, 384
Cryptococcus neoformans, 384
HIV/AIDS patients, 403
Cryptococcus/cryptococcosis, 384, 384f
HIV-related, 401, 403
prophylaxis, 406b
Cryptogenic cirrhosis, 961
Cryptogenic eosinophilic pneumonia, 713b
Cryptogenic fibrosing alveolitis *see* Pulmonary fibrosis, idiopathic
Cryptogenic organising pneumonia (COP), 708b
Cryptorchidism, 759
Cryptosporidia/cryptosporidiosis, 309b, 369, 888
HIV/AIDS patients, 399b, 399f
Crystal formation, 223, 468, 522b, 1086–1087
Crystal shedding, 1086f
Crystal-associated disease, 1086–1092, 1086b, 1086f
Crystalloids, 855b, 1011b
CSF *see* Cerebrospinal fluid
CSS *see* Churg-Strauss syndrome
CT *see* Cognitive therapy
CT (computed tomography)
adrenal adenoma, 781f
angiography, 469, 537, 537f, 1236f
aortic dissection, 606f
brain, 1156b
abscess, 1208f
intracerebral haemorrhage, 1239f, 1246
metastases, 1214f
cancer diagnosis, 269, 269f
cerebral abscess, 1208f
gastrointestinal tract, 846, 847b, 847f
colorectal cancer, 915f
pancreatic cancer, 896f
pancreatic necrosis, 892f
pancreatic pseudocyst, 891f
pancreatitis, 894f
goitre, 753f
Graves' disease, 750f
head, 1156b
hepatobiliary disease, 930–931, 931f, 956f, 970f, 983f
hepatocellular carcinoma, 967f
high-resolution, 651
lymphoma, 1043f
musculoskeletal disease, 1065
neuro-endocrine tumour, 785f
neurological disease, 1149b
brain tumours, 1180b
cerebral abscess, 1208
cerebrovascular disease, 1150f
epilepsy, 1182b
meningitis, 1203
stroke, 1235f, 1239f, 1240b, 1241f
viral encephalitis, 1206
phaeochromocytoma, 782f
pulmonary angiography, 722, 723f
renal disease, 469, 970f
respiratory disease, 650–651, 651f
aspergilloma, 698f
bronchiectasis, 679f
hypersensitivity pneumonitis, 720f
interstitial lung disease, 709f
pleural thickening, 718f
pulmonary fibrosis, 709f
rheumatic disease, 696b, 712f
spine, 1221f
spiral, 1149
Cullen's sign, 890–891
Culture
blood, 140f
stool, 307
Cupulolithiasis, 1186
CURB score, 685b
Curettage
cancer, 281
skin disease, 1268
Cushing's disease, 773
management, 776
Cushing's syndrome, 773–776
aetiology, 773, 773b
classification, 773b
clinical features, 773–774, 773f
hirsutism, 763b
investigations, 774–776, 774f
management, 776
Cutaneous larva migrans (CLM), 375–376, 375f
CVP *see* Central venous pressure
CVS *see* Chorionic villus sampling
CX *see* Circumflex artery
Cyanide poisoning, 209b
Cyanosis, 1158b
congenital heart disease, 631
Cyclic citrullinated peptide, antibodies to, 1067
Cyclical vomiting syndrome, 877
Cyclin-dependent kinases (CDKs), 263
Cyclizine, 290b
Cyclo-oxygenase (COX), 1078, 1078f
Cyclo-oxygenase (COX) inhibitors, 1019b
Cyclopenthiazide, 611

Cyclophosphamide, 266b
  adverse reactions
  blood disorders
    autoimmune haemolysis
    non-Hodgkin's lymphoma, 1045
  bronchial carcinoma, 704
  Churg-Strauss syndrome, 1118
  glomerulonephritis, 500–501
  immunosuppression, 1017
  leukaemias, 1040, 1041b, 1045
  myositis, 1115
  neuromyelitis optica, 1193
  pemphigus, 1294
  rheumatic disease, 1101b
  SLE, 520, 1112
  vasculitis, 519, 520b, 1118
  warm autoimmune haemolysis, 1030
Cyclops spp., 375
Cyclospora cayetanensis, 369
Cyclospora infections, 369
Cyclosporiasis, 369
Cylindromatosis enzyme, 48–49
Cypermethrin, 224b
Cyproterone acetate, 765b
  acne, 1267, 1282
  alopecia, 1297
  prostate cancer, 518
Cystathionine β-synthase deficiency, 449
Cystectomy, 517
Cysteine, 114b
  stones, 507b
Cystic fibrosis (CF), 680–681, 895, 981
  adolescents, 681b
  bronchiectasis, 680–681
  clinical features, 680–681, 680f
  complications, 680b
  genetics/inheritance, 58b, 680–681
  management, 681, 681b
    gene therapy, 681
Cystic fibrosis transmembrane conductance regulator (CFTR), 48
Cystic kidney diseases, 505–507
Cysticercosis, 379f, 380
Cystinosis, 521, 794b
Cystinuria, 509–510
Cystitis, 513b
Cystoscopy, 517
Cystourethrography, micturating, reflex nephropathy, 505f
Cysts
  Baker's (popliteal), 1076b, 1098
    ruptured, 1098
  choledochal, 981, 981f
  colloid, 1212b–1213b
  hepatic, 380–381
  hydatid, liver, 380–381, 956–957, 956f
Cytarabine (Ara-C)
  acute leukaemia, 1037b
  chronic myeloid leukaemia, 1040
Cytochrome bc1 complex, 46b
Cytochrome c oxidase, 46b
Cytochrome P450, 22
Cytogenetic analysis, 269
Cytokeratin, as tumour marker, 268
Cytokine receptor deficiencies, 79
Cytokines, 74
  asthma, 667
  cancer, 265
  deficiencies, 79
  immune response regulation, 74b
  pro-inflammatory, 82, 1121
Cytomegalovirus (CMV) infection, 317b, 321–322
  bone marrow transplants, 1017b
  hepatitis, 955
  HIV/AIDS patients
    encephalitis, 402
    prophylaxis, 406b
    retinitis, 404
  liver transplant patients
  polyradiculitis, 404
  in pregnancy, 314b
  prophylaxis, 406b
  stem cell transplantation, 1017b
Cytopathic hypoxia, 185
Cytosine, 42
Cytoskeleton, 47–48
Cytotoxic drugs *see* Chemotherapy; and names of specific drugs
Cytotoxin-associated gene (cagA), 872f

D
D-dimers
  pulmonary embolism, 722
  reference values, 1312b
  venous thromboembolism, 722
d4T *see* Stavudine
Dabigatran etexilate, indications, 567, 1018b
Dacarbazine, Hodgkin's disease, 1043
Dactylitis, 1109f
Dalfopristin, 151b, 159
Dandruff, 1284
Dantrolene, 249
Dantron, 917b
Dapsone, 1268
  adverse reactions, 158
  with chlorproguanil (Lapdap), 356
  dermatitis herpetiformis, 855
  erythema nodosum, 1303
  haemolysis from, 1031
  leprosy, 349b
  linear IgA disease, 1294
  malaria, 356
  neutropenia, 1005b
  Pneumocystis jirovecii pneumonia, 406
  poisoning, 209b, 212
  prophylactic, 153b
  pyoderma gangrenosum, 1299
Dapsone syndrome, 158
Daptomycin, 151b, 159
  mechanism of action, 150b
Darunavir, 407b
Daunorubicin, acute leukaemia, 1037b
DCCT (Diabetes Control and Complications Trial), 827
DDAVP *see* Desmopressin
ddI *see* Didanosine
DDT, 224b, 1048b
de Musset's sign, 623b
De novo mutations, 59
De Quervain's tenosynovitis, 1075
De Quervain's thyroiditis, 751–752
'Dead-in-bed syndrome', 815
Deafness, 1173
  Alport's syndrome, 502
  gentamicin-induced, 27b
  Lassa fever, 325b
  Paget's disease, 1129
  Pendred's syndrome, 744f
  quinine toxicity, 215
  rubella, 315b
  salicylate overdose, 212, 615
Death and dying, 284f, 290–292
  advance directives, 171, 291
  brainstem death, 203
  care in, 291, 291b
  diagnosis, 291
  ethical issues, 291–292
  talking about, 290–291
  see also Brain death; Palliative care; Sudden death
Debrisoquine, 69
DEC *see* Diethylcarbamazine
Decision making *see* Clinical decision making
Declaration of Geneva, 11
Decompression, musculoskeletal disease, 1133
Decompression illness
  aviators, 107
  divers, 109, 109b
Deep venous thrombosis (DVT) *see* Venous thrombosis/thromboembolism
DEET (diethyltoluamide), malaria prevention, 358
Defecation
  disorders of *see* Constipation; Diarrhoea
  obstructed, 850
Defensins, 843
Defibrillation, 557, 577
  external, 577
  implantable cardiac defibrillator
    heart failure, 553, 553f
    hypertrophic cardiomyopathy, 638
    ventricular arrhythmias, 579, 579b
  myocardial infarction, 557
  public access, 558
Dehydration
  cerebral, hypernatraemia, 439
  cholera, 344
  diabetics, 804
  gastric outlet obstruction, 875–876
  heat illness, 104f, 106
  intestinal resection, 885b
  see also Water, body, depletion
Dehydroepiandrosterone (DHEA), 778
Déjerine-Klumpke paralysis, 1225b
Deletions, 55, 56b
Delirium, 250, 1161
  cognitive impairment, 114
  critically ill patients, 203
  diagnosis, 174b
  older people, 173–175, 173b
  prevalence, 232b
  terminal illness, 290
Delirium tremens (DTs), 253
Delta virus *see* Hepatitis D virus
Delusional disorders, 248, 248b
Delusional parasitosis, 245
Delusional perception, 247–248
Delusions, 234, 236–237
  differential diagnosis, 237
  schizophrenia, 237
Demeclocycline, 438–439
Dementia, 250–251
  aetiology, 250, 250b
  alcoholic, 253
  fronto-temporal, 252, 252f
  HIV-associated, 402–404
  investigations, 251, 251b
  Lewy body, 252
  management, 251–252
  vascular, 250b
  see also Alzheimer's disease
Demography, older people, 168, 168f
Demyelinating polyneuropathy
  acute inflammatory *see* Guillain-Barré syndrome
  chronic, 1225
Demyelination
  acute disseminated encephalomyelitis, 1192–1193
  Guillain-Barré syndrome, 1224–1225, 1225b
  multiple sclerosis, 1188–1192
  transverse myelitis, 1193, 1193b
  vitamin B_{12} deficiency, 129, 1024b
Dendritic cells, 74, 1141
Dendritic ulcers, 326
Dengue haemorrhagic fever, 309b, 322–323, 322b–323b, 322f, 325b
  incubation period, 145b, 310b, 322b, 325b
  pregnancy, 314b
Denosumab, osteoporosis, 1123b
Dense deposit disease, 501
Dental caries, fluoride and, 132
Dentatorubral-pallidoluysian atrophy (DRPLA), 65, 1199b
  genetics, 56b
Deontological ethics, 10, 13
Deoxycoformycin, 1041
11-Deoxycorticosterone, 782
11-Deoxycorticosterone-secreting adrenal tumour, 780b
Depolarisation, cardiac muscle, 529–530
Depression, 235, 243–244
  aetiology, 243
  alcohol and, 253
  assessment, self-poisoning and delusions and hallucinations, 234, 236–237
  diagnosis, 243
  differential diagnosis, 235
  management, 243–244
  see also Antidepressants
  manic (bipolar disorder), 243–245
  and medical illness, 244b
  negative cognitive triad, 241b
  older people, 238b
  in palliative care patients, 290
  post-partum, 257
  prevalence, 232b
  prognosis, 243–244
  stroke patients, 1243b
  symptoms, 235b
  unipolar, 243
Depressive adjustment disorder, 235
Dermatitis
  chronic actinic, 1260b
  exfoliative, 1304b
  herpetiformis, 272, 882, 1293b, 1294
  seborrhoeic, HIV/AIDS, 397
  see also Eczema
Dermatobia hominis, 381
Dermatofibroma, 1275
Dermatographism, 90, 1092–1093
Dermatomyositis/polymyositis, 1091b, 1114–1115, 1194b, 1300–1301
  cancer patients, 271b, 272
  nails in, 1115
  photoaggravation, 1298f
  respiratory complications, 712b, 1073
Dermatophytes/dermatophyte infection, 1279f
  nails in, 1279f
  see also specific infections
Dermatoscopy, 1255, 1256f
Dermatosis, acquired reactive perforating, 1303
Dermis, 1252
Dermoscopy, 1255
Des-aspargate-arginine vasopressin *see* Desmopressin
Desensitisation, 20–21
Desmin, 48
Desmoid tumours, 911–912, 911b
Desmopressin (DDAVP), diabetes insipidus, 794–795
Desmosomes, 1252
Desquamative interstitial pneumonia (DIP), 708b
Detrusor muscle, 466
  failure, 473
  overactivity, 473b
Detrusor-sphincter dyssynergia, 1174
Developing countries
  bladder stones, 507
  diabetic ketoacidosis, 811–812
  epilepsy, 1178–1179
  health-care provision, 9
  peptic ulcer, 850
  tetanus, 1209–1210
  tuberculosis, 696
Devic's disease, 1193

DEXA (dual energy X-ray absorptiometry)
bone mineral density, 760, 1065–1066
hyperparathyroidism, 769
musculoskeletal disease, 1066f
osteoporosis, 172, 1122
Dexamethasone
adjunctive, bacterial meningitis, 1204b
altitude illness, 107
brain tumours, 274, 1214
equivalent dose, 776b
gastrointestinal obstruction, 290
high-altitude cerebral oedema, 107
meningitis, 1204b
pain management, 288b
spinal cord compression, 272–273, 273b
thyrotoxicosis, 742–743
Dexamethasone suppression test (DST)
Cushing's syndrome/disease, 117, 775
hirsutism, 763–764
Dexamfetamine, 1187
Dextran, 1304b
Dextropropoxyphene, 217b
poisoning, 217b, 219
Dextrose, 433b
hypoglycaemia, 216, 357b
DFMO *see* Eflornithine
DHA *see* Docosahexaenoic acid
Di George syndrome, 80
genetics, 56b
Diabetes Control and Complications Trial (DCCT), 827
Diabetes insipidus, 794–795
causes, 794b
cranial (central), 787b, 794b
nephrogenic, 794b
Diabetes mellitus, 797–836
acromegaly, 806
acute myocardial infarction, 818
adolescents, 818, 818b
aetiology and pathogenesis, 802–807, 803f
air travel and, 108
atherosclerotic vascular disease and, 581, 826–827
bronzed diabetes, 972
cardiovascular disease risk prediction, 811
children, 818
classification, 807b, 809–810
clinical examination, 798f, 809–810
complications, 820, 826–835, 826b
pathophysiology, 827–828
prevention, 827–828
see also specific complications
cystic fibrosis and, 680b, 681
driving and, 810b
functional anatomy/physiology, 800–807
gestational, 807b
hyperglycaemic hyperosmolar state, 814, 814b
hypertension and, 810–811
investigations/diagnosis, 807–811, 809b
older people, 806b
latent autoimmune diabetes in adults, 810
long-term supervision, 811
management, 810–811, 820–826
alcohol intake, 821
dietary, 820–821, 820b
exercise, 821
goals, 811
insulin, 824–826, 824b
older people, 828b
oral hypoglycaemic drugs, 821–824
prevention of complications, 827–828
review, 811b
risk factors, 828
transplantation, 826
weight control, 821
maturity onset diabetes of the young (MODY), 807b
morbidity, 826b
mortality, 826b
musculoskeletal manifestations, 1133
nephropathy *see* Diabetic nephropathy
older people, 806b
patient education, 810
pregnancy and, 807b, 817–818
presenting problems, 808–820
prevalence, 800f
renal involvement, 519–520
surgery and, 818–820, 819b, 819f
type 1, 802–804
aetiology and pathogenesis, 803, 803f
clinical features, 809b
environmental factors, 804
genetic predisposition, 803–804
glycaemic control, 827b
HLA associations, 803–804
metabolic disturbance, 804, 804f
risk factors, 803b
sibling risk, 68b, 803b
type 2, 802–803, 805–806
aetiology and pathogenesis, 805–806, 805f
blood pressure control, 811, 811b
clinical features, 809b
environmental factors, 806
genetic predisposition, 806
glycaemic control, 827b
insulin resistance, 805
management, 811, 822b, 822f
metabolic disturbance, 806
multiple risk intervention, 831b
prevention of complications, 827–828
risk factors, 115b, 116f, 806b
vascular disease, 602, 602b, 826–827, 827f
visual loss, 830
Diabetic amyotrophy, 832
Diabetic foot, 602b, 833–835, 834b, 834f
Diabetic ketoacidosis, 804, 811–814, 812b
adolescents, 818b
clinical features, 812, 812b
investigations, 812–813
management, 813–814, 813b
pathogenesis, 812–814
pregnancy, 818
Diabetic microangiopathy, 826–827
Diabetic nephropathy, 830–831, 830b, 830f
pregnancy and, 818
Diabetic neuropathy, 799, 831–833, 832b–833b, 834f
Diabetic retinopathy, 799, 799f, 828–830, 829f
pregnancy and, 818
risk factors, 828b
Diagnosis, 33
interview, 4
investigations, 4–7
see also individual conditions
Diagnostic and Statistical Manual, American Psychiatric Association (DSM-IV) (4th ed)
Dialyser fluid, hypersensitivity to, 492b
Dialysis
amyloidosis associated with, 86b
gastrointestinal, 210
hyperkalaemia, 442–443
peritoneal, 492
poisoning, 207–208, 211
renal
AKI, 483, 491
CRF, 491
older people, 491b
SLE, 520
see also Haemodialysis
3,4-Diaminopyridine, Lambert-Eaton myasthenic syndrome, 1227–1228
Diamorphine
myocardial infarction, 593–594
palliative care, 287, 291
Diaphragm
acquired disorders, 731
congenital disorders, 731
diseases, 731
eventration, 731
Diarrhoea, 857
acute, 306–308, 857
assessment of patient, 306–308
causes, 306b
differential diagnosis, 306b
food poisoning and, 306
management, 307–308
after peptic ulcer surgery, 875
amoebic dysentery, 367–368
antibiotic-associated, 138b, 308
bloody, 897b, 899
cholera, 344
chronic/relapsing, 857, 857b
diabetic, 832b–833b
faecal incontinence, 918, 918b, 1175
haemolytic uraemic syndrome
HIV/AIDS patients, 399–400, 399b
infective, 306–308
older people, 306b
inflammatory bowel disease, 899
irritable bowel syndrome, 907–908
malabsorption, 857–858
small bowel disease, 857b
traveller's, 310–311, 311b
viral, 306b
Zollinger-Ellison syndrome, 876
Diascopy, 1255
Diastematomyelia, 1222b
Diastolic dysfunction, 546b
Diathermy
bladder cancer, 517
cervical cancer, 281
endometrial cancer, 281
gastrointestinal bleeding, 848f
rectal papillomas, 378
Diazepam
acute poisoning, 218, 220, 222
adverse reactions, 26b
alcohol withdrawal, 253–254
convulsions, 220, 357b
disturbed behaviour, 237–238, 291
drug interactions, 28
in renal/hepatic disease, 36b
status epilepticus, 1159b
terminal agitation, 291
Diazoxide, 785
hypertrichosis, 1297, 1304b
Dibenzodiazepines, 249b
Dibenzothiazepines, 249b
DIC *see* Disseminated intravascular coagulation
Dichromate, 1285b
Diclofenac, 288b, 1079b, 1266
actinic keratosis, 1266, 1271
adjuvant analgesia, 288b
and gastrointestinal bleeding, 1079b
hepatotoxicity, 971
renal colic, 509
Didanosine (ddI), 403
Dieldrin, 224b
Dietary supplements, 123
Diethylcarbamazine (DEC), 163, 373
Diethylenepenta-acetic acid (DTPA), indium-labelled, 851b, 896
Dietitian, 2b
Dietl's crisis, 471
Diet(s)
cancer and, 266b, 913b
cholesterol levels and, 113, 114b, 451
cystic fibrosis, 681
diabetes
management, 820–821, 820b
type 2, 806
diverticulosis and, 916
dyslipidaemia management, 456
elimination, 868, 887
gallstones and, 981
gastric cancer risk, 878
gluten-free, 880–882
high-fibre, 916–917
hospital patients, 122–123
inflammatory bowel disease management, 904–905
irritable bowel syndrome management, 908–909
low-carbohydrate, 118b
low-fat, 118b
low-protein
chronic renal failure, 488
obesity, 118b
multiple sclerosis management, 1192
refeeding, 122b
renal failure
AKI, 483
chronic, 488
starvation, 118–119
stone disease, 507b
vegan, 114, 1025
very low calorie, 118–119
vitamin B_{12} deficiency, 1025
weight reduction, 118–119, 118b
Diffuse idiopathic skeletal hyperostosis (DISH), 1133–1134, 1134f
Diffuse infiltrative lymphocytosis syndrome (DILS), 404, 404f
Diffuse parenchymal lung disease (DPLD), 706–711
classification, 707f
diagnosis, 706b
investigations, 708, 708b
DiGeorge syndrome, 80, 629–630, 770
Digestion, 841–843
malabsorption, 857–858, 857b, 858f
Digital subtraction angiography (DSA), 601–602
Digitalis, adverse reactions, 26b
Digoxin
adverse reactions, 26b
arrhythmias, 575b, 576–577
atrial fibrillation, 565–566, 596
atrial flutter, 564
drug interactions, 28b
effect of old age, 36b
heart failure, 553
mitral valve disease, 618, 620b
plasma concentrations, 39b, 209b
pulmonary hypertension, 725
therapeutic monitoring, 39b
toxicity/poisoning, 209b, 215, 577b
Digoxin-specific antibody fragments (F(ab)), 215
Dihydrocodeine, 286
malignant disease, 286
musculoskeletal disease, 1078
poisoning, 217b
Dihydropyridines
angina, 586–587, 594
hypertension, 612, 613b
overdose, 214
see also individual drugs

1,25-Dihydroxycholecalciferol, 766
hypoparathyroidism, 770–771
osteoporosis, 1125
reference values, venous blood, 1310b
1,25-Dihydroxyvitamin D, 464–466, 486–488
Diiodotyrosine (DIT), 738b
Diloxanide furoate, 164, 368
Diltiazem
angina, 586–587, 587b
unstable, 594
aortic dissection, 607
arrhythmias, 574f, 576
atrial fibrillation, 536–537
hypertension, 612
skin reactions, 1304b
Diltiazem cream, anal fissure, 919
Dilute Russell viper venom time (DRVVT), 1055
2,3-Dimercapto-propane sulphonate (DMPS), 224b
2,3-Dimercaptosuccinic acid (DMSA), 224b
technetium-labelled (99mTc-DMSA), 471
DIP *see* Desquamative interstitial pneumonia
Diphencyprone, 1278–1279
Diphenoxylate, 308, 883
Diphenylbutylpiperidines, 249b
2,3-Diphosphoglycerate (DPG), 994–995
Diphtheria, 138b, 345–346, 345b
chemoprophylaxis, 153b
immunisation, 346
incubation period, 145b, 345
laryngeal obstruction, 345, 728
Diphyllobothrium latum, 378
DIPJs (distal interphalangeal joints), psoriatic arthritis, 1108, 1109f
Diplopia, 1169–1170
diabetics, 832
Graves' disease, 735b, 750f
intracranial hypertension, 1217–1218
myasthenia gravis, 1226
Dipyridamole
platelet inhibition, 1050
stroke prevention, 1245b, 1245f
Directly observed therapy (DOT), tuberculosis, 695
Dirofilaria immitis, 375
Disability
critically ill patients, 189
International Classification of Functioning and Disability, 176b
older people, 170
Disability-adjusted life years (DALY), 9
Discoid eczema, 1284
Discs, intervertebral *see* Intervertebral discs
Disease-modifying antirheumatic drugs (DMARDs)
osteoarthritis, 1086
psoriatic arthritis, 1109
reactive arthritis, 1108
rheumatoid arthritis, 1101b, 1102
DISH *see* Diffuse idiopathic skeletal hyperostosis
Disopyramide
arrhythmias, 574, 575b
cardiomyopathy, 638
vasovagal syncope, 555–556
Disseminated intravascular coagulation (DIC), 201, 496, 1000, 1055–1056, 1056b
Dissociative (conversion) disorder, 246, 246b
Distal interphalangeal joints (DIPJs), psoriatic arthritis, 1108, 1109f
Distribution, 22
interactions, 28
volume of distribution, 22
Disturbed behaviour, 237–238, 237f
Disulfiram, 254
DIT *see* Diidotyrosine
Dithranol, 1265–1266
Diuretics
adverse reactions, 26b, 176b, 436, 436b
ascites, 940
clinical use, 435–436
dosage regimen, 35b
drug interactions, 28b
heart failure, 551, 552f
hypertension, 611, 613b
loop, mechanisms of action, 19–20, 435
mitral regurgitation, 620b
mode of action, 434–435
obliterative cardiomyopathy, 638
oedema, 434–436
osmotic, 435
potassium-sparing, 435, 551
resistance, 436
skin reactions, 1304b
tricuspid regurgitation, 625
see also Thiazides
Diverticulitis, acute, 862
Diverticulosis, 916–917, 916f
bleeding, 916
jejunal, 847f
Diving effects/illness, 109–110, 109b
Dizziness, 1157–1159, 1158f
older people, 173, 1158b
DMARDs *see* Disease-modifying antirheumatic drugs
DMPS *see* 2,3-Dimercapto-propane sulphonate
DMSA *see* 2,3-Dimercaptosuccinic acid
DNA, 42
analysis, neurological disease, 1153
copy number, 62
microarrays, 62
mitochondrial (mtDNA), 169
nuclear chromosomal, 168
probes, 62f, 696
proviral, 391–392
repair/repair enzymes, 50, 55–56
replication, 49
sequence analysis, 61f
transcription, 42–43
DNAase, recombinant human, cystic fibrosis, 681b
Dobutamine, circulatory effects, 191b
Docosahexaenoic acid (DHA), 113, 458
Doctor-patient relationship, 2–4, 3f
communication, 4b
difficulties in, 2–4
ethical issues, 9–13
Doctors, 2b
duties of, 3b
Docusate, 917b
Döhle bodies, 1050
Dolorplus pain scale, 285
Dominant negative mutations, 58
Domperidone, 1177
Donath-Landsteiner antibody, 1031
Donepezil, 252
Donovan bodies, 363
Donovanosis, 424b
Dopamine, low-dose, AKI, 482b
Dopamine agonists
acromegaly, 793
Parkinson's disease, 1197, 1197b
pregnancy, 792
prolactinoma, 791–792, 791b
and renal dysfunction, 522b
restless legs syndrome, 1187–1188
Dopamine antagonists
gastroparesis, 833b
and prolactin concentrations, 790–791
Dopamine dysregulation syndrome, 1196–1197
Dopexamine, circulatory effects
Doppler echocardiography, 536–537, 536f
aortic dissection, 606–607, 606f
atrial septal defect, 633f
colour flow Doppler, 536f, 606f
interventricular septum rupture, 597
valvular heart disease, 536f, 613–614, 617b, 617f, 619f, 621b, 623f
Doppler ultrasound
haemorrhoids, 918–919
hepatobiliary disease, 930, 976
leg ulcers, 1262
mitral stenosis, 617f
oesophageal, cardiac output monitoring, 187, 187f
renal, 480b–481b
venous thromboembolism, 722
Doripenem, 154b
Dose-response curves, 19–20, 19f
Dosulepin, 244b
DOT *see* Directly observed therapy, tuberculosis
Double duct sign, 986
Double vision *see* Diplopia
Down's syndrome (trisomy 21)
genetics, 56b
screening, 63b
Doxapram, 665, 678
Doxazosin, 612, 782
Doxorubicin
bronchial carcinoma, 704
cardiotoxicity, 639b
hepatocellular carcinoma, 968
liposomal, ovarian cancer, 280–281
non-Hodgkin's lymphoma, 1045
Doxycycline, 151b
anthrax, 347
bacillary angiomatosis, HIV/AIDS patients, 398
brucellosis, 334b
cholera, 345
filariasis, 373
leptospirosis, 338
louse-borne relapsing fever, 336
Lyme disease, 336
malaria, 356
melioidosis, 340
onchocerciasis, 374
plague, 339
Q fever, 352
reactive arthritis, 1108
relapsing fever, 336
rickettsial fevers, 352
skin eruptions, 1303f
skin infections, 1267
STIs
chlamydial infection, 423b
granuloma inguinale, 424b
lymphogranuloma venereum, 424b
syphilis, 421
Whipple's disease, 884
DPG *see* 2,3-Diphosphoglycerate
DPLD *see* Diffuse parenchymal lung disease
DPP-4 inhibitors, 822b, 824
Dracunculiasis (guinea worm), 375
Dracunculus medinensis, 375
Drainage
intercostal tube, 663, 730, 730f
postural, bronchiectasis, 679
DRESS, 1304b
Dressings, 1266, 1266b
Dressler's syndrome, 597
Dribble, post-micturition, 473
Drinking, problem, 100, 100f, 240, 252–254
Driving
diabetes and, 810b
epileptics, 1183b
Dronedarone, 565–566, 575b, 576
Drowning/near-drowning, 108, 108b, 109f
DRPLA *see* Dentato-rubro-pallidoluysian atrophy
Drug eruptions, 1289, 1303–1305, 1303b, 1303f
blisters, 1258, 1258b
clinical patterns, 1304b
diagnosis, 1305b
fixed, 1304b
maculopapular, 1289, 1304b
photosensitive, 1260b
rash, 398, 1257b
Drug history, 26b
Drug misuse, 240, 240b, 254–255
ecthyma, 1276–1277
hepatitis transmission, 955, 955b
infective endocarditis, 625
injecting drug users
Clostridium novyi, 299–300
compartment syndrome, 299–300
fever, 299–301, 300f
injection site infection, 299–301, 300f
polydrug misuse, 254
psychosis, 248
septic arthritis, 1094
spinal epidural abscess, 1209
stroke, 1242b
tetanus, 1209–1210
Drug resistance, 20
Drug therapy
adverse reactions, number needed to treat (NNT), 32, 1244b
balance of benefit to harm, 10, 33b
best evidence, 9
choice of, 33–34, 33b
clinical trials, 32, 32f
dosage regimen, 34
duration, 18b
evidence-based medicine, 32, 32f
frequency of administration, 23f
monitoring, 36, 39–40, 39b
odds ratio, 32f
older people, 36b
patient information, 35b
stopping, 36
timing of, 35b
topical, 21–22, 1264–1266, 1265b
see also Prescribing
Drug-related disorders
anaphylaxis/anaphylactoid reactions, 92b
aplastic anaemia, 1048b
asthma, 667–668
coagulopathy, 1051b
diabetes mellitus, 807b
dyskinesia, 249b
eosinophilia, 158
gynaecomastia, 762b
haemolysis, 1029b
heparin-induced, thrombocytopenia, 991
hyperpigmentation, 1296b
hyperprolactinaemia, 790b
leukaemia, 1035b
liver, 930b, 970–972, 971b
lungs, 714, 714b
lupus, 1068b, 1132b
musculoskeletal system, 1132b
gout, 1132b
osteomalacia, 1126b
osteoporosis, 1121b
nausea and vomiting, 290
neutropenia, 1005b
obesity, 117b
oesophagitis, 868
parkinsonism, 1166b, 1198
peripheral neuropathy, 403

photosensitivity, 1260b, 1304b
psychosis, 248b
renal, 480b, 483, 522–523, 522b
respiratory system, 708b, 714b
skin, 1304b
tardive dyskinesia, 26, 249b, 877
thrombocytopenia, 1007b
thyrotoxicosis, 742f
tremor, 1200b
see also Drug eruptions
Drugs
absorption/systemic availability, 21–22
adverse reactions, 24–28, 26b
classification, 25–27, 27b
dose-related, 20
inter-individual variation, 23–24, 24b
older people, 175–176, 176b
pharmacovigilance, 27–28
risk factors, 26b
TREND analysis, 27b
controlled, prescription, 29b, 31
development, 30–31, 30b
discovery, 30–31
distribution, 22
dosage regimen, 34
alteration in special circumstances, 36–37
repeated dose, 23, 23f
timing, 35b
dose-response curves, 19–20, 19f
efficacy, 19–20, 19f
excretion, 22
formulations
older people, 36b
prescription/nomenclature and, 26b, 29b
interactions, 28–29, 28b
avoidance of, 29
mechanisms, 28–29
pharmaceutical, 28b
pharmacodynamic, 28b
pharmacokinetic, 28b
licensing, 31
management of use, 31–33
marketing, 31
mechanisms of action *see individual drugs*
metabolism, 22
drug interactions and, 28–29
genetic influences, 24b
interactions, 28–29
older people, 36b
of misuse, 216–219
older people, 36b
overdose/poisoning, 212–216
drugs of misuse, 216–219
plasma concentrations, 39–40, 39b
potency, 20
prescribing *see* Prescribing
route of administration, 21–22, 34b
topical, 21–22
toxicity, 24
treatment endpoints, 39
DRVVT *see* Dilute Russell viper venom time
Dry drowning, 108
DSA *see* Digital subtraction angiography
DSM-IV, 232
DST *see* Dexamethasone suppression test
DTPA *see* Diethylenepenta-acetic acid
DTs *see* Delirium tremens
Dual energy X-ray absorptiometry *see* DEXA
Dubin-Johnson syndrome, 937b
Duchenne muscular dystrophy, 54b, 1228b
inheritance, 1228b
Ductopenia, 970–971
Ductus arteriosus, persistent, 631, 631f
closure device, 632
incidence, 630b
with reversed shunting, 632
Dukes classification of tumours, 914f
Duloxetine, pain management, 288b
Dumping syndrome, 875
Duodenal switch, 119b
Duodenal ulcers, 868b, 872–876
management, 874–875
surgery, 874–875, 874b
Duodenogastro-oesophageal reflux, 866–867
Duodenum, functional anatomy, 840f
Duplications, 55–56, 57f
Dupuytren's contracture/disease, 1133–1134
cirrhosis, 944
diabetes, 799b
Duroziez's sign, 623b
Dusts, lung disease and, 719–720, 719b
Dutasteride, 515
Duties of doctor, 3b
DVT *see* Deep venous thrombosis
Dwarfism
Laron, 786b
zinc deficiency, 131–132
DXA *see* DEXA
Dying *see* Death and dying
Dysaesthesia, 658b
multiple sclerosis, 1192b
Dysarthria, 1168–1169, 1173–1174
causes, 1169b
Dysbetalipoproteinaemia, 455
Dysdiadochokinesis, 1145
Dysentery
amoebic, 367–368
bacillary, 145b, 345
management, 345
Shigella, reactive arthritis and, 345
Dysexecutive syndrome, 1175
Dysgraphia, 1167
Dyshormonogenesis, congenital thyroid disease, 755–756
Dyslexia, 1167
Dyslipidaemia
diabetes, 805, 809
role of statins, 811
type 2, 805, 810
management, 456–458
pregnancy, 434
Dysmetria, 1145
ocular, 1171
Dysmorphic syndromes, 66
Dyspepsia, 852
alarm features, 852b
causes, 852b
functional, 876–877
gallstone, 982–983
investigation, 853f, 876
non-ulcer, 907
Dysphagia, 399, 851, 1173–1174
causes
bronchial carcinoma, 701
oesophageal cancer, 270b
oesophageal dysmotility, 850
gastro-oesophageal reflux, 865–868, 865f
investigation, 851, 852f
stroke patients, 1242–1243
Dysphasia, 1168–1169
Dysphonia, 1168
Dyspnoea *see* Breathlessness
Dysthymia, 243
Dystonia, 1166–1167, 1166b, 1200
poisoning, 211b
Dystrophia myotonica, 250b, 1172b
Dysuria, 471

E

E-cadherin gene, mutations, 878
E3 ligases, 46
Ears
examination, critically ill patients, 200b
freezing injuries, 105
infections of, 108, 314, 332b, 346
squamous cell carcinoma, 1271
Eastern Cooperative Oncology Group (ECOG) performance scale, 268, 268b
Eating disorders, 255–256, 256b
Ebola virus disease, 324, 325b
Ebstein's anomaly, 635b
EBV *see* Epstein-Barr virus
Ecchymosis, 1007
definition, 1251b
Eccrine glands, 1254
ECF *see* Extracellular fluid
ECF (epirubicin, cisplatin and 5-fluorouracil), 879
ECG (electrocardiography), 532–534, 533f
acute coronary syndromes, 541f–542f, 591
AKI, 480b
ambulatory (Holter monitoring), 534
angina, 584–585
aortic dissection, 606–607
aortic regurgitation, 624b
aortic stenosis, 622f
artificial pacemaker, 578f
atrial ectopic beats, 564f
atrial fibrillation, 565f
atrial flutter, 564f
AV block, 571f–572f, 572b
AV nodal re-entrant tachycardia, 568f
cardiac cycle, 561f
cardiac tamponade, 545–546
critically ill patients, 185–187
endocarditis, 628
exercise (stress), 529f, 534, 567f, 584f
hyperkalaemia, 440f
hypokalaemia, 440f
left ventricular hypertrophy, 622f
mitral stenosis, 617
myocardial infarction, 534, 592–593, 592f–593f
myocardial ischaemia, 534
pacemaker, 578f
pericarditis, 639, 640f
potassium balance disorders, 440f
pulmonary embolism, 721b, 722
reading, 533b
sinoatrial disease, 563f
standard 12-lead, 532–534, 533b
supraventricular tachycardia, 567f
syncope, 555–556, 555f
tachyarrhythmias, 567f
torsades de pointes, 571f
tricyclic antidepressant poisoning, 213f
ventricular ectopic beats, 569f
ventricular fibrillation, 557
ventricular tachycardia, 570f
Wolff-Parkinson-White syndrome, 568f
Echinocandins, 160, 160b
Echinococcus granulosus, 309b, 312b, 378, 380–381, 956–957
life cycle, 380f
Echocardiography (ECHO), 536–537
angina, 593
aortic dissection, 606f
aortic stenosis, 622f
atrial septal defect, 633f
cardiac tamponade, 545–546
critically ill patients, 187
Doppler, 536–537, 536f
ventricular septal defect, 634
endocarditis, 627–628
four-chamber view, 536f
heart failure, 549
hypertrophic cardiomyopathy, 638
indications, 536b
left ventricular hypertrophy, 632
mitral regurgitation, 619f
myocardial infarction, 593
myocarditis, 636
papillary muscle rupture, 597
pericardial effusion, 640f
pulmonary embolism, 723
stress, 537, 554
tetralogy of Fallot, 635
three-dimensional, 537
transoesophageal, 187, 537
two-dimensional, 536
valvular disease
aortic, 621, 624
mitral, 617–618
tricuspid, 624
ventricular aneurysm, 597–598
Echovirus, 319, 326–327
ECOG (Eastern Cooperative Oncology Group) performance scale, 268
Econazole, 160b, 417b
Economics, 9
cost-effectiveness of treatment, 32, 32b
health care resources, 9
medicine in low-resource settings, 9
screening programmes, 7b
Ecstasy (drug), 217–218
ECT *see* Electroconvulsive therapy
Ecthyma, 1276–1277
Ectoparasites, 381
Ectopia lentis, 449
Ectopic beats
atrial, 564, 564f
ventricular, 569, 569f
Ectopic pregnancy, 418, 423
Ectothrix, 1280
Eczema, 1283–1286
allergic contact, 1284–1286, 1285f
asteatotic, 1285
atopic, 1283–1284, 1284f
complications, 1284b
diagnosis, 1284b
management, 1286
pruritus, 1284, 1285b
rash, 1257b, 1284b
classification, 1283b
clinical morphology, 1283b
discoid, 1284
gravitational (stasis), 1254, 1286
investigation, 1285
irritant, 1284, 1286
nails in, 1298
management, 1285–1286
pruritus, 1258–1260, 1258b–1259b
seborrhoeic, 1284, 1286
HIV/AIDS, 397
Eczema herpeticum, 326, 326f
Eczema vaccinatum, 327
Edrophonium bromide, myasthenia gravis diagnosis, 1226
EDTA (ethylenediaminetetraacetic acid) clearance, 466b
Education
allergy, 90–91, 92b
asthma, 673
diabetes, 810
fibromyalgia, 1093–1094
food allergy, 888
heart failure, 550, 550b
hypoglycaemia, 816
infection control, 145b
insulin therapy, 810
leprosy, 350
musculoskeletal disease, 1077, 1078b
low back pain, 1073
osteoarthritis, 1085
public health issues, 345
Edwards' syndrome (trisomy 18), genetics, 56b

EEG (electroencephalography), 1151
dementia, 250
epilepsy, 1151, 1152f
hepatic encephalopathy, 942
sleep disorders, 1148, 1151
viral encephalitis, 1206
EFAs *see* Essential fatty acids
Efavirenz, 407b, 409
Efficacy, 19–20
Eflornithine creams, 764
Eflornithine (DFMO), trypanosomiasis, 164, 359b, 360
EHEC (entero-haemorrhagic *Escherichia coli*), 306, 343
Ehlers-Danlos syndrome, 1050
Ehrlichia chaffeensis, 334
Ehrlichiosis, 334
Eicosapentaenoic acid (EPA), 113, 458
EIEC (entero-invasive *Escherichia coli*)
Eikenella spp., 626
Eisenmenger's syndrome, 553, 631, 665–666
Ejaculatory failure, 1175
Ekbom's (restless leg) syndrome, 485–486, 1187–1188, 1188b
Elastase, faecal, 851b, 1311b
Elastin, 66
Elated mood *see* Mania
Elation, 235–236
Elbow pain, 1075, 1075b
Elderly *see* Older people
Elderly Mobility Scale, 177
Electrocardiography *see* ECG
Electroconvulsive therapy (ECT), 241
Electrodes, ion selective, 428b
Electrodessication, warts, 1278–1279
Electroencephalography *see* EEG
Electrofulguration, 426
Electrolyte balance, 429–430, 429b
assessment, in hospitalised patients, 434b
in renal failure
AKI, 480b, 482–483
chronic, 488
Electrolytes
absorption/secretion, 842–843, 843f
depletion, diabetic ketoacidosis, 812
distribution, 429, 429f
investigations, 429–430
normal distribution, 429
reference values, venous blood, 1308b
renal disease, 485
see also Bicarbonate; Chloride; Potassium; Sodium
Electromagnetic spectrum, 1261f
Electromyography *see* EMG (electromyography)
Electron microscopy, 139
cancer diagnosis, 269
sexually transmitted infections, 424
Electrophoresis, 428b
Elephantiasis, 372
non-filarial, 372
Elimination, 22–23
kinetics, 22–23, 23f
ELISA, 141–142, 142f
Clostridium difficile, 343–344
dengue fever, 323
hydatid cysts, 381, 956–957
leishmaniasis, 363–364
leptospirosis, 338
Lyme disease, 335
lymphatic filiarisis, 373
schistosomiasis, 378
strongyloidiasis, 370
Elliptocytes, 994
Elliptocytosis, hereditary, 1028
Embolism
acute limb ischaemia, 603, 603b
arterial gas, 109
during dialysis, 492b
myocardial infarction, 597
pulmonary *see* Pulmonary embolism/ thromboembolism
EMDR *see* Eye movement desensitisation and reprocessing
Emery-Dreyfuss muscular dystrophy, 1228b
EMG (electromyography), 1068, 1152
motor neuron disease, 1201
Emollients, 1264
erythroderma, 1264
pruritus, 1260
in pregnancy, 1259b
psoriasis, 1289b
Emphysema, 647
CT imaging, 675f
lung transplantation, 665–666, 665b
pathology, 674f
respiratory function abnormalities, 653b
Employment, sheltered, 249
Empyema, 662–663, 663b, 663f
subdural, 1209
tuberculous, 691f
Empyema necessitans, 662
Emtricitabine, 153b, 407b
Enalapril
heart failure, 552b
hypertension, 611
myocardial infarction, 599
Encephalitis
brainstem, 1206
CMV, 402
extrapyramidal, 1194b
limbic, 1194b
viral, 1205–1206
herpes simplex virus, 319
Japanese B, 328, 1205
mumps, 319
Nipah virus, 328
tick-borne, 309b
West Nile, 328, 1205
Encephalitozoon bieneusi, 399b
Encephalitozoon intestinalis, 399b
Encephalomyelitis
acute disseminated, 1192–1193
cancer-related, 272
multifocal, 1194b
Encephalomyopathy, mitochondrial neurogastrointestinal (MNGIE), 1229b
Encephalopathy
hepatic (portasystemic), 923b, 941–942, 941b
acute hepatic failure, 932
clinical grading, 933b
HIV-associated, 402
HSV, 326
hypertensive, 609
mitochondrial, 1199b, 1229b
transmissible spongiform, 329, 1211
Wernicke's, 128
End of life decisions, 291–292
Endocarditis
bartonellosis, 352
gonococcal, 422
infective, 625–629
for detailed entry see Infective endocarditis
Libman-Sacks, 1111
mitral valve, 618
Q fever, 352
Endocrine axes, 736f–737f
Endocrine diseases, 733–796
classification, 737b
clinical examination/ presentation, 734f–735f, 735b
genetic testing, 62b
investigation, 737, 737b
musculoskeletal manifestations, 1132–1133, 1133f
pathology, 736
presentation, 737–738, 738b
pruritus, 1259b
Endocrine function, chronic renal failure, 485
Endocrine glands, functional anatomy and physiology, 736
Endocrine therapy, prostate cancer, 518
Endocrine tumours, pancreatic, 896
Endocytosis, 48
Endometrial adhesions, 759
Endometrial cancer, 281
treatment, 281
Endometriosis, 919–920
Endophthalmitis, *Candida*
Endoplasmic reticulum (ER), 44–45
Endorphins, 288
Endoscopic retrograde cholangiopancreatography *see* ERCP
Endoscopy, 846–849
abdominal pain, 863
achalasia, 869
capsule, 848, 849f
corrosive oesophagitis, 224b, 868
double balloon, 848, 849b
dysphagia, 851
gastric cancer, 878
gastric outlet obstruction, 875–876
inflammatory bowel disease, 901
obscure major bleeding, 857f
oesophageal cancer, 870f–871f
oesophageal candidiasis, 399f
oesophageal varices, 946
older people, 850b
peptic ulcer, 873
pharyngeal pouch, 868
respiratory tract, 651–652
therapeutic
gastrointestinal haemorrhage, 848f, 855
oesophageal disease, 863
pancreatitis, 892
uses, 848f
upper gastrointestinal, 846, 848b, 855b
wireless capsule, 849b, 849f
Endosulfan, 224b
Endothelial cells
liver, 925
tumours, 1131b
Endothelin antagonists, 725
Endothelins, 547f
endothelin-1, 531, 547, 925f
Endothelium, 531–532
Endothrix, 1280
Endotoxin, 138
Endotracheal intubation, critically ill patients, 194, 194b
Energy
expenditure, 101, 111f
decreased, 121b
intake, 111f, 118
decreased, 121b
production, 45–46
requirements, 114b
Energy balance, 110–112, 111f
disorders of, 115–124
effects of alteration
older people, 122b
regulation of, 110–112, 112f
and reproduction, 112f
Energy therapies, 15
Energy-yielding nutrients, 110, 112–114, 124–132
WHO recommendations, 114b
Engerix, 955
Enophthalmos, 701
Entacapone, Parkinson's disease, 1197
Entactogens, 217–218
Entamoeba histolytica, 305, 308, 309b, 957
life cycle, 368f
liver abscess, 367
see also Amoebiasis
Entecavir, 161b, 162, 953, 953b
Enteral administration, 21
Enteral tube feeding, 123
Enteric fevers, 339–340
Enteric nervous system, 844–845
Enteritis, radiation, 885–886, 885b
Entero-haemorrhagic *Escherichia coli* (EHEC), 306, 343
Enterobacter spp., 137f, 151b
Enterobacteriaceae, 136f–137f
Enterobius vermicularis (threadworm), 371, 371f
Enterococci, endocarditis, 332b, 626b
Enterococcus faecalis, 137f, 151b, 332b
Enterococcus faecium, 137f, 151b, 332b
Enterocytes, 450–451
Enterohepatic circulation, 22
Enterokinase, 842
Enteropathic arthritis, 1109
Enteropathy, protein-losing, 886, 886b
Enteroscopy *see* Endoscopy
Enterovirus 71, 328
Enteroviruses, 326–327
respiratory infection, 328
Enthesis, 1063–1064
Enthesitis, 1108
Enthesopathy
gluteal, 1075b
knee, 1076b
Entrapment neuropathy, 1224, 1224b
Entropion, 353
Envenomation, 207–208, 207b, 207f, 224–230, 225b
diagnosis, 227–228
follow-up, 230
local effects, 226, 226b
management, 226–230, 229b
systemic effects, 226, 226b
Environment
early, and psychiatric disorders, 233
interactions of people with, 98
Environmental diseases, 100–110
air travel, 107–108
alcohol, 100, 100f
atmospheric pollution, 102
extremes of temperature, 103–106, 103b
high altitude, 106–108, 106f
infections, 133–164, 293–386
obesity, 101
poisoning, 223
poverty and affluence, 101–102, 101b
radiation exposure, 102–103, 102b
smoking, 100–101
under water, 108–110
Environmental factors in disease, 97–132
allergy, 89
asthma, 666
atopic eczema, 1283–1284
cancer, 266–267, 266b
diabetes mellitus
type 1, 804
type 2, 806
inflammatory bowel disease, 897
investigations, 99
cause and effect, 99
incidence and prevalence, 99, 99b
time, person and place, 99
nutrition, 110–115, 110f
older people, 102b
osteoporosis, 1121b
psychiatric disorders, 233

Environmental health effects, 98–99, 98f
Enzyme-linked immunosorbent assay *see* ELISA
Enzymes
drugs acting on, 19b
pancreatic
chronic pancreatitis, 894
cystic fibrosis management, 681
plasma, myocardial infarction, 593
Eosinophil chemotactic factor, 89b
Eosinophilia, 1005
atopy, 90
causes, 1004b
parasite infections, 312b
heart disease, 638
helminthic infections, 312b
investigation, 312b
pulmonary, drug-induced, 714b
tropical, 311–312, 312b, 373
Eosinophilic airway inflammation, 669
Eosinophilic gastroenteritis, 887
Eosinophilic granuloma, 1131b
Eosinophilic oesophagitis, 868
Eosinophilic pneumonia, 708, 713
Eosinophils, 995, 1004f
asthma, 669
count, 1312b
EPA *see* Eicosapentaenoic acid
EPEC (enteropathogenic *Escherichia coli*)
Ependymal cells, 1140–1141
Ependymoma, spine, 1215
Ephelides, 1274
Epidemiology, descriptive, 99b
Epidermal growth factor receptor, 263
Epidermal necrolysis, toxic, 1292, 1292b, 1292f, 1304b
Epidermis, 1252–1254, 1253f
Epidermolysis bullosa, 1292b
acquisita, 1293b, 1294–1295
dystrophic, 1269–1270, 1292b
junctional, 1292b
simplex, 48
Epidermophyton floccosum, 1279–1280
Epididymo-orchitis, 319, 513b
Epigenetic inheritance, 52f, 53, 54b
Epiglottitis, acute, 657
Epilepsy, 1178–1186
adolescents, 1185b
classification, 1179b
cysticercosis, 380
driving regulations, 1183b
genetics, 56b
investigations, 1182, 1182b
brain imaging, 1182b
EEG, 1151, 1152f
management, 1182–1185
anticonvulsant drugs, 1183–1184, 1183b–1184b
first aid, 1183b
lifestyle advice, 1183
monitoring, 1184
surgery, 1184
myoclonic epilepsy with ragged red fibres, 46b, 1199b, 1229b
older people, 1185b
pathophysiology, 1179–1186, 1179f
pregnancy/oral contraception, 1184–1185, 1185b
prognosis, 1183b, 1185
seizure types, 1180–1181
absence, 1181
atonic, 1181
clonic, 1181
focal, 1180, 1180b
myoclonic, 1181
tonic, 1181
tonic-clonic, 1180–1181, 1181b
temporal lobe, 235b, 237, 248
trigger factors, 1180b
Epilepsy syndromes, 1181–1182, 1181b–1182b
Epileptic spasms, 1181
Epimysium, 1063–1064
Epinephrine *see* Adrenaline
Epiphysis, 1060
femoral, 1081
Epirubicin, 879
Episcleritis, rheumatoid arthritis, 1099
Epistaxis
cirrhosis, 1017b
dengue fever, 323
granulomatosis with polyangiitis, 1118
leptospirosis, 337
systemic vasculitis, 1116b
Epithelial membrane antigen (EMA), as tumour marker, 268
Eplerenone
heart failure, 551
mineralocorticoid excess, 781
myocardial infarction, 599
Epley manoeuvre, 1186
Epo *see* Erythropoietin
Epoprostenol *see* Prostacyclin
Epoxy resin, 1285b
EPs *see* Evoked potentials
Epstein-Barr virus (EBV), 317b
cancer and, 266b, 405b
complications, 320, 321b
hepatitis, 948
infectious mononucleosis, 320, 320b
primary CNS lymphoma, 303
Eptifibatide, platelet inhibition, 997
Epworth sleepiness scale, 726b, 1187
ER *see* Endoplasmic reticulum
Erb-Duchenne paralysis, 1225b
ERCP (endoscopic retrograde cholangiopancreatography), 849, 850b, 931, 931f
cholangiocarcinoma, 986f
cholangitis, 966, 985, 985f
cholecystitis, 984
choledocholithiasis, 984f
pancreatic cancer, 895
pancreatitis, acute, 892
Erectile dysfunction, 436b, 474, 474b, 1175
diabetics, 833
haemochromatosis, 972
multiple sclerosis, 1192
Ergocalciferol, 1127
Ergotamine, 1177
Erlotinib, 279, 704
Erosion
cartilage/bone, 1064
skin, definition, 1251b
Ertapenem, 151b, 154b
Erysipelas, 1277, 1277f
Erythema
annular, 1303
drug-induced, 1303b
palmar, 253b, 740, 741b, 922f, 943
pressure sores, 1300
Erythema ab igne, 741b, 892–893
Erythema infectiosum, 316b
Erythema marginatum, 615
Erythema migrans, 335f
Erythema multiforme, 1260b, 1302–1303, 1302b, 1302f, 1304b
Erythema nodosum, 1303, 1303b
Erythema nodosum leprosum, 349
Erythrasma, 1278
Erythroblasts, 994
Erythrocyte sedimentation rate (ESR), 84–85
De Quervain's thyroiditis, 751
older people, 1001b
pneumonia, 684b
reference values, 1312b
rheumatic disease, 1097b
unexplained raised, 84b, 85
weight loss in HIV, 396
Erythrocytes *see* Red cells
Erythrocytosis, 1003b
Erythroderma, 1264
Erythroid cells, 992
Erythroid nests, 992f
Erythromycin, 151b
acne, 1282
bartonellosis, 352–353
cellulitis/erysipelas, 1277
diphtheria, 346
erythrasma, 1278
impetigo, 1276
Lyme disease, 335
pneumonia, 685b
in pregnancy, 154b
prophylactic, 153b
relapsing fever, 336
rheumatic fever, 615–616
rosacea, 1283
skin infections, 1267
STIs
chancroid, 424b
chlamydial infection, 423b
granuloma inguinale, 424b
lymphogranuloma venereum, 424b
syphilis, 421
tetanus, 1210
Erythronychia, 1298
Erythropoiesis
impairment in erythrovirus infection, 1028
ineffective, 1024
Erythropoietic porphyria, congenital, 460b
Erythropoietic protoporphyria, 460b
Erythropoietin (Epo), 992–994
chronic renal failure, 485b
ectopic production, 271b
inappropriate secretion, 1003–1004
myelodysplastic syndrome, 1041
recombinant human, chronic renal failure, 488
renal adenocarcinoma, 516
Erythropoietin (Epo) receptor, 49b
Erythrovirus *see* Parvovirus B19
Eschar
anthrax, 346
rickettsial, 350
scrub typhus, 313f, 350
Escherichia coli, 134, 137f, 138b, 304b
bacterial meningitis, 1202b
entero-aggregative (EAEC), 343
entero-haemorrhagic (EHEC), 306, 343
entero-invasive (EIEC), 342
enteropathogenic (EPEC), 343
enterotoxigenic (ETEC), 342–343
food poisoning, 306, 342–343
spontaneous bacterial peritonitis, 941, 941b
verocytotoxigenic (VTEC), 343f, 496
Escitalopram, 244b
Espundia, 366–367
ESR *see* Erythrocyte sedimentation rate
Essential fatty acids (EFAs), deficiency, 113
Essential tremor, 1166b, 1199
ESWL *see* Extracorporeal shock wave lithotripsy
Etanercept, 1103b
ETEC (enterotoxigenic *Escherichia coli*), 342–343
Ethambutol
adverse reactions, 694b
Mycobacterium avium complex, 406b
opportunistic mycobacterial infection, 406b
and peripheral neuropathy, 1223b
tuberculosis, 693, 694b
Ethanol
pharmacokinetics, 25b
poisoning, 209b
reference values, 1310b
see also Alcohol
Ethical analysis, 12–13, 13b
Ethics, 9–13
artificial nutritional support, 124, 124b
clinical, 10–11
types of problem, 11–12, 12f
definition, 14b
deontological, 10, 13
end of life decisions, 291–292
genetic testing, 9–10
public health, 10
research, 10
situation, 10
teleological, 10, 13
virtue, 10
Ethosuximide, 1182b, 1184b
Ethylene glycol poisoning, 209b, 222–223, 222f
Ethylenediaminetetraacetic acid (EDTA) clearance, 466b
Etidronate
osteoporosis, 1123
Paget's disease, 1129, 1130b
Etodolac, 1079b
Etoposide
acute leukaemia, 1037b
bronchial carcinoma, 704
Etoricoxib, 1079b
Etravirine, 407b
ETT *see* Exercise testing
Eukaryotes, 135
Eumycetoma, 382
Eunuchoid habitus, 759
Euphoria, 235–236
Euthanasia, 292
Evidence-based medicine, 8, 8b
drug therapy, 32, 32f
Evoked potentials, 1152–1153
multiple sclerosis, 1190b
visual, 1153f
Evolutionary selection, 58
Ewing's sarcoma, 1131b
Examination, clinical *see individual body systems*
Exanthem subitum, 316
Exanthems
drug-induced, 1304b
enteroviral, 319
viral, 314–319
Exchange transfusion
hyperparasitaemia, 357
malaria, 357
megaloblastic anaemia, 1026
sickle-cell disease, 1033
Excoriation, definition, 1251b
Excretion, 22
Exenatide, 824
Exercise ECG, 534, 534b
Exercise testing
angina, 584–585, 584f
COPD, 675
myocardial infarction, 534b
respiratory disease, 654
Exercise(s)
arrhythmias and, 534b
asthma and, 668f
atherosclerotic vascular disease and, 581
chest pain and, 540
COPD, 676
diabetes, 821
headache and, 1178, 1178b
heart disease and, 584f
hypoglycaemia and, 810
and hypotension, 637–638
and insulin sensitivity, 810

musculoskeletal disease management, 1077–1078, 1078b
ankylosing spondylitis, 1107
fibromyalgia, 1094
osteoarthritis, 1085
Exertion headache, 1178, 1178b
Exons, 54f
Exophthalmos, Graves' disease, 735b, 741b
Extracellular fluid (ECF), 429
volume overload, 434
Extracorporeal membrane oxygenation therapy (ECMO), 196
Extracorporeal shock wave lithotripsy (ESWL), 985
Extractable nuclear antigens, antibodies to, 1067–1068
Extrapyramidal encephalitis, 1194b
Extrapyramidal gait, 1168
Extrapyramidal system, 1145
Extrasystoles, 564, 569
Extrinsic allergic alveolitis (EAA) *see* Hypersensitivity pneumonitis
Eye disorders
in diabetes, 799, 799f, 828–830, 829f
granulomatosis with polyangiitis, 1118f
Graves' disease, 735b, 741b
HIV/AIDS, 404
leprosy, 348–349
Eye movement desensitisation and reprocessing (EMDR), 242
Eyelid disorders, dermatomyositis, 1115f
Eyes
diabetes mellitus *see* Diabetic retinopathy
examination, diabetes mellitus, 799b
rheumatoid arthritis, 1099
Ezetimibe, 434

F

Fabry's disease, 433–434
Face
angioedema, 93f
frostbite, 105
hemifacial spasm, 1200
numbness, 1157
skin disease *see individual conditions*
superior vena cava obstruction, 273
Facial (7th cranial) nerve
palsy, 1163
tests, 1139b
Facial pain, 1156–1157
Facial warts, 1278
Facial weakness, 1163
Facioscapulohumeral dystrophy, 1228b
Factitious disorders, 247
Factitious fever, 298b
Factor II, 1051b
Factor IX, 1053
concentrates, 1053
deficiency, 1053
haemophilia B, 1053
Factor V, 997
Leiden variant, 1001b, 1009b, 1055
stroke, 1242b
Factor VII, 999–1000
deficiency, 1007, 1054
Factor VIII
antibodies, 1053
concentrates, 1051–1052
virus transmission, 1053
deficiency, 1051b
haemophilia A, 1051–1052
inhibitor bypassing activity (FEIBA), 1053
Factor X, deficiency, 1007, 1051b, 1054
Factor Xa, 1018–1019
Factor XI, deficiency, 1054
Factor XIII, 998f
deficiency, 1007, 1054
Faecal analysis, 1311b
Faecal antigen test, *Helicobacter pylori* infection, 856
Faecal continence, 844
Faecal impaction, 917
Faecal incontinence, 918, 918b, 1175
Faecal occult blood (FOB) testing, 916, 916b
Faints *see* Syncope
Fallot's sign, 635
Fallot's spells, 635
Falls
older people, 172–173, 172b
prevention, 172–173, 173b
Famciclovir
herpesvirus infection, 161–162, 161b, 318b
genital, 424–425
Familial adenomatous polyposis (FAP), 67, 267b, 910f–911f, 911–912, 911b
Familial cancer syndromes, 66–67
Familial hypercholesterolaemia, 48, 454b
Familial hypocalciuric hypercalcaemia, 767, 770
Familial Mediterranean fever (FMF), 85
Familial polyposis coli, 64
Family history, 60
allergic disease, 89
atherosclerotic vascular disease
genetic disease, 64
hypercholesterolaemia, 453–455
immune deficiency, 79b
melanoma, 1272–1273
ovarian cancer, 280
psoriasis, 1286
psychiatric disorders and, 234b
vitiligo, 1295
Family therapy, eating disorders, 255–256
Family tree *see* Pedigree
Famine, 120–121
Fanconi anaemia, 267b
Fanconi syndrome, 510
Fanconi's syndrome, 446
Fansidar, malaria, 163, 356
FAP *see* Familial adenomatous polyposis
Farmer's lung, 719b
Fasciculations, 221b, 223b–224b, 229b, 1139b, 1162b
Fasciculi, 1063–1064
Fascioliasis/*Fasciola hepatica*, 309b, 312b, 379b, 984
Fast
prolonged
hypoglycaemia diagnosis
lipids after
Fat, 113, 113f
body
distribution, 115–116
see also Obesity
diabetic diet, 821
dietary
energy provided by, 110
recommended intake, 114b
digestion/absorption, 842f, 850–851
malabsorption, small bowel disease, 883–884
normal metabolism, 800–802, 801f
Fatal familial insomnia, 329b, 1211
Fatigue
cancer patients, 271b
chronic fatigue syndrome, 246
fibromyalgia, 1093
multiple sclerosis, 1192b
primary biliary cirrhosis, 964
rheumatoid arthritis, 1098
Fatty acids
dietary, 114b
essential, 113
n-3, 434
non-esterified ('free') *see* Free fatty acids
polyunsaturated, 113f
trans, 113
transport, 45–46, 45f
Fatty liver
alcoholic, 958, 958b
microvesicular, 971, 978
non-alcoholic, 959–961, 960f
pregnancy, 978
Favism, 308, 1029b
FBC *see* Full blood count
FDPs *see* Fibrin degradation products
Febrile response, 138
Febuxostat, 1089
Feeding
enteral (tube), 123
cystic fibrosis, 681
pancreatitis, 892
short bowel syndrome, 885
malnutrition management, 121
parenteral, 123–124
Feet *see* Foot/feet
FEIBA, 1053
Feline spongiform encephalopathy (FSE), 1211
Felty's syndrome, 1100b
Femoral neck fractures, 1071
Femoral stretch test, 1073
Fentanyl, transdermal, 287
Ferritin
adult-onset Still's disease, 1104
anaemia of chronic disease, 1023b
haemochromatosis, 972
iron deficiency anaemia, 1023, 1023b
megaloblastic anaemia, 1024b
older people, 1034b
reference values, 1312b
Ferrous gluconate, 1023
Ferrous sulphate, 1023
Festination, 172b, 1168
Fetal circulation, 630f
Fetor hepaticus, 933–934
FEV_1 *see* Forced expiratory volume
Fever(s), 295–303, 297f
accompanying features, 295–296
cancer patients, 271
clinical examination, 296
injecting drug users, 299–301, 300f
patients in/from tropics, 309b
definition, 296
factitious, 298b
febrile response, as defence mechanism, 138
haemorrhagic *see* Haemorrhagic fevers
history-taking, 295b
injecting drug users, 299–301, 300f
returning travellers, 309b
HIV/AIDS, 396
immunocompromised host, 301–302
in/from tropics, 309–310, 309b–310b
injecting drug user, 299–301, 300f
investigations, 296
injecting drug users, 301, 301f
management, 296
injecting drug users, 301
neutropenic, 302, 302b
cancer patients, 274
older people, 296b
post-transplantation, 302–303, 302b
rashes and, 295b
recurrent, 295–296
symptoms and signs, 296
of unknown origin, 296–299
aetiology, 298b
clinical assessment, 296–298
investigations, 298–299, 299b
older people, 296b
prognosis, 299
Fexofenadine, 1267
FFAs *see* Free fatty acids
FFP *see* Fresh frozen plasma
FGF *see* Fibroblast growth factor
Fibrates
dysbetalipoproteinaemia management, 458
hyperlipidaemia management, 434, 458
muscle pain, 1077b, 1132b
Fibre, dietary, 113
Fibrin, 265f, 625, 996f–997f
Fibrin degradation products (FDPs), 201, 998f, 1000
Fibrinogen, 82
concentration, 1000b
deficiency, 1000b
reference values, 1312b
Fibrinoid necrosis, 609
Fibrinolysis, 531–532
Fibroblast growth factor (FGF), 271b
Fibroblasts, tumours, 1131b
Fibrodysplasia ossificans progressiva, 1091b
Fibrolamellar hepatocellular carcinoma, 969
Fibroma, 1131b
Fibromuscular dysplasia, renal artery stenosis, 494
Fibromyalgia, 1092–1094, 1092f–1093f, 1093b
investigations, 1093b
prevalence, 1060b
SLE, 1110
Fibrosarcoma, 1131b
Fibrosing alveolitis
cryptogenic *see* Pulmonary fibrosis, idiopathic
dyspnoea, 543b, 656b
in inflammatory arthritis, 1070b
systemic sclerosis, 1113
Fibrous/fibrocartilaginous joints, 1062
Fidaxomycin, 344
Fifth disease, 316b
Fight or flight response, 1254
Filaggrin, 1252
Filaments, intermediate, 48
Filariases, 309b, 312b, 372–375, 372b
incubation period, 310b
lymphatic, 372–373
Finasteride, 515, 765b
alopecia, 1297
Fine needle aspiration, thyroid nodules, 747
Fingers
clubbing, 644f
asbestosis, 718–719
lung cancer, 271, 701
osteoarthritis, 1083f
rheumatoid arthritis, 1098f
triggering, 799b, 1134
Fingolimod, 1192b
Finkelstein's sign, 1075
First-order kinetics, 22
First-pass metabolism, 21
Fish
allergy, 93b
ciguatera fish poisoning, 308
minerals in, 131b
scombrotoxic fish poisoning, 308
venom, 225b, 229b
vitamins in, 125b
Fish eye disease, 455–456, 456b
FISH (fluorescent in situ hybridisation)
Fish oils, 113, 125b
Fissure
anal, 919
skin, definition, 1251b

Fistulae
anorectal, 919
inflammatory bowel disease, 900, 905
tracheo-oesophageal, 728
see also different types
Fitz-Hugh–Curtis syndrome, 919
Flapping tremor (asterixis), 923b
Flat feet, 1098
Flaviviruses, 322–323
Flavonoids, 129
Fleas, 309b
bartonellosis, 352b
plague, 338–339
typhus, 351–352, 351b
Flecainide, 565–566, 568, 574, 575b
Flora, normal, 136–137, 137f
Flucloxacillin, 151b, 154b
cerebral abscess, 1208b
hepatotoxicity, 971
impetigo, 1276
infective endocarditis, 301, 628, 628b
pneumonia, 685b
septic arthritis, 1095b
staphylococcal infections, 301, 329–331
skin/soft tissue, 1267
Fluconazole, 159, 160b
acute leukaemia patients, 1038
candidiasis, 383
genital, 417b
HIV/AIDS patients, 398–399
cryptococcal infections, HIV-related, 403, 406b
cutaneous leishmaniasis, 367
paracoccidioidomycosis, 386
in pregnancy, 154b
prophylaxis, 406b
skin disease, 1267
Flucytosine, cryptococcal infections, 403
Fludarabine
chronic lymphocytic leukaemia, 1040
Waldenstrom's macroglobulinaemia, 1045
Fludrocortisone
adrenal insufficiency, 779, 779b
postural hypotension, 555–556
Fluid balance
assessment, hospitalised patients, 434b
heat exhaustion, 106
renal failure
acute, 483
chronic, 488
Fluid intake, 307
AKI, 482b
and polyuria, 472b
stone disease, 507b
urinary tract infection, 513b
Fluid loss
bullous skin disorders
diabetic ketoacidosis, 812
diarrhoeal illness, 307
see also Dehydration
Fluid replacement
acute diarrhoea, 307
bacillary dysentery, 345
cholera, 344–345
critically ill patients, 1011b
decompression illness, 110
diabetic ketoacidosis, 814
diving-related illness, 110
food poisoning, 301, 308
heat illness, 106
hospitalised patients, 434b
hyperglycaemic hyperosmolar state, 814b
intensive care unit, 199
intravenous
acute severe asthma, 672
decompression illness, 110
hypovolaemia, 433–434, 433b
older people, 813b
pneumonia, 685
short bowel syndrome, 885
sodium depletion, 433
Fluid resuscitation, 185, 189, 331–332, 1011b
Flukes (trematodes), 376–378
liver, 266b, 312b, 378
lung, 312b
Flumazenil, 217
Fluocinolone acetonide, 1265b
Fluorescent in situ hybridisation (FISH), 62f
Fluoride, 132
dietary sources, 131b
and osteomalacia, 1126b
poisoning, 132
RNI, 131b
Fluorimetry, 428b
5-Fluorocytosine, 160, 160b
Fluoroquinolones, 157, 157b
enteric fever, 340
leprosy, 350
plague, 338–339
skin reactions, 1304b
tuberculosis, 694
Fluorosis, 223
5-Fluorouracil (5-FU), 879
cancer therapy, 276
carcinoid tumour, 889
colorectal cancer, 915
gastric cancer, 879b
premalignant skin tumours, 1266, 1270b
Fluoxetine, 244b
bulimia, 256
fibromyalgia, 1094
Flupentixol, 249b
Flutamide, 765b
Fluticasone, 1265b
Fluvoxamine, 244b
FMF *see* Familial Mediterranean fever
Foamy macrophages, 514, 883
FOB *see* Faecal occult blood testing
Focal nodular hyperplasia (FNH), liver, 970
Focal segmental glomerulosclerosis (FSGS)
Folate antagonists, 158
Folate (folic acid), 129, 1025–1026
absorption, 1025
biochemical assessment of status, 126b
deficiency, 129, 1025–1026, 1025b
coeliac disease, 881
investigation, 1025b
management, 1026
myelofibrosis, 1048–1049
pregnancy, 1022b
dietary sources, 125b
haemolytic anaemia, 1028
prevention of neural tube defects, 125b, 129
reference values, 1312b
RNI, 125b
supplements
hereditary spherocytosis, 1028
periconceptual, 125b
tropical sprue, 882
Folate synthesis inhibitors, 163
Folinic acid
colorectal cancer, 915
toxoplasmosis, 362, 402
Follicle-stimulating hormone (FSH)
deficiency, 787b
reference range, 1309b
Follicular carcinoma, thyroid, 740b, 754
Folliculitis, 1276–1277
pruritic, 1259b
Fomepizole, 223
Fondaparinux, 1001b, 1019b
Fonsecaea, 382–383
Fonsecaea compacta, 381
Fonsecaea pedrosoi, 381
Food allergy, 888
Food hygiene, 147, 148f
Food intolerance, 887–888
irritable bowel syndrome, 907–909
Food poisoning
Bacillus cereus, 306, 341
Clostridium perfringens, 342
Escherichia coli, 306, 342–343
foods associated with, 307b
and gastroenteritis, 306b
listeriosis, 339
management, 307–308
non-infectious causes, 306b, 308
staphylococcal, 341
Foods
diabetic, 804
glycaemic index, 804
Foot drop, 172b, 1168
Foot/feet
arthritis, 1098
Charcot, 835
claw, 1076
cold injury (trench/immersion foot), 105
diabetic, 833–835, 834b, 834f
examination
blood disorders
diabetes, 799b, 799f
flat, 1098
pain, 1076
ulcer, 834–835
Forced expiratory volume (FEV_1), 653b
COPD, 675, 675b
older people, 648b
Forced expiratory volume/vital capacity (FEV_1/VC) ratio, 653b
COPD, 675, 675b
Forced vital capacity (FVC), 653b
Foreign bodies
inhalation, 655f
larynx, 728
Forest plot, 32f
Formication, 254
Formoterol, asthma, 670–671
Fortification spectra, 1170
Foscarnet
CMV infection, 322
herpesvirus infection, 161b, 162
Fosphenytoin, status epilepticus, 1159b
Fournier's gangrene, 305
Fractures, 1071
fragility, 1071b
high-energy, 1071b
hip, preventive measures, 172–173, 173b
investigation, 1071, 1071b
osteoporotic, 1121f, 1123b
prevention, 172–173, 173b
pain, 1071
pathological, 1071b
recurrent, 1125
repair, 1080b
stress (fatigue), 1071b
vertebral, 1071b
Fragile site mental retardation (FRAXE), genetics, 56b
Fragile X syndrome, 66
genetics, 56b
Fragile X tremor ataxia syndrome, 1199b
Frailty, 169–170, 170b
Frameshift mutations, 55
Francisella tularensis, 340
FRAXE *see* Fragile site mental retardation
FRC *see* Functional residual capacity
Freckles, 1274
Free fatty acids (FFAs), 113, 113f, 802
diabetes, 801f, 802, 804f
Free radicals, 82–83, 127, 957–958
Frequency of micturition, 472
Fresh frozen plasma (FFP), 1012b
Fried Frailty score, 170b
Friedreich's ataxia, 1199b
genetics/inheritance, 56b
Froin's syndrome, 1221
Frontal lobes, 1142
functions, 1142b
effects of damage, 1142b
Fronto-temporal dementia, 252, 252f
Frostbite, 105, 105f
Frosted branch angiitis, 404
Frozen shoulder, 1074–1075
Fructose, 112–113, 113b
Fructose intolerance, inherited, 510
FSE *see* Feline spongiform encephalopathy
FSH *see* Follicle-stimulating hormone
FTC *see* Emtricitabine
5-FU *see* 5-Fluorouracil
Full blood count (FBC) *see* Blood count
Fumarates, 1268
Fumes, lung disease and, 717
Functional disorder, 876–877, 1175–1176, 1176b
Functional residual capacity (FRC), 647
Functional somatic syndromes, 236
Fungal infections, 135, 381–386, 382f
antifungal agents, 159–160, 160b, 1267
diabetes, 799b, 824
endocarditis, 626, 626b
HIV/AIDS related, 398–399
HSCT, 302b
immune deficiency and, 78b
nervous system, 1201b
respiratory, 697–699
skin, 1279–1280, 1279f
identification, 1280
scalp, 1280
subcutaneous, 381–383
superficial, 381
systemic, 383–386
see also individual infections
Funnel chest, 731
Funny turns *see* Blackouts
Furosemide
adverse reactions, 26b
ascites, 940
heart failure, 551
hyperkalaemia, 443b
hypertension, 611
mechanism of action, 435
mode of action, 435
oedema, 478
prescription, 38b
and renal disease, 522b
route of administration, 34b
skin reactions, 1304b
Furuncles, 1277
Fusarium/fusariosis, 384, 384f
Fusidic acid, 159
impetigo, 1266
Fusobacterium spp., 137f, 151b
Fusobacterium necrophorum, 687
Fusobacterium ulcerans, 313b
Futile treatment, 291
FVC *see* Forced vital capacity

G
G-CSF *see* Granulocyte colony stimulating factor
G6PD *see* Glucose-6-phosphate dehydrogenase deficiency
GABA
hepatic encephalopathy, 941–942
role in epilepsy, 1179
Gabapentin
abdominal pain, 863
adjuvant analgesia, 288b
epilepsy, 1184b
fibromyalgia, 1094
multiple sclerosis, 1192b
neuropathic pain, 288b
post-herpetic neuralgia, 319

shingles, 319
somatoform pain disorder, 233
GAD antibodies *see* Glutamic acid decarboxylase antibodies
Gain-of-function mutations, 58
Gait
diabetic neuropathy, 831–832
examination, 1059–1060, 1139b
shuffling/festination, 172b, 1168
stamping, 172b, 1168
waddling, 172b
Gait disorders, 172b, 1168
Parkinson's disease, 1196b
unsteadiness, 173
see also specific gaits
Galactorrhoea, 790–791
Galactosaemia, 449–450
Galactose, 449, 842
Galactose-1-phosphate uridylyltransferase gene (GALT), 449
Galantamine, 252
Gallbladder, 926
adenomyomatosis, 988
cholecystitis, 983–984
cholesterolosis, 986–988
disease in older people, 988b
porcelain, 983
strawberry, 987–988
tumours, 985–986
Gallstone ileus, 983
Gallstones, 981–983, 982b–983b
cholesterol, 982
hereditary spherocytosis
pancreatitis, 890
pigment, 982, 982b
in pregnancy, 977
ultrasound, 930, 930f
GALT, 449
Gambiense trypanosomiasis, 359
incubation period, 145b
Gametogenesis, 50f
Gamma butyrolactone, 218
Gamma rays, 102b, 470
γ-aminobutyric acid *see* GABA
γ-glutamyl transferase (GGT)
plasma
alcohol misuse, 240
drugs causing increase, 929b
liver function test, 928–929
reference values, venous blood, 1310b
γ-hydroxybutyrate (GHB), 218
Gammaglobulin, Kawasaki disease, 1116
Gammopathy, monoclonal, of uncertain significance (MGUS; monoclonal gammopathy unclassified; MGu; benign monoclonal gammopathy), 1045
Ganciclovir
CMV infection, 322
HIV-related, 404
transplant patients, 95, 302–303, 1017b
exanthem subitum, 316
herpesvirus infection, 161b, 162
Gangliosidosis, GM2, 451b
Gangrene
Fournier's, 305
gas, 305
synergistic, 305
Gap junctions, 47f, 48
Gas exchange, lungs, 646–647, 647f
Gas gangrene, 305
chemoprophylaxis, 153b
Gas transfer factor
for carbon monoxide (TLco), 653b
measurements, 653
Gas-bloat syndrome, 867–868
Gastrectomy
gastric cancer, 879
gastric outlet obstruction, 875–876
partial
anaemia after, 851
and gastric cancer, 878b
gastric ulcer, 874–875
gastritis, 871b
peptic ulcer, 856
sleeve, 119b, 120f
vitamin B deficiency, 1025
Gastric acid secretion, 841, 841f
Zollinger-Ellison syndrome, 876
Gastric aspiration, 210
Gastric band surgery, 119b
Gastric bypass surgery, 119b
Gastric emptying test, 850, 851b
Gastric inhibitory polypeptide (GIP), 846b
Gastric intrinsic factor, 871–872, 1024–1025
Gastric lavage, 210, 210b
Gastric outlet obstruction, 875–876, 875b
Gastric surgery, anaemia and, 875
Gastric volvulus, 867
Gastrin, 841, 846b
reference range, 1309b
Zollinger-Ellison syndrome, 876
Gastrinomas, 785b
Gastritis, 871–872, 871b
bile reflux, 871b, 875
Helicobacter pylori infection
Gastro-oesophageal reflux disease, 865–868, 865f
and asthma, 866b
older people, 868b
Gastroenteritis
acute, 306–308
management, 307–308
anthrax, 303
bacterial, 342, 342b
causes, 306b
differential diagnosis, 307b
eosinophilic, 887
food poisoning *see* Food poisoning
viral, 327–328
Gastroenteropathy, allergic, 888
Gastroenterostomy, 875–876
Gastrointestinal bleeding, 853–857
acute upper gastrointestinal haemorrhage, 853–856
causes, 854f
endoscopic therapy, 852b, 855
management, 855b
Blatchford score, 854b
liver disease, 942
lower gastrointestinal tract, 856, 856b
NSAIDs and, 873, 1021–1022
occult, 856–857
signs, 855f
unknown cause, 856, 857f
Gastrointestinal decontamination in poisoning, 210, 210b
Gastrointestinal function, 24b
Gastrointestinal obstruction, 290
Gastrointestinal peptide, 801–802
Gastrointestinal stromal tumour (GIST), 870, 880
Gastrointestinal tract
absorption from, 21
biopsy
inflammatory bowel disease, 901
small bowel in coeliac disease, 881
clinical examination, 838f, 839b
diseases/disorders, 783b
chest pain, 540
critically ill patients, 198
endocrine, 782–785
functional, 876–877, 1175–1176, 1176b
HIV-related, 399–400
investigation, 845–851
presenting problems, 851–863
protozoal, 367–369
systemic sclerosis, 1113
tuberculosis, 691
see also Gastroenteritis
function
control of, 844–845
tests, 850, 851b
functional anatomy, 840–844
hormones, 845, 846b
infections *see* Infection(s), gastrointestinal tract
obstruction, 290, 862
see also individual parts
Gastroparesis, 877
Gastropathy, congestive, 948
Gastrostomy, percutaneous endoscopic, 123, 123f
Gatifloxacin, meningitis, 1204b
Gaucher's disease, 46, 433–434
Gaussian distribution *see* Normal distribution/range
Gaze palsy, 1148b
GBM *see* Glomerular basement membrane
GCA *see* Giant cell arteritis
GCK *see* Glucokinase
GCS *see* Glasgow Coma Scale
Gefitinib, 279, 704
Gegenhalten, 1175
Gels, 1265b
Gemcitabine, pancreatic cancer, 895
Gender
alcoholic liver disease and, 957
pharmacokinetics and, 24b
Gene promoter, 42, 43f
Gene testing, 63
Gene therapy, 31b, 69
cystic fibrosis, 681
General anaesthetics, 18–19, 577, 651–652
General Assessment of Locomotor System (GALS), 1059–1060
General Medical Council (UK), 2
duties of registered doctor, 3b
General paralysis of insane, 1209b
Generalised anxiety, 241b, 243
Genes, 42–43
mutations *see* Mutations
oncogenes, 59
Genetic counselling, 67–68, 67b
older people, 64b
Genetic disease(s), 44f, 46b, 50–60
categories of, 64–67
chromosomal, 56b
constitutional, 58–59
gene identification, 63
inheritance patterns, 51–53
investigations, 60–64, 62b
monogenic, 68f
older people, 64b
polygenic, 68f
presenting problems, 64
risk calculation, 53
skin manifestations, 1302
somatic, 59–60
spectrum of, 68f
Genetic factors, 41–70
adverse drug reactions, 26
ageing, 168
alcohol misuse, 252
alcoholic liver disease, 957, 960f
Alzheimer's disease, 251–252
aortic aneurysm, 603
asthma, 666
atopic eczema, 1283–1284
autoimmune disease, 87b
cancer, 262–267, 912
diabetes mellitus
type 1, 803–804
type 2, 806
HIV/AIDS, 395
hypertension, 607
inflammatory bowel disease, 897b
multiple sclerosis, 1188
osteoarthritis, 1081
osteoporosis, 1120
Paget's disease, 1129
Parkinson's disease, 1194–1195
PCOS, 764
prostate cancer, 517
psychiatric disorders, 232–233
puberty onset, 758
rheumatoid arthritis, 1096
SLE, 1110
Genetic screening, 64
Genetic testing, 1153
cardiomyopathy, 638
in children, 63
colorectal cancer, 913
complex disease, 69
cystic fibrosis, 680
ethical issues, 9–10
familial adenomatous polyposis, 912
multiple endocrine neoplasia, 795
neurological disease, 1153
Peutz-Jeghers syndrome, 912
phaeochromocytoma, 781
predictive, 64
Huntington's disease, 64b
prenatal, 62–63, 63b
Genetic variants, 53–57
consequences of, 57–58, 58b
evolutionary selection, 58
Genetics
complex disease, 68–69
twin studies, 68
Genital cancer, HIV-related, 405
Genital itch/rash, 415, 416b
Genital lumps
men, 416–417
women, 418
Genital ulcers
men, 415–416, 416f
women, 418
Genitourinary tuberculosis, 692
Genome, 42
Genome-wide association studies, 63
Genome-wide linkage analysis, 63
Genomic imprinting, 52f, 53
Genotype, 68f
Gentamicin
brucellosis, 334b
cerebral abscess, 1208b
dosing, 157, 157f
drug interactions, 27b
infective endocarditis, 301, 628, 628b
liver abscess, 956
meningitis, 1204b
neutropenic sepsis, 1001
plague, 338–339
prophylactic, 153b
renal toxicity, 35b, 479–481
septic arthritis, 1094–1095
therapeutic monitoring, 39b
tularaemia, 340
urinary tract infection, 513b
Geriatric medicine, 165–177
assessment, 166f, 170–171, 170b
presenting problems, 171–176
see also Ageing; Older people
German measles *see* Rubella
Gerstmann-Sträussler-Scheinker syndrome, 329b, 1211
Gestational diabetes mellitus, 807b, 817, 817b
Get up and go test, 167f
GFR *see* Glomerular filtration rate
GGT *see* γ-Glutamyl transferase
GH *see* Growth hormone
GHB *see* γ-Hydroxybutyrate; Glycated haemoglobin
Ghon focus/complex, 688–689
Ghrelin, 841, 846b
GHRH *see* Growth hormone-releasing hormone
Giant cell arteritis, 1117–1118
Giant cell arteritis (GCA), 1117–1118
management, 1117–1118, 1118b

Giant cell tumour, 1131b
Giardia lamblia (*intestinalis*) infection, 311, 368–369
Giardiasis, 309b, 368–369
Gigantism, 792
Gilbert's syndrome/disease, 936, 937b, 974–975
Gingivitis, 398
GIP *see* Gastric inhibitory polypeptide
GISA *see* Glycopeptide intermediate *Staphylococcus aureus*
GIST *see* Gastrointestinal stromal tumour
Gitelman's syndrome, 441, 510
Glandular fever (infectious mononucleosis), 320, 320b, 321f
Glanzmann's thrombasthenia, 1050
Glasgow alcoholic hepatitis score, 959b
Glasgow Coma Scale (GCS), 198–199, 208, 1159–1160, 1160b
Glasgow criteria for prognosis in acute pancreatitis, 890b
Glatiramer acetate, 1191, 1192b
Glibenclamide, 823
Gliclazide, 823
Glioblastoma multiforme, 1213
Glioma, 1215
  spine, 1222b
Gliosis, 828, 829f
Glipizide, 216, 823
Gliptins *see* DPP-4 inhibitors
Glitazones *see* Thiazolidinediones
Global warming, 102
Glomerular basement membrane (GBM)
  Alport's syndrome, 502, 502f
  anti-GBM (Goodpasture's disease), 499b–500b, 713–714
  thin GBM disease, 502
Glomerular disease, 480b–481b, 497–502, 497f
  drug-related, 522b
  histopathology, 498f
  inherited, 502
  pregnancy, 520–521
Glomerular filtration rate (GFR), 466–468
  assessment, 466b–467b
  renal failure
    acute, 483b
    chronic, 467b, 468, 484
Glomerulonephritis, 498–502
  crescentic, 487b, 501–502
    drug-induced, 522b
  focal segmental (necrotising), 499b–500b
    drug-induced, 522b
  membranous, 499b–500b, 500
  mesangiocapillary (membranoproliferative) (MCGN; MPGN), 499b–500b, 501
  minimal change, 498–500, 499b–500b
  nephrotic syndrome, 475b, 476–478
  post-infection, 499b–500b, 501
  rapidly progressive, 501–502
  SLE, 1111
Glomerulosclerosis
  focal segmental (FSGS), 500
  nodular diabetic, 830f
Glomerulus, 464
Glossitis, 990f
  atrophic, 838f
Glossopharyngeal (9th cranial) nerve, tests, 1139b
Gloves and socks syndrome, 316b
GLP *see* Glucagon-like peptide
GLP-1 receptor antagonists, 822b, 823–824
Glucagon
  cardiotoxic drug poisoning, 214–215
  famine, 121
  hypoglycaemia, 357b
  hypotension, 214
  type 2 diabetes, 806
Glucagon-like peptide (GLP), 119, 801–802
Glucagonomas, 785b
Glucocorticoid therapy, 776–777
  adrenal insufficiency, 779, 779b
  adverse reactions, 776
  advice to patients, 777b
  congenital adrenal hyperplasia, 763b, 782
  dosage regimen, 35b
  older people, 779b
  prescription, 38b
  withdrawal, 776–777
  see also Corticosteroids; Hydrocortisone; Prednisolone
Glucocorticoids, 772–773
  bone remodelling, 1062b
  excess, 772b
    see also Cushing's syndrome
  insufficiency, 778b
  measurement, 777–778
Glucokinase (GCK), 817
Gluconeogenesis, 926
Glucosamine, musculoskeletal disease, 1086
Glucose
  blood
    diabetes, 800, 807–808
    fasting, 807b
    impaired fasting glucose, 809b
    normal metabolism, 800–802, 801f
    reference values, 1310b
    stroke patients, 1243b
    see also Hyperglycaemia; Hypoglycaemia
  cerebrospinal fluid, 1311b
  hypoglycaemia management, 816
  impaired tolerance, 169f, 455, 754b, 1310b
  intravenous
    hyperkalemia, 443b
    porphyria, 460
  urinary, 807
Glucose tolerance, impaired, 800, 809b
Glucose tolerance test
  oral, 809b
Glucose-6-phosphate dehydrogenase (G6PD) deficiency, 1029, 1029b
Glucuronic acid, 995
Glue sniffing, 254, 1048b
GLUT 4 transporter, 801
Glutamate, 49, 114b, 251–252
Glutamic acid decarboxylase (GAD) antibodies, 1194b
Glutaminase, 444
Glutamine, 54f, 801f
Glutathione, 126b, 212
Gluteal enthesopathy, 1075b
Gluten, coeliac disease, 880–882
Gluten-free diet, 880–882
Glycaemic control
  critically ill patients, 198
  diabetes, 827–828, 827b
    adolescents, 818b
    older people, 828b
    pregnancy, 817–818
    retinopathy prevention, 828–829
    self-assessment, 807, 810–811
Glycaemic index of foods, 112–113
Glycated haemoglobin (GHb), 808, 808b, 811f, 1310b
Glycation, 808
Glyceryl trinitrate (GTN)
  angina, 586, 586b
    unstable, 594
  circulatory effects, 183
  dosage regimen, 35b
  duration of action, 586b
  intravenous, malignant hypertension, 612
  ointment, anal fissure, 919
  patches, 1075
  pulmonary oedema, 550
  route of administration, 34b
  sublingual, 586, 594
Glycine, 114b
Glycogen, 73–74, 111–112
Glycogen storage diseases (GSD), 450, 450b
Glycols, poisoning, 222–223
Glycopeptide intermediate *Staphylococcus aureus* (GISA), 151, 152f
Glycopeptide-resistant enterococci (GRE), 151b
Glycopeptides, 157–158
  mechanism of action, 150b
  in pregnancy, 154b
Glycoprotein IIb/IIIa inhibitors, 594b, 1019b, 1050
Glycoprotein intrinsic factor, 841
Glycosaminoglycans, 1062–1063
Glycosidases, 1063
Glycosides *see* Digoxin
Glycosuria, 471–472, 804
  alimentary (lag storage), 741b
  diabetes mellitus, 807
  Fanconi syndrome, 510
  hypernatraemia, 439b
  leg ulcers, 1262
  older people, 806b
  pregnancy, 817
  renal, 510
Glycylcyclines, 154b, 158
GM-CSF *see* Granulocyte macrophage colony stimulating factor
Gnathostomiasis, 309b
GnRH *see* Gonadotrophin-releasing hormone
Goitre
  breathlessness in, 657f
  endemic, 131
  Hashimoto's thyroiditis, 751
  multinodular, 741b, 753–754, 753f
    retrosternal, 753, 753f
    toxic, 754
  simple diffuse, 753, 753f
  thyrotoxicosis, 745–746
Gold
  adverse effects on kidney, 522b
  intramuscular
    adverse reactions, 711, 1005b, 1048b
    rheumatic disease, 1101b, 1102
  oral, asthma, 671
  skin reactions, 1290, 1304b
Golf, 1075b
Golfer's elbow, 1075
Golgi apparatus, 44–45
Golimumab, 1103b
Gonadectomy, prophylactic, 766
Gonadotrophin deficiency, 789
Gonadotrophin-releasing hormone (GnRH), 737f, 757
  deficiency, 787b
  infertility treatment, 762
Gonadotrophin-releasing hormone (GnRH) analogues, 460, 518
  and osteoporosis, 1120, 1121b
  prostate cancer, 518
Gonococcal infection, disseminated (DGI), 422, 1094
Gonococcal urethritis, 415
Gonorrhoea, 422–423
  arthritis, 422
  incubation period, 145b, 422
  management, 422b–423b
  pharyngeal, 422
  urethritis, 415
Good medical practice, 1–16
  clinical audit, 15, 15b, 15f
  clinical decision-making, 7–9
  communication, 4
  doctor-patient relationship, 2–4, 3f
    difficulties in, 2–4
  evidence-based medicine, 8, 8b
  guidelines and protocols, 8–9
  investigations, 4–7
  personal and professional development, 14–15, 14b, 14f
  risk estimation/communication, 7, 7f
Goodpasture's syndrome, 499b–500b, 713–714
Gorlin syndrome, 267b
Goserelin, 278, 518
Gottron's papules, 1115
Gout, 1087–1090
  drug-induced, 1132b
  older people, 1090b
  pressure erosions, 1067b
  prevalence, 1060b
  tophaceous, 1088–1089, 1088f
GRACE score, 591f, 598
Graft-versus-host disease (GVHD), 1290
  stem cell transplantation, 1018
  transfusion-associated, 1014
Graham Steell murmur, 625
Granulocyte colony stimulating factor (G-CSF), 992–993
Granulocyte macrophage colony stimulating factor (GM-CSF), 715b, 992–993
Granulocytes
  count, 1312b
  formation, 993f
Granuloma annulare, 1301
Granuloma inguinale, 424b
Granulomas
  leprosy, 347
  sarcoidosis, 709–710
  schistosomiasis, 376
  tuberculous, 689f
Granulomatosis with polyangiitis (Wegener's granulomatosis), 713, 1118, 1118f
Granulomatous disease, chronic, 79
Granzymes, 75–76
Grapefruit juice, drug interactions, 28b
Graves' disease, 747–751
  management, 748–749
  ophthalmopathy, 735f, 739b, 750–751, 750f
  thyroid autoantibodies, 741b
  thyrotoxicosis, 740, 740b, 747–750, 748f
Gravitational (stasis) eczema, 1254, 1286
Grays (Gy), 103
Greenhouse gases, 102
Grenz (Bucky) ray therapy, 1269
Grey baby syndrome, 154b
Grey Turner's sign, 890–891
Grief reaction, 242
Griseofulvin, 160, 160b
  onchomycosis, 1280
Groin injection sites, febrile drug user, 299
Growth factors, 48
  asthma, 667
  atherosclerosis, 579–580
  cancer, 263, 263f
  haematopoiesis, 993f
Growth failure, 49, 906
Growth hormone (GH), 736, 737f
  deficiency, 766, 787b
  hypersecretion, 787, 792–793
  hypopituitarism treatment, 789
  reference range, 1309b
  resistance, 786b
  secretion tests, 788b

Growth hormone-releasing hormone (GHRH), 737f
Growth retardation
congenital heart disease and, 631
eating disorders, 255–256, 256b
glycogen storage diseases, 450, 450b
intrauterine, 314b, 355, 749
GSD *see* Glycogen storage diseases
GTN *see* Glyceryl trinitrate
Guanine, 42
Guidelines for treatment, 8–9
Guillain-Barré syndrome, 1224–1225, 1225b
Guinea worm (dracunculiasis), 375
Gumma, 420
Gums
Kaposi's sarcoma, 398f
scurvy, 130f
Gums, dietary, 113b
Gut, hormones, 845, 846b
GVHD *see* Graft-versus-host disease
Gynaecomastia, 762–763, 762b, 781, 943–944

H
HAART *see* Antiretroviral therapy
HACE *see* High-altitude, cerebral oedema
HACEK group bacteria, endocarditis, 626, 626b
HAE *see* Hereditary angioedema
Haem
biosynthetic pathway, 459f
synthesis disorders, 458–460
Haemagglutination test, 340
Haemagogus spp., yellow fever, 323
Haemangioblastoma, 267b, 1216
Haemangioma, 1131b, 1274
liver, 970, 970f
Haemarthrosis, 1069
Haematemesis, 854
Haematocrit, 1003, 1312b
Haematological disorders *see* Blood diseases
Haematological function, older people, 1001b
Haematological investigations *see* Blood tests
Haematological tests *see* Blood tests
Haematological values, 1312b
Haematomas
intracerebral, 1218
muscle, haemophilia, 1051
stroke patients, 1239, 1242b, 1246
subdural, 1218
subungual, 1298, 1298f
Haematopoiesis, 992–994
extramedullary, 1006
Haematopoietic stem cell transplantation (HSCT), 1017–1018
acute leukaemia, 1037f, 1038
allogeneic, 1017–1018, 1017b
aplastic anaemia, 1048
autologous, 1018
β-thalassaemia, 1034b
chronic myeloid leukaemia, 1040
fever after, 302–303
infection in, 1017b
myelodysplastic syndrome, 1041
myelofibrosis, 1049
myeloma, 1047b
non-Hodgkin's lymphoma, 1044–1045
Haematopoietic stem cells, 992–994, 993f
Haematuria, 474–476, 475f
dipstick-negative, 475b
dipstick-positive, 474b
investigations, 476f
'loin pain', 471
and malignancy, 475b
Haemochromatosis, 131, 972–973
causes, 972b
hereditary, 972–973
inheritance, 58b
investigations, 972, 973f
liver function tests, 930b
musculoskeletal manifestations, 1133
secondary, 972b, 973
Haemodiafiltration, 492
Haemodialysis, 490–491, 490f–491f
AKI, 483
chronic renal failure, 491
complications, 489b, 492b
intermittent, 491
poisoning, 207–208, 211
Haemofiltration, 490f, 491–492
AKD, 483
continuous venovenous, 491–492
pumped venovenous, 197–198
Haemoglobin, 994–995
abnormal, 1031–1032, 1034
full blood count, 1312b
glycated, 808, 808b, 811f, 1310b
high, 1003–1004
mean cell (MCH), 1312b
oxygen dissociation curve, 183f
reference values, 1312b
Haemoglobin A, 1032–1033
Haemoglobin C, 1031–1032
Haemoglobin C disease, 1034
Haemoglobin D, 1031–1032
Haemoglobin E, 1031–1032
Haemoglobin F, 994–995, 1033
Haemoglobin H disease, 1034–1035
Haemoglobin S, 1031–1033
Haemoglobin SC disease, 1034
Haemoglobinopathies, 1031–1035, 1032f
genetic testing, 62b
Haemoglobinuria, 474b
march, 1031
paroxysmal cold, 420
paroxysmal nocturnal, 1031
Haemolysis
autoimmune, 1029–1030
blood transfusion reaction, 1016f
drug-induced, 1031, 1303b
extravascular, 1027–1029
intravascular, 1026–1027, 1026b, 1031
malaria, 357b
Haemolytic anaemia, 1026–1031, 1026b, 1027f
alloimmune, 1031
autoimmune, 1029–1031
microangiopathic, 1031
non-immune, 1031
Haemolytic crisis, 1028
Haemolytic disease of the newborn (HDN), 1014
Haemolytic uraemic syndrome (HUS), 138b, 468, 495–496
Haemoperfusion, poisoning, 211, 211b
Haemopexin, 1026–1027
Haemophilia, 1052f
haematomas, 1051
inheritance, 1051
Haemophilia A, 1051–1053, 1051b
Haemophilia B (Christmas disease), 1053
Haemophilus spp., 137f
Haemophilus ducreyi, 424b
Haemophilus influenzae, 151b
bacterial meningitis, 1202b, 1204b
immunisation, 149b
immunocompromised patients, 78b
pneumonia, 401, 687
Haemoptysis, 658–659, 659b
bronchial carcinoma, 700
bronchiectasis, 678
COPD, 674
Haemorrhage
cancer-related, 270b
during dialysis, 492b
intracerebral, 1238f–1239f, 1239
retinal, 107, 609, 609f
splinter, 1070b, 1298
subarachnoid, 1246–1247
see also Bleeding
Haemorrhagic fevers
dengue, 309b, 322–323, 322b–323b, 322f, 325b
with renal syndrome (Hantan fever), 325b
viral, 309b, 311f, 324–325
Haemorrhagic papilloedema
Haemorrhoids, 918–919
Haemosiderin, 927, 976
Haemosiderosis, 130
idiopathic pulmonary, 715b
Haemostasis, 996–997, 996f–997f
disorders, 1049–1050
older people, 1056b
Haemothorax, 661
Hair
disorders, 1264, 1296–1297
excess, 763–764, 1297
follicles, 1252–1253
growth cycle, 1253
loss *see* Alopecia
Hair pluck test, 1280
Hairy cell leukaemia, 1041
Hallpike manoeuvre, 1167b, 1186
Hallucinations, 237
differential diagnosis, 237
drug misuse, 20b, 217b
hypnagogic, 237
hypnopompic, 237
schizophrenia, 237, 247–248
visual, 248
Hallucinogens, 254
Hallucinosis, alcoholic, 253
Hallux valgus, 1076
Haloperidol, 249b
adverse reactions, 26b
delirium, 174–175, 203
disturbed behaviour, 237–238
nausea and vomiting, 290b, 291
older people, 237–238
poisoning, 216
schizophrenia, 249b
terminal agitation, 290
Halothane, 87, 933f
Hamartomas
adrenal, 779
lung, 704b
small intestine, 888
Hand, foot and mouth disease, 326–327
Handicap, mental, 66
Hands
examination
blood disorders, 990f
cancer, 260f
cardiovascular disease, 526f
diabetes, 799b
diabetes mellitus, 798f
endocrine disease, 734f
gastrointestinal disease, 838f
infectious disease, 294f
liver and biliary disease, 922f
older people, 166f
renal/urinary tract disease, 462f–463f
respiratory disease, 644f
rheumatic disease, 1058f
skin disease, 1250f
hygiene, infection control, 145–146, 146f
osteoarthritis, 1083f
pain, 1075
psoriatic arthritis, 1109f
rheumatoid arthritis, 1098f
washing, 146f
Hantan fever, 325b
Hantavirus, 337
HAPE *see* High altitude, pulmonary oedema
Haploinsufficiency, 766
Haplotypes, 63, 803–804
Haptoglobins, 1312b
Hard metal disease, 718
Hartmann's procedure, 862
Hartmann's solution, 433b
hypovolaemia, 433b
Hartnup's disease, 128
Hasenclever prognostic index, 1043b
Hashimoto's thyroiditis, 751
HAV *see* Hepatitis A virus
Haversian system, 1062b
Hay fever, 94, 1283
Hayflick limit, 50
HBV *see* Hepatitis B virus
HCG *see* Human chorionic gonadotrophin
Hct *see* Haematocrit
HCV *see* Hepatitis C virus
HDL *see* High-density lipoproteins
HDN *see* Haemolytic disease of the newborn
HDV *see* Hepatitis D virus
Head
examination
diabetes, 799b
endocrine disease, 734f
imaging, 1149–1150, 1150f
injury, 1218
Head lice, 1281
Head and neck
cancer, 262f, 281–282, 282b
examination, gastrointestinal disease, 838f
Headache, 1156–1157, 1176–1178
analgesic, 1176
brain tumour, 1213
cluster, 1177, 1178b
exertion, 1178
fever and, 83f, 295
heat stroke, 106
medication overuse, 1177
meningitis
bacterial, 1202–1204, 1202b, 1203f
viral, 1201–1202
migraine *see* Migraine
morning, in respiratory failure, 657
paroxysmal, 1178b
post-ictal, 1158b
raised ICP, 285b
red flag symptoms, 1157b
and sexual activity, 1178
stroke, 1237
subarachnoid haemorrhage, 1246
syndromes, 1156b
tension-type, 1176
see also specific types
Heaf test, 695b, 695f
Health care
integrated, 16
low-resource settings, 9
resources, fair allocation, 9
Health care-acquired infections, 145–147, 145b, 146f
Clostridium difficile, 304b, 343–344, 344f
control, 146f
MRSA, 134, 330–331
multidrug-resistant tuberculosis, 696
pneumonia, 685–687
risk factors, 146f
Hearing disturbance *see* Deafness
Heart
anatomy, 528–530, 528f–529f
arrhythmias *see* Arrhythmias
auscultation, 527b
blood flow, 528f, 530–531
catheterisation, 538–539, 538f
chambers, 529f
dilatation, 535
conduction system, 529–530, 529f
endothelial function, 531–532
imaging, 537
nerve supply, 530

physiology, 530–532
Starling's Law, 182, 530, 547f
transplantation, 553
tumours, 639
valves
prosthetic, 546b
replacement, 629
see also Valvular heart disease
see also Cardiac
Heart beats
ectopic
atrial, 564, 564f
ventricular, 569, 569f
see also Palpitation
Heart block
atrioventricular, 571–573, 571f–572f, 572b
bifascicular, 573
bundle branch blocks, 573, 573b
complete, 572b
hemiblock, 573
Heart disease
congenital, 629–636, 629b–630b
adult, 635–636, 635b
coronary, 583–600
hepatic damage, 976–977
HIV-related, 405
hypertension and, 609
quantification of risk, 609–610
investigations, 532–539
ischaemic *see* Ischaemic heart disease
New York Heart Association functional classification, 539b
pregnancy, 631, 631b
presentation throughout life, 629b
presenting problems, 539–562
rheumatic, 614–616
rheumatoid arthritis, 1099
risks of non-cardiac surgery, 600, 600b
structural, (pre-)syncope, 555
valvular, 546, 613–629
for detailed entry see Valvular heart disease
see also names of specific conditions
Heart failure, 546–553
acute, 548
acute left, 548
breathlessness, 543
acute-on-chronic, 548
aortic regurgitation, 527b, 623–624, 623b, 623f
biventricular, 548
cardiac resynchronisation therapy, 579, 579b
cardiomyopathy, 636–638
chest X-ray, 550, 550f
chronic, 548–549
breathlessness, 543–544
chronic constrictive pericarditis, 641, 641b
clinical assessment, 548–549
compensated, 548
complications, 549
congestive, older people, 551b
diastolic and systolic dysfunction, 548
heart transplantation, 553
high-output, 548
implantable defibrillator, 553, 553f
investigations, 549–550
left-sided, 548, 549f
acute, 543, 548
liver damage in, 549
management, 550–553, 550b, 551f
drug therapy, 550–553
mechanisms, 546b, 547f
myocardial infarction *see* Myocardial infarction
neurohormonal activation, 547f
pathophysiology, 547–550, 547f, 583b
pleural effusion, 662b
precipitating factors, 548b
revascularisation, 553
rheumatic fever, 614–616, 614f
right-sided, 548, 549f
types, 548
ventricular assist devices, 553
ventricular ectopic beats, 569, 569f
ventricular septal defect, 633–634, 634f
Heart murmurs, 560–562
for detailed entry see Murmurs
Heart rate
control, 191, 566
disorders, 562–579
respiration effects, 532b
Heart rhythm
control, 191, 566
disorders *see* Arrhythmias
Heart sounds
abnormal, 560–562, 560b
aortic stenosis, 562b, 620
atrial myxoma, 639
atrial septal defect, 633
cardiac cycle, 561f
mitral regurgitation, 562b, 610b
mitral stenosis, 617, 617f
normal, 560b
pulmonary stenosis, 625
ventricular septal defect, 562b
Heart transplantation, 553
Heart valves
common infecting organisms, 626b
haemolysis, 1031
mechanical, 629, 629b
see also Valvular heart disease; *and names of individual valves*
Heart-lung transplantation, 665–666
Heartburn, 852–853
Heat cramps, 106
Heat exhaustion, 106
Heat stroke, 106
Heat syncope, 106
Heat-related illness, 105–106
Heavy metals
adverse effects on kidney, 446b
poisoning, 308
Heberden's nodes, 1083f
Height, measurement of, 114–115
Heimlich manoeuvre, 728
Heinz bodies, 1031
Helicobacter pylori
diagnosis of infection, 873b
eradication therapy, 874, 874b
adverse reactions, 874b
indications, 874b
gastric cancer, 266b
gastric lymphoma, 879
gastritis, 871
peptic ulcer and, 872–873
Helium dilution technique, 675
Heller's operation, 869
HELLP syndrome, 978
Helminthic infections, 135, 369–381, 369b
drug therapy, 162–163
eosinophilia and, 312b
nervous system, 1164–1165
soil-transmitted, 312b
treatment, 162–163
Hemicellulose, 113b
Hemicranias, paroxysmal, 1178b
Hemifacial spasm, 1200
Hemiparesis, 1117, 1119
Hemiplegic gait, 172b
Henderson-Hasselbalch equation, 443, 444f
Hendra virus, 144f, 328
Henoch-Schönlein purpura (HSP), 501, 1119
Heparin, 1018–1019
acute limb ischaemia, 603
angina, unstable, 594b
atrial fibrillation, 566
indications, 1018b
low molecular weight, 1019
diabetic ketoacidosis, 813b
pulmonary embolism, 618
venous thromboembolism, 1010–1011, 1019
mechanism of action, 1018–1019
monitoring, 1000–1001
pulmonary embolism, 618
standard (unfractionated), 1018–1019
stroke, 1244
venous thromboembolism, 723, 1010–1011
prophylaxis, 599
Heparin-induced thrombocytopenia (HIT), 1019
Hepatic, *see also* Liver
Hepatic acinus, 924f
Hepatic artery disease, 975
Hepatic decompensation, 944
Hepatic encephalopathy, 923b, 941–942, 941b
clinical grading, 933b
Hepatic failure *see* Liver failure
Hepatic fibrosis, 925f
congenital, 945f
drug-induced, 972
histology, 943f
non-invasive markers, 932
pathogenesis, 925f
schistosomiasis, 377–378
Hepatic hydrothorax, 939
Hepatic osteodystrophy, 963
Hepatic veins, outflow obstruction, 976
Hepatic venous disease, 976–977
Hepatic venous pressure, 943
Hepatitis
acute, drug-induced, 971b
alcoholic, 958, 958b
autoimmune, 930b, 962–963, 962b, 965
cholestatic, 971b
drug-induced, 971b
interface, 962
ischaemic, 198
neonatal, 974
viral *see* Viral hepatitis
Hepatitis A virus (HAV), 309b, 949–950, 949b
antigen, 949
immunisation, 149b
haemophiliacs, 1051–1052
incubation period, 145b, 310b
investigations, 949
management, 949–950
older people, 980b
in pregnancy, 977
prevention, 949b
transmission, 949b
sexual, 426
Hepatitis B virus (HBV), 949b, 950–954, 950f
acute liver failure, 950
antigens, 950–952, 951b, 952f
chronic infection, 951b
HBeAg-negative, 951b, 951f
natural history, 951f
hepatocellular carcinoma, 967
HIV/AIDS patients, 400
immunisation/prevention, 954, 954b
HIV/AIDS patients, 407
incubation period, 145b, 310b
investigations, 950–952, 952b
liver function tests, 930b
management, 952–953
pregnancy, 314b
prevention *see* Immunisation above
transmission, 950b
blood products, 1011–1012
sexual, 426
viral load, 952, 952f
Hepatitis C virus (HCV), 949b, 954–955
antigens, 954
chronic infection, 955b
hepatocellular carcinoma, 967
HIV/AIDS patients, 400
investigations, 954–955
liver function tests, 930b
management, 955, 955b
prevention, 955
prognosis, 955
transmission
blood products, 1011–1012
sexual, 426
Hepatitis D virus (HDV), 949b, 954
antigen, 954
vertical transmission, 954
Hepatitis E virus (HEV), 949b, 955
Hepato-renal disease, 519
Hepatocellular carcinoma, 967–969
fibrolamellar, 969
haemochromatosis, 967–968
older people, 980b
Hepatocellular jaundice, 936–937
Hepatocerebral degeneration
Hepatocytes, 924–925, 925f
necrosis, 971
Hepatomegaly, 938
Budd-Chiari syndrome, 976
cirrhosis, 943
heart failure, 624
Hepatopulmonary syndrome, 975–976
Hepatorenal failure/syndrome, 940–941
Hepcidin, 130–131
HER2 receptor, 268
Herbal medicine, pain management, 288
Herceptin *see* Transtuzumab
Herd immunity, 149
Hereditary angioedema (HAE), 93b, 93f, 94
Hereditary haemorrhagic telangiectasia (HHT), 1007, 1049
Hereditary non-polyposis colon (colorectal) cancer (HNPCC), 67, 267b
Heredity *see* Genetic factors; Inheritance
Hernia
diaphragmatic, 731
hiatus, 865, 865b, 865f
Heroin misuse, 219
Herpangina, 327
Herpes labialis, 326f
Herpes simplex virus (HSV), 325–326
acute leukaemia, 1038
cutaneous, 326f
eczema, 326, 326f
encephalitis, 1205–1206
genital, 416b, 418b, 423–425, 424f
pregnancy, 425
treatment, 318b
HIV infection/AIDS, 397
HSV 1/2, 325–326
liver failure, 934b
in pregnancy, 314b, 414b
recurrent, 326
stem cell transplantation, 1017b
treatment, 318b
Herpes zoster, 295f, 317f, 318–319, 1157, 1207
facial pain, 1157
HIV infection/AIDS, 397
treatment, 318b
Herpesviruses
HIV infection/AIDS, 387
treatment, 161–162, 161b
Hers disease, 450b
HEV (hepatitis E virus), 949b, 955
HFE protein, 972
HHT *see* Hereditary haemorrhagic telangiectasia

HHV *see* Human herpes virus
5-HIAA *see* 5-Hydroxyindole-acetic acid
Hiatus hernia, 865, 865b, 865f
Hibernating myocardium, 537, 584b
Hibernian fever, 85
Hidebound chest, 713
HIDS *see* Hyper IgD syndrome
Hierarchy of systems, 98b
High altitude
  effects/illness, 106f, 107
    cerebral oedema (HACE), 107
    pulmonary oedema (HAPE), 107
High dependency care *see* Critical care
High-density lipoproteins (HDL), 1310b
High-frequency oscillatory ventilation (HFOV), 196
Highly active antiretroviral therapy *see* Antiretroviral therapy
Hip
  fractures, preventive measures, 172–173, 173b
  osteoarthritis, 1084, 1084f
  pain, 1075, 1075b, 1075f
  tendinitis, 1075b
Hip circumference, 115
Hip protectors, 1122
Hippocampus, 1142–1143
Hirschsprung's disease, 917–918
Hirsutism, 763–764, 1297
  causes, 763b
  congenital adrenal hyperplasia, 763b, 782
  polycystic ovarian syndrome, 764–765
His bundle, 529–530
Histamine, 841
Histamine H2-antagonists
  functional dyspepsia, 877
  gastro-oesophageal reflux, 867, 868f
  stress ulcers, 198
  urticaria, 1291
Histidine, 114b
Histiocytosis, Langerhans cell (histiocytosis X), 715b
Histoplasma capsulatum, 304b, 385
Histoplasma duboisii, 385
Histoplasmosis, 385–386
HIT *see* Heparin-induced thrombocytopenia
HIV cholangiopathy, 400
HIV infection/AIDS, 387–410
  associated conditions, 395, 395b
    cardiac disease, 405
    dementia, 402–404
    eyes, 404
    fever, 396
    gastrointestinal, 399–400, 909
    haematological, 404–405
    hepatobiliary, 400, 955
    leishmaniasis, 364–365
    lymphadenopathy, 395–396
    mucocutaneous disease, 396–398, 397b
    musculoskeletal, 1095b
    neoplastic, 405, 405b
    nervous system, 402–404
    oral, 398
    renal disease, 405
    respiratory, 400–401, 400b, 401f
    rheumatological, 404
    tuberculosis, 396, 400–401, 401f, 696
    weight loss, 396, 396f
  asymptomatic, 395
  CD4 counts, 393–394, 395b
  chemoprophylaxis, 153b, 406–407, 406b
  children, 393
  classification, 389b
  clinical examination, 388f
  counselling, 393b
  diagnosis, 392–393
  epidemiology, 390–391, 390f
  immunisation of HIV-infected persons, 407
  immunology, 391–392, 394f
  investigation/tests, 393b
  life cycle, 392f
  management/treatment
    antiretroviral drugs, 407–410
    complications, 408–409
    drug resistance, 408
    efficacy, 408
  natural history, 394–395
  older people, 410b
  opportunistic infections
    prophylaxis, 405–407, 406b
    see also associated conditions above
  pregnancy, 314b, 409–410
  presenting problems, 395–405, 1259b
  prophylaxis, 410, 410b
    opportunistic infections, 405–407, 406b
    perinatal, 409
    post-exposure, 410
    vaccines, 407
  staging, 389b, 394–395
  testing for, 393b, 412
  transmission, 390–391, 390b–391b
    blood products, 391b
    prevention, 410
  viral load, 394
  virology, 391–392
HIV-associated nephropathy (HIVAN), 405
Hives, 1290
  for detailed entry see Urticaria
HLA antigens, 75, 78
  diabetes mellitus, 803–804
  sclerosing cholangitis, 965
  transplant rejection, 94–95
HLA-B, 25b
  HIV/AIDS, 409
  juvenile idiopathic arthritis, 1104b
  spondarthritides, 1104
HMG CoA reductase enzyme inhibitors *see* Statins
HNPCC *see* Hereditary non-polyposis colon/colorectal cancer
Hoarseness
  chronic, causes, 727
  laryngeal disorders, 727
  laryngeal paralysis, 727
  psychogenic, 728
HOCM *see* Hypertrophic obstructive cardiomyopathy
Hodgkin's disease, 1042–1043, 1042f–1043f
  classification, 1042b
  epidemiology/aetiology, 1042b
  HIV-associated, 405, 405b
  prognosis, 1043b
  staging, 1042b
Holmes-Adie syndrome, 1172b
Holter monitoring, 534
Homeopathy, pain management, 288
Homeostasis, 100
Homocystinuria, 449
Homozygosity, 53
Honeycomb lung, 709f
Hookworm, 312b
  ancylostomiasis, 369–370, 370f
  dog, 375–376
Hoover's sign, 1163
Hormone replacement therapy (HRT)
  hypopituitarism, 789
  osteoporosis, 1123b, 1124–1125
  post-menopausal women, 760b, 766b
  secondary amenorrhoea, 760
Hormone therapy
  malignant disease, 278
  skin disease, 1267
Hormones
  actions *see individual hormones*
  ectopic production by tumours, 271, 271b
  gastrointestinal tract, 845, 846b
  reference range, 1309b
Horner's syndrome, 1172b, 1172f
  bronchial carcinoma, 701
Hospital CURB-65 system, 683f
Hospital-acquired infections *see* Nosocomial infections
Hospitals
  prescribing in, 37
  undernutrition in, 115–120, 122f
Host-pathogen interaction, 134, 137–138
Hot tub lung, 720
House dust mites, 666–667, 1255, 1283
Howell-Jolly bodies, 999f
HPOA *see* Hypertrophic pulmonary osteoarthropathy
HPV *see* Human papillomavirus
HRT *see* Hormone replacement therapy
HSCT *see* Haematopoietic stem cell transplantation
β-HSD *see* β-Hydroxysteroid dehydrogenase
HSP (Henoch-Schönlein purpura), 1119
HSV *see* Herpes simplex virus
HTLV *see* Human T-cell lymphotropic virus
Human chorionic gonadotrophin (hCG)
  infertility, 762
  pregnancy testing, 282, 756b, 759–760
  as tumour marker, 268, 270b
Human herpesvirus 6 (HHV6), 316, 317b
Human herpesvirus 7 (HHV7), 316, 317b
Human herpesvirus 8 (HHV8), 326
Human immunodeficiency virus *see* HIV
Human leucocyte antigens *see* HLA
Human papillomavirus (HPV)
  anogenital, 425–426
  cancer and, 267
  HIV infection/AIDS, 405b
  in pregnancy, 414b
  vaccines, 149, 425, 425b
Human T-cell lymphotropic virus (HTLV), 311, 328–329
Humidifier fever, 719b, 720
Hunter's syndrome, 433–434
Huntington's disease, 65, 1198
  genetic testing, 64, 64b, 1153
  genetics, 56b
  inheritance, 232–233, 250b
  juvenile, 1198
Hurler's syndrome, 433–434
HUS *see* Haemolytic uraemic syndrome
Hutchinson's sign, 1273
Hyaluronan, intra-articular injection, 1086
Hydatid cysts, liver, 380–381, 956–957, 956f
Hydatid disease, 380–381, 380f
  alveolar, 380–381
Hydralazine
  hypertension, 612
    malignant, 612
  and lupus syndrome, 1132b
  pharmacokinetics, 25b
  skin reactions, 1304b
Hydration
  dying patients, 291–292
  intravenous, acute leukaemia patients, 1001
  stroke patients, 1243b
  see also Fluid replacement
Hydroa vacciniforme, 1260b
Hydrocephalus, 1216–1217, 1217f
  causes, 1217b
  dementia, 250b
  normal pressure, 1217
  obstructive, 1173b, 1205
Hydrocortisone
  adrenal insufficiency, 779, 779b
  anaphylaxis, 92b
  asthma, 672
  eczema, 1285–1286
  equivalent dose, 776b
  hypopituitarism, 788–789
  inflammatory bowel disease, 903b, 904
  laryngeal obstruction, 728
  potency and strength, 1265b
  sexually transmitted infections
  topical, 1265b
  see also Cortisol
Hydrocortisone sodium succinate, 728
Hydrogen ions
  acid-base disorders, 429b
    diabetic ketoacidosis, 812
  arterial blood, 664b, 1308b
  critically ill patients, 187
Hydromorphone, 287
Hydronephrosis, 377, 481, 510–511
Hydrophobia, 1206
Hydrops fetalis, 316b
Hydrotherapy, 1080
Hydrothorax, hepatic, 939
Hydroxyapatite crystals, deposition, 1062, 1091
Hydroxycarbamide, 1268
  essential thrombocythaemia, 1049
  leukaemia, 1039–1040
  myeloproliferative disorders, 1049
  sickle-cell disease, 1033
Hydroxychloroquine
  adverse reactions, 1101b
  rheumatic disease, 1101b, 1102
  skin reactions, 1304b
  SLE, 1112
  Whipple's disease, 884
1α-Hydroxycholecalciferol (alfacalcidol), 770–771
Hydroxycobalamin *see* Vitamin B_{12}
5-Hydroxyindole-acetic acid (5-HIAA), 1311b
11β-Hydroxylase deficiency, 607b
17α-Hydroxylase deficiency, 607b
21-Hydroxylase deficiency, 782
11β-Hydroxysteroid dehydrogenase (β-HSD), 772, 772f
  deficiency, 607b
5-Hydroxytryptamine (5-HT) *see* Serotonin
25-Hydroxyvitamin D (25(OH)D), 1066b
Hyfrecation, 426
Hygiene hypothesis, 89
Hyoscine butylbromide, 290b, 291
Hyper IgD syndrome (HIDS), 85
Hyperacusis, 1163
Hyperaesthesia
  dengue fever, 322b
  diabetic neuropathy, 831–832
  herpes simplex, 326
Hyperaldosteronism
  diabetes type 1, 804
  glucorticoid suppressible, 607b, 780
  primary, 780–781, 780b
  secondary, 780b
Hyperalgesia, 285b
  fibromyalgia, 1093
Hyperalphalipoproteinaemia, 455
Hyperbilirubinaemia
  congenital non-haemolytic, 937b
  critically ill patients, 198
  see also Jaundice
Hypercalcaemia, 767–769
  cancer patients, 271b, 273, 273b
  causes, 767b

differential diagnosis, 768b
familial hypocalciuric, 767, 770
hyperparathyroidism and, 770–771, 770b
malignant, 767
multiple myeloma, 1046f
sarcoidosis, 711
Hypercapnia, respiratory failure, 192
Hypercarotenosis, 127
Hypercholesterolaemia, 453–455, 454b
atherosclerotic vascular disease risk, 581
biliary cirrhosis, 963–964
familial, 453–455, 455b
management, 456–457
nephrotic syndrome, 477b
polygenic, 453
secondary, 453b
Hypercoagulability, and nephrotic syndrome, 477b
Hypercortisolism, 773b
Hyperemesis gravidarum, 756b
Hyperglycaemia
acute myocardial infarction, 818
clinical assessment, 809–810
critical illness, 198
diabetes mellitus, 799, 808–811
type 1, 803–804
type 2, 806
diabetic ketoacidosis, 804, 811–814, 812b
drugs to reduce, 821–824
fasting, 809b
pancreatitis, 891b
pregnancy, 817–818
stress, 809
symptoms, 809–810, 809b
Hyperglycaemic hyperosmolar state, 814, 814b
Hyperinsulinaemia, 809b, 815
fetal, 817
Hyperkalaemia, 442–443, 443b, 443f
chronic interstitial nephritis, 504
diabetic nephropathy, 814
heart failure, 549
periodic paralysis, 1230b
renal failure
AKI, 482
chronic, 488
Hyperkeratosis, subungual, 1108
Hyperketonaemia, 802
Hyperlipidaemia, 454f
classification, 454b
familial combined, 454b, 455
management, 456–458, 457f, 598
older people, 458b
mixed, 454b, 455, 458
remnant, 455
secondary, 453b
Hypermagnesaemia, 448
Hypermelanosis, 1296
Hypermobility, 1134, 1134b
Hypernatraemia, 439, 439b
older people, 439, 439b
Hyperostosis, diffuse idiopathic skeletal, 1133–1134, 1134f
Hyperparasitaemia, malaria, 357b
Hyperparathyroidism, 769–770, 769b, 770f
chronic renal failure, 486–487
hypercalcaemia and *see* Hypercalcaemia
older people, 770b
pain, 769
Hyperphosphataemia, 449
chronic renal failure, 486–487
Hyperpigmentation, 1296
Hyperprolactinaemia, 790–791, 790b
chronic renal failure, 485
'disconnection', 774
Hyperpyrexia
malaria, 357b
malignant, 51–53
Hypersensitive carotid sinus syndrome (HCSS), 556
Hypersensitivity
allergic rhinitis, 725
Gell and Coombs classification, 88b
patch tests, 1255
prick tests, 1255
reactions to drugs, 25b
type I, 87, 88b, 89f
type II, 87, 88b
type III, 87, 88b
type IV, 87, 88b
Hypersensitivity pneumonitis, 719–720, 720f
Hypersensitivity responses, 83
Hypersomnolence, 1187, 1187b
idiopathic, 727
Hypersplenism
brucellosis, 333
and leucopenia, 929
portal hypertension, 945b
and thrombocytopenia, 946
Hypertension, 607–613
aetiology, 607–613
atherosclerosis and, 551
cardiovascular disease and, 609
quantification of risk, 609–610
cocaine misuse, 218
definition, 607b
diabetes mellitus, 810–811
essential, 607
examination, 608
history, 608
intracranial, 1217–1218
investigations, 609, 610b
malignant (accelerated phase), 497, 497f, 609
AKI, 480b–481b
emergency treatment, 612
management, 609–613
antihypertensive drugs, 610b, 611–612
British Hypertension Society guidelines, 611f
newly-diagnosed hypertension, 607–608
non-drug therapy, 610
quantification of cardiovascular risk, 609–610
refractory hypertension, 612–613
treatment targets, 610, 611b
older people, 610b
portal, 945–948, 945b, 945f
portopulmonary, 976
pre-eclampsia and, 521, 521b
pulmonary *see* Pulmonary hypertension
renal disease, 478
AKI, 480b–481b
chronic, 484
polycystic, 505–507
reflux nephropathy, 504–505
renal artery stenosis, 494–495, 494b–495b, 495f
secondary, 607b
target organ damage, 608–609, 609b, 609f
venous, 1262
white coat, 608
Hyperthermia
malignant, 1230b
organophosphate poisoning, 224b
Hyperthyroidism *see* Thyrotoxicosis
Hypertrichosis, 1297
drug-induced, 1304b
Hypertriglyceridaemia, 454b, 455
familial, 454b, 455
management, 457–458
secondary, 453b
Hypertrophic obstructive cardiomyopathy (HOCM), 554f, 561, 637, 1159
Hypertrophic pulmonary osteoarthropathy (HPOA), 701
Hyperuricaemia, 1087
asymptomatic, 1087
gout, 1087b
Hyperventilation
panic disorder, 243
psychogenic, 246
and respiratory alkalosis, 447
Hyperviscosity syndrome, 1045
Hypervolaemia
CVP, 183f
with hypernatraemia, 439b
with hyponatraemia, 433b, 437b
Hypnic jerks, 1167
Hypnotics
dosage regimen, 35b
effect of old age, 36b
Hypoadrenalism, tuberculosis, 696
Hypoalbuminaemia, 768b
nephrotic syndrome, 477b
Hypobetalipoproteinaemia, 455–456
Hypocalcaemia, 768–769
differential diagnosis, 768b
ethylene glycol poisoning, 222
and hypomagnesaemia, 448
hypoparathyroidism and, 770
management, 769b
pancreatitis, 891b
renal failure
acute, 482–483
chronic, 486–488
Hypochlorhydria
anaemia and, 1025
and small bowel bacterial overgrowth, 872–873
Hypochlorous ions, 73
Hypochondriacal disorder, 245
Hypofibrinogenaemia, 1000b, 1051b
Hypogammaglobulinaemia, 81
Hypoglossal (12th cranial) nerve, tests, 1139b
Hypoglycaemia
awareness of, 815–816
causes, 815b
diabetics, 814–816
drug-induced, 823, 825, 825b
exercise-induced, 815
malaria, 357b
management, 816, 816b
nocturnal, 815
older people, 784b
prevention, 816, 816b
risk factors, 815b
spontaneous, 783–784, 783f, 814–815
symptoms, 815b
Hypogonadism, 758b
hypergonadotrophic, 759
hypogonadotrophic, 759–760
male, 760–762
Hypokalaemia, 440–442, 440f–441f
chloroquine poisoning, 215
heart failure, 549
hyperaldosteronism, 780
mineralocorticoid excess, 781
periodic paralysis, 1230b
Hypomagnesaemia, 448, 448b, 768b
management, 769b
Hypomania, 244–245
Hypomimia, 1196b
Hyponatraemia, 437–439, 437f, 929
adrenal insufficiency, 777, 778b
brain in, 437f
causes, 437b
depletional, 437–438
differential diagnosis, 438b
dilutional, 437b, 438
acute renal failure, 482–483
ecstasy/amphetamine misuse, 218
with euvolaemia, 437b, 438
heart failure, 549
with hypervolaemia, 433b, 437b
hypopituitarism, 787–788
with hypovolaemia, 433b, 437–438, 437b
older people, 176b, 439, 439b
Hypoparathyroidism, 768b, 770–771
Hypophosphataemia, 448–449, 449b
rickets/osteomalacia, 1066b, 1128
Hypophosphatasia, 1128
Hypopigmentation, 1295–1296
Hypopituitarism, 787–789
clinical assessment, 787–788, 788f
investigation, 787b, 788
management, 788–789
Hyposmia, 1169
Hypotension
dialysis, 492b
poisoning, 211b
postural, 554, 556
hypopituitarism, 787–788
management, 172
older people, 36b
renal disease, 479
shock, 83
Hypothalamus, 785–795, 786f, 1143
diseases
classification, 786b
investigation, 786–787, 787b
older people, 795b
presenting problems, 787–791
functional anatomy and physiology, 786–787
thermoregulation, 103–104
tumours, 790b
Hypothermia, 104–105, 104f
cold water immersion, 108
older people, 104b
Hypothyroidism, 743–745
autoimmune, 741b, 743b
causes, 743b
clinical features, 740b, 743
congenital, 755
iatrogenic, 743b
investigations, 743
laboratory abnormalities, 741b
management, 743–745, 744f
musculoskeletal manifestations, 1132
with normal thyroid function tests, 745
obesity, 759
older people, 755b
pregnancy, 745, 756b
primary
causes, 743b
clinical features, 743
investigations, 743
management, 743–745
secondary, 743b
spontaneous atrophic, 743b
subclinical, 746
transient, 743
transient thyroiditis, 743b
Hypoventilation, alveolar, 191, 665
Hypovolaemia
AKI, 197
with hypernatraemia, 439b
with hyponatraemia, 433b, 437–438, 437b
right atrial pressure, 185
shock, 74b
Hypovolaemic shock, 83, 190
CVP, 183f
Hypoxaemia, 106f
acute, 191
circulatory collapse, 191b
cirrhosis, 943
high-altitude pulmonary oedema, 107
near-drowning accidents, 108
respiratory failure, 191
Hypoxia
altitude illness/air travel, 107
cytopathic, 185
pancreatitis, 891b
respiratory failure, 664b
Hypromellose, 1114

Hysterectomy, cancer treatment, 280–281
Hysteria, 1210

I
Ibandronate, osteoporosis, 1123b
IBD *see* Inflammatory bowel disease
IBS *see* Irritable bowel syndrome
Ibuprofen, 1079b
adverse reactions, 26b
and gastroduodenal bleeding, 1079b
ICAM-1, 531–532
ICD *see* Implantable cardiac defibrillator
ICD-10 *see* International Classification of Disease-10
Ice cream headache, 1178b
Ice pick headache, 1178b
ICF *see* Intracellular fluid
Ichthyosis, 350, 1252
ICP *see* Intracranial pressure
Idiopathic thrombocytopenic purpura (ITP), 1050
IDL *see* Intermediate-density lipoproteins
If channel antagonists, angina, 587
Ifosfamide, 446b
Ig *see* Immunoglobulin
IGF *see* Insulin-like growth factor
IGF-BP3 *see* Insulin-like growth factor binding protein
IgG4-associated cholangitis, 966, 988
IGT *see* Impaired glucose tolerance
IL *see* Interleukin
Ileal resection, 850, 884f
Ileus
gallstones, 983
meconium, 895
paralytic, 890–892
Illusions, 234
Iloprost, 603
Imaging
cardiovascular system, 535–538
epilepsy, 1182b
gastrointestinal tract, 845–851, 847b
hepatobiliary disease, 930–931, 961
musculoskeletal disease, 1064–1066
nervous system/brain, 1149–1150, 1149b, 1235–1236, 1235f–1236f, 1241–1242
renal tract, 468–471
respiratory tract, 649–651
see also Radiology; *and individual imaging techniques*
Imatinib, 279
acute leukaemia, 1037b
chronic myeloid leukaemia, 1039–1040
GIST, 880
Imidazoles, 159, 160b
topical, 1266
Imipenem, 154b
melioidosis, 340
Imipramine, 244b
bladder dysfunction, 1175b
irritable bowel syndrome, 909
Imiprothrin, 224b
Imiquimod, 1266
anogenital warts, 426
lentigo maligna, 1273
molluscum contagiosum, 1279
skin cancer, 1270–1271
viral warts, 1278–1279
Immersion foot, 105
Immotile cilia syndrome, 678b
Immune deficiency, 78–82
adaptive immunity, 80–82
combined B/T-lymphocyte, 80
common variable (CVID), 81
genetic testing, 62b
older people, 82b
presenting problems, 79
secondary, 82, 82b
severe combined, 80
T-cell, 78b, 80, 80f
warning signs, 79b
see also HIV infection/AIDS
Immune reconstitution inflammatory syndrome (IRIS), 138, 408–409
Immune response modifiers, 1266
Immune responses
adaptive (acquired), 76–78
cytokines, 74b
innate, 72–76
lower airway defence, 648
Immune senescence, 82
Immune surveillance, 1269–1270
Immune system
adaptive (acquired), 76–78, 76f
deficiencies, 80–82
diabetes type 1, 804
functional anatomy and physiology, 72–78
innate, 72–76
regulation, 927–928
Immunisation, 148–149
antibody deficiencies, 81–82
chickenpox, 318
cholera, 345
diphtheria, 346
Haemophilus influenzae, 149b, 1051–1052
HIV/AIDS patients, 407
influenza, 320
HIV/AIDS patients, 407
meningococcal infection, 1203–1204
mumps, 319
plague, 339
pneumococcal, 346
poliomyelitis, 1207
rabies, 1206
rubella, 315
tetanus, 1210
tick-borne encephalitis, 309b
transplant recipients, 95
tuberculosis, 696
typhoid, 340
varicella, 318
viral hepatitis, 954b
haemophiliacs, 1051–1052
HIV/AIDS patients, 407
whooping cough (pertussis), 149b
yellow fever, 324
see also Vaccines/Vaccination
Immunity
adaptive, 76–78
cellular, 78
HIV infection/AIDS, 390
humoral, 77–78
Immunoblot test, 141–142
innate, 843
Immunoblot test, 141–142
Immunochromatographic tests, 142
Immunocompromised host, fever in, 301–302
Immunodiffusion, 142
Immunofluorescence, 142
amoebiasis, 368
anti-endomysial antibodies, 881
glomerular disease, 498f
leishmaniasis, 363
plague, 338
skin samples, 1294f
Immunoglobulin(s), 77–78, 1011
antiRhD (anti-D), 1014
in glomerulonephritis, 499b–500b
intravenous
Guillain-Barré syndrome, 1225b
myasthenia gravis, 1227b
myositis, 1115
thrombocytopenia, 405, 1050
toxic epidermal necrolysis, 1292b
toxic shock syndrome, 331
in multiple myeloma, 1046b
prophylactic, 149b
reference values, venous blood, 1310b
structure, 77f
thyroid-stimulating, 747–748
Immunoglobulin A (IgA), 77b
deficiency, selective, 81
dermatitis herpetiformis, 1294
linear IgA disease, 1293b, 1294
nephropathy, 499b–500b, 500–501
reference values, venous blood, 1310b
Immunoglobulin D (IgD), 77b
hyper IgD syndrome, 85
Immunoglobulin E (IgE), 77b
antibodies, 89
reference values, 1310b
specific IgE tests, 90, 1255
total serum, 90
Immunoglobulin G (IgG), 77b
anti-HBc, 952b
anti-HDV, 954
cerebrospinal fluid, 1311b
functional IgG antibody deficiency, 81
reference values, 1310b
rubella-specific, 315
Immunoglobulin M (IgM), 77b
anti-HBc, 929, 952f
anti-HDV, 954
cold agglutinin disease, 1030–1031
reference values, 1310b
Immunohistochemistry, tumour identification, 268
Immunological memory, 77–78
Immunological tests, 141–143, 1153
antibody-independent, 142–143
hepatobiliary disease, 929–930
renal disease, 468
respiratory disease, 652
Immunological tolerance, 86–87
Immunomodulation, 1267–1268
Immunophenotyping, 998, 1035–1036
Immunoproliferative small intestinal disease (IPSID), 889
Immunosuppressants
autoimmune hepatitis, 962–963
HSCT, 1018
multiple sclerosis, 1191–1192, 1192b
myasthenia gravis, 1227b
skin disease, 1267–1268
see also individual drugs
Immunosuppression
autoimmune hepatitis, 963b
complications of, 95–96
SLE, 1112
transplant patients, 96b
liver transplantation, 979
Immunotherapy
allergy, 90–91, 91b
cancer, 278
myasthenia gravis, 1227b
Impaired glucose tolerance (IGT), 169f, 455, 754b, 1310b
Impetigo, 1275–1276, 1275f
bullous, 1258b, 1276
Implantable cardiac defibrillator (ICD)
heart failure, 553, 553f
hypertrophic cardiomyopathy, 638
ventricular arrhythmias, 579, 579b, 599
Impotence *see* Erectile dysfunction
Inborn errors of metabolism, 64–65
genetic testing, 62b
intoxicating, 64–65
mitochondrial disorders, 65, 1229, 1229b
storage disorders, 65
Incapacity, 291
Incidence of disease, 99, 99b
Incident pain, 285b
Incidentaloma, 737b, 779
Inclusion body myositis, 1115
Incontinence
faecal, 918, 918b, 1175
stroke patients, 1243b
urinary, 472–474, 1174
neurogenic bladder, 1174
older people, 175, 175f, 473b
overflow, 473, 1174
stress, 473
urge, 473, 1174
incremental cost-effectiveness ratio (ICER), 32
Incretin effect, 801–802, 802f
Incretin-based therapies, 822b, 823–824
Incubation period, infections, 310b
Indigestion *see* Dyspepsia
Indometacin, 1079b
diabetes insipidus, 795
gastrointestinal bleeding, 1079b
paroxysmal headache prevention, 1178
pericarditis, 639
persistent ductus arteriosus, 632
skin reactions, 1304b
Indoramin, 612
Infection(s), 133–164, 293–386
adolescents, 313, 313b
agents of, 134–135, 134b
bacterial, 329–353
gastrointestinal, 341–345
with neurological involvement, 347, 1202–1204, 1202b
respiratory, 345–347
skin, 329–333
soft tissue, 329–333
systemic, 333–341
bone, 329–333
central venous catheters, 303–304
chain of infection, 134f
chlamydial, 353, 423
chronic renal failure, 477b
clinical examination, 294f
common infecting organisms, 151b
constitutive barriers to, 72–76
control, 145–149
critically ill patients, 200b
definition, 134, 184b
deliberate release, 145
emerging/re-emerging disease, 143, 144f
endemic disease, 143
epidemiology, 143–145
fungal *see* Fungal infections
gastrointestinal tract
bacterial infections, 341–345
inflammatory bowel disease, 903b
oesophagus, 868
oral cavity, 864
protozoal, 367–369
small intestine, 888
tests, 849–850
viral, 327–328
glomerulonephritis and, 499b–500b, 501
haematological disorders, 1008
health care-acquired *see* Health care-acquired infections
helminthic, 369–381
history-taking, 295b
hospital-acquired, 685–687
host-pathogen interaction, 134, 137–138
HSCT, 1017b
incubation periods, 145b, 310b
injecting drug users, 299–301, 300f
joints, 1094–1096
neuropathic (Charcot), 833–835
older people, 1094b
kidney, 511–514
tuberculosis, 514, 692

liver, 948–957
microbiological investigations, 138–143, 139b
culture, 140–141
direct detection, 139–140, 139b
immunological tests, 141–143
microbiological sampling, 139b
mycobacterial, 135, 347–350
myocardial, 636
nervous system, 1201–1211, 1201b
normal flora, 136–137, 137f
opportunistic
HIV/AIDS patients, 405–407, 406b
mycobacterial, 696, 696b
outbreaks, 147
reporting, 148b
terminology, 148b
pathogenesis, 138
pericardial *see* Pericarditis
periods of infectivity, 144b
post-operative *see individual infections*
in pregnancy, 313, 314b
presenting problems, 296–313
prevention, 145–149
protozoal, 353–369
recurrent, 78b, 79
reservoirs, 143–144
animal, 144
environmental, 144
human, 143
respiratory tract
asthma and, 667
cystic fibrosis, 681
fungal, 697–699
older people, 686b
pneumonia, 658b, 682–688
rheumatoid disease, 713
SARS, 682–683
upper, 681–682
rickettsial, 350–352, 351b
sexually transmitted *see* Sexually transmitted infections
skin *see* Skin infections
starvation-associated, 121b
stem cell transplantation, 1017b
stroke patients, 1243b
transmission, 144, 147b
blood transfusion, 1014–1015
treatment, 149–164, 151b
tropical, 308–313
urinary tract, 511–514
older people, 512b
stroke patients, 1243b
VUR and, 511b
viral *see* Viral infections
wound *see* Wound infections
Infectious mononucleosis, 320, 320b, 321f
Infective endocarditis, 625–629
acute, 626
bartonellosis, 352–353, 352b
diagnosis, 627b
injecting drug users, 625
management, 628, 628b
older people, 626b
pathophysiology, 625–629, 626b
post-operative, 626–627
prevention, 628–629
subacute, 626
symptoms, 626–627, 627f
Inferior petrosal sinus sampling, 774f
Inferior vena cava, 464, 515–516, 516f
Infertility, 761–762, 761b
hypogonadism, 762
polycystic ovary syndrome, 762, 764b
Infestations, skin, 1275–1281
Inflammation
acute, 82–83, 83f
cancer, 265–266
chronic, 83
investigations, 83–85
local, 184–185
presenting problems, 85
resolution, 82–83
systemic, 185
Inflammatory bowel disease (IBD), 897–907
childhood, 906
clinical features, 899–900
complications, 900–901, 901f–902f
differential diagnosis, 900, 900b
disease distribution, 898f
investigations, 901–902
management, 902–905, 903b
metabolic bone disease, 907
microscopic colitis and, 907
monitoring, 904b
pathophysiology, 897–907, 898b, 898f
perianal, 860, 919
pregnancy, 906–907, 906b
Inflammatory myopathy, 1117b
Inflammatory response, 82–86
asthma, 669
pathophysiology, 184–185
terminology, 184b
Infliximab
inflammatory bowel disease, 903b, 904, 905b
psoriasis, 1289b
rheumatoid arthritis, 1103b
skin reactions, 1304b
Influenza, 319–320
avian, 320
chemoprophylaxis, 153b
epidemic, 138
immunisation, 149b
HIV/AIDS patients, 407
older people, 686b
incubation period, 145b, 310b
swine, 320
treatment, 161b, 162, 320
Influenza-like illness, 1123–1124
Information provision
genetic diseases, 67–68
for informed consent, 10–11
on risk, 7, 7f
truth-telling, 10
Informed consent, 10–11
Infrapatellar bursitis, 1076b
Infrared radiation, 1257b
Inhalation fever, 719b, 720
Inhalational administration, 21–22
Inheritance, 51–53
autosomal dominant, 51–53
autosomal recessive, 53
epigenetic, 52f, 53, 54b
mitochondrial, 53
pedigrees, 51f
X-linked, 53
Inherited diseases *see* Genetic diseases
Inhibin, 737f, 756f
INO *see* Internuclear ophthalmoplegia
Inorganic micronutrients, 130–132
INR *see* International Normalised Ratio
Insect bites, 308–309, 309b
Insect stings, allergic reactions, 94
Insecticides
carbamate, 222
organophosphorus, 220–222, 220b, 221f
pyrethroid, 224b
Insertions, 55
Insight, 234
Insomnia
fatal familial, 329b, 1211
sporadic fatal, 329b
Insulin
adverse reactions, 26b
deficiency, type 1 diabetes, 799
diabetic ketoacidosis, 813
ectopic production, 271b
hypoglycaemia, 810, 810b
manufacture and formulation, 824–826
metabolic actions, 801b, 801f
metabolism, chronic renal failure
reference range, 1309b
secretion, 802f
Insulin receptor, 49b
Insulin resistance, 821
polycystic ovarian syndrome, 764b
in pregnancy, 817
type 2 diabetes, 799, 805
Insulin resistance (metabolic) syndrome (syndrome X), 589, 805
Insulin secretagogues *see* Oral hypoglycaemics
Insulin therapy
adverse reactions, 825b
delivery (systems), 826
diabetes mellitus, 822b, 824–826, 824b
hypoglycaemia and, 810, 810b
myocardial infarction, 818
patient education, 810
regimens, 825, 825f
subcutaneous, 824–825
surgical patients, 818–820
diabetic ketoacidosis, 813
injection sites, 799b
injection technique, 824b
preparations, 825
Insulin tolerance test, 789b
Insulin-like growth factor binding protein (IGF-BP3), 737f
Insulin-like growth factor (IGF), 737f, 786, 925f
Insulinomas, 785b
Insulitis, 803, 803f
Integrase, 391
Integrase inhibitors, 407b
Integrated health care, 16
Integrative medicine, 446
Intellectual abilities, assessment, 234
Intensive care units (ICUs) *see* Critical care
Intention tremor, 1145
Intercostal tube drainage, 663, 730, 730f
Interferon
cancer therapy, 785
leukaemia, 1039b
pegylated, 954b
renal adenocarcinoma, 516
viral hepatitis, 954b, 955
HIV/AIDS patients, 400
warts, 1278–1279
see also specific interferons
Interferon-α, 74b, 162
chronic myeloid leukaemia, 1039–1040
hepatitis B, 161b, 162, 953
hepatitis C, 161b, 162, 955
malignant melanoma, 278
pegylated, 161b, 955b
polycythaemia rubra vera, 1049
Interferon-β, multiple sclerosis, 1191b–1192b
Interferon-γ, 74b, 1266
in coeliac disease, 880f
pulmonary fibrosis, 709
release tests, 142–143, 695, 695f
Interindividual variation in drug response, 23–24, 24b
Interleukin (IL)
bone remodelling, 1062b
immune response, 74b
renal adenocarcinoma, 516
Intermediate filaments, 48
Intermediate syndrome, organophosphate poisoning, 222
Intermediate-density lipoproteins (IDL), 451
Intermittent claudication, 601
Intermittent clean self-catheterisation (ISC), 474, 1174b
Intermittent positive pressure ventilation (IPPV), 195f, 482
International Association for the Study of Pain (IASP), 284
International Classification of Disease-10 (ICD-10), 232
International Classification of Functioning and Disability, 176b
International Normalised Ratio (INR), 926–927, 1000
International Prostate Symptom Score (IPPS), 514b
International system of units, 1308
Internuclear ophthalmoplegia (INO), 1190b
Interpersonal therapy (IPT), 242
Interphalangeal joints (IPJs)
distal, psoriatic arthritis, 1108, 1109f
osteoarthritis, 1083f
rheumatoid arthritis, 1098f
Interstitial cells of Cajal, 845
Interstitial lung disease, 706–714
diagnosis/investigation, 707f
drug-induced, 714b
older people, 714b
rare, 715b
Interstitial nephritis *see* Nephritis, interstitial
Interstitial pneumonia, 709
desquamative, 708b
acute, 708b
idiopathic, 706–709, 708b
lymphocytic, 708b
usual, 708b, 709f
Interstitial pneumonitis
lymphocytic, 401, 404
usual, 709f
Intertrigo, 381, 1280
Interventricular septal rupture, 597
Intervertebral discs, 1062
degeneration, 1218
herniation, 1219–1220
intra-articular, 1063
prolapsed, 541b, 659b, 1073, 1220, 1220b
Interviewing patient, 4b
Intestines *see* Colon; Gut; Small intestine
Intra-articular discs, 1063
Intra-epidermal carcinoma *see* Bowen's disease
Intracellular fluid (ICF), 429
Intracerebral haemorrhage, 1238f–1239f, 1239
causes, 1239b
Intracranial hypertension
idiopathic, 1217–1218
pain, 285b
Intracranial mass lesions, 1211–1218, 1212b
Intracranial pressure (ICP)
control, 199, 199b
raised, 1212–1213, 1212b, 1213f
headache, 285b
Intramuscular administration, 21
Intranasal administration, 21
Intraretinal microvascular abnormalities (IRMA), 829f
Intravenous administration, 21
Intravenous immunoglobulin (IVIgG) *see* Immunoglobulin(s), intravenous
Intravenous urography (IVU), 470, 470f
medullary sponge kidney, 507f
renal colic, 508
renal stones, 508f
retroperitoneal fibrosis, 511
stone disease, 508f
stress incontinence, 473–474

Intrinsic factor, gastric, 871–872, 1024–1025
Introns, 43f
Intubation
critically ill patients, 194, 194b
endotracheal, 194, 194b
nasogastric, 879b
Investigations, 4–7
normal distribution/range, 5, 5f
predictive value, 6
screening, 6–7
sensitivity and specificity, 5–6, 6b, 6f
Involuntary movements, 1145
Iodide, 738
Iodine, 131
deficiency, 131, 752
dietary sources, 131b
radioactive
and fetal hypothyroidism, 750
thyroid cancer, 754b
thyrotoxicosis, 741–742, 749
RNI, 131b
Iodine-induced thyroid dysfunction, 752
Iodoquinol, 164
Iomeara spp., 309b
Ion channels, drugs acting on, 19b, 47f
Ion-exchange resins, 442–443, 443b
Ionising radiation, 102–103, 102b
Ipecacuanha, 210
IPJs *see* Interphalangeal joints
IPPS *see* International Prostate Symptom Score
IPPV *see* Intermittent positive pressure ventilation
Ipratropium bromide
asthma, 560
COPD, 675
IPSID *see* Immunoproliferative small intestinal disease
IPT *see* Interpersonal therapy
Irbesartan, 611–612
Irinotecan, 857
IRMA *see* Intraretinal microvascular abnormalities
Iron, 130–131
absorption/uptake/distribution, 130–131, 1022, 1022f
deficiency, 131, 1001–1002, 1021–1023
alimentary tract disorders, 867
ancylostomiasis, 310
older people, 1034b
pregnancy, 1022b
dietary sources, 131b
overload, 131
haemochromatosis, 131, 972–973
plasma, iron deficiency anaemia, 1023
poisoning, 209b, 216
reference values, 1312b
RNI, 131b
supplements
congestive gastropathy, 928
and constipation, 860b
pregnancy, 1022b
total iron binding capacity, 1023
Iron oxide, 717b
Irritable bowel syndrome (IBS), 907–909
diagnosis, 907b–908b
diarrhoea, 907–908
management, 908–909, 908f, 909b
Irritant eczema, 1284
management, 1286
ISC *see* Intermittent self-catheterisation
Ischaemia
acute limb, 603, 603b
cerebral, 199b, 572, 1046f
critical limb, 601–602, 601f
gastrointestinal tract, 909–910
liver, 975
lower limbs, 580, 601b
myocardial *see* Myocardial ischaemia
splanchnic, 198
Ischaemic heart disease
chest pain, 539f–540f
hierarchy of systems, 98b
sibling risk, 67b
thyroxine replacement, 744–745
Ischaemic hepatitis, 198
Ischaemic nephropathy, 494
Ischaemic pain, 285b
Ischaemic penumbra, 1239
Ischiogluteal bursitis, 1075b
Islet cells
antibodies, type 1 diabetes, 803
transplantation, 826
Isocyanates, lung disease and, 715b
Isolation, 147b
Isoleucine, 114b
Isoniazid
adverse reactions, 694b
hepatotoxicity, 154b, 971b
multiple sclerosis, 1192b
overdose, 224b
and peripheral neuropathy, 1223b
pharmacokinetics, 25b
poisoning, 224b
prophylactic, 153b
and pyridoxine deficiency, 129
resistance, 151–152
skin reactions, 1304b
tuberculosis
HIV/AIDS patients, 406–407, 407b
prophylaxis, 406–407, 407b
treatment, 693, 694b
Isoprenaline, 214–215
AV block, 572–573
torsades de pointes, 571
Isosorbide dinitrate, 586b
Isosorbide mononitrate, 586b
Isospora infections
HIV/AIDS patients, 399b, 406b
prophylaxis, 406b
Isotretinoin (13-cis-retinoic acid), 37b, 1267
Ispaghula husk, 908f, 916–917
Itch *see* Pruritus
ITP *see* Idiopathic thrombocytopenic purpura
Itraconazole, 159–160, 160b
acute leukaemia patients, 1038
aspergillosis, 699
blastomycosis, 386
chromoblastomycosis, 381–382
cutaneous leishmaniasis, 367
fungal infections, 159–160
histoplasmosis, 385–386
mycetoma, 382
onychomycosis, 1280
P. marneffei infection, 385–386
prophylactic, 153b, 1038
skin disease, 1267
sporotrichosis, 383
Ivabradine
angina, 587
heart failure, 552
Ivermectin
helminthic infections, 163, 371
filariases, 373–374
scabies, 1280–1281
IVU *see* Intravenous urography

J
Jaccoud's arthropathy, 1110
Japanese B encephalitis, 328, 1205
Jarisch-Herxheimer reaction (JHR), 335, 338, 421–422
Jaundice, 936–938, 936b
acute liver failure, 932–934, 932b–933b
alcoholic liver disease, 958, 958b
cholestatic, 936b–937b, 937–938
cirrhosis, 943b
cytomegalovirus, 321
heart failure, 549
hepatocellular, 936–937
intensive care unit, 198
investigations, 938f
leptospirosis, 337
obstructive, 937–938, 937b
pancreatic tumours, 895
pancreatitis, 891b, 892, 893b
pre-hepatic, 936
primary biliary cirrhosis, 963
see also Hyperbilirubinaemia
JC virus, 402
Jehovah's Witnesses, 11
Jejunum
coeliac disease *see* Coeliac disease
hormones of, 846b
short bowel syndrome, 885b
Jellyfish, 228b
JIA *see* Juvenile idiopathic arthritis
Jiggers, 381
Jod-Basedow effect, 752
Joint capsule, 1063
Joint disease
crystal-associated, 1086–1092, 1086b, 1086f
infection, 1094–1096
tuberculosis, 691–692
tumours, 1131–1132, 1131b
see also Arthritis; Arthropathy
Joints, 1062–1063, 1062b
aspiration, 1064
bleeding into, 1006, 1051
examination
blood disorders, 990f
febrile patient, 294f
older people, 166f
fibrocartilaginous, 1062
fibrous/fibrocartilaginous, 1062
haemophilia, 1051
hands, diabetes, 799b
hypermobility, 1134, 1134b
infection, 1094–1096
neuropathic (Charcot), 833–835
older people, 1094b
pain, 902f, 1097
prosthetic, infection, 1094, 1094b
protection, 1078
replacement, osteoarthritis, 1086
surgery, 1086
synovial, 1062–1063, 1063f
osteoarthritis, 1085
types of, 1062b
Jugular venous pressure, 548
respiration effects, 532b
Jugular venous pulse (JVP)
ascites, 923b
examination, 527b
pulmonary hypertension, 724
tricuspid valve disease, 624–625
Junin virus, 325b
Justice, 11
Juvenile absence epilepsy, 1182b
Juvenile idiopathic arthritis (JIA), 1103–1104, 1104b
adolescents, 1104b
Juvenile myoclonic epilepsy, 1182b
JVP *see* Jugular venous pulse

K
Kala-azar (visceral leishmaniasis), 362–365
HIV co-infection, 364–365
incubation period, 310b
post-kala-azar dermal leishmaniasis, 365
Kallmann's syndrome, 759
Kaposi's sarcoma, 397–398, 398f
HHV8 and, 317b, 326
treatment, 398
Kartagener's syndrome, 648
Karyotype analysis, 57f
Kashin-Beck disease, 1084–1085
Katayama fever, 312b–313b
Kawasaki disease, 1116
Kayser-Fleischer rings, 974
Kco (transfer coefficient for carbon monoxide), 653b
KDIGO criteria, 481b
Kearns-Sayre syndrome, 1199b, 1229b
Keloids, 1264–1265
Kennedy disease, 65
Keratan sulphate, 1062–1063
Keratinocytes, 1252
Keratins, 48, 1252
Keratoacanthoma, 1272, 1272f
Keratoconjunctivitis sicca
rheumatoid arthritis, 1099
Sjögren's syndrome, 1114
Keratoderma blennorrhagica, 1108
Keratolysis, pitted, 1278
Keratomalacia, 127
Keratosis, actinic, 1266, 1271, 1271f
Kerion, 1280
Kernig's sign, 1201
Kerosene poisoning, 224b
Keshan's disease, 132
Ketamine, 288b
Ketoacidosis, diabetic, 804, 811–814
Ketoconazole, 159, 160b
Cushing's syndrome, 776
cutaneous leishmaniasis, 367
mycetoma, 382
paracoccidioidomycosis, 386
shampoo, 1280
skin disease, 1267
systemic fungal infections
Ketogenesis, 801b, 801f
Ketolides, 156
Ketone bodies, 801f, 802
testing for, 807
Ketones
blood, 808, 808b
urine, 807–808
Ketonuria, 807–808
Ketoprofen, 1079b
Kidney disease *see* Nephropathy; Renal disease
Kidneys, 461–523
acid-base balance control, 444
clinical examination, 462f–463f
congenital abnormalities, 510–511
cystic disease, 505–507
drugs and, 522–523, 522b
duplex, 510
functional anatomy, 464–466, 465f
functions, 24b
tests, 466–471
imaging, 468–471
infections, 511–514
tuberculosis, 514, 692
medullary sponge, 506, 507f
potassium handling, 440, 440f
pregnancy, 520–521, 520b
single, 510
sodium handling, 430–432, 430f
stones, 507–510, 507b
clinical features, 507–510
investigations, 507, 508b
management, 509–510, 509b, 509f
pathophysiology, 507–510
prevention, 509b
systemic conditions affecting, 519–520
transplantation, 482b, 492–494
contraindications, 493b
cystic disease, 506
diabetics, 826, 831
SLE, 520
tumours, 515–519
inherited, 519
urothelial, 516–517, 517f
water handling, 436–437
see also Renal
Kimmelstiel-Wilson nodule, 830f
Kinases, cyclin-dependent, 263
Klebsiella spp., 137f, 512
Klebsiella granulomatis, 424b
Klebsiella oxytoca, 308
Klebsiella pneumoniae infection, 687

Klinefelter's syndrome, 766
  genetics, 56b
Knee
  osteoarthritis, 1083–1084, 1083f
  pain, 1075–1076, 1076b
  rheumatoid arthritis, 1098
Knudsen two-hit hypothesis, 59–60
Köbner phenomenon, 1289–1290, 1290f
Koch's postulates, 99, 134b, 346
Koilonychia, 1298, 1298f
Koplik's spots, 314, 315f
Korsakoff's syndrome/psychosis, 128, 1162
Krebs (citric acid) cycle, 128
Krukenberg tumour, 878
Kupffer cells, 74, 927
Kuru, 329b, 1211
Kussmaul respiration, 484
Kussmaul's sign, 545b
Kwashiorkor, 120–121
Kyasanur forest disease, 309b, 324, 325b
Kyphoplasty, 1080b, 1125, 1125b
Kyphoscoliosis, 644f
  thoracic, 731
Kyphosis, 114–115, 166f, 692f
  ankylosing spondylitis, 1105

L

L-dopa *see* Levodopa
Labetalol
  aortic dissection, 607
  hypertension, 612
    malignant, 612
Laboratory investigations, biochemical, 428–429, 428b
Laboratory values, 1308
Labyrinthitis, 1186
Lactase deficiency, 887
Lactate
  blood, measurement in critically ill patients, 187
  reference values, venous blood, 1310b
Lactate dehydrogenase (LDH)
  AKI, 480b
  empyema, 663
  hypothyroidism, 741b
  megaloblastic anaemia, 1003f, 1024b
  pancreatitis, 890b
  pleural effusion, 275–276
  reference values, venous blood, 1310b
Lactation, nutrition in, 125b
Lactic acidosis, 445
  diabetics, 823
Lactitol, 917b
Lactobacillus spp., 137f
Lactoferrin, 1068
Lactose, refeeding diet, 122b
Lactose hydrogen (H2) breath test, 851b
Lactose intolerance, 112–113, 887–888
Lactulose, 917b
  hepatic encephalopathy management, 942
  hydrogen breath test, 883
  variceal bleeding, 946b
Lacunar infarctions, 1174b, 1237
Lacunar syndrome, 1241f
LAD *see* Left anterior descending artery
LADA *see* Latent autoimmune diabetes in adults
Lambert-Eaton myasthenic syndrome (LEMS), 271b, 272, 1194b, 1227–1228, 1227f
Lamina densa, 1252
Lamina lucida, 1252
Laminins, 48
Lamivudine (3TC), 407b
  resistance, 408
  viral hepatitis, 161b, 162, 953
    HIV/AIDS patients, 400
Lamotrigine, 1184b
  skin reactions, 1304b
Langerhans cell histiocytosis, 715b
Langerhans cells, 1252
Language
  disorders, 1170b
  spoken, 4, 19
Lanreotide, 793
Laparoscopy
  ascites, 940
  infertility, 762
  lower abdominal pain, 418
  pyrexia of unknown origin, 298–299
  tuberculosis, 691
Lapdap, 356
Laron dwarfism, 786b
Larva currens, 370
Larva migrans
  cutaneous, 375–376, 375f
  visceral, 311–312
Laryngeal nerve, recurrent, palsy, 748b, 753
Laryngitis
  acid, 680
  chronic, 727, 727b
  cough, 654–655, 654b
Laryngoscopy, 651, 727
Larynx
  obstruction, 728, 728b
  paralysis, 727
Lasègue's sign, 1219
Laser therapy
  benign prostatic hyperplasia, 515
  bleeding control, 848f
  bronchial carcinoma, 704
  carbon dioxide, 1269
  colorectal cancer, 915
  diabetic retinopathy, 828
  hereditary haemorrhagic telangiectasia, 1049
  hypertrichosis, 1297
  oesophageal carcinoma, 871
  rosacea, 1283
  skin disease, 1269
Lassa fever, 324, 325b
  incubation period, 145b, 325b
Latent autoimmune diabetes in adults (LADA), 810
Latex agglutination test, 383
Lavage
  bronchoalveolar, 711
  gastric, 210, 210b
Law *see* Legal issues
Lawrence-Moon-Biedl syndrome, 116
Laxatives, 917b
  body packers, 219, 219f
  misuse, 917
LBBB *see* Left bundle branch block
LCAT *see* Lecithin cholesterol acyl transferase
LDH *see* Lactate dehydrogenase
LDL *see* Low-density lipoprotein
Lead
  poisoning, 224b
  reference values, venous blood, 1310b
Lead pipe rigidity, 1145
Leão, spreading depression of, 1176–1177
Learning difficulties, 66
  congenital heart disease and, 631
Leber's hereditary optic neuropathy, 1229
Lecithin cholesterol acyl transferase (LCAT), 452
  deficiency, 455–456, 456b
Lectin
  mannose-binding
    deficiency, 79
    pathway, 75f
  pathway, 75
Leflunomide, 1101b, 1102
Left anterior descending artery (LAD)
  coronary circulation, 529f
  occlusion, 538f
  stenosis, 538f
Left atrial dilatation, 535, 566–567
Left bundle branch block (LBBB), 573, 573b
Left main coronary artery, 529f
  occlusion, 529, 589b
Left ventricular dilatation, 535, 618–619
Left ventricular function, 598
Left ventricular hypertrophy, 622f
Legal issues, 13–14
  artificial nutritional support, 124, 124b
  definition of law, 14b
  psychiatry, 257
Legionella spp., 148b, 153b, 310b
Legionella pneumophila infection, 139, 151b
Legs
  examination
    cardiovascular disease, 526f
    diabetes mellitus, 798f, 799b
    endocrine disease, 734f
    febrile injecting drug user, 300f
    HIV/AIDS, 388f
    liver and biliary disease, 922f
    musculoskeletal disease, 1058f
  oedema, 478
  restless, 485–486, 1187–1188, 1188b
  ulcers, 1262–1263, 1262b
    arterial, 1263
    tropical, 333
    venous, 1263, 1263f
  see also Foot
Leigh's syndrome, 46, 1199b
Leishman-Donovan bodies (amastigotes), 363f
Leishmania, 362
  life cycle, 362f–363f
  Viannia subgenus, 366–367
Leishmania aethiopica, 366b
Leishmania amazonensis, 366
Leishmania brasiliensis, 366f
Leishmania chagasi, 362–363
Leishmania donovani, 362–363
Leishmania guyanensis, 366
Leishmania infantum, 362–363, 366f
Leishmania major, 366b, 366f
Leishmania mexicana, 366, 366f
Leishmania tropica, 366b, 366f
Leishmaniasis, 309b, 362–367
  cutaneous, 365–366, 366b, 366f
    incubation period, 145b, 310b
  HIV co-infection, 364–365
  mucosal, 366–367
  post-kala-azar dermal, 365
  transmission, 362
  visceral (kala-azar), 362–365, 363f
    HIV co-infection, 364–365
    incubation period, 145b, 310b
Leishmanin antigen skin test (LST), 367
Lemierre's syndrome, 687
LEMS *see* Lambert-Eaton myasthenic syndrome
Lens opacification, diabetics, 830
Lentigines, 1274
Lentigo maligna, 1273
Leprosy, 347–350, 347f
  borderline, 349
  clinical features, 347–349, 348b, 348f
  control, 350
  epidemiology/transmission, 347
  incubation period, 145b, 347
  investigations, 349
  lepromatous, 348b, 349
  management, 349–350, 349b
  multibacillary, 349b
  pathogenesis, 347
  paucibacillary, 349b
  prevention, 350
  prevention of disability
  prognosis, 350
  pure neural, 349
  reactions in, 349, 349b
  tuberculoid, 348b, 349
Leptin, 110–111
Leptosphaera senegalensis, 382
Leptospira interrogans, 336
Leptospirosis, 309b, 336–338, 337f
  aseptic meningitis, 337
  bacteraemic, 337
  icteric (Weil's disease), 337
  pulmonary syndrome, 337
Lesch-Nyhan syndrome, 1088
Leucine, 114b
Leucocyte adhesion deficiencies, 79
Leucocytes *see* White cells
Leucocytosis, 1005
  hepatobiliary disease, 929, 956
  neutrophil *see* Neutrophilia
Leucoencephalopathy, progressive multifocal, 402, 402f, 1207
Leucoerythroblastic anaemia, 1048–1049
Leuconychia, striate, 1297
Leucopenia, 1004–1005
  hepatobiliary disease, 929
  respiratory disease, 686, 689–690
Leucoplakia *see* Leukoplakia
Leukaemias, 1035–1041
  acute, 1036–1039
    infection in, 1038
    investigations, 1036, 1036f
    management, 1036–1038, 1037b, 1037f
    prognosis, 1038–1039, 1038b
  acute lymphoblastic, 1036f, 1038
  acute myeloid, 1036f
  acute promyelocytic, 1036b, 1039
  aetiology, 1035–1036
  chronic lymphocytic, 1040–1041, 1040b–1041b
  chronic myeloid, 1039–1040
    genetics, 1039
  epidemiology, 1035–1036
  hairy cell, 1041
  HSCT, 1038
  incidence, 262f
  prolymphocytic, 1041
  risk factors, 1035b
  T-cell, 1035b
  terminology/classification, 1035–1036, 1036b
Leukoplakia, oral hairy, 398
Leukotriene receptor antagonists, asthma, 669–671, 670f
Leukotrienes, 75, 89b
Levetiracetam, 1182b, 1184b
  in pregnancy, 1185b
Levodopa
  adverse reactions
    chorea, 1167b
    dark urine, 475b
  Parkinson's disease, 1196
Levofloxacin, 151b, 157b
  plague, 338–339
Levomepromazine, 290b, 291
Lewy body dementia, 252
Leydig cell tumours, 758b
LFTs *see* Liver function tests
LGV *see* Lymphogranuloma venereum
LH *see* Luteinising hormone
Li-Fraumeni syndrome, 67, 267b
Libman-Sacks endocarditis, 1111
Lice, 309b, 1281
  bartonellosis, 352b
  body, 1281
  head, 1281
  pubic, 1281
  relapsing fever, 336, 336f
  typhus fever, 351, 351b
Lichen planus, 1289–1290, 1290f
  nails in, 1289–1290, 1298
  rash, 416b, 1257b
  vulval pain/itch, 418b

Lichen sclerosus, 416b, 418b
Lichen simplex, 1285
Liddle's syndrome, 441
Lidocaine
 arrhythmias, 570, 574, 575b
 effect of old age, 36b
 in renal/hepatic disease, 36b
Life course, 98–99, 102b
Life expectancy, 168, 168b
Life support
 advanced, 558–559, 559f
 basic, 558, 558f
 cardiac arrest, 558–559
Lifestyle changes
 chronic renal failure, 488
 dyslipidaemia management, 456, 458
 hypertension management, 534
 musculoskeletal disorders, 1077–1078
 myocardial infarction, 598
 obesity, 118
Lifestyle factors
 ageing, 169
 atherosclerotic vascular disease
 cancer, 260–262
 diabetes mellitus, 811b, 820–821
 weight reduction, 821
Ligaments, 1063
Ligand assay, 428b
Lightheadedness *see* Presyncope
Lignocaine *see* Lidocaine
Limb girdle dystrophy, 1228b
Limbic encephalitis, 1194b
Limbic system, 1143
Limbs
 lower *see* Legs
 upper *see* Arms
Linagliptin, 824
Lincomycin, 156
Lincosamides, 156
 mechanism of action, 150b
Lindane, 224b
Linear accelerators, 850
Linear IgA disease, 1293b, 1294
Linezolid, 151b, 159
 pneumonia, 686
 in pregnancy, 154b
Linitis plastica, 878
Linoleic acid, 113
Linolenic acid, 113
LIP *see* Lymphocytic interstitial pneumonia
Lipaemia retinalis, 454f
Lipase, 844b
Lipid emulsion therapy, 211
Lipid peroxidation, 169
Lipid-lowering therapy
 chronic renal disease, 488, 488b
 coronary heart disease, 588
  myocardial infarction, 598
 diabetes mellitus, 811
 dyslipidaemia, 456
 see also individual drugs
Lipids
 blood
  diabetes, 801b, 805, 809
  disorders of, 450–458
 and cardiovascular disease, 452–453
 complex, disorders of metabolism, 450
 dietary, 450–452, 452f
 endogenous, 451–452, 452f
 lowering, chronic renal failure, 488, 488b
 measurement, 453
 metabolism, 450–453, 926
  disorders of, 450, 451b, 1229b
  effects of insulin, 801b
 plasma, target levels, 456
 transport, 452f
 see also Fat
Lipodermatosclerosis, 1263
Lipodystrophy, 409, 409f
Lipohypertrophy, 799f
Lipolysis, 111–112
Lipomas
 skin, 1275
 small intestine, 888
Lipoprotein lipase, 450–451, 452f
 deficiency, 454b
Lipoproteins
 and cardiovascular disease *see* Atherosclerosis
 disorders of, 450–458
 high-density (HDL), 1310b
 intermediate-density (IDL), 451
 low-density (LDL), 48, 451
 structure, 451f
 very low-density (VLDL), 451
Liquid nitrogen cryotherapy *see* Cryotherapy
Liquorice misuse/excess intake, 441
Liraglutide, 824
Lisch nodule, 1216b
Lisinopril
 heart failure, 552b
 hypertension, 611
Listeria monocytogenes
 bacterial meningitis, 1202b, 1204b
 listeriosis, 339
Listeriosis, 339
 in pregnancy, 314b, 339
Lisuride, Parkinson's disease, 1197b
Lithium, 241b
 bipolar disorder, 245
 cluster headache, 1177
 dilution, cardiac output measurement, 187
 drug interactions, 28b, 29
 effect of renal insufficiency, 36b
 and hypothyroidism, 743b
 nephrotoxicity, 446b, 504b, 522b
 plasma concentrations, 39b
 poisoning, 209b, 214
 in pregnancy, 256b
 prescribing, 38b
 skin reactions, 1304b
 teratogenesis, 245
 therapeutic monitoring, 39b
Lithotripsy, 985
Livedo reticularis, 1111f
Liver
 abnormal size, 923b, 938b
  see also Hepatomegaly
 abscess, 956–957, 956b, 970
  amoebic, 368, 957
  older people, 980b
  pyogenic, 936, 956
 biopsy, 931–932, 931b
  hepatocellular carcinoma, 968
  non-alcoholic fatty liver disease, 961
 blood supply, 924f, 925–926
 cells *see* Hepatocytes
 critically ill patients, 198
 cysts, 380–381
 drugs and, 970–972
 fatty
  alcoholic, 958, 958b
  microvesicular, 971, 978
  non-alcoholic, 959–961, 960f
  pregnancy, 978
 fibrosis, 971b, 972
  congenital, 981
 functional anatomy/physiology, 924–928
 functions, 926–928, 926f
 HIV infection and, 400
 ischaemia, 975
 nodular regenerative hyperplasia, 977
 paracetamol-induced damage, 212, 934b
 resection, 968
 'shock', 198
 structure, 924, 924f
 transplantation, 978–980
  acute liver failure, 934–935
  alcoholic liver disease, 959
  Budd-Chiari syndrome, 976
  cirrhosis, 978b
  complications, 979
  hepatic encephalopathy, 942
  hepatitis, 955
  hepatocellular carcinoma, 968
  indications/contraindications, 978–979, 978b, 979f
  living donors, 979
  orthotopic, 966
  primary biliary cirrhosis, 964
  prognosis, 979–980
  sclerosing cholangitis, 966
  split, 979
  viral hepatitis, 953
  Wilson's disease, 974
 see also Hepatic
Liver capsule pain, 285b
Liver disease, 921–988
 abdominal signs, 923
 acute, 932f
 alcoholic, 957–959
  fatty, 959–961
  liver function tests, 930b
  older people, 980b
 autoimmune, 961–966
 bleeding, 1054
 chronic, 929b, 932f
 cirrhosis *see* Cirrhosis
 clinical examination, 922f, 923b
 cystic/fibropolycystic, 970
 decompensated, 944
 drug-induced, 930b, 970–972
 effect on drug dosages, 24b, 36b
 HIV-related, 400, 955
 hydatid cysts, 380–381, 956–957, 956f
 infections, 948–957
 inherited, 972–975
 investigation, 928–932, 928b
 older people, 980b
 pregnancy, 977–978
 prescribing in, 35b, 36
 presenting problems, 932–942, 932b
 pruritus, 1259b
 renal involvement, 519
 tumours, 966–970
  benign, 970
  incidence, 262f
  malignant, 967–969
  metastatic, 274–275
  secondary, 969
 vascular, 971, 975–977
 see also specific diseases
Liver failure
 acute, 932–935, 932f
  adverse prognostic criteria, 934b
  causes, 932f–933f, 933–935
  classification, 933b
  complications, 934b
  investigations, 934, 934b
  management, 934–935, 934b
 chronic, 932b, 932f, 944b
 effect on drug dosages, 24b, 36b
 hepatic encephalopathy, 933b
Liver flukes, 266b, 312b, 378
Liver function, 24b
Liver function tests (LFTs), 928–929, 930b
 abnormal, 935–936, 936b
  asymptomatic, 935f
  HIV infection, 956b
 alcoholic liver disease, 929b
 biliary obstruction, 929b
 gastrointestinal bleeding, 850
 hepatitis, 929b, 955
 non-alcoholic fatty liver disease, 961
 in pregnancy, 977b
LMWH (low molecular weight heparin) *see* Heparin, low molecular weight
Loa loa, 312b, 372b, 373
Loading dose, 23
Locked-in syndrome, 1161
Lockjaw, 1210
Locus heterogeneity, 59
LoD score, 63
Lofexidine, 255
Löfgren's syndrome, 710–711
Loiasis, 312b, 373–374
Loin pain, 471
Lomotil, 903b
Long QT syndrome, 571, 571b
Loop of Henle, 431, 464–466
Looser's zones, 1127, 1127f
Loperamide
 faecal incontinence, 918
 inflammatory bowel disease, 903b
 and intussusception, 308
 irritable bowel syndrome, 908f
 radiation enteritis, 886
 short bowel syndrome, 885
 small bowel bacterial overgrowth, 883
Lopinavir, 407b
 prophylactic, 153b
Loratadine, 725, 1291
Lorazepam
 disturbed behaviour, 237f
 dyspnoea, 289
 epilepsy, 1159b
 palliative care, 289
Loricrin, 1252
Losartan, 552b
Loss-of-function (LOF) mutations, 58
Lotions, 1265b
Low back pain
 causes, 1072b
 clinical features, 1073b
 investigations, 1062–1063
 management, 1074b
 mechanical, 1073b
 radicular, 1073b
Low birth weight, and disease susceptibility, 99
Low molecular weight heparin *see* Heparin, low molecular weight
Low-density lipoprotein (LDL), 48, 451
Low-resource settings, 9
Lower limbs
 acute ischaemia, 580, 601b
 chronic arterial disease, 600–602, 601b
 examination, diabetes mellitus, 798f, 799b
 see also Foot; Leg
LSD *see* Lysergic acid diethylamide
LST *see* Leishmanin antigen skin test
Lubiprostone, 909
Lujo virus, 324
Lumbar canal stenosis, 1220
Lumbar disc herniation, 1219–1220
Lumbar puncture, 1153–1154
 meningitis, 1202–1203, 1205
 stroke, 1236
 viral encephalitis, 1206
Lumbar root compression, 1219b
Lumbosacral plexopathy, 1226
Lumefantrine, malaria, 163, 356
Lumps, skin, 1256–1257
Lung cancer, 699–706, 699b
 aetiology, 266b, 267, 699
 finger clubbing, 271
 incidence, 262f
 metastatic, 274
 mortality, 700f
 occupational, 720
 older people, 730b
 pleural effusion, 662b
 secondary tumours, 704–705
 staging, 702–703
 see also Bronchial carcinoma
Lung disease
 alveolar
  alveolitis *see* Alveolitis
  microlithiasis, 715b
  proteinosis, 714b–715b

diffuse parenchymal, 706–711
drug-induced, 714, 714b
dust exposure and, 719–720, 719b
fibrosis *see* Pulmonary fibrosis
HIV-related, 400–401
infections, 681–699
interstitial, 706–714
for detailed entry see Interstitial lung disease
rare, 715b
investigations, 649–654
obstructive, 666–681
older people, 677b
occupational, 715–721
presenting problems, 654–666
radiotherapy-induced, 714
rheumatoid arthritis, 1099
tumours, 699–706, 699b
secondary, 704–705
see also Bronchial carcinoma
vascular, 721–725
Lung flukes, 312b
Lung function monitoring, ventilated patients, 188, 188f
Lung function tests *see* Pulmonary function tests
Lung injury, transfusion-associated (TRALI), 1014
Lung(s)
abscess, 109f, 297f
anatomy, 646f–647f
biopsy
bronchial carcinoma, 702
interstitial disease, 706–707
pleural effusion, 661
cavitation, 650b
collapse
bronchial obstruction and, 650f
upper lobe, 644f
consolidation, 650b
defences, 648–649, 648f
fibrosis *see* Pulmonary fibrosis
gas exchange, 646–647, 647f
irradiation damage, 714
mechanics, 647–649
near-drowning victims, 108
shrinking, 712, 712b
transplantation, 665–666, 665b
volumes, measurement, 653
Lupus, drug-induced, 1132b, 1304b
Lupus anticoagulant, 999–1000
Lupus erythematosus
cutaneous, 1260b, 1300
bullous, 1293b
systemic *see* Systemic lupus erythematosus
Lupus nephritis, 499b–500b
Lupus pernio, 710f, 711
Luteinising hormone (LH)
deficiency, 787b
reference range, 1309b
Lyme borreliosis (disease), 309b, 334–336, 335f, 1209
myopericarditis, 335
Lymecycline, 1267
Lymph nodes, 76, 76f
biopsy, 1042f
diphtheria, 345
examination, 261b
cancer, 260f–261f
trypanosomiasis, 359
tuberculosis, 690–691
Lymphadenopathy, 991b, 1005–1006
causes, 1005b
HIV-associated, 395–396
persistent generalised, 232b, 388f, 395–396
rheumatoid arthritis, 1099–1100
Lymphangiectasia, intestinal, 887
Lymphangioleiomyomatosis, 715b
Lymphangitic carcinomatosis, 705
Lymphatic filariasis, 372–373
Lymphatics, 77
Lymphocytes, 992f, 995–996, 1004f
count, 1312b
older people, 1001b
see also B lymphocytes; T lymphocytes
Lymphocytic interstitial pneumonia (LIP), 708b
Lymphocytosis, 1005
causes, 1004b
infectious mononucleosis, 310b, 320
Lymphogranuloma venereum (LGV), 424b
Lymphoic interstitial pneumonitis, 401
Lymphoid organs, 76–78
Lymphoid tissue
gastrointestinal tract, 266b, 843–844
mucosa-associated (MALT), 76
Lymphomas, 1041–1045
B cell, 879–880, 1272
CNS, HIV-associated, 402–403, 403f
cutaneous, 1272
gastric, 879–880
gastrointestinal tract, 889
HIV-associated, 395–396, 395b, 402–403, 403f, 405
Hodgkin's disease, 405b, 1042–1043
MALT, 266b, 1043
mantle cell, 1043
non-Hodgkin's, 262f, 1043–1045, 1044b, 1044f
primary CNS, 1192
T cell, 1043
cutaneous, 1264
enteropathy-associated, 882
thyroid, 755
treatment, 1044–1045
Lymphopenia, 1004–1005
causes, 1004b
HIV infection, 393–394
sarcoidosis, 711
Lymphoproliferative syndrome, autoimmune, 80
Lyonisation, 1029, 1051
Lysergic acid diethylamide (LSD), 218
Lysine, 114b
Lysolecithin, 983
Lysosomal storage diseases, 450, 451b
Lysosomes, 433–434
Lysozyme, 72–73

M

M-CSF *see* Macrophage colony stimulating factor
M-proteins *see* Monoclonal proteins
MAC (*Mycobacterium avium* complex)
McArdle's disease, 450b
McCune-Albright syndrome, 59, 1131
Machado-Joseph disease, 65
genetics, 56b
Machupo virus, 325b
Macrocytosis, 999f, 1021f
Macroglobulinaemia, Waldenström's, 1045
Macrolides, 151b, 156
mechanism of action, 150b
Macronutrients *see* Energy-yielding nutrients
Macrophage colony stimulating factor (M-CSF), 992–993, 993f
Macrophages, 74
alveolar, 385, 711
foamy, 514, 883
functions of, 74b
gastrointestinal tract, 843–844
Macroprolactin, 791
Macroprolactinaemia, 790b, 791
Macroprolactinoma, 789–791
Macules
ash leaf, 1302f
café au lait, 1216f
definition, 1251b
Maculopathy, diabetic, 830
Maddrey's score, 959
Madopar, 1196
Madura foot, 382
Madurella grisea, 382
Madurella mycetomatis, 382
Magic (hallucinogenic) mushrooms, 254
Magnesium, 132
cardiotoxic drug poisoning, 215
dietary sources, 131b
intravenous
acute severe asthma, 672
arrhythmias, 191
tetany, 769b
torsades de pointes, 211b
metabolism, disorders of, 429b, 447–448
refeeding diet, 122b
reference values, venous blood, 1310b
RNI, 131b
Magnesium ammonium phosphate stones, 507b
Magnesium chloride, 448
Magnesium salts, 448, 917b
Magnesium sulphate
asthma, 672f
hypomagnesaemia, 448
pre-eclampsia, 521
ventricular tachycardia, 211b
Magnetic resonance angiography (MRA)
nervous system, 1149b
renal artery stenosis, 494–495, 495f
stroke, 1240b
urinary tract disease, 469–470
Magnetic resonance cholangiopancreatography *see* MRCP
Magnetic resonance imaging *see* MRI
Magnetic stimulation, 1153
Magnifying glass, skin examination, 1254–1256
Main d'accoucheur, 768
Main en lorgnette, 1108
Major histocompatibility complex, 803–804, 1096, 1286
Malabsorption, 857–858, 857b, 858f
after gastric resection, 850
after ileal resection, 884
biliary cirrhosis, 964
chronic pancreatitis, 894
cystic fibrosis, 681
disorders causing, 880–882
investigation, 858, 858f, 859b
iron deficiency anaemia, 1022
older people, 883b
pathophysiology, 858
Maladie de Roger, 634
Malar flush, 526f
Malar rash, 1110f
Malaria, 304b, 309b, 353–358
algid, 357b
cerebral, 357b
chemoprophylaxis, 153b, 357–358
clinical features, 355, 356f
complications, 357b
distribution, 353f
drug-resistant, 353, 356
exchange transfusion, 357
haemolysis, 357
incubation period, 145b, 310b, 354
investigations, 355
pathogenesis, 354–355
pathology, 354–355
in pregnancy, 314b
prevention, 357–358, 358b
sickle-cell anaemia, 1032
treatment, 163, 356–357
Malarone, 356
Malassezia spp., 137f
Malassezia furfur, 1280
Malathion
louse infestation, 1281
scabies, 1280–1281
Malignant disease *see* Cancer
Malignant hyperpyrexia, 51–53
Malingering, 247
Mallory-Weiss syndrome, 253b, 541b, 659b
Mallory-Weiss tears, 854f
Mallory's hyaline, 958b
Malnutrition
hospital patients, 122–124, 122f
see also Undernutrition
MALT lymphomas, 266b, 1043
MALT (mucosa-associated lymphoid tissue), 843–844
Malt worker's lung, 719b
Mammalian target of rapamycin *see* mTOR
Mammary artery grafts, 588
Mammography, 279, 762–763, 912
Manganese, 132
Mania, 235–236, 244–245
Manipulation, 15
low back pain, 1073
Mannitol, 197
as osmotic diuretic, 199b, 435
Mannose-binding lectin deficiency
Mansonella perstans, 312b, 372b, 375
Mansonella streptocerca, 372b
Mantle cell lymphoma, 1043
Mantoux test, 695b
MAOIs *see* Monoamine oxidase inhibitors
MAP *see* Mean arterial pressure
Maple bark stripper's lung, 719b
Marasmus, 120–121
Maraviroc, 407b
Marburg disease, 324, 325b
March haemoglobulinuria, 1031
Marche à petits pas, 172b, 1168
Marcus Gunn pupil, 1172b
Marfan's syndrome, 603–604
cardiovascular system
aortic aneurysm, 604f
aortic dissection, 605, 605b
mitral valve prolapse, 618
congenital defects, 629–630
joint hypermobility, 1134
mutation, 58, 603–604
Marine envenoming/poisoning, 228b–229b
Marjolin's ulcer, 1095–1096, 1263
MARS *see* Molecular adsorbent recirculating system
Mass spectroscopy, 428b
inductively coupled, 428b
Mast cells, 75
allergy, 89b
tryptase measurement, 90
Mastectomy, 280
prophylactic, 67
Matrix metalloproteinases, 580
Mayaro virus, 329, 1095
MC4R *see* Melanocortin receptor mutations
MCGN *see* Mesangiocapillary glomerulonephritis
MCH *see* Mean cell haemoglobin
MCU *see* Micturating cystourethrography
MCV *see* Mean cell volume
MDMA *see* Ecstasy
MDS *see* Myelodysplastic syndrome
Mean arterial pressure (MAP), 185, 607
Mean cell haemoglobin (MCH), 1312b
Mean cell volume (MCV), 998, 999f
alcohol misuse, 240, 929
anaemia, 1021f
reference values, 1312b

Measles, 314–315, 315f
incubation period, 145b, 310b, 314
period of infectivity, 144b
pregnancy, 314b
rash, 315f
subacute sclerosing panencephalitis and, 314
Mebendazole
helminthic infections, 162, 370–372, 375
hydatid cysts, 957
Meckel's diverticulum, 851b, 887
bleeding from, 856b
Meckel's scan, 851b
Meconium ileus, 895
Medial fibroplasia, 494
Medial longitudinal fasciculus (MLF), 1146
Median nerve
entrapment, 1224b
palsy, 832
Mediastinoscopy, 706
Mediastinum, 705f
assessment, 651–652
tumours, 705–706, 705b, 706f
Medical ethics *see* Ethics
Medical interview, 4b
Medical law *see* Legal issues
Medical practice *see* Good medical practice
Medically unexplained somatic symptoms, 236, 236b, 236f
general management, 246–247, 246b
older people, 238b
Medication errors, 29–30
causes, 30b, 30f
response to, 29–30
types of, 29b
Medication overuse headache, 1177
Medicines management, 30–32
Medroxyprogesterone, 760
Medullary cystic kidney disease, 506–507
Medullary sponge kidney disease, 506, 507f
Medulloblastoma, 911–912
Mefenamic acid, overdose, 213
Mefloquine, malaria, 356
Megacolon, 918
toxic, 900
Megakaryoblasts, 993f, 996–997
Megakaryocytes, 992f–993f
Megaloblastic anaemia, 1024–1026
clinical features, 1024b
investigations, 1024b
management, 1026
Megaloblastic crisis, 1028
Megaureter, 510
Megestrol, cancer cachexia, 290
Meglitinides, 822b, 823
Meglumine antimoniate, 164, 364
Meiosis, 50–51, 50f
Meissner's plexus, 845
Melaena, 854
Melanocortin receptor (MC4R) mutations, 116
Melanocytes, 1252
Melanocytic naevus (mole), 1274–1275, 1275f
Melanoma, 1272–1274
ABCDE rule, 1257b
acral lentiginous, 1273
amelanotic, 269
diagnosis, 1257b
epidemiology, 267b
incidence, 262f
lentigo maligna, 1273
management, 1273–1274, 1274b
nodular, 1273
subungual, 1273
superficial spreading, 1273, 1273f
Melanoptysis, 716–717
Melanosis coli, 917
Melarsoprol, trypanosomiasis, 164, 359b, 360
MELAS, 1199b, 1229b
MELD (Model for End-stage Liver Disease), 944–945, 944b, 978b
Meleney's gangrene, 305b
Melioidosis, 340
Meloxicam, 1079b
Melphalan, 266b, 1047
Memantine, 251
Membrane attack complex, 75, 75f
Membranoproliferative glomerulonephritis (MPGN), 499b–500b, 501
Membranous nephropathy, 497f, 522b
Memory, 1142–1143
Alzheimer's disease, 252
assessment, 234
disorders of, 246, 1142b
long-term, 234, 252
loss, 250–251, 402
short-term, 234, 253
MEN *see* Multiple endocrine neoplasia
Ménétrier's disease, 872
Ménière's disease, 1186
MENIN, 795
Meningioma, 1215
Meningism, 1201
Meningitis, 1201–1205
aseptic, 337, 1205
bacterial, 1202–1204, 1202b, 1203f
cerebrospinal fluid in, 1203
prevention, 1203–1204, 1204b
treatment, 1204b
causes, 1202b
Coccidioides, 1202b
cryptococcal, 403, 1205
fungal, 1205
headache, 1202–1203
herpes simplex, 326
HIV/AIDS patients, 403
immunisation, 1203–1204
Listeria, 1202b
malignant, 1205
mumps, 319
protozoa and parasites, 1205
recurrent aseptic, 1205
tuberculous, 403, 1204–1205, 1205b
cerebrospinal fluid in, 1205
viral, 1201–1202
cerebrospinal fluid in, 1202
Meningococcal infection, 151b, 304b
chemoprophylaxis, 153b
immunisation, 1203–1204
incubation period, 145b, 310b
meningitis, 1202–1204, 1202b, 1204b
prevention, 1203–1204
rash, 1203
treatment, 1204b
see also Meningitis
Meningococcal septicaemia, 295f, 1203b
Meningoencephalitis, 321
Menopause, 757
male, 766b
premature, 759
Menorrhagia, 1004
Menstruation, 757f
Mental handicap, 66
Mental State Examination, 233–234
Mental test, older people, 234
Menthol, topical, 1260
Mepacrine, hyperpigmentation from, 1296b
Meptazinol, 1078
Meralgia paraesthetica, 1224b
Mercaptopurine
acute leukaemia, 1037b
inflammatory bowel disease, 903b
Mercury
adverse effects on kidney, 446b, 499b–500b
poisoning, 210b, 446b
Merkel cells, 1252
Meropenem, 151b, 154b, 155f
melioidosis, 340
neutropenic fever, 274
nocardiosis, 341
pneumonia, 686
in pregnancy, 154b
MERRF (myoclonic epilepsy with ragged red fibres), 1199b, 1229b
Mesalazine
contraindication, renal insufficiency, 502b
inflammatory bowel disease, 860, 900–901, 903b
Mesangiocapillary glomerulonephritis (MCGN), 499b–500b, 501
Mesenteric ischaemia, chronic, 910
Mesna, 1112
Mesothelioma, 262f, 719
Meta-iodobenzyl guanidine (MIBG) scintigraphy, 781
Metabolic acidosis, 445–446, 445b
acute mountain sickness, 107
critically ill patients, 183f
diabetic ketoacidosis, 812
differential diagnosis, 658b
hypothermia, 104–105
malaria, 357b
near-drowning, 108
poisoning, 209b
renal failure
acute, 479
chronic, 484
renal replacement therapy, 197b
starvation, 121
Metabolic alkalosis, 445b, 446–447, 447f
Metabolic disorders
musculoskeletal manifestations, 1132–1133
skin manifestations, 1301–1302
Metabolic (insulin resistance) syndrome, 589, 805
obesity and, 115b
Metabolic myopathies, 1229–1230
Metabolic rate, critically ill patients, 201b
Metabolism, 22
first-pass, 21
interactions, 28–29
phase I, 22
phase II, 22
Metadrenalines, 1310b
Metalloproteinases, 264f, 580
Metamyelocytes, 993f, 995
Metapneumovirus, 328
Metastasis *see various cancer types*
Metatarsophalangeal (MTP) joint pain, 1070f
Metavir scoring system, hepatitis C, 955
Metered-dose inhalers, 670f
Metformin, 821–822, 822b
acidosis, 209b, 216
effect of renal impairment, 36b
mechanism of action, 822–823
overdose, 209b, 216
polycystic ovary syndrome, 764
in pregnancy, 817
in renal/hepatic disease, 36b
Methadone
chronic pain management, 287
misuse, 217b, 219
withdrawal, 20b
Methaemoglobin, 209b
Methanol poisoning, 209b, 211b, 222–223
Methicillin *see* Meticillin
Methimazole, 749
Methionine, 114b, 212
Methotrexate, 1267
acute leukaemia, 1037b
drug interactions, 28b
eczema, 1267
hepatotoxicity, 36b, 971b
inflammatory bowel disease, 860, 897b, 903b
musculoskeletal disorders, 712
myositis, 1115
psoriatic arthritis, 1109
rheumatoid arthritis, 1101b, 1102
vasculitis, 1117–1118
pregnancy, 906b, 1101b
psoriasis, 1267, 1289b
renal toxicity, 36b
and respiratory disease, 714b
sarcoidosis, 711
SLE, 1110
Methyl-phenyl-tetrahydropyridine (MPTP), parkinsonism and, 1195b
Methylbenzethonium chloride, 367
Methylcellulose, 750–751, 917b
3,4-Methylenedioxy-methamphetamine (MDMA) *see* Ecstasy
Methylphenidate, 1187
Methylprednisolone
acute disseminated encephalomyelitis, 1193
Graves' disease, 750–751
histoplasmosis, 385–386
inflammatory bowel disease, 904, 904b
liver transplant patients, 979
multiple sclerosis, 1191b
myositis, 1115
P. marneffei infection, 385–386
rheumatic disease, 1102
SLE, 1112
transverse myelitis, 1193
Methysergide
cluster headache, 1177
nephrotoxicity, 511
and respiratory disease, 714b
Meticillin, 154b
Meticillin-resistant *Staphylococcus aureus* (MRSA), 330–331
Metoclopramide
critically ill patients, 198
and hyperprolactinaemia, 790b
mechanism of action, 290b
myocardial infarction, 593–594
nausea and vomiting, 290b, 1177
overdose, 211b
Metoprolol, 575b
angina, 586
unstable, 594
arrhythmias, 576
hypertension, 612
Metronidazole, 151b, 158
amoebiasis, 368
balanitis, 416b
cerebral abscess, 1208b
cholecystitis, 984
choledocholithiasis, 985
Clostridium difficile infection, 344
diverticulitis, 916–917
gas gangrene, 305
genital infections, 417b
giardiasis, 369
Helicobacter pylori eradication, 874
inflammatory bowel disease, 860
liver abscess, 368, 956
necrotising fasciitis, 305
neutropenic fever, 274
and peripheral neuropathy, 1223b
PID, 418
pneumonia, 687
in pregnancy, 154b
prophylactic, 153b
rosacea, 1258
small bowel bacterial overgrowth, 883
tetanus, 1210b
tropical ulcer, 333
Metyrapone, 776, 777b
Mevalonate kinase deficiency, 85
Mexiletine, 574, 575b

MGUS see Monoclonal gammopathy of uncertain significance
MI see Myocardial infarction
MIBG see Meta-iodobenzyl guanidine (MIGB) scintigraphy
Micafungin, 160b
Micelles, mixed, 841–842
Miconazole, 160b, 1267
erythrasma, 1278
Microalbuminuria, 476–477
diabetes mellitus, 831, 831b
Microaneurysms, retinal, 609
Microangiopathy, diabetic, 826–827
Microarray analysis, 62
Microbiome, 136
Microcytosis, 999f, 1021f
Microdeletion syndromes, 55
Microglia, 1140–1141
β-2-Microglobulin, as tumour marker, 270b
Microlithiasis, alveolar, 715b
Microorganisms
culture, 140–141
detection of components, 139–140
detection of whole organisms, 139
host response, 134, 137–138
MicroRNA (miRNA), 413
Microsatellite repeats, 55
Microscopic polyangiitis (MPA), 1118
Microscopy
bright field, 139
dark field, 139
electron, 139
epiluminescence, 1255
Microsomal ethanol-oxidising system (MEOS), 957–958
Microsporidia, HIV/AIDS patients, 399b
Microsporum audouinii, 1280
Microsporum canis, 1279f, 1280
Micturating cystourethrography (MCU), reflex nephropathy, 505f
Micturition
cycle, 466
disorders of
benign prostatic hyperplasia, 472, 514–515
incontinence see Incontinence, urinary
frequency, 472
mechanisms, 466
Mid-axillary line (MAL), 730
Midazolam, 237f
terminal agitation, 291
Midges, filariases, 375
Miglitol, 823
Migraine, 1176–1177
stroke risk, 1177
visual disturbance, 1170
Migrainous neuralgia, 1177, 1178b
Migrating motor complexes (MMC), 845
Milk, cow's, type 1 diabetes and, 804
Milk alkali syndrome, 130
Milk intolerance, 93b, 1284b
Millard-Gubler syndrome, 1148b
Miller Fisher syndrome, 1224–1225
Miltefosine, 364
Milwaukee shoulder syndrome, 1091b, 1092
Mind-body interactions, 15
Mineralocorticoid receptor, 435
Mineralocorticoid receptor antagonists, 781
Mineralocorticoids, 772–773, 779
excess, 780b
insufficiency, 778b
measurement, 778
Minerals, storage, 927
Mini-mental state examination (MMSE), 234
Mini-tracheostomy, 194
Minimal change nephropathy, 498–500
drug-induced, 522b
Minimally conscious states, 1161, 1161b
Minimum bactericidal concentration (MBC), 143
Minimum inhibitory concentration (MIC), 143
Minocycline
acne, 1267
hyperpigmentation from, 1267, 1296b
leprosy, 349b
skin reactions, 1304b
Minoxidil
alopecia, 1297
hypertension, 612
skin reactions, 1304b
Mirizzi's syndrome, 984
Mirtazepine, 244b, 290
Misoprostol, 1079
Missense mutations, 54f, 58
MIT see Monoiodotyrosine
Mites
house dust, 666–667, 1255, 1283
typhus, 350
Mitochondria, 45–46, 45f
Mitochondrial disorders, 65, 1229, 1229b
Mitochondrial DNA, 169
Mitochondrial inheritance, 53
Mitochondrial myopathy, enchephalopathy, lactic acidosis and stroke-like episodes see MELAS
mitochondrial neurogastrointestinal encephalomyopathy (MNGIE), 1229b
Mitomycin/mitomycin C, 517, 714b
Mitosis see Cell division
Mitotane, 776
Mitotic spindle poisons, 261b
Mitoxantrone, 1191, 1192b
acute leukaemia, 1037b
Mitral regurgitation, 618–620, 618b, 619f
clinical features, 618–619, 618b
heart murmurs, 562b
investigations, 619, 619b
Mitral stenosis, 616–618, 617f
clinical features, 616–617, 616b
investigations, 617, 617b
chest X-ray, 535f
management, 618
Mitral valve
balloon valvuloplasty, 618, 618b
chronic rheumatic heart disease, 616
cleft, 632–633
endocarditis, 618
prolapse (floppy valve), 618
pain, 541
repair, 619–620
replacement, 618
Mixed connective tissue disease, 1091b, 1092, 1113–1114
Mixed venous oxygen saturation, 184
MLF see Medial longitudinal fasciculus
MMC see Migrating motor complex
MMR vaccine, 319
MMSE see Mini-mental state examination
Mobitz types I and II AV blocks, 571, 572f
Moclobemide, 244b
Modafinil, 1187, 1192b
MODS see Multiple organ dysfunction syndrome
MODY see Maturity onset diabetes in the young
MOF see Multiple organ failure
Moh's surgery, 1268
Mole, 1274–1275, 1275f
Molecular adsorbent recirculating system (MARS), 964
Molecular biology, 42–50
Molecular diagnostics, 428b
Molecular medicine, 69–70
molecular mimicry, 87
Mollaret's syndrome, 1205
Molluscum contagiosum, 327f, 426, 426f, 1279, 1279f
HIV/AIDS patients, 388f, 397b
Mometasone, 1265b
Monday fever, 716
Monge's disease, 107
Monitoring
in critically ill patients
circulation, 185–187
respiratory function, 187–188
drug therapy, 36, 39–40, 39b
Monkeypox, 327
Monoamine oxidase inhibitors (MAOIs), 241b, 244, 244b
drug interactions, 28b
Parkinson's disease, 1197
Monoarthritis, acute, 1069, 1069b
Monobactams, 154b, 156
Monoclonal antibody therapy, 31b
allergy, 91
cancer, 279–280, 915
diabetic retinopathy, 829
haemolytic uraemic syndrome, 496
leukaemias, 1039, 1041b
multiple sclerosis, 1037, 1192b
osteoporosis, 1124
psoriasis, 1268
Monoclonal gammopathy of uncertain significance (MGUS; monocolonal gammopathy unclassified; MGu; benign monoclonal gammopathy), 1045
Monoclonal proteins, 1045
Monocytes, 74, 995, 1004f
count, 1312b
Monocytosis, 1004b
Monofilament testing, 799b
Monoiodotyrosine (MIT), 739f
Mononeuritis multiplex, 1224
Mononeuropathy
diabetes mellitus, 832
multifocal, 1224b
Monosodium urate monohydrate (MSUM) crystals, 1064f, 1086b, 1087
Monospot test, 321
Montelukast, asthma, 671
Mood, 1148
assessment, psychiatric interview, 234
Mood (affective) disorders, 243–245
bipolar, 243–245
depression see Depression
Mood-stabilising drugs, 241b
Moral dilemma, 11–12
Moral reasoning (ethical analysis), 12–13, 13b
Moraxella spp., 136f
Moraxella catarrhalis, 137f
Morphine
adverse reactions, 26b–27b, 287, 287b
critically ill patients, 202
misuse, 219
myocardial infarction, 593–594
palliative care, 289, 291
pharmacogenetics, 25b
renal colic, 509
in renal/hepatic disease, 36b
route of administration, 34b
Morphoea, 1300
Morquio's syndrome, 433–434
Mortality ratios, standardised (SMRs)
Morton's neuroma, 1076
Mosaic warts, 1278
Mosquitoes, 309b
filariasis, 372
malaria, 353–358
virus transmission, 144
Motilin, 846b
Motor disorders
diabetes, 826b
see also Diabetic neuropathy
Motor neuron disease, 1162b, 1194b, 1200–1201, 1200b, 1222b
Motor neurons
lesions, 1162b, 1163f
lower, 1144–1145
upper, 1145
Motor neuropathy, 1194b
Motor system, 1144–1145, 1144f
Mountain sickness
acute, 107
chronic, 107
Mouth
diseases of, 863–864
examination
blood disorders, 990f
cardiovascular disease, 526f
respiratory disease, 644f
older people, 864b
oral allergy syndrome, 860
ulcers
Behçet's syndrome, 1119
SLE, 1111
see also Oral
Movement disorders, 1165–1167, 1166b, 1194–1198
involuntary movements, 1145
see also *names of specific disorders*
Moxifloxacin, 157b
meningitis, 1204b
MPA see Microscopic polyangiitis
MPGN see Membranoproliferative glomerulonephritis
MPTP see Methyl-phenyltetrahydropyridine
MRA see Magnetic resonance angiography
MRCP (magnetic resonance cholangiopancreatography), 848–849, 931, 931f
cholangiocarcinoma, 931f
pancreatic cancer, 895
pancreatitis, 892
primary sclerosing cholangitis, 966
MRI (magnetic resonance imaging)
cancer diagnosis, 269
cardiovascular system, 537–538, 538f
aortic dissection, 606f
coarctation of aorta, 632f
craniopharyngoma, 794f
endocrine disease
macroprolactinoma, 792f
pituitary gland, 786f
gastrointestinal tract, 846, 847b, 847f
inflammatory bowel disease, 900f
hepatobiliary disease, 930–931, 931f, 970f
haemangioma, 970f
hepatocellular carcinoma, 967–968
musculoskeletal disease, 1065, 1065f
sacroiliitis, 1107f
neurological disease, 1149b
brain tumours, 1180b–1181b
epilepsy, 1182b
hydrocephalus, 1217f
spinal cord compression, 1221f
stroke, 1235f
viral encephalitis, 1206
pelvic abscess, 847f
renal disease, 469–470, 506f
spine, 1222f
MRSA (meticillin-resistant *Staphylococcus aureus*), 134, 151b, 330–331, 687

MSA *see* Multiple systems atrophy
MSUM *see* Monosodium urate monohydrate (MSUM) crystals
mTOR inhibitors, 785b
MTP *see* Metatarsophalangeal (MTP) joint pain
Mucociliary escalator, 648f
Mucocutaneous disease, HIV-related, 396–398, 397b
Mucopolysaccharidosis, 433–434
Mucor spp., 384
Mucormycosis, 699
Mucosa-associated lymphoid tissue (MALT), 76
Mucous membranes *see individual organ systems*
Mucous patches, syphilis, 419–420
Multidisciplinary team, 2b, 167, 177
Multifocal encephalomyelitis, 1194b
Multifocal neuropathy, 1224, 1224b
Multiple endocrine neoplasia (MEN), 795, 795b
  genetic testing, 63
  genetics/inheritance, 267b
Multiple myeloma, 84b, 262f, 1046–1048, 1046b–1047b, 1046f
Multiple organ dysfunction syndrome (MODS), 184b
Multiple organ failure (MOF)
  AKI, 478
  critically ill patients, 184, 184b
  pancreatitis, 892b
Multiple sclerosis, 1188–1192
  cerebrospinal fluid in, 1188
  clinical features, 1189–1190, 1189b–1190b, 1189f
  investigations, 1150f, 1190, 1190b, 1191f
  Macdonald criteria, 1189b
  management, 1191–1192
    of complications, 1192, 1192b
    complications, 1192, 1192b
    disease-modifying treatments, 1191–1192, 1192b
  pathophysiology, 1188–1189, 1188f
  post-transverse myelitis, 1193b
  pregnancy, 1192b
  sibling risk, 68b
Multiple systems atrophy (MSA), 1198
Mumps, 306b, 319
  immunisation, 319
  incubation period, 145b, 310b, 319
  period of infectivity, 144b
  testicular swelling, 319
Münchausen's syndrome, 247
Mupirocin, impetigo, 1276
Murmurs, 560–562
  aortic regurgitation, 527b, 623–624, 623b, 623f
  aortic stenosis, 527b, 562b, 620–623, 621f
  atrial septal defect, 632–633, 633f
  ausculatory evaluation, 560–562, 561b
  Austin Flint, 623–624
  benign, 560b, 562b
  cardiac, 560–562
  carditis, 614–615
  Carey Coombs, 614–615
  coarctation of aorta, 632, 632f
  continuous, 562
  diastolic, 561–562
  Graham Steell, 625
  mitral regurgitation, 562b, 618–620, 618b, 619f
  mitral stenosis, 616–618, 617f
  persistent ductus arteriosus, 631, 631f
  pulmonary stenosis, 625
  systolic, 561, 562b
  tetralogy of Fallot, 634–635, 634f
  timing and pattern, 561f
  tricuspid stenosis, 624
  ventricular septal defect, 562b
Murphy's sign, 984
Muscle
  biopsy, 1068
    myositis, 1115f
  contraction, 1144, 1152
  haematomas, 1051
  pain, 1076, 1077b
    drug-induced, 1132b
    infections, 295
  sensory changes, diabetes *see* Diabetic neuropathy
  skeletal, 1063–1064
Muscle diseases, 1228–1230, 1228b
  acquired, 1230, 1230b
  chronic renal failure, 485–486
  drug-induced, 1132b
  genetic testing, 62b
  heart muscle, 636–639
  inherited, 1229–1230, 1229b
  metabolic, 1229–1230
  proximal myotonic myopathy, 1228b
  see also specific conditions
Muscle fibre, 531f
Muscle relaxants, 202–203
Muscle weakness/wasting, 1076, 1077b
  diabetes, 831–832
  rheumatoid arthritis, 1098
  systemic sclerosis, 1113
  see also Dermatomyositis/polymyositis; Myositis
Muscular atrophy
  motor neuron disease, 1200b
  spinal, 1201
Muscular dystrophies, 1228–1230, 1228b
  inheritance, 1228b
  see also specific types
Musculoskeletal chest pain, 541
Musculoskeletal disease, 1057–1135
  anatomy and physiology, 1060–1064, 1060f
  clinical examination, 1058f
  drug-induced, 1077b
  investigation, 1064–1068
  management, 1077–1081, 1077b
  in pregnancy, 1101b, 1121
  presenting problems, 1069–1076
  prevalence, 1060b
  systemic illness and, 1132–1133
  see also individual conditions
Musculoskeletal manifestations, 1132–1133
Musculoskeletal system
  anatomy and physiology, 1060–1064, 1060f
  clinical examination, 1138f
  drug-induced effects, 1126b
  manifestations of diseases in other systems, 1132–1133
  tumours of, 1131–1132
Mushrooms
  'magic' (hallucinogenic), 254
  poisoning, 503–504
Mutation(s)
  de novo, 59
  dominant negative, 58
  duplications, 55–56, 57f
  frameshift, 54f, 55
  gain-of-function, 58
  inheritance, 51–53
  insertions and deletions, 55, 56b
  loss-of-function (LOF), 58
  missense, 54f, 58
  nonsense, 54f
  null, 58
  oncogenesis, 54b
  point, 53
  somatic, 59
  splice site, 55f
  tandem repeat, 55, 56b
  triple repeat, 56b
Myalgia, 1076, 1077b
  drug-induced, 1132b
  infections, 295
  see also Polymyalgia rheumatica
Myasthenia gravis, 1194b, 1226–1227, 1227f
  diplopia, 1226
  drug-induced, 1132b
  weakness, 1226
Myasthenic crisis, 1226–1227
Mycetoma, 382
  intracavitary
Mycobacteria, 135, 347–350
  atypical, cystic fibrosis, 681
  opportunistic infection, 696, 696b
Mycobacterium abscessus, 696
Mycobacterium avium complex (MAC), 304b, 396, 407, 696b
  prophylaxis, 406b
Mycobacterium chelonei, 696b
Mycobacterium fortuitum, 696b
Mycobacterium genavense, 696b
Mycobacterium haemophilum, 696b
Mycobacterium kansasii, 696, 696b
Mycobacterium leprae, 134, 141, 347, 696b
  see also Leprosy
Mycobacterium malmoense, 696b
Mycobacterium marinum, 696b
Mycobacterium tuberculosis, 141, 304b
  bacterial meningitis, 1202b
  bone infection, 691–692
  see also Tuberculosis
Mycobacterium ulcerans, 333, 696b
Mycobacterium xenopi, 696, 696b
Mycology, 1255
Mycophenolate mofetil, 96b
  ANCA-associated vasculitis, 1118
  autoimmune hepatitis, 962–963
  myasthenia gravis, 1227b
  myositis, 1115
  psoriasis, 1268, 1289b
  SLE, 1112
  vasculitis, 1118
Mycoplasma spp., 156
Mycoplasma pneumoniae, 682–683
  cold agglutination, 1031
Mycoses *see* Fungal infections
Mycosis fungoides (cutaneous T-cell lymphoma), 1272
Myelin sheaths, 438, 1140–1141
Myelinolysis, 438
Myelitis, 319
  transverse, 1193, 1193b, 1222b
Myeloblasts, 993f
Myelocytes, 992f–993f, 995
Myelodysplasia, 159, 298–299, 1001b
Myelodysplastic syndrome (MDS), 1041, 1041b
Myelofibrosis, 1048–1049
Myelography, spine, 1073, 1149b
Myeloma
  AKI, 480b–481b
  hypercalcaemia, 271b
  multiple, 84b, 262f, 1046–1048, 1046b–1047b, 1046f
Myelopathy, 1194b
  cervical spondylotic, 1219
  HIV-related, 403–404
  vacuolar, 403–404
Myeloperoxidase, 520
Myeloproliferative disorders, 1048–1049
Myelosuppression, drug-induced, 277, 1101b, 1267
Myiasis, 381
Myocardial cells *see* Myocytes
Myocardial contractility
  critically ill patients, 183
  improving, 191
Myocardial contraction, 530, 531f
Myocardial infarction (MI)
  acute, 590b
    haemodynamic subsets, 545b
  atrioventricular block, 572–573
  clinical features, 583b, 590–593, 590b
  cocaine-induced, 218
  complications, 596–598
  definition, 590b
  diabetics, 818
  diagnosis, 591
  expansion, 597
  and hyperglycaemia, 818
  investigations, 592–593, 598
    ECG, 534, 592–593
  management
    early, 593–596
    late, 598–600, 598b
  older people, 599b
  pain, 590
  painless (silent), 590–591
  prognosis, 599–600
  rehabilitation, 598–599
  risk factors, 591, 591f, 598
  risks of non-cardiac surgery, 600, 600b
  secondary prevention, 599
  shock, 545
  time course, 590f
  ventricular ectopic beats, 569, 569f
Myocardial ischaemia
  cocaine-induced, 218
  ECG, 534, 584f
  myocardial infarction, 596–598
Myocardial perfusion imaging, 539, 585, 585f
Myocardial stunning, 190, 545
Myocarditis, 636
  acute, 636
  chronic, 636
  fulminant, 636
  pain, 541
Myocardium
  diseases, 636–639
    specific, 638–639, 639b
  hibernating, 537
    oxygen supply and demand, 584b
Myoclonic epilepsy with ragged red fibres (MERFF), 46b, 1199b, 1229b
Myoclonus, 1166b, 1167
Myocytes, 531f
Myofibrils, 1063
Myoglobin, 543
  urinary, 301, 474–475
Myoglobulinuria, 474b
Myonecrosis, clostridial, 305, 305b
Myopathic gait, 1168
Myopathy *see* Muscle diseases
Myophosphorylase deficiency (McArdle's disease), 450b
Myosin, 530, 531f, 1063
Myositis
  drug-induced, 1132b
  inclusion body, 1115
  systemic sclerosis, 1113
  see also Dermatomyositis/polymyositis
Myotonia, potassium-aggravated, 1230b
Myotonia congenita, 1230b
Myotonic dystrophy, 1228b
  genetics/inheritance, 56b, 1228b
Myxoedema
  coma, 745
  Graves' disease, 751
Myxoma, atrial, 639

N

N-acetylcysteine (NAC) *see* Acetylcysteine
Nabumetone, 1079b
NAD (nicotinamide adenine dinucleotide), 45f, 128, 957
NADH dehydrogenase, 46b
Nadolol
  arrhythmias, 574–576
  thyrotoxicosis, 741–742
  variceal bleeding, 946

NADP/NADPH (nicotinamide adenine dinucleotide phosphate), 73
NADPH oxidase enzyme complex, 73
Naegleria fowleri, 309b
Naevus
  blue, 1275
  melanocytic (mole), 1274–1275, 1275f
  spider, 922f, 962, 975–976
Nafcillin, 154b
NAFLD *see* Non-alcoholic fatty liver disease
Nail fold disorders *see* Nails
Nails, 1254
  abnormalities, 1264, 1297–1299
  arthritis, 1070b
  in congenital disease, 1299
  examination, 1250f
  fungal infections, 398, 1280
  lichen planus, 1289–1290, 1298
  normal variants, 1297
  psoriasis, 1108–1109, 1287f, 1288
  in systemic disease, 1298, 1298f
  trauma, 1297–1298
  whitening, 1298
Na,K-activated ATPase (sodium-potassium pump), 429
Nalidixic acid, 157b
  in pregnancy, 154b
  skin reactions, 1304b
Naloxone, 219, 287b
  adverse reactions, 28
  drug interactions, 28b
Naltrexone
  primary biliary cirrhosis, 964
  pruritus, 964
Naproxen, 1079b
Narcolepsy, 1187, 1187b
NASH *see* Non-alcoholic steatohepatitis
Nasogastric tube, 879b
Nasopharynx, diseases, 725
Natalizumab, 1192, 1192b
Nateglinide, 823
National Institute for Health and Clinical Excellence (NICE), 9
Natriuretic peptide *see* Atrial natriuretic peptide; Brain natriuretic peptide
Natural killer (NK) cells, 75–76
Nausea
  mechanisms, 852
  palliative care, 289–290, 289f
Necator americanus, 312b, 369
Neck
  Casal's necklace, 128, 128f
  examination
    diabetes, 798f
    endocrine disease, 734f
    neurological disease, 1138f
  pain, 1060b, 1074, 1074b
  stiffness, 302
  see also Head and neck
Necrobiosis lipoidica, 1301, 1301f
Necrosis, 50, 262
Necrotising enteritis, 342
Necrotising fasciitis, 305, 305f
Necrotising pancreatitis, 891–892, 892f
Necrotising soft tissue infections, 305, 305b
Nefopam, 1078
Negligence, definition, 14b
Neisseria spp., 136f–137f
Neisseria gonorrhoeae, 151b, 421–422
  in pregnancy, 314b, 414b
  see also Gonorrhoea
Neisseria meningitidis see Meningococcal infection
Nelson's syndrome, 1296
Nematodes, 369b
  intestinal, 369–372
  tissue-dwelling, 372–375
  zoonotic, 375–376
Neomycin
  allergy, 1285b
  and vitamin B_{12} deficiency, 129
Neostigmine, 918
Nephelometry, 428b
Nephrectomy, 505, 514
Nephritic syndrome, 475, 475b
Nephritis
  crescentic, 487b, 501–502
  drug-induced, 504b, 522b
  interstitial, 480b–481b
    acute, 502–503, 502b
    chronic, 503–504
  lupus, 499b–500b
  post-streptococcal, 501
Nephrocalcinosis, 507, 522b
Nephrogenic sclerosing fibrosis, 469b
Nephron, 464
  segments, 430–432, 431f
Nephronophthis, 506–507
Nephropathy
  analgesic, 514
  Balkan, 503–504
  diabetic, 830–831, 830b, 830f
    pregnancy and, 818
  HIV-associated, 405
  IgA, 499b–500b, 500–501
  ischaemic, 494
  membranous, 497f, 522b
  minimal change, 498–500
    drug-induced, 522b
  reflux, 504–505
  salt-losing, 504, 859f
  sickle-cell, 505
  see also Renal disease
Nephrotic syndrome, 475b, 476–478
Nephroureterectomy, 517
Nerve agents, organophosphorus, 220–222, 220b, 221f
Nerve biopsy, 1154–1155
Nerve conduction studies, 1151–1152, 1153f
Nerve root diseases *see* Radiculopathy
Nerve root lesions, 1164–1165
Nerve root pain, 1073b
Nervous impulse, 1141, 1141f
Nervous system
  anatomy and physiology, 1140–1148, 1141f
  cells, 1140–1141, 1140f
  clinical examination, 1138f
    older people, 1139b
  in gastrointestinal function, 844–845
  see also Autonomic nervous system: Peripheral nervous system
Nervous system diseases, 1137–1230
  cerebrovascular disease *see specific conditions*
  clinical examination, 1138f, 1139b
  cranial nerves, 1139b
  diagnosis, 1155b
  emergencies, 1140b
  genetic, 65
  HIV-related, 402–404
  infections, 1201–1211, 1201b
  intracranial/raised intracranial pressure, 1212–1213, 1212b, 1213f
  investigations, 1149–1155
  lesion localisation, 1148, 1156b
  neuromuscular junction, 1226–1228
  paraneoplastic, 271–272, 272b, 1193, 1194b, 1216
  peripheral nervous system, 1223–1226
  presenting problems, 1155–1175, 1155b
  spine/spinal cord, 1218–1222
  symptom evolution, 1156b
  see also Neuropathy; *and specific conditions*
Nettle rash *see* Urticaria
Neural tube defects (NTD), prevention with folic acid, 125b, 129
Neuralgia
  migrainous, 1177, 1178b
  post-herpetic, 319, 1157
  trigeminal, 1157, 1178
Neuralgic amyotrophy, 1223b, 1226
Neuraminidase inhibitors, 320
Neurasthenia, 232b, 246
Neuro-endocrine tumours (NETs), pancreatic, 784–785, 785b, 785f
Neuro-inflammatory diseases, 1188–1193
Neuroacanthocytosis, 1167b
Neurodegenerative diseases, 1194–1201
Neurofibroma, 1213b, 1221f
Neurofibromatosis, 715b, 1216, 1216b, 1216f
  and cancer predisposition, 267b
  inheritance, 267b, 1216
Neurofibromin, 51–53
Neurogenic shock, 190
Neuroglycopenia, 815
Neuroimaging, 1149–1150, 1149b, 1235–1236, 1235f–1236f, 1241–1242
  see also specific modalities
Neuroleptic malignant syndrome, 249
Neuroleptics *see* Antipsychotics
Neurological disease *see* Nervous system diseases
Neurological failure, 198–200
Neuroma
  acoustic, 1215–1216
  Morton's, 1076
Neuromuscular junction disorders, 1226–1228
Neuromyelitis optica, 1193
Neuromyotonia, 1194b
Neuronectomy, multiple sclerosis, 1192b
Neurons, motor *see* Motor neurons
Neuropathic pain, 285, 285b, 1165
  management, 285b, 288b
Neuropathy, 1223
  ataxia and retinitis pigmentosa (NARP), 1229b
  autonomic, 832, 832b–833b
  axonal, 1224
  chronic renal failure, 485–486
  critical illness, 200
  demyelinating, 1225
    see also Guillain-Barré syndrome
  diabetic, 799, 831–833, 832b–833b, 834f
  entrapment, 1224, 1224b
  focal (mononeuropathy), 832
  generalised (polyneuropathy), 1223b, 1224
  hereditary *see* Charcot-Marie-Tooth disease
  leg ulceration, 1263
  motor, 1194b
    multifocal motor, 1224
  multifocal, 1224, 1224b
  optic, 1229
  organophosphate-induced, 222
  peripheral, 1223b
    cancer-related, 272
    diabetic, 826–827, 826b
    drug-related, 403
    HIV-related, 403
    leprosy, 348
    rheumatoid arthritis, 1099
    sensorimotor, 403
  sensory, 1194b
    diabetes mellitus, 799, 831–833, 832b–833b, 834f
  see also Mononeuropathy; Polyneuropathy
Neuropeptides, 47f, 89
Neurosyphilis, 420, 1209, 1209b
Neurotoxic envenoming, 226
Neurotransmission/neurotransmitters, 1141f
  psychiatric disorders, 233
Neutral variants, 58
Neutrons, 102–103
Neutropenia, 1004
  causes, 1004b
  drug-induced, 1005b
  fever in, 274, 302, 302b
  HIV/AIDS, 405
Neutropenic fever, 274
Neutrophil chemotactic factor, 89b
Neutrophilia, 1005
  asthma, 667–668
  causes, 1004b
Neutrophilic dermatoses, 1299
Neutrophils, 72–74, 992f–993f, 995, 1004f
  asthma, 667–668
  count, 1312b
  function and dysfunction, 73f
  older people, 1001b
  toxic granulation, 72–73
Nevirapine, 407b
  in pregnancy, 409
  resistance, 408
NHL (non-Hodgkin's lymphoma) *see* Lymphoma
Niacin (nicotinic acid; vitamin B_3), 128–129
  deficiency, 128–129, 128f
  dietary sources, 125b
  hyperlipidaemia, 434
  RNI, 125b
  toxicity, 129
Nicardipine, angina, 587b
Nickel hypersensitivity, 88b, 1284–1285
Niclosamide, 163
Nicorandil, 587, 864b
Nicotinamide *see* Niacin
Nicotinamide adenine dinucleotide (NAD), 45f, 128, 957
Nicotinamide adenine dinucleotide phosphate (NADP/NADPH), 73
Nicotine replacement therapy, 101b
Nicotinic acid *see* Niacin
Niemann-Pick disease, 433–434
Nifedipine
  altitude illness, 107
  angina, 586–587, 587b
    unstable, 594
  aortic regurgitation, 624
  effect of old age, 36b
  hypertension, 612
  and neutropenia, 1005b
  oesophageal disorders, 869
  older people, 36b
  Raynaud's disease, 602–603
  sphincter of Oddi dysfunction, 987
Nifurtimox, trypanosomiasis, 164, 360
Night blindness, 127
Night sweats, 295–296
Night terrors, 1175
Nightmares, 1175
Nikolsky sign, 1294
Nimodipine, subarachnoid haemorrhage, 1246–1247
Nipah virus, 328
NIPPV *see* Non-invasive positive pressure ventilation
Nitazoxanide, 164, 368–369
Nitrates
  angina, 586, 594
  duration of action, 586b
  heart failure, 552
  long-acting, prescription
  oesophageal disorders, 541, 869
  pulmonary oedema, 550

Nitric oxide (NO), 82, 185, 466, 530–531
anal fissure, 919
in hepatopulmonary syndrome, 975–976
respiratory support, 196
Nitrites, 209b, 512
Nitrofurantoin, 159
and pulmonary eosinophilia, 713b–714b
urinary tract infection, 513b
Nitrogen narcosis, 109
Nitroimidazoles, 158
mechanism of action, 150b
Nitroprusside *see* Sodium nitroprusside
Nitroprusside reaction, 807
Nitrosamines, diabetogenic effect, 804
'Nits', 1281
NK *see* Natural killer (NK) cells
NMDA blockers, pain management, 288b
NMDA (N-methyl-D-aspartate), dementia, 252
NNRTIs *see* Non-nucleoside reverse transcriptase inhibitors
NNTB *see* Number needed to treat for benefit
NNTH *see* Number needed to treat for harm to occur
NO *see* Nitric oxide
Nocardia, 382
pneumonia, 401
Nocardiosis, 341
Nociceptive pain, 285
Nocturia, 472
Nodules
hepatic, 942–943, 943f
pulmonary, 660, 660b
cryptococcosis, 384
lung metastases, 274
rheumatoid, 712
rheumatoid
lung, 712, 712f
subcutaneous, 1097
skin, definition, 1251b
thyroid, 735f, 740
Non-alcoholic fatty liver disease (NAFLD), 926, 944b, 959–961, 960f
clinical features, 961
investigations, 961
liver function tests, 930b
pathophysiology, 960–961
Non-alcoholic steatohepatitis (NASH), 960f, 961, 971b
Non-compliance, 35
Non-epileptic attack disorder (pseudoseizures), 1159, 1185–1186
Non-Hodgkin's lymphoma *see* Lymphoma, non-Hodgkin's
Non-invasive positive pressure ventilation (NIPPV), 550, 678b
Non-maleficence, 11
Non-nucleoside reverse transcriptase inhibitors (NNRTIs), 407–408, 407b
adverse reactions, 409
Non-specific interstitial pneumonia (NSIP), 708b
Non-specific urethritis (NSU), 415, 1107
Non-starch polysaccharides (NSPs; dietary fibre), 113
Non-steroidal anti-inflammatory drugs *see* NSAIDs
Nonsense mutations, 54f
Noradrenaline, 772
circulatory effects, 191b
Noradrenergic re-uptake inhibitors, 241b, 244b
Norepinephrine *see* Noradrenaline
Norfloxacin, 157b
prophylactic, spontaneous bacterial peritonitis, 941
urinary tract infection, 512
Normal distribution/range, 5, 5f
Normetadrenaline, 1311b
Normoblasts, 994, 999f
Norovirus, 327
Nortriptyline, pharmacokinetics, 25b
Norwalk agent, 327
Nosocomial (health care-acquired) infections
Clostridium difficile, 304b, 343–344, 344f
control, 145b
MRSA, 134, 151b, 330–331, 687
pneumonia, 685–687
Notification
cholera, 344
diphtheria, 345
food poisoning, 341
Legionella pneumonia, 685
partner, STIs, 415, 421
plague, 338
whooping cough, 682
Novice-expert shift, 14b
NRTIs *see* Nucleoside reverse transcriptase inhibitors
NSAIDs, 286
adjuvant analgesia, 288b
adverse reactions, 26b, 176b, 1079b
gastrointestinal bleeding, 873, 1021–1022
renal, 522
asthma association, 667–668
cancer cachexia, 290
contraindication
cirrhosis, 971b
renal insufficiency, 483
diabetes insipidus, 795
drug interactions, 28b
effect of old age, 36b
effect on renal function, 481b
hepatotoxicity, 971b
low back pain, 1073
musculoskeletal disorders, 1078–1079, 1078f, 1079b
ankylosing spondylitis, 1107
gout, 1089
osteoarthritis, 1085
psoriatic arthritis, 1109
reactive arthritis, 1108
SLE, 1111–1112
pancreatitis, 894
and peptic ulcer, 856
poisoning, 213
recommendations for use, 1079b
in renal/hepatic disease, 36b
sarcoidosis, 711
skin reactions, 1304b
small intestinal toxicity, 887
topical, 1079–1080
use in older people, 1079b
NSIP *see* Non-specific interstitial pneumonia
NSPs *see* Non-starch polysaccharides
NSU *see* Non-specific urethritis
Nuclear antigens, extractable, antibodies to, 468
Nucleic acid amplification tests (NAAT), 139–140, 141f, 415
Nucleocytoplasmic asynchrony, 1024
Nucleoside reverse transcriptase inhibitors (NRTIs), 392f, 407b
adverse reactions, 409
resistance to, 408
Nucleosomes, 42
Nucleotide substitutions, 53, 54f
Null mutations, 58
Number connection test, 923f
Number needed to treat for benefit (NNTB), 32
Number needed to treat for harm to occur (NNTH), 32
Numbness, 1164–1165
Nutcracker oesophagus, 869
Nutrients
energy-yielding (macronutrients), 110, 112–114
recommended intakes, 125b
inorganic, 130–132
Nutrition, 110–115, 110f
alcoholic liver disease, 959
critical illness, 198
cystic fibrosis, 681
enteral/parenteral *see* Feeding
overnutrition, 111–112
physiology, 110–114
pregnancy and lactation, 125b
stroke patients, 1243b
undernutrition, 111–112, 120–124
Nutritional status, 114–115
Nutritional support
artificial
acute pancreatitis, 892b
Crohn's disease, 904–905
legal and ethical aspects, 124, 124b
hospital patients, 122–124
see also Feeding, parenteral
Nutritional therapy, inflammatory bowel disease, 904–905
Nystagmus, 1145, 1171
balance disorders, 1186f
gaze-evoked, 1171
Nystatin, 160b
candidiasis, 160, 864

O

OA *see* Osteoarthritis
Obesity, 101, 115–120
abdominal, 115–116
aetiology, 116–117, 116b
assessment, 117
asthma and, 666
atherosclerotic vascular disease and, 116f, 581
body fat distribution, 115–116
complications, 115–116, 115b
diabetes, 116f
management, 117, 821
type 2, 806
increasing prevalence of, 116, 116b
management, 117–120, 118f
diet, 118–119, 118b
drugs, 119
lifestyle advice, 118
surgery, 119–120, 119b, 120f
musculoskeletal disease, 1078
non-alcoholic fatty liver disease, 960
polycystic ovarian syndrome, 764b
reversible causes, 117, 117b
susceptibility to, 116
Obesogenic environment, 116b
Obidoxime, 221
Obsessive-compulsive disorder (OCD), 243
Obstructive shock, 190
Occipital lobes, 1143
disorders, 1170b
functions, 1142b
effects of damage, 1142b
Occupational diseases/disorders
cancer, 266b
cramps, 1200
HIV infection/AIDS, 391b, 410
respiratory, 715–716
asthma, 666–667, 669, 715–716, 715b, 716f
dust-related, 717b, 719–720, 719b
lung cancer, 720
pneumonia, 720–721
Occupational therapist, 2b
Occupational therapy
musculoskeletal disorders, 1080
Parkinson's disease, 1198
OCD (obsessive-compulsive disorder), 243
Ochrobactrum spp., 720
Octopus, blue-ringed, 225b
Octreotide
acromegaly, 793
carcinoid tumours, 761b
gastrointestinal obstruction, 290
scintigraphy, 785f
short bowel syndrome, 885
Zollinger-Ellison syndrome, 876
Ocular dysmetria, 1171
Ocular pain, 1157
Oculomotor (3rd cranial) nerve
damage to, 1171b
palsies, 1172b
tests, 1139b
Oculopharyngeal dystrophy, 1228b
Odds ratio, drug therapy, 32f
Odynophagia, 270b, 399
Oedema, 478
ascites, 478
causes, 478b
cerebral *see* Cerebral oedema
cytotoxic, 1237
dependent, 602b, 832b
famine, 120–121
generalised, 363
legs, 478
nephrotic syndrome, 475b, 476–478
peripheral
differential diagnosis, 549b
heart failure, 549b
sodium retention, 434, 435f
pitting, 478
pulmonary *see* Pulmonary oedema
OER *see* Oxygen extraction ratio
Oesophageal candidiasis, HIV/AIDS patients, 399, 399f
Oesophageal cytomegalovirus infection, HIV/AIDS patients, 399
Oesophageal variceal bleeding, 942, 942f, 945
management, 947f
Oesophagitis, 868
CMV, HIV infection/AIDS, 399
eosinophilic, 868
reflux, 866, 866f
systemic sclerosis, 1113
Oesophagus
Barrett's (columnar lined), 866–867, 866f
carcinoma and, 866–867
diseases, 865–871
achalasia, 868–869, 869f
benign stricture, 867, 870, 870b
high-grade dysplasia, 867
motility disorders, 868–870
reflux, 865–868, 865f
tumours, 262f, 870–871
functional anatomy, 840–841, 840f
motility, 850
nutcracker, 869
pain, 541
perforation, 871
transection, varices, 928
Oestradiol, 1309b
Oestrogen
anti-androgen therapy, 765b
bone remodelling, 1062b
deficiency, 760b
hepatotoxicity, 971b
receptors, 268
Oestrogen replacement therapy
delayed puberty, 759
secondary amenorrhoea, 760
Turner's syndrome, 766
Ofloxacin, 157b
leprosy, 349b
PID, 418
STIs
chlamydial infection, 423b
gonorrhoea, 422b

Ogilvie's syndrome, 918, 918b
OGTT *see* Oral glucose tolerance test
OI *see* Osteogenesis imperfecta
Ointments, 1265b
Olanzapine
 bipolar disorder, 245
 schizophrenia, 249b
Older people
 AKI, 483b
 anaemia, 1034b
 antimicrobial therapy, 154b
 blackouts, 172
 blood disorders, 1047b
 blood tests, 1001b
 cancer, 271b
 cardiovascular disease
  angina, 595b
  aortic stenosis, 622b
  atherosclerosis, 602b
  atrial fibrillation, 566b
  congestive heart failure, 551b
  hypertension, 610b
  infective endocarditis, 626b
  myocardial infarction, 599b
 clinical assessment, 166f
 comorbidities, 170
 critically ill, 204b
 delirium, 173–175, 173b–174b
 demography, 168, 168f
 diabetes mellitus, 806b
  management, 828b
 dizziness, 173, 1158b
 drug therapy, 175–176
  adverse drug reactions, 175–176, 176b
  polypharmacy, 176b
 endocrine system
  adrenal glands, 779b
  gonadal function, 766b
  parathyroid glands, 770b
  pituitary and hypothalamus, 795b
  thyroid gland, 755b
 energy balance, 122b
 environmental factors in disease, 102b
 falls, 172–173, 172b
 fever, 296b
 frailty in, 170, 170b
 gastrointestinal disorders
  acute abdominal pain, 862b
  constipation, 918b
  endoscopy, 850b
  GORD, 868b
  infectious diarrhoea, 306b
  malabsorption, 883b
  peptic ulcer, 875b
 genetic disease and counselling, 64b
 geriatric assessment, 166–168
 haematological function, 1001b
 haematological malignancy, 1047b
 haemostasis and thrombosis, 1008–1011
 HIV/AIDS, 410b
 hyperlipidaemia management, 458b
 hypernatraemia, 439, 439b
 hypoglycaemia, 784b
 hyponatraemia, 439, 439b
 immune deficiency, 82b
 incontinence, 175, 175f, 473b
 investigation, 170–171
  Comprehensive Geriatric Assessment, 170, 170b
  decisions on, 170–171
 liver disease, 980b
 musculoskeletal disorders
  bone infection, 1094b
  gout, 1090b
  osteoarthritis, 1085b
  osteomalacia, 1125–1126
  osteoporosis, 1124b
  Paget's disease, 1128–1129
  rheumatoid arthritis, 1097–1098
 neurological disease/disorders
  acute confusional state, 473b
  dizziness, 173, 1158b
  epilepsy, 1185b
  examination, 234
  Parkinson's disease, 1166b, 1194–1198
  visual loss, 1169–1170
 NSAID use, 1079b
 oral health, 864b
 pharmacokinetics in, 24b
 physical examination, 167
 podiatry, 177
 poisoning/drug overdose, 208b
 postural hypotension, 36b
 prescribing in, 36b
 presenting problems, 171–176
 psychiatric disorders, 238b
 rehabilitation, 176–177
 renal replacement therapy, 491b
 respiratory disease
  COPD, 677b
  infections, 686b
  influenza vaccine, 320
  interstitial lung disease, 714b
  lung cancer, 730b
  pleural disease, 730b
  thromboembolic disease, 724b
 respiratory function, 648b
 sedation, 174–175
 skin changes, 1254b
 social assessment, 167
 thermoregulation, 104b
 urinary tract infection, 512b
 vitamin deficiency, 127b
Oleander poisoning, 215
Olecranon bursitis, 1075b, 1099f
Olfactory (1st cranial) nerve, tests, 1139b
Olfactory loss, 1169
Oligoarthritis, 1104, 1104b
 associated extra-articular features
 asymmetrical inflammatory, 1108
Oligoclonal bands, 1154
Oligodendrocytes, 1140–1141
Oligodendroglioma, 1213b
Oligopeptides, 842
Oliguria, 471–472
 critically ill patients, 197
Olsalazine, 903b
Omalizumab, 91
Omega3 fatty acids, 113
Omeprazole
 drug interactions, 28, 28b
 H. pylori eradication, 874
 renal toxicity, 479–481
Onchocerca volvulus, 372b, 374
 life cycle, 374f
Onchocerciasis (river blindness), 312b, 374–375
Onchocercoma, 374
Oncogenes, 59
Oncogenesis, 54b
Oncology *see* Cancer
Onychogryphosis, 1297
Onycholysis, psoriasis, 1287f
Onychomycosis, 398, 1280
O'Nyong-nyong virus, 329, 1095
Oophoritis, mumps, 319
Open reading frames (ORFs), 43
OPG *see* Osteoprotegerin
Ophthalmia neonatorum
 chlamydial, 314b, 423
 gonococcal, 314b, 422f
Ophthalmopathy, Graves' disease, 735f, 739b, 742f, 750–751, 750f, 779b
Ophthalmoplegia, chronic progressive external, 1229b
Opiates/opioids
 adverse reactions, 26b, 176b, 287, 287b
 drug interactions, 28b
 effect of renal insufficiency, 36b
 misuse, 219, 254
  management, 219
 myocardial infarction, 593–594
 myths about, 286b
 older people, 176b
 osteoarthritis, 1085
 pain management, palliative care, 286
 pancreatitis, 894
 poisoning, 217b, 219
 in respiratory failure, 664
 sedation and analgesia, 202
 withdrawal symptoms, 20b, 254
Opisthorchiasis/*Opisthorchis felineus*, 312b, 379b
Opisthotonus, 1210
Opsoclonus-myoclonus, 1194b
Opsonins/opsonisation, 73f
Optic (2nd cranial) nerve
 disorders, 1170b
 tests, 1139b
Optic atrophy, 1173, 1173f
Optic chiasm, disorders, 1170b
Optic disc disorders, 1170b
 oedema *see* Papilloedema
 swelling, 1173b
Optic neuritis, 1170b, 1194b
 multiple sclerosis, 1190b
 onchocerciasis, 374
 and transverse myelitis (neuromyelitis optica), 1193
Optic neuropathy, Leber's hereditary, 1229
OptiMal, 357
OPV (oral polio vaccine), 1207
Oral administration, 21
Oral allergy syndrome, 860
Oral cancer, 864, 864b
Oral cavity, organisms in, 137f
Oral contraception/contraceptives
 acne treatment, 1282
 drug interactions, 155, 694
 in epilepsy, 1183–1184, 1185b
 and hypertension, 607b
 and migraine, 1176–1177
 and porphyria, 459
 skin reactions, 1304b
 and venous thrombosis, 1009b, 1247b
Oral disease, HIV-related, 398
Oral glucose tolerance test (OGTT), 809b
Oral hairy leukoplakia, 398
Oral hypoglycaemics, 821–824, 822b
 poisoning, 216
Oral rehydration solution (ORS), 307b
Orbit, imaging, 1149–1150, 1150f
Orchitis, mumps, 319
Orf, 1279
Organ donation, 96
Organelles, intracellular, 47f, 1238f
Organochlorine poisoning, 224b
Organophosphate-induced delayed polyneuropathy (OPIDN), 222
Organophosphorus compounds, poisoning, 220–222, 220b, 221f
Oriental sore *see* Leishmaniasis, cutaneous
Oriental spotted fever, 351b
Orientation, assessment, 234
Orlistat, 119, 119f
Ornidazole, 368
Oropharynx examination
 HIV/AIDS, 388f
 infectious diseases, 294f
Oroya fever, 352, 352b
Orphenadrine, Parkinson's disease, 1197
ORS *see* Oral rehydration solution
Orthopnoea, 543, 655
Orthoses, 1080
Oscillopsia, 1171
Oseltamivir, 153b, 161b, 162, 320
Osgood-Schlatter disease, 1076b
Osler's nodes, 626
Osmolal gap, poisoning, 209b
Osmolality, 1310b
 hyponatraemia, 437
 refeeding diet, 122b
Osmolarity, 814, 1310b
Osmotic agents, 30
Osmotic diuretics, 435
Osteitis fibrosa
 chronic renal failure, 486–487
 hyperparathyroidism, 769
Osteoarthritis (OA; osteoarthrosis), 1081–1086
 BCP crystal deposition, 1086b
 clinical features, 1082–1085, 1082b
 early-onset, 1084–1085, 1084b
 erosive, 1085
 investigations, 1085
 management, 1085–1086, 1085b
 nodal generalised, 1082–1083, 1082b, 1083f
 older people, 1085b
 pathophysiology, 1081–1082, 1082f
 prevalence, 1060b
 radiology, 1073b
 risk factors, 1081f
 see also specific sites
Osteoarthropathy, hypertrophic pulmonary, 701
Osteoblasts, 1061
 bone remodelling, 1061f
 tumours, 1131b
Osteochondritis
 dissecans, 1075–1076
 Osgood-Schlatter disease, 1076b
 Scheuermann's, 1130–1131
Osteochondroma, 1131b
Osteoclasts, 1061
 bone remodelling, 1061f
 osteopetrosis, 1131
 Paget's disease, 1129
Osteocytes, 1061
Osteodystrophy
 hepatic, 963
 renal, 486f
Osteogenesis imperfecta (OI), 62b, 1131
Osteogenic sarcoma, 66–67
Osteoid, 486f, 1061f
Osteoid osteoma, 1131b
Osteolysis, 1064b, 1095
Osteoma, osteoid, 1131b
Osteomalacia, 1125–1128
 after gastric resection, 851
 biochemical abnormalities, 1066b
 bone biopsy, 1127
 causes, 1126b, 1128
 chronic renal failure, 486–487
 drug-induced, 1132b
 hypophosphataemic, 1128
 older people, 1125–1126
 pain, 1125–1126
 renal, 1128
 vitamin D-deficient, 127
Osteomyelitis, 1095–1096
Osteonecrosis, 1130
 drug-induced, 1123–1124, 1132b
 pain, 1130
Osteopathy *see* Bone diseases
Osteopenia
 biliary cirrhosis, 964
 fractures in, 1071
 hyperparathyroidism, 769
 radiographic, 1127
Osteopetrosis, 1131
Osteophytes, 1064, 1219
Osteoporosis, 1120–1125
 after gastric resection, 851
 biochemical abnormalities, 1066b
 bone mineral density measurement, 1122b
 chronic renal failure, 486–487
 and coeliac disease, 881–882

drug-induced, 1123b, 1132b
corticosteroids, 1120–1121
fractures, 1121f, 1123b
inflammatory bowel disease, 907
management, 1122–1125
men, 1120
older people, 1124b
post-menopausal, 766b, 1120
pregnancy-associated, 1121
prevalence, 1060b
primary biliary cirrhosis, 963–964
secondary, 1121b
Osteoprotegerin (OPG), 1062b
Osteosarcoma, 1132
Paget's disease, 1129
Osteosclerosis
osteoarthritis, 1081–1082, 1084f
Paget's disease, 1129
Osteotomy, 1080b
Ostium primum defect, 632–633
Otitis media, 108, 314, 332b, 346
Ovarian cancer, 280–281
incidence, 262f
investigations, 280
pathogenesis, 280–281
treatment, 280–281
Ovaries
failure, 759
oophoritis, 319
polycystic, 760, 764–765, 764b, 764f
Overflow incontinence, 175, 473, 1174
Overnutrition, response to, 111–112
Ovulation, 762
Oxacillin, 154b
Oxalate, 1311b
Oxazolidinones, mechanism of action, 150b
Oxcarbazepine, 1184b
Oxidative stress, 893f, 958f, 960, 1028–1029
Oximes, 221
Oximetry, 653–654
asthma, 672–673
Oxycodone, 287
Oxygen
arterial blood (PaO_2), 1308b
cascade, 182f
consumption, 184
oxygen delivery and, 184
delivery, 182
content, 182f–183f, 183–184
flow, 182–183
global, 184
regional distribution, 182
toxicity, 193
transport, 182, 183f
Oxygen dissociation curve *see* Oxyhaemoglobin dissociation curve
Oxygen extraction ratio (OER), 184
Oxygen saturation (SpO_2), 1308b
at altitude, 106f
critically ill patients, 187–188
sleep apnoea/hypopnoea syndrome, 726f
sudden changes in, 187b
Oxygen therapy
air passengers, 108
altitude illness, 107
asthma, 672
carbon monoxide poisoning, 220
COPD, 676–677
critically ill patients, 193
decompression illness, 110
gastrointestinal haemorrhage, 855
hyperbaric, carbon monoxide poisoning, 220
long-term, COPD, 676–677
organophosphorus poisoning, 221
pneumonia, 684–685
pulmonary embolism, 723
respiratory failure, 665
toxic effects, 193
Oxyhaemoglobin dissociation curve, 182f–183f, 183–184, 995f
at altitude, 106f
Oxytetracycline
acne, 1267, 1282
rosacea, 1283

P

P gene, 1295
Pabrinex, 128, 253–254
Pacemaker syndrome, 578
Pacemakers *see* Cardiac pacemakers
Pachyonychia congenita, 1299
Pacing
AV block, 573
dual-chamber, 578f
tachyarrhythmias, 564, 571
transcutaneous, 578
see also Cardiac pacemakers
Packed cell volume (PCV), 1312b
Paclitaxel, 280–281, 587–588
PAD *see* Peripheral arterial disease
Paget's disease, 1091b
biochemical abnormalities, 1066b
management, 1129, 1130b
older people, 1128
pain, 1129
radionuclide bone scan, 1129f
PAI *see* Plasminogen activator inhibitor
Pain, 1147, 1147f
abdominal *see* Abdominal pain
acute, management, 286
assessment, 285–286
bone, 285b
bronchial carcinoma
chest *see* Angina; Chest pain
classification, 285
components, 286f
examination, 285–286
facial, 1156–1157
fibromyalgia, 1093
abnormal processing, 1092–1093
headache, 1156–1157, 1176–1178
hepatobiliary disease
cholecystitis, 983–984
choledocholithiasis, 983–985
gallstones, 982
incident, 285b
investigations, 286
ischaemic, 285b
joints, 1074–1076
see also names of specific joints
liver capsule, 285b
loin, 471
low back *see* Low back pain
measurement, 285
mechanisms, 285
muscle, 1076, 1077b
musculoskeletal, 1071b, 1074–1076
management *see individual conditions*
neck, 1060b, 1074, 1074b
neuropathic, 285, 285b, 288b, 1165
nociceptive, 285
ocular, 1157
osteoarthritis, 1082
hip, 1084
pancreatic cancer, 895
perception, 285, 1147f
pleural *see* Pleural pain
psychological aspects, 285
radicular, 1072f, 1073b
rating scales, 285
renal colic, 507–510
somatoform disorder, 245–247
wrist, 1075
see also specific conditions
Pain management/treatment, 286–288
acute pain, 286
cancer, 286
non-pharmacological, 288
palliative care, 284–288
pharmacological, 286–288
see also Analgesia; Analgesics
Pain pathway, 285
PAL *see* Physical activity level
Palliative care, 283–292
chronic renal failure, 550
COPD, 284, 677
dying phase, 290–292
gastric cancer, 879
presenting problems, 284–290
anxiety and depression, 290
breathlessness, 289
cough, 289
delirium and terminal agitation, 290
gastrointestinal obstruction, 290
nausea and vomiting, 289–290, 289f
pain, 284–288
weight loss and weakness, 290
Palmar erythema, 734f, 740, 922f, 943
Palmitate, 981–982
Palmoplantar pustulosis, 1288
Palpation
abdomen, 839b
precordium, 527b
respiratory disease, 644–646
Palpitations, 243, 556–557, 556b, 556f
Pamidronate
bone metastases, 275
hypercalcaemia, 273
Paget's disease, 1129, 1130b
polyostotic fibrous dysplasia, 1131
PAN (polyarteritis nodosa), 1117
Pancoast's syndrome, 701
Pancolitis, 897–898
Pancreas, 844
annular, 894
congenital abnormalities, 894–895
diabetes mellitus, 799, 803
type 2, 806
diseases of, 889–896
divisum, 894
endocrine, 782–785
diseases, 783–784, 783b
function tests, 851b
structure and function, 802f, 844f
transplantation, 826
tumours, 895–896, 896f
endocrine, 896
incidence, 262f
Pancreatic enzymes, 844b
cystic fibrosis management, 681
Pancreatic exocrine insufficiency, 1025
Pancreatic polypeptide, 112f, 802f
Pancreatic pseudocyst, 891f
Pancreatic rests, 880
Pancreaticoduodenectomy, 986
Pancreatitis, 889–896
acute, 768b, 889–892
complications, 891b, 892f
management, 892
nutritional support, 892b
pathophysiology, 890–892, 890b, 890f
pleural effusion, 662b
prognosis, 890b
autoimmune, 894
chronic, 892–894
causes, 893b
complications, 893b
investigations, 893, 893b, 894f
management, 894
pathophysiology, 893f
hereditary, 895, 971b
necrotising, 891–892, 892f
risk, hyperlipidaemia and, 454f
Pancreolauryl test, 851b
Pancytopenia, 363, 1008, 1008b
Panic disorder, 243
Pannus, 1096
Panton-Valentine leukocidin, 687, 1277
Papilla of Vater, 937
Papillary carcinoma, thyroid, 754
Papillary muscle rupture, 597
Papillary necrosis *see* Renal papillary necrosis
Papillary renal cell cancer syndrome, 267b
Papilloedema, 1173, 1173f
haemorrhagic, 734f
Papilloma, basal cell, 1274, 1274f
Papillomaviruses, 1278–1279
see also Human papillomavirus
Papular pruritic eruption, 398
Papular urticaria, 374
Papule, definition, 1251b
Papulosquamous eruptions, 1257–1258
Para-aminosalicylic acid (PAS), skin reactions, 1304b
Parabens, 1285b
Paracentesis, ascites, 940
Paracetamol, 286
adverse reactions, 27b
dosage regimen, 35b
fever, 296
hepatotoxicity, 933, 933f
migraine, 1177
musculoskeletal disorders, 1078, 1103b
nephrotoxicity, 481b, 522b
osteoarthritis, 1085
palliative care, 286
pleural pain, 685
poisoning, 209b, 212
acute liver failure and, 212, 934b
antidotes, 212, 212f
upper respiratory tract infection
Paracoccidioidomycosis, 386
Paracoccidioides brasiliensis, 386
Paraesthesia, 657, 1164–1165
diabetic neuropathy, 832
peripheral neuropathies, 1224b
Paraganglioma, 781–782
Paragonimiasis, 309b
Paragonimus spp., 163
Paragonimus westermani, 312b
Parainfluenza viruses, 328
Paraldehyde
disturbed behaviour, 237f
poisoning, 209b
Paralytic ileus, 890–892
Paralytic shellfish toxin, 308
Paramyotonia congenita, 1230b
Paramyxoviruses, 328
Paraneoplastic disease, neurological, 271–272, 272b, 1193, 1194b, 1216
Paraparesis, 328–329, 403–404, 1168
Paraphasia, 1169
Paraphenylenediamine, 1285b
Paraplegia, hereditary spastic, 1222b
Parapneumonic effusion, 661
Paraproteinaemias, 1045–1048
Paraproteins, 1025, 1044
Paraquat poisoning, 224b
Parasitic infections
and cancer, 266b
eosinophilia, 312b
HIV/AIDS patients, 399
nervous system, 1201b
see also specific infections
Parasitosis, delusional, 245
Parasomnias, 1187–1188
non-REM, 1187
Parathyroid glands, 766–771
diseases
classification, 767b
presenting problems, 767–769
functional anatomy and physiology, 766–767
older people, 770b

Parathyroid hormone (PTH), 767b, 770–771
bone remodelling, 1062b
hyperparathyroidism, 769b
osteoporosis, 1123b, 1124
reference range, 1309b
rickets/osteomalacia, 1127
serum, bone disease, 1066b
Parathyroid hormone-related protein, ectopic production, 271b
Parathyroidectomy, 488, 770
Paratyphoid fever, 339–340
Parenteral administration, 21
Parenteral nutrition, 123–124
total *see* Total parenteral nutrition
Parietal lobes, 1142
disorders, 1170b
functions, 1142b
effects of damage, 1142b
Parinaud's syndrome, 1148b
Parkinsonism, 1198
drug-induced, 249b, 1195b
see also specific syndromes
Parkinson's disease, 1166b, 1194–1198
causes, 1195b
clinical features, 1195, 1196b
non-motor symptoms, 1195
investigations, 1195–1196, 1196f
management, 1196–1198, 1197b
surgery, 1197
pathophysiology, 1195, 1195f
tremor, 1166b
Paromomycin, 164, 364, 368
Paronychia, 1297
Parotitis, 319, 864
Paroxetine, 244b
drug interactions, 28b
Paroxysmal cold haemoglobinuria, 420
Paroxysmal nocturnal haemoglobinuria, 1031
Partial agonists, 18
Partial anterior circulation syndrome (PACS), 1241f
Partial thromboplastin time with kaolin (PTTK), 999–1000
Parvovirus B19, 315–316, 316b, 316f
and aplastic crisis, 1028, 1032
arthropathy, 316b
pregnancy, 314b
red cell aplasia, 404–405
Past-pointing, 1145
Pastes, 1265b
Pastia's sign, 331, 332f
Pastoral care, 2b
Patau's syndrome (trisomy 13), genetics, 56b
Patch, definition, 1251b
Patch tests, 1285
hypersensitivity, 1255
Paterson-Kelly syndrome, 870
Pathergy reaction, 1119
Pathogens
host-pathogen interaction, 134, 137–138
successful, 137–138
transmission, 134f
Pathway medicine, 70
Patients
autonomy, 10–11
relationship with doctor, 2–4, 3f
communication, 4b
difficulties in, 2–4
ethical issues, 9–13
Pauciarticular disease *see* Oligoarthritis
Paul-Bunnell test, 321
PAVMs *see* Pulmonary arteriovenous malformations
PAWP *see* Pulmonary artery wedge pressure
PCI *see* Percutaneous coronary intervention
PCNSL *see* Primary CNS lymphoma
PCOS *see* Polycystic ovarian syndrome
PCP *see Pneumocystis jirovecii*
PCR *see* Polymerase chain reaction
PCT *see* Porphyria cutanea tarda
PCV *see* Packed cell volume; Pressure controlled ventilation
PDB *see* Paget's disease
PDT *see* Photodynamic therapy
PE *see* Plasma exchange
Peak expiratory flow (PEF)
asthma, 668f, 672f
dyspnoea, 657
home monitoring, 652
morning dipping, 668f
Peak flow meters, 652, 668
Peanut allergy, 94
PECAM-1, 531–532
Pectins, 113b
Pectus carinatum (pigeon chest), 731
Pectus excavatum (funnel chest), 731
Pediculus humanus, 336
Pediculus humanus capitis, 1281
Pedigree, genetic information, 60
PEEP *see* Positive end-expiratory pressure
PEF *see* Peak expiratory flow
PEG *see* Percutaneous endoscopic gastrostomy
Pegloticase, 1090
Pegvisomant, 793
Pegylated interferons, 161b, 954b–955b
Pellagra, 128–129, 128f, 1260b
Pelvi-ureteric junction obstruction, 510–511
Pelvic floor exercises, faecal incontinence, 918
Pelvic inflammatory disease (PID), 418
Pemphigoid, bullous, 1292–1293, 1293b, 1294f
Pemphigoid gestationis, 1259b, 1293b
Pemphigus, 1294
paraneoplastic, 272
Pemphigus foliaceus, 1293b
Pemphigus vulgaris, 1293b
Penciclovir, herpesvirus infection, 161–162, 161b
Pendred's syndrome, 739f
Pendrin, 739f
Penetrance, genetic, 51–53
Penicillamine
adverse reactions
aplastic anaemia, 1048b
muscle weakness, 1077b, 1132b
nephrotoxicity, 522b
neutropenia, 1005b
oral ulceration, 864b
pharmacokinetics, 25b
pyridoxine deficiency, 129
and respiratory disease, 714b
rheumatic disease, 1101b, 1102
skin reactions, 1290, 1304b
Wilson's disease, 974
Penicillin(s), 151b, 154b, 155
adverse reactions, 26, 27b
neutropenia, 1005b
pulmonary eosinophilia, 714b
allergy, 93b
anthrax, 347
cellulitis, 1277
diphtheria, 346
endocarditis, 628
leptospirosis, 338
listeriosis, 339
meningitis, 1203
nephrotoxicity, 522b
neurosyphilis, 1209
penicillinase-resistant, 155
in pregnancy, 154b
prophylactic, 79, 153b
resistance, 151
rheumatic fever, 615–616
sickle-cell disease, 1033
skin reactions, 1303b–1304b
syphilis, 421
tetanus, 1210b
tropical ulcer, 333
urinary tract infection, 512
see also Benzylpenicillin; Procaine penicillin
Penicillium marneffei, 385
Penile erection, 474
see also Erectile dysfunction
Penis, 466
Pentamidine
adverse reactions, 164
leishmaniasis, 364
Pneumocystis jirovecii pneumonia, 164
prophylactic, 153b
trypanosomiasis, 164, 359b
Pentavalent antimonials, 164
Pentoxifylline
alcoholic liver disease, 959, 959b
frostbite, 105
Pepper-pot skull, 769
Pepsin, 841–842
Pepsinogen, 841
Peptic ulcer, 872–876
complications, 875–876
management
adjunctive drug therapy, 874
surgery, 874–875
NSAID-induced, 873
older people, 875b
perforation, 862–863, 875
Zollinger-Ellison syndrome, 876
Peptide YY, 846b
Peptides, antimicrobial, 72
Peptostreptococcus spp., 332b
Perception(s)
abnormal, 234, 1167
delusional, 248, 248b
Percussion
abdomen, 839b
respiratory disease, 644–646
Percutaneous ablation, hepatocellular carcinoma, 968
Percutaneous coronary intervention (PCI)
angina, 587–588, 587b–588b, 587f
myocardial infarction, 595, 595f, 596b, 599
vs. CABG, 589b
Percutaneous endoscopic gastrostomy (PEG), 123, 123f
Percutaneous transhepatic cholangiography (PTC), 931
Perforin, 75–76
Pergolide, Parkinson's disease, 1197b
Pericardial aspiration, 640
Pericardial (cardiac) tamponade, 532, 545–546, 545b, 640
Pericardial disease, 639–641
Pericardial effusion, 261b, 640, 640f
tuberculous, 691
Pericardial friction rub, 562, 614–615
Pericardiocentesis, 640
Pericarditis
acute, 639–641
chronic renal failure, 483
constrictive, chronic, 641, 641b
myocardial infarction, 597
pain, 541
rheumatoid arthritis, 1099
tuberculous, 640
Perimysium, 1063–1064
Perinephric abscess, 512
Periodic fever syndromes, 85, 1135
Periodic limb movement syndrome, 1188
Periodic paralysis
hyperkalaemic, 1230b
hypokalaemic, 1230b
Periostitis, 420, 648
Peripheral arterial disease (PAD), 600–603, 600b
best medical therapy, 601b
Peripheral nerves
diseases, 1223–1226
lesions, 1164
Peripheral nervous system
motor, 1144
paraneoplastic disorders, 1194b
sensory, 1144
Peripheral neuropathy, 1223b
cancer-related, 272
diabetic, 826–827, 826b
drug-related, 403
HIV-related, 403
leprosy, 348
rheumatoid arthritis, 1099
sensorimotor, 403
Peripheral oedema
differential diagnosis, 549b
heart failure, 549b
sodium retention, 434, 435f
Peristalsis, 845
Peritoneal cavity, tumours, 919
Peritoneal dialysis, 490f, 492
automated, 492
continuous ambulatory (CAPD), 492
problems, 493b
Peritoneo-venous shunt, ascites, 940
Peritonitis, 919
CAPD, 489b
spontaneous bacterial, 941, 941b
tuberculous, 691
Permethrin
louse infestation, 1281
malaria prevention, 358
scabies, 1280–1281
Pernicious anaemia, 1025
Peroxisome proliferator activated receptor (PPAR) α, 434
Peroxisomes, 47
Persistent generalised lymphadenopathy (PGL), 395
Personal and professional development (PPD), 14–15, 14b, 14f
Personality, 1148
atherosclerotic vascular disease and, 581
and psychiatric disorders, 233
Personality disorder(s), 255, 1175
prevalence, 232b
Pertussis *see* Whooping cough
Pes cavus, 1076
Pes planus, 1098
Pesticides, 219–223
PET *see* Positron emission tomography
Petechiae, 1007, 1007f
definition, 1251b
Pethidine, 287
renal colic, 509
Petit mal, 1179
Petroleum distillates, poisoning, 224b
Pets
and allergic rhinitis, 725
and asthma, 666–667
opportunistic infection in HIV/AIDS, 406
Peutz-Jeghers syndrome, 267b, 911b, 912, 912f
Peyer's patches, 76, 843–844
PGL *see* Persistent generalised lymphadenopathy
pH monitoring
gastro-oesophageal reflux, 850
hyperglycaemic hyperosmolar state, 814
Phaeochromocytoma, 781–782, 781b, 782f
Phaeohyphomycosis, 382–383
Phagocyte deficiencies, 78b, 79
Phagocytes, 72–74

Phagocytosis, 73f
Phagolysosomes, 73
Pharmacist, 2b
Pharmacodynamics, 18–21, 18f, 25b
dose-response curves, 19–20, 19f
drug targets, 18–19, 19f
mechanisms of action, 18–19
Pharmacogenomics, 69
Pharmacokinetics, 18f, 21–23, 21f
absorption, 21–22
distribution, 22
drug interactions, 24b–25b
elimination, 22–23
patient-specific factors, 23–24, 24b
in pregnancy, 37b
repeated dose regimens, 23, 23f
Pharmacovigilance, 27–28
Pharyngeal pouch, 868
Pharyngitis, 681
infectious mononucleosis, 320
rheumatic fever, 614
Phenelzine, 244b
Phenobarbital
effect of old age, 36b
epilepsy, 1184b
poisoning, 211b
status epilepticus, 1159b
Phenothiazines, 241b
hyperpigmentation from, 1296b
schizophrenia, 249b
skin reactions, 1304b
Phenotype, 68f
Phenoxybenzamine, 769
Phenoxymethylpenicillin, 154b
anthrax, 347
prophylactic, 153b
rheumatic fever, 615
Phentolamine, phaeochromocytoma, 782
Phenylalanine, 114b
Phenylbutazone
aplastic anaemia, 1048b
pulmonary eosinophilia, 713b
Phenylketonuria, 449
genetic investigations, 64, 67b
Phenytoin
adverse reactions, 27b
ataxia, 1199b
drug interactions, 28b
epilepsy, 1184b
multiple sclerosis, 1192b
and peripheral neuropathy, 1223b
pharmacokinetics, 23
plasma concentrations, 39b
poisoning, 224b
prescribing, 38b
in renal/hepatic disease, 36b
skin reactions, 1304b
status epilepticus, 1159b
therapeutic monitoring, 39b
Phialophora verrucosa, 381
Philadelphia (Ph) chromosome, 1039
Phobias, 243
Phosphate
accumulation (hyperphosphataemia), 449
AKI, 480b
deficiency (hypophosphataemia), 130, 448–449, 449b, 1066b, 1128
enema, 917b, 946b
metabolism, 448
disorders of, 429b, 448–449
reference values
urine, 1311b
venous blood, 1310b
serum, bone disease, 1066b
supplements, 1128
see also Hyperphosphataemia; Hypophosphataemia
Phosphenes, 1170
Phosphodiesterase inhibitors
anticoagulation, 1019b
erectile dysfunction, 474
pulmonary hypertension, 725
Phospholipase A, 49b, 138
Phospholipids, 160, 450
Phosphorus, 130
deficiency, 130
dietary sources, 131b
radioactive
polycythaemia, 1049
thrombocythaemia, 1049
RNI, 131b
see also Phosphate
Photochemotherapy, 1266–1267
psoriatic arthritis, 1109
Photocoagulation
laser, 830
retinal, 829–830
Photodynamic therapy (PDT), 848f, 1269
cholangiocarcinoma, 986
oesophagitis, 849
oral cancer, 864
skin cancer, 1270b
Photopatch testing, skin disease, 1255
Photosensitivity, 1260–1262, 1260b, 1260f
drug-induced, 1260b, 1304b
porphyria, 1260b
Phototesting, skin disease, 1255–1256
Phototherapy, 1266–1267
atopic eczema, 1286
cutaneous lymphoma, 1272
pruritus, 1260
psoriasis, 1289b
vitiligo, 1295
Phrenic nerve paralysis, 702b, 705b
Phrygian cap, 988
Physical activity level (PAL), 111f
Physiotherapist, 2b
Physiotherapy
aspergillosis, 697
bronchiectasis, 679
cervical spondylosis, 1219
cystic fibrosis, 681
fractures, 1071
headache, 1176
leprosy, 350
low back pain, 1073
multiple sclerosis, 1160
muscular dystrophies, 1228–1229
musculoskeletal disorders, 1080
pain management, 288
palliative care, 288
Parkinson's disease, 1198
pneumonia, 686–687
stress incontinence, 474
stroke, 1243b
Phytoestrogens, 129
Pick's disease, 252f
PID *see* Pelvic inflammatory disease
Pigbel, 342
Pigeon chest, 731
Pigmentation
disorders of, 1295–1296
drug-induced, 1183b
Pigmented villonodular synovitis, 1134
Piles (haemorrhoids), 918–919
Pimecrolimus, 1266
Pimozide, 249b
Pineal tumours, 1213b
'Pink puffers', 674–675
Pinta, 333, 333b
Pioglitazone, 823
Piperacillin, 154b
neutropenic fever, 274
Piperacillin-tazobactam, 151b
necrotising fasciitis, 305
neutropenic fever, 302
Piperazine, 163, 371
Piroxicam, 1079b
PIs *see* Protease inhibitors
Pituitary apoplexy, 789
Pituitary gland, 785–795, 786f
diseases
anterior pituitary hormone deficiency, 787b
classification, 786b
investigation, 786–787, 787b
older people, 795b
presenting problems, 787–791
tumours *see* Pituitary tumours
functional anatomy and physiology, 786–787
Pituitary hormones, 736
Pituitary tumours, 789–790, 1215
clinical assessment, 789
Cushing's syndrome, 790b
investigations, 789
treatment, 789–790, 790b
visual field defect, 764b
Pityriasis lichenoides chronica, 1289
Pityriasis rosea, 1289
rash, 1257b
Pityriasis rubra pilaris, 1264
Pityriasis versicolor, 1257b, 1280
PKD *see* Polycystic kidney disease, autosomal dominant
Plague, 309b, 338–339, 338f
bubonic, 338
immunisation, 339
pneumonic, 338
septicaemic, 338
Plane warts, 1278
Plant toxins, 308
Plantar fasciitis, 1107–1108
Plantar warts, 1278
Plaques
amyloid, 251–252
atheromatous, 496, 580
pleural, 714b, 718, 718f
skin
definition, 1251b
erythematous, 1257b, 1279
Plasma
fresh frozen, 1012b
osmolarity, 814
virus-inactivated, 1012b, 1014–1015
viscosity, 85
Plasma derivatives, 1011
Plasma exchange (PE)
glomerulonephritis, 501–502
Guillain-Barré syndrome, 1225b
myasthenia gravis, 1227b
peripheral neuropathies, 1225
pre-renal transplant, 492–493
systemic vasculitis, 520
thrombotic thrombocytopenic purpura, 1056
Plasma membrane *see* Cell membrane
Plasmapheresis, 95, 964
Plasmin, 998f
Plasminogen, 265f
Plasminogen activator inhibitor (PAI), 998f
Plasmodium falciparum infection, 353, 354f, 355b
chloroquine resistance, 353
clinical features, 355, 356f
complications, 357b
intravascular haemolysis, 1031
diagnosis, 355
management, 356–357
Plasmodium malariae infection, 353, 355, 355b
Plasmodium ovale infection, 353, 355, 355b
Plasmodium spp., life cycle, 354, 354f, 355b
Plasmodium vivax infection, 353, 355, 355b
Platelet-activating factor, in allergy, 89b
Platelet-derived growth factor (PDGF), 263–264
Platelets, 996–997
concentrate, 1012b
count, 1000b
high, 1008
low, 1007–1008
disorders, functional, 1050
formation, 993f
function, assessment, 1000
reference values, 1312b
structure, 997, 998f
transfusions
acute leukaemia, 1001, 1037b
myelodysplastic syndrome, 1041
platelet functional disorders, 1050
thrombocytopenia, 1008
Platinum-based chemotherapy, 280–281, 704
Plethysmography, 653
Pleural aspiration, 661
Pleural biopsy, 661
bronchial carcinoma, 662b
tuberculosis, 668
Pleural disease, 728–730
asbestos-related, 718, 718f
bronchoscopy, 652
drug-induced, 714b
older people, 730b
Pleural effusion, 661–663
aortic dissection, 606–607, 606f
causes, 661b–662b
connective tissue disorders
febrile injecting drug user
heart failure, 549f, 662b
malignant, 261b, 275–276, 275b, 662b, 702b
oedema, 478
pancreatitis, 662b
rheumatoid disease, 662b, 712
signs, 644–646
SLE, 662b
tuberculosis, 662b, 689f, 691f
Pleural pain
aspergillosis, 698
bronchial obstruction, 701
empyema, 663b
pneumonia, 685
Pleural plaques, 718, 718f
Pleural rub, 560
Pleural thickening, 718, 718f
Pleurisy
asbestos-related, 718
connective tissue disorders, 1111
tuberculous, 681b
Pleurodesis
bronchial carcinoma, 704
pneumothorax, 730
Plexopathy, 1223
brachial, 1225–1226
lumbosacral, 1226
Plumboporphyria, 460b
Plummer-Vinson syndrome, 870
Pluripotent stem cells, 69–70
PMFL *see* Progressive multifocal leucoencephalopathy
PMNs *see* Polymorphonuclear cells
PMR *see* Polymyalgia rheumatica
Pneumatosis cystoides intestinalis, 920
Pneumococcus *see Streptococcus pneumoniae*
Pneumoconiosis, 716–718
Pneumocystis carinii see Pneumocystis jirovecii
Pneumocystis jirovecii pneumonia
acute leukaemia, 1038
chemoprophylaxis, 153b
HIV/AIDS patients, 400, 400b, 401f
HSCT, 1017b
immunocompromised patients, 687–688, 688b
prophylaxis, 406b
stem cell transplantation, 1017b
Pneumocytes, 646–647
Pneumonia, 658b, 682–688
aspirational, 687
malaria, 357b
bacterial, 401
clinical features, 683, 686

community-acquired, 682–685, 683b
complications, 685b
cryptogenic organising (bronchiolitis obliterans), 708b
differential diagnosis, 683b
eosinophilic, 708, 713
HIV/AIDS patients, 401
hospital-acquired (nosocomial), 685–687
in immunocompromised patient, 687–688, 688b
interstitial, 709
acute, 708b
desquamative, 708b
idiopathic, 706–709, 708b
lymphocytic, 708b
usual, 708b, 709f
investigations, 684, 684b, 686
ITU referral, 685b
lobar, 682, 684f
management, 684–686
antibiotic therapy, 685, 685b
middle lobe, signs, 644–646
necrotising, 138b
occupational, 720–721
Pneumocystis jiroveci see Pneumocystis jirovecii pneumonia
predisposing factors, 682b
prevention, 685–687
suppurative, 687, 687b
tuberculous, 690
viral, 319–320, 706b
Pneumonic plague, 338
Pneumonitis
hypersensitivity, 719–720, 720f
interstitial
lymphocytic, 401, 404
usual, 709f
radiation, 714
Pneumothorax, 645f, 728–730
after permanent pacing, 579
age distribution, 729f
air travel after, 108, 730
barotrauma, 109
classification, 729b
pain, 540, 729
signs, 644–646
spontaneous, 729f
management, 730f
older people, 730b
recurrent, 730
tension, 558, 664, 729
POCT *see* Point-of-care testing
Podiatry
diabetics, 834
older people, 177
Podocytes, 464
Podophyllin, 1279
Podophyllotoxin, 425
Poikilocytes, teardrop, 1048–1049
Point mutations, 53
Point-of-care testing (POCT), 428
Poiseuille's Law, 530–531
Poisoning, 205–230
acute, 208
approach to patients, 208–212
assessment and investigations, 209
chemicals and pesticides, 219–223
clinical features, 207f
complications, 211b
drugs, 212–216
of misuse, 216–219
envenomation, 207–208, 207b, 207f, 224–230, 225b–226b, 226f
environmental, 223
evaluation, 206f
external decontamination, 208f
history taking, 206
laboratory screening, 209b
low toxicity substances, 209b
management, 210–212
antidotes, 212
gastrointestinal decontamination, 210, 210b
haemodialysis/haemoperfusion, 211, 211b
lipid emulsion therapy, 211
supportive care, 212
urinary alkalinisation, 210–211
in old age, 208b
psychiatric assessment, 210
substances involved, 208b
triage and resuscitation, 208
see also Food poisoning; Venoms
Poliomyelitis, 1207
immunisation, 1207
incubation period, 145b, 1207
Pollens, 90–91, 1255, 1283
Pollution, atmospheric, 102
PolyA tail, 43, 43f
Polyangiitis
with granulomatosis (Wegener's granulomatosis), 713
microscopic, 1118
Polyarteritis nodosa (PAN), 1117
Polyarthritis, 1069–1071, 1069b, 1104b
associated extra-articular features, 1070b
joint involvement, 1070f
symmetrical, 1108
Polychondritis, relapsing, 1119
Polychromasia, 994
Polycystic kidney disease (PKD), autosomal dominant, 62b
Polycystic ovarian syndrome (PCOS), 760, 764–765, 764b, 764f
acne, 764b
hirsutism, 763b
Polycythaemia, 107, 271b, 464–466, 516
Polycythaemia rubra vera (PRV), 1049
Polydipsia, 738b
diabetes insipidus, 794
hypercalcaemia, 767
hyponatraemia, 438
Polyenes, 160, 160b
Polyethylene glycol, 895, 917
Polymerase chain reaction (PCR), 139–140
acute leukaemia, 1039–1040
genetic diseases, 60–62, 60f–61f
herpes simplex virus, 415, 1154
leishmaniasis, 367
meningitis, 1203f
pertussis, 682
viral haemorrhagic fever, 303b
viral hepatitis, 950
Whipple's disease, 884
Polymorphic eruption of pregnancy, 1259b
Polymorphic light eruption, 1260b
Polymorphisms, 58
restriction fragment length, 693
single nucleotide, 63
Polymorphonuclear cells (PMNs), 154, 1205
Polymyalgia rheumatica (PMR), 1117–1118
conditions mimicking, 1117b
management, 1117–1118
prevalence, 1060b
Polymyositis *see* Dermatomyositis/polymyositis
Polyneuropathy, 1223b, 1224
acute axonal, 1223b
acute inflammatory, demyelinating *see* Guillain-Barré syndrome
chronic, 1225
chronic axonal, 1223b
critical illness, 200
demyelinating, 1223b, 1225
organophosphate-induced delayed, 222
sensorimotor, 1194b
symmetrical sensory, diabetics, 831–832
Polyostotic fibrous dysplasia, 1131
Polypectomy, colonoscopic, colonic polyps, 848f, 910
Polypeptides, 842, 844b
Polypharmacy, older people, 176b
Polyposis, juvenile, 911b, 912
Polyposis syndromes, 910–912, 911b
see also Familial adenomatous polyposis
Polyps
colonic, 910–916
gastric, 911b
small bowel, 911b
Polyradiculitis, CMV, 404
Polysaccharides
non-starch (dietary fibre), 113b
starch, 113b
Polyuria, 472, 472b, 738b
diabetes insipidus, 794
hyperaldosteronism, 780
hypercalcaemia, 767
Pompe disease, 450b
Pompholyx, 1285
Poncet's arthropathy, 692
Popcorn worker's lung, 718
Popliteal cysts *see* Baker's cysts
Popliteal nerve palsy, 832, 1099
Population health, 98f
Porcelain gallbladder, 983
Porphyria cutanea tarda (PCT), 460b, 1301, 1302f
Porphyrias, 458–460, 459f, 475b
acute intermittent, 460b
congenital erythropoietic, 460b
erythropoietic protoporphyria, 460b
hereditary coproporphyria, 460b
photosensitivity, 1260b
plumboporphyria, 460b
skin lesions, 1301–1302
variegate, 450b, 459f
Porphyrins, 460b
Portal circulation, 464
Portal hypertension, 945–948
classification, 945f
complications, 945b
Portal venous pressure, 946
reduction, 946
Portal venous thrombosis, 975
Portopulmonary hypertension, 976
Portosystemic encephalopathy *see* Hepatic encephalopathy
Portosystemic shunts, 928, 945, 948
Posaconazole, 160, 160b
aspergillosis, 698–699
chromoblastomycosis, 381–382
coccidioidomycosis, 386
fusariosis, 384–385
mucormycosis, 699
mycetoma, 382
prophylactic, 153b
Positive end-expiratory pressure (PEEP), 195b
Positron emission tomography (PET)
cancer diagnosis, 269, 269f
gastrointestinal tract, 847b
lymphoma, 1043
myocardial, 539
nervous system, 1149b
respiratory disease, 651, 651f
Post-cholecystectomy syndrome, 986–987, 987b
Post-herpetic neuralgia, 319, 1157
Post-myocardial infarction syndrome, 597
Post-partum 'blues', 256
Post-partum thyroiditis, 752, 756b
Post-traumatic stress disorder (PTSD), 242
Posterior circulation stroke (POCS), 1241f
Posterior descending artery, 529
Postural drainage, bronchiectasis, 679
Postural hypotension, 554, 556
hypopituitarism, 787–788, 788f
management, 556
older people, 36b
peripheral neuropathy, 832b–833b, 1223
renal dysfunction, 479
Posture
examination, 1139b
Parkinson's disease, 1196b, 1198
Potassium, 132
channelopathies, 1230b
daily requirements, 433b
depletion, diabetic ketoacidosis, 814
dietary sources, 131b
disorders of balance, 429b–430b, 439–443
intake, chronic renal failure, 488
refeeding diet, 122b
reference values
urine, 1311b
venous blood, 1308b
renal handling, 440, 440f
replacement, 813b
RNI, 131b
ROMK channel, 431
supplements, 447, 672
see also Hyperkalaemia; Hypokalaemia
Potassium channel activators, angina, 587
Potassium chloride
diabetic ketoacidosis, 813b
hypokalaemia, 442
Potassium iodide
erythema nodosum, 585
Graves' disease, 749
sporotrichosis, 383
Potassium perchlorate, 752
Potassium permanganate, 1263
Potassium phosphate, 449
Potency, 20
Pott's disease, 691–692
Poverty, health consequences, 101–102, 101b
Poxviruses, 327
PPAR-α/γ agonists *see* Thiazolidinediones
PPD *see* Personal and professional development
Practice guidance, 14b
Practolol, nephrotoxicity, 522b
Prader-Willi syndrome, 116
genetics, 54b, 56b
Pralidoxime, 221
Pramipexole, Parkinson's disease, 1197b
Prasugrel, 1019b
Prayer sign, 798f
Praziquantel, 163
cysticercosis, 380
hydatid disease, 381
liver flukes, 163, 312
schistosomiasis, 378
Prazosin, 230, 612, 782
Pre-eclampsia, 521, 521b
Pre-implantation genetic testing, 62–63
Pre-patellar bursitis, 1076b
Prednisolone
autoimmune hepatitis, 962–963
blood disorders
acute leukaemia, 1037b
autoimmune haemolysis, 1030
myeloma, 1047
non-Hodgkin's lymphoma, 1045
thrombocytopenia, 1050
bullous pemphigoid, 1294b
cysticercosis, 380

dosage interval, 35b
eosinophilic gastroenteritis, 887
Epstein-Barr virus, 321
equivalent dose, 776b
filariases, 374
Graves' ophthalmopathy, 750–751
histoplasmosis, 385–386
inflammatory bowel disease, 860, 903b
leprosy reactions, 349b
liver transplant patients, 979
musculoskeletal disorders
giant cell arteritis, 1117–1118
myositis, 1115
polymyositis, 1115
rheumatoid arthritis, 1102
SLE, 1111–1112
onchocerciasis, 374
and osteoporosis, 1120–1121
pericarditis, 640
renal disease
acute interstitial nephritis, 503
glomerulonephritis, 499b–500b
lupus nephritis, 499b–500b
respiratory diseases
aspergillosis, 697
asthma, 650
chronic eosinophilic pneumonia, 713
COPD, 678
hypersensitivity pneumonitis, 720
interstitial lung disease, 709
sarcoidosis, 711
rheumatic fever, 615
syphilis, 421–422
thyroiditis, 748b, 752
trypanosomiasis, 360
tuberculous pericarditis
Pregabalin, 1184b
herpes zoster, 397
pain management, 288b
Pregnancy
air travel, 108
allergy, 94b
antimicrobial agents in, 154b
asthma, 671b
autoimmune disease, 94b
cholestasis, 977–978, 1259b
congenital heart disease and, 631, 631b
cytomegalovirus infection, 314b
diabetes and, 807b, 817–818
dopamine agonist therapy, 792
dyslipidaemia, 458b
ectopic, 418, 423
folate deficiency/supplements, 125b
genetic testing, 62–63, 63b
glycosuria, 817
haematological physiology, 1022b
HELLP syndrome, 978
HIV treatment in, 409–410
hyperemesis gravidarum, 756b
hypothyroidism, 745
infections in, 313, 314b
inflammatory bowel disease, 906–907, 906b
kidneys in, 520–521, 520b
listeriosis, 314b, 339
liver disease, 977–978
malaria, 314b
management, 358b
prophylaxis, 358b
Marfan's syndrome, 603–604
neurological disease
epilepsy, 1184–1185, 1185b
multiple sclerosis, 1192b
nutrition, 125b
osteoporosis, 1121
pituitary tumours, 792
pre-eclampsia, 521, 521b
prenatal genetic testing, 62–63, 63b
prescribing in, 36–37, 37b
pruritus, 1259b
psychiatric illness, 256–257, 256b
renal disease, 520–521
rhesus D negative women, 1014b
rheumatic disease, 1101b
rubella in, 314b
STIs, 414, 414b
anogenital warts, 421, 425
genital herpes, 425
syphilis, 421
thyroid disease, 743–745, 756b
toxaemia, 978
toxoplasmosis, 314b, 362
venous thromboembolism, 723b
Preload, 182–183, 547
heart failure, 551
increasing, 191, 547f
Premature beats, 564, 569
Prenatal genetic testing, 62–63, 63b
Prescribing, 18b, 33–40
abbreviations, 38b
choice of drug, 33–34, 33b
controlled drugs, 31
decision-making, 33–36
dosage regimen, 34
drug doses, 34
hepatic disease, 36, 36b
high-risk moments, 38b
hospitals, 37
junior doctors, 29
medication errors, 29–30, 29b–30b, 30f
monitoring effects, 36, 39–40, 39b
older people, 36b
patient involvement, 34–35, 35b
pregnancy and breastfeeding, 36–37, 37b
primary care, 37–39
renal disease, 36, 36b
stopping therapy, 36
topical drugs, 21–22, 1264–1266, 1265b
writing, 35, 37–39, 38b
Pressure controlled ventilation (PCV), 183
Pressure sores, 1299–1300
stroke patients, 1243b
Pressure support ventilation (PSV), 195f
Pressure-controlled ventilation (PCV), 183
Presyncope
cardiac, 554–556, 555b
differential diagnosis, 554–556, 554f
investigations, 555f
Prevalence of disease, 99, 99b
Preventive medicine, 100
Prevotella spp., 137f
Prick tests, hypersensitivity, 1255
Primaquine, malaria, 357
Primary CNS lymphoma (PCNSL), 402–403, 403f
Primary complex of Ranke, 688–689
Primidone, 1184b
Prion diseases, 250b, 329b, 1211
see also Transmissible spongiform encephalopathies
Prions, 134–135, 329, 1211
Priority-setting, 11
Pro-carboxypeptidases, 844b
Pro-drugs, 22
Pro-elastase, 844b
Pro-insulin, 802f
Probenecid
gonorrhoea, 422b
gout, 1089–1090
neurosyphilis, 1209
Probiotics, 908–909
Problem-solving therapy, 241, 242b
Procainamide
and lupus syndrome, 1132b
and neutropenia, 1005b
pharmacokinetics, 25b
Procaine penicillin
neurosyphilis, 1209
reaction to, 422
relapsing fever, 336
syphilis, 421
Procarbazine, 714b
Procarboxypeptidases, 842
Prochlorperazine, 877, 1186
Proctitis, 278
management, 886
men who have sex with men, 417
Proctocolitis, radiation, 885–886, 885b
Proctography, defecating, 918
Proctoscopy, 422
Proctosigmoiditis, 898f
Procyclidine, 205, 237–238
Progenitor cells, 992f
Progeria *see* Werner's syndrome
Progesterones, reference range, 1309b
Progestogens
in cancer treatment, 278
hormone replacement therapy, 760, 1124–1125
and sebum secretion, 1281
secondary amenorrhoea, 764
Progressive multifocal leucoencephalopathy (PMFL), 402, 402f, 1207
Progressive supranuclear palsy, 1198
Proguanil, 163
malaria, 163, 356
pharmacokinetics, 25b
Prokaryotes, 135
Prolactin
plasma/serum levels, 791
reference range, 1309b
Prolactinoma, 790b–791b, 791–792, 792f
Proline, 114b
Prolymphocytic leukaemia, 1041
Promastigotes, 362
Promyelocytes, 993f
Propafenone, 565–566, 574, 575b
Propantheline, 1226–1227
Propionibacterium spp., 137f, 1281
Propranolol
anxiety disorder, 243
arrhythmias, 574–576
congestive gastropathy, 948
effect of old age, 36b
endocrine disease
thyrotoxic crisis, 742–743
thyrotoxicosis, 741–742
older people, 36b
phaeochromocytoma, 782
in renal/hepatic disease, 36b
variceal bleeding, 946, 946b
Proptosis, Graves' disease, 741b, 756b
Propylthiouracil, 748b, 749–750
Prosody, 1146
Prostacyclin (epoprostenol)
endothelial function, 531
haemostasis, 996f–997f
pulmonary hypertension, 725
secondary Raynaud's phenomenon, 603
Prostaglandins
allergy, 75, 89b
over-production, 1132
pulmonary hypertension, 725
and renal blood flow, 522
prostaglandin E, and finger clubbing, 271
Prostaglandin E1, erectile dysfunction, 474
Prostaglandin E2, febrile response, 138
Prostate, 466
benign hyperplasia, 472, 514–515
incontinence and, 473
biopsy, 518
International Prostate Symptom Score, 514b
Prostate cancer, 517–518
incidence, 262f
inheritance, 267b
management, 518, 518b
screening, 518
staging, 518
Prostate-specific antigen (PSA), 268, 270b, 515, 761
Prostatic acid phosphatase, 268
Prostatitis, 515
bacterial, antibiotic therapy, 513b
Protamine sulphate, 1019
Protease inhibitors (PIs), 407b, 955
Proteases, 673f, 842, 842f
26S Proteasomes, 46
Protein binding, 22, 1020
Protein C
activated, 1001b
inflammation, 185
in pregnancy, 1022b
deficiency, 1054–1055
pregnancy, 1022b
Protein S
deficiency, 1054–1055
pregnancy, 1022b
Protein-losing enteropathy, 886, 886b
Proteinosis, alveolar, 714b–715b
Proteins, 114, 169
acute phase, 82
Bence Jones, 477–478
biliary transport, 927f
cell membrane, 47–48
cerebrospinal fluid, 1311b
cholesterol ester transfer, 452
degradation, 46–47
dietary
energy provided by, 110
recommended intake, 114b
digestion, 842, 843f
HFE, 972
IGF-BP3, 737f
monoclonal, 1045
plasma, 926, 995, 1025
production, 44–45
refeeding diet, 122b
reference values
urine, 1311b
venous blood, 1310b
restriction
chronic renal failure, 488
hepatic encephalopathy, 942
urea cycle disorders, 64–65
synthesis, 43
Tamm-Horsfall, 476
urinary, 807
Proteinuria, 476–478, 487–488
Bence Jones, 477–478
diabetic nephropathy, 807, 830–831
investigations, 476b, 477–478, 477f
orthostatic, 476
pregnancy, 978
tubular, 477
Proteoglycans, 1062
Proteus spp., 137f
bacterial meningitis, 1202b
urinary tract infection, 512
Prothrombin G20210A, 1055
Prothrombin time (PT), 926–927, 999–1000, 1000b
disseminated intravascular coagulation, 1056b
gastrointestinal bleeding, 850
liver disease, 929, 931b
acute liver failure, 934b
alcoholic liver disease, 959b
reference values, 1312b
Proto-oncogenes, 59–60, 69
Protocols, 9
Proton pump, 841
Proton pump inhibitors
GORD, 867, 868f
nephrotoxicity, 502b

peptic ulcer/dyspepsia, bleeding peptic ulcers, 198
skin reactions, 1304b
variceal bleeding, 856b
Protoporphyria, erythropoietic, 460b
Protozoal infections, 135, 353–369
blood and tissue parasites, 353–362
gastrointestinal, 367–369
immune deficiency and, 78b
nervous system, 1201b
Proximal myotonic myopathy, 1228b
Prozone phenomenon, 420–421
Prucalopride, 909
Prurigo
actinic, 1260b
gestationis, 1259b
Pruritus, 1258–1260, 1258b–1259b
in cancer patients, 272
HIV-associated, 398
pregnancy, 1259b
primary biliary cirrhosis, 964
sclerosing cholangitis, 965–966
Pruritus ani, 919, 919b
Pruritus vulvae, 418b, 809–810
PRV *see* Polycythaemia rubra vera
PSA *see* Prostate-specific antigen
Pseudo-Cushing's syndrome, 773b
Pseudo-dementia, 1162
Pseudo-hallucinations, 237
Pseudo-puberty, precocious, 782
Pseudobulbar palsy, 1174b
Pseudocyst, pancreatic, 891f
Pseudofractures, 1127, 1127f
Pseudogout, 1090–1092
Pseudohypoparathyroidism, 768b, 770–771
Pseudomonas spp.
cerebral abscess, 1208b
drug resistance, 152f
health care-associated infections, 146f
osteomyelitis, 1095
respiratory infection
bronchiectasis, 679
cystic fibrosis, 680–681
pneumonia, 685–686
urinary tract infection, 512
urinary tract infection, 512
Pseudomonas aeruginosa, 151b, 304b
bronchiectasis, 678–679
cystic fibrosis, 681b
pneumonia, 401
sepsis, 304b
Pseudomonas fluorescens, 303–304
Pseudoporphyria, 1260b, 1304b
Pseudopseudohypoparathyroidism, 770
Pseudoseizures, 1159
Psilocybin, 254, 308
Psittacosis, incubation period, 145b
Psoralens, 1266–1267
hyperpigmentation from, 1296b
skin reactions, 1304b
see also PUVA
Psoriasis, 1286–1289
aetiology, 1286–1287
clinical features, 1287–1288, 1287f
erythrodermic, 1287f, 1288
exacerbating factors, 1286b
guttate, 1287f, 1288
histology, 1287f
inheritance, 1286
investigations, 1288, 1288b
management/treatment, 1288–1289, 1288b–1289b
nails in, 1287f, 1288
pathogenesis, 1286–1287
plaque, 1287f, 1288
pustular, 1287f, 1288
rash, 1257b
Psoriatic arthritis, 1104b, 1108–1109, 1109f
erosions, 1109
PSV *see* Pressure support ventilation
Psychiatric disorders, 231–257, 1175
aetiology, 232–233, 233b
biological, 232–233
psychological/behavioural, 233
social/environmental, 233
classification, 232, 232b
diagnosis, 233–234
Mental State Examination, 233–234
psychiatric interview, 233–234, 234b
emergencies, 238b
epidemiology, 232, 232b
genetics, 232–233
HIV-related, 404
law and, 257
older people, 238b
organic, 238b
patient's understanding ('insight'), 234
physical illness and, 232
presenting problems, 234–240
prevalence, 232b
psychological factors in medical illness, 240, 240b
puerperal, 256–257, 256b
self-poisoning and, 210
stress-related, 233, 242
treatments, 240–242
biological, 240–241
psychological, 241–242
social interventions, 242
see also specific disorders
Psychodynamic psychotherapy, 241–242
Psychogenic attacks (pseudoseizures), 1159
Psychogenic pruritus, 1259b
Psychological factors
angina, 585
erectile dysfunction, 833
fibromyalgia, 1092f
irritable bowel syndrome, 909
low back pain, 1072–1073
in medical illness, 240, 240b
migraine, 1176–1177
non-ulcer dyspepsia, 877
pain, 286f
psoriasis, 1286b
psychiatric disorders, 240
Psychological treatment/psychotherapy, 241–242
adjustment disorder, 242
alcohol misuse, 254
eating disorders, 256
erectile dysfunction, 474
general (supportive), 241–242
interpersonal, 242
pain management, 288
psychodynamic (interpretative), 241–242
see also specific therapies
Psychopathic (antisocial) personality disorder, 255
Psychosis
affective, 245
organic, 248
prevalence, 232b
puerperal, 257
Psychotherapy *see* Psychological treatment/Psychotherapy
Psychotropic drugs, 241b
adverse reactions, 1005b
PT *see* Prothrombin time
PTC *see* Percutaneous transhepatic cholangiography
PTH *see* Parathyroid hormone
Pthirus pubis, 416b
Ptosis, 701, 1171, 1172b
PTSD *see* Post-traumatic stress disorder
PTTK *see* Partial thromboplastin time with kaolin
Puberty, delayed, 758–759, 758b
Pubic lice, 1281
Public health, 98
ethics, 10
Puerperal psychiatric disorders, 256–257, 256b
Pulmonary abscess, 687
Pulmonary angiography, 723
CT, 722, 723f
Pulmonary arteriovenous malformations (PAVMs), 1049
Pulmonary artery, cannulation/catheterisation, critically ill patients, 185–186, 186f
Pulmonary artery pressure, 539, 617b
Pulmonary artery wedge pressure (PAWP), 186f
mitral regurgitation, 619
monitoring, 185–186
myocardial infarction, 545
portopulmonary hypertension, 976
Pulmonary atresia, 635b
Pulmonary circulation, 648, 651
Pulmonary embolism/thromboembolism, 658b, 721–724
acute, 545
and atrial fibrillation, 565
clinical features, 721–724, 721b, 722f
critically ill patients, 192b
heart failure, 548
investigations, 722–723, 722f
management, 723–724
anticoagulants, 723
thrombolytic therapy, 723
pain, 540, 541b
prognosis, 724
stroke patients, 1243b
Pulmonary eosinophilia, 713–714, 713b
drug-induced, 714b
tropical, 713
Pulmonary fibrosis, 644–646
idiopathic, 707–709, 709f
older people, 714b
respiratory function abnormalities, 644–646, 653b
rheumatoid arthritis, 712b, 1099
sarcoidosis, 711b
SLE, 712, 712b
systemic sclerosis, 712b, 713
Pulmonary function tests, 653f
asthma, 653b
bronchitis, 653b
COPD, 675, 675b
emphysema, 653b
pulmonary fibrosis, 644–646, 653b
Pulmonary hypertension, 724–725
classification, 724b
congenital heart disease, 631
mitral stenosis, 616
primary, 724
pulmonary regurgitation, 625
systemic sclerosis, 1113
Pulmonary infarction, pleural effusion, 662b
Pulmonary nodules, 660, 660b
clinical/radiographic features, 660b
cryptococcosis, 384
follow-up, 661b
lung metastases, 274
rheumatoid, 712
Pulmonary oedema, 658b
AKI, 482, 482f
chest X-ray, 482f
drug-induced, 714b
heart failure, 550f
high altitude, 107
malaria, 357b
management, 550
near-drowning, 108
non-cardiogenic, 714b
papillary muscle rupture, 597
renal artery stenosis, 494
sputum, 644f
symptoms, 657
Pulmonary plethora, 633
Pulmonary regurgitation, 625
Pulmonary stenosis, 625
incidence, 630b
Pulmonary syndrome, leptospirosis, 337
Pulmonary–renal syndrome, 519
Pulse oximetry, 192b
Pulseless electrical activity, 557–558
Pulses, cardiovascular disease, 526f, 527b
Pulsus paradoxus, 532
Punch-drunk syndrome, 250b
PUO *see* Pyrexia of unknown origin
Pupillary abnormalities, 1172, 1172b
autonomic neuropathy, 832b
critically ill patients, 189, 198–199
Graves' ophthalmopathy, 735b
neurosyphilis, 1209
older people, 1064b
Purines, 1087f
Purkinje network, 529–530
Purpura
definition, 1251b
drug-induced, 1304b
Henoch-Schönlein, 501, 1119
idiopathic thrombocytopenic (ITP)
non-thrombocytopenic, 1007b
petechial, 1007, 1007f
pinch, 1302
senile, 1056b
thrombotic thrombocytopenic, 1056
Pustule, definition, 1251b
Pustuloderma, drug-induced, 1304b
Pustulosis
acute generalised exanthematous, 1304b
drug-induced, 1304b
palmoplantar, 1288
PUVA, 1266
granuloma annulare, 1301
lichen planus, 1290
necrobiosis lipoidica, 1301
psoriasis, 1289b
psoriatic arthritis, 1109
vitiligo, 1295
Pyelography, 470
retrograde, 470f
Pyelonephritis
acute, 513–514
antibiotic therapy, 513b
chronic, 504–505
emphysematous, 514
pregnancy, 520
Pyeloplasty, 510–511
Pyloroplasty, 856
Pyoderma gangrenosum, 1299, 1299f
Pyonephrosis, 509
Pyopneumothorax, 662–663
Pyramidal gait, 1168
Pyrantel pamoate, 163, 371
Pyrazinamide
adverse reactions, 694b
tuberculosis, 693, 694b
tuberculous meningitis, 1205
Pyrethroid insecticide poisoning, 224b
Pyrexia *see* Fever
Pyrexia of unknown origin (PUO)
biopsy, 299b
bone marrow, 298–299
laparoscopy, 298–299
older people, 296b
see also Fever
Pyridostigmine, 1226–1228
Pyridoxal, 126, 126b
Pyridoxamine, 126

Pyridoxine (vitamin B_6), 129
biochemical assessment of status, 126b
deficiency, 129
dietary sources, 125b
excess, 129
and peripheral neuropathy, 1223b
RNI, 125b
supplements, 129
tuberculosis, 694b
Pyrimethamine
malaria, 356
toxoplasmosis, 362
HIV-related, 402
Pyrimethamine/sulfadoxine *see* Fansidar
Pyrimidine 5′ nucleotidase deficiency, 1029
Pyrin, 85
Pyrophosphate arthritis, 1086b
Pyruvate kinase deficiency, 1029
Pyuria, sterile, 505

Q
Q fever, 309b, 352
endocarditis, 352, 626
Quality of life, 102b
Quality-adjusted life years (QALY), 9, 32
Questions, medical interview, 4b
Quetiapine
bipolar disorder, 245
schizophrenia, 249b
Quinagolide, prolactinoma, 791b
Quincke's sign, 623b
Quinidine
arrhythmias, 574
malaria, 356–357
and neutropenia, 1005b
poisoning, 211b
Quinine
babesiosis, 358
malaria, 163, 356–357
poisoning, 215
skin reactions, 1304b
Quinolones, 157, 157b
adverse reactions, 157
mechanism of action, 150b
pharmacokinetics, 157
in pregnancy, 154b
prophylactic, spontaneous bacterial peritonitis, 941
skin reactions, 1304b
see also Fluoroquinolones
Quinupristin, 151b, 159

R
R protein, 1024–1025
RA *see* Rheumatoid arthritis
Rabies, 309b, 1206
immunisation, 1206
incubation period, 145b, 1206
prophylaxis, 1206
Radial nerve, entrapment, 1224b
Radial pulse, 632
respiratory disease, 644f
Radiation(s)
dose and exposure, 103
effects of exposure, 103
enteritis, 885–886, 885b
infrared, 1257b
ionising, 102–103, 102b
management of exposure, 103
mutagenic effects, 266b
natural background, 103
non-ionising, 67, 102
pneumonitis, 714
proctocolitis, 885–886, 885b
ultraviolet *see* Ultraviolet radiation
Radicular pain, 1072f, 1073b
Radiculography, 1149b
Radiculopathy, 1218–1223, 1226
cervical spondylotic, 1218–1219
HIV-related, 403–404
Radioallergosorbent test (RAST), 90
Radiofemoral delay, 630f
Radiofrequency ablation
arrhythmias, 576b, 577f
cardiovascular disease, 577–578
GORD, 867
liver metastases, 274–275
renal adenocarcinoma, 516
Radiography *see* X-rays
Radioiodine
multinodular goitre, 754
thyroid cancer, 754b
thyrotoxicosis, 733, 748b
Radioisotope imaging *see* Radionuclide imaging
Radioisotope tests, gastroenterology, 850–851, 851b
Radioisotopes
cancer treatment, 278
exposure to, 103
Radiology *see* CT; MRI; X-rays
Radionuclide (radioisotope) imaging
bone, 1063f, 1065
cardiovascular, 539
nervous system, 1149b
Paget's disease, 1129f
renal disease, 470–471, 471f
Radiotherapy, 277–278
acromegaly, 790b, 793
adverse reactions, 277f, 278
blood disorders
chronic lymphocytic leukaemia, 1040
Hodgkin's disease, 1043
multiple myeloma, 1047
non-Hodgkin's lymphoma, 1044–1045
brain tumours, 1215
breast cancer, 280
bronchial carcinoma, 703–704
colorectal cancer, 915
conformal, 278
continuous hyperfractionated accelerated (CHART), 703
endometrial cancer, 281
fractionation, 278
late effects, 796, 1035b
lung damage, 714
mesothelioma, 719
oesophageal cancer, 870–871
oral cancer, 864
pain management, 288
palliative, 288
pituitary tumours, 792–793
prolactinoma, 792
prostate cancer, 518
skin cancer, 1269, 1271
Radon, lung cancer and, 660b
Raloxifene, osteoporosis, 1123b, 1124–1125
Raltegravir, 407b
Ramichloridiium mackenzei
Ramipril
heart failure, 552b
hypertension, 611
myocardial infarction, 599
Ramsay Hunt syndrome, 319
Randomised clinical trials (RCTs), 8b
Ranitidine
and neutropenia, 1005b
stress ulcer prophylaxis, 198
urticaria, 1291
RANK (receptor activator of nuclear κB), 49b
RANKL (receptor activator of nuclear κB ligand), 1062, 1062b
Rapid immunochromatographic tests, 338
Rapid plasma reagin (RPR) test, 420–421
Rapidly progressive glomerulonephritis (RPGN), 471–472, 501–502
Rasagiline, Parkinson's disease, 1197
Rashes, 398, 1257–1258, 1257b
atopic eczema, 1257b, 1284b
butterfly (malar), 1110f
chickenpox, 317, 317f
clinical features, 1257b
dengue, 322b
dermatitis herpetiformis, 1294
dermatomyositis, 1115
distribution, 1257
drug eruption, 398, 1257b, 1303f
erythema migrans, 335f
erythematous, 1293
erythrovirus, 316f
in fever, 295b
genital, 415, 416b
haemorrhagic, 351b
hand, foot and mouth disease, 326–327
herpes simplex, 326f
HIV-associated, 397b, 398, 409
infectious mononucleosis, 321f
lichen planus, 416b, 1257b
Lyme borreliosis (disease), 335f
macular/maculopapular, 351b
measles, 315f
meningococcal infection, 1203
morbilliform, 351b
petechiae, 1007, 1007f
photosensitivity, 1260f
pityriasis rosea, 1257b
pityriasis versicolor, 1257b
post-kala-azar leishmaniasis, 365f
psoriasiform, 1257b, 1304b
psoriasis, 1257b
purpura *see* Purpura
rheumatic fever, 614
rubella, 315
scaly, 1257b
scarlet fever, 332f
shingles, 317f
SLE, 1110f
syphilis, 1257b
tinea corporis, 1257b
toxic shock syndrome, 1276
tropical diseases, 313b
typhoid, 339
typhus, 350–351
urticarial, 1291f
vesicular, 397
RAST (radioallergosorbent test), 90
Rat bite fever, 313f
Raynaud's phenomenon/disease/syndrome, 602–603, 1110, 1110f, 1113
treatment, 1113
RB-ILD *see* Respiratory bronchiolitis-interstitial lung disease
RBBB *see* Right bundle branch block
RCA *see* Right coronary artery
Re-entry, 562f
Reactive airways dysfunction syndrome, 716
Reactive arthritis, 1107–1108, 1107b
Reaven's syndrome *see* Insulin resistance syndrome
Receiver operating characteristic (ROC) curve, 6f
Receptor activator of nuclear κB *see* RANK
Receptor activator of nuclear κB ligand *see* RANKL
Receptor diseases, 44f
Receptors
B-cell, 77
cell membrane, 48–49
drugs acting on, 19b
Recombinant human DNAase (rhDNAase), cystic fibrosis, 681b
Recombinant human erythropoietin, chronic renal failure, 488
Recombinant tissue plasminogen activator (rt-PA), stroke, 1244, 1244b
Recompression, 110
Rectal administration, 21
Rectal examination, 839b
gastrointestinal disease, 860
prostate, 511, 515, 517–518
Rectum, 845f
disorders of, 910–920
neurological disease, 1175
tumours, 910–916
see also Anorectal; Colorectal cancer
Red cell enzymopathies, 1028–1029
Red cell membrane
defects, 1027–1028
structure, 994, 994f
Red cells, 994–995
agglutination, cold, 1030–1031
anaemia, 1021f
aplasia, 1032
blood film examination, 999f
concentrate, 1012b
count, 1312b
destruction, 995
effects of malaria, 354–355
formation, 993f, 994
fragments, 999f
haemolytic anaemia, 1026–1031, 1026b, 1027f
lifespan, 994, 1312b
nucleated, 999f
sickled *see* Sickle-cell anaemia/disease
structure and functions, 994–995, 994f
transfusion, 1011b
(in)compatibility, 1012–1014
Red hepatisation, 682
Red man reaction, 158
5α-Reductase inhibitors, 515, 765b
Reduviid bugs, 309b
Reed-Sternberg cells, 1042f
Refeeding diet, 122b
Refeeding syndrome, 124
Reference nutrient intake, 124
Reference range, 5, 5f
Reflex sympathetic dystrophy, 1130, 1130f
Reflex(es)
Bezold-Jarisch, 555–556
cough, 654
diabetes, 831–832
stretch, 1144, 1174
tendon, root values, 1139b
Reflux
bile, 875
duodenogastro-oesophageal, 866–867
gastro-oesophageal, 865–868, 865f
Reflux nephropathy, 504–505
Regenerative medicine, 69–70
Regurgitation, 852–853
aortic, 527b, 623–624, 623b, 623f
chest X-ray, 535f
clinical features, 623–624, 623b
investigations, 624, 624b
mitral, 618–620, 618b, 619f
clinical features, 618–619, 618b
heart murmurs, 562b
investigations, 619, 619b
Rehabilitation
leprosy, 350
myocardial infarction, 598–599
older people, 176–177, 176b–177b
schizophrenia, 249
stroke, 1242–1243
Rehydration *see* Fluid replacement
Reiter's cells, 1108
Reiter's disease/syndrome *see* Reactive arthritis
Relapsing fevers
louse-borne, 336, 336f
tick-borne, 336
REM sleep behaviour disorder, 1187

Renal, *see also* Kidneys
Renal arteriography/venography, 470
Renal artery stenosis, 494–495, 494b–495b, 495f
Renal biopsy, 471, 471b
Renal colic, 507–510
Renal dialysis *see* Dialysis, renal
Renal disease, 461–523
adolescents, 521, 521b
atheroembolic, 469b, 496
chronic, 483–488
pruritus, 484
stages of, 467b
in connective tissue disease
Henoch-Schönlein purpura, 1119
SLE, 1111
systemic sclerosis, 1113
cystic, 505–507
adult polycystic kidney disease, 505–507
autosomal dominant polycystic disease, 62b
medullary, 506–507
diabetics *see* Diabetic nephropathy
drug-induced, 522–523
drug-related, 522–523, 522b
genetic testing, 62b
glomerular, 480b–481b, 497–502, 497f
HIV-related, 405
hypertension and, 609
infections, 511–514
investigation, 466–471
pregnancy, 520–521
prescribing in, 36–37, 36b, 523
presenting problems, 471–478
signs, 485f
tuberculosis, 692
tubulo-interstitial, 502–505
tumours/cancer, 262f
vascular, 494–497
see also Nephropathy
Renal failure
acute *see* Acute kidney injury
ascites, 940
bleeding, 1054
chronic, 483–488, 768b
causes, 484b
interstitial, 503–504
management, 487–488
osteodystrophy, 486f
osteomalacia, 1126b
referral, 487b
renal replacement therapy, 491
screening tests, 483–484
critically ill patients, 197–198, 197b
cystic disease *see* Renal disease, cystic
diabetics, 830
end-stage, 484b
heart failure, 549
hepatic cirrhosis, 944
investigations, 487, 487b
pregnancy, 520–521
pruritus, 1259b
pyelonephritis *see* Pyelonephritis
SLE, 1111
Renal function, 24b
Renal function tests, 466–471
Renal infarction, acute, 495
Renal insufficiency, effect on drug dosages, 36b
Renal osteodystrophy, 1066b
Renal papillary necrosis, 505
and NSAID ingestion, 522b
pyelonephritis and, 514
Renal pelvis
obstruction at, 469f, 472, 510–511
pyelonephritis, 513
stone in, 507–508
tumours, 515–516
Renal replacement therapy, 488–494, 490f
AKI, 483
chronic renal failure, 488–494
critically ill patients, 197–198, 197b
older people, 491b
preparation for, 489
see also specific types
Renal tract
obstruction, 483
see also specific areas
Renal transplantation *see* Kidney, transplantation
Renal tubular acidosis (RTA), 446, 446b
Renal tubules, 464–466, 465f
acute necrosis *see* Acute tubular necrosis
collecting ducts, 432, 464–466
distal, 431–432
isolated defects, 510
loop of Henle, 431, 464–466
proximal, 430–431
Renin, 432, 772
activity, venous blood, 1309b
hyperaldosteronism *see* Hyperaldosteronism
Renin-angiotensin-aldosterone system, 432, 432f
in hypertension, 608
hypokalaemia, 440–441
stimulation of, 547
Repaglinide, 216, 823
Repeated dose regimens, 23, 23f
Reperfusion therapy, myocardial infarction, 594–596
Replicative immortality, 264
Reproductive diseases
classification, 758b
presenting problems, 758–764
see also specific conditions
Reproductive system, 756–766
female, 757, 757f
male, 756f, 757
older people, 766b
Research ethics, 10
Residual volume (RV), 653b
Resins
bile acid sequestering, 434
ion-exchange, 442–443, 443b
Resistance, vascular *see* Vascular resistance
Resistin, 115–116
Respect for persons and autonomy, 10–11
Respiration
Cheyne-Stokes, 544
haemodynamic effects, 532, 532b
Kussmaul, 484
see also Breathing
Respiratory acidosis, 445b, 447
Respiratory alkalosis, 445b, 447
respiratory bronchiolitis-interstitial lung disease (RB-ILD), 708b
Respiratory burst, 73
Respiratory chain complexes, 46b
Respiratory disease, 643–732
air travel and, 108
chest pain, 658
common infecting organisms, 688b
drug-induced, 714, 714b
HIV-related, 400–401
investigations, 649–654
physical signs, 644–646
presenting problems, 654–666
tumours, 699–706
Respiratory distress syndrome, acute *see* Acute respiratory distress syndrome
Respiratory failure, 663–666
assessment, 192b
blood gases in, 664b
critically ill patients, 191–197, 192b
home ventilation, 665
management, 664
pathophysiology, 663–664
type I, 651–652, 664
type II, 664–666, 664b
Respiratory function
monitoring, critically ill patients, 187–188
older people, 648b
tests, 652–654, 653b, 653f
Respiratory infections, 681–699
asthma and, 667
bacterial, 345–347
cystic fibrosis, 681
fungal, 697–699
HIV-related, 400–401
older people, 686b
pneumonia, 682–688
rheumatoid disease, 712
SARS, 310b, 682–683
stroke patients, 1243b
upper respiratory tract, 681–682
viral, 328
Respiratory rate, 195b
Respiratory support
critically ill patients, 193–197
non-invasive, 193–194, 193f
weaning from, 183, 194
Respiratory syncytial virus (RSV), 146f, 328
Respiratory system
applied anatomy and physiology, 646–649, 646f
clinical examination, 644–646
common infecting organisms, 688b
infections *see* Respiratory infections
older people, 648b
tumours, 699–706
Restless legs syndrome, 485–486, 1187–1188, 1188b
Restraint, disturbed patients, 238
Restriction fragment length polymorphisms (RFPLs), 693
Resuscitation
allergic reaction, 90
cardiopulmonary, 204b
critically ill patient, 188–189
drowning, 108
fluid, 185, 189, 331–332, 1011b
gastrointestinal haemorrhage, 855
hypothermia, 105
poisoning, 208
Resynchronisation therapy, cardiac, 553
RET proto-oncogene, 795
Reteplase (rPA), 595
Reticular formation, brainstem, 1144f
Reticulin, 530–531, 1048–1049
Reticulocytes, 993f
reference values, 1312b
Reticulocytosis, 994
Retina
degeneration, 1194b
detachment, 828, 1170
microaneurysms, 609
visual field loss, 1170b
Retinal haemorrhage
high-altitude, 107
hypertension, 609, 609f
see also Diabetic retinopathy
Retinal pigment epithelium, congenital hypertrophy, 911–912, 911b
Retinitis
cytomegalovirus, 388f
HIV-related, 404
Retinitis pigmentosa, 886, 1199b
Retinoblastoma, 66–67, 267b
Retinochoroiditis, toxoplasmosis, 361f
all-trans-Retinoic acid, 1266
13-cis-Retinoic acid (isotretinoin), 37b, 1267
Retinoids, 126, 1267
acne vulgaris, 1282
adverse reactions, 1267
skin reactions, 1304b
and hyperlipidaemia, 455
in pregnancy, 37b
psoriasis, 1289b
psoriatic arthritis, 1109
retinol *see* Vitamin A
warts, 1278–1279
Retinopathy
cancer-related, 272
diabetic, 799f, 828–830, 828b, 829f
pregnancy and, 818
hypertensive, 609, 609b, 609f
Retroperitoneal fibrosis, 511
drug-induced, 522b
Retroviruses, 134–135, 328–329
and leukaemia, 1035b
see also HIV infection/AIDS
Reverse transcriptase inhibitors
non-nucleoside, 407–409, 407b
nucleoside, 392f, 407b, 408–409
Reverse transcriptase (RT), 162, 391
Reversibility test, 668f
Reye's syndrome, 319–320
RF *see* Rheumatoid factor
RFPLs *see* Restriction fragment length polymorphisms
Rhabdomyolysis, 106, 442, 456
Rhabdoviruses, 1206
Rhesus D blood group, 1014, 1014b
Rheumatic fever, 614–616, 614f
chemoprophylaxis, 153b, 615–616
investigations, 615b
Jones criteria, 614b, 614f
respiratory complications, 712b
Rheumatic heart disease, 614–616
chronic, 616
Rheumatoid arthritis (RA), 1096–1103
clinical features, 1097–1100, 1098f–1099f
cardiopulmonary involvement, 1099
cutaneous and vascular, 1098–1099
erosions, 1097f
extra-articular, 1098–1100, 1098b
neurological complications, 1099, 1099f
ocular involvement, 1099
connective tissue disorders, 712b
diagnostic criteria, 1097b
HLA associations, 1096
investigations, 1100, 1100b, 1100f
management, 1100–1103
biological therapy, 1102–1103
corticosteroids, 1102
DMARDs, 1102
surgery, 1103
older people, 1097–1098
pathophysiology, 1096–1097, 1097f
polymyalgia, 1097–1098
pregnancy, 1101b
prevalence, 1060b, 1096
Rheumatoid disease
HIV-related, 404
pleural effusion, 662b
respiratory involvement, 662b, 712, 712f
Rheumatoid factor (RF), 1067, 1067b
Rheumatoid nodules
lung, 712, 712f
subcutaneous, 1097
Rheumatology *see* Musculoskeletal disease
Rhinitis, allergic (vasomotor), 725
Rhinocladiella mackenziei, 382–383
Rhinosinusitis, 682
Rhinoviruses, 328
Rhizomucor spp., 384

Rhizopus spp., 384
Rhodesiense trypanosomiasis, 359
Rhodococcus equi, 401
Rhodopsin, 49
Rib fractures, 730b
Ribavirin
  hepatitis C, 161b, 162, 955
  Lassa fever, 325, 325b
  viral haemorrhagic fevers, 325
  viral hepatitis, 955
    HIV/AIDS patients, 400
Riboflavin (vitamin B_2), 128
  biochemical assessment of status, 126b
  deficiency, 128
  dietary sources, 125b
  RNI, 125b
Ribonuclear protein, antibodies to, 1067–1068
Ribonucleic acid *see* RNA
Ribosomes, 43f
Ribozymes, 295
Richmond Agitation Sedation Scale (RASS), 202b
Richter's transformation, 1040–1041
Rickets, 127, 1125–1128
  biochemical abnormalities, 1066b
  causes, 1126b
  hypophosphataemic, 1066b, 1128
  renal, 1128
  vitamin D-resistant, 1128
Rickettsial fevers, 350–352, 351b
Rickety rosary, 1126–1127
Riedel's thyroiditis, 755
Rifampicin, 151b
  adverse reactions, 694, 694b
  bartonellosis, 352–353
  brucellosis, 334b
  Buruli ulcer, 333
  dark urine, 475b, 694
  drug interactions, 28
  endocarditis, 628, 628b
  hepatotoxicity, 36b, 971b
  HIV/AIDS patients
  infective endocarditis, 628
  leprosy, 349b, 350
  meningitis, 1204b
  nocardiosis, 341
  pneumonia, 685b
  primary biliary cirrhosis, 964
  prophylactic, 153b
  pruritus, 964
  Q fever, 352
  resistance, 151–152, 693
  rickettsial fevers, 352
  tuberculosis, 693, 694b
Rifamycin, mechanism of action, 150b
Rifaximin, 909, 942
RIFLE criteria, 481b
Rift Valley fever, 325b
Right atrial pressure (RAP), critically ill patients, 179
Right bundle branch block (RBBB), 533b, 560b, 571, 573, 573f
  atrial septal defect, 633
  causes, 573b
Right coronary artery (RCA), 529, 529f
  bypass graft, 588f
  occlusion, 595f
Right ventricle, 528f, 630f
Right ventricular cardiomyopathy, arrhythmogenic, 637f, 638
Right ventricular dilatation, 535, 624, 624b
Rigidity
  cog wheel, 1145
  lead pipe, 1145
  Parkinson's disease, 1196b
  tetanus, 1210
Rigors, 295–296
Riluzole, amyotrophic lateral sclerosis, 1201b
Rimantadine, 161b, 162
Rimonabant, 119
Ringer-lactate, 344–345
Ringworm, 1279
Risedronate
  osteoporosis, 1123, 1123b
  Paget's disease, 1129, 1130b
Risk
  attributable, 99b
  cause and effect, 99
  estimation and communication, 7, 7f
  relative, 99b
  susceptibility to, 102b
Risk measurement, 99
  descriptive epidemiology, 99b
  genetic diseases, 68f
Risperidone
  bipolar disorder, 245
  schizophrenia, 249b
Risus sardonicus, 1210
Ritonavir, 153b
Rituximab, 278
  ANCA-associated vasculitis, 520b, 1118
  chronic lymphocytic leukaemia, 1041b
  rheumatoid arthritis, 1103, 1103b
Rivaroxaban, indications, 567, 1018b
Rivastigmine
  Alzheimer's disease, 252
  Parkinson-associated dementia, 1196
River blindness (onchocerciasis), 374–375
RNA
  degradation, 43–44
  editing, 43–44
  messenger (mRNA), 42
  microRNA (miRNA), 43–44
  mtRNA, 45–46
  ncRNA, 43–44
  ribosomal (rRNA), 43–44
  splicing, 43–44
  synthesis, 43f
  transfer (tRNA), 43–45
RNA polymerase II, 42
RNI *see* Reference nutrient intake
Robertsonian translocations, 57f
Rocky Mountain spotted fever, 350, 351b
Rodent ulcer, 1270
Rodenticide poisoning, 224b
Roflumethiazide, 611
Rokitansky–Aschoff sinuses, 988
Romaña's sign, 360
Romberg test, 1138f
Ropinirole, Parkinson's disease, 1197b
Rosacea, 1260b, 1283, 1283f
Roseola infantum, 316
Rosiglitazone, 823, 1121
Ross River virus, 329, 1095
Rotator cuff lesions, 1074–1075, 1074b
Rotavirus, 327–328
Rotigotine, Parkinson's disease, 1197b
Rotor's syndrome, 937b
Roundworm (*Ascaris lumbricoides*), 312b, 371
Roux-en-Y gastric bypass, 119b
rPA *see* Reteplase
RPGN *see* Rapidly progressive glomerulonephritis
RPR *see* Rapid plasma reagin test
RSV *see* Respiratory syncytial virus
RT *see* Reverse transcriptase
rt-PA *see* Recombinant tissue plasminogen activator
RTA *see* Renal tubular acidosis
Rubber allergy, 1284–1285
Rubella (German measles), 315
  arthritis, 1095
  congenital malformations and, 315b
  immunisation, 315
  incubation period, 145b, 310b, 315
  maternal infection, 314b
  period of infectivity, 144b, 315
Rubeosis iridis, 828
'Rum fits', 253
Russell's sign, 256
Ruxolitinib, 1049
RV *see* Residual volume
Ryanodine receptor channelopathies, 1230b

S

SA node *see* Sinoatrial node
Sabin-Feldman dye test, 361–362
Saccades, 1171
Sacroiliitis
  and ankylosing spondylitis, 1105–1106, 1106b
  in brucellosis, 334f
  and inflammatory bowel disease, 902f
  inflammatory joint disease, 1107f
  pain, 1070f
St John's wort, drug interactions, 28b
St Vitus dance, 615
Salbutamol
  COPD, 21–22, 675
  dosage regimen, 35b
  drug interactions, 28b
  hyperkalaemia, 443b
  palliative care, 289
  scombrotoxic fish poisoning, 308
Salicylate
  plasma concentration, 213
  poisoning, 209b, 212–213
  skin reactions, 1304b
Salicylic acid
  molluscum contagiosum, 1279
  warts, 1278b
Saline
  composition, 433b
  gastroenteritis, 307
  heat cramps, 106
  hypercalcaemia, 273
  hyperkalaemia, 443b
  hypernatraemia, 439
  hyperphosphataemia, 449
  hypertonic, 652
  hypovolaemia, 433b
  isotonic, 814
Salivary glands
  diseases of, 863–864
  enlargement, 864b
Salmeterol
  asthma, 670–671
  COPD, 675
Salmonella
  food poisoning/gastroenteritis, 342, 342b
  HIV/AIDS patients, 406
Salmonella enteritidis, 342
Salmonella paratyphi, 339
Salmonella typhi, 151b, 339
Salmonella typhimurium, 342
Salmonellosis, 309b
Salt *see* Sodium
Salt-losing nephropathy, 504, 859f
Salt-wasting disease, 782
Sand fleas, 381
Sandflies, 309b
  bartonellosis, 352b
  leishmaniasis, 362
Sandhoff's disease, 451b
Sanfilippo's syndrome, 433–434
Saphenous vein grafts, 588
SAPS *see* Simplified Acute Physiology Score
SARA *see* Sexually acquired reactive arthropathy
Sarcoidosis
  lung, 709–711, 710f
  management, 711, 711b
  musculoskeletal manifestations, 1132
  presentation, 710b
  skin lesions, 1301
  systemic involvement, 710f
Sarcoma
  Ewing's, 1131b
  osteogenic, 66–67
  see also Kaposi's sarcoma
Sarcomere, cardiac, 530
Sarcoptes scabiei, 1280
SARS *see* Severe acute respiratory syndrome
Sausage digit, 1109f
Saxagliptin, 824
Saxitoxin, 308
Saxophone player's lung, 719b
SBP *see* Spontaneous bacterial peritonitis
Scabies, 1280–1281, 1280f
  HIV/AIDS, 397b
  Norwegian, 1280–1281
  pruritus, 1280
Scaling, 1251b
Scalp
  fungal infections, 1280
  head lice, 1281
  psoriasis, 1288
  ringworm, 1279
  tinea capitis, 1280
Scapula, winging, 1138f
Scarlet fever
  incubation period, 145b, 310b
  period of infectivity, 144b
  streptococcal, 331, 332f
Scars, definition, 1251b
Scedosporium apiospermum, 382
SCF *see* Stem cell factor
Schatzki ring, 870
Scheuermann's osteochondritis, 1130–1131
Schilling test, 1025
Schirmer tear test, 1114
Schistosoma, 376f
Schistosoma haematobium, 376–377, 377b, 378f
Schistosoma intercalatum, 376–378
Schistosoma japonicum, 376–378, 377b
Schistosoma mansoni, 376–377, 377b
Schistosoma mekongi, 376–378
Schistosomiasis, 309b, 312b, 376–378
  geographical distribution, 377f
  incubation period, 310b
  pathology, 377b
Schizoaffective disorder, 245
Schizophrenia, 247–249
  acute, 247
  aetiology, 247–249
  diagnosis, 245, 247–248
  differential diagnosis, 248, 248b
  genetic factors, 232–233
  management, 241b, 248–249
  prognosis, 249
  Schmidt's syndrome, 796, 796b
  sibling risk, 68b
  symptoms, 248b
    auditory hallucinations, 237
    thought disorder, 234
Schmidt's syndrome, 796, 796b
Schumm's test, 1026–1027
Schwann cells, 1140–1141
Sciatica, 1219
Scintigraphy
  meta-iodobenzyl guanidine, 781
  musculoskeletal disease, 1065
  neuro-endocrine tumours, 785f
  thyroid, 746
  see also Radionuclide (radioisotope) imaging
SCLE *see* Subacute cutaneous lupus erythematosus
Scleritis, rheumatoid arthritis, 1099
Sclerodactyly, 1112
Scleroderma *see* Systemic sclerosis
Scleromalacia, rheumatoid arthritis, 1099

Sclerosing bone dysplasia, 1131
Sclerosing cholangitis
  liver function tests, 930b
  primary, 965–966, 966f, 980b
    diseases associated with, 965b
  secondary, 965, 965b
Sclerosis, systemic *see* Systemic sclerosis
Sclerosteosis, 1131
Sclerostin, 1062b
Sclerotherapy, variceal bleeding, 928
Sclerotic bodies, 381–383
Scombrotoxic fish poisoning, 308
Scorpion stings, 227b, 229b
Scotoma, 1170b, 1172b
Screening, 6–7
  aortic aneurysms, 605b
  cancer
    breast cancer, 271b, 279
    cervical cancer, 281
    colorectal, 916
    prostate cancer, 518
  chronic liver disease, 928, 929b
  ciliary dysfunction syndrome, 679
  cost-effectiveness, 7b
  cystic fibrosis, 58b, 680–681
  cystic kidney disease, 506
  diabetes, 807
  diabetic nephropathy, 831, 831b
  diabetic retinopathy, 829
  Down's syndrome (trisomy 21), 63b
  genetic, 64
  hepatocellular carcinoma, 968
  microalbuminuria, 831b
  poisoning, 209b
Scrub typhus, 350–351, 351b
Scurvy, 129, 130b, 1050
Sebaceous glands, 1253–1254
Sebocytes, 1253–1254
Seborrhoeic eczema/dermatitis, 1284
  HIV/AIDS, 397
  management, 1286
Seborrhoeic warts, 1274, 1274f
Sebum, 1253–1254
  acne vulgaris, 1281
Secretin, 846b
Sedation
  aggressive behaviour, 237–238
  critically ill patients, 202–203, 202b
  older people, 174–175
Sedative misuse, 217b, 254–255, 254b
Sedatives, effect of old age, 36b
75SeHCAT test, 851b
Seizures, 1159
  alcohol withdrawal, 20b
  brain tumour, 1213
  cocaine-induced, 217b
  distinction from syncope, 1158b
  epilepsy *see* Epilepsy
  malaria, 357b
  poisoning, 211b
  stroke patients, 1237
Selectins, 531–532
Selective noradrenaline reuptake inhibitors (SNRIs), poisoning, 214
Selective oestrogen receptor modulators (SERMs), 1124–1125
Selective serotonin re-uptake inhibitors (SSRIs), 244, 244b
  poisoning, 214
  withdrawal symptoms, 20b
Selectivity, 18
Selegiline, Parkinson's disease, 1197
Selenium, 132, 738
  deficiency, 132
  dietary sources, 131b
  excess, 132
  Graves' ophthalmopathy, 751b
  RNI, 131b
Selenium sulphide shampoo, 397
Selenosis, 130
Self-harm (SH), 238–240
  older people, 238b
  patient assessment, 239b, 239f
  see also Drugs, overdose/poisoning
Sellar tumours, 789
Seminoma, 270b
Senescence *see* Age/ageing; Older people
Sengstaken-Blakemore tube, 928, 947f
Senna, 475b, 917b
Sensorimotor polyneuropathy, 1194b
Sensory ataxia, 1209b
Sensory disturbances, 1164–1165, 1164f
  diabetes *see* Diabetic neuropathy
Sensory neuropathy, 1194b
Sensory system examination, 1138f
Sentinel lymph node biopsy, 1274
Sentinel pile, 919
Sepsis, 83, 190, 200–201, 304–305
  AKI, 479f, 480b, 483
  causes, 304b
  definition, 184b
  hyperdynamic, 183
  management, 201, 201b
  meningococcal, 295f, 1203b
  musculoskeletal disease
    see also individual conditions
  neutropenic, 274
  renal transplant patients, 493
  risk factors, 200b
Sepsis syndrome, 548
Septic arthritis, 1094–1095
  emergency management, 1095b
  synovial fluid analysis, 1094
Septic shock, 83
  circulatory effects, 185
  definition, 184b
  treatment/management, 201
Septicaemia, meningococcal, 1203b
Septicaemic plague, 338
Sequestration crisis, 1032
SERMs *see* Selective oestrogen receptor modulators
Seroconversion, 141
Serology, 141
  AKI, 480b
  eosinophilia, 312b
  gastrointestinal infection, 850
  Helicobacter pylori infection, 850
  pyrexia of unknown origin, 299b, 310b
  respiratory disease, 652
  viral hepatitis, 950–952
Seronegative spondarthritis, 1060b
Serotonin (5-hydroxytryptamine, 5-HT), 289f, 755
  excess in irritable bowel syndrome, 907
Serotonin agonists, irritable bowel syndrome, 907
Serotonin selective (specific) re-uptake inhibitors (SSRIs), 214, 244
  adverse reactions, 176b
  overdose, 214
Serotonin syndrome, 213b, 244
Serotonin-noradrenaline reuptake inhibitors (SNRIs), 241b, 244b
Serratia spp., 136f
Serratia marscescens
Sertraline, 244b
Serum sickness, 88b
  antivenins, 230
  diphtheria antitoxin, 346
  schistosomiasis, 377b
Severe acute respiratory syndrome (SARS), 682–683
  incubation period, 310b
Severe combined immune deficiency, 80
Sex chromosomes, 42
  abnormalities, 50–51
  see also X chromosome; Y chromosome
Sex hormone replacement therapy *see* Hormone replacement therapy
Sex hormones, *see individual hormones*
Sexual activity, and headache, 1178
Sexual dysfunction, 1174–1175
  diabetics, 833
  see also Erectile dysfunction
Sexually acquired reactive arthropathy (SARA), 423
Sexually transmitted infections (STIs), 411–426
  approach to patients, 414–415, 414b
  bacterial, 419–423
  children, 414–415
  clinical examination
    men, 413–414
    women, 412
  contact tracing (partner notification), 419
  HIV testing, 412
  investigations
    men, 412b
    women, 413b
  management goals, 413b
  men who have sex with men, 412b, 417
  in pregnancy, 414, 414b
  presenting problems
    men, 415–417, 415f
    women, 417–419
  prevention, 419
  those at particular risk, 413b
  viral, 423–426
  see also specific STIs
Sézary syndrome, 1264
SGLT2 inhibitors, 822b, 824
SH *see* Standard heparin
SH (self-harm) *see* Self-harm
Shagreen patches, 1302
Shampoo
  ketoconazole, 1280
  selenium sulphide, 397
Sheehan's syndrome, 787b, 789
Shellfish toxin, paralytic, 308
Sheltered accommodation, 249
Sheltered employment, 249
Shigella
  diarrhoea, 306, 399
  dysentery/shigellosis, 345
    reactive arthritis and, 345
Shingles *see* Herpes zoster
Shivering, 103b, 104f
Shock, 190–191
  anaphylactic, 190
  assessment and complications, 190
  cardiogenic, 190
  clinical features, 181b
  dengue shock syndrome, 322
  early, 191
  hypovolaemic, 190
  late, 191
  malaria, 357b
  management, 190–191, 191b
  neurogenic, 190
  obstructive, 190
  septic *see* Septic shock
  toxic shock syndrome, 295f, 331–332, 331f
'Shock' liver, 198
Short bowel syndrome, 884–885, 884b–885b
Short stature
  Turner's syndrome, 754b, 766
  see also Dwarfism; Growth retardation
Shoulder
  frozen (capsulitis), 1074–1075
  pain, 1074–1075, 1074b, 1074f
    stroke patients, 1243b
  tendinitis, 1074b, 1074f
Shrinking lungs, 712, 712b
Shuffling gait, 172b, 1168
Shunts
  arteriovenous, 548, 631
  Blalock-Taussig, 635
  intracardiac, 539, 560
  left-to-right, 535–536, 561–562, 597, 631
  peritoneo-venous, 940
  persistent ductus arteriosus, 631, 631f
  portosystemic, 928
  reversed, 632
  right-to-left, 631
  TIPSS, 931, 940, 947f–948f
SI units, 1308
SIADH *see* Syndrome of inappropriate secretion of ADH
Siberian tick typhus, 351b
Sibutramine, 119
Sick euthyroidism, 746
Sick sinus syndrome, 563–564, 563b, 563f, 575b
Sickle chest syndrome, 1032
Sickle-cell anaemia/disease, 1032–1034, 1033f
  inheritance, 1032
  nephropathy, 505
Sickle-cell trait, 1032
Siderosis, 717b, 718
Sieverts (Sv), 103
Sigmoidoscopy, 848
  amoebiasis, 368
  Clostridium difficile infection, 344
  colorectal cancer, 916
  familial adenomatous polyposis, 912
  inflammatory bowel disease, 899b
  irritable bowel syndrome, 908
  schistosomiasis, 378
Sildenafil, 474, 725
Silicosis, 717, 717b, 717f
Silicotuberculosis, 717
Simplified Acute Physiology Score (SAPS), 204
Simulium spp., onchocerciasis, 374
SIMV *see* Synchronised intermittent mandatory ventilation
Simvastatin
  chronic renal disease, 488b
  dosage interval, 35b
  drug history, 26b
  effect of hepatic impairment
  prescribing, 38b
  stroke prevention, 1245f
Sindbis virus, 329
Sinemet, 1196
Single nucleotide polymorphisms (SNPs; snips), 63
Single photon emission tomography (SPECT), 1149
Sinoatrial disease, 563–564, 563b, 563f, 575b
Sinoatrial (SA) node, 529–530, 529f
  rhythms, 563–564
Sinus, definition, 1251b
Sinus bradycardia, 563, 563b
  ECG, 563f
  myocardial infarction, 590–591
Sinus rhythms, 563
Sinus tachycardia, 563, 563b
Sinusitis, 682
Sipple's syndrome, 795b
SIRS (systemic inflammatory response syndrome), 190, 304
  definition, 184b
  pancreatitis, 891b
Sister Joseph's nodule, 280
Sitagliptin, 824

Sitosterolaemia, 455–456, 456b
Situation ethics, 10
Sixth disease, 316
Sjögren's syndrome, 84b, 1114, 1114b
  secondary, 1099
Skeletal muscle, 1063–1064
Skin
  anatomy and physiology, 1252–1254
  antisepsis, 147b
  biopsy, 1255, 1268
  blood supply, 1254
  cancer manifestations, 267b, 272
  changes in older people, 1254b
  epidermal appendages, 1252–1254
  examination
    cancer, 261b
    diabetes, 798–800
    endocrine disease, 734f
    gastrointestinal disease, 838f
    infectious disease, 295f
    renal/urinary tract disease, 462f–463f
  functions, 1254, 1254b
  infestations, 1275–1281
  microbiology, 1255
  nerves, 1254
  rheumatic fever, 614f
  in systemic disease, 1299b
  temperature, critically ill patients, 187
  tumours, malignant *see* Skin cancer
Skin cancer, 1269–1275
  changing mole and, 1274–1275
  non-melanoma, 1266, 1270–1274, 1270b
  pathogenesis, 1269–1270
  see also names of specific tumours
Skin diseases/disorders, 1249–1305
  acute skin failure, 1264
  clinical examination, 1250–1252, 1251b
  colour abnormalities, 1263
  diagnosis/investigations, 1254–1256
  in general medicine, 1299–1305
  genetic *see specific disorders*
  HIV-related, 396–398
  infections *see* Skin infections
  leishmaniasis
    cutaneous, 365–366, 366b, 366f
    post-kala-azar, 365, 365f
  leprosy, 347–350
  presenting problems, 1256–1264
  SLE, 1110
  systemic sclerosis, 1112–1113
  terminology, 1251b
  treatment
    surgical, 1268
    systemic, 1267–1268
    topical, 1264–1266, 1265b
  tropical diseases, 304b, 312–313, 313b
  tumours *see* Skin cancer
Skin grafts, vitiligo, 1295
Skin infections, 295b, 305, 1275–1281
  bacterial, 1275–1278
  diabetes, 809, 833
  fungal, 1279–1280
  tropics, 312–313, 313b, 313f
  viral, 1278–1279
Skin snips, 312b
Skin tags, 1275
Skin tests
  asthma, 669
  patch tests, 1255, 1285
  prick tests, 90
  respiratory disease, 652
    tuberculosis, 695, 695b, 695f
Skinfold thickness, 115
Slapped cheek syndrome, 315–316, 316f
SLE *see* Systemic lupus erythematosus
Sleep, 1148
Sleep apnoea/hypopnoea syndrome, 726–727, 726f
Sleep disorders, 1187–1188
Sleep disturbance, 1175
  fibromyalgia, 1092
Sleep paralysis, 1175
Sleepiness
  Epworth scale, 726b, 1187
  persistent, differential diagnosis, 727b
  see also Somnolence
Sleeping sickness (African trypanosomiasis), 309b, 358–360, 359f
Sleeve gastrectomy, 119b
Small interfering RNA (siRNA), 31b
Small intestine
  bacterial overgrowth, 882–883, 882b
  biopsy, coeliac disease, 881, 881f
  chronic pseudo-obstruction, 886, 886b
  Crohn's disease *see* Crohn's disease
  diseases/disorders, 880–889
    coeliac disease *see* Coeliac disease
    vitamin B_{12} deficiency *see* Vitamin B_{12}, deficiency
  functional anatomy, 841–844, 841f
  immunoproliferative disease, 889
  infections, 888
  ischaemia, 909–910
  motility disorders, 886
  obstruction, 862
  older people, 883b
  protective function, 843–844, 844f
  radiation enteritis, 885–886, 885b
  resection, 884–885
  transplantation, 885
  tumours, 888–889
  ulceration, 887, 887b
Small-vessel vasculitis, 496
Smallpox, 327
Smell, disturbance of, 1169
Smith–Magenis syndrome, genetics, 56b
Smoking
  atherosclerotic vascular disease, 581
  and autoimmune disease, 87
  and bone mineral density, 1120
  and cardiovascular risk, 582f
  cessation, 101b
  cocaine, 218
  COPD, 675b, 676f
  effects on health, 100–101
  Graves' disease and, 748
  and idiopathic pulmonary fibrosis, 708b
  lung cancer and, 266b, 267
  myocardial infarction, management, 598
  older people, 169, 527b
  passive, 98f, 100
  peptic ulcers and, 873
  pharmacokinetics and, 24b
  rheumatoid arthritis and, 1096
Snail track ulcers, 419–420
Snake bites, 225–226, 225b, 227b–229b
Snoring, 726
SNPs *see* Single-nucleotide polymorphisms
Social factors
  atherosclerotic disease, 581
  psychiatric disorders, 233
Social isolation, 233
Social worker, 2b
Sodium, 132
  channelopathies, 1230b
  daily requirements, 433b
  depletion, 432–434, 433b
  diabetic diet, 821
  dietary sources, 131b
  disorders of, 429b–430b, 430–436
    presenting problems, 432–434
  excess/retention, 434, 434b, 435f
    drugs and, 940b
    renal retention, 476
  intake, chronic renal failure, 488
  reabsorption, 464
  refeeding diet, 122b
  reference values
    urine, 1311b
    venous blood, 1308b
  renal handling, 430–432, 430f
  renal retention, 477b
  restriction, ascites, 940
  retention, 940b
  RNI, 131b
  transport regulation, 432, 432f
  see also Hypernatraemia; Hyponatremia
Sodium aurothiomalate (gold), 1102
Sodium bicarbonate
  diabetic ketoacidosis, 812
  drug interactions, 28b
  renal failure
    AKI, 482b
    chronic, 488
  salicylate poisoning, 213
  urinary alkalinisation, 210
Sodium calcium edetate, 224b
Sodium chloride
  dietary, 132
  see also Saline
Sodium cromoglicate, 90
  allergic rhinitis, 725
  eosinophilic gastroenteritis, 887
  food allergy, 888
Sodium ipodate, 742–743
Sodium nitroprusside
  aortic dissection, 607
  hypertension, 612
  phaeochromocytoma, 782
Sodium phosphate, 448–449
Sodium stibogluconate, 164, 364
Sodium valproate, 241b
  bipolar disorder, 245
  epilepsy, 1182b, 1184b
    in pregnancy, 1185b
  hepatotoxicity, 978b
  migraine prevention, 1177
  and neutropenia, 1005b
  poisoning, 209b, 224b
  sodium retention, 940b
  status epilepticus, 1159b
Sodium-potassium pump *see* Na,K-activated ATPase
Soft tissue infections, 305
  bacterial, 332b
  clostridial, 305
  necrotising, 305, 305b, 305f
Soft tissue release, 1080b
Solar urticaria, 1260b
Solitary rectal ulcer syndrome, 919
Solvent inhalation, 254
Somatic disorders, medically unexplained *see* Somatic symptoms
Somatic mutations, 59
Somatic symptoms, medically unexplained, 236, 236b, 236f, 238b
Somatic syndromes, functional, 236, 236b
Somatisation disorder, 236b, 245
Somatoform autonomic dysfunction, 246
Somatoform disorders, 245–247
  prevalence, 232b
Somatoform pain disorder, 246
Somatosensory system, 1146–1148, 1147f
Somatostatin, 841, 846b
Somatostatin analogues
  acromegaly, 793
  see also specific drugs
Somatostatin receptor scan (SRS), 851b
Somatostatinomas, 785b
Somnolence
  daytime, 726
  idiopathic hypersomnolence, 727
Sorafenib, 968–969
Sorbitol, 888
Sotalol, 575b
  arrhythmias, 576
South American botfly, 381
Space of Disse, 925
Space-occupying lesions, 402–403
Sparganosis, 381
Spastic catch, 1145
Spastic paraplegia, hereditary, 1222b
Spasticity, 1145
Specialist nurse, 2b
SPECT *see* Single photon emission tomography
Spectinomycin, 151b, 159, 422b
Spectrin, 994f, 1028
Spectrophotometry, 428b
Spectroscopy, mass, 428b
Speech and language therapist, 2b
Speech therapy in Parkinson's disease, 1198
Speech/speech disorders, 1146, 1146f, 1168–1169, 1169f
  assessment, psychiatric interview, 233
  stroke, 1236
Spermatogenesis, 756f
Spherocytes, 994, 999f
Spherocytosis, hereditary, 1028
Sphincter of Oddi, 926
  dysfunction, 987, 987b
Sphincterotomy
  biliary, 848f, 985
  endoscopic, 983b, 987, 988b
  pancreatic, 987
Sphincters
  anal, 473, 845f
  bladder, 272, 466
  control, 1148
  neurological deficit, 272b
  urethral, 136–137, 473
Sphygmomanometry, 608
Spider bites, 228b
Spider naevi, 922f, 962, 975–976
Spider telangiectasia, 943
Spina bifida, 1222b
Spinal cord, 1144
  compression, 1220–1222, 1220b–1221b
    cancer patients, 272
    cauda equina syndrome, 1073b
    cervical, 1218f, 1221f
    lumbar, 1155–1175, 1219b
    thoracic, 1221b
  degeneration, vitamin B_{12} deficiency and, 1024b
  disorders, 1218–1222
    intrinsic, 1222, 1222b
  lesions
    bladder dysfunction, 1156b, 1175b
    sensory loss, 1164f, 1165
  tumours, 1220b
Spinal epidural abscess, 1209
Spinal muscular atrophies, 1201
  inheritance, 58b
Spinal muscular atrophy, 1201
Spinal root lesions *see* Radiculopathy
Spinal stenosis, 1220
Spine
  bamboo, 1105–1106, 1107f
  cervical
    disorders, 1218–1219
    epidural abscess, 1209
    imaging, 1150, 1151f
    spondylosis, 1218–1219
    spondylotic myelopathy, 1219

spondylotic radiculopathy, 1218–1219
subluxation, 1099, 1099f
lumbar
disorders, 1219–1220
imaging, 1150, 1151f
see also Lumbar
osteoarthritis, 1084
thoracic, imaging, 1150, 1151f
tuberculosis, 693
Spinobulbar muscular atrophy, 56b
Spinocerebellar ataxia, 65, 1199b
genetics, 56b
Spiramycin, toxoplasmosis, 362
Spirillum minus, 313b
Spirometry
asthma, 668
COPD, 675b
Spironolactone, 765b
adverse reactions, gynaecomastia, 940
ascites, 940
heart failure, 551
mineralocorticoid excess, 781
Splanchnic ischaemia, 198
Splanchnic vasodilatation, 939
Spleen, 76
clinical examination, 991b
enlarged see Splenomegaly
see also Haematopoiesis
Splenectomy, 1028b
autoimmune haemolysis, 1030
chronic lymphocytic leukaemia, 1040
hereditary spherocytosis, 1028
myelofibrosis, 1049
thrombocytopenia, 1050
Splenomegaly, 1006
causes, 1006b
chronic myeloid leukaemia, 1039
portal hypertension, 945
primary biliary cirrhosis, 963–964
see also specific conditions
Splice site mutations, 55f
Splicing, 43–44, 43f
Splinter haemorrhage, 1070b, 1298
Splints, 1080
Spondarthritis, seronegative, 1060b
Spondylitis
ankylosing *see* Ankylosing spondylitis
inflammatory, 1105b
psoriatic, 1114
Spondyloarthropathies, seronegative, 1104–1109, 1105b
Spondylolisthesis, 1133
Spondylolysis, 1133
Spondylosis
cervical, 1218f
lumbar, 1219–1220
Spondylotic myelopathy, cervical, 1219
Spondylotic radiculopathy, cervical, 1218–1219
Spongiosis, 1283
Spontaneous bacterial peritonitis (SBP), 941, 941b
Sporadic fatal insomnia, 329b
Sporothrix schenckii, 383
Sporotrichosis, 383
Sporozoites, malaria, 354
Spreading depression of Leão, 1176–1177
Sputum, 644f
bronchial carcinoma, 703f
bronchiectasis, 678
cytology, 652
investigations, 652
pneumonia, 683
pulmonary oedema, 644f
Squamous cell carcinoma
oesophagus, 870b
skin, 1271, 1271f
SRS *see* Somatostatin receptor scan
SSPE *see* Subacute sclerosing panencephalitis
SSRIs *see* Serotonin selective (specific) re-uptake inhibitors
SSSS *see* Staphylococcal infections, scalded skin syndrome)
Stamping gait, 172b, 1168
Standard Early Warning System (SEWS), 181b
Standard heparin (SH), 1018–1019
Stannosis, 717b, 718
Staphylococcal infections
bone and joint, 329–331
endocarditis, 624b, 625
food poisoning, 341
pneumonia, 682–683
scalded skin syndrome, 1276, 1276f
skin, 329–331
soft tissue, 332b
toxic shock syndrome, 331, 331f
urinary tract, 512
see also specific infections
Staphylococcus aureus, 137f, 138b, 151b, 304b
acute leukaemia, 1001
bacterial meningitis, 1202b
cannula-related infection, 330f
cystic fibrosis, 681
eczema, 1284b
endocarditis, 625, 626b
folliculitis, 1276–1277
food poisoning, 306, 341
glycopeptide intermediate, 330–331
HIV/AIDS, 401
immunocompromised patients, 78b, 688b
impetigo, 1275
infections caused by, 330f
meningitis, 1202b
meticillin-resistant *see* MRSA
pneumonia
bacterial, 401
community-acquired, 682–683, 683b
hospital-acquired, 687
septic arthritis, 1094
skin and soft tissue infections, 329, 330f
vancomycin-resistant, 330–331
wound infections, 330, 330f
Staphylococcus caprae, 329
Staphylococcus epidermidis
endocarditis, 626
skin and soft tissue infections, 329
urinary tract infection, 512
Staphylococcus intermedius, 329
Staphylococcus lugdensis, 329
Staphylococcus saprophyticus, 329
Staphylococcus schleiferi, 329
Starches
dietary, 112, 113b
hydrolysis, 842
resistant, 113, 344–345
Starling's Law, 182, 530, 547f
Starvation, 120–121
infections associated with, 121b
Statins
acute limb ischaemia, 603
atherosclerotic disease prevention, 583b
diabetic dyslipidaemia, 811, 831b
dosage regimen, 35b
drug reactions, 1303b
hepatotoxicity, 971b
hyperlipidaemia, 434, 457b
familial, 455b
in older people, 458b
hypertension, 613
and myalgia, 1132b
myocardial infarction prevention, 39
NAFLD, 961
and peripheral neuropathy, 1077b
pharmacodynamics, 25b
renal artery stenosis, 495
stroke prevention, 1245b
Statistics, 7
reference ranges, 1307–1308
risk, 7b
Status epilepticus, 1159, 1159b, 1185
Stavudine (d4T), 396f, 403, 409f
Steady state, 23
Steatohepatitis, non-alcoholic (NASH), 960f, 961, 971b
Steatorrhoea
cystic fibrosis, 680
malabsorption, 964
pancreatitis, 892–893
small bowel disorders, 883, 885
Steatosis, 959–960, 971
Stellate cells, 845
hepatic fibrosis, 843f
pancreatic, 893f
Stem cell factor (SCF), 992–993
Stem cells
diabetes treatment, 826
haematopoietic *see* Haematopoietic stem cells
plasticity, 993–994
pluripotent, 69–70
therapeutic use, 31b
Stenotrophomonas maltophilia, 146f, 681
Stents/stenting
aortic dissection, 606f
bronchial carcinoma, 704
colorectal cancer, 915f
coronary artery, 496f
drug-eluting, 587–588
endobronchial, 704
oesophageal carcinoma, 871
pancreatic cancer, 895
pancreatitis, 894b
percutaneous coronary intervention, 587
renal artery, 470
renal artery stenosis, 495b
superior vena cava obstruction, 273
thrombosis, 590b
tracheal, 728
ureteric, 511
Stercobilin, 927
Stercobilinogen, 927
Steroids
anabolic, 970
synthesis of, 772f
see also Corticosteroids
Stevens–Johnson syndrome, 398
Stiff-person syndrome, 1194b
Still's disease
adult-onset, 1104
see also Juvenile idiopathic arthritis
Stimulant misuse, 217–218, 217b, 254
Stings
insect, 94
scorpion, 227b, 229b
see also Envenomation
STIs *see* Sexually transmitted infections
Stockings, compression, 556
Stokes-Adams attacks, 572
Stomach
diseases, 871–880
emptying, 850, 851b
defective, 866
erosions, 854f
functional anatomy, 840f
outlet obstruction, 875–876, 875b
surgery *see* Surgery, gastrointestinal
tumours/carcinoma, 877–880, 877f, 878b
after gastric resection, 846
incidence, 262f
ulcers, 872–876
watermelon, 1113
see also Gastric
Stomatitis
angular, 128, 838–840, 899–900
herpetic, 326f
Stones *see* Calculi (stones)
Stool cultures, 849
Storage disorders, 65
Stratum corneum, 1252
Strawberry gallbladder, 987–988
Strawberry tongue, 331, 332f
Streptococcal infections
bone and joint, 331–332, 332b
endocarditis, 626b
in pregnancy, 314b
rheumatic fever, 614–616, 614f
skin, 331–332, 332b
toxic shock syndrome, 295f, 331–332
urinary tract, 499b–500b
glomerulonephritis, 501
infection, 512
Streptococci, 136f
α-haemolytic, 136f
anaerobic, 300
β-haemolytic, 136f
group A, 305
group B, 314b
meningitis, 1202
Streptococcus agalactiae, 332b
Streptococcus anginosus, 137f
Streptococcus bovis, 332b
endocarditis, 303
Streptococcus constellatus, 137f
Streptococcus intermedius, 137f
Streptococcus lugdenensis, 626
Streptococcus milleri, 625
Streptococcus mitis, 332b
Streptococcus mutans, 332b
Streptococcus pneumoniae (pneumococcus), 137f, 151b, 304b, 332b, 346, 687
bacterial meningitis, 1202b, 1204b
endocarditis, 625
immunisation, 346
pneumonia, 401, 682, 682f
Streptococcus pyogenes, 137f, 151b, 332b
endocarditis, 625
pneumonia, 687
Streptococcus salivarius, 332b
Streptococcus sanguis, 332b
Streptococcus suis, bacterial meningitis, 1204b
Streptococcus viridans endocarditis, 625
Streptogramins, 159
mechanism of action, 150b
Streptokinase, Budd-Chiari syndrome, 976
Streptomyces, 382
Streptomycin
adverse reactions, 694b
Buruli ulcer, 333
infective endocarditis, 628b
nocardiosis, 341
plague, 338–339
tuberculosis, 693
HIV/AIDS patients
tularaemia, 340
Stress
acute reaction, 242
adjustment disorder, 242
atherosclerotic vascular disease and
diabetes and, 809, 812
oxidative, 893f, 958f, 960, 1028–1029
post-traumatic stress disorder, 242
psychiatric disorders and, 233, 242
Stress incontinence, 175, 473
Stress testing
echocardiography, 537, 554
exercise ECG, 529f, 534, 567f, 584f
Stressors, 233
Stretch reflex, 1144, 1174

Stria
corticosteroid-induced, 1265f
definition, 1251b
Strictures, endoscopic techniques for management *see* Endoscopy
Stridor
bronchial carcinoma, 701
connective tissue disorders, 712b
cough, 654, 654b
hypocalcaemia, 768
laryngeal obstruction, 728
tracheal obstruction, 657f, 728
String test, 369
Stroke, 1231–1247
anatomy and physiology, 1234–1235, 1234f–1235f
clinical assessment, 1232f–1233f, 1233b
clinical classification, 1234f
clinical features, 1232f, 1236–1237, 1239–1240, 1240b, 1241f
ataxia, 1237
coma, 1237
headache, 1237
seizure, 1237
speech disturbance, 1236
visual deficit, 1237
visuo-spatial dysfunction, 1237
weakness, 1236
completed, 1240
complications, 1243b
differential diagnosis, 1240b
HIV/AIDS patients, 403
investigations, 1235–1236, 1240–1242, 1240b, 1242b
blood tests, 1236
cardiovascular, 1236, 1242
lumbar puncture, 1236
neuroimaging, 1235–1236, 1235f, 1241–1242, 1242b
vascular imaging, 1235–1236, 1236f, 1242
management, 1242–1246, 1243b–1244b
aspirin, 1244
carotid endarterectomy/angioplasty, 1244–1246
coagulation abnormalities, 1244
heparin, 1244
supportive care, 1242–1244
thrombolysis, 1244
pathophysiology, 1237–1239
cerebral infarction, 1237–1239, 1238f
intracerebral haemorrhage, 1238f–1239f, 1239, 1239b
progressing (in evolution), 1240
risk factors, 1237b, 1241
atrial fibrillation, 567b
hypertension, 609–610
management, 1244
migraine, 1177
secondary prevention, 1245f
Stroke mimics, 1240b
Stroke units, 1243b
Stroke volume, 190, 530
Stroke work, ventricular, 183
Strongyloides hyperinfection syndrome, 370
Strongyloides stercoralis, 304b, 309b, 312b, 370
Strongyloidiasis, 312b, 370–371, 370b
Strontium ranelate, osteoporosis, 1123b, 1124
Struvite stones, 507
Subacromial bursitis, 1074b
Subacute cutaneous lupus erythematosus (SCLE), 1110
Subacute sclerosing panencephalitis (SSPE), 314, 1207
Subarachnoid haemorrhage, 1246–1247
clinical features, 1246
investigations, 1246, 1246f
management, 1246–1247
see also Stroke
Subcalcaneal bursitis, 1076
Subclavian steal, 602
Subcutaneous administration, 21
Subdural empyema, 1209
Subdural haematoma, 1218
Sublingual administration, 21
Substance misuse, 240, 240b, 254–255
see also Drug misuse
Substance P, 1079–1080, 1092–1093
Subungual melanoma, 1273
Succinate dehydrogenase, 46b
Sucralfate, 851
Sudden death
athletes, 638
cardiac causes, 557–560, 557b, 583b
hypertrophic cardiomyopathy, 638, 638b
raised ICP, 1212
Sugars
dietary, 113b
recommended intake, 114b
Suicide
assisted, 9–10
attempted, 238–239
poisoning *see* Poisoning
depression and, 235
older people, 238b
risk/risk factors, 235b
see also Self-harm
Sulfadiazine
prophylactic, 153b
rheumatic fever, 615–616
toxoplasmosis, 362
HIV-related, 402
Sulfadoxine, 158
and neutropenia, 1005b
Sulfadoxine-pyrimethamine *see* Fansidar
Sulfamethoxazole, melioidosis, 340
Sulfasalazine
ankylosing spondylitis, 1107
haemolysis from, 1031
inflammatory bowel disease, 860, 903b
and pulmonary eosinophilia, 713b
rheumatic disease, 1101b, 1102
Sulfinpyrazone, gout, 1089–1090
Sulindac, 911–912
Sulphonamides
mechanism of action, 150b
in pregnancy, 154b
skin reactions, 1304b
Sulphonylureas, 822b, 823
effect of hepatic impairment, 36b
effect of renal insufficiency, 36b
hypoglycaemia and, 783f, 810
skin reactions, 1304b
and weight gain, 117b
Sulphur, 132
Sulpiride, 249b
Sumatriptan, migraine, 1177
Sunbeds, and skin cancer, 1269b
Sunburn, 1260f
SUNCT, 1178, 1178b
Sunitinib, 516, 785
Sunlight, 1260
sensitivity to, 1260, 1286b
skin cancer and, 1272–1273
Sunscreens, 1262
albinism, 1296
photosensitivity, 1261–1262
protection levels, 1262
role in skin cancer, 1270b
vitiligo, 1295
Superior vena cava, 260f, 528f, 630f
malignant invasion, 705b
obstruction, 186b
malignant, 260f, 261b, 273, 273b, 701
thrombosis, 940
Superior vena cava syndrome, 604
Superoxide dismutase, 82, 1200
Supranuclear palsy, progressive, 1198
Supraventricular tachycardia, 567–569, 567f
Suramin, trypanosomiasis, 164, 359, 359b
Surfactant, 108, 192, 646–647
Surgery
acute abdomen, 861–863
bariatric, 119–120, 119b, 120f
brain tumours, 1214–1215
cancer, 276
cardiac risk, 600, 600b
cholecystitis, 984
dermatological, 1268
diabetes and, 818–820, 819b, 819f
endocrine disease
Cushing's syndrome/disease
hyperparathyroidism, 488, 770
epilepsy, 1184
gastrointestinal
achalasia, 869
chemoprophylaxis, 153b
colorectal cancer, 915
gastric cancer, 879
inflammatory bowel disease, 905–906
peptic ulcer, 874–875, 874b
upper acute haemorrhage, 856
haemophiliacs, 1051
infective endocarditis, 628, 629b
musculoskeletal disorders, 1080, 1080b
osteoarthritis, 1086
osteoporosis, 1125
rheumatoid arthritis, 1103
obesity, 119–120, 119b, 120f
Parkinson's disease, 1197
pituitary tumours, 789–790, 792
portosystemic shunt, 928
prostatic disease, 518
respiratory disease
bronchial carcinoma, 703
bronchiectasis, 679
COPD, 677
tuberculosis, 694
solid tumours *see individual tumour types*
stone disease, 985
valve replacement, 629
Surrogate endpoints, 39
Suxamethonium
allergy, 92b
pharmacokinetics, 25b
Swabs, bacterial/viral *see various conditions*
Swallowing, difficulty in *see* Dysphagia
Swan neck deformity of fingers, 1098, 1098f
Sweat glands, 1254
Sweating
excessive, 295–296
diabetic neuropathy, 833b
Swine influenza, 320
Sydenham's chorea (St Vitus dance), 615
Sympathetic nervous system
activation, 547
sodium transport regulation, 432
Synacthen test (ACTH stimulation test), 778b
Synaptic transmission, 1141
Synchronised intermittent mandatory ventilation (SIMV), 183, 195f
Syncope, 554–556, 1159
aortic stenosis, 620
cardiac, 554–555, 555b, 1159
congenital heart disease, 631
differential diagnosis, 554–556, 554f, 1158b
gastrointestinal haemorrhage, 854b
heat, 106
investigations, 555f
neurocardiogenic, 554–556
older people, 172
situational, 555
vasovagal, 555–556, 555b
Syndesmophytes, 1064, 1064b
Syndrome of inappropriate secretion of ADH (SIADH), 438b
cancer patients, 271b
Syndrome X *see* Insulin resistance syndrome
Synergistic gangrene, 305, 305b
Synovectomy, 1080b
medical (radiation), 1134
rheumatoid arthritis, 1080b, 1103
Synovial biopsy, 1068
Synovial fluid, 1063, 1064f
gout, 1089
pseudogout, 1090–1092
septic arthritis, 1094
Synovial joints, 1062–1063
structure, 1063f
Synovial membrane, 1063
Synoviocytes, 1063
Synovitis
acute (pseudogout), 1090–1092
pigmented villonodular, 1134
rheumatoid arthritis, 1100
seronegative spondarthritis, 1060b
Synovium, 1063
loose bodies, 1064
needle trauma, 1064
osteoarthritis, 1082
Syphilis, 332, 419–422
acquired, 419–420, 419f
benign tertiary, 420
cardiovascular, 420
classification, 419b
congenital, 420–422, 421b
dementia, 420, 1209, 1209b
early, 419–420
HIV/AIDS, 402–403
investigations, 420–421, 421b
late, 420
latent, 420
management, 421–422
neurosyphilis, 420, 1209, 1209b
in pregnancy, 314b, 421
primary, 419
quaternary, 420
secondary, 419–420, 1257b
treatment reactions, 421–422
Syringomyelia, 1133, 1133f, 1165, 1222b
Systemic inflammatory response syndrome *see* SIRS
Systemic lupus erythematosus (SLE), 1109–1112
autoantibodies, 1110
clinical features, 1110–1111
management, 1111–1112
pathophysiology, 1110–1112
pleural effusion, 662b, 1111
renal involvement, 520, 1111
respiratory complications, 712, 712b, 1111
sibling risk, 68b
Systemic sclerosis, AKI, 480b–481b
Systemic sclerosis (scleroderma), 1091b, 1112–1113, 1300
diffuse, 1112
oesophagitis, 1113
renal involvement, 496, 1113
respiratory complications, 712b, 713, 1113
small bowel disease, 1113
Systolic dysfunction, 535

T

T lymphocytes (T cells), 78
combined B/T lymphocyte deficiencies, 80
cytotoxic (CD8+), 78

deficiencies, 78b, 80, 80f
gastrointestinal tract, 843–844
helper (CD4+), 78, 394f
HIV infection/AIDS, 391–392
hypersensitivity pneumonitis, 720
liver, 925f
lymphoma, 1043
cutaneous, 1264
enteropathy-associated, 882
multiple sclerosis, 1188
skin, 1252
psoriasis, 1287f
T3 *see* Triiodothyronine
T4 *see* Thyroxine
Tabes dorsalis, 1209b
Tachyarrhythmias
atrial, 564–567
ventricular, 569–571, 570b, 570f
Tachycardia
atrial, 564
AV nodal re-entry, 567–569, 568f
Wolff-Parkinson-White syndrome, 568–569, 568f
orthrodromic, 568f
sinus, 563, 563b
supraventricular, 567–569, 567f
ventricular, 569–570, 570b, 570f
Tachyphylaxis, 20
Tacrolimus, 96b
eczema, 1266
myositis, 1115
nephrotoxicity, 522b
thrombocytopenia, 1050
transplant patients, 96b
liver transplant, 979
lung transplant, 666
Tactoids, 1032
Taenia asiatica, 378–379
Taenia echinococcus, 309b, 312b, 378, 380–381
Taenia saginata, 312b, 378–379
Taenia solium, 309b, 312b, 378–379
life cycle, 379f
Takayasu's disease, 1116
Tamm-Horsfall protein, 476
Tamoxifen
breast cancer, 280, 280b
desmoid tumour, 911–912
gynaecomastia, 763
hepatotoxicity, 971
retroperitoneal fibrosis, 511
Tamponade
balloon, variceal bleeding, 928, 947f
cardiac/pericardial, 532, 545–546, 545b, 640
Tamsulosin, 515
Tandem repeat mutations, 55, 56b
Tangier disease, 455–456, 456b
Tapeworms (cestodes), 312b, 378–381
Tar preparations, psoriasis, 1289b
Tardive dyskinesia, 248
drug-induced, 26, 249b, 877
Target cells, 999f
Tarsal tunnel syndrome, 1099
Tarui disease, 450b
Tay-Sachs disease, 451b
Tazobactam *see* Piperacillin-tazobactam
TBG *see* Thyroxine-binding globulin
TBNA *see* Transbronchial needle aspiration
TBW *see* Total body water
3TC *see* Lamivudine
TCAs *see* Tricyclic antidepressants
Teardrop poikilocytes, 1048–1049
Teichopsia, 1170
Teicoplanin, 151b, 157–158
adverse reactions, 158
neutropenic fever, 274
pharmacokinetics, 158
Telangiectasia
definition, 1251b
hereditary haemorrhagic, 1007, 1049
spider, liver disease, 943
Telaprevir, 161b, 162, 955
Telbivudine, 161b, 162, 953b
Teleological ethics, 10, 13
Teletherapy, 277
Telithromycin, 156
Telomerase, 264
Telomeres, 168–169
Temperature
body, 103
cold injury, 105, 105f
extremes of, 103–106
heat-related illness, 105–106
hypothermia, 104–105, 104b, 104f
peripheral/skin, circulation monitoring, 187
stroke patients, 1243b
thermoregulation, 103–104, 103b
Temporal artery biopsy, 1068
pyrexia of unknown origin, 299b
Temporal coning, 1212–1213, 1212f
Temporal lobes, 1142–1143
disorders, 1170b
functions, 1142b
effects of damage, 1142b
Tendinitis
Achilles, 1107–1108
hip, 1075b
shoulder, 1074b, 1074f
Tendon reflexes, root values, 1139b
Tendons
repair, 1080b
transfer, 1080b
xanthomas, 454f, 455
Tenecteplase (TNK), 595
Tennis elbow, 1075b
Tenofovir, 153b, 407b
hepatitis B, 161b, 162, 953, 953b
Tenosynovectomy, 1080
Tenosynovitis, 1075
De Quervain's, 1075
flexor (trigger finger), 1134
psoriatic arthritis, 1108
SLE, 1110
TENS (transcutaneous electrical nerve stimulation), 288
Tensilon test, 1226
Tension-type headache, 1176
Teratogens, 27, 37b
Terbinafine, 160, 160b
chromoblastomycosis, 381–382
onychomycosis, 1280
skin disease, 1267
skin reactions, 1304b
sporotrichosis, 383
Terbutaline
asthma, 669
COPD, 675
Terfenadine, drug interactions, 28b
Teriparatide, 1124
Terlipressin, 940–941, 946
Terminal agitation, 290
Terminal illness *see* Palliative care
Terrorism *see* Bioterrorism
Testis
epididymo-orchitis, 319
undescended, 759
Testosterone
bone remodelling, 1062b
deficiency, osteoporosis, 1120
reference range, 1309b
Testosterone therapy
delayed puberty, 759
hypogonadism, 761, 761b
osteoporosis, 1124–1125
Tests *see* Investigations
Tetanus, 138b, 1209–1210, 1210b
chemoprophylaxis, 1210
prevention/immunisation, 1210
wound, 1210
Tetany, 768
Tetrabenazine, 1195b, 1198
Tetracosactide test (ACTH stimulation test), 778b
Tetracycline(s), 151b, 158
adverse reactions, 158
bartonellosis, 352–353
cholera, 345
dosage regimen, 35b
drug interactions, 28b
hepatotoxicity, 971
mechanism of action, 150b
pharmacokinetics, 158
plague, 338–339
in pregnancy, 37b, 154b
relapsing fever, 336
rickettsial fevers, 352
skin reactions, 1260b, 1304b
small bowel bacterial overgrowth, 883
trachoma, 353
tropical sprue, 882
Tetralogy of Fallot, 634–635, 634f
acyanotic, 635
incidence, 630b
Tetraparesis, 1099, 1162b
TF *see* Tissue factor
TFPI *see* Tissue factor pathway inhibitor
Tg (thyroglobulin) *see* Thyroglobin
TG (triglyceride) *see* Triglyceride
TGF-β, 724, 925f
Thalamus, 1143
Thalassaemias, 1032, 1034–1035
Thalidomide
Behçet's syndrome, 1119
leprosy reactions, 349b
myeloma, 1047
and peripheral neuropathy, 1223b
sarcoidosis, 711
teratogenesis, 1047
Thallium poisoning, 308
Thanatophoric dysplasia, 59
Theophylline
asthma, 670f, 671
COPD, 676
effect of old age, 36b
plasma concentrations, 39b
poisoning, 209b, 224b
prescription, 38b
therapeutic monitoring, 39b
Therapeutic drug monitoring, 36, 39–40, 39b, 154
Therapeutic efficacy, 19–20
Therapeutic goals, 33
Therapeutic index, 19f, 20
Therapeutic privilege, 10
Thermodilution, cardiac output measurement, 539
Thermogenesis, diet-induced, 110, 111f
Thermoregulation, 103–104, 103b
older people, 104b
Thermotherapy, benign prostatic hyperplasia, 515
Thiabendazole, 163
Thiamin pyrophosphate (TPP), 127–128
Thiamin (vitamin B_1), 127–128, 253–254
biochemical assessment of status, 126b
deficiency, 128
dietary sources, 125b
RNI, 125b
Thiazides
adverse reactions, 436b
diabetes insipidus, 795
hypertension, 611, 613b
and hyponatraemia, 437b, 439b
mode of action, 435
skin reactions, 1260b, 1304b
Thiazolidinediones, 822b, 823
non-alcoholic fatty liver disease, 961
and osteoporosis, 1121
polycystic ovary syndrome, 764
Thienobenzodiazepines, 249b
Thiopurine methyltransferase, 903b
Thiopurines, inflammatory bowel disease, 903b
Thioxanthenes, 249b
Thirst
diabetes insipidus, 794–795
water balance disorders, 433b
Thomsen's disease, 1230b
Thoracic aortic aneurysms, 604
Thoracic duct obstruction, pleural effusion, 662b
Thoracic kyphoscoliosis, 731
Thoracic outlet syndrome, 1225b
Thorax, examination, respiratory disease, 645f
Thought, passivity of, 247–248
Thought content, assessment, 234
Threadworm (*Enterobius vermicularis*), 371, 371f
Threonine, 114b
Throat, sore *see* Laryngitis; Pharyngitis
Thrombasthenia, Glanzmann's, 1050
Thrombin, 996f–998f
Thrombin inhibitors, 1019b
Thromboangiitis obliterans, 603–605
Thrombocythaemia, essential, 1049
Thrombocytopenia, 1007–1008, 1050
causes, 1007b
heparin-induced (HIT), 1019
hepatobiliary disease, 929
HIV/AIDS, 394, 405
older people, 1056b
Thrombocytopenic purpura
idiopathic, 1050
thrombotic, 496, 1056
Thrombocytosis, 1008
causes, 1008b
clonal, 1008b
leukaemia, 1039
reactive, 1008b
rheumatoid arthritis, 1099–1100
Thromboembolism
atrial fibrillation, 566–567
heart failure, 549
older people, 1056b
pulmonary *see* Pulmonary embolism/thromboembolism
venous *see* Venous thrombosis/thromboembolism
Thrombolytic therapy
myocardial infarction, 595–596
pulmonary embolism, 723
relative contraindications, 596b
stroke, 1244
Thrombophilia, investigation, 1001b
Thrombopoietin (Tpo), 992–993
Thrombosis
acute limb ischaemia, 603, 603b
older people, 1056b
venous *see* Venous thrombosis/thromboembolism
Thrombospondin, 264
Thrombotic disorders, 1001, 1054–1056
Thrombotic thrombocytopenic purpura (TTP), 496, 1056
Thromboxanes
allergy, 89b
thromboxane A, 113, 996f–997f
Thrush, 381
oral, 864
Thumb, Z deformity, 1128
Thymectomy, myasthenia gravis, 1227b
Thymine, 42
Thymus, 76
Thyroglobulin antibodies, 741b
Thyroglobulin (Tg), 738, 739f
as tumour marker, 270b
Thyroid autoantibodies, 741b
Thyroid disease
autoimmune, 743b, 747–751
classification, 738b

clinical features, 741b
congenital, 755–756
investigations, 738–740
iodine-associated, 752
malignant *see* Thyroid neoplasia
pregnancy, 756b
presenting problems, 740–747
Thyroid function tests
asymptomatic abnormal results, 745–746
hypothyroidism, 739b
interpretation, 739b
obese patients, 117
pregnancy, 745
thyrotoxicosis, 739b
and thyroxine therapy, 743–744
transient thyroiditis, 743b
Thyroid gland, 738–756
enlargement, 746–747, 746b
see also Goitre
examination, 735b
functional anatomy/physiology, 738–740, 739f
in old age, 755b
scintigraphy, 746
ultrasound, 747
Thyroid hormones, 738–740, 739f
bone remodelling, 1062b
dyshormonogenesis, 744f
in pregnancy, 745
replacement
hypopituitarism, 788–789
hypothyroidism, 743–745
neonates, 749–750
resistance, 756
Thyroid neoplasia, 754–755, 754b
anaplastic carcinoma and lymphoma, 755
differentiated carcinoma, 754–755
medullary carcinoma, 755
toxic adenoma, 754
Thyroid nodule, solitary, 746
Thyroid peroxidase antibodies, 741b
Thyroid storm, 742–743
Thyroid-stimulating hormone (TSH; thyrotrophin), 736, 738–740
deficiency, hypopituitarism, 787b
reference range, 1309b
Thyroid-stimulating hormone-receptor antibodies (TRAb), 741b, 747–748
Thyroid-stimulating immunoglobulins, 747–748
Thyroidectomy
and hypoparathyroidism, 743b
partial/subtotal, Graves' disease, 748b, 749
prophylactic, 63, 795
thyroid cancer, 754–755
Thyroiditis
Hashimoto's, 751
post-partum, 752, 756b
Riedel's, 755
subacute (de Quervain's), 751–752
transient, 741b, 751–752
Thyrotoxic crisis, 742–743
Thyrotoxicosis, 740–743
amiodarone and, 740b, 742f, 752
atrial fibrillation, 742
causes, 740b
clinical features, 740, 741b
differential diagnosis, 742f
factitious, 740–741
goitre, 740, 740b
Graves' disease, 740, 740b, 747–750, 748f
management, 748–749, 748b
investigations, 740–741
iodine-associated, 740b
laboratory abnormalities, 741b
low-uptake, 740–741
management, 741–743
musculoskeletal manifestations, 1132
neonatal, 749–750
older people, 755b
pregnancy, 749–750, 756b
subclinical, 739b, 742, 745–746
T3:T4 ratio, 740–741
toxic adenoma, 742f, 754
Thyrotrophin *see* Thyroid-stimulating hormone
Thyrotrophin-releasing hormone (TRH), 737f, 738–740
Thyrotrophin-releasing hormone (TRH) receptor, 49b
Thyroxine (T4), 737f, 738, 739f
dose adjustments, 745b
hypothyroidism management, 743–744
Hashimoto's thyroiditis, 751
ischaemic heart disease patients, 744–745
reference range, 1309b
therapeutic monitoring, 39b
Thyroxine-binding globulin (TBG), 738
Tiagabine, 1184b
TIAs *see* Transient ischaemic attacks
TIBC *see* Total iron binding capacity
Tibial compartment syndrome, anterior, 1135
Tibolone, osteoporosis, 1123b, 1124–1125
Tic douloureux, 1178
Ticarcillin, 154b
Tick-borne diseases, 309b
babesiosis, 358
encephalitis, 309b
Lyme disease, 309b, 334–336, 335f, 1209
relapsing fever, 336
rickettsial/typhus, 350–352, 351b
tularaemia, 340
viral haemorrhagic fevers, 309b, 311f, 324–325
Tics, 1166b, 1167
Tidal volume, 195b
Tietze's syndrome, 541b, 659b
Tigecycline, 151b, 158
Tiludronate, Paget's disease, 1129, 1130b
Tin oxide, 717b
Tinea capitis, 1280
Tinea corporis, 1279
rash, 1257b
Tinea cruris, 1279
Tinea incognito, 1279f
Tinea pedis, 1279–1280
Tinidazole, 158, 368
Tiotropium bromide, 675
TIPSS (transjugular intrahepatic portasystemic shunts), 931, 940, 947f–948f
Tirofiban
myocardial infarction, 594
platelet inhibition, 594, 997
Tissue factor pathway inhibitor (TFPI), 185
Tissue factor (TF), 185, 265f
Tissue plasminogen activator (tPA), 595
recombinant, stroke, 1244b
Tizanidine, 1192b
TLC *see* Total lung capacity
TLCO (gas transfer factor for carbon monoxide), 653b
TNF *see* Tumour necrosis factor
TNF-receptor-associated proteins (TRAFs), 48–49, 48f
TNFR1 receptor, 49b
TNK *see* Tenecteplase
TNM classification of tumours, 268b
Tobramycin
cystic fibrosis, 681b
dosing interval, 153b
Tocilizumab, 1103, 1103b
Tocopherol *see* Vitamin E
Toes
cock-up deformities, 1098
ingrowing toenails, 1297
Tolbutamide, 216
Tolcapone, Parkinson's disease, 1197
Tolerance, 20
Toll-like receptors, 843
Tolterodine, 175f, 1175b
Tongue
biting, 1158b
strawberry, 331, 332f
Tonsillar coning, 1212–1213, 1213f
Tonsillitis, 321
membranous, 345b
streptococcal, 331
Tonsils, 76f, 345
Tophi, gout, 1088–1089, 1088f
Topical administration, 21–22, 1264–1266, 1265b
Topiramate, 1184b
idiopathic intracranial hypertension, 1218
Topotecan, 280–281
Torsades de pointes, 570–571, 571b, 571f
Torticollis, 1166–1167, 1200
Total anterior circulation syndrome (TACS), 1241f
Total body water (TBW), 429
Total iron binding capacity (TIBC), 1023
Total lung capacity (TLC), 653b
Total parenteral nutrition (TPN)
acute pancreatitis, 892b
gastroparesis, 877
short bowel syndrome, 885
Tourette's syndrome, 1166b, 1167
Toxaemia, pregnancy, 978
Toxic epidermal necrolysis, 1292, 1292b, 1292f, 1304b
Toxic megacolon, 900
Toxic shock syndrome (TSS), 138b, 1276
staphylococcal, 331, 331f
streptococcal, 295f, 331–332
Toxins
bacterial, 138b, 1209–1211
botulinum toxin *see* Botulinum toxin
chemical, 308
ciguatera fish poisoning, 308
scombrotoxic fish poisoning, 308
shellfish, 308
food poisoning, 308
gastrointestinal decontamination, 210
marine sources, 308
plant, 308
renal effects, 197
routes of exposure, 208f
venoms, 225
Toxocara canis, 312b
Toxocariasis, 312b
Toxoplasma gondii, 361
HIV-related, 402
life cycle, 361f
Toxoplasmosis, 361–362
acquired, 361
cerebral, HIV-related, 402, 403f
congenital, 361
pregnancy, 314b, 362
prophylaxis, 406b
tPA *see* Tissue plasminogen activator
TPN *see* Total parenteral nutrition
Tpo *see* Thrombopoietin
TPP *see* Thiamin pyrophosphate
TRAb *see* TSH-receptor antibodies
Trace elements, absorption, 843
Trachea, obstruction, 728
Tracheal intubation *see* Endotracheal intubation
Tracheitis, 654b
Tracheo-oesophageal fistula, 728
Tracheostomy, 194, 195b
Trachoma, 353, 353f
Trachyonychia, 1298
TRAFs *see* TNF-receptor-associated proteins
Tramadol, 1078
Tranexamic acid, 1050
Tranquillisers, effect of old age, 36b
Transaminases *see* Aminotransferases
Transaminitis, 198
Transarterial chemo-embolisation (TACE), hepatocellular carcinoma, 968
Transbronchial needle aspiration (TBNA), 651
Transcobalamin II, 1024–1025
Transcription, DNA, 42–43
Transcription factor diseases, 44f
Transcription factors, 42
Transcutaneous nerve stimulation *see* TENS
Transcutaneous PCO_2, 188
Transdermal administration, 21
Transfer coefficient for carbon monoxide (KCO), 653b
Transference, 241–242
Transferrin, 1023
older people, 1034b
reduced levels, 1023
saturation, 972, 1312b
Transforming growth factor (TGF)-α, 263
Transforming growth factor (TGF)-β, 1049
Transient ischaemic attacks (TIAs), 1240
sensory loss, 1164
visual loss, 1170
see also Stroke
Transjugular intrahepatic portasystemic shunts (TIPSS), 931, 940, 947f–948f
Translation, 44–45
Translocations
chromosomes, 57f, 879–880, 1044
Robertsonian, 57f
Transmissible spongiform encephalopathies (TSEs), 329, 1211
Transplantation, 94–96
bone marrow *see* Haematopoietic stem cell transplantation
complications of immunosuppression, 95–96
graft rejection, 94–95, 95b
heart, 553
heart-lung, 665–666
islet cells, 826
kidney *see* Kidneys, transplantation
liver *see* Liver, transplantation
living donors, 96
lung, 665–666, 665b
organ donation, 96
pancreas, 826
pre-transplant investigations, 95
small intestine, 885
stem cell *see* Stem cells, transplantation
Transposition of great arteries, 635b
incidence, 630b
Transrectal ultrasound scan (TRUS) of prostate, 515
Transurethral resection of prostate (TURP), 515
Transverse myelitis, 1193, 1193b, 1222b
Tranylcypromine, 244b
TRAPS *see* Tumour necrosis factor-associated periodic syndrome
Trastuzumab, 279, 879
Trauma
head, 1218
psychiatric disorders, 242
Travellers
eosinophilia
fever in, 309–310, 309b–310b

health needs, 309b
immunisations, 309b
incubation times and illnesses, 310b
Traveller's diarrhoea, 310–311, 311b
Treadmill testing, 534
Trefoil factor family, 841
Trematodes *see* Flukes
Tremor, 1165–1166, 1166b, 1199
causes/characteristics, 1166b
drug-induced, 1200b
dystonic, 1166b
essential, 1166b, 1199
flapping (asterixis), 923b
functional, 1166b
intention, 1145
Parkinson's disease, 1166b, 1196b
resting, 1163
Trench fever, 352
Trench foot, 105
Treponema pallidum, 151b, 414b, 415, 418
see also Syphilis
Treponema pertenue, 332
Treponema vincentii, 333
Treponemal (specific) antibody tests, 421b
Treponematoses, 332–333
endemic, 332–333
see also Syphilis
Tretinoin, acne, 1282
TRH *see* Thyrotrophin-releasing hormone
Triamcinolone, 864, 1102, 1282
Triamterene, 435
Triatoma infestans, 360
Triazoles, 159–160, 160b
Tricalcium phosphate, 1091
Tricarboxylic acid (Krebs) cycle, 128
Trichiasis, 353
Trichinella spiralis, 312b, 375
Trichinosis (trichinellosis), 375
Trichloroacetic acid, 1279
Trichomonas vaginalis, 415
Trichomoniasis, genital, 417b
Trichophyton interdigitale, 1279–1280, 1279f
Trichophyton mentagrophytes, 1279–1280
Trichophyton rubrum, 1279, 1279f
Trichophyton tonsurans, 1280
Trichophyton verrucosum, 1280
Trichuris trichiura (whipworm), 371–372
Triclabendazole, 379b
Tricuspid regurgitation, 624–625, 624b
Tricuspid stenosis, 624
Tricuspid valve
atresia, 635b
balloon valvuloplasty, 624
repair/replacement, 625
Tricyclic antidepressants (TCAs), 241b, 244, 244b
irritable bowel syndrome, 909
pain management, 288b
poisoning, 209b, 213–214
Trientine dihydrochloride, Wilson's disease, 974
Trigeminal (5th cranial) nerve, tests, 1139b
Trigeminal neuralgia, 1157, 1178
Trigger finger (flexor tenosynovitis), 1134
diabetes, 799b
Triglycerides
measurement, 453
reference values, venous blood, 1310b
Trihexyphenidyl, Parkinson's disease, 1197
Triiodothyronine (T3), 121, 737f, 739f
myxoedema coma management, 745
reference range, 1309b
Trimethoprim
adverse reactions, 158
brucellosis, 334b
mechanism of action, 150b
melioidosis, 340
in pregnancy, 154b, 334b
urinary tract infection, 513b
Trimethoprim/sulfamethoxazole *see* Co-trimoxazole
Triple X syndrome, 56b
Triplet repeat disorders, 65
Triptans, 21, 1177
Trismus, 1210
Trisomy 13 (Patau's syndrome), 56b
Trisomy 18 (Edwards' syndrome), 56b
Trisomy 21 (Down's syndrome)
genetics, 56b
screening, 63b
Trochanteric bursitis, 1075b, 1075f
Trochlear (4th cranial) nerve, 1139b
damage to, 1171b
Troisier's sign, 878
Tropheryma whipplei, 134, 141, 883
Tropical diseases, 308–313
diarrhoea, 310–311, 311b
eosinophilia, 311–312, 312b
fever and, 309–310, 309b–310b
patterns in tropical countries
skin, 304b, 312–313, 313b
see also names of specific diseases
Tropical pulmonary eosinophilia, 713
Tropical sprue, 882
Tropical ulcer, 333
Tropomyosin, 530
Troponins, 535
acute coronary syndromes, 600b
reference values, venous blood, 1310b
Trousseau's sign, 447, 768
Truncus arteriosus, 629
TRUS (transrectal ultrasound scan) of prostate, 515
Truth-telling, 10
Trypanosoma brucei gambiense, 359
Trypanosoma brucei rhodesiense, 359
Trypanosoma cruzi, 868–869
Trypanosomiasis
African (sleeping sickness), 309b, 358–360, 359f
American (Chagas disease), 309b, 360–361
incubation period, 145b
treatment, 163–164
Trypsin, 842
Trypsinogen, 844b
Tryptase, 1310b
Tryptophan, 114b
TSEs *see* Transmissible spongiform encephalopathies
Tsetse fly, 309b
TSH *see* Thyroid-stimulating hormone
TSS *see* Toxic shock syndrome
TTP *see* Thrombotic thrombocytopenic purpura
Tube drainage, intercostal, 663, 730, 730f
Tube feeding *see* Feeding, enteral
Tuberculin test, tuberculosis, 662b, 690–691, 697
Tuberculoma, 403
Tuberculosis, 688–696
abdominal, 691, 888
bone and joints, 1096
chemoprophylaxis, 153b
HIV/AIDS patients, 406
clinical features, 689–690, 689f, 690b–691b
complications, 691b
diagnosis, 692–693, 693b, 693f
drug resistance, 696, 696b
empyema, 691f
epidemiology, 688–696
extra-pulmonary, 690–692, 692f
fever, 396
HIV-related, 396, 400–401, 401f, 696
prevention, 406
immunisation, 696
incubation period, 145b, 310b
latent, 695
management, 693–694, 694b
directly observed therapy, 695
HIV/AIDS patients, 401
meningitis *see* Tuberculous meningitis
miliary, 689–690
cryptic, 690b
multi-drug resistant, 696
natural history, 690b
older people, 686b
pathology/pathogenesis, 688–689
pleural effusion, 662b, 691f
post-primary pulmonary, 690
prevalence, 689f
prevention, 694–696
prognosis, 696
progressive, 688–689, 690b
pulmonary, 662b, 689, 689f, 691b
renal/urinary tract, 514, 692
risk factors, 690b
spinal cord, 693
Tuberculous meningitis, 1204–1205, 1205b
Tuberculous pericarditis, 640
Tuberculous peritonitis, 691
Tuberous sclerosis, 1302
pulmonary, 715b
Tubular necrosis, acute *see* Acute tubular necrosis
Tubulins, 48
Tubulo-interstitial diseases, 502–505
Tularaemia, 309b, 340
Tumbu fly, 381
Tumour lysis syndrome, 449
Tumour markers, 269, 270b
prostate cancer, 268, 270b, 515, 761
Tumour necrosis factor α (TNF-α), 74b
bone remodelling, 1062b
rheumatoid arthritis, 1097f
Tumour necrosis factor (TNF), receptor, 48f
Tumour necrosis factor-associated periodic syndrome (TRAPS), 85
Tumour suppressor genes, 59
Tumours
HIV-related, 405
malignant *see* Cancer
neuro-endocrine, 784–785, 785b, 785f
see also Cancer; *and specific types and sites*
Tunga penetrans, 381
Tungiasis, 381
Turbidimetry, 428b
Turcot's syndrome, 911–912
Turner's syndrome, 765–766, 765f
genetics, 56b
TURP *see* Transurethral resection of prostate
Twisting points *see* Torsade de pointes
Typhoid fever, 339–340, 339b
complications, 340b
immunisation, 340
incubation period, 145b, 310b
Typhus fever, 309b, 350–352
endemic, 351–352, 351b
epidemic, 351, 351b
incubation period, 310b
scrub typhus, 350–351, 351b
Tyrosine, 114b, 739f
Tyrosine kinase, receptor, 47f, 49b, 1005
Tyrosine kinase inhibitors, 785b, 1039b
TZD drugs *see* Thiazolidinediones

U
Ubiquitin, 46
UDCA *see* Ursodeoxycholic acid
UIP *see* Usual interstitial pneumonia
UK Prospective Diabetes Study (UKPDS), 821–822, 828
Ulcerative colitis
arthritis
and cancer, 266b
childhood, 906
clinical features, 899, 899b
comparison with Crohn's disease, 897b
complications, 900–901, 901f–902f
differential diagnosis, 900b
investigations, 901–902
management, 904b
medical, 903–904
surgical, 905–906, 905b
pathophysiology, 897–898, 899f
pregnancy, 906–907, 906b
sclerosing cholangitis and, 965
Ulcers, 270b
amoebic, 367, 368f
aphthous, 863–864, 864b
Buruli, 333
Chiclero's, 366
dendritic, 326
digital, 1113
foot, diabetics, 834–835
genital
men, 415–416, 416f
women, 418
leg, 1262–1263, 1262b, 1262f–1263f
leishmaniasis, 366f
leprosy, 347–348
Marjolin's, 1095–1096, 1263
mouth, 398
neuropathic, 834f
oesophageal, 868
oral, 1111, 1119
peptic *see* Peptic ulcers
rodent, 1270
skin
definition, 1251b
leg ulcers, 1262–1263
small intestine, 887, 887b
solitary rectal ulcer syndrome, 919
tropical, 333
Ulnar nerve
entrapment, 1080b, 1099, 1224b
palsy, 832
Ultrafiltration, 430, 464
failure, 493b
Ultrasound
cancer diagnosis, 269
Doppler *see* Doppler ultrasound
echocardiography *see* Echocardiography
endocrine disease
polycystic ovary, 764f
thyroid gland, 747
endoscopic, 985f
gastrointestinal tract, 846, 847b, 847f
oesophageal cancer, 871f
pancreatitis, 891
hepatobiliary disease, 930, 930f
cholangitis, 985f
gallstones, 847f, 930f
NAFLD, 961
hepatocellular carcinoma, 967–968
musculoskeletal disease, 1065
synovitis, 1065f
nervous system, 1149b
prenatal, 63b
renal, 468–469, 469f, 480b
renal artery stenosis, 494–495

respiratory disease, 651, 663f
pleural disease/pleural effusion, 663f
Ultraviolet radiation (UVR), 102, 1269
photosensitivity, 1260, 1260f
psoriasis, 1289b
ultraviolet B, 1289b
PUVA *see* PUVA
skin cancer and, 266b
ultraviolet A, 1266
ultraviolet B, 1266, 1289b
Wood's light, 1255
Undernutrition, 111–112, 120–124
causes, 121b
classification, 120b
in hospital, 122–124, 122f
response to, 111–112
Upper limb, chronic arterial disease, 602
Uracil, 43
Uraemia
haemolytic uraemic syndrome, 138b, 468, 495–496
see also Renal failure
Urea, 430b
AKI, 480b
blood levels, 1308b
reference values
urine, 1311b
venous blood, 1308b
Urea breath tests, 851b
Helicobacter pylori infection, 850–851
Urea and electrolytes (U&Es) test, 430b
gastrointestinal bleeding, 855
Ureidopenicillins, 154b
Ureter, 466
colic, 507–508
diseases of, 510–511
ectopic, 510
megaureter, 510
obstruction, 508f
stones, 507–508
Ureteropyelogram, retrograde, 517
Ureterovaginal fistula, 473
Urethral discharge, 415, 415f
Urethral syndrome, 511–512
Urethritis
chlamydial, 415, 1104, 1108
gonococcal, 415
non-specific, 415, 1107
reactive arthritis, 1107
subclinical, 416b
Urge incontinence, 175, 473, 1174
Uric acid (urate)
crystals, 507b
gout, 1087
lowering, 1089b
pool, 1087f
raised, 1087b
reference values
urine, 1311b
venous blood, 1310b
Uricosuric drugs, 1089–1090
Urinalysis, 468
AKI, 480b
reference values, 1311b
Urinary diversion, 517
Urinary incontinence *see* Incontinence
Urinary tract
calculi, 507–510
clinical examination, 462–464
collecting system
diseases, 510–511
imaging, 469f–470f
congenital abnormalities, 510–511
tumours, 515–519
Urinary tract disease
investigation, 466–471
presenting problems, 471–478
Urinary tract infection (UTI), 511–514
clinical features, 511–512
investigation, 512, 512b
management, 512, 513b
older people, 512b
pathophysiology, 511, 511b
prophylaxis, 513b
recurrent, 512–513
risk factors, 511b
stroke patients, 1243b
tuberculosis, 692
vesico-ureteric reflux and, 511b
Urine
alkalinisation, 210–211
black, 1026–1027
microscopy, 463b, 480b
output measurement, critically ill patients, 187
red/dark, 475b
retention
acute, 514–515
benign prostatic hyperplasia, 472, 514–515
chronic, 515
volume, 471–472
see also Anuria; Oliguria
Urine testing
diabetes, 807–808
glycaemic control assessment, 811
Urobilin, 927
Urobilinogen, 927
Urography, intravenous *see* Intravenous urography
Urokinase, 265f, 998f
Urothelial tumours, 516–517, 517f
Ursodeoxycholic acid (UDCA)
gallstones, 983b
primary biliary cirrhosis, 964, 964b
Urticaria (nettle rash; hives), 1290–1291, 1290b, 1291f
drug-induced, 1291, 1304b
papular, 374
pathogenesis, 1291f
solar, 1260b
Ustekinumab, 1109
Usual interstitial pneumonia (UIP), 708b, 709f
Uterine tumours, 262f
Uterocele, 510
UTI *see* Urinary tract infection
Uveitis
acute anterior, ankylosing spondylitis, 1105
brucellosis, 334f
HTLV-1-associated, 328–329
immune recovery, 404
reactive arthritis, 1108
treatment, 338
Weil's disease, 337
UVR *see* Ultraviolet radiation

V

vacA *see* Vacuolating cytotoxin
Vaccines/vaccination, 148–149, 149b
anthrax, 149b
antibody deficiencies, 81–82
BCG, 696
chickenpox, 318
cholera, 345
COPD patients, 676f, 677
diphtheria, 346
guidelines, 149b
Haemophilus influenzae, 149b
hepatitis, 149b, 1051–1052
HIV, 410
in HIV/AIDS patients, 407
human papillomavirus, 425, 425b
influenza, 320
HIV/AIDS patients, 407
older people, 320
Japanese B encephalitis, 328
leprosy, 350
Lyme disease, 336
malaria, 358
meningococcal infection, 1203–1204
MMR, 319
mumps, 319
plague, 339
pneumococcal pneumonia, 346
poliomyelitis, 1207
rabies, 1206
rotavirus, 327–328
rubella, 315
tetanus, 1210
tick-borne encephalitis, 309b
typhoid, 340
use of, 149
varicella, 318
viral hepatitis, 954b
whooping cough (pertussis), 149b
yellow fever, 324
see also Immunisation
Vaccinia virus, 327
Vacuolating cytotoxin (vacA), 873f
VAD *see* Ventricular assist devices
Vagina
discharge, 417–419, 417b, 417f
see also Vulvovaginal conditions
Vaginosis, bacterial, 417, 417b, 417f
Vagotomy, peptic ulcer, 875
Vagus (10th cranial) nerve, tests, 1139b
Valaciclovir
herpes simplex infection, 318b
herpes virus infection, 161–162, 161b
genital, 424–425
Valganciclovir
CMV, 322, 406b
herpesvirus infection, 161b, 406b
Valine, 114b
Valproate *see* Sodium valproate
Valsartan
heart failure, 552b
hypertension, 611–612
myocardial infarction, 599
Valves of Heister, 926
Valvular heart disease, 546, 613–629
causes, 546b, 614b
infective endocarditis, 625–629
prevention, 628–629
rheumatic, 614–616
risks of non-cardiac surgery, 600, 600b
valve replacement, 629
see also names of individual valves and diseases
Valvuloplasty
aortic, 621–623
mitral, 618, 618b
Van Buchem's disease, 1131
Vancomycin, 151b, 157–158
acute leukaemia, 1001
adverse reactions, 158
Clostridium difficile infection, 344
infective endocarditis, 301, 628
meningitis, 1204b
neutropenic sepsis, 274
pharmacokinetics, 158
respiratory disease, 686
skin reactions, 1304b
therapeutic monitoring, 39b
toxic shock syndrome, 331
Vancomycin-resistant *Staphylococcus aureus* (VRSA), 330–331
Vandetanib, 755
Vanishing bile duct syndrome, 966, 980
Variability of disease, 99
Variceal bleeding, 942, 942f
cirrhosis, 942, 942f
management, 946–948, 946b, 947f
portal hypertension, 945
prevention, 946, 946b, 948b
Variceal ligation, 848f
Varicella, pneumonia, 650b
Varicella zoster virus immunoglobulin (VZIG), 318, 318b
Varicella zoster virus (VZV), 317b, 317f
HIV infection/AIDS, 404
HSCT, 1017b
immunisation, 149b, 318
pregnancy, 314b
stem cell transplantation, 1017b
treatment, 317b–318b
Varices
gastrointestinal haemorrhage, 942
oesophageal, 942, 942f, 945
rectal, 945
Varicose veins, 1262–1263
Variegate porphyria, 450b, 459f
Variola, 327
Vascular dementia, 250b
Vascular disease, 600–613
atherosclerotic *see* Atherosclerosis
diabetics, 602, 602b, 826–827, 827f
diffuse, 250
liver, 975–977
peripheral, 600–603, 600b
pulmonary, 721–725
renal, 494–497
Vascular endothelial growth factor (VEGF), 264
Vascular imaging, 1235–1236, 1236f, 1242
Vascular malformations, gastrointestinal haemorrhage, 849f
Vascular resistance
portal hypertension, 945
in pregnancy, 520
pulmonary, 548, 553, 616, 630f
systemic, 201, 530–531
Vasculitis, 1115–1119, 1116f, 1299
ANCA-associated, 1118
cerebral, 1174b, 1190
cryoglobulinaemic, 1119
cutaneous, 680b
drug-induced, 1132b, 1304b
leg ulceration, 1263
renal arteries, 494
rheumatoid arthritis, 1098–1099
small-vessel, 496
systemic, 1116b, 1117f
renal involvement, 519–520
urticarial, 1290
see also individual conditions
Vaso-occlusive crisis, 1032–1033
Vasoactive drugs, circulatory effects, 191b
Vasoactive intestinal polypeptide (VIP), 846b
Vasodilatation, 190
splanchnic, 939
Vasodilators
angina, 589
heart failure, 552
hypertension, 612
myocardial infarction, 545b
valvular heart disease, 619–620
Vasomotor rhinitis, 725
Vasopressin *see* Antidiuretic hormone
VC *see* Vital capacity
VDRL *see* Venereal Diseases Research Laboratory test
VDRR *see* Vitamin D-resistant rickets
Vegans, 114
vitamin B deficiency, 1025
Velocardiofacial syndrome, 56b, 66
Venae cavae, 528, 528f
see also Inferior vena cava; Superior vena cava
Venereal Diseases Research Laboratory (VDRL) test, 251b, 420–421
Venesection
haemochromatosis, 972–973
polycythaemia rubra vera, 1049
Venlafaxine, 244b
Veno-occlusive disease, liver, 976
Venography
cerebral, 1247
hepatic portal, 931, 976
venous thrombosis, 1010, 1247

Venomous animals, 225–226, 225b, 227b, 229b
Venoms, 225
  effects, 225b
  insect, allergy to, 94
  marine animals, 228b
  scorpions, 227b, 229b
  snakes, 225–226, 225b, 227b–229b
  spiders, 228b
  see also Envenomation
Venous disease
  cerebral, 1247
  leg ulcers, 1263, 1263f
Venous hypertension, 1262
Venous pulse
  distinction from arterial pulse, 527b
  jugular, 527b
Venous thrombosis/ thromboembolism (VTE), 721–724, 1008–1011
  air travellers, 108
  at high altitude, 107
  causes, 1009f
  clinical features, 721–724, 721b, 1008–1011
  investigation, 722–723, 1010, 1010f
  management, 723–724, 1010–1011, 1011b
    anticoagulants, 723
    caval filters, 724
    thrombolytic therapy, 723
  older people, 724b
  predisposing factors, 1009b
  pregnancy, 723b
  prevention, 1020–1021, 1020b
  prognosis, 724
  retinal vein, 609f
  risk factors, 721b
  stroke patients, 1243b
  Wells score, 1010b
Ventilation
  mechanical (artificial), 195f
    advanced strategies, 196
    ARDS, 196b
    asthma, 672
    conditions requiring, 194b
    COPD, 678b
    critically ill patients, 194, 194b
    envenomation, 230
    high-frequency oscillatory, 196
    mandatory modes, 195–196
    prone, 196
    respiratory failure
    settings, 195, 195b
    withdrawal, 183, 196–197, 197b
  non-invasive, 194, 195f
    COPD exacerbations, 678, 678b
    non-invasive positive pressure ventilation
  respiratory failure, 665
Ventilation-perfusion mismatch, 648
  older people, 648b
Ventilation-perfusion (V/Q) lung scanning, pulmonary embolism, 722
Ventricles
  heart, 534f
  see also Left ventricle; Right ventricle
Ventricular aneurysm, 597–598
Ventricular assist devices (VAD), 553
Ventricular contractility, reduced, 546b
Ventricular ectopic beats, 569, 569f
Ventricular fibrillation (VF)
  cardiac arrest, 557, 557f
  myocardial infarction, 596
Ventricular inflow obstruction, 546b
Ventricular outflow obstruction, 546b
Ventricular remodelling, 597–598, 597f
Ventricular rupture, 597
Ventricular septal defect, 633–634, 634f
  heart murmurs, 562b
  incidence, 630b
  tetralogy of Fallot, 634–635, 634f
Ventricular tachyarrhythmias, 569–571
Ventricular tachycardia (VT), 569–570, 570b, 570f
  poisoning, 211b
  pulseless, 557–558
Ventricular volume overload, 546b
Ventriculitis, 1205
Ventriculography, left, 538–539
VER *see* Visual evoked responses
Verapamil
  angina, 586–587, 587b, 594
  aortic dissection, 607
  arrhythmias, 565–566, 575b, 576
  cluster headache, 1177
  hypertension, 612
  tachyarrhythmias
    atrial fibrillation, 565–566
    atrial flutter, 564
Verbal rating scale for pain, 285
Verocytotoxigenic *Escherichia coli* (VTEC), 343f, 496
Verotoxin, 495–496
Verrucae, 1278
Verruga peruana, 352, 352b
Vertebral fracture, 1071b
Vertebroplasty, 1080b, 1125, 1125b
Vertigo, 173, 1157, 1167–1168
  benign paroxysmal positional, 1186, 1186f
Very low-density lipoproteins (VLDL), 451
Vesicle, definition, 1251b
Vesico-ureteric reflux (VUR), 505f
Vesicovaginal fistula, 473
vestibular disorders, 1186
Vestibular failure, acute, 1186
Vestibular neuronitis, 853f, 1158f
Vestibulitis, 418b
Vestibulocochlear (8th cranial) nerve, tests, 1139b
VF *see* Ventricular fibrillation
Vibrio cholerae, 138b, 306, 344
Vibrio parahaemolyticus, 345
Vibrio vulnificus, 305
Vildagliptin, 824
Villi, intestinal, atrophy, 881b
Vimentin, 48
Vinblastine, Hodgkin's disease, 1043
Vinca alkaloids *see* Vinblastine; Vincristine
Vincristine
  bronchial carcinoma, 704
  leukaemia, 1037b
  non-Hodgkin's lymphoma, 1045
  and peripheral neuropathy, 1223b
VIP *see* Vasoactive intestinal polypeptide
Viper venom time, dilute Russell, 1055
VIPomas, 785b
Viral arthritis, 1095
Viral haemorrhagic fevers, 309b, 311f, 324–325
Viral hepatitis, 948–955
  causes, 948b
  complications, 949b
  HIV-related, 400
  icteric, 955
  immunisation, 954b
    haemophiliacs, 1051–1052
    HIV/AIDS patients, 407
  non-A, non-B, 954
  non-A, non-B, non-C (NANBNC), 955
  transmission, 950b
    blood products, 1011–1012
    sexual, 426
  treatment, 161b, 162
  see also under individual hepatitis viruses
Viral infections, 314–329
  antiviral agents, 161, 161b, 1267
    see also Antiretroviral drugs
  arthritis, 1095
  and cancer, 266b
  diabetes type 1 and, 804
  gastrointestinal, 327–328
  haemorrhagic fevers, 324–325, 325b
  immune deficiency and, 78b
  nervous system
    encephalitis, 1205–1206
    meningitis, 1201–1202
  with neurological involvement, 328–329
  respiratory tract, 328
    pneumonia, 319–320, 706b
    upper, 681–682
  with rheumatological involvement, 329
  sexually transmitted, 423–426
    see also specific infections
  skin, 325–327, 1278–1279
    HIV/AIDS, 397
  systemic
    with exanthem, 314–319
    without exanthem, 319–325
  TSEs, 329, 1211
  see also specific infections/infectious diseases
Viral load
  hepatitis B, 951f
  HIV, 393–394, 408
Viral warts *see* Warts, viral
Virchow's gland, 838f
Virilisation, 763, 1282
Virions, HIV, 391
Virtue ethics, 10
Viruses, 134–135
  bioterrorism, 145
  incubation periods, 310b
  life cycle, 135f
  oncogenic, HIV/AIDS, 391–392
Vision
  diabetics, 828
  double (diplopia), 1169–1170
  loss
    diabetics, 828
    leprosy, 348–349
    older people, 166f
    quinine overdose, 215
    see also Blindness
Visual analogue rating scale for pain, 285
Visual disorders, 1169–1173
  giant cell arteritis, 1117
  granulomatosis with polyangiitis, 1118f
  Graves' disease, 735f, 739b, 750–751, 750f
  positive visual phenomena, 1170
  stroke, 1237
Visual evoked responses (VER), 1153f
Visual field defect, 1170b
  pituitary tumours, 764b
Visual fields, examination by confrontation, 735f
Visual Infusion Phlebitis score, 330b
Visual loss, 1169–1170
Visual pathways, 1145–1146, 1145f–1146f
Visuo-spatial dysfunction, 1237
Vital capacity (VC), 648b, 653f
  forced (FVC), 653b
Vitamins, 124–130
  absorption, 843
  biochemical assessment of status, 126b
  deficiencies, 124–126
    older people, 127b
  dietary sources, 125b
  excess, 127
  fat-soluble, 126–127
  reference nutrient intake, 125b
  storage, 927
  water-soluble, 127–129
  see also specific vitamins
Vitamin A (retinol), 126–127
  biochemical assessment of status, 126b
  deficiency, 126f, 127
  dietary sources, 125b
  excess, 127
  RNI, 125b
  supplements, 127
  toxicity, 127
Vitamin B_1 *see* Thiamin
Vitamin B_2 *see* Riboflavin
Vitamin B_3 *see* Niacin
Vitamin B_6 *see* Pyridoxine
Vitamin B_{12} (cobalamin), 129
  absorption, 1024–1025
  biochemical assessment of status, 126b
  deficiency, 1024–1025, 1222b
    causes, 1025
    management, 1026
    neurological consequences, 129, 1024b, 1223b
    older people, 127b
    pregnancy, 1022b
    small bowel disease, 1025
  dietary sources, 125b
  older people, 127b
  reference values, 1312b
  RNI, 125b
Vitamin C (ascorbic acid), 129
  biochemical assessment of status, 126b
  deficiency, 129, 130b, 1050
  dietary sources, 125b
  RNI, 125b
Vitamin D, 127
  biochemical assessment of status, 126b
  deficiency, 127, 768b, 1126–1127
    older people, 127b
    reference range, 1310b
    rickets/osteomalacia management, 1127
  dietary sources, 125b
  excess, 127
  metabolism, 127, 1127f
  osteoporosis, 1123b, 1124
  reference values, venous blood, 1310b
  RNI, 125b, 127
  supplements, stone disease and
Vitamin D analogues, hypoparathyroidism, 770–771
Vitamin D and calcium supplements, osteoporosis prophylaxis, 1124
Vitamin D-deficient osteomalacia, 1126–1127
Vitamin D-resistant rickets (VDRR), 1128
Vitamin E, 127
  biochemical assessment of status, 126b
  deficiency, 127
  dietary sources, 125b
  RNI, 125b
Vitamin K, 127
  antagonists, 1019b
  anticoagulant poisoning, 224b
  biochemical assessment of status, 126b
  blood coagulation, 127
  deficiency, 127
  dietary sources, 125b
  RNI, 125b
  supplements, epilepsy in pregnancy, 1185b
Vitiligo, 272, 777, 1295, 1295f
Vitrectomy, 830

VLDL *see* Very low-density lipoproteins
Voiding *see* Micturition
Volume of distribution, 22
Vomiting, 853
  causes, 306b, 853f
  cyclical vomiting syndrome, 877
  palliative care, 289–290, 289f
  peptic ulcer, 875–876
  psychogenic, 877
Von Gierke disease, 450b
Von Hippel-Lindau disease/ syndrome, 267b, 1216
Von Willebrand disease, 1053–1054, 1053b
Von Willebrand factor, 1053
Voriconazole, 160, 160b
  acute leukaemia patients, 1001
  aspergillosis, 698–699
  candidiasis, 383
  fusariosis, 384
  mycetoma, 382
  neutropenic fever, 274
  paracoccidioidomycosis, 386
VRSA *see* Vancomycin-resistant *Staphylococcus aureus*
VT *see* Ventricular tachycardia
VTE *see* Venous thromboembolism
VTEC *see* Verocytotoxigenic *Escherichia coli*
Vulva
  chronic pain, 418–419, 418b
  pruritus, 418–419, 418b
  schistosomal papilloma, 377
Vulvodynia, 418b
VUR *see* Vesico-ureteric reflux
VZV *see* Varicella zoster virus

W
Waddling gait, 172b
Waist circumference, 115, 117
Waldenström's macroglobulinaemia, 1045
Wallenberg's syndrome, 1148b
Warfarin, 1019–1020
  adverse reactions, 176b, 1020
  antiphospholipid syndrome, 1055
  atrial fibrillation, 567b, 594, 742
  drug interactions, 28b
  indications, 1018b
  monitoring, 1000
  older people, 36b, 566b, 724b
  overdose, 224b
  pharmacokinetics, 25b
  in pregnancy, 37b, 723b
  pulmonary embolism, 723
  SLE, 1112
  stroke prevention, 1245f
  venous thromboembolism, 723, 1004, 1011b
    in pregnancy, 723b
Warfarin-like rodenticides, 224b
Warm autoimmune haemolysis, 1029–1030
Warts
  seborrhoeic, 397
  viral, 1278–1279, 1278f
    (ano)genital, 425–426
Water
  absorption/secretion, 842–843, 843f
  daily requirements, 433b
  depletion, 432–434, 433b
    see also Dehydration
  disorders of balance, 429–430, 429b, 436–439
  distribution, 428b, 429
  excess, 434b
  inhalation, 108
  investigations, 429–430
  reabsorption, 884–885
  renal handling, 436–437
  restriction, ascites, 940
  total body (TBW), 429
Water deprivation test, 795b
Waterbrash, 866
Watermelon stomach, 1113
Wax baths, 1080
WBC *see* White cells
Weakness, 1162–1163, 1162b
  facial, 1163
  limb, 1228b
  muscle, 1076, 1077b
  palliative care, 290
  stroke, 1236
Weal, definition, 1251b
Weber's syndrome, 1148, 1148b
Wegener's granulomatosis *see* Granulomatosis with polyangiitis
Weight gain, 117b
  see also Obesity
Weight loss, 859–860
  after gastric resection, 875
  anorexia nervosa, 255–256, 256b, 1121
  cancer patients, 271, 271b
  causes, 121b, 859f, 860b
  diabetes, 804, 806
  HIV/AIDS, 396, 396f
  investigations, 860
  palliative care, 290
  pancreatitis, 892–893
  rheumatoid arthritis, 1098
Weight reduction
  diabetics, 821
  diets, 118–119, 118b
  musculoskeletal disease, 1078
  obesity, 117–120
Weil-Felix reaction, 142
Weil's disease, 337
Wells scoring system, venous thrombosis, 1010b
Wenckebach's phenomenon, 572f
Werner's syndrome, 50, 795b
Wernicke-Korsakoff disease/ syndrome, 253
  prevention, 253–254
Wernicke's aphasia, 1169f
Wernicke's area, 1142–1143, 1146
Wernicke's encephalopathy, 128
West Nile encephalitis, 328, 1205
West Nile virus, 328
Western blot test, 141–142
WG *see* Wegener's granulomatosis
Wheeze, asthma, 667
Whipple's disease, 883–884, 883b
Whipple's triad, 783, 783f
Whipworm (*Trichuris trichiura*), 371–372
White cells, 995–996
  count, 1026b
    acute fever without localising signs, 310b
    differential, 1312b
    high *see* Leucocytosis
    low *see* Leucopenia
    viral hepatitis, 948–949
  formation, 995
  polymorphonuclear *see* Neutrophils
  reference values, 1312b
  structure and function, 999f
White spirit, poisoning, 224b
Whiteheads, 1281
Whitlow, herpetic, 326f
WHO *see* World Health Organization
Whole bowel irrigation, 210, 210b
Whooping cough (pertussis), 682
  chemoprophylaxis, 153b
  immunisation, 149b
  incubation period, 145b, 310b
  period of infectivity, 144b
Wickham's striae, 1289–1290
Williams syndrome, 66
  genetics, 56b
Wills, living, 171
Wilms' tumour, 267b
Wilson's disease, 132, 973–974
  inheritance, 973
  investigations, 974
  liver disease, 973
  liver function tests, 930b
  neurological aspects, 974, 1198
Windkessel effect, 530
Winterbottom's sign, 359
Withdrawal effects, 20–21, 20b
Wolbachia spp., 372
Wolff-Parkinson-White (WPW) syndrome, 568–569, 568f
Wood's light, 1255
World Health Organization (WHO)
  analgesic ladder, 286–287, 287f
  ICD-10, 232
  macronutrient recommendations, 114b
  refeeding diet, 122b
Worms *see* Helminthic infections; and specific types of infection
Wound dressings, 1266, 1266b
Wound infections
  staphylococcal, 330, 330f
  tetanus, 1210
WPW syndrome *see* Wolff-Parkinson-White (WPW) syndrome
Wrist
  fracture, 1120f
  pain, 1075
Writer's cramp, 1166–1167
Wuchereria bancrofti, 312b, 372, 372b, 372f, 713

X
X chromosome, 50–51
  abnormalities *see individual conditions*
  inactivation disorders, 54b
  mutations, 53
  see also X-linked
X-linked diseases
  haemophilia A, 1051–1053
  hypophosphataemic rickets (XLH), 1128
X-linked inheritance, 53
X-linked mental handicap (XLMH), 66
X-rays
  ankylosing spondylitis, 1106f
  body packers, 219f
  brain tumours, 1215
  cancer diagnosis, 269
  cardiovascular system *see* Chest radiography/X-ray
  Charcot foot, 834f
  chest *see* Chest radiography/X-ray
  gastrointestinal disease, 845–846, 847b, 847f
    achalasia, 869f
    contrast studies, 846
    inflammatory bowel disease, 901–902, 901f
  hepatobiliary disease, 948f
  hyperparathyroidism, 769–770
  musculoskeletal disorders, 1064, 1064b
    algodystrophy, 1130f
    ankylosing spondylitis, 1106f
    bone fractures, 1071, 1120f
    bony metastases, 275
    Charcot joint, 1133f
    chondrocalcinosis, 1090f
    gout, 1067b, 1089f
    osteoarthritis, 1083f–1084f
    osteomalacia, 1127f
    osteoporosis, 1120f
    osteosarcoma, 1132
    Paget's disease, 1129f
    reactive arthritis, 1108
    supraspinatus tendon calcification, 1091f
  nervous system, 1149b, 1150f
  properties, 102b
  renal, 62b
  respiratory system *see* Chest radiography/X-ray
  skull, 1150f
  spine, 1134f, 1151f, 1220
  see also DEXA
Xa inhibitors, 1019b
Xanthelasma
  biliary disease, 937b
  hyperlipidaemia, 454f
Xanthomas, 1302
  biliary cirrhosis, 963–964
  hyperlipidaemia, 454f
  tendon, 454f, 455
Xanthomatosis, cerebrotendinous, 456b
Xeroderma pigmentosum (XP), 67, 267b, 1260b
Xerophthalmia, 127
Xerostomia, 1114
XLH *see* X-linked hypophosphataemic rickets

Y
Y chromosomes, 50–51
  microdeletions, 761
Yaws, 332–333, 333b
Yellow Card scheme, 27
Yellow fever, 322f, 323–324, 325b
  immunisation, 324
  incubation period, 325b
Yersinia enterocolitica, 344
Yersinia pestis, 304b, 338
Young's syndrome, 648

Z
Zanamivir, 161b, 162, 320
Zellweger's syndrome, 47
Zero-order kinetics, 23
Zidovudine (ZDV), 407b
  adverse reactions, 409
    anaemia, 404–405
    lipodystrophy, 409f
    neutropenia, 405, 1005b
  effect of renal insufficiency
  HIV/AIDS, 407, 407b
  muscle pain/weakness, 1077b
  onychomycosis, 398
Zinc, 131–132
  deficiency, 131–132
  dietary sources, 131b
  refeeding diet, 122b
  reference values
    urine, 1311b
    venous blood, 1310b
  RNI, 131b
Zinc phosphide poisoning, 223
Zinc therapy, Wilson's disease, 974
Zoledronate
  osteoporosis, 1123b, 1125
  Paget's disease, 1129, 1130b
Zollinger-Ellison syndrome, 876
Zoonoses
  transmission, 144
  viral haemorrhagic fevers, 324–325
Zoster sine herpete, 318